T

10 0465021 5

reference

FOR
REFERENCE
ONLY

KU-050-608

WITHDRAWN

Endocrinology

Volume 1

Endocrinology

FIFTH EDITION

Senior Editors

Leslie J. DeGroot, MD
Professor of Medicine (Research)
Brown University
Providence, Rhode Island
Professor of Medicine, Emeritus
University of Chicago
Chicago, Illinois

J. Larry Jameson, MD, PhD
Irving S. Cutter Professor and Chairman
Department of Medicine
Northwestern University Feinberg School of
    Medicine
Chicago, Illinois

Section Editors

David de Kretser, AO, FAA, FTSE, MD, FRACP
Director, Monash Insitute of Medical
    Research
Monash University
Monash Medical Centre
Clayton, Victoria
Australia

Ashley B. Grossman, BA, BSc, MD, FRCP, F Med Sci
Professor of Neuroendocrinology
Barts and the London School of Medicine
    and Dentistry
Queen Mary, University of London
Honorary Consultant Physician
St. Bartholomew's Hospital
London, United Kingdom

John C. Marshall, MD, PhD
Andrew D. Hart Professor of Medicine
Director, Center for Research in Reproduction
University of Virginia School of Medicine
Charlottesville, Virginia

Shlomo Melmed, MD
Senior Vice President, Academic Affairs
Director, Burns and Allen Research Institute
Associate Dean, UCLA School of Medicine
Cedars-Sinai Medical Center
Los Angeles, California

John T. Potts, Jr, MD
Jackson Distinguished Professor of Clinical
    Medicine
Department of Medicine
Harvard Medical School
Physician-in Chief Emeritus,
Department of Medicine
Massachusetts General Hospital
Boston, Massachusetts

Gordon C. Weir, MD
Head, Section on Islet Transplantation
    and Cell Biology
Diabetes Research and Wellness
    Foundation Chair
Joslin Diabetes Center
Professor of Medicine
Harvard Medical School
Boston, Massachusetts

University of Nottingham
at Derby Library

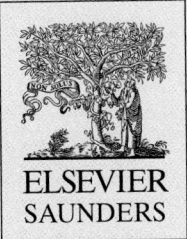

ELSEVIER
SAUNDERS

ELSEVIER
SAUNDERS

Elsevier
1600 John F. Kennedy Blvd.
Ste 1800
Philadelphia, PA 19103-2899

ENDOCRINOLOGY

Part number 9-9976-3674-0 (vol 1)
Part number 9-9976-3675-9 (vol 2)
Part number 9-9976-3676-7 (vol 3)
ISBN 0-7216-0376-9 (set)

Copyright © 2006, 2001, 1995, 1989, 1979, Elsevier Inc. All rights reserved.

No part of this publication may be reproduced or transmitted in any form or by any means, electronic or mechanical, including photocopying, recording, or any information storage and retrieval system, without permission in writing from the publisher. Permissions may be sought directly from Elsevier's Health Sciences Rights Department in Philadelphia, PA, USA: phone: (+1) 215 239 3804, fax: (+1) 215 239 3805, e-mail: healthpermissions@elsevier.com. You may also complete your request on-line via the Elsevier homepage (http://www.elsevier.com), by selecting 'Customer Support' and then 'Obtaining Permissions'.

NOTICE

Knowledge and best practice in this field are constantly changing. As new research and experience broaden our knowledge, changes in practice, treatment and drug therapy may become necessary or appropriate. Readers are advised to check the most current information provided (i) on procedures featured or (ii) by the manufacturer of each product to be administered, to verify the recommended dose or formula, the method and duration of administration, and contraindications. It is the responsibility of the practitioner, relying on their own experience and knowledge of the patient, to make diagnoses, to determine dosages and the best treatment for each individual patient, and to take all appropriate safety precautions. To the fullest extent of the law, neither the Publisher nor the Editors/Authors assume any liability for any injury and/or damage to persons or property arising out of or related to any use of the material contained in this book.

Previous editions copyrighted 2001, 1995, 1989, 1979 by Elsevier Inc.

Library of Congress Cataloging-in-Publication Data

Endocrinology / senior editors, Leslie J. DeGroot, J. Larry Jameson; section editors,
    David de Krester . . . [et al.].— 5th ed.
        p. ; cm.
Includes bibliographical references and index.
    ISBN 0-7216-0376-9 (set)
        1. Endocrine glands—Diseases. 2. Endocrinology. I. DeGroot, Leslie J. II. Jameson, J. Larry.
    [DNLM: 1. Endocrine Diseases. 2. Endocrine Glands. 3. Hormones. WK 140 E5585 2005]
    RC648.E458 2005 2006
    616.4—dc22

                                                                    2004051091

University of Nottingham
at Derby Library

100465 0215

Acquisitions Editor: Rebecca Schmidt Gaertner
Developmental Editor: Jennifer Shreiner
Project Manager: Mary Stermel

Printed in the United States of America

Last digit is the print number: 9 8 7 6 5 4 3 2 1

Working together to grow
libraries in developing countries
www.elsevier.com | www.bookaid.org | www.sabre.org

ELSEVIER   BOOK AID International   Sabre Foundation

Contributors

Lloyd Paul Aiello, MD, PhD
Associate Director, Beetham Eye Institute
Joslin Diabetes Center;

Director, Section Eye Research
Joslin Diabetes Center;

Associate Professor of Ophthalmology
Harvard Medical Center
Boston, Massachusetts
Diabetic Eye Disease

Carolyn A. Allan, MBBS(Hons), DRCOG, FRACP
Clinical Research Fellow
Male Reproduction Group
Prince Henry's Institute of Medical Research
Clayton, Victoria, Australia
Androgen Deficiency Disorders

Nobuyuki Amino, MD
Kuma Hospital
Center for Excellence in Thyroid Care
Chuo-ku
Kobe, Japan
Chronic (Hashimoto's) Thyroiditis

Marianne S. Anderson, MD
Assistant Professor
Pediatrics
University of Colorado Health Sciences Center
Aurora, Colorado
Fuel Homeostasis in the Fetus and Neonate

Josephine Arendt, PhD, FRCPath
Professor of Endocrinology, Emeritus
School of Biomedical and Molecular Sciences
University of Surrey
Guildford, Surrey, United Kingdom
*The Pineal Gland: Basic Physiology and Clinical
Implications*

Richard J. Auchus, MD, PhD
Assistant Professor
Internal Medicine/Endocrinology and Metabolism
University of Texas Southwestern Medical School;

Staff Endocrinologist
Internal Medicine
Zale Lipshy University Hospital/St. Paul University Hospital;

Staff Endocrinologist
Internal Medicine
Veterans' Administration Hospitals of North Texas
Dallas, Texas
*The Principles, Pathways, and Enzymes of Human
Steroidogenesis*

Joseph Avruch, MD
Professor, Medicine
Harvard Medical School;
Physician and Chief, Diabetes Unit
Medical Services
Massachusetts General Hospital;

Member
Department of Molecular Biology
Massachusetts General Hospital
Boston, Massachusetts
Hormone Signaling via Tyrosine Kinase Receptors

Lloyd Axelrod, MD
Associate Professor of Medicine
Department of Medicine
Harvard Medical School;

Physician and Chief of the James Howard Means Firm
Medical Services
Massachusetts General Hospital
Boston, Massachusetts
Glucocorticoid Therapy

Eric S. Bachman, MD, PhD
Senior Research Fellow
Pharmacology Division
Merck Research Laboratories
Boston, Massachusetts
Appetite Regulation and Thermogenesis

Rebecca S. Bahn, MD
Professor of Medicine
Mayo Clinic College of Medicine,
Consultant in Endocrinology, Mayo Clinic
Department of Internal Medicine, Mayo Clinic
Rochester, Minnesota
Graves' Ophthalmopathy

H. W. Gordon Baker, MD, PhD, FRACP
Professor, Department of Obstetrics and Gynaecology
  (Royal Women's Hospital)
University of Melbourne
Melbourne IVF
Melbourne, Victoria, Australia
Clinical Management of Male Infertility

Stephen G. Ball, MD
BHF Heart Research Centre (Clinical)
Leeds General Infirmary
Leeds, United Kingdom
*Vasopressin, Diabetes Insipidus, and Syndrome of Inappropriate
Antidiuresis*

Randall B. Barnes, MD
Associate Professor
Department of Obstetrics and Gynecology
University of Chicago Pritzker School of Medicine;

Attending Physician
Chicago Lying-in Hospital
Chicago, Illinois
Hyperandrogenism, Hirsutism, and the Polycystic Ovary Syndrome

Peter H. Baylis, BSc, MD, FRCP, FMedSci
Pro-Vice-Chancellor, Faculty of Medical Sciences
University of Newcastle upon Tyne;

Consultant Endocrinologist, Endocrinology Unit
Newcastle Hospital NHS Trust
Newcastle upon Tyne, United Kingdom
*Vasopressin, Diabetes Insipidus, and Syndrome of Inappropriate
Antidiuresis*

Paolo Beck-Peccoz, MD
Professor of Endocrinology
Institute of Endocrine Sciences
University of Milan
Ospedale Maggiore IRCCS
Milan, Italy
*TSH-Producing Adenomas
Resistance to Thyroid Hormone*

Graeme I. Bell, PhD
Professor of Biochemistry and Molecular Biology
Medicine and Human Genetics
University of Chicago
Chicago, Illinois
  *Chemistry and Biosynthesis of the Islet Hormones: Insulin, Islet
  Amyloid Polypeptide (Amylin), Glucagon, Somatostatin,
  and Pancreatic Polypeptide*

Norman H. Bell, MD
Distinguished University Professor of Medicine
Medical University of South Carolina;

Attending Physician
Medical University Hospital
Charleston, South Carolina
  Disorders of Calcification: Osteomalacia and Rickets

Laura Berman, LCSW, PhD
Clinical Assistant Professor
Northwestern University;

Director
Berman Center
Chicago, Illinois
  Female Sexual Dysfunction

Vikas Bhalla, MD
Division of Cardiology
Department of Medicine
Veterans Affairs Medical Center and University of California, San
  Diego
San Diego, California
  Neurohormonal Alterations in Heart Failure

Meenakshi A. Bhalla, MD
Division of Cardiology
Department of Medicine
Veterans Affairs Medical Center
  and University of California, San Diego
San Diego, California
  Neurohormonal Alterations in Heart Failure

Shalender Bhasin, MD
Professor of Medicine,
Chief, Section of Endocrinology
Boston University School of Medicine;

Chief, Section of Endocrinology
Evans Department of Medicine
Boston Medical Center
Boston, Massachusetts
  Sexual Dysfunction in Men

Neil A. Bhowmick, PhD
Assistant Professor
Urologic Surgery and Cancer Biology
Vanderbilt University
Nashville, Tennessee
  Endocrinology of the Prostate and Benign Prostatic Hyperplasia

John P. Bilezikian, MD
Professor of Medicine and Pharmacology
Department of Medicine
College of Physicians and Surgeons, Columbia University;

Chief, Division of Endocrinology,
Director, Metabolic Bone Diseases Unit
Department of Medicine
New York Presbyterian Hospital
New York, New York
  Primary Hyperparathyroidism

Stephen R. Bloom, MA, MD, DSc, FRCP, FRCPath, FMedSci
Head of Division of Investigative Science
Metabolic Medicine
Imperial College London;

Professor of Medicine
Pathology and Therapy Services
Hammersmith Hospitals NHS Trust
London, United Kingdom
  Gastrointestinal Hormones and Tumor Syndromes

Jeffrey A. Bluestone, MD
A.W. and Mary Margaret Distinguished Professor
UCSF Diabetes Center
University of California San Francisco
San Francisco, California
  Immunologic Mechanisms Causing Autoimmune Endocrine Disease

Manfred Blum, MD, FACP
Professor of Medicine and Radiology,
Director of the Nuclear Endocrine Laboratory
Medicine and Radiology
NYU School of Medicine;

Attending Physician
Tisch Hospital of NYU Medical Center;

Attending Physician
Bellevue Hospital
New York, New York
  Thyroid Imaging

Steen J. Bonnema, MD, PhD
Associate Professor
Endocrinological Research Unit, Institute of Clinical Research
University of Southern Denmark;

Associate Professor, Staff Specialist
Department of Endocrinology and Metabolism
Odense University Hospital
Odense, Denmark
  Multinodular Goiter

Roger Bouillon, MD, PhD, FRCP
Laboratory of Experimental Medicine and Endocrinology
Katholieke Univeriteit Leuven
Leuven, Belgium
  *Vitamin D: From Photosynthesis, Metabolism, and Action to Clinical
  Applications*

Andrew J. M. Boulton, MD, DSc(Hon), FRCP
Professor of Medicine
Academic Division of Medicine
University of Manchester;

Consultant Physician
Manchester Royal Infirmary
Manchester, United Kingdom;

Professor of Medicine
Division of Endocrinology
University of Miami
Miami, Florida
  Diabetes Mellitus: Neuropathy

Glenn D. Braunstein, MD
Professor of Medicine
The David Geffen School of Medicine at UCLA;

Chairman, Department of Medicine
The James R. Klinenberg, MD Chair in Medicine
Department of Medicine
Cedars-Sinai Medical Center
Los Angeles, California
  Hypothalamic Syndromes

F. Richard Bringhurst, MD
Associate Professor
Medicine
Harvard Medical School;

Physician
Massachusetts General Hospital
Boston, Massachusetts
  Regulation of Calcium and Phosphate Homeostasis

Arthur E. Broadus, MD, PhD
Professor
Internal Medicine, Section of Endocrinology
Yale University School of Medicine
New Haven, Connecticut
  Malignancy-Associated Hypercalcemia

Marcello D. Bronstein, MD
Associate Professor of Medicine
Department of Internal Medicine
University of Sao Paulo Medical School;

Chief, Neuroendocrine Unit
Division of Endocrinology and Metabolism
Department of Internal Medicine
Hospital das Clinicas, University of Sao Paulo Medical School
Sao Paulo, Brazil
  Disorders of Prolactin Secretion and Prolactinomas

Edward M. Brown, MD
Professor of Medicine
Department of Medicine
Harvard Medical School;

Senior Physician
Endocrine-Hypertension Division, Department of Medicine
Brigham and Women's Hospital
Boston, Massachusetts
  Parathyroid Hormone and Parathyroid Hormone–Related Peptide in the Regulation of Calcium Homeostasis and Bone Development
  Familial Hypocalciuric Hypercalcemia and Other Disorders Due to Calcium-Sensing Receptor Mutations

Chuong Bui, MD
Resident, Department of Radiology
University of Michigan Medical Center
Ann Arbor, Michigan
  Adrenal Gland Imaging

Henry B. Burch, MD, FACP, FACE
Chair, Endocrinology Division
Department of Medicine
Uniformed Services University of the Health Sciences
Bethesda, Maryland;

Chief
Endocrinology, Diabetes, and Metabolism Service
Walter Reed Army Medical Center
Washington, DC
  Graves' Ophthalmopathy

Henry G. Burger, AO, FAA, MD, BS, FRCP, FRACP, FCP (SA), FRCOG, FRANZCOG
Professor
Faculty of Medicine
Monash University;

Professor
Prince Henry's Institute of Medical Research at Monash Medical Centre
Melbourne, Victoria, Australia
  Gonadal Peptides: Inhibins, Activins, Follistatin, Müllerian-Inhibiting Substance (Antimüllerian Hormone)

John B. Buse, MD, PhD
Chief, Division of General Medicine and Clinical Epidemiology
Director, Diabetes Care Center
University of North Carolina School of Medicine;

Director, Diabetes Care Center
UNC Health Care
Chapel Hill, North Carolina
  Management of Type 2 Diabetes Mellitus

Peter C. Butler, MD
Professor of Medicine
Larry L. Hillblom Islet Research Center
David Geffen School of Medicine at UCLA;

Director
Larry L. Hillblom Islet Research Center
David Geffen School of Medicine at UCLA
Los Angeles, California
  Insulin Secretion

Paolo Cappabianca, MD
Professor and Chairman of Neurological Surgery
Department of Neurological Sciences, Division of Neurosurgery
Università degli Studi di Napoli Federico II
Naples, Italy
  Pituitary Surgery

Esther Carlton, CLS
Project Manager, Clinical Correlations Department
Quest Diagnostics Nichols Institute
San Juan Capistrano, California
  Endocrine Testing

Jose F. Caro, MD
Professor of Medicine
Indiana University School of Medicine;

Vice President, Endocrine Research and Clinical Investigation
Lilly Research Laboratories
Eli Lilly and Company
Indianapolis, Indiana
  Obesity: The Problem and Its Management

Don H. Catlin, MD
Professor, Molecular and Medical Pharmacology
University of California, Los Angeles;

Professor, Molecular and Medical Pharmacology
David Geffen School of Medicine at UCLA;

Director
UCLA Olympic Analytical Laboratory
University of California, Los Angeles
Los Angeles, California
  Anabolic Steroids

Francesco Cavagnini, MD
Head
Chair of Endocrinology
University of Milan;

Chief
Department of Endocrinology
Istituto Auxologico Italiano, Ospedale San Luca, IRCCS
Milan, Italy
  Adrenal Causes of Hypercortisolism

Jerry Cavallerano, PhD
Assistant to the Director
Beetham Eye Institute
Joslin Diabetes Center
Boston, Massachusetts
  Diabetic Eye Disease

Luigi Maria Cavallo, MD, PhD
Staff Neurosurgeon
Department of Neurological Sciences, Division of Neurosurgery
Università degli Studi di Napoli Federico II
Naples, Italy
Pituitary Surgery

John R. G. Challis, PhD, DSc, FIBiol, FRCOG, FRSC
Vice-President
Research and Associate Provost;

Professor
Physiology, Ob/Gyn, Medicine
University of Toronto
Toronto, Ontario, Canada
Endocrinology of Parturition

Shu J. Chan, PhD
Associate Professor of Biochemistry and Molecular Biology
University of Chicago Pritzker School of Medicine;

Senior Research Associate
Howard Hughes Medical Institute
Chicago, Illinois
Chemistry and Biosynthesis of the Islet Hormones: Insulin, Islet Amyloid Polypeptide (Amylin), Glucagon, Somatostatin, and Pancreatic Polypeptide

Roland D. Chapurlat, MD, PhD
Assistant Professor
Rheumatology
Université Claude Bernard;

Assistant Professor
Rheumatology and Bone Diseases
Hôpital E Herriot;

Assistant Professor
Unit 403
INSERM
Lyon, France
Osteoporosis

V. Krishna Chatterjee, BMBCh, FRCP
Professor of Endocrinology
Department of Medicine
University of Cambridge;

Honorary Consultant Physician
Department of Diabetes and Endocrinology
Addenbrooke's Hospital
Cambridge, United Kingdom
Resistance to Thyroid Hormone
Adrenarche and Adrenopause

Luca Chiovato, MD, PhD
Professor of Endocrinology
Internal Medicine and Medical Therapy
University of Pavia;

Head, Unit of Internal Medicine and Endocrinology
Fondazione Salvatore Maugeri I.R.C.C.S
Pavia, Italy
Graves' Disease

Kyung J. Cho, MD, FACR
William Martell Professor of Radiology
University of Michigan Medical Center
Ann Arbor, Michigan
Adrenal Gland Imaging

Daniel Christophe, PhD
Research Director FNRS
IRIBHM-IBMM
Université Libre de Bruxelles
Charleroi (Gosselies), Belgium
Thyroid Regulatory Factors

George P. Chrousos, MD
Pediatrics
Athens University
Athens, Greece
Interactions of the Endocrine and Immune Systems

John A. Cidlowski, PhD
Chief
Laboratory of Signal Transduction
National Institute of Environmental Health Science
National Institutes of Health
Research Triangle Park, North Carolina
Glucocorticoid Receptors and Their Mechanisms of Action

Adrian J. L. Clark, DSc FRCP
Professor
Department of Endocrinology
Barts and the London, Queen Mary, University of London
London, United Kingdom
Adrenal Insufficiency

David R. Clemmons, MD
Kenan Professor of Medicine
Internal Medicine
University of North Carolina School of Medicine;

Attending Physician
Internal Medicine
University of North Carolina Hospitals
Chapel Hill, North Carolina
Insulin-like Growth Factor 1 and Its Binding Proteins

Jack W. Coburn, MD[†]
Formerly, Adjunct Professor of Medicine
UCLA School of Medicine
University of California, Los Angeles;

Formerly, Staff Physician
VA West Los Angeles Medical Center
Los Angeles, California
The Renal Osteodystrophies

P. Conton, MD
Department of Medical and Surgical Sciences
OU of Endocrinology
University of Padova
Azienda Ospedaliera di Padova
Padova, Italy
Adrenal Cancer

Georges Copinschi, MD, PhD
Professor Emeritus of Endocrinology
Laboratory of Physiology
Faculty of Medicine, Université Libre de Bruxelles;

Formerly Chief
Division of Endocrinology
Hôpital Universitaire Saint-Pierre;

Formerly Chairman
Department of Medicine
Hôpital Universitaire Saint-Pierre
Brussels, Belgium
Endocrine and Other Biologic Rhythms

C. Hamish Courtney, MD, MRCP
Consultant Physician
Regional Centre for Diabetes and Endocrinology
Royal Victoria Hospital
Belfast, Ireland
Type 2 Diabetes Mellitus: Etiology, Pathogenesis, and Natural History

[†]Deceased

Vincent L. Cryns, MD
Associate Professor
Departments of Medicine and Cell and Molecular Biology
Feinberg School of Medicine, Northwestern University;

Attending Physician
Department of Medicine
Northwestern Memorial Hospital
Chicago, Illinois
  Cell Division, Differentiation, Senescence, and Death

Gerald R. Cunha, PhD
Professor
Anatomy, Urology and Obstetrics and Gynecology
University of California
San Francisco, California
  Endocrinology of the Prostate and Benign Prostatic Hyperplasia

Gary C. Curhan, MD, ScD
Associate Professor of Medicine
Department of Medicine
Harvard Medical School;

Renal Division, Department of Medicine
Brigham and Women's Hospital;

Associate Professor of Epidemiology
Harvard School of Public Health
Boston, Massachusetts
  Nephrolithiasis

Leona Cuttler, MD
Professor, Pediatrics
Case Western Reserve University;

Chief, Endocrinology, Diabetes, and Metabolism
Pediatrics
Rainbow Babies and Children's Hospital
Cleveland, Ohio
  Somatic Growth and Maturation

Jamie Dananberg, MD
Executive Director
Exploratory and Program Medical
Lilly Research Laboratories, Eli Lilly and Co.
Indianapolis, Indiana
  Obesity: The Problem and Its Management

Mehul T. Dattani, FRCP, MD
Reader in Paediatric Endocrinology
Biochemistry, Endocrinology, and Metabolism
Institute of Child Health London;

Consultant in Paediatric Endocrinology
Endocrinology
Great Ormond Street Children's Hospital;

Consultant in Paediatric Endocrinology
Adolescent Endocrinology
Middlesex Hospital
London, United Kingdom
  Growth Hormone Deficiency in Children

Marlyse A. Debrincat
Division of Cancer and Haematology
The Walter and Eliza Hall Institute of Medical Research
Parkville, Victoria, Australia
  Hormone Signaling via Cytokine Receptors

Oreste de Divitiis, MD
Associate Professor of Neurosurgery
Department of Neurological Sciences, Division of Neurosurgery
Università degli Studi di Napoli Federico II
Naples, Italy
  Pituitary Surgery

Mario De Felice, MD
Senior Scientist
Laboratory of Animal Genetics
Stazione Zoologica Anton Dohrn
Naples, Italy
  Anatomy and Development of the Thyroid

Ralph A. DeFronzo, MD
Professor of Medicine; Chief, Diabetes Division
University of Texas Health Science Center
San Antonio, Texas
  Regulation of Intermediatory Metabolism during Fasting and Feeding

Leslie J. DeGroot, MD
Professor of Medicine (Research)
Brown University
Providence, Rhode Island;

Professor of Medicine, Emeritus
University of Chicago
Chicago, Illinois
  Endocrinology: Impact on Science and Medicine
  Nonthyroidal Illness Syndrome
  Thyroid Neoplasia

David de Kretser, AO, FAA, FTSE, MD, FRACP
Director, Monash Institute of Medical Research
Monash University
Monash Medical Centre
Clayton, Victoria, Australia
  Gonadal Peptides: Inhibins, Activins, Follistatin, Müllerian-Inhibiting
    Substance (Antimüllerian Hormone)
  Functional Morphology of the Testis

Pierre D. Delmas, MD, PhD
Professor of Medicine
Claude Bernard University of Lyon;

Chief of Department, Rheumatology
Hôpital E. Herriot;

Director, Research Unit 403 (Pathophysiology of Osteoporosis)
INSERM
Lyon, France;

President, International Osteoporosis Foundation
Nyon, Switzerland
  Osteoporosis

Paul Devroey, PhD
AZ-Vrije Universiteit Brussel
Centre for Reproductive Medicine
Brussels, Belgium
  Ovulation Induction and Assisted Reproduction

Roberto Di Lauro, MD
Full Professor of Human Genetics
University of Naples Frederico II Medical School;

Head, Laboratory of Biochemistry and Molecular Biology
Stazione Zoologica Anton Dohrn
Naples, Italy
  Anatomy and Development of the Thyroid

Ruben Diaz, MD, PhD
Instructor in Pediatrics
Harvard Medical School;

Assistant in Medicine
Endocrinology
Children's Hospital Boston
Boston, Massachusetts
  Familial Hypocalciuric Hypercalcemia and Other Disorders Due to
    Calcium-Sensing Receptor Mutations

Sean F. Dinneen, MD, FACP, FRCPI
Consultant Diabetologist
Addenbrooke's Hospital
Cambridge, United Kingdom
  Classification and Diagnosis of Diabetes Mellitus

Annemarie A. Donjacour
Assistant Research Anatomist
University of California at San Francisco
San Francisco, California
Endocrinology of the Prostate and Benign Prostatic Hyperplasia

Daniel J. Drucker, MD
Director, Banting and Best Diabetes
Professor of Medicine
University of Toronto;

Staff Physician
Toronto General Hospital
Toronto, Ontario, Canada
Glucagon and the Glucagon-like Peptides

Jacques E. Dumont, MD, PhD
Founding Director
Institute of Interdisciplinary Research (IRIBHM)
University of Brussels
Brussels, Belgium
Thyroid Regulatory Factors

Christopher R. W. Edwards, MD, FRCP, FRCPEd, FRSE, FMedSci
Professor, Vice-Chancellor
University of Newcastle upon Tyne
Newcastle upon Tyne, United Kingdom
Primary Mineralocorticoid Excess Syndromes

David A. Ehrmann, MD
Professor of Medicine and Associate Director
The University of Chicago General Clinical Research Center
The University of Chicago
Chicago, Illinois
Hyperandrogenism, Hirsutism, and the Polycystic Ovary Syndrome

Graeme Eisenhofer, PhD
Staff Scientist
Clinical Neurocardiology Section, National Institutes of
   Neurological Disorders and Stroke
National Institutes of Health
Bethesda, Maryland
Pheochromocytoma

Ilia J. Elenkov, MD
Division of Rheumatology
Immunology, and Allergy
Georgetown University Medical Center
Washington, DC
Interactions of the Endocrine and Immune Systems

Gregory F. Erickson, PhD
Professor
Reproductive Medicine
University of California, San Diego
La Jolla, California
Folliculogenesis, Ovulation, and Luteogenesis

Barbro Eriksson, MD, PhD
Professor, Department of Medical Sciences
Senior Consultant, Department of Endocrine Oncology
University Hospital Uppsala
Uppsala, Sweden
Carcinoid Syndrome

Eric A. Espiner, MBChB, MD, FRACP, FRS (NC)
Emeritus Professor, Medicine
Christ Church School of Medicine and Health Sciences
Christ Church, New Zealand
Hormones of the Cardiovascular System

Victoria Esser, PhD
Associate Professor, Internal Medicine
University of Texas Southwestern Medical Center at Dallas
Dallas, Texas
Ketoacidosis and Hyperosmolar Coma

Erica A. Eugster, MD
Associate Professor of Clinical Pediatrics, School of Medicine
Indiana University;

Director, Section of Pediatric Endocrinology/Diabetology
Riley Hospital for Children
Indianapolis, Indiana
Precocious Puberty
Delayed Puberty

I. Sadaf Farooqi, MD
Department of Medicine and Clinical Biochemistry
University of Cambridge
Adderbrooke's Hospital
Cambridge, United Kingdom
Genetic Syndromes Associated with Obesity

Bart C. J. M. Fauser, MD, PhD
Department of Reproductive Medicine
University of Medical Center Utrecht
Utrecht, The Netherlands
Female Subfertility: Evaluation and Management

Eleuterio Ferrannini, MD
Professor, Department of Internal Medicine
University of Pisa
Pisa, Italy
Regulation of Intermediatory Metabolism during Fasting and Feeding

David M. Findlay, PhD
Associate Professor, Orthopaedics and Trauma
The University of Adelaide;

Member, Hanson Institute
Adelaide, South Australia, Australia
Calcitonin

Joel S. Finkelstein, MD
Associate Professor of Medicine
Harvard Medical School;

Associate Physician, Department of Medicine
Massachusetts General Hospital
Boston, Massachusetts
Medical Management of Hypercalcemia

Delbert A. Fisher, MD
Professor of Pediatrics and Medicine Emeritus
UCLA School of Medicine;

VP Science and Innovation
Quest Diagnostics Incorporated
San Juan Capistrano, California
Fetal and Neonatal Endocrinology
Endocrine Testing

Susan J. Fisher, PhD
Professor, Cell and Tissue Biology
University of California, San Francisco
San Francisco, California
*Implantation and Placental Physiology in Early Human Pregnancy:
The Role of the Maternal Decidua and the Trophoblast*

Jeffrey S. Flier, MD
George C. Reisman Professor of Medicine
Harvard Medical Center;

Chief Academic Officer, Research
Beth Israel Deaconess Medical School;

Harvard Faculty Dean for Academic Programs
Beth Israel Deaconess Medical Center
Boston, Massachusetts
Syndromes of Insulin Resistance and Mutant Insulin

Maguelone G. Forest, MD, PhD
Directeur de Recherche à Titre Exceptionnel, Professor Emeritus
Hôpital Debrousse
INSERM
Lyon, Rhône, France
Diagnosis and Treatment of Disorders of Sexual Development

Daniel W. Foster, MD
John Denis McGarry, PhD Distinguished Chair in Diabetes and
  Metabolic Research
Department of Internal Medicine
The University of Texas Southwestern Medical School
Dallas, Texas
  Ketoacidosis and Hyperosmolar Coma

Aaron L. Friedman, MD
Professor and Chair, Department of Pediatrics
University of Wisconsin School of Medicine
Madison, Wisconsin
  Hormonal Regulation of Electrolyte and Water Metabolism

Eli A. Friedman, MD, FACP, FRCP (London)
Distinguished Teaching Professor of Medicine
Chief, Renal Disease Division
Department of Medicine
Downstate Medical Center;

Director, Nephrology, Department of Medicine
Kings County Hospital Center
Brooklyn, New York
  Diabetic Nephropathy

Mark Frydenberg, MBBS, FRACS (Urol)
Chairman of the Department of Urology
Monash Medical Centre;

Clinical Associate Professor, Department of Surgery
Clinical Director of the Centre of Urological Research
Monash Institute of Reproduction and Development
Monash University
Clayton, Victoria, Australia
  Endocrinology of Prostate Cancer

Peter J. Fuller, MBBS, BMedSc(Hons), PhD, FRACP
Professorial Fellow, Medicine and Biochemistry
  and Molecular Biology
Monash University
Melbourne, Victoria, Australia;

Director, Endocrinology
Southern Health;

NHMRC Senior Principal Research Fellow
Prince Henry's Institute of Medical Research
Clayton, Victoria, Australia
  Aldosterone: Secretion and Action

John W. Funder, MD, PhD, FRACP
Professor, Medicine
Monash University;

Prince Henry's Institute of Medical
Monash Medical Center
Clayton, Victoria, Australia
  Essential Hypertension and Endocrine Hypertension

Dana Gaddy, PhD
Associate Professor, Physiology and Biophysics
University of Arkansas for Medical Sciences
Little Rock, Arkansas
  Hormone Signaling via Serine Kinase Receptors

Robert F. Gagel, MD
Professor of Medicine and Division Head
Division of Internal Medicine
University of Texas Health Science Center;

Professor of Medicine and Division Head
Division of Internal Medicine
MD Anderson Cancer Center
Houston, Texas
  Multiple Endocrine Neoplasia Type 2

Jason L. Gaglia, MD
Clinical Fellow, Department of Medicine
Harvard Medical School;

Clinical Fellow, Endocrinology, Diabetes, and Metabolism
Beth Israel Deaconess Medical Center;

Clinical Fellow, Adult Diabetes
Joslin Diabetes Center
Boston, Massachusetts
  Pancreatic and Islet Transplantation

David Galton, MD, FRCP
Professor, Human Metabolism and Genetics
Wolfson Institute of Preventive Medicine;

Hon. Consultant, Metabolism and Genetics
St. Bartholomew's Hospital;

Consultant Physician, Diabetes and Metabolism
London Medical Center
London, United Kingdom
  Diabetes, Lipids, and Atherosclerosis

Thomas J. Gardella, PhD
Associate Professor, Medicine
Harvard Medical School;

Associate Professor, Medicine, Endocrine Unit
Massachusetts General Hospital
Boston, Massachusetts
  *Parathyroid Hormone and Parathyroid Hormone–Related Peptide in the
  Regulation of Calcium Homeostasis and Bone Development*

Bruce D. Gaylinn, PhD
Research Assistant Professor
Internal Medicine Division of Endocrinology
University of Virginia Health System
Charlottesville, Virginia
  *Growth Hormone–Releasing Hormone, Ghrelin, and Growth Hormone
  Secretagogues*

Harry K. Genant, MD
Professor, Emeritus
Radiology, Medicine and Orthopaedic Surgery;
Executive Director, Osteoporosis and Arthritis Research Group
Department of Radiology
University of California, San Francisco;

Chairman, Emeritus and Member, Board of Directors, Synarc, Inc.
San Francisco, California
  Bone Density and Imaging of Osteoporosis

Hans Gerber, MD
Privatdozent, University of Bern School of Medicine;

Head of Division, Department of Clinical Chemistry
University Hospital
Inselspital
Bern, Switzerland
  Multinodular Goiter

John E. Gerich, MD
Professor of Medicine
University of Rochester;

Endocrine Attending
Strong Memorial Hospital
Rochester, New York
  Hypoglycemia

Michael S. German, PhD
Professor, Medicine and Diabetes Center
University of California, San Francisco
San Francisco, California
  Development of the Endocrine Pancreas

Marvin C. Gershengorn, MD
Director, Division of Intramural Research
National Institute of Diabetes and Digestive and Kidney
  Diseases, NIH
Bethesda, Maryland
  Second Messenger Signaling Pathways: Phospholipids and Calcium

Mohammad A. Ghatei, MD
Department of Metabolic Medicine
Imperial College School of Medicine
London, United Kingdom
  Gastrointestinal Hormones and Tumor Syndromes

William Gibb, PhD
Professor, Obstetrics and Gynecology, and Cellular and Molecular
  Medicine
University of Ottawa
Ottawa, Ontario, Canada
  Endocrinology of Parturition

Lisa K. Gilliam, MD, PhD
Senior Fellow, Medicine
University of Washington Medical Center
Seattle, Washington
  Type 1 (Insulin-dependent) Diabetes Mellitus:
  Etiology, Pathogenesis, and Natural History

Monica Girotra, MD
Clinical Fellow in Endocrinology
College of Physicians and Surgeons, Columbia University;

Clinical Fellow in Endocrinology
New York-Presbyterian Hospital
New York, New York
  Immunologic Mechanisms Causing Autoimmune Endocrine Disease

Linda C. Giudice, MD, PhD
Stanley McCormick Memorial Professor
Obstetrics and Gynecology
Stanford University School of Medicine;

Physician, Obstetrics and Gynecology
Stanford University Hospital;

Chief, Division of Reproductive Endocrinology and Infertility
Stanford University Hospital and Clinics;

Associate Chair of Research
Department of Obstetrics and Gynecology
Stanford University
Stanford, California
  Endometriosis
  Implantation and Placental Physiology in Early Human Pregnancy:
  The Role of the Maternal Decidua and the Trophoblast

Anna Glasier, BSc, MD, FRCOG, MFFP
Director, Family Planning and Well Woman Services
Lothian Primary Care NHS Trust;

Senior Lecturer, Department of Obstetrics and Gynaecology
University of Edinburgh
Edinburgh, Scotland
  Contraception

Francis H. Glorieux, MD, PhD
Professor, Surgery, Pediatrics and Human Genetics
McGill University;

Director of Research, Shriners Hospital for Children
Montreal, Canada
  Genetic Defects in Vitamin D Metabolism and Action

Steven R. Goldring, MD
Professor of Medicine, Harvard Medical School;

Chief of Rheumatology
Beth Israel Deaconess Medical Center;

Chief of Rheumatology
New England Baptist Hospital
Boston, Massachusetts
  Disorders of Calcification: Osteomalacia and Rickets

Javier González-Maeso, PhD
Research Associate, Department of Neurology
Mount Sinai School of Medicine
New York, New York
  Hormone Signaling via G Protein-Coupled Receptors

Theodore L. Goodfriend, MD
Professor Emeritus, Medicine and Pharmacology
University of Wisconsin Medical School;

Associate Chief of Staff for Research
Wm. S. Middleton Memorial Veterans Hospital
Madison, Wisconsin
  Hormonal Regulation of Electrolyte and Water Metabolism

Louis J. G. Gooren, MD
Professor of Endocrinology
Vrije Universiteit Medical Center
Amsterdam, The Netherlands
  Gender Identity and Sexual Behavior

William J. Gradishar, MD
Associate Professor of Medicine
Division of Hematology and Oncology
Northwestern University; Northwestern Memorial Hospital;

Director Breast Medical Oncology
Robert H. Lurie Comprehensive Cancer Center
Chicago, Illinois
  Endocrine Management of Breast Cancer

Karen A. Gregerson, PhD
Associate Professor of Physiology
College of Pharmacy, Division of Pharmaceutical Sciences
University of Cincinnati
Cincinnati, Ohio
  Prolactin

Milton D. Gross, MD
Professor, Radiology and Internal Medicine
University of Michigan Medical School
Ann Arbor, Michigan;

Director/Chief
Nuclear Medicine and Radiation Safety Service
Department of Veterans Affairs Health System
Ann Arbor, Michigan and Washington, DC (field-based)
  Adrenal Gland Imaging

Ashley B. Grossman, BA, BSc, MD, FRCP, F Med Sci
Professer of Neuroendocrinology
Barts and the London School of Medicine and Dentistry
Queen Mary, University of London
Honorary Consultant Physician
St. Bartholomew's Hospital
London, United Kingdom
  Cushing's Syndrome
  Adrenal Insufficiency

Valeria C. Guimarães, MD
Institute of Biological Sciences
Federal University of Minas Geiras (ICB-UFMG)
Belo Horizonte-MG, Brazil;

Unité de Recherches Laitières et de Génétique Appliquée,
Institut National de la Recherche Agronomique, Domaine
  de Vilvert
Cedex, France
  Subacute and Riedel's Thyroiditis

Mark Gurnell, BSc(Hons), MBBS, MRCP(UK), PhD
University Lecturer, Medicine, University of Cambridge;

Honorary Consultant Physician
Endocrinology and Diabetes Mellitus
Addenbrooke's Hospital
Cambridge, United Kingdom
  Resistance to Thyroid Hormone

Joel F. Habener, MD
Professor, Medicine
Harvard Medical School;

Chief
Laboratory of Molecular Endocrinology
Massachusetts General Hospital;

Investigator
Howard Hughes Medical Institute
Boston, Massachusetts
  The Cyclic AMP Second Messenger Signaling Pathway

Charles B. Hammond, MD
E.C. Hamblen Professor
Department of Obstetrics and Gynecology
Duke University Medical Center
Durham, North Carolina
  Gestational Trophoblastic Neoplasms

David J. Handelsman, MB, BS, PhD, FRACP
Professor of Reproductive Endocrinology and Andrology
Director, ANZAC Research Institute
Head, Andrology Department, Concord Hospital
ANZAC Research Institute
University of Sydney
Sydney, NSW, Australia
  Androgen Action and Pharmacologic Uses
  Male Contraception

John B. Hanks, MD
C. Bruce Morton Professor and Chief
Division of General Surgery
University of Virginia Health System
Charlottesville, Virginia
  Adrenal Surgery

Shun-ichi Harada, MD
Senior Research Fellow
Molecular Endocrinology/Bone Biology
Merck Research Laboratories
West Point, Pennsylvania
  Bone Development and Remodeling

William W. Hay, Jr, MD
Professor, Pediatrics
Scientific Director, Perinatal Research Center
University of Colorado Health Sciences Center
Aurora, Colorado;

Director, Neonatal Clinical Research Center (NIH – Pediatric GCRC)
University of Colorado School of Medicine and The Children's
  Hospital
Denver, Colorado
  Fuel Homeostasis in the Fetus and Neonate

Simon W. Hayward, PhD
Assistant Professor
Urologic Surgery and Cancer Biology
Vanderbilt University Medical Center
Nashville, Tennessee
  Endocrinology of the Prostate and Benign Prostatic Hyperplasia

David Heber, MD, PhD
Professor of Medicine, Department of Medicine
David Geffen School of Medicine at UCLA;

Director, Department of Medicine
UCLA Center for Human Nutrition
Los Angeles, California
  Starvation and Parenteral Nutrition

Matthias Hebrok, PhD
Assistant Professor in Residence
Diabetes Center and Department of Medicine
University of California, San Francisco (UCSF)
San Francisco, California
  Development of the Endocrine Pancreas

Laszlo Hegedüs, MD, DMSc
Professor, Department of Endocrinology and Metabolism
Odense University;

Head of Department
Department of Endocrinology and Metabolism
Odense University Hospital
Odense, Denmark
  Multinodular Goiter

Wayne J. G. Hellstrom, MD, FACS
Chief, Section of Andrology and Male Infertility
Department of Urology
Tulane University School of Medicine
New Orleans, Louisiana
  Sexual Dysfunction in Men

Georg Hennemann, MD, PhD, FRCP, FRCP(E)
Professor of Medicine and Endocrinology
Medical Faculty
Erasmus University
Rotterdam, The Netherlands
  Autonomously Functioning Thyroid Nodules and Other Causes
  of Thyrotoxicosis

Kevan C. Herold, MD
Associate Professor of Medicine
College of Physicians and Surgeons
Columbia University
New York, New York
  Immunologic Mechanisms Causing Autoimmune Endocrine Disease

Yoh Hidaka, MD
Associate Professor, Laboratory Medicine
Osaka University Graduate School of Medicine
Suita, Osaka, Japan
  Chronic (Hashimoto's) Thyroiditis

Douglas J. Hilton, PhD
Division of Cancer and Haematology
The Walter and Eliza Hall Institute of Medical Research
Parkville, Victoria, Australia
  Hormone Signaling via Cytokine Receptors

Peter C. Hindmarsh, BSc, MD, FRCP, FRCPCH
Professor of Paediatric Endocrinology
Institute of Child Health
University College London;

Hon Consultant in Paediatric Endocrinology
London Centre for Paediatric Endocrinology and Metabolism
Great Ormond Street Hospital for Children
London, United Kingdom
  Growth Hormone Deficiency in Children

Patricia M. Hinkle, PhD
Professor, Pharmacology and Physiology
University of Rochester Medical Center
Rochester, New York
  Second Messenger Signaling Pathways: Phospholipids and Calcium

Clement K. M. Ho, MBBS, DRCOG, PhD
Clinical Biochemistry
Royal Infirmary of Edinburgh
Edinburgh, Scotland
  Ovarian Hormone Synthesis

Ken K. Y. Ho, FRACP, MD
Professor, Medicine
University of New South Wales;

Head, Endocrinology
St. Vincent's Hospital;

Head, Pituitary Research Unit
Garvan Institute of Medical Research
Sydney, NSW, Australia
  Growth Hormone Deficiency in Adults

Ana O. Hoff, MD
Assistant Professor of Medicine
Endocrine Neoplasia and Hormonal Disorders
University of Texas
MD Anderson Cancer Center
Houston, Texas
  Multiple Endocrine Neoplasia Type 2

Anthony N. Hollenberg, MD
Associate Professor, Medicine
Harvard Medical School;

Chief, Thyroid Unit
Division of Endocrinology
Beth Israel Deaconess Medical Center
Boston, Massachusetts
  Mechanisms of Thyroid Hormone Action

Nelson D. Horseman, PhD
Professor of Molecular and Cellular Physiology
Department of Molecular and Cellular Physiology
University of Cincinnati
Cincinnati, Ohio
  Prolactin

Ieuan A. Hughes, MD
Department of Paediatrics
University of Cambridge
Addenbrooke's Hospital
Cambridge, United Kingdom
  Adrenarche and Adrenopause

Hero K. Hussain, MD
Siemens Medical Systems/RSNA Fellow
Department of Radiology
University of Michigan Health System
Ann Arbor, Michigan
  Adrenal Gland Imaging

John M. Hutson, MD, FRACS, FAAP(Hon)
Professor of Paediatric Surgery, Paediatrics
University of Melbourne;

Director, General Surgery
Royal Children's Hospital;

Associate Director, Clinical Research
Murdoch Childrens Research Institute
Melbourne, Victoria, Australia
  Cryptorchidism and Hypospadias

Peter Illingworth MB, MD(Hon), FRANZCOG
Associate Professor, Obstetrics and Gynaecology
University of Sydney;

Director of Reproductive Medicine
Westmead Hospital
Sydney, NSW, Australia
  Amenorrhea, Anovulation, and Dysfunctional Uterine Bleeding

J. Larry Jameson, MD, PhD
Irving S. Cutter Professor and Chairman
Department of Medicine
Northwestern University Feinberg School of Medicine
Chicago, Illinois
  Endocrinology: Impact on Science and Medicine
  Applications of Genetics in Endocrinology
  Mechanisms of Thyroid Hormone Action
  Endocrinology of Sexual Maturation

Michael Jergas, MD
Assistant Professor of Radiology
Teaching Hospital at the University of Cologne;

Director, Department of Radiology
St. Katharinen-Hospital
Frechen, Germany
  Bone Density and Imaging of Osteoporosis

V. Craig Jordan, OBE, PhD, DSc
Vice President and Research Director for Medical Sciences
Alfred G. Knutson Chair of Cancer Research
Fox Chase Cancer Center
Philadelphia, Pennsylvania
  Endocrine Management of Breast Cancer

Nathalie Josso
Institut Paris-Sud sur les Cytokines
Université Paris-Sud;

Attaché, Service d' Endocrinologie Pédiatrique
Hôpital Saint Vincent-de-Paul;

Directeur de Recherches, Unité 493
Institut National de la Santé et de la Recherche Médicale
Paris, France
  Embryology and Control of Fetal Sex Differentiation

Andreas Jöstel, MD
Clinical Research Fellow
Department of Endocrinology
Christie Hospital
Manchester, United Kingdom
  Hypopituitarism

Harald Jüppner, MD
Associate Professor of Pediatrics
Harvard Medical School;

Associate Pediatrician
Endocrine Unit and Pediatric Nephrology Unit
Massachusetts General Hospital
Boston, Massachusetts
  Parathyroid Hormone and Parathyroid Hormone–Related Peptide in
    the Regulation of Calcium Homeostasis and Bone Development
  Genetic Disorders of Calcium Homeostasis Caused by Abnormal
    Regulation of Parathyroid Hormone Secretion or Responsiveness

Ursula B. Kaiser, MD
Associate Professor of Medicine
Harvard Medical School;

Associate Physician and Director
Neuroendocrine Program
Department of Medicine
Brigham and Women's Hospital
Boston, Massachusetts
  Gonadotropin-Releasing Hormone and Gonadotropins

Edwin L. Kaplan, MD
Professor, Surgery
The University of Chicago, Pritzker School of Medicine;

Professor, Surgery
The University of Chicago Hospitals
Chicago, Illinois
  Surgery of the Thyroid

Jeffrey A. Kalish, MD
General Surgery Resident
Boston Medical Center
Boston, Massachusetts
  Diabetic Foot and Vascular Complications

Gerard Karsenty, MD, PhD
Professor, Molecular and Human Genetics
Baylor College of Medicine
Houston, Texas
  Genetic Analysis of Skeleton Physiology

Rasa Kazlauskaite, MD
Assistant Professor
Department of Medicine
Division of Endocrinology
Rush University
John H. Stroger, Jr. Hospital of Cook County
Chicago, Illinois
  Thyroid-Stimulating Hormone and Regulation of the Thyroid Axis

Gary L. Keeney, MD
Assistant Professor, Mayo Medical School;

Consultant
Department of Laboratory Medicine and Pathology
Division of Anatomic Pathology
Mayo Clinic
Rochester, Minnesota
Ovarian Tumors with Endocrine Manifestations

Harry Keiser, MD
Scientist Emeritus, Attending Physician
The Clinical Center
National Institutes of Health
Bethesda, Maryland
Pheochromocytoma

Ruth A. Keri, PhD
Assistant Professor
Department of Pharmacology;

Assistant Professor
Division of General Medical Sciences, Oncology
Case Western Reserve University School of Medicine
Cleveland, Ohio
Transgenic and Genetic Animal Models

Jeffrey B. Kerr, PhD
Department of Anatomy and Cell Biology
Faculty of Medicine
Monash University
Melbourne, Victoria, Australia
Functional Morphology of the Testis

Paul Kim, MD
System Director
Department of Endocrinology
Geisinger Health System
Danville, Pennsylvania
Thyroid Hormone Formation

Ronald Klein, MD, MPH
Professor, University of Wisconsin
Ophthalmology and Visual Sciences
Medical School
Madison, Wisconsin
Diabetic Eye Disease

David L. Kleinberg, MD
Professor, Medicine
Director, Neuroendocrine Unit
New York University School of Medicine;

Attending, Medicine
New York University Medical Center
New York, New York
Endocrinology of Lactation

Meyer Knobel, MD
Thyroid Unit, Division of Endocrinology
University of Sao Paulo Medical School
Sao Paulo, Brazil
Iodine Deficiency Disorders

Isaac S. Kohane, MD, PhD
Associate Professor, Pediatrics
Harvard Medical School;

Director, Informatics Program
Children's Hospital;

Director, Harvard Partners Center for Genetics and Genomics
Brigham and Women's Hospital;

Henderson Professor
Health Sciences and Technology
Harvard University-Massachusetts Institute of Technology
Boston, Massachusetts
Genomics and Proteomics

Efstratios M. Kolibianakis, MD, PhD
Consultant, Centre for Reproductive Medicine
Dutch Speaking Brussels Free University
Brussels, Belgium
Ovulation Induction and Assisted Reproduction

John J. Kopchick, PhD
Goll-Ohio Professor of Molecular Biology
Edison Biotechnology Institute;

Professor of Molecular Biology
Department of Biomedical Sciences
College of Osteopathic Medicine, Ohio University
Athens, Ohio
Growth Hormone

Peter Kopp, MD
Associate Professor, Associate Division Chief for Education
Division of Endocrinology, Metabolism and Molecular Medicine
Feinberg School of Medicine, Northwestern University
Chicago, Illinois
Applications of Genetics in Endocrinology

Kenneth S. Korach, MD
Chief, Laboratory of Reproductive and Developmental Toxicology
Director, Environmental Disease & Medicine Program
Division of Intramural Research
National Institute of Environmental Health Sciences, NIH
Research Triangle Park, North Carolina
Environmental Agents and the Reproductive System

Márta Korbonits, MD, PhD
MRC Clinician Scientist
Senior Lecturer in Endocrinology
Department of Endocrinology
St. Bartholomew's Hospital
London, United Kingdom
Growth Hormone–Releasing Hormone, Ghrelin, and Growth Hormone Secretagogues

Melvyn Korobkin, MD
Professor, Department of Radiology
University of Michigan
Ann Arbor, Michigan
Adrenal Gland Imaging

Stephen M. Krane, MD
Persis, Cyrus and Marlow B. Harrison Distinguished Professor of Medicine
Harvard Medical School;

Physician
Massachusetts General Hospital
Boston, Massachusetts
Disorders of Calcification: Osteomalacia and Rickets

Henry M. Kronenberg, MD
Professor of Medicine, Harvard Medical School;

Chief, Endocrine Unit
Massachusetts General Hospital
Boston, Massachusetts
Parathyroid Hormone and Parathyroid Hormone–Related Peptide in the Regulation of Calcium Homeostasis and Bone Development

Wendy Kuohung, MD
Assistant Professor, Department of Obstetrics and Gynecology
Boston University School of Medicine;

Associate Physician of the Research Staff
Department of Medicine, Division of Endocrinology, Diabetes, and Hypertension
Brigham and Women's Hospital;

Visiting Assistant Professor
Harvard Medical School
Boston, Massachusetts
Gonadotropin-Releasing Hormone and Gonadotropins

John M. Kyriakis, PhD
Professor, Medicine
Tufts University School of Medicine;

Investigator, Molecular Cardiology Research Institute
Tufts-New England Medical Center
Boston, Massachusetts
Map Kinase and Growth Factor Signaling Pathways

Ruth B. Lathi, MD
Clinical Assistant Professor
Division of Reproductive Endocrinology and Infertility
Department of Obstetrics & Gynecology
Stanford University School of Medicine
Stanford, California
Implantation and Placental Physiology in Early Human Pregnancy: The Role of the Maternal Decidua and the Trophoblast

Joop S. E. Laven, MD, PhD
Senior Lecturer
Obstetrics and Gynecology, Division of Reproductive Medicine;

Senior Consultant OBGYN, Subspecialist Reproductive Medicine
Obstetrics and Gynecology, Division of Reproductive Medicine
Erasmus Medical Center
Rotterdam, The Netherlands
Female Subfertility: Evaluation and Management

Diana L. Learoyd, MD
Molecular Genetics Unit
Kolling Institute of Medical Research (DLL, MM, BGR);

Departments of Endocrinology (DLL, BGR) and Surgery (AIG, LWD)
Royal North Shore Hospital and University of Sydney
Sydney, NSW, Australia;

Department of Surgery
Karolinska Hospital (JZ)
Stockholm, Sweden
Medullary Thyroid Carcinoma

Harold E. Lebovitz, MD, FACE
Professor of Medicine
State University of New York Health Science Center at Brooklyn
Brooklyn, New York
Hyperglycemia Secondary to Nondiabetic Conditions and Therapies

Benjamin Z. Leder, MD
Assistant Professor of Medicine
Harvard Medical School;

Endocrine Unit
Massachusetts General Hospital
Boston, Massachusetts
Regulation of Calcium and Phosphate Homeostasis

Colin A. Leech, PhD
Laboratory of Molecular Endocrinology
Massachusetts General Hospital
Boston, Massachusetts
The Cyclic AMP Second Messenger Signaling Pathway

Åke Lernmark, Med. Dr.
Robert H. Williams Professor of Medicine
University of Washington
Seattle, Washington;

Adjunct Professor of Experimental Diabetes
Clinical Medicine
University Hospital MAS
Malmö, Sweden
Type 1 (Insulin-dependent) Diabetes Mellitus: Etiology, Pathogenesis, and Natural History

Michael A. Levine, MD
Chairman, Department of Pediatrics
Cleveland Clinic Lerner College of Medicine of Case Western Reserve University;

Physician-in-Chief
The Children's Hospital
The Cleveland Clinic Foundation
Cleveland, Ohio;

Visiting Professor, Department of Pediatric
The Johns Hopkins University School of Medicine
Baltimore, Maryland
Hypoparathyroidism and Pseudohypoparathyroidism

David M. Levy, MD, FRCP
Consultant Physician, Diabetes & Endocrinology
Gillian Hanson Centre for Diabetes & Endocrinology
Whipps Cross University Hospital;

London Diabetes & Lipid Centre
London, United Kingdom
Diabetes, Lipids, and Atherosclerosis

Laura J. Lewis-Tuffin, PhD
Laboratory of Signal Transduction
National Institute of Environmental Health Sciences, NIH, HHS
Research Triangle Park, North Carolina
Glucocorticoid Receptors and Their Mechanisms of Action

Jonathan Lindzey, PhD
Assistant Professor, Department of Biology
University of South Florida
Tampa, Florida
Environmental Agents and the Reproductive System

Ling Choo LIM, MBBS, MMed, MRCP(UK)
Associate Consultant, Division of Endocrinology
Alexandra Hospital
Singapore
Medullary Thyroid Carcinoma

Catherine Ann Lissett, MBChB, MRCP
Department of Endocrinology
Christie Hospital
Manchester, United Kingdom
Hypopituitarism

Frank W. LoGerfo, MD
William V. McDermott Professor of Surgery
Harvard Medical School;

Chief, Division of Vascular and Endovascular Surgery
Beth Israel Deaconess Medical Center
Boston, Massachusetts
Diabetic Foot and Vascular Complications

B. Macino, MD
Molecular Targeting Unit
Department of Experimental Oncology
Istituto Nazionale Tumori
Milan, Italy
Adrenal Cancer

Noel K. Maclaren, M.D.
Director, Research Institute for Children
Harahan, Louisiana
Autoimmune Polyglandular Syndromes

Carine Maenhaut, PhD
Assistant Professor, IRIBHM
Free University of Brussels
Brussels, Belgium
Thyroid Regulatory Factors

Alan Maisel, MD
Professor of Medicine
University of California, San Diego;

Director, Coronary Care Unit and Heart Failure Program
San Diego, California
Neurohormonal Alterations in Heart Failure

Carl D. Malchoff, MD, PhD
Associate Professor, Medicine
University of Connecticut Health Center
Farmington, Connecticut
Generalized Glucocorticoid Resistance

Diana M. Malchoff, PhD
Assistant Professor, Medicine
University of Connecticut Health Center
Farmington, Connecticut
Generalized Glucocorticoid Resistance

Rayaz A. Malik, BSc, MSc, MB.ChB, MRCP, PhD
Senior Lecturer, Medicine
University of Manchester;

Consultant Physician
Manchester Royal Infirmary
Manchester, United Kingdom
Diabetes Mellitus: Neuropathy

Susan J. Mandel, MD, MPH
Associate Professor of Medicine and Radiology
Division of Endocrinology, Diabetes, and Metabolism
University of Pennsylvania School of Medicine;

Associate Chief for Clinical Affairs
Division of Endocrinology, Diabetes, and Metabolism
Hospital of the University of Pennsylvania
Philadelphia, Pennsylvania
Diagnosis and Treatment of Thyroid Disease during Pregnancy

F. Mantero, MD, PhD
Professor of Endocrinology
Department of Medical and Surgical Sciences
University of Padua;

Director, Division of Endocrinology
University Hospital
Padua, Italy
Adrenal Cancer

Christos Mantzoros, MD, DSc
Associate Professor in Internal Medicine
Division of Endocrinology, Diabetes, and Metabolism
Harvard Medical School
Boston, Massachusetts
Syndromes of Insulin Resistance and Mutant Insulin

Eleftheria Maratos-Flier, MD
Associate Professor of Medicine
Harvard Medical School;

Division of Endocrinology
Beth Israel Deaconess Medical Center
Boston, Massachusetts
Appetite Regulation and Thermogenesis

Michele Marinò, MD
Assistant Professor, Endocrinology
University of Pisa
Pisa, Italy
Graves' Disease

John C. Marshall, MD, PhD
Andrew D. Hart Professor of Medicine
Director, Center for Research in Reproduction
University of Virginia School of Medicine
Charlottesville, Virginia
Regulation of Gonadotropin Synthesis and Secretion
Hormonal Regulation of the Menstrual Cycle and Mechanisms of Ovulation

T. John Martin, MD, DSc, FRS
Emeritus Professor, Medicine
University of Melbourne;

John Holt Fellow
St. Vincent's Institute of Medical Research
Melbourne, Australia
Calcitonin

Thomas F. J. Martin, PhD
Professor of Biochemistry
University of Wisconsin
Madison, Wisconsin
Control of Hormone Secretion

Christopher J. Mathias, PhD, FMedSci
Clinical Professor
Division of Neurosciences and Mental Health, Medicine
Imperial College
London, United Kingdom
Orthostatic Hypotension and Orthostatic Intolerance

Neil J. McKenna, MD
Department of Molecular and Cellular Biology
Baylor College of Medicine
Houston, Texas
Nuclear Receptors: Structure, Function, and Cofactors

Robert I. McLachlan, MD, PhD
Professor, Obstetrics and Gynecology
Monash University;

Deputy Director, Endocrinology
Monash Medical Centre;

Director of Clinical Research
Prince Henry's Institute of Medical Research
Clayton, Victoria, Australia
Androgen Deficiency Disorders

Michael J. McPhaul, MD
Professor
Department of Internal Medicine/Endocrinology and Metabolism
University of Texas Southwestern Medical Center
Dallas, Texas
Mutations That Alter Androgen Receptor Function: Androgen Insensitivity and Related Disorders

Geraldo Medeiros-Neto, MD, FACP
Professor of Endocrinology
Department of Clinical Medicine
University of Sao Paulo Medical School;

Chief of Thyroid Unit
Division of Endocrinology
Department of Clinical Medicine
Hospital Das Clinicas
Sao Paulo Medical School
Sao Paulo, Brazil
Iodine Deficiency Disorders

Juris J. Meier, MD
Research Fellow
Larry L. Hillblom Islet Research Center
University of California, Los Angeles
Los Angeles, California
Insulin Secretion

Shlomo Melmed, MD
Senior Vice President, Academic Affairs
Director, Burns and Allen Research Institute
Associate Dean, UCLA School of Medicine
Cedars-Sinai Medical Center
Los Angeles, California
Evaluation of Pituitary Masses
Acromegaly

Boyd E. Metzger, MD
Tom D. Spies Professor
Northwestern University Feinberg School of Medicine;

Attending Physician
Northwestern Memorial Hospital
Chicago, Illinois
Diabetes Mellitus and Pregnancy

Walter L. Miller, MD
Professor, Pediatrics
University of California, San Francisco;

Chief of Endocrinology
University of California, San Francisco Children's Hospital
San Francisco, California
The Principles, Pathways, and Enzymes of Human Steroidogenesis

Mark E. Molitch, MD
Professor of Medicine
Division of Endocrinology, Metabolism & Molecular Medicine
Department of Medicine
Northwestern University Feinberg School of Medicine;

Attending Physician
Northwestern Memorial Hospital
Chicago, Illinois
Hormonal Changes and Endocrine Testing in Pregnancy

David D. Moore, PhD
Professor, Molecular and Cellular Biology
Baylor College of Medicine
Houston, Texas
Nuclear Receptors: Structure, Function, and Cofactors

Damian G. Morris, MBBS, BSc, MRCP
Department of Endocrinology
St. Bartholomew's and the Royal London School of Medicine and Dentistry
London, United Kingdom
Cushing's Syndrome

Allan Munck, PhD
Third Century Professor of Physiology, Emeritus
Physiology
Dartmouth Medical School
Lebanon, New Hampshire
Glucocorticoid Physiology

Monzur Murshed, PhD
Postdoctoral Associate
Molecular and Human Genetics
Baylor College of Medicine
Houston, Texas
Genetic Analysis of Skeleton Physiology

Anikó Náray-Fejes-Tóth, MD
Professor of Physiology
Dartmouth Medical School
Lebanon, New Hampshire
Glucocorticoid Physiology

Ralf Nass, MD
Research Associate
University of Virginia School of Medicine
Charlottesville, Virginia
Growth Hormone–Releasing Hormone, Ghrelin, and Growth Hormone Secretagogues

David M. Nathan, MD
Professor, Medicine
Harvard Medical School;

Director, Diabetes Center and General Clinical Research Center
Massachusetts General Hospital
Boston, Massachusetts
Diabetes Control and Long-term Complications

Maria I. New, MD
Professor of Pediatrics
Director, Adrenal Steroid Disorders Program
Attending Pediatrician, Department of Pediatrics
Mount Sinai School of Medicine
New York, New York
Defects of Adrenal Steroidogenesis

Lynnette K. Nieman, MD
Senior Investigator
Pediatric and Reproductive Endocrinology Branch, NICHD
National Institutes of Health
Bethesda, Maryland
Cushing's Syndrome

John H. Nilson, PhD
Edward R. Meyer Distinguished Professor Director
School of Molecular Biosciences
Washington State University
Pullman, Washington
Hormones and Gene Expression: Basic Principles

Christopher F. Njeh, MSc, PhD, CPhys
Assistant Adjunct Professor, Physics
California State University;

Senior Medical Physicist
Radiation Oncology
Saint Agnes Medical Center
Fresno, California
Bone Density and Imaging of Osteoporosis

Jeffrey A. Norton, MD
Professor of Surgery, Chief of Surgical Oncology
Stanford University;

Surgery
Stanford University Hospital
Stanford, California
Surgical Management of Hyperparathyroidism

Kjell Öberg, MD, PhD
Medical Faculty
Department of Medical Sciences
Uppsala University;

Department of Endocrine Oncology
University Hospital
Uppsala, Sweden
Carcinoid Syndrome

William D. Odell, MD, PhD, MACP
Emeritus Professor of Medicine and Physiology
University of Utah School of Medicine
Salt Lake City, Utah
Endocrinology of Sexual Maturation

Jerrold M. Olefsky, MD
Professor of Medicine
Department of Medicine
University of California, San Diego;

Associate Dean for Scientific Affairs
School of Medicine
University of California, San Diego
La Jolla, California
Type 2 Diabetes Mellitus: Etiology, Pathogenesis, and Natural History

Stephen O'Rahilly, MD, FRS
Professor of Clinical Biochemistry and Medicine
Clinical Biochemistry
University of Cambridge;

Honorary Consultant
Diabetes and Endocrinology
Addenbrooke's Hospital
Cambridge, United Kingdom
Genetic Syndromes Associated with Obesity

Karel Pacak, MD, PhD, DSc
Chief, Unit on Clinical Neuroendocrinology
Pediatric and Reproductive Endocrinology Branch
National Institute of Child Health and Human Development
National Institutes of Health
Bethesda, Maryland
  Pheochromocytoma

Furio Pacini, MD
Professor of Endocrinology
Internal Medicine, Endocrinology and Metabolism
Sienna, Italy
  Thyroid Neoplasia

Samuel Parry, MD
Assistant Professor
Obstetrics and Gynecology
University of Pennsylvania
Philadelphia, Pennsylvania
  Placental Hormones

Francesca Pecori Giraldi, MD
Researcher
Chair of Endocrinology
University of Milan;

Staff Physician
Department of Endocrinology
Istituto Auxologico Italiano, Ospedale San Luca, IRCCS
Milan, Italy
  Adrenal Causes of Hypercortisolism

Luca Persani, MD, PhD
Associate Professor
Institute of Endocrine Science
University of Milan;

Head, Laboratory of Experimental Endocrinology
IRCCS Instituto Auxologico Italiano
Milan, Italy
  TSH-Producing Adenomas

Ora Hirsch Pescovitz, MD
Executive Associate Dean for Research Affairs
Edwin Letzer Professor of Pediatrics
Professor of Cellular and Integrative Physiology
School of Medicine
Indiana University;

President and CEO
Riley Hospital for Children
Indianapolis, Indiana
  Precocious Puberty
  Delayed Puberty

Richard L. Phelps, MD
Assistant Clinical Professor of Medicine
Northwestern University Medical School;

Attending Physician
Northwestern Memorial Hospital
Chicago, Illinois
  Diabetes Mellitus and Pregnancy

Aldo Pinchera, PhD
Department of Endocrinology
University of Pisa
Cisanello Hospital
Pisa, Italy
  Graves' Disease

John T. Potts, Jr., MD
Jackson Distinguished Professor of Clinical Medicine
Department of Medicine
Harvard Medical School;

Physician-in-Chief Emeritus
Department of Medicine
Massachusetts General Hospital
Boston, Massachusetts
  Parathyroid Hormone and Parathyroid Hormone–Related Peptide in the Regulation of Calcium Homeostasis and Bone Development
  Medical Management of Hypercalcemia

Lisa P. Purdy, MD, CM, MPH
Assistant Professor of Medicine
University of Rochester School of Medicine and Dentistry;

Attending Physician
Genesee Hospital
Rochester General Hospital
Strong Memorial Hospital
Rochester, New York
  Diabetes Mellitus and Pregnancy

Charmian A. Quigley, MBBS
Assistant Professor
Indiana University School of Medicine
Indiana University;

Senior Clinical Research Physician
Endocrinology
Lilly Research Laboratories
Indianapolis, Indiana
  Genetic Basis of Gonadal and Genital Development

Marcus O. Quinkler, MD
Clinical Endocrinology, Department of Medicine
Charité Campus Mitte
Berlin, Germany
  Mineralocorticoid Deficiency

Christine Campion Quirk, PhD
Assistant Professor
Medical Sciences Program
Indiana University School of Medicine
Bloomington, Indiana
  Hormones and Gene Expression: Basic Principles

Miriam T. Rademaker, MD
Christchurch School of Medicine
Christchurch, New Zealand
  Hormones of the Cardiovascular System

Ewa Rajpert-De Meyts, MD, PhD
Senior Scientist
Deparment of Growth and Reproduction
Copenhagen University Hospital (Rigshopitalet)
Copenhagen, Denmark
  Testicular Tumors with Endocrine Manifestations

Valerie Anne Randall, PhD
Professor of Biomedical Sciences
The University of Bradford
Bradford, United Kingdom
  Physiology and Pathophysiology of Androgenetic Alopecia

Eric Ravussin, PhD
Professor, Human Physiology
Pennington Biomedical Research Center
Louisiana State University
Baton Rouge, Louisiana
  Role of the Adipocyte in Metabolism and Endocrine Function

David W. Ray
Senior Lecturer in Medicine
Centre for Molecular Medicine and Endocrine Sciences Research
    Group
University of Manchester;

Consultant in Endocrinology
Manchester Royal Infirmary
Manchester, United Kingdom
    Ectopic Hormone Syndromes

Nancy E. Reame, MSN, PhD, FAAN
The Rhetaugh Graves Dumas Professor of Nursing
School of Nursing;

Research Scientist
Reproductive Sciences Program
Department of Obstetrics-Gynecology
The University of Michigan
Franklin, Michigan
    Premenstrual Syndrome

Samuel Refetoff, PhD
Professor of Medicine, Pediatrics, Genetics
University of Chicago
Chicago, Illinois
    Diagnostic Tests of the Thyroid

Ravi Retnakaran, MD, MSc, FRCPC
Endocrinology Fellow
Division of Endocrinology and Metabolism
University of Toronto;

Endocrinology Fellow
Leadership Sinai Centre for Diabetes
Mount Sinai Hospital
Toronto, Ontario, Canada
    Treatment of Type 1 Diabetes Mellitus in Adults

Rodolfo Rey, MD, PhD
Centro de Investigaciones en Reproducción
Department of Histology, Cell Biology, Embryology and Genetics
School of Medicine, University of Buenos Aires;

Centro do Investigaciones Endocrinológicas (CONICET)
Hospital de Niños R. Gutiérrez
Buenos Aires, Argentina
    Embryology and Control of Fetal Sex Differentiation

Gail P. Risbridger, PhD
Professor and Associate Director
Monash Institute of Reproduction and Development
Monash University
Clayton, Victoria, Australia
    Endocrinology of Prostate Cancer

Robert A. Rizza, MD
Earl and Arlene McDonough Professor of Medicine
Division of Endocrinology, Diabetes, Metabolism and Nutrition
Mayo School of Medicine
Rochester, Minnesota
    Classification and Diagnosis of Diabetes Mellitus

Bruce G. Robinson, MD
Professor
Royal North Shore Hospital
University of Sydney
Syndey, NSW, Australia
    Medullary Thyroid Carcinoma

Gideon A. Rodan, MD, PhD
Adjunct Professor
Biochemistry and Biophysics
University of Pennsylvania
Philadelphia, Pennsylvania
    Bone Development and Remodeling

Pierre P. Roger, MD
Department of Endocrinology and Reproductive Diseases
Assistance Publique-Hopitaux de Paris
Centre Hospitalier d'Universite Bicetre
Le Kremlin-Bicetre, France.
    Thyroid Regulatory Factors

Michael G. Rosenfeld, PhD
Professor of Medicine
Endocrinology and Metabolism
University of California, San Diego
La Jolla, California
    Development of the Pituitary

Robert L. Rosenfield, MD
Professor, Pediatrics and Medicine
The University of Chicago Pritzker School of Medicine;

Pediatric Endocrinologist
The University of Chicago Comer Children's Hospital
Chicago, Illinois
    Somatic Growth and Maturation
    Hyperandrogenism, Hirsutism, and the Polycystic Ovary Syndrome

Peter Rotwein, MD
Professor and Chair
Department of Biochemistry and Molecular Biology;

Director, Molecular Medicine Division
Department of Medicine
Oregon Health and Science University
Portland, Oregon
    Peptide Growth Factors Other than Insulin-like Growth Factors
    or Cytokines

Arthur H. Rubenstein, MD
Dean
Mount Sinai School of Medicine
New York, New York
    Chemistry and Biosynthesis of the Islet Hormones: Insulin,
    Islet Amyloid Polypeptide (Amylin), Glucagon, Somatostatin, and
    Pancreatic Polypeptide

Robert T. Rubin, MD, PhD
Professor, Psychiatry and Biobehavioral Sciences
David Geffen School of Medicine at UCLA;

Chair, Department of Psychiatry
Veterans Affairs Greater Los Angeles Healthcare System
Los Angeles, California
    Anorexia Nervosa, Bulimia Nervosa, and Other Eating Disorders

Neil Ruderman, MD, DPhil
Professor of Medicine, Physiology, and Biophysics
Boston University School of Medicine;

Director, Diabetes Unit
Boston Medical Center
Boston, Massachusetts
    The Metabolic Syndrome

Irma H. Russo, MD, FCAP, FASCP
Adjunct Professor of Pathology and Cell Biology
Jefferson Medical College
Thomas Jefferson University;

Chief, Molecular Endocrinology Section
Breast Cancer Research Laboratory
Department of Pathology;
Active Staff
Department of Surgical Oncology
American Oncologic Hospital;
Member, Medical Science Division
Fox Chase Cancer Center
Philadelphia, Pennsylvania
    Hormonal Control of Breast Development

Jose Russo, MD
Professor of Pathology and Laboratory Medicine
Jefferson School of Medicine;

American Oncology Hospital, Pathology
Director, Breast Cancer and the Environment Research Center
Fox Chase Cancer Center;
Philadelphia, Pennsylvania
Hormonal Control of Breast Development

Isidro B. Salusky, MD
Professor of Pediatrics
Director, Pediatric Dialysis Program
Director, General Clinical Research
David Geffen School of Medicine at UCLA
Los Angeles, California;

Treasurer, International Pediatric Nephrology Association (IPNA)
Freibrug, Germany
The Renal Osteodystrophies

Richard J. Santen, MD
Professor of Internal Medicine
Department of Internal Medicine
Division of Endocrinology and Metabolism
University of Virginia Health System
Charlottesville, Virginia
Hormonal Control of Breast Development
Benign Breast Disorders
Gynecomastia

Nanette Santoro, MD
Professor and Director
Division of Reproductive Endocrinology and Infertility
Albert Einstein College of Medicine
Bronx, New York
Mechanisms of Menopause and the Menopausal Transition

Stuart C. Sealfon, MD
Saunders Professor of Neurology
Mount Sinai School of Medicine
New York, New York
Hormone Signaling via G Protein-Coupled Receptors

Patrick M. Sexton, PhD
Senior Research Fellow, Molecular Pharmacology
Howard Florey Institute
The University of Melbourne
South Carlton, Victoria, Australia
Calcitonin

Stephen Michael Shalet, BSc, MBBS, MD, FRCP
Professor of Medicine (Endocrinology)
University of Manchester;

Head of Department, Endocrinology
Christie Hospital
Manchester, England
Hypopituitarism

Yoram Shenker, MD
Associate Professor, Medicine
University of Wisconsin;

Staff Physician
University of Wisconsin;

Chief, Section of Endocrinology
William S. Middleton Memorial VA Hospital
Madison, Wisconsin
Hormonal Regulation of Electrolyte and Water Metabolism

Gerald I. Shulman, MD, PhD
Professor of Medicine and Cellular and Molecular Physiology
Internal Medicine
Yale School of Medicine;

Doctor
Endocrinology
Yale New Haven Hospital
New Haven, Connecticut
The Metabolic Syndrome

Alison Silverberg, MD
Albert Einstein College of Medicine
Division of Reproductive Endocrinology
Bronx, New York
Mechanisms of Menopause and the Menopausal Transition

Shonni J. Silverberg, MD
Professor of Clinical Medicine
Columbia University, College of Physicians and Surgeons;

Attending, Division of Endocrinology
New York Presbyterian Hospital
New York, New York
Primary Hyperparathyroidism

Frederick R. Singer, MD
Clinical Professor of Medicine
David Geffen School of Medicine
Los Angeles, California;

Director, Endocrine/Bone Disease Program
John Wayne Cancer Institute
Santa Monica, California
Paget's Disease of Bone

Niels E. Skakkebœk, MD, DSc
Professor
University of Copenhagen;

Head, Department of Growth and Reproduction
Copenhagen University Hospital (Rigshospitalet)
Copenhagen, Denmark
Testicular Tumors with Endocrine Manifestations

Carolyn L. Smith, PhD
Associate Professor
Molecular and Cellular Biology
Baylor College of Medicine
Houston, Texas
Estrogen and Progesterone Action

Steven R. Smith, MD
Associate Professor
Chief, Inpatient Unit
Experimental Endocrinology
Pennington Biomedical Research Center
Baton Rouge, Louisianna
Role of the Adipocyte in Metabolism and Endocrine Function

Peter J. Snyder, MD
Professor of Medicine
University of Pennsylvania
Philadelphia, Pennsylvania
Gonadotroph and Other Clinically Nonfunctioning Pituitary Adenomas

John T. Soper, MD
Professor, Department of Obstetrics and Gynecology
Duke University Medical Center
Durham, North Carolina
Gestational Trophoblastic Neoplasms

Richard Stanhope, MD, FRCP
Honorary Senior Lecturer
Department of Biochemistry, Endocrinology and Metabolism
Institute of Child Health;

Consultant Paediatric Endocrinologist
Department of Endocrinology
Great Ormond Street Hospital for Children;

Consultant Paediatric Endocrinologist
Department of Adolescent Endocrinology
University College Hospital;

Consultant Paediatric Endocrinologist
Department of Paediatrics
The Portland Hospital for Women and Children
London, United Kingdom
*Evaluation and Management of Childhood Hypothalamic and
Pituitary Tumors*

René St-Arnaud, PhD
Associate Professor
Medicine, Surgery, and Human Genetics
McGill University;

Scientist, Genetics Unit
Shriners Hospital for Children
Montreal, Quebec, Canada
Genetic Defects in Vitamin D Metabolism and Action

Donald L. St. Germain, MD
Professor, Medicine and Physiology
Dartmouth Medical School
Lebanon, New Hampshire
Thyroid Hormone Metabolism

Donald F. Steiner, MD
Professor, Biochemistry and Molecular Biology
The University of Chicago;

Senior Investigator
Howard Hughes Medical Institute
Chicago, Illinois
*Chemistry and Biosynthesis of the Islet Hormones: Insulin, Islet
Amyloid Polypeptide (Amylin), Glucagon, Somatostatin, and
Pancreatic Polypeptide*

Andrew F. Stewart, MD
Professor and Chief
Division of Endocrinology and Metabolism
University of Pittsburgh School of Medicine
Pittsburgh, Pennsylvania
Malignancy-Associated Hypercalcemia

Paul M. Stewart, MD
Professor of Medicine
University of Birmingham
Queen Elizabeth Hospital
Birmingham, United Kingdom
Mineralocorticoid Deficiency

Jim Stockigt, MD, FRACP, FRCPA
Professor of Medicine
Monash University;

Senior Endocrinologist
Ewen Downie Metabolic Unit
Alfred Hospital;

Consultant Endocrinologist
Epworth Hospital
Melbourne, Australia
Thyroid Hormone Binding and Variants of Transport Proteins

Michael Stowasser, MBBS, FRACP, PhD
Associate Professor
Hypertension Unit, Department of Medicine
University of Queensland;

Director, Hypertension Unit
Princess Alexandra Hospital;

Director, Hypertension Unit
Greenslopes Hospital
Brisbane, Queensland, Australia
Primary Mineralocorticoid Excess Syndromes

Jerome F. Strauss, III, MD, PhD
The Luigi Mastroianni Jr. Professor and Director
Center for Research on Reproduction and Women's Health
University of Pennsylvania;

Associate Chairman
Department of Obstetrics and Gynecology
University of Pennsylvania Health System
Philadelphia, Pennsylvania
Ovarian Hormone Synthesis
Placental Hormones

Lillian M. Swiersz, MD
Departments of Gynecology and Obstetrics and Radiation Biology
Stanford University
Stanford, California
Endometriosis

Mariusz W. Szkudlinski, MD, PhD
Vice President for Research and Development
Trophogen, Inc
Rockville, Maryland
Thyroid-Stimulating Hormone and Regulation of the Thyroid Axis

Shahrad Taheri BSc, MSc, PhD, MB, BS, MRCP
Lecturer in Medicine and Endocrinology
Henry Wellcome Laboratories for Integrative Neuroscience and
  Endocrinology
University of Bristol;

Lecturer in Medicine and Endocrinology
Diabetes and Endocrinology
Bristol Royal Infirmary;

Lecturer in Medicine and Endocrinology
Diabetes and Endocrinology
Southmead Hospital
Bristol, United Kingdom
Gastrointestinal Hormones and Tumor Syndromes

Rajesh V. Thakker, MD, FRCP, FRCPath, FMedSci
May Professor of Medicine
Nuffield Department of Medicine
University of Oxford
Oxford, Oxon, United Kingdom
*Genetic Disorders of Calcium Homeostasis Caused by Abnormal
  Regulation of Parathyroid Hormone Secretion or Responsiveness
Multiple Endocrine Neoplasia Type 1*

Axel A. Thomson, PhD
Programme Leader, MRC Human Reproductive Sciences Unit
Edinburgh, Scotland
Endocrinology of the Prostate and Benign Prostatic Hyperplasia

Michael O. Thorner, MB, BS, DSc
Henry B. Mulholland Professor and Chair
Internal Medicine
University of Virginia School of Medicine
Charlottesville, Virginia
*Growth Hormone–Releasing Hormone, Ghrelin, and Growth Hormone
Secretagogues*

Jorma Toppari, MD, PhD
Professor, Departments of Physiology and Pediatrics
University of Turku
Turku, Finland
Testicular Tumors with Endocrine Manifestations

Cristina Traggiai, MD
Department of Paediatrics
Institute G. Gaslini
Genoa, Italy
Evaluation and Management of Childhood Hypothalamic and Pituitary Tumors

Greet Van den Berghe, MD, PhD
Professor of Medicine
Faculty of Medicine
Catholic University of Leuven;

Director, Department of Intensive Care
University Hospital Gasthuisberg-Catholic University of Leuven
Leuven, Belgium
Endocrine Aspects of Critical Care Medicine

Eve Van Cauter, PhD
Department of Medicine
The University of Chicago
Chicago, Illinois
Endocrine and Other Biologic Rhythms

André C. Van Steirteghem, MD, PhD
Professor, Embryology and Genetics
Vrije Universiteit Brussel (VUB);

Co-Director, Centre for Reproductive Medicine
Academisch Ziekenhuis VUB
Brussels, Belgium
Ovulation Induction and Assisted Reproduction

Gilbert Vassart, MD, PhD
Institut de Recherche Interdisciplinaire en Biologie Humaine et
  Moléculaire
Université Libre de Bruxelles
Campus Erasme;

Department of Medical Genetics
Université Libre de Bruxelles
Hôpital Erasme
Brussels, Belgium
Thyroid Regulatory Factors
Thyroid-Stimulating Hormone Receptor Mutations

Jan J. M. de Vijlder, MSc, PhD
Professor of Biochemistry
University of Amsterdam;

Emma Children's Hospital
Academic Medical Center
Amsterdam, The Netherlands
Genetic Defects in Thyroid Hormone Synthesis and Action: Defects in Thyroid Hormone Synthesis

Thomas Vulsma, MD, PhD, MSc
Associate Professor of Pediatric Endocrinology
University of Amsterdam;

Pediatric Endocrinologist
Emma Children's Hospital
Academic Medical Center
Amsterdam, The Netherlands
Genetic Defects in Thyroid Hormone Synthesis and Action: Defects in Thyroid Hormone Synthesis

Michael P. Wajnrajch, MD
Assistant Professor of Pediatrics
Department of Pediatrics
Division of Pediatric Endocrinology
Weill Medical College of Cornell University;

Visiting Associate Research Scientist
Department of Pediatrics
Division of Molecular Genetics
Columbia University College of Physicians and Surgeons
New York, New York
Defects of Adrenal Steroidogenesis

Kathleen E. Walsh, DO, MS
Assistant Clinical Professor, School of Medicine
University of Wisconsin-Madison
Madison, Wisconsin;

Emergency Medicine Physician, The Monroe Clinic
Monroe, Wisconsin
Female Sexual Dysfunction

Anthony P. Weetman, MD, DSc
Professor of Medicine and Dean
School of Medicine and Biomedical Sciences
University of Sheffield;

Honorary Consultant Endocrinologist
Sheffield Teaching Hospitals
Sheffield, United Kingdom
Autoimmune Thyroid Disease

Nancy L. Weigel, PhD
Professor, Molecular and Cellular Biology
Baylor College of Medicine
Houston, Texas
Estrogen and Progesterone Action

David A. Weinstein, MD, MMSc
Instructor in Pediatrics, Harvard Medical School;

Director, Glycogen Storage Disease Program
Division of Endocrinology
Children's Hospital Boston
Boston, Massachusetts
Management of Diabetes in Children

Bruce D. Weintraub, MD
Chief Operating Officer, Chief Scientific Officer
Trophogen Inc.
Rockville, Maryland
Thyroid-Stimulating Hormone and Regulation of the Thyroid Axis

Gordon C. Weir, MD
Head, Section on Islet Transplantation and Cell Biology
Diabetes Research and Wellness Foundation Chair
Joslin Diabetes Center;

Professor of Medicine
Harvard Medical School
Boston, Massachusetts
Pancreatic and Islet Transplantation

Roy E. Weiss, MD, PhD, FACP
Professor of Medicine, Program Director
General Clinical Research Center
University of Chicago, Pritzker School of Medicine
Chicago, Illinois
Diagnostic Tests of the Thyroid

Katherine Wesseling, MD
Fellow, Pediatrics, Division of Nephrology
University of California at Los Angeles;

Doctor, Pediatric Nephrology
Mattel Children's Hospital, UCLA
Los Angeles, California
The Renal Osteodystrophies

Anne White, PhD
Professor, Endocrine Sciences
University of Manchester
Manchester, United Kingdom
Adrenocorticotropic Hormone

Morris F. White, PhD
Principal Investigator
Harvard Medical School
Joslin Diabetes Center
Boston, Massachusetts
The Molecular Basis of Insulin Action

Wilmar M. Wiersinga, MD
Professor of Endocrinology
Endocrinology Metabolism
Academic Medical Center, University of Amsterdam;

Professor and Doctor
Department of Endocrinology and Metabolism
Academic Medical Center
Amsterdam, The Netherlands
Hypothyroidism and Myxedema Coma

Joseph I. Wolfsdorf, MB, BCh
Associate Professor, Pediatrics
Harvard Medical School
Boston, Massachusetts;

Director, Diabetes Program
Associate Chief, Division of Endocrinology
Department of Medicine
Children's Hospital Boston
Boston, Massachusetts
Management of Diabetes in Children

Yalemzewd Woredekal, MD
Assistant Professor of Medicine
Medicine Renal Division
SUNY-Downstate Medical Center;

Medical Director of Dialysis Service
Medicine Renal Division
Kings County Hospital Center
Brooklyn, New York
Diabetic Nephropathy

Sharon Y. Wu, MD
Fellow, Section of Endocrinology
Department of Medicine
University of Chicago
Chicago, Illinois
Diagnostic Tests of the Thyroid

Wei Wu, PhD
Assistant Project Scientist
University of California at San Diego
La Jolla, California
Development of the Pituitary

Run Yu
Fellow, Cedars-Sinai Research Institute
University of California Los Angeles School of Medicine;

Fellow, Division of Endocrinology, Diabetes, and Metabolism
Cedars-Sinai Medical Center
Los Angeles, California
Cell Division, Differentiation, Senescence, and Death

Bernard Zinman, MDCM, FRCPC, FACP
Professor of Medicine
University of Toronto;

Director
Leadership Sinai Centre for Diabetes
Mount Sinai Hospital;

Senior Scientist
Samuel Lunenfeld Research Institute
Mount Sinai Hospital
Toronto, Ontario, Canada
Treatment of Type 1 Diabetes Mellitus in Adults

Preface

The origins of the fifth edition of *Endocrinology* go back nearly 40 years, which is a long time in the history of contemporary textbooks, although obviously a mere step in the march of medical history. In 1966, John B. Stanbury, MD, who had just successfully published a new and important text called "The Metabolic Basis of Inherited Disease," suggested that a similar approach to endocrinology would be useful. The idea was to develop a book that combined basic mechanisms with diagnosis and management of endocrine diseases, in sharp contrast to the quite clinically oriented texts then available. The idea took root, but a very long gestation followed.

George Cahill and David Kipnis were instrumental in nurturing the concept, but it finally took nine editors and years of work to bring the first edition to press in 1979. The second edition followed in 1989, third edition in 1995, and fourth edition in 2001. Of the original editors, Leslie J. DeGroot, John C. Marshall, and John T. Potts have persisted through each edition. Gordon M. Besser, Don H. Nelson, William D. Odell, Arthur Rubenstein, Emil Steinberger, Henry G. Burger, and D. Lynn Loriaux made immense contributions to these earlier editions. We proudly add Gordon C. Weir, Ashley B. Grossman, and David de Kretser to the masthead of the fifth edition. The authors include more than 300 experts from all over the globe, reflecting the international contributions to the science of endocrinology.

Our goals, as stated in the first edition, remain unchanged. We want our text to provide a complete, contemporary source of basic and clinical aspects of endocrinology. Our book is directed to serious students of endocrinology—a group that includes undergraduates, residents, fellows, and practicing physicians, as well as researchers.

The goals we sought to achieve in 1966 are as crucial today as they were then: to review basic knowledge of endocrine physiology and biochemistry in a complete and up-to-date manner; to provide a thorough clinical discussion of each topic; to integrate the basic and clinical material around human endocrinology; to make clear the integration of the endocrine system in a gland-by-gland manner, as well as the important multi-hormonal integration in endocrine function; and to have our presentation made by the most accomplished endocrinologists in the world.

We recognize the enormous transformation in the use of medical information. Readers, especially those in training, desire instant access to information on the internet. Powerful search engines can track down even the most obscure facts within seconds. While this strategy is valuable for locating snippets of information, it often lacks context and depth. Thus, while great effort and cost are necessary to prepare a multi-authored book, such texts remain important because an expert synthesizes the daunting body of available information. A growing number of students are rediscovering the value of well-written chapters as a means to gain a deep understanding of a topic.

The best of both worlds is a living text that is continuously updated and designed to complement other forms of electronically available information. That is why the fifth edition is available as a hardcover text and on the internet. The online e-dition will be updated regularly with a particular focus on ground-breaking studies. The e-dition also provides a means to keep diagnostic and treatment guidelines updated between editions.

In closing, the editors express their deep gratitude to the authors who once again have provided very readable chapters filled with carefully organized medical information. It is their dedication to teaching that makes our book valuable to readers.

Leslie J. DeGroot, MD

Larry Jameson, MD

Contents

A complete index appears at the end of each volume.

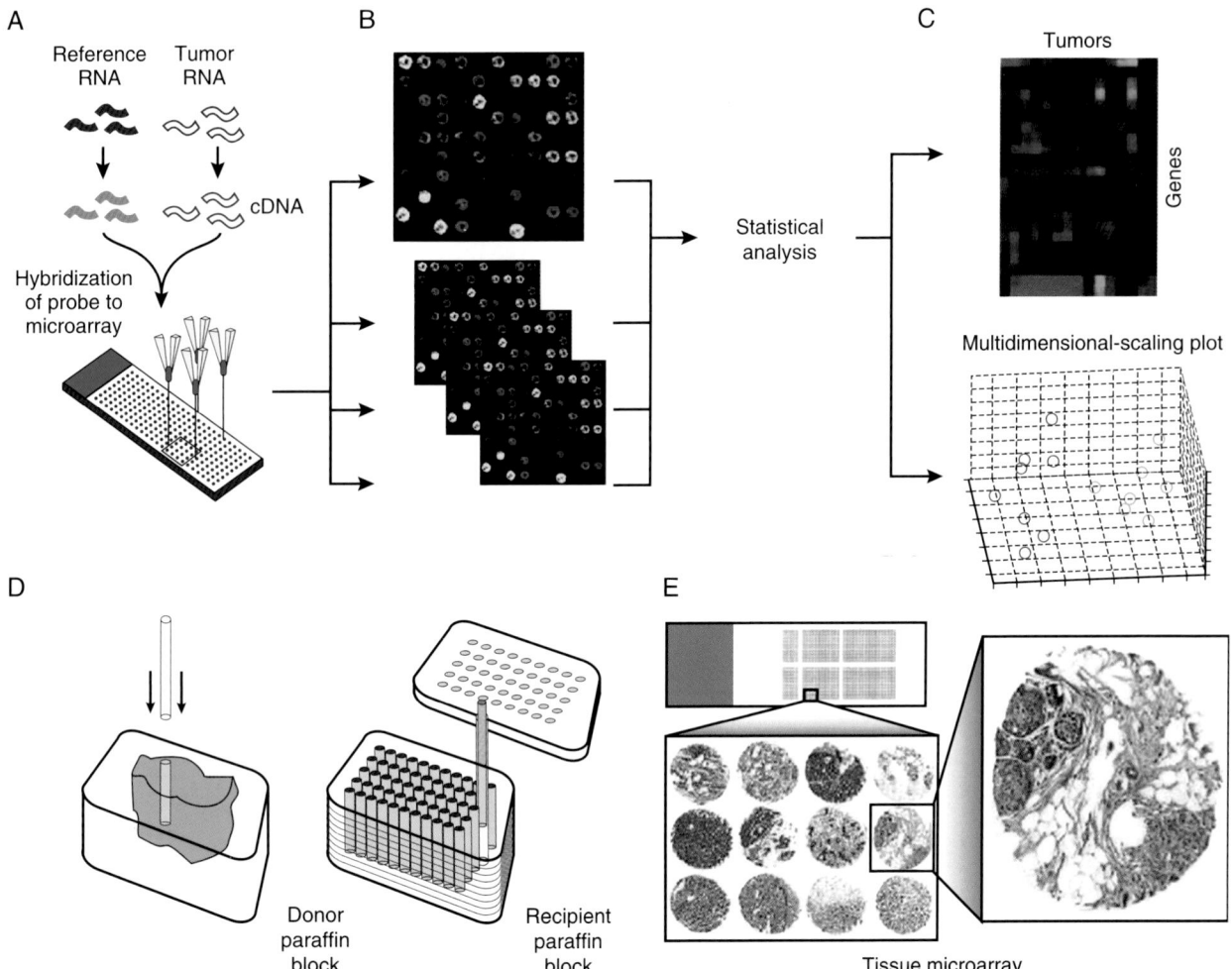

Figure 4-3 Robotically spotted microarray hybridized to two samples, each stained with two colored dyes. An overview of procedures for preparing and analyzing complementary DNA (cDNA) microarrays and breast-tumor tissue. **Panel A:** Reference RNA and tumor RNA are labeled by reverse transcription with different fluorescent dyes (green for the reference cells and red for the tumor cells) and hybridized to a cDNA microarray containing robotically printed cDNA clones. **Panel B:** The slides are scanned with a confocal laser scanning microscope, and color images are generated for each hybridization with RNA from the tumor and reference cells. Genes upregulated in the tumors appear red, whereas those with decreased expression appear green. Genes with similar levels of expression in the two samples appear yellow. Genes of interest are selected on the basis of the differences in the level of expression by known tumor classes (e.g., BRCA1-mutation-positive and BRCA2-mutation-positive). Bioinformatics analysis determines whether these differences in the gene-expression profiles are greater than would be expected by chance. **Panel C:** The differences in the patterns of gene expression between tumor classes can be portrayed in the form of a color-coded plot, and the relations between tumors can be portrayed in the form of a multidimensional-scaling plot. Tumors with similar gene-expression profiles cluster close to one another in the multidimensional-scaling plot. **Panel D:** Particular genes of interest can be further studied through the use of a large number of arrayed, paraffin-embedded tumor specimens, referred to as tissue microarrays. **Panel E:** Immunohistochemical analyses of hundreds or thousands of these arrayed biopsy specimens can be performed in order to extend the microarray findings.

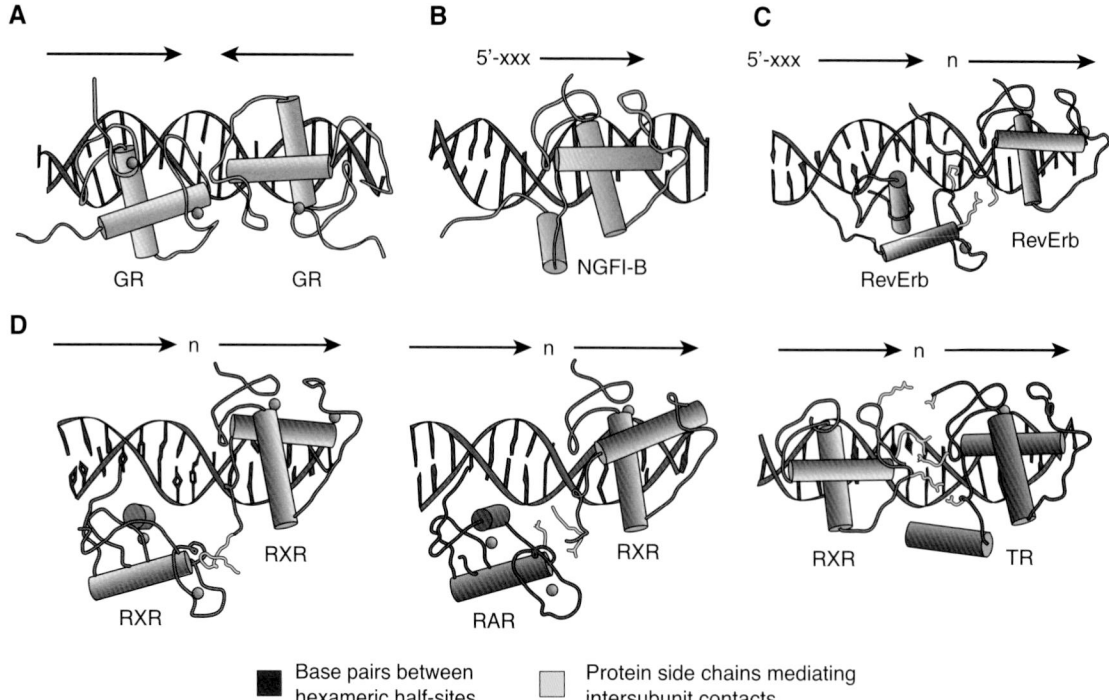

Figure 15-2 Structures of complexes between receptor DNA-binding domains and their cognate DNA-response elements. **A,** GR homodimer bound to an inverted element with a 3-base-pair spacer (IR-3). **B,** NGFI-B bound to its extended monomeric site. **C,** RevErb homodimer bound to an extended direct repeat element with a 2-base-pair spacer (DR-2) and **D,** RXR as a homodimer bound to a DR-1 element, RAR/RXR on a DR-1 element and TR/RXR heterodimer bound to a DR-4 site. Note that RXR binds only at the upstream half-site on the DR-4 HRE with TR, and only at the downstream half-site on the DR-1 with RAR. Cylinders indicate helices, base pairs between the hexameric half-sites are shown in red, and protein side chains mediating intersubunit contacts are shown in yellow. (Reproduced with permission from Khorasanizadeh S, Rastinejad F: Nuclear-receptor interactions on DNA-response elements. Trends Biochem Sci 26:384–390, 2001.)

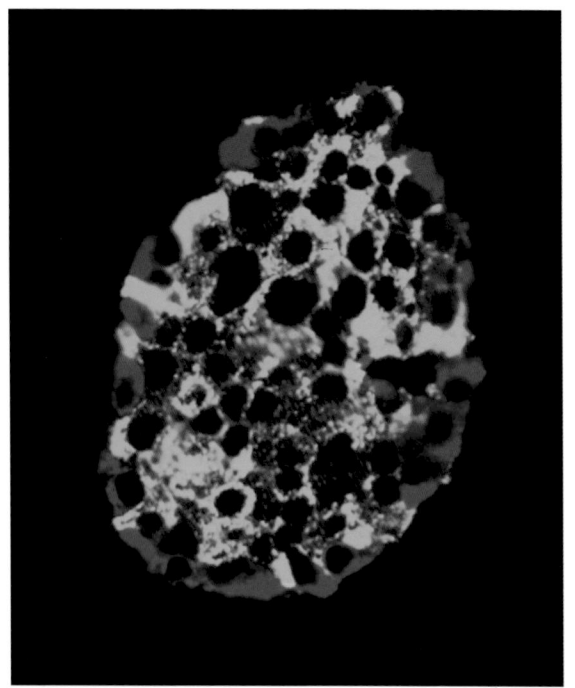

Figure 49-1 A human islet of Langerhans stained by immunofluoresence for insulin (green) and glucagons (blue).

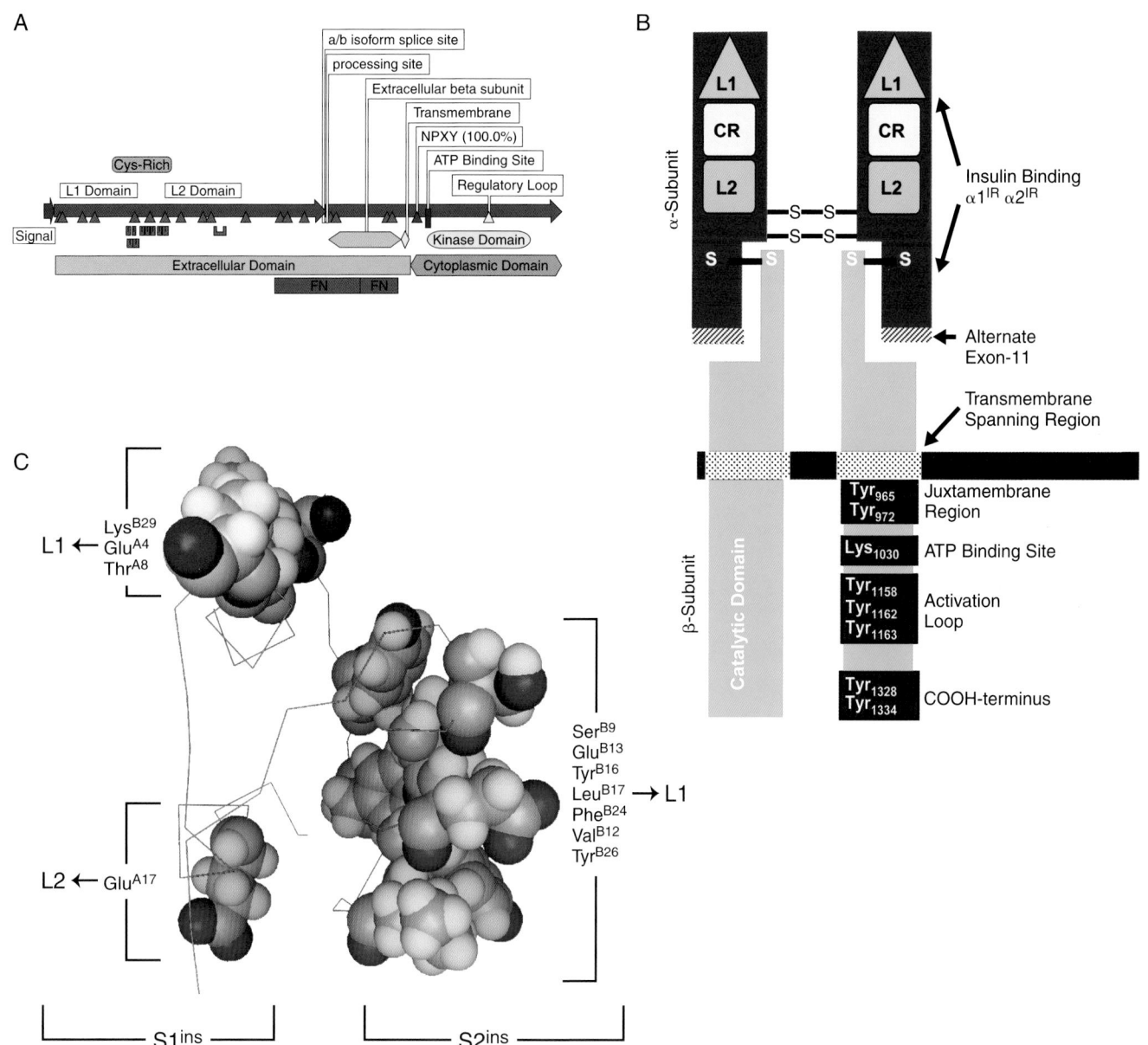

Figure 50-2 Structure of insulin and the insulin receptor. **A,** A linear diagram of the insulin receptor precursor showing the relative position of important landmarks in the a subunit, the ligand contact points L1 and L2, the cysteine-rich region (Cys-rich), disulfide bonds (⊔), glycosylation sites (▲) the IRa/IRb splice site, the processing site between the α subunit and the β subunit, and important landmarks in the β subunit, the extracellular region, the hydrophobic transmembrane region, the PTB recognition motif, the ATP binding site, and the regulatory loop (A loop) in the kinase domain. **B,** A diagram of the insulin receptor extracellular, transmembrane, and intracellular components composed of two extracellular α subunits and two β subunits that contain. The holoreceptor is joined by disulfide bonds between cysteine residues in the extracellular α and β subunits as well as by noncovalent interactions. The a subunit contains several regions that contribute to insulin binding, including the L1 and L2 regions separated by a cysteine-rich region, and a 12-amino acid alternatively spliced region encoded by exon-11. The β subunit contains a tyrosine kinase catalytic domain with an ATP-binding site and a number of tyrosine phosphorylation sites including those in the juxtamembrane, activation loop, and COOH-terminal regions. **C,** The insulin diagram shows the amino acids that compose the two surfaces of the insulin molecule (S1^{ins} and S2^{ins}) and the amino acids that interact with the L1 and L2 regions of the insulin receptor.

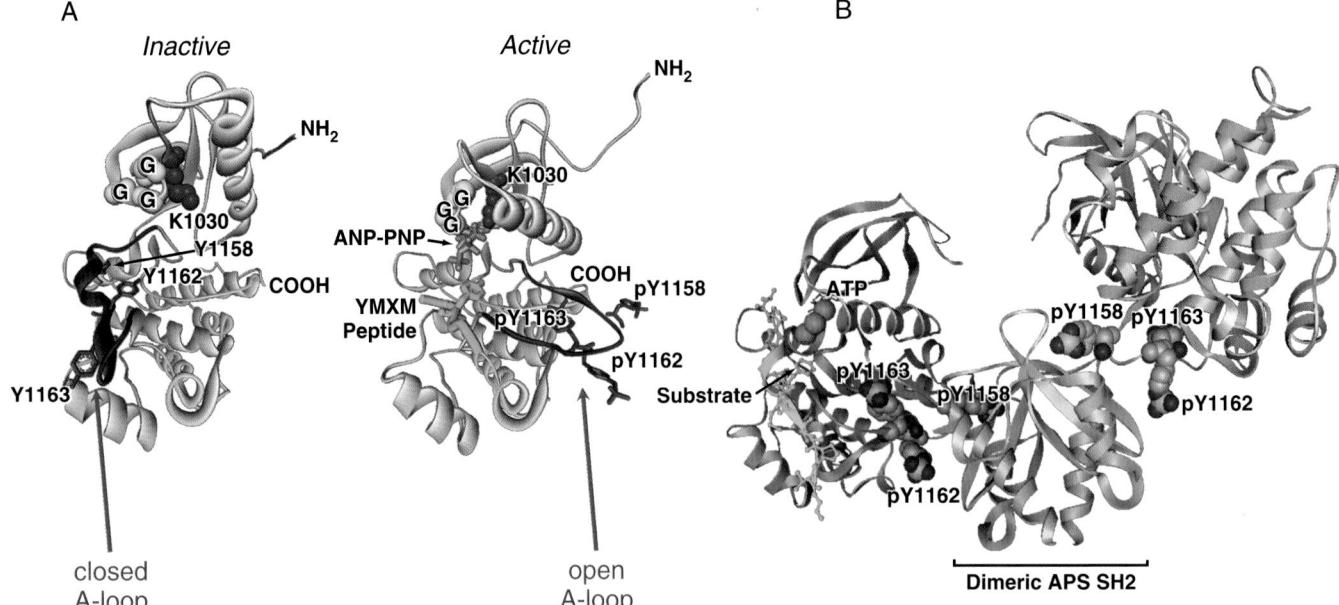

Figure 50-3 The role of insulin receptor autophosphorylation. **A,** Structure of the insulin receptor activation loop shown as ribbon diagrams of the kinase domain of the insulin receptor along with the side chains of important amino acids, including the three glycine residues and K1030 that comprise the ATP-binding site. The activation loop (A loop) is shown in red; the three activation loop tyrosine residues (Y1158, Y1162, and Y1163) are shown with their side chains. In the inactive, unphosphorylated state *(left panel)*, the activation loop blocks access by potential substrates. Following phosphorylation *(right panel)*, however, the activation loop moves, allowing substrates such as YMXM peptides of the IRS-proteins (shown in green) to access the active site. **B,** A structural representation of the binding of dimeric APS SH2 domains to the phosphorylated A loop of the insulin receptor. These structure were based on published coordinates.[83,86,90]

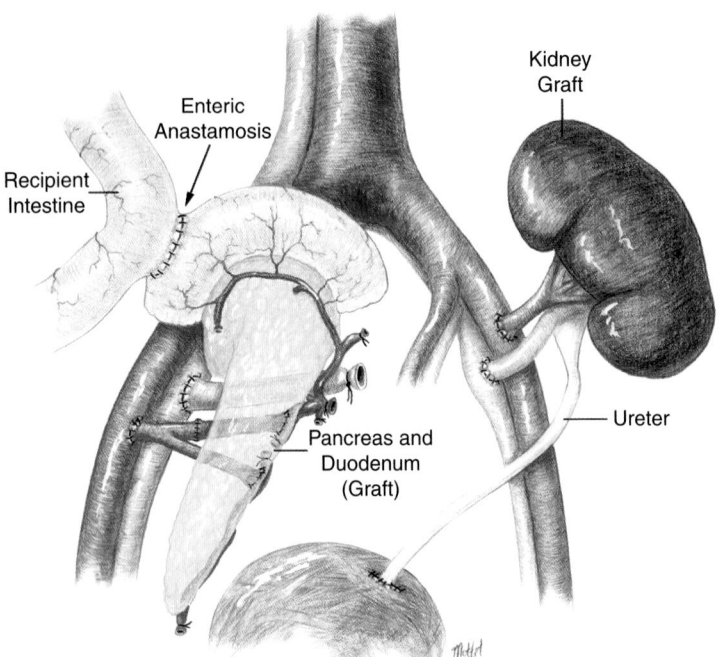

Figure 65-1 Combined pancreas and kidney transplant. Digestive juices of the pancreas are drained into the intestine via an enteric anastomosis between the donor duodenum and the recipient ileum. Venous outflow can be either into the portal vein or to the peripheral circulation via the iliac vein as shown. (Drawing courtesy of Dr. David Sutherland.)

PRINCIPLES OF HORMONE ACTION

Endocrinology: Impact on Science and Medicine

J. Larry Jameson and Leslie J. DeGroot

DEFINITION AND SCOPE OF ENDOCRINOLOGY

HISTORICAL PERSPECTIVES

PRINCIPLES OF HORMONE ACTION
Hormone Biosynthesis and Secretion
Feedback Regulation
Paracrine and Autocrine Regulation
Hormonal Rhythms and Pulsatility
Hormone Transport and Degradation

HORMONE ACTION THROUGH RECEPTORS
Membrane Receptors
Nuclear Receptors

ROLE OF THE CLINICAL ENDOCRINOLOGIST

MAJOR UNSOLVED PROBLEMS

DEFINITION AND SCOPE OF ENDOCRINOLOGY

The term *endocrine* was coined by Starling to contrast the actions of hormones secreted internally (endocrine) with those secreted externally (exocrine) or into a lumen, such as the gastrointestinal tract.[1] This terminology continues today but makes the specialty somewhat opaque to the general public, who are more familiar with the term *hormone* or with particular disorders of the endocrine system. The term *hormone* is derived from the Greek verb *hormao*, meaning "to set in motion." This phrase captures the dynamic properties of hormones and their ability to elicit a cascade of physiologic responses by acting on specific target tissues. Reminiscent of Newton's third law of motion, "For every action, there is an equal and opposite reaction," hormone action is typically counteracted by physiologic responses that restore the system to equilibrium.

The major physiologic processes controlled by hormones include (1) growth and maturation, (2) intermediary metabolism, and (3) reproduction. However, the clinical specialty of endocrinology is most clearly delineated by diseases that afflict the classic glands: hypothalamus, pituitary, thyroid, parathyroid, pancreatic islets, adrenal gland, testis, and ovary. In various parts of the world, additional clinical disorders, such as hypertension, nutrition, obesity, osteoporosis, and hyperlipidemia, also fall within the scope of endocrinology.

The basic science of endocrinology has evolved from studies of hormone action. Concepts of receptors, intracellular signaling, and many aspects of transcriptional regulation remain an essential component of the field. Endocrinology is ultimately the study of intercellular communication. In some cases, the communication occurs within the same tissue, as exemplified by autocrine and paracrine actions of insulin-like growth factor-1 (IGF-1). More classically, hormones mediate communication between organs, as exemplified by the actions of parathyroid hormone (PTH) on bone or kidney. In this era of genomics and proteomics, the traditional lines that separate endocrinology from other physiologic disciplines are becoming blurred. Erythropoietin is a classic hormone. Because it is produced by the kidney and regulates erythrocyte production, erythropoietin's clinical role is primarily in nephrology and hematology. Similarly, blood cell–stimulating factors such as granulocyte colony-stimulating factor (G-CSF) are studied and used by hematologists and oncologists. The receptors for colony-stimulating growth factors, such as G-CSF and granulocyte-macrophage colony-stimulating factor, are members of a superfamily that includes the growth hormone (GH) and prolactin (PRL) receptors. These receptors share similar intracellular signaling systems, including the JAK-STAT pathways. Growth factors with more pleomorphic functions, such as cytokines, are being investigated and used in almost every specialty.

Principles of endocrinology are readily transferable to other clinical disciplines. For example, hormones play a crucial role in blood pressure maintenance, intravascular volume regulation, and peripheral vascular resistance tone in the cardiovascular system. Angiotensin II, catecholamines, endothelins, and other vasoactive substances act via specific receptors to mediate dynamic changes in vascular tone. The heart produces hormones, such as atrial natriuretic peptide, in response to volume overload, resulting in compensatory natriuresis. The gastrointestinal tract is a remarkably rich source of peptide hormones, such as ghrelin, gastrin, cholecystokinin, secretin, and vasoactive intestinal peptide, among many others. Some of these factors, such as ghrelin and cholecystokinin, modulate appetite in addition to local actions in the gastrointestinal tract; others, such as gastrin and secretin act mainly in the gastrointestinal tract to induce physiologic responses to meals.

With the discovery of new hormones (e.g., parathyroid hormone–related peptide, leptin, ghrelin, activin, atrial/brain natriuretic peptide), the scope of investigative and clinical endocrinology continues to expand. In addition, many areas of traditional endocrinology have been "spun off" and transformed into other disciplines. For example, while hypothalamic regulation of the pituitary remains a core element of endocrinology, neuroendocrinology is rapidly becoming a separate discipline. Similarly, calcium regulation has functionally linked to bone metabolism. Some bone disorders, such as osteoporosis or rickets, are treated mainly by endocrinologists, whereas others, such as renal osteodystrophy or phosphate wasting disorders, are often managed by nephrologists. Reproductive endocrinology has become a subspecialty of gynecology and urology, primarily because of invasive procedures needed to evaluate and treat infertility. Ovulation induction protocols and various forms of assisted reproductive technology are increasingly used to manage infertility, which affects 10% to 15% of reproductive-age couples. Intracytoplasmic sperm injection has revolutionized the approach to male infertility. Common endocrine diseases, such as autoimmune thyroid disease and type 1 diabetes mellitus, are caused by abnormal regulation of immune surveillance and tolerance. Less common diseases, such as polyglandular failure, Addison's disease, and lymphocytic hypophysitis, also have an immunologic basis. Although immunology is an independent discipline, the interface with endocrinology is important for understanding the pathogenesis of these disorders. Cytokines and interleukins have profound effects on the functions of the pituitary, adrenal, thyroid, and gonads. Thus, the boundaries of endocrinology change constantly, spawning new disciplines and expanding into new scientific realms.

HISTORICAL PERSPECTIVES

Although concepts of fertility and reproduction can be traced to ancient times, most of our current understanding of endocrinology evolved during the last 150 years.[2] The structures of the major glands and ducts were initially captured in drawings by Renaissance anatomists and artists. The publication of *De Humani Corporis Fabrica* in 1543 by Vesalius provided a turning point in studies of human anatomy. Fallopio, also of the Padova school, published *Observationes Anatomicae* in 1561, which included a detailed description of the "slender and narrow seminal passage that arises from the horn of the uterus."

A timeline for selected advances in endocrinology is depicted in Figure 1-1. Berthold recorded the physiologic consequences of castration in 1849. He demonstrated that castration of a cock caused regression of secondary sex characteristics and mating behavior. Transplantation of the testes into the abdominal cavity restored these features, proving a role for the gonads in sexual differentiation and illustrating basic principles of hormone withdrawal and replacement. In 1855, Claude Bernard noted that the liver produced two secretions, an external secretion (bile) and an internal secretion (glucose), which passed directly into the circulation. This concept was later extended by Bayliss and Starling, who discovered that secretin, a substance extracted

from duodenal mucosa, induced pancreatic exocrine secretion after intravenous injection. This observation distinguished the properties of circulating hormones from physiologic reflexes mediated by the nervous system.

In the late 1800s, the clinical manifestations of many endocrine disorders were described. The Report on Myxedema by the Clinical Society of London in 1888 is a remarkable example of the power of astute clinical observation. In addition to recognizing that the adult disorder of myxedema shared certain clinical features of cretinism,[3] a tenuous connection to thyroid gland dysfunction was proposed. The plates shown in Figure 1-2 illustrate some of the clinical manifestations of hypothyroidism described by William Ord, who coined the term *myxedema* (mucinous edema).[4] Several years later, George Murray tested the role of the thyroid gland in myxedema by demonstrating that repeated subcutaneous injections of sheep thyroid extract corrected the disorder.[5] This was probably the first example of successful hormone replacement and spawned parallel efforts for other glandular diseases. By the turn of the century, the clinical manifestations of Graves' disease, acromegaly, Addison's disease, diabetes mellitus, and pheochromocytoma were well established. Hormone isolation and replacement strategies became a major research effort, culminating in the characterization of corticosteroids, thyroid hormones, and sex steroids. The history of endocrinology is replete with colorful renditions of hormone isolation and discovery. A recurring theme is teamwork and parallel observations by different teams working on the same problem, a testimony to the impact of scientific communication and the need for technology to drive advances.

The discovery of insulin in 1921 has been chronicled extensively and is a true inflection point in endocrinology.[6] The pancreatic islets form clusters that are embedded within the exocrine pancreas. Early experiments in dogs by Minkowski[7] demonstrated that pancreatectomy caused diabetes, demonstrating the pancreas as the organ responsible for regulating

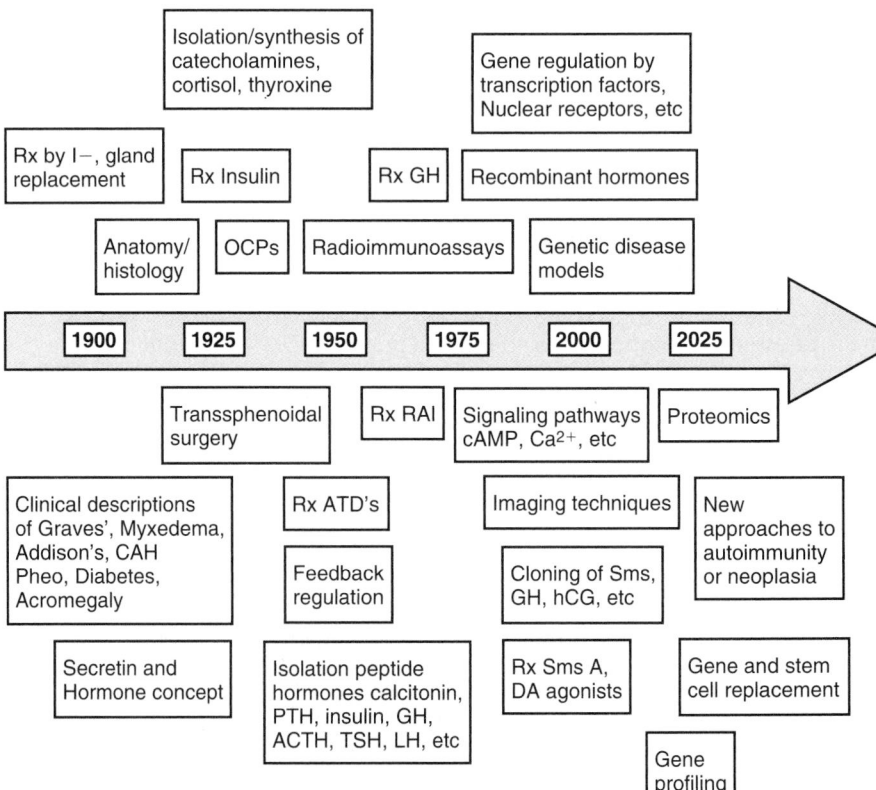

Timeline of Endocrinology

Figure 1-1 Timeline of selected advances in endocrinology. I–, iodine; CAH, congenital adrenal hyperplasia; Pheo, pheocromocytoma; Rx, treatment; ATD's, antithyroid drugs; OCPs, oral contraceptive pills; Sms A, somatostatin analogues; DA, dopamine; RAI, radioactive iodine.

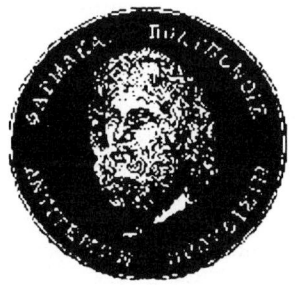

REPORT

OF A

COMMITTEE OF THE CLINICAL SOCIETY OF LONDON

NOMINATED DECEMBER 14, 1883

TO INVESTIGATE THE SUBJECT OF

MYXEDEMA

SUPPLEMENT TO VOLUME THE TWENTY-FIRST

LONDON:
LONGMANS, GREEN, AND CO.
1888.

A

General Society Report on Myxedema (1888)

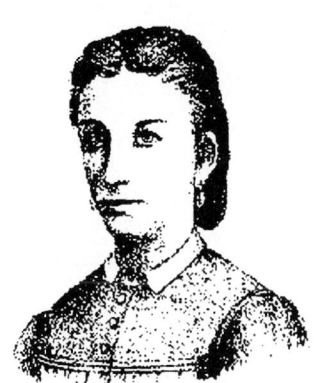

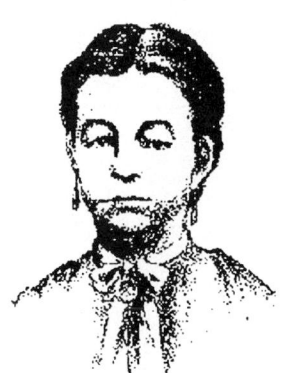

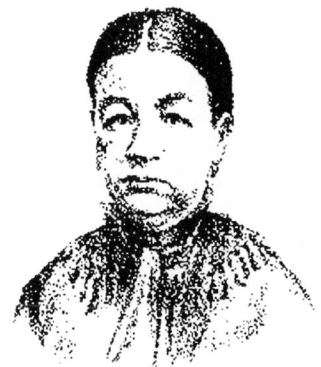

Plate 1   **Plate 2**   **Plate 3**

From Photographs   *Danielsson&Co., lith*

B

Figure 1-2 **A,** Cover page from the 1888 Society of London Report on Myxoedema. **B,** Clinical manifestations of myxedema. Plates taken from serial photographs of a woman with untreated hypothyroidism. Plate 1: Age 21, before onset of myxedema; Plate 2: Age 28, showing early features of myxedema; Plate 3: Age 32, illustrating overt features of myxedema. (Source: Clinical Society of London Report on Myxedema. Boston: Francis A. Countway Library of Medicine, 1888. Photographs originally published in Ord WM: On myxoedema, a term proposed to be applied to an essential condition in the "cretinoid" affection occasionally observed in middle-aged women. Medico-chirurgical Trans 1978:61:57–78.)

glucose. Banting and Best set out to isolate insulin, a process that was greatly aided by the expertise of Collip, a protein chemist who isolated several other peptide hormones, including parathyroid hormone.[8,9] Despite erratic initial results in diabetic dogs, Banting and Best soon achieved unequivocal success using partially purified insulin. At the time of insulin isolation, children with type 1 diabetes had no treatment options aside from starvation therapy, which could not prevent their ultimate demise from hyperglycemia and ketoacidosis. The initial insulin treatment results were stunningly successful, with immediate benefits soon followed by the ability to achieve long-term management using repeated insulin injections (Fig. 1-3). This dramatic treatment strategy was stymied initially by the limited supply of purified insulin, a problem that was ultimately solved by the development of recombinant human insulin. In this current era, pancreas and islet transplantation represent alternative treatment approaches. However, limited human donor tissue and complications of immunosuppression have restricted the use of transplantation to patients with severe type 1 diabetes. There is hope, however, that stem cell biology or the ability to regenerate pancreatic islet β cells, might overcome these limitations.

Recognition that the hypothalamus produces a variety of pituitary regulatory factors was a major advance. In addition to establishing a link between the brain and the "master gland," the hypothalamic-pituitary system underscored the critical importance of anatomic proximity and vascular delivery for the regulation of hormone action. It is now appreciated that discrete pulses of hypothalamic gonadotropin-releasing hormone (GnRH), growth hormone releasing hormone (GHRH), thyrotropin-releasing hormone (TRH), and corticotropin-releasing hormone (CRH) act locally on the pituitary and exert little, if any, physiologic effects at more distal sites in the body.

Following the isolation of many steroid and peptide hormones during the first half of the twentieth century, a conceptual framework was outlined for mechanisms of hormone action. For peptide hormones, Sutherland established the idea of a second messenger system in which a hormone binds to a membrane receptor, thereby activating intracellular second messenger pathways such as cyclic adenosine monophosphate (cAMP).[10] For steroid and thyroid hormones, Tata established the concept of hormone action at the nuclear level, acting via intracellular receptors that altered gene expression, which in turn caused changes in protein levels.[11] The development of the radioimmunoassay (RIA) by Berson and Yalow revolutionized endocrine physiology and diagnosis by allowing accurate measurements of minute amounts of circulating hormones.[12] The impact of RIAs on physiology, endocrinology, and clinical medicine cannot be overemphasized. RIAs and related assays are now used routinely for almost all hormone measurements and have replaced many less sensitive chemical methods and bioassays. RIAs were once the province of specialty endocrine labs but have gradually become automated and integrated into clinical pathology labs.

Important advances in therapeutic modalities have accompanied our improved understanding of endocrine diseases. Hormone replacement strategies have been refined along with advances in surgical approaches for endocrine tumors. Many hormone excess syndromes are primarily managed surgically, including transsphenoidal surgery for pituitary tumors or excision of parathyroid, adrenal, and pancreatic tumors. Many glandular surgeries are now performed using minimally invasive techniques, such as laparoscopy or video-assisted resection through very small incisions. In addition to hormonal replacements, important medical therapies that have been developed include the use of radioactive iodine[13] and antithyroid drugs[14] for hyperthyroidism, bromocriptine for prolactinomas and acromegaly,[15] oral hypoglycemics for

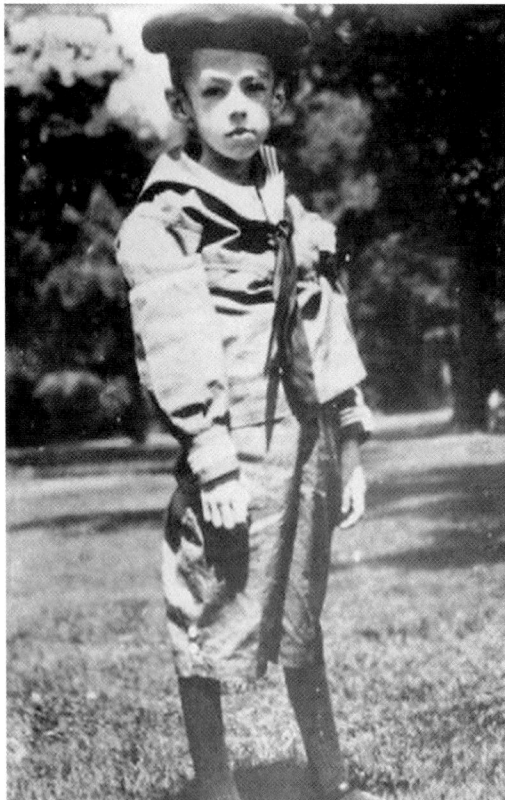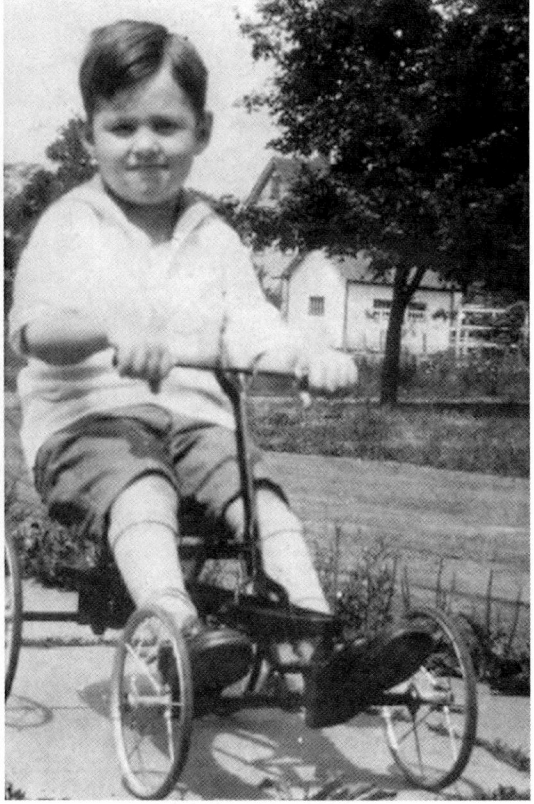

Figure 1-3 Treatment of type 1 diabetes mellitus with insulin. Teddy Ryder was one of the first patients treated by Dr. Banting. After undergoing "starvation treatment," **(left panel)** which was the only therapy available at the time, he began insulin treatment at age 5 (July 10, 1922) **(right panel)**. One year later (July 10, 1923), he is seen "cured." Teddy Ryder lived to age 76. (Source: Adapted with permission from the University of Toronto Libraries Discovery and Early Development of Insulin online collection, *http://digital.library.utoronto.ca/insulin/*.)

diabetes,[16] gonadal steroids as contraceptives,[17] and somatostatin analogues for acromegaly and tumors of the gastrointestinal tract.[18]

In recent years, the tools of molecular genetics have dramatically accelerated our understanding of endocrinology. DNA sequences encoding hormones such as somatostatin,[19] growth hormone,[20] insulin,[21] and chorionic gonadotropin[22] were among the first human cDNAs cloned. Recombinant DNA techniques are now routinely used to identify new hormones and receptors and to elucidate hormone function.

Hormone genes have provided important models for understanding mechanisms of transcriptional regulation. Hormones are typically expressed in a cell-specific manner (e.g., growth hormone, thyroglobulin), providing prototypes for identifying transcription factors (e.g., Pit-1, TTF-1) that restrict expression to particular cells or tissues. Hormone-regulated pathways have provided experimental variables that can be switched on or off, thereby revealing highly regulated target genes that can be used as experimental models. Thus, studies of the cAMP signaling system have unraveled the protein kinase A cascade and transcription factor targets, such as cAMP response element binding protein (CREB) (Chapter 12). Nuclear receptor pathways have been particularly illuminating. In addition to identifying target genes regulated by hormones such as estrogen, glucocorticoid, or thyroid hormone, detailed analyses of these pathways have helped to define how DNA binding specificity is encoded in promoters and how transcription factors suppress or enhance gene expression by recruiting corepressor or coactivator complexes (Chapter 15). Transcription by nuclear receptors is arguably the best understood paradigm for how transcription factors initiate transcription, assemble a transcription complex, and renew the process to ensure multiple rounds of RNA synthesis. The genetic basis of several hundred endocrine disorders has been determined by using molecular biological approaches, and these tests are increasingly being used in clinical practice (Chapter 6).

In addition to technical advances such as RIAs and recombinant DNA technology, endocrinology has contributed disproportionately to pivotal conceptual advances in science and medicine. Almost every aspect of physiology is tied to rhythms. The endocrine system has provided models for rapid rhythms such as luteinizing hormone (LH) or GH pulsatility, circadian rhythms such as cortisol or vasopressin production, and longer rhythms such as the menstrual cycle or bone remodeling. Concepts of hormone-receptor interaction and second messengers established signal transduction paradigms that proliferated into innumerable signaling networks. Polypeptide precursors, such as pro-opiomelanocortin (POMC), preproglucagon, and others, established pathways for protein processing, transport, and secretion. Studies of growth factors helped to refine concepts of autocrine and paracrine action, which can be viewed as an extension of classic endocrine action. Hormone replacement formed the foundation for the use of biologic agents such as factor VIII, G-CSF, and erythropoietin. The genetic basis of cancer has been elucidated by studies of the multiple endocrine neoplasia syndromes, types I and II.

PRINCIPLES OF HORMONE ACTION

The principles of hormone action include fundamental concepts such as hormone biosynthesis and secretion, feedback regulation, hormone-receptor binding, and initiation of intracellular signaling. These principles are broadly applicable and can be applied to the physiology of other subspecialties.

HORMONE BIOSYNTHESIS AND SECRETION

Hormones can be divided into five major classes: (1) amino acid derivatives such as dopamine, catecholamines, and thyroid hormone; (2) small neuropeptides such as GnRH, TRH, somatostatin, and vasopressin; (3) large proteins such as insulin, LH, and PTH produced by classic endocrine glands; (4) steroid hormones such as cortisol and estrogen that are synthesized from cholesterol-based precursors; and (5) vitamin derivatives such as retinoids (vitamin A) and vitamin D. As a rule, amino acid derivatives and peptide hormones interact with cell-surface membrane receptors. Steroids, thyroid hormones, vitamin D, and retinoids are lipid soluble and interact with intracellular nuclear receptors.

Many peptide hormones are produced from precursor polypeptides. Characteristic signal or leader sequences target these peptides for extracellular transport via secretory granules. Some precursors, such as the POMC or preproglucagon, encode multiple biologically active peptides that are generated by specific processing enzymes; other precursors, such as preproPTH, preproinsulin, and vasopressin, encode single hormones that are excised from larger proteins. The secretion of peptide hormones is tightly controlled by intracellular signals that regulate vesicle transport and fusion with the plasma membrane, resulting in hormone release into the extracellular milieu (Chapter 7). Steroid hormones such as progesterone, cortisol, and testosterone are synthesized from cholesterol derivatives by a series of enzymatic steps. These enzymes are expressed specifically in steroidogenic tissues such as the adrenal gland and gonads. Their enzymatic activities are regulated in response to trophic hormones such as adrenocorticotropic hormone (ACTH), LH, or follicle-stimulating hormone (FSH). Thyroid hormone is produced by modifications (iodination) of tyrosines in thyroglobulin. Vitamin D and retinoic acid are derived in part from dietary sources but can also be generated and activated by endogenous synthetic pathways.

FEEDBACK REGULATION

The elucidation of negative feedback has had a profound impact on endocrinology. This principle holds that hormones have a particular set point that is controlled by downregulating stimulatory pathways when the set point is exceeded, and upregulating stimulatory pathways when hormone levels fall below the set point. Probably every hormone is regulated in this manner, although the regulatory pathways might not be immediately evident for new hormones. These regulatory loops are well illustrated by the major hypothalamic-pituitary-hormone axes and include both stimulatory (e.g., TRH stimulates thyroid-stimulating hormone (TSH); TSH stimulates T4/T3 production) and inhibitory components (e.g., T4/T3 suppress TRH and TSH) (Fig. 1-4). Feedback regulation also occurs for endocrine systems that do not involve the pituitary gland. For example, calcium feeds back to inhibit PTH, glucose inhibits insulin secretion, and leptin acts on hypothalamic pathways to suppress appetite. While these feedback mechanisms oversimplify the complex physiologic pathways that regulate hormone levels, they provide useful insight into endocrine testing paradigms. For example, hypothyroidism is characterized by elevated TSH, an appropriate physiologic response to deficient thyroid hormone levels. Dexamethasone suppression of the CRH/ACTH axis is used to diagnose Cushing's disease, which is characterized by impaired negative feedback regulation. A deficient adrenal response to exogenous ACTH is used to document primary adrenal insufficiency.

PARACRINE AND AUTOCRINE REGULATION

Whereas feedback mechanisms control many classic endocrine pathways, local regulatory systems, often involving growth factors, play critical roles in all tissues (Fig. 1-5). Paracrine regulation refers to factors released by one cell that act on an adjacent cell in the same tissue. For example,

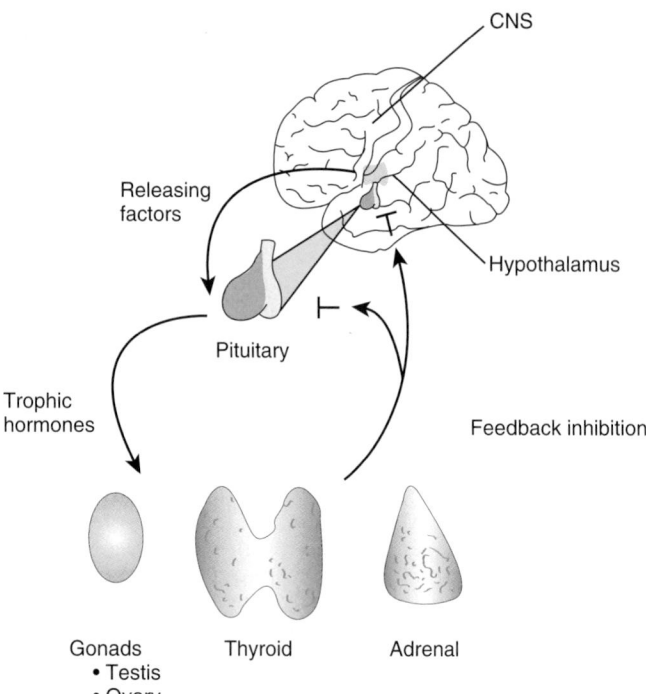

Figure 1-4 Feedback regulation of the hypothalamic-pituitary axis.

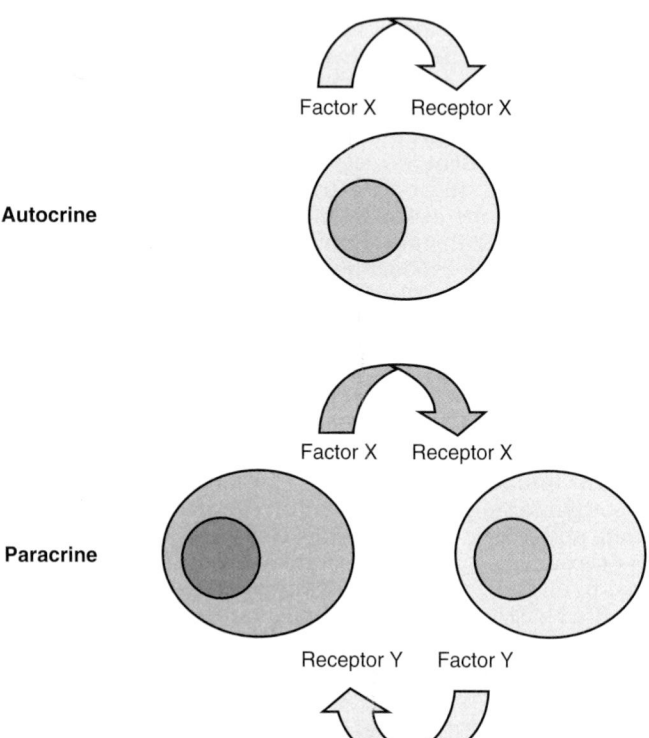

Figure 1-5 Autocrine and paracrine regulation. Many growth factors act locally to regulate cell growth, differentiation, and function. Autocrine regulation describes the action of a factor that acts on the same cell, whereas paracrine regulation describes a circumstance in which the product of one cell acts on different cell type.

somatostatin secretion by pancreatic islet delta cells inhibits insulin secretion from nearby β cells. The oocyte produces growth and differentiation factor-9 (GDF-9), which acts on adjacent granulosa cells to stimulate the transition of primary follicles to secondary follicles. The anatomic relationships of cells have an important influence on paracrine regulation. Seminiferous tubules are exposed to a very high testosterone concentration from the interstitial Leydig cell compartment. On the other hand, the Sertoli cell product, androgen-binding protein (ABP), helps to retain high local testosterone concentrations. Activin exerts paracrine effects in the pituitary, where it stimulates FSH production. However, activin also exerts biological activity in many other tissues, perhaps explaining why it is regulated locally and neutralized by binding proteins such as follistatin. Autocrine regulation describes the action of a factor on the same cell from which it is produced. IGF-1 acts on many cells that produce it, including chondrocytes, breast epithelium, and gonadal cells. Intracrine regulation refers to effects within a cell. The term is not commonly used but captures the important concept that many signaling and enzymatic pathways are influenced by other pathways or by substrate or product concentrations. For example, HMG-CoA reductase, the rate-limiting enzyme in cholesterol biosynthesis, is inhibited by the end product, cholesterol.

HORMONAL RHYTHMS AND PULSATILITY

Hormonal rhythms are used to adapt to environmental changes, such as seasons of the year, the daily light-dark cycle, sleep, meals, and stress. In many species, reproduction is seasonal, presumably a mechanism to ensure survival of the offspring. In the extreme northern and southern hemispheres, calcium absorption and bone remodeling decline during winter, when vitamin D production is reduced. The human menstrual cycle is repeated on average every 28 days, reflecting the time required for follicular maturation and ovulation. In some species, estrus cycles are intimately linked to mating behavior induced by behavioral cues and the production of pheromones. Essentially all pituitary hormone rhythms are entrained to sleep and the circadian cycle, which in turn is dictated by sunlight exposure. The hypothalamic-pituitary-adrenal (HPA) axis, for example, exhibits characteristic peaks of ACTH and cortisol production before dawn and a nadir between late afternoon and midnight. Recognition of these rhythms is important for endocrine testing and treatment. Patients with Cushing's syndrome exhibit inappropriately increased midnight cortisol levels. The HPA axis is more susceptible to suppression by glucocorticoids administered at night because they blunt the early morning rise of ACTH. Understanding this diurnal rhythm provides the basis for more physiologic hormone replacement by using larger glucocorticoid doses in the morning than in the afternoon.

Many peptide hormones are secreted in discrete pulses, often reflecting regulation by the nervous system. For example, hypothalamic GnRH induces LH pulses once every 1 to 2 hours. Intermittent hypothalamic GnRH pulses are required to maintain pituitary gonadotrope sensitivity, whereas continuous GnRH exposure causes desensitization. This feature of gonadotropin regulation is the basis for using long-acting GnRH agonists to treat central precocious puberty or to decrease testosterone levels in the management of prostate cancer.

The pulsatile nature of hormone secretion and the rhythmic pattern of hormone production have important implications for the measurement of circulating hormone levels, as levels can change dramatically over several hours. For some hormones, integrated markers have been developed to circumvent hormonal fluctuations. For example, a 24-hour collection of urinary free cortisol integrates cortisol production throughout a diurnal cycle. IGF-1 provides a relatively stable biologic marker of GH action. HbA1c is used as an index of long-term (weeks to months) circulating blood glucose, which is covalently linked to hemoglobin in a concentration-dependent manner.

HORMONE TRANSPORT AND DEGRADATION

The level of a hormone is determined by its rate of secretion and its circulating half-life. After protein biosynthesis and precursor processing, peptide hormones are stored in secretory granules. These granules undergo progressive maturation and sequential translocation before arriving at the plasma membrane for imminent release into the circulation. The stimulus for hormone secretion is typically a releasing factor or neural signal that induces rapid changes in intracellular calcium concentration, which leads to secretory granule fusion with the plasma membrane and releases its contents into the extracellular environment and blood stream. In contrast, steroid hormones usually diffuse into the circulation as they are synthesized. Thus, their secretion closely mirrors rates of synthesis. For example, ACTH and LH induce steroidogenesis by stimulating the activity of *st*eroidogenic *a*cute *r*egulatory (StAR) protein, which transports cholesterol into the mitochondrion. In parallel, ACTH and LH stimulate other rate-limiting steps in the steroidogenic pathway such as the cholesterol side-chain cleavage enzyme (CYP11A1).

Hormone-binding proteins can affect the volume of distribution, level of unbound or "free hormone," and rates of hormone clearance. Most steroid hormones and many peptide hormones circulate in association with binding proteins. T4 and T3 bind to thyroxine-binding globulin (TBG), albumin, and thyroxine-binding prealbumin (TBPA). Similarly, cortisol binds to cortisol-binding globulin (CBG), and androgens and estrogens bind to sex hormone–binding globulin (SHBG). IGF-1 and IGF-2 bind to multiple IGF-binding proteins (IGFBPs). GH interacts with GH-binding protein (GHBP), a circulating fragment of the GH receptor extracellular domain. Abnormal binding proteins can significantly alter total hormone concentrations but usually have little clinical consequence, as the regulatory feedback systems respond to unbound hormone levels. For example, TBG deficiency greatly reduces total thyroid hormone levels, but the free concentrations of T4 and T3 remain normal. Liver disease and medications can also influence binding protein levels (e.g., estrogen increases TBG). Nonetheless, these abnormalities can create diagnostic confusion, and some alterations (e.g., increased SHBG) may shift ratios of hormones (e.g., testosterone, estradiol) that bind with different affinities.

Knowledge of hormone half-life is important for achieving physiologic hormone replacement, as the frequency of dosing and the time required to reach steady state are determined by rates of hormone decay. T4, for example, has a half-life of about 7 days. Consequently, more than 1 month is required to reach a new steady state, and single daily doses are sufficient to achieve constant hormone levels. T3, in contrast, has a half-life of about 1 day. Its administration is associated with more dynamic serum levels, and it must be administered two to three times per day to generate more constant blood levels. Synthetic glucocorticoids vary widely in their half-lives. Analogues with a longer half-life (e.g., dexamethasone) are associated with greater suppression of the HPA axis. Most protein hormones (e.g., ACTH, GH, PRL, PTH, LH) have relatively short half-lives (<20 minutes), leading to sharp peaks of secretion and decay. These dynamic hormone fluctuations must be considered in analyzing hormone levels, which may vary widely over short time intervals and between patient visits. Although frequent hormone sampling can trace these pulses, this is not practical outside of a research setting. In some instances, clinicians elect to pool several samples to obtain a more representative hormone level. Rapid hormone decay is useful in certain clinical settings. Because PTH has a short half-life, intraoperative PTH can be used to confirm successful removal of a parathyroid adenoma. This is particularly valuable diagnostically when there is a possibility of multicentric disease or parathyroid hyperplasia, as occurs with multiple endocrine neoplasia or renal insufficiency.

HORMONE ACTION THROUGH RECEPTORS

Hormone receptors can be divided broadly into membrane receptors and nuclear receptors. Membrane receptors primarily bind peptide hormones and small molecules that cannot traverse the plasma membrane (e.g., catecholamines, dopamine). Nuclear receptors bind small, lipid-soluble molecules that diffuse or are transported across the cell membrane (e.g., thyroid hormone, steroids, vitamin D). Hormones bind to both classes of receptors with specificity and high affinity. These characteristics are often described by Scatchard plots, which allow estimation of equilibrium dissociation constants (K_d) and maximum binding (B_{max}) (Fig. 1-6).

Binding affinity generally coincides with the concentration of circulating hormones and is typically in the subnanomolar range. Receptor occupancy at any given moment is a function of hormone concentration and the receptor's affinity for the hormone. Receptor numbers vary greatly in different target tissues, providing one of the major determinants of specific cellular responses to circulating hormones. For example, ACTH receptors are located almost exclusively in the adrenal cortex, and FSH receptors are found only in the gonads. In contrast, insulin and thyroid hormone receptors are widely distributed, reflecting the need for metabolic responses in all tissues. Tissue-specific knockouts of insulin receptors have revealed distinct metabolic actions of insulin in various tissues.[23] For example, deletion in muscle causes increased free fatty acids and adipose tissue, whereas insulin receptor deletion in adipose tissue reduces fat mass and enhances insulin sensitivity. Deletion of the receptor in pancreatic islet β cells impairs insulin secretion, apparently because of reduced islet cell mass.[24]

MEMBRANE RECEPTORS

Membrane receptors can be divided into several major groups (Fig. 1-7): (1) seven transmembrane *domain* G protein–coupled receptors (GPCRs), (2) tyrosine kinase receptors, (3) cytokine receptors, and (4) transforming growth factor beta (TGF-β) family serine kinase receptors. There are several hundred GPCRs (Chapter 11). They bind a broad array of hormones, including large proteins (e.g., TSH, PTH), small peptides (e.g., TRH, somatostatin), catecholamines (epinephrine, dopamine), and even minerals (e.g., calcium). These receptors possess seven transmembrane-spanning regions composed of hydrophobic ahelical domains that are connected by extracellular and intracellular loops. After the receptor binds a hormone, these transmembrane domains undergo conformational changes that alter interactions with intracellular G proteins. The G proteins provide a link to intracellular signaling pathways such as adenyl cyclase, phospholipase C, and others. G proteins form a heterotrimeric complex that is composed of various Gα and Gβ–γ subunits. The a subunit contains the guanine nucleotide-binding site and hydrolyzes GTP to GDP. Ga is active when GTP is bound and inactive after hydrolysis to GDP. The β–γ subunits modulate the activity of the a subunit and mediate their own effector-signaling pathways. A variety of endocrinopathies result from G protein mutations or from mutations in receptors that modify their interactions with G proteins. For example, McCune-Albright syndrome is caused by somatic mutations in Ga that prevent GTP hydrolysis, thereby causing constitutive activation of the Ga-signaling pathway. Selected mutations in the transmembrane domains of GPCRs can

Saturation Plot

Scatchard Plot

Y-axis: Bound Labeled Hormone (nM)

Total binding

Rt

Specific binding

Nonspecific binding

X-axis: Free Labeled Hormone (nM)

Y-axis: Bound/Free

$$[RS] = \frac{[R_t][S]}{K_d + [S]}$$

$$\text{Slope} = -\frac{1}{K_d}$$

Rt

X-axis: Bound Hormone (nM)

Figure 1-6 Plots of ligand-receptor interactions. **Left panel,** Theoretical equilibrium saturation plot. As increasing amounts of labeled hormone are added, the amount of receptor-bound hormone increases until the binding sites are saturated (total binding). The addition of a large amount of unlabeled hormone allows determination of nonspecific or unsaturable binding. The hormone concentration at which half-maximal binding occurs provides a measure of binding affinity. **Right panel,** Theoretical Scatchard plot. The X-axis represents specific binding, and the Y-axis denotes specific binding divided by free radioligand concentration. Maximal binding is estimated by the X-intercept (B_{max}) and the dissociation constant (K_d) is estimated as the negative reciprocal of the slope.

mimic hormone-induced conformational changes, leading to activation of G proteins independent of hormone binding. This type of mutation in the TSH receptor accounts for a significant fraction of solitary autonomously functioning thyroid nodules. Activating mutations in the LH receptor cause LH-independent precocious puberty in boys.

Tyrosine kinase receptors transmit signals for insulin and a variety of growth factors, such as IGF-1, epidermal growth factor, platelet-derived growth factor, and fibroblast growth factor (Chapter 8). Ligand binding induces autophosphorylation, leading to interactions with intracellular adaptor proteins such as Shc and insulin receptor substrates (IRS). Depending on the receptor and adaptor complexes, one or more kinases are activated including the Raf-Ras-MAPK and the Akt/protein kinase B pathways (Chapter 14). The tyrosine kinase receptors play a prominent role in cell growth and differentiation, as well as intermediary metabolism.

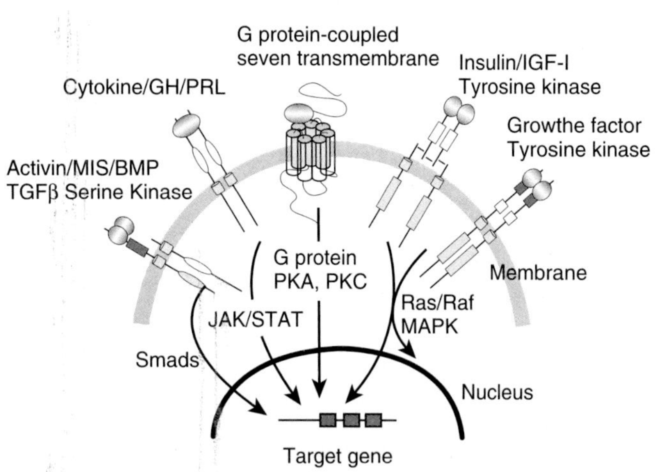

The GH and PRL receptors belong to the cytokine receptor family (Chapter 9). Ligand binding induces receptor interactions with intracellular kinases such as the Janus kinases (JAKs), which phosphorylate members of the signal transduction and activators of transcription (STAT) family, and other signaling pathways (Ras, PI3-K, MAPK). The activated STAT proteins translocate to the nucleus and stimulate expression of target genes.

The TGF-β receptor family mediate the actions of TGF-βs, activins, Müllerian inhibiting substance (MIS, also known as anti-Müllerian hormone), and bone morphogenic proteins (Chapter 10). This receptor family consists of type I and II subunits, which undergo autophosphorylation after ligand binding. The phosphorylated receptors bind intracellular Smads (named for a fusion of terms for *Caenorhabditis elegans* sma + mammalian mad). Like the STAT proteins, the Smads serve a dual role of transducing the receptor signal and acting as transcription factors.

NUCLEAR RECEPTORS

The nuclear receptor superfamily can be divided into receptors with known ligands (type I and II) and so-called orphan nuclear receptors, for which ligands have not been identified or might not exist (Chapter 15). Type I nuclear receptors include classic steroid receptors (e.g., glucocorticoid, estrogen, progesterone, androgen, mineralocorticoid) that bind to DNA as homodimers. Type II nuclear receptors bind to DNA as heterodimers, typically using the retinoid X receptor as a partner. Type II receptors bind a variety of molecules, including thyroid hormones, vitamin D, retinoic acid, and bile acids. Many orphan receptors bind DNA as monomers. Nuclear receptors have a highly conserved central zinc-finger DNA binding domain (Fig. 1-8). The carboxyterminal domain is more variable and includes a ligand-binding pocket, dimerization surfaces, and transcription-activating motifs. The aminoterminal domain varies greatly in length and in some receptors contains transcription-activating domains.

Nuclear receptors act primarily by altering rates of gene transcription, although there is growing evidence for interactions with other cellular signaling pathways, such as the mitogen-activated protein kinase (MAPK) pathway. Hormone binding induces conformational changes that induce receptor

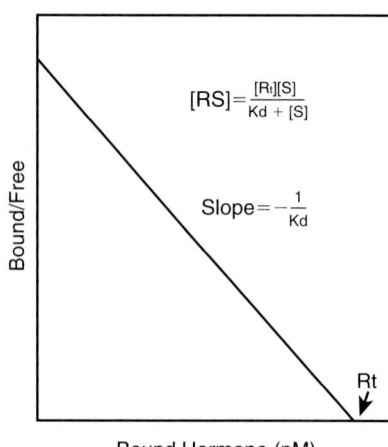

Figure 1-7 Membrane receptors. Classes of membrane receptors can be defined on the basis of structural similarities and signaling pathways. The figure depicts major classes of membrane receptors, although these categories are somewhat arbitrary. Each of these receptor classes is described in separate chapters. (Source: Adapted with permission from Harrison's Principles of Internal Medicine, 15th Edition, McGraw-Hill, 2001.)

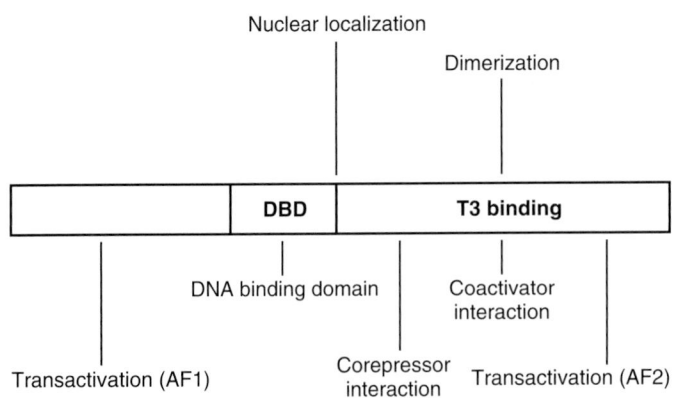

Figure 1-8 Nuclear receptor structure. The central zinc-finger DNA binding domain is highly conserved among nuclear receptors. The carboxyterminus includes regions involved in ligand binding, transcriptional repression and activation, and dimerization. The aminoterminus is highly variable in length and, for some receptors, contains transcriptional regulatory sequences.

interactions with transcriptional cofactors. For type I receptors, ligand binding creates a bend in the extreme carboxyterminus (AF-2 domain) such that a hydrophobic cleft is created, providing a docking site for coactivators (e.g., steroid receptor coactivators, SRCs). For type II receptors, hormone binding induces similar conformational changes. However, in the absence of hormone, corepressors are bound and silence gene transcription. Hormone binding induces the dissociation corepressors and the recruitment of coactivators (Fig. 1-9). Consequently, gene expression can shift from being silenced in the absence of hormone to being stimulated in the presence of hormone.

ROLE OF THE CLINICAL ENDOCRINOLOGIST

Clinicians are attracted to the field of endocrinology because it integrates physiology, biochemistry, and cell signaling with patient care. The fact that many endocrine disorders are amenable to cure or effective treatment also makes the practice of endocrinology especially satisfying.

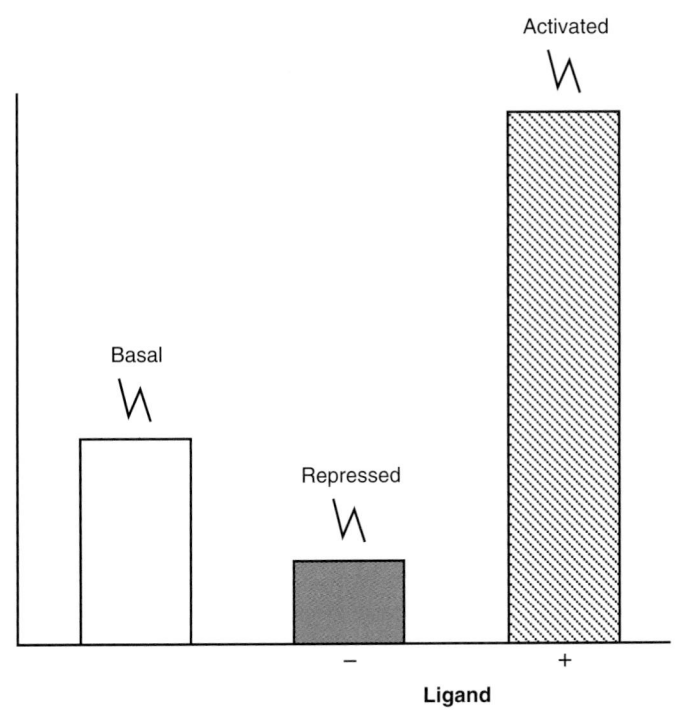

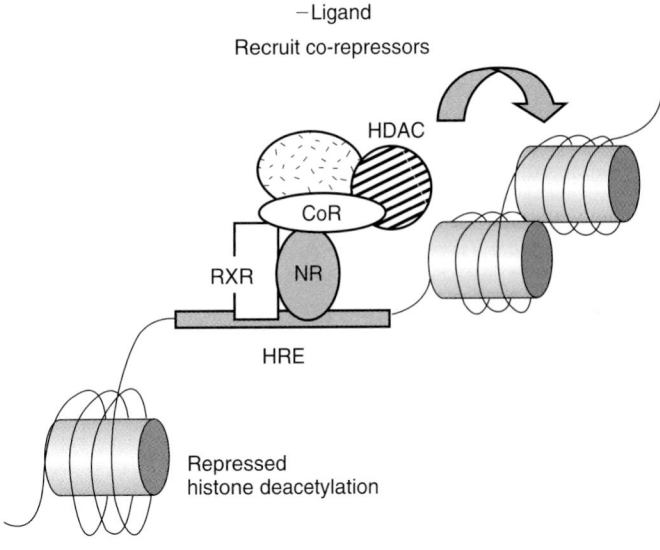

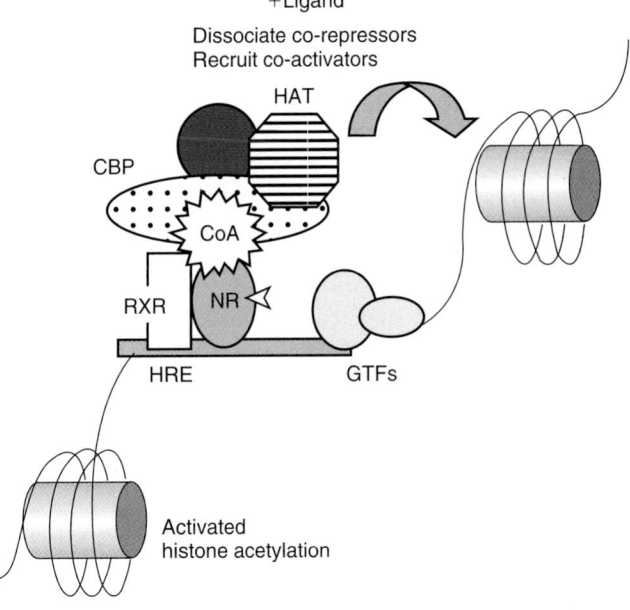

Figure 1-9 Pathways of nuclear receptor transcriptional repression and activation. Nuclear receptors act primarily by altering rates of gene transcription. Many nuclear receptors, particularly type II receptors, cause transcriptional repression or silencing in the absence of ligand. After ligand binding, repression is relieved, and transcription is stimulated above the basal state. Although the exact mechanism of transcriptional repression or activation is variable, the model shown here illustrates ligand-induced relief of repression by corepressors (CoR), followed by the recruitment of coactivators (CoA). Many CoR complexes possess histone deacetylase activity, which is thought to induce gene silencing. CoA complexes possess histone acetylase activity, which induces changes in chromatin structure that facilitate the recruitment of additional transcriptional activators, which ultimately stimulate RNA polymerase. (Abbreviations: NR, nuclear receptor; RXR, retinoid X receptor; GTFs, general transcription factors; HRE, hormone response element; HDAC, histone deacetylase; HAT, histone acetyl transferase; CBP, CREB-binding protein.)

As medicine becomes more specialized, physician roles are changing. Many general medicine inpatient services are now managed by hospitalists, who work in conjunction with primary care physicians and consultants. Inpatient length of stay continues to fall, and this setting is now rarely used for extensive endocrine evaluation and testing. In fact, many endocrine pathways are perturbed by the stress associated with acute illness or hospitalization (e.g., sick euthyroid; false-positive dexamethasone suppression tests). These changes have resulted in a shift of an endocrinologist's activity to the outpatient setting.

Clinical endocrinologists serve three main roles: (1) as consultants for patients who present with clinical endocrine conundrums that stretch the knowledge base and expertise of general internists or physicians in nonmedical specialties; (2) to provide specific short-term services for the treatment of endocrine disorders such as Graves' disease, management of a thyroid nodule, or evaluation and treatment of hyperparathyroidism; and (3) for chronic management of challenging disorders such as brittle diabetes mellitus, congenital adrenal hyperplasia, or hypocalcemia. For many years, endocrinologists developed and performed specialized tests, including radioimmunoassays. In addition to performing appropriate stimulation or suppression protocols, special expertise was required to run and interpret these hormone assays. However, sensitive immunoradiometric assays, such as those for TSH, PTH, and most other hormones, are now commercially available. In some countries, these changes have impacted reimbursement, since hormone testing was generating revenue and compensated for other services, such as diabetic education. In the United States, endocrinologists are currently reimbursed primarily on the basis of evaluation and management coding, which takes into account the diagnosis and complexity of the evaluation. Endocrine procedures include thyroid aspiration biopsies, bone density measurements, and radioiodine treatment. However, there is wide institutional variation in who performs these procedures.

In addition to these classical roles, clinicians often make important contributions by recognizing new diseases or variants of old themes. For example, thyroid hormone resistance, lack of the GH receptor, and leptin deficiency states were identified in clinical practice. Often this role is played by the physician who sees patients and is involved in research: the clinical investigator.

Although practices vary considerably, the most common disorders seen by most endocrinologists are diabetes mellitus, thyroid disorders, metabolic bone disease, pituitary disorders, and reproductive abnormalities and infertility.[25] Pediatric endocrinologists also see a large number of patients with growth deficiency, pubertal delay, and a variety of inherited endocrine diseases such as congenital adrenal hyperplasia and Turner's syndrome. Many academic centers have begun structuring multidisciplinary clinics for the management of diabetes mellitus, pituitary tumors, and thyroid nodules.[26]

Increasingly, the clinical challenge is to identify endocrine disorders at their earliest stages, before clinical manifestations are obvious. Terms such as *subclinical hypothyroidism*, *impaired glucose tolerance*, and *incidental adrenal or pituitary adenoma* have crept into our vocabulary and have changed our approach to patients. Similarly, endocrine disorders such as osteoporosis, hyperparathyroidism, hypertension, or hyperlipidemia rarely present with specific symptoms or signs. Because the clinical features of subclinical endocrine disorders are subtle or absent, laboratory testing takes on added importance as we attempt to diagnose more subtle forms of disease.

The practice of endocrinology is strongly influenced by available treatment options. Many new drugs have been discovered and approved during the last decade. Type 2 diabetes can now be treated by using drugs that influence insulin sensitivity (thiazolidinediones, metformin) and with agents that enhance insulin release (sulfonylureas, repaglinide). Insulin derivatives with altered pharmacokinetics (lispro, insulin glargine) facilitate intensive blood glucose control with reduced risk of hypoglycemia. Bisphosphonates provide a novel mechanism for inhibiting osteoclast function and are widely used to treat osteoporosis and hypercalcemia. PTH analogues are being used to stimulate osteoblast function to enhance bone mass. Medical therapy of prolactinomas with dopamine agonists established a new paradigm for nonsurgical management of pituitary tumors. More recently, somatostatin analogues have been developed, including depot formulations, for adjunctive or primary treatment of acromegaly. Pegvisomant is a novel GH analogue that blocks the GH receptor and is highly efficacious for reducing IGF-1 levels in patients with acromegaly. A variety of new formulations are available for delivering sex steroids. These include estrogen and testosterone patches. Testosterone gels and gum patches are also available. Building on the observation that tamoxifen exhibits mixed agonist/antagonist activity in various tissues, an active search is under way for additional selective estrogen receptor modulators (e.g., raloxifene) that exhibit unique profiles of estrogen action. It is expected that similar drugs might be identified for androgen, glucocorticoid, thyroid, and other nuclear receptors. Inhibitors of enzymes such as aromatase (anastrozole, letrozole) and 5α-reductase (finasteride) allow selective reduction of steroid levels. The potential for producing recombinant hormones has been fully realized, providing unlimited supplies of uncontaminated hormones or their derivatives. Examples of recombinant hormones in general use include insulin, GH, TSH, LH, and FSH. There is now great interest in the activities and clinical use of a variety of others, including leptin, GLP 1-37, YY 3-36, ghrelin, and others.

MAJOR UNSOLVED PROBLEMS

Despite many impressive advances in endocrinology, a surprising number of fundamental problems remain incompletely solved. Although it is not possible to review all of these, it is provocative to identify a few, if only as a matter of perspective.

What is the basis of variability in normal ranges of hormones? The normal range for most hormones is remarkably broad. Testosterone, for example, varies between 300 and 1000 ng/dL, and total T4 varies between 4 and 12 ng/dL. However, for any given individual, hormone levels are relatively constant, suggesting a defined set point. Some of this variability results from pulsatile or rhythmic hormone secretion. In some cases, variations in plasma-binding proteins account for variability. It seems likely that tissue responses, mediated by receptors and signaling pathways, may also define set points. From a practical perspective, the wide normal ranges create challenges for determining when there are subtle changes in hormone levels for a particular individual.

How should we optimally deliver hormone replacement? We currently have reasonable hormone replacements for each glandular deficiency syndrome. However, in no case does hormone replacement perfectly recapitulate normal physiology. In type 1 diabetes, ideal insulin replacement would always maintain euglycemia without hypoglycemia. Thyroid hormone replacement, because of its relatively long half-life, approximates physiologic replacement, at least as assessed by TSH levels. Nonetheless, there is ongoing controversy about the need to replace T3 as well as T4. Glucocorticoid replacement is notoriously challenging, and patients often exhibit mild cushingoid features to avoid adrenal insufficiency. Ideally, we would use a physiologic marker, analogous to TSH, to assess adequate adrenal replacement. Similar issues exist for sex steroid replacement. GH replacement in GH hormone–deficient children rarely completely corrects height or even growth velocity. This might reflect relatively late diagnosis, or we might not have optimized hormone administration such that it mimics physiologic GH secretion or integrated actions with other hormones such as sex steroids. There are many possible solutions to these challenges, including modified hormones and new formulations to alter absorption or pharmacokinetics. In addition, careful clinical studies will be needed to correlate the physiologic effects of various hormone regimens.

How can osteoporosis be prevented? Currently, osteoporosis is identified after a fracture or on the basis of markedly reduced bone density. Treatment strategies can prevent further bone loss or induce modest increases in bone mass. Clearly, it would be preferable to generate greater maximum bone mass early in life and to identify those who are at risk for accelerated bone loss.

What causes common autoimmune endocrinopathies such as type 1 diabetes mellitus, Hashimoto's thyroiditis, Graves' disease, and Addison's disease? Treatments are available for these disorders, but they are not directed at the underlying autoimmune process. If effective treatments could prevent, interrupt, or suppress the autoimmune process without significant side effects, the lifelong consequences of these disorders might be avoided. For autoimmune diseases associated with significant morbidity, such as type 1 diabetes, strategies directed toward immune tolerance should be considered, even if they are associated with moderate risk of complications or side effects.

What causes nodularity in endocrine glands? One or more nodules develop in the thyroid, pituitary, and adrenal glands in about 25% of patients when assessed at autopsy or using sensitive techniques such as ultrasound or magnetic resonance imaging. The detection of "incidentalomas" is becoming commonplace as imaging methods are more widely used. Although these nodules are rarely malignant, they may produce excess hormones. Rarely, somatic mutations are found in nodules, and these may cause clonal expansion. More commonly, the nodules are polyclonal, and the causes are unknown. Understanding this process is likely to provide fundamental insight into neoplasia and create novel treatment approaches.

What regulates the onset of puberty? The reproductive axis is activated during fetal life, when high levels of gonadotropins are produced. Soon after birth, gonadotropins are suppressed, in part because of exquisite sensitivity of the hypothalamic-pituitary axis to sex steroid feedback. The pathways and mechanisms that regulate the suppression and reawakening of the reproductive axis remain incompletely defined despite the fundamental importance of this process. Like many other complex endocrine pathways, it is likely that genetic models, created in mice or identified in humans, will help to unravel the steps that control puberty.[24]

What regulates appetite and energy expenditure set points? The current obesity epidemic underscores the importance of understanding these metabolic processes to develop risk profiles and new treatments. The hypothalamic control of appetite is gradually being dissected, largely on the basis of mutations associated with severe, early-onset obesity (e.g., MC4R, leptin receptor).[27] These and other receptors are potential targets for drugs that suppress appetite and/or increase energy expenditure.

As we look at the last 150 years of endocrinology and consider likely advances over the next decade, there is every reason to expect the pace of discovery to accelerate. Many advances have been driven by new technologies such as RIAs, recombinant DNA technology, and imaging. Current technology focuses on genomics, proteomics, nanotechnology, bioinformatics, and the use of computerized information systems in clinical practice. As scientists and clinicians, we will harness these and other technologies to tackle the many unanswered questions that remain in endocrinology.

REFERENCES

1. Bayliss WM, Starling EH: The mechanism of pancreatic secretion. J Physiol 28:325–353, 1902.
2. Medvei VC: A History of Endocrinology. Hingham, MA, MTP Press, 1982.
3. Clinical Society of London: Report on myxoedema. Boston, Francis A. Countway Library of Medicine, 1888.
4. Ord WM: On myxoedema, a term proposed to be applied to an essential condition in the "cretinoid" affection occasionally observed in middle-aged women. Medico-chirurgical Trans 61:57–78, 1978.
5. Murray G: Note on the treatment of myxoedema by hypodermic injections of an extract of the thyroid gland of a sheep. Br Med J 2:796–797, 1891.
6. Bliss M: The Discovery of Insulin. Chicago, The University of Chicago Press, 1982.
7. Von Mering J, Minkowski O: Diabetes mellitus nach pankreas extirpation. Arch Exp Path Pharmakol 26:371–387, 1890.
8. Collip JB: The original method as used for the isolation of insulin in semi pure form for the treatment of the first clinical cases. J Biol Chem 55:50–51, 1923.
9. Collip JB: The extraction of a parathyroid hormone that will prevent or control parathyroid tetany and which regulates the level of blood calcium. J Biol Chem 63:395–438, 1925.
10. Sutherland EW, Oye I, Butcher RW: The action of epinephrine and the role of the adenyl cyclase system in hormone action. Recent Prog Horm Res 21:623–646, 1965.
11. Tata JR, Widnell CC: Ribonucleic acid synthesis during the early action of thyroid hormone. Biochem J 98:604–620, 1966.
12. Berson SA, Yalow RS: Radioimmunoassays of peptide hormones in plasma. N Engl J Med 277:640–647, 1967.
13. Means JH: Historical background of the use of radioactive iodine in medicine. N Engl J Med 252:936–940, 1955.
14. Astwood EB: Treatment of hyperthyroidism with thiourea. J Am Med Assoc 122:78–81, 1943.
15. Thorner MO, McNeilly AS, Hagan C, Besser GM: Long-term treatment of galactorrhoea and hypogonadism with bromocriptine. Br Med J 2:419–422, 1974.
16. Loubatieres A: These Doctorat No. 86. Sci naturelles. Montpellier, France, Montpellier, 1946.
17. Pincus G: Control of conception by hormonal steroids. Science 153:493–500, 1966.
18. Lamberts SW, Uitterlinden P, Verschoor L, et al: Long-term treatment of acromegaly with the somatostatin analogue SMS 201-995. N Engl J Med 313:1576–1580, 1985.
19. Itakura K, Hirose T, Crea R, et al: Expression in Escherichia coli of a chemically synthesized gene for the hormone somatostatin. Science 198:1056–1063, 1977.
20. Seeburg PH, Shine J, Martial JA, et al: Nucleotide sequence and amplification in bacteria of structural gene for rat growth hormone. Nature 270:486–494, 1977.
21. Ullrich A, Shine J, Chirgwin J, et al: Rat insulin genes: Construction of plasmids containing the coding sequences. Science 196:1313–1319, 1977.
22. Fiddes JC, Goodman HM: Isolation, cloning and sequence analysis of the cDNA for the alpha-subunit of human chorionic gonadotropin. Nature 281:351–356, 1979.
23. Minokoshi Y, Kahn CR, Kahn BB: Tissue-specific ablation of the GLUT4 glucose transporter or the insulin receptor challenges assumptions about insulin action and glucose homeostasis. J Biol Chem 278:33609–33612, 2003.

24. Beier D, Dluhy RG: Bench and bedside: The G protein-coupled receptor GPR54 and puberty. N Engl J Med 349:1589–1592, 2003.
25. Brennan MD, Miner KM, Rizza RA: The Mayo Clinic. J Clin Endocrinol Metab 83:3427–3434, 1988.
26. Biller BMK, Swearingen B, Zervas NT, Klibanski A: A decade of the Massachusetts General Hospital neuroendocrine clinical center. J Clin Endocrinol Metab 82:1668–1674, 1997.
27. List JF, Habener JF: Defective melanocortin 4 receptors in hyperphagia and morbid obesity. N Engl J Med 348:1160–1163, 2003.

GENOMICS AND ENDOCRINOLOGY

Hormones and Gene Expression: Basic Principles

Christine Campion Quirk and John H. Nilson

OVERVIEW

Synthesis of hormones and other biologically active substances requires gene expression. Peptide and polypeptide hormones are encoded directly by a gene(s), whereas biogenic amines and steroid hormones are indirect products of several genes that provide enzymes necessary for their biosynthesis. In some instances, more than one peptide hormone can be derived from the expression of a single gene, further underscoring the complexity of their synthesis. Furthermore, ensuring synthesis of the right amount of hormone at the right time requires that gene expression be regulated. Finally, hormones also regulate gene expression. This includes expression of non-hormone-encoding genes as well as genes that encode hormones. Some hormones even exert an autologous feedback on their own cognate gene. Because the regulation of gene expression plays such a pivotal role in the synthesis of hormones and their subsequent action, it is fitting that this chapter will focus largely on the basic principles underlying this process. However, we would be remiss if we omitted a brief description of the effects that polypeptide and peptide hormones have on protein secretion. Thus, in considering both the synthesis and action of hormones, we propose extending the term *gene expression* to include the entire process required for production of a biologically active substance that acts at a distance.

THE CENTRAL DOGMA OF MOLECULAR BIOLOGY REVISITED

Expression of genes encoding proteins follows the central dogma of molecular biology that was first outlined by Francis Crick.[1–3] This dogma states that genetic information is stored in the cell as DNA, a macromolecule that serves as a template for its own replication. When this genetic information is expressed in a cell, it flows unidirectionally from DNA to messenger RNA (mRNA) (transcription) to protein (translation). However, it has become clear that the scope of this process is far more complicated than was envisioned by its early proponents.

As we will describe in more detail later (see the section entitled "Transcription: Creating the Template for Protein Synthesis"), the first transfer of genetic information occurs in the nucleus, where a gene residing within the chromatin mass undergoes transcription and yields a large precursor RNA, historically referred to as heterogenous nuclear RNA (hnRNA).[3] This large precursor undergoes 5', 3', and internal modifications to generate the mature form of mRNA that is transported from the nucleus to the cytoplasm (see the section entitled "Posttranscriptional Modification of mRNA"). The second transfer of genetic information occurs in the cytoplasm, where the mature mRNA interacts with ribosomes and other protein synthetic machinery to encode a protein through the process of translation (see the section entitled "Translation: Regulated Protein Biosynthesis"). During translation, several ribosomes, composed of structural RNAs and associated proteins, produce a convoy of nascent polypeptide chains as they move in 5' to 3' direction along the mRNA template. This complex structure, designated the polyribosome, resides either freely in the cytoplasm or tightly attached to the endoplasmic reticulum (ER), which transmits the nascent polypeptide chains down a path that typically leads to their secretion from the cell. For polypeptide hormones, this vectorial transport is an essential component of their synthetic life cycle.

In short, gene expression begins when structural changes in chromatin are activated, allowing for the initiation of gene transcription, processing of the emergent RNA transcript, transport of mature RNA to the cytoplasm, and translation of the encoded polypeptide. It is important to note that a translated protein may require posttranslational modifications before it acquires normal biologic activity (see the section entitled "Posttranslational Modifications"). The ensuing sections will highlight additional conceptual details for each of these aspects of gene expression and protein biosynthesis and will summarize how hormones function to regulate each stage.

CHEMICAL NATURE OF DNA AND ITS RELATIONSHIP TO CHROMATIN

While DNA was first discovered to be a component of chromosomes in 1869,[3] the simple composition of nucleic acids actually misled investigators into believing that they were a purely structural component of the chromosome and that proteins accounted for cell specificity. The idea that DNA may be the genetic material was spawned by studies performed by Frederick Griffith in 1928.[1,3–5] Griffith observed that heat-killed pathogenic bacteria had the capacity to transform live nonpathogenic bacteria into pathogenic organisms. On transformation, the once nonvirulent bacteria acquired the appearance of pathogenic bacteria. In 1944, Avery and colleagues chemically identified this "transforming factor" as DNA.[1,3,5,6] However, this information was not broadly received by the scientific community, as many believed that the "genetic protein" was overlooked in the experiments. It was not until 1952 that Hershey and Chase firmly identified DNA as the genetic material.[1,3,5,7] They accomplished this by infecting *Escherichia coli* with bacteriophage in which DNA was radiolabeled with ^{32}P and protein with ^{35}S. They found that only radioactive DNA entered the infected *E. coli*. Additionally, the radiolabeled parental DNA was identified in the progeny phage that was expelled from the infected cells.

Even before DNA was determined to be the genetic material, scientists had begun to characterize the chemical makeup of the molecule. Each polynucleotide chain contains a "random" array of four different nucleobases representing two chemical classes, pyrimidines [cytosine (C) and thymine (T)] and purines [adenine (A) and guanine (G)] (Fig. 2-1). Each base contains a pentose sugar moiety (deoxyribose) and a phosphate group. Each base links to the deoxyribose through a N1 glycosidic bond to form a nucleoside. The 5' carbon of the pentose ring of the deoxyribonucleoside links to the phosphate through a phosphodiester bond to form a deoxyribonucleotide. The backbone of a polynucleotide chain forms by linking the 5' phosphate group of one nucleotide to the 3' hydroxyl of the deoxyribose ring of the adjacent nucleotide, allowing the nitrogenous bases to protrude. Two polynucleotide chains run in opposite directions to form a right-handed double helix structure with hydrogen bonding between complementary nitrogenous base pairs where A always pairs with T, and G pairs with C.[1-3,5]

The DNA from an individual haploid human cell contains approximately 3×10^9 base pairs,[1] totaling a length of 2 meters if extended end to end. Since the nucleus of a eukaryotic cell is less that 10 μm in diameter, fitting long linear DNA into this small space requires several ordered steps of compaction. In a sense, compaction is initially achieved through segmentation of DNA into series of discrete fragments with each length of DNA forming the backbone of the chromosome, the ultimate compacted form of DNA. The second level of compaction occurs as the long fragmented strands of DNA begin to wrap around a class of highly basic proteins referred to as histones. DNA wraps around a protein octamer consisting of two copies each of four core histone proteins (H3, H4, H2A, and H2B) (see Fig. 2-1)[1-3,5,8] The surface of the histone octamer contains two left-hand turns of DNA that span 146 base pairs (bp).[2,5,9] This complex of DNA and histones defines a nucleosome, a series of structures that are linked by DNA that enters or leaves the core particle. The length of DNA that links two nucleosomes varies between 8 and 114 bp and itself is complexed with another histone (H1).[1,5,8,10] The ordered periodicity of histone octamers can be visualized by electron microscopy and yields a classic "beads on a string" appearance. Ultimately, nucleosomes become covered by nonhistone chromosomal proteins, the largest and best characterized group of which are the high-mobility group proteins.[5,8,11,12] This ternary complex of DNA, histone proteins, and nonhistone proteins, defines chromatin, which is the basic unit of genetic material found in transcriptionally active, nondividing cells.

Although chromatin is essential for the compaction of the eukaryotic genome, it creates a formidable obstacle between the gene expression machinery and DNA regulatory elements. In fact, the topologic problem becomes even more complex as the so-called "beads on a string" become more compacted. Histone H1 proteins are responsible for packing nucleosomes on each other to form solenoid structures (see Fig. 2-1),[2,5,10] higher-order arrays in which DNA is further condensed to

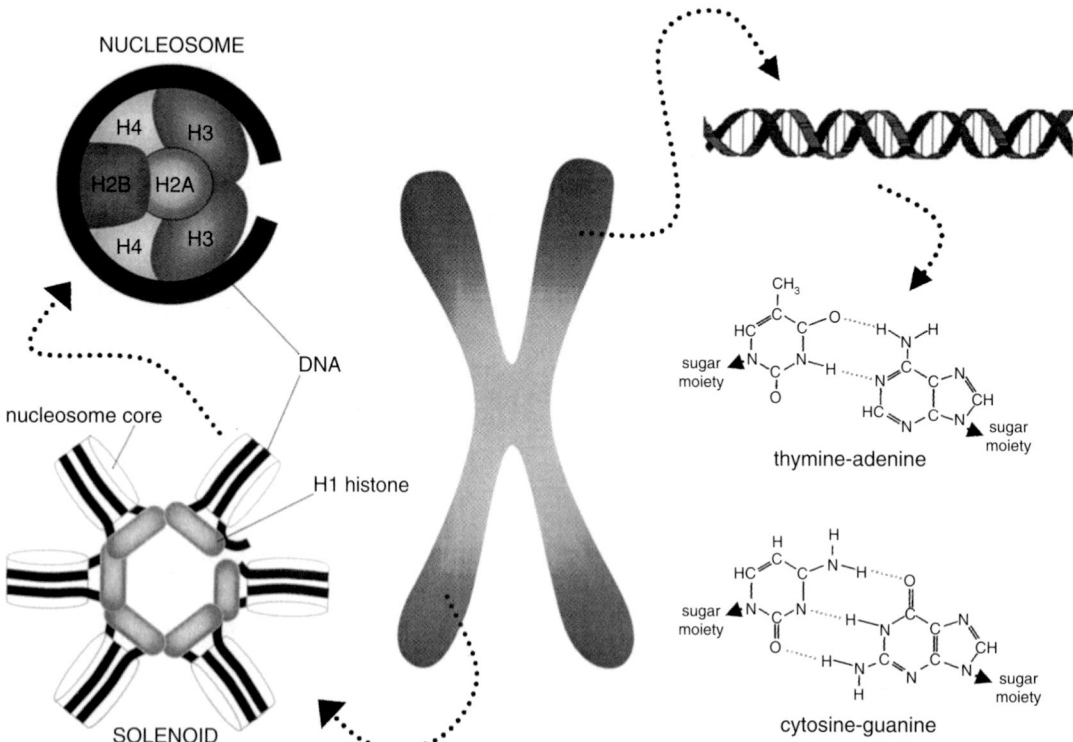

Figure 2-1 Chemical structure of DNA and its relationship to chromatin. The most basic unit of the chromosome is DNA, which is composed of polynucleotide chains made up of four different nucleobases: thymine, adenine, cytosine, and guanine. Each polynucleotide chain runs in opposite directions to form a right-handed double helical structure with hydrogen bonding between complementary base pairs, where adenine always pairs with thymine and guanine always pairs with cytosine. This double helix is compacted by wrapping around a protein octamer consisting of two copies each of four core histone proteins (H3, H4, H2A, and H2B) forming a nucleosome. Nucleosomes are further condensed via another histone (H1), which links flanking DNA that enters and leaves the core particle and functions to pack nucleosomes on each other to form solenoid structures.

form euchromatin. Heterochromatin is the highly compacted form of chromatin that makes DNA sequences structurally inaccessible to the transcription machinery, resulting in functionally inactive genes. In fact, chromosomes represent the culminating form of compaction. These are transcriptionally inactive, transient structures that occur only during a unique temporal period of the cell cycle that leads ultimately to DNA replication and cell division.[13]

A striking example of heterochromatinization that correlates with gene inactivation is the nuclear structure called the Barr body. All female mammals have evolved a mechanism to permanently inactivate one of the two X chromosomes that are present in virtually all somatic cells to achieve dosage equivalence of gene products of the X chromosome between males and females.[14] During this process, which is known as X inactivation, one of the X chromosomes is highly condensed to form a distinct structure known as the Barr body.[2] Hypoacetylation of histone H4 moieties is necessary for maintenance of X inactivation. Additionally, it appears that hypermethylation stabilizes the inactive X chromosome. Studies have shown that genes on the inactive X chromosome can be reactivated by preventing methylation of the DNA.

In sum, nucleosomes may be randomly or very specifically located over the bulk of chromosomal DNA and provide an important conceptual framework for fully understanding how hormones regulate gene transcription. The structure of chromatin is dynamic, with the state of the nucleosome core playing a pivotal role in governing the transcriptional competence of the targeted genes. Consequently, acetylation (associated with activation) and deacetylation (associated with repression) of histone proteins represent important steps that must be accommodated in a mechanistic model that defines hormone action.[5] We will explore this issue in greater detail later in the chapter (see the section entitled "Hormonal Control of Gene Expression and Protein Biosynthesis").

FUNCTIONAL ANATOMY OF A GENE

Within the vast amount of DNA from each eukaryotic cell, approximately 30,000 genes can be found per haploid genome. Although Gregor Mendel called them particulate factors instead of genes in 1865,[1] he clearly characterized their essential attributes. Strictly defined, a gene is the region of DNA transcribed by RNA polymerase.[1,5] This definition holds for both prokaryotes and eukaryotes. In prokaryotes, however, the gene is colinear with respect to the transcribed

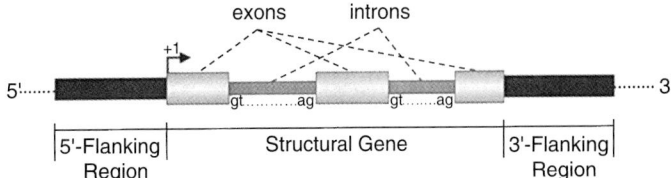

Figure 2-2 Functional anatomy of a gene. Regions of the structural gene that are retained in mature mRNA are known as exons, while the intervening sequences that are excised are called introns. The 5' and 3' sequences of all introns are conserved, encoding the splice donor (gt) and splice acceptor (ag), respectively. The region immediately upstream of the first transcribed nucleotide is referred to as the 5'-flanking region while the portion of the gene that is located downstream of the structural gene is referred to as the 3'-flanking region. The gene promoter is typically located in the 5'-flanking region, allowing for the correct initiation and efficiency of transcription. The nucleotide where transcription begins is designated +1.

mRNA, whereas in eukaryotes, colinearity is often lacking. Regions of the transcribed gene found in mature mRNA are referred to as exons, short for expressed regions of DNA (Fig. 2-2). The precursor hnRNA exons are interrupted by intervening sequences (introns) that are excised as the nascent transcript is processed to its mature form. Steps involved in RNA processing are explored in more detail below.

The region immediately upstream of the first transcribed nucleotide is referred to as the 5'-flanking region (see Fig. 2-2).[1,2,5] Within this region lies the promoter, which contains all the information necessary for specifying the correct initiation of transcription and regulates the efficiency of transcription. Typically, the nucleotide where transcription begins is designated +1. Consequently, most portions of a promoter are denoted by a negative numbering system of nucleotides, indicating the upstream positioning of the domain. Achieving accurate initiation of transcription is essential for ensuring constancy of the reading frame used for translation of the transcribed mRNA. Modulating the efficiency of transcription gives cells the capacity to produce more or less protein as the need arises.

Since a gene is typically defined as the region transcribed by RNA polymerase, all transcribed regions downstream of the +1 nucleotide fall within this functional domain. Most genes encoding mRNA (those transcribed by RNA polymerase II) begin with a purine, either A or G (Fig. 2-3). However, defining the end of a gene transcribed by RNA polymerase II is

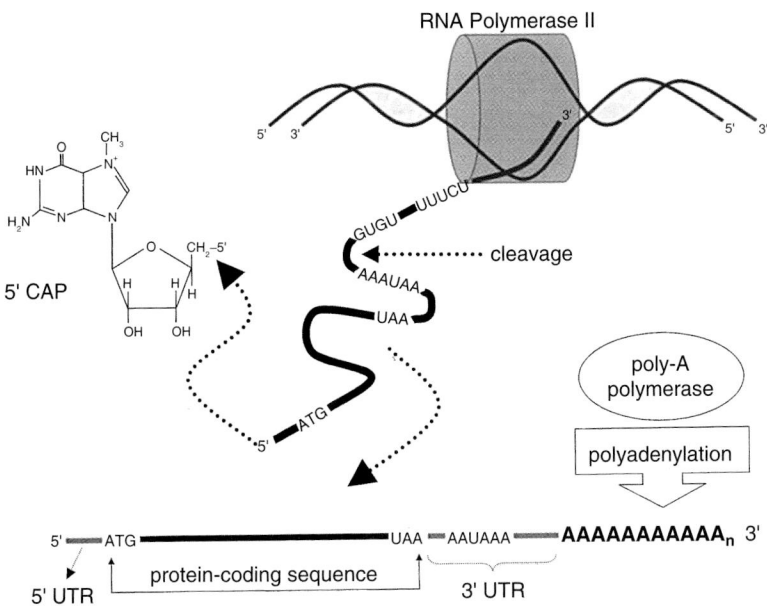

Figure 2-3 Transcription by RNA polymerase II creates the template for protein synthesis. Messenger RNA is the single-stranded molecule that transfers the genetic information from DNA in the nucleus to the cytoplasm, where proteins are translated. Mature mRNA is "capped" by addition of 7-methylguanosine to the 5' end through a triphosphate linkage formed between its 5'-hydroxyl and the 5'-hydroxyl of the terminal residue in the untranslated region (5' UTR) of the initial transcript. The 3' ends of growing transcripts are cleaved between the polyadenylation sequence and sequences rich in guanine and uracil found in the 3' untranslated region (3' UTR). Following this cleavage event, poly-A polymerase enzyme adds 200 to 250 adenine residues. Both modifications of the mRNA confer mRNA stability, translational efficiency, and play a role in exportation of the mature mRNA from the nucleus to the cytoplasm.

more problematic. Unlike prokaryotic genes, there is no fixed site that specifies termination of transcription.[1] Instead, a posttranscriptional processing event, addition of a homopolymeric tail of adenine nucleotides (poly A) signifies the end of the precursor hnRNA that will be further processed to generate mature mRNA.[1–3,5,15] The enzyme that specifies polyadenylation, poly A polymerase, recognizes a specific hexameric sequence (AATAAA) and then cleaves the precursor mRNA approximately 29 bp downstream with resulting 3'-OH group used as the substrate for subsequent addition of approximately 200 to 250 adenine residues.[1,3,15] The region of the gene that extends beyond the site of polyadenylation is referred to as the 3'-flanking region.

In most mRNAs transcribed by RNA polymerase II, the start codon that specifies the beginning of the translation reading frame (ATG) is located between 5 and 100 bp downstream from the 5'-end of the transcribed mRNA.[1,3] Thus, the region between the 5'-end of the mRNA and the translation start site is referred to as the 5'-untranslated region. Similarly, the codon that defines the end of the translation reading frame (UAG, UAA, or UGA) is usually followed by a relatively long run of nucleotides before reaching the hexanucleotide sequence that defines the site for polyadenylation (see Fig. 2-3). This region is referred to as the 3'-untranslated region.

The processing of the precursor mRNA (hnRNA) will be described in more detail in a subsequent section (see the section entitled "Posttranscriptional Modification of mRNA"). However, before we treat this subject, it is useful to note that the functional significance of introns remains unclear. One important clue stems from the observation that some mRNAs can undergo alternative processing. When this occurs, a specific transcribed segment can either be retained and act as an exon or can be excised and act as an intron. Introns that can act as exons when retained contain long open reading frames that encode a polypeptide fragment. The unique duality of this type of intron (the capacity to act as translation reading frame when retained) may allow for the shuffling of functional units to create families of related products from a single gene.[1,3] Additionally, certain intronic sequences in lower eukaryotes have been shown to contain open reading frames that encode proteins involved with either DNA or RNA metabolism; including endonucleases, reverse transcriptases, and maturases.[1] These "parasitic genes" have the intrinsic capacity to remove themselves from the nascent host transcript that surrounds them. This excision process is known as self-splicing or autosplicing.[1]

FUNCTIONAL ANATOMY OF THE PROMOTER-REGULATORY REGION

In general, a promoter contains two functional domains. The core region of the promoter is defined as the minimal 5'-flanking region that is required for accurate initiation of transcription. The second promoter domain usually resides immediately upstream and contains one to several regulatory elements that regulate the level of transcription in various cell types and in response to extracellular signals. Since these elements are physically linked to the gene they regulate, they are referred to as *cis*-acting regulatory elements. However, the functionality of these elements emerges only on the binding of a specific transcription factor that is almost always encoded by a different gene. Hence, *cis*-acting elements bind *trans*-acting factors.

Transcription factors are modular and contain at least two functional domains: one that binds specifically to a given *cis*-acting element and one that directly or indirectly either influences correct initiation or modulates the efficiency of transcription. The boundaries of *cis*-acting elements are defined by the region of DNA that is actually contacted by the DNA-

binding domain of a specific *trans*-acting factor and are usually less than 20 bp in length.[1,2] Frequently, they contain a core recognition sequence of 8 to 10 bp that is often palindromic,[1,2] reflecting twofold symmetry of transcription factor binding as dimers composed of the same subunit (homodimers) or different subunits (heterodimers).

The core promoter usually consists of an initiator element (Inr) that encompasses the transcription start site and a TATA box that is typically located 25 to 35 bp upstream of the transcription start site in higher eukaryotes and binds TATA-binding protein (TBP) (Fig. 2-4).[16,17] TBP is a key component of transcription factor (TF) IID, the only general transcription factor to bind DNA in a sequence-specific manner.[3,5,16] TBP binds in the minor groove of the DNA double helix and forms the foundation of the preinitiation complex. Native TFIID is a large multi-subunit protein (>700 kDa) consisting of TBP and at least eight TATA-associated factors (TAFs).[16,17]

Once TFIID binds, several other general transcription factors follow in an ordered succession, forming an extremely large core transcription complex (see Fig. 2-4). TFIIA, composed of three subunits (14, 19, and 34 kDa), binds TFIID and DNA upstream of TBP, although this event is not DNA sequence-specific.[2,5,16] TFIIA stabilizes TFIID and causes a conformational change in TBP that may displace a negative component in the native TFIID.[16] TFIIB, a single 35-kDa subunit, binds to and stabilizes the TFIID-IIA complex. TFIIF, consisting of two polypeptides (30 and 74 kDa), forms a molecular bridge with TFIIB between RNA polymerase II (Pol II) and TBP.[5,16] Both TFIIB and TFIIF appear to function in start site selection. RNA polymerase II consists of 10 polypeptides,

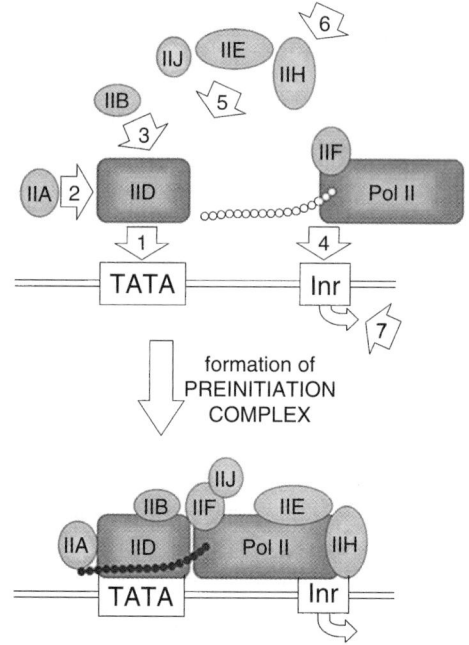

Figure 2-4 Assembly of the basal transcription machinery. The first step in formation of the preinitiation complex is the recognition and binding of TFIID (TBP plus 8 TAFs) to the TATA box. The second step consists of the coupling of TFIIA to TFIID, stimulating and stabilizing TFIID binding. The third step involves TFIIB binding to either TFIID or the TFIID/TFIIA complex. Fourth is the association of the unphosphorylated form of RNA polymerase II (Pol IIA) with the growing complex. The fifth step consists of the sequential binding of TFIIE, TFIIH, and TFIIJ to form the preinitiation complex. The sixth step involves the enzymatic activities of TFIIH allowing the phosphorylation of RNA polymerase II (Pol IIO), melting of the DNA duplex at the transcription start site, and the release of TFIIE, TFIIB, and two subunits of TFIIH. Finally, TFIIA and TFIID remain bound to the promoter, while Pol IIO, TFIIF, and one subunit of TFIIH move to form the elongation complex.

ranging in size from 10 to 240 kDa, the largest of which contains an unusual C-terminal domain (CTD) that is extensively phosphorylated.[16,18] The unphosphorylated form of Pol II (Pol IIA) preferentially associates with the committed complex relative to the phosphorylated form (Pol IIO). TFIIE, which functions as a tetramer (two copies each of 34 and 56 kDa subunits), binds TBP, TFIIF, Pol IIA, and TFIIH, the next protein to bind the growing complex.[19] TFIIH (at least eight subunits totaling 200 to 300 kDa) is the only general transcription factor to show catalytic activity, including CTD kinase activity that is regulated by TFIIE.[16,19] Additionally, TFIIH appears to function as a helicase and a DNA-dependent ATPase.[16,19] TFIIJ is the last factor to enter the preinitiation complex. Although it is known that TFIIJ is required, the function of this factor has not been characterized. It is the formation of this core transcription complex that determines the accurate initiation of transcription.

Although TFIID is capable of recognizing several nonconsensus TATA sequences, some promoters clearly lack a TATA box.[2,20] This is especially true for promoters in some housekeeping genes such as the gene encoding an enzyme that catalyzes the formation of adenosine monophosphate from adenine and phosphoribosylpyrophosphate.[1] This protein acts as a salvage enzyme for recycling of adenine into nucleic acids. Preinitiation complex assembly on these TATA-less promoters is mediated through the Inr, the consensus sequence of which is pyrimidine-pyrimidine-**A**-N-T/A-pyrimidine-pyrimidine, A being the transcription start site at +1.[20] In these cases, Pol II recognizes and binds the Inr directly and nucleates the binding of the other factors in the preinitiation complex.[21]

One to several *cis*-acting elements are located in close proximity and 5′ to the TATA box (Fig. 2-5). These accessory elements set the basal transcriptional tone of the promoter by increasing the efficiency of transcription. The *trans*-acting factors that bind these elements are generally ubiquitous, including Sp1 and NF-Y, which bind GC-rich regions and CCAAT boxes, respectively.[1,2,22] The binding of these factors

to DNA results in protein-protein interactions with the basal transcription machinery to increase or decrease transcription in a non-tissue-specific manner. Given the ubiquitous presence of factors such as Sp1 and NF-Y, it is not surprising that their corresponding *cis* elements are located on promoters of many genes, including housekeeping genes that provide basic functions needed for maintenance of all cell types.

Given their close proximity and direct interaction with the core transcriptional machinery, accessory elements are position- and orientation-dependent. This is in contrast to enhancers, another class of promoter regulatory elements (see Fig. 2-5), which are located farther upstream from 100 bp to several thousand base pairs or even within 3′ to the gene they regulate.[1-3,5] When assayed for activity by attachment to a heterologous core promoter, activities of enhancers display considerable distance, orientation, and position independence. Nevertheless, the *trans*-acting factors that bind this class of regulatory elements must also make contact with the core transcriptional machinery. Although the distance between an enhancer and TATA box may be considerable, this contact may occur through looping of the DNA.[1-3]

Enhancers represent a broad class of elements that are capable of binding a variety of transcriptional factors. Some of these are tissue- or cell-specific and thus confer this property to the promoter they regulate. In addition to increasing transcription, enhancers can also repress transcription, depending on the nature of the protein they bind. While some enhancers act alone, others are represented by tightly packed arrays of *cis*-acting elements and are designated as composite enhancers.[1] In fact, it is not uncommon to find that tissue- or cell-specific expression is determined by the concerted action of composite enhancers that bind both ubiquitous and tissue- or cell-specific proteins.

In addition to housing elements that determine basal transcriptional tone and spatially restricted expression, promoter regulatory regions also contain *cis*-acting elements that confer responsiveness to a wide variety of homeostatic agents, such as hormones, and to an equally wide array of environmental cues and insults. These elements are referred to as response elements. Like the elements noted above, response elements can bind proteins that are either ubiquitous or relatively cell-type specific. One such inducible factor, presumably activated by stress, is the heat shock transcription factor (HSTF) that binds heat shock elements (HSEs).[1] Normally, this factor exists in cells but is inactive. When cells are insulted by a sudden increase in temperature, HSTF becomes active and binds HSEs located in the promoters of genes that encode proteins. This aids in cell survival at higher temperatures. An explanation about how hormones bind response elements and either induce or repress transcription of the genes they regulate will be explored later (see the section entitled "Hormonal Control of Gene Expression and Protein Biosynthesis").

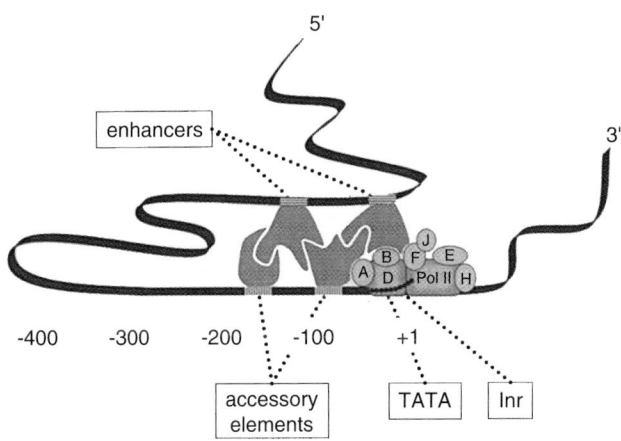

Figure 2-5 Functional anatomy of the promoter-regulatory region. The core region of the promoter, defined as the minimal 5′-flanking region required for accurate initiation of transcription, is typically made up of the initiator element (Inr), which encompasses the transcription start site, and a TATA box. The second domain resides in close proximity to the core promoter and contains one to several accessory elements that modulate the efficiency of transcription. Enhancers are another class of promoter regulatory elements that are usually located further upstream from the gene to which they regulate. Contact between *trans*-acting factors that bind enhancers, accessory elements, and the basal transcription machinery occurs through looping of the DNA. All transcription factors that bind regulatory elements contain a domain that binds specifically to a given *cis*-acting element and another domain that directly or indirectly influences transcription.

TRANSCRIPTION: CREATING THE TEMPLATE FOR PROTEIN SYNTHESIS

Although DNA is the genetic material, it does not function as the scaffold for protein synthesis. Messenger RNA is the single-stranded intermediate molecule that transfers the genetic information from DNA in the nucleus to the cytoplasm, where it serves as a template in the formation of polypeptides. RNA is quite similar in structure to DNA; in fact, a single strand of RNA can even form a double-stranded hybrid helix with a DNA strand. One minor difference between RNA and DNA involves the pentose sugar of RNA.[1,2] It contains an additional hydroxyl group (ribose as opposed to deoxyribose). In addition, uracil (U) replaces T in RNA. Despite these subtle differences, organisms have evolved mechanisms allowing for a smooth transition from DNA to RNA through transcription.

Transcription is the first step in which genetic information is converted from DNA into RNA and proteins. It is also the major point at which gene expression is regulated. A eukaryotic gene can be classified on the basis of the enzyme that drives its transcription. RNA polymerases are multi-subunit enzymes that synthesize RNA using a DNA template. The most active of the RNA polymerases is RNA polymerase I, which resides in the nucleolus and is responsible for transcribing genes encoding ribosomal RNA (rRNA), a major component of ribosomes.[1,3,5] RNA polymerase II, or Pol II, as was mentioned previously, is also a highly active nuclear enzyme that is responsible for synthesizing hnRNA, a precursor to mRNA.[1,3,5] The final RNA polymerase, RNA polymerase III, transcribes transfer RNA (tRNA), an adapter molecule involved in translation. This chapter will remain focused on genes whose expression is transcribed by Pol II.

POSTTRANSCRIPTIONAL MODIFICATION OF mRNA

During synthesis, immature mRNAs are covalently modified at both their 5' and 3' ends (see Fig. 2-3). Almost immediately following initiation of precursor mRNA synthesis, the 5' end of the molecule is "capped" by addition of a methylated guanosine.[1,3,5] 7-Methylguanosine is attached through a triphosphate linkage formed between its 5'-hydroxyl and the 5'-hydroxyl of the terminal residue in the initial transcript. This cap plays a role in nuclear transport of the mRNA. Additionally, the 5' cap is essential for most mRNA translation, because it facilitates binding of the translation machinery to the 5' end of the mRNA.[1,3] This modification also protects the fragile mRNA from degradation as the unique 5' to 5' phosphodiester bond of the cap makes it intrinsically resistant to general ribonucleases.[23]

The 3' ends of growing transcripts are cleaved at a point 10 to 30 bases downstream of the polyadenylation signal sequence, AAUAAA (see Fig. 2-3). This sequence is found in nearly all eukaryotic mRNAs and is one of the most conserved elements known.[1,3,5,15,24] Other elements, containing GUGU and UUUCU sequences, are located 20 to 40 bases downstream of the cleavage site. Immediately following cleavage of the nascent transcript, poly-A polymerase enzyme adds 200 to 250 adenylate residues.[1,24] Like the 5' cap, this modification confers mRNA stability, promotes mRNA translational efficiency, and plays a role in mature mRNA export from the nucleus to the cytoplasm.[1,3,24]

Many mRNA precursors in the nucleus are much larger than their cytoplasmic mRNA counterparts associated with ribosomes. Excision of the intronic, or noncoding, sequences (Fig. 2-6) is the most significant modification that mRNA undergoes before the mature form is transported to the cytoplasm. Each intron contains conserved sequences at the 5' and 3' ends, known as the splice donor (GU) and acceptor (AG), respectively.[1,3,5] An array of small ribonucleoproteins and associated nuclear proteins form a complex known as the spliceosome, which recognizes the ends of the intron and brings them together.[1,3,5] The immature mRNA is cleaved immediately upstream of the splice donor at the 5' end of the intron, and the terminal G covalently links to an A found near a pyrimidine-rich region that precedes the splice acceptor, forming a lariat structure.[1,3,5] The lariat is cleaved immediately downstream of the splice acceptor, and the intron is rapidly degraded while the adjacent two exons are joined together.

Alternative splicing of precursor mRNAs is a common mechanism whereby cells exploit the splicing mechanism to generate multiple related proteins from a single gene.[25] Once thought to be an exception to the rule (one gene, one protein), alternative splicing is now estimated to occur in at least 1 of every 20 genes.[25] One example of a single gene that

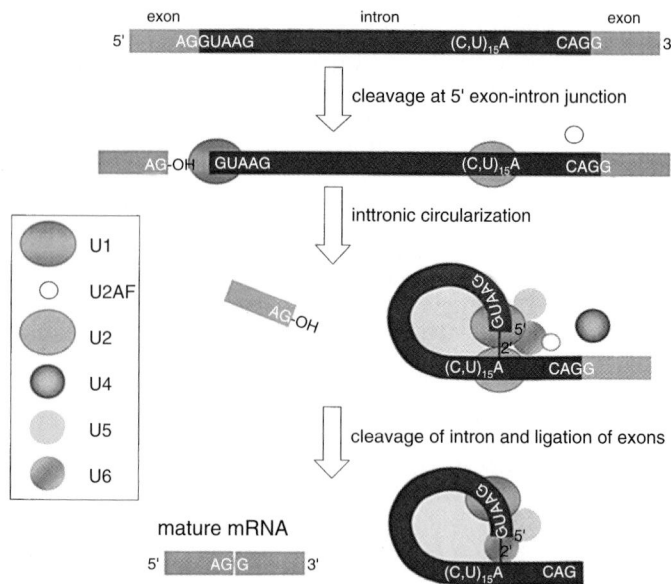

Figure 2-6   Splicing is a posttranscriptional modification of mRNA. Splicing involves the excision of intronic sequences from the mRNA before the mature form is transported to the cytoplasm. Immature mRNA is cleaved immediately upstream of the splice donor (GU) at the 5' end of the intron and the terminal G nucleotide covalently links to an A residue found near a pyrimidine-rich region near the 3' end of the intron, forming a lariat structure. A large array of small ribonucleoproteins and associated nuclear proteins identified in the box to the left form a complex known as the spliceosome, which recognizes the ends of the intron and brings them together. This lariat is cleaved immediately downstream of the splice acceptor (AG), and the adjacent two exons are joined together while the intron is degraded.

is alternatively spliced is α-tropomyosin, which encodes seven tissue-specific variants of the muscle protein that associates with actin in the rat.[3,5] This gene consists of "constitutive" exons that are found in all transcripts of the gene, "cell-specific" exons that appear only in transcripts produced in certain tissues, and exons that show variable expression. The mechanism of splice site selection and the interaction between multiple *cis*-acting elements and corresponding protein factors during these alternative splicing events remain to be determined. Another type of alternative processing involves the inclusion or removal of various intronic sequences. Such is the case for the bovine growth hormone gene, in which the last intronic sequence may be retained in a fraction of mRNA and transported to the nucleus, allowing for production of a variant form of the hormone.[26–29] Additionally, the use of alternative polyadenylation signals from a single transcript increases the diversity of its biologic responses, as with the hormone calcitonin, which is produced in the thyroid gland, and calcitonin gene-related peptide, which is produced in the hypothalamus.[2,24,27,30,31] Both hormones are the products of a single gene that undergo alternative processing and polyadenylation of its RNA transcript.

TRANSLATION: REGULATED PROTEIN BIOSYNTHESIS

Once a mature mRNA has been transported from the nucleus to the cytoplasm by unknown mechanisms, it becomes an integral part of protein synthesis. Nucleotides now carry the genetic message that determines the specific amino acid sequence composing a protein. Each amino acid is represented in the mRNA by a sequence of triplet nucleotides called codons, which are arranged in a contiguous reading frame. The first codon, or "start" codon, in mRNA is usually AUG. It encodes methionine and is most often used to initiate translation. The 3' end of the reading frame contains one or more specific "stop" codons, serving as signals to terminate extension of the polypeptide chain.[2]

Amino acids are delivered to the mRNA via an adapter molecule, the cloverleaf-shaped tRNA. Each tRNA contains a trinucleotide sequence, an anticodon, complementary to the codon sequence of the amino acid to which it is covalently linked. The anticodon allows each tRNA to recognize the appropriate codon sequence in the mRNA through complementary base pairing, which occurs in conjunction with ribosomes. Ribosomes are compact ribonucleoproteins, comprising two subunits (40S and 60S) whose mass consists primarily of rRNAs that control the recognition between a codon of mRNA and the anticodon of tRNA.[1] Protein synthesis requires synchronized involvement of all the above-listed RNA species and is generally considered in three stages: initiation, elongation, and termination, each of which will be considered further.

To initiate eukaryotic protein synthesis, the ribosome must first bind to the mRNA, forming the initiation complex and delivering the first amino acid. This step usually determines the rate of synthesis of a given protein.[1,3] Binding of the ribosome 40S subunit to the mRNA requires the presence of methionine-tRNA as well as several initiation factors, including proteins that recognize the 5' methylated cap on mRNA. Once bound, the 40S subunit migrates along the mRNA until it identifies the start codon, as well as a conserved sequence around the initiation codon, GCC(A/G)CCAUGG.[1,3,5] When the 40S subunit is joined by the 60S subunit, ribosome binding is stabilized at the initiation site.

The elongation phase of protein synthesis begins once the complete ribosome is formed at the start codon. Ribosomes have two sites for tRNA binding. Peptidyl-tRNA, the most recent addition to the nascent polypeptide chain, occupies the P, or donor, site, and aminoacyl-tRNA, the next amino acid to be added, enters the A, or acceptor, site.[1,5] Constituents of the ribosomal 60S subunit catalyze peptide bond formation when the polypeptide chain carried by the peptidyl-tRNA is transferred to the amino acid carried by the aminoacyl-tRNA. After the bond forms, a deacetylated tRNA devoid of an amino acid occupies the P site, and a peptidyl-tRNA now occupies the A site, while the peptide chain has increased in length by one amino acid. The ribosome translocates, advancing three nucleotides and moving the deacetylated tRNA out of the ribosome by expelling it directly into the cytosol, and the new peptidyl-tRNA moves into the P site, while the next codon lies in the A site, waiting for the appropriate aminoacyl-tRNA to enter. An elongation factor mediates entry of the next aminoacyl-tRNA to the A site.[1,5]

The final stage of translation is termination, which encompasses the steps necessary to release the completed polypeptide chain from tRNA and allow for dissociation of the ribosome from mRNA. Three stop or termination codons, UAG, UAA, and UGA, known as amber, ochre, and opal, respectively, do not encode an amino acid but function to end protein synthesis.[3,5] These codons are recognized directly by protein factors that signal the termination of protein synthesis, which involves the release of the completed polypeptide from the last tRNA. This reaction is analogous to the peptidyl-tRNA transfer, except that water enters instead of the aminoacyl-tRNA. The ribosome is also released from mRNA owing to a conformational change, but the complex set of accessory factors involved has not yet been identified.[1]

POSTTRANSLATIONAL MODIFICATIONS

Many secreted peptide hormones are biosynthesized as larger precursor species.[5,31] These precursor species are converted by proteolytic processing to a final hormone, as is the case for the biosynthesis of parathyroid hormone (PTH). Pre-pro-PTH, an initial product of synthesis on the ribosomes, is converted to pro-PTH during polypeptide transport into the cisterna of the rough ER. The function of the "pre-" sequence that is cleaved is to facilitate the insertion of the nascent peptide into the membrane of the rough ER. The resulting pro-PTH is further cleaved by another specific peptidase to form PTH, the mature form of the hormone, which is packaged into secretory granules in the parathyroid gland.[27]

As was previously mentioned, alternative splicing allows an exception to the "one gene, one protein" rule, a part of the central dogma of molecular biology, as more than one transcript can be derived from a single gene. Another exception to this rule is found in the pathway of gene expression and protein biosynthesis; that is, alternative protein processing, a process by which a single gene is transcribed into a single mRNA and translated into a large precursor protein molecule that is fragmented into several functional units. Pro-opiomelanocortin (POMC) undergoes this type of posttranslational processing.

Corticotroph cells of the anterior lobe, melanotroph cells of the intermediate lobe of the pituitary gland, as well as specific loci of the brain, synthesize the precursor glycoprotein molecule known as POMC. However, processing of the propolyhormone varies depending on its cellular site. In the anterior lobe, the majority of POMC is processed to adrenocorticotropic hormone (ACTH), β-lipotropin, γ-lipotropin, and β-endorphin.[27,31] Processing of POMC is different in the intermediate lobe of the pituitary gland, where peptide bonds in the ACTH sequence are broken to produce mainly α-melanocyte-stimulating hormone (α-MSH) and a corticotropin-like peptide called CLIP. In the brain, the major products are ACTH, β-endorphin, and α-MSH.[27,31]

Many newly synthesized polypeptides undergo major modifications as they mature to functional proteins: formation of disulfide bonds; protein folding, including possible formation of multichain proteins; proteolytic cleavage; as well as addition and modification of carbohydrates, phosphates, and lipids. All of these events are regulated functions, although the magnitude of their importance is variable.[31]

REGULATED SECRETION OF PROTEINS

Translation occurs free in the cytosol unless there is a signal sequence that directs its synthesis elsewhere. The sequence of many proteins begins with approximately 20 amino acids that function as a signal sequence, targeting the protein to its proper destination within the cell. For example, the signal sequence of secretory proteins, which is comprised mostly of hydrophobic amino acids, is bound by a complex of ribonucleoproteins, called the signal recognition particle (SRP) that directs ribosome attachment to an SRP receptor site on the cytosolic face of the ER. As the newly synthesized protein enters the cisternal space of the ER, a complex of five proteins (i.e., the signal peptidase) cleaves off this signal sequence as translation of the protein continues. In essence, the cell utilizes signal sequences as a general mechanism to dispatch proteins to specific sites.[1,5,27,31]

Many proteins leave the ER wrapped in transport vesicles, budded from the transitional ER, to the *cis* face of the Golgi apparatus, which modifies and/or stores proteins until they are eventually shipped to the cell surface or other destinations. Mature proteins exit the *trans* faces of Golgi within the lumen of budding membranous vesicles that eventually fuse with the plasma membrane, allowing for protein secretion.[1,31] The stored polypeptides remain in these vesicles, the secretory granules, until the appropriate extracellular signals (e.g., interaction of a hormone with cellular membrane receptors) produce secondary and tertiary messengers that trigger the release of such stored proteins (Chapter 7). Such signals may activate specific intracellular kinases that phosphorylate other proteins within the cell, which then interact with the secretory granules to participate in release of their stored contents.[1,27,31] These intracellular signals will be discussed in the following section (see the section entitled "Hormonal Control of Gene Expression and Protein Biosynthesis") and in subsequent chapters (Chapters 8 through 14).

HORMONAL CONTROL OF GENE EXPRESSION AND PROTEIN BIOSYNTHESIS

From this general overview of information flow of the gene to the secretory granule during polypeptide biosynthesis, it is clear that there are multiple potential sites of hormone regulation. However, only the regulation of the initiation of transcription is common to all hormones. For example, polypeptide hormones regulate transcription and secretion. In contrast, steroid hormones generally regulate transcription but not protein secretion. Therefore, this section will focus on this one property that is common to the action of all hormones.

All hormones act on distant cellular targets.[31] To regulate transcription, hormones must transduce their signals from outside the cell to the nucleus and ultimately to a set of specific gene targets (Fig. 2-7). All hormone-responsive cells must harbor a receptor that is specific for the incoming hormone. Additionally, all hormone-responsive genes must contain a specific hormone response element (RE) that binds a cognate DNA-binding protein. Transcription factors that interpret the hormone signal can be regarded as a subclass of DNA-binding proteins that regulate transcription. Thus, they contain at least two modular domains shared by all transcriptional factors: a DNA-binding domain and a domain required for transcriptional activation.

All polypeptide and peptide hormones, along with some biogenic amines such as epinephrine and norepinephrine, bind receptors that reside on the cell surface (see Fig. 2-7).[31] Since these hormones cannot enter cells to initiate their biologic actions, they instead rely on an indirect mechanism for communicating with their hormone-responsive DNA-binding proteins. The signal transduction event begins when this class of hormones binds their cell-surface receptors with great specificity and high affinity. Binding induces a conformational change in the receptor that converts it from an inactive to active state.[1,2,5] The activated receptor directly or indirectly activates or inhibits a cascade of molecular effectors that culminates in the posttranscriptional activation of a specific hormone-responsive DNA-binding protein.

There are four general classes of cell-surface hormone receptors (see Chapters 8 through 11). The first types of cell-surface receptors are in fact effectors, since binding of agonist directly activates the effector function.[31,32] Enzymatic function is activated when the ligand binds to the receptor, as exemplified by the epidermal growth factor and insulin receptors, which are tyrosine kinases.[31,32] However, cytokine receptors, such as the growth hormone and prolactin receptors, do not have intrinsic kinase activity but can activate intracellular kinases.[32] Another family of receptors with intrinsic enzymatic activity on ligand binding is the serine/ threonine kinase receptor class, which binds transforming growth factor-β and related proteins.[32]

There are also activated receptors that couple through guanosine triphosphate (GTP)-binding regulatory proteins to activate effectors. These receptors, known as G protein–coupled receptors, include receptors for epinephrine, thyroid-stimulating hormone, and glucagon.[31,32] These membrane receptors, when bound by agonist, lead to increases in intracellular second messengers, such as adenosine 3′,5′-monophosphate (cylic adenosine monophosphate [cAMP]), phosphoinositides, diacylglycerol, and calcium.[32] This signaling triggers serine kinase

cascades and phosphorylation of resident nuclear transcription factors, leading to activation and/or inhibition of gene transcription.

Generally, DNA-binding proteins that transduce signals from polypeptide hormones retain their binding specificity in the absence of hormone. Thus, signal transduction along this pathway generally involves a series of kinases that lead to the phosphorylation and subsequent activation of the target transcription factor. Examples of hormone-responsive DNA-binding proteins include members of the b-Zip family of transcription factors: cAMP response element binding protein (CREB) and c-Jun/c-Fos in the protein kinase A and C signaling systems, respectively.[5,33,34]

Though necessary, activation of the transcription factor is often not sufficient for subsequent transduction of a signal that requires communication with components of the downstream core transcription complex. A large nuclear "integrator" provides the bridge serving to functionally integrate the signal from the hormone-responsive transcription factor to the basal transcription complex (see Fig. 2-7). One of these integrators, known as CREB-binding protein (CBP), belongs to a distinct subclass of transcription factors, known as coactivators, that do not bind directly to DNA but bind to other proteins that bind DNA.[35] CBP was originally identified as a coactivator of the transcription factor CREB. However, CBP and its homologue p300 have multiple domains that are capable of interacting with the transactivation domains from several different hormone-responsive DNA-binding proteins. In fact, an array of transcription factors are able to form stable physical complexes with, and respond to the coactivating properties of, CBP/p300, including CREB, MyoD, c-Jun, c-Fos, c-Myb, NF-κB, nuclear receptors, and numerous others.[35,36] The p300 and CBP integrators bind multiple factors simultaneously with their protein-binding domains and assist in the "recruitment" of basal transcription machinery as well as other coactivators. CBP/p300 also has domains that are required for interacting with members of the core-transcription complex.

Multiple coactivators have been identified, including the integrator, defined as a protein that interacts with the DNA-bound transcription factors and the basal transcription machinery, forming a functional connection between the two to enhance transcription.[36–38] Besides this bridging function, CBP/p300 has intrinsic histone acetyltransferase activity and the capacity to interact with extrinsic histone acetyltransferases.[9,35–37,39] As histones become hyperacetylated, they dissociate from DNA and generate a more open chromatin structure that allows for increased transcription.[5,9,40] In addition to these critical roles, CBP/p300 can also acetylate transcription factors directly, which may result in stimulation of their DNA-binding activity. Indeed, a rich network of communication encompassing various signaling pathways results in abundant molecular cross-talk. Additionally, increasing evidence indicates that this integrator molecule appears to transduce signals from virtually all steroid and polypeptide hormones studied to date.

In contrast to polypeptide hormones, steroids are hydrophobic molecules that usually circulate in the serum bound with low affinity to nonspecific carrier proteins. Because steroid hormones are lipophilic, free hormone can easily diffuse through the cellular membrane and bind with high affinity to intracellular nuclear receptors that are, themselves, transcription factors (see Fig. 2-7).[31,36] These nuclear receptors are members of a superfamily of functionally and structurally related transcription factors that have a third domain required for ligand-specific binding (LBD). Indeed, steroid hormone receptors were among the first transcription factors to be cloned and characterized. Members of this superfamily include receptors for steroid hormones, such as estrogen, androgens, progesterone, glucocorticoids, and aldosterone, as well as hormonal forms of vitamins A and D,

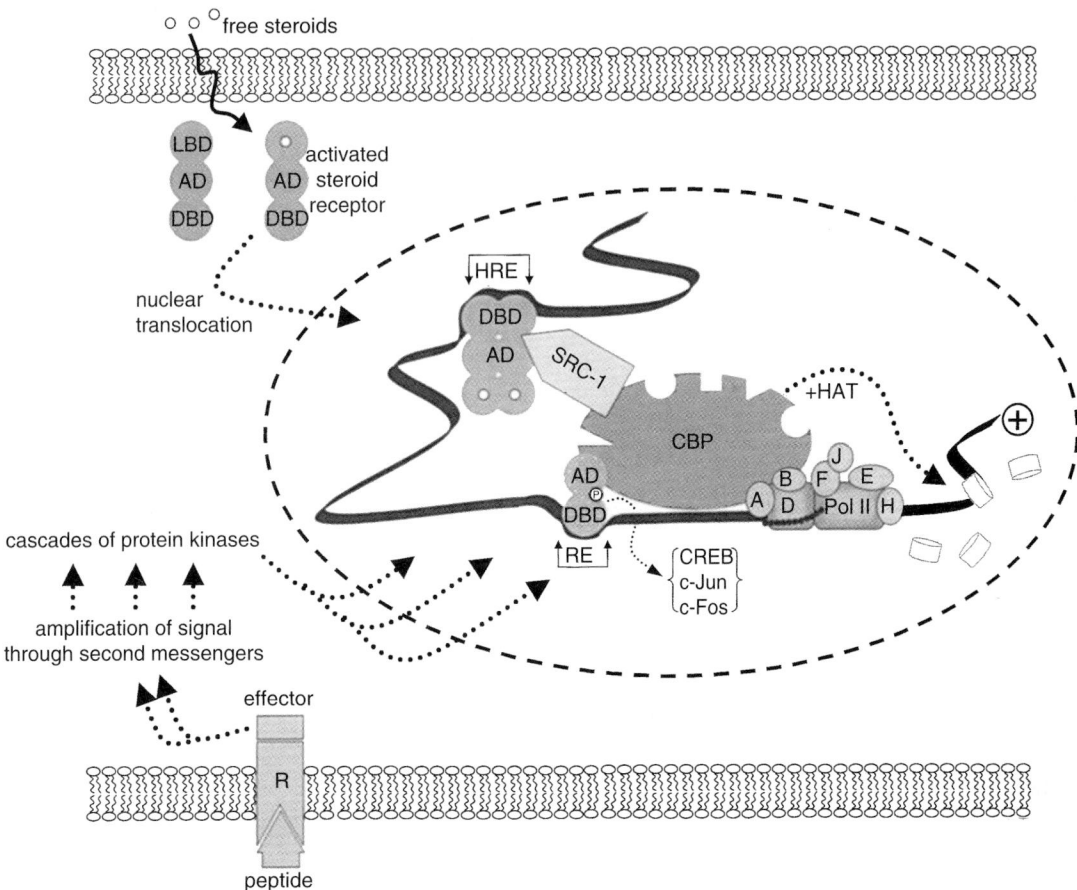

Figure 2-7 Steroid and peptide hormone control of gene expression. Free steroid hormones diffuse through the cellular membrane and associate with the ligand-binding domain (LBD) of intracellular nuclear receptors found in the cytoplasm, causing phosphorylation of the receptor, dissociation of several receptor-associated proteins, and exposure of a cysteine-rich zinc-finger DNA-binding domain (DBD). This "activated" receptor, which is itself a transcription factor, translocates to the nucleus and binds specifically to its cognate hormone response element (HRE). The transcription factor typically associates with the CBP integrator indirectly via an additional coactivator, such as steroid coactivator-1 (SRC-1), that binds both the activation domain (AD) of the steroid receptor and a glutamine-rich region in CBP. In contrast, some steroid hormones function through the binding of corepressors, which interact with extrinsic factors, including histone deacetylases that function to tighten the chromatin structure, providing a barrier to transcription by making nucleosomes more stable. Peptide hormones, on the other hand, bind receptors (R) located on the cell surface, inducing a conformational change in the receptor that converts it to an active state. This starts a signal transduction cascade, culminating in the posttranscriptional activation of a specific hormone-responsive DNA-binding protein, which binds to specific response elements (RE) in the 5'-flanking region of the promoter from the hormonally responsive gene. The CBP integrator has intrinsic histone acetyltransferase (HAT) activity, which acts to relieve the nucleosome barrier to transcription, providing the bridge to functionally integrate the signal from the transcription factor to the basal transcription complex.

thyroid hormone, and others, many of which have not yet been identified.[31,36]

Unlike the DNA-binding proteins that transduce the signal from polypeptide hormones, most of the members of the nuclear receptor family reside in the cytosol in the absence of hormone (see Fig. 2-7). Initiation of the hormone response is triggered on the noncovalent, reversible association of the steroid receptor with its ligand.[5,31,38,41] Generally, steroid receptors become phosphorylated, and several receptor-associated proteins, including heat shock protein 90, are dissociated.[42] This "activated" receptor translocates to the nucleus via a nuclear localization signal.[5,31] A cysteine-rich zinc-finger DNA-binding domain permits the ligand-occupied steroid receptor to bind specifically to its cognate hormone RE.[5,31,41]

As will be discussed in more detail in a subsequent chapter (see Chapter 15), nuclear receptors can be subclassified according to the sequence and spatial relationship of the *cis*-acting elements to which they bind. These steroid hormone REs are organized as two partially palindromic half-sites that are separated by a specific number of nucleotides.[36,41] For example, the consensus glucocorticoid (G) RE is AGAACAnnnTGTTCT, where the three "n" bases can be any nucleotide but the spacing is invariant. The configuration of

other hormone REs is quite similar to that of the GRE, but slight variations in sequence, orientation, and spacing between the half-sites allows for specificity of receptor binding. Alteration of these sequences may result in loss of hormonal responsiveness.

In contrast to the hormone-responsive DNA-binding proteins that mediate the action of polypeptide hormones, ligand-occupied steroid receptors, although capable of interacting directly with the integrator CBP molecule, typically exhibit an indirect interaction through the bridging of additional cofactors (see Fig. 2-7).[36,37] These nuclear receptor coactivator proteins, which functionally link the hormone-responsive DNA-binding protein to the integrator, do not bind directly to DNA but instead bind specifically to the trans-activation domains of the hormone-responsive DNA-binding proteins and to specific domains found within CBP.[36,38] The yeast two-hybrid system and Far Western blotting have been used to identify several cofactor proteins that interact with members of the nuclear receptor superfamily.[37,38] The first functional coactivator, the steroid receptor coactivator-1 (SRC-1), appears to be a general enhancer of transactivation of steroid hormone–dependent target genes.[36,38] Subsequently, many more coactivators have been identified, including other

SRC family members[43,44] and TRAPs/DRIPs.[45,46] CBP functionally interacts with the steroid hormone receptor coactivators to synergistically enhance transcription of steroid hormone–responsive genes.

The activity of some members of the nuclear receptor superfamily is not regulated by coactivators but rather is regulated through relief of tonic inhibition by corepressors.[37] For example, in the absence of thyroid hormone, thyroid hormone receptors repress transcription of many genes; and in the presence of thyroid hormone, thyroid hormone receptors activate transcription of those same genes.[38,47,48] In the unliganded state, thyroid hormone receptors interact with one of several corepressor proteins. These proteins interact with extrinsic factors, including histone deacetylases, which function to tighten chromatin structure; thus, nucleosomes become more stable and provide a barrier to transcription. The binding of thyroid hormone to the thyroid hormone receptor elicits a conformational change that causes the release of the corepressor and recruitment of coactivator proteins.

Although the mechanism by which steroid and peptide hormones ultimately regulate transcription is similar, polypeptides work through second messengers, while generally, steroid hormones directly activate the target DNA-binding receptors (see Fig. 2-7). Consequently, much higher concentrations of steroid hormones are required to achieve a transcriptional response, since there is no amplification of the hormonal signal. For example, a single polypeptide hormone can interact with a receptor on the cell surface. Each activated receptor in turn can interact with several downstream effectors. Each activated effector generates a large number of second messengers, which activate protein kinases. Each protein kinase may phosphorylate and thereby activate other enzymes, producing a large number of product molecules and contributing to the cellular response. Many of these intracellular signaling pathways are illustrated in Chapters 12 through 14. In contrast, each steroid receptor must be bound by ligand to elicit the active conformation of each individual *trans*-acting factor.

It has long been suspected that many steroids have another mechanism of action, as some rapid responses cannot be explained by intracellular receptors functioning as transcription factors.[49] One exception to the genomic actions of steroid receptors and their family members that has recently been uncovered is the existence of cell-surface estrogen receptors that have been shown to stimulate intracellular signaling events on ligand binding.[50] This suggests that estrogen can function much like peptide hormones at cell-surface receptors and that estrogen may perform transcription-independent functions.[51]

Although focus has been directed to events occurring at the gene transcriptional level, it is evident that other sites of the protein synthesis pathway may be points at which hormone regulation may occur. For example, estrogen has been shown to stabilize chicken liver vitellogenin mRNAs, and prolactin has been shown to increase the half-life of casein mRNAs in breast tissue. RNA splicing may also be hormonally regulated. In addition to tissue-specific RNA-splicing events that have already been described, it is possible that such processes are hormonally regulated, not only to yield different mRNAs by alternative exon and polyadenylation site choice, but also to alter the expression of one *versus* another mRNA by alternative promoter choice. In addition, it is possible that transcription elongation and termination may be other foci for hormonal regulation. Furthermore, translation and protein processing are also likely to be hormonally regulated.

FUNCTIONAL GENOMICS

It has been stated that we have entered the third technologic revolution. Great advances have been made with the passing of the Industrial and Computer Revolutions. The next great era, the Genomics Revolution, is upon us.[52] The term *genome*, first used by Hans Winkler in 1920, was created by merging the words *gene*s and chromo*some*s and refers to an organism's complete set of chromosomes and their genes.[53] The term *genomics* was coined much later, in 1986, by Thomas Roderick, to describe the scientific discipline of mapping, sequencing, and analyzing genomes and was consequently the namesake for a scientific journal that was initiated at that time, *Genomics*.[53,54] In essence, the goal of genomics is to make biologic and functional sense of raw genetic information.

Structural genomics represents an initial phase of genomic analysis that is the construction of a high resolution genetic map of an organism. The Human Genome Project (HGP), which emerged in 1990, was a coordinated effort to characterize all human genetic material by determining the complete sequence of the human genome. The year 2003, which commemorated the fiftieth anniversary of the discovery of the double-helical structure of DNA,[55–57] marked another landmark event: completion of a high-quality, comprehensive sequence of the human genome.[58] With completion of the genetic map, 30,000 protein-encoding genes have been identified, making up only 1% to 2% of the 3 billion base pairs of DNA in the human genome.[58] Further information pertaining to the HGP can be accessed via the National Human Genome Research Institute at http://www.nhgri.nih.gov/.

Already, the field of genomics has expanded from the mapping and sequencing of the human and other genomes, to include an emphasis on genome function,[54] allowing for a better understanding of the function of human genes and their roles in health and disease.[59] In fact, technology and resources promoted by the HGP have made a profound impact on biomedical research and promise to revolutionize the wider spectrum of biologic research and clinical medicine. Increasingly detailed genome maps have aided researchers in seeking genes associated with many genetic conditions, including myotonic dystrophy, fragile X syndrome, neurofibromatosis types 1 and 2, inherited colon cancer, Alzheimer's disease, and familial breast cancer.

More than 2000 transcription factors are encoded in the human genome.[32] Mutations in transcription factors have been associated with numerous genetic endocrine disorders. Hence, it is not surprising that the HGP, by identifying thousands of new genes, many of which encode transcription factors, will ultimately provide the building blocks necessary to identify the causes of many genetic diseases. Additionally, in connection with the shift to functional genomics, the study of gene expression involved with genetic disorders has become invaluable, as important therapeutic strategies are based on an understanding of how the promoter regulatory elements drive or inhibit expression of specific genes.

While the complete sequencing of an organism's genome is an amazing accomplishment, it pales in comparison to the task that awaits scientists who must put meaning to these base pairs.[53] Functional genomics makes use of the vast amount of information provided by structural genomics to develop experimental approaches to assess gene function and has been defined as the continuum from a gene's physical structure to its role in the context of the biology of the whole organism.[59,60] The "new science" that is functional, or physiologic, genomics has been among us for many years, although its name was coined only a few years ago, corresponding with the HGP initiative.

The field of functional genomics has focused on elucidating the function of proteins encoded by genes that have been identified, and to understand the pathways in which these genes participate.[61] The concept of one gene causing one phenotype is rapidly giving way to the appreciation that many human diseases are genetically complex with the phenotype reflecting the combined contribution of many genes. In fact there is growing appreciation that any perturbation of a cell has a global impact affecting the expression of many genes that ultimately define the homeostatic response. To approach analysis of this complex biology, the field of functional genomics can be subdivided into two complementary approaches: measurement of transcriptomes and proteomes. Transcriptome refers to all the mRNAs expressed by a specific cell in a given physiologic state. This type of measurement is accomplished by using a genomewide array of specific DNA probes.[62–65] Similarly, a proteome describes all the proteins associated with a specific physiologic state.[66–68] Resolving these complex mixtures of proteins can be accomplished via two-dimensional gel electrophoresis and mass spectrometry using a procedure known as mass profiling.[66–69] Even with these emerging subdisciplines, there is a growing awareness for the need to develop mathematic models and other bioinformatic tools. This will allow contributions of kinetic parameters that govern biologic processes to be included in the analysis of transcriptomes and proteomes. In short, phenotypes are the net result of complex interactions and rate processes that occur among members of a specific pathway.

Rapid progress in genome science and a glimpse into its potential applications have spurred observers to predict that mathematically based biology, bioinformatics, will be the foremost science of the twenty-first century.[70] Technology and resources generated by the HGP and other genomics research are already having a major impact on research across the life sciences. On the horizon is a new era of molecular medicine characterized less by treating symptoms and more by looking to the most fundamental causes of disease.[70] Rapid and more specific diagnostic tests will make earlier treatment of countless maladies possible. Medical researchers also will be able to devise novel therapeutic regimens based on new classes of drugs, immunotherapy techniques, avoidance of environmental conditions that may trigger disease, and possible augmentation or even replacement of defective genes through gene therapy.[60,70]

REFERENCES

1. Lewin BM: Genes, vol VI. New York, Oxford University Press, 1997.
2. Darnell J, Lodish H, Baltimore D: Molecular Cell Biology, 2nd ed. New York, Scientific American Books, 1990.
3. Watson JD, Gilman M, Witkowski J, Zoller M: Recombinant DNA, 2nd ed. New York, Scientific American Books, 1992.
4. Griffith F: The significance of *pneumococcal* types. J Hyg 27:113–159, 1928.
5. Zubay G: Biochemistry, 3rd ed. Dubuque, IA, Wm C Brown Communications 1993.
6. Avery OT, MacLeod CM, McCarty M: Studies on the chemical nature of the substance inducing transformation of *pneumococcal* types. J Exp Med 98:451–460, 1944.
7. Hershey AD, Chase M: Independent functions of viral protein and nucleic acid in growth of bacteriophage. J Gen Physiol 36:39–56, 1952.
8. Wolffe AP, Kurumizaka H: The nucleosome: A powerful regulator of transcription. Prog Nucleic Acid Res Mol Biol 61:379–422, 1998.
9. Workman JL, Kingston RE: Alteration of nucleosome structure as a mechanism of transcriptional regulation. Annu Rev Biochem 67:545–579, 1998.
10. Laybourn PJ, Kadonaga JT: Role of nucleosomal cores and histone H1 in regulation of transcription by RNA polymerase II. Science 254:238–245, 1991.
11. Bustin M, Reeves R: High-mobility-group chromosomal proteins: Architectural components that facilitate chromatin function. Prog Nucleic Acid Res Mol Biol 54:35–100, 1996.
12. Goodwin G: The high mobility group protein, HMGI-C. Int J Biochem Cell Biol 30:761–766, 1998.
13. Wolffe AP: Packaging principle: How DNA methylation and histone acetylation control the transcriptional activity of chromatin. J Exp Zool 282:239–244, 1998.
14. Kay GF: Xist and X chromosome inactivation. Mol Cell Endocrinol 140:71–76, 1998.

15. Barabino SM, Keller W: Last but not least: Regulated poly(A) tail formation. Cell 99:9–11, 1999.
16. Orphanides G, Lagrange T, Reinberg D: The general transcription factors of RNA polymerase II. Genes Dev 10:2657–2683, 1996.
17. Barberis A, Gaudreau L: Recruitment of the RNA polymerase II holoenzyme and its implications in gene regulation. Biol Chem 379:1397–1405, 1998.
18. Corden JL: Tails of RNA polymerase II. Trends Biochem Sci 15:383–387, 1990.
19. Goodrich JA, Tjian R: Transcription factors IIE and IIH and ATP hydrolysis direct promoter clearance by RNA polymerase II. Cell 77:145–156, 1994.
20. Zenzie-Gregory B, Khachi A, Garraway IP, Smale ST: Mechanism of initiator-mediated transcription: Evidence for a functional interaction between the TATA-binding protein and DNA in the absence of a specific recognition sequence. Mol Cell Biol 13:3841–3849, 1993.
21. Colgan J, Manley JL: TFIID can be rate limiting in vivo for TATA-containing, but not TATA-lacking, RNA polymerase II promoters. Genes Dev 6:304–315, 1992.
22. Maity SN, de Crombrugghe B: Role of the CCAAT-binding protein CBF/NF-Y in transcription. Trends Biochem Sci 23:174–178, 1998.
23. Sachs AB: Messenger RNA degradation in eukaryotes. Cell 74:413–421, 1993.
24. Colgan DF, Manley JL: Mechanism and regulation of mRNA polyadenylation. Genes Dev 11:2755–2766, 1997.
25. Sharp PA: Split genes and RNA splicing. Cell 77:805–815, 1994.
26. Edens A, Talamantes F: Alternative processing of growth hormone receptor transcripts. Endocr Rev 19:559–582, 1998.
27. Norman AW, Litwack G: Hormones, 2nd ed. San Diego, Academic Press, 1997.
28. Stallings-Mann ML, Ludwiczak RL, Klinger KW, Rottman F: Alternative splicing of exon 3 of the human growth hormone receptor is the result of an unusual genetic polymorphism. Proc

Natl Acad Sci U S A 93:12394–12399, 1996.
29. Hampson RK, Rottman FM: Alternative processing of bovine growth hormone mRNA: Nonsplicing of the final intron predicts a high molecular weight variant of bovine growth hormone. Proc Natl Acad Sci U S A 84:2673–2677, 1987.
30. Lou H, Gagel RF: Alternative RNA processing: Its role in regulating expression of calcitonin/calcitonin gene-related peptide. J Endocrinol 156:401–405, 1998.
31. Baulieu E-E, Kelley P: Hormones: From Molecules to Disease. New York, Chapman and Hall, 1990.
32. Brivanlou AH, Darnell JE Jr: Signal transduction and the control of gene expression. Science 295:813–818, 2002.
33. Habener JF: Cyclic AMP response element binding proteins: A cornucopia of transcription factors. Mol Endocrinol 4:1087–1094, 1990.
34. Tamai KT, Monaco L, Nantel F, et al: Coupling signalling pathways to transcriptional control: Nuclear factors responsive to cAMP. Recent Prog Horm Res 52:121–139, 1997.
35. Goldman PS, Tran VK, Goodman RH: The multifunctional role of the co-activator CBP in transcriptional regulation. Recent Prog Horm Res 52:103–119, 1997.
36. Giguere V: Orphan nuclear receptors: From gene to function. Endocr Rev 20:689–725, 1999.
37. Jenster G: Coactivators and corepressors as mediators of nuclear receptor function: An update. Mol Cell Endocrinol 143:1–7, 1998.
38. Shibata H, Spencer TE, Onate SA, et al: Role of co-activators and co-repressors in the mechanism of steroid/thyroid receptor action. Recent Prog Horm Res 52:141–164, 1997.
39. Utley RT, Ikeda K, Grant PA, et al: Transcriptional activators direct histone acetyltransferase complexes to nucleosomes. Nature 394:498–502, 1998.

40. Kadonaga JT: Eukaryotic transcription: An interlaced network of transcription factors and chromatin-modifying machines. Cell 92:307–313, 1998.

41. Freedman LP: Anatomy of the steroid receptor zinc finger region. Endocr Rev 13:129–145, 1992.

42. McDonnell DP, Norris JD: Connections and regulation of the human estrogen receptor. Science 296:1642–1644, 2002.

43. McKenna NJ, O'Malley BW: Minireview: Nuclear receptor coactivators: An update. Endocrinology 143:2461–2465, 2002.

44. Liao L, Kuang SQ, Yuan Y, et al: Molecular structure and biological function of the cancer-amplified nuclear receptor coactivator SRC-3/AIB1. J Steroid Biochem Mol Biol 83:3–14, 2003.

45. Fondell JD, Ge H, Roeder RG: Ligand induction of a transcriptionally active thyroid hormone receptor coactivator complex. Proc Natl Acad Sci U S A 93:8329–8333, 1996.

46. Rachez C, Suldan Z, Ward J, et al: A novel protein complex that interacts with the vitamin D3 receptor in a ligand-dependent manner and enhances VDR transactivation in a cell-free system. Genes Dev 12:1787–1800, 1998.

47. Koenig RJ: Thyroid hormone receptor coactivators and corepressors. Thyroid 8:703–713, 1998.

48. Apriletti JW, Ribeiro RC, Wagner RL, et al: Molecular and structural biology of thyroid hormone receptors. Clin Exp Pharmacol Physiol Suppl 25:S2–S11, 1998.

49. Moggs JG, Orphanides G: Estrogen receptors: Orchestrators of pleiotropic cellular responses. EMBO Rep 2:775–781, 2001.

50. Ho KJ, Liao JK: Nonnuclear actions of estrogen. Arterioscler Thromb Vasc Biol 22:1952–1961, 2002.

51. Kelly MJ, Levin ER: Rapid actions of plasma membrane estrogen receptors. Trends Endocrinol Metab 12:152–156, 2001.

52. Abelson PH: A third technological revolution. Science 279:2019, 1998.

53. McKusick VA: Genomics: Structural and functional studies of genomes. Genomics 45:244–249, 1997.

54. Hieter P, Boguski M: Functional genomics: It's all how you read it. Science 278:601–602, 1997.

55. Watson JD, Crick FH: Molecular structure of nucleic acids: A structure for deoxyribose nucleic acid. Nature 171:737–738, 1953.

56. Wilkins MHF, Stokes AR, Wilson HR: Molecular structure of deoxypentose nucleic acids. Nature 171:738–740, 1953.

57. Franklin RE, Gosling RG: Molecular configuration in sodium thymonucleate. Nature 171:740–741, 1953.

58. Collins FS, Green ED, Guttmacher AE, Guyer MS: A vision for the future of genomics research. Nature 422:835–847, 2003.

59. Woychik RP, Klebig ML, Justice MJ, et al: Functional genomics in the post-genome era. Mutat Res 400:3–14, 1998.

60. Cowley AW Jr: The Banbury Conference. Genomics to physiology and beyond: How do we get there? Physiologist 40:205–211, 1997.

61. Borrebaeck CA: Tapping the potential of molecular libraries in functional genomics. Immunol Today 19:524–527, 1998.

62. Kozian DH, Kirschbaum BJ: Comparative gene-expression analysis. Trends Biotechnol 17:73–78, 1999.

63. Brent R: Functional genomics: Learning to think about gene expression data. Curr Biol 9:R338–R341, 1999.

64. Lipshutz RJ, Fodor SP, Gingeras TR, Lockhart DJ: High density synthetic oligonucleotide arrays. Nat Genet 21:20–24, 1999.

65. Schena M, Heller RA, Theriault TP, et al: Microarrays: Biotechnology's discovery platform for functional genomics. Trends Biotechnol 16:301–306, 1998.

66. Dove A: Proteomics: Translating genomics into products? Nat Biotechnol 17:233–236, 1999.

67. Hochstrasser DF: Proteome in perspective. Clin Chem Lab Med 36:825–836, 1998.

68. Blackstock WP, Weir MP: Proteomics: Quantitative and physical mapping of cellular proteins. Trends Biotechnol 17:121–127, 1999.

69. Lopez MF: Proteome analysis. I: Gene products are where the biological action is. J Chromatogr B Biomed Sci Appl 722:191–202, 1999.

70. Bailey JE: Lessons from metabolic engineering for functional genomics and drug discovery. Nat Biotechnol 17:616–618, 1999.

Cell Division, Differentiation, Senescence, and Death

Run Yu and Vincent L. Cryns

INTRODUCTION

Despite the seemingly infinite intracellular protein-protein interactions and signaling pathways, each cell has only a limited number of fates: it can divide, differentiate, permanently growth arrest (senescence), or die (apoptosis). These fundamental cellular processes are essential for the normal development and function of multicellular organisms, and they play an important role in maintaining homeostasis in response to a variety of stress stimuli. Cell division is the process by which one cell faithfully replicates its DNA and divides the duplicated DNA equally between two daughter cells. Cell differentiation is the process by which a stem cell acquires the specialized features of a given cell type. Both senescence (irreversible growth arrest) and apoptosis (cell death) are homeostatic responses to diverse stress stimuli (oncogenes, DNA damage, or cellular aging) that potentially lead to uncontrolled cell division and cancer. These fundamental cellular processes are carefully executed by highly conserved genetic programs. Given their central role in normal development, function, and homeostasis, defects in any one of these processes can lead to disease.

CELL DIVISION AND THE CELL-CYCLE MACHINERY

Cell division is a ubiquitous process largely conserved throughout evolution. Cell division was first observed by light microscopy in the late 1800s.[1] Insights into mechanisms governing cell division were first proposed in the 1950s, and fundamental concepts of the cell cycle were established in the 1960s.[2] Current understanding of cell division is based on microscopic, genetic, biochemical, and molecular biology studies. Cell division is accomplished through a series of predictable, sequential stages (the cell cycle) that results in a parent cell dividing into two daughter cells containing genetic information identical to that of the parent cell.[2-4] The essential goal is to synthesize an exact DNA copy and to partition the DNA equally into two daughter cells. Each cell cycle is subdivided into five phases: G_0, G_1, S, G_2, and M (Fig. 3-1). The M (*mitosis*) phase is readily apparent by light microscopy by virtue of the striking chromosome condensation and separation that occur. In contrast, G_0, G_1, S, and G_2 (collectively called *interphase*) cannot be distinguished by light

microscopy. DNA replication that defines S (*synthesis*) phase can be identified by incorporation of bromodeoxyuridine (BrdU) or radioactively labeled thymidine. G_0 and G_1 (*gap*) phases precede S phase, and G_2 follows S phase before mitosis onset.

Although cells in G_0 are functionally active, they are quiescent in terms of proliferation. At any given time, most adult solid tissue cells are in the G_0 phase. Even in pituitary adenomas, about 80% of cells are in G_0.[5] During G_1, the cell prepares for DNA synthesis. Proteins (especially enzymes) required for DNA synthesis are transcribed, translated, and targeted to their correct subcellular localization. In addition, raw materials required for DNA synthesis (four deoxyribonucleoside triphosphates: adenosine [dATP], guanosine [dGTP], thymidine [dTTP], and cytidine [dCTP]) also are stored. DNA is synthesized during S phase.[2-4] During G_2, the newly synthesized DNA is packaged into chromatin, and the cell also prepares for mitosis. M phase is further divided into prophase, prometaphase, metaphase, anaphase, and telophase by light microscopy.[6,7] Prophase starts as chromosomes condense and become visible by microscopy and ends with nuclear envelope breakdown. Chromosomes become attached to mitotic spindles during prometaphase, and metaphase begins with alignment of chromosomes at the equatorial plate. Anaphase is initiated by separation of sister chromatids and the concomitant shortening of mitotic spindles. During telophase, chromosomes begin to decondense and fuse to form a new nucleus, the nuclear envelope is reformed, and cytokinesis (separation of cytoplasm) occurs. It was recently proposed that mitosis also can be staged as five functional "transitions" between G_2 and the next interphase.[7]

The conserved cell-cycle machinery that regulates cell division has been studied in a variety of model organisms. The Nobel Prize in Physiology or Medicine in 2001 was awarded to Hartwell, Hunt, and Nurse for their pioneering work on cyclins and cyclin-dependent kinases (CDKs). Cyclins, CDKs, and CDK inhibitors (CKIs) are the core components of the cell-cycle apparatus.[8-10] Levels of cyclin protein expression oscillate during the cell cycle because of their regulated proteolysis by the ubiquitin-proteasome system.[8-10] Cyclins bind and activate CDKs, which are kinases that phosphorylate and modify the functions of key proteins required for cell-cycle progression. More than 10 mammalian cyclins and about 10 mammalian CDKs have been identified, and their differential expression and activity at precise stages of the cell-cycle

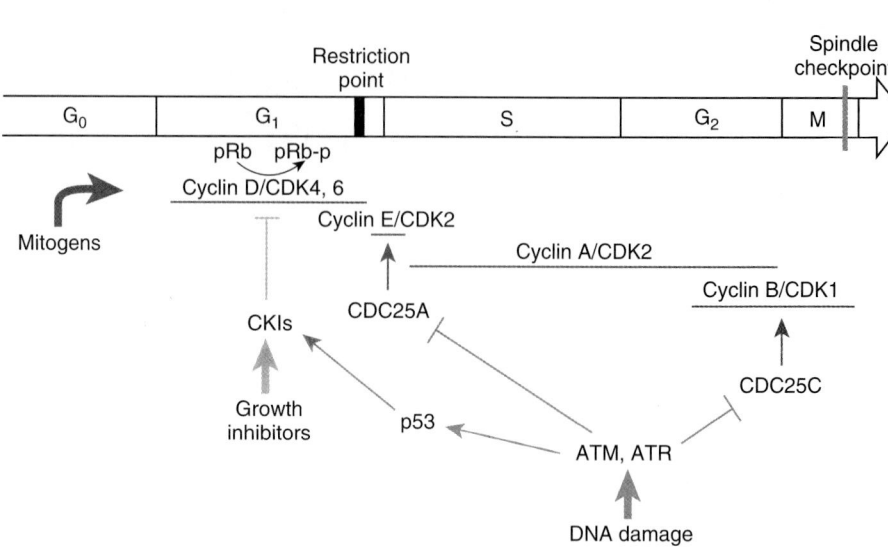

Figure 3-1 Schematic illustration of the cell cycle and its regulation. Each cell cycle has five sequential phases: G_0, G_1, S, G_2, and M. After completion of M phase, two daughter cells undergo similar cell-cycle phases to divide further. For most eukaryotic cells, the parental cell is incorporated into the daughter cells and no longer exists after each cell cycle. The cell cycle is propelled forward by orderly, phase-dependent expression of cyclin and cyclin-dependent kinases (CDKs) in response to mitogens, which are no longer required after the restriction point in late G_1 phase. Cyclin-dependent kinase inhibitors (CKIs) are activated by extracellular and intracellular signals and inhibit CDK4 and CDK6. Checkpoints provide the quality control for the cell cycle. Both CDKs and CKIs are effectors for DNA damage checkpoint. *Arrow* denotes activation, whereas *perpendicular line* denotes inhibition. This is a simplified presentation to depict the principle of cell-cycle regulation. See text for details.

orchestrate its orderly progression (see Fig. 3-1).[8–10] For example, when cells in the G_0 phase are stimulated by growth factors, D-type cyclins are first induced. Cyclin D then binds and activates CDK4 and CDK6, the primary target of which is the retinoblastoma tumor-suppressor gene product (pRb).[11–13] Hypophosphorylated pRb binds to and inhibits E2F family transcription factors, which are required for progression through G_1.[14,15] However, hyperphosphorylation of pRb by cyclin D-CDK4/CDK6 dissociates E2F from pRb, thereby activating E2F and allowing cell-cycle progression. Although mitogen withdrawal during early G_1 returns cells to G_0, cell-cycle progression will continue if mitogens are withdrawn after a "restriction point" in late G_1.[16] Cyclin E expression occurs at the G_1-to-S transition; cyclin E binds to CDK2 and initiates DNA synthesis.[17] Cyclin A is induced in S phase; it also binds to CDK2 (after cyclin E is degraded) and supports DNA synthesis.[18] It is not clear how CDK2 regulates DNA synthesis. Cyclin B levels gradually increase in G_2 and M, and translocation of cyclin B and its partner CDK1 to the nucleus irreversibly destines the cell to mitosis.[19] The cyclin B-CDK1 complex is the key component of the M phase–promoting factor (MPF). Although the specific mechanism for MPF to initiate and maintain mitosis status remains uncertain, it was recently shown that CDK1 has numerous targets that include proteins involved in CDK1 regulation, DNA synthesis, mitosis, spindle assembly, and actin polarization.[19,20] Cell cycle–dependent destruction of cyclin B and other mitotic proteins such as securin (see later) is critical for mitotic exit.[7,21]

CKI proteins inhibit CDKs, and structurally and functionally different CKI families include: the INK4 family (including p16INK4a, p15INK4b, p18INK4c, and p19INK4d) and the Cip/Kip family (including p21Cip1, p27Kip1, and p57Kip2).[22–24] CKIs cause G_1 arrest in response to extracellular and intracellular antiproliferative signals, and CKIs are regulated mostly at the expression level.[22–24] For example, p15INK4b is upregulated by transforming growth factor (TGF)-β, and p21Cip1 is upregulated by p53, a checkpoint effector (see later).[25,26] The INK4 family of CKIs disrupts the association of cyclin D and CDK4 and CDK6, thereby inhibiting G_1 progression, whereas the Cip/Kip family has a broader inhibitory range.[22–24,27] For example, p21Cip1 inhibits CDK2, CDK3, CDK4, as well as CDK6 by interfering with CDK phosphorylation rather than affecting cyclin binding.[27] Importantly, CKIs frequently function as tumor suppressors, and reduced or absent expression of CKIs is commonly encountered in tumors.[22–24,27]

The cell cycle can be viewed as an assembly line in which the successful execution of any given step depends on the perfect execution of the previous step. Abnormalities at any step result in defective and potentially harmful cell products. Cell-cycle checkpoints act to ensure quality control and integrity of the cell cycle.[8,28,29] The checkpoint mechanism is composed of a sensor, a transducer, and effectors, all of which are protein based.[8] When the checkpoint senses that appropriate criteria are not met, the transducer is activated and relays the signal to effector proteins required to correct the problem. Checkpoint activation induces cell-cycle arrest at that specific step, and the cell cycle is allowed to progress only after checkpoint criteria are satisfied. Numerous checkpoints have been identified throughout the cell cycle, and the best characterized are the DNA damage checkpoint and spindle checkpoint.[8,28,29] DNA damage threatens genetic integrity, and DNA requires repair for further cell-cycle progression to proceed. For the DNA damage checkpoint, which functions mostly in the G_1, S, and G_2 phases, sensors have yet to be identified, but transducers include the ataxia telangiectasia mutated (ATM) and ATM-related (ATR) proteins. Effectors are DNA damage-repair enzymes, transcription factors, and CDK and CKIs, such as BRCA1, p53, Cdc25C, and Cdc25A (see Fig. 3-1).[28,30] The spindle checkpoint prevents premature sister chromatid separation and consequent aneuploidy (abnormal numbers of chromosomes or chromosome segments). Again the molecular sensors for this checkpoint have not been identified, although they sense unattached kinetochores (the structures that attach spindles to centromeres). Mad and Bub proteins function as transducers, and the effector is the anaphase-promoting complex (discussed later).[29] The tumor suppressor p53 functions as a checkpoint effector and causes G_1/S or G_2/M block in response to a variety of cellular insults including DNA damage, and p53 also may contribute to the spindle checkpoint.[31]

REGULATION OF CELL DIVISION AND ABNORMAL CELL DIVISION

Cell division is influenced by a number of humoral factors including hormones or growth factors that act as endocrine, paracrine, and autocrine signals. Signal transduction from these humoral factors ultimately leads to changes in CDK and CKI expression levels and characteristics.[32] Insulin-like growth factor I (IGF-I), estrogen, and thyroid-stimulating hormone (TSH) stimulate cell division.[33–35] Both IGF-I and TSH induce cyclin D expression by increasing cyclin D messenger RNA (mRNA) transcription and activating cyclic adenosine monophosphate (cAMP), respectively.[36,37] Estrogen promotes cell proliferation by inhibiting p21^{Cip1} through multiple mechanisms, such as changing p21^{Cip1} subcellular localization away from cyclin E/CDK2 and forming different cyclin E/CDK2 complexes with reduced or no affinity for p21^{Cip1}.[32,38,39] In contrast, activin and glucocorticoids inhibit cell proliferation.[40,41] Glucocorticoids induce p21^{Cip1} mRNA transcription and increase p21^{Cip1} binding to CDK4, resulting in G$_1$ cell-cycle arrest.[42]

Oncogenes may deregulate the cell cycle, resulting in unrestrained proliferation and ultimately in tumor formation. In pituitary tumors, two prominent oncogenes are cyclin D1 and securin (originally termed PTTG, pituitary tumor transforming gene).[43] Securin regulates M phase by ensuring the equal partitioning of duplicated sister chromatids.[7,43] Mitotic spindles are attached to chromosomes at prometaphase and exert traction, but chromosomes are not separated because of chromatid bonding by cohesin proteins that hold sister chromatids together.[44,45] The cohesin protein complex comprises four subunits: SMC1, SMC2 (both bind to chromosomes), SCC1/RAD21, and SCC3/SA (both bind to SMC1 or SMC2). At the metaphase-to-anaphase transition, the cohesion component SCC1/RAD21 is cleaved by an enzyme termed *separase*, and this cleavage is essential for chromatid separation that initiates anaphase.[46,47] Separase is distantly related to caspases, cell-death proteases discussed later in this chapter.[48] To avoid premature chromatid separation, separase function is inhibited by its binding partner, securin.[49,50] When the spindle checkpoint is satisfied, an anaphase-promoting complex degrades securin, thus activating separase and allowing sister chromatid separation.[51,52] Securin was first identified as PTTG, which is overexpressed in pituitary tumors.[49,53] PTTG overexpression transforms fibroblasts, inhibits chromatid separation, and results in aneuploidy, demonstrating that mitosis disruption can result in tumorigenesis (Fig. 3-2).[54,55]

CELL DIFFERENTIATION

Cell differentiation was originally observed by zoologists in the late 1800s, and in 1945, the first experimental identification of stem cells, which have the capacity to proliferate indefinitely and to differentiate into other cell types, occurred.[56] In embryos, cell differentiation is an intrinsic component of development.[57–59] Stem cells proliferate, migrate, and establish contact with other cells, and simultaneously differentiate into specific cell types. In the adult, cell differentiation functions to maintain the pool of cells comprising tissue-specific functions (such as pancreatic β cells or blood cells). In this section, the major concepts underlying stem cells and cell differentiation are discussed.

STEM CELLS

In adult tissues, most cells are terminally differentiated and generally cannot further differentiate. In contrast, stem cells have the capacity to proliferate indefinitely and to differentiate into other cell types (*plasticity*) (Figs. 3-3 and 3-4).[60–63] Stem cells possess different potentials to differentiate.[62] Totipotent cells (i.e., the fertilized oocyte) can give rise to the whole embryo and part of the placenta. Pluripotent cells (i.e., embryonic stem cells) can form all the cells composing the embryo. Multipotential cells (e.g., hemopoietic stem cells) can differentiate into a limited range of cells. Unipotential cells (e.g., epidermal stem cells) give rise to only one type of cell. Because the DNA sequence in the genome remains constant through differentiation, differences between a stem cell and a differentiated cell are due to epigenetic modifications of the genome such as programmed DNA methylation.[57,60–64] Stem cells possess a unique gene-expression profile and are maintained in a favorable microenvironment milieu composed of differentiated cells and extracellular matrix

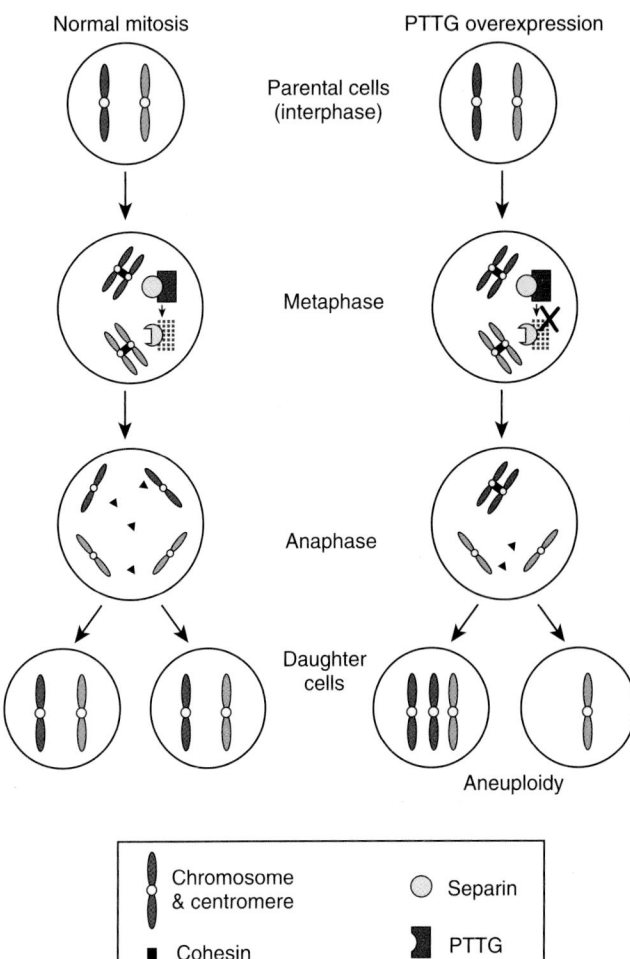

Figure 3-2 Schematic diagram of securin function and aneuploidy. **Left,** Normal mitosis. Pituitary tumor transforming gene (PTTG) is a mammalian securin which maintains binding of sister chromatids during mitosis. During mitosis, sister chromatids are bound with cohesins. PTTG inhibits separin, an enzyme that regulates cohesin degradation. At the end of metaphase, securin is degraded by an anaphase-promoting complex, releasing tonic separin inhibition, which in turn mediates degradation of cohesins that hold sister chromatids together. In this manner, sister chromatids are separated equally into daughter cells. **Right,** Mitosis in cells overexpressing PTTG. PTTG overexpression may render sister chromatid separation difficult and result in aneuploidy.

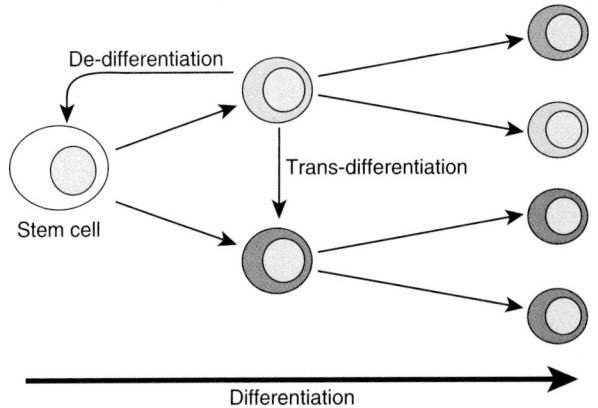

Figure 3-3 Cell differentiation. Cell differentiation is depicted as changing cytoplasmic colors in the cytoplasm, whereas the cell nucleus maintains identical genetic materials for all progeny. See text for details.

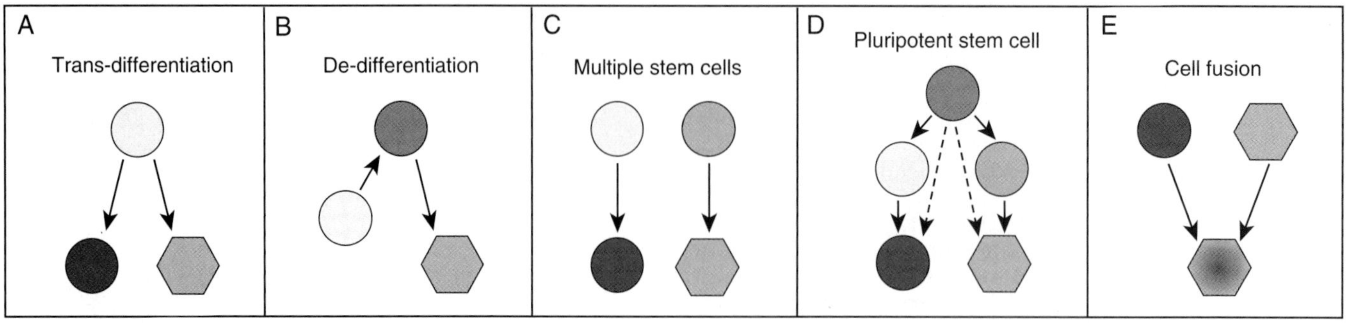

Figure 3-4   Potential mechanisms for adult stem cell plasticity. Multipotential (tissue-specific) stem cells are represented as *orange* or *green ovals*, pluripotent stem cells (embryonic) as *blue ovals*, and differentiated cells of the orange lineage as *red ovals* and of the green lineage as *green hexagons*. See text for details. (From Wagers AJ, Weissman IL: Plasticity of stem cells. Cell 116:639–648, 2004, with permission.)

for nourishment and support.[65,66] In adult mammals, such unique niches exist in the testis, ovary, gut crypt, and skin.[62,66] In practical terms, stem cell markers are used to isolate these cells from differentiated cells. For example, hematopoietic stem cells are positive for CD34 and Thy-1 but negative for CD10, 14, 15, 16, 18, or 20.[60] No endocrine stem cell markers have yet been identified.

Stem Cell Differentiation
Because stem cells possess a genetic content similar to that of terminally differentiated cells, two fundamental questions arise. The first is how a stem cell differentiates into a specific cell type. The second question is the converse of the first: how does a differentiated cell regain the "stemness" of a stem cell? For a cell to differentiate, it must first exhibit the characteristics of a stem cell. Extracellular signals then trigger the expression of specific transcription factors and differential gene expression (see Fig. 3-3).[57–59,65] The cell with the new gene-expression profile continues to be exposed to extracellular signals and undergoes further changes in gene expression. Initial cell differentiation during embryonic development is intricately linked to organogenesis. For example, both pancreatic β cells and pituitary endocrine cells are formed concurrent with the formation of the pancreas and pituitary organs, respectively.[58,59] Once progenitor cells are formed, specific transcription-factor and growth-factor expression commits the cells to specific cell types. In the pituitary gland, Pit-1 expression induces differentiation into somatotrophs, lactotrophs, and thyrotrophs, whereas GATA-2 expression induces cells to differentiate into gonadotrophs.[59] In a well-characterized in vitro system, mouse preadipocytes differentiate into adipocytes with added fetal bovine serum, insulin, dexamethasone, and methylisobutylxanthine, which result in differential expression of the PPARγ and C/EBPα transcription factors that are critical for the adipocyte phenotype.[67,68]

Although it has long been held that cell differentiation is irreversible, this dogma has recently been challenged. De-differentiation refers to the process by which a more differentiated cell reverts and becomes less differentiated, whereas trans-differentiation refers to the process by which a multipotential cell committed to one cell type is reprogrammed to give rise to other cell types (e.g., hematopoietic stem cells differentiating into muscle cells).[63,69,70] Although no clinically relevant studies used de-differentiation, some experiments have demonstrated that bone marrow cells may give rise to skeletal muscle, myocardial, hepatic, and brain cells.[62,71–73] The validity of such trans-differentiation claims is being challenged. For instance, multipotential cells can differentiate into different cell types by fusing with pluripotent cells, rather than by bona fide trans-differentiation.[71,72] In addition, contamination of donor tissue with other stem cells can occur.[73] De-differentiation and trans-differentiation are likely mediated by mechanisms similar to those of

differentiation: extrinsic signals that result in differential gene expression.

Stem Cell Therapy
The capacity of stem cells to proliferate and differentiate into various human cell types brings hope for potential therapies based on stem cell transplantation. Bone marrow transplantation is an excellent example of such therapy. The general procedure of stem cell therapy includes three steps: (1) procurement of stem cells, (2) in vitro stem cell proliferation, and (3) infusion of stem cells to the appropriate organs.[74] The most challenging task is procurement of stem cells because of our limited understanding of stem cell biology.[63] In principle, at least three ways are known to obtain stem cells (see Fig. 3-4). First, multipotential and unipotential cells can be directly isolated ex vivo (e.g., bone marrow stem cells).[60] Second, multipotential stem cells may be trans-differentiated to form other multipotential cells (e.g., trans-differentiation of bone marrow stem cells to neuronal stem cells).[70,73] Last, embryonic stem cells (pluripotent) can be engineered potentially to form any cell type.[61] More research is needed to determine which approach will be most productive. Few ethical concerns exist regarding the first and second approaches. However, the third approach is the subject of ethical debate, especially as the donor cells are derived from human embryos; currently federal funds are available only for research using preexisting embryonic stem cell lines.[75] Considerable controversy surrounds these restrictions.[76,77]

Unlike bone marrow, which contains numerous hemopoietic stem cells, endocrine cells usually do not proliferate rapidly, and rigorously defined endocrine stem cells have not been identified. Use of stem cell therapy for treating endocrine diseases remains largely theoretical. Stem cell therapy for diabetes would have an enormous clinical impact because diabetes has a high prevalence, significant comorbidities, inconvenience of replacement medication (subcutaneous insulin injection and blood glucose monitoring), and the paucity of islet cells available for islet cell transplantation.[78] Nestin appears to be expressed on pancreatic stem cell surfaces and may facilitate isolation of such stem cells.[79] A bone marrow pool of pancreatic stem cells also may be available for use.[80] Endoderm cells can be coaxed into pancreatic stem cells; for example, chick embryonic gut endoderm cells give rise to insulin-producing cells when cocultured with gut mesodermal cells.[81] These research accomplishments suggest that stem cell therapy may be a viable strategy to treat a number of diseases.

CELLULAR SENESCENCE: ESCAPING CELL DIVISION

As discussed in the previous sections, cell division plays a critical role in development and in tissue renewal, but the proliferative capacity of most cell types is limited. Indeed, most cells undergo a finite number of cell divisions in culture and then irreversibly growth arrest and permanently exit the cell cycle by a process known as replicative senescence.[82-84] More recently, it has become clear that cells also irreversibly exit the cell cycle in response to a variety of stress stimuli (e.g., oncogene activation, oxidative stess, and DNA damage). This latter process shares many of the features of replicative senescence and has been termed *stress-induced* or *premature senescence*. Regardless of the initiating event, senescent cells have a characteristic morphology (large and flattened shape) and a distinctive gene-expression profile (discussed later) that results in permanent cell-cycle arrest and other functional alterations. In this section, we present evidence that cellular senescence (replicative or stress-induced) is a genetically regulated safeguard activated by diverse stimuli that protects cells from unrestrained proliferation, thereby suppressing tumor formation.

REPLICATIVE SENESCENCE: TELOMERE EROSION

Replicative senescence is a response to the progressive shortening of telomeres, the protective structures that cap chromosome ends (repetitive DNA and associated proteins) and prevent chromosomes from fusing at these ends.[82-84] During each round of cell division, the DNA replication machinery fail to copy 50 to 200 base pairs of telomeric DNA thereby resulting in a small but steady erosion of telomeres. When telomeric structures have eroded to a critical point, resulting in their dysfunction (poorly understood at present but not simply a matter of telomeric length), replicative senescence is triggered to prevent further disintegration of telomeres, which could ultimately lead to chromosomal fusion and instability, a hallmark of cancer. Indeed, such critically eroded telomeres mimic damaged DNA and induce the activation of the p53 tumor-suppressor gene product, which halts proliferation in response to DNA damage.[84,85] As a "guardian of the genome," p53 is a key effector of senescence (both replicative and stress-induced), cell-cycle arrest, and apoptosis.[82-84,86] Telomerase synthesizes telomeres and is made up of RNA and protein components. Until recently, only cancer cells and some germ cells were thought to express telomerase. However, recent findings indicate that telomerase is transiently expressed in normal human fibroblasts during S phase.[87] In contrast to cancer cells, which constitutively express telomerase and escape replicative senescence, transient expression of telomerase during S phase does not prevent telomere erosion but plays an important, yet-to-be characterized role in cell proliferation.

STRESS-INDUCED SENESCENCE: THWARTING ONCOGENES AND DNA DAMAGE

Before the onset of replicative senescence, cells respond to diverse, potentially oncogenic stimuli (e.g., oncogene activation, reactive oxygen species, and agents that damage or modify DNA) by undergoing "premature" senescence. Although these cells do not have shortened telomeres, and telomerase does not prevent oncogene-induced senescence, prematurely senescent cells are strikingly similar to those that have undergone replicative senescence, in terms of both their cellular phenotype and their gene-expression patterns.[82-84,88] As is the case with replicative senescence, senescence induced by oncogenic Ras also is mediated by p53 and by cyclin-dependent kinase inhibitors such as p16[INK4a] (discussed later).[89] In this way, stress-induced senescence provides an important tumor-suppressive function by derailing the mitogenic actions of oncogenic stimuli.

CELLULAR SENESCENCE: P53 AND RB TUMOR SUPPRESSORS LEAD THE WAY

Given the tumor-protective effects of cellular senescence, it is not surprising that tumor-suppressor genes, such as p53 and RB, play critical roles in the induction of both types of cellular senescence (Fig. 3-5).[82-84] p53 is activated in senescent cells by a number of mechanisms, including via the induction of the tumor-suppressor gene product ARF (p14[ARF] in humans and p19[ARF] in mice).[90,91] ARF stabilizes the p53 protein by antagonizing MDM2/HDM2, a p53-binding protein that induces the degradation of p53 via the ubiquitin-proteasome pathway.[92] Conversely, the RB tumor-suppressor gene product is maintained in its active, hypophosphorylated state in senescent cells through the induction of a second tumor-suppressor gene in the ARF locus, called p16[INK4a], a cyclin-dependent kinase inhibitor that prevents cyclin D-CDKs from phosphorylating and inactivating RB.[89,92] Active RB inhibits cell-cycle progression through the G_1/S transition by binding and sequestering E2F family members, which are required for the expression of proteins critical for S phase. Mitogen-activated protein (MAP) kinases and the putative tumor suppressor promyelocytic leukemia (PML) have been implicated in the induction of ARF and p16[INK4a] during cellular senescence.[93,94] In this way, sustained activation of the p53 and RB

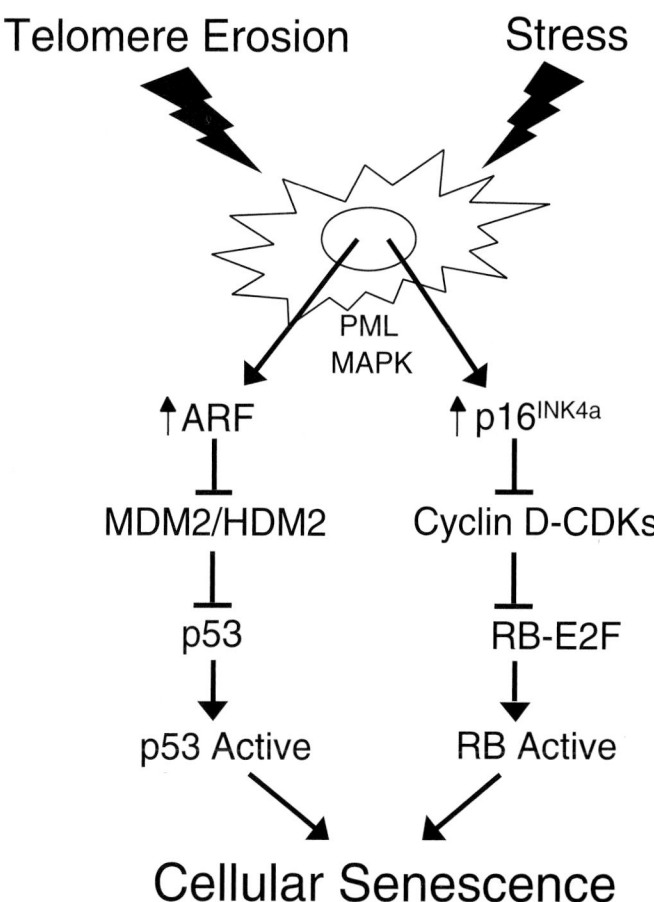

Figure 3-5 Regulation of cellular senescence by p53 and RB tumor-suppressor gene products. Cells respond to proliferation-dependent erosion/dysfunction of telomeres or stress (e.g., DNA damage or oncogene activation) by inducing the expression of ARF and p16[INK4a]. The induction of ARF and p16[INK4a] is mediated by promyelocytic leukemia (PML), tumor-suppressor protein, and mitogen-activated protein kinases (MAPK). ARF activates p53 by inhibiting MDM2/HDM2, a protein that promotes the proteasomal destruction of p53. p16[INK4a] maintains RB in its active, hypophosporylated state (with E2F bound) by inhibiting cyclin D-CDK complexes, which normally phosphorylate and inactivate RB.

tumor-suppressor gene products permanently growth arrests senescent cells. Finally, the importance of the ARF and p16[INK4a] pathways in suppressing tumors is underscored by their frequent inactivation in cancer.[92]

APOPTOSIS: A GENETIC PROGRAM FOR CELL DEATH

The fourth and final fate available to cells is apoptosis or programmed cell death. All cells in multicellular organisms are genetically programmed to respond to diverse stimuli (e.g., developmental signals, tissue injury, or growth factor withdrawal) by committing suicide.[95] During development, cells that are redundant or no longer useful are removed by apoptosis, whereas in the adult, irreparably damaged or dangerous cells, such as nascent cancer cells, are eradicated by this process. In the endocrine system, the atresia of ovarian follicles, regression of the corpus luteum, and sloughing of the endometrium that occur with each menstrual cycle are all executed by apoptosis.[96,97] Consequently, derangements in apoptosis play a fundamental role in the pathogenesis of many diseases.[98,99] Apoptotic cells are readily identified (and distinguished from necrotic cells) by a number of stereotypical morphologic changes, including plasma membrane blebbing, chromatin condensation, and reduction of cytoplasmic volume.[100] These events are soon followed by the systematic disassembly of the nucleus and cytoplasm, the fragmentation of genomic DNA between nucleosomes (resulting in DNA "ladders"), the packaging of cellular debris into "apoptotic bodies," and their inconspicuous disposal within neighboring cells without provoking an inflammatory response.[100,101] These stereotypical changes culminating in the death of the cell are triggered by the activation of the apoptotic cell-death machinery that has been remarkably conserved from nematodes to humans.[102] A key component of this apparatus is a family of cell-death proteases called caspases, which execute the apoptotic cell-death signal by proteolyzing intracellular proteins.[103,104] In this final section, we examine the cell-death machinery in detail and explore the contribution of defects in apoptotic cell-death pathways to endocrine diseases.

CASPASES: CONSERVED CELL-DEATH PROTEASES

Caspases are a novel and conserved family of proteases that were first identified by virtue of their sequence homology to the *Caenorhabditis elegans* cell-death gene, *ced-3*.[105,106] Several key aspects of their function are indicated by the caspase name: **c**ysteine prote**ases** that cleave protein substrates at **asp**artic acid (Asp) residues. At present, 11 human caspases have been identified and differ somewhat in their substrate specificities determined by the three amino acids aminoterminal to the Asp residue at the caspase cleavage site.[103,104] Caspases are expressed in all tissues as proenzymes or zymogens with little proteolytic activity, an intrinsic safeguard against adventitious caspase activation and apoptosis. Procaspases contain an amino-terminal prodomain (which inhibits its protease activity but targets procaspases to other molecules), a large subunit and small subunit; each of these domains is separated by one or more Asp residues. Procaspases (except for caspase-9, discussed later) are activated by proteolytic cleavage at these Asp residues, which removes the inhibitory prodomain and produces a heterodimer of one large and small subunit. Active caspases are tetrameric structures formed by the dimerization of two heterodimers.[107,108]

As we shall see later in this chapter, caspases are arranged in a proteolytic cascade in which upstream initiator procaspases are recruited and activated by distinct cellular caspase-activating complexes, and these active initiator caspases then cleave and activate downstream effector caspases.[103,104] This caspase cascade is an efficient mechanism to amplify protease activation, because each active protease can activate multiple zymogens, which when activated can, in turn, activate multiple additional zymogens, and so on. The effector caspases, then, execute the cell-death signal by (1) cleaving and activating proapoptotic proteins (e.g., procaspases and several kinases such as MEKK-1 and PKCδ); (2) cleaving and inactivating antiapoptotic proteins (e.g., Bcl-2 and Bcl-x$_L$); or (3) cleaving and dismantling cytoskeletal proteins (e.g., the nuclear lamins, cytokeratins and actin).[103,109–115] Perhaps the most compelling evidence for the essential role of caspases in the execution of apoptosis comes from the observed apoptotic defects in caspase knockout mice. For instance, mice with homozygous deletion of caspase-9 die in utero and have grossly enlarged and abnormal brains because of insufficient apoptosis during brain development; thymocytes derived from these mice are resistant to apoptosis induced by DNA damage or dexamethasone.[116] In contrast, caspase-8–deficient mice also die in utero and have abnormal cardiac muscle development; fibroblasts derived from these mice are resistant to apoptosis induced by tumor necrosis factor (TNF)-α and related cytokines.[117] These findings underscore that caspases are critical effectors of apoptosis in vivo.

APOPTOTIC CELL DEATH PATHWAYS: TWO ROADS TO CASPASE ACTIVATION

For a cell to undergo apoptosis, caspase zymogens must be activated. Two principal caspase-activating pathways have been described. They use different molecular machinery and cellular compartments to recruit and activate distinct initiator caspases.[103,104] These intrinsic (mitochondrial) and extrinsic (death receptor) caspase-activating pathways are outlined in Figure 3-6. The intrinsic pathway is activated by most apoptotic stimuli, including a variety of cellular stresses such as DNA damage, hypoxia, and growth factor withdrawal. The mitochondria play a critical role in this pathway by releasing a number of proapoptotic molecules including cytochrome *c* into the cytosol in response to apoptotic stimuli.[118,119] Although the proximal events leading to the mitochondrial release of cytochrome *c* are poorly understood (recent studies suggest a role for caspase-2),[120] the proapoptotic Bcl-2 family members (e.g., Bax, BID, and Bak) promote cytochrome *c* release, whereas the antiapoptotic Bcl-2 family members (e.g., Bcl-2 and Bcl-x$_L$) suppress cytochrome *c* release.[119,121–125] These Bcl-2 family members are either permanently or transiently associated with the mitochondrial outer membrane. Cytosolic cytochrome *c* binds to Apaf-1 and triggers its assembly into a large multimeric complex termed the *apoptosome*, which recruits procaspase-9 and promotes its activation by inducing a conformational change in the zymogen.[126,127] Active initiator caspase-9 then cleaves and activates downstream effector caspases (e.g., caspase-3, -6, and -7). In addition to cytochrome *c*, mitochondria also release several other proapoptotic molecules in response to apoptotic stimuli, including Smac/DIABLO and Omi (which promote caspase activation by displacing endogenous caspase inhibitors called inhibitor of apoptosis proteins [IAPs] from caspases) and apoptosis-inducing factor (AIF, which induces caspase-independent cell death).[128–131]

The extrinsic pathway is activated by cytokines of the TNF-α family (e.g., TNF-α, Fas ligand, and tumor necrosis factor α–related apoptosis-inducing ligand [TRAIL]).[132] These cytokines bind to their specific cell-surface receptors, collectively termed *death receptors* because they signal apoptosis via a conserved cytoplasmic *death domain*. The death domain–containing adaptor protein FADD is recruited to cytokine-bound receptors via homotypic death domain protein-protein interactions.[133] FADD then recruits procaspases-8 and -10 to the death-receptor complex by virtue of a second protein-interaction domain (the death effector domain) common to both FADD and the prodomains of

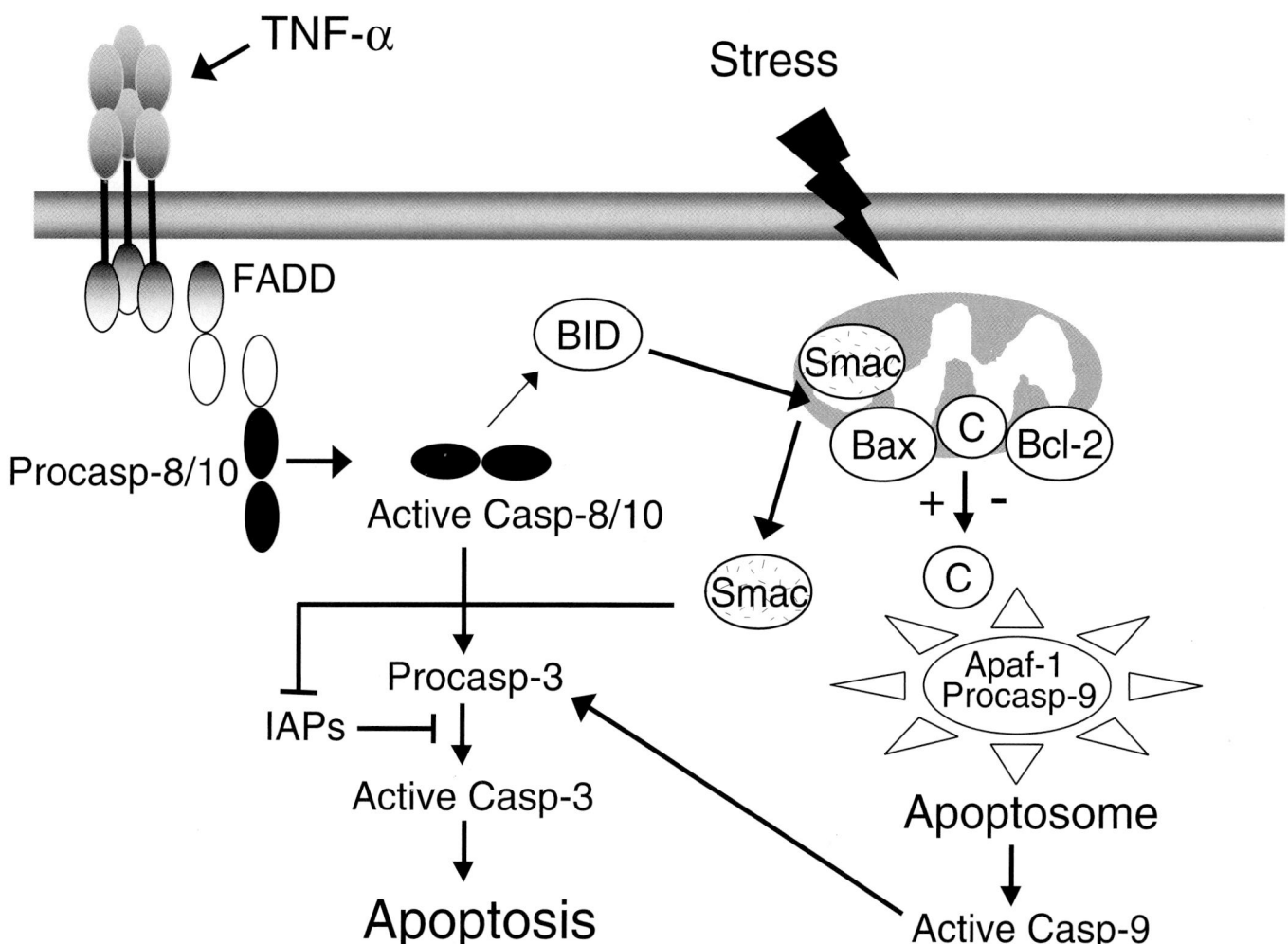

Figure 3-6   The extrinsic and intrinsic apoptotic pathways of caspase activation. The extrinsic pathway **(left)** is activated by cytokines of the TNF-α family (e.g., TNF-α, tumor necrosis factor α–related apoptosis-inducing ligand [TRAIL], and Fas ligand), which bind to cell-surface death receptors. Cytokine-bound death receptors recruit the adaptor protein FADD and subsequently procaspases-8 and -10, which leads to their activation. Active caspase-8/10 cleaves and activates the effector caspase-3 directly or indirectly via proteolysis of BID and activation of the intrinsic or mitochondrial pathway **(right)**. In this latter pathway, stress stimuli such as DNA damage or growth-factor deprivation trigger the mitochondrial release of cytochrome *c* and Smac; this release is promoted by proapoptotic Bcl-2 family members (e.g., Bax and BID) and inhibited by antiapoptotic Bcl-2 family members (e.g., Bcl-2). Cytochrome *c*, Apaf-1, and procaspase-9 form a multimeric cytoplasmic complex (apoptosome) that activates caspase-9, which then proteolytically activates procaspase-3. Cytosolic Smac promotes apoptosis by inhibiting inhibitor of apoptosis proteins (IAPs), endogenous caspase-3 inhibitors. Together with other executioner caspases, active caspase-3 induces apoptosis by proteolyzing a number of cellular proteins.

procaspases-8 and -10.[134–136] The "induced proximity" of multiple procaspases-8 and -10 in the death-receptor signaling complex promotes the proteolytic activation of these initiator caspases by increasing the likelihood of an intermolecular cleavage event.[137] Active caspase-8 or -10 either directly cleaves and activates effector caspases (-3, -6 and -7) or indirectly activate these caspases by cleaving the proapoptotic Bcl-2 family member BID.[122,123,138] Once cleaved, BID moves from the cytoplasm to the mitochondria and induces cytochrome c release, setting into motion the various events described in the previous paragraph, which culminate in activation of effector caspases. In this way, the extrinsic pathway uses the mitochondria (intrinsic pathway) to amplify caspase activation, an important functional interaction between these pathways.

To prevent accidental caspase activation and cell death, each of these pathways is negatively regulated by multiple molecules acting at many different steps. As noted, the antiapoptotic Bcl-2 family members (e.g., Bcl-2 and Bcl-x$_L$) suppress the release of cytochrome c (and other proapoptotic molecules) from the mitochondria.[124,125] In addition, several heat shock proteins bind to components of the apoptosome to prevent assembly of this caspase-9 activating complex: Hsp70 and Hsp90 bind to Apaf-1, whereas Hsp27 binds to cytochrome c.[139–141] In the extrinsic pathway, a truncated caspase-8–like molecule (FLIP), which lacks protease activity, functions as a dominant negative inhibitor by interfering with the recruitment of procaspase-8 to death receptors.[142] Finally, several molecules that directly inhibit active effector caspases or disrupt their activation by initiator caspases have been described, including XIAP and the small heat shock protein αB-crystallin.[143,144] Hence the expression levels of these apoptosis inhibitors greatly influences the cellular threshold for apoptosis induction.

DYSREGULATED APOPTOSIS IN SELECTED ENDOCRINE DISEASES

Because apoptosis plays a critical role in normal development and in maintaining homeostasis, derangements in apoptosis resulting in either too much or too little cell death invariably lead to disease.[98,99] Moreover, the core apoptotic cell-death machinery that regulates caspase activation is used by all cell types in response to diverse apoptotic stimuli, thereby making it a valuable molecular framework to examine disease pathogenesis. For instance, diseases with excess apoptosis are characterized by inappropriate caspase activation, as a result of either sustained injury or reduced activity of the cellular antagonists to caspase activation (e.g., XIAP, FLIP, and Bcl-2). In contrast, diseases with insufficient apoptosis (i.e., apoptosis resistance) are characterized by inadequate activation of caspases, as a result of loss of caspases or caspase-activating molecules or enhanced activity of caspase antagonists. Finally, the conserved apoptotic cell-death machinery provides a number of potential drug targets to regulate apoptosis therapeutically, an area of intense interest in academia and in the private sector. In the remainder of this chapter, we examine the contribution of the apoptotic cell-death machinery to selected endocrine diseases.

DIABETES

Before the onset of clinically overt disease, type 2 diabetes mellitus is characterized by insulin resistance leading to a compensatory increase in β-cell mass and insulin secretion that maintains normoglycemia.[145] However, β-cell failure due to decreased β-cell mass ultimately leads to hyperglycemia. Data from animal models indicate that this reduction in β-cell mass is mediated, at least in part, by apoptosis of β cells.[146] Several potential mechanisms of β-cell apoptosis in type 2 diabetes have been postulated. Hyperglycemia itself has been shown to induce apoptosis in cultured human islets, at least in part, by reducing the expression of FLIP (a caspase-8 antagonist) and increasing the expression of Fas (the death receptor for Fas ligand), two components of the extrinsic death-receptor pathway.[147,148] Indeed, human islets from type 2 diabetic patients were observed to have diminished FLIP levels and increased Fas levels compared with those in nondiabetic controls. Such alterations in type 2 diabetic patients would also likely sensitize β cells to cytokine-induced apoptosis. The elevated circulating free fatty acids in type 2 diabetics also have been implicated in β-cell apoptosis.[149] A third potential inducer of β-cell apoptosis in this disease is amylin or islet amyloid polypeptide, an amyloidogenic peptide that accumulates in the islets of type 2 diabetic patients.[150] Like the related β-amyloid implicated in neuronal death in Alzheimer's disease, oligomerized amylin induces caspase activation and β-cell apoptosis in cultured islet cells.[151,152] In addition, transgenic expression of amylin induces amylin deposition in islets, β-cell apoptosis, and type 2 diabetes in a subset of transgenic mice (gender, diet, and body weight influence phenotypic outcomes).[153–155] In contrast, type 1 diabetes mellitus is caused by the autoimmune destruction of islets and absolute insulin deficiency.[156] A critical event in the pathogenesis of type 1 diabetes (and other autoimmune diseases) is a defect in the apoptotic destruction of autoreactive T-cell clones during development (negative selection).[157] Recent studies in the nonobese diabetic (NOD) mouse model of this disease indicate that NOD thymocytes fail to undergo negative selection because FLIP is abnormally induced by T cell–receptor stimulation, thereby rendering NOD thymocytes resistant to Fas-induced apoptosis.[158] Although the evidence from human studies is limited, these findings suggest that dysregulated apoptosis likely plays an important role in the pathogenesis of both type 1 and type 2 diabetes.

THYROID DISEASE

Alterations in the extrinsic death-receptor pathway have been implicated in a number of thyroid diseases.[159] The expression of Fas ligand and Fas are both increased in thyrocytes from patients with Hashimoto's thyroiditis and Graves' disease.[160,161] In Hashimoto's thyroiditis, these alterations are coupled with diminished expression of Bcl-2 in thyrocytes, thereby resulting in increased cytokine-induced apoptosis and destruction of thyrocytes.[160] In contrast, Graves' disease thyrocytes have increased expression of the antiapoptotic proteins FLIP and Bcl-x$_L$.[161] These antiapoptotic proteins inhibit cytokine-induced apoptosis in Graves' disease and allow sustained thyroid stimulation by TSH-receptor autoantibodies. Furthermore, thyroid carcinomas, like other human cancers, are often resistant to apoptosis by virtue of defects in the apoptotic machinery (e.g., enhanced expression of Bcl-2 or diminished expression of FADD), thereby limiting the efficacy of cancer therapies.[162,163] In thyroid cancer, an urgent need exists to develop therapies for radioiodine-resistant differentiated thyroid carcinomas and for anaplastic carcinomas; these carcinomas are resistant to conventional chemotherapeutic drugs.[164] One especially promising agent is TNF-related apoptosis-inducing ligand (TRAIL or Apo2L), which preferentially induces apoptosis in transformed cells.[165] TRAIL activates the extrinsic pathway by binding to its death receptors DR4 and DR5. TRAIL has been demonstrated to have broad antitumor activity in vitro and in vivo and to lack systemic toxicity in primates.[166] Moreover, human thyroid carcinomas and cell lines (including some anaplastic carcinomas) commonly express DR4 and DR5 and are often sensitive to TRAIL-induced apoptosis in vitro (either alone or in combination with other agents).[167,168] These findings indicate that the death-receptor apoptotic pathway contributes broadly to the pathogenesis of thyroid disease, and they suggest that TRAIL may be a novel proapoptotic therapy for thyroid cancer.

Acknowledgment
The authors thank Dr. Shlomo Melmed for critical reading of the sections on cell division and differentiation of this chapter.

REFERENCES

1. Amos B: Lessons from the history of light microscopy. Nat Cell Biol 2:E151–E152, 2000.
2. Nurse P: A long twentieth century of the cell cycle and beyond. Cell 100:71–78, 2000.
3. Nasmyth K: Putting the cell cycle in order. Science 274:1643–1645, 1996.
4. Sherr CJ: Cancer cell cycles. Science 274:1672–1677, 1996.
5. Tsanaclis AM, Brem SS, Gately S, et al: Statin immunolocalization in human brain tumors: Detection of noncycling cells using a novel marker of cell quiescence. Cancer 68:786–792, 1991.
6. Rieder CL, Khodjakov A: Mitosis through the microscope: Advances in seeing inside live dividing cells. Science 300:91–96, 2003.
7. Pines J, Rieder CL: Re-staging mitosis: A contemporary view of mitotic progression. Nat Cell Biol 3:E3–E6, 2001.
8. Elledge SJ: Cell cycle checkpoints: preventing an identity crisis. Science 274:1664–1672, 1996.
9. Johnson DG, Walker CL: Cyclins and cell cycle checkpoints. Annu Rev Pharmacol Toxicol 39:295–312, 1999.
10. Nurse P: Cyclin-dependent kinases and cell cycle control. Nobel Lect, 2001.
11. Hunter T, Pines P: Cyclins and cancer. II: Cyclin D and CDK inhibitors come of age. Cell 79:573–582, 1994.
12. Motokura T, Arnold A: Cyclin D and oncogenesis. Curr Opin Genet Dev 3:5–10, 1993.
13. Sherr CJ: D-type cyclins. Trends Biochem Sci 20:187–190, 1995.

14. Nevins JR, Leone G, DeGregori J, et al: Role of the Rb/E2F pathway in cell growth control. J Cell Physiol 173:233–236, 1997.

15. Harbour JW, Dean DC: Rb function in cell-cycle regulation and apoptosis. Nat Cell Biol 2:E65–E67, 2000.

16. Pardee AB: G1 events and regulation of cell proliferation. Science 246:603–608, 1989.

17. Keyomarsi K, Herliczek TW: The role of cyclin E in cell proliferation, development and cancer. Prog Cell Cycle Res 3:171–191, 1997.

18. Yam CH, Fung TK, Poon RY: Cyclin A in cell cycle control and cancer. Cell Mol Life Sci 59:1317–1326, 2002.

19. Porter LA, Donoghue DJ: Cyclin B1 and CDK1: nuclear localization and upstream regulators. Prog Cell Cycle Res 5:335–347, 2003.

20. Ubersax JA, Woodbury EL, Quang PN, et al: Targets of the cyclin-dependent kinase Cdk1. Nature 425:859–864, 2003.

21. Hershko A: Mechanisms and regulation of the degradation of cyclin B. Philos Trans R Soc Lond B Biol Sci 354:1571–1575, 1999.

22. Sherr CJ, Roberts JM: Inhibitors of mammalian G1 cyclin-dependent kinases. Genes Dev 9:1149–1163, 1995.

23. Peter M: The regulation of cyclin-dependent kinase inhibitors (CKIs). Prog Cell Cycle Res 3:99–108, 1997.

24. Ruas M, Peters G: The p16INK4a/CDKN2A tumor suppressor and its relatives. Biochim Biophys Acta 1378:F115–F1177, 1998.

25. Hannon GJ, Beach D: p15INK4B is a potential effector of TGF-beta-induced cell cycle arrest. Nature 371:257–261, 1994.

26. el-Deiry WS, Tokino T, Velculescu VE, et al: WAF1, a potential mediator of p53 tumor suppression. Cell 75:817–825, 1993.

27. Gartel AL, Serfas MS, Tyner AL: p21: Negative regulator of the cell cycle. Proc Soc Exp Biol Med 213:138–149, 1996.

28. Zhou BB, Elledge SJ: The DNA damage response: Putting checkpoints in perspective. Nature 408:433–439, 2000.

29. Yu H: Regulation of APC-Cdc20 by the spindle checkpoint. Curr Opin Cell Biol 14:706–714, 2002.

30. Zhao H, Watkins JL, Piwnica-Worms H: Disruption of the checkpoint kinase 1/cell division cycle 25A pathway abrogates ionizing radiation-induced S and G2 checkpoints. Proc Natl Acad Sci U S A 99:14795–14800, 2002.

31. Agarwal ML, Taylor WR, Chernov MV, et al: The p53 network. J Biol Chem 273:1–4, 1998.

32. Pestell RG, Albanese C, Reutens AT, et al: The cyclins and cyclin-dependent kinase inhibitors in hormonal regulation of proliferation and differentiation. Endocr Rev 20:501–534, 1999.

33. Monzavi R, Cohen P: IGFs and IGFBPs: role in health and disease. Best Pract Res Clin Endocrinol Metab 16:433–447, 2002.

34. Dickson RB, Stancel GM: Estrogen receptor-mediated processes in normal and cancer cells. J Natl Cancer Inst 27:135–145, 2000.

35. Kimura T, Van Keymeulen A, Golstein J, et al: Regulation of thyroid cell proliferation by TSH and other factors: A critical evaluation of in vitro models. Endocr Rev 22:631–656, 2001.

36. Furlanetto RW, Harwell SE, Frick KK: Insulin-like growth factor-I induces cyclin-D1 expression in MG63 human osteosarcoma cells in vitro. Mol Endocrinol 8:510–517, 1994.

37. Yamamoto K, Hirai A, Ban T, et al: Thyrotropin induces G1 cyclin expression and accelerates G1 phase after insulin-like growth factor I stimulation in FRTL-5 cells. Endocrinology 137:2036–2042, 1996.

38. Planas-Silva MD, Weinberg RA: Estrogen-dependent cyclin E-cdk2 activation through p21 redistribution. Mol Cell Biol 17:4059–4069, 1997.

39. Prall OW, Sarcevic B, Musgrove EA, et al: Estrogen-induced activation of Cdk4 and Cdk2 during G1-S phase progression is accompanied by increased cyclin D1 expression and decreased cyclin-dependent kinase inhibitor association with cyclin E-Cdk2. J Biol Chem 272:10882–10894, 1997.

40. Ying SY, Zhang Z. Furst B, et al: Activins and activin receptors in cell growth. Proc Soc Exp Biol Med 214:114–122, 1997.

41. Baxter JD: Mechanisms of glucocorticoid inhibition of growth. Kidney Int 14:330–333, 1978.

42. Ramalingam A, Hirai A, Thompson EA: Glucocorticoid inhibition of fibroblast proliferation and regulation of the cyclin kinase inhibitor p21Cip1. Mol Endocrinol 11:577–586, 1997.

43. Yu R, Melmed S: Oncogene activation in pituitary tumors. Brain Pathol 11:328–341, 2001.

44. Nasmyth K, Peters JM, Uhlmann F: Splitting the chromosome: Cutting the ties that bind sister chromatids. Science 288:1379–1385, 2000.

45. Lee JY, Orr-Weaver TL: The molecular basis of sister-chromatid cohesion. Annu Rev Cell Dev Biol 17:753–777, 2001.

46. Waizenegger IC, Hauf S, Meinke A, et al: Two distinct pathways remove mammalian cohesin from chromosome arms in prophase and from centromeres in anaphase. Cell 103:399–410, 2000.

47. Hauf S, Waizenegger IC, Peters JM: Cohesin cleavage by separase required for anaphase and cytokinesis in human cells. Science 293:1320–1323, 2001.

48. Uhlmann F, Wernic D, Poupart MA, et al: Cleavage of cohesin by the CD clan protease separin triggers anaphase in yeast. Cell 103:375–386, 2000.

49. Zou H, McGarry TJ, Bernal T, et al: Identification of a vertebrate sister-chromatid separation inhibitor involved in transformation and tumorigenesis. Science 285:418–422, 1999.

50. Waizenegger I, Gimenez-Abian JF, Wernic D, et al: Regulation of human separase by securin binding and autocleavage. Curr Biol 12:1368–1378, 2002.

51. Zur A, Brandeis M: Securin degradation is mediated by fzy and fzr and is required for complete chromatid separation but not for cytokinesis. EMBO J 20:792–801, 2001.

52. Hagting A, Den Elzen N, Vodermaier HC et al: Human securin proteolysis is controlled by the spindle checkpoint and reveals when the APC/C switches from activation by Cdc20 to Cdh1. J Cell Biol 157:1125–1137, 2002.

53. Zhang X, Horwitz GA, Heaney AP, et al: Pituitary tumor transforming gene (PTTG) expression in pituitary adenomas. J Clin Endocrinol Metab 84:761–767, 1999.

54. Zhang X, Horwitz GA, Prezant TR, et al: Structure, expression, and function of human pituitary tumor-transforming gene (PTTG). Mol Endocrinol 13:156–166, 1999.

55. Yu R, Lu W, Chen J, et al: Overexpressed pituitary tumor transforming gene (PTTG) causes aneuploidy in live human cells. Endocrinology 144:4991–4998, 2003.

56. Di Berardino MA: Animal cloning: The route to new genomics in agriculture and medicine. Differentiation 68:67–83, 2001.

57. Reik W, Dean W, Walter J: Epigenetic reprogramming in mammalian development. Science 293:1089–1093, 2001.

58. Edlund H: Factors controlling pancreatic cell differentiation and function. Diabetologia 44:1071–1079, 2001.

59. Scully KM, Rosenfeld MG: Pituitary development: regulatory codes in mammalian organogenesis. Science 295:2231–2235, 2002.

60. Weissman IL: Translating stem and progenitor cell biology to the clinic: Barriers and opportunities. Science 287:1442–1446, 2000.

61. Donovan PJ, Gearhart J: The end of the beginning of pluripotent stem cells. Nature 414:92–97, 2001.

62. Preston SL, Alison MR, Forbes SJ, et al: The new stem cell biology: Something for everyone. Mol Pathol 56:86–96, 2003.

63. Wagers AJ, Weissman IL: Plasticity of stem cells. Cell 116:639–648, 2004.

64. Surani MA: Reprogramming of genome function through epigenetic inheritance. Nature 414:122–128, 2001.

65. Ramalho-Santos M, Yoon S, Matsuzaki Y, et al: "Stemness": Transcriptional profiling of embryonic and adult stem cells. Science 298:597–600, 2002.

66. Spradling A, Drummond-Barbosa D, Kai T: Stem cells find their niche. Nature 414:98–104, 2001.

67. Student AK, Hsu RY, Lane MD: Induction of fatty acid synthetase synthesis in differentiating 3T3-L1 preadipocytes. J Biol Chem 255:4745–4750, 1980.

68. MacDougald OA, Lane MD: Transcriptional regulation of gene expression during adipocyte differentiation. Annu Rev Biochem 64:345–373, 1995.

69. Uriel J: Cancer, retrodifferentiation, and the myth of Faust. Cancer Res 36:4269–4275, 1976.

70. Weissman IL, Anderson DJ, Gage F: Stem and progenitor cells: Origins, phenotypes, lineage commitments, and transdifferentiations. Annu Rev Cell Dev Biol 17:387–403, 2001.

71. Ying QL, Nichols J, Evans EP, et al: Changing potency by spontaneous fusion. Nature 416:545–548, 2002.

72. Terada N, Hamazaki T, Oka M, et al: Bone marrow cells adopt the phenotype of other cells by spontaneous cell fusion. Nature 416:542–545, 2002.

73. Alison MR, Poulsom R, Otto WR, et al: Plastic adult stem cells: Will they graduate from the school of hard knocks? J Cell Sci 116:599–603, 2003.

74. Bianco P, Robey PG: Stem cells in tissue engineering. Nature 414:118–121, 2001.

75. Daley GQ: Cloning and stem cells: Handicapping the political and scientific debates. N Engl J Med 349:211–212, 2003.

76. Eliot Marshall: The business of stem cells. Science 287:1419–1421, 2000.

77. Donald Kennedy: Stem cells: Still here, still waiting. Science 300:865, 2003.

78. Shapiro AMJ, Lakey JRT, Ryan EA, et al: Islet transplantation in seven patients with type 1 diabetes mellitus using a glucocorticoid-free immunosuppressive regimen. N Engl J Med 343:230–238, 2000.

79. Zulewski H, Abraham EJ, Gerlach MJ, et al: Multipotential nestin-positive stem cells isolated from adult pancreatic islets differentiate ex vivo into pancreatic endocrine, exocrine, and hepatic phenotypes. Diabetes 50:521–533, 2001.

80. Ianus A, Holz GG, Theise ND, et al: In vivo derivation of glucose-competent pancreatic endocrine cells from bone marrow without evidence of cell fusion. J Clin Invest 111:843–850, 2003.

81. Kumar M, Jordan N, Melton D, et al: Signals from lateral plate mesoderm instruct endoderm toward a pancreatic fate. Dev Biol 259:109–122, 2003.

82. Campisi J: Cellular senescence as a tumor-suppressor mechanism. Trends Cell Biol 11:S27–S31, 2001.

83. Lundberg AS, Hahn WC, Gupta P, Weinberg RA: Genes involved in senescence and immortalization. Curr Opin Cell Biol 12:705–709, 2000.

84. Serrano M, Blasco MA: Putting the stress on senescence. Curr Opin Cell Biol 13:748–753, 2001.

85. Chin L, Artandi SE, Shen Q, et al: p53 deficiency rescues the adverse effects of telomere loss and cooperates with telomere dysfunction to accelerate carcinogenesis. Cell 97:527–538, 1999.

86. Vogelstein B, Lane D, Levine AJ: Surfing the p53 network. Nature 408:307–310, 2000.

87. Masutomi K, Yu EY, Khurts S, et al: Telomerase maintains telomere structure in normal human cells. Cell 114:241–253, 2003.

88. Wei S, Sedivy JM: Expression of catalytically active telomerase does not prevent premature senescence caused by overexpression of oncogenic Ha-Ras in normal human fibroblasts. Cancer Res 59:1539–1543, 1999.

89. Serrano M, Lin AW, McCurrach ME, et al: Oncogenic ras provokes premature cell senescence associated with accumulation of p53 and p16INK4a. Cell 88:593–602, 1997.

90. Palmero I, Pantoja C, Serrano M: p19ARF links the tumour suppressor p53 to Ras. Nature 395:125–126, 1998.

91. Lin AW, Lowe SW: Oncogenic ras activates the ARF-p53 pathway to suppress epithelial cell transformation. Proc Natl Acad Sci U S A 98:5025–5030, 2001.

92. Sherr CJ, McCormick F: The RB and p53 pathways in cancer. Cancer Cell 2:103–112, 2002.

93. Lin AW, Barradas M, Stone JC, et al: Premature senescence involving p53 and p16 is activated in response to constitutive MEK/MAPK mitogenic signaling. Genes Dev 12:3008–3019, 1998.

94. Ferbeyre G, de Stanchina E, Querido E, et al: PML is induced by oncogenic ras and promotes premature senescence. Genes Dev 14:2015–2027, 2000.

95. Steller H: Mechanisms and genes of cellular suicide. Science 267:1445–1449, 1995.

96. Pru JK, Tilly JL: Programmed cell death in the ovary: Insights and future prospects using genetic technologies. Mol Endocrinol 15:845–853, 2001.

97. Kokawa K, Shikone T, Nakano R: Apoptosis in the human uterine endometrium during the menstrual cycle. J Clin Endocrinol Metab 81:4144–4147, 1996.

98. Thompson CB: Apoptosis in the pathogenesis and treatment of disease. Science 267:1456–1462, 1995.

99. Talanian RV, Brady KD, Cryns VL: Caspases as targets for anti-inflammatory and anti-apoptotic drug discovery. J Med Chem 43:3351–3371, 2000.

100. Kerr JFR, Wyllie AH, Currie AR: Apoptosis: A basic biological phenomenon with wide-ranging implication in tissue kinetics. Br J Cancer 26:239–257, 1972.

101. Wyllie AH, Morris RG, Smith AL, Dunlop D: Chromatin cleavage in apoptosis: Association with condensed chromatin morphology and dependence on macromolecular synthesis. J Pathol 142:66–77, 1984.

102. Meier P, Finch A, Evan G: Apoptosis in development. Nature 407:796–801, 2000.

103. Cryns V, Yuan J: Proteases to die for. Genes Dev 12:1551–1570, 1998.

104. Thornberry NA, Lazebnik Y: Caspases: Enemies within. Science 281:1312–1316, 1998.

105. Yuan J, Shaham S, Ledoux S, et al: The C. elegans cell death gene ced-3 encodes a protein similar to mammalian interleukin-1b-converting enzyme. Cell 75:641–652, 1993.

106. Alnemri ES, Livingston DJ, Nicholson DW, et al: Human ICE/CED-3 protease nomenclature. Cell 87:171, 1996.

107. Walker NPC, Talanian RV, Brady KD, et al: Crystal structure of the cysteine protease interleukin-1B-converting enzyme: a (p20/p10)$_2$ homodimer. Cell 78:343–352, 1994.

108. Rotonda J, Nicholson DW, Fazil KM, et al: The three-dimensional structure of apopain/CPP32, a key mediator of apoptosis. Nature Struct Biol 3:619–625, 1996.

109. Cardone MH, Salvesen GS, Widmann C, et al: The regulation of anoikis: MEKK-1 activation requires cleavage by caspases. Cell 90:315–323, 1997.

110. Emoto Y, Manome Y, Meinhardt G, et al: Proteolytic activation of protein kinase C d by an ICE-like protease in apoptotic cells. EMBO J 14:6148–6156, 1995.

111. Cheng EHY, Kirsch DG, Clem RJ, et al: Conversion of Bcl-2 to a Bax-like death effector by caspases. Science 278:1966–1968, 1997.

112. Clem R, Cheng E, Karp C, et al: Modulation of cell death by Bcl-X$_L$ through caspase interaction. Proc Natl Acad Sci U S A 95:554–559, 1998.

113. Lazebnik YA, Takahashi A, Moir RD, et al: Studies of the lamin proteinase reveal multiple parallel biochemical pathways during apoptotic execution. Proc Natl Acad Sci U S A 92:9042–9046, 1995.

114. Caulín C, Salvesen GS, Oshima RG: Caspase cleavage of keratin 18 and reorganization of intermediate filaments during epithelial cell apoptosis. J Cell Biol 138:1379–1394, 1997.

115. Kayalar C, Örd T, Testa MP, et al: Cleavage of actin by interleukin 1b-converting enzyme to reverse DNase I inhibition. Proc Natl Acad Sci U S A 93:2234–2238, 1996.

116. Hakem R, Hakem A, Duncan GS, et al. Differential requirement for caspase 9 in apoptotic pathways in vivo. Cell 94:339–352, 1998.

117. Varfolomeev EE, Schuchmann M, Luria V, et al: Targeted disruption of the mouse caspase 8 gene ablates cell death induction by the TNF receptors, Fas/Apo1, and DR3 and is lethal prenatally. Immunity 9:267–276, 1998.

118. Liu X, Kim CN, Yang J, et al: Induction of apoptotic program in cell-free extracts: Requirement for dATP and cytochrome c. Cell 86:147–157, 1996.

119. Green DR, Reed JC: Mitochondria and apoptosis. Science 281:1309–1311, 1998.

120. Lassus P, Opitz-Araya X, Lazebnik Y: Requirement for caspase-2 in stress-induced apoptosis before mitochondrial permeabilization. Science 297:1352–1354, 2002.

121. Wei, MC, Zong, WX, Cheng EH, et al: Proapoptotic BAX and BAK: A requisite gateway to mitochondrial dysfunction and death. Science 292:727–730, 2001.

122. Li H, Zhu H, Xu CJ, Yuan J: Cleavage of BID by caspase 8 mediates the mitochondrial damage in the Fas pathway of apoptosis. Cell 94:491–501, 1998.

123. Luo X, Budihardjo I, Zou H, et al: Bid, a Bcl2 interacting protein, mediates cytochrome c release from mitochondria in response to activation of cell surface death receptors. Cell 94:481–490, 1998.

124. Kluck R, Bossy-Wetzel E, Green DR, Newmeyer DD: The release of cytochrome c from mitochondria: A primary site for Bcl-2 regulation of apoptosis. Science 275:1132–1136, 1997.

125. Yang J, Liu X, Bhalla K, et al: Prevention of apoptosis by Bcl-2: Release of cytochrome c from mitochondria blocked. Science 275:1129–1132, 1997.

126. Li P, Nijhawan D, Budihardjo I, et al: Cytochrome c and dATP-dependent formation of apaf-1/caspase-9 complex initiates an apoptotic protease cascade. Cell 91:479–489, 1997.

127. Rodriguez J, Lazebnik Y: Caspase-9 and APAF-1 form an active holoenzyme. Genes Dev 13:3179–3184, 1999.

128. Du C, Fang M, Li Y, Li L, Wang X: Smac, a mitochondrial protein that promotes cytochrome c-dependent caspase activation by eliminating IAP inhibition. Cell 102:33–42, 2000.

129. Verhagen AM, Ekert PG, Pakusch M, et al: Identification of DIABLO, a mammalian protein that promotes apoptosis by binding to and antagonizing IAP proteins. Cell 102:43–53, 2000.

130. Hegde R, Srinivasula SM, Zhang Z, et al: Identification of Omi/HtrA2 as a mitochondrial apoptotic serine protease that disrupts inhibitor of apoptosis protein-caspase interaction. J Biol Chem 277:432–438, 2002.

131. Joza N, Susin SA, Daugas E, et al: Essential role of the mitochondrial apoptosis-inducing factor in programmed cell death. Nature 410:549–554, 2001.

132. Ashkenazi A, Dixit VM: Apoptosis control by death and decoy receptors. Curr Opin Cell Biol 11:255–260, 1999.

133. Chinnaiyan AM, O'Rourke K, Tewari M, Dixit VM: FADD, a novel death domain-containing protein, interacts with the death domain of Fas and initiates apoptosis. Cell 81:505–512, 1995.

134. Boldin MP, Goncharov TM, Goltsev YV, Wallach D: Involvement of MACH, a novel MORT1/FADD-interacting protease, in Fas/APO-1- and TNF receptor-induced cell death. Cell 85:803–815, 1996.

135. Muzio M, Chinnaiyan AM, Kischkel FC, et al: FLICE, a novel FADD-homologous ICE/CED-3-like protease, is recruited to the CD95

(Fas/APO-1) death-inducing signaling complex. Cell 85:817–827, 1996.

136. Fernandes-Alnemri T, Armstrong RC, Krebs J, et al: In vitro activation of CPP32 and Mch3 by Mch4, a novel apoptotic cysteine protease containing two FADD-like domains. Proc Natl Acad Sci U S A 93:7464–7469, 1996.

137. Muzio M, Stockwell BR, Salvesen GS, Dixit VM: An induced proximity model for caspase-8 activation. J Biol Chem 273:2926–2930, 1998.

138. Muzio M, Salvesen GS, Dixit VM: FLICE induced apoptosis in a cell-free system: Cleavage of caspase zymogens. J Biol Chem 272:2952–2956, 1997.

139. Beere HM, Wolf BB, Cain K, et al: Heat-shock protein 70 inhibits apoptosis by preventing recruitment of procaspase-9 to the Apaf-1 apoptosome. Nat Cell Biol 2:469–475, 2000.

140. Pandey P, Saleh A, Nakazawa A, et al: Negative regulation of cytochrome c-mediated oligomerization of Apaf-1 and activation of procaspase-9 by heat shock protein 90. EMBO J 19:4310–4322, 2000.

141. Bruey JM, Ducasse C, Bonniaud P, et al: Hsp27 negatively regulates cell death by interacting with cytochrome c. Nat Cell Biol 2:645–652, 2000.

142. Irmler M, Thome M, Hahne M, et al: Inhibition of death receptor signals by cellular FLIP. Nature 388:190–195, 1997.

143. Deveraux QL, Takahashi R, Salvesen GS, Reed JC: X-linked IAP is a direct inhibitor of cell-death proteases. Nature 388:300–304, 1997.

144. Kamradt MC, Chen F, Cryns VL: The small heat shock protein aB-crystallin negatively regulates cytochrome c- and caspase-8-dependent activation of caspase-3 by inhibiting its autoproteolytic maturation. J Biol Chem 276:16059–16063, 2001.

145. Bell GI, Polonsky KS: Diabetes mellitus and genetically programmed defects in b-cell function. Nature 414:788–791, 2001.

146. Pick A, Clark J, Kubstrup C, et al: Role of apoptosis in failure of β-cell mass compensation for insulin resistance and beta-cell defects in the male Zucker diabetic fatty rat. Diabetes 47:358–364, 1998.

147. Maedler K, Fontana A, Ris F, et al: FLIP switches Fas-mediated glucose signaling in human pancreatic beta cells from apoptosis to cell replication. Proc Natl Acad Sci U S A 99:8236–8241, 2002.

148. Maedler K, Spinas GA, Lehmann R, et al: Glucose induces beta-cell apoptosis via upregulation of the Fas receptor in human islets. Diabetes 50:1683–1690, 2001.

149. Shimabukuro M, Zhou YT, Levi M, Unger RH: Fatty acid-induced β cell apoptosis: A link between obesity and diabetes. Proc Natl Acad Sci U S A 95:2498–2502, 1998.

150. Hoppener JW, Ahren B, Lips CJ: Islet amyloid and type 2 diabetes mellitus. N Engl J Med 343:411–419, 2000.

151. Lorenzo A, Razzaboni B, Weir GC, Yankner BA: Pancreatic islet cell toxicity of amylin associated with type-2 diabetes mellitus. Nature 368:756–760, 1994.

152. Zhang S, Liu J, Dragunow M, Cooper GJ: Fibrillogenic amylin evokes islet b-cell apoptosis through linked activation of a caspase cascade and JNK1. J Biol Chem 278:52810–52819, 2003.

153. Verchere CB, D'Alessio DA, Palmiter RD, et al: Islet amyloid formation associated with hyperglycemia in transgenic mice with pancreatic beta cell expression of human islet amyloid polypeptide. Proc Natl Acad Sci U S A 93:3492–3496, 1996.

154. Janson J, Soeller WC, Roche PC, et al: Spontaneous diabetes mellitus in transgenic mice expressing human islet amyloid polypeptide. Proc Natl Acad Sci U S A 93:7283–7288, 1996.

155. Butler AE, Janson J, Soeller WC, Butler PC: Increased b-cell apoptosis prevents adaptive increase in b-cell mass in mouse model of type 2 diabetes: Evidence for role of islet amyloid formation rather than direct action of amyloid. Diabetes 52:2304–2314, 2003.

156. Atkinson MA, Eisenbarth GS: Type 1 diabetes: New perspectives on disease pathogenesis and treatment. Lancet 358:221–229, 2001.

157. Kuhtreiber WM, Hayashi T, Dale EA, Faustman DL: Central role of defective apoptosis in autoimmunity. J Mol Endocrinol 31:373–399, 2003.

158. Kishimoto H, Sprent J: A defect in central tolerance in NOD mice. Nat Immunol 2:1025–1031, 2001.

159. Mitsiades N, Poulaki V, Mitsiades CS, et al: Apoptosis induced by FasL and TRAIL/Apo2L in the pathogenesis of thyroid diseases. Trends Endocrinol Metab 12:384–390, 2001.

160. Mitsiades N, Poulaki V, Kotoula V, et al: Fas/Fas ligand up-regulation and Bcl-2 down-regulation may be significant in the pathogenesis of Hashimoto's thyroiditis. J Clin Endocrinol Metab 83:2199–2203, 1998.

161. Stassi G, Di Liberto D, Todaro M, et al: Control of target cell survival in thyroid autoimmunity by T helper cytokines via regulation of apoptotic proteins. Nat Immunol 1:483–488, 2000.

162. Pilotti S, Collini P, Rilke F, et al: Bcl-2 protein expression in carcinomas originating from the follicular epithelium of the thyroid gland. J Pathol 172:337–342, 1994.

163. Tourneur L, Mistou S, Michiels FM, et al: Loss of FADD protein expression results in a biased Fas-signaling pathway and correlates with the development of tumoral status in thyroid follicular cells. Oncogene 22:2795–2804, 2003.

164. Braga-Basaria M, Ringel MD: Clinical review 158: Beyond radioiodine: A review of potential new therapeutic approaches for thyroid cancer. J Clin Endocrinol Metab 88:1947–1960, 2003.

165. LeBlanc HN, Ashkenazi A: Apo2L/TRAIL and its death and decoy receptors. Cell Death Differ 10:66–75, 2003.

166. Ashkenazi A, Pai RC, Fong S, et al: Safety and antitumor activity of recombinant soluble Apo2 ligand. J Clin Invest 104:155–162, 1999.

167. Ahmad M, Shi Y: TRAIL-induced apoptosis of thyroid cancer cells: Potential for therapeutic intervention. Oncogene 19:3363–3371, 2000.

168. Mitsiades N, Poulaki V, Tseleni-Balafouta S, et al: Thyroid carcinoma cells are resistant to FAS-mediated apoptosis but sensitive to tumor necrosis factor-related apoptosis-inducing ligand. Cancer Res 60:4122–4129, 2000.

Genomics and Proteomics

Isaac S. Kohane

INTRODUCTION

Measurement of gene and protein expression has a long history in the investigation of endocrine mechanisms and endocrine diseases. Indeed, it can be argued that it was a protein discovery, of insulin, in 1921 that launched the modern era of endocrinology. So why is it that there is so much tumult and excitement about current methods of protein and RNA measurement? Simply put, the ability to measure rapidly the individual molecules making up a significant fraction of the entire transcriptome and proteome of a specified cell or tissue qualitatively changes the way that scientific questions are posed, data are analyzed, and systems are modeled. Furthermore, the computational requirements of these massively parallel data, both in storage and in analysis, have required the development of a new breed of multidisciplinary team well versed in the biologic and computational sciences. This chapter is intended to serve as a broad introduction to the application of proteomics and genomics to biomedical research and practice and endocrinology in particular. It is written very much in the present so that readers may judge for themselves whether the currently available technologies and analytic techniques fit well with the questions and hypotheses of interest.

THE SINGULAR SUCCESS OF MICROARRAYS

It is telling that perhaps the most influential paper in functional genomics was that published by Alizadeh and colleagues in *Nature* in 2000.[1] By the timeline of this discipline, it is a classical paper and one that has not launched a thousand ships but tens of thousands of chips. To understand why that is does not require understanding the details of expression microarray analysis that follow later in this chapter. Rather, it only requires an appreciation of the quantum change in insights provided by this experiment as will be described. Beforehand, it should be noted that this experiment pertains to large B-cell lymphoma, a malignancy and not an endocrine disorder. As will be explained subsequently, cancer research was the first to benefit from functional genomics, primarily because cancer is a disease in which the

affected tissue is all too clear and, in most cases, surgically removed, and in which transcriptional disorders are very close to the etiologic root of the disease. Subsequently, as genomic techniques have become more refined and cost effective, significant comprehensive contributions have been made in endocrinology.

To return to this classical piece of research, it studied a group of patients with large B-cell lymphoma and the gene expression profiles of their malignancy. The latter means that the expression of over 10,000 genes was measured for each patient's sample. These data were then sorted in such a way (see discussion in the section on unsupervised clustering later in this chapter) that samples with similar expression profiles would be grouped together, as shown in Figure 4-1A. In this figure, commonly called a *dendrogram,* each row represents a gene and each column a sample. The visual shorthand used is that the redder the color, the higher the level of gene expression relative to a control RNA mixture, and the greener the color, the more downregulated the gene is with respect to a control. Figure 4-1A shows samples with similar patterns of green and red (i.e., similar expression profiles) grouped together. The investigators at that time recognized that there seemed to be two major groups in the data with distinct expression profiles, without having any additional information about the patients. Once they went back to the clinical data regarding these same patients, it became apparent that there was an important difference between the two groups of patients that could have only been determined after the fact, many years after their diagnosis: their mortality. Shown in Figure 4-1B are the Kaplan-Meier survival curves corresponding to the two groups of patients identified by gene expression profile. Shown on the X-axis is the number of years of survival, shown on the Y-axis is the probability of survival. What should be clear is that these two groups of patients have significantly different survival curves. On the publication of this research it became abundantly clear that there were four new large opportunities that had become immediately available:

- A new diagnosis had been identified where previously the diagnosis of B-cell lymphoma in this group of patients was a monolithic one and variations in presentation could not be used for further meaningful classification.

Figure 4-1 Redefining Large B-cell lymphoma by genomic profile. **Left,** A dendrogram constructed across the samples of B-cell lymphoma, using an unsupervised technique. The top branch essentially defines an even split between the category "GC B-like DLBCL" and "Activated B-like DLBCL," but this distinction was never before made clinically. **Right,** Kaplan-Meier survival curves of the patients from whom the samples were obtained. Patients whose cancer matched the "Activated B-like DLBCL" gene expression profile had a significantly worse prognosis. DLBCL, diffuse large B-cell lymphoma; GC, guanine-cytosine.

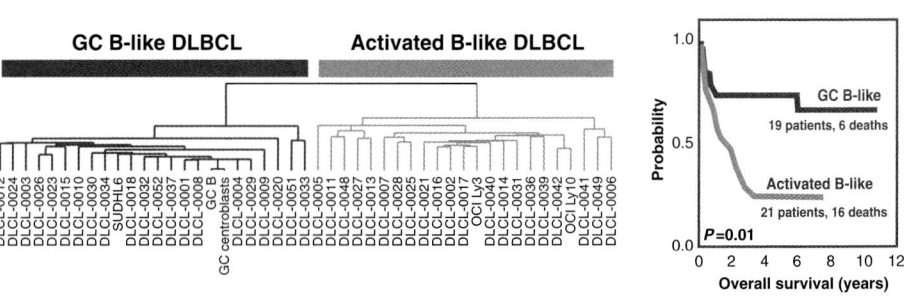

- A new prognosis had been developed. Where previously, variations in outcome were ascribed post hoc, if at all, to individual variation of unknown origin, this result pointed the way to a biologic, data-driven process by which outcome could be predicted. Concretely, a patient with a gene expression profile that resembled that of the high-risk group in Figure 4-1*B* could be informed of a very different set of risks and expectations than a patient with an expression profile similar to the low-risk group. It was understood that this step would require considerable validation before practicing this form of genomic prognostication, but nonetheless the direction was clear.

- A new therapeutic opportunity presented itself. Even if new chemotherapeutic agents were not developed, the change in prognostic knowledge changes the therapeutic decision-making process. A patient in a cohort that is likely to be dead within 2 years has a different risk profile than a cohort with better than 50% long-term survival. Therefore, the aggressiveness with which available chemotherapeutics are used may differ. Additionally, the cellular profile of groups of these patients (e.g. "activated B cell") based on the gene expression cluster to which they "belong" suggests a variety of specific and novel therapies.

- Several new research opportunities presented themselves. What was it about the patients that placed them in one or the other risk groups? This was not clear, but with the measurement of a significant fraction of the total number of human mRNA transcripts (the "transcriptome") it was and remains a good bet that these measurements might provide important clues or hypotheses to test.

This was a remarkable set of results for a very modestly scaled clinical research effort. Instead of the hundreds or thousands of patients typically used for establishing clinical outcomes, this study used fewer than 100 patients. For this and the reasons already stated, it served to inspire a large number of clinical researchers to apply these techniques to their own areas of interest and expertise.

How did this come about? The past 7 years have seen an astounding confluence of disparate technologies, such as robotics, fluorescence detection, photolithography, and the human genome project, so that in the present day, biologists can routinely use RNA expression microarray detection technologies to increase greatly the data known about cells in various states. With currently available commercial tools, a single experiment using RNA expression detection microarrays can now provide systematic quantitative information on the expression of 60,000 unique RNAs within cells in any given state. cDNA and oligonucleotide microarray technology can not only be used to determine, classify, and prognosticate disease states, but can also be used to analyze complex systems, such as traits with multigenic origins or those linked to the environment.[2] They can be used in time series to measure how a particular intervention[3,4] may start a transcriptional

program, that is, change the expression of large numbers of genes in a reproducible pattern determined by inherent genetic regulatory networks. Whereas the former applications resemble the kinds of classification efforts that endocrinologists have applied to samples such as thyroid biopsies, the latter efforts are analogous to the dynamic and provocative testing that has been part of the endocrinologist's armamentarium for the past 50-plus years. By virtue of comprehensive measurement rather than targeted measurements, however, these novel technologies do not fit well into the usual scientific method employed by endocrinologists.

The ability to measure such expression affords an opportunity to reduce our dependence on a priori knowledge (or biases) and allow the organism's biology to point us in potentially fruitful investigational directions. That is, much of the current mission of bioinformatics and functional genomics is a hypothesis-generating effort, which, if carefully crafted, can then lead to a highly productive set of investigations using more conventional hypothesis-driven research. Thoughtless or poorly controlled instances of such measurements can unfortunately be characterized as "fishing expeditions" and not provide the high-yield hypotheses that have resulted from the more successful functional genomic experiments.

Gene expression detecting microarrays are notable not because they can uniquely measure gene expression. There have certainly been many technologies that have allowed for the quantitative or semiquantitative measurement of gene expression for well over 3 decades. What distinguishes gene expression detection microarrays (and other genome-scale technologies) is that they are able to measure tens of thousands of genes at a time, and it is this quantitative change of the scale of gene measurement that has led to a qualitative change in our understanding of gene regulation. It is in this context that is worth defining what constitutes a microarray. One important reason to do this is that it can help explain why microarray technology has been so successful for gene expression, whereas the dozens of other efforts that have also used the term *microarray* are unlikely to be successful, at least in the near future. At a higher level of abstractions, the following pragmatic desiderata define microarrays:

- Low cost: The cost should be such that at least hundreds of samples be measurable within a typical National Institutes of Health investigator-initiated grant (NIH RO1) budget.
- Commodity level workflow: The microarray should be commoditized such that a routine set of procedures requiring no scientific judgment can be performed using standard equipment to obtain the needed measurement.
- Automation: The process of data acquisition should be completely automated so that after the biomaterial—whether it is protein, RNA, or DNA—is loaded into the analytic pipeline, most of the steps are fully automated and those that are not automated can be done by a nonspecialized technician.

- Form factor: The equipment required should easily fit into a standard laboratory bench format and not require its own room.
- Translational friendliness: A clinical investigator should not have to understand molecular biology techniques to be able to provide the necessary materials for the acquisition of the microarray data.
- Identifiability: All items identified by the microarray technology, whether they are proteins or RNA species, should be automatically identified against standard reference nomenclatures.
- High throughput: Hundreds of patient samples can be processed within days so that large cohorts of patients can be studied within a year.
- Commodity level priced infrastructure: The technology equipment and budget should be available to most biologic and clinical investigational laboratories.
- Massively parallel measurements of the relevant analytes: That is, the members of transcriptome, the members of the proteome, the metabolome, or any other comprehensive measure of molecular physiology.

By 2001, largely due to the technological and marketing success of Affymetrix (Santa Clara, CA), expression microarray technology had reached the maturity by which it could qualify fully for the microarray definition stated here. Although excellent science was previously conducted with microarrays, they did not meet all these criteria and it is only when they did that the full measure of the success of this technology was achieved. In contrast, as we will see, proteomic technology has yet to achieve similar growth and applicability precisely because it does not meet the desiderata.

PRAGMATICS OF GENE EXPRESSION MICROARRAYS

The gene expression assaying technology discussed in this section is RNA detection microarrays, variously known as DNA chips, biochips, or, simply, chips. It is easiest to think of the utility of microarrays in functional genomics as a five-step process.

1. Probe: The biochemical agent that finds or complements a specific sequence of DNA, RNA, or protein from a test sample.[5] It can include pieces of cDNA amplified from a vector stored within a bacterial clone, oligonucleotides synthesized in a fluid medium, oligonucleotides built on a solid phase base pair-by-base pair, or nucleotide fragments of a chromosome. This can be extended to incorporate the database of expressed sequence tags (ESTs) for serial analysis of gene expression (SAGE).
2. Array: The method for placing the probes on a medium or platform. Current techniques include robotic spotting, electric guidance, photolithography, piezo-electricity, fiber optics, and microbeads. This step also specifies the type of medium involved, such as glass slides, nylon meshes, silicon, nitrocellulose, membranes, gels, and beads.
3. Sample probe: The mechanism for preparing RNA from test samples. Total RNA may be used, or messenger RNA (mRNA) may be selected using a poly-deoxythymidine (poly-dT) to bind the poly-adenine (poly-A) tail. Alternatively, mRNA may be copied into cDNA, using labeled nucleotides or biotinylated nucleotides.

Assay: How is the signal of gene expression being transduced into something more easily measurable? For the microarrays in common use, gene expression is transduced into hybridization. For SAGE, gene expression is transduced into oligonucleotides via restriction enzymes and ligation. For polymerase chain reaction (PCR), gene expression is transduced into amplified pieces of cDNA.

Readout: How is the transduced signal going to be measured? How is information about the signal represented? For the microarrays in common use, hybridization is typically measured either by using one or two colored dyes or by using radioactive labels. For SAGE, the constructed oligonucleotides are measured through sequencing. For PCR, the amplified pieces of cDNA can be measured using gel electrophoresis.

For the microarrays in common use, one typically starts by taking a specific biologic tissue or system of interest, extracting its mRNA, and making a fluorescence-tagged cDNA copy of this mRNA. This tagged cDNA copy, typically called the *sample probe*, is then hybridized to a slide containing a grid or array of single-strand cDNAs called *probes*, which have been built or placed in specific locations on this grid (see Table 4-1 for alternative terminology). Similar to the general hybridization principles behind Southern or Northern blots, a sample probe will only hybridize with its complementary probe. Fluorescence is typically added to the sample probe in one of two ways: (1) fluorescent nucleotide bases are used when making the cDNA copy of the RNA; or (2) biotinylated nucleotides are first incorporated, followed by an application of fluorescence-labeled streptavidin, which will bind to the biotin. Depending on manufacturer-specific protocols, the probe-sample probe-hybridization process on a microarray typically occurs over several hours. All unhybridized sample probes are then washed off and the microarray is lit under laser light and scanned using laser confocal microscopy analogous to the phosphor imager in the traditional blot procedures. A digital image scanner records the brightness level at each grid location on the microarray corresponding to particular RNA species.

Studies have demonstrated that the brightness level is correlated with the absolute amount of RNA in the original same, and by extension, the expression level of the gene associated with this RNA.[6] A single microarray experiment is often thought of, erroneously, as many Northern blots simultaneously performed for as many different mRNA species as there are probes on a microarray. Note that the amount of total RNA required for a typical Northern blot is more than sufficient for one microarray experiment in the current technologies. This analogy breaks down, however, in that only a single hybridization condition (e.g., temperature, time) is used in hybridizing all N assays and, unless the probes are carefully chosen, this may not be the optimal condition for the assay of all RNA species.

A prominent characteristic of microarray technologies is that they enable the comprehensive measurement of the expression level of many genes simultaneously on a common substrate. In this regard, typical applications of microarrays include the comprehensive quantification of RNA expression profiles of a system under different experimental conditions, or expression profile comparisons of two systems under one or several conditions. The former embraces the comparison of expression profiles of a system under a control and a test condition, whereas the latter includes contrasts between different strains of organisms, as for instance between a normal

Table 4-1	Common Probe Nomenclature	
	Immobilized Nucleic Acid	Free Nucleic Acid on Microarray Surface That Is Being Interrogated
General microarray	Probe	Sample Probe
Robotically spotted microarray	Probe	Probe
Affymetrix microarray	Probe	Target

(e.g., wild-type) and a constructed (e.g., knockout) organism. Another intriguing use of microarrays is to compare expression levels between neighboring cells within the same microscopic field.[7] Aside from their widespread utility in functional genomics, oligonucleotide microarrays have also been used for single nucleotide polymorphism (SNP) analysis since many probe SNPs can be placed on the microarray for comprehensive parallel SNP detection; in much the same way, one can also perform DNA sequence analysis. These latter DNA-measurement rather than RNA-measurement techniques are not within the scope of this chapter, however.

Almost all gene expression technologies have performance factors that depend critically on the general validity of certain fundamental biologic assumptions, outlined as follows.

There is a close correspondence between mRNA transcription and its associated protein translation. As noted by Brown and Botstein,[8] one would ideally like to measure the final products of every gene, such as proteins, or even better, the biochemical activity of these products, which is more directly related to biologic functionality. Such quantitation would provide a link between chemical DNA bases at microscopic levels with biologic aspects that are manifest at macroscopic scales, such as phenotype and physiology. There is no practical generic tool to do this yet, however. The assumption that there is a principle of parsimony—akin to Hamilton's principle of least action in the physical sciences—which drives the close relationship between gene expression and biologic function was most clearly articulated in the work of Brown and Botstein.[8]

The second reason for using DNA microarrays to study gene expression on a genomic scale is the tight connection between the function of a gene product and its expression pattern. As a rule, each gene is expressed in the specific cells and under the specific conditions in which its product makes a contribution to fitness. Just as natural selection has precisely tuned the biochemical properties of the gene product, so it has tuned the regulatory properties that govern when, where, and in what quanity the product is made. The logic of natural selection, as well as experimental evidence, provides part of the basis for our belief that there is a sensible link between the expression pattern and the function of its gene product. Thirty years of molecular biology have provided numerous examples of genes that function under specific conditions and whose expression is tightly restricted to those conditions. Biologists can quickly find exceptions to this assumption. For example, proteins that make up the cellular matrix can considerably outlast the lifetime of their associated mRNA or, conversely, they may be metabolized or degraded much more rapidly than the mRNA from which they were transcribed. Nevertheless, the initial successes in the applications of gene expression microarrays in investigations of expression and function suggest that this assumption holds true more frequently than not.

All mRNA transcripts have similar life spans. Again, there are several well-known exceptions. For instance, we know that the length of the 3' poly-adenine (poly-A) tail of an mRNA appears to be related to its stability. Furthermore, there are examples of mRNA that have longer- or shorter-term stability within specific cells or after its transcriptional event such as dystrophin mRNA from patients with certain types of muscular dystrophies. As a tangential comment on temporal effects: probe-sample probe-hybridization rate is known to be a function of the guanine-cytosine (GC) content of a transcript. In general, this rate is proportional to GC richness, a consideration that goes into microarray design when the mRNA being measured has considerable variation in GC content.

All cellular activities and responses are programmed by transcriptional events. At a meta-systems level, this assumption may indeed be true, but in terms of direct mechanistic coupling, there exist many examples in which external stimuli cause changes in the biochemical program within the cell without engaging the transcriptional machinery. Figure 4-2 is an illustration of a response of free intracellular calcium to aldosterone exposure. Aldosterone is a steroid hormone that typically acts through binding with receptors that are translocated to the nucleus and then initiate or modify a transcriptional program. Here, the time scale of the acute response suggests a non-genomic mechanism. In other words, the response does not require transcriptional activation. This example demonstrates how a molecule that usually works via modulation of transcription (i.e., steroid hormones) may also affect bioprocesses at the non-genomic level. There is also a much larger class of biologic processes that do not primarily operate at the transcriptional level. These include muscular contraction, nerve excitation, and hormonal release. Eventually, all these events will cause some change in transcriptional activity, for example, replenishing stores of neurotransmitters, but the patterns of gene expression would probably not reveal the control processes that govern them at the sub-genomic time scale.

There are presently two types of chip technologies in common usage: robotically spotted and oligonucleotide microarrays. It is important to note that these two microarray technologies are the very earliest and are currently the most widely used. Several competing technologies are emerging that may prove to be more cost effective, reliable, and versatile, but most of them fall within the bounds of these two most popular microarray technologies.

ROBOTICALLY SPOTTED MICROARRAYS

Robotically spotted microarrays (Fig. 4-3), specifically the robotically spotted cDNA glass slide, were introduced into common use at Stanford University and first described by Mark Schena and colleagues in 1995.[6] These are also known as cDNA microarrays.

In making the array, a robotic spotter mechanically picks up specific cDNA sequences, typically amplified from vectors in bacterial clones using polymerase chain reaction, from separate physical containers and deposits them in specific locations in the grid on the glass slide to create specific probes. Each cDNA drop should ideally be equal in quantity. This fabrication approach epitomizes the do-it-yourself tendency in microarray measurement, even though there are several commercial ready-to-use versions available. The frequently home-grown quality of these arrays has led to the production of

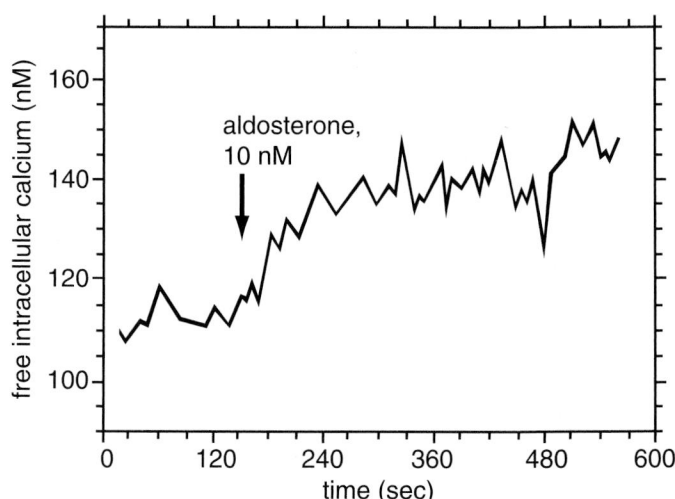

Figure 4-2 The non-genomic time scale response in aldosterone exposure. The response (in seconds) shown here is much faster than any known receptor-to-transcription response that is typical of steroid hormone actions via nuclear receptors.

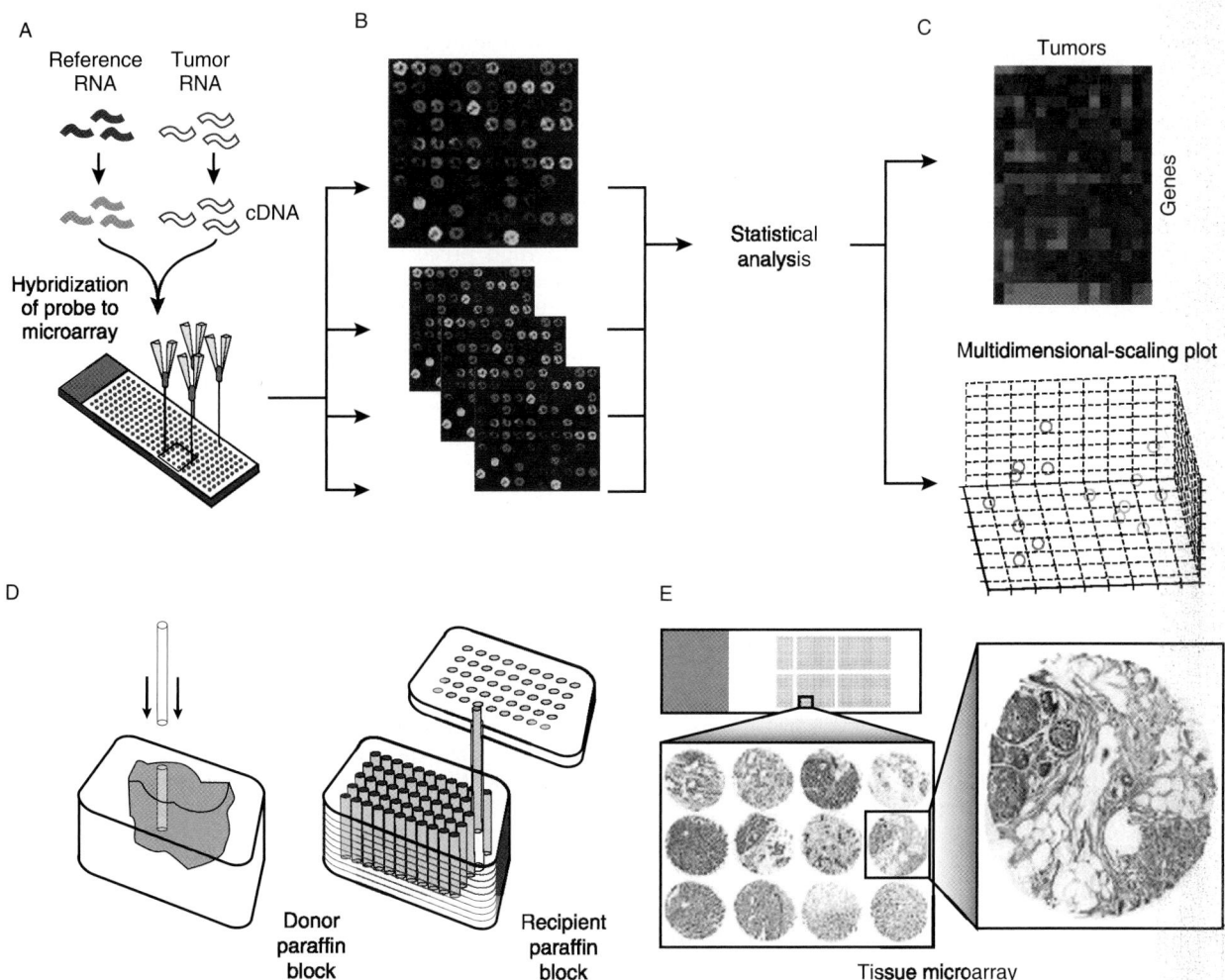

Figure 4-3 Robotically spotted microarray hybridized to two samples, each stained with two colored dyes. An overview of procedures for preparing and analyzing complementary DNA (cDNA) microarrays and breast-tumor tissue. **Panel A:** Reference RNA and tumor RNA are labeled by reverse transcription with different fluorescent dyes (green for the reference cells and red for the tumor cells) and hybridized to a cDNA microarray containing robotically printed cDNA clones. **Panel B:** The slides are scanned with a confocal laser scanning microscope, and color images are generated for each hybridization with RNA from the tumor and reference cells. Genes upregulated in the tumors appear red, whereas those with decreased expression appear green. Genes with similar levels of expression in the two samples appear yellow. Genes of interest are selected on the basis of the differences in the level of expression by known tumor classes (e.g., BRCA1-mutation-positive and BRCA2-mutation-positive). Bioinformatics analysis determines whether these differences in the gene-expression profiles are greater than would be expected by chance. **Panel C:** The differences in the patterns of gene expression between tumor classes can be portrayed in the form of a color-coded plot, and the relations between tumors can be portrayed in the form of a multidimensional-scaling plot. Tumors with similar gene-expression profiles cluster close to one another in the multidimensional-scaling plot. **Panel D:** Particular genes of interest can be further studied through the use of a large number of arrayed, paraffin-embedded tumor specimens, referred to as *tissue microarrays*. **Panel E:** Immunohistochemical analyses of hundreds or thousands of these arrayed biopsy specimens can be performed in order to extend the microarray findings. (See Color Plate.)

highly localized and customized microarrays that pose specific challenges in the dual tasks of background noise reduction and foreground RNA signal amplification during subsequent data analysis stages. Designer-definable parameters exist to control spot-basing size, the amount of time for drying, as well as experimental parameters concerning the glass slide material to be used. In practice, mastering this "home-brewed" approach can easily take up to a year even in a competent molecular biology laboratory.

There are several advantages and disadvantages in using a robotically spotted microarray.

The first advantage is customizability. A large subsequence (~2×10^3 base pairs long) complementary to the actual sequence that is to be probed is laid down on the chip by the designer who has full control over the species of probes that are to be used. This means, for example, that if one wishes to make customized chips for a specific purpose, such as for probing the expression of specific RNA in certain cell types,

one can design a layout and can direct a robotic spotter to make these microarrays. The setup cost for this approach is on the order of US$20,000; detailed guidelines may be found at the Brown laboratory microarray website (*http://cmgm. stanford.edu/pbrown/mguide/index.html*). Additionally, several companies sell robotic spotters–arrayer units. Glass slides are available from a variety of vendors specifically for microarray construction. Commercial aspects in the manufacture of such chips appear to be expanding. The notable disadvantage with greater customizability is that it may lead to more possibilities for errors. For instance, poor quality control or nonuniformity in the construction of different species probes, such as nonuniformity in spot-basing size, will complicate the subsequent analysis and interpretation of the resulting chip data.

The second advantage of robotically spotted microarrays is that larger pieces, or entire cDNAs, are placed on the chip, thus reducing the likelihood of nonspecific hybridization of labeled sample probes to the probe that was laid on the chip. Typically, a designer who wishes to have a particular gene probe on a chip will create a clone with 5 and 3 end of that particular gene of interest. These cDNA's substrings of the original gene are on the order of 100 to 200 base pairs long. A distinct weakness here is that even though a long probing subsequence ensures a sufficiently confident representative substring of the original gene, it does not mean that hybridization conditions will be fully and equally optimized for all species of cDNA subsequences. As we have noted earlier, probe-sample probe-hybridization rate is known to vary depending on the GC content of a transcript.

The third advantage is that RNA from two different samples (typically a test and a control condition) can be hybridized onto a common cDNA microarray substrate at the same time. The two separate RNA samples are typically labeled with different fluorescent dyes, such as Cy3 and Cy5. The two-dye system allows for the excitation of the microarray by laser light at two different frequencies and thus the image of hybridized RNA abundance can be scanned for both colors (corresponding to distinct samples) separately. Since the hybridization conditions, and thus the brightness, of any one spot is not the same as another spot, the individual signals are not typically used separately. Instead, the calculated signal is the ratio or fold difference in the brightness of the hybridized RNA of one sample versus another, specifically the intensity of Cy3 versus Cy5, that is, [(Cy3)/(Cy5)]. If a background intensity for each color is measured and controlled for, the ratio becomes [(Cy3–Cy3 background)/(Cy5–Cy5 background)]. This, in turn, provides a measure of relative abundance of the RNA from one sample with respect to the RNA from another sample, and hence the relative expression level of the corresponding gene in the samples. On the other hand, it has been shown that not all cDNA sample probe sequences label symmetrically with Cy3 and Cy5,[9] and paired dye-swapping experiments are performed (i.e., if the first hybridization is control (Cy3) versus test (Cy5), then switch dyes for second hybridization). If the labeling was symmetric, then the plot of $(Cy3)/(Cy5)_{Hybridization\ 1}$ versus $(Cy5)/(Cy3)^{-1}_{Hybridization\ 2}$ for every probe would be line of slope one through the origin.

Increasingly, rather than using cDNA, robotic spotters are being used for oligonucleotide microarrays. These are arrays that use the two-dye methods described, but employ probe sequences (typically shorter than 80 bases) designed to hybridize with a specific portion of each gene. These have many of the benefits and disadvantages of the photolithographically constructed microarrays, described in the next section, and, at the time of this writing, may be more cost effective, although they require an experienced technical staff.

In summary, each robotically spotted microarray experiment has its own built-in control, and results are given in terms of fold change or difference from a control situation. The measurement of absolute quantities and variations are more challenging in this technology, however.

PHOTOLITHOGRAPHIC MICROARRAYS

The second popular class of microarrays in use has been notably developed and marketed by Affymetrix. Currently, over 1.5×10^6 many oligonucleotides of length 25 base pairs each, called *25-mers*, are selectively constructed in a grid. These oligonucleotide chips, or oligochips, are constructed using a photolithographic masking technique, similar to the process that is used in microelectronics and integrated circuits fabrication, first described by Fodor and colleagues in 1991.[10] Currently, these commercially available microarrays are not produced individually, but instead are made in parallel. An entire wafer (containing between 40 and 400 microarrays) is constructed, tested, then broken apart to create the individual microarrays. At this time, commercially produced oligochips

exist that are disease as well as species specific, such as rat neurobiology and yeast genome arrays, and custom microarrays can be ordered with a 4-week turnaround or less.

The manufacturing technique for an Affymetrix oligochip is markedly different from the more mechanical process of making robotically spotted arrays. Each wafer starts out as an empty glass slide. On this, 25-mer probes are built base by base by placing single DNA bases on the foundation, then on top of a preceding base. These are constructed in parallel with high precision by selectively masking and unmasking specific coordinates of the array, and exposing the entire ensemble to ultraviolet light in between separately laying on the bases—adenines (A), thymines (T), guanines (G), and cytosines (C). Each applied photolithographic mask generates different areas of photodeprotection on the solid glass substrate. The combination of these masks with an intervening chemical coupling step allows the incorporation of additional nucleotides into existing strands only where desired. This entire process is known as light-directed oligonucleotide synthesis.

One advantage of the oligonucleotide microarray is that its higher density of probe pairs allows for more genes to be screened or assayed on a single chip, as compared to robotically spotted arrays. Consequently, there is less need for a priori restrictions on the number of genes that are to be scanned. A disadvantage is that the current technology only allows for, at most, one experiment to be run on a single chip at any one time. Thus, for example, one does not obtain meaningful data from placing the control sample and test probes on an oligonucleotide microarray simultaneously; instead, these two samples are measured on two separate oligochips. This means, in turn, that one typically has to apply a suitable normalization transformation across separate microarray data sets (i.e., interarray) at the subsequent data analysis stage in order to make meaningful comparisons of reported expression changes from a control to a test condition. Additionally, if a scientist is interested in studying a specific species for which no appropriate oligochip exists, then this technology is not presently available. Oligochips are not as easily customizable at the user's end as robotically spotted microarrays are.

Since each probe is limited to 25 base pairs in length, a question immediately arises as to how each gene can be screened uniquely using only 25 base pairs. For each gene that needs to be represented, or whose expression needs to be measured on Affymetrix's oligochip, a set of 16 to 20 25-mers are chosen that uniquely represent that particular gene, and would hybridize under the same general conditions. The Affymetrix literature calls the sample probe to be interrogated by cDNA probes on its microarray, the *target*. Every set of *perfect match* (PM) probes for an mRNA has a corresponding set of *mismatch* (MM) probes. An MM probe is constructed from the same nucleotide sequence as its PM probe partner, except that the middle (usually the 13th) base pair has been switched to result in an alphabet mismatch. For example, the following two 25-mers may be associated PM-MM probes to assay for the sample probe in Figure 4-4.

The combination of a PM and its associated MM oligonucleotide probe is called a *probe pair*. There are two principal

Probe on chip   PM : ATCGACTGATGC**A**TGCATCCATCAT
                 MM : ATCGACTGATGC**C**TGCATCCATCAT

Sample probe   TAGCTGACTACG**T**ACGTAGGTAGTA

Figure 4-4 Probe pair (MM and PM) designed to test for the sample probe (lowest in the figure). MM, mismatch; PM, perfect match.

reasons for the use of MM probes. First, at low concentrations of the target or sample probe when the PM probes have already reached their lower limit of sensitivity, the MM probes display greater sensitivity to changes in concentration. Second, MM probes are thought to bind to nonspecific sequences at the same rate as the PM probes. Thus, MM probes serve as an internal control for background nonspecific hybridization. Depending on the total RNA sample, however, it could turn out that the PM probe is already highly specific and the MM probes are simply binding to differently specific labeled subsequences in the sample. One has to be careful to distinguish between nonspecific hybridization and differently specific hybridization regarding the use of MM probe data. This explains, in part, the number of competing analytic programs that claim to perform best in translating PM and MM values into expression levels (Fig. 4-5).

For target preparation, sufficient amounts of sample probe are first synthesized by reverse transcribing the total RNA using an oligo-deoxythymidine (oligo-dT) primer containing a T7 polymerase site for 5' to 3' transcription. Amplification and labeling of the cDNA sample probe is achieved by carrying out an in vitro transcription reaction in the presence of biotinylated deoxynucleotide triphosphate (dNTP), resulting in the linear amplification of the cDNA population (approximately 30- to 100-fold). This linearity assumption becomes increasingly weak with decreasing quantities of total RNA and increasing number of amplification cycles. The biotin-labeled cRNA probe generated from the sample is then hybridized to the oligonucleotide arrays, followed by binding to a streptavidin-conjugated fluorescent marker. Laser excitation of the hybridized sample, confocal microscopy, and image acquisition by a optical scanner is performed. This results in an image file in which each oligonucleotide species is represented by a small rectangular area (~50 μm²), called the *probe cell*, which is itself composed of several image pixels, each occupying an area from 3 to 24 μm² (Fig. 4-6).

The image file is processed so that the recorded intensity of the appropriate pixels in a probe cell are stored in a .cel file, which therefore reports a measure of hybridization per contiguous oligonucleotide surface on the microarray. The .cel files are then processed to provide aggregate measures of expression for each *probe set*, the collection of probe pairs that are designed to measure a single RNA gene product. These probe sets are referred to by an Affymetrix accession number that is, in turn, linked to a Genbank identifier (and thereby usually to a single gene).

Much controversy surrounds the best way to calculate the aggregate measure of expression over a probe set from these .cel files[11,12] using publicly available packages such as dCHIP or the algorithms developed by Affymetrix (the Microarray Array Suite or MAS 5.0). Since the latter is used most frequently (because it is available by default with the Affymetrix data acquisition system), it is outlined here. As described by Hubbell and colleagues,[13] the measure of expression they selected was designed to: (1) capture the difference in the hybridization of the perfect match probe cells versus the mismatch probe cells, (2) always return a nonnegative value, and (3) be relatively insensitive to outlier values. Using the MM probes as a measure of stray (nonspecific) hybridization signals, these are subtracted from the PM probe intensities and then log-transformed. The Tukey biweight[14] is then applied to the log-transformed intensities to provide a robust estimate of intensity, relatively insensitive up to 50% outlier values. MM probes that have higher intensities than the PM probes are replaced with several different estimates, all guaranteed to be less than that of the perfect match probes. In addition to this measure of aggregate intensity for each probe set, MAS 5.0 also provides a "detection" measure calculated from a measure of the contrast between PM and MM probe cells, which is reported as *P* value (i.e., lower values are more significant and represent a more reliable measure). Furthermore, the *P* values are binned into three bins: the lowest *P* values are scored as *present*, the highest *P* values as *absent*, and the ones in the middle as *marginal*. The boundaries between these bins can be adjusted by the user. In summary, for each probe set, MAS 5.0 returns three measures: a measure of expression intensity, a *P* value for that measure, and a present/marginal/absent call. These measures are then used in multichip comparisons and calculations as described later in this chapter.

PROTEOMICS VERSUS GENOMICS

There is a good deal of enthusiasm at the present about the emerging discipline of proteomics. The promise of proteomics is that we will be able to measure, in a similarly comprehensive and parallel fashion to RNA microarray measurements, the concentrations of proteins present in a particular cellular system The assumption underlying RNA expression microarray measurements is that, by capturing the patterns of expression management, we will capture the basic regulatory rhythms of the cell. Although this assumption may hold at times and has done remarkably well in helping biologists elucidate some fundamental biology and in classifying clinical phenomena, there are several persuasive reasons why this assumption should not always hold. First, we know that most of the effector molecules in cellular metabolism are proteins. To the extent that the timing of protein synthesis and the half-life of proteins is not closely coupled to that of RNA expression, the assumption that RNA levels are representative does not hold. Nonetheless, in proteomics, we are bedeviled by a new set of assumptions of that are equally problematic and challenging. Assuming that we have high reproducibility

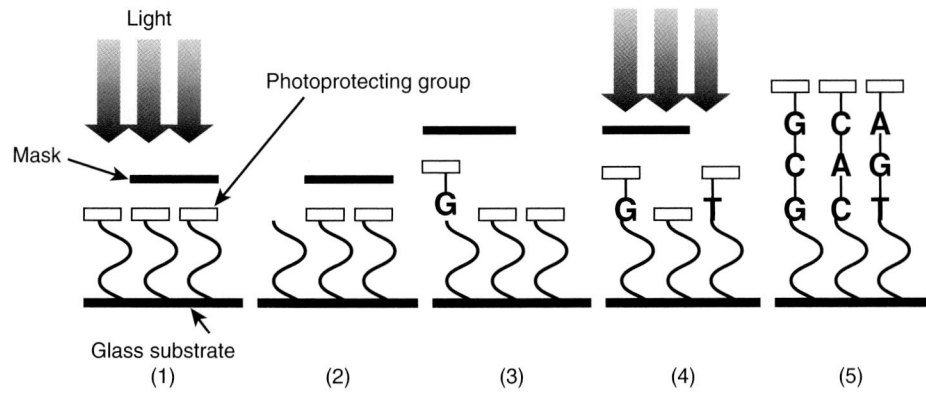

Figure 4-5 The photolithographic construction of microarrays. Synthesized high-density oligonucleotide microarray manufacturing with photolithography. Using selective masks, photo-labile protecting groups are light-activated for DNA synthesis (1, 2), photoprotected DNA bases are added and coupled to the intended coordinates (3). This cycle is repeated (4) with the appropriate masks to allow for controlled parallel synthesis of oligonucleotide chains in all coordinates on the array (5).

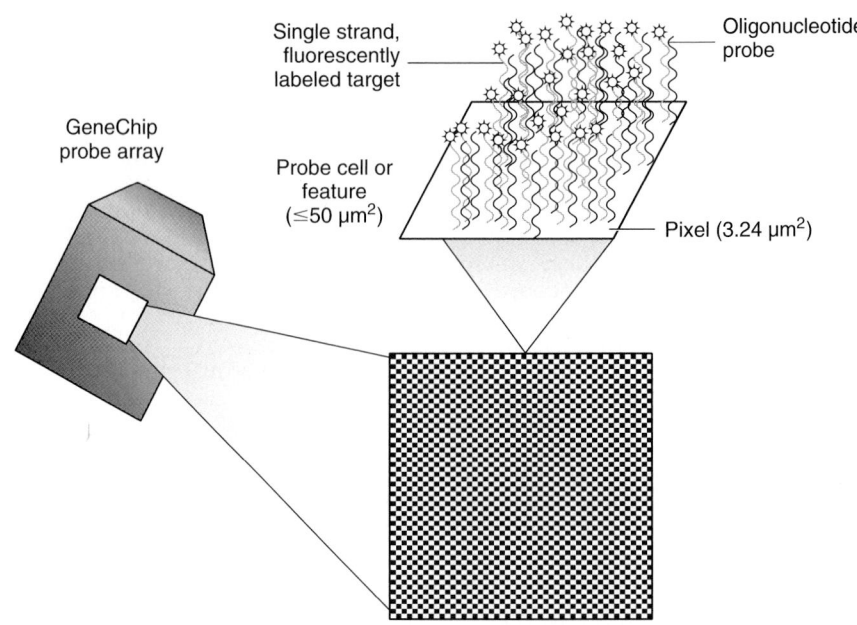

Figure 4-6 Probe cell image.

and compact systems for assessing the concentration of tens of thousands of proteins, we face the following challenges:

- Similar concentrations do not imply coregulation. Given that proteins have greatly different half-lives, even within a single cell (e.g., a structural protein in a bone osteoblast and a parathyroid hormone receptor in the same cell), then the concentrations of protein molecules in a cell may only remotely reflect joint regulation. This problem also haunts the analysis of RNA expression microarray data because of the wide range of stability/degradation rate of mRNA.
- Conversely, repeatedly different concentrations of two proteins may imply coregulation or interactions. At any given sampling time, the two proteins could have quite variable concentrations and different mutual relationships. Yet, there is nothing about this to preclude important functional interactions between these proteins.
- Protein activity has functions that are localized. Unlike transcription of genes which occurs within the nucleus, protein activity has very distinct and heterogeneous functional significance in different parts of the cellular compartments, and, therefore, an essential part of understanding protein function and regulation from proteomic data will require detailed localization to subcompartments of organelles in order to be meaningful.

These challenges of proteomics will eventually be addressed by novel ways of looking at protein activity over time and in different spatial locations. Nonetheless, at the present, the basic mechanism for cheaply and reliably obtaining large numbers of parallel measurements of protein activity has yet to be worked out and industrialized, so that these developments are likely not to occur on a large scale for at least 2 to 4 years. When these challenges have been resolved, then the arrays of proteomic data will be amenable to the same techniques of analysis as described in this chapter for RNA microarray data sets. At present, proteomics lacks the kind of prismatic successful clinical study that is represented by the B-cell lymphoma study described previously, although some important first studies are being performed, as will be described here.

Proteomics are not the monolithic entity that gene-expression functional genomics are. As the preamble here suggests, there are many kinds of proteomics with their own

techniques, research communities, and, increasingly, their own names, such as phosphoproteomics[15] and interactomics.[16]

This chapter focuses on the most common types of proteomics: *descriptive proteomics*, those in which protein presence is assayed and those in which protein quantity is assayed. In this context, just as the goal of RNA expression microarrays is to measure the entirety of the transcriptome, the principal goal of proteomics is to identify systematically every protein expressed in all cells or tissues in humans and other organisms. This includes the wide variety of posttranslational modifications and localizations. Currently, the state of the art involves multiple, often laborious steps requiring expert laboratory technicians rather than the "commodity" level expertise required by RNA expression microarrays. The technology for proteomic analyses integrates separation science for the separation of proteins and peptides, analytical science for the identification and quantification of the analytes, and bioinformatics for data management and analysis. In its most common form, the technology involves the combination of high-resolution 2-dimensional gel electrophoresis (2DE), using isoelectric focusing/SDS-PAGE gel, for the separation, detection, and quantification of individual proteins present in a complex sample with mass spectrometry and sequence database searching for the identification of the separated proteins. A simplified view of the steps of this overall method is schematically illustrated in Figure 4-7.

Figure 4-7 illustrates the separation of a protein extract using 2-dimensional gel electrophoresis. Individual spots are selected and removed from the gel and the spots' peptide contents trypsin-digested and further separated through high-performance liquid chromatography (HPLC). The eluted peptides are run through the mass spectrometer and the spectra obtained are compared to the mass-charge ratios (m/z) theoretically matching a particular peptide. A set of such theoretical matches may allow the unambiguous identification of the protein in question. This process becomes more complex in more recent technologies where the proteins are not completely fragmented.

The first part of this process, 2DE, has a long history[17] of small-scale successes that preceded those of the genomic revolution by 20 years but was then overshadowed by the industrialization of genome sequencing and subsequently by gene expression profiling. The early proteomics efforts were hobbled by several, then unsolved technical problems, but also by the far larger size of the proteome as compared to the genome

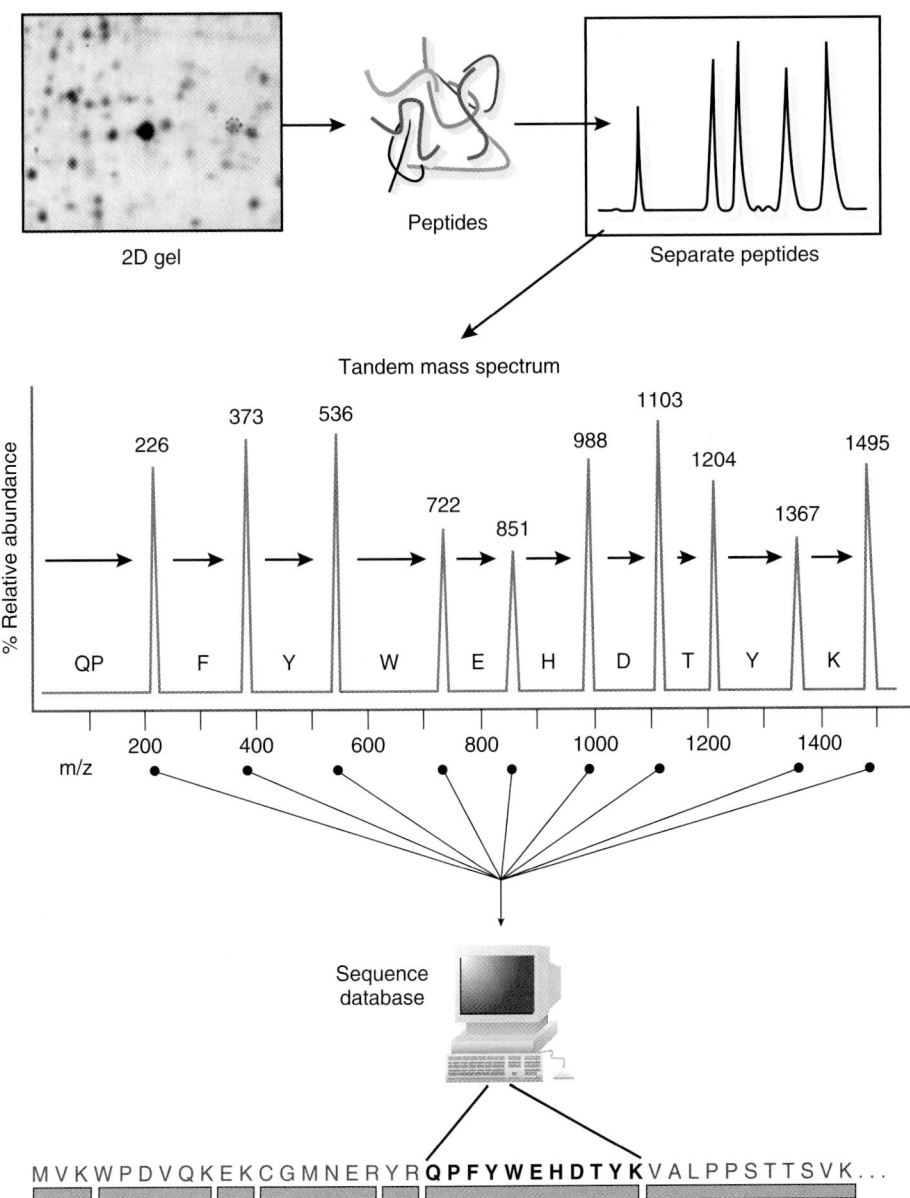

2D gel

Peptides

Separate peptides

Tandem mass spectrum

Sequence database

MVKWPDVQKEKCGMNERYR **QPFYWEHDTYK** VALPPSTTSVK...

Sequence and protein identified

Figure 4-7 Sketch of isoelectric focusing combined with mass-spectrometry for protein identification. (From Gygi SP, Abersold R: Mass spectometry and proteonomics. Curr Opin Chem Biol 4:489–494, 2000.)

or transcriptome (if one includes all the protein products and their posttranslational modifications). The steady but incremental improvements in 2DE (new fluorescent staining methods have provided higher sensitivity and larger dynamic range and increased resolution by expanding the pI range of the first dimension [zoom gels and prefractionation of complex protein samples before 2DE]) and the standardization of the 2DE methodology (including partial automation and more robust and reproducible image processing of the gels) have made productivity much higher than was previously possible. Controversy remains as to whether 2DE performs adequately to measure the entire proteome. Gygi and colleagues,[18] for example, note that without pre-enrichment, 2DE misses low-abundance proteins, very large and very small proteins, or very basic or very acidic proteins. Nonetheless, these challenges are being addressed and it seems likely, in the absence of a viable alternative, that 2DE will remain a persistent first step in proteomics in the near future.

It is the coupling of mass-spectrometry to 2DE, essentially the addition of another, even higher throughput dimension of separation (the mass/charge ratio, m/z) that has rekindled the vision of a comprehensive index of the human proteome

and the feasibility of comparing the proteome across disease states.

The bioinformatics challenges posed by proteomics just in the basic data acquisition stage are staggering. The spectra of m/z peaks per sample can generate hundreds of megabytes of data. "Merely" assigning a set of peaks to a protein identity has created a secondary industry of commercial and free software (e.g., Mascot; see Ref. 19) that heuristically match these spectra to growing protein identity databases.

Even at this date, no single mass-spectrometry configuration has the necessary resolution, specificity, and sensitivity across the entire dynamic range to meet all measurement needs of the proteome. In part, this is because of the broad nature of such needs, ranging from detecting a phosphorylation difference on a large protein to detecting small, low-abundance peptides. As a result there has been a proliferation of mass-spectrometry technologies—matrix-assisted laser desorption ionization (MALDI) time-of-flight (TOF),[20] hybrid quadrupole-time-of-flight (Q-TOF),[21] MALDI TOF-TOF,[22] and surface-enhanced laser surface-enhanced laser (SELDI)-TOF[23,24]—all with a different set of optimizations. The experienced shopper of consumer electronics will recognize that such proliferation of technologies and acronyms is evidence that (1) none of the technologies is clearly dominant, and (2) it will be much better and much cheaper very soon and what you bought this year will be obsolete next year.

QUANTITATION

Inspired by the success of RNA expression microarrays, proteomics technologists have turned to the challenge of quantitative proteomics or, more specifically, measures of relative protein abundance (differential protein expression) across tissues or pathophysiologic states. The first approach taken was one which would be quite familiar to classically trained endocrinologists, the use of a stable isotope as a dilution measure or point of reference. A reference tissue or organism is cultured/grown in conditions such that that one or more isotopes (e.g., ^2H, ^{13}C, ^{15}N) are taken up and incorporated into the proteins of the reference sample. The test or comparison organism/tissue is simply exposed to the common, abundant isotopes. The protein extracts from test and reference sample are mixed and, because the proteins from both sources are chemically identical, it is assumed that they behave the same during isolation, ionization, and other analytic procedures. But, because the test and reference samples are shifted with respect to one another by mass, their relative signals and, therefore, abundance can be estimated. This form of protein quantification has not been widely adopted because of several additional technical challenges: (1) The mass shift for any given protein is not predictable and, therefore, an additional identification step has to precede the quantification, and (2) many tissues are not amenable to this approach for practical reasons (e.g., human tissues). Consequently, more recent efforts have been focused on tagging proteins under different conditions with a different defined tag, after the fact (after extraction from tissue). The most popular of these at the time of this writing is isotope-coded affinity tag (ICAT).

The ICAT procedure is summarized in Figure 4-8A. It starts with a tagging molecule that has a moiety that specifically reacts with a portion of the peptide/protein molecule, most commonly, the thiol group in cysteine residues. Each tagging molecule also has an affinity tag (typically, biotin) that can subsequently be detected in chromatography. Finally, each tag exists in two forms, a heavy and a light form, depending on which stable isotopes were used to make the linker portion of the tagging molecule, as shown in Figure 4-8. After sample material is obtained from two tissues or tissue states, the proteins are extracted and labeled with the tagging molecule. These protein extracts are then combined and trypsinized, the proteins bound to the ICAT label are then picked up in an affinity procedure (typically HPLC), and the output of the affinity procedure is fed into a mass spectrometer. The mass spectrometer reveals twin peaks offset by the mass of the tagging molecule(s) and thereby the relative abundance of each tagged protein in the two source tissues/tissue states. These same tagged proteins can then be identified using standard mass-spectrometry sequencing methods.

Limitations of the ICAT approach include the change of mass caused by the entire tagging molecule. This change has to be accounted for when the standard algorithms and software packages (like the aforementioned Mascot) are used to

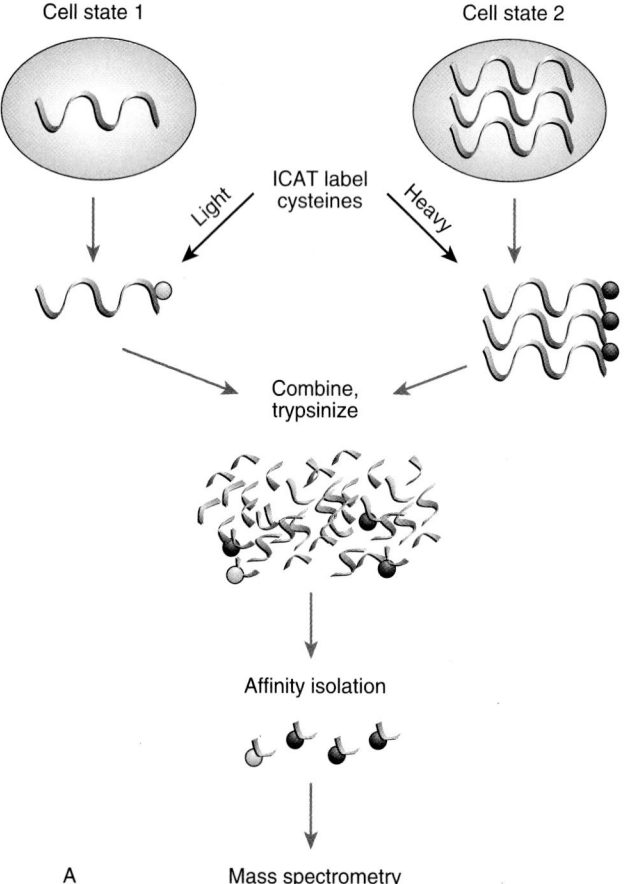

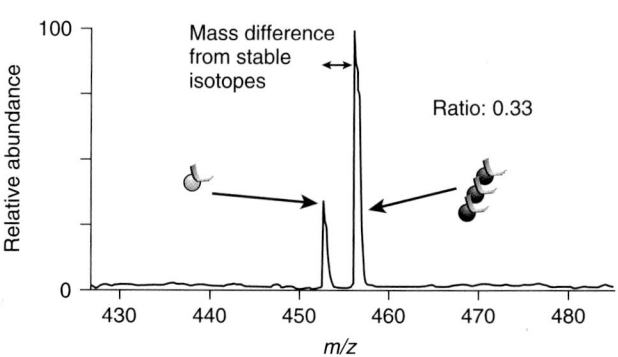

Quantitate relative protein levels by measuring peak ratios

Mass difference from stable isotopes

Ratio: 0.33

Relative abundance

430 440 450 460 470 480

m/z

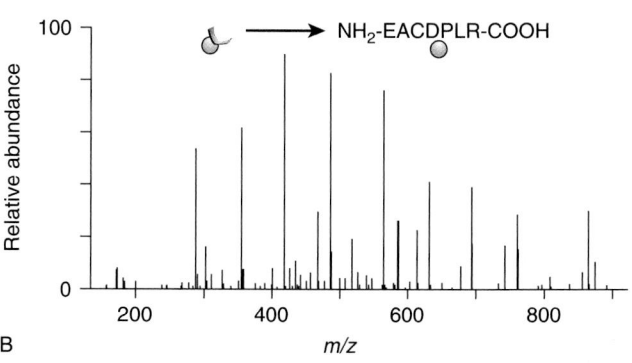

Identify peptide by sequence information (MS/MS scan)

NH₂-EACDPLR-COOH

Relative abundance

200 400 600 800

m/z

Figure 4-8 **A,** ICAT approach to differentiated protein expression. Proteins from two different states, tissues, or diseases are extracted. The cysteine residues are labeled with the ICAT reagent using a different isotope on the ICAT reagent for each state. Samples are then combined and digested and analyzed by HPLC coupled to a mass spectrometer. **B,** The ratio of the ion intensities corresponding to the proteins labeled with different isotopes (in the ICAT reagent) corresponds to the relative abundance of these proteins. Tandem mass spectroscopy is then used to unambiguously identify the proteins corresponding to the peaks of interest. (From Gygi SP, Abersold R: Mass spectrometry and proteonomics. Curr Opin Chem Biol 4:489–494, 2000.)

match m/z profiles to proteins/peptides. Also, not all proteins have cysteine residues and, furthermore, the ICAT procedure is laborious, complex, and less efficient than other techniques under development (see Ref. 25). Again, like many other high-throughput proteomic techniques, quantification is still under rapid development and a standardized platform for quantification, comparable to the microarrays of gene expression, has yet to be developed. If we revisit the definition of microarrays earlier in this chapter, it becomes clear that many of the properties that have made gene expression microarrays such a useful and successful adjunct to biomedical research have yet to be realized in proteomics. This is most clearly demonstrated by the small number of clinical proteomic studies used to conduct the kind of new disease classification operation described for B-cell lymphoma at the beginning of this chapter. Even when these studies are done (e.g., for classification of serum samples of patients with ovarian cancer[26]), they have been greeted with far more controversy[27–29] than the early genomic microarray studies.

WHY DO PROTEOMICS AND FUNCTIONAL GENOMICS REQUIRE NEW ANALYTIC TECHNIQUES?

A first look at a typical gene expression or proteomics study might cause a quantitatively trained scientist or even a biologically trained scientist to ask the following, quite legitimate question: Why is this field not amenable to standard biostatistical techniques? After all, the goal is to understand the relationship between multiple variables (i.e., RNA or protein expression) and the mechanisms that the relationships reveal (i.e., pathophysiology), and there has been a long history of the development of biostatistical techniques to analyze large studies with large numbers of cases with many variables to elucidate precisely this kind of question.

Conventional epidemiologic studies ask questions such as: What risk factors are associated with heart disease? Does smoking cause disease? On the surface, these questions seem similar to many of those posed regarding genetic risk factors for acute and chronic disease. Yet, a review of the bioinformatics/functional genomics literature from the past 5 years reveals that most of the analyses have been performed using techniques borrowed from the computational sciences, and machine-learning communities in particular. Why is this? Is there a reason other than disciplinary parochialism?

If we examine Figure 4-9, we see the fundamental difference between a typical epidemiologic/clinical study and a typical genomic study. A high-quality clinical study will involve thousands to tens of thousands of patients, as in the Nurses' Health Study[30] or the Framingham Heart Study,[31] and the analysis of tens or even hundreds of variables. In contrast, in a typical genomic study, there are only tens or, exceptionally, hundreds of cases, each with tens of thousands of measured variables.

Initially, the low number of cases may have been due to the high cost of the microarrays (in 1999, around several thousand dollars per microarray; in 2004, in the low hundreds), but, increasingly, the scarcity of cases in a typical functional genomic study relates to the scarcity of appropriate biologic samples. Since these experiments involve the measurement of gene expression, a particular tissue (e.g., brain, muscle, fat) has to be obtained under the right conditions. This is in distinction to genomic DNA samples where most blood samples will suffice. (Proteomic studies have the same analytic challenges, but the cost-to-sample tradeoffs are less clear because of the earlier stage of development of this technology.)

Especially in human populations, suitable tissue samples are relatively scarce. Even though there are only tens of cases, each case involves the measurements of tens of thousands of variables corresponding to the expression of tens of thousands of genes measurable with microarray technology. The result of the large number of variables compared to the number of cases is that we have highly underdetermined systems. That is, these are measurements of very high dimensionality (on the order of tens of thousands), but we are only providing a small number of cases to explore this high-dimensional space. Another way to say this is that there are many, many ways in which the variables being measured could be interrelated mechanistically, based on the relatively small number of observations. Due to this high dimensionality and the underdetermined nature of these systems, standard biostatistical techniques do not hold up well because many of the assumptions that underlie conventional biostatistical techniques do not hold. In fairness, there has been quite a lot of research by statisticians on the analysis of underdetermined systems of high dimensionality. This work has just not found its way into mainstream biomedical study until recently.

THE INVESTIGATIONAL PIPELINE IN THE FUNCTIONAL GENOMIC AND PROTEOMIC ERA

Although it is typically the case that a functional genomic or proteomic experiment is not hypothesis driven, the more successful research efforts are question driven. The questions range from "Is gene regulation of oxidative phosphorylation altered in type 2 diabetes mellitus?" to "What gene expression signatures best predict diabetic retinopathy in individuals with adequate glycemic control" to "Which genes participate in circadian rhythmicity in the suprachiasmatic nucleus of the hypothalamus?" This crucial step is only the first one of a series of steps, often described as the functional genomic pipeline, and outlined in Figure 4-10. The remainder of the pipeline is summarized here to guide the investigator and also to frame the methodological challenges:

- Selection of the right tissue: Experiments in functional genomics require selection of the functionally relevant tissue or cell type. In certain experiments, such as those using blood and solid cancers, the functionally relevant tissue is clear. In other analyses, the functionally relevant tissue is not so easily ascertainable or acquirable. For example, the clinical phenotype seen in type 2 diabetes mellitus, or insulin resistance, involves the coordinated physiologic dysfunction of several organs and cell types, including liver, muscle, and fat cells. Schizophrenia involves a higher-order brain dysfunction, but brain cells are not easily accessible in humans. For some common diseases, such as hypertension, the functionally relevant tissue may not be known. A successful pipeline involves collaboration with a source of tissue, such as a surgical

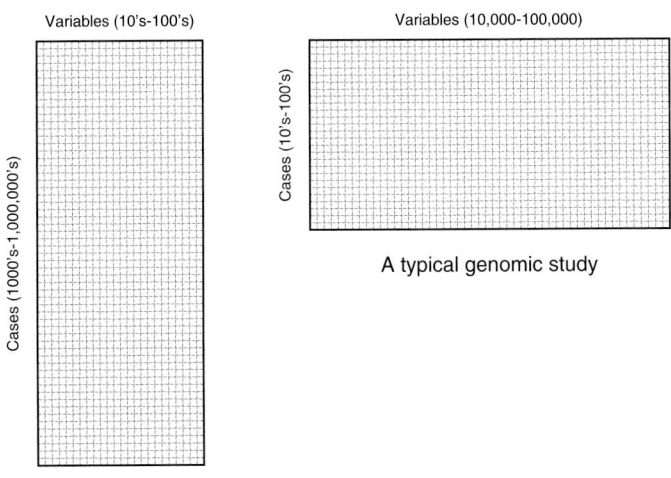

Variables (10's-100's)

Cases (1000's-1,000,000's)

A typical clinical study

Variables (10,000-100,000)

Cases (10's-100's)

A typical genomic study

Figure 4-9 Major differences between classical clinical/epidemiologic studies and genomic or proteomic studies.

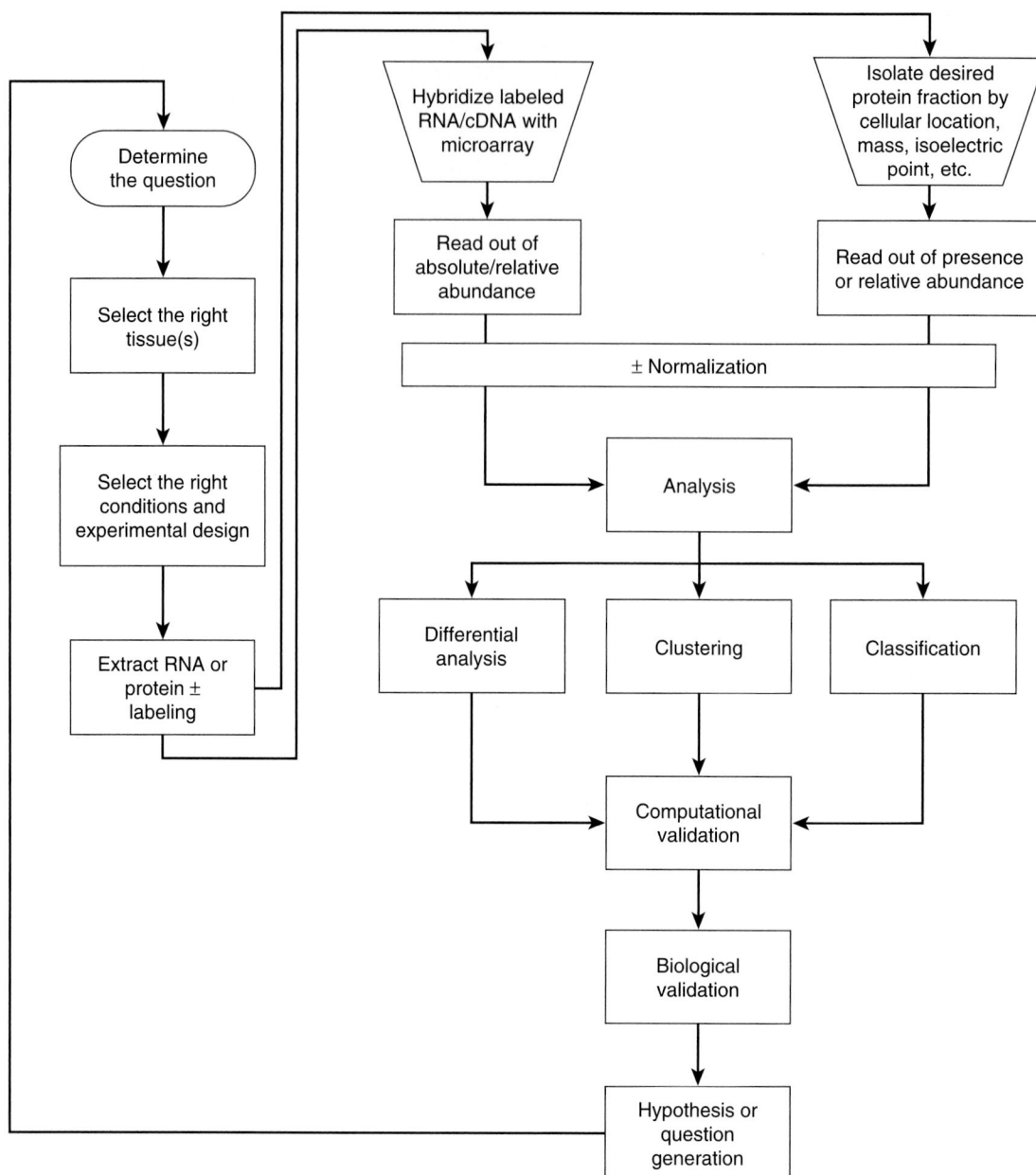

Figure 4-10   Overall flow of the genomic/proteomic pipeline.

team, a laboratory with biologically interesting animals, or a laboratory with cell lines of interest.

- Right conditions: Even if the appropriate tissue is selected from the organism of interest, the conditions under which the tissue is obtained (e.g., number of hours post mortem) can determine whether or not the investigation is successful. An insulin-sensitive tissue such as skeletal muscle will have a different characteristic metabolic and expression profile depending on the glucose and insulin concentrations before the extraction of RNA. The time of day will influence the expression of genes in all tissues that have endogenous circadian rhythms or processes that can be entrained by physiologic clocks. Awareness of these issues and cooperation from a surgeon, pathologist, or technician responsible for obtaining the tissue is therefore an essential component to the success of the functional genomic pipeline. In truth, any competent endocrinologist should be fully conversant with these experimental design considerations. It remains the case that because microarrays or proteomics apparently commodify the parallel measurement of thousands of analytes instead of the usual handful, many of

these important physiologic considerations were omitted in the majority of experiments in the first 5 years of broad availability of microarray technologies. These are only some of the issues involved in experimental design. Others include: (1) whether the experimental design is to determine the natural classes of samples, (2) whether the experimental design is to compare two or more conditions, or (3) whether a predictor for a clinical state is being sought. These three most common classes of question are touched on in subsequent sections. Readers interested in more details on functional genomic or proteomic experimental design are referred to one of several recent books.[32,33]

- Extract RNA/protein, with or without labeling, hybridized to microarray or loaded into the 2DE mass-spectrometry system: Each of these steps in this "wet" component of a functional genomics/proteomics pipeline is susceptible to operator error and is a potential source of poor or noisy measurements. The RNA extracted may be of poor quality, conditions under which the protein samples were conserved were variable, the hybridization conditions (e.g., the room temperature) may vary, and the settings of the scanner that produces the digital image of the microarray may vary from one scan to another. Industrialization and standardization of these hybridization and extraction components has been the focus of the more successful and high-quality functional genomic and proteomic efforts. It is perhaps not glamorous, but no analytic technique can overcome poor performance in this step.

- Readout of the raw data on abundance (absolute or relative) and/or presence of proteins or RNA: Depending on the particular experimental setup, this step can be numbingly arduous. Quality control of the data or identification of the RNA or protein to which a given measured value corresponds is close to fully automated in commodity microarray systems and much less so in individually tweaked, state-of-the-art proteomics instrumentation.
- Normalization: Often, before any further analysis is performed, the raw data from each experiment in a set of experiments is adjusted so that the data are more comparable within a set. This highly controversial step is discussed later in its own subsection.
- Differential expression: This most common analytic step is also often the most poorly done. As described in its own subsection, the large numbers of gene products measured lead all too many investigators to overinterpret the very noisy data generated by these high-throughput modalities.
- Clustering and classification: These "dry" components of the pipeline are often thought to be what bioinformatics is about. In fact, it may be that this stage, with the algorithmic analysis of a proteomic or gene expression study to detect biologically or clinically meaningful patterns or associations, is the only time a bioinformatician is involved. This can be an expensive mistake and there is good reason to involve the bioinformaticians from the very first step in this pipeline.
- Computational validation: As will be elaborated in this chapter, there are many reasons to perform bioinformatics analyses on functional genomics data sets, and many methods that can be used. One unique problem with these types of data sets is that they are "short and wide," meaning that many characteristics/variables are measured on relatively few samples. This makes it all too easy for apparently significant and interesting findings to be obtained by chance. To avoid being misled, some computational validation is required immediately after the bioinformatics analysis so that computationally sound but biologically spurious or improbable hypotheses are screened out. The principal motivation for the screening out of spurious or improbable hypotheses is the efforts that follow. Each hypothesis generated that passes the computational validation step must be validated in a biologic laboratory. Some laboratories may wish (and may have the resources) to pursue many hypotheses and can tolerate the eventual refutation of large numbers of false-positive hypotheses. Other biologic laboratories may only be able to validate a few. An ideal computation validation does not merely provide a "yes" or "no" answer as to potential validity of a hypothesis, but instead provides a continuum of validation, or a receiver-operating characteristic curve. With such a curve, the biologist can select the desired point of sensitivity or specificity and true and false negatives and positives.
- Biologic validation: Most biologic questions will not be answered using microarrays. Instead, the most likely outcome from a functional genomics analysis is the next biologic question to ask. As hypotheses are generated from bioinformatics analyses, biologic validation is crucial in verifying these hypotheses. This verification may include, for instance, making sure a particular set of genes is truly expressed at the proper time and place as hypothesized,

using conventional biologic techniques such as Northern blotting and in situ hybridization or scale cell-line-based overexpression and knockdown experiments all the way up to whole organismal models.
- Asking the next question: The entire pipeline is of necessity a highly iterative process. By measuring so many gene products simultaneously, further hypotheses pertaining to multiple regulatory systems are going to develop in the course of answering the first question.

In most settings, all of these steps, from asking the germane question to acquisition of source material to microarray construction to bioinformatics analysis to biologic verification, cannot be performed by a single group or laboratory. A successful functional genomics/proteomics pipeline brings together resources from many disciplines and with varied backgrounds.

NORMALIZATION

If you take a photograph of a friend on two different occasions but at the same angle and distance, the two resulting pictures may well differ due to different exposure time and different lighting conditions, among other possible variables. If you want to determine whether your friend has changed between the two pictures, however, perhaps in skin tone or the amount of freckling, then one reasonable approach would be to try to adjust the images after the fact, using an image processing program such as Adobe Photoshop to make the two pictures more alike and potentially more comparable. For example, you might adjust the contrast and the brightness of the two photos to be closer to one another or adjust the distribution of red, green, and blue colors so that they are again more similar to one another. In other words, you would normalize the two photographs so that they are more similar, in the hope that you would then be able to detect more clearly the features that are different between the two photographs. This is the essence of the process of normalizing a large number of measurements taken at one time and comparing them to another set of measurements obtained at another time, whether this is done using expression microarray technology or quantitative proteomic measurement techniques. It is important to recognize that any normalization technique runs the risk of obscuring essential differences between the two data sets, that is, of obscuring a difference that might be biologically relevant in the process of making data sets more similar. To return to the original analogy: If the two photographs of your friend are manipulated with a particular set of filters, they may end up looking very similar, but you may also not be able to determine whether your friend has, in fact, substantially changed between the two photographs. This illustrates the tension deriving from any normalization method: the intent to make the two data sets more comparable while preserving their essential differences. Some methods may be more successful than others for particular kinds of data distributions, but there are likely always to be other contexts in which they obscure important biologic differences. Notwithstanding, there are some methodologists who argue that *any* kind of normalization procedure obscures the true biologic differences measured and that normalization of any sort is, in fact, decreasing the amount of information obtainable from a study.

With these caveats in mind, the two most popular normalization methods are outlined here. Linear regression is based on the assumption that the change of intensity that will make two microarrays more comparable is going to be linear, and lowess normalization operates on the assumption that there are nonlinear effects that must be compensated for (e.g., saturation of expression measurements at higher levels of expression). It should be noted, however, there are literally dozens of alternative published normalization methods, each claiming improved relative performance.

Linear Regression

The discussion here focuses first on the assumptions that are correctable by linear transformations. If a x_i and y_i denote the reported expression intensity (of gene i in the duplicate experiments B_1 and B_2, respectively), with i = 1, . . . , N, where N = 13,179 is the total number of unique probes on the Mu11K Affymetrix chip set, for example. In this discussion, B_1 is the designated reference data set. Often, however, the reference data set is picked on the basis of which one was thought to have the best quality (e.g., of the RNA extracted).

Now, consider for the moment a hypothetical situation where chip B_2 has a systematic error in relation to its (reference) duplicate B_1 such that the expression level for every gene i, x_i in B_1 is remeasured or reproduced in the B_2 experiment as $y_i = a_1x_i + a_0$ for some real constants a_0 and a_1. A global linear shift of this kind could arise, for instance, if chip B_2 were scanned at a different uniform ambient brightness from chip B_1. Physically, a_1 is the magnification or dilation factor and a_0 is the translation factor. A linear regression line through a scatter plot of x_i versus y_i would then look like a line of slope a_1 with its vertical or Y-intercept at a_0. Clearly, if chips B_1 and B_2 were ideal duplicates, then the points (x_i, y_i) would be aligned on a line of slope one through the origin (without scatter).

Knowing the values a_1 and a_0 (from having calculated the linear regression), the transformation $y'_i = (y_i - a_0)/(a_1)$ will correct this systematic difference in B_2 with respect to B_1 so that a plot of x_i versus y'_i is a line of slope one through the origin (0,0). So, in summary, this linear transformation for any number of chips, in regard to a reference chip or experiment, is to calculate the slope and intercept using linear regression and then to use these, as described, to rotate and alter the slope and intercept of each of the nonreference chips/experiments, so that they have a slope of 1 with respect to the reference chip and an intercept of (0,0).

Lowess Normalization

If you plot the ratio of two sets of measurements (e.g., of Cy3-labeled RNA versus Cy5-labeled RNA) against the product of the same measurements, then, if the conditions and imaging on both sets of measurements were identical, you would expect to see a straight horizontal line. Instead, you will often see a curving line, as shown in Figure 4-11. There have been a number of proposed techniques to normalize such nonlinear relationships, but, in essence, all of them involve performing mathematical operations essentially to straighten out the curve. Unlike linear regression, which makes the assumption that the "curve" is a straight

line, most of these methods attempt to minimize any assumptions regarding the shape of the curve. This is often necessary because there are a number of effects on the distribution of expression values that are not obvious or precisely quantifiable after the fact. The most widely used of these nonlinear curve-fitting procedures is for the loess (aka lowess) curve.

The lowess curve-fitting function attempts drawing a smooth curve through a scatter diagram. The smooth curve is drawn in such a way as to ensure that the curve indeed be smooth (as opposed to oscillated wildly about the data) and that, locally, the curve minimizes the variance of the residuals or prediction error (analogously to the minimization of residuals in linear regression).

Replotting the points with respect to this curve, as if it were a straight line, results in the plot shown in Figure 4-12.[34] This is the corresponding operation to subtracting the intercept and dividing by the slope for the linear regression method. Again as in our original analogy with respect to our photographs, the investigator should be aware that making two microarrays similar may also hide true biologic differences in the data.

DIFFERENTIAL EXPRESSION ANALYSIS

In routine, pre-genomic endocrine investigations, a question that is often asked is: How does a hormone serum level change from one condition to another? For example, what is the 8:00 A.M. average serum cortisol level in nonobese versus obese subjects? Similarly, the comparison of the entire transcriptome or proteome across two conditions is the most frequently performed analysis in gene expression and proteomics. Questions often asked in endocrine genomic studies include:

- Which genes are differentially expressed between two tissues such as brown fat and white fat?[35]
- What is the difference in gene expression between the same muscle tissue exposed to a different dose of insulin?[36]
- What is the difference in expression of the adipose tissue of mice with diet-induced obesity versus nonobese mice?[37]

If these questions are answered by a researcher using a single microarray for each of the two conditions (i.e., two microarrays per question), the analysis is as straightforward as it is limited. All that can be done is to divide the value of the expression of each gene in one condition by the expression value of that same gene in the other condition. The ratios of

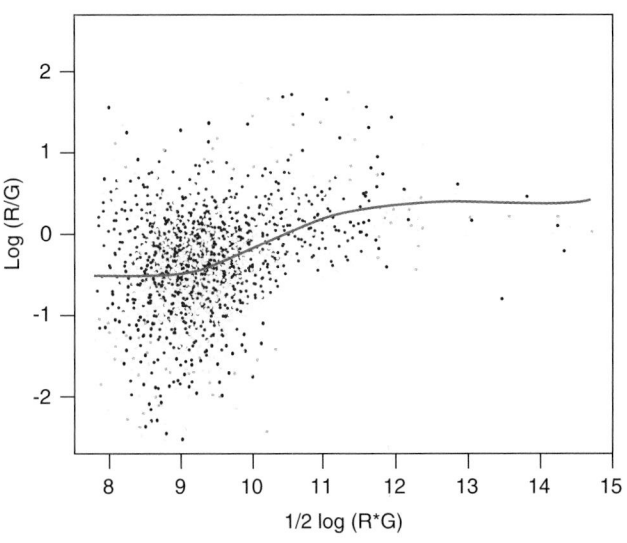

Figure 4-11   Before loess normalization.

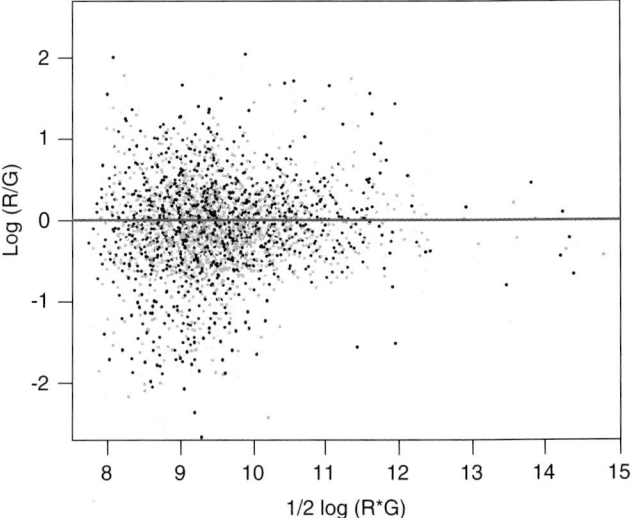

Figure 4-12   After loess normalization.

each gene's expression value can then be reviewed, typically sorted from highest to lowest. This parsimonious use of microarrays, not uncommon today, does not account for the measurement variation that is omnipresent in all analogue measurement techniques including gene expression. To estimate the measurement error, multiple replicates for each condition must be obtained. Early in the development of microarray technology, the variance in the quality of the arrays was such that the same hybridization "cocktail" (i.e., the same extracted RNA) was used for multiple arrays (i.e., technical replicates) to estimate variance due to the arrays. Currently, the quality of many of the commercial arrays is such that RNA from different samples is used for each microarray hybridization (i.e., biologic replicates). This still begs the question: How are the replicate measurements used to obtain a more robust measure of differential expression across conditions?

In the late 1990s and in the first couple of years of the millennium, the standard of care with multiple replicate experiments was to pick an arbitrary threshold for the amount for which a gene would have to change to have it considered significant. For example, if the average of any gene was up threefold or down threefold across a set of conditions, it was considered significant and reportable. As shown in Figure 4-13, at different expression levels, these kinds of arbitrary thresholds determined different numbers of differentially expressed genes (i.e., true-positive and false-positive rates varied with expression level). In response to the obvious arbitrariness of this approach and the increasing number of poorly produced studies, a number of more rigorous measures for differential expression have been developed. There are now literally dozens of published alternate methods for performing differential expression analysis and the interested reader is invited to peruse any one of the cited textbooks[32,33,38] for further details. The focus here is on the most used cited and perhaps most useful one, although this is certainly debatable. Before proceeding, however, the reader should be aware of some limitations and desiderata that are important in the use of any of these methodologies.

First, microarrays are very noisy and it is inevitable that even with substantial numbers of repeated samples there will always be one or more genes that are either falsely labeled as differentially regulated (i.e., a false positive) or falsely labeled as having no differential expression when it indeed could be found to be differentially expressed by more rigorous means (i.e., a false negative).

Second, there are many more genes in a microarray than we intuitively understand. This means that we are often underappreciative of how many false positives can be obtained in even a high-specificity experiment. It is common for seasoned endocrinology researchers to spot a gene a long way down the list of differentially expressed genes that they know for a fact is differentially expressed under the conditions tested. Consequently, they are surprised and nonplussed when a

given statistical test describes this particular gene and many other interesting ones as not being differentially expressed. What is underappreciated is how many hundreds of genes would have to be included as being differentially expressed if the genes identified by these investigators were included and how many of these would prove to be false positives. Specifically, the difficulty and cost of wading through hundreds of genes putatively differentially expressed, where very few of them might in fact truly be differentially expressed, is initially not appreciated. Given that even the simplest validation steps such as real-time polymerase chain reaction (RT-PCR) would take hundreds of days if performed on all these potential false positives, it becomes clear why several biotech companies and pharmaceutical companies have become disenchanted by the use of microarray technology. Even they found a large number of false positives too costly with respect to their available resources.

Finally, the great challenge of differential gene expression analysis is what Nir Friedman (in personal communication with the author) characterized as gene staring syndrome (GSS). Simply put, given the wealth of the number of genes present on the microarray, the multiplicity of the roles of many genes, and, furthermore, the creativity of biologic investigators, it is all too easy to take any of these lists and come up with an apparently coherent story of why a particular list of genes was, in fact, differentially expressed. Gene staring syndrome is all too common and again points to the need for rigorous analyses of the data.

Applying a traditional test of the difference of means of two groups, such as the Student's T test, is problematic for a number of reasons. First among these is that the P values obtained would have to be corrected for multiple hypothesis testing. Second, the traditional correction for multiple hypothesis testing such as the Bonferroni correction is unnecessarily stringent and therefore would unnecessarily decrease the sensitivity of the differential analysis in order to achieve a desired specificity. In 1995, Hochberg and Benjamini[39] developed a procedure for controlling the false discovery rate. The false discovery rate can be described as how many false positives are found in a list of genes said to be differentially expressed. By controlling the false discovery rate, an investigator can specify how many false leads to follow up. The most popular automated method available for differential analysis of gene expression in microarrays that addresses false discovery was described by Tusher and colleagues[40] and implemented in a program called Significant Analysis of Microarrays (SAM). In essence, SAM works very much like a T test, with the following differences:

- The difference between the means is calculated as for a T test, but with a correction factor applied that improves the performance of this measure for data sets with small numbers of microarrays.
- Hundreds of permutations of the data are performed and the aforementioned difference between the means is recalculated across the two conditions. This allows a direct estimate of the likelihood that such a difference could be obtained by chance and thereby provides a built-in correction for multiple hypotheses testing without an unnecessarily direct or unnecessarily naive correction. Furthermore, an ordering of these genes by this score allows a list of genes to be generated with a predictable false discovery rate. Best of all for the purposes of the investigator, this program is freely available to academic researchers at *http://www-stat.stanford.edu/~tibs/SAM/*.

To be clear, this is only one of several differential analysis algorithms and, in the rapidly moving field of functional genomics, it is likely that one or more of the new generation of differential analysis algorithms, particularly the Bayesian calculators that take into account the distributional properties of microarray measurements, may ultimately provide superior performance and, therefore, greater usefulness.

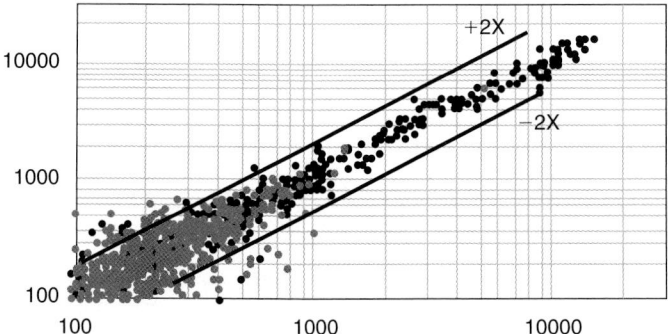

Figure 4-13 Using twofold thresholds for determining differential expression.

CLUSTERING AND CLASSIFICATION

There is a central underlying assumption in all gene-clustering techniques for expression analysis. Simply put, the assumption is that genes that appear to be expressed in similar patterns are in fact mechanistically related. Furthermore, the corollary to this assumption is that, although genes may distantly affect the function of other gene products, they fall into groups of more tightly regulated mechanisms. For instance, the genes that govern chromosome function or meiosis may be more tightly linked to each other than they are to the genes involved with another function, such as apoptosis. This has been the basis of our collective experience in biologic investigations in the past century: that there are groups of proteins that interact more closely than others. Often, they have been organized into pathways such as glycolysis, Kreb's cycle, and other metabolic pathways in which the gene products called enzymes have to work in concert. Other more obvious functional clusters are those of structural proteins that have to come together in a conserved and reproducible fashion in order to serve their purpose, whether they are the components of the ribosomal unit or the histoproteins that are essential for the maintenance of the structure of chromatin. On this basis, if we can find genes whose expression patterns approximate one another, we can possibly impute that they are functionally clustered together; that is, they have function that is related.

Several important caveats are worth noting here. First of all, it remains unclear just how discrete the functional groupings of gene function are in the cellular apparatus. It may be that individual gene products have so many different roles under different circumstances that several of them partake of essential roles in significantly different functions. The second caveat is that the term *functionally related* is itself ill specified. If the pattern of expression of one gene is similar to that of another, it could signify all kinds of relationships ranging from "two genes having gene products that physically interact," to "one gene encoding a transcriptional factor for the other gene," to "two genes having different functions but similar promoter sequences," to "two genes both with promoter sequences bound by repressors which are 'knocked off' when a nuclear receptor is activated, even though the two genes have widely disparate functions." Of course, there is a level of abstraction at which all genes are functionally related in their role to keep the cell alive and produce whatever components are needed for the rest of the organism. But below this level of abstraction, there are many alternate and, by their nature, sloppy definitions of clustering. Therefore, we should be somewhat wary of the claim that similarity in expression corresponds to similarity in function. Nonetheless, it is a useful starting point for many analyses of a genome whose function remains, by and large, unknown at this time. Additionally, the question of what constitutes similar expression pattern is itself poorly defined, or at least has multiple alternate definitions. For example, similarity could mean having similar patterns of change over time. It could mean similar absolute levels of expression at any given point in time, or it could mean perfectly opposite but well-choreographed patterns of expression. The similarity measure chosen for looking at patterns of expression influences the kind of functional clusters that we expect.

SUPERVISED VERSUS UNSUPERVISED LEARNING

The analyses of gene expression are qualitatively different from those of traditional biostatistics: The data sets are of high dimensionality and, yet, the number of cases is relatively small. Consequently, the number of solutions that could explain the observed behavior is quite large. For this reason, the machine-learning community has recognized the potential role for their techniques specifically designed to explore high-dimensional spaces (such as those of voice or face recognition) and have also recognized the enormous need to apply these techniques to genomic data sets.

Two useful broad categorizations of the techniques used by the machine-learning community are *supervised learning techniques* and *unsupervised learning techniques*. These are also commonly known as classification techniques and clustering techniques, respectively. The two techniques are easily distinguished by the presence of external labels of cases. For example, labeling a tissue as obtained from a patient with glucose intolerance or diabetes mellitus is needed before applying a supervised learning technique, to create a method to learn those combinations of variables that predict/determine those labels. In an unsupervised learning task, such as finding those genes that are coregulated across all the samples, the organization/clustering of the variables operates independently of any external labels. The kinds of variables (also known as *features*, in the jargon of the machine-learning community) that characterize each case in a data set can be quite varied. Each case can include measures of clinical outcome, gene expression, gene sequence, drug exposure, proteomic measurements, or any other discrete or continuous variable believed to be relevant to the case.

What kinds of questions are answered by the two types of machine learning? In supervised learning, the goal is typically to obtain a set of variables (e.g., expressed genes as measured on a microarray) on the basis of which one can reliably make the diagnosis of the patient, predict future outcome, predict future response to pharmacologic intervention, or categorize that patient, tissue, or animal as part of a class of interest. In unsupervised learning, the typical application is either to find a completely novel cluster of genes with putative common (but previously unknown) function or, more commonly, to obtain a cluster or group of genes that appear to have similar patterns of expression to a gene (i.e., they fall into the same cluster) already known to have an important well-defined function. The goal is to find more details about the mechanism by which the known gene works and to find other genes involved in that same mechanism to obtain a more complete view of a particular cellular physiology or, in the case of pharmacologically oriented research, other possible therapeutic targets. Although the distinct goals of supervised versus unsupervised machine-learning techniques may appear rather obvious, it is important to be aware of their implications for study design. For example, an analyst may be asked to find classifiers between different states of glucose tolerance (as was done in the case of Mootha and colleagues,[41] described later). The lists of genes that reliably divide the two states may have little to do, however, with the actual pathophysiologic causes of the diabetes and may not represent any particular close relationship of those genes and function. Why might this be? It is quite possible that small amounts of change of some gene products, such as transcriptional activators and genes, may cause large downstream changes in gene expression. That is, with only a subtle change, an important upstream gene may cause dramatic changes in the expression in several pathways that are functionally only distantly related but are highly influenced by the same upstream gene. When applying a classification algorithm directly on the gene expression levels, the algorithm will naturally identify those genes that change the most between the two or more states being classified. That is, a study design geared toward the application of a supervised learning technique may generate a useful artifact for classification, diagnosis, or even prognosis, but it will not necessarily lead to valuable insights into the biology underlying the classes obtained.

Let us consider the more general cases in which gene expression values are not the only data type. A given case can include several thousand gene expression measurements, but also several hundred phenotypic measurements such as blood pressure, a laboratory value, or the response to a hormonal supplementation regimen. Here again, a clustering algorithm can be used to find those features most tightly coupled in the observed data. When designing an experiment that includes the various data types, it is worthwhile to think ahead of time whether some kinds of features are more likely to cluster together, separately from the genomic data. That is, after application of a clustering algorithm, the data set may reveal relationships between the non-genomic variables that are much more significant and stronger than any of those that involve gene expression or sequence. Although that is not necessarily a bad outcome, it will not help the investigator who is trying to understand the particular contribution of genetic regulation to the observed phenomenon. As an example, if one looks at the effect of thousands of drugs on several cancer cell lines, then it should not be surprising if these drug effects are most tightly clustered around groups of pharmaceutical agents that were derived from one another through combinatorial chemistry. Similarly, phenotypic features that are highly interdependent, such as height and weight, will cluster together. The strength of these obvious clusters will often dominate those of heterogeneous clusters that contain phenotypic measurements as well as gene expression measurements. This suggests that careful feature reduction to include only those features that are nonredundant and only truly independent phenotypic measures for each case should be employed. The reader interested in systematic approaches to feature reduction is referred to the excellent text by Sholom Weiss.[42]

Because the wide range of techniques developed for both supervised and unsupervised learning fall considerably beyond the scope of this chapter, they are only mentioned and referenced in the list to follow.

UNSUPERVISED LEARNING

Analysis to look for characteristics in the data set, without a priori input on cases or genes.

Feature determination: Determine genes with interesting properties, without specifically looking for a specific pattern.

Principle component analysis and singular value decomposition: Determine genes explaining the majority of the mathematical variance in the data set.[43–47]

Cluster determination: Determine groups of genes or samples with similar patterns of gene expression.

Nearest neighbor clustering: The number of clusters is decided first, the boundaries of the clusters are calculated, then each gene is assigned to a single cluster.[48]

Agglomerative clustering: Bottom-up method, where clusters start as empty, then genes are successively added to the existing clusters.

Dendrogram algorithm: Groups are defined as sub-trees in phylogenetic-type tree, created by comprehensively measuring a pairwise metric, such as the correlation coefficient.[46]

Two-dimensional dendrograms: Both genes and samples are clustered separately.

Divisive or partitional clustering: Top-down method, where large clusters are successively broken into smaller ones, until each subcluster contains only one gene.

Matrix incision tree[49]

Two-way clustering binary tree[50]

Coupled two-way clustering[51]

Cluster affinity search technique[52]

Gene shaving[53]

Network determination: Determine networks of gene-gene or gene-phenotype interactions

Bayesian networks[54]

Hybrid petri networks[55]

Boolean regulatory networks[56–60]

Relevance networks: Determine associations between features (genes, phenotypic measures, or samples).[2,61,62]

SUPERVISED LEARNING

Analysis to determine ways of accurately splitting into or predicting groups of samples or disease based on external (typically, expert-provided) labels.

Single feature or sample determination: Find genes or samples that match a particular a priori pattern.

Naive Bayes classifier[63,64]

Naive Bayes global relevance[65]

Multiple-feature determination: Find combinations of genes that match a particular a priori pattern.

Decision trees: Use the training set of genes or samples to construct a decision tree to help classify test samples or test genes; typically uses entropy as the classification measure.[66]

Support vector machines: First, take the set of measured genes, then create a richer feature set with combinations of genes, then find a hyperplane that linearly separates groups of samples in this larger multidimensional space.[64,67,68]

Tree harvesting[69]

Boosting[48]

ANNOTATION

Whether the analysis involves clustering or classification or a differential analysis, after all that effort, the net result is a list of accession numbers and expression values. The accession numbers refer to either a cDNA clone or a set of oligonucleotides in the case of the Affymetrix microarray platform. These cDNAs/oligonucleotides, in turn, correspond to a stretch of expressed sequence, which usually identifies a particular gene. The manufacturer of the clone sets or microarrays provide translation tables and software facilities to convert the accession numbers to gene names and locuslink IDs, and Gene IDs (Gene IDs are the durable unique names for genes that are maintained by the National Center for Biotechnology Information (NCBI) at *http://www.ncbi.nlm. nih.gov/entrez/query.fcgi?db=gene*).

Even after identifying the gene names and identifier numbers, most researchers would be nonplussed. This is a marked contrast to a typical endocrinology investigation in which most, if not all, of the analytes are well known and characterized. Because of the comprehensive nature of modern microarray technology, the entire transcriptome may be measured and, consequently, most of the genes and gene products measured will be unfamiliar to the endocrinologist, even though they clearly have some relevant activity in the experiment devised by the endocrinologist. In 2001 or earlier, the laborious part of any functional genomic experiment began with the determination of the biologic significance of the upregulation or downregulation of each of the particular genes in the specified aforementioned list. This typically required a search in PubMed (*http://www.ncbi.nlm. nih.gov*) to determine, from a review of the literature, the processes in which that gene was known to be involved. This formed the basis for a verbose argument of the biologic mechanism explaining why a particular gene coclustered with other genes. Fortunately, this challenge of gene annotation became widely recognized around the turn of the millennium and resulted in several efforts to generate compendia of gene annotations, some in the commercial sector and some in the public sector. Perhaps the single most successful such effort was led by Michael Ashburner.[70] The resulting compendium, called the Gene Ontology (or more commonly, simply GO), provides three kinds of annotations for genes, each organized in its own hierarchy, as follows:

1. A description of *molecular function*: This describes the biochemical activity of the entity, such as whether it is a transcriptional factor, a transporter, or an enzyme, without making any further commitments as to where the function occurs or whether the function occurs as part of a larger biochemical process.
2. The *cellular component* within which gene products are located: This provides a localization of a gene product's molecular function, such as the ribosome, the nucleosome, or the mitochondrion. Localization can help determine whether a purported function could occur through direct physical interaction between gene products or as a result of an indirect mechanism.
3. The *biologic process* implemented by the gene products: Biologic process refers to a higher-order process, such as pyrimidine metabolism, protein translation, or signal transduction.

A view of a portion of the third hierarchy, the process hierarchy, is shown in Figure 4-14.

A set of tools to browse this gene etiology is available at *http://geneontology.org*, which allows the investigator to determine at a glance the processes, biochemical function, and locations of every annotated gene. Further, as a matter of convenience, these tools allow entire lists of genes to be submitted en masse. Useful as such an annotation may be, it is misleading, as it can lead all too easily, yet again, to the aforementioned GSS. It is not that difficult to come up with a plausible but often incorrect biologic story to justify why this list of genes was generated or how this list of genes supports a particular hypothesis. One way that gene staring syndrome may lead investigators is through them having no sense of how likely it is that the gene annotations would have been generated by chance. For example, cell cycle, proteome synthesis, DNA synthesis, and other common cellular functions are highly represented as annotations in the gene ontology, due to their importance and complexity. Therefore, based on random chance alone, any set of genes would include large numbers of genes annotated with these functions. It was this realization that led to an understanding that what investigators were really asking for was what processes are remarkable or characteristic of the genes obtained in a particular list and, similarly, what is the biochemical function or cellular location by which they are characterized. One way to respond to this question is to ask how overrepresented is a particular annotation with respect to its frequency in its entire gene ontology. For example, an annotation such as cell cycle, which is of high frequency in the gene, would have to be a considerably larger fraction of the genes in the list compared to a much less frequent gene annotation such as angiogenesis. Again, at *http://geneontology.org* there are several relevant tools, such as DAVID (available from the National Institute of Allergy and Infectious Diseases [NIAID]) and Mappfinder (from the University of California at San Francisco).

CASE HISTORY: OVERCOMING THE TYRANNY OF DATA WITH KNOWLEDGE

For endocrinologists, perhaps one of the most disconcerting and dismaying aspects of early functional genomics was that it appeared to be wholly data driven and not at all knowledge driven. Solely by measuring gene expression comprehensively across the transcriptome and then applying rigorous statistical analysis, one could discover which gene was truly involved in any set of conditions. In that context, knowledge of pathways and a lifetime of experience in understanding how a particular endocrinologic system might operate did not appear to have significant value. This knowledge-free approach, and the not infrequent conceit on the part of computational experts that they could solve a number of biologic questions without a detailed knowledge of biology, was disconcerting. Of course, this was wrong, as was well illustrated by the following study.

Mootha and his colleagues[41] were interested in understanding what gene expression dysregulation exists in patients with type 2 diabetes, insulin resistance, or adult-onset diabetes mellitus. They obtained muscle samples from three groups of individuals, those with a normal excursion in their glucose

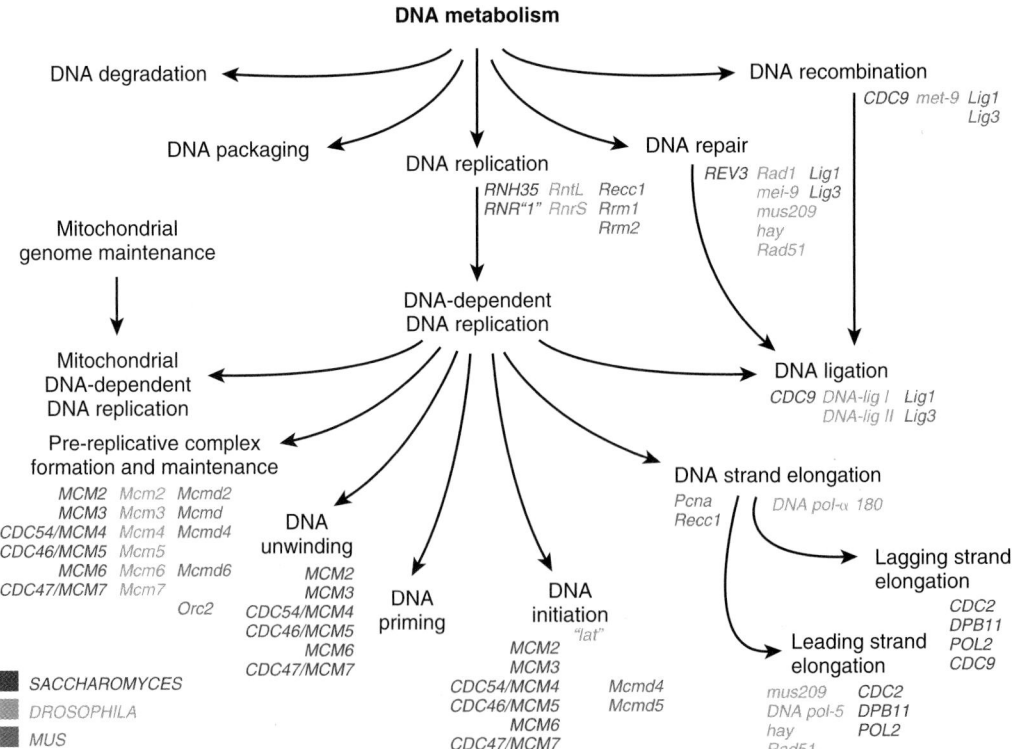

Figure 4-14 Sample process hierarchy from Gene Ontology (GO). (From Ashburner M, Ball CA, Blake JA, et al: Gene ontology: Tool for the unification of biology. The Gene Ontology Consortium. Nat Genet 25:25–29, 2000.)

levels after a standard oral load of glucose (NGT), those with impaired glucose tolerance (IGT) as measured by an increased rise in the glucose levels, and those with type 2 diabetes (DM2) who met the criteria of type 2 diabetes per the American Diabetes Association.

When a differential analysis was attempted using the SAM package previously mentioned in this chapter, the investigators were unable to find any genes that were significantly differentially expressed between NGT and IGT, between IGT and DM2, or, for that matter, between NGT and DM2. That is, if there were any genes that were differentially expressed, the changes were so subtle as to make them indistinguishable from the variation due to measurement error. It was at this juncture that a fundamental endocrinologic insight was invaluable. Although individual genes might not be differentially expressed in a statistically discernable fashion, an entire metabolic pathway might indeed be systematically perturbed in a pathophysiologic condition such as type 2 diabetes. Therefore, as a whole, the genes that function as members of this pathway would be distinguishable from the nonpathologic state. With this insight, the analysis became relatively straightforward. The list of genes measured by microarrays was sorted or ordered by the genes' differential expression across two conditions, such as between NGT and IGT. For example, at the top of the list was the gene that was most upregulated in IGT versus NGT and at the bottom of the list was the gene that was most downregulated in IGT versus NGT. For each pathway that the investigators were interested in (and therefore had previously compiled several lists of gene [gene sets], each corresponding to a different pathway, process, or group of genes of interest), the genes that were members of this pathway were highlighted or labeled on the sorted list of genes just described. It then had to be determined if the members of the pathway, heretofore referred to as the gene set, were distributed in a nonrandom fashion across the list of genes, that is, if all or part of that gene set grouped together anywhere along the spectrum of upregulation-downregulation of expression between the two conditions. At the risk of laboring the obvious, if all or part of the gene sets clumped together in any part of the order of the list of the entire genes measured by microarray, then this might be evidence of systematic perturbation of the pathway represented by that gene set in the investigated conditions, in this example, IGT or DM2.

To determine whether the observed clumpiness of the genes in a gene set was unusual or what one might expect from chance, the investigators permuted or scrambled the genes in the data set and determined how clumpy the gene set was in the permuted data. By repeating the permutation procedure 1000 times, they would obtain a quantitative estimate of how unlikely the observed clumpiness was to be due to chance. For example, if in only 9 out of 1000 permutations did the clumpiness of the gene set exceed that of the gene set against the original data, then the P value of 0.009 would be estimated. This procedure would then be done for all the gene sets under consideration and the gene set with the lowest P value for the data set would be posited to be the most likely pathway perturbed across the two conditions. There are several ways that clumpiness can be calculated. In this study, the investigators chose the Kolmagarov-Smirnoff (KS) test. The details of the KS test are not relevant here; the reader is welcome to read more about it in the article. In this instance, of the 149 gene sets that the investigators evaluated, the top scoring one was a set of genes involved in oxidative phosphorylation. This was intriguing in two ways. First of all, if the differential analysis was repeated as shown in Figure 4-15, but the genes known to be members of the oxidative phosphorylation gene set were highlighted, then we can see that, although none of the genes exceeded the boundaries of noisy variation across the two conditions, they do systematically show up on the lower side of the diagonal 45-degree line. That is, most of the genes are downregulated

even though, on average, they were downregulated by considerably less than twofold. This is a change in expression level, which typically is not reliably ascertainable on a single gene-by-gene basis. The second intriguing aspect of this investigation was that it supported and confirmed other investigations suggesting that the processes of oxidative phosphorylation were downregulated in type 2 diabetes and that, as the authors were able to investigate further, the transcriptional coactivator peroxisome-proliferator-activated receptor-γ co-activator alpha (PGC1-α) is an important determinant of the downregulation in this process. The overall gene set enrichment analysis procedure is diagrammed in Figure 4-16, but the central point can be succinctly stated in one sentence: Understanding how a process is regulated or the pathway involved in a process enables far more information to be extracted from genomic and proteomic experiments than does statistical analysis alone. This suggests that as the functional genomic and proteomic "revolutions" move forward, endocrine knowledge will become more and not less important in analyzing the data in a high-throughput genome-wide fashion.

CASE HISTORY: WHOLE-TRANSCRIPTOME VIEWS OF PATHOPHYSIOLOGY

Microarrays and proteomic tests are still used largely as a high-throughput method of measuring or comparing the expression of one gene at a time across several physiologic or pathologic conditions. The preceding case history, regarding the elaboration of the members of the oxidative phosphorylation pathway in type 2 diabetes, exemplifies how looking at a concerted pattern of a set of genes rather than individual gene measurements provides far more significant biologic insight. In the following case history, the value of entire global patterns of the expression is motivated. In particular, this case demonstrates the value of understanding system dynamics in exploring pathophysiology. The use of dynamics, particularly in provocative testing, is well known to endocrinologists, but the simultaneous examination of 10,000 or more variables over time is quite foreign to them. This example begins in the domain of cancer, but then extends to endocrinology to demonstrate the broad ramifications of comprehensive measurements of the transcriptome or proteome in the study and practice of endocrinology.

In 2002, Zhao and colleagues[71] reported on a microarray study of genes expressed in the developing cerebellum of the mouse. In this study, several genes coding for proteins potentially implicated in controlling the proliferation and differentiation of the cerebellum were identified. Among these were genes controlled by a secreted protein, sonic hedgehog (Shh). The relevance to human disease included the knowledge that the elements of the Shh pathway, such as the patched (ptch) gene product were involved in human malignancy, particularly medulloblastoma, the most common pediatric central nervous system tumor. Further, mouse models such as the ptch +/− heterozygote demonstrated, in about 20% of the mice, tumors resembling the histology of human medulloblastoma. For this reason, Kho and colleagues[72] noted a paper that appeared in *Nature* in 2002 by Pomeroy and colleagues[73] describing the gene expression profiles of human with medulloblastoma. Since the tissues that Pomeroy and colleagues studied were obtained from surgical biopsies of the cerebellum, it seemed that some form of comparison between the gene expression patterns of these cerebellar malignancies and the developing cerebellum would be of interest.

At this early stage in the functional genomic revolution, some of the techniques discussed here may not be part of the common currency of investigators, so they are spelled out in somewhat more detail than may be required in the near future. The first step was to determine which genes expressed in the human tumors are homologous to those in the mouse

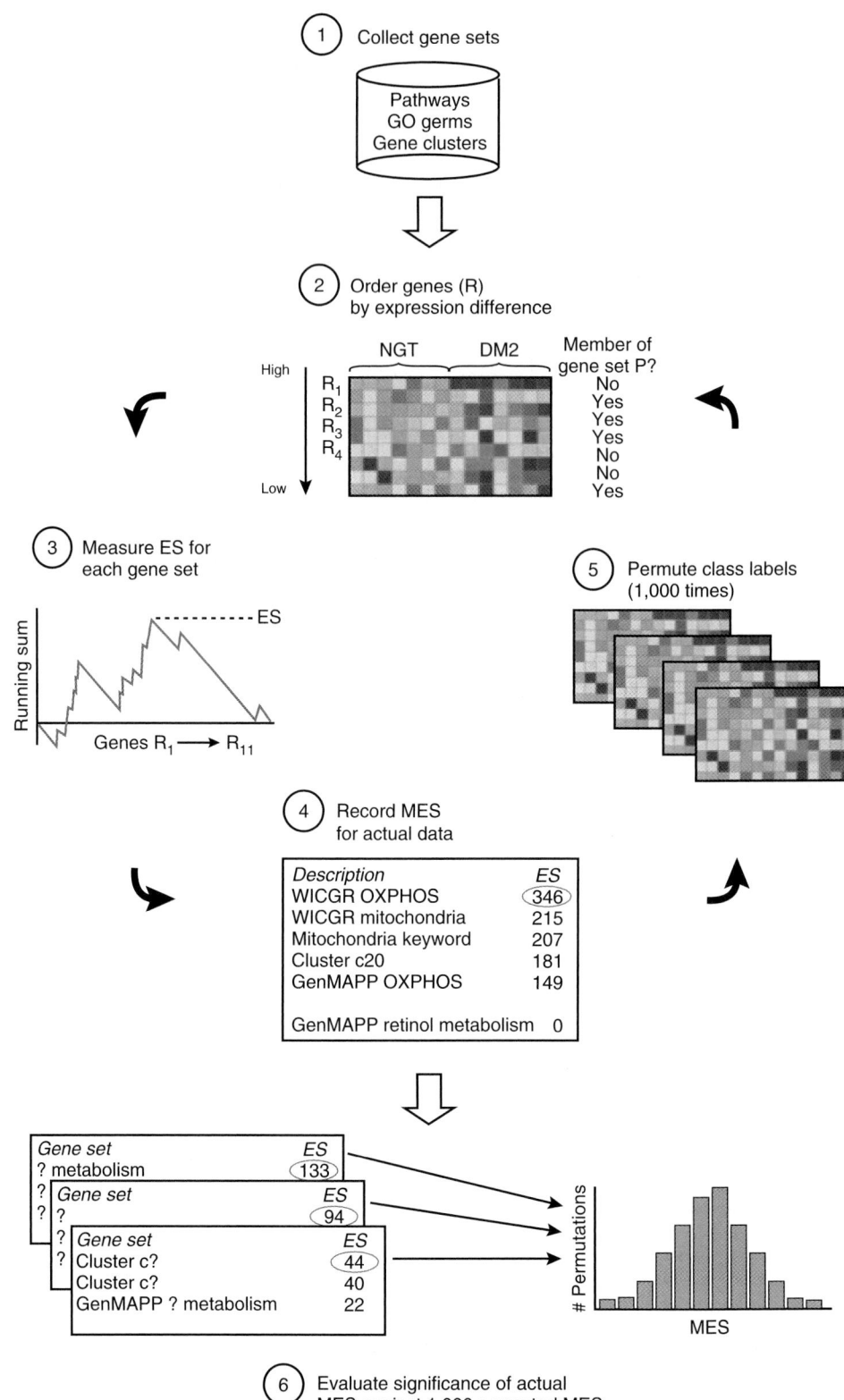

① Collect gene sets

Pathways
GO germs
Gene clusters

② Order genes (R)
by expression difference

	NGT	DM2	Member of gene set P?
High			
R₁			No
R₂			Yes
R₃			Yes
			Yes
R₄			No
			No
Low			Yes

③ Measure ES for each gene set

Running sum — ES
Genes $R_1 \longrightarrow R_{11}$

⑤ Permute class labels (1,000 times)

④ Record MES for actual data

Description	ES
WICGR OXPHOS	346
WICGR mitochondria	215
Mitochondria keyword	207
Cluster c20	181
GenMAPP OXPHOS	149
GenMAPP retinol metabolism	0

Gene set	ES
? metabolism	133

Gene set	ES
?	94

Gene set	ES
Cluster c?	44
Cluster c?	40
GenMAPP ? metabolism	22

Permutations
MES

⑥ Evaluate significance of actual MES against 1,000 permuted MES

Figure 4-15 Overall bias in the expression of genes involved in oxidative phosphorylation. (From Mootha VK, Lindgren CM, Eriksson KF, et al: PGC-1 alpha-responsive genes involved in oxidative phosphorylation are coordinately downregulated in human diabetes. Nat Genet 34:267–273, 2003.

models. Fortunately, the National Center for Biotechnology Information (NCBI) has maintained a resource called Homologene (available at *http://www.nlm.nih.gov*), which allows the determination of homologues across multiple species. As the mouse cerebellar expression measurements were performed on one Affymetrix platform (mu11k), and the human medulloblastoma measurements were made on another (HuFL), only a subset of those homologues could be studied: the homologues that are present on both microarray platforms. This constitutes a total of 2552 genes.

To obtain an overall view of the pattern of gene expression, the gene expression measurements across the multiple time-points of cerebellar development in the mouse were plotted along their two first principal components. Without burdening the reader with the details of principal component analysis, the nature of this analysis is to transform the data linearly so that a new set of axes are identified where the first axis captures the maximal variation of the data and the second axis is perpendicular (orthogonal) to the first and captures the second-most variance of the data. The third axis captures the

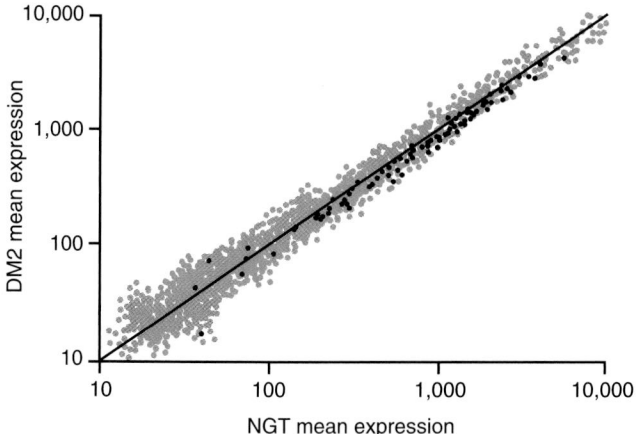

Figure 4-16 Overall gene set enrichment procedure.

third-most variance and is orthogonal to first two axes, and so on. This is illustrated in Figure 4-17B, where selected genes are show in their original axes (time course and expression value), and Figure 4-17A, where they are shown plotted on the first two principal component along with an egg-shaped cloud (called the "egg-gram") of dots, where each dot represents the coordinate of one of the mouse genes in the first two principal component axes.

Note that the first principal component, plotted along the X-axis, represents the dimension of maximal variation in the developmental time series, and the second component, the Y-axis, is the axis with the second-most variance. By plotting the time course of genes picked from the left side of the graph and genes from the right side of the graph, it can be quickly determined that the genes on the left correspond to genes that are upregulated early in cerebellar development

(cerebellar early mouse partition, or CEMP), whereas these on the right are upregulated late (cerebellar late mouse partition, or CLMP). This is illustrated in Figure 4-17B, where the time courses of sample genes from each of these two halves are plotted. Note that the left hand of the graph corresponds to the genes where the first principal component value is less than 0 and the genes on the right half are where the values of the first principal component are positive or greater than 0. This impression is further reinforced by graphs in Figure 4-17C and D, which show the time of maximal expression for the genes that had a first principal component value that was less than 0 and greater than 0, respectively. All that this analysis shows is that the first principal component captures the large variance in the transcriptome that occurs with development.

This analysis becomes a lot more interesting when one plots the homologues of the upregulated and downregulated human medulloblastoma genes onto the prior principal component analysis or "egg-gram." That is, the genes that are upregulated in medulloblastoma fall into the early period of mouse cerebellar development (CEMP) and, conversely, the genes that are downregulated in human medulloblastoma relative to normal human cerebellar samples fall into the late period of mouse cerebellar development (CLMP). In case this was not visually compelling, the odds ratio of this very biased segregation of upregulation and downregulation is 7.19, with a χ^2 of 62.59 and P value that is less than 0.0001.

Although it may be interesting that the upregulation and downregulation of human medulloblastoma genes cosegregates with the early and late development of the mouse cerebellum, does this pattern generalize to other tissues? Fortunately, it is the nature of the functional genomics culture that many data sets have been made publicly available, particularly through the NCBI's gene expression omnibus (GEO) database. One such data set is a mouse lung development data set and the other is a squamous-cell carcinoma data set, and exactly the same analysis as previously described

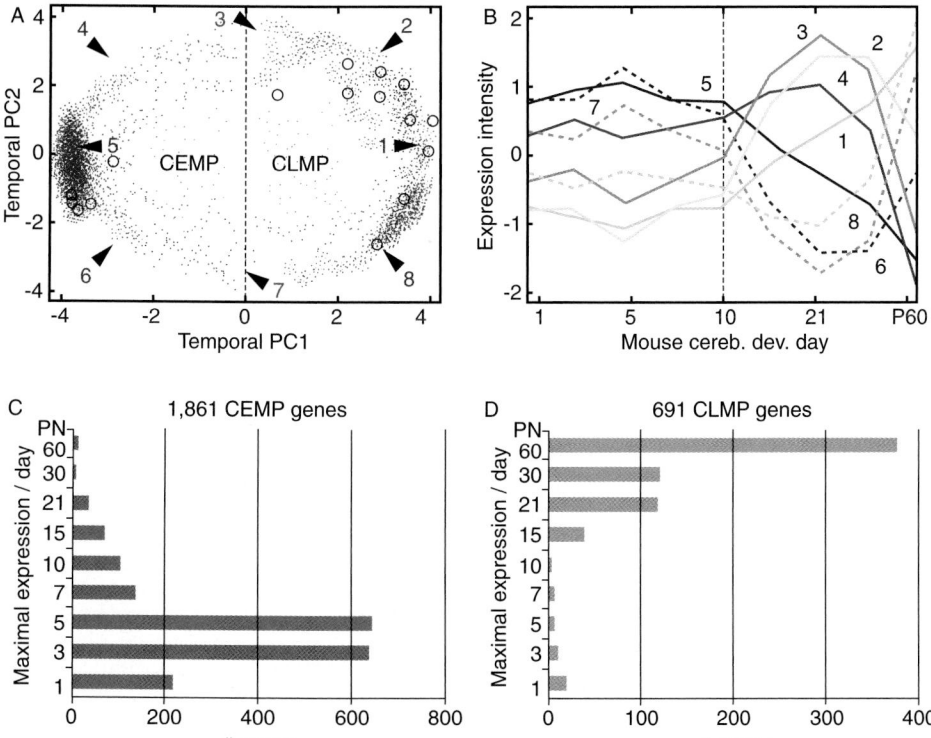

Figure 4-17 Principal component and time series analysis of mouse cerebellar expression in development.

can be performed, with the results shown in Figure 4-18. Figure 4-18 shows the projection of those genes in the human squamous-cell lung carcinoma line; those upregulated with respect to nonmalignant lung tissue are noted with X's on the left and those downregulated with triangles on the right. As before, the upregulated genes are overrepresented in the early phase of development and the downregulated genes in the carcinoma are in the late phase of development. This demonstrates that the functional pattern of upregulation of the tumor in regard to the early chronology of the development of the cognate tissue in the mouse model does hold in multiple tissues. Nevertheless, all that we might be seeing here is an elaborate way to mark cell proliferation and, therefore, to demonstrate that this is not the case. In Figure 4-19A, the mouse developmental lung times series is shown and, instead of mapping the genes upregulated and downregulated in human squamous-cell lung carcinoma, the genes upregulated and downregulated in human medulloblastoma are plotted. Conversely, in Figure 4-19B, the upregulated and downregulated genes of human squamous-cell lung carcinoma are projected against a background of mouse cerebellum. In this case, the segregation is no longer statistically significant. That is, there is not a systematic bias of upregulated and downregulated genes in the human tumors to the early and late phases of mouse development, respectively, and, therefore, the previously noted phenomenon is a cognate tissue-specific sign of a developmental program.

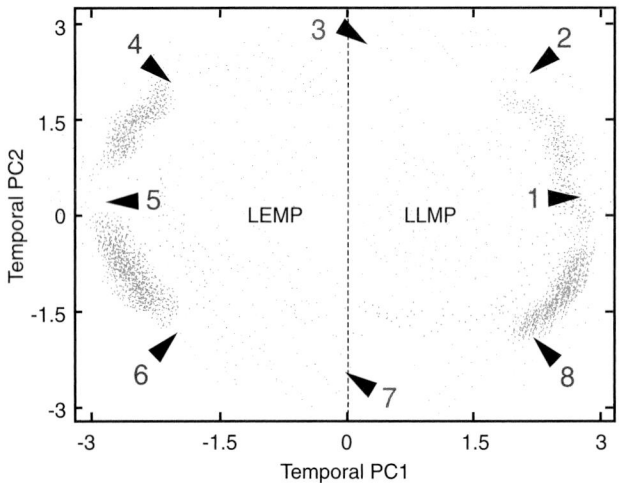

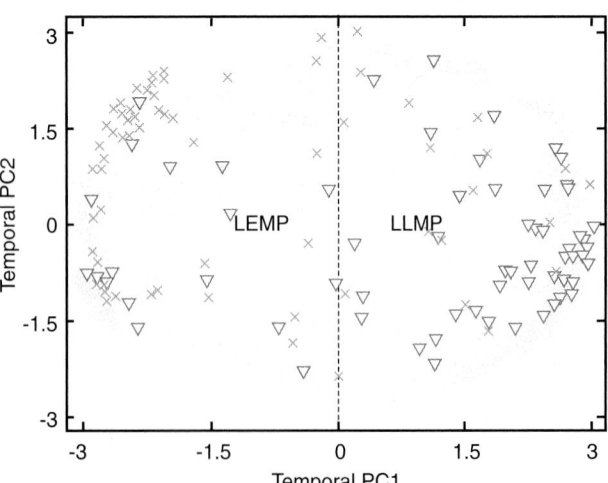

Figure 4-18 Lung cancer mapped onto the developing mouse lung.

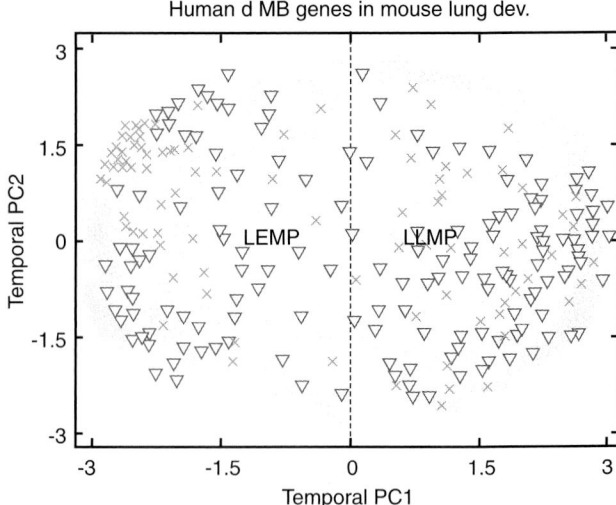

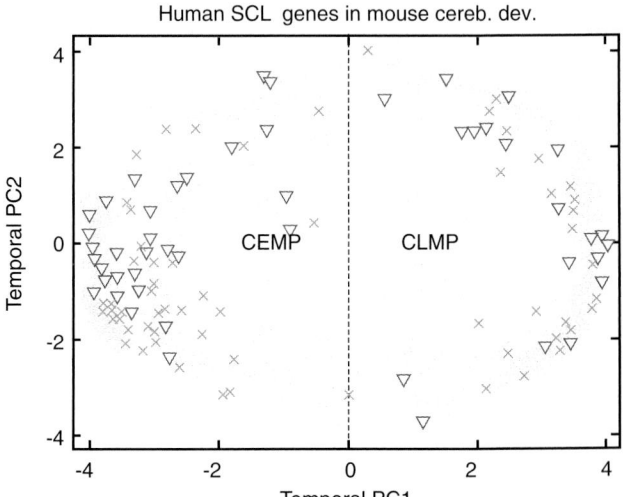

Figure 4-19 Projecting human cancer genes onto noncognate tissues.

So far, the analysis has been looking at the data from the perspective of the genes. If we now look at the principal components in terms of the samples themselves, then we get an analysis shown in Figure 4-20. In Figure 4-20A, mouse developmental samples are shown as circles and the human samples as X's. Figure 4-20B shows the day of mouse cerebellar development to which these various human tumor samples are most similar. This figure shows that the medulloblastoma samples resemble the early developmental phase of the mouse and the normal human sample resembles the later development and, most interestingly, the metastatic tumors are the closet to day 5 of the mouse development.

This analysis demonstrates several items of importance, first in the context of oncology and then for endocrinology. This analysis revisits an old idea with the quantitation and the precision of the genomic era. Lobstein in 1829 and Cohnheim in 1887[74] were amongst the first to theorize the similarities between human embryogenesis and the biology of tumor cancer cells. Indeed, the brain tumor classification system of Bailey and Cushing articulated in 1926,[75] from which all the modern taxonomies of central nervous system malignancy derive, emphasizes the histologic resemblance to cells of the developing central nervous system. In that sense, the foregoing analysis only adds precision and quantitation to an old idea. In doing so, however, it performs several functions. It allows greater precision in diagnostic staging and it also provides insight (and poses additional questions) into the

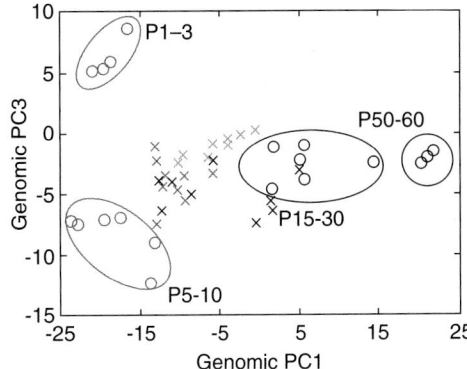 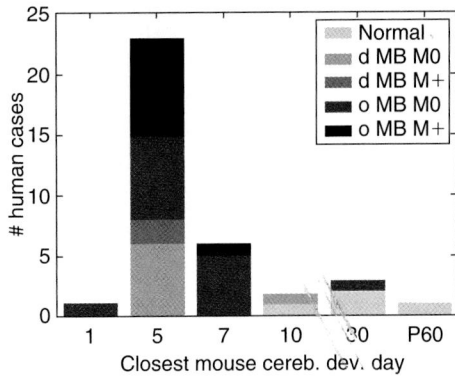

Figure 4-20 Human samples and mouse samples in principal component space.

biologic processes that may characterize tumors. For example, as noted, the metastatic human medulloblastoma samples most resemble day 5 of mouse cerebellar development, approximately the time of maximal cellular migration in the mouse cerebellum. This then poses the question: Which set of genes are most responsible for the metastatic samples resembling day 5 of development and do they have known or potential roles in cellular motility? By contrast, the large B-cell lymphoma study by Alizadeh and colleagues,[1] provided as motivation at the beginning of this chapter, was based on a purely computational clustering of gene expression profiles, and two subsequent studies of lymphoma developed quite different lists of prognostic genes.[76,77] By using the developmental framework as a means of grading the biology of these cancers, this kind of functional genomic analysis may provide a more robust biologic underpinning to the eventual prognoses than a purely statistical analysis.

From an endocrinologic perspective, there are several immediately relevant classes of investigations that can benefit from the whole-transcriptome, multivariate style of analysis (as opposed to the classical single gene or oligogenic styles of analysis):

- Most obviously, several endocrinologic pathophysiologic processes can be evaluated for a developmental component. Just as was done in this example for cancer vis-à-vis development in a murine model, the corresponding analysis can be done for bone disease and bone development, for example. Several public data sets are available to allow investigators to explore the potential yield of such experiments in silico before attempting their own "wet" experimentation. More generally, this kind of analysis can be performed for any endocrinologic process to determine how a particular disease state (e.g., type 1 diabetes) relates to a dynamic process (e.g., islet cell development).

- The appropriateness of various mouse models for human diseases can be evaluated in this kind of framework so that, for example, adipose tissue of different mouse models of obesity can be plotted in the same multivariate space as the gene expression profile of human adipose tissue samples. This would allow a quantitative determination of which of these mouse models are more reflective of the pathophysiology at the whole transcriptome level of obesity in humans. This may avoid the problems of mouse models that appear to be phenocopies of human disease, but in which the underlying cellular molecular pathophysiology is not as close as some other mouse models might be to that human disease.

- Finally, the prior analysis can be used to take well-known pathways such as the hypothalamic-pituitary-adrenal axis and examine all the genes involved in this well-established hormonal axis in a variety of systems. For example, as shown in an enlargement of the detail of the proceeding cerebellar expression of the mouse cerebellar expression time series (Fig. 4-21), several of these well-known "endocrine" genes are significantly expressed in a controlled manner in this organ system.

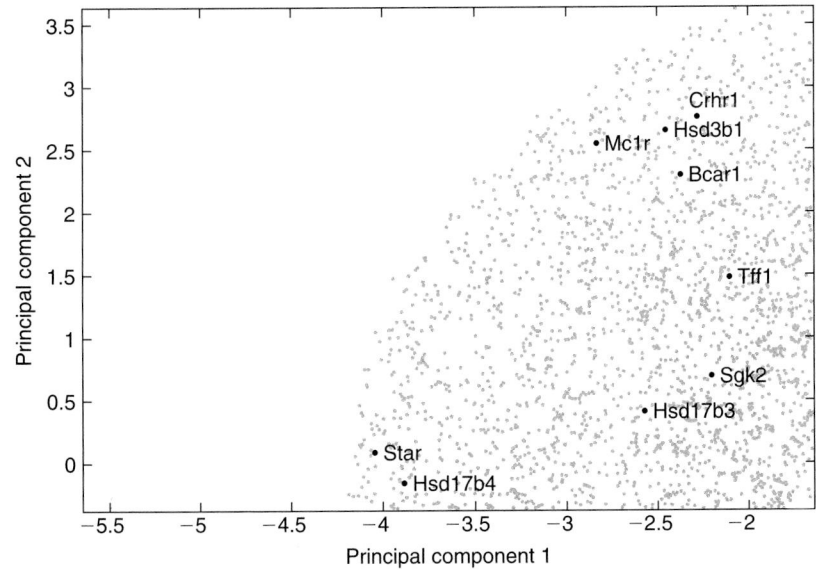

Figure 4-21 Genes of the hypothalamic-pituitary-adrenal (HPA) axis expressed during cerebellar development.

The last point is perhaps the most important consequence of the genomic and proteomic revolution. Increasingly, through the comprehensive measurements of all genes at the protein and RNA level in multiple tissues, we can anticipate that many genes previously thought to be essentially and only involved in our classical hormonal internal organ communication networks are in fact also critical components of multiple intracellular processes. Indeed, casual perusal of the Gene Expression Omnibus at the NCBI (which all readers should do at least once) will reveal that: (1) the latest generation of microarrays measure all the known "endocrine" genes, and (2) these endocrine genes are expressed at significant levels in a regulated fashion across multiple tissues and diseases not classically thought to be relevant to endocrinology. Perhaps this is not surprising; the classical endocrine formulation has already expanded to include paracrine and autocrine effects of signaling molecules. It is in this perspective that genomics and proteomics are likely to broaden considerably the range of biologic processes covered by the endocrine discipline. In turn, this will require the education of endocrinology to have a more expansive embrace over the molecular sciences as well as the computational ones. Although this is a daunting challenge, endocrine training programs have already shown themselves to be leaders in these two areas.

ENDOCRINE PROTEOMIC AND GENOMICS CHALLENGES FOR THE NEAR FUTURE

In conclusion, it should be clear from this chapter that endocrinology is only now beginning to leverage the massively parallel data measurements of the genomic and proteomic era. As a community, we have not yet created the framework that will enable us to generalize our hard-won understanding of the pathophysiologic regulation of control through signaling molecules in this new era. In this spirit, the following goals are left as a challenge to a new generation of investigational endocrinologists:

1. Multiorgan tracking of metabolic disease: Simultaneous and comprehensive measurements of RNA and protein expression in multiple tissues to provide the intellectual and data substrate for an integrative view of metabolic disease.
2. Unification of linkage studies with expression and proteomics: Expression and proteomic studies are only beginning[78] to be mined for their import to clarify some long-standing linkage peaks for a variety of endocrine diseases.
3. Measurement of the dynamics posttranslational "omics": Glycosylation and phosphorylation. So much of endocrinology is depending on posttranslational modifications of proteins and specific localizations of these proteins within cells that, until we can comprehensively and accurately measure the changes in posttranslational modification and translocation, our ability to adequately model whole-cell endocrinology will be significantly limited.
4. Whole-animal protein and gene tracking using noninvasive imaging: Measurements of the genome and proteome by extracting tissue and then processing the tissue to obtain proteins and RNA are fundamentally limiting in allowing the study of the dynamics in vivo of endocrine regulation. Imaging techniques that allow multiple RNAs and/or proteins to be measured in a whole living animal are only now being developed,[79,80] but are likely to become important tools for dynamic endocrine testing in model organisms within the decade.

REFERENCES

1. Alizadeh AA, Eisen MB, Davis RE, et al: Distinct types of diffuse large B-cell lymphoma identified by gene expression profiling. Nature 403:503–511, 2000.
2. Butte AJ, Tamayo P, Slonim D, et al: Discovering functional relationships between RNA expression and chemotherapeutic susceptibility using relevance networks [in process citation]. Proc Natl Acad Sci U S A 97:12182–12186, 2000.
3. Spellman PT, Sherlock G, Zhang MQ, et al: Comprehensive identification of cell cycle-regulated genes of the yeast Saccharomyces cerevisiae by microarray hybridization. Mol Biol Cell 9:3273–3297, 1998.
4. Iyer VR, Eisen MB, Ross DT, et al: The transcriptional program in the response of human fibroblasts to serum [see comments]. Science 283:83–87, 1999.
5. Anonymous: The chip challenge. Nat Genet 21:61–62, 1999.
6. Schena M, Shalon D, Davis RW, Brown PO: Quantitative monitoring of gene expression patterns with a complementary DNA microarray. Science 270:467–470, 1995.
7. Luo L, Salunga RC, Guo H, et al: Gene expression profiles of laser-captured adjacent neuronal subtypes. Nat Med 5:117–122, 1999.
8. Brown PO, Botstein D: Exploring the new world of the genome with DNA microarrays. Nat Genet 21(Suppl 1):33–37, 1999.
9. Kerr M, Martin M, Churchill G: Analysis of variance for gene expression microarray data. J Comput Biol 7:819–837, 2000.
10. Fodor SP, Read JL, Pirrung MC, et al: Light-directed, spatially addressable parallel chemical synthesis. Science 251:767–773, 1991.
11. Rajagopalan D: A comparison of statistical methods for analysis of high density oligonucleotide array data. Bioinformatics 19:1469–1476, 2003.
12. Lemon WJ, Liyanarachchi S, You M: A high performance test of differential gene expression for oligonucleotide arrays. Genome Biol 4:R67, 2003.
13. Hubbell E, Liu WM, Mei R: Robust estimators for expression analysis. Bioinformatics 18:1585–1592, 2002.
14. Hoaglin DC, Mosteller F, Tukey JW: Understanding Robust and Exploratory Data Analysis. New York, John Wiley & Sons, 2000.
15. Oda Y, Nagasu T, Chait BT: Enrichment analysis of phosphorylated proteins as a tool for probing the phosphoproteome. Nat Biotechnol 19:379–382, 2001.
16. Li S, Armstrong CM, Bertin N, et al: A map of the interactome network of the metazoan C. elegans. Science 303:540–543, 2004.
17. Anderson NG, Matheson A, Anderson NL: Back to the future: The human protein index (HPI) and the agenda for post-proteomic biology. Proteomics 1:3–12, 2001.
18. Gygi SP, Rist B, Aebersold R: Measuring gene expression by quantitative proteome analysis. Curr Opin Biotechnol 11:396–401, 2000.
19. Perkins DN, Pappin DJ, Creasy DM, Cottrell JS: Probability-based protein identification by searching sequence databases using mass spectrometry data. Electrophoresis 20:3551–3567, 1999.
20. Yates JR III: Mass spectrometry and the age of the proteome. J Mass Spectrom 33:1–19, 1998.
21. Michalet S, Favreau P, Stocklin R: Profiling and in vivo quantification of proteins by high resolution mass spectrometry: The example of goserelin, an analogue of luteinizing hormone-releasing hormone. Clin Chem Lab Med 41:1589–1598, 2003.
22. Medzihradszky KF, Campbell JM, Baldwin MA, et al: The characteristics of peptide collision-induced dissociation using a high-performance MALDI-TOF/TOF tandem mass spectrometer. Anal Chem 72:552–558, 2000.
23. Merchant M, Weinberger SR: Recent advancements in surface-enhanced laser desorption/ionization-time of flight-mass spectrometry. Electrophoresis 21:1164–1177, 2000.
24. Seibert V, Wiesner A, Buschmann T, Meuer J: Surface-enhanced laser

desorption ionization time-of-flight mass spectrometry (SELDI TOF-MS) and ProteinChip technology in proteomics research. Pathol Res Pract 200:83–94, 2004.

25. Zhou H, Ranish JA, Watts JD, Aebersold R: Quantitative proteome analysis by solid-phase isotope tagging and mass spectrometry. Nat Biotechnol 19:512, 2002.

26. Petricoin EF, Ardekani AM, Hitt BA, et al: Use of proteomic patterns in serum to identify ovarian cancer. Lancet 359:572–577, 2002.

27. Sorace JM, Zhan M: A data review and re-assessment of ovarian cancer serum proteomic profiling. BMC Bioinformatics 4:24, 2003.

28. Diamandis EP: Analysis of serum proteomic patterns for early cancer diagnosis: Drawing attention to potential problems. J Natl Cancer Inst 96:353–356, 2004.

29. Diamandis EP: OvaCheck: Doubts voiced soon after publication. Nature 430:611, 2004.

30. Belanger C, Hennekens C, Rosner B, Speizer F: The Nurses' Health Study. Am J Nurs 78:1039–1040, 1978.

31. Dawber T, Meadors G, Moore F: The Framingham Study: Epidemiological approaches to heart disease. Am J Public Health 41:279–286, 1951.

32. Speed TP: Statistical Analysis of Gene Expression Microarray Data. Boca Raton, FL, Chapman & Hall/CRC, 2003.

33. Kohane IS, Kho AT, Butte AJ: Microarrays for an Integrative Genomics. Cambridge, MA, MIT Press, 2003.

34. Kauhanen H, Komi PV, Hakkinen K: Standardization and validation of the body weight adjustment regression equations in Olympic weightlifting. J Strength Cond Res 16:58–74, 2002.

35. Unami A, Shinohara Y, Kajimoto K, Baba Y: Comparison of gene expression profiles between white and brown adipose tissues of rat by microarray analysis. Biochem Pharmacol 67:555–564, 2004.

36. Sreekumar R, Halvatsiotis P, Schimke JC, Nair KS: Gene expression profile in skeletal muscle of type 2 diabetes and the effect of insulin treatment. Diabetes 51:1913–1920, 2002.

37. Moraes RC, Blondet A, Birkenkamp-Demtroeder K, et al: Study of the alteration of gene expression in adipose tissue of diet-induced obese mice by microarray and reverse transcription-polymerase chain reaction analyses. Endocrinology 144:4773–4782, 2003.

38. Dræghici S: Data Analysis Tools for DNA Microarrays. Boca Raton, FL, Chapman & Hall/CRC, 2003.

39. Hochberg Y, Benjamini Y: Controlling the false discovery rate: A practical and powerful approach to multiple testing. J R Stat Soc 57:289–300, 1995.

40. Tusher VG, Tibshirani R, Chu G: Significance analysis of microarrays applied to the ionizing radiation response. Proc Natl Acad Sci U S A 98:5116–5121, 2001.

41. Mootha VK, Lindgren CM, Eriksson KF, et al: PGC-1alpha-responsive genes involved in oxidative phosphorylation are coordinately downregulated in human diabetes. Nat Genet 34:267–273, 2003.

42. Weiss SM, Indurkhya N: Predictive Data Mining: A Practical Guide. San Francisco, Morgan Kaufmann, 1997.

43. Raychaudhuri S, Stuart JM, Altman RB: Principal components analysis to summarize microarray experiments: Application to sporulation time series. Pac Symp Biocomput 455–466, 2000.

44. Alter O, Brown PO, Botstein D: Singular value decomposition for genome-wide expression data processing and modeling. Proc Natl Acad Sci U S A 97:10101–10106, 2000.

45. Hilsenbeck SG, Friedrichs WE, Schiff R, et al: Statistical analysis of array expression data as applied to the problem of tamoxifen resistance. J Natl Cancer Inst 91:453–459, 1999.

46. Wen X, Fuhrman S, Michaels GS, et al: Large-scale temporal gene expression mapping of central nervous system development. Proc Natl Acad Sci U S A 95:334–339, 1998.

47. Fiehn O, Kopka J, Dormann P, et al: Metabolite profiling for plant functional genomics. Nat Biotechnol 18:1157–1161, 2000.

48. Ben-Dor A, Bruhn L, Friedman N, et al: Tissue classification with gene expression profiles. J Comput Biol 7:559–583, 2000.

49. Kim JH, Ohno-Machado L, Kohane IS: Unsupervised learning from complex data: The matrix incision tree algorithm. Pac Symp Biocomput 30–41, 2001.

50. Alon U, Barkai N, Notterman DA, et al: Broad patterns of gene expression revealed by clustering analysis of tumor and normal colon tissues probed by oligonucleotide arrays. Proc Natl Acad Sci U S A 96:6745–6750, 1999.

51. Getz G, Levine E, Domany E: Coupled two-way clustering analysis of gene microarray data. Proc Natl Acad Sci U S A 97:12079–12084, 2000.

52. Ben-Dor A, Shamir R, Yakhini Z: Clustering gene expression patterns. J Comput Biol 6:281–297, 1999.

53. Hastie T, Tibshirani R, Eisen MB, et al: "Gene shaving" as a method for identifying distinct sets of genes with similar expression patterns. Genome Biol 1:RESEARCH0003, 2000.

54. Friedman N, Linial M, Nachman I, Pe'er D: Using Bayesian networks to analyze expression data. J Comput Biol 7:601–620, 2000.

55. Matsuno H, Doi A, Nagasaki M, Miyano S: Hybrid Petri net representation of gene regulatory network. Pac Symp Biocomput 341–352, 2000.

56. Liang S, Fuhrman S, Somogyi R: Reveal, a general reverse engineering algorithm for inference of genetic network architectures. Pac Symp Biocomput 18–29, 1998.

57. Wuensche A: Genomic regulation modeled as a network with basins of attraction. Pac Symp Biocomput 89–102, 1998.

58. Szallasi Z, Liang S: Modeling the normal and neoplastic cell cycle with "realistic Boolean genetic networks": Their application for understanding carcinogenesis and assessing therapeutic strategies. Pac Symp Biocomput 66–76, 1998.

59. Akutsu T, Miyano S, Kuhara S: Algorithms for identifying Boolean networks and related biologic networks based on matrix multiplication and fingerprint function. J Comput Biol 7:331–343, 2000.

60. Akutsu T, Miyano S, Kuhara S: Inferring qualitative relations in genetic networks and metabolic pathways. Bioinformatics 16:727–734, 2000.

61. Butte A, Kohane I: Mutual information relevance networks: Functional genomic clustering using pairwise entropy measurements. Pac Symp Biocom 418–429, 2000.

62. Butte A, Kohane IS: Unsupervised knowledge discovery in medical databases using relevance networks. Annu Symp Proc 711–715, 1999.

63. Ben-Dor A, Friedman N, Yakhini Z: Tissue classification with gene expression profiles. ACM 31–38, 1999.

64. Chow ML, Moler EJ, Mian IS: Identifying marker genes in transcription profiling data using a mixture of feature relevance experts. Physiol Genomics 5:99–111, 2001.

65. Moler EJ, Radisky DC, Mian IS: Integrating naive Bayes models and external knowledge to examine copper and iron homeostasis in S. cerevisiae. Physiol Genomics 4:127–135, 2000.

66. Dietterich TG: Approximate statistical tests for comparing supervised classification learning algorithms. Neural Comput 10:1895–1923, 1998.

67. Furey TS, Cristianini N, Duffy N, et al: Support vector machine classification and validation of cancer tissue samples using microarray expression data. Bioinformatics 16:906–914, 2000.

68. Brown MP, Grundy WN, Lin D, et al: Knowledge-based analysis of microarray gene expression data by using support vector machines. Proc Natl Acad Sci U S A 97:262–267, 2000.

69. Hastie T, Tibshirani R, Botstein D, Brown P: Supervised harvesting of expression trees. Genome Biol 2:RESEARCH0003, 2001.

70. Ashburner M, Ball CA, Blake JA, et al: Gene ontology: Tool for the unification of biology. The Gene Ontology Consortium. Nat Genet 25:25–29, 2000.

71. Zhao Q, Kho A, Kenney AM, et al: Identification of genes expressed with temporal-spatial restriction to developing cerebellar neuron precursors by a functional genomic approach. Proc Natl Acad Sci U S A 99:5704–5709, 2002.

72. Kho AT, Zhao Q, Cai Z, et al: Conserved mechanisms across development and tumorigenesis revealed by a mouse development perspective of human cancers. Genes Dev 18:629–640, 2004.

73. Pomeroy SL, Tamayo P, Gaasenbeek M, et al: Prediction of central nervous system embryonal tumour outcome based on gene expression. Nature 415:436–442, 2002.

74. Rather J: The Genesis of Cancer: A Study in the History of Ideas. Baltimore, Johns Hopkins University Press, 1978.

75. Bailey P, Cushing H: Classification of the Tumors of the Glioma Group on Histogenetic Basis with a Correlated Study of Prognosis. Philadelphia, Lippincott, 1926.

76. Shipp MA, Ross KN, Tamayo P, et al: Diffuse large B-cell lymphoma outcome prediction by gene-expression profiling and supervised machine learning. Nat Med 8:68–74, 2002.

77. Rosenwald A, Wright G, Chan WC, et al: The use of molecular profiling to predict survival after chemotherapy for diffuse large-B-cell lymphoma. N Engl J Med 346:1937–1947, 2002.

78. Mootha VK, Lepage P, Miller K, et al: Identification of a gene causing human cytochrome c oxidase deficiency by integrative genomics. Proc Natl Acad Sci U S A 100:605–610, 2003.

79. Wu JC, Chen IY, Wang Y, et al: Molecular imaging of the kinetics of vascular endothelial growth factor gene expression in ischemic myocardium. Circulation 110:685–691, 2004.

80. Ponomarev V, Doubrovin M, Serganova I, et al: A novel triple-modality reporter gene for whole-body fluorescent, bioluminescent, and nuclear noninvasive imaging. Eur J Nucl Med Mol Imaging 31:740–751, 2004.

Transgenic and Genetic Animal Models

Ruth A. Keri

INTRODUCTION

In the early 1900s, Clarence Cook Little began the first genetic studies on the inheritance of coat color in mice. With his development of the first inbred strain of mice (DBA),[1] Little became convinced that genetic experiments in mice would lead to novel insights regarding the basis of human development and disease. Indeed, as more inbred strains of mice were developed, it became clear that individual strains had differing susceptibilities to a number of diseases that had human counterparts, such as cancer, infertility, obesity, and growth insufficiency, to name a few. These experiments constituted the first genetic manipulations of a species that would become the mammalian model of choice for many human diseases. In addition to the decided advantage of our knowledge of mouse genetics that stemmed from these early studies, the small size and short generation time of mice have made them an indispensable research model for mammalian biology.

While selective breeding gave rise to several diverse mouse models of human disease, the advent of recombinant DNA technology, married with murine embryology, led to the first gene-specific alterations in the mouse genome in the early 1980s.[2-6] This was the dawn of transgenic mouse technology. Fueled by the rapid pace of sequencing of the human and mouse genomes, the use of this technology has become widespread, spanning all areas of mammalian biology. In this chapter, the two main approaches for manipulating the mouse genome are discussed. While both involve insertion of novel DNA sequences into the genome, the first approach relies on random integration of DNA fragments, while the second involves homologous recombination of new fragments with regions of the endogenous genome.

RANDOM INTEGRATION OF FOREIGN DNA INTO THE MOUSE GENOME

The first gene-specific manipulations of the mouse genome involved random insertion of heterologous sequences, or transgenes, into the genome.[2] Following the first proof-of-principle studies demonstrating that these heterologous sequences could be stably integrated into the genome and were heritable,[4,7-9] focus quickly shifted toward restricting expression of foreign genes to specific target organs or cell types.[3,5,6,9] This foreign DNA can take many forms; however, all transgenic mice that are made with this approach have one thing in common: Their goal is to express a specific protein in a selective set of cells. This can involve expression of an innocuous reporter gene, overexpression or misexpression of an endogenous protein, expression of a mutant protein, or expression of an inherently toxic protein. The general principles for producing and analyzing transgenic mice with randomly inserted transgenes will be discussed, followed by specific experimental paradigms that utilize this technology.

GENERAL PRINCIPLES

Transgene Construction

Transgene composition is driven by desired function. Three main components are required (Fig. 5-1A). These include the promoter, the gene to be expressed in the mice, and a polyadenylation signal sequence. Since transgenes become integrated into the germ line of mice, they are incorporated into all cells of subsequent progeny. To confer expression to a subset of cells within the organism, cell-specific promoters are typically utilized (see Chapter 2 for a discussion of eukaryotic promoters). These promoters are linked to the 5′ end of an expression cassette that contains the coding sequence for the gene of interest fused to a eukaryotic polyadenylation signal sequence. The polyadenylation signal can be the cognate sequence from the core gene, or it can be obtained from heterologous genes such as bovine growth hormone. The choice is usually governed by whether the cloned source of the structural gene contains a resident polyadenylation site. Transgenes are also frequently engineered to contain introns of either the gene to be expressed or introns from heterologous genes such as the SV40 small T antigen gene or the β-globin gene. The global importance of including an intron into the transgene cassette requires further study. While several investigators have shown that the presence of an intron generally facilitated transgene expression, all of these studies utilized a limited number of transgenes,[10-15] making global conclusions about their importance difficult. However, as a result of these studies, most transgene constructs designed today include either an intrinsic or heterologous intron.

Pronuclear Injection and Founder Animals

Once a transgene has been produced using molecular biology techniques, it must be inserted into the mouse genome. Random insertion of DNA into mice typically involves the use of pronuclear microinjection of transgene cassettes (Fig. 5-1B). Young female mice are superovulated and mated. Prior to the fusion of the male and female pronuclei, the fertilized oocytes

A

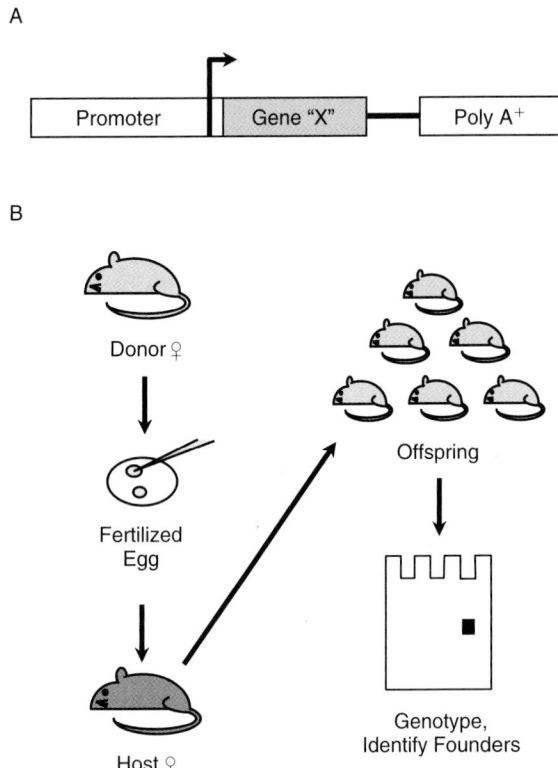

B

Donor ♀

Fertilized Egg

Host ♀

Offspring

Genotype, Identify Founders

Figure 5-1 Construction of transgenic mice by pronuclear injection. **A,** Transgenes typically have the following features: a promoter that directs expression of a gene with appropriate temporal and spatial patterning, that is, the coding sequence of the transgene should be expressed in the correct tissues within the desired developmental time frame; a coding sequence that can encode a physiologically relevant protein or a reporter protein (Gene "X"); and a polyadenylation sequence (Poly A+). High-level expression can be facilitated by the inclusion of an intron (thin line). **B,** Fertilized oocytes are collected from superovulated female mice. The male pronucleus of these embryos is injected with DNA. The embryos are placed back into a recipient, pseudopregnant female. Progeny are then screened for presence or absence of the transgene.

are collected. Small volumes of a dilute DNA solution are injected into the male pronucleus with the expectation that some of the introduced DNA molecules will randomly integrate into the genome of the subsequent embryo. The injected oocytes are returned to a pseudopregnant female mouse that is obtained by mating with a vasectomized male. Pseudopregnant females are required because the uterus must be hormonally primed to receive and nourish the growing embryo. Depending on the strain, mouse pups are typically born 19 to 20 days following introduction of the manipulated embryos into the pseudopregnant recipient mother.

Pups that are born after embryo transfer are genotyped to determine which animals have the transgene stably integrated into their genome. Depending on the skill of the microinjector and the quality of the source transgene DNA, 10% to 30% of the offspring will be transgenic. Each transgenic pup is the result of an independent integration event of the transgene DNA into the genome. The transgenic offspring are termed *founder* animals because each houses a distinct integration site that can be utilized to generate a unique line of mice. If the DNA causes an embryonically lethal phenotype, significantly fewer that 10% of the offspring will be transgenic. For example, expression of a proapoptotic protein within the two cell embryo may actually kill that embryo. As a result, no transgenic mice would be born.

Integration of the DNA into the genome of the embryo is a relatively rare event; therefore, most animals will harbor the

transgene at a single site within the genome. Transgenes typically integrate in tandem arrays ranging from one to a few hundred copies of the transgene.[16] If integration of the transgene occurred before the first cell division, the resulting transgenic mouse will have a uniform genetic composition in all cells. If, on the other hand, integration occurred after the first cell division, a mosaic mouse will result. Depending on the lineage of the cells that incorporated the DNA, the mouse might or might not have the transgene in the specific cells of interest. Mosaic mice can represent up to 30% of the transgenic progeny obtained from any one set of microinjections (personal observations). Thus, while the founder mice can be used experimentally, a large number of animals are necessary to rule out experimental outcomes that may simply be due to mosaicism. More typically, transgenic lines of mice are developed from the founder animals. This involves breeding the transgenic founders and analyzing their progeny. In contrast to the founder mice, all cells within the progeny will be genetically uniform.

Genotyping and Pedigree Analyses

Once offspring are obtained from transgenic founder mice, they are genotyped by either PCR or Southern blotting. Pedigree analyses can then be performed (Fig. 5-2). If the transgene DNA integrated into one position within the genome and this event occurred prior to the first cell division, inheritance of the transgene should follow a Mendelian pattern for a single, dominant, hemiallele. In particular, approximately 50% of the progeny from the transgenic founder should also be transgenic.[17] In contrast, if integration occurred later in the development of the embryo, the transgene may only contribute to a small portion of the germ line. If so, significantly less that the expected 50% of the progeny will be transgenic. Lastly, in some cases, transgenes can integrate into multiple sites within the genome of an individual embryo. If so, considerably more than 50% of the progeny will be transgenic. In this case, offspring from this founder represent multiple lines of mice. These multiple lines can be separated by breeding and segregating progeny according to integration site. Once progeny with one integration site are identified, these can subsequently be bred to produce individual lines of mice.

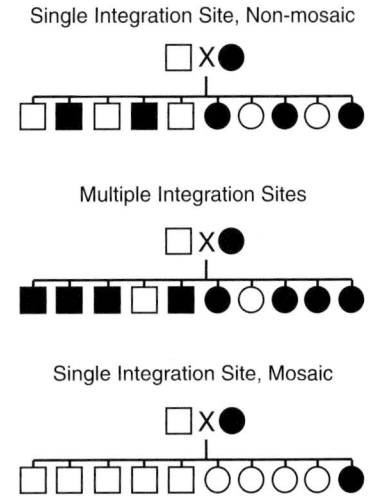

Figure 5-2 Pedigree analysis of progeny from transgenic founders. *Squares* represent males, and *circles* represent females. *Black shapes* designate transgenic animals. If more than 50% of the progeny from a transgenic founder are transgenic, this may be indicative of multiple integrations of the transgene. In contrast, if fewer than 50% of the progeny are transgenic, this is suggestive of mosaicism in the transgenic founder.

Position Variegation

Integration of the transgene is a random event. Thus, the transgene can reside either in euchromatin (actively transcribed regions of the genome) or in heterochromatin (transcriptionally silent regions of the chromatin). In either case, the transgene will follow the appropriate inheritance pattern. However, if the transgene is incorporated into heterochromatic regions, it will be expressed minimally, if at all. In contrast, if the transgene integrated into euchromatin, it could be integrated within a gene or in intergenic regions. Depending on the proximity of the transgene to an endogenous gene and the strength of the endogenous gene's promoter regulatory regions, control of transgene expression may be affected. Hence, the impact of integration into euchromatin can range from no expression to inappropriate expression in the wrong tissue type.

In addition to regulating tissue-specificity, integration position also strongly modulates the absolute level of transgene expression. Indeed, position effects play a more profound role in regulating transgene expression levels than the number of transgene molecules that have been integrated.[17] While one might intuitively expect that the number of integrated molecules of the transgene would dictate expression level, transgene expression is almost always unrelated to copy number. As an extreme example, one integration site may contain 100 tandem copies of the transgene but fail to be expressed owing to its residence in heterochromatin. In contrast, a single integrated molecule in euchromatin may display robust expression resulting from residence near a highly expressed endogenous gene. As such, transgenes are typically described as "integration-site dependent and copy-number independent." To compensate for positional variegation, some studies have taken advantage of homologous recombination techniques to insert various versions of a transgene into the same position within the genome.[18–21] Others have utilized so-called boundary or insulator elements.[22–25] These are regions of genes that inhibit the formation of heterochromatin and thus guard against the intrusion of unwanted regulatory processes associated with the adjacent chromatin environment.[22]

Insertional Mutagenesis

Since transgene integration is a random event, it can occur within endogenous genes and alter the function of those genes. Unless a gene displays haploinsufficiency, insertional mutations in one allele of the gene will not impact the physiology of the transgenic animals. However, if homozygous animals are generated by intercrossing hemizygous mice from the same line, the homozygous transgenic progeny will now lack functional allele of the disrupted gene. Depending on the gene's normal function, the impact of this mutation on the physiology of the animal could range from being inconsequential to causing embryonic lethality. Insertional events give rise to obvious or "visible" phenotypes in approximately 5% to 10% of all transgenic mouse lines.[26]

Although insertional mutagenesis is typically not the desired outcome of developing new transgenic mouse lines, mice with insertional mutations can be highly informative. In particular, these mutations may occur in previously uncharacterized genes or in genes that have not yet been mutated in the context of a whole animal. In addition, the phenotypes accompanying the insertional mutations may mimic human genetic diseases. If so, this equates to the development of a novel animal model that can be used to assess the genetic basis of such diseases. Furthermore, identification of the affected endogenous gene is straightforward because the transgene serves as a molecular beacon for identifying corresponding clones of the gene within a genomic library from the mutant mouse.[26] Thus, the endogenous gene, and the phenotype induced by its disruption, can be rapidly evaluated with this approach. However, an important factor to consider is that the newly identified gene probably plays little, if any, role in the initial biologic question that was being asked when the transgenic mouse was first developed.

The generation of random insertional mutants has been so effective in identifying and characterizing unknown genes that large-scale mutagenesis initiatives have been developed.[27–29] The explicit goal of these studies is to saturate the genome with mutations that will allow the discovery of novel genes and phenotypes.[28] Such programs typically couple embryonic stem cell technology with retroviral trapping vectors to allow rapid isolation of genomic sequences that have undergone insertional mutagenesis.[27–30] To facilitate identification of functional genes rather than insertions in the vast sea of intergenic DNA, reporter constructs lacking intrinsic promoter regulatory regions are often used. As a result, reporter gene expression is detected only when the transgene has integrated downstream of a functional promoter (i.e., within a functional gene). Only mice with detectable transgene expression are further evaluated. In addition, expression patterns of the transgene are indicative of the cells and/or tissues that normally express the endogenous, disrupted gene. Depending on the composition of the transgene, these approaches can be referred to as "promoter-trap," "gene-trap," or "enhancer-trap."[30–32] The outcome is largely the same—endogenous genes can be disrupted by an easily monitored insertion of heterologous DNA.

PROMOTER ANALYSES

One of the first applications of transgenic mouse technology was the in vivo assessment of tissue-specific promoter regulatory elements. Early studies showed that selected promoters could induce transgene expression in the same tissue sites that expressed the promoter's corresponding endogenous gene.[33–37] While identification and analyses of promoter regulatory elements had previously been confined to transfections of immortalized cell lines, transgenic technology permitted a more robust analysis within a physiologic and developmental context. Similar to in vitro transfection analyses, the level of activity of the reporter protein is a direct reflection of promoter function. Often, results from studies identifying promoter regulatory elements in transgenic mice paralleled those from in vitro culture studies. Nevertheless, numerous transgenic studies have also refuted data obtained in vitro. In most cases, small regulatory regions that are sufficient for expression in cultured cells are insufficient to direct high level, tissue-specific expression in mice.[38–45] This difference has largely been attributed to the absence of chromatin regulatory domains within the transgenes which, in contrast to transiently transfected genes, reside within a chromatin environment. Alternatively, the intricate developmental processes at play in the transgenic mouse may necessitate more robust transcriptional regulatory elements for initial activation of the gene than cells in culture that are typically locked in a specific developmental stage.

Reporter Genes

Intrinsic to performing promoter analyses in transgenic animals is the selection of an appropriate reporter gene. Expression of reporter genes, ideally, should have little to no impact on the physiology of the transgenic animal. This permits an analysis of promoter regulation in the context of normal physiology in which the only permutation is the introduction of an innocuous transgene. In some contexts, a biologically active reporter such as growth hormone has been used.[46,47] This resulted in excessively large mice with a spectrum of pathologies that ranged from hyperinsulinemia to infertility.[48]

Selection of reporter genes is based on the desired analytical end point. Many early studies utilized the bacterial chloramphenicol acetyl transferase (CAT) reporter gene. The CAT enzyme can be sensitively assayed with low background;

however, the quality of antibodies to this enzyme has generally been poor. Thus, most assays evaluating CAT levels involve the production of tissue lysates. This precludes any analysis of cell-specific expression within the evaluated tissue. Similar limitations apply when using the firefly luciferase gene as a reporter, that is, high sensitivity with low background that is largely limited to a soluble assay. The bacterial β-galactosidase (β-gal) gene also provides a useful soluble assay with slightly lower sensitivity but permits evaluation of expression on a per cell basis. Tissue sections are incubated with a chromogenic substrate for the enzyme such as X-gal. Cells expressing the β-galactosidase enzyme produce a blue precipitate in the presence of this substrate. While useful for histologic assessment of tissues, there are limitations to this approach. In particular, cryosections are required because the heat associated with the paraffin embedding process will denature the enzyme. It is also difficult to perform immunohistochemistry in combination with the β-galactosidase staining. Furthermore, fixed sections are used, which prevents imaging of live cells within the section of tissue.

Another reporter gene encoding green fluorescent protein (GFP), isolated from the jellyfish *Aequorea victoria*, does not suffer from some of the limitations of these other reporter genes. Although use of native GFP in mammals was limited by thermal instability and low-level fluorescence intensity, mutants have subsequently been developed that have the same advantages as the β-gal reporter gene.[49] In addition, the GFP assay appears to be more sensitive than the colorimetric assay that is used to quantify β-gal, suggesting that it may be a better choice as a reporter gene.[50] A further advantage of GFP is that it does not require an exogenous substrate or enzymatic reaction. Only a microscope capable of viewing fluorescent objects is necessary. Importantly, GFP is compatible with immunohistochemistry protocols and can also be used to study living cells expressing the reporter gene.[51–53]

"Indicator" Strains of Mice

In addition to facilitating the dissection of promoter regulatory elements in transgenic mice, reporter genes can also be used to measure the activity of specific transcription factors. This typically involves the construction of a transgene containing a minimal promoter such as the truncated herpes simplex virus thymidine kinase (HSV-TK) promoter that has the potential to be activated in all cell types in the mouse throughout development into adulthood. Upstream of the minimal promoter, multimers of response elements (enhancers) for a specific transcription factor are added. This entire promoter regulatory cassette is then linked to a reporter gene such as β-gal. Activation of the transcription factor that binds to the enhancer element will then increase expression of the reporter gene. This approach is used to follow the activity of a specific transcription factor in question.

Two different indicator strains have been developed to follow estrogen receptor function. One of these involves the use of two estrogen response elements (EREs) upstream of the HSV-TK minimal promoter driving expression of the luciferase reporter gene.[54] To prevent untoward effects of the chromatin environment, insulator elements were also added. In the other indicator strain, three copies of an ERE were placed upstream of the HSV-TK promoter, which directed expression of the β-gal reporter.[55] No insulator elements were added to this vector. Expression of the respective reporter genes in these strains of mice is responsive to estrogenic compounds indicating that the ERE in the transgenes is accurately reporting activation of the estrogen receptor. Most important, patterns of expression and activation of the transgenes are unique for distinct tissues, indicating tissue-specific activity of ER and/or its coregulators.[54,55] These mouse models should facilitate the in vivo assessment of novel selective estrogen receptor modulators (SERMs) as well as permit future analyses of estrogen receptor mechanisms of action using

in vivo imaging[56] (see below). Similar approaches have been developed to monitor activity of the retinoic acid receptor,[57] cyclic adenosine monophosphate (cAMP) response element–binding protein (CREB),[58] nuclear factor-κB (NF-κB),[59] and the Wnt/β-catenin canonical pathway[60] as well as several other transcription factors.

In Vivo Imaging

A new and exciting application of transgenic technology has arisen from the recent marriage between luciferase reporter genes and extremely sensitive optical imaging devices. The combination of these technologies has provided the capability to visualize transgene activity within the context of the living animal. Cells or tissues expressing luciferase can be detected with a cooled, charge-coupled device (CCD) camera following intraperitoneal or intravenous injection of the fluorogenic substrate luciferin.[61] Luciferin is widely distributed in the body and can cross the blood-brain and placental barriers; also, the light produced by luciferase enzymatic reaction is relatively resistant to scattering and absorption by tissues within the mouse. Thus, any cells that express luciferase in the presence of luciferin will emit light that can be detected by the CCD camera.

In vivo imaging will likely enjoy extensive use in future assessments of transgenic mouse models. For example, in vivo imaging using the luciferase reporter gene can be used in indicator strains of mice, allowing whole animal appraisal of transcription factor activation.[56,62] In addition, luciferase imaging technology has been used to identify small pituitary tumors within the living animal.[63] Such approaches may help to eliminate the broad-scale evaluation of large numbers of mice that is currently required to identify early tumorigenic events in a number of cancer models. Furthermore, evaluation of novel chemotherapeutics will be greatly enhanced by the ability to rapidly detect and quantify molecular changes in tumors within treated animals.[63] Last, *in vivo* imaging has been used to noninvasively follow apoptosis in response to tumor necrosis factor α-related apoptosis-inducing ligand (TRAIL) using a caspase-sensitive luciferase fusion protein.[64] This should have broad ranging impact on the experimental evaluation of models of human diseases that have significant imbalances of apoptotic processes such as cancer, neurodegenerative diseases, and acquired immunodeficiency syndrome (AIDS).[64]

CELL-SPECIFIC ABLATION AND TUMORIGENESIS

Cell-Specific Ablation

While the discovery of tissue-specific promoter activity in transgenic mice permitted rigorous evaluation of promoter regulatory regions, it also led to the realization that these promoters could be used to mediate selective expression of proteins in individual cell types. Targeted expression of toxic gene products to specific cells with the intention of ablating these cell types can be used to address their roles in tissue development as well as cell fates. Genes encoding two toxins have been widely used: diphtheria toxin A (DT-A) chain or HSV-TK. The A subunit of diphtheria toxin adenosine diphosphate (ADP)-ribosylates elongation factor 2 (EF2), subsequently preventing protein synthesis. DT-A is extraordinarily potent; as little as one molecule is sufficient for cell lethality.[65] Thus, once the transgene promoter is activated, cells expressing the transgene will be killed. This effect is cell autonomous because internalization of DT-A into adjacent cells requires the DT-B protein subunit, which is not endogenously expressed.[66] Early studies using this approach facilitated the development of cell lineage models for the development of the anterior pituitary.[67] This approach has also been used to selectively eliminate specific cell types in a number of tissues relevant to endocrinology including the pancreas,[66,68] adipose tissue,[69,70] and pituitary.[67,71–73]

DT-A encoding transgenes have been useful for cell lineage assessments; however, the extreme toxicity of this agent limits its utility.[74] In particular, cells that initially activate the promoter are immediately killed, truncating any analysis of cell fate at the primary cell's initial decision to activate the promoter being used. Additionally, any "leaky" expression of the transgene in heterologous cells also leads to their lethality. If the promoter is active at a low level early in embryogenesis, it is possible that all transgenic mice will be lost to embryonic lethality. Thus, inducible or conditional ablation, such as that afforded by HSV-TK, is now preferred over the immediate cell death that occurs on activation of the DT-A transgenes. HSV-TK expression in cells is benign in the absence of nucleoside analogues such as acyclovir or ganciclovir, which act as chain-terminating agents in DNA synthesis.[75] In the absence of HSV-TK, these prodrugs have minimal toxicity,[75] whereas in the presence of HSV-TK, they become incorporated into the DNA of replicating cells, causing fatal DNA damage. The timing of cell ablation can thus be regulated by modulating when the animals are treated with these drugs. While this approach has been used for assessment of cell lineage and function in endocrine systems,[76–81] limitations such as inherent toxicity to spermatids[82] and low potency have restricted its general use.

A recent modification of the diphtheria toxin approach has been described that takes advantage of the 10^5-fold lower affinity of the murine receptor for diphtheria toxin B chain (HB-EGF) when compared to the affinity of the human receptor.[83] Transgene constructs contain the human HB-EGF receptor under control of a cell-specific promoter. Transgenic mice are then treated with intact diphtheria toxin (i.e., with both A and B subunits). Only cells that express the human HB-EGF receptor will internalize diphtheria toxin and die as a result. This allows temporal control of cell ablation with a potent toxin and should prove more beneficial than either the HSV-TK or DT-A approaches that were used previously.[74] Such conditional cell ablation approaches not only will be useful for addressing cell lineage questions but also will facilitate the development of disease models in which selective cell loss is observed such as heart disease,[84] hepatitis,[83] and neural degeneration.[85]

Cell-Specific Tumorigenesis

While elimination of cell types using toxigenes can provide useful information regarding cell lineage and specification, unrestrained growth of cell populations using oncogenes can generate insight concerning tumorigenic mechanisms as well as lead to the development of valuable in vitro cell culture models. The ability to selectively induce tumors in transgenic mice was first observed with mice harboring the simian virus 40 (SV40) early region genes and enhancers.[86] These mice routinely developed tumors in the choroid plexus by 6 months of age. Shortly thereafter, it was shown that overexpression of the c-myc proto-oncogene under the control of a mammary gland selective promoter caused mammary adenocarcinomas.[87] The oncogenic region of the SV40 genome encoding the Large T-antigen has been used to create a vast array of endocrinologically relevant tumor models including those arising in the pancreas,[88] adrenal gland,[89] prostate,[90] mammary gland,[91] thyroid,[92] ovary,[93] testes,[93] and pituitary,[94,95] as well as many others.

In addition to providing useful tumor models, selective targeting of an oncogene to a particular tissue permits development of novel cell lines. Tumors arising from these tissues can be isolated and cultured to produce transformed cell lines, facilitating in vitro studies. Furthermore, tumors can be induced at different developmental stages of the tissue, allowing the production of cell lines that represent distinct functional end points. For example, an array of cell lines has been developed using promoters from the different anterior pituitary hormone genes to "capture" cells within distinct developmental windows as a result of transformation and, hence, loss of further differentiation.[94,96] Although developmental

selection is desired in some cases, it is often advantageous to transform mature, differentiated cells. This can be accomplished with a temperature-sensitive form of SV40 T antigen that has low activity at 37°C (i.e., the body temperature of the mouse) but is fully active at 33°C.[97] Thus, tumors generally do not form in vivo, but tissues harvested from transgenic mice will give rise to immortalized cells when cultured at the permissive temperature.

CONDITIONAL EXPRESSION OF TRANSGENES

Thus far, we have focused on transgenes that are under the control of naturally occurring promoter regulatory elements. While the use of such promoters allows appropriate temporal and spatial expression of transgenes, it also has fundamental limitations. Specifically, there is no way for the investigator to tightly control the timing of transgene expression. If the transgene promoter is active during embryogenesis, expression of the transgene may fundamentally alter the physiology of the adult animal. In this case, it is unclear whether pathologic changes in the adult are cell autonomous (i.e., the result of transgene expression in the cell type of interest in the adult) or cell nonautonomous (i.e., the result of early expression in undesired cells that alters the global biology of the organism). Hence, the phenotype of the transgenic mouse represents a summation of all processes affected by transgene expression. It is also possible that expression of a selected transgene may cause considerable toxicity. If so, the adults might have a shortened life span or might be infertile, limiting the ability to generate lines of mice and reducing the numbers of experimental animals that can be produced. To circumvent these limitations, conditional expression systems have been developed in which the researcher has the ability to dictate when transgene expression is activated or repressed.

Site-Specific Recombination

One approach for regulating transgene expression employs nonmammalian recombinases from the family of site-specific integrases. Both Cre recombinase, from bacteriophage P1, and Flp integrase, from *Saccharomyces cerevisiae*, have been used. Variant forms of these proteins are active in mammalian cells, and they require no additional cellular proteins for activity. Both recognize 34 base pair (bp) sequences ("loxP" sites for Cre and "FRT" sites for Flp) in the genome as sites for recombination.[98–100] Depending on the orientation of the recognition sequences, these enzymes can delete, invert, duplicate, or translocate intervening regions of DNA.[101] Regions of DNA that are flanked by loxP sequences (or "floxed") in the same orientation will be deleted following recombinase-mediated recombination.

Using appropriate promoters, expression of either Cre or Flp can be directed specifically to the cell types of interest in transgenic mice.[102–104] These proteins will induce a recombination event at any recognition sequences that occur within the genome. Since the wild-type genome of the mouse lacks complete recognition sequences for either Cre or Flp, they are benign in normal cells.[102] The recognition sequences can be introduced into the mouse genome in the form of a second transgene that remains dormant until activated by a recombination event. Dormant transgenes can be designed with a strong "stop" sequence in the transcribed region of the transgene (i.e., downstream of the promoter) that terminates transcription or translation (Fig. 5-3),[102,105,106] or they can have intervening genes such as those encoding β-galactosidase.[103] Both prevent translation of the downstream expression cassette. Transgenic mice harboring either the recombinase or the dormant transgene alone are normal. However, when the two lines of mice are mated, a population of cells within bitransgenic progeny will contain the dormant transgene as well as express the Cre recombinase. As a result, in these cells the stop sequence will be excised from the dormant transgene,

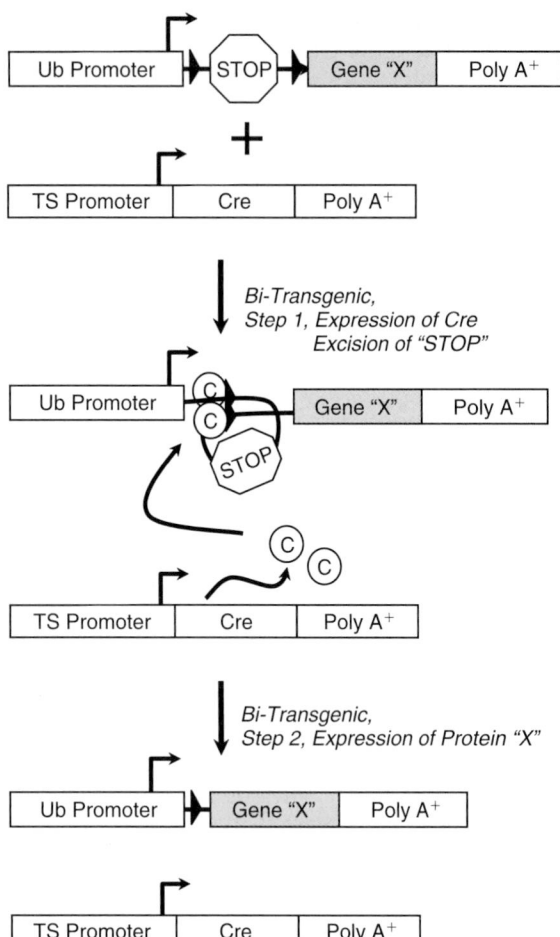

Figure 5-3 Cre-mediated induction of transgene expression. Bitransgenic mice are developed containing a transgene with the gene to be studied (Gene "X") under control of a ubiquitous (Ub) promoter. Inserted between the promoter and the coding sequence is a strong STOP sequence that inhibits translation of the mRNA. This sequence is flanked by *loxP* sequences (*black triangle*). The second transgene encodes the Cre recombinase under control of a tissue-specific (TS) promoter. Once the Cre recombinase is expressed, it will excise any intervening sequences between two *loxP* sequences that are in the same orientation.

thus producing an active expression cassette. This is an irreversible event that permanently changes the genome of the cells expressing Cre recombinase as well as all progeny derived from these precursor cells. This approach was originally used with a quiescent transgene containing the SV40 large T antigen (T-Ag) to induce tumor formation in the mouse lens. Exquisite control of T-Ag was evident because none of the mice harboring the dormant transgene developed tumors, whereas all bitransgenic mice did.[102]

Cell-specific recombination can also be used to irreversibly "mark" cells within a specific cell lineage using a similar bitransgenic approach. The first transgene contains a quiescent β-gal reporter gene. The second transgene expresses Cre recombinase under the control of a cell-specific, transiently active promoter. In bitransgenic mice, cells that activate this promoter at any time will induce a recombination event that irreversibly activates β-gal expression. This genetic change will persist in the parental cells and their progeny even after many subsequent cell divisions and differentiation events. Using this approach, one can follow cell lineages from precursor cells capable of expressing the Cre transgene through adulthood.[107–110]

Ligand-Regulated Transgene Expression

Using the Cre or Flp recombination systems relies on the use of tissue-specific promoters to dictate site-specific recombination in a particular cell type. The timing of the recombination event depends on when the promoter used to direct expression of the recombinase is activated. In many cases, it would be advantageous to restrict expression to a specified time period that might not be capitulated by a naturally occurring promoter. Drug-inducible systems have been developed to accomplish temporal regulation of transgene expression. While a number of systems exist, they all involve at least two transgenes. The first is an "effector" transgene that directs expression of a ligand-regulated transcription factor to the tissue of interest using an appropriate promoter. The second is a "target" transgene that utilizes a minimal promoter regulated by this transcription factor to control expression of a protein of interest.[111] An optimal drug-inducible system has the following properties: specificity (the transcription factor is regulated only by the exogenous ligand), noninterference (neither the ligand nor the transcription factor should have an impact on normal cellular physiology), inducibility and dose-dependency (activation of expression and the absolute levels of expression should be tightly regulated by the ligand), bioavailability (the ligand should be freely accessible to all sites in the body, including having the ability to cross the blood-brain and placental-fetal barriers), and reversibility (expression should rapidly return to baseline with the loss of ligand).[101,111,112] The most commonly used systems employ modified versions of the tetracycline repressor (tetR) from bacteria,[113–115] the ecdysone receptor (EcR) from *Drosophila*,[116] or the Gal4 transactivator from yeast fused to the ligand-binding domain of the progesterone receptor.[117] Here, we will discuss only those systems employing the tetR because they are the most widely utilized to date.

In *Escherichia coli*, the tetR binds to 19-bp DNA sequences (*tetO* elements) within the tetracycline resistance operon. On binding tetracycline, the repressor can no longer bind to DNA. Dissociation of the repressor from the *tet* operon permits subsequent transcription. Two versions of the tetracycline regulatory system have been developed for use in mammalian cells: "tet-off" and "tet-on" (Fig. 5-4). Both utilize a fusion protein consisting of a form of the tetR linked to the transactivation domain of VP16, a viral transcription factor,

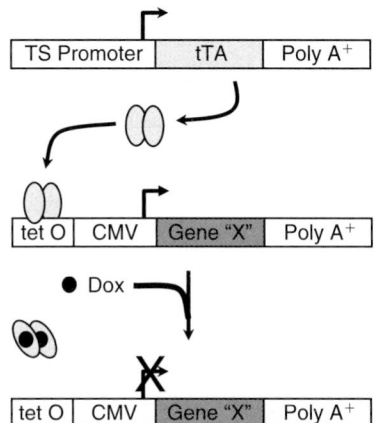

Figure 5-4 Inducible expression of transgenes. Shown is the Tet-Off system. Bitransgenic mice are required. One transgene encodes the gene to be studied (Gene "X") under control of a CMV minimal promoter with Tet operator sequences (tet O). The CMV promoter is active when the modified tet repressor (tTA) is bound to the tet O sequences. On treatment with doxycycline (*black circle*), the tet repressor undergoes a conformational change and dissociates from DNA. The loss of tTA binding causes a loss of CMV promoter activity.

In the tet-off system, addition of the strong transactivation domain from VP16 converts the tetR into a transcriptional activator, called tTA. The tTA protein can bind to and activate transgenes that are engineered to contain *tetO* elements within the promoter regulatory region. Treatment with a tetracycline analogue, doxycycline, inhibits binding of tTA to DNA, hence terminating transcription.[114] This approach is called tet-off because transcription ceases with the addition of doxycycline. Two primary limitations have been described that diminish the utility of the tet-off system. These include highly variable regulation of target genes with unacceptable leakiness of the target gene (i.e., the target remains active in the presence of doxycycline). In addition, this system requires that animals be treated with doxycycline at all times when repression of target gene expression is desired, which can become cumbersome.

To address these limitations, the tet-on system was developed. Mutations were engineered into the tetR portion of the tTA protein (reverse tTA or rtTA) that promote binding to, rather than dissociation from, DNA with the addition of doxycyline.[115] This system requires treatment with doxycycline only when target transgene expression is desired. In addition, the target tends to have very low levels of expression in the absence of doxycycline.

As a result of these and many other creative transgenic approaches, investigators now have the ability to dictate when, where, and how much transgenic mRNA and protein will be expressed. Coupling regulated expression with the use of novel transgenic proteins has greatly advanced our understanding of how these proteins function throughout development in a model organism and have spawned the creation of countless models of human disease.

HOMOLOGOUS RECOMBINATION OF FOREIGN DNA INTO THE MOUSE GENOME

Transgenic techniques have been developed to address a wide array of physiologic and pathologic problems, but many questions require complete suppression of an endogenous gene's activity. Although antisense and RNA interference approaches hold some promise for the removal of mRNA corresponding to the gene of interest, results thus far have been variable and seldom culminate in the elimination of all protein product derived from that gene.[118–120] As with any transgene, expression of most RNA-targeting transgenes will be highly variable owing to position variegation (see above). Even within a specific tissue, all cells might not express a transgene in the same way, which may generate numerous phenotypic outcomes. Thus, the most unambiguous tool that can be used to eliminate activity of a gene is disruption of that gene by homologous recombination to generate knockout mice. This approach was made possible by the development of two technologies: establishment of pluripotent embryonic stem (ES) cell lines with the ability to contribute to all cell lineages within the developing mouse, including the germ line,[121–123] and the creation of molecular tools that permitted selection and identification of cells that had undergone homologous recombination.[124–127]

GENERAL PRINCIPLES

Homologous Recombination Requirements
Homologous recombination requires the development of targeting vectors that have the following features: long homologous stretches of DNA (up to several thousand base pairs) from the gene to be disrupted and selectable markers. The long regions of homologous DNA allow alignment of the targeting DNA with the endogenous gene sequence, while the selectable markers permit identification of cells that have undergone the recombination event.

Selectable Markers
The first mouse harboring a selectable disruption of an endogenous gene was reported in 1987.[128] Creation of this mouse involved random mutagenesis of the murine genome in ES cells infected with retroviral vectors. Cells that harbored a disruption of the hypoxanthine-guanosine phosphoribosyl transferase (HPRT) gene were identified by their ability to grow in thioguanine-containing media, which kills cells with an intact HPRT locus. The HPRT gene is on the X chromosome. Since ES cells are derived from male embryos, mutagenesis of a single allele results in an HPRT-deficient cell line.[129] Selection using thioguanine was critical for identifying cells that had undergone disruption of the HPRT gene.

While the HPRT gene was a useful target for demonstrating the power of selected mutagenesis, this approach was possible only because of the selective pressure that could be placed on cells harboring mutant HPRT alleles. Unfortunately, selection tools that will readily identify cells that have undergone targeted disruption of most genes of interest are not available. In fact, many genes are not even expressed within ES cells. Thus, selectable markers are required to identify cells that have undergone homologous recombination within the target gene even if this disruption causes no change in the biology of the ES cell. In addition, rather than utilizing random mutagenesis as described above, DNA targeting vectors are employed to act as homing agents to mediate disruptions of specific genes in the genome. In most cases, targeting vectors are constructed that permit a positive/negative selection strategy (Fig. 5-5).

Positive selection will identify any cells that have incorporated foreign DNA into the genome. Typically, this foreign DNA contains an expression cassette for either the neomycin or hygromycin resistance gene. Treatment of normal cells with either G418 or hygromycin, respectively, will result in lethality; however, cells that express the appropriate resistance gene will grow normally in the presence of the otherwise lethal drug. This selection step eliminates all cells that have not undergone an insertional event of the targeting DNA.

Positive selection identifies cells that have incorporated the foreign DNA cassette into their genome; however, because random integration is much more efficient than insertion by homologous recombination,[126] most of the surviving cells will have integrated the DNA randomly.[130] Since the underlying purpose of this approach is disruption of a specific gene, another selection method is necessary to eliminate all cells that have undergone random insertion of the targeting DNA. This involves the use of a negative selection expression cassette encoding HSV-TK. Recall that treating cells expressing HSV-TK with ganciclovir will block DNA synthesis and, hence, replication (see the section entitled "Cell-Specific Ablation"). In the targeting vector, the HSV-TK expression cassette is placed outside of the regions of homology with the endogenous gene. Random insertion of DNA occurs via the ends of the DNA, incorporating the entire vector. Thus, randomly inserted DNA will usually include the HSV-TK expression cassette. In contrast, with homologous recombination, crossover events occur within the regions of homology between the targeting vector and the endogenous gene; thus, the HSV-TK gene will be excised.[131] Treating cells with ganciclovir will discriminate between those that have undergone random insertion versus homologous recombination because those cells retaining the HSV-TK cassette will be eliminated. Addition of negative selection can increase the efficiency of identifying cells that have undergone targeted disruption by up to 2000-fold.[132]

Targeting Vectors
Expression cassettes encoding selectable markers are an essential component of targeting vectors. To direct appropriate expression of the selection genes, these cassettes include promoters that are active in the ES cells and, often, a heterologous

A

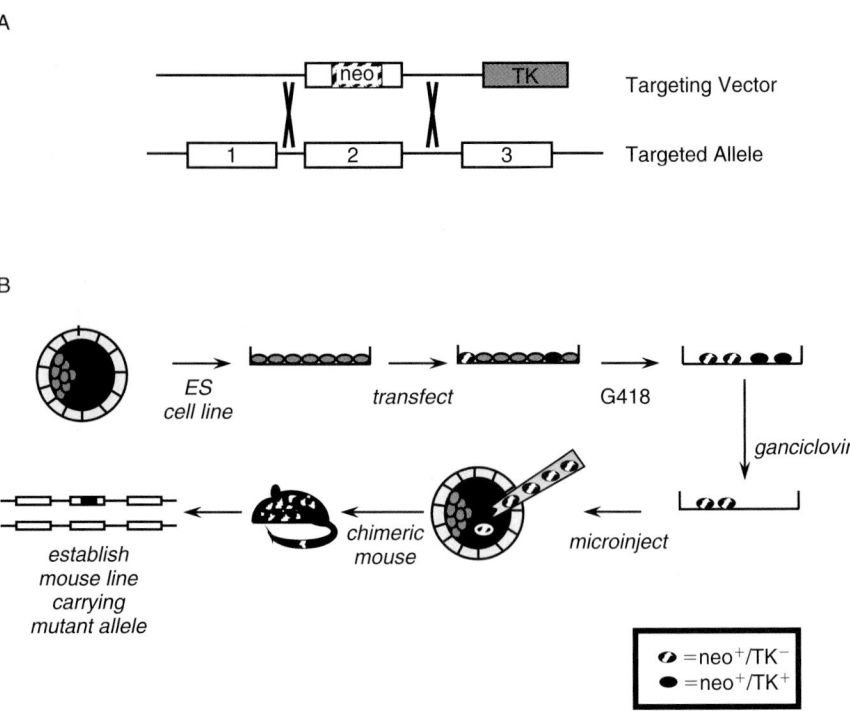

Figure 5-5 Construction of knockout mice. **A,** Targeting vectors are constructed to induce homologous recombination in ES cells. These vectors have several thousand base pairs of sequence identical to the gene to be disrupted. Typically, a positive selectable marker, such as the neomycin resistance gene (neo), is placed within a critical exon. A negative selectable marker such as the HSV-TK gene is place at one end of the targeting vector. Areas of homologous recombination are indicated by "X." Numbered white boxes are exons. **B,** Embryonic stem cell lines are derived from the inner cell mass of blastocysts. These cells are transfected with the targeting vector. Incorporation of the targeting vector is assessed by screening for G418 (neomycin) resistance. Homologous recombinants must have lost the HSV-TK allele; hence, these are identified by the ability to grow on ganciclovir. Once the homologous recombination is confirmed by Southern blot analyses, the heterozygous ES cells are injected into new blastocysts. They become part of the inner cell mass and give rise to chimeric mice. These mice are then bred to wild-type animals to generate heterozygous progeny.

polyadenylation signal. Targeting constructs are usually designed with the intention of replacing or disrupting the coding sequence of the target gene with the positive selection cassette. Typically, an exon within the target gene containing the start site of translation or one encoding an essential domain of the encoded protein is targeted. Significant lengths of genomic regions homologous to the gene being targeted flank the positive selection cassette; thus, it is essential that a large genomic clone containing the sequence to be disrupted be obtained before a targeting vector can be produced. It is the homologous sequences that promote recombination. Rates of homologous recombination increase as the length of homologous sequences increases up to about 10 Kbp, the minimal length of homology being about 500 bp.[133,134] In addition to length, recombination efficiency can also be affected by the source of the homologous gene sequences used to produce the targeting vector. DNA that is isogenic to the ES cell line is generally more efficient than DNA sequences collected from alternate mouse strains.[134,135] This type of targeting vector is known as a replacement or Ω-type vector, meaning that the targeting vector will actually replace a region of the genome upon homologous recombination.[130,136–138] The arms of the Ω represent the homologous gene sequences, while the loop represents the inserted selection cassette that replaces a portion of the endogenous gene. Insertion vectors (O-type) are used much less frequently. With this type of vector, plasmid DNA is added to the genome, resulting in duplication of a small region of the gene of interest.[139]

Targeting vectors are linearized and are usually introduced into ES cells by electroporation. Following a brief recovery period, the cells are selected for neomycin and ganciclovir resistance. Clones are isolated, expanded, and characterized.

Genetic Screens of Modified ES Cells
Multiple genetic screens must be performed on the ES cell clones following selection and expansion. This includes confirming that homologous recombination has occurred and usually involves Southern blot analyses using probes to the endogenous locus. While all clones that are capable of growing under the positive/negative selection conditions should have undergone an accurate recombination, this is often not

the case. If random insertion occurred but the HSV-TK cassette was lost, these cells would grow in the selection medium.[139] Thus, it is critical that the targeted allele be evaluated to confirm the anticipated recombination event. In addition to screening for appropriate recombination, the chromosomal integrity of the modified cell lines should be confirmed. Since ES cells are maintained in culture, it is inevitable that they will eventually accumulate genetic changes.[140] To ensure the use of cells that lack gross chromosomal changes, karyotype analysis is used as a screening tool.[140] These approaches should lead to the identification of euploid cells that are heterozygous for the disrupted gene and can then be used to produce chimeric animals.

Production of Chimeric Mice
Following confirmation of the genetic composition of the manipulated ES cells, the cells are used to produce chimeric mice that are derived from two cell lineages: one that includes descendents of the manipulated ES cells and another corresponding to the host embryo. The different sources of the cells are readily identified in the chimeric mouse because the ES cells have distinct coat color alleles from the donor blastocyst. Chimeras are produced either by direct microinjection of ES cells into blastocysts or by aggregating the ES cells with eight cell embryos.[141] In both cases, the ES cells become part of the inner cell mass of the blastocyst and ultimately contribute to most lineages within the resulting fetus. Since the parental ES cells are totipotent, the injected cells should retain the ability to contribute to all cell lineages. Chimeric mice are primarily used for production of a second generation of animals that are genetically uniform; therefore, it is of primary importance that the manipulated stem cell line contributes to the germ line of the chimeric mouse. Chimeric animals in which the ES cells have not contributed specifically to the formation of germ cells are not useful for generation of a knockout mouse line. To rapidly assess the ability of the ES cells to contribute to the germ line, coat color of the progeny is used as a marker. It is also important to note that most ES cell lines have a male, XY, genotype.[142] Thus, only male chimeras will be capable of generating offspring harboring the targeted mutation.

Generation of Knockout Animals

Once progeny are obtained from chimeric mice, they must be genotyped to determine which animals harbor a mutant allele of the targeted gene. These mice will be heterozygous for the disrupted allele. The number of progeny from the chimeric animal that have the disrupted allele will depend on the degree to which the ES cell line contributed to the germ line of the chimera. Male and female heterozygous mice that are obtained are subsequently crossed to generate progeny that are homozygous for the null allele.

If the targeted gene is not essential for life, inheritance of the disrupted allele should follow Mendelian inheritance patterns. Progeny from heterozygous matings should occur in the following ratios: one fourth homozygous for the wild-type allele, one half heterozygous for the wild-type and null allele, and one fourth homozygous for the null allele. With sufficiently large numbers of animals, any skewing of these ratios is suggestive of a lethal phenotype resulting from loss of one or more alleles of the targeted gene. An absence of homozygous null animals indicates that deficiency of the targeted allele induces lethality whereas a reduction in heterozygote numbers may imply haploinsufficiency. Whether the loss of one or more alleles causes embryonic or postnatal lethality can be readily assessed by counting the number of pups that are born versus the number that survive to weaning.

Once a population of homozygous mice has been identified, studies evaluating the importance of the disrupted allele can be accomplished. Experiments evaluating knockout animals must always be performed with appropriate control mice. This usually involves the use of wild-type littermates. If loss of a single allele does not cause a noticeable phenotype, the heterozygous animals may also be used as controls. Below, we will discuss the importance of genetic background in defining phenotypic consequences of genetic manipulations in mice. The use of age-matched wild-type littermates as controls is important to avoid erroneously attributing phenotypic differences that are caused by genetic strain composition to the function of the disrupted gene.

CONDITIONAL GENE TARGETING

In studying knockout animals, it cannot be overemphasized that the resultant phenotype is a conglomeration of all cellular changes that occurred as a consequence of the gene disruption. Owing to the fundamental changes in homeostasis that may occur, interpretations regarding the cell-autonomous function of a gene can be problematic. This is particularly true in the endocrine system, where target tissues are often reliant on multiple inputs from various organs. In addition, if a disrupted allele is essential for life, analysis of the function of this gene can be studied only up to the point of this vital stage. Last, compensatory changes in the expression or activity of similar protein family members may obscure a phenotype. For these reasons, site-specific, or conditional, gene targeting was developed.

The most common approach for developing mice with tissue-specific gene disruptions utilizes a variation of the Cre/lox recombination system that was described earlier.[143] Rather than using Cre recombinase to activate a randomly integrated transgene, it can be used to inactivate an endogenous gene that is engineered to contain loxP sequences surrounding a critical portion of the gene, such as the first coding exon. As is shown in Figure 5-6, the loxP sites are arranged in the same orientation, hence leading to excision of the sequence residing between the sites when encountered by Cre recombinase. To circumvent any impact on gene function prior to the Cre-mediated excision, the loxP sites are usually inserted into introns or into the 5' or 3' flanking regions of genes.[111] Thus, the targeted gene should function normally until the recombination event occurs. Recombination will occur only where Cre recombinase is expressed. Thus, using a tissue-specific promoter to direct expression of Cre will lead to recombination only in the tissues where this promoter is active. For example, SF1 is an orphan nuclear receptor that is expressed in adrenal, gonads, hypothalamus, and pituitary. To determine the specific pituitary role of SF1, this gene was floxed, and mice harboring this allele were crossed with mice

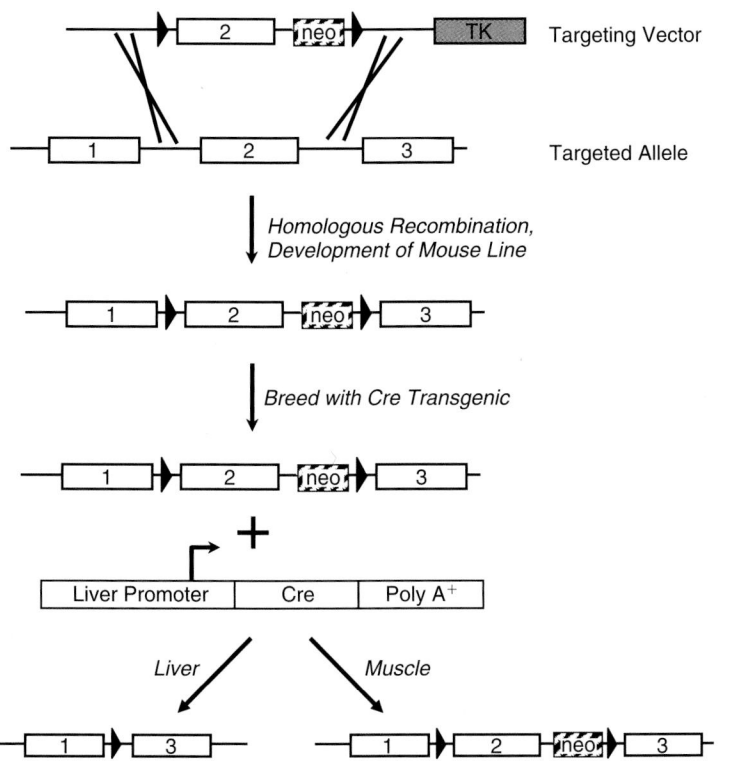

Figure 5-6 Cre-mediated tissue-specific knockout. A targeting vector is constructed as described in Figure 5-5 with a few modifications. The positive selectable marker (neo) is placed within an intron (*thin line*), hence not disrupting the function of the gene but allowing appropriate selection in ES cells. In addition, two loxP sequences (*black triangles*) are added that flank the region to be removed in future mice. Using approaches previously described, chimeric mice are obtained, and lines are generated. These mice are then crossed with another transgenic mouse line that contains a Cre-encoding transgene under control of a tissue-specific promoter (e.g., liver). Liver cells will undergo recombination and remove sequences between the loxP sequences, while other cells such as muscle will have normal gene function. Numbered white boxes are exons.

that express Cre only in gonadotropes. This allowed definitive assessment of the gonadotrope autonomous function of SF1.[144]

Introduction of *loxP* sites into the gene of interest requires the development of a targeting construct similar to that used for the conventional homologous recombination approach. Significant regions of sequence that are identical to the targeted gene are necessary; however, here the small, 34 bp *loxP* sequences are also included. These short sequences should have minimal impact on recombination efficiency. Selectable markers are also a necessary component of the targeting vector. In this case, the positive selection cassette (e.g., neo[r]) can be placed in a noncoding region of the gene to avoid altering the function of the gene prior to Cre recombination. Alternatively, one can ensure that the selectable marker will not alter the function of the targeted gene, by flanking the marker cassette with *loxP* sites. The cassette can then be excised by short-term Cre expression in ES cells following transient transfection with a Cre expression vector.[143] Following this transfection paradigm, it is necessary to assess clones for loss of the selection cassette but maintenance of the *loxP* sequences within the targeted gene.

Disruption of all gene function in a particular cell type requires that homozygous mice are obtained that have the *floxed* gene at both alleles. These mice must also harbor a randomly integrated transgene that expresses Cre solely in the desired cell type. Complete recombination in the majority of cells of interest is often necessary for development of an interpretable phenotypic change.[105,111] Unfortunately, recombination of both alleles in all target cells can be difficult to achieve due to variable Cre expression or positional effects on the *floxed* alleles in the genome.[145] One tactic to circumvent this problem is the use of a combined approach that utilizes a traditional disruption of one allele and a conditional, Cre-mediated, disruption of the second allele. Hence, obtaining a complete knockout in the cells of interest requires only a single recombination event within each cell.

One of the key limitations of conditional approaches is the reliance on a limited number of cell-specific promoters that generate high level Cre expression in the desired cell type. In many cases, the temporal regulation of such promoters might not correspond to the preferred timing of the recombination event. For example, one might wish to determine the role of a gene in the adult testes. However, if the only available cell type–specific promoter is active in these cells during embryonic development, the recombination event will occur long before adulthood. To circumvent this issue, a number of modifications have been made to the Cre recombinase that permits ligand-mediated activation.[146-149] Of note, fusion proteins between Cre and either the estrogen receptor or progesterone receptor ligand-binding domains have been used in transgenic mice.[150-153] The ligand-binding domains for these receptors amass heat shock protein complexes that cloak the Cre recombinase in the absence of ligand. Once ligands such as tamoxifen or mifepristone are present, the heat shock proteins are shed, and active Cre enzyme is revealed. This allows inhibition of Cre activity, and hence recombination, until the desired time point at which the transgenic mice are treated with the appropriate ligand. Similar approaches have been described that involve tetR regulation of Cre expression.[154,155]

KNOCK-INS

Complete removal of a gene permits assessment of global gene or protein function. While somewhat informative, this approach does not allow evaluation of the precise mechanisms of action of a particular protein. Identification of specific physiologic roles is particularly important for proteins that may have dual functions. Furthermore, it is often desirable to assess the physiologic/pathologic significance of individual protein domains or even single amino acids within a protein. Last, in the case of multiple, highly conserved, protein family members, it is often useful to determine their extent of functional redundancy. As was mentioned above, selective disruption of a single gene in mice may result in the absence of a discernable phenotype due to overlapping functions of members of the same protein family. Although studies examining molecular functions or redundancy can be performed in cell culture systems, the physiologic function would still remain untested. Knock-in mice, which have undergone specific gene replacement of an endogenous locus, have been used extensively to address these types of questions within whole organisms. This can lead to generation of a gene with a point mutation, replacement of murine genes with their human counterparts ("humanized" mice), or replacement of one gene family member with another member.

Three approaches have been used to develop knock-in transgenics. These include the "hit and run" or "in-out" strategy,[156,157] the "tag and exchange" approach,[158,159] and recombinase-mediated cassette exchange (RMCE).[160,161] All involve two rounds of recombination within embryonic stem cells and selection steps to identify ES clones with the appropriate genetic composition. The unifying theme is the use of targeting vectors containing positive and negative selection cassettes, such as the neomycin resistance and HSV-TK genes previously described for a traditional knockout targeting vector. In contrast to the traditional targeting cassette that contains the negative selectable marker (HSV-TK) outside the region targeted for recombination, both cassettes are placed within the targeted region of the locus. In addition to the selection cassettes, a mutant form (typically with a point mutation) of the targeted allele is present in the targeting vector. The vectors are introduced into the ES cells, which then undergo selection for the presence of the neomycin resistance gene by growth in G418 containing media. The "tag and exchange" and "in-out" approaches then require the addition of another vector or intrachromosomal recombination, respectively, for production of the desired mutant allele. Owing to their inefficiency and labor intensive nature, both approaches have been replaced by recombinase-mediated cassette exchange (RMCE; Fig. 5-7) and will not be discussed further in this chapter. RMCE involves modification of the targeting construct to contain *loxP* sequences flanking the selection cassettes. Following selection for the presence of the neomycin resistance gene with G418, ES cells are genetically screened for the presence of the targeting vector within the desired location in the genome. Once homologous recombinants are identified, they are transiently transfected with a vector that expresses the Cre recombinase. The Cre recombinase will excise any sequence residing between the *loxP* sites, that is, the selection cassettes. Following transfection, growth in ganciclovir is used to select cells that have lost the HSV-TK cassette. This ultimately results in the modest modification of the targeted allele with nearly complete absence of sequences from the selection cassette. Only a single *loxP* sequence remains. The vector can be constructed such that this remaining sequence resides in an intron, minimizing its impact on the targeted allele.

The Cre recombinase-mediated approach for constructing knock-ins was first used to evaluate regulatory regions of the IgH locus[160] immediately followed by the development of mice that express humanized antibodies.[161] Since that time, a number of knock-in mouse strains have been constructed. This approach has many advantages over traditional transgenics, which overexpress a gene of interest. These include maintenance of appropriate expression patterns of the gene (because the mutant form of the gene is under control of the endogenous promoter) as well as permitting analyses of function on a genetic background deficient for the wild-type gene.[162-166] In addition, complete replacement of related genes can be performed, which permit expression of one gene

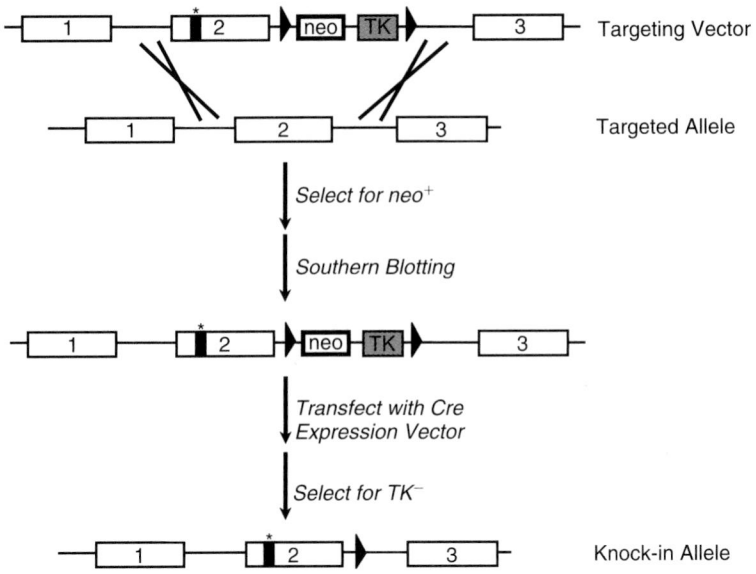

Figure 5-7 Recombinase-mediated cassette exchange (RMCE) to construct knock-in mice. A targeting vector is constructed as in Figure 5-5 with modifications. In this case, the positive (neo) and negative (HSKTK) selectable markers are in the same position in a region that does not disrupt the targeted gene. These are flanked *by loxP* sequences for later removal of the selection cassettes. A point mutation is placed in the desired position of the targeted gene (*asterisk*). Following transfection into ES cells, the cells are selected for growth on G418, indicating that the cells have integrated the targeting vector. Clones of ES cells are then screened by Southern blotting to identify those that have undergone homologous recombination. These cells are then transfected with a Cre expression vector and screened for growth on ganciclovir. Only those cells that have lost the selection cassette will grow. These cells are then used for injection into blastocysts.

family member under control of another family member's promoter regulatory region.[167–169] Last, "humanized" mice have been developed that harbor the human form of a specific gene in the murine locus.[170–172]

THE IMPORTANCE OF GENETICS

Although the production and analysis of transgenic and knockout/knock-in mice has revolutionized our ability to assess the functional roles of individual genes within complex organisms, one last caveat should be considered whenever interpretations regarding phenotypic consequences are made using such models. Specifically, the complex genetic nature of such organisms can contribute to the phenotypes observed and, in some cases, can actually be the underlying cause of a particular phenotype. It has long been acknowledged that phenotypes of knockout mice represent the combination of phenotypes due to the loss of the targeted gene as well as any compensatory changes that may have occurred as a result of the gene disruption. Hence, phenotypes are ultimately due to the overall genetic composition of the animals. As a result, the same genetic disruption in two distinct inbred strains of mice can cause vastly disparate phenotypes due to the differences in genetic background that harbor the disrupted gene. This was first reported when mice deficient for the epidermal growth factor receptor (EGFR) were developed by using targeted disruption (i.e., knockout) techniques. Mice that lack a functional EGFR allele displayed a wide range of phenotypes that depended on the genetic strain of mice used for propagation of the line and production of null animals.[173,174]

Thanks to individuals like Clarence Cook Little, many inbred strains of mice are available for use. The unique features of the various strains have been beneficial for the development of model systems of human disease and have facilitated identification of the genetic basis of a host of phenotypic traits; however, the sheer abundance of distinct strains has also led to the introduction of genetic complexity into the realm of transgenic/knockout technology. Transgenic mice are usually constructed in F1 hybrid strains such as C57BL/6 X SJL owing to the ability of hybrid embryos to withstand the pronuclear injection procedure. In contrast, production of knockout animals typically occurs in the 129 strain, since it is the source of easily manipulated ES cell lines. Given the low fecundity of the 129 strain, the disrupted allele is usually moved into another genetic background, such as C57BL/6, to facilitate production of a line of animals. As a result, most transgenic and knockout animals exist in hybrid mouse strains. Use of multiple strains

generates two confounding issues that must be kept in mind when interpreting data: epistasis and "hitchhiking" genes.

EPISTASIS

Although nontransgenic littermates are often considered genetically matched with their transgenic counterparts, this is generally not the case when using hybrid strains. When transgenic or knockout mice from one strain are crossed with another strain, the resultant F1 progeny are genetically identical and heterozygous at each gene, with one allele for each gene being derived from the newly introduced strain. In the case of a heterozygous knockout strain, the progeny are then intercrossed to generate homozygous null animals. As a result of meiotic recombination, subsequent progeny display considerable genetic diversity; each gene is represented by alleles from one, the other, or both strains of mice. Many of these alleles may contribute to the phenotype of the transgenic/knockout mice. The interaction of multiple genes to generate a unique phenotype is known as epistasis. Care must be used in the interpretation of phenotypes from genetically manipulated mice. While it is tempting to conclude that the observed phenotype is the sole consequence of the targeted genetic manipulation, it is more accurate to suggest that the phenotype is a combinatorial consequence of the genetic background as well as the genetic manipulation. Indeed, phenotypes of genetically manipulated mice can vary dramatically depending on the mouse strain.[173–177] The issues of genetic background influences on the phenotype of knockout mice can be minimized by producing congenic mice through many consecutive backcrosses with the mouse strain of choice. As a result, most genes will be identical among the knockout and control animals, thereby minimizing the contributions of numerous, unique genetic backgrounds to the phenotype. It is important to note that while genetic background can be considered a confounding variable, these differences can also be used as an avenue to identify and clone "modifier" genes: those genes that affect the ultimate phenotypic consequence of the original genetic manipulation. Identifying modifier genes generates considerable novel insight into the mechanisms involved in establishment of the phenotype.[178–180]

HITCHHIKING GENES

Even when congenic strains of mice are developed, the genes flanking the integration site of the transgene or the site of homologous recombination will seldom undergo recombination resulting in linkage disequilibrium. That is, the DNA sequences that are in close proximity to the transgene or targeted allele will correspond to the parental strain of mice used for the original genetic manipulation. Even after 12 generations of backcrossing, approximately 1% of the genome will correspond to the parental alleles. Depending on the density of genes surrounding the integration site, hundreds of genes could have the allelic configuration of the parental strain.[177,181] These genes are known as "hitchhiking" genes because they are carried along with the integration site through each subsequent generation.[181] It is important to note that these genes could have a profound impact on the phenotype of the resultant animal. In the extreme case, the phenotype of resulting mice could be due simply to placing these allelic variants into the background of the congenic strain and have nothing to do with the transgene or knockout allele.[182]

Avoiding the issue of "hitchhiking" genes in transgenic mice is relatively simple: Multiple lines of mice can be generated, each with a unique integration site. If the phenotype is consistent across all integration sites, it is due to the transgene. Addressing this issue in knockout animals is more difficult. Several approaches have been suggested, which range in level of difficulty and expense.[176,177,181] One obvious approach is to test Koch's postulate directly: If disruption of a gene causes a phenotype, can the phenotype be reversed by replacing the gene? In this case, transgenic mice are made that express the gene in all cell types. These mice are then bred with the knockout strain. If the transgene rescues the phenotype, hitchhiking genes are not responsible. Alternatively, control mice can be constructed that have a genetic marker inserted into the same position as the targeting construct. The marker would be developed in a way that it would not disrupt the endogenous gene. In this case, the phenotypes of the null mice would then be compared to the marker-containing mice. Any differences in phenotypes would then be attributable to the null allele. Last, and most economical, is the development of conditional knockout animals, in which the gene is disrupted only upon induction of a recombinase. In this case, mice with and without excision of the allele can be compared. A phenotypic change would again be attributable to the null allele rather than to the integration site.

SUMMARY

The development and use of transgenic and knockout animals permit the assessment of gene function in whole animal systems. These technologies have revolutionized our interpretations of biologic functions of hundreds of genes and will continue to reveal novel pathways and functions. It is now feasible to perform many cell biologic studies in mice that were once possible only in cell culture systems. With this expanded capability, the numbers of genetically manipulated mice continue to rise at an exponential rate, making formation of appropriate databases for cataloguing the phenotypes of these animals essential. The Jackson Laboratory has generated such a database (Tbase). This is complemented by efforts of the NIH with the Online Inheritance in Man (OMIM) database. We anticipate that in the coming years, continued transgenic research will lead to unprecedented growth in our understanding of mammalian genetics and biology, revealing novel insights into human development and disease.

Acknowledgment
The author would like to thank Erin L. Milliken, Jonathan D. Mosley, and John H. Nilson for thoughtful discussions regarding the content of this chapter.

REFERENCES

1. Crow JF: C.C. Little, cancer, and inbred mice. Genetics 161:1357–1361, 2002.
2. Gordon JW, Scangos GA, Plotkin DJ, et al: Genetic transformation of mouse embryos by microinjection of purified DNA. Proc Natl Acad Sci U S A 77:7380–7384, 1980.
3. Brinster RL, Chen HY, Trumbauer ME, et al: Somatic expression of herpes thymidine kinase in mice following injection of a fusion gene into eggs. Cell 27:223–231, 1981.
4. Constantini F, Lacy E: Introduction of a rabbit β-globin gene into the mouse germ line. Nature 294:92–94, 1981.
5. Wagner TE, Hoppe PC, Jollick JD, et al: Microinjection of a rabbit b-globin gene in zygotes and its subsequent expression in adult mice and their offspring. Proc Natl Acad Sci U S A 78:6376–6380, 1981.
6. Wagner EF, Stewart TA, Mintz B: The human β-globin gene and a functional thymidine kinase gene in developing mice. Proc Natl Acad Sci U S A 78:5016–5020, 1981.
7. Gordon JW, Ruddle FH: Integration and stable germ line transmission of genes injected into mouse pronuclei. Science 214:1244–1246, 1981.
8. Stewart TA, Wagner EF, Mintz B: Human β-globin gene sequences injected into mouse eggs, retained in adults, and transmitted to progeny. Science 217:1046–1048, 1982.
9. Palmiter RD, Chen HY, Brinster RL: Differential regulation of metallothionein-thymidine kinase fusion genes in transgenic mice and their offspring. Cell 29:701–710, 1982.
10. Brinster RL, Allen JM, Behringer RR, et al: Introns increase transcriptional efficiency in transgenic mice. Proc Natl Acad Sci U S A 85:836–840, 1988.
11. Choi T, Huang M, Gorman C, Jaenisch R: A generic intron increases gene expression in transgenic mice. Mol Cell Biol 11:3070–3074, 1991.
12. Kriegler M: Assembly of enhancers, promoters, and splice signals to control expression of transferred genes. Methods Enzymol 185:512–527, 1990.
13. Lozano G, Levine AJ: Tissue-specific expression of p53 in transgenic mice is regulated by intron sequences. Mol Carcinog 4:3–9, 1991.
14. Palmiter RD, Sandgren EP, Avarbock MR, et al: Heterologous introns can enhance expression of transgenes in mice. Proc Natl Acad Sci U S A 88:478–482, 1991.
15. Whitelaw CB, Archibald AL, Harris S, et al: Targeting expression to the mammary gland: Intronic sequences can enhance the efficiency of gene expression in transgenic mice. Transgenic Res 1:3–13, 1991.
16. Palmiter RD, Brinster RL: Germ line transformation of mice. Ann Rev Genet 20:465–499, 1986.
17. Palmiter RD, Brinster RL: Transgenic Mice. Cell 41:343–345, 1985.
18. Bronson SK, Plaehn EG, Kluckman KD, et al: Single-copy transgenic mice with chosen site integration. Proc Natl Acad Sci U S A 93:9067–9072, 1996.
19. Cvetkovic B, Yang B, Williamson RA, Sigmund CD: Appropriate tissue- and cell-specific expression of a single copy human angiotensinogen transgene specifically targeted upstream of the HPRT locus by homologous recombination. J Biol Chem 275:1073–1078, 2000.
20. Evans V, Hatzopoulos A, Aird WC, et al: Targeting the Hprt locus in mice reveals differential regulation of Tie2 gene expression in the endothelium. Physiol Genomics 2:67–75, 2000.
21. Wallace H, Ansell R, Clark J, McWhir J: Preselection of integration site imparts repeatable transgene expression. Nucleic Acids Res 28:1455–1464, 2000.
22. Zhan H-C, Liu D-P, Liang C-C: Insulator: from chromatin domain boundary to gene regulation. Hum Genet 109:471–478, 2001.
23. Potts W, Tucker D, Wood H, Martin C: Chicken beta-globin 5'HS4 insulators to reduce variability in transgenic founder mice. Biochem Biophys Res Comm 273:1015–1018, 2000.
24. Guglielmi L, LeBert M, Truffinet V, et al: Insulators to improve the expression of a 3(')IgH LCR-driven reporter gene in transgenic mouse models. Biochem

Biophys Res Comm 307:466–467, 2003.

25. Frazar TF, Weisbein JL, Anderson SM, et al: Variegated expression from the murine band 3 (AE1) promoter in transgenic mice is associated with mRNA transcript initiation at upstream start sites and can be suppressed by the addition of the chicken beta-globin 5′ HS4 insulator element. Mol Cell Biol 23:4753–4763, 2003.

26. Meisler MH: Insertional mutation of "classical" and novel genes in transgenic mice. Trends Genet 8:341–349, 1992.

27. Friedrich G, Soriano P: Promoter traps in embryonic stem cells: A genetic screen to identify and mutate developmental genes in mice. Genes Dev 5:1513–1523, 1991.

28. Hansen J, Floss T, Van Sloun P, et al: A large-scale gene-driven mutagenesis approach for the functional analysis of the mouse genome. Proc Natl Acad Sci U S A 100:9918–9922, 2003.

29. von Melchner H, DeGregori JV, Rayburn H, et al: Selective disruption of genes expressed in totipotent embryonal stem cells. Genes Dev 6:919–927, 1992.

30. Stanford WL, Cohn JB, Cordes SP: Gene-trap mutagenesis: Past, present and beyond. Nat Rev Genet 2:756–768, 2001.

31. Evans MJ: Gene trapping: A preface. Dev Dyn 212:167–169, 1998.

32. Cecconi F, Meyer BI: Gene trap: A way to identify novel genes and unravel their biological function. FEBS Lett 480:63–71, 2000.

33. Swift GH, Hammer RE, MacDonald RJ, Brinster RL: Tissue-specific expression of the rat pancreatic elastase I gene in transgenic mice. Cell 38:639–646, 1984.

34. Townes TM, Lingrel JB, Chen HY, et al: Erythroid-specific expression of human beta-globin genes in transgenic mice. EMBO J 4:1715–1723, 1985.

35. Khillan JS, Schmidt A, Overbeek PA, et al: Developmental and tissue-specific expression directed by the alpha 2 type I collagen promoter in transgenic mice. Proc Natl Acad Sci U S A 83:725–729, 1986.

36. Overbeek PA, Chepelinsky AB, Khillan JS, et al: Lens-specific expression and developmental regulation of bacterial chloramphenicol acetyltransferase gene driven by the murine alpha A-crystallin promoter in transgenic mice. Proc Natl Acad Sci U S A 82:7815–7819, 1985.

37. Ornitz DM, Palmiter RD, Hammer RE, et al: Specific expression of an elastase-human growth hormone fusion gene in pancreatic acinar cells of transgenic mice. Nature 313:600–602, 1985.

38. Quirk CC, Lozada KL, Keri RA, Nilson JH: A single Pitx1 binding site is essential for activity of the LHb promoter in transgenic mice. Mol Endocrinol 15:734–746, 2001.

39. Graves RA, Tontonoz P, Ross SR, Spiegelman BM: Identification of a potent adipocyte-specific enhancer: Involvement of an NF-1-like factor. Genes Dev 5:428–437, 1991.

40. Ross SR, Graves RA, Greenstein A, et al: A fat-specific enhancer is the primary determinant of gene expression for adipocyte P2 in vivo. Proc Natl Acad Sci U S A 87:9590–9584, 1990.

41. Halmekyto M, Alhonen L, Wahlfors J, et al: Position-independent, aberrant expression of the human ornithine decarboxylase gene in transgenic mice. Biochem Biophys Res Comm 180:262–267, 1991.

42. Forrester WC, Fernandez LA, Grosschedl R: Nuclear matrix attachment regions antagonize methylation-dependent repression of long-range enhancer-promoter interactions. Genes Dev 13:3003–3014, 1999.

43. Ray MK, Magdaleno SW, Finegold MJ, DeMayo F: cis-acting elements involved in the regulatio of mouse Clara cell-specific 10-kDa protein gene: In vitro and in vivo analysis. J Biol Chem 270:2689–2694, 1995.

44. Cakouros D, Cockerill PN, Bert AG, et al: A NF-kB/Sp1 region is essential for chromatin remodeling and correct transcription of a human granulocyte-macrophage colony-stimulating factor transgene. J Immunol 167:302–310, 2001.

45. Bennani-Baiti IM, Asa SL, Song D, et al: DNase I hypersensitive sites I and II of the human growth hormone locus control region are a major developmental activator of somatotrope gene expression. Proc Natl Acad Sci U S A 95:10655–10660, 1998.

46. Palmiter RD, Brinster RL, Hammer RE, et al: Dramatic growth of mice that develop from eggs microinjected with metallothionein-growth hormone fusion genes. Nature 300:611–615, 1982.

47. Palmiter RD, Norstedt G, Gelinas RE, et al: Metallothionein-human GH fusion genes stimulate growth of mice. Science 222:809–814, 1983.

48. Bartke A, Chandrashekar V, Turyn C, et al: Effects of growth hormone overexpression and growth hormone resistance on neuroendocrine and reproductive functions in transgenic and knock-out mice. Proc Soc Exp Biol Med 222:113–123, 1999.

49. Hadjantonakis AK, Nagy A: The color of mice: in the light of GFP-variant reporters. Histochem Cell Biol 115:49–58, 2001.

50. Chiocchetti A, Tolosano E, Hirsch E, et al: Green fluorescent protein as a reporter of gene expression in transgenic mice. Biochim Biophys Acta 1352:193–202, 1997.

51. Hadjantonakis A-K, Dickinson ME, Fraser SE, Papaioannou VE: Technicolor transgenics: Imaging tools for functional genomics in the mouse. Nat Rev Genet 4:613–625, 2003.

52. Takada T, Iida K, Awaji T, et al: Selective production of transgenic mice using green fluorescent protein as a marker. Nat Biotechnol 15:458–461, 1997.

53. Ikawa M, Kominami K, Yoshimura Y, et al: A rapid and non-invasive selection of transgenic embryos before implantation using green fluorescent protein (GFP). FEBS Lett 375:125–128, 1995.

54. Ciana P, Di Luccio G, Belcredito S, et al: Engineering of a mouse for the in vivo profiling of estrogen receptor activity. Mol Endocrinol 15:1104–1113, 2001.

55. Nagel SC, Hagelbarger JL, McDonnell DP: Development of an ER action mouse for the study of estrogens, selective ER modulators (SERMs), and xenobiotics. Endocrinol 142:4721–4728, 2001.

56. Ciana P, Raviscioni M, Mussi P, et al: In vivo imaging of transcriptionally active estrogen receptors. Nat Med 9:82–86, 2003.

57. Balkan W, Colbert M, Bock C, Linney E: Transgenic indicator mice for studying activated retinoic acid receptors during development. Proc Natl Acad Sci U S A 89:3347–3351, 1992.

58. Impey A, Smith DM, Obrietan K, et al: Stimulation of cAMP response element (CRE)-mediated transcription during contextual learning. Nat Neurosci 1:595–601, 1998.

59. Schmidt-Ullrich R, Memet S, Lilienbaum A, et al: NF-kB activity in transgenic mice: developmental regulation and tissue specificity. Development 122:2117–2128, 1996.

60. DasGupta R, Fuchs E: Multiple roles for activated LEF/TCF transcription complexes during hair follicle development and differentiation. Development 126:4557–4568, 1999.

61. Contag CH, Bachmann MH: Advances in in vivo bioluminescence imaging of gene expression. Annu Rev Biomed Eng 4:235–260, 2002.

62. Carlson H, Moskaug JO, Fromm SH, Blomhoff R: In vivo imaging of NF-kB activity. J Immunol 168:1441–1446, 2002.

63. Vooijs M, Jonkers J, Lyons S, Berns A: Noninvasive imaging of spontaneous retinoblastoma pathway-dependent tumors in mice. Cancer Res 62:1862–1867, 2002.

64. Laxman B, Hall DE, Bhojani MS, et al: Noninvasive real-time imaging of apoptosis. Proc Natl Acad Sci U S A 99:16551–16555, 2002.

65. Yamaizumi M, Mekada E, Uchida T, Okada Y: One molecule of diptheria toxin fragment A introduced into a cell can kill the cell. Cell 15:245–250, 1978.

66. Palmiter RD, Behringer RR, Quaife CJ, et al: Cell lineage ablation in transgenic mice by cell-specific expression of a toxin gene. Cell 50:435–443, 1987.

67. Behringer RR, Mathews LS, Palmiter RD, Brinster RL: Dwarf mice produced by genetic ablation of growth hormone-expressing cells. Genes Dev 2:453–461, 1988.

68. Herrera P–L, Huarte J, Zufferey R, et al: Ablation of islet endocrine cells by targeted expression of hormone-promoter-driven toxigenes. Proc Natl Acad Sci U S A 91:12999–13003, 1994.

69. Ross SR, Graves RA, Spiegelman BM: Targeted expression of a toxin gene to

adipose tissue: Transgenic mice resistant to obesity. Genes Dev 7:1318–1324, 1993.

70. Lowell BB, S-Susulic V, Hamann A, et al: Development of obesity in transgenic mice after genetic ablation of brown adipose tissue. Nature 366:740–742, 1993.

71. Burrows HL, Birkmeier TS, Seasholtz AF, Camper SA: Targeted ablation of cells in the pituitary primordia of transgenic mice. Mol Endocrinol 10:1467–1477, 1996.

72. Kendall SK, Saunders TL, Jin L, et al: Targeted ablation of pituitary gonadotropes in transgenic mice. Mol Endocrinol 5:2025–2036, 1991.

73. Kendall SK, Samuelson LC, Saunders TL, et al: Targeted disruption of the pituitary glycoprotein hormone alpha-subunit produces hypogonadal and hypothyroid mice. Genes Dev 9:2007–2019, 1995.

74. Palmiter R: Interrogation by toxin. Nat Biotechnol 19:731–732, 2001.

75. Heyman RA, Borrelli E, Lesley J, et al: Thymidine kinase obliteration: creation of transgenic mice with controlled immune deficiency. Proc Natl Acad Sci U S A 86:2698–2702, 1989.

76. Zhou Y, Unterweld EM, Ho A, et al: Ablation of pituitary pro-opiomelaocortin (POMC) cells produces alterations in hypothalamic POMC mRNA levels and midbrain mu opiod receptor binding in a conditional transgenic mouse model. J Neuroendocrinol 13:808–817, 2001.

77. Allen RG, Carey C, Parker JD, et al: Targeted ablation of pituitary pre-proopiomelanocortin cells by herpes simplex virus-1 thymidine kinase differentially regulates mRNA encoding the adrenocorticotropin receptor and aldosterone synthase in the mouse adrenal gland. Mol Endocrinol 9:1005–1016, 1995.

78. Markkula M, Kananen K, Paukku T, et al: Induced ablation of gonadotropins in transgenic mice expressing Herpes simplex virus thymidine kinase under the FSH b-subunit promoter. Mol Cell Endocrinol 108:1–9, 1995.

79. Wallace H, Ledent C, Vassart G, et al: Specific ablation of thyroid follicle cells in adult transgenic mice. Endocrinology 129:3217–3226, 1991.

80. Rindi G, Ratineau C, Ronco A, et al: Targeted ablation of secretin-producing cells in transgenic mice reveals a common differentiation pathway with multiple enteroendocrine cell lineages in the small intestine. Development 126:4149–4156, 1999.

81. Mikola MK, Rahman NA, Paukku TH, et al: Gonadal tumors of mice double transgenic for inhibin-alpha promoter-driven simian virus 40 T-antigen and herpes simplex virus thymidine kinase are sensitive to ganciclovir treatment. J Endocrinol 170:79–90, 2001.

82. Braun RE, Lo D, Pinkert CA, et al: Infertility in male transgenic mice: Disruption of sperm development by HSV-tk expression in postmeiotic germ cells. Biol Reprod 43:684–693, 1990.

83. Saito M, Iwawaki T, Taya C, et al: Diphtheria toxin receptor-mediated conditional and targeted cell ablation in transgenic mice. Nat Biotechnol 19:746–750, 2001.

84. Lee P, Morley G, Huang Q, et al: Conditional lineage ablation to model human diseases. Proc Natl Acad Sci U S A 95:11371–11376, 1998.

85. Kobayashi K, Morita S, Sawada H, et al: Immunotoxin-mediated conditional disruption of specific neurons in transgenic mice. Proc Natl Acad Sci U S A 92:1132–1136, 1995.

86. Brinster RL, Chen HY, Messing A, et al: Transgenic mice harboring SV40 T-antigen genes develop characteristic brain tumors. Cell 37:367–379, 1984.

87. Stewart TA, Pattengale PK, Leder P: Spontaneous mammary adenocarcinomas in transgenic mice that carry and express MTV/myc fusion genes. Cell 38:627–637, 1984.

88. Hanahan D: Heritable formation of pancreatic beta-cell tumours in transgenic mice expressing recombinant insulin/simian virus 40 oncogenes. Nature 315:115–122, 1985.

89. Mellon SH, Miller WL, Bair SR, et al: Steroidogenic adrenocortical cell lines produced by genetically targeted tumorigenesis in transgenic mice. Mol Endocrinol 8:97–108, 1994.

90. Greenberg N, DeMayo F, Finegold MJ, et al: Prostate cancer in a transgenic mouse. Proc Natl Acad Sci U S A 92:3439–3443, 1995.

91. Tzeng YJ, Guhl E, Graessmann M, Graessmann A: Breast cancer formation in transgenic animals induced by the whey acidic protein SV40 T antigen (WAP-SV-T) hybrid gene. Oncogene 8:1965–1971, 1993.

92. Ledent C, Dumont J, Vassar G, Parmentier M: Thyroid adenocarcinomas secondary to tissue-specific expression of simian virus-40 large T-antigen in transgenic mice. Endocrinology 129:1391–1401, 1991.

93. Kananen K, Markkula M, Rainio E, et al: Gonadal tumorigenesis in transgenic mice bearing the mouse inhibin alpha-subunit promoter/simian virus T-antigen fusion gene: Characterization of ovarian tumors and establishment of gonadotropin-responsive granulosa cell lines. Mol Endocrinol 9:616–627, 1995.

94. Windle JJ, Weiner RI, Mellon PL: Cell lines of the pituitary gonadotrope lineage derived by targeted oncogenesis in transgenic mice. Mol Endocrinol 4:597–603, 1990.

95. Lew D, Brady H, Klausing K, et al: GHF-1-promoter-targeted immortalization of a somatotrophic progenitor cell results in dwarfism in transgenic mice. Genes Dev 7:683–693, 1993.

96. Alarid ET, Windle JJ, Whyte DB, Mellon PL: Immortalization of pituitary cells at discrete stages of development by directed oncogenesis in transgenic mice. Development 122:3319–3329, 1996.

97. Jat PS, Noble MD, Ataliotis P, et al: Direct derivation of conditionally immortal cell lines from an H-2Kb-tsA58 transgenic mouse. Proc Natl Acad Sci U S A 88:5096–5100, 1991.

98. Shimshek DR, Kim J, Hubner MR, et al: Codon-improved Cre recombinase (iCre) expression in the mouse. Genesis 32:19–26, 2002.

99. Rodriguez CI, Buccholz F, Galloway J, et al: High efficiency deleter mice show that FLPe is an alternative to Cre-loxP. Nat Genet 25:139–140, 2000.

100. Buchholz F, Angrand PO, Stewart AF: Improved properties of FLP recombinase evolved by cycling mutagenesis. Nat Biotechnol 16:657–662, 1998.

101. Ryding ADS, Sharp MGF, Mullins JJ: Conditional transgenic technologies. J Endocrinol 171:1–14, 2001.

102. Lakso M, Sauer B, Mosinger B Jr, et al: Targeted oncogene activation by site-specific recombination in transgenic mice. Proc Natl Acad Sci U S A 89:6232–6236, 1992.

103. Orban PC, Chui D, Marth JD: Tissue- and site-specific DNA recombination in transgenic mice. Proc Natl Acad Sci U S A 89:6861–6865, 1992.

104. Dymecki SM: Flp recombinase promotes site-specific DNA recombination in embryonic stem cells and transgenic mice. Proc Natl Acad Sci USA 93:6191–6196, 1996.

105. Sauer B: Inducible gene targeting in mice using the Cre/lox system. Methods 14:381–392, 1998.

106. Isaka F, Ishibashi M, Taki W, et al: Ectopic expression of the bHLH gene Math1 disturbs neural development. Eur J Neurosci 11:2582–2588, 1999.

107. Herrera PL, Orci L, Vassalli JD: Two transgenic approaches to define the cell lineages in endocrine pancreas development. Mol Cell Endocrinol 140:45–50, 1998.

108. Wagner KU, Boulanger CA, Henry MD, et al: An adjunct mammary epithelial cell population in parous females: Its role in functional adaptation and tissue renewal. Development 129:1377–1386, 2002.

109. Yamauchi Y, Abe K, Mantani A, et al: A novel transgenic technique that allows specific marking of the neural crest cell lineage in mice. Dev Biol 212:191–203, 1999.

110. Zinyk DL, Mercer EH, Harris E, et al: Fate mapping of the mouse midbrain-hindbrain constriction using a site-specific recombination system. Curr Biol 8:665–668, 1998.

111. Lewandowski M: Conditional control of gene expression in the mouse. Nature Rev Genet 2:743–755, 2001.

112. Saez E, No D, West A, Evans RM: Inducible gene expression in mammalian cells and transgenic mice. Curr Opin Biotechnol 8:608–616, 1997.

113. Furth PA, St-Onge L, Boger H, et al: Temporal control of gene expression in transgenic mice by a tetracycline-responsive promoter. Proc Natl Acad Sci USA 91:9302–9306, 1994.

114. Gossen M, Bujard H: Tight control of gene expression in mammalian cells by tetracycline-responsive promoters. Proc Natl Acad Sci U S A 89:5547–5551, 1992.

115. Gossen M, Freundlieb S, Bender G, et al: Transcriptional activation by tetracyclines in mammalian cells. Science 268:1766–1769, 1995.

116. No D, Yao TP, Evans RM: Ecdysone-inducible gene expression in mammalian cells and transgenic mice. Proc Natl Acad Sci U S A 3346:3351, 1996.

117. Wang XJ, Liefer KM, Tsai S, et al: Development of gene-switch transgenic mice that inducibly express transforming growth factor b1 in the epidermis. Proc Natl Acad Sci U S A 96:8483–8488, 1999.

118. Hasuwa H, Kaseda K, Einarsdottir T, Okabe M: Small interfering RNA and gene silencing in transgenic mice and rats. FEBS Lett 532:227–230, 2002.

119. Lenferink AEG, Magoon J, Pepin M-C, et al: Expression of a TGF-b type II receptor antisense RNA impairs TGF-b1 signaling in vitro and promotes mammary gland differentiation in vivo. Int J Cancer 107:919–928, 2003.

120. Shinagawa T, Ishii S: Generation of Ski-knockdown mice by expressing a long double-strand RNA from an RNA polymerase II promoter. Genes Dev 17:1340–1345, 2003.

121. Bradley A, Evans M, Kaufman MH, Robertson E: Formation of germ-line chimaeras from embryo-derived teratocarcinoma cell lines. Nature 309:255–256, 1984.

122. Evans MJ, Kaufman MH: Establishment in culture of pluripotential cells from mouse embryos. Nature 292:154–156, 1981.

123. Martin GR: Isolation of a pluripotent cell line from early mouse embryos cultured in medium conditioned by teratocarcinoma stem cells. Proc Natl Acad Sci U S A 78:7634–7638, 1981.

124. Koller BH, Hagemann LJ, Doetschman T, et al: Germ-line transmission of a planned alteration made in a hypoxanthine phosphoribosyltransferase gene by homologous recombination in embryonic stem cells. Proc Natl Acad Sci U S A 86:8927–8931, 1989.

125. Smithies O, Gregg RG, Boggs SS, et al: Insertion of DNA sequences into the human chromosomal beta-globin locus by homologous recombination. Nature 317:230–234, 1985.

126. Thomas KR, Capecchi MR: Site-directed mutagenesis by gene targeting in mouse embryo-derived stem cells. Cell 51:503–512, 1987.

127. Thompson S, Clarke AR, Pow AM, et al: Germ line transmission and expression of a corrected HPRT gene produced by gene targeting in embryonic stem cells. Cell 56:313–321, 1989.

128. Kuehn MR, Bradley A, Robertson EJ, Evans MJ: A potential animal model for Lesch-Nyhan syndrome through introduction of HPRT mutations into mice. Nature 326:295–298, 1987.

129. Capecchi MR: Altering the genome by homolgous recombination. Science 244:1288–1292, 1989.

130. Bronson SK, Smithies O: Altering mice by homologous recombination using embryonic stem cells. J Biol Chem 269:27155–27158, 1994.

131. Capecchi MR: The new mouse genetics: altering the genome by gene targeting. Trends Genet 5:70–76, 1989.

132. Mansour SL, Thomas KR, Capecchi MR: Disruption of the proto-oncogene int-2 in mouse embryo-derived stem cells: A general strategy for targeting mutations to non-selectable genes. Nature 336:348–352, 1988.

133. Hasty P, Rivera-Perez J, Bradley A: The length of homology required for gene targeting in embryonic stem cells. Mol Cell Biol 11:5586–5591, 1991.

134. Deng C, Capecchi MR: Reexamination of gene targeting frequency as a function of the extent of homology between the targeting vector and the target locus. Mol Cell Biol 12:3365–3371, 1992.

135. te Riele H, Maandag ER, Berns A: Highly efficient gene targeting in embryonic stem cells through homologous recombination with isogenic DNA constructs. Proc Natl Acad Sci U S A 89:5128–5132, 1992.

136. Hasty P, Rivera-Perez J, Chang C, Bradley A: Target frequency and integration pattern for insertion and replacement vectors in embryonic stem cells. Mol Cell Biol 11:4509–4517, 1991.

137. Muller U: Ten years of gene targeting: targeted mouse mutants, from vector design to phenotype analysis. Mech Dev 82:3–21, 1999.

138. Thomas KR, Deng C, Capecchi MR: High-fidelity gene targeting in embryonic stem cells by using sequence replacement vectors. Mol Cell Biol 12:2919–2923, 1992.

139. Galli-Taliadoros LA, Sedgwick JD, Wood SA, Korner H: Gene knock-out technology: A methodological overview for the interested novice. J Immunol Methods 181:1–15, 1995.

140. Longo L, Bygrave A, Grosveld FG, Pandolfi PP: The chromosome make-up of mouse embryonic stem cells is predictive of somatic and germ cell chimaerism. Transgenic Res 6:321–328, 1997.

141. Rani PU, Khillan JS: A simple and convenient method for preparing chimeric animals from embryonic stem (ES) cells. Transgenic Res 12:739–741, 2003.

142. Stewart CL: Production of chimeras between embryonic stem cells and embryos. Methods Enzymol 225:823–855, 1993.

143. Gu H, Marth JD, Orban PC, et al: Deletion of a DNA polymerase b-gene segment in T cells using cell type-specific gene targeting. Science 265:103–106, 1994.

144. Zhao L, Bakke M, Krimkevich Y, et al: Steroidogenic factor 1 (SF1) is essential for pituitary gonadotrope function. Development 128:147–154, 2001.

145. Vooijs M, Jonkers J, Berns A: A highly efficient ligand-regulated Cre recombinase mouse lines shows that LoxP recombination is position dependent. EMBO J 2:292–297, 2001.

146. Zhang Y, Riesterer C, Ayrall AM, et al: Inducible site-directed recombination in mouse embryonic stem cells. Nucleic Acids Res 15:543–548, 1996.

147. Wunderlich FT, Wildner H, Rajewsky K, Edenhofer F: New variants of inducible Cre recombinase: A novel mutant of Cre-PR fusion protein exhibits enhanced sensitivity and an expanded range of inducibility. Nucleic Acids Res 29:E47, 2001.

148. Brocard J, Feil R, Chambon P, Metzger D: A chimeric Cre recombinase inducible by synthetic, but not by natural ligands of the glucocorticoid receptor. Nucleic Acids Res 26:4086–4090, 1998.

149. Metzger D, Clifford J, Chiba H, Chambon P: Conditional site-specific recombination in mammalitan cells using a ligand-dependent chimeric Cre recombinase. Proc Natl Acad Sci U S A 92:6991–6995, 1995.

150. Pierson TM, Wang Y, DeMayo FJ, et al: Regulable expression of inhibin A in wild type and inhibin a null mice. Mol Endocrinol 14:1075–1085, 2000.

151. Feil R, Brocard J, Mascrez B, et al: Ligand-activated site-specific recombination in mice. Proc Natl Acad Sci U S A 93:10887–10890, 1996.

152. Kellendock C, Tronche F, Casanova E, et al: Inducible site-specific recombination in the brain. J Mol Biol 285:175–182, 1999.

153. Imai T, Jiang M, Chambon P, Metzger D: Impaired adipogenesis and lipolysis in the mouse upon selective ablation of the retinoid X receptor alpha mediated by a tamoxifen-inducible chimeric Cre recombinase (Cre-ERT2) in adipocytes. Proc Natl Acad Sci U S A 98:224–228, 2001.

154. Saam JR, Gordon JI: Inducible gene knock-outs in the small intestine and colonic epithelium. J Biol Chem 274:38071–38082, 1999.

155. Mucenski ML, Wert SE, Nation JM, et al: β-catenin is required for specification of proximal/distal cell fate during lung morphogenesis. J Biol Chem 278:40231–40238, 2003.

156. Hasty P, Ramirez-Solis R, Krumlauf R, Bradley A: Introduction of a subtle mutation into the Hox-2.6 locus in embryonic stem cells. Nature 350:243–246, 1991.

157. Valancius V, Smithies O: Testing an "in-out" targeting procedure for

making subtle genomic modifications in mouse embryonic stem cells. Mol Cell Biol 11:1402–1408, 1991.

158. Askew GR, Doetschman T, Lingrel JB: Site directed point mutations in embryonic stem cells: A: gene-targeting tag-and-exchange strategy. Mol Cell Biol 13:4115–4124, 1993.

159. Stacey A, Schnieke A, McWhir J, et al: Use of double replacement gene targeting to replace the murine a-lactalbumin gene with its human counterpart in embryonic stem cells and mice. Mol Cell Biol 14:1009–1016, 1994.

160. Gu H, Zou YR, Rajewsky K: Independent control of immunoglobulin switch recombination at individual switch regions evidenced through Cre-loxP-mediated gene targeting. Cell 73:1155–1164, 1993.

161. Zou YR, Muller W, Gu H, Rajewsky K: Cre-loxP-mediated gene replacement: a mouse strain producing humanized antibodies. Curr Biol 4:1099–1103, 1994.

162. Jakacka M, Ito M, Martinson F, et al: An estrogen receptor (ER)alpha deoxyribonucleic acid-binding domain knock-in mutation provides evidence for nonclassical ER pathway signaling in vivo. Mol Endocrinol 16:2188–2201, 2002.

163. Kissel H, Timokhina I, Hardy MP, et al: Point mutation in kit receptor tyrosine kinase reveals essential roles for kit signaling in spermatogenesis and oogenesis without affecting other kit responses. EMBO J 1312:1326, 2000.

164. Amsterdam A, Kannan K, Givol D, et al: Apoptosis of granulosa cells and female infertility in achodroplastic mice expressing mutant fibroblast growth factor receptor 3 G374R. Mol Endocrinol 15:1610–1623, 2001.

165. Sotillo R, Dubus P, Martin J, et al: Wide spectrum of tumors in knock-in mice carrying a Cdk4 protein insensitive to INK4 inhibitors. EMBO J 20:6637–6647, 2001.

166. Reichardt HM, Kaestner KH, Tuckermann J, et al: DNA binding of the glucocorticoid receptor is not essential for survival. Cell 93:531–541, 1998.

167. Alcolea S, Jarry-Guichard T, de Bakker J, et al: Replacement of connexin 40 by connexin 45 in the mouse: Impact on cardiac electrical conduction. Circ Res 94:100–109, 2004.

168. Geng Y, Whoriskey W, Park MY, et al: Rescue of cyclin D1 deficiency by knockin cyclin E. Cell 97:767–777, 1999.

169. Wang Y, Schnegelsberg PN, Dausman J, Jaenisch R: Functional redundancy of the muscle–specific transcription factors Myf5 and myogenin. Nature 379:823–825, 1996.

170. Kitamoto T, Nakamura K, Nakao K, et al: Humanized prion protein knock-in by Cre-induced site-specific recombination in mouse. Biochem Biophys Res Comm 222:742–747, 1996.

171. Moriguchi T, Motohashi H, Hosoya T, et al: Distinct response to dioxin in an arylhydrocarbon receptor (AHR)-humanized mouse. Proc Natl Acad Sci U S A 100:5652–5657, 2003.

172. Liu Z, Hergenhahn M, Schmeiser HH, et al: Human tumor p53 mutations are selected for in mouse embryonic fibrobalsts harboring a humanized p53 gene. Proc Natl Acad Sci U S A 101:2963–2968, 2004.

173. Threadgill DW, Dlugosz AA, Hansen LA, et al: Targeted disruption of mouse EGF receptor: Effect of genetic background on mutant phenotype. Science 269:230–234, 1995.

174. Sibilia M, Wagner EF: Strain-dependent epithelial defects in mice lacking the EGF receptor. Science 269:234–238, 1995.

175. Keri RA, Lozada KL, Abdul-Karim FW, Nadeau JHaNJH: Luteinizing hormone induction of ovarian tumors: Oligogenic differences between mouse strains dictates tumor disposition. Proc Natl Acad Sci U S A 97:383–387, 2000.

176. Lariviere WR, Chesler EJ, Mogil JS: Transgenic studies of pain and analgesia: Mutation or background genotype? J Pharm Exp Ther 297:467–473, 2001.

177. Lathe R: Mice, gene targeting and behavior: More than just genetic background. Trends Neurosci 19:183–186, 1996.

178. MacPhee M, Chepenik KP, Liddell RA, et al: The secretory phospholipase A2 gene is a candidate for the Mom1 locus, a major modifier of ApcMin-induced intestinal neoplasia. Cell 81:957–966, 1995.

179. Tang Y, McKinnon ML, Leong LM, et al: Genetic modifiers interact with maternal determinants in vascular development of Tgfb1$^{-/-}$ mice. Hum Mol Genet 12:1579–1589, 2003.

180. Hide T, Hatakeyama J, Kimura-Yoshida C, et al: Genetic modifiers of otocephalic phenotypes in Otx2 heterozygous mutant mice. Development 129:4347–4357, 2002.

181. Gerlai R: Gene-targeting studies of mammalian behavior: Is it the mutation of the background genotype? Trends Neurosci 19:177–181, 1996.

182. Kelly MA, Rubenstein M, Phillips TJ, et al: Locomotor activity in D2 dopamine receptor-deficient mice is determined by gene dosage, genetic background, and developmental adaptations. J Neurosci 18:3470–3479, 1998.

Applications of Genetics in Endocrinology

J. Larry Jameson and Peter Kopp

THE HUMAN GENOME

Coinciding with the 50th anniversary of the description of the DNA double helix by Watson and Crick in 1953, the Human Genome Project (HGP) completed the sequencing of the entire human genome in 2003.[1] Current efforts, often designated as "postgenomic" disciplines, are now increasingly focusing on functional genomics, that is, comprehensive analyses of gene transcripts (transcriptomics), the translated proteins (proteomics), and metabolites (metabolomics) (see Chapter 4).[2] In addition, the field of bioinformatics is undergoing a significant development with the aim of integrating data generated by functional genomics and developing a more comprehensive understanding of biologic processes (systems biology).[3]

Advances in molecular biology were essential for this impressive development in biologic sciences. Therefore, these concepts and techniques are key elements for an understanding of genetics, (patho)physiology, cell biology, and biochemistry, and a basic understanding of these approaches is therefore relevant for clinicians as well as scientists engaged in laboratory investigation. A recurring theme throughout this book is the synergism derived by combining information from traditional studies focusing on clinical pathophysiology with new insights from molecular biology. This is illustrated, for example, by inherited endocrine disorders like multiple endocrine neoplasia type 1 and 2 (MEN1 and -2) (see Chapters 191 and 192) or pseudohypoparathyroidism and its variants (see Chapter 82).

In addition to providing a new means for the diagnosis of inherited disorders, the identification of mutations in endocrine genes also enhances our understanding of pathophysiology.[4] Mutations have been described at multiple different steps in the pathways of hormone action. There are now examples of mutations in hormones themselves, hormone receptors, second messenger signaling pathways, and the transcription factors that transduce hormone signals. Genetic testing is available for a rapidly growing number of

monogenic disorders and one can predict continued rapid advances in this field.

With the completion of the human genome sequence, many aspects of gene cloning, which were covered in the previous edition of this chapter,[5] have lost their importance. Several comprehensive databases now provide easy access to nucleotide and polypeptide sequences. These electronic resources are linked to multiple other databases, and they contain tools for the analysis of sequences and structures. Published guidelines facilitate the use of these increasingly important and rapidly evolving databases (Table 6-1).[6]

The HGP was launched in 1990 and its impact on all areas of medicine, including endocrinology, is profound.[2,7–10] Due to the complexity and size of the human genome, which consists of about 3 billion base pairs (bp) of DNA per haploid genome contained in the 23 chromosomes, initial emphasis was placed on the development of genetic and physical maps. The *genetic map* localizes heritable traits or DNA markers relative to other loci on the same chromosome (Fig. 6-1). It is established by assessing how frequently two markers are inherited together, that is, *linked*, by linkage studies. Distances of the genetic map are expressed in recombination units (centimorgans, cM). One cM corresponds to a recombination frequency of 1% between two loci and corresponds to approximately 1 megabase pairs (Mb) of DNA. *Physical maps* indicate the position of a DNA sequence in absolute values (see Fig. 6-1). After cloning of DNA fragments, unique DNA sequences can serve as landmarks for arranging overlapping cloned DNA fragments in the same order as they occur in the genome. These overlapping clones allow the characterization of contiguous DNA sequences (*contigs*). This approach led to high-resolution physical maps by cloning the whole genome into overlapping fragments. The complete DNA sequence of each chromosome provides the highest resolution physical map. The human genome is estimated to contain about 30,000 to 40,000 *genes*. They account for about 15% of the whole genome. Much of the DNA does not encode expressed genes and is thought to be important for regulatory and structural functions (see Fig. 6-1). The number of genes is

Table 6-1 Selected Databases

Site	Content	URL
National Center for Biotechnology Information (NCBI)	Access to genomic databases, PubMed, OMIM Links to educational online resources Information for the use of genomic databases	*http://www.ncbi.nlm.nih.gov/*
Online Mendelian Inheritance in Man (OMIM)	Catalogue of human genetic disorders	*http://www.ncbi.nlm.nih.gov/omim/*
European Bioinformatics Institute (EBI)	Access to genomic databases and tools for the analysis of sequences and structures	*http://www.ebi.ac.uk*
National Human Genome Research Institute	Information about the human genome sequence, genomes of other organisms, and genomic research	*http://www.genome.gov/*
American College of Medical Genetics	Access to databases relevant for the diagnosis, treatment, and prevention of genetic disease	*http://www.acmg.net/*
GeneTests.GeneClinics	Directory of laboratories offering genetic testing	*http://www.genetests.org/*
National Organization for Rare Disorders	Catalogue of rare disorders, including clinical presentation, diagnostic evaluation, and treatment	*http://www.rarediseases.org/*

smaller than the original predictions of 70,000 to 100,000 genes, which were based on assumptions derived from protein diversity. This observation emphasizes that *alternative splicing* of genes and the use of alternative promoters are important mechanisms generating protein diversity (see Chapter 2).

From its very beginning, the development of ethical, legal, and social issues were important components of the HGP.[11]

The remarkably rapid discovery of new disease-causing genes and the advances in genetic testing continue to raise ethical and financial questions concerning the use of genetic techniques in medicine. For example, the discovery of the *BRCA1* and *BRCA2* genes, which predispose to breast and ovarian cancer, have enhanced our understanding of familial forms of these cancers. It remains unclear, however, how to use genetic testing in potentially affected individuals and

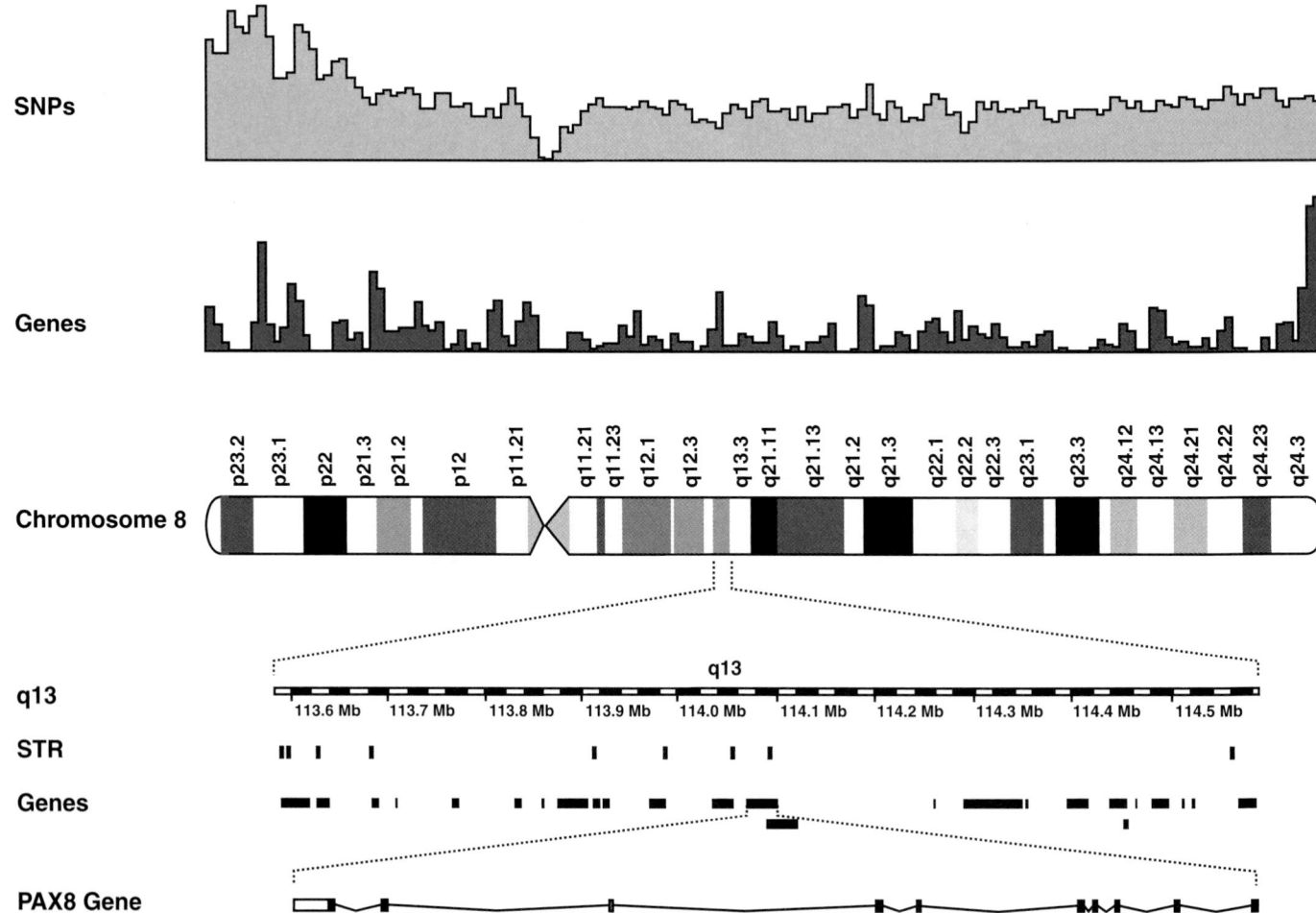

Figure 6-1 Genes and polymorphic marker density of chromosome 8. The relative numbers of genes and SNPs are shown above chromosome 8. The microsatellite markers (short tandem repeats, STRs) and genes located within band q13 are shown below the chromosome. SNPs and microsatellites are essential for linkage and association studies. The gene structure of one of the genes in band 13, the paired box transcription factor PAX8, indicates that it consists of 10 exons. Alternative splicing of these exons generates multiple variants of PAX8.

family members. Breast cancer is a common disease and mutations in the *BRCA* genes account for relatively few cases. Thus, the absence of mutation does not eliminate the risk of breast cancer and, at present, it remains unclear how the presence of a mutation should be used in patient management. Should prophylactic mastectomy be performed, or should genetically susceptible individuals only undergo more intensive screening? What are the implications for insurability, employment, childbearing, and interpersonal relationships? The answers to these questions require additional clinical investigation, further development of legislative policies to prevent discrimination, and greater availability of genetic counseling.[11] On the other hand, the discovery of the *MEN2* gene has provided a useful strategy for identifying affected individuals with this highly penetrant autosomal-dominant disorder. In this case, unaffected individuals can be spared screening for pheochromocytoma, medullary thyroid cancer, and hyperparathyroidism. In carriers of a *RET* gene mutation, prophylactic thyroidectomy in early childhood reduces the risk for development of medullary thyroid cancer (see Chapter 192). Thus, the discoveries resulting from the HGP are only the beginning of a much larger effort to apply this new information.

CATEGORIES OF GENETIC DISORDERS

Although many disorders are transmitted according to traditional Mendelian rules, it is now clear that a variety of different mechanisms can lead to genetic diseases (Table 6-2). Fundamental principles of genetic transmission are summarized briefly here, and additional information is available in other sources.[12-14]

Disorders of chromosome number or structure were among the first to be recognized because they can be detected using cytogenetic techniques. In endocrinology, disorders of the sex chromosomes including Klinefelter syndrome (XXY) and Turner's syndrome (XO) are particularly relevant.

Molecular cytogenetics, in particular the advent of fluorescent in situ hybridization (FISH), has led to the identification of more subtle chromosome abnormalities such as microdeletions. The inheritance of either two maternal or paternal chromosomes, so called *uniparental disomy*, can be associated with endocrine disorders if it involves an autosome that is imprinted (see later).

Mendelian disorders are caused by mutations in single genes. Information about many of these genetic disorders is available in the OMIM (Online Mendelian Inheritance in Man) database (see Table 6-1). The patterns of Mendelian transmission are now part of classical genetic teaching and include autosomal-recessive, autosomal-dominant, and X-linked disorders (Fig. 6-2). The transmission of genes or traits is typically depicted in family trees or pedigrees. Analysis of the pattern of transmission, particularly in large families with multiple generations, can be invaluable for predicting the mode of inheritance. This information is useful for genetic counseling and it often narrows the differential diagnosis, particularly when mutations in several different genes can give rise to similar phenotypes (nonallelic or locus heterogeneity). For example, neurohypophyseal diabetes insipidus caused by mutations in the *AVP-NPII* gene is typically transmitted as an autosomal disorder.[15] In rare cases, it can, however, be recessive.[16] The nephrogenic form of diabetes insipidus can be X-linked due to mutations in the AVPR2 receptor, whereas mutations in aquaporin 2 are associated with a recessive or a dominant inheritance.[17] For this reason, when dealing with a genetic disorder, it is important to obtain a detailed family history, often from several different family members. This information can then be combined with laboratory and genetic testing to arrive at an accurate diagnosis.

AUTOSOMAL-DOMINANT DISORDERS

Diseases inherited in an autosomal-dominant manner are typically characterized by the presence of one mutant allele and a normal allele on the other chromosome. A single mutant allele is sufficient to cause the disorder. In some instances, such as nonautoimmune familial hyperthyroidism, the gene is dominant because the mutations in the thyroid-stimulating hormone receptor (TSHR) are constitutively active[18] (see Chapter 111). In other cases, such as thyroid hormone resistance, the mutant gene acts in a dominant-negative manner to antagonize the function of the normal, wild-type gene[19,20] (see Chapter 114). Mutations in one allele may be associated with haploinsufficiency, a situation in which a single normal copy provides insufficient protein to assure normal function. Haploinsufficiency is a frequent mechanism of disease associated with mutations in transcription factors,[21] or rate-limiting enzymes.

In MEN1, a germ-line mutation in the tumor suppressor gene *menin* is transmitted in a dominant manner[22] (see Chapter 191). If the second allele is inactivated by a somatic mutation, this will lead to neoplastic growth (*Knudson hypothesis* or *two-hit model*). Whereas the defective allele in the germ line is transmitted in a dominant way, the tumorigenic mechanism results from a recessive loss of the tumor suppressor gene in affected tissues. Thus, the mechanisms by which genes act in a dominant manner are highly variable, even though they share similar features of transmission. In dominant disorders, the probability that an offspring will inherit the mutant gene is 50% and individuals can be affected in each generation (see Fig. 6-2A). The disease does not occur in the offspring of unaffected individuals. Males and females are affected with equal frequency.

AUTOSOMAL-RECESSIVE DISORDERS

In an autosomal-recessive disease, both parents of an affected individual are obligate heterozygotes (see Fig. 6-2B). The affected individual, who can be of either sex, can be homozygous

Table 6-2 Mechanisms of Transmission of Genetic Endocrine Diseases

Transmission	Example of Endocrine Disorder	
	Gene	Disorder
Chromosomal	XXY Multiple genes	Klinefelter syndrome
Autosomal recessive	CYP21 (21-hydroxylase)	Congenital adrenal hyperplasia
Autosomal dominant	CASR (Calcium-sensing receptor)	Familial benign hypocalciuric hypercalcemia
X-linked	KAL1 (Kallmann)	Kallmann's syndrome
Y-linked	SRY (Testis determining factor)	XY sex-reversal
Autosomal-dominant Knudson two-hit model	MEN1 (Menin)	Multiple endocrine neoplasia type 1
Mitochondrial	tRNA (Leu-UUR)	Diabetes-deafness syndrome
Mosaic	GNAS1 (G$_s$α)	McCune-Albright syndrome
Somatic	TSHR (TSH receptor)	Autonomous thyroid nodules
Imprinting	GNAS1 (G$_s$α)	Albright hereditary osteodystrophy
Multigenic	Multiple genes	Type 2 diabetes mellitus

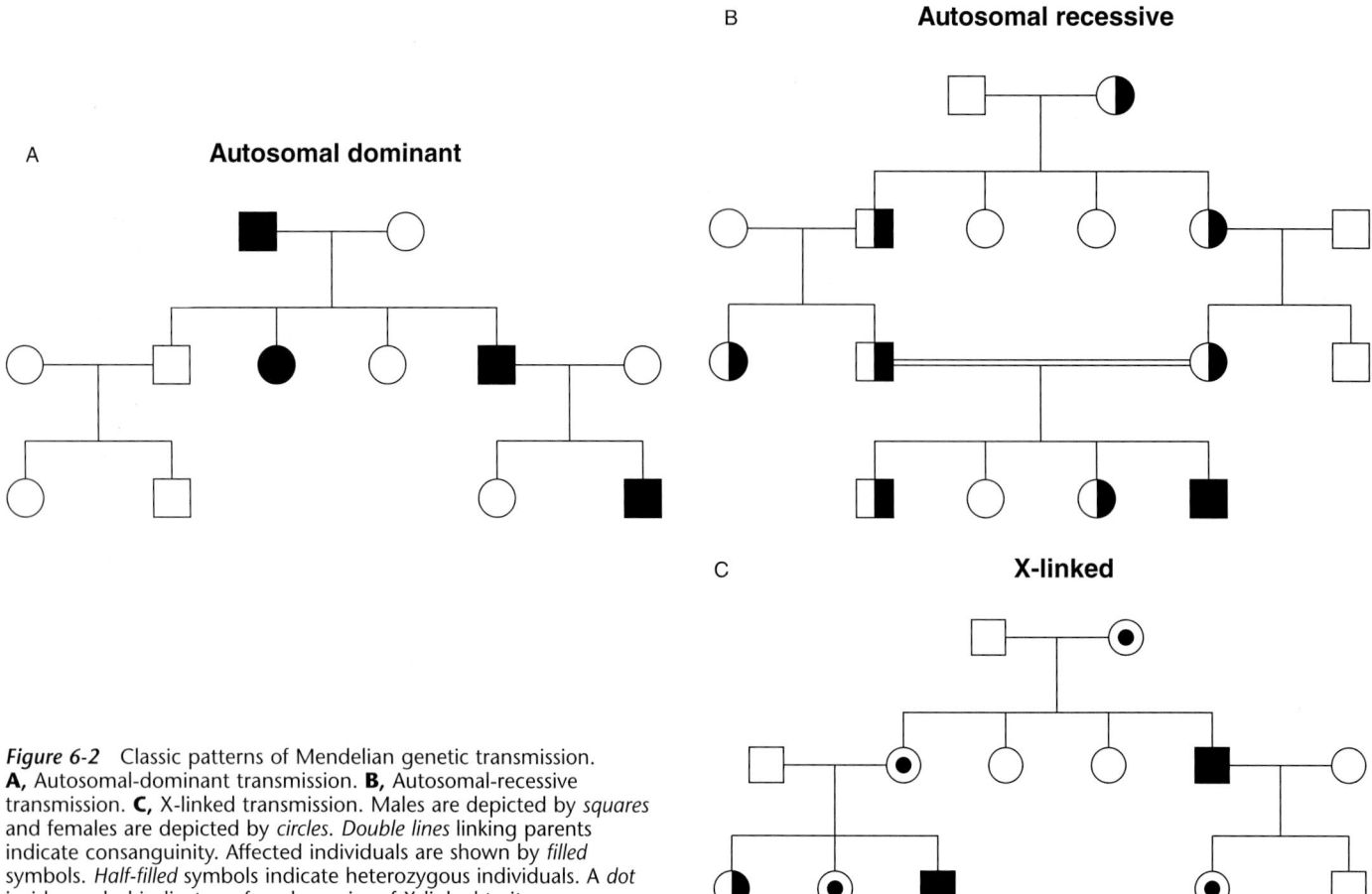

Figure 6-2 Classic patterns of Mendelian genetic transmission. **A,** Autosomal-dominant transmission. **B,** Autosomal-recessive transmission. **C,** X-linked transmission. Males are depicted by *squares* and females are depicted by *circles*. *Double lines* linking parents indicate consanguinity. Affected individuals are shown by *filled symbols*. *Half-filled symbols* indicate heterozygous individuals. A *dot* inside symbol indicates a female carrier of X-linked traits.

(inherit two copies of the same mutation) or inherit distinct mutations in each copy of the gene (compound heterozygote). Heterozygous carriers of a defective gene do not usually display phenotypic features of the disease. When both parents are heterozygous for a mutation, their offspring have a 25% chance of inheriting a normal genotype, a 50% probability of a heterozygous state, and a 25% risk of disease. If one parent is heterozygous and one is homozygous, the probability of disease increases to 50% for each child and the pedigree analysis may mimic that of autosomal-dominant inheritance (*pseudodominance*). Most cases of homozygous mutations occur in situations of parental consanguinity or in isolated populations in which the gene pool is small. The likelihood of compound heterozygous mutations depends on the gene frequency in the population for each of the mutations, which is usually very low. Congenital adrenal hyperplasia caused by mutations in 21-hydroxylase is representative of autosomal-recessive disorders (see Chapter 124). There are many distinct mutations in the *21-hydroxylase* gene (*CYP21*), and the prevalence of these mutations is high enough ($\approx$1/100 in most populations) that it is not unlikely for unrelated parents to be heterozygous. As a result, a child that inherits two distinct mutations in 21-hydroxylase will be affected with the disorder. Depending on the degree to which the mutation affects enzyme function, a range of phenotypic severity can be seen in different individuals.

X-LINKED DISORDERS

A daughter always inherits her father's X chromosome together with one of the two maternal X chromosomes. A son inherits one of the maternal X chromosomes and the Y chromosome from his father. Thus, there is no father-to-son transmission in X-linked inheritance and all daughters of an affected male are obligate carriers of the mutant allele (see Fig. 6-2C). Because males have only one X chromosome, they are hemizygous for a mutant allele, and are therefore more likely to develop the mutant phenotype. In females, the expression of X-chromosomal genes is influenced by X-chromosome inactivation, which leads to random inactivation of most genes on one of the two copies. Occasionally, predominant X-inactivation of the normal allele can result in a partial phenotype in females carrying an X-lined trait, for example, nephrogenic diabetes insipidus caused by AVPR2 mutations.[17]

Several endocrine disorders including Kallmann's syndrome, adrenal hypoplasia congenita, adrenal leukodystrophy, nephrogenic diabetes insipidus, androgen insensitivity, and hypophosphatemic vitamin D–resistant rickets are transmitted in an X-linked manner. As expected from the aforementioned mechanism of X-linked transmission, these disorders are much more common in males than females.

Y-LINKED DISORDERS

Only a few genes are known on the Y chromosome and there are few Y-linked disorders. One of the Y-chromosomal genes, the sex-region determining Y gene (SRY), which encodes the testis-determining factor (TDF), can cause XY sex-reversal when mutated.[23] Alternatively, translocation of the SRY gene to the X chromosome can cause an XX male phenotype. Another group of genes on the Y chromosome includes the highly repetitive *DAZ* genes that are important for spermatogenesis. (Micro)deletions of these genes, often transmitted as a new germ-line mutation, are an important cause of azoospermia and male infertility.[24,25]

RELATIONSHIP BETWEEN GENOTYPE AND PHENOTYPE IN GENETIC DISORDERS

Variations in the clinical phenotype in inherited disorders are common and can be explained by various mechanisms. *Allelic heterogeneity* indicates that multiple different mutations can occur in the same gene. In some instances there is a clear genotype-phenotype correlation between a specific allele and the phenotype. Certain mutations can completely inactivate a protein, whereas others retain partial function. For example, the phenotype of androgen insensitivity includes a wide spectrum of disorders that ranges from severe resistance and testicular feminization to partial resistance in Reifenstein syndrome.[26] Allelic heterogeneity is often a problem for genetic testing because it requires one to examine the entire gene to exclude a mutation definitively.

Nonallelic or *locus heterogeneity* designates a situation in which a similar disease phenotype results from mutations in different genes. For example, the nephrogenic forms of diabetes insipidus can be caused by mutations in the X-chromosomal AVPR2 receptor gene, whereas mutations in the aquaporin 2 (AQP2) gene cause either autosomal-recessive or -dominant nephrogenic diabetes insipidus.[17] Nonallelic heterogeneity can pose problems for genetic testing since different genes may have to be considered along with the possibility of allelic heterogeneity in each of the candidate genes.

A phenotype not caused by inheritance of a mutated gene that is identical or similar to a genetic trait is called a *phenocopy*. For example, goiter may be the consequence of defects in thyroid hormone synthesis or it can be the consequence of nutritional iodide deficiency.[27]

Sometimes there are marked phenotypic differences in individuals carrying the same mutation. If some individuals harboring the mutation fail to express the phenotype, the trait is said to display *incomplete penetrance. Expressivity* is used to describe the phenotypic spectrum in the individuals with the disorder. Expressivity is thus dependent on penetrance. The phenotypic variation leading to incomplete penetrance and variable expressivity can be explained by environmental factors, modifier genes, or gender. Incomplete penetrance in some individuals leads to skipping of generations and can confound pedigree analysis. Variable expressivity and penetrance illustrate that genetic and/or environmental factors may influence "simple" Mendelian traits, as well as playing a role in complex genetic disorders that involve multiple genes. This has practical relevance for genetic counseling, because one cannot always predict the course of disease, even when the mutation is known.

Aside from mutations in the sex chromosomes, some diseases are expressed in a sex-limited manner because of the differential function of the gene product in males and females. For example, gain-of-function mutations in the luteinizing hormone (LH) receptor cause dominant male-limited precocious puberty in boys because activation of the receptor induces testosterone production in the testis, whereas it is functionally silent in the immature ovary.[28]

VARIATIONS IN SIMPLE MENDELIAN INHERITANCE PATTERNS

Many diseases display a familial clustering without having a clear pattern of classical Mendelian inheritance (see Table 6-2). This applies to the *complex disorders*, which underlie the pathogenesis of many congenital defects and major healthcare problems such as type 2 diabetes mellitus, hypertension, obesity, osteoporosis, heart disease, and psychiatric disorders.

These disorders are thought to involve multiple different genes, each of which contributes partially to the disease phenotype. Since the contribution of any one of these genes is usually relatively weak, they are difficult to localize using classical genetic linkage approaches in large pedigrees. Therefore, the genetic analysis of complex disorders often relies, at least initially, on large population-based *association* studies.[29,30] In this approach, one can search for genetic variants that occur with increased frequency in affected individuals. Alternatively, one can search for genetic variants that occur more often in affected sib-pairs versus the population at large. These analyses are challenging because of the large number of individuals who need to be studied (several hundreds to thousands). In addition, the entire genome must be searched for candidate genetic markers associated with the disease. Since many different genes (and environmental events) contribute to the pathogenesis of these disorders, this type of gene search is most successful when one can identify specific sub-phenotypes that are likely to be caused by a relatively small number of genes. The sib-pair approach has been used successfully for the identification of genetic loci associated with type 1 diabetes mellitus.[30] Although several different genes confer some degree of risk, the major histocompatibility locus on chromosome 6 is a particularly strong risk factor that predisposes to this and other autoimmune diseases.[30,31]

Each mitochondrion contains several copies of a circular chromosome, which encodes proteins that are part of the respiratory chain, and transfer and ribosomal RNAs. The mitochondrial genome does not recombine and is transmitted exclusively through the maternal line, as all mitochondria reside within the oocyte cytoplasm. Thus, mitochondrial disorders are only transmitted from mother to offspring, and males and females are affected equally. Mitochondrial disorders typically have complex clinical features that often involve muscle and brain because of the high dependence of these tissues on oxidative phosphorylation. Moreover, these disorders often have endocrine manifestations. For example, the maternally transmitted diabetes-deafness syndrome is due to mutations in the mitochondrial gene encoding the tRNA for leucine.[32]

In addition to the inactivation of one of the two X chromosomes in females (X-inactivation), gene inactivation also occurs on selected chromosomal regions of autosomes.[33] This phenomenon, referred to as *genomic imprinting*, leads to preferential expression of an allele depending on its parental origin and can influence the expression of certain genetic diseases. The classical example involves the Prader-Willi syndrome and the Angelman's syndrome, which are caused by genes located on the short arm of chromosome 15. In the Prader-Willi syndrome, deletions are found exclusively on the paternally derived chromosome. Alternatively, Prader-Willi syndrome may be caused by the inheritance of two maternal copies of chromosome 15, that is, maternal uniparental disomy 15. In contrast, patients with Angelman's syndrome have deletions in the same region of chromosome 15, but they occur only on the maternally derived chromosome, or they have paternal uniparental disomy 15.[34] Genomic imprinting is also involved in the various clinical presentations associated with mutations in the *GNAS1* gene encoding the stimulatory $G_s\alpha$ subunit (see Chapter 82).[35,36] Heterozygous loss-of-function mutations in the *GNAS1* gene lead to Albright hereditary osteodystrophy (AHO). Paternal transmission of *GNAS1* mutations leads to the AHO phenotype alone (*pseudo*pseudohypoparathyroidism) (Fig. 6-3), whereas maternal transmission leads to AHO in combination with resistance to hormones such as parathyroid hormone (PTH), thyroid-stimulating hormone (TSH), and gonadotropins, all of which stimulate G protein 7 transmembrane receptors (pseudohypoparathyroidism type IA). These phenotypic differences are due to a tissue-specific imprinting of the *GNAS1* gene, which is expressed primarily from the maternal allele in

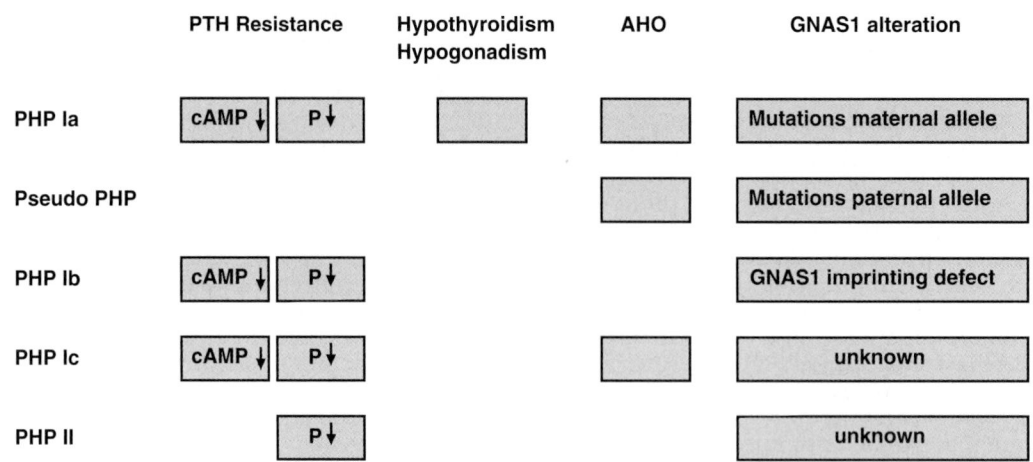

Figure 6-3 Effects of imprinting of the *GNAS1* gene. The *GNAS1* gene encodes the stimulatory $G_s\alpha$ subunit. Inactivating mutations cause Albright hereditary osteodystrophy (AHO). Maternal transmission leads to AHO in combination with resistance to hormones such as parathyroid hormone (PTH), thyroid-stimulating hormone (TSH), and gonadotropins, all of which stimulate G protein 7 transmembrane receptors (pseudohypoparathyroidism type IA, PHP IA). Paternal transmission of *GNAS1* mutations leads to the AHO phenotype alone (*pseudo*pseudohypoparathyroidism). These phenotypic differences are due to a tissue-specific imprinting of the *GNAS1* gene, which is expressed primarily from the maternal allele in tissues such as the thyroid, gonadtropes, and the proximal renal tubule. In most other tissues, the *GNAS1* gene is expressed biallelically. In patients with isolated renal resistance to PTH (PHP IB), an imprinting defect of the *GNAS1* gene results in decreased $G_s\alpha$ expression in the proximal renal tubules (see Ref. 36). The molecular basis of PHP IC and PHP II remain to be elucidated. cAMP, cyclic adenosine monophosphate; p, phosphorus.

tissues such as the thyroid, gonadtropes, and the proximal renal tubule. In most other tissues, the *GNAS1* gene is expressed biallelically. In patients with isolated renal resistance to PTH (pseudohypoparathyroidism type IB), an imprinting defect of the *GNAS1* gene results in decreased $G_s\alpha$ expression in the proximal renal tubules.[36]

Mosaicism refers to the presence of two or more cell lines in an individual that differ in their genotype. Mosaicism can result from a mutation that occurs during embryogenesis or later in development. The developmental stage at which the defect arises will determine whether germ cells or only somatic cells are involved. Somatic mosaicism is characterized by a patchy distribution of somatic cells containing a mutation. For example, activating mutations that occur in the $G_s\alpha$ subunit early in development cause the McCune-Albright syndrome.[37] The clinical phenotype, which can include ovarian cysts that secrete sex steroids and cause precocious puberty, polyostotic fibrous dysplasia, café-au-lait skin pigmentation, pituitary adenomas, and hypersecreting autonomous thyroid nodules, varies depending on the tissue distribution of the mutation.

Somatic mutations also play an important role in various forms of neoplasia.[38] When somatic mutations enhance cell proliferation or prolong cell survival, they can be associated with the clonal expansion of the cell population and the development of tumors. Activating mutations in the TSHR or $G_s\alpha$ can cause autonomously functioning thyroid nodules (see later). In inherited cancer syndromes in which the "first hit" has already been transmitted in the germ line, somatic mutations in the second allele of the involved tumor suppressor genes play an important role (two-hit model). Multiple endocrine neoplasia type 1 provides an example of such a disorder.

Trinucleotide repeats are found in several genes and their number varies among healthy individuals (polymorphic variants). For example, the number of CAG nucleotide repeats found in the first exon of the androgen receptor (AR) gene is lowest in African-Americans, intermediate in Caucasians, and highest in Asians.[39] An increase in the number of repeats above a certain critical threshold is associated, however, with the X-linked form of spinal and bulbar muscular atrophy, and

partial androgen resistance (SBMA or Kennedy syndrome).[40] Several other trinucleotide disorders are frequently associated with endocrine features. For example, male patients with dystrophia myotonica frequently present with hypogonadism,[41] and the risk for developing diabetes mellitus correlates with the length of the nucleotide repeat expansion in patients with Friedreich's ataxia.[42]

PRINCIPLES OF GENETIC LINKAGE AND ASSOCIATION

Genetic linkage refers to the fact that genes are physically attached to one another along the length of the chromosome. Consequently, two genes that are close together on a chromosome are usually transmitted together, unless a recombination event separates them. Recombination, which occurs during meiosis, is useful for purposes of mapping genes, because it provides a landmark that delineates borders for the location of a gene. The odds of a crossover, or recombination event, are proportionate to the distance that separates them. Thus, genes that are far apart are more likely to be separated by a recombination event than genes that are close together. These features make it possible, given large pedigrees or populations, to calculate the genetic distance between two genes. A centiMorgan (cM) is defined as a recombination frequency between two loci of 1% and corresponds to about 1 Mb of DNA (see Fig. 6-1).

Linkage is usually expressed as a logarithm of the odds (lod) score, which is a ratio that reflects the probability that the disease and marker loci are linked rather than unlinked.[43] Positive numbers favor linkage and negative scores support nonlinkage. Lod scores of +3 are generally accepted as supporting linkage, whereas a score of −2 is consistent with the absence of linkage. When candidate genetic regions have been identified by linkage, more detailed analyses can be performed using additional markers, or if the region is small enough, one can attempt to identify the disease gene among the many genes present within a particular locus.

The presence of polymorphic variation in DNA is essential for linkage studies. Genetic variation provides a means to distinguish the maternal and paternal chromosomes in an individual, as well as providing markers of different regions along the chromosomes. Historically, these polymorphisms consisted of restriction fragment length polymorphisms (RFLPs), in which nucleotide sequence variation altered the presence of specific restriction sites in DNA. Thus, when combined with Southern blot analysis, RFLPs allow one to track the transmission of genes within a pedigree. Although principles of RFLP analysis are useful for understanding disease transmission and gene mapping, the technique has been supplanted by other means of polymorphic analysis. In particular, short tandem repeats (STRs) or microsatellites, consisting of highly repetitive 2, 3, or 4 bp sequences, are now used for linkage studies (Fig. 6-4). The human genome project has generated high-density maps of STRs throughout the entire genome (see Fig. 6-1). The technique is performed using polymerase chain reaction (PCR) and can be automated. In a similar manner, maps of single nucleotide polymorphisms (SNPs) are also being generated. In addition to their greater frequency (≈1 in 300 bp), the SNPs are amenable to analyses using DNA chips, providing a promising means for rapid analysis of genetic variation and linkage.

An example of using STRs to examine linkage within a pedigree is shown in Figure 6-5. In this case, two heterozygous, related parents have transmitted an autosomal-recessive disorder. A series of STRs on the short arm of the chromosome are used to track transmission of this chromosomal region within the family. Note that a recombination event distinguishes the shared chromosomes (*b* and *c*) of the parents. Two of their children are affected with the disorder. A group of closely linked markers that are inherited together is referred to as a haplotype. They each inherit the *b/c* haplotype and are homozygous for the markers 115-134-122. Although this pattern does not prove linkage, it is consistent with a disease gene within this region of the chromosome. Additional studies would be necessary to confirm linkage in an expanded version of the pedigree or using other families with the same disorder.

Allelic association designates a significantly increased or decreased frequency of an allele with a disease. This can be due to a true biologic association or *linkage dysequilibrium*, that is, association due to close linkage. Association studies compare a population of affected individuals with a control population, for example, affected individuals and matched controls, or affected and unaffected siblings.[29] Allelic association studies are useful for identifying susceptibility genes in complex disorders. For example, association studies have revealed a role for the HLA region, the insulin VNTR (variable number of tandem repeats), and the *CTLA4* (cytotoxic T-lymphocyte associated 4) gene in diabetes mellitus type 1 (see Chapter 55). In diabetes mellitus type 2, associations have been established between a variant in PPAR-γs and the genes encoding the sulfonylurea receptor (SUR1, KIR6.2).[30]

METHODS USED TO DETECT GENE DELETIONS AND POINT MUTATIONS

Mutations, any change in the primary nucleotide sequence, are structurally diverse. They can affect one (point mutations) or a few nucleotides, consist of gross numeric or structural alterations in individual genes or chromosomes, or involve the entire genome. Mutations may be located in regulatory regions, introns, or exons. Point mutations occurring in the coding region may lead to amino acid substitutions (missense mutations), premature stop codons (nonsense mutation), or frameshifts, or they can be silent. Mutations in introns can introduce or destroy sequences that are important for proper splicing of the precursor RNA to the mature mRNA.

PCR Amplification

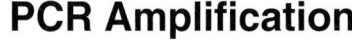

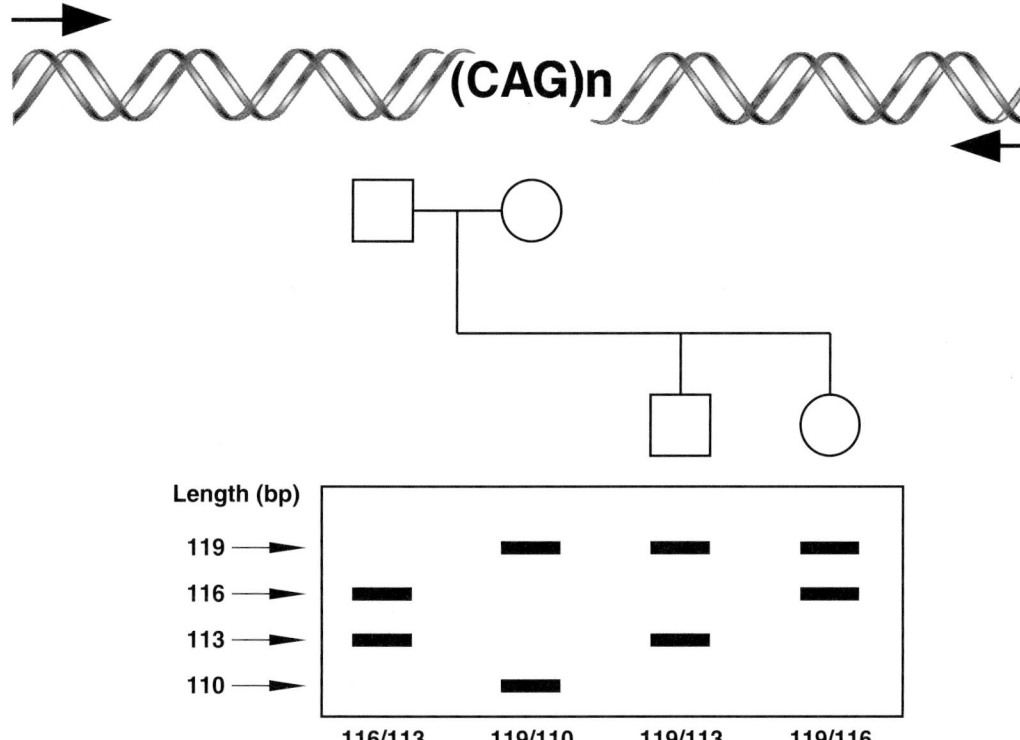

Figure 6-4 Polymerase chain reaction (PCR) amplification of polymorphic short tandem repeat markers. Polymorphic di-, tri-, and tetra-nucleotide short tandem repeats, or microsatellites, are common in the human genome. These regions are very useful for tracking chromosomal segregation within pedigrees and for mapping genes. If PCR primers are placed on either side of these repeats, the resulting fragments will vary in length, depending on the number of copies of the repeats. When an individual is heterozygous (the allele on each chromosome harbors a different number of repeats), two distinct PCR products are generated that can be resolved by electrophoresis. The genotype, at this locus, of each individual in the pedigree can therefore be determined based on the length of the marker they inherit.

Chromosome

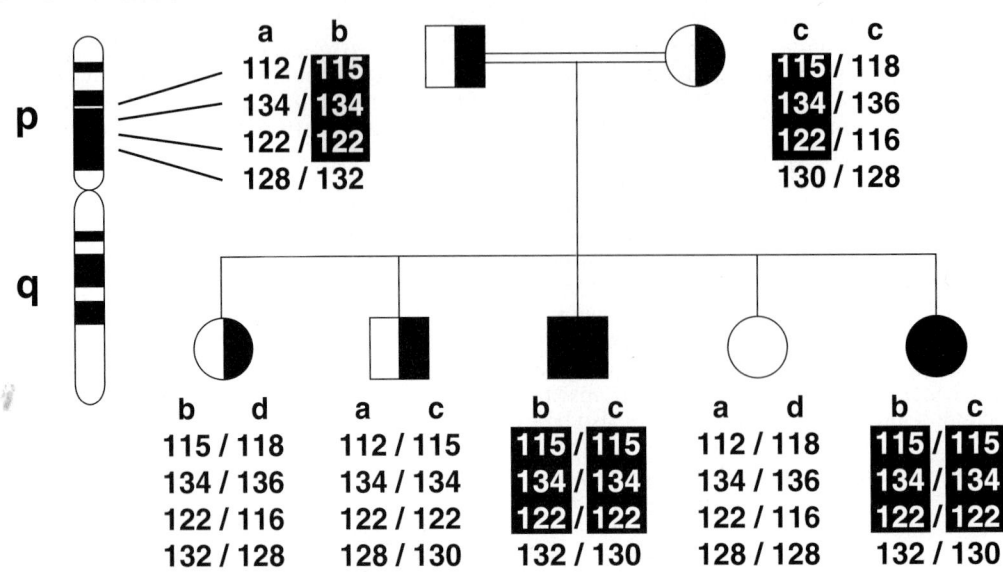

Figure 6-5 Linkage analysis using short tandem repeat markers. Short tandem repeats (STRs) can be used to track the transmission of genes within a pedigree (see Fig. 6-4). In the pedigree shown, two heterozygous parents, who are first cousins, have transmitted a disease gene to several progeny. A series of STR markers, located on the short arm (p) of a chromosome, are used to determine the haplotype of various members of the family. Note that the parents are heterozygous for most of the markers, but are homozygous for others (e.g., 134/134). Nevertheless, because a panel of markers is used, one can readily ascertain the pattern of chromosomal segregation. In addition, recombination events on the parental chromosome *b* and the maternal chromosome *c*, are apparent because their haplotypes differ between the third and fourth markers. Shaded regions indicate homozygous, shared haplotypes in the affected children. Although these data are not sufficient to prove linkage, they are consistent with this region of the genome being involved in the disease. Additional studies of this region in other pedigrees could be used to support, or refute, the possibility of linkage. Studies of additional families might also identify recombination events that would narrow the disease locus further, ultimately allowing the cloning of a responsible gene.

Recombinant DNA approaches that are used to investigate a particular disorder are usually based on clues derived from its clinical and pathophysiologic characteristics, which, in some cases, allow one to predict the gene that harbors a defect (Table 6-3). For example, it is reasonable to postulate that selective growth hormone (GH) deficiency in several members of a family might be due to a defect in the gene encoding GH,

GH releasing hormone (GHRH), or the GHRH receptor (GHRHR). In other cases, however, there are no obvious candidate genes. For example, in the multiple endocrine neoplasia syndromes, it was difficult to predict a gene that causes proliferation of selected lineages of endocrine cells. In this case, the most expeditious approach was to localize chromosomal regions carrying markers associated with the disease phenotype (see earlier). After candidate genes were identified, they could be analyzed for mutations in affected patients to verify that they cause the disorder. A summary of techniques that are used to identify different types of mutations are listed in Table 6-4.

USE OF SOUTHERN BLOTS TO ANALYZE GENE STRUCTURE

After identification of a disease gene, a number of different types of molecular techniques are available for defining specific mutations. To define the gross structure of the gene, a useful first approach is to use Southern blot analyses to detect large gene deletions or rearrangements (Fig. 6-6).[44] In this method, genomic DNA is digested with one or more restriction endonucleases creating an array of DNA fragments that are separated according to length using agarose gel electrophoresis. After transfer of the DNA fragments to a membrane, a radiolabeled probe that is specific for the gene of interest is hybridized to the DNA on the membrane. Under appropriate conditions of hybridization stringency, the probe will only detect the few DNA fragments that are complementary in sequence. Gene deletions would be detected as absent fragments or by fragments with reduced size. Gene rearrangements result in complex patterns of DNA fragments with increased and/or decreased lengths. If the gene appears to be intact when analyzed using multiple restriction enzymes, a single base mutation or a small deletion that alters the final

Table 6-3 Approach to Patient with a Suspected Genetic Disease
Detailed clinical characterization
Establish phenotypes and heterogeneity
Consider possible candidate genes based on phenotype
Are there major deletions or rearrangements?
Cytogenetics or FISH
Southern blot analyses
Disorders caused by an unknown gene
Linkage by short tandem repeats (STRs) or single nucleotide
polymorphisms (SNPs)
Cloning of candidate genes
Small deletions or point mutations
Screen for mutations by SSCP, DGGE, D-HPLC
Screen for mutations by direct DNA sequencing
Does the mutation alter a known function of the protein?
In vitro analyses of mutant proteins
In vivo and transgenic analyses of mutant proteins
Therapeutic implications
Genetic counseling
Other interventions based on nature of the mutation

DGGE, denaturing gradient gel electrophoresis; D-HPLC, denaturing high-performance liquid chromatography; SSCP, single-stranded conformational polymorphism.

Table 6-4 Molecular Genetic Diagnostic Procedures

Method	Gene Deletions	Gene Rearrangements	Loss of Heterozygosity	Linkage	Point Mutations
Cytogenetics		+	+		
FISH	+	+	+		
Southern blot	+	+			
RFLP			+	+	
VNTR			+	+	
PCR	+	+	+	+	+
Direct DNA sequencing					+
RNase cleavage					+
OSH					+
DGGE					+
SSCP					+
D-HPLC					+
Mass-spectrometry					+

DGGE, denaturing gradient gel electrophoresis; D-HPLC, denaturing high-performance liquid chromatography; FISH, fluorescent in situ hybridization; OSH, oligonucleotide specific hybridization; PCR, polymerase chain reaction; RFLP, restriction fragment length polymorphism; SSCP, single-stranded conformational polymorphism; VNTR, variable number tandem repeat.

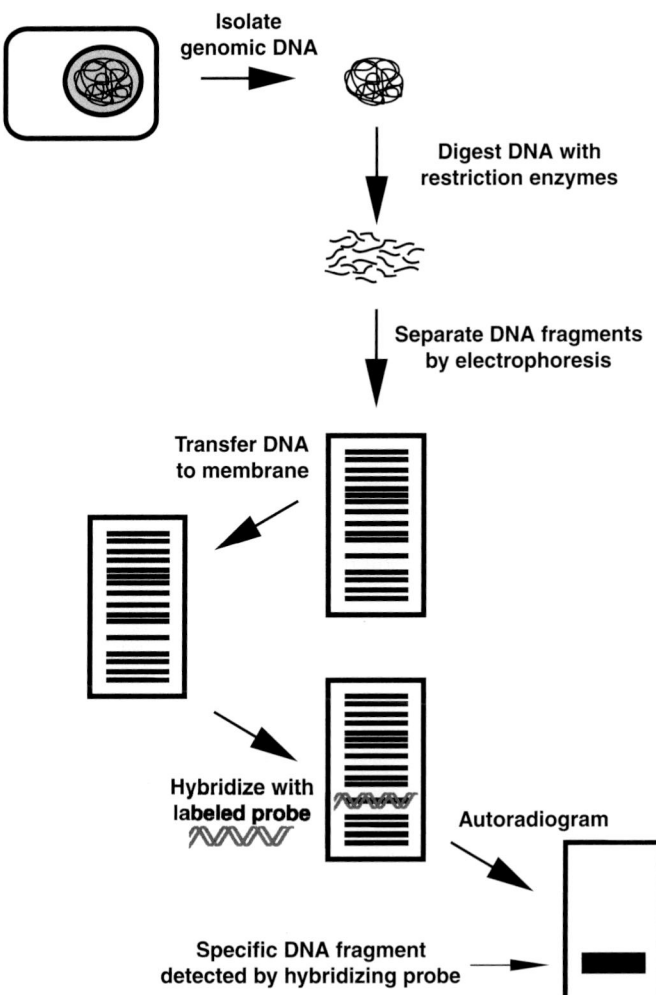

Figure 6-6 Southern blot method. The Southern blot is used to analyze gene structure. Genomic DNA is isolated and digested into an array of fragments using restriction enzymes. The DNA is separated according to length by agarose gel electrophoresis and transferred to a membrane. The immobilized DNA is hybridized with a radiolabeled probe, which only binds to its complementary sequence. Specific hybridizing bands are detected by autoradiography.

Labels in figure: Isolate genomic DNA; Digest DNA with restriction enzymes; Separate DNA fragments by electrophoresis; Transfer DNA to membrane; Hybridize with labeled probe; Autoradiogram; Specific DNA fragment detected by hybridizing probe

protein product is more likely than a gross alteration in gene structure.

THE POLYMERASE CHAIN REACTION AND DETECTION OF POINT MUTATIONS

The polymerase chain reaction (PCR) has greatly improved the efficiency of detecting single base changes by allowing rapid amplification and analyses of a particular gene or a portion of the gene (Fig. 6-7).[45] The PCR technique is a very powerful tool for molecular diagnostics for the following reasons. First, the dramatic amplification of DNA allows diagnostic analyses using very small amounts of initial starting tissue. Sufficient DNA for PCR is routinely extracted from lymphocytes or from cells present in saliva, hair, amniotic fluid, chorionic villi, or other accessible tissue sources. Second, because PCR uses short synthetic oligonucleotides to prime the reaction, it can be readily applied to any known sequence. PCR is also essential for linkage studies because highly polymorphic sequences (microsatellites and SNPs) can easily be amplified.[46]

In many cases, the PCR is the starting point for more detailed characterization of a mutation. In early studies to identify a specific mutation, the PCR product is often used for DNA sequencing to establish the location and base change that is present in the gene. Because the amount of DNA provided by PCR is relatively large, it is usually not difficult to subclone the amplified DNA fragment into a plasmid to allow subsequent DNA sequencing. Alternatively, automated DNA sequencing methods allow direct sequencing of the DNA fragment without an intervening subcloning step.[47] In addition, direct sequencing has the advantage that the sequence analysis is based on a large population of amplified DNA molecules rather than individual clones that may contain PCR-generated sequence errors (occur in ≈1/3000 bases). Direct DNA sequencing of the PCR product also has the advantage that a heterozygous mutation can be detected by the presence of two different nucleotides at the mutant position.

After characterization of specific mutations, several techniques allow more rapid screening for the mutation in other family members or patients. In some methods, the critical regions of a gene can be screened for mutations by detecting altered mobility during gel electrophoresis. In denaturing gradient gel electrophoresis (DGGE), the PCR primers contain a long stretch of Gs and Cs that anneal to create a "GC clamp."[48] In this manner, the double-stranded DNA can be partially melted during electrophoresis, but will be clamped at the end because of the relatively high melting temperature of G-C bonds (three hydrogen bonds for G-C versus two

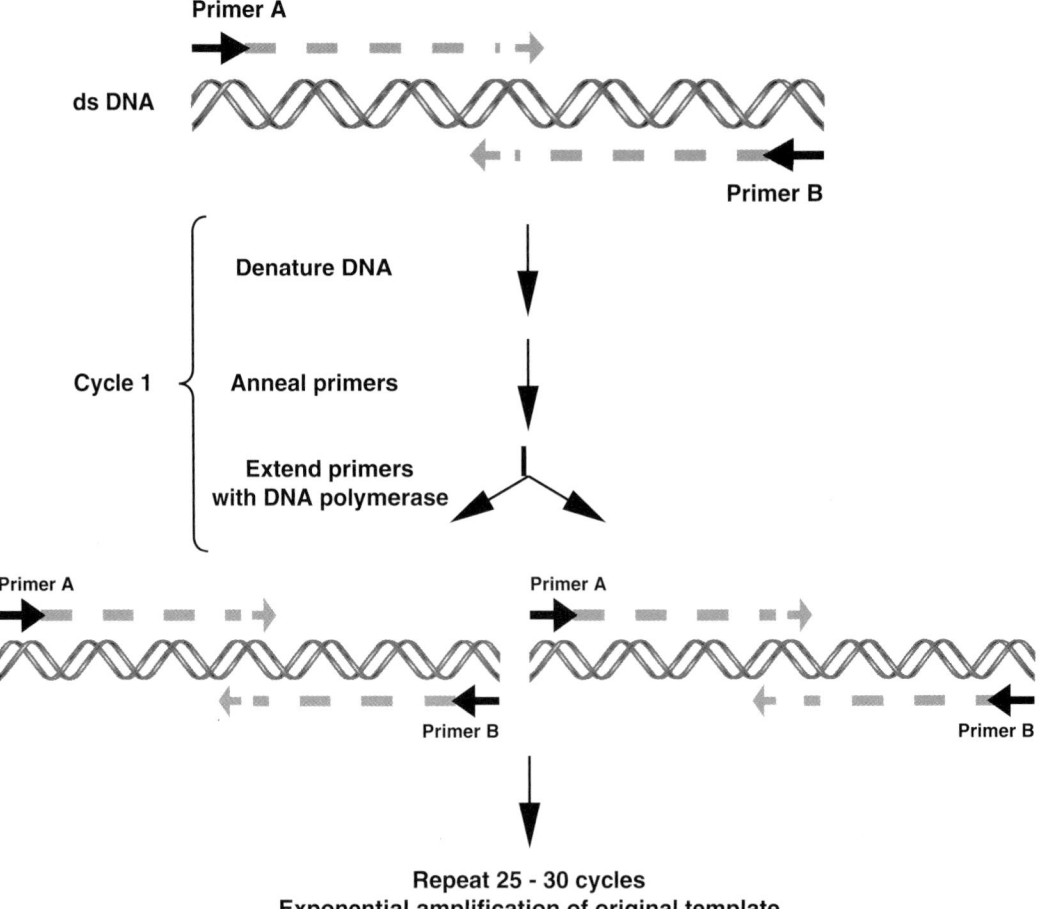

Figure 6-7 The polymerase chain reaction (PCR). In the initial cycle of PCR, the double-stranded DNA template is heat-denatured to allow primers A and B to anneal and initiate synthesis of a new copy of each strand of DNA. Because Taq polymerase is heat stable, the reaction mixture can be immediately subjected to another round of denaturation and new DNA synthesis. In each cycle of PCR, the number of DNA molecules is doubled, resulting in a rapid expansion in the amount of DNA as the cycle number progresses. In a typical reaction or 25 to 30 cycles, the amount of DNA is theoretically amplified by several million-fold. PCR has broad applications including DNA diagnostics from small amounts of tissue, quantitative mRNA analysis, cloning, construction of plasmids, and site-directed mutagenesis.

for A-T). Consequently, the GC clamp emphasizes differences in melting temperatures that result from sequence mismatches caused by mutations. If a mutation is present, a mismatch with the wild-type sequence lowers the melting point of the DNA hybrid resulting in strand separation and altered mobility in the gel. A similar technique, referred to as single-strand conformational polymorphism (SSCP), is based on the property that mutations will cause altered conformation and mobility of single-stranded DNA during nondenaturing electrophoresis.[49] Both DGGE and SSCP can be applied to PCR products to screen large regions of a gene for mutations or to screen large numbers of patients in separate reactions. At present, SSCP appears to be more readily applied to a wide array of sequences. Both of these methods require that the reaction conditions be established rigorously to avoid false-negative results. It should also be noted that polymorphisms appear as mutations until further characterized. Denaturing high-performance liquid chromatography (DHPLC) and mass-spectrometry technology is increasingly used for the detection of point mutations or SNPs, as well as small deletions and insertions.[50,51]

After a particular mutation has been identified, oligonucleotide specific hybridization (OSH) can be useful to establish whether this nucleotide change is present in other family members or in unrelated patients.[52] For example, specific mutations have been identified that cause constitutive activation of the guanosine triphosphate (GTP)-binding *ras* and $G_s\alpha$ proteins that are involved in cellular signaling. These mutations prevent GTP hydrolysis, which is necessary to inactivate signaling by these proteins. In the case of the *ras* genes (*H-ras, K-ras, N-ras*), mutations in two different regions of the proteins (codons 12/13 or codon 61) cause constitutive activation. Further adaptation of this hybridization technique

has led to the development of microarray DNA sequencing chips.[53]

Mutations often eliminate, or generate, restriction enzyme sites. Thus, another useful strategy for screening for specific mutations is to amplify the relevant region of a gene by PCR and then test the pattern of restriction enzyme digestion. If a mutation does not create a new restriction site, it is usually possible to generate a new site by inserting a base pair change in the PCR primer, near the mutation site, to create a unique digestion pattern. Because restriction enzymes are very specific and easy to use, this strategy is a powerful and inexpensive means to screen for known mutations. Lastly, if the specific mutation is known, allele-specific primers permit to amplify the wild-type and/or the mutant allele.

FUNCTIONAL STUDIES OF MUTANT HORMONES AND RECEPTORS

Identification of a DNA sequence alteration is not sufficient to establish that it is responsible for the disease phenotype. First, nucleotide substitutions could represent polymorphisms or DNA sequence variations that occur in the population as a whole. If the base change occurs in the coding sequence, but does not alter an amino acid, it is most likely a polymorphism. Occasionally, a seemingly silent mutation may affect mRNA stability or splicing mechanisms.[54] If a mutation results in an alteration of the amino acid sequence, it is still possible that the amino acid substitution is "physiologically silent" and doesn't significantly alter protein function. One approach for addressing the issue of polymorphisms is to screen a large number of normal individuals (e.g., 100) for the putative mutation. If the amino acid substitution is found in normal individuals, it is, by definition, a polymorphism, although it may have subtle functional consequences. Substitution of codons that are highly conserved across species (presumably implying functional importance) have a higher chance of being mutations than amino acids that are more variable in different species. Finally, mutations tend to be "linked" to the disease phenotype when examined in several family members, whereas polymorphisms should sort randomly unless they are located close to the disease locus. Although these determinations of polymorphisms are not entirely reliable, they are of practical importance because the next steps of assessing the functional importance of a "candidate mutation" can require significant experimental effort.

Assuming there is evidence against a polymorphism, it is almost always possible using recombinant techniques to assess the effect of a mutation in a functional assay. As illustrated in Figure 6-8, recombinant mutant and wild-type proteins can be expressed and subjected to a variety of functional assays. In the example shown, expression of mutant LH-β allows it to be assessed for its ability to form an α-β heterodimer, to undergo glycosylation, to bind to its receptor, and to activate receptor signaling pathways.[55] Mutant enzymes such as 21-hydroxylase can be analyzed for their ability to bind substrate or to carry out catalysis.[56] Mutant receptors like the insulin receptor have been subjected to an array of functional tests including insulin binding, receptor autophosphorylation, receptor internalization, and receptor stability.[57] Likewise, G protein–coupled receptors (GPCRs) containing activating or inactivating mutations can be tested for their

LHβ gene

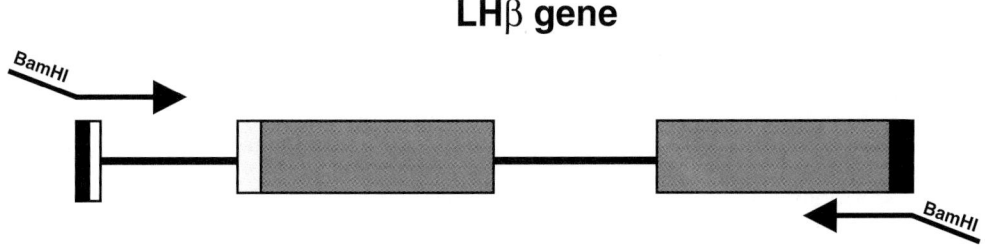

PCR amplify mutant and wild-type LHβ genes

Subclone into an eukaryotic expression vector

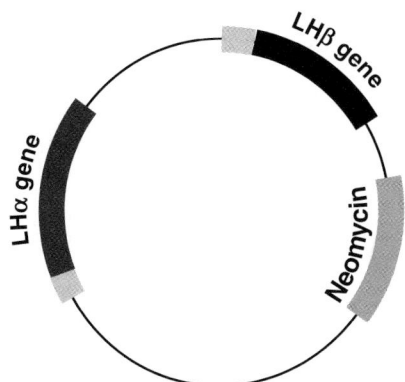

Transfect into eukaryotic cell lines

Select for Neomycin resistance

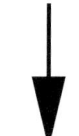

Assay recombinant LH
RIA
Bioassay
Structure-function

Figure 6-8 Expression of recombinant hormones to verify the biological effect of a mutation. The ability to express recombinant hormones or receptors is an important strategy for testing the effects of putative disease-causing mutations. A variety of expression systems are available including *E. coli*, baculovirus, vaccinia virus, and mammalian cells. The choice of expression system is dictated by a variety of issues including characteristics of the protein, desired production level, and the nature of the bioassay that will be used. A strategy for producing recombinant luteinizing hormone (LH) is illustrated for the purpose of analyzing the functional consequences of mutations in the *LH-β* gene (see Ref. 55). The *LH-β* gene is amplified by the polymerase chain reaction (PCR) from genomic DNA and inserted into a eukaryotic expression vector. The presence of a viral long terminal repeat (LTR) provides a strong promoter to drive expression in transfected mammalian cell lines. Because LH is a heterodimer containing an α and β subunit, the vector is designed to contain a copy of the α gene to allow the genes to be coexpressed from the same plasmid. A third gene encoding neomycin resistance allows selection and isolation of clonal cell lines that have been successfully transfected with the expression vector. Secreted LH can be analyzed by structural methods and for its functional properties. This approach allows delineation of hormone domains important for α-β subunit dimerization, receptor binding, and receptor activation. RIA, radioimmunoassay.

abilities to bind hormones and to signal through second messenger pathways.[18,28,58] Nuclear receptors, such as the thyroid hormone receptor, can be analyzed not only for their ability to bind thyroid hormone and DNA target sequences, but also for their capacity to function as transcription factors in transient gene expression assays.[59] These types of studies not only establish whether a given mutation is of functional importance, but also provide insight into protein structure-function and hormone action. In many instances, these "experiments of nature" provide rapid identification of critical functional domains because identification of the mutations is biased by the presence of a recognizable clinical phenotype.

OVERVIEW OF INHERITED ENDOCRINE DISORDERS

The technical aspects of the foregoing discussion of recombinant DNA methodology sometimes raise questions concerning how such techniques are useful to the practicing endocrinologist. In large measure, molecular biology has already transformed the practice of endocrinology and will continue to do so.[4] In addition to improving our understanding of hormone and receptor structure-function, these techniques have allowed the production of large quantities of recombinant insulin, growth hormone, gonadotropins, thyrotropin, and erythropoietin, among others. For many monogenic disorders, molecular testing is now available and has a growing impact on clinical management. The current

"postgenomic" disciplines will undoubtedly lead to the identification of unknown molecules involved in endocrine systems, and provide novel insights into metabolic networks.[60]

The presentation of a few "case studies" in the use of these procedures, coupled with an overview of recent progress in the molecular basis of endocrine diseases, emphasizes the impact and role of these methods in clinical practice.

Several hundred endocrine disorders exhibit an inheritance pattern suggestive of a primary gene defect (see OMIM database).[61,62] Gene mutations have now been identified in many of these disorders (Table 6-5). Some common themes emerge from the relatively small number of mutations that have been described to date. First, the phenotypic variability that characterizes many endocrine diseases is often reflected in genetic heterogeneity. Some clinical phenotypes that were previously thought to represent distinct diseases can now be interpreted as manifestations of different types of mutations within a single gene. For example, the clinical variants of congenital adrenal hyperplasia can be attributed to distinct mutations in 21-hydroxylase or other enzymes involved in steroid biosynthesis.[56] Second, the propensity of certain genes to be frequent targets for mutations may be explained in part by gene structure and organization. Genes such as *growth hormone* that have been duplicated to form gene clusters are predisposed to undergo recombination and deletion.[63,64] Third, although many of the mutations reported initially have been associated with severely affected patients, it is now obvious that mutations with less severe consequences can result in a

Table 6-5 Examples of Genetic Endocrine Diseases

Endocrine Mutation	Disorder	Mode of Inheritance	Chromosome Location	Types of Mutation	Reference
HORMONE MUTATIONS					
Insulin	Hyperproinsulinemia	AR	11p15.5	P	73
Growth hormone	Dwarfism	AR, AD	17q22-q24	D, P	64
Pro-opiomelanocortin (POMC)	Adrenal insufficiency; obesity	AR	2p23.3	P	85
Parathyroid hormone (PTH)	Hypoparathyroidism	AD	11p15.3-15.1	P	74
Thyroid-stimulating hormone (TSH)	TSH deficiency; hypothyroidism	AR	1p22	D, P	79
Thyroglobulin	Hypothyroidism; Goiter	AR	8q24.2-q24.3	P	221
Luteinizing hormone (LH)	LH deficiency; hypogonadism	AR	19q13.32	P	55
Follicle-stimulating hormone (FSH)	FSH deficiency; hypogonadism	AR	11p13	P	81
Vasopressin/neurophysin II	Neurohypophyseal diabetes insipidus (DI)	AD	20p12.21	P	75
Antimüllerian hormone	Retained müllerian ducts	AR	19p13.3-p13.2	P	231
Leptin	Obesity	AR	7q31.3	P	84
BINDING PROTEIN MUTATIONS					
Thyroxine-binding globulin (TBG)	Euthyroid hypothyroxinemia	XL	Xq21-22	D, P	87
Transthyretin	Euthyroid hyperthyroximemia	AD	18q11.2-12.1	P	93
Albumin	Euthyroid hyperthyroximemia	AD	4q11-q13	P	90
MEMBRANE RECEPTOR MUTATIONS					
Insulin receptor	Insulin resistance	AR, AD	19p13.3-13	P	57
GnRH receptor	Hypogonadotropic hypogonadism	AR	4q21.2	P	104
GHRH receptor	GH deficiency	AR	7p15-p14	P	66
TRH receptor	Hypothalamic hypothyroidism	AR	8q23	P	232
Growth hormone (GH) receptor	Laron dwarfism	AR	5p13-p12	P	95
TSH receptor (inactive)	TSH resistance	AR	14q31	P	111
TSH receptor (activating)	Hyperthyroidism	AD, S	14q31	P	58
LH receptor (inactive)	Hypogonadism	AR	2p21	P	233
LH receptor (activating)	Male precocious puberty	AD, S	2p21	P	28
FSH receptor (inactivating)	Ovarian failure; ↓ spermatog.	AR	2p21-p16	P	117
PTH receptor (inactivating)	Blomstrand chondrodysplasia	AR	3p22-p21.1	P	234
PTH receptor (activating)	Jansen chondrodysplasia	AD	3p22-p21.1	P	107
ACTH receptor	Adrenal insufficiency	AR	18p11.2	P	235
Vasopressin V2 receptor	Nephrogenic DI	XL	Xq27-q28	P	100
Calcium receptor (inactive)	Hypocalciuric hypercalcemia	AD, AR	3q21-q24	P	119
Calcium receptor (activating)	Hypoparathyroidism	AD	3q21-q24	P	108
AMH receptor	Retained müllerian ducts	AR	12q13	P	236
Leptin receptor	Obesity	AR	1p31	P	237
Melanocortin 4 receptor	Obesity	AD	18q22	P	238
NUCLEAR RECEPTOR MUTATIONS					
Vitamin D	Type II Vit-D resistant rickets	AR	12q12-q14	P	136
Thyroid hormone	Thyroid hormone resistance	AD	3p24.3	P, D	239
Glucocorticoid	Glucocorticoid resistance	AR	5q31	P	138

Table 6-5 Examples of Genetic Endocrine Diseases—*cont'd*

Endocrine Mutation	Disorder	Mode of Inheritance	Chromosome Location	Types of Mutation	Reference
NUCLEAR RECEPTOR MUTATIONS—*cont'd*					
Mineralocorticoid	Pseudohypoaldosteronism type 1	AD	4q31.1	P	240
Androgen	Androgen resistance	XL, S	Xcen-q13	P, D	241
Estrogen	Estrogen resistance	AR, S	6p25.1	P	139
PPAR-γ2	Obesity; insulin resistance	AD	3p25	P	242
Steroidogenic factor 1	XY sex-reversal; adrenal insuffic.	AD	9q33	P	144
DAX1	Adrenal hypoplasia congenita	XL	Xp21.3-p21.2	P, D	146
SIGNAL PATHWAY MUTATIONS					
Ras P21	Tumorigenesis	S	20q12-13.2	P	243
G$_s$α	Acromegaly	S	20q12-13.2	P	120
G$_s$α	Albright osteodystrophy	AD, imprinting	20q12-13.2	P	124
G$_s$α	McCune-Albright	Mosaic	20q12-13.2	P	37
Giα	Tumorigenesis	S	3p21	P	120
PTTG (pit tumor transf. gene)	Pituitary tumors	S	5q33	Overexpression	244
p53	Tumorigenesis	S	17p13	D, P	245
Retinoblastoma	Tumorigenesis	S	13q14	D, P	246
PRAD1 (Cyclin D1)	Tumorigenesis	S	11q13	Translocation	127
PTC (papillary thyroid carcin.)	Tumorigenesis	S	10q11-q12	Translocation	183
BRCA1	Breast, ovarian Ca	AD, S	17q21	P, D	247
BRCA2	Breast, ovarian Ca	AD, S	13q12.3	P, D	248
TRANSCRIPTION FACTOR MUTATIONS					
HNF 1α	MODY 3	AD	12q24.2	P	249
HNF 1β	MODY 5	AD	17cen-q21.3	P	250
Insulin promoter factor 1	MODY 4	AD	13q12.1	P	171
Pit1	GH, PRL (prolactin), TSH deficiency	AR, AD	3p11	D, P	160
Prop1	GH, PRL, TSH, LH, FSH deficiency	AR	5q	P	161
Thyroid transcription factor 1	Congenital hypothyroidism	Unknown	14q13	Underexpression	251
Thyroid transcription factor 2	Congenital hypothyroidism	AR	9q22	P	166
PAX-8	Congenital hypothyroidism	AR	2q12-q14	P	167
SRY translocation	XX male	XL	Ypter	Translocation	152
SRY mutation	XY female	YL	Ypter	P	252
SOX-9	XY female; campomelic dysplasia	AD	17q24.3-q25.1	P	149
Wilms' tumor	Frasier syndrome; Denys-Drash	AD	11p13	P	150
DAZ (RNA-binding protein)	Azoospermia	YL	Yq11	D	24
ENDOCRINE SYNDROMES					
Kallmann	Hypogonadotropic hypogonadism	XL, AR, AD	Xp22.3	D, P, Translocation	253
Prader-Willi	Hypogonadism, obesity	AD; imprint	15q11	D	254
Von Hippel-Lindau	Pheochromocytoma; renal Ca	AD	3p26-p25	D, P	255
MEN1	Neoplasia: Pituitary, pancreas, parathyroid	AD	11q13	P	22
MEN2 (ret mutations)	Neoplasia: Parathyroid, pheochromocytoma medullary thyroid carcinoma (MTC)	AD	10q11.2	P	181
MEN2B	MEN2 and neurofibromas	AD	10q11.2	P	182
Carney complex	Cushing's; acromegaly, myxomas	AD	2p16	Unknown	203
Pendred syndrome	Goiter; deafness	AR	7q31	P, D	199
DiGeorge syndrome	Hypoparathyroidism; cardiac abn.	AD	22q11	D	256
Prohormone convertase 1	ACTH, GnRH, insulin deficiency	AR	5q15-q21	P	257
Polyglandular failure type 1	Polyglandular failure	AR	21q22.3	P	202
ENZYME AND CHANNEL MUTATIONS					
Glucokinase	MODY 2	AD	7p15-p13	P	172
Sulfonylurea receptor	Nesidioblastosis	AR	11p15.1-p14	P	227
Potassium channel KCNJ11	Nesidioblastosis	AR	11p15.1	P	228
Sodium iodide symporter	Goiter, hypothyroidism	AR	19p12-13.2	P	258
Thyroid peroxidase	Goiter, hypothyroidism	AR	2pter-12	P	219
21-hydroxylase	Congenital adrenal hyperplasia (CAH), androgen excess	AR	6p21	P, D	56
17α-hydroxylase	Androgen deficiency, hypertension (HTN)	AR	10q24.3	P	209
17,20-lyase activity	XY ambiguous genitalia	AR	10q24.3	P	210
11β-hydroxylase	Androgen excess, HTN	AR	8q21	P	208
3β-hydroxysteroid dehydrog.	CAH; Androgen deficiency	AR	1p13.1	P	211
Steroidogenic acute regulatory	Lipoid CAH	AR	8p11.2	P	213
5α-reductase type 2	Male pseudohermaphroditism	AR	2p23	D, P	215
Aldosterone synthase	Glucocorticoid, remediable HTN	AD	8q21	D, Translocation	217
Amiloride sensitive Na channel	Liddle syndrome; HTN	AD	16p13-p12	P	259
Aquaporin 2	Nephrogenic DI	AR	12q13	P	102
PHEX	Hypophos, Vit-D resistant rickets	XL	Xp22.2-p22.1	P	225
1α-hydroxylase	Type I Vit-D resistant rickets	AR	12q14	P	224
MCT8	Elevated T3, TSH Quadriplegia, hypotonia, mental retardation	XL	Xq13.2	D, P	230

AD, autosomal dominant; AR, autosomal recessive; D, deletion; P, point mutation; S, somatic cell mutation; XL, X-linked; YL, Y-linked. Representative references are provided. Many endocrine disorders are not listed, including a large number of metabolic disorders. The interested reader is referred to additional Refs. 4 and 260.

more subtle phenotype and there is often a phenotypic spectrum. For example, the phenotype of androgen insensitivity includes a spectrum of disorders that ranges from severe resistance in the case of testicular feminization to milder resistance in Reifenstein syndrome and other syndromes of mild androgen resistance associated with gynecomastia and infertility.[26] These disorders are each caused by mutations in the androgen receptor, but the mutations result in different degrees of receptor dysfunction. In some cases, the receptor is deleted or mutated in a manner that it is completely inactive. In other examples, mutations perturb the amount or stability of the receptor, causing partial resistance. Phenotypic variation can also be ascribed to environmental influences and/or the action of other genes, so called *modifier genes*. A further extension of this concept is that genetic polymorphisms (DNA sequence variants) in the normal population cause subtle differences in hormone or receptor activity, thereby constituting part of the basis for the variability that is seen in the normal range of hormone levels and activity.

Because a staggering number of mutations in different endocrine genes have already been reached,[4] it is not practical to describe each of these disorders in a comprehensive manner. The interested reader is referred to individual chapters and to the references in Table 6-5. In addition, many of these disorders can be found in the OMIM or at the human gene mutation database (see Table 6-1). It is, nevertheless, useful to provide an overview of mutations that occur at different steps in endocrine pathways to illustrate the breadth and heterogeneous nature of disorders caused by gene defects.

HORMONE MUTATIONS

One might have expected that mutations in hormones would represent a common molecular basis for endocrine disorders. This does not appear to be the case, however. For the most part, causes of hormone deficiency syndromes remain enigmatic. For example, growth hormone deficiency rarely involves deletions or mutations in the *growth hormone* gene.[65] Rather, most cases can be attributed to an inherited or acquired hypothalamic defect that could involve GHRH, the GHRH producing neuron, the GHRH receptor, or one of the regulatory pathways that control GHRH secretion. Attempts to attribute GH deficiency to GHRH mutations have not been successful, and most patients respond to exogenous GHRH, implying that GHRH and GHRH receptor mutations[66] may also be uncommon. In some respects, GH deficiency is reminiscent of idiopathic hypogonadotropic hypogonadism, which is not due to a *GnRH* (gonadotropin-releasing hormone) gene defect, but rather to a defect in genes (*KAL1, FGFR1*) that control migration of the GnRH producing neurons.[67,68]

The *GH* gene is a member of a large gene cluster that also includes a GH variant gene as well as several structurally related *chorionic somatomammotropin* genes and pseudogenes (highly homologous but functionally inactive relatives of a normal gene). Because such gene clusters contain multiple homologous DNA sequences arranged in tandem, they are particularly prone to undergoing recombination, leading to gene duplication or deletion. It has been proposed that mispairing of areas with sequence homology can lead to unequal crossover during meiosis, with resultant gene duplication on one chromosome and gene deletion on the other chromosome.[64,69] In autosomal-recessive isolated GH deficiency IA (IGHD IA), deletions of the *GH* gene represent one of the best-studied hormone mutations[63,70] (see Chapter 37). Southern blot analyses of DNA from affected children demonstrate homozygous deletions of the *GH* gene, consistent with the autosomal-recessive inheritance pattern for transmission. Recessive point mutations in the *GH* gene lead to IGHD IB. More recently, autosomal-dominant mutations in the *GH* gene

have been described (IGHD II). In these cases, the mutation generates a misfolded protein that aggregates with the normal GH protein, thus exerting a dominant-negative effect.[71,72] These complexes may also be toxic to somatotrope cells.

Other mutations in hormones are listed in Table 6-5. The mutations in preproinsulin prevent processing of the preproinsulin precursor molecule, causing secretion of biologically inactive insulin molecules.[73] A mutation in the signal sequence of PTH causes hypoparathyroidism, even when only one of the two *PTH* genes is affected.[74] It has been shown that this mutation interferes with hormone transport and processing, leading to the hypothesis that the mutant molecule could interfere with the transport of other cellular proteins, including the normal PTH protein. Most mutations in the *AVP-NPII* gene, which encodes vasopressin and neurophysin, appear to be somewhat analogous to the PTH mutation. An autosomal-dominant form of diabetes insipidus is caused by heterozygous mutations in the signal peptide or the neurophysin moiety of the AVP-NPII precursor protein.[75] These amino acid changes in the signal sequence and the carboxyterminal vasopressin carrier protein neurophysin suggest that abnormalities in protein processing may prevent vasopressin synthesis or result in cellular toxicity. In vitro studies demonstrate abnormal processing and cellular toxicity of the mutant forms of vasopressin,[15,76] and mice carrying one mutated allele show progressive loss of arginine-vasopressin (AVP)-producing neurons relative to oxytocin-producing neurons,[77] explaining the delayed onset of the disease.[78] Very rarely, mutations lead to amino acid substitutions in the AVP moiety. In this case, the disease is inherited in a recessive manner.[16]

Homozygous mutations in the *TSH-β* gene cause hypothyroidism. One TSH-β subunit mutation defines a region of the molecule that is required for heterodimerization with the α subunit,[79] whereas others either truncate the protein or interfere with its biological activity.[80] An LHβ subunit mutation defines a region that is critical for binding to the LH receptor.[55] Interestingly, follicle-stimulating hormone-beta (FSH-β) mutations have different phenotypes in males and females. They cause primary ovarian failure in females because of a defect in follicular maturation and estrogen synthesis.[81,82] In males, FSH-β mutations do not impair virilization or testosterone production, but they cause variable impairment of spermatogenesis.[83] *Leptin* mutations, initially described in murine models of obesity, have now been identified in humans.[84] Unexpectedly, mutations in *POMC* not only cause adrenal insufficiency, but also lead to obesity because of a role for α-melanocyte-stimulating hormone (MSH) in appetite control[85] (see Chapter 44). In these and other autosomal-recessive disorders, there is an opportunity to examine the effect of a "gene knockout" in humans. Thus, elimination of functional hormones such as GH, LH, FSH, or TSH allows one to attribute specific physiologic roles to the hormone, which may be difficult to discern in normal individuals. For example, complete elimination of LH, with retention of normal FSH, allows the functions of these hormones to be distinguished. Creation of gene knockouts and knockins by homologous recombination in mice, or transgenic overexpression, allows the creation of animal models for studying hormone and receptor function (see Chapter 5).

BINDING PROTEIN MUTATIONS

The binding protein mutations cause little in the way of clinical disease, but if not recognized, they often lead to unnecessary treatment. As shown in Table 6-5, these defects are predominantly confined to proteins that bind thyroid hormone (see Chapter 113). Thyroxine-binding globulin (TBG) is the major thyroid hormone transport protein in the serum. Abnormalities in its production are not rare, occurring in approximately 1 in 2500 male births.[86] Complete TBG deficiency is X-linked and is clinically apparent in males who are euthyroid but have very low levels of thyroid hormone in the serum. They are often mistakenly treated for hypothyroidism. Although large deletions of the *TBG* gene have not been found,[87] a number of different point mutations cause functional loss of TBG, either by alterations in protein structure or glycosylation.[86] TBG excess is most commonly due to effects of drugs or hormones, although familial cases with amplification of the *TBG* gene have been reported.[88] In the latter situation, the total TBG and thyroxine levels are elevated threefold to fivefold in hemizygote males, and twofold to threefold in heterozygote females.

In addition to TBG, thyroid hormone binds to albumin and transthyretin (TTR). Familial dysalbuminemic hyperthyroxinemia (FDH) is an autosomal-dominant condition in which albumin has an increased affinity for thyroid hormone.[89] Most cases are caused by a mutation in codon 218, in which there is replacement of Arg by His[90] or Pro.[91] It is characterized by elevated levels of total thyroxine (T_4) and normal levels of free T_4 and TSH. Another form of the disorder causes a selective increase in triiodothyronine (T_3) binding.[92] The presence of abnormal binding proteins can be detected using electrophoretic analyses of serum thyroid hormone binding proteins or, now, by mutational analyses. Occasionally, TTR can be overproduced by pancreatic endocrine tumors, or mutant forms may have increased affinity for T_4.[93] The impact of TTR mutations on T_4 affinity is variable and can be normal, decreased, or increased. Many of them are associated with an autosomal-dominant form of amyloidosis, affecting predominantly the peripheral nervous system and the heart.[94]

MEMBRANE RECEPTOR MUTATIONS

In Laron-type dwarfism, a receptor or postreceptor defect had been proposed because growth hormone levels were high, insulin-like growth factor (IGF) levels were low, and patients failed to respond to growth hormone therapy. Consistent with this prediction, a number of different point mutations have now been identified in the GH receptor.[95,96] Such hormone resistance is characteristic of many receptor mutations,[97] although alterations in signaling pathways can result in a similar phenotype (e.g., pseudohypoparathyroidism).

Mutations in the insulin receptor have been characterized in patients with severe insulin resistance. Multiple missense and nonsense mutations have been described in different regions of the receptor, causing different insulin resistance phenotypes such as leprechaunism, the Rabson-Mendenhall syndrome, and type A insulin resistance.[57,98] The mechanisms of insulin receptor inactivation and their relationship to the above syndromes and others are summarized in Chapter 58.

The X-linked form of vasopressin resistance has now been attributed to mutations in the *vasopressin 2 (V2)* receptor gene on the long arm of the X chromosome.[99-101] There are many different vasopressin receptor mutations, reflecting allelic heterogeneity.[17] A similar phenotype (nephrogenic diabetes insipidus) can be caused, however, by recessive or dominant mutations in the *aquaporin 2* gene,[102,103] providing an example of nonallelic heterogeneity.

In recent years, mutations have been defined in most peptide hormone receptors. For the most part, the phenotypes are predictable based on the known function of the hormone pathway. Several exceptions merit emphasis, however. For example, some GnRH receptor mutations only partially alter its function.[104] Consequently, patients may exhibit an LH response to pharmacologic doses of exogenous GnRH, whereas they do not respond normally to lower levels of endogenous GnRH. These patients usually present with idiopathic hypogonadism. GHRHR mutations cause severe GH deficiency, even though other releasing factors theoretically might compensate for the defect.[105]

Among the most important revelations in recent years is the finding that a subset of mutations in GPCRs can cause constitutive activation of receptor function, whereas other mutations cause loss of function. This phenomenon was first recognized in adrenergic receptors, in which certain mutations in the sixth transmembrane domain were found to cause constitutive activation of cyclic adenosine monophosphate (cAMP) signaling, in the absence of added ligand.[106] The ability of mutations to activate GPCRs has had a tremendous impact in the field of endocrinology. Based on the idea that activating mutations of GPCR could mimic the effects of hormone excess, phenotypes for activating mutations have now been identified in the TSHR,[58] LH receptor (LHR),[28] PTH receptor (PTHR),[107] and calcium receptor (CaR).[108]

Constitutively active mutations in the TSHR are characteristic of this class of mutations. The activating mutations in the TSHR were first identified in autonomously functioning thyroid nodules.[58] In this case, somatic mutations occur in the thyroid follicular cell that are not present in the germ line. These mutations cause an increase in basal production of cAMP by the receptor, indicating that it couples to $G_s\alpha$ in the absence of TSH. Because the TSHR mediates thyroid cell growth as well as function, the mutant receptor leads to the clonal expansion of cells harboring the mutation, ultimately resulting in a clinically apparent "hot" nodule. In addition to somatic mutations, activating TSHR mutations can also occur as de novo germ-line mutations causing congenital hyperthyroidism.[109] Or, they can be transmitted as an autosomal-dominant disorder, since a mutation in one allele is sufficient to cause hyperfunction.[18] The locations of these activating mutations delineate residues in the TSHR that play a critical role in G protein coupling, either because they are involved directly, or more likely, because they play a structural role to maintain the receptor in an inactive state.[110] Homozygous inactivating mutations in the TSH receptor cause resistance to TSH.[111,112] In these patients, the phenotype encompasses a wide spectrum, ranging from isolated TSH elevation to severe hypothyroidism, and there is a clear correlation between genotype and phenotype. Some of the mutations inactivate the receptor only partially, whereas others completely destroy its function (see Chapter 111).

Activating mutations in the LHR cause familial male-limited precocious puberty.[28] The autonomous function of the LHR induces testosterone production in the absence of LH (prepubertally), causing virilization in boys. Interestingly, females with the mutations exhibit no phenotypic abnormalities, presumably because autonomous function of the LHR in the ovary does not significantly alter steroidogenesis, since the receptor is only expressed as follicles mature and are normally exposed to high levels of LH. For this reason, pedigrees with LHR mutations exhibit an autosomal-dominant pattern of transmission, but only males are affected. Analogous mutations in the FSH receptor (FSHR) appear to be rare,[113] or perhaps do not cause a phenotype that is readily recognized. Homozygous inactivating mutations in the LHR cause Leydig cell hypoplasia and pseudohermaphroditism in males[114,115] and primary amenorrhea in females.[116] Homozygous inactivating mutations in the FSHR cause primary ovarian failure in females[117] and impaired spermatogenesis in males.[117]

The cloning of a GPCR that binds calcium provided unexpected insights into mechanisms of calcium handling.[118] The identification of this receptor led to a molecular basis for familial hypocalciuric hypercalcemia (FHH), which is caused by inactivating mutations,[119] as well as one of the familial causes of hypoparathyroidism.[108] The heterozygous inactivating mutations cause calcium resistance, resulting in increased PTH and a new set point for calcium feedback. On the other hand, activating mutations of the calcium receptor mimic the effects of calcium, leading to suppression of PTH and low calcium levels. Activating mutations in the PTHR cause severe skeletal abnormalities (Jansen's metaphyseal chondrodysplasia), as well as hypercalcemia, because autonomous function of the receptor is present from early development.[107]

SIGNALING PATHWAY MUTATIONS

Mutations at several steps along signaling pathways can alter hormone action or contribute to tumorigenesis. As noted previously, there is now evidence that somatic mutations in membrane receptors, such as the TSH receptor, can lead to constitutive activation of downstream signaling pathways, resulting in altered cell growth.[58] Mutations in G proteins have been described in several different types of endocrine neoplasia.[120] For example, mutations in the $G_s\alpha$ subunit have been identified in somatotroph adenomas, either at codon 201 or 227.[121] Both of these mutations inhibit GTP hydrolysis and thereby cause constitutive activation of the $G_s\alpha$ subunit. Activation of $G_s\alpha$ in this cell type stimulates adenylyl cyclase, leading to elevated cAMP levels, a situation that mimics GHRH stimulation. As a result, the $G_s\alpha$ mutation causes excess GH secretion and contributes to abnormal cell growth as well. $G_s\alpha$ mutations are found in approximately 30% to 40% of somatotrope adenomas.[122] Importantly, these mutations are somatic rather than inherited, as evidenced by the fact that G proteins from other tissues do not contain the amino acid substitution. $G_s\alpha$ mutations have also been identified in autonomous thyroid adenomas.[120] It is interesting to note that $G_s\alpha$ mutations identical to those described in somatotroph adenomas also occur in McCune-Albright syndrome.[37] In McCune-Albright, the mutations occur early in development and lead to mosaicism, explaining the pleiotropic but variable manifestations in the bone, the endocrine system, and the skin. Mutations in the regulatory subunit of protein kinase A (PRKAR1A), which is further downstream in the same signaling pathway, form the molecular basis of Carney complex 1 (see discussion to follow).

Albright hereditary osteodystrophy (AHO) is also caused by a $G_s\alpha$ mutation, although, in this case, the mutation eliminates $G_s\alpha$ function rather than causing constitutive activity.[123] AHO is characterized by short stature, obesity, and skeletal abnormalities. Because the GNAS1 gene encoding $G_s\alpha$ is imprinted, the phenotype varies depending on whether the mutated allele is inherited from the mother or the father (see Fig. 6-3). If the mutation is on the paternal allele, the phenotype is restricted to AHO. In instances where the mutation is on the maternal allele, the phenotype also includes resistance to several $G_s\alpha$ protein–coupled hormones such as PTH, TSH, LH, and FSH because the GNAS1 gene is expressed from the maternal allele in these tissues.[36,124,125] In patients with isolated renal resistance to PTH (pseudohypoparathyroidism type IB), an imprinting defect leads to decreased $G_s\alpha$ expression in the proximal renal tubule.

A novel mechanism for tumorigenesis has been provided by studies of parathyroid adenomas. A subset of parathyroid tumors were found to contain rearrangements of the PTH gene.[126] Analysis of the translocation revealed that the PTH promoter was fused to a member of the cyclin D family.[127] The translocation involves an intrachromosomal rearrangement on chromosome 11. The fusion gene is referred to as PRAD for parathyroid adenomatosis. Because cyclins regulate progression through the cell cycle, it is likely that overexpression of cyclin D1 from the PTH promoter, rather than from its native promoter, causes abnormal regulation of the parathyroid cell.

Endocrine neoplasms are providing important models for the identification of new oncogenes as well as the steps involved in the progression of tumors from the benign to the malignant phenotype. Because many oncogenes involve alterations of cellular signaling pathways that have been well characterized in hormone-secreting cells, it is likely that endocrine tumors will continue to provide important models for the pathophysiology of neoplasia.

NUCLEAR RECEPTOR MUTATIONS

In addition to mutations in membrane receptors (e.g., LH resistance), hormone resistance syndromes also occur as a consequence of defects in nuclear receptors (i.e., resistance to thyroid hormone). The syndrome of resistance to thyroid hormone (RTH) is representative of nuclear receptor resistance syndromes, but it also illustrates some unique aspects of a disease that is inherited in a dominant manner (see Chapter 114). RTH was first described by Refetoff and colleagues,[128] and is characterized by elevated circulating levels of free thyroid hormone, inappropriately normal or increased levels of TSH, and a spectrum of clinical manifestations that can include signs of hypothyroidism in combination with features of thyrotoxicosis. Two thyroid hormone receptor genes, designated TR-α and TR-β, encode highly homologous proteins with different tissue distributions. Genetic analyses show linkage between the RTH syndrome and the TR-β receptor gene locus.[19,129] This observation has been confirmed by sequencing β-receptor genes in multiple different families with this disorder. In the families that have a dominant mode of transmission, affected individuals have mutations in one allele of the TR-β receptor together with a second normal allele.[130,131] Interestingly, these and additional mutations are clustered in three discrete regions in the carboxy-terminal ligand-binding domain of the receptor. The mutant receptors bind hormone with reduced affinity or they have defects in hormone-dependent transcriptional activation. Consequently, their ability to modulate target gene expression is impaired.[132] Because the affected individuals possess a second normal β-receptor allele and two normal α-receptor alleles, the mutant receptor has been proposed to inhibit the activity of normal receptors. In support of this concept, the receptor mutants have been shown to block the action of the wild-type receptors in transient gene expression assays, probably by binding to DNA target sites where the mutant receptors function as antagonists.[133] It is also notable that the mutant receptors retain the ability to bind transcriptional corepressors.[134] Thus, once bound to DNA target sites, they act as repressors of these target genes.

Mutations have also been identified in several other members of the nuclear hormone receptor family. Syndromes of androgen resistance represent one of the more common and well-studied receptor defects.[26] These disorders exhibit sex-linked transmission, consistent with the location of the androgen receptor on the X chromosome. The androgen receptor gene has now been sequenced in a relatively large number of affected individuals, although primarily those with severe forms of resistance.[26] Many mutations result in premature termination codons, although gene deletions and single amino acid substitutions have also been found. No clinical effects of the heterozygous condition have been noted in females with androgen receptor mutations. In female carriers of the mutation, X-inactivation would likely allow expression of only one of the receptor alleles within a given cell, and the dominant-negative activity seen with the thyroid hormone receptor may not be possible.

Hypocalcemic vitamin-D resistant rickets (HVDRR) is a rare inherited form of rickets that is unresponsive to treatment with 1,25-dihydroxyvitamin D.[135,136] The disease has a recessive pattern of inheritance and most cases have involved consanguineous families. A variety of mutations have been identified in different kindreds including amino acid substitutions in the zinc-finger DNA-binding domains, as well as nonsense mutations that cause premature termination. The naturally occurring mutations in the vitamin D receptor have been useful for providing insights into the biologic role of vitamin D in skin differentiation, hair growth, and lymphocyte function.[136,137]

In familial glucocorticoid resistance, serum concentrations of cortisol and cortisol production rates are elevated without the characteristic clinical manifestations of glucocorticoid excess. Adrenocorticotropic hormone (ACTH) levels are inappropriately increased, indicating reduced feedback inhibition at the level of the hypothalamic-pituitary adrenal axis. Because ACTH also stimulates adrenal androgens and mineralocorticoids, precocious puberty and hypertension can comprise features of this syndrome. An autosomal-codominant mode of inheritance has been suggested in view of the fact that heterozygotes are mildly affected.[138] Mutations in the mineralocorticoid receptor cause a form of pseudohypoaldosteronism type I, which is characterized by neonatal renal salt wasting with dehydration, hypotension, hyperkalemia, and metabolic acidosis, despite elevated aldosterone levels. It is transmitted in an autosomal-dominant manner and is less severe than the homozygous form of pseudohypoaldosteronism, which is caused by homozygous mutations in the amiloride-sensitive epithelial sodium channel.

A homozygous estrogen receptor α mutation has been described in a male.[139] In addition to reduced estrogen action on the hypothalamic-pituitary-gonadal axis, it impaired fusion of the epiphyses, leading to increased linear growth. Estrogen receptor variants and mutations have been described in breast cancers, although a role in pathogenesis has not been clearly defined.[140,141]

Mutations in orphan nuclear receptors also cause endocrine disorders. Steroidogenic factor-1 (SF-1) controls adrenal and gonadal development and is expressed in the ventromedial hypothalamus and pituitary gonadotropes.[142] SF-1 also regulates the expression of a wide array of steroidogenic enzyme genes.[143] A heterozygous mutation in SF-1 has been demonstrated in an XY individual with adrenal insufficiency and complete male-to-female sex reversal.[144] The orphan nuclear receptor DAX1 is expressed in the same distribution as SF-1, and inhibits its transcriptional activity.[145] DAX1 is located on the X chromosome and mutations cause X-linked adrenal hypoplasia congenita (AHC), which is characterized by adrenal insufficiency and hypogonadotropic hypogonadism.[146]

TRANSCRIPTION FACTOR MUTATIONS

One of the final steps in hormone action involves effects on gene expression, mediated via transcription factors. In principle, the nuclear hormone receptors could be classified as transcription factors and described under this category. Because transcription factors are often expressed in various tissues, it is not uncommon to observe a syndromic phenotype. Mechanistically, monoallelic mutations in transcription factors often cause haploinsufficiency, and biallelic mutations may result in a more severe phenotype.[21] Not surprisingly, some of the other transcription factor mutations involve developmental pathways. Elucidation of mutations in the SRY gene provides a dramatic example of one these developmental mutations.[23] The Y chromosome determines male sex by virtue of encoding the testis-determining factor (TDF). In the absence of a Y chromosome, ovaries form, and the female phenotype develops. The SRY gene was located by examining rare cases of phenotypic females with an XY genotype. It was hypothesized that these individuals might have deleted or mutated SRY genes on the Y chromosome. The sex-determining region on the short arm of the Y chromosome was delineated by mapping large deletions or translocations of the Y chromosome that were associated with a female phenotype. Three lines of evidence support the view that SRY is the primary testis-determining gene. First, in XY females

who do not have a large deletions of the Y chromosome, mutations are found in SRY that are not present in their fathers.[23] Second, there is a deletion in the mouse homologue of SRY in sex-reversed mice.[147] Third, expression of SRY in transgenic mice is sufficient to induce testis development in XX mice.[148] Although these data indicate that SRY is the critical gene for an early step in male sex determination, it is likely that SRY is only one of several developmental switches that initiate a cascade of sex-specific gene expression. As noted, mutations in SF-1 also preclude normal testis development in XY individuals. SOX9[149] and WT1[150] mutations also impair testis development.

XX males have been shown to have translocations of Y chromosome–specific sequences onto the pseudoautosomal region of the X chromosome.[151,152] These translocated Y chromosome sequences contain SRY. Sterility in XX males may reflect the presence of two X chromosomes (analogous to the situation in Klinefelter syndrome) or the absence of additional Y chromosome sequences that are required for fertility.

The pituitary-specific transcription factor (Pit-1) was first identified based on its binding to multiple sites in the growth hormone and prolactin promoters.[153,154] Pit-1 expression is restricted to the pituitary gland and the protein is found only in somatotropes, lactotropes, and thyrotropes.[155] Pit-1 mutations have been identified in several strains of mice that have specific deficits of GH, prolactin (PRL), and TSH.[156] These data confirm a central role for Pit-1 in the development of these cell types and/or the expression of these genes. Similar patterns of pituitary hormone deficiencies have been described in humans with mutations in PIT1 (POU1F1).[157] Interestingly, different PIT1 mutations result in autosomal-recessive[158,159] and autosomal-dominant[160] inheritance patterns, suggesting that the distinct mutations have different effects on PIT1 function. The recessive mutation inactivates PIT1, whereas the dominant disorder involves a dominant negative mutation analogous to that for the thyroid hormone receptor. Another pituitary transcription factor, PROP1, which acts upstream of PIT1 during pituitary development, causes a more severe form of pituitary hormone deficiency that includes GH, PRL, and TSH, and occasionally also ACTH.[161] Recessive mutations in LHX3, a LIM homeodomain transcription factor, also cause combined pituitary hormone deficiency (CPHD) of all anterior pituitary hormones with the exception of ACTH. In addition, these patients have a rigid cervical spine and a limited ability to rotate the head.[162] A syndromic form of CPHD associated with septo-optic dysplasia can be caused by homozygous mutations in HESX1 (RPX), a member of the paired-like class of homeobox transcription factors.[163] A similar phenotype was observed in Hesx1-/-mice. Interestingly, a small proportion of the mice heterozygous for a Hesx1 null allele also had a milder form of septo-optic dysplasia. This prompted further screening of patients presenting with a wide spectrum of congenital pituitary dysfunctions and a subset of these patients was indeed found to be heterozygous for HESX1 mutations.[164] Heterozygous HESX1 mutations result in various constellations of pituitary hormone deficiencies and the phenotype is variable among family members with the same mutation.

Like transcription factors involved in pituitary development, the discovery of factors involved in thyroid gland development has provided insight into the molecular basis of thyroid dysgenesis. Thyroid transcription factor 1 (TTF1/NKX2.1), thyroid transcription factor 2 (TTF2/FOXE1), and paired homeobox 8 (PAX8) each play a key role in thyroid gland development.[165] These factors are, therefore, candidates for genetic causes of thyroid agenesis, hypoplasia, and ectopy. Although several cases of mutations have been reported, the incidence of mutations in these developmental transcription factors appears to be relatively low.[166–169] Remarkably, heterozygous mutations in TTF1 only lead to transient congenital hypothyroidism, but, consistent with a role of this transcription factor in brain and lung development, the patients present with neurologic alterations (choreoathetosis, mental retardation) and neonatal distress.[168,169] Biallelic mutations in TTF1 result in a syndromic form of thyroid dysgenesis associated with cleft palate, choanal atresia, bifid epiglottis, and spiky hair (Bamforth-Lazarus syndrome).[166] Monoallelic mutations in PAX8 cause thyroid hypoplasia and hypothyroidism,[167] but the penetrance of these mutations is incomplete.[170]

A genetic pathway that involves transcription factors causes several forms of maturity-onset diabetes of the young (MODY). Presently, six different types of MODY are recognized. They share in common an autosomal-dominant mode of transmission and late-onset nonketotic form of diabetes mellitus of variable severity. MODY 1 is caused by mutations in *hepatocyte nuclear receptor-4α (HNF-4α)*, which is a member of the steroid/thyroid nuclear receptor superfamily. It is expressed in the liver, but also in the kidney, intestine, and pancreatic islets. HNF-4α controls the expression of a wide variety of genes, including *HNF-1α* (which causes MODY 3). It is involved in the expression of hepatocyte genes as well as certain islet genes, including *insulin*. Mutations have also been described in HNF-1β, which is structurally related to HNF-1α. HNF-1β can form homodimers or heterodimers with HNF-1α. MODY 4 is caused by mutations in insulin promoter factor-1 (IPF-1), which is a homeobox transcription factor, also referred to as STF-1 or IDX-1. It controls development of the pancreas. Homozygous mutations cause pancreatic agenesis, whereas heterozygous mutations cause diabetes.[171] MODY 2 was the first form of MODY to be characterized at the genetic level. In contrast to the other forms of MODY, it is not caused by a transcription factor mutation. Rather, it results from mutations in glucokinase, an enzyme that phosphorylates glucose to glucose-6-phosphate.[172] This reaction plays a key role in glucose-sensing by the pancreatic β cell. As a result of glucokinase mutations, increased glucose levels are required to elicit insulin secretory responses. Lastly, MODY 6 is caused by mutations in the basic helix-loop-helix transcription factor NEUROD, which is involved in the regulation of the insulin promoter.[173]

ENDOCRINE SYNDROMES

Multiple endocrine neoplasia syndromes have long been recognized as autosomal-dominant disorders that predispose to endocrine tumor development. Both syndromes are associated with hyperplasia and adenomas of the parathyroid glands. MEN1, however, is also characterized by adenomas of the pituitary and pancreas (see Chapter 191), whereas MEN2 is associated with adrenal (pheochromocytomas) and thyroid C-cell (medullary carcinoma) neoplasia (see Chapter 192).

The MEN syndromes represent good examples of the experimental approaches that are required to identify and characterize unknown genes that cause well-characterized syndromes. A critical first step is to determine the chromosome on which a candidate *MEN* gene resides. Subsequently, the position of the disease-causing gene can be more precisely mapped in relation to known genes and other DNA markers on that chromosome. For MEN1 and -2, candidate genes were mapped to chromosomes 11 and 10, respectively, using linkage analyses.[174,175] The *MEN1* locus was found to be near *PYGM*, the muscle phosphorylase gene, which is known to be located on chromosome 11, band q13.[174,176] After a long search, and a tribute to the power of modern genomics, the gene for *MEN1* was identified within this locus.[22] The protein menin is localized in the nucleus and involved in transcriptional regulation by interacting with multiple transcription factors.[177] It acts like a classic tumor suppressor gene, as inactivating mutations are found in the germ line of most families with the disorder. Subsequently, the second copy of

the gene is deleted or mutated in tumor tissue, apparently because of acquired "second hits" or somatic mutations.[178] This scenario is analogous to the two-hit model for loss of function of the *retinoblastoma* gene, a well-characterized example of a tumor suppressor gene.[179]

Unlike MEN1, loss of heterozygosity is not seen at the *MEN2* locus on chromosome 10, suggesting a different pathophysiology for MEN2.[180] In the case of MEN2, affected individuals often have thyroid C-cell hyperplasia in childhood before the development of medullary thyroid carcinoma. This observation is consistent with a model in which the *MEN2* gene predisposes to hyperplastic growth with a second and perhaps distinct somatic mutation leading to tumorigenesis and clonal proliferation. Mutations in the *RET* protooncogene, a putative tyrosine kinase receptor, have been identified as the cause of MEN2A.[181] In several MEN2 kindreds, distinct *RET* mutations were found in a cluster of cysteines located at the juncture of the extracellular and transmembrane domains of the protein. These mutations appear to induce receptor dimerization, leading to constitutive function. Distinct mutations, in the tyrosine kinase domain of the RET receptor, cause MEN2B.[182] Interestingly, rearrangements of *RET* had previously been identified in papillary thyroid carcinoma (PTC), leading to its designation as a PTC oncogene.[183,184] Identification of *MEN2* gene carriers is particularly important since prophylactic thyroidectomy can be performed at an early age before developing medullary thyroid carcinoma and intense endocrine screening permits early detection of pheochromocytomas, whereas individuals without the mutation do not require further testing (see Chapter 192).

Kallmann's syndrome or idiopathic hypogonadotropic hypogonadism (IHH) associated with anosmia is an inherited disorder that is caused by GnRH deficiency. Several different inheritance patterns have been described, including autosomal recessive, X-linked, and autosomal dominant with incomplete penetrance.[185–187] In contrast to an animal model of this disorder (the hypogonadal mouse) in which there is a *GnRH* gene deletion,[188] all IHH patients examined to date appear to have an intact *GnRH* gene.[189] Furthermore, the sequence of the *GnRH* gene in several different individuals with IHH has been shown to be normal.[190,191] Thus, it appears that IHH in the human, unlike the hypogonadal mouse model, may involve defects in the processes that regulate development of GnRH-producing neurons or expression of the *GnRH* gene, rather than defects in the gene itself.[192,193] Genetic linkage studies provided evidence for a candidate gene on the short arm of the X chromosome (Xp22.3) in patients with the X-linked form of Kallmann's syndrome,[194,195] and mutations in the *KAL1* gene were found in several individuals with the syndrome.[192,193] Coupled with the finding that GnRH neurons migrate into the hypothalamus from the olfactory placode,[192,196] the product of the *KAL1* gene, anosmin 1, appears to be involved in the migration of the GnRH neurons, as well as development of the olfactory tract.[197] These observations are consistent with a model in which a defect in this gene causes Kallmann's syndrome and might account for some of its phenotypic variants, in that different degrees of developmental aberrations in neuronal migration could lead to isolated anosmia, IHH, or both. The autosomal-dominant form of Kallmann's syndrome is caused by mutations in the FGFR1.[68] Anosmin 1 is thought to be involved in fibroblast growth factor (FGF) signaling. Recessive mutations in G protein–coupled receptor 54 (GPR54) cause delayed puberty and IHH by blocking a step upstream of the GnRH pulse generator.[197a] Causes of other forms of IHH, including autosomal-recessive and autosomal-dominant forms, remain to be described.[187]

Pendred syndrome is an autosomal-recessive disorder characterized by goiter, defective organification of iodine, and deafness that is caused by a malformation of the endolymphatic system and the cochlea. The genetic defect in Pendred syndrome was determined by genetic linkage studies in consanguineous families.[198,199] The use of short tandem repeat markers throughout the genome identified a region on chromosome 7q31 in which affected individuals were homozygous for a series of the microsatellite markers. Because the same region was localized in several different pedigrees, genes within this locus were cloned and screened for mutations leading to the identification of the *PDS/SCL26A4* gene,[199] which encodes an iodide and chloride transporter.[200]

Autoimmune polyendocrinopathy-candidiasis-ectodermal dystrophy (APECED) is an autosomal-recessive syndrome that causes polyglandular failure syndrome type 1.[201] The disorder usually presents in childhood and is characterized by autoimmune destruction of several tissues including the parathyroids, adrenal cortex, gonads, pancreatic β cells, gastric parietal cells, and the thyroid gland. As implied by its name, other features include chronic mucocutaneous candidiasis, dystrophy of the dental enamel and nails, alopecia, vitiligo, and keratinopathy. Although the spectrum of clinical features is variable, the most common presentation includes hypoparathyroidism, adrenal insufficiency, and mucocutaneous candidiasis. Linkage analysis localized the gene for *APECED* to chromosome 21q22.3. Subsequently, the gene, designated *AIRE* (for autoimmune regulator), was cloned and found to encode a 545–amino acid transcription factor that is expressed in the thymus, lymph nodes, and fetal liver.[202]

Carney complex is an autosomal-dominant syndrome characterized by multiple neoplasias, including myxomas at various sites, endocrine tumors, and lentiginosis. Common endocrine manifestations include Cushing's syndrome, caused by pigmented nodular adrenal hyperplasia and acromegaly caused by pituitary tumors. Linkage analysis using short tandem repeat markers has localized two candidate regions on chromosome 17q23-24 and 2p16 indicating locus heterogeneity.[203] The Carney complex 1 gene on chromosome 17 encodes the regulatory subunit of the protein kinase A (PRKAR1A)[204]; the gene on chromosome 2 remains to be identified.

DEFECTS IN HORMONE SYNTHESIS

Because hormone biosynthesis and metabolism require an intricate series of steps, it is not surprising that multiple defects occur in several hormonogenic systems such as steroid and thyroid hormone synthesis. Distinct clinical syndromes may arise depending on the involved step and the severity of the mutation.

Congenital adrenal hyperplasia (CAH) is caused by mutations in several genes, most commonly, 21-hydroxylase (*CYP21*) (see Chapter 124).[205] 21-Hydroxylase is responsible for conversion of progesterone to corticosterone in the mineralocorticoid pathway and for conversion of 17-hydroxyprogesterone to 11-deoxycortisol in the glucocorticoid pathway. Because of decreased cortisol production, excess ACTH is secreted, leading to stimulation of the adrenal gland and overproduction of precursor steroids, including adrenal androgens. Deficiency of 21-hydoxylase encompasses a broad phenotypic spectrum. The severe classic form occurs in approximately 1/5000 to 1/20,000 births; less severe nonclassic forms occur as frequently as 1/30 to 1/100 births in certain ethnic groups. In females affected with the classic form of the disease, hypersecretion of adrenal androgens during fetal development causes ambiguous external genitalia, whereas in males the classic form is usually recognized because of severe salt wasting and glucocorticoid deficiency. In the nonclassic form, prenatal virilization does not occur, but virilization of variable severity occurs postnatally.

Many of the earlier clinical observations regarding CAH are now well explained by the molecular basis for the disease.[56] The 21-hydroxylase locus is on the short arm of chromosome 6, adjacent to the HLA locus, explaining previous findings that HLA typing was useful for predicting disease

risk (the HLA locus is tightly linked to the 21-hydroxylase locus). There are two *21-hydroxylase* genes, A and B. The *21A* gene is a functionally inactive pseudogene, whereas the adjacent *21B* gene is the active copy. The *21-hydroxylase* genes appear to have been duplicated along with the adjacent *C4A* and *C4B* complement genes. A large number of different types of deletions and point mutations of the *21B* gene have been described. Large deletions and rearrangements probably occur in 10% to 20% of cases. On the other hand, small deletions and point mutations are relatively common. Interestingly, many of the mutations in the *21B* gene correspond to sequences in the inactive *21A* gene. These data have been interpreted as evidence for *gene conversion*, a mechanism in which sequences from the adjacent *21A* gene are substituted for sequences in *21B*, probably as a consequence of chromatid mispairing coupled with a DNA repair mechanism. The inheritance of CAH is autosomal recessive. Heterozygotes are clinically unaffected. Biochemical testing is unreliable in detecting heterozygous carriers, whereas genetic testing provides an accurate answer for purposes of genetic counseling. The classic form of the disease is due to large deletions or severe mutations of both *21B* alleles, whereas the nonclassic form of the disease is caused by one of several combinations of severe and mildly affected *21B* alleles. Thus, the variability in clinical phenotype is partly the consequence of a high degree of heterogeneity at the genetic level. Prenatal testing for CAH is now possible using genotyping of the *CYP21* gene.[206,207] It is important to recognize the disorder during the first trimester in a female fetus, since the administration of glucocorticoids can avoid prenatal virilization.

Mutations in the *11β-hydroxylase* and *17α-hydroxylase* genes are also classified under congenital adrenal hyperplasia because impaired production of cortisol causes elevation of ACTH and, consequently, adrenal stimulation. Mutations in 11β-hydroxylase cause androgen excess and virilization, but are distinguished clinically from 21-hydroxylase mutations by mineralocorticoid excess, which causes hypertension in about two thirds of patients.[208] By contrast, defects in 17α-hydroxylase cause sex steroid deficiency with overproduction of mineralocorticoids, resulting in hypertension and hypokalemia. Recognition of mutations in the *P-450c17* gene led to the finding that a single protein had two different enzymatic activities (17α-hydroxylase and 17,20 lyase) that were previously thought to represent different proteins.[209,210] Mutations in 3β-hydroxysteroid dehydrogenase are a relative rare cause of CAH.[211] Because the block in steroid synthesis occurs early in the pathway of steroid synthesis, it is also associated with androgen deficiency.

A critical step in steroid synthesis actually involves the transport of cholesterol into the mitochondrion by steroidogenic acute regulatory protein (StAR).[212] Mutations in StAR cause lipoid CAH, which is characterized by large, lipid-filled adrenal glands and gonads.[213] The discovery of this protein has provided important new insights into how steroidogenesis is rapidly modulated by hormones such as ACTH and LH.

The 5α-reductases type I and II convert testosterone to dihydrotestosterone, an androgen that plays an important role in the development of male external genitalia. Defects in the enzyme 5α-reductase type II (SRD5A2), the major enzyme in genital tissue, result in a complex phenotype of male pseudohermaphroditism.[214] These individuals have an XY karyotype and are born with ambiguous genitalia characterized as pseudovaginal perineoscrotal hypospadias. At puberty, there is masculinization with good muscle development and enlargement of the phallus, but the prostate remains small and beard growth is scanty. In some cultures where the prevalence of the disease is high, affected individuals are raised as girls, but change gender identity at puberty.[214] As with 21-hydroxylase deficiency, a number of different sites in the enzyme are mutated in different families and many affected individuals are compound heterozygotes.[215,216]

Glucocorticoid remediable hypertension (GRA) is characterized by high levels of abnormal adrenal steroids, 18-oxocortisol and 18-hydroxycortisol, and a variable degree of hyperaldosteronism. Because production of these steroids occurs in a region of the adrenal cortex that is under the control of ACTH, their production is reduced by administration of glucocorticoids. This disorder is caused by an unusual gene rearrangement.[217] The genes encoding aldosterone synthetase and steroid 11β-hydroxylase are arranged in tandem on chromosome 8q. Aldosterone synthetase is expressed in the zona glomerulosa, where it is involved in aldosterone production, whereas 11β-hydroxylase is expressed in the ACTH-dependent zona fasciculata, as well as in the zona glomerulosa. These two genes are 95% identical, predisposing to gene duplication by unequal crossing over. Because the fusion gene contains the regulatory regions of 11β-hydroxylase and the coding sequence of aldosterone synthetase, the latter enzyme is subjected to an abnormal pattern of expression in the ACTH-dependent zone of the adrenal gland, resulting in overproduction of mineralocorticoids.

Defects in thyroid hormone synthesis are characterized by hypothyroidism and, if untreated, by goiter, due to stimulation of the gland by TSH. Defects in thyroid hormone synthesis are typically recessive. Normal iodide uptake at the basolateral membrane by the perchlorate-sensitive Na^+/I^- symporter (NIS) is a rate-limiting step in thyroid hormone synthesis, and several homozygous or compound heterozygous mutations have been identified in individuals with hypothyroidism associated with impaired iodide uptake.[218] Efflux of iodide at the apical membrane of thyroid follicular cells is, at least in part, mediated by pendrin (SCL26A4).[199] Mutations in pendrin cause Pendred syndrome and, as a consequence of the impaired organification of iodide, some patients present with congenital hypothyroidism under conditions of low nutritional iodide intake.[199] Thyroperoxidase (TPO), a glycosylated hemoprotein located at the apical membrane facing the follicular lumen, iodinates tyrosine residues in thyroglobulin (TG), and the coupling of iodinated tyrosines generates T_4 and T_3. TPO defects are among the most frequent causes of inborn errors of thyroid hormone synthesis.[219] Monoallelic mutations in the oxidoreductase THOX2, which is important for the synthesis of hydrogen peroxide, lead to mild transient hypotyroidism, whereas biallelic THOX2 mutations are associated with a severe phenotype.[220] Recessive mutations in the *TG* gene, an unusually large gene spanning more than 300 kb and containing 48 exons, have been reported in a number of animal models and human patients.[221] In many instances, the mutated TG protein is retained in the endoplasmic reticulum, resulting in a classical endoplasmic reticulum storage disease (ERSD). Nonsense mutations in the *TG* gene also illustrate the phenomenon of

nonsense-mediated altered splicing.[222] Mutations introducing a premature stop codon are predicted to result in a truncated protein with at least a partial loss of function. There are, however, instances in which altered splicing removes the exon harboring the premature stop codon, resulting in sufficient amounts of a functional transcript and protein.[223] Several mechanisms have been proposed to explain nonsense-mediated altered splicing. They include removal of the altered exon by nuclear scanning, nonsense-mediated mRNA decay of the mutant transcript in combination with translation of small amounts of exon-skipped isoforms, disruption of the secondary structure leading to exon excision, and disruption of exonic splicing enhancers by the premature stop codon.[222]

Type I vitamin D–dependent rickets (also known as pseudovitamin D–deficient rickets) is caused by mutations in the enzyme, 1α-hydroxylase, which converts 25-vitamin D_3 to its more active metabolite, 1α,25-hydroxyvitamin D_3.[224] In this disorder, patients have low concentrations of 1α,25-hydroxyvitamin D_3 and normal or elevated concentrations of the precursor, 25-vitamin D_3. They can be treated with physiologic doses of 1α,25-hydroxyvitamin D_3. An X-linked form of rickets is referred to as hypophosphatemic (XLH) vitamin D–resistant rickets, a misnomer because the patients are not vitamin-D resistant. XLH is caused by mutations in the *PHEX* gene, which is thought to metabolize a putative phosphate-regulating hormone called phosphatonin.[225,226]

DEFECTS IN CHANNELS

Closure of adenosine triphosphate (ATP)–sensitive potassium channels in pancreatic islet β cells initiates a cascade of events that, in turn, lead to insulin secretion. Potassium currents are reconstituted by the inward rectifier Kir6.2 and the sulfonylurea receptor (SUR), a member of the ATP-binding cassette superfamily. Homozygous mutations in either SUR[227] or Kir6.2 can cause persistent hyperinsulinemic hypoglycemia of infancy (PHHI; nesidioblastosis).[228]

Cellular uptake of thyroid hormones is, at least in part, mediated by channels.[229] Point mutations and deletions in the X-chromosomal *MCT8* gene have been identified in several male patients presenting with elevated T_3 and TSH levels and a severe neurologic phenotype that includes mental retardation, spastic quadriplegia, hypotonia rotary nystagmus, and impaired gaze and hearing.[230] Heterozygous females have discrete thyroid hormone abnormalities, but no neurologic alterations. The abnormal T_3 elevation may be due to impaired uptake into cells such as neurons and differs from severe hypothyroidism. It remains unclear whether MCT8 transports other amino acid derivatives that could be involved in the development of the complex phenotype.

REFERENCES

1. Waterston RH, Lindblad-Toh K, Birney E, et al: Initial sequencing and comparative analysis of the mouse genome. Nature 420:520–562, 2002.
2. Collins FS, Green ED, Guttmacher AE, Guyer MS: A vision for the future of genomics research. Nature 422:835–847, 2003.
3. Stein LD: Integrating biological databases. Nat Rev Genet 4:337–345, 2003.
4. Jameson JL: Principles of Molecular Medicine. Totowa, NJ, Humana Press, 1998.
5. Jameson JL: Application of molecular biology and genetics in endocrinology. In DeGroot LJ,

Jameson JL (eds): Endocrinology, 4th ed. Philadelphia, WB Saunders, 2001, pp 143–166.
6. Wolfsberg T, Wetterstrand K, Guyer M, et al: A user's guide to the human genome. Nat Genet 32:1–79, 2002.
7. Collins FS, Patrinos A, Jordan E, et al: New goals for the U.S. Human Genome Project: 1998–2003. Science 282:682–689, 1998.
8. Jameson JL: The human genome project. In Jameson JL (ed): Principles of Molecular Medicine. Totowa, NJ, Humana Press, 1998, pp 59–64.
9. Guttmacher AE, Collins FS: Genomic medicine: A primer. N Engl J Med 347:1512–1520, 2002.

10. Guttmacher AE, Collins FS: Welcome to the genomic era. N Engl J Med 349:996–998, 2003.
11. Clayton EW: Ethical, legal, and social implications of genomic medicine. N Engl J Med 349:562–569, 2003.
12. Beaudet AL: Genetics and disease. In Fauci AS, Braunwald E, Isselbacher KJ, et al (eds): Harrison's Principles of Internal Medicine, 14th ed. New York, McGraw-Hill, 1998, pp 365–394.
13. Kopp P, Jameson JL: Transmission of human genetic disease. In Jameson JL (ed): Principles of Molecular Medicine. Totowa, NJ, Humana Press, 1998, pp 43–58.

14. Jameson JL, Kopp P: Principles of human genetics. In Braunwald E, Fauci AS, Kasper DL, et al (eds): Harrison's Principles of Internal Medicine, 16th ed. New York, McGraw-Hill, 2004 (in press).

15. Ito M, Jameson JL: Molecular basis of autosomal dominant neurohypophyseal diabetes insipidus: Cellular toxicity caused by the accumulation of mutant vasopressin precursors within the endoplasmic reticulum. J Clin Invest 99:1897–1905, 1997.

16. Willcutts MD, Felner E, White PC: Autosomal recessive familial neurohypophyseal diabetes insipidus with continued secretion of mutant weakly active vasopressin. Hum Mol Genet 8:1303–1307, 1999.

17. Morello JP, Bichet DG: Nephrogenic diabetes insipidus. Annu Rev Physiol 63:607–630, 2001.

18. Duprez L, Parma J, Van Sande J, et al: Germline mutations in the thyrotropin receptor gene cause non-autoimmune autosomal dominant hyperthyroidism. Nat Genet 7:396–401, 1994.

19. Refetoff S, Weiss RE, Usala SJ: The syndromes of resistance to thyroid hormone. Endocr Rev 14:348–399, 1993.

20. Chatterjee VKK, Clifton-Bligh RJ, Gurnell M: Thyroid hormone resistance. In Jameson JL (ed): Hormone Resistance Syndromes. Totowa, NJ, Humana Press, 1999, pp 145–164.

21. Seidman JG, Seidman C: Transcription factor haploinsufficiency: When half a loaf is not enough. J Clin Invest 109:451–455, 2002.

22. Chandrasekharappa SC, Guru SC, Manickam P, et al: Positional cloning of the gene for multiple endocrine neoplasia-type 1. Science 276:404–407, 1997.

23. Berta P, Hawkins JR, Sinclair AH, et al: Genetic evidence equating SRY and the testis-determining factor. Nature 348:448–450, 1990.

24. Reijo R, Lee TY, Salo P, et al: Diverse spermatogenic defects in humans caused by Y chromosome deletions encompassing a novel RNA-binding protein gene. Nat Genet 10:383–393, 1995.

25. Fox MS, Reijo Pera RA: Male infertility, genetic analysis of the DAZ genes on the human Y chromosome and genetic analysis of DNA repair. Mol Cell Endocrinol 184:41–49, 2001.

26. McPhaul MJ, Marcelli M, Zoppi S, et al: Genetic basis of endocrine disease. 4. The spectrum of mutations in the androgen receptor gene that causes androgen resistance. J Clin Endocrinol Metab 76:17–23, 1993.

27. Kopp P, Arseven OK, Sabacan L, et al: Phenocopies for deafness and goiter development in a large inbred Brazilian kindred with Pendred's syndrome associated with a novel mutation in the PDS gene. J Clin Endocrinol Metab 84:336–341, 1999.

28. Shenker A, Laue L, Kosugi S, et al: A constitutively activating mutation of the luteinizing hormone receptor in familial male precocious puberty. Nature 365:652–654, 1993.

29. Haines J, Pericak-Vance M: Approaches to Gene Mapping in Complex Human Diseases. New York, Wiley-Liss, 1998.

30. Florez JC, Hirschhorn J, Altshuler D: The inherited basis of diabetes mellitus: Implications for the genetic analysis of complex traits. Annu Rev Genomics Hum Genet 4:257–291, 2003.

31. Davies JL, Kawaguchi Y, Bennett ST, et al: A genome-wide search for human type 1 diabetes susceptibility genes. Nature 371:130–136, 1994.

32. van den Ouweland JM, Lemkes HH, Trembath RC, et al: Maternally inherited diabetes and deafness is a distinct subtype of diabetes and associates with a single point mutation in the mitochondrial tRNA(Leu[UUR]) gene. Diabetes 43:746–751, 1994.

33. Wilkins JF, Haig D: What good is genomic imprinting: The function of parent-specific gene expression. Nat Rev Genet 4:359–368, 2003.

34. Goldstone AP: Prader-Willi syndrome: advances in genetics, pathophysiology and treatment. Trends Endocrinol Metab 15:12–20, 2004.

35. Peters J, Wroe SF, Wells CA, et al: A cluster of oppositely imprinted transcripts at the Gnas locus in the distal imprinting region of mouse chromosome 2. Proc Natl Acad Sci U S A 96:3830–3835, 1999.

36. Weinstein LS, Yu S, Warner DR, Liu J: Endocrine manifestations of stimulatory G protein alpha-subunit mutations and the role of genomic imprinting. Endocr Rev 22:675–705, 2001.

37. Weinstein LS, Shenker A, Gejman PV, et al: Activating mutations of the stimulatory G protein in the McCune-Albright syndrome. N Engl J Med 325:1688–1695, 1991.

38. Balmain A, Gray J, Ponder B: The genetics and genomics of cancer. Nat Genet 33:238–244, 2003.

39. Edwards A, Hammond HA, Jin L, et al: Genetic variation at five trimeric and tetrameric tandem repeat loci in four human population groups. Genomics 12:241–253, 1992.

40. Dejager S, Bry-Gauillard H, Bruckert E, et al: A comprehensive endocrine description of Kennedy's disease revealing androgen insensitivity linked to CAG repeat length. J Clin Endocrinol Metab 87:3893–3901, 2002.

41. Mastrogiacomo I, Pagani E, Novelli G, et al: Male hypogonadism in myotonic dystrophy is related to (CTG)n triplet mutation. J Endocrinol Invest 17:381–383, 1994.

42. Pandolfo M: Friedreich's ataxia: Clinical aspects and pathogenesis. Semin Neurol 19:311–321, 1999.

43. Ott J: Estimation of the recombination fraction in human pedigrees: Efficient computation of the likelihood for human linkage studies. Am J Hum Genet 26:588–597, 1974.

44. Southern EM: Detection of specific sequences among DNA fragments separated by gel electrophoresis. J Mol Biol 98:503–517, 1975.

45. Saiki RK, Gelfand DH, Stoffel S, et al: Primer-directed enzymatic amplifcation of DNA with a thermostable DNA polymerase. Science 239:487–491, 1988.

46. Nakamura Y, Leppert M, O'Connell P, et al: Variable number of tandem repeat (VNTR) markers for human gene mapping. Science 235:1616–1622, 1987.

47. Zhang X, Kousoulas KG: Direct sequencing of PCR-amplified high GC DNA. Biotechniques 14:376–377, 1993.

48. Top B: A simple method to attach a universal 50-bp GC-clamp to PCR fragments used for mutation analysis by DGGE. PCR Methods Appl 2:83–85, 1992.

49. Poduslo SE, Dean M, Kolch U, O'Brien SJ: Detecting high-resolution polymorphisms in human coding loci by combining PCR and single-strand conformation polymorphism (SSCP) analysis. Am J Hum Genet 49:106–111, 1991.

50. Lilleberg SL: In-depth mutation and SNP discovery using DHPLC gene scanning. Curr Opin Drug Discov Devel 6:237–252, 2003.

51. Kim S, Ruparel HD, Gilliam TC, Ju J: Digital genotyping using molecular affinity and mass spectrometry. Nat Rev Genet 4:1001–1008, 2003.

52. Verlaan-de Vries M, Bogaard ME, van den Elst H, et al: A dot-blot screening procedure for mutated ras oncogenes using synthetic oligodeoxynucleotides. Gene 50:313–320, 1986.

53. Hacia JG, Collins FS: Mutational analysis using oligonucleotide microarrays. J Med Genet 36:730–736, 1999.

54. Mankodi A, Ashizawa T: Echo of silence: Silent mutations, RNA splicing, and neuromuscular diseases. Neurology 61:1330–1331, 2003.

55. Weiss J, Axelrod L, Whitcomb RW, et al: Hypogonadism caused by a single amino acid substitution in the a-subunit of luteinizing hormone. N Engl J Med 326:179–183, 1991.

56. White PC, New MI: Genetic basis of endocrine disease 2: Congenital adrenal hyperplasia due to 21-hydroxylase deficiency. J Clin Endocrinol Metab 74:6–11, 1992.

57. Taylor SI, Cama A, Accili D, et al: Genetic basis of endocrine disease. 1. Molecular genetics of insulin resistant diabetes mellitus. J Clin Endocrinol Metab 73:1158–1163, 1991.

58. Parma J, Duprez L, Van Sande J, et al: Somatic mutations in the thyrotropin receptor gene cause hyperfunctioning thyroid adenomas. Nature 365:649–651, 1993.

59. Jameson JL: Thyroid hormone resistance: Pathophysiology at the molecular level. J Clin Endocrinol Metab 74:708–711, 1992.

60. Papin JA, Price ND, Wiback SJ, et al: Metabolic pathways in the post-genome era. Trends Biochem Sci 28:250–258, 2003.

61. McKusick VA: Mendelian Inheritance in Man. Baltimore, Johns Hopkins University Press, 1988.

62. Hamosh A, Scott AF, Amberger J, et al: Online Mendelian Inheritance in Man (OMIM). Hum Mutat 15:57–61, 2000.

63. Vnencak JCL, Phillips JA III, Chen EY, Seeburg PH: Molecular basis of human growth hormone gene deletions. Proc Natl Acad Sci U S A 85:5615–5619, 1988.

64. Vnencak JCL, Phillips JA: Hot spots for growth hormone gene deletions in homologous regions outside of Alu repeats. Science 250:1745–1748, 1990.

65. Rogol AD, Blizzard RM, Foley T Jr, et al: Growth hormone releasing hormone and growth hormone: Genetic studies in familial growth hormone deficiency. Pediatr Res 19:489–492, 1985.

66. Wajnrajch MP, Gertner JM, Harbison MD, et al: Nonsense mutation in the human growth hormone-releasing hormone receptor causes growth failure analogous to the little (lit) mouse. Nat Genet 12:88–90, 1996.

67. Franco B, Guioli S, Pragliola A, et al: A gene deleted in Kallmann's syndrome shares homology with neural cell adhesion and axonal path-finding molecules. Nature 353:529–536, 1991.

68. Dode C, Levilliers J, Dupont J, et al: Loss-of-function mutations in FGFR1 cause autosomal dominant Kallmann syndrome. Nat Genet 33:463–465, 2003.

69. Vnencak JCL, Phillips JA III, Wang DF: Use of polymerase chain reaction in detection of growth hormone gene deletions. J Clin Endocrinol Metab 70:1550–1553, 1990.

70. Moseley CT, Orenstein MD, Phillips JA III: GH gene deletions and IGHD type IA. Rev Endocr Metab Disord 3:339–346, 2002.

71. Cogan JD, Prince MA, Lekhakula S, et al: A novel mechanism of aberrant pre-mRNA splicing in humans. Hum Mol Genet 6:909–912, 1997.

72. Cogan JD, Ramel B, Lehto M, et al: A recurring dominant negative mutation causes autosomal dominant growth hormone deficiency: A clinical research center study. J Clin Endocrinol Metab 80:3591–3595, 1995.

73. Steiner DF, Tager HS, Chan SJ, et al: Lessons learned from molecular biology of insulin-gene mutations. Diabetes Care 13:600–609, 1990.

74. Arnold A, Horst SA, Gardella TJ, et al: Mutation of the signal peptide-encoding region of the preproparathyroid hormone gene in familial isolated hypoparathyroidism. J Clin Invest 86:1084–1087, 1990.

75. Ito M, Mori Y, Oiso Y, Saito H: A single base substitution in the coding region for neurophysin II associated with familial central diabetes insipidus. J Clin Invest 87:725–728, 1991.

76. Ito M, Yu RN, Ito M, Jameson JL: Mutant vasopressin precursors that cause autosomal dominant neurohypophyseal diabetes insipidus retain dimerization and impair the secretion of wild-type proteins. J Biol Chem 274:9029–9037, 1999.

77. Russell TA, Ito M, Yu RN, et al: A murine model of autosomal dominant neurohypophyseal diabetes insipidus reveals progressive loss of vasopressin-producing neurons. J Clin Invest 112:1697–1706, 2003.

78. McLeod JF, Kovacs L, Gaskill MB, et al: Familial neurohypophyseal diabetes insipidus associated with a signal peptide mutation. J Clin Endocrinol Metab 77:599A–599G, 1993.

79. Hayashizaki Y, Hiraoka Y, Endo Y, et al: Thyroid-stimulating hormone (TSH) deficiency caused by a single base substitution in the CAGYC region of the beta-subunit. EMBO J 8:2291–2296, 1989.

80. Dacou-Voutetakis C, Feltquate DM, Drakopoulou M, et al: Familial hypothyroidism caused by a nonsense mutation in the thyroid-stimulating hormone beta-subunit gene. Am J Hum Genet 46:988–993, 1990.

81. Matthews CH, Borgato S, Beck-Peccoz P, et al: Primary amenorrhoea and infertility due to a mutation in the beta-subunit of follicle-stimulating hormone. Nat Genet 5:83–86, 1993.

82. Layman LC, Lee EJ, Peak DB, et al: Delayed puberty and hypogonadism caused by mutations in the follicle-stimulating hormone beta-subunit gene. N Engl J Med 337:607–611, 1997.

83. Phillip M, Arbelle JE, Segev Y, Parvari R: Male hypogonadism due to a mutation in the gene for the beta-subunit of follicle-stimulating hormone. N Engl J Med 338:1729–1732, 1998.

84. Montague CT, Farooqi IS, Whitehead JP, et al: Congenital leptin deficiency is associated with severe early-onset obesity in humans. Nature 387:903–908, 1997.

85. Krude H, Biebermann H, Luck W, et al: Severe early-onset obesity, adrenal insufficiency and red hair pigmentation caused by POMC mutations in humans. Nat Genet 19:155–157, 1998.

86. Mori Y, Seino S, Takeda K, et al: A mutation causing reduced biological activity and stability of thyroxine-binding globulin probably as a result of abnormal glycosylation of the molecule. Mol Endocrinol 3:575–579, 1989.

87. Mori Y, Refetoff S, Flink IL, et al: Detection of the thyroxine-binding globulin (TBG) gene in six unrelated families with complete TBG deficiency. J Clin Endocrinol Metab 67:727–733, 1988.

88. Mori Y, Miura Y, Takeuchi H, et al: Gene amplification as a cause of inherited thyroxine-binding globulin excess in two Japanese families. J Clin Endocrinol Metab 80:3758–3762, 1995.

89. Yeo PP, Yabu Y, Etzkorn JR, et al: A four generation study of familial dysalbuminemic hyperthyroxinemia: Diagnosis in the presence of an acquired excess of thyroxine-binding globulin. J Endocrinol Invest 10:33–38, 1987.

90. Sunthornthepvarakul T, Angkeow P, Weiss RE, et al: An identical missense mutation in the albumin gene results in familial dysalbuminemic hyperthyroxinemia in 8 unrelated families. Biochem Biophys Res Commun 202:781–787, 1994.

91. Wada N, Chiba H, Shimizu C, et al: A novel missense mutation in codon 218 of the albumin gene in a distinct phenotype of familial dysalbuminemic hyperthyroxinemia in a Japanese kindred. J Clin Endocrinol Metab 82:3246–3250, 1997.

92. Sunthornthepvarakul T, Likitmaskul S, Ngowngarmratana S, et al: Familial dysalbuminemic hypertriiodothyroninemia: A new, dominantly inherited albumin defect. J Clin Endocrinol Metab 83:1448–1454, 1998.

93. Moses AC, Rosen HN, Moller DE, et al: A point mutation in transthyretin increases affinity for thyroxine and produces euthyroid hyperthyroxinemia. J Clin Invest 86:2025–2033, 1990.

94. Saraiva MJ: Transthyretin mutations in hyperthyroxinemia and amyloid diseases. Hum Mutat 17:493–503, 2001.

95. Amselem S, Sobrier ML, Duquesnoy P, et al: Recurrent nonsense mutations in the growth hormone receptor from patients with Laron dwarfism. J Clin Invest 87:1098–1102, 1991.

96. Laron Z: Laron syndrome: Primary growth hormone resistance. In Jameson JL (ed): Hormone Resistance Syndromes. Totowa, NJ, Humana Press, 1999, pp 17–38.

97. Jameson JL: Hormone Resistance Syndromes. Totowa, NJ, Humana Press, 1999.

98. Taylor SI, Arioglu E: Diabetes mellitus: Insulin resistance. In Jameson JL (ed): Hormone Resistance Syndromes. Totowa, NJ, Humana Press, 1999, pp 165–184.

99. Merendino J Jr, Speigel AM, Crawford JD, et al: Brief report: A mutation in the vasopressin V2-receptor gene in a kindred with X-linked nephrogenic diabetes insipidus. N Engl J Med 328:1538–1541, 1993.

100. Holtzman EJ, Harris H Jr, Kolakowski L Jr, et al: Brief report: A molecular defect in the vasopressin V2-receptor gene causing nephrogenic diabetes insipidus. N Engl J Med 328:1534–1537, 1993.

101. Lightman SL: Molecular insights into diabetes insipidus. N Engl J Med 328:1562–1563, 1993.

102. Deen PM, Verdijk MA, Knoers NV, et al: Requirement of human renal water channel aquaporin-2 for vasopressin-dependent concentration of urine. Science 264:92–95, 1994.

103. Mulders SM, Bichet DG, Rijss JP, et al: An aquaporin-2 water channel mutant which causes autosomal dominant nephrogenic diabetes insipidus is retained in the Golgi complex. J Clin Invest 102:57–66, 1998.

104. de Roux N, Young J, Misrahi M, et al: A family with hypogonadotropic hypogonadism and mutations in the gonadotropin-releasing hormone receptor. N Engl J Med 337:1597–1602, 1997.

105. Baumann G: Dwarfism: GHRH resistance. In Jameson JL (ed): Hormone Resistance Syndromes. Totowa, NJ, Humana Press, 1999, pp 1–16.

106. Kjelsberg MA, Cotecchia S, Ostrowski J, et al: Constitutive activation of the alpha 1B-adrenergic receptor by all amino acid substitutions at a single site: Evidence for a region which constrains receptor activation. J Biol Chem 267:1430–1433, 1992.

107. Schipani E, Kruse K, Juppner H: A constitutively active mutant PTH-PTHrP receptor in Jansen-type metaphyseal chondrodysplasia. Science 268:98–100, 1995.

108. Pollak MR, Brown EM, Estep HL, et al: Autosomal dominant hypocalcaemia caused by a Ca(2+)-sensing receptor gene mutation. Nat Genet 8:303–307, 1994.

109. Kopp P, van Sande J, Parma J, et al: Brief report: Congenital hyperthyroidism caused by a mutation in the thyrotropin-receptor gene. N Engl J Med 332:150–154, 1995.

110. Vassart G: New pathophysiological mechanisms for hyperthyroidism. Horm Res 48:47–50, 1997.

111. Sunthornthepvarakui T, Gottschalk ME, Hayashi Y, Refetoff S: Brief report: Resistance to thyrotropin caused by mutations in the thyrotropin-receptor gene. N Engl J Med 332:155–160, 1995.

112. Abramowicz MJ, Duprez L, Parma J, et al: Familial congenital hypothyroidism due to inactivating mutation of the thyrotropin receptor causing profound hypoplasia of the thyroid gland. J Clin Invest 99:3018–3024, 1997.

113. Gromoll J, Simoni M, Nieschlag E: An activating mutation of the follicle-stimulating hormone receptor autonomously sustains spermatogenesis in a hypophysectomized man. J Clin Endocrinol Metab 81:1367–1370, 1996.

114. Kremer H, Kraaij R, Toledo SP, et al: Male pseudohermaphroditism due to a homozygous missense mutation of the luteinizing hormone receptor gene. Nat Genet 9:160–164, 1995.

115. Latronico AC, Anasti J, Arnhold IJ, et al: Brief report: testicular and ovarian resistance to luteinizing hormone caused by inactivating mutations of the luteinizing hormone-receptor gene. N Engl J Med 334:507–512, 1996.

116. Toledo SP, Brunner HG, Kraaij R, et al: An inactivating mutation of the luteinizing hormone receptor causes amenorrhea in a 46,XX female. J Clin Endocrinol Metab 81:3850–3854, 1996.

117. Aittomaki K, Lucena JL, Pakarinen P, et al: Mutation in the follicle-stimulating hormone receptor gene causes hereditary hypergonadotropic ovarian failure. Cell 82:959–968, 1995.

118. Brown EM, Gamba G, Riccardi D, et al: Cloning and characterization of an extracellular Ca(2+)-sensing receptor from bovine parathyroid. Nature 366:575–580, 1993.

119. Pollak MR, Brown EM, Chou YH, et al: Mutations in the human Ca(2+)-sensing receptor gene cause familial hypocalciuric hypercalcemia and neonatal severe hyperparathyroidism. Cell 75:1297–1303, 1993.

120. Lyons J, Landis CA, Harsh G, et al: Two G protein oncogenes in human endocrine tumors. Science 249:655–659, 1990.

121. Landis CA, Masters SB, Spada A, et al: GTPase inhibiting mutations activate the alpha chain of Gs and stimulate adenylyl cyclase in human pituitary tumours. Nature 340:692–696, 1989.

122. Spada A, Arosio M, Bochicchio D, et al: Clinical, biochemical, and morphological correlates in patients bearing growth hormone-secreting pituitary tumors with or without constitutively active adenylyl cyclase. J Clin Endocrinol Metab 71:1421–1426, 1990.

123. Al-Zahrani A, Levine MA, Schwindinger WF: Pseudohypoparathyroidism. In Jameson JL (ed): Hormone Resistance Syndromes. Totowa, NJ, Humana Press, 1999, pp 39–58.

124. Patten JL, Johns DR, Valle D, et al: Mutation in the gene encoding the stimulatory G protein of adenylate cyclase in Albright's hereditary osteodystrophy. N Engl J Med 322:1412–1419, 1990.

125. Weinstein LS, Gejman PV, Friedman E, et al: Mutations of the Gs alpha-subunit gene in Albright hereditary osteodystrophy detected by denaturing gradient gel electrophoresis. Proc Natl Acad Sci U S A 87:8287–8290, 1990.

126. Arnold A, Kim HG, Gaz RD, et al: Molecular cloning and chromosomal mapping of DNA rearranged with the parathyroid hormone gene in a parathyroid adenoma. J Clin Invest 83:2034–2040, 1989.

127. Motokura T, Bloom T, Kim HG, et al: A novel cyclin encoded by a bcl1-linked candidate oncogene. Nature 350:512–515, 1991.

128. Refetoff S, DeWind LT, DeGroot LJ: Familial syndrome combining deaf-mutism, stuppled epiphyses, goiter and abnormally high PBI: Possible target organ refractoriness to thyroid hormone. J Clin Endocrinol Metab 27:279–294, 1967.

129. Usala SJ, Weintraub BD: Thyroid hormone resistance syndromes. Trends Endocrinol Metab 2:140–144, 1991.

130. Sakurai A, Takeda K, Ain K, et al: Generalized resistance to thyroid hormone associated with a mutation in the ligand-binding domain of the human thyroid hormone receptor beta. Proc Natl Acad Sci U S A 86:8977–8981, 1989.

131. Usala SJ, Tennyson GE, Bale AE, et al: A base mutation of the C-erbA beta thyroid hormone receptor in a kindred with generalized thyroid hormone resistance: Molecular heterogeneity in two other kindreds. J Clin Invest 85:93–100, 1990.

132. Chatterjee VK, Nagaya T, Madison LD, et al: Thyroid hormone resistance syndrome: Inhibition of normal receptor function by mutant thyroid hormone receptors. J Clin Invest 87:1977–1984, 1991.

133. Nagaya T, Madison LD, Jameson JL: Thyroid hormone receptor mutants that cause resistance to thyroid hormone: Evidence for receptor competition for DNA sequences in target genes. J Biol Chem 267:13014–13019, 1992.

134. Tagami T, Jameson JL: Nuclear corepressors enhance the dominant negative activity of mutant receptors that cause resistance to thyroid hormone. Endocrinology 139:640–650, 1998.

135. Hughes MR, Malloy PJ, Kieback DG, et al: Point mutations in the human vitamin D receptor gene associated with hypocalcemic rickets. Science 242:1702–1705, 1988.

136. Malloy PJ, Hochberg Z, Tiosano D, et al: The molecular basis of hereditary 1,25-dihydroxyvitamin D3 resistant rickets in seven related families. J Clin Invest 86:2071–2079, 1990.

137. Feldman D, Malloy PJ: Hereditary 1,25-dihydroxyvitamin D resistant rickets: Molecular basis and implications for the role of 1,25(OH)2D3 in normal physiology. Mol Cell Endocrinol 72:C57–62, 1990.

138. Hurley DM, Accili D, Stratakis CA, et al: Point mutation causing a single amino acid substitution in the hormone binding domain of the glucocorticoid receptor in familial glucocorticoid resistance. J Clin Invest 87:680–686, 1991.

139. Smith EP, Boyd J, Frank GR, et al: Estrogen resistance caused by a mutation in the estrogen-receptor gene in a man. N Engl J Med 331:1056–1061, 1994.

140. McGuire WL, Chamness GC, Fuqua SA: The importance of normal and abnormal estrogen receptor in breast cancer. Cancer Surv 14:31–40, 1992.

141. Fuqua SA, Chamness GC, McGuire WL: Estrogen receptor mutations in breast cancer. J Cell Biochem 51:135–139, 1993.

142. Luo X, Ikeda Y, Parker KL: A cell-specific nuclear receptor is essential for adrenal and gonadal development and sexual differentiation. Cell 77:481–490, 1994.

143. Parker KL, Schimmer BP: Steroidogenic factor 1: A key determinant of endocrine development and function. Endocr Rev 18:361–377, 1997.

144. Achermann JC, Ito M, Hindmarsh PC, Jameson JL: A mutation in the gene encoding steroidogenic factor-1 causes XY sex reversal and adrenal failure in humans. Nat Genet 22:125–126, 1999.

145. Ito M, Yu R, Jameson JL: DAX-1 inhibits SF-1-mediated transactivation via a carboxy-terminal domain that is deleted in adrenal hypoplasia congenita. Mol Cell Biol 17:1476–1483, 1997.

146. Muscatelli F, Strom TM, Walker AP, et al: Mutations in the DAX-1 gene give rise to both X-linked adrenal hypoplasia congenita and hypogonadotropic hypogonadism. Nature 372:672–676, 1994.

147. Gubbay J, Collignon J, Koopman P, et al: A gene mapping to the sex-determining region of the mouse Y chromosome is a member of a novel family of embryonically expressed genes. Nature 346:245–250, 1990.

148. Koopman P, Gubbay J, Vivian N, et al: Male development of chromosomally female mice transgenic for Sry. Nature 351:117–121, 1991.

149. Foster JW, Dominguez-Steglich MA, Guioli S, et al: Campomelic dysplasia and autosomal sex reversal caused by mutations in an SRY-related gene. Nature 372:525–530, 1994.

150. Pelletier J, Bruening W, Kashtan CE, et al: Germline mutations in the Wilms' tumor suppressor gene are associated with abnormal urogenital development in Denys-Drash syndrome. Cell 67:437–447, 1991.

151. Petit C, de la Chapelle A, Levilliers J, et al: An abnormal terminal X-Y interchange accounts for most but not all cases of human XX maleness. Cell 49:595–602, 1987.

152. Page DC, Brown LG, De la Chappelle A: Exchange of terminal portions of X- and Y-chromosomal short arms in human XX males. Nature 328:437–440, 1987.

153. Ingraham HA, Chen RP, Mangalam HJ, et al: A tissue-specific transcription factor containing a homeodomain specifies a pituitary phenotype. Cell 55:519–529, 1988.

154. Castrillo JL, Bodner M, Karin M: Purification of growth hormone-specific transcription factor GHF-1 containing homeobox. Science 243:814–817, 1989.

155. Simmons DM, Voss JW, Ingraham HA, et al: Pituitary cell phenotypes involve cell-specific Pit-1 mRNA translation and synergistic interactions with other classes of transcription factors. Genes Dev 4:695–711, 1990.

156. Li S, Crenshaw EB, Rawson EJ, et al: Dwarf locus mutants lacking three pituitary cell types result from mutations in the POU-domain gene pit-1. Nature 347:528–533, 1990.

157. Wit JM, Drayer NM, Jansen M, et al: Total deficiency of growth hormone and prolactin, and partial deficiency of thyroid stimulating hormone in two Dutch families: A new variant of hereditary pituitary deficiency. Horm Res 32:170–177, 1989.

158. Pfaffle RW, DiMattia GE, Parks JS, et al: Mutation of the POU-specific domain of Pit-1 and hypopituitarism without pituitary hypoplasia. Science 257:1118–1121, 1992.

159. Tatsumi K, Miyai K, Notomi T, et al: Cretinism with combined hormone deficiency caused by a mutation in the PIT1 gene. Nat Genet 1:56–58, 1992.

160. Radovick S, Nations M, Du Y, et al: A mutation in the POU-homeodomain of Pit-1 responsible for combined pituitary hormone deficiency. Science 257:1115–1118, 1992.

161. Wu W, Cogan JD, Pfaffle RW, et al: Mutations in PROP1 cause familial combined pituitary hormone deficiency. Nat Genet 18:147–149, 1998.

162. Netchine I, Sobrier ML, Krude H, et al: Mutations in LHX3 result in a new syndrome revealed by combined pituitary hormone deficiency. Nat Genet 25:182–186, 2000.

163. Dattani MT, Martinez-Barbera JP, Thomas PQ, et al: Mutations in the homeobox gene HESX1/Hesx1 associated with septo-optic dysplasia in human and mouse. Nat Genet 19:125–133, 1998.

164. Thomas PQ, Dattani MT, Brickman JM, et al: Heterozygous HESX1 mutations associated with isolated congenital pituitary hypoplasia and septo-optic dysplasia. Hum Mol Genet 10:39–45, 2001.

165. Missero C, Cobellis G, De Felice M, Di Lauro R: Molecular events involved in differentiation of thyroid follicular cells. Mol Cell Endocrinol 140:37–43, 1998.

166. Clifton-Bligh RJ, Wentworth JM, Heinz P, et al: Mutation of the gene encoding human TTF-2 associated with thyroid agenesis, cleft palate and choanal atresia. Nat Genet 19:399–401, 1998.

167. Macchia PE, Lapi P, Krude H, et al: PAX8 mutations associated with congenital hypothyroidism caused by thyroid dysgenesis. Nat Genet 19:83–86, 1998.

168. Pohlenz J, Dumitrescu A, Zundel D, et al: Partial deficiency of thyroid transcription factor 1 produces predominantly neurological defects in humans and mice. J Clin Invest 109:469–473, 2002.

169. Krude H, Schutz B, Biebermann H, et al: Choreoathetosis, hypothyroidism, and pulmonary alterations due to human NKX2-1 haploinsufficiency. J Clin Invest 109:475–480, 2002.

170. Congdon T, Nguyen LQ, Nogueira CR, et al: A novel mutation (Q40P) in PAX8 associated with congenital hypothyroidism and thyroid hypoplasia: Evidence for phenotypic variability in mother and child. J Clin Endocrinol Metab 86:3962–3967, 2001.

171. Stoffers DA, Ferrer J, Clarke WL, Habener JF: Early-onset type-II diabetes mellitus (MODY4) linked to IPF1. Nat Genet 17:138–139, 1997.

172. Froguel P, Zouali H, Vionnet N, et al: Familial hyperglycemia due to mutations in glucokinase: Definition of a subtype of diabetes mellitus. N Engl J Med 328:697–702, 1993.

173. Malecki MT, Jhala US, Antonellis A, et al: Mutations in NEUROD1 are associated with the development of type 2 diabetes mellitus. Nat Genet 23:323–328, 1999.

174. Larsson C, Skogseid B, Oberg K, et al: Multiple endocrine neoplasia type 1 gene maps to chromosome 11 and is lost in insulinoma. Nature 332:85–87, 1988.

175. Mathew CG, Chin KS, Easton DF, et al: A linked genetic marker for multiple endocrine neoplasia type 2A on chromosome 10. Nature 328:527–528, 1987.

176. Bystrom C, Larsson C, Blomberg C, et al: Localization of the MEN1 gene to a small region within chromosome 11q13 by deletion mapping in tumors. Proc Natl Acad Sci U S A 87:1968–1972, 1990.

177. Agarwal SK, Lee Burns A, Sukhodolets KE, et al: Molecular pathology of the MEN1 gene. Ann N Y Acad Sci 1014:189–198, 2004.

178. Marx S, Spiegel AM, Skarulis MC, et al: Multiple endocrine neoplasia type 1: Clinical and genetic topics. Ann Intern Med 129:484–494, 1998.

179. Friend SH, Bernards R, Rogelj S, et al: A human DNA segment with properties of the gene that predisposes to retinoblastoma and osteosarcoma. Nature 323:643–646, 1986.

180. Kidd KK, Simpson NE: Search for the gene for multiple endocrine neoplasia type 2A. Recent Prog Horm Res 46:305–341, 1990.

181. Mulligan LM, Kwok JBJ, Healey CS, et al: Germ-line mutations of the RET proto-oncogene in multiple endocrine neoplasia type 2A. Nature 363:458–460, 1993.

182. Carlson KM, Dou S, Chi D, et al: Single missense mutation in the tyrosine kinase catalytic domain of the RET protooncogene is associated with multiple endocrine neoplasia type 2B. Proc Natl Acad Sci U S A 91:1579–1583, 1994.

183. Fusco A, Grieco M, Santoro M, et al: A new oncogene in human thyroid papillary carcinomas and their lymph-nodal metastases. Nature 328:170–172, 1987.

184. Grieco M, Santoro M, Berlingieri MT, et al: PTC is a novel rearranged form of the ret proto-oncogene and is frequently detected in vivo in human thyroid papillary carcinomas. Cell 60:557–563, 1990.

185. Santen RJ, Paulsen CA: Hypogonadotropic eunuchoidism. I. Clinical study of the mode of inheritance. J Clin Endocrinol Metab 36:47–54, 1973.

186. White BJ, Rogol AD, Brown KS, et al: The syndrome of anosmia with hypogonadotropic hypogonadism: A genetic study of 18 new families and

a review. Am J Med Genet 15:417–435, 1983.
187. Waldstreicher J, Seminara SB, Jameson JL, et al: The genetic and clinical heterogeneity of gonadotropin-releasing hormone deficiency in the human. J Clin Endocrinol Metab 81:4388–4395, 1996.
188. Capecchi MR: Mouse genetics: YACs to the rescue. Nature 362:205–206, 1993.
189. Weiss J, Crowley WF, Jameson JL: Structure of the GnRH gene in patients with idiopathic hypogonadotropic hypogonadism. J Clin Endocrinol Metab 69:299–303, 1989.
190. Nakayama Y, Wondisford FE, Lash RW, et al: Analysis of gonadotropin-releasing hormone gene structure in families with familial central precocious puberty and idiopathic hypogonadotropic hypogonadism. J Clin Endocrinol Metab 70:1233–1238, 1990.
191. Weiss J, Adams E, Whitcomb RW, et al: Normal sequence of the GnRH gene in patients with idiopathic hypogonadotropic hypogonadism. Biol Repro 45:743–747, 1991.
192. Schwanzel-Fukuda M, Bick D, Pfaff DW: Luteinizing hormone-releasing hormone (LHRH)-expressing cells do not migrate normally in an inherited hypogonadal (Kallmann) syndrome. Brain Res Mol Brain Res 6:311–326, 1989.
193. Crowley WF, Jameson JL: Clinical counterpoint: Gonadotropin-releasing hormone deficiency: Perspectives from clinical investigation. Endocr Rev 13:635–640, 1993.
194. Ballabio A, Bardoni B, Carrozzo R, et al: Contiguous gene syndromes due to deletions in the distal short arm of the human X chromosome. Proc Natl Acad Sci U S A 86:10001–10005, 1989.
195. Meitinger T, Heye B, Petit C, et al: Definitive localization of X-linked Kallman syndrome (hypogonadotropic hypogonadism and anosmia) to Xp22.3: Close linkage to the hypervariable repeat sequence CRI-S232. Am J Hum Genet 47:664–669, 1990.
196. Wray S, Nieburgs A, Elkabes S: Spatiotemporal cell expression of luteinizing hormone-releasing hormone in the prenatal mouse: Evidence for an embryonic origin in the olfactory placode. Brain Res Dev Brain Res 46:309–318, 1989.
197. Bick D, Curry CJ, McGill JR, et al: Male infant with ichthyosis, Kallmann syndrome, chondrodysplasia punctata, and an Xp chromosome deletion. Am J Med Genet 33:100–107, 1989.
197a. Seminara SB, Messager S, Chatzidaki EE, et al: The GPR54 gene as a regulator of puberty. N Engl J Med 349:1614–1627, 2003.
198. Gausden E, Coyle B, Armour JA, et al: Pendred syndrome: Evidence for genetic homogeneity and further refinement of linkage. J Med Genet 34:126–129, 1997.
199. Everett LA, Glaser B, Beck JC, et al: Pendred syndrome is caused by mutations in a putative sulphate transporter gene (PDS). Nat Genet 17:411–422, 1997.
200. Scott DA, Wang R, Kreman TM, et al: The Pendred syndrome gene encodes a chloride-iodide transport protein. Nat Genet 21:440–443, 1999.
201. Eisenbarth GS, Gottlieb PA: Autoimmune polyendocrine syndromes. N Engl J Med 350:2068–2079, 2004.
202. Nagamine K, Peterson P, Scott HS, et al: Positional cloning of the APECED gene. Nat Genet 17:393–398, 1997.
203. Stratakis CA, Carney JA, Lin JP, et al: Carney complex, a familial multiple neoplasia and lentiginosis syndrome: Analysis of 11 kindreds and linkage to the short arm of chromosome 2. J Clin Invest 97:699–705, 1996.
204. Kirschner LS, Carney JA, Pack SD, et al: Mutations of the gene encoding the protein kinase A type I-alpha regulatory subunit in patients with the Carney complex. Nat Genet 26:89–92, 2000.
205. New MI: Basic and clinical aspects of congenital adrenal hyperplasia. J Steroid Biochem 27:1–7, 1987.
206. Speiser PW, Laforgia N, Kato K, et al: First trimester prenatal treatment and molecular genetic diagnosis of congenital adrenal hyperplasia (21-hydroxylase deficiency). J Clin Endocrinol Metab 70:838–848, 1990.
207. Pang S, Pollack MS, Marshall RN, Immken L: Prenatal treatment of congenital adrenal hyperplasia due to 21-hydroxylase deficiency. N Engl J Med 322:111–115, 1990.
208. White PC, Dupont J, New MI, et al: A mutation in CYP11B1 (Arg-448—His) associated with steroid 11 beta-hydroxylase deficiency in Jews of Moroccan origin. J Clin Invest 87:1664–1667, 1991.
209. Kagimoto K, Waterman MR, Kagimoto M, et al: Identification of a common molecular basis for combined 17 alpha-hydroxylase/17,20-lyase deficiency in two Mennonite families. Hum Genet 82:285–286, 1989.
210. Geller DH, Auchus RJ, Mendonca BB, Miller WL: The genetic and functional basis of isolated 17,20-lyase deficiency. Nat Genet 17:201–205, 1997.
211. Rheaume E, Simard J, Morel Y, et al: Congenital adrenal hyperplasia due to point mutations in the type II 3 beta-hydroxysteroid dehydrogenase gene. Nat Genet 1:239–245, 1992.
212. Stocco DM: A review of the characteristics of the protein required for the acute regulation of steroid hormone biosynthesis: The case for the steroidogenic acute regulatory (StAR) protein. Proc Soc Exp Biol Med 217:123–129, 1998.
213. Bose HS, Sugawara T, Strauss JF III, Miller WL: The pathophysiology and genetics of congenital lipoid adrenal hyperplasia. International Congenital Lipoid Adrenal Hyperplasia Consortium. N Engl J Med 335:1870–1878, 1996.
214. Imperato-McGinley J, Gautier T, Peterson RE, Shackleton C: The prevalence of 5 alpha-reductase deficiency in children with ambiguous genitalia in the Dominican Republic. J Urol 136:867–873, 1986.
215. Thigpen AE, Davis DL, Milatovich A, et al: Molecular genetics of steroid 5 alpha-reductase 2 deficiency. J Clin Invest 90:799–809, 1992.
216. Thigpen AE, Davis DL, Gautier T, et al: Brief report: The molecular basis of steroid 5 alpha-reductase deficiency in a large Dominican kindred. N Engl J Med 327:1216–1219, 1992.
217. Lifton RP, Dluhy RG, Powers M, et al: A chimaeric 11 beta-hydroxylase/aldosterone synthase gene causes glucocorticoid-remediable aldosteronism and human hypertension. Nature 355:262–265, 1992.
218. Dohan O, De la Vieja A, Paroder V, et al: The sodium/iodide symporter (NIS): characterization, regulation, and medical significance. Endocr Rev 24:48–77, 2003.
219. Abramowicz MJ, Targovnik HM, Varela V, et al: Identification of a mutation in the coding sequence of the human thyroid peroxidase gene causing congenital goiter. J Clin Invest 90:1200–1204, 1992.
220. Moreno JC, Bikker H, Kempers MJ, et al: Inactivating mutations in the gene for thyroid oxidase 2 (THOX2) and congenital hypothyroidism. N Engl J Med 347:95–102, 2002.
221. Ieiri T, Cochaux P, Targovnik HM, et al: A 3′ splice site mutation in the thyroglobulin gene responsible for congenital goiter with hypothyroidism. J Clin Invest 88:1901–1905, 1991.
222. Cartegni L, Chew SL, Krainer AR: Listening to silence and understanding nonsense: Exonic mutations that affect splicing. Nat Rev Genet 3:285–298, 2002.
223. Ricketts MH, Simons MJ, Parma J, et al: A nonsense mutation causes hereditary goitre in the Afrikander cattle and unmasks alternative splicing of thyroglobulin transcripts. Proc Natl Acad Sci U S A 84:3181–3184, 1987.
224. Kitanaka S, Takeyama K, Murayama A, et al: Inactivating mutations in the 25-hydroxyvitamin D3 1alpha-hydroxylase gene in patients with pseudovitamin D-deficiency rickets. N Engl J Med 338:653–661, 1998.
225. A gene (PEX) with homologies to endopeptidases is mutated in patients with X-linked hypophosphatemic rickets. The HYP Consortium. Nat Genet 11:130–136, 1995.
226. Quarles LD, Drezner MK: Pathophysiology of X-linked hypophosphatemia, tumor-induced osteomalacia, and autosomal dominant hypophosphatemia: A perPHEXing problem. J Clin Endocrinol Metab 86:494–496, 2001.

227. Thomas PM, Cote GJ, Wohllk N, et al: Mutations in the sulfonylurea receptor gene in familial persistent hyperinsulinemic hypoglycemia of infancy. Science 268:426–429, 1995.

228. Thomas P, Ye Y, Lightner E: Mutation of the pancreatic islet inward rectifier Kir6.2 also leads to familial persistent hyperinsulinemic hypoglycemia of infancy. Hum Mol Genet 5:1809–1812, 1996.

229. Friesema EC, Ganguly S, Abdalla A, et al: Identification of monocarboxylate transporter 8 as a specific thyroid hormone transporter. J Biol Chem 278:40128–40135, 2003.

230. Dumitrescu AM, Liao XH, Best TB, et al: A novel syndrome combining thyroid and neurological abnormalities is associated with mutations in a monocarboxylate transporter gene. Am J Hum Genet 74:168–175, 2004.

231. Knebelmann B, Boussin L, Guerrier D, et al: Anti-Mullerian hormone Bruxelles: A nonsense mutation associated with the persistent Mullerian duct syndrome. Proc Natl Acad Sci U S A 88:3767–3771, 1991.

232. Collu R, Tang J, Castagne J, et al: A novel mechanism for isolated central hypothyroidism: Inactivating mutations in the thyrotropin-releasing hormone receptor gene. J Clin Endocrinol Metab 82:1561–1565, 1997.

233. Laue L, Wu SM, Kudo M, et al: A nonsense mutation of the human luteinizing hormone receptor gene in Leydig cell hypoplasia. Hum Mol Genet 4:1429–1433, 1995.

234. Zhang P, Jobert AS, Couvineau A, Silve C: A homozygous inactivating mutation in the parathyroid hormone/parathyroid hormone-related peptide receptor causing Blomstrand chondrodysplasia. J Clin Endocrinol Metab 83:3365–3368, 1998.

235. Clark AJ, McLoughlin L, Grossman A: Familial glucocorticoid deficiency associated with point mutation in the adrenocorticotropin receptor. Lancet 341:461–462, 1993.

236. Imbeaud S, Faure E, Lamarre I, et al: Insensitivity to anti-mullerian hormone due to a mutation in the human anti-mullerian hormone receptor. Nat Genet 11:382–388, 1995.

237. Clement K, Vaisse C, Lahlou N, et al: A mutation in the human leptin receptor gene causes obesity and pituitary dysfunction. Nature 392:398–401, 1998.

238. Yeo GS, Farooqi IS, Aminian S, et al: A frameshift mutation in MC4R associated with dominantly inherited human obesity. Nat Genet 20:111–112, 1998.

239. Weiss RE, Refetoff S: Thyroid hormone resistance. Annu Rev Med 43:363–375, 1992.

240. Geller DS, Rodriguez-Soriano J, Vallo Boado A, et al: Mutations in the mineralocorticoid receptor gene cause autosomal dominant pseudohypoaldosteronism type I. Nat Genet 19:279–281, 1998.

241. Zoppi S, Marcelli M, Deslypere JP, et al: Amino acid substitutions in the DNA-binding domain of the human androgen receptor are a frequent cause of receptor-binding positive androgen resistance. Mol Endocrinol 6:409–415, 1992.

242. Deeb SS, Fajas L, Nemoto M, et al: A Pro12Ala substitution in PPARgamma2 associated with decreased receptor activity, lower body mass index and improved insulin sensitivity. Nat Genet 20:284–287, 1998.

243. Bos JL: ras Oncogenes in human cancer: A review. Cancer Res 49:4682–4689, 1989.

244. Zhang X, Horwitz GA, Heaney AP, et al: Pituitary tumor transforming gene (PTTG) expression in pituitary adenomas. J Clin Endocrinol Metab 84:761–767, 1999.

245. Vogelstein B, Kinzler KW: p53 Function and dysfunction. Cell 70:523–526, 1992.

246. Weinberg RA: Tumor suppressor genes. Science 254:1138–1146, 1991.

247. Castilla LH, Couch FJ, Erdos MR, et al: Mutations in the BRCA1 gene in families with early-onset breast and ovarian cancer. Nat Genet 8:387–391, 1994.

248. Weber BH, Brohm M, Stec I, et al: A somatic truncating mutation in BRCA2 in a sporadic breast tumor. Am J Hum Genet 59:962–964, 1996.

249. Yamagata K, Oda N, Kaisaki PJ, et al: Mutations in the hepatocyte nuclear factor-1alpha gene in maturity-onset diabetes of the young (MODY3). Nature 384:455–458, 1996.

250. Horikawa Y, Iwasaki N, Hara M, et al: Mutation in hepatocyte nuclear factor-1 beta gene (TCF2) associated with MODY. Nat Genet 17:384–385, 1997.

251. Acebron A, Aza-Blanc P, Rossi DL, et al: Congenital human thyroglobulin defect due to low expression of the thyroid-specific transcription factor TTF-1. J Clin Invest 96:781–785, 1995.

252. Jager RJ, Anvret M, Hall K, Scherer G: A human XY female with a frame shift mutation in the candidate testis-determining gene SRY. Nature 348:452–454, 1990.

253. Bick D, Franco B, Sherins RJ, et al: Brief report: Intragenic deletion of the KALIG-1 gene in Kallmann's syndrome. N Engl J Med 326:1752–1755, 1992.

254. Nicholls RD, Knoll JH, Butler MG, et al: Genetic imprinting suggested by maternal heterodisomy in nondeletion Prader-Willi syndrome. Nature 342:281–285, 1989.

255. Latif F, Tory K, Gnarra J, et al: Identification of the von Hippel-Lindau disease tumor suppressor gene. Science 260:1317–1320, 1993.

256. Wilson DI, Cross IE, Goodship JA, et al: DiGeorge syndrome with isolated aortic coarctation and isolated ventricular septal defect in three sibs with a 22q11 deletion of maternal origin. Br Heart J 66:308–312, 1991.

257. Jackson RS, Creemers JW, Ohagi S, et al: Obesity and impaired prohormone processing associated with mutations in the human prohormone convertase 1 gene. Nat Genet 16:303–306, 1997.

258. Fujiwara H, Tatsumi K, Miki K, et al: Congenital hypothyroidism caused by a mutation in the Na+/I-symporter. Nat Genet 16:124–125, 1997.

259. Hansson JH, Schild L, Lu Y, et al: A de novo missense mutation of the beta subunit of the epithelial sodium channel causes hypertension and Liddle syndrome, identifying a proline-rich segment critical for regulation of channel activity. Proc Natl Acad Sci U S A 92:11495–11499, 1995.

260. Scriver CR, Beaudet AL, Sly WS, Valle D: The Metabolic and Molecular Basis of Inherited Disease, 7th ed. New York, McGraw-Hill, 1995.

MECHANISMS OF ENDOCRINE SIGNALING AND RESPONSE

Control of Hormone Secretion

Thomas F. J. Martin

MORPHOLOGY OF PEPTIDE HORMONE-SECRETING
ENDOCRINE CELLS AND THE REGULATED
SECRETORY PATHWAY

SYNTHESIS, PROCESSING, AND SORTING
OF PREPROHORMONE PRECURSORS

COMPOSITION OF MATURE SECRETORY GRANULES

SEQUENTIAL STAGES OF THE REGULATED
SECRETORY PATHWAY

ESSENTIAL PROTEIN MACHINERY FOR DENSE-CORE
GRANULE EXOCYTOSIS

REGULATION OF EXOCYTOSIS BY CALCIUM

MODULATION OF CALCIUM-DEPENDENT HORMONE
SECRETION BY PROTEIN KINASE C

MORPHOLOGY OF PEPTIDE HORMONE-SECRETING ENDOCRINE CELLS AND THE REGULATED SECRETORY PATHWAY

Like other cell types (e.g., acinar pancreatic) dedicated to the synthesis of secretory proteins, peptide hormone-secreting endocrine cells are endowed with an abundant rough endoplasmic reticulum (ER), a stack of Golgi cisternae, and an array of dense-core secretory granules, all of which are components of an anterograde pathway for conveying secretory proteins to the extracellular space (Fig. 7-1). Classic morphologic and autoradiographic studies established the sequence for trafficking of secretory proteins, which consists of their initial synthesis in the ER, segregation into the ER cisternal space, intracellular transport to the Golgi stacks, concentration in Golgi-derived secretory granules (or dense-core vesicles), intracellular storage of granules, and, finally, granule discharge and protein secretion by exocytosis upon cellular activation.[1] Proteins synthesized on bound polyribosomes in the ER have several cellular destinations, with critical protein-targeting events occurring in late Golgi cisternae or the *trans*-Golgi network (TGN), where proteins are sorted to the endosome-lysosomal system or to the cell surface.[2] Multiple post-Golgi pathways mediate protein transport from the Golgi to the plasma membrane and extracellular space.[3,4] All cells continuously replenish plasma membrane proteins and export proteins to the extracellular space via constitutive secretory pathways with the use of several types of small (40 to 100 nm) clear Golgi-derived transport vesicles or tubulovesicular elements that translocate to and fuse with the plasma membrane.[4] Delivery of secreted proteins to the extracellular space by the constitutive pathway is rapid[5] (half-life of about 20 minutes), and protein secretion is rate-limited by the biosynthetic rates of the proteins rather than by regulated trafficking steps within the pathway.

In contrast, specialized secretory cells such as peptide hormone-secreting endocrine cells contain an additional pathway from the TGN to the cell surface, known as the regulated secretory pathway (see Fig. 7-1), that allows the acute regulated export of high concentrations of secretory proteins.[5] In this pathway, proteins are sorted to dense-core vesicles or secretory granules that form by budding from the TGN with condensed luminal contents.[5,6] Newly formed immature secretory granules may fuse during maturation in some endocrine cells.[7,8] In addition, the immature secretory granules that form undergo further maturation during which clathrin-coated vesicles bud from the immature granule and

sort out excess membrane and soluble contents for constitutive-like secretion or recycling to the endosomal and Golgi compartment[9–11] (see Fig. 7-1). At this stage, initially missorted proteins (lysosomal enzymes) or Golgi constituents (e.g., furin, synaptotagmin4, VAMP4, syntaxin6) are sorted from immature granules to provide fusion-competent mature secretory granules.[11–14]

Mature granules are stored in the cytoplasm for considerable periods ($t_{1/2}$> 10 hours) in the absence of stimulation,[5,6] which enables endocrine cells to accumulate secretory products over an integrated period of biosynthetic activity. Endocrine cells accumulate a large number of secretory granules (Fig. 7-2), which can constitute 10% to 20% of the cellular volume, that are filled with high (millimolar) peptide concentrations.[15] Secretory granules discharge their contents only when an appropriate physiologic stimulus to the cell activates exocytotic fusion of the granule with the plasma membrane (discussed later), a process that is rapid (seconds to minutes) and mediated through rises in cytoplasmic calcium levels initiated through signal transduction events.[16] Thus, an accumulated biosynthetic cargo can be rapidly discharged into the bloodstream at relatively high concentrations. The large size and condensed state of the contents of dense-core secretory granules are probably features of a specialized branch of the secretory pathway that coevolved with the development of an expanded circulatory system and the need to deliver adequate concentrations of signaling peptides into the bloodstream.

SYNTHESIS, PROCESSING, AND SORTING OF PREPROHORMONE PRECURSORS

Secretory peptide precursors contain an N-terminal leader or signal peptide sequence to direct their synthesis in the ER and vectorial transfer into the cisternae of the ER-Golgi pathway[17] (see Fig. 7-1). After transfer from the ER to the Golgi, most peptide hormone and neuropeptide precursors exist as prohormones from which multiple peptides are excised by proteolytic processing at sites usually marked by pairs of basic amino acid residues.[18–20] The endoproteases responsible for precursor maturation belong to a prohormone convertase (PC) family of serine proteases related to bacterial subtilisin, which has several members[20] (furin, PACE4, PC1, PC2, PC4, PC6A/B, LPC). PC1 and PC2, whose expression is restricted to tissues of neuroendocrine lineage, undergo sorting to dense-core vesicles formed in the TGN and are considered to be the

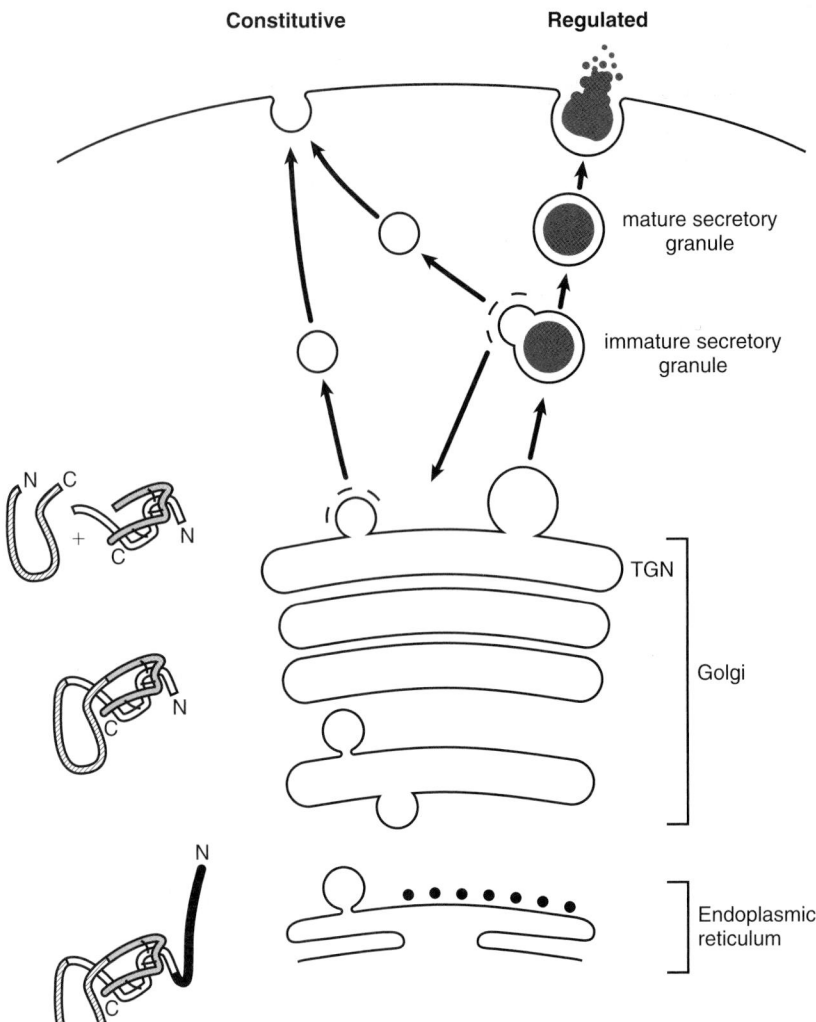

Figure 7-1 Schematic diagram of the anterograde secretory pathway in a peptide hormone-secreting endocrine cell. Secretory proteins synthesized in the endoplasmic reticulum (ER) are transported to and through Golgi stacks by vesicular transport. Within the *trans*-Golgi network (TGN), proteins are sorted to either constitutive or regulated secretory pathways. Immature secretory granules formed in the TGN are subject to additional sorting events during which clathrin-coated vesicles *(dashes)* divert constitutive membrane and soluble proteins back into the constitutive secretory pathway or to endosomes or Golgi. During exocytosis, mature secretory granules fuse with the plasma membrane, which is activated by increases in cytoplasmic calcium levels. Processing intermediates for a prepropeptide (such as preproinsulin) secreted by the regulated pathway are shown on the left and include cleavage of the N-terminal signal sequence *(filled)* in the ER and cleavage of the proregion *(stippled)* in the TGN-immature secretory granule stage.

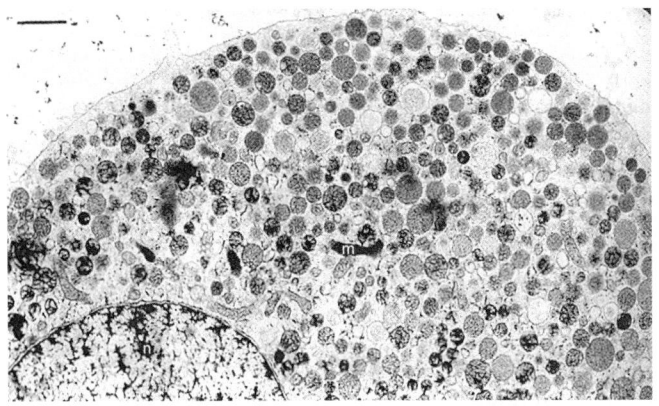

Figure 7-2 Transmission electron micrograph of a bovine adrenal medullary chromaffin cell prepared by cryofixation. Pleomorphic dense-core secretory granules with a mean diameter of 356 ± 91 (SD) nm are dispersed throughout the cytoplasm. Of the approximately 22,000 granules per cell, very few (~500) are in close proximity to the plasma membrane, possibly in a docked state. The scale bar corresponds to 1 μm. (From Plattner H, Artalejo AR, Neher E: Ultrastructural organization of bovine chromaffin cell cortex—analysis by cryofixation and morphometry of aspects pertinent to exocytosis. J Cell Biol 139:1709–1717, 1997.)

proteases essential for the initial proteolytic maturation of neuropeptide and peptide hormone precursors.[18–20] Although proteolytic cleavage of hormonal precursors may be initiated in the TGN,[21] most of the cleavage occurs after entry into immature granules[22] in the low-pH, high-calcium environment required for optimal PC activity (see Fig. 7-1). Mature secretory granules contain a "cocktail" of multiple peptides derived from a prohormone precursor that is discharged upon exocytosis, and the multiple bioactive peptides can exert concerted physiologic regulation.[19,21,23] Sorting events in the immature granule also result in constitutive-like secretion of some of the peptide products (such as the C peptide of proinsulin).[10,24] In some instances, mature peptides from a common precursor are segregated into distinct secretory granules, which may involve initial proteolysis before sorting in the TGN.[13] Production of distinct dense-core vesicles (e.g., those for prolactin and growth hormone in mammosomatotrophs) can also occur for proteins that are separate gene products.[25]

The biogenesis of immature secretory granules is closely linked to the condensation and sorting of prohormones in the TGN.[1,2,6,9,19,21] Cellular mechanisms used for sorting to the regulated pathway appear to be common to neural, endocrine, and probably exocrine cell types as inferred from the finding that peptide hormone precursors, as well as pancreatic prozymogens expressed by DNA transfection, are properly sorted to the regulated pathway in neuroendocrine and exocrine cells.[5,6] Because in many cases expressed protein chimeras containing prohormone sequences are properly targeted to the regulated secretory pathway in neuroendocrine cells, it is thought that prohormonal precursors share consensual features that provide sorting information. The nature of the putative sorting signal is not entirely clear.[5,6,9,11,26–29] Studies indicate that precursors for adrenocorticotropic hormone, enkephalins, and insulin may contain a sorting signal that consists of similarly spaced acidic and hydrophobic residues on the surface of an amphipathic loop.[30,31] This region was reported to interact with carboxypeptidase E, a hormone-processing enzyme that is membrane associated in regulated granules and that was proposed to be a sorting signal receptor.[30–32] Controversial aspects of this model have recently been discussed.[24,33] An alternative, sorting-by-condensation model proposes that sorting in the TGN is mediated by the protein aggregation that is promoted at the low-pH and high-calcium concentration in the TGN cisternae.[5,6,34,35] Chromogranin B, an acidic granule protein ubiquitously expressed in neuroendocrine cells, aggregates under these conditions and also associates with membranes via a disulfide-bonded loop region of the protein that is required for proper targeting to regulated granules.[27,28] Some evidence suggests that aggregation of chromogranin proteins in the TGN may suffice to promote the biogenesis of dense-core vesicles, although the mechanism is unclear.[36–38] The general property of regulated (e.g., growth hormone, prolactin, follicle-stimulating hormone, PC2) but not constitutive (e.g., IgGs, albumin) secretory proteins to self-aggregate, as well as to aggregate heterophilically[39] and to associate with membranes[20,40] under TGN luminal conditions, provides the basis for the sorting-by-condensation model, which envisions prohormonal aggregates sorting away from constitutive secretory proteins by associating with specific membrane domains in the TGN.[35] An alternative version of this model suggests that these features of regulated secretory proteins dictate their retention in immature granules during post-Golgi sorting events that remove constitutive proteins from immature granules.[9,10] Targeting transmembrane proteins to regulated granules, in contrast, appears to require the cytoplasmic regions of these proteins, which interact with cytosolic protein factors.[41,42]

For vesicle budding at several sites in the anterograde secretory pathway, transmembrane proteins link cargo in the vesicle lumen to the cytosolic components (e.g., coat proteins) required for vesicle formation, which provides a mechanism for coupling vesicle generation with content filling.[43–45] It is unclear whether similar events occur during the formation of secretory granules in the TGN because potential cargo receptors and protein coats have not been identified. However, aspects of immature granule biogenesis in the TGN have been elucidated by studies of cell-free budding reactions.[46–53] Granule formation in vitro requires adenosine triphosphate (ATP) and cytosolic protein factors. One of the required cytosolic factors is phosphatidylinositol transfer protein (PITP), which interacts with membrane phosphatidylinositol and to a lesser extent with phosphatidylcholine. PITP may alter the phospholipid composition of the Golgi membrane to facilitate budding[54] or may promote the phosphorylation of phosphatidylinositol by a lipid kinase.[48,55] The latter could account for the ATP dependence of vesicle formation. Phosphorylated inositides such as phosphatidylinositol mono- or bisphosphate (PIP or PIP_2) are known to regulate membrane events by promoting protein (e.g., coat or cytoskeletal) recruitment to membranes[56] or by serving as essential cofactors for membrane enzymes such as phospholipase D,[57] which converts phosphatidylcholine to phosphatidic acid (see Chapter 13). The small guanosine triphosphate (GTP)-binding protein ARF1 (ADP [adenosine diphosphate] ribosylation factor), which is required for recruitment of coat protein to generate other Golgi-derived transport vesicles,[44] is also required for secretory granule formation.[50] ARF1 may function by recruiting an unidentified coat protein or cytoskeletal constituents or by regulating the activity of a

PIP_2-dependent phospholipase D.[51–53] Overall, the TGN-budding process that generates immature granules resembles other vesicle-budding events in their requirement for GTP-binding proteins and factors that alter membrane phospholipids.[57] Immature secretory granules that form contain a type II PI 4-kinase and PIP, which may be required for subsequent maturation or priming events in preparation for fusion at the plasma membrane.[58,59]

COMPOSITION OF MATURE SECRETORY GRANULES

Mature secretory granules in endocrine and neural cells consist of a membrane bilayer surrounding an electron-opaque dense core that consists of condensed secretory materials such as peptide hormones, granin proteins, and processing enzymes. In some endocrine cells, such as β cells in the islets of Langerhans, the contents are crystalline and consist of insulin hexamers chelated by zinc.[60] Proteolytic processing of proinsulin in the immature granule is required to form this crystalline deposit in some species.[61] Dense-core vesicles vary widely in properties from one endocrine cell type to another and range in size from 50 nm in the sympathetic nervous system, to 200 nm in pituitary corticotrophs and gonadotrophs, and up to 1000 nm in pituitary mammotrophs or neurohypophyseal cells.

Mature secretory granules engage in multiple cellular functions, including vectorial transport of small molecules into the luminal space (nucleotides, divalent cations, protons, and neurotransmitters), translocation of the granules through the cytoplasm and their anchorage to cytoskeletal elements, docking of the granules at the plasma membrane, and their calcium-dependent exocytotic fusion at the plasma membrane. These functions would require an array of organelle-specific proteins exposed on the cytoplasmic face of the granule. Analyses of purified secretory granules have been undertaken to identify proteins that participate in aspects of the granule life cycle. The chromaffin granules of adrenal medullary tissue are best studied (see Fig. 7-2), although granules purified from anterior and posterior pituitary or from pancreatic islet cells have also been analyzed to a lesser extent.[62,63] Individual adrenal chromaffin cells contain 10,000 to 30,000 granules with a mean diameter of 350 nm,[64–66] which has enabled extensive purification at yields of 2 to 3 mg per bovine adrenal gland.[65]

The adrenal chromaffin granule possesses a number of general features likely to be representative of other secretory granules. Chromaffin granules consist of approximately 20% lipid and about 42% protein (percent dry weight). The membrane of the chromaffin granule exhibits a lipid composition similar to that of other cellular membranes but is notable for its relatively high cholesterol content, which is characteristic of late Golgi-derived membranes.[67] In addition, a surprisingly high concentration of lysophosphatidylcholine is present, which has also been reported for exocrine tissue granules but not for pituitary granules and synaptic vesicles.[67] Thus, a high lysophospholipid content does not appear to be essential for a common granule function such as exocytotic fusion, but the precise role of lysophospholipids in granules is not known. Chromaffin (and other) granules contain, like many cellular membranes, 2% to 5% phosphatidylinositol, a phospholipid that is an essential precursor for the formation of PIP_2, which is required in membrane fusion mechanisms (discussed later).

Although the characterization of chromaffin granule proteins was anticipated to identify constituents that mediate general functions of dense-core vesicles, including exocytosis, it instead revealed specialized constituents unique to the function of these catecholaminergic and peptidergic granules.[66] Composition of chromaffin granule protein is dominated by abundant proteins that catalyze catecholamine synthesis or the posttranslational processing of neuropeptides.

About 75% of the protein is soluble in the lumen. Luminal contents are dominated by a family of acidic, heat-stable glycoproteins, the granins (chromogranin A and secretogranins I and II), and their proteolytic products. Granins may function in the aggregative sorting of peptide hormone precursors to the regulated pathway (discussed previously) and are general constituents of neuroendocrine secretory granules from the parathyroid, pituitary, thyroid, and pancreas, as well as sympathetic neurons.[68] Granins are also precursors for a variety of bioactive peptides such as pancreastatin, vasostatin, parastatin (derived from chromogranin A), and secretoneurin (derived from secretogranin II).[35,64–66] Other chromaffin granule luminal proteins are glycoproteins (glycoprotein III), neuropeptides (enkephalins and neuropeptide Y), and enzymes for catecholamine synthesis (dopamine β-monooxygenase), neuropeptide proteolytic cleavage (carboxypeptidase E/H, PC1, and PC2), and peptide amidation (peptidylglycine α-monooxygenase). The dense core of chromaffin granules observed by transmission electron microscopy is attributed to the high luminal content of granin proteins and neuropeptides in the millimolar concentration range.[65–66] Small-molecular-weight constituents are also abundant and consist of catecholamines (~0.6 M), ATP (~0.15 M), ascorbic acid (~0.02 M), and calcium (~0.02 M). Other endocrine dense-core vesicles contain high concentrations of ATP and calcium.[69]

The membrane protein composition of chromaffin granules is dominated by membrane-bound dopamine β-monooxygenase and cytochrome b_{561}, both dedicated constituents that function in the oxidation of dopamine to norepinephrine.[66] Other membrane proteins found in lesser abundance are the subunits of the chromaffin granule proton pump (H(+)-ATPase), lysosome-associated membrane proteins (LAMP-1 and LAMP-2), and neuropeptide-processing enzymes that are present in soluble and membrane-anchored forms (PC1, PC2, carboxypeptidase E/H, peptidylglycine α-monooxygenase).[64] Molecular cloning with subsequent immunochemical detection also identified catecholamine transporters (vesicular monoamine transporters VMAT1 and VMAT2) as chromaffin granule membrane constituents.[70]

A large number of more minor but functionally important membrane protein constituents have been identified immunochemically on chromaffin granules by using antibodies to proteins initially discovered on the compositionally simpler neuronal small clear synaptic vesicles (see Fig. 7-6). Several of these proteins, which are also found on other neural and endocrine dense-core vesicles,[71] function in regulated exocytosis (synaptotagmin, synaptobrevin/VAMP [vesicle-associated membrane protein], Rab3A, cysteine string proteins). Proteins with putative regulatory roles (G_o) or of unknown function (SV2, synaptophysin) have also been identified.[72,73] A variety of Rab proteins (Rab3a, Rab27a) and putative Rab-binding effector proteins (rabphilin, Slac2c/MyRIP, Slp4a/granuphilin) are present on granules as are proteins that mediate actin-based granule translocation such as myosin V.[74–77] Additional membrane constituents detected by activity include K^+ channels,[78] N-type Ca^{2+} channels,[79] and a phosphatidylinositol 4-kinase.[80]

SEQUENTIAL STAGES OF THE REGULATED SECRETORY PATHWAY

In most endocrine cells, the majority of dense-core vesicles are cytoplasmic, with only a small portion in direct contact with the plasma membrane in a docked state (see Fig. 7-2). Dense-core vesicles undergo rapid translocation from their site of biogenesis in the TGN to sites in the cortical cytoskeleton, which occurs by kinesin-mediated movement on microtubules followed by myosin V-catalyzed transport via actin filaments.[81,82] The basis for docking of granules at the plasma

membrane, which immobilizes them,[83] is unclear. The most recently arrived granules that dock at the plasma membrane are used for exocytosis in preference to older granules, which are largely cytoplasmic.[84] Peptide hormone secretion upon cellular activation is believed to proceed by the rapid exocytotic fusion of a portion of the docked granules (release-ready pool), which are subsequently replenished by recruitment of granules to the plasma membrane from a cytoplasmic recruitment pool.[85,86] Thus, current views suggest a sequential pathway in which granules transit through recruitment, docking, and exocytotic fusion steps (Fig. 7-3). Evidence for the sequential model is provided by rapid kinetic studies of exocytosis by patch clamp electrophysiologic methods, in which increases in membrane capacitance reflect expansion of the surface membrane area after exocytosis,[87,88] and from amperometry studies, which use carbon fiber electrodes to detect secreted oxidizable granule constituents such as catecholamines.[89] Capacitance increases and amperometric spikes from single granule fusion events have been detected in adrenal chromaffin and other secretory cell types.[87–90] Combining these techniques in a single pipette revealed that content release can occur during transient reversible fusion of the granule with the plasma membrane.[90] Cellular activation to elevate cytoplasmic calcium levels results in multiphasic increases in secretion (Fig. 7-4) that consist of at least two components, an ultrafast (or exocytotic burst) component within the first 100 msec, followed by a slower component over the ensuing 1 to 10 seconds. These components of exocytosis are interpreted to represent the sequential fusion of secretory granules in a docked release-ready state, followed by fusion of granules that require recruitment into the release-ready pool.[87–91] The size of the exocytotic burst or release-ready pool (corresponding to 100 to 300 granules in chromaffin cells) is smaller than the number of morphologically detected docked granules (500 to 1000 granules in chromaffin cells; see Fig. 7-2), thus indicating that docked granules may exist in several functional states.[83,87,92] The release-ready pool represents a very small fraction of the cellular granule complement of 10,000 to 30,000.[65] Under physiologic stimulation conditions (i.e., splanchnic nerve stimulation), catecholamine secretion corresponding to 1% to 2% of the adrenal pool is mobilized, which indicates that the docked pool of granules in a release-ready pool is sufficient to mediate physiologic responses with short latency.[93] Similar fractional release during physiologic stimulation is commonly observed in other endocrine tissues.[94]

Recent technical developments have allowed the study of secretory granule movement in living neuroendocrine cells (Fig. 7-5). Fusion proteins consisting of prohormone peptides with green fluorescent protein at the carboxyl terminus undergo proper sorting to dense-core vesicles when expressed in neuroendocrine cells.[95,96] Confocal fluorescence, or evanescent-wave microscopy, has enabled the tracking of individual granules during their cytoplasmic translocation, docking at the plasma membrane, and exocytosis.[83,95–97] Granule movement to the plasma membrane is a directed process that occurs at speeds of approximately 50 nm/sec, followed by immobilization at the plasma membrane by a presumed docking process that either occasionally reverses or culminates in exocytosis if calcium levels are elevated.[83,96,97] New granules move to the plasma membrane and replenish the pool of docked granules within several minutes.[77] Sustained stimulated secretion entails a cytoplasmic pool of mobile granules.[95] Previous biochemical studies had implicated an actin cytoskeleton as a barrier to the plasma membrane recruitment of granules, but recent work indicates that granule recruitment to the plasma membrane is likely actin-mediated via myosin V, an actin-based motor that is present on secretory granules.[77,81,82,86,98]

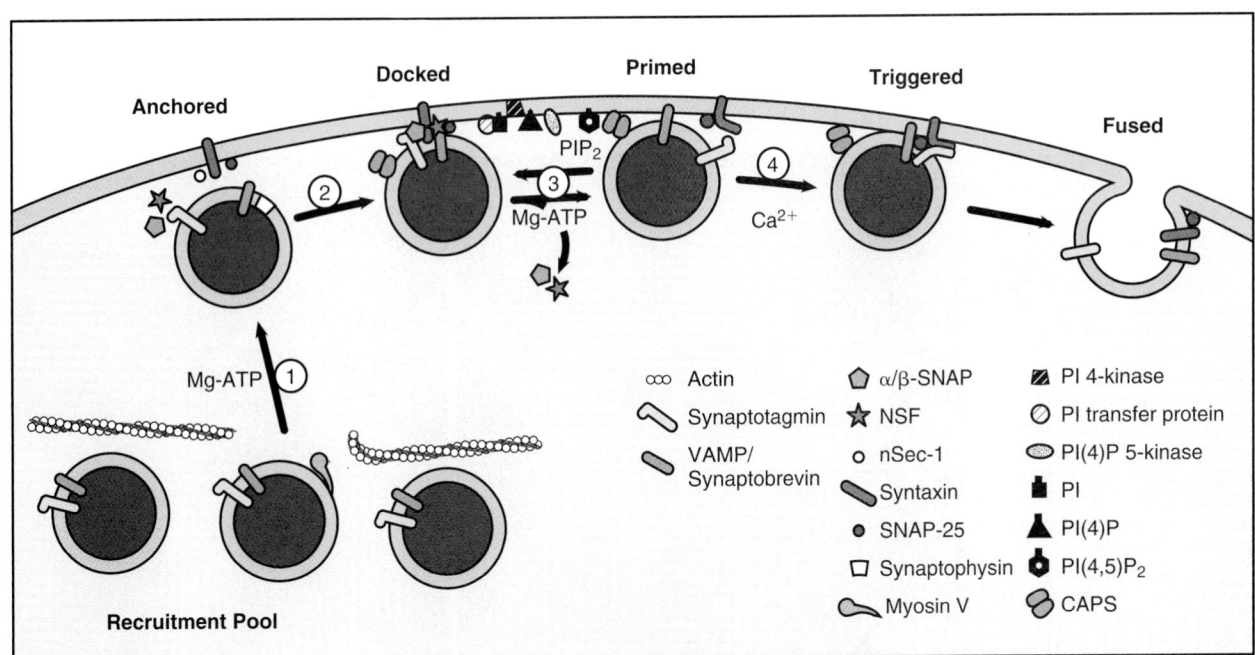

Figure 7-3 Late stages of dense-core vesicle exocytosis. The diagram depicts several stages that secretory granules transit before fusion with the plasma membrane. **1,** A recruitment pool of granules associated with cytoskeletal elements is recruited to the plasma membrane. **2,** Granules are anchored close to and docked at the plasma membrane by mechanisms that remain to be clarified. **3,** An ATP-dependent priming process involving the action of NSF on SNARE proteins and the synthesis of phosphatidylinositol 4,5-bisphosphate (PIP2) is required for granules to attain competence for calcium-triggered fusion. **4,** Calcium elevations to the 1 to 30 µM range trigger fusion in a process that requires SNARE proteins, synaptotagmin, and CAPS. Inset and symbols refer to several proteins essential at these stages of dense-core vesicle exocytosis. (From Martin TFJ: Stages of regulated exocytosis. Trends Cell Biol 7:271–276, 1997.)

ESSENTIAL PROTEIN MACHINERY FOR DENSE-CORE GRANULE EXOCYTOSIS

Regulated dense-core vesicle exocytosis is mediated by protein machinery that is the neuroendocrine counterpart of a universal core apparatus generally involved in membrane fusion events.[99-102] The key neuroendocrine proteins are the SNARE (*soluble NSF [N-ethylmaleimide-sensitive factor] attachment protein receptor*, or SNAP receptor) proteins syntaxin 1, SNAP-25, and synaptobrevin/VAMP2. Synaptobrevin/VAMP was initially identified[101,102] as a brain synaptic vesicle and *Torpedo* cholinergic vesicle protein of approximately 18 kDa that spans the vesicle membrane with a short luminal C-terminal tail (Fig. 7-6). It is ubiquitously expressed in endocrine secretory tissues and localizes to large dense-core and small clear synaptic vesicles.[71] Syntaxin 1 was identified as a plasma membrane protein of around 35 kDa in a complex with synaptic vesicle proteins, and it has a membrane topology similar to that of synaptobrevin/VAMP.[101] SNAP-25 (synapse-associated protein of ~25 kDa) was discovered as a synapse-specific protein of 25 kDa by subtractive screening for brain-specific

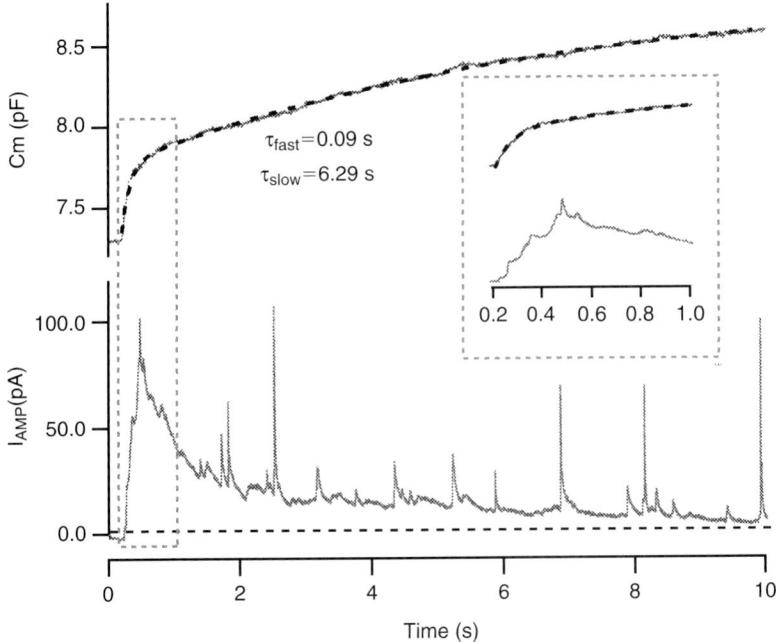

Figure 7-4 Multiple kinetic components of dense-core vesicle exocytosis in chromaffin cells. Capacitance measurements with a patch clamp pipette in the whole-cell configuration *(upper trace)* and amperometric current determinations with a carbon fiber electrode *(lower trace)* were obtained simultaneously from a bovine adrenal medullary cell that was stimulated by elevating calcium levels to 27 µM by flash photolysis with a photolabile calcium chelator. A rapid (exocytotic burst) component exhibiting a time constant of 0.09 seconds and a slow component with a time constant of 6.29 seconds were detected. (From Xu T, Binz T, Niemann H, Neher E: Multiple kinetic components of exocytosis distinguished by neurotoxin sensitivity. Nat Neurosci 1:192–200, 1998.)

Figure 7-5 Exocytosis of chromaffin granules recorded by evanescent-wave fluorescence microscopy. Bovine adrenal medullary cells were loaded with acridine orange, an acidophilic dye, to render chromaffin granules fluorescent. Total internal reflection fluorescence microscopy was used to visualize granules in an optical section representing about 300 nm from the cell surface. Images were captured before *(left)* and after *(right)* 2 minutes of depolarization with high K+, during which numerous granules close to the cell surface underwent exocytosis. (Reprinted by permission from Steyer JA, Horstmann H, Almers W: Transport, docking and exocytosis of single secretory granules in live chromaffin cells. Nature 388:474–478, 1997. Copyright © MacMillan Magazines Ltd.)

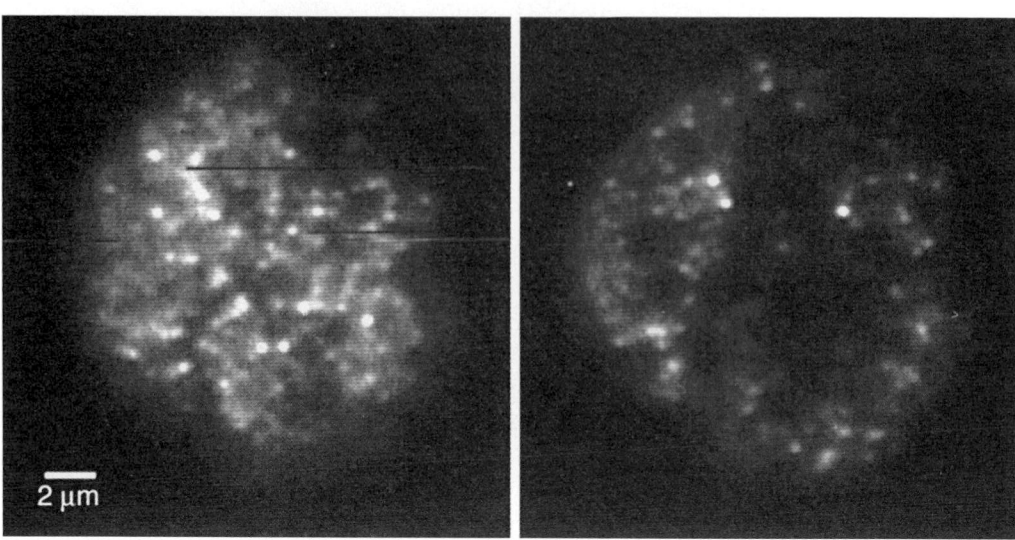

2 μm

cDNAs.[103] The plasma membrane association of SNAP-25 is mediated by palmitoylation at four central cysteine residues. The central importance of SNARE proteins for calcium-dependent synaptic vesicle exocytosis is indicated by the finding that these three proteins constitute the major, if not exclusive, substrates for clostridial neurotoxins,[104,105] which are highly specific proteases that enter nerve cells by receptor-mediated endocytosis. Eight members of this bacterial neurotoxin family act to proteolytically cleave the three SNARE proteins at seven distinct cleavage sites (Table 7-1), which results in strong inhibition of neurotransmitter release. The neuroendocrine SNARE proteins were also identified as components of a 20S protein complex isolated by affinity chromatography of brain detergent extracts on immobilized NSF plus SNAP.[106] This observation linked the general role of NSF and SNAP proteins in membrane fusion to the function of neural proteins involved in synaptic vesicle exocytosis.[100]

The neuronal SNARE proteins exhibit an expression pattern that is not restricted to neurons, and virtually all peptide hormone-secreting endocrine tissues that have been examined express syntaxin 1, SNAP-25, and synaptobrevin/VAMP2.[71] It is important to note that regulated peptide hormone secretion in all instances in which it has been examined is strongly inhibited by clostridial neurotoxins.[91,99,107] The neurotoxins need to be introduced into endocrine cells by cell permeabilization, microinjection, patch clamp pipette, or transfection methods because endocrine cells lack receptors that mediate endocytic uptake of the toxins.[105,106] Inhibition of stimulated peptide hormone secretion by clostridial neurotoxins provides compelling evidence that regulated exocytosis in endocrine cells is a SNARE protein-dependent process.

SNARE proteins self-assemble into heterotrimeric complexes that are extremely stable.[108,109] Structural studies of the central portion of the SNARE complex (Fig. 7-7) revealed that it consists of a four-helix bundle containing α-helical regions in parallel register contributed by each of the SNARE proteins, one each from the C-terminal segment of syntaxin 1 and the central region of synaptobrevin/VAMP and one each from the N- and C-terminal regions of SNAP-25.[110]

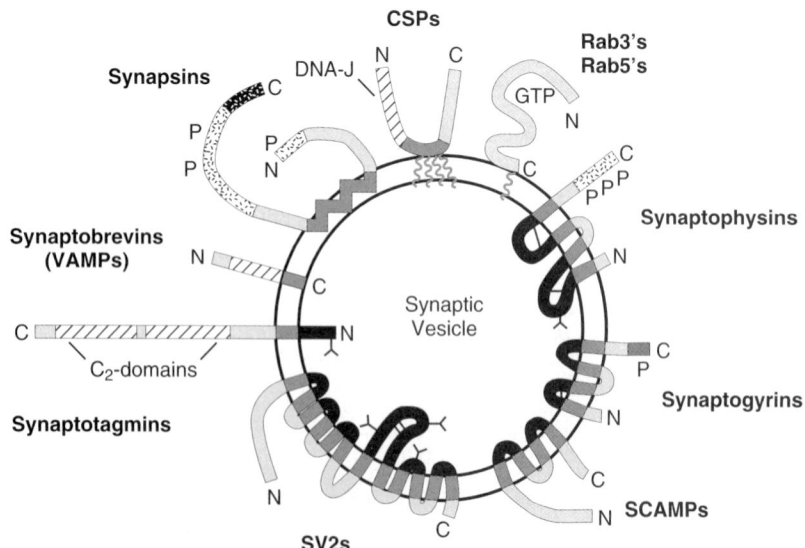

Figure 7-6 Membrane proteins associated with brain synaptic vesicles. Some of the characterized organelle-specific membrane proteins associated with synaptic vesicles are summarized in the figure. P indicates phosphorylation sites, and N or C refers to the N- or C-terminus of the proteins. Synaptic vesicles are compositionally simpler than dense-core vesicles. Many of these proteins have also been identified on dense-core vesicles with the exception of synapsins and synaptogyrins. (Reprinted by permission from Sudhof TC: The synaptic vesicle cycle: A cascade of protein-protein interactions. Nature 375:645–653, 1995. Copyright © MacMillan Magazines Ltd.)

Table 7-1	Clostridial Neurotoxin Substrates	
Botulinum serotype D		
Synaptobrevin 2/VAMP2		
Glin197-Arg198		
Toxin	**Substrate**	**Cleavage Site**
Tetanus	Synaptobrevin/VAMP	Gln76-Phe77
Botulinum serotype B	Synaptobrevin/VAMP	Gln76-Phe77
Botulinum serotype D	Synaptobrevin/VAMP	Lys59-Leu60
Botulinum serotype F	Synaptobrevin/VAMP	Gln58-Lys59
Botulinum serotype G	Synaptobrevin/VAMP	Ala81-Ala82
Botulinum serotype A	SNAP-25	Gln197-Arg198
Botulinum serotype E	SNAP-25	Arg180-Ile181
Botulinum serotype C	Syntaxin	Lys253-Ala254
SNAP-25	Arg198-Ala199	

SNAP, soluble NSF (*N*-ethylmaleimide-sensitive factor) attachment protein; VAMP, vesicle-associated membrane protein.
Data from Montecucco C, Schiavo G: Tetanus and botulism neurotoxins: A new group of zinc proteases. Trends Biochem Sci 18:324–329, 1993 and Niemann H, Blasi J, Jahn R: Clostridial neurotoxins: New tools for dissecting exocytosis. Trends Cell Biol 4:179–185, 1994.

Complexes of SNAREs that form in *trans* across vesicle and plasma membranes are considered to be key mediators of vesicle fusion in regulated exocytosis (Fig. 7-8). The self-assembly properties of the SNARE proteins in vitro,[108,109] the specificity of their binding interactions,[110,111] and their distribution on either vesicles or the plasma membrane originally led to a proposed role for SNARE complexes in vesicle-plasma membrane docking interactions,[100,101,106,108] but this hypothesis has not been supported by subsequent toxin inhibition or genetic SNARE deletion studies.[112] Moreover, there is direct experimental support in neuroendocrine cells for an essential role of SNARE proteins after secretory granule docking.[86,107] Current evidence rather indicates a direct role for SNARE complexes in membrane fusion reactions based on the ability of proteoliposomes containing syntaxin and SNAP-25 to fuse with synaptobrevin/VAMP liposomes.[113–118] The formation of SNARE helix bundles contributed by the proteins in *trans* mediate the close apposition of membrane bilayers to drive bilayer mixing and fusion (see Fig. 7-8).

An additional set of biochemical reactions are essential for late steps in regulated dense-core vesicle exocytosis that precede fusion, which are termed *priming*[119,120] (see Fig. 7-3). ATP is required for the regulated secretion of hormones,[86,87,91] and multiple roles for ATP-dependent processes in the secretory granule exocytotic pathway have been described.[89] Granules proceed through an ATP-dependent priming step before calcium-triggered exocytosis.[121] Although this step involves in part the action of ATPase NSF on SNARE complexes,[122] it has also been found to involve ATP acting as a substrate for phospholipid phosphorylation reactions.[123,124] Phosphatidylinositol undergoes conversion to PI-4-P and PI-4,5-P_2 catalyzed sequentially by a membrane-bound phosphatidylinositol 4-kinase and by a soluble PIP 5-kinase[86,124] (see Fig. 7-3). PI-4,5-P_2 may be synthesized to serve a signaling role on the plasma membrane for recruitment or activation of proteins for calcium-triggered fusion reactions.[56] ATP-dependent priming involving the synthesis of PIP_2 is required for dense-core vesicle exocytosis, but whether it is essential for synaptic vesicle exocytosis is unclear.[125,126] One potential mechanism by which PIP_2 has been proposed to act is by activating Ca^{2+}-dependent activator protein in secretion (CAPS), a neural/endocrine-specific PIP_2-binding protein that is required for the calcium-triggered exocytosis of dense-core vesicles.[127,128] CAPS is required for dense-core vesicle but not synaptic vesicle exocytosis,[128–130] and this protein may play a role in mediating contact between dense-core vesicles and the plasma membrane.[86,131] Studies in pancreatic β cells indicate that priming reactions involving PIP_2 synthesis and CAPS activation are regulated by ADP, which may function as a metabolic sensor in the β cell for insulin secretion.[59,132]

REGULATION OF EXOCYTOSIS BY CALCIUM

The neuronal SNARE proteins that are essential for regulated exocytosis are the neuroendocrine counterparts of a protein superfamily whose members are required for membrane trafficking and fusion reactions in the constitutive secretory pathway.[100,101] Unregulated constitutive secretion in the yeast *Saccharomyces cerevisiae* uses homologues of synaptobrevin/VAMP (SNC1/2), syntaxin 1 (SSO1/2), and SNAP-25 (SEC9).[101] A unique feature of neural synaptic vesicle and endocrine dense-core vesicle exocytosis is its regulation mediated by cytoplasmic calcium increases[85,86,102,133] (see Chapter 13).

As studied in permeable neuroendocrine cells, regulated dense-core vesicle exocytosis is completely calcium dependent and activated by calcium ion concentrations in the micromolar range.[133] The basal hormone secretion in intact endocrine cells that is detected in the absence of secretagogues, which is mediated by exocytosis of dense-core vesicles rather than by constitutive vesicles,[134] probably arises from excursions of cytoplasmic calcium that exceeds the threshold for activating exocytosis.

Although numerous mechanistic similarities can be found between the dense-core vesicle-mediated release of peptide hormones and biogenic amines in neuroendocrine cells and the synaptic vesicle-mediated release of neurotransmitters such as acetylcholine and glutamate in nerve cells, these two processes have significant differences in their physiologic regulation[99,129,130] Dense-core vesicle exocytosis exhibits a longer latency (~10 msec) between calcium entry and fusion than does synaptic vesicle exocytosis, in which latencies shorter

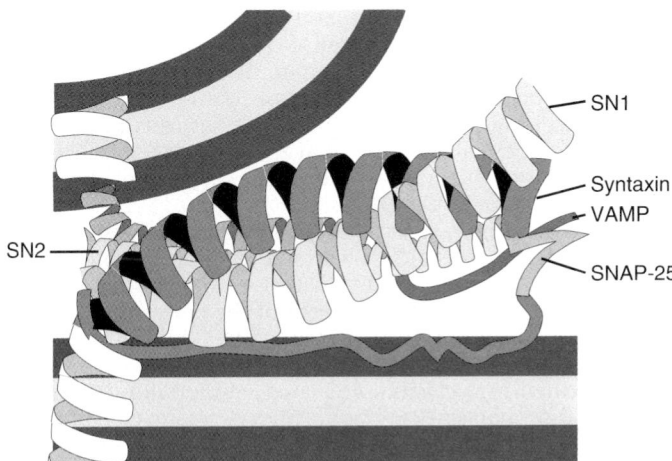

Figure 7-7 Structure of the neuronal SNARE protein complex. The structure of a protease-resistant core derived from heterotrimeric complexes of syntaxin 1, SNAP-25, and synaptobrevin/VAMP was solved by radiographic crystallography.[92] The figure reproduced here provides a hypothetical structure of the membrane-associated complex. The structure is a four-helix bundle consisting of helical regions in parallel register. Whereas syntaxin and synaptobrevin/VAMP each contribute a helical region, SNAP-25 contributes N-terminal (SN1) and C-terminal (SN2) regions connected by a linker region. (Figure modified from modification from Sutton RB, Fasshauer D, Jahn R, Brunger AT: Crystal structure of a SNARE complex involved in synaptic exocytosis at 2.4A resolution. Nature 395:347–353, 1998.)

Figure 7-8 Hypothetical model of SNARE protein-mediated fusion. SNARE protein complexes shown in Figure 7-7 are thought to be essential for vesicle fusion. A potential mechanism for the role of SNARE complexes in promoting vesicle fusion is depicted in this figure. Heterodimers of syntaxin and SNAP-25 on the plasma membrane are shown progressively "zippering" with synaptobrevin/VAMP on the vesicle to form a four-helix bundle. SNARE complex formation promotes the close apposition of membrane bilayers such that calcium, acting through synaptotagmin (not shown), triggers the final transition to bilayer fusion. (Reprinted by permission from Jahn R, Hanson PI: SNAREs line up in a new environment. Nature 393:14–15, 1998. Copyright © MacMillan Magazines Ltd.)

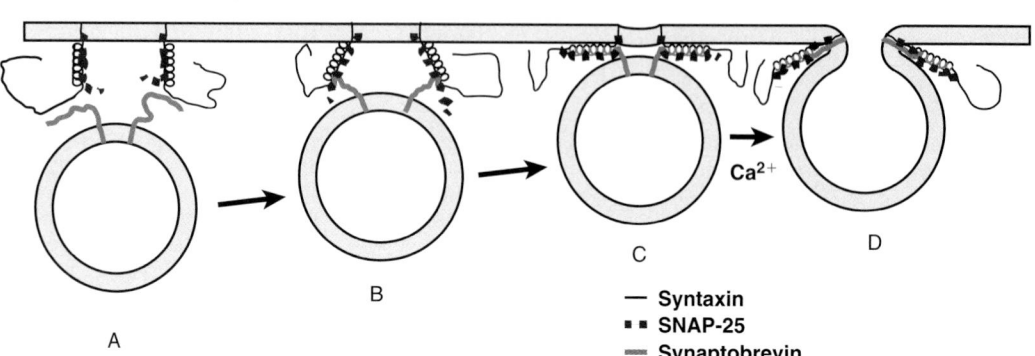

— Syntaxin
■■ SNAP-25
━ Synaptobrevin

than 1 msec have been reported.[85,89] Most of the delay between calcium entry through calcium channels and hormone release is attributed to the diffusion delay for calcium because of a lack of colocalization of dense-core vesicles and calcium channels.[135] Conversely, the short latency observed for evoked neurotransmitter release is thought to involve SNARE protein-mediated tethering of synaptic vesicles to calcium channels.[136,137] In addition to differences in latencies, dense-core granule exocytosis is triggered by calcium concentrations that are considerably lower (1 to 30 μM) than those reached in close proximity to open calcium channels, which is estimated to be several 100 μM.[85,99,112,133,138,139] At some synapses, but not others,[140,141] synaptic vesicle exocytosis requires these very high calcium concentrations.[115] Dense-core vesicle exocytosis is also triggered by cytoplasmic calcium rises resulting from inositol triphosphate-induced mobilization from the ER, which have been estimated to be lower than 5 μM even at cisternal sites close to granules.[142]

Regulation of the dense-core granule exocytotic pathway by calcium occurs at multiple sites, including granule recruitment, exocytosis, fusion pore dilation, and endocytic membrane retrieval. Release-ready granules are depleted by strong stimulation, and replenishment of the release-ready pool occurs within approximately 1 minute after depletion.[85,143] Rates of pool replenishment depend on cytoplasmic calcium at concentrations lower than the threshold for exocytosis.[144] Although the molecular basis for calcium-dependent pool replenishment is unknown, it may be mediated in part through calcium activation of protein kinase C.[143,145]

Calcium regulation of exocytosis has been proposed to be mediated by the synaptotagmins, a protein family not expressed in yeast whose members are abundant secretory vesicle C2 domain-containing proteins that bind calcium ions.[102,146] Genetic studies in *Drosophila*, *Caenorhabditis elegans*, and mice have demonstrated an essential role for synaptotagmin I in evoked rapid synchronous neurotransmitter release via synaptic vesicle exocytosis, and mutations that affect calcium-dependent properties of synaptotagmin I correspondingly affect probabilities of synaptic vesicle fusion.[101,111,147] The burst but not the sustained component of dense-core vesicle exocytosis was reduced in chromaffin cells from synaptotagmin I knockout mice.[148] Synaptotagmins exhibit calcium-dependent interactions with the plasma

membrane SNARE proteins syntaxin 1 and SNAP-25 and are found in biochemically isolated heterotrimeric SNARE complexes,[108] so it has been suggested that synaptotagmins could directly mediate the calcium triggering of SNARE complex-dependent membrane fusion.[102,149–154] Alternatively, calcium-dependent interactions of synaptotagmins with membrane phospholipids may help drive membrane fusion.[149]

The molecular basis for differences in the calcium sensitivity of vesicle exocytosis is unclear. Multiple synaptotagmin isoforms that differ in apparent calcium sensitivity are present on different classes of vesicles and it has been suggested that distinct isoforms may dictate different calcium sensitivities.[146] For example, synaptotagmins I and II exhibit apparent low-affinity calcium binding compared to the higher affinity binding by synaptotagmins III and VII.[146] The composition of synaptotagmin isoforms on dense-core vesicles, which may contribute to the calcium sensitivity of exocytosis, has been established only for catecholamine-secreting PC12 cells and insulin-secreting β-cell lines.[149,155–157] Other calcium-binding proteins such as rabphilin,[158] CAPS,[127] and the SNARE complex itself[110] may mediate aspects of the calcium regulation of priming or fusion in exocytosis.

After fusion, the rate of dilation of the fusion pore is regulated by calcium levels.[159] Recent studies indicate that synaptotagmin proteins participate in fusion pore formation and dilation.[160] Beyond fusion, retrieval of the dense-core granule membrane by endocytosis is stimulated by calcium in a calmodulin-dependent process.[161] In synaptic vesicle endocytosis, calcineurin, a calcium-activated, calmodulin-dependent protein phosphatase that dephosphorylates several proteins (dynamin, amphiphysin, synaptojanin) involved in endocytosis, is a major locus of calcium regulation.[162,163] A similar mechanism may underlie calcium regulation of endocytic retrieval of the dense-core granule membrane, whose components are trafficked back to the Golgi.[2]

Imaging of dense-core vesicles containing fluorescent soluble or membrane-bound constituents has revealed diverse modes of granule fusion that may differentially release small and large luminal molecules (Fig. 7-9). In pancreatic β cells, the release of an islet amyloid peptide-green fluorescent protein was substantially (1 to 10 s) delayed beyond initial fusion pore formation.[164] In PC12 cells, a large luminal constituent (tPA) was retained in the granule while a smaller peptide

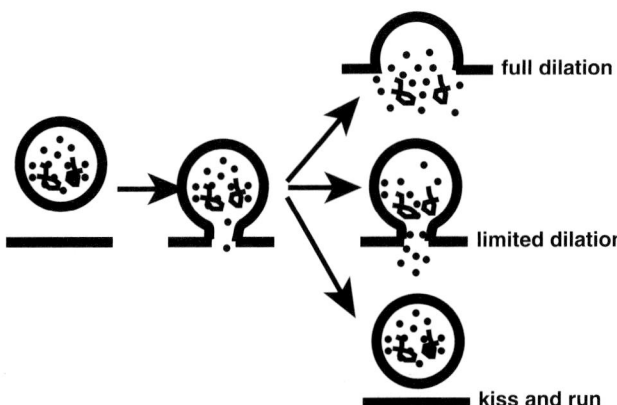

Figure 7-9 Diverse modes of fusion pore dilation. Membrane fusion generates a pore that connects the lumen of the vesicle with the extracellular space. Three modes of fusion pore opening have been detected. The fusion pore rapidly reseals (kiss and run), opens to a limited extent and persists for variable times followed by closure (limited dilation), or fully dilates (full dilation). The secretion of low-molecular-weight constituents such as monoamines *(small closed circles)* would occur earlier and to a greater extent than larger peptide hormones *(curved lines)* dependent on the degree of fusion pore dilation, the size of the constituent, and its solubility within the matrix of the granule.

(NPY) was released quickly.[165] In several reported studies, dense-core vesicles exhibited at least three modes of exocytosis: full merger with the plasma membrane and complete fusion pore dilation[166]; limited but long-term fusion pore opening followed by fusion pore closure[165]; or transient fusion pore opening with rapid closure ("kiss and run").[165,167,168] This indicates that exocytosis can result in the differential release of granule constituents depending on their size and rate of solubilization from the luminal matrix. Monoamines such as norepinephrine may be released by some granule fusion events without accompanying peptide hormone release. Thus, the fusion pore machinery is an important site for physiologic regulation of hormone secretion.

MODULATION OF CALCIUM-DEPENDENT HORMONE SECRETION BY PROTEIN KINASE C

Because the proximal regulator of dense-core granule exocytosis is cytoplasmic calcium, receptor mechanisms that mobilize intracellular calcium through inositol triphosphate generation or that promote calcium influx will correspondingly influence the rates of hormone secretion (see Chapter 13). However, other signal transduction pathways exert significant modulatory effects on calcium-dependent hormone secretion. In virtually all endocrine cells that have been examined, phorbol ester activators of protein kinase C enhance hormone secretion.[169] In some cases, phorbol ester stimulation of hormone secretion may be indirect and mediated

through ion channel regulation that alters calcium entry.[170] However, stimulatory effects of phorbol esters are also seen at sites distal to calcium entry. In some cases, phorbol ester stimulation is observed at a low resting cytoplasmic calcium concentration[171,172]; in other cases, phorbol ester treatment synergistically enhances the stimulation of secretion by cytoplasmic calcium elevation.[173,174] Although phorbol ester-binding proteins other than protein kinase C (e.g., Munc-13 protein) may mediate some of the actions of phorbol esters (discussed later), a stimulatory role for protein kinase C on exocytosis has been directly demonstrated in studies of calcium-dependent hormone secretion in permeable neuroendocrine cells.[175,176]

Protein kinase C regulates hormone secretion at several sites in the exocytotic pathway. Strong enhancing effects of phorbol esters on constitutive secretion have been reported and attributed to steps in the secretory pathway between the ER and Golgi or at vesicle-budding reactions in the TGN.[177–179] Stimulation of rate-limiting steps early in the secretory pathway alters the transit of proteins to both the regulated and constitutive secretory pathways (see Fig. 7-1). In addition, protein kinase C activation stimulates steps in the regulated pathway close to exocytosis. Phorbol ester treatment was shown to enhance the recruitment and docking of dense-core vesicles in chromaffin and PC12 cells.[145,180–182] In addition, the direct stimulation of calcium-dependent exocytosis by protein kinase C at a postdocking step has been observed in permeable neuroendocrine cells.[175]

Many protein substrates for protein kinase C have been identified in endocrine cells, but protein substrates that mediate the stimulatory effects of protein kinase C on hormone secretion or exocytosis remain elusive.[183–185] Of identified proteins that function at a late step in regulated exocytosis, two (Munc18 and SNAP-25) have been shown to be direct substrates for protein kinase C-mediated phosphorylation.[186,187] SNAP-25 is phosphorylated by protein kinase C at Ser187[188] and phosphomimetic SNAP-25 mutations were reported to enhance secretory granule recruitment in chromaffin cells.[181] Mild effects of phosphomimetic mutations at protein kinase C phosphorylation sites in Munc18 on the kinetics of exocytosis have also been reported.[189] Neither of these fully accounts for the stimulatory effects of protein kinase C activation on secretion, which indicates that other relevant protein substrates remain to be identified.

The stimulatory effects of phorbol esters on secretion via dense-core vesicles appear to be mediated by both protein kinase C-dependent and -independent mechanisms.[182] Munc13 contains a β-phorbol ester-binding C1 domain that has been shown to mediate the augmentation of neurotransmitter release via synaptic vesicle exocytosis by phorbol esters.[190] It is unclear whether endogenous Munc13-dependent mechanisms mediate some of the phorbol ester stimulation of hormone secretion in endocrine cells. It has been shown that overexpressed Munc13 modulates dense-core vesicle exocytosis, but a role for the endogenous protein remains to be examined.[191,192]

REFERENCES

1. Palade G: Intracellular aspects of the process of protein synthesis. Science 189:347–358, 1975.

2. Farquhar MG: Multiple pathways of exocytosis, endocytosis, and membrane recycling: Validation of a Golgi route. Fed Proc 42:2407–2413, 1983.

3. Griffiths G, Simons K: The *trans*-Golgi network: Sorting at the exit site of the Golgi complex. Science 234:438–443, 1986.

4. Traub LM, Kornfeld S: The *trans*-Golgi network: A late secretory sorting station. Curr Opin Cell Biol 9:527–533, 1997.

5. Kelly RB: Pathways of protein secretion in eukaryotes. Science 230:25–32, 1985.

6. Burgess TL, Kelly RB: Constitutive and regulated secretion of proteins. Annu Rev Cell Biol 3:243–293, 1987.

7. Tooze SA, Flatmark T, Tooze J, Huttner WB: Characterization of the immature secretory granule, an intermediate in granule biogenesis. J Cell Biol 115:1491–1503, 1991.

8. Wendler F, Page L, Urbe S, Tooze SA: Homotypic fusion of immature secretory granules during maturation requires syntaxin 6. Mol Biol Cell 12:1699–1709, 2001.

9. Arvan P, Castle D: Sorting and storage during secretory granule biogenesis: Looking backward and looking forward. Biochem J 332:593–610, 1998.

10. Arvan P, Kuliawat R, Prabakaran D, et al: Protein discharge from immature secretory granules displays both regulated and constitutive characteristics. J Biol Chem 266:14171–14174, 1991.

11. Dittie A, Thomas L, Thomas G, Tooze SA: Interaction of furin in immature secretory granules from neuroendocrine cells with AP-1 adaptor complex is modulated by casein kinase II phosphorylation. EMBO J 16:4859–4870, 1997.

12. Eaton BA, Haugwitz M, Lau D, Moore HP: Biogenesis of regulated exocytic carriers in neuroendocrine cells. J Neurosci 20:7334–7344, 2000.

13. Kuliawat R, Klumperman J, Ludwig T, Arvan P: Differential sorting of lysosomal enzymes out of the regulated secretory pathway in pancreatic beta cells. J Cell Biol 137:595–608, 1997.

14. Klumperman J, Kuliawat R, Griffith JM, et al: Mannose 6-phosphate receptors are sorted from immature secretory granules via adaptor protein AP-1, clathrin, and syntaxin 6-positive vesicles. J Cell Biol 141:359–371, 1998.

15. Phillips JH, Pryde JG: The chromaffin granule: A model system for the study of hormone and neurotransmitters. Ann N Y Acad Sci 493:27–42, 1987.

16. Rubin RP: Calcium and Cellular Secretion. New York, Plenum, 1982.

17. Schatz G, Dobberstein B: Common principles of protein translocation across membranes. Science 271:1519–1526, 1996.

18. Rouille Y, Duguay SJ, Lund K, et al: Proteolytic processing mechanisms in the biosynthesis of neuroendocrine peptides: The subtilisin-like proprotein convertases. Front Neuroendocrinol 16:322–361, 1995.

19. Halban PA, Irminger J-C: Sorting and processing of secretory proteins. Biochem J 299:1–18, 1994.

20. Creemers JWM, Jackson RS, Hutton JC: Molecular and cellular regulation of prohormone processing. Semin Cell Dev Biol 9:3–10, 1998.

21. Jung LJ, Scheller RH: Peptide processing and targeting in the neuronal secretory pathway. Science 251:1330–1335, 1991.

22. Orci L, Ravazzola M, Storch MJ, et al: Proteolytic maturation of insulin is a post-Golgi event which occurs in acidifying clathrin-coated secretory vesicles. Cell 49:865–868, 1987.

23. Eipper BA, Mains RE: Structure and biosynthesis of pro-adrenocorticotropin/endorphin and related peptides. Endocr Rev 1:1–27, 1980.

24. Arvan P, Halban PA: Sorting ourselves out: Seeking consensus on trafficking in the beta cell. Traffic 5:53–61, 2004.

25. Hashimoto S, Fumagalli G, Zanini A, Meldolesi J: Sorting of three secretory proteins to distinct secretory granules in acidophilic cells of cow anterior pituitary. J Cell Biol 105:1579–1586, 1987.

26. Natori S, Huttner WB: Chromogranin B promotes sorting to the regulated secretory pathway of processing intermediates derived from a peptide hormone precursor. Proc Natl Acad Sci U S A 93:4431–4436, 1996.

27. Thiele C, Huttner WB: The disulfide-bonded loop of chromogranins, which is essential for sorting to secretory granules, mediates homodimerization. J Biol Chem 273:1223–1231, 1998.

28. Kromer A, Glombik MM, Huttner WB, Gerdes HH: Essential role of the disulfide-bonded loop of chromogranin B for sorting to secretory granules is revealed by expression of a deletion mutant in the absence of endogenous granin synthesis. J Cell Biol 140:1331–1346, 1998.

29. Kelly RB: Storage and release of neurotransmitters. Cell 72:43–53, 1993.

30. Cool DR, Normant E, Shen F-S, et al: Carboxypeptidase E is a regulated secretory pathway sorting receptor: Genetic obliteration leads to endocrine disorders in Cpe(fat) mice. Cell 88:73–83, 1997.

31. Cool DR, Loh PY: Carboxypeptidase E is a sorting receptor for prohormones: Binding and kinetic studies. Mol Cell Endocrinol 139:7–13, 1998.

32. Dhanvantari S, Shen FS, Adams T, et al: Disruption of a receptor-mediated mechanism for intracellular sorting of proinsulin in familial hyperproinsulinemia. Mol Endocrinol 17:1856–1867, 2003.

33. Thiele C, Gerdes HH, Huttner WB: Protein secretion: Puzzling receptors. Curr Biol 7:R496–R500, 1997.

34. Chanat E, Huttner WB: Milieu-induced selective aggregation of regulated secretory proteins in the trans-Golgi network. J Cell Biol 115:1505–1519, 1991.

35. Huttner WB, Natori S: Helper proteins for neuroendocrine secretion. Curr Biol 5:242–245, 1995.

36. Huh YH, Jeon SH, Yoo SH: Chromogranin B-induced secretory granule biogenesis: Comparison with the similar role of chromogranin B. J Biol Chem 278:40581–40589, 2003.

37. Kim T, Tao-Cheng J, Eiden LE, Loh YP: Chromogranin A, an on/off switch controlling dense-core secretory granule biogenesis. Cell 106:499–509, 2001.

38. Day R, Gorr SU: Secretory granule biogenesis and chromogranin A: Master gene, on/off switch or assembly factor? Trends Endocrinol Metab 14:10–13, 2003.

39. Colomer V, Kicska GA, Rindler MJ: Secretory granule content proteins and the luminal domains of granule membrane proteins aggregate in vitro at mildly acidic pH. J Biol Chem 271:48–55, 1996.

40. Sheenan KIJ, Taylor NA, Docherty K: Calcium- and pH-dependent aggregation and membrane association of the precursor of the prohormone convertase PC2. J Biol Chem 269:18646–18650, 1994.

41. Alam MR, Johnson RC, Darlington DN, et al: Kalirin, a cytosolic protein with spectrin-like and GDP/GTP exchange factor-like domains that interacts with peptidylglycine alpha-amidating monooxygenase, an integral membrane peptide processing enzyme. J Biol Chem 272:12667–12675, 1997.

42. Disdier M, Morrissey JH, Fugate RD, et al: Cytoplasmic domain of P selectin contains the signal for sorting into the regulated secretory pathway. Mol Biol Cell 3:309–321, 1992.

43. Marcusson EG, Horazdovsky BF, Cereghino JL, et al: The sorting receptor for yeast vacuolar carboxypeptidase Y is encoded by the VPS10 gene. Cell 77:579–586, 1994.

44. Rothman JE, Wieland FT: Protein sorting by transport vesicles. Science 272:227–234, 1996.

45. Kuehn MJ, Herrmann JM, Schekman R: COPII-cargo interactions direct protein sorting into ER-derived transport vesicles. Nature 391:187–190, 1998.

46. Tooze SA, Huttner WB: Cell-free protein sorting to the regulated and constitutive secretory pathways. Cell 60:837–847, 1990.

47. Tooze SA, Weiss U, Huttner WB: Requirement for GTP hydrolysis in the formation of secretory vesicles. Nature 347:207–208, 1990.

48. Ohashi M, DeVries KJ, Frank R, et al: A role for the phosphatidylinositol transfer protein in secretory vesicle formation. Nature 377:544–547, 1995.

49. Chen Y-G, Shields D: ADP-ribosylation factor-1 stimulates formation of nascent secretory vesicles from the trans-Golgi network of endocrine cells. J Biol Chem 271:297–300, 1996.

50. Barr FA, Huttner WB: A role for ADP-ribosylation factor 1, but not COP I, in secretory vesicle biogenesis from the trans-Golgi network. FEBS Lett 384:65–70, 1996.

51. Chen Y-G, Siddhanta A, Austin CD, et al: Phospholipase D stimulates release of nascent secretory vesicles from the trans-Golgi network. J Cell Biol 138:495–504, 1997.

52. Siddhanta A, Shields D: Secretory vesicle budding from the trans-Golgi network is mediated by phosphatidic acid levels. J Biol Chem 273:17995–17998, 1998.

53. Tuscher O, Lorra C, Bouma B, et al: Cooperativity of phosphatidylinositol transfer protein and phospholipase D in secretory vesicle formation from the TGN-phosphoinositides as a common denominator? FEBS Lett 419:271–275, 1997.

54. Simon J-P, Morimoto T, Bankaitis VA, et al: An essential role for the phosphatidylinositol transfer protein in the scission of coatomer-coated vesicles from the *trans*-Golgi network. Proc Natl Acad Sci U S A 95:11181–11186, 1998.

55. Martin TFJ: New directions for phosphatidylinositol transfer. Curr Biol 5:990–992, 1995.

56. Martin TFJ: Phosphoinositide lipids as signaling molecules: Common themes for signal transduction, cytoskeletal regulation and membrane trafficking. Annu Rev Cell Dev Biol 14:231–264, 1998.

57. Roth MG, Sternweis PC: The role of lipid signaling in constitutive membrane traffic. Curr Opin Cell Biol 9:519–526, 1997.

58. Panaretou C, Tooze SA: Regulation and recruitment of phosphatidylinositol 4-kinase on immature secretory granules is independent of ADP-ribosylation factor 1. Biochem J 363:289–295, 2002.

59. Olsen HL, Hoy M, Zhang W, et al: Phosphatidylinositol 4-kinase serves as a metabolic sensor and regulates priming of secretory granules in pancreatic β cells. Proc Natl Acad Sci U S A 100:5187–5192, 2003.

60. Greider MH, Howell SL, Lacy PE: Isolation and properties of secretory granules from rat islets of Langerhans. Ultrastructure of the beta granule. J Cell Biol 41:162–168, 1969.

61. Naggert JK, Fricker LD, Varlamov O, et al: Hyperproinsulinemia in obese fat/fat mice associated with a carboxypeptidase E mutation which reduces enzyme activity. Nat Genet 10:135–142, 1995.

62. Pelletier G, Labrie F: Anterior pituitary secretory granules. In Poisner AM, Trifaro JM (eds): The Secretory Granule. New York, Elsevier, 1982, pp 173–209.

63. Howell SL, Tyhurst M: The insulin storage granule. In Poisner AM, Trifaro JM (eds): The Secretory Granule. New York, Elsevier, 1982, pp 155–172.

64. Apps DK: Membrane and soluble proteins of adrenal chromaffin granules. Semin Cell Dev Biol 8:121–131, 1997.

65. Winkler H, Carmichael SW: The chromaffin granule. In Poisner L, Trifaro JM (eds): The Secretory Granule. New York, Elsevier, 1982, pp 3–79.

66. Winkler H: Membrane composition of adrenergic large and small dense core vesicles and of synaptic vesicles: Consequences for their biogenesis. Neurochem Res 8:921–932, 1997.

67. Westhead EW: Lipid composition and orientation in secretory vesicles. Ann N Y Acad Sci 493:92–100, 1987.

68. Wiedenmann B, Huttner WB: Synaptophysin and chromogranins/secretogranins— widespread constituents of distinct types of neuroendocrine vesicles and new tools in tumor diagnosis. Virchows Arch 58:95–121, 1989.

69. Howell SL, Montague W, Tyhurst M: Calcium distribution in islets of Langerhans: A study of calcium concentrations and of calcium accumulation in B cell organelles. J Cell Sci 19:395–409, 1975.

70. Liu Y, Schweitzer ES, Nirenberg MJ, et al: Preferential localization of vesicular monoamine transporter to dense core vesicles in PC12 cells. J Cell Biol 127:1419–1433, 1994.

71. Martin TFJ: Mechanisms of protein secretion in endocrine and exocrine cells. Vitam Horm 54:207–226, 1998.

72. Gasman S, Chasserot-Golaz S, Hubert P, et al: Identification of a potential effector pathway for the trimeric G_0 protein associated with secretory granules. J Biol Chem 273:16913–16920, 1998.

73. Caumont A-S, Galas M-C, Vitale N, et al: Regulated exocytosis in chromaffin cells—translocation of ARF6 stimulates a plasma membrane-associated phospholipase D. J Biol Chem 273:1373–1379, 1998.

74. Izumi T, Gomi H, Kasai K, et al: The roles of Rab27 and its effectors in the regulated secretory pathway. Cell Struct Funct 28:465–474, 2003.

75. Waselle L, Coppola T, Fukuda M, et al: Involvement of the Rab27 binding protein Slac2c/MyRIP in insulin exocytosis. Mol Biol Cell 14:4103–4113, 2003.

76. Fukuda M: Slp4-a/granuphilin-a inhibits dense-core vesicle exocytosis through interaction with the GDP-bound form of Rab27A in PC12 cells. J Biol Chem 278:15390–15396, 2003.

77. Rose SD, Lejen T, Casaletti L, et al: Myosins II and V in chromaffin cells: Myosin V is a chromaffin vesicle molecular motor involved in secretion. J Neurochem 85:287–298, 2003.

78. Arispe N, De Mazancourt P, Rojas E: Direct control of a large conductance K⁺ selective channel by G proteins in adrenal chromaffin granule membranes. J Membr Biol 147:109–119, 1995.

79. Passafaro M, Rosa P, Sala C, et al: N-type Ca²⁺ channels are present in secretory granules and are transiently translocated to the plasma membrane during regulated exocytosis. J Biol Chem 271:30096–30104, 1996.

80. Phillips JH: Phosphatidylinositol kinase—a component of the chromaffin granule membrane. Biochem J 136:579–587, 1973.

81. Desnos C, Schonn JS, Huet S, et al: Rab27A and its effector MyRIP link secretory granules to F-actin and control their motion towards release sites. J Cell Biol 163:559–570, 2003.

82. Rudolf R, Kogel T, Kuznetsov SA: Myosin Va facilitates the distribution of secretory granules in the F-actin rich cortex of PC12 cells. J Cell Sci 116:1339–1348, 2003.

83. Steyer JA, Horstmann H, Almers W: Transport, docking and exocytosis of single secretory granules in live chromaffin cells. Nature 388:474–478, 1997.

84. Duncan RR, Greaves J, Wiegand UK, et al: Functional and spatial segregation of secretory vesicle pools according to vesicle age. Nature 422:176–180, 2003.

85. Neher E: Vesicle pools and calcium microdomains: New tools for understanding their roles in neurotransmitter release. Neuron 20:389–399, 1998.

86. Martin TFJ: Stages of regulated exocytosis. Trends Cell Biol 7:271–276, 1997.

87. Parsons TD, Coorssen JR, Horstmann H, Almers W: Docked granules, the exocytic burst, and the need for ATP hydrolysis in endocrine cells. Neuron 15:1085–1096, 1995.

88. Neher E, Zucker RS: Multiple calcium-dependent processes related to secretion in bovine chromaffin cells. Neuron 10:21–30, 1993.

89. Chow RH, von Ruden L, Neher E: Delay in vesicle fusion revealed by electrochemical monitoring of single secretory events in adrenal chromaffin cells. Nature 356:60–63, 1992.

90. Albillos A, Dernick G, Horstmann H, et al: The exocytotic event in chromaffin cells revealed by patch amperometry. Nature 389:509–512, 1997.

91. Xu T, Binz T, Niemann H, Neher E: Multiple kinetic components of exocytosis distinguished by neurotoxin sensitivity. Nat Neurosci 1:192–200, 1998.

92. Plattner H, Artalejo AR, Neher E: Ultrastructural organization of bovine chromaffin cell cortex-analysis by cryofixation and morphometry of aspects pertinent to exocytosis. J Cell Biol 139:1709–1717, 1997.

93. Blaschko H, Comline RS, Schneider FH, et al: Secretion of a chromaffin granule protein chromogranin from the adrenal gland after splanchnic stimulation. Nature 215:58–59, 1967.

94. Levine R: Mechanisms of insulin secretion. N Engl J Med 283:522–526, 1970.

95. Burke NV, Han W, Li D, et al: Neuronal peptide release is limited by secretory granule mobility. Neuron 19:1095–1102, 1997.

96. Lang T, Wacker I, Steyer J, et al: Ca²⁺ triggered peptide secretion in single cells imaged with green fluorescent protein and evanescent-wave microscopy. Neuron 18:857–863, 1997.

97. Oheim M, Loerke D, Stuhmer W, Chow RH: The last few seconds in the life of a secretory granule: Docking, dynamics and fusion visualized by total internal reflection fluorescence microscopy (TIRFM). Eur Biophys J 27:83–98, 1998.

98. Burgoyne RD: Control of exocytosis in adrenal chromaffin cells. Biochim Biophys Acta 1071:174–202, 1991.

99. Martin TFJ: The molecular machinery for fast and slow neurosecretion. Curr Opin Neurobiol 4:626–632, 1994.

100. Rothman JE: Mechanisms of intracellular protein transport. Nature 372:55–63, 1994.

101. Bennett MK, Scheller RH: A molecular description of synaptic vesicle membrane trafficking. Annu Rev Biochem 63:63–100, 1994.

102. Sudhof TC: The synaptic vesicle cycle: A cascade of protein-protein interactions. Nature 375:645–653, 1995.

103. Bark IC, Wilson MC: Regulated vesicular fusion in neurons: Snapping together the details. Proc Natl Acad Sci U S A 91:4621–4624, 1994.

104. Montecucco C, Schiavo G: Tetanus and botulism neurotoxins: A new group of zinc proteases. Trends Biochem Sci 18:324–329, 1993.

105. Niemann H, Blasi J, Jahn R: Clostridial neurotoxins: New tools for dissecting exocytosis. Trends Cell Biol 4:179–185, 1994.

106. Sollner T, Whiteheart SW, Brunner M, et al: SNAP receptors implicated in vesicle targeting and fusion. Nature 362:318–324, 1993.

107. Banerjee J, Kowalchyk JA, DasGupta BR, Martin TFJ: SNAP-25 is required for a late postdocking step in calcium-dependent exocytosis. J Biol Chem 271:20227–20230, 1996.

108. Sollner T, Bennett MK, Whiteheart SW, et al: A protein assembly-disassembly pathway in vitro that may correspond to sequential steps of synaptic vesicle docking, activation and fusion. Cell 75:409–418, 1993.

109. Hayashi T, McMahon H, Yamasaki S, et al: Synaptic vesicle membrane fusion complex: Action of clostridial neurotoxins on assembly. EMBO J 13:5051–5061, 1994.

110. 9Sutton RB, Fasshauer D, Jahn R, Brunger AT: Crystal structure of a SNARE complex involved in synaptic exocytosis at 2.4A resolution. Nature 395:347–353, 1998.

111. Bennett MK: SNAREs and the specificity of transport vesicle targeting. Curr Opin Cell Biol 7:581–586, 1995.

112. Augustine GJ, Burns ME, DeBello WM, et al: Exocytosis: Proteins and perturbations. Annu Rev Pharmacol Toxicol 36:659–701, 1996.

113. Hanson P, Heuser J, Jahn R: Neurotransmitter release—four years of SNARE complexes. Curr Opin Neurobiol 7:310–315, 1997.

114. Jahn R, Hanson PI: SNAREs line up in a new environment. Nature 393:14–15, 1998.

115. Weis WI, Scheller RH: SNARE the rod, coil the complex. Nature 395:328–329, 1998.

116. Rizo J, Sudhof TC: Mechanics of membrane fusion. Nat Struct Biol 5:839–842, 1998.

117. Weber T, Zemelman, McNew JA, et al: SNAREpins: Minimal machinery for membrane fusion. Cell 92:759–772, 1998.

118. Mahal LK, Sequeira SM, Gureasko JM, Sollner TH: Calcium-independent stimulation of membrane fusion and SNAREpin formation by synaptotagmin I. J Cell Biol 158:273–282, 2002.

119. Klenchin VA, Martin TF: Priming in exocytosis: Attaining fusion-competence after vesicle docking. Biochimie 82:399–407, 2000.

120. Rettig J, Neher E: Emerging roles of presynaptic proteins in Ca^{2+} triggered exocytosis. Science 298:781–785, 2002.

121. Hay JC, Martin TFJ: Resolution of regulated secretion into sequential MgATP-dependent and calcium-dependent stages mediated by distinct cytosolic proteins. J Cell Biol 119:139–151, 1992.

122. Banerjee J, Barry VA, DasGupta BR, Martin TFJ: N-ethylmaleimide-sensitive factor acts at a prefusion ATP-dependent step in calcium-activated exocytosis. J Biol Chem 271:20223–20226, 1996.

123. Hay JC, Martin TFJ: Phosphatidylinositol transfer protein required for ATP-dependent priming of calcium-activated secretion. Nature 366:572–575, 1993.

124. Hay JC, Fisette PL, Jenkins GH, et al: ATP-dependent inositide phosphorylation required for calcium-activated secretion. Nature 374:173–177, 1995.

125. Khvotchev M, Sudhof TC: Newly synthesized phosphatidylinositol phosphates are required for synaptic norepinephrine but not glutamate or γ-aminobutyric acid release. J Biol Chem 273:21451–21454, 1998.

126. Wiedemann C, Schafer T, Burger MM, Sihra TS: An essential role for a small synaptic vesicle-associated phosphatidylinositol

127. Ann K, Kowalchyk JA, Loyet KM, Martin TFJ: Novel calcium binding protein (CAPS) related to UNC-31 required for calcium-activated exocytosis. J Biol Chem 272:19637–19640, 1997.

128. Loyet KM, Kowalchyk JA, Chaudhary A, et al: Specific binding of PIP_2 to CAPS, a potential phosphoinositide effector protein for regulated exocytosis. J Biol Chem 273:8337–8343, 1998.

129. Berwin B, Floor E, Martin TFJ: CAPS (mammalian UNC-31) protein localizes to membranes involved in dense-core vesicle exocytosis. Neuron 21:137–145, 1998.

130. Tandon A, Bannykh S, Kowalchyk JA, et al: Differential regulation of exocytosis by calcium and CAPS in semi-intact synaptosomes. Neuron 21:147–154, 1998.

131. Grishanin RN, Klenchin VA, Loyet KM, et al: Membrane association domains in CAPS mediate plasma membrane and dense-core vesicle binding required for Ca^{2+} dependent exocytosis. J Biol Chem 277:22025–22034, 2002.

132. Lang J: PIPs and pools in insulin secretion. Trends Endocrinol Metab 14:297–299, 2003.

133. Burgoyne RD, Morgan A: Calcium and secretory-vesicle dynamics. Trends Neurosci 18:191–196, 1995.

134. Varro A, Nemeth J, Dickinson CJ, et al: Discrimination between constitutive secretion and basal secretion from the regulated secretory pathway in GH3 cells. Biochim Biophys Acta 1313:101–105, 1996.

135. Chow RH, Klingauf J, Heinemann C, et al: Mechanisms determining the time course of secretion in neuroendocrine cells. Neuron 16:369–376, 1996.

136. Sheng Z-H, Rettig J, Cook T, Catterall WA: Calcium-dependent interaction of N-type calcium channels with the synaptic core complex. Nature 379:451–454, 1996.

137. Mochida S, Sheng Z-H, Baker C, et al: Inhibition of neurotransmission by peptides containing the synaptic protein interaction site of N-type calcium channels. Neuron 17:781–788, 1996.

138. Heidelberger R, Heinemann C, Neher E, Matthews G: Calcium dependence of the rate of exocytosis in a synaptic terminal. Nature 371:513–515, 1994.

139. Augustine GJ, Santamaria F, Tanaka K: Local calcium signaling in neurons. Neuron 40:331–346, 2003.

140. Schneggenburger R, Neher E: Intracellular calcium dependence of transmitter release rates at a fast central synapse. Nature 406:889–893, 2000.

141. Bollmann JH, Sakmann B, Borst JG: Calcium sensitivity of glutamate release in a calyx-type terminal. Science 289:953–957, 2000.

142. Tse FW, Tse A, Hille B, et al: Local calcium release from internal stores controls exocytosis in pituitary gonadotrophs. Neuron 18:121–132, 1997.

143. Smith C, Moser T, Xu T, Neher E: Cytosolic calcium acts by two separate pathways to modulate the supply of release-competent vesicles in chromaffin cells. Neuron 20:1243–1253, 1998.

144. von Ruden L, Neher E: A Ca^{2+} dependent early step in the release of catecholamines from adrenal chromaffin cells. Science 262:1061–1065, 1993.

145. Gills KD, Mossner R, Neher E: Protein kinase enhances exocytosis from chromaffin cells by increasing the size of the readily releasable pool of secretory granules. Neuron 16:1209–1220, 1996.

146. Sudhof TC, Rizo J: Synaptotagmins: C2-domain proteins that regulate membrane traffic. Neuron 17:379–388, 1996.

147. Fernandez-Chacon R, Konigstorfer A, Gerber SH: Synaptotagmin I functions as a calcium regulator of release probability. Nature 410:41–49, 2001.

148. Voets T, Toonen RF, Brian EC, et al: Intracellular calcium dependence of large dense-core vesicle exocytosis in the absence of synaptotagmin I. Proc Natl Acad Sci U S A 98:11680–11685, 2001.

149. Sudhof TC: Synaptotagmins: Why so many? J Biol Chem 277:7629–7632, 2002.

150. Chapman ER: Synaptotagmin: A Ca^{2+} sensor that triggers exocytosis? Nature Rev Mol Cell Biol 3:1–11, 2002.

151. Gerona RR, Larsen EC, Kowalchyk JA, Martin TF: The C terminus of SNAP25 is essential for Ca^{2+} dependent binding of synaptotagmin to SNARE complexes. J Biol Chem 275:6328–6336, 2000.

152. Davis AF, Bai J, Fasshauer D, et al: Kinetics of synaptotagmin responses to Ca^{2+} and assembly with the core SNARE complex onto membranes. Neuron 24:363–376, 1999.

153. Bai J, Wang C-T, Richards DA, et al: Fusion pore dynamics are regulated by synaptotagmin-t SNARE interactions. Neuron 41:929–942, 2004.

154. Zhang X, Kim-Miller MJ, Fukuda M, et al: Ca^{2+}, dependent synaptotagmin binding to SNAP25 is essential for Ca^{2+}, triggered exocytosis. Neuron 34:599–611, 2002.

155. Fukuda M, Kowalchyk JA, Zhang X, et al: Synaptotagmin IX regulates Ca^{2+} dependent secretion in PC12 cells. J Biol Chem 277:4601–4604, 2002.

156. Tucker WC, Edwardson JM, Bai J, et al: Identification of synaptotagmin effectors via acute inhibition of secretion from cracked PC12 cells. J Cell Biol 162:199–209, 2003.

157. Gut A, Kiraly CE, Fukuda M, et al: Expression and localization of synaptotagmin isoforms in endocrine β cells: Their function in insulin exocytosis. J Cell Sci 114:1709–1716, 2001.

158. Chung S-H, Takai Y, Holz RW: Evidence that the Rab3a-binding protein Rabphilin enhances regulated secretion. J Biol Chem 270:16714–16718, 1995.

159. Scepek S, Coorssen J, Lindau M: Fusion pore expansion in horse eosinophils is modulated by calcium and protein kinase C via distinct mechanisms. EMBO J 17:4340–4345, 1998.

160. Wang C-T, Grishanin R, Earles CA, et al: Synaptotagmin modulation of fusion pore kinetics in regulated exocytosis of dense-core vesicles. Science 294:1111–1115, 2001.

161. Artalejo CR, Elhamdani A, Palfrey HC: Calmodulin is the divalent cation receptor for rapid endocytosis, but not exocytosis, in adrenal chromaffin cells. Neuron 16:195–205, 1996.

162. Marks B, McMahon HT: Calcium triggers calcineurin-dependent synaptic vesicle recycling in mammalian nerve terminals. Curr Biol 8:740–749, 1998.

163. Slepnev VI, Ochoa G-C, Butler MH, et al: Role of phosphorylation in regulation of the assembly of endocytic coat complexes. Science 281:821–824, 1998.

164. Barg S, Olofsson CS, Schriever-Abein J, et al: Delay between fusion pore opening and peptide release from large dense-core vesicles in neuroendocrine cells. Neuron 33:287–299, 2002.

165. Taraska JW, Perrais D, Ohara-Imaizumi M, et al: Secretory granules are recaptured largely intact after stimulated exocytosis in cultured endocrine cells. Proc Natl Acad Sci U S A 100:2070–2075, 2003.

166. Takahashi N, Kishimoto T, Nemoto T, et al: Fusion pore dynamics and insulin granule exocytosis in the pancreatic islet. Science 297:1349–1352, 2002.

167. Tsuboi T, Rutter GA: Multiple forms of kiss and run exocytosis revealed by evanescent wave microscopy. Curr Biol 13:563–567, 2003.

168. Holroyd P, Lang T, Wenzel D, et al: Imaging direct dynamin-dependent recapture of fusing secretory granules on plasma membrane lawns from PC12 cells. Proc Natl Acad Sci U S A 99:16806–16811, 2002.

169. Nishizuka Y: Intracellular signaling by hydrolysis of phospholipids and activation of protein kinase C. Science 258:607–614, 1992.

170. Conn PJ, Sweatt JD: Protein kinase C in the nervous system. In Kuo JF (ed): Protein Kinase C. Oxford, Oxford University Press, 1994, pp 199–235.

171. Knight DE, Baker PF: The phorbol ester TPA increases the affinity of exocytosis for calcium ions in "leaky" adrenal medullary cells. FEBS Lett 160:98–100, 1983.

172. Billiard J, Koh D-S, Babcock DF, Hille B: Protein kinase C as a signal for exocytosis. Proc Natl Acad Sci U S A 94:12192–12197, 1997.

173. Yamanishi J, Takai K, Kaibuchi K, et al: Synergistic functions of phorbol ester and calcium in serotonin release from human platelets. Biochem Biophys Res Commun 112:778–786, 1983.

174. Ronning SA, Martin TFJ: Characterization of phorbol ester- and diacylglycerol-stimulated secretion in permeable GH_3 pituitary cells. J Biol Chem 261:7840–7845, 1986.

175. Nishizaki T, Walent JH, Kowalchyk JA, Martin TFJ: A key role for a 145 kD cytosolic protein in the stimulation of calcium-dependent secretion by protein kinase C. J Biol Chem 267:23972–23981, 1992.

176. Naor Z, Dan-Cohen H, Hermon J, Limor R: Induction of exocytosis in permeabilized pituitary cells by alpha- and beta-type protein kinase C. Proc Natl Acad Sci U S A 86:4501–4504, 1989.

177. Luini A, DeMatteis MA: Receptor-mediated regulation of constitutive secretion. Trends Cell Biol 3:290–292, 1993.

178. Westermann P, Knoblich M, Maier O, et al: Protein kinase C bound to the Golgi apparatus supports the formation of constitutive transport vesicles. J Biol Chem 320:651–658, 1996.

179. Simon JP, Ivanov IE, Shopsin B, et al: The in vitro generation of post-Golgi vesicles carrying viral envelope glycoproteins requires an ARF-like GTP-binding protein and a protein kinase C associated with the Golgi apparatus. J Biol Chem 271:16952–16961, 1996.

180. Yang Y, Udayasankar S, Dunning J, et al: A highly Ca^{2+} sensitive pool of vesicles is regulated by protein kinase C in adrenal chromaffin cells. Proc Natl Acad Sci U S A 99:17060–17065, 2002.

181. Nagy G, Matti U, Nehring RB, et al: Protein kinase C-dependent phosphorylation of synaptosome-associated protein of 25 kD at Ser 187 potentiates vesicle recruitment. J Neurosci 22:9278–9286, 2002.

182. Shoji-Kasai Y, Itakura M, Kataoka M, et al: Protein kinase C-mediated translocation of secretory vesicles to plasma membrane and enhancement of neurotransmitter release from PC12 cells. Eur J Neurosci 15:1390–1394, 2002.

183. Pocotte SL, Frye RA, Senter RA, et al: Effects of phorbol ester on catecholamine secretion and protein phosphorylation in adrenal medullary cell cultures. Proc Natl Acad Sci U S A 82:930–934, 1985.

184. Drust DS, Martin TFJ: Thyrotropin-releasing hormone rapidly activates protein phosphorylation in GH_3 pituitary cells by a lipid-linked, protein kinase C-mediated pathway. J Biol Chem 259:14520–14530, 1984.

185. Morgan A, Burgoyne RD: Interaction between protein kinase C and exo I and its relevance to exocytosis in permeabilized adrenal chromaffin cells. Biochem J 286:807–811, 1992.

186. Fujita Y, Sasaki T, Fukui, et al: Phosphorylation of Munc-18/n-Sec1/rbSec1 by protein kinase C. J Biol Chem 271:7265–7268, 1996.

187. Shimazaki Y, Nishiki T, Omori A, et al: Phosphorylation of 25 kD synaptosome-associated protein. J Biol Chem 271:14548–14553, 1996.

188. Iwasaki S, Kataoka M, Sekiguchi M, et al: Two distinct mechanisms underlie the stimulation of neurotransmitter release by phorbol esters in clonal rat pheochromocytoma PC12 cells. J Biochem (Tokyo) 128:407–414, 2000.

189. Barclay JW, Craig TJ, Fisher RJ, et al: Phosphorylation of Munc18 by protein kinase C regulates the kinetics

of exocytosis. J Biol Chem 278:10538–10545, 2003.

190. Rhee JS, Betz A, Pyott S, et al: Beta phorbol ester- and diacylglycerol-induced augmentation of transmitter release is mediated by Munc13 and not by PKC. Cell 108:121–133, 2002.

191. Ashery U, Varoqueaux F, Voets T, et al: Munc13-1 acts as a priming factor for large dense-core vesicles in bovine chromaffin cells. EMBO J 19:3586–3596, 2000.

192. Sheu L, Pasyk EA, Ji J, et al: Regulation of insulin exocytosis by Munc13-1. J Biol Chem 278:27556–27563, 2003.

Hormone Signaling via Tyrosine Kinase Receptors

Joseph Avruch

RECEPTOR TYROSINE KINASES

Protein phosphorylation, reciprocally regulated by protein kinases and protein phosphatases, is the dominant posttranslational modification employed for rapid reversible control of intracellular protein function. The vast majority of protein phosphorylation occurs on the hydroxyl amino acid residues serine and threonine, with less than 1% recovered on tyrosine. Despite this low abundance, protein tyrosine phosphorylation plays a crucial role in cellular regulation. Phosphotyrosine does not occur in prokaryotes, and tyrosine-specific protein kinases are not evident in the *Saccharomyces cerevisiae* (a yeast) genome. Yeast protein tyrosine-specific phosphatases, however, do exist; these enzymes apparently act to reverse tyrosine phosphorylations catalyzed by so-called dual-specificity kinases, a minor class of protein kinases (e.g., MAP kinase kinases and MKKs, discussed later and in Chapter 14) capable of phosphorylating both Ser/Thr and tyrosine residues concomitantly on their substrates. The earliest evidence of tyrosine-specific protein phosphorylation is in the cellular slime mold, *Dictyostelium discoideum*, a probable precursor of the animal and fungal phyla. Protein kinase catalytic domain sequences are first observed in the earliest multicellular forms of the animal phyla, that is, sponges and hydra. These observations, together with the pivotal role of tyrosine phosphorylation in mammalian cellular differentiation, point to the probable emergence of tyrosine-specific protein kinases at the dawn of metazoan evolution, concomitant with the development of multicellular animals containing differentiated cell types.

Tyrosine-specific protein kinases are classified into two major groups, the receptor tyrosine kinases (RTKs) and the nonreceptor tyrosine kinases (Table 8-1). The former are transmembrane proteins whose extracellular segment contains a ligand-binding domain, a single transmembrane segment followed by an intracellular extension that contains the tyrosine kinase catalytic domain (Fig. 8-1). Catalytic activity is normally controlled by the occupancy of the extracellular ligand-binding domain, with activation resulting from ligand-induced apposition of the RTK polypeptides as homo- or heterodimers. The nonreceptor tyrosine kinases are entirely intracellular, mostly cytoplasmic proteins whose catalytic activity is regulated through protein-protein interactions, usually at the plasma membrane (Fig. 8-2). Both classes of protein tyrosine kinases participate in signal transduction pathways that specify cell differentiation and/or proliferation with the former outcome predominant in vivo and proliferation most evident when examined in a tissue culture setting using immortalized cells. An exception is the insulin receptor, which acts primarily to control cellular fuel metabolism from minute to minute.

The RTKs, by virtue of their regulation by extracellular ligands such as insulin, polypeptide growth factors, and other cell surface and extracellular matrix proteins, are perched at the apex of cellular signaling pathways, whereas the intracellular tyrosine kinases act as one of several signal generators downstream of these and other receptors. This chapter focuses on the receptor tyrosine kinases, including their structure, general mechanism of activation/deactivation, the signal transduction pathways most relevant to their action, their reciprocal interactions with other signaling pathways, mechanisms for downregulation/desensitization, and their role in disease, particularly of the endocrine system.

HISTORY

The work that led to the discovery of RTKs arose from the effort to understand the biochemical basis for the transforming activity of acutely transforming oncogenic retroviruses such as the Rous sarcoma virus (RSV), a tumor virus of chickens. Earlier work had shown that RSV encoded only a few (4 to 5) genes, only one of which, named v-Src, appeared to be both indispensable to cellular transformation and lacking other known function (e.g., envelope protein, reverse transcriptase, etc.). This viral gene came to be considered the oncogene, and the protein product, pp60 v-Src, as the transforming agent. In 1978,[1] having succeeded in obtaining a polyclonal antibody to pp60 v-Src, it was shown that immunoprecipitates of this antigen, incubated in vitro in the presence of γ^{32}-ATP, catalyzed the transfer of ^{32}P onto the Ig heavy chain, indicating that a protein kinase activity had been precipitated by this antibody, which was perhaps attributable to the pp60 v-Src itself. Subsequently, a subset of transforming antigens were

Table 8-1	Protein Tyrosine Kinases	

RECEPTOR TYROSINE KINASES

Epidermal growth factor receptor family
  EGF receptor c-ErbB
  ErbB2 Neu HER2
  ErbB3 HER3
  ErbB4 HER4 Tyro2

Insulin receptor family
  Insulin receptor
    IGF-1 receptor
  Insulin receptor-related kinase
    IRR
    c-Ros
  Ltk
  Alk

Hepatic growth factor (HGF) receptor family
  HGF receptor Met
  Ron
  c-Sea

Vascular endothelial growth factor receptor family
  VEGF receptor (Flt1)
  VEGF receptor (Flk1)
  KDR
  Flt4

Eph family
  EphA1 (Eph)
  EphA2 (Eck/Sek2/Myk2)
  EphA3 (Hek/Cek4/Mek4/Tyro4)
  EphA4 (Sek1/Cek8/Hek8/Tyro1)
  EphA5 (Cek7/Bsk/Hek7/Ehk1/Rek7)
  EphA6 (Ehk2)
  EphA7 (Hek11/Mdk1/Ehk3/Ebk)
  EphA8 (Eek/Ptk4)
  EphB1 (Elk/Cek6/Net)
  EphB2 (Cek5/Nuk/Erk/Sek3/Tyro5/Hek5)
  EphB3 (Hek2/Cek10/Sek4/Mdk5/Tyro6)
  EphB4 (Myk1/Htk/Hek5)
  EphB5 (Cek9)
  EphB6 (Mep)

Fibroblast growth factor receptor family
  FGF receptor-1 (Flg/Cek1)
  FGF receptor-2 (Bek/K-Sam Cek3)
  FGF receptor-3
  FGF receptor-4

Nerve growth factor receptor family
  NGF receptor (Trk)
  BDNF/NT-3/NT-4/5 receptor (TrkB)
  NT-3 receptor (TrkC)

Platelet-derived growth factor receptor family
  PDGF receptor α *patch* locus
  PDGF receptor β
  CSF-1 receptor (c-Fms)
  SCF receptor (c-Kit) (*W* locus)
  Flk2/Flt3

Ror family
  Ror1
  Ror2

DDr family
  DDR (Nep/Cak)
  TKT/Tyro10

Axl family
  Axl (UFO/Ark/Tyro7)
  Rse (Brt/Sky/Tif/Tyro3)
  Dtk/Etk2
  Mer (c-Eyk/Nyk/Tyr12)

Tie family
  Tie
  Tek/Tie2

Ret family
  Klg
  Ryk (Nyk-r/Voik)
  MuSK (Nsk2)

NONRECEPTOR TYROSINE KINASES

Src family
  c-Src
  c-Yes
  Fyn
  Yrk
  Lck
  Lyn
  c-Fgr
  Blk
  Hck

Csk family
  Csk (Cyl)
  Ctk (Hyl/Matk/Ntk/Lsk/Batk)

Abl family
  c-Abl
  Arg

Fes/Fps family
  c-Fes/Fps
  Fer

Twin SH2 domain family
  Zap 70
  Syk
    Ack
    AckII

Src family related
  Frk/Rak (Mkk3)
  Brk (Sik)
  Srm
  Sad
  Lyk

Btk family
  Btk (Atk/Bpk/Emb)
  Itk (Tsk/Emt)
  Tec
  Bmx (Etk)
  Txk (Rlk)

Janus kinase family
  JAK1
  JAK2
  JAK3
  Tyk2

Fak family
  Fak
  Pyk2

Ack family

---

shown to possess such protein kinase activity. This immediately implied that transformation could be a result of inappropriate phosphorylation of cellular proteins. This view was strongly supported by the discovery that pp60 v-Src catalyzed the phosphorylation of a novel target—protein tyrosine residues. In 1979, Eckhart and colleagues,[2] characterizing the amino acid residue phosphorylated in vitro on polyoma virus middle T antigen, noted that the ^{32}P-amino acid recovered in acid hydrolysates ^{32}P-labeled middle T antigen did not migrate on electrophoresis exactly with a phosphothreonine standard, as had been reported for pp60 v-Src; by changing the pH of the electrophoresis buffer from 1.9 to 3.5, an entirely clean separation of the ^{32}P-amino acid from the P-Thr standard was obtained, indicating that the residue phosphorylated on polyoma middle T antigen was novel. The identity of the novel phosphoamino acid generated in vitro on middle T antigen, as well as by RSV[3] and the[4] oncoproteins, was rapidly shown to be phosphotyrosine, a known but uncharacterized amino acid derivative. Thus, these transforming proteins were associated with a tyrosine-specific protein kinase activity.

Contemporaneously, Stanley Cohen, who was first to purify the polypeptide epidermal growth factor (EGF), was attempting to detect and isolate the EGF receptor (EGFR). Using radioiodated EGF polypeptide, Cohen surveyed cell lines for receptor abundance and identified a human epidermoid carcinoma cell line (A431) that expressed greater than 10^6 EGFR/cell; addition of EGF to membrane vesicles from these cells stimulated overall ^{32}P incorporation from γP^{32}-ATP into the membrane proteins severalfold. Further work showed that the EGF-binding activity and EGF-stimulated autokinase activities copurified. The EGF receptor, purified as a 180-kDa polypeptide, proved to be the dominant substrate for the EGF-stimulated membrane phosphorylation reaction. Moreover, using the newly modified conditions for phosphoamino acid separation, Cohen showed that the amino acid modified by EGF-stimulated phosphorylation was not threonine, as originally concluded, but tyrosine.[5]

These findings established the EGFR as the first receptor tyrosine kinase and provided the first link between the biochemical function of retroviral transforming proteins and human growth factor receptors. In 1982, the receptors for insulin[6] and for the growth factors, insulin-like growth factor-1 (IGF-1) and platelet-derived growth factor (PDGF),[7] were shown to possess analogous ligand-activated tyrosine kinase activity. The identification in 1983 of the v-sis oncogene as a transduced form of the *PDGF (B)* gene[8,9] and the discovery in 1984 that the *v-erb-B* oncogene[10] molecular sequence was closely related to that of the EGFR served to reinforce the conceptual link between receptor tyrosine kinases and cellular growth regulation. By 1990, a large number of RTKs assignable to several subfamilies had been identified.

THE RECEPTOR TYROSINE KINASE SUBFAMILIES

The RTKs are all type 1 membrane proteins, with large aminoterminal extracellular ligand-binding domains, a single membrane spanning segment, and an intracellular extension encompassing the catalytic domain (see Fig. 8-1). The structure of RTK extracellular domains varies greatly across subfamilies, reflecting the broad diversity of interacting ligands. The RTK polypeptides are monomeric proteins, with the exception of the insulin and hepatic growth factor receptor subfamilies; here the receptors are synthesized as a single polypeptide chain and cotranslationally cleaved into two subunits, which become covalently linked through disulfide bonds. The insulin receptor α/β heterodimer then undergoes a further oligomerization by the formation of disulfide bonds between two α subunits, which is the aminoterminal, extracellular, ligand-binding component, to form a covalent βααβ

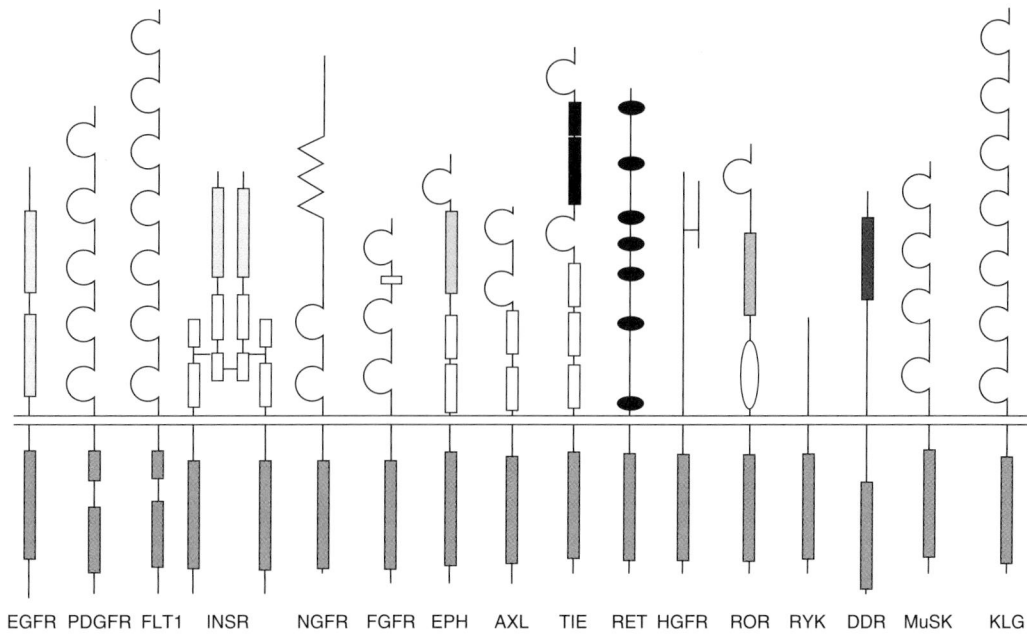

EGFR PDGFR FLT1 INSR NGFR FGFR EPH AXL TIE RET HGFR ROR RYK DDR MuSK KLG

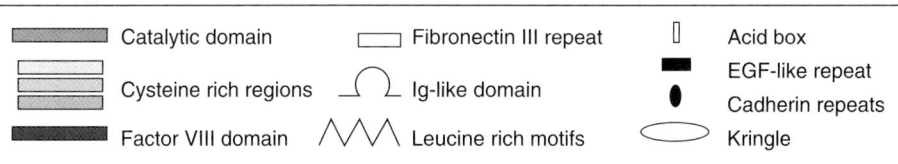

Catalytic domain	Fibronectin III repeat	Acid box
Cysteine rich regions	Ig-like domain	EGF-like repeat
Factor VIII domain	Leucine rich motifs	Cadherin repeats / Kringle

Figure 8-1 Schematic structures of receptor protein-tyrosine kinase families. (From Hunter T: The Croonian Lecture, 1997. Phil Trans Roy Soc Lond B 353:587, 1997.)

tetramer; only the β subunit spans the membrane and contains the tyrosine kinase domain. RTK catalytic domains approximately 260 amino acids long all exhibit nearly 30% amino acid sequence identity and, in turn, exhibit the conserved features of the protein kinase superfamily. With the completion of the human genome, it appears that 90 of the 518 protein kinases are tyrosine-specific, based on catalytic domain sequence homology, which can be subdivided into 31 subfamilies based on catalytic domain amino acid sequence alignments.[11]

LIGAND BINDING

A large and compelling body of data indicate that ligand binding causes dimerization of two RTK polypeptides, or in the case of the preassembled IR (βααβ) structure, ligand promotes an even more intimate coupling between the two αβ half-receptors.[12–16] Importantly, this ligand-induced dimerization is indispensable to the ability of ligand to activate the kinase catalytic function. Mutations in the RTK or ligand that inhibit dimerization prevent ligand-dependent kinase activation, and a variety of mutations or gene translocations that cause ligand-independent dimerization of the kinase domain are sufficient to cause ligand-independent kinase activation. As regards the mechanisms underlying dimerization, several are now directly established. Growth hormone provided the first example of a monomeric ligand that has two binding surfaces and dimerizes two receptor polypeptides. In the ErbB/EGFR family, although the ligand has two separate contact surfaces for the receptor, both are contacting different sites on the same receptor polypeptide, and dimerization is driven by the exposure of the receptor dimerization interface, a conformation that is stabilized by ligand binding.[17] Ligand-induced RTK dimerization is often caused by a ligand that is itself a dimer; that is, PDGF and colony-stimulating factor-1 (CSF-1) are disulfide linked dimers, whereas c-kit-ligand/stem

cell factor is a noncovalent dimer. PDGF occurs as a homo- or heterodimer of A and/or B chains; the PDGF A chain binds only to the α isoform of the PDGFR, whereas the PDGF B chain binds with high affinity to both the PDGFR α and β isoforms. Thus, PDGF AA will dimerize and activate only PDGFR αα dimers, PDGF AB activates αα and αβ PDGFR dimers, whereas PDGF BB dimerizes and activates all three possible PDGFR dimers.[15] A more complex, hybrid mechanism is exemplified by fibroblast growth factor (FGF), wherein residues from both the ligand and receptor participate in dimerization. In addition, the receptor contains a binding site for heparin sulfate, which is occluded in the ligand-free state. In the presence of FGF, heparin sulfate bridges fibroblast growth factor receptors (FGFRs) to stabilize and activate the oligomers (Fig. 8-3).

The EGF/EGFR (ErbB) family are important proproliferative elements in many human cancers through activating mutations, overexpression, or autocrine autostimulation. A diverse array of ligand/receptor dimers is available in this family (Fig. 8-4).[18] Invertebrates (e.g., *Drosophila* and *C. elegans*) exhibit one ErbB homologue, and four ligands are known for the *Drosophila* EGFR homologue (DER); three are activating ligands, including one membrane-bound TGF-α homologue (Gurken), a second TGF-α homologue that acts as a soluble ligand after proteolytic cleavage from a membrane precursor (Spitz), and a third, conventional secreted polypeptide (vein) homologous to the mammalian ErbB3/4 ligand neuregulin.[19,20] A fourth ligand, Argos, appears to be a diffusible inhibitory DER ligand whose expression is activated by DER signaling. Four ErbB RTK isoforms have been identified in mammalian systems and at least a dozen high-affinity ligands, with K_D in the nM range. The expanded mammalian ErbB family consists of ErbB1, the EGFR, which binds at least six distinct ligands with high affinity (EGF, TGF-α, amphiregulin, betacellulin, heparin-binding EGF, and epiregulin); ErbB2, for which no high-affinity ligand (i.e., K_D in the nM range) is known; ErbB3, which binds strongly to the neuregulins and less avidly to

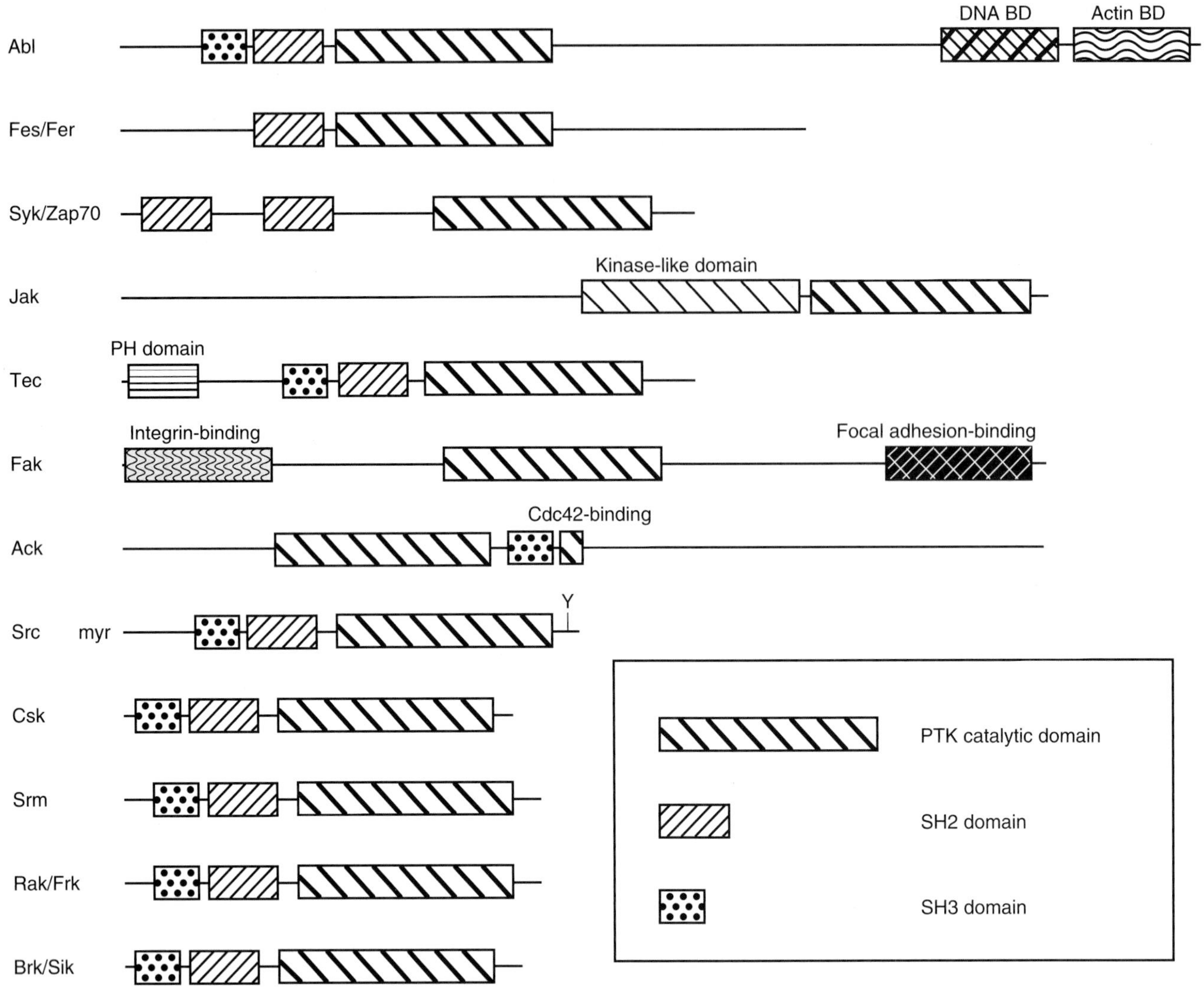

Figure 8-2   Schematic structures of nonreceptor protein tyrosine kinase (PTK) families. (From Hunter T: The Croonian Lecture, 1997. Phil Trans Roy Soc Lond B 353:586, 1997.)

EGF, betacellulin, and epiregulin, but lacks kinase activity completely due to amino acid sequence variation at a number of catalytic domain residues otherwise highly conserved among the protein kinase superfamily; and ErbB4, which has ligand-binding properties similar to ErbB3 but contains a catalytically competent kinase domain. Among those ligands where the question of valency has been examined, specifically EGF, TGF-α, and neuregulin, considerable evidence indicates that these ligand polypeptides each contain two

topologically distinct binding sites that bind to different regions on the RTK surface. ErbB2, although lacking high-affinity binding sites for any known ligand, is readily coprecipitated as a heterodimer with the other ErbB isoforms in a ligand-dependent manner and often in preference to the generation of ErbB1, ErbB3, or ErbB4 homodimers (Fig. 8-5). In this manner, ErbB2, despite its lack of a high-affinity binding site, functions as a potent and preferred coreceptor.[18] The ErbB2/3 heterodimer, for example, generates a very potent

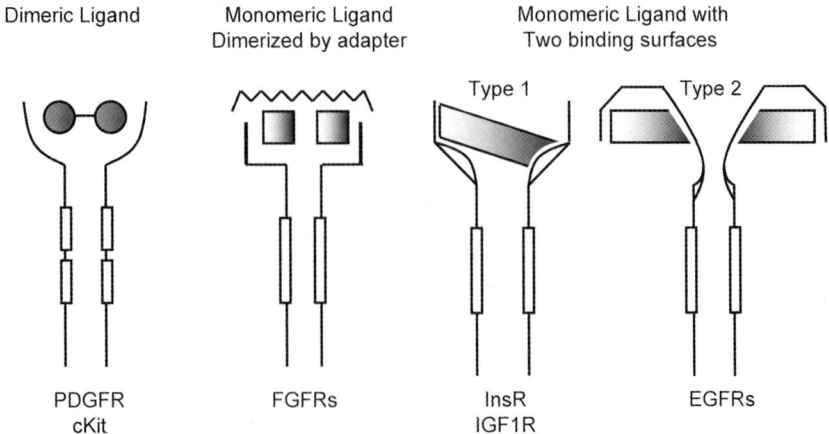

Figure 8-3   Differing modes of ligand-induced dimerization of receptor protein-tyrosine kinases.

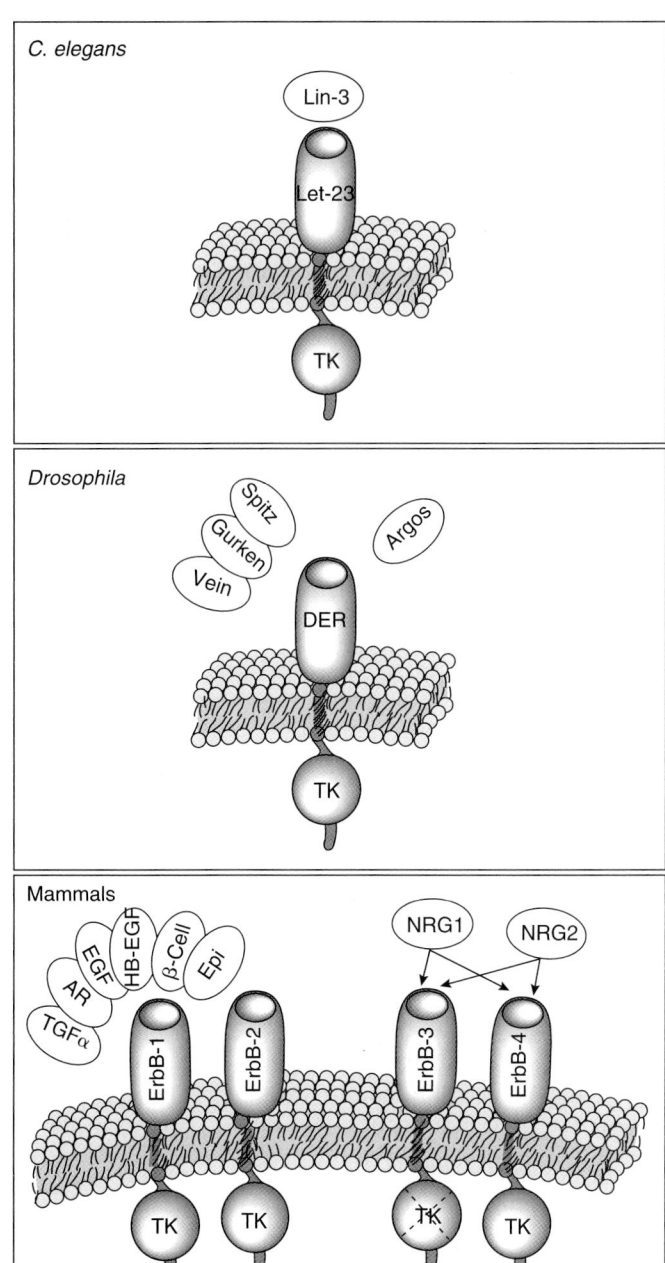

Figure 8-4 The evolution of EGF-related ligands and receptors. (From Tzahar E, Yarden Y: The ErbB-2/HER2 oncogenic receptor of adenocarcinomas: From orphanhood to multiple stromal ligands. Biochim Biophys Acta 1377:M25–M37, 1998.)

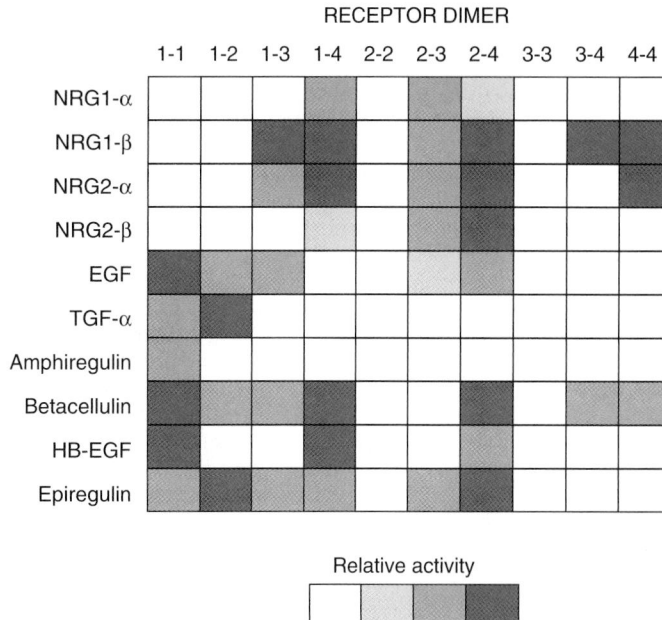

Figure 8-5 ErbB specificity of EGF-like ligands. Each column represents one of ten possible dimeric complexes of ErbB proteins. The extent of response to various ligands *(horizontal rows)* is shown by boxes: Black indicates a potent response and white stands for no response. Responses that are either detectable at high ligand concentration or require extreme receptor overexpression are shown as light gray or dark gray boxes. Note that ErbB3 homodimers bind all forms of neuregulin (NRG), but their response is defective due to an inactive kinase domain. NRG, neuregulin; EGF, epidermal growth factor; TGF-α, transforming growth factor α; HB-EGF, heparin-binding EGF-like growth factor. (From Tzahar E, Yarden Y: The ErbB-2/HER2 oncogenic receptor of adenocarcinomas: From orphanhood to multiple stromal ligands. Biochim Biophys Acta 1377:M25–M37, 1998.)

and prolonged signal even though the ErbB3 dimer half is catalytically inactive. It is likely that all of the EGF-like ligands are bivalent (except perhaps the inhibitory ligand, Argos).

The first definitive information concerning the structure of an RTK extracellular domain and its interaction with ligand was achieved for the EGF receptor family[17]; at this time, seven crystal structures are known, encompassing ErbB1 through ErbB3 extracellular domains. The structure of a deglycosylated form of the 621 amino acid extracellular portion of ErbB3 is composed of four domains; domains I and III contain a series of beta sheets arranged in a helical or "solenoid" structure, whereas domains II and IV are cysteine disulfide-rich. A striking feature is the presence of a loop extending from domain II to contact domain IV, creating a fairly large interaction surface.[21] Cross-linking studies had shown that EGF binds through separate surfaces to domains I and III; however, the

distance between the residues involved on these separate domains is no less than 60Å, whereas the longest distance that can be bridged by EGF is 30Å. Based on the knowledge that deletion of domain IV increases affinity for EGF by 20- to 40-fold, it is proposed that the native receptor resonates between the "tethered" low-affinity state revealed in the ligand-and-free ErbB3 (1 through 621) crystal (and also in a nonactivated form of the ErbB1/EGFR extracellular domain[22]) and a high-affinity, "extended" state that permits the apposition of domains I and III to an extent sufficient to enable EGF binding, which in turn locks in this "activated" conformation. The dramatic rearrangement of the domain relationships from a tethered to an extended form engendered/stabilized by ligand binding was shown directly in a structure of ErbB1/EGFR extracellular domain bound to TGF-α.[23] An essential feature of this extended, ligand-bound state is the availability of receptor residues that participate in dimerization, including those on the domain II loop, which is now free to seek a dimer partner. Critically, dimerization is mediated entirely by receptor residues, and the ligand does not participate directly but only through its ability to reorient receptor structure. The ErbB2 structure is unique in several respects.[24] First, the sequence of the domain II loop is altered in a manner that would predict a lack of interaction between domains II and IV and this is borne out in the crystal structure. Rather, the unliganded ErbB2 extracellular segment exhibits an extended conformation wherein domain I contacts domain III directly, mimicking the effect of ligand activation. Thus, the ligand-binding site of ErbB2 is occluded by endogenous receptor sequences, accounting both for the lack of identified ErbB2 ligands and the "activated" behavior of this receptor;

although homodimerization is weak, ErbB2 dimerization surfaces are available for heterodimerization in the absence of ligand.

The insulin receptor is synthesized as a single polypeptide chain and is processed by proteolysis into α and β subunits.[25] The α subunit is entirely extracellular and contains the ligand-binding site. The three aminoterminal domains of the α subunit resemble those in the ErbB family and are successively Leu-rich (L1), Cys-rich (CR), and Leu-rich (L2); these are followed by two fibronectin III domains. The second FnIII domain is interrupted by an insert encoded in exon 10 followed by an alternately spliced short exon 11, followed by the α-β cleavage site. The first FnIII domain and the exon 10 insert contain the inter-alpha disulfide linkages. The presence of the 12 amino acids encoded by exon 11 (in the B isoform) significantly alters ligand binding; both isoforms bind insulin with similar affinity, but the A isoform, predominant in fetal life, binds IGF-1 and IGF-2 with much higher affinity than does the B isoform.[26] This feature confers on the insulin receptor (IR) its modest role in the determination of fetal growth, inasmuch as the IGFs are the dominant growth factors in prenatal life. The β subunit contains an extracellular extension comprised of the continuation of the insert and the interrupted second FnIII domain and a third FnIII domain that is linked to the α subunit by a single disulfide bond. Thereafter follows a transmembrane segment and the intracellular portion, encompassing a 50-residue juxtamembrane region, the kinase catalytic domain, and a 100-residue noncatalytic tail.

Recent evidence suggests that insulin is also a bivalent ligand for the IR, providing two surfaces that each bind to a distinct site on the IR α subunit, one with high affinity and the other with low affinity.[27] The optimal apposition (i.e., for kinase activation) of two IR αβ halves is achieved when a single insulin molecule is bound to the high-affinity site on one α subunit and to the low-affinity site on the other α, that is, a stoichiometry of one insulin per βααβ receptor assembly. This model explains some longstanding anomalies in insulin action, such as the occurrence of diminished IR signaling at very high insulin concentrations. Presumably, large excesses of insulin (>10(−7)M, never achieved in vivo) enable binding of two (or perhaps more) insulins per βααβ assembly, each to the high-affinity site, which results in a receptor configuration that is less productive for kinase activation.[28] No high-resolution structure of the insulin-IR interaction is as yet available. A scanning transmission EM image of the IR has been resolved at 20Å[29] and is proposed to show a ligand-binding tunnel sufficient to bind a single insulin molecule, whose A-chain aminoterminus binds electrostatically to the L1/L2 of one α subunit, whereas the B-chain carboxyterminus interacts hydrophobically with the L1 and CR domains of the other α subunit.

Interestingly, despite the 49% identity in amino acid sequence and great similarity in three-dimensional (3-D) structures between insulin and IGF-1[30] as well as the considerable amino acid sequence identity in the α subunits of the IR and IGF-1R, and particularly the very high conservation in the placement of cysteine residues and N-linked glycosylation sites in the two α subunits, each receptor nevertheless binds the cognate ligand with about 100-fold higher affinity than the other ligand. Moreover, insulin binding to the IR exhibits negative cooperativity (i.e., binding of the first insulin to the $(\alpha_2\beta_2)$ receptor inhibits the binding of a second insulin molecule to the same receptor) that is actually less pronounced at very high insulin concentrations, whereas IGF-1 binding to the IGF-1R exhibits a more straightforward negative cooperativity. In view of these differences, the finding that insulin and IGF-1 bind to very different sites on their respective receptors, in part through different ligand surface domains, is not entirely surprising.[31] High-affinity IGF-1 binding to the IGF-1R is crucially dependent on the integrity of the IGF-1R cysteine-rich domain; swapping this segment

from the IGF-1R into the IR confers high affinity for IGF-1 but does not abrogate high-affinity insulin binding, whereas the reciprocal swap (IR CRD into the IGF-1R) gives a chimera incapable of high-affinity binding to either ligand. In contrast, high-affinity insulin binding requires specific IRα residues in the aminoterminal L1 domain (IR amino acids 38 through 68), and if amino acids found at these IR sites crucial to high-affinity insulin binding are introduced into the homologous sites on the IGF-1R, high-affinity binding of insulin is conferred without the loss of high-affinity IGF-1 binding. Mapping the IGF-1 structure onto the STEM picture of the IR reveals that the D domain of IGF-1 (a carboxyterminal extension not present in insulin) creates a marked steric hindrance as compared to insulin.[28] The structure of the aminoterminal three domains (L1/CR/L2) of the IGF-1R have been solved,[32] and although this segment does not bind ligand, substituting this structure into the IR model provided by STEM allows some rationalization of the poor binding of insulin to the IGF-1R. Heterodimers of the IR and IGF-1 receptors (IR (βα)-(αβ) IGF-1R) occur; these chimeric receptors show a highly preferential activation by IGF-1 as compared to insulin, comparable to the IGF-1R. The in vivo abundance and physiologic relevance of such obligate IR/IGF-1R heterodimers is unclear.

Another mechanism of ligand-induced RTK heterodimer is presented by the FGFR family.[33,34] Early work had established that heparin or heparan sulfate proteglycans were critical for FGF signaling; FGF freed of traces of heparin-like molecules is unable to activate FGFRs. Heparin is a linear, highly sulfated polysaccharide that binds FGF through a minimum tetrasaccharide unit; a heparin decasaccharide unit will bind two FGF molecules and is thus the minimal unit capable of "dimerizing" the FGF ligand (see Fig. 8-3). Conventional heparin and heparan sulfate proteglycans can bind many molecules of FGF. A crystal structure of the FGF-FGFR complex shows that heparin makes many contacts both with the ligand and the receptor, as well as with adjacent FGF-FGFR complexes.[33] Heparin analogues that bind a single FGF molecule (e.g., tetrasaccharide units) block FGF signaling by failing to stabilize adequately the FGF-FGFR assembly as well as by preventing FGFR dimerization, whereas heparin decasaccharide enables FGF-induced receptor activation.[35,36] At least 12 FGF variants and 4 FGFR isoforms are known, each capable of binding heparin; thus, the diversification of ligand-receptor pairs created by heparin is very substantial.

The sufficiency of FGFR dimerization for signaling is graphically illustrated by a variety of autosomal-dominant human chondrodysplasias, skeletal dysplasias, and craniostenosis disorders that are caused by activating mutations of FGFRs. These include the Crouzon, Pfeiffer, Jackson-Weiss, and Apert syndromes, each attributable to mutations in FGFR2,[37-39] and achondroplasia, hypochondrophasia, and thanatophoric dysplasia, each due to mutations in FGFR3.[40] A majority of these mutations are found in the Cys-rich Ig-like region of the receptor extracellular domain, resulting in the creation of an unpaired Cys residue (by either the mutational loss or gain of a Cys residue). The generation of an extracellular unpaired Cys promotes intermolecular disulfide formation and ligand-independent receptor dimerization.[41] A few mutations appear to cause intermolecular disulfide formation without altering the number of Cys residues, presumably by reconfiguring the Cys-rich domain so as to interfere with the normal intramolecular disulfide formation.

The RET tyrosine kinase is an important regulator of the differentiation of a subset of cells of neural crest origin. The targeted disruption of the murine *RET* gene causes a severe defect in the development of the enteric nervous system and absent or rudimentary kidneys and ureters.[42] The RET extracellular domain contains two centrally located cadherin-like repeats and a Cys-rich region immediately before the transmembrane segment.[43] The ligands known to activate *RET* are the secreted proteins, glial-derived neurotrophic factor

(GDNF), bitemin, neurturin, and persephin, members of the TGF-β superfamily. As with RET deletion, GDNF knockout results in the absence of enteric neurons and renal agenesis. These ligands activate RET indirectly through their binding to one of a family of glycosylphosphatidylinositol-linked membrane proteins known as *GDNF-Receptorα* (GFRα1-4); the complex of GRFα:ligand:RET is the active signaling unit.[44,45] The encoding of a ligand-binding subunit on a different gene than that encoding the tyrosine kinase domain is exceptional among the transmembrane tyrosine kinases, but it is the usual situation with the hematopoietic growth factor (including growth hormone, prolactin, etc.) and cytokine (e.g., IL-2, interferons, etc.) receptors; the latter classes of receptor generally consist of a transmembrane ligand-binding subunit with a short, noncatalytic intracellular segment encoded by genes distinct from those that encode the intracellular tyrosine kinase polypeptides, which are entirely cytoplasmic, "nonreceptor" tyrosine kinases, mostly of the JAK or Src subfamilies (see Chapter 9).

RET is of special interest in endocrinology because germ line–activating mutations in RET account for the multiple endocrine neoplasia syndromes, type IIA (MEN-IIA, medullary thyroid carcinoma, pheochromocytoma, and parathyroid hyperplasia) (see Chapter 194),[42,46] and type IIB (MEN-II, medullary thyroid carcinoma, pheochromocytoma, buccal neuromas, hyperganglionosis of the hindgut) and the familial medullary thyroid cancer (FMTC) syndrome,[42,47,48] whereas inactivating mutations of *RET* cause 15% to 20% of familial colonic aganglionosis (Hirschsprung's disease).[49,50] In addition, sporadic cases of papillary thyroid cancer containing rearranged *RET* oncogenes have been reported.[51–53] *RET* is encoded by a large (approximately 60 Kb) gene composed of at least 21 exons expressing a large variety of alternatively spliced mRNAs specifying at least 10 different polypeptides (Fig. 8-6). The mutations that underlie aganglionosis (i.e., loss of function) are missense, nonsense, and frameshift mutations (nearly 50 thus far), which are distributed randomly along the gene. By contrast, the activating mutations of MEN-IIA/FMTC are overwhelmingly (>85%) clustered in exons 10 and 11, which encode the Cys-rich region of the extracellular domain, and nearly all are missense mutations that result in the elimination of a Cys, thereby creating an unpaired extracellular Cys, intermolecular disulfide formation, and RET dimerization and activation. The clinical syndrome correlates with the specific Cys residue mutated; 80% of MEN-IIA involve the loss of Cys 634, with the remainder attributable to loss of Cys 609, 611, and scattered other residues. Approximately 50% of FMTC families exhibit mutations at Cys 618 or 620. The basis for this correlation appears to arise primarily from the proclivity of each of these mutations to promote intermolecular disulfide formation, which determines the abundance of RET dimers, and thus the extent of RET activation. The Cys 634 mutation (MEN-IIA) generates more kinase activation than do the Cys 618/620 mutations (FMTC), when the mutant recombinant RET is examined at comparable polypeptide expression on the same cellular background. A few MEN-IIA families with loss-of-Cys mutations (e.g., at 609, 618, or 620) also exhibit colonic aganglionosis; conversely, some families with aganglionosis due to RET mutations typical of MEN-IIA show no clinical features of MEN-IIA. How the same RET mutation results in activation of endocrine cells and involution of enteric ganglion cells is not currently understood. Conceivably, in addition to promoting dimerization, these Cys mutations may also impair RET maturation and delivery to the surface, and the relative expression of the mutant RET may differ in the two cell backgrounds.[54]

Interestingly, *RET* was originally discovered as a *re*arranged oncogene through the transfection of DNA from a human T-cell lymphoma into murine fibroblasts. Subsequent studies, however, reveal that *RET* has been activated by *re*arrangement during *t*ransfection rather than in the original tumor's DNA. Nevertheless, spontaneous or radiation-induced *RET* gene translocations are identified in about 10% to 40% of human papillary thyroid carcinoma (RET/PTC genes) and illustrate another mechanism of aberrant RET dimerization. These translocations fuse new open reading frames to the region on Chr10 upstream of the RET tyrosine kinase domain. The three different fusion partners (PTC genes) identified thus far include the gene encoding the R1α regulatory (cAMP binding) subunit of the cAMP-dependent protein kinase (PTC II) and the genes encoding proteins of unknown function, H4 (PTC I) and ELL1 (PTC III). The R1α sequences fused aminoterminal to the RET a tyrosine kinase domain include the R1α dimerization domain, thus providing a ready explanation for kinase activation.[52] The MEN-IIB syndrome is *not* due to mutations in the RET Cys-rich domain and is not associated with RET dimerization, but it is due to a novel mutation in the RET

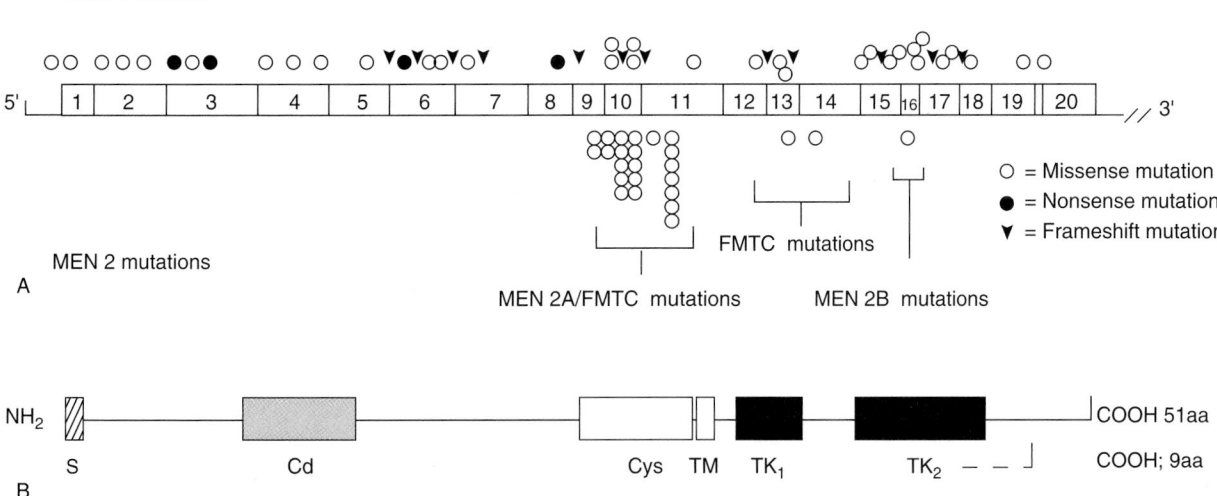

Figure 8-6 **A,** Different types of mutation of the RET proto-oncogene found in HSCR (*above diagram*) and in MEN-II syndromes (*below diagram*), represented with respect to the RET exons. **B,** The corresponding structural features of the RET receptor tyrosine kinase are indicated: S, signal sequence; Cd, cadherin-like domain; TM, transmembrane domain; Cys, cysteine-rich domain; TK1 and TK2, tyrosine kinase domains. (From Edery P, Eng C, Munnick A, et al: RET in human development and oncogenesis. Bioessays 19:389–395, 1997. Copyright © 1997. Reprinted by permission of John Wiley & Sons, Inc.)

catalytic domain that increases intrinsic activity and probably alters substrate specificity (discussed later).[55]

The largest RTK subfamily, the EPH receptors,[56] are involved in axonal guidance in development and interact with a family of membrane protein ligands called ephrins, which are expressed either as GPI-linked membrane proteins or as transmembrane polypeptides with short intracellular tails. Membrane-attached RTK ligands are not susceptible to internalization by the target cell bearing the RTK and consequently produce sustained and potent RTK activation, as compared to the cleaved, soluble form of the same ligand. As to the functional importance of prolonged RTK stimulation, a variety of experiments indicate that several hours' engagement of RTK by ligand is important to entrain DNA synthesis. The greater mitogenic potency of cell-associated ligand over the soluble ligand has also been well shown for the c-kit ligand (stem cell factor), CSF-1, and several of the ErbB ligands. The mitogenic potency of various mutant insulins, for example, correlates closely with their rate of dissociation (K_D) from the IR (slower dissociation is more mitogenic) rather than with the rate of association (K_D) or overall affinity.[29] As regards the biologic importance of membrane-bound ligands for the EPH RTKs, soluble versions of ephrins appear completely incapable of EPH RTK activation. The sustained nature of the ephrin-EPH interaction is probably critical for spatial localization and continuous axonal guidance during axon or cell migration. In addition, the EPH RTKs appear to be capable of transmitting a signal through the ephrin ligand into the cytoplasm of the ligand-bearing cell; thus, a soluble form of the extracellular domain of the EphB2 RTK is capable of inducing tyrosine phosphorylation of the intracellular tail of the ephrin B1 or B2 transmembrane ligands. Moreover, deletion of the entire EphB2 RTK gene produces substantial defects in axonal connections that are not reproduced by deletion of only the TK domain.[56]

Among the other RTK subfamilies listed in Table 8-1, few have had extensive analysis of ligand-binding properties and ligand uncovered, some of which may introduce paradigms not yet encountered in the several well-studied subfamilies reviewed here. In addition, structural analysis of ligand-RTK domains is eagerly anticipated because this information should provide a great impetus to drug development.

KINASE ACTIVATION

Immediately after the transmembrane segment, the intracellular extension of RTKs contains a noncatalytic segment of 50 to 100 amino acids followed by the tyrosine kinase domain (usually 250 to 280 amino acids), which in some subfamilies (e.g., PDGFR, FLT1) is interrupted by a short nonconserved noncatalytic segment of variable length; the catalytic domain is followed by a noncatalytic carboxyterminal tail, which usually contains several tyrosine autophosphorylation sites (see Fig. 8-1). Given that receptor dimerization is indispensable for ligand activation of the kinase function, how precisely is activation brought about? The solution of several protein kinase catalytic domain crystal structures has revealed that the 3-D organization of these enzymes shares a common framework, as would be expected from 11 clusters (subdomains) of highly conserved amino acid sequence distributed through the catalytic domains, as first described by Hanks and Hunter.[57] All Ser/Thr and Tyr protein kinases examined thus far exhibit a bilobed architecture,[58] with a smaller upper lobe, primarily responsible for binding ATP, connected by a single polypeptide strand to a larger lower lobe, which is primarily responsible for peptide substrate binding. Catalysis (phosphotransfer) occurs in the cleft between the lobes; ATP is bound with its base moiety lodged deeply in the cleft and the (poly)peptide substrate is bound along the surface of the lower lobe, with the substrate phosphoacceptor site positioned toward the cleft. An active kinase conformation requires an optimal

degree of apposition between the two lobes, as well as access of ATP and the protein substrate to the crucial kinase residues lining the cleft between the lobes. Both factors (i.e., lobe apposition and substrate access) are strongly determined by the position of a peptide segment in the lower lobe located between catalytic subdomains VII and VIII and flanked by the conserved residues DFG and APE; this segment, generally called the "activation loop" or A loop, forms part of the border between the lower and upper lobes. Many but not all kinases require phosphorylation of one or more residues on this loop to attain optimal positioning of the two lobes and/or to enable substrate access. In some instances, as with the kinase A catalytic subunit, the activation loop phosphorylation occurs in a constitutive manner immediately posttranslation and is an unregulated step in the structural maturation of the kinase polypeptide.[58] In a majority of instances, however, phosphorylation of the activation loop occurs posttranslationally in a regulated manner and provides a major mechanism for the control of the activity of both Ser/Thr and tyrosine-specific protein kinases. Among the RTKs, the regulatory role of A loop phosphorylation was first demonstrated for the IR[59] and is now known to occur in response to ligand binding and dimerization for many RTK subfamilies (e.g., the FGFRs, HGFR, Trks, etc.).[60] In the case of the IR, binding of insulin promotes a concerted phosphorylation of at least 6 of the 13 tyrosine residues on the IR β subunit intracellular extension, including a set of three tyrosines (1146/50/51) situated on the activation loop[59,61]; the phosphorylation of these 3 tyrosines corresponds closely with the acquisition of the capacity of the IR to phosphorylate exogenous peptide/protein substrates.[62,63] The other tyrosine autophosphorylation sites, one in the juxtamembrane segment (Tyr960) and two in the carboxyterminal tail (Tyr1314, Tyr1322), although not concerned with activation of kinase catalytic function, play an important role in signaling through different mechanisms (discussed later). Once phosphorylation of the activation loop occurs, kinase activity persists despite removal of insulin from the ligand-binding site, and RTK deactivation requires an A loop tyrosine dephosphorylation. Mutagenesis of the A loop tyrosines shows that, in addition to the importance of their phosphorylation in insulin-induced kinase activation, these tyrosine residues in their unphosphorylated state are also crucial to the maintenance of basal, inactive state of the kinase, as mutation to Phe also gives a significant increase in ligand-independent kinase activity.[64] The molecular basis for these features was revealed by comparison of the structures of the IR catalytic domain in the unphosphorylated[65] and in the triply phosphorylated[66] active state, as solved by radiographic crystallography (Fig. 8-7). The unphosphorylated IR kinase exhibits a relatively open bilobed structure, with the side chain of A loop Tyr1150 lodged in the active site much as "*pseudo*substrate" and hydrogen bonded to the catalytic base, Asp1120. Nevertheless, although positioned in the active site, IR Tyr1150 fails to undergo cis-autophosphorylation because the ATP site is occluded, both by the proximal portion of the unphosphorylated activation loop (G1140 M1141) and by the side chain of Tyr1150 which extends into the hydrophobic pocket usually occupied by the adenine ring of ATP. Phosphorylation of Tyr1146/50/51 results in a major rearrangement of the A loop, disoccluding both the ATP binding site and active site. Moreover, the specificity of the IR for tyrosine was illuminated, in part, by a cocrystal of triply phosphorylated active IR kinase with a synthetic tyrosine peptide substrate, which showed clearly that the hydroxyl group of a serine or threonine inserted into the peptide in place of the substrate tyrosine would be unable to reach the active site. The FGFR also undergoes activation through a ligand-dependent phosphorylation at the tandem tyrosines (Tyr653/654) within the A loop and illustrates a second, perhaps more general mechanism of RTK activation (see Fig. 8-2). In contrast to the

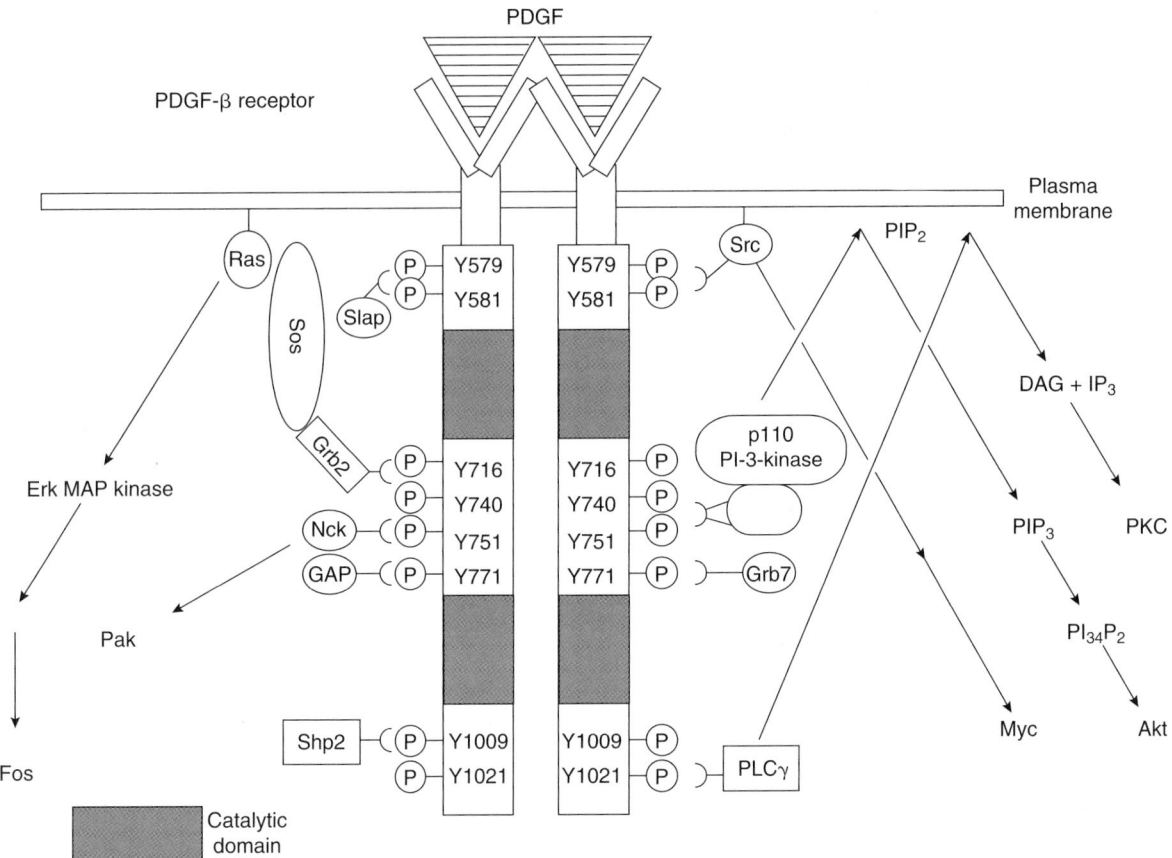

Figure 8-7   Platelet-derived growth factor (PDGF) receptor protein-tyrosine kinase signaling pathways. (From Hunter T: The Croonian Lecture, 1997. Phil Trans Roy Soc Lond B 353:588, 1997.)

IR, the unphosphorylated FGFR activation loop does not obstruct ATP binding or the active sites, but rather appears to preempt peptide substrate binding by the presence of FGFR residues R661 and P663 near the putative substrate binding pocket.[67]

How does ligand binding promote A loop phosphorylation?[60] Abundant evidence indicates that the ligand-induced dimerization enables one kinase domain to catalyze phosphorylation of the opposing kinase domain's A loop. Although certain genetically engineered RTK mutants can be shown to catalyze dimer-independent, cis-autophosphorylation, this does not occur in the context of ligand-induced RTK autophosphorylation. It is entirely clear, for example, that an IRαβ half receptor, despite well-preserved insulin-binding capacity, is unable to catalyze insulin-stimulated tyrosine autophosphorylation if reassembly into an αβ2 structure is prevented. Moreover, the ability of one receptor dimeric assembly (e.g., an IRα2β2) to catalyze an intermolecular phosphorylation of another receptor dimer appears negligible. The significance of this intradimer transphosphorylation mechanism to the signaling capacity of RTKs depends heavily on whether the RTK forms a fixed, covalent dimer (i.e., the IR subfamily) and whether the ability of the RTK to signal arises primarily from its ability to phosphorylate exogenous protein substrates (also true of the IR subfamily) or from its ability to catalyze its own autophosphorylation (as is the case for EGFR/PDGFR and most RTKs). In the case of the IR, dimers that contain one catalytically active RTK with a kinase-dead RTK mutant exhibit a greatly inhibited signaling ability because the normal RTK peptide will fail to undergo transphosphorylation by the inactive partner (and thus will remain unable to phosphorylate exogenous substrates), and the kinase inactive RTK, despite its tyrosine phosphorylation by the nonmutant partner, is unable to signal. This "dominant inhibitory" phenotype may be ameliorated by diminished expression of the mutant receptor (e.g., due to accelerated degradation) as compared to wild type. Nevertheless, clinically evident insulin resistance has been observed in the setting of heterozygous inactivating mutations of the IR.[68] Conversely, RTKs such as those in the ErbB/EGFR family, whose kinase activation does not require A loop phosphorylation, are not covalent dimers and, most important, signal primarily through tyrosine autophosphorylation rather than by substrate phosphorylation (discussed later), experience little or no impairment in signaling potency when coexpressed with kinase inactive EGFRs. This is well illustrated by ErbB3, an RTK isoform whose wild-type polypeptide is intrinsically kinase inactive, but which nevertheless functions as a potent signal generator when coexpressed with a compatible dimer partner whose kinase domain is active (see Fig. 8-5).[18] Other examples are the RTKs related to the avian RTK Klg, such as the human colon carcinoma kinase 4 (CCK-4).[69] The catalytic domain of these RTKs contains an alanine (Ala) in place of an indispensable asparagine (Asp) in a highly conserved catalytic motif, a substitution known to render the kinase catalytically inactive. Whether CCK-4 acts as a coreceptor capable of unique signal generation or as a signal attenuator is not yet known. This assignment will require examination of these "inactive" kinases in their native contexts because the experimental format employed and the impact of potential dimer partners can strongly bias the conclusion reached. By example, overexpression of kinase-dead EGFRs in the absence of a detectable active ErbB isoform is still able to confer a weak, partial response to added EGF (e.g., activation of MAPK), where none was evident prior to overexpression of recombinant, kinase-dead EGFRs. This appears to be attributable to the association of the kinase-dead EGFRs with nonreceptor tyrosine kinases; when the RTKs are dimerized by ligand, the nonreceptor TKs catalyze modest tyrosine phosphorylation of the kinase-negative EGFR polypeptide.

An A-loop-independent mode of autoinhibition is illustrated by the EphB2 receptor, wherein the juxtamembrane segment contacts the catalytic domain in a manner that prohibits kinase activity.[70] Ligand-induced autophosphorylation of two tyrosines within the juxtamembrane segment promotes its displacement from the catalytic domain, enabling the latter to phosphorylate exogenous substrates.

As to the mechanism of ligand-induced kinase activation for those RTKs that do not require activation loop autophosphorylation, little direct information is available. It is clear from the structures of the unphosphorylated IR and FGFR TK domains that the activation loops are relatively mobile and that a distribution of different A loop conformations exists, among which are some that would allow access of polypeptide substrate and consequent substrate Tyr phosphorylation. It is suggested that for RTKs activated by dimerization without A loop phosphorylation like the EGFR, the conformation of the A loop is sufficient to prevent significant as autophosphorylation unless a substrate is imposed through the ligand-induced dimerization. Presumably, these RTKs, monomers in the absence of ligand, experience few random collisions and may therefore tolerate a somewhat more open kinase domain configuration and a rather modest autoinhibitory mechanism, whereas the IR is a preassembled, covalent dimer that in the absence of ligand requires an extensive autoinhibitory apparatus to prevent autophosphorylation of the A loop.[60] Consistent with this view is the observation that overexpression of native ErbB2 or EGFR, as occurs commonly in malignancies, is itself sufficient to engender substantial kinase activation.

The critical importance of protein tyrosine phosphatases (PTPs) in maintaining the low RTK activity of the ligand-free state should be emphasized. Addition of general tyrosine phosphatase inhibitors (such as vanadate) to cells in the absence of ligand will allow a slow accumulation of RTK tyrosine phosphorylation that over several hours will cause substantial and ultimately full RTK activation. Thus, PTPs are constitutively active at a level sufficient to overcome the ligand-free activity of RTKs (and, in general, nonreceptor PTKs). Conversely, overexpression of RTKs, as is easily accomplished experimentally or as occurs spontaneously with the RTK gene amplification seen in malignancies such as breast cancer, readily results in significant signaling in the absence of ligand, demonstrating the intrinsic leakiness of the RTK autoinhibitory mechanisms and the importance of the balance between basal cellular PTPase and total RTK abundance in signal generation.[18,19,71] The impact of RTK overexpression is greatly enhanced if it is also associated with even a small increase in ligand-independent activity. Thus, a mutant, truncated EGFR is found to be amplified in many cases of glioblastoma multiforme. The truncation deletes the ligand-binding domain, abrogating ligand-induced activation and resulting in a kinase whose activity is greatly diminished compared with that of the ligand-activated wild-type EGFR. Nevertheless, truncation also results in a small increase in ligand-independent activity, which is constitutive. Moreover, the truncated receptors are retained at the cell surface and these features combined with substantial overexpression results in the creation of a potent oncogene.

Mutations within the kinase catalytic domain are most often associated with loss of function either due to premature termination or major structural disorganization, resulting in misfolding and accelerated degradation. Missense mutations that are relatively conservative may nevertheless still disrupt the structure necessary for optimal binding of ATP or polypeptide substrate or for the optimal alignment of these substrates at the active site in an arrangement that permits phosphotransfer. Occasionally, however, catalytic domain mutations may disrupt the autoinhibitory mechanisms and promote activation and/or alter the determinants for protein substrate binding. Thus, a patient with the fatal skeletal

disorder thanatophoric dysplasia exhibited a mutation in FGFR3 that substituted an acidic residue (Lys660-Glu) immediately following the double tyrosine autophosphorylation sites in the FGFR3 A loop, resulting in ligand-independent activation. Activating A-loop mutations have also been observed in c-kit (in a mast cell leukemia) and HGFR (in a human renal papillary carcinoma). The activating mutation of *RET* (Met918→Thr, ATG→ACG) seen in 95% of MEN-IIB and in 30% to 40% of sporadic medullary thyroid cancers involves a residue situated in catalytic subdomain VIII, distal to the activation loop, in a region that in protein (Ser/Thr) kinases is known to influence substrate selectivity (see Fig. 8-6). Although Met918 is well conserved among RTKs, the homologous site in most nonreceptor TKs is usually Thr. Studies using synthetic peptide substrates have shown that the wild-type *RET* favors peptides resembling those optimal for the EGFR and other RTKs, whereas the mutant *RET* (Thr918) selects peptide substrates more like those chosen by the nonreceptor tyrosine kinases, Src and Abl.[55] It is tempting to relate this change in RET substrate specificity to the different clinical picture engendered by RET (Met918 Thr), for example, MEN-IIB compared with that seen with *RET* activation by dimerization (i.e., MEN-IIA).

THE MECHANISM OF RTK SIGNALING

THE IDENTIFICATION OF RTK TARGETS

Progress in understanding the signaling mechanisms employed by this receptor family advanced only slightly during the 1980s.[10] Although the RTKs showed vigorous phosphotransferase activity in vitro, the abundance of phosphotyrosine in intact cells was very low, and endogenous RTK substrates were hard to find. Even in RSV transformed cells, which contained a mutant, constitutively active retroviral tyrosine kinase transforming protein, the abundance of phosphotyrosine was less than 0.1% that of P-Ser plus P-Thr. In such cells many of the proteins found to have P-Tyr proved to be abundant proteins (e.g., enolase or LDH) phosphorylated incidentally to a trivial stoichiometry (<0.1 mole P/mole protein). The development of polyclonal[72] and subsequently monoclonal antibodies reactive selectively with phosphotyrosine greatly accelerated the detection and isolation of physiologic RTK substrates. Using immunoblotting and immunoprecipitation, it was shown that there was an array of proteins whose P-Tyr content was increased by activation of the RTK. Subsequently, it was shown that receptors that lack intrinsic PTK activity but that are capable of promoting cell proliferation or differentiation also promote protein tyrosine phosphorylation in the "appropriate" cell backgrounds. Nevertheless, it was repeatedly observed that the RTK polypeptides themselves were among the most prominent Tyr P proteins detected in such experiments. The findings presented a paradox, namely, how was signal transmission occurring if the dominant substrate for the RTK was the RTK itself?

Complementary experiments employing immunoprecipitation of the RTKs (EGF, PDGF, CSFRs) from ligand-stimulated cells showed that many of the same polypeptide bands detected in antiphosphotyrosine immunoprecipitates were also recovered in anti-RTK immunoprecipitates. Labeling of cells with ^{35}S-methionine, to tag the polypeptide backbones rather than phosphate groups, revealed that many of the proteins that coprecipitated with the RTKs were seen only after ligand stimulation. Thus, it emerged that ligand activation of many RTKs (but not all, e.g., not IR or IGF-1R) resulted in the assembly on the receptor of a set of polypeptides, of which the majority exhibited some tyrosine phosphorylation. Several of these polypeptides were isolated, cloned, and functionally identified; among the first was a phospholipase C (PLC) enzyme, the γ isoform.[73,74] Inasmuch as the products of the PLC-γ reaction (i.e., diacylglycerol and inositol triphosphate) were already well recognized as signaling molecules, the identification of PLC-γ as one of the proteins recruited to (at least some) RTKs consequent to receptor activation supported the view that activated RTKs were capable of recruiting intracellular signal generators. PLC-γ was subsequently shown to undergo receptor-catalyzed tyrosine phosphorylation, with a further increase in catalytic activity, providing one of the first examples of positive regulation of enzyme catalytic activity through tyrosine phosphorylation in trans (as distinct from the IR and cSrc autoactivating tyrosine autophosphorylations). Other RTK-associated polypeptides identified were a 120-kDa polypeptide that contained a GTPase activating domain (GAP) for Ras near its carboxyterminus, the c-Src kinase polypeptide, and several noncatalytic polypeptides, most notably an 85-kDa protein later shown to be a noncatalytic subunit of the lipid kinase, Ptd Ins-3'-OH kinase (PI-3 kinase). This enzyme had been discovered as a phosphatidylinositide (Ptd Ins) kinase of novel specificity (3'-OH) associated with the polyoma middle T antigen, a viral transforming protein.[75] The Ptd Ins (3,4,5)P product is now known to be a membrane lipid signaling molecule (discussed later).

RECRUITMENT OF RTK TARGETS

How do the ligand-activated RTKs recruit these candidate signaling molecules to associate with the receptor? The first important clue was provided by experiments directed at understanding the functional significance of a novel feature of the PDGFR kinase domain, whose structure is interrupted by a noncatalytic segment ("kinase insert") that contains several candidate tyrosine autophosphorylation sites, and which is not conserved among other RTKs (Fig. 8-8). Deletion of this segment, or conversion of two of these Tyr residues to phenylalanine (Phe), abolished the mitogenic function of the PDGFR as effectively as did inactivation of the PDGFR kinase ATP-binding site. In contrast to the PDGFR kinase-negative mutant, the PDGFR kinase-insert deletion (KI) mutant exhibited a vigorous tyrosine phosphotranferase activity, continued autophosphorylation at other tyrosine residues, and an unimpaired ability to activate PLCγ in response to PDGF. Most important, after PDGF binding, the immunoprecipitates of the PDGFR KI mutant lacked one of the major receptor-associated polypeptides; the p85 polypeptide (i.e., the noncatalytic subunit of the PI-3 kinase) was selectively absent and this correlated with a lack of receptor-associated PI-3 kinase activity.[76] These observations, in addition to indicating the importance of the PI-3 kinase activity to the mitogenic action of the PDGFR, provided the first evidence that specific receptor-associated signaling proteins bound to the receptor in a manner that depended on specific, individual receptor phosphotyrosine residues.[77,78] Conclusive evidence for this idea was the demonstration that synthetic peptides as short as five amino acids with a sequence based on the PDGFR KI segment were capable of selectively displacing the p85 polypeptide from activated receptors; such displacement depended on the

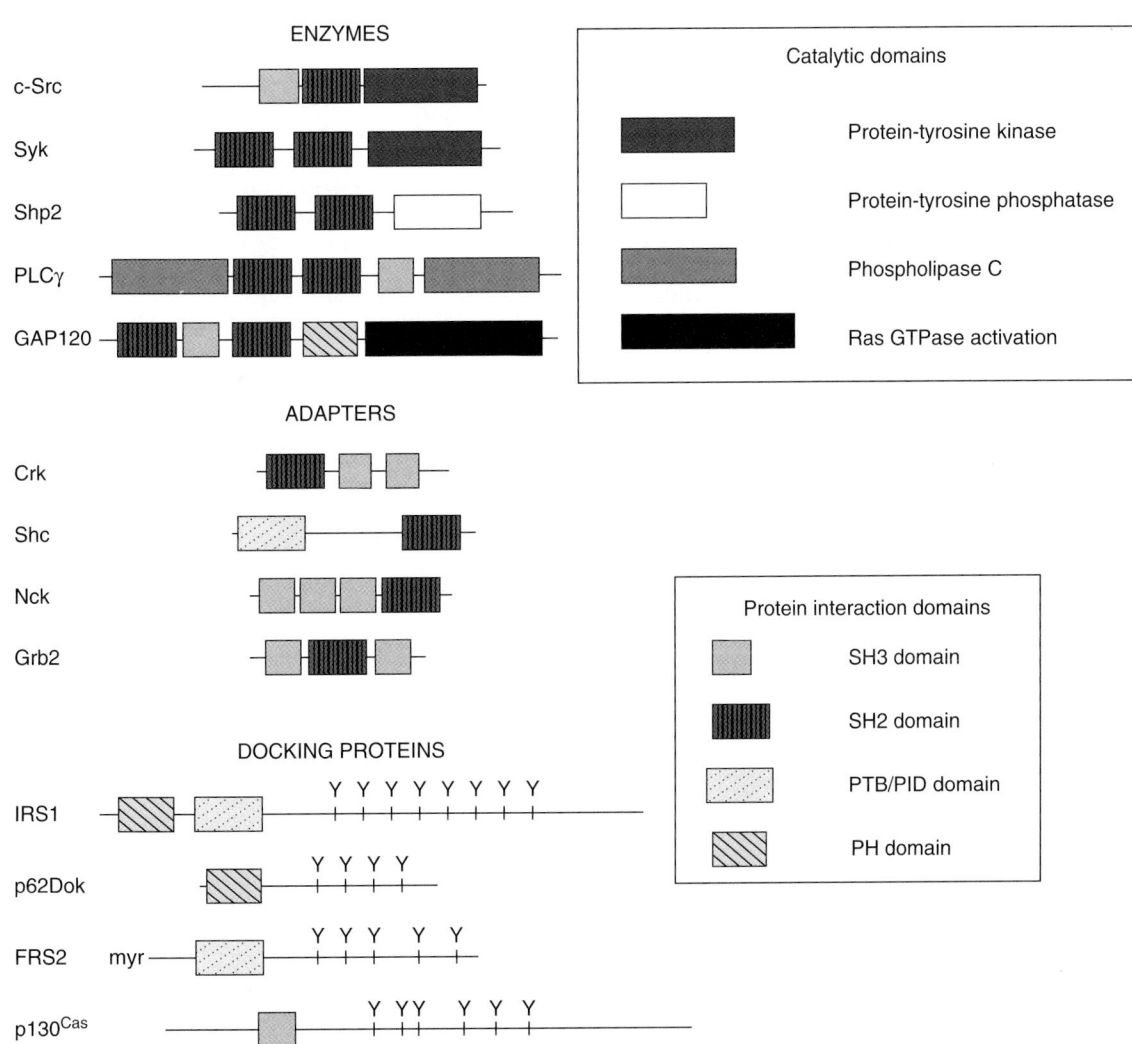

Figure 8-8 Schematic structures of representative enzyme and adaptor targets for signaling protein tyrosine kinases. (From Hunter T: The Croonian Lecture, 1997. Phil Trans Roy Soc Lond B 353:589, 1997.)

presence of a phosphotyrosine on the peptide and on preservation of the specific amino acid sequence immediately surrounding the P-Tyr, especially to the carboxyterminal side.[78,79] The PDGFR is unique in that its various phosphotyrosine sites show little overlap in their ability to bind different polypeptide targets; other RTKs (e.g., the EGFR) exhibit substantial overlap in the specificity of their P-Tyr sites with regard to the binding of receptor-associated signaling polypeptides. Nevertheless, conversion of 5 to 6 EGFR Tyr autophosphorylation sites to Phe results in a marked impairment in the signaling function of the EGFR as well as the PDGFR, despite a well-maintained receptor tyrosine kinase activity.

SH2 DOMAINS

Given that signaling proteins assemble on active RTKs by binding at or near specific Tyr P autophosphorylation sites and that this assemblage is important to the efficiency of signaling to downstream targets (at least for the PDGFR/EGFR/CSF-1R), what enables the phosphotyrosine specific binding of the RTK associated-signaling proteins? It is now known that these polypeptides each contain domains capable of binding specifically to short peptide segments that contain a Tyr-P residue (Fig. 8-9). The first of these domains to be identified was characterized by Pawson and colleagues, who analyzed a set of mutations of the v-Fps tyrosine kinase located outside of the catalytic domain that markedly impaired or rendered temperature-sensitive the transforming activity or altered the host range of v-Fps, without much effect on its catalytic activity measured in vitro.[80] They noted that these mutations tended to cluster in regions that, like the catalytic domain, were well conserved in amino acid sequence among all the Src family kinases. They identified two such conserved domains, which they named Src homology (SH) domains 2 and 3 (with the catalytic domain representing SH domain 1), and suggested that the SH2 and SH3 domains might function in vivo to assist in substrate selection and/or direct the kinases to specific locations in the cells. The molecular cloning of PLC-γ[81] and p120 Ras-GAP,[82] two RTK-associated signaling proteins, provided the first examples of enzymes other than nonreceptor tyrosine kinases that contained SH2 and SH3 domains. The cloning of the retroviral oncogene v-Crk revealed the first example of a polypeptide that was composed entirely of SH2 and SH3 domains, lacking a catalytic domain.[83] Nonetheless, immunoprecipitates of the v-Crk polypeptide from transformed cells were heavily decorated by tyrosine-phosphorylated proteins and by an associated tyrosine kinase activity. It was soon appreciated that essentially all

of the RTK-associated proteins (p120 Ras-GAP, PLC-γ, c-Src, the p85 subunit of PI-3 kinase, etc.) contain at least one SH2 domain and often an SH3 domain.[84] Expression cloning with the multiply (tyrosine) phosphorylated, noncatalytic carboxyterminal tail of the EGFR as a hybridization probe yielded more than a dozen polypeptides that bound only to the tyrosine-phosphorylated form of the EGFR tail; these polypeptides, named "growth factor receptor–binding" (Grb) proteins each contains one or more SH2 domains. The specific biochemical function of SH2 domains was established by the demonstration that recombinant SH2 domains per se were capable of binding directly to activated, tyrosine-phosphorylated receptors, in a manner entirely dependent on prior RTK tyrosine autophosphorylation, as well as to short phosphotyrosine-containing synthetic peptide modeled on the sequence surrounding RTK tyrosine surrounding autophosphorylation sites.[85,86] Peptide binding to SH2 domains absolutely requires phosphotyrosine and is strongly influenced by identity of the four to five amino acids immediately carboxyterminal to the phosphotyrosine.[87]

The proteins that contain SH2 domains can be classified into two groups, depending on the presence of a catalytic domain; those lacking catalytic function are presumed to serve as adaptors. A catalogue of SH2 adaptor proteins is shown in Table 8-2; the mode of action of two important examples, the p85 subunit of the PI-3 kinases and Grb-2, are discussed later in this chapter.

PTB/PID DOMAINS

A second type of TyrP-binding domain was identified through the analysis of the proto-oncogene *Shc*, which contains a single carboxyterminal SH2 domain and is phosphorylated at a single tyrosine by many RTKs, which creates an excellent binding site for the adaptor Grb-2 (see Fig. 8-9). Thus, *Shc* can bind through its SH2 domain to an activated RTK, undergo tyrosine phosphorylation, recruit Grb-2/SOS, and promote Ras activation (discussed later). Surprisingly, it was observed that despite deletion of its SH2 domain, Shc still bound to some proteins in a phosphotyrosine-dependent manner.[88,89] The novel Shc phosphotyrosine-specific binding was mediated by an aminoterminal segment whose primary sequence proved to be conserved among several other proteins (e.g., IRS-1) and are now known as the phosphotyrosine-binding (PTB) or phosphotyrosine-interacting domains (PID). Like SH2 domain, PTB/PID domains exhibit the ability to bind to phosphotyrosine-containing peptides, but with a specificity distinct from SH2 domains, in that PTB/PID domains bind the

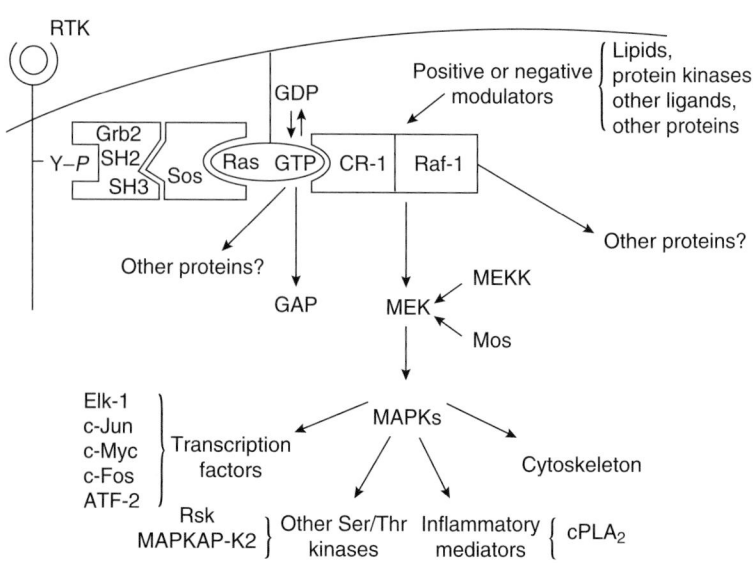

Figure 8-9 Model for receptor tyrosine kinase signal transduction through the Ras-activated protein kinase cascade. Activation of an RTK leads to its phosphorylation on tyrosine residues (*Y-P*), which allows the receptor to interact with SH2 domain–containing proteins, such as Grb2. In turn, Grb2 binds to an adaptor protein, SOS (son of sevenless), which recruits Ras to the receptor. Ras recruits Raf to the complex, allowing Raf activation and providing a means of activating the MAPK cascade. MAPKAP-K2, MAPK-activated protein kinase 2; cPLA2, cytoplasmic phospholipase A2. (From Avruch J, Zhang ZF, Kyriakis J: Raf meets Ras: Completing the framework of a signal transduction pathway. Trends Biochem Sci 19:279–283, 1994.)

Table 8-2 Representative SH2 Domain–Containing Proteins

Substrates	Targets
Enzymes	
PLC-γ_1 and PLC-γ_2 (PI-specific phospholipase)	SH2 (2), SH3, split PHD
GAP 120 (Ras GTPase activator)	SH2, SH3, PHD
Src family PTKs	SH2, SH3
Zap 70/Syk family PTKs	SH2 (2)
Shp1 (PTP1c/SH-PTP1/HC-PTP)	SH2 (2)
Shp2 (PTP1D/SH-PTP2/SYP)	SH2 (2)
PI-3 kinase p85 (p110 regulatory subunit)	SH2 (2), SH3
Ship (inositol polyphosphate-5'-phosphatase)	SH2
Vav (and Vav2) (Rho/Rac/Cdc42 GEF)	SH2, SH3, PHD
Adaptors	
Shc and (ShcB and ShcC) Shb	SH2, PTB
Nck	SH2, SH3 (3)
Crk (and CrkL)	SH2, SH3 (2)
Lnk	SH2
Slp76	SH2
Slap (negative regulator)	SH3, SH2
Grb2 (and Grap)	SH2, SH3 (2) (not phosphorylated)
Structural proteins	
Talin (focal adhesion)	SH2
Others	
STAT1–STAT5 (transcription factors)	SH2, SH3
Grb7 (Ras GAP related)	SH2, PHD
Grb10	SH2, PHD

GAP, guanosine triphosphatase (GTPase)-activating protein; GEF, guanine nucleotide exchange factor; Grb2, growth factor receptor-binding protein-2; PHD, pleckstrin homology domain; PI, phosphatidylinositol; PLC, phospholipase C; PTK, protein tyrosine kinase; PTP, protein tyrosine phosphatase; SH2, Src homology-2; STAT, signal transducer and activator of transcription.

motif NPXY(P), with additional specificity provided by hydrophobic residues situated 5 to 8 residues aminoterminal to the phosphotyrosine.[90] The NPXY sequence, which is found in IR, EGFR, Trk, polyoma middle T antigen, and others, can also serve as a protein-interacting surface in the absence of phosphorylation for a different set of polypeptides, which function primarily in membrane protein sorting and localization.

TYR P DOCKING PROTEINS: THE IR/IGF-1R SYSTEM

The paradigms developed from the study of the PDGFR and EGFR did not appear directly relevant to signaling from the IR and IGF-1R because despite robust autophosphorylation, few signaling molecules coprecipitate with these receptors, save for a modest and inconsistent recovery of PI-3 kinase activity. Mutation of the IR A loop Tyr residues abolishes insulin-regulated signaling but does not completely abolish IR signaling, inasmuch as these mutations increase somewhat the basal, insulin-independent receptor kinase activity.[64] However, mutation of IR-Tyr960, an NPXY motif situated in the juxtamembrane segment aminoterminal to the IR catalytic domain, essentially abolishes the IR signaling function in vivo, although causing no impairment in the IR kinase activity in vitro or in the IR autophosphorylation at other sites.[91] This null phenotype was accompanied by the disappearance in vivo of the insulin-stimulated tyrosine phosphorylation of a 180-kDa polypeptide, the dominant insulin-stimulated TyrP-containing polypeptide in all cell backgrounds. This protein was molecularly cloned and named insulin receptor substrate 1 (IRS-1); the structure of IRS-1 suggested a specific model for IR signaling[92] (see Fig. 8-9). The aminoterminal one third of IRS-1 contains a pleckstrin

homology (PH) domain followed by a phosphotyrosine-binding (PTB) domain, which together mediate the binding of IRS-1 to the activated IR at the NPEY(P)960 site. The carboxyterminal two thirds of IRS-1 contains at least 16 tyrosine phosphorylation sites, most of which can be phosphorylated by the IR in vivo and in vitro, and which provide an array of TyrP-containing motifs that enable the binding of SH2 domain-containing proteins such as p85, Grb-2, Nck, and so on, proteins that bind directly to other RTKs, such as the EGFR. The identification of IRS-1 was followed by IRS-2 (similar in size and overall structure to IRS-1), IRS-3 (about 60 kDa), and IRS-4.[93] Evidence that these IR substrates are critical for IR/IGF-1R signaling in vivo is provided by the phenotypes of mice whose IRS genes have been deleted. Mice with a homozygous deletion of both IRS-1 alleles are about one half the size of wild-type mice and are moderately insulin resistant but rarely hyperglycemic.[94] IRS-2-"knockout" mice are 80% of wild-type size and insulin resistant, and they ultimately develop hyperglycemia at a high frequency because the compensatory β cell hyperplasia that occurs in IRS-1-knockout mice does not occur in IRS-2-knockouts, who instead exhibit a reduced β cell mass.[95] Interestingly, whereas heterozygous deletion of either the IR or IRS-1 has no phenotype, a double heterozygote mouse IR-IRS-1⁻ develops profound insulin resistance and hyperglycemia.[96] These features establish the crucial role of the IRS family in the signaling function of the insulin and IGF-1 receptors in vivo.

Although initially considered to be relatively specific substrates for the IR and IGF-1 receptors, it is now clear that a variety of hematopoietic and cytokine receptors (including the receptors for interferons, IL-4 and GH) acting through recruitment of the Janus family of nonreceptor tyrosine kinases (JAKs) can also cause IRS tyrosine phosphorylation and therefore signal via insulin-like, RTK-activated pathways.[93] Moreover, although the EGFR has no ability to phosphorylate IRS-1-4, an analogous protein, called GAB-1, can be multiply phosphorylated by both the IR and EGFR so as to provide a platform apart from the EGFR polypeptide for multiple SH2-containing proteins.[97] Drosophila genetics first identified "daughter of sevenless" (DOS), a PH domain-containing protein that, like IRS-1 and GAB-1, has many tyrosine phosphorylation sites, but unlike IRS and GAB-1, it is a substrate for the EGFR but not (apparently) for the IR. Other docking proteins are shown in Figure 8-9. Thus, it appears that most RTKs employ substrate docking proteins analogous in function to the IRS polypeptides, although the specific contribution of these docking proteins to signal generation, compared with the RTK autophosphorylation sites, remains to be determined. Docking proteins presumably allow for great diversification and wide cellular localization of the RTK signal, comparable to that available to diffusible ligands such as cAMP and Ca²⁺. Interestingly, the Drosophila and C. elegans insulin receptor homologues exhibit carboxyterminal extensions that encode multiple additional tyrosine phosphorylation sites not observed in the mammalian counterparts, which may therefore enable the invertebrate IRs to function as docking sites, whereas this has evolved to a separate function in mammals. This evolution may reflect some further divergence in function not as yet elucidated. Nevertheless, as is true of the mammalian IR, the Drosophila insulin receptor expressed in mammalian cells will not support insulin-stimulated mitogenesis without the coexpression of IRS-1, despite the presence of the additional carboxyterminal TyrP sites.[98]

SPECIFICITY DETERMINANTS IN RTK SIGNALING

The structure of several SH2 domains has been solved, both unliganded and complexed with TyrP-containing peptides; the SH2 domain is a compact globular structure that contains a bipartite binding site for the tyrosine phosphopeptide.[86] The phosphotyrosine residue itself sits in a pocket lined by basic residues, including an invariant arginine (Arg) conserved in all SH2 domains. The crucial binding energy is provided by this site, as unphosphorylated peptides of the same sequence exhibit a two-log lower affinity. In addition, a second, immediately adjacent binding surface enables specific accommodation of the amino acids immediately carboxyterminal to the phosphotyrosine. Studies with synthetic peptides indicate that the binding site for these carboxyterminal sequences fall into several broad categories.[99] The most common SH2 subtype, found in nearly all nonreceptor tyrosine kinases, preferentially accommodates amino acids with hydrophilic side chains at the (TyrP) +1 and +2 positions and a small hydrophobic residue at +3. Another common type of SH2 exhibits a long hydrophobic groove extending from the Tyr(P)-binding pocket that can accommodate up to five hydrophobic amino acids. The disparate preferences of various SH2 domains for the +1 residue is determined largely by a single amino acid on the fourth β strand of the SH2 domain; a Tyr or Phe at the fifth residue on this strand confers a preference for smaller hydrophilic residues at the Tyr(P) +1 position, whereas an Ile or Cys at this site in the SH2 domain leads to a preference for hydrophobic residues at the Tyr(P) +1 position (Table 8-3). A comparison of the binding preferences of SH2 domains to the specificity determinants of tyrosine kinases reveals several informative patterns (Table 8-4). Although each tyrosine kinase exhibits a relatively distinct amino acid sequence preference for synthetic peptides substrates, all protein-tyrosine kinases select peptides with hydrophobic residues at +3; this, in turn, is consistent with the binding preferences of all SH2 domains. In addition, the nonreceptor TKs (e.g., Src, Lck), all of which contain SH2 domains themselves, prefer to phosphorylate peptides that contain, at the Tyr(P) positions +1 and +2, amino acids with small neutral (glycine [Gly], Ala) or acidic (glutamic acid [Glu]) side chains. Thus, the specificity of these kinases corresponds closely with the binding preferences of their endogenous SH2 domains. In contrast, the RTKs prefer to phosphorylate peptides that contain multiple hydrophobic amino acids at +1 through +4, as well as multiple acidic residues at the −1 to −3 positions. This pattern corresponds best with the binding specificity of the SH2 domains found on p85, PLC-γ, and SH-PTP2, targets known to bind consistently to activated RTKs. These general correlations accommodate exceptions and considerable variation. Thus, the binding specificity of the Grb-2 SH2 domain is determined primarily by a preference for N at the +2 residue, allowing Grb-2 to accommodate a wide range of amino acids at +1 and +3, which probably accounts in part for the ubiquitous recruitment of Grb-2. Moreover, many activated RTKs recruit nonreceptor TKs, which bind through their SH2 domains to RTK autophosphorylation sites whose sequence matches more closely the binding specificity of the nonreceptor TK SH2 domain than the RTK specificity toward peptide substrates. This reflects a broadening of RTK specificity when catalyzing autophosphorylation, presumably due to the imposed proximity of an intramolecular substrate. The effect of proximity on RTK substrate selection is recreated when protein substrate becomes bound to the autophosphorylated RTK through its SH2, PTB, or perhaps PH domains; the RTK is then capable of catalyzing a multiple, processive substrate phosphorylation, including the phosphorylation of sites that would be unfavorable in a conventional bimolecular reaction. Thus, in contrast to most Ser/Thr protein kinases, the intrinsic specificity of the RTK kinase domain is greatly modified by the associations imposed by the high-affinity binding of proteins through their SH2 and PTB domains.

Despite the differences in the specificity of individual RTKs for tyrosine-containing motifs as well as in the binding of SH2 domains to P-tyrosine–containing motifs defined previously, ligand stimulation of different RTKs in cell culture results in the activation of a common set of signal transduction pathways, described in part later, and often a similar cellular phenotype (e.g., proliferation). The question therefore arises as to mechanisms operative in vivo by which activation of different RTKs on a single cell or activation of the same RTK in different cells results in different phenotypic outcomes. Several general answers have emerged. One factor is that the intensity and duration of RTK activation influences the identity and intensity of the downstream pathways activated. Thus, the mechanisms that terminate RTK signaling (i.e., PTPase activities, ubiquitin-mediated RTK degradation, transcriptional upregulation of feedback inhibitors) all serve to refine the nature of the cellular response. A second factor is simply the identity of the available downstream targets and effectors, a feature defined by the pattern of gene expression established

Table 8-3 **Phosphopeptide Motifs for SH2 Domains***

Group	SH2 Domain	Y(P) + 1	Y(P) + 2	Y(P) + 3	βD5
1A	Src	E	E	I	Y
	Fyn	E	E		Y
	Lck	E	E	I	Y
	Fgr	E	E	I/V	Y
	Lyn				Y
	Yes				Y
	Hck				Y
	D-Src				Y
1B	Syk C	Q/T/E	E/Q/T	L	Y
	Syk N	T	T	I/L/M	Y
	ZAP70 C				Y
	Tec			Y	
	Atk			Y	
	Itk			Y	
	Abl	E	N	P	Y
	Arg				Y
	Csk	T	N	M/R	Y
	Crk	D	H	P	Y
	Nck	D	E	P	F
	Fes/Fps	E	—	V/I	F
	ZAP70 N				
	Sem5	L/V	N	V/P	F
	D-Grb2	Y	N		F
	Grb2	QY	N	Y	F
	GAP C				F
	GAP N				F
	Tensin	E	N	F/I/V	F
	3BP2	E	N	—	Y
2	Vav	M	E	P	T
3	P85α N	M/I/V/E	—	M	I
	p85β N				I
	p85α C	M/L/I		M	C
	p85β C				C
	PLC-γ1 C	V/I	I/L	P/I/V	C
	PLC-γ2 C				C
	PLC-γ1 N	L/I/V	E/D	L/I/V	C
	PLC-γ2 N				C
	SHPTP1 N	F	—	F	I
	SHPTP2 N	I/V	—	V/I	I
	Csw N				I
	SHPTP1 C				I
	Shc	E/I	—	I/L/M	L
4	Shb	T	T	L	M
	SHPTP2 C				V
	Csw C			V	
	STATs			A?S?	

*Columns Y(P) + 1, 2, and 3 comprise the first, second, and third residues C-terminal to phosphotyrosine of the optimal phosphopeptide selected by each SH2 domain (e.g., Y(P)YEEI for Src SH2). The far-right column indicates the residue at the βD5 position of the SH2 domain. Strength of selection varies; see original for details. A hyphen indicates no selection. Motifs not yet determined or not submitted for publication are left blank. C or N in the first column designates the C-or N-terminal SH2 domain.
SH2, Src homology-2.
Adapted from Songyang Z, Cantley LC: Recognition and specificity in protein tyrosine kinase-mediated signaling. TIBS 20:470–475, 1995.

Table 8-4 Optimal Substrate Sequences Recognized by Different Protein Tyrosine Kinases*

	Substrate Sequence at Position								
	−4	−3	−2	−1	0	+1	+2	+3	+4
Tyrosine kinases									
c-Fps/Fes	E	E	E	I	Y	E	E	I	E
Middle T antigen/c-Src	D	E	E	I	Y	G/E	E	F	F
v-Src	E	E	E	I	Y	G/E	E	F	D
Lck	X	E	X	I	Y	G	V	F	F
c-Abl	A†	X	V	I	Y	A	A	P	F
EGF receptor	E	E	E	E	Y	F	E	L	V
PDGF receptor	E	E	E	E	Y	V	F	I	X
FGF receptor	A†	E	E	E	Y	F	F	L	F
Insulin receptor	X	E	E	E	Y	M	M	M	M

*Relative importance of substrate residues for selection by the protein-tyrosine kinases varies; see original for details. Consistent with known phosphorylation sites of receptor protein tyrosine kinases (PTKs), these kinases favorably phosphorylated peptides with the general motif Tyr-hydrophobic-x-hydrophobic. This motif, once phosphorylated, is predicted to bind proteins containing group III SH2 (Src homology-2) domains (see Table 8–3). In contrast, the SH2-containing PTKs preferentially phosphorylate peptides with the motif Tyr-hydrophilic-hydrophilic-hydrophobic. Sites phosphorylated by these PTKs are predicted to bind proteins with group I SH2 domains (see Table 8–3). These results suggest that the binding sites of individual SH2 domains and PTKs have converged on overlapping selectivities to maintain specificity in downstream signaling.
†Partially caused by lag from the previous sequencing cycle.
EGF, epidermal growth factor; FGF, fibroblast growth factor; PDGF, platelet-derived growth factor.
Adapted from Songyang Z, Cantley LC: Recognition and specificity in protein tyrosine kinase-mediated signaling. TIBS 20:470–475, 1995.

prior to RTK activation. This undoubtedly is the major factor through which a single RTK entrains tissue-specific patterns of cellular differentiation. A third factor involves cell-specific coreceptors that serve both to restrict RTK activation in a cell-specific manner and to amplify and diversify the downstream responses in the target cell. An example is provided by the Met receptor, which uses the integrin α6β4, the semaphorin 4D-binding transmembrane protein plexin B1, and the hyaluronate receptor CD44 (splicing variant that contains exon 6) as tissue-specific coreceptors, each necessary in its specific cell for the ability of hepatic growth factor (HGF) activation of Met to generate the motility and branching morphogenesis responses characteristic of HGF action in vivo.[100] Although relatively limited information is available, it appears that integrins commonly play a coreceptor role for RTKs, as reported for the VEGFR-2, ErbB, and IR/IGF-1R subfamilies. Other mechanisms that underlie the specificity of RTK signaling in vivo undoubtedly remain to be uncovered.

SIGNAL TRANSMISSION THROUGH THE CELL

The net output of RTK-mediated tyrosine phosphorylation and SH2/PTB domain recruitment is to activate a set of secondary intracellular signal generators, among which four major types are well understood. These include the STAT transcriptional regulatory proteins[101] and three enzymatic proteins: PLC-γ, PI-3 kinase, and the guanyl nucleotide exchangers for small GTPases, especially those acting on Ras. Each of these elements generates one or more secondary signals, each of which entrains multiple separate signal transduction pathways extending to all compartments of the cell. Clearly, SH2 domain proteins of still uncharacterized function are known that may yet be shown to regulate novel signaling pathways; a plausible working hypothesis is that each of the already known but uncharacterized RTK targets as well as those yet to be uncovered will be found to function in a critical manner in vivo downstream of one or more RTKs in one or

more cells, at one or more times in development or during adult life. Nevertheless, based on a variety of genetic and biochemical data, it is possible at present to identify several of the known secondary signals, specifically the small GTP-binding protein Ras and the products of the PI-3 kinase, as indispensable outputs for cellular differentiation and mitogenesis. This conclusion is strongly supported by the identification of the apical two members of each of these two pathways, namely Ras/Raf[102] and PI-3 kinase/Akt,[103–105] as spontaneously occurring, dominant transforming oncogenes. Thus, any of these four elements, converted to a constitutively active state, is sufficient to drive "susceptible" but otherwise normal cells into a state that exhibits at least some properties of an oncogenically transformed cell (e.g., immortality, increased growth rate, loss of growth inhibition on cell-cell contact, loss of dependence on matrix attachment for survival and growth, etc.). In addition, the tumor suppressor gene, PTEN/MMAC, inactivated in many breast cancers, as well as in 60% to70% of advanced prostate cancers and glioblastoma multiforme,[106] has been identified as a Ptd Ins 3′-phosphatase, that is, the key degradative enzyme for 3′-OH phosphorylated Ptd inositides.[107] In addition to their capacity for promoting mitogenesis, the genes encoding each of these polypeptides have been identified as crucial determinants in a variety of developmental programs in C. elegans and Drosophila. Thus, the ability of RTKs to promote the accumulation of Ras-GTP and PIP3 is central to their characteristic biologic actions. Both of these responses are initiated by the recruitment of an enzyme polypeptide (i.e., a Ras-specific guanyl nucleotide exchanger or a Ptd Ins 3′-OH kinase) to an RTK-generated phosphotyrosine motif through an SH2 domain–containing adaptor protein (i.e., Grb-2 or p85, respectively). The Ras-GTP and PIP3 signals, although chemically different, function in an analogous manner; they, like the RTKs themselves, represent membrane-bound signals that attract an array of effectors through specific, high-affinity binding. Once recruited to the membrane, these effectors, which are mostly protein (Ser/Thr) kinases and guanyl nucleotide exchangers for other small GTPases, become activated and convey the message downstream into all cellular compartments, to the proteins that mediate the ultimate enzymatic, structural, synthetic, and degradative functions required for the final biologic response.

THE RTK-RAS SIGNAL TRANSDUCTION PATHWAY

The first RTK-initiated pathway to be unraveled was that underlying the activation of Ras and the mechanism of Ras action. Ras is the progenitor of a superfamily of small GTPase proteins, which now number more than 60 and encompass four subfamilies: Ras, Rho, Rabs, and Arfs.[108] These proteins serve as GTP-dependent timers that interact with and initiate the activation of target proteins in a GTP-dependent reaction. The three Ras genes (giving four polypeptides: Harvey, Kirsten-a, Kirsten-b, and N-Ras) encode very similar polypeptides of approximately 190 amino acids, which must be anchored to the inner surface of the plasma membrane for biologic activity. Membrane attachment is initiated by the attachment of a hydrophobic C-15 farnesyl (Ha-Ras, N-Ras) or C20 geranylgeranyl group (Ki-Ras4b) to a cysteine, four amino acids from the Ras carboxyterminus, through a thioether linkage. This prenylation reaction is followed by cleavage of the C-terminal three amino acids and methylation of the C-terminal carboxyl group. These modifications greatly increase the hydrophobicity of the Ras polypeptide and for Ki Ras, which contains a polybasic segment (6 lysine) just N-terminal to the prenylation site, are sufficient to confer constitutive binding to the inner surface of the plasma membrane. Ha-Ras, lacking a carboxyterminal polybasic segment, requires a further hydrophobic modification, which is accomplished by the attachment of two palmitate thioesters to each of two cysteines just upstream of the prenylation. Ras is a GTPase that operates in a cyclic fashion, binding GTP (whose cytoplasmic concentration is 10-fold higher than that of guanosine diphosphate [GDP]), hydrolyzing this to GDP, releasing GDP, and rebinding GTP. The intrinsic Ras GTPase activity is very low, but it can be accelerated over 1000-fold by Ras-specific GTPase-activating proteins (GAPs), which thereby deactivate Ras. In the presence of a GAP, the dissociation of GDP becomes the rate-limiting step in the overall GTPase cycle, and catalytic proteins exist, first identified in yeast, that accelerate the release of bound guanyl nucleotide and are thus guanyl nucleotide exchange factors (GNEFs). Given the much higher cytosolic concentrations of GTP over GDP, GNEF action favors Ras occupancy by GTP in vivo. Although first encountered in mutant form as a retroviral transforming gene, Ras gained wide notice from its discovery in mutant form as the first human dominant oncogene, that is, the gene responsible for the transformation of cultured murine fibro-blasts caused by the introduction of DNA from human tumors. The mutations in Ras found to confer oncogenic capacity are generally those that inactivate the intrinsic GTPase and its ability to be stimulated by GAPs; a few activating mutations result from an increase in the rate of spontaneous guanyl nucleotide dissociation, mimicking the effect of GNEF action. The oncogenic behavior of such mutations established that Ras is active, or promitogenic, when bound to GTP.

Identification of the link between the RTK and Ras activation required elucidation of the TyrP adaptor protein Grb-2, a 25-kDa polypeptide composed of an SH2 domain flanked by two SH3 domains (see Fig. 8-8).[86,108] Mutations in the gene encoding the *C. elegans* homologue of Grb-2 (called SEM-5) inhibit cellular (vulval) differentiation downstream of the gene encoding an EGFR homologue (Let23); this defect can be overcome by an activated Ras gene. *Drosophila* photoreceptor cell development, a process known to be regulated by an RTK (sevenless), is also dependent on *Drk*, the fly homologue of SEM-5 and Grb-2, and on Ras. Another *Drosophila* gene named *SOS* (son of sevenless) is necessary for photoreceptor development and by genetic epistasis appears to function downstream of the sevenless RTK but upstream of Ras; *SOS* encodes a polypeptide that contains an N-terminal PH domain, a centrally located catalytic domain homologous to the Ras guanyl nucleotide exchange enzymes first characterized in yeast, and a proline-rich carboxyterminal segment. Thus, genetic evidence provided the first indication that cellular development was directed by the ability of an RTK to promote GTP-charging (i.e., activation) of the Ras GTPase. The biochemical operation of the steps between the RTK and Ras was established by work in both insect and mammalian cells, showing that Grb-2, through its SH3 domains (discussed later), associates with the carboxyterminal proline-rich segment of the SOS protein, and the complex of Grb-2/mSOS is recruited to the activated, tyrosine-phosphorylated RTK through the Grb-2 SH2 domain; however, the SOS PH domain is also necessary for effective membrane association and Ras activation. Together these N- and C-terminal noncatalytic segments ensure that SOS is positioned to enable Ras-GTP charging. The recruitment of Grb-2 directly to the RTK is only one of several pathways by which Grb-2/mSOS is recruited to the plasma membrane. The proto-oncogene *Shc* is a particularly versatile TyrP adaptor, containing an aminoterminal PTB domain and a carboxyterminal SH2 domain. The Shc SH2 domain is recruited to the vast majority of activated RTKs and nonreceptor TKs, which thereupon catalyze Shc tyrosine phosphorylation creating an excellent binding site for the Grb-2 SH2 domain. Another Grb-2 partner is the SH2 domain–containing intracellular tyrosine phosphatase, SH-PTP2; once recruited to an RTK, SH PTP2, like Shc, undergoes a tyrosine phosphorylation that creates an effective Grb-2 binding site. While it is counterintuitive for a PTP to serve as a positive element in RTK signaling, genetic evidence indicates that loss of the *Drosophila* SH-PTP2 homologue, Corkscrew (CSW), impairs DER signaling in a

manner that can be bypassed by active Ras. Thus, numerous pathways have evolved that enable RTKs to recruit Ras to an active state. In addition, SOS is only one of several types of Ras-specific guanyl nucleotide exchangers; Ras-specific RTK-independent guanyl nucleotide exchangers exist (primarily expressed in the central nervous system [CNS]) that are regulated directly by Ca^{++} and diacylglycerol, and indirectly by heterotrimeric GTPases acting through nonreceptor tyrosine kinases.[109]

A comparison of the crystal structures of Ras bound to GDP or to GTP shows that only two Ras loops adopt a different configuration depending on which nucleotide is bound—one loop involves amino acids 32 through 40, and the second, amino acids 60 through 72; these segments are therefore named switch 1 and 2, respectively. An extensive analysis of the effect of site-specific mutations on the ability of mutant active (GTPase-deficient) Ras to transform fibroblasts revealed that alterations in the switch 1 loop greatly impaired transforming ability. The importance of the switch 1 loop for transformation, together with its selective GTP-dependent reconfiguration, suggested strongly that the switch 1 loop is (part of) the Ras "effector" domain, that is, the Ras segment that mediates the GTP-dependent interaction with the proteins that act as "effectors" of Ras transforming action.[110] This prediction was verified with the discovery that cRaf-1, a proto-oncogene protein (Ser/Thr) kinase, binds selectively to Ras in a GTP-dependent manner through the Ras effector loop.[111] The Raf kinase contains an aminoterminal noncatalytic regulatory domain and a carboxyterminal kinase catalytic domain; deletion of the Raf regulatory domain produces an oncogenic, constitutively active kinase. As Raf is an RTK-regulated protein kinase, the Raf regulatory domain must have two functions; in unstimulated cells, it must act to suppress the kinase domain, whereas with RTK stimulation, the Raf regulatory domain must serve as the receptor for the activating upstream signal. This activating signal is the Ras-GTP complex itself. The Raf aminoterminal regulatory domain contains a segment of about 100 amino acids that binds directly to the Ras effector loop with high affinity (K_DnM) in a reaction that is essentially completely GTP-dependent.[112] Immediately carboxyterminal to this Raf segment is a Cys-His rich, zinc-binding (so-called zinc-finger) structure (homologous to those found in the PKCs) that mediates a second, lower affinity, GTP-independent-binding interaction with a second Ras epitope, distinct from the effector loop.[113,114] This second binding step between the Raf zinc finger and Ras is absolutely required to convert Raf to an active state,[115] a process that also requires the active participation of 14-3-3 proteins and the (serine) phosphorylation of Raf by a still unknown protein kinase.[116] This second-site Ras-Raf binding interaction confers a crucial additional specificity, inasmuch as other Ras-like proteins contain an effector loop sequence identical to that of Ras enabling the binding of Raf; however, as they fail to engage in a productive second-site interaction, they are unable to support cRaf activation in vivo. Once activated, Raf then serves as the immediate upstream activator of the MAPKK[117] and thus the MAPK pathway (see Chapter 14).

Several proteins other than Raf are known to bind to Ras in a GTP-dependent manner and are thus candidates to serve, like Raf, as Ras effectors. The best supported among these candidates are the three p110 polypeptides that serve as the type 1A PI-3 kinase catalytic subunits and a family of three guanyl nucleotide exchangers that act on the Ras-related small GTPase known as Ral.[118] Little is known at present concerning the biologic consequences of Ral activation. As regards the PI-3 kinase, the importance of Ras-GTP for the full activation of the type 1A subfamily is now well established. Mutations in the p110 polypeptides that impair their ability to bind to Ras-GTP substantially decrease their activation in vivo by RTKs[119]; conversely, mutations in the RTKs that diminish the activation of Ras also impair the activation of PI-3 kinase, to some degree.[120] Nevertheless, Ras-GTP plays only a secondary role in the regulation of the PI-3 kinase. The affinity of p110 for Ras-GTP is 100-fold lower than for Raf[121]; whereas Raf is recruited to the membrane entirely through its high-affinity binding to Ras-GTP, the p110 PI-3 kinase polypeptides are recruited to the membrane through their p85 adaptor subunits, independent of Ras-GTP, and interact with Ras effectively only after the p85-mediated recruitment. The contribution of other candidate Ras-GTP effectors (e.g., MEKK1, NORE 1, AF-6, etc.) to the biologic responses caused by activated Ras is not yet known. It is presumed that the elucidation of the biochemical function of the substantial number of candidate Ras effectors will ultimately be required to achieve a full understanding of the mechanism of Ras action.

THE RTK-PI-3 KINASE SIGNAL TRANSDUCTION PATHWAY

PI-3 kinases were first encountered as PI kinases of novel specificity that coprecipitated with polyoma middle T antigen (a viral transforming protein) and appeared to copurify with an 85-kDa polypeptide.[75] A similar p85 polypeptide and PI kinase activity were found to coprecipitate with a variety of activated RTKs,[122] and the p85 was ultimately isolated and cloned from this source. Independently, purification of a hepatic PI-3 kinase yielded a p85/p110 heterodimer, and the p85 polypeptide was shown to be the noncatalytic adaptor subunit of the PI-3 kinase (Figs. 8-10 and 8-11). This adaptor protein (p85α) has an N-terminal SH3 domain, followed by a segment with substantial homology to the C-terminal portion of the Bcr gene product (a GAP for Rho family GTPases) that is flanked by proline-rich sequences on both sides. The C-terminal half of p85α contains two SH2 domains separated by a segment that binds tightly to the aminoterminus of a p110 PI kinase catalytic subunit. Three other splice variants of this gene are described: p85α1, p55α, and p50α. The p85α1 variant is nearly identical to p85α, whereas the shorter isoforms lack the SH3, first proline-rich sequence, and the BCR domain, with p55α containing a novel 32 amino acid N-terminus immediately before the second proline-rich segment, that is lacking in p50α, which is otherwise identical. Two related genes encode p85β and p55γ, which are architecturally identical to p85α and p55α, respectively. Each of these SH2-adaptor proteins contains a functional inter SH2 segment that binds to a p110 catalytic subunit. PI-3 kinases catalytic subunits that bind to this family of adaptor have been classified as type 1A, and three closely related type 1A p110s are known: α, β, and δ; each contains an N-terminal segment that binds to the adaptor protein, a Ras-binding domain, a

noncatalytic domain conserved among all PI-4 kinase and PI-3 kinases (the PIK domain), and a C-terminal lipid kinase catalytic domain. When TyrP-containing synthetic peptides bind to a p85/p110 heterodimer, the lipid kinase activity is increased severalfold. However, if both SH2 domains are simultaneously ligated, either by a multiply phosphorylated receptor polypeptide or by a single synthetic peptide containing two TyrP motifs, the catalytic activity of the p110 lipid kinase is activated to an extent that greatly exceeds that caused by a peptide containing a single phosphotyrosine. Thus, the binding of the p85 subunit to the RTK brings the p85/p110 lipid kinase to the membrane, in contiguity to its PI substrate, and the simultaneous engagement of the two SH2 domains (per se, without p85 tyrosine phosphorylation) strongly activates PI-3 kinase catalytic function. The recruitment of the p85/p110 heterodimer to the membrane contributes in one further way to the activation of the lipid kinase: Membrane association facilitates a relatively low affinity but specific interaction of p110 with Ras-GTP, as described previously. This interaction enables optimal activation of the p110 lipid kinase, inasmuch as mutations in the p110 Ras-binding domain or in the RTK sites critical to Ras activation substantially diminish the ability of the RTK to activate PI-3 kinase, despite the integrity of the RTK sites that mediate p85 SH2 binding. The type 1A PI-3 kinases can phosphorylate PI, PI-4 P and PI-4,5 P_2 comparably in vitro but appear to use PI-4,5 P_2 preferentially in vivo[123–125] (Fig. 8-12). The catalytic function of type 1A PI-3 kinases is inhibited somewhat specifically by low concentrations of the drugs wortmannin (<0.1 μM) and Ly294002 (<10 μM), which therefore are useful probes. The class 1B PI-3 kinase catalytic subunits have similar substrate specificity but different regulatory properties; thus, p110γ does not bind to the p85/p50/p55 class of SH2 domain–containing adaptors nor to Ras-GTP, but rather to a p101 adaptor. The p101/p110γ complex is activated by the βγ subunits of heterotrimeric GTPases.

Ptd Ins 4 P and 4,5 P_2 are minor but constitutive components of cell membranes; Ptd Ins 4,5 P_2 content is regulated by the activity of PLC isozymes (which catalyze hydrolysis to Ins 1,4,5 P_3 and DAG) and by PI-4 kinases, which convert PI to PI-4 P and PI-4,5 P_2. The 3'-OH phosphorylated Ptd Ins appear only with activation of PI-3 kinase and are maximally present at no more than 10% the level of Ptd Ins 4,5 P_2. The 3'-OH-phosphorylated Ptd Ins derivatives are not susceptible to phospholipase (PL-C/PL-D) action and are catabolized by 5'-OH- and 3'-OH-specific phosphatases. Overexpression of PTEN, a 3'-OH Ptd Ins polyphosphate phosphatase, markedly interferes with insulin signaling; however, homozygous deletion of the PTEN gene in

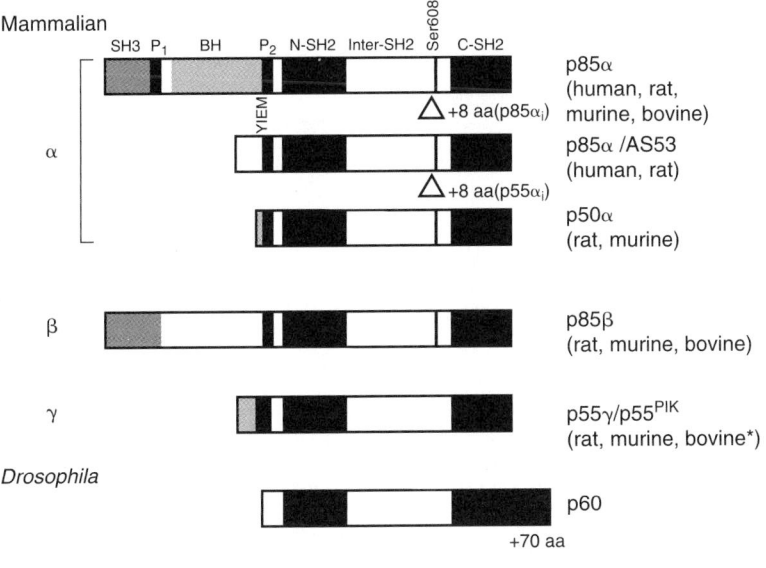

Figure 8-10 Overview of the different adaptor subunits for class IA phosphoinositide 3-kinases. P, Pro-rich region; BH, bcr homology region. p50α and p55α (also known as p85/AS53) are splice variants of p85α, whereas p85β and p55γ (also indicated as p55(PIK)) are encoded by different genes. Triangles indicate further splice insertions in p85α and p55α (here named p85αi and p55αi). Possible regulatory phosphorylation sites are indicated as Ser608 and YIEM. GenBank/EMBL accession numbers are as follows: p85α (human, M61906; bovine, M61745; mouse, M60651, U50413; rat, D64045), p50α (mouse, U50414; rat, U50412), p55α (human, U49349; rat, D64048), p85β (bovine, M61746; rat, D64046), p55γ (mouse, S79169; rat, D64047), p60 (*Drosophila melanogaster*, Y12498). *Bovine p55γ. (From Vanhaesebroeck B, Leevers SJ, Panayotou G, et al: Phosphoinositide 3-kinases: A conserved family of signal transducers. Trends Biochem Sci 22:267–272, 1997.)

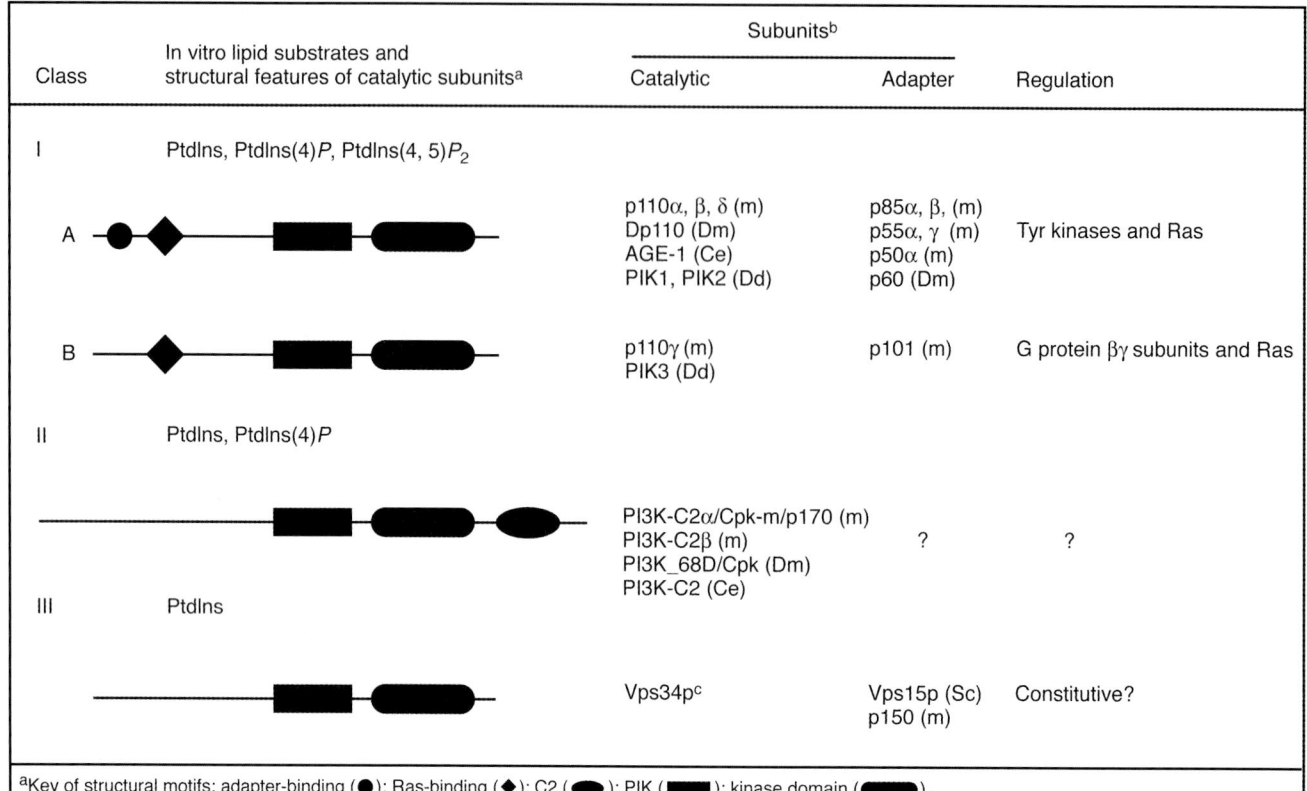

| Class | In vitro lipid substrates and structural features of catalytic subunits[a] | Subunits[b] | | Regulation |
		Catalytic	Adapter	
I	PtdIns, PtdIns(4)P, PtdIns(4, 5)P_2			
A		p110α, β, δ (m) Dp110 (Dm) AGE-1 (Ce) PIK1, PIK2 (Dd)	p85α, β, (m) p55α, γ (m) p50α (m) p60 (Dm)	Tyr kinases and Ras
B		p110γ (m) PIK3 (Dd)	p101 (m)	G protein βγ subunits and Ras
II	PtdIns, PtdIns(4)P	PI3K-C2α/Cpk-m/p170 (m) PI3K-C2β (m) PI3K_68D/Cpk (Dm) PI3K-C2 (Ce)	?	?
III	PtdIns	Vps34p[c]	Vps15p (Sc) p150 (m)	Constitutive?

[a]Key of structural motifs: adapter-binding (●); Ras-binding (◆); C2 (⬭); PIK (▬); kinase domain (▬).
[b]For the proteins other than those derived from yeast, fruit fly and mammals, no biochemical proof of PI3K lipid kinase activity is available. These enzymes have been allocated to a particular class of PI3K mainly based on primary sequence homology of the core kinase domain[5]. The abbreviations used are: m, mammalian; Ce, *Caenorhabditis elegans*; Dd, *Dictyostelium discoideum*; Dm, *Drosophila melanogaster*; Sc, *Saccharomyces cerevisiae*. The GenBank/EMBL accession numbers for class I and II catalytic subunits are: *mammalia*: p110α (human: Z29090, HSU79143; mouse: U03279; bovine: M93252), p110β (human: S67334), p110γ (human: X83368; pig Y10743), p110δ (human: Y10055, U57843, U86587; mouse, U86453), PI3K-C2α (human: Y13367), Cpk-m (also known as p170) (mouse: U52193; U55772), PI3K-C2β (Y13892, Y11312) - *D. melanogaster*: Dp110 (Y09070), PI3K_68D (also known as Cpk) (X92892; U52192)—*C. elegans*: age-1 (U56101), putative C2-domain containing PI3K (on cosmid Z69660)—*D. discoideum*: PIK1 (U23476), PIK2 (U23477) and PIK3
[c]The prototype of the class III PI3Ks is the *S. cerevisiae* protein Vps34p (X53531). Vps34p homologues from other species are not shown individually. They are: human PI3K (Z46973); *D. melanogaster*, PI3K_59F (X99912); *D. discoideum*, PIK5 (U23480); and the Vps34p-related PI3Ks from *Schizosaccharomyces pombe* (U32583), Soybean (L29770), *Arabidopsis thaliana* (U10669) and *C. elegans* (Y12543).

Figure 8-11 A classification of phosphoinosotide 3-kinase (PI-3-K) family members. (From Vanhaesebroeck B, Leevers SJ, Panayotou G, et al: Phosphoinositide 3-kinases: A conserved family of signal transducers. Trends Biochem Sci 22:267–272, 1997.)

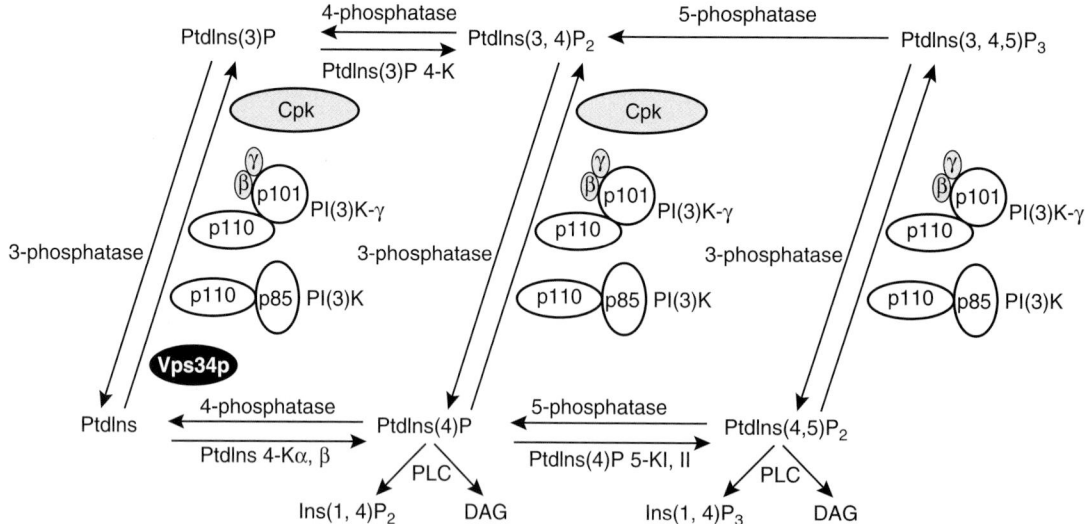

Figure 8-12 Pathways for phosphoinositide synthesis. The enzymes that synthesize the various phosphoinositides are indicated. Three classes of PI-3-K enzymes exist: the class I enzymes (p110) can use phosphatidylinositide (PtdIns), PtdIns,4 or (PtdIns4,52) as substrates; class II enzymes (Cpk) phosphorylate PtdIns and PtdIns,4 and class III enzymes (Vps34p) can only phosphorylate PtdIns. (PtdIns4,52) is of particular importance: Hydrolysis by phosphoinositide-specific phospholipase C (PLC) generates the two second messengers, diacylglycerol (DAG) and (Ins1,4,53), and phosphorylation by PI-3-K generates the putative second messenger (PtdIns3,4,53). (PtdIns3,42) can be generated through the phosphorylation of (PtdIns4) by a PI-3-K (Cpk, C2 domain–containing PI-3-K), as well as by dephosphorylation of (PtdIns3,4,53). In mammalian cells, D3 phosphoinositides are degraded by phosphatases that convert them back to PtdIns, PtdIns,4 or (PtdIns4,52). (From Toker A, Cantley LC: Signaling through the lipid products of phosphoinositide-3-OH kinase. Nature 387:673, 1997.)

mice results in a tumor-prone state, rather than dramatic alterations in metabolism.[126] This is consistent with the tumor suppressor phenotype of PTEN loss in man (i.e., the Cowden and Bannayan-Riley-Ruvalcaba syndromes), wherein germline transmission of heterozygous PTEN allelic inactivation results in proclivity to multiple tumor types. By contrast, mice homozygous for the deletion of the gene encoding SHIP2, an SH2 domain-containing 5′-OH Ptd Ins polyphosphate phosphatase, exhibit a marked increase in insulin sensitivity and spontaneous neonatal hypoglycemia; SHIP2 is thus a potent negative regulator of insulin signaling.[127] Both the SHIP2 and PTEN loss-of-function phenotypes are explicable by a failure of negative regulation along RTK-activated PI-3 kinase pathways; however, it is not clear why SHIP2 inactivation selectively upregulates PI-kinase signaling downstream of the IR as opposed to other, proproliferative RTKs.

The class II PI-3 kinases are 170-kDa polypeptides distinguished by a carboxyterminal C2 domain, homologous to the sequences in PKCs that mediate Ca^{2+}-sensitive phospholipid (PS and PI) binding. In contrast to class 1A and 1B enzymes, class II PI-3 kinases are not known to be recruited to receptors or GTPases and are insensitive to the inhibitors wortmannin and LY294002. Class III PI-3 kinases exhibit a substrate specificity distinct from the class 1A, 1B, and II enzymes acting only on Ptd Ins and not on PI-4 P or PI-4,5 P_2. Class III enzymes are homologous in structure and specificity to the yeast PI-3 kinase, VPS 34p, which functions in vesicle trafficking, osmoregulation, and endocytosis; no evidence for RTK regulation exists for the mammalian class III PI-3 kinases. The downstream effectors of Ptd Ins 3,4,5 P_3 include a subset of the many proteins that contain PH domains (discussed later) or other polyphosphatidylinositide-binding domains (e.g., atypical PKCs). Genetic evidence points to the Ptd Ins 3,4,5 P_3–binding protein (Ser/Thr) kinases, PKB, and its A loop kinase, PDK1, as central effectors, as well as a large family of GNEFs (the Dbl family) for the Rho subfamily (RHO, Rac, Cdc42) of small GTPases. In *Drosophila*, the lethality of PTEN deletion is abrogated by introduction of a point mutation into the PH domain of PKB that inhibits the ability of PKB to bind Ptd Ins 3,4,5 P_3. Moreover, genetic evidence identifies PI-3 kinase PDK1 and PKB as crucial downstream targets of the *C. elegans* IR/IGF-1R homologue.[128,129] A further discussion of the Ptd Ins 3,4,5 P_3–regulated protein kinases (i.e., PDK1, PKBs, p70 S6 kinase, GSK3, etc.) can be found in Chapter 13.

OTHER PROTEIN-PROTEIN INTERACTION DOMAINS RELEVANT TO RTK SIGNALING

Pleckstrin Homology Domains

Pleckstrin homology (PH) domains, named after pleckstrin, the major PKC substrate of platelets, are found in both catalytic and noncatalytic proteins and are among the most ubiquitous motifs encountered in signal transduction proteins[130,131] (Table 8-5). PH domains are roughly 100 to 120 amino acids long and although relatively divergent in primary sequence, exhibit a well-conserved three-dimensional architecture that is very similar to that of PTB/PID domains.[132,133] A similar domain was detected in a noncatalytic region of the β-adrenergic receptor kinase (βARK) that was shown to mediate membrane binding of the kinase to the βγ subunits of heterotrimeric G-proteins; the optimal βγ-binding region of βARK extends, however, carboxyterminal to the borders of a canonical PH domain.[134,135] Isolated recombinant PH domains of the two guanyl nucleotide exchangers mSOS and Dbl (specific for Ras and the Rho subfamily, respectively) as well as from IRS-1 also bind directly to βγ with high affinity (K_D of 20 to 45 nM); nevertheless, little evidence exists for βγ as a physiologic ligand except for βARK.[136] Much more evidence favors the likelihood that polyphosphorylated inosites (i.e., Ptd Ins-4,5 P_2; 3,4,5 P_3; and 3,4 P_2), as well as the free inositol polyphosphates (Ins 1,4,5 P_3; Ins 1,3,4,5 P_4)

are physiologic ligands for PH domains.[137,138] Some PH domains (e.g., that from β spectrin, gelsolin, etc.) bind Ptd 4,5 P_2 and Ptd Ins 3,4,5 P_3 with comparable avidity, whereas the PH domains of other proteins exhibit a substantial preference for Ptd Ins 3,4,5 P_3 over Ptd Ins 4,5 P_2; examples of the latter include the nonreceptor B-cell Tyr kinase, BTK; the serine kinase PKB/Akt; and the guanyl nucleotide exchange proteins, SOS (Ras-specific) and *T*-cell lymphoma *i*nvasion *a*nd *m*etastasis protein (TIAM, a Rac-specific member of the Db1 family). These polypeptides are likely to be specifically recruited to the membrane by the activation of PI-3 kinase and synthesis of Ptd Ins 3,4,5 P_3, whereas proteins whose PH domains exhibit comparable affinity for Ptd Ins 4,5 P_2 and 3,4,5 P_3 are likely to be associated primarily with more abundant PI-4,5 P_2. Such proteins may be constitutively membrane-associated and perhaps released or untethered by activation of PLC, both because of a local decrease in Ptd Ins 4,5 P_2 content as well as by the generation of the competing soluble ligands, Ins 1,4,5 P_3 and especially by the higher polyphosphoinositols (e.g., Ins P_4 and Ins P_5). The very similar structure of PH and PTB domains suggested that PTB domains might represent a subclass of PH domains capable of phosphotyrosine as well as phospholipid binding. The ability of Ptd Ins 4,5 P_2 to displace the autophosphorylated EGFR from the PTB domain of Shc is consistent with this idea.

Perhaps the most striking of evidence for the functional importance of PH domains in signaling is Bruton's X-linked agammaglobulinemia, where a point mutation of the B-cell tyrosine kinase BTK in a conserved PH domain Arg residue involved in Ptd Ins-phosphate binding is the mutation responsible for a substantial subset of families.[125] The ability of IRS-1 to undergo insulin-stimulated tyrosine phosphorylation in vivo is abolished by mutation or deletion of the IRS-1 PH domain, despite the presence of an intact IRS PTB domain.[139] Mutation in the PH domain of the Dbl oncogene abolishes its transforming activity despite an unimpaired Rac GEF activity.[140] Thus, PH domains are major targets for the signals generated by PI-3 kinase and are regulated as well by the PLC hydrolysis of Ptd Ins 4,5 P_2.

At least two other polypeptide domains in addition to PH domains have been shown to bind selectively to 3′-OH-phosphorylated Ptd Ins derivatives.[141] Thus, FVYE domains bind exclusively to monophosphorylated Ptd Ins 3P, a lipid involved primarily in vesicle transport, whose abundance is increased by insulin. Phox homology (PX) domains bind to Ptd Ins-3P, −3,4 P_2, −3 5 P_2, −4,5 P_2, and possibly Ptd Ins 3,4,5 P_3. A diverse array of domains have been shown to bind Ptd Ins 4,5 P_2 including FERM, ANTH, ENTH, AP-2a, and others.

SH3 WW and EVH-1, Polyproline-Binding Domains

SH3 domains[86,142,143] are compact globular domains of about 60 amino acids that bind with μM K_D to short, proline-rich motifs of the minimal type, XPXXPX; this motif, which binds as a left-handed helix with three amino acids per turn, can bind to the SH3 domain in either direction (i.e., N→ C or C→N) by fitting into two adjacent hydrophobic pockets, one for each XP pair. Further specificity is conferred by the interaction between the amino acids flanking the PXXP with adjacent SH3 domain residues (Fig. 8-13). The relatively low affinity of these domains for ligands points to their operation primarily in intramolecular interactions, as illustrated by the role of the Src SH3 domain in maintaining Src in an inactive state through an intramolecular interaction. The ability of SH3 domains to couple effectively in intermolecular interactions probably depends on the presence of multiple SH3 domains on a single polypeptide (e.g., as in Grb-2, Nck, Crk) or on the forced proximity to a polyproline sequence induced by a higher affinity protein-protein interaction, mediated by, for example, an SH2 domain on the same protein.

WW domains contain 38 to 40 amino acids and are named for the conserved tryptophans located 20 to 22 amino acids

Table 8-5 **Mammalian Proteins Containing Pleckstrin Homology Domains**

Serine/threonine kinases

β-ARK1	β-Adrenergic receptor kinase type 1
β-ARK2	β-Adrenergic receptor kinase type 2
AktI/Rac-α/PKB	AKT8 retrovirus proto-oncogene, related to A and C kinase, protein kinase B
AktII/Rac-β/PKB	AKT8 retrovirus proto-oncogene, related to A and C kinase, protein kinase B
PKCμ	Protein kinase C, unique isoform
Bcr	Breakpoint cluster region gene

Tyrosine kinases

Tec	Tyrosine kinase expressed in hepatocellular carcinoma
BTK (Atk, Bpk, Emb)	B cell tyrosine kinase, a.k.a. Bruton's tyrosine kinase for Bruton's XLA (see text)
Itk (Tsk, Emt)	Interleukin-2–inducible T cell tyrosine kinase
Bmx	Bone marrow-expressed tyrosine kinase

Regulators of small G proteins

Ras-GAP	GTPase activator protein for the Ras family of small G proteins
Ras-GRF (2)	Guanine nucleotide–releasing factor for the Ras family of small G proteins
GAP1[IP4BP]	GTPase activator protein for the Ras family, inositol (1,3,4,5) tetraphosphate-binding protein
SOS1	Son of sevenless is required for development of the seventh ommatidial cell in Drosophila retina
SOS2	Grb2 binding, Ras and probably also Rac/Rho activating
HUMORF3__1	Human open reading frame. Hypothetical Ras-GAP protein
Vav	DNA from human esophageal carcinomas[*]
Dbl	Diffuse B cell lymphoma
Dbs	Dbl's big sister; close relative of Dbl (see above)
Ect2	Epithelial cell transforming
Ost	Truncated protein associated with osteosarcoma
Bcr	Breakpoint cluster region gene in Philadelphia chromosome
Abr	Active Bcr (see above) related gene
Lbc	Lymphoid blast crisis gene
Lfc	Lbc's first cousin; very close relative of Lbc (see above)
Tim	Transforming immortalized mammary gene
Tiam-1 (2)[†]	T lymphocyte invasion and metastasis; mRNA upregulated in metastatic cells
FGD-1 (2)	Faciogenital dysplasia causative gene

Endocytotic GTPases

Dynamin-1	GTPase involved in endocytotic vesicle formation, brain
Dynamin-2	GTPase involved in endocytotic vesicle formation, general
Dynamin T	GTPase involved in endocytotic vesicle formation, testes

Adaptors

IRS-1	Insulin receptor substrate-1, tyrosine-phosphorylated by the insulin receptor
IRS-2	Insulin receptor substrate-2, tyrosine-phosphorylated by the insulin receptor
Grb7	Growth factor receptor–binding protein-7
Grb10	Growth factor receptor–binding protein-10
3BP2	SH3 domain binding protein, binds certain SH3 domains in vitro

Cytoskeletal-associated molecules

Spectrin βIεII	Major component of erythrocyte membranous cytoskeleton
Fodrin/spectrin βIIεII	Major component of neuron membranous cytoskeleton
Kif1a/Unc104	Neuronal kinesin family homologue
hSEC7	Human homologue of yeast protein involved in vascular secretion
Syntrophin-α/DAP59 (2)	Dystrophin associated protein, molecular weight of 59 kDa
Synthrophin-β (2)	Syntrophin = protein neighbor of dystrophin
AFAP-110, AFAP-120 (2)	Actin filament–associated proteins, 110 and 120 kDa
Pleckstrin (2)	Platelet and leukocyte C-kinase substrate; major platelet PKC substrate

Lipid-associated enzymes

Phospholipase C-β$_1$	Isotype of PLC, N-terminal PH domain
Phospholipase C-β$_2$	Isotype of PLC, N-terminal PH domain
Phospholipase C-β$_3$	Isotype of PLC, N-terminal PH domain
Phospholipase C-β$_4$	Isotype of PLC, N-terminal PH domain
Phospholipase C-γ$_1$ (2)	Isotypes contain 2 PH domains, 2 SH2 domains, and 1 SH3 domain
Phospholipase C-γ$_2$ (2)	Isotypes contain 2 PH domains, 2 SH2 domains, and 1 SH3 domain
Phospholipase C-δ$_1$	PIP$_2$, IP$_3$, and membrane binding mediated by N-terminal PH domain
Phospholipase C-δ$_2$	PIP$_2$, IP$_3$, and membrane binding mediated by N-terminal PH domain
Phospholipase C-δ$_3$	PIP$_2$, IP$_3$, and membrane binding mediated by N-terminal PH domain
PI-3 kinase-γ	Adds 3-phosphate to phosphoinositides
PI-4 kinase	Adds 4-phosphate to phosphoinositides

Unknown

IGBP	Interferon-γ–binding protein
Eps8	EGF receptor pathway substrate protein
Mig2	Migration–inducing gene
OSBP	Oxysterol-binding protein; involved in cellular response to oxysterols
HUMORFV__1	Human open reading frame, hypothetic protein
HUMORA5__1	Human open reading frame, hypothetic protein
LL5	Named after discoverer, ubiquitous protein

In some cases, alternative transcripts of these proteins do not contain PH domains (e.g., βIIεII and βIεI spectrin). Many proteins with PH domains (e.g., Tec/Btk-family, β-ARK family, Kif1a/Unc104, PKCμ, dynamins) are closely related to proteins lacking PH domains (e.g., Src family, rhodopsin kinase, Kif1b, other PKCs, Mx proteins). PH domains have been described in a PI-4 kinase and somewhat less convincing examples have been claimed for eps8, an epidermal growth factor receptor tyrosine kinase substrate, and GAP1[IP4BP], a human Ras-GAP protein that also binds PI-3,4,5-P. Allocation of proteins to particular classes is in many cases tentative. Proteins with (2) after their name contain two PH domains. In many cases, the acronyms contain useful information about the source or properties of the protein and are therefore given here.

[*]An exception is Vav, which is Hebrew for 6. The Vav gene was the sixth oncogene isolated by Katzav and colleagues.

[†]The C-terminal PH domain in Tiam-1 is the only one thus known that lacks the conserved Trp residue in the C-terminal (presumably α-helical) region, instead having a Phe. Assuming that this substitution has no functional consequence, we can conclude that no single amino acid in the PH domain is absolutely conserved.

EGF, epidermal growth factor; IP$_3$, inositol 1,4,5-triphosphate; PIP$_2$, phosphatidylinositol 4,5-bisphosphate; XLA, X-linked agammaglobulinemia.

From Shaw G: The pleckstrin homology domain: An intriguing multifunctional protein module. Bioessays 18:35–46, 1996. Copyright © 1996. Reprinted by permission of John Wiley & Sons, Inc.

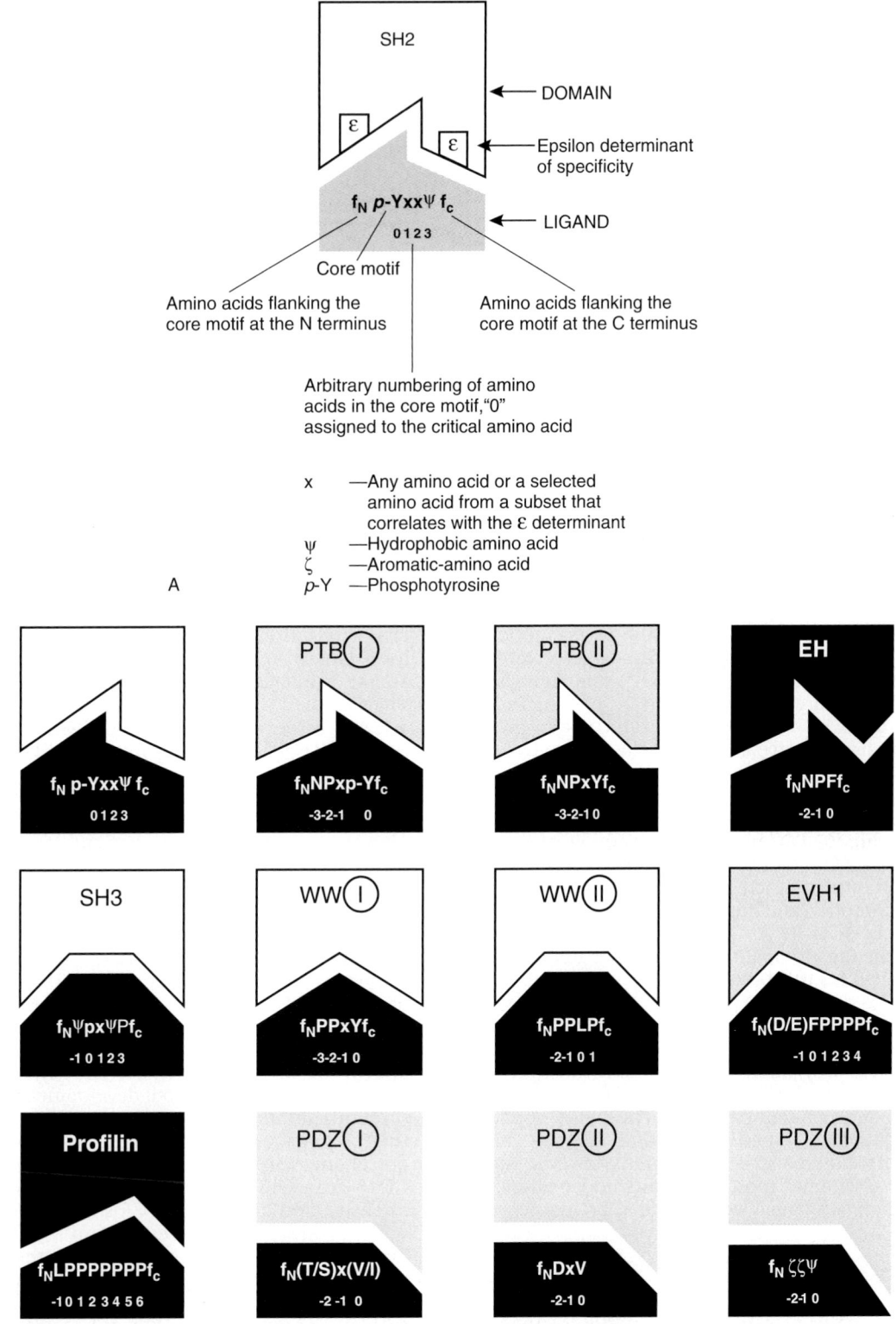

Figure 8-13 **A,** Formalization of terms to describe protein-protein interaction mediated by modules using the SH2 domain and its ligand as an example. **B,** Modular protein domains and core sequences of their dognate ligands. SH2 and a subgroup of PTB domains recognize phosphotyrosine in the context of specific sequences. Another subgroup of PT domains and the EH domain bind ligands with NP x Y and NPF cores, respectively. SH3, WW, and EVH1 domains and EVH1 domains bind proline-rich sequences. Profilin also recognizes polyprolines (a minimum of six to eight prolines). Profilin is both a protein domain and an independent, functional protein of 13- to 15-kDa molecular mass. PDZ domains evolved to recognize motifs at the C-terminal ends of proteins. Many more intracellular and extracellular modular protein domains have been identified. However, their ligands are as yet unknown, and significant portions of the newly described modules so far seem to be confined to a limited number of specialized proteins. (From Sudol M: From Src homology domains to other signaling modules: Proposal of the 'protein recognition code'. Oncogene 17:1469–1474, 1998.)

apart. Initial studies defined two general core-binding motifs, PPXY and PPLP, with additional amino- and carboxyterminal flanking residues on the peptide providing further affinity and specificity. WW domains are not *psuedo*symmetrical like SH3 domains, but they do exhibit overlap with SH3 domains in the ability to bind PPLP-containing substrates. More recent studies[144] of the WW domains of the prolyl isomerase PIN1 and the ubiquitin ligase Nedd4 have shown clearly that these WW domains bind preferentially to P-Ser/P Thr–containing sequences, probably involving (Ser/Thr) Pro motifs. Thus, in analogy with SH2 and PTB domains in P-Tyr binding, WW domains (and 14-3-3 proteins) bind to short peptide segments containing P-Ser/P-Thr with a specificity yet to be fully defined. The actin-binding protein, profilin, also contains a polyproline-binding domain and the profilin-binding proteins VASP and Mena exhibit a conserved domain, called EVH1, that binds another polyproline motif. The SH3, EVH$_1$, and profilin polyproline-binding domains are not recruited in a regulated manner as occurs with SH2 domains; however, phosphorylation within the polyproline regions, either by tyrosine kinases (e.g., at PPXY) or by proline-directed Ser/Thr kinases (at [S/T] P motifs), as well as competition with polyphosphoinositides may negatively regulate these protein-protein interactions. Conversely, proline-directed (Ser/Thr) kinases may generate binding sites for proteins that contain WW domains.

PDZ Domains

These domains were first identified in the postsynaptic density protein, *PSD*-95, the *Drosophila* Discs-large septate protein, and the tight junction protein ZO-1, and thus labeled PDZ. Such domains are now known to be present in more than 100 proteins.[145] PDZ domains bind other proteins through a specific sequence at the protein carboxyterminus, ending in Leu, Ile, or Val (see Fig. 8-13). These partners are thus available either to be modified by the catalytic domain of the PDZ-containing protein or to act selectively at the cellular locus bearing the PDZ proteins. An example of the latter is InaD, a *Drosophila* noncatalytic protein that contains multiple PDZ domains, each capable of binding a protein involved in phototransduction (e.g., the Ca$^+$ channel Trp, PLCβ, PKC). Loss of InaD greatly impairs light-induced responses despite the unimpaired expression of all the catalytic elements required for this process.

The picture of the early steps in RTK signaling developed here emphasizes the importance of phosphotyrosine-initiated protein-protein interactions in collecting multiple effectors, colocalizing them with their activators and substrates, and thereby initiating the wide distribution of the RTK signal down multiple independent pathways. The ability of protein-protein associations to speed up and/or spatially restrict signaling events should also be considered; however, the features of these assemblies most important under physiologic circumstances remain largely conjectural at present.

TERMINATION OF THE RTK SIGNAL

A variety of mechanisms exist for termination of the signal initiated by ligand binding to the RTK (e.g., ligand dissociation from the cell surface receptor; internalization of the ligand-receptor complex into an endosomal compartment, endosomal acidification, ligand dissociation followed by ligand degradation; recyling of RTK to the cell surface or degradation of RTK in parallel with the ligand; tyrosine-specific dephosphorylation of the RTK and other early mediators; and Ser/Thr phosphorylation of the RTK and other early mediators in a feedback manner by downstream Ser/Thr kinases or by "cross-talk" from antagonistic signal transduction pathways). The ability of pharmacologic inhibition of PTPases and noninternalizable RTK ligands to greatly increase

RTK signal intensity and duration has established beyond question the importance of tyrosine phosphatase and receptor-mediated endocytosis in signal termination. The contribution of RTK target serine phosphorylation to the termination and downregulation of RTK-activated tyrosine phosphorylation under physiologic condition has received most attention in regard to the negative regulation of IRS targets of the IR/IGF-1R.

PROTEIN TYROSINE PHOSPHATASES

First discovered in 1988,[146] these enzymes are now nearly as numerous as the protein-tyrosine kinases and like the tyrosine kinases, the PTPs can be classified into transmembrane and intracellular types[147,148] (Fig. 8-14). The type 1 transmembrane (receptor-like) RPTPases can be classified into seven or more subfamilies that, like the RTKs, display widely divergent extracellular extensions but more uniform intracellular domains. A distinctive feature of all but one RPTPase subfamily is the presence of two tandem catalytic domains, with the membrane-proximal domain contributing all, or nearly all, of the catalytic activity. As purified from cells, both RPTPases and intracellular PTPases exhibit very high catalytic activity, with turnover numbers (using model phosphotyrosine peptide as protein substrates) that far exceed those of the tyrosine kinases. Although some RPTP subfamilies have been shown to form homotypic transcellular associations, the identification of RPTP ligands has proceeded slowly. Consequently, the characterization of the effects of native ligands on PTP activity is largely unknown. The replacement of the extracellular and transmembrane domain of the T-cell PTP, CD45, with those of the EGF receptor does not impair the measured PTP activity; however, addition of EGF and consequent dimerization results in a marked inhibition of PTP activity.[16] The crystal structure of the membrane proximal PTP domain of RPTP α shows the domains to adopt a symmetrical dimeric configuration, wherein a wedge-shaped loop just N-terminal to the phosphatase domain is inserted into the catalytic site of the other PTP monomer. Based on these observations, a reasonable inference is that RPTP activity may be negatively regulated by ligand in a manner precisely opposite to the ligand activation of RTKs (i.e., ligand-induced dimerization of the RPTP induces inhibition of the catalytic function). CD45 activity is crucial to T-cell receptor (TCR) signaling by virtue of its ability to dephosphorylate the C-terminal autoinhibitory tyrosine phosphorylation site of the cSrc-family PTKs (e.g., fyn, lyn, etc.). The extracellular domain of CD 45 is known to undergo extensive modification by alternative mRNA splicing during T-cell development, a process that may substantially alter the binding specificity and/or affinity of the EC domain and thereby modify RPTP activity, even without changes in ligand availability. In turn, changes in the CD45 extracellular domain may greatly modify the sensitivity, intensity, and duration of TCR signaling.

The nonreceptor PTPases contain a variety of noncatalytic targeting domains that tether them to the nucleus, cytoskeleton, ER, and so on. Of particular interest are those intracellular PTPases that contain protein-protein interaction domains such as SH2 domains.[148] Thus, the intracellular PTP, SHPTP 1, and SHPTP 2 each contain a pair of SH2 domains in their N-terminal half followed by a single C-terminal PTP domain. These PTP are recruited to activated RTKs/nonreceptor RTKs through the PTP SH2 domains. Genetic evidence indicates that as expected, SHPTP1 is a negative regulatory element in the hematopoietic system. Surprisingly, however, SHPTP2 (and its *Drosophila* homologue, corkscrew, CSW) appear to function as positive regulators in RTK signaling; loss of CSW gene function impairs RTK signaling. The basis for this apparently paradoxical response is uncertain, although once recruited to the RTK, SHPTP2 can undergo an RTK-catalyzed phosphorylation that creates a strong site for the Grb-2 SH2

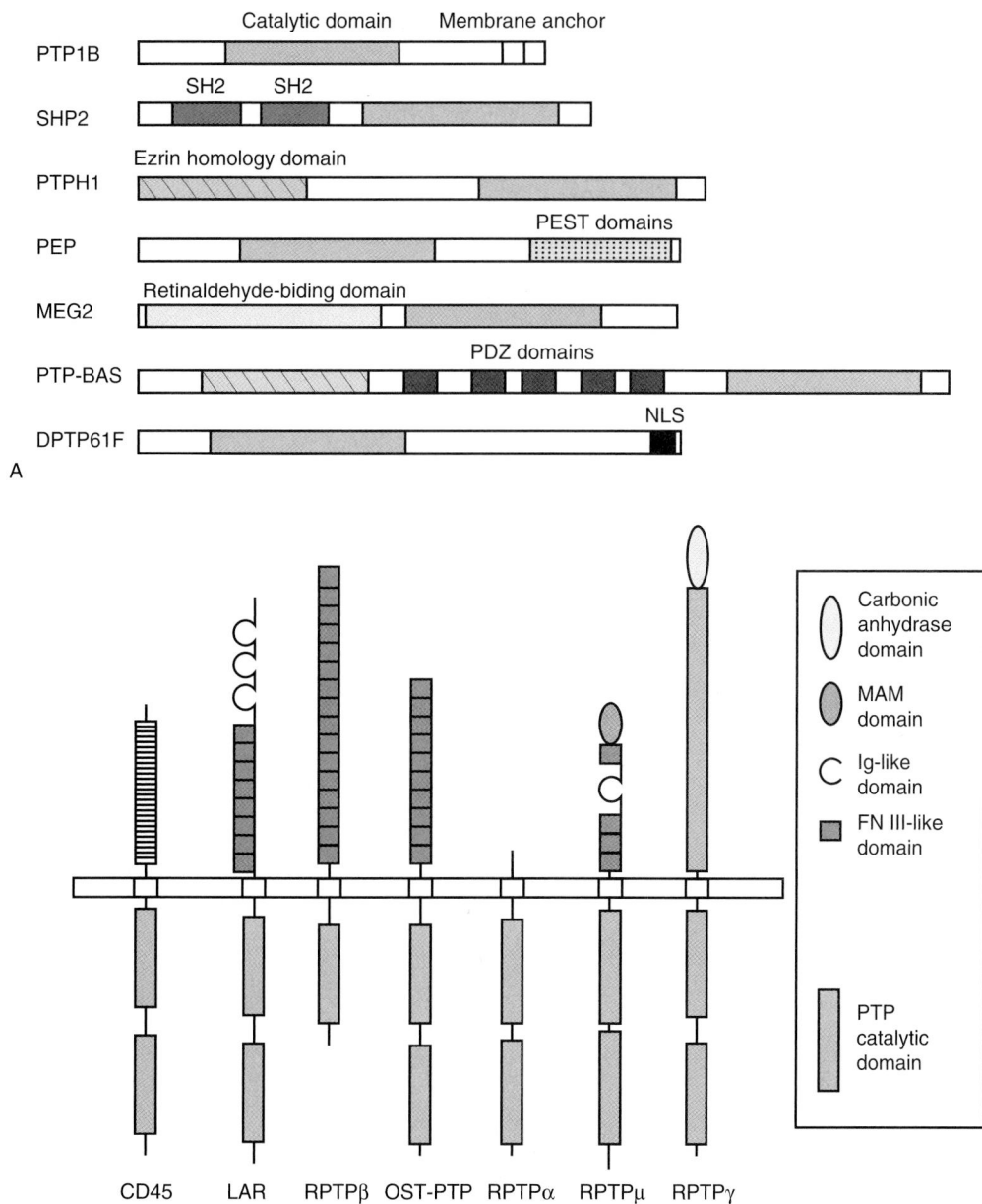

Figure 8-14 Schematic structures of non-receptor-**(A)** and receptor-like **(B)** protein tyrosine phosphatase families. (From Hunter T: The Croonian Lecture, 1997. Phil Trans Roy Soc Lond B 353:597, 1997.)

domain, enabling recruitment of SOS and activation of Ras. Phosphotyrosine-containing synthetic peptides stimulate SHPTP2 catalytic activity and a structural explanation is provided by the finding that in unliganded SHPTPase, a segment of the N-terminal SH2 domain is wedged into the catalytic site; the binding of a TyrP-containing substrate to the SH2 domain may therefore disocclude the catalytic site. Whether the catalytic activity of other intracellular PTP is subject to dynamic regulation or is constitutively available at crucial intracellular sites remains uncertain. A frequent mechanism for the pathologic inactivation of tyrosine phosphatase in vivo arises from the presence of a critical, highly reactive cysteine residue at the catalytic site of all PTPs. This residue is especially susceptible to oxidation by reactive oxygen intermediates, resulting in PTP inactivation. Such a mechanism has been claimed to underlie the increase in RTK-mediated tyrosine phosphorylation engendered by UV irradiation and ionizing radiation, as these responses can be suppressed by antioxidants.[149] Surprisingly, the identification of PTPs as tumor suppressor genes in the context of human tumors has not emerged, reflecting perhaps the substantial redundancy

and high catalytic efficiency of these enzymes. In contrast, the homozygous deletion of the gene encoding the endoplasmic reticulum-based PTPase 1B results in mice that exhibit a substantial increase in insulin sensitivity and a resistance to the development of both diet-induced obesity and insulin resistance.[150] The increase in insulin sensitivity reflects increased tyrosine phosphorylation and kinase activity of the insulin receptor, whereas the resistance to diet-induced obesity may be related primarily to enhanced signaling through the hypothalamic leptin receptor/JAK kinase pathway.[151] In cell culture, PTP1B acts on the EGFR and PDGFR, and while this effect is evident in vivo, other compensatory mechanisms make up for the lack of PTP1B action on the latter RTKs so as to maintain their output within a homeostatic range. The interaction of the IR with PTP1B occurs in the ER after ligand-induced internalization, but it is also evident immediately upon IR biosynthesis.[152] The surprisingly selective negative regulatory action of PTP1B on the IR and LeptinR systems in vivo has made PTP1B a favored target for the development of drugs for the treatment of obesity and type 2 diabetes.[153]

RECEPTOR INTERNALIZATION AND RECEPTOR/TARGET DEGRADATION

Receptor-mediated endocytosis is a complex process of general importance in the biology of all surface receptors, whose mechanisms and regulation continue to be under active investigation. RTK internalization and recycling is a constitutive process that, depending on RTK, is accelerated by ligand to varying extents and is the major route for ligand removal in vivo.[154,155] This process is best shown for the insulin/IR interaction, where abundant evidence indicates that receptor-mediated endocytosis is the primary and dominant physiologic pathway for insulin clearance in vivo. The internalization of the IR is considerably accelerated by insulin; the insulin is largely degraded, but the bulk of IR recycles to the PM, freed of ligand, so that the ligand-induced fall in steady-state surface IR content is modest. By contrast, high levels of EGF can promote a nearly complete clearance of EGFR from the cell surface, due in part to a relative resistance of EGF to acid-induced dissociation from the EGFR, resulting in diversion of the EGFR from recycling endosomes into late endosomes and lysosomes, and consequent EGFR degradation. TGF-α in contrast, dissociates readily from the EGFR at low pH and is associated with much less EGFR degradation. Receptor internalization occurs through clathrin-coated pits, and ligand strongly promotes clustering in the pits. The signals for RTK internalization reside on the intracellular segment of the RTK and are predominantly tyrosine-based motifs either NPXY or YXX φ (hydrophobic); internalization involves the interaction of the tyrosine motif with one or more adaptor protein (AP) complexes. Having entered an early endosome, the decision regarding receptor recycling versus degradation involves a complex interplay between the pH-dependent dissociation of ligand and interaction of the RTK with a variety of other proteins, such as exins (which bind through EH domains to NPF motifs) and RTK targets. Among the latter is the proto-oncogene c-Cbl, an RTK substrate that associates with the EGFR in endosomes and promotes EGFR ubiquitination and degradation by proteosomal and lysosomal pathways[156]; Cbl itself is now recognized as a ubiquitin ligase. The Grb7,10, 14 family of proteins bind through an SH2 domain to phosphotyrosine residues on several activated RTKs and interfere directly in RTK-catalyzed tyrosine phosphorylation in vivo and in vitro.[157] Nevertheless, recent data indicates that at least for the IGF-1R, it is the ability of Grb10 to recruit the ubiquitin ligase NEDD4 to the receptor that accounts for Grb10's negative regulatory effects on IGF-1 signaling in vivo. In a similar manner, the suppressor of cytokine signaling, or SOCs, polypeptides, SH2 domain–containing proteins discovered as inhibitors of JAK-STAT signaling, function as negative regulators by competition for critical phosphotyrosine sites and through their ability to bind and recruit the Elongin B/C ubiquitin ligase complex to target effectors for proteosomal degradation.[158]

RECEPTOR/TARGET INHIBITION BY SERINE/THREONINE PHOSPHORYLATION

Insulin resistance is a prevalent condition, associated with type 2 diabetes as well as with the type 2 diabetes precursor state known as the *metabolic syndrome*. Consequently, the mechanisms underlying the impedance to insulin signaling in these circumstances have been vigorously sought. Essentially all of insulin's downstream responses are blunted, largely in parallel, suggesting that a major defect lies high in the insulin signaling pathway, that is, somewhere between the IR itself and activation of the type 1A PI-3 kinase. Although IR numbers are often diminished, the magnitude of this deficit is far short of that necessary to explain the defective downstream responses, and direct measurements in vitro of the kinase-specific activity of IR purified from the muscle or other sources from insulin-resistant subjects have generally been indistinguishable from that of IR from insulin-sensitive subjects. In contrast, defects in insulin-stimulated tyrosine phosphorylation of IRS polypeptides and in the total and IRS-associated activity of PI-3 kinase have been consistently observed in insulin-resistant states.[159] Early studies in vitro indicated that treatment of cultured cells with protein Ser/Thr phosphatase inhibitors reduced insulin-stimulated IRS tyrosine phosphorylation and glucose transport with altering IR tyrosine autophosphorylation. Subsequent studies have established that a wide variety of perturbations known to cause insulin resistance in vivo (e.g., the inflammatory cytokine TNF-α, high ambient FFA levels and high concentrations of insulin itself) engender increased IRS Ser/Thr phosphorylation, decreased insulin-stimulated IRS tyrosine phosphorylation, and association with PI-3 kinase. A significant number of in vivo studies in mice and humans have recapitulated these findings and pointed to the ability of phosphorylation at a number of IRS-1 Ser/Thr residues (e.g., catalyzed by a variety of protein Ser/Thr kinases (e.g., JNK/SAPK, erk/MAPK, mTOR, etc.) to inhibit insulin-stimulated IRS tyrosine phosphorylation and/or PI-3 kinase docking and to accelerate IRS-1 degradation.[160,161] The generality of Ser/Thr phosphorylation as a negative regulatory mechanism in other RTK pathways remains to be explored.

REFERENCES

1. Collett MS, Erikson RL: Protein kinase activity associated with the avian sarcoma virus src gene product. Proc Natl Acad Sci U S A 75:2021–2024, 1978.
2. Eckhart W, Hutchinson MA, Hunter T: An activity phosphorylating tyrosine in polyoma T antigen immunoprecipitates. Cell 18:925–933, 1979.
3. Collett MS, Purchio AF, Erikson RL: An activity phosphorylating tyrosine in polyoma T antigen immunoprecipitates. Nature 285:167–169, 1980.
4. Witte ON, Dasgupta A, Baltimore D: Abelson murine leukaemia virus protein is phosphorylated in vitro to form phosphotyrosine. Nature 283:826–831, 1980.
5. Ushiro H, Cohen S: Identification of phosphotyrosine as a product of epidermal growth factor-activated protein kinase in A-431 cell membranes. J Biol Chem 2555:8363–8365, 1980.
6. Kasuga M, Karlsson FA, Kahn CR: Insulin stimulates the phosphorylation of the 95,000-dalton subunit of its own receptor. Science 215:185–187, 1982.
7. Ek B, Westermork B, Warteson A, Heldin CH: Stimulation of tyrosine-specific phosphorylation by platelet-derived growth factor. Nature 295:419–420, 1982.
8. Doolittle RF, Hinkapillar MW, Hood LE, et al: Simian sarcoma virus onc gene, v-sis, is derived from the gene (or genes) encoding a platelet-derived growth factor. Science 221:275–277, 1983.
9. Waterfield MD, Scrace GT, Whittle N, et al: Platelet-derived growth factor is structurally related to the putative transforming protein p28sis of simian sarcoma virus. Nature 304:35–39, 1983.
10. Ullrich A, Coussens L, Hayflick JS, et al: Human epidermal growth factor receptor cDNA sequence and aberrant expression of the amplified gene in A431 epidermoid carcinoma cells. Nature 309:418–425, 1984.
11. Manning G, Whyte DB, Martinez R, et al: The protein kinase complement of the human genome. Science 298:1912–1934, 2002.
12. Ullrich A, Schlessinger J: Signal transduction by receptors with tyrosine kinase activity. Cell 61:203–212, 1990.
13. Fantl WJ, Johnson DE, Williams LT: Signaling by receptor tyrosine kinases. Annu Rev Biochem 62:453–481, 1993.
14. van der Geer P, Hunter T, Lundberg RA: Receptor protein-tyrosine kinases and their signal transduction pathways. Ann Rev Cell Biol 10:251–337, 1994.

15. Heldin C-H: Dimerization of cell surface receptors in signal transduction. Cell 80:213–223, 1995.
16. Weiss A, Schlessinger J: Switching signals on or off by receptor dimerization. Cell 94:277–280, 1998.
17. Burgess AW, Cho H-S, Elgenbrot C, et al: An open-and-shut case? Recent insights into the activation of EGF/ErbB receptors. Mol Cell 12:541–552, 2003.
18. Tzahar E, Yarden Y: The ErbB-2/HER2 oncogenic receptor of adenocarcinomas: From orphanhood to multiple stromal ligands. Biochem Biophys Acta 1377:25–37, 1988.
19. Alroy I, Yarden Y: The ErbB signaling network in embryogenesis and oncogenesis: Signal diversification through combinatorial ligand-receptor interactions. FEBS Lett 410:83–86, 1997.
20. Perrimon N, Perkins LA: There must be 50 ways to rule the signal: The case of the Drosophila EGF receptor. Cell 89:13–16, 1997.
21. Cho Y-S, Leahy DJ: Structure of the extracellular region of HER3 reveals an interdomain Tether. Science 297:1330–1333, 2002.
22. Ferguson KM, Berger MB, Mendrola JM, et al: EGF activates its receptor by removing interactions that autoinhibit ectodomain dimerization. Mol Cell 2:507–517, 2003.
23. Garrett TP, McKern NM, Elleman LM, et al: Crystal structure of a truncated epidermal growth factor receptor extracellular domain bound to transforming grown factor alpha. Cell 110:763–773, 2002.
24. Garrett TP, McKern NM, et al: The crystal structure of a truncated ErbB2 ectodomain reveals an active conformation, poised to interact with other ErbB receptors. Mol Cell 2:495–505, 2003.
25. Lee J, Pilch PF: The insulin receptor: Structure, function and signaling. Am J Physiol 266:C319–C334, 1994.
26. Frasca F, Pandini G, Scalia P, et al: Insulin receptor isoform A, a newly recognized, high-affinity insulin-like gr receptor in fetal and cancer cells. Mol Cell Biol 5:3278–3288, 1999.
27. De Meyts P, Whittaker J: Structural biology of insulin and IGF1 receptors: Implications for drug design. Nature Rev 1:769–783, 2002.
28. DeMeyts P, Urso B, Christofferson CT, Shymko RM: Mechanism of insulin and IGF-1 activation and signal transduction specificity. Ann N Y Acad Sci 766:388–401, 1995.
29. Yip CC, Ottensmeyer: Three-dimensional structural interactions of insulin and its receptor. J Biol Chem 27:27329–27332, 2003.
30. McInnes C, Sykes BD: Growth factor receptors: Structure, mechanism, and drug discovery. Biopolymers 43:339–366, 1997.
31. Blakesley VA, Scrimgeour A, Esposito D, LeRoith D: Signaling via the insulin-like growth factor-I receptor: Does it differ from insulin receptor signaling. Cytokine & Growth Factor Rev 153–159, 1996.

32. Garrett TP, McKern NM, Lou M, et al: Crystal structure of the first three domains of the type-1 insulin-like growth factor receptor. Nature 394:395–399, 1998.
33. Slessenger J, Plotnikov AN, Ibrahimi OA, et al: Crystal structure of a teranary FGF-FGFR-heparin complex reveals a dual role of rheparin in FGFR binding and dimerization. Mol Cell 3:743–750, 2000.
34. Plotnikov AN, Schlessinger J, Hubbard SR, Mohammadi M: Structural basis for FGF receptor dimerization and activation. Cell 98:641–650, 1999.
35. Moy FJ, Safran M, Seddon AP, et al: Properly oriented heparin-decasaccharide-induced dimers are the biologically active form of basic fibroblast growth factor. Biochem 36:4782–4791, 1997.
36. DiGabriele AD, Lax I, Chen DI, et al: Structure of a heparin-linked biologically active dimer of fibroblast growth factor. Nature 393:812–817, 1998.
37. Mangasarian K, Li Y, Mansukhani A, Basilico C: Mutation associated with Crouszon syndrome causes ligand-independent dimerization and activation of FGF receptor-2. J Cell Physiol 172:117–125, 1997.
38. Steinberger D, Vriend G, Mulliken JB, Muller U: The mutations in FGFR2-associated craniosynostoses are clustered in five structural elements of immunoglobulin-like domain III of the receptor. Hum Genet 102:145–150, 1998.
39. Robertson SC, Meyer AN, Hart KC, et al: Activating mutations in the extracellular domain in the fibroblast growth factor receptor 2 function by disruption of the disulfide bond in the third immunoglobulin-like domain. Proc Natl Acad Sci U S A 95:4567–4572, 1998.
40. Horton WA: Fibroblast growth factor receptor 3 and the human chondrodysplasias. Curr Opin Pediatr 9:437–442, 1997.
41. Neilson KM, Friesel R: Ligand-independent activation of fibroblast growth factor receptors by point mutations in the extracellular, transmembrane, and kinase domain. J Biol Chem 271:25049–25057, 1996.
42. Donis-Keller H, et al: Mutations in the Ret proto-oncogene are associated with MEN 2A and FMTC. Hum Mol Genet 7:851–856, 1993.
43. Edery P, Eng C, Munnich A, Lyonnet S: RET in human development and oncogenesis. Bioessays 19:389–395, 1997.
44. Jing S, Wen D, Yu Y, et al: GDNF induced activation of the Ret protein tyrosine kinase is mediated by GDNFR-alpha, a novel receptor for GDNF. Cell 85:1113–1124, 1996
45. Enokido Y, de Sauvage F, Hongo J-A, et al: GFRα-4 and the tyrosine kinase Ret form a functional receptor complex for persephin. Curr Biol 8:1019–1022, 1998.

46. Mulligan LM, Kwok JB, Healy CS, et al: Germ-Line mutations of the Ret proto-oncogene in multiple endocrine neoplasia type 2A. Nature 363:458–460, 1993.
47. Hostra RMW, Landsuater RM, Ceccherini I, et al: A mutation in the Ret proto-oncogene associated with endocrine neoplasia type 2B and sporadic medullary thyroid carcinoma. Nature 367:375–376, 1994.
48. Carlson KM, Dou S, Chi D, et al: Single missense mutation in the tyrosine kinase catalytic domain of the Ret proto-oncogene is associated with multiple endocrine neoplasia Type 2B. Proc Natl Acad Sci U S A 91:1579–1583, 1994.
49. Romeo G, Ronchetto P, Luo Y, et al: Point mutations affecting the tyrosine kinase domain of the Ret proto-oncogene in Hirschsprung's disease. Nature 367:377–378, 1994.
50. Edery P, Lyonnet S, Mulligan LM, et al: Mutations of the Ret proto-oncogene in Hirschsprung's disease. Nature 367:378–380, 1994.
51. Grieco M, Santoro M, Berlingieri MT, et al: PTC is a novel rearranged form of the Ret proto-oncogene and is frequently detected in vivo in human thyroid papillary carcinomas. Cell 60:557–563, 1990.
52. Bongarzone I, Monzini N, Borrello MG, et al: Molecular characterization of a thyroid tumor-specific transforming sequence formed by the fusion of Ret tyrosine-kinase and the regulatory subunit RI alpha of cyclic AMP protein kinaseA. Mol Cell Biol 13:358–366, 1993.
53. Santoro M, Dathan NA, Berlingieri MT, et al: Molecular characterization of Ret/PTC3: A novel rearranged version of the Ret proto-oncogene in a human thyroid papillary carcinoma. Oncogene 9:509–516, 1994.
54. Pelet A, Geneste O, Edery P, et al: Various mechanisms cause RET-mediated signaling defects in Hirschsprung's disease. J Clin Invest 101:1415–1423, 1998.
55. Songyang Z, Carraway KL III, Eck MJ, et al: Catalytic specificity of protein tyrosine kinases is critical for selective signaling. Nature 373:536–539, 1995.
56. Chang HW, Aoki M, Fruman D, et al: Transformation of chicken cells by the gene encoding the catalytic subunit of PI 3-kinase. Science 276:1848–1850, 1997.
57. Hanks SK, Hunter T: Protein kinases 6. The eukaryotic protein kinase superfamily: Kinase (catalytic) domain structure and classification. FASEB J 9:576–596, 1995.
58. Knighton DR, Zheng J, Ten Eyck LF, et al: Crystal structure of the catalytic subunit of cyclic adenosine monophosphate-dependent protein kinase. Science 253:407–414, 1991.
59. Tornqvist HE, Pierce MW, Frackelton AR, et al: Identification of insulin receptor tyrosine residues autophosphorylated in vitro. J Biol Chem 262:10212–10219, 1987.

60. Hubbard SR, Mohammadi M, Schlessinger J: Autoregulatory mechanisms in protein-tyrosine kinases. J Biol Chem 273:11987–11990, 1998.

61. Tornqvist HE, Gunsalus JR, Nemenoff RA, et al: Identification of the insulin receptor tyrosine residues undergoing insulin-stimulated phosphorylation in intact rat hepatoma cells. J Biol Chem 263:350–359, 1988.

62. Rosen OM, Herrera R, Olowe Y, et al: Phosphorylation activates the insulin receptor tyrosine protein kinase. Proc Natl Acad Sci U S A 80:3237–3240, 1983.

63. Tornqvist HE, Avruch J: Relationship of site-specific beta subunit tyrosine autophosphorylation to insulin activation of the insulin receptor (tyrosine) protein kinase activity. J Biol Chem 263:4593–4601, 1988.

64. Ellis L, Clauser E, Morgan DO, et al: Replacement of insulin receptor tyrosine residues 1162 and 1163 compromises insulin-stimulated kinase activity and uptake of 2-deoxyglucose. Cell 45:721–732, 1986.

65. Hubbard SR, Wei L, Ellis L, Hendrickson WA: Crystal structure of the tyrosine kinase domain of the human insulin receptor. Nature 372:746–754, 1994.

66. Hubbard SR: Crystal structure of the activated insulin receptor tyrosine kinase in complex with peptide substrate and ATP analog. EMBO J 16:5572–5581, 1997.

67. Mohammadi M, Schlessinger J, Hubbard SR: Structure of the FGF receptor tyrosine kinase domain reveals a novel autoinhibitory mechanism. Cell 86:577–587, 1996.

68. Taylor SI: Molecular mechanisms of insulin resistance. Diabetes 41:1473–1490, 1992.

69. Mossie K, Jallal B, Alves F, et al: Colon carcinoma kinase-4 defines a new subclass of the receptor tyrosine kinase family. Oncogene 11:2179–2184, 1995.

70. Wybenga-Groot LE, Baskin B, Ong SH, et al: Structural basis for autoinhibition of the Ephb2 receptor tyrosine kinase by the unphosphorylated juxtamembrane region. Cell 106:745–757, 2001

71. Kolibaba KS, Druker BJ: Protein tyrosine kinases and cancer. Biochem Biophys Acta 1333:217–248, 1997.

72. Ross AH, Baltimore D, Eisen HN: Phosphotyrosine-containing proteins isolated by affinity chromatography with antibodies to a synthetic hapten. Nature 294:654–656, 1981.

73. Margolis B, Rhee SG, Felder S, et al: EGF induces tyrosine phosphorylation of phospholipase C-II: A potential mechanism for EGF receptor signaling. Cell 57:1101–1107, 1989.

74. Meisenhelder J, Suh PG, Rhee SG, Hunter T: Phospholipase C-gamma is a substrate for the PDGF and EGF receptor protein-tyrosine kinases in vivo and in vitro. Cell 57:1109–1122, 1989.

75. Whitman M, Downes CP, Keeler M, et al: Type I phosphatidylinositol kinase makes a novel inositol phospholipid, phosphatidylinisitol-3-phosphate. Nature 332:644–646, 1988.

76. Coughlin SR, Escobedo JA, Williams LT: Role of phosphatidylinositol kinase in PDGF receptor signal transduction. Science 243:1191–1194, 1989.

77. Kazlauskas A, Cooper JA: Phosphorylation of the PDGF receptor beta subunit creates a tight binding site for phosphatidylinositol 3 kinase. EMBO J 9:3279–3286, 1990.

78. Fantl WJ, Escobedo JA, Martin GA, et al: Distinct phosphotyrosines on a growth factor receptor bind to specific molecules that mediate different signaling pathways. Cell 69:413–423, 1992.

79. Escobedo JA, Kaplan DR, Kavanaugh WM, et al: A phosphatidylinositol-3 kinase binds to platelet-derived growth factor receptors through a specific receptor sequence containing phosphotyrosine. Mol Cell Biol 11:1125–1132, 1991.

80. Sadowski I, Stone JC, Pawson T: A noncatalytic domain conserved among cytoplasmic protein-tyrosine kinases modifies the kinase function and transforming activity of Fujinami sarcoma virus P130gag-fps. Mol Cell Biol 6:4396–4408, 1986.

81. Rhee SG, Choi KD: Regulation of inositol phospholipid-specific phospholipase C isozymes. J Biol Chem 267:12393–12396, 1992.

82. Bollag G, McCormick F: Regulators and effectors of ras proteins. Ann Rev of Cell Biol 7:601–632, 1991.

83. Mayer BJ, Hamaguchi M, Hanafusa H: A novel viral oncogene with structural similarity to phospholipase C. Nature 332:272–275, 1988.

84. Matsuda M, Mayer BJ, Fukui Y, Hanafusa H: Binding of transforming protein, P47gag-crk, to a broad range of phosphotyrosine-containing proteins. Science 248:1537–1539, 1990.

85. Koch CA, Anderson D, Moran MF, et al: SH2 and SH3 domains: Elements that control interactions of cytoplasmic signaling proteins. Science 252:668–674, 1991.

86. Pawson T: Protein modules and signaling networks. Nature 373:573–580, 1995.

87. Songyang Z, Shoelson SE, Chaudhurl M, et al: SH2 domains recognize specific phosphopeptide sequences. Cell 72:767–778, 1993.

88. Kavanaugh WM, Williams LT: An alternative to SH2 domains for binding tyrosine-phosphorylated proteins. Science 266:1862–1865, 1994.

89. Blaikie P, Immanuel D, Wu J, et al: A region in Shc distinct from the SH2 domain can bind tyrosine-phosphorylated growth factor receptors. J Biol Chem 269:32031–32034, 1994.

90. van der Geer P, Pawson T: The PTB domain. TIBS 20:277–280, 1995.

91. White MF, Livingston JN, Backer JM, et al: Mutation of the insulin receptor at tyrosine 960 inhibits signal transmission but does not affect its tyrosine kinase activity. Cell 54:641–649, 1988.

92. Sun XJ, Rothenberg P, Kahn CR, et al: Structure of the insulin receptor substrate IRS-1 defines a unique signal transduction protein. Nature 382:73–77, 1991.

93. Yenush L, White MF: The IRS-signaling system during insulin and cytokine action. Bioassays 19:491–500, 1997.

94. Araki E, Lipes MA, Patti ME, et al: Alternative pathway of insulin signaling in mice with targeted disruption of the IRS-1 gene. Nature 372:186–190, 1994.

95. Withers DJ, Gutierrez JS, Towery H, et al: Disruption of IRS-2 causes type 2 diabetes in mice. Nature 391:900–904, 1998.

96. Bruning JC, Winnay J, Bonner-Weir S, et al: Development of a novel polygenic model of NIDDM in mice heterozygous for IR and IRS-1 null alleles. Cell 88:561–572, 1997.

97. Holgado-Madruga M, Emlet DR, Moscatello DK, et al: A Grb2-associated docking protein in EGF- and insulin-receptor signaling. Nature 379:560–556, 1996.

98. Yenush L, Fernandez R, Myers MG Jr, et al: The *Drosophila* insulin receptor activates multiple signaling pathways but requires insulin receptor substrate proteins for DNA synthesis. Mol Cell Biol 16:2509–2517, 1996.

99. Songyang Z, Cantley L: Recognition and specificity in protein tyrosine kinase-mediated signaling. TIBS 20:470–475, 1995.

100. Bertotti A, Comoglio PM: Tyrosine kinase signal specificity: Lessons from the HGF receptor. Trends Biochem Sci 10:527–533, 2003.

101. Darnell JE Jr: STATs and gene regulation. Science 277:1630–1635, 1997.

102. Bos JL: Ras oncogenes in human cancer: A review [published erratum appears in Cancer Res 1990 Feb 15;50(4)352.] Cancer Research 49(17):4682–4689, 1989.

103. Jiminez C, Jones DR, Rodriquez-Viciana P, et al: Identification and characterization of a new oncogene derived from the regulatory subunit of phosphoinositide 3-kinase. EMBO J 17:743–753, 1998.

104. Chang HW, Aoki M, Fruman D, et al: Transformation of chicken cells by the gene encoding the catalytic subunit of PI 3-kinase. Science 276:1848–1850, 1997.

105. Staal SP: Molecular cloning of the akt oncogene and its human homologues AKT1 and AKT2: Amplification of AKT1 in a primary human gastric adenocarcinoma. Proc Natl Acad Sci U S A 84:5034–5037, 1987.

106. Li J, Yen C, Liaw D, et al: *PTEN*, a putative protein tyrosine

phosphatase gene mutated in human brain, breast, and prostate cancer. Science 275:1943–1947, 1997.

107. Maehama T, Dixon JE: The tumor suppressor, PTEN/MMAC1, dephosphorylates the lipid second messenger, phosphatidylinositol 3,4,5-trisphosphate. J Biol Chem 273:13375–13378, 1998.

108. Bos JL: Ras-like GTPases. Biochim Biophys Acta 1333:19–31, 1997.

109. Schlessinger J: How receptor tyrosine kinases activate Ras. TIBS 18:273–275, 1993.

110. Marshall MS: The effector interactions of p21ras. TIBS 18:250–255, 1993.

111. Avruch J, Zhang X-F, Kyriakis JM: Ras meets Raf. TIBS 19:279–283, 1994.

112. Chuang E, Barnard D, Hettich L, et al: Critical binding and regulatory interactions between Ras and Raf occur through a small, stable N-terminal domain of Raf and specific Ras effector residues. Mol Cell Biol 14:5318–5325, 1994.

113. Hu CD, Kariya K, Tamada M, et al: Cysteine-rich region of Raf-1 interacts with activator domain of post-translationally modified Ha-Ras. J Biol Chem 270(51):30274–30277, 1995.

114. Luo Z, Diaz B, Marshall MS, Avruch J: An intact raf zinc finger is required for optimal binding to processed ras and for ras-dependent raf activation in situ. Mol Cell Biol 17:46–53, 1997.

115. Mineo C, Anderson RG, White M: Physical association with Ras enhances activation of membrane-bound Raf (Raf CAAX). J Biol Chem 272:10345–10348, 1997.

116. Tzivion G, Luo Z, Avruch J: A dimeric 14-3-3 protein is an essential cofactor for Raf kinase activity. Nature 394:88–92, 1998.

117. Kyriakis JM, App H, Zhang XF, et al: Raf-1 activates MAP kinase-kinase. Nature 358:417–421, 1992.

118. Malumbreas M, Pellicer A: Ras pathways to cell cycle control and cell transformation. Frontiers Biosci 3:d887–d912, 1998.

119. Rodriquez-Viciana , Warne PH, Vanhaesebroeck B, et al: Activation of phosphoinositide 3-kinase by interaction with Ras and by point mutation. EMBO J 15:2442–2451, 1996.

120. Klinghoffer RA, Duckworth B, Valius M, et al: Platelet-derived growth factor-dependent activation of phosphatidylinositol 3-kinase is regulated by receptor binding of SH2-domain-containing proteins which influence Ras activity. Mol Cell Biol 16:5905–5914, 1996.

121. Rodriquez-Viciana, Warne PH, Dhand R, et al: Phosphatidylinositol-3-OH kinase as a direct target of Ras. Nature 370:527–532, 1994.

122. Courtneidge SA, Heber A: An 85 kd protein complexed with middle T antigen and pp60c-src: A possible phosphatidylinositol kinase. Cell 50:1031–1037, 1987.

123. Vanhaesebroeck B, Leevers SJ, Panayotou G, Waterfield MD: Phosphoinositide 3-kinases: A conserved family of signal transducers. TIBS 22:267–272, 1997.

124. Shepherd PR, Withers DJ, Siddle K: Phosphoinositide 3-kinase: The key switch mechanism in insulin signaling. Biochem J 333:471–490, 1998.

125. Toker A, Cantley L: Signaling through the lipid products of phosphoinositide-3-OH kinase. Nature 387:673–676, 1997.

126. Sulis ML, Parsons R: PTEN: From pathology to biology. Trends Cell Biol 13:478–483, 2003.

127. Clement S, Krause U, Desmendt F, et al: The lipid phosphatase SHIP controls insulin sensitivity. Nature 409:92–97, 2001.

128. Morris JZ, Tissenbaum HA, Ruvkun G: A phosphatidylinositol-3-OH kinase family member regulating longevity and diapause in *caenorhabditis elegans*. Nature 382:536–539, 1996.

129. Kimura KD, Tissenbaum HA, Liu Y, Ruvkun G: daf-2, and insulin receptor-like gene that regulates longevity and diapause in *caenorhabditis elegans*. Science 277:942–946, 1997.

130. Mayer BJ, Ren R, Clark KL, Baltimore D: A putative modular domain present in diverse signaling proteins. Cell 73:629–630, 1993.

131. Haslam RJ, Koide HB, Hemmings BA: Pleckstrin domain homology. Nature 363:309–310, 1993.

132. Lemmon MA, Ferguson KM, Schlessinger J: PH domains: Diverse sequences with a common fold recruit signaling molecules to the cell surface. Cell 85:621–624, 1996.

133. Shaw S: The pleckstrin homology domain: An intriguing multifunctional protein module. Bioessays 18:35–46, 1996.

134. Touhara K, Inglese J, Pitcher JA, et al: Binding of G protein βγ-subunits to pleckstrin homology domains. J Biol Chem 269:10217–10220, 1994.

135. Pitcher JA, Touhara K, Payne SE, Lefkowitz, RJ: Pleckstrin homology domain-mediated membrane association and activation of the β-adrenergic receptor kinase requires coordinate interaction with Gβγ subunits and lipid. J Biol Chem 270:11707–11710, 1995.

136. Mahadevan D, Thanki N, Singh J, et al: Structural studies on the PH domains of Dbl, SOS1 IRS-1 and βARK1 and their differential binding to Gβγ subunits. Biochem 34:9111–9117, 1995.

137. Harlan JE, Hajduk PH, Yoon H-S, Feslk SW: Pleckstrin homology domains bind to phsophatidylinositol-4,-bisphosphate. Nature 371:168–170, 1994.

138. Rameh LE, Arvidsson A-K, Carraway KL III, et al: A comparative analysis of the phosphoinositide binding specificity of pleckstrin homology domains. J Biol Chem 272:22059–22066, 1997.

139. Voliovitch H, Schindler DG, Hadari YR, et al: Tyrosine phosphorylation of insulin receptor substrate-1 in vivo depends upon the presence of its pleckstrin homology region. J Biol Chem 270:18083–18087, 1995.

140. Zheng Y, Zangrilli D, Cerione RA, Eva A: The pleckstrin homology domain mediates transformation by oncogenic Dbl through specific intracellular targeting. J Biol Chem 271:19017–19020, 1996.

141. Lemmon MA: Phosphoinositide recognition domains. Traffic 4:201–213, 2003.

142. Pawson T, Scott JD: Signaling through scaffold, anchoring, and adaptor proteins. Science 278:2075–2080, 1997.

143. Sudol M: From Src homology domains to other signaling modules: Proposal of the "protein recognition code." Oncogene 17:1469–1474, 1998.

144. Lu P-J, Zhou XZ, Shen M, KP Lu: Function of WW domains as phosphoserine- or phosphothreonine-binding modules. Science 283:1325–1328, 1999.

145. Ponting CP, Phillips C, Davies KE, Blake DJ: PDZ domains: Targeting signaling molecules to sub-membranous sites. Bioessays 19:469–479, 1997.

146. Tonks NK, Diltz CD, Fischer EH: Purification of the major protein-tyrosine-phosphatases of human placenta. J Biol Chem 263(14):722–730, 1988.

147. Denu JM, Stuckey JA, Saper MA, Dixon JE: Form and function in protein dephosphorylation. Cell 87:361–364, 1996.

148. Streuli M: Protein tyrosine phosphatases in signaling. Curr Opin Cell Biol 8:182–188, 1996.

149. Weiss UF, Daub H, Ullrich A: Novel mechanisms of RTK signal generation. Curr Opin Genet & Dev 7:80–86, 1997.

150. Elchebly M, Payette P, Michaliszyn E, et al: Increased insulin sensitivity and obesity resistance in mice lacking the prote-phosphatase-1B gene. Science 283:1544–1548, 1999.

151. Zabolotny JM, Bence-Hanulec KK, Stricker-Krongrad A, et al: PTP1B regulates leptin signal transduction in vivo. Dev Cell 4:489–495, 2002.

152. Boute N, Boubekeur S, Lacasa D, Issad T: Dynamics of the interaction between the insulin receptor and protein tyrosine-phosphatase 1B in living cells. EMBO reports 4:313–319, 2003.

153. Johnson TO, Ermolieff J, Jirousek MR: Protein tyrosine phosphatase 1B inhibitors for diabetes. Nat Rev Drug Discov 1:696–709, 2002.

154. Vieira AV, Lamaze C, Schmid SL: Control of EGF receptor signaling by clathrin-mediated endocytosis. Science 274:2086–2089, 1996.

155. Mukherjee S, Ghosh RN, Maxfield FR: Endocytosis Physiol Rev 77:759–803, 1997.

156. Levkowitz G, an H, Zamir E, et al: c-Cbl/Sli-1 regulates endocytic sorting

and ubiquitination of the epidermal growth factor receptor. Genes & Dev 12:3663–3674, 1998.

157. Morrione A: Crb10 adapter protein as regulator of insulin-like growth factor receptor signaling. J Cell Phys 197:307–311, 2003.

158. Kile BT, Schulman BA, Alexander WS, et al: The SOCS box: A tale of destruction and degradation. Trends Biochem Sci 27:235–241, 2002.

159. Petersen KF, Shulman GI: Pathogenesis of skeletal muscle insulin resistance in type 2 diabetes mellitus. Am J Cardiol 90:11G–18G, 2002.

160. White MF: IRS proteins and the common path to diabetes. Am J Physiol Endocrinol Metab 283:E413–E422, 2002.

161. Johnston AM, Pirola L, Van Obberghen E: Molecular mechanisms of insulin receptor substrate protein-mediated modulation of insulin signaling. FEBS Lett 546:32–36, 2003.

Hormone Signaling via Cytokine Receptors

Marlyse A. Debrincat and Douglas J. Hilton

INTRODUCTION AND HISTORY

Cytokines (from the Greek *kytos* meaning cell and *kinein* to move) are secreted proteins that function as potent mediators in important biologic processes, such as development, fertility, lactation, hematopoiesis, and immunity.[1] In 1957, the discovery of the first cytokine, interferon, was described.[2] This heralded several decades of research and isolation of a diverse array of cytokines. The mechanisms by which cytokines act began to be clarified in the 1980s and 1990s by the molecular cloning of cytokine receptors and signaling proteins.[3,4] Cytokines initiate cell communication by binding to specific cell surface receptors. Signals received by the receptor's signal-transducing subunit are transmitted to downstream target proteins through the recruitment of cytoplasmic proteins. A series of protein-protein interactions, phosphorylation events, and DNA binding results in a modulation of gene expression and subsequent biologic response by the target cell.[3,4]

Cytokines share many of their characteristic properties with other groups of protein mediators, such as hormones. It is difficult to distinguish between these two groups. However, one difference is that classic hormones are produced by specialized cells; for example, growth hormone is produced by the anterior pituitary. In contrast, cytokines are usually produced by less specialized cells, and it is common for several unrelated cell types to produce the same cytokine. Despite their differences, cytokines and hormones function as extracellular signaling molecules with fundamentally similar mechanisms of action. This is highlighted by common structural features found in both cytokine and hormone receptors (i.e., IL-2, IL-3, IL-4, IL-5, IL-6, IL-7, GM-CSF, G-CSF, erythropoietin, prolactin, and growth hormone).[3–8] For the purposes of this chapter, the term *cytokine* will be used to describe secreted proteins, including hormones, that utilize cytokine receptors for signaling.

Cell surface receptors may be classified on the basis of sequence similarity, structural motifs, and biochemical function. At least five families of receptors have been identified (Fig. 9-1). This chapter focuses on cell signaling via receptors that utilize the Janus kinase (JAK) and signal transducer and activator (STAT) signal transduction pathway, namely, the hemopoietin/interferon or class I/II cytokine receptor family. The class I/II cytokine receptor family is characterized by their conserved amino acid residues within the receptor extracellular domains.[9,10] The features of these cytokine receptors, their signaling pathways, and their regulatory mechanisms are outlined below.

THE HEMOPOIETIN/INTERFERON (CLASS I AND II) CYTOKINE RECEPTORS

CLASS I CYTOKINE RECEPTORS

There are over 20 known receptors that share features with cytokine receptors designated as class I. These include receptors for growth hormone (GH), erythropoietin (EPO), prolactin (PRL), granulocyte colony-stimulating factor (G-CSF), several of the interleukins (IL-2 -IL-7, IL-9, IL-11, IL-13, and IL-15), thrombopoietin (TPO), leukemia inhibitory factor (LIF), ciliary neurotrophic factor (CNTF), oncostatin M (OSM), and leptin[1] (Fig. 9-2).

FEATURES OF CLASS I RECEPTORS

Class I cytokine receptors are transmembrane proteins generally composed of a cytokine-specific binding subunit and one or more signal-transducing subunit(s) with limited (14% to 44%) primary amino acid sequence identity (Box 9-1).[11] These receptors lack intrinsic kinase activity. The extracellular domain contains one or two hemopoietin receptor or cytokine-binding domains (CBD) typically composed of two fibronectin type III–like modules, each consisting of approximately 100 amino acids.[12–14] Both modules contain seven anti-parallel β-strands folded together to form barrel-like structures. The hemopoietin domain is also characterized by conserved cysteine and tryptophan residues at the N-terminal CBD and a tryptophan-serine-X-tryptophan-serine (W-S-X-W-S) motif at the C-terminal CBD (where X refers to a nonconserved amino acid residue). The W-S-X-W-S motif appears to stabilize the receptor by forming many contacts with adjacent β-strands.[15,16]

All receptor chains have a single transmembrane domain of 22 to 28 amino acids, which is followed by a **membrane proximal domain,** a critical region involved in receptor/JAK interaction. This domain typically contains the conserved box 1 and box 2 motifs.[17] The box 1 motif is composed of eight proline residues and determines the specificity of JAK association and activation. Several cytokine receptors, such as those for prolactin, growth hormone, and erythropoietin,

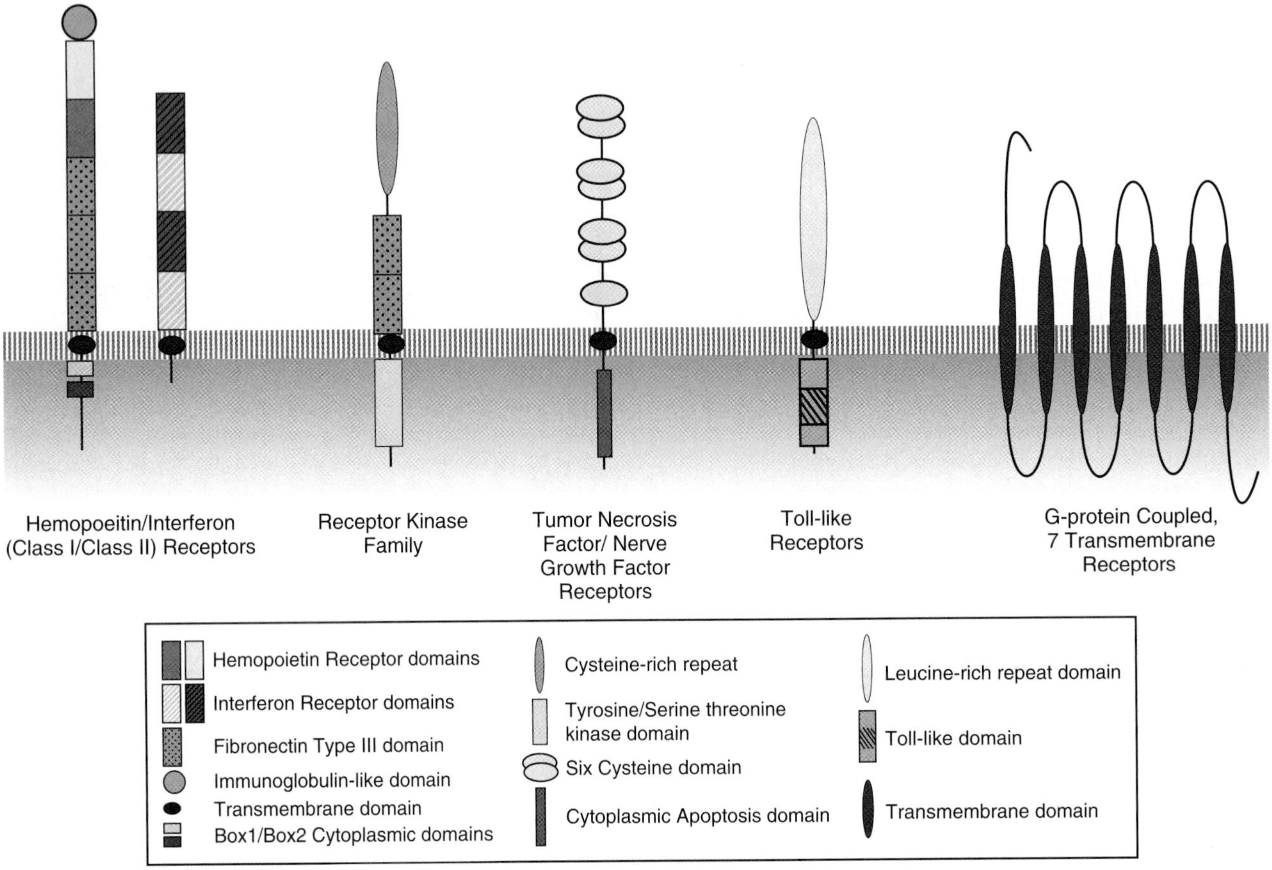

Figure 9-1 Schematic view of receptor families.

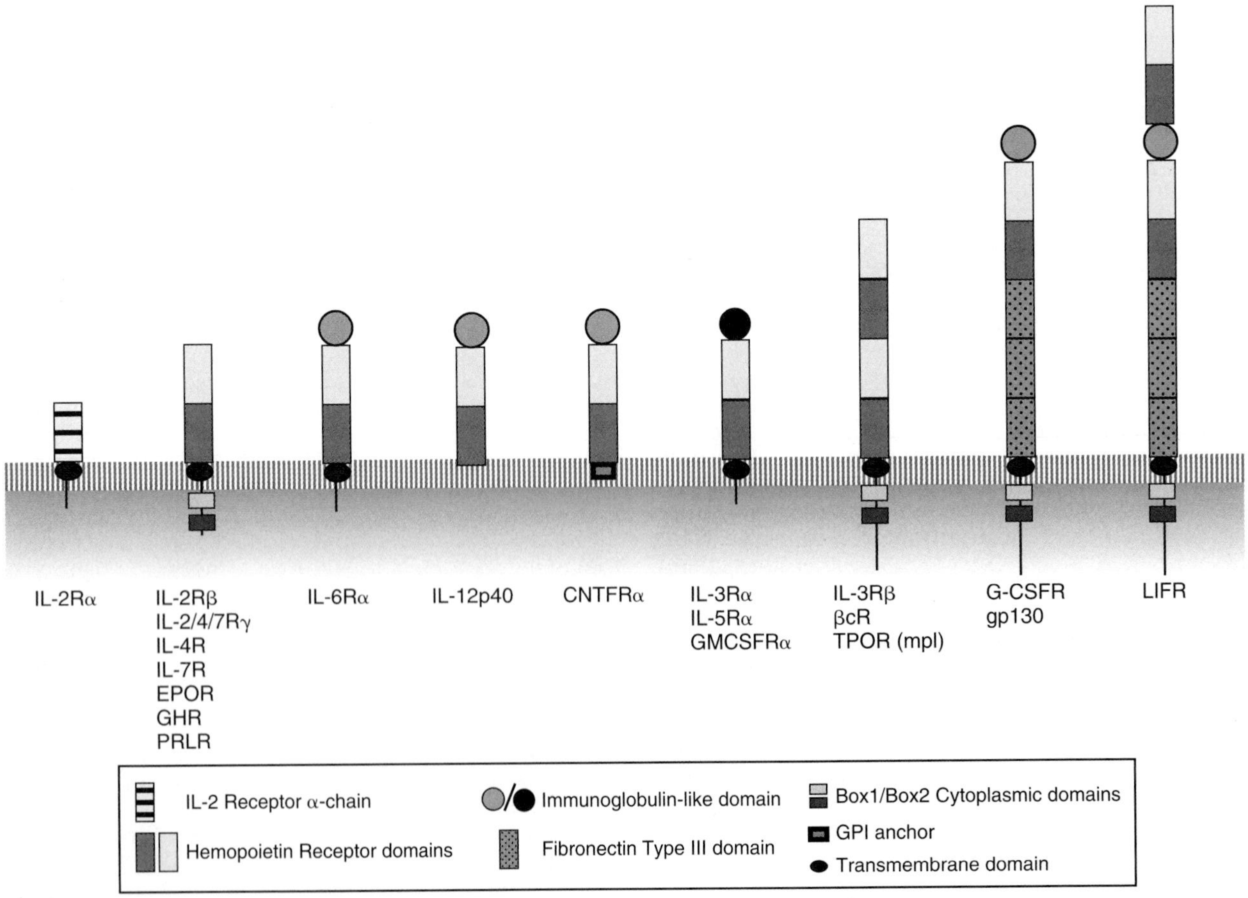

Figure 9-2 Schematic view of class I receptors.

Box 9-1   Summary of Class I Cytokine Receptor Features

1. A single membrane pass receptor made up of homodimers or heterodimer/oligomeric assemblies
2. Two or more fibronectin III domains
3. Two pairs of cysteine residues and a conserved tryptophan adjacent to the cysteine in the N-terminal region
4. An extracellular tryptophan-serine-X-tryptophan-serine (W-S-X-W-S) motif or equivalent
5. No intrinsic enzymatic activity
6. Two conserved membrane proximal sequences in the cytoplasmic domain, referred to as box 1 and box 2.
7. Ligands share a similar four-α-helical bundle structure.[1]

utilize the box 1 motif for interaction with JAK2 (reviewed in Ref. 18). Receptors that lack a classic box 1 motif, such as the IL-2 receptor γc chain, can still activate JAKs. These receptors use alternate sites within the membrane proximal region.[1,18] Box 2 is conserved in only about half the members of the class I receptor family; it comprises a cluster of hydrophobic amino acids, followed by negatively charged residues, and ends with one or two positively charged amino acids.[14]

To add to the complexity of cytokine receptors, some receptors that are designated as class I comprise more than one type of receptor. These include receptors that lack transmembrane and cytoplasmic domains. Such receptors, described as soluble, have been implicated in both the enhancement and reduction of biologic effects mediated by their cognate cytokine. For example, the IL-13-binding protein, or IL-13Rα2, is structurally distinct from the originally identified cell surface IL-13 receptor component , IL-13Rα1. IL-13Rα2 was shown to act as a potent inhibitor of IL-13 binding, demonstrating a possible in vivo role in the modulation of IL-13-mediated responses.[19] Another example is IL-12, which is composed of two covalently linked polypeptide chains defined as p35 and p40. The p35 subunit shares homology to cytokines, while the p40 subunit is a soluble receptor-like subunit that displays many of the hallmarks of class I receptors. Other soluble receptors that

belong to the hemopoietin family include the α chains of the IL-2, IL-7, IL-9, GM-CSF, and LIF receptors as well as the NR6 receptor.[20,21]

CLASS II CYTOKINE RECEPTORS

The interferon or class II receptor family consists of at least 12 members (Fig. 9-3; Box 9-2). These receptors display some structural similarities to the class I receptors, for example, conserved cysteine residues and include receptors for type 1 (interferon-α, IFN-β, IFN-κ, and IFN-ω) and type 2 (IFN-γ) IFNs as well as IL-10. Other IL-10-related cytokines also utilize class II–designated receptors, such as IL-19, IL-20, IL-22/IL-TIF, IL-24 (MDA-7), and IL-26 (AKK-155).[22] The majority of class II receptor family members are classic transmembrane proteins that heterodimerize to form high-affinity binding sites for class II cytokines. The interactions between class II cytokines and their receptors can be quite complex. For example, one cytokine can bind to different receptor complexes, while that one particular receptor complex can bind to several cytokines, as is observed in the case of type I IFNs.[23] Overall, functional data on the class II cytokines and receptors reveal that they are essentially involved in the regulation of inflammatory and antiviral responses. For example, type 1 IFNs, IL-28, and IL-29 mediate antiviral responses through STAT2 activation, while IL-10 and IFN-γ have anti- or proinflammatory activities. Mice that are deficient in these factors are generally viable and fertile and show a phenotype only when challenged with pathogens (reviewed in Ref. 22).

The two remaining members of the class II receptor family show distinct characteristics. The tissue factor receptor appears to possess the structural characteristics of a cytokine receptor but does not bind any cytokine. Instead, it serves as a receptor for coagulation factor V11a.[24] The IL-22-binding protein has a typical class II cytokine-binding domain but no transmembrane and cytoplasmic domains. The absence of these domains indicates that it is a soluble receptor, which might act as either a cytokine carrier molecule or a cytokine antagonist in vivo.[25-28]

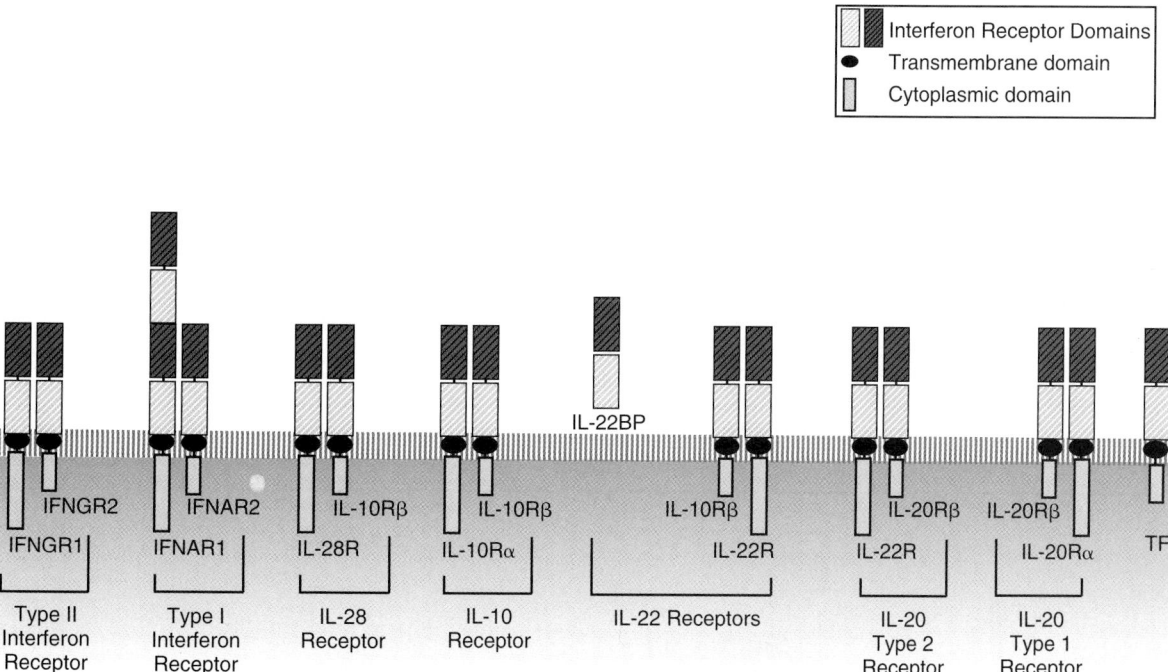

Figure 9-3   Class II receptor complexes. The II cytokine receptor family of 11 transmembrane proteins and 1 soluble protein. There are IFNGR1, IFNGR2, IFNAR1, IFNAR2, IL-10Rα, IL-10Rβ, IL-20Rα, IL-20Rβ, IL-22R, IL-28R, TF, and IL-22BP. These proteins form heterodimeric complexes (as shown above) to create binding sites for class II cytokines.

Box 9-2   Summary of Class II Cytokine Receptor Features

1. Consist of 1 soluble and 11 transmembrane proteins (20% to 30% amino acid identity in their extracellular domain). Receptors associate as heterodimers including common chains.
2. Two fibronectin type III domains (except IFNαR1 which has 4)
3. Conserved cysteine sequence (different position from class I receptors)
4. No tryptophan-serine-X-tryptophan-serine (W-S-X-W-S) motif
5. No intrinsic enzymatic activity
6. Ligands have a common six-α-helical structure. Can be monomers or homodimers and share 20% to 30% amino acid identity
7. Roles in antiviral and inflammatory responses

CLASS I/CLASS II CYTOKINE RECEPTORS SUBTYPES

Cytokines binding to class I/class II receptors often share receptor subunits but have a unique subunit that imparts specificity for the binding of a particular cytokine (Fig. 9-4). An example of this is the IL-2R system, in which IL-2 binds to a complex of IL-2Rα, IL-2Rβ, and IL-2Rγ and the IL-2Rγ chain is shared with IL-4, IL-7, IL-9, and IL-15. IL-15 also uses the IL-2Rβ chain. This feature may explain both the specificity and redundancy of some cytokines and gives rise to an additional level of receptor classification based on the cytokines with which they interact.[1,4,29-31]

The main subtypes of the cytokine receptor family are:

1. the gp130 family
2. the IL-2 (γc) receptor family
3. the IL-3 (βc) receptor family
4. the single-chain (homodimeric) receptor family
5. the interferon receptor family

Further detail relating to class 1/class II cytokine receptor subtypes is described in Table 9-1.

THE JAK-STAT PATHWAY

Cytokines mediate biologic responses in target cells by inducing receptor dimerization and activating intracellular signal transduction proteins. Although cytokines are able to activate many signaling pathways, including the JAK/STAT, Raf/MEK/ERK, and P13K/Akt pathways, this section will focus on the **JAK-STAT pathway**. The JAK-STAT pathway is integral in cell signaling by cytokines whose receptors are members of the cytokine receptor class I/II family. This pathway influences normal cell survival and growth mechanisms and was initially identified in a genetic screen to determine signaling molecules required for the interferon-induced transcription of known target genes. The JAK-STAT pathway represents a rapid signaling system and lends specificity to the signals that are induced by the different cytokines.

The JAK-STAT pathway is initiated by the binding of a cytokine to its receptor. On cytokine stimulation, receptors undergo dimerization, thereby inducing the juxtaposition of JAKs associated to the box 1 sequence of the receptor. JAKs are then activated by transphosphorylation. In turn, the activated JAKs phosphorylate multiple target proteins, including tyrosine residues in the cytoplasmic domains of the receptor and receptor-associated STAT monomers. The STAT monomers then form homodimers or heterodimers via reciprocal phosphotyrosine-SH2 domain interactions. These transcription factors translocate to the nucleus, where they bind to a specific DNA sequence adjacent to target genes. The transcription of a wide range of genes is initiated in this way (Fig. 9-5).[3,18,32-35]

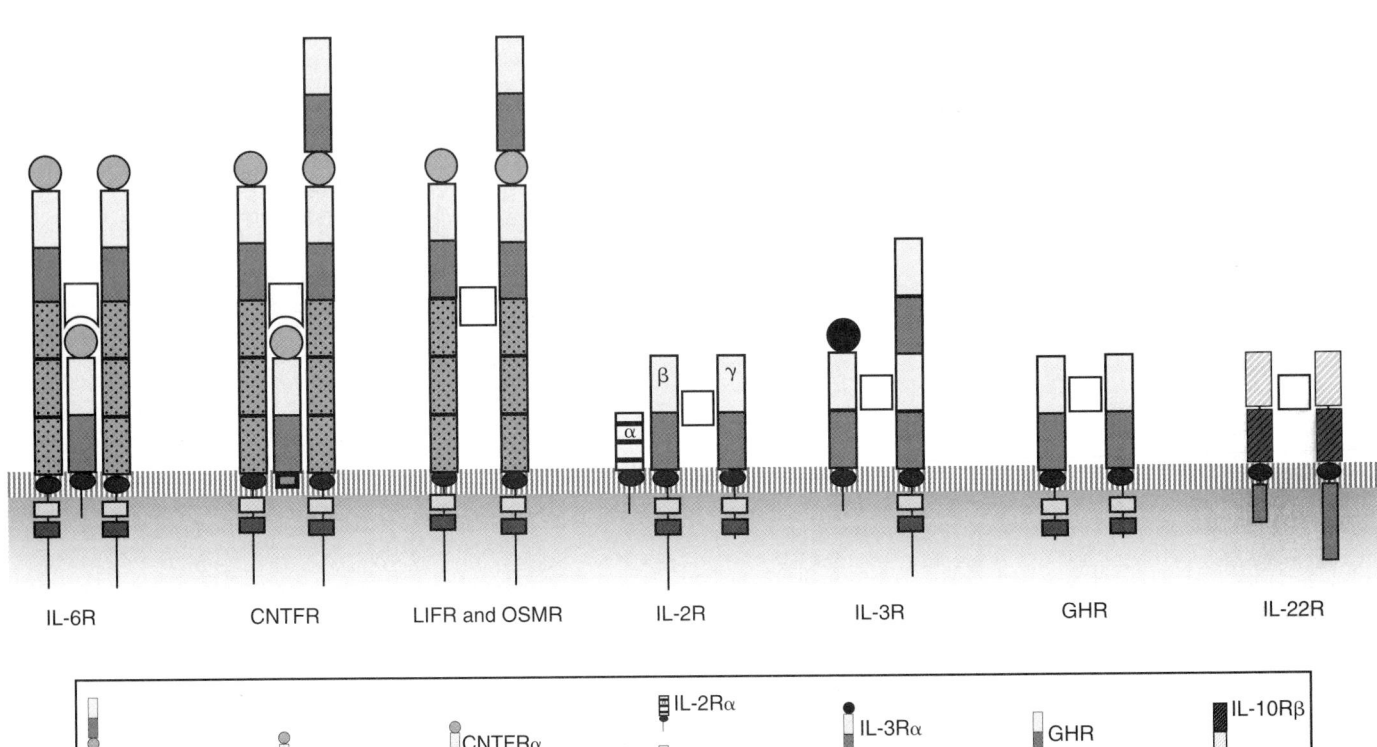

Figure 9-4 Examples of shared receptor subunits.

Table 9-1 Cytokine-Specific JAK and STAT Activation

Ligands	Signaling Molecules	
CLASS I CYTOKINES	JAKs	STATs
(i) gp130 family		
IL-6	JAK1, JAK2, TYK2	STAT3, STAT1
IL-11	JAK1, JAK2, TYK2	STAT3, STAT2
LIF	JAK1, JAK2, TYK2	STAT3, STAT5
OSM	JAK1, JAK2, TYK2	STAT3, STAT3
Leptin	JAK2	STAT1, STAT3, STAT5, STAT6
CNTF	JAK1, JAK2, TYK2	STAT3, STAT4
CT-1	JAK2	STAT1, STAT3, STAT5, STAT6
IL-12	JAK1, JAK2, TYK2	STAT3
IL-23	JAK2, TYK2	STAT1, STAT3, STAT4, STAT5
G-CSF	JAK1, JAK2	STAT3
(ii) IL-2 (γc) family		
IL-2	JAK1, JAK3	STAT5, STAT3
IL-4	JAK1, JAK3	STAT6
IL-7	JAK1, JAK3	STAT5, STAT3, STAT1
IL-9	JAK1, JAK3	STAT5, STAT3
IL-13	JAK1, JAK2, TYK2	STAT6, STAT3
IL-15	JAK1, JAK3	STAT5, STAT3, STAT1
IL-21	JAK1, JAK3	STAT5, STAT3, STAT1
(iii) IL-3 (βc) family		
IL-3	JAK2	STAT5, STAT3
IL-5	JAK2	STAT5, STAT3, STAT1
GM-CSF	JAK2	STAT5
(iv) Single-chain (homodimeric) family		
GH	JAK2	STAT5
PRL	JAK2	STAT5
EPO	JAK2	STAT5
TPO	JAK2	STAT5
CLASS II CYTOKINES		
(v) Interferon family		
IFN-α, IFN-β	JAK1, TYK2	STAT1, STAT2, STAT3, STAT4, STAT5
IFN-γ	JAK1, JAK2	STAT1, STAT
IL-10	JAK1, TYK2	STAT3
IL-19	?	STAT3
IL-20	?	STAT3
IL-22	JAK1, TYK2	STAT1, STAT3, STAT5

JANUS KINASES

Four mammalian JAKs have been identified: JAK1, JAK2, JAK3, and TYK2, with TYK2 (tyrosine kinase 2) the first to be discovered. Initially, these proteins along with several other tyrosine kinases were grouped by using the acronym JAK ("just another kinase"). However, sequencing studies revealed that JAK1, JAK2, JAK3, and TYK2 differed from other tyrosine kinases by the presence of an additional kinase domain (described later in this section). Thus, to differentiate between the other classes, these proteins were renamed Janus kinases in reference to a mythologic two-faced Roman god of gates and doorways (reviewed in Ref. 36).

The JAKs are relatively large kinases of approximately 1000 amino acids with molecular weights of about 120 to 130 kDa. Their transcripts range from 4.4 to 5.4 kb in length. JAK2 has two transcripts, while JAK3 has multiple spliced forms, one with an absent catalytic domain.[35] JAK1, JAK2, and TYK2 are ubiquitously expressed, whereas JAK3 shows a more restricted profile, primarily with expression in lymphoid cells.[35,37]

The genomic organization of the murine and human JAKs has been determined. The murine genes reside on chromosomes 4 (JAK1), 19 (JAK2), 8 (JAK3), and 9 (TYK2).[38,36] In humans, JAK1 is located on chromosome 1p31.3,[39] JAK2

has been mapped to chromosome 9p24, and JAK3 and TYK2 are both located on chromosome 19, mapping to 19p13.1 and 19p13.2, respectively.[39-41]

STRUCTURE AND FUNCTION OF JAKs

The Janus family of protein tyrosine kinases possesses a unique feature: dual kinase domains (JH1 and JH2), of which only the JH1 domain is catalytically active. The JH2 or pseudo-kinase domain shares considerable homology to JH1 but lacks critical amino acids required for kinase activity. The JH2 domain appears to have a regulatory function, as this domain is essential for a normal kinase activity.[36] Studies have shown, for instance, that in a growth hormone receptor/JAK chimera, deletion of the JH2 domain led to more robust signaling, indicating that the JH2 domain may serve to inhibit JAK activity. Both domains are located at the C-terminus of the protein. In addition, there are several other regions of sequence similarity within the 600 N-terminal amino acids residues, which have been defined as JAK homology (JH) domains (JH3 to JH7). Given the many interactions involving JAKs, it is possible that these domains may facilitate key functions such as interactions with other proteins and recruitment of substrates (Fig. 9-6).

The N-terminal region of JAK proteins constitutes a FERM (Four-point-one, Ezrin, Radixin, Moesin) domain, which is a known protein-protein interaction motif.[42,43] Many studies indicate that the N-terminus region is crucial for cytokine receptor association. This was first demonstrated for the interaction of JAK2 with the erythropoietin and growth hormone receptors, where deletions or mutations in the N-terminal region eliminated binding.[44,45] Another example, which supports the importance of the JAK N-terminus in binding to cytokine receptors, involves JAK3. It is known that mutations in the γc chain are responsible for X-linked severe combined immunodeficiency syndrome (SCID), a condition characterized by an absence of T-lymphocytes and natural killer (NK) cells.[46] Since JAK3 selectively associates with the γc chain of the IL-2 receptor, it was hypothesized that a mutation in JAK3 may also lead to some form of SCID. Subsequently, several patients with autosomal-recessive SCID were identified with JAK3 mutations.[47-50] Cacalano and colleagues later identified one of the mutations as a single amino acid substitution in the N-terminus JH7 domain of JAK3 in a patient with autosomal-recessive SCID.[50]

SIGNAL TRANSDUCERS AND ACTIVATORS OF TRANSCRIPTION

STATs were first discovered in interferon-signaling pathways.[51-53] Seven mammalian STAT proteins have since been identified: STAT1–STAT4, two isoforms of STAT5 (STAT5a and STAT5b), and STAT6. STAT1, 3, 4, 5a, and 5b are 750 to 795 amino acids long, while STAT2 and STAT6 are longer at approximately 850 amino acids.[54,55] In the absence of specific receptor stimulation, STAT proteins are inactive and are localized to the cytoplasm of unstimulated target cells.

STATs are organized in clusters on three chromosomes, suggesting a common ancestral origin. STAT1 and STAT4 are located on mouse chromosome 1 (equivalent to human chromosome 2 bands q12 to q13); STAT2 and STAT6 on mouse chromosome 10 (human chromosome 17, bands q11.1 to q22), and STAT3, STAT5a; and STAT5b on mouse chromosome 11 (human chromosome 12, bands q13 to q14.1).[54,55]

STRUCTURE AND FUNCTION OF STATs

STATs contain several domains, including a conserved N-terminal domain, a DNA-binding domain, a putative SH3-like domain, an SH2 domain, and a C-terminal transcriptional activation domain.[56] Other domains include coiled-coil and linker domains (Fig. 9-7).

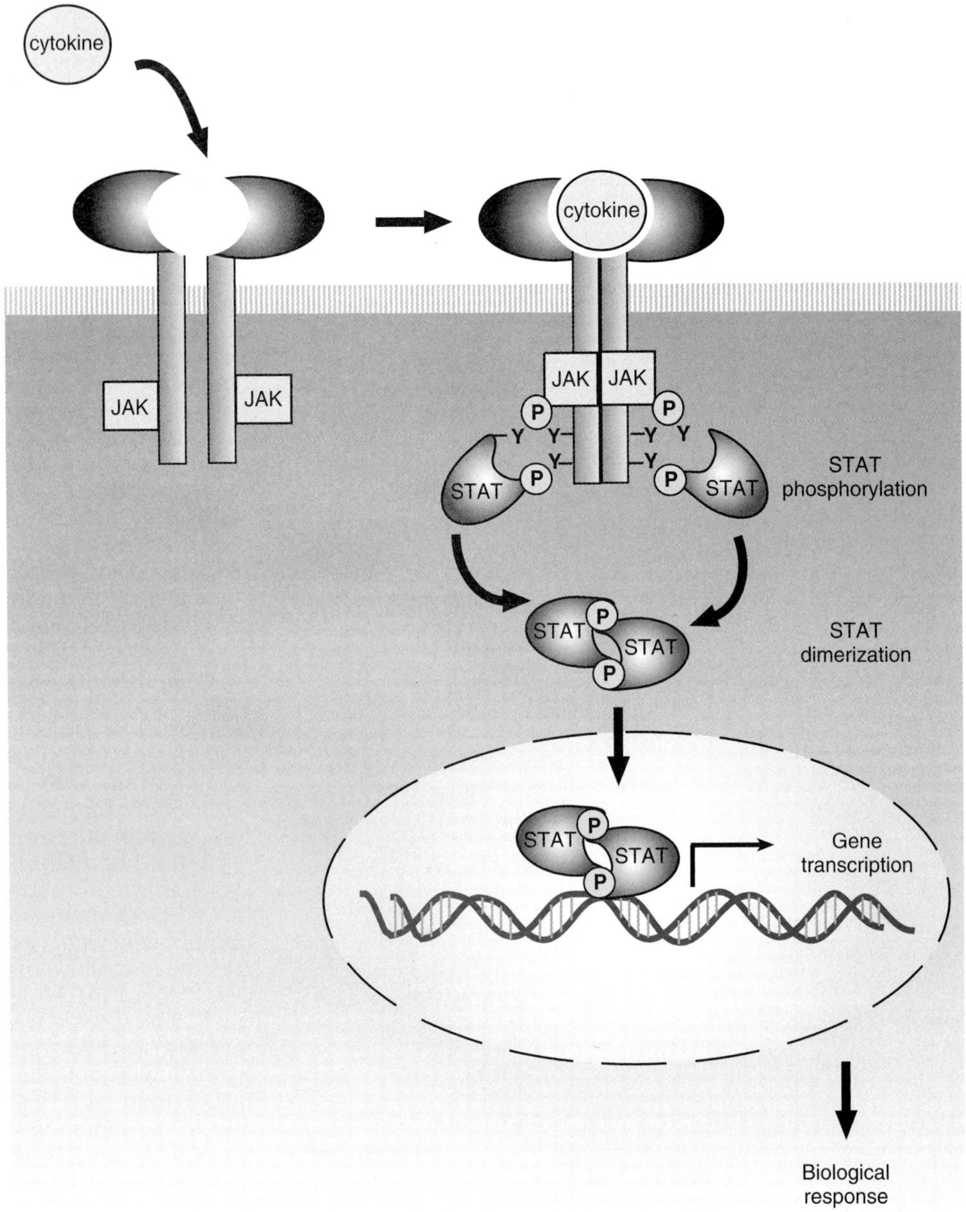

Figure 9-5   The JAK-STAT signaling pathway. The JAK-STAT signaling pathway is initiated upon the binding of a cytokine to its receptor at the cell surface. This causes receptor dimerization to occur and brings receptor-associated JAKs into close proximity. The JAKs become activated and phosphorylate (P) the receptor, creating docking sites for STATs, which are also phosphorylated by JAKs. Activated STATs dimerize and translocate to the nucleus, where they stimulate the transcription of cytokine-responsive genes, resulting in an appropriate biologic response to the cytokine.

Figure 9-6   The domain structure of JAKs. The structural domains in the JAK kinase family are referred to as the JAK homology regions (JH1 to JH7). The JH1 domain is the kinase domain, and the kinase-like (pseudo-kinase) domain is the JH2 domain. The JHI domain harbors conserved tyrosine residues. The remainder of the homology domains are represented but have undefined functions. Association with cytokine receptors is thought to be through the N-terminus of the JAKs.

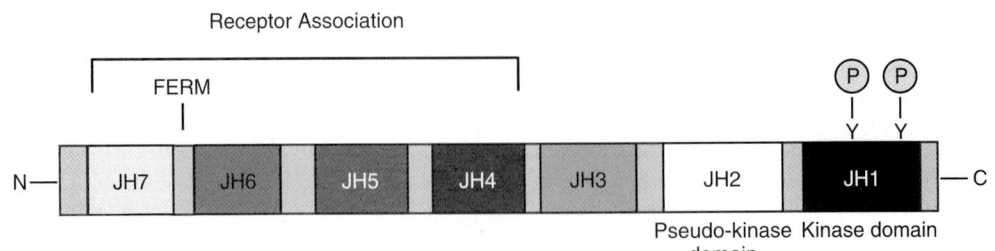

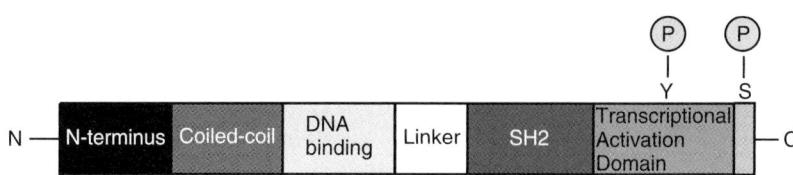

Figure 9-7 The domain structure of STATs. The STAT proteins comprise conserved motifs, such as the DNA-biding domain, a putative SH3-like domain (linker), and SH2 domain and a transcriptional activation domain. This domain, along with conserved tyrosine (Y) and serine (S) residues reside at the C-terminal of the proteins. The activity of STATs can be regulated by protein modification, including tyrosine and serine phosphorylation.

The conserved **N-terminus** of STAT proteins is functionally critical, as deletions in this region eliminate the ability of STATs to be phosphorylated.[18] The N-terminus enables the polymerization of STAT dimers and has been implicated in a number of protein-protein interactions affecting transcription. The N-terminal of STAT is also involved in regulating STAT activity via tyrosine dephosphorylation.[57] Following this region is a central **DNA-binding domain** located between amino acids 400 and 500.[58] This highly conserved region is the site through which most STATs bind to a semi-palindromic DNA motif, TTNCNNNAA (some variation may occur). This motif was originally identified as a GAS element, for IFNγ-activated sequences, based on the sequence recognized by IFNγ-induced STAT1 homodimers. Other STATs recognize and bind to similar DNA sequences.[18,58,59] Adjacent to the DNA-binding domain is the **SH3 domain**. This domain is the least conserved, and the function of this domain is far from clear.

In contrast, the conserved **SH2 domain** is essential in STAT signaling. In the context of the JAK-STAT signal transduction pathway, the SH2 domain provides a site for STAT proteins to dock to tyrosine phosphorylated receptor subunits. It is important to note that each STAT protein possesses slightly different SH2 domains, which recognize distinct phosphorylated receptor motifs, conferring a level of specificity (see Table 9-1). Furthermore, the subsequent dimerization of STAT molecules is also dependent on this domain; STAT dimers are formed on the basis of the interaction between the SH2 domain on one STAT molecule and the phosphorylated C-terminal tyrosine on another. Finally, STAT proteins may also interact with other proteins through their SH2 domains; however, the importance of these interactions are still being investigated.[36]

At their C-terminal tail, all STATs possess a conserved **tyrosine residue**. This is a phosphorylation site that regulates the dimerization of STATs. On phosphorylation, the tyrosine residue mediates STAT dimerization by binding to the SH2 domain of a reciprocal STAT molecule (as described above). Additionally, a second phosphorylation site in the C-terminal domain, a **serine residue**, is present in all STATs, with the exception of STAT2 and STAT6. In response to cytokine stimulation, STAT1, STAT3, STAT4, and STAT5 become serine phosphorylated at a conserved site near the transcriptional activation domain.[60] Mutation of the serine residue has been shown to decrease transcriptional activation and gene regulation, although this is not consistently observed.[61] Finally, MAP kinase proteins and stimuli other than cytokines also play roles in STAT serine phosphorylation, suggesting the possibility for cross-talk between different receptors and pathways.[60]

ROLES OF JAKs AND STATs IN VIVO

The crucial role the JAKs and STATs play in signaling are highlighted by the phenotypes of mice and humans containing mutated genes. Targeted genes in mice have provided valuable insights into their respective physiologic roles in response to cytokines. For example, deletions in JAK1 causes a perinatal lethal phenotype and immunologic defects,[62] targeted deletion of JAK2 results in an embryonic lethal phenotype,[63,64] highlighting its importance in early development, especially red blood cell formation, while JAK3 knockout

mice display immunologic deficiencies that resemble those seen in human SCID patients.[65–68]

In a similar manner, murine models demonstrated that STAT isoforms are key mediators in cytokine receptor–specific signaling such as STAT1 in IFN-γ,[69] STAT2 for immune response associated with type 1 IFNs,[70] STAT3 during embryonic development,[71] STAT4 for IL-12 action,[72] STAT5 for IL-2 signaling and mammary gland function,[73–75] and STAT6 in IL-4-dependent response.[76] The various phenotypes of these mice and the signaling of various cytokines affected are described in Table 9-2.

NEGATIVE REGULATION OF THE JAK-STAT PATHWAY

The JAK-STAT pathway is controlled by both positive and negative regulatory mechanisms at multiple levels, including JAK activation, trafficking of STAT factors, and negative feedback loops. These mechanisms serve to modify the specificity, intensity, and duration of signals transduced from the cytokine receptor at the cell membrane to transcription elements of genes in the nucleus, ultimately preventing aberrant activation of downstream signals and inappropriate gene expression.

Negative regulation of the JAK-STAT pathway is accomplished by various mechanisms (Fig. 9-8) including cytokines such as transforming growth factor betas (TGF-β) and IL-10 that affect secretion of key cytokines, soluble cytokine receptors that reduce the availability of cytokine to bind cell surface receptors,[77,78] and receptor internalization and degradation, which limit the period of cytokine receptor activation.[79] Attenuation is also achieved by feedback inhibitors of the cytokine response, including protein tyrosine phosphatases, protein inhibitors of activated STAT proteins, and the suppressors of cytokine-signaling proteins.[57,80–84]

PROTEIN TYROSINE PHOSPHATASES

Protein tyrosine phosphatases (PTPs) regulate the kinase activities of tyrosine kinases such as the JAKs by dephosphorylating critical tyrosine residues involved in catalytic function. Several studies have demonstrated the regulatory roles that PTPs such as **SHP1, SHP2, CD45, protein tyrosine phosphatase 1B (PTP1B),** and **T-cell protein tyrosine phosphatase (TCPTP)** play in JAK-STAT signaling. The importance of these PTPs in cytokine-signaling regulation has been has been further supported by gene-targeting studies.[57]

SHP1 and SHP2 are SH2-domain containing phosphatases. SHP1 is predominantly expressed in hematopoietic cells, whereas SHP2 is more widely expressed. SHP1 has been shown to associate with a number of receptors, including the EPO receptor. A mutation in receptor tyrosine motifs that recruit SHP1 to the EPO receptor resulted in prolonged EPO-induced JAK2 autophosphorylation, indicating that SHP1 may be involved in the dephosphorylation of JAK2.[85] SHP1 is also involved in the dephosphorylation of JAK1, as is SHP2, where SHP2−/− fibroblasts exhibited elevated levels of JAK1 tyrosine phosphorylation following IFN-γ stimulation.[86,87]

CD45, a transmembrane phosphatase, is highly expressed on hematopoietic cells and has a role in T- and B-cell receptor signaling (reviewed in Ref. 88). CD45 can directly bind

Table 9-2 Phenotypes of Mice Deficient for JAKs and STATs

Gene	Cytokine(s) Affected	Phenotype of Gene Deletion
JAK		
JAK1	IFN-α/β, -γ, IL-10, and cytokines using γc gp130 chain	Perinatal lethal, defects in lymphoid development
JAK2	IFN-γ, EPO	Embryonic lethal (E12.5), failure of erythropoiesis
JAK3	IL-2, IL-4, IL-7, IL-19, IL-15	SCID, increased apoptosis
TYK2	IFN-α/β, -γ, and IL-12	Hypersensitivity to pathogens
STAT		
STAT1	IFN-α/β, -γ	Highly susceptible to viral and bacterial infections
STAT2	IFN-α/β	Susceptible to viral infections
STAT3	IL-2, IL-6, IL-7, IL-9, IL-10, IL-11, IL-15, IL-21 EGF, OSM, G-CSF, TPO, LIF, GH	Embryonic lethal (E7.5) due to failure in mesoderm formation Impaired responses to pathogens, cell-survival defects Impaired T-cell proliferation Impaired anti-inflammatory responses
STAT4	IL-12	Defects in T-cell differentiation, increased susceptibility to pathogens
STAT5a	IL-2, IL-3, IL-5, IL-7, IL-9, IL-15, G-CSF, GM-CSF, EPO, TPO, GH, PRL	Defects in mammary gland development and lactogenesis Defects in T-cell and macrophage proliferation
STAT5b	GH, IL-2, and IL-15	Defects in NK cell activity, growth in males
STAT5a/5b	as for STAT5a and STAT5b	Female infertility, fetal anemia Defects in T-cell proliferation and absent NK cells
STAT6	IL-4, IL-13	Impaired B- and T-cell proliferation, defects in Th2 differentiation and IgE class switch

Source: Refs. 32, 55–57.

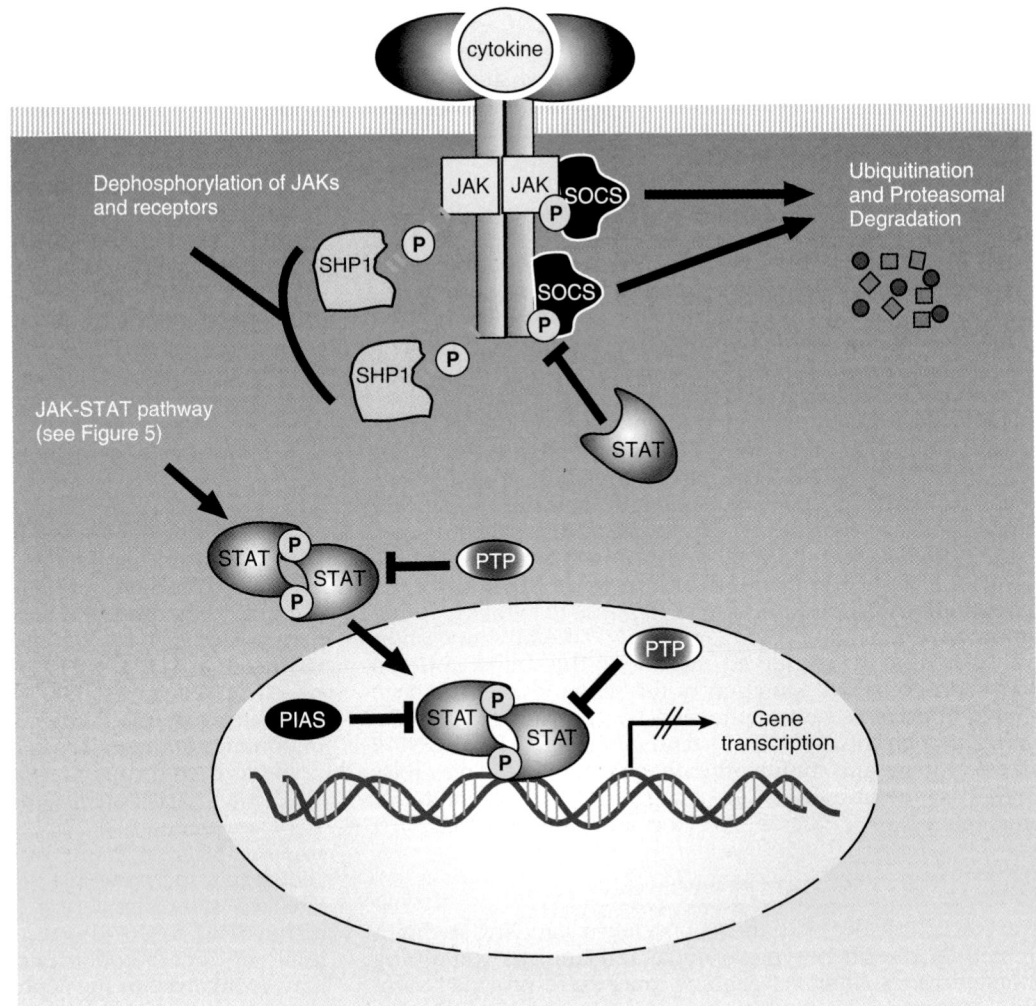

Figure 9-8 Negative regulation of the JAK-STAT-signaling pathway. The JAK-STAT pathway is regulated at many levels. JAKs can be negatively regulated by protein tyrosine phosphatases (PTPs) such as SHP-1. SHP-1 is constitutively expressed and can dephosphorylate activated JAKs or receptors. Suppressor of cytokine signaling (SOCS) proteins are induced in response to cytokine signaling and inhibit JAK activity by binding directly to JAKs, competing with STATs for phosphorylated binding sites on receptors and by targeting bound signaling components for proteasomal degradation. STATs are negatively regulated by PTPs in the cytoplasm and the nucleus as well as by protein inhibitor of activated STAT (PIAS) proteins. PIAS proteins also constitutively expressed interact with STATs in response to cytokine stimulation and inhibit transcriptional activity of STATs through distinct mechanisms.

and dephosphorylate all JAKs, and enhanced JAK phosphorylation can be observed in CD45-deficient cells.[89] The phosphatases PTP1B and TCPTP have also been suggested to dephosphorylate JAKs.[90] PTP1B associates with JAK2 and TYK2 and has been implicated in the negative regulation of leptin signaling by targeting JAK2,[91,92] while TCPTP can dephosphorylate JAK1 and JAK3.[93]

The regulation of the JAK-STAT pathway by PTPs is not limited to their interactions with JAKs. PTPs may also influence STAT activity in the cytoplasm and the nucleus. For example, SHP2 can interact with and directly dephosphorylate cytoplasmic STAT5.[94,95] SHP2-mediated dephosphorylation of STAT1 at both the serine and tyrosine residues has also been indicated. Furthermore, overexpression systems have implied a role for PTB1B in the dephosphorylation of STAT5.[96] Studies in this area continue in order to understand the precise actions of PTPs on JAKs and STATs.

PROTEIN INHIBITORS OF ACTIVATED STATs

Another regulatory mechanism of the JAK-STAT pathway involves the **protein inhibitor of activated STATs (PIAS) protein family.** The PIAS family comprises four members (PIAS1, PIAS3, PIASx, and PIASy) that share a highly conserved RING-finger-like zinc-binding domain. PIAS1 was first identified in a yeast two-hybrid screen to determine STAT interacting proteins and was later shown to inhibit STAT1 activation by directly associating with dimeric STATs, thus disrupting DNA binding.[97] PIAS3 regulates STAT4 activation in a similar manner. However, the mechanism by which PIASy and PIASx inhibits activation of STAT1 and STAT4, respectively, differs from PIAS1 and PIAS3.[97,98] PIASy inhibits STAT1 activity without affecting its DNA-binding activity,[99] while PIASx acts as a transcriptional corepressor of STAT4.[100]

Recently, several interesting experiments have introduced a new player: the ubiquitin-like protein modifier SUMO1. In a yeast two-hybrid screen for proteins that interact with SUMO1, the *Saccharomyces cerevisiae* protein Siz1p was identified.[101] This protein contains a similar conserved RING domain seen in the PIAS family, hinting that PIAS proteins could function as E3 SUMO ligases in mammals.[102] Since this discovery, E3 SUMO ligase activity has been demonstrated for all members of the PIAS family, with STATs one of the many targets identified. PIAS1, PIAS3, and PIASx have been reported to sumoylate STAT1 at a site that is in close proximity to a tyrosine phosphorylated by JAKs; however, how sumoylation inhibits STAT1 activation is not yet understood.[103,104]

REGULATION OF THE JAK-STAT PATHWAY BY THE SUPPRESSOR OF CYTOKINE SIGNALING PROTEINS

The **suppressor of cytokine signaling (SOCS)** proteins function as part of a classical negative feedback loop, attenuating cytokine action through inhibition of the JAK-STAT signal transduction pathway.[105] The SOCS family of proteins has eight members: CIS (cytokine-inducible SH2 domain protein) and SOCS1 to SOCS7.[84,106] The SOCS proteins are structurally characterized by an N-terminal region, a central SH2 domain, and a conserved C-terminal motif of approximately 40 amino acids, termed the *SOCS box*. These SOCS proteins are generally expressed at low levels in unstimulated cells and become rapidly induced by a wide range of cytokines such as LIF, GH, PRL, leptin, interleukins, and other growth factors.[80]

SOCS proteins inhibit cytokine signaling through distinct mechanisms. Structural and functional analyses have shown that the SOCS proteins directly interact with activated JAKs and cytokine receptors through their N-terminal and SH2 domains, inhibiting signal transduction. For example, the SH2 domain of SOCS1 binds directly to tyrosine-phosphorylated JAKs, resulting in the direct inhibition of JAK activity, whereas the inhibition of signaling by SOCS2, SOCS3, and CIS involves binding to phosphorylated cytokine receptors.[107,108]

Finally, the involvement of SOCS proteins in the degradation of signaling proteins and receptors through the ubiquitin-proteasome pathway has also been suggested. This degradation pathway is mediated via the SOCS box.[109] The SOCS box binds elongin C, which in turn associates with a complex consisting of elongin B, a cullin family member, and a RING-finger protein called Roc-1 or Rbx-1. This protein complex constitutes an E3 ubiquitin ligase termed the *ECS* (elongin C-cullin-SOCS box), which together with a ubiquitin-activating enzyme (E1) and a ubiquitin-conjugating enzyme (E2) facilitates the polyubiquitination of proteins bound to the SH2 domain of SOCS family members.[109–111] It has been suggested by several groups that the SOCS box functions as an adaptor, linking specific protein-protein interaction domains to generic components of the ubiquitin ligase machinery. This results in the polyubiquitination and proteasomal degradation of bound signaling proteins.[112,113]

Genetic manipulation of the mouse has shown the crucial role that some of the SOCS proteins play in negatively regulating cytokine-mediated signaling. For example, SOCS1$^{-/-}$ mice display increased sensitivity to IFN-γ and prolonged STAT activation. Consequently, mice die at 3 weeks of age from a complex disease characterized by lymphopenia, fatty degeneration of the liver, and macrophage infiltration of major organs. The lethality is due to excessive production of and response to IFN-γ, as mice lacking both SOCS1 and IFN-γ are healthy.[114] SOCS2$^{-/-}$ mice are significantly larger than their wild-type littermates, most probably owing to enhanced signaling by growth hormone and insulin-like growth factor 1. Thus, a role for SOCS2 in postnatal growth is likely.[115] Finally, ablation of SOCS3 results in embryonic lethality between E12 and E14 from severe erythrocytosis and placental insufficiency.[116,117] To overcome this lethality, SOCS3 conditionally deleted mice were generated. In conditionally targeted cells, a prolonged activation of STAT1 and STAT3 was observed, suggesting that SOCS3 is important for attenuating IL-6-mediated signaling.[118–120]

CONCLUSIONS

A vast array of cytokines exert their biologic effects by binding to cytokine receptors and activating one of the major pathways involved in cytokine signaling: the JAK-STAT pathway. As has been described, the JAK-STAT pathway is composed of various components that allow for the rapid transduction of signals mediated on the binding of a cytokine to its receptor. Normal biologic responses elicited by cytokines are dependent on effective regulatory mechanisms that control JAK-STAT signaling. It has been shown that disruptions involving these mechanisms leads to serious pathologies. Finally, while the JAK-STAT pathway has been the focus of this chapter, cytokines also operate in many other signaling pathways. It is therefore important to determine how JAK-STAT signals are integrated with signals from other pathways downstream of cytokine receptors. Scientific studies continue in this dynamic area of research; dissecting the complexities of cytokine signaling is required to more completely understand the molecular basis of cytokine action and to develop potential strategies to overcome various disease states that may arise from aberrant cytokine signaling.

Acknowledgments
Research in the authors' laboratory is supported by the Australian National Health and Medical Research Council, Canberra, Australia; the Anti-Cancer Council of Victoria, Melbourne, Australia; the Australian Federal Government Cooperative Research Centers Program, Australia; and the AMRAD Corporation, Melbourne, Australia. M. Debrincat is a recipient of a Dora Lush Postgraduate Award from the Australian National Health and Medical Research Council.

REFERENCES

1. Nicola NA: Guidebook to Cytokines and Their Receptors. New York, Oxford University Press, 1994.
2. Isaacs A, Lindenmann J: Virus interference. I: The interferon. Proc R Soc Lond B Biol Sci 147:258–267, 1957.
3. Ihle JN: Cytokine receptor signalling. Nature 377:591–594, 1995.
4. Kishimoto T, Taga T, Akira S: Cytokine signal transduction. Cell 76:253–262, 1994.
5. Bazan JF: A novel family of growth factor receptors: A common binding domain in the growth hormone, prolactin, erythropoietin and IL-6 receptors, and the p75 IL-2 receptor beta-chain. Biochem Biophys Res Commun 164:788–795, 1989.
6. D'Andrea AD, Fasman GD, Lodish HF: Erythropoietin receptor and interleukin-2 receptor beta chain: A new receptor family. Cell 58:1023, 1989.
7. Gearing DP, King JA, Gough NM, Nicola NA: Expression cloning of a receptor for human granulocyte-macrophage colony-stimulating factor. EMBO J 8:3667–3676, 1989.
8. Taga T, Kishimoto T: Signaling mechanisms through cytokine receptors that share signal transducing receptor components. Curr Opin Immunol 7:17–23, 1995.
9. Bazan JF: Structural design and molecular evolution of a cytokine receptor superfamily. Proc Natl Acad Sci U S A 87:6934–6938, 1990.
10. Thoreau E, Petridou B, Kelly PA, et al: Structural symmetry of the extracellular domain of the cytokine/growth hormone/prolactin receptor family and interferon receptors revealed by hydrophobic cluster analysis. FEBS Lett 282:26–31, 1991.
11. Waters MJ, Shang CA, Behncken SN, et al: Growth hormone as a cytokine. Clin Exp Pharmacol Physiol 26:760–764, 1999.
12. Barry SC, Korpelainen E, Sun Q, et al: Roles of the N and C terminal domains of the interleukin-3 receptor alpha chain in receptor function. Blood 89:842–852, 1997.
13. Patthy L: Homology of a domain of the growth hormone/prolactin receptor family with type III modules of fibronectin. Cell 61:13–14, 1990.
14. Moutoussamy S, Kelly PA, Finidori J: Growth-hormone-receptor and cytokine-receptor-family signaling. Eur J Biochem 255:1–11, 1998.
15. de Vos AM, Ultsch M, Kossiakoff AA: Human growth hormone and extracellular domain of its receptor: Crystal structure of the complex. Science 255:306–312, 1992.
16. Yawata H, Yasukawa K, Natsuka S, et al: Structure-function analysis of human IL-6 receptor: Dissociation of amino acid residues required for IL-6-binding and for IL-6 signal transduction through gp130. EMBO J 12:1705–1712, 1993.
17. Murakami M, Narazaki M, Hibi M, et al: Critical cytoplasmic region of the interleukin 6 signal transducer gp130 is conserved in the cytokine receptor family. Proc Natl Acad Sci U S A 88:11349–1153, 1991.
18. Rane SG, Reddy EP: JAKs, STATs and Src kinases in hematopoiesis. Oncogene 21:3334–3358, 2002.
19. Zhang JG, Hilton DJ, Willson TA, et al: Identification, purification, and characterization of a soluble interleukin (IL)-13-binding protein: Evidence that it is distinct from the cloned Il-13 receptor and Il-4 receptor alpha-chains. J Biol Chem 272:9474–9480, 1997.
20. Heaney ML, Golde DW: Soluble cytokine receptors. Blood 87:847–857, 1996.
21. Alexander WS, Rakar S, Robb L, et al: Suckling defect in mice lacking the soluble haemopoietin receptor NR6. Curr Biol 9:605–608, 1999.
22. Renauld JC: Class II cytokine receptors and their ligands: Key antiviral and inflammatory modulators. Nat Rev Immunol 3:667–676, 2003.
23. Lewerenz M, Mogensen KE, Uze G: Shared receptor components but distinct complexes for alpha and beta interferons. J Mol Biol 282:585–599, 1998.
24. Riewald M, Ruf W: Orchestration of coagulation protease signaling by tissue factor. Trends Cardiovasc Med 12:149–154, 2002.
25. Dumoutier L, Lejeune D, Colau D, Renauld JC: Cloning and characterization of IL-22 binding protein, a natural antagonist of IL-10-related T cell-derived inducible factor/IL-22. J Immunol 166:7090–7095, 2001.
26. Kotenko SV, Izotova LS, Mirochnitchenko OV, et al: Identification, cloning, and characterization of a novel soluble receptor that binds IL-22 and neutralizes its activity. J Immunol 166:7096–7103, 2001.
27. Xu W, Presnell SR, Parrish-Novak J, et al: A soluble class II cytokine receptor, IL-22RA2, is a naturally occurring IL-22 antagonist. Proc Natl Acad Sci U S A 98:9511–9516, 2001.
28. Gruenberg BH, Schoenemeyer A, Weiss B, et al: A novel, soluble homologue of the human IL-10 receptor with preferential expression in placenta. Genes Immunol 2:329–334, 2001.
29. Stahl N, Yancopoulos GD: The alphas, betas, and kinases of cytokine receptor complexes. Cell 74:587–590, 1993.
30. Taniguchi T: Cytokine signaling through nonreceptor protein tyrosine kinases. Science 268:251–255, 1995.
31. Hunter T: Signal transduction. Cytokine connections. Nature 366:114–116, 1993.
32. Liu KD, Gaffen SL, Goldsmith MA: JAK/STAT signaling by cytokine receptors. Curr Opin Immunol 10:271–278, 1998.
33. Imada K, Leonard WJ: The Jak-STAT pathway. Mol Immunol 37:1–11, 2000.
34. Aaronson DS, Horvath CM: A road map for those who know JAK-STAT. Science 296:1653–1655, 2002.
35. Leonard WJ, O'Shea JJ: Jaks and STATs: Biological implications. Annu Rev Immunol 16:293–322, 1998.
36. Rane SG, Reddy EP: Janus kinases: Components of multiple signaling pathways. Oncogene 19:5662–5679, 2000.
37. Verbsky JW, Bach EA, Fang YF, et al: Expression of Janus kinase 3 in human endothelial and other non-lymphoid and non-myeloid cells. J Biol Chem 271:13976–13980, 1996.
38. Kono DH, Owens DG, Wechsler AR: Jak3 maps to chromosome 8. Mamm Genome 7:476–477, 1996.
39. Pritchard MA, Baker E, Callen DF, et al: Two members of the JAK family of protein tyrosine kinases map to chromosomes 1p31.3 and 9p24. Mamm Genome 3:36–38, 1992.
40. Kumar A, Toscani A, Rane S, Reddy EP: Structural organization and chromosomal mapping of JAK3 locus. Oncogene 13:2009–2014, 1996.
41. Firmbach-Kraft I, Byers M, Shows T, et al: tyk2, prototype of a novel class of non-receptor tyrosine kinase genes. Oncogene 5:1329–1336, 1990.
42. Girault JA, Labesse G, Mornon JP, Callebaut I: Janus kinases and focal adhesion kinases play in the 4.1 band: A superfamily of band 4.1 domains important for cell structure and signal transduction. Mol Med 4:751–769, 1998.
43. Gadina M, Hilton D, Johnston JA, et al: Signaling by Type I and II cytokine receptors: Ten years after. Curr Opin Immunol 13:363–373, 2001.
44. Witthuhn BA, Quelle FW, Silvennoinen O, et al: JAK2 associates with the erythropoietin receptor and is tyrosine phosphorylated and activated following stimulation with erythropoietin. Cell 74:227–236, 1993.
45. Argetsinger LS, Campbell GS, Yang X, et al: Identification of JAK2 as a growth hormone receptor-associated tyrosine kinase. Cell 74:237–244, 1993.
46. O'Shea JJ, Notarangelo LD, Johnston JA, Candotti F: Advances in the understanding of cytokine signal transduction: The role of Jaks and STATs in immunoregulation and the pathogenesis of immunodeficiency. J Clin Immunol 17:431–447, 1997.
47. Candotti F, Oakes SA, Johnston JA, et al: Structural and functional basis for JAK3-deficient severe combined immunodeficiency. Blood 90:3996–4003, 1997.
48. Russell SM, Tayebi N, Nakajima H, et al: Mutation of Jak3 in a patient with SCID: essential role of Jak3 in lymphoid development. Science 270:797–800, 1995.
49. Macchi P, Villa A, Giliani S, et al: Mutations of Jak-3 gene in patients with autosomal severe combined immune deficiency (SCID). Nature 377:65–68, 1995.

50. Cacalano NA, Migone TS, Bazan F, et al: Autosomal SCID caused by a point mutation in the N-terminus of Jak3: Mapping of the Jak3-receptor interaction domain. EMBO J 18:1549–1558, 1999.

51. Darnell JE Jr, Kerr IM, Stark GR: Jak-STAT pathways and transcriptional activation in response to IFNs and other extracellular signaling proteins. Science 264:1415–1421, 1994.

52. Sadowski HB, Shuai K, Darnell JE Jr, Gilman MZ: A common nuclear signal transduction pathway activated by growth factor and cytokine receptors. Science 261:1739–1744, 1993.

53. Shuai K, Stark GR, Kerr IM, Darnell JE Jr: A single phosphotyrosine residue of Stat91 required for gene activation by interferon-gamma. Science 261:1744–1746, 1993.

54. Darnell JE Jr: STATs and gene regulation. Science 277:1630–1635, 1997.

55. Takeda K, Akira S: STAT family of transcription factors in cytokine-mediated biological responses. Cytokine Growth Factor Rev 11:199–207, 2000.

56. Benekli M, Baer MR, Baumann H, Wetzler M: Signal transducer and activator of transcription proteins in leukemias. Blood 101:2940–2954, 2003.

57. Shuai K, Liu B: Regulation of JAK-STAT signalling in the immune system. Nat Rev Immunol 3:900–911, 2003.

58. Horvath CM, Wen Z, Darnell JE Jr: A STAT protein domain that determines DNA sequence recognition suggests a novel DNA-binding domain. Genes Dev 9:984–994, 1995.

59. Xu X, Sun YL, Hoey T: Cooperative DNA binding and sequence-selective recognition conferred by the STAT amino-terminal domain. Science 273:794–797, 1996.

60. Decker T, Kovarik P: Serine phosphorylation of STATs. Oncogene 19:2628–26237, 2000.

61. Kovarik P, Mangold M, Ramsauer K, et al: Specificity of signaling by STAT1 depends on SH2 and C-terminal domains that regulate Ser727 phosphorylation, differentially affecting specific target gene expression. EMBO J 20:91–100, 2001.

62. Rodig SJ, Meraz MA, White JM, et al: Disruption of the Jak1 gene demonstrates obligatory and nonredundant roles of the Jaks in cytokine-induced biologic responses. Cell 93:373–383, 1998.

63. Neubauer H, Cumano A, Muller M, et al: Jak2 deficiency defines an essential developmental checkpoint in definitive hematopoiesis. Cell 93:397–409, 1998.

64. Parganas E, Wang D, Stravopodis D, et al: Jak2 is essential for signaling through a variety of cytokine receptors. Cell 93:385–395, 1998.

65. Park SY, Saijo K, Takahashi T, et al: Developmental defects of lymphoid cells in Jak3 kinase-deficient mice. Immunity 3:771–782, 1995.

66. Thomis DC, Gurniak CB, Tivol E, et al: Defects in B lymphocyte maturation and T lymphocyte activation in mice lacking Jak3. Science 270:794–797, 1995.

67. Nosaka T, van Deursen JM, Tripp RA, et al: Defective lymphoid development in mice lacking Jak3. Science 270:800–802, 1995.

68. Russell SM, Tayebi N, Nakajima H, et al: Mutation of Jak3 in a patient with SCID: Essential role of Jak3 in lymphoid development. Science 270:797–800, 1995.

69. Durbin JE, Hackenmiller R, Simon MC, Levy DE: Targeted disruption of the mouse Stat1 gene results in compromised innate immunity to viral disease. Cell 84:443–450, 1996.

70. Park C, Li S, Cha E, Schindler C: Immune response in Stat2 knockout mice. Immunity 13:795–804, 2000.

71. Takeda K, Noguchi K, Shi W, et al: Targeted disruption of the mouse Stat3 gene leads to early embryonic lethality. Proc Natl Acad Sci U S A 94:3801–3804, 1997.

72. Kaplan MH, Sun YL, Hoey T, Grusby MJ: Impaired IL-12 responses and enhanced development of Th2 cells in Stat4-deficient mice. Nature 382:174–177, 1996.

73. Moriggl R, Topham DJ, Teglund S, et al: Stat5 is required for IL-2-induced cell cycle progression of peripheral T cells. Immunity 10:249–259, 1999.

74. Liu X, Robinson GW, Wagner KU, et al: Stat5a is mandatory for adult mammary gland development and lactogenesis. Genes Dev 11:179–186, 1997.

75. Udy GB, Towers RP, Snell RG, et al: Requirement of STAT5b for sexual dimorphism of body growth rates and liver gene expression. Proc Natl Acad Sci U S A 94:7239–7244, 1997.

76. Takeda K, Tanaka T, Shi W, et al: Essential role of Stat6 in IL-4 signalling. Nature 380:627–630, 1996.

77. Romano M, Sironi M, Toniatti C, et al: Role of IL-6 and its soluble receptor in induction of chemokines and leukocyte recruitment. Immunity 6:315–325, 1997.

78. Jostock T, Mullberg J, Ozbek S, et al: Soluble gp130 is the natural inhibitor of soluble interleukin-6 receptor transsignaling responses. Eur J Biochem 268:160–167, 2001.

79. Aarts LH, Roovers O, Ward AC, Touw IP: Receptor activation and 2 distinct COOH-terminal motifs control G-CSF receptor distribution and internalization kinetics. Blood 103:571–579, 2004.

80. Greenhalgh CJ, Hilton DJ: Negative regulation of cytokine signaling. J Leukoc Biol 70:348–356, 2001.

81. Wormald S, Hilton DJ: Inhibitors of cytokine signal transduction. J Biol Chem 279:821–824, 2004.

82. Nicola NA, Greenhalgh CJ: The suppressors of cytokine signaling (SOCS) proteins: Important feedback inhibitors of cytokine action. Exp Hematol 28:1105–1112, 2000.

83. Yoshimura A: The CIS/JAB family: Novel negative regulators of JAK signaling pathways. Leukemia 12:1851–1857, 1998.

84. Hilton DJ: Negative regulators of cytokine signal transduction. Cell Mol Life Sci 55:1568–1577, 1999.

85. Klingmuller U, Lorenz U, Cantley LC, et al: Specific recruitment of SH-PTP1 to the erythropoietin receptor causes inactivation of JAK2 and termination of proliferative signals. Cell 80:729–738, 1995.

86. David M, Chen HE, Goelz S, et al: Differential regulation of the alpha/beta interferon-stimulated Jak/Stat pathway by the SH2 domain-containing tyrosine phosphatase SHPTP1. Mol Cell Biol 15:7050–7058, 1995.

87. You M, Yu DH, Feng GS: Shp-2 tyrosine phosphatase functions as a negative regulator of the interferon-stimulated Jak/STAT pathway. Mol Cell Biol 19:2416–2424, 1999.

88. Alexander DR: The CD45 tyrosine phosphatase: A positive and negative regulator of immune cell function. Semin Immunol 12:349–359, 2000.

89. Irie–Sasaki J, Sasaki T, Matsumoto W, et al: CD45 is a JAK phosphatase and negatively regulates cytokine receptor signalling. Nature 409:349–354, 2001.

90. Neel BG, Tonks NK: Protein tyrosine phosphatases in signal transduction. Curr Opin Cell Biol 9:193–204, 1997.

91. Myers MP, Andersen JN, Cheng A, et al: TYK2 and JAK2 are substrates of protein-tyrosine phosphatase 1B. J Biol Chem 276:47771–47774, 2001.

92. Cheng A, Uetani N, Simoncic PD, et al: Attenuation of leptin action and regulation of obesity by protein tyrosine phosphatase 1B. Dev Cell 2:497–503, 2002.

93. Simoncic PD, Lee-Loy A, Barber DL, et al: The T cell protein tyrosine phosphatase is a negative regulator of janus family kinases 1 and 3. Curr Biol 12:446–453, 2002.

94. Chen Y, Wen R, Yang S, et al: Identification of Shp-2 as a Stat5A phosphatase. J Biol Chem 278:16520–16527, 2003.

95. Chughtai N, Schimchowitsch S, Lebrun JJ, Ali S: Prolactin induces SHP-2 association with Stat5, nuclear translocation, and binding to the beta-casein gene promoter in mammary cells. J Biol Chem 277:31107–31114, 2002.

96. Aoki N, Matsuda T: A cytosolic protein-tyrosine phosphatase PTP1B specifically dephosphorylates and deactivates prolactin-activated STAT5a and STAT5b. J Biol Chem 275:39718–39726, 2000.

97. Liu B, Liao J, Rao X, et al: Inhibition of Stat1-mediated gene activation by PIAS1. Proc Natl Acad Sci U S A 95:10626–10631, 1998.

98. Chung CD, Liao J, Liu B, et al: Specific inhibition of Stat3 signal transduction by PIAS3. Science 278:1803–1805, 1997.

99. Liu B, Gross M, ten Hoeve J, Shuai K: A transcriptional corepressor of Stat1 with an essential LXXLL signature motif. Proc Natl Acad Sci U S A 98:3203–3207, 2001.
100. Arora T, Liu B, He H, et al: PIASx is a transcriptional co-repressor of signal transducer and activator of transcription 4. J Biol Chem 278:21327–21330, 2003.
101. Takahashi Y, Toh-e A, Kikuchi Y: A novel factor required for the SUMO1/Smt3 conjugation of yeast septins. Gene 275:223–231, 2001.
102. Johnson ES, Gupta AA: An E3-like factor that promotes SUMO conjugation to the yeast septins. Cell 106:735–744, 2001.
103. Rogers RS, Horvath CM, Matunis MJ: SUMO modification of STAT1 and its role in PIAS-mediated inhibition of gene activation. J Biol Chem 278:30091–30097, 2003.
104. Ungureanu D, Vanhatupa S, Kotaja N, et al: PIAS proteins promote SUMO-1 conjugation to STAT1. Blood 102:3311–3313, 2003.
105. Alexander WS: Suppressors of cytokine signalling (SOCS) in the immune system. Nat Rev Immunol 2:410–416, 2002.
106. Hilton DJ, Richardson RT, Alexander WS, et al: Twenty proteins containing a C-terminal SOCS box form five structural classes. Proc Natl Acad Sci U S A 95:114–119, 1998.

107. Nicholson SE, Willson TA, Farley A, et al: Mutational analyses of the SOCS proteins suggest a dual domain requirement but distinct mechanisms for inhibition of LIF and IL-6 signal transduction. EMBO J 18:375–385, 1999.
108. Sasaki A, Yasukawa H, Shouda T, et al: CIS3/SOCS-3 suppresses erythropoietin (EPO) signaling by binding the EPO receptor and JAK2. J Biol Chem 275:29338–29347, 2000.
109. Kile BT, Schulman BA, Alexander WS, et al: The SOCS box: A tale of destruction and degradation. Trends Biochem Sci 27:235–241, 2002.
110. Zhang JG, Farley A, Nicholson SE, et al: The conserved SOCS box motif in suppressors of cytokine signaling binds to elongins B and C and may couple bound proteins to proteasomal degradation. Proc Natl Acad Sci U S A 96:2071–2076, 1999.
111. Kamura T, Sato S, Haque D, et al: The Elongin BC complex interacts with the conserved SOCS-box motif present in members of the SOCS, ras, WD-40 repeat, and ankyrin repeat families. Genes Dev 12:3872–3881, 1998.
112. De Sepulveda P, Ilangumaran S, Rottapel R: Suppressor of cytokine signaling-1 inhibits VAV function through protein degradation. J Biol Chem 275:14005–14008, 2000.
113. Kamizono S, Hanada T, Yasukawa H, et al: The SOCS box of SOCS-1

accelerates ubiquitin-dependent proteolysis of TEL-JAK2. J Biol Chem 276:12530–12538, 2001.
114. Alexander WS, Starr R, Fenner JE, et al: SOCS1 is a critical inhibitor of interferon gamma signaling and prevents the potentially fatal neonatal actions of this cytokine. Cell 98:597–608, 1999.
115. Metcalf D, Greenhalgh CJ, Viney E, et al: Gigantism in mice lacking suppressor of cytokine signalling-2. Nature 405:1069–1073, 2000.
116. Marine JC, McKay C, Wang D, et al: SOCS3 is essential in the regulation of fetal liver erythropoiesis. Cell 98:617–627, 1999.
117. Roberts AW, Robb L, Rakar S, et al: Placental defects and embryonic lethality in mice lacking suppressor of cytokine signaling 3. Proc Natl Acad Sci U S A 98:9324–9329, 2001.
118. Croker BA, Krebs DL, Zhang JG, et al: SOCS3 negatively regulates IL-6 signaling in vivo. Nat Immunol 4:540–545, 2003.
119. Yasukawa H, Ohishi M, Mori H, et al: IL-6 induces an anti-inflammatory response in the absence of SOCS3 in macrophages. Nat Immunol 4:551–556, 2003.
120. Lang R, Pauleau AL, Parganas E, et al: SOCS3 regulates the plasticity of gp130 signaling. Nat Immunol 4:546–550, 2003.

Hormone Signaling via Serine Kinase Receptors

Dana Gaddy

INTRODUCTION

Numerous hormones and growth factors initiate cellular signaling by direct or indirect stimulation of protein kinase activity, as discussed in Chapters 8, 9, and 11 through 14. The receptor serine kinases (RSKs) represent one of the most recently characterized classes of transmembrane signaling systems that use membrane-associated kinases. Like the receptor tyrosine kinases (RTKs), these receptors bind an extracellular factor at the cell membrane and directly activate protein kinases.

The RSK family encompasses receptors for transforming growth factor-β (TGF-β) and related proteins. TGF-β and related factors signal through a heteromeric complex of transmembrane receptors with intrinsic protein serine/threonine kinase activity. Conceptually, the design of this RSK signaling system shares substantial similarity with both the RTK (Chapter 8) and Janus kinase (JK)/signal transduction and activators of transcription (STAT) (Chapter 9) signaling systems.

HISTORY

The founding member of the superfamily, TGF-β1, was originally identified as a regulator of mesenchymal and epithelial cell growth.[1,2] Activins were identified as endocrine regulators of pituitary function (reviewed in Ref. 3) and, independently, as erythroid differentiation inducers,[4] as well as stimulators of mesoderm development in frogs.[5] Bone morphogenic proteins (BMPs) were initially identified as bone repair factors[6] but have been more recently shown to be involved in the regulation of reproductive function as well.[7]

Unlike the RTKs, which bind to their family of ligands as homodimers, specific binding of each [^{125}I]-labeled ligand in the TGF-β superfamily to responsive cells resulted in the labeling of two species of approximately 50 and 75 kilodalton, known as the type I and type II receptors. Although the identification of the first RTK activity was reported in 1980 (see Chapter 8; Ref. 8), another 10 years passed before identification of the first high-affinity binding receptor moiety that signaled by one of the members of the TGF-β superfamily, activin.[9] This receptor, ActRII, represented the type II approximately 75-kilodalton [^{125}I]-activin A–binding species. Subsequently, molecular cloning yielded genes encoding two type II receptors (ActRII and ActRIIB) and at least two type I receptors (ALK2 and ALK4) for activin.[10] As with the superfamily of structurally related ligands, the activin receptors are members of a larger family of RSKs, which include type I and type II receptors for TGF-β, BMPs, and the *Drosophila* protein, decapentaplegic.

LIGANDS AND BIOLOGICAL EFFECTS

The TGF-β superfamily includes more than 30 peptide growth factors[11–14] that regulate a broad range of cellular functions, including proliferation, cell differentiation, immune surveillance, extracellular matrix secretion and cell adhesion, apoptosis, and specification of developmental fate[15–17]; detailed discussion of the functions of activin, inhibin, and the more distantly related MIS is found in Chapter 143. Ligands within the superfamily are disulfide-linked dimers; both homodimers and heterodimers are known. In mammals, the study of TGF-β–related molecules has focused on control of sexual development and function (müllerian-inhibiting substance [MIS], inhibin, activin, and BMPs), pituitary hormone production (activin and inhibin), and the creation and maintenance of bones and cartilage (activin, BMPs, and growth and differentiation factors [GDFs]). In addition, TGF-β ligands play important roles in the induction of growth arrest through cell-cycle inhibition and stimulation of apoptosis. These activities can be exerted by classic delivery of the factor to its target tissue from a distant site of production via the circulation (endocrine), by local action on neighboring cells (paracrine), or by stimulation of the same cell that produced and secreted the factor (autocrine). Insight into the mechanisms of pleiotropy and redundancy for TGF-β–related factors has been gained through signal-transduction studies in a variety of cell types. Together, it is clear that the panoply of actions regulated by these factors is critical for normal growth and homeostasis. Abnormal signaling arising from mutations in individual components of the pathway described in this chapter leads to significant developmental defects, pathophysiology, clinical syndromes, cancers, and diseases in a wide variety of tissues (reviewed in Refs. 12 and 18).

RECEPTORS

STRUCTURES AND BINDING PROPERTIES OF TYPE II AND TYPE I RECEPTORS

The holoreceptor complex for TGF-β–related factors contains proteins from each of the two subfamilies of RSKs. In mammals, five type II receptors and eight type I receptors have been identified that transduce signals for activin, TGF-β, BMP2/4, BMP7/OP-1 (osteogenic, protein-1), MIS, and GDF-5.[1,19–21] Most receptor complexes bind several ligands, and several type I receptors form combinatorial interactions with type II receptors, thus creating signal diversity (Table 10-1; reviewed in Refs. 12, 22–24).

The RSKs contain an extracellular ligand-binding domain, a single membrane-spanning region, and a cytoplasmic kinase domain with serine-threonine phosphorylation specificity (Fig. 10-1). Several structural features distinguish the type I and type II receptors. They share conserved cysteine residues in their extracellular domains; the three-dimensional structure of the extracellular domain of a type II activin receptor indicates that these cysteines probably direct all the members of this family to adopt a common fold.[25] Type I and type II receptors possess distinct kinase domain sequences with less than 50% sequence identity. The type I receptors contain a unique, approximately 30-amino acid juxtamembrane sequence called the glycine/serine-rich (GS) domain that contains serine and threonine residues whose phosphorylation by type II receptors is essential for signal propagation.[26–28] The three-dimensional structure of the kinase domain of the type I TGF-β receptor suggests that phosphorylation of GS domain residues places the kinase in an enzymatically active conformation.[29] In general, the type II receptor confers ligand-binding specificity, whereas the type I receptor, in combination with the type II receptor, transmits the phosphorylation signal.

For TGF-β and activin signaling, ligands bind to type II receptors in the absence of type I receptors; however, type I receptors bind ligands only in the presence of type II receptors, creating

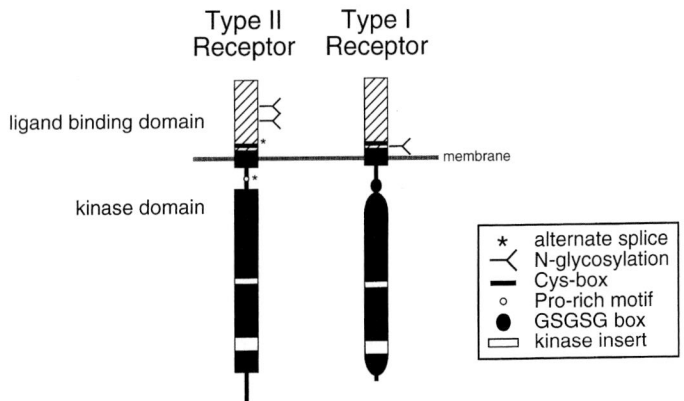

Figure 10-1 Schematic diagram of type I and type II receptor serine kinases. Specific features are indicated.

a sequential binding interaction. In contrast to the receptor requirements for activin and TGF-β binding, BMPs bind with low affinity to BMP type I or type II receptors individually. High-affinity BMP binding and signaling are observed only when both receptor types are presented together in a cooperative manner.[21,30,31] Thus, BMPs 2, 4, and 7 and GDF5 bind weakly to the type II receptor BMPR-II expressed alone[32–35] and to the type I receptors BMPR-IA or BMPR-IB expressed alone.[30,31] ActR-II and -IIB are true activin receptors that bind BMP poorly, if at all. However, ActR-II and -IIB can bind BMPs 2 and 7 in cooperation with BMPR-IA or BMPR-IB.[36] Several different combinations of type I and type II receptors are possible for each ligand (see Table 10-1), some of which result in signal diversity for each ligand.[12] For example, BMP2 can stimulate the differentiation of pluripotent stromal cells to an adipogenic lineage by signaling through BMPRII-BMPRIA and

Table 10-1 Mammalian Transforming Growth Factor-β Family Members, Their Receptors, Signaling Molecules, and Their Antagonists

| Ligand Subfamily | Receptors | | R-Smad | Antagonist/Trap |
	Type II	Type I		
TGF-β	TβRII	ALK5	Smad2	Decorin
			Smad3	Biglycan
		ALK1	Smad1	α₂M
Activin	ActRII	ALK4	Smad2	α₂M
	ActRIIB		Smad3	Cerberus
				Follistatin
BMP2/4	BMPRII	ALK3	Smad1	Cerberus, Chordin
	ActRII	ALK4	Smad5	Gremlin, Noggin
		ALK6	Smad8	Dan
BMP7 (OP1)	BMPRII	ALK2	Smad1	Cerberus, Chordin
	ActRII	ALK3	Smad5	Gremlin, Noggin
	ActRIIB	ALK6	Smad8	Dan
GDF5	BMPRII	ALK6	Smad1	Cerberus, Chordin
	ActRII		Smad5	Gremlin, Noggin
	ActRIIB		Smad8	Dan
MIS	MIS-RII	ALK2	Smad8	ND
Nodal	ActRIIB	ALK4	Smad2	ND
		ALK7	Smad3	

TGF-β, transforming growth factor-β; BMP, bone morphogenic protein; GDF, growth and differentiation factor; OP-1, osteogenic protein-1; MIS, müllerian-inhibiting substance; ALK, activin-like kinase; α₂M, α₂-macroglobulin; ND, not determined.[26,73,129]

can stimulate differentiation to an osteoblastic lineage through BMPRII-BMPRIB signaling in murine cells.[37]

CORECEPTORS FOR TRANSFORMING GROWTH FACTOR-β SUPERFAMILY LIGANDS

Receptors I and II are both necessary and sufficient to generate a transmembrane signal for most members of the TGF-β superfamily; however, other cell-surface-binding proteins have been described that may not be RSKs. TGF-β binds to a type III non–kinase domain-containing receptor called betaglycan with a core size of 130 kilodalton, which can either facilitate or modulate TGF-β binding to type I/II receptors.[38,39]

A related proteoglycan to betaglycan, endoglin, a dimer of disulfide-linked 95-kilodalton subunits,[40,41] also binds TGF-β as well as activin and BMPs.[42] Although its role in signaling remains unclear, the overexpression of endoglin antagonizes several cellular responses to TGF-β1, whereas its downregulation potentiates cellular responses to TGF-β1.[43] In addition, endoglin appears to be necessary for cardiogenesis,[44] and mutations in endoglin are associated with hereditary hemorrhagic telangiectasia type 1.[45]

INHIBIN-RECEPTOR INTERACTIONS

More recently, betaglycan has been identified as a coreceptor that binds inhibin and increases the affinity of inhibin for the type II activin receptors.[46] The specificity of betaglycan binding to inhibin and TGF-β is conferred through two independent ligand-binding regions of the betaglycan ectodomain. The inhibin-binding domain is located in the carboxy-terminal uromodulin-related region. Both the uromodulin-related region and the amino-terminal endoglin-related region are capable of binding TGF-β2 at higher affinity than TGF-β1. However, only the endoglin-related region increases the TGF-β2 labeling of the type II receptor, serving the TGF-β "presentation to the type II receptor" function.[47] The inhibin-betaglycan interaction with ActRII/ActRIIB appears to sequester the type II receptors, thereby providing a mechanism whereby inhibin acts as a competitive antagonist by competing with activin for access to the type II receptors. Interestingly, the complex formed between the inhibins, ActRIIA, and betaglycan was resistant to disruption by activin A, whereas activin A potently competed for inhibin binding to ActRIIB2 and betaglycan.[48] Thus, inhibin isoforms have different affinities for the activin type II receptors but bind betaglycan with high affinity. A similar mechanism has been reported for inhibin-betaglycan interaction with BMPRII,[49] providing a mechanism by which inhibin may antagonize a variety of activin and BMP responses, depending on which ligand and receptor combination is present in a given cell type.[48,50] However, betaglycan may not be required to mediate all of the effects of inhibin. At least some of the inhibin antagonism in liver cells is based in part on dominant negative interaction of the shared β subunit of inhibin with activin receptors.[51] However, inhibin-specific binding to betaglycan-associated complexes in testis cell lines have identified additional moieties of approximately 145 and 95 kilodaltons. These data suggest that the high-affinity binding complex for inhibin A found in these cells may consist of betaglycan and several other proteins of unknown identity, and together may represent the putative inhibin-receptor complex.[52]

Identification of the glycosyl-phosphatidylinositol (GPI)-anchored 120-kilodalton inhibin-binding protein, InhBP/p120, suggested the involvement of another non-RSK molecule in inhibin signaling.[53] However, p120 may not directly bind inhibins but may interact with the activin type IB receptor, ALK4, and participate in the inhibin B antagonism of activin signaling.[54] However, InhBP/p120 mutant male

and female mice were viable and fertile and showed no alterations in follicle-stimulating hormone (FSH) synthesis or secretion or in ovarian or testicular function, which suggests that this binding protein is not essential for inhibin signaling.[55]

GLIAL CELL LINE–DERIVED NEUROTROPHIC FACTOR/RECEPTOR INTERACTIONS

Finally, the glial cell line–derived neurotrophic factor (GDNF) family of ligands (GDNF, neurturin, artemin, and persephin) are distant members of the TGF-β superfamily that are unique in their mode of non-RSK signaling. The GDNF ligands activate intracellular signaling cascades via a heterodimeric receptor complex containing the tyrosine kinase Ret and a specific GPI-linked-binding protein, the GDNF family receptor alpha (GFRα).[56] The GDNF-GFRα complex binds to and stimulates autophosphorylation of Ret. Alternatively, a preassociated complex between GFRα and Ret could form the binding site for the GDNF family ligand. GFRα1, GFRα2, GFRα3, and GFRα4 are the physiological coreceptors for GDNF, neurturin, artemin, and persephin, respectively.[13] Interestingly, in many neuronal systems, TGF-β itself is required as a cofactor for GDNF family ligand signaling.[13]

DOWNSTREAM SIGNALING CASCADE

The mechanism of activation of RSKs has been characterized for TGF-β, activin, and BMP signaling (Fig. 10-2, steps 1 to 4; reviewed in Refs. 12 and 26). The general signaling mechanism is initiated by high-affinity binding of the ligand to the constitutively phosphorylated type II receptor and formation of the ligand-RI-RII complex. The type II receptor kinase then phosphorylates the catalytically inactive type I receptor cytoplasmic domain, at least in part at the GS site.[29] Once phosphorylated and activated, the type I receptor phosphorylates substrate proteins, which transmit the signal to the nucleus. Although several type I–interacting proteins have been described, the Smads (see later) are the primary molecules known to be activated by type I receptor–mediated phosphorylation and transmit the ligand-dependent signal to the nucleus to alter gene transcription.

The RSK model resembles the JAK/STAT signal-transduction pathway for cytokine receptors described in the previous chapter. In RSK signaling, the type I receptor corresponds to the JAK, and the Smads correspond to the STATs. As with cytokine signaling, these proteins manifest diversity through different combinatorial associations between type II and type I receptors, as well as through different type I–Smad interactions. Pathway redundancy can be achieved by multiple ligands using similar receptors or activating similar Smads.

INTRACELLULAR SIGNAL MEDIATORS

Smads

Activation of the Smads is a central cytoplasmic event in TGF-β superfamily signaling.[12,57,58] The Smads are so named as a contraction of the first identified members of this class of signaling proteins, Sma (from *Caenorhabditis elegans*[59]) and Mad (from *Drosophila melanogaster*[60]). Alignment of Smad sequences reveals strongly conserved domains in the amino and carboxy termini (termed *Mad homology [MH] domains*), separated by a central linker region (Fig. 10-3). Such analysis suggests a division into three subgroups of Smads, the receptor-regulated Smads (R-Smads), the common mediator Smads (Co-Smads), and the inhibitory Smads (I-Smads). The AR-Smads are Smad2 and Smad3, which are phosphorylated specifically by TGF-β and activin receptors. The BR-Smads are Smad1, Smad5, and Smad8, which are activated specifically

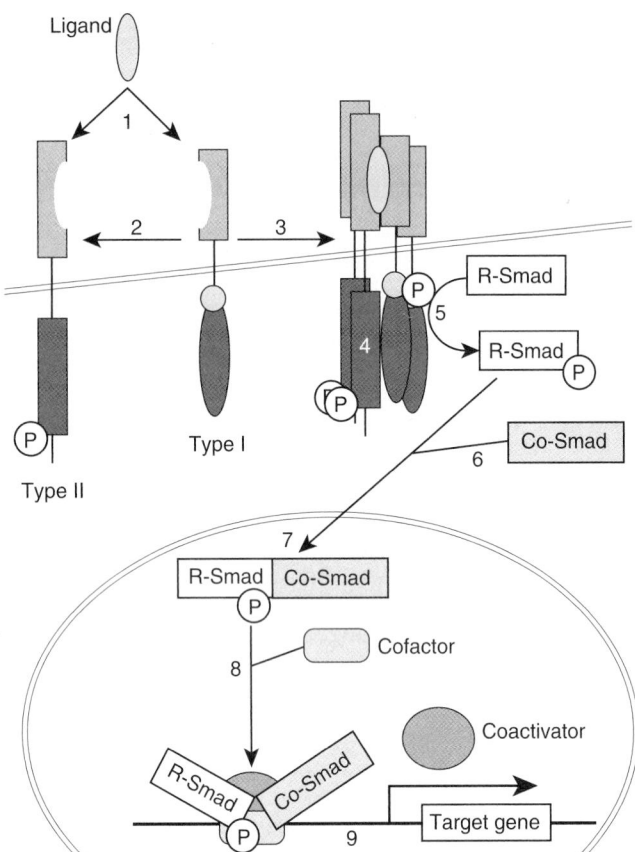

Figure 10-2 Overview of SMAD signaling via ligands of the transforming growth factor (TGF)-β superfamily. Binding of a TGF-β family member to its type II receptor (**1**) in concert with a type I receptor (**2**) occurs sequentially for the binding of activin and TGF-β ligands and occurs coordinately for bone morphogenic protein (BMP) ligands. In either case, this interaction leads to formation of a heterotetrameric receptor complex (**3**) and phosphorylation of the type I receptor in the GS box by the kinase domain of the type II receptor (**4**). Once activated, the type I receptor subsequently phosphorylates selective receptor-regulated SMADs (R-Smad) (**5**), which facilitates the R-SMAD protein association with the Co-Smad, Smad4 (**6**), and subsequent translocation to the nucleus (**7**). In the nucleus, the SMAD complex associates with several DNA-binding cofactors (**8**) that include cognate transcription factors that themselves bind DNA or that will interact with Smads on a Smad-binding element (SBE), and coregulators (activators or repressors) that will either enhance or suppress the rate of transcription on targets genes (**9**).

in response to BMP 2/4/7 or MIS stimulation (see Table 10-1[12,57,58]). Specific sequences in the carboxyl domain serve to restrict Smad interaction with the type I receptors.[61] Once phosphorylated in the C-terminal SSXS motif, the R-Smad then associates with a member of the second group, the Co-Smad, to allow nuclear translocation and facilitation of TGF-β, activin, or BMP responses (see Fig. 10-2, steps 5 to 7[62,63]). Finally, the third group of Smads are the I-Smads, Smad6 and Smad7. These inhibitory Smads lack the SSXS phosphorylation motif of the R-SMADs and act primarily as competitors for binding of the pathway-restricted Smads to activated receptors[64–67] or, to a lesser extent, Smad4.[68] However, I-SMADs also block RSK signaling through interaction with type I receptors, preventing R-SMAD binding, and targeting the receptor for internalization and degradation (Fig. 10-4).[65,69]

Additional signal suppression occurs through modification of the R-Smads. Between the MH1 and MH2 domains of the R-Smads is a linker region of variable sequence and length (see Fig. 10-3). Phosphorylation of the linker region in R-Smads

can be stimulated by mitogen-activated protein kinase (MAPK) through the activation of RTK ligands, such as epidermal growth factor (EGF) and fibroblast growth factor (FGF). Linker-region phosphorylation of Smad1 at cognate MAPK sites prevents nuclear localization of the Smad1-Smad4 complex and blocks BMP signaling.[70] Similar MAPK-mediated phosphorylation and nuclear exclusion of other R-Smads may provide an explanation for the antagonism between FGF ligands and BMPs during development,[71] as well as in the ability of hyperactive RAS/MAPK activity to override normal TGF-β-mediated growth inhibition.[72]

A summary of Smad activation and function is shown in Figure 10-2. The expression of cell-specific repertoires of a limited number of type II and type I receptors and Smads allows convergence and redundancy of effects of ligands within the TGF-β superfamily. However, intracellularly, Smads interact with various proteins, including transcriptional enhancers and repressors, to confer a wide variety of biologic activities in multiple cell types in response to a given ligand within the TGF-β superfamily. As shown in Figure 10-3, in addition to transcription regulators and coregulators (described in more detail later), R-Smads also interact with other cellular proteins, which aid in signal transmission (e.g., nuclear import proteins), inhibit their activity (e.g., calmodulin), and facilitate downregulation of the signal through proteosomal degradation of signal components (e.g., Smurf).[12,73–75]

Smad REGULATION OF GENE TRANSCRIPTION

Smads directly bind DNA and induce or repress transcriptional responses through cooperative binding with other transcription factors.[76,77] A consensus Smad-binding core element (SBE), AGAC, is found in several TGF-β-inducible and activin-inducible promoters that bind to Smad complexes.[78] Smads activate transcription in response to ligand either alone or through functional cooperation with other transcription factors, which themselves also bind to DNA. Interaction of Smad2 with FAST-1 (forkhead activin signal transducer) or FAST-2 is required for activin-dependent Smad2/4-mediated transcription from the *Mix.2* (mesoderm inducer) and *goosecoid* promoters, respectively.[79–81] Similarly, Smads 3 and 4 cooperate with TFE3 (transcription factor μE3) to induce TGF-β-dependent transcription from the *plasminogen activator inhibitor-1 (PAI-1)* promoter.[82] TGF-β-inducible transcription via adaptor protein 1 (AP-1) sites also can be achieved through Smad3 interaction with c-*Jun* and c-*Fos* to form a multiprotein complex with Smad4.[78,83] Interaction of Smads and members of the AP-1 transcription factor family provides one example of a plethora of converging signaling pathways.[76] Others are described later, exemplified by the R-Smad binding partners listed in Figure 10-3.

Interestingly, Smad2 and Smad3 are not functionally equivalent. Smad3, but not Smad2, participates in ligand-dependent DNA binding to SBEs in both the *PAI-1*[84] and *JunB*[85] promoters. The lack of Smad2 binding to DNA is due to a sequence insert in the DNA-binding region of Smad2 that is not present in Smad3; this insert probably interferes with DNA recognition.[86,87] Conversely, Smad2 and Smad3 have opposing functions in transcriptional activation of the *goosecoid* promoter.[80] More recently, ornithine decarboxylase antizyme (OAZ) was identified as a zinc-finger transcription factor that acts as a DNA-binding cofactor that associates with an activated Smad1-Smad4 complex. OAZ and Smads are required for efficient binding to a BMP-response element containing an OAZ-binding site as well as a CAGAC SBE on the homeobox gene, *Xvent-2*, to enhance gene transcription.[88]

Smads also interact with transcriptional cofactors from other signaling pathways and induce either enhancement or inhibition of Smad-dependent responses (see Fig. 10-4). Among the first identified, the transcriptional coactivators CBP (cyclic adenosine monophosphate [cAMP] response ele-

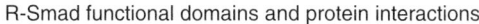

R-Smad functional domains and protein interactions

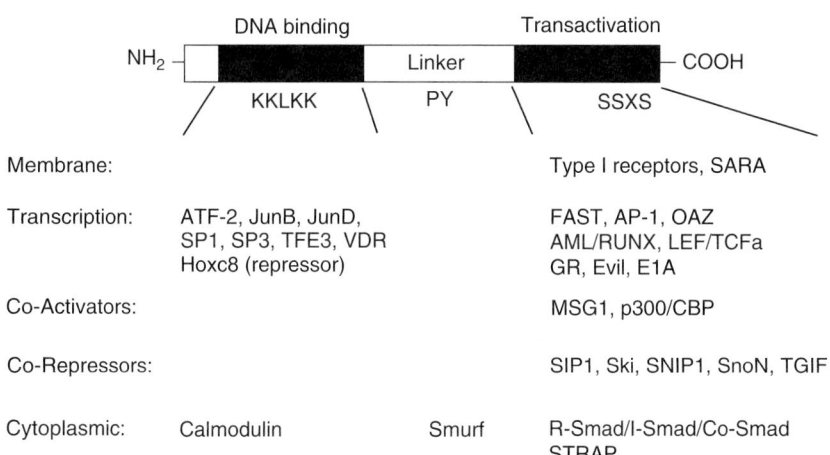

	DNA binding		Linker		Transactivation	
NH$_2$						COOH
	KKLKK		PY		SSXS	

Membrane:			Type I receptors, SARA	
Transcription:	ATF-2, JunB, JunD, SP1, SP3, TFE3, VDR Hoxc8 (repressor)		FAST, AP-1, OAZ AML/RUNX, LEF/TCFa GR, Evil, E1A	
Co-Activators:			MSG1, p300/CBP	
Co-Repressors:			SIP1, Ski, SNIP1, SnoN, TGIF	
Cytoplasmic:	Calmodulin	Smurf	R-Smad/I-Smad/Co-Smad STRAP	
Nuclear import:	Nuclear importin-β		Nup214, Nup153	

Figure 10-3 Schematic diagram of R-Smad functional domains and the proteins that interact with those domains. Examples of plasma membrane components, transcription factors, coactivators, corepressors, cytoplasmic proteins, and proteins involved in nuclear importation are listed under the domain of the R-Smad with which each protein is known to interact. Other cytoplasmic proteins also interact with R-Smads, although the sites of interaction have not yet been determined: tubulin[152]; β-catenin[106]; TAK1[137]; ARIP1[120]; whose interaction sites on the R-Smad molecules have been identified. AML, acute myeloid leukemia; ATF-2, activating transcription factor-2; AP-1, activator protein-1; CBP, CREB-binding protein; Co-Smad, common mediator Smad4; CREB, cAMP-responsive element binding protein; E1A, early region 1A; Evi-1, ectopic viral integration site-1; FAST, forkhead activin signal transducer; GR, glucocorticoid receptor; Hoxc-8, homeobox gene c-8; I-Smad, inhibitory Smad; Lef1/Tcf, lymphoid enhancer binding factor 1/T cell-specific factor; MH, mad homology domain; MSG1, melanocyte-specific gene 1; Nup, nucleoporin; OAZ, Olf-1/EBF associated zinc-finger; R-Smad, pathway restricted Smad; Runx, runt-related gene; SARA, Smad anchor for receptor activation; Ski, Sloan-Kettering avian retrovirus; SnoN, ski-related novel gene; Smurf, Smad ubiquitination regulatory factor; SNIP-1, Smad nuclear interacting protein 1; SP, specificity protein; STRAP, serine-threonine kinase receptor-associated protein; TAK1, TGF-β-activated kinase 1; TFE3, transcription factor E3; TGIF, TGF-β-interacting factor; VDR, vitamin D receptor. Selected references describing interactions of R-Smads with proteins listed in this table include ATF-2[153]; Jun/c–Fos[83]; calmodulin[75]; E1A[154]; Evi-1[155]; FAST[80,156]; GR[157]; Hoxc-8[158,159]; β-importin[146]; junB and junD[160]; Lef1/Tcf[104]; MSG1[93]; Nup214 and Nup153[147,148]; OAZ[88]; p300/CBP[90,161]; Runx/AML[99–101]; SARA[142]; SIP1[162]; Ski[107,108]; Smads (reviewed in Refs. 22 and 163); SnoN[109]; Smurf[164,165]; SNIP1[166]; SP1[102,103]; STRAP[116]; TAK1[137]; TFE3[82]; TGIF[167]; type I receptors (reviewed in Refs. 22 and 163); and VDR.[95]

ment [CREB] binding protein) and p300 interact with and enhance the transcriptional activity of Smads after Smad phosphorylation.[89–92] CBP and p300 modify chromatin organization and may serve to bridge specific transcription factors, such as CREB, AP-1, STATs, nuclear factor-kappa B (NF-κB), p53, and steroid/nuclear receptors, with components of the basal transcriptional apparatus.[89] More recently, it was shown that nuclear MSG1, which does not itself bind DNA, enhances Smad-mediated transcription in a manner dependent on p300/CBP.[93] Thus, the identification of Smads as transcription factors that bind p300/CBP provides a mechanism whereby integration of signals from multiple ligands can occur. Smad3 also cooperates with activated vitamin D receptors to enhance the transcription of vitamin D–regulated genes, which explains, in part, the known cross-talk between the TGF-β and vitamin D signaling pathways.[94–96]

Recently, the list of Smad-binding transcription factor partners whose integrative interactions modulate downstream gene expression has greatly expanded to include cell lineage–specific and pathway-specific transcription factors, other coactivators, and several transcriptional repressors (Fig. 10-3; reviewed in Refs. 12 and 97). For example, in addition to AP-1 and activating transcription factor 2 (ATF-2), Smads 1 to 4 also interact with several members of the runt-domain–containing family of transcription factors (AML/CBF/Runx), suggesting that the Runx-Smad interactions play important roles in hematopoiesis, osteoblastogenesis, and chondrogenesis.[98–101] Interaction of R-Smads with Sp1 and Sp3 results in modulation of *p15 (Ink4b)* and *p21 (Waf1/Cip1)* transcription,[102,103] providing a mechanism by which increased expression of cyclin-dependent kinase inhibitors can lead to growth inhibition.

Finally, Smads have been demonstrated to interact physically with LEF1/TCF transcription factors, which normally mediate Wnt signaling.[104] Moreover, specific DNA-binding sites in the *Xenopus twin* promoter have demonstrated synergistic activation by the TGF-β and Wnt pathways, which may have important signaling-interaction implications during development.[105] Interestingly, TGF-β-dependent activation of LEF1/TCF target genes was shown to occur independent of β-catenin, an essential component of the Wnt signaling pathway.[105]

Conversely, β-catenin does appear to play a role in TGF-β-regulated loss of cell-cell contact and disassembly of adherens junctions in kidney proximal tubule cells.[106] Immunoprecipitation experiments demonstrated colocalization of E-cadherin, β-catenin, and TβRII in unstimulated cells. In response to TGF-β1 stimulation, TβRII dissociated from the adherens protein and β-catenin, leaving β-catenin free to associate with Smad3 and Smad4.[106] These data suggest a dual role for the Wnt/β-catenin pathway in mediating TGF-β regulation of cell contact and gene transcription.

Several transcriptional repressors have been found to bind Smads, such as Ski, its related protein, SnoN, and TG-interacting factor (TGIF).[107–109] These repressors interact with Smads 2, 3, and 4 in the nucleus. They compete with the transcriptional coactivators (p300/CBP) and recruit histone deacetylases to the Smad complex, resulting in transcriptional repression (see Fig. 10-4; reviewed in Refs. 73 and 110).

Together, these DNA-binding Smad cofactors provide several levels of specificity to a Smad-dependent transcriptional response. By specifically interacting with only one

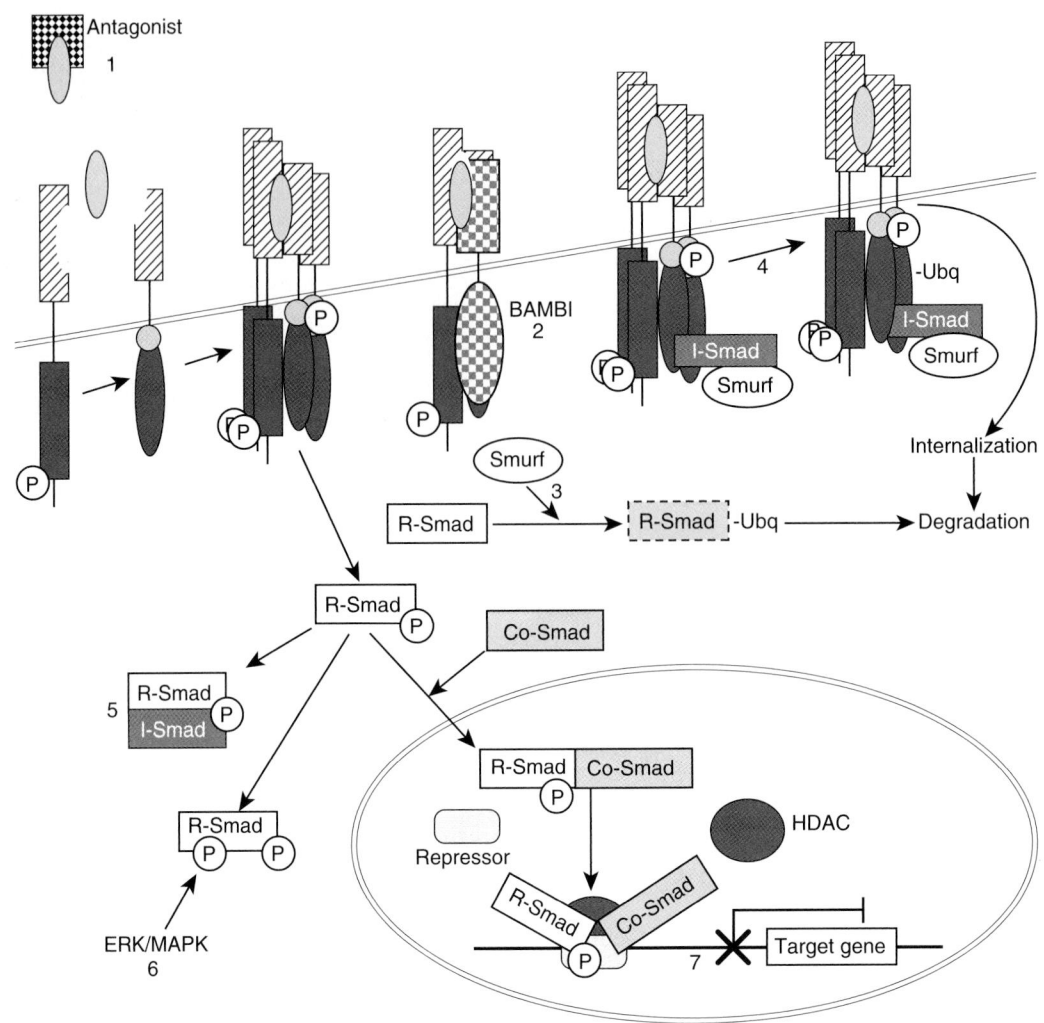

Figure 10-4 Overview of sites of downregulation of receptor serine kinase signaling. Selective soluble extracellular antagonists **(1)** soak up ligand and prevent interaction with the receptor complex. BAMBI **(2)**, an ALK-like receptor lacking a kinase domain acts as a pseudoreceptor to block ligand-type II downstream signaling. Unactivated R-Smads are ubiquitinated by the E3-ubiquitin ligases (Smurf, **3**), and targeted for proteosomal degradation. Smurf also is recruited to the receptor complex by I-Smads **(4)**, facilitating ubiquitination of the type I receptor and its internalization in calveolin vesicles, and leading to proteosomal degradation. Signaling through phosphorylated R-Smads can be blocked by **(5)** binding of the R-Smad to I-Smad, thus preventing interaction with Co-Smad and nuclear translocation, or **(6)**, further phosphorylation in the linker region by an ERK/MAPK that has been activated by another pathway, preventing nuclear import. The transcriptional activity of the nuclear phosphorylated R-Smad/Co-Smad complex can be blocked by binding of corepressors and histone deacetylases to the Smad complex on DNA **(7)**.

class of R-Smad, transcription factors can ensure pathway specificity. By binding to target genes that contain the SBE and selective ligand-specific enhancers (i.e., BMP response element [BRE] or activin response elements), the transcription factors can confer target gene specificity within the given ligand-activated pathways. Finally, coordinate cell-specific expression of the transcription factors, the R-Smads, and the receptors for which the Smads are activated will restrict transcriptional response that can be mediated by the cofactor. Together, these mechanisms underlie the specificity and the wide variety of biologic actions of the many TGF-β superfamily ligands.

OTHER SIGNAL MEDIATORS

Several cytoplasmic proteins have been identified that interact with the kinase domain of type I and type II receptors, thereby modulating their downstream aspects of RSK-initiated signaling. TAK1 (TGF-β–activated kinase-1), a protein involved in the JNK (c-*Jun* NH$_2$-terminal kinase) and p38/MPK2 pathways,[111] is a TGF-β or BMP-activated MAPK that can regulate a TGF-β-responsive promoter.[112,113] TRIP-1 (TGF-β receptor–interacting protein-1) binds and becomes phosphorylated by TβR-II. The interaction requires a functional TβR-II kinase and leads to suppression of the TGF-β-induced PAI-1 transcriptional response, but not TGF-β-induced cyclin A response.[114,115]

The WD domain–containing protein STRAP can associate with TβR-I and TβR-II. STRAP and the inhibitory Smad7

synergistically block TGF-β-mediated transcriptional activation.[116,117] TβR-I-associated protein-1 (TRAP-1) interacts specifically with the activated TβR-I. However, its functional role in TGF-β signaling is unclear.[118] A TRAP-1-like protein (TLP) has been shown to associate with both active and kinase-deficient TGF-β and activin type II receptors, but interacts with the common-mediator Smad4 only in the presence of TGF-β or activin signaling, suggesting its function as a selective chaperone of activated AR-Smads.[119]

Activin receptors also interact with additional proteins. ARIP-1 has been identified as a type II activin receptor interacting protein, which binds to both ActRII and to Smad3 via the PDZ domain in the ARIP-1 molecule.[120] Overexpression of ARIP1 in neural cells indicates that ARIP1 has a significant role in assembling activin signaling molecules at specific subcellular sites and in regulating signal transduction in neuronal cells.[120]

REGULATION OF RECEPTOR SERINE KINASE SIGNALING

The magnitude of the RSK signal is subject to extensive regulation, at multiple subcellular sites of action in the pathway (examples summarized in Fig. 10-4), which is similar to that of the cytokine receptors. One notable difference is the characterization of several soluble, extracellular ligand-binding proteins that antagonize signaling through RSKs. Local expression of these ligand family–specific antagonists and less-specific ligand traps provides an additional level of signaling control (see Table 10-1 and Fig. 10-4, mechanism 1).

ACTIVIN ANTAGONISTS

Follistatin suppresses several activin-induced functions[121,122] (see Chapter 143 for more information). Follistatin also antagonizes the effects of inhibin, BMP7 (OP-1),[36] and BMP11,[123] although at higher concentrations than needed to neutralize activin. This result is consistent with the ability of BMP7 and inhibin to bind and signal through both type II and type I activin receptors.[124] However, follistatin has not been reported to bind BMP2/4 directly, and it does not neutralize the effects of TGF-β1, even at 3000-fold molar excess.[36] A follistatin-like protein, follistatin-related gene (FLRG), binds activins and BMPs and controls their functions extracellularly. However, the mode of association of follistatin and FLRG with activins and their expression patterns are different, suggesting the distinct functions of follistatin and FLRG in vivo.[125]

BMP ANTAGONISTS

In contrast to follistatin and FLRG, other secreted proteins bind and neutralize BMPs but not activin (see Table 10-1). Noggin binds with high affinity (K_d of 19 pmol/L) to BMP2/4 and prevents interaction with cognate receptors; noggin binds to BMP7 less tightly and not at all to TGF-β or activin, even at nanomolar concentrations.[126] A second BMP4-binding antagonist, chordin, binds specifically to BMP4 (K_d of 3 pmol/L) but not to activin or TGF-β.[127] Other identified antagonists include gremlin and Cerberus.[128] Cerberus blocks signaling by BMPs, as well as by activin- and nodal-like members of the TGF-β superfamily.[128] In addition, cerberus functions as a multivalent growth factor antagonist in the extracellular space; it binds to nodal, BMP, and Wnt proteins via independent sites.[127] The fact that these antagonists are usually expressed in the same local environment as the ligands and that they antagonize suggests a mechanism whereby ligand-dependent effects can be limited by the secretion of a specific antagonist that can act to sequester extracellular ligand in the absence of receptor signaling.[129]

SIGNAL DOWNREGULATION VIA CELL SURFACE RECEPTORS AND INTERACTING PROTEINS

Once ligand is available to interact with its specific receptor, several mechanisms exist at the plasma membrane to limit downstream signal transmission. At the receptor level, the immunophilin FKBP12 (FK506-binding protein-12) binds to all type I receptors tested and inhibits RSK signaling in the absence of ligand.[130,131] Furthermore, during TGF-β signaling, clathrin-dependent internalization of an activated type I–type II TGF-β receptor complex occurs within minutes of ligand stimulation.[132] Optimal endocytosis and subsequent downregulation of the heteromeric TGF-β receptor requires kinase activity of the type II but not the type I receptor.[132] Studies of TGF-β receptor downregulation in murine osteoblastic cells also implicated focal adhesion kinase (FAK) activation and its diverse downstream signals in this process.[133] Thus, additional levels of limiting or extending TGF-β signaling may be achieved through modulation of receptor downregulation in response to ligand stimulation.

Another level of receptor downregulation occurs via BAMBI (see Fig. 10-4, mechanism 2), a type I pseudoreceptor whose expression is regulated by TGF-β family members.[134] BAMBI is a pseudoreceptor related to the TGF-β-family type I receptors but lacking an intracellular kinase domain. BAMBI stably associates with TGF-β-family receptors and inhibits BMP and activin as well as TGF-β signaling by preventing the formation of productive type II–type I ligand-receptor complexes.[134]

INHIBITORY Smads AND CYTOPLASMIC PROTEINS

Accumulating evidence supports the presence of a negative feedback loop through which activation of Smad-dependent signaling induces expression of the inhibitory Smads, Smad6 and Smad7.[65,68,135] The inhibitory Smads block TGF-β-, activin-, and BMP-dependent responses either by inactivating ligand-bound receptors or by interfering with intracellular Smad-dependent reactions.[65,66,68,69,117,136] In addition, regulated expression of the I-Smads is a key mechanism by which other pathways can modulate the extent of R-SMAD-activated activity.[137,138] I-Smad expression can be induced in response to EGF in lung tumor cells, representing additional cross-talk between TGF-β and other signaling pathways.[139] Interferon (IFN)-γ induces the expression of Smad7, an antagonistic Smad, which prevents the interaction of Smad3 with the type I TGF-β receptor to prevent TGF-β signaling. These data provide a transmodulation mechanism between the JAK/STAT and the Smad signaling pathways whereby a cell can integrate signals from cytokines as well as TGF-β ligands.[140] Together, the I-Smads play important roles in providing convergence of signaling with other pathways, as well as an important negative-feedback mechanism to limit the signal being induced by cognate TGF-β superfamily ligands.

A membrane-anchored Smad-binding protein, SARA (Smad anchor for receptor activation) serves to bind quiescent Smads. SARA localizes Smad2 to specific subcellular endosomes containing EEA1 in the cell that are near TGF-β receptors for ligand-dependent activation.[141,142] Disruption of this localization inhibits TGF-β-induced Smad2 nuclear translocation,[141] which normally occurs after SARA dissociation from Smad2 to allow complex formation with Smad4 and subsequent signaling.[142] These results indicate that traffic of the TGF-β receptor into the endosome enables TGF-β signaling, revealing an additional potential level of signaling regulation by limiting expression or proper subcellular localization of SARA or both.

Smad NUCLEOPLASMIC SHUTTLING

As indicated earlier, ligand-receptor activation results in R-Smad phosphorylation, subsequent release from the receptor, movement away from the cell membrane, and partnering with the Co-Smad. The R-Smad/Co-Smad complex then enters the nucleus via a presumptive nuclear localization sequence (NLS; KKLKK) residing in the MH1 domain of the R-Smad, located next to the DNA-binding motif β-hairpin. The NLS appears to mediate nuclear import when the Smad1 and Smad3 are phosphorylated[143-145] by binding to importin-β but not to importin-α.[143,146]

Alternatively, import and export of Smad2 and Smad3 has been demonstrated to occur by direct interaction of the MH2 domain of Smad2 and 3 with Nup214 and Nup153, nucleoporins of the nuclear pore complex.[147,148] Thus, Smads can be imported without the aid of importins, originally considered to be required as chaperones for nuclear entry. Nuclear export of Smad2 and Smad3 also occurs without the aid of the general export factor Crm-1, again by directly contacting the nucleoporins.[148] Together, the direct import/export of R-Smads through the nuclear pore complex provides a continuous nucleoplasmic shuttling mechanism to regulate the amount of R-Smads available for receptor activation in the cytoplasm or DNA binding and gene regulation in the nucleus or both.[148,149]

Finally, nucleoplasmic shuttling of Smad4 is slightly different. Smad4 accumulates in the nucleus through its association with activated R-Smads.[81,150] In addition, Smad4 can enter the nucleus in the absence of R-Smads. Smad4 is aided by an additional basic residue (Arg81) in the β-hairpin near the KKLKK nuclear localization sequence in the MH1 domain sequence described earlier.[151] Evidence also suggests that Smad4 interacts with the nucleoporin, Nup214.[148] However, although a surface hydrophobic corridor within the MH2 domain of R-Smads is sufficient for association with CAN/Nup214 and nuclear import, Smad4 nuclear import through Nup214 requires additional structural elements present only in the full-length Smad4.[148] Together, these observations are consistent with initial models in which R-Smad phosphorylation by the type I receptor drives the nuclear translocation of the activated Smad complex. However, it is evident from these studies that both the R-Smads and Smad4 are continually engaged in dynamic nucleocytoplasmic shuttling that is regulated by a variety of pathways and importation/exportation proteins, resulting in exquisite regulation of eventual RSK signaling output.

DIRECT SIGNALING TO THE NUCLEUS

A notable aspect of each of these systems is the activation of latent cytoplasmic transcription factors through direct phosphorylation by growth factor receptors at the cell membrane. Other well-characterized transcription factors that become activated in response to extracellular factors (for example, CREB and AP-1) do so as the result of a multiple-step enzymatic pathway, providing a greater amplification of a response initiated by ligand binding to a limited receptor pool at the cell surface. In contrast, for Smad signaling, it appears that the flow of information from the receptor to the nucleus is brief and direct, with amplification limited to the receptor kinases themselves. The simplicity of the pathway suggests a coarse level of regulation. However, because it is critical to limit transcriptional regulation in the absence of ligand-receptor activation, the rate-limiting step with the greatest sensitivity to regulation may need to be the concentration and localization of R-Smads in the cytoplasm in the absence of ligand, which then ensures the proper level of gene expression. In addition to this regulation of availability of Smads to DNA, several additional pathways exist within each signaling compartment of the RSK pathway itself to downregulate or limit the signal (extracellular antagonists, pseudoreceptors, I-Smads, corepressors), as well as mechanisms to receive input from other pathways (e.g., vitamin D_3 receptor [VDR], IFN, RTK) that also restrict and downregulate the extent of Smad signaling.

SUMMARY

Although the several signaling networks discussed in this and previous chapters involve direct activation of protein kinases at the cell membrane, virtually all the components of those pathways are distinct. Nevertheless, the pathways have striking similarities in the kinds of reactions involved and in the manner in which they are organized. Of particular note is the characteristic pleiotropy and redundancy present in both systems. Each pathway is used by a large number of extracellular factors that influence a diverse set of biologic responses, but that diversity is achieved through the use of a relatively limited number of receptors and signaling molecules. Use of multimeric components allows cells to increase greatly the repertoire of responses stimulated by a small group of factors as a result of different combinatorial possibilities. Despite significant progress in unraveling the basic pathways of RSK signaling, significant challenges remain in elucidating the mechanisms controlling specificity at each level that result in the formation of distinct combinations of signaling complexes that exert their actions in response to a given ligand.

Acknowledgment
I acknowledge the contributions of Lawrence S. Mathews in preparation of the previous edition of this chapter, of which a portion is retained in the current edition.

REFERENCES

1. Massague J, Heino J, Laiho M: Mechanisms in TGF-beta action. Ciba Found Symp 157:51–59; discussion 59–65, 1991.
2. Roberts AB, Sporn MB: Transforming growth factors. Cancer Surv 4:683–705, 1985.
3. Bernard DJ, Chapman SC, Woodruff TK: Mechanisms of inhibin signal transduction. Recent Prog Horm Res 56:417–450, 2001.
4. Ying SY: Inhibins, activins and follistatins. J Steroid Biochem Mol Biol 33:705–713, 1989.
5. Thomsen G, Woolf T, Whitman M, et al: Activins are expressed early in *Xenopus* embryogenesis and can induce axial mesoderm and anterior structures. Cell 63:485–493, 1990.
6. Wozney JM: The bone morphogenetic protein family and osteogenesis. Mol Reprod Dev 32:160–167, 1992.
7. Shimasaki S, Moore RK, Otsuka F, Erickson GF: The bone morphogenetic protein system in mammalian reproduction. Endocr Rev 25:72–101, 2004.
8. Ushiro H, Cohen S: Identification of phosphotyrosine as a product of epidermal growth factor-activated protein kinase in A-431 cell membranes. J Biol Chem 255:8363–8365, 1980.
9. Mathews LS, Vale WW: Expression cloning of an activin receptor, a predicted transmembrane serine kinase. Cell 65:973–982, 1991.
10. Zimmerman CM, Mathews LS: Activin receptors: Cellular signalling by receptor serine kinases. Biochem Soc Symp 62:25–38, 1996.
11. Cheifetz S: BMP receptors in limb and tooth formation. Crit Rev Oral Biol Med 10:182–198, 1999.
12. Miyazono K, Kusanagi K, Inoue H: Divergence and convergence of TGF-beta/BMP signaling. J Cell Physiol 187:265–276, 2001.
13. Saarma M: GDNF: A stranger in the TGF-beta superfamily? Eur J Biochem 267:6968–6971, 2000.
14. Shimasaki S, Moore RK, Erickson GF, Otsuka F: The role of bone morphogenetic proteins in ovarian function. Reprod Suppl 61:323–337, 2003.
15. Moses HL, Serra R: Regulation of differentiation by TGF-beta. Curr Opin Genet Dev 6:581–586, 1996.
16. Roberts AB, Sporn MB: Physiological actions and clinical applications of transforming growth factor-beta (TGF-beta). Growth Factors 8:1–9, 1993.
17. Wall NA, Hogan BL: TGF-beta related genes in development. Curr Opin Genet Dev 4:517–522, 1994.
18. Miyazono K: TGF-beta/SMAD signaling and its involvement in tumor progression. Biol Pharm Bull 23:1125–1130, 2000.
19. Josso N, di Clemente N: Serine/threonine kinase receptors and ligands. Curr Opin Genet Dev 7:371–377, 1997.
20. Mathews LS: Activin receptors and cellular signaling by the receptor serine kinase family. Endocr Rev 15:310–325, 1994.
21. Yamashita H, Ten Dijke P, Heldin CH, Miyazono K: Bone morphogenetic protein receptors. Bone 19:569–574, 1996.
22. Itoh S, Itoh F, Goumans MJ, Ten Dijke P: Signaling of transforming growth factor-beta family members through Smad proteins. Eur J Biochem 267:6954–6967, 2000.
23. Massague J, Weis-Garcia F: Serine/threonine kinase receptors: Mediators of transforming growth factor beta family signals. Cancer Surv 27:41–64, 1996.
24. Miyazono K: Signal transduction by bone morphogenetic protein receptors: Functional roles of Smad proteins. Bone 25:91–93, 1999.
25. Greenwald J, Fischer WH, Vale WW, Choe S: Three-finger toxin fold for the extracellular ligand-binding domain of the type II activin receptor serine kinase. Nat Struct Biol 6:18–22, 1999.

26. Massague J: TGF-beta signal transduction. Annu Rev Biochem 67:753–791, 1998.

27. Willis SA, Zimmerman CM, Li LI, Mathews LS: Formation and activation by phosphorylation of activin receptor complexes. Mol Endocrinol 10:367–379, 1996.

28. Wrana JL, Attisano L, Wieser R, et al: Mechanism of activation of the TGF-beta receptor. Nature 370:341–347, 1994.

29. Huse, M, Chen YG, Massague J, Kuriyan J: Crystal structure of the cytoplasmic domain of the type I TGF beta receptor in complex with FKBP12. Cell 96:425–436, 1999.

30. Koenig BB, Cook JS, Wolsing DH, et al: Characterization and cloning of a receptor for BMP-2 and BMP-4 from NIH 3T3 cells. Mol Cell Biol 14:5961–3974, 1994.

31. ten Dijke P, Yamashita H, Sampath TK, et al: Identification of type I receptors for osteogenic protein-1 and bone morphogenetic protein-4. J Biol Chem 269:16985–16988, 1994.

32. Liu F, Ventura F, Doody J, Massague J: Human type II receptor for bone morphogenic proteins (BMPs): Extension of the two-kinase receptor model to the BMPs. Mol Cell Biol 15:3479–3486, 1995.

33. Nishitoh H, Ichijo H, Kimura M, et al: Identification of type I and type II serine/threonine kinase receptors for growth/differentiation factor-5. J Biol Chem 271:21345–21352, 1996.

34. Nohno T, Ishikawa T, Saito T, et al: Identification of a human type II receptor for bone morphogenetic protein-4 that forms differential heteromeric complexes with bone morphogenetic protein type I receptors. J Biol Chem 270:22522–22526, 1995.

35. Rosenzweig BL, Imamura T, Okadome T, et al: Cloning and characterization of a human type II receptor for bone morphogenetic proteins. Proc Natl Acad Sci U S A 92:7632–7636, 1995.

36. Yamashita H, ten Dijke P, Huylebroeck D, et al: Osteogenic protein-1 binds to activin type II receptors and induces certain activin-like effects. J Cell Biol 130:217–226, 1995.

37. Chen D, Ji X, Harris MA, et al: Differential roles for bone morphogenetic protein (BMP) receptor type IB and IA in differentiation and specification of mesenchymal precursor cells to osteoblast and adipocyte lineages. J Cell Biol 142:295–305, 1998.

38. Lopez-Casillas F, Payne HM, Andres JL, Massague J: Betaglycan can act as a dual modulator of TGF-beta access to signaling receptors: Mapping of ligand binding and GAG attachment sites. J Cell Biol 124:557–568, 1994.

39. Lopez-Casillas F, Wrana JL, Massague J: Betaglycan presents ligand to the TGF beta signaling receptor. Cell 73:1435–1444, 1993.

40. Cheifetz S, Bellon T, Cales C, et al: Endoglin is a component of the transforming growth factor-beta receptor system in human endothelial cells. J Biol Chem 267:19027–19030, 1992.

41. Yamashita H, Ichijo H, Grimsby S, et al: Endoglin forms a heteromeric complex with the signaling receptors for transforming growth factor-beta. J Biol Chem 269:1995–2001, 1994.

42. Barbara NP, Wrana JL, Letarte M: Endoglin is an accessory protein that interacts with the signaling receptor complex of multiple members of the transforming growth factor-beta superfamily. J Biol Chem 274:584–594, 1999.

43. Fonsatti E, Altomonte M, Arslan P, Maio M: Endoglin (CD105): A target for anti-angiogenetic cancer therapy. Curr Drug Targets 4:291–296, 2003.

44. Pece N, Vera S, Cymerman U, et al: Mutant endoglin in hereditary hemorrhagic telangiectasia type 1 is transiently expressed intracellularly and is not a dominant negative. J Clin Invest 100:2568–2579, 1997.

45. van den Driesche S, Mummery CL, Westermann CJ: Hereditary hemorrhagic telangiectasia: An update on transforming growth factor beta signaling in vasculogenesis and angiogenesis. Cardiovasc Res 58:20–31, 2003.

46. Lewis KA, Gray PC, Blount AL, et al: Betaglycan binds inhibin and can mediate functional antagonism of activin signalling. Nature 404:411–414, 2000.

47. Esparza-Lopez J, Montiel JL, Vilchis-Landeros MM, et al: Ligand binding and functional properties of betaglycan, a co-receptor of the transforming growth factor-beta superfamily: Specialized binding regions for transforming growth factor-beta and inhibin. Am J Biol Chem 2768:14588–14596, 2001.

48. Chapman SC, Bernard DJ, Jelen J, Woodruff JK: Properties of inhibin binding to betaglycan, InhBP/p120 and the activin type II receptors. Mol Cell Endocrinol 196:79–93, 2002.

49. Wiater E, Vale W: Inhibin is an antagonist of bone morphogenetic protein signaling. J Biol Chem 278:7934–7941, 2003.

50. Gaddy-Kurten D, Coker JK, Abe E, et al: Inhibin suppresses and activin stimulates osteoblastogenesis and osteoclastogenesis in murine bone marrow cultures. Endocrinology 143:74–83, 2002.

51. Xu J, McKeehan K, Matsuzaki K, McKeehan WL: Inhibin antagonizes inhibition of liver cell growth by activin by a dominant-negative mechanism. J Biol Chem 270:6308–6313, 1995.

52. Harrison CA, Farnworth PG, Chan KL, et al: Identification of specific inhibin A-binding proteins on mouse Leydig (TM3) and sertoli (TM4) cell lines. Endocrinology 142:1393–1402, 2001.

53. Chong H, Pangas SA, Bernard DJ, et al: Structure and expression of a membrane component of the inhibin receptor system. Endocrinology 141:2600–2607, 2000.

54. Chapman SC, Woodruff TK: Modulation of activin signal transduction by inhibin B and inhibin-binding protein (INhBP). Mol Endocrinol 15:668–679, 2001.

55. Bernard DJ, Burns KH, Haupt B, et al: Normal reproductive function in InhBP/p120-deficient mice. Mol Cell Biol 23:4882–4891, 2003.

56. Robertson K, Mason I: The GDNF-RET signalling partnership. Trends Genet 13:1–3, 1997.

57. Miyazawa K, Shinozaki M, Hara T, et al: Two major Smad pathways in TGF-beta superfamily signalling. Genes Cells 7:1191–1204, 2002.

58. Nishimura R, Hata K, Ikeda F, et al: The role of Smads in BMP signaling. Front Biosci 8:s275–s284, 2003.

59. Savage C, Das P, Finelli AL, et al: Caenorhabditis elegans genes sma-2, sma-3, and sma-4 define a conserved family of transforming growth factor beta pathway components. Proc Natl Acad Sci U S A 93:790–794, 1996.

60. Sekelsky JJ, Newfeld SJ, Raftery LA, et al: Genetic characterization and cloning of mothers against dpp, a gene required for decapentaplegic function in Drosophila melanogaster. Genetics 139:1347–1358, 1995.

61. Lo RS, Chen YG, Shi Y, et al: The L3 loop: A structural motif determining specific interactions between SMAD proteins and TGF-beta receptors. EMBO J 17:996–1005, 1998.

62. Lagna G, Hata A, Hemmati-Brivanlou A, Massague J: Partnership between DPC4 and SMAD proteins in TGF-beta signalling pathways. Nature 383:832–8326, 1996.

63. Zhang Y, Feng X, We R, Derynck R: Receptor-associated Mad homologues synergize as effectors of the TGF-beta response. Nature 383:168–172, 1996.

64. Ebara S, Nakayama K: Mechanism for the action of bone morphogenetic proteins and regulation of their activity. Spine 27(16 Suppl 1):S10–S15, 2002.

65. Hayashi H, et al: The MAD-related protein Smad7 associates with the TGFbeta receptor and functions as an antagonist of TGFbeta signaling. Cell 89:1165–1173, 1997.

66. Imamura T, Takase M, Nishihara A, et al: Smad6 inhibits signalling by the TGF-beta superfamily. Nature 389:622–626, 1997.

67. Zhu HJ, Burgess AW: Regulation of transforming growth factor-beta signaling. Mol Cell Biol Res Commun 4:321–330, 2001.

68. Hata A, Lagna G, Massague J, Hemmati-Brivanlou A: Smad6 inhibits BMP/Smad1 signaling by specifically competing with the Smad4 tumor suppressor. Genes Dev 12:186–197, 1998.

69. Ebisawa T, Fukuchi M, Murakami G, et al: Smurf1 interacts with transforming growth factor-beta type I receptor through Smad7 and induces

receptor degradation. J Biol Chem 276:12477–12480, 2001.

70. Kretzschmar M, Doody J, Massague J: Opposing BMP and EGF signalling pathways converge on the TGF-beta family mediator Smad1. Nature 389:618–622, 1997.

71. Pera EM, Ikeda A, Eivers E, De Robertis EM: Integration of IGF, FGF, and anti-BMP signals via Smad1 phosphorylation in neural induction. Genes Dev 17:3023–3028, 2003.

72. Kretzschmar M, Doody J, Timokhina I, Massague J: A mechanism of repression of TGFbeta/ Smad signaling by oncogenic Ras. Genes Dev 13:804–816, 1999.

73. Miyazono K: Positive and negative regulation of TGF-beta signaling. J Cell Sci 113:1101–1109, 2000.

74. Shi Y, Massague J: Mechanisms of TGF-beta signaling from cell membrane to the nucleus. Cell 113:685–700, 2003.

75. Zimmerman CM, Kariapper MS, Mathews LS: Smad proteins physically interact with calmodulin. J Biol Chem 273:677–680, 1998.

76. Massague J, Wotton D: Transcriptional control by the TGF-beta/Smad signaling system. EMBO J 19:1745–1754, 2000.

77. Wotton D, Massague J: Smad transcriptional corepressors in TGF beta family signaling. Curr Top Microbiol Immunol 254:145–164, 2001.

78. Derynck R, Zhang Y, Feng XH: Smads: Transcriptional activators of TGF-beta responses. Cell 95:737–740, 1998.

79. Chen X, Rubock MJ, Whitman M: A transcriptional partner for MAD proteins in TGF-beta signalling. Nature 383:691–696, 1996.

80. Labbe E, Silvestri C, Hoodless PA, et al: Smad2 and Smad3 positively and negatively regulate TGF beta-dependent transcription through the forkhead DNA-binding protein FAST2. Mol Cell 2:109–120, 1998.

81. Liu F, Pouponnot C, Massague J: Dual role of the Smad4/DPC4 tumor suppressor in TGFbeta-inducible transcriptional complexes. Genes Dev 11:3157–3167, 1997.

82. Hua X, Liu X, Ansari DO, Lodish HF: Synergistic cooperation of TFE3 and smad proteins in TGF-beta-induced transcription of the plasminogen activator inhibitor-1 gene. Genes Dev 1219:3084–3095, 1998.

83. Zhang Y, Feng XH, Derynck R: Smad3 and Smad4 cooperate with c-Jun/c-Fos to mediate TGF-beta-induced transcription [published erratum appears in Nature 396:491, 1998]. Nature 394:909–913, 1998.

84. Dennler S, Itoh S, Vivien D, et al: Direct binding of Smad3 and Smad4 to critical TGF beta-inducible elements in the promoter of human plasminogen activator inhibitor-type 1 gene. EMBO J 17:3091–3100, 1998.

85. Jonk LJ, Itoh S, Heldin CH, et al: Identification and functional characterization of a Smad binding element (SBE) in the JunB promoter that acts as a transforming growth

factor-beta, activin, and bone morphogenetic protein-inducible enhancer. J Biol Chem 273:21145–21152, 1998.

86. Shi Y, Wang YF, Jayaraman L, et al: Crystal structure of a Smad MH1 domain bound to DNA: Insights on DNA binding in TGF-beta signaling. Cell 94:585–594, 1998.

87. Yagi K, Goto D, Hamamoto T, et al: Alternatively spliced variant of Smad2 lacking exon 3: Comparison with wild-type Smad2 and Smad3. J Biol Chem 274:703–709, 1999.

88. Hata A, Seoane J, Lagna G, et al: OAZ uses distinct DNA- and protein-binding zinc fingers in separate BMP-Smad and Olf signaling pathways. Cell 100:229–240, 2000.

89. Janknecht R, Wells NJ, Hunter T: TGF-beta-stimulated cooperation of smad proteins with the coactivators CBP/p300. Genes Dev 12:2114–2119, 1998.

90. Nishihara A, Hanai JI, Okamoto N, et al: Role of p300, a transcriptional coactivator, in signalling of TGF-beta. Genes Cells 3:613–623, 1998.

91. Pouponnot C, Jayaraman L, Massague J: Physical and functional interaction of SMADs and p300/CBP. J Biol Chem 273:22865–22868, 1998.

92. Shen X, Hu PP, Liberati NT, et al: TGF-beta-induced phosphorylation of Smad3 regulates its interaction with coactivator p300/CREB-binding protein. Mol Biol Cell 9:3309–3319, 1998.

93. Yahata T, de Caestecker MP, Lechleider RJ, et al: The MSG1 non-DNA-binding transactivator binds to the p300/CBP coactivators, enhancing their functional link to the Smad transcription factors. J Biol Chem 275:8825–8834, 2000.

94. Takeshita A, Imai K, Kato S, et al: 1alpha,25-dehydroxyvitamin D3 synergism toward transforming growth factor-beta1-induced AP-1 transcriptional activity in mouse osteoblastic cells via its nuclear receptor. J Biol Chem 273:14738–14744, 1998.

95. Yanagisawa J, Kitagawa H, Fuse H, et al: Convergence of transforming growth factor-beta and vitamin D signaling pathways on SMAD transcriptional coactivators. Science 283:1317–1321, 1999.

96. Yang L, Yang J, Venkateswarlu S, et al: Autocrine TGFbeta signaling mediates vitamin D$_3$ analog-induced growth inhibition in breast cells. J Cell Physiol 188:383–393, 2001.

97. Attisano L, Tuen Lee, Hoeflich S: The Smads. Genome Biol 2:3010, 2001.

98. Franceschi RT, Xiao G: Regulation of the osteoblast-specific transcription factor, Runx2: responsiveness to multiple signal transduction pathways. J Cell Biochem 88:446–454, 2003.

99. Hanai J, Chen LF, Kanno T, et al: Interaction and functional cooperation of PEBP2/CBF with Smads: Synergistic induction of the immunoglobulin

germline C alpha promoter. J Biol Chem 274:31577–31582, 1999.

100. Lee KS, Hong SH, Bae SC: Both the Smad and p38 MAPK pathways play a crucial role in Runx2 expression following induction by transforming growth factor-beta and bone morphogenetic protein. Oncogene 21:7156–7163, 2002.

101. Pardali E, Xie XQ, Tsapogas P, et al: Smad and AML proteins synergistically confer transforming growth beta1 responsiveness to human germ-line IgA genes. J Biol Chem 275:3552–3560, 2000.

102. Feng XH, Lin X, Derynck R: Smad2, Smad3 and Smad4 cooperate with Sp1 to induce p15(Ink4B) transcription in response to TGF-beta. EMBO J 19:5178–5193, 2000.

103. Pardali K, Kurisaki A, Moren A, et al: Role of Smad proteins and transcription factor Sp1 in p21(Waf1/Cip1) regulation by transforming growth factor-beta. J Biol Chem 275:29244–29256, 2000.

104. Labbe E, Letamendia A, Attisano L: Association of Smads with lymphoid enhancer binding factor 1/T cell-specific factor mediates cooperative signaling by the transforming growth factor-beta and wnt pathways. Proc Natl Acad Sci U S A 97:8358–8363, 2000.

105. Letamendia A, Labbe E, Attisano L: Transcriptional regulation by Smads: crosstalk between the TGF-beta and Wnt pathways. J Bone Joint Surg Am 83(Suppl 1):S31–S39, 2001.

106. Tian YC, Phillips AO: Interaction between the transforming growth factor-beta type II receptor/Smad pathway and beta-catenin during transforming growth factor-beta1-mediated adherens junction disassembly. Am J Pathol 160:1619–1628, 2002.

107. Akiyoshi S, Inoue H, Hanai J, et al: c-Ski acts as a transcriptional co-repressor in transforming growth factor-beta signaling through interaction with Smads. J Biol Chem 274:35269–35277, 1999.

108. Luo K, Stroschein SL, Wang W, et al: The Ski oncoprotein interacts with the Smad proteins to repress TGFbeta signaling. Genes Dev 13:2196–2206, 1999.

109. Stroschein SL, Wang W, Zhou S, et al: Negative feedback regulation of TGF-beta signaling by the SnoN oncoprotein. Science 286:771–774, 1999.

110. Massague J, Chen YG: Controlling TGF-beta signaling. Genes Dev 14:627–644, 2000.

111. Moriguchi T, Kuroyanagi N, Yamaguchi K, et al: A novel kinase cascade mediated by mitogen-activated protein kinase kinase 6 and MKK3. J Biol Chem 271:13675–13679, 1996.

112. Shibuya H, Iwata H, Masuyama N, et al: Role of TAK1 and TAB1 in BMP signaling in early *Xenopus*

development. EMBO J 17:1019–1028, 1998.

113. Yamaguchi K, Shirakabe T, Shibuya H, et al: Identification of a member of the MAPKKK family as a potential mediator of TGF-β signal transduction. Science 270:2008–2011, 1995.

114. Chen RH, Miettinen PJ, Maruoka EM, et al: A WD-domain protein that is associated with and phosphorylated by the type II TGF-beta receptor. Nature 377:548–552, 1995.

115. Choy L, Derynck R: The type II transforming growth factor (TGF)-beta receptor-interacting protein TRIP-1 acts as a modulator of the TGF-beta response. J Biol Chem 273:31455–31462, 1998.

116. Datta PK, Chytil A, Gorska AE, Moses HL: Identification of STRAP: A novel WD domain protein in transforming growth factor-beta signaling. J Biol Chem 273:34671–34674, 1998.

117. Datta PK, Moses HL: STRAP and Smad7 synergize in the inhibition of transforming growth factor beta signaling. Mol Cell Biol 20:3157–3167, 2000.

118. Charng MJ, Zhang D, Kinnunen P, Schneider MD: A novel protein distinguishes between quiescent and activated forms of the type I transforming growth factor beta receptor. J Biol Chem 273:9365–9368, 1998.

119. Felici A, Wurthner JU, Parks WT, et al: TLP, a novel modulator of TGF-beta signaling, has opposite effects on Smad2- and Smad3-dependent signaling. EMBO J 22:4465–4477, 2003.

120. Shoji H, Tsuchida K, Kishi H, et al: Identification and characterization of a PDZ protein that interacts with activin type II receptors. J Biol Chem 275:5485–5492, 2000.

121. DePaolo LV, Bicsak TA, Erickson GF, et al: Follestatin and activin: A potential intrinsic regulatory system within diverse tissues [published erratum appears in Proc Soc Exp Biol Med 1992 Jul;200(3):447]. Proc Soc Exp Biol Med 198:500–512, 1991.

122. Mather JP, Moore A, Li RH: Activins, inhibins, and follistatins: Further thoughts on a growing family of regulators. Proc Soc Exp Biol Med 215:209–222, 1997.

123. Gamer LW, Wolfman NM, Celeste AJ, et al: A novel BMP expressed in developing mouse limb, spinal cord, and tail bud is a potent mesoderm inducer in Xenopus embryos. Dev Biol 208:222–232, 1999.

124. Macias-Silva M, Hoodless PA, Tang SJ, et al: Specific activation of Smad1 signaling pathways by the BMP7 type I receptor, ALK2. J Biol Chem 273:25628–25636, 1998.

125. Tsuchida K, Matsuzaki T, Yamakawa N, et al: Cellular and extracellular control of activin function by novel regulatory molecules. Mol Cell Endocrinol 180:25–31, 2001.

126. Zimmerman LB, De Jesús-Escobar JM, Harland RM: The Spemann organizer signal noggin binds and inactivates bone morphogenetic protein 4. Cell 86:599–606, 1996.

127. Piccolo S, Agius E, Leyns L, et al: The head inducer Cerberus is a multifunctional antagonist of Nodal, BMP and Wnt signals. Nature 397:707–710, 1999.

128. Hsu DR, Economides AN, Wang X, et al: The Xenopus dorsalizing factor Gremlin identifies a novel family of secreted proteins that antagonize BMP activities. Mol Cell 1:673–683, 1998.

129. Piek E, Heldin CH, Ten Dijke P: Specificity, diversity, and regulation in TGF-beta superfamily signaling. FASEB J 13:2105–2124, 1999.

130. Chen YG, Liu F, Massague J: Mechanism of TGFbeta receptor inhibition by FKBP12. EMBO J 16:3866–3876, 1997.

131. Wang TW, Li BY, Danielson PD, et al: The immunophilin FKBP12 functions as a common inhibitor of the TGFβ family type I receptors. Cell 86:435–444, 1996.

132. Anders RA, Dore JJ Jr, Arline SL, et al: Differential requirement for type I and type II transforming growth factor beta receptor kinase activity in ligand-mediated receptor endocytosis. J Biol Chem 273:23118–23125, 1998.

133. Takeuchi Y, Suzawa M, Kikuchi T, et al: Differentiation and transforming growth factor-beta receptor down-regulation by collagen-alpha2beta1 integrin interaction is mediated by focal adhesion kinase and its downstream signals in murine osteoblastic cells. J Biol Chem 272:29309–29316, 1997.

134. Onichtchouk D, Chen YG, Dosch R, et al: Silencing of TGF-beta signalling by the pseudoreceptor BAMBI. Nature 401:480–485, 1999.

135. Nakao A, et al: Identification of Smad7, a TGFbeta-inducible antagonist of TGF-beta signalling [see comments]. Nature 389:631–635, 1997.

136. Kitamura K, Aota S, Sakamoto R, et al: Smad7 selectively interferes with different pathways of activin signaling and inhibits erythroid leukemia cell differentiation. Blood 95:3371–3379, 2000.

137. Kimura N, Matsuo R, Shibuya H, et al: BMP2-induced apoptosis is mediated by activation of the TAK1-p38 kinase pathway that is negatively regulated by Smad6. J Biol Chem 275:17647–17652, 2000.

138. Yanagi Y, Suzawa M, Kawabata M, et al: Positive and negative modulation of vitamin D receptor function by transforming growth factor-beta signaling through smad proteins. J Biol Chem 274:12971–12974, 1999.

139. Afrakhte M, Moren A, Jossan S, et al: Induction of inhibitory Smad6 and Smad7 mRNA by TGF-beta family members. Biochem Biophys Res Commun 249:505–511, 1998.

140. Ulloa L, Doody J, Massague J: Inhibition of transforming growth factor-beta/SMAD signalling by the interferon-gamma/STAT pathway [In Process Citation]. Nature 397:710–713, 1999.

141. Hayes S, Chawla A, Corvera S: TGF beta receptor internalization into EEA1-enriched early endosomes: role in signaling to Smad2. J Cell Biol 158:1239–1249, 2002.

142. Tsukazaki T, Chiang TA, Davison AF, et al: SARA, a FYVE domain protein that recruits Smad2 to the TGFbeta receptor. Cell 95:779–791, 1998.

143. Kurisaki A, Kose S, Yoneda Y, et al: Transforming growth factor-beta induces nuclear import of Smad3 in an importin-beta1 and Ran-dependent manner. Mol Biol Cell 12:1079–1091, 2001.

144. Xiao Z, Liu X, Henis YI, Lodish HF: A distinct nuclear localization signal in the N terminus of Smad 3 determines its ligand-induced nuclear translocation. Proc Natl Acad Sci U S A 97:7853–7858, 2000.

145. Xiao Z, Watson N, Rodriguez C, Lodish HF: Nucleocytoplasmic shuttling of Smad1 conferred by its nuclear localization and nuclear export signals. J Biol Chem 276:39404–39410, 2001.

146. Xiao Z, Liu X, Lodish HF: Importin beta mediates nuclear translocation of Smad 3. J Biol Chem 275:23425–23428, 2000.

147. Xu L, Alarcon C, Col S, Massague J: Distinct domain utilization by Smad3 and Smad4 for nucleoporin interaction and nuclear import. J Biol Chem 278:42569–42577, 2003.

148. Xu L, Kang Y, Col S, Massague J: Smad2 nucleocytoplasmic shuttling by nucleoporins CAN/Nup214 and Nup153 feeds TGFbeta signaling complexes in the cytoplasm and nucleus. Mol Cell 10:271–282, 2002.

149. Inman GJ, Nicolas FJ, Hill C: Nucleocytoplasmic shuttling of Smads 2, 3, and 4 permits sensing of TGF-beta receptor activity. Mol Cell 10:283–294, 2002.

150. Watanabe M, Masuyama N, Fukuda M, Nishida E: Regulation of intracellular dynamics of Smad4 by its leucine-rich nuclear export signal. EMBO Rep 1:176–182, 2000.

151. Xiao Z, Latek R, Lodish HF: An extended bipartite nuclear localization signal in Smad4 is required for its nuclear import and transcriptional activity. Oncogene 22:1057–1069, 2003.

152. Dong C, Li Z, Alvarez R Jr, et al: Microtubule binding to Smads may regulate TGF beta activity. Mol Cell 5:27–34, 2000.

153. Sano Y, Harada J, Tashiro S, et al: ATF-2 is a common nuclear target of Smad and TAK1 pathways in transforming growth factor-beta signaling. J Biol Chem 274:8949–8957, 1999.

154. Nishihara A, Hanai J, Imamura T, et al: E1A inhibits transforming growth

factor-beta signaling through binding to Smad proteins. J Biol Chem 274:28716–28723, 1999.

155. Kurokawa M, Mitani K, Irie K, et al: The oncoprotein Evi-1 represses TGF-beta signalling by inhibiting Smad3. Nature 394:92–96, 1998.

156. Chen X, Weisberg E, Fridmacher V, et al: Smad4 and FAST-1 in the assembly of activin-responsive factor. Nature 389:85–89, 1997.

157. Song CZ, Tian X, Gelehrter TD: Glucocorticoid receptor inhibits transforming growth factor-beta signaling by directly targeting the transcriptional activation function of Smad3. Proc Natl Acad Sci U S A 96:11776–11781, 1999.

158. Shi X, Yang X, Chen D, et al: Smad1 interacts with homeobox DNA-binding proteins in bone morphogenetic protein signaling. J Biol Chem 274:13711–13717, 1999.

159. Yang X, Ji X, Shi X, Cao X: Smad1 domains interacting with Hoxc-8 induce osteoblast differentiation. J Biol Chem 275:1065–1072, 2000.

160. Liberati NT, Datto MB, Frederick JP, et al: Smads bind directly to the Jun family of AP-1 transcription factors. Proc Natl Acad Sci U S A 96:4844–4849, 1999.

161. Feng XH, Zhang Y, Wu RY, Derynck R: The tumor suppressor Smad4/DPC4 and transcriptional adaptor CBP/p300 are coactivators for smad3 in TGF-beta-induced transcriptional activation. Genes Dev 12:2153–2163, 1998.

162. Verschueren K: SIP1, a novel zinc finger/homeodomain repressor, interacts with Smad proteins and binds to 5'-CACCT sequences in candidate target genes. J Biol Chem 274:20489–20498, 1999.

163. Kawabata M, Imamura T, Miyazono K: Signal transduction by bone morphogenetic proteins. Cytokine Growth Factor Rev 9:49–61, 1998.

164. Lin X, Liang M, Feng XH: Smurf2 is a ubiquitin E3 ligase mediating proteasome-dependent degradation of Smad2 in transforming growth factor-beta signaling. J Biol Chem 275:36818–36822, 2000.

165. Zhu H, Kavsak P, Abdollah S, et al: A SMAD ubiquitin ligase targets the BMP pathway and affects embryonic pattern formation. Nature 400:687–693, 1999.

166. Kim RH, et al: A novel smad nuclear interacting protein, SNIP1, suppresses p300-dependent TGF-beta signal transduction. Genes Dev 14:1605–1616, 2000.

167. Wotton D, Lo RS, Lee S, Massague J: A Smad transcriptional corepressor. Cell 97:29–39, 1999.

Hormone Signaling via G Protein–Coupled Receptors

Javier González-Maeso and Stuart C. Sealfon

INTRODUCTION

The function of multicellular organisms requires that the various cell types having specialized biologic functions respond in a specific manner to diverse stimuli to maintain physiologic homeostasis. The extracellular mediators that modulate and coordinate cellular activity include hormones, neurotransmitters, small peptides and proteins, ions, and lipids, as well as sensory stimuli such as odorants, pheromones, and light. These mediators act through receptors to elicit characteristic cellular responses.

The earliest formulation of the modern concept of receptors is found in Erhlich's "side-chain theory" of the immune response. His statement, "*corpora non agunt nisi fixata*" (agents cannot act unless they are bound) embodies the principle of receptor biology.[1] The term *receptive substance* was first coined by Langley[2] nearly a century ago to describe the cellular sites of interaction responsible for neuromuscular transmission.

Traditionally, receptors have been classified according to the agonist or mediator to which they respond. The first example of receptor classification, proposed by Dale[3] in 1914, distinguished the nicotinic and muscarinic acetylcholine receptors based on the differing effects of the plant alkaloids nicotine and muscarine at receptor subtypes activated by the neurotransmitter acetylcholine. More recently, receptors have been distinguished according to their general effector mechanisms. This functional classification recognizes at least three general types of cell-surface receptors: ion-channel receptors, enzyme-associated receptors, and G protein–coupled receptors (GPCRs).[4,5]

GPCRs share a characteristic topology consisting of seven α-helical transmembrane (TM) spans.[6–9] The utility of this structural template is evident from its wide evolutionary conservation. Members of the largest rhodopsin-like GPCR family can be found in slime mold,[10] yeast,[11] plants,[12] protozoa, and the earliest diploblastic metazoa.[13,14] A topologically similar seven-TM structure also is found in the prokaryotic light-driven proton pump bacteriorhodopsin from *Halobacterium halobium*,[15,16] although its amino acid sequence does not resemble that found in GPCRs in higher organisms. The rhodopsin family of GPCRs has several thousand members in the human genome, making it one of the largest gene families known.[17,18] This class of GPCRs represents approximately 1% to 5% of total cellular protein.[19,20]

GPCRs owe their name to their effector interaction with heterotrimeric (α, β, and γ subunits) G proteins.[21–23] The mechanism by which GPCRs transduce extracellular stimuli into cellular responses was initially attributed entirely to the stimulation of G protein dissociation into G_α and $G_{\beta\gamma}$ subunits, both of which can modulate the activity of downstream effectors.[24] More recently, diverse effector mechanisms for heptahelical receptors that are independent of heterotrimeric G proteins have been identified.[25] GPCRs interact with a variety of proteins in addition to signal mediators, including GPCR regulatory proteins,[26] multidomain scaffolding proteins, and chaperone molecules.[27] The signaling and specificity of GPCRs also can be influenced by GPCR homo- and heterodimerization[28] and by biochemical signal-transduction switching.[20] The large number of GPCRs and the plethora of GPCR signaling and modulatory mechanisms provide the specificity and flexibility in controlling cellular targeting and cellular response required for endocrine physiology.

CLASSIFICATION OF G PROTEIN-COUPLED RECEPTORS

The term *GPCR* refers to diverse heptahelical proteins that are known either to mediate signaling via heterotrimeric G proteins or to have homologous sequences to receptors that signal via G proteins. The first GPCRs that were cloned in the mid-1980s were the visual pigment opsin[29] and the β-adrenergic receptor.[30] Since then, the sequences of hundreds of pharmacologically distinct GPCRs have been identified.[31] Attempts to classify GPCRs according to their effects on signal transduction alone were unsatisfactory because of the difficulty of classifying receptors that signal through more than one type of G protein or through mechanisms independent of heterotrimeric G proteins.[25] Classification schemes have therefore relied predominantly on GPCR structure, as reflected in the predicted amino acid sequence. Among GPCRs, several families can be distinguished that have conserved amino acid sequence motifs within families but no discernable sequence similarities between families.[23,32]

All GPCRs contain seven hydrophobic α-helical TM spans connected by alternative intracellular and extracellular loops. The amino terminus of GPCRs is located on the extracellular side, and the carboxy terminus, on the intracellular side (Fig. 11-1). GPCRs have been divided into as many as six classes.[5,23,33,34] The most widely used classification of neurotransmitter/hormone receptors has been endorsed by the International Union of Pharmacology (IUPHAR).[35] The three major subclasses (Table 11-1) include the rhodopsin-like receptors (subclass I), the glucagon-related receptors (subclass II), and metabotropic glutamate-related receptors (subclass III). Two minor unrelated receptor classes for fungal pheromones are subclass IV (STE2-like receptors) and subclass V (STE3-like receptors). *Dictyostelium discoideum* cyclic adenosine monophosphate (cAMP) receptors make up yet another minor, unique group of GPCRs (subclass VI). Other putative subclasses such as frizzled and smoothened receptors, *Drosophila* odorant receptors, nematode chemoreceptors, and vomeronasal receptors, as well as the unclassified orphans GPCRs, also have been proposed.[36] A different classification scheme has been developed by using bioinformatics analysis of receptor sequences that segregates GPCRs in five main families identified as glutamate, rhodopsin, adhesion, frizzled/taste2, and secretin.[37]

Subclass I rhodopsin-like receptors, which form the largest GPCR subgroup, include receptors having a wide diversity of agonists, including light, neurotransmitters, and glycoprotein hormones.[38] Subclass I contains receptors for 31 agonist families (see Table 11-1), with each family including as many as 13 members (serotonin receptors). The separate receptors are all encoded on different genes. Functionally distinct isoforms of the dopamine D_2 receptor are generated by alternative exon splicing.[39,40]

The overall sequence homology among subclass I receptors is low, restricted to several highly conserved amino acids located mostly in the cytoplasmic half of the TM core (see Fig. 11-1). Mutagenesis experiments suggest that many of these highly conserved amino acids contribute to protein stability and to the conformational changes that mediate recep-

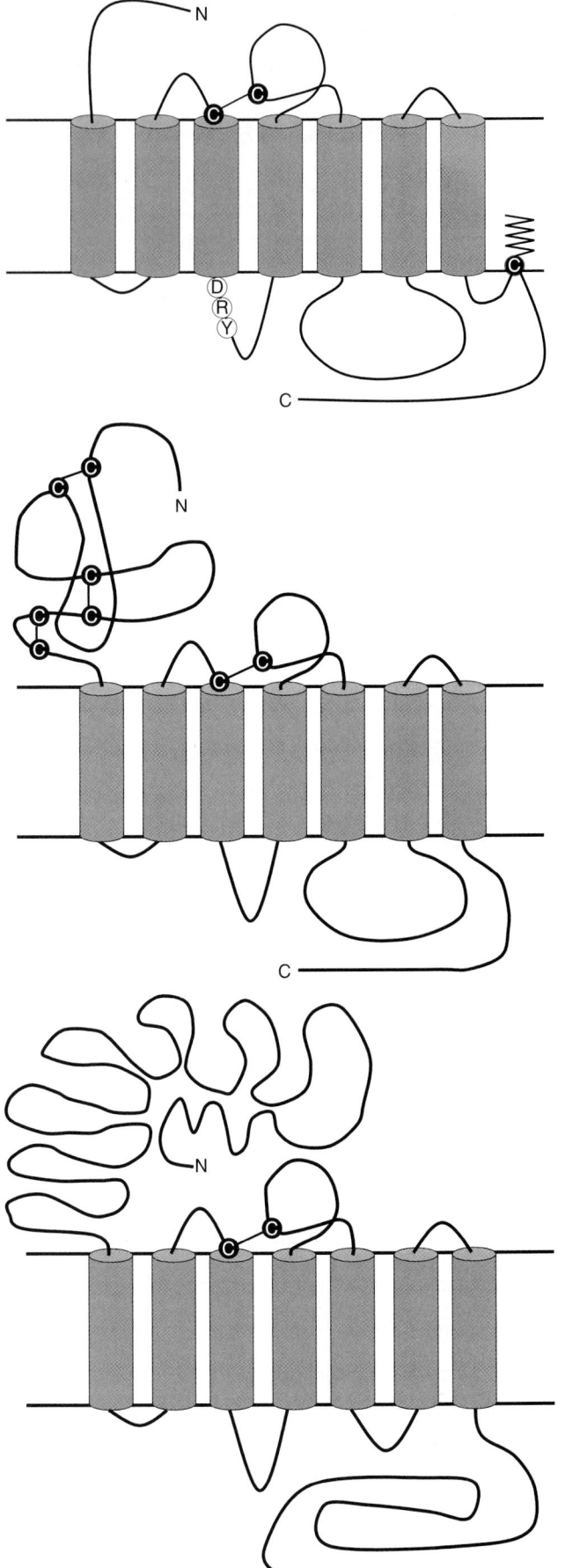

Figure 11-1 Schematic of G protein–coupled receptor (GPCR) structures. **Top,** A subclass I rhodopsin/neurotransmitter GPCR. **Middle,** A subclass II glucagons-related receptor. **Bottom,** A subclass III metabotropic glutamate-related receptor.

Table 11-1 Classification and G Protein–Coupling Preference of GPCRs[31,34]

GPCR Subclass	Ligand Structure	Family	Receptor Type	G Protein–Coupling Preference	Refs.
I. RHODOPSIN-LIKE	11-*cis*-retinal	Rhodopsin	Rhodopsin color opsins	G_t	155
	Various	Olfactory	OLF	G_{olf}	332
	Various	Gustatory	GUS	G_{gust}	333
	Biogenic amines	Acetylcholine	Muscarinic $M_{1,3,5}$	$G_{q/11}$	334
			Muscarinic $M_{2,4}$	$G_{i/o}$	335
		Adrenoceptors	$\alpha_{1A,1B,1D}$	$G_{q/11}$	335
			$\alpha_{2A,2B,2C}$	$G_{i/o}$	
			$\beta_{1,2,3}$	G_s	
		Dopamine	$D_{1,5}$	G_s	63
			$D_{2,3,4}$	$G_{i/o}$	
		Histamine	H_1	$G_{q/11}$	336
			H_2	G_s	
			H_3	$G_{i/o}$?	337,338
		Serotonin	$5HT_{1A,B,D,E,F}$	$G_{i/o}$	
			$5HT_{2A,B,C}$	$G_{q/11}$	
			$5HT_{4,6,7}$	G_s	
			$5ht_{5A,5B}$	?	
	Peptides	Angiotensin	AT_1	$G_{q/11}$	339
			AT_2	$G_{i/o}$?	
		Apelin	APJ	$G_{i/o}$	340
		Bradykinin	$B_{1,2}$	$G_{q/11}$	341
		Chemokines	CCR1-10	$G_{i/o}$	342,343
			CXCR1-6		
		Cholecystokinin	CCK1,2	$G_{q/11}$	344
		Endothelin	$ET_{A,B}$	$G_{q/11}$	345,346
		Galanin	GAL1	$G_{q/11}$	347
		Gonadotropin-releasing hormone	GnRH	$G_{q/11}$	62
		Melatonin	MT_1, MT_2	$G_{i/o}$	34,348
			MT_3	$G_{q/11}$?	
		Melanocortin	MC_{1-5}	G_s	349
		Neuropeptide Y	Y_{1-5}	$G_{i/o}$	350
		Oxytocin	OT	$G_{q/11}$	351
		Opioid	μ, δ, κ	$G_{i/o}$	352
		Somatostatin	SST_{1-5}	$G_{i/o}$	353
		Thyrotropin-releasing hormone	TRH	$G_{q/11}$	354
		Vasopressin	$V_{1a,1b}$	$G_{q/11}$	355
			V_2	G_s	
	Proteinases	Proteinase-activated	$PAR_{1,3,4}$ (thrombin-activated)	$G_{q/11}$/$G_{i/o}$	356,357
			PAR_2 (trypsin-like proteases-activated)	$G_{q/11}$/$G_{i/o}$	
	Lipids	Cannabinoid	$CB_{1,2}$	$G_{i/o}$	358
		Lysophospholipid	LPA_{1-3}	$G_{q/11}$/$G_{i/o}$	359,360
			$S1P_{1-5}$	$G_{q/11}$/$G_{i/o}$	
		Prostanoid	DP, EP_2, IP	G_s	361
			$EP_{3,4}$	$G_{i/o}$	
			EP_1, FP, TP	$G_{q/11}$	362
		Leukotriene and lipoxin	$BTL_{1,2}$	$G_{q/11}$	362
			$CysLT_{1,2}$	$G_{q/11}$	
			Lipoxin ALX	$G_{q/11}$	
	Nucleotide-like	Adenosine	$A_{1,3}$	$G_{i/o}$	363
			$A_{2A,2B}$	G_s	
		Purinoreceptors	$P2Y_{1,2,4,6,11}$	$G_{q/11}$	364
II. GLUCAGON-LIKE	Peptides	Calcitonin	$CGRP_{\alpha,\beta}$	G_s	365
			$AM_{1,2,3}$	G_s	
			$AMY_{1,2}$	G_s	
			CT	G_s	366
		Corticotropin-releasing factor	CRF_1, $CRF_{2(a),(b),(c)}$	G_s	
			Urocortin 1, 2, 3	G_q?	45
		Glucagon	GHRH	G_s	
			GIP	G_s	
			Glucagon	G_s	
			GLP-1, GLP-2	G_s	
			Secretin	G_s	
		Parathyroid hormone	$PTH_{1,2}$	G_s	367
		Vasoactive intestinal peptide and pituitary adenylate cyclase-activating polypeptide	PAC_1	G_s	
			$VPAC_{1,2}$		

Continued

Table 11-1 Classification and G Protein–coupling Preference of GPCRs[31,34]—cont'd

GPCR Subclass	Ligand Structure	Family	Receptor Type	G Protein–Coupling Preference	Refs.
III. METABOTROPIC GLUTAMATE-LIKE	Ions	Calcium sensor	CaS	$G_{q/11}$	368
	Amino acids	γ-Aminobutyric acid	$GABA_{B1}$ $GABA_{B2}$	$G_{i/o}$	50
		Metabotropic glutamate	$mGlu_{1,5}$ $mGlu_{2-4,6-8}$	$G_{q/11}$ $G_{i/o}$	48

tor activation.[41–44] The only residue that is conserved among all subclass I receptors is an arginine in the Asp-Arg-Tyr motif at the cytoplasmic side of TM helix 3.[32] Two cysteine residues in the second and third extracellular loops, which are conserved in most GPCRs, form a disulfide bridge that has been implicated in the packing and stabilization of the TM bundle (see Fig. 11-1).

The glucagon-like receptors (subclass II) include a relatively small group of peptide receptors that are expressed in endocrine cells of the pancreas and gastrointestinal epithelium and in specialized neurons in the brain (see Table 11-1).[45] Glucagon, glucagon-like peptide-1, glucagon-like peptide-2, glucose-dependent insulinotropic peptide, growth hormone–releasing hormone, and secretin are structurally related peptides that exert their actions through glucagon-like subclass II receptors.[45] Except for the disulfide bridge between the second and third extracellular loops, subclass II receptors do not contain any of the conserved structural features characterizing subclass I receptors, such as the Asp-Arg-Tyr motif. These receptors share a relatively large amino terminus extracellular domain (~100 residues) containing several cysteines that form a network of disulfide bridges.[46,47]

The metabotropic glutamate-like receptors (subclass III) are characterized by an extremely long amino terminus extracellular domain (~500 to 600 residues) that is implicated in ligand binding. This subclass include the metabotropic glutamate (mGlu) receptors,[48] the calcium-sensing receptors,[49] the γ-aminobutyric acid (GABA_B) receptor,[50] the vomeronasal mammalian pheromone receptors,[51] and putative taste receptors.[52] Except for a disulfide bridge between extracellular loops 2 and 3, subclass III receptors do not share any conserved residues with subclasses I and II.

STRUCTURAL FEATURES OF G PROTEIN–COUPLED RECEPTORS

GPCRs have an extracellular amino terminus; seven α-helical TM spans, which form the TM core; three extracellular loops; three intracellular loops; and an intracellular carboxy terminus (see Fig. 11-1). Each of the seven TM spans is generally composed of 20 to 27 amino acids. In different GPCRs, the amino terminus (7 to 595 amino acids), loops (5 to 230 amino acids), and carboxy terminus (12 to 359 amino acids) vary considerably in length.

The conserved GPCR sequences are largely contained within the hydrophobic TM domains.[7,32,53] To facilitate comparisons of corresponding residues among different class I receptors, several numbering schemes have been developed. The Schwartz and Baldwin numbering schemes are similar.[54,55] In these schemes, the most conserved residues in each helix are numbered according to their predicted relative position in a standard helix of 26 amino acids.[54,55] A given residue is then described by the helix in which it is located (I to VII) followed by a number indicating its position in the helix. For example, II.9 corresponds to residue number nine in TM span two. One limitation in this approach, which leads to differences between the two related systems, is that the beginning of the helix cannot be unequivocally assigned. In the

Ballesteros numbering scheme,[56] the most conserved amino acid in each TM span is given the arbitrary number 50, and each amino acid is numbered according to its position relative to this conserved residue. For example, 4.57 indicates a residue located in TM span four, seven residues toward the carboxy terminus from Trp(4.50), the most conserved amino acid in helix four. In this chapter, the residues are indicated according to the Ballesteros numbering.[56] Thus, the index residues in each of the TMs of bovine rhodopsin are Asn1.50, Asp2.50, Arg3.50, Trp4.50, Pro5.50, Pro6.60, and Pro7.50. All of these are highly conserved among rhodopsin-like GPCRs, and therefore this approach allows unambiguous alignment of the TM spans of these receptors.

What advantages are conferred by this widely adopted seven-TM template?[57] An odd number of TM spans places the amino and carboxy termini at opposite membrane surfaces. This allows ligand binding and receptor glycosylation at the amino terminus and phosphorylation and palmitoylation at the carboxy terminus (see later). We can speculate that seven TM spans may be the minimum necessary to form a stable yet flexible TM core, with sufficient size and versatility to offer the specificity, regulatory mechanisms, and contact sites for G proteins and other signaling molecules.

The first crystal structure of any GPCR, the structure of bovine rhodopsin, has been solved at 2.8-Å resolution.[58] The determination of the structure of rhodopsin at atomic resolution represents a milestone in the study of GPCRs and TM signaling.[59,60] The crystal structure of rhodopsin[58] confirmed the existence of seven TM helices (Fig. 11-2). The seven TM segments are arranged as a closed loop in a clockwise direction for TM1 to TM7, as viewed from the intracellular surface. A fourth intracellular loop is anchored by palmitoyl groups attached to a pair of cysteine residues, forming an eighth cytoplasmic amphiphilic helix that lies along the surface of the cell membrane.[61] Sequence conservation[32] suggests a similar helical structure (H8) among other subclass I GPCRs.

Within the inner leaflet of the plasma membrane, TM4 and TM6 are perpendicular to the lipid bilayer plane, whereas TM1, TM2, TM3, and TM5 have a lateral tilt, and TM7 is kinked inward in the center (see Fig. 11-2). In this arrangement, the core comprises primarily TM1, TM2, TM3, TM5, TM6, and TM7, whereas TM1 and TM4 are peripherally located.[62,63] The inner sections of TM2 and TM3 are nearly parallel, and both helices form a nucleus for packing the other TM helices. The TM helices are slightly longer on the exofacial side and shorter on the endofacial side than had been predicted from earlier cryo-electron microscopy studies.[55] A network of hydrogen bonds forms in the middle of the heptahelical core, thus constraining rhodopsin in the ground state. This network is mediated in part by the side chains of the highly conserved Asn(1.50)-Asp(2.50) pair in helices I and II (see Fig. 11-2), and Trp(4.50) in helix IV. The cytoplasmic side of the helical core is organized mainly by hydrophobic interactions. These interactions are arranged in two layers parallel to the lipid bilayer. One of the layers overlies the hydrogen-bond network in the middle of the heptahelical core described earlier, and the other surrounds the highly conserved E(D)RY (3.49 to 3.51) motif (see Fig. 11-2).

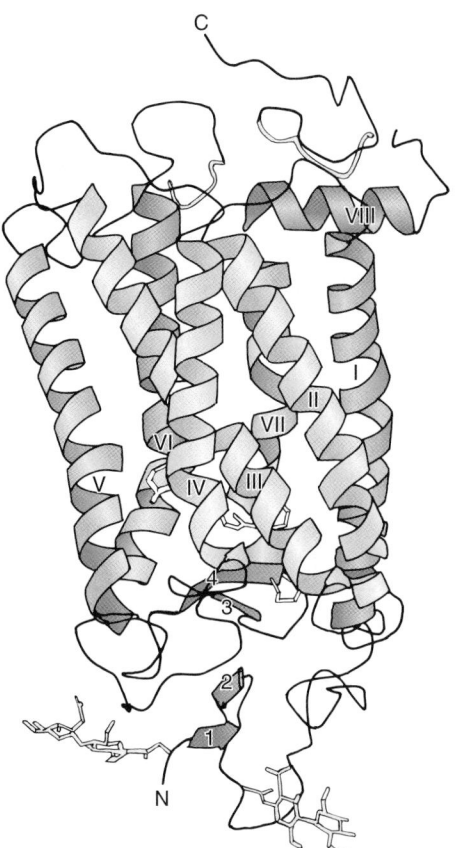

Figure 11-2 Ribbon drawing of the crystal structure of rhodopsin in a plane parallel to the membrane. The top is intracellular, and the bottom is extracellular. N and C, amino and carboxy termini, respectively. Roman numerals, helices. (Adapted from Palczewski K, Kumasaka T, Hori T, et al: Crystal structure of rhodopsin: A G protein-coupled receptor. Science 289:739–745, 2000, with permission.)

The intracellular loops of rhodopsin extend from the TM core. The boundaries of the loops determined from the crystal structure correspond to the predictions from spin-labeling studies of cysteine-substitution mutants.[64–66] The helical structure of the cytoplasmic region of the fourth intracellular loop is of particular interest. This region had been implicated in G protein coupling by studies using synthetic peptides.[67] The presence of a helical structure for this domain was previously proposed based on nuclear magnetic resonance (NMR) spectroscopy of the β-adrenergic receptor.[68] It also was proposed that a family of peptides called *mastoparans*, which present amphiphilic helical structure and can activate G proteins by mimicking the structure of this GPCR domain.[69]

The extracellular loops of rhodopsin are folded around two β-sheets (see Fig. 11-2), confirming early predictions of a compact domain.[70] The first pair of antiparallel strands is located in the amino terminus, forming a typical β-sheet running almost parallel to the plasma membrane. Because of wide sequence divergence, this is unlikely to be a general feature of GPCRs. The second β-sheet, which is positioned over TM3 by a highly conserved disulfide bond, may have homologues in most of class I rhodopsin-like receptors. The functional role of this unusual structure is not yet known.

Recent comparisons of the rhodopsin structure with the results of previous experimental approaches suggest very similar overall structures within class I GPCRs.[71,72] Several of the highly unusual structural features in rhodopsin also are present in aminergic GPCRs. Therefore, rhodopsin and its crystal structure provides a good framework for approximating the three-dimensional structure of other subclass I GPCRs.[71,72]

POSTTRANSLATIONAL MODIFICATIONS

GLYCOSYLATION

In common with most membrane proteins, the majority of GPCRs have at least one glycosylation site in their N-terminal domain.[73] A few GPCRs, such as the α_{2B}-adrenoceptor, lack identifiable glycosylation sites.[74] In glycosylated GPCRs, high mannose, complex or hybrid oligosaccharides are linked to the Asn side chain (N-linked glycosylation) in a multistep process.[75]

The first step of N-glycosylation is the cotranslational transfer of $Glc_3Man_9GlcNAc_2$ from the lipid carrier dolichol pyrophosphate oligosaccharide onto the nascent protein by oligosaccharide transferase, a process that occurs in the lumen of the rough endoplasmic reticulum.[73] All types of N-linked glycans share a common pentasaccharide core structure. The glycan is attached to the Asn residue in the Asn-Xxx-Thr/Ser consensus sequence. This consensus sequence must be correctly oriented and accessible for glycosylation to occur. Not all consensus sites are glycosylated.

As the glycoprotein is processed through the smooth endoplasmic reticulum and the Golgi apparatus, the oligosaccharide is trimmed and elaborated. The initial step of this processing is the removal of the three glucosyl residues, which results in a high-mannose-type chain. Complex oligosaccharides contain additions to the core glycan, which include galactosyl, fucosyl, sialyl, and GlcNAc residues.

The functional significance of glycosylation differs in individual GPCRs. The oligosaccharide moieties are important for the expression and stability of the gonadotropin-releasing hormone (GnRH) and V_{1a} receptors but do not contribute to high-affinity agonist interaction. Likewise, glycan chains are essential for correct folding and trafficking of the vasoactive intestinal peptide ($VPAC_1$) receptor, the thyrotropin-releasing hormone (TRH) receptor, and the follicle-stimulating hormone (FSH) receptor. For some GPCRs, including somatostatin, β_2-adrenergic, TRH, and gastrin-releasing peptide receptors, glycosylation is important for high-affinity ligand binding and also may contribute to receptor/G protein coupling. For many GPCRs, however, glycosylation has no known function. This latter group includes oxytocin, histamine H_2, M_2 muscarinic acetylcholine, neurokinin $(NK)_1$, bombesin BB_1, adenosine A_{2a}, and angiotensin AT_2 receptors. Although N-linked glycosylation of GPCRs is almost universal, its influence on the mature protein properties are variable and unpredictable.

PALMITOYLATION

Covalent lipid modifications anchor numerous signaling proteins to the cytoplasmic face of the plasma membrane. These modifications mediate protein-membrane and protein-protein interactions and are often essential for function.[76–78] Protein fatty acylation occurs either through amide linkages (N-acylation) or thioester linkages (S-acylation). N-Acylation occurs on the amino-terminal glycine residue after removal of the initiator methionine by a methionyl-aminopeptidase. S-acylation occurs on cysteine residues through a thioester linkage in a wide variety of sequence contexts. Palmitate is the most commonly used S-linked fatty acid. This posttranslational process is usually referred to as protein palmitoylation. However, other fatty acids can be incorporated into cellular proteins by a thio-ester linkage, including myristate, stearate, and arachidonate.

Palmitoylation is a posttranslational modification restricted to a small subset of cellular proteins, among which proteins involved in signal transduction are prevalent. This thioesterification of cysteine residues by palmitate is distinguished from other lipid modifications by its reversibility.[79] Indeed, in contrast to myristoyl and prenyl moieties that are added cotranslationally and generally remain attached to the proteins until protein degradation, the protein-bound palmitate is added posttranslationally. Moreover, the palmitoylation state of several proteins is dynamically regulated. In particular, biologic regulation of the palmitoylation state of the G proteins and of their cognate receptors has been demonstrated.

Many GPCRs have been shown to be palmitoylated at cysteine residues in the intracellular C-terminal tail,[76,77,80,81] including rhodopsin, β_2- and α_2-adrenoceptors, luteinizing hormone (LH)/chorionic gonadotropin, endothelin ET_A and ET_B, and vasopressin V_2 receptors. The 5-HT_{1A} and 5-HT_{1B} serotonin, dopamine D_1 and D_2, and $mGlu_4$ receptors also have been reported to be palmitoylated; however, the actual sites of palmitoylation for these receptors have not been demonstrated. A mutant μ-opioid receptor with its two cysteines in the carboxy terminus replaced was still palmitoylated, suggesting that palmitoylation of this receptor must occur at another position.[82]

Palmitoylation serves to enhance the association of cytosolic proteins with the membrane. Palmitoylation of GPCRs anchors the C-terminal tail to the plasma membrane, creating in essence a fourth intracellular loop. The elimination of palmitoylation sites attenuated G protein coupling of β_2-adrenoceptors, endothelin ET_B, and somatostatin SST_5 receptors.[80] Initial activation of the β_2-adrenoceptor promotes rapid depalmitoylation of both the receptor and the G_α G protein subunit, and sustained activation prevents palmitoylation from occurring. Palmitoylation has been found to be obligatory for ligand-promoted extracellular signal-regulated kinase (ERK)/mitogen-activated protein kinase (MAPK) activation by the endothelin (ET) receptor.[83] However, for many GPCRs, palmitoylation is not essential for receptor–G protein coupling.[80]

The palmitoylation state of the receptor governs internalization by regulating the accessibility of receptor to the arrestin-mediated internalization pathway.[79] Thus, desensitization of the β_2-adrenoceptor and the LH receptor proceeds through a palmitoylated, hyperphosphorylated state. The β_2-adrenoceptor contains a cAMP-dependent protein kinase consensus sequence in the close vicinity of the palmitoylation site. It is possible that reduced palmitoylation of the β_2-adrenoceptor exposes the cAMP-dependent protein kinase site and causes constitutive desensitization of this receptor.

DIVERSITY OF RECEPTOR-LIGAND BINDING

Different GPCRs have evolved varying molecular mechanisms for interacting with specific agonists.[57] This structural diversity superimposed on a common seven-TM spans template reflects the conservation of an efficient protein structure for signal transduction across a membrane and the need to distinguish diverse activating ligands as different as a photon of light and a 40-kilodalton protein.[19]

In general, GPCRs are activated by receptor-specific ligands that bind to their extracellular or TM domains. Rhodopsin is unique in the activation of the receptor by the ligand. Its ligand, 11-*cis*-retinal, is coupled via a protonated Schiff's base to the aldehyde moiety of retinal and the ε-amine of Lys7.43.[84] This 11-*cis*-retinylidene moiety acts as an inverse agonist and prevents spontaneous activation of the receptor. The protonated Schiff's base forms a salt bridge with Glu3.28 located at the boundary between TM3 and the first extracellular loop, thus bringing TM3 and TM7 into apposition. In rhodopsin, the chromophore is completely buried inside the protein, with no accessibility to the aqueous or membrane environment. Photon absorption switches retinal from the 11-*cis* to the all-*trans*-retinylidene conformation, which neutralizes the salt bridge between the protonated Schiff's base and Glu3.28 and activates the receptor.[85]

The simplest mechanism for a ligand to use to activate a receptor is to bind the TM core. The protonated amine present in all biogenic amines (i.e., adrenaline, noradrenaline, dopamine, histamine, serotonin, and acetylcholine) makes a direct contact with Asp3.32, a residue conserved in all aminergic receptors.[86] This Asp is essential for neurotransmitter binding but not for signal generation. In certain aminergic receptors, this interaction with the protonated amine is shared with the residue 3.36.[87,88] In catecholamine receptors, the catechol ring of the ligand has been found to dock in the pocket between TM5 and TM6. In some neurotransmitter receptors, the *meta*- and *para*-hydroxy groups of the catecholamine agonists hydrogen bind Ser5.42 and Ser5.46, respectively.[86] The cluster of aromatic residues of TM6 is highly conserved among aminergic GPCRs and includes Trp6.48, Phe/Trp6.51, and Phe6.52. These residues have been implicated in ligand binding in many aminergic receptors.[86]

The amino acids that are conserved in neurotransmitter GPCRs that contribute to ligand interaction cannot account for the pharmacologic differences between receptor subtypes. However, in a number of receptors, single residues that differ among related receptor subtypes have been shown to mediate pharmacologic specificity. For example, the residue at position 7.39 contributes to the specificity of different receptors such as α_2- and β_2-adrenoceptors[89] and 5-HT_{1A} and 5-HT_{1B} serotonin receptors.[86,90]

Peptide hormone receptors for short peptide ligands such as formyl receptor or gonadotropin-releasing hormone receptor (3 and 10 residues, respectively) complex with the peptide ligand through interactions involving both extracellular loops and the TM core.[62] Peptide hormone receptors with larger peptide agonists such as glucagon, parathyroid hormone, or calcitonin (30 to 40 amino acids) use both the amino terminus and the extracellular loops to generate high-affinity ligand binding.[91]

Receptors for thrombin and other proteases are activated by proteolysis of the amino terminus.[92,93] The protease ligand thrombin specifically recognizes an amino acid sequence in the amino terminus of the receptor and cleaves it. The new shorter amino terminus revealed by proteolysis functions as a tethered ligand that binds intramolecularly and activates the receptor.

The glycoprotein hormones, which include LH, FSH, chorionic gonadotropin, and thyroid stimulating hormone, are the largest (30 to 40 kilodaltons) and most complex GPCR agonists. These ligands are heterodimers that contain a common α subunit and a hormone-specific β subunit. The initial high-affinity binding site of these receptors is located in their large (300 to 400 residues) amino terminus domains.

The metabotropic glutamate subclass of GPCRs is characterized by a large extracellular domain similar to bacterial periplasmic-binding proteins that contains the agonist binding site.[48] The three-dimensional crystal structure of this domain has been solved for the metabotropic glutamate receptor type 1.[94] This so-called *Venus flytrap module* consists of two lobes separated by a large cleft in which agonists bind. Another feature of subclass III receptors is that they all form dimers, either homodimers[94] or heterodimers.[95]

The $GABA_B$ receptors are constitutive heterodimers (see later) and represent a novel principle of receptor processing and signal transduction, in that two nonfunctional seven α-helical TM span proteins associate to form a functional G protein–coupled receptor.[96–99]

MECHANISM OF RECEPTOR ACTIVATION

The most widely accepted pharmacologic model to explain GPCR activation is the ternary complex model.[100] This model has been extended to explain the observation that, under certain conditions, several GPCRs can activate G proteins in the absence of agonists.[101,102] The extended ternary complex model[102] proposes that the receptor exists in an equilibrium between two conformational states: the inactive (R) and the active (R*) state. In the absence of agonists, the basal level of activity of the receptor is determined by the equilibrium between R and R*. The efficacy of ligands is thought to be dependent on their ability to shift the equilibrium between these two states.[103,104] Whereas most properties of GPCRs can be explained by the extended ternary complex model, other models have been proposed.[105]

When receptors are heterologously expressed in cell lines, many receptors show spontaneous activity in the absence of agonist. Consistent with the predictions of the extended ternary complex model,[102] inverse agonist ligands have been identified that are able to decrease the basal level of activity of the receptors.[106,107] Many ligands that were previously considered antagonists have been found to suppress this basal level of signaling and are now considered inverse agonists. According to the model, full and partial agonists bind R* with higher affinity than R, shifting the equilibrium to the activated state, whereas inverse agonists bind R with higher affinity, shifting the equilibrium to the inactive state.

The inactive state is stabilized by several intramolecular interactions, such as the salt bridge stabilizing TM3 and TM7 in rhodopsin. Similar stabilizing interactions have been suggested in the angiotensin AT_1 receptor and the α_{1B}-adrenoceptor.[23] Various point mutations in many GPCRs have been found to increase the basal agonist-independent activity of the receptors.[23,108,109] As described later, some of these activating mutations contribute to several endocrine diseases. The constraining intramolecular interactions are proposed to be released on activation (or by specific mutations), causing key sequences to be exposed to the G protein.[21] This hypothesis is supported by the observation that a mutation causing constitutive activation on the β_2-adrenoceptor is associated with a marked structural instability and enhanced conformational flexibility.[110]

Although the high-resolution structure of rhodopsin shows only the inactivated state of the receptor,[58] data from crosslinking and site-directed spin labeling,[59,111] together with the x-ray diffraction data, suggest that activation by light opens a cleft at the cytoplasmic end of the helix bundle.[85] TM7, which contains the protonated Schiff's base linkage with the chromophore, and TM3 and 6 are critical to the activation of GPCRs.[112,113] Photoisomerization of the chromophore neutralizes the salt bridge between the protonated Schiff's base and its counterion Glu3.28 in TM3 (see earlier). This salt bridge corresponds to a similar ionic interaction formed between norepinephrine and an acidic side chain (3.32) in adrenergic receptors.[114] TM7 is kinked at a highly conserved proline residue. This region of TM7 is stabilized by many interhelical constraints,[44,58] including the salt bridge between the protonated Schiff's base and Glu3.28, and an interaction with a kinked region in TM6 containing the conserved Pro6.50. Therefore, once the salt bridge is lost, a set of hydrogen bonds among TM7, TM1, and TM2 would no longer remain. These changes rearrange the TMs, especially TM2, TM6, and TM7, leading to the receptor activation.

Isomerization from 11-*cis* to the all-*trans*-retinylidene induces a large displacement of the C13 methyl group. This group interacts with Trp6.48 in the ground state, and after photoisomerization, the indole ring is able to rotate during the activation process.[115] Trp6.48 is highly conserved among GPCRs, and the binding of a ligand could induce the movement of TM7 through its indole ring.

The conformational changes described earlier lead to the rearrangement of the cytoplasmic side of the GPCR, allowing receptor–G protein coupling. One of the proposed key events in the activation process among subclass I GPCRs involves the protonation of the Asp3.49 in the highly conserved Asp-Arg-Tyr motif at the cytoplasmic side of TM3. This "protonation hypothesis" has been supported by experiments showing that charge-neutralizing mutations, which mimic the unprotonated state of the aspartic acid, cause constitutive activation of receptor subtypes such as α_{1B}-adrenoceptor and the β_2-adrenoceptors.[23,116] The experimental data have been supported by molecular modeling and computational simulations. Thus, the so-called *arginine-cage model*[116] proposed that Arg3.50 forms an ionic interaction with Arg3.49 in the inactive state of the receptor. During receptor activation, Asp3.49 becomes protonated, and the Arg3.50 side chain is released. The conserved bulky side chain of Ile3.54 restricts the positioning of the arginine side chain, promoting a rearrangement that characterizes the active state of the receptor.

The interaction between the 3.49 and 3.50 residues is observed in the crystal structure of rhodopsin.[58] In addition, the guanidinium group of Arg3.50 interacts with the polar side chains of the cytoplasmic side of TM6. These arrangements support the previous conclusions that protonation of the acidic group of Asp3.49 and movement of the cytoplasmic side of TM6 are critical for receptor activation.

RECEPTOR–G PROTEIN COUPLING AND SELECTIVITY

Although many GPCRs have been found to also couple by G protein–independent mechanisms,[25] the interaction with heterotrimeric G proteins is the major signaling mechanism of these proteins.[21,22,117] G protein activation modulates classic downstream effectors, such as adenylate cyclases,[118] phospholipases,[119] and ionic channels,[120] through well-characterized molecular mechanisms.[121–123]

HETEROTRIMERIC G PROTEINS

G proteins were described for the first time in the 1970s by Rodbell[124,125] and Gilman.[126] The "nucleotide binding protein necessary to reconstitute the stimulation of adenylate cyclase" was first purified by Gilman's laboratory.[127]

Two main families of signal transduction–related proteins that bind and hydrolyze guanine nucleotides have been described, monomeric G proteins (small G proteins) and heterotrimeric G proteins.[128,129] Monomeric G proteins are approximately 200 amino acids in size. They are implicated in biologic processes, such as the cell cycle, protein secretion, or intracellular vesicular interaction, and present certain structural similarities with heterotrimeric G proteins.[129,130] Heterotrimeric G proteins have three subunits (α, β, and γ). The β and γ subunits form a dimer that does not dissociate under physiologic conditions. Heterotrimeric G proteins are soluble intracellular proteins that may associate with the plasma membrane through covalent attachment of fatty acids.[131] The G_α subunit may be either myristoylated or palmitoylated, and the G_γ subunit either farnesylated or geranylgeranylated.

G proteins are classified according to the G_α subunit present in the heterotrimeric complex. Mammals have more than 20 different α subunit subtypes encoded on 17 genes. Some subtypes are different isoforms.[132–134] The G_α subunits form four different families ($G_{\alpha s}$, $G_{\alpha i}$, $G_{\alpha q}$, and $G_{\alpha 12}$) based on the degree of homology of the primary structure (Table 11-2). These subtype sequences are highly conserved across different species. In this regard, no differences are found in the amino acidic sequences between mouse and human $G_{\alpha s}$.[133]

Except for the G proteins that are expressed in sensory organs ($G_{\alpha t}$, $G_{\alpha g}$, and $G_{\alpha olf}$), and certain subtypes found mainly in hematopoietic ($G_{\alpha 16}$) or nervous ($G_{\alpha o}$) cells, most α subunits are ubiquitous. Moreover, each cellular type generally expresses four or five different α subunits.[135] The G proteins can be expressed at high concentration in certain tissues. Thus, in brain, $G_{\alpha o}$ may represent 1% to 2% of the total membrane protein.[136]

Table 11-2   Classification and Properties of G_α Proteins

Family/Subunit	Mass (kDa × 10⁻³)	% Amino Acid Identity	Toxin	Tissue Distribution	Example of Receptor	Effectors
G_s						
$\alpha_{S(S)}$	44.2	—	CTX	Ubiquitous	β-Adrenoceptor	↑ Adenylate cyclase
						↑ Ca²⁺ channels
$\alpha_{S(L)}$	45.7	—	CTX	Ubiquitous		↓ Na²⁺ channels
α_{olf}	44.7	88	CTX	Olfactory neuroepithelium	Olfactory	↑ Adenylate cyclase
G_i						
α_{i1}	40.3	—	PTX	Nearly ubiquitous	α₂-Adrenoceptor	↑ K⁺ channels
α_{i2}	40.5	88	PTX	Ubiquitous		↓ Ca²⁺ channels
α_{i3}	40.5	94	PTX	Nearly ubiquitous		↓ Adenylate cyclase
α_{OA}	40.0	73	PTX	Brain, others	α₂-Adrenoceptor	
α_{OB}	40.1	73	PTX	Brain, others		
α_{t1}	40.0	68	CTX, PTX	Retinal rods	Rhodopsin	↑ cGMP-specific phosphodiesterase
α_{t2}	40.1	68	CTX, PTX	Retinal cones	Cone opsin	
α_{g}	40.5	67	CTX, PTX	Taste buds	Gustatory	Depending on the taste
α_{z}	40.9	60		Brain, adrenal plateles	Muscarinic M₂	↓ Adenylate cyclase
G_q						
α_{q}	42	—		Nearly ubiquitous	Serotonin 5-HT₂ₐ	↑ Phospholipase Cβ
α_{11}	42	88		Nearly ubiquitous		
α_{14}	41.5	79		Lung, kidney, liver	Opioid receptor like	
α_{15}	43	57		B cells, myeloid cell	Carbachol	↑ Phospholipase Cβ
α_{16}	43.5	58		T cells, myeloid cell	Opioid receptor like	↑ Phospholipase Cβ
G_{12}						
α_{12}	44	—		Ubiquitous	α₁-Adrenoceptor	↑ Phospholipase C
α_{13}	44	67		Ubiquitous	Serotonin 5-HT₂c	↑ Phospholipase D

cGMP, cyclic guanosine monophosphate; CTX, cholera toxin; PTX, pertussis toxin.

Six different subtypes of G_β subunits (35 to 39 kilodaltons), encoded by six different genes, have been reported in mammals.[137] Twelve different G_γ subunits, which are encoded on 12 different genes, show a high heterogeneity.[138] Although in theory these protein subtypes could form 72 different $G_{\beta\gamma}$ dimers, not all the combinations are expressed in vivo.

The potential functional importance of such $G_{\beta\gamma}$ diversity is not yet understood. Most $G_{\beta\gamma}$ dimers (except for $\beta_1\gamma_1$ expressed in the retina) appear to exhibit similar functional properties. However, studies showing a specific βγ subtype requirement for the cholinergic acetylcholine muscarinic M₁ receptor to activate phospholipase C (PLC) suggest that βγ interactions are not completely interchangeable.[139]

The high-resolution structure of the heterotrimeric G proteins G_t and G_i show the overall shape of the guanosine diphosphate (GDP)-bound heterotrimer and the residues on the surface that can interact with other proteins.[140,141] The α subunit contains three domains.[129] The guanosine triphosphatase (GTPase) domain is highly conserved and has structural features in common with monomeric G proteins.[128,129] The nucleotide-binding pocket, as well as sites for binding the receptor, effector, and $G_{\beta\gamma}$ are located within the GTPase domain. The helical domain surrounds the nucleotide-binding pocket and has been proposed to increase the affinity of GTP binding,[142] act as a tethered GTPase-activating protein (GAP; see later),[143] and participate in effector recognition.[144] The third domain is the amino terminus of the G_α subunit, which forms an α-helix.[129,145]

The tertiary structure of the β subunit consists of two domains.[146] The amino-terminal domain forms an α-helix of about 20 amino acids. The carboxy-terminal domain G_β contains the so-called β-propeller fold, formed by seven antiparallel β-sheets. This motif is formed by a class of repeating sequences (WD) also found in a variety of other proteins, many of them unrelated to members of the G_β family.[147,148]

The γ subunit contains two α-helices connected by a 4-amino acid loop. In the $G_{\beta\gamma}$ dimer, the amino terminals of G_β and G_γ show helix-helix interactions, and the carboxy terminal of G_γ is embedded on one surface of the toroidal G_β subunit. This structure explains the stability of the $G_{\beta\gamma}$ dimer.[129]

The G proteins undergo a cyclic activation and deactivation process, which transmits the signal from receptor to effector (Fig. 11-3).[24,149,150] When an agonist activates the GPCR, the GDP-bound $G_{\alpha\beta\gamma}$ heterotrimer interacts with the receptor, and the α subunits decrease the affinity for GDP. Because the concentration of GTP is higher than that of GDP in the cytoplasm,[134,151] GDP is displaced by GTP in the nucleotide-binding pocket. Once GTP is bound, the now active α subunit dissociates both from the receptor and $G_{\beta\gamma}$. This active state of the G_α persists until its intrinsic Mg²⁺-dependent GTPase activity hydrolyzes GTP to GDP.[22] All isoforms of G_α are GTPases, but the intrinsic rate of GTP hydrolysis varies from one type to another.[152,153] Once GTP is cleaved to GDP, the G_α and $G_{\beta\gamma}$ reassociate and become inactive until stimulated by a receptor (see Fig. 11-3).

The original hypothesis about the G protein–mediated signal transduction was that GTP-bound G_α subunits were able to activate effectors, whereas $G_{\beta\gamma}$ dimers were only negative modulators.[24] Thus, release of free $G_{\beta\gamma}$ from a high expressed G protein such as G_i can deactivate other stimulatory G_α subunits such as $G_{\alpha s}$. This view changed with the discovery that $G_{\beta\gamma}$, as well as G_{α}, could positively regulate effectors such as K⁺ channels.[137,154]

MOLECULAR BASIS OF RECEPTOR/G PROTEIN COUPLING

Although many aspects of the structural principles of GPCR activation can be inferred from structural studies and the inactive state structure of rhodopsin,[85,155] confirmation awaits the high-resolution structure of an active state GPCR–G protein complex. Studies performed with receptor chimeras, deletions, and site-directed mutants provide insight into the GPCR regions involved in G protein coupling.[22,33,156]

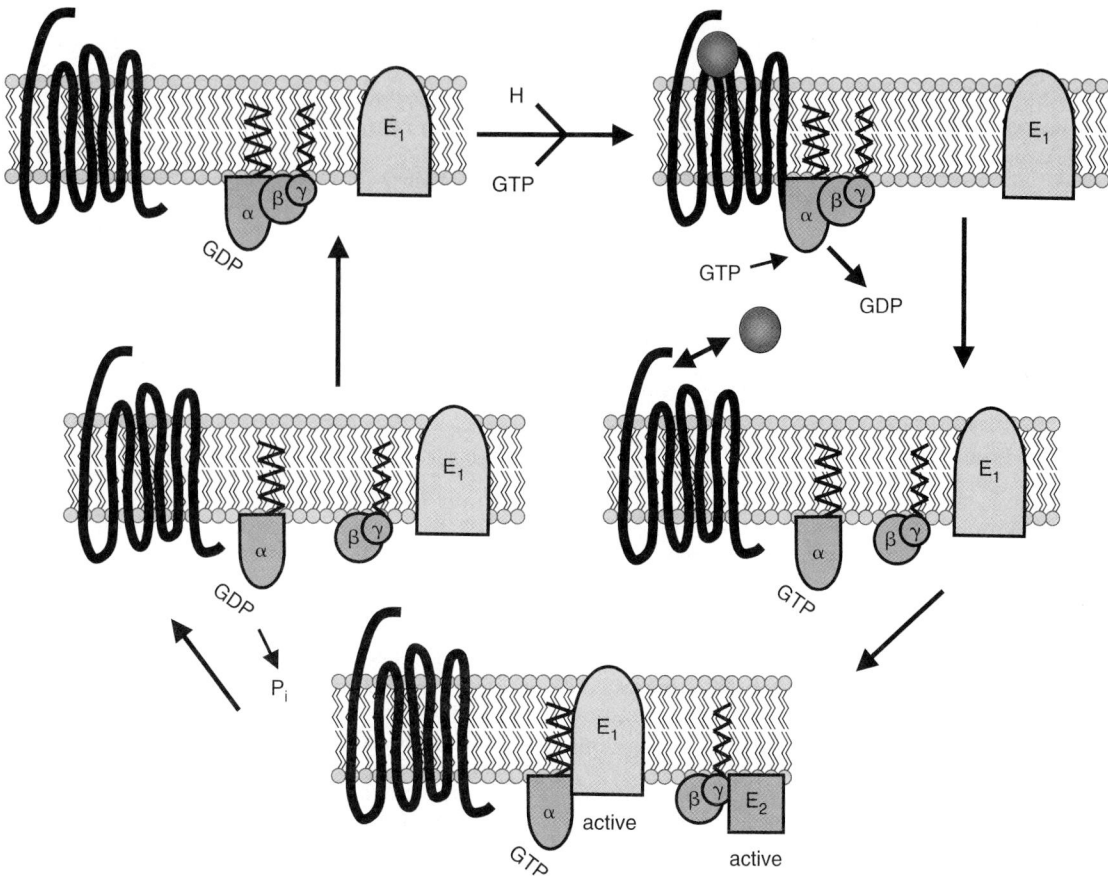

Figure 11-3 G protein cycle. In the inactive state, the heterotrimeric guanosine diphosphate (GDP)-bound G protein is associated with the receptor **(top right)**. Activation of the receptor leads to guanosine triphosphate (GTP)/GDP exchange in the G_α subunit, dissociation of the G_α and $G_{\beta\gamma}$ subunits from the receptor and each other, and interaction with signaling effector proteins (E_1,E_2). The intrinsic GTPase activity of G_α regenerates the GDP-bound G_α subunit, which reassociates with $G_{\beta\gamma}$ and the receptor, completing the cycle.

Most GPCRs can recognize and activate only a limited set of the many structurally similar G proteins (as defined by their α subunits) expressed in a cell.[33] Based on this G protein–coupling preference, GPCRs can be broadly subdivided into $G_{i/o}$-, G_s-, and $G_{q/11}$-coupled receptors (see Table 11-1). Although it has been reported that several GPCR subtypes can activate $G_{12/13}$ proteins, receptors that preferentially activate $G_{12/13}$ proteins have not yet been indentified.[157]

As discussed earlier, receptor activation is likely to involve a cleft opening at the cytoplasmic receptor surface, which enables the receptor to expose previously buried residues critical for G protein recognition and activation. All GPCR intracellular loops have been implicated in receptor–G protein specificity.[158–160]

The length of the intracellular loop 1 is highly conserved among GPCRs, suggesting an important structural role in G protein coupling. Several studies have shown that the structural integrity of the intracellular loop 1 is critical for receptor–G protein coupling.[33] However, it remains to be determined whether these residues are in direct contact with the G protein or indirect conformational effects are exerted by intracellular loop 1 on the accessibility of other regions (such as intracellular loops 2 and 3), which can directly interact with the G protein.

Mutational studies on several subclass I GPCRs have demonstrated that replacement of the arginine residue within the highly conserved DRY motif at the amino terminus of the intracellular loop 2 (see earlier) abolishes or drastically reduces G protein coupling.[161,162] However, charge-conserving mutations result in only modest reduction of receptor function.[162] These results suggest that the conserved arginine residue interacts with an electron-rich site on the G protein. In this regard, both *N*-formyl peptide receptor[163] and rhodopsin[164] have been shown to be unable to associate physically with G proteins when the conserved arginine residue was mutated. Thus, this arginine residue has been proposed to represent the primary trigger for the release of GDP from the receptor–G protein complex.[165]

The intracellular loop 2 has been implicated in the regulation of receptor–G protein coupling selectivity by using GPCR chimeras. Several studies have reported that substitution of the intracellular loop 2 (alone or together with other intracellular receptor regions such as the intracellular loop 3 or the carboxy terminus) from a donor receptor into a functionally different receptor can confer on the receptor chimera the G protein–coupling profile of the donor receptor.[33] In this context, the intracellular loop 3 also has been involved in receptor–G protein–coupling selectivity. However, it is usually not sufficient for controlling all the coupling characteristics of a particular receptor. Thus, detailed mutational analysis of different muscarinic receptors (M_1 to M_5) have identified single amino acids, primarily hydrophobic or noncharged, within the intracellular loop 3 playing a key role in determining receptor–G protein–coupling selectivity in conjunction with residues present in the intracellular loop 2.

As discussed earlier, the helical structure of the carboxy terminus forming a fourth intracellular loop is one of the most striking findings of the high-resolution structure of rhodopsin.[58] Receptor-truncation studies have reported that removal of the carboxy terminus usually produces functionally inactive receptors. Moreover, some of these truncated receptors, such as vasopressin V_2 receptors,[166] have been shown to be retained intracellularly. Biochemical studies with short peptides corresponding to intracellular loop 4 support the direct involvement of this region in G protein coupling.[167] The carboxy terminus of the GPCRs also has been implicated in interactions with a plethora of other proteins that participate in the trafficking, targeting, and signaling of the receptor (see later).[168]

REGULATION OF RECEPTOR–G PROTEIN COUPLING BY RNA EDITING

It has been demonstrated that the messenger RNA (mRNA) for serotonin 5-HT$_{2C}$ receptor is posttranscriptionally modified.[169] The mRNA sequences encoding adenosine are converted to inosines by the action of dsRNA adenosine deaminases. This editing generates multiple receptor isoforms, some of which have been found to differ in their signaling properties. It has been demonstrated that in rat brain, at least seven 5-HT$_{2C}$ receptor isoforms show distinct anatomic distributions.[169] In human brain, 14 different 5-HT$_{2C}$ receptor isoforms involving editing of the second intracellular loop have been reported.[170]

The generation of different 5-HT$_{2C}$ receptor isoforms in several brain regions may control specific cellular responses. In this regard, both receptor–G protein coupling[171,172] and receptor activation of effectors[173,174] have been reported to differ for edited 5-HT$_{2C}$ receptor isoforms. Moreover, the conformation of the 5-HT$_{2C}$ receptor isoforms studied by computer structural approaches suggests that the edited second intracellular loops would differ structurally.[175] RNA editing also has been found to regulate 5-HT$_{2C}$ receptor transactivation of the small G protein RhoA.[176] 5-HT$_{2C}$ receptor isoforms also differ in their desensitization and trafficking.[177]

EFFECT OF POSTTRANSLATIONAL MODIFICATIONS ON RECEPTOR–G PROTEIN–COUPLING SELECTIVITY

The selectivity of receptor–G protein coupling has been shown to be regulated by receptor phosphorylation.[33,178] Activation of the β$_2$-adrenoceptor stimulates an increase of intracellular cAMP via activation of G$_s$ proteins, as well as activation of protein kinase A (PKA) and stimulation of MAPK through a pathway involving G$_i$ proteins. Studies with mutant β$_2$-adrenoceptors lacking PKA phosphorylation sites have shown that receptor-mediated activation of G$_i$ proteins is dependent on the phosphorylation of the β$_2$-adrenoceptor by PKA.[179] As receptor phosphorylation by PKA decreases the coupling efficiency of the β$_2$-adrenoceptor to G$_s$ proteins, phosphorylation represents a switch mechanism for regulating G protein–coupling selectivity.

As we discussed earlier, many GPCRs have a conserved cysteine residue in their carboxy terminus that may be covalently modified by palmitic acid.[76,77] Some receptors, such as endothelin receptor, have been shown to regulate G protein–coupling selectivity by this palmitoylation (see earlier).

REGULATORS OF G PROTEIN–SIGNALING PROTEINS

The rate of inactivation of G proteins by intrinsic GTP hydrolysis is augmented by regulator of G protein–signaling (RGS) proteins.[180–182] RGS proteins are a family of highly diverse proteins that share a conserved 120-amino acid domain (RGS domain). The RGS domain binds directly to the activated G$_α$-GTP subunits and acts as a GAP. Thus, RGS proteins accelerate GTP hydrolysis, attenuating or modulating hormone and neurotransmitter receptor-mediated responses (Fig. 11-4).

More than 20 different RGSs have been described in mammals; they can be grouped into five subfamilies (RZ, R4, R7, R12, and RA) based on sequence similarities (Table 11-3).[181] Several G protein effectors and regulators such as G protein–coupled receptor kinase (GRK), PLC-β, RhoGEF, or cyclic guanosine monophosphate (cGMP) phosphodiesterase also display GAP activity and have domains distantly related to the RGS domain (see Table 11-3). The globular and mostly helical structure of the RGS domain has been solved by x-ray crystallography in the RGS4-G$_{αi1}$ complex.[183]

RGS proteins also have been implicated in the modulation of adenylate cyclase, MAPK, IP$_3$/Ca^{2+} signaling, K$^+$ conductance, and visual signaling.[184] Larger RGS domain–containing

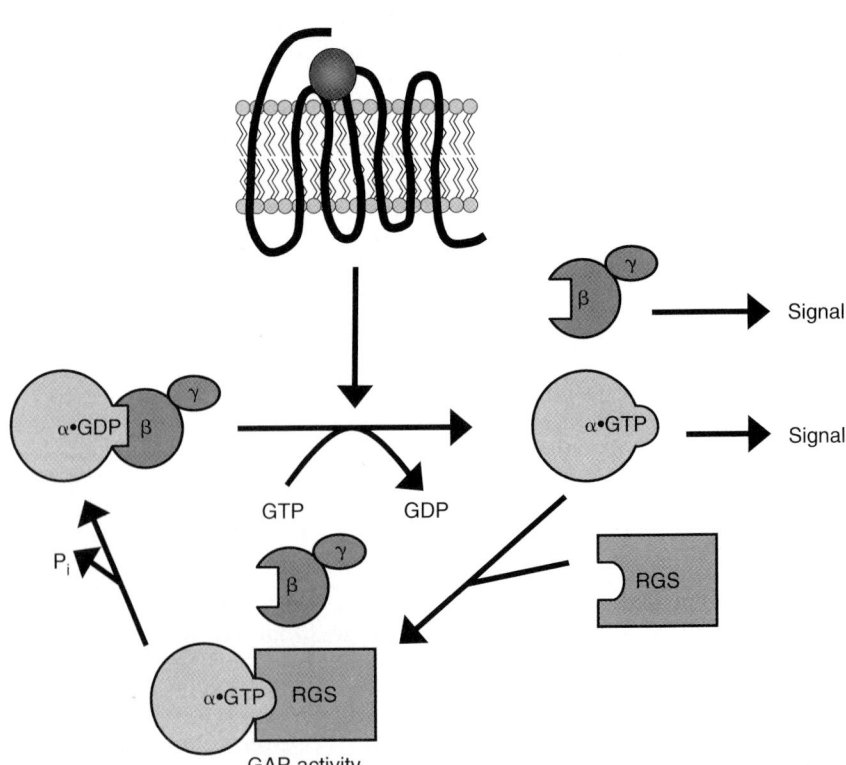

Figure 11-4 Schematic illustrating the role of regulator of G protein–signaling (RGS) proteins in accelerating the guanosine triphosphatase (GTPase) activity and inactivation of active G$_α$ subunits. GAP, GTPase-activating protein.

Table 11-3 Classification and Characteristics of Regulators of G Protein Signaling (RGS) proteins

Family	RGS	G_α Class Targeted by RGS	% Amino Acid Identity
RZ subfamily	RGS19 (GAIP)	G_i, G_q	—
	RGS17 (RGS-Z2)	G_i, (G_z)	81%
	RGS20 (RGS-Z1)	G_i, (G_z)	85%
R4 subfamily	RGS4	G_i, G_q	—
	RGS1	G_i, G_q	66%
	RGS2 (G0S8)	G_q > G_i	68%
	RGS3	G_i, G_q	76%
	RGS5	G_i, G_q	73%
	RGS8	G_i	76%
	RGS13	ND	62%
	RGS16	G_i, G_q	68%
	RGS18	G_i, G_q	65%
R7 subfamily	RGS9	G_i	—
	RGS6	G_i (G_o)	57%
	RGS7	G_i (G_o > G_{i2} > G_{i1})	59%
	RGS11	G_i (G_o)	72%
R12 subfamily	RGS12	G_i	—
	RGS10	G_i	67%
	RGS14	G_i	74%
RA subfamily	Axin	ND	—
	Axil	ND	73%
GEF subfamily	P115-RhoGEF	G_{12}	—
	PDZ-RhoGEF	G_{12}	47%
	LARG	G_{12}	58%
GRK subfamily	GRK2	G_q	—
	GRK1	ND	41%
	GRK3	ND	83%
	GRK4	ND	42%
	GRK5	ND	42%
	GRK6	ND	38%
	GRK7	ND	29%
SNX subfamily	SNX13 (RGS-PX1)	G_s	—
	SNX14	ND	38%
	SNX25	ND	43%
D-AKAP2	D-AKAP2	ND	—

proteins have additional domains that are likely to contribute to cellular functions in addition to attenuating G protein activation.[180] For example, the guanine-nucleotide-exchange factor for the monomeric small G protein RhoA (RhoGEF) induces the GTP for GDP interchange in the small G protein and contains an RGS domain. When RhoGEF binds the receptor-activated $G_{\alpha13}$, the GEF activity of RhoGEF increases, leading to RhoA activation and the modulation of several downstream effectors.[185]

Most of the RGS proteins are predicted to be cytosolic and are recruited to the plasma membrane by activated G_α subunits.[186] RGS proteins are widely expressed, and many tissues express multiple RGS proteins. Mechanisms identified that contribute to the selectivity of RGS proteins for specific GPCR signaling pathways are their cell-type expression and intracellular localization,[187] the timing of their expression, and the presence of other domains outside of the RGS domain that interact with other signaling proteins.[181,182] The central, specific, and diverse signaling effects of RGS proteins make them important potential targets for drug development.[188]

ACTIVATORS OF G PROTEIN SIGNALING

The activation of heterotrimeric G proteins in the absence of involvement of a typical heptahelical GPCR has been described. Three activators of G protein signaling (AGS) proteins have been identified by using a functional screen based on the pheromone response pathway in *Saccaromyces cerevisiae*.[189] AGS proteins could provide novel mechanisms for input to G protein–signaling pathways.[189–191]

G PROTEIN–COUPLED RECEPTORS SIGNALING NETWORKS

In the classic model of GPCR signaling, receptor activation induces dissociation of heterotrimeric G proteins into α and βγ subunits. These subunits sequentially activate effector molecules, including second-messenger systems, such as adenylate cyclases[118] or phospholipases,[119] and ion channels.[120] These linear pathways lead to the modulation of various well-characterized cellular responses (see Table 11-2, Fig. 11-3).[121–123] However, the number of identified effectors is considerably smaller than the large number of GPCRs. Because most of the cells express multiple types of GPCRs that signal through a relatively limited number of effectors, it is not surprising that the signal processing involves cross-regulation among the different signaling pathways. Moreover, the discovery of new GPCR-activated heterotrimeric G protein–independent signaling pathways demonstrates that the classic paradigm of linear G protein–signaling pathways represents only part of a more complex receptor-regulated signaling system.

MULTIPLE G PROTEIN COUPLING

Although specific GPCRs preferentially activate one class of G protein (see Table 11-1), many individual receptors have the potential to couple to several G protein classes.[20] One of the first examples of promiscuous GPCR coupling with G proteins was the finding that the α_2-adrenoceptor can activate or suppress adenylate cyclase activity through G_s or $G_{i/o}$ depending on the level of agonist concentration.[192] Studies using specific antibodies against different G_α subunits have shown examples of receptor that interact largely with G proteins from one class,[193,194] as well as receptors that interact with more than one type of G protein.[195–197] Promiscuous coupling also has been found by using receptor–G protein fusion proteins, in which a given G_α subunit is fused to the carboxy terminus of the receptor.[198] The TRH receptor shows a remarkable degree of coupling diversity, being able to activate all four major classes of G proteins.[157] Many studies showing promiscuous receptor coupling have been performed in recombinant expression systems. Notably, the receptor–G protein–coupling profile can vary between different cell lines[199] and may depend on the level of receptor expression.[200] Moreover, the relative stoichiometry of receptor, G proteins, and intracellular effectors in recombinant expression systems may not represent the cell in which the receptor is normally found.[201] Indeed, modifying the stoichiometry of the components within the receptor–G protein complex has been shown to alter the potency and the efficacy of agonists eliciting cellular responses.[202,203] These observations raise the question of whether promiscuity in receptor–G protein coupling is a physiologic property of GPCRs or a biochemical artifact. However, some studies have reported promiscuous GPCRs in experimental systems in which the receptor is constitutively expressed.[157,197]

Thus, although receptor promiscuity at the G protein level remains controversial,[20,204] several lines of evidence support the view that for many subtypes of GPCRs, simultaneous functional coupling with distinct unrelated G proteins can occur, providing a cellular mechanism for modulation of multiple signaling pathways by a single receptor.

AGONIST-SPECIFIC TRAFFICKING OF RECEPTOR SIGNALING

The concept of "signaling-selective agonism" or "agonist trafficking of receptor signals" proposes that different drugs acting at the same receptor may differentially activate the distinct transduction pathways coupled to that receptor.[104,205,206] According to the extended ternary complex for

GPCR activation (see earlier), agonists achieve their physiologic effects by complexing with the receptors and altering the relative distribution of the inactive (R) and active (R*) conformers.[102] Therefore, it was generally proposed that the receptor exist in two different conformations, active and inactive,[207] that differ in their ability to activate G proteins. This pharmacologic model is sufficient to explain the physiologic properties of agonists, partial agonists, inverse agonists, and antagonists.[102]

However, the demonstration that a single receptor subtype may activate different G proteins[208] led to the proposal that multiple active conformational states of the receptor may exist.[209] In this three-state or multistate model, distinct active conformations of the receptor are involved in the activation of distinct G proteins. Recent studies have confirmed that GPCRs assume distributions among multiple active and inactive conformers,[44,210] and these multiple active conformational states of the receptor have been shown differentially to bind distinct receptor agonists.[211,212] According to these findings, agonists could stabilize distinct activated receptor conformations that preferentially activate specific signaling pathways. Supporting evidence for agonist trafficking of receptor signals has been obtained in both in vitro experiments with heterologous receptor expression[20,213–215] and murine models in vivo.[215] Interestingly, G protein–independent pathways (see later) also have been reported to be differentially activated by distinct agonists activating dopamine D_2 receptors.[214] Agonist trafficking of receptor signals also has been found in nature. Thus, the glycosylated and nonglycosylated varieties of FSH have been found to activate differentially the effector enzymes coupled to the FSH receptor.[216]

The pharmacologic concept of agonist trafficking of receptor signals and the identification of clinical drugs that show signal trafficking[214] suggest that new drugs can be rationally designed specifically to activate particular signaling pathways.[206] Therefore, if some drugs induce unwanted side effects by activation of several signaling pathways coupled to a particular receptor subtype, these side effects could potentially be reduced by developing drugs that direct signaling preferentially toward the desired pathways.

MEMBRANE MICRODOMAINS AND G PROTEIN–COUPLED RECEPTOR SIGNALING

Many of the mathematical approaches to study the cellular and physiologic responses elicited by GPCR activation assume random collisions between proteins that diffuse freely in the plasma membrane. However, numerous observations have reported that different GPCRs coupling to the same G protein in a single cell can activate different cellular responses.[217] The classic random mixing model cannot readily account for these observations. Stoichiometric analysis of the overall cellular expression of components of signal-transduction pathways may be an overly simplistic approach, because such analysis fails to account for the compartmentation of molecules in cells.[203,218] Therefore, the compartmentalization of receptor and effector molecules in specialized microdomains of the plasma membrane is an important determinant of receptor signaling.[217,219–221]

Caveolae are microdomains of the plasma membrane enriched in specific proteins (caveolins) and lipids (cholesterol, sphingolipids).[222] Several GPCRs have been localized in caveolae or caveolin-rich cellular fractions together with many signaling proteins such as G proteins, adenylyl cyclase, protein kinase C, or MAPK.[217] The recruitment of GPCRs on agonist activation into caveolae may enhance efficient coupling of the receptor to more than one effector system[223,224] and enable a more rapid and specific transduction of the extracellular stimuli to the intracellular signaling molecules. An alternative effect is that the caveolae structure may hold signaling molecules in their inactive state until they are activated and translocate out of the microdomain.[225]

CROSS-TALK BETWEEN G PROTEIN–COUPLED RECEPTORS

Under physiologic conditions, stimulation of a particular GPCR subtype results in activation of signaling pathways that can modulate pathways activated by other GPCR subtypes.[121,208,226,227] GPCR signaling networks presumably play a role in fine-tuning the strength and duration of cellular responses. Activation of a GPCR can either amplify or inhibit the signaling pathway activated by another GPCR.[228] For example, activation of PLC by purinergic $P2Y_2$ receptors via G_q proteins specifically inhibits the cAMP synthesis stimulated by β-adrenoceptors via G_s proteins.[229] Cross-talk between G_s- and G_q-coupled receptors also has been described. Thus, besides the stimulation of inositol phosphates metabolism, G_q protein activation also can potentiate the G_s-mediated stimulation of adenylate cyclase activity. This potentiation may be mediated by PKC, as the $α_1$-adrenoceptor potentiation of the $β_2$-adrenoceptor stimulation of adenylate cyclase activity is blocked by PKC inhibitors.[230]

The signaling pathways activated by GPCRs, in addition to modulating other GPCR-signaling pathways, also affect the signaling of other structural classes of receptors. GPCR signaling may be modulated by receptor tyrosine kinase–mediated phosphorylation. Several GPCRs have conserved tyrosine residues that, when phosphorylated, are putative binding sites for a number of proteins such as Src, Shc, or Grb2, involved in receptor tyrosine kinase–signaling pathways. For example, the dopamine D_2 receptor agonist bromocriptine induces a robust protection against apoptosis induced by oxidative stress in PC12 cells through a signaling pathway involving Akt.[214] The dopamine D_2 receptor forms a signaling complex with the epidermal growth factor receptor and c-Src that is augmented by bromocriptine, suggesting cross-talk between the GPCR and the receptor tyrosine kinase in mediating the activation of Akt.[231] Receptor tyrosine kinases also have been reported to phosphorylate several GPCRs.[232,233] Epidermal growth factor receptors can be transactivated by stimulation of a number of GPCRs, including dopamine, GnRH, bradykinin, angiotensin, thrombin, lysophosphatidic acid (LPA), bombesin, endothelin, and muscarinic acetylcholine receptors.[227]

Stimulation of GPCRs also may result in cross-talk regulation of downstream signaling pathways.[227,228] For example, bombesin and vasopressin (acting at G_q-coupled receptors) have been shown to act synergistically with a number of growth factors to augment growth.[228]

G PROTEIN–COUPLED RECEPTOR–INTERACTING PROTEINS

A wide variety of proteins in addition to G proteins, GRKs, and arrestins have been found to interact directly with GPCRs.[26,27,168,234] Numerous proteins involved in cellular signaling contain protein-protein interacting domains that have been implicated in the specificity, selectivity, and time course of signaling.[27,234] These include Src homology 2 (SH2) and SH3, pleckstrin homology, postsynaptic density protein (PSD95), disc large-zona occludens (PDZ), and Ena/VASP (EVH) domains. The biologic functions of these GPCR-interacting proteins include targeting GPCRs to specific subcellular compartments, clustering receptors with specific effectors, and allosteric regulation of GPCRs.[26,27,168,234]

RECEPTOR ACTIVITY–MODIFYING PROTEINS

Receptor activity–modifying proteins (RAMPs) can modulate the expression or phenotype or both of some calcitonin-related GPCRs (see Table 11-1).[235,236] RAMP1 was discovered through attempts to clone the calcitonin gene-related peptide (CGRP) receptor. Human RAMP1 is a 148-amino acid protein with a large extracellular amino-terminal domain, a single predicted TM-spanning domain, and a short cytoplasmic domain.[237] Two related proteins, RAMP2 and RAMP3, have been identified. The interaction of specific RAMPs with GPCRs has been found to contribute to receptor trafficking to the membrane, alter receptor glycosylation, and modify a receptor's pharmacologic profile.

For the calcitonin receptor–like receptor (CRLR), coexpression with RAMPs is required for transport of the receptor to the plasma membrane. Unlike CRLR, the calcitonin (CT) receptor does not require a RAMP for cell-surface expression.[235] However, CT receptors, like CRLRs, cause the cell-surface translocation of RAMP1. In addition to inducing cell-surface translocation of the receptor, RAMP1 alters the terminal glycosylation of CRLR.[237] Coimmunoprecipitation studies using tagged protein demonstrate that RAMP1 directly complexes to both the immature and mature forms of CRLR, with RAMP remaining stably complexed with the mature form of CRLR at the cell surface. Neither RAMP2 nor RAMP3 changes the glycosylation pattern of CRLR, leading to speculation that the RAMP1-induced changes in CRLR glycosylation may be important in conferring the CGRP-receptor phenotype.

RAMPs may contribute to the structure of the ligand-binding pocket by direct cell-surface RAMP-receptor interaction.[236] The CRLR-RAMP complex is maintained during agonist-induced receptor internalization, with complexes targeted primarily to the lysosomal-degradation pathway rather than being recycled to the plasma membrane. Thus, RAMPs and receptors exist in stable cell-surface complexes that are maintained after agonist binding, suggesting that receptor-RAMP association is important for exhibition of altered receptor phenotype.

HOMER FAMILY PROTEINS

The so-called *Homer* is a protein family that contains an EHV1 domain. The EHV1 domain of Homer interacts with a proline-rich motif (PPXXFR) called the Homer ligand. This Homer ligand is present in the carboxy terminus of the group I metabotropic glutamate receptors (mGlu1 and mGlu5 receptors).[238] Homer 1a is an immediate-early gene protein upregulated in the hippocampus by seizure-induced neuronal activation, whereas all other genes encoding Homer proteins are constitutively expressed.[239] With the exception of Homer 1a, Homer proteins express a carboxy-terminal coiled-coil domain, allowing these proteins to form homo- and heterodimers.[239]

Homer proteins have been implicated in the trafficking of group I metabotropic glutamate receptors to the plasma membrane. Homer 1b retains these receptors in the endoplasmic reticulum, whereas Homer 1a is involved in the insertion of the mature receptor into the plasma membrane.[240] Once the metabotropic glutamate receptor is expressed at the cell surface, Homer 1a is not stably associated with the receptor. In contrast, Homer 1c interacts with group I metabotropic glutamate receptors at the plasma membrane. mGlu-Homer interactions have been proposed to regulate agonist-independent receptor activity.[241]

Homer proteins have been shown to interact with Shank,[242] a protein present in the N-methyl-D-aspartate (NMDA) glutamate receptor–associated postsynaptic density complex. This may contribute to synergism between metabotropic and NMDA glutamate receptors in modulating intracellular Ca^{2+} concentrations.[242]

Homer ligand is also present in the intracellular inositol 1,4,5-triphosphate receptors (IP_3R). Homer proteins have been reported to couple group I metabotropic glutamate receptors to endoplasmic reticulum–associated IP_3R by Homer protein dimers formed through the interaction of the coiled-coil domains.[243] Phosphoinositide 3 kinase enhancer (PIKE) is a GTPase that activates phosphoinositide 3 kinase (PI 3-kinase). It has been found that activation of group I metabotropic glutamate receptors induces the formation of receptor-Homer-PIKE complexes, leading to the activation of PI 3-kinase and preventing neuronal apoptosis.[244]

G PROTEIN–INDEPENDENT SIGNALING BY G PROTEIN–COUPLED RECEPTORS

Several cellular responses to activation of GPCRs are not mediated by G protein activation.[25,245,246] As described later, arrestins bind to phosphorylated GPCRs to induce receptor uncoupling from heterotrimeric G proteins. β-Arrestin also can function as an adaptor protein that associates the tyrosine kinase Src (through SH3-domain interactions) to the signaling protein complex of the $β_2$-adrenoceptor.[247] The recruitment of Src to the $β_2$-adrenoceptor leads to the activation of MAPK signaling cascade.[247] Thus, the agonist-activated receptor is phosphorylated by G protein–receptor kinases, leading to its interacting with arrestin and its uncoupling from G proteins. The receptor is then targeted to clathrin-coated pits, to which Src is recruited, leading to activation of the MAPK signaling pathway. Small G proteins in the ARF/Rho A family have been implicated in the activation of phospholipase D by several GPCRs.[248] The activation of parathyroid hormone receptor inhibits Na^+-H^+ exchange via an increase of cytoplasmic cAMP and activation of PKA. The Na^+-H^+ exchanger regulatory factor (NHERF) inhibits renal Na^+-H^+ exchangers (NHEs) in a PKA-dependent manner, leading to the inhibition of the ionic exchange. In contrast, agonist activation of $β_2$-adrenoceptor, which also induces cAMP-dependent PKA activation, activates Na^+-H^+ exchange. The molecular mechanism of this $β_2$-adrenoceptor signaling pathway is the presence in the C-terminal tail of the receptor of a PDZ consensus-binding site (Asp-Ser/Thr-Xxx-Leu), which directly binds the PDZ domain of NHERF.[249] Thus, NHERF colocalizes with activated $β_2$-adrenoceptors in the plasma membrane. When $β_2$-adrenoceptors are activated, the receptor competes with NHE for NHERF binding, alleviating the inhibition of NHE.[249]

The SH2 domain–containing adaptor protein Grb2 has been reported to associate with $β_2$-adrenoceptors after tyrosine phosphorylation.[250] The skeletal muscle 5-HT_{2A} serotonin receptors also have been found to activate a G protein–independent pathway. In response to serotonin, 5-HT_{2A} serotonin receptors induce the autophosphorylation of Jak2, followed by the tyrosine phosphorylation of STAT3 (signal transducers and activators of transcription). The receptor, Jak2, and STAT3 are physically associated.[251] Although G protein activation is a key event in GPCR signaling, GPCR signaling through mechanisms independent of classic heterotrimeric G proteins serves an important role in the signal transduction of these receptors.

G PROTEIN–COUPLED RECEPTOR DIMERIZATION

A range of approaches have provided evidence that GPCRs can exist both as homo- and heterodimer complexes,[28,234,252,253] or even form larger oligomers.[254] Studies have shown that GPCRs can form heterodimers not only with closely related receptor subtypes, but also with more distant GPCRs, and even members of other protein families. Thus, the formation of homo- and heterodimers has emerged as an important aspect of the functional modulation of several GPCRs types, such as adenosine,[255] dopamine,[256] muscarinic,[257] opioid,[258] and serotonin[259] receptors (Table 11-4).

EXPERIMENTAL APPROACHES TO STUDY RECEPTOR DIMERIZATION

Several approaches have been used to identify GPCR dimerization.[260] Pharmacologic methods provided the first evidence

Table 11-4 G Protein–Coupled Receptor Dimerization

Receptor	Constitutive or Ligand-Induced	Effects of Ligands
β_2-Adrenoceptor	Constitutive	Agonist increases dimerization
Dopamine D_2	Constitutive	No effect of agonist
mGlu5	Constitutive	Not tested
δ-Opioid	Constitutive	Agonist decreases dimerization
Calcium sensor	Constitutive	Not tested
Muscarinic M_3	Constitutive	No effect of agonist
$GABA_B$	Constitutive	No applicable
δ-, k-Opioid	Constitutive	Not tested
SST_5	Ligand-induced	Agonist increases dimerization
SST_2	Constitutive	Not tested
SST_3	Constitutive	Not tested
Adenosine A_1, dopamine D_1 heterodimer	Constitutive	Dopamine agonist decreases dimerization
δ-, μ-Opioid	Constitutive	Not tested
Angiotensin AT_1, bradykinin B_2 heterodimer	Constitutive	Not tested
δ-Opioid, β_2-adrenoceptor heterodimer	Constitutive	Agonist increases dimerization
β_2-adrenoceptor	Constitutive	Not tested
δ-Opioid	Constitutive	No effect of ligands
TRH	Constitutive	Agonist increases dimerization
GnRH	Ligand-induced	No basal dimerization. Agonist increases dimerization
SST_5, dopamine D_2 heterodimer	Ligand-induced	No basal dimerization. Agonist and antagonist increase dimerization
CCR5	Ligand-induced	No basal dimerization. Both antibody and agonist increase dimerization
CCR2	Ligand-induced	No basal dimerization. Both antibody and agonist increase dimerization
CXCR4	Ligand-induced	Agonist increases dimerization
mGlu1	Constitutive	Agonist induces change of conformation

for existence of physical interactions between receptors.[261] More recently, the homodimerization of the dopamine D_2 receptor has been reported by using radioligand-binding approaches.[262] Functional complementation of receptor chimeras also suggested that GPCRs might form functional dimers.[257]

Differential epitope tagging of the receptors followed by immunoprecipitation and Western blotting has been used to reveal interactions between two GPCR monomers. Thus coexpression of HA- and Myc-tagged β_2-adrenoceptors, HA immunoreactivity was detected in fractions immunoprecipitated with the anti-Myc antibody, suggesting intermolecular interactions between the two differentially tagged receptors.[263] Similar coimmunoprecipitation approaches have shown the existence of dimers for several GPCR subtypes, such as opioid receptors; V_2 vasopressin receptors; $mGlu_5$; CCR2 receptors; M_1, M_2, and M_3 muscarinic receptors; and histamine H_2 receptors.[252]

To investigate the existence of GPCR dimers in living cells, biophysical methods, such as fluorescence resonance energy transfer (FRET) and bioluminescence resonance energy transfer (BRET), have been used to assess protein-protein interactions.[264] BRET assays quantify the energy transfer from the light emitted by the catalytic degradation of colenterazine by luciferase (from *Renilla luciferans*) to the acceptor green fluorescent protein (GFP) from *Aequoera victoria*. Excitation of GFP is detectable only when donor and acceptor proteins are located within 50 Å of each other. Thus, cotransfection with both fusion constructs (GPCR-luciferase and GPCR-GFP) has shown homodimerization of the β_2-adrenoceptors,[265] TRH receptors, and δ-opioid receptors, and heterodimerization of δ-opioid receptors with β_2-adrenoceptors.[252] FRET between fluorescently conjugated antibodies detecting differentially epitope-tagged receptors has been used to detect homodimers of SST5-somatostatin[266] and δ-opioid receptors[267] in whole cells. The modification of the FRET technique, photobleaching FRET (pbFRET), measures the slowing of the photobleaching of

the donor by the presence of the acceptor.[266] This approach has demonstrated heterodimerization of dopamine D_2 and SST5 somatostatin receptors.[268]

CONSTITUTIVE AND LIGAND-INDUCED G PROTEIN–COUPLED RECEPTOR DIMERIZATION

Three patterns of receptor dimerization are observed (see Table 11-4): (1) dimers are detected under basal conditions that are unchanged by agonist; (2) dimers are detected under basal conditions, but agonists modulate their levels; and (3) dimerization requires the presence of agonist.[28] Thus, agonists have been found to increase (β_2-adrenoceptor homodimerization), decrease (dopamine D_1–adenosine A_1 receptor heterodimerization), or have no effect (κ-opioid and muscarinic M_3 receptor homodimerization)[253] on the levels of dimers (see Table 11-4). The heterodimerization of the dopamine D_2 and somatostatin SST_5 receptors was detected only in the presence of either somatostatin or dopamine.[268]

IMPLICATION OF DIMERIZATION IN RECEPTOR FUNCTION

The effect of dimerization on signal transduction is not certain for most GPCRs. Thus, although increasing evidence supports the hypothesis that receptor dimerization may be important for GPCR function,[253] whether dynamic regulation of dimers is involved in receptor activity is not resolved.[28,253] However, some examples support the role of GPCR dimerization in signal transduction, such as the $GABA_B$ receptor, which requires the heterodimerization of two nonfunctional GPCRs (GB1 and GB2) for the expression of functional $GABA_B$ receptors in the cell surface.[95]

GB1 was initially identified by expression cloning.[269] However, the agonist affinity for cloned GB1 receptors was significantly lower than that of native receptors. Furthermore, GB1 failed to produce a functional $GABA_B$ receptor at the cell surface.[270] An explanation for these findings was then provided by the discovery that the GABA$_B$ receptor exists as a heterodimer, with a companion protein (GB2) linked in a 1:1 stoichiometry to the GB1 through coiled-coil domains at C termini.[96–99] Coexpression of GB1 and GB2 proteins results in the functional expression of GABA$_B$ receptor in plasma membrane, exhibiting a pharmacologic profile equivalent to wild-type GABA$_B$ receptors in brain.[99,271,272] Thus, although the GB1 subunit has been implicated in ligand binding,[273–276] the GB2 terminus has been implicated in G protein coupling of the receptor.[277,278]

Additional evidence supporting the role of dimerization has been provided by reports showing that a peptide derived from the proposed dimerization interface of the β$_2$-adrenoceptor can inhibit both dimerization and receptor-stimulated adenylyl cyclase activity.[263] In this regard, the resolution of the crystal structure of rhodopsin[58] provides indirect information about GPCR dimerization. The size of the intracellular surface exposed to the cytoplasm is too small to account for the simultaneous interaction with both α and βγ subunits of the G proteins. Because it is well accepted that this simultaneous interaction is necessary for receptor functionality, this could suggest that a receptor dimer is required for the complete and productive interaction with a single G protein.[253]

STRUCTURE OF G PROTEIN–COUPLED RECEPTOR DIMERS

Although the high-resolution structure adopted by GPCR dimers is still not resolved, indirect approaches have provided three different mechanisms of interaction between the two GPCRs within the dimer: disulphide bond formation, carboxy-terminus coiled-coil interaction, and TM spans interaction.[253,279]

The recently solved structure of the amino terminus ligand-binding domain of the mGlu1 receptor provides the only available data on the three-dimensional structure of GPCR dimers.[94] The crystal structure presents a disulfide bridge connecting the two protomers. Similarly, disulfide bonding within the amino terminus domains of mGlu5 and the calcium-sensing receptor has been reported to be important for covalent dimerization. Cysteines located in the second and third extracellular loops of the M$_3$ muscarinic receptor also have been involved in the dimerization of this receptor subtype.[258] However, these disulfide bonds are not the only points of contact, and noncovalent interactions have been proposed.[253]

The involvement of noncovalent interactions between the TM domains was first proposed for the β$_2$-adrenoceptor.[263] Thus, glycine and leucine residues located within the sixth TM span have been suggested as part of the dimerization interface of this receptor.[263] Computational studies support the involvement of TM helices 5 and 6 in the dimerization interface, proposing two alternative three-dimensional models, the so-called *domain-swapped* and *contact-dimer* configurations, that could describe GPCR dimers.[279,280]

The coassembly of two nonfunctional GPCRs, GB1 and GB2, is required for the expression of functional GABA$_B$ receptors.[95] Yeast two-hybrid screens proposed coiled-coil domains within the carboxy terminus of GB1 and GB2 as a molecular mechanism for GABA$_B$ receptor heterodimerization.[99] The carboxy terminus of the δ-opioid receptor also has been implicated in receptor dimerization.[252]

MECHANISMS OF G PROTEIN–COUPLED RECEPTOR DESENSITIZATION

One component of homeostasis in endocrine systems is the rapid attenuation of many cellular responses with continuous receptor stimulation. Functional receptor desensitization has several molecular mechanisms, including the uncoupling of the receptor from heterotrimeric G proteins, endocytosis of cell-surface receptors, and reduced responsiveness of postreceptor signaling elements.[281–284] The time frames over which these processes occur range from seconds for receptor uncoupling, minutes for endocytosis, to hours for receptor degradation.

UNCOUPLING OF RECEPTORS FROM G PROTEINS

Many GPCRs are rapidly desensitized through phosphorylation by intracellular kinases. Two types of receptor uncoupling can be distinguished based on the molecular mechanism. Homologous receptor uncoupling is mediated by agonist-dependent activation of the same receptor, whereas heterologous receptor uncoupling is caused by activation of a different receptor type.[281] Homologous and heterologous receptor uncoupling are mediated by GRKs and second messenger–dependent protein kinases, respectively.

Both second messenger–dependent protein kinases (such as PKA or PKC) and GRKs phosphorylate serine and threonine residues within the intracellular loops and carboxy-terminus domains of GPCRs. GRKs recognize the active receptor conformation and therefore selectively phosphorylate agonist-activated receptors. Receptor phosphorylation by GRKs promotes the binding of arrestins, which sterically uncouple the receptor from G proteins. The phosphorylation of GPCRs by second messenger–dependent protein kinases do not depend on the activation state of the receptor.

Second messenger–dependent protein kinases are activated by the signal transduction–mediated increases in the intracellular concentration of second messengers, such as cAMP and diacylglycerol, and catalyze the phosphorylation of downstream signaling proteins. These kinases also phosphorylate GPCRs as a feedback regulatory mechanism that contributes to receptor uncoupling. For example, PKC activation leads to the phosphorylation and desensitization of many G$_i$- and G$_q$-coupled receptors.[285,286] Notably, the activation of at least one receptor, the GABA$_B$ receptor, is enhanced by PKA phosphorylation.[287] As described earlier, receptor phosphorylation by PKA also has been implicated in the regulation of the G protein–coupling specificity.[178]

Seven GRKs that vary in size from 62 to 80 kilodaltons have been identified (Table 11-5).[288–290] The seven members of the GRK family show homologous structures with an amino terminus containing an RGS-like domain implicated in the recognition of the receptor, a central catalytic domain, and a carboxy-terminus domain involved in the targeting of the kinase to the plasma membrane. According to sequence and functional homology, the GRK family can be subdivided into three different groups: GRK1 (rhodopsin kinase) and GRK7; GRK2 (formerly β-adrenoceptor kinase 1, βARK1) and GRK3 (formerly β-adrenoceptor kinase 2, βARK2); and GRK4, GRK5, and GRK6. GRK1 is expressed almost exclusively in the eye. GRK2 and GRK3 are widely distributed and phosphorylate a wide range of GPCRs. In studies using genetically modified mice,[291,292] it has been reported that eliminating expression of GRK2 leads to embryonic lethality. Eliminating GRK3 impairs odorant-receptor desensitization, and eliminating GRK5 reduces muscarinic-receptor desensitization. Eliminating GRK6 enhancing the responses to dopaminergic psychostimulants. The expression of GRK4 is limited to the testis, whereas GRK7 is expressed in the eye and may specifically regulate cone opsins.[291]

In unstimulated cells, GRK1-3 are located in the cytoplasm and directed to bind their substrates in response to agonist activation of the GPCRs. The light-induced translocation of GRK1 to the plasma membrane is facilitated by the posttranslational farnesylation of its carboxy terminus. GRK2 and GRK3 are not farnesylated, and the translocation of these kinases to the plasma membrane is regulated by their association with G$_{βγ}$ subunits.[289] This association between GRK2 and GRK3 and the βγ subunits of the heterotrimeric G proteins is

Table 11-5 G Protein–Coupled Receptor Kinases (GRKs)

Subtype	Alternative Name	Membrane Association	Tissue Distribution	Features/Regulation
GRK1	Rhodopsin kinase	Farnesylation	Retina	Autophosphorylation
GRK2	βARK1	$G_{\beta\gamma}$, Acidic phospholipid	Ubiquitous	Pleckstrin homology domain, PKC, calmodulin
GRK3	βARK2	$G_{\beta\gamma}$, Acidic phospholipid	Ubiquitous	Pleckstrin homology domain
GRK4	IT-11	Palmitoylation	Testis	Four splice variants
GRK5		Phospholipid binding	Ubiquitous	Autophosphorylation, PKC, calmodulin
GRK6		Palmitoylation	Ubiquitous	Calmodulin
GRK7		Geranylgeranylation	Retina	

PKC, phosphokinase C.

mediated by a 125-amino acid $\beta\gamma$ subunit–binding domain located in the carboxy terminus of the kinase. The targeting of GRK2 and GRK3 to the plasma membrane has been reported to be modulated by the binding of phosphatidylinositol 4,5-bisphosphate to the carboxy terminus of the kinases. Moreover, the kinase activity of GRK2 toward GPCRs has been shown to be decreased by MAPK and increased by PKC or c-Src phosphorylation of the kinase, respectively.[282]

In the absence of agonist activation of GPCRs, GRK4, GRK5, and GRK6 are preferentially located at the plasma membrane. Both GRK4 and GRK6 are palmitoylated at cysteine residues,[293] which most likely is responsible for their plasma membrane localization and increases the kinase activity of GRK6 for β_2-adrenoceptors.[293] The association of GRK5 with the plasma membrane has been proposed to be mediated by electrostatic interactions between a basic amino acid domain within the carboxy terminus of the kinase and plasma membrane phospholipids.[294] The activity of GRK5 is modulated by PKC, Ca^{2+}-calmodulin, and/or phospholipid metabolism.[289]

Several GPCRs have been shown to be phosphorylated by GRKs after agonist activation, including rhodopsin; β_2-adrenergic; M_1, M_2, and M_3 muscarinic cholinergic; α_2-adrenergic; angiotensin$_{1A}$; substance P; prostaglandin E_1; somatostatin; and olfactory receptors.[289,290] Although GRKs are able to phosphorylate multiple receptors in vitro, specificities of the kinases for different GPCR substrates have been observed.[290,295] GRKs phosphorylate GPCRs at serine and threonine residues located within either the third intracellular loop or the carboxy-terminus domains. Although some amino acid sequences (such as Glu/Asp-Xxx-Ser) were initially identified as phosphorylation consensus sites for GRK1-3,[281] and the localization of acidic amino acids proximal to the phosphorylation site seems to favor GRK2-mediated phosphorylation,[296] no general GRK phosphorylation consensus motifs have yet been identified.[282]

The phosphorylation of either rhodopsin or the β_2-adrenoceptor by GRKs was not sufficient for inactivation. An additional component or "arresting agent" was required. The first arrestin was identified in retinal rods.[297] Four members of the arrestin gene family have been identified.[291,292,298] Two arrestins, visual arrestin and cone arrestin, are expressed almost exclusively in the retina and regulate rhodopsin function. The β-arrestins, β-arrestin 1 and β-arrestin 2, are widely expressed proteins with the highest levels of expression in the brain and spleen.[298]

Phosphorylation of GPCRs by GRKs promotes the binding of arrestins to the receptor, which sterically interferes with G protein coupling.[291] Therefore, arrestins play a critical role in homologous receptor desensitization. Arrestins preferentially bind to agonist-activated and GRK-phosphorylated GPCRs rather than to second messenger–dependent protein kinase–phosphorylated or –nonphosphorylated receptors.[282]

Mutagenesis studies[282] and the high-resolution three-dimensional crystal structure of arrestin[299] revealed that visual arrestin has two major domains, an amino-terminus domain and a carboxy-terminus domain, that each form seven-stranded β sandwich structures. The amino-terminus domain contains the receptor activation–recognition region. A secondary receptor-binding region is located within the carboxy-terminus domain. A phosphate sensor region is located in the linker between the two major domains.[298]

The physiological importance of β arrestins is indicated from experiments performed in β-arrestin null mutant mice, which have exaggerated responses to β-adrenoceptor agonists. Homozygous β-arrestin 2 null mutant animals show a dramatic potentiation and prolongation of the analgesic effects induced by morphine, suggesting impaired μ-opioid receptor desensitization.[300]

Binding of arrestins to phosphorylated receptors induces GPCR uncoupling from G proteins and facilitates agonist-promoted endocytosis of many GPCRs. However, arrestins have been recently reported to function as signaling adapters or intermediates that recruit other key molecules to the GPCR signaling complex.[247] These scaffolding properties of arrestins were discussed earlier.

ENDOCYTOSIS AND INTERNALIZATION OF G PROTEIN–COUPLED RECEPTORS

Several mechanisms influence the cellular distribution of GPCRs.[281,282,284] De novo synthesized receptors reach the plasma membrane from the Golgi complex. In unstimulated cells, the rate of receptor endocytosis from the cell surface into endosomes is relatively slow. In the presence of an agonist, this endocytic rate is dramatically increased. Once the GPCRs have been internalized, they can either be recycled back to the plasma membrane or directed to lysosomes for degradation (Fig. 11-5). Therefore, the loss of receptor number at the cell surface is determined by the relative rates of endocytosis and recycling.[284] Long-term exposure to the agonist (hours or days) may cause receptor downregulation, a loss in the total receptor number due to agonist-induced endocytosis, and subsequent degradation.

The generation and expression of fusion proteins containing modified forms of the GFP have provided insight into the kinetics and regulation of protein distribution and trafficking in intact living cells.[301] Ligand-induced GPCR endocytosis has been monitored in real time after expression of forms of GPCRs with GFP attached to their C-terminal tails.[302,303]

A role of GRK-mediated phosphorylation and β-arrestin binding in facilitating GPCR endocytosis has been found for several receptors.[282] However, some examples have been reported in which GRK-mediated phosphorylation is not absolutely necessary for receptor endocytosis.[304] The predominant pathway for agonist-induced receptor endocytosis is through clathrin-coated pits.[305] Clathrin is a major component of coated vesicles that are implicated in protein transport. The heavy and light chains of clathrin form a triskelion, the main structural element of clathrin coats (see Fig. 11-5). β-Arrestins act as adaptors that link the receptors to the clathrin-coated pits. Both β-arrestin 1 and β-arrestin 2 directly interact with at least two components of the endocytic

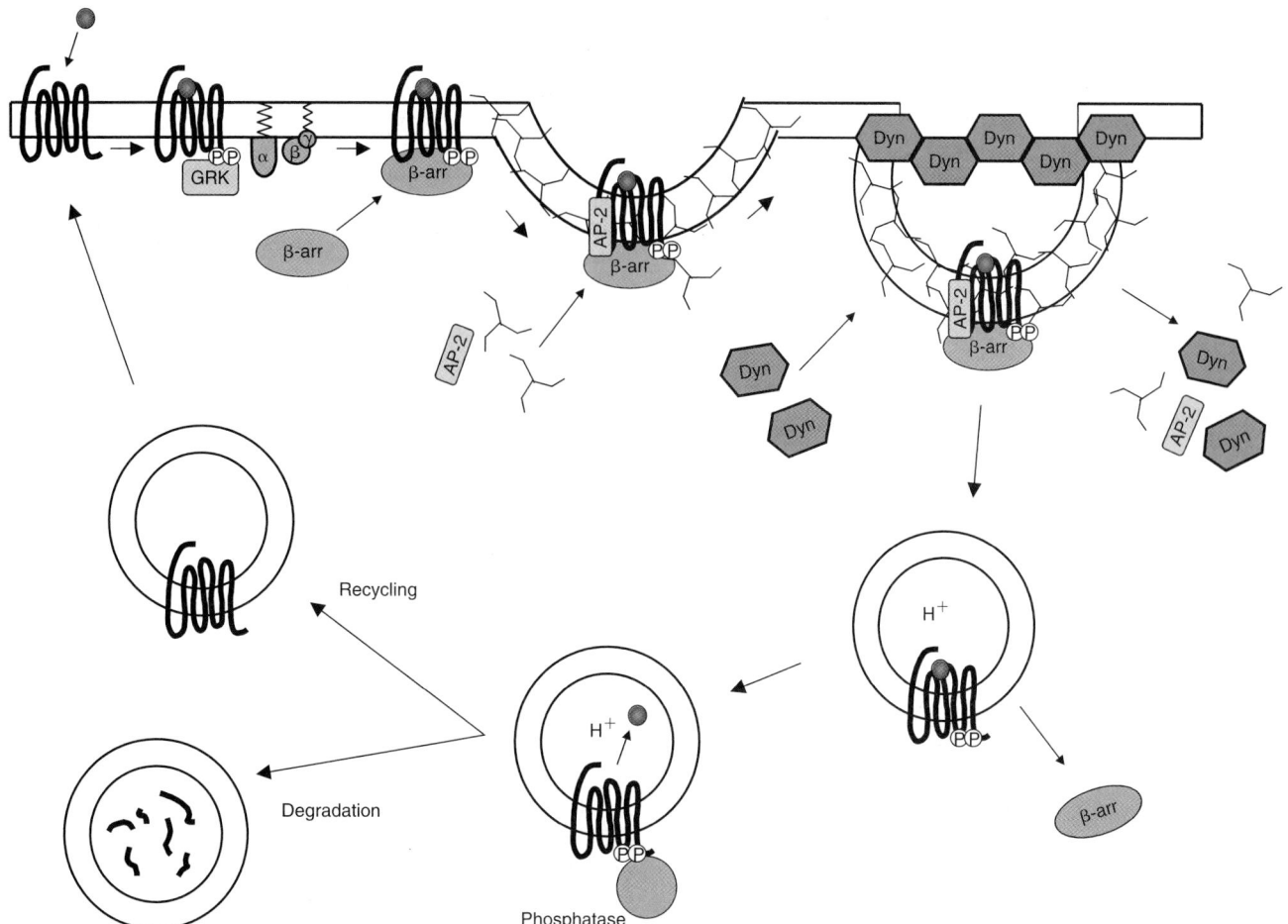

Figure 11-5 G protein–coupled receptor endocytosis. After endocytosis in clathrin-coated vesicles, the receptors are either recycled back to the plasma membrane or degraded.

machinery, clathrin and the β_2-adaptin subunit of the adaptor protein (AP)-2 complex. The AP-2 complex is a heterotetrameric complex formed by subunits called *adaptins*.[291] The formation of this endocytic protein complex leads to endocytosis of the receptors to acidic endosomes, where they are either dephosphorylated and recycled to the plasma membrane or degraded in lysosomes. The clathrin-coated vesicles are pinched off from the plasma membrane by the large GTPase dynamin (see Fig. 11-5).[306] Although endocytosis through clathrin-coated pits has been reported for many different GCPR subtypes,[282] a caveolin-dependent mechanism, which is independent of both clathrin and β-arrestin, also has been described.[307]

The rhodopsin-like (subclass I) and the glucagon-like (subclass II) receptors have different endocytic patterns. Subclass I GPCRs, such as the β_2-adrenoceptor, preferentially internalize through a β-arrestin 2 mechanism. The receptor-β-arrestin interaction is transient for this GPCR subclass, and β-arrestin does not colocalize with the receptor in the endosome. Conversely, subclass II GPCRs, such as the angiotensin AT_{1A} receptor, internalize either through β-arrestin 1 or β-arrestin 2. The receptor-β-arrestin interaction is stabler, and receptor and β-arrestin colocalize in the endosome.[308]

Individual drugs may differ in their effects on the regulation of a particular GPCR subtype. In this regard, it has been reported that the highly addictive opioid drug morphine does not induce desensitization or endocytosis of μ-opioid receptors, whereas the opioid peptide D-Ala2, *N*-McPhe4, Gly5-ol]enkephalin (DAMGO) promotes the rapid desensitization and endocytosis of μ-opioid receptors.[309] The absence of μ-opioid receptor desensitization at the level of G protein

coupling also has been reported in postmortem human brains of opioid addicts.[310] Therefore, the deficiency of certain opioid drugs to induce receptor desensitization and endocytosis has been related to the mechanisms of tolerance and addiction, suggesting a role for receptor endocytosis in the mechanisms of opioid drug action and addiction.[309,311]

GPCR internalization was originally considered to be a primary mechanism of receptor desensitization. Thus, by depleting the plasma membrane of receptors that are available to interact with hormones or neurotransmitters, GPCR endocytosis and internalization may contribute to desensitization. However, it has been reported that pharmacologic agents that block GPCR internalization do not alter the desensitization profile of β_2-adrenoceptors[312] or muscarinic receptors.[313] Moreover, it has been observed that internalization plays a role in the resensitization of GPCR responsiveness.[313,314] The mechanisms involved in resensitization of the sequestered receptor include dissociation of the ligand in acidified endosomes, dephosphorylation of the receptor, dissociation of arrestins, and recycling of the receptor to the plasma membrane. A specific GPCR-associated sorting protein (GASP) that binds to the carboxy terminus of δ-opioid receptors has been implicated in the lysosomal sorting and functional downregulation of GPCRs.[315]

DOWNREGULATION OF G PROTEIN–COUPLED RECEPTORS

Receptor downregulation is characterized by a decrease in the total receptor number in the cell due to endocytosis and subsequent degradation of the receptors caused by long-term exposure to agonists (see Fig. 11-5). Several efficient mechanisms exist in vivo to remove hormones and neuro-transmitters from the extracellular fluid, such as transporters or degrading enzymes.[281] Therefore, it is probably rare that a cell is continuously exposed to agonists under physiologic conditions. However, long-term agonist exposure may occur under pathologic circumstances such as uncontrolled secretion of hormones from tumors. Downregulation also is an important cellular mechanism during prolonged administration of therapeutic drugs. Although the molecular mechanisms of receptor downregulation are not completely understood, both enhanced receptor degradation and reduced synthesis have been implicated.

G PROTEIN–COUPLED RECEPTOR UBIQUITINATION

Protein ubiquitination was originally identified as a process implicated in degradation by the proteasome. However, it has been found that the ubiquitination of several activated cell-surface receptors induces internalization, followed by receptor degradation in lysosomes.[316] For the GPCRs, ubiquitination has been reported for rhodopsin,[317] opioid receptors,[318] β_2-adrenergic receptors,[319] and V$_2$ vasopressin receptors.[320]

The proteasome is formed by a central cylinder with multiple distinct protease domains and by two large protein complexes bound to the bases of the central cylinder, which are implicated in the recognition and regulation of substrates. Proteasomes act on proteins that have been marked by the covalent attachment of ubiquitin by the sequential action of three enzymes.[316] Thus, the glycine residue located at the C terminus of ubiquitin is activated by the formation of a thioester bond with an ubiquitin-activated enzyme (E1). Activated ubiquitin is then transferred to the ubiquitin-carrying enzyme (E2). The final step is performed by an ubiquitin protein ligase (E3), which links the C terminal of ubiquitin to a lysine of the substrate protein.

Ubiquitination of β_2-adrenergic receptors has been implicated in their internalization and degradation.[319] It has been reported that the ubiquitination of the β_2-adrenergic receptor requires its agonist-dependent phosphorylation, followed by interaction with β-arrestin 2. β-Arrestin acts as an adapter protein to bring an E3 ligase to the activated receptor. The Mdm2 protein functions as a ligase to ubiquitinate β-arrestin after agonist stimulation. The ubiquitination of β-arrestin catalyzed by Mdm2 contributes to β_2-adrenergic receptor internalization. Thus, receptor internalization is inhibited in Mdm2-null cells. β-Arrestin also is processed by ubiquitination, although the kinetics of its processing is more rapid than that of the receptor.[319]

G PROTEIN–COUPLED RECEPTOR SIGNALING AND DISEASE

Altered GPCR signaling contributes to the pathophysiology of many diseases.[321–325] Among the 100 most commonly prescribed medications, one fourth act at GPCRs.[326] The alterations causing abnormal signal transduction may originate at the different levels in the signal-transduction process. Thus, reduced or increased level of expression of the receptor, impaired activation, and alterations in the desensitization processes have implicated in several human diseases. In addition, a large number of endocrine diseases and diseases of other systems are caused by hereditary or acquired mutations of G proteins and GPCRs that modulate GPCR signaling.

PROLONGATION OR INACTIVATION OF G PROTEIN–COUPLED RECEPTOR SIGNALING

As described earlier, after activation by a GPCR, G protein signaling is terminated by intrinsic G_α GTP hydrolysis (see

Fig. 11-3). Several diseases are caused by alterations in this process, causing excessive or prolonged G protein signaling.

Cholera is produced by *Vibrio cholerae* infection, producing intestinal excretion of water and salts. The cholera toxin generated by *V. cholerae* causes adenosine diphosphate (ADP)-ribosylation of an arginine located in the nucleotide-binding pocket of the $G_{\alpha s}$ subunit blocking the GTP hydrolyzation. This covalent modification causes prolonged G protein activation, resulting in high levels of cAMP in the mucous intestinal cells and secretory diarrhea. A similar toxin produced by certain strains of *Escherichia coli* causes travelers' diarrhea.

The first $G_{\alpha s}$ oncogenic mutation was described in pituitary tumors in patients with acromegaly. This *gsp* (G stimulatory protein) oncogene results in $G_{\alpha s}$ subunits with a mutation in the same arginine that is the target of choleric toxin. The *gsp* mutation leads to prolonged activation of adenylate cyclase and excessive production and release of growth hormone.[327] G protein *gsp* mutations also have been found in McCune-Albright syndrome, leading to autonomous hyperfunctioning of several endocrine systems. The mutations in McCune-Albright syndrome originate in early development, leading to a mosaic pattern of expression and diverse symptoms.[328]

Pseudohypoparathyroidism types I and Ib and congenital night blindness can result from mutations causing inactivation of specific G proteins. Pseudohypoparathyroidism type I results from an inactivating mutation in one allele of $G_{\alpha s}$, resulting in reduced responsiveness to parathyroid hormone. Whooping cough is caused by *Bordetella pertussis* infection in the tracheobronchial tree. The pertussis toxin induces an ADP-ribosylation of the $G_{\alpha i/o}$ in a cysteine residue located in the GPCR coupling region that interferes with signaling from the receptor to G protein.[129] Pseudohypoparathyroidism type Ia results from a mutation of arginine 231 of $G_{\alpha s}$, a different target from that of cholera toxin.

A single temperature-sensitive mutation at position 366 in $G_{\alpha s}$ contributes simultaneously to two diseases.[324] At normal body temperature, the mutation decreases the activity of $G_{\alpha s}$, causing pseudohypoparathyroidism type Ia. However, in the testes, which are cooler, this mutation causes a receptor-independent increased activity leading to testotoxicosis.

G PROTEIN–COUPLED RECEPTOR MUTATIONS

Loss-of-function mutations are usually inherited as recessive genetic traits. Color blindness was the first disorder shown to be caused by a defective GPCR. Opsins are activated by light of a particular spectral bandwidth and couple to cone transducin (G_t), which modulates cGMP phosphodiesterase activity. A variety of mutations in cone opsin genes that include point mutations and deletions have been found to cause color blindness. In X-linked nephrogenic diabetes insipidus, numerous different loss-of-function mutations in the V$_2$ vasopressin receptor have been found that cause renal resistance to the antidiuretic action of the hormone. One missense mutation in a residue in the second intracellular loop creates a receptor that binds vasopressin normally but is incapable of stimulating G_s. In familial glucocorticoid deficiency caused by adrenocorticotropic hormone (ACTH) resistance, point mutations that disrupt function of the ACTH receptor also have been found. Mutations in the Ca^{2+} receptors have been identified in familial hypocalciuric hypercalcemia.

Several naturally occurring mutations have been identified that cause diseases by resulting in receptors that signal constitutively, in the absence of agonist. A mutation of Lys296 that leads to constitutive activation of rhodopsin is one cause of autosomal-dominant retinitis pigmentosa. Hyperfunctioning thyroid adenomas have been found to contain activating mutations in the thyrotropin receptor. An activating mutation of the FSH receptor has been found to sustain spermatogenesis after hypophysectomy.[329] Familial male precocious puberty can be caused by a single activating mutation in TM6 of the luteinizing hormone receptor that results in spontaneous receptor activity.[330]

A mutation in the high-affinity binding site of the thyrotropin-stimulating hormone receptor has been identified as a cause of familial gestational hyperthyroidism.[331] The altered receptor can be activated by chorionic gonadotropin as well as its native agonist, thyrotropin-stimulating hormone.

Elevated levels of chorionic gonadotropin during pregnancy lead to unregulated activation of the thyrotropin-stimulating hormone receptor, resulting in clinical hyperthyroidism occurring only during pregnancy.

Acknowledgment

We thank the National Institutes of Health for grant support of our studies of GnRH receptor structure and signaling.

REFERENCES

1. Erhlich P: Chemotheraputics: Scientific principles, methods and results. Lancet 2:445–451, 1913.
2. Langley JN: On the contraction of muscle, chiefly in relation to the presence of "receptive" substances. J Physiol 39:235–295, 1909.
3. Dale HH: The action of certain esters and ethers of choline and their relation to muscarine. J Pharmacol Exp Ther 6:147–190, 1914.
4. Neubig RR, Thomsen WJ: How does a key fit a flexible lock? Structure and dynamics in receptor function. Bioessays 11:136–141, 1989.
5. IUPHAR 1998: The IUPHAR Compendium of Receptor Characterization and Classification, 1st ed. London, IUPHAR Media, 1988.
6. Pierce KL, Premont RT, Lefkowitz RJ: Seven-transmembrane receptors. Nat Rev Mol Cell Biol 3:639–650, 2002.
7. Strader CD, Fong TM, Graziano MP, et al: The family of G-protein-coupled receptors. FASEB J 9:745–754, 1995.
8. Lefkowitz RJ: The superfamily of heptahelical receptors. Nat Cell Biol 2:E133–E136, 2000.
9. Ubarretxena-Belandia I, Engelman DM: Helical membrane proteins: Diversity of functions in the context of simple architecture. Curr Opin Struct Biol 11:370–376, 2001.
10. Devreotes PN: G protein-linked signaling pathways control the developmental program of *Dictyostelium*. Neuron 12:235–241, 1994.
11. Dohlman HG, Thorner J, Caron MG, et al: Model systems for the study of seven-transmembrane-segment receptors. Annu Rev Biochem 60:653–688, 1991.
12. Plakidou-Dymock S, Dymock D, Hooley R: A higher plant seven-transmembrane receptor that influences sensitivity to cytokinins. Curr Biol 8:315–324, 1998.
13. Vernier P, Cardinaud B, Valdenaire O, et al: An evolutionary view of drug-receptor interaction: The bioamine receptor family. Trends Pharmacol Sci 16:375–381, 1995.
14. New DC, Wong JT: The evidence for G-protein-coupled receptors and heterotrimeric G proteins in protozoa and ancestral metazoa. Biol Signals Recept 7:98–108, 1998.
15. Lanyi JK, Luecke H: Bacteriorhodopsin. Curr Opin Struct Biol 11:415–419, 2001.
16. Ovchinnikov Yu A: Rhodopsin and bacteriorhodopsin: Structure-function relationships. FEBS Lett 148:179–191, 1982.
17. Lander ES, Linton LM, Birren B, et al: Initial sequencing and analysis of the human genome. Nature 409:860–921, 2001.
18. Venter JC, Adams MD, Myers EW, et al: The sequence of the human genome. Science 291:1304–1351, 2001.
19. Bockaert J, Pin JP: Molecular tinkering of G protein-coupled receptors: An evolutionary success. EMBO J 18:1723–1729, 1999.
20. Hermans E: Biochemical and pharmacological control of the multiplicity of coupling at G-protein-coupled receptors. Pharmacol Ther 99:25–44, 2003.
21. Hamm HE: The many faces of G protein signaling. J Biol Chem 273:669–672, 1998.
22. Bourne HR: How receptors talk to trimeric G proteins. Curr Opin Cell Biol 9:134–142, 1997.
23. Gether U: Uncovering molecular mechanisms involved in activation of G protein-coupled receptors. Endocr Rev 21:90–113, 2000.
24. Gilman AG: G proteins: Transducers of receptor-generated signals. Annu Rev Biochem 56:615–649, 1987.
25. Brzostowski JA, Kimmel AR: Signaling at zero G: G-protein-indepenent functions for 7-TM receptor. Trends Biochem Sci 26:291–297, 2001.
26. Brady AE, Limbird LE: G protein-coupled receptor interacting proteins: Emerging roles in localization and signal transduction. Cell Signal 14:297–309, 2002.
27. Kreienkamp HJ: Organisation of G-protein-coupled receptor signalling complexes by scaffolding proteins. Curr Opin Pharmacol 2:581–586, 2002.
28. Angers S, Salahpour A, Bouvier M: Dimerization: an emerging concept for G protein-coupled receptor ontogeny and function. Annu Rev Pharmacol Toxicol 42:409–435, 2002.
29. Nathans J, Hogness DS: Isolation, sequence analysis, and intron-exon arrangement of the gene encoding bovine rhodopsin. Cell 34:807–814, 1983.
30. Dixon RA, Kobilka BK, Strader DJ, et al: Cloning of the gene and cDNA for mammalian beta-adrenergic receptor and homology with rhodopsin. Nature 321:75–79, 1986.
31. Horn F, Weare J, Beukers MW, et al: GPCRDB: an information system for G protein-coupled receptors. Nucleic Acids Res 26:275–279, 1998.
32. Probst WC, Snyder LA, Schuster DI, et al: Sequence alignment of the G-protein coupled receptor superfamily. DNA Cell Biol 11:1–20, 1992.
33. Wess J: Molecular basis of receptor/G-protein-coupling selectivity. Pharmacol Ther 80:231–264, 1998.
34. IUPHAR: IUPHAR Receptor Database. www.iuphar.org
35. Humphrey PP, Barnard EA: International Union of Pharmacology. XIX: The IUPHAR receptor code: A proposal for an alphanumeric classification system. Pharmacol Rev 50:271–277, 1998.
36. Lee DK, George SR, Evans JF, et al: Orphan G protein-coupled receptors in the CNS. Curr Opin Pharmacol 1:31–39, 2001.
37. Fredriksson R, Lagerstrom MC, Lundin LG, et al: The G-protein-coupled receptors in the human genome form five main families: Phylogenetic analysis, paralogon groups, and fingerprints. Mol Pharmacol 63:1256–1272, 2003.
38. Karasinska JM, George SR, O'Dowd BF: Family 1 G protein-coupled receptor function in the CNS: Insights from gene knockout mice. Brain Res Rev 41:125–152, 2003.
39. Giros B, Sokoloff P, Martres MP, et al: Alternative splicing directs the expression of two D2 dopamine receptor isoforms. Nature 342:923–926, 1989.
40. Usiello A, Baik JH, Rouge-Pont F, et al: Distinct functions of the two isoforms of dopamine D2 receptors. Nature 408:199–203, 2000.
41. Baldwin JM: Structure and function of receptors coupled to G proteins. Curr Opin Cell Biol 6:180–190, 1994.
42. Parnot C, Miserey-Lenkei S, Bardin S, et al: Lessons from constitutively active mutants of G protein-coupled receptors. Trends Endocrinol Metab 13:336–343, 2002.
43. Kitanovic S, Yuen T, Flanagan CA, et al: Insertional mutagenesis of the arginine cage domain of the gonadotropin-releasing hormone receptor. Mol Endocrinol 15:390–397, 2001.
44. Prioleau C, Visiers I, Ebersole BJ, et al: Conserved helix 7 tyrosine acts as a multistate conformational switch in the 5HT2C receptor: Identification of a novel "locked-on" phenotype and double revertant mutations. J Biol Chem 277:36577–36584, 2002.
45. Mayo KE, Miller LJ, Bataille D, et al: International Union of Pharmacology XXXV: The glucagon receptor family. Pharmacol Rev 55:167–194, 2003.

46. Ulrich CD 2nd, Holtmann M, Miller LJ: Secretin and vasoactive intestinal peptide receptors: Members of a unique family of G protein-coupled receptors. Gastroenterology 114:382–397, 1998.

47. Laburthe M, Couvineau A, Gaudin P, et al: Receptors for VIP, PACAP, secretin, GRF, glucagon, GLP-1, and other members of their new family of G protein-linked receptors: Structure-function relationship with special reference to the human VIP-1 receptor. Ann N Y Acad Sci 805:94–109; discussion 110–111, 1996.

48. Conn PJ, Pin JP: Pharmacology and functions of metabotropic glutamate receptors. Annu Rev Pharmacol Toxicol 37:205–237, 1997.

49. Brown EM, Gamba G, Riccardi D, et al: Cloning and characterization of an extracellular Ca(2+)-sensing receptor from bovine parathyroid. Nature 366:575–580, 1993.

50. Bowery NG, Bettler B, Froestl W, et al: International Union of Pharmacology. XXXIII: Mammalian gamma-aminobutyric acid(B) receptors: structure and function. Pharmacol Rev 54:247–264, 2002.

51. Herrada G, Dulac C: A novel family of putative pheromone receptors in mammals with a topographically organized and sexually dimorphic distribution. Cell 90:763–773, 1997.

52. Hoon MA, Adler E, Lindemeier J, et al: Putative mammalian taste receptors: A class of taste-specific GPCRs with distinct topographic selectivity. Cell 96:541–551, 1999.

53. Strader CD, Fong TM, Tota MR, et al: Structure and function of G protein-coupled receptors. Annu Rev Biochem 63:101–132, 1994.

54. Schwartz T, Gether U, Schambye H, et al: Molecular mechanism of action of non-peptide ligands for peptide receptors. Curr Pharm Design 1:325–342, 1995.

55. Baldwin JM, Schertler GF, Unger VM: An alpha-carbon template for the transmembrane helices in the rhodopsin family of G-protein-coupled receptors. J Mol Biol 272:144–164, 1997.

56. Ballesteros JA, Weinstein H: Integrated methods for the construction of three-dimensional models and computational probing of structure-function relations in G protein coupled receptors. Methods Neurosci 25:366–428,1995.

57. Ji TH, Grossmann M, Ji I: G protein-coupled receptors, I: Diversity of receptor-ligand interactions. J Biol Chem 273:17299–17302, 1998.

58. Palczewski K, Kumasaka T, Hori T, et al: Crystal structure of rhodopsin: A G protein-coupled receptor. Science 289:739–745, 2000.

59. Menon ST, Han M, Sakmar TP: Rhodopsin: Structural basis of molecular physiology. Physiol Rev 81:1659–1688, 2001.

60. Filipek S, Teller DC, Palczewski K, et al: The crystallographic model of rhodopsin and its use in studies of other G protein-coupled receptors. Annu Rev Biophys Biomol Struct 32:375–397, 2003.

61. Ovchinnikov Yu A, Abdulaev NG, Bogachuk AS: Two adjacent cysteine residues in the C-terminal cytoplasmic fragment of bovine rhodopsin are palmitoylated. FEBS Lett 230:1–5, 1988.

62. Sealfon SC, Weinstein H, Millar RP: Molecular mechanisms of ligand interaction with the gonadotropin-releasing hormone receptor. Endocr Rev 18:180–205, 1997.

63. Sealfon SC, Olanow CW: Dopamine receptors: From structure to behavior. Trends Neurosci 23:S34–S40, 2000.

64. Altenbach C, Yang K, Farrens DL, et al: Structural features and light-dependent changes in the cytoplasmic interhelical E-F loop region of rhodopsin: A site-directed spin-labeling study. Biochemistry 35:12470–12478, 1996.

65. Farahbakhsh ZT, Ridge KD, Khorana HG, et al: Mapping light-dependent structural changes in the cytoplasmic loop connecting helices C and D in rhodopsin: A site-directed spin labeling study. Biochemistry 34:8812–8819, 1995.

66. Klein-Seetharaman J, Hwa J, Cai K, et al: Single-cysteine substitution mutants at amino acid positions 55-75, the sequence connecting the cytoplasmic ends of helices I and II in rhodopsin: Reactivity of the sulfhydryl groups and their derivatives identifies a tertiary structure that changes upon light-activation. Biochemistry 38:7938–7944, 1999.

67. Konig B, Arendt A, McDowell JH, et al: Three cytoplasmic loops of rhodopsin interact with transducin. Proc Natl Acad Sci U S A 86:6878–6882, 1989.

68. Jung H, Windhaber R, Palm D, et al: Conformation of a beta-adrenoceptor-derived signal transducing peptide as inferred by circular dichroism and 1H NMR spectroscopy. Biochemistry 35:6399–6405, 1996.

69. Odagaki Y, Nishi N, Koyama T: Receptor-mediated and receptor-independent activation of G-proteins in rat brain membranes. Life Sci 62:1537–1541, 1998.

70. Doi T, Molday RS, Khorana HG: Role of the intradiscal domain in rhodopsin assembly and function. Proc Natl Acad Sci U S A 87:4991–4995, 1990.

71. Ballesteros JA, Shi L, Javitch JA: Structural mimicry in G protein-coupled receptors: implications of the high-resolution structure of rhodopsin for structure-function analysis of rhodopsin-like receptors. Mol Pharmacol 60:1–19, 2001.

72. Lu ZL, Saldanha JW, Hulme EC: Seven-transmembrane receptors: crystals clarify. Trends Pharmacol Sci 23:140–146, 2002.

73. Wheatley M, Hawtin SR: Glycosylation of G-protein-coupled receptors for hormones central to normal reproductive functioning: Its occurrence and role. Hum Reprod Update 5:356–364, 1999.

74. Libert F, Parmentier M, Lefort A, et al: Selective amplification and cloning of four new members of the G protein-coupled receptor family. Science 244:569–572, 1989.

75. Kornfeld R, Kornfeld S: Assembly of asparagine-linked oligosaccharides. Annu Rev Biochem 54:631–664, 1985.

76. Bouvier M, Chidiac P, Hebert TE, et al: Dynamic palmitoylation of G-protein-coupled receptors in eukaryotic cells. Methods Enzymol 250:300–314, 1995.

77. Ross EM: Protein modification: Palmitoylation in G-protein signaling pathways. Curr Biol 5:107–109, 1995.

78. Dunphy JT, Linder ME: Signalling functions of protein palmitoylation. Biochim Biophys Acta 1436:245–261, 1998.

79. Loisel TP, Ansanay H, Adam L, et al: Activation of the beta(2)-adrenergic receptor-Galpha(s) complex leads to rapid depalmitoylation and inhibition of repalmitoylation of both the receptor and Galpha(s). J Biol Chem 274:31014–31019, 1999.

80. Jin H, Xie Z, George SR, et al: Palmitoylation occurs at cysteine 347 and cysteine 351 of the dopamine D(1) receptor. Eur J Pharmacol 386:305–312, 1999.

81. Hawtin SR, Tobin AB, Patel S, et al: Palmitoylation of the vasopressin V1a receptor reveals different conformational requirements for signaling, agonist-induced receptor phosphorylation, and sequestration. J Biol Chem 276:38139–38146, 2001.

82. Chen C, Shahabi V, Xu W, et al: Palmitoylation of the rat mu opioid receptor. FEBS Lett 441:148–152, 1998.

83. Cramer H, Schmenger K, Heinrich K, et al: Coupling of endothelin receptors to the ERK/MAP kinase pathway: Roles of palmitoylation and G(alpha)q. Eur J Biochem 268:5449–5459, 2001.

84. Sakmar TP: Structure of rhodopsin and the superfamily of seven-helical receptors: The same and not the same. Curr Opin Cell Biol 14:189–195, 2002.

85. Meng EC, Bourne HR: Receptor activation: What does the rhodopsin structure tell us? Trends Pharmacol Sci 22:587–593, 2001.

86. Shi L, Javitch JA: The binding site of aminergic G protein-coupled receptors: The transmembrane segments and second extracellular loop. Annu Rev Pharmacol Toxicol 42:437–467, 2002.

87. Almaula N, Ebersole BJ, Zhang D, et al: Mapping the binding site pocket of the serotonin 5-hydroxytryptamine2A receptor: Ser3.36(159) provides a second interaction site for the protonated amine of serotonin but not of lysergic acid diethylamide or bufotenin. J Biol Chem 271:14672–14675, 1996.

88. Ebersole BJ, Visiers I, Weinstein H, et al: Molecular basis of partial agonism: Orientation of indoleamine ligands in the binding pocket of the human serotonin 5-HT2A receptor determines relative efficacy. Mol Pharmacol 63:36–43, 2003.

89. Suryanarayana S, Daunt DA, Von Zastrow M, et al: A point mutation in the seventh hydrophobic domain of the alpha 2 adrenergic receptor increases its affinity for a family of beta receptor antagonists. J Biol Chem 266:15488–15492, 1991.

90. Oksenberg D, Marsters SA, O'Dowd BF, et al: A single amino-acid difference confers major pharmacological variation between human and rodent 5-HT1B receptors. Nature 360:161–163, 1992.

91. Stroop SD, Nakamuta H, Kuestner RE, et al: Determinants for calcitonin analog interaction with the calcitonin receptor N-terminus and transmembrane-loop regions. Endocrinology 137:4752–4756, 1996.

92. Vollenweider FX, Vollenweider-Scherpenhuyzen MF, Babler A, et al: Psilocybin induces schizophrenia-like psychosis in humans via a serotonin-2 agonist action. Neuroreport 9:3897–3902, 1998.

93. Nanevicz T, Wang L, Chen M, et al: Thrombin receptor activating mutations: Alteration of an extracellular agonist recognition domain causes constitutive signaling. J Biol Chem 271:702–706, 1996.

94. Kunishima N, Shimada Y, Tsuji Y, et al: Structural basis of glutamate recognition by a dimeric metabotropic glutamate receptor. Nature 407:971–977, 2000.

95. Bowery NG, Enna SJ: gamma-aminobutyric acid(B) receptors: First of the functional metabotropic heterodimers. J Pharmacol Exp Ther 292:2–7, 2000.

96. Jones KA, Borowsky B, Tamm JA, et al: GABA(B) receptors function as a heteromeric assembly of the subunits GABA(B)R1 and GABA(B)R2. Nature 396:674–679, 1998.

97. Kaupmann K, Malitschek B, Schuler V, et al: GABA(B)-receptor subtypes assemble into functional heteromeric complexes. Nature 396:683–687, 1998.

98. Kuner R, Kohr G, Grunewald S, et al: Role of heteromer formation in GABAB receptor function. Science 283:74–77, 1999.

99. White JH, Wise A, Main MJ, et al: Heterodimerization is required for the formation of a functional GABA(B) receptor. Nature 396:679–682, 1998.

100. De Lean A, Stadel JM, Lefkowitz RJ: A ternary complex model explains the agonist-specific binding properties of the adenylate cyclase-coupled beta-adrenergic receptor. J Biol Chem 255:7108–7117, 1980.

101. Samama P, Cotecchia S, Costa T, et al: A mutation-induced activated state of the beta 2-adrenergic receptor: Extending the ternary complex model. J Biol Chem 268:4625–4636, 1993.

102. Lefkowitz RJ, Cotecchia S, Samama P, et al: Constitutive activity of receptors coupled to guanine nucleotide regulatory proteins. Trends Pharmacol Sci 14:303–307, 1993.

103. Kenakin T: Drug efficacy at G protein-coupled receptors. Annu Rev Pharmacol Toxicol 42:349–379, 2002.

104. Kenakin T: Agonist-receptor efficacy, II: Agonist trafficking of receptor signals. Trends Pharmacol Sci 16:232–238, 1995.

105. Weiss JM, Morgan PH, Lutz MW, et al: The cubic ternary complex receptor-occupancy model, III: Resurrecting efficacy. J Theor Biol 181:381–397, 1996.

106. Strange PG: Mechanisms of inverse agonism at G-protein-coupled receptors. Trends Pharmacol Sci 23:89–95, 2002.

107. de Ligt RA, Kourounakis AP, Ijzerman AP: Inverse agonism at G protein-coupled receptors: (Patho)physiological relevance and implications for drug discovery. Br J Pharmacol 130:1–12, 2000.

108. Gether U, Kobilka BK: G protein-coupled receptors, II: Mechanism of agonist activation. J Biol Chem 273:17979–17982, 1998.

109. Decaillot FM, Befort K, Filliol D, et al: Opioid receptor random mutagenesis reveals a mechanism for G protein-coupled receptor activation. Nat Struct Biol 10:629–636, 2003.

110. Gether U, Ballesteros JA, Seifert R, et al: Structural instability of a constitutively active G protein-coupled receptor: Agonist-independent activation due to conformational flexibility. J Biol Chem 272:2587–2590, 1997.

111. Okada T, Palczewski K: Crystal structure of rhodopsin: Implications for vision and beyond. Curr Opin Struct Biol 11:420–426, 2001.

112. Gether U, Lin S, Ghanouni P, et al: Agonists induce conformational changes in transmembrane domains III and VI of the beta2 adrenoceptor. EMBO J 16:6737–6747, 1997.

113. Befort K, Zilliox C, Filliol D, et al: Constitutive activation of the delta opioid receptor by mutations in transmembrane domains III and VII. J Biol Chem 274:18574–18581, 1999.

114. Porter JE, Perez DM: Characteristics for a salt-bridge switch mutation of the alpha(1b) adrenergic receptor: Altered pharmacology and rescue of constitutive activity. J Biol Chem 274:34535–34538, 1999.

115. Lin SW, Sakmar TP: Specific tryptophan UV-absorbance changes are probes of the transition of rhodopsin to its active state. Biochemistry 35:11149–11159, 1996.

116. Ballesteros J, Kitanovic S, Guarnieri F, et al: Functional microdomains in G-protein-coupled receptors: The conserved arginine-cage motif in the gonadotropin-releasing hormone receptor. J Biol Chem 273:10445–10453, 1998.

117. Birnbaumer L, Abramowitz J, Brown AM: Receptor-effector coupling by G proteins. Biochim Biophys Acta 1031:163–224, 1990.

118. Hanoune J, Defer N: Regulation and role of adenylyl cyclase isoforms. Annu Rev Pharmacol Toxicol 41:145–174, 2001.

119. James SR, Downes CP: Structural and mechanistic features of phospholipases C: Effectors of inositol phospholipid-mediated signal transduction. Cell Signal 9:329–336, 1997.

120. Dascal N: Ion-channel regulation by G proteins. Trends Endocrinol Metab 12:391–398, 2001.

121. Neves SR, Ram PT, Iyengar R: G protein pathways. Science 296:1636–1639, 2002.

122. Gomperts BD: Signal Transduction. Academic Press, San Diego, 2002.

123. Siegel GJ: Basic Neurochemistry. Philadelphia, Lippincott Williams & Wilkins, 1999.

124. Rodbell M, Krans HM, Pohl SL, et al: The glucagon-sensitive adenyl cyclase system in plasma membranes of rat liver, IV: Effects of guanylnucleotides on binding of 125I-glucagon. J Biol Chem 246:1872–1876, 1971.

125. Lin MC, Nicosia S, Lad PM, et al: Effects of GTP on binding of (3H) glucagon to receptors in rat hepatic plasma membranes. J Biol Chem 252:2790–2792, 1977.

126. Maguire ME, Van Arsdale PM, Gilman AG: An agonist-specific effect of guanine nucleotides on binding to the beta adrenergic receptor. Mol Pharmacol 12:335–339, 1976.

127. Northup JK, Sternweis PC, Smigel MD, et al: Purification of the regulatory component of adenylate cyclase. Proc Natl Acad Sci U S A 77:6516–6520, 1980.

128. Bourne HR, Sanders DA, McCormick F: The GTPase superfamily: Conserved structure and molecular mechanism. Nature 349:117–127, 1991.

129. Sprang SR: G protein mechanisms: Insights from structural analysis. Annu Rev Biochem 66:639–678, 1997.

130. Macara IG, Lounsbury KM, Richards SA, et al: The Ras superfamily of GTPases. FASEB J 10:625–630, 1996.

131. Wedegaertner PB, Wilson PT, Bourne HR: Lipid modifications of trimeric G proteins. J Biol Chem 270:503–506, 1995.

132. Kaziro Y, Itoh H, Kozasa T, et al: Structure and function of signal-transducing GTP-binding proteins. Annu Rev Biochem 60:349–400, 1991.

133. Simon IM, Strathmann MP, Gautam N: Diversity of G proteins in signal transduction. Science 252:802–808, 1991.

134. Neer EJ: Heterotrimeric G proteins: Organizers of transmembrane signals. Cell 80:249–257, 1995.

135. Neer EJ: G proteins: Critical control points for transmembrane signals. Protein Sci 3:3–14, 1994.

136. Hepler JR, Gilman AG: G proteins. Trends Biochem Sci 17:383–387, 1992.

137. Clapham DE, Neer EJ: G protein beta gamma subunits. Annu Rev Pharmacol Toxicol 37:167–203, 1997.

138. Cali JJ, Balcueva EA, Rybalkin I, et al: Selective tissue distribution of G protein gamma subunits, including a new form of the gamma subunits identified by cDNA cloning. J Biol Chem 267:24023–24027, 1992.

139. Dippel E, Kalkbrenner F, Wittig B, et al: A heterotrimeric G protein complex couples the muscarinic m1 receptor to phospholipase C-beta. Proc Natl Acad Sci U S A 93:1391–1396, 1996.

140. Wall MA, Coleman DE, Lee E, et al: The structure of the G protein heterotrimer Gi alpha 1 beta 1 gamma 2. Cell 83:1047–1058, 1995.

141. Lambright DG, Sondek J, Bohm A, et al: The 2.0 A crystal structure of a heterotrimeric G protein. Nature 379:311–319, 1996.

142. Noel JP, Hamm HE, Sigler PB: The 2.2 A crystal structure of transducin-alpha complexed with GTP gamma S. Nature 366:654–663, 1993.

143. Markby DW, Onrust R, Bourne HR: Separate GTP binding and GTPase activating domains of a G alpha subunit. Science 262:1895–1901, 1993.

144. Mixon MB, Lee E, Coleman DE, et al: Tertiary and quaternary structural changes in Gi alpha 1 induced by GTP hydrolysis. Science 270:954–960, 1995.

145. Sprang SR: G proteins, effectors and GAPs: Structure and mechanism. Curr Opin Struct Biol 7:849–856, 1997.

146. Sondek J, Bohm A, Lambright DG, et al: Crystal structure of a G-protein beta gamma dimer at 2.1A resolution. Nature 379:369–374, 1996.

147. Murzin AG: Structural principles for the propeller assembly of beta-sheets: The preference for seven-fold symmetry. Proteins 14:191–201, 1992.

148. Neer EJ, Schmidt CJ, Nambudripad R, et al: The ancient regulatory-protein family of WD-repeat proteins. Nature 371:297–300, 1994.

149. Birnbaumer L: G proteins in signal transduction. Annu Rev Pharmacol Toxicol 30:675–705, 1990.

150. Taylor CW: The role of G proteins in transmembrane signalling. Biochem J 272:1–13, 1990.

151. Clapham DE: The G-protein nanomachine. Nature 379:297–299, 1996.

152. Linder ME, Ewald DA, Miller RJ, et al: Purification and characterization of Go alpha and three types of Gi alpha after expression in Escherichia coli. J Biol Chem 265:8243–8251, 1990.

153. Carty DJ, Padrell E, Codina J, et al: Distinct guanine nucleotide binding and release properties of the three Gi proteins. J Biol Chem 265:6268–6273, 1990.

154. Logothetis DE, Kurachi Y, Galper J, et al: The beta gamma subunits of GTP-binding proteins activate the muscarinic K+ channel in heart. Nature 325:321–326, 1987.

155. Filipek S, Stenkamp RE, Teller DC, et al: G protein-coupled receptor rhodopsin: A prospectus. Annu Rev Physiol 65:851–879, 2003.

156. Neubig RR: Specificity of receptor-G protein coupling: Protein structure and cellular determinants. Semin Neurosci 9:189–197, 1998.

157. Laugwitz KL, Allgeier A, Offermanns S, et al: The human thyrotropin receptor: A heptahelical receptor capable of stimulating members of all four G protein families. Proc Natl Acad Sci U S A 93:116–120, 1996.

158. Wong SK, Ross EM: Chimeric muscarinic cholinergic:beta-adrenergic receptors that are functionally promiscuous among G proteins. J Biol Chem 269:18968–18976, 1994.

159. Strader CD, Sigal IS, Dixon RA: Structural basis of beta-adrenergic receptor function. FASEB J 3:1825–1832, 1989.

160. Takagi Y, Ninomiya H, Sakamoto A, et al: Structural basis of G protein specificity of human endothelin receptors: A study with endothelinA/B chimeras. J Biol Chem 270:10072–10078, 1995.

161. Zhu SZ, Wang SZ, Hu J, et al: An arginine residue conserved in most G protein-coupled receptors is essential for the function of the m1 muscarinic receptor. Mol Pharmacol 45:517–523, 1994.

162. Jones PG, Curtis CA, Hulme EC: The function of a highly-conserved arginine residue in activation of the muscarinic M1 receptor. Eur J Pharmacol 288:251–257, 1995.

163. Prossnitz ER, Schreiber RE, Bokoch GM, et al: Binding of low affinity N-formyl peptide receptors to G protein: Characterization of a novel inactive receptor intermediate. J Biol Chem 270:10686–10694, 1995.

164. Ernst OP, Hofmann KP, Sakmar TP: Characterization of rhodopsin mutants that bind transducin but fail to induce GTP nucleotide uptake: Classification of mutant pigments by fluorescence, nucleotide release, and flash-induced light-scattering assays. J Biol Chem 270:10580–10586, 1995.

165. Acharya S, Karnik SS: Modulation of GDP release from transducin by the conserved Glu134-Arg135 sequence in rhodopsin. J Biol Chem 271:25406–25411, 1996.

166. Wenkert D, Schoneberg T, Merendino JJ Jr, et al: Functional characterization of five V2 vasopressin receptor gene mutations. Mol Cell Endocrinol 124:43–50, 1996.

167. Merkouris M, Dragatsis I, Megaritis G, et al: Identification of the critical domains of the delta-opioid receptor involved in G protein coupling using site-specific synthetic peptides. Mol Pharmacol 50:985–993, 1996.

168. Bockaert J, Marin P, Dumuis A, et al: The "magic tail" of G protein-coupled receptors: An anchorage for functional protein networks. FEBS Lett 546:65–72, 2003.

169. Burns CM, Chu H, Rueter SM, et al: Regulation of serotonin-2C receptor G-protein coupling by RNA editing. Nature 387:303–308, 1997.

170. Fitzgerald LW, Iyer G, Conklin DS, et al: Messenger RNA editing of the human serotonin 5-HT(2C) receptor. Neuropsychopharmacology 21(Suppl)1:S82–S90, 1999.

171. Wang Q, O'Brien PJ, Chen CX, et al: Altered G protein-coupling functions of RNA editing isoform and splicing variant serotonin2C receptors. J Neurochem 74:1290–1300, 2000.

172. Price RD, Weiner DM, Chang MS, et al: RNA editing of the human serotonin 5-HT2C receptor alters receptor-mediated activation of G13 protein. J Biol Chem 276:44663–44668, 2001.

173. Berg KA, Cropper JD, Niswender CM, et al: RNA-editing of the 5-HT(2C) receptor alters agonist-receptor-effector coupling specificity. Br J Pharmacol 134:386–392, 2001.

174. Price RD, Sanders-Bush E: RNA editing of the human serotonin 5-HT(2C) receptor delays agonist-stimulated calcium release. Mol Pharmacol 58:859–862, 2000.

175. Visiers I, Hassan SA, Weinstein H: Differences in conformational properties of the second intracellular loop (IL2) in 5HT(2C) receptors modified by RNA editing can account for G protein coupling efficiency. Protein Eng 14:409–414, 2001.

176. McGrew L, Price RD, Hackler E, et al: RNA editing of the human serotonin 5-HT2C receptor disrupts transactivation of the small G-protein RhoA. Mol Pharmacol 65:252–256, 2004.

177. Marion S, Weiner DM, Caron MG: RNA editing induces variation in desensitization and trafficking of 5-hydroxytryptamine 2c receptor isoforms. J Biol Chem 279:2945–2954, 2004.

178. Lefkowitz RJ, Pierce KL, Luttrell LM: Dancing with different partners: Protein kinase A phosphorylation of seven membrane-spanning receptors regulates their G protein-coupling specificity. Mol Pharmacol 62:971–974, 2002.

179. Daaka Y, Luttrell LM, Lefkowitz RJ: Switching of the coupling of the beta2-adrenergic receptor to different G proteins by protein kinase A. Nature 390:88–91, 1997.

180. Neubig RR, Siderovski DP: Regulators of G-protein signalling as new central nervous system drug targets. Nat Rev Drug Discov 1:187–197, 2002.

181. Ross EM, Wilkie TM: GTPase-activating proteins for heterotrimeric G proteins: Regulators of G protein signaling (RGS) and RGS-like proteins. Annu Rev Biochem 69:795–827, 2000.

182. De Vries L, Zheng B, Fischer T, et al: The regulator of G protein signaling family. Annu Rev Pharmacol Toxicol 40:235–271, 2000.

183. Tesmer JJ, Berman DM, Gilman AG, et al: Structure of RGS4 bound to AlF4-activated G(i alpha1): Stabilization of the transition state for GTP hydrolysis. Cell 89:251–261, 1997.

184. Hepler JR: Emerging roles for RGS proteins in cell signalling. Trends Pharmacol Sci 20:376–382, 1999.

185. Hart MJ, Jiang X, Kozasa T, et al: Direct stimulation of the guanine nucleotide exchange activity of p115 RhoGEF by Galpha13. Science 280:2112–2114, 1998.

186. Druey KM, Sullivan BM, Brown D, et al: Expression of GTPase-deficient Gialpha2 results in translocation of cytoplasmic RGS4 to the plasma membrane. J Biol Chem 273:18405–18410, 1998.

187. Gold SJ, Ni YG, Dohlman HG, et al: Regulators of G-protein signaling (RGS) proteins: region-specific expression of nine subtypes in rat brain. J Neurosci 17:8024–8037, 1997.

188. Zhong H, Neubig RR: Regulator of G protein signaling proteins: Novel multifunctional drug targets. J Pharmacol Exp Ther 297:837–845, 2001.

189. Takesono A, Cismowski MJ, Ribas C, et al: Receptor-independent activators of heterotrimeric G-protein signaling pathways. J Biol Chem 274:33202–33205, 1999.

190. Cismowski MJ, Takesono A, Bernard ML, et al: Receptor-independent activators of heterotrimeric G-proteins. Life Sci 68:2301–2308, 2001.

191. Cismowski MJ, Takesono A, Ma C, et al: Genetic screens in yeast to identify mammalian nonreceptor modulators of G-protein signaling. Nat Biotechnol 17:878–883, 1999.

192. Eason MG, Kurose H, Holt BD, et al: Simultaneous coupling of alpha 2-adrenergic receptors to two G-proteins with opposing effects: Subtype-selective coupling of alpha 2C10, alpha 2C4, and alpha 2C2 adrenergic receptors to Gi and Gs. J Biol Chem 267:15795–15801, 1992.

193. Chalecka-Franaszek E, Weems HB, Crowder AT, et al: Immunoprecipitation of high-affinity, guanine nucleotide-sensitive, solubilized mu-opioid receptors from rat brain: Coimmunoprecipitation of the G proteins G(alpha o), G(alpha i1), and G(alpha i3). J Neurochem 74:1068–1078, 2000.

194. Odagaki Y, Koyama T: Identification of g alpha subtype(s) involved in gamma-aminobutyric acid(B) receptor-mediated high-affinity guanosine triphosphatase activity in rat cerebral cortical membranes. Neurosci Lett 297:137–141, 2001.

195. Herrlich A, Kuhn B, Grosse R, et al: Involvement of Gs and Gi proteins in dual coupling of the luteinizing hormone receptor to adenylyl cyclase and phospholipase C. J Biol Chem 271:16764–16772, 1996.

196. Brydon L, Roka F, Petit L, et al: Dual signaling of human Mel1a melatonin receptors via G(i2), G(i3), and G(q/11) proteins. Mol Endocrinol 13:2025–2038, 1999.

197. Jin LQ, Wang HY, Friedman E: Stimulated D(1) dopamine receptors couple to multiple Galpha proteins in different brain regions. J Neurochem 78:981–990, 2001.

198. Milligan G, Rees S: Chimaeric G alpha proteins: Their potential use in drug discovery. Trends Pharmacol Sci 20:118–124, 1999.

199. Selkirk JV, Price GW, Nahorski SR, et al: Cell type-specific differences in the coupling of recombinant mGlu1alpha receptors to endogenous G protein sub-populations. Neuropharmacology 40:645–656, 2001.

200. Cordeaux Y, Briddon SJ, Megson AE, et al: Influence of receptor number on functional responses elicited by agonists acting at the human adenosine A(1) receptor: Evidence for signaling pathway-dependent changes in agonist potency and relative intrinsic activity. Mol Pharmacol 58:1075–1084, 2000.

201. Kenakin T: Differences between natural and recombinant G protein-coupled receptor systems with varying receptor/G protein stoichiometry. Trends Pharmacol Sci 18:456–464, 1997.

202. Jakubik J, Haga T, Tucek S: Effects of an agonist, allosteric modulator, and antagonist on guanosine-gamma-[35S]thiotriphosphate binding to liposomes with varying muscarinic receptor/G0 protein stoichiometry. Mol Pharmacol 54:899–906, 1998.

203. Gonzalez-Maeso J, Rodriguez-Puertas R, Meana JJ: Quantitative stoichiometry of G-proteins activated by mu-opioid receptors in postmortem human brain. Eur J Pharmacol 452:21–33, 2002.

204. Grosse R, Schmid A, Schoneberg T, et al: Gonadotropin-releasing hormone receptor initiates multiple signaling pathways by exclusively coupling to G(q/11) proteins. J Biol Chem 275:9193–9200, 2000.

205. Kenakin T: Agonist-specific receptor conformations. Trends Pharmacol Sci 18:416–417, 1997.

206. Kenakin T: Ligand-selective receptor conformations revisited: The promise and the problem. Trends Pharmacol Sci 24:346–354, 2003.

207. Leff P: The two-state model of receptor activation. Trends Pharmacol Sci 16:89–97, 1995.

208. Jordan JD, Landau EM, Iyengar R: Signaling networks: The origins of cellular multitasking. Cell 103:193–200, 2000.

209. Leff P, Scaramellini C, Law C, et al: A three-state receptor model of agonist action. Trends Pharmacol Sci 18: 355–362, 1997.

210. Peleg G, Ghanouni P, Kobilka BK, et al: Single-molecule spectroscopy of the beta(2) adrenergic receptor: Observation of conformational substates in a membrane protein. Proc Natl Acad Sci U S A 98:8469–8474, 2001.

211. Zhang D, Weinstein H: Signal transduction by a 5-HT2 receptor: A mechanistic hypothesis from molecular dynamics simulations of the three-dimensional model of the receptor complexed to ligands. J Med Chem 36:934–938, 1993.

212. Lopez-Gimenez JF, Villazon M, Brea J, et al: Multiple conformations of native and recombinant human 5-hydroxytryptamine(2a) receptors are labeled by agonists and discriminated by antagonists. Mol Pharmacol 60:690–699, 2001.

213. Berg KA, Maayani S, Goldfarb J, et al: Effector pathway-dependent relative efficacy at serotonin type 2A and 2C receptors: Evidence for agonist-directed trafficking of receptor stimulus. Mol Pharmacol 54:94–104, 1998.

214. Nair VD, Sealfon SC: Agonist specific transactivation of phosphoinositide 3-kinase signaling pathway mediated by the dopamine D2 receptor. J Biol Chem 278:47053–47061, 2003.

215. Gonzalez-Maeso J, Yuen T, Ebersole BJ, et al: Transcriptome fingerprints distinguish hallucinogenic and nonhallucinogenic 5-hydroxytryptamine 2A receptor agonist effects in mouse somatosensory cortex. J Neurosci 23:8836–8843, 2003.

216. Arey BJ, Stevis PE, Deecher DC, et al: Induction of promiscuous G protein coupling of the follicle-stimulating hormone (FSH) receptor: A novel mechanism for transducing pleiotropic actions of FSH isoforms. Mol Endocrinol 11:517–526, 1997.

217. Ostrom RS: New determinants of receptor-effector coupling: Trafficking and compartmentation in membrane microdomains. Mol Pharmacol 61:473–476, 2002.

218. Remmers AE, Clark MJ, Alt A, et al: Activation of G protein by opioid receptors: Role of receptor number and G-protein concentration. Eur J Pharmacol 396:67–75, 2000.

219. Neubig RR: Membrane organization in G-protein mechanisms. FASEB J 8:939–946, 1994.

220. Strange PG: G-protein coupled receptors: Conformations and states. Biochem Pharmacol 58:1081–1088, 1999.

221. Ostrom RS, Post SR, Insel PA: Stoichiometry and compartmentation in G protein-coupled receptor signaling: Implications for therapeutic interventions involving G(s). J Pharmacol Exp Ther 294:407–412, 2000.

222. Anderson RG: The caveolae membrane system. Annu Rev Biochem 67:199–225, 1998.

223. Okamoto T, Schlegel A, Scherer PE, et al: Caveolins, a family of scaffolding proteins for organizing "preassembled signaling complexes" at the plasma membrane. J Biol Chem 273:5419–5422, 1998.

224. Sabourin T, Bastien L, Bachvarov DR, et al: Agonist-induced translocation of the kinin B(1) receptor to caveolae-related rafts. Mol Pharmacol 61:546–553, 2002.

225. Schlegel A, Volonte D, Engelman JA, et al: Crowded little caves: Structure and function of caveolae. Cell Signal 10:457–463, 1998.

226. Bhalla US, Iyengar R: Emergent properties of networks of biological signaling pathways. Science 283:381–387, 1999.

227. Hur EM, Kim KT: G protein-coupled receptor signalling and cross-talk: Achieving rapidity and specificity. Cell Signal 14:397–405, 2002.

228. Selbie LA, Hill SJ: G protein-coupled-receptor cross-talk: The fine-tuning of multiple receptor-signalling pathways. Trends Pharmacol Sci 19:87–93, 1998.

229. Suh BC, Kim JS, Namgung U, et al: Selective inhibition of beta(2)-adrenergic receptor-mediated cAMP generation by activation of the P2Y(2) receptor in mouse pineal gland tumor cells. J Neurochem 77:1475–1485, 2001.

230. Ho AK, Chik CL, Klein DC: Effects of protein kinase inhibitor (1-(5-isoquinolinesulfonyl)-2-methylpiperazine (H7) on protein kinase C activity and adrenergic stimulation of cAMP and cGMP in rat pinealocytes. Biochem Pharmacol 37:1015–1020, 1988.

231. Nair VD, Olanow CW, Sealfon SC: Activation of phosphoinositide 3-kinase by D2 receptor prevents apoptosis in dopaminergic cell lines. Biochem J 373:25–32, 2003.

232. Karoor V, Baltensperger K, Paul H, et al: Phosphorylation of tyrosyl residues 350/354 of the beta-adrenergic receptor is obligatory for counterregulatory effects of insulin. J Biol Chem 270:25305–25308, 1995.

233. Baltensperger K, Karoor V, Paul H, et al: The beta-adrenergic receptor is a substrate for the insulin receptor tyrosine kinase. J Biol Chem 271:1061–1064, 1996.

234. Milligan G, White JH: Protein-protein interactions at G-protein-coupled receptors. Trends Pharmacol Sci 22:513–518, 2001.

235. Sexton PM, Albiston A, Morfis M, et al: Receptor activity modifying proteins. Cell Signal 13:73–83, 2001.

236. Foord SM, Marshall FH: RAMPs: Accessory proteins for seven transmembrane domain receptors. Trends Pharmacol Sci 20:184–187, 1999.

237. McLatchie LM, Fraser NJ, Main MJ, et al: RAMPs regulate the transport and ligand specificity of the calcitonin-receptor-like receptor. Nature 393:333–339, 1998.

238. Brakeman PR, Lanahan AA, O'Brien R, et al: Homer: A protein that selectively binds metabotropic glutamate receptors. Nature 386:284–288, 1997.

239. Xiao B, Tu JC, Petralia RS, et al: Homer regulates the association of group 1 metabotropic glutamate receptors with multivalent complexes of homer-related, synaptic proteins. Neuron 21:707–716, 1998.

240. Roche KW, Tu JC, Petralia RS, et al: Homer 1b regulates the trafficking of group I metabotropic glutamate receptors. J Biol Chem 274:25953–25957, 1999.

241. Ango F, Prezeau L, Muller T, et al: Agonist-independent activation of metabotropic glutamate receptors by the intracellular protein Homer. Nature 411:962–965, 2001.

242. Tu JC, Xiao B, Naisbitt S, et al: Coupling of mGluR/Homer and PSD-95 complexes by the Shank family of postsynaptic density proteins. Neuron 23:583–592, 1999.

243. Tu JC, Xiao B, Yuan JP, et al: Homer binds a novel proline-rich motif and links group 1 metabotropic glutamate receptors with IP3 receptors. Neuron 21:717–726, 1998.

244. Rong R, Ahn JY, Huang H, et al: PI3 kinase enhancer-Homer complex couples mGluRI to PI3 kinase, preventing neuronal apoptosis. Nat Neurosci 6:1153–1161, 2003.

245. Hall RA, Premont RT, Lefkowitz RJ: Heptahelical receptor signaling: Beyond the G protein paradigm. J Cell Biol 145:927–932, 1999.

246. Heuss C, Gerber U: G-protein-independent signaling by G-protein-coupled receptors. Trends Neurosci 23:469–475, 2000.

247. Luttrell LM, Ferguson SS, Daaka Y, et al: Beta-arrestin-dependent formation of beta2 adrenergic receptor-Src protein kinase complexes. Science 283:655–661, 1999.

248. Mitchell R, McCulloch D, Lutz E, et al: Rhodopsin-family receptors associate with small G proteins to activate phospholipase D. Nature 392:411–414, 1998.

249. Hall RA, Premont RT, Chow CW, et al: The beta2-adrenergic receptor interacts with the Na+/H+-exchanger regulatory factor to control Na+/H+ exchange. Nature 392:626–630, 1998.

250. Karoor V, Wang L, Wang HY, et al: Insulin stimulates sequestration of beta-adrenergic receptors and enhanced association of beta-adrenergic receptors with Grb2 via tyrosine 350. J Biol Chem 273:33035–33041, 1998.

251. Guillet-Deniau I, Burnol AF, Girard J: Identification and localization of a skeletal muscle serotonin 5-HT2A receptor coupled to the Jak/STAT pathway. J Biol Chem 272:14825–14829, 1997.

252. Rios CD, Jordan BA, Gomes I, et al: G-protein-coupled receptor dimerization: Modulation of receptor function. Pharmacol Ther 92:71–87, 2001.

253. Bouvier M: Oligomerization of G-protein-coupled transmitter receptors. Nat Rev Neurosci 2:274–286, 2001.

254. Ongun Onaran H, Gurdal H: Ligand efficacy and affinity in an interacting 7TM receptor model. Trends Pharmacol Sci 20:274–278, 1999.

255. Franco R, Ferre S, Agnati L, et al: Evidence for adenosine/dopamine receptor interactions: Indications for heteromerization. Neuropsychopharmacology 23:S50–S59, 2000.

256. Ng GY, O'Dowd BF, Lee SP, et al: Dopamine D2 receptor dimers and receptor-blocking peptides. Biochem Biophys Res Commun 227:200–204, 1996.

257. Maggio R, Vogel Z, Wess J: Coexpression studies with mutant muscarinic/adrenergic receptors provide evidence for intermolecular "cross-talk" between G-protein-linked receptors. Proc Natl Acad Sci U S A 90:3103–3107, 1993.

258. Jordan BA, Devi LA: G-protein-coupled receptor heterodimerization modulates receptor function. Nature 399:697–700, 1999.

259. Lee SP, Xie Z, Varghese G, et al: Oligomerization of dopamine and serotonin receptors. Neuropsychopharmacology 23:S32–S40, 2000.

260. Gomes I, Filipovska J, Jordan BA, et al: Oligomerization of opioid receptors. Methods 27:358–365, 2002.

261. Limbird LE, Lefkowitz RJ: Negative cooperativity among beta-adrenergic receptors in frog erythrocyte membranes. J Biol Chem 251:5007–5014, 1976.

262. Armstrong D, Strange PG: Dopamine D2 receptor dimer formation: Evidence from ligand binding. J Biol Chem 276:22621–22629, 2001.

263. Hebert TE, Moffett S, Morello JP, et al: A peptide derived from a beta2-adrenergic receptor transmembrane domain inhibits both receptor dimerization and activation. J Biol Chem 271:16384–16392, 1996.

264. Boute N, Jockers R, Issad T: The use of resonance energy transfer in high-throughput screening: BRET versus FRET. Trends Pharmacol Sci 23:351–354, 2002.

265. Angers S, Salahpour A, Joly E, et al: Detection of beta 2-adrenergic receptor dimerization in living cells using bioluminescence resonance energy transfer (BRET). Proc Natl Acad Sci U S A 97:3684–3689, 2000.

266. Rocheville M, Lange DC, Kumar U, et al: Subtypes of the somatostatin receptor assemble as functional homo- and heterodimers. J Biol Chem 275:7862–7869, 2000.

267. McVey M, Ramsay D, Kellett E, et al: Monitoring receptor oligomerization using time-resolved fluorescence resonance energy transfer and bioluminescence resonance energy transfer: The human delta-opioid receptor displays constitutive oligomerization at the cell surface, which is not regulated by receptor

occupancy. J Biol Chem 276:14092–14099, 2001.

268. Rocheville M, Lange DC, Kumar U, et al: Receptors for dopamine and somatostatin: Formation of hetero-oligomers with enhanced functional activity. Science 288:154–157, 2000.

269. Kaupmann K, Huggel K, Heid J, et al: Expression cloning of GABA(B) receptors uncovers similarity to metabotropic glutamate receptors. Nature 386:239–246, 1997.

270. Couve A, Filippov AK, Connolly CN, et al: Intracellular retention of recombinant GABAB receptors. J Biol Chem 273:26361–26367, 1998.

271. Couve A, Moss SJ, Pangalos MN: GABAB receptors: A new paradigm in G protein signaling. Mol Cell Neurosci 16:296–312, 2000.

272. Billinton A, Ige AO, Bolam JP, et al: Advances in the molecular understanding of GABA(B) receptors. Trends Neurosci 24:277–282, 2001.

273. Malitschek B, Schweizer C, Keir M, et al: The N-terminal domain of gamma-aminobutyric acid(B) receptors is sufficient to specify agonist and antagonist binding. Mol Pharmacol 56:448–454, 1999.

274. Galvez T, Duthey B, Kniazeff J, et al: Allosteric interactions between GB1 and GB2 subunits are required for optimal GABA(B) receptor function. EMBO J 20:2152–2159, 2001.

275. Galvez T, Prezeau L, Milioti G, et al: Mapping the agonist-binding site of GABAB type 1 subunit sheds light on the activation process of GABAB receptors. J Biol Chem 275:41166–41174, 2000.

276. Margeta-Mitrovic M, Jan YN, Jan LY: Function of GB1 and GB2 subunits in G protein coupling of GABA(B) receptors. Proc Natl Acad Sci U S A 98:14649–14654, 2001.

277. Margeta-Mitrovic M, Jan YN, Jan LY: Ligand-induced signal transduction within heterodimeric GABA(B) receptor. Proc Natl Acad Sci U S A 98:14643–14648, 2001.

278. Robbins MJ, Calver AR, Filippov AK, et al: GABA(B2) is essential for G-protein coupling of the GABA(B) receptor heterodimer. J Neurosci 21:8043–8052, 2001.

279. Gouldson PR, Higgs C, Smith RE, et al: Dimerization and domain swapping in G-protein-coupled receptors: A computational study. Neuropsychopharmacology 23:S60–S77, 2000.

280. Filizola M, Weinstein H: Structural models for dimerization of G-protein coupled receptors: The opioid receptor homodimers. Biopolymers 66:317–325, 2002.

281. Bohm SK, Grady EF, Bunnett NW: Regulatory mechanisms that modulate signalling by G-protein-coupled receptors. Biochem J 322:1–18, 1997.

282. Ferguson SS: Evolving concepts in G protein-coupled receptor endocytosis: The role in receptor desensitization and signaling. Pharmacol Rev 53:1–24, 2001.

283. Tsao P, Cao T, von Zastrow M: Role of endocytosis in mediating downregulation of G-protein-coupled receptors. Trends Pharmacol Sci 22:91–96, 2001.

284. Koenig JA, Edwardson JM: Endocytosis and recycling of G protein-coupled receptors. Trends Pharmacol Sci 18:276–287, 1997.

285. Diviani D, Lattion AL, Cotecchia S: Characterization of the phosphorylation sites involved in G protein-coupled receptor kinase- and protein kinase C-mediated desensitization of the alpha1B-adrenergic receptor. J Biol Chem 272:28712–28719, 1997.

286. Liang M, Eason MG, Jewell-Motz EA, et al: Phosphorylation and functional desensitization of the alpha2A-adrenergic receptor by protein kinase C. Mol Pharmacol 54:44–49, 1998.

287. Couve A, Thomas P, Calver AR, et al: Cyclic AMP-dependent protein kinase phosphorylation facilitates GABA(B) receptor-effector coupling. Nat Neurosci 5:415–424, 2002.

288. Lefkowitz RJ: G protein-coupled receptors, III: New roles for receptor kinases and beta-arrestins in receptor signaling and desensitization. J Biol Chem 273:18677–18680, 1998.

289. Krupnick JG, Benovic JL: The role of receptor kinases and arrestins in G protein-coupled receptor regulation. Annu Rev Pharmacol Toxicol 38:289–319, 1998.

290. Pitcher JA, Freedman NJ, Lefkowitz RJ: G protein-coupled receptor kinases. Annu Rev Biochem 67:653–692, 1998.

291. Pierce KL, Lefkowitz RJ: Classical and new roles of beta-arrestins in the regulation of G-protein-coupled receptors. Nat Rev Neurosci 2:727–733, 2001.

292. Kohout TA, Lefkowitz RJ: Regulation of G protein-coupled receptor kinases and arrestins during receptor desensitization. Mol Pharmacol 63:9–18, 2003.

293. Stoffel RH, Inglese J, Macrae AD, et al: Palmitoylation increases the kinase activity of the G protein-coupled receptor kinase, GRK6. Biochemistry 37:16053–16059, 1998.

294. Premont RT, Koch WJ, Inglese J, et al: Identification, purification, and characterization of GRK5: A member of the family of G protein-coupled receptor kinases. J Biol Chem 269:6832–6841, 1994.

295. Oppermann M, Diverse-Pierluissi M, Drazner MH, et al: Monoclonal antibodies reveal receptor specificity among G-protein-coupled receptor kinases. Proc Natl Acad Sci U S A 93:7649–7654, 1996.

296. Chen CY, Dion SB, Kim CM, et al: Beta-adrenergic receptor kinase: Agonist-dependent receptor binding promotes kinase activation. J Biol Chem 268:7825–7831, 1993.

297. Pfister C, Chabre M, Plouet J, et al: Retinal S antigen identified as the 48K protein regulating light-dependent phosphodiesterase in rods. Science 228:891–893, 1985.

298. Luttrell LM, Lefkowitz RJ: The role of beta-arrestins in the termination and transduction of G-protein-coupled receptor signals. J Cell Sci 115:455–465, 2002.

299. Hirsch JA, Schubert C, Gurevich VV, et al: The 2.8 A crystal structure of visual arrestin: A model for arrestin's regulation. Cell 97:257–269, 1999.

300. Bohn LM, Lefkowitz RJ, Caron MG: Differential mechanisms of morphine antinociceptive tolerance revealed in (beta)arrestin-2 knock-out mice. J Neurosci 22:10494–10500, 2002.

301. Kallal L, Benovic JL: Using green fluorescent proteins to study G-protein-coupled receptor localization and trafficking. Trends Pharmacol Sci 21:175–180, 2000.

302. McLean AJ, Bevan N, Rees S, et al: Visualizing differences in ligand regulation of wild-type and constitutively active mutant beta(2)-adrenoceptor-green fluorescent protein fusion proteins. Mol Pharmacol 56:1182–1191, 1999.

303. Gonzalez-Maeso J, Wise A, Green A, et al: Agonist-induced desensitization and endocytosis of heterodimeric GABA(B) receptors in CHO-K1 cells. Eur J Pharmacol 481:15–23, 2003.

304. Ferguson SS, Menard L, Barak LS, et al: Role of phosphorylation in agonist-promoted beta 2-adrenergic receptor sequestration: Rescue of a sequestration-defective mutant receptor by beta ARK1. J Biol Chem 270:24782–24789, 1995.

305. Ferguson SS, Downey WE 3rd, Colapietro AM, et al: Role of beta-arrestin in mediating agonist-promoted G protein-coupled receptor internalization. Science 271:363–366, 1996.

306. Damke H, Baba T, Warnock DE, et al: Induction of mutant dynamin specifically blocks endocytic coated vesicle formation. J Cell Biol 127:915–934, 1994.

307. Chun M, Liyanage UK, Lisanti MP, et al: Signal transduction of a G protein-coupled receptor in caveolae: Colocalization of endothelin and its receptor with caveolin. Proc Natl Acad Sci U S A 91:11728–11732, 1994.

308. Oakley RH, Laporte SA, Holt JA, et al: Association of beta-arrestin with G protein-coupled receptors during clathrin-mediated endocytosis dictates the profile of receptor resensitization. J Biol Chem 274:32248–32257, 1999.

309. Whistler JL, Chuang HH, Chu P, et al: Functional dissociation of mu opioid receptor signaling and endocytosis: Implications for the biology of opiate tolerance and addiction. Neuron 23:737–746, 1999.

310. Meana JJ, Gonzalez-Maeso J, Garcia-Sevilla JA, et al: mu-opioid receptor and alpha2-adrenoceptor agonist stimulation of [35S]GTPgammaS binding to G-proteins in postmortem brains of opioid addicts. Mol Psychiatry 5:308–315, 2000.

311. He L, Fong J, von Zastrow M, et al: Regulation of opioid receptor trafficking and morphine tolerance by receptor oligomerization. Cell 108:271–282, 2002.

312. Pippig S, Andexinger S, Lohse MJ: Sequestration and recycling of beta 2-adrenergic receptors permit receptor resensitization. Mol Pharmacol 47:666–676, 1995.

313. Szekeres PG, Koenig JA, Edwardson JM: Involvement of receptor cycling and receptor reserve in resensitization of muscarinic responses in SH-SY5Y human neuroblastoma cells. J Neurochem 70:1694–1703, 1998.

314. Zhang J, Barak LS, Winkler KE, et al: A central role for beta-arrestins and clathrin-coated vesicle-mediated endocytosis in beta2-adrenergic receptor resensitization: Differential regulation of receptor resensitization in two distinct cell types. J Biol Chem 272:27005–27014, 1997.

315. Whistler JL, Enquist J, Marley A, et al: Modulation of postendocytic sorting of G protein-coupled receptors. Science 297:615–620, 2002.

316. Hershko A, Ciechanover A: The ubiquitin system. Annu Rev Biochem 67:425–479, 1998.

317. Obin MS, Jahngen-Hodge J, Nowell T, et al: Ubiquitinylation and ubiquitin-dependent proteolysis in vertebrate photoreceptors (rod outer segments): Evidence for ubiquitinylation of Gt and rhodopsin. J Biol Chem 271:14473–14484, 1996.

318. Chaturvedi K, Bandari P, Chinen N, et al: Proteasome involvement in agonist-induced down-regulation of mu and delta opioid receptors. J Biol Chem 276:12345–12355, 2001.

319. Shenoy SK, McDonald PH, Kohout TA, et al: Regulation of receptor fate by ubiquitination of activated beta 2-adrenergic receptor and beta-arrestin. Science 294:1307–1313, 2001.

320. Martin NP, Lefkowitz RJ, Shenoy SK: Regulation of V2 vasopressin receptor degradation by agonist-promoted ubiquitination. J Biol Chem 278:45954–45959, 2003.

321. Coughlin SR: Expanding horizons for receptors coupled to G proteins: Diversity and disease. Curr Opin Cell Biol 6:191–197, 1994.

322. Spiegel AM: Defects in G protein-coupled signal transduction in human disease. Annu Rev Physiol 58:143–170, 1996.

323. Spiegel AM: Hormone resistance caused by mutations in G proteins and G protein-coupled receptors. J Pediatr Endocrinol Metab 12(Suppl 1):303–309, 1999.

324. Farfel Z, Bourne HR, Iiri T: The expanding spectrum of G protein diseases. N Engl J Med 340:1012–1020, 1999.

325. Iiri T, Farfel Z, Bourne HR: G-protein diseases furnish a model for the turn-on switch. Nature 394:35–38, 1998.

326. Flower DR: Modelling G-protein-coupled receptors for drug design. Biochim Biophys Acta 1422:207–234, 1999.

327. Vallar L, Spada A, Giannattasio G: Altered Gs and adenylate cyclase activity in human GH-secreting pituitary adenomas. Nature 330:566–568, 1987.

328. Weinstein LS, Shenker A, Gejman PV, et al: Activating mutations of the stimulatory G protein in the McCune-Albright syndrome. N Engl J Med 325:1688–1695, 1991.

329. Gromoll J, Simoni M, Nieschlag E: An activating mutation of the follicle-stimulating hormone receptor autonomously sustains spermatogenesis in a hypophysectomized man. J Clin Endocrinol Metab 81:1367–1370, 1996.

330. Shenker A, Laue L, Kosugi S, et al: A constitutively activating mutation of the luteinizing hormone receptor in familial male precocious puberty. Nature 365:652–654, 1993.

331. Rodien P, Bremont C, Sanson ML, et al: Familial gestational hyperthyroidism caused by a mutant thyrotropin receptor hypersensitive to human chorionic gonadotropin. N Engl J Med 339:1823–1826, 1998.

332. Dryer L, Berghard A: Odorant receptors: A plethora of G-protein-coupled receptors. Trends Pharmacol Sci 20:413–417, 1999.

333. Robertson HM: Taste: Independent origins of chemoreception coding systems? Curr Biol 11:R560–R562, 2001.

334. Caulfield MP, Birdsall NJ: International Union of Pharmacology, XVII: Classification of muscarinic acetylcholine receptors. Pharmacol Rev 50:279–290, 1998.

335. Bylund DB, Eikenberg DC, Hieble JP, et al: International Union of Pharmacology: Nomenclature of adrenoceptors. Pharmacol Rev 46:121–136, 1994.

336. Hill SJ, Ganellin CR, Timmerman H, et al: International Union of Pharmacology, XIII: Classification of histamine receptors. Pharmacol Rev 49:253–278, 1997.

337. Hoyer D, Clarke DE, Fozard JR, et al: International Union of Pharmacology classification of receptors for 5-hydroxytryptamine (serotonin). Pharmacol Rev 46:157–203, 1994.

338. Barnes NM, Sharp T: A review of central 5-HT receptors and their function. Neuropharmacology 38:1083–1152, 1999.

339. de Gasparo M, Catt KJ, Inagami T, et al: International Union of Pharmacology, XXIII: The angiotensin II receptors. Pharmacol Rev 52:415–472, 2000.

340. Medhurst AD, Jennings CA, Robbins MJ, et al: Pharmacological and immunohistochemical characterization of the APJ receptor and its endogenous ligand apelin. J Neurochem 84:1162–1172, 2003.

341. Regoli D, Nsa Allogho S, Rizzi A, et al: Bradykinin receptors and their antagonists. Eur J Pharmacol 348:1–10, 1998.

342. Murphy PM, Baggiolini M, Charo IF, et al: International Union of Pharmacology. XXII: Nomenclature for chemokine receptors. Pharmacol Rev 52:145–176, 2000.

343. Murphy PM: International Union of Pharmacology, XXX: Update on chemokine receptor nomenclature. Pharmacol Rev 54:227–229, 2002.

344. Noble F, Wank SA, Crawley JN, et al: International Union of Pharmacology, XXI: Structure, distribution, and functions of cholecystokinin receptors. Pharmacol Rev 51:745–781, 1999.

345. Masaki T, Vane JR, Vanhoutte PM: International Union of Pharmacology: Nomenclature of endothelin receptors. Pharmacol Rev 46:137–142, 1994.

346. Davenport AP: International Union of Pharmacology, XXIX: Update on endothelin receptor nomenclature. Pharmacol Rev 54:219–226, 2002.

347. Branchek TA, Smith KE, Gerald C, et al: Galanin receptor subtypes. Trends Pharmacol Sci 21:109–117, 2000.

348. Witt-Enderby PA, Bennett J, Jarzynka MJ, et al: Melatonin receptors and their regulation: Biochemical and structural mechanisms. Life Sci 72:2183–2189, 2003.

349. Adan RA, Gispen WH: Brain melanocortin receptors: From cloning to function. Peptides 18:1279–1287, 1997.

350. Michel MC, Beck-Sickinger A, Cox H, et al: XVI. International Union of Pharmacology: Recommendations for the nomenclature of neuropeptide Y, peptide YY, and pancreatic polypeptide receptors. Pharmacol Rev 50:143–150, 1998.

351. Zingg HH, Laporte SA: The oxytocin receptor. Trends Endocrinol Metab 14:222–227, 2003.

352. Dhawan BN, Cesselin F, Raghubir R, et al: International Union of Pharmacology, XII: Classification of opioid receptors. Pharmacol Rev 48:567–592, 1996.

353. Moller LN, Stidsen CE, Hartmann B, et al: Somatostatin receptors. Biochim Biophys Acta 1616:1–84, 2003.

354. Wilber JF, Xu AH: The thyrotropin-releasing hormone gene 1998: Cloning, characterization, and transcriptional regulation in the central nervous system, heart, and testis. Thyroid 8:897–901, 1998.

355. Birnbaumer M: Vasopressin receptors. Trends Endocrinol Metab 11:406–410, 2000.

356. Hollenberg MD, Compton SJ: International Union of Pharmacology, XXVIII: Proteinase-activated receptors. Pharmacol Rev 54:203–217, 2002.

357. Trejo J: Protease-activated receptors: New concepts in regulation of G protein-coupled receptor signaling and trafficking. J Pharmacol Exp Ther 307:437–442, 2003.

358. Howlett AC, Barth F, Bonner TI, et al: International Union of Pharmacology, XXVII: Classification of cannabinoid receptors. Pharmacol Rev 54:161–202, 2002.

359. Chun J, Goetzl EJ, Hla T, et al: International Union of Pharmacology, XXXIV: Lysophospholipid receptor nomenclature. Pharmacol Rev 54:265–269, 2002.

360. Yu N, Lariosa-Willingham KD, Lin FF, et al: Characterization of lysophosphatidic acid and sphingosine-1-phosphate-mediated signal transduction in rat cortical oligodendrocytes. Glia 45:17–27, 2004.

361. Coleman RA, Smith WL, Narumiya S: International Union of Pharmacology: Classification of prostanoid receptors: Properties, distribution, and structure of the receptors and their subtypes. Pharmacol Rev 46:205–229, 1994.

362. Brink C, Dahlen SE, Drazen J, et al: International Union of Pharmacology XXXVII: Nomenclature for leukotriene and lipoxin receptors. Pharmacol Rev 55:195–227, 2003.

363. Fredholm BB, AP IJ, Jacobson KA, et al: International Union of Pharmacology, XXV: Nomenclature and classification of adenosine receptors. Pharmacol Rev 53:527–552, 2001.

364. Fredholm BB, Abbracchio MP, Burnstock G, et al: Nomenclature and classification of purinoceptors. Pharmacol Rev 46:143–156, 1994.

365. Poyner DR, Sexton PM, Marshall I, et al: International Union of Pharmacology XXXII: The mammalian calcitonin gene-related peptides, adrenomedullin, amylin, and calcitonin receptors. Pharmacol Rev 54:233–246, 2002.

366. Hauger RL, Grigoriadis DE, Dallman MF, et al: International Union of Pharmacology, XXXVI: Current status of the nomenclature for receptors for corticotropin-releasing factor and their ligands. Pharmacol Rev 55:21–26, 2003.

367. Harmar AJ, Arimura A, Gozes I, et al: International Union of Pharmacology, XVIII: Nomenclature of receptors for vasoactive intestinal peptide and pituitary adenylate cyclase-activating polypeptide. Pharmacol Rev 50:265–270, 1998.

368. Hofer AM, Brown EM: Extracellular calcium sensing and signalling. Nat Rev Mol Cell Biol 4:530–538, 2003.

The Cyclic AMP Second Messenger Signaling Pathway

Joel F. Habener and Colin A. Leech

INTRODUCTION

The discovery of the cyclic adenosine monophosphate (cAMP) second messenger signaling pathway made a major impact in understanding how growth, development, and metabolism of cells is regulated in response to environmental cues. Studies that led to an elucidation of the mechanisms involved in the important cAMP-directed signaling pathway have spanned over 5 decades. The historical aspects of the key research discoveries are reviewed briefly. Lessons can be learned by appreciating the conceptualization and experimentation that systematically led to further conclusions, modifications of hypotheses, and additional experimentation carried out by the pioneers of the cAMP signaling pathway. Four Nobel prizes have been awarded for discoveries linked to this pathway: first to Car and Gerti Cori for their discovery of glucagon phosphorylase; then to Earl Sutherland for the discovery of cAMP; then to Edmund Fischer and Edwin Krebs for their discoveries of protein kinase A; and to Alfred Gilman and Martin Rodbell for their discoveries of G proteins in cAMP signaling. Several excellent reviews of various aspects of the cAMP-dependent signaling system have appeared.[1–16]

HISTORICAL PERSPECTIVES

In the early 1940s, the Coris established the basic biochemistry of glycogenolysis by the identification of the key enzymes of glycogen metabolism, namely, glycogen phosphorylase, phosphoglucomutase, and glucose-6-phosphatase.[17] Most importantly, they demonstrated that glycogen breakdown is stimulated by the hormones glucagon and epinephrine. A key finding was that glycogen phosphorylase was interconvertible from an inactive form (phosphorylase b) to an active form (phosphorylase a), a discovery for which the Coris were jointly awarded the Nobel Prize in 1951. These pioneering studies were further pursued by Sutherland and his coworkers, who, using broken liver cell preparations, showed that glucagon and epinephrine stimulated the activity of glycogen phosphorylase, a rate-limiting step in the conversion of glycogen to glucose.[18] Further, they demonstrated that

although the hormonally responsive enzymatic activity resided in the particulate fraction, the generation of activity required the re-addition of the soluble fraction contained in the broken cell preparation.[19] These seminal observations led Sutherland to the isolation and identification of the essential factor in the soluble fraction as an adenine ribonucleotide, subsequently established to be 3′,5′ cAMP.[20] The work of this group of investigators culminated in the isolation and characterization of adenylyl cyclase and phosphodiesterase, the two key enzymes responsible for the synthesis and degradation of cAMP, respectively. Identification of cAMP was an essential step for the consequent conceptualization of the second messenger hypothesis by which hormones, acting on receptors located on the cell surface, lead to the synthesis of the second messenger (cAMP), which, in turn, regulates cellular activity. This concept provided a model to explain how extracellular signals, such as hormones, can transduce their informational cues to the interior of the cell. For this series of brilliant discoveries, Sutherland was awarded the Nobel Prize in 1971.

During the time that Sutherland and his coworkers were characterizing adenylyl cyclase and phosphodiesterase, Fischer and Krebs pursued further the identification of the targets in the signal transduction pathway on which cAMP exerts its effects. In the late 1950s, they discovered that the activity of glycogen phosphorylase is altered by a reversible phosphorylation mediated by phosphorylase kinase and opposing phosphatases, and that the phosphorylation required cAMP.[11,21,22] In 1968, the laboratories of Krebs and Greengard independently isolated the enzyme responsible for the activation of phosphorylase kinase.[23,24] The enzyme was called phosphorylase kinase kinase because it phosphorylated phosphorylase kinase. However, it was soon discovered to be the key enzyme activated by cAMP and was renamed cAMP-dependent protein kinase A (cPK, PKA), because of its widespread importance in the phosphorylation of many substrate proteins other than phosphorylase kinase.[11] As discussed later, PKA is a heterotetrameric protein consisting of two regulatory and two catalytic subunits. cAMP binds to the regulatory subunit and thereby relieves inhibition of the catalytic subunit by releasing the activated catalytic subunit from the inactive complex with the regulatory subunit. The catalytic subunit is then free to phosphorylate specifically certain serine and threonine residues in proteins whose functions are regulated by PKA. Krebs and Fischer shared the Nobel Prize in 1992 for their seminal work on this critically important pathway of phosphorylation (and dephosphorylation) initiated by cAMP-dependent PKA.

THE PLEIOTROPIC ACTIONS OF cAMP

The cellular actions of cAMP are numerous (Fig. 12-1). Notably, most of the actions of cAMP are mediated by PKA. Two exceptions are that cAMP binds to and directly regulates the activity of cyclic nucleotide-gated ion channels[25–27] and cAMP also activates guanine nucleotide exchange factors that have diverse functions, which are reviewed later.[28] cAMP, via its actions on PKA, activates certain enzymes and inactivates others. For example, phosphorylase kinase[11] and type II PKA[7,8] are activated, and glycogen synthase is inactivated by PKA[11] (see later discussion). Certain receptors, for example, β-adrenergic receptors[29,30] and ion channels, for example, cystic fibrosis transmembrane conductance regulator (CFTR),[31] are regulated by phosphorylation by PKA. In addition, the structural proteins tubulin[32] and microtubule-associated proteins[33] are modified by PKA-induced phosphorylation. An important function of PKA is the phosphorylation and consequent activation of nuclear transcription factors that bind to cAMP response enhancer elements of many genes. These proteins are known variously as cAMP response element binding proteins (CREBs) or activating transcription factors (ATFs).[34–36] PKA also stimulates glucocorticoid receptor-mediated gene transcription, but this effect of PKA may be indirect via the phosphorylation of an intermediate factor.[37] The regulatory subunit of PKA is a homologue of the prokaryotic catabolite activating protein,[38] and the regulatory subunit has been shown by fluorescence assays to bind DNA in vitro.[39] There is, however, as yet no clear evidence to support a functional role for the regulatory subunit in animal cells apart from its important actions as an inhibitor of the catalytic subunit.

The mechanism by which phosphorylation activates or inactivates the biologic functions of a protein most often involves a change in the conformation or folding of the protein.[39,40] The change in conformation is considered allosteric when the change in the shape of the protein occurs at a distance from the site that is phosphorylated by a specific protein kinase, for example, by PKA. Examples of the involvement of

PKA in the allosteric regulation of protein activities are discussed in more detail later in this chapter.

COMPONENTS OF THE cAMP-DEPENDENT CELLULAR SIGNALING PATHWAY

The cAMP-dependent signaling pathway consists of several intermolecular interactions leading to the generation of an active catalytic subunit of PKA capable of phosphorylating target sites on protein substrates. A generalized overall schematic illustration of this pathway is given in Figure 12-2. The detailed molecular mechanisms at work in the cascade of molecular interactions have yet to be completely elucidated. However, some interpretations can be made regarding how the individual components of the pathway are linked together.

MODEL OF ACTIVATION OF PKA BY cAMP

The initiating event in the pathway of cAMP-dependent signaling is the binding of a hormone (ligand) to its receptor. This type of interaction appears to be a crucial first step in the signaling cascade, resulting in the eventual formation of cAMP. The binding of the hormone ligand to its receptor, which occurs specifically and with a high affinity (in the range of nanomolar concentrations of ligand), results in a change in the conformation of the receptor reflected within the transmembrane and cytoplasmic domains. The second step in the signaling cascade is the receptor-directed conversion of an associated guanine nucleotide-binding protein (G protein) from an inactive to an active form. The cycling of G protein from an inactive to an active state and back to inactive form is described in greater detail later in reference to the model shown in Figure 12-3. The activated, guanosine triphosphate (GTP)-bound, G protein α-subunit, $G_s\alpha$, activates the enzyme adenylyl cyclase, referred to earlier, leading to the conversion of ATP to 3'5' cyclic AMP. The degradation of cAMP to 5' AMP is effected by phosphodiesterase enzymes (see Fig. 12-2). The key role of cAMP is to bind to the regulatory subunits of the inactive heterotetrameric complex of protein kinase A, thereby eliciting an allosteric change in the complex, resulting in the liberation of the active catalytic subunits from the inactive complex. The catalytic subunits, once freed from their regulatory subunits, are available to phosphorylate sites on protein substrates, resulting in the modification of the biologic actions of the proteins (see Fig. 12-2).

Pleiotropic Actions of cAMP Second Messenger

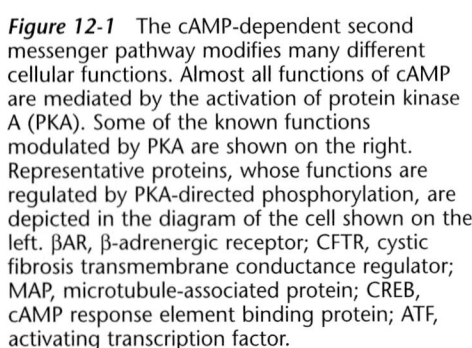

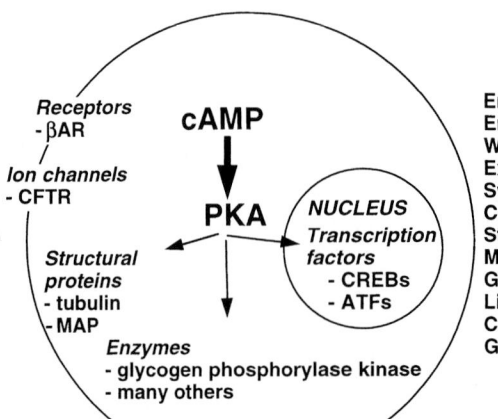

Figure 12-1   The cAMP-dependent second messenger pathway modifies many different cellular functions. Almost all functions of cAMP are mediated by the activation of protein kinase A (PKA). Some of the known functions modulated by PKA are shown on the right. Representative proteins, whose functions are regulated by PKA-directed phosphorylation, are depicted in the diagram of the cell shown on the left. βAR, β-adrenergic receptor; CFTR, cystic fibrosis transmembrane conductance regulator; MAP, microtubule-associated protein; CREB, cAMP response element binding protein; ATF, activating transcription factor.

Cyclic AMP -Dependent Signal Transduction Pathway

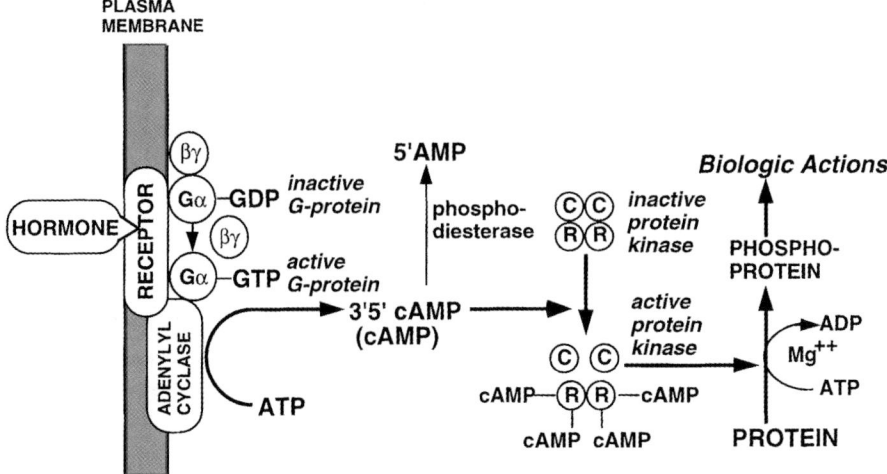

Figure 12-2   cAMP-dependent signal transduction pathway. The diagram depicts the essential components of the cellular signaling pathway mediated by the second messenger cAMP. The "first" messenger or activator is the hormone/receptor/G protein complex. The "second" messenger effector is cAMP. The "third" messenger is the protein kinase A that phosphorylates critical protein substrates, resulting in the generation of the final bioactive "fourth" messenger. See text for a more detailed explanation.

A more detailed explanation of the cAMP-stimulated activation of PKA is given later in this chapter.

THE G PROTEIN CYCLE

The coupling of G proteins is of critical importance in transmitting the signal generated by hormone receptor interactions to the formation of cAMP (see Fig. 12-3). The G proteins consist of complex families of α, β, and γ subunits that in the inactive state form heterotrimeric complexes with guanosine diphosphate (GDP) bound to the α subunit.[13,41-44] Much attention has been focused on the regulatory functions of the α subunit, various isotypes of which can be either stimulatory or inhibitory.

Binding of a ligand to its receptor effects a conformational change in the receptor and its associated G protein, leading to the exchange of GTP for GDP and concomitant dissociation of the GTP-bound α subunit from the $\beta\gamma$ subunit dimeric complex. This GTP-activated G_α then binds to adenylyl cyclase to either activate or inhibit the enzyme, depending on

whether the type of G_α is stimulatory ($G_{\alpha s}$) or inhibitory ($G_{\alpha i}$). The extent of activated adenylyl cyclase formed depends on the relative amounts of active stimulatory or inhibitory G_α subunits present in a given location within the cell at a given time. The pharmacologic distinction between the actions of stimulatory and inhibitory G proteins has been facilitated by the use of two bacterial toxins that adenosine diphosphate (ADP) ribosylate G_α subunits. Cholera toxin activates $G_{\alpha s}$ and pertussis toxin inhibits $G_{\alpha i}$ and $G_{\alpha o}$ (other), a G protein enriched in brain but whose functions are poorly understood. The use of nonhydrolyzable analogues of GTP, such as GPP(NH)P and GTPγS, has also been of great value in dissecting the G protein pathways. These GTP analogues constitutively activate G_α proteins because they cannot be hydrolyzed to GDP.

Following the activation of adenylyl cyclase, the G proteins return to the inactive state. GTP is hydrolyzed to GDP by the intrinsic GTPase activity contained in the G_α subunit. G_α dissociates from adenylyl cyclase and the $\beta\gamma$ subunits reassociate with the α subunit. It is unknown to what extent the inactivation of G protein is due to the hydrolysis of GTP to GDP or to the reassociation of the α and $\beta\gamma$ subunits. It also appears that the $\beta\gamma$ complex may control certain effectors directly. It has been proposed that $\beta\gamma$ can inhibit adenylate cyclase directly or indirectly through interactions with calmodulin. Studies in vitro have shown that $\beta\gamma$ inhibits type I adenylyl cyclase and stimulates the type II enzyme, whereas $G_{\alpha s}$ stimulates both enzyme isotypes.[45] In addition, $\beta\gamma$ regulate the activities of K$^+$ channels[46,47] and certain isotypes of phospholipase C.[48,49] The inhibitory or stimulatory actions of $\beta\gamma$ appear to reside in the particular isotype of the γ subunit involved. The unraveling of the complex interactions of the G protein subunits is at the forefront of molecular and cellular research.

Investigators are just now beginning to understand the complex nature of the G proteins. In addition to the G_s and G_i heterotrimeric complexes, there are G_q and G_o complexes that are coupled to phospholipid/Ca^{2+} and brain-specific pathways of signal transduction, respectively. Specific G protein isotypes exist in the retina (G_t) and the olfactory epithelium (G_{olf}). Sixteen or more isotypes of G_α and at least 16 isotypes of the G_β (5) and G_γ (8) subunit have been identified by sequencing of cloned recombinant cDNAs.[13] Many of the primary transcripts derived from the subunit genes are alternatively spliced, resulting in the formation of mRNAs that encode yet additional isoforms of the subunit proteins.[13] The precise functions of most of the large number of G protein subunit isoforms are unknown because, at present, they are proteins identified only by recombinant DNA cloning technology; investigators are in search of their cellular functions.

G Protein Cycle

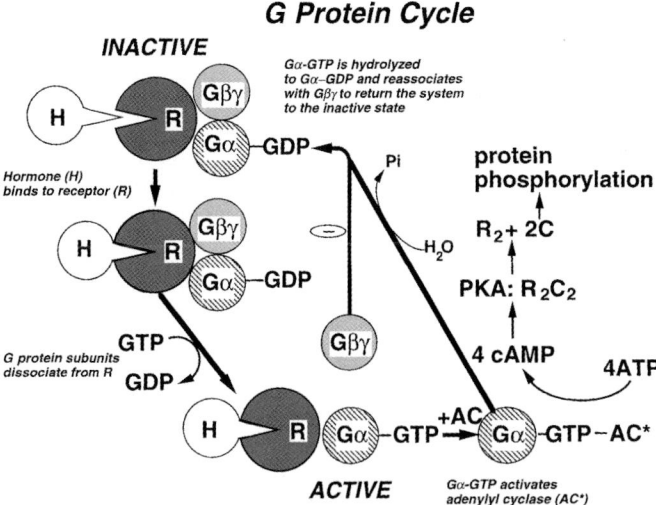

Figure 12-3   The guanine nucleotide-binding protein (G protein) cycle. The diagram is a more detailed depiction of the G protein function shown in Figure 12-2. The G_α subunit can be either stimulatory ($G_{\alpha s}$) or inhibitory ($G_{\alpha i}$), depending on the isotype of the subunit involved. The activated G_α-GTP complex modulates the activity of adenylyl cyclase leading to the activation of protein kinase A and the resultant phosphorylation of key protein substrates that manifest the cellular response. G_α-GTP is inactivated by hydrolysis of GTP to GDP by the intrinsic GTPase activities of the G_α subunit.

An additional important function, however, of the class of G proteins that has been shown to couple to receptors is to regulate ion channels. G_s directly modulates the activity of voltage-dependent calcium channels, and evidence has been presented supporting a role for the pertussis-sensitive G_i and G_o in the coupling of receptors of a variety of hormones and neurotransmitters to potassium and calcium channels,[50] resulting in either stimulatory or inhibitory control, depending on the type of channel affected.[51,52] Further, the receptor-coupled and channel-coupled G proteins represent merely a subfamily of a much larger family of GTP-binding proteins involved in such diverse functions as the control of protein synthesis, for example, elongation factor (EF-Tu), protein translocation across membranes, and ADP ribosylation factors (ARFs).[41] In addition, there exists an entire complex family of small GTP-binding proteins known as the Ras proteins involved in growth and differentiation, regulation of adenylyl cyclase, vesicular transport, and many other functions that have yet to be defined.[41]

Genetic mutations in $G_s\alpha$ (GNAS1) manifest in a variety of human endocrine diseases, as a consequence of loss-of-function of the actions of $G_s\alpha$.[53,54] Over 40 loss-of-function mutations have been identified that contribute predominantly to phenotypes of pseudohypoparathyroidism, so-called Albright heredity osteodystrophy, in which there exists a resistance to the actions of parathyroid hormone. Such mutations in $G_s\alpha$ may also impair the actions of hormones other than parathyroid hormone, such as thyrotropin-stimulating hormone and gonadotropin-stimulating hormones, indicating that loss-of-function mutations in $G_s\alpha$ contribute to complex trait, polygenic disorders, as well as monogenic disease. Mutations in GNAS1 that result in gain-of-function known as gsp (G_s protein) oncogenic mutations, also occur and are less frequent than loss-of-function mutations. These mutations, resulting in constitutive overactivity of cAMP signaling, lead to neoplasia of endocrine organs, such as pituitary, thyroid, and adrenal adenomas, Leydig cell tumors of the ovary, and the McCune-Albright syndrome that affects functions not only of endocrine glands (gonads, pituitary, thyroid, adrenal cortex) but also melanocytes (café-au-lait hyperpigmentation) and bone (polyostotic fibrous dysplasia). Screening studies indicate that 30% to 40% of growth hormone secreting adenomas harbor gsp mutations, the most common of which is a cysteine for arginine substitution at amino acid 201 of $G_s\alpha$. The variable disease phenotypes associated with mutations in $G_s\alpha$ is because they are somatic and not germ-line mutations occurring as an early postzygotic event. The time of occurrence of the mutations in GNAS1 determines the nature and extent of disease. Late occurring mutations result in focal disease, such as pituitary or thyroid adenomas, whereas very early mutations manifest in more widespread disease such as McCune-Albright syndrome. It is curious that given the ubiquitous presence of $G_s\alpha$ and $G_s\alpha$-coupled receptors throughout all organs of the body, mutations in them are overwhelmingly reflected in endocrine and neuroendocrine organs. Such a circumstance may indicate that cAMP signaling has evolved to be particularly critical in the development and regulation of endocrine systems.

THE ADENYLYL CYCLASES

The adenylyl cyclases consist of a diverse family of membrane-associated enzymes of which at least nine distinct isotypes have been identified.[55–57] The distribution of the various enzyme isotypes amongst different tissues is highly variable. Most tissues contain several different isotypes, but in many tissues, one or more of the isotypes are absent.

The structures of the adenylyl cyclases are remarkable inasmuch as they consist of two alternating hydrophobic and hydrophilic domains (Fig. 12-4).[55,58] The hydrophobic

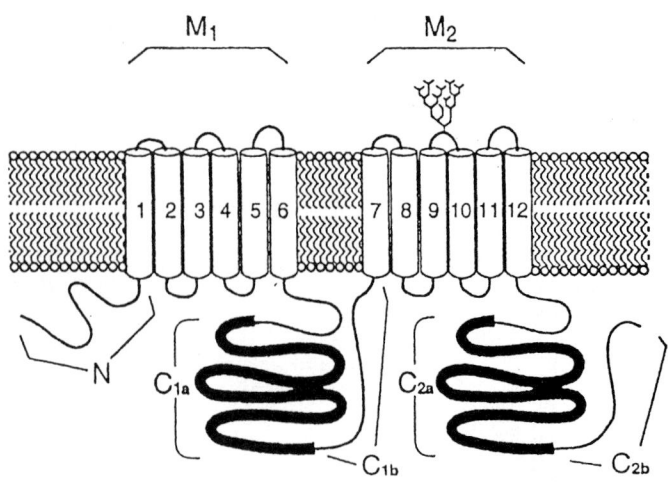

Figure 12-4 Diagram of the cellular location and orientation of adenylyl cyclase predicted from its primary amino acid sequence. The cyclase contains two symmetrical regions that span the plasma membrane six times (M_1 and M_2). Two large cytoplasmic loops (C_{1a} / C_{1b} and C_{2a} and C_{2b}) share sequence similarities with guanylyl cyclase (black).

domains contain six membrane-spanning domains, and the cytoplasmic hydrophilic domains each contain 250 residues that are homologous to the putative catalytic domains of the guanylyl cyclases. This overall structure of adenylyl cyclase is similar to those of the glucose transporters and to the P glycoprotein, the product of the multi-drug resistance gene. This structure suggests that, in addition to its catalytic function of converting ATP to cAMP, the enzyme serves as the transporter that exports cAMP from the cell. The disposal of cAMP appears to involve two mechanisms: degradation by phosphodiesterase in the cell and transport out of the cell. Both mechanisms may, in turn, be regulated as a means for titrating the amount of cAMP available in the cell during the time that the catalytic activity of the enzyme is turned on by the active G protein, G_α-GTP. The differences in functions of the various isoforms of the adenylyl cyclases have not yet been completely determined. However, it is now appreciated that most, if not all, of the nine different adenylyl cyclases are multiply regulated.[59] Both Ca^{2+} and the phospholipase C signaling pathways are implicated in the regulation of adenylyl cyclase activities.[55,59] For example, Ca^{2+} calmodulin kinases II and IV inhibit the adenylyl cyclases types III and I, respectively. Ca^{2+} calmodulin activates type II adenylyl cyclase.[55] In general, Mn^{2+} activates and Ca^{2+} inhibits activities of all the adenylyl cyclase isotypes. The G protein subunits also regulate the adenylyl cyclases. $G_s\alpha$ activates all isotypes (I–IX), whereas Giα inhibits specifically isotypes V and VI. Gβγ activates several of the adenylyl cyclases, but is relatively specific for activating the type II isotype.

A relatively new concept has arisen regarding the cellular compartmentalization of the components involved in cAMP signaling. The activation of cAMP signaling by a ligand binding to a G protein–coupled receptor does not flood the entire cytoplasm of the cell with cAMP. Rather, the molecules involved in signal transduction are located in distinct intracellular compartments, such as specialized plasma membrane-derived vesicles, known as caveoli or "lipid rafts." Upon exposure to a ligand, G protein–coupled receptors coalesce in the plasma membrane in association with G proteins, adenylyl cyclase, and other receptor regulators, such as A-kinase anchoring proteins, form a localized signal transduction complex. The reader is referred to an excellent review describing the compartmentalization of the adenylyl cyclases.[56] The cAMP signaling pathway is spatially segregated and oriented in cells in response to the initiation of signaling by extracellular receptor ligands.

STRUCTURES OF THE R AND C SUBUNITS OF PROTEIN KINASE A

The heterotetrameric complex that constitutes the holoenzyme of PKA consists of two catalytic and two regulatory subunits.[6-8,60] Thus far, three isotypes have been identified for the catalytic subunit (C_α, C_β, C_γ), apparent molecular weights (Mr) = 40,800, and two types for the regulatory subunit (RI, RII), each of which has two isotypes (RI_α, RI_β, RII_α, RII_β), Mrs of 92,000–108,000 (Table 12-1). The sequences of both the catalytic and the regulatory subunits are highly conserved. For example, the amino acid sequences of C_α and C_β are 93% identical. The C_γ subunit is somewhat less well conserved; 79% and 83% identical to C_α and C_β, respectively.[7] Conservation of the sequences among the four regulatory subunits is, likewise, quite high. As discussed later in more detail, certain of the various types and isotypes of subunits have distinct subcellular distributions and functions.

THE CATALYTIC SUBUNITS

The catalytic subunit contains a region that is highly conserved in the catalytic core of many different protein kinases. This region contains several motifs involved in ATP-binding, substrate recognition, and phosphotransfer (Fig. 12-5). The structure of C_α has been partially solved by x-ray crystallography both with and without a bound pseudosubstrate, so that the relevant contacts between ATP, Mg^{2+}, and substrate are relatively well understood.[61,62]

The ATP-binding fold resides in the amino-terminal region and contains a glycine loop motif GXGXXG followed carboxy proximal by a lysine (K-72) and an acidic residue, glutamic acid (E-91), common to a variety of proteins that bind nucleotides. The glycine loop, lysine-72, glutamic acid-91, and aspartic acid-184 are all involved in the coordinate binding of Mg^{2+}-ATP. For reasons yet unknown, Mg^{2+}-ATP binds more tightly to the catalytic subunit when complexed with the type I, as opposed to the type II, regulatory subunit.

The catalytic subunit of PKA phosphorylates serines or threonines in protein substrates when the serine or threonine is located in a motif RRXS/TY (where X and Y are usually hydrophobic amino acids) that is accessible to the kinase on the surface of the protein substrate. The catalytic subunit can also bind to (but cannot phosphorylate) pseudosubstrate motifs in which the serine or threonine are replaced by any other amino acid. Both phosphorylatable (RII) substrates and pseudosubstrates (RI) are present in the regulatory subunits and serve as so-called autoinhibitory domains (see Fig. 12-5 and Table 12-2).[63] In addition to the regulatory subunits, the catalytic subunits can be inhibited by endogenous cellular proteins known as protein kinase inhibitors (PKIs). At least four isoforms of PKIs have been cloned from skeletal muscle and testis, all of which contain a pseudosubstrate site for interaction with the catalytic subunits of PKA.[64] The PKIs are described in more detail later in this chapter.

The substrate recognition domain overlaps the Mg^{2+} ATP-binding and R subunit-binding regions and appears to consist of a hydrophobic pocket in which key acidic residues such as glutamic acids-170, -322, and -346, (E-170, E-322, E-346) form

Subunits of Protein Kinase-A

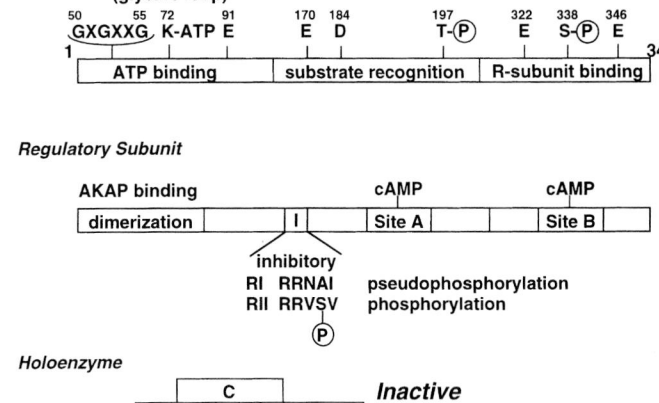

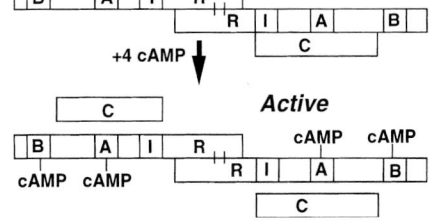

Figure 12-5 Diagrammatic representations of the catalytic and regulatory subunits of protein kinase A. Shown are the catalytic subunit (*upper*), regulatory subunit (*middle*), and the holoenzyme (*lower*) consisting of the heterotetrameric complex of catalytic and regulatory subunits (*lower*). The holoenzyme is depicted in both the inactive, fully complexed form, and the active, dissociated form. As is described in detail in the text, the catalytic subunit consists of three (overlapping) domains responsible for the binding of mg^{2+}-ATP, recognition of and binding to substrate, and binding to dimerization with the regulatory (R) subunit. The regulatory subunits consist of dimerization domains that also function as sites for binding to anchoring proteins (AKAPs), domains that serve as inhibitory domains, and two cAMP-binding sites designated as sites A and B.

ionic interactions with one of the arginines in the substrate recognition motif RRXS/TY. Threonine-197 is phosphorylated and the negatively charged phosphothreonine seems to likewise potentiate interaction with the positively charged arginines in substrate recognition motifs. The R subunit-binding domain is not yet clearly delineated but appears to involve the carboxyl-terminal region of the catalytic subunit, as well as an inhibitory region. The catalytic subunits undergo at least two types of posttranslational modifications, phosphorylations[65] and myristylation[66] at the amino terminus, the functional consequences of which are entirely unknown.

THE REGULATORY SUBUNITS

The structures of the regulatory subunits are highly asymmetrical proteins of apparent Mrs ranging from 92,000 to 108,000 and consist of functionally distinct domains (see Fig. 12-5). The amino-terminal domain is responsible for protein-protein interactions, that is, dimerization of the two R subunits, binding to the catalytic subunit, and binding to anchoring proteins that target the inactive holoenzyme to specific subcellular locations. The carboxyl-terminal domain consists of two tandem repeated sequences that bind cAMP and thereby allosterically regulate the affinity of association of the R with the C subunit (see following discussion).

The two regulatory subunits form antiparallel dimers through binding interactions at the amino-terminal regions

Table 12-1	Cyclic Adenosine Monophosphate-Dependent Protein Kinase A Heterotetrameric Complex
Subunits	2 Regulatory (R)
	2 Catalytic (C)
Isoforms	R: RI_α, RI_β, RII_α, RII_β
	C: C_α, C_β, C_γ

Table 12-2   Pseudosubstrate and Autoinhibitor Sequences in Protein Kinase A

							R	G	A	I	S		A	E	V
atRI$_\alpha$	K	G	R	R	—	R	R	G	A	I	S		A	E	V
RI$_\beta$	K	A	R	R	—	R	R	G	C	V	S		A	E	V
RII$_\alpha$	P	G	R	F	D	R	R	V	S*	V	C		A	E	T
RII$_\beta$	I	N	R	F	T	R	R	A	S*	V	C		A	E	A
PKI	S	G	R	T	G	R	R	N	A	I	H		D	I	L
Consensus	X	X	R	X	X	R	R	R	X	X	X	X	A	E	X
Phosphorylation motif							R	R	X		S*/T*	Y			

*Serines or threonines phosphorylated by protein kinase A.
PKI, protein kinase inhibitor.

of the promoters. The RI subunits are covalently crosslinked by two disulfide linkages between cysteines, Cys16 and Cys37. Dimerization of the RII subunits, however, does not involve covalent linkages. Rather, the dimerization of RII involves strong noncovalent interactions of β-sheetlike secondary structure contained within the first 30 amino acids of the RII subunits. The contrast in the biochemical mechanisms of dimer formation between RI and RII subunits may reflect important differences in the biologic functions of the RI and RII subunit isotypes. The type II regulatory subunit differs from the type I subunit in several respects. The autophosphorylation of RII by the catalytic subunits facilitates its release from the catalytic subunit. The phosphorylated type II holoenzyme dissociates at a lower concentration of cAMP than dephosphorylated holoenzyme. Unlike RI, RII is located in particulate fractions of cells and readily binds to membrane-located anchoring proteins, A kinase anchoring proteins.[7,67-69] In addition, RII associates much more tightly with the catalytic subunits compared with RI, and much higher concentrations of cAMP are required to effect the allosteric change in conformation necessary to release the catalytic from the regulatory subunits.

In addition to the "autophosphorylation" of the type II regulatory subunit by the catalytic subunit of PKA, both the type I and II regulatory subunits are phosphorylated by protein kinases other than PKA. The biologic relevance, however, of the phosphorylations is unknown. RI$_\alpha$ is phosphorylated by cyclic guanosine monophosphate (cGMP)-dependent protein kinase, but requires the presence of cAMP. Both isotypes of the RII subunit (RII$_\alpha$ and RII$_\beta$) are phosphorylated by the synergistic actions of the processive protein kinases, glycogen synthase kinase-3 and casein kinase II (CK II).[70] Although the functional significance of these multiple phosphorylations is unclear, it seems certain that they represent important posttranslational modifications of the subunits that, in some way, alter their biologic functions.

ALLOSTERIC REGULATION OF THE ACTIVATION OF PKA BY cAMP

Each regulatory subunit monomer contains two high affinity cAMP-binding sites, termed A and B, located in the carboxyl-terminal region of the subunit.[7,8] The domain A and B regions share sequence similarities and probably arose by gene duplications. Analyses of the kinetics of dissociation of the catalytic subunit from the regulatory subunit in response to cAMP indicate that the binding of cAMP to sites A and B of the holoenzyme shows positive cooperativeness. cAMP first binds to site B on the regulatory subunit leading to a partial conformational change in R that loosens its association with C, rendering site A more accessible for binding of a second molecule of cAMP. Occupancy of both sites A and B by cAMP results in the complete dissociation of the catalytic subunits from the heterotetrameric enzyme complex.

The A and B sites have different exchange rates for cAMP: Site A has a faster rate of cAMP dissociation than does site B.

Further, sites A and B have different binding preferences for cAMP analogues. Site A preferentially binds N-6 and C-6 substituted cAMP analogues, such as dibutryl cAMP, whereas site B prefers C-8 substituted analogues such as 8-bromo-cAMP or 8-chlorophenylthio-cAMP.[71] In addition, there are differences in the preferential selectivities of cAMP analogues between the type I and type II regulatory subunits.[71] Certain of the analogues bind more tightly to sites A or B of RI than RII and vice versa. These differences in the relative potencies and selectivities of cAMP analogues for RI versus RII further indicate that the biologic roles of the subunits must differ significantly.

Two particularly useful analogues of cAMP have been developed, of which one is an agonist (Sp-cAMP) and the other an antagonist (Rp-cAMP) for the activation of PKA.[72] The analogues contain alterations of the two exocyclic oxygens. The two chiral isomers of 3',5'-monophosphothioate contain sulfur at either the equatorial (Rp) or axial (Sp) position. Rp-cAMP is the first bona fide cAMP antagonist, and its actions can be compared directly with the Sp-cAMP agonist.

FUNCTIONS OF THE ISOTYPES OF R AND C SUBUNITS OF PKA

As discussed earlier, compared with the extensive complexities of the isotypes of the G proteins and adenylyl cyclases, the isoforms of the PKA subunits appear to be relatively limited in numbers. There are two major types of regulatory subunits, RI and RII, each of which has two subtypes: RI$_\alpha$, RI$_\beta$, RII$_\alpha$, and RII$_\beta$. Three isotypes of the catalytic subunit have been identified so far: C$_\alpha$, C$_\beta$, and C$_\gamma$. The differences in functions of the various isotypes of the subunits are not fully understood. Their relative expression, however, appears to depend on the type of tissue involved, and they differ in their distributions among different subcellular compartments. In general, the α isotypes RI$_\alpha$, RII$_\alpha$, and C$_\alpha$ are expressed uniformly in a wide variety of tissues, whereas the expression of the β isotypes RI$_\beta$, RII$_\beta$, and C$_\beta$ is more restricted to brain and neuroendocrine and endocrine tissues.[7] The RI$_\alpha$ and RI$_\beta$ subunits are located in the cytoplasm and soluble fractions of broken cell preparations in contrast to RII$_\alpha$ and RII$_\beta$, which are in the particulate, membranous fraction. A substantial fraction of RII$_\beta$ has been localized to the nucleus and perinuclear regions, suggesting a special role for this subunit in the targeting of the associated catalytic subunit close to substrate sites for phosphorylation in the nucleus.[73]

In particular, the RII subunits associate with high affinities with A-kinase anchoring proteins that are located at specific sites within the cell and are proposed to target the PKA holoenzyme to specific subcellular locations by binding to the RII subunits.[74,75] No distinctions have been made between the substrate recognition properties or actions of C$_\alpha$ and C$_\beta$. However, C$_\gamma$ apparently has a higher affinity for histone than for kemptide, LRRASLG, the high-affinity standard substrate for phosphorylation by C$_\alpha$ and C$_\beta$.[76] Further, the activity of C$_\gamma$ is not inhibited by the protein kinase inhibitor peptide (5-24amide), which is widely used as a PKA-specific inhibitor. The expression of C_γ appears to be restricted to the testis, from which a unique testis inhibitor isoform has been cloned.[77] It is possible that C_γ may have novel kinase activities distinct from those of C_α and C_β, and that by analogy subtle differences in functions of C_α and C_β exist also, but have not yet been discovered. For example, certain A-kinase anchoring proteins target PKA next to ion channels to facilitate phosphorylation and modulation of various ion channels.[78]

REGULATION OF SUBUNIT GENE EXPRESSION, STABILITY, TRANSLOCATION, AND REASSOCIATION

The complexities of the interactions, regulation, and even autoregulation of the expression of the subunits of PKA are only now beginning to be understood. The regulation of the expression of many of the subunits in a specific phenotype of cell under a certain circumstance can involve changes in gene transcription, RNA processing and export from the nucleus, mRNA stability, translocation, and protein stability. In spite of the complexities of the regulation some generalizations can be made. First, free subunits are less stable than the subunits in the intact holoenzyme complex, that is, the free subunits are more susceptible to proteolysis compared to the bound subunits. Second, the type II regulatory subunit (RII) binds catalytic subunits more tightly than does RI. Higher cellular levels of cAMP are required to dissociate RII from C than RI from C. Thus, at relatively low levels of cAMP, RI will preferentially dissociate and be susceptible to degradation. Third, in certain cells, such as Sertoli cells of the testis, sustained high levels of cAMP increases RII_β subunit by increasing the half-lives of both RII_β mRNA and protein, whereas mRNAs for RI_α, RII_α, and C_α are increased only twofold to fourfold.[79] Fourth, it is likely that the induction of mRNA for certain of the subunits, for example, RI_α, involves increased gene transcription mediated by activation of cAMP-responsive transcription factors, such as CREB, whose transcriptional transactivational activity is stimulated by phosphorylation by C_α or C_β (discussed later). PhosphoCREB stimulates the transcription of many genes by binding to cAMP response elements located in their promoters.[34,36,80]

Increased RII_β can serve as a "trap" to inactivate C. For example, overexpression of C_α programmed by an expression plasmid transfected into rat pheochromocytoma cells results in a 50-fold enhanced stimulation of a cotransfected reporter plasmid consisting of the vasoactive intestinal peptide promoter containing a cAMP-response element and the chloramphenicol acetyltransferase gene.[81] Cotransfection, however, with an expression plasmid encoding the RII_β subunit, inhibits stimulation by the C_α subunit to 10% of control levels.[81] Because RII_β associates more tightly to C subunits than does RI_α or RI_β, all free C subunits will be complexed with RII_β, resulting in the liberation of RI subunits, which are then degraded. Thus, increased RII_β levels not only lower levels of C subunits but also lower levels of RI subunits.

Paradoxically, in some circumstances, RII_β can also stimulate or restore cAMP-dependent gene transcription.[82] The cAMP-unresponsive pheochromocytoma cell line, A126-1B2, is incapable of activating a transfected somatostatin gene promoter containing a cAMP response element. However, cotransfection of a vector expressing the RII_β, but not RII_α or RI_α, subunit restores cAMP responsivity of the transcription driven by the somatostatin gene promoter. Although the role of RII_β in the restoration of cAMP-responsive transcription is unknown, it is possible that RII_β may target the catalytic subunit in a holoenzyme complex to the nucleus or to a perinuclear location.[73] Activation of PKA by cAMP releases catalytic subunit, which phosphorylates and activates nuclear transcription factor CREB. Localization of RII to the perinuclear Golgi apparatus has been demonstrated by immunocytochemical techniques.[73] It seems unlikely that RII has a direct role in the activation of transcription, but

such a possibility cannot be totally discarded. Evidence has been presented that RII can bind to cAMP-response elements.[83]

The type I regulatory subunit of PKA can also inhibit the transcription of cAMP responsive genes.[84] Several liver-specific genes are transcriptionally regulated by cAMP-dependent mechanisms likely involving CREBs. In the course of carrying out studies of cell fusions between hepatocytes and fibroblasts, extinction of the transcription of the hepatic genes was observed.[84] By genetic and recombinant DNA approaches, the gene encoding the tissue specific extinguisher was isolated and shown to be RI_α.[84] Further analyses revealed that in hepatic cells RI_α levels are unusually low but are at normal levels in most other tissues, including fibroblasts. Thus, fusion of fibroblasts to hepatocytes introduced RI_α into the hepatocyte, thereby binding C subunit and preventing phosphorylation of CREBs necessary for the activation of the transcription of the liver-specific genes. It appears that the regulation of both the translocation and the activities of the PKA subunit isotypes play a major role in the cAMP-dependent signal transduction pathway.

THE PROTEIN KINASE INHIBITORS

In addition to the inhibitory actions of the regulatory subunits, the catalytic subunits are also inhibited by the actions of a family of endogenous cellular proteins, distinct in structure from the regulatory subunits, known as PKIs. The PKIs are increasingly recognized as important components in the regulation of the cAMP-signaling pathway. The PKIs are unique novel molecules inasmuch as they are small 71–76 amino acids resembling peptide ligands, and inhibit cAMP signaling by at least two mechanisms: direct pseudosubstrate inhibition, a mechanism similar to that of the $RI\alpha$ and β subunits, and by the active export of catalytic subunit (C) from the nucleus to the cytoplasm.

The PKI inhibitory activity was first reported in 1965 as a heat stabile, protease-sensitive component of rabbit skeletal muscle extracts.[85] Subsequently, the cloning and structural characterization revealed at least three isoforms of PKI: $PKI\alpha$, $PKI\beta1$, and $PKI\gamma$.[86] The α, β, and γ isoforms are encoded by separate genes in the mouse. The evolutionary duplication and maintenance of the expression of different isoforms of PKI attest to the potential importance of their functions in cellular metabolism.

The tissue distributions of the three PKI isoforms are quite different. At the mRNA level, $PKI\alpha$ is expressed predominantly in brain, heart, and skeletal muscle. $PKI\beta$ expression is mostly restricted to testis, and $PKI\gamma$ is widely expressed at relatively high levels in all tissues tested. $PKI\gamma$ was discovered only recently.[86] Before the discovery of $PKI\gamma$, it was estimated that the amount of $PKI\alpha$ in the heart was only sufficient to inhibit 20% of total C subunits.[87] The contribution of the newly discovered widely distributed γ isoform of PKI can now account for inhibition of approximately 50% of C subunits.

Structural-functional studies of the PKIs have established two distinct mechanisms by which they inhibit the steps in the cAMP-signaling pathway. A pseudosubstrate domain, consisting of the sequence RTGRRNA, is located at residues 16–23 in the amino-terminal region of the PKIs and a demonstrated nuclear export signal sequence (NES) L-XL-XXL-XHy is highly conserved at residues 37–49 (Fig. 12-6).[88,89]

The pseudosubstrate and NES domains act together in the attenuation phase of the burst-attenuation kinetics of cAMP signaling responses within cells and the partitioning of C between the cytoplasm and the nucleus. Upon activation of a cell, such as by a ligand binding to a cAMP-coupled receptor, the catalytic subunit (C) is released from the inhibitory regulatory subunit (R; burst phase). Although the C subunit is 40 kilodaltons, just at the upper size limit required to pass through nuclear pores, it is generally believed that after

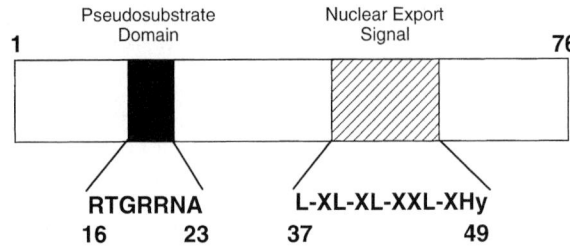

Figure 12-6 Diagram of a protein kinase A inhibitor showing locations of the two known functional domains, pseudosubstrate and nuclear export signal. Numbers indicate amino acid sequence positions. The amino acids are given in the single letter designations; X, any amino acid; Hy, a hydrophobic amino acid.

release from R, C can passively diffuse into the nucleus where it phosphorylates and activates transcription factors, such as CREB, specifically stimulating gene transcription.[90] PKI is freely capable of entering the nucleus where it tethers to C via its pseudosubstrate domain forming a C:PKI complex. The NES domain of PKI is then activated by ATP and a temperature-dependent mechanism[91] involving the formation of a complex among PKI, C, and the proteins CRM1[92] (exportin) and Ran.[93] This results in the shuttling of C:PKI out of the nucleus back into the cytoplasm where GTPase-activating proteins bind and stimulate the hydrolysis of Ran-bound GTP causing the complex to dissociate. Then C recombines with R subunits to form inactive holoenzyme and to restore cAMP regulation to the cell. Thus, with respect to its nuclear functions, the burst of cAMP signaling activity within the nucleus is attenuated by the export of C subunit back into the cytoplasm. Further attenuation of the nuclear cAMP response is accomplished by phosphatases that dephosphorylate CREB and other cAMP-responsive transcription factors (Fig. 12-7).

Notably, the NES is not essential per se for the inhibition of cAMP-mediated gene expression. In experiments in which C subunit was epitope-tagged and transfected to cells, C distributed evenly between cytoplasm and nucleus. Cotransfection of either PKI or R subunit inhibited nuclear localization and gene expression. A mutated PKI lacking the NES still inhibited gene expression but not the nuclear accumulation of C, indicating that the NES and nuclear export is not essential for inhibition of gene expression. These findings suggest that the function of the NES to export C subunit out of the nucleus back into the cytoplasm may not be so much to inhibit C activity but rather to recycle C back into holoen-

zyme in the cytoplasm. By this means, C is available to phosphorylate cytoplasmic as well as nuclear proteins upon the initiation of another cycle of cAMP signaling.

At least two isoforms of PKI β-70 have been identified: PKI β-78 and PKI β-105. The 78 amino acid PKI arises by the usage of an alternative translational initiation site and the 105 amino acid isoform is a result of alternative RNA splicing. Of note, the PKI β-105 is a dual specificity PKI isoform that inhibits both cAMP-dependent protein kinase (PKA) and cGMP-dependent protein kinase (PKG).[94] Mice with germ-line disruptions in the PK1α or PKIβ genes, or both genes (double knockout) are viable, fertile, and without obvious physiologic defects.[95] PKIs are involved in embryo development in organizing left-right axis formation,[96] inhibition of pancreatic cancer cell growth,[97] and the inhibition of long-lasting synaptic potentiation in hippacampal neurons.[98]

CROSS-TALK OF cAMP WITH OTHER SIGNALING PATHWAYS

The cAMP-dependent signaling pathway is frequently coupled to, and works in concert with, other cellular signaling pathways.[99,100] Such pathways include: (1) the phospholipase C-mediated production of the second messengers diacylglycerol and inositol trisphosphate that activate protein kinase C and intracellular receptors responsible for the mobilization of ionic calcium from intracellular stores, respectively[101,102]; (2) the calcium-calmodulin kinases[103]; and (3) the receptor tyrosine-kinases that include the insulin, epidermal growth factor, insulin-like growth factor, and platelet-derived growth factor receptors,[104,105] among others.[106,107]

Cross-talk among the different signaling pathways can occur by at least two mechanisms involving either intermolecular or intramolecular phosphorylation cascades. A classic example of an intermolecular cascade is the activation of an isoform of type II PKA in which the catalytic subunit "autophosphorylates" the regulatory subunit and thereby is at least partially responsible for the activation of the catalytic subunit (discussed later). Active PKA then phosphorylates and activates phosphorylase kinase, which in turn phosphorylates and activates glycogen phosphorylase, the key enzyme in converting glycogen to glucose-1-phosphate. Intramolecular phosphorylation cascades involve multisite and hierarchical protein phosphorylation by the participation of several so-called "processive" kinases that act synergistically with other kinases by successive phosphorylations of closely adjacent sites on the same protein.[70,108] For example, glycogen synthase is regulated (inactivated) by such a cascade in which an initial phosphory-

Figure 12-7 Schematic diagram of a cell showing cycling of protein kinase A inhibitor (PKI) and catalytic subunit of PKA (C), between cytoplasm and nucleus. PKI and C enter the nucleus by passive diffusion and form an inhibitory complex along with Ran and CRM1, preventing phosphorylation (P) and activation of cAMP response element binding protein (CREB). The PKI/C/Ran/CRM1 complex is actively exported out of the nucleus to the cytoplasm. Such export is dependent on the presence of the nuclear export signal in PKI (see Fig. 12-6). After reentering the cytoplasm, PKI is liberated from the complex by the actions of GTPase on Ran, thereby allowing PKI to enter the nucleus and begin another cycle of translocation.

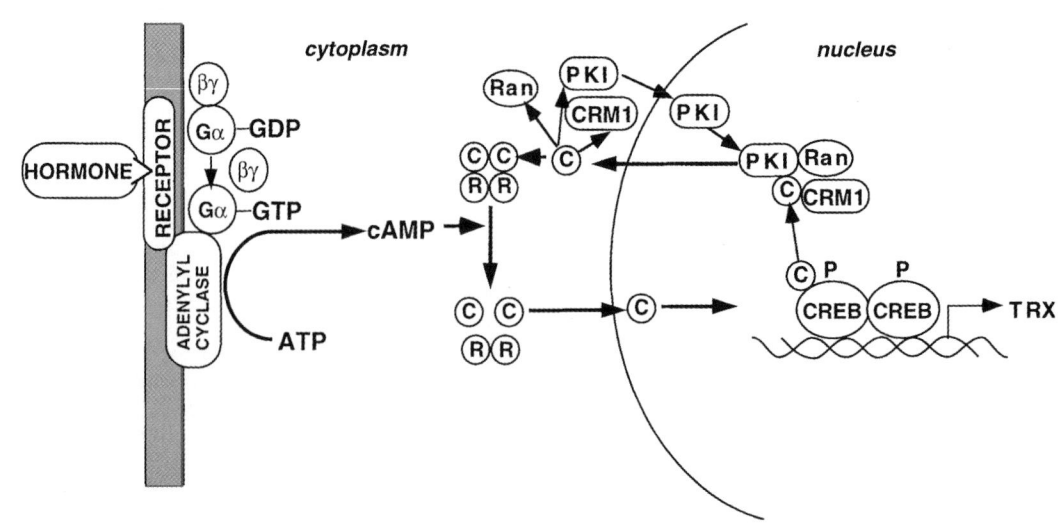

lation by PKA (the primary kinase) is required for phosphorylation on a close-by serine or threonine by casein kinase isotype I. CK I and CK II preferentially phosphorylate serines or threonines in proteins that contain acidic amino acids within two to three residues amino-proximal (CK I) or carboxy-proximal (CK II) to the serine or threonine that is phosphorylated. The phosphorylation of a serine, threonine (or tyrosine) converts a neutral or hydrophobic amino acid to a negatively charged amino acid because of the highly negative charge imparted by the phosphate. To fully inactivate glycogen synthase, yet another intramolecular processive phosphorylation by CK II, followed by a secondary phosphorylation by glycogen synthase kinase-3 is required.[109] The intricacies of the signaling pathways involved in the activation of these multiple kinases are not fully understood. However, a potent activator of CK II is the activated (ligand-bound) epidermal growth factor-receptor kinase, a finding pointing to a cross-talk of signaling pathways between a receptor-tyrosine kinase and cAMP-dependent protein kinase.[110]

The actions of cAMP on cellular proliferation and differentiation have been controversial.[16,111] In some cell culture systems, cAMP signaling inhibits proliferation and promotes differentiation.[112] In other types of cells, cAMP stimulates proliferation.[113] Although the mechanisms involved in the control of cell proliferation and differentiation are highly complex, the mitogen-activated protein kinase (MAPK) signaling pathway is generally believed to be a critical determinant in governing the cell division cycle.[114] Activation of the MAPK pathway promotes cellular proliferation and conversely, inhibition of the MAPK pathway slows down or arrests proliferation. The MAPK pathway consists of a wide variety of factors that are only partially understood. A working model of this complex MAPK pathway includes in order of signaling: a growth factor ligand, a receptor (typically a tyrosine kinase receptor), guanine nucleotide-binding protein (Ras), a MAP kinase kinase kinase (Raf), a MAP kinase kinase, MAP kinase, and a transcription factor (Fos, Myc, CREB) that activates the promoter of genes involved in the control of the cell division cycle.[115,116] Until recently, the reasons for these differing actions of cAMP signaling amongst different cell types cultured in different environments of growth factors have been largely unknown.

It now appears likely that cAMP signaling "cross-talks" with the MAPK signaling pathway by at least two distinct mechanisms: one mechanism inhibits and another mechanism stimulates the MAPK pathway (Fig. 12-8). Both the inhibitory and activatory cAMP signaling act on Ras in the MAPK pathway, although by quite different mechanisms. Phosphorylation of Raf-1 by PKA inhibits its translocation and consequent activation by Ras.[112] In contrast, PKA is not involved in the activation of MAPK signaling. Rather, cAMP binds to and activates a cAMP-regulated guanine nucleotide exchange factor (cAMP-GEF).[117] Ras is a member of an extensive family of so-called small G proteins that serve as signal switches early in the MAPK and other signaling pathways.[118–121] In the GTP-bound form Ras is active and in the GDP form it is inactive. GEFs including cAMP-GEF convert GDP to GTP on Ras and thusly activate Ras. Ras is then inactivated by the actions of GTPases.[122]

The discovery of cAMP-GEFs was made only recently.[117] Two distinct gene products have been identified and there likely are many more awaiting their discovery. Notably, there are also GEFs with binding sites for diacylglycerol and for calcium.[117,123] Thus, at least three major second messenger systems (cAMP, diacylglycerol, and calcium) are coupled to Ras and Ras-like protein signaling, thereby providing direct mechanisms for transducing second messenger input to GEF output. The kinase-independent actions of cAMP are further discussed in the following section.

KINASE-INDEPENDENT CELLULAR ACTIONS OF cAMP

cAMP-REGULATED GUANINE NUCLEOTIDE EXCHANGE FACTORS

cAMP-GEFs, also known as exchange protein activated by cAMP (EPAC), are nonkinase effectors of cAMP signaling that activate the small Ras-like GTPases Rap1 and Rap2, and also interact with other proteins, described in the next section.[28,124] There are currently two known related isoforms of EPAC: EPAC 1 and EPAC 2. EPAC 1 has a single cAMP-binding domain whereas EPAC 2 has a second, N-terminal, domain and also a Ras-association domain.[28] The activation of Rap by

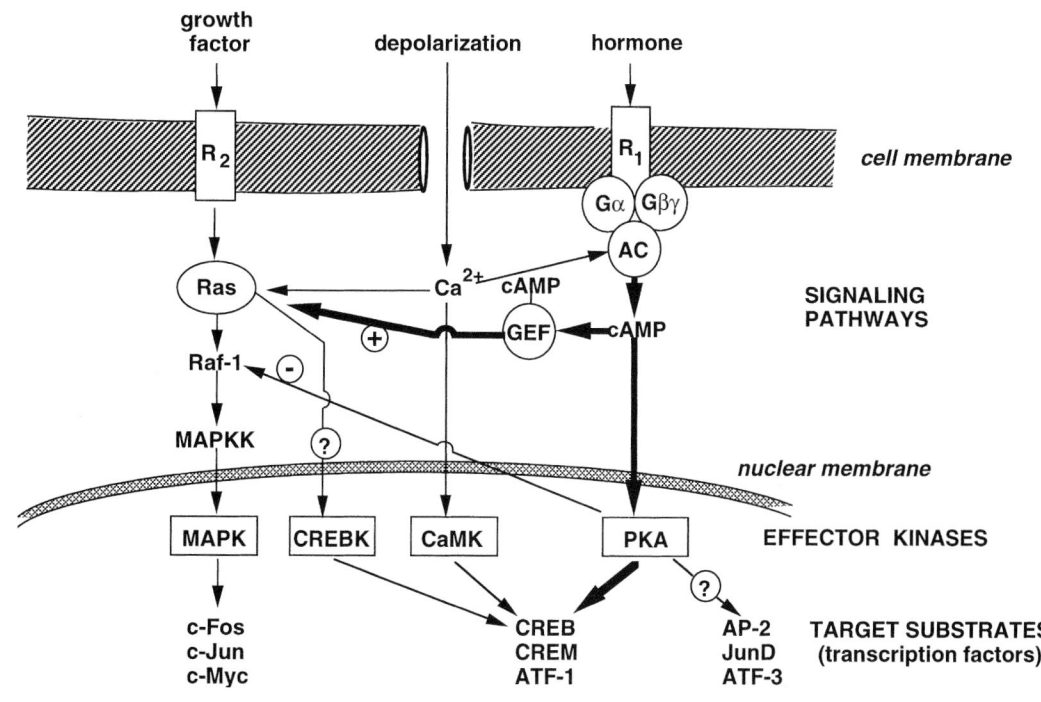

Figure 12-8 Model diagram depicting the newly discovered potential signal transduction pathway by which cAMP not only activates protein kinase A (PKA), but also binds to the cAMP family of guanine nucleotide exchange factor proteins (GEF) and thereby activates Ras-like proteins in the mitogen activated pathways (MAP). Thus, the cAMP signaling pathway is more versatile than previously considered. Activation by cAMP of PKA leads to cellular differentiation, whereas activation of cAMP binding proteins, such as GEFs, leads to the stimulation of cell proliferation.

EPAC is well-established but the downstream signaling remains controversial. Some studies suggest that Rap activates B-Raf and the MEK/Erk pathway[124] whereas others, using the EPAC-specific cAMP analogue, 8-(4-chloro-phenylthio)-2′-O-methyl adenosine-3′-5′-cyclic monophosphate (8-pCPT-2′-O-Me-cAMP), suggest that EPAC/Rap does not regulate Erk signaling and are consistent with PKA-mediated effects.[125] However, the availability of 8-pCPT-2′-O-Me-cAMP is enabling a more clear definition of the role of EPAC independent of PKA activation.

EPAC-induced Rap1 activation has been implicated in the regulation of integrins and cell adhesion. Rap1 regulates several integrin isoforms but the underlying signaling pathway is not known.[126] The regulation of integrins by EPAC/Rap1 is also controversial as the effect of phosphodiesterases on cAMP levels and integrin-dependent cell adhesion is reported to be PKA-mediated in REF52 cells.[127] Alternatively, cAMP-dependent integrin function in retinal neurons appears to be independent of both PKA and EPAC, suggesting a novel cAMP-signaling pathway.[128] Thus, EPAC/Rap signaling requires further investigation to clearly define their downstream effectors and cellular actions.

EPAC 2 is an important effector of the potentiation of glucose-induced insulin secretion by the incretin hormone glucagon-like peptide-1.[129] This potentiation is mediated, in part, by direct effects on exocytosis through an interaction of EPAC 2 with Rim 2, a Rab 3–interacting protein that is believed to play a role in regulating the fusion of secretory vesicles with the plasma membrane.[130] EPAC 2 also appears to regulate intracellular Ca^{2+} release from ryanodine-sensitive stores, in addition to PKA-sensitive release from inositol trisphosphate (IP3)-gated stores. Both EPAC 2– and PKA-mediated release of Ca^{2+} from ryanodine- and IP3-gated stores appear to stimulate mitochondrial adenosine triphosphate (ATP) production that may be an important effector of the potentiation of insulin secretion.[131,132] EPAC has also been implicated at the neuromuscular junction in the potentiation of transmitter release through a process called temporal synaptic tagging.[133] However, the role of EPAC in synaptic tagging has not been fully elucidated.

A role for EPAC in the recruitment of T-type (Ca_v3) calcium channels in chromaffin cells has been reported.[134] These cells normally express Ca_v3 channels weakly but after exposure of the cells to cAMP analogues, including 8-pCPT-2′-O-Me-cAMP, the density of Ca_v3 channels increases. This was suggested as a mechanism whereby autocrine activation of β-adrenoceptors could increase secretory activity in response to sustained sympathetic stimulation. The signaling mechanism controlling this increased channel synthesis is not known but is specific for Ca_v3 channels and does not affect Ca_v1 and 2 channels.[134]

CYCLIC NUCLEOTIDE-GATED CHANNELS

Cyclic nucleotide-gated (CNG) channels can be broadly divided into two subgroups. One group is ligand-gated and shows little or no voltage-dependent activation, although the open probability of the ligand-gated channel may be voltage-dependent (CNG channels). The second group is activated by hyperpolarization and this voltage-dependent gating is modified by cyclic nucleotide-binding (hyperpolarization and cyclic nucleotide [HCN]-gated channels).

CNG channels were first identified in rod photoreceptors where they are activated by cGMP to produce the dark current.[135] It is now known that these channels are formed by a tetrameric complex of three CNGA1 subunits and one CNGB1 subunit.[136,137] There are currently six known proteins in the CNG family from vertebrates, CNGA1–4 and CNGB1 and 3. CNGA1–3 (but not CNGA4) subunits form functional channels when expressed alone and the CNGA4/CNGB subunits modify the channel properties.[135,138] CNGA1 and CNGB1 form channels in the rod photoreceptors while CNGA3 and CNGB3 form cone photoreceptor channels and these rod and cone channels are preferentially gated by cGMP. CNG channels in olfactory neurons are formed by three subunits, CNGA2, CNGA4, and an alternatively spliced form of CNGB1 (CNGB1b) and are equally sensitive to cGMP and cAMP.[135,139]

CNG channel subunits contain cyclic nucleotide-binding domains (CNBDs) that are homologous to those in PKA, PKG, and the *Escherichia coli* catabolite gene activator protein (CAP). Channel activation occurs following ligand-binding to each subunit and the open probability of the channel increases with the number of ligand molecules bound.[140,141] The CNBD of CAP contains a β-sheet and two α-helices (called B- and C-helices). Mutagenesis studies have identified several amino acids in the CNBD that play an important role in regulating channel function, with two being particularly noteworthy. One is T560 in the β-sheet of CNGA1; mutations at this site decrease the affinity for cGMP with little effect on cAMP binding. The second is D604 in the C-helix where a D604M mutation reverses the ligand specificity so the mutant channels are preferentially activated by cAMP.[135]

There are four known HCN channel proteins in mammals, HCN1–4.[138,142] An additional protein, MinK-related peptide-1 (MiRP1), modulates expression and activation properties of HCN1 and HCN2 in oocytes and may form a β subunit for these channels.[143] However, other studies failed to show an effect of MiRP1 on HCN4 or HCN4-1 tandem channels expressed in HEK 293 cells[144] and the role of MiRP1 in HCN channel function remains to be fully elucidated.

HCN channels are formed as a complex that can be either homotetrameric or heterotetrameric.[145] These heterotetramers can be formed by several combinations of HCN subunits with the apparent exception of the HCN2/3 combination.[146] Each HCN subunit contains a CNBD in its C-terminal tail that is similar to the CNBD in CNG channels. The binding of cAMP to these domains produces a positive shift in the voltage activation range of the channels and in their rate of activation. HCN2 and HCN4 show a marked cAMP-dependent shift in activation range whereas HCN1 shows only a small change.[138,142,147] Given that all the HCN isoforms contain a CNBD, this leads to the question of why HCN2 and HCN4, but not HCN1, are sensitive to cAMP. This question was addressed by Wainger and colleagues,[148] whom constructed deletion mutants in the C-terminal tail of the channels. It was shown that deletion of the CNBD in HCN2 produced effects that were similar to, or greater than, the effect of adding cAMP, whereas a similar deletion in HCN1 had only a small effect, similar to the effect of cAMP. From these observations, it was concluded that the CNBD of HCN2 inhibits activation of the channel with greater efficacy than the CNBD of HCN1, but that in each case, cAMP relieves inhibition by the CNBD.[148] Thus, the differential sensitivity to cAMP seems to result from differences in channel conformation, rather than differences in cAMP binding to the CNBD.

The best known physiologic role of the HCN channels is in the generation of pacemaker currents in heart and neuronal cells where changes in cAMP levels modulate the firing rate of these cells.[149] Thyroid hormone also increases the expression of HCN2 in heart cells that may underlie the effect of thyroid state on heart rate[150] as an additional mechanism to changes in cAMP. HCN channels also play a role in setting the membrane potential of some cells and also regulate synaptic function.[149] In taste cells, HCN channels are activated by extracellular protons and an additional role of HCN channels appears to be in the transduction of sour taste.[151]

REPRESENTATIVE CELLULAR ACTIONS OF cAMP-DEPENDENT PROTEIN KINASE A

The targets for the biologic actions of cAMP mediated by PKA are multiple. In almost every instance, phosphorylation of a protein substrate results in a change in the biologic activity of the protein, either stimulatory or inhibitory. Phosphorylation evokes crucial changes in the conformation of the proteins, often by allosteric mechanisms. Four representative examples of how PKA-directed phosphorylation regulates the activities of proteins are given in the following sections: an enzyme, glycogen phosphorylase; a receptor, β-adrenergic receptor (β-AR); an ion channel, the CFTR, which is a chloride channel; and a DNA-binding transcription factor, CREB.

GLYCOGEN PHOSPHORYLASE

As discussed earlier, glycogen phosphorylase was important historically as the model protein for investigations that led to defining the important roles of cAMP and phosphorylation in the transmission of hormone action to modulation of the biologic activity of a protein.[11,18] In the 1940s, it was recognized that glycogen phosphorylase existed in both active (phosphorylase a) and inactive (phosphorylase b) forms.[17] Subsequent studies of the phosphorylation of glycogen phosphorylase in both skeletal muscle and liver showed that phosphorylase b was activated to phosphorylase a by a phosphorylase kinase and inactivated by a phosphorylase phosphatase.

$$ATP \rightarrow ADP$$
$$kinase$$

Phosphorylase b ⇌ Phosphorylase a
(inactive)   (active)

$$phosphatase$$
$$Pi \leftarrow H_2O$$

Next, it was demonstrated that the activity of phosphorylase kinase was reversible, and although the kinase was capable of autophosphorylation, its activation was mediated by phosphorylation by yet another kinase, phosphorylase kinase kinase, subsequently renamed cAMP-dependent PKA (Fig. 12-9).[11]

The enzymatic cycle of glycogen breakdown represents a classic example of regulation by successive phosphorylations, a so-called kinase cascade. PKA activates phosphorylase kinase that then activates glycogen phosphorylase. In addition, both a negative and a positive counter-regulatory phosphorylation are effected by PKA. Phosphorylations initiated by PKA but followed by an additional phosphorylation by the processive kinase, CK I, inhibit glycogen synthase, the biosynthetic enzyme in the cycle (see Fig. 12-6). Phosphorylation by PKA

activates a phosphatase-inhibitor protein resulting in inhibition of protein phosphatase, thereby enhancing the PKA-mediated phosphorylation.[152] The complexity of the regulation of phosphorylase kinase is reviewed in Brushia and Walsh.[153]

β-ADRENERGIC RECEPTOR

New findings on the novel mechanisms of signaling by the β-adrenergic receptors is provided in several reviews of the subject.[154–157] The mechanism of the rapid agonist-induced desensitization of the β-adrenergic receptor appears to involve phosphorylations by PKA and an additional cAMP-independent protein kinase known as β-adrenergic receptor kinase (BARK), a member of the G protein–coupled receptor kinase (GRK) family (Fig. 12-10).[29,30,158,159] These phosphorylations are important for the rapid desensitization that occurs within 30 minutes after the receptor is occupied by ligand. The rapid phase of receptor desensitization is to be distinguished from the slow desensitization that takes place during longer (several hours) periods of exposure to ligand.[29] The rapid desensitization is reversible, does not require ongoing protein synthesis, and almost certainly involves an "uncoupling" of the receptor to G protein (see following discussion). In contrast, the slow desensitization results from sequestration and internalization of the receptor, and recovery requires new protein synthesis.

The mechanisms of the desensitization appear to be distinct for the two different kinases; phosphorylation by PKA occurs at low (nanomolar) and by BARK at high (micromolar) concentrations of ligand. BARK was discovered by analyses of the β-adrenergic receptor expressed in two distinct mutant S49 mouse lymphosarcoma cell lines.[29] The CYC− mutant line lacks G protein ($G_s\alpha$) and the Kin− mutant line lacks PKA. In both cell lines, rapid desensitization occurred (albeit somewhat less than in wild-type cells), pointing to the existence of a relevant kinase other than PKA. The agonist-induced desensitization of receptors can be either homologous or heterologous. In the former, the agonist specifically desensitizes the distinct receptors that are occupied. In the latter, a liganded receptor desensitizes other distinctly different receptors on the cell surface.

BARK appears to induce homologous and PKA heterologous desensitization of the β-adrenergic receptor.[29] Although the reasons for the dependence of these two kinases on different

Enzymatic Cycle of Glycogen Breakdown

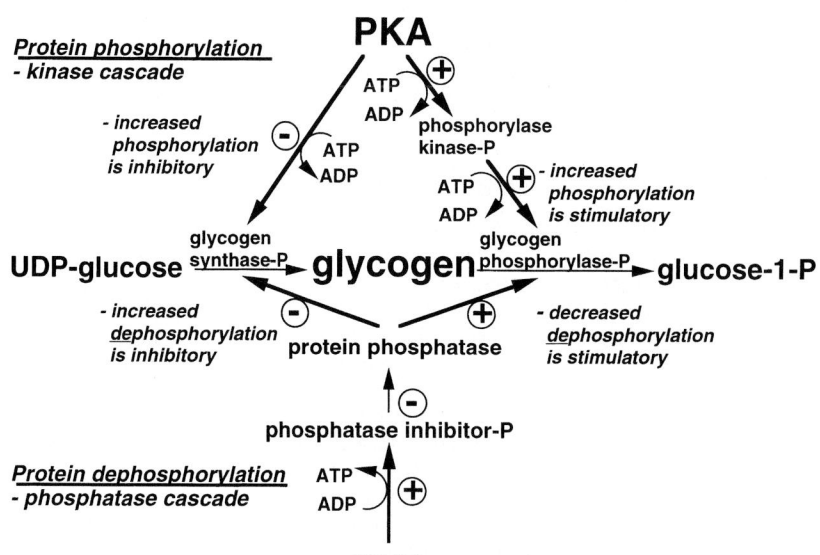

Figure 12-9   The enzymatic cycle of glycogen breakdown (conversion of glycogen to glucose). Phosphorylations of key enzymes in the cycle by cAMP-dependent protein kinase A (PKA) regulate the formation of glucose (glucose-1-phosphate) by the breakdown of glycogen in muscle tissue. PKA stimulates by phosphorylation of the activity of the enzyme phosphorylase kinase which, in turn, phosphorylates and activates glycogen phosphorylase. At the same time, PKA phosphorylates and so inactivates the glycogen synthetic enzyme, glycogen synthase. Protein phosphatases (protein ptase) provide counter-regulatory influences imposed by the protein kinases. Further, phosphatase inhibitor proteins (ptase-inhibitor) and protein kinase A proteins (PKI) modulate the phosphorylation-dependence cascade of regulation and counter-regulation of the enzymes involved in glycogen breakdown.

Human β₂-Adrenergic Receptor

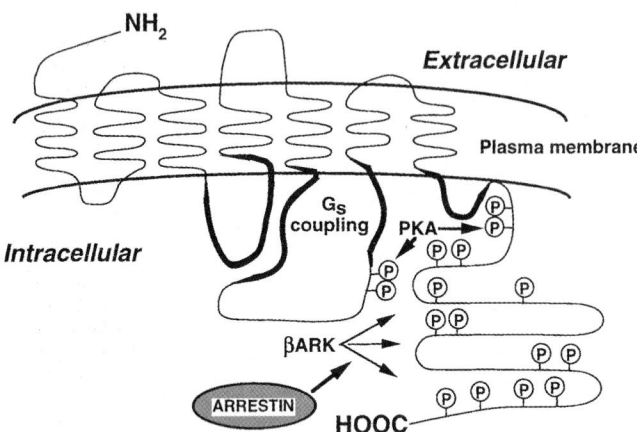

Figure 12-10 The human β₂-adrenergic receptor (β₂–AR). The structure of the amino acid sequence of β–AR was determined by cloning the cDNA encoding the receptor. The model shown is deduced from the structure of the receptor, as well as from analyses of the perturbations in function induced by mutations introduced into the receptor. The β-AR is a member of a large family of receptors that are coupled to G proteins. It consists of seven membrane-spanning segments and three cytoplasmic domains that are believed to be involved in the interactions of the receptor with G proteins (highlighted by the thickened lines). The cytoplasmic domains are phosphorylated by both protein kinase A (PKA) and a β-adrenergic receptor kinase (BARK). The phosphorylations mediate, in some way, the desensitization or uncoupling of the receptor from the G proteins (see text). Arrestin is a protein that is involved in the modulation of phosphorylations by PKA and BARK.

concentrations of agonist are not known, it appears that a functionally significant level of phosphorylation of the receptor by BARK occurs only when a substantial number of receptors in a cell are occupied by agonist. The physiologic implications of this circumstance are unknown. It has been proposed that the PKA-mediated desensitization may be tuned to receptors that respond to low concentrations of circulating hormones, whereas the BARK-induced desensitization occurs in locally acting paracrine or autocrine systems, such as receptors located at nerve synapses where concentrations of agonist are relatively high.[29]

That agonist-induced rapid desensitization of the β-adrenergic receptor involves phosphorylation by either PKA or BARK was shown in reconstitution experiments using isolated receptors incorporated into phospholipid vesicles.[160] Receptors prepared from desensitized cells or from cells that had not been treated with agonist and were phosphorylated in vitro with either PKA or BARK were all resistant to desensitization. Evidence that the phosphorylation of the receptor uncouples it from $G_s\alpha$ was likewise shown in reconstitution experiments in which phosphorylation of the receptor by PKA or BARK attenuated agonist-induced GTPase activity.[86,161] A small GTP-binding protein, Ras homologue enriched in striatum (Rhes), may also play a role in uncoupling the β₂-adrenergic receptor from G protein activation.[162] The cloning of the β-adrenergic receptor has allowed analyses of the effects of mutations in the receptor on its function. The serines and threonines that are phosphorylated by PKA and BARK reside in the third cytoplasmic loop and the cytoplasmic C-terminal tail of the receptor (see Fig. 12-10). PKA phosphorylates at least two sites, one in the cytoplasmic loop and the other in the tail, whereas BARK phosphorylates several sites, all of which reside in the tail. The integrity of both the loop and the tail have been shown to be important in the coupling of the G protein to the receptor. Mutations of the sites for phosphorylation by either PKA or BARK reduced the level of

phosphorylation of the receptor and the agonist-induced desensitization by 50% of the wild-type receptor.[29] Mutations of both PKA and BARK sites extinguished phosphorylation and markedly attenuated desensitization.

It should be noted that activation of PKA does not always induce receptor desensitization. The desensitization and internalization of metabotropic glutamate receptors 1a and 1b is inhibited by PKA through a mechanism that involves a decreased ability of glutamate to stimulate association of these receptors with GRK2 and arrestin.[163]

The mechanisms by which phosphorylation of the β-adrenergic receptor result in the uncoupling of the G protein from the receptor are not yet understood. At least two mechanisms have been proposed, however, and are under investigation: phosphorylation-induced modification of amphipathic α-helices in the receptor and inhibition of G protein receptor coupling by an effector protein, arrestin.[29] Amphipathic α-helices are well known to be structured motifs in proteins that are used in protein-protein interactions. The introduction of a highly negatively charged phosphoserine in place of a neutral serine residue may in some way perturb the helicity and/or amphipathy of the helix, thereby impairing interaction with the G protein. Arrestin is a protein that has been proposed to competitively inhibit the interaction of G protein with the receptor.[164] It was first identified as an inhibitor of the interaction of transducin, a retinal G protein, to phosphorylated rhodopsin.[165] Later, a cDNA encoding a homologue of retinal arrestin was cloned from a bovine brain library. The brain and retinal arrestins are 59% identical in their amino acid sequences. Further, when the brain and retinal arrestins, prepared by cDNA-directed expression and isolation from COS-7 cells, were tested in a reconstitution assay containing G_s and β-adrenergic receptor phosphorylated by BARK, the brain arrestin was much more effective than the retinal arrestin in facilitating desensitization. Conversely, the retinal arrestin was more effective than the brain arrestin in reversing the light activation of the rhodopsin receptor.[29] Thus, it seems likely that the arrestins are important regulatory effectors whose actions are integrated with both the PKA and BARK phosphorylations of the receptors and the interactions of G proteins with the receptors.

Aberrant regulation of GRKs may have pathophysiologic relevance in a number of disease states. Overexpression of GRKs has been shown in patients with heart failure[166] and in those with cystic fibrosis.[167] Furthermore, transgenic mice overexpressing BARK1/GRK2 exhibit cardiac failure that can be rescued by expression of a peptide that contains the Gβγ binding domain of GRK2 and interferes with the membrane translocation of the kinase.[166] Similarly, small peptides derived from the catalytic domain of GRK2 and GRK3 can ameliorate diabetes in several animal models of this disease.[168] Thus, changes in the GRK-mediated regulation of GPCR function may be a useful therapeutic target for several disease states.

THE CYSTIC FIBROSIS TRANSMEMBRANE CONDUCTANCE REGULATOR

The CFTR is a regulated chloride channel located in the apical membranes of secretory epithelia.[31] The channel regulates the transepithelial secretion of chloride. cDNAs and genes encoding the channel have been cloned.[169] It is now determined that mutations in the gene impair the normal functioning of the channel and cause the inborn error of metabolism known as cystic fibrosis.[170] Defective secretion of chloride and accompanying water leads to increased viscosity of epithelial cell secretions, culminating in the development of impaired airway and gastrointestinal functions. The mutations in the CFTR gene result in the synthesis of defective CFTR chloride channels that do not open in response to intracellular signaling pathways. Several reviews summarize the most recent findings on how CFTR channels function and misfunction when mutated.[171-174]

Activation of the CFTR (opening of the channel) is mediated by phosphorylation by PKA and is enhanced by the binding of ATP at two sites located on the cytoplasmic face of the channel. cAMP-dependent signaling is crucial for the activation (opening) of the CFTR channel. It has been shown that cAMP agonists increase the permeability of apical membranes to chloride of normal epithelia but not epithelia of patients with cystic fibrosis.[175]

The CFTR chloride channel is composed of five distinct domains: two transmembrane spanning domains, each of which spans the membrane six times and forms the pore that conducts the chloride ions; two nucleotide-binding domains that regulate the channel by binding and/or hydrolysis of ATP; and an R-domain phosphorylated on at least four serines by PKA (Fig. 12-11).[31,169] These serines in the R-domain are phosphorylated by PKA in vitro and by cAMP agonists in vivo.[170] Furthermore, mutation of the serines to alanines results in a loss of channel activation, and mutational deletion of the R-domain results in a constitutively active channel that is only partially responsive to increases in cAMP. The dephosphorylation of the serines phosphorylated by PKA appears to involve protein phosphatase 2A and not phosphatases 1 or 2B.[176] Evidence has been presented that the R-domain may also be phosphorylated by both calcium-dependent and calcium-independent isotypes of protein kinase C.

Activation of CFTR chloride channels also requires ATP; once phosphorylated by PKA, the channels require cytosolic ATP to open. The ATP binds to single sites on each of the nucleotide-binding domains (see Fig. 12-11). Notably, the nonhydrolyzable analogue of ATP, ATPγS does not open CFTR channels, whereas the hydrolyzable analogues ATP>GTP>CTP (order of potency) reversibly open the channels phosphorylated by PKA. Thus, both phosphorylation of the R-domain and binding of ATP to the nucleotide binding domains are required to fully activate (open) the channels.

These observations on the effects of phosphorylation and ATP binding on the function of the CFTR have led to the proposal of a model to explain how the channel might work.[31,169] The membrane spanning domains constitute a hollow cylinder with a central pore or channel created by 12 α-helical structures inserted transversely through the membrane (see Fig. 12-11). The nucleotide-binding domains, located on the cytoplasmic face adjacent to the opening of the channel, change conformation upon binding of ATP so as to enlarge the "diameter" of the pore. In the unphosphorylated state, the R-domain, presumed to be globular in shape, "plugs" the pore and, when phosphorylated (by PKA), is repelled from the region of the opening (perhaps by electrostatic forces), thereby opening the pore to allow the passage of chloride ions through the channel.

Phosphorylation by cAMP-dependent PKA is clearly an important step in the regulation of the activity CFTR chloride

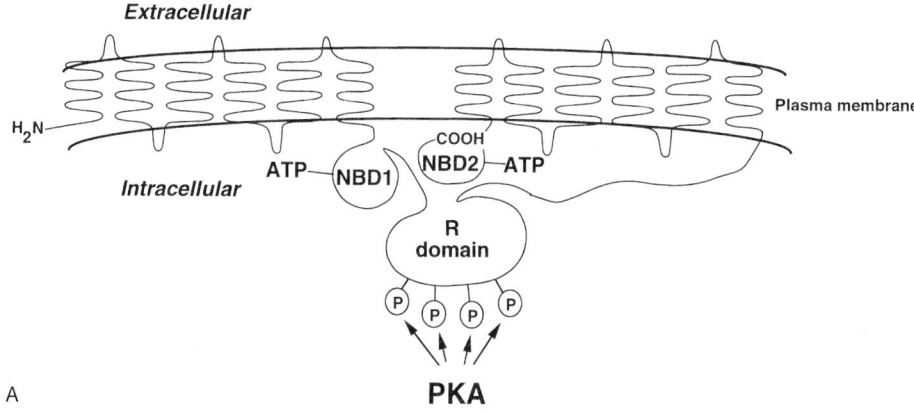

Cystic Fibrosis Transmembrane Conductance Regulator

A

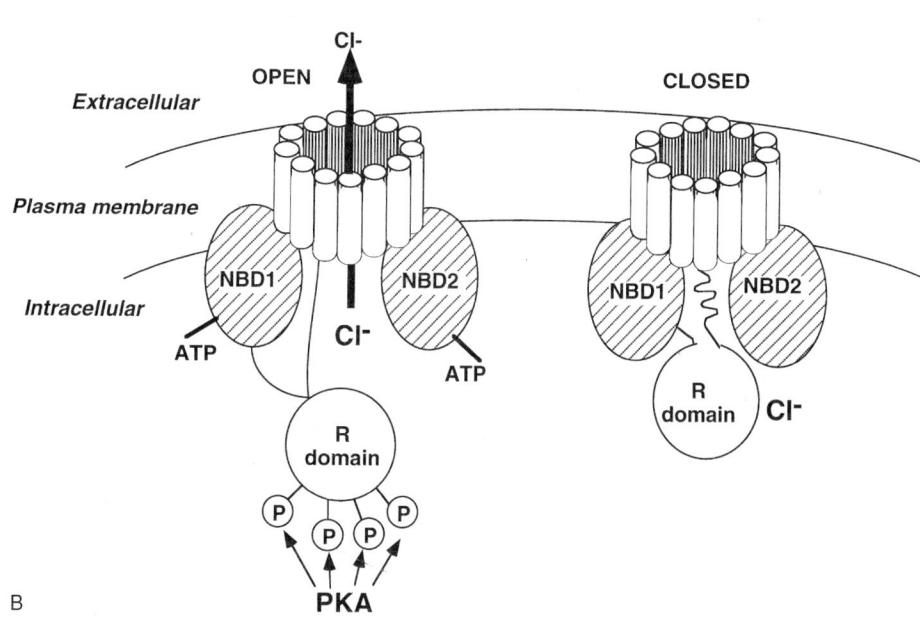

B

Figure 12-11 Models of the cystic fibrosis transmembrane conductance regulator (CFTR), a chloride channel whose defective functioning causes the disease cystic fibrosis. **A,** Overall topography of the CFTR. The channel spans the plasma membrane twelve times and thereby forms a 12-sided cylinder creating the pore through which chloride ions flow as shown schematically in **B.** The two nucleotide binding domains (NBD1 and NBD2) located on the cytoplasmic face of the channel bind ATP and as such are believed to conformationally widen the channel opening. The globular regulatory domain (R-domain) is phosphorylated on at least four sites by cAMP-dependent protein kinase A (PKA). It has been proposed that in the unphosphorylated state, the R-domain plugs the pore of the channel and thereby closes the channel. When phosphorylated, the R-domain is repelled by electrostatic forces away from the channel pore and thereby opens the channel, allowing for export of chloride ions from the inside to the outside of the cell.

channel. It is highly likely that PKA is of tantamount importance in the regulation of many other ion channels as well. Evidence has been presented suggesting a role of PKA in the modulation of the activity of ATP-sensitive potassium channels on pancreatic β cells, again in concert with the binding and/or hydrolysis of ATP.[177,178]

ACTIVATION OF GENE TRANSCRIPTION BY PROTEIN KINASE A

A major discovery has been the identification of DNA-binding proteins whose transcriptional functions are activated by phosphorylation by PKA.[34–36,179–181] These proteins bind specific DNA elements located in the promoters of many genes. These elements, and the DNA-binding proteins that interact with them, are referred to as cAMP response elements (CREs) and CREBs, respectively.[34–36] The term *activating transcription factor* (ATF) is also used to describe proteins that bind to CREs because the nomenclature derived from virologic research in which viral proteins activate cellular proteins that bind to CREs.[34] Not all ATFs mediate cAMP responses. A representative example of the role of PKA and CREB in the regulation of proinsulin gene transcription in pancreatic beta cells is shown in Figure 12-12.[182]

The CREB DNA-binding protein, and its structurally closely related homologues cAMP response element modulator (CREM) and ATF-1, have all been cloned. Numerous isoforms of CREB and CREM exist that arise by way of the alternative splicing of exons.[35,183–185] The structural components responsible for the functions of CREB and CREM have been characterized in considerable detail. These proteins are members of a subfamily of a large superfamily of DNA-binding proteins known collectively as the bZIP proteins, so named because of the similar structures of their DNA-binding domains that consist of a basic region (b) involved in recognition and binding to DNA and a leucine zipper (ZIP), a coiled-coil structure with heptad repeats of leucines responsible for dimerization[36] (Fig. 12-13). Additional information is contained in several reviews on CREB and bZIP proteins.[34–36,186]

The transcriptional activities of CREB and the proteins that most closely resemble it in their structures are intensely regulated by the cAMP-dependent signaling pathway and appear to be unique in this regard. Given that the bZIP transcriptional proteins now identified constitute a large family, members of which compete for binding to their enhancer DNAs, it is understandable that nature would evolve only a limited set of these proteins for activation by cAMP-dependent protein kinase A, with the other proteins responsive to other non-cAMP-directed pathways. Thus, as far as is known, CREB, CREM, and ATF-1 represent the final communicative link in the regulation of gene expression in response to the activation of cAMP-dependent signaling systems.[36]

The primary amino acid sequences of the bZIP proteins diverge considerably outside their DNA-binding and dimerization domains, that is, their domains that activate transcription (transactivation) have evolved so as to mediate signal transduction, each factor in response to distinct stimuli. For example, of the known bZIP transcription factors, only CREB, CREM, and ATF-1 are activated upon phosphorylation by cAMP-dependent PKA, and also in some circumstances CREB is activated by calcium-calmodulin kinase.[187,188] By contrast, the protein kinase C (PKC) signal transduction pathway regulates the phosphorylation of the Jun-Fos (AP-1) complex.[107] Consistent with the role of CREB in the cAMP pathway, there is a consensus site, RRPSY (A-kinase box), also known as the kinase-inducible domain (KID), for phosphorylation by PKA at serine 119 in CREB327 and at the corresponding serine 133 in CREB341 (see Fig. 12-13). The two CREB isoforms differ by an alternatively spliced exon of 14 amino acids. The identical A-kinase box, RRPSY, is present in the corresponding location in CREM and ATF-1. The PKA site in CREB is surrounded by a cluster of potential phosphorylated serine and threonine residues (KID or phosphorylation, P-Box) over a stretch of about 50 residues. Consensus sites for potential phosphorylations by PKC, CK II, and glycogen synthase kinase-3 reside in the P-Box. The protein kinases CK II and glycogen synthase kinase-3 are known to be processive or hierarchical kinases, inasmuch as phosphorylation of one site facilitates the successive phosphorylation of adjacent sites.[70] Phosphorylation of the PKA site may trigger a cascade of phosphorylations by the other kinases (see Fig. 12-13). Studies have shown that phosphorylation of the PKA site (serine 119) is essential for the activation of CREB.[189] However,

Figure 12-12 Hypothetic model of a pancreatic β cell showing opposing actions of the hormones glucagon-like peptide-1(7–37) and galanin in the regulation of the cAMP-dependent signaling pathway. The receptor for GLP-1(7–37) is coupled to a stimulatory G protein (G_s), whereas the receptor for galanin is coupled to an inhibitory G protein (G_i) See Figure 5-3. Thus, the extent of activation of adenylyl cyclase (AC) is a result of the relative levels of G_s and G_i. The final response in the signaling pathway is the activation of the DNA-binding transcription factor CREB that binds to cAMP-response elements located in the promoters of genes such as the proinsulin gene, and thereby stimulates transcription of the gene. The pharmacologic agents cholera toxin (CT) and pertussis toxin (PT) activate G_s and G_i, respectively. Forskolin directly stimulates the activity of adenyl cyclase. Isobutylmethyl-xanthine (IBMX) inhibits phosphodiesterase (PDE) and 8-br-cAMP is a cell permeable cAMP agonist. AKAP, A-kinase anchoring protein (see text).

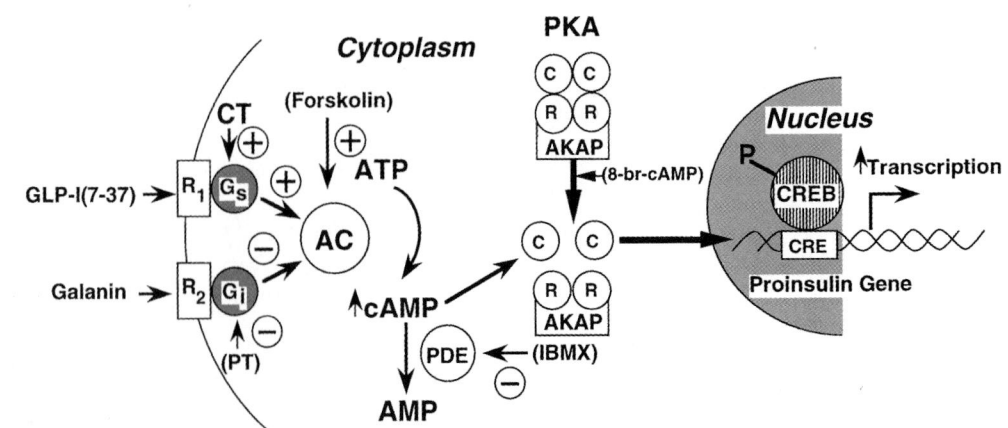

cAMP Response Element Binding Protein (CREB)

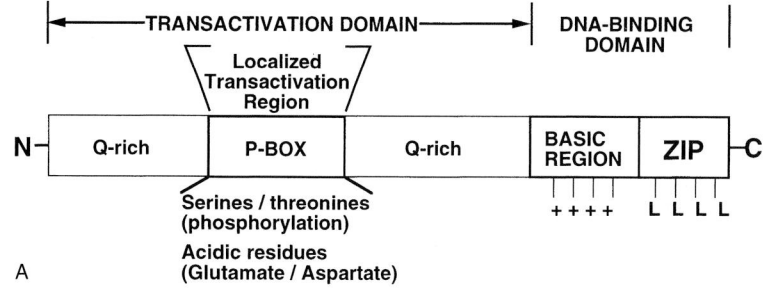

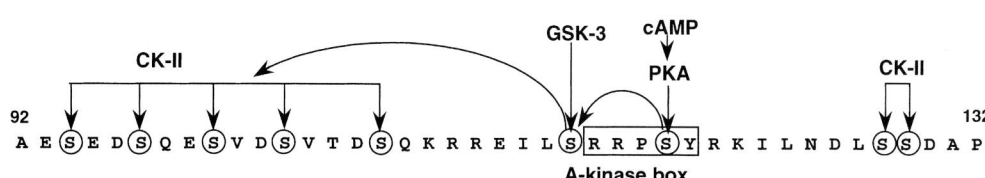

Figure 12-13 Diagram of the structure of CREB, cAMP response element binding protein. **A,** CREB belongs to the superfamily of transcription factors known as the bZIP proteins, so named because the DNA-binding region consists of a basic region (b) responsible for DNA recognition and a leucine zipper coiled-coil (ZIP) involved in dimerization. **B,** The transcriptional transactivation domain of CREB consists of a region of approximately 50 residues and contains multiple sites that are phosphorylated by protein kinases among the most important of which is cAMP-dependent protein kinase

phosphorylation of the serine 119 of CREB327 or the corresponding serine 133 in CREB341 is necessary, but not sufficient to generate the transactivation functions of CREB. Sequences located carboxy-proximal to serine 119 are required to confer transcriptional transactivation functions of CREB.[190] Phosphorylation of the P-Box may allosterically alter CREB to reveal the protein conformational structure required for transcriptional transactivation.[190] It has been proposed that the regions involved in transactivation are the glutamine-rich regions that flank the KID.[190,191] Furthermore, this model predicts that this allosteric effect would be potentiated by the insertion of the alternatively spliced 14 amino acids that constitute the difference between CREB327 and CREB341.[192] Whether or not, however, these extra 14 amino acids enhance the transactivation of CREB341 over CREB327 is uncertain. In addition to the KID, which is crucial for transcriptional transactivation, evidence has been presented that the additional spliced 14 amino acids are important for transactivation in some but not all cell lines.[184,190–192]

The importance in vivo of the requirement for phosphorylation of CREB by PKA to generate its transactivational functions was shown by Struthers and colleagues,[193] who produced dwarfism in transgenic mice expressing a CREB with a serine to alanine substitution mutation at the site (residue serine 133) phosphorylated by PKA. The transgene consisted of the promoter of the rat growth hormone gene fused to the coding sequence of the point-mutated CREB. Thus, expression of the mutated CREB was directed to the somatotrophs of the pituitary during development. Because the mutated CREB still dimerized with wild-type CREB and bound to CREs but could not transactivate gene transcription, the mutated CREB competed the actions of wild-type CREB, resulting in atrophied pituitary glands deficient in somatotrophs and the production of growth hormone. Because CREB proteins are expressed at relatively high levels in testis,[186] it would be interesting to learn the effects on mice that have been rendered transgenic with mutation CREB Ser 133 Ala under the regulation of testes-specific promoters.

Notably, in certain circumstances CREB appears to activate gene transcription independent of its phosphorylation by PKA. In the pancreatic islet cell line, Tu6, both wild-type CREB and CREB with a mutation in the PKA-regulated Ser 133 phosphorylation site of a somatostatin CRE-reporter plasmid, activate transcription equally in the presence of cAMP-activated PKA.[194] In this case, the activation of transcription

of the CRE required a second promoter element, which appears to bind an islet cell factor Isl-1. Thus, in the absence of phosphorylation by PKA, CREB may activate transcription via other nonphosphorylation-dependent mechanisms. CREB also has been reported to lack transactivational activity on somatostatin and vasoactive intestinal peptide-CRE reporters in undifferentiated F9 embryonal carcinoma cells, however, in differentiated cells, this is not the case.[195] Both undifferentiated and differentiated cells appeared to contain equivalent amounts of functionally active PKA, suggesting the possibility that an inhibitor of CREB transactivation is present in the undifferentiated cells. Because the state of phosphorylation of CREB in undifferentiated versus differentiated cells was not examined in these studies, the mechanisms for the inhibition remains unknown.

Whereas most research on the regulation of CREB transactivation has been directed toward mechanisms involving protein kinases, relatively little is known about phosphatase-mediated inactivation of CREB. Recently, however, Hagiwara and colleagues[196] have provided compelling evidence that protein phosphatase-1 (PP-1) selectively dephosphorylates the serine 133 in CREB341 (serine 119 in CREB327) and correspondingly attenuates the transactivational activity of CREB. Although both PP-1 and PP-2A will dephosphorylate this site in CREB, examination of the relative inhibition constants of PP-1 and PP-2A for the phosphatase inhibitor okadaic acid, IC_{50} of 20 nM and 0.2 nM, respectively, strongly suggests that PP-1 is the relevant phosphatase in vivo.[196] Further, the PP-1-specific phosphatase inhibitor protein-1 (IP-1) abrogated the activity of PP-1. Thus, an interesting model for regulation is proposed because the activity of IP-1 depends on phosphorylation by either PKA or calcium-calmodulin kinase. In this model, activation of PKA by cAMP would result in the phosphorylation and activation of CREB and IP-I, the latter leading to the inhibition of PP-1.

The effects of phosphorylation on the dimerization and DNA-binding of CREB are less certain than the effects on transactivation. Yamamoto and colleagues[197] originally reported that phosphorylation of a partially purified CREB or CREB-like protein by PKC, but not PKA, enhanced dimerization and binding to a CRE. The studies, however, relied on analyses of the effects of phosphorylation on the transition of CREB from a monomer to a dimer as assessed by binding to a CRE-containing oligonucleotide using an electrophoretic mobility shift assay. Because it is now generally believed that bZIP proteins including CREB bind to DNA only as dimers and not as monomers, these observations of Yamamoto and colleagues[197] may have to be reinterpreted in a different light. Nichols and colleagues[198] provided evidence that phosphorylation of CREB by PKA enhances binding to asymmetrical CREs such as the CRE in the tyrosine amino transferase gene (TGACGCAG), but not to symmetrical CREs such as those found in the promoters of the somatostatin (TGACGTCA) gene. These observations are interesting because they indicate that phosphorylation of a site approximately 150 amino acids distant from the bZIP DNA-binding domain can influence binding. Such a mechanism must involve a phosphorylation-induced folding or stabilization of CREB. Such effects of phosphorylation on distant sites have also been observed for the transcription factors jun, myb, and SRF. The binding of CREB to CREs may also be enhanced by phosphorylation through a non-cAMP-dependent signaling pathway. TGF-β induces phosphorylation of CREB or a CREB-like protein resulting in increased binding to a fibronectin gene CRE and collagenase gene tetraphorbol acetate-response element.[199] The studies suggest that the CREB-like protein binds to these DNA elements as a heterodimer with a Fos-like protein, but the identity of the DNA-binding complex remains to be determined.

SUMMARY

The cAMP-dependent signal transduction pathway is one of several such signaling pathways whose function is to convey information from the environment outside of cells to the complex metabolic activities that take place within the cell. Many actions of cAMP are conveyed by way of its activation of the enzyme, cAMP-dependent PKA. The inactive holoenzyme is a heterotetrameric complex consisting of two regulatory and two catalytic subunits. The allosteric regulator cAMP binds to two sites on each of the two regulatory subunits, thereby dissociating the two catalytic subunits from the complex. The free catalytic subunits bind Mg^{2+}-ATP and are phosphotransferases that phosphorylate protein substrates on serines and threonines in the sequence motif RRXS/T. Two isoforms of the regulatory subunit have been identified (RI and RII), each of which has two isotypes (RI_α, RI_β, RII_α, RII_β). Three isotypes of the catalytic subunit are known (C_α, C_β, C_γ). The RI and RII isoforms are located predominantly either in the cytoplasm and associated with membranous organelles, respectively. The α isotypes are distributed ubiquitously in mostly all tissue types, whereas the β isotypes appears to be restricted to brain, endocrine glands, and testes. The RII subunits are targeted to specific subcellular locations by binding to A-kinase anchoring proteins, perhaps to bring the catalytic subunits in close proximity to their substrates. Functional differences among the three catalytic subunits have not yet been found, except that C_γ is enriched in testis and phosphorylates substrates with other than the standard motif. The relative cellular levels of subunits of PKA are autoregulated in a complex manner at levels of gene transcription, subunit mRNA, and protein stability and subunit interactions. Phosphorylations by PKA of substrate proteins such as enzymes, receptors, ion channels, and DNA-binding transcription factors alter the conformation and thereby the functional activities of the proteins.

Other cellular effects of cAMP are mediated by proteins that directly bind cAMP but do not function as kinases. The best known examples of these kinase-independent effectors are the CNG channels that regulate cell excitability, and the GEFs whose actions are only beginning to be elucidated.

Acknowledgments
We thank George Holz, Mario Vallejo, and Christopher Miller for helpful suggestions and Melissa Fannon for preparation of the chapter. J.F.H. is an Investigator with the Howard Hughes Medical Institute.

REFERENCES

1. Skalhegg BS, Tasken K: Specificity in the cAMP/PKA signaling pathway. Differential expression, regulation, and subcellular localization of subunits of PKA. Front Biosci 5:D678–D693, 2000.
2. Richards JS: New signaling pathways for hormones and cyclic adenosine 3′,5′-monophosphate action in endocrine cells. Mol Endocrinol 15(2):209–218, 2001.
3. Schwartz JH: The many dimensions of cAMP signaling. Proc Natl Acad Sci U S A 98(24):13482–13484, 2001.
4. Chin KV, et al: Reinventing the wheel of cyclic AMP: Novel mechanisms of cAMP signaling. Ann N Y Acad Sci 968:49–64, 2002.
5. Tasken K, et al: PKAI as a potential target for therapeutic intervention. Drug News Perspect 13(1):12–18, 2000.
6. Edelman AM, Blumenthal DK, Krebs EG: Protein serine/threonine kinases. Annu Rev Biochem 56:567–613, 1987.
7. Scott JD: Cyclic nucleotide-dependent protein kinases. Pharmacol Ther 50(1):123–145, 1991.
8. Taylor SS, Buechler JA, Yonemoto W: cAMP-dependent protein kinase: Framework for a diverse family of regulatory enzymes. Annu Rev Biochem 59:971–1005, 1990.
9. Taylor SS: cAMP-dependent protein kinase. Model for an enzyme family. J Biol Chem 264(15):8443–8446, 1989.
10. Harper JF, et al: Compartmentation of second messenger action: Immunocytochemical and biochemical evidence. Vitam Horm 42:197–252, 1985.
11. Krebs EG: The Albert Lasker Medical Awards. Role of the cyclic AMP-dependent protein kinase in signal transduction. JAMA 262(13):1815–1818, 1989.
12. Hanks SK, Quinn AM, Hunter T: The protein kinase family: Conserved features and deduced phylogeny of the catalytic domains. Science 241(4861):42–52, 1988.
13. Gilman AG: The Albert Lasker Medical Awards. G proteins and regulation of adenylyl cyclase. JAMA 262(13):1819–1825, 1989.
14. Daniel PB, Walker WH, Habener JF: Cyclic AMP signaling and gene regulation. Annu Rev Nutr 18:353–383, 1998.
15. Sassone-Corsi P: Coupling gene expression to cAMP signalling: Role of CREB and CREM. Int J Biochem Cell Biol 30(1):27–38, 1998.
16. Walsh DA, Van Patten SM: Multiple pathway signal transduction by the cAMP-dependent protein kinase. FASEB J 8(15):1227–1236, 1994.
17. Cori CF, Cori CT: The enzymatic conversion of phosphorylase a to b. J Biol Chem 158:321–345, 1945.
18. Sutherland EW: Studies on the mechanism of hormone action. Science 177(47):401–408, 1972.
19. Berthet J, Rall TW, Sutherland EW: The relationship of epinephrine and glucagon to liver phosphorylase. IV. Effect of epinephrine and glucagon on the reactivation of phosphorylase in liver homogenates. J Biol Chem 224(1):463–475, 1957.
20. Sutherland EW, Rall TW: Fractionation and characterization of a cyclic adenine ribonucleotide formed by tissue particles. J Biol Chem 232(2):1077–1091, 1958.
21. Krebs EG, Graves DJ, Fischer EH: Factors affecting the activity of muscle phosphorylase b kinase. J Biol Chem 234:2867–2873, 1959.
22. Fischer EH, Krebs EG: Conversion of phosphorylase b to phosphorylase a in muscle extracts. J Biol Chem 216(1):121–132, 1955.
23. Kuo JF, Greengard P: An adenosine 3′,5′-monophosphate-dependent protein kinase from Escherichia coli. J Biol Chem 244(12):3417–3419, 1969.
24. Walsh DA, Perkins JP, Krebs EG: An adenosine 3′,5′-monophosphate-dependant protein kinase from rabbit skeletal muscle. J Biol Chem 243(13):3763–3765, 1968.
25. Nakamura T, Gold GH: A cyclic nucleotide-gated conductance in

olfactory receptor cilia. Nature 325(6103):442–444, 1987.

26. Pedarzani P, Storm JF: Protein kinase A-independent modulation of ion channels in the brain by cyclic AMP. Proc Natl Acad Sci U S A 92(25):11716–11720, 1995.

27. Zufall F, Shepherd GM, Barnstable CJ: Cyclic nucleotide gated channels as regulators of CNS development and plasticity. Curr Opin Neurobiol 7(3): 404–412, 1997.

28. Bos JL: Epac: A new cAMP target and new avenues in cAMP research. Nat Rev Mol Cell Biol 4(9):733–738, 2003.

29. Hausdorff WP, Caron MG, Lefkowitz RJ: Turning off the signal: Desensitization of beta-adrenergic receptor function. FASEB J 4(11):2881–2889, 1990.

30. Okamoto T, et al: Identification of a Gs activator region of the beta 2-adrenergic receptor that is autoregulated via protein kinase A-dependent phosphorylation. Cell 67(4):723–730, 1991.

31. Collins FS: Cystic fibrosis: Molecular biology and therapeutic implications. Science 256(5058):774–779, 1992.

32. Sandoval IV, Cuatrecasas P: Opposing effects of cyclic AMP and cyclic GMP on protein phosphorylation in tubulin preparations. Nature 262(5568):511–514, 1976.

33. Lohmann SM, et al: High-affinity binding of the regulatory subunit (RII) of cAMP-dependent protein kinase to microtubule-associated and other cellular proteins. Proc Natl Acad Sci U S A 81(21):6723–6727, 1984.

34. Habener JF: Cyclic AMP response element binding proteins: A cornucopia of transcription factors. Mol Endocrinol 4(8):1087–1094, 1990.

35. Meyer TE, Habener JF: Cyclic AMP response element binding protein CREB and modulator protein CREM are products of distinct genes. Nucleic Acids Res 20(22):6106, 1992.

36. Meyer TE, Habener JF: Cyclic adenosine 3′,5′-monophosphate response element binding protein (CREB) and related transcription-activating deoxyribonucleic acid-binding proteins. Endocr Rev 14(3):269–290, 1993.

37. Rangarajan PN, Umesono K, Evans RM: Modulation of glucocorticoid receptor function by protein kinase A. Mol Endocrinol 6(9):1451–1457, 1992.

38. Weber IT, et al: Predicted structures of cAMP binding domains of type I and II regulatory subunits of cAMP-dependent protein kinase. Biochemistry 26(2):343–351, 1987.

39. Johnson LN, Barford D: Glycogen phosphorylase: The structural basis of the allosteric response and comparison with other allosteric proteins. J Biol Chem 265(5):2409–2412, 1990.

40. Sprang SR, et al: Structural changes in glycogen phosphorylase induced by phosphorylation. Nature 336(6196):215–221, 1988.

41. Bourne HR, Sanders DA, McCormick F: The GTPase superfamily: Conserved

structure and molecular mechanism. Nature 349(6305):117–127, 1991.

42. Birnbaumer L: Transduction of receptor signal into modulation of effector activity by G proteins: The first 20 years or so. FASEB J 4(14):3178–3188, 1990.

43. Johnson GL, Dhanasekaran N: The G-protein family and their interaction with receptors. Endocr Rev 10(3):317–331, 1989.

44. Neer EJ, Clapham DE: Roles of G protein subunits in transmembrane signalling. Nature 333(6169):129–134, 1988.

45. Taussig R, Quarmby LM, Gilman AG: Regulation of purified type I and type II adenylylcyclases by G protein beta gamma subunits. J Biol Chem 268(1):9–12, 1993.

46. Peng L, et al: Critical determinants of the G protein gamma subunits in the Gbetagamma stimulation of G protein-activated inwardly rectifying potassium (GIRK) channel activity. J Biol Chem 278(50):50203–50211, 2003.

47. Zhao Q, et al: Interaction of G protein beta subunit with inward rectifier K(+) channel Kir3. Mol Pharmacol 64(5):1085–1091, 2003.

48. Uezono Y, et al: Involvement of G protein {beta}{gamma} subunits in diverse signaling induced by Gi/o-coupled receptors: Study using the Xenopus oocyte expression system. Am J Physiol Cell Physiol 287(4): C885–C894, 2004.

49. Wing MR, Bourdon DM, Harden TK: PLC-epsilon: A shared effector protein in Ras-, Rho-, and G alpha beta gamma-mediated signaling. Mol Interv 3(5):273–280, 2003.

50. Holz GGT, Rane SG, Dunlap K: GTP-binding proteins mediate transmitter inhibition of voltage-dependent calcium channels. Nature 319(6055):670–672, 1986.

51. Hescheler J, et al: The GTP-binding protein, Go, regulates neuronal calcium channels. Nature 325(6103):445–447, 1987.

52. Yatani A, et al: Direct activation of mammalian atrial muscarinic potassium channels by GTP regulatory protein Gk. Science 235(4785):207–211, 1987.

53. Lania A, Mantovani G, Spada A: G protein mutations in endocrine diseases. Eur J Endocrinol 145(5):543–559, 2001.

54. Spiegel AM, Weinstein LS: Inherited diseases involving g proteins and g protein-coupled receptors. Annu Rev Med 55:27–39, 2004.

55. Hurley JH: Structure, mechanism, and regulation of mammalian adenylyl cyclase. J Biol Chem 274(12):7599–7602, 1999.

56. Cooper DM: Regulation and organization of adenylyl cyclases and cAMP. Biochem J 75(Pt 3):517–529, 2003.

57. Hanoune J, Defer N: Regulation and role of adenylyl cyclase isoforms. Annu Rev Pharmacol Toxicol 41:145–174, 2001.

58. Taussig R, Gilman AG: Mammalian membrane-bound adenylyl cyclases. J Biol Chem 270(1):1–4, 1995.

59. Cooper DM, Mons N, Karpen JW: Adenylyl cyclases and the interaction between calcium and cAMP signalling. Nature 374(6521):421–424, 1995.

60. Taylor SS, et al: PKA: A portrait of protein kinase dynamics. Biochim Biophys Acta 1697(1–2):259–269, 2004.

61. Knighton DR, et al: Crystal structure of the catalytic subunit of cyclic adenosine monophosphate-dependent protein kinase. Science 253(5018):407–414, 1991.

62. Knighton DR, et al: Structure of a peptide inhibitor bound to the catalytic subunit of cyclic adenosine monophosphate-dependent protein kinase. Science 253(5018):414–420, 1991.

63. Soderling TR: Protein kinases. Regulation by autoinhibitory domains. J Biol Chem 265(4):1823–1826, 1990.

64. Van Patten SM, et al: The alpha- and beta-isoforms of the inhibitor protein of the 3′,5′-cyclic adenosine monophosphate-dependent protein kinase: Characteristics and tissue- and developmental-specific expression. Mol Endocrinol 6(12):2114–2122, 1992.

65. Toner-Webb J, et al: Autophosphorylation of the catalytic subunit of cAMP-dependent protein kinase. J Biol Chem 267(35):25174–25180, 1992.

66. Clegg CH, et al: A mutation in the catalytic subunit of protein kinase A prevents myristylation but does not inhibit biological activity. J Biol Chem 264(33):20140–20146, 1989.

67. Alto N, et al: Intracellular targeting of protein kinases and phosphatases. Diabetes 51 (Suppl 3):S385–S388, 2002.

68. Carnegie GK, Scott JD: A-kinase anchoring proteins and neuronal signaling mechanisms. Genes Dev 17(13):1557–1568, 2003.

69. Malbon CC, Tao J, Wang HY: AKAPs (A-kinase anchoring proteins) and molecules that compose their G-protein-coupled receptor signalling complexes. Biochem J 379(Pt 1):1–9, 2004.

70. Roach PJ: Multisite and hierarchal protein phosphorylation. J Biol Chem 266(22):14139–14142, 1991.

71. Ally S, et al: Selective modulation of protein kinase isozymes by the site-selective analog 8-chloroadenosine 3′,5′-cyclic monophosphate provides a biological means for control of human colon cancer cell growth. Proc Natl Acad Sci U S A 85(17):6319–6322, 1988.

72. Rothermel JD, et al: Inhibition of glycogenolysis in isolated rat hepatocytes by the Rp diastereomer of adenosine cyclic 3′,5′-phosphorothioate. J Biol Chem 258(20):12125–12128, 1983.

73. Nigg EA, et al: Cyclic-AMP-dependent protein kinase type II is associated with the Golgi complex and with centrosomes. Cell 41(3):1039–1051, 1985.

74. Carr DW, et al: Interaction of the regulatory subunit (RII) of cAMP-dependent protein kinase with RII-anchoring proteins occurs through an amphipathic helix binding motif. J Biol Chem 266(22):14188–14192, 1991.

75. Colledge M, Scott JD: AKAPs: From structure to function. Trends Cell Biol 9(6):216–221, 1999.

76. Beebe SJ, et al: The C gamma subunit is a unique isozyme of the cAMP-dependent protein kinase. J Biol Chem 267(35):25505–25512, 1992.

77. Van Patten SM, et al: Molecular cloning of a rat testis form of the inhibitor protein of cAMP-dependent protein kinase. Proc Natl Acad Sci U S A 88(12):5383–5387, 1991.

78. Gray PC, Scott JD, Catterall WA: Regulation of ion channels by cAMP-dependent protein kinase and A-kinase anchoring proteins. Curr Opin Neurobiol 8(3):330–334, 1998.

79. Knutsen HK, et al: Inhibitors of RNA and protein synthesis stabilize messenger RNA for the RII beta subunit of protein kinase A in different cellular compartments. Biochem Biophys Res Commun 183(2):632–639, 1992.

80. Mayr B, Montminy M: Transcriptional regulation by the phosphorylation-dependent factor CREB. Nat Rev Mol Cell Biol 2(8):599–609, 2001.

81. Buchler W, et al: Regulation of gene expression by transfected subunits of cAMP-dependent protein kinase. Eur J Biochem 188(2):253–259, 1990.

82. Tortora G, Cho-Chung YS: Type II regulatory subunit of protein kinase restores cAMP-dependent transcription in a cAMP-unresponsive cell line. J Biol Chem 265(30):18067–18070, 1990.

83. Wu JC, Wang JH: Sequence-selective DNA binding to the regulatory subunit of cAMP-dependent protein kinase. J Biol Chem 264(17):9989–9993, 1989.

84. Jones KW, et al: Subtractive hybridization cloning of a tissue-specific extinguisher: TSE1 encodes a regulatory subunit of protein kinase A. Cell 66(5):861–872, 1991.

85. Posner JB, et al: The assay of adenosine-3′,5′-phosphate in skeletal muscle. Biochemistry 28:1040–1044, 1964.

86. Collins SP, Uhler MD: Characterization of PKIgamma, a novel isoform of the protein kinase inhibitor of cAMP-dependent protein kinase. J Biol Chem 272(29):18169–18178, 1997.

87. Walsh DA, Ashby CD: Protein kinases: Aspects of their regulation and diversity. Recent Prog Horm Res 29:329–359, 1973.

88. Wiley JC, et al: Role of regulatory subunits and protein kinase inhibitor (PKI) in determining nuclear localization and activity of the catalytic subunit of protein kinase A. J Biol Chem 274(10):6381–6387, 1999.

89. Wen W, et al: Identification of a signal for rapid export of proteins from the nucleus. Cell 82(3):463–473, 1995.

90. Harootunian AT, et al: Movement of the free catalytic subunit of cAMP-dependent protein kinase into and out of the nucleus can be explained by diffusion. Mol Biol Cell 4(10):993–1002, 1993.

91. Fantozzi DA, et al: Thermostable inhibitor of cAMP-dependent protein kinase enhances the rate of export of the kinase catalytic subunit from the nucleus. J Biol Chem 269(4):2676–2686, 1994.

92. Fornerod M, et al: CRM1 is an export receptor for leucine-rich nuclear export signals. Cell 90(6):1051–1060, 1997.

93. Ohno M, Fornerod M, Mattaj IW: Nucleocytoplasmic transport: The last 200 nanometers. Cell 92(3):327–336, 1998.

94. Kumar P, Walsh DA: A dual-specificity isoform of the protein kinase inhibitor PKI produced by alternate gene splicing. Biochem J 362(Pt 3):533–537, 2002.

95. Belyamani M, Gangolli EA, Idzerda RL: Reproductive function in protein kinase inhibitor-deficient mice. Mol Cell Biol 21(12):3959–3963, 2001.

96. Kawakami M, Nakanishi N: The role of an endogenous PKA inhibitor, PKIalpha, in organizing left-right axis formation. Development 128(13):2509–2515, 2001.

97. Farrow B, et al: Inhibition of pancreatic cancer cell growth and induction of apoptosis with novel therapies directed against protein kinase A. Surgery 134(2):197–205, 2003.

98. Duffy SN, Nguyen PV: Postsynaptic application of a peptide inhibitor of cAMP-dependent protein kinase blocks expression of long-lasting synaptic potentiation in hippocampal neurons. J Neurosci 23(4):1142–1150, 2003.

99. Robinson-White A, Stratakis CA: Protein kinase A signaling: "Cross-talk" with other pathways in endocrine cells. Ann N Y Acad Sci 968:256–270, 2002.

100. Stork PJ, Schmitt JM: Crosstalk between cAMP and MAP kinase signaling in the regulation of cell proliferation. Trends Cell Biol 12(6):258–266, 2002.

101. Berridge MJ: Inositol trisphosphate and calcium signalling. Nature 361(6410):315–325, 1993.

102. Nishizuka Y: The role of protein kinase C in cell surface signal transduction and tumour promotion. Nature 308(5961):693–698, 1984.

103. Schulman H, Lou LL: Multifunctional Ca2+/calmodulin-dependent protein kinase: Domain structure and regulation. Trends Biochem Sci 14(2):62–66, 1989.

104. Hunter T, Cooper JA: Protein-tyrosine kinases. Annu Rev Biochem 54:897–930, 1985.

105. Blackshear PJ, Nairn AC, Kuo JF: Protein kinases 1988: A current perspective. FASEB J 2(14):2957–2969, 1988.

106. Karin M: Signal transduction from cell surface to nucleus in development and disease. FASEB J 6(8):2581–2590, 1992.

107. Hunter T, Karin M: The regulation of transcription by phosphorylation. Cell 70(3):375–387, 1992.

108. Roach PJ: Control of glycogen synthase by hierarchal protein phosphorylation. FASEB J 4(12):2961–2968, 1990.

109. Woodgett JR: A common denominator linking glycogen metabolism, nuclear oncogenes and development. Trends Biochem Sci 16(5):177–181, 1991.

110. Ackerman P, Glover CV, Osheroff N: Stimulation of casein kinase II by epidermal growth factor: Relationship between the physiological activity of the kinase and the phosphorylation state of its beta subunit. Proc Natl Acad Sci U S A 87(2):821–825, 1990.

111. Dumont JE, Jauniaux JC, Roger PP: The cyclic AMP-mediated stimulation of cell proliferation. Trends Biochem Sci 14(2):67–71, 1989.

112. Burgering BM, Bos JL: Regulation of Ras-mediated signalling: More than one way to skin a cat. Trends Biochem Sci 20(1):18–22, 1995.

113. Cook SJ, McCormick F: Inhibition by cAMP of Ras-dependent activation of Raf. Science 262(5136):1069–1072, 1993.

114. Cobb MH, Goldsmith EJ: How MAP kinases are regulated. J Biol Chem 270(25):14843–14846, 1995.

115. Pierrat B, et al: RSK-B, a novel ribosomal S6 kinase family member, is a CREB kinase under dominant control of p38alpha mitogen-activated protein kinase (p38alphaMAPK). J Biol Chem 273(45):29661–29671, 1998.

116. Tan Y, et al: FGF and stress regulate CREB and ATF-1 via a pathway involving p38 MAP kinase and MAPKAP kinase-2. EMBO J 15(17):4629–4642, 1996.

117. Kawasaki H, et al: A family of cAMP-binding proteins that directly activate Rap1. Science 282(5397):2275–2279, 1998.

118. Boguski MS, McCormick F: Proteins regulating Ras and its relatives. Nature 366(6456):643–654, 1993.

119. Singh LP, Aroor AR, Wahba AJ: Translational control of eukaryotic gene expression. Role of the guanine nucleotide exchange factor and chain initiation factor-2. Enzyme Protein 48(2):61–80, 1994.

120. Quilliam LA, et al: Guanine nucleotide exchange factors: Activators of the Ras superfamily of proteins. Bioessays 17:395–404, 1995.

121. Overbeck AF, et al: Guanine nucleotide exchange factors: Activators of Ras superfamily proteins. Mol Reprod Dev 42(4):468–476, 1995.

122. Franke B, Akkerman JW, Bos JL: Rapid Ca2+-mediated activation of Rap1 in human platelets. EMBO J 16(2):252–259, 1997.

123. Ebinu JO, et al: RasGRP, a Ras guanyl nucleotide-releasing protein with calcium- and diacylglycerol-binding motifs. Science 280(5366):1082–1086, 1998.

124. Springett GM, Kawasaki H, Spriggs DR: Non-kinase second-messenger signaling: New pathways with new promise. Bioessays 26(7):730–738, 2004.

125. Enserink JM, et al: A novel Epac-specific cAMP analogue demonstrates independent regulation of Rap1 and ERK. Nat Cell Biol 4(11):901–906, 2002.

126. Bos JL, et al: The role of Rap1 in integrin-mediated cell adhesion. Biochem Soc Trans 31(Pt 1):83–86, 2003.

127. Fleming YM, Frame MC, Houslay MD: PDE4-regulated cAMP degradation controls the assembly of integrin-dependent actin adhesion structures and REF52 cell migration. J Cell Sci 117(Pt 11):2377–2388, 2004.

128. Ivins JK, Parry MK, Long DA: A novel cAMP-dependent pathway activates neuronal integrin function in retinal neurons. J Neurosci 24(5):1212–1216, 2004.

129. Holz G: Epac: A new cAMP-binding protein in support of glucagon-like peptide-1 receptor-mediated signal transduction in the pancreatic beta-cell. Diabetes 53(1):5–13, 2004.

130. Ozaki N, et al: cAMP-GEFII is a direct target of cAMP in regulated exocytosis. Nat Cell Biol 2(11):805–811, 2000.

131. Kang G, et al: Epac-selective cAMP analog 8-pCPT-2′-O-Me-cAMP as a stimulus for Ca2+induced Ca2+ release and exocytosis in pancreatic beta-cells. J Biol Chem 278(10):8279–8285, 2003.

132. Tsuboi T, et al: Glucagon-like peptide-1 mobilizes intracellular Ca2+ and stimulates mitochondrial ATP synthesis in pancreatic MIN6 beta-cells. Biochem J 369(Pt 2):287–299, 2003.

133. Zhong N, Zucker RS: Roles of Ca2+, hyperpolarization and cyclic nucleotide-activated channel activation, and actin in temporal synaptic tagging. J Neurosci 24(17):4205–4212, 2004.

134. Novara M: Exposure to cAMP and beta-adrenergic stimulation recruits Ca(V)3 T-type channels in rat chromaffin cells through Epac cAMP-receptor proteins. J Physiol 558(Pt 2):433–449, 2004.

135. Matulef K, Zagotta WN: Cyclic nucleotide-gated ion channels. Annu Rev Cell Dev Biol 19:23–44, 2003.

136. Zhong H, et al: The heteromeric cyclic nucleotide-gated channel adopts a 3A:1B stoichiometry. Nature 420(6912):193–198, 2002.

137. Zhong HJ, Lai J, Yau KW: Selective heteromeric assembly of cyclic nucleotide-gated channels. Proc Natl Acad Sci U S A 100(9):5509–5513, 2003.

138. Hofmann F, Biel M, Kaupp UB: International Union of Pharmacology. XLII. Compendium of voltage-gated ion channels: Cyclic nucleotide-modulated channels. Pharmacol Rev 55(4):587–589, 2003.

139. Bonigk W, et al: The native rat olfactory cyclic nucleotide-gated channel is composed of three distinct subunits. J Neurosci 19(13):5332–5347, 1999.

140. Ruiz ML, Karpen JW: Single cyclic nucleotide-gated channels locked in different ligand-bound states. Nature 389(6649):389–392, 1997.

141. Karpen JW, Ruiz M: Ion channels: Does each subunit do something on its own? Trends Biochem Sci 27(8):402–409, 2002.

142. Kaupp UB, Seifert R: Molecular diversity of pacemaker ion channels. Annu Rev Physiol 63:235–257, 2001.

143. Yu H, et al: MinK-related peptide 1: A beta subunit for the HCN ion channel subunit family enhances expression and speeds activation. Circ Res 88(12):E84–E87, 2001.

144. Altomare C, et al: Heteromeric HCN1-HCN4 channels: A comparison with native pacemaker channels from the rabbit sinoatrial node. J Physiol 549(Pt 2):347–359, 2003.

145. Xue T, Marban E, Li RA: Dominant-negative suppression of HCN1- and HCN2-encoded pacemaker currents by an engineered HCN1 construct: Insights into structure-function relationships and multimerization. Circ Res 90(12):1267–1273, 2002.

146. Much B, et al: Role of subunit heteromerization and N-linked glycosylation in the formation of functional hyperpolarization-activated cyclic nucleotide-gated channels. J Biol Chem 278(44):43781-43786, 2003.

147. Ludwig A, et al: Structure and function of cardiac pacemaker channels. Cell Physiol Biochem 9(4–5):179–186, 1999.

148. Wainger BJ, et al: Molecular mechanism of cAMP modulation of HCN pacemaker channels. Nature 411(6839):805–810, 2001.

149. Robinson RB, Siegelbaum SA: Hyperpolarization-activated cation currents: From molecules to physiological function. Annu Rev Physiol 65:453–480, 2003.

150. Pachucki J, Burmeister LA, Larsen PR: Thyroid hormone regulates hyperpolarization-activated cyclic nucleotide-gated channel (HCN2) mRNA in the rat heart. Circ Res 85(6):498–503, 1999.

151. Stevens DR, et al: Hyperpolarization-activated channels HCN1 and HCN4 mediate responses to sour stimuli. Nature 413(6856):631–635, 2001.

152. Cohen P, Cohen PT: Protein phosphatases come of age. J Biol Chem 264(36):21435–21438, 1989.

153. Brushia RJ, Walsh DA: Phosphorylase kinase: The complexity of its regulation is reflected in the complexity of its structure. Front Biosci 4:D618–D641, 1999.

154. Ma YC, Huang XY: Novel signaling pathway through the beta-adrenergic receptor. Trends Cardiovasc Med 12(1):46–49, 2002.

155. Liggett SB: Update on current concepts of the molecular basis of beta2-adrenergic receptor signaling. J Allergy Clin Immunol 110(6 Suppl):S223–S227, 2002.

156. Skeberdis VA: Structure and function of beta3-adrenergic receptors. Medicina (Kaunas) 40(5):407–413, 2004.

157. Hall RA: Beta-adrenergic receptors and their interacting proteins. Semin Cell Dev Biol 15(3):281–288, 2004.

158. Penela P, Ribas C, Mayor F Jr: Mechanisms of regulation of the expression and function of G protein-coupled receptor kinases. Cell Signal 15(11):973–981, 2003.

159. Penn RB, Pronin AN, Benovic JL: Regulation of G protein-coupled receptor kinases. Trends Cardiovasc Med 10(2):81–89, 2000.

160. Hausdorff WP, et al: Phosphorylation sites on two domains of the beta 2-adrenergic receptor are involved in distinct pathways of receptor desensitization. J Biol Chem 264(21):12657–12665, 1989.

161. Sibley DR, et al: Regulation of transmembrane signaling by receptor phosphorylation. Cell 48(6):913–922, 1987.

162. Vargiu P, et al: The small GTP-binding protein, Rhes, regulates signal transduction from G protein-coupled receptors. Oncogene 23(2):559–568, 2004.

163. Mundell SJ, et al: Activation of cyclic AMP-dependent protein kinase inhibits the desensitization and internalization of metabotropic glutamate receptors 1a and 1b. Mol Pharmacol 65(6):1507–1516, 2004.

164. Benovic JL, et al: Functional desensitization of the isolated beta-adrenergic receptor by the beta-adrenergic receptor kinase: Potential role of an analog of the retinal protein arrestin (48-kDa protein). Proc Natl Acad Sci U S A 84(24):8879–8882, 1987.

165. Wilden U, Hall SW, Kuhn H: Phosphodiesterase activation by photoexcited rhodopsin is quenched when rhodopsin is phosphorylated and binds the intrinsic 48-kDa protein of rod outer segments. Proc Natl Acad Sci U S A 83(5):1174–1178, 1986.

166. Iaccarino G, Koch WJ: Transgenic mice targeting the heart unveil G protein-coupled receptor kinases as therapeutic targets. Assay Drug Dev Technol 1(2):347–355, 2003.

167. Mak JC, et al: Increased expression of G protein-coupled receptor kinases in cystic fibrosis lung. Eur J Pharmacol 436(3):165–172, 2002.

168. Anis Y, et al: Antidiabetic effect of novel modulating peptides of G-protein-coupled kinase in experimental models of diabetes. Diabetologia 47(7):1232–1244, 2004.

169. Cheng SH, et al: Phosphorylation of the R domain by cAMP-dependent protein kinase regulates the CFTR chloride channel. Cell 66(5):1027–1036, 1991.

170. Anderson MP, et al: Nucleoside triphosphates are required to open the CFTR chloride channel. Cell 67(4):775–784, 1991.
171. Kunzelmann K, Schreiber R: CFTR, a regulator of channels. J Membr Biol 168(1):1-8, 1999.
172. Peters KW, et al: Mechanisms underlying regulated CFTR trafficking. Med Clin North Am 84(3):633–640, ix–x, 2000.
173. Bradbury NA: cAMP signaling cascades and CFTR: Is there more to learn? Pflugers Arch 443 (Suppl 1):S85–S91, 2001.
174. Kunzelmann K: The cystic fibrosis transmembrane conductance regulator and its function in epithelial transport. Rev Physiol Biochem Pharmacol 137:1–70, 1999.
175. Riordan JR, et al: Identification of the cystic fibrosis gene: Cloning and characterization of complementary DNA. Science 245(4922):1066–1073, 1989.
176. Berger HA, Travis SM, Welsh MJ: Regulation of the cystic fibrosis transmembrane conductance regulator Cl-channel by specific protein kinases and protein phosphatases. J Biol Chem 268(3):2037–2047, 1993.
177. Holz GG, Habener JF: Signal transduction crosstalk in the endocrine system: Pancreatic beta-cells and the glucose competence concept. Trends Biochem Sci 17(10):388–393, 1992.
178. Holz GGT, Kuhtreiber WM, Habener JF: Pancreatic beta-cells are rendered glucose-competent by the insulinotropic hormone glucagon-like peptide-1(7-37). Nature 361(6410):362–365, 1993.
179. Montminy MR, Gonzalez GA, Yamamoto KK: Regulation of cAMP-inducible genes by CREB. Trends Neurosci 13(5):184–188, 1990.
180. Lamprecht R: CREB: A message to remember. Cell Mol Life Sci 55(4):554–563, 1999.
181. Andrisani OM: CREB-mediated transcriptional control. Crit Rev Eukaryot Gene Expr 9(1):19–32, 1999.
182. Fehmann HC, Habener JF: Galanin inhibits proinsulin gene expression stimulated by the insulinotropic hormone glucagon-like peptide-I(7-37) in mouse insulinoma beta TC-1 cells. Endocrinology 130(5):2890–2896, 1992.
183. Hoeffler JP, et al: Cyclic AMP-responsive DNA-binding protein: Structure based on a cloned placental cDNA. Science 242(4884):1430–1433, 1988.
184. Gonzalez GA, Montminy MR: Cyclic AMP stimulates somatostatin gene transcription by phosphorylation of CREB at serine 133. Cell 59(4):675–680, 1989.
185. Foulkes NS, et al: Developmental switch of CREM function during spermatogenesis: From antagonist to activator. Nature 355(6355):80–84, 1992.
186. de Groot RP, Sassone-Corsi P: Hormonal control of gene expression: Multiplicity and versatility of cyclic adenosine 3',5'-monophosphate-responsive nuclear regulators. Mol Endocrinol 7(2):145–153, 1993.
187. Dash PK, et al: cAMP response element-binding protein is activated by Ca2+/calmodulin—as well as cAMP-dependent protein kinase. Proc Natl Acad Sci U S A 88(11):5061–5065, 1991.
188. Sheng M, Thompson MA, Greenberg ME: CREB: A Ca(2+)-regulated transcription factor phosphorylated by calmodulin-dependent kinases. Science 252(5011):1427–1430, 1991.
189. Gonzalez GA, et al: A cluster of phosphorylation sites on the cyclic AMP-regulated nuclear factor CREB predicted by its sequence. Nature 337(6209):749–752, 1989.
190. Gonzalez GA, et al: Characterization of motifs which are critical for activity of the cyclic AMP-responsive transcription factor CREB. Mol Cell Biol 11(3):1306–1312, 1991.
191. Lamph WW, et al: Negative and positive regulation by transcription factor cAMP response element-binding protein is modulated by phosphorylation. Proc Natl Acad Sci U S A 87(11):4320–4324, 1990.
192. Yamamoto KK, et al: Characterization of a bipartite activator domain in transcription factor CREB. Cell 60(4):611–617, 1990.
193. Struthers RS, et al: Somatotroph hypoplasia and dwarfism in transgenic mice expressing a non-phosphorylatable CREB mutant. Nature 350(6319):622–624, 1991.
194. Leonard J, et al: The LIM family transcription factor Isl-1 requires cAMP response element binding protein to promote somatostatin expression in pancreatic islet cells. Proc Natl Acad Sci U S A 89(14):6247–6251, 1992.
195. Masson N, et al: Cyclic AMP response element-binding protein and the catalytic subunit of protein kinase A are present in F9 embryonal carcinoma cells but are unable to activate the somatostatin promoter. Mol Cell Biol 12(3):1096–1106, 1992.
196. Hagiwara M, et al: Transcriptional attenuation following cAMP induction requires PP-1-mediated dephosphorylation of CREB. Cell 70(1):105–113, 1992.
197. Yamamoto KK, et al: Phosphorylation-induced binding and transcriptional efficacy of nuclear factor CREB. Nature 334(6182):494–498, 1988.
198. Nichols M, et al: Phosphorylation of CREB affects its binding to high and low affinity sites: Implications for cAMP induced gene transcription. EMBO J 11(9):3337-3346, 1992.
199. Kramer IM, et al: TGF-beta 1 induces phosphorylation of the cyclic AMP responsive element binding protein in ML-CCl64 cells. EMBO J 10(5):1083–1089, 1991.

Second Messenger Signaling Pathways: Phospholipids and Calcium

Marvin C. Gershengorn and Patricia M. Hinkle

PHOSPHOINOSITIDES
    Phosphoinositide-Specific Phospholipase C
    Receptor Activation of PPI-PLC
    Phosphoinositide Metabolism

CALCIUM SIGNALING
    I-1,4,5-P$_3$ Mobilization of Calcium
    Receptor Activation of Calcium Influx
    Receptor-Mediated Changes in [Ca^{2+}]$_i$

1,2-Dag and Protein Kinase C
Activation of Phospholipase D
Activation of Phospholipase A2

3-PHOSPHOINOSITIDES

INTERACTIONS BETWEEN SIGNALING PATHWAYS

CONCLUDING REMARKS

Extracellular regulatory molecules, such as hormones, neurotransmitters, and growth factors, interact with cells by binding to specific cell-surface receptors. As a result of this interaction, the receptor may be activated to lead to the generation of second messenger molecules intracellularly. A ubiquitous second messenger system utilizes the hydrolysis of phosphoinositides (PPIs), phospholipids that contain the sugar *myo*-inositol as the polar head group. The primary PPI hydrolyzed is phosphatidylinositol 4,5-bisphosphate (PI(4,5)P$_2$) by a phospholipase C (PLC) to generate two molecules that serve as second messengers: inositol-1,4,5-trisphosphate (I-1,4,5-P$_3$) and 1,2-diacylglycerol (1,2-DAG).[1,2] In addition, PI(4,5)P$_2$ (and PI and PI(4)P) is a substrate for phosphoinositide 3-kinase (PI 3-kinase) that generates PI(3,4,5)P$_3$ (and PI(3)P and PI(3,4)P$_2$), which are docking sites for proteins with lipid-binding motifs. Closely related to the actions of these messengers are changes in the concentration of free (or ionized) calcium in the cytoplasm ([Ca^{2+}]$_i$). Because the same signaling pathway is used in many different cell types to stimulate distinct responses, for example, secretion from endocrine cells and contraction of smooth muscle cells, it is evident that there are cell-specific factors that are required to elicit the final responses. The major aim of this chapter is to discuss the mechanisms by which these second messengers are generated, regulated, and metabolized and their proximate effects. The more distal steps that lead to specific cellular responses will not be discussed.

PHOSPHOINOSITIDES

PPIs, or inositol lipids, are composed of a glycerol backbone containing fatty acyl groups at the 1- and 2-positions and a phosphate group coupled via a phosphodiester linkage at the 3-position to *myo*-inositol (Fig. 13-1). The *myo*-inositol head group may have additional phosphates, usually at the 4-position or the 4- and 5-positions. A subclass of PPIs has been described that contains a phosphate at the 3-position of *myo*-inositol (see the section entitled "3-Phosphoinositides"). PPIs are minor lipids in cells constituting on average 5% to 10% of the total phospholipid. Phosphatidylinositol (PI) is the parent lipid and is phosphorylated by a specific enzyme, PI 4-kinase, to yield PI 4-monophosphate (PI(4)P), which is in turn phosphorylated by PI(4)P5-kinase to PI(4,5)P$_2$. PI, PI(4)P, and PI(4,5)P$_2$ can be phosphorylated at the 3-position by PI 3-kinase. There are lipid phosphatases within cells that dephosphorylate PI(4)P and PI(4,5)P$_2$ to PI. Specific enzymes that dephosphorylate 3-phosphoinositides at the 3-position

are present also. These phosphatases are active and limit the levels of polyphosphorylated PIs in unstimulated cells. PI accounts for 85% to 95% of PPIs, whereas PI(4,5)P$_2$, which is the primary phosphoinositide substrate in cells for second messenger generation, constitutes only 2% to 3%. An agonist, such as a hormone, binds to its receptor, which in turn activates a PPI-specific phospholipase C (PPI-PLC) that hydrolyzes PI(4,5)P$_2$ to I-1,4,5-P$_3$ and 1,2-DAG. I-1,4,5-P$_3$ is water-soluble; it is released into the cytoplasm and diffuses away from the membrane, whereas 1,2-DAG remains membrane-bound. I-1,4,5-P$_3$ leads to release of Ca^{2+} from intracellular stores into the cytoplasm and elevates cytoplasmic free Ca^{2+} concentration ([Ca^{2+}]$_i$), and 1,2-DAG activates protein kinase C (PKC).

It is noteworthy that PI(4,5)P$_2$ has been found to bind to AKAP79, a multivalent anchoring protein that binds several protein kinases and phosphatases,[3] and to several cytoskeletal proteins, such as ezrin.[4] Therefore, PI(4,5)P$_2$ appears to play a role in signal transduction as an anchoring protein in addition to being a substrate for second messenger generation. 3-Phosphoinositides are not substrates for PPI-PLC but are important in signal transduction because they serve to anchor signaling proteins to cellular membranes (see the section entitled "3-Phosphoinositides").

PHOSPHOINOSITIDE-SPECIFIC PHOSPHOLIPASE C

Enzymes that hydrolyze phospholipids at the 3-position phosphodiester bond of the glycerol backbone are phospholipases C.[5] When PI(4,5)P$_2$ is the substrate, PLC action leads to the formation of I-1,4,5-P$_3$ and 1,2-DAG (Fig. 13-2). Because of its well-established role in signaling, I-1,4,5-P$_3$ is often referred to simply as IP$_3$. PPI-PLC is a subfamily of PLC that acts specifically on inositol-containing lipids and does not hydrolyze other phospholipids, such as phosphatidylcholine. There are multiple families of PPI-specific PLCs, referred to as PLCβ, PLCγ, PLCδ, and PLCζ.[6–8] Each PLC family comprises several closely related members, encoded by distinct genes that share a high degree of sequence identity. The PLCs are single polypeptide chains that carry out the same enzymatic reaction, share high sequence homology in their catalytic domains, and appear to utilize the same mechanism of catalysis.[8] PLCs in the β, γ, and δ families also contain a PH (pleckstrin homology) domain[9] and a C2 domain[10] involved in phospholipid binding. Other regions of the various PLCs differ markedly in structure. There are important differences in how the various classes of PLCs are regulated.

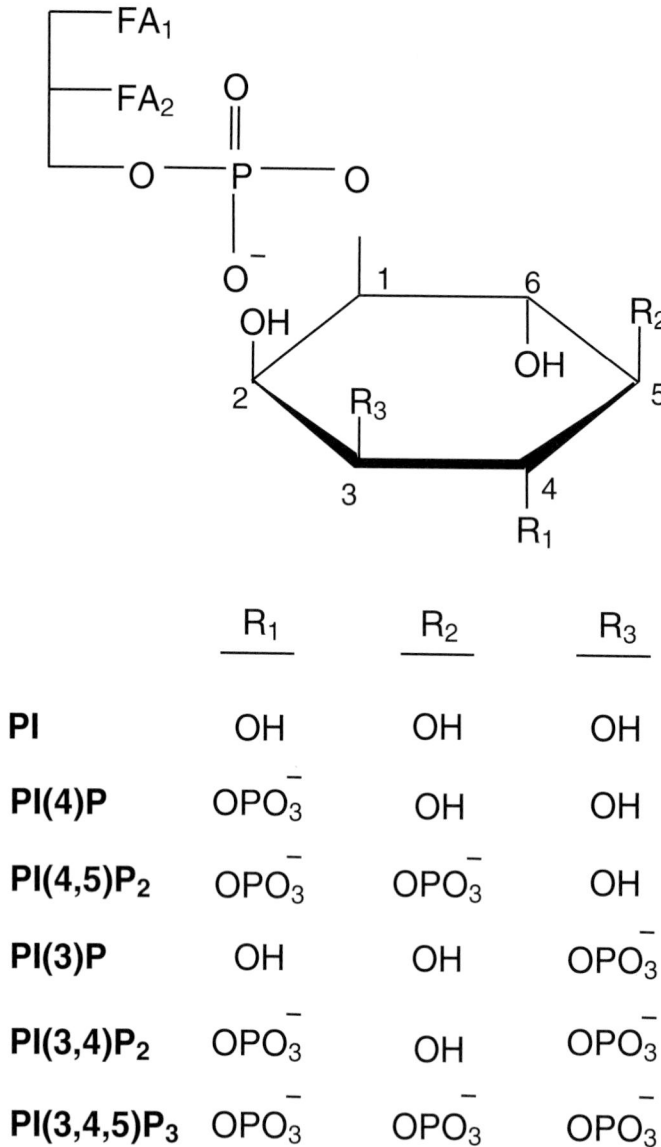

	R_1	R_2	R_3
PI	OH	OH	OH
PI(4)P	OPO_3^-	OH	OH
PI(4,5)P$_2$	OPO_3^-	OPO_3^-	OH
PI(3)P	OH	OH	OPO_3^-
PI(3,4)P$_2$	OPO_3^-	OH	OPO_3^-
PI(3,4,5)P$_3$	OPO_3^-	OPO_3^-	OPO_3^-

Figure 13-1 Structures of the major phosphoinositides. The glycerol backbone is esterified at positions 1 and 2 to fatty acids FA$_1$ and FA$_2$, respectively. FA$_1$ is usually a saturated fatty acid, whereas FA$_2$ may be arachidonic acid. The phosphate head group is coupled to *myo*-inositol at the 3-position of glycerol. PI, phosphatidylinositol; PI(4)P, phosphatidylinositol 4-monophosphate; PI(4,5)P$_2$, phosphatidylinositol 4,5-bisphosphate; PI(3)P, phosphatidylinositol 3-monophosphate; PI(3,4)P$_2$, phosphatidylinositol 3,4-bisphosphate; PI(3,4,5)P$_3$, phosphatidylinositol 3,4,5-trisphosphate.

PI(4,5)P$_2$ is the primary substrate for the PPI-specific PLCs in vivo, although these enzymes also catalyze hydrolysis of PI and PI(4)P in vitro and may do so in vivo in some cell types. PPIs that are phosphorylated at the 3-position of the *myo*-inositol head group, such as PI(3,4,5)P$_3$, the product of PI 3-kinase, are not substrates for PPI-specific PLCs. In cells, enzymes in the PLCβ and PLCγ families are regulated primarily by activation of G protein–coupled receptors and tyrosine kinase pathways, respectively (see below), whereas the PLCδs appear to have a different mechanism of regulation. PLCδ is activated by calcium ion and PLCε by the monomeric small G proteins, including ras. The newly discovered PLCζ appears to play a critical role in fertilization. PLCγs contain two src homology domains, SH2 and SH3, which mediate binding to certain phosphorylated tyrosine residues and proline-rich regions, respectively. The binding of PLCγs to phosphotyrosines

docks them at activated tyrosine kinases, where they are consequently phosphorylated on key tyrosine residues and thereby activated. PLCβs lack SH2 domains and are not activated by tyrosine phosphorylation, but they interact with and are activated by either the activated α subunits of the Gq family or with G protein βγ subunits.

RECEPTOR ACTIVATION OF PPI-PLC

The general features of signal transduction by G protein–coupled receptors, and of the heterotrimeric G proteins, are discussed in Chapter 11. In most cell types, hormones that activate the phosphoinositide pathway via G protein–coupled receptors activate members of the Gq family, and the responses are not blocked by prior treatment with pertussis toxin.[11] An exception to this generalization, as discussed below, occurs especially with cells of hematopoietic lineage. Figure 13-3 illustrates the two mechanisms by which G protein–coupled receptors activate PPI-PLCs. Members of the Gq family, including Gq, G11, G14, and G16, activate PLCβs. The active α subunits of each of these G proteins can stimulate PLCβ activity in vitro and the α subunits are believed to be primarily responsible for PLC activation in vivo. An unusual feature of this pathway is the ability of PLCβ to act as a GAP, or GTPase-activating protein, for Gαq. The effector itself helps to terminate signaling by promoting the conversion of the active Gαq-GTP to the inactive Gαq-GDP, which reassociates with Gβγ. PLCβ1 and β3, which are widely expressed, and PLCβ4, which is present at high levels in some neuronal tissues and retina, are strongly stimulated by the activated α subunits of Gq family members. PLCβ2, which is found primarily in hematopoietic cells, is only weakly activated by Gαq or guanine nucleotides such as GTPγS, a poorly hydrolyzable analogue of GTP that activates α subunits. Gβγ has been shown to activate several of the PLCβs in the order PLCβ3 > PLCβ2 > PLCβ1. In hematopoietic cells, activation of phosphoinositide turnover usually results from the activation of receptors coupled to Gi and Go and is blocked by pertussis toxin, which adenosine diphosphate (ADP)-ribosylates the α subunits of Gi and Go and inhibits interaction with receptors. The α subunits of Gi and Go do not affect the activity of any PLC, but the βγ subunits activate PLCβ2. Although the concentrations of Gβγ that are needed to activate PLCβ2 are quite high, Gi and Go are generally present at high enough concentrations to account for responses via pertussis toxin sensitive pathways. Gβγ also activates PLCβ3, and increased hydrolysis of PI(4,5)P$_2$ is sometimes observed in nonhematopoietic cells, such as fibroblasts and smooth muscle cells, following activation of receptors coupled to Gi and Go.

PLCγs, in contrast to PLCβs, have been shown to associate with and be activated by activated tyrosine kinases. As is discussed in Chapter 8, receptors for numerous growth factors, including epidermal growth factor, platelet-derived growth factor, and fibroblast growth factor, are themselves tyrosine kinases that carry out autophosphorylation or transphosphorylation following agonist binding. Once phosphorylated, specific tyrosines in these growth factor receptors serve as binding sites for the SH2 domains of PLCγ. PLCγ is itself a substrate for the tyrosine kinase. Once it has docked at the kinase, PLCγ becomes phosphorylated on specific tyrosines, which increases its enzyme activity. Activation of nonreceptor (intracellular) tyrosine kinases can lead to activation of PLCγ by a similar mechanism. In this way, PLCγ can be activated by cytokines that activate kinases in the JAK/STAT pathway and by hormones that activate tyrosine kinases such as src. Once PLCγ is activated, it carries out the same reaction as PLCβ and activates the same downstream pathways.

PHOSPHOINOSITIDE METABOLISM

After hydrolysis of PI(4,5)P$_2$, both I-1,4,5-P$_3$ and 1,2-DAG serve as intracellular messengers and then are rapidly

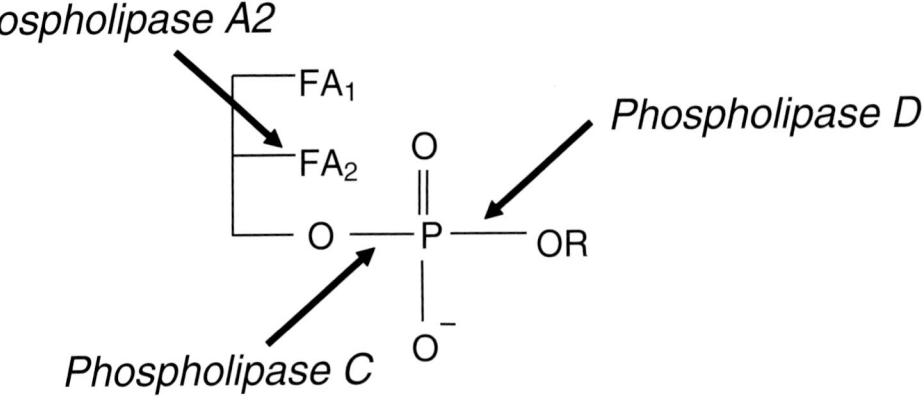

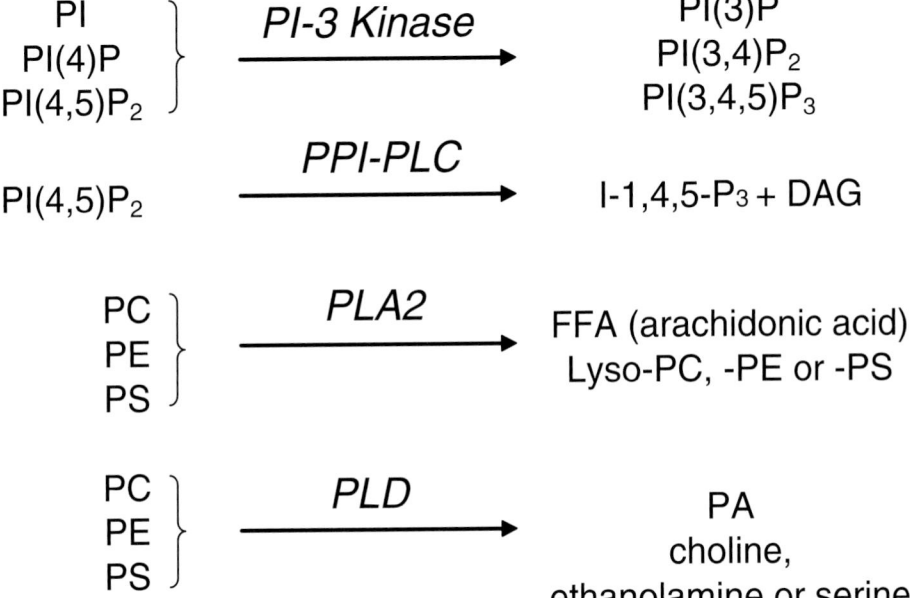

Figure 13-2 Enzymatic reactions modifying phospholipids. The sites of phospholipid hydrolysis are indicated by arrows. FA_1, fatty acid at position 1; FA_2, fatty acid at position 2; PPI-PLC, phosphoinositide-specific phospholipase C; PLD, phospholipase D; PLA2, phospholipase A2; $I-1,4,5-P_3$, inositol-1,4,5-trisphosphate; DAG, 1,2-diacylglycerol; PC, phosphatidylcholine; PE, phosphatidylethanolamine; PS, phosphatidylserine; FFA, free fatty acid; lyso-PE, PC, or PS, lysophospholipids; PA, phosphatidic acid. The fatty acid that is most often released by PLA2 is arachidonic acid. Reactions catalyzed by phosphatidylinositol-3-kinase (PI-3 kinase) are also shown.

metabolized. $I-1,4,5-P_3$ undergoes a series of metabolic conversions that generate a large number of inositol phosphate derivatives. $I-1,4,5-P_3$ can be hydrolyzed by a series of phosphatases to *myo*-inositol, or it can be phosphorylated by a specific kinase to inositol-1,3,4,5-tetrakisphosphate ($I-1,3,4,5-P_4$). Although it has not been proved, some investigators think that $I-1,3,4,5-P_4$ is biologically active and can influence cellular Ca^{2+} homeostasis. $I-1,3,4,5-P_4$ can be dephosphorylated to inositol-1,3,4-trisphosphate ($I-1,3,4-P_3$), which does not affect Ca^{2+} fluxes and can be converted by successive dephosphorylations to *myo*-inositol. Alternatively, $I-1,3,4,5-P_4$ can be phosphorylated to inositol pentakisphosphate (IP_5) and possibly to inositol hexakisphosphate (IP_6). It is not known whether IP_5 or IP_6 has second messenger activity. Thus, $I-1,4,5-P_3$ is metabolized in a series of dephosphorylation reactions that constitute a degradative pathway, whereas phosphorylation of $I-1,4,5-P_3$ may be an activating pathway.

1,2-DAG may be phosphorylated by 1,2-DAG kinase to phosphatidic acid (PA). 1,2-DAG and PA are central intermediates in the synthesis of many cellular phospholipids. PA, which may be an important signaling molecule itself, as discussed below, can be condensed with cytidine triphosphate (CTP) to form CDP-diacylglycerol (CDP-DAG), a reaction catalyzed by PA: cytidylyl transferase. CDP-DAG and *myo*-inositol are utilized by PI synthase to form PI; cytidine monophosphate (CMP) is a by-product of this reaction. PI synthase is the only

enzyme that is specific for the synthesis of PI. PI may then be successively phosphorylated to PI(4)P and $PI(4,5)P_2$ by PI 4-kinase and PI(4)P 5-kinase, respectively.

During stimulation of PPI hydrolysis, there is increased synthesis of PI, PI(4)P, and $PI(4,5)P_2$ to replenish the pool of $PI(4,5)P_2$ that would otherwise be rapidly depleted.[12] For example, the amount of inositol phosphates that is formed in cells during a 15-minute stimulation by agonist can be the equivalent of 10 times the original content of $PI(4,5)P_2$. Therefore, during agonist stimulation, there is a marked activation of PI synthase and of the PI 4-kinase and PI(4)P 5-kinase. The mechanism(s) through which synthesis of these lipids is increased has not been conclusively demonstrated. There is no evidence of direct activation of the synthetic enzymes by the receptor or by the second messengers that are generated. A mechanism for activation of PI synthase has been proposed[13]; however, data supporting it have been obtained in only a few cell types. This hypothesis is based on the observation that PI inhibits the activity of PI synthase, a phenomenon that has been termed *product inhibition*. It was proposed that during agonist-stimulated hydrolysis of PPIs and synthesis of PI(4)P and $PI(4,5)P_2$, the decrease in the level of PI releases the PI synthase from product inhibition and increases its activity. A similar mechanism does not account for the increase in the activities of the PPI kinases because there is only a transient decrease in PI(4)P or $PI(4,5)P_2$ during

G Protein-Coupled Receptors

Receptor Tyrosine Kinase

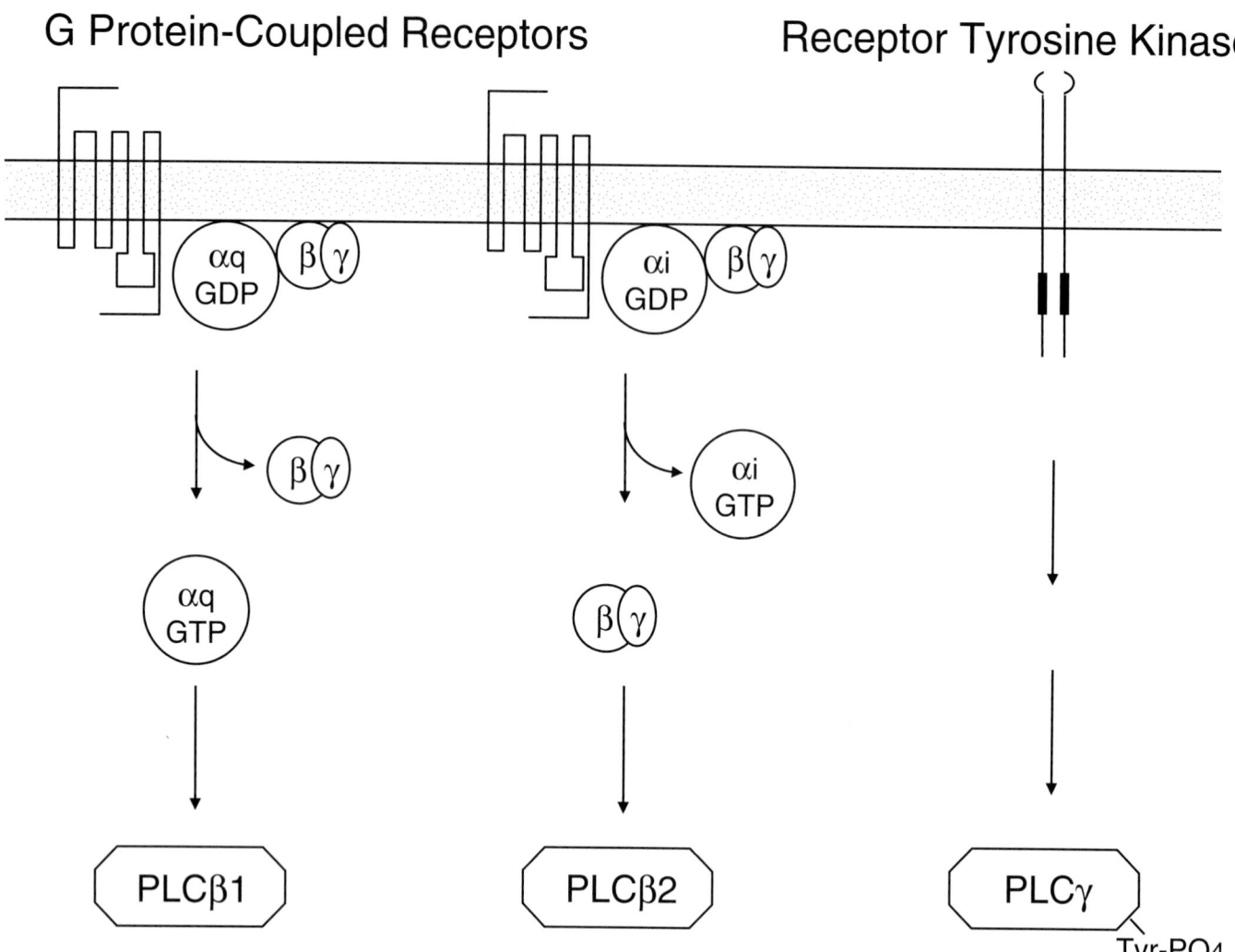

Figure 13-3   Receptor activation of phosphoinositide-specific phospholipase C (PPI-PLC). G protein–coupled receptor activation of PI(4,5)P$_2$ hydrolysis may proceed via two pathways. Receptor may couple to a member of the Gq subfamily of G proteins, leading to exchange of GTP for GDP on the αq subunit and αq-GTP in turn activates PPI-PLCβ1. Another receptor may couple to a member of the Gi subfamily leading to exchange of GTP for GDP on the αi subunit and release of βγ that in turn activates PPI-PLCβ2. Receptor tyrosine kinase autophosphorylates, binds (binds PPI-PLCγ1 via an SH2 domain), and phosphorylates PPI-PLCγ1, thereby activating PPI-PLCγ1.

stimulation. Another circumstance in which PI synthesis can be diminished in some cell types in tissue culture is when they are deprived of the precursor, *myo*-inositol. This situation does not seem to be operative in the intact animal or human because the levels of *myo*-inositol in blood do not vary widely enough to affect PI synthesis under normal physiologic conditions. It has been suggested, however, that *myo*-inositol depletion may occur in patients with diabetes mellitus[14] or that intracellular *myo*-inositol depletion could occur in cells of the central nervous system in patients who are receiving lithium therapy for bipolar disorder.[15] Lithium may deplete cellular *myo*-inositol by inhibiting several of the phosphatases that dephosphorylate the inositol polyphosphates.

The principal cellular site of synthesis of PI appears to be within the endoplasmic reticulum, but there is evidence that it also occurs in the plasma membrane.[16] Phosphorylation of PI to PI(4)P and then to PI(4,5)P$_2$ occurs predominantly in the plasma membrane. Because the majority of PPI hydrolysis occurs at the cell-surface membrane, PI that is synthesized within the endoplasmic reticulum would have to be transferred to the plasma membrane. Transport proteins for phospholipids have been found, and recent evidence is consistent with a role for these proteins in PPI signaling.[17] However, it is not clear whether these proteins bind and transfer PI from the endoplasmic reticulum to the plasma membrane or participate

in membrane cycling from the endoplasmic reticulum to the plasma membrane. Receptor activation stimulates internalization (or endocytosis) and recycling (or retroendocytosis) of receptors[18] and may stimulate exocytosis in secretory cells. It is noteworthy that PI transfer proteins are involved in exocytosis also.[19] These movements of membrane-delimited vesicles from within the cell to the cell surface could serve to replenish some of the PI that is lost secondary to PPI hydrolysis. PI synthesis within the plasma membrane could be activated also. Phosphoinositides of the PI-PLC cycle has also been found in the nucleus, where a role in DNA repair, transcription, and RNA metabolism has been suggested.[20,21]

CALCIUM SIGNALING

Regulated changes in intracellular Ca^{2+} mediate many critical processes, including secretion, contraction, and transcription.[22,23] Therefore, it is clear that events that lead to changes in the intracellular free Ca^{2+} concentration, [Ca^{2+}]$_i$, constitute an important signaling mechanism for diverse cellular functions. The [Ca^{2+}]$_i$ in unstimulated cells is approximately 100 nanomolar (1×10^{-7} M), which is about 10,000-fold lower than the ambient extracellular free Ca^{2+} concentration (Fig. 13-4). The low concentration of Ca^{2+} in the cytoplasm is

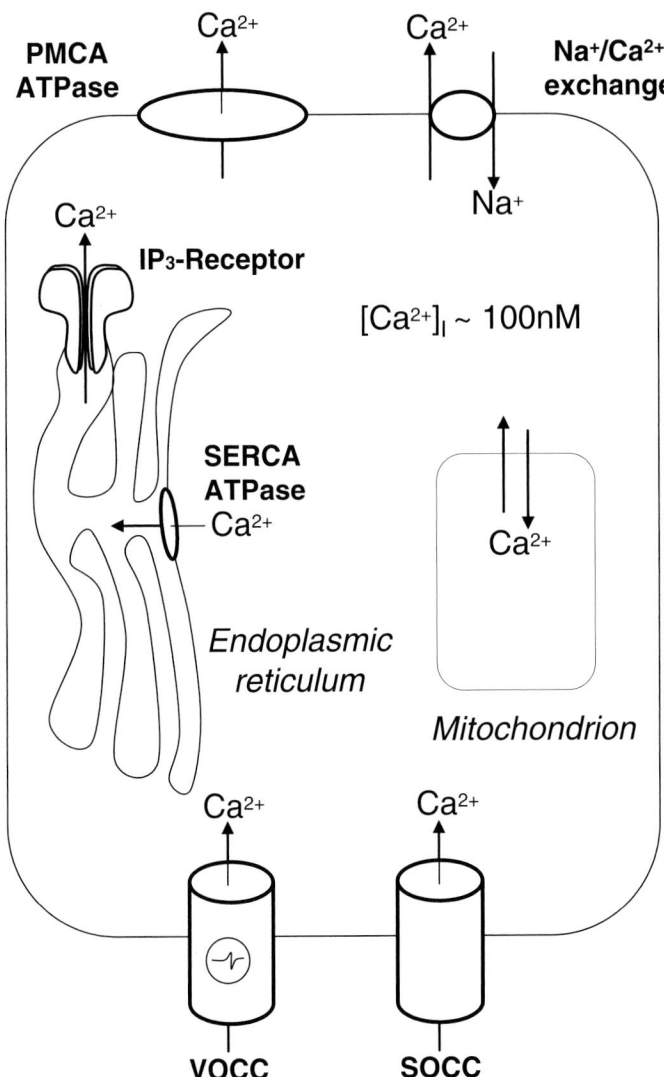

Figure 13-4 Schematic depiction of a cell illustrating mechanisms of regulation of intracellular ionized calcium. The concentration of ionized, or free, intracellular Ca^{2+} ($[Ca^{2+}]_i$) in the unstimulated cell is approximately 100 nM. The plasma membrane contains $Ca^{2+}Mg^{2+}$ ATPases, or plasma membrane "Ca^{2+} pumps," and Na^+Ca^{2+} antiporters that extrude Ca^{2+} from the cell as well as voltage-operated calcium channels (VOCCs) and store-operated Ca^{2+} channels (SOCCs), through which Ca^{2+} can enter the cell. VOCCs are present in excitable cells. The endoplasmic or sarcoplasmic reticulum contains $Ca^{2+}Mg^{2+}$ ATPases, which are different from those present in the plasma membrane and allow sequestration of Ca^{2+} and I-1,4,5-P_3-sensitive (I-1,4,5-P_3 receptor, IP_3-R) and I-1,4,5-P_3-insensitive mechanisms to allow for mobilization of Ca^{2+}. The mitochondria sequester calcium by less well-defined mechanisms.

maintained by the concerted effects of a number of cellular processes that limit the influx of extracellular Ca^{2+} and cause active removal of Ca^{2+} into the extracellular space or into cellular organelles. Cellular membranes are highly impermeable to Ca^{2+}. Ca^{2+} can flow into the cell through ion channels in the plasma membrane; these are predominantly inactive (or "closed") in unstimulated cells. In some cells, especially excitable cells such as neurons and neuroendocrine cells, voltage-operated Ca^{2+} channels (VOCCs) can exhibit brief spontaneous activations leading to "Ca^{2+} spikes" that allow significant basal Ca^{2+} influx. VOCCs in the plasma membrane can be activated (or "opened") by depolarization to permit a large Ca^{2+} influx as Ca^{2+} flows down its electrochemical gradient. Ca^{2+} is pumped out of the cell, against a gradient, by two

energy-dependent processes. The plasma membrane contains a Ca^{2+} pump, a Ca^{2+}-Mg^{2+} ATPase (PMCA for plasma membrane Ca^{2+} ATPase) that uses ATP directly to move Ca^{2+} across the plasma membrane. There are four known plasma membrane Ca^{2+} pumps and multiple splice variants of these, which differ in their modes of regulation and tissue expression.[24] Cytoplasmic Ca^{2+} can also be moved across the plasma membrane by the Na^+-Ca^{2+} exchanger, which is dependent on the Na^+ gradient established by the Na^+-K^+ ATPase and can operate in either direction.

Within the cell, several organelles sequester Ca^{2+} from the cytoplasm and thereby contribute to the maintenance of a low $[Ca^{2+}]_i$. The major organelles that are involved in this process are the endoplasmic reticulum[25] and mitochondria.[26] The lumen of the endoplasmic reticulum maintains a much higher Ca^{2+} concentration than the cytoplasm. The concentration of free Ca^{2+} in the endoplasmic reticulum is not known with certainty but is estimated at 0.1 to 1 mM, far above the typical cytoplasmic level of 100 nM. An adenosine triphosphate (ATP)-driven Ca^{2+} pump, the SERCA (for sarco/endoplasmic reticulum Ca^{2+} ATPase), sequesters Ca^{2+} in the endoplasmic reticulum. The SERCA pumps in the endoplasmic reticulum are distinct from the Ca^{2+} pumps in the plasma membrane and can be selectively inhibited by drugs such as the irreversible inhibitor thapsigargin. Ca^{2+} in the endoplasmic reticulum can be released into the cytoplasm in response to $I(1,4,5)P_3$ when hormones activate PPI-PLCs, as described below. The I-1,4, 5-P_3-sensitive Ca^{2+} stores can also be depleted experimentally by thapsigargin. Because there is a spontaneous leak of Ca^{2+} from the endoplasmic reticulum, blockade of the SERCA pump leads to a gradual depletion of the Ca^{2+} stores, preventing agonist-activated responses.

Mitochondria also contain a high total concentration of Ca^{2+}. Mitochondria were traditionally viewed as low-affinity, high-capacity buffers for Ca^{2+} that protect the cell against very large increases in $[Ca^{2+}]_i$. However, recent work has shown that mitochondrial Ca^{2+} concentrations change in response to agonists that mobilize Ca^{2+} from the endoplasmic reticulum and that mitochondrial Ca^{2+} oscillates along with cytoplasmic Ca^{2+}.[26,27] Mitochondria can be found at the mouth of Ca^{2+} release channels. These results suggest that mitochondria may play an active role in shaping the spatiotemporal pattern of Ca^{2+} signals[28]. Thus, $[Ca^{2+}]_i$ can rise either through entry of extracellular Ca^{2+} via the plasma membrane or through release of Ca^{2+} from intracellular stores. Elevations from either source are usually from 0.1 to 10 micromolar (1×10^{-7}M to 10^{-5}M) and may take the form of oscillations or of sustained changes (see below).

A central aspect of Ca^{2+} signaling is that changes in $[Ca^{2+}]_i$ are translated into changes in cellular function through a number of specific, Ca^{2+}-binding regulatory proteins or protein subunits. On binding Ca^{2+}, these proteins undergo conformational changes that regulate their activity. For example, in skeletal muscle cells, Ca^{2+} binds to troponin C and stimulates contraction. Calmodulin is a ubiquitous Ca^{2+}-binding protein[29] that regulates a number of processes, including macromolecular synthesis, secretion, cytoskeletal function, carbohydrate metabolism, and ion transport. The activity of a calmodulin target protein is altered when Ca^{2+}-calmodulin binds to its calmodulin-binding domain or, much less often, when free calmodulin binds. Ca^{2+}-calmodulin complexes bind to and activate several enzymes. Activation by Ca^{2+}-calmodulin complexes of some enzymes leads directly to the response, for example, activation of Ca^{2+}-Mg^{2+} ATPase leads to Ca^{2+} transport. Ca^{2+}-calmodulin complexes also activate a number of protein kinases that in turn phosphorylate other regulatory proteins on serine and threonine residues.[30] Some of these Ca^{2+}-calmodulin-dependent protein kinases, such as myosin light chain kinase (which regulates cytoskeletal function) and phosphorylase kinase (which regulates carbohydrate metabolism), phosphorylate a limited number of proteins and regulate specific processes. An important family of Ca^{2+}-calmodulin-dependent multifunctional protein kinases called CaM kinases phosphorylate a broad array of proteins and may mediate many of the more diverse actions caused by elevation of $[Ca^{2+}]_i$, for example, regulation of gene transcription, protein synthesis, and secretion in many different cells. Thus, subsequent to the elevation of $[Ca^{2+}]_i$, Ca^{2+} binds to regulatory proteins, which in turn amplify and propagate the signal by activating a number of enzymes that activate other distal steps in the signaling cascade.

I-1,4,5-P_3 MOBILIZATION OF CALCIUM

Agonist stimulation of $PI(4,5)P_2$ hydrolysis leads to a rapid formation of I-1,4,5-P_3 that causes an elevation of $[Ca^{2+}]_i$ within seconds.[31] I-1,4,5-P_3 is generated on the intracellular side of the plasma membrane and very rapidly diffuses in the cytoplasm to bind to receptors on localized regions of the endoplasmic reticulum. The I-1,4,5-P_3 receptors, called simply IP_3 receptors, are Ca^{2+} channels.[32] When I-1,4,5-P_3 binds to an IP_3 receptor, the IP_3 receptor undergoes a conformational change that causes the channel to open and allows the downhill flow of Ca^{2+} from the lumen of the endoplasmic reticulum into the cytoplasm.[33]

The IP_3 receptor is a glycosylated homotetramer composed of four noncovalently bound subunits with single subunit molecular weights of over 300,000.[34] Three different genes encoding IP_3 receptors have been identified to date, and splice variants exist.[35] The type I IP_3 receptor is ubiquitously expressed, whereas the type II and III receptors are less widely distributed. Each of the subunits contains six membrane-spanning segments, such that both the amino and carboxyl termini are facing the cytoplasm. The four subunits form a single central transmembrane pore through which Ca^{2+} flows.

I-1,4,5-P_3 binding to the IP_3 receptor regulates opening of the calcium channel. The kinetics of channel regulation are complex, and the number of I-1,4,5-P_3 molecules binding to the tetrameric receptor and the rate of binding are both important. It is also well documented that the concentration of Ca^{2+} on the cytoplasmic side of the membrane regulates channel opening by I-1,4,5-P_3.[36] The type I IP_3 receptor exhibits a biphasic dependence on Ca^{2+}, such that I-1,4,5-P_3 becomes more effective at opening the channel as cytoplasmic Ca^{2+} rises and then less effective as cytoplasmic Ca^{2+} reaches high concentrations. This regulation is thought to underlie oscillatory Ca^{2+} responses in nonexcitable cells.[37] The IP_3 receptor can be viewed as a coincidence detector that is activated by a simultaneous rise in I-1,4,5-P_3 and Ca^{2+}. IP_3 receptors are also regulated by phosphorylation and a variety of calcium binding proteins.[38]

There is sequence homology between the IP_3 receptors and the skeletal muscle ryanodine receptor, a calcium channel in the muscle sarcoplasmic reticulum that is involved in stimulus-contraction coupling.[39] Like the IP_3 receptor, the ryanodine receptor comes in multiple types and is a large, four-subunit channel with the bulk of the protein on the cytoplasmic side. The ryanodine receptor is regulated by changes in the Ca^{2+} concentration and also by cyclic ADP ribose and phosphorylation. The ryanodine receptor is responsible for calcium-induced calcium release in muscle cells and in some other cell types, including pancreatic β cells. Calcium-induced calcium release can sustain a Ca^{2+} response or generate Ca^{2+} oscillations stimulated by agonists that signal via PPI hydrolysis (see below).

RECEPTOR ACTIVATION OF CALCIUM INFLUX

Cell surface calcium channels can be viewed as pores in the plasma membrane that, when opened, permit the rapid influx of a large number of Ca^{2+} ions down an electrochemical gradient. Ca^{2+} channels have been divided into two large classes:

VOCCs and non-voltage-operated Ca^{2+} channels.[40] The latter class includes channels regulated by depletion of intracellular Ca^{2+} stores termed *store-operated Ca^{2+} channels* (SOCCs).[41,42]

Much more is known about the structures and pharmacology of VOCCs than of SOCCs. Multiple subtypes of VOCCs have been described in different tissues, including T, L, N, P/Q, and R channels. In general, the different types of VOCCs display differences in the membrane potential (or voltage) at which they are activated and the magnitude and duration of their conductances. Two important subtypes of VOCCs have been named on the basis of these properties: the L-type (long-lasting) and T-type (transient) channels. Dihydropyridine drugs such as nifedipine, benzothiazepines such as diltiazem, and diphenylalkylamines such as verapamil are three classes of highly effective and relatively selective inhibitors of L-type calcium channels.

L-channels play a critical role in regulating the function of excitable endocrine tissues. For example, in the anterior pituitary gland, agonists such as thyrotropin-releasing hormone (TRH) and gonadotropin-releasing hormone (GnRH) that act via G protein–coupled receptors initiate a Ca^{2+} transient through the phosphoinositide pathway described above and also cause a gradual membrane depolarization, which leads to an influx of Ca^{2+} through L-channels.[43] Ca^{2+} influx through these VOCCs is essential for hormone secretion and transcriptional activation. In the β cells of the pancreas, glucose metabolism leads to increased concentrations of ATP. ATP inhibits an ATP-regulated potassium channel and thereby depolarizes the cell, also leading to increased influx of Ca^{2+} through L-type Ca^{2+} channels. Conversely, hormones such as somatostatin and dopamine can hyperpolarize pituitary cells by activating certain potassium channels, leading to reduced influx of extracellular Ca^{2+}. VOCCs can also be regulated as a consequence of second messenger formation. For example, in cardiac myocytes, activation of the β-adrenergic receptor leads to generation of cyclic adenosine monophosphate (cAMP) that activates cAMP-dependent protein kinase (protein kinase A), which phosphorylates the L-type Ca^{2+} channel. Phosphorylation of the L-channel does not in itself activate the channel; rather, it increases the Ca^{2+} flux when the channel is activated by depolarization.

It has been recognized for some time that Ca^{2+} influx across the plasma membrane increases when Ca^{2+} stores in the endoplasmic reticulum become depleted. This phenomenon is often referred to as capacitative Ca^{2+} entry.[44] This Ca^{2+} influx takes place through distinct Ca^{2+} channels that are not regulated by voltage. Store-operated Ca^{2+} channels, or SOCCs, are regulated by the Ca^{2+} content of intracellular stores. These channels open in response to severe depletion of intracellular Ca^{2+} pools, which can be brought about either by high concentrations of an agonist that depletes stores by activating IP_3 receptors or by drugs like thapsigargin that deplete stores by preventing Ca^{2+} sequestration.[45] It is not known how a decline in Ca^{2+} in the lumen of the endoplasmic reticulum signals to the plasma membrane to activate SOCCs. The mechanism may involve a diffusible messenger, a physical coupling, or fusion of a vesicle containing the store-operated channel. Ca^{2+} currents that are activated by depletion of intracellular Ca^{2+} stores, termed I_{CRAC}, have been characterized in electrophysiologic experiments, but the molecules that make up the channel remain elusive. Several of the mammalian homologues of the *Drosophila melanogaster* TRP (transient receptor potential) channels have some of the characteristics expected of SOCCs[46] but do not appear to have the requisite calcium selectivity.[47] The store-operated Ca^{2+} entry described above occurs only in response to very high concentrations of agonists that cause severe store depletion. Ca^{2+} influx also occurs when cells are stimulated with low, physiologic concentrations of agonists, even though intracellular stores are not emptied. One of the established pathways for Ca^{2+} entry that is promoted by low concentrations of agonists is a channel that has not been identified but is known to be stimulated by arachidonic acid.[48] As is described below, arachidonic acid is formed by phospholipase A2 (PLA2), which is activated by many signaling pathways.

Regulated Ca^{2+} influx can occur not only through the VOCCs and SOCCs described above, but also through several cell surface receptors that are themselves cation channels. The gating of these receptor-operated channels and influx of cations are activated by agonist binding. Nicotinic acetylcholine receptors, N-methyl-D-aspartate glutamate receptors, and some 5-hydroxytrypamine and ATP receptors are cation channels. These are primarily monovalent cation channels, but they also allow some Ca^{2+} influx.

RECEPTOR-MEDIATED CHANGES IN $[Ca^{2+}]_i$

This section describes the changes in $[Ca^{2+}]_i$ that result from agonist action. Techniques for monitoring $[Ca^{2+}]_i$, which use intracellularly trapped, fluorescent Ca^{2+}-sensing dyes such as fura2, indo1, and fluo3, allow $[Ca^{2+}]_i$ in individual cells to be measured on a rapid time scale. Both spatial and temporal aspects of Ca^{2+} signaling shape the cell's response. Agonist activation of PLC leads to an increase in I-1,4,5-P_3, and I-1,4,5-P_3 releases Ca^{2+} from intracellular stores via the IP_3 receptors. In many cell types, Ca^{2+} spikes, or waves, are initiated in specific parts of the cell. Such subcellular specificity in Ca^{2+} signaling can occur if either plasma membrane receptors or I-1,4,5-P_3 receptors are spatially restricted.

The temporal pattern of $[Ca^{2+}]_i$ responses generally depends on the concentration of agonist (Fig. 13-5). When G protein–coupled receptors linked to PLCβ are activated with low concentrations of agonist, Ca^{2+} oscillations often result. Transient, moderate increases in $[Ca^{2+}]_i$ occur anywhere from every few seconds to every few minutes. At low concentrations of agonist, there is often great heterogeneity in the response patterns of individual cells. The frequency of $[Ca^{2+}]_i$ oscillations tends to increase as the agonist concentration is raised. Both the amplitude and the frequency of $[Ca^{2+}]_i$ oscillations are decoded by the cell and translated into highly regulated responses. One of the calmodulin-dependent kinases, CaM kinase II, has properties that make it a strong candidate for a protein that responds to the frequency of $[Ca^{2+}]_i$ transients.[49] In most cases, however, it is not known how the information encoded by the frequency and amplitude of $[Ca^{2+}]_i$ transients is translated into downstream responses.[50] Oscillatory changes in $[Ca^{2+}]_i$ can occur in both excitable and nonexcitable cells. $[Ca^{2+}]_i$ oscillations that result from a cyclic release of Ca^{2+} from intracellular stores have been termed *cytosolic oscillations*, and these are often sustained without extracellular Ca^{2+}. In excitable cells, agonists can initiate an I-1,4,5-P_3-induced release of intracellular Ca^{2+} and also increase action potential frequency. During depolarizations, Ca^{2+} enters via VOCCs, and spikes in $[Ca^{2+}]_i$ result. At very high concentrations of agonist, $[Ca^{2+}]_i$ usually increases in a spike/plateau pattern, in which $[Ca^{2+}]_i$ rises to a high level but quickly declines to a lower plateau phase. The initial $[Ca^{2+}]_i$ response, which is due to I-1,4,5-P_3-induced release of Ca^{2+}, is independent of extracellular Ca^{2+}. In some cell types, which contain both I-1,4,5-P_3 and ryanodine receptors, Ca^{2+}-induced Ca^{2+} release may follow I-1,4,5-P_3-induced Ca^{2+} release and amplify the early $[Ca^{2+}]_i$ response. Many factors combine to limit the duration of the initial $[Ca^{2+}]_i$ spike, including desensitization of receptor signaling, depletion of intracellular Ca^{2+} stores, and active extrusion of Ca^{2+} from the cytoplasm by the plasma membrane Ca^{2+} pump and uptake into endoplasmic reticulum and mitochondria. The plateau phase of a spike/plateau response often results from the influx of Ca^{2+} through SOCCs and/or VOCCs, and it is dependent on extracellular Ca^{2+}. Both the spike and sustained increases in $[Ca^{2+}]_i$ may be critical for cellular responses such as changes in secretion or transcription.

1,2-DAG AND PROTEIN KINASE C

The other limb of the PPI pathway is activated by 1,2-DAG. 1,2-DAG, in combination with phosphatidylserine (PS) and, depending on the isoenzyme subtype (see below), with or without an elevation of $[Ca^{2+}]_i$, activates phospholipid-dependent PKC.[51] PKC in turn phosphorylates a number of regulatory proteins, leading to more distal effects such as stimulation of secretion and of transcription. In unstimulated cells, the level of 1,2-DAG in membranes is very low, but 1,2-DAG accumulates transiently in response to an agonist. Agonists that activate $PI(4,5)P_2$ hydrolysis cause a transient translocation of some isoforms of PKC to the plasma membrane within seconds.

PKC phosphorylates serine and threonine residues in protein substrates but does not phosphorylate tyrosine residues. The PKC family contains multiple structurally related isoenzymes, divided into what are called conventional, novel, and atypical PKCs.[52,53] The conventional PKCs have in their N-terminal regions a C2 domain that binds both Ca^{2+} and phospholipids,[10] and these enzymes (PKC α, β, and γ) are activated by Ca^{2+} and by phorbol esters in vitro. Phorbol esters, such as phorbol myristate acetate (12-O-tetradecanoylphorbol-13-acetate), are potent tumor promoters that can mimic 1,2-DAG. The novel PKCs (PKC ε, η, δ, and θ) lack a typical C2 domain and are activated by phorbol esters but not by Ca^{2+}. The atypical PKCs (PKC ζ and τ) are not stimulated by Ca^{2+} or by phorbol esters but are activated by binding to PI-3Ps at the membrane. The Ca^{2+}-dependent PKC isoenzymes may require involvement of both limbs of the PPI pathway for activation in vivo, whereas the Ca^{2+}-independent isoenzymes apparently require 1,2-DAG alone. Sometimes receptor-activated phospholipases hydrolyze phospholipids other than PPIs to generate 1,2-DAG without forming I-1,4,5-P_3 or stimulating increases in $[Ca^{2+}]_i$. Activation of different PKC isoenzymes in vivo may lead to distinct cellular responses. The different isoenzymes of PKC have similar substrate specificity but differ in their intracellular localization, which results in a high degree of specificity. PKCs are often found in association with cytoskeletal elements, and localization of individual types of PKC is thought to occur because they bind to specific targeting proteins. There is good evidence for association of individual isoenzymes of PKC to proteins that are substrates and to anchoring proteins (RACKs, or receptors for activated C kinase) that are not phosphorylated by activated PKC.[54]

An important proximate effect of activation of PKC is one of negative feedback to inhibit PPI signaling, which has been observed in several cell types.[55] This effect, which can be mediated by phosphorylation of a receptor or PPI-PLC, can

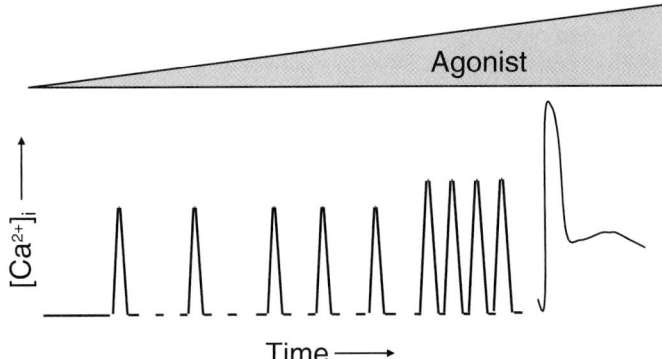

Figure 13-5 Examples of calcium responses to an agonist for a receptor coupled to PPI-PLC activation. Low concentrations cause oscillations in $[Ca^{2+}]_i$ that increase in frequency as the concentration is raised. High concentrations typically cause a spike/plateau response.

inhibit continued activation of the PPI-PLC and thereby limit the response. Activation of PKC has also been found to inhibit Ca^{2+} influx by phosphorylation of Ca^{2+} channels. The more distal effects of activation of PKC, which are primarily mediated by phosphorylation of regulatory proteins, include stimulation of secretion from endocrine, exocrine, and blood cells; of steroidogenesis in adrenal and Leydig cells; of lipogenesis in adipocytes; of glycogenolysis in hepatocytes; and of contraction of smooth muscle cells. PKC is also a mediator of cellular growth and proliferation and may be abnormally activated in some forms of tumorigenesis.[56]

ACTIVATION OF PHOSPHOLIPASE D

The major substrate for phospholipase D (PLD)[57] is phosphatidylcholine and, as is shown in Figure 13-2, hydrolysis of phosphatidylcholine by PLD leads to formation of choline and phosphatidic acid. Activation of PLD is complex, and many agonists that activate PLCs also activate PLD.[58] Interestingly, $PI(4,5)P_2$ strongly activates PLD. In addition, PLD is activated by some G proteins acting through a member of the Rho family of small monomeric G proteins, by another small monomeric G protein ARF, and by PKC in a manner that does not depend on its kinase activity. Activation of PLD changes the localized lipid milieu, decreasing the localized concentration of the neutral phosphatidylcholine while increasing the localized concentration of the acidic phosphatidic acid. Because choline is abundant, it seems unlikely that it plays a signaling role. There is growing evidence that changes in the lipid composition caused by PLD may have important localized effects on processes such as vesicle budding.[58,59]

ACTIVATION OF PHOSPHOLIPASE A2

As is shown in Figure 13-2, PLA2[60–62] releases the fatty acyl group from the sn-2 position of the glycerol backbone. The PLA2 family contains secreted, low-molecular-weight forms that are not thought to be hormonally regulated and two classes of cytoplasmic phospholipase A2s, the Ca^{2+}-dependent forms (cPLA2s), which are widely expressed, and the Ca^{2+}-independent forms, which are more restricted.[61] The well-studied Ca^{2+}-sensitive PLA2s require Ca^{2+} for binding to membranes rather than for catalysis. cPLA2s are strongly activated by a specific phosphorylation carried out by ERK1/2, the final enzyme in the classical MAP kinase cascade. These cPLA2s are activated by many of the same agonists that stimulate $PI(4,5)P_2$ hydrolysis. Since $PI(4,5)P_2$ is the preferred substrate of cytoplasmic PLA2, arachidonic acid is released when the enzyme is activated. Arachidonic acid has signaling activity by itself and serves as a precursor for eicosanoids, including those made via the cyclooxygenase pathway (prostaglandins, prostacyclins, and thromboxanes) and those made by the lipoxygenase pathway (leukotrienes).

3-PHOSPHOINOSITIDES

An enzyme activity that adds a phosphate group to the D-3 position of PI (PI 3-kinase) was discovered[63] and shown to form 3-phosphoinositides ($PI(3)P$, $PI(3,4)P_2$, and $PI(3,4,5)P_3$) in mammalian cells. The D-3 lipids constitute only a small fraction of total phosphoinositides.[64] 3-Phosphoinositides are not substrates for PPI-PLC and, therefore, are not precursors for second messenger formation. Nevertheless, they appear to play important roles in regulation of many cellular processes, including vesicle trafficking, adhesion, actin rearrangement, proliferation, and survival.[65] Rapid activation of PI 3-kinase leading to the synthesis of, in particular, $PI(3,4,5)P_3$ occurs following cell stimulation by a number of extracellular regulatory factors, including growth factors that signal via

tyrosine kinase receptors (see Chapter 8) and hormones that signal via G proteins (see Chapter 11).[66]

PI 3-kinases make up a family of enzymes that exhibit different activities to phosphorylate PI, $PI(4)P$, or $PI(4,5)P_2$[67] and that exhibit different modes of regulation.[68] The class I enzymes can phosphorylate PI, $PI(4)P$, and $PI(4,5)P_2$; the class II enzymes phosphorylate PI and $PI(4)P$; and class III enzymes phosphorylate PI only. Class I PI 3-kinases are heterodimers composed of an adapter/regulatory subunit and a catalytic subunit. Class Ia PI 3-kinases contain adapter subunits that have src homology (SH2) domains, which bind phosphorylated Tyr residues and are thereby linked to Tyr kinase–signaling pathways. Class Ib PI 3-kinases are activated by βγ subunits of heterotrimeric G proteins and are thereby linked to G protein–signaling pathways. Both type 1a and type 1b enzymes also interact with Ras proteins in a GTP-dependent manner, and this interaction may contribute to the regulation of PI 3-kinase activity or localize the enzyme to the plasma membrane, or both. Class II PI 3-kinases, which do not appear to have a regulatory subunit associated with them, bind lipid in a calcium-dependent manner, but whether this enzyme is activated in an extracellular regulatory factor-mediated pathway is not known. Class III PI 3-kinase appears to be primarily involved in intracellular membrane trafficking and vesicle morphogenesis.

Accumulating evidence has led to the idea that phospholipid products of PI 3-kinases, in particular $PI(3,4,5)P_3$, are involved in signal transduction pathways because these lipids interact with proteins of these cascades. It has been postulated that 3-phosphoinositides localize proteins to macromolecular complexes that are needed to propagate a signal along the transduction pathway, to affect the activities of these proteins, or both. Two domains within some of these proteins, pleckstrin homology (PH)[9] and C2 domains,[10] bind D-3 phosphoinositides and appear to be responsible for these interactions. A number of proteins bind to 3-phosphoinositides and function downstream of PI 3-kinases in signaling pathways. Three pathways appear to have PI 3-kinase upstream of different Ser/Thr protein kinases: Akt/protein kinase B (PKB), which appears to be important for cell survival and gluconeogenesis; p70(S6k), which plays a role in progression of cells through the cell cycle; and atypical PKC, which is important in signal transduction through the $PI(4,5)P_2$ pathway (see above). However, the physiologic relevance of activating PKC through PI 3-kinases has not been established.

Critical roles for $PI(3,4,5)P_3$, $PI(3,4)P_2$, and $PI(4,5)P_2$ within the plasma membrane in membrane retrieval and insertion during exocytosis and endocytosis, and of $PI(3)P$ within endosomes in the trafficking and recycling of intracellular vesicles has recently begun to be elucidated.[69] These phosphoinositides accomplish these functions by binding a large array of proteins involved in these processes.

As with other intracellular mediators of signal transduction, the levels of 3-phosphoinositides are tightly controlled not only by the activities of their synthetic enzymes but also by degradative enzymes. There are specific phosphatases that catalyze the dephosphorylation of these lipids. One of these that specifically dephosphorylates at the D-3 position is PTEN (MMAC1).[70] This lipid phosphatase was first discovered as a candidate tumor suppressor gene and has been shown to mediate cell survival in a $PI(3,4,5)P_3$-dependent manner.[71] Thus, 3-phosphoinositides, in particular $PI(3,4,5)P_3$, are important intracellular mediators of proliferation and programmed death (apoptosis) and of vesicle trafficking in mammalian cells.

INTERACTIONS BETWEEN SIGNALING PATHWAYS

It is important to consider that agonist stimulation of the PPI-signaling cascade often occurs in a physiologic setting in which the cell is receiving input from multiple extracellular regulatory factors. The cell integrates these several stimuli, and different responses are elicited depending on the number and types of agonists and their respective signaling mechanisms. One type of interaction at the PPI-signaling cascade may involve activation of two G protein–coupled receptors. Both receptors may use the same G protein and activate the same PPI-PLC, or one receptor may signal through Gq, so that the α_q subunit would activate PPI-PLCβ1, and the other may signal via Gi, so that the βγ subunit would activate PPI-PLCβ2 or β3. Another type of interaction may occur when a G protein–coupled receptor activates PPI-PLCβ and a receptor for a growth factor (see Chapter 8), which contains intrinsic protein tyrosine kinase activity, activates PPI hydrolysis by phosphorylating PPI-PLCγ.[72]

In another circumstance, several signaling pathways may be activated simultaneously by the same agonist or by different agonists. It is now clear that several of the hormones, neurotransmitters, and growth factors that activate the I-1,4,5-P_3/1,2-DAG/Ca^{2+}-signaling pathway activate other pathways concomitantly. This may occur because a cell expresses more than one receptor (or receptor subtype) that can bind a given agonist. For example, adrenergic agonists can bind to different G protein–coupled receptors that can activate PPI hydrolysis (α-1 receptors) or stimulate (β receptors) or inhibit (α-2 receptors) adenylyl cyclase by coupling to different G proteins.[73] Alternatively, a single receptor can couple to two different G proteins and regulate two different signaling pathways.[74] The advent of molecular cloning techniques has made it possible to transfect a cell with a specific receptor and distinguish whether a single receptor can activate more than one G protein. For example, activation of the m2 muscarinic receptor causes marked inhibition of adenylyl cyclase and weak stimulation of PPI hydrolysis[75] by interacting with Gi and Gq, respectively, whereas binding of agonist to the receptor for thyroid-stimulating hormone (thyrotropin, TSH) simultaneously stimulates adenylyl cyclase and PPI hydrolysis, apparently by activating Gs and Gq, respectively.[76] The physiologic significance of dual coupling is unclear, because one pathway is usually activated at much lower agonist concentrations than the other.

When the same signaling pathway is activated by two or more receptors or when two or more transduction cascades are activated simultaneously, cellular response(s) to a single pathway can be varied. Two (or more) distinct pathways can affect the same response in an additive, synergistic, or antagonistic fashion owing to interactions at one or several steps in the signaling cascade. For example, secretion from the anterior pituitary gland can be stimulated by elevations of either $[Ca^{2+}]_i$ or cAMP.[77] In prolactin-secreting cells, TRH stimulates prolactin secretion by activating the PPI-signaling cascade, whereas vasoactive intestinal peptide (VIP) stimulates prolactin secretion by elevating cAMP. When TRH and VIP are added simultaneously, stimulation of prolactin secretion is approximately additive. Angiotensin II (AII), like TRH, stimulates prolactin secretion by activating the PPI signaling cascade. When both TRH and AII are added simultaneously,

stimulation of prolactin secretion is not fully additive. If cells are exposed to TRH before addition of AII, stimulation of prolactin secretion by AII is attenuated. This diminished response to AII may be caused by feedback inhibition caused by TRH, which might be mediated by PKC-mediated phosphorylation of the AII receptor or G protein (see Chapter 11), or of PPI-PLC (see above). Attenuation of the response to TRH is also observed when pituitary cells are stimulated persistently by TRH.[78,79] This attenuation of response to agonist has been termed *desensitization*.[80] Desensitization caused during persistent or repeated stimulation by the same agonist is called homologous desensitization, whereas desensitization of response to one agonist caused by a different agonist is called heterologous desensitization. The molecular mechanisms of homologous and heterologous desensitization are different.

Cross-talk between insulin signaling via activation of its receptor tyrosine kinase and G protein–coupled receptor signaling has been shown.[65] Insulin receptor phosphorylation leads to binding of insulin receptor substrate-1 that stimulates PI-3-kinase, forming 3-phosphoinositides causing activation of phosphoinositide-dependent kinase-1 and activation of Akt/protein kinase B that phosphorylates the β-adrenergic receptor on serine and tyrosine residues. These phosphorylations modulate the function of the β-adrenergic receptor.[81]

Thus, cellular responses are varied not only by which agonists are acting at a given time, but also by the regulatory factors to which a cell has been previously exposed. These interactions, for example, among hormones, neurotransmitters, and growth factors, are common and are responsible for the differences observed in the actions of these extracellular regulatory factors under different physiologic and pathophysiologic conditions.

CONCLUDING REMARKS

A fundamental aspect of cell regulation is that different extracellular regulatory molecules in a single cell can elicit specific responses using the same signal transduction pathway. For receptors that signal through phospholipid hydrolysis, specificity is in part the result of the interactions among the three intracellular messengers—I-1,4,5-P_3, 1,2-DAG, and Ca^{2+}—and the effects of PI(4,5)P_2 and PI(3,4,5)P_3 serving as anchoring proteins. These molecules interact in positive and negative ways to modulate initiation and propagation of the signaling cascade. Because different receptors cause distinct patterns of generation of second messengers, distinct interactions occur, and varied responses are elicited. This contrasts with another ubiquitous signaling system, adenylyl cyclase–cAMP, in which a single messenger is generated. Thus, signaling via phospholipid hydrolysis appears to generate a broader range of specific responses than can be elicited by receptors that signal via cAMP. Moreover, the variety of cellular responses that are elicited through the PPI-PLC signal transduction pathway is greatly expanded through interactions with other signaling pathways.

REFERENCES

1. Berridge MJ, Irvine RF: Inositol phosphates and cell signalling. Nature 341:197–205, 1989.
2. Majerus PW, Ross TS, Cunningham TW, et al: Recent insights in phosphatidylinositol signaling. Cell 63:459–465, 1990.
3. Lester LB, Scott JD: Anchoring and scaffold proteins for kinases and phosphatases. Recent Prog Horm Res 52:409–429, 1997.
4. Heiska L, Alfthan K, Gronholm M, et al: Association of ezrin with intercellular adhesion molecule-1 and -2 (ICAM-1 and ICAM-2): Regulation by phosphatidylinositol -4,5-bisphosphate. J Biol Chem 273:21893–21900, 1998.
5. Rhee SG: Regulation of phosphoinositide-specific phospholipase C. Annu Rev Biochem 70:281–312, 2001.
6. Rhee SG, Bae YS: Regulation of phosphoinositide-specific phospholipase C isozymes. J Biol Chem 272:15045–15048, 1997.
7. Singer WD, Brown HA, Sternweis PC: Regulation of eukaryotic phosphatidylinositol-specific phospholipase C and phospholipase D. Annu Rev Biochem 66:475–509, 1997.
8. Katan M: Families of phosphoinositide-specific phospholipase C: Structure and

function. Biochim Biophys Acta Lipids Lipid Metab 1436:5–17, 1998.

9. Lemmon MA, Ferguson KA: Pleckstrin homology domains. Curr Top Microbiol Immunol 228:39–74, 1998.

10. Rizo J, Sudhof TC: C_2-domains, structure and function of a universal Ca^{2+}-binding domain. J Biol Chem 273:15879–15882, 1998.

11. Exton JH: Cell signalling through guanine-nucleotide-binding regulatory proteins (G proteins) and phospholipases. Eur J Biochem 243:10–20, 1997.

12. Monaco ME, Gershengorn MC: Subcellular organization of receptor-mediated phosphoinositide turnover. Endocr Rev 13:707–718, 1992.

13. Imai A, Gershengorn MC: Regulation by phosphatidylinositol of rat pituitary plasma membrane and endoplasmic reticulum phosphatidylinositol synthase activities: A mechanism for activation of phosphoinositide resynthesis during cell stimulation. J Biol Chem 262:6457–6459, 1987.

14. Zhu X, Eichberg J: A *myo*-inositol pool utilized for phosphatidylinositol synthesis is depleted in sciatic nerve from rats with streptozotocin-induced diabetes. Proc Natl Acad Sci U S A 87:9818–9822, 1990.

15. Berridge MJ, Downes CP, Hanley MR: Neural and developmental actions of lithium: A unifying hypothesis. Cell 59:411–419, 1989.

16. Imai A, Gershengorn MC: Independent phosphatidylinositol synthesis in pituitary plasma membrane and endoplasmic reticulum. Nature 325:726–728, 1987.

17. Sur C, Mallorga PJ, Wittmann M, et al: N-desmethylclozapine, an allosteric agonist at muscarinic 1 receptor, potentiates N-methyl-D-aspartate receptor activity. Proc Natl Acad Sci U S A 100:13674–13679, 2003.

18. Goldstein JL, Brown MS, Anderson RGW, et al: Receptor-mediated endocytosis: Concepts emerging from the LDL receptor system. Annu Rev Cell Biol 1:1–39, 1985.

19. Hay JC, Fisette PL, Jenkins GH, et al: ATP-dependent inositide phosphorylation required for Ca^{2+}-activated secretion. Nature 374:173–177, 1995.

20. Marinissen MJ, Servitja JM, Offermanns S, et al: Thrombin protease-activated receptor-1 signals through G_q- and G_{13}-initiated MAPK cascades regulating c-Jun expression to induce cell transformation. J Biol Chem 278:46814–46825, 2003.

21. Marino MJ, Williams DL Jr, O'Brien JA, et al: Allosteric modulation of group III metabotropic glutamate receptor 4: A potential approach to Parkinson's disease treatment. Proc Natl Acad Sci U S A 100:13668–13673, 2003.

22. Berridge MJ: Elementary and global aspects of calcium signaling. J Physiol (Lond) 499:291–306, 1997.

23. Berridge MJ, Bootman MD, Roderick HL: Calcium signalling: Dynamics homeostasis and remodelling. Nat Rev Mol Cell Biol 4:517–529, 2003.

24. Carafoli E: Plasma membrane calcium pump: Structure, function and relationships. Basic Res Card 92(Suppl 1):59–61, 1997.

25. Meldolesi J, Pozzan T: The endoplasmic reticulum Ca^{2+} store: A view from the lumen. Trends Biochem Sci 23:10–14, 1998.

26. Gunter TE, Buntinas L, Sparagna GC, Gunter KK: The Ca^{2+} transport mechanisms of mitochondria and Ca^{2+} uptake from physiological-type Ca^{2+} transients. Biochim Biophys Acta 1366:5–15, 1998.

27. Rizzuto R, Simpson AW, Brini M, Pozzan T: Rapid changes of mitochondrial Ca^{2+} revealed by specifically targeted recombinant aequorin. Nature 358:325–327, 1992.

28. Parekh AB: Mitochondrial regulation of intracellular Ca2+ signaling: More than just simple Ca2+ buffers. News Physiol Sci 18:252–256, 2003.

29. Klee CB, Crouch TH, Richman PG: Calmodulin. Annu Rev Biochem 49:489–515, 1980.

30. Heist EK, Schulman H: The role of Ca^{2+}/calmodulin-dependent protein kinases within the nucleus. Cell Calcium 23:103–114, 1998.

31. Berridge MJ: Inositol trisphosphate as a second messenger in signal transduction. Ann N Y Acad Sci 494:39–51, 1987.

32. Joseph SK: The inositol triphosphate receptor family. Cell Signal 8:1–7, 1996.

33. Ferris CD, Snyder SH: Inositol 1,4,5-trisphosphate-activated calcium channels. Annu Rev Physiol 54:469–488, 1992.

34. Wilcox RA, Primrose WU, Nahorski SR, Challiss RAJ: New developments in the molecular pharmacology of the *myo*-inositol 1,4,5-trisphosphate receptor. Trends Pharmacol Sci 19:467–475, 1998.

35. Taylor CW, Traynor D: Calcium and inositol trisphosphate receptors. J Membr Biol 145:109–118, 1995.

36. Ehrlich BE, Kaftan E, Bezprozvannaya S, Bezprozvanny I: The pharmacology of intracellular Ca^{2+}-release channels. Trends Pharmacol Sci 15:145–149, 1994.

37. Berridge MJ: Inositol trisphosphate and calcium signaling. Ann N Y Acad Sci 766:31–43, 1995.

38. Haynes LP, Tepikin AV, Burgoyne RD: Calcium-binding protein 1 is an inhibitor of agonist-evoked, inositol 1,4,5-trisphosphate-mediated calcium signaling. J Biol Chem 279:547–555, 2004.

39. Franzini-Armstrong C, Protasi F: Ryanodine receptors of striated muscles: A complex channel capable of multiple interactions. Physiol Rev 77:699–729, 1997.

40. Jones SW: Overview of voltage-dependent calcium channels. J Bioenerg Biomembr 30:299–312, 1998.

41. Thomas D, Kim HY, Hanley MR: Capacitative calcium influx. Vitam Horm 54:97–119, 1998.

42. Bootman MD, Berridge MJ: The elemental principles of calcium signaling. Cell 83:675–678, 1995.

43. Stojilkovic SS, Catt K: Calcium oscillations in anterior pituitary cells. Endocr Rev 13:256–280, 1992.

44. Putney JW Jr: The capacitative model for receptor-activated calcium entry. Adv Pharmacol 22:251–269, 1991.

45. Parekh AB, Penner R: Store depletion and calcium influx. Physiol Rev 77:901–930, 1997.

46. Zhu X, Birnbaumer L: Calcium channels formed by mammalian Trp homologues. News Physiol Sci 13:211–217, 1998.

47. Clapham DE: TRP channels as cellular sensors. Nature 426:517–524, 2003.

48. Shuttleworth TJ, Mignen O: Calcium entry and the control of calcium oscillations. Biochem Soc Trans 31:916–919, 2003.

49. De Koninck P, Schulman H: Sensitivity of CaM kinase II to the frequency of Ca^{2+} oscillations. Science 279:227–230, 1998.

50. Berridge MJ: Calcium signalling and cell proliferation. BioEssays 17:491–500, 1995.

51. Nishizuka Y: Protein kinase C and lipid signaling for sustained cellular responses. FASEB J 9:484–496, 1995.

52. Mellor H, Parker PJ: The extended protein kinase C superfamily. Biochem J 332:281–292, 1998.

53. Newton AC: Regulation of protein kinase C. Curr Opin Cell Biol 9:161–167, 1997.

54. Mochly-Rosen D, Gordon AS: Anchoring proteins for protein kinase C: A means for isozyme selectivity. FASEB J 12:35–42, 1998.

55. Chuang TT, Iacovelli L, Sallese M, De Blasi A: G protein-coupled receptors: Heterologous regulation of homologous desensitization and its implications. Trends Pharmacol Sci 17:416–421, 1996.

56. Weinstein IB, Kahn SM, O'Driscoll K, et al: The role of protein kinase C in signal transduction, growth control and lipid metabolism. Adv Exp Med Biol 400A:313–321, 1997.

57. Cockcroft S: Phospholipase D: Regulation by GTPases and protein kinase C and physiological relevance. Prog Lipid Res 35:345–370, 1997.

58. Exton JH: New developments in phospholipase D. J Biol Chem 272:15579–15582, 1997.

59. Hodgkin MN, Pettitt TR, Martin A, et al: Diacylglycerols and phosphatidates: Which molecular species are intracellular messengers? Trends Biochem Sci 23:200–204, 1998.

60. Balsinde J, Dennis EA: Function and inhibition of intracellular calcium-independent phospholipase A_2. J Biol Chem 272:16069–16072, 1997.

61. Leslie CC: Properties and regulation of cytosolic phospholipase A_2. J Biol Chem 272:16709–16712, 1997.

62. Balsinde J, Winstead MV, Dennis EA: Phospholipase A(2) regulation of arachidonic acid mobilization. FEBS Lett 531:2–6, 2002.

63. Whitman M, Downes CP, Keeler M, et al: Type I phosphatidylinositol kinase makes a novel inositol phospholipid, phosphatidylinositol-3-phosphate. Nature 332:644–646, 1988.

64. Traynor-Kaplan AE, Harris AL, Thompson BL, et al: An inositol tetrakisphosphate-containing phospholipid in activated neutrophils. Nature 334:353–356, 1988.

65. Shenoy SK, Lefkowitz RJ: Multifaceted roles of β-arrestins in the regulation of seven-membrane-spanning receptor trafficking and signalling. Biochem J 375:503–515, 2003.

66. Shepherd PR, Withers DJ, Siddle K: Phosphoinositide 3-kinase: The key switch mechanism in insulin signalling. Biochem J 333:471–490, 1998.

67. Snir M, Kehat I, Gepstein A, et al: Assessment of the ultrastructural and proliferative properties of human embryonic stem cell-derived cardiomyocytes. Am J Physiol Heart Circ Physiol 285:H2355–H2363, 2003.

68. Vanhaesebroeck B, Leevers SJ, Panayotou G, Waterfield MD: Phosphoinositide 3-kinases: A conserved family of signal transducers. Trends Biochem Sci 22:267–272, 1997.

69. Canals M, Marcellino D, Fanelli F, et al: Adenosine A$_{2A}$-dopamine D2 receptor-receptor heteromerization: Qualitative and quantitative assessment by fluorescence and bioluminescence energy transfer. J Biol Chem 278:46741–46749, 2003.

70. Maehama T, Dixon JE: The tumor suppressor, PTEN/MMAC1, dephosphorylates the lipid second messenger phosphatidylinositol 3,4,5-trisphosphate. J Biol Chem 273:13375–13378, 1998.

71. Stambolic V, Suzuki A, de la Pompa JL, et al: Negative regulation of PKB/Akt-dependent cell survival by the tumor suppressor PTEN. Cell 95:29–39, 1998.

72. Selbie LA, Hill SJ: G protein-coupled-receptor cross-talk: The fine-tuning of multiple receptor-signalling pathways. Trends Pharmacol Sci 19:87–93, 1998.

73. Dohlman HG, Thorner J, Caron MG, Lefkowitz RJ: Model systems for the study of seven-transmembrane-segment receptors. Annu Rev Biochem 60:653–688, 1991.

74. Strader CD, Fong TM, Tota MR, et al: Structure and function of G protein-coupled receptors. Annu Rev Biochem 63:101–132, 1994.

75. Hosey MM: Diversity of structure, signaling and regulation within the family of muscarinic cholinergic receptors. FASEB J 6:845–852, 1992.

76. Vassart G, Desarnaud F, Duprez L, et al: The G protein-coupled receptor family and one of its members the TSH receptor. Ann N Y Acad Sci 766:23–30, 1995.

77. Mason WT, Rawlings SR, Cobbett P, et al: Control of secretion in anterior pituitary cells: Linking ion channels, messengers and exocytosis. J Exp Biol 139:287–316, 1988.

78. Perlman JH: Gershengorn MC: Thyrotropin-releasing hormone stimulation of phosphoinositide hydrolysis desensitizes: Evidence against mediation by protein kinase C or calcium. Endocrinology 129:2679–2686, 1991.

79. Yu R, Hinkle PM: Desensitization of thyrotropin-releasing hormone receptor-mediated responses involves multiple steps. J Biol Chem 272:28301–28307, 1997.

80. Lefkowitz RJ, Cotecchia S, Kjelsberg MA, et al: Adrenergic receptors: Recent insights into their mechanism of activation and desensitization. Adv Second Messenger Phosphoprotein Res 28:1–9, 1993.

81. Doronin S, Wang HY, Malbon CC: Insulin stimulates phosphorylation of the β2-adrenergic receptor by the insulin receptor, creating a potent feedback inhibitor of its tyrosine kinase. J Biol Chem 277:10698–10703, 2002.

Map Kinase and Growth Factor Signaling Pathways

John M. Kyriakis

Since the discovery of protein phosphorylation over 40 years ago, the mechanisms by which extracellular stimuli regulate protein phosphorylation have been the subject of intense interest. From the vantage point of the endocrinologist, protein kinase signaling pathways represent the primary means by which hormones such as insulin, acting at the cell surface can generate pleiotrophic intracellular responses. Protein tyrosine kinases and their mechanisms of signal transduction have been discussed in Chapter 8. This chapter will focus on protein-serine/threonine kinase cascades, the phosphatidyl inositol-3′-OH-kinase (PI 3-kinase) and Ras mitogen-activated protein kinase (MAPK) pathway, in particular, that are activated by receptors coupled to tyrosine kinases. Recent studies of protein kinase signaling mediated by stress and inflammatory cytokines of the tumor necrosis factor (TNF) family, along with the integration of these pathways and hormone-regulated pathways will also be discussed.

GENERAL THEMES

It is often an initial impression that protein phosphorylation, catalyzed by protein-tyrosine (Tyr) or serine/threonine (Ser/Thr) kinases, activates biochemical processes while dephosphorylation, catalyzed by Tyr or Ser/Thr phosphatases, inactivates these processes. This assumption is an erroneous oversimplification. Regulation of cellular processes by protein phosphoryation can take two forms: While many biochemical processes are activated by phosphorylation, protein translation and some transcriptional responses are examples; many are activated by dephosphorylation—insulin activation of glycogen synthase is a major example. Many protein kinase signaling pathways are complex and involve several protein

kinases arrayed in a multi-tiered manner. Often, there is considerable apparent redundancy in these pathways, and conversely, individual component elements often participate in several signaling pathways.

This chapter will deal with a subset of insulin, mitogen, and stress-activated Ser/Thr kinases and their regulation of cellular physiology. Accordingly, a few words on protein Ser/Thr kinase structure are warranted. The overall structure of all protein kinases (Ser/Thr, Tyr, or dual specificity) is well conserved and, in 1987, Hanks and colleagues aligned the sequences of all known protein kinases and identified 11 protein kinase subdomains (referred to with the Roman numerals I–XI).[1] Of note, subdomain VIII is critically important to the regulation of many protein kinases. This domain, referred to as the activation loop, often contains sites of regulatory phosphorylation, catalyzed by upstream protein kinases.[2]

All protein kinases share a bilobed structure. The two lobes are oriented such that protein kinase catalysis occurs in the cleft between the two protein kinase lobes. For protein kinases that are activated by phosphorylation (the MAPKs are examples), the regulatory phosphorylation is thought to reorient the two lobes so as to bring them into a conformation optimal for catalyzing the phosphotransfer reaction.[2,3]

INITIAL STEPS IN INSULIN AND MITOGEN SIGNALING

The receptors for insulin as well as many mitogens and hormones are either ligand-activated protein-tyrosine kinases or are functionally coupled to tyrosine kinases. This insulin/mitogen-activated Tyr phosphorylation is followed by a quantitatively much larger wave of Ser/Thr phosphorylation[4,5]; recent research has begun to dissect the mechanisms by which receptor tyrosine kinases couple to Ser/Thr kinases.

The activation of the insulin, as well as other Tyr kinase receptors is discussed in further detail in Chapter 8, as is the recruitment by the insulin receptor of insulin receptor substrate (IRS) proteins. The regulation and function of pleckstrin homology (PH), Src homology (SH)-2, phosphotyrosine binding (PTB), and SH-3 domains is also discussed in Chapter 8. With regard to the activation of Ser/Thr protein kinase pathways by mitogen receptors, among the most important SH2-containing polypeptides that bind to Tyr phosphorylated mitogen receptors and insulin receptor substrates are the 85-kilodalton regulatory subunit of PI 3-kinase (p85) and growth factor receptor binding protein 2 (GRB2).[5]

PI 3-Kinase

PI 3-kinases are a family of heterodimeric lipid kinases that phosphorylate the 3′ hydroxyl group of inositol phospholipids, including phosphatidyl inositol (PtdIns)-4,5 bisphosphate (tdIns-4,5-P_2) and phosphatidyl inositol-4 phosphate (tdIns-4-P_2) thereby generating PtdIns-3,4,5,P_3 and PtdIns-3,4-P_2, respectively (Fig. 14-1).[6] The trisphosphorylated PI is thought to be the most biologically active 3′ phosphoinositide. 3′-Phosphorylated inositol lipids are believed to serve as second messengers; however, their functions are not completely understood.

Accumulating evidence suggests that at least one function of 3′-phosphorylated inositol lipids is to bind proteins containing certain subsets of PH domains (see Chapter 8) thereby recruiting or tethering such proteins to the plasma membrane. This binding may serve to nucleate proteins at the membrane and allow for the regulation of signaling.[6] This sort of lipid-dependent protein recruitment is thought to be critical for regulation of the PKB/Akt and p70 S6 kinase pathways (discussed later).

The PI 3-kinases regulated by insulin and mitogens consist of an 85-kilodalton regulatory subunit (p85) and a 110-kilodalton catalytic subunit (p110). A related 60-kilodalton regulatory subunit has also been identified. p85 is an adapter molecule that couples p110 to phosphotyrosine-containing polypeptides (see Chapter 8).[6]

Growth Factor Receptor Binding-2

Growth factor receptor binding-2 (GRB-2) is another adapter molecule with the configuration SH3-SH2-SH3 (see Chapter 8). Perhaps the best characterized effector for GRB-2 is mammalian son of sevenless, a guanine nucleotide exchange fac-

tor required for the activation of the Ras proto-oncoprotein.[4] The regulation of Ras and Ras regulation of MAPKs will be discussed later.

INSULIN AND MITOGEN ACTIVATION OF Ser/Thr PHOSPHORYLATION I

GENERAL CONSIDERATIONS

The activation of Ser/Thr kinases by insulin was initially unexpected. This is because among the first polypeptides shown to be regulated by insulin in a phosphorylation-dependent manner was glycogen synthase (GS); this regulation involved dephosphorylation. Inactive GS is phosphorylated at up to seven sites: 1, 2, 3a, 3b, 3c, 4, and 5. Sites 3a–c, and 4 reside near the GS carboxyl terminus. Insulin stimulates the glucose-6-phosphate-independent activation of GS by fostering GS dephosphorylation—primarily of sites 2, 3a–c, and, to a lesser extent, 4. GS is phosphorylated and inactivated by protein kinases that are active in the resting cell such as casein kinase II and glycogen synthase kinase-3 (GSK3; Fig. 14-2A; also see Fig. 14-7), which phosphorylate sites 2, 3a–c, and 4.[4,7,8]

GS is also inactivated, albeit to a slightly lesser extent, by agonists that elevate cyclic adenosine monophosphate (cAMP) and activate the cAMP-dependent protein kinase A cascade, which culminates in the phosphorylation of sites 1 and 2 (see Fig. 14-2A and Chapter 12). The protein kinase A pathway can be antagonized by insulin; and the opposing effects of insulin and cAMP agonists on GS phosphorylation led to the view that insulin's primary effect on Ser/Thr phosphorylation would be to promote dephosphorylation.[4,7–9] This view came into question with the identification of several polypeptides that undergo rapid insulin-stimulated Ser/Thr phosphorylation in vivo. Most prominent among these was S6, a protein of the 40S small ribosomal subunit.[10,11] The identification of insulin-stimulated Ser/Thr phosphorylation led to a reassessment of the effect of insulin and other receptor Tyr kinases on protein phosphorylation. It is now accepted that the major mode of insulin action is to promote protein phosphorylation. The remainder of this section and later sections will focus on two of the major mechanisms of insulin and mitogen-stimulated protein Ser/Thr phosphorylation: protein Ser/Thr kinases activated by PI 3-kinase and the Ras-MAPK pathway.

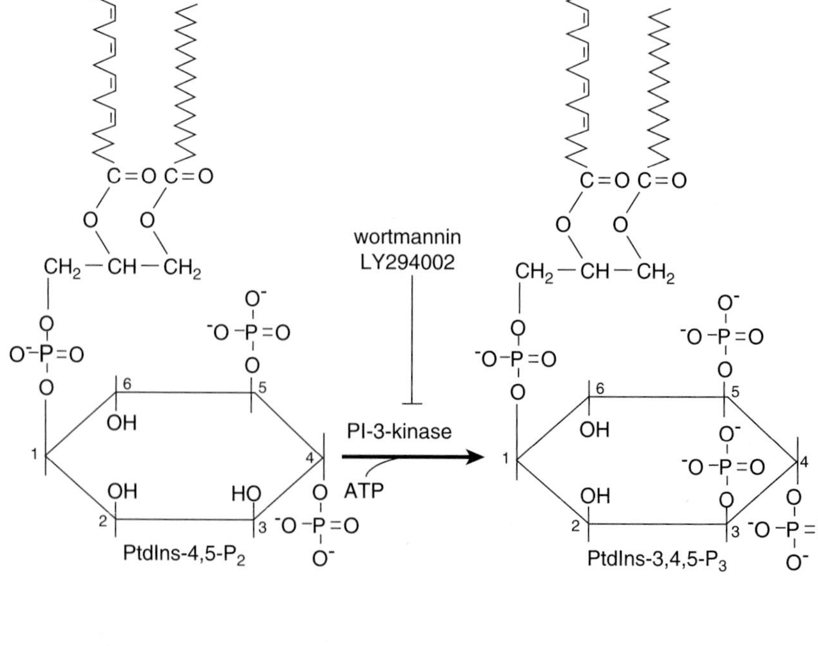

Figure 14-1 Reaction catalyzed by PI 3-kinase. Only phosphorylation of PI 4,5,P_2 is shown, although PI-4-P is also a substrate. Inhibition by the fungal toxin wortmannin and the synthetic inhibitor LY294002 is indicated.

PROTEIN KINASE B/Akt

The effectors of PI 3-kinase are likely to be important in insulin regulation of metabolism. For example, insulin-resistant Native American (Pima) individuals manifest defective insulin activation of protein kinase signaling pathways that are regulated through PI 3-kinase, specifically GS activation and activation of p70 S6 kinase.[5]

The Ser/Thr kinase protein kinase B (PKB)/Akt is a critical element that links PI 3-kinase with several downstream effectors. PKB/Akt is the normal cellular homologue of the oncoprotein encoded by v-akt of the acutely transforming retrovirus AKT8. PKB/Akt is activated by a wide variety of stimuli including insulin, mitogens, and stresses. The activation of PKB/Akt by insulin and mitogens (but not stress) requires PI 3-kinase inasmuch as blocking PI 3-kinase with the fungal toxin wortmannin or with the synthetic inhibitor LY294002 completely abrogates recruitment of PKB/Akt by these stimuli. In addition, dominant inhibitory mutants of the p85 adapter subunit of PI 3-kinase can block mitogen activation of PKB/Akt and constitutively active mutants of the p110 subunit of PI 3-kinase are sufficient to induce activation of PKB/Akt in the absence of extracellular stimuli.[12]

Four PKB family members (α, $\beta1$, $\beta2$, and γ) have been identified. All are comprised of an N-terminal regulatory region containing a PH domain, and a C-terminal kinase domain; the structure of PKBα is shown in Fig. 14-2A. The role of the PH domain in the in vivo activation of PKB has recently been characterized. The products of PI 3-kinase activity, PI $3,4,5,P_3$ and PI $3,4,P_2$ bind with high affinity to the PH domain of PKB/Akt. The binding of PI $3,4,5,P_3$ does not activate PKB/Akt directly. Instead, the function of PI lipid binding is to mediate the translocation of PKB/Akt from the cytosol to the membrane. This translocation/lipid binding appears to be necessary in order to present PKB/Akt to upstream activating kinases (discussed in a later section).[12]

ROLE OF PKB/Akt SUBSTRATES IN METABOLIC REGULATION

PKBs/Akts phosphorylate Ser/Thr residues that reside within the basic amino acid rich consensus Arg-Lys-Arg-X-Arg-Thr-Tyr-Ser(P)-Phe-Gly (X is any amino acid, P indicates phosphorylation).[13] Kinases of the PKB/Akt family have a wide variety of substrates that reveal roles in metabolic control and in the inhibition of programmed cell death (apoptosis). These include GSK3 and the cardiac isoform of 6-phosphofructo-2-kinase (PFK2), some forkhead superfamily transcription factors, the mitochondrial apoptosis inducer Bad, the proapoptotic protease caspase-9, apoptosis signal-regulating kinase-1 (ASK1), and others (see Figs. 14-2A and B).[14] These functions for PKB/Akt are illustrated in Figure 14-2B; however, we will limit this discussion to PKB/Akt substrates implicated in metabolic regulation. Figure 14-2C is a summary diagram of the aspects of carbohydrate metabolism regulated by PKB/Akt alone or in conjunction with other signaling pathways including MAPKs (discussed later).

GSK3

As noted earlier, inactive GS is phosphorylated at up to seven sites. Sites 2, 3a–c, and 4 are dephosphorylated in response to insulin.[4,7,8] GSK3s comprise a highly conserved family of Ser/Thr kinases that are among the major protein kinases involved in the phosphorylation and inactivation of GS.[15–17] In the absence of insulin, GSK3 is active and phosphorylates sites 3a–c and 4 on the GS polypeptide (but not site 2 which is phosphorylated by many kinases including phosphorylase a, protein kinase A, and phosphorylase b kinase) thereby contributing to GS inactivation (see Fig. 14-2A–C). GSK3 phosphorylation of GS is described as processive or hierarchical. Thus, phosphorylation of GS by GSK3 requires prior phosphorylation of site 5 by casein kinase II. This creates a GSK3

docking site, recruiting GSK3 to the GS polypeptide. GSK3 then phosphorylates GS at a Ser residue amino terminal to site 5, thereby creating a new GSK3-binding motif with the sequence Ser-X-X-X-Ser(P) (X is any amino acid and P indicates phosphorylation). This enables the next phosphorylation creating another Ser-X-X-X-Ser(P) motif.[14,17]

GSK3 also has an important role in the regulation of protein synthesis (see Fig. 14-2B). Eukaryotic initiation factor 2 (eIF-2) is a GTPase required for the recruitment of the initiator tRNA to the 40S ribosome. As with all cellular regulator GTPases (discussed later), eIF-2 is active in the GTP-bound state and is inactive in the GDP-bound state. eIF-2 is activated by a multisubunit guanine nucleotide exchange factor (GEF), eIF-2B, which promotes the exchange of bound guanosine diphosphate (GDP) for guanosine triphosphate (GTP). The ϵ subunit of eIF-2B is phosphorylated (at Ser540) and inhibited by GSK3.[14,18] PKB/Akt-mediated inhibition of GSK3 (discussed later), therefore, reverses GSK3's contribution to suppression of eIF-2B function, thereby promoting enhanced protein synthesis.[14,18]

GSK3 has several additional physiologic functions. In particular, GSK3 can phosphorylate c-Jun, a component of the activator protein-1 transcription factor, at a site just amino terminal to the c-Jun DNA-binding domain (at Thr231, Thr239, Ser243, and Ser249). This phosphorylation inhibits DNA binding and inactivates activator protein-1 activity (see Figs. 14-2B, 14-12B, and 14-13A).[19]

GSK3 is phosphorylated at a single Ser residue (Ser21 in the GSK3-α isoform and Ser9 in GSK3-β) and inactivated in response to mitogens and insulin.[5,20] By this process, proteins that are phosphorylated by GSK3 in resting cells, such as GS eIF-2Bϵ, c-Jun, and others, are rapidly dephosphorylated by constitutively active Ser/Thr phosphatases. Several kinases, most notably, p70 S6 kinase and ribosomal S6 kinase-1 have been implicated as GSK3 kinases in vitro; however, PKB/Akt is likely the most physiologically relevant insulin-activated GSK3 kinase (see Fig. 14-2B and C).[5,20]

PFK2

Insulin rapidly stimulates glycolysis in cardiomyocytes via activation of cardiac PFK2 (the Pasteur effect). This process involves phosphorylation of the PFK2 polypeptide at Ser466 and Ser483.[21] Phosphorylation of these sites can be catalyzed by several insulin-stimulated kinases including PKB/Akt (see Fig. 14-2B and C) and p70 S6 kinase (which are effectors of PI 3-kinase), and Rsk, a Ras-MAPK effector.[21]

Forkhead Transcription Factors

The forkhead family of transcription factors is a large group of winged helix transcription factors a subset of which (the FOXO group) are PKB/Akt substrates.[22] FOXO group forkhead transcription factors bind to the consensus DNA sequence TTGTTTAC.[22] As with many PKB/Akt substrates, phosphorylation of FOXO transcription factors (at Thr32, Ser253, and Ser315 for FOXO3a, the principal FOXO transcription factor thought to be involved in metabolic regulation) is inhibitory. Phosphorylation enables binding to the FOXO polypeptide of 14-3-3 proteins.[22] 14-3-3s comprise a large class of abundant cytosolic polypeptides that can simultaneously homodimerize and heterodimerize with a wide array of signaling proteins in a regulatory manner. 14-3-3 proteins require prior phosphorylation of their target proteins within the consensus motif Arg-Ser(P)-X-X-Ser-Pro (X is any amino acid and P indicates phosphorylation) for binding.[23] The binding of 14-3-3s to FOXO transcription factors both prevents nuclear import and potentiates nuclear export, thereby blocking FOXO-mediated gene expression.[22] Among the genes thought to be regulated by FOXO proteins is that encoding phosphoenolpyruvate carboxykinase (PEPCK). PEPCK is the rate-limiting enzyme in gluconeogenesis, a process potently inhibited by insulin. pepck expression is dramatically and rapidly blunted by insulin; there is evidence that this inhibition

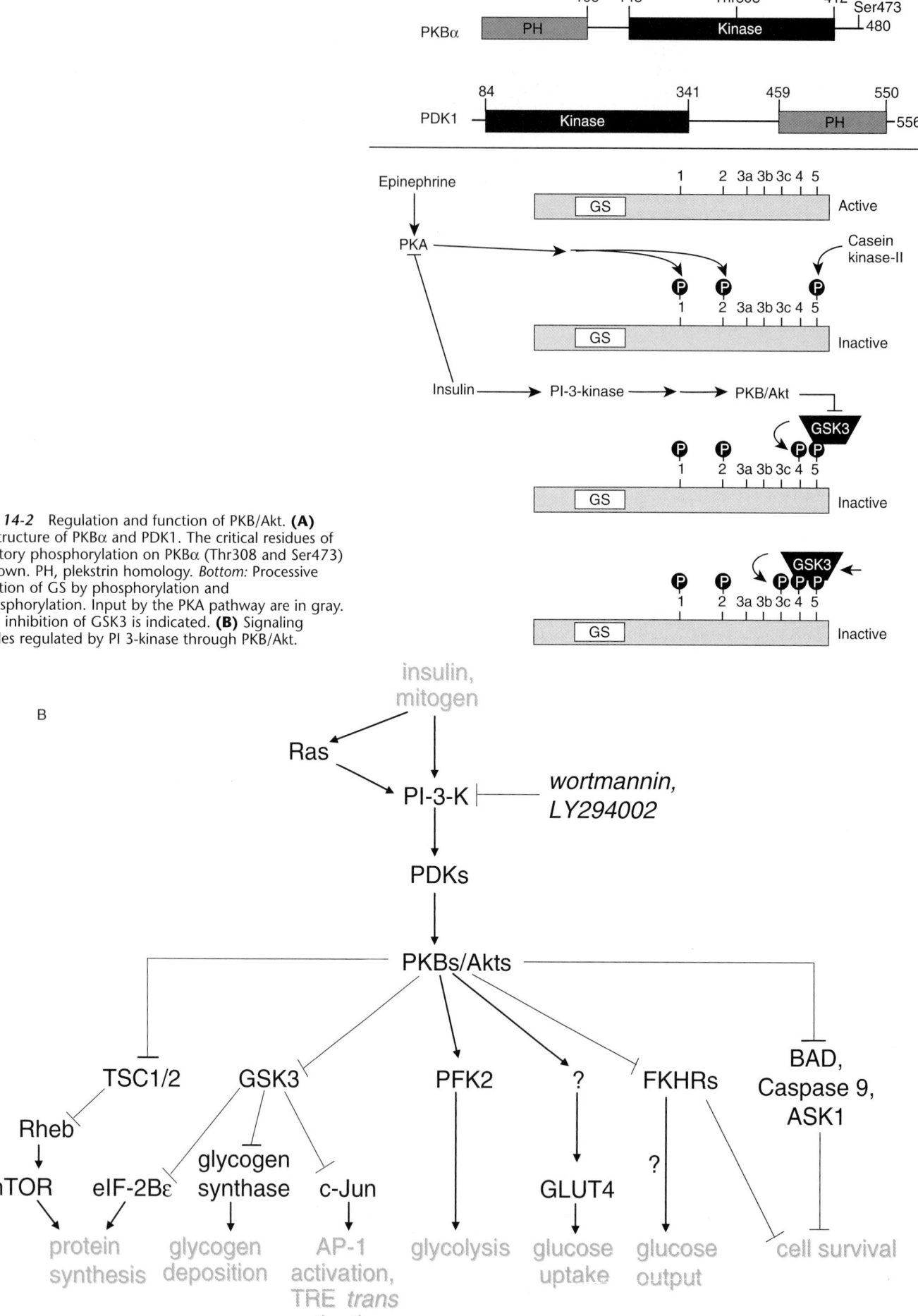

Figure 14-2 Regulation and function of PKB/Akt. **(A)** *Top:* Structure of PKBα and PDK1. The critical residues of regulatory phosphorylation on PKBα (Thr308 and Ser473) are shown. PH, plekstrin homology. *Bottom:* Processive regulation of GS by phosphorylation and dephosphorylation. Input by the PKA pathway are in gray. Insulin inhibition of GSK3 is indicated. **(B)** Signaling cascades regulated by PI 3-kinase through PKB/Akt.

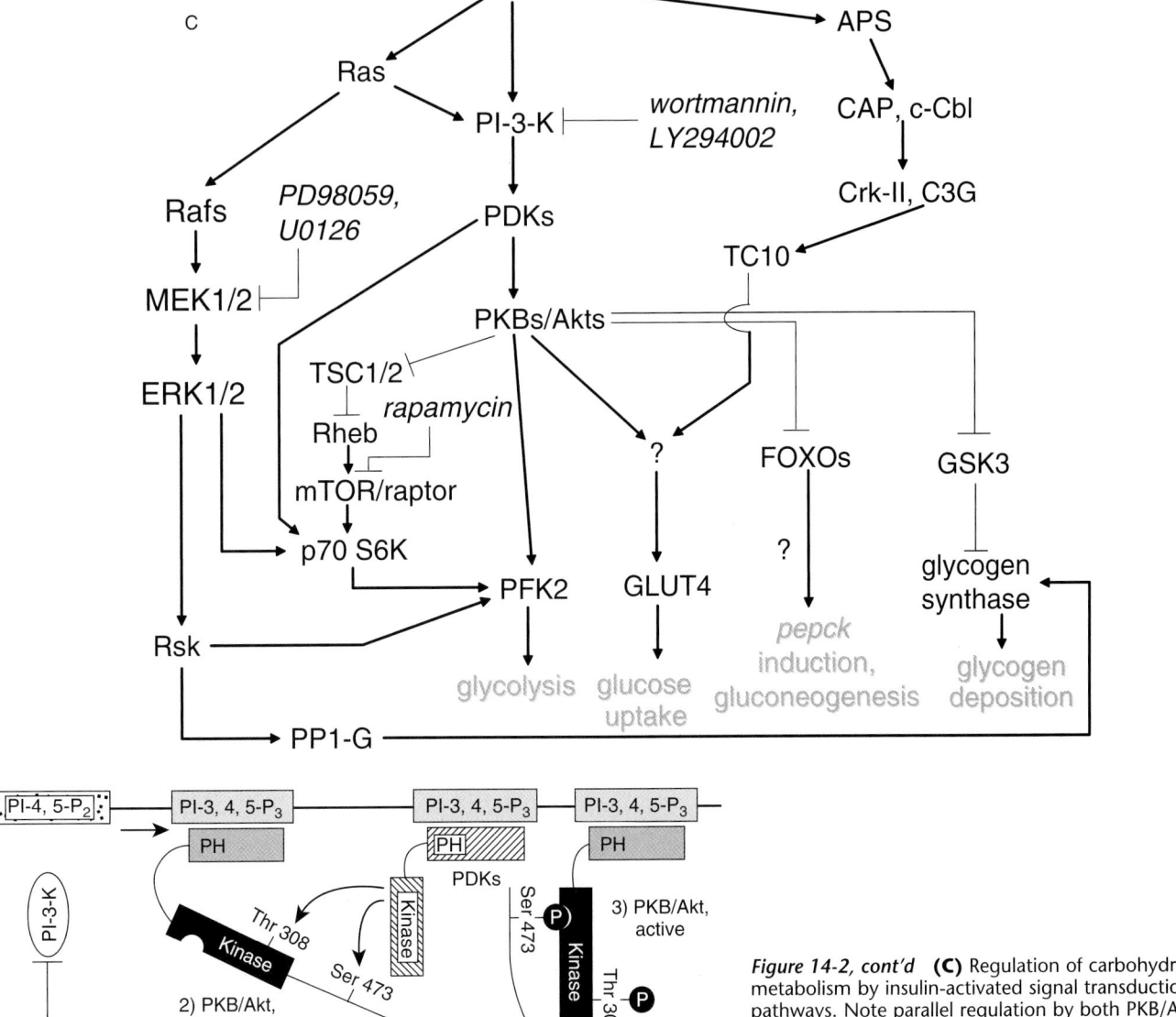

Figure 14-2, cont'd   **(C)** Regulation of carbohydrate metabolism by insulin-activated signal transduction pathways. Note parallel regulation by both PKB/Akt and Ras/MAPK, as well as Crk-II. **(D)** Three step, substrate-directed activation of PKB/Akt by PDK1. Wortmannin inhibits this process by preventing generation of PI 3,4,5,P$_3$ to which PKB/Akt must bind in order permit phosphorylation of Thr308. The black circle with the white P indicates phosphorylation. Note that PKB/Akt assumes an active conformation upon the binding of phospho-Ser473 to the conserved binding pocket in the kinase domain. Compare this to p70 and Rsk activation, both of which share this mode of regulation (see Figs. 14-3*B* and 14-6*B*).

requires elements in the *pepck* promoter that bind forkhead transcription factors.[24] Overexpression experiments indicate that FOXO3a is involved in insulin-regulated *pepck* expression; however, this has not been demonstrated for the endogenous protein (see Fig. 14-2*B* and *C*).[24]

Insulin-Stimulated Glucose Transport

Insulin stimulation of glucose transport is responsible for most physiologically relevant glucose disposal. Still, in spite of the clear physiologic importance of glucose uptake regulation to understanding insulin action and the pathophysiology of type 2 diabetes, this process remains poorly understood. Insulin-stimulated glucose transport appears to

require PI 3-kinase inasmuch as this process can be inhibited with the PI 3-kinase inhibitor wortmannin.[5,12] There is some evidence that PKB/Akt can relay signals from PI 3-kinase to the glucose transport machinery; thus, dominant inhibitory PKB/Akt constructs can also inhibit insulin activation of glucose transport and constitutively active PKB/Akt constructs can activate glucose uptake in the absence of insulin.[5,12]

Most importantly, however, gene disruption studies in mice indicate that PKBβ/Akt2 is the major PKB isoform responsible for physiologic glucose homeostasis.[25] Thus, disruption of *pkbβ/akt2* produces a phenotype remarkably similar to key features of type 2 diabetes-impaired glucose disposal, insulin-resistant hepatic gluconeogenesis.[25] PKBβ/Akt2 binds GLUT4, and this interaction may be important to the direct control of GLUT4 translocation.[5,12,14] However, aside from studies indicating that PKBβ/Akt2 can phosphorylate polypeptides that associate with GLUT4 complexes in coimmunoprecipitation studies, a clear picture of how PKBβ/Akt2 regulates glucose uptake remains elusive.

By contrast, *pkbα/akt1*-deficient mice display no obvious metabolic defects indicative of insulin resistance. Instead, these mice appear small at birth, suggesting that PKBα/Akt1 plays a role in regulating cell growth/cell size.[26] These effects may be mediated by PKBα/Akt1 regulation of protein translation (see Figs. 14-2B and 14-4A). As indicated above, PKB/Akt has been shown to phosphorylate and inhibit GSK3 and its suppression of eIF-2B activity.[18] In addition, as will be discussed later, PKB/Akt has been implicated in the control, by insulin and mitogens, of protein synthesis, through the inhibition of the tuberous sclerosis proteins tuberin and hamartin (TSC1/2).

Other signaling pathways emanating from the insulin receptor may also participate in regulating glucose uptake (see Fig. 14-2C). Insulin activation of glucose uptake requires the redistribution of GLUT4 from the cytosol to the membrane— a process in which the actin cytoskeleton likely plays an important role. Recent studies indicate that a protein complex consisting of the c-Cbl adapter protein and c-Cbl-associated protein (CAP) is recruited to the autophosphorylated insulin receptor by binding to a third protein, adapter protein with PH and SH2 domains (APS); this third protein binds through its SH2 domain to the Tyr phosphorylated insulin receptor independently of the IRS proteins. Once at the membrane, CAP-Cbl undergoes Tyr phosphorylation by the insulin receptor (a reaction of unclear significance) and recruits additional polypeptides—specifically, a GEF (C3G coupled with the adapter protein Crk II), along with the Ras superfamily GTPase TC10. As with eIF-2, Ras and all regulatory GTPases, Crk II-mediated loading of TC10 with GTP, activates TC10 signaling. Active TC10 has been implicated in the rearrangement of the actin cytoskeleton, by a process that is not fully understood. Transfection/overexpression experiments indicate that this mechanism contributes in an as yet incompletely understood manner to insulin activation of glucose uptake.[27]

REGULATION OF PKB/Akt BY PDKs

Of the three PKB/Akt isoforms, the regulation of PKBα/Akt1 has been the most extensively studied. In response to mitogen or insulin treatment, PKBα/Akt1 undergoes rapid phosphorylation at Thr308 in the protein kinase domain activation loop (subdomain VIII) and Ser473 in the C-terminal tail.[28] Ser473 lies within a hydrophobic motif (Phe-Pro-Gln-Phe-Ser473-Tyr) that is conserved among several protein kinases.[29] These include p70 S6 kinase and Rsk. The phosphorylation of PKB/Akt by upstream kinases leads to conformational changes that involve the binding of phospho-Ser473 to a specific binding region that, for PKBα/Akt1, spans residues 141–228. As with the hydrophobic phosphoacceptor motif, amino acids 141–228 of PKBα/Akt1 comprise an evolutionarily conserved motif present in several other protein kinases including 3-phosphoinositide-dependent kinase 1 (PDK1 amino acids 73–160—PDK1 does not, however, possess a hydrophobic phosphoacceptor motif), p70 S6 kinase and Rsk. This binding event is pivotal to the establishment of an active conformation (see Fig. 14-2D).[29]

In vivo, phosphorylation of PKB/Akt Thr308/Ser473 requires the activity of PI 3-kinase and can be blocked by PI 3-kinase inhibitors such as wortmannin (see Fig. 14-2A).[12,28] In vitro biochemical dissection of the mechanism of activation of PKB/Akt by phosphorylation indicates that the role of PI 3-kinase-derived PI lipids in PKB/Akt activation is complex.

PDK1 was originally identified as a Ser/Thr kinase that could specifically phosphoryate Thr308 of PKB/Akt. PDK1 contains an N-terminal protein kinase domain that is in the same general protein kinase family as that of PKB/Akt itself. At the PDK1 C terminus is a PH domain that can bind 3'-inositol lipids (see Fig. 14-2A). PDK1 alone can catalyze a 30-fold activation of recombinant PKB/Akt in vitro, in a reaction that absolutely requires 3'-phosphorylated inositol lipids, PI 3, 4, 5, and P3 in particular (see Fig. 14-2D).[12,30,31]

It appears that a major component of 3'-phosphoinositide-dependent activation of PKB/Akt by PDK1 is substrate-directed; in other words, PDK1 intrinsic activity does not appear to increase upon binding PI lipids. Instead, the binding of PI lipids to PKB/Akt renders Thr308 of PKB/Akt available for PDK1-dependent phosphorylation (see Fig. 14-2D). Thus, deletion of the PKB/Akt PH domain results in a modest elevation of PKB/Akt activity and permits lipid-independent PDK1 activation of PKB/Akt, suggesting that the PH domain restricts access of Thr308 and lipid binding reverses this inhibition and makes PKB/Akt a better PDK1 substrate. Moreover, PDK1, when purified or immunoprecipitated from resting or stimulated cells appears to be constitutively active and does not undergo further activation in response to mitogens or insulin, suggesting that much of the regulation of PDK1 involves gating access to PKB/Akt phosphoacceptor sites rather than alterations in PDK1 activity per se.[12,30,31]

The identity of the kinase responsible for PKB/Akt Ser473 phosphorylation has yet to be established. Inasmuch as phosphorylation of Ser473 in vivo requires PI 3-kinase products, it has been proposed that the Ser473 kinase, while possessing a substrate selectivity targeted toward Ser473, is at least superficially similar to PDK1.[12,32] Indeed, the sequences of several protein kinases similar to PDK1 have been deposited in various databases[12,32]; and, accordingly, the Ser473 kinase has been tentatively designated PDK2.

p70 S6 KINASE

As was noted previously, phosphorylation of the 40S small ribosomal subunit protein S6 was among the first insulin- and mitogen-stimulated Ser/Thr phosphorylation events to be identified.[10,11] While the physiologic significance of this phosphorylation was initially unclear, S6 phosphorylation served as a distal marker that could be used as a means of dissecting signal transduction pathways recruited by insulin and growth factors.

Ribosomal S6 kinase (Rsk, also called mitogen-activated protein kinase-activated protein kinase-1; MAPKAP-K1), the first enzyme with S6 kinase activity to be purified and cloned, was isolated from *Xenopus* oocytes arrested in the first meiotic prophase, following treatment of the oocytes with insulin or progesterone.[4,5,33,34] Subsequent analysis revealed that Rsk, while representing the dominant S6 kinase in oocytes, was not the major S6 kinase activated by insulin or mitogens in somatic cells, although Rsk is expressed in somatic cells.[5,34,35] Rsk is a component of the Ras-MAPK pathway and will be discussed in a later section.

Purification of the mammalian somatic cell S6 kinase revealed an enzyme with an apparent molecular weight of 70-kilodaltons upon SDS polyacrylamide gel electrophoresis, hence the name p70 S6 kinase (p70). Copurifying with the 70-kilodalton polypeptide was an 85-kilodalton species.[4,5,36] Molecular cloning has identified two p70 genes: p70α and p70β.[4,5,37,38] The mRNAs transcribed from either the α or β gene contain two alternative translational start sites. The more 5' start sites give rise to the 85-kilodalton polypeptides while the more 3' sites give rise to the 70-kilodalton polypeptides. The 85-kilodalton polypeptides each contain an amino-terminal nuclear localization signal. Consequently, these longer p70 polypeptides reside exclusively in the nucleus. Sequence analysis of the p70α and β cDNAs predicts proteins of 55–60 kilodaltons; therefore, the 70- and 85-kilodalton apparent molecular weights indicate that these proteins migrate aberrantly on SDS gels.[4,5,37,38]

p70 S6 KINASE SUBSTRATES

The best characterized substrates for p70 (Fig. 14-3A) suggest that p70 is intimately involved in the regulation of protein synthesis and, possibly, gene expression. In addition, p70 may regulate key metabolic pathways in response to insulin.

Ribosomal S6

The S6 protein of the 40S small ribosomal subunit is the major p70 substrate. The sites phosphorylated on rat S6 reside in a cluster at the C terminus of the polypeptide (Ser235, Ser236, Ser240, Ser244, and Ser247). Both purified and recombinant p70 can phosphorylate all five sites on ribosomal S6. Importantly, p70 preferentially phosphorylates these sites when S6 is in the context of 40S ribosomal subunits. By contrast, other kinases such as protein kinases C and A, while able to phosphorylate synthetic peptides containing the phospho-acceptor sites of S6, cannot appreciably phosphorylate S6 as part of an intact 40S subunit.[4,5]

The physiologic role of p70 was obscure until it was observed that the immunosuppressant macrolide rapamycin (also called sirolimus or Rapamune), a potent inhibitor of p70 activation in vivo, could selectively block the insulin and mitogen-stimulated translation of 5′ terminal oligopyrimidine (TOP) mRNAs—a subset of mRNAs containing a polypyrimidine tract immediately C terminal to the N^7-methylguanosine cap (see Fig. 14-3A).[5,39,40] Serum-stimulated increases in protein synthesis usually occur at the level of ini-

tiation and correlate with a rapid recruitment of 80S ribosomes onto actively translating polysomes. Thus, upon serum stimulation, there is a relative increase in the number of actively translating polysomes. Most mRNAs redistribute to polysomes of the same size following insulin or mitogen stimulation; in other words, there are simply more of the same size polysomes present upon stimulation with insulin or mitogen. However, 5′TOP mRNAs redistribute to larger polysomes (i.e., ones with more ribosomes) following insulin or mitogen stimulation; thus, initiation of translation from 5′TOP mRNAs is markedly enhanced by insulin or growth factors, even against an overall agonist-stimulated increase in protein translation. A significant proportion of 5′TOP mRNAs encode proteins that are involved in the translation process itself such as the translational elongation factor eEF-1α, and most ribosomal proteins; insulin is known to increase preferentially the translation of these polypeptides. Thus, increased translation of these mRNAs in response to insulin and mitogen serves to further increase protein synthesis in response to extracellular stimuli (see Fig. 14-4A).[39,41]

As will be discussed later, rapamycin does not act directly on p70, but acts instead to inhibit p70 activation by upstream activators. The mechanism by which p70 might regulate translation of 5′TOP mRNAs remains unclear. It has been proposed that S6 phosphorylation allows for the enhanced binding of the 40S subunit to 5′TOP mRNAs, perhaps through a process involving additional cytosolic polypeptides.[39,41] The ability of p70 to influence 5′TOP mRNA translation coincides in vivo with an additional insulin and mitogen-regulated signaling pathway that acts on the general translational mechanism to enhance overall protein synthesis (see Fig. 14-4A and B).

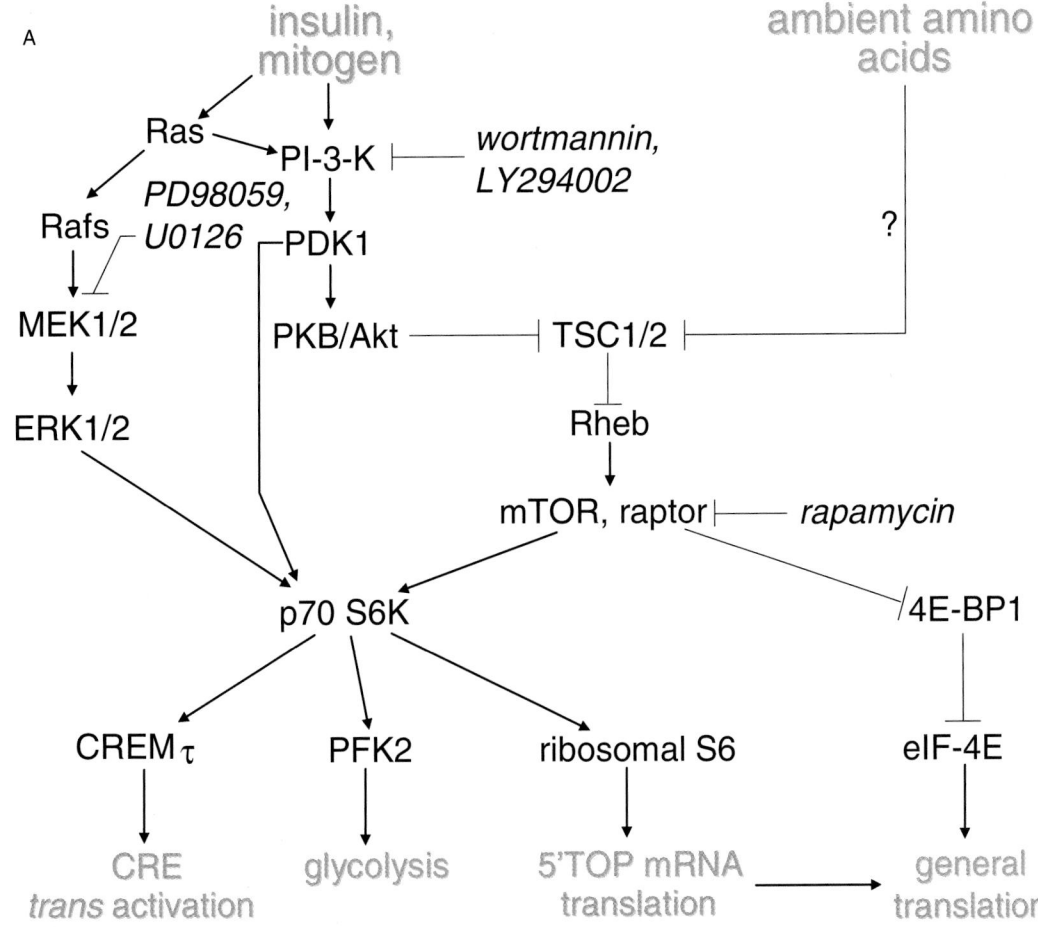

Figure 14-3 Regulation and function of p70 S6 kinase. **(A)** Signaling pathways regulated by Ras, PI 3-kinase, and mTOR through the p70 S6 kinase. Targets of inhibition by wortmannin, LY294002, rapamycin, and the MEK inhibitors PD98059 and U0126 are shown. **(B)** Multistep regulation of p70 S6 kinase. MAPKs and mTOR mediate initial phosphorylations that permit phosphorylation of Thr412 by an unknown kinase. As is indicated, phosphorylation of Thr412 gates phosphorylation, by PDK1, of Thr252. This gating is probably due to the conformational changes incurred upon the binding of phospho-Thr412 to the conserved binding pocket in the p70 kinase domain (see Figs. 14-2B and 14-6B for similar mechanisms governing regulation of PKB/Akt and Rsk, respectively). The black circle with the white P indicates phosphorylation.

Continued

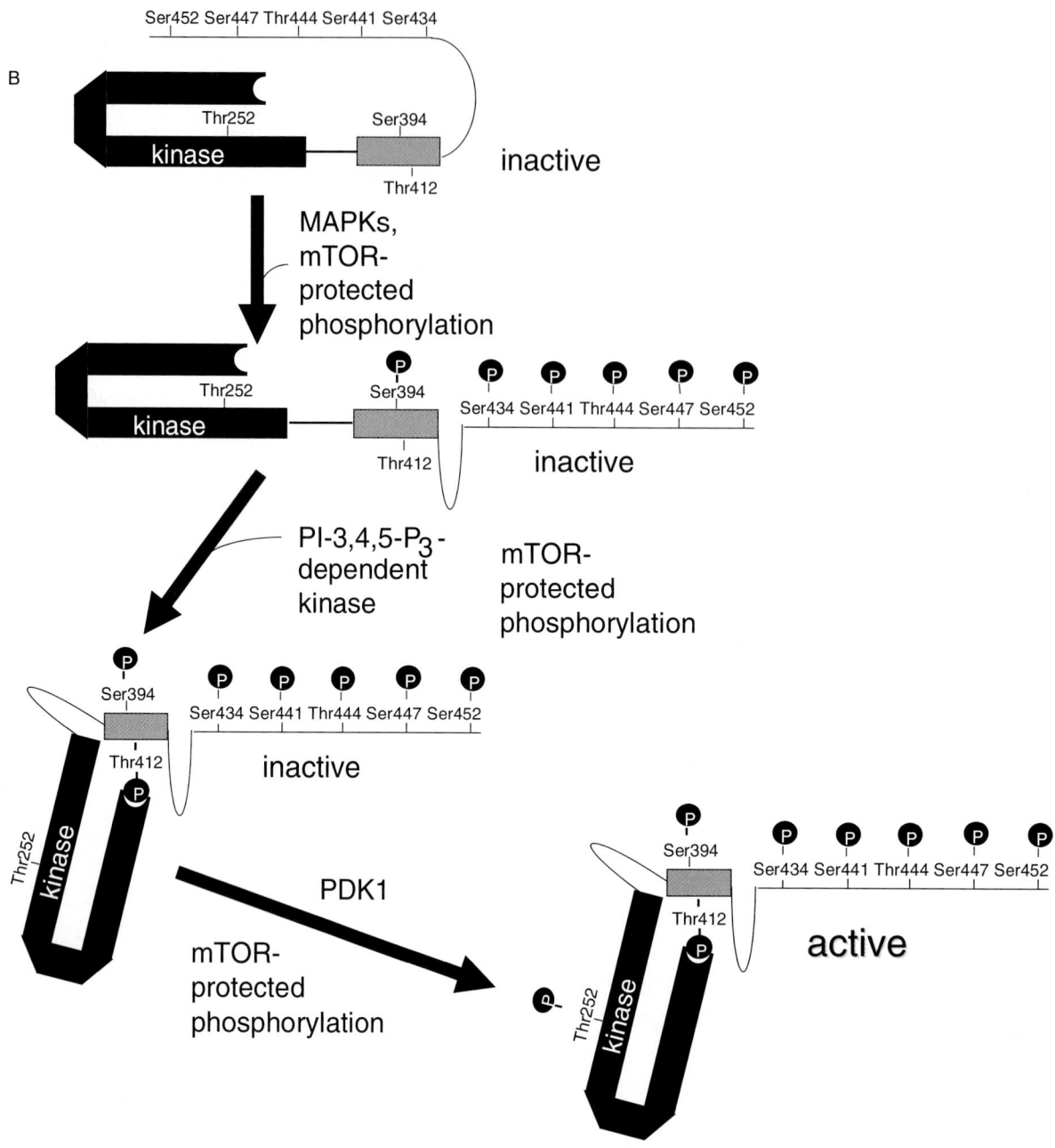

Figure 14-3, cont'd.

Cyclic Adenosine Monophosphate Response Element Modulator

Transcriptional mechanisms activated by cAMP, mitogen, and stress pathways are mediated in part by the cAMP-response element (CRE)-binding proteins (CREB)/activating transcription factors (ATFs), a subgroup of the basic-leucine zipper (bZIP) family of transcription factors. bZIP transcription factors contain a stretch of basic amino acids followed by a leucine zipper. This domain is required for bZIP transcription factor dimerization, a process that is important for regulation and function. In response to elevations in cAMP, CREB/ATFs can *trans* activate genes containing a CRE (see Chapter 12).[42,43] In partnership with c-Jun, some ATFs can also *trans* activate CREs and thyroid hormone response elements (TREs) in response to stress or other stimuli. CRE modulator (CREM) is a CREB/ATF family member that is important to the regulation of gene expression in response to mitogenic and neuroendocrine stimuli. The *crem* gene encodes a large number of polypeptides that arise from alternative promoter usage, differential hnRNA splicing and the presence of alternate translational start sites on several of the resulting mRNAs. The heterogeneous population of CREM proteins includes transcriptional repressors, such as CREMα, β, and γ that arise from alternate splicing to remove glutamine-rich *trans* activation domains, and S-CREM, which is generated from an alternative initiation codon and gives rise to a protein lacking phospho-acceptor sites.[44–47] mRNAs encoding additional CREM repressors can also be transcribed from an alternative, intronic, cAMP-inducible promoter. These transcripts, referred to as inducible cAMP early repressors encode truncated CREM

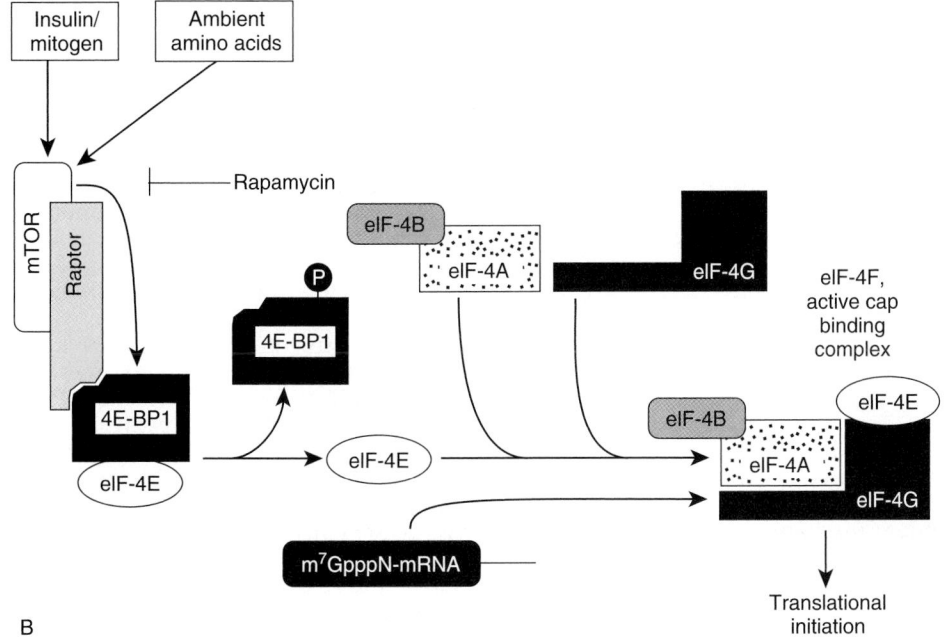

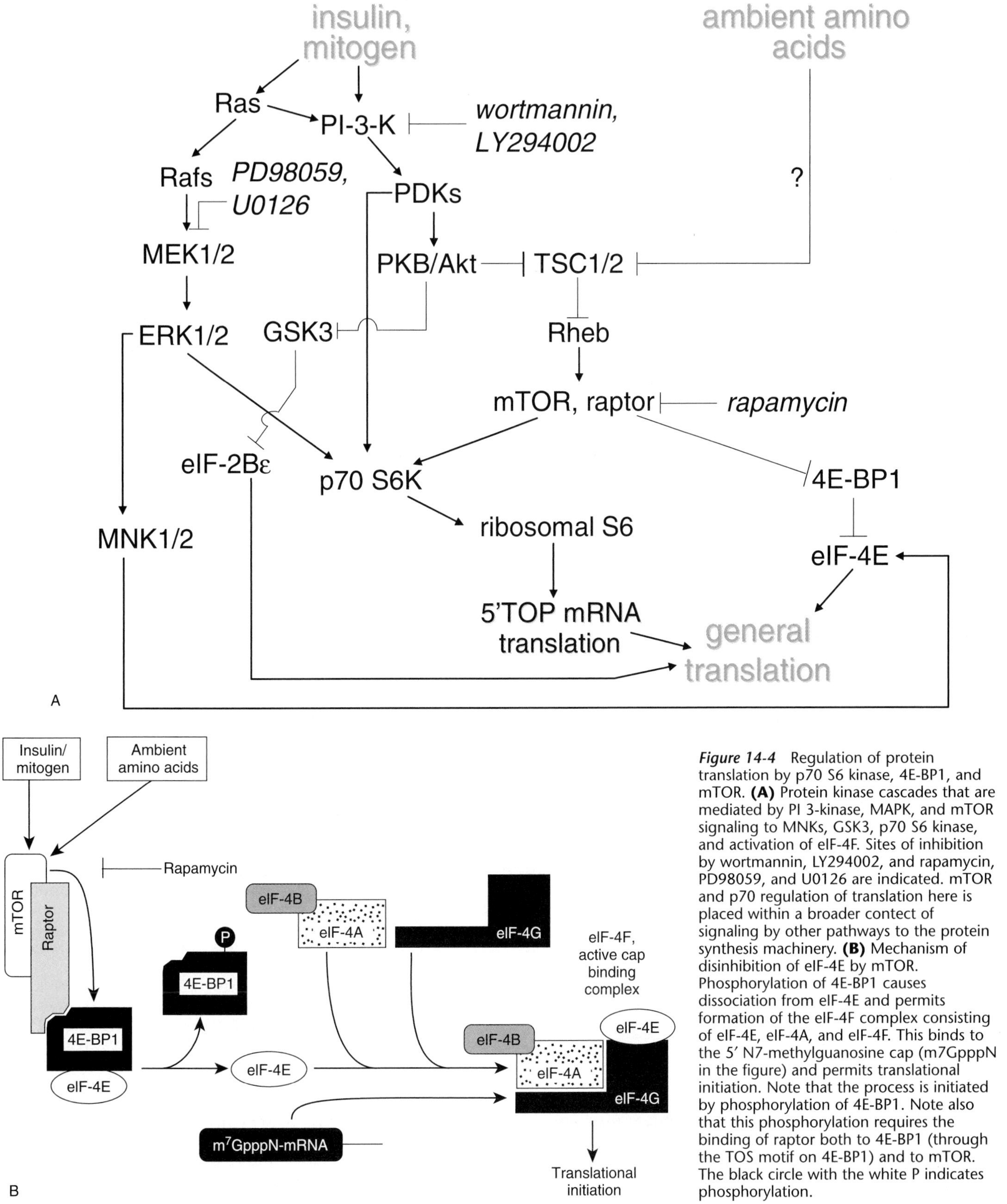

A

B

Figure 14-4 Regulation of protein translation by p70 S6 kinase, 4E-BP1, and mTOR. **(A)** Protein kinase cascades that are mediated by PI 3-kinase, MAPK, and mTOR signaling to MNKs, GSK3, p70 S6 kinase, and activation of eIF-4F. Sites of inhibition by wortmannin, LY294002, and rapamycin, PD98059, and U0126 are indicated. mTOR and p70 regulation of translation here is placed within a broader contect of signaling by other pathways to the protein synthesis machinery. **(B)** Mechanism of disinhibition of eIF-4E by mTOR. Phosphorylation of 4E-BP1 causes dissociation from eIF-4E and permits formation of the eIF-4F complex consisting of eIF-4E, eIF-4A, and eIF-4F. This binds to the 5′ N7-methylguanosine cap (m7GpppN in the figure) and permits translational initiation. Note that the process is initiated by phosphorylation of 4E-BP1. Note also that this phosphorylation requires the binding of raptor both to 4E-BP1 (through the TOS motif on 4E-BP1) and to mTOR. The black circle with the white P indicates phosphorylation.

polypeptides containing only the bZIP domains and are potent repressors of cAMP- and CREB-mediated gene expression (see Chapter 12).[48]

The *crem* gene also encodes transcriptional activators containing one (CREMτ1 or CREMτ2) or both (CREMτ) glutamine-rich *trans* activation domains.[48] Expression of CREMτ is particularly prevalent in male germ cells. There, expression is developmentally regulated by follicle-stimulating hormone during spermatogenesis.[49] CREMτ is rapidly phosphorylated at Ser117 by PKA, a reaction that activates CREMτ *trans* activation function, implicating CREMτ in cAMP-mediated gene expression. In addition, CREMτ Ser117 is a target for Ca/calmodulin-dependent kinases and PKC, suggesting that multiple signaling pathways can activate CREMτ.[50]

Mitogens and serum can also stimulate CREMτ phosphorylation at Ser117 under conditions wherein p70 is activated. This phosphorylation is completely inhibited by rapamycin and can be recapitulated in vitro with purified p70. From these results, it can be concluded that p70 represents the major mechanism by which insulin and mitogens regulate CREMτ. p70 phosphorylation of CREMτ has no effect on DNA binding. Coexpression of a GAL4-CAT reporter, p70, and a GAL4-CREM fusion protein indicates that p70 enhances the *trans* activating activity of CREMτ (see Fig. 14-3A).[51]

PFK2

The insulin-stimulated phosphorylation of cardiac PFK2, and the ramifications of this phosphorylation to metabolic regulation were discussed previously. In addition to PKB/Akt, p70 can phosphorylate PFK2 at the activating sites (see Fig. 14-3A).[21]

Requirement for PI 3-Kinase Activity through PDK Enzymes

That p70 was regulated by Ser/Thr phosphorylation was evident when it was observed that the kinase undergoes rapid Ser/Thr phosphorylation upon insulin and mitogen stimulation, and that this phosphorylation correlates with activation. Moreover, treatment of p70 with Ser/Thr-specific phosphatases rapidly deactivates p70 in a reaction accompanied by dephosphorylation of the p70 polypeptide.[4,36]

The mechanism by which p70 is activated by upstream phosphorylation is exceedingly complex and still incompletely understood. p70 undergoes regulatory phosphorylation in three domains: (1) several sites in a C-terminal pseudosubstrate autoinhibitory domain (Ser434, Ser441, Thr444, Ser447, Ser452); (2) two sites in a short motif immediately C terminal to the catalytic domain, referred to as the catalytic domain extension (Ser394, Thr412); and (3) a site in the activating loop of the kinase domain (Thr252; see Fig. 14-3B).[5] Phosphorylation of these sites is hierarchical with phosphorylation of some sites gating the phosphorylation of other sites. Moreover, these phosphorylations are subject to regulation by several different pathways.

Phosphorylation of the pseudosubstrate autoinhibitory domain of p70, in response to insulin and mitogens, is likely mediated primarily by proline-directed Ser/Thr kinases including MAP kinases, insofar as these kinases represent the major peaks of autoinhibitory domain kinase activity detectable upon fractionation, over several chromatographic steps, of insulin-stimulated cell extracts.[5,52] However, phosphorylation of these sites alone is insufficient to activate p70 in vitro. Moreover, deletion of the autoinhibitory domain (ΔCT104) does not result in a constitutively active p70 mutant and, in fact, the ΔCT104 construct can still be activated by mitogen and insulin in vivo. Current evidence suggests that phosphorylation of the MAPK sites is necessary to render p70 capable of undergoing phosphorylation at the sites within the catalytic domain and the catalytic domain extension (see Fig. 14-3B).[5]

The activation of p70 in vivo can be inhibited by wortmannin and rapamycin. Phosphorylation of Thr412 and Thr252 is wortmannin sensitive, indicating that these sites are phosphorylated by a PI 3-kinase-dependent mechanism.[5] PDK1 can phosphorylate Thr252 and likely contributes to the activation of p70 in vivo inasmuch as coexpression of PDK1 and p70ΔCT104 results in a substantial elevation in basal p70 activity and dominant inhibitory mutant constructs of PDK1 can block the activation of p70 by mitogen. However, PDK1 phosphorylation of p70 requires prior phosphorylation of the p70 polypeptide by additional upstream kinases. Thus, PDK1 cannot phosphorylate inactive, unphosphorylated full length p70 in vitro. Deletion of the autoinhibitory domain results in a p70 construct that can still be activated in vivo by coexpressed PDK1; however, this construct also cannot be activated by PDK1 in vitro (see Fig. 14-3B).[5,53]

Phosphorylation of Thr252 by PDK1 requires prior phosphorylation of Thr412. The identity of the T412 kinase is unknown.[5,52,53] Thr412 lies in a hydrophobic phosphoacceptor motif similar to that surrounding Ser473 of PKBα/Akt1.[29] A hydrophobic phosphoacceptor-binding pocket similar to PKB amino acids 141–228 spans p70 amino acids 82–173.[29] Phosphorylation of Thr412 is likely to result in the binding of the phosphoThr412 hydrophobic phosphoacceptor motif to the amino acids 82–173 binding pocket. The consequent conformational change probably enables PDK1 phosphorylation, and contributes to the ultimate active conformation of the p70 polypeptide (see Fig. 14-3B).[5,29,53]

Mutagenesis of p70ΔCT104 Thr412 to an acidic residue (Asp), a mutation that mimics the charge of phosphorylation, results in a modest (~5–10-fold) elevation of basal p70 activity and renders the mutant construct capable of being activated in vitro by PDK1.[5,53] To summarize thus far, p70 is regulated by MAPK-catalyzed phosphorylation of the autoinhibitory domain sites.[5,52,53] This phosphorylation is then thought to permit PI 3-kinase-dependent phosphorylation of Thr412. Once these sites are phosphorylated, PDK1 phosphorylates Thr252. Whereas phosphorylation by PDK1 of Thr 252 alone (on the p70ΔCT104/Asp412 mutant) results in approximately 15-fold activation of p70, dual Thr 412 and Thr 252 phosphorylation of wild type p70 results in synergistic (>200-fold) activation of p70 (see Fig. 14-3B).[53]

Although the phosphorylation of Thr412 and Thr252 of p70 are wortmannin sensitive, the specific role of PI lipids in the regulation of p70 is uncertain. In contrast to the activation of PKB/Akt by PDK1, activation of P70ΔCT104/Asp412 by PDK1 is unaffected by PI $3,4,5,P_3$ in vitro. It is possible that p70 phosphorylation by the Thr412 kinase is PI lipid-dependent, a situation that would, by virtue of the gating function of Thr412 phosphorylation, make PDK1 phosphorylation of Thr252 PI-lipid dependent in vivo (see Fig. 14-3B).[33]

REGULATION OF p70 S6 KINASE BY mTOR

Rapamycin is a macrolide immunosuppressant that potently inhibits T-cell activation and can block eukaryotic cell cycle progression at G1/S. Rapamycin strongly and selectively inhibits activation of p70 in vivo and has no effect on the MAPK Rsk or PI 3-kinase PKB/Akt pathways. Rapamycin does not directly bind or inhibit p70 in vitro.[25,44,54-56]

Rapamycin exerts its effects by binding to a small polypeptide, FK506 binding protein-12 (FKBP12). Interestingly, as its name suggests, FKBP12 is also a target for another immunosuppressant, FK506. Complexes of FKBP12-FK506 can bind and inhibit the calcium-dependent protein phosphatase calcineurin; this inhibition accounts for most of the biologic effects of FK506.[54]

Rapamycin and FK506 are structurally related, sharing a similar FKBP12-binding interface. Outside of this interface, however, the structures differ. Therefore, whereas FKBP12 can bind both FK506 and rapamycin, FKBP12-rapamycin complexes neither bind nor inhibit calcineurin.[54] Potential targets of rapamycin (TORs) were first identified in the budding yeast *Saccharomyces cerevisiae* as mutant alleles that conferred rapamycin resistance. Yeast *TOR1* and *TOR2* consist of a kinase domain that is distantly related to the PI 3-kinase p110 subunit; however, recent studies indicate that TOR polypeptides are Ser/Thr protein kinases.[57,58] The kinase domain is preceded by a very large amino-terminal domain.

This domain includes a 1200-amino acid N-terminal Huntingtin elongation factor-3-regulatory subunit A of phosphatase 2A and Tor2p (HEAT) repeat region, followed by an FRAP-ATM-TTRAP (FAT) domain and an FKBP-rapamycin binding domain (FRB) domain. Immediately carboxyl terminal to the kinase domain is an FAT–carboxy-terminal domain (FATC) similar in sequence to the FAT domain.[57,58] It is likely that these noncatalytic regions participate in binding proteins that collaborate with TOR to regulate protein synthesis.

Mammalian TOR (mTOR, also called rapamycin and FKBP12 target, RAFT, and FKBP-rapamycin-associated protein, FRAP) was identified by biochemical purification as a polypeptide that could bind immobilized FKBP12-rapamycin. mTOR cannot bind FKBP12 in the absence of rapamycin, nor can rapamycin directly bind mTOR. mTOR contains kinase and noncatalytic regions that are strikingly homologous to those of TOR1p and TOR2p. As with TOR1p/2p, the kinase domain of mTOR catalyzes protein phosphorylation, but is distantly related to PI 3-kinase p110.[58–60]

The inhibition of mTOR by rapamycin accounts for the lion's share of the effects of this drug in the clinic. Of note, rapamycin is an excellent and well-tolerated immunosuppressant. It also is a potent inhibitor of cell-cycle progression; and cardiovascular stents impregnated with rapamycin are dramatically effective at preventing restenosis after balloon angioplasty. Finally, the cell-cycle inhibitory effects of rapamycin highlight the considerable promise of this drug as an anticancer agent.[58]

mTOR is presumed to be at least partially active in resting cells, given that the protein undergoes no apparent stimulation consequent to insulin treatment (see later discussion of mTOR regulation); nevertheless, coexpression of mTOR and p70 results in little or no p70 activation in vivo.[60,61] However, if the cell culture medium is depleted of amino acids, mTOR activity is dramatically inhibited. In addition, under low amino acid conditions, p70 is no longer responsive to mitogen and no longer undergoes phosphorylation at Thr412, the site whose phosphorylation is repressed both by wortmannin and rapamycin (see Figs. 14-3B and 14-4A).[61] Thus, it appears that mTOR is a sensor for ambient amino acids, a role fitting for a component of a pathway implicated in the regulation of protein synthesis.

The exact function of mTOR in the regulation of p70 remains to be established unambiguously. Rapamycin blocks phosphorylation of p70 Thr252 and Thr412, sites that are phosphorylated in a PI 3-kinase-dependent manner (see Fig. 14-3B).[5,53] The mechanism of this inhibition is unclear. Immunoprecipitates of mTOR can catalyze the phosphorylation p70 in vitro at Thr412, one of the rapamycin-sensitive sites[61,62]; however, the stoichiometry of this phosphorylation is unknown. It remains to be determined if this phosphorylation is catalyzed directly or by an mTOR-associated kinase. In particular, a p70 mutant, Δ2-46/ΔCT104, is entirely resistant to rapamycin yet remains mitogen responsive and inhibited by wortmannin. Moreover, insulin stimulates the phosphorylation of Δ2-46/ΔCT104 at Thr412 in the presence of rapamycin, indicating that inhibition of mTOR by rapamycin does not result in inhibition of Thr412 kinase activity.[5,61] For now, it is plausible to propose that Thr412 is phosphorylated by a PI lipid-dependent kinase distinct from mTOR, and that mTOR inhibits a phosphatase selective for phosphorylated Thr412.[5] Having said this, phosphorylation of p70 by mTOR, coupled with phosphorylation of 4E-BP1 are reasonable in vitro methods for assessing mTOR activity; and these approaches have been used extensively to study mTOR regulation.

mTOR AND GENERAL PROTEIN SYNTHESIS

Figure 14-4A illustrates insulin/mitogen regulation of protein synthesis and includes mechanisms regulated by mTOR, GSK3, and MAPKs. As was mentioned previously, insulin and mitogens stimulate an increase in the synthesis of proteins required for progression through the cell cycle. The p70 pathway contributes to this increase by enhancing the translation of 5′TOP mRNAs. In addition to regulating the p70 pathway (and therefore 5′TOP mRNA translation), mTOR directly regulates general protein synthesis through the disinhibition of the eukaryotic initiation factor-4E (eIF-4E), a component of the multisubunit translational initiating complex eIF-4F (see Fig. 14-4A and B).[63–65]

Cellular mRNAs contain a 5′ cap structure, the N^7-methylguanosine cap. Efficient translation of proteins is dependent on the binding of eIF-4F to the methylguanosine cap. The binding of eIF-4F to mRNA is thought to result in a relaxation of mRNA secondary structure, thereby facilitating the binding of the 40S small ribosomal subunit. eIF-4F is a hetero oligomer that consists of eIF-4A, an RNA helicase that acts in collaboration with eIF-4B, and RNA-binding protein, to unwind mRNA thereby allowing for ribosome binding. The eIF-4F complex also contains eIF-4G, a multifunctional scaffolding protein that binds eIF-4A, eIF-4B, and the final eIF-4F component, eIF-4E. The ability of eIF-4F to bind to the 5′ cap is dictated by the association between eIF-4E and eIF-4G. This association is thought to recruit the remaining eIF-4F subunits and foster the formation of a complete eIF-4F complex capable of binding to the 5′ cap (see Fig. 14-4B).[64,65]

The eIF-4E to eIF-4G interaction is negatively regulated by the translational repressor protein 4E-binding protein 1 (4E-BP1 also called phosphorylated heat- and acid-stable protein regulated by insulin, PHAS-I). 4E-BP1 is rapidly phosphorylated at Ser64 in response to insulin and mitogens; and this phosphorylation results in the dissociation of 4E-BP1 from eIF-4E.[63–65] In vivo, the phosphorylation of 4E-BP1 is completely inhibited by rapamycin; and immunoprecipitates of mTOR can directly phosphorylate 4E-BP1 at Ser64, when 4E-BP1 is bound to eIF-4E, and promote the dissociation of the 4E-BP1–eIF-4E complex. This, in turn, fosters formation of the eIF-4F complex (see Fig. 14-4B).[63] One remaining conundrum is the observation that mTOR is constitutively active in resting cells maintained in medium replete with amino acids whereas 4E-BP1 phosphorylation is clearly insulin stimulated. It is conceivable that a 4E-BP1 kinase, activated by insulin through mTOR-dependent and -independent mechanisms, coimmunoprecipitates with mTOR.

Inasmuch as rapamycin can completely block insulin/mitogen activation of protein translation, mTOR regulation of translation represents a key step in translational control. However, the mTOR > 4E-BP1 mechanism is not the only way in which eIF-4F is regulated by insulin and mitogens. eIF-4E, itself, is also directly phosphorylated by insulin/mitogen- and stress-activated protein kinases. This phosphorylation is discussed in a later section.

REGULATION OF TRANSLATION AND THE PKB PATHWAY

Several recent papers have identified polypeptides that are critical for coupling mTOR to the phosphorylation of p70 and 4E-BP1, and to the regulation of mTOR by extracellular stimuli. Regulatory associated protein of mTOR (raptor) is an evolutionarily conserved 150-kilodalton polypeptide that binds mTOR and is required for mTOR regulation of p70 S6 kinase and 4E-BP1 (see Fig. 14-4A and B).[66,67] Raptor contains several potential protein-protein interaction motifs including an amino-terminal raptor N-terminal conserved motif, as well as three HEAT and seven WD40 repeat motifs. The HEAT repeats of mTOR are necessary for binding raptor. Conversely, both the HEAT and raptor N-terminal conserved motifs on raptor appear important for mTOR binding.[66,67] The binding of raptor to mTOR substantially increases the ability of mTOR to phosphorylate 4E-BP1 and p70 in vitro, and silencing of raptor gene expression blunts insulin activation of p70 and 4E-BP1 phosphorylation in vivo.[66,67] Taken together, these results indicate that raptor is an essential mTOR-binding partner.

How does raptor couple mTOR to its effectors? As noted previously, deletion of amino acids 2–46 renders p70 resistant to rapamycin; however, the polypeptide is still phosphorylated in response to mitogen at sites that, in the wild type enzyme, are phosphorylated in a rapamycin-inhibitable manner.[5,61] Deletion of a larger segment of p70 (amino acids 1–53) completely abrogates activation of p70 in vivo.[68,69] Taken together, these results indicate that the amino terminus of p70 is critical to regulation by mTOR. Examination of the sequences of the p70 amino terminus and 4E-BP1 revealed a conserved 5-amino acid motif, termed the *Tor signaling (TOS) motif* (Phe-Asp-Ile-Asp-Leu in p70, Phe-Glu-Met-Asp-Ile in 4E-BP1).[68,69] Mutagenesis of the phenylalanine residue in this motif, be it in p70 or 4E-BP1, completely prevents phosphorylation of rapamycin-sensitive sites.[68-71] Raptor not only binds mTOR but it binds p70 and 4E-BP1; and the TOS motif on both p70 and 4E-BP1 is required for binding raptor (see Fig. 14-4B). By binding both mTOR and its effectors, raptor permits efficient coupling of mTOR to downstream target proteins.[68-71]

mTOR regulation has been difficult to dissect due to the high apparent constitutive activity of the protein isolated from cells cultured in an amino acid–rich medium. However, as noted previously, depletion of amino acids inactivates mTOR.[60,61] Moreover, wortmannin, an inhibitor of PI 3-kinase, reduces the phosphorylation of sites on p70 whose phosphorylation is also rapamycin-inhibitable. This latter observation suggested a link between mTOR and the PI 3-kinase pathway. Recent evidence indicates that mTOR is regulated in part by the PI 3-kinase pathway.

Tuberous sclerosis is an autosomal-dominant syndrome that predisposes afflicted individuals to the development of hamartomas, and, albeit rarely, malignant cancers, especially of the brain, skin, kidneys, and heart. Tuberous sclerosis occurs due to loss of function mutations in one of two genes: *Tsc1* or *Tsc2*, which encode the proteins hamartin (130 kDa) and tuberin (180 kDa), respectively. There are few clear structural features in either polypeptide, other than a domain in tuberin homologous to GTPase-activating proteins (GAPs). Hamartin and tuberin form a tight complex in vivo and in vitro.[72]

The GAP-like motif in tuberin suggested that the hamartin-tuberin complex might function to stimulate the inactivating GTPase activity of small, monomeric GTP-binding proteins. However, it was genetic studies of *Drosophila* that revealed the function of the hamartin-tuberin complex. As in mammals, the *Drosophila* PI 3-kinase > PKB/Akt pathway is critical in the regulation of protein synthesis and cell size. Genetic epistasis studies of *Drosophila* placed the hamartin-tuberin complex downstream of PKB/Akt and upstream of p70 S6K.[72] Biochemical studies of mammalian tuberin revealed it to be a substrate for PKBα/Akt1 with phosphorylation at Ser924 and Thr1518 triggering tuberin's insulin-dependent dissociation from hamartin (see Figs. 14-2C, 14-3B, and 14-4A).[73,74] As with *Drosophila*, mammalian *Tsc1*–/– or *Tsc2*–/– cells display elevated constitutive protein synthesis and increased size. From these studies, it was concluded that PKB/Akt functioned to promote increases in cell size by phosphorylating and inactivating the hamartin-tuberin complex.[72-74]

In cultured mammalian or *Drosophila* cells, disruption of either *Tsc1* or *Tsc2* leads to constitutive, but rapamycin-inhibitable activation of p70 and phosphorylation of 4E-BP1, consistent with the idea that the activation of mTOR function involves suppression of the hamartin tuberin complex.[72-74] Additional genetic epistasis studies of *Drosophila* revealed that inactivating mutations in *ras homologue expressed in brain* (*rheb*) were able to rescue ablation of *Tsc1* or *Tsc2*.[75-77] Rheb is an evolutionarily conserved member of the Ras superfamily of monomeric GTPases. As such, Rheb is active in the GTP-bound state and inactive in the GDP-bound state. Rheb, itself, has very weak intrinsic GTPase activity; and it was recently shown that tuberin was a GAP specific for Rheb (see Figs. 14-2C, 14-3B, and 14-4A).[72,78] Moreover, genetic studies of both mammalian and *Drosophila* cells indicate that Rheb is required for in vivo TOR activity.[72,75-78]

These results suggest a pathway wherein insulin recruitment of the PI 3-kinase pathway triggers PKB/Akt-dependent phosphorylation of tuberin. This results in dissociation from hamartin and inactivation of tuberin's GAP activity. In turn, Rheb is derepressed and contributes to maintenance of mTOR activity (see Fig. 14-4A). mTOR functions at least in part by binding raptor. Raptor, then, delivers mTOR's effectors (p70 and 4E-BP1), which also bind to raptor through their TOS motifs. Ultimately, p70 and 4E-BP1 are phosphorylated at key regulatory sites (4E-BP1 directly by mTOR, p70 by an as yet incompletely characterized process), thereby enhancing overall protein synthesis (see Fig. 14-4A and B).[66-78]

INSULIN AND MITOGEN ACTIVATION OF Ser/Thr PHOSPHORYLATION II

THE MAP3K > MEK > MAPK CORE SIGNALING MODULE

Mitogen-activated protein kinase (MAPK) signal transduction pathways are among the most widespread mechanisms of cellular regulation. All eukaryotic cells possess multiple MAPK pathways, each of which is preferentially recruited by distinct sets of stimuli, thereby allowing the cell to respond in parallel to multiple divergent inputs. Mammalian MAPK pathways can be recruited by a wide variety of different stimuli ranging from hormones such as insulin and growth hormone, to mitogens (i.e., epidermal growth factor [EGF], platelet-derived growth factor [PDGF], fibroblast growth factor [FGF]), vasoactive peptides (angiotensin II, endothelin), inflammatory cytokines of the TNF family, and environmental stresses, such as osmotic shock, ionizing radiation, and ischemic injury.[79-83]

All MAPK pathways consist of a central three-tiered "core signaling module" wherein MAPKs are activated by concomitant Thr and Tyr phosphorylation catalyzed by a family of dual specificity kinases referred to as MAPK/extracellular signal-regulated kinase (ERK) kinases (MEKs or MKKs). MEKs, in turn, are regulated by Ser/Thr phosphorylation catalyzed by several protein kinases collectively referred to as MAPK-kinase-kinases (MAP3Ks; Fig. 14-5A). The core signaling modules are themselves regulated by a divergent variety of upstream activators and inhibitors including GTPases of the Ras superfamily and adapter proteins coupled to cytokine receptors.[79-83]

The notion of multiple parallel MAPK signaling cascades was first appreciated from studies of simple eukaryotes such as the budding yeast *S. cerevisiae*. To date, six *S. cerevisiae* MAPK signaling pathways have been identified.[79] Several features of yeast signaling pathways are relevant to the understanding of mammalian signaling, and these features illustrate general properties of MAPK signaling modules (see Fig. 14-5B).

Signaling Components with More Than One Biological Function

There are instances wherein individual elements can function in more than one pathway, for example, the MAP3K Ste11p functions as part of the mating pheromone response pathway and the osmosensing pathway (see Fig. 14-5B).[84]

Pathway Segregation by Scaffolding Proteins

Some yeast signaling pathways include distinct scaffolding proteins that bind several components in a specific signaling pathway and act to segregate these components so as to maintain pathway integrity and efficiency. Alternatively, in some MAPK pathways, the signaling components themselves possess intrinsic scaffolding properties. Thus, Ste5p of the yeast mating pheromone pathway is a scaffolding protein that selectively binds an MAP3K (Ste11p), an MEK (Ste7p), and an MAPK (Fus3p) and couples them to upstream activators.[79,85] Therefore, although Ste11p can function in both the mating and osmosensing pathways, it selectively activates different MEKs in each pathway: Ste7p for the mating pathway and Pbs2p for the osmosensing pathway. This selectivity is due, in part, to the fact that Ste5p maintains signaling pathway

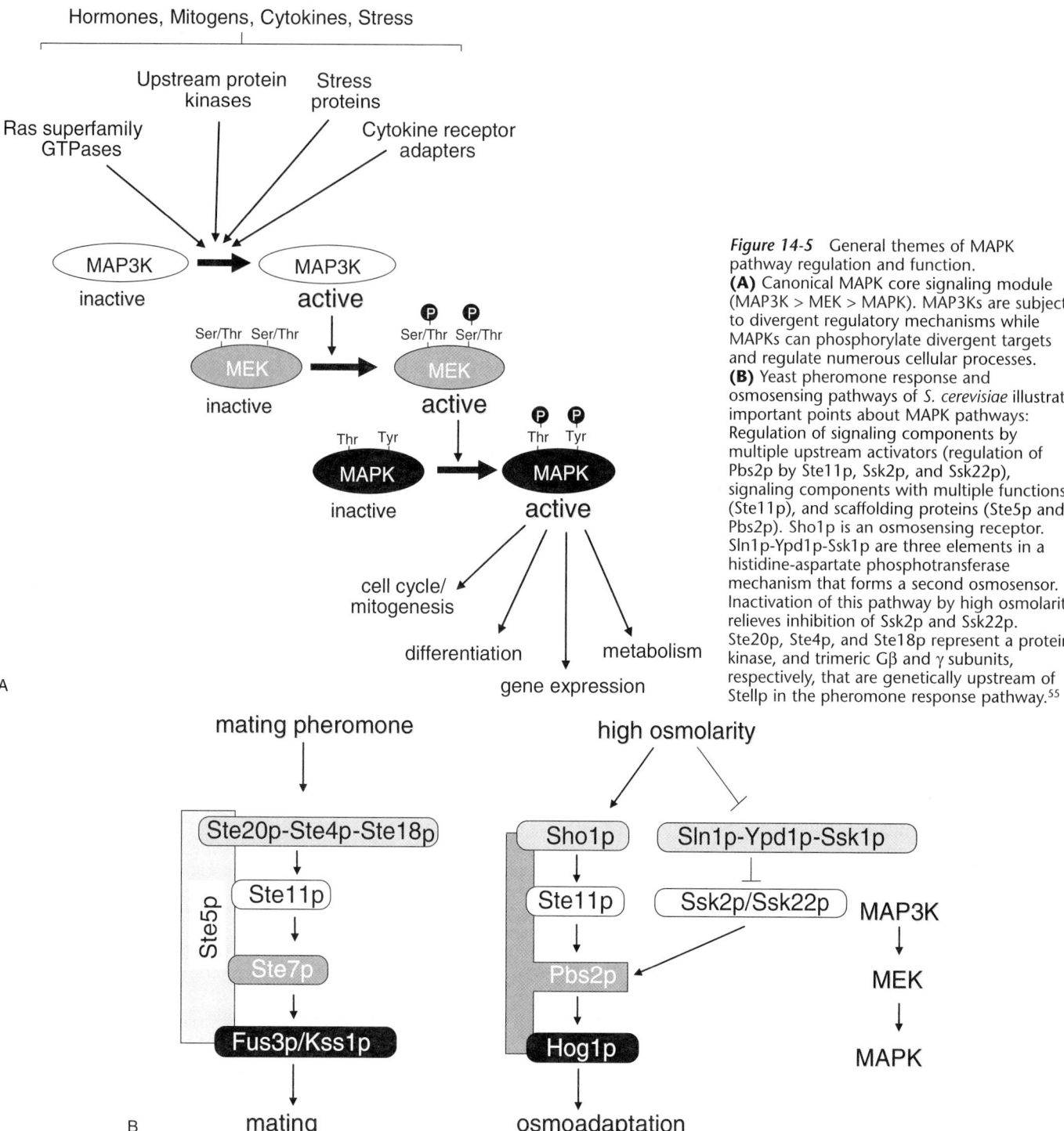

Figure 14-5 General themes of MAPK pathway regulation and function. **(A)** Canonical MAPK core signaling module (MAP3K > MEK > MAPK). MAP3Ks are subject to divergent regulatory mechanisms while MAPKs can phosphorylate divergent targets and regulate numerous cellular processes. **(B)** Yeast pheromone response and osmosensing pathways of *S. cerevisiae* illustrate important points about MAPK pathways: Regulation of signaling components by multiple upstream activators (regulation of Pbs2p by Ste11p, Ssk2p, and Ssk22p), signaling components with multiple functions (Ste11p), and scaffolding proteins (Ste5p and Pbs2p). Sho1p is an osmosensing receptor. Sln1p-Ypd1p-Ssk1p are three elements in a histidine-aspartate phosphotransferase mechanism that forms a second osmosensor. Inactivation of this pathway by high osmolarity relieves inhibition of Ssk2p and Ssk22p. Ste20p, Ste4p, and Ste18p represent a protein kinase, and trimeric Gβ and γ subunits, respectively, that are genetically upstream of Ste11p in the pheromone response pathway.[55]

specificity by binding selectively Ste7p and not Pbs2p.[79] Conversely, Pbs2p, in addition to serving as an MEK, acts as a scaffold protein, selectively binding Ste11p and the osmosensing MAPK Hog1p. Pbs2p does not bind Fus3p; thus, Pbs2p maintains signaling pathway integrity by interacting specifically with Hog1p and not with Fus3p or Kss1p (see Fig. 14-5*B*).[84]

Redundancy of Signaling Components
There are examples of signaling elements in yeast MAPK that can be activated by several upstream components, often in response to the same class of stimulus. Thus, as part of the osmosensing pathway, the MEK Pbs2p can not only be acti-

vated by the MAP3K Ste11p, but it can also be activated by two additional osmosensing MAP3Ks: Ssk2p and Ssk22p (see Fig. 14-5*B*).[79,84]

Regulation of Signaling Specificity by Docking Domains
In vitro assays using peptide substrates indicate that the MAPKs are "proline-directed"—phosphorylating Ser/Thr residues followed immediately by Pro residues. However, kinetic analysis revealed these peptides to be relatively low affinity substrates. Moreover, in numerous instances, different MAPKs could phosphorylate the peptides apparently indiscriminately.[81,82] How, then, do MAPKs achieve physiologic specificity? While scaffold proteins are one such

mechanism, it is clear that in a broader sense MAPK signaling specificity and affinity are determined by docking domains on both MAPK regulators and effectors. These docking motifs permit high affinity, specific protein-protein interactions that confer signaling fidelity and efficiency.[86–88]

THE Ras > MAPK PATHWAY

General Considerations

The first mammalian MAPK was detected as an insulin-stimulated 40–44 kilodalton Ser/Thr kinase that could phosphorylate microtubule-associated protein 2. The name MAPK stemmed from the observation that this kinase was activated not only by insulin but by a wide variety of mitogens that couple to Tyr kinases. Activation of the insulin-stimulated MAPK is rapid, preceding activation of other known mitogen-activated Ser/Thr kinases, suggesting a proximal role in signal transduction; this MAPK can, in fact, phosphorylate and activate another insulin-activated kinase, Rsk (Fig. 14-6).[4,5]

Molecular cloning of the insulin- and mitogen-stimulated MAPKs revealed 44- and 42-kilodalton protein Ser/Thr kinases. These cDNAs were designated, respectively, ERK-1 and ERK-2 (Table 14-1). Structural analysis of the ERK-1 and ERK-2 sequences revealed a striking homology to *S. cerevisiae* Fus3p and Kss1p, kinases of the yeast mating pheromone pathway (see Fig. 14-5B).[4,79] This was the first indication of the conservation of MAPK pathways.

SUBSTRATES OF ERK-1 AND ERK-2

ERK-1 and ERK-2 phosphorylate and activate both transcription factors and other protein kinases. These physiologic substrates serve to illustrate the importance of MAPKs in cellular physiology (see Fig. 14-6A).

Rsk was the first insulin-stimulated protein kinase with S6 phosphorylating activity to be purified and cloned.[4,33,34] As was shown previously, however, in spite of its name, Rsk does not represent the physiologic S6 kinase activated by insulin and mitogens in somatic cells.[25] At least three Rsk isoforms have been cloned and they have a distinct molecular structure in that each possesses two complete protein kinase domains (see Fig. 14-6B).[4,34] Both domains are necessary for Rsk regulation and function.

Rsk is thought to be important in insulin and mitogen regulation of glycogen metabolism. GSK3 can phosphorylate GS at sites 3a–c and 4; however, site 2 is not phosphorylated by GSK3, and insulin-stimulated dephosphorylation of GS involves dephosphorylation primarily of sites 2 and 3a–c. Thus, insulin-mediated inhibition of GSK3 cannot account for all of insulin's action on GS (Fig. 14-7).

Rsk phosphorylation of the G subunit of phosphatase-1 represents a mechanism by which MAPK pathways, in conjunction with the PI 3-kinase > GSK3 pathway, can regulate skeletal muscle GS activation (see Fig. 14-7). PP-1G is a skeletal muscle polypeptide that binds protein phosphat-1 (PP-1) in a reversible fashion and interacts constitutively with the glycogen granule. Of note, GS is constitutively associated with skeletal muscle glycogen granules. PP-1G can be phosphorylated at two sites referred to as sites 1 and 2. PP-1G site 2 is a substrate for cAMP-dependent protein kinase. Dephosphorylation of PP-1G site 2 promotes the association of PP-1 with PP-1G.[4,16] Phosphorylation of PP-1G site 1 by Rsk substantially enhances the rate at which PP-1 dephosphorylates GS. By this process, PP-1 is targeted, in an insulin-stimulated manner, to GS and can dephosphorylate (at GS sites 3a–c) and activate GS (see Fig. 14-7).[4,89] It should be noted that this mechanism is specific for skeletal muscle inasmuch as PP-1G is a muscle-specific protein. Whether or not analogous mechanisms exist in other tissues is unclear.

Thus, in response to insulin and mitogens, both the PI 3-kinase and MAPK pathways can potentially regulate GS.

Which pathway, then, is the dominant mechanism of GS activation? This question has not yet been answered unambiguously; however, studies using pharmacologic inhibitors of the MAPK pathway (the Parke-Davis compound PD98059) or the PI 3-kinase pathway (wortmannin) suggest that whether or not the MAPK or PI 3-kinase pathway is dominant in GS activation may depend on the stimulus. Thus, inhibition of the PI 3-kinase pathway strongly blocks insulin activation of GS, suggesting that the PI 3-kinase > GSK3 mechanism is the preferential pathway for GS activation by insulin. By contrast, EGF activation of GS is substantially blocked on inhibition of the MAPK > MAPKAP-K1-Rsk mechanism, suggesting that the MAPKs are more important in EGF regulation of GS.[4,5]

Rsk, once activated by insulin or mitogens, can be completely inactivated with protein Ser/Thr phosphatases. Both ERK-1 and ERK-2 can phosphorylate and activate phosphatase-inactivated Rsk. That ERK-1 and ERK-2 are physiologically relevant Rsk kinases is evidenced by the observation that the ERKs are activated in vivo prior to Rsk activation, and high-resolution column chromatography and other methods have revealed that ERK-1 and -2 represent major insulin and mitogen-activated Rsk kinases.[4,5,81] More recently, it has been demonstrated that PDK1 also contributes to Rsk activation.[90]

The mechanism by which the ERKs and PDK1 activate Rsk is complex (see Fig. 14-6B). ERKs activate the C-terminal catalytic domain by phosphorylating Thr574 and participate in the activation of the N-terminal catalytic domain by phosphorylating Ser364. The activated carboxyl-terminal catalytic domain then phosphorylates Ser381 (*trans* autophosphorylation).

Thr574, Ser364, and Ser381 all lie within the subdomain VIII activation loops.[91] Rsk Ser381 also resides within a hydrophobic phosphoacceptor motif similar to that present in PKB and p70.[29] As with PDK1, PKB, and p70, a corresponding conserved binding pocket for the Ser381 hydrophobic phosphoacceptor motif (amino acids 53–142 for Rsk1) resides within the amino-terminal kinase domain.[29] Phosphorylation of Ser381 serves two purposes. First, it creates an interaction site for the hydrophobic phosphoacceptor domain binding pocket of PDK1.[29] Consequently, PDK1 binds the phosphorylated Rsk hydrophobic phosphoacceptor domain and phosphorylates Rsk at Ser222 (see Fig. 14-6B),[29,90] the final phosphorylation event required for full activation of Rsk. Interestingly, following this phosphorylation, PDK1 dissociates, and the phospho-Ser/hydrophobic domain binding pocket of Rsk1 itself binds to phospho-Ser381, and Rsk thereby assumes an active conformation (see Fig. 14-6B).[29] It is the amino-terminal kinase domain that is likely responsible for phosphorylation of Rsk substrates.[91]

MNKs

While dissociation of 4E-BP1 is likely the rate limiting step in the regulation of formation of a functional eIF-4F complex, eIF-4E itself also undergoes a regulatory phosphorylation at Ser209 in response to both insulin/mitogen and environmental stress.[65,92] This phosphorylation is thought to increase the affinity of eIF-4E for the 5' cap, and both crystallographic and biochemical data indicate that phosphorylated eIF-4E is preferentially associated with the 5' cap (see Figs. 14-4 and 14-6A). MAPK interacting kinases (MNKs)-1 and -2 are two closely related kinases that are the physiologically relevant eIF-4E Ser209 kinases. As the name implies, MNKs associate in vivo with MAPKs and are in vitro and in vivo MAPK substrates. MNKs are phosphorylated and activated both by ERKs 1/2 (in response to insulin and mitogens) and by the p38 MAPKs (in response to stress, discussed later).[92]

Elk1

One of the earliest transcriptional events known to occur in response to mitogen is the induction of c-*fos* expression. c-*fos* is a bZIP transcription factor that, together with c-Jun,

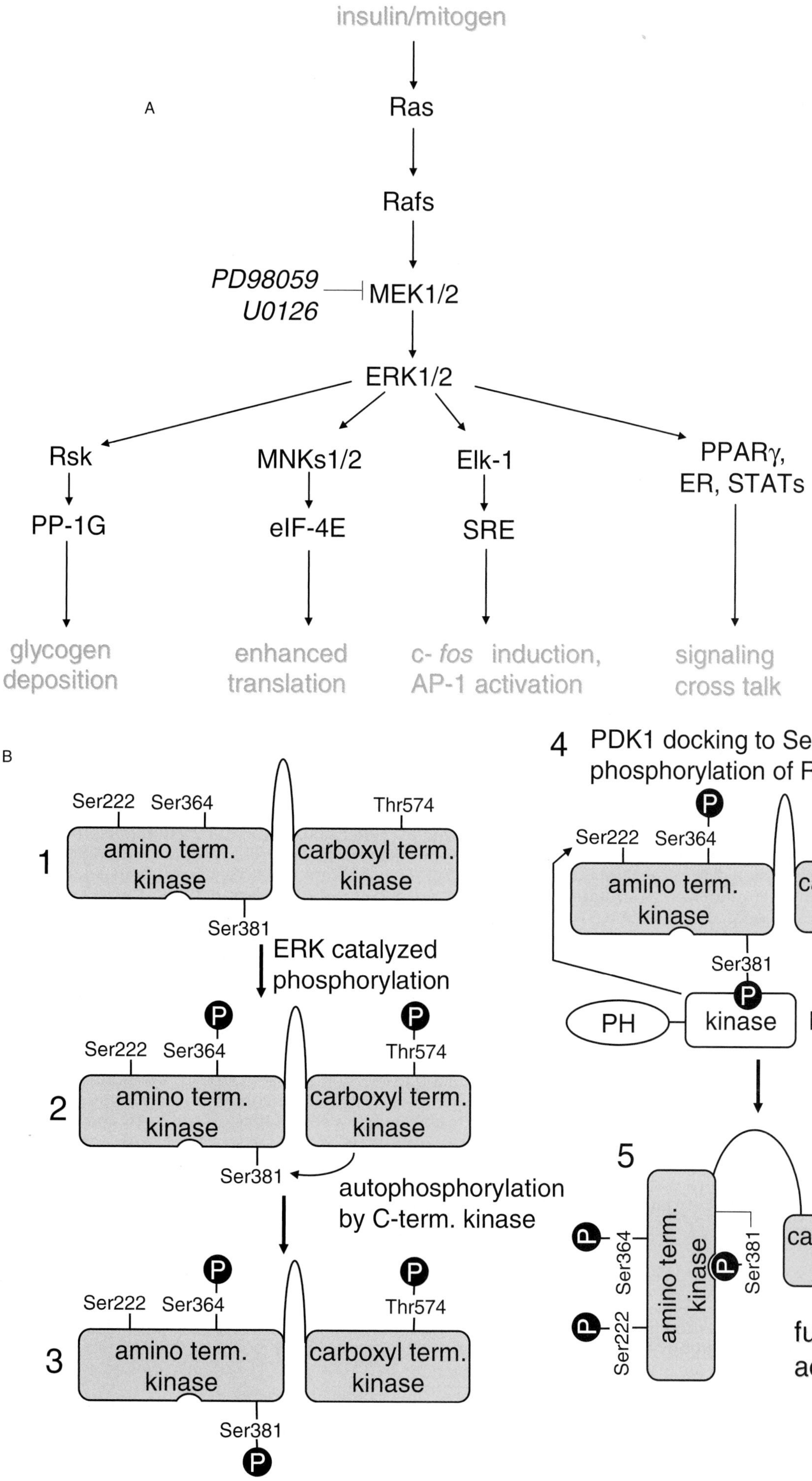

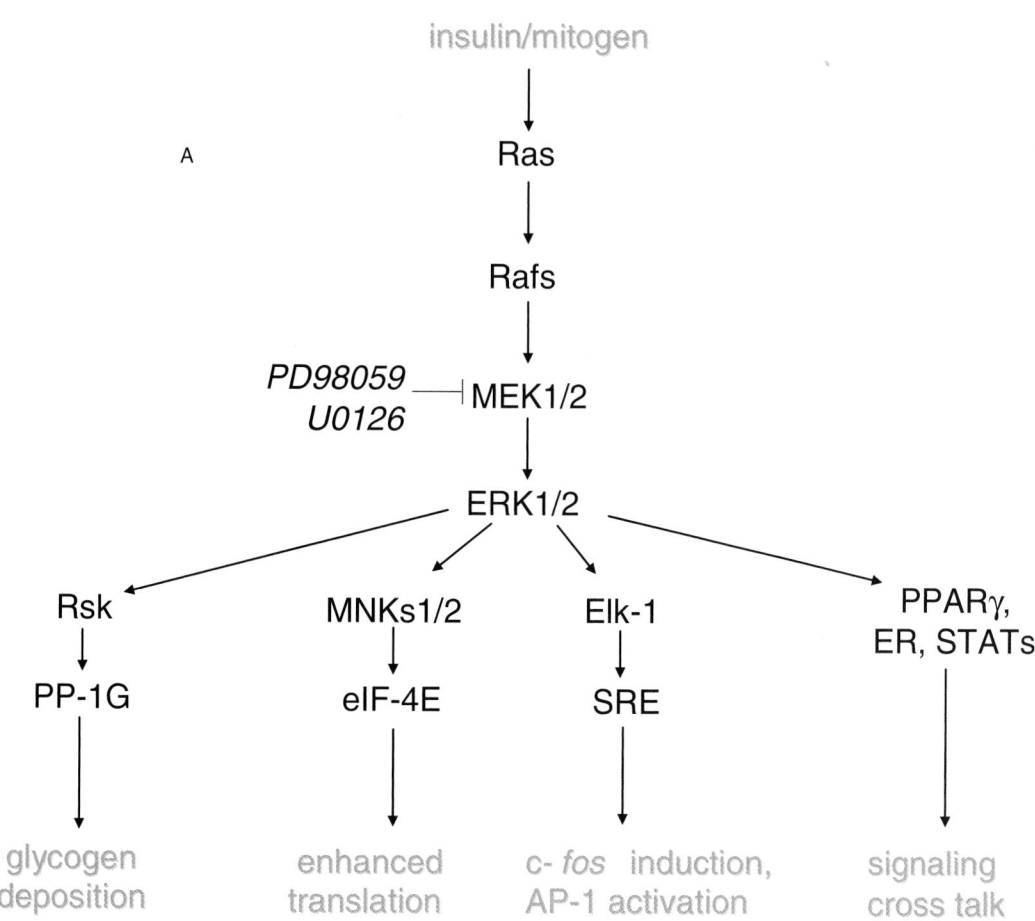

insulin/mitogen

A

Ras

Rafs

PD98059
U0126 ──| MEK1/2

ERK1/2

Rsk   MNKs1/2   Elk-1   PPARγ,
                                             ER, STATs

PP-1G   eIF-4E   SRE

glycogen   enhanced   c-fos induction,   signaling
deposition   translation   AP-1 activation   cross talk

Figure 14-6 Major signaling pathways activated via ERKs −1 and −2. **(A)** Regulation of Rsk, MNKs (see Fig. 14-4*A*), Elk-1, and nuclear receptors by ERK-dependent mechanisms. The effects of PD98059 and U0126 are indicated. **(B)** Mechanism of activation of Rsk by ERKs1/2. ERK phosphorylation of the C-terminal catalytic domain at Thr574 and the N-terminal catalytic domain at Ser364 is followed by *trans* autophosphorylation (the C-terminal catalytic domain phosphorylates Ser381 of the N-terminal catalytic domain). Phosphorylation of Ser381 triggers the binding of phospho-Ser381 to the conserved phosphoacceptor/hydrophobic binding motif in PDK1. PDK1 then phosphorylates Rsk Ser222. PDK1 then dissociates and phospho-Ser381 of Rsk then binds to the conserved phosphoacceptor/hydrophobic binding motif in the amino-terminal kinase domain, resulting in an active conformation (see Figs. 14-2*D* and 14-3*B* for similar mechanisms involved in the regulation of, respectively, PKB/Akt and p70).

B

1   Ser222   Ser364   Thr574
    amino term.   carboxyl term.
    kinase   kinase
             Ser381

ERK catalyzed phosphorylation

2   Ser222   Ser364 (P)   (P) Thr574
    amino term.   carboxyl term.
    kinase   kinase
             Ser381

autophosphorylation by C-term. kinase

3   Ser222   Ser364 (P)   (P) Thr574
    amino term.   carboxyl term.
    kinase   kinase
             Ser381 (P)

4 PDK1 docking to Ser381 and phosphorylation of Rsk Ser222

    Ser222 (P) Ser364   (P) Thr574
    amino term.   carboxyl term.
    kinase   kinase
             Ser381
    PH — kinase (P) PDK1

5   (P) Ser364   amino term. kinase (P) Ser381   (P) Thr574
    (P) Ser222   carboxyl term. kinase

    fully active

251

Table 14-1 **Table 14-1** MAPK Nomenclature

Name	Alternate Names	Human Genome Designation	Human Genome mRNA Accession Number
MAPKS			
ERK-1	p44-MAPK	MAPK3	XM055766
ERK-2	p42-MAPK	MAPK1	NM138957
JNK1	SAPK-γ, SAPK1c	MAPK8	NM002750
JNK2	SAPK-α, SAPK1a	MAPK9	NM002752
JNK3	SAPK-β, SAPK1b	MAPK10	NM138980
p38α	SAPK2a, CSBP1	MAPK14	NM001315
p38β	SAPK2b	MAPK11	NM002751
p38γ	SAPK3	MAPK12	NM002969
p38δ	SAPK4	MAPK13	NM002754
MEKS			
MEK1	MAPKK1, MKK1	MAP2K1	NM002755
MEK2	MAPKK2, MKK2	MAP2K2	NM030622
MKK4	SEK1, JNK kinase (JNKK)-1, MEK4, SAPK-kinase (SKK)-1	MAP2K4	NM003010
MKK7	JNKK2, MEK7, SKK4	MAP2K7	NM145185
MKK3	MEK3, SKK2	MAP2K3	NM145109
MKK6	MEK6, SKK3	MAP2K6	NM002758

Nomenclature for mammalian MAPKs. Included are all accepted nomenclatures commonly used in the primary literature; however, not all of these are included in the text.

comprises one form of the activator protein-1 transcription factor.[93] Activator protein-1 regulation is quite complex; and serum or growth factor induction of c-*fos* is one mechanism for activator protein-1 activation. Elevated levels of c-*fos* polypeptide correlate well with elevations in activator protein-1 *trans* activating activity.[93,94]

The *fos* promoter contains a *cis* acting element, the serum response element that mediates the recruitment of transcription factors which induce *fos* expression. The serum response element binds a heterodimeric transcription factor containing two polypeptides, the serum response factor and the ternary complex factor.

Ternary complex factors comprise a family of Ets domain transcription factors that includes Elk1 and Sap1. The regulation of Elk1 by MAPKs has been characterized extensively. Activation of ERK-1 and ERK-2 (and, indeed, all MAPKs) coincides with the translocation of a portion of the ERK1/2 pool to the nucleus (Fig 14-8; see Fig. 14-6A), thereby enabling phosphorylation of nuclear substrates.[5,93,94] ERK-1 and ERK-2, as well as JNKs can phosphorylate two critical residues in the Elk1 C terminus (Ser383, Ser389). This enhances the binding of Elk1 to the serum response factor and thereby elevates *trans* activation at the serum response element. In a similar vein, p38s can phosphorylate Sap1a. By this process, MAPKs contribute to c-*fos* induction (see Fig. 14-8).[82,93]

CROSS-TALK BETWEEN THE ERK AND OTHER SIGNALING PATHWAYS THAT REGULATE TRANSCRIPTION

Several important nuclear hormone receptors and transcription factors activated dominantly by signaling pathways outside the insulin/mitogen pathways discussed herein are also substrates of the ERK pathway (see Fig. 14-6A). Phosphorylation by the ERKs influences the activity of these transcription factors and allows for insulin/mitogen modulation of nuclear hormone receptor signaling.

Peroxisome proliferator-activated receptor-γ

Peroxisome proliferator-activated receptor-γ (PPAR-γ) is a member of the nuclear hormone receptor family that includes the steroid hormone receptors (see Chapter 15). PPAR-γ is expressed primarily in adipose tissue and binds several compounds including synthetic antidiabetic thiazolidinediones and 15-deoxy-$\Delta^{12,14}$prostaglandin J_2. Binding of these compounds activates the *trans* activating function of PPAR-γ, resulting in a powerful adipogenic response. PPAR-γ-mediated adipogenesis can be inhibited on contemporaneous administration of serum or growth factors such as platelet-derived growth factor. Insulin has a more complicated role in the development of adipose cells, serving as either a growth or differentiation factor depending on the specific cell type. Preadipocytes express few of insulin receptors, but generally undergo adipogenesis in response to insulin or insulin-like growth factor 1 and growth, in response to mitogens such as platelet-derived growth factor. By contrast, mature, differentiated adipocytes express large numbers of insulin receptors and undergo lipogenesis in response to insulin (as a result of the ability of insulin to activate lipogenic enzymes and stimulate GLUT4-mediated glucose transport).

Rat fibroblasts programmed to express large numbers of insulin receptors (Rat-IR-fibroblasts) respond to insulin with cell growth; however, expression of PPAR-γ in NIH3T3 fibroblasts (NIH-PPAR-γ cells) will result in insulin stimulation of adipogenesis. Mitogen treatment of NIH-PPAR-γ cells stimulates the phosphorylation of Ser112 of PPAR-γ, resulting in inhibition of PPAR-γ *trans* activating activity and adipogenesis. ERKs-1/2 can phosphorylate Ser112 of PPAR-γ; and inhibition of ERK activity blocks mitogenic inhibition of PPAR-γ-induced adipogenesis.[95]

Estrogen Receptor

The estrogen receptor is a member of the nuclear hormone receptor superfamily (see Chapter 15). Maximal activation of the estrogen receptor requires not only the binding of estrogen, but the phosphorylation of Ser118 in the amino-terminal AF-1 domain (see Chapter 15). This phosphorylation is catalyzed by ERK-1 and ERK-2 and is stimulated in vivo by EGF, insulin-like growth factor 1, and transforming alleles of *ras* (see Fig. 14-6A).[96] From a clinical standpoint, this finding is particularly important inasmuch as the physiologic responses to estrogen and other steroid hormones often require the collaboration of polypeptide growth factors; the regulation of the estrogen receptor by the ERKs indicates a convergence of steroid hormone and mitogen action. In addition, many breast cancers that require estrogen for viability also manifest genetic amplification of the *ras* proto-oncogene.

STATs

The signal transduction and activators of transcription (STAT) are a family of SH2 domain-containing transcription factors that are activated by a wide variety of mitogens and cytokines including EGF, platelet-derived growth factor, interleukin-6, interferon-γ growth hormone, and the antilipogenic hormone leptin. Many of these agonists (interleukin-6, growth hormone, and leptin, in particular) act through a common signaling receptor subunit, gp130, which couples to specific agonist-binding receptor subunits. Recruitment of the STAT requires agonist activation of the Janus kinase family of Tyr kinases. Janus kinases phosphorylate the STAT at Tyr residues. Tyr phosphorylation of STAT results in dimerization, mediated by the binding of P-Tyr on one STAT to the SH2 domain on its partner. STAT dimerization is followed by nuclear translocation and *trans* activation of STAT-responsive genes, which contain a consensus interferon-γ activation site (GAS, consensus ATTTCCCCGAAAT). However, in addition to Tyr phosphorylation, STAT also require ERK-catalyzed Ser phosphorylation for maximal *trans* activating function (see Fig. 14-6A).[97]

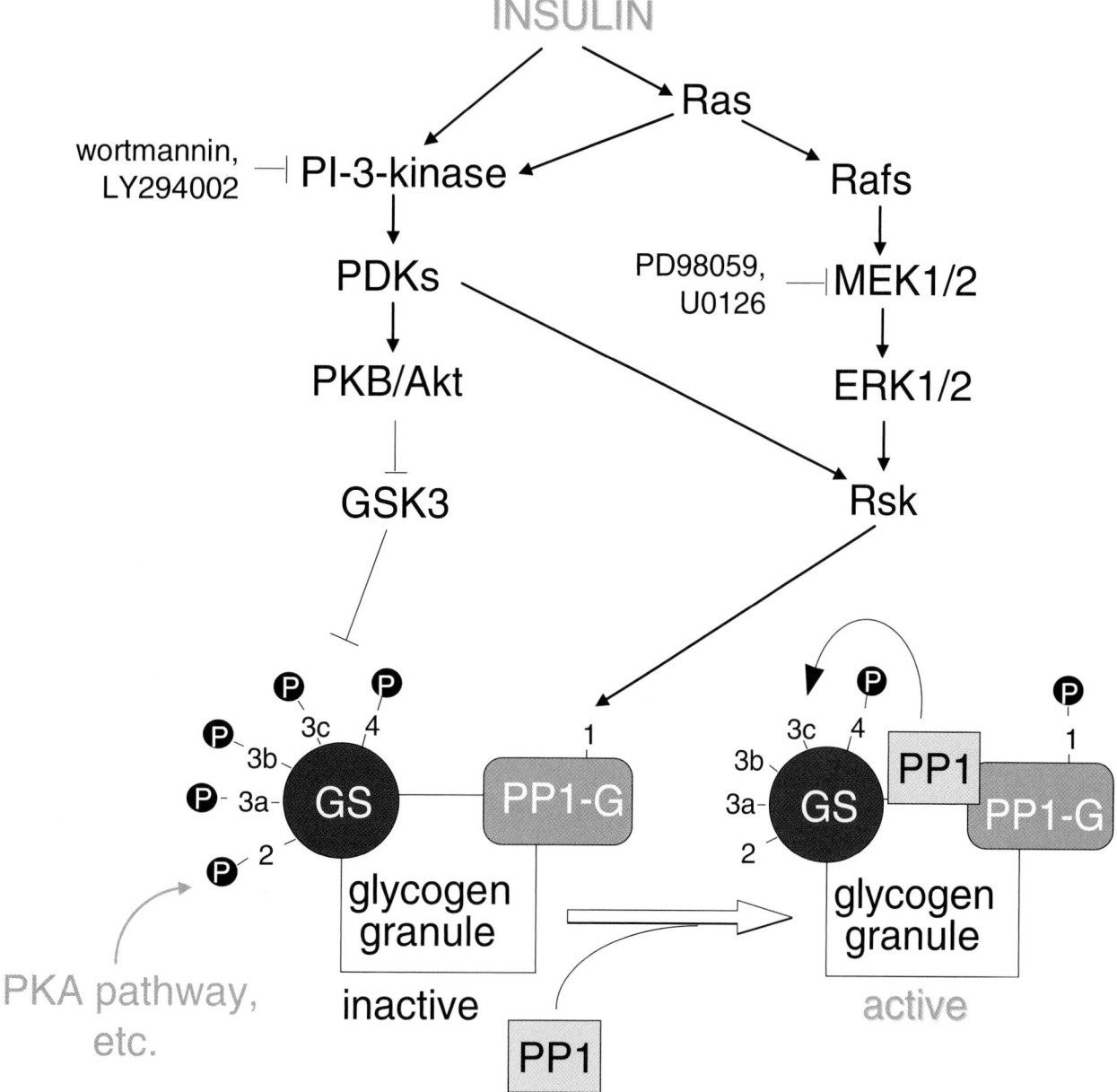

Figure 14-7 Insulin regulation of dephosphorylation and activation of skeletal muscle GS by the PKB/Akt > GSK3 and MAPK > Rsk mechanisms. PKB/Akt inhibits GSK3, thereby preventing its inhibitory phosphorylation of GS sites 3a–c and 4. Rsk phosphorylates the PP1 glycogen targeting subunit (PP1-G) accelerating the rate at which it dephosphorylates sites 2 and 3a–c. Targets of inhibition by wortmannin, LY294002, PD98059, and U0126 are indicated.

REGULATION OF ERK-1 AND ERK-2 BY MAPK/ERK KINASES 1 AND 2

Partial purification of ERK-2 from ^{32}P-labeled, insulin-stimulated cells revealed that upon insulin stimulation, ERK-1 underwent concomitant Tyr and Thr phosphorylation. It was subsequently demonstrated that ERK-2 could be inactivated with Tyr-specific protein phosphatases, which selectively dephosphorylate the P-Tyr, and with Ser/Thr-specific phosphatases, which selectively dephosphorylate the P-Thr. These results indicated that ERK-2 required concomitant Tyr and Thr phosphorylation for activity. The sites of phosphorylation were mapped to Thr183 and Tyr185, sites located in the activation loop of subdomain VIII of the catalytic domain (Fig. 14-9).[4,5,81]

The existence of a MAPK "activator" was first demonstrated by fractionating cytosolic extracts of EGF-treated cells on ion exchange columns and assaying the fractions for an activity that could activate ERK-1 and/or ERK-2 in vitro. It was observed that a single broad peak of activity could catalyze the concomitant Tyr and Thr phosphorylation and activation of ERK-1 and ERK-2. Purification and molecular cloning of this activity revealed a family of novel dual specificity (Thr/Tyr) protein kinases termed variously *MAPK-kinases-1 and -2* (MAPKKs-1 and -2 or MEKs-1 and -2).[4,5,81]

As with ERK-1 and ERK-2, MEK-1 and MEK-2 share a remarkable homology with kinases from lower eukaryotes. Thus, Fus3p and Kss1p, MAPKs of the *S. cerevisiae* mating pheromone response pathway, are regulated in vivo by a MEK homologue, Ste7p. Likewise, Hog1p, a MAPK of the *S. cerevisiae* osmosensing pathway, is activated by the MEK Pbs2p (see Fig. 14-5B).[4,5,79,81]

MEK-1 can be inhibited by two highly specific pharmacologic agents: PD98059 and U0126. PD98059 prevents MEK-1 phosphorylation by Rafs. U0126 does not prevent phosphorylation of MEK-1 by upstream activators, but instead

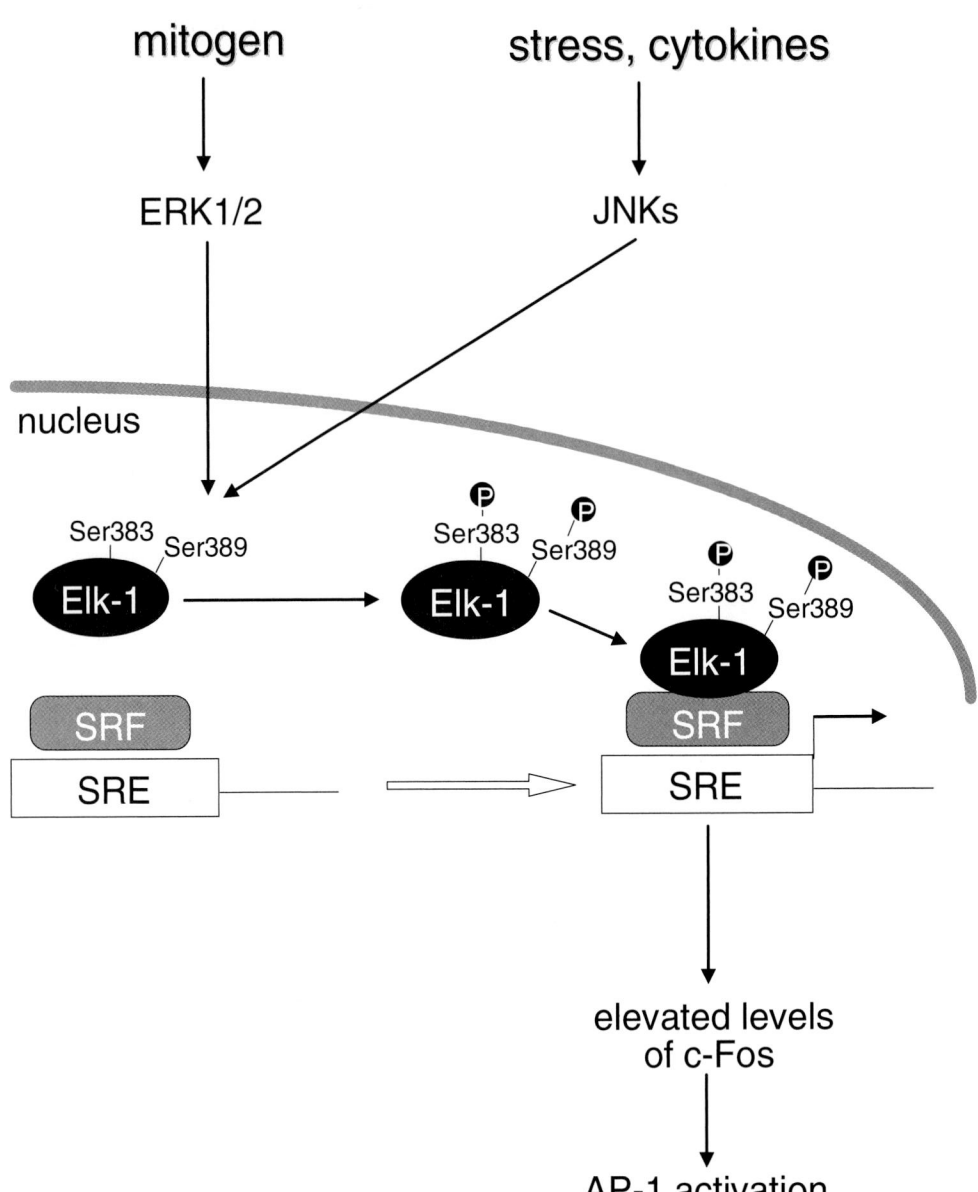

Figure 14-8 Coordinate regulation of Elk1 and the SRE by MAPKs (ERKs and JNKs). MAPKs phosphorylate Elk1 at Ser383 and Ser389. This fosters enhanced binding to SRF which, in turn, promotes trans activation of the SRE. The resulting elevations in c-*fos* expression contribute to AP-1 activation.

restrains MEK-1 in an inactive conformation, preventing its signaling to downstream elements. Both of these compounds have been used extensively to identify pathways in which the ERKs play a dominant role.[98]

MEK-1 AND MEK-2

Any notions of a swift completion of the characterization of the ERK pathway were dashed when it was shown that MEK-1 and MEK-2 were inactivated not by Tyr phosphatases but by Ser/Thr phosphatases. Thus, at least one Ser/Thr kinase lay between MEK-1 and MEK-2 and receptor Tyr kinases (see Fig. 14-9).[4,5,81]

Raf-1 is the normal cellular homologue of v-*raf*, an acutely transforming oncogene that encodes a Ser/Thr protein kinase (Fig. 14-10A). Raf-1 is one of a small family of related Ser/Thr kinases, A-Raf, B-Raf, and Raf-1, all of which share similar structural properties.[4,5,81] Several observations pointed to the possibility that the Rafs were upstream of ERK-1 and ERK-2. First, some v-*raf*-transformed cells manifest constitutively active ERK-1 and ERK-2. Second, expression of dominant inhibitory constructs of Raf-1 could block induction of activator protein-1 in response to mitogens. As was noted previously, activator protein-1 can be regulated in part by the ERK pathway via Elk1/serum response factor induction of c-*fos*.[4,5,81,93] However, there remained the possibility that Raf-1 was not upstream of the ERKs, a hypothesis based on the observation that not all *raf*-transformed cells displayed constitutive MAPK activation. Moreover, yeast studies had identified protein kinases homologous to *STE11* as MEK activators (see Fig. 14-5B).[4,5,79,81] Although mammalian kinases homologous to *STE11* have been identified (e.g., MEK-kinase-1, MEKK1) the sequence of Raf-1 has no significant homology to *STE11* outside the regions shared by all protein kinases.[4,5,79,81]

The placement of Raf-1 as a direct upstream activator of MEK-1 and MEK-2 was established with the observation that upon phosphatase inactivation, purified MEK could be phosphorylated and reactivated by purified, oncogenic Raf-1.[4,5,81,99] It was subsequently shown that endogenous Raf-1 activity toward MEK-1 was stably activated by insulin and mitogens. Detailed analysis of Raf-1 phosphorylation of MEK-1 indicated that MEK-1 was phosphorylated at Ser 218 and 222. Again,

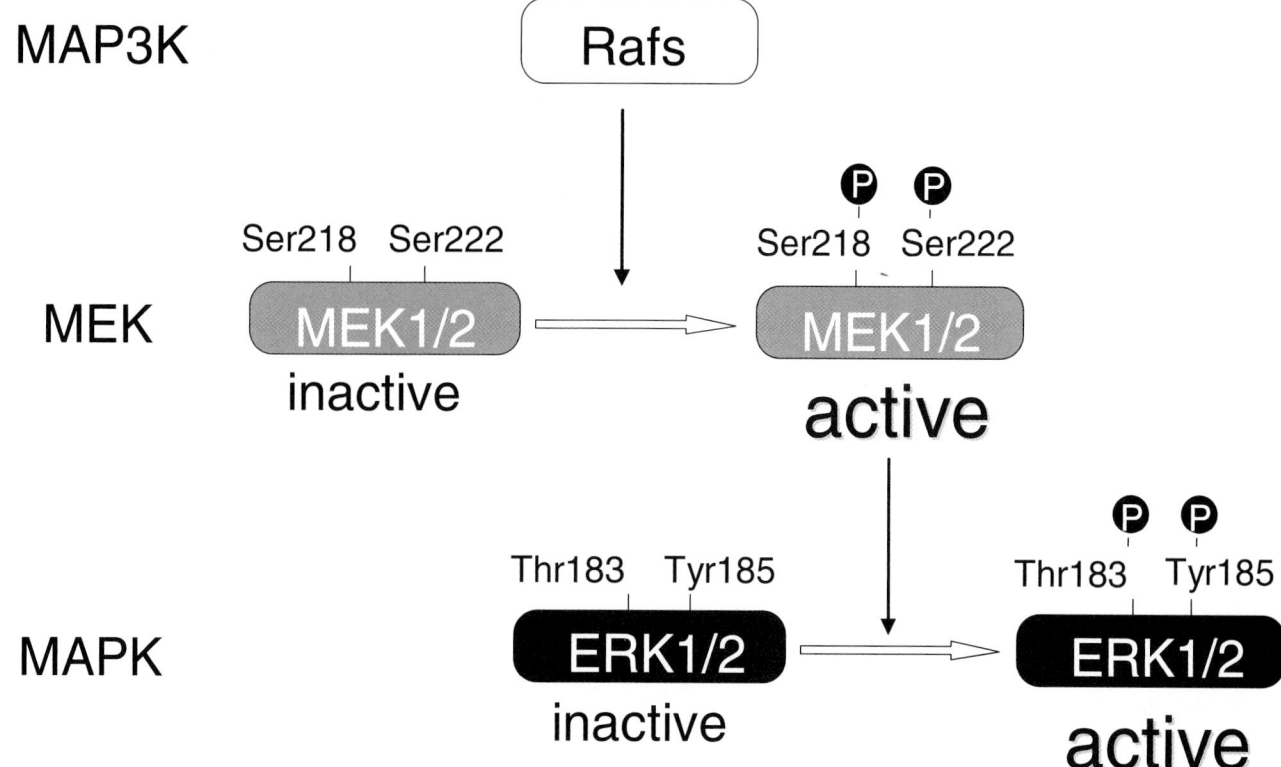

Figure 14-9   The Raf ➤ ERK three-tiered MAPK core signaling module. The black circle with a white P indicates phosphorylation.

these residues lie within the activation loop of subdomain VIII of the catalytic domain (see Fig. 14-9).[4,5,81,99]

It has since been shown that all three Raf polypeptides can phosphorylate and activate MEK-1 and MEK-2 in vitro and in transfected cells. However, recent genetic knockout studies have identified specific functions for the endogenous forms of the different Raf family kinases. These studies reveal that while of the three Raf family members Raf-1 regulation and function have been most extensively characterized, disruption of *B-raf* has the most profound effect on mitogen activation of the ERK pathway. Consistent with this, a large percentage of human melanomas, as well as some colon tumors bear activating mutations in *B-raf*.[100–104]

Ras

Activating mutations in the *ras* proto-oncogenes, especially *Ki-ras*, are present in at least 30% of human cancers. Accordingly, the role of Ras proteins in mitogenic signaling has attracted widespread interest. Three *ras* genes are present in the human genome: *Ha-ras*, *Ki-ras*, and *N-ras*. These comprise a subfamily, the Ras subfamily, of a large superfamily of small monomeric GTPases referred to as the Ras superfamily (Fig. 14-11A).[4,5,80,81,105–107]

Ras superfamily proteins are molecular switches that relay signals from receptor complexes to downstream effectors. All Ras proteins bind the guanine nucleotides GTP and GDP and possess a slow, intrinsic GTPase activity. Ras proteins are competent to signal downstream when they are GTP bound. GDP-bound Ras proteins are inactive (see Fig. 14-11B).[4,5,80,81,105–107]

The members of the Ras superfamily also share a common structural configuration (see Fig. 14-11A). At the N terminus is a GTP-binding domain, followed by the effector loop, a domain that binds downstream effector proteins. There are also two switch domains (switches I and II), which undergo conformational changes upon exchanging GDP for GTP.

The switch I domain overlaps considerably with the effector loop, while the switch II domain contains residues important to Ras GTPase activity (see Fig. 14-11A). Crystallographic studies indicate that GTP binding causes conformational changes that render switch I accessible to effector proteins. At the extreme C terminus of mature Ras family proteins is the CAAX domain, a region of posttranslational modification: prenylation (farnesylation in the case of the Ras subfamily, and geranylgeranylation in the case of the Rho subfamily) and, in the case of Ha-Ras, palmitoylation. These lipid modifications localize Ras proteins to the inner leaflet of the plasma membrane and are essential for Ras protein function, one of the major roles of Ras superfamily proteins is to recruit effector proteins to the plasma membrane.[4,5,80,81,105–107]

Activation of Ras superfamily proteins is catalyzed by GEFs (see Chapter 8). These proteins act to accelerate the dissociation of GDP (see Fig. 14-11B). Inasmuch as GTP is in excess in the cytosol, GDP dissociation is quickly followed by GTP binding and activation of the Ras protein signaling capacity.[4,6,56,71] Inactivation of Ras superfamily proteins is catalyzed by GTPase-activating proteins (GAPs). These act to accelerate the rate of Ras protein GTPase activity. By extension, then, GTPase-deficient mutants of Ras proteins, such as Val12-Ras, are constitutively active and oncogenic. Conversely, Ras superfamily proteins, such as Asn17-Ras, that cannot exchange GDP for GTP if overexpressed, can titer out or sequester GEFs and prevent activation of endogenous, wild-type Ras proteins.[4,5,56,71]

That Ki- or Ha-Ras were involved in insulin and mitogen signaling, and, in particular, activation of the ERKs, became clear as a consequence of several independent lines of investigation. First, either ectopic expression or scrape loading of cells with Val12-Ha-Ras resulted in activation of the ERKs. Furthermore, addition of active, GTP-loaded Val12-Ha-Ras to cell extracts could trigger ERK activation. In addition, several genetic models of tyrosine kinase signaling, in particular the

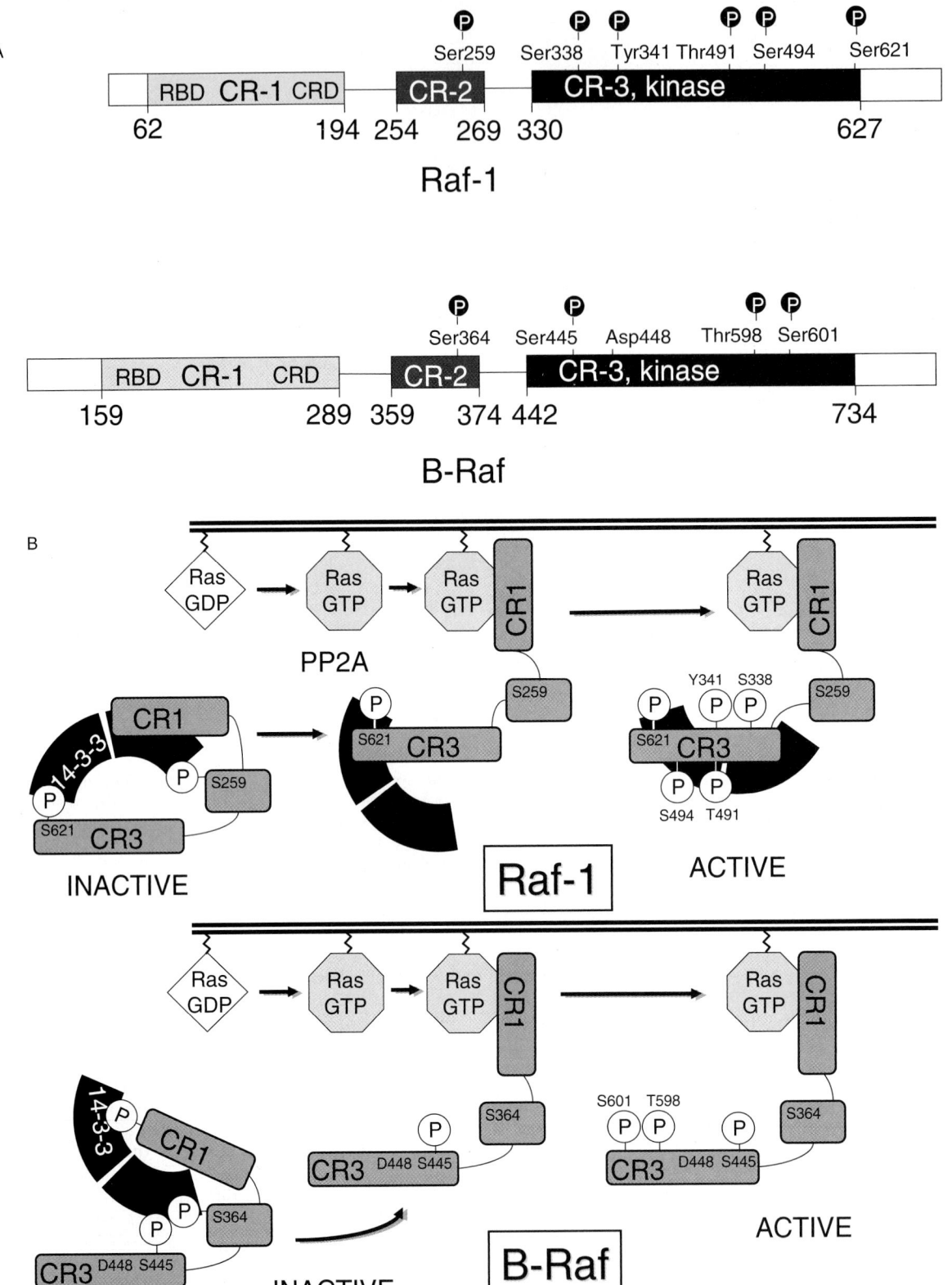

Figure 14-10   Structure and regulation of Raf-1. **(A)** Structures of Raf-1 and B-Raf. Phosphorylated residues are indicated with the black circle with a white P. CR, conserved region; RBD, canonical Ras-binding domain—this region binds the Ras effector loop; CRD, zinc-finger domain that contributes to binding the Ras C terminus. **(B)** Hypothetical models of Raf-1 and B-Raf regulation based on current evidence. For both Rafs, activation commences upon binding (through the Raf CR1) to GTP-Ras. In resting cells, Raf-1 is held in an inactive conformation by a dimer of 14-3-3ζ, which interacts with phosphorylated Ser621 and Ser259. Binding of Ras triggers phosphatase-2A-catalyzed dephosphorylation of Ser259 and consequent displacement of the 14-3-3ζ dimer from Ser259. This may expose additional phosphorylation sites. These sites are phosphorylated by PAK (Ser338), Src (Tyr341), and an unknown kinase (Thr491, Ser494). Ras may also fosters Raf-1 oligomerization which is, in addition to phosphorylation, important to Raf regulation. The phosphorylation of Raf reorients the binding of the 14-3-3ζ such that it now interacts with one of the newly phosphorylated sites. This results in a stable, active conformation. B-Raf activation is somewhat simpler inasmuch as S445 (analogous to Raf-1 Ser338) is constitutively phosphorylated and the negative charge on Asp448 (analogous to Raf-1 Tyr341) mimicks phosphorylation. For B-Raf, displacement/reorientation of 14-3-3 is also a consequence of Ras-dependent phosphorylation (of Ser364, which is analogous to Raf-1 Ser259). Activation of B-Raf also absolutely requires phosphorylation, by an as yet unknown kinase of Thr598 and Ser601 (analogous to Raf-1, Thr491, and Ser494).

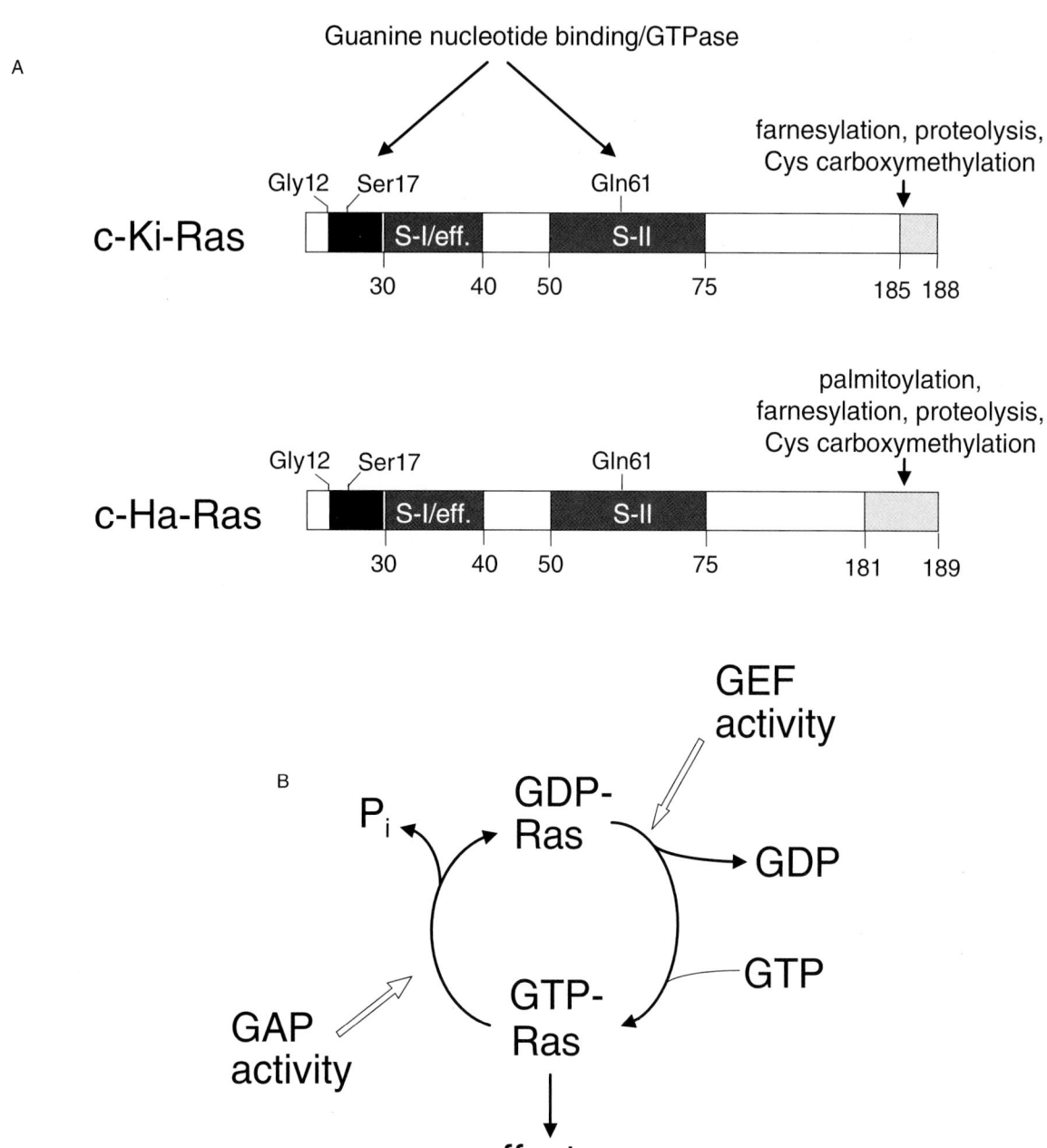

Figure 14-11 Regulation of signaling by Ras superfamily GTPases. **(A)** Schematic structures of Ki- and Ha-Ras. Residues essential to guanine nucleotide binding and GTPase activity (Gly12, Ser17, and Gln61) are indicated. S1, switch-1 domain; S2, switch-2 domain; P, prenylation/palmytoylation domain. Amino acid numbers are indicated. **(B)** The cycle of activation/inactivation of Ras superfamily proteins. Ras is shown here as the canonical example. Regulation of other Ras superfamily GTPases (i.e., Rheb and the Rho subfamily) proceeds in a similar manner.

sevenless Tyr kinase pathway of *Drosophila* photoreceptor development and the vulval induction pathway in the nematode worm *Caenorhabditis elegans*, implicated Ras as a downstream effector of receptor Tyr kinases. Finally, ectopic overexpression of dominant inhibitory Asn17-Ha-Ras could effectively block activation of the ERKs by mitogens and insulin, suggesting that Ras was downstream of mitogen receptors in mammalian cells.[4,5,80,81,105] Curiously, however, gene disruption studies indicate that, at least in mice, Ha-Ras has does not play a prominent role in mitogen activation of ERK. By contrast, disruption of *ki-ras* is embryonic, lethal, and severely impairs mitogen activation of ERK—a finding consistent with the prevalence of *ki-ras* mutations in cancer.[108]

GTP-Ras activates the ERK pathway by directly binding and promoting the activation of Raf family kinases (see Fig. 14-10*B*). The identification of Rafs as direct effectors for GTP-loaded Ras came from biochemical and genetic studies, which showed that the two polypeptides could interact in vivo and in vitro.[4,5,109] Raf polypeptides consist of three conserved domains: a carboxyl-terminal kinase domain (conserved region 3, CR-3), CR-2, a Ser/Thr-rich hinge domain, and CR-1, an amino-terminal regulatory domain that contains a canonical Ras-binding domain and, a zinc-finger motif (see Fig. 14-10*A*). The interaction of Ras and Raf-1 is mediated by two interactions: a high-affinity GTP-dependent interaction between the Raf CR-1 Ras-binding domain and the Ras effector loop, and a low-affinity GTP-independent interaction between the Ras CAAX motif and the zinc-finger region of Raf CR-1 (see Fig. 14-10B).[5,110]

The binding of Rafs to Ras is insufficient for Raf activation; the exact mechanism of Raf activation has not been elucidated completely. However, it is apparent that Ras, by recruiting Rafs to the plasma membrane, fosters Raf phosphorylation and oligomerization, both of which appear necessary for Raf activation.[4,5,110–112] The regulation of Raf-1 has been the most extensively characterized. Current evidence suggests that Raf-1 is maintained in an inactive state by interactions with a dimeric form of the protein 14-3-3ζ.[45,110,113] Inactive Raf-1 is phosphorylated at Ser259 and Ser621. P-Ser259 and P-Ser621 bind a homodimer of 14-3-3ζ.

Ser259 is phosphorylated by PKB/Akt, and dephosphorylation, catalyzed by protein phosphatase-2A, requires binding to GTP-Ras. This dephosphorylation triggers the displacement of the 14-3-3ζ dimer from P-Ser259, leaving the 14-3-3ζ bound only to P-Ser621. The free end of the 14-3-3 dimer, which had dissociated from Ser259, then binds to an as yet unidentified phosphacceptor site, contributing to a stable, active Raf-1 conformation (see Fig. 14-10B).[5,110,113]

Activation of Raf-1 also requires phosphorylation at Tyr341 and Ser338. The former is probably catalyzed by the Src nonreceptor Tyr kinase. Ser338 phosphorylation is likely catalyzed by Ser/Thr kinases of the p21-activated kinase family, a group of kinases regulated by Rac and Cdc42, members of the Rho group of the Ras superfamily.[5,81,110]

In addition, Raf-1 is phosphorylated, in a Ras-dependent manner, at two sites (Thr491 and Ser494) in the activation loop (subdomain VIII) of the kinase domain (CR-3).[110,114] Phosphorylation of these sites is required for activity. The kinase required for this phosphorylation is unknown. Finally, activation of Raf-1 requires signal-dependent oligomerization. Whether or not this oligomerization is directly Ras dependent is still controversial.[111,112]

What is known about B-Raf regulation indicates that it resembles Raf-1 activation superficially, but is in many ways simpler (see Fig. 14-10B).[110] Inactive B-Raf is also bound to 14-3-3, and is phosphorylated at Ser364, a residue analogous to Raf-1 Ser259. The binding of B-Raf to GTP-Ras is accompanied by dephosphorylation of Ser364 and, apparently, the relief of 14-3-3-mediated inhibition, although how this occurs is still nebulous.[110] B-Raf Ser445 is analogous to Raf-1 Ser338; however, this residue is constitutively phosphorylated and is apparently not a p21-activated kinase target. B-Raf Asp448 is analogous to Tyr341 of Raf-1. The negative charge of Asp448 mimics the charge of phosphorylation, obviating the need for phosphorylation at this site.[110,115] Because of the constitutive phosphorylation of Ser364, and the preexisting negative charge of Asp448, B-Raf has considerably higher basal activity than Raf-1. Critical to B-Raf activation, however, is phosphorylation at Thr598 and Ser601, sites analogous to Thr491 and Ser494 of Raf-1.[114,116] As was mentioned above, mutations in B-Raf are common in melanomas and in colon cancers. Mutation of B-Raf Val599 to Glu is the most common mutation observed for B-Raf. By mimicking the phosphorylation at positions 598 and 601, this mutation elevates substantially the activity of B-Raf.[104]

COLLABORATIVE ACTIVATION OF PI 3-KINASE BY p85 AND Ras

As was mentioned previously, the activity of PI 3-kinase can be increased in vitro and in vivo upon binding of the p85 subunit SH2 domains to P-Tyr residues on receptor Tyr kinases, nonreceptor Tyr kinases, or IRS proteins. While this activation is significant, further activation of PI 3-kinase incurred upon binding GTP-Ras.[117] The impact of this mechanism of activation is most apparent in ras-transformed cells. Thus, coexpression of V12-Ras and PI 3-kinase results in substantial PI 3-kinase activation in the absence of mitogen. Ras binds in a

GTP-dependent and p85 subunit-independent manner to the p110 catalytic subunit of PI 3-kinase. Lysine 227 of the α isoform of p110 appears to be critical for the Ras-PI 3-kinase interaction, and mutation of this residue results in a construct that can no longer be activated by Ras. This construct can still be activated by the P-Tyr-p85 interaction, however.[117,118] Therefore, Ras is a crucial regulator not only of the MAPK pathway, but of signaling to PI 3-kinase.

JNK, P38, AND NUCLEAR FACTOR-κB PATHWAYS

GENERAL CONSIDERATIONS

The cellular and physiologic responses to inflammation are central to the pathology of a number of important conditions including atherosclerosis, endotoxin shock, arthritis, inflammatory bowel disease, and diabetes. It has become clear that parallel mammalian MAPK pathways exist and that these, in conjunction with the nuclear factor-κB (NF-κB) pathway, are pivotal to the inflammatory response. From the point of view of the endocrinologist, an understanding of these mechanisms is critical inasmuch as many inflammatory conditions are treated with steroids or steroid analogues, the efficacy of which is often dubious.

Several components of stress-activated MAPK pathways can interact antagonistically with the targets of steroidal anti-inflammatory pharmaceuticals; the mutual antagonism of these steroids and stress signaling pathways probably forms the basis of steroidal anti-inflammatory action. As mammalian stress-activated signaling pathways are elucidated, it is becoming clear that these pathways will be important novel targets for anti-inflammatory therapies. Finally, recent genetic evidence indicates that stress-activated MAPK pathways may be involved in the pathophysiology of type 2 diabetes.

MAMMALIAN STRESS-ACTIVATED MAPKs

The existence of multiple MAPK pathways in yeast (see Fig. 14-5B) was an indication that mammalian cells possessed analogous signaling mechanisms. Indeed, indications that mammalian cells had several MAPK pathways came shortly after the identification of the ERKs.[79,81,82] The protein synthesis inhibitor cycloheximide, when administrated to rats, can elicit the in vivo activation of ribosomal S6 phosphorylation; in fact, this strategy was used to activate p70 S6 kinase in vivo prior to purification.[4,36] That cycloheximide could recruit p70 led to the notion that several protein kinase signaling pathways might be activated by cycloheximide. This hypothesis was proved correct when it was demonstrated that injection of cycloheximide into rats activated a Ser/Thr kinase activity that could be inactivated with Tyr or Ser/Thr phosphatases, indicating that, like the ERKs, this kinase required concomitant Tyr and Ser/Thr phosphorylation for activity. This novel MAPK was initially referred to as p54 because the purified kinase was observed to migrate at 54 kilodaltons on SDS polyacrylamide gels.[4,5,81,82,119,120] The substrate specificity of this kinase differed from that of the ERKs. In particular, p54 was unable to activate Rsk in vitro under conditions wherein ERK-mediated activation of Rsk (see Fig. 14-6B) was observed. More importantly, p54 was able to phosphorylate the c-Jun transcription factor at two sites (Ser 63 and Ser73) implicated in regulation of c-Jun and activator protein-1 trans activation function (see Fig. 14-13B).[4,81,82,119–121] Immunoprecipitation of endogenous p54 from extracts of cells subjected to various treatments revealed that in most cells, p54 was, in many but not all instances, not strongly activated by insulin or polypeptide mitogens. By contrast, p54 was vigorously activated by environmental stresses, such as heat shock, ionizing radiation, oxidant stress, DNA damaging chemicals such as topoisomerase inhibitors and alkylating agents, reperfusion injury, mechanical shear stress, and, of course, protein synthesis inhibitors. In addition, p54 could be activated by vasoactive peptides (endothelin and angiotensin II) and inflammatory cytokines of the TNF family (TNF, interleukin-1, CD40 ligand, CD27 ligand, Fas ligand, etc.).[81-83,122,123] p54 has since been renamed and the nomenclature of this family of kinases is somewhat confusing (see Table 14-1). Two systems are generally accepted: c-Jun-NH$_2$-terminal kinase (JNK) in reference to the phosphorylation by these kinases of the c-Jun amino-terminal *trans* activation domain (see Fig. 14-13B); and stress-activated protein kinase (SAPK) in reference to the regulation of these kinases by environmental stress and inflammation. Molecular cloning of JNK revealed a family of at least three genes (see Table 14-1): JNK1, JNK2, and JNK3. Like the ERKs, each of these contains a characteristic phosphoacceptor loop in subdomain VIII of the protein kinase catalytic domain. The ERK sequence is Thr183-Glu-Tyr185, while that of the JNKs is Thr183-Pro-Tyr185. The JNK genes are further diversified into up to 12 polypeptides by differential hnRNA splicing.[81,82,122,123]

The p38 MAPKs represent a third mammalian MAPK family. p38 was originally described as a 38-kilodalton polypeptide that underwent Tyr phosphorylation in response to endotoxin treatment and osmotic shock. p38 was purified by anti-phosphotyrosine immunoaffinity chromatography, and cDNA cloning revealed that p38 was the mammalian MAPK homologue most closely related to *HOG1*, the osmosensing MAPK of *S. cerevisiae* (see Fig. 14-5B). Most notably, the p38s like Hog1p contain the phosphoacceptor sequence Thr-Gly-Tyr.[79,124] Of particular interest, p38 was also independently purified as a polypeptide that could bind to a class of experimental pyridinyl-imidazole anti-inflammatory drugs, the cytokine suppressive anti-inflammatory drugs (CSAIDs).

The CSAIDs are best exemplified by two compounds, SB203580 and SB202190, both of which are quite specific and are widely used to study p38 function, but neither of which is currently in clinical development (although novel derivatives of the CSAIDs are in clinical trials as anti-inflammatories). The CSAIDs were originally characterized as compounds that could inhibit the transcriptional induction of TNF and interleukin-1 during endotoxin shock. As we shall see, the basis for these compounds efficacy as anti-inflammatory agents was their ability to bind and directly inhibit a subset of the p38s, thereby blocking p38-mediated activation of activator protein-1, a *trans* acting factor crucial to TNF and interleukin-1 induction.[98,125] Like the JNKs, the p38s are a family of kinases. Four p38 genes have been described thus far (see Table 14-1): p38α (also called CSAIDs binding protein and, somewhat confusingly, SAPK2a), p38β (also called SAPK2b and ERK6), p38γ (also called SAPK3), and p38δ (also called SAPK4). Interestingly, only p38α and p38β are inhibited by SB203580 and SB202190. p38γ and p38δ are completely unaffected by these drugs in vitro or in transfected cells.[82,124-127] In further similarity with the JNKs, the p38s are preferentially activated in vivo by environmental stresses and inflammatory cytokines and are relatively poorly activated by insulin and growth factors. In almost all instances, the same stimuli that recruit the JNKs also recruit the p38s. One exception is ischemia-reperfusion. JNKs are selectively activated during reperfusion whereas the p38s are activated during ischemia and remain active during reperfusion. The basis for this difference is unknown.[82,124-127]

JNK AND p38 SUBSTRATES

As with the ERKs, the JNKs and p38s phosphorylate both transcription factors and other protein kinases (Fig. 14-12). These reactions are important to the inflammatory response. Mitogen-activated protein kinase-activated protein kinases: MAPKAP kinase-2 (MAPKAP-K2) and the structurally related MAPKAP-K3 (also called three pathway regulated kinase or 3PK) are a small family of Ser/Thr kinases that consist of an amino-terminal regulatory domain and a carboxyl-terminal kinase domain. Along with p38-regulated and activated kinase (PRAK, see next section), MAPKAP-K2 and MAPKAP-K3 phosphorylate the small heat shock protein Hsp27[128-134]; however, gene disruption studies indicate that MAPKAP-K2 is a major, although not sole, Hsp27 kinase activated during sepsis.[135] Non-phosphorylated Hsp27 normally exists in high-molecular-weight aggregates that serve as molecular chaperones. Phosphorylation of Hsp27 by MAPKAP kinase-2 and -3 at Ser15, Ser78, Ser82, and Ser90 coincides with the dissociation of Hsp27 into monomers and dimers, and its redistribution to the actin cytoskeleton.[132] In peroxide-treated human umbilical vein endothelial cells, redistribution of Hsp27 may participate in eliciting the reorganization of F-actin into stress fibers, thereby affecting cell motility.[132,133] MAPKAP-K2 and -K3 catalyzed phosphorylation of Hsp27 at Ser90 appears necessary for this process and mutation of Ser90 to Ala prevents stimulus-induced changes in Hsp27 oligomerization.[133]

Like p38, MAPKAP-K2 is activated by stresses and inflammatory cytokines. MAPKAP-K2 is phosphorylated and activated in vitro and in vivo by p38α and p38β (but not by p38γ or p38δ). Activation of MAPKAP-K2 is a multistep process (see Fig. 14-12A).[82,136] Phosphorylation of Thr25, catalyzed by p38α and p38β, gates subsequent p38 catalyzed phosphorylation of Thr222 and Ser272 in the kinase activation loop. An additional autophosphorylation at Thr334 then results in activation of MAPKAP-K2. Consistent with regulation by p38α and p38β, MAPKAP-K2 activation and Hsp27 phosphorylation are inhibited by CSAIDs.[136]

Disruption of murine *mapkap-k2* indicates an important role for this kinase in the sepsis response. *mapkap-k2* −/− mice are resistant to lipopolysaccharide (LPS) endotoxin toxicity, showing substantially reduced LPS-stimulated production, by macrophages from the knockout mice, of TNF.[135] The production of TNF by LPS-stimulated macrophages is regulated at multiple levels by MAPKs. The *tnf* promoter contains activator protein-1 sites, enabling MAPK-mediated transcriptional induction.[81,82] In addition, the TNF mRNA contains several AU-rich elements. AU-rich elements are present in mRNAs that are highly unstable and subject to signal-induced stabilization. Finally, TNF can also enhance translation of the TNF mRNA. Disruption of *mapkap-k2* has no effect on *tnf* transcription, mRNA stabilization, or on the process of secretion. It is believed, therefore, that p38α and β, through MAPKAP-K2, modulate TNF mRNA translation or some other posttranscriptional process, although the underlying mechanism is still not understood.[135]

MAPKAP-K3 can also phosphorylate Hsp27[130,131]; although the physiologic significance of this is somewhat unclear given that disruption of *mapkap-k2* reduces substantially (but not completely) LPS-stimulated Hsp27 phosphorylation; and PRAK also exhibits Hsp27 phosphorylating activity.[134,135] As with MAPKAP-K2, endogenous MAPKAP-K3 is activated primarily by stresses and inflammatory cytokines; and in a manner that can be completely inhibited with CSAIDs, suggesting that p38α and/or p38β are the major MAPKAP-K3 kinases in vivo.[130,131]

PRAK

PRAK is an approximately 50-kilodalton Ser/Thr kinase with a similar overall structure to MAPKAP-K2, -K3, and the MNKs (see next section).[134] Thus, PRAK consists of an amino-terminal regulatory domain and a carboxyl-terminal kinase domain. As with MAPKAP-K2 and -K3, PRAK is activated selectively in response to stress and inflammatory cytokines and is not detectably activated by mitogens.[134] PRAK is phosphorylated at Thr182 in the kinase domain subdomain VIII activation loop and activated in vivo and in vitro by p38α and p38β. Consistent with this, PRAK activation can be blocked

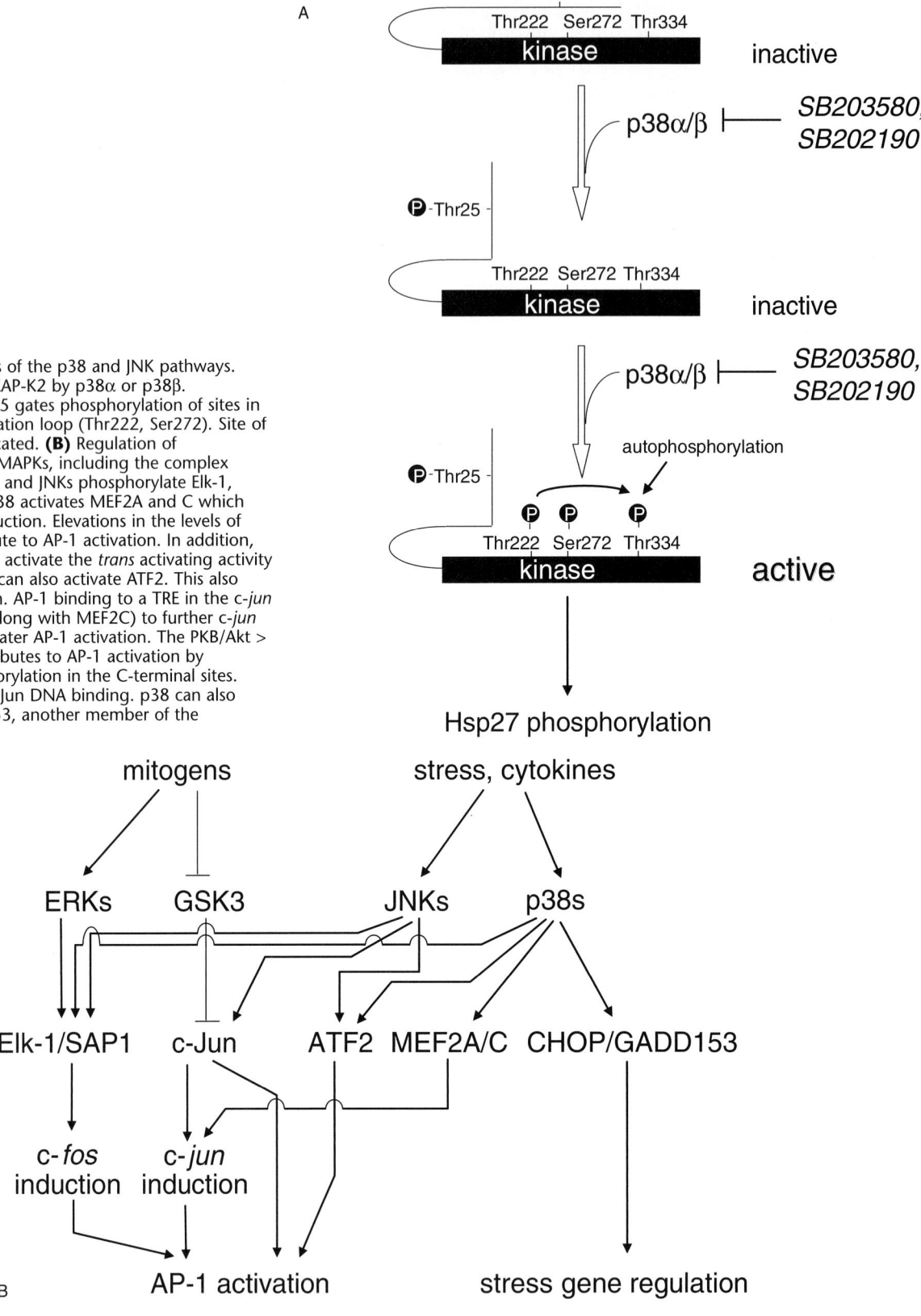

Figure 14-12 Functions of the p38 and JNK pathways. **(A)** Regulation of MAPKAP-K2 by p38α or p38β. Phosphorylation of Thr25 gates phosphorylation of sites in the kinase domain activation loop (Thr222, Ser272). Site of action of CSAIDs is indicated. **(B)** Regulation of transcription factors by MAPKs, including the complex regulation of AP-1. ERKs and JNKs phosphorylate Elk-1, elevating c-Fos levels. p38 activates MEF2A and C which contributes to c-*jun* induction. Elevations in the levels of c-Fos and c-Jun contribute to AP-1 activation. In addition, JNKs phosphorylate and activate the *trans* activating activity of c-Jun and ATF2. p38 can also activate ATF2. This also results in AP-1 activation. AP-1 binding to a TRE in the c-*jun* promoter contributes (along with MEF2C) to further c-*jun* induction, and even greater AP-1 activation. The PKB/Akt > GSK3 mechanism contributes to AP-1 activation by inhibiting c-Jun phosphorylation in the C-terminal sites. This fosters enhanced c-Jun DNA binding. p38 can also activate CHOP/GADD153, another member of the CREB/ATF family

with SB203580.[134] Once activated, PRAK can phosphorylate Hsp27 at the physiologically relevant sites. However, while disruption of *mapkap-k2* reduces substantially LPS-stimulated Hsp27 phosphorylation (indicating that MAPKAP-K2 is a relevant Hsp27 kinase), the fact that both MAPKAP-K3 and PRAK can phosphorylate Hsp27 in vitro and in transfected cells[130,131,134] makes the relative contribution of MAPKAP-K3 and PRAK to agonist-stimulated Hsp27 phosphorylation unclear.[134]

MNKs

The p38s can phosphorylate and activate MNK-1 and -2 in response to stress and cytokines.[92] Thus, the MNKs, as with activator protein-1 are a site of integration of stress and mitogenic signaling. The regulation and function of the MNKs was discussed earlier.

CHOP/GADD153

CREB homologous protein (CHOP)/growth arrest and DNA damage-153 (GADD153) is a CREB/ATF family member that is transcriptionally induced in response to genotoxic and inflammatory stresses (see Chapter 12). These stimuli can also activate the transcriptional regulatory functions of CHOP/GADD153 through agonist-induced phosphorylation of Ser78 and Ser81. CHOP/GADD153 acts as a transcriptional repressor of certain cAMP-regulated genes and a transcriptional activator of stress-induced genes. Recruitment of CHOP/GADD153 correlates with cell-cycle arrest at G1/S. This cell-cycle arrest is an important consequence of DNA damage inasmuch as it allows for DNA repair prior to DNA replication thereby preserving genomic integrity. p38α can phosphorylate CHOP/GADD153 at Ser78 and Ser81 in vivo and in vitro and is a likely regulator of CHOP/GADD153 function (see Fig. 14-12B).[137]

Activator Protein-1 (AP-1)

The JNKs and p38s are the dominant Ser/Thr kinases responsible for the recruitment of the activator protein-1 (AP-1) transcription factor in response to environmental stresses and inflammatory stimuli (see Fig. 14-12B).[4,5,81,82] AP-1 is comprised of bZIP transcription factors—typically c-Jun, JunD, along with members of the c-fos (usually c-Fos), and ATF (usually ATF2) families. ATFs are a subgroup of the CREB family (see Chapter 12).[42,43,93,94] All bZIP transcription factors contain leucine zippers that enable homodimerization and heterodimerization, and AP-1 components are organized into Jun-Jun, Jun-Fos, or Jun-ATF dimmers.[94]

The presence of Jun family members enables AP-1 to bind to cis acting elements containing the tetradecanoyl phorbol myristate acetate response element (consensus sequence: TGAC/GTCA).[42,43,94] AP-1 heterodimers containing ATF transcription factors can also bind to the CRE (Chapter 12). AP-1 is an important trans activator of a number of stress responsive genes including the genes for interleukins-1 and -2 and TNF. In addition, AP-1 participates in the transcriptional induction of cell adhesion proteins important to inflammation including E selectin.[94]

Activation of AP-1 involves both the direct phosphorylation/dephosphorylation of AP-1 components, as well as the phosphorylation and activation of transcription factors that induce elevated expression of c-jun or c-fos. Both events can be activated independently by several pathways.[94] Phosphorylation of c-Jun or ATF2 within their trans activation domains correlates well with enhanced trans activating activity (Fig. 14-13; see Fig. 14-12B).[94] The JNKs can phosphorylate the c-Jun trans activating domain at Ser63 and Ser73. These residues are phosphorylated in vivo under conditions wherein the JNKs are activated and depletion of JNK from cell extracts removes all stress-activated c-Jun kinase. Thus, JNKs appear to be the dominant kinases responsible for c-Jun phosphorylation.[122,123,138] JunD is also phosphorylated by JNKs, albeit less effectively than is c-Jun. This phosphorylation occurs at Ser90 and Ser100, a region of the JunD trans activation domain similar to the phosphoacceptor domain of c-Jun (see Figs. 14-13A and B).[139]

Both the JNKs and p38s can phosphorylate ATF2 at Thr69 and Ser71 in the trans activation domain. Again, these residues are phosphorylated under circumstances when the JNKs and/or p38s are activated (see Figs. 14-12B and 14-13B), and phosphorylation of ATF2 activates its trans activating activity. Whether the JNKs or p38s represent the dominant ATF2 kinases depends on the cell type and stimulus used. During reperfusion of ischemic kidney, for example, the JNKs are the only detectable ATF2 kinases. By contrast, in response to interleukin-1, the p38s are the major ATF2 kinases activated in KB keratinocytes.[126,127,140]

The JNKs and p38s also contribute to AP-1 activation by stimulating the transcription of genes encoding AP-1 components. Thus, the JNKs can phosphorylate Elk-1 at Ser383 and Ser389, the same sites phosphorylated by the ERKs. The p38s phosphorylate the related ternary complex factor Sap1a. As is discussed previously, this phosphorylation results in activation of the serum response factor and induction of c-fos expression (see Fig. 14-8). In addition, the p38s can phosphorylate at Thr293 and Thr300, and activate the trans activating activity of the transcription factors myocyte enhancer factor 2A and 2C (MEF-2A and -2C). A cis element for MEF-2A and -2C resides in the promoter for c-jun; thus, p38 activation can contribute to induction of c-jun expression (see Fig. 14-12B). The c-Jun promoter also contains a consensus activator protein-1 site and can therefore be autoregulated by elements that activate AP-1.[82,93,94,141,142]

REGULATION OF ACTIVATOR PROTEIN-1

How does the complex regulation of activator protein-1 constituent transcription factors translate into the recruitment of

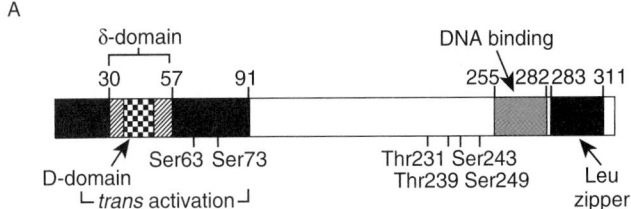

Figure 14-13 Mechanistic characteristics of the regulation of AP-1 by MAPKs. **(A)** Schematic structure of c-Jun. Note that the D domain of c-Jun (AAs 58–78, which lie within the δ domain [AAs 30–57]) is considerably distal from the sites of phosphorylation (Ser63 and Ser73). The C-terminal GSK3 phosphorylation sites near the DNA-binding domain are also indicated. **(B)** Comparison of Jun family phosphoacceptor motifs D and DEF domains of MAPK activators (MKK7) and effectors (see Table 14-2). Phosphorylated residues are underlined, single letter amino acid code is used; gaps are introduced to optimize alignment. Note that JunB contains two potential phosphorylation sites; however, these are not followed by Pro. MAPKs are proline-directed and therefore, JunB cannot undergo JNK-catalyzed phosphorylation. Note also that JunD contains a putative D domain, which although superficially similar to that of c-Jun and JunB, is significantly shorter and does not conform to the consensus. Thus, JunD cannot interact strongly with JNK.

Continued

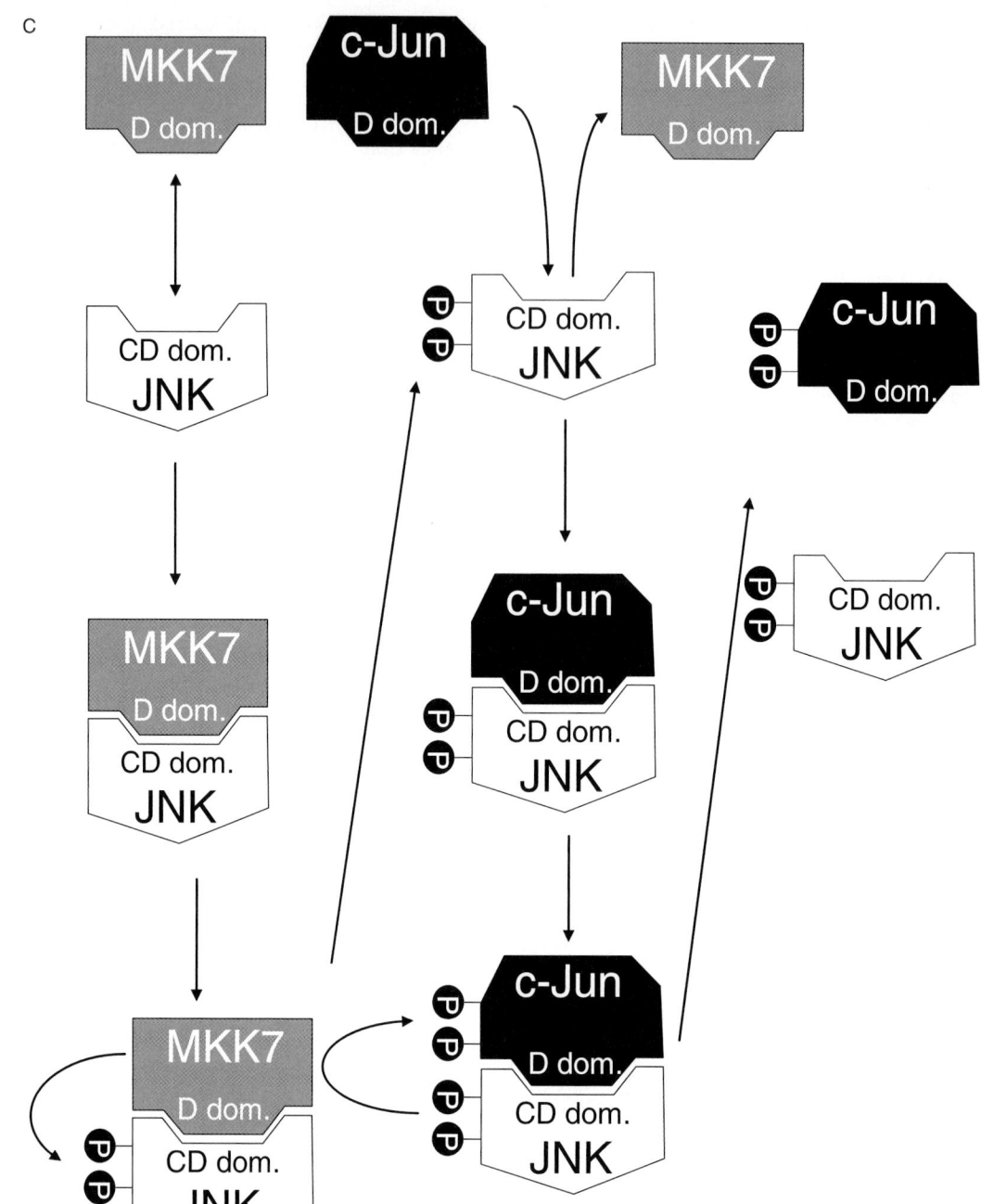

Figure 14-13, cont'd **(C)**
Schematic illustration of how D domain CD domain interactions mediate the specific activation of JNK by MKK7 and the specific phosphorylation of c-Jun by JNK. See also Fig. 14-14B for how these interactions combine with scaffold proteins to provide for exquisite MAPK signaling specificity.

Continued

AP-1 by extracellular stimuli? The facets of AP-1 regulation, activation of constituent transcription factor expression, and direct phosphorylation/ activation of constituent transcription factors can be independently regulated by several pathways.[94] Thus, mitogenic stimuli, which preferentially recruit the ERKs (and inhibit GSK3 via PKB/Akt) will preferentially activate AP-1, respectively, through enhancement of expression of AP-1 components (e.g., via ERK phosphorylation of Elk-1, resulting in c-*fos* expression) and through the relief of GSK3-mediated inhibition of c-Jun DNA binding (see Fig. 14-12B).[4,5,19,81,82,93,94,122,123]

By contrast, stresses and inflammatory cytokines such as TNF, which preferentially activate the JNKs and p38s, can recruit AP-1 through the direct phosphorylation of AP-1 components (c-Jun by JNKs and ATF2 by both JNKs and p38s). However, stress pathways can also promote enhanced expression of AP-1 components through recruitment of Elk-1

(mediated by JNK phosphorylation), which results in elevated c-*fos* expression, and through p38-catalyzed phosphorylation of myocyte enhancer factor-2C (MEF-2C). Both MEF-2C and AP-1 itself can bind and *trans* activate the promoter for c-Jun.[4,5,81,82,93,94,122,123,140–142] Stresses can also modestly recruit PKB/Akt, which can inhibit GSK3 thereby blocking its negative regulation of c-Jun DNA binding (see Fig. 14-13D).[12,19]

Finally, the c-Jun promoter contains an AP-1 site; thus, c-*jun* expression can be autoregulated by any pathway that activates AP-1 (see Fig. 14-12B).[94]

DOCKING DOMAINS

MAPKs and their effectors and activators contain discrete regions that confer specific high-affinity interactions that, in conjunction with scaffold proteins, ensure signaling fidelity and efficiency. Two types of docking domains on MAPK

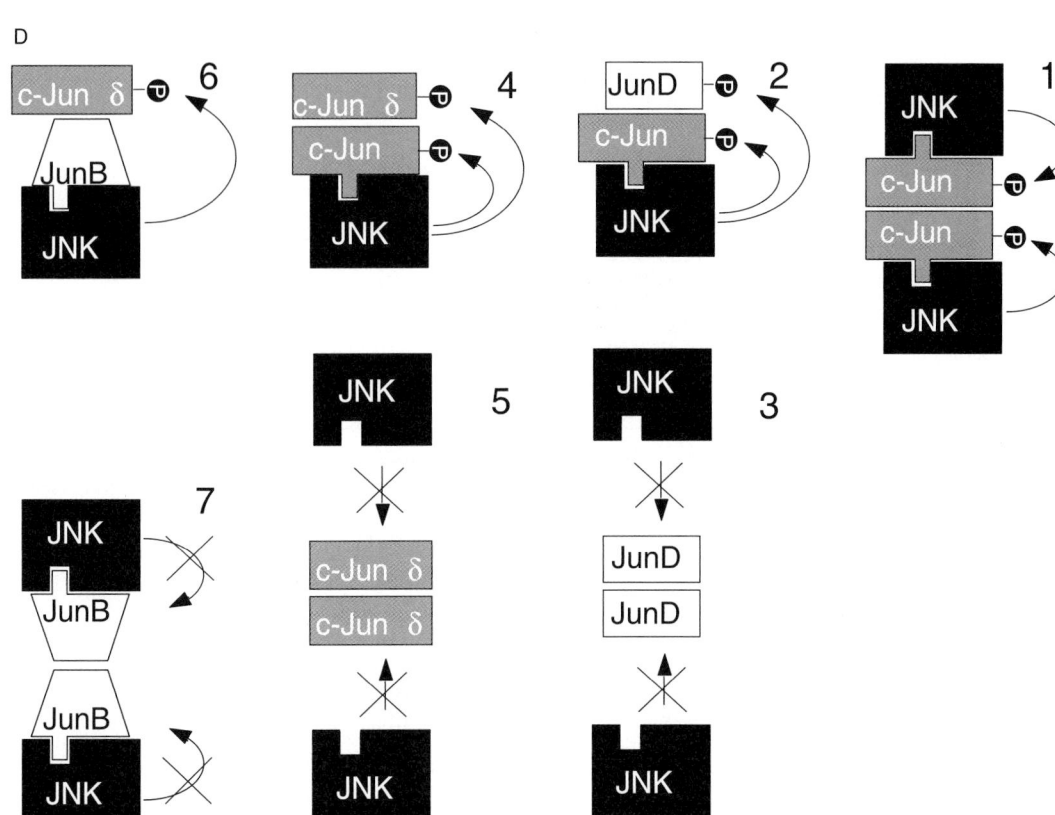

D

Figure 14-13, cont'd **(D)** Phosphorylation of Jun family members by JNKs involves both the presence of a JNK-binding site (D-domains in this instance), JNK proline-directed phosphorylation sites and the ability of Jun family members to dimerize. Thus, in **(1)** JNK bound to c-Jun dimers can phosphorylate the canonical proline-directed sites. In **(2)**, JunD heterodimerizes with c-Jun which, in turn, binds JNK. In this scheme, both proteins, which have phosphoacceptor sites for JNK are phosphorylated. Whereas in **(3)** JunD homodimers cannot bind JNK and undergo JNK-catalyzed phosphorylation, in spite of the presence of phosphoacceptor sites. Similarly, in **(5)** deletion of the δ domain (c-JunΔδ in the figure) from c-Jun abrogates JNK binding and, accordingly, phosphorylation; however, if c-JunΔδ heterodimerizes with a Jun partner with an intact JNK-binding pocket (such as wild type c-Jun in **[4]** or JunB in **[6]**), it can be phosphorylated by JNK bound to the wild type c-Jun or JunB. Finally, in **(7)**, although JunB can bind JNK, it cannot be phosphorylated due to a lack of suitable proline-directed phosphoacceptor sites.

effectors have been identified: docking domains (referred to as D-domains) and Phe-X-Phe-Pro (DEF) domains (see Fig. 14-13A and B; Table 14-2).[86–88] D-domains share a common overall consensus sequence Lys-X-X-$^{\text{Arg}}/_{\text{Lys}}$-X-X-X-X-Leu-X-$^{\text{Leu}}/_{\text{Ile}}$ (X is any amino acid). As is shown in Figure 14-13B and Table 14-2, D-domains or a variation of the D-domain in which the Leu-X-Ile motif is not present, can be found in a number of MAPK substrates and upstream activators. In some instances, the Leu-X-$^{\text{Leu}}/_{\text{Ile}}$ is replaced with three hydrophobic residues (see Fig. 14-13B and Table 14-2).[87,88] D-domains bind to a region of MAPKs, the common docking domain (referred to as the CD domain), located in the substrate binding loop of the kinase domain between domains IX and X.[86–88] Table 14-2 indicates several representative CD motifs. Of note, while D-domains are relatively rich in basic residues, the CD motifs are rich in acidic residues, and it has been proposed that the D-domain MAPK interaction is electrostatic.[86–88] Figure 14-13C shows how D-domains are thought to function in the activation (by MKK7) and downstream signaling of JNK.

DEF domains include a conserved Phe-X-$^{\text{Phe}}/_{\text{Tyr}}$-Pro stretch that is critical for MAPK binding (see Fig. 14-13B).[87,88] Some MAPK substrates (e.g., Elk-1) contain both D- and DEF domains. Mutagenesis studies indicate that for such proteins both domains are necessary to confer signaling specificity and efficiency.[87,88] The D-domain on c-Jun lies between residues 30 and 50, well away from Ser63 and Ser73, the sites of phosphorylation (13A). This binding site lies within the so-called δ domain (amino acids 30–57), a hydrophobic region initially implicated in the regulation of c-Jun oncogenicity due to its deletion in oncogenic v-Jun (for this rea-

son, v-Jun is not a JNK substrate) (see Fig. 14-13A and B)[4,5,82,86–88,138,139] The D-domain is responsible for the high specificity of c-Jun for JNK. However, the presence of the D-domain, coupled with the ability of c-Jun to heterodimerize with other members of the Jun family enables the JNKs to phosphorylate other AP-1 constituents in vivo that, as monomers or homodimers, ordinarily are poor JNK substrates (see Fig. 14-13D).[4,5,82,86–88,138,139] Thus, while JunD possesses a phosphoacceptor region, its putative D-domain is shorter than that of c-Jun, and differs substantially in sequence (see Fig. 14-13B). As a consequence, JunD binds JNK poorly. Accordingly, JunD is not ordinarily a JNK substrate in vitro; however, when heterodimerized with c-Jun, JunD can undergo JNK-catalyzed phosphorylation and activation in vivo and in vitro (see Fig. 14-13B and D).[139] JunB, by contrast, possesses a functional D-domain and binds JNK well (see Fig. 14-13B). However, JunB does not possess the proline-directed phosphoacceptor sites that are prerequisite for JNK phosphorylation. Thus, JunB can bind JNK, but is not phosphorylated in vivo or in vitro by JNK. However, JunB can heterodimerize with c-Jun mutants missing the δ domain and foster JNK phosphorylation of these mutants. Interestingly, JunB can function as a negative regulator of c-Jun (see Fig. 14-13B and D).[139]

MEKs AND MAP3Ks UPSTREAM OF THE JNKs AND p38s

As with the ERK pathway and all MAPK pathways, the p38 and JNK pathways are organized into three tiered MAP3K > MEK > MAPK core signaling modules.[81,82] Two MEKs have

Table 14-2 MAPK Effector/Activator Docking Domains (D-domains) and MAPK Common Docking (CD) Motifs

DOCKING DOMAINS

Type of Protein with Docking Domains	Examples	MAPK Docking Site Sequence	Target MAPK(s)
MKK	MEK1	MP**KKK**PTPIQLNPNP	ERK
	MKK6	S**K**G**KKR**NPGL**K**IP	p38
	MKK7	EA**RR**IDLNLDISP	JNK
MAPK-activated protein kinase	Rsk1	SSILAQ**RRVRK**LPSTTL	ERK
	MSK1	**K**APLA**KRRK**M**KK**TSTSTE	ERK, p38α/β
	MAPKAP-K2	NPLLL**KRRKKA**RALEAAA	p38α/β

COMMON DOCKING MOTIFS

MAPK	Common Docking Domain Sequence
ERK1	333YY**DPTDE**PV341
ERK2	314YY**DPSDE**PI322
p38α	311YH**DPDDE**PV319
p38β	319YH**DPEDE**PE327
p38γ	314LH**DTEDE**PQ322
p38δ	311FR**DTEEETE**319
JNK1	324WY**DPSEAE**A332
JNK2	324WY**DPAEAE**A332
JNK3	362WY**DPAEVE**A370

Representative D-domains that bind specific CD domains on complementary MAPKs (not a comprehensive list—for review see Fig. 13B.[87,88] Note the preponderance of basic residues (**bold**) in the docking site sequences. Also, note that both MAPK regulators (MKKs for example) and MAPK effectors (MAPK-activated protein kinases for example) contain MAPK-binding D-domains that bind MADK CD domains. Representative common docking domain sequences (for a review see Refs. 87 and 88. Note the positions and overall frequency of acidic residues (**bold**) and the conservation of sequence within different MAPK groups. This sequence conservation probably contributes to the selectivity of MAPKs for specific activators/effectors.

been identified as activators of p38, MAP-kinase-kinase (MKK)3 and MKK6[81,82,143,144] Likewise, the JNKs are activated by two MEKs: MKK4 and MKK7 (Fig. 14-14A; see Table 14-1).[81,82,143–147] Biochemical and genetic studies indicate that in spite of the fact that the JNKs and p38s each are activated by multiple MEKs, the functions of these MEKs are not entirely redundant. MKK4 and MKK7 have considerably overlapping substrate specificity; however, gene disruption studies indicate that MKK7 is significantly more sensitive to activation by inflammatory cytokines while MKK4 is preferentially recruited by physical stresses, such as hyperosmolar stress and protein synthesis inhibition.[81,82,145–149] However, these genetic studies do not take into account biochemical features of the MKK4 and MKK7 enzymes—features which indicate that these kinases are really both required for all stimuli to activate the JNKs.[149,150] Thus, while MKK4 is not strongly activated by TNF, disruption of *mkk4* indicates that it is absolutely required for TNF activation of JNK.[149] This is because MKK4, although a priori a dual specificity kinase, preferentially phosphorylates JNKs at the regulatory Tyr (Tyr187). Conversely, MKK7, although robustly activated by TNF, preferentially phosphorylates JNKs at the regulatory Thr (Thr185) and only weakly phosphorylates the regulatory Tyr.[150] Accordingly, in vitro and probably in vivo, both kinases are required for full JNK activation.[149,150] MKK3 and MKK6 differ more substantially in their substrate selectivity. MKK3 preferentially activates p38α and p38β while MKK6 can activate strongly all known p38 isoforms. Similarly, MKK3 appears to be more restricted with regard to activation by upstream stimuli. Whereas MKK6 is activated by all known p38 activators, MKK3, like MKK4, is more strongly activated by physical and chemical stresses.[151,152]

A somewhat daunting array of diverse MAP3Ks has been implicated in the regulation of the JNKs and p38s (see Fig. 14-14A). This diversity is consistent with the heterogeneous nature of the stimuli that recruit the JNKs and p38s. The MEK-kinases (MEKKs 1–4) are mammalian homologues of *S. cerevisiae* Ste11p, a MAP3K that regulates both the yeast mating pheromone and osmosensing pathways (see Figs. 14-5B; Fig. 14-14A).[79,82,153–157]

MEKK1 can directly and strongly activate MKK4 and is predominantly JNK specific; however, under certain circumstances it can weakly activate MEK1 and the ERKs.[82,153,154,158–160] Gene disruption studies indicate that MEKK1 is recruited primarily by environmental stresses (microtubule poisons such as taxol and nocodazole) and, to a lesser extent, proinflammatory cytokines and polypeptide mitogens. MEKK1 cannot recruit the p38 pathway.[82,153,154,158–160] In transfection/overexpression experiments, MEKK2 and MEKK3 can activate the JNK (via MKK4), p38 (via MKK3 and MKK6), and ERK (via MEK1) pathways (see Fig. 14-14A).[155] Gene disruption studies indicate that MEKK3 can also recruit NF-κB and is required for NF-κB activation by TNF.[161] However, it is not known how MEKK3 couples to the NF-κB pathway. Disruption of murine *mekk3* indicates that it is required also for normal heart development, although the molecular basis for this requirement is still unclear.[162] Moreover, genetic data linking MEKK2 and MEKK3 to the recruitment of MAPKs by specific extracellular stimuli are still somewhat nebulous; although MEKK2 may be recruited by engagement of the T-cell receptor.[163] MEKK4 (also called MAP 3 kinase-1, MTK1) can activate both the JNK and p38 pathways with equal potency in vivo and can activate MKKs 4, 3, and 6 in vitro and in vivo.[82,156,157] Again, definitive genetic evidence indicating a functional role for MEKK4 in known MAPK pathways is not yet available, although MEKK4 has been linked to recruitment of the JNKs and p38s by genotoxic stresses.[164]

In addition to the MEKKs, other protein kinase families manifest MAP3K activity. ASK1 is recruited by cytokines to activate the JNKs and p38s (via their cognate MEKs). Gene disruption studies suggest that ASK1 couples TNF to sustained, oxidant-dependent JNK and p38 activation.[165,166] TGF-β-activated kinase-1 (TAK1) was originally identified as a MAP3K that, via activation of MKKs 3–7, coupled TGF-β to the JNKs and p38s.[167,168] Recent biochemical studies of the mammalian enzyme, and genetic data from *Drosophila* indicate, however, that TAK1 lies downstream of proinflammatory cytokines that couple to TRAF6-interleukin-1, in particular, and is important not only in MAPK activation but in recruitment of NF-κB as well.[169–171] Tpl-2, the product of the *cot* proto-oncogene, can, in overexpression experiments,

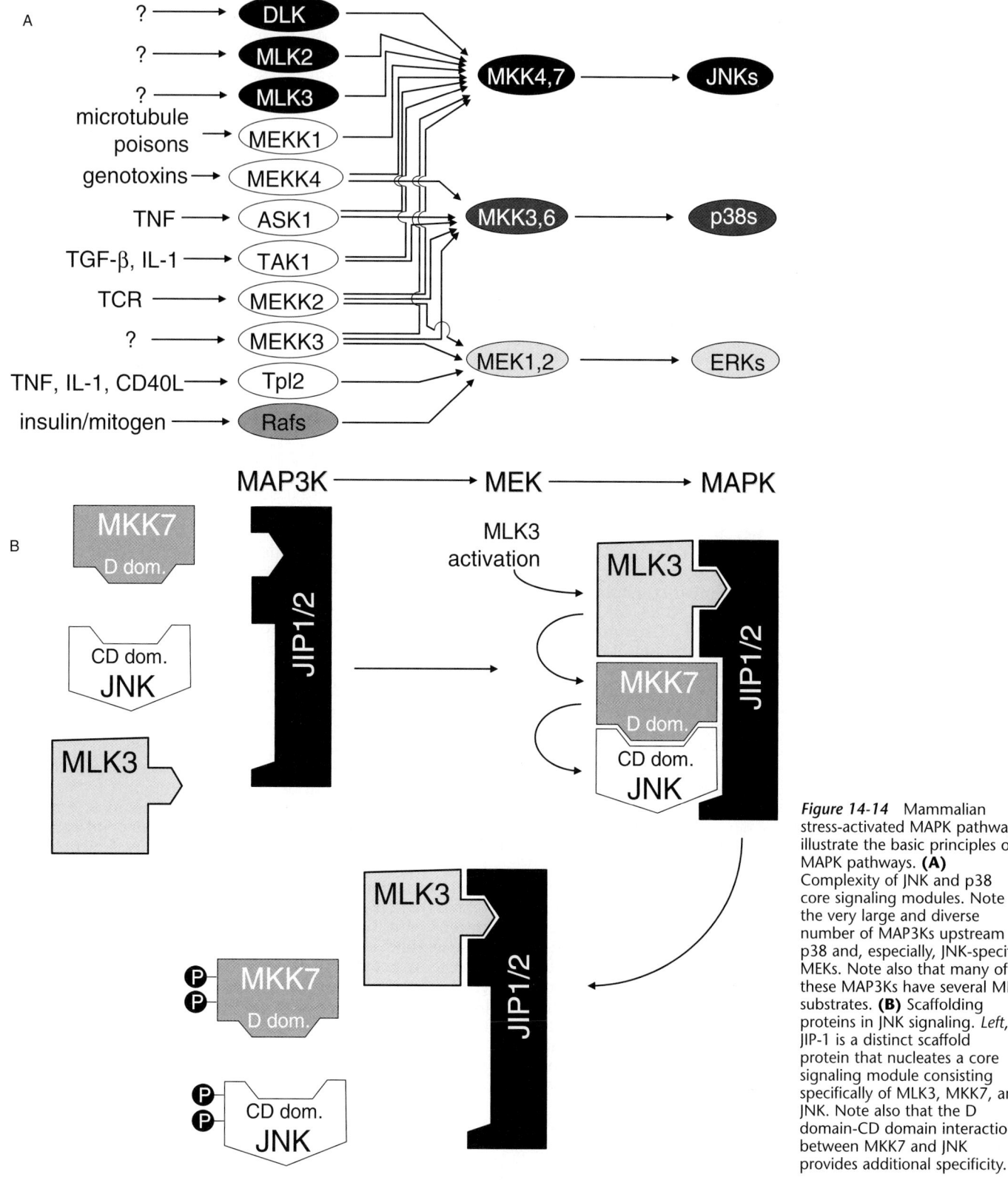

Figure 14-14 Mammalian stress-activated MAPK pathways illustrate the basic principles of MAPK pathways. **(A)** Complexity of JNK and p38 core signaling modules. Note the very large and diverse number of MAP3Ks upstream of p38 and, especially, JNK-specific MEKs. Note also that many of these MAP3Ks have several MEK substrates. **(B)** Scaffolding proteins in JNK signaling. *Left*, JIP-1 is a distinct scaffold protein that nucleates a core signaling module consisting specifically of MLK3, MKK7, and JNK. Note also that the D domain-CD domain interaction between MKK7 and JNK provides additional specificity.

recruit both the JNK and ERK pathways by activating MKK4 and MEK1, respectively[82,172]; however, gene disruption studies indicate that murine Tpl-2 is required only for ERK activation by proinflammatory cytokines.[173] Mixed lineage kinases (MLKs) are also MAP3Ks. These kinases bear structural homology to both Ser/Thr and Tyr kinases and also contain leucine zippers and SH3-binding sites, as well as, in the case of MLK2 and MLK3, SH3 domains. MLKs are comparatively JNK-specific, selectively activating MKK4 and MKK7 (see Fig. 14-14A), although some can also recruit MKK3 and MKK6 and, consequently, the p38s.[82,174-176]

STRESS-ACTIVATED MAPK CORE SIGNALING MODULES

An earlier section described four overarching principles of MAPK pathways that are apparent from an examination of yeast signaling: (1) many MAPK signaling components have more than one biochemical/biologic function; (2) MAPK pathway components are often segregated by proteins with scaffolding properties; these scaffold proteins may be either distinct or may be intrinsic to the signaling kinases themselves; (3) individual MAPK pathway elements are often subject to regulation by several divergent upstream activators (see Fig. 14-5B)[79]; and (4) specific docking sites on MAPKs, their substrates, and effectors mediate high-affinity interactions that ensure signaling fidelity and efficiency. Mammalian stress signaling pathways possess all of these properties.

With regard to signaling components with more than one function (or target), as we have seen, several MAP3Ks can impinge on more than one MAPK pathway. Thus, for example, ASK1 can activate both the JNKs and p38s, while MEKK2 can activate both the ERK and JNK pathways. Similarly, elements in mammalian stress-activated MAPK pathways can be activated by multiple mechanisms. Thus, MKK4 is a substrate for several MAP3Ks including the MLKs, all of the MEKKs, ASK1, TAK1, and Tpl2. Similarly, p38 is a substrate for MKK3 and MKK6 while JNKs are activated by MKK7 and MKK4 (see Fig. 14-14A).[81,82] Having said this, with regard to mammalian MAP3K signaling, much of the available data are from transfection/overexpression experiments. Thus, pending definitive genetic data, caution is warranted in designating signaling components as truly promiscuous in vivo.

Mammalian MAPK pathway scaffold proteins are only beginning to be identified. JNK interacting proteins (JIPs) 1, 2, and 3 are novel mammalian scaffold proteins that are thought to regulate specific JNK activation pathways.[177-180] For example, JIPs 1 and 2 are highly similar structurally and form complexes in vivo and in vitro with MLK3, MKK7, and JNK (see Fig. 14-14B).[177-179] JIP1 consists of a C-terminal SH3 domain (a D-domain, amino acids 491–600), an N-terminal JNK-binding site (amino acids 143–163), and an intermediate domain with several SH3-binding motifs. The MLK3-JIP1 interaction is mediated by the JIP1 SH3 domain and any of several SH3-binding sites on MLK3. MKK7 interacts with the middle segment of JIP1 (amino acids 283–571).[177,178] JIP1 is highly expressed in the brain, and recent gene disruption studies indicate that murine *jip1* is required for JNK activation by excitotoxic or anoxic stresses.[181] The specific biologic functions of JIPs 2 and 3 remain to be determined. As with the *S. cerevisiae* MEK Pbs2p (see Fig. 14-5B), MKK4 possesses intrinsic scaffold properties. Thus, the N terminus (amino acids 1–77) of inactive, dephosphorylated MKK4 can specifically bind one of its upstream activators, MEKK1. Upon phosphorylation and activation of MKK4, the MKK4-MEKK1 complex dissociates and MKK4 forms a second specific complex, with JNK, mediated by the JNK CD domain and a D-domain in the MKK4 amino terminus, near the MEKK1-binding domain. Upon activation of JNK, this second complex dissociates. The intrinsic scaffold properties of MKK4, therefore, enable it to form specific, sequential dynamic complexes with both an upstream activator and a substrate.[81,82] As noted earlier, the interactions between MAPKs, their effectors, and substrates are mediated by docking and DEF domains.[86-88]

REGULATION OF THE JNKs AND p38s BY Rho FAMILY GTPases

While considerable progress has been made in the identification of MEKs and MAP3Ks that recruit the JNKs and p38s, elucidation of the molecular mechanisms of MAP3K regulation has been difficult and little is known of the physiologic function and coupling to cell-surface receptors of stress-regulated MAP3Ks. However, as with the Ras-ERK pathway, there is accumulating evidence that Ras superfamily GTPases regulate the JNKs and p38s. Thus, GTPases of the Rho subfamily of the Ras superfamily have been implicated in JNK and p38 regulation. The Rho subfamily is comprised in mammals of the Rho (RhoA–E), Rac (Rac1 and -2), and Cdc42 (Cdc42Hs, G25K, and

Tc10) subgroups. As with other members of the Ras superfamily, Rho subfamily GTPases are active in the GTP-bound state and inactive in the GDP-bound state (see Fig. 14-10B). Activation of Rho subfamily GTPases is mediated by GEFs homologous to the proto-oncogene *dbl*. GAPs selective for the Rho subfamily have also been identified.[183] Constitutively active, GTPase-deficient forms of Rac1 and Cdc42Hs can activate both the JNKs and p38s in cotransfection experiments. Ras itself can, in some instances, recruit the JNKs, and it appears that Rac1 mediates the activation of JNK by transforming alleles of *ras*, and in response to mitogens such as EGF.[184-189] Aside from this, the stimuli that recruit Rac1 and Cdc42Hs remain unidentified. Most, but not all, effectors for Rac1 and Cdc42Hs contain a Cdc42-Rac interaction and binding (CRIB) domain to which the GTP-loaded Rac and Cdc42 bind. Several potent SAPK/p38 activators can also bind Rac1 and Cdc42Hs in a GTP-dependent manner including MEKK1, MEKK4, MLK2, and MLK3, and MEKK4, MLK2, and MLK3 possess Cdc42-Rac interaction and binding domains. However, the role of Rac1 or Cdc42Hs in the regulation of these MAP3Ks is unclear.[56,187-189]

NUCLEAR FACTOR-κB PATHWAY

The transcription factor NF-κB, like AP-1, the JNKs, and p38s is regulated by environmental stresses and inflammatory cytokines of the TNF family. In most cell types, NF-κB is composed of a heterodimer of the Rel family transcription factor subunits p50 (50-kDa) and p65 (65-kDa) that is sequestered in the cytosol by inhibitory polypeptides of the inhibitor of κB (IκB) family (IκB-α, β, ε, p100, p105; see Fig. 14-5B).[190] IκBs mask the nuclear localization signals of Rel proteins, thereby preventing NF-κB nuclear translocation. Activation of NF-κB requires the signal-induced phosphorylation of Ser residues on IκB proteins (Ser32 and Ser36 of IκBα or Ser19 and Ser23 of IκBβ). This phosphorylation promotes the further covalent modification of IκB (primarily at Lys21 in IκBα) with the 7-kilodalton polypeptide ubiquitin (Ub), a tag that, among other things, recruits the 26S proteasome, a supramolecular complex with proteolytic activity.[190-192] Ubiquitination, itself, requires three activities: E1 Ub activating enzyme, E2 Ub conjugating enzyme, and E3 Ub ligase. E1 recruits and activates Ub through formation of a thioester bond between the C terminus of Ub and a Cys residue on E1 itself. The activated Ub is then *trans* esterified to a conserved Cys on E2. The E3 ligase interacts with both E2 and the target protein, facilitating transfer of the Ub to the target protein. Poly-Ub chains are thus assembled on target proteins.[191,192] E3 recognition of target proteins is often highly regulated, occurring only under certain physiologic circumstances and frequently requiring additional posttranslational modifications of the target protein.[191,192] In the case of IκB, the relevant E3 ligase, a complex of β-transducin repeat-containing protein-1 (β-TrCP1), Skp1, Cul1, and Roc1, only recognizes phosphorylated IκB polypeptides.[190,193] With the degradation of IκB, NF-κB/Rel, is free to migrate to the nucleus where it *trans* activates genes that contain the κB enhancer *cis*-acting element (consensus: GGGACTTCC).[190] NF-κB is a pivotal transcription factor in the inflammatory response. Thus, for example, in addition to its important role in the *trans* activation of the immunoglobulin κ-light chain, NF-κB is required for full induction of interleukin-2 and E-selectin in response to inflammatory signals.[190] Genes induced by NF-κB also exert a powerful antiapoptotic effect that often trumps proapoptotic signaling. Thus, while TNF can recruit elements of the apoptotic machinery, in most instances, TNF does not trigger apoptosis due to robust, coincident activation of NF-κB.[190]

Initial gel filtration isolates of a protein complex with IκB kinase (IKK) activity selective for Ser32/36 of IκBα suggested a massive oligomer (~700–900-kDa).[190,194,195] Present evidence indicates that the catalytic nucleus of the IKK complex consists of three subunits. IκB phosphorylation is catalyzed by either of two protein kinase subunits: IKK-α and IKK-β also called IKK1 and IKK2, respectively. Both kinases are highly selective for the phosphoacceptor sites on IκBα and -β, and even substitution of Thr for the Ser residues is not tolerated.[194–198] A third subunit, IKK-γ (also called NF-κB essential modulator) is devoid of apparent catalytic activity, but can interact in vivo with IKK-β and is required for proper regulation of the IKK complex in vivo (Fig. 14-15).[199,200] The IKK subunits can form higher order oligomers in vivo. IKK-β can interact in vivo and in vitro with itself and with IKK-α. IKK-α can also homodimerize (see Fig. 14-15B).[196–200] IKK-α and -β share approximately 50% homology; both consist of an amino-terminal kinase domain, a leucine (Leu) zipper, and a C-terminal helix-loop-helix motif.[194–198] Likewise, the IKK-γ primary sequence contains an N-terminal helix-loop-helix domain and a C-terminal leucine zipper (see Fig. 14-15A).[199,200] Deletion of the Leu zipper from either kinase subunit abrogates IKK-α/β homodimerization or heterodimerization.[195–198] Thus, it appears that the Leu zippers are critical for dimerization of the IKK kinase subunits. IKK-γ itself can form homodimers, and can heterodimerize with IKK-β, and the Leu zipper appears necessary for both functions, as well as for IKK-γ biologic activity.[199,200] Functionally speaking, however, biochemical studies indicate that the intact IKK complex consists of an oligomer of IKK-α, IKK-β, and IKK-γ with a stoichiometry of 1:1:1 (see Fig. 14-15B).[190] Genetic studies have revealed specific functional roles for the IKK subunits. The human gene for IKKγ is located on the X chromosome. X-linked recessive anhidrotic ectodermal dysplasia with immunodeficiency (EDA-ID), as well as incontinentia pigmenti, are sex-linked

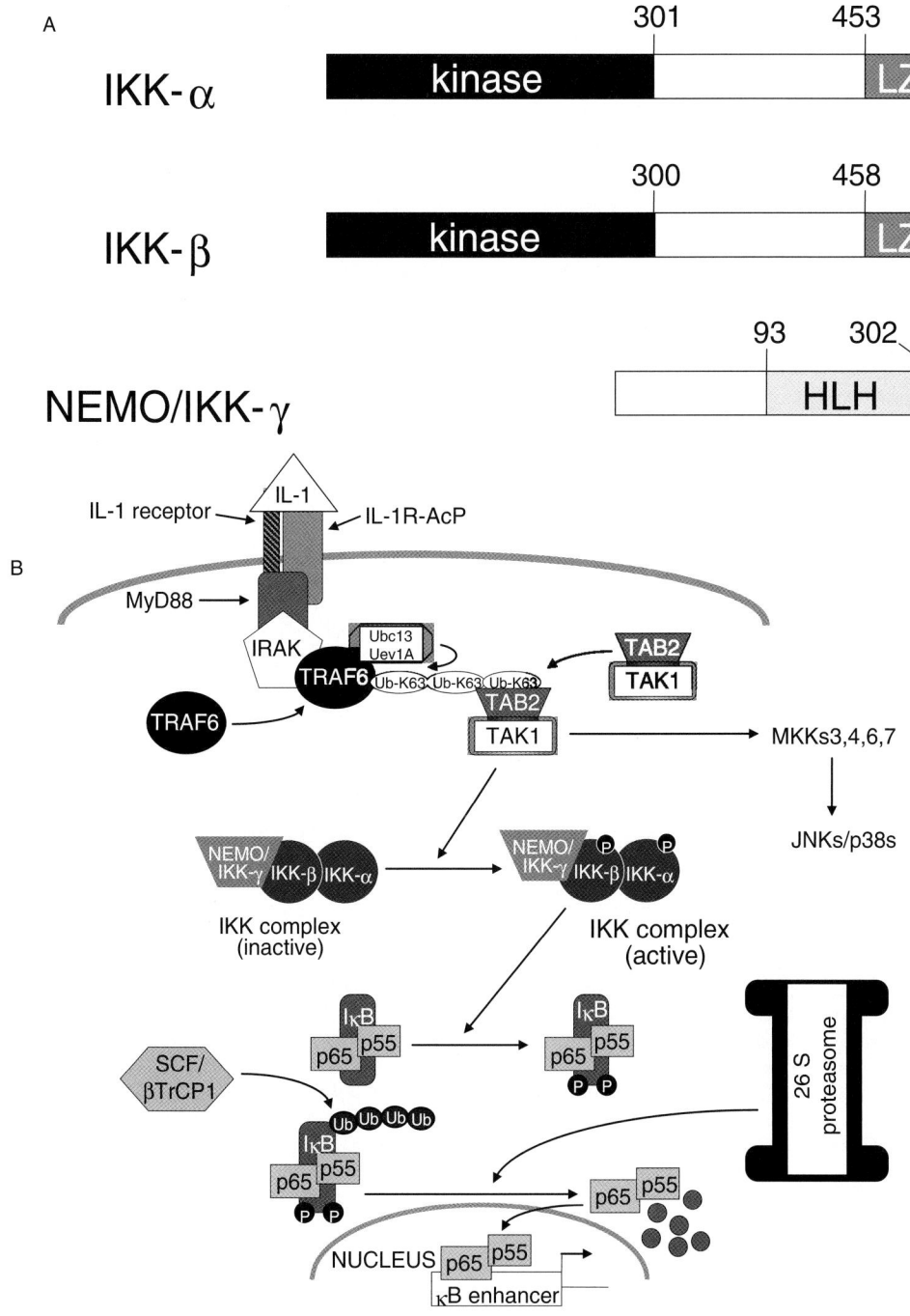

Figure 14-15 The NF-κB signaling pathway. (A) Schematic structures of the IKK catalytic core. HLH, helix-loop-helix domain; LZ, leucine zipper. Amino acid numbers are indicated. (B) Regulation by IL-1 of IκB phosphorylation as well as JNK and p38 is initiated by a novel form of ubiquitination. IL-1 signaling is initiated by agonist-induced oligomerization of the receptor with the IL-1 receptor accessory protein (IL-1R-AcP in the figure). This recruits intracellular adapter proteins, MyD88 and IL-1 receptor-associated kinase (IRAK). IRAK, in turn, recruits TRAF6 polypeptides, likely resulting in TRAF6 oligomerization of the membrane. This leads to E1 and Ubc13/Uev1A recruitment and consequent autoubiquitination of TRAF6. The poly-Ub chains are linked through Ub-Lys63. The CUE domain protein TAB2, a regulatory subunit of the MAP3K TAK1, binds the Ub-Lys63-linked poly-Ub chains on TRAF6, resulting in TAK1 activation and phosphorylation and activation of the IKK complex as well as MEKs upstream of the JNKs and p38s. IKK phosphorylates IκB triggering its ubiquitination (through Lys48-linked chains) in a process that requires β-TrCP1. Consequent proteasome degradation of IκB frees NF-κB to migrate to the nucleus and trans activate target genes, many of which act to suppress apoptosis and promote inflammation.

disorders that have been linked to loss of function mutations in IKK-γ.[201] Individuals with these conditions manifest impaired NF-κB activation in response to proinflammatory cytokines, highlighting the key role for IKK-γ in this process.[201] Interestingly, disruption of murine *ikk-α*, while embryonically lethal, has little or no effect on cytokine (TNF) recruitment of murine embryonic fibroblast NF-κB. Instead, these animals display a severe dermal phenotype in which the epidermis is pathologically thickened, impairing limb growth.[202,203] By contrast, disruption of *ikk-β* also results in early embryonic lethality. In this instance, lethality is accompanied by massive hepatic apoptosis. Cells derived from these animals show no TNF activation of NF-κB.[204,205] Of note, these cells are exquisitely sensitive to TNF-induced apoptosis.[204,205] This finding is consistent with earlier studies indicating that NF-κB confers resistance to apoptosis by recruiting genes that inhibit apoptotic pathways.

The IKK complex is regulated by phosphorylation. Both IKK-α and IKK-β require phosphorylation within their kinase activation loops for activity.[206] Gene disruption studies indicate that MEKK3 is required for TNF activation of the IKK complex[161]; however, biochemical mechanistic studies remain to be performed that would implicate MEKK3 as an IKK kinase. A series of elegant studies has implicated TAK1 as a major direct upstream activator of IKK recruited by interleukin-1.[170,171] These findings are discussed in the next section.

SIGNALING THROUGH THE TNFR FAMILY

The TNF receptor (TNFR) family includes TNFR1, TNFR2, the interleukin-1 and lymphotoxin-β receptors, cluster of differentiation (CD) 27, CD30, CD40, Fas, receptor activator of NF-κB (also called osteoprotegerin ligand or TNF-related activation-induced cytokine), Ox40, the p75 neurotrophin receptor, and others.[83,207] Upon binding ligand, these receptors can elicit a wide variety of inflammatory responses and are critical to immune cell development, innate and acquired immunity, as well as the pathogenesis of a number of diseases such as arthritis, type 2 diabetes, and septic shock. Accordingly, this family of receptors is among the most important activators of the JNKs, p38s, and NF-κB. Many ligands of the TNF family are homotrimeric and initiate responses by binding to cell-surface receptors. Receptors for TNF family cytokines are themselves preformed trimers, and ligand binding triggers a conformational change in the trimers that leads to the recruitment of intracellular effector proteins.[208] Some, but not all, of these receptors contain an intracellular death domain. Death domains, so-named for their role in promoting apoptosis, mediate homotypic and heterotypic protein-protein interactions and are critical for nucleating receptor-effector complexes and implementing several signaling programs.[83] Signal transduction by TNF has been characterized in some detail, although the picture is far from complete. TNF homotrimers bind to one of two receptors: TNFR1 (55–60-kDa) or TNFR2 (75–80-kDa). TNFR1 contains a death domain.[59] Upon binding TNF, the TNFR1 death domain binds the adapter protein TNFR-associated death domain protein (TRADD). TRADD, in turn, associates with TNFR-associated factor (TRAF) 2, a member of the TRAF family, and with receptor interacting protein (RIP), a death domain-containing Ser/Thr kinase. RIP can also bind TRAF2 and, accordingly, TNF treatment is thought to result in the formation of a TRADD-RIP-TRAF2 complex.[83,209–214] The TRAFs and RIP represent key adapter proteins in the regulation of the JNKs, p38s, and NF-κB. Six TRAFs (TRAFs 1–6) have been identified. Transient overexpression of TRAFs 1, 2, 3, 5, and 6 results in potent activation of NF-κB, while overexpression of TRAFs 2, 5, and 6 results in JNK and p38 activation.[82,83] Gene disruption studies indicate that murine TRAF2 is required for TNF activation of JNK and is necessary for optimal TNF activation of NF-κB.[215,216] On the other hand, disruption of murine

RIP completely abrogates TNF activation of NF-κB, suggesting that RIP is critical for coupling TNF to NF-κB.[217,218] Disruption of murine *traf6*, by contrast, impairs substantially interleukin-1, CD40L, receptor activator of NF-κB, and endotoxin activation of both JNK and NF-κB. These mice manifest severe osteopetrosis, suggesting that TRAF6 (probably as a consequence of receptor activator of NF-κB recruitment) positively regulates osteoclastogenesis.[218]

The molecular basis by which interleukin-1, through TRAF6, couples to JNK and NF-κB has been elucidated biochemically (see Fig. 14-15B). The results indicate a signaling pathway mediated by a novel form or protein ubiquitination. Poly-Ub chains are most commonly linked through either Ub-Lys48 or Lys63. Poly-Ub chains linked through Ub Lys48 typically confer recruitment of the proteasome, with consequent degradation of the ubiquitinated target protein. Until recently, few functions for Lys63-linked poly-Ub were known.[191,192,219] TRAF6 is an E3 Ub ligase and can activate IKK in vitro, and in vivo in response to interleukin-1, only in the presence of a complex of the ubiquitin activating protein E1 and an E2 ubiquitin conjugating enzyme complex consisting of the proteins Ubc13 and Uev1A (see Fig. 14-15B).[170,171] TRAF6, in the presence of Uev1A/Ubc13 and E1, autoubiquitinates, generating poly-Ub chains linked through Ub Lys63. These poly-Ub chains do not lead to proteasomal degradation. Instead, they function in a manner similar to phosphotyrosine (see Chapter 8), specifically, they serve to recruit proteins with coupling of ubiquitin conjugation to endoplasmic reticulum (CUE) degradation domains.[170,171] TAK1-associated-binding protein 2 is an obligate regulatory subunit of the MAP3K TAK1.[82] TAK1-associated-binding protein has a CUE domain and consequently, TAK1-TAK1-associated-binding protein 2 heterodimers bind polyubiquitinated TRAF6 (see Fig. 14-15B).[170,171] TAK1 recruited in this manner is activated and then phosphorylates and activates both the IKK complex and MEKs upstream of the JNKs and p38s.[170,171]

TNF ACTIVATION OF JNK; JNK AND TYPE 2 DIABETES

The interplay between stress and hormonal signaling mechanisms is becoming more established. It is evident that stress pathways can often influence the magnitude of both insulin and steroid hormone function. This section and the following section will describe some of what is known. The reader should then begin to appreciate the possibility that stress pathways may provide attractive targets for therapeutics. In addition, considerations of the ramifications of endocrine therapies need to consider the effects of stress signaling on these therapies (and vice versa).

Obesity and type 2 diabetes are associated with a chronic inflammation that includes abnormally elevated levels of proinflammatory cytokines (especially TNF). These abnormalities appear to originate in adipose tissue, which can produce substantial levels of TNF.[220,221] Free fatty acids are also implicated in the pathophysiology of obesity and insulin resistance.[222] Both TNF and free fatty acids can trigger activation of the JNK pathway.[223] Evidence has emerged that JNK, possibly in conjunction with other MAPKs, can directly contribute to insulin resistance.

First, activation of ERK, JNK, and p38 can inhibit insulin signaling in cultured 3T3-L1 adipocytes, albeit by different mechanisms. Constitutive activation of ERK results in suppression of insulin receptor, as well as IRS1 and IRS2 expression. Activation of p38 modestly reduces IRS1 an IRS2, but not insulin receptor expression (see Chapter 8). Activation of JNK profoundly reduces insulin receptor Tyr phosphorylation of IRS1 and IRS2.[224–226]

The effects of JNK on insulin signaling can be traced at least, in part, to direct JNK-catalyzed phosphorylation of IRS1 at Ser307. Ser307 resides near the IRS1 phosphotyrosine-binding domain (see Chapter 8). This phosphorylation strongly reduces insulin-stimulated IRS1 Tyr phosphorylation and suppresses the recruitment by insulin of key downstream targets such as PI 3-kinase, which are coupled to metabolic regulation. Mutagenesis of IRS1 Ser307 to Ala abrogates, in Chinese hamster ovary cells, TNF-mediated inhibition of JNK activation, suggesting that among the MAPKs, it is JNK that functions most prominently to inhibit insulin signaling.[226]

Recent genetic evidence makes a compelling argument that JNK is indeed physiologically relevant to obesity-induced insulin resistance. In both dietary (mice fed a high-fat diet) and genetic (*ob/ob* mice) models of obesity, constitutive elevations in JNK activity occur in several insulin-responsive tissues (liver, fat, and skeletal muscle).[227] When *jnk1−/−*, but not *jnk2−/−* mice were fed a high-fat diet, weight gain was significantly reduced, as compared to wild type controls, indicating that JNK1 is important in mediating weight gain in response to elevated dietary fat. This reduced weight gain coincided with reduced adiposity (adipocyte size) and total body fat.[227] No difference was observed in plasma triglyceride, cholesterol, or free fatty acid concentrations, indicating that lipid metabolism, food intake, and absorption were not affected by disruption of *jnk1*.[227] The *jnk1−/−* mice had an improved balance in the levels of hormones implicated in insulin sensitivity. Thus, the ratio of 30-kilodalton adipocyte complement-related protein (ACRP30)/adiponectin concentration (a measure of the endocrine regulation of fatty acid oxidation) was higher in the *jnk1−/−* mice, while resistin (a hormone implicated in insulin resistance) levels were lower. Consistent with this, normal mice fed a high-fat diet developed mild hyperglycemia, while *jnk1−/−* mice had significantly lower blood glucose under identical dietary conditions. Moreover, the obese wild type, but not the *jnk1−/−* mice, also developed hyperinsulinemia and the *jnk1−/−* mice fared better in intraperitoneal insulin and glucose tolerance tests.[227] *ob/ob* mice develop spontaneous obesity and type 2 diabetes. Crossing *ob/ob* mice with *jnk1−/−* mice to produce combination *jnk1−/−/ob/ob* mice resulted in animals with a significantly reduced extent of weight gain as compared to *ob/ob* mice. Furthermore, the *jnk1−/−/ob/ob* mice also exhibited reduced hyperinsulinemia and hyperglycemia. It is interesting to note that all of the metabolic effects of the *jnk1* deletion coincided with a reduced constitutive phosphorylation of IRS1 at Ser307. Thus, JNK1 but not JNK2 (the reasons for this difference are unknown) appears to play an important role in the development of obesity-induced insulin resistance, possibly through direct inhibition of IRS recruitment.[227]

ANTAGONISM BETWEEN GLUCOCORTICOID RECEPTORS AND JNK > ACTIVATOR PROTEIN-1

It has been known for some time that glucocorticoids are potent anti-inflammatory agents. Similarly, the ability of inflammatory mediators to inhibit the actions of glucocorticoids is well known and is discussed in Chapter 15 and Part 9. The glucocorticoid receptor (GR) is a member of the steroid receptor superfamily (see Chapter 15). The basis for the mutual antagonism of glucocorticoids and inflammation was unclear until it was observed that AP-1 and the GR could block each other's transcriptional activity.[228–230] The presence of c-Jun prevents the association of the GR with the GRE; similarly, the presence of the GR blocks AP-1 association with the TRE. This antagonism is not due to a dislodging of GR or AP-1 already bound to DNA, nor is it due to covalent modifications of either the GR or Fos-Jun per se (notably glucocorticoids do not affect Jun phosphorylation). Instead, this inhibitory activity is due to a direct interaction between the DNA-binding domain of c-Jun and the DNA-binding domain of the GR that prevents subsequent DNA binding by either transcription factor.[228–230]

Recently, an additional level of GR/JNK pathway antagonism was elucidated. Glucocorticoids trigger the dissociation of JNK from MKK7 in vitro by promoting the formation of a GR-JNK complex. This interaction strongly represses JNK activation by TNF in the presence of glucocorticoids. Interestingly, the GR-JNK complex can still translocate into the nucleus. In the nucleus, the complex binds to AP-1 but because the JNK is inactive, AP-1 is not recruited.[231] These phenomena indicate that stress-regulated MAPK pathways and steroid receptor pathways share an intimate cross-talk at the molecular level and should not be considered as independent entities when contemplating existing therapeutic options or designing new ones.

UNIFYING THEMES AND CONCLUSIONS

This chapter has discussed some of what is known about how polypeptide hormones such as insulin, as well as environmental and organismal stress mechanisms, recruit protein Ser/Thr kinases to affect changes in cellular physiology. There are several general themes that emerge from the findings covered.

Subdomain VIII of the kinase domain is often critical to regulation PKB/Akt, Rsk, p70, MAPKAP-K2, all of the MAPKs, and all of the MEKs are regulated at least, in part, by phosphorylation within the kinase domain activation loop in subdomain VIII. Thus, phosphorylation within this region is a common theme in Ser/Thr kinase regulation.

Ras superfamily GTPases are critical signaling intermediates It is clear that the ERK pathway (through Ras) and the JNK and p38 pathways (through Rac1 and Cdc42Hs, as well as Ras in some instances) rely heavily on Ras family proteins to relay signals from activated receptors to MAP3Ks. In addition, PI 3-kinase also requires Ras for optimal activation by insulin and mitogens.

Signaling pathways often are multi-tiered All MAPK pathways proceed through three-tiered core signaling pathways. In addition, the PKB/Akt and p70 S6 kinase pathways require multiple upstream protein kinases for regulation. In the case of the MAPK pathways, the core signaling modules can activate additional distal protein kinases (Rsk and MAPKAP-K2). Moreover, each tier in MAPK pathways is apparently occupied by multiple homologues (especially at the MEK and MAP3K level). The significance of this complexity is unclear; however, it likely permits the regulation of these pathways by multiple, often divergent inputs (e.g., stimuli as varied as TNF and hyperosmolarity can activate JNK). In addition, this complexity permits kinases at each level to influence multiple effectors (thus, PKB/Akt can regulate both GSK3 and p70 S6 kinase). Multi-tiered protein kinase cascades also allow for catalytic amplification at each level, rendering these pathways exquisitely sensitive to external stimuli.

Pathway cross-talk requires consideration of signal integration As we have seen, individual effectors can be influenced by divergent agonistic and antagonistic stimuli. Thus, the ERKs can influence nonmitogenic signaling pathways such as those involving PPAR-γ, the ER, and the STATs. AP-1 can be activated through mitogen-Elk-1 induction of c-*fos* expression, TNF, or stress activation of c-Jun *trans* activation function (as well as c-Jun and p38-MEF2C induction of c-*jun* expression), and antagonism by glucocorticoids and GSK3. Similarly, insulin and cAMP agonists can, through p70 S6 kinase and PKA, respectively, activate CREMτ function. Conversely, insulin and cAMP are antagonistic regulators of GS. Thus, as more of these signaling pathways are elucidated, conventional and novel treatment strategies will have to consider the effects of novel therapeutics on multiple pathways that could be affected by drugs that "apparently" target a single signaling constituent.

REFERENCES

1. Hanks SK, Quinn MA, Hunter T: The protein kinase family: Conserved features and deduced phylogeny of the catalytic domains. Science 241:42–52, 1988.
2. Knighton DR, Zheng J, Ten Eyck LF, et al: Crystal structure of the catalytic subunit of cyclic adenosine monophosphate-dependent protein kinase. Science 253:407–414, 1991.
3. Zhang F, Strand A, Robbins D, et al: Atomic structure of the MAP kinase ERK2 at 2.3 A resolution. Nature 367:704–711, 1994.
4. Kyriakis JM, Avruch J: S6 kinases and MAP kinases: Sequential intermediates in insulin/mitogen-activated protein kinase cascades. In Woodgett JR (ed): Protein Kinases: Frontiers in Molecular Biology. Oxford, Oxford University Press, 1994, p 85.
5. Avruch J: Insulin signal transduction through protein kinase cascades. Mol Cell Biochem 182:31–48, 1998.
6. Carpenter CL, Cantley LC: Phosphoinositide kinases. Curr Opin Cell Biol 8:153–158, 1996.
7. Cohen P: Muscle glycogen synthase. In Boyer P, Krebs EG (eds): The Enzymes. New York, Academic Press, 1988, p 461.
8. Larner J: Insulin signalling mechanisms—lessons from the old testament of glycogen metabolism and from the new testament of molecular biology. Diabetes 37:262–282, 1988.
9. Krebs EG: Protein kinases. Curr Topics Cell Reg 5:99–120, 1972.
10. Avruch J, Witters LA, Alexander MC, et al: The effect of insulin and glucagon on the phosphorylation of hepatic cytoplasmic peptides. J Biol Chem 253:4754–4762, 1978.
11. Haselbacher GK, Humbel RE, Thomas G: Insulin-like growth factors, insulin or serum increase phosphorylation of ribolomal S6 during transition of stationaary chick embryo fibroblasts in early G1 phase of the cell cycle. FEBS Lett 100:185–191, 1979.
12. Downward J: Mechanisms and consequences of activation of protein kinase B/Akt. Curr Opin Cell Biol 10:262–267, 1998.
13. Obata T, Yaffe MB, Leparc GG, et al: Peptide and protein library screening defines optimal substrate motifs for AKT/PKB. J Biol Chem 275:36108–36115, 2000.
14. Whiteman EL, Cho H, Birnbaum MJ: Role of Akt/protein kinase B in metabolism. Trends Endocrinol 13:444–451, 2002.
15. Embi N, Rylatt DB, Cohen P: Glycogen synthase kinase-3 from rabbit skeletal muscle. Separation from cyclic-AMP-dependent protein kinase and phosphorylase kinase. Eur J Biochem 107:519–527, 1980.
16. Parker PJ, Embi N, Caudwell FB, et al: Glycogen synthase from rabbit skeletal muscle. State of phosphorylation of the seven phosphoserine residues in vivo in the presence and absence of adrenaline. Eur J Biochem 124:47–55, 1982.
17. Roach PJ: Multisite and heirarchical protein phosphorylation. J Biol Chem 266:14139–14142, 1991.
18. Wang X, Paulin FE, Campbell LE, et al: Eukaryotic initiation factor 2B: Identification of multiple phosphorylation sites in the ε-subunit and their functions in vivo. EMBO J 20:4349–4359, 2001.
19. Boyle WJ, Smeal T, Defize LHK, et al: Activation of protein kinase C decreases phosphorylation of c-jun at sites that negatively regulate its DNA binding activity. Cell 64:573–584, 1991.
20. Cross DAE, Alessi DR, Cohen P, et al: Inhibition of glycogen synthase kinase-3 by insulin mediated by protein kinase B. Nature 378:785–789, 1995.
21. Deprez J, Vertommen D, Alessi DR, et al: Phosphorylation and activation of heart phosphofructo-2-kinase by protein kinase B and other protein kinases of the insulin signaling cascades. J Biol Chem 272:17269–17275, 1997.
22. Burgering BMT, Kops GJPL: Cell cycle and death control: Long live forkheads. Trends Biochem Sci 27:352–360, 2002.
23. Muslin AJ, Tanner JW, Allen PM, et al: Interaction of 14-3-3 with signaling proteins is mediated by the recognition of phosphoserine. Cell 84:889–897, 1996.
24. Hall RK, Yamasaki T, Kucera T, et al: Regulation of phosphoenolpyruvate carboxykinase and insulin-like growth factor-binding protein-1 gene expresion by insulin. The role of winged helix/forkhead proteins. J Biol Chem 275:30169–30175, 2000.
25. Cho H, Mu J, Kim JK, et al: Insulin resistance and a diabetes mellitus-like syndrome in mice lacking the protein kinase Akt2 (PKBβ). Science 292:1728–1731, 2001.
26. Cho H, Thorvaldsen JL, Chu Q, et al: Akt1/PKBα is required for normal growth but dispensable for maintenance of glucose homeostasis in mice. J Biol Chem 276:38349–38352, 2001.
27. Chiang SH, Baumann CA, Kanzaki M, et al: Insulin-stimulated GLUT4 translocation requires the CAP-dependent activation of TC10. Nature 410:944–948, 2001.
28. Alessi DR, Andjelkovic M, Caudwell B, et al: Mechanism of activation of protein kinase B by insulin and IGF-1. EMBO J 15:6541–6551, 1996.
29. Frödin M, Antal TL, Dümmler BA, et al: A phosphoserine/threonine-binding pocket in AGC kinases and PDK1 mediates activation by hydrophobic motif phosphorylation. EMBO J 21:5396–5407, 2002.
30. Alessi DR, James SR, Downes CP, et al: Characterization of a 3-phosphoinositide-dependent protein kinases which phosphorylates and activates protein kinase Bα. Curr Biol 7:261–269, 1997.
31. Alessi DR, Deak M, Casamayor A, et al: 3-phosphoinositide-dependent protein kinase-1 (PDK1): Structural and cunctional homology with the Drosophila DSTPK61 kinase. Curr Biol 7:776–789, 1997.
32. Stephens L, Anderson K, Stokoe D, et al: Protein kinase B kinases that mediate phosphatidylinositol 3,4,5-trisphosphate-dependent activation of protein kinase B. Science 279:710–714, 1998.
33. Erikson E, Maller JL: Purification and characterization of a protein kinase from Xenopus eggs highly specific for ribosomal protein S6. J Biol Chem 261:350–355, 1986.
34. Alcorta DA, Crews CM, Sweet LJ, et al: Homologs of Xenopus laevis ribosomal S6 kinase. Mol Cell Biol 9:3850–3859, 1989.
35. Calvo V, Crews CM, Vik TA, et al: Interleukin 2 stimulation of p70 S6 kinase activity is inhibited by the immunosuppressant rapamycin. Proc Natl Acad Sci U S A 89:7571–7575, 1992.
36. Price DJ, Nemenoff RA, Avruch J: Purification of hepatic S6 kinase from cycloheximide-treated rats. J Biol Chem 264:13825–13833, 1989.
37. Banerjee P, Ahmad MF, Grove JR, et al: Molecular structure of a major insulin/mitogen-activated 70-kDa S6 protein kinase. Proc Natl Acad Sci U S A 87:8550–8554, 1990.
38. Gout I, Minami T, Hara K, et al: Molecular cloning and characterization of a novel p70 S6 kinase, p70 S6 kinase-β, containing a proline-rich region. J Biol Chem 273:30061–30064, 1998.
39. Jeffries HBJ, Reinhard C, Kozma SC, et al: Rapamycin selectively represses translation of the "polypyrimidine tract" mRNA family. Proc Natl Acad Sci U S A 91:4441–4445, 1994.
40. Jeffries HBJ, Fumagalli S, Dennis PB, et al: Rapamycin suppresses 5′TOP mRNA translation through inhibition of p70 S6k. EMBO J 16:3693–3704, 1997.
41. Jeffries HBJ, Thomas G: Ribosomal protein S6 phosphorylation and signal transduction. In Hershey JWB, Mathews MB, Sonenberg N (eds): Translational Control. New York, Cold Spring Harbor, Cold Spring Harbor Press, 1996, p 389.
42. Habener JF: Cyclic AMP-response element binding proteins: Acornucopia of transcription factors. Mol Endocrinol 4:1087–1094, 1990.
43. de Groot RP, Sassone-Corsi P: Hormonal control of gene expression: Multiplicity and versatility of cyclic adenosine 3′,5′-monophosphate-responsive nuclear regulators. Mol Endocrinol 7:145–153, 1993.

44. Foulkes NS, Borelli E, Sassone-Corsi P: CREM gene: Use of alternative DNA binding domains generates multiple antagonists of cAMP-induced transcription. Cell 64:739–749, 1991.

45. Foulkes NS, Mellström B, Benusiglio E, et al: Developmental switch of CREM function during spermatogenesis from antagonist to activator. Nature 355:80–84, 1992.

46. Laoide BM, Foulkes NS, Schlotter F, et al: The functional diversity of CREM is determined by its modular structure. EMBO J 12:1179–1191, 1993.

47. Delmas V, Laoide BM, Masquilier D, et al: Alternative usage of initiation codons in mRNA encoding the cAMP-responsive element modulator (CREM) gene generates regulators with opposite functions. Proc Natl Acad Sci U S A 89:4226–4230, 1992.

48. Molina CA, Foulkes NS, Lalli E, et al: Inducibility and negative autoregulation of CREM: An alternaitve promoter directs the expression of ICER, an early response repressor. Cell 75:875–886, 1993.

49. Foulkes NS, Schlotter F, Pevet P, et al: Pituitary hormone FSH directs the CREM functional switch during spermatogenesis. Nature 362:264–267, 1993.

50. de Groot RP, den Hertog J, Vandenheede JR, et al: Multiple and cooperative phosphorylation events regulate the CREM activator function. EMBO J 12:3903–3911, 1993.

51. de Groot RP, Ballou LM, Sassone-Corsi P: Positive regulation of the cAMP-responsive activator CREM by the p70 S6 kinase: An alternative route to mitogen-induced gene expression. Cell 79:81–91, 1994.

52. Mukhopadhyay NK, Price DJ, Kyriakis JM, et al: An array of insulin-activated, proline-directed (Ser/Thr) protein kinases phosphorylate the p70 S6 kinase. J Biol Chem 267:3325–3335, 1992.

53. Alessi DR, Kozloski MT, Weng QP, et al: 3-phosphoinositide-dependent protein kinase 1 (PDK1) phosphorylates and activates the p70 S6 kinase in vivo and in vitro. Curr Biol 8:69–81, 1997.

54. Schreiber SL, Crabtree GR: The mechanism of action of cyclosporin A and FK506. Immunol Today 13:136–142, 1992.

55. Chung J, Kuo CJ, Crabtree GR, et al: Rapamycin FKBP specifically blocks growth-dependent activation of signaling by the 70 kd S6 protein kinase. Cell 69:1227–1236, 1992.

56. Kuo CJ, Chung J, Fiorentino DF, et al: Rapamycin selectively inhibits interleukin-2 activation of p70 S6 kinase. Nature 358:70–73, 1992.

57. Heitman J, Movva NR, Hall MN: Targets for cell cycle arrest by the immunosuppressive agent rapamycin in yeast. Science 253:905–909, 1991.

58. Gingras AC, Raught B, Sonenberg N: Regulation of translation initiation by FRAP/mTOR. Genes Dev 15:807–826, 2001.

59. Brown EJ, Alberts MW, Shin TB, et al: A mammalian protein targeted by G1-arresting rapamycin-receptor complex. Nature 369:756–758, 1994.

60. Brown EJ, Beal PA, Keith CT, et al: Control of p70 S6 kinase by kinase activity of FRAP in vivo. Nature 377:441–446, 1995.

61. Hara K, Yonezawa K, Weng QP, et al: Amino acid sufficiency and mTOR regulate p70 S6 kinase and eIF-4E BP1 through a common effector mechanism. J Biol Chem 273:14484–14494, 1998.

62. Burnett PE, Barrow RK, Cohen NA, et al: RAFT1 phosphorylation of the translational regulators p70 S6 kinase and 4E-BP1. Proc Natl Acad Sci U S A 95:1432–1437, 1998.

63. Brunn GJ, Hudson CC, Sekulic A, et al: Phosphorylation of the translational repressor PHAS-I by the mammalian target of rapamycin. Science 277:99–101, 1997.

64. Pause A, Belsham GJ, Gingras A-C, et al: Insulin-dependent stimulation of protein synthesis by phosphorylation of a regulator of 5'-cap function. Nature 371:762–767, 1994.

65. Sonenberg N, Gingras A-C: The mRNA 5' cap-binding protein eIF4E and control of cell growth. Curr Opin Cell Biol 10:268–275, 1998.

66. Kim D-H, Sarbassov DD, Alik SM, et al: mTOR interacts with raptor to form a nutrient-sensitive complex that signals to the cell growth machinery. Cell 110:163–175, 2002.

67. Hara K, Maruki Y, Long X, et al: Raptor, a binding partner of target of rapamycin (TOR), mediates TOR action. Cell 110:177–189, 2002.

68. Schalm SS, Blenis J: Identification of a conserved motif required for mTOR signaling. Curr Biol 12:632–639, 2002.

69. Schalm SS, Fingar DC, Sabatini DM, et al: TOS motif-mediated raptor binding regulates 4E-BP1 multisite phosphorylation and function. Curr Biol 13:797–806, 2003.

70. Nojima H, Tokunaga C, Eguchi S, et al: The mammalian target of rapamycin (mTOR) partner, raptor, binds the mTOR substrates p70 S6 kinase and 4E-BP1 through their TOR signaling (TOS) motif. J Biol Chem 278:15461–15464, 2003.

71. Choi KM, McMahon LP, Lawrence JC Jr: Two motifs in the translational repressor PHAS-I required for efficeint phosphorylation by mammalian target of rapamycin and for recognition by raptor. J Biol Chem 278:19667–19673, 2003.

72. Kwiatkowski DJ: Tuberous sclerosis: From tubers to mTOR. Ann Hum Genet 67:87–96, 2003.

73. Manning BD, Tee AR, Logsdon MN, et al: Identification of the tuberous sclerosis complex-2 tumor suppressor gene product tuberin as a target of the phosphoinositide 3-kinase/akt pathway. Mol Cell 10:151–162, 2002.

74. Inoki K, Li Y, Zhu T, et al: TSC2 is phosphorylated and inhibited by Akt and suppresses mTOR signalling. Nat Cell Biol 4:648–657, 2002.

75. Stocker H, Radimerski T, Schindelholz B, et al: Rheb is an essential regulator of S6K in controlling cell growth in Drosophila. Nat Cell Biol 5:559–565, 2003.

76. Saucedo LJ, Gao X, Chiarelli DA, et al: Rheb promotes cell growth as a component of the insulin/TOR signalling network. Nat Cell Biol 5:566–571, 2003.

77. Garami A, Zwartkruis FJT, Nobukuni T, et al: Insulin activation of Rheb, a mediator of mTOR/S6K/4E-BP signaling is inhibited by TSC1 and 2. Mol Cell 11:1457–1466, 2003.

78. Tee AR, Manning BD, Roux PP, et al: Tuberous sclerosis complex gene products, tuberin and hamartin, comtrol mTOR signaling by acting as a GTPase-activating protein toward Rheb. Curr Biol 13:1259–1268, 2003.

79. Herskowitz I: MAP kinase pathways in yeast: For mating and more. Cell 80:187–197, 1995.

80. Marshall CJ: Specificity of receptor tyrosine kinase signaling: Transient versus sustained extracellular signal regulated kinase activation. Cell 80:179–185, 1995.

81. Kyriakis JM: Mammalian MAP kinase pathways. In Woodgett JR (ed): Protein Kinase Functions. Oxford, Oxford University Press, 2000, p 40.

82. Kyriakis JM, Avruch J: Mammalian mitogen-activated protein kinase pathways activated by stress and inflammation. Physiol Rev 81:807–869, 2001.

83. Arch RH, Gedrich RW, Thompson CB: Tumor necrosis factor receptor-associated factors (TRAFs)—a family of adapter proteins that regulates life and death. Genes Dev 12:2821–2830, 1998.

84. Posas F, Saito H: Osmotic activation of the HOG MAPK pathway via Ste11p MAPKKK: Scaffold role of Pbs2p MAPKK. Science 276:1702–1705, 1997.

85. Choi K-Y, Satterberg B, Lyons DM, et al: Ste5 tethers multiple protein kinases in the MAP kinase cascade required for mating in S. cerevisiae. Cell 78:499–512, 1994.

86. Tanoue T, Adachi M, Moriguchi T, et al: A conserved docking motif in MAP kinases common to substrates, activators and regulators. Nat Cell Biol 2:110–116, 2000.

87. Tanoue T, Nishida E: Docking interactions in the mitogen-activated protein kinase cascades. Pharmacol Ther 93:193–202, 2002.

88. Biondi RM, Nebreda AR: Signalling specificity of Ser/Thr protein kinases through docking site-mediated interactions. Biochem J 372:1–13, 2003.

89. Dent P, Lavoinne A, Nakielny S, et al: The molecular mechanism by which insulin stimulates glycogen systhesis in mammalian skeletal mucscle. Nature 348:302–308, 1990.

90. Richards SA, Fu J, Romanelli A, et al: Ribosomal S6 kinase 1 (RSK1) activation requires signals dependent on and independent of the MAP kinase ERK. Curr Biol 9:810–820, 1999.

91. Dalby KN, Morrice N, Caudwell FB, et al: Identification of regulatory phosphorylation sites in mitogen-activated protein kinase (MAPK)-activated protein kinase-1a/p90rsk that are inducible by MAPK. J Biol Chem 273:1496–1505, 1998.

92. Waskiewicz AJ, Flynn A, Proud CG, et al: Mitogen-activated protein kinases activate the serine/threonine kinases Mnk1 and Mnk2. EMBO J 16:1909–1920, 1997.

93. Treisman R: Regulation of transcription by MAP kinase cascades. Curr Opin Cell Biol 8:205–215, 1996.

94. Karin M, Liu Z-g, Zandi E: AP-1 function and regulation. Curr Opin Cell Biol 9:240–246, 1997.

95. Hu E, Kim JB, Sarraf P: Inhibition of adipogenesis through MAP kinase-mediated phosphorylation of PPAR. Science 274:2100–2103, 1996.

96. Kato S, Endo H, Matsuhiro Y, et al: Activation of the estrogen receptor through phosphorylation by mitogen-activated protein kinase. Science 270:1491–1494, 1995.

97. Zhang X, Blenis J, Li H-C, et al: Requirement of serine phosphorylation for formation of STAT promoter complexes. Science 267:1900–1994, 1995.

98. Davies SP, Reddy H, Caivano M, et al: Specificity and mechanism of action of some commonly used protein kinase inhibitors. Biochem J 351:95–105, 2000.

99. Kyriakis JM, App H, Zhang X-F, et al: Raf-1 activates MAP kinase-kinase. Nature 358:417–421, 1992.

100. Huser M, Luckett J, Chiloeches A, et al: MEK kinase activity is not necessary for Raf-1 function. EMBO J 20:1940–1951, 2001.

101. Mikula M, Schreiber M, Husak Z, et al: Embryonic lethality and fetal liver apoptosis in mice lacking the c-raf-1 gene. EMBO J 20:1952–1962, 2001.

102. Wojnowski L, Zimmer AM, Beck TW, et al: Endothelial apoptosis in Braf-deficient mice. Nat Genet 16:293–297, 1997.

103. Wojnowski L, Stancato LF, Larner AC, et al: Overlapping and specific functions of Braf and Craf-1 proto-oncogenes during mouse embryogenesis. Mech Dev 91:97–104, 2000.

104. Davies H, Bignell GR, Cox C, et al: Mutations of the BRAF gene in human cancer. Nature 417:949–954, 2000.

105. Avruch J, Zhang X-f, Kyriakis JM: Raf meets Ras: Completing the framework of a signal transduction pathway. Trends Biochem Sci 19:279–283, 1994.

106. McCormick F: Activators and effectors of ras p21 proteins. Curr Opin Genet Dev 4:71–76, 1994.

107. McCormick F, Wittinghofer A: Interactions between Ras proteins and their effectors. Curr Opin Biotechnol 7:449–456, 1996.

108. Bar-Sagi D: A ras by any other name. Mol Cell Biol 21:1441–1443, 2001.

109. Zhang X-f, Settleman J, Kyriakis JM, et al: Normal and oncogenic p21ras bind to the amino-terminal regulatory domain of c-Raf-1. Nature 364:308–313, 1993.

110. Mercer KE, Pritchard CA: Raf proteins and cancer: B-Raf is identified as a mutational target. Biochim Biophys Acta 1653:25–40, 2003.

111. Luo Z, Tzivion G, Belshaw PJ, et al: Oligomerization activates c-Raf-1 through a Ras-dependent mechanism. Nature 383:181–184, 1996.

112. Farrar MA, Alberola-Ila J: Perlmutter RM: Activation of the Raf-1 kinase cascade by coumermycin-induced dimerization. Nature 383:178–181, 1996.

113. Tzivion G, Luo Z, Avruch J: A dimeric 14-3-3 protein is an essential cofactor for Raf kinase activity. Nature 394:88–92, 1998.

114. Chong H, Lee J, Guan K-L: Positive and negative regulation of Raf kinase activity and function by phosphorylation. EMBO J 20:3716–3727, 2001.

115. Mason CS, Springer CJ, Cooper RG, et al: Serine and tyrosine phosphorylations cooperate in Raf-1, but not B-Raf activation. EMBO J 18:2137–2148, 1999.

116. Zhang B-H, Guan K-L: Activation of B-Raf kinase requires phosphorylation of the conserved residues Thr598 and Ser601. EMBO J 19:5429–5539, 2000

117. Rodriguez-Viciana P, Warne PH, Dhand R, et al: Phosphatidyl-3-OH kinase as a direct target for Ras. Nature 370:527–532, 1994

118. Rodriguez-Viciana P, Warne PH, Vanhaesebroeck B, et al: Activation of phosphoinositide 3-kinase by interaction with Ras and by point mutation. EMBO J 15:2442–2451, 1996

119. Kyriakis JM, Avruch J: pp54 MAP-2 kinase. A novel serine/threonine protein kinase regulated by phosphorylation and stimulated by poly-L-lysine. J Biol Chem 265:17355–17363, 1990

120. Kyriakis JM, Brautigan DL, Ingebritsen TS, et al: pp54 microtubule-associated protein-2 kinase requires both tyrosine and serine/threonine phosphorylation for activity. J Biol Chem 266:10043–10046, 1991

121. Pulverer BJ, Kyriakis JM, Avruch J, et al: Phosphorylation of c-jun mediated by MAP kinases. Nature 353:670–674, 1991.

122. Kyriakis JM, Banerjee P, Nikolakaki E, et al: The stress-activated protein kinase subfamily of c-Jun kinases. Nature 369:156–160, 1994.

123. Dérijard B, Hibi M, Wu I-H, et al: JNK1: A protein kinase stimulated by UV light and Ha-Ras that binds and phosphorylates the c-Jun transactivation domain. Cell 76:1025–1037, 1994.

124. Han J, Lee J-D, Bibbs L, et al: A MAP kinase targeted by endotoxin and hyperosmolarity in mammalian cells. Science 265:808–811, 1994.

125. Lee JC, Laydon JT, McDonnell PC, et al: A protein kinase involved in the regulation of inflammatory cytokine biosynthesis. Nature 273:739–746, 1994.

126. Mertens S, Craxton M, Goedert M: SAP kinase-3, a new member of the family of mammalian stress-activated protein kinases. FEBS Lett 383:273–276, 1996.

127. Goedert M, Cuenda A, Craxton M, et al: Activation of the novel stress-activated protein kinase SAPK4 by cytokines and cellular stresses is mediated by SKK3 (MKK6); comparison of its substrate specificity with that of other SAP kinases. EMBO J 16:3563–3571, 1997.

128. Stokoe D, Campbell DG, Nakielny S, et al: MAPKAP kinase-2; a novel protein kinase activated by mitogen-activated protein kinase. EMBO J 11:3985–3994, 1992.

129. Stokoe D, Engel K, Campbell DG, et al: Identification of MAPKAP kinase 2 as a major enzyme responsible for the phosphorylation of the small mammalian heat shock proteins. FEBS Lett 313:307–313, 1992.

130. McLaughlin MM, Kumar S, McDonnell PC, et al: Identification of mitogen-activated protein (MAP) kinase-activated protein kinase-3, a novel substrate of CSBP p38 MAP kinase. J Biol Chem 271:8488–8492, 1996.

131. Sithanandam G, Latif F, Smola U, et al: 3pK, a new mitogen-activated protein kinase-activated protein kinase located in the small cell lung cancer tumor suppressor gene region. Mol Cell Biol 16:868–876, 1996 [published erratum appears in Mol Cell Biol 16:1880, 1996].

132. Huot J, Houle F, Marceau F, et al: Oxidative stress-induced actin reorganization mediated by the p38 mitogen-activated protein kinase/heat shock protein 27 pathway in vascular endothelial cells. Circ Res 80:383–392, 1997.

133. Lambert H, Charette SJ, Bernier AF, et al: HSP27 multimerization mediated by phosphorylation-sensitive intermolecular interactions at the amino terminus. J Biol Chem 274:9378–9385, 1999.

134. New L, Jiang Y, Zhao M, et al: PRAK, a novel protein kinase regulated by the p38 MAP kinase. EMBO J 17:3372–3384, 1998.

135. Kotlyarov A, Neininger C, Schubert R, et al: MAPKAP kinase 2 is essential for LPS-induced TNF-α biosynthesis. Nat Cell Biol 1:94–97, 1999.

136. Ben-Levy R, Leighton IA, Doza YN, et al: Identification of novel phosphorylation sites required for activation of MAPKAP kinase-2. EMBO J 14:5920–5930, 1995.

137. Wang XZ, Ron D: Stress-induced phosphorylation adn activation of the transcription factor CHOP (GADD153) by p38 MAP kinase. Science 272:1347–1349, 1996.

138. Dai T, Rubie E, Franklin CC, et al: Stress-activated protein kinases bind directly to the delta domain of c-jun in resting cells: Implications for repression of c-jun function. Oncogene 10:849–855, 1995.

139. Kallunki T, Deng T, Hibi M, et al: c-Jun can recruit JNK to phosphorylate dimerization partners via specific docking interactions. Cell 87:929–939, 1996.

140. Gupta S, Campbell D, Dérijard B, et al: Transcription factor ATF2 regulation by the JNK signal transduction pathway. Science 267:389–393, 1995.

141. Han J, Jiang Y, Li Z, et al: MEF2C participates in inflammatory responses via p38-mediated activation. Nature 386:563–566, 1997.

142. Zhao M, New L, Kravchenko VV, et al: Regulation of the MEF2 family of transcription factors by p38. Mol Cell Biol 19:21–30, 1999.

143. Dérijard B, Raingeaud J, Barrett T, et al: Independent human MAP kinase signal transduction pathways defined by MEK and MKK isoforms. Science 267:682–685, 1995.

144. Raingeaud J, Whitmarsh AJ, Barett T, et al: MKK3- and MKK6-regulated gene expression is mediated by the p38 mitogen-activated protein kinase signal transduction pathway. Mol Cell Biol 16:1247–1255, 1996.

145. Sánchez I, Hughes RT, Mayer BJ, et al: Role of SAPK/ERK kinase-1 in the stress-activated pathway regulating transcription factor c-Jun. Nature 372:794–798, 1994.

146. Tournier C, Whitmarsh AJ, Cavanagh J, et al: Mitogen-activated protein kinase kinase 7 is an activator of the c-Jun NH$_2$-terminal kinase. Proc Natl Acad Sci U S A 94:7337–7342, 1997.

147. Holland PM, Suzanne M, Campbell JS, et al: MKK7 is a stress-activated mitogen-activated protein kinase kinase functionally related to hemopterous. J Biol Chem 272:24994–24998, 1997.

148. Nishina H, Fischer KD, Radvanyi L, et al: Stress signalling kinase Sek1 protects thymocytes from apoptosis mediated by CD95 and CD3. Nature 385:350–353, 1997.

149. Ganiatsas S, Kwee L, Fujiwara Y, et al: SEK1 deficiency reveals mitogen-activated protein kinase cascade crossregulation and leads to abnormal hepatogenesis. Proc Natl Acad Sci U S A 95:6881–6886, 1998.

150. Lawler S, Fleming Y, Goedert M, et al: Synergistic activation of SAPK1/JNK1 by two MAP kinase kinases in vitro. Curr Biol 8:1387–1390, 1998.

151. Cuenda A, Alonso G, Morrice N, et al: Purification and cDNA cloning of SAPKK3, the major activator of RK/p38 in stress- and cytokine-stimulated monocytes and epithelial cells. EMBO J 15:4156–4164, 1996.

152. Meier R, Rouse J, Cuenda A, et al: Cellular stresses and cytokines activate multiple mitogen-activated-protein kinase kinase homologues in PC12 and KB cells. Eur J Biochem 236:796–805, 1996.

153. Lange-Carter CA, Pleiman C, Gardner AM, et al: A divergence in the MAP kinase regulatory network defined by MEK kinase and Raf. Science 260:315–319, 1993.

154. Xu S, Robbins DJ, Christerson LB, et al: Cloning of Rat MEK kinase 1 cDNA reveals an endogenous membrane-associated 195-kDa protein with a large regulatory domain. Proc Natl Acad Sci U S A 93:5291–5295, 1996.

155. Blank JL, Gerwins P, Elliot EM, et al: Molecular cloning of mitogen activated protein/ERK kinase kinases (MEKK) 2 and 3. J Biol Chem 271:5361–5368, 1996.

156. Gerwins P, Blank JL, Johnson GL: Cloning of a novel mitogen-activated protein kinase-kinase-kinase, MEKK4, that selectively regulates the c-Jun amino terminal kinase pathway. J Biol Chem 272:8288–8295, 1997.

157. Takekawa M, Posas F, Saito H: A human homolog of the yeast Ssk2/Ssk22 MAP kinase kinase kinases, MTK1, mediates stress-induced activation of the p38 and JNK pathways. EMBO J 16:4973–4982, 1997.

158. Yan M, Dai T, Deak JC, et al: Activation of stress-activated protein kinase by MEKK1 phosphorylation of its activator SEK1. Nature 372:798–800, 1994.

159. Yujiri T, Sather S, Fanger GR, et al: Role of MEKK1 in cell survival and activation of JNK and ERK pathways defined by targeted gene disruption. Science 282:1911–1914, 1998.

160. Xia Y, Makris C, Su B, et al: MEK kinase 1 is critically required for c-Jun N-terminal kinase activation by proinflammatory stimuli and growth factor-induced cell migration. Proc Natl Acad Sci U S A 97:5243–5248, 2000.

161. Yang J, Lin Y, Guo Z, et al: The essential role of MEKK3 in TNF-induced NF-κB activation. Nat Immunol 2:620–624, 2000.

162. Yang J, Boerm M, McCarthy M, et al: Mekk3 is essential for early embryonic cardiovascular development. Nat Genet 24:309–313, 2000.

163. Schaefer B, Ware MF, Marrack P, et al: Live cell fluorescence imaging of T cell MEKK2: Redistribution and activation in response to antigen stimulation of the T cell receptor. Immunity 11:411–421, 1999.

164. Takekawa M, Saito H: A family of stress-inducible GADD45-like proteins mediate activation of the stress-responsive MTK1/MEKK4 MAPKKK. Cell 95:521–530, 1998.

165. Ichijo H, Nishida E, Irie K, et al: Induction of apoptosis by ASK1, a mammalian MAPKKK that activates JNK and p38 signaling pathways. Science 275:90–94, 1997.

166. Tobiume K, Matsuzawa A, Takahashi T, et al: ASK1 is required for sustained activations of JNK/p38 MAP kinases and apoptosis. EMBO Rep 2:222–228, 2001.

167. Yamaguchi K, Shirakabi K, Shibuya H, et al: Identification of a member of the MAPKKK family as a potential mediator of TGF-β signal transduction. Science 270:2008–2011, 1995.

168. Moriguchi T, Kuroyanagi N, Yamaguchi K, et al: A novel kinase cascade mediated by mitogen-activated protein kinase kinase 6 and MKK3. J Biol Chem 271:13675–13679, 1996.

169. Vidal S, Khush RS, Leulier F, et al: Mutations in the Drosophila dTAK1 gene reveal a conserved function for MAPKKKs in the control of rel/NF-κB-dependent innate immune responses. Genes Dev 15:1900–1912, 2001.

170. Deng L, Wang C, Spencer E, et al: Activation of the IκB kinase complex by TRAF6 requires a dimeric ubiquitin-conjugating enzyme complex and a unique polyubiquitin chain. Cell 103:351–361, 2000.

171. Wang C, Deng L, Hong M, et al: TAK1 is a ubiquitin-dependent kinase of MKK and IKK. Nature 412:346–351, 2001.

172. Salmerón A, Ahmad TB, Carlile GW, et al: Activation of MEK-1 and SEK-1 by Tpl-2 proto oncoprotein, a novel MAP kinase kinase kinase. EMBO J 15:817–826, 1996.

173. Dumitru CD, Ceci, JD, Tsatsanis C, et al: TNF-α induction by LPS is regulated posttranscriptionally via a TPL2/ERK-dependent pathway. Cell 103:1071–1083, 2000.

174. Rana A, Gallo K, Godowski P, et al: The mixed lineage protein kinase SPRK phosphorylates and activates the stress-activated protein kinase activator, SEK1. J Biol Chem 271:19025–19028, 1996.

175. Hirai S-i, Katoh M, Terada M, et al: MST/MLK2, a member of the mixed lineage kinase family, directly phosphorylates and activates SEK1, an activator of c-Jun N-terminal kinase/stress-activated protein kinase. J Biol Chem 272:15167–15173, 1997.

176. Fan G, Merritt SE, Kortenjann M, et al: Dual leucine zipper-bearing kinase (DLK) activates p46SAPK and p38mapk but not ERK2. J Biol Chem 271:24788–24793, 1996.

177. Dickens M, Rogers JS, Cavanagh J, et al: A cytoplasmic inhibitor of the JNK signal transduction pathway. Science 277:693–696, 1997.

178. Whitmarsh AJ, Cavanagh J, Tournier C, et al: A mammalian scaffold complex that selectively mediates MAP kinase activation. Science 281:1671–1674, 1998.

179. Yasuda J, Whitmarsh AJ, Cavanagh J, et al: The JIP group of mitogen-activated protein kinase scaffold proteins. Mol Cell Biol 19:7245–7254, 1999.

180. Kelkar N, Gupta S, Dickens M, et al: Interaction of a mitogen-activated protein kinase signaling module with the neuronal protein JIP3. Mol Cell Biol 20:1030–1043, 2000.

181. Whitmarsh AJ, Kuan CY, Kennedy NJ, et al: Requirement of the JIP1 scaffold protein for stress-induced JNK activation. Genes Dev 15:2421–2432, 2001.

182. Xia Y, Wu Z, Su B, et al: JNKK1 organizes a MAP kinase module through specific and sequential interactions with upstream and downstream components mediated by its amino-terminal extension. Genes Dev 12:3369–3381, 1998.

183. Van Aelst L, D'souza-Schorey C: Rho GTPases and signaling networks. Genes Dev 11:2295–2322, 1997.

184. Coso OA, Chiarello M, Yu J-C, et al: The small GTP binding proteins Rac1 and Cdc42 regulated the activity of the JNK/SAPK signaling pathway. Cell 81:1137–1146, 1995.

185. Minden A, Lin A, Claret F-X, et al: Selective activation of the JNK signaling cascade and c-Jun transcriptional activity by the small GTPases Rac and Cdc42Hs. Cell 81:1147–1157, 1995.

186. Bagrodia S, Dérijard B, Davis RJ, et al: Cdc42 and PAK-mediated signaling leads to Jun kinase and p38 mitogen-activated protein kinase activation. J Biol Chem 270:27995–27998, 1995.

187. Burbelo PD, Drechsel D, Hall A: A conserved binding motif defines numerous candidate target proteins for both Cdc42 and Rac GTPases. J Biol Chem 270:29071–29074, 1995.

188. Tapon N, Nagata K, Lamarche N, et al: A new Rac target POSH is an SH3-containing scaffold protein involved in the JNK and NF-κB signalling pathways. EMBO J 17:1395–1404, 1998.

189. Nagata K, Puls A, Futter C, et al: The MAP kinase kinase kinase MLK2 co-localizes with activated JNK along microtubules and associates with kinesin superfamily motor KIF3. EMBO J 17:149–158, 1998.

190. Rothwarf DM, Karin M: The NF-κB activation pathway: A paradigm in information transfer from membrane to nucleus. Science STKE 1999; *www.stke.org/cgi/content/full/OC_sigtrans; 1999/5/re1.*

191. Hochstrasser M: Ubiquitin-dependent protein degradation. Annu Rev Genet 30:405–439, 1996.

192. Pickart C: Mechanisms underlying ubiquitination. Annu Rev Biochem 70:503–533, 2001.

193. Yaron A, Hatsubai A, Davis M, et al: Identification of the receptor component of the IκBα-ubiquitin ligase. Nature 396:590–594, 1998.

194. Régnier CH, Song HY, Gao X, et al: Identification and characterization of an IκB kinase. Cell 90:373–383, 1997.

195. DiDonato JA, Mayakawa M, Rothwarf DM, et al: A cytokine-responsive IκB kinase that activates the transcription factor NF-κB. Nature 388:548–554, 1997.

196. Zandi E, Rothwarf DM, Delhase M, et al: The IκB kinase complex (IKK) contains two kinase subunits, IKK-α and IKK-β, necessary for IκB phosphorylation and NF-κB activation. Cell 91:243–252, 1997.

197. Woronicz JD, Gao X, Cao Z, et al: IκB kinase-β-NF-κB activation and complex formation with IκB kinase-α and NIK. Science 278:866–869, 1997.

198. Mercurio F, Zhu HY, Murray BW, et al: IKK-1 and IKK-2-cytokine-activated IκB kinases essential for NF-κB activation. Science 278:860–866, 1997.

199. Yamaoka S, Courtois G, Bessia C, et al: Complementation cloning of NEMO, a component of the IκB kinase complex essential for NF-κB activation. Cell 93:1231–1240, 1998.

200. Rothwarf DM, Zandi E, Natoli G, et al: IKK-γ is an essential regulatory subunit of the IκB kinase complex. Nature 395:297–300, 1998.

201. Courtois G, Smahi A, Israel A: NEMO/IKKγ: linking NF-κB to human disease. Trends Mol Med 7:427–430, 2001.

202. Takeda K, Takeuchi O, Tsujimur, T, et al: Limb and skin abnormalities in mice lacking IKKα. Science 284:313–316, 1999.

203. Hu Y, Baun V, Delhase M, et al: Abnormal morphogenesis byt intact IKK activation in mice lacking the IKKα subunit of IκB kinase. Science 284:316–320, 1999.

204. Li Q, Van Antwerp D, Mercurio F, et al: Severe liver degeneration in mice lacking the IκB kinase 2 gene. Science 284:321–325, 1999.

205. Tanaka M, Fuentes ME, Yamaguchi K, et al: Embryonic lethality, liver degeneration, and impaired NF-κB activation in IKK-β-deficient mice. Immunity 10:421–429, 1999.

206. Delhase M, Hayakawa M, Chen Y, et al: Positive and negative regulation of IκB kinase activity through IKKβ subunit phosphorylation. Science 284:309–313, 1999.

207. Smith CA, Farrah T, Goodwin RG: The TNF receptor superfamily of cellular and viral proteins: Activation, costimulation and death. Cell 76:959–962, 1994.

208. Chan FKM, Chun HJ, Zheng LA: Domain in TNF receptors that mediates ligand-independent receptor assembly and signaling. Science 288:2351–2354, 2000.

209. Chen G, Goeddel DV: TNF-R1 signaling: A beautiful pathway. Science 296:1634–1635, 2002.

210. Hsu H, Xiong J, Goeddel DV: The TNF receptor-1-associated protein TRADD signals cell death and NF-κB activation. Cell 81:495–504, 1995.

211. Hsu H, Shu H-B, Pan M-G, et al: TRADD-TRAF2 and TRADD-FADD interactions define two distinct TNF receptor 1 signal transduction pathways. Cell 84:299–308, 1996.

212. Stanger BZ, Leder P, Lee T-H, et al: RIP: A novel protein containing a death domain that interacts with Fas/APO-1 (CD95) in yeast and causes cell death. Cell 81:513–523, 1995.

213. Hsu H, Huang J, Shu H-B, et al: TNF-dependent recruitment of the protein kinase RIP to the TNF receptor-1 signaling complex. Immunity 4:387–396, 1996.

214. Liu Z-g, Hsu H, Goeddel DV, et al: Dissection of TNF receptor-1 effector functions: JNK activation is not linked to apoptosis while NF-κB activation prevents cell death. Cell 87:565–576, 1996.

215. Lee SY, Reichlin A, Santana A, et al: TRAF2 is essential for JNK but not NF-κB activation and regulates lymphocyte proliferation and survival. Immunity 7:703–713, 1997.

216. Yeh W-C, Shahinian A, Speiser D, et al: Early lethality, functional NF-κB activation, and increased sensitivity to TNF-induced cell death in TRAF2-deficient mice. Immunity 7:715–725, 1997.

217. Kelliher MA, Grimm S, Ishida Y, et al: The death domain kinase RIP mediates the TNF-induced NF-κB signal. Immunity 8:297–303, 1998.

218. Lomaga MA, Yeh W-C, Sarosi I, et al: TRAF6 deficiency results in osteopetrosis and defective interleukin-1, CD40, and LPS signaling. Genes Dev 13:1015–1024, 1999.

219. Hofmann RM, Pickart CM: Noncanonical MMS2-encoded ubiquitin-conjugating enzyme functions in assembly of novel polyubiquitin chains for DNA repair. Cell 96:645–653, 1999.

220. Sethi JK, Hotamisligil GS: The role of TNF alpha in adipocyte metabolism. Semin Cell Dev Biol 10:19–29, 1999.

221. Uysal KT, Wiesbrock SM, Marino MW, et al: Protection from obesity-induced insulin resistance in mice lacking TNF-function. Nature 389:610–614, 1997.

222. Hotamisligil GS, Spiegelman BM: Diabetes Mellitus. Philadelphia,Williams & Wilkins, 2000, pp 651–658.

223. Rizzo MT, Leaver AH, Yu WM, et al: Arachidonic acid induces mobilization of calcium stores and s-Jun gene expression: evidence that intracellular

calcium release is associated with c-Jun activation. Prostaglandins Leukot Essent Fatty Acids 60:187–198, 1999.

224. Fujishiro M, Gotoh Y, Katagiri H, et al: Three mitogen-activated protein kinases inhibit insulin signaling by different mechanisms in 3T3-L1 adipocytes. Mol Endocrinol 17:487–497, 2001.

225. Hotamisligil GS, Peraldi P, Budavari A, et al: IRS-1-mediated inhibition of insulin receptor tyrosine kinase activity in TNF- and obesity-induced insulin resistance. Science 271:665–668, 1996.

226. Aguirre V, Uchida T, Yenush L, et al: The Jun NH_2-terminal kinase promotes insulin resistance during association with insulin receptor substrate-1 and phosphorylation of Ser(307) J Biol Chem 275:9047–9054, 2000.

227. Hirosumi J, Tuncman G, Chang L, et al: A central role for JNK in obesity and insulin resistance. Nature 420:333–336, 2002.

228. Jonat C, Rahnsdorf HJ, Park K-K, et al: Antitumor promotion and antiinflammation: Down-modulation of AP-1 (Fos/Jun) activity by glucocorticoid hormone. Cell 62:1189–1204, 1990.

229. Yang-Yen H-F, Chambard J-C, Sun Y-L, et al: Transcription interference between c-Jun and the glucocorticoid receptor: Mutual inhibition of DNA binding due to direct protein-protein interaction. Cell 62:1205–1215, 1990.

230. Schüle R, Rangarajan P, Kliewer S, et al: Functional antagonism between oncoprotein c-Jun and the glucocorticoid receptor. Cell 62:1217–1226, 1990.

231. Bruna A, Nicolàs M, Muñoz A, et al: Glucocorticoid receptor-JNK interaction mediates inhibition of the JNK pathway by glucocorticoids. EMBO J 22:6035–6044, 2003.

Nuclear Receptors: Structure, Function, and Cofactors

Neil J. McKenna and David D. Moore

THE SUPERFAMILY OF NUCLEAR RECEPTORS

THE CLASSIC NUCLEAR RECEPTORS

Receptor proteins transmit information to the cell by sensing the presence (or absence) of their cognate ligand. This transmission process often involves complex, multi-step pathways. The nuclear hormone receptors are a superfamily of transcription factors that short-circuit this process, eliciting biologic responses by directly increasing or repressing the expression of appropriate target genes in response to the binding of specific hormonal or other ligands.

The human genome encodes at least 48 nuclear hormone receptors (Table 15-1). The first member of this superfamily was also the first receptor of any type to be characterized. Jensen and colleagues discovered the estrogen receptor in an early application of radioactive tracers to biology.[1] Subsequent work by many laboratories identified specific receptors for a number of other relatively low-molecular-weight hydrophobic hormones and signaling molecules, including other steroids, thyroid hormone, and all trans-retinoic acid.

An important insight into the function of these receptors was the demonstration by O'Malley and colleagues that steroid hormones directly regulate expression of specific mRNAs.[2] Another key step was the cloning and characterization of the cDNA encoding the glucocorticoid receptor (GR) by the laboratories of Yamamoto, Gustaffson,[3] and Evans.[4] This immediately revealed at least a small family of receptor proteins, based on the striking similarity of the GR sequence to that of the cellular proto-oncogene c-erb-A. c-erb-A was, thus, the first of what is now a much larger group of orphan receptors—members of the superfamily that do not have identified ligands. The rapid subsequent isolation of cDNA clones encoding additional steroid receptors,[5–7] followed later by an unexpected second estrogen receptor isoform, ER-β,[8] highlighted the importance of the structurally conserved DNA-binding and ligand-binding domains shared by the family members, as described later.

The scope of the superfamily increased with the identification of c-erb-A as the thyroid hormone receptor TR-α,[9,10] which was soon joined by its closely related TR-β isoform. Similarly, another orphan identified as a receptor for all trans-retinoic acid (RAR-α)[11,12] was joined by RAR-β and RAR-γ isoforms.

The retinoid X receptors (RXR-α, -β, and -γ) were first described as being activated by an unknown analog of all trans-retinoic acid that was later identified as 9-cis-retinoic acid (9-cis-RA).[13] Although the physiologic importance of 9-cis-RA remains somewhat uncertain, this was the first use of an orphan nuclear receptor to identify a novel endogenous signaling molecule.

The endocrine and physiologic functions of steroids and thyroid hormone are described in depth in other chapters. This chapter reviews the functions of the newer members of the superfamily and the general molecular mechanisms of nuclear receptor function. An online resource for information on nuclear receptors and their cofactors (*www.nursa.org*) is maintained by the Nuclear Receptor Signaling Atlas group.

THE NEW NUCLEAR RECEPTORS

The aforementioned examples of previously unknown nuclear receptors motivated the isolation and characterization of many additional orphan receptors in many laboratories. Many were independently isolated and received several names. Those in most common usage are employed here and in Table 15-1, which also lists systematic names introduced to reduce confusion.

The results with the classic receptors suggested that the members of this rapidly expanding orphan group would have analogous hormonal ligands, combining potent biologic regulatory effects with specific high-affinity receptor binding. In contrast, many of the ligands for the new receptors are endogenous compounds or metabolites that had not generally been associated with direct transcriptional regulatory functions. The normal concentrations of these compounds are much higher than the classic hormones and their affinity for their cognate receptors is correspondingly lower. This contrasts with earlier predictions, but makes sense in retrospect since it allows appropriate signaling responses to variations around the physiologic concentrations of the ligands. The relatively low affinity is often associated with relatively low specificity, thereby allowing groups of compounds much more structurally diverse than conventional hormones to target a single receptor.

PPARs

The peroxisome-proliferator-activated receptor (PPAR-α) was the first receptor associated with such ligands. PPAR-α was initially described as a potential mediator of the hypolipidemic effects of fibrate drugs.[14] This linkage was consistent with the prediction that new receptor ligands should have potent biologic effects. However, the concerns at the time that fibrates and other initially identified PPAR-α ligands are active only at

Table 15-1 Nuclear Hormone Receptor Subgroups

Conventional Receptors	
Classical	**New**
STEROID	**FATTY ACID**
ER-α, -β (NR3A1, 2)	PPAR-α, -δ, -γ (NR1C1-3)
PR (NR3C3)	
AR (NR3C4)	**CHOLESTEROL/BILE ACID**
GR (NR3C1)	LXR-α, -β (NR1H3, 2)
MR (NR3C2)	FXR (NR1H4)
VDR (NR1I1)	
THYROID	**XENOBIOTIC**
TR-α, -β (NR1A1, 2)	PXR (NR1I2), CAR (NR1I3)
RETINOID	
RAR-α, -β, -γ (NR1B1-3)	
RXR-α, RXR-β, RXR-γ (NR2B1-3)	

Orphan Receptors
ERR-α, -β, -γ (NR3B1-3)*
COUP-TFI, II (NR2F1, 2), ear2 (NF2F6)
HNF4-α (NF2A1), HNF4-γ (NR2A2)
SF-1, LRH-1 (NR5A1, 2)
NGF-IB, Nurr1, Nor1 (NR4A1-3)
RevErbA-α, RevErbA-β (NR1D1, 2)
ROR-α, -β, -γ (NR1F1-3)
TR-2, TR-4, (NR 2C1-2),
TLX (NR2E1)
PNR (NR2E3)
GCNF-1 (NR6A1)
SHP (NR0B2)
DAX-1 (NR0B1)

*Synthetic inverse agonist ligands identified. Conventional and orphan receptors are listed based on ligand-binding properties. Many of the nuclear receptors have a number of different names and/or different isoforms generated by alternate splicing or promoter utilization, but only a single commonly used name is included here for each. Closely related receptors are grouped together. See www.nursa.org, or www.enslyon.fr/LBMC/laudet/NucRec/nomenclature_table.html for more comprehensive lists and GenBank access numbers. The standardized nomenclature for the nuclear receptors uses NR followed by a three character code based on evolutionary relatedness, and the standard name is indicated in parentheses for each family member.

relatively high concentrations were heightened when fatty acids were proposed to be the endogenous ligands for PPAR-α[15] and later the additional PPAR-γ and PPAR-δ isoforms (the mammalian PPAR-δ is sometimes referred to as PPAR-β but that name originally belonged to a *Xenopus* isoform). As described later, however, this proposal was strongly supported by structural studies showing that fatty acids can occupy the ligand-binding pockets of the PPARs, which are unusually capacious relative to those of the classic receptors with their high-affinity ligands.[16]

As described in more detail in Chapter 53, it is now clear that PPAR-α functions in the liver to stimulate fatty acid oxidation and PPAR-γ functions in fat cells to promote adipogenesis and expression of fat-specific genes.[17] Importantly, PPAR-γ is the target for the antidiabetic effects of the recently introduced thiazolidinedione (or glitazone) drugs. PPAR-γ also functions in macrophages to promote the return of cholesterol to the liver via the reverse transport pathway.[18] The function of PPAR-δ, which is much more broadly expressed than the other isoforms, is less clear. However, intriguing recent results suggest that PPAR-δ agonists may be therapeutically useful in treatment of hyperlipidemia and possibly other metabolic problems.[19]

LXRs

In addition to these fatty acid activated receptors, a number of former orphans are activated by nonsteroidal cholesterol metabolites. The first of these was liver X receptor (LXR-α), which is activated by hydroxylated cholesterol derivatives called oxysterols.[20] In agreement with its expression in the liver and the identification of these compounds as potential regulators of the expression of proteins involved in cholesterol homeostasis, LXR-α knockout mice showed a profound defect in cholesterol metabolism.[21] Although normal mice are able to manage high levels of dietary cholesterol, the LXR-α knockouts are unable to metabolize and eliminate excess cholesterol, which accumulates in the liver. The closely related LXR-β isoform is also activated by oxysterols and is expressed in a number of tissues, including the liver, but the phenotype of the LXR-α knockout animals demonstrates that LXR-β is unable to fully compensate for the loss of the former isoform.

The phenotype of the LXR-α knockout raised the possibility that LXR agonists could be useful in treatment of hypercholesterolemia. Unfortunately, synthetic LXR agonists significantly increase triglyceride levels in rodent models.[22] This undesirable side effect is associated with the induction of the transcription factor SREBP-1c, which promotes fatty acid synthesis. However, pharmacologic studies demonstrate that LXRs also function with PPAR-γ in the process of reverse cholesterol transport from the periphery to the liver.[23] Thus, LXR agonists may have beneficial effects in both the liver and the periphery if their effects on triglycerides can be circumvented.

FXR

Farnesoid X receptor (FXR) is another former orphan that functions in cholesterol homeostasis. It is activated by bile acids,[24-26] downstream metabolites of cholesterol that are produced in high amounts in the liver and are essential for absorption of dietary lipids. Despite their efficient reabsorption in the gut, release of both bile acids and cholesterol from the liver in bile is the major pathway of cholesterol elimination from the body. The potential function of FXR in bile acid and cholesterol homeostasis is supported by results with knockout animals, which show significant defects in these processes.[27] These abnormalities include the inability to appropriately downregulate hepatic bile acid biosynthesis and uptake in response to increased bile acid levels. This suggests that FXR functions to protect against elevated bile acid levels, which can cause severe hepatotoxicity, and recent results with synthetic FXR agonists show protective effects in rodent models of cholestasis.[28]

Like the cholesterol efflux from macrophages, the FXR-mediated negative regulation of bile acid production is apparently also a consequence of a nuclear receptor cascade. In this case, bile acid activation of FXR results in increased expression of an unusual orphan receptor named short heterodimer partner (SHP), which lacks a DNA-binding domain and functions to inhibit transactivation by other nuclear receptors. Another orphan receptor, LRH-1 (also known as FTF), is both particularly sensitive to this repression and essential for the expression of the rate-limiting enzyme in bile acid biosynthesis, encoded by the *Cyp7A1* gene. Thus, the induction of FXR by bile acids results in decreased *Cyp7A1* expression via a pathway dependent on both SHP and LRH-1.[29,30]

FXR regulates the expression of many other genes in the liver and intestine and, like the LXRs, is a potential therapeutic target for treatment of dyslipidemias. In particular, FXR agonists decrease elevated levels of serum triglycerides in rodents via a process that appears to reflect decreased production of very-low-density lipoproteins by the liver.[31] As with the synthetic LXR agonists, it remains unclear whether these effects are also observed in humans.

CAR and PXR

Constitutive androstane receptor (CAR) and pregnane X receptor (PXR) are two closely related receptors that are evolutionarily related to LXR-α, LXR-β, and FXR. They are also expressed in the liver and function to regulate metabolic pathways.

It has been known for millenia that exposure to small amounts of harmful agents can sometimes produce resistance to their effects. Pharmacologists have known for decades that high levels of particular drugs and other foreign compounds, collectively termed *xenobiotics*, induce the expression of a number of cytochrome P450 and other drug-metabolizing enzymes in the liver.[32] This is generally considered a beneficial response that protects against potentially toxic compounds. In some cases, however, the induction of such enzymes can increase production of toxic metabolites. The activation of drug metabolism by one agent can also lead to clinically significant drug-drug interactions in which the clearance of coadministered drugs is increased and their effectiveness is correspondingly decreased.

CAR and PXR are promiscuous receptors that are activated by many structurally diverse compounds and mediate their ability to induce such responses.[33,34] An unusual feature of these xenobiotic receptors is the relatively low evolutionary conservation of amino acid sequences of their ligand-binding domains. This results in highly variable responses to different sets of agonist ligands in different species, which resolves the previously puzzling discrepancies in drug metabolism. For example, human PXR is potently activated by the antibiotic rifampicin, a well-known inducer of the broad-spectrum drug-metabolizing enzyme Cyp3A4 in humans, but it has no such effect on either mouse PXR or mouse liver.[35]

The functions of PXR and CAR are overlapping, but not identical, at the levels of both their activators and the genes they regulate. Among a number of previously defined pharmacologic effects, PXR mediates the paradoxical ability of a series of both steroids and steroid receptor antagonists, collectively termed *catatoxic steroids*, to induce drug metabolism.[35] The barbiturate drug phenobarbital induces a characteristic xenobiotic response that centers on Cyp2b enzymes and is mediated by CAR, which also directs similar responses to other "phenobarbital-like" inducers.[36] Some agents, such as the antifungal drug clotrimazole, can activate both xenobiotic receptors. Their effects on target genes also overlap, and both can induce expression of a series of cytochrome P450 and other broad-specificity drug-metabolizing enzymes and transporters.

Interestingly, the xenobiotic receptors are also activated by potentially deleterious endogenous compounds. Hydrophobic bile acids are particularly toxic but they can be detoxified by the same enzymes induced by xenobiotics. Thus, prior activation of either CAR or PXR can completely block their toxic effects in mouse models.[37,38] Because both receptors can be activated by elevated levels of bile acids, it is likely that they exert protective effects in cholestasis that complement those of FXR. In addition, phenobarbital has been known for many years to increase hepatic bilirubin clearance in patients. Recent studies indicate that this effect is mediated by CAR and suggest that it is a potential therapeutic target in jaundice.[39]

THE ORPHAN NUCLEAR RECEPTORS

Much less is known about those members of the nuclear receptor superfamily that remain orphans. In several cases, however, key insights from knockouts or other sources that have revealed potential impacts on endocrine or metabolic pathways will be briefly outlined here. Recent reviews detail the intriguing developmental and other functions that have emerged for other superfamily members.[40–45]

SF-1

In contrast to the isolation of many of the orphans using molecular cloning approaches such as low-stringency hybridization, steroidogenic factor-1 (SF-1) was first identified based on its ability to coordinately activate their expression of genes encoding steroid hydroxylases by binding a series of

related sites in their promoters.[46] Also, unlike the majority of nuclear receptors that bind DNA as dimers, SF-1 belongs to the smaller group that binds as monomers. Like many other orphans, however, SF-1 functions as an apparently constitutive transcriptional activator.

The function of SF-1 in regulation of adrenal steroidogenesis was significantly expanded by the observation that the loss of SF-1 function in mice resulted in the absence of adrenals, gonads, and the ventromedial hypothalamus, as well as male-to-female sex reversal of internal and external genitalia.[47] As recently reviewed,[48] SF-1 is, thus, a key regulator of the development of important endocrine tissues.

HNF-4

Hepatocyte nuclear factor-4α (HNF-4α) is another orphan originally identified based on its ability to recognize specific sites, in this case in various promoters active in the liver.[49] It binds these elements as a homodimer. Additional studies revealed that it is also expressed in the kidney, intestine, and pancreas, particularly the insulin-producing β cells. A wide variety of target genes have been identified, including genes involved with fatty acid and cholesterol metabolism, glucose metabolism, urea biosynthesis, and liver differentiation.[50] HNF-4α null mouse embryos die at a very early stage of development. The heterozygotes do not show an obvious phenotype, but in humans heterozygous loss of HNF-4α results in defective pancreatic β cell function and a characteristic syndrome called mature-onset diabetes of the young (MODY).[51] HNF-4α is MODY1; heterozygous loss of function of several other nonreceptor transcription factors that function in the β cell results in a similar phenotype.

SHP and DAX-1

Small heterodimer partner (SHP) and dosage-sensitive sex reversal adrenal hypoplasia congenita critical region on the X chromosome (DAX-1) are unique orphan receptors that lack a nuclear receptor DNA-binding domain. SHP can interact directly with a number of other nuclear receptors and inhibit their ability to activate transcription.[52] As noted previously, results with SHP knockouts supported a specific role proposed for SHP in an FXR-dependent pathway for negative feedback regulation of bile acid biosynthesis. Interestingly, there are apparently additional, redundant mechanisms for this process, since SHP null mice do show the expected loss of repression in response to a synthetic FXR agonist, but largely maintain the repressive effect of high levels of dietary bile acids.[29,30]

In contrast to SHP, which consists solely of a ligand-binding domain, DAX-1 includes an additional N-terminal domain.[53] This domain has been associated with various DNA-binding activities, but the significance of this potential function remains uncertain. Loss of function of the human DAX-1 gene causes an X-linked form of adrenal hypoplasia congenita that is associated with hypogonadotropic hypogonadism.[53] Like SHP, DAX-1 functions as a transcriptional repressor and it is thought that loss of this repression function accounts for this phenotype. The transcriptional targets of DAX-1 remain unknown but several lines of evidence, including direct interaction and similar patterns of expression, suggest that it modulates SF-1 function.[54]

NUCLEAR RECEPTOR STRUCTURE

Comparison of the initial steroid receptor sequences with each other and c-erb-A revealed two conserved segments that were soon identified as separate functional modules for binding specific DNA sequences and hormones. They are referred to as the DNA-binding domain (DBD) and ligand-binding domain (LBD) and, as shown in Figure 15-1, are separated by a nonconserved linker segment of variable length. The DBD is often preceded by an N-terminal segment that can be

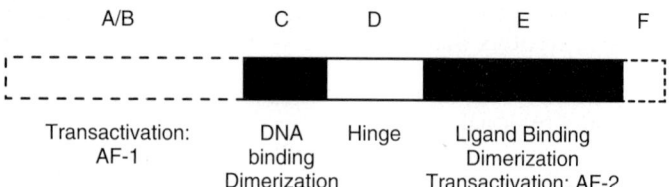

Figure 15-1 Modular structure of nuclear hormone receptors. The most highly conserved domain is the DNA-binding domain, DBD, followed by the ligand-binding domain, LBD. The domains are sometimes also referred to by their alphabetic designations. Functions of the domains are indicated. The N-terminal or A/B domain is highly variable in length and sequence and is not present in some receptors. The F domain is present in only a limited number of receptors and is also not conserved in sequence. Its functions have generally not been well characterized, but it is thought to modulate transactivation in some cases.

relatively large but is not conserved, even among isoforms of the same receptor. Particularly for the steroid receptors, this N-terminal or A/B domain has intrinsic transcriptional activation function. This activity, referred to as activation function 1 (AF-1), is distinct from the ligand-dependent activation function of the LBD, called AF-2, though the two often function coordinately.

A more limited number of receptors have short C-terminal extensions (F domain) after the LBD. These are often dispensable for basic transcriptional regulation but may have modulatory functions.

DNA-BINDING DOMAINS

The DNA-binding sites recognized by the receptors are called hormone response elements (HREs), and are present in pro-moters and regulatory regions of receptor target genes. Nuclear hormone receptors bind three different types of response elements. Except for the estrogen receptors (ERs), the steroid receptors function as homodimers and recognize two copies of a hexameric sequence related to the consensus 5' AGAACA 3', which are separated by 3 base pairs and arranged as a head-to-head inverted repeat. More than a dozen of the other nuclear receptor family members bind DNA as heterodimers with the RXRs; nearly all are either classic receptors (TRs, RARs, VDR) or new receptors (PPARs, LXRs, FXR, CAR, PXR). Surprisingly, the RXRs, their heterodimer partners, the ERs, and nearly all of the orphan receptors recognize hexameric motifs related to a consensus, 5' AGGTCA 3,' which is similar to that bound by the other steroid receptors. Most of these complexes bind as dimers, but several orphan receptors can bind the same hexameric consensus element as monomers. In this mode, a C-terminal extension of the DBD makes additional base-specific contacts upstream of the hexamer, with different receptors recognizing different sequences. The structures of homodimeric, heterodimeric, and monomeric receptor–DNA complexes are shown in Figure 15-2.

The ability of the vast majority of the receptors to recognize the AGGTCA consensus creates an obvious specificity problem that is addressed, in part, by variations in the spacing and arrangement of the two hexameric binding sites. For example, TR/RXR heterodimers recognize direct repeats of this hexamer separated by 4 base pairs, while RAR/RXR and VDR/RXR heterodimers prefer 5-base-pair and 3-base-pair spacers, respectively.[55] These rules are not absolute, since the receptor complexes are remarkably flexible and can often bind multiple types of elements. TR/RXR complexes, for example, can also bind head-to-head inverted repeats of the hexamer with no spacer, as well as tail-to-tail or everted repeats separated by 6 base pairs. Based on the diversity of sites for a single receptor complex and the large number of receptors, it is not surprising

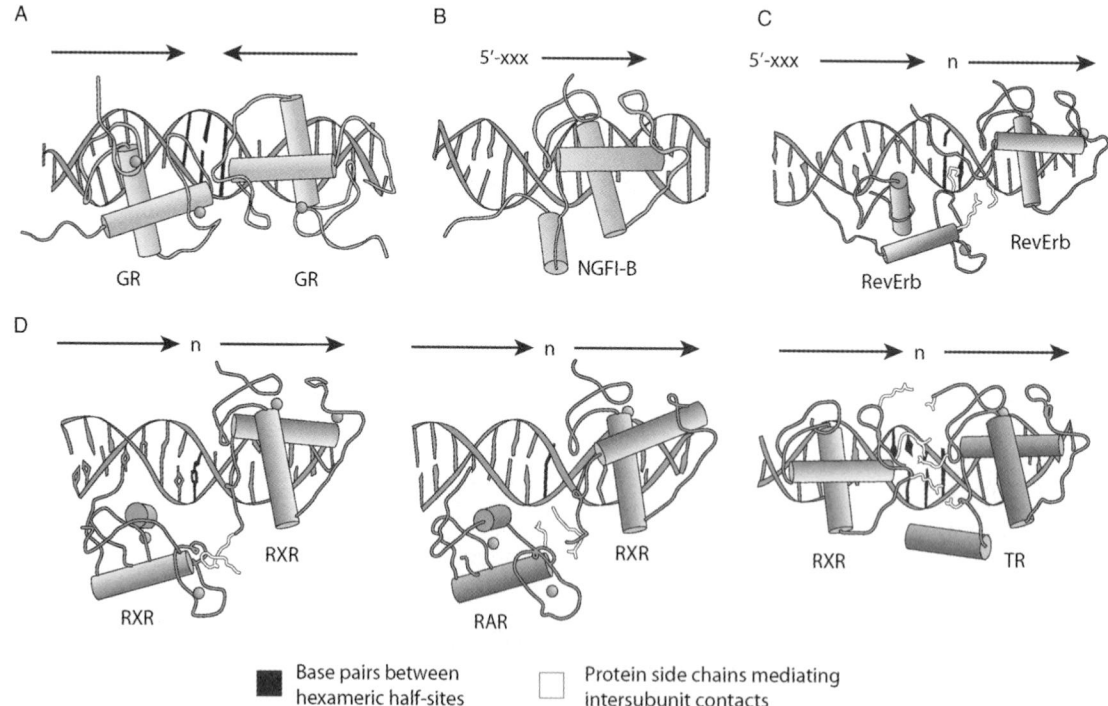

Figure 15-2 Structures of complexes between receptor DNA-binding domains and their cognate DNA-response elements. **A,** GR homodimer bound to an inverted element with a 3-base-pair spacer (IR-3). **B,** NGFI-B bound to its extended monomeric site. **C,** RevErb homodimer bound to an extended direct repeat element with a 2-base-pair spacer (DR-2) and **D,** RXR as a homodimer bound to a DR-1 element, RAR/RXR on a DR-1 element and TR/RXR heterodimer bound to a DR-4 site. Note that RXR binds only at the upstream half-site on the DR-4 HRE with TR, and only at the downstream half-site on the DR-1 with RAR. Cylinders indicate helices, base pairs between the hexameric half-sites are shown in red, and protein side chains mediating intersubunit contacts are shown in yellow. (Reproduced with permission from Khorasanizadeh S, Rastinejad F: Nuclear-receptor interactions on DNA-response elements. Trends Biochem Sci 26:384–390, 2001.) (See Color Plate.)

that a particular element can often be recognized by multiple receptor complexes. Although they are not well defined, additional mechanisms such as cell- and tissue-specific expression of receptors and cofactors, as well as differential interactions with other transcription factors, must allow specific receptors to appropriately regulate their target genes.

No complete structures are available for any receptor, despite extensive efforts, but high-resolution x-ray crystal structures have been solved for complexes of DBDs with their response elements and also LBDs with or without various ligands and/or cofactor peptides. The DBDs are primarily α-helical, compact units of 66 to 68 amino acids that fold around two Zn[++] ions, each of which is coordinated by four invariant cysteine residues. The receptor DBDs are frequently described as "zinc fingers," but this is not strictly accurate since they are folded together in a single unit and are not functionally independent.

As shown in Figure 15-2 and recently reviewed,[56] the structures of appropriate DBDs and response elements provide detailed information on the distinct modes of binding. For the homodimeric steroid receptors, the structures reveal specific head-to-head protein-protein contacts that lock the two DBDs in position to bind the two inverted hexamers.[57] Since the hexamers are separated by approximately one turn of the double helix, the two monomers bind the same face of the helix. A similar mode of binding is evident from the structures of some of the RXR complexes, but different head-to-tail contacts with RXR position the various partners appropriately and allow the complexes to recognize different direct-repeat-response elements.[58]

Like many other transcription factors, specific DNA contacts are made by residues present in short α helices. The highly conserved but distinct sequences of the primary recognition helix, termed the *P-box*,[59] account for the ability of the steroid receptors and the other members of the superfamily to bind the two distinct hexameric consensus sites. The receptors that bind as monomers also use two helices to make specific DNA contacts, with the additional helix coming from the C-terminal extension of the conserved DBD.[60]

LIGAND-BINDING DOMAINS

In addition to binding ligand, LBDs function in receptor dimerization and transcriptional activation. The molecular mechanisms for all of these functions have been revealed by numerous x-ray crystal structures of LBDs. Despite a rather low degree of primary sequence conservation across the superfamily, the overall LBD structure is highly conserved and is typically described as an antiparallel three-layered sandwich of 12 α helices. In the conventional receptors, a portion of the middle layer is missing, creating a pocket for the ligand, which, by convention, is considered the lower portion of the structure.

The structures of the ligand-occupied steroid, thyroid hormone, and retinoic acid receptors are quite consistent with the high affinity and specificity of their ligands. The hormone fits very tightly into the pocket, making multiple favorable contacts with the residues that line it. Importantly, ligand binding results in appropriate positioning of the C-terminal helix 12, which forms a hydrophobic cleft with portions of helices 3, 4, and 5. This surface is the binding site for the large number of transcriptional coactivators that mediate nuclear receptor transactivation of gene expression, and allosteric modulation of the structure of helix 12 is the molecular mechanism for the modulation of the AF-2 transcriptional activation function of the LBD by ligand (Figure 15-3).

The contact between activated nuclear receptors (NRs) and coactivators is mediated primarily by a surprisingly short conserved element found in most coactivators, the LXXLL motif or NR-box.[61] The conserved leucine residues of the

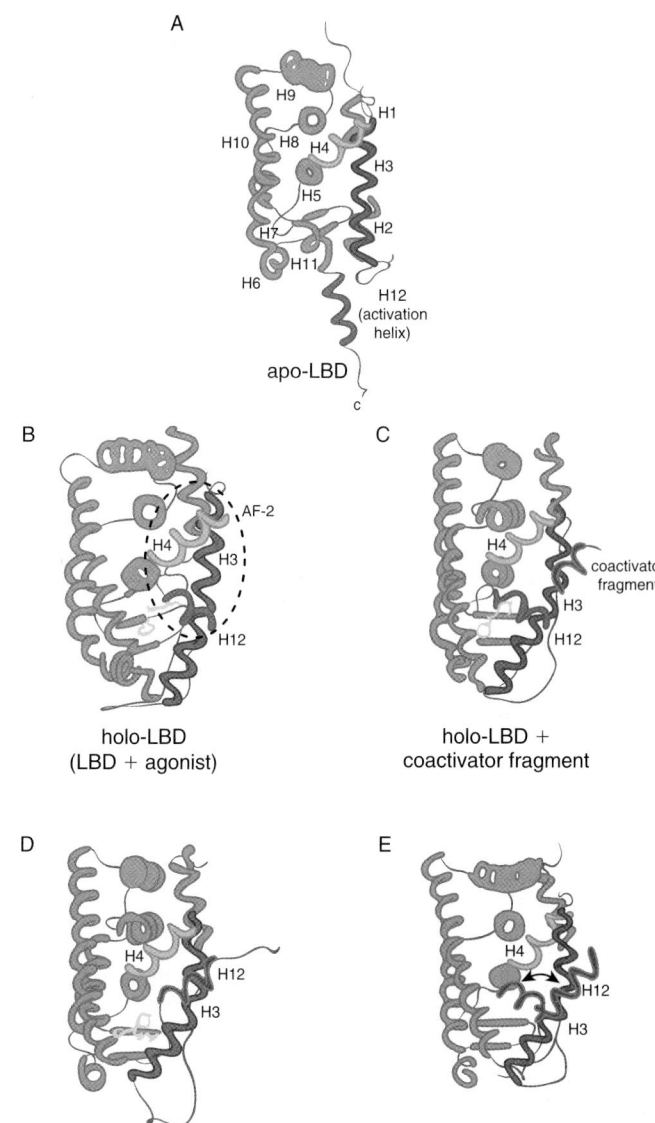

Figure 15-3 Diagrams of LBDs of representative NRs. Protein, green; helix 3, blue; helix 4, pink; ligands, yellow; helix 12, red; LXXLL motif of coactivators, violet. Helices are numbered 1 to 12 as reported for the first NR structure, RXR. **A,** The apo-form of RXR, the binding site of which is not accessible to ligand (PDB entry code 1lbd). **B,** 8pThe binary complex of RAR and all trans-retinoic acid in the transcriptionally active form (PDB entry code 2lbd). **C,** The ternary complex of ER, distilbestrol, and a fragment of the coactivator GRIP, which contains the LXXLL motif (PDB entry code 3erd). This structure represents the transcriptionally active form of NRs and indicates the binding site of coactivators. **D,** The binary complex of ER and the selective ER modulator tamoxifen (PDB entry code 3ert). This structure represents a transcriptionally inactive form of NRs where helix 12 is located in the binding site of coactivators. **E,** The binary complex of ER and the partial agonist genistein (PDB entry code 1qkm). In the crystal structure, helix 12 is located in the coactivator-binding groove. Helix 12 as observed in the transcriptionally active form of NRs is superimposed in order to illustrate the alternative positioning of helix 12 in complexes of NRs with partial agonists as underlined by the double pointed arrow. (Reproduced with permission from Steinmetz AC, Renaud JP, Moras D: Binding of ligands and activation of transcription by nuclear receptors. Annu Rev Biophys Biomol Struct 30:329–359, 2001.)

coactivator NR-box are found on the same face of an amphipathic helix and fit into the hydrophobic cleft. Coactivator binding is also supported by charge-based interactions between conserved receptor residues and the helical backbone of the coactivator motif that are referred to as the "charge clamp."[61]

Agonist ligands often stabilize the appropriate position of helix 12 by hydrogen bonding or other direct interactions. In contrast, antagonist ligands force it to adopt alternate conformations that do not allow coactivator binding. In examples such as 4-hydroxytamoxifen, a portion of the antagonist extends into the space where helix 12 would be found in an activated receptor and displaces it.[62] This helix is also amphipathic and the hydrophobic face can fold back onto the receptor surface to occupy the remainder of the coactivator cleft. As with the agonists, antagonists can also disrupt the AF-2 structure by less direct means.

In contrast to this hand-in-glove mode of binding for the classic receptors, the ligand-binding pocket can be much bigger than the ligands for the new receptors. For example, eicosapentaenoic acid occupies only a fraction of the ligand pocket of PPAR-δ, with the acyl side chain adopting two quite different structures that are each supported by weak hydrophobic interactions with distinct residues that line the pocket.[16] Based on this, it is not surprising that many different fatty acids can bind PPAR-δ and the other isoforms with similar affinities, or that ligands such as the synthetic thiazolidinediones fill the PPAR-γ pocket more completely and bind with much higher affinity and specificity. As with the conventional hormone receptors, both low affinity and high affinity agonists for the more promiscuous receptors function to stabilize the active conformation of helix 12.

Crystal structures have revealed unexpected features of the LBDs of orphan receptors. In some cases, unexpected constituents have been observed in the ligand-binding pocket. The fatty acids in the HNF-4α pocket[63,64] and the cholesterol in the retinoid-related orphan receptor α (ROR-α) pocket[65] presumably bound to and stabilized them in the E. coli host used to express the crystallized LBDs. Particularly for HNF-4α, studies indicate that the fatty acids are essentially permanent occupants of the cavity that do not modulate receptor function and may be more analogous to the Zn^{++} atoms in the DBD than to conventional ligands.

In the LRH-1 structure, the AF-2 surface is in the active conformation but the pocket is empty.[66] It is likely that endogenous ligands will be identified for this orphan and its close relative SF-1. In contrast, the potential pocket of Nurr1 is fully occupied by bulky amino acid side chains.[67] It has been speculated that this may actually be the primordial LBD structure, particularly since apparently ligand-independent orphan receptors are the most highly conserved superfamily members in distantly related species.[68] The HNF-4α structure suggests that the transition to hormone responsiveness may have begun with the mutation of a bulky side chain in the hydrophobic core to a smaller residue, resulting in a pocket that could have been occupied initially by structural ligands.

Crystal structures also reveal the basis for the dimerization function of the LBDs. Parallel contacts between helix 10 in each monomer form the primary interface, with additional contacts made between helix 7, the loop between helices 8 and 9 on one side, and between helix 9 and the N-terminus of helix 10 on the other. Steroid receptors and RXR homodimers are symmetric, but this symmetry is slightly disrupted in the RXR heterodimers. A recent analysis suggests that all receptors can be identified as homodimerizing or heterodimerizing based on only a few differentially conserved LBD residues that affect this interface.[69] However, the structure of the GR LBD indicates that it uses a quite different dimerization strategy based on interactions between beta-sheets.[70]

REGULATION OF GENE EXPRESSION BY NUCLEAR RECEPTORS

BASIC COACTIVATORS

Soon after the existence of limiting transcriptional cofactors was first suggested by studies in yeast, evidence for their function in nuclear receptor transactivation was provided by competitive effects between receptors or with receptors and other transcription factors. The demonstration of hormone-dependent recruitment of specific proteins to the activated estrogen receptor[61,71] was followed by the isolation of cDNAs encoding ligand receptor interacting proteins in many laboratories. Functional studies confirmed that such ligand-dependent receptor interactors can act as coactivators to support hormone-dependent transcriptional activation.

Two primary aspects of the multi-step process of transcriptional activation are: (1) counteracting the inherent repressive effects of the packaging of genes into chromatin, and (2) recruiting RNA polymerase and the basal transcriptional apparatus to the promoter. The theme that has emerged is that binding of a ligand-activated receptor to an appropriate target gene results in the recruitment of a surprisingly large number of multi-protein complexes that mediate these effects via a variety of enzymatic activities.

DNA packed into chromatin is obviously less accessible than free DNA, and chromatin plays a dominant repressive role in the basal activity of genes in eukaryotic cells. As shown in Figure 15-4, recruitment of complexes designed to overcome this constraint is thought to be an early step in receptor-dependent transcriptional activation. Among the best characterized of these are a series of multi-protein complexes that contain one of two ATPase subunits, called BRG1 and brahma, which are related to the yeast protein SNF2. They are referred to as SWI/SNF complexes based on similarities to the complex originally described in yeast. Both the yeast and mammalian complexes use the energy from adenosine triphosphate (ATP) hydrolysis to remodel nucleosomes, rendering them more accessible to transcription factors.[72] In at least some cases, their function is essential for nuclear receptor transactivation.[73]

Local regulation of histone-histone and histone-DNA interactions is also mediated by the three members of the steroid receptor coactivator (SRC)/p160 family, which were among the first NR coactivators identified. These large proteins, which have received many names (SRC-1/NCoA-1; GRIP-1/TIF2/SRC-2; and p/CIP/ACTR/AIB-1/RAC-3/TRAM-1/SRC-3), contain a number of shared domains.[74] These include both a central region containing repeating LxxLL NR-boxes and an intrinsic histone acetyltransferase activity. The repressive transcriptional effect of histones is due, in part, to electrostatic contacts between their positively charged lysine side chains and negatively charged DNA phosphate groups. By acetylating histone lysine residues, SRC family members can disrupt these inhibitory interactions.

CREB-binding protein and its close relative p300 are other well-characterized NR coactivators that function in multi-protein complexes with the SRC/p160 family members.[74] These even larger multifunctional proteins are referred to as transcriptional integrators based on their ability to mediate transactivation by many other transcription factors in addition to nuclear receptors. They are apparently recruited to nuclear receptor target genes via their direct interactions with the SRC/p160 proteins and their potent intrinsic acetyltransferase activities may play a predominant role in the receptor-dependent histone acetylation.

A third prominent coactivator complex called TRAP or DRIP based on its functional interactions with the TRs or VDR was initially identified in biochemical screens for proteins recruited by activated thyroid hormone receptor[75] and vitamin D receptor (VDR).[76] Subsequent studies showed that

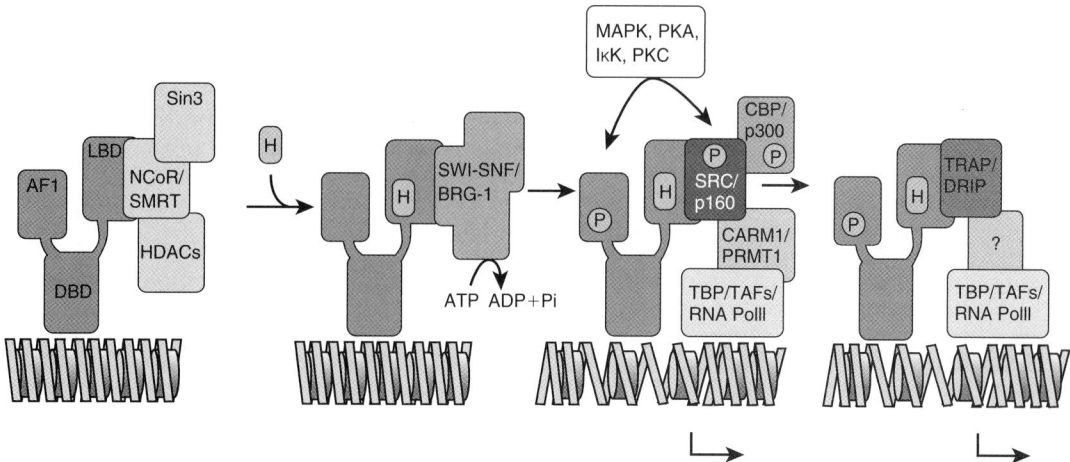

Figure 15-4 Model of combinatorial NR-mediated transcriptional initiation. Initial binding of ligand results in dissociation of corepressors and recruitment of SWI/SNF chromatin remodeling machines to modify chromatin domains. Binding of SRCs and CBP results in local acetyltransferase activity and disruption of local nucleosomal structure. Kinase-mediated signaling pathways may communicate directly with NR-regulated promoters. AF-1 phosphorylation might serve to further consolidate ligand-dependent NR-SRC interactions or to recruit SRCs directly to the promoter in the absence of ligand. TRAP/DRIP directly contacts components of the basal transcription machinery to effect transcriptional initiation, and certain TAFs may afford some additional input into promoter-specific NR transcription. The extent of overlap in binding of complexes to the promoter is currently unclear. Local coactivator requirements may vary, for example, a promoter in a readily accessible chromatin context may not require significant chromatin remodeling or histone acetyltransferase activity for assembly of a preinitiation complex. (Reproduced with permission from McKenna NJ, O'Malley BW: Combinatorial control of gene expression by nuclear receptors and coregulators. Cell 108:465–474, 2002.)

TRAP/DRIP contains a single subunit with NR-boxes that contact nuclear receptors, as well as other subunits that are targets for other transcription factors. A number of the TRAP/DRIP subunits complex are also components of the large RNA polymerase II holoenzyme complex; it is thought that the TRAP/DRIP complex functions at a later stage in the activation process to contact the basal transcriptional machinery and directly contribute to the recruitment of RNA polymerase II (see Fig. 15-3).

Nuclear receptors can recruit a number of additional chromatin remodeling complexes, particularly those associated with other histone modifications such as lysine methylation. The potential complexity of this process is exemplified by the recent description of a complex that contains both the histone methyltransferase CARM1 and components of the SWI/SNF complex, including the ATPase BRG1.[77] It is apparent from this and many other examples that various subunits with distinct functions and intrinsic enzymatic activities can join together in different complexes that are stable enough to be isolated by biochemical strategies, but also quite dynamic in the cell.

This is consistent with the surprisingly rapid intranuclear movement of the receptors and their cofactors. Analysis of individual promoters indicates that receptors recruit different cofactor complexes at different times, with individual complexes cycling in and out over time scales of minutes after hormone addition.[78] Recent imaging studies of live cells suggest that the shuttling process may be even more rapid, with steroid receptors and coactivators occupying their HREs for only seconds before being displaced.[79]

SELECTIVE COACTIVATORS

Remarkably, current estimates suggest that the number of coactivators exceeds the number of nuclear receptors by at least three-fold (see www.nursa.org/ for an up-to-date catalog of coactivators). Thus, the basic transcription activation functions just outlined are by no means the only activities of the myriad proteins recruited to the DNA by the nuclear receptors. These functions are still emerging and only two primary aspects will be outlined here. The first is effects of coactivators

on steps in the complex process of gene expression that lie outside of transcriptional initiation. Recent results indicate that proteins recruited to the promoter by nuclear receptors can affect both the rate by which RNA polymerase transcribes the target gene and the nature of the spliced mRNAs produced from the transcript. Thus, receptor interaction with both positive[80] and negative[81] modulators of transcriptional elongation has been reported to stimulate or inhibit gene expression, respectively. A larger number of reports describe effects of several nuclear receptor coactivators on either splicing efficiency or the differential generation of alternative spliced products.[82,83] Alternative splicing accounts for the expression of more than 100,000 proteins from the approximately 30,000 genes in the human genome, and the alternate products can have quite different functions. While the generality and importance of the effects of nuclear receptors on this process remain to be established, the impact of hormonal modulation of the final product of gene expression may rival that of the modulation of the amount of gene expression.

Another possible rationale for the existence of multiple coactivators is specific effects on particular target genes or tissues. One could imagine a cofactor expressed in only a limited number of cells or tissues that would mediate specific effects on appropriate receptor target genes. Although there are not many examples of such coactivator-dependent specificity, PPAR gamma coactivator-1α (PGC-1α) provides a particularly interesting one. Originally identified as a coactivator for PPAR-γ, it is now clear that it can stimulate transactivation by other nuclear receptors and, importantly, NRF-1 and NFR-2, transcription factors that regulate expression of genes in mitochondrial biogenesis.[84] The remarkably potent induction of expression of PGC-1α in brown adipose tissue in response to cold stress results in a dramatic increase in heat production, which is due to both increased number of mitochondria and nuclear receptor–dependent expression of the mitochondrial energy uncoupling protein UCP-1.[85] Regulation of PGC-1α levels also modulates energy balance and metabolism in other contexts, including the fasting liver, where its increased expression promotes expression of nuclear receptor target genes required for gluconeogenesis, such as phosphenolpyruvate carboxy kinase.[86]

COREPRESSORS

A much more limited number of corepressors interact with unliganded aporeceptors and, in some cases, antagonist-bound receptors, to mediate their transcriptional repressive effects. In many ways, the molecular mechanisms of this repression mirror the manner in which coactivators effect transcriptional activation. The best characterized nuclear receptor corepressors are two very large, related proteins, nuclear receptor corepressor (NCoR)[87] and silencing mediator for thyroid and retinoid receptors (SMRT),[88] which bind the same surface of the LBD as the coactivators when the C-terminal helix 12 is displaced from the active conformation. Like the coactivators, the corepressors contain multiple copies of a short amphipathic helical motif called the "CoRNR box" that contacts this surface.[89] Corepressors also are functionally analogous to coactivators in that their opposite transcriptional effects are a consequence of an inverse effect on histone acetylation. Neither NCoR nor SMRT possesses intrinsic histone deacetylase activity, but both are components of multi-protein complexes that include such activities.

TRANSREPRESSION

It is well known that nuclear receptor ligands repress expression of many target genes. Prominent examples described in more detail elsewhere are the negative feedback regulation of the expression of pro-opiomelanocortin (POMC) and corticotrophin-releasing hormone by glucocorticoids, and of the two thyroid-stimulating hormone subunits (TSH-α and TSH-β) by thyroid hormone.

Although these and other negative targets have been extensively studied, no clear single mechanism has emerged. One common pathway involves the inhibition of the positive effects of other transcription factors by ligand-activated receptors, resulting in a net decrease in gene expression. The details of this inhibition are not well understood. However, it often relies on protein-protein interactions and does not require specific DNA binding by the activated receptors. In some contexts, coactivators such as SRC-2/Grip1 somehow exert negative, rather than positive, effects when recruited to the complex of GR and another transcription factor.[90] As noted later in the section on cross-talk, the transcription factors inhibited by the nuclear receptors, including AP-1 and NF-κB, are, themselves, often the mediators of other signaling pathways.

In a different mechanism, it is hypothesized that binding of the activated receptor to unusual negative HREs in some of the repressed genes results in allosteric effects that somehow alter receptor function. For example, the negative glucocorticoid response element in the POMC gene is thought to sequentially bind a GR homodimer to one side of the helix followed by binding a monomer to the other side.[91] However, it is not clear why this results in the observed hormone-dependent repression, and other mechanisms, including inhibition of the positive effects of the orphan receptor Nur77 by the activated GR,[92] are thought to contribute to the potent repression of pituitary POMC expression by glucocorticoids.

SELECTIVE LIGANDS

An individual LxxLL motif or NR-box in a particular coactivator has the potential to bind each of the nuclear receptors, but the affinities of these interactions are quite variable. Based on the different functions and activities of the different coactivators, the responses elicited by binding an agonist to a receptor in any given cell will be a complex function of the level of expression of individual coactivators in that cell and their inherent affinity for the activated receptor. Importantly, this affinity is very sensitive to even small differences in agonist structure. This was clearly demonstrated by studies using a number of LxxLL peptides individually selected for their ability to bind ER-α activated by different agonists, which revealed that each compound recruited a different subset of peptides.[93] Thus, in contrast to the overall conservation and rigidity of the structures of the activated receptors that might be expected from the x-ray crystallography results, even closely related compounds can have different effects on LBD structure that can result in recruitment of distinct coactivators.

Recruitment of distinct subsets of coactivators is a primary mechanism for the selective biologic effects of various synthetic nuclear receptor ligands that are collectively referred to as *selective receptor modulators*. As described in more detail in Chapter 152 and recently reviewed,[94] such effects were first characterized for the estrogen receptors and have been particularly well studied for selective estrogen receptor modulators, such as tamoxifen, which was originally thought to be a receptor antagonist but was later shown to have agonist estrogenic effects in target tissues such as bone. These initially enigmatic effects are a consequence of the ability of the tamoxifen-bound ERs to appropriately homodimerize and bind DNA. This results in transcriptional activation in tissues that contain coactivators able to mediate the ligand-independent effects of the divergent AF-1 domains. As described previously, tamoxifen binding actively disrupts the ER-α AF-2 surface, so in cells that lack AF-1 coactivators but contain the general AF-2 specific coactivators, tamoxifen blocks estrogenic effects by competing with the hormone for LBD binding.

The selective effects of distinct ligands on nuclear receptor function in different cells are by no means limited to the steroid receptors. The apparently more flexible receptors with relatively low affinity for their endogenous ligands may be even more susceptible to such effects. Several PPAR-γ agonists with differential impact on AF-2 coactivator recruitment and distinct biologic activities have been described. For example, one PPAR-γ specific non-thiazolidinedione agonist with differential effects on coactivator recruitment was reported to retain beneficial effects on insulin sensitivity but to lack adipogenic effects.[95]

A variety of very powerful tools including molecular modeling, combinatorial chemistry, and high-throughput screening are available to identify and characterize selective receptor modulators. Thus, it seems possible in principle to identify specific ligands that "dial in" desirable therapeutic effects by promoting recruitment of particular coactivators and "dial out" undesirable side effects by blocking the recruitment of others. Substantial effort is being invested in this topic for a number of nuclear receptor targets. At the present time, however, the daunting complexity of cofactor function precludes rational design of compounds with desirable properties or even the development of high-throughput assays to identify them. In the future, the combination of insights into the function of multiple coactivators with large-scale genomic/proteomic analysis of their detailed expression patterns may allow the development of more effective strategies.

NUCLEAR RECEPTOR CROSS-TALK WITH OTHER SIGNALING PATHWAYS

The ability of the nuclear hormone receptors to bind specific DNA sequences and directly regulate transcription has long been considered their primary function. Substantial and increasing evidence indicates that they also act via several other mechanisms.

One pathway not far removed from the primary mechanism involves functional interactions with other transcription factors. In the simplest case, the positive transcriptional effects of a nuclear receptor bound to an HRE can synergize with those of other nearby transcription factors. Receptors can apparently also exert less direct positive effects by binding to other DNA-bound transcription factors. For example, ER-α binding to several different common transcription factors, including AP-1 and SP1, can indirectly recruit the receptor to DNA and confer estrogen responsiveness to a number of different promoters.[96] Such positive effects are dependent on both cell and promoter contexts and are not observed for every binding site of the potential ER-α targets. The basis for these differences and the degree to which such pathways contribute to effects of other nuclear receptors is not clear.

Studies with GR indicate that an analogous, but opposite, pathway of mutual functional antagonism with AP-1 and other proinflammatory transcription factors is a major component of glucocorticoid effects. Mutation of the dimerization interface of the GR DNA-binding domain prevents homodimer binding to normal HREs, but does not prevent such functional antagonism. Mice lacking GR function completely are not viable, but mice homozygous for such a dimerization mutant have a much less severe phenotype and retain the anti-inflammatory effects ascribed to the inhibition of AP-1 activity.[97] A number of other receptors including ER-β also show mutual antagonism with AP-1, but the functional significance of such effects remains to be determined.

Another major pathway of cross-talk initiates at the membrane. It has been known for many years that nuclear receptor ligands can exert effects on membrane-based kinase signaling pathways that are too rapid to be accounted for by primary transcriptional regulatory effects. Such effects are referred to as non-genomic and have been described for a number of nuclear receptor ligands, including steroids, vitamin D, and thyroid hormone. More recently, it has become clear that the nuclear receptors (misnamed in this instance) are also found at the membranes and can directly mediate these effects.[98] This is perhaps best characterized at the molecular level for the ERs, which can activate both G proteins and the epidermal growth factor receptor at the membrane.[99] Such direct stimulation of growth factor–dependent protein kinase pathways may contribute to the proliferative effects of estrogen in the mammary gland.[100]

Of course, it is also possible that membrane-dependent effects of steroids or other nuclear receptor ligands could be mediated by distinct classes of receptors. Recent results have identified a novel G-protein-coupled receptor as a potential mediator of the rapid effects of progestins on maturation of fish oocytes.[101] A number of close relatives of this receptor found in mammalian genomes[102] could obviously contribute to membrane signaling pathways for progestins or other steroids.

In addition to being upstream of protein kinase pathways, nuclear receptors and their cofactors are also among their downstream targets. Indeed, studies to date indicate that essentially all nuclear receptors are phosphoproteins, and it is likely that the same will be the case for cofactors. As recently reviewed for the progesterone receptor, for example, the levels of receptor phosphorylation, are often sensitive to the presence or absence of ligand and also to activation of growth factor and other signaling pathways.[103] In several cases, kinase-dependent signaling pathways are able to activate nuclear receptors in the absence of their ligand.[104,105] However, there are frequently multiple sites for phosphorylation, and effects on transactivation can be either positive or negative. Recent results demonstrate that kinase pathways can have powerful and selective effects on coactivator function.[106] Thus, the only general conclusion is that phosphorylation can have a major impact on receptor signaling pathways.

REFERENCES

1. Jensen EV, DeSombre ER: Mechanism of action of the female sex hormones. Annu Rev Biochem 41:203–230, 1972.

2. Rosenfeld GC, Comstock JP, Means AR, et al: Estrogen-induced synthesis of ovalbumin messenger RNA and its translation in a cell-free system. Biochem Biophys Res Commun 46:1695–1703, 1972.

3. Miesfeld R, Okret S, Wikstrom AC, et al: Characterization of a steroid hormone receptor gene and mRNA in wild-type and mutant cells. Nature 312:779–781, 1984.

4. Weinberger C, Hollenberg SM, Rosenfeld MG, et al: Domain structure of human glucocorticoid receptor and its relationship to the v-erb-A oncogene product. Nature 318:670–672, 1985.

5. Green S, Walter P, Kumar V, et al: Human oestrogen receptor cDNA: Sequence, expression and homology to v-erb-A. Nature 320:134–139, 1986.

6. Jeltsch JM, Krozowski Z, Quirin-Stricker C, et al: Cloning of the chicken progesterone receptor. Proc Natl Acad Sci U S A 83:5424–5428, 1986.

7. Conneely OM, Sullivan WP, Toft DO, et al: Molecular cloning of the chicken progesterone receptor. Science 233:767–770, 1986.

8. Kuiper GG, Enmark E, Pelto-Huikko M, et al: Cloning of a novel receptor expressed in rat prostate and ovary. Proc Natl Acad Sci U S A 93:5925–5930, 1996.

9. Sap J, Munoz A, Damm K, et al: The c-erb-A protein is a high-affinity receptor for thyroid hormone. Nature 324:635–640, 1986.

10. Weinberger C, Thompson CC, Ong ES, et al: The c-erbA gene encodes a thyroid hormone receptor. Nature 324:641–646, 1986.

11. Giguere V, Ong ES, Segui P, et al: Identification of a receptor for the morphogen retinoic acid. Nature 330:624–629, 1987.

12. Petkovich M., Brand NJ, Krust A, et al: A human retinoic acid receptor which belongs to the family of nuclear receptors. Nature 330:444–450, 1987.

13. Mangelsdorf DJ, Borgmeyer U, Heyman RA, et al: Characterization of three RXR genes that mediate the action of 9-cis retinoic acid. Genes Dev 6:329–344, 1992.

14. Issemann I, Green S: Activation of a member of the steroid hormone receptor superfamily by peroxisome proliferators. Nature 347:645–650, 1990.

15. Gottlicher M, Widmark E, Li Q, et al: Fatty acids activate a chimera of the clofibric acid–activated receptor and the glucocorticoid receptor. Proc Natl Acad Sci U S A 89:4653–4657, 1992.

16. Xu HE, Lambert MH, Montana VG, et al: Molecular recognition of fatty acids by peroxisome proliferator–activated receptors. Mol Cell 3:397–403, 1999.

17. Kersten S, Desvergne B, Wahli W: Roles of PPARs in health and disease. Nature 405:421–424, 2000.

18. Chawla A, Boisvert WA, Lee CH, et al: A PPAR gamma-LXR-ABCA1 pathway in macrophages is involved in cholesterol efflux and atherogenesis. Mol Cell 7:161–171, 2001.

19. Oliver WR Jr, Shenk JL, Snaith MR, et al: A selective peroxisome proliferator–activated receptor delta agonist promotes reverse cholesterol transport. Proc Natl Acad Sci U S A 98:5306–5311, 2001.

20. Janowski BA, Willy PJ, Devi TR, et al: An oxysterol signalling pathway mediated by the nuclear receptor LXR-alpha. Nature 383:728–731, 1996.

21. Peet DJ, Turley SD, Ma W, et al: Cholesterol and bile acid metabolism are impaired in mice lacking the nuclear oxysterol receptor LXR alpha. Cell 93:693–704, 1998.

22. Schultz JR, Tu H, Luk A, et al: Role of LXRs in control of lipogenesis. Genes Dev 14: 2831–2838, 2000.

23. Tangirala RK, Bischoff ED, Joseph SB, et al: Identification of macrophage liver X receptors as inhibitors of atherosclerosis. Proc Natl Acad Sci U S A 99:11896–11901, 2002.

24. Parks DJ, Blanchard SG, Bledsoe RK, et al: Bile acids: Natural ligands for an orphan nuclear receptor. Science 284:1365–1368, 1999.

25. Makishima M, Okamoto AY, Repa JJ, et al: Identification of a nuclear receptor for bile acids. Science 284:1362–1365, 1999.

26. Wang H, Chen J, Hollister K, et al: Endogenous bile acids are ligands for the nuclear receptor FXR/BAR. Mol Cell 3:543–553, 1999.

27. Sinal CJ, Tohkin M, Miyata M, et al: Targeted disruption of the nuclear receptor FXR/BAR impairs bile acid and lipid homeostasis. Cell 102:731–744, 2000.

28. Liu Y, Binz J, Numerick MJ, et al: Hepatoprotection by the farnesoid X receptor agonist GW4064 in rat models of intra- and extrahepatic cholestasis. J Clin Invest 112:1678–1687, 2003.

29. Wang L, Lee Y-K, Bundman D, et al: Redundant pathways for negative feedback regulation of bile acid production. Dev Cell 2:721–723, 2002.

30. Kerr TA, Saeki S, Schneider M, et al: Loss of nuclear receptor SHP impairs but does not eliminate negative feedback regulation of bile acid synthesis. Dev Cell 2:713–720, 2002.

31. Watanabe M, Houten SM, Wang L, et al: Bile acids lower triglyceride levels via a pathway involving FXR, SHP, and SREBP-1c. J Clin Invest 113:1408–1418, 2004.

32. Waxman DJ: P450 gene induction by structurally diverse xenochemicals: Central role of nuclear receptors CAR, PXR, and PPAR. Arch Biochem Biophys 369:11–23, 1999.

33. Honkakoski P, Sueyoshi T, Negishi M: Drug-activated nuclear receptors CAR and PXR. Ann Med 35:172–182, 2003.

34. Willson TM, Kliewer SA: PXR, CAR and drug metabolism. Nat Rev Drug Discov 1:259–266, 2002.

35. Xie W, Barwick JL, Downes M, et al: Humanized xenobiotic response in mice expressing nuclear receptor SXR. Nature 406:435–439, 2000.

36. Wei P, Zhang J, Egan-Hafley M, et al: The nuclear receptor CAR mediates specific xenobiotic induction of drug metabolism. Nature 407:920–923, 2000.

37. Staudinger JL, Goodwin B, Jones SA, et al: The nuclear receptor PXR is a lithocholic acid sensor that protects against liver toxicity. Proc Natl Acad Sci U S A 98:3369–3374, 2001.

38. Zhang J, Huang W, Qatanani M, et al: The constitutive androstane receptor and pregnane X receptor function coordinately to prevent bile acid–induced hepatotoxicity. J Biol Chem 2004.

39. Huang W, Zhang J, Chua SS, et al: Induction of bilirubin clearance by the constitutive androstane receptor (CAR). Proc Natl Acad Sci U S A 100:4156–4161, 2003.

40. Giguere V: Orphan nuclear receptors: From gene to function. Endocr Rev 20:689–725, 1999.

41. Sladek R, Giguere V: Orphan nuclear receptors: An emerging family of metabolic regulators. Adv Pharmacol 47:23–87, 2000.

42. Cooney AJ, Lee CT, Lin SC, et al: Physiological function of the orphans GCNF and COUP-TF. Trends Endocrinol Metab 12:247–251, 2001.

43. Giguere V: To ERR in the estrogen pathway. Trends Endocrinol Metab 13:220–225, 2002.

44. Alvarez JD, Sehgal A: REV-ving up the clock. Dev Cell 3:150–152, 2002.

45. Wallen A, Perlmann T: Transcriptional control of dopamine neuron development. Ann N Y Acad Sci 991:48–60, 2003.

46. Lala DS, Rice DA, Parker KL: Steroidogenic factor I, a key regulator of steroidogenic enzyme expression, is the mouse homolog of fushi-tarazu factor I. Mol Endocrinol 6:1249–1258, 1992.

47. Luo X, Ikeda Y, Parker KL: A cell-specific nuclear receptor is essential for adrenal and gonadal development and sexual differentiation. Cell 77:481–490, 1994.

48. Parker KL, Rice DA, Lala DS, et al: Steroidogenic factor 1: An essential mediator of endocrine development. Recent Prog Horm Res 57:19–36, 2002.

49. Sladek FM, Zhong W, Lai E, et al: Liver-enriched transcription factor HNF-4 is a novel member of the steroid hormone receptor superfamily. Genes Dev 4:2353–2365, 1990.

50. Watt AJ, Garrison WD, Duncan SA: HNF4: A central regulator of hepatocyte differentiation and function. Hepatology 37:1249–1253, 2003.

51. Yamagata K, Furuta H, Oda N, et al: Mutations in the hepatocyte nuclear factor-4alpha gene in maturity-onset diabetes of the young (MODY1) [see comments]. Nature 384:458–460, 996.

52. Seol W, Choi HS, Moore DD: An orphan nuclear hormone receptor that lacks a DNA binding domain and heterodimerizes with other receptors. Science 272:1336–1339, 1996.

53. Zanaria E, Muscatelli F, Bardoni B, et al: An unusual member of the nuclear hormone receptor superfamily responsible for X-linked adrenal hypoplasia congenita. Nature 372:635–641, 1994.

54. Ito M, Yu R, Jameson JL: DAX-1 inhibits SF-1-mediated transactivation via a carboxy-terminal domain that is deleted in adrenal hypoplasia congenita. Mol Cell Biol 17:1476–1483, 1997.

55. Umesono K, Murakami KK, Thompson CC, et al: Direct repeats as selective response elements for the thyroid hormone, retinoic acid, and vitamin D receptors. Cell 65:1255–1266, 1991.

56. Khorasanizadeh S, Rastinejad F: Nuclear-receptor interactions on DNA-response elements. Trends Biochem Sci 26:384–390, 2001.

57. Luisi BF, Xu W-X, Otwinowski Z, et al: Crystallographic analysis of the interaction of the glucocorticoid receptor with DNA. Nature 352:497–505, 1991.

58. Rastinejad F, Perlmann T, Evans RM, et al: Structural determinants of nuclear receptor assembly on DNA direct repeats. Nature 375:203–211, 1995.

59. Umesono K, Evans RM: Determinants of target gene specificity for steroid/thyroid hormone receptors. Cell 57:1139–1146, 1989.

60. Zhao Q, Khorasanizadeh S, Miyoshi Y, et al: Structural elements of an orphan nuclear receptor-DNA complex. Mol Cell 1:849–861, 1998.

61. Cavailles V, Dauvois S, Danielian PS, et al: Interaction of proteins with transcriptionally active estrogen receptors. Proc Natl Acad Sci U S A 91:10009–10013, 1994.

62. Shiau AK, Barstad D, Loria PM, et al: The structural basis of estrogen receptor/coactivator recognition and the antagonism of this interaction by tamoxifen. Cell 95:927–937, 1998.

63. Wisely GB, Miller AB, Davis RG, et al: Hepatocyte nuclear factor 4 is a transcription factor that constitutively binds fatty acids. Structure (Camb) 10:1225–1234, 2002.

64. Dhe-Paganon S, Duda K, Iwamoto M, et al: Crystal structure of the HNF4 alpha ligand binding domain in complex with endogenous fatty acid ligand. J Biol Chem 277:37973–37976, 2002.

65. Kallen JA, Schlaeppi JM, Bitsch F, et al: X-ray structure of the hRORalpha LBD at 1.63 A: structural and functional data that cholesterol or a cholesterol derivative is the natural ligand of RORalpha. Structure (Camb) 10:1697–1707, 2002.

66. Sablin EP, Krylova IN, Fletterick RJ, et al: Structural basis for ligand-independent activation of the orphan nuclear receptor LRH-1. Mol Cell 11:1575–1585, 2003.

67. Wang Z, Benoit G, Liu J, et al: Structure and function of Nurr1 identifies a class of ligand-independent nuclear receptors. Nature 423:555–560, 2003.

68. Escriva H, Delaunay F, Laudet V: Ligand binding and nuclear receptor evolution. Bioessays 22:717–727, 2000.

69. Brelivet Y, Kammerer S, Rochel N, et al: Signature of the oligomeric behaviour of nuclear receptors at the sequence and structural level. EMBO Rep 5:423–429, 2004.

70. Bledsoe RK, Montana VG, Stanley TB, et al: Crystal structure of the glucocorticoid receptor ligand binding domain reveals a novel mode of receptor dimerization and coactivator recognition. Cell 110:93–105, 2002.

71. Halachmi S, Marden E, Martin G, et al: Estrogen receptor-associated proteins: Possible mediators of hormone-induced transcription. Science 264:1455–1458, 1994.

72. Lusser A, Kadonaga JT: Chromatin remodeling by ATP-dependent molecular machines. Bioessays 25:1192–1200, 2003.

73. Trotter KW, Archer TK: Reconstitution of glucocorticoid receptor-dependent transcription in vivo. Mol Cell Biol 24:3347–3358, 2004.

74. McKenna NJ, O'Malley BW: Combinatorial control of gene

expression by nuclear receptors and coregulators. Cell 108:465–474, 2002.

75. Fondell JD, Ge H, Roeder RG: Ligand induction of a transcriptionally active thyroid hormone receptor coactivator complex. Proc Natl Acad Sci U S A 93:8329–8333, 1996.

76. Rachez C, Suldan Z, Ward J, et al: A novel protein complex that interacts with the vitamin D3 receptor in a ligand-dependent manner and enhances VDR transactivation in a cell-free system. Genes Dev 12:1787–1800, 1998.

77. Xu W, Cho H, Kadam S, et al: A methylation-mediator complex in hormone signaling. Genes Dev 18:144–156, 2004.

78. Shang Y, Hu X, DiRenzo J, et al: Cofactor dynamics and sufficiency in estrogen receptor–regulated transcription. Cell 103:843–852, 2000.

79. Nagaich AK, Walker DA, Wolford R, et al: Rapid periodic binding and displacement of the glucocorticoid receptor during chromatin remodeling. Mol Cell 14:163–174, 2004.

80. Lee DK, Duan HO, Chang C: Androgen receptor interacts with the positive elongation factor P-TEFb and enhances the efficiency of transcriptional elongation. J Biol Chem 276:9978–9984, 2001.

81. Aiyar SE, Sun JL, Blair AL, et al: Attenuation of estrogen receptor alpha-mediated transcription through estrogen-stimulated recruitment of a negative elongation factor. Genes Dev 18:2134–2146, 2004.

82. Monsalve M, Wu Z, Adelmant G, et al: Direct coupling of transcription and mRNA processing through the thermogenic coactivator PGC-1. Mol Cell 6:307–316, 2000.

83. Auboeuf D, Honig A, Berget SM, et al: Coordinate regulation of transcription and splicing by steroid receptor coregulators. Science 298:416–419, 2002.

84. Puigserver P, Spiegelman BM: Peroxisome proliferator-activated receptor-gamma coactivator 1 alpha (PGC-1 alpha): Transcriptional coactivator and metabolic regulator. Endocr Rev 24:78–90, 2003.

85. Puigserver P, Wu Z, Park CW, et al: A cold-inducible coactivator of nuclear

receptors linked to adaptive thermogenesis. Cell 92:829–839, 1998.

86. Yoon JC, Puigserver P, Chen G, et al: Control of hepatic gluconeogenesis through the transcriptional coactivator PGC-1. Nature 413:131–138, 2001.

87. Horlein AJ, Naar AM, Heinzel T, et al: Ligand-independent repression by the thyroid hormone receptor mediated by a nuclear receptor co-repressor. Nature 377:397–404, 1995.

88. Chen JD, Evans RM: A transcriptional co-repressor that interacts with nuclear hormone receptors. Nature 377:454–457, 1995.

89. Hu X, Lazar MA: The CoRNR motif controls the recruitment of corepressors by nuclear hormone receptors. Nature 402:93–96, 1999.

90. Rogatsky I, Luecke HF, Leitman DC, et al: Alternate surfaces of transcriptional coregulator GRIP1 function in different glucocorticoid receptor activation and repression contexts. Proc Natl Acad Sci U S A 99:16701–16706, 2002.

91. Drouin J, Sun YL, Chamberland M, et al: Novel glucocorticoid receptor complex with DNA element of the hormone-repressed POMC gene. Embo J 12:145–156, 1993.

92. Philips A, Maira M, Mullick A, et al: Antagonism between Nur77 and glucocorticoid receptor for control of transcription. Mol Cell Biol 17:5952–5959, 1997.

93. Paige LA, Christensen DJ, Gron H, et al: Estrogen receptor (ER) modulators each induce distinct conformational changes in ER alpha and ER beta. Proc Natl Acad Sci U S A 96:3999–4004, 1999.

94. Smith CL, O'Malley BW: Coregulator function: A key to understanding tissue specificity of selective receptor modulators. Endocr Rev 25:45–71, 2004.

95. Rocchi S, Picard F, Vamecq J, et al: A unique PPARgamma ligand with potent insulin-sensitizing yet weak adipogenic activity. Mol Cell 8:737–747, 2001.

96. Barkhem T, Nilsson S, Gustafsson JA: Molecular mechanisms, physiological consequences and pharmacological implications of estrogen receptor

action. Am J Pharmacogenomics 4:19–28, 2004.

97. Wintermantel TM, Berger S, Greiner EF, et al: Genetic dissection of corticosteroid receptor function in mice. Horm Metab Res 36:387–391, 2004.

98. Boonyaratanakornkit V, Edwards DP: Receptor mechanisms of rapid extranuclear signalling initiated by steroid hormones. Essays Biochem 40:105–120, 2004.

99. Levin ER: Bidirectional signaling between the estrogen receptor and the epidermal growth factor receptor. Mol Endocrinol 17:309–317, 2003.

100. Osborne CK, Schiff R: Growth factor receptor cross-talk with estrogen receptor as a mechanism for tamoxifen resistance in breast cancer. Breast 12:362–367, 2003.

101. Zhu Y, Rice CD, Pang Y, et al: Cloning, expression, and characterization of a membrane progestin receptor and evidence it is an intermediary in meiotic maturation of fish oocytes. Proc Natl Acad Sci U S A 100:2231–2236, 2003.

102. Zhu Y, Bond J, Thomas P: Identification, classification, and partial characterization of genes in humans and other vertebrates homologous to a fish membrane progestin receptor. Proc Natl Acad Sci U S A 100:2237–2242, 2003.

103. Lange CA: Making sense of cross-talk between steroid hormone receptors and intracellular signaling pathways: Who will have the last word? Mol Endocrinol 18:269–278, 2004.

104. Mani SK, Allen JM, Clark JH, et al: Convergent pathways for steroid hormone– and neurotransmitter-induced rat sexual behavior. Science 265:1246–1249, 1994.

105. Weigel NL, Zhang Y: Ligand-independent activation of steroid hormone receptors. J Mol Med 76:469–479, 1998.

106. Wu RC, Qin J, Yi P, et al: Selective phosphorylations of the SRC-3/AIB1 coactivator integrate genomic responses to multiple cellular signaling pathways. Mol Cell 15:937–949, 2004.

NEUROENDOCRINOLOGY AND PITUITARY DISEASE

Development of the Pituitary

Wei Wu and Michael G. Rosenfeld

INTRODUCTION

Advancement in genetics and molecular techniques has significantly increased our understanding of mechanisms underlying the development of the pituitary gland. The pituitary gland serves as an intermediary between the brain and the peripheral systems. By means of multiple feedback control mechanisms, the pituitary gland integrates incoming signals from the peripheral and central nervous systems and responds with regulation of production and secretion of critical regulatory hormones to target organs. The pituitary gland facilitates many critical functions including metabolism, growth, reproduction, circadian rhythm, and stress responses. The functional regulation of gene transcription, pituitary hormone synthesis and secretion, and hormone cell proliferation is critical to homeostasis.

ANATOMY AND HISTOLOGY

The pituitary gland, also termed *hypophysis*, situates in a depression on the upper surface on the sphenoid bone, the *sella turcica*. The hypophysis consists of two major components, the adenohypophysis and the neurohypophysis. The neurohypophysis is of neuronal origin and can be divided into the posterior lobe, or *pars nervosa*, consisting mainly of terminal processes of infundibulum derived from hypothalamic neurons, and the infundibulum, which consists of an elongated infundibular stem and the median eminence. The adenohypophysis can be divided into the intermediate lobe, or *pars intermedia*, which exists in most animals and in the human fetus although less prominent in the mature human pituitary gland, the *pars tuberalis*, and the anterior lobe, or *pars distalis*. The *pars tuberalis* extends up along the anterior and lateral aspects of the infundibular to constitute the pituitary, or hypophyseal, stalk. The glandular adenohypophysis, particularly the anterior lobe, is composed of functionally distinct cell types and is the primary site of endocrine action.

Functional anterior pituitary contains five main cell types: somatotrope cells produce growth hormone (GH) and regulate linear growth and metabolism; lactotrope cells produce prolactin (PRL), which regulates milk production in females;

thyrotrope cells produce thyroid-stimulating hormone (TSH), which controls the secretion of thyroid hormone from the thyroid gland; gonadotrope cells produce gonadotropins (follicle-stimulating hormone, FSH, and luteinizing hormone, LH), which regulate reproductive development and function; and corticotrope cells produce adrenocorticotropic hormone (ACTH), a product of precursor pro-opiomelanocortin (POMC) cleaved by proteolytic processing, which regulates metabolic function through stimulation of glucocorticoid synthesis in the adrenal cortex. TSH, LH, and FSH are heterodimeric glycoproteins consisting of a common alpha subunit (αGSU) and a specific beta subunit. In adult pituitary, GH-producing somatotrope cells occupy most of the gland, which weighs less than 1 gram in humans. The size of the pituitary gland and the proliferation of each pituitary cell type are regulated according to physiologic conditions indicated by feedback regulation.[1]

These five anterior pituitary cell types are present at birth (Table 16-1). Initial expression of distinct pituitary hormone genes marks the terminal differentiation events of the cell types, which derive from a seemingly common primordia and are the results of internal programming of the pituitary as well as a consequence of its interaction with surrounding organs during development. Evidence suggests the internal programming is dictated by the expression of transcriptional regulators, including a cascade of homeodomain transcription factors, and additional cell type–restricted transcription factors. The mechanisms that control the temporal and spatial expression of these transcription factors include diffusible signals from developing hypothalamus at the dorsal aspect and factors from surrounding structures. These spatially distributed signals and gradients of signaling molecules are critical in establishing positional pituitary cell type commitment events.[2,3] Disruption of these apparently evolutionarily conserved events underlying proper development of the pituitary gland can result in morphologic abbreviation and pituitary dysfunction. Through analysis of the expression of pituitary hormone genes in human cases of hypopituitarism, as well as in genetic models of pituitary defects, particularly in mouse models of pituitary dwarfism, a significant amount of knowledge has been accumulated regarding the molecular mechanisms underlying proper development of the pituitary gland.

Table 16-1 Onset of Adenohypophyseal Hormone Expression

Hormone	Human (weeks)	Mouse (dpc)	Chick (dpc)	Zebrafish (hpf)
GH	8	15.5	4.5	42
FSH/LH	8	16	4	—
ACTH	8	2.5	7	24
TSHβ	13	13.3	6.5	42
PRL	13	17.5	6	22

dpc, days post coitus; hpf, hours post fertilization

PITUITARY DEVELOPMENT

ORIGIN

Phylogenetic studies in several vertebrate species lead to the conclusion that the pituitary gland arises from oral epithelia. Fate-mapping experiments conducted in these animal species trace the origination of pituitary gland back to the neural plate. In studies of grafting quail-chick chimeras, the origin of the pituitary had been localized to the midline of the anterior neural ridge. By means of surgical ablation performed in chick embryos, the rostral ridge of the neural plate has been identified as the source of cells that give rise to pituitary tissue.[4-6] In amphibians, tracing experiments have confirmed the neural origin of pituitary gland[7,8] and similar conclusions have been reached about zebrafish.[9,10] More recently, by focalized application of a carbocyanin dye DiI into the rostral end of the neural plate at the open neurula stage (9.5 days post coitus) in rats, labeled cells could be identified in Rathke's pouch and they could develop into the secretory cells of the adenohypophysis in 7 additional days.[11] Thus, evidence indicates that the anterior neural ridge is the origin of Rathke's pouch, which eventually gives rise to cells of the pituitary gland. Subsequent to the folding of the embryonic head, the anterior neural ridge is displaced ventrally to form the portion of the oral epithelium, later giving rise to the roof of the mouth and additional structures including the pituitary gland. Consistent findings in many species make it apparent that the process of pituitary development is, for the most part, evolutionarily conserved from lower vertebrates to higher mammals.

ONTOGENY

In humans, the anterior lobe of the pituitary gland originates from an invagination of the stomodeal epithelium, termed Rathke's pouch.[12] The stomodeal epithelium that contains the pituitary primordium is formed by third fetal week. The invagination of stomodeal epithelium occurs dorsally to form Rathke's pouch by the fourth week, and the formation of Rathke's pouch is complete and disconnected from the oral epithelium by the end of the sixth week of fetal life.[13] In parallel, the hypothalamus is the first region of the forebrain to differentiate. From 4 weeks, the hypothalamic sulcus, chiasmatic plate, and mammillary bodies are recognizable. These two organs, hypothalamus and pituitary, develop interdependently.[14]

Similar to the ontogeny observed in humans, Rathke's pouch in mice is derived from an anlage that arises as an upgrowth from lining of the oral cavity's roof. At its earliest stage, the murine pituitary primordium is defined as an intimate point of contact between the neural ectoderm and the oral roof ectoderm on embryonic day 8.5 post coitus (e8.5), which marks the first event in the pituitary's development. Organogenesis of the adenohypophysis begins as the cells of the pituitary placode in the oral ectoderm thicken and invaginate to form the nascent pituitary. This anlage can be seen in the e9.5 mouse embryo, located rostrally to the oropharyngeal membrane. The arising of the epithelial layer from the roof of the mouth gives off a cone-shaped intrusion dorsally as the Rathke's pouch, or adenohypophyseal pouch. Before the formation, a developmentally important molecular marker, Sonic hedgehog (Shh), is expressed uniformly in the oral epithelial layer. The expression of Shh is excluded before the intrusion of pituitary anlagen can occur in the e9 mouse embryo.[15] The Rathke's pouch thickens as development proceeds and elongates dorsally relative to the oral cavity by the stomodia-adenohypophyseal channel. By e10.5 in the mouse, Rathke's pouch has formed as a rudimentary structure and separated from ventral pharyngeal epithelium (Fig. 16-1).

At the time Rathke's pouch is pinched off at e11 in mice, the first round of accelerated mitotic activity is initiated in the anlagen.[16,17] In the ensuing patterning period, mitotic activity is observed most prominently in the rostral part of Rathke's pouch, with several buds emerging and enveloping areas of vascularized mesenchyme. Progenitors of the hormone-secreting cell types arise from the ventral proliferation of cells and this region of rostral Rathke's pouch eventually gives rise to the anterior lobe, or the *pars distalis*. The dorsal aspects of Rathke's pouch, in contact with the descending infundibulum processes and rostroventrally with the hypophyseal cleft, remain thin and form the intermediate lobe, or the *pars intermedia*. Anterior pituitary cell types are initially positionally determined as they emerge from proliferation zones,[15,18] with the somatotrope/lactotrope cells arising caudomedially and gonadotrope cells more rostroventrally, corticotrope cells ventrally, and melanotrope cells dorsally (see Fig. 16-1). This pattern of pituitary development is generally similar in most mammals.

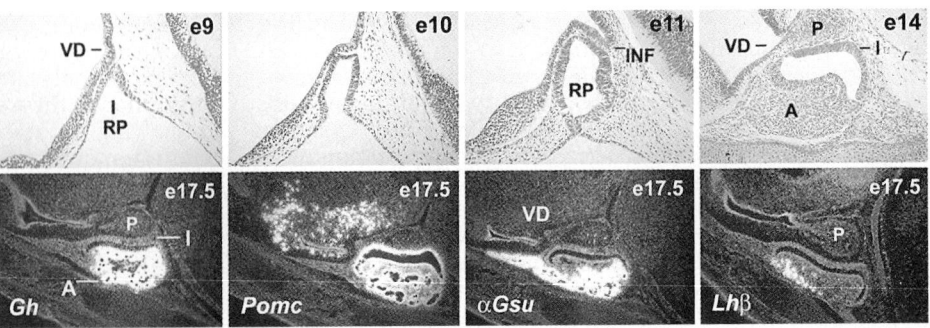

Figure 16-1 Ontogeny of Rathke's pouch (RP) formation and expression of pituitary hormone genes in mouse. **Upper:** Hematoxylin and eosin-stained mid-sagittal sections with nostril to the left, revealing the formation of RP during development. RP is derived from an anlage that arises as an upgrowth from the lining of the roof of the oral cavity and thickens as development proceeds. By e11, RP loses ventral connections with the pharyngeal epithelial. Nascent anterior pituitary (A) cells are derived from asymmetric division of RP epithelial cells. **Lower:** Mid-sagittal sections depicting domains of expression of pituitary hormone genes at e17.5 by in situ hybridization. Signal of *Gh* gene is dorsally located compare to that of αGSU and *Lhβ*. e, embryonic day; VD, ventral diencephalons; P, posterior lobe; I, intermediate lobe; INF, infundibulum.

CELL LINEAGE DETERMINATION

Endocrine pituitary cell types in the adenohypophysis are derived from a single population of cells. The initial expression of pituitary hormone genes marking the terminal differentiation events of individual cell types occurs in a sequential manner. In mice, *Pomc* gene expression emerges as the first pituitary marker at e11.5 and can be detected in the anterior pituitary by e13.5. However, the fate of cells that will give rise to those five different anterior pituitary cell types is determined prior to the initial pituitary *Pomc* expression. In tissue culture experiments where pituitary anlagen were taken and placed in a culture away from the influence of the diencephalons, pituitary anlagen taken at e11 were capable of generating cells expressing all five anterior pituitary hormone genes, while anlagen taken at e9.5 required additional growth factors, with the exception of corticotrope, which always differentiates regardless of the culture medium.[19] Critical events have occurred at the time that pituitary anlagen become committed to become pituitary precursors, with the subsequent expression of pituitary genes that become regulated in a cell autonomous fashion.[20] The timing of this commitment event is coincidental with the formation of Rathke's pouch.

As an anlage, Rathke's pouch is the source of all endocrine pituitary cell types. In mice, after the initial appearance of corticotrope, expression of *Gh* gene can be detected by e15.5, followed by *thyrotropins, gonadotropins,* and *Prl*. Gene expressions of all anterior pituitary hormones are detectable by e17.5, with the exception of *Prl*, which can be consistently seen by the time of birth (e19 in the mouse) (see Fig. 16-1). Another early marker of Rathke's pouch is *αGsu*, and the transcripts are detected throughout Rathke's pouch by e9,[21] although confined to the rostral tip of the anterior lobe by e12.5, and are ultimately restricted to thyrotrope and gonadotrope from late gestation through adulthood. Following proliferation and early organ expansion, a series of different cell types arise in a distinct spatial and temporal fashion. Table 16-1 provides a time line of the initial expression of pituitary hormone genes in several species.

TRANSCRIPTION FACTORS AND PITUITARY DEVELOPMENT

Parallel to the sequential emergence of pituitary cell types, a series of homeodomain family transcription factors are expressed as the adenohypophysis is becoming committed. With improved molecular genetic techniques, functional studies of these transcription factors in animal models, particularly in mouse models, have established molecular mechanisms underlying development of the pituitary gland. The expression profiles of *Hesx1, Lhx3, Lhx4, Prop1,* and *Pit1* homeodomain factors, in addition to the expressions of *Tpit/Tbx19* and *gli2*, dictate the commitment, determination, and differentiation events of the pituitary gland. These genes were initially studied in animal model systems that arose either from naturally occurring mutations or were created by reverse genetic techniques. Without exception, phenotypes observed in each animal model system are also observed in human cases with defects in the corresponding orthologous genes (Table 16-2). The phenotypes observed in human cases range from single pituitary hormone deficiency to combined pituitary hormone deficiency (CPHD) affecting several pituitary hormones in addition to GH. Study of the development of the pituitary gland serves as a model of progressive restriction in gene expression, and the pituitary gland has become a prototypic model organ system to study organogenesis, cell type determination, and differentiation.

PIT1 GENE

The *PIT1* gene (POU domain, class 1, transcription factor 1 *[POU1F1]*) encodes a 33-kD, 291 amino acid transcriptional activator that is capable of DNA binding and transactivation, and it was initially isolated by its ability to bind to the responsive element of the *GH* gene promoter.[22,23] *PIT1* is expressed exclusively in the pituitary gland. In mice, the initial expression of the *Pit1* gene transcripts can be detected by e13.5, exclusively in the anterior ventral pituitary (Fig. 16-2). The expression of *Pit1* persists in adults and colocalizes with expression of *Gh, Prl,* and *Tshβ* genes. Further studies revealed that the product of the *Pit1* is capable of binding to responsive elements in the promoters of the *Gh* gene,[24] the growth hormone–releasing hormone receptor *(Ghrhr)* gene,[25] the *Prl* gene,[26] and the *Tshβ* gene. The Pit1 protein is also capable of binding to the responsive elements of the *Pit1* gene itself[27] and is required for the continued transcription of the *Pit1* gene.[28] The structure of the *Pit1* gene is evolutionarily conserved and is found in mouse, human, and all other vertebrate animals examined, although *Pit1* may play diverse functional roles in different physiologic pathways in individual species.

Animal Model

Snell mice[29] are a well-studied animal model of pituitary function, which arises from a spontaneous single nucleotide mutation in the *Pit1* gene that results in the substitution of W261C in the homeodomain, rendering the mutant gene product incapable of DNA binding, and hence unable to activate potential target genes.[30] Mice heterozygous for this mutation are phenotypically normal. The homozygous offspring of this mutation are dwarf and infertile, and they exhibit loss of three pituitary hormone cell types, Gh, Prl, and Tshβ; whereas the gonadotrope and corticotrope cells are unaffected, suggesting that the *Pit1* is required for terminal differentiation of the somatotrope, lactotrope, and thyrotrope cell types. In the *Pit1Snell* animal model where the *Pit1* gene is functionally defective, the initial activation of the *Pit1* is unaffected, while the later transcription of the *Pit1* gene is altered, resulting in the failed expression of the *Pit1* in the adult animal and a dwarf phenotype.[30,31] The *Pit1* lineage can

Table 16-2 Transcription Factors in Pituitary Hormone Deficiency

Human				Model System	
Gene	Chr.	Inheritance	Hormone Deficiency	Mutation	Pituitary Phenotype
PIT1	3p11	Recessive/dominant	GH, PRL, and variable TSH	*Snell*	Gh, Prl, and Tsh
PROP1	5q35	Recessive	GH, PRL, TSH, FSH/LH, and ACTH	*Ames*	Gh, Prl, Tsh, and Fsh/Lh
LHX3	9q34	Recessive	GH, PRL, TSH, and FSH/LH	K.O.	Gh, Prl, Tsh, and Fsh/Lh
LHX4	1q25	Dominant	GH, TSH, and ACTH	K.O.	Reduction of all anterior cell types
HESX1	3p21	Recessive/dominant	Variable hormone deficiency	K.O.	Pouch bifurcations, pituitary absence
TBX19	1q23	Recessive	POMC	K.O.	Pituitary Pomc transdifferentiation
GLI2	2q14	Dominant	Variable hormone deficiency	*yot-too*	Transdifferentiation into a lens

Chr., chromosome location; K.O., targeted deletion in mouse; *yot-too*, zebrafish *gli2* mutant

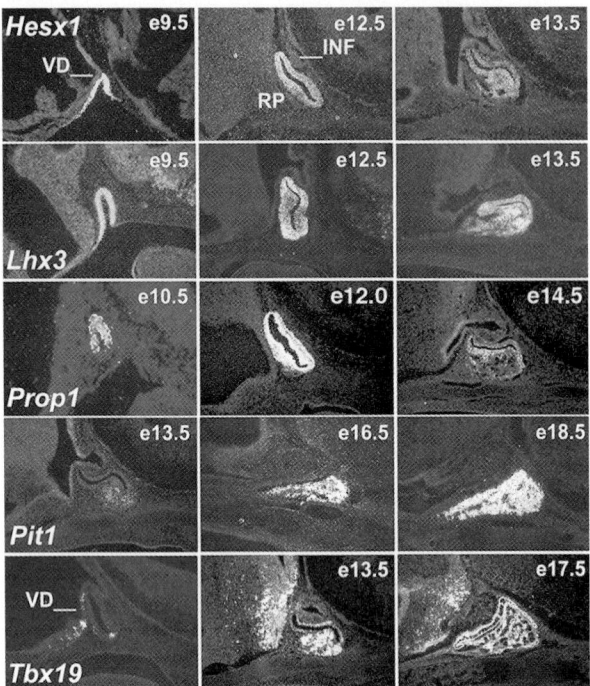

Figure 16-2 Expression of selected transcription factors in pituitary development by *in situ* hybridization. Expression of *Hesx1* and *Lhx3* are detected in Rathke's pouch at mouse embryonic stage e9.5 and are maintained at e12.5, after which *Hesx1* expression is rapidly extinguished while *Lhx3* continue to be expressed. *Prop1* expression initiates at e10.5, reaches maximum intensity at e12.5, and attenuates at e14.5. *Pit1* expression initiates at e13.5 and is maintained throughout pituitary development and adulthood. Initial *Tbx19* expression can be observed in the ventral Rathke's pouch and ventral diencephalons at e11.5, and its expression is maintained.

be converted to alternative fates before e17.5 but exhibits a cell-autonomous commitment after e17.5, when *Pit1* gene regulation shifts from a *Pit1*-independent early enhancer to a *Pit1*-autoregulated later enhancer.[32] *Pit1^Jackson* is a second mouse model with a defect in the *Pit1* gene. The genomic structure of the *Pit1* gene, located on chromosome 16, is grossly rearranged in mutant *Pit1^Jackson* mice, with a phenotype very similar or identical to that of the *Pit1^Snell* mice.[30] In addition, *Pit1* mutations result in decreased activity of the *insulin/IGF1* pathway, which may result in physiologic homeostasis consequences that favor longevity.[33,34]

Related Diseases

The human *PIT1* gene has been mapped to chromosome 3. Lesions in *PIT1* have been identified as an etiology of CPHD (see Table 16-2). Initial study has revealed a homozygous nonsense mutation R172X in the *PIT1* gene in a patient of consanguineous parents with cretinism due to deficiency of GH, PRL, and TSH.[35] Many cases of CPHD with *PIT1* defects have since been reported. It appears that the inheritance of *PIT1* mutations in humans is complex, ranging from autosomal recessive to autosomal dominant to imprinting with variable phenotypic penetrance.[36] Pituitary gonadotropins and corticotropins are normal in *PIT1*-defective patients. Deficiency of GH is consistently observed in all *PIT1* patients, and deficiency for PRL is observed in most patients, whereas the TSH deficiency usually has a delayed onset and incomplete penetrance (see Table 16-2). Different backgrounds may be the major contributing factor to the TSH phenotypic variation. Alternatively, however, there exists an embryonic population of thyrotrope termed *rostral tip thyrotrope*. The expression of this embryonic TSH is not *Pit1* dependent, and consequently it may be a contributing element to the TSH phenotypic

variation observed in the *PIT1* patients. The presentation of patients with *PIT1* disorders varies considerably. At infancy, they usually have a protruding forehead, depressed facial structures, and a saddled nose, although CPHD is generally not diagnosed until growth retardation becomes obvious due to the deficiencies of GH and thyroid hormone.[37,38]

Mechanism

The modular structure of the Pit1 protein can be divided into the transactivation and the DNA-binding domains. The transcriptional activation domain is located in the first 80 amino acids, followed by a POU DNA-binding domain at the C terminus. The POU domain is further divided into a 75-amino acid POU-specific domain, which is conserved among various POU domain proteins, and a 60-amino acid POU homeodomain with a linker region between them. The POU homeodomain by itself is sufficient for low-affinity DNA binding, although both POU-specific domain and POU homeodomain are required for specific high-affinity DNA binding of the *Pit1* responsive elements. Pit1 protein is able to bind as a monomer in solution to the consensus (A/T)(A/T)TATNCAT site, where N may be any nucleotide; in most cases, however, Pit1 binds DNA as a dimer.[39] Analysis of data derived from a cocrystal study of the Pit1 protein and the Prl proximal promoter Pit1-binding element reveals that the Pit1 protein binds to DNA in a parallel dimer form.[40,41] Pit1 protein wraps around the DNA molecule with the POU-specific domain and the POU homeodomain binding to the DNA molecule in a perpendicular angle in opposite orientation. The POU-specific domain of one Pit1 molecule interacts with the C terminus of the POU homeodomain of the other Pit1 molecule in a dual composition. In addition, the spacing between the DNA contacts made by the POU-specific domain and the POU homeodomain of each monomer is critical. Compared to the Pit1 binding site in the Prl minimum promoter sequences, two additional base pairs spacing are needed to direct restricted *Gh* gene transcription based on elements of two Pit1 binding sites on the proximal promoter of rat *Gh* locus.[28,42]

This dimerization interface is a "hot spot" for debilitating mutations. In the *Pit1^Snell* mice, a G-to-T mutation results (W261C) in the third helix of the POU homeodomain, eliminating its DNA-binding ability by altering the contact point of the mutant gene product with the major groove of the responsive elements, causing a dwarf phenotype in an autosomal-recessive fashion. Similarly, several mutations observed in human cases could affect the stability and specificity of this protein-DNA interface.[43,44]

As a transcription factor, Pit1 exerts its effects as a component of a transcriptional complex, regulated by coactivator and repressor elements. The Pit1 POU domain can associate with coactivator complex of CBP/p300 and P/CAF, both of which possess histone acetylase activity. N-CoR, acting as a corepressor, can bind to the homeodomain of Pit1 and actively suppresses transactivation by Pit1, and this suppression depends on Sin3, SAP30, and histone deacetylase. Thus, the transcriptional activity of Pit1 may be regulated by the competing binding of complexes mediating either acetylation or deacetylation events, resulting in activation or repression, respectively.[45]

In addition to *Pit1*, the determination of individual pituitary cell types may require other molecules. The estrogen receptor has been implicated in synergistic activation of the *Prl* gene.[46,47] Members of the *ETS* family of transcription factors can bind to the Pit1 binding sites in the Prl promoter and mediate signals from growth factors and the Ras/mitogen-activated protein kinase pathway.[48] The transcription factor *Gata2* appears to be required for the formation of both thyrotrope and gonadotrope cells, and the presence of Pit1 represses the gonadotropic phenotype and promotes the thyrotrope phenotype. Pit1 can inhibit binding of Gata2 to cognate DNA sites important for generation of the gonadotrope phenotype. In contrast, Pit1 leads to synergistic activation with Gata2 on promoters that contain both Pit1 and Gata2 sites, such as the thyrotrope-specific TSH_β promoter.[49]

PROP1 *GENE*

PROP1 (Prophet of Pit-1) is a homeodomain-containing transcription factor that is capable of binding to its cognate DNA site and activating its target genes. The expression pattern of the *Prop1* gene has been examined in mice and is detected only in Rathke's pouch. *Prop1* expression is detected initially at e10 in the mouse, when the structure of Rathke's pouch has been established. The expression initially is observed dorsally but subsequently involves most cells in the Rathke's pouch. Expression of *Prop1* reaches a maximum level of intensity at e12 in Rathke's pouch, with the signal diminishing by e14.5[50] (see Figs. 16-2 and 16-3). The expression of the *Prop1* gene is required for the activation of the downstream *Pit1* gene.[51,52] The integrity of *PROP1* is necessary for full-scale manifestation of pituitary gonadotrope cells, as well as the generation of somatotrope, lactotrope, and thyrotrope cells (see Fig. 16-3). Mutations in the *PROP1* gene have been identified as the leading cause of familial CPHD, resulting in short stature as a consequence.

Animal Model

The *Prop1* gene was initially identified by a positional cloning strategy in the naturally occurring *Ames* mouse mutant. The mutant *Prop1* allele at the *Prop1^Ames* locus harbors a point mutation that results in a single amino acid substitution (S83P) in the second helix of the homeodomain, causing altered progression of nascent pituitary gland and subsequent failed expression of *Pit1*.[50] Phenotypes of the *Prop1^Ames* mice

are transmitted in an autosomal-recessive fashion; heterozygous mutant mice are normal. Homozygous mutant mice are born grossly normal but develop a proportional dwarfism by the time of weaning.[53] The adult mutant mice are about half the size of the wild-type animals. The *Prop1^Ames* mutation caused dysmorphogenesis of Rathke's pouch at e12.5, with convolution of the lumen and a failure of expression of the *Pit1* lineage. The appearance of gonadotrope was delayed, but corticotrope appeared as expected. In contrast to the complete absence of somatotrope, lactotrope, and thyrotrope cells in the *Pit1^Snell* mouse, the *Prop1^Ames* mouse pituitary gland contains a small number (<1%)[51,54] of the normal complement of somatotrope cells as well as a few lactotrope and thyrotrope cells.[54] *Prop1^Ames* dwarf mice live twice as long as their wild-type littermates.[55]

Related Diseases

The human *PROP1* coding region has three exons separated by two introns and maps to chromosome 5q34. The *PROP1* gene encodes a polypeptide of 226 amino acids and contains a short N terminus, a 60-amino acid homeodomain, and a transactivating C terminus. Compared to the mouse homologue, the human PROP1 homeodomain is highly conserved with only two amino acid substitutions.

Initial reports identified mutations in the human *PROP1* gene in patients with short stature in several families. Direct sequencing of polymerase chain reaction (PCR) products of the *PROP1* gene revealed that all the affected patients were harboring mutations in both alleles of the *PROP1* gene and their parents were heterozygous for the respective mutations, suggesting that the mutations in the *PROP1* gene act in an autosomal-recessive manner, causing CPHD in these patients. All of the affected individuals in this study failed to respond to

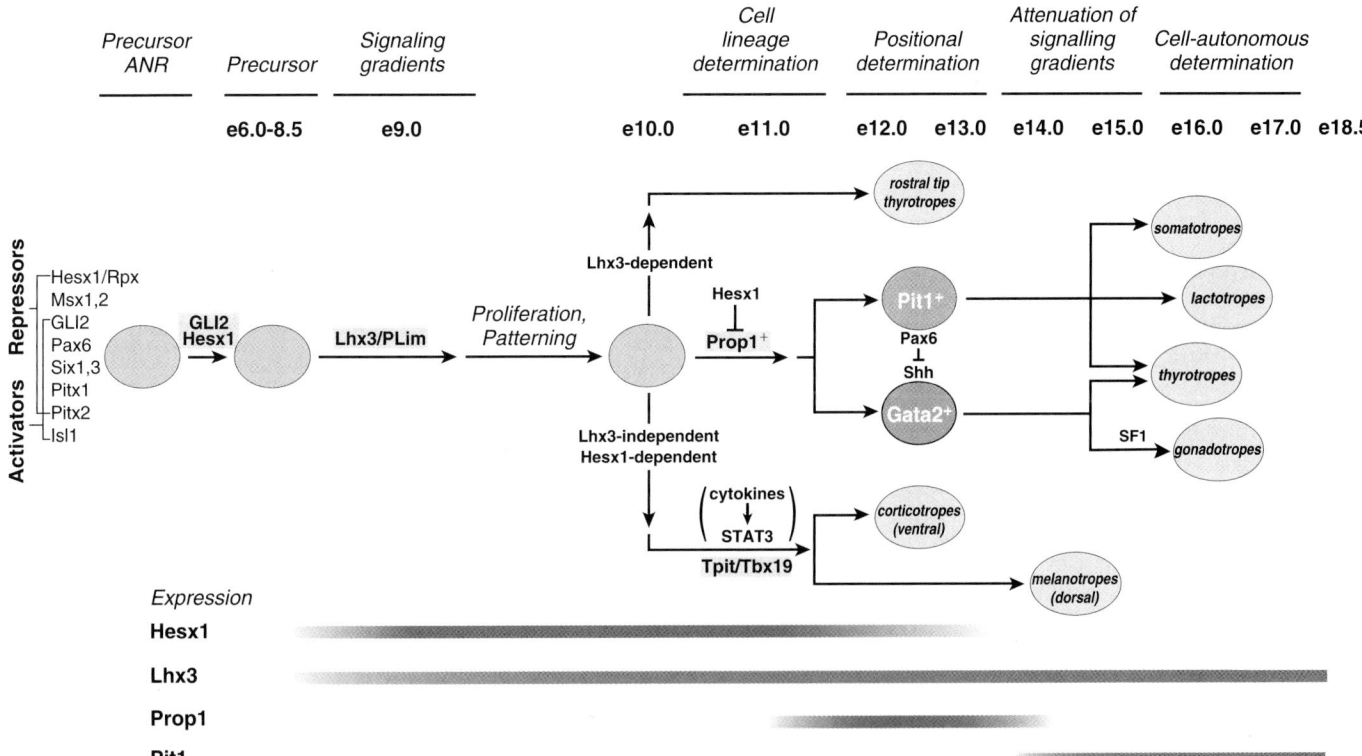

Figure 16-3 Roles of pituitary expressed transcription factors in cell lineage determination. Pituitary cells are derived from a single population of primordial cell originating from anterior neuronal ridge (ANR), and several transcription factors, including Gli2 and Hesx1, are required for the commitment events. Precursor cell types are committed to the pituitary fate through the induction of Lhx3 expression. Prop1 is required for the asymmetric ventral proliferation and determination of at least four cell types. Pit1 is required for the cell fate determination of somatotropes, lactotropes, and thyrotropes. Tbx19 is required for the cell fate determination of corticotropes and melanotropes. (Modified from Scully KM, Rosenfeld MG: Pituitary development: Regulatory codes in mammalian organogenesis. Science 295:2231–2235, 2002.)

GHRH, thyrotropin-releasing hormone, and LH-releasing hormone stimulation, suggesting a defect in hormone-secreting cells of the pituitary gland.[56] Subsequent reports have revealed that *PROP1* mutation is a common cause of familial CPHD. These alternations in the *PROP1* gene range from point mutation to deletions, affecting structure and integrity in the homeodomain of the *PROP1* gene. A 2-bp A301G302 deletion, leading to a frame-shift and the loss of DNA-binding homeodomain and C-terminal transactivation domain of the PROP1 gene product, is the most frequently encountered mutation among these *PROP1* patients, representing a mutational "hot spot."[57] Individuals with various *PROP1* mutations invariably display severe deficiencies for pituitary gonadotropins in addition to the defects of GH, PRL, and TSH. In human cases with *PROP1* mutations, many adult patients express ACTH at a normal level; however, there are reported cases with a late onset of corticotropin deficiency (see Table 16-2). The expression of ACTH phenotypes is highly heterogeneous; differences in genetic background in these patients may contribute to the discrepancy of this phenotype.[58,59]

Mechanism

The Prop1 gene product exerts its actions through binding to the responsive elements of target genes, with the helix-turn-helix motif of the homeodomain providing the contact point for protein-DNA interactions. The fact that most of the naturally occurring mutations of the *Prop1* gene are located in the homeodomain suggests that the Prop1 homeodomain is critical for *Prop1* function.

In the *Prop1^Ames* mice, examination of mutant Rathke's pouch revealed severe dysmorphogenesis but the pituitary precursor cells were generated initially. The precursor cells of Rathke's pouch failed to migrate to form the nascent pituitary gland, leading to failed expression of a late pituitary differentiation marker, the *Pit1* gene. However, proliferation of the mutant precursor cells in the *Ames* mice continued, resulting in a normal-sized pituitary glands.[50] Later, persistent expression of *Prop1* under control of the αGsu promoter caused decreased gonadotrope differentiation and increased adenomatous hyperplasia,[60] indicating that properly extinguishing *Prop1* also may be an important later step in paired-like homeodomain-mediated organogenesis. Subtractive hybridization suggests that *Prop1* may play a role in the *Wnt* signaling that is intrinsic to the developing gland at this time.[61]

Phenotypic comparisons have been made between the *PROP1*-defective patient and the *Prop1* mutant *Prop1^Ames* mouse. The deficiencies of GH, PRL, and TSH are consistently observed in both species. All the patients with the *PROP1* mutations eventually develop the gonadotropin deficiency in their adult lives. In the *Prop1^Ames* mice, the expression of gonadotropin is observed at birth, but the level of expression of the gonadotropin is reduced to one quarter of that of the wild-type animals.[50] The expression of *Acth* is apparent during development in the *Prop1^Ames* mouse pituitary, and the level of ACTH in the blood is normal in adults. In human *PROP1* patients, cortisol levels are normal at birth, but some of the patients develop cortisol deficiency later in life.[62–64] The *Prop1* mutation may affect all the major cell types in the anterior pituitary gland, including the gonadotrope and the corticotrope (see Table 16-2).

HESX1 *GENE*

HESX1 (homeodomain gene expressed in ES cells) is a paired-class homeodomain transcription factor that is capable of binding to its cognate DNA site and regulating its target genes. Mutations in the *HESX1* gene have been identified in septo-optic dysplasia and CPHD. In mice, the earliest expression of the *Hesx1* gene can be detected at the embryonic stem cell stage. High levels of expression can be detected in the ectoderm, subsequently at the anterior extreme of the rostral

neural folds, and finally restricted to the ventral diencephalons and to the thickened layer of oral ectoderm, which will give rise to the Rathke's pouch at e9.0 in the mouse.[65,66] *Hesx1* gene expression can be observed for 2 more days but only in the Rathke's pouch with diminishing intensity at a time that coincides with the rise of *Prop1* gene expression (see Figs. 16-2 and 16-3). In humans, strong expression of *HESX1* in Rathke's pouch can be detected in a 7-week-old embryo. Hesx1 is the earliest molecular marker for the definitive pituitary primordium.

Animal Model

The mouse *Hesx1* gene is located on chromosome 14, and targeted deletion of *Hesx1* resulted in mice that exhibit variable anterior central nervous system defects with reduced prosencephalon and defective olfactory development.[67] *Hesx1* mutants also have defects in the pituitary gland with bifurcations in the Rathke's pouch in most cases. By e12.5, multiple oral ectoderm invaginations reflecting pituitary glands are observed in most *Hesx1* embryos. Between e13.5 and e15.5, *Hesx1* mutants are characterized by a dramatic cellular overproliferation of all the hormone-producing cell types, leading to a failure of the underlying mesenchyme to condense and form the sphenoid cartilage that separates the pituitary from the oral cavity. In the late stages of pituitary development, the terminal differentiation of the hormone-producing cell types appear normal in most *Hesx1* mutants, with overexpression of αGsu, *Tshβ*, *Gh*, *Pomc*, and *Pit1* by e16.5. Earlier in development, there is a delay in the onset of *Pomc* expression both in Rathke's pouch and in the developing hypothalamus at e12.5, and there also appears to be a dual induction of αGsu expression on both the rostral and caudal sides of Rathke's pouch. Strikingly, in occasional *Hesx1* gene–deleted mice, the initial thickening of oral ectoderm and minimal activation of *Lhx3* are observed at e12.5, but the embryos exhibit a complete arrest of pituitary development and the pituitary gland is absent by e18.5. The discrepancy of incomplete phenotype penetrance in *Hesx1* mutants is likely influenced by the actions of the linked modifier genes.[68,69]

Related Diseases

The human *HESX1* gene contains four exons separated by three introns, and it maps to chromosome 3p21. The *HESX1* gene encodes a highly conserved polypeptide of 185 amino acids with a 60-amino acid homeodomain at its C terminus. Initial analyses of the *HESX1* mutations carried out in kindreds with septo-optic dysplasia, identified a nucleotide transition that resulted in the substitution of R160C (in the third helix of the homeodomain) in two children with CPHD, born to a highly consanguineous family. Magnetic resonance imaging revealed ectopic/undescended posterior pituitary associated with a hypoplastic anterior lobe in these two affected siblings.[67] None of the heterozygote parents exhibited features of septo-optic dysplasia, consistent with an autosomal-recessive inheritance. To date, five additional mutations (Q6H, S170L, T181A, I26T, and 306/307InsAG-X) have been found in the coding region of the *HESX1* gene. These five mutations are all found in heterozygous form and are associated with variable phenotypes including hypopituitarism ranging from isolated GH deficiency to CPHD. It is clear from these reported cases that mutation in the *HESX1* gene can cause pituitary hormone deficiency with variable phenotypes and with incomplete penetrance.[70]

Mechanism

The Hesx1 gene product can bind to either dimer or monomer DNA sites with high affinity in transient transfection assays.[71,72] Modular structure analysis revealed that in addition to the DNA-binding homeodomain, Hesx1 contains two sequences in the N terminus; one is similar to the *eh1* motif found in *Drosophila engrailed*[73] and one is similar to the WRPW motif found in several helix-loop-helix proteins,[74] both of which are capable of recruiting the *Groucho* class of corepressors.[75,76] Both the N-terminal and homeodomain regions of Hesx1 can independently act as repressors. Hesx1 is a strong transcriptional repressor that acts by recruiting the mSin3A/B, HDACs 1 and 2, and the Brg1 complexes to its homeodomain and the TLE corepressor to its eh1 domain. The strong association between Tle1 and Hesx1 is mediated by a highly conserved helical motif (FXLXXIL) present in the Hesx1 N terminus, which can also be found in Nkx, Six, and certain Pax homeodomain factors' family members.[77] These recruitments are required and sufficient for the repressive actions of Hesx1 *in vivo*. Forced persistent expression of *Hesx1* and *Tle1* resulted in the loss of the *Pit1* lineage and a *Prop1^Ames*-like dysmorphogenesis while the expression of *Prop1* and *Pomc* remained. The mutation in human *HESX1* (R160C) has a dominant negative effect both *in vitro* and *in vivo*. This dominant negative activity requires the eh1 repression domain, which is also required for full-length recombinant Hesx1 dimerization in solution. This dominant transcription repressor activity may help to explain the heterozygous phenotypes observed in *HESX1* patients.[71]

Hesx1 and Prop1 share a conserved DNA-recognition site. The repression domain in Hesx1 can suppress the transcription activation activity of Prop1. The Hesx1 repressor can heterodimerize with Prop1 and can bind to the palindromic site as homodimers or heterodimers, with Prop1 acting as an activator and Hesx1 as a repressor, to inhibit Prop1 activation function. The expression of *Prop1* is elevated in *Hesx1*-mutant mice, suggesting not only that *Hesx1* can repress *Prop1* activation function but also that it is required for proper *Prop1* expression.[68] Forced early expression of *Prop1* to the uncommitted oral ectoderm blocks the formation of Rathke's pouch, which results in absence of the anterior pituitary gland with no initial induction of *Lhx3* expression, demonstrating that premature expression of *Prop1* can block the pituitary organogenesis that phenocopies the effects of *Hesx1*-gene deletion,[15] in contrast to the *Hesx1/TLE1* transgenic mouse with a *Prop1^Ames*-like phenotype, suggesting that the antagonistic repressor complex can suppress *Prop1* activation.[68] The sequential repression and activation of a common set of regulatory genes may prove to be an underlying strategy in the temporal code of pituitary organ development, with initial repression required for organ commitment and proliferation and subsequent activation required for commitment of specific cell lineages.

LHX3 *AND* LHX4 *GENES*

LHX3 (LIM homeo box gene 3) is a LIM-type homeodomain transcription factor. In addition to a C-terminus homeodomain, Lhx3 contains two tandem repeats of LIM zinc-binding motifs, each composed of 50 to 60 amino acids with a conserved pattern of cysteine and histidine residues that form a pair of zinc fingers, separated by a linker of 2 amino acids. Expression analysis revealed that mouse *Lhx3* mRNA can be detected in the developing nervous system and accumulates in the Rathke's pouch beginning at e9.5 (see Fig. 16-2). *Lhx3* remains expressed in the entire pouch and its expression is maintained through e15.5; the expression is particularly strong in the anterior and intermediate lobes of the adult pituitary. In addition, *Lhx3* is expressed bilaterally along the spinal cord and the hindbrain at early stages of development.[78]

Lhx4 (LIM homeodomain gene 4) is structurally closely related to *Lhx3*. The *Lhx* gene gamily consists of at least 12 members; many of them are expressed in the pituitary during development including *Isl1*, *Isl2*, *Lhx2*, *Lhx3*, and *Lhx4*. *Lhx3* and *Lhx4* have been genetically defined as required elements for both the early stages of pituitary determination and the later differentiation of pituitary cell types. By *in situ* hybridization, *Lhx4* gene is found to be expressed transiently in ventrolateral regions of the neural tube and hindbrain in the developing mouse. During pituitary development, *Lhx4* is expressed throughout the invaginating Rathke's pouch at e9.5. At e12.5, *Lhx4* expression becomes restricted to the future anterior lobe of the pituitary gland, and by e15.5, *Lhx4* expression diminishes. In the adult pituitary, *Lhx4* is found in the anterior and intermediate lobes at a much lower level than that of *Lhx3*.[79]

Animal Model

Employing a reverse genetic approach, mice with a targeted disruption in the *Lhx3* gene were generated. Mice heterozygous for the mutation are apparently normal and fertile, whereas homozygous individuals are stillborn or expire within 24 hours of birth. In these homozygous mice, the hindbrain, spinal cord, and pineal gland are grossly normal, as is the posterior lobe of the pituitary, but the anterior and intermediate lobes of the pituitary are absent. During embryonic development, the mutant animal exhibits a lack of growth in Rathke's pouch, and pituitary gland development does not progress beyond the Rathke's pouch stage. With the exception of residual corticotrope, other anterior pituitary cell types are absent, indicating that *Lhx3* is required for the appearance of the somatotrope, lactotrope, thyrotrope, and gonadotrope cell types.[80]

Mice homozygous for the targeted deletion of *Lhx4* gene exhibit an early postnatal death from a failure of pulmonary maturation.[81] *Lhx4*-deleted mice have a well-formed Rathke's pouch but display incomplete pituitary development following this stage, and the differentiation of pituitary cell types is perturbed. Consequently, by e12.5, there exists a miniature Rathke's pouch and by e14.5, the nascent pituitary structure has progressed to a larger pouch, but the anterior lobe is discernible only as a slight thickening in the ventral region. This hypocellularity of the anterior lobe is caused by failure of pituitary precursor cells to survive; large numbers of apoptotic cells are evident throughout the pituitary primordia of *Lhx4*-mutant mice at e12.5.[82] In later gestation stages, Rathke's pouch is hypoplastic with an enlarged lumen resulting from reduced proliferation of the precursors, and the anterior lobe of the pituitary is reduced in size. Expression analyses have revealed residual amounts of Lh- and Gnrhr-positive cells at e18.5. Thus, *Lhx4* is not required for specification of gonadotrope cells, but it does support the expansion of the cell population. Similarly, all five anterior pituitary-specific cell lineages are present in the *Lhx4*-mutant pituitary, but in dramatically reduced numbers. By contrast, the intermediate lobe melanotrope cells are undisturbed.

Mice with double deletion of *Lhx3* and *Lhx4* demonstrated that both genes direct formation of the pituitary gland.[83] The early formation of the Rathke's pouch rudiment from pituitary primordium does not depend entirely on the function of either *Lhx3* or *Lhx4* alone, but together these genes redundantly control the formation of the definitive pouch. *Lhx3* also controls a subsequent step of pituitary fate commitment, and in these early stages, *Lhx4* appears to act upstream of the *Lhx3* and *Isl1* genes and is required for expansion of Rathke's pouch. Therefore, *Lhx3* and *Lhx4* dictate pituitary gland identity by controlling decision points of organogenesis and regulation of the proliferation and differentiation of pituitary-specific cell lineages.

Related Diseases

Human *LHX3* shares high degree of homology with its mouse orthologue, exhibiting 94% identity at the amino acid level. *LHX3* is located on human chromosome 9q34 and spans a genomic fragment of at least 6 kb that includes 6 exons.[84,85] In a candidate-gene screen based on pituitary phenotypes observed in a recessive lethal mutation in mice, two mutations in the *LHX3* gene were identified in two unrelated consanguineous pedigrees that display CPHD.[86] In one family, affected individuals are homozygous for a Y116C mutation located in the highly conserved LIM2 domain of LHX3, a domain critical for protein-protein interactions. In the second family, affected individuals are homozygous for a 23-base-pair deletion in an intragenic region, predicting a severely truncated protein that lacks the entire homeodomain and rendering it incapable of DNA binding. *LHX3*-defective patients have deficiencies in GH, TSH, PRL, FSH, and LH, but they display intact levels of ACTH, similar to the endocrine profiles observed in *PROP1* patients (see Table 16-2). In addition, these *LHX3*-defective patients displayed a rigid cervical spine that restricted their head rotation. This unique feature facilitates differential diagnosis.

The human *LHX4* gene encodes a 390-amino acid protein that contains two LIM domains and a homeodomain that shares 99% sequence identity with its mouse orthologue. Genomic analysis revealed that the human *LHX4* gene contains 6 exons and is mapped to chromosome 1q25.[87] In a large consanguineous pedigree of three generations, a G-to-C substitution in the intron preceding exon 5 of *LHX4* generates a mutant protein with perturbed homeodomain, which affects its DNA-binding function. Patients with this disease have short stature with CPHD, which affects GH, thyroxine, and cortisol, as well as cerebellar defects and abnormalities of the sella turcica. This mutant allele is transmitted in a dominant fashion, affecting only the maternal side of the kindred with a high phenotypic penetrance.[87]

Mechanism

LIM homeodomain proteins are transcription factors and exert their effects by regulating target gene expression. Lhx3 binds with high affinity to AT-rich DNA sequences (including minor groove interaction) and bend the DNA molecule to an angle of 62° in a model system.[88] Lhx3 can activate the regulatory regions of pituitary genes, including *αGsu*, *Prl*, *Tshβ*, and *Pit1*. *Lhx3* expression is partially regulated by the *Lhx4* gene during pituitary development. At e12.5, only a few cells express *Lhx3* in the dorsal-most aspect of the pouch in the *Lhx4* mutants. However, the normal pattern of *Lhx3* expression, including the dorsal-ventral gradient, is established in *Lhx4* mutants by e14.5.[82]

Genetic analysis revealed that *Lhx4* interacts with *Prop1* to stimulate anterior pituitary lobe expansion. Neither gene is essential for initiating corticotrope specification. However, no *Pomc* or *αGsu* expression is detected in double-mutant mice at e14.5, suggesting that *Prop1* and *Lhx4* have overlapping roles in corticotrope and gonadotrope development.[82] In *Hesx1*-deleted mutants the expression domains of *Lhx3* and *Prop1* are increased, as well as those of *Fgf8* and *Fgf10* in the infundibulum, which has expanded rostrally.[68] These findings indicate that *Hesx1* is required for maintaining the proper expression of *Fgfs*, consistent with the notion that *Lhx3* expression can be regulated by FGF signaling.

The etiology of CPHD is heterogeneous. Mutations in the *PROP1* gene are the major cause of CPHD, accountable for about 60% of the familial cases examined. Mutations in the *PIT1*, *HESX1*, *LHX3*, *LHX4*, and others are also responsible for this condition. Although the phenotypes of these patients are somewhat grossly similar, their pituitary endocrine profiles are distinctive, which can facilitate diagnosis of the types of CPHD.

TBX19 *GENE*

TPIT/TBX19 is a T-box transcription factor family member (the T-box in the mouse *T* [*Brachyury*] gene) that encodes a 448-amino acid protein.[89] Functional identification of *Tbx19*, also known as *Tpit*, was established after the observation of elements in a critical *cis*-acting sequence in the *POMC* promoter.[90] Transcripts of *Tpit/Tbx19* can be found only in the anterior and intermediate pituitary and brain (see Fig. 16-2)[90,91]; *TBX19* is specifically required for continued *Pomc* transcription.[90]

Animal Model

Mice with targeted disruption of the *Tpit/Tbx19* gene have been generated. Mice heterozygous for the mutation are apparently normal. Adult mice homozygous for the mutation have very few Acth-positive cells in the pituitary, although the initial expression of *Pomc* gene is undisturbed at the Rathke's pouch stages. These cells are born in normal quantities in mutants but are lost or fail to expand appropriately, suggesting *Tpit/Tbx19* is not required for corticotrope cell commitment but is later important for *Pomc* lineage differentiation. The intermediate lobe melanotropes in mutant mice are populated by gonadotrope and some Pit1-independent thyrotrope, also indicating that *Tpit/Tbx19* normally represses pituitary gonadotrope differentiation.[92,93]

Related Diseases

The human *TBX19* gene shares 94% amino acid identity with that of mouse *Tbx19* and maps to chromosome 1q23-q24. A case of isolated ACTH deficiency was identified in a consanguineous family with a nonsense mutation C-to-T transition in exon 6 in *TBX19*, resulting in a truncated gene product (R286X). The transmission of this mutation appears to be recessive. In another case of isolated ACTH deficiency, a heterozygous C-to-T transition in exon 2 of the *TBX19* gene was identified, resulting in a conserved amino acid S128F mutation, suggesting a dominant negative inheritance.[90] *TBX19* defects result in POMC deficiency in both humans and mice, establishing *TBX19* as the gene required for effective *POMC* expression *in vivo*.[92,93]

Mechanism

Tbx19 is a transcriptional regulator, recognizing target genes through its T-box DNA-binding domain. In response to signals elicited by the hypothalamic hormone corticotrope-releasing hormone, Tbx19 functions as an activator of transcription by recruiting SRC/p160 coactivators to its cognate DNA target in the *Pomc* promoter.[94] Tbx19 can synergize with orphan nuclear receptor NGFI-B, serving as part of the transcription regulatory complex on the *Pomc* promoter in response to hormonal stimulation.[95] Transgenic expression of *Tbx19* in non-Pomc producing regions of the pituitary gland can cause ectopic *Pomc* expression[90] and *Tbx19* is an inhibitor of *αGsu* expression in rostral tip cells, gonadotrope, and thyrotrope, and of *Tshβ* production in caudomedial thyrotrope.[91] *Tbx19* deficiency is permissive for trans-differentiation of cells normally destined to be corticotrope and melanotrope into alternative cell fates, namely, gonadotrope and rostral tip thyrotrope, suggesting a determinative role of *Tbx19* in cell lineage specification. *Tbx19* defects have no effect on differentiation of *Pit1*-dependent cell lineages (see Fig. 16-3 and Table 16-2).[92,93]

GLI2 *GENE*

The *GLI* genes (GLI-Kruppel family member 2) were named because of amplification observed in gliomas of the brain. Sequencing of *GLI* cDNA clones indicated the presence of 5 tandem zinc fingers connected by conserved histidine-cysteine links, a motif found in the *Kruppel* family of zinc-finger genes. In both humans and mice, three closely related *GLI* genes, *Gli1*, *Gli2*, and *Gli3*,[96] have been implicated in the signal transduction of the secreted glycoprotein Shh. At embryonic stages, *Gli2* is expressed throughout the neural plate, in the floor plate, in the telencephalon and the midline of the diencephalons, and in the dermomyotome.[97] Gli2 has been characterized as a transcription factor and demonstrated to bind targeted DNA sequences through its zinc-finger motifs.

Animal Model

Gli2-mutant mice die at birth with severe skeletal and neural defects.[98–100] In *Gli2*-mutant mouse embryos,[101] the development of Rathke's pouch appears normal. Mice with simultaneous inactivation of both *Gli1* and *Gli2* have very severe defects in the development of pituitary gland; about half of these mutants completely lack a Rathke's pouch at e12.5. In these mutants, the domains of expression of *Shh* and *Nkx2.1* are abnormal, and the loss of Shh signaling boundary in the oral ectoderm could be a cause of this defect.[102]

Mutation in the zebrafish *gli2* gene interferes with hedgehog (Hh) signaling during embryogenesis in the *yot-too* (*yot*) mutant. The alleles of *yot* contain nonsense mutations that result in carboxy-terminally truncated protein products. In addition to causing defects in midline development, *yot* mutations disrupt anterior pituitary formation and cause ectopic lens formation.[103] It is also worth noting that in a recessive polarity mutation in chicken *talpid*,[3] Rathke's pouch is abnormal or almost absent in homozygous embryos, and in some cases ectopic lenses are produced in the corresponding region of the head, providing the possibility of transformation of adenohypophysis anlage into lens.[104]

Related Diseases
GLI2 encodes a protein of 1258 amino acids, belongs to the C2H2-type zinc-finger protein subclass of the GLI family, and maps to 2q14. In a screen of 390 patients with holoprosencephaly, seven heterozygous sequence variations in *GLI2* are found. Three mutations (2274del1, W113X, R168X) in the *GLI2* resulted in severe prematurely truncated gene products. One pedigree harbors a mutation (IVS5 + 1G > 5) that would affect the proper splicing events of exon 5, resulting in truncation or termination affecting the zinc-finger DNA-binding domain. Although phenotypic penetrance is variable, the principal features among these patients are associated with pituitary anomalies and holoprosencephaly.[105] Results from analyses of the phenotypes in these pedigrees are consistent with autosomal-dominant transmission of these traits.

Mechanism
There are multiple Gli proteins in vertebrates; three each in the mouse and in the human, displaying highly similar DNA-binding zinc fingers, with these proteins exhibiting distinctive and overlapping regulatory activities in the mediation of Shh signaling. Genetic analyses in model systems have revealed that the Gli2 protein has both activation and repression functions. The C-terminally truncated Gli2 proteins, observed both in human cases and in zebrafish mutations, act as repressor proteins.[106] Such repressor forms of Gli2 protein are capable of exerting a dominant negative effect on gene activation by normal Gli1 or Gli2 proteins. Gli2 normally acts predominantly as a transcriptional activator of *Shh* target genes. *Gli2* is downstream of *Shh*, as *Shh* and *Gli2* double mutants have the same phenotype as the *Shh* mutants.[107] In a knock-in approach, replacing *Gli2* with its homologue *Gli1*, a known transcription activator, results in normal development. This experiment suggests that the mouse *Gli1* and *Gli2* may have redundant functions in mediating *Shh* signaling during development, and that *Gli1* may compensate the loss of *Gli2* in *Gli2*-mutant mouse models. Evidence of transdifferentiation of the adenohypophysis into a lens in *yot* mutants and severe pituitary phenotypes in mouse *Gli1*- and *Gli2*-double mutant, as well as in human cases, support the notion that Shh signaling is necessary for initial commitment of the Rathke's pouch and early steps in pituitary formation.

Gli2 is an upstream regulator of *Lhx3* (see Fig. 16-3). One consequence of the *Gli2* defect in *yot*-mutant embryos was the absence of *Lhx3* expression in the anterior part of the adenohypophysis anlage.[108] In the mouse, absence of *Lhx3* results in failure of development of Rathke's pouch into the adenohypophysis. However, *Lhx3* mutation alone is not sufficient to cause transdifferentiation into the lens from the adenohypophysis anlage as observed in *gli2*-truncated *yot* mutant.

OTHER TRANSCRIPTION FACTORS
Transcription factors act as activators and repressors and are expressed in a coordinated fashion, mediating organogenesis and cell type specification in the pituitary gland (see Fig. 16-3). During the early commitment stage, the expressions of *Pitx1/2* and *Hesx1* are found in the anterior neural plate stages and in the invagination of Rathke's pouch. *Lhx3* is expressed on e9.5 in the nascent RP and is required for initial organ commitment and growth[80] and for cell proliferation together with *Lhx4*.[82] *Prop1* appears on e10.5 and is required for determination of four ventral cell types, including the *Pit1*-dependent lineages (somatotrope, lactotrope, and thyrotrope) and gonadotrope.[50,56] Sequential expression of this cascade of homeodomain genes represents a model system of transcription control of organogenesis and cell type determination and differentiation in mammals. Phenotypic comparisons in these pituitary loci in both mice and humans suggest that the developmental pathways in determination of the pituitary gland are highly conserved.

Some of these factors expressed transiently in the Rathke's pouch, and their reduced expression is likely to be required for the progression of specific cell types, as evident in the *Prop1^Ames* mutant where the temporal patterns of *Hesx1*, *Prop1*, and *Brn4* gene expression are extended. As the lineage-determining transcription factor Pit1 appears, certain transcription factors that characterize earlier stages of development are gradually eliminated, including *Hesx1*, *Pfrk*,[15] *GATA-3*,[49] *Pax6*,[109] and *Brn4*.[110]

In addition to the genes mentioned here, the list of pituitary-expressed transcription factors implicated in the developing pituitary gland is growing. Several families of factors, including homeodomain (Isl1, Isl2, Oct1, Otx1, Pax6, Pitx1, Pitx2, Pitx3, Six1, Six3, and Six6), zinc-finger (Krox24, Gli1, Gata2, Nzf1, Sp1, Sp3, Zfhep, and Zn16), nuclear receptor (T3R, SF1, ERα, ERβ, and Dax), basic HLH domain (AP2, NeuroD, Mash1, Nhlh2, and Math) and other (AP1, Ets1, Foxl2, CBf, Cp1, Rb, Men1, Preb, and Tef) proteins have been implicated (see reviews in Refs. 20, 111, and 112). Pitx1 and Pitx2 represent two of the bicoid-related Pitx homeodomain transcription factors. They display distinct but overlapping patterns of expression and are critical in the development of several organs including the pituitary, with *Pitx1* required for the gonadotrope, thyrotrope, and *Pomc* gene expression[113,114] and *Pitx2* required for the earliest phases of pituitary development for the patterning and proliferation events within Rathke's pouch.[115–117] Multiple members of the Six family (*Six1*, *Six6*, *Six2*, and *Six3*) are also expressed in the pituitary. *Six6*, acting as a strong tissue-specific repressor in association with dachshund (Dach) corepressors, directly represses cyclin-dependent kinase inhibitors including the *p27^Kip1* promoter and regulates early progenitor cell proliferation in retinogenesis and pituitary development.[118] *Six1* exhibits synergistic genetic interactions with the *eyes absent* (*Eya*) family of protein phosphatases and is required to regulate genes that encode growth control and modulating precursor cell proliferation. The phosphatase activity of Eya converts the function of Six1-Dach from repression to activation, causing transcriptional activation through recruitment of coactivators.[119] Evidence suggests that *Six3* acts upstream of the *Wnt* pathway, and deletion of *Six3* in mice resulted in failure of development of the ventral diencephalons and, consequently, the development of pituitary.[120] *Gata2* is involved in establishing molecular memory of signaling gradients during pituitary development in conjunction with *Pit1*, and loss of *Gata2* is associated with failure to differentiate into gonadotrope.[49,116] The orphan nuclear receptor steroidogenic factor 1, Sf1, is essential for pituitary gonadotrope.[121]

Although pituitary cell types in the adult anterior lobe do not appear to be stratified, initial appearance of these cell types follows a ventral-dorsal pattern. With the Rathke's pouch cleft as the dorsal reference, *Gh*, *Prl*, and *Tsh* of *Pit1* lineages are located dorsally, whereas gonadotrope cells appear ventrally. Several transcription factors display vertical gradients, including *Pax6*, which exhibits a dorsal to ventral expression gradient; *Pax6*-mutant mice exhibit an increased number of ventral thyrotrope and gonadotrope, at the expense of the more dorsal somatotrope and lactotrope cell types.[109] Thus, *Pax6* may functionally oppose Shh signaling to specify a dorsal rather than ventral cell fate. Another pituitary transcription factor displaying an initial dorsal-ventral gradient is *Prop1* (see Fig. 16-2). *Prop1*-mutant mice lose dorsal cell types of the *Pit1* lineage, while ventral cell types of corticotrope and gonadotrope are less affected.

The induction of expression of transcription factors in spatially overlapping patterns in the developing pituitary may act as a molecular memory of prior signals in the positional determination of specific cell types. The signaling pathways that dictate expression patterns of transcription factor are the focus of current research application, with several classes of early morphogenic gradients of broadly expressed signaling molecules likely to be critical elements of pituitary cell type determination and differentiation.

SIGNALING PATHWAYS IN PITUITARY DEVELOPMENT

Vertebrate organogenesis events are coordinated through the interplay of highly organized signaling pathways and these developmental signaling systems have proved to be remarkably conserved throughout evolution.[122] Extrinsic signals, in the form of secreted morphogens, create local environments for organ patterning and progenitor cell type determination. These signals are interpreted through the functions of cell type–restricted transcriptional regulators, resulting in various intrinsic or cell-autonomous determination events. Numerous extrinsic signaling molecules have been implicated, including members of the HH, transforming growth factor-beta (TGF$_\beta$)/bone morphogenic protein (BMP), Wingless/Wnt, and fibroblast growth factor (FGF) superfamilies, as well as others (see review in Ref. 123).

Influenced by the growth of the forebrain structures, the midline anterior neural ridge cells ultimately responsible for the origin of the pituitary gland are displaced and eventually become located immediately ventral to the diencephalons. The initial extrinsic signaling of murine pituitary development requires signals from both the ventral diencephalon and the oral ectoderm. Organogenesis of the anterior pituitary gland begins at e9 in mouse, as the cells of the anterior pituitary placode in the oral ectoderm thicken and invaginate to form the nascent pituitary of Rathke's pouch.[19] *Shh*, seemingly uniformly expressed in the oral epithelia at the time, is excluded from the pituitary placode prior to the initiation of the invagination.[124] The presumptive ventral diencephalon provides Bmp4, the first known dorsal signal required for the initial formation of Rathke's pouch.[18] Immediately following formation, the dorsal portion of Rathke's pouch directly contacts the midline ventral diencephalon, which evaginates on e10 and acts as a key organizing center for the patterning and commitment of Rathke's pouch. Opposing dorsal Fgfs/Bmp4 and ventral Shh/Bmp2 gradients provide positional and proliferative signals to the pituitary progenitor field, acting to positionally establish cell types through the induction of overlapping patterns of transcription factor expression.[15,18] Initial proliferation and determination is controlled by sequential cascades of exogenously and endogenously restricted combinatorial signaling, with subsequent attenuation of specific signal events required for establishment of the cellular environment permissive for terminal differentiation (Figs. 16-4 and 16-5).[2]

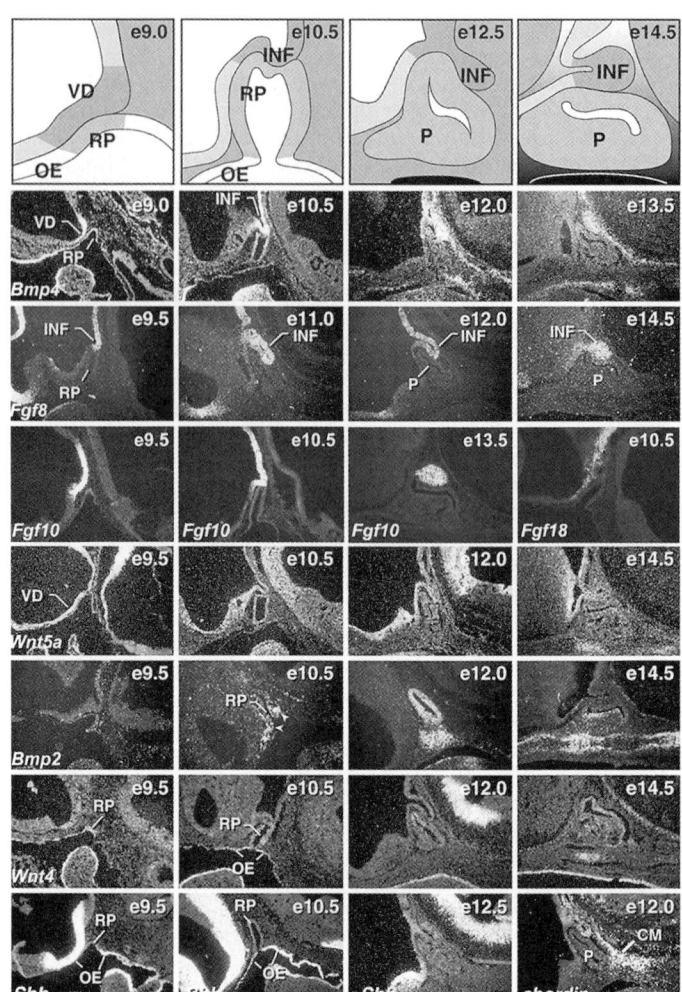

Figure 16-4 Signaling molecules expressed in the early phases of pituitary organogenesis detected by *in situ* hybridization. Schematic representation of different stages of pituitary development *(top)*. An initially uniform oral ectoderm (oe) makes contact with the overlying neural epithelium (ne) by e9.0 in the mouse, with *Sonic hedgehog (Shh)* becoming excluded from the region that forms Rathke's pouch. The infundibulum epithelium of the ventral diencephalons expresses *Bmp4, Fgf8, Fgf10, Fgf18,* and *Wnt5a,* while *Bmp2* is expressed within Rathke's pouch at the *Shh* restriction boundary and within the ventral mesenchyme. The BMP antagonist chordin is expressed in the caudal mesenchyme adjacent to Rathke's pouch. (Modified from Treier M, Gleiberman AS, O'Connell SM, et al: Multistep signaling requirements for pituitary organogenesis *in vivo.* Genes Dev 12:1691–1704, 1998.)

SONIC HEDGEHOGS

Shh, one of three vertebrate homologues of the *Drosophila*-secreted protein *hh*, plays a crucial role in defining the border between the anterior and posterior compartments in the imaginal disk.[125] It is expressed in Hensen's node, the floor plate of the neural tube, the posterior of the limb buds, and throughout the notochord. *Shh* has been implicated as the key inductive signal in patterning of the ventral neural tube,[126,127] the anterior-posterior limb axis,[128] and the ventral somites.[129] The mouse, zebrafish, and human *Shh* homologues are highly conserved,[130] suggesting conserved functional properties. The human *SHH* gene encodes a predicted protein that is 92.4% identical to its mouse homologue and is mapped to chromosome 7q. Many *SHH* mutations, including nonsense and missense, deletions, and insertion mutations, are identified throughout the gene in patients with holoprosencephaly, the most common forebrain defect in humans.

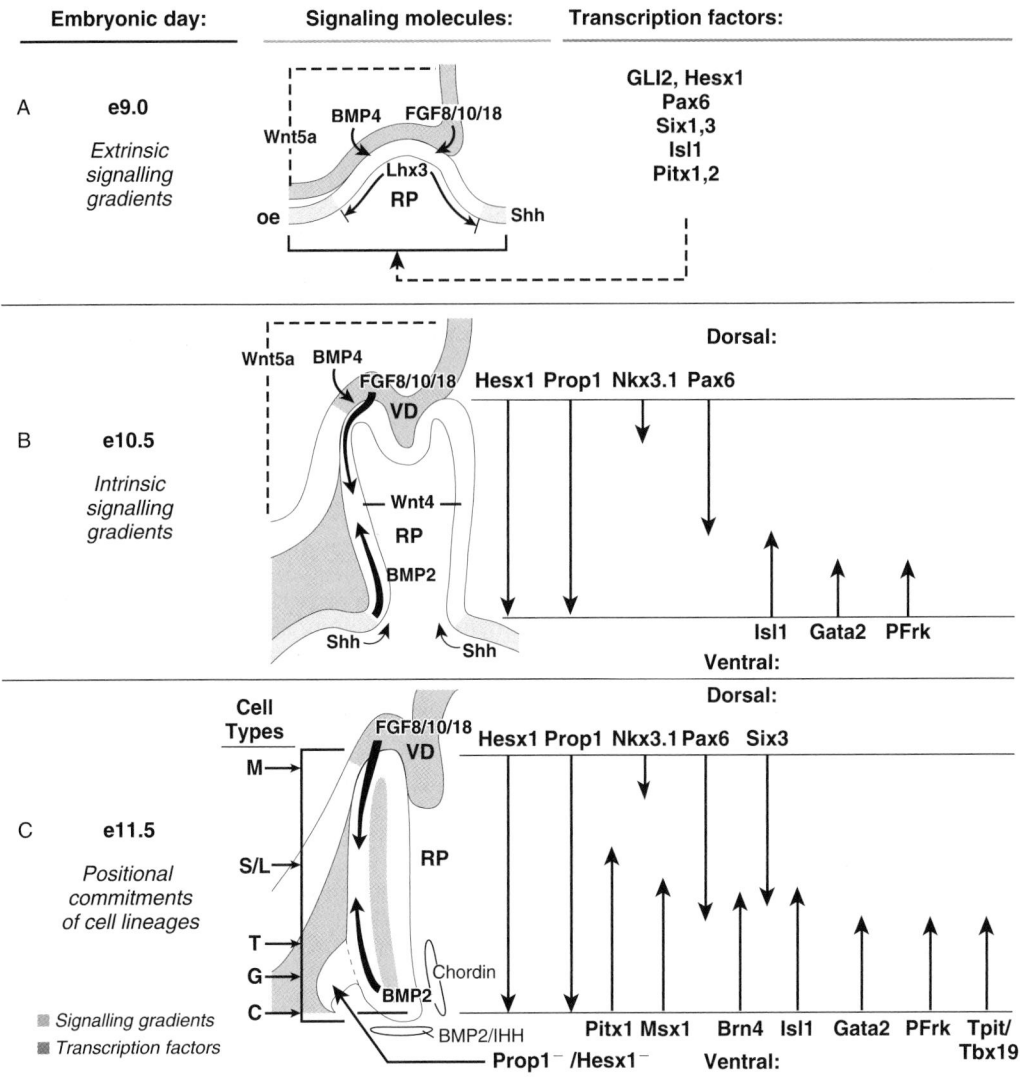

Figure 16-5 Model for the progression of pituitary cell lineages in response to extrinsic and intrinsic signals. Primordial-cell types derived from the anterior neural ridge are committed to the pituitary fate through the induction of Lhx3 expression, which may require the combinatorial actions of Fgfs, Bmp4, and Shh, Bmp4 suppresses the expression of Shh to create a Shh-nonexpressing zone. When Rathke's pouch has formed by e11, Fgf8 expressed in the infundibulum functions antagonistically to Bmp2, resulting in ventrodorsal Bmp and dorsoventral Fgf activity gradients in Rathke's pouch. This leads to the induction of several temporally and spatially restricted transcription factors. (Modified from Scully KM, Rosenfeld MG: Pituitary development: Regulatory codes in mammalian organogenesis. Science 295:2231–2235, 2002.)

Mouse mutants homozygous for a disrupted *Shh* gene revealed defects in the establishment of maintenance of midline structures such as the notochord and floor plate, and cyclopia.[131] In mice, *Shh* is expressed in ventral diencephalons and throughout the oral ectoderm on e8 but is excluded from the invaginating Rathke's pouch, thereby creating a potential molecular compartment boundary within the oral ectoderm. Transgenic overexpression of *hedgehog-interacting protein* (*HIP*), which acts to attenuate *Hh* function, specifically blocks *Hh* signaling in the oral ectoderm and Rathke's pouch within the head region, affecting both proliferation and cell type determination, and this results in an absence of ventral cell type markers in Rathke's pouch.[124] By contrast, a gain-of-function transgenic approach to overexpress *Shh* in Rathke's pouch results in a phenotype of the expansion of ventral cell types, with modified levels of *Lhx3* gene expression. This phenotype is consistent with results derived from an animal cap explant culture with banded hh in *Xenopus laevis*, in which the expression domains of pituitary-restricted factor *hesx1*[65,132] are expanded, supporting a role for *Shh* signaling in control of proliferative events in pituitary development.[9]

The secreted protein Hh binds to a 12-transmembrane receptor protein Patched and regulates obligatory mediators of the signal transduction, members of the *Gli* transcription factor. In *gli2*[yot] mutants, the rostral expression domains (analogous to the ventral domains in mice) of pituitary-specific transcription factors such as *lim3* (*Lhx3*) and *six3* are lost, and other pituitary-restricted factors such as *nk 2.2* are

absent.[108,133] This observation is consistent with the sequential and cooperative interaction that *Bmps* and *Hh* exert in limb and neural-tube development[134] that *Shh* acts to induce the expression of *Bmps*. Overexpression of *Shh* in zebrafish results in expanded adenohypophyseal expression of *lhx3*, expansion of *nk2.2* into the posterior adenohypophysis, and an increase in Prl- and somatolactin-secreting cells. In addition, *Hh* signaling is necessary between 10 and 15 hours post fertilization for induction of the zebrafish adenohypophysis, a time when *shh* is expressed only in adjacent neural tissue. These results suggest multiple and distinct roles for *Hh* signaling in the formation of the vertebrate pituitary gland and also suggest that *Hh* signaling from neural ectoderm of ventral diencephalons is necessary for induction and functional patterning of the vertebrate pituitary gland.[133]

FIBROBLAST GROWTH FACTORS

The fibroblast growth factor family contains 22 genes and can further be divided into six subfamilies according to sequence similarities. Members of each subfamily tend to share biochemical and functional properties and are expressed in specific spatial and developmental patterns.[135] Functions of *Fgfs* are mediated by four distinct Fgf-receptor tyrosine kinase molecules, and the specificity for each Fgf is achieved through alternative mRNA splicing.[136] Fgf activity and specificity are further regulated by heparan sulfate oligosaccharides with tissue-specific modifications, in a form of trimolecular complex with receptors.[137,138] The *Fgf* system plays significant roles in many biological events including pattern formation in many tissues during vertebrate embryogenesis. Several members of the *Fgf* family are expressed in the infundibulum and provide proliferative and positional cues to Rathke's pouch (see Fig. 16-4). *Fgf8* and *Fgf10* are expressed in a temporally and spatially overlapping manner within the infundibulum as an evagination of ventral diencephalons and makes direct contact with the dorsal portion of Rathke's pouch following *Bmp4* induction.

Fgf10-deficient mice have complete truncation of the fore and hind limbs and no lung.[139] In mice null for the *Fgfr2 (IIIb)* isoform, which presumably would abolish *Fgf* signaling including that of *Fgf10*,[140] Rathke's pouch forms but rapidly undergoes apoptosis with the pituitary becoming completely absent by e14.5, suggesting a critical role in *Fgf10* signaling for the continued proliferation of the pouch ectoderm. *Fgf8* and *Fgf10* appear to play critical roles in the early patterning and proliferation events in pituitary organogenesis.

Fgf8 is expressed in the primitive streak of the gastrulating mouse embryo, as well as in the visceral endoderm. Mice null for *Fgf8* lack all embryonic mesoderm- and endoderm-derived structures and do not survive beyond e9.5.[141,142] In mice null for a homeodomain gene *Nkx2.1*, which is normally expressed in the ventral diencephalons but not in the Rathke's pouch, *Fgf8* fails to be expressed in the ventral diencephalons, leading to a loss of the infundibulum and consequently a loss of *Lhx3* expression in the Rathke's pouch and the loss of all three lobes of the pituitary gland.[143] In transgenic mice misexpressing *Fgf8* in the ventral regions of the pituitary under control of the regulatory sequences for the *αGSU* gene, most ventral and intermediate cell types are absent with dysmorphogenesis of Rathke's pouch and hyperplasia of corticotrope and melanotropes observed, consistent with a role in the positional determination of dorsally arising pituitary cell types and pituitary progenitor cells.[15] In mice null for *Hesx1*, the most severely affected embryos exhibit a complete arrest of pituitary development after the initial induction of *Lhx3* on e9.5, with *Fgf8* and *Fgf10* ectopically expressed in the oral ectoderm to mirror the normal expression in the overlying neural ectoderm. In *Hesx1* mutants with less severe pituitary defects, *Fgf* expression is abnormally extended rostrally, causing formation of multiple Rathke's pouches. This is potentially significant because transgenic misexpression of *Fgf8* in the oral ectoderm well before the initial invagination of Rathke's pouch produces an identical blockage of pouch formation, and *Hesx1* fails to be expressed in the *Lhx3*-positive rudiment that does form in the transgenic embryos. Thus, the dynamic interplay between boundaries of *Hesx* and *Fgf8/10* expression[68] could suggest a model of reciprocal feedback regulation. This is in keeping with the role of *Fgfs* in committing oral ectoderm to the Rathke's pouch fate (see Fig. 16-5).[143] These genetic data, in conjunction with tissue culture evidence, where the infundibulum is both required and sufficient for the induction of *Lhx3* gene expression in cultured pouch and infundibulum activity can be replaced with Fgf8 or Fgf2, suggest an instructive role for *Fgf8* signaling in pituitary development.[2]

TRANSFORMIONG GROWTH FACTORS AND BMPs

The transforming growth factor-beta superfamily of secreted signaling molecules, which includes several Bmps, has been demonstrated to play critical roles in patterning and cell type specification in several species.[144] During the early stages of pituitary development, *Bmp4* is expressed in the ventral diencephalons as the infundibulum makes direct contact with Rathke's pouch at e9.0 (see Fig. 16-4). Functional evidence with dual explants culture of embryonic diencephalons and Rathke's pouch suggests that Bmp4 is one of the early signaling factors required for the initial commitment of a subpopulation of oral ectodermal cells to form the pituitary gland.[15,18] Deletion of the *Bmp4* gene causes embryonic death at about e10, in which the initial invagination of Rathke's pouch fails to occur.[143] Similarly, driven by the regulatory sequences of the *Pitx1* gene to target the *Bmp2/4* antagonist *Noggin* expression to the oral ectoderm including the Rathke's pouch, pituitary development is arrested at e10 with a failure of the ventral proliferation of cells from the pouch beginning at e11.5 and an absence of pituitary cell types.[18] The phenotype observed in genetic models of the *Bmp4* signaling pathway is similar to the phenotype observed in mice with a targeted disruption of the *Lhx3* gene critical for the determination of most pituitary cell types,[80] suggesting a requirement of *Bmp4* signaling for the continued organ development after pouch formation. Together with the ventral diencephalic *Fgfs*, *Bmp4* is required for initial pituitary commitment and for continued cell proliferation and progression.

Expression of *Bmp2* is initially detected at the ventral boundary between Rathke's pouch and *Shh*, intrinsic to the pouch in the most ventral aspect of the invaginating gland at e9.5, and in a ventral-dorsal gradient at e10.5 (see Fig. 16-4).[15] *Bmp2* expression expands throughout the pouch by e12.5. *Bmp2* expression is also detected in the ventral juxtapituitary mesenchyme, along with *Bmp2/4* antagonist *chordin* in the caudal mesenchyme (see Fig. 16-4), potentially serving to maintain a ventrodorsal Bmp2 gradient. After the closure of Rathke's pouch, *Bmp2* is expressed in mesenchyme adjacent to the pituitary cells expressing ventrally the transcription factors *Gata2*, *Isl1*, and *P-Frk* as well as the hormone subunit *αGsu*.[2] Overexpression of *Bmp2/4* under the control of *αGsu* regulatory elements in ventral mouse pituitary leads to a dorsal expansion of the ventral lineage markers *Isl1* and *Msx1* with induction of *Gata2* gene expression.[15] Similarly, cultivation of Rathke's pouch explants in Bmp2 is sufficient for the induction of *Isl1* and *αGsu* expression.[18] Proper expression of *Bmp2* is therefore critical for progression of pituitary cell types, whereas overexpression of *Bmp2* in vivo prevents terminal differentiation. These studies suggest pouch-intrinsic and ventral signals including Bmp2 contribute to the establishment of the positional identity of ventral pituitary cell types of thyrotrope and gonadotrope marked by *αGsu* expression.

OPPOSING BMPs AND FGFs SIGNALING GRADIENTS

Analogous to the combinatorial signal regulation in organogenesis observed in many organs, physically opposing dorsal-to-ventral Fgf8/10/18 and ventral-to-dorsal Bmp2 gradients appear to be associated with the positional determination of specific pituitary cell types.[145] The ability of the infundibulum or *Fgfs* to induce *Lhx3* gene expression correlates with the restricted expression of the *Bmp2*-induced genes *Isl1* and *αGsu* distal to the source of the *Fgf* signaling.[18] The ability of ventralized expression of *Fgf8* to prevent the appearance of ventral cell types *in vivo* can be attributed to the inhibition of ventral *Bmp2* signaling.[15] Conversely, while cultivation of Rathke's pouch with Bmp2/4 initiates the expression of the ventral markers *Isl1* and *αGsu*, it inhibits the expression of more dorsal cell type markers such as Acth *in vitro*[18] and *Pit1 in vivo*.[15] Thus, antagonistic and opposing dorsal-to-ventral Fgf8 and ventral-to-dorsal Bmp2 gradients appear to be associated with the positional determination of dorsal and ventral cell types.[2,145]

WNTs

The *Wnt* proto-oncogene family contains at least 19 known members.[146] As classical morphogens, the *Wnt* family of signaling molecules induces various cellular responses from proliferation to cell fate determination and differentiation.[147,148] The canonic *Wnt* pathway stated that Wnt ligands bind to the

Frizzled family of seven-transmembrane domain receptors, leading to the stabilization and accumulation of β-catenin, which interacts with members of the TCF/LEF family of DNA-binding transcription factors and changes them from repressors to activators of transcription primarily by displacing the groucho/Tle corepressor[149,150] to influence target gene expression.[151]

In *Pitx2*-deficient mice, mutant embryos fail to survive to term and develop arrest of early determination events in anterior pituitary gland.[115,152-155] Pitx2 has been demonstrated to be acting downstream of the *Wnt* signal, and *Lef1* and β-catenin have been demonstrated to physically occupy the *Pitx2* promoter in the context of a pituitary cell line. *Pitx2*-mutant pituitary glands contained decreased numbers of proliferating cells, while transgenic overexpression of *Pitx2* in the anterior pituitary led to increased cell numbers.[154] In a subtraction expression profiling analysis of *Porp1^Ames*-mutant pituitary, several members of the *Wnt* signaling pathway are identified including the *frizzled2* receptor, *Apc*, β-catenin, *groucho*, and *Tcf7l2*.[61] This genetic evidence suggests critical roles for the *Wnt* pathway in pituitary cellular proliferation and probably in cell type determination and differentiation.

Several *Wnt*-signaling molecules are expressed during the development of pituitary, *Wnt4* is expressed in the ventral diencephalon, and *Wnt5a* is expressed in the cells of Rathke's pouch (see Fig. 16-4). In *Wnt4*-mutant mice, the pituitary is mildly hypocellular, with the ventral cell types showing normal differentiation but incomplete expansion. Additionally, cultivation of Rathke's pouch with Wnt5a and Bmp4 can induce expression of the early cell type marker αGsu.[15] Thus, *Wnts* and *BMPs* may act in synergy to expand pituitary cell lineages and induce cell determination programs.

OTHER POTENTIAL MORPHOGENETIC FACTORS

Extrinsically derived signals that possibly affect Rathke's pouch arising from ventral mesenchyme beneath the developing pituitary gland include *Indian Hedgehog (IHH)*, *Wnt4*, and *Bmp2*; whereas caudal mesenchyme is a source of a *Chordin* signal capable of opposing the function of *Bmp2*.[156] In addition, little is known about the contribution of cytokines, despite the potent ability of cytokines such as leukemia inhibitory factor (LIF) to maintain mouse embryonic stem cells in an undifferentiated state. A potential role for Lif in pituitary development investigated in pituitary-derived cell lines is that Lif can activate synthesis of *Acth* in combination with the hypothalamic peptide corticotropin-releasing hormone.[157] In transgenic animals that express *Lif* under control of αGsu regulatory information, most cell types fail to properly differentiate, and the pituitary is characterized by the formation of ciliated cysts of Rathke's pouch and corticotrope hyperplasia,[158] suggesting that LIF may contribute to the identity establishment of dorsal-cell phenotypes.

In addition to the dorsal and ventral structures, another organizer signaling center, the notochord, is located just posterior to the developing pituitary gland. The proximity of these two structures, albeit from different origins, suggests a role for the notochord in the initial invagination of Rathke's pouch, as indicated by tissue explant experiments.[19]

Pituitary development research in the past decade has defined a model (see Fig. 16-5) that encompasses the signaling mechanisms governing the early and late aspects of pituitary development. A series of signaling molecules from multiple organizing centers appears to coordinate the commitment, early patterning, proliferation, and positional determination of six hormone-producing pituitary cell types. The *Shh* system defines a boundary for the initial appearance of pituitary anlagen. Secretion of Bmp4 from the ventral diencephalons appears to be required for the initial pituitary organ commitment, with subsequent opposing and antagonistic dorsal Fgf8 and ventral Bmp2 gradients governing the patterning and positional determination of cell types through the induction of overlapping patterns of transcription factor gene expression. The establishment of these distinct expression patterns allows the positional determination of pituitary cell types long before the cell-type-specific terminal differentiation markers appear.

HORMONE RECEPTORS

GROWTH HORMONE–RELEASING HORMONE RECEPTOR

Hypothalamic growth hormone–releasing hormone (GHRH) plays a pivotal role in the regulation of GH synthesis and secretion, acting through the pituitary GH cell specific GHRHR (GHRH receptor). Human *GHRHR* gene encodes a 423-amino acid belongs to seven putative transmembrane domains secretin family of G protein–coupled receptors. The *GHRHR* gene contains at lease 10 exons and is mapped to 7p15-p14.[159] GH secretion is regulated by GHRH and somatostatin interaction and is released in 10 to 20 pulses in a 24-hour cycle.

Mutations in the *GHRHR* cause isolated GH deficiency (IGHD) type IB. Since the initial discovery,[160] several mutations ranging from point mutation in the coding region, to the promoter of the *GHRHR* gene, and to the intron-exon boundary have been identified as affecting gene function as well as transcription and splicing. The phenotypes of affected individuals are consistent with IGHD with marked growth failure and are highly penetrant, and mutations in the *GHRHR* cause a significant percentage of IGHD type IB.[161]

A point mutation in the *Ghrhr* that alters Asp60 to Gly is the cause of the *little (lit)* mouse, characterized by a hypoplastic anterior pituitary gland with a significantly reduced number of Gh cells and consequently a dwarf phenotype. Analysis of mutant pituitary revealed spatially distinct proliferate zones of Gh-producing stem cells and mature somatotropes.[162,163] Ghrh binds to Ghrhr that interacts with the heterotrimeric G proteins to stimulate the production of cyclic adenosine monophosphate (cAMP) by adenylyl cyclase, while somatostatin binds to surface receptors that interact with G_i to inhibit the production of cAMP. Developmentally, the two populations of the Gh-containing cell, a stem cell population and a mature cell expressing Ghrhr that is capable of responding to Ghrh stimulation, exemplify a common strategy for regulating cellular proliferation in other mammalian organs. Both *Gh* and *Ghrhr* genes depend on functional *Pit1* gene product and fail to express in *Pit1*-defective dwarf mouse pituitary.[162] A *GH* target, *IGFI* is expressed in somatotrope, and *IGFI receptors* are expressed in most somatotrope and some corticotrope in the mouse pituitary gland. *Igf1* expression in somatotrope is regulated by pituitary *Gh* and, in turn, suppresses *Gh* expression and stimulates *Pomc* expression at the transcriptional level.[164]

OTHER HORMONE RECEPTORS

Thyrotropin-releasing hormone receptor (TRHR) is a G protein–coupled receptor that activates the inositol phospholipid-calcium-protein kinase C transduction pathway upon the binding of TRH. The *TRHR* gene is expressed in the thyrotrope cells of the anterior pituitary. One case of heterozygous mutations in the TRHR is reported in a patient with isolated central hypothyroidism.[165]

Gonadotropin-releasing hormone receptor (GNRHR) is a member of the G protein–coupled, Ca^{2+}-dependent family of receptors. Located on the cell surface of pituitary gonadotrope, GNRHR transduces signals from GNRH and modulates the synthesis and secretion of *LH* and *FSH*. The human *GNRHR* gene encodes a 328-amino acid protein and is mapped to 4q21. After initial discovery of mutations of the *GNRHR* gene,[166] several reports have followed identifying mutations in the *GRHR* gene as the cause of isolated hypogonadotropic hypogonadism.[167]

SUMMARY

Coordinated regulation of cell type determination, differentiation, and cell proliferation, is a central feature in development of all organs. Organogenesis is controlled by sequential and spatially distributed morphogens of four major families of signaling molecules including the WNT, SHH, TGF/BMP, and FGF.[133,145] The distal targets of regulatory signaling pathways are cell-autonomous transcription regulators including many tissue-restricted transcription factors, which act to mediate crucial steps in organogenesis, and the downstream effects of the signaling pathways result in the preprogramming of target cells. Pituitary development has become a model system ideal for the demonstration of the principles underlying organogenesis (see Fig. 16-5).

Continued advancement in genomic and genetic applications, particularly genome-based mutagenesis screens in mice and in nonmurine model organisms, will identify novel genes and pathways that influence the signaling and cell-determination events. Biochemical approaches, including proteomics techniques, will define the signaling-induced alterations in protein-protein interactions and phosphorylation/methylation/acetylation essential to these events. The description of developmental events leading to the formation of the pituitary gland will be described increasingly in molecular terms as the molecular mechanisms being elucidated. (See also the comprehensive recent reviews of pituitary development in Refs. 2, 3, 20, and 168–170.)

Acknowledgments

We apologize to our colleagues whose contributions could not be cited based on the limitation of references in this format, which also precluded detailed discussions of the impact of receptor systems in development of the pituitary gland. We thank R. McEvilly and K. Japsen for critical readings. M.G.R. is an investigator with the Howard Hughes Medical Institute and is supported by grants from the NIH.

REFERENCES

1. Melmed S: Mechanisms for pituitary tumorigenesis: The plastic pituitary. J Clin Invest 112:1603–1618, 2003.
2. Rosenfeld MG, Briata P, Dasen J, et al: Multistep signaling and transcriptional requirements for pituitary organogenesis *in vivo*. Recent Prog Horm Res 55:1–13; discussion 13–14, 2000.
3. Savage JJ, Yaden B, Kiratipranon P, et al: Transcriptional control during mammalian anterior pituitary development. Gene 319:1–319, 2003.
4. Takor TT, Pearse AG: Neuroectodermal origin of avian hypothalamo-hypophyseal complex: The role of the ventral neural ridge. J Embryol Exp Morphol 34:311–325, 1975.
5. Levy NB, Andrew A, Rawdon BB, et al: Is there a ventral neural ridge in chick embryos? Implications for the origin of adenohypophyseal and other APUD cells. J Embryol Exp Morphol 57:71–78, 1980.
6. elAmraoui A, Dubois PM: Experimental evidence for the early commitment of the presumptive adenohypophysis. Neuroendocrinology 58:609–615, 1993.
7. Eagleson GW, Jenks BG, Van Overbeeke AP: The pituitary adrenocorticotropes originate from neural ridge tissue in *Xenopus laevis*. J Embryol Exp Morphol 95:1–14, 1986.
8. Eagleson GW, Harris WA: Mapping of the presumptive brain regions in the neural plate of *Xenopus laevis*. J Neurobiol 21:427–440, 1990.
9. Herzog W, Zeng X, Lele Z, et al: Adenohypophysis formation in the zebrafish and its dependence on Sonic hedgehog. Dev Biol 254:36–49, 2003.
10. Liu NA, Huang H, Yang Z, et al: Pituitary corticotroph ontogeny and regulation in transgenic zebrafish. Mol Endocrinol 17:959–966, 2003.
11. Kouki T, Imai H, Aoto K, et al: Developmental origin of the rat adenohypophysis prior to the formation of Rathke's pouch. Development 128:959–963, 2001.
12. Rathke H: Ueber die Entstehung der glandula pititaria. Arch Anat Physio Wissen Med:482–485, 1838.
13. Ikeda H, Suzuki J, Sasano N, et al: The development and morphogenesis of the human pituitary gland. Anat Embryol (Berl) 327–336, 1988.
14. Treier M, Rosenfeld MG: The hypothalamic-pituitary axis: Codevelopment of two organs. Curr Opin Cell Biol 8:833–843, 1996.
15. Treier M, Gleiberman AS, O'Connell SM, et al: Multistep signaling requirements for pituitary organogenesis *in vivo*. Genes Dev 12:1691–1704, 1998.
16. Ikeda H, Yoshimoto T: Developmental changes in proliferative activity of cells of the murine Rathke's pouch. Cell Tissue Res 263:41–47, 1991.
17. Han KS, Iwai-Liao Y, Higashi Y: Early organogenesis and cell contacts in the proliferating hypophysis of the developing mouse. Okajimas Folia Anat Jpn 75:97–109, 1998.
18. Ericson J, Norlin S, Jessell TM, et al: Integrated FGF and BMP signaling controls the progression of progenitor cell differentiation and the emergence of pattern in the embryonic anterior pituitary. Development 125:1005–1015, 1998.
19. Gleiberman AS, Fedtsova NG, Rosenfeld MG: Tissue interactions in the induction of anterior pituitary: Role of the ventral diencephalon, mesenchyme, and notochord. Dev Biol 213:340–353, 1999.
20. Dasen JS, Rosenfeld MG: Signaling and transcriptional mechanisms in pituitary development. Annu Rev Neurosci 24:327–355, 2001.
21. Kendall SK, Gordon DF, Birkmeier TS, et al: Enhancer-mediated high level expression of mouse pituitary glycoprotein hormone alpha-subunit transgene in thyrotropes, gonadotropes, and developing pituitary gland. Mol Endocrinol 8:1420–1433, 1994.
22. Ingraham HA, Chen RP, Mangalam HJ, et al: A tissue-specific transcription factor containing a homeodomain specifies a pituitary phenotype. Cell 55:519–529, 1988.
23. Bodner M, Castrillo JL, Theill LE, et al: The pituitary-specific transcription factor GHF-1 is a homeobox-containing protein. Cell 55:505–518, 1988.
24. Mangalam HJ, Albert VR, Ingraham HA, et al: A pituitary POU domain protein, Pit-1, activates both growth hormone and prolactin promoters transcriptionally. Genes Dev 3:946–958, 1989.
25. Lin C, Lin SC, Chang CP, et al: Pit-1-dependent expression of the receptor for growth hormone releasing factor mediates pituitary cell growth. Nature 360:765–768, 1992.
26. Crenshaw EB 3rd, Kalla K, Simmons DM, et al: Cell-specific expression of the prolactin gene in transgenic mice is controlled by synergistic interactions between promoter and enhancer elements. Genes Dev 3:959–972, 1989.
27. Chen RP, Ingraham HA, Treacy MN, et al: Autoregulation of pit-1 gene expression mediated by two *cis*-active promoter elements. Nature 346:583–586, 1990.
28. Rosenfeld MG, Wu W, Ryan A: POU homeodomain proteins in human diseases. In: Wiley Encyclopedia of Molecular Medicine. Wiley, 2002, p 2557.
29. Snell GD: Dwarf, a new Mendelian recessive character of the house mouse. Proc Natl Acad Sci 15:733–734, 1929.
30. Li S, Crenshaw EB 3rd, Rawson EJ, et al: Dwarf locus mutants lacking three pituitary cell types result from mutations in the POU-domain gene pit-1. Nature 347:528–533, 1990.

31. Camper SA, Saunders TL, Katz RW, et al: The Pit-1 transcription factor gene is a candidate for the murine *Snell* dwarf mutation. Genomics 8:586–590, 1990.

32. Rhodes SJ, Chen R, DiMattia GE, et al: A tissue-specific enhancer confers Pit-1-dependent morphogen inducibility and autoregulation on the pit-1 gene. Genes Dev 7:913–932, 1993.

33. Flurkey K, Papaconstantinou J, Miller RA, et al: Lifespan extension and delayed immune and collagen aging in mutant mice with defects in growth hormone production. Proc Natl Acad Sci U S A 98:6736–6741, 2001.

34. Bartke A, Brown-Borg H, Mattison J, et al: Prolonged longevity of hypopituitary dwarf mice. Exp Gerontol 36:21–28, 2001.

35. Tatsumi K, Miyai K, Notomi T, et al: Cretinism with combined hormone deficiency caused by a mutation in the PIT1 gene. Nat Genet 1:56–58, 1992.

36. Parks JS, Brown MR, Hurley DL, et al: Heritable disorders of pituitary development. J Clin Endocrinol Metab 84:4362–4370, 1999.

37. Pfaffle RW, Blankenstein O, Wuller S, et al: Combined pituitary hormone deficiency: Role of Pit-1 and Prop-1. Acta Paediatr Suppl 88:33–41, 1999.

38. Wu W, Anderson B, Rosenfeld MG: PIT1 transcription factor and diseases. In Creighton TE (ed): Wiley Encyclopedia of Molecular Medicine. New York, Wiley, 2002, p 2501.

39. Holloway JM, Szeto DP, Scully KM, et al: Pit-1 binding to specific DNA sites as a monomer or dimer determines gene-specific use of a tyrosine-dependent synergy domain. Genes Dev 9:1992–2006, 1995.

40. Jacobson EM, Li P, Leon-del-Rio A, et al: Structure of Pit-1 POU domain bound to DNA as a dimer: Unexpected arrangement and flexibility. Genes Dev 11:198–212, 1997.

41. Jacobson EM, Li P, Rosenfeld MG, et al: Crystallization and preliminary X-ray analysis of Pit-1 POU domain complexed to a 28 base pair DNA element. Proteins 24:263–265, 1996.

42. Scully KM, Jacobson EM, Jepsen K, et al: Allosteric effects of Pit-1 DNA sites on long-term repression in cell type specification. Science 290:1127–1131, 2000.

43. Cohen LE, Wondisford FE, Salvatoni A, et al: A "hot spot" in the Pit-1 gene responsible for combined pituitary hormone deficiency: Clinical and molecular correlates. J Clin Endocrinol Metab 80:679–684, 1995.

44. Andersen B, Rosenfeld MG: POU domain factors in the neuroendocrine system: Lessons from developmental biology provide insights into human disease. Endocr Rev 22:2–35, 2001.

45. Xu L, Lavinsky RM, Dasen JS, et al: Signal-specific co-activator domain requirements for Pit-1 activation. Nature 395:301–306, 1998.

46. Simmons DM, Voss JW, Ingraham HA, et al: Pituitary cell phenotypes involve cell-specific Pit-1 mRNA translation and synergistic interactions with other classes of transcription factors. Genes Dev 4:695–711, 1990.

47. Day RN, Koike S, Sakai M, et al: Both Pit-1 and the estrogen receptor are required for estrogen responsiveness of the rat prolactin gene. Mol Endocrinol 4:1964–1971, 1990.

48. Bradford AP, Conrad KE, Wasylyk C, et al: Functional interaction of c-Ets-1 and GHF-1/Pit-1 mediates Ras activation of pituitary-specific gene expression: Mapping of the essential c-Ets-1 domain. Mol Cell Biol 15:2849–2857, 1995.

49. Dasen JS, O'Connell SM, Flynn SE, et al: Reciprocal interactions of Pit1 and GATA2 mediate signaling gradient-induced determination of pituitary cell types. Cell 97:587–598, 1999.

50. Sornson MW, Wu W, Dasen JS, et al: Pituitary lineage determination by the Prophet of Pit-1 homeodomain factor defective in Ames dwarfism. Nature 384:327–333, 1996.

51. Andersen B, Pearse RV 2nd, Jenne K, et al: The Ames dwarf gene is required for Pit-1 gene activation. Dev Biol 172:495–503, 1995.

52. Gage PJ, Roller ML, Saunders TL, et al: Anterior pituitary cells defective in the cell-autonomous factor, df, undergo cell lineage specification but not expansion. Development 122:151–160, 1996.

53. Buckwalter MS, Katz RW, Camper SA: Localization of the panhypopituitary dwarf mutation (df) on mouse chromosome 11 in an intersubspecific backcross. Genomics 10:515–526, 1991.

54. Gage PJ, Lossie AC, Scarlett LM, et al: *Ames* dwarf mice exhibit somatotrope commitment but lack growth hormone-releasing factor response. Endocrinology 136:1161–1167, 1995.

55. Brown-Borg HM, Borg KE, Meliska CJ, et al: Dwarf mice and the ageing process. Nature 384:33, 1996.

56. Wu W, Cogan JD, Pfaffle RW, et al: Mutations in PROP1 cause familial combined pituitary hormone deficiency. Nat Genet 18:147–149, 1998.

57. Deladoey J, Fluck C, Buyukgebiz A, et al: "Hot spot" in the PROP1 gene responsible for combined pituitary hormone deficiency. J Clin Endocrinol Metab 84:1645–1650, 1999.

58. Mody S, Brown MR, Park JS: The spectrum of hypopituitarism caused by PROP1 mutations. Best Pract Res Clin Endocrinol Metab 16:421–431, 2002.

59. Wu W, Rosenfeld MG: PROP1 Gene. In Creighton TE (ed): Wiley Encyclopedia of Molecular Medicine. New York, Wiley, 2002, p 2597.

60. Cushman LJ, Watkins-Chow DE, Brinkmeier ML, et al: Persistent Prop1 expression delays gonadotrope differentiation and enhances pituitary tumor susceptibility. Hum Mol Genet 10:1141–1153, 2001.

61. Douglas KR, Brinkmeier ML, Kennell JA, et al: Identification of members of the Wnt signaling pathway in the embryonic pituitary gland. Mamm Genome 12:843–851, 2001.

62. Pernasetti F, Toledo SP, Vasilyev VV, et al: Impaired adrenocorticotropin-adrenal axis in combined pituitary hormone deficiency caused by a two-base pair deletion (301-302delAG) in the prophet of Pit-1 gene. J Clin Endocrinol Metab 85:390–397, 2000.

63. Agarwal G, Bhatia V, Cook S, et al: Adrenocorticotropin deficiency in combined pituitary hormone deficiency patients homozygous for a novel PROP1 deletion. J Clin Endocrinol Metab 85:4556–4561, 2000.

64. Lamesch C, Neumann S, Pfaffle R, et al: Adrenocorticotrope deficiency with clinical evidence for late onset in combined pituitary hormone deficiency caused by a homozygous 301–302delAG mutation of the PROP1 gene. Pituitary 5:163–168, 2002.

65. Hermesz E, Mackem S, Mahon KA: Rpx: A novel anterior-restricted homeobox gene progressively activated in the prechordal plate, anterior neural plate and Rathke's pouch of the mouse embryo. Development 122:41–52, 1996.

66. Thomas P, Beddington R: Anterior primitive endoderm may be responsible for patterning the anterior neural plate in the mouse embryo. Curr Biol 6:1487–1496, 1996.

67. Dattani MT, Martinez-Barbera JP, Thomas PQ, et al: Mutations in the homeobox gene HESX1/Hesx1 associated with septo-optic dysplasia in human and mouse. Nat Genet 19:125–133, 1998.

68. Dasen JS, Barbera JP, Herman TS, et al: Temporal regulation of a paired-like homeodomain repressor/TLE corepressor complex and a related activator is required for pituitary organogenesis. Genes Dev 15:3193–3207, 2001.

69. Thomas PQ, Dattani MT, Brickman JM, et al: Heterozygous HESX1 mutations associated with isolated congenital pituitary hypoplasia and septo-optic dysplasia. Hum Mol Genet 10:39–45, 2001.

70. Woods K, Dattani MT: Transcription factors involved in disorders of forebrain and pituitary development. In Epstein J, Wynshaw-Boris AJ (eds): Inborn Errors of Development: The Molecular Basis of Clinical Disorders on Morphogenesis. New York, Oxford University Press, 2004, p 540.

71. Brickman JM, Clements M, Tyrell R, et al: Molecular effects of novel mutations in Hesx1/HESX1 associated with human pituitary disorders. Development 128:5189–5199, 2001.

72. Quirk J, Brown P: Hesx1 homeodomain protein represses transcription as a monomer and antagonises transactivation of specific sites as a homodimer. J Mol Endocrinol 28:193–205, 2002.

73. Smith ST, Jaynes JB: A conserved region of engrailed, shared among all en-, gsc-, Nk1-, Nk2- and msh-class homeoproteins, mediates active transcriptional repression in vivo. Development 122:3141–3150, 1996.

74. Paroush Z, Finley, RL J., Kidd T, et al: Groucho is required for Drosophila neurogenesis, segmentation, and sex determination and interacts directly with hairy-related bHLH proteins. Cell 79:805–815, 1994.

75. Jimenez G, Paroush Z, Ish-Horowicz D: Groucho acts as a corepressor for a subset of negative regulators, including Hairy and Engrailed. Genes Dev 11:3072–3082, 1997.

76. Tolkunova EN, Fujioka M, Kobayashi M, et al: Two distinct types of repression domain in engrailed: One interacts with the Groucho corepressor and is preferentially active on integrated target genes. Mol Cell Biol 18:2804–2814, 1998.

77. Eberhard D, Jimenez G, Heavey B, et al: Transcriptional repression by Pax5 (BSAP) through interaction with corepressors of the Groucho family. EMBO J 19:2292–2303, 2000.

78. Zhadanov AB, Bertuzzi S, Taira M, et al: Expression pattern of the murine LIM class homeobox gene Lhx3 in subsets of neural and neuroendocrine tissues. Dev Dyn 202:354–364, 1995.

79. Li H, Witte DP, Branford WW, et al: Gsh-4 encodes a LIM-type homeodomain, is expressed in the developing central nervous system and is required for early postnatal survival. EMBO J 13:2876–2885, 1994.

80. Sheng HZ, Zhadanov AB, Mosinger B Jr, et al: Specification of pituitary cell lineages by the LIM homeobox gene Lhx3. Science 272:1004–1007, 1996.

81. Li H, Zeitler PS, Valerius MT, et al: Gsh-1, an orphan Hox gene, is required for normal pituitary development. EMBO J 15:714–724, 1996.

82. Raetzman LT, Ward R, Camper SA: Lhx4 and Prop1 are required for cell survival and expansion of the pituitary primordia. Development 129:4229–4239, 2002.

83. Sheng HZ, Moriyama K, Yamashita T, et al: Multistep control of pituitary organogenesis. Science 278:1809–1812, 1997.

84. Sloop, KW, Showalter AD, Von Kap-Herr C, et al: Analysis of the human LHX3 neuroendocrine transcription factor gene and mapping to the subtelomeric region of chromosome 9. Gene 245:237–243, 2000.

85. Schmitt S, Biason-Lauber A, Betts D, et al: Genomic structure, chromosomal localization, and expression pattern of the human LIM-homeobox3 (LHX 3) gene. Biochem Biophys Res Commun 274:49–56, 2000.

86. Netchine I, Sobrier ML, Krude H, et al: Mutations in LHX3 result in a new syndrome revealed by combined pituitary hormone deficiency. Nat Genet 25:182–186, 2000.

87. Machinis K, Pantel J, Netchine I, et al: Syndromic short stature in patients with a germline mutation in the LIM homeobox LHX4. Am J Hum Genet 69:961–968, 2001.

88. Sloop KW, Dwyer CJ, Rhodes SJ: An isoform-specific inhibitory domain regulates the LHX3 LIM homeodomain factor holoprotein and the production of a functional alternate translation form. J Biol Chem 276:36311–36319, 2001.

89. Yi CH, Terrett JA, Li QY, et al: Identification, mapping, and phylogenomic analysis of four new human members of the T-box gene family: EOMES, TBX6, TBX18, and TBX19. Genomics 55:10–20, 1999.

90. Lamolet B, Pulichino AM, Lamonerie T, et al: A pituitary cell-restricted T box factor, Tpit, activates POMC transcription in cooperation with Pitx homeoproteins. Cell 104:849–859, 2001.

91. Liu J, Lin C, Gleiberman A, et al: Tbx19, a tissue-selective regulator of POMC gene expression. Proc Natl Acad Sci U S A 98:8674–8679, 2001.

92. Pulichino AM, Vallette-Kasic S, Couture C, et al: Human and mouse TPIT gene mutations cause early onset pituitary ACTH deficiency. Genes Dev 17:711–716, 2003.

93. Pulichino AM, Vallette-Kasic S, Tsai JP, et al: Tpit determines alternate fates during pituitary cell differentiation. Genes Dev 17:738–747, 2003.

94. Maira M, Couture C, Le Martelot G, et al: The T-box factor Tpit recruits SRC/p160 coactivators and mediates hormone action. J Biol Chem 278:46523–46532, 2003.

95. Maira M, Martens C, Batsche E, et al: Dimer-specific potentiation of NGFI-B (Nur77) transcriptional activity by the protein kinase A pathway and AF-1-dependent coactivator recruitment. Mol Cell Biol 23:763–776, 2003.

96. Ruppert JM, Kinzler KW, Wong AJ, et al: The GLI-Kruppel family of human genes. Mol Cell Biol 8:3104–3113, 1988.

97. Hui CC, Slusarski D, Platt KA, et al: Expression of three mouse homologs of the Drosophila segment polarity gene cubitus interruptus, Gli, Gli-2, and Gli-3, in ectoderm- and mesoderm-derived tissues suggests multiple roles during postimplantation development. Dev Biol 162:402–413, 1994.

98. Mo R, Freer AM, Zinyk DL, et al: Specific and redundant functions of Gli2 and Gli3 zinc finger genes in skeletal patterning and development. Development 124:113–123, 1997.

99. Motoyama J, Liu J, Mo R, et al: Essential function of Gli2 and Gli3 in the formation of lung, trachea and oesophagus. Nat Genet 20:54–57, 1998.

100. Mill P, Mo R, Fu H, et al: Sonic hedgehog-dependent activation of Gli2 is essential for embryonic hair follicle development. Genes Dev 17:282–294, 2003.

101. Ding Q, Motoyama J, Gasca S, et al: Diminished Sonic hedgehog signaling and lack of floor plate differentiation in Gli2 mutant mice. Development 125:2533–2543, 1998.

102. Park HL, Bai C, Platt KA, et al: Mouse Gli1 mutants are viable but have defects in SHH signaling in combination with a Gli2 mutation. Development 127:1593–1605, 2000.

103. Karlstrom RO, Talbot WS, Schier AF: Comparative synteny cloning of zebrafish you-too: Mutations in the Hedgehog target gli2 affect ventral forebrain patterning. Genes Dev 13:388–393, 1999.

104. Ede DA, Kelly WA: Developmental Abnormalities in the head region of the talpid mutant of the fowl. J Embryol Exp Morphol 12:161–182, 1964.

105. Roessler E, Du YZ, Mullor JL, et al: Loss-of-function mutations in the human GLI2 gene are associated with pituitary anomalies and holoprosencephaly-like features. Proc Natl Acad Sci U S A 100:134241342–9, 2003.

106. Sasaki H, Nishizaki Y, Hui C, et al: Regulation of Gli2 and Gli3 activities by an amino-terminal repression domain: Implication of Gli2 and Gli3 as primary mediators of Shh signaling. Development 126:3915–3924, 1999.

107. Bai CB, Auerbach W, Lee JS, et al: Gli2, but not Gli1, is required for initial Shh signaling and ectopic activation of the Shh pathway. Development 129:4753–4761, 2002.

108. Kondoh H, Uchikawa M, Yoda H, et al: Zebrafish mutations in Gli-mediated hedgehog signaling lead to lens transdifferentiation from the adenohypophysis anlage. Mech Dev 96:165–174, 2000.

109. Kioussi C, O'Connell SL, St-Onge L, et al: Pax6 is essential for establishing ventral-dorsal cell boundaries in pituitary gland development. Proc Natl Acad Sci U S A 96:14378–14382, 1999.

110. Rosenfeld MG, Bach I, Erkman L, et al: Transcriptional control of cell phenotypes in the neuroendocrine system. Recent Prog Horm Res 51:217–238; discussion 238–239, 1996.

111. Cushman LJ, Showalter AD, Rhodes SJ: Genetic defects in the development and function of the anterior pituitary gland. Ann Med 34:179–191, 2002.

112. Cohen LE, Radovick S: Other transcription factors and hypopituitarism. Rev Endocr Metab Disord 3:301–311, 2002.

113. Szeto DP, Rodriguez-Esteban C, Ryan AK, et al: Role of the bicoid-related homeodomain factor Pitx1 in specifying hindlimb morphogenesis and pituitary development. Genes Dev 13:484–494, 1999.

114. Marcil A, Dumontier E, Chamberland M, et al: Pitx1 and Pitx2 are required for development of hindlimb buds. Development 130:45–55, 2003.

115. Lin CR, Kioussi C, O'Connell S, et al: Pitx2 regulates lung asymmetry, cardiac positioning and pituitary and tooth

morphogenesis. Nature 401:279–282, 1999.

116. Suh H, Gage PJ, Drouin J, et al: *Pitx2* is required at multiple stages of pituitary organogenesis: Pituitary primordium formation and cell specification. Development 129:329–337, 2002.

117. Semina EV, Reiter R, Leysens NJ, et al: Cloning and characterization of a novel bicoid-related homeobox transcription factor gene, RIEG, involved in Rieger syndrome. Nat Genet 14:392–399, 1996.

118. Li X, Perissi V, Liu F, et al: Tissue-specific regulation of retinal and pituitary precursor cell proliferation. Science 297:1180–1183, 2002.

119. Li X, Oghi KA, Zhang J, et al: Eya protein phosphatase activity regulates *Six1*-Dach-Eya transcriptional effects in mammalian organogenesis. Nature 426:247–254, 2003.

120. Lagutin OV, Zhu CC, Kobayashi D, et al: *Six3* repression of Wnt signaling in the anterior neuroectoderm is essential for vertebrate forebrain development. Genes Dev 17:368–379, 2003.

121. Zhao L, Bakke M, Krimkevich Y, et al: Steroidogenic factor 1 (SF1) is essential for pituitary gonadotrope function. Development 128:147–154, 2001.

122. Edlund T, Jessell TM: Progression from extrinsic to intrinsic signaling in cell fate specification: A view from the nervous system. Cell 96:211–224, 1999.

123. Hogan BL: Morphogenesis. Cell 96:225–233, 1999.

124. Treier M, O'Connell S, Gleiberman A, et al: Hedgehog signaling is required for pituitary gland development. Development 128:377–386, 2001.

125. Dahmann C, Basler K: Compartment boundaries: At the edge of development. Trends Genet 15:320–326, 1999.

126. Echelard Y, Epstein DJ, St-Jacques B, et al: Sonic hedgehog, a member of a family of putative signaling molecules, is implicated in the regulation of CNS polarity. Cell 75:1417–1430, 1993.

127. Roelink H, Augsburger A, Heemskerk J, et al: Floor plate and motor neuron induction by vhh-1, a vertebrate homolog of hedgehog expressed by the notochord. Cell 76:761–775, 1994.

128. Riddle RD, Johnson RL, Laufer E, et al: Sonic hedgehog mediates the polarizing activity of the ZPA. Cell 75:1401–1416, 1993.

129. Johnson RL, Laufer E, Riddle RD, et al: Ectopic expression of Sonic hedgehog alters dorsal-ventral patterning of somites. Cell 79:1165–1173, 1994.

130. Marigo V, Roberts DJ, Lee SM, et al: Cloning, expression, and chromosomal location of SHH and IHH: Two human homologues of the Drosophila segment polarity gene hedgehog. Genomics 28:44–51, 1995.

131. Chiang C, Litingtung Y, Lee E, et al: Cyclopia and defective axial patterning in mice lacking Sonic hedgehog gene function. Nature 383:407–413, 1996.

132. Thomas PQ, Rathjen PD: HES-1, a novel homeobox gene expressed by murine embryonic stem cell, identifies a new class of homeobox genes. Nucleic Acid Res 11:5840, 1992.

133. Sbrogna JL, Barresi MJ, Karlstrom RO: Multiple roles for Hedgehog signaling in zebrafish pituitary development. Dev Biol 254:19–35, 2003.

134. Laufer E, Nelson CE, Johnson RL, et al: Sonic hedgehog and Fgf-4 act through a signaling cascade and feedback loop to integrate growth and patterning of the developing limb bud. Cell 79:993–1003, 1994.

135. Ornitz DM, Itoh N: Fibroblast growth factors. Genome Biol 2:3005, 2001.

136. Johnson DE, Williams LT: Structural and functional diversity in the FGF receptor multigene family. Adv Cancer Res 60:1–41, 1993.

137. Rapraeger AC, Krufka A, Olwin BB: Requirement of heparan sulfate for bFGF-mediated fibroblast growth and myoblast differentiation. Science 252:1705–1708, 1991.

138. Allen BL, Rapraeger AC: Spatial and temporal expression of heparan sulfate in mouse development regulates FGF and FGF receptor assembly. J Cell Biol 163:637–648, 2003.

139. Min H, Danilenko DM, Scully SA, et al: Fgf-10 is required for both limb and lung development and exhibits striking functional similarity to Drosophila branchless. Genes Dev 12:3156–3161, 1998.

140. De Moerlooze L, Spencer-Dene B, Revest J, et al: An important role for the IIIb isoform of fibroblast growth factor receptor 2 (FGFR2) in mesenchymal-epithelial signalling during mouse organogenesis. Development 127:483–492, 2000.

141. Meyers EN, Lewandoski M, Martin GR: An Fgf8 mutant allelic series generated by Cre- and Flp-mediated recombination. Nat Genet 18:136–141, 1998.

142. Chi CL, Martinez S, Wurst W, et al: The isthmic organizer signal FGF8 is required for cell survival in the prospective midbrain and cerebellum. Development 130:2633–2644, 2003.

143. Takuma N, Sheng HZ, Furuta Y, et al: Formation of Rathke's pouch requires dual induction from the diencephalon. Development 125:4835–4840, 1998.

144. Zhao G: Consequences of knocking out BMP signaling in the mouse. Genesis 35:43–56, 2003.

145. Ohkubo Y, Chiang C, Rubenstein JL: Coordinate regulation and synergistic actions of BMP4, SHH and FGF8 in the rostral prosencephalon regulate morphogenesis of the telencephalic and optic vesicles. Neuroscience 111:1–17, 2002.

146. Miller JR: The Wnts. Genome Biol 3:3001, 2002.

147. Nusse R, Rulifson E, Fish M, et al: Interactions between wingless and frizzled molecules in Drosophila. Ernst Schering Res Found Workshop:1–11, 2000.

148. Muroyama Y, Fujihara M, Ikeya M, et al: Wnt signaling plays an essential role in neuronal specification of the dorsal spinal cord. Genes Dev 16:548–553, 2002.

149. Fisher AL, Caudy M: Groucho proteins: Transcriptional corepressors for specific subsets of DNA-binding transcription factors in vertebrates and invertebrates. Genes Dev 12:1931–1940, 1998.

150. Eastman Q, Grosschedl R: Regulation of LEF-1/TCF transcription factors by Wnt and other signals. Curr Opin Cell Biol 11:233–240, 1999.

151. Boutros M, Mihaly J, Bouwmeester T, et al: Signaling specificity by Frizzled receptors in Drosophila. Science 288:1825–1828, 2000.

152. Briata P, Ilengo C, Corte G, et al: The Wnt/beta-catenin—>Pitx2 pathway controls the turnover of Pitx2 and other unstable mRNAs. Mol Cell 12:1201–1211, 2003.

153. Gage PJ, Suh H, Camper SA: Dosage requirement of Pitx2 for development of multiple organs. Development 126:4643–4651, 1999.

154. Kioussi C, Briata P, Baek SH, et al: Identification of a Wnt/Dvl/beta-Catenin—> Pitx2 pathway mediating cell-type-specific proliferation during development. Cell 111:673–685, 2002.

155. Liu W, Selever J, Lu MF, et al: Genetic dissection of Pitx2 in craniofacial development uncovers new functions in branchial arch morphogenesis, late aspects of tooth morphogenesis and cell migration. Development 130:6375–6385, 2003.

156. Anderson RM, Lawrence AR, Stottmann RW, et al: Chordin and noggin promote organizing centers of forebrain development in the mouse. Development 129:4975–4987, 2002.

157. Bousquet C, Ray DW, Melmed S: A common pro-opiomelanocortin-binding element mediates leukemia inhibitory factor and corticotropin-releasing hormone transcriptional synergy. J Biol Chem 272:10551–10557, 1997.

158. Yano H, Readhead C, Nakashima M, et al: Pituitary-directed leukemia inhibitory factor transgene causes Cushing's syndrome: Neuro-immune-endocrine modulation of pituitary development. Mol Endocrinol 12:1708–1720, 1998.

159. Gaylinn BD, von Kap-Herr C, Golden WL, et al: Assignment of the human growth hormone-releasing hormone receptor gene (GHRHR) to 7p14 by in situ hybridization. Genomics 19:193–195, 1994.

160. Wajnrajch MP, Gertner JM, Harbison MD, et al: Nonsense mutation in the human growth hormone-releasing hormone receptor causes growth failure analogous to the little (lit) mouse. Nat Genet 12:88–90, 1996.

161. Salvatori R, Fan X, Phillips JA 3rd, et al: Three new mutations in the gene

for the growth hormone (gh)-releasing hormone receptor in familial isolated gh deficiency type ib. J Clin Endocrinol Metab 86:273–279, 2001.

162. Lin SC, Lin CR, Gukovsky I, et al: Molecular basis of the little mouse phenotype and implications for cell type-specific growth. Nature 364:208–213, 1993.

163. Godfrey P, Rahal JO, Beamer WG, et al: GHRH receptor of little mice contains a missense mutation in the extracellular domain that disrupts receptor function. Nat Genet 4:227–232, 1993.

164. Honda J, Manabe Y, Matsumura R, et al: IGF-I regulates pro-opiomelanocortin and GH gene expression in the mouse pituitary gland. J Endocrinol 178:71–82, 2003.

165. Collu R: Genetic aspects of central hypothyroidism. J Endocrinol Invest 23:125–134, 2000.

166. de Roux N, Young J, Misrahi M, et al: A family with hypogonadotropic hypogonadism and mutations in the gonadotropin-releasing hormone receptor. N Engl J Med 337:1597–1602, 1997.

167. Silveira LF, MacColl GS, Bouloux PM: Hypogonadotropic hypogonadism. Semin Reprod Med 20:327–338, 2002.

168. Scully KM, Rosenfeld MG: Pituitary development: Regulatory codes in mammalian organogenesis. Science 295:2231–2235, 2002.

169. Cohen LE, Radovick S: Molecular basis of combined pituitary hormone deficiencies. Endocr Rev 23:431–442, 2002.

170. Cushman LJ, Camper SA: Molecular basis of pituitary dysfunction in mouse and human. Mamm Genome 12:485–494, 2001.

Prolactin

Nelson D. Horseman and Karen A. Gregerson

Prolactin (PRL) was the first of the pituitary hormones to be biochemically identified and purified,[1,2] and hyperprolactinemia caused by hormone-secreting tumors is the most common human pituitary disease. Only recently, however, have the physiology and biochemistry of prolactin actions yielded to contemporary analytic methods to reveal a biology that is at once elegantly simple and sublimely complex. PRL has been identified in the pituitary glands of members of all vertebrate classes, and it has diverse effects on osmoregulation, metabolism, reproduction, metamorphosis, migratory behavior, parental behavior, and lactation.[3-6] In most species, especially mammals, PRL has a specialized role in the postmating phase of reproduction. The predominant mammalian actions of PRL are stimulation of lactation and maternal behavior, and inhibition of reproductive function. Associated with the specialization of PRL in mammals, novel genes that encode placentally derived lactogens have evolved. PRL does not perform any indispensable function for the survival of the individual, but gestation and lactation lie at the core of the mammalian life cycle, and they place extreme demands on physiology. Adaptations in the control of PRL secretion and its physiologic actions have therefore been integral to the biology of all mammals, and abnormalities of PRL secretion are a relatively common cause of endocrine disease. The deepening understanding of PRL actions on both physiologic and molecular levels has facilitated improved therapeutic approaches to diseases of PRL secretion and has opened opportunities to use the physiology of PRL and lactation in new ways.

THE EVOLUTIONARY BIOLOGY OF PROLACTIN

THE PROLACTIN FAMILY

PRL and growth hormone (GH) are related at the primary amino acid sequence level.[7] PRL has been identified in all of the vertebrate classes, and it has been inferred that the PRL and GH genes arose from a duplication of an ancestral gene at least 400 million years ago, at about the time of the origin of vertebrates.[8]

Deeper relationships with other hormones are less certain, but erythropoietin shares substantial primary sequence similarity, as well as three-dimensional structural features with PRL and GH, suggesting that all three of these hormones share an ancient common ancestry. In addition to PRL and GH, which have been conserved in all vertebrate lineages, a wide variety of derivative genes have appeared in specific vertebrate groups by duplication of either the PRL or GH gene. The most familiar of these are the various mammalian placental lactogens.[9,10]

PLACENTAL LACTOGENS

Placental lactogens (PLs) are synthesized during pregnancy in most, but not all, eutherian mammals. Species that apparently do not produce any placental lactogens are distributed among many mammalian families and include familiar species such as pigs, horses, and dogs.[11] Primates (including humans) synthesize a PL that is encoded by a gene duplicated within the GH locus.[8] The GH locus in humans encompasses five genes spanning a region of about 50 kb on the long arm (q22–24) of chromosome 17. This locus includes two PL or, preferably, chorionic somatomammotropin (CS) genes (hCS-A and hCS-B). The CS-A and CS-B genes, though slightly divergent at the nucleotide sequence level, encode identical proteins, and the genes are coexpressed in the placenta during gestation. In nonprimates (e.g., rodents, ruminants), the PLs have descended evolutionarily from duplications of the PRL gene.[8] Multiple PL genes and nonlactogenic PRL-like genes have evolved from PRL. In mice, placental lactogen-I (PL-I) is synthesized early during gestation, appearing immediately after implantation. PL-I expression is extinguished at about mid-gestation and replaced by PL-II. Both of the mouse PL genes are synthesized in trophoblast giant cells. In species that synthesize PLs, including humans, the major stimulus to mammary gland development during pregnancy is presumably from PLs, rather than pituitary PRL. PL levels generally rise in correlation with placental growth, and their secretion is controlled by both positive and negative regulators.[12] The loss of PLs and placental steroids at parturition is accompanied by elevation of pituitary PRL secretion, and a corresponding shift to pituitary-dominated regulation of mammary gland function during lactation. The importance of this shift is that pituitary PRL is strongly regulated by a suckling-induced neuroendocrine reflex, which allows nursing activity to determine directly the lactational stimulus to the mammary glands.

NONLACTOGENIC PROLACTIN RELATIVES

Nonlactogenic members of the PRL gene family are synthesized by the placenta of nonprimates. Although the physiologic activities of these PRL-related proteins have not been established, the expression patterns for some of these proteins are tightly regulated during gestation,[10] and this has been interpreted to indicate that the proteins are functionally important. In mice and rats, there are at least five nonlactogenic PRL-like proteins (PLP-A through PLP-E). In addition, mice synthesize two proteins, named proliferin and proliferin-related protein, which have been proposed to act as regulators of angiogenesis.[13] Nonlactogenic PRL-like protein genes have also been extensively characterized in cattle.[14] One curious feature of the PRL-like gene family is the apparently rapid evolutionary divergence of members of this family. These proteins generally share less than 25% sequence identity with PRL, but all share two pairs of cysteine residues that are conserved throughout the PRL and GH superfamily.[10] Information regarding receptors for the nonlactogenic PRL-related proteins is scant. Proliferin binds to the mannose-6-phosphate insulin-like growth factor 2 (IGF-2) receptor.[15]

EXTRAPITUITARY PROLACTIN

Many mammalian tissues, including the human mammary gland and uterine decidua, express the PRL gene. In addition, various tissues metabolize PRL to alternative forms that may be biologically active. PRL is synthesized by both the decidua and the uterine myometrium in humans.[16] High concentrations of PRL are present in the amniotic fluid; this can be traced to both decidually synthesized hormone and plasma PRL that is transported across the placenta into the amniotic fluid. The synthesis of human PRL in extrapituitary sites is controlled by a promoter that is distinct from the pituitary PRL promoter. Human extrapituitary PRL messenger RNA (mRNA) has a distinct 5' untranslated sequence corresponding to an additional exon (exon 1A)[17] (Fig. 17-1). Exon 1A and the promoter elements associated with it are located about 8000 base pairs (bp) distal to the initiation site for pituitary PRL transcription. In rodents, the evidence for a distinct extrapituitary PRL promoter is less certain than in the human. It is conceivable that rodents use other mechanisms, such as growth factors that control the conventional pituitary PRL promoter, to provide for regulation of PRL synthesis in extrapituitary tissues. The mammary gland is an important site of PRL synthesis and secretion. PRL is present in significant concentrations in milk, and milk PRL is absorbed by the neonatal gut and causes changes in the maturation of the hypothalamic neuroendocrine system.[18] Pituitary PRL is transported out of the circulation, across the mammary epithelium, and into the alveolar lumen, and locally synthesized PRL is secreted into milk.[16] To date, there are no disease states that have been connected to dysregulation of extrapituitary PRL secretion. The lack of any clear proofs that there are symptoms caused by either hypersecretion of extrapituitary PRL, say, from a PRL-secreting ectopic tumor or from loss of extrapituitary PRL gene expression, makes it difficult to surmise the normal functional roles of extrapituitary PRL in humans. It has been suggested that locally synthesized PRL in the mammary gland might act as a growth factor for both normal breast epithelium and breast cancer cells.[19]

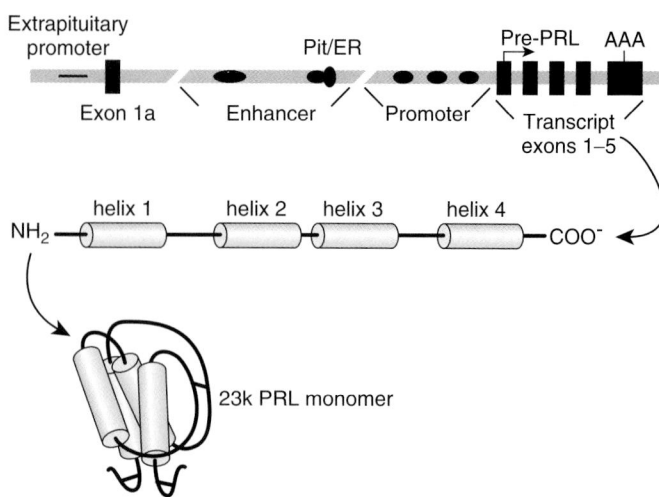

Figure 17-1 Biosynthesis of prolactin (PRL). The PRL gene is depicted at the top of the figure as consisting of five exons (*black rectangles*) encoding the structural gene for preprolactin (pre-PRL). The translation start site in exon 1 is marked by an *arrow*, and the polyadenylation site in exon 5 is marked AAA. The region labeled promoter includes multiple binding sites for the pituitary-specific transcription factor-1 (Pit-1, *black ellipses*), but only three are depicted in the diagram. The line that depicts the DNA sequence is broken by two interruptions to indicate that the upstream regulatory regions are separated from the promoter by several thousand base pairs. A distal regulatory region (enhancer) includes binding sites for Pit-1 and other factors, including a complex site that binds both Pit-1 and the estrogen receptor (Pit/ER). Exon 1a is transcribed in extrapituitary tissues, and is controlled by a distinct "extrapituitary promoter." After transcription and translation, the PRL protein consists of four α-helical regions, which are labeled helix 1 through 4, and intervening β-strand regions. The protein spontaneously folds into a globular structure in which three disulfide bridges connect β-strand regions, and this mature structure is depicted as the 23k PRL monomer.

THE BIOCHEMISTRY OF PROLACTIN

Human PRL is synthesized as a prehormone that is encoded by a mRNA with an open reading frame of 684 bases. The native gene for PRL is divided into five exons, and the initiation site for translation is in exon 1[20] (see Fig. 17-1). Preprolactin (pre-PRL) is 227 amino acids in length, with a deduced molecular weight of nearly 26,000. Cleaving the signal peptide from the N-terminus of pre-PRL results in a mature polypeptide that is 199 residues in length and has a molecular weight of nearly 23,000 (23k PRL). On the basis of the fact that the bacterially synthesized recombinant 23k PRL monomer binds to the PRL receptor (PRL-R) and transduces functional signals, it is clear that no additional modifications are essential for the core functions of PRL. PRL folds itself into a tertiary structure that includes three intrachain disulfide bridges, two of which are conserved in all members of the PRL-GH family, and one, linking residues 4 and 11 in the N-terminus, which is unique to PRL and its closest relatives.[7] Four α-helical domains in PRL are arranged so that helices 1 and 2 run antiparallel to helices 3 and 4. This general molecular architecture of PRL has been conserved with GH and other homologous proteins and also has evolved independently in several families of cytokines.[21] The convergent evolution of hormone and cytokine ligand architecture has apparently been driven by the properties of receptors that bind these hormones and transduce signals to the intracellular space.

A variety of biochemical variants of 23k PRL, which appear to have altered functions, have been identified. PRL has a tendency to aggregate and form intermolecular disulfide bridges spontaneously when in solution at high concentrations.

High-molecular-weight variants (sometimes referred to as "big" PRLs) may arise by virtue of multimerization, glycosylation, or cross-linking with other proteins. Only a small fraction of human PRL is glycosylated, whereas in some other species, such as swine, glycosylated PRL represents a large portion of both pituitary and plasma hormone.[22] Glycosylation may alter the relative potency of PRL either by changing its receptor-binding characteristics or by modifying its pharmacokinetic properties in the animal (plasma half-life, partitioning between plasma and interstitial compartments, etc.). PRL is metabolized by tissue uptake and by proteolysis in the circulation or in cells. Proteolysis also produces a 16-kDa PRL fragment that has been proposed to have antiangiogenic bioactivity.[23]

Phosphorylated PRL has reduced potency in standard bioassays, and it antagonizes the actions of the predominant unphosphorylated form.[24] Actions of kinases or phosphatases in either the pituitary or individual target tissues may have an important effect on the bioactivity of PRL *in vivo*.

THE ONTOGENY AND PHYSIOLOGY OF PRPLACTIN SECRETION

DEVELOPMENT OF LACTOTROPHS

PRL is synthesized by lactotrophs, which are acidophilic cells that represent 20% to 50% of the anterior pituitary cell population. The lactotrophs are the last of the pituitary cell types to fully differentiate and, coincidentally, the most likely to give rise to pituitary adenomas. Pituitary PRL mRNA synthesis begins at 12 weeks in human gestation, and is preceded by GH synthesis by at least 4 weeks.[8,25] In rodents the pattern is similar, with the GH gene being expressed several days before PRL, with dual-functioning somatolactotrophs being observed before fully differentiated lactotrophs.[26] The control of pituitary development and lactotroph differentiation depends on the orchestrated expression of a series of intrinsic, tissue-specific regulatory molecules that act as "molecular switches" to induce the sequence of developmental changes leading up to full pituitary differentiation. Many of the intrinsic factors that have been implicated in pituitary development are evolutionarily related to "homeotic mutation" genes, which were first identified by their dramatic effects on development in fruit flies.[25] Some genetic diseases of the pituitary, pituitary tumors, and physiologic states of hormone deficiency or excess can be attributed to dysfunctions of these regulatory molecules.

The homeobox transcription factors are a diverse class of developmental regulatory proteins that share sequence similarities in their DNA-binding regions and are sequentially activated during organogenesis. Two pituitary homeobox proteins (Ptx1 and Ptx2) are expressed in multiple anterior (head and face) tissues prior to the development of Rathke's pouch and continue to be expressed in some differentiated pituitary cells. Rathke's pouch homeobox protein (Rpx) is expressed first in neural structures associated with the head region and then in Rathke's pouch. During the formation of Rathke's pouch, a subgroup of LIM-related homeobox proteins are synthesized (P-LIM, Lhx3, and Lhx4), and these genes continue to be expressed in specific regions of the pituitary throughout life. Properly timed extinction of expression is, for certain genes, as important during development as is their appropriate induction. Rpx must be turned off after Rathke's pouch has been formed so that genes that are specific to later stages of pituitary differentiation can be turned on. The transcription factor that downregulates Rpx expression is PROP-1 (Prophet of Pit-1). PROP-1 turns off Rpx and turns on Pit-1, leading to differentiation of some of the hormone-producing cells of the pituitary gland, including lactotrophs.[27]

Pit-1 is essential for differentiation of both PRL- and GH-secreting cells, hence its alternative name, GH factor-1 (GHF-1).[28] An early-developing subpopulation of thyrotrophs is also dependent on Pit-1. The Pit-1 protein shares close sequence similarity with two other transcription factors within regions referred to as the POU (*Pit, Oct, Unc*)-specific domain, and the POU-homeodomain.[29] Pit-1 expression in the developing pituitary gland precedes the synthesis of hormones and is necessary for the expression of GH, PRL, and thyroid-stimulating hormone (TSH) in fetal pituitaries. Variant forms of Pit-1 are encoded by alternatively spliced mRNAs and may differentially control expression of individual hormones. Pit-1 binds not only to DNA sequences in the GH, PRL, and TSH genes, but also to autoregulatory sites in the Pit-1 promoter. Autoactivation of Pit-1 transcription is one means of preserving phenotypic stability in differentiated pituitary cells. The factors that act after Pit-1 to drive the differentiation of lactotrophs from somatotroph progenitors are not known. Estrogen receptors synergize with Pit-1 to induce PRL, but not GH, gene expression. Estrogen may therefore be one of the factors that drives the ultimate differentiation of lactotrophs.[30-33]

Several extrinsic factors are involved in lactotroph differentiation. Estrogen is an important positive regulator of lactotroph development. Lactotrophs are greater in number and contain more PRL per cell in females during their reproductive years. Estrogen acts directly on lactotrophs to stimulate PRL synthesis and cell proliferation. Estrogen-induced galanin secretion from lactotrophs is an important mediator of these estrogen actions[34,35] and involves signaling through the classic estrogen receptor isoform alpha (ERα).[36] Paracrine factors produced by other anterior pituitary cell types include basic fibroblast growth factor (B-FGF or FGF-2), which has a specific positive stimulatory effect on lactotrophs. Likewise, epidermal growth factor (EGF) stimulates lactotrophs and may act as a developmental regulatory factor as well as a physiologic stimulator of PRL secretion.[37,38] As will be presented in subsequent sections, the same factors that drive vectorial differentiation of pituitary cells can participate in regulating the tides of hormone secretion on a physiologic time scale and in disorders of hormone secretion.

REGULATION OF PITUITARY PROLACTIN SYNTHESIS AND SECRETION

In mammals, PRL secretion is normally restrained by the action of dopamine (DA), which is secreted from the hypothalamus.[39] While the levels of other pituitary hormones are modulated by inhibitory secretagogues such as somatostatin, PRL is the only such hormone that is secreted at unrestrained high levels when completely isolated from the positive trophic influences of the hypothalamus. This unconventional situation is unique to mammals. The control of PRL secretion in birds and other nonmammals is more conventional in the sense that positively acting secretagogues are the predominant regulators of PRL secretion.[40,41] Lactotrophs are excitable cells in that they display spontaneous membrane depolarizations associated with calcium ion influx, and their resting membrane potential is influenced by neurotransmitters and peptide neuromodulators.

The normal secretory pattern of PRL is a series of daily pulses, occurring every 2 to 3 hours, which vary in amplitude so that the bulk of the hormone is secreted during rapid eye movement (REM) sleep. REM sleep is the dominant organizer in men and nonparous women and occurs mostly during the latter half of the sleep phase. Thus, the highest levels of PRL generally occur during the night in humans.[42] In nocturnal rodents, the relationship to the light cycle is reversed, so higher PRL secretion occurs during the daytime, which is the inactive phase. It is unclear how REM and PRL secretion are linked. Infusion of PRL increases REM activity in the electroencephalogram (EEG),[43,44] suggesting that it is PRL that induces REM sleep and not vice versa.

In lactating women, suckling is a potent stimulator of PRL secretion. This classic neuroendocrine reflex originates with the stimulation of sensory nerve endings in the nipple and is transmitted via the spinal cord and brain stem, ultimately to the hypothalamus. Stress and sexual orgasm are also potent stimulators of PRL secretion. Stress-induced PRL secretion varies with the duration, degree, and modality of the stressor. The relative contributions of PRL-releasing (PRF) and PRL-inhibiting factors to these PRL secretory events remain controversial.

DOPAMINE

As was mentioned earlier, the major regulatory input to lactotrophs is inhibitory, provided in the form of DA produced within the hypothalamus. The primary PRL-regulating DA neurons are the tuberoinfundibular dopaminergic (TIDA) cells, which have their cell bodies in the arcuate nucleus of the hypothalamus, and they release DA in the median eminence and pituitary stalk (Fig. 17-2). A secondary tuberohypophysial dopaminergic system has cell bodies in the rostral caudate and paraventricular nuclei, and these neurons release DA in the posterior pituitary.[39] The type 2 isoforms (D_2) of the DA receptor mediate the direct inhibitory actions of DA on PRL secretion, synthesis, and cell proliferation. Targeted disruption of the D_2 receptor in mice leads to a phenotype of PRL hypersecretion and lactotroph proliferation.[45]

Dopamine is synthesized by a two-step reaction in which tyrosine conversion to levodopa is catalyzed by tyrosine hydroxylase, and levodopa is converted to DA by the action of aromatic amine decarboxylase. As is the case for catecholamine synthesis in other cells, the momentary rate of DA synthesis in the TIDA neurons is determined by the activity of tyrosine hydroxylase. The negative feedback mechanism for controlling PRL release is to increase tyrosine hydroxylase activity in the TIDA neurons, thereby increasing the amount of DA available for release from the median eminence. PRL receptors are located in both the arcuate nucleus (site of the TIDA perikarya) and the median eminence.[46] Therefore, circulating PRL may feed back on TIDA neurons at their terminals, which lay outside the blood-brain barrier, or systemic

PRL may enter the cerebrospinal fluid via the choroid plexus. The choroid plexus expresses high levels of a short isoform of the PRL-R, which may serve to transport PRL across the blood-brain barrier. Levels of PRL in the cerebrospinal fluid reflect changes of PRL in the systemic circulation.[47] Isolated PRL deficiency resulting from targeted gene disruption in the mouse results in decreased DA in the median eminence but does not affect DA levels in other regions of the hypothalamus.[48]

Activation of D_2 receptors in lactotrophs has at least two main actions that result in inhibition of PRL. D_2 receptors are members of the heptahelical G protein–coupled receptor superfamily, and they activate the α_i subunits, which leads to inhibition of cyclic adenosine monophosphate (cAMP) synthesis.[39] In addition, D_2 receptors activate a G protein–coupled, inwardly rectifying potassium channel, which instantaneously causes hyperpolarization of the lactotroph membrane and closes voltage-gated calcium channels.[49] Cytoplasmic calcium levels fall because of decreased influx of extracellular calcium, and the reduction in cytosolic free calcium decreases the exocytosis of secretory vesicles.

Dopamine-induced membrane hyperpolarization opposes the actions of some stimulatory factors such as thyrotropin-releasing hormone (TRH), which acts predominantly to increase influx of extracellular calcium by depolarizing the lactotroph membrane. Inhibition of cAMP by DA also opposes the actions of stimulatory factors such as vasoactive intestinal peptide (VIP), which acts via a positive effect on cAMP. This action decreases PRL release in the short to intermediate term. Second, because cAMP is mitogenic in lactotrophs, as well as other pituitary cells, activation of G_i signaling by DA is antimitogenic. Lactotroph proliferation is important for physiologic elevation of PRL release during lactation. The proliferative action of cAMP on lactotrophs is understood to be an important promoter of pituitary tumor growth, thereby contributing to pathologic hyperprolactinemia.[27]

Other hypothalamic factors, as well as DA, and local pituitary peptides can inhibit PRL secretion. Somatostatin inhibits PRL secretion and acts through both cAMP-dependent and independent mechanisms.[50] Calcitonin has also been shown to inhibit PRL secretion and may be secreted from the hypothalamus.[51] Endothelin-1 is produced by lactotrophs and inhibits PRL secretion, and transforming growth factor-β1 can act as a paracrine inhibitor of PRL.[52,53] The biologic significance of these factors in pituitary development and physiology has not yet been established.

PROLACTIN-RELEASING FACTORS

A wide variety of stimulatory PRL secretagogues have been identified over the years, and it is likely that additional PRFs will be identified in the future. The known stimulators of PRL secretion include, but are not limited to, steroids (estrogen[54]), hypothalamic peptides (TRH, VIP, oxytocin,[55,56] pituitary adenylate cyclase activating peptide [PACAP],[57] and galanin[58]), and local pituitary factors (growth factors such as EGF[59] and FGF-2[60], angiotensin II,[61] and, again, PACAP[62] and galanin[34]).

TRH is a potent and rapid stimulator of PRL release in vitro via a set of calcium-mediated pathways activated by a G_q-coupled receptor. However, the relative contribution of TRH to physiologic control of lactotrophs is not clear. VIP acts through cAMP to stimulate PRL synthesis and release on an intermediate to long-term basis. The importance of VIP as a positive lactotrophic factor is supported by two types of evidence. Using antibodies against VIP, the secretion of PRL can be inhibited to a very low level.[39] In addition, VIP appears to be the primary PRF in birds and other nonmammals,[63,64] suggesting that this positive mechanism may have been in place before the evolution of the dopaminergic inhibitory system in mammals. Oxytocin secretion is tightly coupled with PRL secretion during lactation, and both are secreted in response to nipple stimulation. The potential

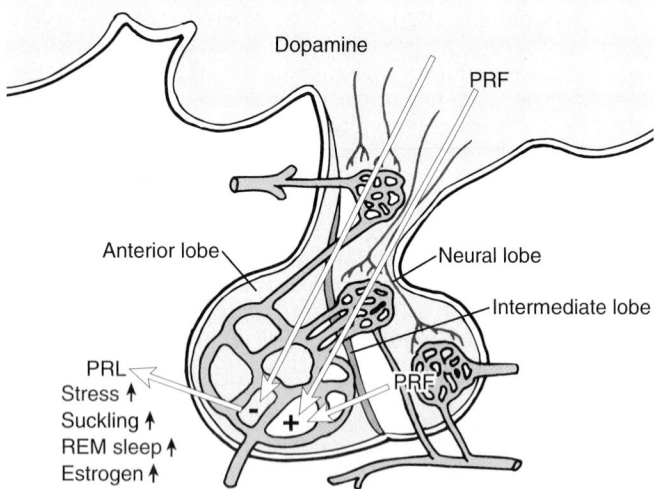

Figure 17-2 Control of pituitary secretion of prolactin (PRL). Dopamine from the hypothalamus is the predominant inhibitory regulator of pituitary PRL secretion. Multiple factors act as PRL-releasing factors (PRF; see text), and these come from both the hypothalamus and the posterior pituitary. Physiologic states that stimulate PRL release are listed on the figure. REM, rapid eye movement.

role of oxytocin as a PRF, given that it can reach the anterior pituitary through the short portal system, has remained controversial. Oxytocin antagonism partially suppresses PRL secretion,[39] so this peptide is likely to provide some portion of the physiologic stimulus for PRL release. PACAP stimulates PRL synthesis and release. Galanin is synthesized in both the pituitary and the hypothalamus. In the pituitary, it colocalizes with PRL in lactotroph secretory granules and acts by autocrine and paracrine mechanisms to stimulate lactotrophs.[34,56]

A putative PRL-releasing peptide (PrRP) from the hypothalamus was identified by searching for ligands that activate an orphan pituitary G protein–coupled receptor. The mature peptide that was identified from bovine hypothalamus is a 20-amino acid molecule and was originally reported to cause rapid secretion of PRL from isolated pituitary cells.[65] However, subsequent studies have failed to confirm that PrRP acts on lactotrophs to stimulate PRL release.[66] Rather, PrRP may act within the hypothalamus to indirectly elevate PRL by inhibiting DA release. Antagonists of serotonin or opioid receptors inhibit PRL secretion under physiologically meaningful stimuli. Conversely, antidepressants that inhibit serotonin reuptake (fluoxetine [Prozac], etc.) increase PRL secretion in humans and laboratory animals. Serotonin and opioids are important indirect regulators of PRL by virtue of their actions on DA and releasing factor secretion in the hypothalamus.

Lactotrophs display a large degree of functional heterogeneity within the anterior pituitary. This heterogeneity is manifested in differences of morphology (i.e., secretory granule size and density), basal hormone release, electrical activity, and response to releasing and inhibiting factors. Assay of hormone release from single cells has revealed not only substantial cell-to-cell variations in function, but also marked temporal variations in a single cell.[67]

Transcription regulators that control the development of the anterior pituitary lactotrophs also participate in controlling PRL synthesis during adult life. Prominent among these factors is the Pit-1 protein. Pit-1 binds to two regions of the human PRL gene, the proximal promoter (within 250 bp of the transcription start) and a distal enhancer (beyond –1300 bp) (see Fig. 17-1). There are multiple Pit-1 binding sites in each of these regions. Transcription regulators such as cAMP and estrogen receptors can control PRL gene expression by influencing Pit-1 activity.[30,54]

PATHOPHYSIOLOGY OF PROLACTIN SECRETION

Normal plasma PRL concentrations in women who are neither pregnant nor lactating range from 4 to <20 ng/mL. In men, the values are, on average, several units lower. Late pregnancy and lactational levels are normally in the range of 100 to 200 ng/mL, the highest levels that occur following active bouts of nursing. PRL is normally measured by radioimmunoassay (RIA). Although glycosylation and other chemical modifications of PRL can affect its immunoreactivity and therefore lead to aberrant RIA results,[22] pathologic levels are generally readily detected by RIA. The original method for bioassay of PRL was by measuring the growth of the pigeon crop sac mucosal epithelium.[68] This method is still occasionally used and is the basis of the international standardization of PRL bioactivity. However, the method has been largely supplanted by a simpler bioassay that takes advantage of the ability of PRL to stimulate the proliferation of Nb2 lymphoma cells in culture.[69]

PROLACTIN DEFICIENCY

When PRL deficiency occurs, it is normally one component of a combined pituitary hormone deficiency. However, a few cases of PRL deficiency without evidence of other pituitary defects have been reported in women. Isolated PRL deficiency results in lactational failure and reproductive difficulty but no other obvious problems.[70-73] No cases of isolated PRL deficiency have been reported in men. These results in a few humans are consistent with the phenotype of mice in which the PRL gene has been disrupted by a targeted mutation. In mice with disruptions of either PRL or its receptor genes, mammary gland development is defective, and the females fail to reproduce, but the males do not have any overt symptoms.[48,74] The concordance of these results from humans and mice is remarkable, given the possible differences between PRL physiology in humans and rodents. One important difference is that progesterone secretion from the rodent corpus luteum requires PRL, but in the human, it does not. This difference in luteal control probably explains why women who have isolated PRL deficiency are merely subfertile[70-73] whereas PRL deficient mouse females were completely infertile.[75,76]

Mice with a targeted mutation of the PRL gene develop pituitary hyperplasia[48] and adenomas[77] that are more severe in females. Mice with targeted disruption of the PRL receptor gene also exhibit this lactotroph hyperplasia and prolactinoma development.[78] The loss of PRL feedback in both these genetic models leads to decreased hypothalamic DA, and the deficiency of DA leads to poorly restrained pituitary growth. It is possible that some "nonfunctional" pituitary adenomas in humans arise by virtue of mutations in the PRL gene, although there is currently no direct evidence of this. Some forms of combined pituitary hormone deficiency have been identified in which PRL, GH, and TSH are hyposecreted as a consequence of mutations in important developmental factors. Familial inheritance of defects in either the Pit-1 gene or PROP-1 results in individuals who fail to develop lactotrophs, somatotrophs, and thyrotrophs, and consequently are dwarfed and hypothyroid, as well as PRL-deficient. Two spontaneous mutations that cause dwarfism in mice have been shown to correspond to these human conditions. In Snell dwarf mice, there is a mutation of the Pit-1 gene, and in Ames dwarfs, the PROP-1 gene is mutated.[27,79,80]

HYPERPROLACTINEMIA

Hypersecretion of PRL is among the most common of pituitary disorders. Medications that elevate PRL secretion, and may cause hyperprolactinemia, include commonly used antiemetics, antipsychotics, antidepressants, and narcotics. These medications alter PRL secretion by antagonizing DA action, or by elevating serotonin or endorphin bioactivity. Reserpine and methyldopa increase PRL secretion as a result of DA depletion. DA receptor antagonists, such as haloperidol and phenylthiazines, increase PRL secretion. Serotonin reuptake inhibitors, such as fluoxetine, elevate serum PRL.[39] It is uncommon for any of these medications to cause clinical signs of hyperprolactinemia because the levels of PRL seldom reach more than 30 to 50 ng/mL with these drugs. One might imagine that there could be subtle hormonal effects after long-term treatments.

Hyperprolactinemia that manifests clinical symptoms is most commonly a consequence of a lactotroph adenoma (see Chapter 25). These tumors may secrete high levels of PRL alone or both PRL and GH. Any intracranial mass or trauma that causes compression or disruption of the pituitary stalk can cause hyperprolactinemia because of the loss of dopaminergic tone from the hypothalamus. Pituitary adenomas have been discovered to be much more common than once believed, with more than 20% of individuals harboring tumors of at least 3 mm at autopsy.[27] Tumors that do not hypersecrete hormones are usually of gonadotroph or lactotroph origin. Some symptoms of prolactinomas may be caused by tumor mass effects. These include visual field defects, associated with pressure on the medial aspect of the optic chiasm, and alterations in temperature regulation, feeding patterns, or other effects secondary to hypothalamic compression. However, effects associated with the physiologic actions of the hormone are the more common presenting symptoms.

Galactorrhea (breast milk secretion in an individual who is not postpartum) and amenorrhea are the result of PRL actions directly on the breast and hypothalamus-pituitary-ovarian axis. In men, galactorrhea and impotence are the most common presenting symptoms of a hypersecreting prolactinoma. The causes of impotence in hyperprolactinemia, whether hormonal or neurogenic, are unclear. Hyperprolactinemia is treated medically by administration of DA agonists, including bromocriptine and cabergoline, or surgically by resection of the tumor tissue.

PROLACTIN RECEPTORS AND SIGNAL TRANSDUCTION

RECEPTORS

The PRL-R is a member of the type 1 cytokine receptor family,[81] and its nearest relative is the GH receptor. Several hematopoietic cytokine receptors, such as those for erythropoietin, most interleukins, and granulocyte-macrophage colony-stimulating factor, are also very similar to PRL and GH receptors. Other receptors, such as those for the interferons, are members of a broader superfamily of proteins that includes cell adhesion proteins. The features that define the type 1 cytokine receptor family include two signature motifs in the extracellular domain and one in the intracellular domain. Four cysteine residues in the extracellular domain are absolutely conserved among all of the type 1 cytokine receptors, and they form two disulfide bridges that are essential for the proper tertiary folding of the ligand-binding domain. A short sequence, which includes a tandem repeat of tryptophan-serine interrupted by a single amino acid (the WSXWS motif), is the second signature motif in the extracellular domain. This sequence is highly conserved near the base of the extracellular domain, but the function of these residues has not yet been proven with any degree of certainty. The structure of the PRL-R extracellular domain, like that of the GH and other cytokine receptors, has been extensively analyzed by x-ray crystallography, as well as by biochemical methods.[82] This domain comprises two 100-amino acid subdomains, which are structurally related to the type III repeats of fibronectin. Each of the type III subdomains includes a

conserved series of seven β-strands folded into two β-sheets that run in an antiparallel orientation. These type III subdomains are connected by a short, flexible hinge peptide and residues that contact the ligand span this connector to include amino acids in each of the type III subdomains. Across the vertebrate lineages, there is substantial conservation of the major features of the PRL-Rs, with some notable exceptions. In birds (pigeons, chickens), the extracellular domain has duplicated and diverged, and in cattle, the distal C-terminus has been truncated, eliminating a tyrosine residue that is conserved in other lineages (Fig. 17-3). Neither of these evolutionary changes appears to have functional significance.[83,84]

Within the intracellular region of the PRL-R an 8-amino acid proline-rich motif, referred to as box 1, is the third conserved signature motif that characterizes type 1 cytokine receptors. These amino acids interact directly with the tyrosine kinases that are activated on ligand binding to the extracellular domain, and mutations in box 1 completely disable PRL-R signaling.[5] There are multiple PRL-R isoforms that vary in the length and amino acid sequence of the intracellular domain. The long isoform, which has been identified in all species to date, has an intracellular domain that is about 350 amino acids in length. Short isoforms (<100 intracellular residues) have been identified in rodents, humans, and several other mammalian species. The short forms of the PRL-R include box 1 but lack other regions of the intracellular domain that are required for signal transduction. In particular, there are conserved tyrosine residues in the distal portion of the long form of the receptor that are phosphorylated after ligand binding, and these tyrosines are required for normal signal transduction.

Mutations of the conserved tyrosines indicate that there is some degree of functional redundancy among these residues, but at least one of the conserved tyrosines must be present to allow normal receptor signal transduction. A mutant PRL-R isoform in rat Nb2 lymphoma cells has a large deletion between box 1 and the distal conserved tyrosines, and this receptor is able to transduce all of the known signaling functions of the long form. Multiple short isoforms of the PRL-R have been discovered in a variety of mammalian species. The functional significance of the short isoforms is not completely known. Although these could provide for signaling diversity, they may also act as decoy receptors and/or transport molecules. The possibility that the short PRL-R isoforms act as PRL transporters is supported by the observation that

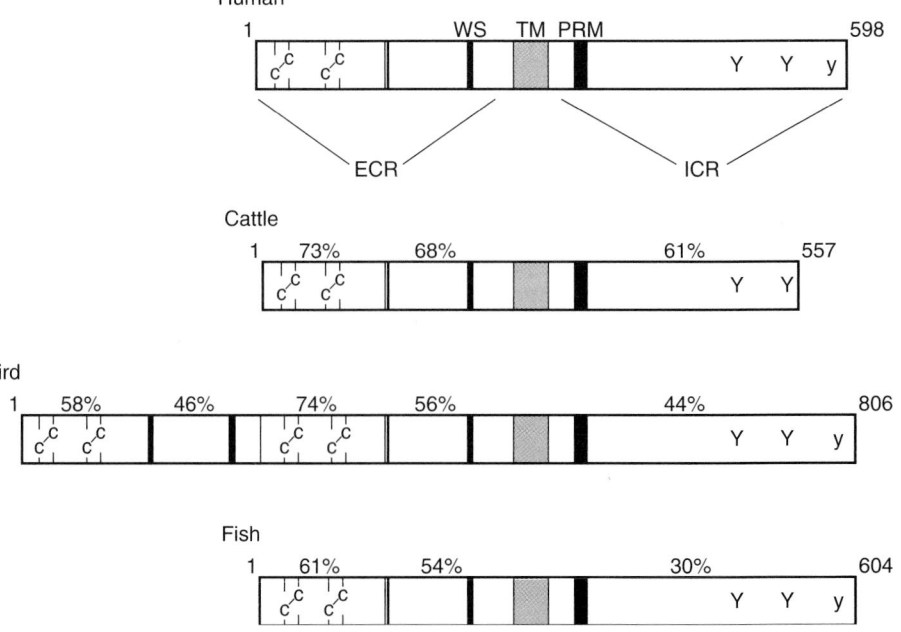

Figure 17-3 Prolactin receptor structure and function. Schematic diagram of the linear sequences of representative prolactin receptors. Pertinent structural features are two pairs of cysteines, the flexible hinge (*double line*), and the WSxWS repeat in the extracellular region (ECR). The transmembrane-spanning sequence (TM) marks the separation between the ECR and the intracellular region (ICR). In the ICR, the conserved motifs are the proline rich box 1 motif (PRM), and conserved tyrosine residues. The uppercase Y indicates ubiquitously conserved tyrosines, and the lowercase y is a tyrosine that is conserved in all known species except cattle. The percentage of identical amino acid residues in each region, compared with the human receptor, is labeled above each receptor.

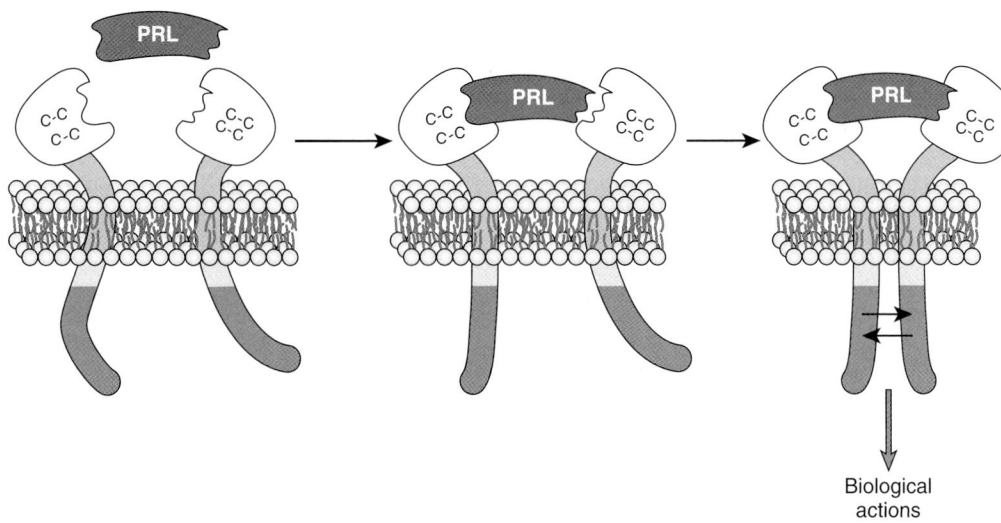

Figure 17-4 Dimerization and conformational changes of the prolactin (PRL) receptor cause activation. Based on studies described in the text, PRL is understood to cause receptor interaction between the receptors and associated proteins, leading to activation of appropriate biologic actions.

the choroid plexus and liver have a preponderance of short-form receptors. The most likely function of the receptors in these tissues is for transporting PRL across membranes. It is also conceivable that short PRL-R isoforms, acting as decoy receptors, in some tissues protect those cells from exaggerated PRL signaling during pregnancy and lactation.

Ligand binding appears to facilitate conformational changes or dimerization of the PRL-Rs as the first step toward signal transduction. The first evidence favoring dimeric receptor interactions as a physiologically important step in PRL signaling was derived from experiments in which antibodies were used to artificially induce receptor dimerization and consequent signaling in PRL-responsive cells. The results from this creative experimental approach were ultimately proved to be correct when hormone-receptor complexes for human GH and PRL receptors were biochemically and crystallographically mapped.[5,82,85,86] The formation of 1:2 complexes of the hormone with its receptor (Fig. 17-4) appears to be the essential first step in the transmission of the biologic signal within target cells. Transcriptional activation requires homodimerization of the long-form PRL-R. Heterodimers of short and long receptors, or short homodimers, do not mediate normal signal transduction.[87]

The PRL-R gene, which is located on the long arm of human chromosome 5 (p13–14), is composed of at least 10 coding exons. Multiple transcripts, reflecting alternative splicing variants and transcription start sites, account for some of the variability in PRL-R structure and tissue distribution.[5]

TYROSINE KINASE ACTIVATION

JAK2 (Janus kinase-2) is a protein kinase that is associated with the PRL-R through binding to the box 1 motif. Its activation is the first intracellular event in a complex, and incompletely understood, web of interactions that mediate PRL effects within its target cells (Fig. 17-5). JAK2 has been shown to be the essential PRL-regulated protein kinase by both biochemical and genetic experiments,[88,89] but this kinase is also essential for signaling by ot' er cytokines.[90] Although it is presumed today that JAK2 binds directly to the PRL-R, it remains possible that another protein could mediate this association. This possibility is raised by the observation that JAK2 is associated with unliganded PRL-Rs, whereas in the case of the GH signaling, where JAK2 is also the important receptor-activated kinase, ligand binding is necessary before the kinase can bind to GH receptor. On ligand-induced dimerization of PRL-Rs,

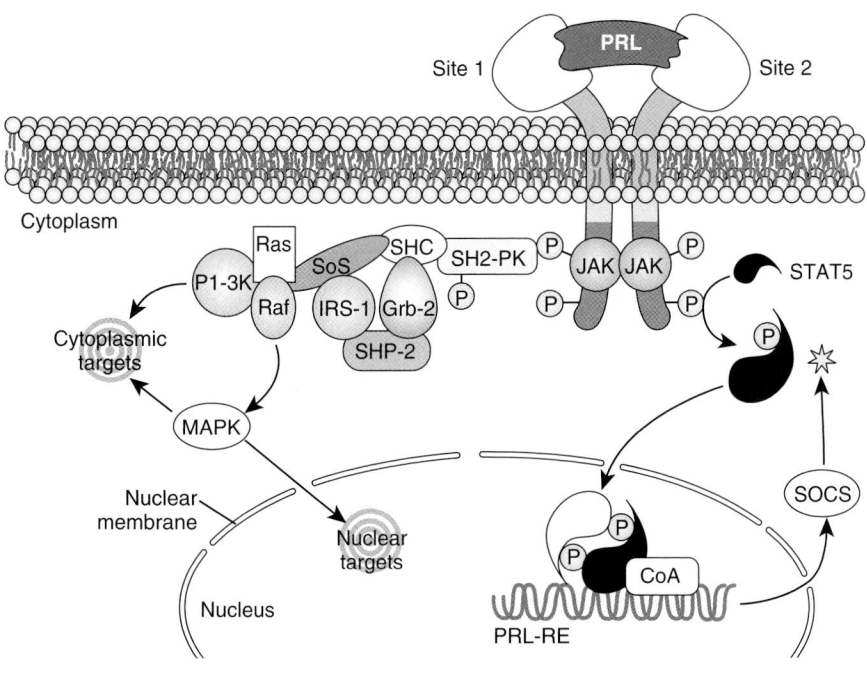

Figure 17-5 Intracellular signal transduction by prolactin (PRL). Janus kinase 2 (JAK2) is associated with the PRL receptor and becomes active after receptor dimerization. A signal transducer and activator of transcription protein (STAT5) is phosphorylated (P), dimerizes, associates with CO-activators (CO-A) and binds to appropriate genes through prolactin response elements (PRL-RE). Activation of the JAK2-STAT5 pathway is inhibited (*asterisk*) by suppressors of cytokine signaling proteins (SOCS). JAK2 also activates other Src-related protein kinases (SH2-PK), and these couple with an array of signaling molecules that can activate cytoplasmic or nuclear target molecules, including mitogen-activated protein kinases (MAPK).

JAK2 phosphorylates specific tyrosine residues on the receptor intracellular domain and autophosphorylates residues within the kinase. These phosphotyrosines serve as docking sites for additional signal transduction proteins. The actions of the kinase are counteracted by multiple tyrosine phosphatases, which rapidly dephosphorylate specific proteins and maintain the steady-state level of tyrosine phosphorylation at a very low level in the absence of hormonal stimulation.

In addition to the signal transduction and activators of transcription (STAT)-dependent events triggered by JAK2 activation, there are other STAT-independent signaling pathways that can be activated when PRL binds to its receptor, as shown in Figure 17-6. Src-family kinases may be involved in PRL signaling by virtue of their ability to couple to multiple signaling intermediates. Phosphotidylinositol-3'-kinase, mitogen-activated protein kinases (MAPKs), and protein kinase C have each been observed to be activated by PRL in some systems.[5] The tyrosine phosphatase short heterodimer partner (SHP)-2 is essential for PRL signaling.[91]

STAT-independent pathways have been proposed for PRL signaling, but the physiologic relevance of such mechanisms is not yet clear. It has been suggested that STAT-independent signaling mediates the mitogenic actions of PRL.[92] This would be consistent with findings in other cytokine-signaling systems, where STAT activation determines certain differentiation-related effector functions, whereas other pathways, such as MAPK activation, are involved in mitogenic signal transduction. However, it is unclear whether this analogy can be extended to PRL. In tissues where PRL has a growth-stimulating action, such as mammary gland or pigeon crop sac, it is not established whether the growth stimulus is direct or is mediated by local synthesis of growth factors other than PRL. The rat Nb2 lymphoma cell line, for which PRL acts as a direct mitogen, expresses a mutated form of the PRL-R, which may transduce an unbalanced set of intracellular signals. The role of specific signal transducers in the proliferative response of Nb2 cells has not yet been established.

TRANSCRIPTIONAL REGULATION

Analysis of PRL-induced genes led, in 1994, to the identification of *cis*-acting elements that bind members of the STAT family of transcription factors.[21,93] PRL-regulated genes were shown to include conserved DNA motifs in their promoter regions, and these sequences bound to STAT proteins.[94] A novel STAT protein (STAT5) was cloned from lactating sheep mammary glands.[95] Mammals synthesize two STAT5 proteins encoded by closely related genes. Genetic studies, making use of targeted gene disruption in mice, have made it clear that both STAT5a and STAT5b are partially responsible for mediating the primary PRL effects in the ovaries and mammary glands. STAT5a is more important in the mammary glands, whereas STAT5b is more important in the ovaries.[96-98] The mouse genetic studies also have revealed a remarkable degree of concordance of the characteristics of animals that lack genes for either the ligand (PRL), its receptor, or the PRL-regulated STAT5 transcription factors.[75,76] The concordance among these studies convincingly demonstrates that the known PRL-R and STAT5 proteins are the primary mediators of the physiologic actions of PRL. There are, however, subtle differences among the various animal models that suggest that the STAT5-dependent mechanism might not be the only component of PRL signaling in mammalian cells. STAT5 is phosphorylated by JAK2 on an essential tyrosine residue in its C terminus.[99] Following its tyrosine phosphorylation, STAT5 dimerizes through interactions between phosphotyrosine and src homology 2 (SH2) domains. Dimeric STAT complexes translocate into the nucleus, where they interact with specific sites in the promoters of PRL-regulated genes, leading to an increase in the rate of transcription of those genes. The exact mechanism by which STAT5 is transported into the nucleus is not known, nor is it known how this inducible transcription factor interacts with the basal transcription machinery during activation of gene expression. There is good evidence that the glucocorticoid receptor (GR) collaborates with STAT5 during milk protein gene induction.[100] This positive interaction depends on occupancy of the GR by its ligand.

STAT activation by PRL is regulated inside the cell by a negative feedback mechanism. CIS (cytokine-inducible SH2 protein), and SOCS (suppressor of cytokine signaling) are members of a class of proteins that are transcriptionally regulated by activated STAT proteins. These proteins feed back on the receptor complex to inhibit the coupling of JAK to either receptor or to STAT.[101]

Whereas STAT5 appears to be the exclusive mediator of the primary physiologic PRL actions in mammals, other STAT proteins, such as STAT1, may be activated in response to PRL in certain pathophysiologic or pharmacologic conditions. In a rat T lymphoma cell line (Nb2), PRL induces the expression of the interferon response factor-1 (IRF-1) gene. This effect of PRL is mediated by STAT1 and, paradoxically, inhibited by STAT5.[102] Although IRF-1 gene regulation is probably not involved in the normal functions of PRL, the regulation of this gene through STAT1 in Nb2 cells provides important lessons regarding the potential derangements in PRL signaling that can mediate pathologic changes. Other experimental models in which the normal pathways of PRL signaling are subverted will provide additional important insights.

THE PHYSIOLOGY AND PATHOPHYSIOLOGY OF PROLACTIN ACTIONS IN MAMMALS

MAMMARY GLANDS

PRL is essential for lactation in all mammals, though the precise temporal dimensions of its actions vary among species. The first step in mammary gland organogenesis is the prenatal establishment of the mammary ductal rudiment. Parathyroid hormone-related peptide (PTHrP) is essential at this first stage of mammary gland development, but PRL is not.[74,76,103] The epithelial rudiment and fat pad grow isometrically until puberty, at which time the epithelial ductal system expands rapidly under the influence of estrogen, GH, and IGF-1.[104,105] During the latter stages of puberty, lobular buds

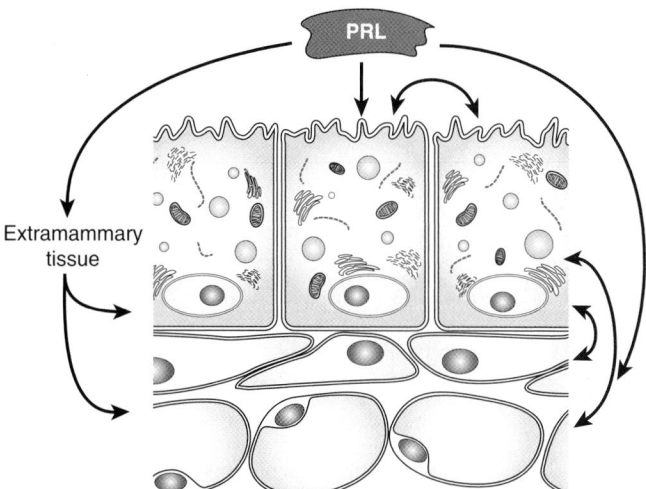

Figure 17-6 Mammary gland regulation by prolactin. Acting directly on mammary epithelial cells, and indirectly through extramammary tissues such as the ovaries and other cells within the mammary glands, prolactin causes growth and functional differentiation of the epithelium. Interactions among the cell types may be either supportive for prolactin-induced functions or homeostatic negative feedbacks.

PRL

Extramammary
tissue

branch off from the ductal system under the influence of PRL and progesterone. As a consequence of the regular cycles of estrous or menstrual hormone surges, the complexity of the mammary ductal branching increases progressively, and the epithelial cells undergo cyclic changes. If the female becomes pregnant before lobule budding and maturation are complete, these processes occur during the first pregnancy. As a general rule, progesterone induces ductal arborization, whereas PRL induces the formation of alveolar progenitors. However, the relative roles of progesterone and PRL in the pubertal development of the mammary glands have not been completely resolved at the organ level, and the genes that are induced by each of these hormones during development are not completely known.

During pregnancy, the lobuloalveolar epithelium undergoes extensive proliferation under the influence of PRL, PLs, progesterone, and local growth factors such as RANK-ligand and IGF-2[106-108] (see Fig. 17-6). During and after parturition, progesterone, estrogen, and PLs fall precipitously, and PRL rises. This combination of hormone changes leads to functional lactogenesis and lactation. The lobuloalveolar epithelium is converted to a secretory phenotype, and the full complement of milk proteins and lactogenic enzymes is synthesized. At the end of lactation, involution of the lobuloalveolar system occurs in response to milk stasis and falling systemic lactogens.[109] According to this scheme of development, PRL and PLs, each of which binds to the PRL-R, act during three stages of mammary gland development: lobule budding during organogenesis, lobuloalveolar expansion during pregnancy, and lactational differentiation after parturition.

Pioneering studies using surgical ablation of endocrine glands and hormone replacement established specific roles for estrogen and GH in ductal development, and for PRL, progesterone, and corticosteroids in lobuloalveolar development and lactogenesis.[110] Transgenic and gene disruption techniques have recently added to our knowledge of hormone actions in mammary gland development *in vivo*. In laboratory mice, complete PRL deficiency results in the arrest of mammary organogenesis at an immature pubertal state. In this arrested developmental state, the epithelial component of the gland consists of a basic ductal system and terminal end buds but none of the structures that are progenitors of the lobuloalveolar system.

PRL induces the differentiation and growth of alveolar progenitor cells from the ductal epithelium.[111,112] This development of alveoli from precursor cells in the ductal epithelium may involve both clonal growth from committed precursors and induction of phenotypic changes in cells that are near specialized "organizer" cells. PRL is also an essential survival factor for lobuloalveolar cells during both pregnancy and lactation.[113-116] During lactation, PRL regulates several secreted milk proteins, including the caseins, lactoglobulin (except in rodents), lactalbumin, and whey acidic protein. Enzymes such as lactose synthetase, lipoprotein lipase, and fatty acid synthase, which are essential for milk synthesis, are induced by PRL in the mammary gland.

FEMALE REPRODUCTIVE TISSUES

PRL has two general types of actions on female reproduction in mammals. First, high levels of PRL inhibit gonadal activity by actions at the hypothalamus, pituitary, and ovary. These antigonadal effects are manifest during lactation in humans and in clinical hyperprolactinemia. Second, PRL is an essential luteotropic hormone in rodents, although not so in humans or most other mammals.

PRL inhibits reproductive function by decreasing the hypothalamic drive for pulsatile luteinizing hormone (LH) secretion,[117,118] inhibiting ovarian folliculogenesis,[119] and inhibiting granulosa cell aromatase activity, which leads to lower estradiol synthesis.[120,121] Elevated DA levels in the hypothala-

mus, secondary to high PRL levels, is one mechanism for the antigonadal effects of PRL. PRL contributes to the breakdown of the corpus luteum in many mammalian species, including humans. In rodents, however, PRL is essential to corpus luteum maintenance in early pregnancy. One of the well-characterized mechanisms of the luteotropic action of PRL is inhibition of 20α-hydroxysteroid dehydrogenase activity.[122] This action prevents the conversion of progesterone to 20α-hydroxyprogesterone and therefore increases progesterone secretion from the corpus luteum.

The maintenance of early pregnancy in rodents depends on the establishment of a stereotypic pattern of twice-daily surges of PRL which are established after coital stimulation of the cervix. In laboratory rodents the luteal phase of the estrous cycle is transient, and implantation cannot occur unless the corpus luteum is maintained by high levels of PRL. The cervical stimulus drives a hypothalamic reflex which alters the secretion of a variety of regulatory factors, including DA, opioids, and various putative PRFs. While it is clear that the diurnal and nocturnal PRL surges in early pregnancy are controlled by different sets of factors,[123] neither the exact circuitry nor the essential hypophysiotropic factors that are responsible for each of the surges are yet known.

Lactational infertility is one consequence of high PRL secretion in women who are breastfeeding. Suckling-induced elevation of PRL can decrease gonadotropin-releasing hormone (GnRH), LH, and estrogen secretion and can cause persistent amenorrhea. If ovulatory cycles occur in women who are breastfeeding, the luteal phase defect caused by luteolytic actions of PRL can prevent conception. Although breastfeeding has been promoted as a natural means of contraception, it is very unreliable for most women. Most studies have pointed out that frequent bouts of nursing, especially during the nighttime, are essential to successful lactational contraception. In some societies, where children sleep with the mother for many months, birth spacing has been strongly influenced by lactational infertility.

MALE REPRODUCTIVE TISSUES

High levels of PRL are inhibitory to male reproductive function, much the same as they are to female function. Common presenting symptoms of human hyperprolactinemia in males are loss of libido and impotence. These symptoms may or may not be associated with galactorrhea. PRL inhibits GnRH and LH secretion in males as well as in females.[124] PRL increases LH and follicle-stimulating hormone receptors in the testis, as well as androgen receptors in the prostate.[125] The antigonadal actions of PRL are the most widely conserved PRL actions among mammals and nonmammalian vertebrates.

Male mice with a targeted disruption of either the PRL gene itself or the PRL-R gene are completely fertile.[75,76] Consistent with this, there are no reports in the literature of human males with isolated PRL deficiency. The prostate gland of PRL-deficient mice is smaller (by about 30%) than that of normal mice, and high levels of PRL cause prostate hyperplasia in mice.[126] PRL secretion may therefore be a contributing factor in human prostate disease, but no data specifically addressing this possibility are yet available.

ION BALANCE AND CALCIUM METABOLISM

PRL is an essential freshwater survival hormone in many species of fish and amphibians, and it has effects on all of the osmoregulatory epithelia in these species. Its actions include decreasing water permeability in the gills and skin and increasing salt reabsorption in the kidney and urinary bladder (which is evolutionarily homologous with the collecting ducts of the mammalian kidney).[3] Similar actions have not been proved in mammals, which is not surprising, since the osmoregulatory challenges facing terrestrial mammals are not at all similar to those confronted by freshwater fishes. PRL does increase the absorption of a variety of minerals in the intestine of mammals,[127] and this effect may be physiologically important during pregnancy and breastfeeding, which place large demands on water and solute homeostasis.

PRL may have important physiologic actions on calcium metabolism in mammals, and these actions directly relate to changes of calcium balance during pregnancy and lactation. In the mammary gland, PRL induces the secretion of PTHrP, which can act as either a local or a systemic effector of calcium homeostasis.[128]

Hyperprolactinemia in humans has been associated with decreased bone density, which is normalized when the elevated PRL levels are corrected medically. Decreased estrogen, due to the antigonadal effects of PRL, may explain part of the bone loss in hyperprolactinemia, but there appears to be a component of bone loss that is due to direct actions of PRL independent of estrogen loss.[129,130] Recent genetic evidence has shown that the PRL-R is essential to normal bone formation and calcium homeostasis.[130] PRL-R-deficient mice displayed reductions in bone mineral density and bone mineral content, as well as a deceleration in the apposition rate for new bone. Plasma total calcium and parathyroid hormone (PTH) were each higher in the receptor-deficient mice. The phenotypic characteristics of bone growth and calcium homeostasis in PRL-R-deficient mice argue that there must be multiple sites of PRL action that influence calcium metabolism, including both direct effects on bone cells and systemic actions on other hormones or carriers.[131] PRL-R mRNA levels are very high in bone during development,[132] and PLs, as well as PRL per se, could contribute to prenatal control of bone growth.

BRAIN AND BEHAVIOR

The vertebrate brain is a target tissue for numerous PRL actions, many of which are related directly to the parental care of offspring. The first evidence that PRL is a brain-regulating hormone was in birds, where systemic or intracranial PRL infusion stimulates behaviors associated with brooding and migration.[3,64] In rats, PRL infusions increase the intensity of parental attendance to offspring or shorten the time required for inexperienced adults to begin showing parental behaviors.[133] Mice that lack the PRL-R are profoundly deficient in maternal behaviors.[134] The neuroanatomic and neurochemical substrates that mediate the PRL-regulated parental behaviors in mammals are not yet known. However, sensory stimuli are clearly important cues for these behaviors and elevated PRL, such as that seen during pregnancy, stimulates neurogenesis in the olfactory lobe of mice.[135]

Whereas stereotypic maternal behavior patterns in animals such as birds, mice, and rats have been quantified and studied objectively, it has not been possible to characterize such behaviors in humans in a way that would allow one to determine whether PRL has a similar role in human parenting. Human PRL increases DA turnover in the nucleus accumbens, corpus striatum, and median eminence, but it decreases DA turnover in the substantia nigra, ventral tegmentum, and cingulate nucleus. It has been proposed that human hyperprolactinemia can be one component of an organic response to psychologic traumas (particularly deprivation from parental attention) and that the behavior patterns associated with high PRL levels (a "maternal subroutine") may be an adaptive psychologic response.[136]

Behavioral actions of PRL that are not directly related to parenting, but may be indirectly supportive, include stimulation of appetite (orexia) and analgesia and increases in REM sleep activity.[7,137–139] The analgesia caused by PRL is blocked by naloxone, indicating that the effect is through an opioid pathway.

HEMATOPOIESIS AND IMMUNOREGULATION

Several laboratories have made a strong case for an important immunoregulatory role of PRL. PRL-Rs are found on a majority of immune precursor and effector cells in each of the major hematopoietic organs (bone marrow, spleen, thymus). PRL can potentiate the growth and effector functions of lymphoid and myeloid cells, and hematopoietic cytokine receptors and signal transducers are closely related to those used by PRL. The Nb2 cell line, grown from an estrogenized male rat lymphoma, is exquisitely sensitive to growth-promoting and antiapoptotic effects of PRL and has been widely used as a model of PRL actions on immune cells.

In humans, PRL secretion is correlated with disease severity in systemic lupus erythematosus, an autoimmune disease that affects primarily women of child-bearing age.[140] In a rat model of immunosuppression following acute hemorrhagic shock, PRL stimulates immune effector cell functions as well as normal cytokine secretion.[141] Whereas PRL can act as a positive stimulus for immune cells when given to animals by injection or to cells in culture, PRL deficiency does not significantly impair immune function or hematopoiesis.[75] Elevated PRL can block lymphocyte apoptosis, and PRL secretion during stress, pregnancy, and lactation may be sufficient to affect immune cells.[142] It is also conceivable that the higher level of PRL secretion in females compared with males is one factor that contributes to a sexual difference in immune responses.

METABOLISM

PRL-Rs are present in the liver, gut, pancreas, and adipose tissue.[5] PRL causes splanchnomegaly (gut growth) and accelerates liver regrowth after partial hepatectomy.[143,144] Bile acid secretion and taurocholate transport in liver are elevated by PRL during lactation.[145] PRL and placental lactogens stimulate growth of pancreatic β cells during pregnancy and lactation. Beta cell proliferation is both a direct response to PLs and PRL[146] and an adaptive response to gestational insulin resistance. In general, the actions of PRL on organs that control whole-body metabolism are consistent with the metabolic alterations that support successful gestation and lactation. Many hormones in addition to PRL contribute to these metabolic adjustments.

Figure 17-7 Prolactin target tissues support parenting. Prolactin has direct effects on both the primary organs associated with parenting (brain and mammary glands) and on a variety of organs that support parenting through secondary physiologic processes.

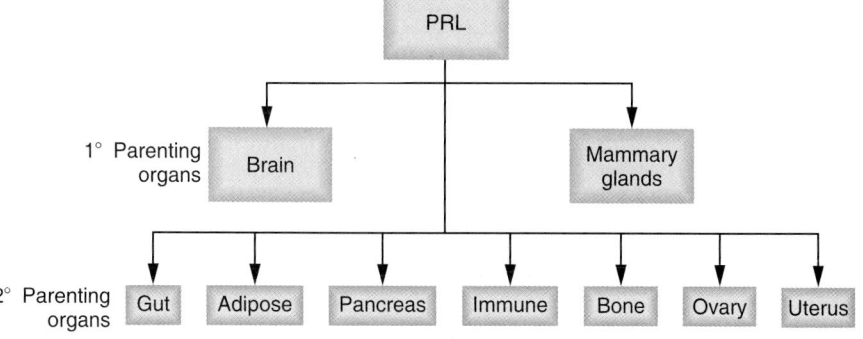

SUMMARY

PRL, along with PLs in many species, plays a central role in ensuring successful reproduction by acting after fertilization to promote a variety of developmental, metabolic, and behavioral adaptations (Fig. 17-7). Hypothalamic DA inhibits PRL secretion and is the dominant PRL regulator in mammals but not in other species. The specialization of the mammalian life cycle to include not only maternal gestation but also postpartum nurturing of offspring has been accompanied by a wide range of physiologic adaptations. Breast milk secretion in mammals, as well as milklike secretions that occur in certain nonmammalian vertebrates, are direct responses to PRL. PRL suppression of gonadal development and sexual drive in both males and females is mediated both centrally and peripherally. The physiologic actions of PRL are pathologically exaggerated in human hyperprolactinemia.

REFERENCES

1. Riddle O, Bates RW, Dykshorn SW: The preparation, identification and assay of prolactin: A hormone of the anterior pituitary. Am J Physiol 105:191, 1933.
2. Stricker P, Grueter F: Action du lobe antérieur de l'hypophyse sur la montée laiteue. C R Seances Soc Biol Fil 99:1978, 1928.
3. Horseman ND: Models of prolactin action in nonmammalian vertebrates. In Rillema JA (ed): Actions of Prolactin on Molecular Processes. Boca Raton, FL, CRC Press, 1987, p 41.
4. Bern HA, Nicoll CS: The comparative endocrinology of prolactin. Recent Prog Horm Res 24:681, 1968.
5. Bole-Feysot C, Goffin V, Edery M, et al: Prolactin (PRL) and its receptor: Actions, signal transduction pathways and phenotypes observed in PRL receptor knockout mice. Endocr Rev 19:225, 1998.
6. Nicoll CS: Physiological actions of prolactin. In Knobil E, Sawyer WH (eds): Handbook of Physiology. Section 7: Endocrinology, Washington, DC, American Physiology Society, 1974, p 253.
7. Li CH: The chemistry of prolactin. In Li CH (ed): Hormonal Proteins and Peptides, vol 8. New York, Academic Press, 1980, p 2.
8. Cooke NE, Liebhaber SA: Molecular biology of the growth hormone-prolactin gene system. Vitam Horm 50:385, 1995.
9. Soares MJ, Faria TN, Roby KF, et al: Pregnancy and the prolactin family of hormones: Coordination of anterior pituitary, uterine, and placental expression. Endocr Rev 12:402, 1991.
10. Soares MJ, Muller H, Orwig KE, et al: Uteroplacental prolactin family and pregnancy. Biol Reprod 58:273, 1998.
11. Talamantes F, Ogren L, Markoff E, et al: Phylogenetic distribution, regulation of secretion, and prolactin-like effects of placental lactogens. Fed Proc 39:2582, 1980.
12. Handwerger S: Clinical counterpoint: The physiology of placental lactogen in human pregnancy. Endocr Rev 12:329, 1991.
13. Jackson D, Volpert OV, Bouck N, et al: Stimulation and inhibition of angiogenesis by placental proliferin and proliferin-related protein. Science 266:1581, 1994.
14. Kessler MA, Schuler LA: Purification and properties of placental prolactin-related protein-I. Placenta 18:29, 1996.
15. Lee SJ, Nathans D: Proliferin secreted by cultured cells binds to mannose 6-phosphate receptors. J Biol Chem 263:3521, 1988.
16. Ben-Jonathan N, Mershon JL, Allen DL, et al: Extrapituitary prolactin: Distribution, regulation, functions, and clinical aspects. Endocr Rev 17:639, 1997.
17. Gellerson B, Dimattia GE, Friesen HG, et al: Prolactin (PRL) mRNA from human decidua differs from pituitary PP mRNA but resembles the IM-9-P3 lymphoblast PRL transcript. Mol Cell Endocrinol 64:127, 1989.
18. Kacsóh B, Veress Z, Tóth BE, et al: Bioactive and immunoreactive variants of prolactin in milk and serum of lactating rats and their pups. J Endocrinol 138:243, 1993.
19. Clevenger CV, Furth PA, Hankinson SE, Schuler LA: The role of prolactin in mammary carcinoma. Endocr Rev 24:1, 2003.
20. Miller WL, Baxter JD, Eberhardt NL: Peptide hormone genes: Structure and evolution. In Krieger DT, Brownstein MJ, Martin JB (eds): Brain Peptides, vol 21, New York, John Wiley, 1983, p 16.
21. Horseman ND, Yu-Lee L-Y: Transcriptional regulation by the helix bundle peptide hormones: GH, PRL, and hematopoietic cytokines. Endocr Rev 15:627, 1994.
22. Sinha YN: Structural variants of prolactin: Occurrence and physiological significance. Endocr Rev 16:354, 1995.
23. Lee H, Struman I, Clapp C, et al: Inhibition of urokinase activity by the antiangiogenic factor 16K prolactin: Activation of plasminogen activator inhibitor 1 expression. Endocrinology 139:3696, 1998.
24. Wang Y-F, Walker AM: Dephosphorylation of standard prolactin produces a more biologically active molecule: Evidence for antagonism between nonphosphorylated and phosphorylated prolactin in the stimulation of Nb2 cell proliferation. Endocrinology 133:2156, 1993.
25. Kenyon C: If birds can fly, why can't we? Homeotic genes and evolution. Cell 78:175, 1994.
26. Frawley SL: Mammosomatotropes: Current status and possible functions. Trends Endocrinol Metab 1:31, 1989.
27. Asa SL, Ezzat S: The cytogenesis and pathogenesis of pituitary adenomas. Endocr Rev 19:798, 1998.
28. Theill LE, Castrillo J-L, Wu D, et al: Dissection of functional domains of the pituitary-specific transcription factor GHF-1. Nature 342:945, 1989.
29. He X, Treacy MN, Simmons DM, et al: Expression of a large family of POU-domain regulatory genes in mammalian brain development. Nature 340:35, 1989.
30. Ingraham HA, Chen R, Mangalam HJ, et al: A tissue-specific transcription factor containing a homeodomain specifies a pituitary phenotype. Cell 55:519, 1988.
31. Simmons DM, Voss JW, Ingraham HA, et al: Pituitary cell phenotypes involve cell-specific Pit-1 mRNA translation and synergistic interactions with other classes of transcription factors. Genes Dev 4:695, 1990.
32. Morris AE, Kloss B, McChesney RE, et al: An alternatively spliced Pit-1 isoform altered in its ability to trans-activate. Nucleic Acids Res 20:1355, 1992.
33. Seyfred MA, Kladde MP, Gorski J: Transcriptional regulation by estrogen of episomal prolactin gene regulatory elements. Mol Endocrinol 3:305, 1989.
34. Cai A, Bowers RC, Moore JPJ, et al: Function of galanin in the anterior pituitary of estrogen-treated Fischer 344 rats: Autocrine and paracrine regulation of prolactin secretion. Endocrinology 139:2452, 1998.
35. Wynick D, Small CJ, Bacon A, et al: Galanin regulates prolactin release and lactotroph proliferation. Proc Natl Acad Sci U S A 95:12671, 1998.
36. Shen ES, Hardenburg JL, Meade EH, et al: Estradiol induces galanin gene expression in the pituitary of the mouse in an estrogen receptor alpha-dependent manner. Endocrinology 140:2628, 1999.
37. Schweppe RE, Frazer-Abel AA, Gutierrez-Hartmann A, et al: Functional components of fibroblast growth factor (FGF) signal transduction in pituitary cells: Identification of FGF response elements in the prolaction gene. J Biol Chem 272:30852, 1997.
38. Zhang K, Kulig E, Jin L, et al: Effects of estrogen and epidermal growth factor on prolactin and Pit-1 mRNA in GH3 cells. Proc Soc Exp Biol Med 202:193, 1993.
39. Ben-Jonathan N: Regulation of prolactin secretion. In Imura H (ed): The Pituitary Gland, 2d ed. New York, Raven Press, 1994, p 261.
40. Lea RW, Vowles DM: Vasoactive intestinal polypeptide stimulates prolactin release in vivo in the ring dove

(Streptopelia risoria). Experentia 42:420, 1986.

41. Lea RW, Talbot RT, Sharp PJ: Passive immunization against chicken vasoactive intestinal polypeptide suppresses plasma prolactin and crop sac development in incubating ring doves. Horm Behav 25:283, 1991.

42. Sassin JF, Frantz AG, Kapen S, et al: The nocturnal rise of human prolactin is dependent upon sleep. J Clin Endocrinol Metab 37:436, 1973.

43. Obál F Jr, Payne L, Kacsóh B, et al: Involvement of prolactin in the REM sleep-promoting activity of systemic vasoactive intestinal peptide (VIP). Brain Res 645:143, 1994.

44. Roky R, Obal F, Valatx J-L, et al: Prolactin and rapid eye movement sleep regulation. Sleep 18:536, 1995.

45. Kelly M, Rubinstein M, Asa S, et al: Pituitary lactotroph hyperplasia and chronic hyperprolactinemia in dopamine D2 receptor-deficient mice. Neuron 19:103, 1997.

46. Pi X, Grattan DR: Expression of prolactin receptor mRNA is increased in the preoptic area of lactating rats. Endocrine 1:91, 1999.

47. Login IS, MacLeod RM: Prolactin in human and rat serum and cerebrospinal fluid. Brain Res 132(3):477, 1977.

48. Steger RW, Chandrashekar V, Zhao W, et al: Neuroendocrine and reproductive functions in male mice with targeted disruption of the prolactin gene. Endocrinology 139:3691, 1998.

49. Gregerson K, Flagg T, Anderson M, et al: Identification of the G-protein-coupled, inward rectifying potassium channel gene products in rat anterior pituitary gland. Endocrinology 142:2820, 2001.

50. Koch BD, Blalock JB, Schonbrunn A: Characterization of the cyclic AMP-independent actions of somatostatin in GH cells: I. An increase in potassium conductance is responsible for both the hyperpolarization and the decrease in intracellular free calcium produced by somatostatin. J Biol Chem 263:216, 1988.

51. Shah GV, Pedchenko V, Stanley S, et al: Calcitonin is a physiological inhibitor of prolactin secretion in ovariectomized female rats. Endocrinology 137:1814, 1996.

52. Kanyicska B, Lerant A, Freeman ME: Endothelin is an autocrine regulator of prolactin secretion. Endocrinology 139:5164, 1998.

53. Sarkar DK, Kim KH, Minami S: Transforming growth factor β-1 messenger RNA and protein expression in the pituitary gland: Its action on prolactin secretion and lactotropic growth. Mol Endocrinol 6:1825, 1992.

54. Seyfred MA, Gorski J: An interaction between the 5′ flanking distal and proximal regulatory domains of the rat prolactin gene is required for transcriptional activation by estrogens. Mol Endocrinol 4:1226, 1990.

55. Yan G-Z, Pan WT, Bancroft C: Thyrotropin-releasing hormone action on the prolactin promoter is mediated by the POU protein Pit-1. Mol Endocrinol 5:535, 1991.

56. Bredow S, Kacsóh B, Obál F Jr, et al: Increase of prolactin mRNA in the rat hypothalamus after intracerebroventricular injection of VIP or PACAP. Brain Res 660:301, 1994.

57. Arbogast LA, Voogt JL: Progesterone suppresses tyrosine hydroxylase messenger ribonucleic acid levels in the arcuate nucleus on proestrus. Endocrinology 135:343, 1994.

58. López FJ, Merchenthaler I, Ching M, et al: Galanin: A hypothalamic-hypophysiotropic hormone modulating reproductive functions. Proc Natl Acad Sci U S A 88:4508, 1991.

59. Pickett CA, Gutierrez-Hartmann A: Ras mediates Src but not epidermal growth factor-receptor tyrosine kinase signaling pathways in GH_4 neuroendocrine cells. Proc Natl Acad Sci U S A 91:8612, 1994.

60. Porter TE, Wiles CD, Frawley LS: Stimulation of lactotrope differentiation *in vitro* by fibroblast growth factor. Endocrinology 134:164, 1994.

61. Aguilera G, Hyde CL, Catt KJ: Angiotensin II receptors and prolactin release in pituitary lactotrophs. Endocrinology 111:1045, 1982.

62. Koves K, Molnar J, Kantor O, et al: New aspects of the neuroendocrine role of PACAP. Ann N Y Acad Sci 805:648, 1996.

63. El Halawani ME, Burke WH, Millam JR, et al: Regulation of prolactin and its role in gallinaceous bird reproduction. J Exp Zool 232:521, 1984.

64. Horseman ND, Buntin JD: Regulation of pigeon crop milk secretions and parental behaviors by prolactin. Annu Rev Nutr 15:213, 1995.

65. Hinuma S, Habata Y, Fujii R, et al: Prolactin-releasing peptide in the brain. Nature 393:272, 1998.

66. Samson WK, Keown C, Samson CK, et al: Prolactin-releasing peptide and its homology RFRP-1 act in hypothalamus but not in anterior pituitary gland to stimulate stress hormone secretion. Endocrine 20:59, 2003.

67. Castano JP, Kineman RD, Frawley LS: Dynamic fluctuations in the secretory activity of individual lactotropes as demonstrated by a modified sequential plaque assay. Endocrinology 135:1747, 1994.

68. Nicoll CS: Bioassay of prolactin. Analysis of the pigeon crop-sac response to local protein injection by objective and quantitative methods. Endocrinology 80:641, 1967.

69. Gout PW, Beer CT, Noble RL: Prolactin-stimulated growth of cell cultures established from malignant Nb rat lymphomas. Cancer Res 40:2433, 1980.

70. Kauppila A, Chatelain P, Kirkinen P, et al: Isolated prolactin deficiency in a woman with puerperal alactogenesis. J Clin Endocrinol Metab 64:309, 1987.

71. Falk RJ: Isolated prolactin deficiency: A case report. Fertil Steril 58:1060, 1992.

72. Douchi T, Nakae M, Yamamoto S, et al: A woman with isolated prolactin deficiency. Acta Obstet Gynecol Scand 80:368, 2001.

73. Zargar AH, Masoodi SR, Laway BA, et al: Familial puerperal alactogenesis: Possibility of a genetically transmitted isolated prolactin deficiency. Br J Obstet Gynaecol 104:629, 1997.

74. Vomachka AJ, Pratt SL, Lockefeer JA, et al: Prolactin gene-disruption arrests mammary gland development and retards T-antigen-induced tumor growth. Oncogene 19:1077, 2000.

75. Horseman ND, Zhao W, Montecino-Rodriguez E, et al: Defective mammopoiesis, but normal hematopoiesis, in mice with a targeted disruption of the prolactin gene. EMBO J 16:6926, 1997.

76. Ormandy C, Camus A, Barra J, et al: Null mutation of the prolactin receptor gene produces multiple reproductive defects in the mouse. Genes Dev 11:167, 1997.

77. Cruz-Soto ME, Scheiber MD, Gregerson KA, et al: Pituitary tumorigenesis in prolactin gene-disrupted mice. Endocrinology 143:4429, 2002.

78. Schuff KG, Hentges ST, Kelly MA, et al: Lack of prolactin receptor signaling in mice results in lactotroph proliferation and prolactinomas by dopamine-dependent and independent mechanisms. J Clin Invest 110:973, 2002.

79. Radovick S, Nations M, Du Y, et al: A mutation in the POU-homeodomain of Pit-1 responsible for combined pituitary hormone deficiency. Science 257:1115, 1992.

80. Voss JW, Rosenfeld MG: Anterior pituitary development: Short tales from dwarf mice. Cell 70:527, 1992.

81. Cosman D, Lyman SD, Idzerda RL, et al: A new cytokine receptor superfamily. Trends Biochem Sci 15:265, 1990.

82. Somers W, Ultsh M, De Vos AM, et al: The x-ray structure of a growth hormone-prolactin receptor complex. Nature 372:478, 1994.

83. Chen X, Horseman ND: Cloning, expression, and mutational analysis of the pigeon prolactin receptor. Endocrinology 135:269, 1994.

84. Schuler LA, Nagel RJ, Gao J, et al: Prolactin receptor heterogeneity in bovine fetal and maternal tissues. Endocrinology 138:3187, 1997.

85. de Vos AM, Ultsch M, Kossiakoff AA: Human growth hormone and extracellular domain of its receptor: Crystal structure of the complex. Science 255:306, 1992.

86. Gertler A, Grosclaude J, Djiane J: Interaction of lactogenic hormones with prolactin receptors. Ann N Y Acad Sci 839:177, 1998.

87. Chang W-P, Clevenger CV: Modulation of growth factor receptor function by isoform heterodimerization. Proc Natl Acad Sci U S A 93:5947, 1996.

88. Campbell GS, Argentsinger LS, Ihle JN, et al: Activation of JAK2 tyrosine kinase by prolactin receptors in Nb2

cells and mouse mammary gland explants. Proc Natl Acad Sci U S A 91:5232, 1994.

89. Gao J, Hughes JP, Auperin B, et al: Interaction among JANUS kinases and the prolactin (PRL) receptor in the regulation of a PRL response element. Mol Endocrinol 10:847, 1995.

90. Parganas E, Wang D, Stravopodis D, et al: Jak2 is essential for signaling through a variety of cytokine receptors. Cell 93:385, 1998.

91. Berchtold S, Volarevic S, Moriggl R, et al: Dominant negative variants of the SHP-2 tyrosine phosphatase inhibit prolactin activation of Jak2 (janus kinase 2) and induction of Stat5 (signal transducer and activator of transcription 5)-dependent transcription. Mol Endocrinol 12:556, 1998.

92. Das R, Vonderhaar BK: Prolactin as a mitogen in mammary cells. J Mammary Gland Biol Neoplasia 2:29, 1997.

93. Darnell JE Jr, Kerr IM, Stark GR: Jak-Stat pathways and transcriptional activation in response to IFNs and other extracellular signaling proteins. Science 264:1415, 1994.

94. Sidis Y, Horseman ND: Prolactin induces rapid p95/p70 tyrosine phosphorylation, and protein binding to GAS-like sites in the $anx\ I_{cp35}$ and c-fos genes. Endocrinology 134:1979, 1994.

95. Wakao H, Gouilleux F, Groner B: Mammary gland factor (MGF) is a novel member of the cytokine regulated transcription factor gene family and confers the prolactin response. EMBO J 13:2182, 1994.

96. Liu X, Robinson GW, Wagner K-U, et al: Stat5a is mandatory for adult mammary gland development and lactogenesis. Genes Dev 11:179, 1997.

97. Udy GB, Towers RP, Snell RG, et al: Requirement of STAT5b for sexual dimorphism of body growth rates and liver gene expression. Proc Natl Acad Sci U S A 94:7239, 1997.

98. Teglund S, McKay C, Schuetz E, et al. Stat5a and Stat5b proteins have essential and nonessential, or redundant, roles in cytokine responses. Cell 93:841, 1998.

99. Gouilleux F, Wakao H, Mundt M, et al: Prolactin induces phosphorylation of tyr694 of Stat5 (MGF), a prerequisite for DNA binding and induction of transcription. EMBO J 13:4361, 1994.

100. Stocklin E, Wissler M, Gouilleux, et al: Functional interactions between Stat5 and the glucocorticoid receptor. Nature 383:726, 1996.

101. Helman D, Sandowski Y, Cohen Y, et al: Cytokine-inducible SH2 protein (CIS3) and Jak2 binding protein (JAB) abolish prolactin receptor-mediated Stat5 signaling. FEBS Lett 441:287, 1998.

102. Luo G, Yu-Lee L-Y: Transcriptional inhibition by Stat5. J Biol Chem 272:26841, 1997.

103. Wysolmerski JJ, Stewart AF: The physiology of parathyroid hormone-related protein: An emerging role as a developmental factor. Annu Rev Physiol 60:431, 1998.

104. Topper YJ, Freeman CS: Multiple hormone interactions in the developmental biology of the mammary gland. Physiol Rev 60:1049, 1980.

105. Kleinberg DL: Early mammary development: Growth hormone and IGF-1. J Mammary Gland Biol Neoplasia 2:49, 1997.

106. Srivastava S, Matsuda M, Hou Z, et al: Receptor activator of NF-kappaB ligand induction via Jak2 and Stat5a in mammary epithelial cells. J Biol Chem 278:46171, 2003.

107. Hovey RC, Harris J, Hadsell DL, et al: Local insulin-like growth factor-II mediates prolactin-induced mammary gland development. Mol Endocrinol 17:460, 2003.

108. Brisken C, Ayyannan A, Nguyen C, et al: IGF-2 is a mediator of prolactin-induced morphogenesis in the breast. Dev Cell 3:877, 2002.

109. Schmitt-Ney M, Happ B, Hofer P, et al: Mammary gland-specific nuclear factor activity is positively regulated by lactogenic hormones and negatively by milk stasis. Mol Endocrinol 6:1988, 1992.

110. Lyons W, Li CH, Johnson RE: Hormonal control of mammary growth and lactation. Recent Prog Horm Res 14:219, 1958.

111. Chepko G, Smith GH: Three division-competent, structurally-distinct cell populations contribute to murine mammary epithelial renewal. Tissue Cell 29:239, 1997.

112. Smith GH: Experimental mammary epithelial morphogenesis in an in vivo model: Evidence for distinct cellular progenitors of the ductal and lobular phenotype. Breast Cancer Res Treat 39:21, 1996.

113. Travers MT, Barber MC, Tonner E, et al: The role of prolactin and growth hormone in the regulation of casein gene expression and mammary cell survival: Relationships to milk synthesis and secretion. Endocrinology 137:1530, 1996.

114. Humphreys RC, Hennighausen L: Signal transducer and activator of transcription 5a influences mammary epithelial cell survival and tumorigenesis. Cell Growth Differ 10:685, 1999.

115. Capuco AV, Li M, Long E, et al: Concurrent pregnancy retads mammary involution: Effects on apoptosis and proliferation of the mammary epithelium after forced weaning of mice. Biol Reprod 66:1471, 2002.

116. Bailey JP, Nieport K, Herbst MP, et al: Prolactin and transforming growth factor-beta signaling exert opposing effects on mammary gland morphogenesis, involution, and the Akt-forkhead pathway. Mol Endocrinol 12:1171, 2004.

117. Sarkar D, Yen S: Hyperprolactinemia decreases the luteinizing hormone releasing hormone concentration in pituitary portal plasma: A possible role for β-endorphin as a mediator. Endocrinology 116:2080, 1985.

118. Cohen-Becker I, Selmanoff M, Wise P: Hyperprolactinemia alters the frequency and amplitude of pulsatile lutenizing hormone secretion in the ovariectomized rat. Neuroendocrinology 42:328, 1986.

119. Larsen J, Bhanu A, Odell W: Prolactin inhibition of pregnant mare's serum stimulated follicle development in the rat ovary. Endocr Res 16:449, 1990.

120. Tsai-Morris C, Ghosh M, Hirshfield A, et al: Inhibition of ovarian aromatase by prolactin in vivo. Biol Reprod 29:342, 1983.

121. Krasnow J, Hickey G, Richards J: Regulation of aromatase mRNA and estradiol biosynthesis in rat ovarian granulosa and luteal cells by prolactin. Mol Endocrinol 4:13, 1990.

122. Albarracin CT, Parmer TG, Duan WR, et al: Identification of a major prolactin-regulated protein as 20α-hydroxysteroid dehydrogenase: Coordinate regulation of its activity, protein content, and messenger ribonucleic acid expression. Endocrinology 134:2453, 1994.

123. Freeman ME, Smith MS, Nazian SJ, et al: Ovarian and hypothalamic control of the daily surges of prolactin secretion during pseudopregnancy. Endocrinology 94:875, 1974.

124. Voogt JL, de Greef WJ, Visser TJ, et al: In vivo release of dopamine, luteinizing hormone-releasing hormone and thyrotropin-releasing hormone in male rats bearing a prolactin-secreting tumor. Neuroendocrinol 46:110, 1987.

125. Bex FJ, Bartke A: Testicular LH binding in the hamster: Modification by photoperiod and prolactin. Endocrinology 100:1223, 1977.

126. Wennbo H, Kindblom J, Isaksson OG, et al: Transgenic mice overexpressing the prolactin gene develop dramatic enlargement of the prostate gland. Endocrinology 138:4410, 1997.

127. Mainoya JR, Bern HA, Regan JW: Influence of ovine prolactin on transport of fluid and sodium chloride by the mammalian intestine and gall bladder. J Endocrinol 63:311, 1974.

128. Ferrari SL, Rizzoli R, Bonjour JP: Parathyroid hormone-related protein production by primary cultures of mammary epithelial cells. J Cell Physiol 150:304, 1992.

129. Klibanski A, Neer RM, Beitins IZ, et al: Decreased bone density in hyperprolactinemic women. N Engl J Med 303:1511, 1980.

130. Klibanski A, Greenspan SL: Increase in bone mass after treatment of hyperprolactinemic amenorrhea. N Engl J Med 315:542, 1986.

131. Clément-Lacroix P, Ormandy C, Lepescheux L, et al: Osteoblasts are a new target for prolactin: Analysis of bone formation in prolactin receptor

knockout mice. Endocrinology 140:96, 1999.

132. Freemark M, Nagano M, Edery M, et al: Prolactin receptor gene expression in the fetal rat. J Endocrinol 144:285, 1995.

133. Bridges RS: The role of lactogenic hormones in maternal behavior in female rats. Acta Paediatr Suppl 397:33, 1994.

134. Lucas BK, Ormandy CJ, Binart N, et al: Null mutation of the prolactin receptor gene produces a defect in maternal behavior. Endocrinology 139:4102, 1998.

135. Shingo T, Gregg C, Enwere E, et al: Pregnancy-stimulated neurogenesis in the adult female forebrain mediated by prolactin. Science 299:117, 2003.

136. Sobrinho LG: The psychogenic effects of prolactin. Acta Endocrinol 129:38, 1993.

137. Buntin JD: Time course and response specificity of prolactin-induced hyperphagia in ring doves. Physiol Behav 45:903, 1989.

138. Sauve D, Woodside B: The effect of central administration of prolactin on food intake in virgin female rats is dose-dependent, occurs in the absence of ovarian hormones and the latency to onset varies with feeding regimen. Brain Res 729:75, 1996.

139. Ramaswamy S, Pillai NP, Bapna JS. Analgesic effect of prolactin: Possible mechanism of action. Eur J Pharmacol 96:171, 1983.

140. Walker SE, Allen SH, McMurray RW: Prolactin and autoimmune disease. Trends Endocrinol Metab 4:147, 1993.

141. Zellweger R, Zhu X-H, Wichmann MW, et al: Prolactin administration following hemorrhagic shock improves macrophage cytokine release capacity and decreases mortality from subsequent sepsis. J Immunol 157:5748, 1996.

142. Krishnan N, Thellin O, Buckley DJ, et al: Prolactin suppresses glucocorticoid-induced apoptosis in vivo. Endocrinology 144:2102, 2003.

143. Bates RW, Riddle O, Lahr EL, et al: Aspects of splanchnomegaly associated with the action of prolactin. Am J Physiol 119:603, 1937.

144. Buckley AR, Crowe PD, Russell DR: Rapid activation of protein kinase C in isolated rat liver nuclei by prolactin, a known hepatic mitogen. Proc Natl Acad Sci U S A 85:8649, 1988.

145. Liu Y, Hyde JF, Vore M: Prolactin regulates maternal bile secretory function post partum. J Pharmacol Exp Ther 261:560, 1992.

146. Brelje TC, Sorenson RL: Role of prolactin versus growth hormone on islet B-cell proliferation in vitro: Implications for pregnancy. Endocrinology 128:45, 1991.

Adrenocorticotropic Hormone

Anne White

INTRODUCTION

Adrenocorticotropic hormone (ACTH) is synthesized as part of the precursor pro-opiomelanocortin (POMC) and as such represents a challenge to endocrinologists in understanding how ACTH is cleaved from the precursor to produce the peptide that acts on the adrenal gland to stimulate the release of adrenal steroids.

This chapter focuses on ACTH in humans and in the first section describes the structure, expression, and regulation of the *POMC* gene, with emphasis on the difference between POMC in the pituitary and POMC in other tissues and tumors. The second section covers ACTH and related peptides and examines the structure of the precursor, how it is processed, and the biologic activity of the different peptides derived from POMC. It is important to understand which peptides are present in the circulation and how differential processing of POMC produces an alternative spectrum of peptides (including precursors and fragments) in different tissues. The impact of the host of factors and mechanisms known to regulate ACTH and related peptides is considered in the context of biologic activity.

The hypothalamic-pituitary-adrenal (HPA) axis (Fig. 18-1) is well recognized for its role in the homeostatic mechanisms regulating the stress response. The hypothalamic secretion of corticotropin-releasing factor stimulates ACTH in the anterior pituitary, which in turn regulates the synthesis of glucocorticoids in the adrenal cortex.

HISTORY

The many important contributions to the understanding of ACTH physiology make it difficult to provide a synopsis. However, the following events are some of the major milestones:

1930—Discovery by Smith that ACTH is a factor produced by the pituitary that maintains the weight of the adrenal cortex
1954—Primary structure of ACTH[1]
1964—Isolation of β-lipotropin pituitary hormone (β-lipotropin)[2]

1975—Peptide with opioid activity isolated from the pituitary and named β-endorphin[3]
1978—Proof that POMC is the common precursor[4]
1979—Nucleotide sequence of POMC[5]
1981—Isolation and sequencing of corticotropin-releasing hormone (CRH)[6]
1992—Cloning of the ACTH receptor[7,7a]
1998—Inherited mutations in POMC associated with early-onset obesity, adrenal insufficiency, and red hair pigmentation[8]

PRO-OPIOMELANOCORTIN GENE

STRUCTURE OF THE POMC GENE

Humans have a single *POMC* gene located on the short arm of chromosome 2 at 2p23 (the mouse and pig have two copies of the gene). The structure of the gene is well conserved and has been characterized in humans,[9–11] as well as in other species.[12] The *POMC* gene consists of three exons interspersed with two large introns (Fig. 18-2). The first exon, which consists of 87 base pairs (bp), contains no coding sequence, and its RNA transcript is thought to act as a leader sequence that binds the ribosome at the start of translation. Exon 2 (152 bp) contains the initiation sequence, a signal sequence that translocates the nascent peptide into the endoplasmic reticulum, and then the N-terminal part of the coding sequence for the POMC peptide. The third exon (835 bp) encodes most of the mature protein, including ACTH,[9–11] the termination codon, and the signal for addition of the poly A tail.

POMC Promoters

POMC contains three identified promoter regions (P1, P2, and P3 in Fig. 18-3) that give rise to RNA transcripts of 1150, 800, and 1350 nucleotides, respectively. P1 is the promoter that gives rise to the mRNA transcript found in corticotrope cells of the anterior pituitary in humans.

Pituitary Promoter P1

This promoter is near the 5′ boundary of exon 1 and generates an RNA transcript consisting of exon 1, exon 2, and part of exon 3 after splicing out of the introns. This arrangement

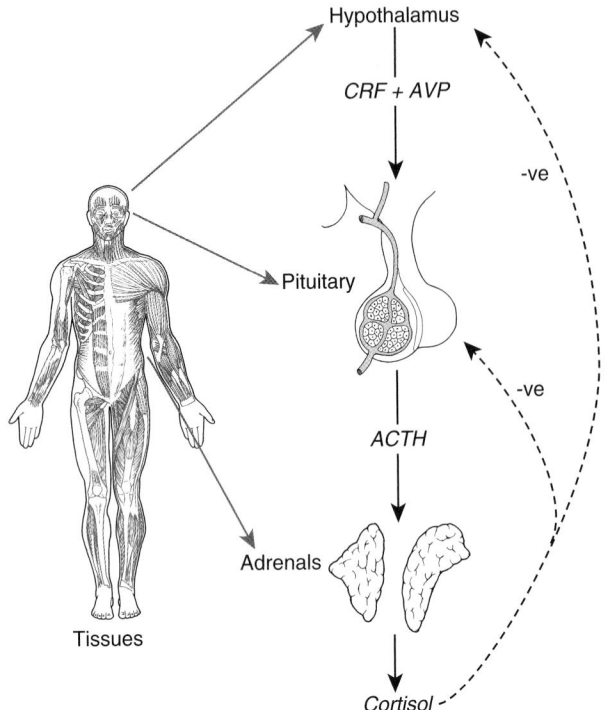

Figure 18-1 Schematic representation of the hypothalamic-pituitary-adrenal axis representing sites of glucocorticoid negative feedback. ACTH, adrenocorticotropic hormone; AVP, arginine-vasopressin; CRF, corticotropin-releasing factor.

would be predicted to give a transcript of 1100 to 1200 nucleotides and this concurs with the size of POMC mRNA from the pituitary, as detected by Northern blotting. This mRNA is also found in the arcuate nucleus of the hypothalamus. Analysis of this promoter has identified a central region at approximately −270 to −290 nucleotides and a distal region at approximately −300 to −370 nucleotides, which are responsible for pituitary-specific expression (discussed later).

Upstream Promoter P3
The upstream promoter, which produces a 1350-nucleotide transcript, lies upstream of the pituitary promoter. Both these promoters should generate the same peptide product because the only relevant translation initiation site is in exon 1.

Downstream Promoter P2
The downstream promoter produces an 800-nucleotide RNA transcript and has been shown in humans and rats to arise from transcription initiation at the 5′ end of exon 3.[13,14] This finding suggests that the promoter is located at the 3′ end of intron 2.[12] Therefore, this transcript could not give rise to a mature POMC molecule and would lack a signal peptide, so its physiologic role is unclear.[15] The smaller POMC transcript is found primarily in peripheral tissues, which indicates that there may be switching to the downstream promoter in peripheral tissues.

Regulatory Sites for Transcription
The *POMC* promoter has a number of elements found in other genes that may contribute to regulation of *POMC* gene transcription. The TATA box is located 27 nucleotides upstream of the initiation site and binds a protein that positions RNA polymerase II on the gene to initiate transcription.

Very little information is available for human *POMC*, but two regions in the rat *POMC* gene[16] confer tissue specificity on the promoter.[13,17-19] These regions are between −320 and −478 bp and between −34 and −166 bp in the rat *POMC* gene. The factors that bind to these regions have not been characterized, but presumably they would be specific to corticotrope cells of the pituitary and binding would be required for *POMC* gene expression.

EXPRESSION OF THE POMC GENE

Pituitary
In humans, expression of POMC is most abundant in the corticotrope cells of the anterior pituitary, and in healthy subjects, these cells are the only ones that express the gene at high levels.[20,21] POMC mRNA expressed in the pituitary has a size of 1100 to 1200 nucleotides, which indicates that it is transcribed under control of the P1 promoter. POMC mRNA is also detected in the intermediate lobe of the pituitary, which is present during fetal life in humans and is found in other species such as the mouse and rat.

Most of the studies have focused on the rat *POMC* gene. Pituitary expression is conferred by the 5′ flanking region of the gene,[14,16-18] but there does not appear to be a specific

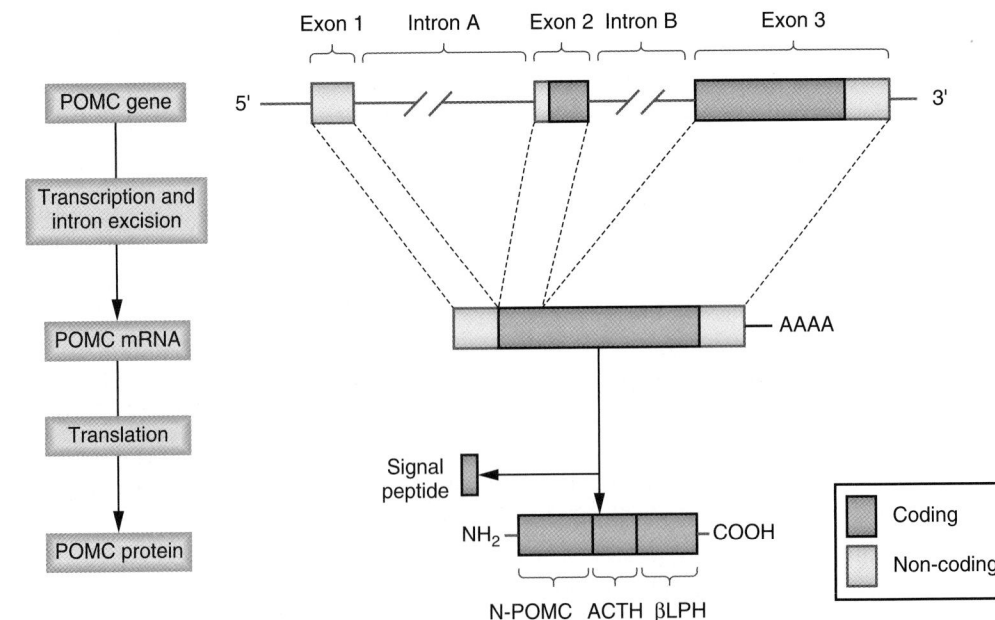

Figure 18-2 Genomic structure of human pro-opiomelanocortin (POMC) with the major spliced product and preprohormone. ACTH, adrenocorticotropic hormone; βLPH, β-lipotropin.

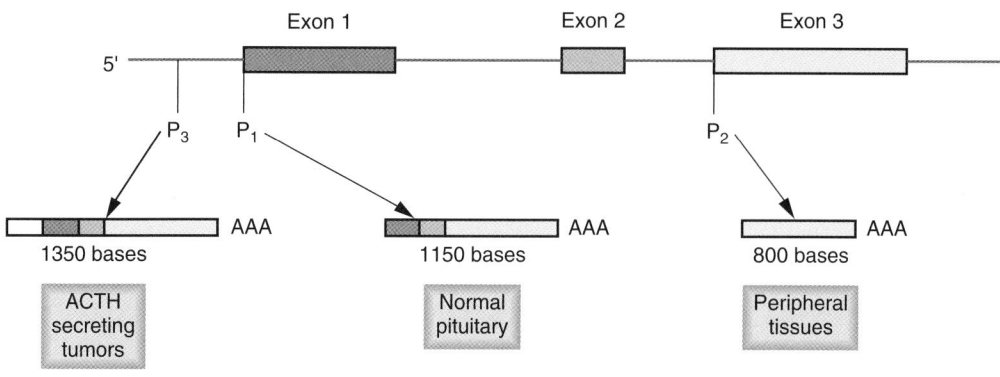

Figure 18-3 Tissue-specific promoter utilization of the human pro-opiomelanocortin (POMC) gene. P1 gives high-level expression of POMC in pituitary tissue. P2 gives low-level expression in numerous extrapituitary tissues. P3 is used in some extrapituitary tumors causing the ectopic adrenocorticotropic hormone (ACTH) syndrome. AAA, polyA tail.

element sufficient to direct high-level transcription, as, for example, in the prolactin gene, where the pituitary-specific transcription factor Pit-1 binds to multiple sites to direct transcription. Rather, in the case of the *POMC* gene, there appears to be a requirement for integrity of the promoter.

The region just 5′ to the start site close to the TATA box confers basal expression and contains the binding sites for PO-B (at −27 nucleotides) and NUR 77 (−67 nucleotides). Further upstream, in the central region of the pituitary promoter there is a response element which binds the homeobox protein Ptx1.[22] During development, Ptx1 plays an important role in corticotrope development and in the development of the anterior pituitary in general.[23] Close to the response element that binds Ptx1, there is a binding site for the T box factor, Tpit, which acts in synergy with Ptx1 and is required for expression of the *POMC* gene and for terminal differentiation of the pituitary corticotrope lineage.[24] Evidence for the role of Tpit comes from Tpit-deficient mice, which represent a model of isolated ACTH deficiency and from humans with Tpit gene mutations, which are associated at high frequency with early-onset isolated ACTH deficiency.[25] The distal region of the pituitary promoter cannot confer activity independently of the central region but does contain a binding site for NeuroD/1A and binds the CUTE (corticotrope upstream transcription element) binding proteins.[26]

Other Tissues

POMC is also expressed, but at a much lower level, in other tissues such as the arcuate nucleus of the hypothalamus, skin, testis, ovary, placenta, duodenum, liver, kidney, adrenal medulla, lung, thymus, and lymphocytes.[14,27–30] POMC mRNA expressed in the hypothalamus has a size of 1100 to 1200 nucleotides, which is similar to that in the pituitary. However, POMC mRNA from extracranial tissues has a size of 800 nucleotides, which suggests that it is derived from transcription initiation at the downstream promoter (P2 in Fig. 18-3) 5′ to exon 3 and thus only includes the coding sequence for exon 3.[29] Therefore, as indicated previously, this transcript could not give rise to mature *POMC* and would lack a signal sequence so its physiological role is unclear.

Pituitary Tumors

Expression of the *POMC* gene in corticotrope adenomas giving rise to pituitary-dependent Cushing's disease appears to be similar to that in the normal pituitary.[31]

Nonpituitary Tumors

Tumors giving rise to the ectopic ACTH syndrome produce a mRNA transcript of 1200 bp, similar to that found in the pituitary, and approximately 20% of tumors express a larger transcript of 1400 to 1500 bp.[31] This larger transcript seems to be initiated from a promoter located at −392 and −432 bp relative to the conventional start site.[32–35] The larger transcript[34]

would still initiate translation from the same site as that used by the pituitary promoter, and thus the POMC peptide would be identical to the pituitary product. Analysis of this domain in the human small cell lung carcinoma cell line DMS-79 showed that it binds the E2F family of trans-acting factors.[36]

The expression of this promoter in the ectopic ACTH syndrome suggests loss of the tight tissue-specific expression. This promoter is embedded in a CpG island, which has been shown to be unmethylated in a number of tumors giving rise to the ectopic ACTH syndrome and in the POMC expressing small cell lung carcinoma cell line, DMS-79.[37] In contrast, the CpG island was methylated in normal nonexpressing tissues, whereas most somatically expressed CpG island promoters are normally unmethylated.[38]

Some tumors not associated with the ectopic ACTH syndrome express the smaller *POMC* mRNA transcript of 800 nucleotides that is found in many normal tissues.[29,35,39] It is probable that these nonneuroendocrine tumors arise from cells that express the short mRNA transcript, and because this short transcript does not give rise to a peptide that is secreted, these tumors would not be expected to release POMC peptides.

REGULATION OF POMC GENE EXPRESSION

Normal Tissues

Numerous factors are known to regulate *POMC* gene expression in the pituitary but perhaps the most important are CRH and glucocorticoids (Fig. 18-4). Expression of the *POMC* gene appears to be predominantly controlled at the level of gene transcription.[40]

Corticotropin-releasing Hormone Stimulation of the POMC Gene
Corticotropin-releasing hormone binds transmembrane receptors on corticotrope cells and stimulates cyclic adenosine monophosphate (cAMP) production and consequently serine phosphorylation of the CREB (cAMP response element binding protein) transcription factor (see Fig. 18-4). Distally, this cascade appears to enhance gene transcription, but the rat *POMC* gene does not harbor a consensus cAMP response element. Further analysis of the *POMC* promoter has identified two DNA elements that appear capable of conferring CRH responsiveness to the gene. One element at 166 nucleotides upstream from the transcription start site binds a protein termed the *CRH response element binding protein*.[41] The second element reported to be CRH responsive is found in the noncoding exon 1 of the rat *POMC* gene.[42] This element shares close homology with a consensus activator protein-1 (AP-1) transcription factor-binding site and indeed appears to bind recombinant AP-1 protein in a sequence-specific manner. CRH causes activation of mitogen-activated protein kinase (MAPK) and induction of the DNA-binding activity of AP-1 in the

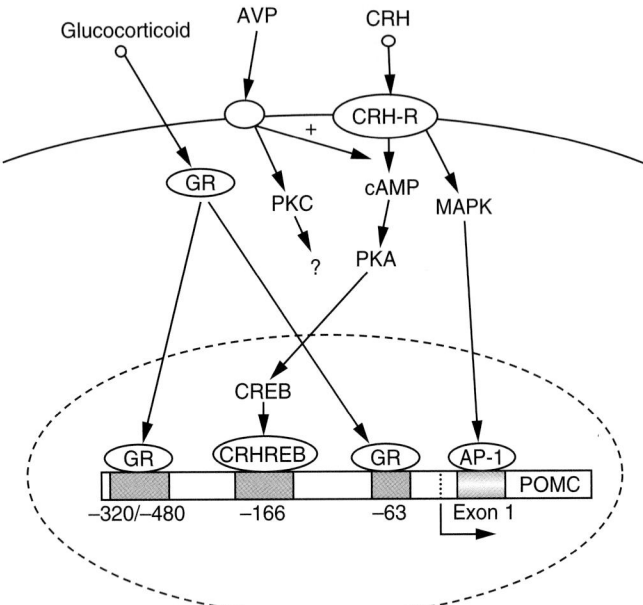

Figure 18-4 Intracellular signaling pathways regulating transcription of the pro-opiomelanocortin (POMC) gene. Through its receptor, corticotropin-releasing hormone (CRH) induces cyclic adenosine monophosphate (cAMP), which activates protein kinase A (PKA) and thereby phosphorylation of cAMP response element-binding protein (CREB) and results in binding of CRH response element-binding protein (CRHREB) to a motif at −166 on the POMC gene. CRH also activates mitogen-activated protein kinase (MAPK) pathways, which ultimately induce activator protein-1 (AP-1) binding to an exon 1 response element. Arginine-vasopressin (AVP) activates cAMP and/or protein kinase C (PKC) pathways, which may also feed into this pathway. Glucocorticoids acting through the glucocorticoid receptor (GR) can repress transcription through two cooperative binding sites.

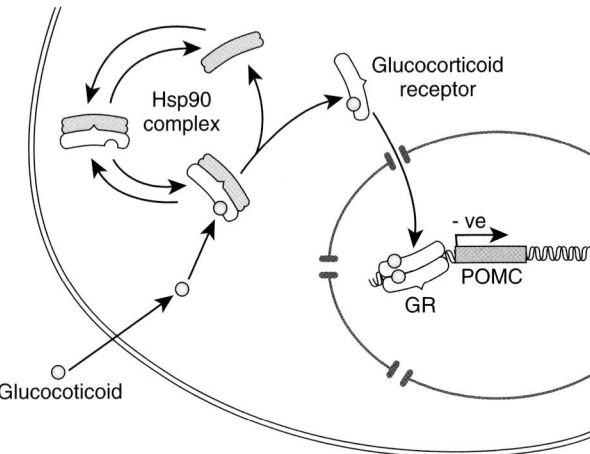

Figure 18-5 Glucocorticoid regulation of pro-opiomelanocortin (POMC). Glucocorticoids activate their receptor (GR) and release it from the heat shock protein (Hsp90) complex, thereby allowing translocation of the GR to the nucleus and binding to the POMC gene.

mouse pituitary corticotrope cell line, AtT20. In addition, the POMC exon 1 element confers both phorbol ester and CRH responsiveness to a heterologous promoter. Therefore, there is considerable evidence for a physiologic role of the MAPK/AP-1 cascade in mediating some actions of CRH.[42–44]

Glucocorticoid Inhibition of the POMC Gene
Glucocorticoids are known to decrease ACTH levels, partly as a result of inhibition of POMC mRNA (see Fig. 18-4), although they also act at the level of translation and antagonize actions of CRH. Considerable evidence indicates that glucocorticoids suppress transcription.[45–49] Glucocorticoids enter the cell where they bind to glucocorticoid receptors complexed to heat shock proteins in the cytoplasm (Fig. 18-5). This results in the translocation of the ligand-bound receptor to the nucleus where it acts as a transcription factor, binding (usually as a dimer with another glucocorticoid receptor) to the promoter region of a gene in order to regulate gene expression. In the pituitary corticotrope, the glucocorticoid receptor mediates inhibition of the POMC gene. The binding sites for glucocorticoid receptors on the human POMC gene have not been identified. However, the rat POMC gene has four sites, although only those at −63 and between −480 and −320[50] are needed in vivo.

The −63-negative glucocorticoid-regulated element overlaps the putative COUP (chicken ovalbumin upstream promoter) box, and it has been suggested that the inhibitory effect may occur by displacement of a stimulatory factor.

This more proximal element is an imperfect palindrome and is thought to bind three glucocorticoid receptor molecules in an unusual trimer formation[51]; it has been suggested that this conformation of receptors on DNA directs repression

of transcription. The glucocorticoid-regulated element further upstream between nucleotides −480 and −320 is required to interact for the full effect of glucocorticoid to be manifested. However, this element has not been fully defined.[50]

Stimulation of the POMC Gene by Arginine Vasopressin
A number of other hypothalamic factors act on the pituitary corticotrope to influence POMC expression; however, their modes of action are less well defined. In particular, arginine-vasopressin (AVP) augments the effect of CRH and can act independently, though rather weakly, to stimulate POMC expression.[20,52,53] The intracellular pathways activated by AVP appear to depend on protein kinase C, but AVP also potentiates the action of CRH on cAMP generation (see Fig. 18-4).

Leukemia Inhibitory Factor Stimulation of the POMC Gene
A number of lines of evidence point to intrapituitary factors as important modulators of corticotrope function. One such factor is the proinflammatory cytokine leukemia inhibitory factor (LIF). This factor has been shown to stimulate the POMC gene through a specific response element that overlaps with the −166-nucleotide CRH response element.[43]

Tumors
Corticotropin-releasing Hormone Regulation of the POMC Gene in Tumors
In general, CRH stimulates POMC expression only in pituitary corticotrope tumors, but a few exceptions occur in ectopic tumors.[54–56] However, it is likely that the increased ACTH stimulation of glucocorticoids will result in inhibition of the CRH gene. Therefore, CRH may not be relevant in POMC-expressing tumors.

Glucocorticoid Regulation of the POMC Gene in Tumors
In pituitary corticotrope cells, expression of the POMC gene is repressed by glucocorticoids, and in pituitary corticotrope tumors, glucocorticoids are able to repress ACTH secretion. In contrast, in extrapituitary tumors, ACTH is characteristically resistant to glucocorticoids.[57] This concept is the basis of the high-dose dexamethasone suppression test used to distinguish pituitary from ectopic sources of ACTH in Cushing's syndrome.

It is intriguing that most extrapituitary tumors are resistant to glucocorticoid inhibition of POMC expression; this suggests that exploration of the mechanisms of this glucocorticoid resistance is of importance, particularly since receptors for glucocorticoids are present on most cells, including malignant cells. To study this, a panel of human small cell lung carcinoma cell lines have been established as models of the ectopic ACTH syndrome.[21,58] These cell lines express the *POMC* gene, and the glucocorticoid receptor has been found to be present.[12,21,59] Significantly, all cell lines studied are resistant to glucocorticoid suppression. To determine whether glucocorticoid signaling was functional, a synthetic, glucocorticoid-responsive gene linked to a chloramphenicol acetyltransferase reporter gene was transfected into the cells. In contrast to the brisk induction of expression in control pituitary cells, none of the human small cell lung carcinoma cells responded to either natural or synthetic glucocorticoids.[59] Thus, resistance of the *POMC* gene to glucocorticoids is only part of the global resistance of these malignant cells to glucocorticoid action. Expression of high concentrations of wild-type glucocorticoid receptor in the cells was sufficient to restore glucocorticoid signaling,[59] and in two of the cell lines, mutations in the endogenous glucocorticoid receptor appeared to cause the resistance.[58,60] However, in a further cell line, even overexpression of wild-type receptor was insufficient to restore glucocorticoid signaling, which suggests that different molecular mechanisms had developed in different tumors to evade glucocorticoid action.[59,61] Because glucocorticoids can inhibit proliferation in some cell types and induce differentiation in others, it is possible that evasion of glucocorticoid signaling confers a survival advantage to the malignant cells. This suggests that POMC expression and ACTH secretion are incidental to the malignant phenotype.

ADRENOCORTICOTROPIC HORMONE AND RELATED PEPTIDES

STRUCTURE OF POMC AND RELATED PEPTIDES

Many bioactive peptides are synthesized from large precursor molecules, and a number of techniques have elucidated the structures of these peptides. Studies have used pulse chase analysis whereby labeled amino acids are incubated with cells to detect the labeled precursors and the peptides derived from them. Subsequently, sequence analysis and cDNA cloning have been important approaches to determine peptide structures. Discovery of the structure and biosynthesis of POMC and ACTH-related peptides and the differences between species is reviewed extensively by Eipper and Mains.[62]

Pro-opiomelanocortin

In 1973, the characterization of high-molecular-weight forms of ACTH in human plasma,[63] in mouse pituitary cells,[64,65] and in human tumors[66] predicted the presence of precursors of ACTH.

Expression of the *POMC* gene leads to synthesis of the preprohormone POMC. This protein undergoes proteolytic cleavage at dibasic amino acid residues, which generates a series of small molecules, including ACTH[62] (Fig. 18-6). Processing of POMC to its constituent peptides varies in a tissue-specific fashion in that both the nature of the processing and the degree of processing varies in different tissues. This results in different groups of peptides being secreted from different tissues, although the exact ratios of the constituent peptides and precursors are still not fully understood.

Adrenocorticotropic Hormone

The ACTH peptide consists of 39 amino acids, is a single polypeptide chain, and has a molecular weight of 4.5 kDa.[67] The N-terminal 12 amino acids are highly conserved between species, thus reflecting the importance of this region for biologic activity. In comparison with the human sequence, ACTH in other mammals has only one or two substitutions, which are in the region of amino acids 24 to 39. In birds,

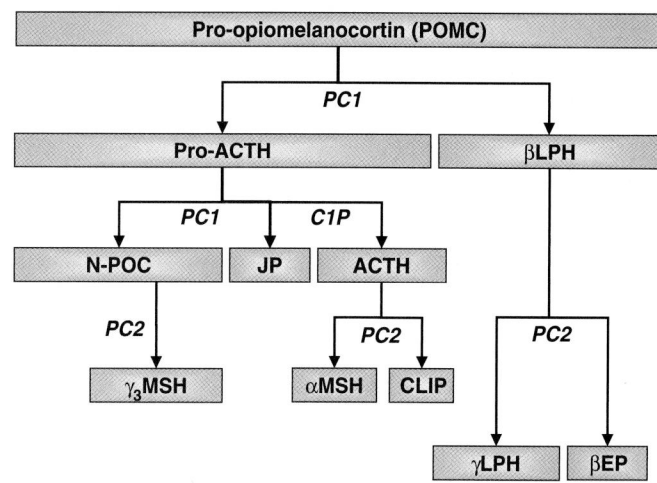

Figure 18-6 Processing of pro-opiomelanocortin (POMC). POMC is cleaved into pro-adrenocorticotropic hormone (pro-ACTH) and β-lipotropin (βLPH). Further processing of pro-ACTH yields ACTH, joining peptide, and *N*-proopiomelanocortin (N-POC), all of which are found in human plasma. Cleavage to smaller fragments occurs in a tissue- and species-specific manner. Shaded boxes represent peptides found in the human circulation. CLIP, corticotropin-like intermediate lobe peptide; EP, endorphin; JP, joining peptide; LPH, lipotropin; MSH, melanocyte-stimulating hormone; PC, prohormone convertase.

amphibians, and fish, although the N-terminal sequence is conserved, the ACTH sequence is more variable, particularly between amino acids 24 and 39. The melanocyte-stimulating hormone (MSH) sequence His-Phe-Arg-Trp is found at ACTH 6-9, and although this sequence is present in β-lipotropin (as β-MSH) and *N*-pro-opiomelanocortin (N-POC) (as γ-MSH), it is thought that the surrounding amino acids influence its specific activity.

α-Melanocyte-stimulating Hormone

α-MSH consists of ACTH 1-13 and is derived from ACTH 1-39 by proteolysis at the C terminal, which is followed by C-terminal amidation and N-terminal acetylation. α-MSH is produced predominantly by melanotroph cells in the intermediate lobe of the pituitary, particularly in species such as the rat and mouse. The adult human pituitary does not have a distinct intermediate lobe and therefore this is not a source of α-MSH in humans. In addition, α-MSH is not thought to be produced in the anterior lobe. However, α-MSH produced by the skin or hypothalamus may access the circulation. Therefore, it is not clear whether α-MSH circulates in humans under normal circumstances.[68–70]

Corticotropin-like Intermediate Lobe Peptide

Corticotropin-like intermediate lobe peptide (CLIP) consists of ACTH 18-39 and is produced during the cleavage that generates α-MSH. Because this process occurs primarily in the intermediate lobe of the pituitary, which is not present in humans, CLIP is not thought to circulate in humans under normal circumstances.

N-Pro-opiomelanocortin

Also called *N*-pro-opiocortin, N-POC (see Fig. 18-6) comes from the N-terminal sequence of POMC, and in humans, it is a 76-amino acid peptide with an MSH sequence in the midregion.[71] The peptide has a tryptophan residue at the N terminus and two disulfide bridges linking cysteines 2 to 24 and 8 to 20, which are thought to be important for the sorting signal that directs POMC to the regulated pathway.[72] N-POC can also undergo *N*-glycosylation at Asn65 and *O*-glycosylation at Thr45.

γ-Melanocyte-Stimulating Hormone

γ_1-MSH is found at position 51 to 62 of human N-POC and has sequence homology with α-MSH. There are C-terminally extended forms of γ_1-MSH, which are called γ_2-MSH (51-63) and γ_3-MSH (51-76).

Joining Peptide

Joining peptide, found between N-POC and ACTH, is a 30-amino acid peptide, amidated at the C terminus. It was isolated from human pituitaries in 1981[71] and has been shown to circulate in humans in the form of homodimers.[73]

β-Lipotropin

β-lipotropin lies at the C terminus of POMC and can be cleaved to γ-lipotropin (which contains the β-MSH sequence at its C terminus) and β-endorphin (see Fig. 18-6). In the human anterior pituitary, cleavage appears to be limited in as much as the main form of this peptide in the human circulation is β-lipotropin with very little β-endorphin.[74,75]

β-Endorphin

This 31-amino acid peptide contains the sequence for met-enkephalin as the first 5 amino acids at its N terminus. β-endorphin can undergo N-acetylation, which is thought to be a tissue-specific effect, and C-terminally truncated peptides have been found such as α-endorphin (β-endorphin 1-16), γ-endorphin (β-endorphin 1-17), and δ-endorphin (β-endorphin 1-27).

PROCESSING PATHWAY AND PROCESSING ENZYMES

Processing

After translation of the mRNA into peptide, a series of processing stages are needed for release of the constituent peptides.[76] The N-terminal signal sequence that is involved in movement of the peptide into the endoplasmic reticulum is no longer required and is removed at an early phase of post-translational modification. Subsequently, POMC undergoes glycosylation and phosphorylation in the Golgi apparatus before transport to secretory vesicles, where it undergoes cleavage into its constituent peptides. The ACTH-related peptides are stored in dense core secretory granules and released from the cell in the regulated secretory pathway (Fig. 18-7).

N-glycosylation and Phosphorylation

These events occur in the Golgi apparatus before cleavage of the peptides. γ-MSH has the sequence Asn-X-Ser, which can be glycosylated on the Asn residue, and in mouse POMC, N-glycosylation of the CLIP sequence can occur. Some evidence indicates phosphorylation of serine 31 in ACTH, although the significance of this finding is unclear.[77]

Processing Enzymes

POMC is cleaved to its constituent peptides by limited proteolysis at pairs of basic amino acids, primarily Lys-Arg and Arg-Arg. The mammalian convertases responsible for this endoproteolytic cleavage are precursor-converting enzymes from the subtilisin/Kex2 serine proteases, which include furin, a protease known to cleave peptides in the constitutive pathway of secretion.[78] Prohormone convertase 1, or PC1 (also called PC3[79]), cleaves POMC preferentially at pairs of basic residues and produces ACTH, β-lipotropin, N-POC, and joining peptide, in the anterior pituitary. PC2 cleaves at different pairs of basic residues and releases smaller peptides such as β-endorphin and α-MSH,[80] as observed in the neurointermediate lobe. This arrangement suggests that these convertases work in a tissue-specific fashion. In addition, they are coregulated with POMC in that PC1 mRNA is regulated by CRH and glucocorticoids in mouse AtT20 cells[81] and bromocriptine decreases PC1 and PC2 mRNA in rat neurointermediate lobe cells.[82]

After cleavage at the dibasic amino acids, several peptides (e.g., ACTH 1-17) have amino acids removed from the C terminus by carboxypeptidase E. Subsequently, α-amidation is catalyzed by peptidylglycine α-amidating monooxygenase, an enzyme that has multiple molecular forms, and/or acetylation occurs by the action of specific acetyltransferases.[83]

PROCESSING IN DIFFERENT TISSUES

POMC processing varies depending on the species and the tissue. Although POMC is expressed primarily in the pituitary, POMC mRNA has been detected in many extrapituitary tissues. However, such detection does not provide evidence that the peptides are synthesized or secreted there. POMC peptides have been detected by immunocytochemistry or radioimmunoassay of human[29] and rat[84] tissue extracts. Whether the POMC peptides produced in extrapituitary tissues reach the circulation is debatable, and it is more likely that they act in an autocrine or paracrine role.

Anterior Pituitary

In the human anterior pituitary, POMC is cleaved to give pro-ACTH, which is then cleaved to ACTH, N-POC, and joining peptide (see Fig. 18-6). Interestingly, the ACTH precursors, POMC and pro-ACTH, are found in the human circulation with ACTH, N-POC, joining peptide, and β-lipotropin.[85] That very little β-endorphin appears to be present indicates that processing of β-lipotropin is minimal (Fig. 18-8). However, reports can be confounded by the fact that in some β-endorphin assays, the antibodies also detect β-lipotropin. In the rat and sheep anterior pituitary, some ACTH is processed to des-acetyl-α-MSH and α-MSH.[83]

Studies in the mouse pituitary tumor cell line, AtT20, suggests that cleavage is sequential, starting with the C terminus of ACTH.[62] However, the same pair of basic amino acids is found between ACTH and β-lipotropin, joining peptide and ACTH, ACTH 1-16 and ACTH 17-39, and γ-lipotropin and β-endorphin. Therefore, the adjacent amino acids and peptide folding must influence the sequential processing.

Intermediate Lobe

In the rodent intermediate lobe, POMC is found in melanotroph cells and undergoes more comprehensive processing to give the smaller fragments α-, β-, and γ-MSH, CLIP, and

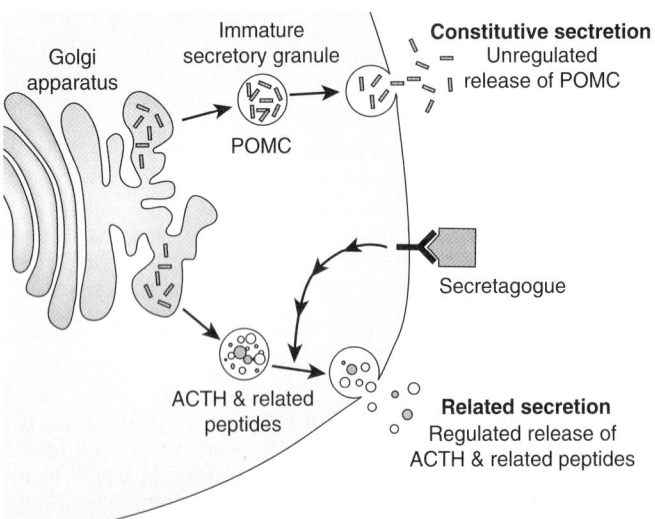

Figure 18-7 Pro-opiomelanocortin (POMC) processing and peptide release from cells. POMC is processed in secretory vesicles, which are released after stimulation by secretagogues.

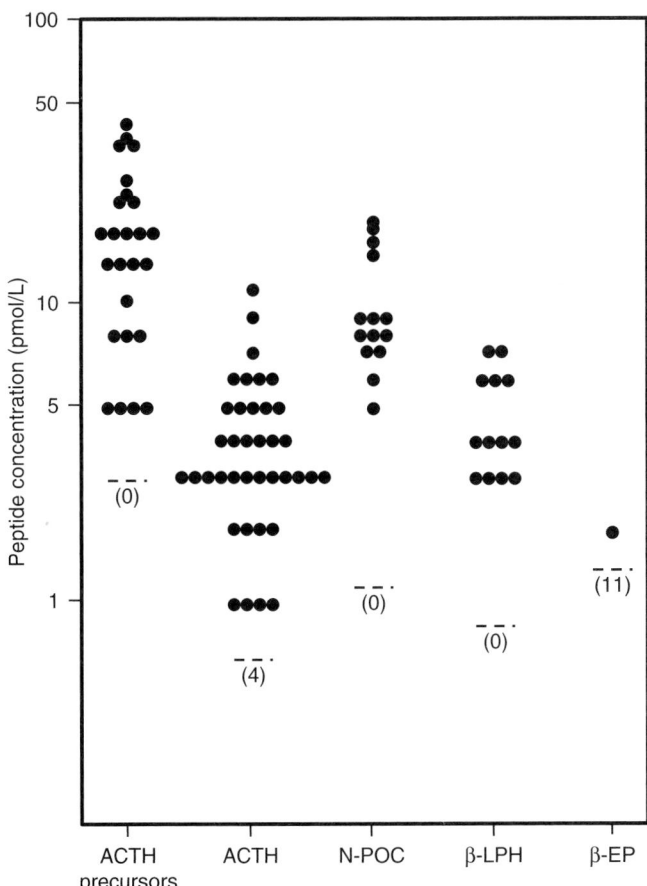

Figure 18-8 Concentrations of adrenocorticotropic hormone (ACTH) precursors and derived peptides in the circulation of normal subjects. EP, endorphin; LPH, lipotropin; N-POC, *N*-pro-opiomelanocortin. (From ref. 85.)

β-endorphin. The protease responsible for this cleavage is PC2. After endopeptidase cleavage, ACTH 1-17 is further modified by an exopeptidase that removes amino acids from the C terminus to give ACTH 1-13. Subsequently, ACTH 1-13 undergoes *N*-acetylation and C-terminal amidation.

Central Nervous System

POMC is produced primarily in the neurons of the hypothalamic arcuate nucleus, where the peptides are central to regulation of food intake and energy balance. POMC is also expressed in the median eminence and the ventromedial border of the third ventricle and much smaller amounts in the tractus solitarius. Processing is different from that in the anterior pituitary, in that smaller peptides characteristic of the neurointermediate lobe are produced.[86] However, most of the studies are limited to the rat hypothalamus. In these extracts, high-performance liquid chromatographic separation of peptides suggests that ACTH is processed to CLIP and that des-acetyl-α-MSH, rather than α-MSH, is detected, thus indicating that N-terminal acetylation is limited. β-Endorphin 1-31 is found in the rat hypothalamus, again suggesting more extensive processing.[83,87]

POMC peptides have also been detected in cerebrospinal fluid (CSF), although whether they originate from the pituitary or hypothalamus is uncertain. Evidence from changes in precursors and ACTH in rat CSF in relation to food intake and obesity suggest that they originate from the hypothalamus.[88] In human CSF, the POMC precursor peptide has been shown to occur at high concentrations and predominates over ACTH when molar ratios are compared.[89] However, several of the POMC peptides can be detected in CSF.[90,91]

Other Tissues

In comparison to the pituitary, other tissues produce very low levels of POMC peptides, with reports in rat tissue extracts of 0.00003% of the levels in the pituitary and no mature ACTH.[29] POMC peptides have been detected in the thyroid, pancreas, gastrointestinal tract, placenta, testis, ovary, adrenal gland, and immune system.[83] POMC peptides are also produced in the skin. α-MSH, the first peptide to be detected, was found, by immunostaining, to predominate in human melanocytes, but ACTH has also been detected in human keratinocytes.[92] A role for POMC peptides in hair pigmentation is also suggested by two patients with inherited mutations in POMC that prevented synthesis of the ACTH/α-MSH region; both patients had red hair pigmentation.[8]

Pituitary Tumors

In patients with pituitary-dependent Cushing's syndrome, the processing of precursors to ACTH appears to be relatively normal as judged by the molar ratios of these peptides in plasma.[75] However, the molar ratio of precursors to ACTH is much higher for corticotrope macroadenomas, thus suggesting that processing is impaired.[93]

Extrapituitary Tumors

Data on tumor extracts suggest that most extrapituitary tumors that cause the ectopic ACTH syndrome do not process the prohormone efficiently. In an early study, analysis of tumor tissue from patients without clinical features of hormone excess identified a high-molecular-weight form of ACTH, and this purified material could be cleaved to mature ACTH (4.5 kDa) by the action of trypsin. The ACTH immunoreactivity was found to have no biologic activity and was assumed to be due to ACTH precursors.[94]

Evidence that processing is impaired in tumors from patients with the ectopic ACTH syndrome also comes from the elevated levels of ACTH precursors in plasma and the high ratio of precursors to ACTH.[75,95] Identification of ACTH precursors predominating in the circulation of patients with clinically apparent Cushing's syndrome suggests that these precursors may have some activity at the ACTH receptor or are processed at the adrenal. Most of these patients had clinically obvious small cell carcinoma of the lung. However, patients with highly differentiated, slowly growing tumors, typically bronchial carcinoids, have lower but nevertheless elevated levels of ACTH precursors.[96] CLIP has also been detected in four tumor extracts from patients with carcinoid tumors,[97] thus suggesting that some tumors may process POMC in the manner of the neurointermediate lobe. It is not yet clear whether the same tumors give rise to increased precursors and smaller fragments or whether processing varies in different tumors.

BIOLOGIC ACTIVITY OF ACTH-RELATED PEPTIDES

ACTH and Its Receptor

The major role of ACTH is to stimulate steroidogenesis in the adrenal cortex, which results in the synthesis and release of cortisol in humans and corticosterone in rodents. In pathologic conditions, it is evident that ACTH can increase the production of adrenal androgens and aldosterone; however, under physiologic situations, these pathways are regulated by other factors. Long-term overexpression of ACTH can cause adrenal cell proliferation,[98,99] although peptides from the N-terminal of POMC have also been implicated in this process. In situations with prolonged ACTH excess such as Nelson's syndrome, Addison's disease, and ectopic ACTH syndrome, skin pigmentation can occur and is thought to be due to ACTH binding through its MSH sequence to melanocortin receptors in the skin, although whether the skin pigmentation results from cleavage of ACTH to MSH peptides is unclear. ACTH receptors are also present on human mononuclear leukocytes and have been identified on other rat and mouse immune cells, which suggests that ACTH may have a role in immune function.

ACTH Receptors and Signaling

The ACTH 1-39 sequence is most potent in stimulating steroidogenesis, but ACTH 1-24 is also known to have full agonist activity in certain systems. It is clear that the ACTH 1-13 sequence is involved in binding and activation, but ACTH 6-24 has been shown to have some steroidogenic activity.

ACTH binds to the melanocortin-2 receptor (MC2R),[100] which has been identified in human adrenal glands[101,102]; there is a suggestion that low-affinity ACTH-binding sites are also present in rat and ovine adrenocortical cells. Binding of ACTH to human receptors requires calcium[101] and occurs with a K_d of approximately 2.0 nmol/L. However, ACTH at 10 pmol/L causes maximal steroidogenesis, and therefore only a small number of the predicted 3500 sites per cell need to be occupied to achieve this activity.

The ACTH receptor is a member of the melanocortin receptor family, all members of which have similar seven-membrane-spanning domains and are G protein coupled.[102] On binding to its receptor, ACTH stimulates cAMP production,[101] and cAMP in turn stimulates a cAMP-dependent protein kinase that activates the steroidogenic pathway. Calcium is also involved in ACTH stimulation of cAMP in human adrenal cells.

Corticostatins, low-molecular-weight inhibitors of ACTH-induced steroidogenesis, are thought to act by preventing ACTH binding to its receptor, although their physiologic role is unclear.

ACTH Effects on the Adrenal

ACTH acts at a number of levels to increase cortisol production. On binding to its receptor, it stimulates lipoprotein uptake, activates hydrolysis of cholesterol, and increases transport of cholesterol to mitochondria. Importantly, ACTH also regulates cholesterol side chain cleavage, which is the rate-limiting step in steroidogenesis and results in the production of pregnenolone. This activity takes place in the inner membrane of the mitochondria and is catalyzed by cytochrome P450 side chain cleavage enzyme.[103]

Longer stimulation by ACTH eventually results in down-regulation of the ACTH receptor, but it is known to cause increased transcription of enzymes in the steroidogenic pathway and can result in adrenal cell proliferation.

α-Melanocyte-Stimulating Hormone

In most mammals, α-MSH is produced in the melanotroph cells of the neurointermediate lobe, but because these cells are absent from the human pituitary, it is unlikely that this peptide has a role as a secreted peptide in humans. In mice, α-MSH acting at the MC-1 receptor, causes changes in coat color, and in frogs, it affects skin pigmentation. It is also thought that locally produced α-MSH peptides stimulate melanogenesis in human skin.[92]

α-MSH-related peptides produced in the arcuate nucleus of the hypothalamus and acting at the MC-4 receptor in the paraventricular nucleus of the hypothalamus are important in the regulation of food intake and energy balance and are the principal mediators of the effects of leptin.[86] The role of POMC peptides is evidenced by a number of inherited deletions in the *POMC* gene that are associated with obesity.[8,104,105]

N-pro-opiomelanocortin and Joining Peptide

N-POC has been reported to potentiate ACTH-induced steroidogenesis in human and rat adrenocortical cells, and it is thought that the γ_3-MSH region, from mid- to C-terminal of N-POC, is responsible for this activity. It has also been shown that N-POC 1-48 and not the γ_3-MSH region stimulates adrenal growth after unilateral adrenalectomy in the rat.[106] Since N-POC circulates intact, it has been proposed that cleavage of N-POC occurs at the adrenal gland and a serine protease capable of cleaving N-POC has been identified in the outer adrenal cortex.[107] In addition, N-POC stimulates the release of aldosterone from human adrenal tumor cells.[108,109]

The role of joining peptide is unclear. It has been suggested that it is the adrenal androgen-stimulating hormone, but subsequently, several reports showed that joining peptide lacks the ability to increase adrenal androgens.[110]

β-Lipotropin and β-endorphin

β-Lipotropin was named because of its lipolytic activity, and it was suggested that the β-MSH sequence in the mid region was responsible for this activity. Subsequently, most studies have concentrated on this peptide as a precursor of β-endorphin.

Data conflict regarding whether β-endorphin circulates in human plasma.[74,85] It may have a more important role when released locally in the brain because, when administered, it has opiate-like analgesic activity associated with the met-enkephalin sequence at its N terminus, and mice lacking β-endorphin exhibit absence of stress-induced analgesia.[111] β-Endorphin has also been shown to affect sexual behavior and learning.

ACTH Precursors

It has proved difficult to get a clear indication of ACTH precursor bioactivity because of problems in obtaining pure preparations of the peptides and the limited availability of bioassays. POMC itself is thought to have little biologic activity,[94] whereas pro-ACTH was shown to be equipotent with ACTH in a rat adrenal cell bioassay or 8% to 33% as potent in a cytochemical ACTH bioassay.[112] Nothing is currently known about the binding of POMC and pro-ACTH to the ACTH receptor (MC2-R) and the other MSH receptors (MC1-R, MC3-R, MC4-R, MC5-R).[113] Because ACTH precursors are present in the circulation at concentrations greater than those of ACTH,[85] it would be valuable to examine the agonist/antagonist activity of the precursors at the human receptors. In patients with hyperpigmentation related to postadrenalectomy Cushing's disease, concentrations of both ACTH and ACTH precursors correlated with pigmentation scores.[114] The interaction of ACTH precursor peptides with the recently cloned receptor MC4-R found exclusively in the brain may also be of interest in as much as concentrations of ACTH precursors in CSF are 100-fold those of ACTH (414 vs. 3.2 pmol/L).[89]

Some information regarding in vivo POMC bioactivity can be gained from clinical studies. If patients with the ectopic ACTH syndrome produce ACTH precursors in preference to ACTH,[75] it must either have biologic activity when present at very high levels or be cleaved to ACTH at the level of the adrenal, as previously suggested.[106]

FACTORS REGULATING SECRETION OF ACTH AND RELATED PEPTIDES

Glucocorticoids

Glucocorticoids exert a classic feedback inhibitory effect on the production of CRH and ACTH. However, the multiple ways they negatively regulate the activity of the HPA axis are not fully understood. Much is known about the molecular mechanisms whereby the glucocorticoid receptor acts as a transcription factor to activate gene transcription but less is known about inhibition of the human *POMC* gene (see section entitled "Regulation of POMC Gene Expression" earlier in chapter) or about the early effects, which must involve nongenomic mechanisms. These interactions have been grouped into fast, intermediate, and slow feedback, based on the timing of the phenomenon.

Fast Feedback

Fast feedback occurs over minutes and is linked to the rate of increase in glucocorticoid concentration. An acute reduction in ACTH release takes place, but fast feedback has no impact on gene expression or peptide synthesis. It appears that the targets of glucocorticoid action are hypothalamic CRH secretion and direct action on the pituitary corticotrope to reduce ACTH release.

Intermediate Feedback

Intermediate feedback occurs over a few hours (typically maximal at 2 hours in vivo) and again appears to be due to acute inhibition of ACTH and CRH release, with no discernible effect on gene transcription or peptide synthesis. Annexin 1 is a key mediator of the inhibitory effects of glucocorticoids over this time frame and since it is produced by the folliculostellate cells in the pituitary, it is probably a paracrine mediator of glucocorticoid action.[115]

Slow Feedback

The slow component depends on the concentration and time of exposure and occurs over days. *POMC* gene transcription and POMC peptide synthesis are reduced, but changes in CRH expression are uncertain and glucocorticoids may also inhibit hypothalamic AVP levels. To effect inhibition of the *POMC* gene, glucocorticoids enter the cell where they bind to the glucocorticoid receptor (GR) in the cytoplasm, which translocates to the nucleus, where it inhibits *POMC* gene transcription (see Fig. 18-5).

In addition, glucocorticoids may act at the hippocampus, where their actions are mediated by both the type I receptor (mineralocorticoid receptor) and the type II receptor (glucocorticoid receptor). It appears that the type I receptor, which has higher affinity for cortisol, is important for mediating feedback at basal cortisol concentrations and that the lower-affinity type II receptor mediates feedback by stress levels of cortisol.

Glucocorticoids also act on *POMC* gene expression in the hypothalamus where they influence food intake and energy balance. However the evidence is controversial, since adrenalectomy has been shown to increase POMC mRNA in rat hypothalamus[116] or to decrease POMC mRNA in the medial basal hypothalamus.[117] Nevertheless, in rodents, adrenalectomy reverses many forms of obesity, suggesting adrenalectomy increases POMC; alternatively, this could be explained by adrenalectomy affecting a number of other related pathways.[118]

Corticotropin-releasing Hormone

Corticotropin-releasing hormone (CRH) is an important physiological activator of ACTH. This is evidenced by mice with inactivating mutations in the *CRH* gene that die at birth with dysplastic lungs, preventable by prenatal maternal glucocorticoids.[119] Thus, CRH activation of ACTH is necessary to provide sufficient glucocorticoids for lung development. Both CRH and AVP are considered important for activation of pituitary ACTH, but CRH is a more potent secretagogue in rat and horse, whereas AVP is thought to be more potent in sheep. In all cases, there is a marked synergism with CRH functioning permissively, while AVP is the main dynamic signal.

CRH stimulates ACTH secretion from dispersed pituitary cells in a sustained manner, initially causing the release of preformed peptide but simultaneously stimulating peptide synthesis (Fig. 18-9). In humans, a biphasic response to exogenous CRH reflects these two mechanisms of action.[120]

The effects of CRH on the levels of ACTH precursors in the human circulation have been examined only during petrosal sinus sampling, which is used as a diagnostic test in patients with suspected Cushing's syndrome. In this test, CRH is given intravenously and ACTH peptides are measured in the

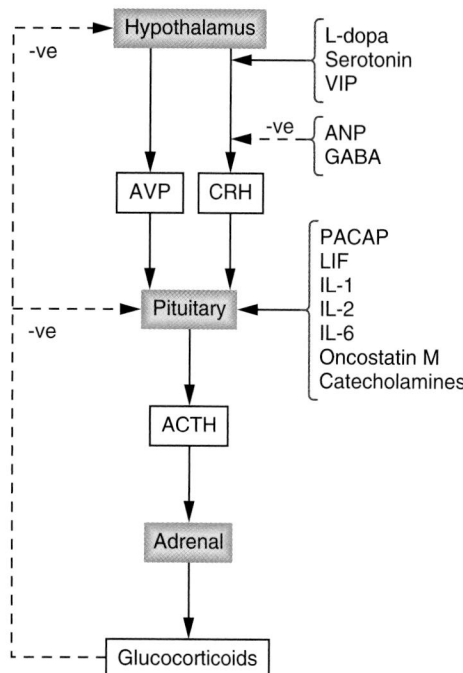

Figure 18-9 Factors regulating pituitary secretion of adrenocorticotropic hormone (ACTH)-related peptides. ANP, atrial natriuretic peptide; AVP, arginine-vasopressin; CRH, corticotropin-releasing hormone; GABA, γ-aminobutyric acid; LIF, leukemia inhibitory factor; PACAP, pituitary adenylate cyclase-activating polypeptide; VIP, vasoactive intestinal polypeptide.

petrosal sinuses draining the pituitary. In this situation, the increase in ACTH is much greater than the increase in precursors, which suggests that CRH is stimulating release of processed ACTH from secretory granules.[85]

Hypothalamic CRH is subject to regulation by multiple afferent signals and in turn influences ACTH release. These signals include upregulation by catecholamines via β- and α_1-adrenoceptors, serotonin (5-HT) acting via the 5-HT1A, 5-HT2A, and 5-HT2C receptors,[121] acetylcholine acting through both muscarinic and nicotinic receptors, and the cytokines interleukin-1 (IL-1) and IL-6, possibly acting by generation of prostaglandins. In addition, CRH expression may be inhibited by glucocorticoids, catecholamines via α_2-receptors, and γ-aminobutyric acid (GABA) released by neuronal input from the hippocampus and amygdala.

Vasopressin

Vasopressin (AVP) is synthesized in the same region of the paraventricular nucleus of the hypothalamus as CRH (see Fig. 18-9). The two peptides are released concurrently from the median eminence into the hypophysial portal system. In addition, AVP reaches portal blood from the supraoptic nucleus. AVP exerts weak, direct stimulation on ACTH release but powerfully synergizes with CRH. In vivo evidence indicates a role for AVP in stress-induced ACTH secretion.[122,123] In contrast to CRH, which acts via protein kinase A, AVP acts by stimulation of protein kinase C. AVP also increases the cAMP response to CRH in isolated pituicytes, which suggests multiple sites of interaction between the two signaling cascades.

Cytokines and Growth Factors

Cytokines are pleiotropic polypeptides released from immune cells in response to inflammation, infection, and tissue injury.[124] Proinflammatory cytokines stimulate the HPA axis in vivo[125] and although some act via CRH, several cytokines including IL-2, interferons, and the gp130 cytokine family

(IL-6, leukemia inhibitory factor, oncostatin M) act at the pituitary.

Interleukin-1

IL-1, α and β, are endogenous pyrogenic proteins induced by bacterial endotoxin. The two forms bind to the same receptor, the IL-1 receptor type 1, and display identical biologic activities. IL-1β is released by several cell types, including activated macrophages and monocytes.

The specifics of the action of IL-1 on ACTH release are controversial. In the intact rat, infusion of human IL-1 increased circulating levels of ACTH, but IL-1 acted at the hypothalamus by stimulating CRH release.[126] However, primary cultures of rat pituitary cells responded to IL-1β by increasing secretion of ACTH.[127] In another study using primary rat pituitary cultures, no effects of acute IL-I administration on POMC gene transcription or ACTH peptide release were observed. Interestingly, chronic treatment of these cultures with either IL-1α or IL-1β exerted weak induction of ACTH release with no effect on POMC mRNA accumulation.[128] An explanation for these divergent results may be that IL-1 modulates the actions of other ACTH secretogogues, including catecholamines.

Interleukin-2

Expression of IL-2 mRNA and IL-2 receptor mRNA was detected in human corticotrope adenoma cells and in mouse pituitary AtT20 cells.[129]

IL-2 enhances POMC gene expression in the pituitary and ACTH secretion in AtT20 cells and primary rat pituitary cultures. IL-2, when administered to human subjects during cancer therapy trials, was found to increase circulating β-endorphin and ACTH levels,[130,131] thus demonstrating a role for IL-2 in activating the HPA axis in vivo.

Interleukin-6

IL-6 is synthesized and secreted by bovine pituitary folliculostellate cells, which do not express pituitary trophic hormones or their precursors in vitro.[132] In addition, cultured primary rat pituitary cells release IL-6 relatively abundantly,[133] and IL-6 is synthesized by both normal human and neoplastic anterior pituitary tissue.[134–136]

In vivo, IL-6 is a potent stimulus of the HPA axis in humans and probably acts at the hypothalamus to stimulate AVP release and subsequent ACTH induction.[137] Because IL-6 is also present in the circulation, especially during inflammatory stress, the relative importance of locally derived versus systemically available IL-6 in pituitary function remains to be determined.[138]

Leukemia Inhibitory Factor

Leukemia inhibitory factor regulates differentiation and development of pituitary corticotropes during ontogenesis and is involved in the HPA response to inflammation. LIF is produced by human pituitary cells and LIF receptors (LIF-Rs) are present in murine AtT20 pituicytes, human fetal corticotropes and somatotrophs, as well as in other functional hormone-producing cells.[139] Pituitary LIF-R mRNA is induced by lipopolysaccharide (LPS) in vivo, although the changes were less pronounced than those observed for LIF mRNA.[140]

LIF acts principally on the pituitary corticotrope, potently inducing POMC gene transcription and enhancing ACTH secretion.[139,141,142] In addition, LIF potentiates the action of CRH to induce ACTH secretion in AtT20 cells.[141] Oncostatin M, a related cytokine with similar receptor signaling, also induces ACTH.[141]

LIF stimulates the JAK/STAT (Janus kinase/signal transducer and activator of transcription) pathway[141] and induces transcription of the POMC gene. It very potently synergizes with CRH to enhance POMC expression[141] but does not induce cAMP or *c-fos*, unlike CRH; therefore, it is likely that their synergy occurs distally. Both signaling cascades involve distal

POMC promoter response elements apposed between –190 and –130 nucleotides upstream of the POMC transcription start site and interact directly on the POMC gene.[43]

Studies of the HPA axis in LIF knockout mice revealed a defect in activation of the axis in response to stress. Circulating ACTH levels are attenuated after fasting in the knockout animals, and chronic replacement by LIF infusion restores HPA responses to levels in wild-type littermates.[143] Interestingly, in mice with a double knockout of LIF and CRH, the POMC response to inflammation was robust and similar to wild-type animals. These animals had increased tumor necrosis factor-alpha (TNF-α), IL-1β, and IL-6, suggesting that increased central proinflammatory cytokines may compensate for the impaired HPA axis function caused by loss of CRH and LIF.[144]

Other Regulatory Factors

L-Dopa and serotonin both increase ACTH secretion by means of neuronal release into the paraventricular nucleus of the hypothalamus.[145–147] Pituitary adenylate cyclase–activating polypeptide (PACAP) and vasoactive intestinal polypeptide (VIP) both enhance ACTH secretion; but while PACAP directly stimulates pituitary ACTH, VIP promotes release of CRH. The role of these two peptides is probably most relevant in regulating HPA responses to inflammatory and cold stressors.[148]

In contrast, GABA inhibits ACTH when released from hippocampal afferents to the hypothalamus by inhibiting release of CRH and AVP.[149] Atrial natriuretic peptide (ANP) has been shown to decrease ACTH secretion and inhibit CRH gene expression. In comparison, opiate receptor agonists inhibit ACTH release probably by effects at the hypothalamic or hippocampal level, although it has been reported that met-enkephalin can directly inhibit corticotrope ACTH release. Oxytocin can inhibit CRH-stimulated ACTH secretion in humans, but in rats, oxytocin stimulates ACTH probably by binding to AVP receptors.

Integrated Control of ACTH Secretion

Three tiers of control subserve the regulation of anterior pituitary hormone secretion (see Figs. 18-9 and 18-10).

Tier 1

Tier 1 consists of central signals from the brain and hypothalamus and includes the hypothalamic release and inhibiting hormones, neurotransmitters, and brain peptides. These molecules traverse the portal venous system in classic endocrine fashion to impinge on their respective distal receptors located on the corticotrope cell surface. These highly differentiated receptors transduce their signals to the cell nucleus, thus determining biosynthesis and ultimate secretion of POMC peptides. The hypothalamic hormones also determine pituitary cell mitotic activity, and, clinically, pathologic oversecretion of these hormones results in pituitary hyperplasia and adenoma formation.

Tier II

The second tier of pituitary control consists of an intra-pituitary network of cytokines. These molecules provide highly specific unique signals to the pituicyte or an overlapping redundancy (e.g., interleukin regulation of ACTH). Furthermore, they may often synergize with hypothalamic hormones (e.g., LIF and CRH).

The pituitary factors invariably have dual functions—regulating cell development and replication and controlling differentiated gene expression. These two functions are often subserved independently and may in fact be discordant (e.g., LIF induces POMC transcription while blocking corticotrope cell proliferation).

Tier III

The third tier of pituitary control is the peripheral target hormone. Clinically, loss of negative feedback inhibition by

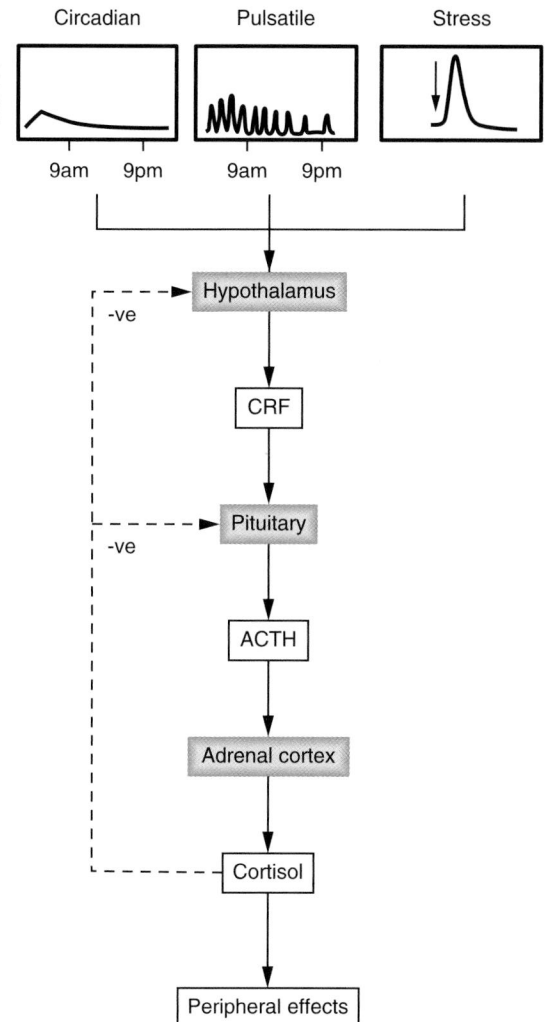

Figure 18-10 Mechanisms regulating pituitary secretion of adrenocorticotropic hormone (ACTH) and related peptides. CRF, corticotropin-releasing factor.

target hormones results in pituitary trophic hormone hypersecretion, hyperplasia, and sometimes adenoma formation, as may be encountered in hypoadrenalism. Peripheral hormones may also directly induce pituitary hormone genes.

MECHANISMS REGULATING SECRETION OF ACTH AND RELATED PEPTIDES

The many factors that regulate secretion of ACTH and related peptides are integrated in the mechanisms that underpin the regulatory processes (see Fig. 18-10). There is a marked circadian rhythm for ACTH and underlying this is a pulsatile release process. However, it is clear that stress responses can be superimposed on these, as can the feedback regulation of cortisol, which downregulates activity. The details of this feedback inhibition are described in the section on glucocorticoid regulation. Studies describe the factors involved in the stress response and feedback regulation, but much less is known about the factors regulating circadian control and pulsatile secretion.

Circadian Rhythmicity
The primary "clock" is located in the suprachiasmatic nucleus. Neuronal afferents from this nucleus feed into the paraventricular nucleus of the hypothalamus and regulate

CRH expression. The circadian rhythm of ACTH is generated by variation in the amplitude of the pulses rather than variation in pulse frequency. Therefore, the amplitude of ACTH pulses during peak secretion is fourfold higher than during the ACTH nadir. Peak levels of ACTH, and concordantly cortisol, are reached at 6:00 A.M., decline during the day to 4:00 P.M., and then further decline to a nadir between 11:00 P.M. and 3:00 A.M. (see Fig. 18-10). The 6:00 A.M. peak is reached after an abrupt increase in ACTH secretion. Although all the circulating POMC peptides show a diurnal variation and peak at the same time, their decline occurs at different rates, probably conferred by different circulatory half-lives and/or variation in extrapituitary processing.

Pulsatility
ACTH is secreted in a pulsatile manner, which is reflected in the pulsatile release of cortisol. However, the analysis of this depends very much on the sampling techniques. In humans, studies have shown 12 to 40 pulses per 24 hours depending on the sampling frequency.[150–152] There are fewer pulses during the nadir of ACTH secretion and there are more pulses, with greater peak amplitude and higher mean level in males.[151] The pulsatility may be a mechanism for overcoming desensitization of the ACTH receptor and may reflect pulsatile release of CRH.

Stress Response
The HPA axis is stimulated by a number of types of stress. These include exercise, acute illness, surgical stress, hemorrhage, and hypoglycemia. Infection, which activates the immune system, causes release of cytokines, which in turn stimulate the HPA axis. This network of interactions between the immune system and the HPA axis provides a mechanism whereby activation of the immune system is inhibited by glucocorticoid feedback on the immune cells leading to the well-recognized immune suppression that limits the overall response. Chronic stress as, for example, in depression also activates the HPA axis but this persistent activation can be attributed to failures in the normal feedback regulatory loops.

In response to stress, peripheral and central signals are integrated by the pituitary to modulate adrenal glucocorticoid production. Several lines of evidence suggest a unifying hypothesis linking hypothalamic releasing factors, activation of peripheral cytokine cascades, and intrapituitary cytokine expression with pituitary-mediated modulation of the systemic inflammatory response.

An acute septic insult provokes a local inflammatory response, with coordinated and sequential activation of a series of proinflammatory cytokines[138,153,154] and neural and bacterial toxin signals that activate the HPA axis.[155] Initially, peripheral activation of local and distal TNF expression is followed by IL-1, IL-6, and LIF.[138] A number of the proinflammatory cytokines exert most, if not all, their activities at the hypothalamus, notably IL-6 acting on hypothalamic AVP[137] and IL-1 and TNF acting on CRH.[126] Others, notably LIF, clearly act at the pituitary.[141,156]

At the hypothalamic level, both circulating and locally derived cytokines enhance expression of CRH and AVP. Hypothalamic LIF mRNA is also upregulated by LPS treatment, a well-recognized model of gram-negative septic shock.[140]

The pituitary is also a site of de novo cytokine synthesis, and thus in addition to the circulating, peripherally derived cytokines, an intrapituitary network of cytokines is established in the acute phase of septic shock. IL-1β and LIF are upregulated by LPS[140,157] and macrophage migration inhibitory factor is acutely released from pituicytes in vitro and in vivo in response to LPS.[158] In addition, intrapituitary IL-6 is upregulated by IL-1.[138,159]

Two opposing pituitary responses to septic shock take place. The first involves cytokines such as IL-6 and LIF, which limit the inflammatory response, whereas the second group is associated with enhanced release of proinflammatory factors and increases the lethality of experimental endotoxemia (macrophage migration inhibitory factor[158]). The former group of cytokines causes activation of the HPA axis and increased glucocorticoid production, thus limiting the extent of the inflammatory response and protecting against lethality. The increase in intrapituitary LIF stimulates POMC expression and strongly potentiates CRH action on the corticotrope.[141,143] The key role of HPA activation in limiting the lethal effects of unrestrained activation of proinflammatory cytokine cascades is underscored by the poor performance of the CRH knockout mouse exposed to endotoxin.[160] IL-1, TNF, and IL-6 have also been shown by some, but not all, studies to exert direct effects on pituitary ACTH secretion.[127,161,162]

A further level of action of the cytokines is to antagonize the negative feedback loop of adrenal glucocorticoids on hypothalamic CRH expression and pituitary POMC secretion.[155] The pattern of acute proinflammatory cytokines induced by septic shock opposes effective glucocorticoid signaling[163,164] in part by activation of the nuclear factor-kappa B (NF-κB) nuclear transcription factor, which inhibits glucocorticoid receptor action.[165–167]

Stress-associated disorders, such as melancholic depression, are characterized by persistent activation of the HPA axis. In this situation, multiple feedback loops activate central CRH pathways, including downregulation of the glucocorticoid receptor, which prevents the normal negative feedback on the HPA axis, resulting in the vicious circle of continued activation of the HPA.[168]

MEASUREMENT OF ACTH AND RELATED PEPTIDES

ACTH and ACTH Precursors
One of the first peptides to be measured by radioimmunoassay, ACTH presented a significant challenge because of the difficulty in generating high-affinity antisera and in labeling ACTH. The development of sensitive immunoradiometric assays for ACTH has improved the reliability of ACTH measurement.[96,169,170] This ability provides many benefits, including improved sensitivity, speed, reproducibility, and parallel results. The high sample throughput and wide working range of these assays make them ideal for measuring samples taken during inferior petrosal sinus sampling, a test that is fast becoming an important component in the diagnosis of pituitary tumors that secrete ACTH.

The assays are based on a labeled monoclonal antibody that usually binds the N-terminal region of ACTH and a solid-phase antibody that recognizes a different sequence in ACTH. Because binding of both antibodies is required to generate a signal, the assay does not recognize α-MSH or CLIP. However, it is not always clear whether current ACTH assays recognize the ACTH precursors. This can have considerable significance because in some clinical situations the use of an assay that is highly specific for ACTH 1-39 may be insufficient or misleading. In one patient with the ectopic ACTH syndrome shown by chromatography to be producing high-molecular-weight ACTH precursors, the ACTH concentration was very low when measured by immunoradiometric assay.[169] To ensure that patients with the ectopic ACTH syndrome are flagged by an ACTH assay, it is important that the ACTH precursors have a high degree of cross-reactivity in the ACTH assay or that a separate specific assay for ACTH precursors be available.

Detection of ACTH precursors in plasma was first demonstrated in normal subjects after stimulation with metyrapone,[171] and it was later observed after insulin-induced hypoglycemia.[172] However, complex chromatographic techniques were required to separate ACTH precursors from ACTH. Clearly, this approach cannot be used for large numbers of patient samples and would not provide a quantitative assessment of the concentrations of ACTH precursors in plasma.

Direct measurement of ACTH precursors was made possible by the development of a two-site immunoradiometric assay for the ACTH precursors POMC and pro-ACTH.[173] The assay is based on a labeled monoclonal antibody that binds within the ACTH region of POMC and a solid-phase antibody that recognizes N-POC (see Fig. 18-6). Because binding of both antibodies is required to generate a signal, the assay does not detect ACTH. With this assay, the concentrations of ACTH precursors in normal subjects were found to be 5 to 40 pmol/L, which is equivalent to or greater than the concentrations of ACTH, N-POC, β-lipotropin, and β-endorphin.[85] Measurement of ACTH precursors in patients with ectopic ACTH syndrome has indicated that the precursors are present at much higher concentrations than is ACTH.[96] A similar approach has been used to measure POMC in aggressive ACTH-secreting tumors.[95,174]

Other POMC-related Peptides
The development of radioimmunoassays and immunoradiometric assays for N-POC, γ-MSH, α-MSH, β-lipotropin, and β-endorphin has proved extremely valuable in understanding the production and action of POMC peptides. The development of specific immunometric assays that distinguish circulating levels of β-lipotropin and β-endorphin has shown that β-lipotropin is the main form in human plasma and that relatively little β-endorphin is secreted.[74] Nevertheless, questions relating to the relative molar ratios of the family of POMC peptides are still unanswered. The relative concentrations of ACTH precursors and ACTH in the circulation will depend not only on regulatory mechanisms influencing expression of the *POMC* gene but also on precursor processing and mechanisms of secretion from the corticotrope cells. Evidence from studies with the mouse corticotrope adenoma cell line AtT20 suggests that in the absence of stimulation, corticotrope cells "leak" newly synthesized POMC.[175] Therefore, the levels of ACTH precursors and constituent peptides in the circulation at any given time could well vary because of the differing regulatory mechanisms.

Acknowledgments
I am grateful to Dr. Robert Oliver for advice and editorial assistance and to Dr. David Ray for coauthorship of the previous edition of this chapter.

REFERENCES

1. Bell PH: Purification and structure of beta-corticotropin. J Am Chem Soc 76:5565–5567, 1954.
2. Li CH: Lipotropin, a new active peptide from pituitary glands. Nature 201:924, 1964.
3. Li CH: Isolation, characterization and opiate activity of beta-endorphin from human pituitary glands. Biochem Biophys Res Commun 72:1542–1547, 1976.
4. Eipper BA, Mains RE: Analysis of the common precursor to corticotropin and endorphin. J Biol Chem 253:5732–5744, 1978.
5. Inoue A, Kita T, Nakamura M, et al: Nucleotide sequence of cloned cDNA for bovine corticotropin-β-lipotropin precursor. Nature 278:423–427, 1979.
6. Vale W, Spiess J, Rivier C, Rivier J: Characterization of a 41-residue ovine hypothalamic peptide that stimulates secretion of corticotropin and beta endorphin. Science 213:1394–1397, 1981.
7. Mountjoy K, Robbins L, Mortrud M, Cone RD: The cloning of a family of genes that encode the melanocortin receptors. Science 257:1248–1251, 1992.
7a. Lefkowitz RJ, Roth J, Pricer W, Pastan I: ACTH receptors in the adrenal: Specific

binding of ACTH-125I and its relation to adenyl cyclase. Proc Natl Acad Sci U S A 65(3):745–752, 1970.

8. Krude H, Biebermann H, Luck W, et al: Severe early-onset obesity, adrenal insufficiency and red hair pigmentation caused by POMC mutations in humans. Nat Genet 19:155–157, 1998.

9. Cochet M, Chang ACY, Cohen SN: Characterisation of the structural gene and putative 5′ regulatory sequences for human proopiomelanocortin. Nature 297:335–339, 1982.

10. Takahashi H, Teranishi Y, Nakanishi S, Numa S: Isolation and structural organisation of the human corticotropin-beta-lipotropin precursor gene. FEBS Lett 135:97–102, 1981.

11. Whitfield PL, Shire J: The human proopiomelanocortin gene: Organisation sequence and interspersion with repetitive DNA. DNA 1:133–143, 1982.

12. White A, Clark AJ, Stewart MF: The synthesis of ACTH and related peptides by tumours. Baillieres Clin Endocrinol Metab 4:1–27, 1990.

13. Jeannotte L, Trifiro MA, Plante RK, et al: Tissue-specific activity of the pro-opiomelanocortin gene promoter. Mol Cell Biol 7:4058–4064, 1987.

14. Jingami H, Nakanishi S, Numa S: Tissue distribution of messenger RNAs coding for opioid peptide precursors and related RNA. Eur J Biochem 142:441–447, 1984.

15. Clark AJ, Lavender PM, Coates P, et al: In vitro and in vivo analysis of the processing and fate of the peptide products of the short proopiomelanocortin mRNA. Mol Endocrinol 4:1737–1743, 1990.

16. Roberts JL, Lundblad JR, Eberwine JH: Hormonal regulation of POMC gene expression in the pituitary. Ann N Y Acad Sci 512:275–285, 1988.

17. Hammer GD, Fairchild-Huntress V, Low MJ: Pituitary specific and hormonally regulated gene expression directed by the rat proopiomelanocortin promoter in transgenic mice. Mol Endocrinol 4:1689–1697, 1990.

18. Therrien M, Drouin J: Cell-specific helix-loop-helix factor required for pituitary expression of the pro-opiomelanocortin gene. Mol Cell Biol 13:2342–2353, 1993.

19. Tremblay Y, Tretjakoff I, Peterson A, et al: Pituitary-specific expression and glucocorticoid regulation of a proopiomelanocortin fusion gene in transgenic mice. Proc Natl Acad Sci U S A 85:8890–8894, 1988.

20. Lundblad JR, Roberts JL: Regulation of proopiomelanocortin gene expression in pituitary. Endocr Rev 9:135–158, 1988.

21. White A, Clark AJ: The cellular and molecular basis of the ectopic ACTH syndrome. Clin Endocrinol 39:131–141, 1993.

22. Lamonerie T, Tremblay JJ, Lanctot C, et al: Ptx1, a bicoid-related homeo box transcription factor involved in transcription of the pro-opiomelanocortin gene. Genes Dev 10:1284–1295, 1996.

23. Drouin J, Lamolet B, Lamonerie T, et al: The PTX family of homeodomain transcription factors during pituitary developments. Mol Cell Endocrinol 140:31–36, 1998.

24. Lamolet B, Pulichino AM, Lamonerie T, et al: A pituitary cell-restricted T box factor, Tpit, activates POMC transcription in cooperation with Pitx homeoproteins. Cell 104:849–859, 2001.

25. Pulichino AM, Vallette-Kasic S, Couture C, et al: Human and mouse TPIT gene mutations cause early onset pituitary ACTH deficiency. Genes Dev 17:711–716, 2003.

26. Poulin G, Turgeon B, Drouin J: NeuroD1/beta2 contributes to cell-specific transcription of the proopiomelanocortin gene. Mol Cell Biol 17:6673–6682, 1997.

27. Buzzetti R, McLoughlin L, Lavender PM, et al: Expression of pro-opiomelanocortin gene and quantification of adrenocorticotropic hormone-like immunoreactivity in human normal peripheral mononuclear cells and lymphoid and myeloid malignancies. J Clin Invest 83:733–737, 1989.

28. Chen C-LC, Chang AC, Krieger DT, Bardin CW: Expression and regulation of pro-opiomelanocortin-like gene in the ovary and placenta: Comparison with the testis. Endocrinology 118:2382–2389, 1986.

29. DeBold CR, Menefee JK, Nicholson WE, Orth DN: Proopiomelanocortin gene is expressed in many normal human tissues and in tumors not associated with ectopic adrenocorticotropin syndrome. Mol Endocrinol 2:862–870, 1988.

30. Lacaze-Masmonteil T, De Keyzer Y, Luton JP, et al: Characterization of proopiomelanocortin transcripts in human nonpituitary tissues. Proc Natl Acad Sci U S A 84:7261–7265, 1987.

31. De Keyzer Y, Bertagna X, Lenne F, et al: Altered proopiomelanocortin gene expression in adrenocorticotropin-producing nonpituitary tumors. Comparative studies with corticotropic adenomas and normal pituitaries. J Clin Invest 76:1892–1898, 1985.

32. De Keyzer Y, Bertagna X, Luton JP, Kahn A: Variable modes of proopiomelanocortin gene transcription in human tumors. Mol Endocrinol 3:215–223, 1989.

33. De Keyzer Y, Rousseau-Merck MF, Luton JP, et al: Pro-opiomelanocortin gene expression in human phaeochromocytomas. J Mol Endocrinol 2:175–181, 1989.

34. Nakai Y, Nakao K: Adrenocorticotropic hormone and related peptides in human tissue. In Black PM, et al (eds): Secretory Tumours of the Pituitary Gland. New York, Raven, 1984, pp 227–243.

35. Texier PL, De Keyzer Y, Lacave R, et al: Proopiomelanocortin gene expression in normal and tumoral human lung. J Clin Endocrinol Metab 73:414–420, 1991.

36. Picon A, Bertagna X, De Keyzer Y: Analysis of the human proopiomelanocortin gene promoter in a small cell lung carcinoma cell line reveals an unusual role for E2F transcription factors. Oncogene 18:2627–2633, 1999.

37. Newell-Price J, King P, Clark AJ: The CpG island promoter of the human proopiomelanocortin gene is methylated in nonexpressing normal tissue and tumors and represses expression. Mol Endocrinol 15:338–348, 2001.

38. Newell-Price J: Proopiomelanocortin gene expression and DNA methylation: Implications for Cushing's syndrome and beyond. J Endocrinol 177:365–372, 2003.

39. DeBold CR, Nicholson WE, Orth DN: Immunoreactive proopiomelanocortin (POMC) peptides and POMC-like messenger ribonucleic acid are present in many rat nonpituitary tissues. Endocrinology 122:2648–2657, 1988.

40. Birnberg NC, Lissitsky J-C, Hinman M, Herbert E: Glucocorticoids regulate proopiomelanocortin gene expression in vivo at the levels of transcription and secretion. Proc Natl Acad Sci U S A 80:6982–6986, 1983.

41. Boutillier AL, Sassone-Corsi P, Loeffler JP: The protooncogene c-fos is induced by corticotropin-releasing factor and stimulates proopiomelanocortin gene transcription in pituitary cells. Mol Endocrinol 5:1301–1310, 1991.

42. Jin WD, Boutillier AL, Glucksman MJ, et al: Characterization of a corticotropin-releasing hormone-responsive element in the rat proopiomelanocortin gene promoter and molecular cloning of its binding protein. Mol Endocrinol 8:1377–1388, 1994.

43. Bousquet C, Ray DW, Melmed S: A common pro-opiomelanocortin-binding element mediates leukemia inhibitory factor and corticotropin-releasing hormone transcriptional synergy. J Biol Chem 272:10551–10557, 1997.

44. Becquet D, Guillaumond F, Bosler O, Francois-Bellan AM: Long-term variations of AP-1 composition after CRH stimulation: consequence on POMC gene regulation. Mol Cell Endocrinol 175:93–100, 2001.

45. Eberwine JH, Jonassen JA, Evinger MJ, Roberts JL: Complex transcriptional regulation by glucocorticoids and corticotropin-releasing hormone of proopiomelanocortin gene expression in rat pituitary cultures. DNA 6:483–492, 1987.

46. Eberwine JH, Roberts JL: Glucocorticoid regulation of pro-opiomelanocortin gene transcription in the rat pituitary. J Biol Chem 259:2166–2170, 1984.

47. Fremeau RT, Lundblad JR, Pritchett DB, et al: Regulation of pro-opiomelanocortin gene transcription in individual cell nuclei. Science 234:1265–1269, 1986.

48. Gagner JP, Drouin J: Opposite regulation of pro-opiomelanocortin gene transcription by glucocorticoids and CRH. Mol Cell Endocrinol 40:25–32, 1985.

49. Israel A, Cohen SN: Hormonally mediated negative regulation of human pro-opiomelanocortin gene expression after transfection into mouse L-cells. Mol Cell Biol 5:2443–2453, 1985.

50. Riegel AT, Lu Y, Remenick J, et al: Proopiomelanocortin gene promoter elements required for constitutive and glucocorticoid-repressed transcription. Mol Endocrinol 5:1973–1982, 1991.

51. Drouin J, Sun YL, Chamberland M, et al: Novel glucocorticoid receptor complex with DNA element of the hormone-repressed POMC gene. EMBO J 12:145–156, 1993.

52. Abou-Samra AB, Harwood JP, Manganiello VC, et al: Phorbol 12-myristate 13-acetate and vasopressin potentiate the effect of corticotropin-releasing factor on cyclic AMP production in rat anterior pituitary cells. Mechanisms of action. J Biol Chem 262:1129–1136, 1987.

53. Smoak B, Deuster P, Rabin D, Chrousos G: Corticotropin releasing hormone is not the sole factor mediating exercise induced adrenocorticotropin release in humans. J Clin Endocrinol Metab 73:302–306, 1991.

54. Kubo M, Nakagawa K, Akikawa K, et al: In vivo and in vitro ACTH response to ovine corticotropin-releasing factor in a bronchial carcinoid from a patient with ectopic ACTH syndrome. Endocrinol Jpn 32:577–581, 1985.

55. Malchoff CD, Orth DN, Abboud C, et al: Ectopic ACTH syndrome caused by a bronchial carcinoid tumor responsive to dexamethasone, metyrapone, and corticotropin-releasing factor. Am J Med 84:760–764, 1988.

56. Suda T, Tozawa F, Dobashi I, et al: Corticotropin-releasing hormone, proopiomelanocortin, and glucocorticoid receptor gene expression in adrenocorticotropin-producing tumors in vitro. J Clin Invest 92:2790–2795, 1993.

57. Liddle GW, Nicholson WE, Island DP, et al: Clinical and laboratory studies of ectopic humoral syndromes. Recent Prog Horm Res 25:283–314, 1969.

58. Gaitan D, DeBold CR, Turney MK, et al: Glucocorticoid receptor structure and function in an adrenocorticotropin-secreting small cell lung cancer. Mol Endocrinol 9:1193–1201, 1995.

59. Ray DW, Littlewood AC, Clark AJ, et al: Human small cell lung cancer cell lines expressing the proopiomelanocortin gene have aberrant glucocorticoid receptor function. J Clin Invest 93:1625–1630, 1994.

60. Ray DW: Molecular mechanisms of glucocorticoid resistance. J Endocrinol 149:1–5, 1996.

61. Ray DW, Davis JR, White A, Clark AJ: Glucocorticoid receptor structure and function in glucocorticoid-resistant small cell lung carcinoma cells. Cancer Res 56:3276–3280, 1996.

62. Eipper BA, Mains RE: Structure and biosynthesis of pro-adrenocorticotropin/endorphin and related peptides. Endocr Rev 1:1–27, 1980.

63. Yalow RS, Berson SA: Characteristics of "big ACTH" in human plasma and pituitary extracts. J Clin Endocrinol Metab 36:415–423, 1973.

64. Eipper BA, Mains RE: High molecular weight forms of adrenocorticotropic hormone in the mouse pituitary and in a mouse pituitary cell line. Biochemistry 14:3836–3844, 1975.

65. Orth DN, Nicholson WE, Mitchell WM, et al: ACTH and MSH production by a single cloned mouse pituitary tumor cell line. Endocrinology 92:385–393, 1973.

66. Lowry PJ, Rees L, Tomlin S, et al: Chemical characterization of ectopic ACTH purified from a malignant thymic carcinoid tumour. J Clin Endocrinol Metab 43:831–835, 1976.

67. Schwyzer R: ACTH: A short introductory review. Ann N Y Acad Sci 297:3–26, 1977.

68. Croughs RJ, Thijssen JH, Mol JA: Absence of detectable immunoreactive alpha melanocyte stimulating hormone in plasma in various types of Cushing's disease. J Endocrinol Invest 14:197–200, 1991.

69. Kortlandt W, De Rotte AA, Arts CJM, et al: Characterization of alpha-MSH-like immunoreactivity in human plasma. Acta Endocrinol (Copenh) 113:175–180, 1986.

70. Nam SY, Kratzsch J, Kim KW, et al: Cerebrospinal fluid and plasma concentrations of leptin, NPY, and alpha-MSH in obese women and their relationship to negative energy balance. J Clin Endocrinol Metab 86:4849–4853, 2001.

71. Seidah NG, Chretien M: Complete amino acid sequence of a human pituitary glycopeptide: An important maturation product of proopiomelanocortin. Proc Natl Acad Sci U S A 78:4236–4240, 1981.

72. Cool DR, Fenger M, Snell CR, Loh YP: Identification of the sorting signal motif within pro-opiomelanocortin for the regulated secretory pathway. J Biol Chem 270:8723–8729, 1995.

73. Bertagna X, Camus F, Lenne F, et al: Human joining peptide: A proopiomelanocortin product secreted as a homodimer. Mol Endocrinol 2:1108–1114, 1988.

74. Gibson S, Crosby SR, White A: Discrimination between beta-endorphin and beta-lipotrophin in human plasma using two-site immunoradiometric assays. Clin Endocrinol 39:445–453, 1993.

75. Stewart PM, Gibson S, Crosby SR, et al: ACTH precursors characterize the ectopic ACTH syndrome. Clin Endocrinol 40:199–204, 1994.

76. Wilson H, White A: Prohormones: Their clinical relevance. Trends Endocrinol Metab 9:396–402, 1998.

77. Mountjoy KG, Wong J: Obesity, diabetes and functions for proopiomelanocortin-derived peptides. Mol Cell Endocrinol 128:171–177, 1996.

78. Steiner DF: The proprotein convertases. Curr Opin Chem Biol 2:31–39, 1998.

79. Thomas L, Leduc R, Thorne BA, et al: Kex2-like endoproteases PC2 and PC3 accurately cleave a model prohormone in mammalian cells: Evidence for a common core of neuroendocrine processing enzymes. Proc Natl Acad Sci U S A 88:5297–5301, 1991.

80. Benjannet S, Rondeau N, Day R, et al: PC1 and PC2 are proprotein convertases capable of cleaving proopiomelanocortin at distinct pairs of basic residues. Proc Natl Acad Sci U S A 88:3564–3568, 1991.

81. Bloomquist BT, Eipper BA, Mains RE: Prohormone-converting enzymes: Regulation and evaluation of function using antisense RNA. Mol Endocrinol 5:2014–2024, 1991.

82. Day R, Schafer MK, Watson SJ, et al: Distribution and regulation of the prohormone convertases PC1 and PC2 in the rat pituitary. Mol Endocrinol 6:485–497, 1992.

83. Smith AI, Funder JW: Proopiomelanocortin processing in the pituitary, central nervous system, and peripheral tissues. Endocr Rev 9:159–179, 1988.

84. Saito E, Odell WD: Corticotropin/lipotropin common precursor-like material in normal rat extrapituitary tissues. Proc Natl Acad Sci U S A 80:3792–3796, 1983.

85. Gibson S, Crosby SR, Stewart MF, et al: Differential release of proopiomelanocortin-derived peptides from the human pituitary: Evidence from a panel of two-site immunoradiometric assays. J Clin Endocrinol Metab 78:835–841, 1994.

86. Pritchard LE, Turnbull AV, White A: Pro-opiomelanocortin processing in the hypothalamus: Impact on melanocortin signalling and obesity. J Endocrinol 172:411–421, 2002.

87. Castro MG, Morrison E: Post-translational processing of proopiomelanocortin in the pituitary and in the brain. Crit Rev Neurobiol 11:35–57, 1997.

88. Pritchard LE, Oliver RL, McLoughlin JD, et al: Proopiomelanocortin-derived peptides in rat cerebrospinal fluid and hypothalamic extracts: Evidence that secretion is regulated with respect to energy balance. Endocrinology 144:760–766, 2003.

89. Tsigos C, Crosby SR, Gibson S, et al: Proopiomelanocortin is the predominant adrenocorticotropin-related peptide in human cerebrospinal fluid. J Clin Endocrinol Metab 76:620–624, 1993.

90. McLoughlin L, Lowry PJ, Ratter SJ, et al: Characterisation of the proopiocortin family of peptides in human cerebrospinal fluid. Neuroendocrinology 32:209–212, 1981.

91. Nakao K, Oki S, Tanaka I: Immunoreactive beta-endorphin and adrenocorticotropin in human cerebrospinal fluid. J Clin Invest 66:1383–1390, 1980.

92. Thody AJ, Graham A: Does alpha-MSH have a role in regulating skin pigmentation in humans? Pigment Cell Res 11:265–274, 1998.

93. Gibson S, Ray DW, Crosby SR, et al: Impaired processing of proopiomelanocortin in corticotroph macroadenomas. J Clin Endocrinol Metab 81:497–502, 1996.

94. Odell WD: Ectopic ACTH syndrome: A misnomer. Endocrinol Metab Clin North Am 20:371–379, 1991.

95. Oliver RL, Davis JR, White A: Characterisation of ACTH related peptides in ectopic Cushing's syndrome. Pituitary 6:119–126, 2003.

96. White A, Gibson S: ACTH precursors: Biological significance and clinical relevance. Clin Endocrinol 48:251–255, 1998.

97. Vieau D, Massias JF, Girard F, et al: Corticotrophin-like intermediary lobe peptide as a marker of alternate pro-opiomelanocortin processing in ACTH-producing non-pituitary tumours. Clin Endocrinol 31:691–700, 1989.

98. Dallman MF, Makara GB, Roberts JL, et al: Corticotrope response to removal of releasing factors and corticosteroids in vivo. Endocrinology 117:2190–2197, 1985.

99. Dallman MF, Akana SF, Cascio CS, et al: Regulation of ACTH secretion: Variations on a theme of B. Recent Prog Horm Res 43:113–173, 1987.

100. Clark AJL: The melanocortin-2 receptor in normal adrenocortical function and familial adrenocorticotrophic hormone resistance. In Cone RD (ed): The Melanocortin Receptors. Totowa, New Jersey, Humana Press, 2000, pp 361–384.

101. Catalano RD, Stuve L, Ramachandran J: Characterization of corticotrophin receptors in human adrenocortical cells. J Clin Endocrinol Metab 62:300–304, 1986.

102. Cone RD, Ly D, Koppula S, et al: The melanocortin receptors: Agonists, antagonists, and the hormonal control of pigmentation. Recent Prog Horm Res 51:287–317, 1996.

103. Miller WL: Molecular biology of steroid hormone synthesis. Endocr Rev 9:295–318, 1988.

104. Krude H, Biebermann H, Gruters A: Mutations in the human proopiomelanocortin gene. Ann N Y Acad Sci 994:233–239, 2003.

105. Challis BG, Pritchard LE, Creemers JW, et al: A missense mutation disrupting a dibasic prohormone processing site in pro-opiomelanocortin (POMC) increases susceptibility to early-onset obesity through a novel molecular mechanism. Hum Mol Genet 11:1997–2004, 2002.

106. Lowry PJ, Silas L, McLean C, et al: Pro-γ-melanocyte-stimulating hormone cleavage in adrenal gland undergoing compensatory growth. Nature 306:70–73, 1983.

107. Bicknell AB, Lomthaisong K, Woods RJ, et al: Characterization of a serine protease that cleaves pro-gamma-melanotropin at the adrenal to stimulate growth. Cell 105:903–912, 2001.

108. Al-Dujaili EAS, Hope J, Estivariz FE, et al: Circulating human pituitary pro-γ-melanotropin enhances the adrenal response to ACTH. Nature 291:156–159, 1981.

109. Rochemont J, Hamelin J: The missing fragment of the pro-sequence of human pro-opiomelanocortin: Sequence and evidence for C-terminal amidation. Biochem Biophys Res Commun 102:710–716, 1981.

110. Robinson P, Bateman A, Mulay S, et al: Isolation and characterization of three forms of joining peptide from adult human pituitaries: Lack of adrenal androgen-stimulating activity. Endocrinology 129:859–867, 1991.

111. Rubinstein M, Mogil JS, Japon M, et al: Absence of opioid stress-induced analgesia in mice lacking beta-endorphin by site-directed mutagenesis. Proc Natl Acad Sci U S A 93:3995–4000, 1996.

112. Ratter SJ, Gillies G, Hope J, et al: Pro-opiocortin related peptides in human pituitary and ectopic ACTH secreting tumours. Clin Endocrinol 18:211–218, 1983.

113. Hruby VJ, Han G: The molecular pharmacology of alpha-melanocyte stimulating hormone. In Cone RD (ed): The Melanocortin Receptors. Totowa, New Jersey, Humana, 2000, pp 239–261.

114. Ray DW, Gibson S, Crosby SR, et al: Elevated levels of adrenocorticotropin (ACTH) precursors in post-adrenalectomy Cushing's disease and their regulation by glucocorticoids. J Clin Endocrinol Metab 80:2430–2436, 1995.

115. Tierney T, Christian HC, Morris JF, et al: Evidence from studies on co-cultures of TtT/GF and AtT20 cells that Annexin 1 acts as a paracrine or juxtacrine mediator of the early inhibitory effects of glucocorticoids on ACTH release. J Neuroendocrinol 15:1134–1143, 2003.

116. Beaulieu S, Gagne B, Barden N: Glucocorticoid regulation of proopiomelanocortin messenger ribonucleic acid content of rat hypothalamus. Mol Endocrinol 2:727–731, 1988.

117. Wardlaw SL, McCarthy KC, Conwell IM: Glucocorticoid regulation of hypothalamic proopiomelanocortin. Neuroendocrinol 67:51–57, 1998.

118. Drazen DL, Wortman MD, Schwartz MW, et al: Adrenalectomy alters the sensitivity of the central nervous system melanocortin system. Diabetes 52:2928–2934, 2003.

119. Venihaki M, Carrigan A, Dikkes P, Majzoub JA: Circadian rise in maternal glucocorticoid prevents pulmonary dysplasia in fetal mice with adrenal insufficiency. Proc Natl Acad Sci U S A 97:7336–7341, 2000.

120. DeBold CR, DeCherney GS, Jackson RV, et al: Effect of synthetic ovine corticotropin-releasing factor: Prolonged duration of action and biphasic response of plasma adrenocorticotropin and cortisol. J Clin Endocrinol Metab 57:294–298, 1983.

121. Jorgensen H, Knigge U, Kjaer A, et al: Serotonergic stimulation of corticotropin-releasing hormone and pro-opiomelanocortin gene expression. J Neuroendocrinol 14:788–795, 2002.

122. Guillaume V, Conte-Devolx B, Magnan E: Effect of chronic active immunization with antiarginine vasopressin on pituitary-adrenal function in sheep. Endocrinology 130:3007–3014, 1992.

123. Whitnall MH: Regulation of the hypothalamic corticotropin-releasing hormone neurosecretory system. Prog Neurobiol 40:573–629, 1993.

124. Ray D, Melmed S: Pituitary cytokine and growth factor expression and action. Endocr Rev 18:206–228, 1997.

125. Turnbull AV, Rivier CL: Regulation of the hypothalamic-pituitary-adrenal axis by cytokines: Actions and mechanisms of action. Physiol Rev 79:1–71, 1999.

126. Sapolsky R, Rivier C, Yamamoto G, et al: Interleukin-I stimulates the secretion of hypothalamic corticotropin-releasing factor. Science 238:522–524, 1987.

127. Bernton EW, Beach JE, Holaday JW, et al: Release of multiple hormones by a direct action of interleukin-1 on pituitary cells. Science 238:652–654, 1987.

128. Suda T, Tozawa F, Ushiyama T: Effects of protein kinase C related adrenocorticotrophin secretogogues and interleukin-I on proopiomelanocortin gene expression in rat anterior pituitary cells. Endocrinology 124:1444–1449, 1989.

129. Arzt E, Stelzer G, Renner U, et al: Interleukin-2 and interleukin-receptor expression in human corticotrophic adenoma and mouse pituitary cell cultures. J Clin Invest 90:1944–1951, 1992.

130. Denicoff KD, Durkin TM, Lotze MT: The neuroendocrine effects of interleukin 2 treatment. Clin Endocrinol Metab 69:402–410, 1989.

131. Lotze MT, Frana LW, Sharrow SO, et al: In vivo administration of purified human interleukin alpha I half-life and immunologic effects of the JURKAT cell-line derived IL-2. J Immunol 134:157–166, 1985.

132. Vankelecom H, Carmeliet P, Van Damme J, et al: Production of interleukin-6 by folliculostellate cells of the anterior pituitary gland in a histiotypic cell aggregate culture system. Neuroendocrinol 49:102–106, 1989.

133. Spangelo BL, MacLeod RM, Isakson PC: Production of interleukin-6 by anterior pituitary cells in-vitro. Endocrinology 126:582–586, 1990.

134. Jones TH, Justice S, Price A, Chapman K: Interleukin-6 secreting human pituitary adenomas in vitro. J Clin Endocrinol Metab 73:207–209, 1991.

135. Jones TH, Daniels M, James RA, et al: Production of bioactive and immunoreactive interleukin-6 (IL-6) and expression of IL-6 messenger ribonucleic acid by human pituitary adenomas. J Clin Endocrinol Metab 78:180–187, 1994.

136. Tsagarakis S, Kontogeorgos G, Giannou P: Interleukin-6, a growth promoting cytokine, is present in human pituitary adenomas: An immunocytochemical study. Clin Endocrinol 37:163–167, 1992.

137. Mastorakos G, Weber JS, Magiakou MA, et al: Hypothalamic-pituitary-adrenal axis activation and stimulation of systemic vasopressin secretion by recombinant interleukin-6 in humans: Potential implications for the syndrome of inappropriate vasopressin secretion. J Clin Endocrinol Metab 79:934–939, 1994.

138. Fong Y, Moldawer LL, Marano M: Endotoxemia elicits increased circulating beta2-IFN/IL-6 in man. J Immunol 142:2321–2324, 1989.

139. Akita S, Webster J, Ren SG, et al: Human and murine pituitary expression of leukemia inhibitory factor: Novel intrapituitary regulation of adrenocorticotrophin synthesis and secretion. J Clin Invest 95:1288–1298, 1995.

140. Wang Z, Ren SG, Melmed S: Hypothalamic and pituitary leukemia inhibitory factor gene expression in vivo: A novel endotoxin-inducible neuro-endocrine interface. Endocrinology 137:2947–2953, 1996.

141. Ray DW, Ren SG, Melmed S: Leukemia inhibitory factor (LIF) stimulates proopiomelanocortin (POMC) expression in a corticotroph cell line. Role of STAT pathway. J Clin Invest 97:1852–1859, 1996.

142. Stefana B, Ray DW, Melmed S: Leukemia inhibitory factor induces differentiation of pituitary corticotroph function: An immuno-neuroendocrine phenotypic switch. Proc Natl Acad Sci U S A 93:12502–12506, 1996.

143. Akita S, Malkin J, Melmed S: Disrupted murine leukemia inhibitory fact (LIF) gene attenuates adrenocorticotrophic hormone (ACTH) secretion. Endocrinology 137:3140–3143, 1996.

144. Kariagina A, Romanenko D, Ren SG, Chesnokova V: Hypothalamic-pituitary cytokine network. Endocrinology 145:104–112, 2004.

145. Elias AN, Valenta LJ, Szekeres AV, Grossman MK: Regulatory role of gamma-aminobutyric acid in pituitary hormone secretion. Psychoneuroendocrinology 7:15–30, 1982.

146. Fish HR, Chernow B, O'Brian JT: Endocrine and neurophysiologic responses of the pituitary to insulin-induced hypoglycemia: A review. Metabolism 35:763–780, 1986.

147. Hornby PJ, Piekut DT: Opiocortin and catecholamine input to CRF-immunoreactive neurons in rat forebrain. Peptides 10:1139–1146, 1989.

148. Nussdorfer GG, Malendowicz LK: Role of VIP, PACAP, and related peptides in the regulation of the hypothalamo-pituitary-adrenal axis. Peptides 19:1443–1467, 1998.

149. Koenig JI: Pituitary gland: Neuropeptides, neurotransmitters and growth factors. Toxicol Pathol 17:256–265, 1989.

150. Desir D, Van Cauter E, Beyloos M, et al: Prolonged pulsatile administration of ovine corticotropin-releasing hormone in normal man. J Clin Endocrinol Metab 63:1292–1299, 1986.

151. Horrocks PM, Jones AF, Ratcliffe WA, et al: Patterns of ACTH and cortisol pulsatility over twenty-four hours in normal males and females. Clin Endocrinol 32:127–134, 1990.

152. Veldhuis JD, Iranmanesh A, Johnson ML, Lizarralde G: Twenty-four-hour rhythms in plasma concentrations of adenohypophyseal hormones are generated by distinct amplitude and/or frequency modulation of underlying pituitary secretory bursts. J Clin Endocrinol Metab 71:1616–1623, 1990.

153. Hesse DG, Tracey KJ, Fong Y: Cytokine appearance in human endotoxemia and primate bacteremia. Surg Gynecol Obstet 166:147–153, 1988.

154. Van Deveter SJH, Buller HR, ten Cate JW, et al: Experimental endotoxemia in humans: Analysis of cytokine release and coagulation, fibrolytic and complement pathways. Blood 76:2500–2526, 1990.

155. Chrousos GP: The hypothalamic-pituitary-adrenal axis and immune-mediated inflammation. N Engl J Med 332:1351–1362, 1995.

156. Ray DW, Stefana B, Zand O, Melmed S: Leukaemia inhibitory factor: A potent modulator of CRH action on pituitary corticotroph cells. Proceedings of the Annual Meeting of the Endocrine Society. San Francisco, Endocrine Society, 1996, p 532.

157. Takao T, Culp SG, De Souza EB: Reciprocal modulation of interleukin 1 beta and interleukin-I receptors by lipopolysaccharide (endotoxin) treatment in the mouse brain-endocrine-immune axis. Endocrinology 132:1497–1504, 1993.

158. Bernhagen J, Calandra T, Mitchell RA, et al: MIF is a pituitary-derived cytokine that potentiates lethal endotoxaemia. Nature 365:756–959, 1993.

159. Yamaguchi M, Matsuzaki N, Hirota K, et al: Interleukin-6 possibly induced by interleukin-1 beta in the pituitary gland stimulates the release of gonadotrophins and prolactin. Acta Endocrinol (Copenh) 122:201–205, 1990.

160. Muglia L, Jacobson L, Dikkes P, Majzoub JA: Corticotrophin-releasing hormone deficiency reveals major fetal but not adult glucocorticoid need. Nature 373:427–432, 1995.

161. Milenkovic L, Rettori V, Snyder GD, et al: Cachectin alters pituitary hormone release by a direct action in vitro. Proc Natl Acad Sci U S A 86:2418–2422, 1989.

162. Spangelo BL, Judd AM, Isakson PC, MacLeod RM: Interleukin-6 stimulates anterior pituitary hormone release in vitro. Endocrinology 125:575–577, 1989.

163. Almawi WY, Lupman ML, Stevens AR, et al: Abrogation of glucocorticoid-mediated inhibition of T cell proliferation by the synergistic actions of IL-6 and IFN-gamma. J Immunol 146:3523–3527, 1991.

164. Kam JC, Szeffer SJ, Surs W, et al: Combination IL-2 and IL-4 reduces glucocorticoid receptor-binding affinity and T cell response to glucocorticoids. J Immunol 151:3460–3466, 1993.

165. Caldenhoven E, Liden J, Wissink S, et al: Negative cross-talk between Re1A and the glucocorticoid receptor: A possible mechanism for the anti-inflammatory action of glucocorticoids. Mol Endocrinol 9:401–412, 1995.

166. Ray A, Prefontaine KE: Physical association and functional antagonism between the p65 subunit of transcription factor NK-kappa B and the glucocorticoid receptor. Proc Natl Acad Sci U S A 91:752–756, 1994.

167. Scheinman RI, Gualberto A, Jewell CM, et al: Characterization of mechanisms involved in transrepression of NF-kappa B by activated glucocorticoid receptors. Mol Cell Biol 15:943–953, 1995.

168. Makino S, Hashimoto K, Gold PW: Multiple feedback mechanisms activating corticotropin-releasing hormone system in the brain during stress. Pharmacol Biochem Behav 73:147–158, 2002.

169. Raff H, Findling JW: A new immunoradiometric assay for corticotropin evaluated in normal subjects and patients with Cushing's syndrome. Clin Chem 35:596–600, 1989.

170. Talbot JA, Kane JW, White A: Analytical and clinical aspects of adrenocorticotrophin determination. Ann Clin Biochem 40:453–471, 2003.

171. Yalow RS, Berson SA: Size heterogeneity of immunoreactive human ACTH in plasma and in extracts of pituitary glands and ACTH-producing thymoma. Biochem Biophys Res Commun 44:439–445, 1971.

172. Hale AC, Besser GM, Rees LH: Characterization of pro-opiomelanocortin-derived peptides in pituitary and ectopic

adrenocorticotrophin-secreting tumours. J Endocrinol 108:49–56, 1986.

173. Crosby SR, Stewart MF, Ratcliffe JG, White A: Direct measurement of the precursors of adrenocorticotropin in human plasma by two-site immunoradiometric assay. J Clin Endocrinol Metab 67:1272–1277, 1988.

174. Raffin-Sanson ML, Massias JF, Dumont C, et al: High plasma proopiomelanocortin in aggressive adrenocorticotropin-secreting tumors. J Clin Endocrinol Metab 81:4272–4277, 1996.

175. Kelly RB: Pathways of protein secretion in eukaryotes. Science 230:25–32, 1985.

Endocrine and Other Biologic Rhythms

Eve Van Cauter and Georges Copinschi

MAJOR MECHANISMS CONTROLLING ENDOCRINE RHYTHMS

A prominent feature of the endocrine system is its high degree of temporal organization. Indeed, far from obeying the concept of "constancy of the internal milieu," circulating hormonal levels undergo pronounced temporal oscillations ranging in period from a few minutes to a year. This intricate temporal organization provides the endocrine system with remarkable flexibility. Not only can specific physiologic processes be turned on and off depending on the presence or absence of a particular hormone, but the precise pattern of hormonal release may provide specific signaling information.

Hormonal variations in the circadian (i.e., approximately once per 24 hours) and ultradian (i.e., once per 1–2 hours) range are ubiquitous in endocrine systems. However, the whole spectrum of endocrine rhythms includes both higher and lower frequency ranges. Indeed, secretory oscillations with periods in the 5- to 15-minute range have been observed for a number of hormones. The menstrual cycle and seasonal rhythms belong to the so-called infradian range, corresponding to periods longer than those of the circadian range.

As schematically illustrated in Figure 19-1, the temporal variability and organization of hormonal concentrations during the 24-hour cycle ultimately result from the activity of two interacting timekeeping mechanisms in the central nervous system: endogenous circadian rhythmicity and sleep-wake homeostasis. Although this dual control was first demonstrated for hormones of the hypothalamic-pituitary axes, a similar regulation appears to apply for other endocrine subsystems. In mammals, endogenous circadian rhythmicity is generated by a pacemaker located in the paired suprachiasmatic nucleus (SCN) of the hypothalamus.[1] Sleep-wake homeostasis is an hourglass-like mechanism relating the amount and quality of sleep to the duration of prior wakefulness.[2] The two major pathways by which circadian rhythmicity and sleep-wake homeostasis affect peripheral endocrine function are the hypothalamic-pituitary axes and the autonomous nervous system.

The first two sections of this chapter provide an overview of current concepts and recent advances in the understanding of circadian rhythmicity and sleep-wake regulation. Conditions of altered or abnormal circadian and/or sleep regulation that have implications for the temporal organization of hormonal release are presented in the third section. General properties, physiologic significance, and medical implications of ultradian rhythmicity are presented in a broad context in the fourth section. Methodologic aspects specific to the study of hormonal rhythms in human subjects are described in the fifth section. The last section summarizes the current state of knowledge of circadian and ultradian endocrine rhythms in health and disease for the major endocrine axes. Due to limitations on the length and scope of this chapter, this review is limited to findings in adults.

CIRCADIAN RHYTHMICITY

General Characteristics
One of the most obvious characteristics of life on earth is the ability of almost all species to change their behavior on a daily or 24-hour basis. A remarkable feature of these daily rhythms is that they are not simply a response to the 24-hour changes in the physical environment imposed by the principles of celestial mechanics, but instead arise from an internal timekeeping system.[1] Under laboratory conditions devoid of any external time-giving cues, it has indeed been found that nearly all 24-hour rhythms continue to be expressed. However, under such constant conditions, the period of the rhythm rarely remains exactly 24 hours but instead is "about" 24 hours, and this is why these rhythms are referred to as circadian, from the Latin *circa diem*, meaning around a day. When a circadian rhythm is expressed in the absence of any 24-hour signals in the external environment, it is said to be "free running." Strictly speaking, a diurnal rhythm should not be referred to as circadian until it has been demonstrated that such a rhythm persists under constant environmental conditions. The purpose of this distinction is to separate those rhythms that are simply a response to 24-hour changes in the

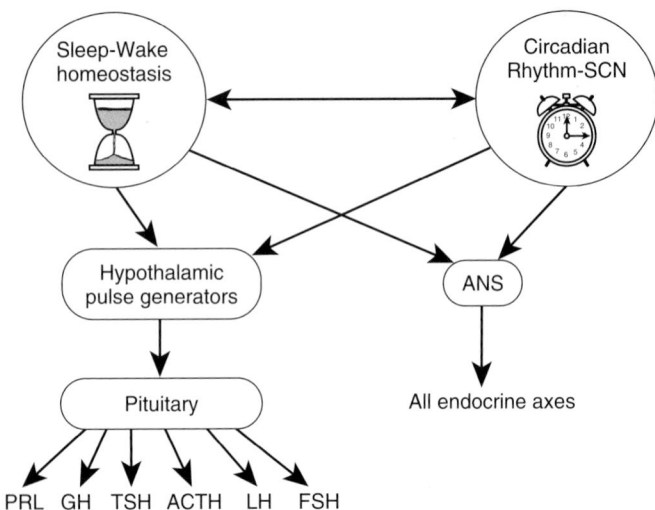

Figure 19-1 Schematic representation of the central mechanisms involved in the control of temporal variations in pituitary hormone secretions over the 24-hour cycle. Sleep-wake homeostasis is an hourglass-like mechanism relating the propensity for deep non–rapid eye movement (NREM) sleep to the amount of prior wakefulness. Circadian rhythmicity is an endogenous nearly 24-hour oscillation generated in the suprachiasmatic nuclei (SCN) of the hypothalamus and transmitted via neural and humoral mechanisms. ACTH, adrenocorticotropic hormone; FSH, follicle-stimulating hormone; GH, growth hormone; LH, luteinizing hormone; PRL, prolactin; TSH, thyroid-stimulating hormone; ANS, autonomous nervous system.

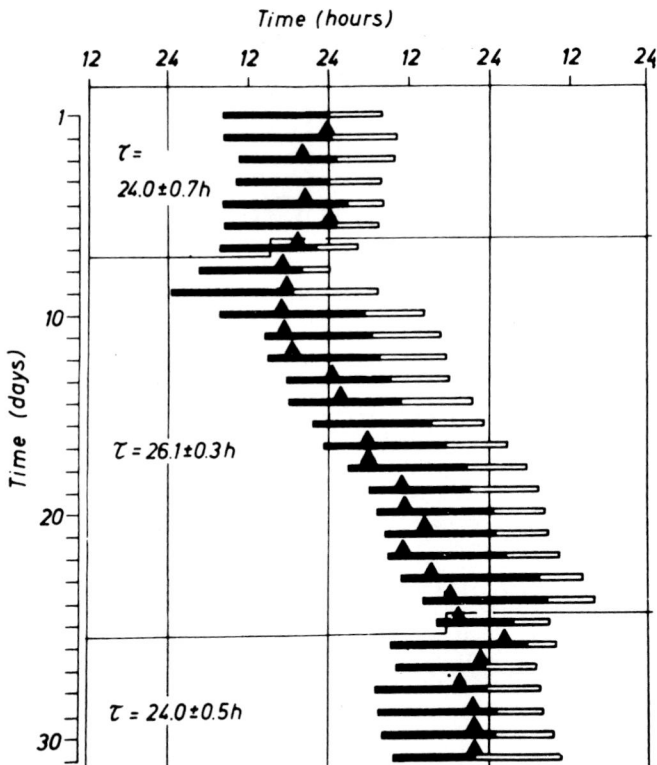

Figure 19-2 Circadian rhythms of wakefulness (solid bars), sleep (open bars), and maximal rectal temperature (triangles) in a human subject who was exposed to the external synchronizing agents for the first and last 7 days and was isolated from all time cues in an underground bunker between days 8 and 24.

environment from those that are endogenous. However, for practical purposes, there is little reason to make a distinction between diurnal and circadian rhythms because almost all diurnal rhythms are largely endogenous. In this chapter, we therefore extend the use of the term *circadian rhythm* to all diurnal variations recurring regularly at a time interval of approximately 24 hours.

An immense variety of circadian rhythms has been observed in humans. Human circadian rhythms have been characterized for blood constituents such as white blood cells, amino acids, phosphorous; innumerable physiologic variables such as body temperature, heart rate, blood pressure, urinary volume; and behavioral parameters such as mood, vigilance, and cognitive performance. There are also rhythms in responsive to various challenges such as drugs and stress. Circadian rhythmicity is maintained when subjects are sleep deprived, when they are starved, or when they receive equal amounts of food at short intervals over the day. The timing of single meals, however, can have effects on the pattern of at least some variables including hormones, and effects of sleep-wake homeostasis can alter the expression of many rhythms, especially those of the endocrine system.

The endogenous nature of human circadian rhythms has been established by experiments in which subjects were isolated with no access to the natural light-dark (LD) cycle and no time cues. Such experiments were first performed in natural caves, then in underground bunkers, and finally in specially designed windowless soundproof apartments. The results of such an experiment, conducted in an artificial underground unit in Germany, are shown in Figure 19-2.[3,4] The rest-activity cycle of the subject is plotted horizontally day by day, and the times of occurrence of the daily maximum of the body temperature cycle are indicated by closed triangles. During the first 7 days of the experiment, the door of the isolation unit was left open and the subjects knew the time of day. The average period (t) of the rest-activity cycle and of the rhythm of body temperature was 24 hours. When, thereafter, the subject lived in complete isolation, both rhythms free-ran but with a mean period of about 26 hours.

The free-running period varies from one individual to another. In humans, free-running periods around 25 hours have been commonly observed under conditions of prolonged temporal isolation.

The Suprachiasmatic Nucleus: A Master Circadian Pacemaker
In mammals, the SCN, that is, two small bilaterally paired nuclei in the anterior hypothalamus immediately above the optic chiasm, functions as the master circadian clock. Under both free-running and entrained conditions, destruction of the SCN in a variety of species leads to the abolishment or the severe disruption of many behavioral and physiologic rhythms. The role of the SCN as the control center for the circadian system, first suggested by lesion studies, was confirmed by studies involving transplantation of the SCN from one animal to another. Indeed, circadian rhythmicity can be restored in adult arrhythmic SCN-lesioned rodents by transplanting fetal SCN tissue into the region of the SCN.[5,6] A number of SCN rhythms persist in vitro, including those of neural firing, vasopressin release, and glucose metabolism.[7,8] Finally, immortalized SCN cells can generate robust rhythms in both glucose uptake and their content of neurotrophins.[8a] It is now clear that the ability of SCN cells to generate a circadian signal does not rely on some inherent network property of many cells acting together: Single SCN cells in culture can generate circadian neural signals.[9] The generation and maintenance of circadian oscillations in the SCN involve a series of clock genes that interact in a complex feedback loop of transcription/translation. (For reviews on the molecular and genetic control of circadian rhythmicity, the reader is referred to Reppert and Weaver.[10])

In recent years, it has been recognized that circadian oscillators are also present in peripheral tissues, in particular in the liver, lung, and skeletal muscle.[11] The oscillations generated by these peripheral clocks appear to dampen after a few cycles when monitored in vitro, although oscillations persisting for more than 20 cycles have been identified in a number of peripheral tissues.[12] It has been suggested that the SCN controls the synchronization of peripheral circadian oscillators,[11] but little is known so far about the mechanisms and extent of the putative control of the SCN over peripheral clocks.[13]

Photic Entrainment of Circadian Rhythms

The fact that the endogenous circadian period observed under constant conditions is not exactly equal to 24 hours implies that changes in the physical environment must synchronize or entrain the internal clock. Otherwise, a clock with a period only a few minutes shorter or longer than 24 hours would soon be totally out of synchrony with the environmental day. Agents that are capable of entraining or synchronizing circadian rhythms are often called zeitgebers, a German neologism meaning time giver.

The LD cycle is the primary agent that synchronizes most circadian rhythms. Thus, in the presence of a 24-hour LD cycle, the period of circadian rhythms exactly matches the period of the LD cycle. In addition to establishing period control, an entraining LD cycle establishes phase control such that specific phases of the circadian rhythm occur at the same time in each cycle. Entrainment is restricted to cycles with periods that are close to 24 hours in duration and, in general, is not possible for LD cycles that are more than a few hours shorter or longer than the endogenous circadian period. If the period of the LD cycle is too short or long for entrainment to occur, the circadian rhythm free-runs. This rigidity of the circadian pacemaker has been used in so-called forced desynchrony studies in which the subjects are maintained on a LD and sleep-wake cycle with a period outside the range of entrainment, such as 20 hours or 28 hours.[14,15] Such protocols have provided estimations of the endogenous period of the human circadian system that are closer to 24 hours (i.e., averaging 24.1 hours) than those obtained in prolonged studies of temporal isolation.[15] The fact that the human endogenous circadian period is probably very close to 24 hours is consistent with the findings of a recent study that showed that a schedule of sleep-wake and LD cycles with very low light intensity during wakefulness is able to maintain entrainment to the 24-hour day but not to a 23.5- or 24.6-hour day.[16]

The eyes are involved in relaying entraining information from the LD cycle to the circadian timing system in mammals via a unique pathway, separate from the visual system, and referred to as the retinohypothalamic tract.[17] At the level of the optic chiasm, retinal projections first enter the brain in the region of the SCN and surrounding hypothalamic areas.[17] The integrity of the primary visual centers of the brain and/or the perception of light is not necessary for entrainment of circadian rhythms by the LD cycle. It has been recently shown that a population of directly light-sensitive retinal ganglionic cells act as brightness detectors and regulate circadian rhythms.[18] Thus, visual light perception is not necessary for circadian light perception, and in some totally blind humans, light exposure is capable of suppressing melatonin levels, indicating that visual blindness should not be equated with circadian blindness.[19] In addition to the retinohypothalamic tract, the SCN also receives retinal information indirectly from the lateral geniculate nucleus (LGN), which receives a direct projection from the retina.[17]

To examine how a zeitgeber such as light influences the circadian system, the organism is maintained in constant conditions and then briefly exposed to the zeitgeber before being returned to constant conditions.[20] The effects of zeitgeber exposure on a phase reference point of an overt circadian rhythm (e.g., onset of locomotor activity, minimum of body temperature) in subsequent cycles is then determined. A plot of the direction and magnitude of the phase shift as a function of the circadian time of zeitgeber exposure is called a phase-response curve (PRC). In the human, light exposure during the late evening and first half of the usual sleep period results in phase delays, whereas light exposure at the end of the usual sleep period and in the early morning results in phase advances. The transition from phase delays to phase advances occurs around the time of the minimum of body temperature, that is, between 4:00 A.M. and 6:00 A.M. in most subjects. The magnitude of the phase shifts is also wavelength dependent, with exposure to short wavelength monochromatic light (shifted to the blue) resulting in much larger shifts than exposure to longer wavelength light of equal photon density.[21] Although differences in amplitude may exist, the general shape and characteristics of the PRC to light pulses are similar for all species. Based on this PRC, appropriate exposure to bright light can accelerate adaptation to shifts such as those occurring in jet lag and shift work. The amplitude of the phase shifts depends on light intensity and duration and the number of consecutive exposures.[22] Exposure to single 3- to 7-hour light pulses results in immediate phase shifts on the order of 1 to 3 hours.[23–25] Repeated exposure for 2 to 3 consecutive days may cause much larger 6- to 12-hour shifts.[26,27] The possible role of the intervening periods of dark/sleep exposure could play a role in enhancing the phase-shifting effects of repeated exposure to light.

Exposure to dark is also able to phase-shift mammalian circadian rhythms. Because under most circumstances, exposure to dark is also associated with changes in activity levels (i.e., increases in activity in nocturnal animals and decreases in activity and/or sleep induction in diurnal animals), it has been unclear whether the phase shifts occurred in response to dark exposure per se or in response to the associated changes in activity levels. A recent study in hamsters has, however, demonstrated resetting of the rhythm of locomotor activity and concomitant downregulation of clock genes after exposure to dark pulses independently of wheel-running activity.[28] In humans, abrupt 8-hour advances or 8-hour delays of the sleep-wake cycle result in immediate 2-hour phase shifts in the same direction.[29,30] Daytime naps of 6 hours duration in total darkness presented over a background of very dim light were found to cause delay shifts when initiated in the morning and advance shifts when initiated in the evening.[31] Naps initiated in the afternoon cause no significant phase shifts.

Nonphotic Zeitgebers

Nonphotic cues (e.g., social and/or behavioral cues) may also cause an alteration of the rest-activity cycle, either by eliciting activity during the normal rest period or preventing activity during the normal active period, resulting in phase shifts of circadian rhythms of activity and of other behavioral, physiologic, and endocrine markers.[32–35] In nocturnal rodents, the PRC to activity-inducing stimuli are approximately 12 hours out of phase with the PRC to light pulses.

How nonphotic information reaches the SCN is still not known, although there is evidence from lesion studies to suggest that a distinct subdivision of the LGN, the intergeniculate leaflet (IGL), may be involved in mediating the effects of activity on the clock.[36] Furthermore, the IGL is the source of the neuropeptide Y (NPY) innervation of the SCN, and the administration of NPY into the SCN area and electrical stimulation of the geniculohypothalamic tract both induce phase shifts in the hamster locomotor activity rhythm that are similar to those induced by activity-inducing stimuli.[36] The LGN/IGL may be a common pathway by which information about the lighting environment and the activity-rest state reaches the circadian clock and may be involved in integrating information from both the external and internal environments. Both the LGN/IGL and the SCN receive a dense serotonergic projection from the midbrain raphe nuclei, and there is now substantial evidence that these projections play a role in both the photic and nonphotic regulation of the mammalian circadian clock.[37]

Nonphotic stimuli may affect human circadian rhythms. Exposure to a single session of 3 hours of moderate-intensity exercise during the usual nighttime period was found to result in phase shifts of markers of circadian phase on the next day, with the direction and magnitude of the phase shifts being dependent on the timing of exercise.[38] Similar findings were obtained with nocturnal exposure to high-intensity 1-hour exercise sessions.[39] Supporting evidence of a zeitgeber effect of exercise was obtained in a field study that found that adaptation to night work could be facilitated by nocturnal exercise.[40] These findings were recently confirmed by a study demonstrating that daily exposure to nighttime exercise facilitates phase delays of circadian melatonin rhythm even when the subjects are maintained in very dim light.[41] Nocturnal exercise of low intensity is also able to phase-delay circadian rhythms in older adults, suggesting that it could be a useful treatment for the adjustment of circadian rhythmicity in older populations.[42]

Another nonphotic agent that has been shown to induce phase shifts in human circadian rhythms is melatonin.[43,44] There are specific neural connections between the master circadian pacemaker and the pineal gland, and the diurnal variation of plasma melatonin levels is driven by the circadian clock.[45] Phase shifts of the central circadian signal induced by changes in the LD cycle will be faithfully reflected in the synchronization of the onset of nocturnal melatonin secretion.[24,46,47] There is evidence that, in turn, the melatonin rhythm feeds back on the clock (where melatonin receptors have been identified) and exerts synchronizing effects.[45] Low doses (0.5 mg) of melatonin on 4 consecutive days cause small (± 30 minutes) phase advances in the late afternoon or evening and may cause phase delays in the early morning.[48] Treatment with melatonin may also ameliorate sleep disorders in totally blind people. Many of these patients have lost both visual and circadian light perception and have free-running rhythms that are not synchronized to environmental cues. Melatonin administration 1 hour before the preferred bedtime is capable of entraining circadian rhythms to a stable phase and of improving sleep quality.[49]

Finally, the timing of feeding, when temporally restricted to a limited window of time, is also a potent synchronizer of peripheral circadian rhythms.[50,51] When food is available ad libitum but only during a restricted time period, SCN rhythms remain synchronized to the LD cycle, whereas peripheral rhythms entrain to the feeding schedule. However, when caloric intake is restricted, central circadian rhythmicity is affected by the feeding rhythm, indicating that the SCN responds to metabolic cues.[50] In support of a role for the SCN in the homeostatic regulation of feeding and energy metabolism is the recent finding that leptin phase-advances the rat SCN circadian clock in vitro.[52]

SLEEP-WAKE REGULATION

General Characteristics
The sleep-wake cycle may be viewed as a 24-hour rhythm partly driven by the circadian pacemaker and partly by the homeostatic regulation of sleep pressure. Sleep itself is an ultradian rhythm because it involves two states of distinct brain activity that are each generated in specific brain regions. The ultradian rhythm of normal sleep is an approximately 90-minute oscillation between non-REM (rapid eye movement) stages and REM stages. In young healthy subjects, this pattern is usually repeated four to six times per night. REM sleep and non-REM sleep are characterized by distinct patterns of both cerebral activity and peripheral activity.

In the normal sequence, sleep onset corresponds to the appearance of the lighter stages of non-REM sleep (i.e., stages

I and II), followed within 10 to 20 minutes by slow-wave sleep (SWS; stages III and IV). These deeper stages of sleep are maintained for nearly 60 minutes in normal young subjects but are usually much shorter (5–10 minutes), if at all present, in older adults. Then, lighter stages of non-REM sleep reappear and the first REM period is initiated. As the night progresses, non-REM sleep becomes more shallow, the duration of REM episodes becomes longer, and the number and duration of awakenings increase. In normal young subjects, approximately 50% of a normal night is spent in stages I and II sleep, 20% in SWS, 25% in REM, and 5% wake. In adults older than 60 years of age, SWS is usually reduced to only 5% to 10% and REM sleep to 10% to 15%, whereas the proportion of time awake may reach 30% of the night.

During deep non-REM sleep, the electroencephalogram (EEG) is synchronized with low-frequency, high-amplitude waveforms, referred to as slow waves or delta waves. During REM sleep, eye movements are present, muscle tone is inhibited, and the EEG resembles that of active waking. During REM sleep, cerebral glucose utilization is similar to that of waking, whereas it is decreased during SWS.

The all-night recording of EEG, muscle tone, and eye movements is called the polysomnogram and is visually scored over 20- or 30-second periods in stages I, II, III, IV, REM, and wake using standardized criteria.[53] This procedure allows the determination of the duration of each sleep stage but does not quantify the intensity of non-REM sleep. In contrast, the quantification of EEG recordings by power spectral analysis provides useful information regarding sleep depth or sleep intensity because spectral analysis is sensitive to the amplitude of the delta waves. Higher amplitude delta waves reflect more intense, deeper sleep, less sensitive to arousal stimuli. Slow-wave activity is spectral EEG power in the low-frequency range (also called delta range; 0.5–4.0 Hz) and is a marker of the intensity of non-REM sleep.

As detailed below, the timing, duration, and architecture of sleep are under the dual control of central circadian rhythmicity and of a homeostatic mechanism relating sleep pressure to the duration of prior wakefulness.

Neuroanatomic Basis of Sleep Regulation
Considerable progress has been made in recent years in the identification of brain structure involved in sleep regulation, particularly for SWS.[54] The hypothalamus has been identified as playing a crucial role in the switch between wakefulness and sleep. The ventrolateral preoptic (VLPO) area of the hypothalamus contains sleep-active neurons that use γ-aminobutyric acid and galanin as neurotransmitters and have much higher firing rates during deep sleep than during wakefulness.[55-57] Lesions of the central cell cluster of the VLPO area drastically reduce slow-wave activity. Neurons of the VLPO area provide GABAergic inhibitory innervation of the major monoamine arousal systems in the brain stem. Reciprocally, there are inhibitory pathways from the monoamine arousal nuclei and the VLPO area. The lateral hypothalamus contains recently identified wake-active neurons that use the peptide orexin as a neurotransmitter.[54] These orexin neurons innervate all components of the ascending arousal system and also project to the VLPO area. REM sleep is primarily regulated by cholinergic nuclei in the pons. However, a role of the extended VLPO area in REM sleep regulation had been suggested by studies showing that this region is selectively activated during REM sleep.[58]

Interactions between Circadian Rhythmicity and Sleep-Wake Homeostasis
There are several features of the interaction between sleep and circadian rhythmicity that appear to be fairly unique to the human species. First, human sleep is generally consolidated in a single 6- to 9-hour period, whereas fragmentation of the

sleep period in several bouts is the rule in the majority of other mammals. Possibly as a result of this consolidation of the sleep period, the wake-sleep transition in humans is associated with physiologic changes that are usually more marked than those observed in animals. For example, the secretion of growth hormone (GH) in normal adults is closely associated with the beginning of the sleep period, whereas the relationship between GH secretory pulses and sleep stages is much less evident in rodents, primates, and dogs. Second, humans are also unique in their capacity to ignore circadian signals and to maintain wakefulness despite an increased pressure to go to sleep. Finally, approximately 25% of human subjects maintained for prolonged periods in temporal isolation have shown behavioral modifications that have not been observed in laboratory animals under constant conditions. These modifications consist of a desynchronization between the sleep-wake cycle and other rhythms, such as those of body temperature and cortisol secretion, which continue to free-run with a circadian period. Under conditions of so-called internal desynchronization, the sleep-wake cycle may be suddenly lengthened to 30 hours and more, whereas the rhythm of body temperature continues to free-run with a circadian period.[3,4] Wakefulness may last more than 30 hours. Remarkably, the subjects are not aware of these drastic changes in their way of living. Instead, most of them believe that they are living on a more or less regular 24-hour schedule. This can be explained by the observation that time perception is profoundly altered: Estimations of 1-hour intervals are positively correlated with the duration of wakefulness.[59] Of particular interest is that the subjects continue to have three meals per "day," irrespective of the actual number of hours that they are awake.[60] The intervals between meals and those between wake-up and breakfast or between dinner and bedtime are stretched or compressed in strong proportionality to the duration of wakefulness.[61] The mechanisms causing spontaneous internal desynchronization are not completely understood.

Detailed analyses of data obtained during temporal isolation and forced desynchrony protocols showed that the timing, duration, and architecture of sleep are partially regulated by circadian rhythmicity.[14,62] Thus, the duration of sleep episodes is correlated with the phase of the circadian rhythm of body temperature and not with the duration of prior wakefulness. Short (i.e., 7–8 hours) sleep episodes occur in free-running conditions when the subject goes to sleep around the minimum of body temperature, whereas long (i.e., 12–14 hours) sleep episodes occur when sleep starts around the maximum of body temperature. Moreover, the distributions of REM sleep and sleep spindle activity are also markedly modulated by circadian timing. In contrast, the hourglass-like mechanism of sleep-wake homeostasis is thought to be largely independent of the circadian system and to involve one or several putative neural sleep factor(s) (factor(s) "S"), which increase(s) during waking and decay(s) exponentially during sleep.[2] This homeostatic mechanism regulates the timing, amount, and intensity of SWS and slow-wave activity. A neuroanatomic basis for the interaction of the homeostatic process and central circadian rhythmicity has been recently identified because the VLPO area receives dense projections from the dorsomedial hypothalamic nucleus, which itself receives direct and indirect projections from the SCN.[63] Based on the human studies described below, it is thought that the SCN generates a waking signal that promotes alertness during the active period. In support of this theory, detailed studies have indicated that rodents and monkeys with SCN lesions have an increased sleep duration.[64,65] A role for the SCN in promoting sleep at other circadian times is suggested by the finding of decreased sleep in a mouse with a mutation of the *Clock* gene.[66]

The dual control of sleep by circadian and homeostatic mechanisms extends to the control of objective and subjective measures of sleep tendency, mood, and vigilance.[67–70] Figure 19-3 shows representative profiles of body temperature, subjective sleepiness (using the Stanford Sleepiness Score), positive affect (using the Profile of Positive and Negative Affect), and performance on a vigilance task in normal young men studied during 40 consecutive hours of continuous wakefulness. Maximal subjective sleepiness coincides with the minimum of body temperature, mood, and performance. Remarkably, despite continued sleep deprivation, subjective fatigue decreased, and mood and performance partially recovered during the daytime hours after nocturnal sleep deprivation, reflecting an interaction of circadian timing with the accumulation of waking time.[68–74] It is currently thought that the circadian clock generates a waking signal that increases from morning to evening and is maximally expressed in the

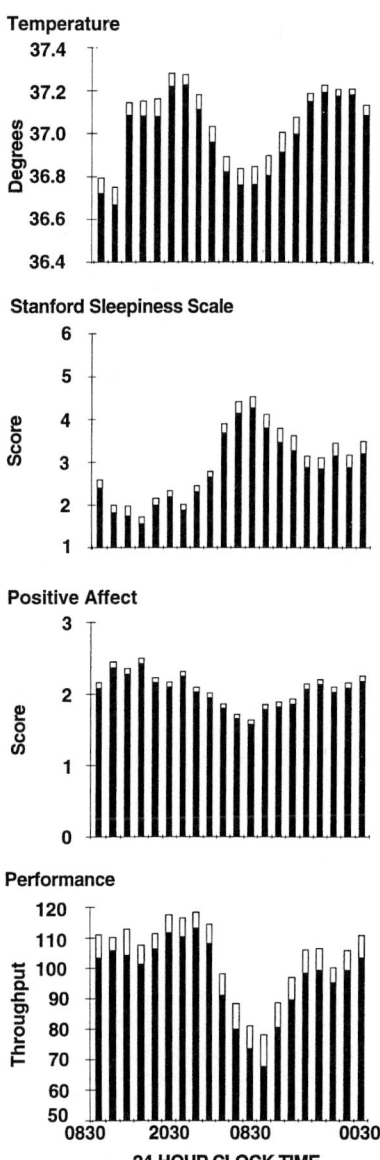

Figure 19-3 Mean profiles of body temperature, subjective sleepiness (using the Stanford Sleepiness Score), positive affect (using the Positive and Negative Affect Scale), and performance on a vigilance task in normal young men studied during 40 consecutive hours of continuous wakefulness at bedrest. Data are represented as mean *(solid bar)* and SEM *(open bar)* for each 2-hour interval.

early evening hours, 1 to 2 hours before the onset of nocturnal melatonin secretion.[69] This circadian waking signal counteracts the buildup of the putative factor "S" underlying the homeostatic process, allowing a high level of alertness throughout the usual waking period to be maintained. Current data from human studies are also compatible with the hypothesis that the SCN also generates a "sleep" signal in the early evening hours.[75]

Circadian rhythmicity and sleep-wake homeostasis also interact to regulate hormonal secretion. These modulatory effects were long thought to be present only in hormones directly dependent of the hypothalamic-pituitary axis. However, it is now clear that modulation by circadian rhythmicity and sleep is also present in other endocrine systems, such as glucose regulation and the renin-angiotensin system.[76,77] The pathways by which circadian rhythmicity, sleep-wake homeostasis, and their interaction modulate hormonal release are largely unknown. As illustrated in Figure 19-1, humoral and/or neural signals originating from the hypothalamic circadian pacemaker and from brain regions involved in sleep regulation affect the activity of the hypothalamic structures responsible for the pulsatile release of neuroendocrine factors that stimulate or inhibit intermittent secretion of pituitary hormones. The autonomic nervous system is another pathway linking the central control of sleep-wake homeostasis and circadian rhythmicity with peripheral endocrine organs. Stimulatory or inhibitory effects of sleep on endocrine release are temporally associated with variations of SWS activity.[78] Theoretically, the modulation of neuroendocrine release by sleep and circadian rhythmicity could be achieved by modulation of pulse amplitude, modulation of pulse frequency, or a combination of both. The data available so far seem to indicate that circadian rhythmicity of pituitary hormonal release is achieved primarily by modulation of pulse amplitude without changes in pulse frequency, whereas sleep-wake and REM-non-REM transitions affect pulse frequency. Pituitary hormones that influence endocrine systems not directly controlled by hypothalamic factors, probably mediate, together with the autonomous nervous system, the modulatory effects of sleep and circadian rhythmicity on these systems (e.g., counterregulatory effects of GH and cortisol on glucose regulation).[77]

To delineate the relative roles of circadian and sleep effects in the temporal organization of hormonal secretion, strategies based on the fact that circadian rhythmicity needs several days to adapt to abrupt shifts of the sleep-wake cycle have been used. Thus, by shifting the sleep times by 8 to 12 hours, masking effects of sleep on circadian inputs are removed and the effects of sleep at an abnormal circadian time are revealed. Figure 19-4 illustrates mean profiles of plasma cortisol, GH, prolactin, and thyrotropin-stimulating hormone (TSH) observed in normal subjects who were studied before and during an abrupt 12-hour shift of the sleep-wake and LD cycle. The study period extended over a 53-hour span and included an 8-hour period of nocturnal sleep, a 28-hour period of continuous wakefulness, and a daytime period of recovery sleep. To eliminate the effects of feeding, fasting, and postural changes, the subjects remained recumbent throughout the study, and the normal meal schedule was replaced by intravenous glucose infusion at a constant rate. As shown in Figure 19-4, this drastic manipulation of sleep had only modest effects on the wave shape of the cortisol profile in sharp contrast to the immediate shift of the GH and prolactin rhythms that followed the shift of the sleep-wake cycle. As is reviewed in subsequent sections, numerous studies have indicated that the control of diurnal rhythms of corticotropic activity is primarily dependent on circadian timing, whereas sleep-wake homeostasis appears to be an important factor in the control of the 24-hour profiles of GH and prolactin.[79] Nevertheless, small modulatory effects of sleep-wake homeostasis on cortisol secretion and, conversely, influences of circadian timing on somatotropic function have been clearly

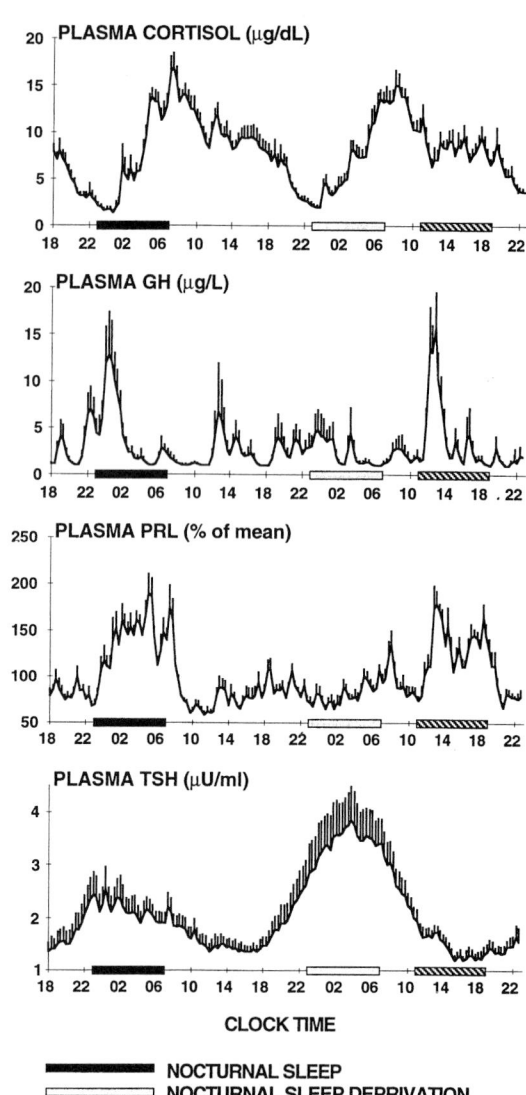

Figure 19-4   From top to bottom: Mean 24-hour profiles of plasma cortisol, growth hormone (GH), prolactin (PRL), and thyroid-stimulating hormone (TSH) in a group of eight normal young men (20–27 years old) studied during a 53-hour period, including 8 hours of nocturnal sleep, 28 hours of sleep deprivation, and 8 hours of daytime sleep. The *vertical line* at each time point represents the SEM. The *solid bars* represent the sleep periods. The *open bars* represent the period of nocturnal sleep deprivation. The *hatched bars* represent the period of daytime sleep. Data were sampled at 20-minute intervals. (From Van Cauter E, Spiegel K: Circadian and sleep control of endocrine secretions. In Turek FW, Zee PC [eds]: Neurobiology of Sleep and Circadian Rhythms, vol 133. New York, Marcel Dekker, 1999, pp 397–426.)

demonstrated.[80] The diurnal variation of TSH levels includes an evening elevation thought to be under circadian control and nocturnal inhibition by sleep-dependent processes, which is clearly demonstrated during sleep deprivation when a large increase in nocturnal TSH level is apparent, as shown in the lower panel of Figure 19-4.[79]

Hormonal profiles are thus easily measurable reflections of central mechanisms of biologic timekeeping. In clinical investigations of conditions of abnormal circadian rhythmicity such as jet lag and in human studies of the effects of exposure to natural or artificial zeitgebers, they are commonly used as markers of the status of the circadian clock and of its interactions with sleep.

CONDITIONS OF ALTERED CIRCADIAN RHYTHMICITY AND SLEEP

AGING

Age-related changes in endocrine, metabolic, and behavioral circadian rhythms have been reported in a variety of species, including humans.[81–83] One of the most prominent changes is a reduction in rhythm amplitude. The overall findings of a study that examined age-related differences in 24-hour endocrine rhythms in healthy male subjects are shown in Figure 19-5.[81] A marked decrease in the nocturnal release of TSH, melatonin, prolactin, and GH was observed in the older volunteers. The amplitude of the cortisol rhythm was decreased in the elderly men, primarily because of an elevation of the nocturnal nadir. A retrospective analysis of poly-graphic sleep recordings and concomitant profiles of plasma GH and cortisol from 149 normal healthy men, ages 16 to 83 years, showed a different rate of aging of SWS and REM sleep[84] (Fig. 19-6). SWS decreased markedly from early adulthood to midlife and was replaced by lighter sleep (stages I and II) without significant increases in sleep fragmentation or decreases in REM sleep. The transition from midlife to late life involved an increase in wake at the expense of both non-REM and REM sleep. The chronology of aging of GH secretion paralleled that of SWS. In contrast, the elevation of evening cortisol levels became significant only after the age of 50 years, when sleep became more fragmented and REM sleep declined.

Other studies have shown that these deficits in the maintenance and depth of nocturnal sleep[85] are paralleled by decreased alertness during the daytime. In both rodents and humans, many circadian rhythms are also advanced under entrained conditions such that specific phase points of the rhythms occur earlier than in young subjects.[81,86] Both amplitude reduction and phase advance of the rhythm of body temperature have been observed in elderly subjects, and these alterations in circadian regulation were closely associated with changes in sleep-wake habits (i.e., earlier bedtimes and wake times).[82]

Age-related changes in the amplitude and/or the phase of circadian rhythms could be due to changes in the inner workings of the master clock, to alterations in the input pathways to the clock, or to factors "downstream" between the circadian clock and the system expressing the rhythm. Some early studies[87,88] reported that the free-running period of various rhythms in rodents is systematically shortened with age, suggesting that the circadian clock itself is altered in advanced age. This concept has been recently confirmed in rats using measurement of Per1-luc expression in transgenic animals.[89] Age-related phase advances of a number of different behavioral and endocrine rhythms are consistent with the hypothesis that the period of the human circadian clock is shorter in the elderly. However, a recent study that measured the free-running period in healthy young and older adults using the forced desynchrony protocol found no age difference.[15] It should be noted, however, that the older individuals who participated in this demanding protocol passed extremely stringent exclusion criteria and may have been more representative of "successful aging" than "normal aging." Moreover, "after effects" of entrainment to the environmental 24-hour period may have obscured the expression of endogenous circadian rhythmicity and the demonstration of age differences. Nevertheless, these very healthy older individuals had marked decreases in sleep consolidation and had greater difficulties sleeping at adverse circadian phases than young subjects. These alterations and the clear advance of the propensity to awaken from sleep are thought to be related to both a reduction in the homeostatic drive to sleep and a reduction in the strength of the circadian signal.[90] In older adults, in contrast to young subjects, there is no significant correlation between the length of the circadian period and the phase angle of entrainment.[91]

Studies in rodents indicate that aging is also associated with a decreased responsiveness to the phase-shifting effects of both photic and nonphotic stimuli. Old hamsters show a decreased response to the phase-shifting effects of low-intensity light pulses.[92] This observation raises the possibility that, in old age, there is either decreased signal transmission of light information to the SCN or that the SCN itself is less responsive to photic stimulation. Similarly, although induction of locomotor activity during a time of normal inactivity can induce pronounced phase shifts in the circadian rhythm of locomotor activity in young animals, in old animals the response is greatly diminished or completely abolished.[93,94] Interestingly, transplantation of fetal SCN tissue into the SCN region of old hamsters with an intact SCN can restore the response to the phase-shifting effects of triazolam on the activity rhythm.[95]

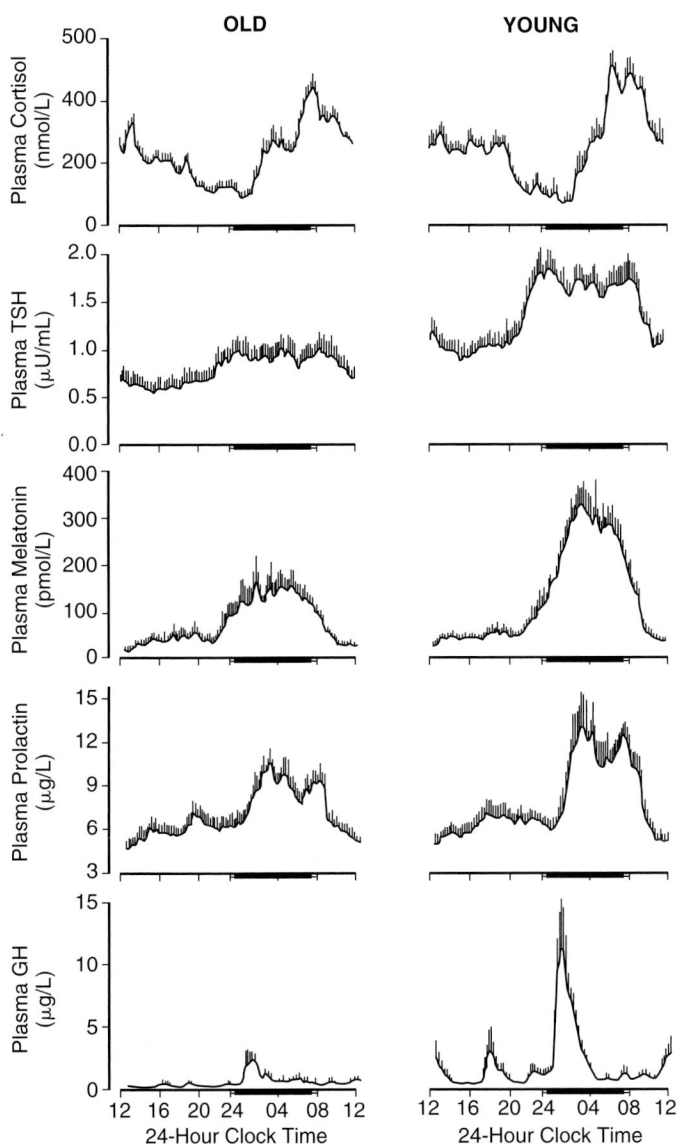

Figure 19-5 **From top to bottom**: Mean 24-hour profiles of plasma cortisol, thyroid-stimulating hormone (TSH), melatonin, prolactin, and growth hormone (GH) levels in old (67–84 years) and young (20–27 years) subjects. Data were sampled at 15-minute intervals. At each time point, the *vertical line* represents the standard error for the group ($N = 8$). The *solid bars* represent the mean sleep period. (From van Coevorden A, Mockel J, Laurent E, et al: Neuroendocrine rhythms and sleep in aging men. Am J Physiol 260:E651–E661, 1991.)

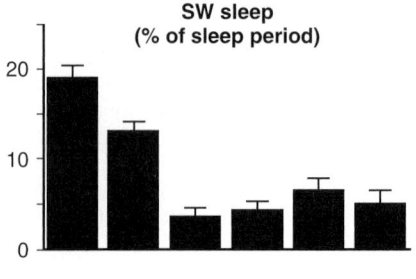

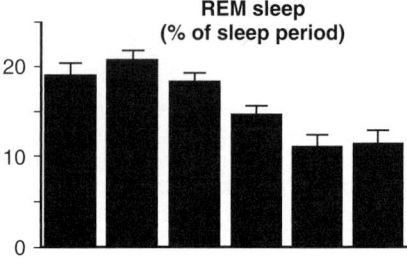

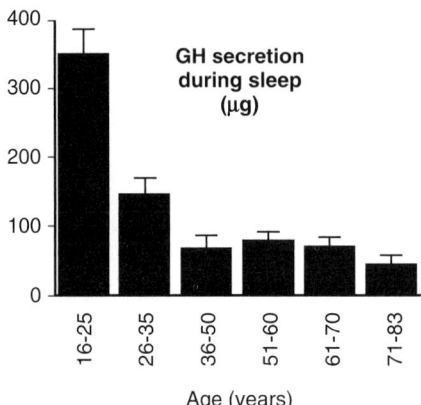

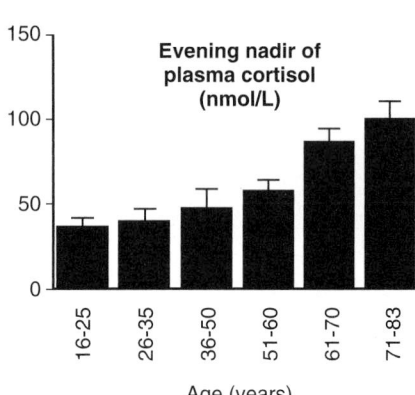

Figure 19-6 **Left,** Slow-wave (SW) sleep and growth hormone (GH) secretion during sleep as a function of age. Note the temporal concomitance between the decrease in SW sleep and GH secretion. **Right,** Rapid eye movement (REM) sleep and level of evening nadir of plasma cortisol as a function of age. Note the temporal concomitance between the decrease in REM sleep and the increase in evening cortisol levels. Values shown are means (± SEM) for each age group. Data were obtained in 149 healthy men, ages 16 to 83 years. (Data from Van Cauter E, Leproult R, Plat L: Age-related changes in slow-wave sleep and relationship with growth hormone and cortisol levels in healthy men. JAMA 284:861–868, 2000.)

Behavioral changes in the elderly may also lead to changes in environmental input to the circadian clock. In older adults, exposure to bright light and social cues, both potential entraining agents, is markedly diminished when compared with young adults.[96-98] Absence of professional constraints, decreased mobility due to illness, and reduced socialization and outdoor activities are all hallmarks of old age. Thus, decreased exposure to environmental stimuli that entrain circadian rhythms could contribute to disruptions in circadian rhythmicity. The use of exposure to bright light and enriched social schedules to reinforce circadian rhythms in older adults and improve nighttime sleep and daytime alertness has proved beneficial in several studies.[99] In elderly insomniacs living in a nursing home with limited exposure to environmental light, supplementary light exposure during the middle of the day significantly increased nocturnal melatonin secretion without circadian phase shifting.[100]

CIRCADIAN MISALIGNMENT

Circadian rhythms provide synchronization with the pronounced periodic fluctuations in the external environment and organize the internal milieu so that there is coordination and synchronization of internal processes. External synchronization is of obvious importance for the survival of the species and ensures that the organism "does the right thing" at the right time of the day. Of equal importance, but perhaps less appreciated, is the fact that the circadian clock system provides internal temporal organization between the myriad of biochemical and physiologic systems in the body. Lack of synchrony within the internal environment may lead to chronic difficulties with serious consequences for the health and well-being of the organism. The physical and mental malaise occurring after rapid travel across time zones (i.e., jet lag syndrome) and the pathologies associated with long-term shift work are assumed to be due in part to an alteration in the normal phase relationships between various internal rhythms. In addition, it has been speculated that alterations of internal phase relationships between rhythms may underlie some forms of affective illness.

Jet Lag

Subjects who travel rapidly across time zones are confronted with a desynchronization between their internal circadian rhythms and the periodicity of the new external environment. Upon arrival, the timings of the LD cycle, social schedule, and meals are abnormally matched to the phase of the physiologic rhythms of the traveler. Associated with this lack of synchronization are symptoms of fatigue, subjective discomfort, sleep disturbances, reduced mental and psychomotor performance, and gastrointestinal disorders.

The rate of adaptation is generally slower for overt rhythms, which are strongly dependent on the circadian system, such as those of cortisol and melatonin secretions, than for those that are markedly modulated by sleep-wake homeostasis, such as prolactin and GH secretions. As a result, during the period of adaptation, abnormal phase relationships between overt rhythms occur. Thus, jet lag syndrome involves not only desynchronization between internal and external rhythms but also a perturbation of internal temporal organization of physiologic functions. Depending on the strength of the zeitgebers, the rate of adaptation can be as low as half an hour per day or as high as 3 hours per day. The rate of adaptation is not constant: Adaptation to a large shift occurs at a faster rate during the first few days and progresses at a slower pace thereafter.[101] The rate of adaptation is also dependent on the direction of the shift, with adaptation occurring generally faster after a delay (i.e., westward) shift than after an advance (i.e., eastward) shift.[101] This eastward-westward difference in the rate of adaptation is believed to be due to the fact that the endogenous circadian period of the human is longer than 24 hours and thus adjustment by delays is more easily achieved than adjustment by advances. There is strong evidence to suggest that reentrainment after a transmeridian flight is facilitated by exposure to bright light at appropriate circadian phases. It is widely believed that adherence to the local social and meal schedule upon arrival will accelerate adaptation to jet lag, but this has not been rigorously demonstrated. Laboratory studies suggest that physical exercise scheduled during the period corresponding to the nighttime before travel will facilitate adaptation to a delay (i.e., westward) shift.[38,39]

Shift Work

Shift work, which is voluntarily accepted by millions of workers, is a major health hazard, involving an increased risk of cardiovascular illness, gastrointestinal disorders, infertility, and insomnia.[102-104] Epidemiologic studies have also indicated that shift work is a risk factor for weight gain.[105] The medical consequences of shift work are associated with chronic misalignment of physiologic circadian rhythms and the rest-activity cycle. In addition, shift work almost invariably results in substantial sleep loss because daytime sleep is generally shorter and more fragmented than nocturnal sleep. Shift work usually creates conditions in which some zeitgebers (e.g., an artificial LD cycle) and additional phase-setting factors such as the rest-activity cycle, are shifted while others remain unaltered (e.g., the natural LD cycle and the routines of family life). Shift workers thus live in a situation of conflicting zeitgebers that almost never allow a complete shift of the circadian system. Indeed, several studies have shown that workers on permanent or rotating night shifts do not adapt to these schedules, even after several years.[106-108] Besides its health implications, this misalignment with the circadian system has important social and economic implications because night work is associated with substantial decrements in performance and vigilance, resulting in diminished productivity and increased accident rates. A number of studies have demonstrated that scheduled exposure to bright light during night work and complete darkness during daytime sleep after night work can accelerate the adjustment to the new schedule and improve nighttime alertness and performance.[109-114]

SLEEP CURTAILMENT

Chronic sleep loss is a hallmark of modern society. "Normal" sleep duration has decreased from approximately 9 hours in 1910 to an average of 7.5 hours today. Many individuals voluntarily choose to curtail their sleep to the shortest amount tolerable to maximize the time available for work and leisure activities. To meet the demands of around-the-clock operations, millions of shift workers sleep on average less than 6 hours per day. Despite the fact that sleep is a major modulator of metabolic and endocrine regulation, the consensus that prevailed until recently was that sleep loss results in increased sleepiness and decreased cognitive performance but has little or no effect on peripheral function. A study that measured metabolic and hormonal parameters in subjects studied during 1 week of sleep restriction (4 hours in bed) and after 1 week of sleep recovery (12 hours in bed) provided evidence to the contrary.[115,116] Figure 19-7 shows the 24-hour profiles of plasma TSH and leptin as well as the profile of the homeostatic model assessment (HOMA) index, an index directly proportional to the product of insulin by glucose concentrations. In the sleep restriction condition, the normal nocturnal TSH rise was strikingly decreased and the overall mean TSH levels were reduced by more than 30%. Differences in TSH profiles between the two conditions were probably related to changes in thyroid hormone concentrations because the free thyroxine index was higher in the sleep restriction condition than in the sleep recovery condition. Mean leptin levels were 20% lower during sleep restriction than during sleep extension and the nocturnal acrophase was reduced by 30%, despite identical amounts of caloric intake and physical activity as well as stable BMI. Inhibition of leptin release due to increased sympathetic nervous outflow is a likely mechanism underlying this decrease of leptin levels during chronic partial sleep loss. Cardiac sympathovagal balance was indeed elevated when the subjects were in the state of sleep debt. The lower panels of Figure 19-7 show that the HOMA index was elevated post-breakfast when the subjects were sleep deprived as compared to fully rested. This observation of an alteration in parameters of glucose tolerance after sleep loss was confirmed by the results of intravenous glucose tolerance testing (upper panels of Figure 19-8) performed on the fifth day of both conditions.[115] The parameters of glucose tolerance measured at the end of the recovery period were in the normal range for young healthy men, but the parameters measured in the state of sleep debt were consistent with a clinically significant impairment of carbohydrate tolerance. Thus, the rate of disappearance of glucose postinjection was nearly 40% slower in the sleep debt condition than after recovery and the acute insulin

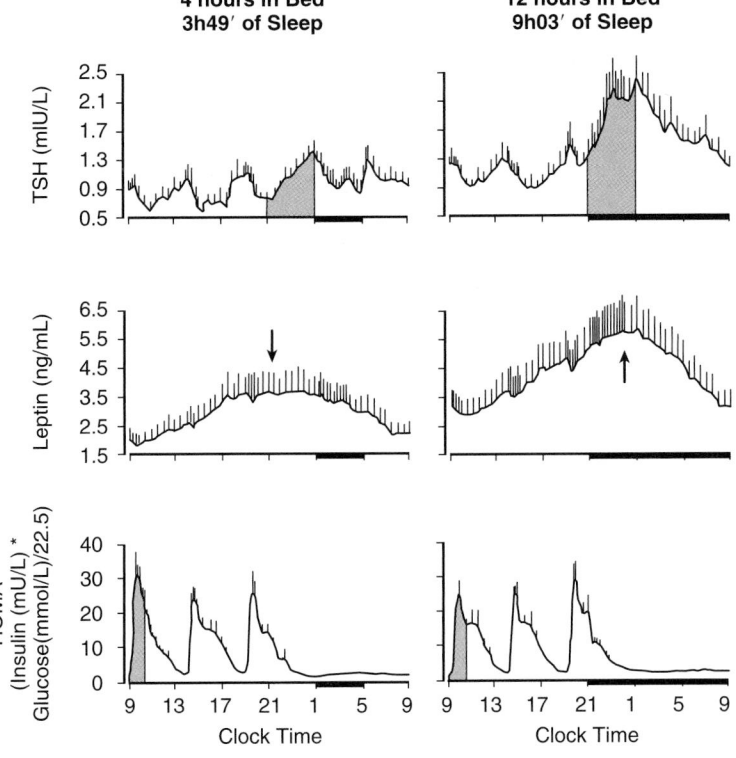

Figure 19-7 Impact of sleep curtailment (4 hours in bed for six nights) and of sleep recovery (12 hours in bed for six nights) on 24-hour profiles of plasma thyroid-stimulating hormone (TSH), plasma leptin, and homeostatic model assessment (HOMA). HOMA was calculated as glucose concentrations (mg/dL) × insulin concentrations (μU/mL)/1.22. (Adapted from Spiegel K, Leproult R, Van Cauter E: Impact of sleep debt on metabolic and endocrine function. Lancet 354:1435–1439, 1999. © The Lancet Ltd., 1999, and from Spiegel K, Leproult R, L'Hermite-Balériaux M, et al: Leptin levels are dependent on sleep duration: Relationships with sympathovagal balance, carbohydrate regulation, cortisol and thyrotropin. J Clin Endocrinol Metab 89:5762–5771, 2004. © The Endocrine Society, 2004.)

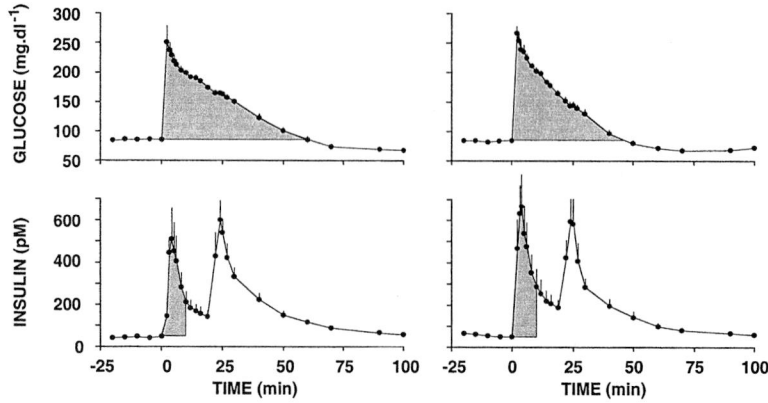

Figure 19-8 **Upper panels,** Impact of a sleep debt (4 hours in bed for 6 nights) on mean (± SEM) profiles of blood glucose and serum insulin during an intravenous glucose tolerance test. In the sleep debt condition, the duration of the glucose response was longer *(shaded area)* and the acute insulin response to glucose *(shaded area)* was lower than after sleep recovery. The rate of disappearance of glucose postinjection was nearly 40% slower in the sleep debt condition than after recovery, indicating a marked decrease in glucose tolerance. **Lower panels,** Impact of a sleep debt on the normal afternoon decrease of cortisol levels, estimated from total plasma concentrations or free saliva levels. The rate of decrease of free cortisol concentrations between 4:00 and 9:00 P.M. was approximately six times slower in the sleep debt condition than in the fully rested state. (Adapted from Spiegel K, Leproult R, Van Cauter E: Impact of sleep debt on metabolic and endocrine function. Lancet 354:1435–1439, 1999. © The Lancet Ltd., 1999.)

response to glucose was reduced by 30%. The lower glucose tolerance appeared to partly reflect diminished non-insulin-dependent glucose utilization, consistent with findings of decreased cerebral glucose utilization in positron emission tomography studies of sleep-deprived subjects. When compared with the fully rested condition, the state of sleep debt was also associated with alterations in cortisol secretion, whether estimated by total cortisol levels in plasma or free cortisol levels in saliva. The primary alteration was an elevation of cortisol concentrations in the afternoon and early evening (see Fig. 19-8, lower panels). This later disturbance, which had been previously observed in conditions of acute total and partial sleep loss,[117] may reflect decreased efficacy of the negative feedback regulation of the hypothalamic-pituitary-adrenal axis. An elevation of plasma cortisol levels in the afternoon and early evening similar to that observed in our subjects in the sleep debt condition has been previously reported in several studies of normal aging[81,118,119] and could promote the development of insulin resistance and memory impairments.[120,121]

The findings from these laboratory studies are consistent with the conclusions of several epidemiologic studies that revealed a negative association between self-reported sleep duration and body mass index.[122–124] A cohort study of women has shown an increased risk of symptomatic diabetes with short sleep.[125]

SLEEP DISORDERS

Sleep-disordered breathing is the most common sleep disorders, and its incidence is rapidly increasing in parallel with the current epidemic of obesity. A few studies have examined pituitary hormonal release in patients with obstructive apnea before and after treatment.[126–129] As expected, the nocturnal release of the two pituitary hormones, which are markedly dependent on sleep (i.e., GH and prolactin), is decreased in untreated apneic subjects. As illustrated in Figure 19-9, treatment with continuous positive airway pressure (CPAP) results in a clear increase in the amount of GH secreted during the first few hours of sleep.[126,128] The effects of CPAP treatment on overnight prolactin secretion are less clear than those seen for GH.[129] Indeed, the total amount of prolactin secreted during the sleep period is not modified, but the frequency of prolactin pulses is restored to values similar to those observed in normal subjects.

Elevated leptin levels have been consistently observed in patients with sleep apnea when compared with weight-matched nonapneic subjects, and there is a positive correlation between the severity of sleep apnea (as assessed by the apnea-hypopnea index) and morning leptin levels.[130–133] Similarly, levels of the soluble leptin receptor are also elevated.[134] Several studies have reported that CPAP treatment

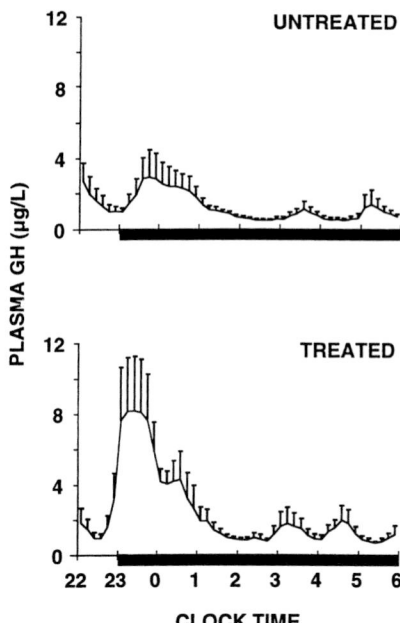

Figure 19-9 Mean profiles of plasma growth hormone (GH) in patients with sleep apnea studied before **(top)** and after **(bottom)** treatment with continuous positive airway pressure. The *vertical line* at each time point represents the standard error of the mean. (Data from Saini et al.[106]) (From Van Cauter E, Spiegel K: Circadian and sleep control of endocrine secretions. In Turek FW, Zee PC [eds]: Neurobiology of Sleep and Circadian Rhythms. New York, Marcel Dekker, 1999, pp 397–426.)

decreases morning leptin levels.[135–138] In several studies, CPAP has also been shown to improve insulin sensitivity and sleep apnea is now recognized as an independent risk factor for insulin resistance.[134,139–143]

Some much less prevalent forms of sleep disorders seem to originate from a disturbance in the circadian system.[144] Delayed sleep-phase insomnia is characterized by a chronic inability to fall asleep at a normal bedtime and to awake in the morning. Nonpharmacologic chronotherapy involving repeated scheduled exposure to bright light is the treatment of choice for this disorder.[145] In contrast, in the advanced sleep-phase syndrome, the timing of the major sleep episode is advanced in relation to normal bedtime, resulting in symptoms of extreme evening sleepiness and early morning awakening. Recent studies have indicated that familial forms of this syndrome could reflect an autosomal-dominant mutation.[146]

ULTRADIAN RHYTHMS

RANGE OF ULTRADIAN RHYTHMS

The term *ultradian* is primarily used to designate rhythms with periods ranging from fractions of hours to several hours. Ultradian oscillations are often less regular and less reproducible than circadian rhythms. In most cases, they appear to represent an optimal functional status within the system in which they occur rather than serve the primary function of a clock, that is, an accurate time measuring device. There is a wide variety of ultradian rhythms. The most prominent are pulsatile hormonal release and the alternating of REM and non-REM stages in sleep. In the human, the approximately 90-minute REM-non-REM cycle is accompanied by similar periodicity of dreaming, penile erections, sympathovagal balance, and breathing. Kleitman[147] has suggested that this ultradian rhythm during sleep was a reflection of a basic rest-activity cycle, which would occur during wakefulness as well. This con-

cept has received some experimental support from a study demonstrating the existence of an ultradian rhythm of brain electrical activity in the frequency range 13 to 35 Hz, an index of central alertness, during waking.[148] Interestingly, pulses of cortisol release were significantly associated with ultradian oscillations in alertness.[148]

Oscillations at frequencies higher than the hourly (i.e., circhoral) range characterizing pulsatile release have been observed for a variety of hormones. In particular, rapid oscillations of insulin secretion with periods in the 10- to 15-minute range have been well characterized in humans,[149,150] monkeys,[151] and dogs.[152]

PROPERTIES AND CLINICAL IMPLICATIONS OF PULSATILE HORMONAL RELEASE

In the endocrine system, ultradian variations have been observed for anterior and posterior pituitary hormones, for hormones under direct pituitary control, and for other endocrine variables such as parathyroid hormone, norepinephrine, plasma renin activity, leptin, and insulin secretion. The interval of recurrence of pulses varies from hormone to hormone and from species to species. The relative importance of pulsatile or oscillatory secretory activity versus tonic release also varies from one axis to the other. For some hormones, secretory activity appears to be entirely pulsatile, with no detectable secretion between pulses. In normal men, evidence suggestive of intermittent secretion without tonic release has been obtained for luteinizing hormone (LH), follicle-stimulating hormone (FSH), GH, and adrenocorticotropic hormone (ACTH).[153–155] For some hormones, pulsatile release is superimposed on a tonic level of secretion or secretion occurs continuously but is increased and decreased in an oscillatory fashion. Pancreatic insulin secretion is a well-established example of this type of ultradian oscillation.[156,157] Evidence of the existence of tonic secretion has also been obtained for pituitary prolactin and TSH release.[153,154]

The pulsatile nature of hormonal release implies that changes well in excess of 100% may occur within less than 1 hour. Therefore, it is necessary to obtain multiple samples to estimate the mean circulating level of many hormones. For many hormones, frequent sampling is also necessary to determine the presence or absence of a circadian rhythm. Therefore, measurement of the cortisol level on only two blood samples taken in the morning (i.e., between 8:00 and 10:00 A.M.) and in the late afternoon (i.e., between 4:00 and 6:00 P.M.) is no longer used to assess the normality of the diurnal variation in the diagnostic workup of Cushing's syndrome.

The physiologic significance of pulsatile hormone secretion was first proven when the essential role of the episodic nature of gonadotropin-releasing hormone (GnRH) release for the normal functioning of the pituitary-ovarian axis was demonstrated.[158] Landmark studies showed that continuous infusions of exogenous GnRH in rhesus monkeys with lesions of the arcuate nucleus, which abolished endogenous GnRH production, inhibited the secretion of LH and FSH. In contrast, the pulsatile administration of the synthetic hypothalamic hormone at a rate of one 6-minute pulse per hour restored normal LH and FSH levels.[158] Furthermore, if the rate of pulse delivery was increased to three pulses per hour or decreased to one pulse every 2 hours, serum LH and FSH levels were partly inhibited. The findings from the early studies on GnRH pulsatility were rapidly applied to the treatment of a variety of disorders of the pituitary-gonadal axis[159] and led the way to the discovery of the functional significance of pulsatility in other endocrine systems. For example, it was found that oscillatory administration of insulin with a period matching that of the normal pulsatility of insulin secretion is more effective in lowering glucose levels than constant infusion.[160]

METHODOLOGIC ASPECTS OF THE STUDY OF ENDOCRINE RHYTHMS

EXPERIMENTAL PROTOCOLS

The majority of investigations of circadian rhythms of hormonal release are based on a transversal design, that is, a group of individuals are studied for a minimum of 24 hours each, following the same experimental protocol. The demonstration of circadian rhythmicity is then based on the observation of consistently reproducible characteristics in the observed set of temporal profiles. The group of subjects should be as homogeneous as possible not only in terms of physical parameters such as age and gender but also in terms of living habits such as sleep-wake cycles, exercise habits, and meal schedules. Subjects who have regular social habits and describe themselves as "good sleepers" should be preferred. Shift workers or subjects having made a transmeridian flight less than 2 months before the experiment should be excluded. Before the beginning of the experiment, the volunteers should be asked to adhere to a standardized schedule of meals and bedtimes for several days to maximize interindividual synchronization. The use of continuous wrist activity recording during the prestudy period is a convenient way to monitor compliance. At least one night of habituation to the laboratory environment and recording procedures should be included. To avoid disruptions of sleep due to the sampling procedure, the catheter should be connected to tubing extending to an adjoining room during the night. Because of the modulatory effects exerted by sleep stages on hormonal release, it is important to obtain polygraphic sleep recordings using standardized methods for recording and scoring. Daytime naps should be avoided. The catheter should be inserted at least 2 hours before the collection of the first sample to avoid possible artifactual effects related to the venepuncture stress. To obtain valid estimations of the circadian parameters, it is necessary to sample at intervals not exceeding 1 hour.

If hormonal profiles are measured as markers of the output of the central circadian oscillator, as is often the case for the 24-hour cortisol profile, direct effects of other factors need to be minimized. Sleep-wake transitions, meals, stressful activity, and postural changes may all be reflected in increases or decreases of hormonal secretion. To eliminate these "masking" effects, experimental protocols usually referred to as "constant routines" have been developed to reliably derive estimates of circadian amplitude and phase from temporal patterns of peripheral hormones and other physiologic variables such as body temperature. "Constant routine" conditions generally involve a regimen of continuous wakefulness, constant recumbent posture, constant illumination, and constant caloric intake either in the form of hourly identical aliquots of liquid diet or solid food or a constant glucose infusion. Although such constant routine conditions have been extensively used in basic studies of human circadian rhythmicity, the sleep deprivation inherent to this protocol is an obvious limitation. The use of circadian markers that are not masked by sleep, meals, and other factors, such as the 24-hour profile of melatonin, has therefore been advocated. Finally, if only circadian phase, and not amplitude, is of interest, measurements of both free cortisol and melatonin levels in saliva during the evening and first half of the night provide a noninvasive way to observe the timings of two neuroendocrine events timed by the circadian clock: the onset of nocturnal melatonin secretion and the onset of the circadian increase of cortisol release.

To characterize episodic hormonal fluctuations, considerations on the total amount of blood withdrawn and the amount of plasma needed to assay the hormones under study are obviously essential to the definition of an adequate sampling protocol. The definition of an optimal sampling protocol thus depends on the type of phenomenon under study. Sampling rates of 1 and 2 minutes will uncover high-frequency, low-amplitude episodic variations superimposed on the slower pulsatile release at intervals of 1 to 2 hours. Sampling rates of 20 and 30 minutes will only detect major pulses lasting more than 1 hour.

PROCEDURES TO QUANTIFY CIRCADIAN VARIATIONS

To determine rhythm parameters in biologic time series, mathematical procedures are necessary. Among the methods proposed for and applied to 24-hour profiles of blood components, the oldest is the Cosinor test.[161] The major disadvantage of this test and of its derivatives is its assumption that the observed profile may be adequately described by a single sinusoidal curve. This assumption is practically never met for biologic rhythms, which are asymmetrical in nature (e.g., the sleep-wake cycle is an 08:16 alternation, not 12:12). Therefore, the Cosinor test generally provides unreliable estimations of rhythm parameters.

Other procedures for the detection and estimation of circadian variation have been based on periodogram calculations or on nonlinear regression procedures.[162,163] These methods provide an adequate description of asymmetric waveshapes. The times of occurrence of the maximum and the minimum of the best-fit curve are often referred to as the acrophase and the nadir, respectively. The amplitude of the rhythm may be estimated as 50% of the difference between the maximum and the minimum of the best-fit curve. With the periodogram procedure, confidence intervals for the amplitude, acrophase, and nadir may be calculated.

PROCEDURES TO QUANTIFY PULSATILE HORMONAL SECRETION

The analysis of pulsatile variations may be considered at two levels.[164] One may wish to define and characterize significant variations in peripheral levels based on estimations on the size of measurement error (i.e., primarily assay error). However, under some circumstances, it is possible to mathematically derive secretory rates from the peripheral concentrations.[165–167] This procedure, often referred to as deconvolution, will often reveal more pulses of secretion than the analysis of peripheral concentrations. It will also more accurately define the temporal limits of each pulse. However, deconvolution involves an amplification of measurement error, with increased risk of false-positive error. Whether examining peripheral concentrations or secretory rates, there are two major approaches to analyzing the episodic fluctuations. The first, and most commonly used, is the time domain analysis, in which the data are plotted against time and pulses are detected and identified. The second is the analysis in the frequency domain, in which amplitude is plotted against frequency or period. The time domain analysis will provide an estimation of pulse frequency, calculated as the total number of pulses detected divided by the duration of the study period. The regularity of pulsatile behavior may be quantified by examining the distribution of interpulse intervals. Alternatively, the issue of regularity of pulsatile behavior may be approached by examining the distribution of spectral power in a frequency domain analysis.[168] Finally, another analytical tool, the approximate entropy has been introduced to quantify the regularity of oscillatory behavior in endocrine and other physiologic time series.[169]

A number of computer algorithms for identification of pulses of hormonal concentration have been proposed. A detailed presentation of the operating principles of each of these procedures is beyond the scope of this chapter. Review articles[170,171] provide comparisons of performance of several pulse detection algorithms. These comparisons have indicated that ULTRA, CLUSTER, and DETECT perform similarly when used with appropriate choices of parameters.[171]

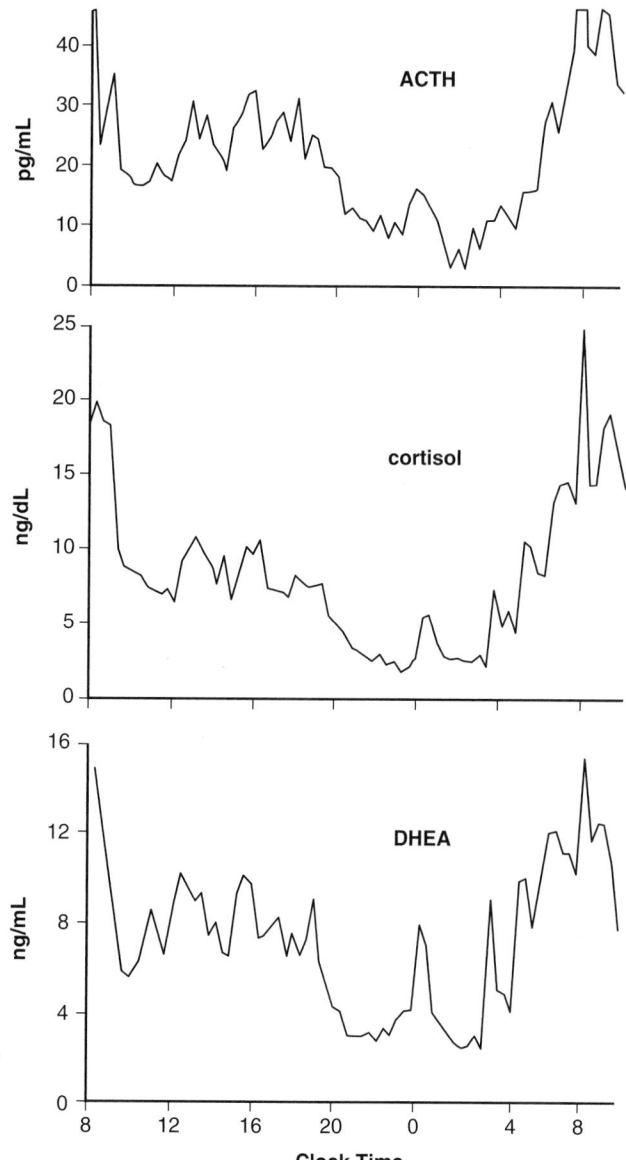

ENDOCRINE RHYTHMS IN HEALTH AND DISEASE

Diurnal and/or ultradian oscillations have been observed in essentially all endocrine systems. An exhaustive review of all such observations is not possible. The following summary of the findings is therefore limited to the various hypothalamic-pituitary axes, parathyroid hormone, hydromineral hormones, glucose and insulin, and hormones involved in appetite regulation.

THE CORTICOTROPIC AXIS

Normal Rhythms of Adrenocorticotropic Hormone and Adrenal Secretions

The temporal organization of the corticotropic axis may be measured peripherally via plasma levels of ACTH and cortisol. The 24-hour profiles of ACTH and cortisol show an early morning maximum, decreasing levels throughout daytime, a quiescent period of minimal secretory activity at around midnight, and an abrupt elevation during late sleep resulting in an early morning maximum. Mathematical derivations of secretory rates from plasma concentrations have suggested that the 24-hour profile of plasma cortisol reflects a succession of secretory pulses of magnitude modulated by a circadian rhythm with no evidence of tonic secretion.[155,172] In normal conditions, the acrophase of the pituitary-adrenal periodicity occurs between 6:00 and 10:00 A.M. With a 15-minute sampling interval, 12 to 18 significant pulses of plasma ACTH and cortisol per 24-hour span can be detected.[173] Circadian and pulsatile variations parallel to those of cortisol have been demonstrated for the plasma levels of several other adrenal steroids, in particular dehydroepiandrosterone.[174] The temporal concomitance of 24-hour profiles of ACTH, cortisol, and dehydroepiandrosterone is illustrated in Figure 19-10.

The 24-hour rhythm of adrenal secretion is primarily dependent on the diurnal pattern of ACTH release. The rhythm in ACTH release results, in turn, from periodic changes in the level of stimulation by corticotropin-releasing hormone. The profiles shown in the upper panels of Figure 19-4 illustrate the remarkable persistence of the cortisol and, by inference, ACTH secretory rhythm when sleep is manipulated. Indeed, the overall wave shape of the profile was not markedly affected by the absence or presence of sleep at an abnormal time of day. Thus, this rhythm is primarily controlled by the circadian pacemaker.

Modulatory effects of sleep-wake homeostasis have, however, been clearly demonstrated. As illustrated in Figure 19-11, sleep onset is consistently associated with a short-term inhibition of cortisol secretion (which may not be detectable when sleep is initiated in the morning, i.e., at the peak of corticotropic activity).[175-178] This inhibitory effect of sleep appears to be related to SWS stages.[179-182] Conversely, as illustrated in Figure 19-11, awakening from sleep is consistently followed by a secretory cortisol pulse.[177,183,184] Under conditions of sleep deprivation, the nadir of cortisol levels is higher (because of the absence of the inhibitory effects of sleep) and the acrophase is lower (because of the absence of the stimulatory action of morning awakening), so that the amplitude of the cortisol circadian variations is reduced by approximately 15%. Transient awakenings interrupting the sleep period consistently trigger pulses of cortisol secretion.[155,179,183] In an analysis of cortisol profiles during nocturnal sleep, it was observed that all transient awakenings interrupting sleep and lasting at least 10 minutes were followed within the next 20 minutes by significant bursts of cortisol secretion.[185] In addition, a temporal coupling of pulses of cortisol secretion and ultradian variations in an EEG marker of alertness has been reported.[148]

Modulatory effects of dark-light transitions have also been demonstrated. Cortisol secretory pulses associated with morning awakening are enhanced by increasing light intensity.[186]

Figure 19-10 Twenty-four hour profiles of plasma adrenocorticotropic hormone (ACTH), cortisol, and dehydroepiandrosterone (DHEA) levels sampled at 20-minute intervals in a healthy young man. Note the temporal concomitance of circadian and pulsatile variations of the three hormones. (Unpublished data kindly provided by Dr. K. Spiegel.)

Moreover, the transition from to darkness to dim light and from dim to bright light may also stimulate cortisol secretion in subjects who are awake at bed rest.[185,187] When dark-light and sleep-wake transitions occur concomitantly, associated cortisol elevations are nearly twice as high as when the final awakening occurs in continuous darkness[185] (see Fig. 19-11). Thus, in usual bedtime schedules, both the sleep-wake and the dark-light transitions amplify the effects of circadian rhythmicity.

Studies of the 24-hour cortisol profile in the course of adaptation to shifts of the sleep-wake cycle have demonstrated that the end of the quiescent period, which coincides with the onset of the early morning increase, takes longer to adjust and appears to be a robust marker of circadian timing. Twin studies have demonstrated that the timing of the nadir is influenced by genetic factors,[188] providing evidence of a genetic control of the human circadian phase. In contrast, the timing of the morning acrophase is more labile and may be influenced by the timing of sleep offset,[184] the transition from

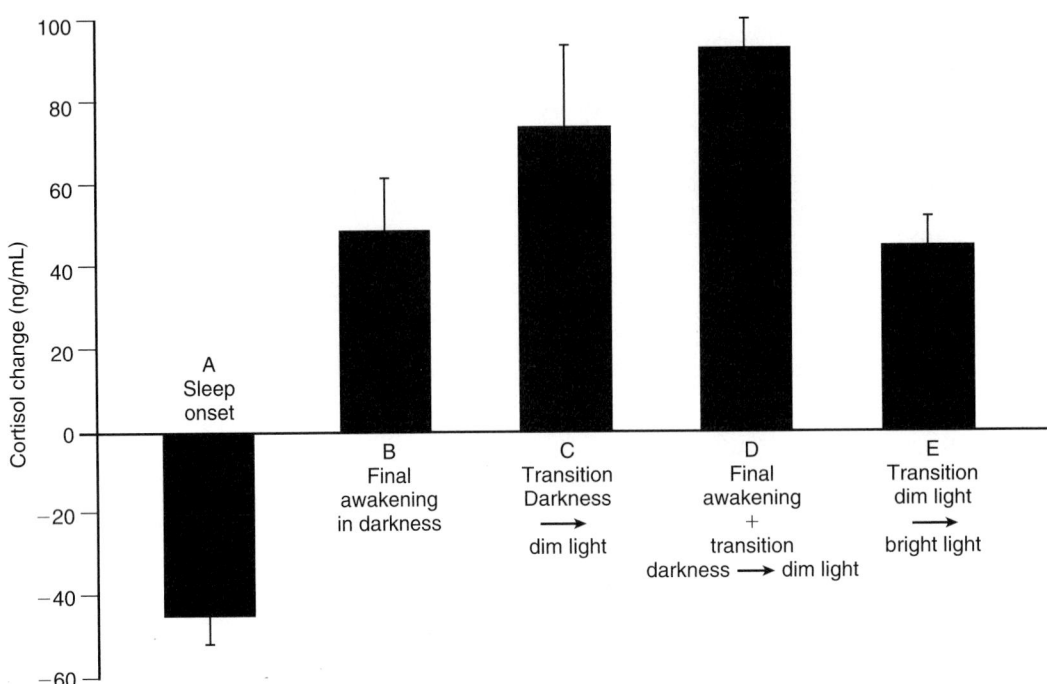

Figure 19-11   Mean (and standard error of the mean) changes in plasma cortisol levels: within 120 minutes after sleep onset at 3:00 P.M. (*n* = 32) **(A)**; within 20-minutes after final spontaneous awakening in darkness (scheduled sleep period 11:00 P.M.–7:00 A.M. or 3:00–11:00 P.M.; in *n* = 10) **(B)**; within 20-minutes after transition from darkness to dim light at 7:00 A.M. or 11:00 P.M. in subjects awake at bed rest (*n* = 10) **(C)**; within 20-minutes after final awakening concomitant with transition from darkness to dim light at 7:00 A.M. or 11:00 P.M. (*n* = 38) **(D)**; within 15 minutes after transition from dim to bright light at 5:00 A.M. in subjects awake at bed rest (*n* = 8) **(E)**. (**A–D,** Data from Caufriez A, Moreno-Reyes R, Leproult R, et al: Immediate effects of an 8-h advance shift of the rest-activity cycle on 24-h profiles of cortisol. Am J Physiol 282:E1147–E1153, 2002; **E,** data from Leproult R, Colecchia EF, L'Hermite-Balériaux M, et al: Transition from dim to bright light in the morning induces an immediate elevation of cortisol levels. J Clin Endocrinol Metab 86:151–157, 2001.)

dark to bright light,[186] and breakfast intake.[189] Finally, anticipation of the expected time of waking has been reported to be associated with an increase in ACTH, but not cortisol, levels during the end of the sleep period.[190]

In addition to the immediate modulatory effects of sleep-wake transitions on ACTH and cortisol levels, nocturnal sleep deprivation, whether partial or total, acute (one night) or semichronic (2 week), results in increased cortisol concentrations on the following evening[115,117] (see Fig. 19-8). Chronic insomnia was also found to be associated with higher cortisol levels throughout the night,[191] but it is unclear whether this relative hypercortisolism resulted from the sleep loss or, alternatively, whether insomnia was induced by the hyperactivity of the corticotropic axis. In any case, sleep loss appears to delay the return to quiescence of the hypothalamic-pituitary-adrenal axis normally occurring in the evening. This suggests that sleep loss, similar to aging, may slow down the rate of recovery of the hypothalamic-pituitary-adrenal axis response after a challenge and could therefore facilitate the development of central and peripheral disturbances associated with glucocorticoid excess, in particular with increased cortisol concentrations at the time of the normal daily nadir, such as memory deficits, insulin resistance, and osteoporosis.[120,192–195]

The circadian rhythm of cortisol persists throughout adulthood and has been observed through the ninth decade.[81,119] In young adults, 24-hour cortisol levels are slightly lower in women than in men, primarily because of lower morning maxima. With aging, evening cortisol levels increase progressively, both in men and women, so that the cortisol nadir is three- to fourfold higher in healthy subjects older than 70 years of age than in young adults. Interestingly, this increase in evening cortisol levels occurs with a chronology similar to that observed for a progressive decrease in the duration of REM sleep[84] (see Fig. 19-6). As a result, older subjects have elevated 24-hour mean cortisol levels and a

reduced amplitude of cortisol variations. In addition, the timing of the nadir is advanced by 1 to 2 hours, indicating that aging is associated with an advance of the circadian phase.[81,119]

In pregnancy, total and, to a much lesser extent, free cortisol levels are elevated, but the circadian pattern of secretion persists, albeit set at a higher level.[196] Interestingly, placental corticotropin-releasing hormone is secreted into the maternal circulation in a pulsatile but not a circadian fashion, and there is no correlation between maternal levels of corticotropin-releasing hormone and ACTH. Remarkably, ACTH and cortisol concentrations remain strongly correlated with each other over time, suggesting that diurnal variation of maternal ACTH is probably driven by another ACTH secretagogue, most likely arginine vasopressin.[197]

Alterations in Disease States
The 24-hour profile of pituitary-adrenal secretion remains largely unaltered in a wide variety of pathologic states. Disease states in which pronounced alterations of the cortisol rhythm have been observed include primarily (1) disorders involving abnormalities in binding and/or metabolism of cortisol, (2) the various forms of Cushing's syndrome, and (3) severe depression.

The relative amplitude of the circadian rhythm and of the episodic fluctuations of cortisol is blunted in patients with liver disease[198] and in those with anorexia nervosa,[199] primarily because of the decreased metabolic clearance of cortisol. In patients with hypothyroidism, the mean level is markedly elevated, and the relative amplitude of the rhythm is therefore dampened.[200] These alterations are thought to be due to both diminished clearance and decreased efficiency of the feedback control. In contrast, in hyperthyroidism, in which cortisol production and peripheral metabolism are increased, episodic pulses are enhanced.[201]

In patients with Cushing's syndrome secondary to adrenal adenoma or ectopic ACTH secretion, the circadian variation of plasma cortisol is invariably absent.[202] In contrast, a low-amplitude circadian variation may persist in pituitary-dependent Cushing's disease. Cortisol pulsatility is blunted in approximately 70% of patients with Cushing's disease, suggesting autonomous tonic secretion of ACTH by a pituitary tumor. However, in approximately 30% of these patients, the magnitude of the pulses is instead enhanced.[203] These hyperpulsatile patterns could be caused by enhanced hypothalamic release of corticotropin-releasing hormone or persistent pituitary responsiveness to corticotropin-releasing hormone. It has also been shown that patients with Cushing's disease secrete ACTH and cortisol jointly more asynchronously than healthy subjects.[204] The left and middle panels of Figure 19-12 compare representative and mean 24-hour cortisol profiles in normal subjects and patients with Cushing's disease.

The absence or even the dampening of cortisol circadian variations in Cushing's syndrome has obvious implications for clinical diagnosis because the time of day when plasma samples are obtained must be taken into account in the evaluation of the result. Differentiation between normal and pathologic levels may actually be greatly improved by adequately selecting the sampling time because the overlap between normal individual values and values in patients with Cushing's syndrome is minimal during a 4-hour interval around midnight.

Hypercortisolism with persistent circadian rhythmicity and increased pulsatility is found in a majority of severely depressed patients.[205-207] This is illustrated in the right panel of Figure 19-12. In these patients, who do not develop the clinical signs of Cushing's syndrome despite the high circulating cortisol levels, the quiescent period of cortisol secretion is shorter and more fragmented and often starts later and ends earlier than in normal subjects of comparable age. These alterations could reflect the impact of sleep disturbances as well as an advance of the circadian phase. When a clinical remission of the depressed state is obtained, the hypercortisolism and the alterations in quiescent period disappear, indicating that these disturbances are state rather than trait dependent.[208]

In posttraumatic stress disorder, some authors have reported that plasma cortisol levels are decreased in the afternoon and/or in the evening and that the amplitude of circadian variations is enhanced.[209-211] Yehuda[210] has suggested that low cortisol levels may represent a risk factor for the development of a stress disorder after exposure to a trauma because similar alterations of the cortisol rhythm were found in healthy subjects who have a parent with posttraumatic stress disorder. In fibromyalgia and chronic fatigue syndrome, cortisol levels have been reported to be low, normal, or elevated,[212-214] depending on the study, but ACTH and cortisol pulsatility were found to be normal.[214] In a well-documented study performed in constant routine conditions, normal circadian variations of plasma cortisol levels were evidenced in women with fibromyalgia.[215] Saliva cortisol levels appear blunted in the early morning in the so-called burnout syndrome.[216]

THE SOMATOTROPIC AXIS

The 24-Hour Profile of Growth Hormone in Normal Subjects

Pituitary secretion of GH is stimulated by hypothalamic GH-releasing hormone and inhibited by somatostatin. In addition, the acylated form of ghrelin, a peptide produced predominantly by the stomach, binds to the GH secretagogue receptor and is therefore another potent endogenous stimulus of GH secretion.[217,218] In normal adult subjects, the 24-hour profile of plasma GH levels consists of stable low levels abruptly interrupted by bursts of secretion. The most reproducible pulse occurs shortly after sleep onset, in association with the first phase of SWS.[219] Other secretory pulses may occur in later sleep and during wakefulness, in the absence of any identifiable stimulus. Studies in young male twins have demonstrated a major genetic effect on GH secretion during waking but not during sleep.[220] In adult men, the sleep-onset GH pulse is generally the largest, and often the only, pulse observed over the 24-hour span. In normally cycling women, the 24-hour GH levels are higher than in age-matched men, daytime pulses are more frequent, and the sleep-associated pulse, although still present in most cases, does not generally account for the majority of the 24-hour GH release.[221] Typical profiles of young men and women are shown in Figure 19-13. Well-documented studies have demonstrated that, in women, the amplitude of GH secretory pulses is correlated with the circulating level of estradiol.[221,222] In normally cycling young women, it was also observed that daytime GH secretion was increased during the luteal phase as compared with the follicular phase and that this elevation correlated positively with plasma levels of progesterone but not estradiol.[223]

Sleep onset will elicit a GH secretory pulse whether sleep is advanced, delayed, interrupted, or fragmented.[219] Thus, as illustrated in Figure 19-4, shifts of the sleep-wake cycle are immediately followed by parallel shifts of the GH rhythm.[219] In night workers, the main GH secretory episode occurs during

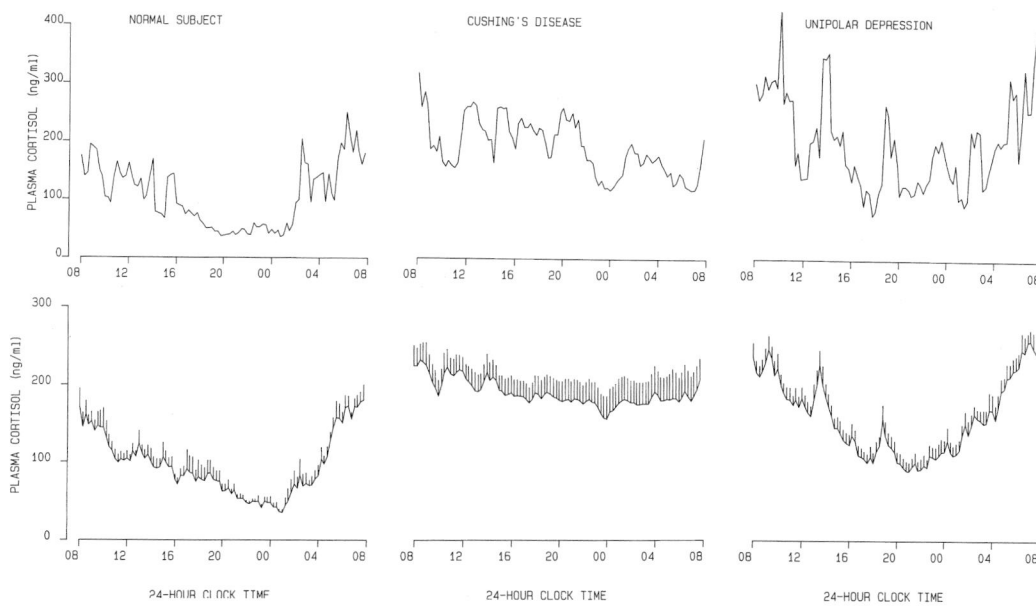

Figure 19-12 Twenty-four-hour profiles of plasma cortisol in normal subjects **(left)**, patients with pituitary Cushing's disease **(middle)**, and patients with major endogenous depression of the unipolar subtype **(right)**. For each condition, a representative example is shown in the top panel and mean profiles from 8 to 10 subjects are shown in the lower panel. In the **lower panel,** the *vertical line* at each time point represents the standard error of the mean. (From Van Cauter E: Physiology and pathology of circadian rhythms. In Edwards CW, Lincoln DW [eds]: Recent Advances in Endocrinology and Metabolism. Edinburgh, Churchill Livingstone, 1989, vol 3, pp 109–134.)

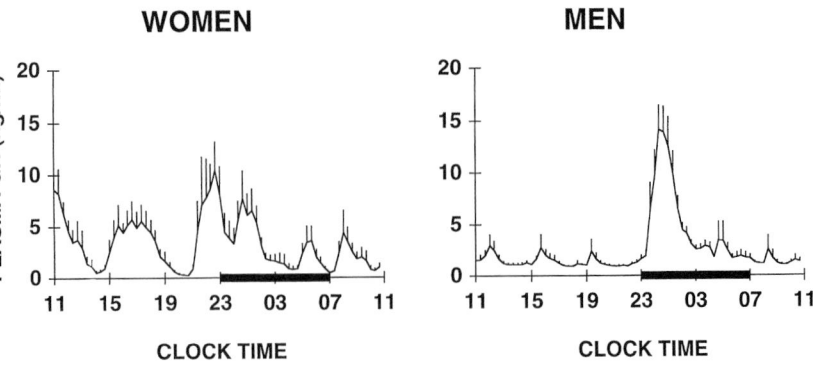

Figure 19-13   Mean (± standard error of the mean) 24-hour plasma growth hormone profiles in nine men (age 18–30 years) and in seven women (age 21–33 years) during the follicular phase. The *solid bars* represent the sleep periods. (Adapted from Van Cauter E, Plat L, Copinschi G: Interrelations between sleep and the somatotropic axis. Sleep 21:533–566, 1998.)

the first half of the shifted sleep period.[108] The release of GH in early sleep is temporally and quantitatively associated with the amount of SWS.[224,225] There is good evidence that the mechanisms underlying the relationship between SWS and GH release involve synchronous activity of at least two different populations of hypothalamic GH-releasing hormone neurons.[226] Indeed, inhibition of endogenous GH-releasing hormone, either by administration of a specific antagonist or immunoneutralization, inhibits sleep as well as GH secretion.[227] Additional evidence for the existence of a robust relationship between SWS activity and GH release is provided by studies using pharmacologic stimulation of SWS. Indeed, enhancement of SWS by oral administration of low doses of γ-hydroxybutyrate, a natural metabolite of γ-aminobutyric acid used in the treatment of narcolepsy,[228] or of ritanserin, a selective 5-HT2 antagonist,[229] results in simultaneous and highly correlated increases in nocturnal GH secretion. Conversely, transient awakenings during sleep inhibit GH secretion.[230] Thus, sleep fragmentation will generally decrease nocturnal GH release.

However, although sleep is clearly the major determinant of GH secretion in humans, there is also evidence of the existence of a circadian modulation of the occurrence and amplitude of GH pulses, reflecting decreased somatostatin inhibitory activity in the evening and during the night.[231] Thus, the major sleep onset–associated GH pulse is caused by a surge of hypothalamic GH-releasing hormone coincident with a circadian period of relative somatostatin disinhibition.[219,227] It is also possible that ghrelin plays a role because the normal 24-hour profile of total ghrelin (i.e., acylated and nonacylated) exhibits a marked nocturnal elevation.[232] Sleep enhances nocturnal plasma ghrelin levels in healthy subjects.[233] Presleep GH pulses, reported by some investigators, in normal subjects[234] could reflect the circadian component of GH secretion.

After a night of total sleep deprivation, a compensatory increase in GH release is observed during the daytime, so that the overall 24-hour secretion is not significantly altered.[235] The mechanisms underlying this compensatory increase might involve decreased somatostatinergic tone and/or elevated ghrelin levels. Semichronic partial sleep restriction is consistently associated with the appearance of a presleep GH pulse.[236]

Aging is associated with dramatic decreases in circulating levels of GH.[81,221] This reduction is achieved by a decrease in amplitude rather than in frequency of GH pulses.[81,237,238] It has also been suggested that the orderliness of GH secretion is decreased in the elderly.[239] As illustrated in Figure 19-6, this age-related GH decrease occurs in an exponential fashion between young adulthood and midlife and follows the same chronology of the decrease in SWS. Despite the persistence of high levels of sex steroids, plasma concentrations and pulsatile secretion rates of GH decrease in midlife to less than half of the values achieved in young adulthood. Thereafter, smaller and more progressive decrements occur from midlife to old age.[84] In the elderly, GH secretory profiles are similar in men and women.[221] The age-related reduction of GH secre-

tion appears to result from increased somatostatin secretion and diminished GH-releasing responsiveness.[240]

Interestingly, during pregnancy, a placental GH variant, which substitutes for pituitary GH to regulate maternal insulin-like growth factor 1 levels,[241] is released in a tonic rather than pulsatile fashion.[242]

Alterations in Disease States

Abnormalities in the 24-hour profile of plasma GH have been reported in a variety of metabolic, endocrine, neurologic, and psychiatric conditions. We briefly describe the major alterations found in those conditions for which the temporal pattern has been defined in detail. There is an inverse relationship between adiposity and GH release that results in a marked suppression of GH levels throughout the 24-hour span in obese subjects. A reduction in pulse frequency, as well as a decrease in GH half-life, has been suggested to underlie the hyposomatotropism of obesity.[243] A normal pattern can be restored after prolonged fasting.[244] In normal-weight subjects, fasting, even for only 1 day, enhances GH secretion via an increase in both pulse amplitude and pulse frequency.[245] In anorexia nervosa, GH pulse amplitude and frequency are increased and the orderliness of GH release is disrupted.[246] Nonobese patients with juvenile or maturity-onset diabetes hypersecrete GH during wakefulness and sleep, primarily because of an increase in amplitude of pulses.[247] This abnormality may disappear when glycemia is strictly controlled.

In functional hypothalamic amenorrhea, the 24-hour mean GH levels are normal, but the pattern of pulsatile GH release is distinctly altered, with a decrease in pulse amplitude, a 40% increase in pulse frequency and a twofold increase in interpulse GH concentrations.[248] In lean women with polycystic ovary syndrome (PCOS), the amplitude, but not the frequency, of GH pulses is increased as compared with body mass index–matched normally cycling controls. In contrast, pulse amplitude is similarly reduced in both obese PCOS and obese controls.[249]

Diurnal and nocturnal episodes of GH secretion are more frequent and of higher amplitude in adult subjects with hyperthyroidism, who have an overall daily GH production rate fourfold greater than normal.[250] Patients with major endogenous depression often have the major nocturnal GH pulse before rather than after sleep onset.[251]

As discussed earlier, the nocturnal GH release is decreased in patients with untreated obstructive apnea.[126–129] Treatment with CPAP results in a clear increase in the amount of GH secreted during the first few hours of sleep.[126,128] In Cushing's disease, there is an inverse relationship between the degree of cortisol hypersecretion and total GH secretion, and the frequency and disorderliness of GH pulses are increased.[252] In acromegaly, GH is hypersecreted throughout the 24-hour span, with a highly irregular pulsatile pattern superimposed over elevated basal levels, indicative of the presence of tonic secretion.[253,254] After pituitary surgery, a normal 24-hour pattern of GH release can be restored in most, but not all, patients.[253,255]

THE LACTOTROPIC AXIS

The 24-Hour Profile of Prolactin in Normal Subjects

Under normal conditions, the 24-hour profile of prolactin levels exhibits minimal levels around noon, a modest increase in the afternoon, followed by a major nocturnal elevation starting shortly after sleep onset and culminating around mid-sleep[256,257] at levels corresponding with an average increase of more than 200% above minimal levels (see Fig. 19-4).[258,259] Episodic pulses occur throughout the 24-hour span, but their amplitude and frequency are higher during the night than the day. Decreased dopaminergic inhibition of prolactin secretion during sleep is likely to be the primary mechanism underlying this nocturnal elevation. Mean prolactin levels, pulse amplitude, and pulse frequency are all higher in normally cycling women than in either postmenopausal women or normal young men.[260] These data indicate that endogenous estrogens play a critical role in the differential regulation of prolactin secretion associated with gender and age. Deconvolution analysis has shown that the prolactin profile reflects both tonic and intermittent release.[154] Twin studies have revealed that genetic factors determine partially the temporal organization of prolactin secretion.[261]

Diurnal prolactin variations are primarily regulated by sleep-wake homeostasis. Sleep onset is invariably associated with an increase in prolactin secretion, irrespective of the time of the day. Thus, as illustrated in Figure 19-4, shifts of the sleep-wake cycle are immediately followed by parallel shifts of the prolactin rhythm,[219] but the amplitude of the prolactin increase may be dampened when associated with daytime sleep compared with nocturnal sleep.[262] Conversely, modest elevations of prolactin levels may occur during waking around the time of the usual sleep onset, particularly in women.[259] Thus, prolactin secretion appears to be modulated by circadian rhythmicity and maximal secretion occurs when sleep and circadian effects are superimposed, that is, at the usual bedtime.[258,259,263] Benzodiazepine (e.g., triazolam) and imidazopyridine (e.g., zolpidem) hypnotics taken at bedtime generally enhance the nocturnal prolactin elevation.[264,265]

A close temporal relationship has been demonstrated between increased prolactin secretion and SWS activity when sleep structure was characterized by power spectral analysis of the EEG.[266] Conversely, prolonged awakenings interrupting sleep are consistently associated with decreasing prolactin concentrations.[266] Thus, shallow and fragmented sleep will generally be associated with a dampening of the nocturnal prolactin increase. This is indeed observed in elderly subjects who have a nearly 50% dampening of the nocturnal prolactin elevation (see Fig. 19-5).[81,267]

During pregnancy, serum prolactin levels rise, but the 24-hour pattern of secretion is maintained, albeit at a higher level. During the postpartum period, prolactin secretory pulses follow suckling episodes and the nocturnal increase, independent of suckling, is only evident once breastfeeding has ceased.[268]

Alterations in Disease States

Absence or blunting of the nocturnal increase of plasma prolactin has been reported in a variety of pathologic states, including uremia and breast cancer in postmenopausal women. In Cushing's disease, prolactin levels are elevated throughout the 24-hour cycle and the relative amplitude of the nighttime increase is reduced.[269] In subjects with insulin-dependent diabetes, the circadian and sleep modulation of prolactin secretion is preserved, but overall levels are markedly diminished.[270] In patients with untreated obstructive apnea, the nocturnal prolactin release is decreased.[129]

In hyperprolactinemia associated with prolactinomas or secondary to functional pituitary stalk disconnection, the number of prolactin pulses is increased and the regularity of the pulsatile pattern is decreased.[271,272] The nocturnal elevation of prolactin may be preserved.[272,273] Selective removal of prolactin-secreting adenomas generally results in the normalization of the prolactin pattern.

Abnormal prolactin profiles have also been reported in a variety of neurologic and psychiatric disorders, including narcolepsy, depression, and schizophrenia.

THE GONADOTROPIC AXIS

Normal Diurnal Profiles of Luteinizing Hormone, Follicle-Stimulating Hormone, Testosterone, and Estradiol

Rhythms in the gonadotropic axis cover a wide range of frequencies, from episodic release in the ultradian range to diurnal rhythmicity and menstrual cycles. These various rhythms interact to provide a coordinated temporal program governing the development of the reproductive axis and its operation at every stage of maturation. The following description of the current state of knowledge in this area will be limited on 24-hour rhythms and their interaction with pulsatile release during adulthood.

Patterns of LH release in adult men exhibit episodic pulses with large interindividual variability.[274] The diurnal variation is dampened or even undetectable. During the sleep period, LH pulses appear to be temporally related to the REM-non-REM cycle.[275] FSH profiles may show some occasional pulses without any diurnal variation. In contrast, a marked diurnal rhythm in circulating testosterone levels is present in young normal men, with minimal levels in the late evening and maximal levels in the early morning.[174,276] In young adult men, the amplitude of the testosterone rhythm averages 25%.[174] With a 15-minute sampling interval, 17 to 18 testosterone pulses per 24-hour span can be detected.[174] Thus, the robust circadian rhythm of plasma testosterone may be partially controlled by factors other than LH. The nocturnal increase of testosterone is temporally linked to the latency of the first REM episode.[277] Experimental sleep fragmentation (schedule allowing 7 minutes of sleep every 20 minutes) resulted in a dampening of the nocturnal testosterone increase, particularly in subjects who did not achieve REM sleep.[278] Diurnal profiles of testosterone are paralleled by inhibin B variations, with peak values in the early morning and nadirs in the late afternoon; significant cross-correlations between inhibin B and testosterone or estradiol, but not between inhibin B and FSH, were detected.[279]

In older men, the amplitude of LH pulses is decreased,[280,281] but their frequency is increased[282] and no significant diurnal pattern can be detected.[283] In contrast, pulsatile FSH secretion is increased in older men.[284] The circadian variation of testosterone is still present, but may be markedly dampened.[276,283] A strong positive correlation has been evidenced between the amplitude of the 24-hour testosterone rhythm and the amount of REM sleep.[285] Pulsatile testosterone secretion is attenuated, suggesting a possible partial desensitization of Leydig cells to LH.[282] The temporal relationship of the sleep-related testosterone increase to REM latency is no longer detectable.[286] In addition, older males secrete LH and testosterone more irregularly and jointly more asynchronously than younger men.[287]

In adult women, the 24-hour variation in plasma LH is markedly modulated by the menstrual cycle.[288,289] Representative profiles are shown in Figure 19-14. In the early follicular phase, LH pulses are large and infrequent and a slowing of the frequency of secretory pulses occurs during sleep. In the mid-follicular phase, pulse amplitude is decreased, pulse frequency is increased, and the frequency modulation of LH pulsatility by sleep is less apparent. Pulse amplitude increases again by the late follicular phase. In the early luteal phase, the pulse amplitude is markedly increased, the pulse frequency is decreased, and nocturnal slowing of pulsatility is again evident. In the mid-luteal phase, pulse amplitude and frequency are decreased and there

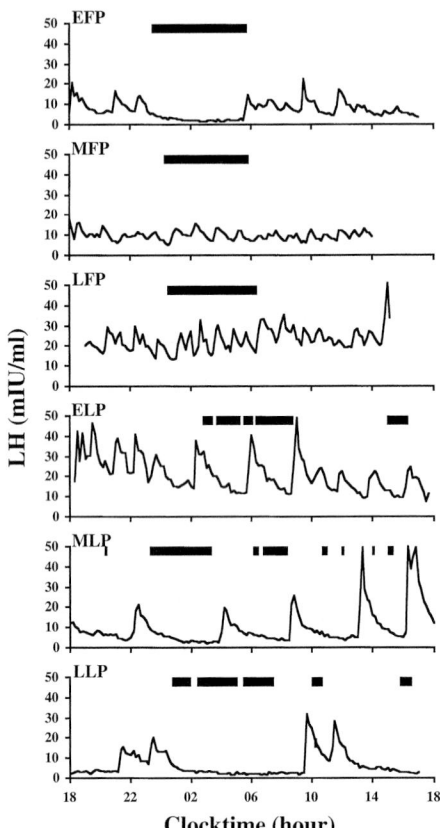

Figure 19-14 Representative 24-hour profiles of plasma luteinizing hormone (LH) in healthy women studied in the early follicular phase (EFP), mid-follicular phase (MFP), late-follicular phase (LFP), early luteal phase (ELP), mid-luteal phase (MLP), and late-luteal phase (LLP). Sleep periods are indicated by *solid bars*. (Adapted from Filicori M, Santoro N, Merriam GR, Crowley WFJ: Characterization of the physiological pattern of episodic gonadotropin secretion throughout the menstrual cycle. J Clin Endocrinol Metab 62:1136–1144, 1986.)

is no modulation by sleep. Both pulse amplitude and frequency further decrease in the late luteal phase. During the luteal-follicular transition, there is a four- to fivefold increase in LH pulse frequency, which accompanies the selective FSH increase necessary for normal folliculogenesis.[290] The apparent inhibitory effect of sleep during the early follicular phase is particularly intriguing because this effect is in the opposite direction from that observed in pubertal girls in whom the sleep period is associated with an increase in LH pulse amplitude and an elevation of overall LH levels. Circulating levels of LH and FSH and LH pulse frequency increase with aging and are higher in normal women older than 40 years of age with regular menstrual cycles than in women younger than age 35. After menopause, gonadotropin levels are elevated but show no consistent circadian pattern.[291]

Alterations in Disease States

Early studies on the 24-hour profile of plasma LH in anorexia nervosa have established the importance of an adequate temporal secretory program in the maintenance of normal reproductive function. In women with amenorrhea secondary to anorexia nervosa, the secretory pattern of LH regresses to the pubertal or prepubertal pattern, with low daytime pulsatility and increased secretion at night.[291] Secretory profiles of LH usually return to normal after weight gain and clinical remission. Short-term fasting was recently shown to suppress pulsatile LH secretion while enhancing its regularity in young, but not older men.[292] States of hyperprolactinemia are associated

with a reduction of LH pulse amplitude and frequency, but normal pulsatile profiles are recovered when prolactin levels are normalized by dopaminergic therapy.[293]

The slowing or absence of pulsatile hypothalamic GnRH release is the underlying cause of ovarian acyclicity in women with functional hypothalamic amenorrhea.[291,294] The reduction appears more marked during the daytime than during sleep, suggesting that the mechanisms involved in this pathologic suppression of pulsatile GnRH release are partially inhibited during sleep.[294] Women afflicted with functional hypothalamic amenorrhea show an approximately 50% reduction in LH pulse frequency and an increase in the LH pulse interval, whereas the integrated plasma LH and FSH concentrations are reduced by 30% to 45%.[248] Decreased LH pulse frequency and amplitude may also be observed in women runners who are normally menstruating,[295] suggesting that exercise-associated amenorrhea is a further development of the alterations in the pattern of GnRH activity seen in eumenorrheic women runners.

Different forms of abnormal temporal organization of the GnRH signal seem involved in the PCOS. In pubertal girls with recent-onset PCOS,[296] the circadian rhythm of LH secretion was found to be out of phase with the sleep-wake cycle so that, in normal pubertal children, LH increased during the night, whereas in patients with PCOS, the LH augmentation occurred during the day. Similar alterations were found in anovulatory healthy adolescent girls at early gynecologic age. Interestingly, these alterations persisted in those of the girls who were still amenorrheic at the late gynecologic age, whereas the diurnal LH variations disappeared in the girls who became ovulatory.[297] Thus, the abnormal circadian timing of the LH rhythm in patients with PCOS might not allow normal ovulatory cycles to develop. In adult patients with PCOS, the amplitude and frequency of LH pulses were consistently found to be increased and overall levels of FSH to be depressed,[249,298,299] suggesting that the excessively rapid GnRH pulsations selectively suppress FSH secretion. A similar defect of abnormally high GnRH frequency seems to underlie luteal phase deficiency. Indeed, studies have shown that, in this condition, LH pulse frequency is increased during the follicular phase, indicating that this temporal alteration may be implicated in the etiology of the condition.[300]

Increased LH pulse frequency and decreased pulse amplitude have also been observed in patients with premenstrual syndrome, and these findings have suggested the possible involvement of opioidergic dysfunction in this condition.[301] Alterations in circadian rhythmicity, consisting of advances in circadian rhythms relative to the timing of the sleep-wake cycle, as well as reduced melatonin levels, have also been found in patients with premenstrual syndrome.[302] These abnormalities may contribute to pathologies associated with premenstrual syndrome, and correcting such circadian disturbances may lead to clinical remission.[302] Patients with late luteal phase dysphoric disorders have abnormally phase-advanced rhythms, and exposure to bright light in the evening, but not in the morning, was effective in inducing a significant reduction in the depression score.[302] Because evening bright light can cause phase delays of circadian rhythms, these results raise the possibility that circadian dysregulation, whether induced by lifestyle, the environment, or the reproductive system itself, may be a common pathogenic factor in mood disorders observed in women.[302]

In the majority of men with idiopathic hypogonadotropic hypogonadism, LH pulses are undetectable.[303] In a small number of patients, an early pubertal pattern, with enhanced pulse amplitude during the nighttime, may be observed.[303] Nocturnal LH and testosterone secretions are decreased in men with untreated obstructive apnea.[304] These alterations are partially corrected during chronic CPAP treatment.[305]

An attenuation of pulsatile LH secretion has been reported in men, but not in women, during both hypo- and hypercortisolism. The authors speculated that this sex difference could be due to a higher level of hypothalamic opioid activity in men.[306] Poorly controlled type 1 diabetes mellitus was found to be associated with decreased amplitude of pulsatile LH secretion.[307]

THE THYROTROPIC AXIS

The 24-Hour Profile of Thyroid-Stimulating Hormone in Normal Subjects

In normal adult men and women, TSH levels are low and relatively stable throughout the daytime and begin to increase in the late afternoon or early evening. Maximal levels occur around the beginning of the sleep period.[182] TSH levels progressively decrease during the later part of sleep, and daytime values resume shortly after morning awakening. Because the onset of the nocturnal increase in TSH occurs well before sleep onset, it is believed to reflect a circadian effect. This 24-hour pattern of TSH levels appears to be generated by frequency as well as amplitude modulation of thyrotropin-releasing hormone (TRH)-driven secretory pulses.[153] Studies involving sleep deprivation and shifts of the sleep-wake cycle have consistently indicated that sleep exerts an inhibitory influence on TSH secretion, and sleep deprivation relieves this inhibition.[182,308] Interestingly, when sleep occurs during the daytime, TSH secretion is not suppressed significantly below normal daytime levels. Profiles of plasma TSH during normal nocturnal sleep, nocturnal sleep deprivation, and daytime sleep are illustrated in the lower panel of Figure 19-4. When the depth of sleep at the habitual time is enhanced by previous sleep deprivation, the inhibition of the nocturnal TSH increase is more pronounced than in basal conditions. Descending slopes of TSH concentrations during sleep are consistently associated with SWS stages, and negative cross-correlations have been found between TSH fluctuations and SWS activity,[309,310] suggesting that SWS is probably the primary determinant of the sleep-associated TSH decrease. Conversely, awakenings are frequently associated with TSH increments.[311] The timing of the TSH evening increase seems to be controlled by circadian rhythmicity and shifts in concordance with the melatonin rhythm after exposure to light or nocturnal exercise.[39]

Circadian and/or sleep-related variations in thyroid hormones are difficult to detect.[312,313] It has been suggested that the nocturnal TSH surge could involve variant TSH molecules with reduced bioactivity. Animal studies indicate that besides the neuroendocrine pathway, the SCN might use neuronal pathways to set the sensitivity of the thyroid gland to TSH and to control the peripheral conversion of thyroxine to triiodothyronine.[314] Under conditions of sleep deprivation, the increased amplitude of the TSH rhythm may result in a detectable increase in plasma triiodothyronine levels, paralleling the nocturnal TSH increase,[311] although negative findings have been also reported.[315] If sleep deprivation is prolonged for a second night, the nocturnal increase in TSH is markedly diminished compared with that occurring during the first night.[315] It is likely that, after the first night of sleep deprivation, the elevated thyroid hormone levels, which persist during the daytime period because of the prolonged half-life of these hormones, limit the subsequent TSH increase. A study involving 64 hours of sleep deprivation demonstrated during the second night of sleep deprivation a nocturnal increase in both triiodothyronine and thyroxine levels, contrasting with the decreases seen during normal sleep.[316] These data suggest that prolonged sleep loss may be associated with an upregulation of the thyroid axis. Consistent findings have been reported in a study of 1 week of partial sleep loss (4 hours in bed per night) in which the nocturnal TSH increase was strikingly decreased, probably secondary to increased levels of thyroid hormones resulting from an initial TSH elevation at the beginning of sleep curtailment (see Fig. 19-7).[115]

Because inhibitory effects of sleep on TSH secretion are time dependent, elevations of plasma TSH levels may occur in conditions of misalignment of sleep and circadian timing. This is illustrated in Figure 19-15, which shows the mean profiles of plasma TSH observed in a group of normal young men in the course of adaptation to simulated jet lag involving an abrupt 8-hour advance of the sleep-wake cycle and the dark period after a 24-hour baseline period.[311] In the course of adaptation, TSH levels increased progressively because nighttime wakefulness was associated with large circadian-dependent TSH elevations, whereas daytime sleep failed to inhibit TSH. As a result, mean TSH levels were more than twofold higher after awakening from the second shifted period than during the same time interval after normal nocturnal sleep. This study indicates that the subjective discomfort and fatigue associated with jet lag may involve a prolonged elevation of a hormonal concentration in the peripheral circulation.

Aging is associated with a progressive decrease in overall TSH secretion (which is achieved by a decrease in amplitude, rather than in frequency, of secretory pulses) and in circulating TSH levels and with a dampening of the amplitude of the circadian variation.[81] In subjects in the seventh and eighth decades, TSH levels are lower than in young adults throughout the 24-hour span, although the difference is more marked during sleep than during the daytime period (see Fig. 19-5). In middle-age subjects, age-related decreases in TSH levels may be evidenced only in response to nocturnal sleep deprivation. Thus, it appears that the TSH secretory capacity decreases progressively with aging.

Alterations in Disease States

A decreased or absent nocturnal increase of TSH has been observed in a wide variety of nonthyroidal illnesses,[317] suggesting that hypothalamic dysregulation will generally affect the circadian TSH surge. This is in contrast to the circadian variation of plasma cortisol, which persists in a wide variety of disease states. The nocturnal TSH surge is diminished or absent in various conditions of hypercortisolism[318] as well as in hyperthyroidism and primary and secondary hypothyroidism.[319,320] In poorly controlled diabetic states, whether insulin dependent or noninsulin dependent, the surge also disappears.[321] Correction of hyperglycemia is associated with a reappearance of the nocturnal elevation.[321] Interestingly,

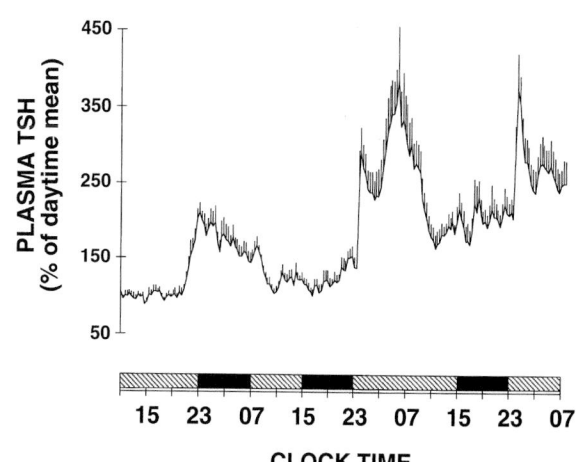

Figure 19-15   Mean (and standard error of the mean) profiles of plasma thyrotropin from eight normal young men who were submitted to an 8-hour advance of the sleep-wake and light-dark cycles. *Solid bars* indicate bedtime periods. (Data from Hirschfeld U, Moreno-Reyes R, Akseki E, et al: Progressive elevation of plasma thyrotropin during adaptation to simulated jet lag: Effects of treatment with bright light or zolpidem. J Clin Endocrinol Metab 81:3270–3277, 1996.)

morning TSH values in the hyperglycemic patients do not differ from those of control subjects, and the TSH response to TRH is only marginally reduced.[321]

PARATHYROID HORMONE

The 24-hour profile of circulating parathyroid hormone (PTH) levels shows a major nocturnal peak occurring around 1:00 to 3:00 A.M. and morning minimal values around 10:00 to 11:00 A.M. This diurnal rhythm persists, albeit dampened, in constant routine conditions.[322] Thus, this rhythm appears to be primarily regulated by the circadian pacemaker but modulated by other factors. Although serum calcium, the major modulator of PTH secretion, may also exhibit diurnal variations, the timing of the maximum was found to be highly variable among individuals and did not have any apparent relation to PTH.[322] An early study suggested that the nocturnal PTH increase was related to SWS,[323] but in more recent studies, shifts of the sleep-wake cycle did not alter the timing of the nocturnal PTH peak.[324] In contrast, this nocturnal rise was completely suppressed after a 4-day fast.[325] Diurnal profiles of circulating PTH levels are temporally related to diurnal variations of urinary calcium and phosphate and are likely to play an important role in the optimization of calcium balance.[322] The nocturnal PTH increase has been reported to be abolished in women with osteoporosis[326] and in primary hyperparathyroidism.[327]

HYDROMINERAL HORMONES

The hormones of the renin-angiotensin-aldosterone system exhibit diurnal variations with higher nocturnal levels. These diurnal variations are primarily regulated by the sleep-wake homeostasis because shifts of the sleep-wake cycle are immediately followed by parallel shifts of hormonal profiles.[76] A close temporal relationship has been evidenced between increases in SWS activity and parallel increases in plasma renin activity and aldosterone levels.[328,329] The nocturnal increase in plasma renin activity and aldosterone levels is markedly blunted by acute total sleep deprivation[330] (Fig. 19-16). In conditions of abnormal sleep architecture (e.g., narcolepsy,

sleeping sickness), disturbances of the REM-non-REM cycle are faithfully reflected in the plasma renin activity temporal pattern.[331]

Vasopressin release is pulsatile but shows no apparent relation to sleep stages.[331] Diurnal variations in plasma levels of atrial natriuretic peptide (ANP) have been evidenced in some, but not all, studies, and the existence of a circadian rhythm of ANP is still matter of controversy.[332]

GLUCOSE TOLERANCE AND INSULIN SECRETION

Diurnal and Ultradian Variations in Normal Subjects
In normal humans, glucose tolerance varies with the time of day. Figure 19-17 shows circadian variations in glucose tolerance to oral glucose, identical meals, intravenous glucose,

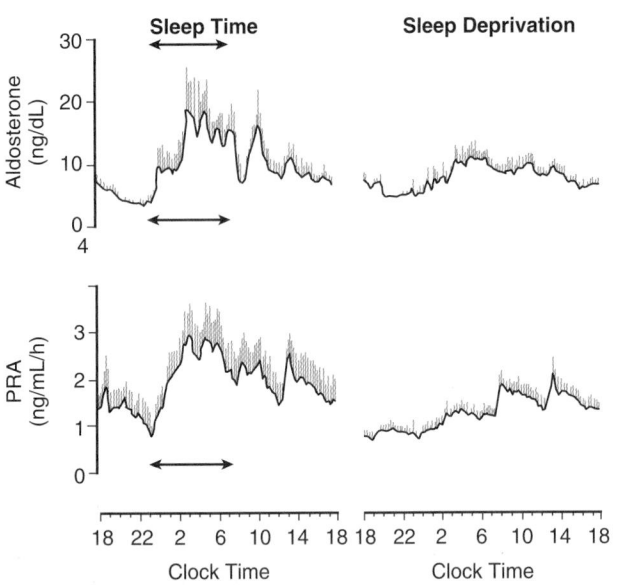

Figure 19-16 Mean (and standard error of the mean) 24-hour profiles of plasma aldosterone and plasma renin activity (PRA) in a group of eight normal young men (21–28 years old) during a period of normal nocturnal sleep and a period of total acute sleep deprivation. (Adapted from Charloux A, Gronfier C, Chapotot F, et al: Sleep deprivation blunts the nighttime increase in aldosterone release in humans. J Sleep Res 10:27–33, 2001.)

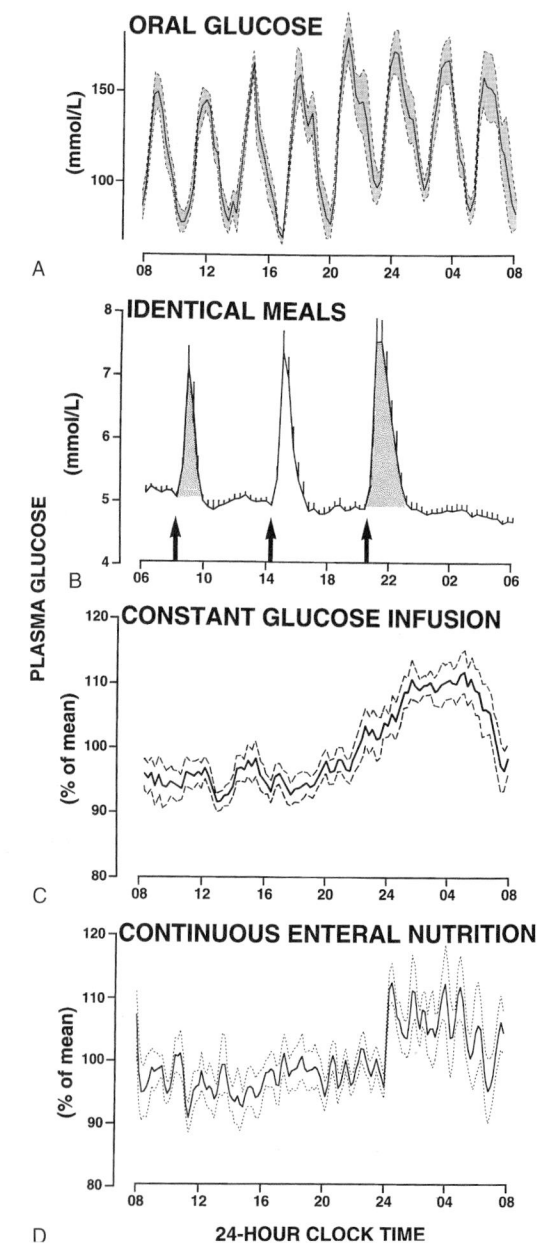

Figure 19-17 Twenty-four hour pattern of plasma glucose changes in response to 50 g oral glucose every 3 hours (A), identical meals (B), constant glucose infusion (C), and continuous enteral nutrition (D) in normal young adults. At each time point, the mean glucose level is shown with the standard error of the mean. (From Van Cauter E, Polonsky KS, Scheen AJ: Roles of circadian rhythmicity and sleep in human glucose regulation. Endocr Rev 18:716–738, 1997.)

and constant glucose infusion. In all four conditions, plasma glucose levels are markedly higher in the evening than the morning.[77] Studies of fasting during nocturnal sleep have consistently observed that, despite the prolonged fasting condition, glucose levels remain stable or decrease only minimally during the night, contrasting with a clear decrease during daytime fasting. Thus, a number of mechanisms operative during nocturnal sleep are likely to maintain stable glucose levels during the overnight fast. Experimental protocols involving intravenous glucose infusion or enteral nutrition while allowing normal nocturnal sleep have shown that glucose tolerance deteriorates further as the evening progresses, reaches a minimum around mid-sleep, and then improves to return to morning levels.[177,333] There is evidence that this diurnal variation in glucose tolerance is partly driven by the wide and highly reproducible diurnal rhythm of plasma cortisol, an important counterregulatory hormone.[77,120,334] Indeed, the diurnal variation in insulin secretion was found to be inversely related to the cortisol rhythm, with a significant correlation of the magnitudes of their morning to evening excursions. Elevations of plasma levels of glucose and insulin after short-term elevations of plasma cortisol are more pronounced in the evening than the morning.[120] Diminished insulin sensitivity and decreased β-cell responsiveness are also involved in reduced glucose tolerance later in the day. Under conditions of constant glucose infusion, sleep-associated increases in glucose were found to correlate with the amount of concomitant GH secreted. Thus, during the first part of the night, decreased glucose tolerance is due to decreased glucose utilization both by peripheral tissues, resulting from muscle relaxation and rapid insulin-like effects of sleep-onset GH secretion, and by the brain, as assessed by imaging studies demonstrating a reduction in glucose uptake during SWS.[335] During the second part of the night, these effects subside as sleep becomes shallow and more fragmented and GH is no longer secreted. Thus, complex interactions of circadian and sleep effects, possibly partly mediated by cortisol and GH, result in a consistent pattern of changes of set point of glucose regulation over the 24-hour period. Consistent with the important modulatory effects of sleep on glucose regulation, chronic sleep loss is associated with marked alterations of parameters of glucose tolerance, as described earlier in the section "Conditions of Altered Circadian Rhythmicity and Sleep."[115] The modulation of glucose regulation by circadian rhythmicity has implications for the postprandial carbohydrate regulation in night workers.[335a]

Human insulin secretion is a complex oscillatory process involving rapid pulses of low amplitude recurring every 10 to 15 minutes superimposed on slower ultradian oscillations with periods in the 90- to 120-minute range.[156,336] The ultradian oscillations are tightly coupled to glucose, with a tendency for glucose pulses to lead insulin pulses by 10 minutes, and have been shown to promote more efficient glucose utilization.[160] They are best seen in conditions in which insulin secretion is stimulated, including ingestion of meal, continuous enteral nutrition, and constant intravenous glucose infusion.[156,333] Under these conditions, their relative amplitude is approximately 50% to 70% for insulin secretory pulses and 20% for plasma glucose. Their amplitude is maximal immediately after a meal, and then it decreases progressively. Moreover, the periodicity of the insulin secretory oscillations can be entrained to the period of an oscillatory glucose infusion,[337] supporting the concept that these ultradian oscillations are generated by the glucose-insulin feedback mechanism.[338] However, ultradian oscillations, but less regular and of lower amplitude, are still present in fasting conditions. Stimulatory effects of sleep on insulin secretion are mediated by an increase in the amplitude of the oscillation.[333] During constant glucose infusion, REM sleep and wake episodes coincide significantly with decreasing levels of glucose and insulin, whereas increasing glucose levels occur during the deeper stages of non-REM sleep.[335]

The rapid 10- to 15-minute pulsations seem to have a different origin than the ultradian oscillations. Indeed, they may appear independently of glucose because they were observed in the isolated perfused pancreas and perifused islets.[156] Rapid insulin pulsations were also observed in perfused human islets.[338a] Insulin administration by pulsatile infusion improves insulin-mediated glucose uptake.[339,340] The frequency, amplitude, and regularity of rapid insulin pulses are decreased in aging.[341]

Alterations in Metabolic Disorders

In obese and diabetic subjects, the diurnal and ultradian variations in glucose regulation are abnormal. In obesity, the morning versus evening difference in glucose tolerance is abolished. Obese adult subjects show no diurnal variation in glucose tolerance, no decline in insulin sensitivity in the afternoon, and only a marginally significant decline in β-cell responsiveness to glucose in the later part of the day.[342] In patients with insulin-dependent diabetes, an increase in glucose levels and/or insulin requirements occurs in a pre–breakfast period ranging from 5:00 to 9:00 A.M. and has been called the "dawn phenomenon."[343] A role for nocturnal GH secretion in the pathogenesis of the dawn phenomenon was demonstrated.[344,345] The observation of a dawn phenomenon in patients with non-insulin-dependent diabetes mellitus under normal dietary conditions has been less consistent. However, prominent late night and early morning elevations in glucose levels and insulin secretion in both normal subjects and patients with diabetes become apparent during prolonged fasting.[346]

Counterregulatory mechanisms that are already deficient in type 1 diabetes are further impaired during sleep compared with wakefulness because autonomic responses to hypoglycemia are reduced during sleep in patients with diabetes. As a result, patients with type 1 diabetes are substantially less likely to be awakened by hypoglycemia than subjects without diabetes.[347]

The rapid and ultradian oscillations of insulin secretion are perturbed in non-insulin-dependent diabetes mellitus and impaired glucose tolerance without hyperglycemia.[156,348,349] The ultradian oscillations, which have an exaggerated amplitude in obese subjects without apparent changes in frequency or pattern of recurrence, are also more irregular and of lower amplitude in subjects with established non-insulin-dependent diabetes mellitus.[156]

HORMONES INVOLVED IN APPETITE REGULATION

Leptin

Leptin, a hormone released by the adipocytes, provides information about energy status to hypothalamic regulatory centers.[350,351] As illustrated in Figure 19-18, plasma leptin levels in normal lean men and women show a robust diurnal rhythm, with minimal values during the daytime and a nocturnal increase with maximal values during early to mid-sleep.[352] The amplitude of the circadian variation averages 25% to 30% of the mean level.[353] Leptin levels reflect cumulative energy balance, with a decrease or increase in response to under- or overfeeding, respectively.[354,355] These changes have been found to be associated with reciprocal changes in hunger.[355] Circulating leptin concentrations are higher and the relative amplitude of their diurnal variation is lower in obese subjects than in normal-weight controls.[353] There are marked gender differences in 24-hour mean leptin levels that are 2- to 10-fold higher in women than in men, regardless of fat mass.[353,356] In anorexia nervosa, as in amenorrheic female athletes, leptin levels are low and diurnal variations are abolished.[357,358] Aging is associated with a dampening of the amplitude of the 24-hour rhythm of plasma leptin and an advance of the nocturnal acrophase.[359] Several studies have

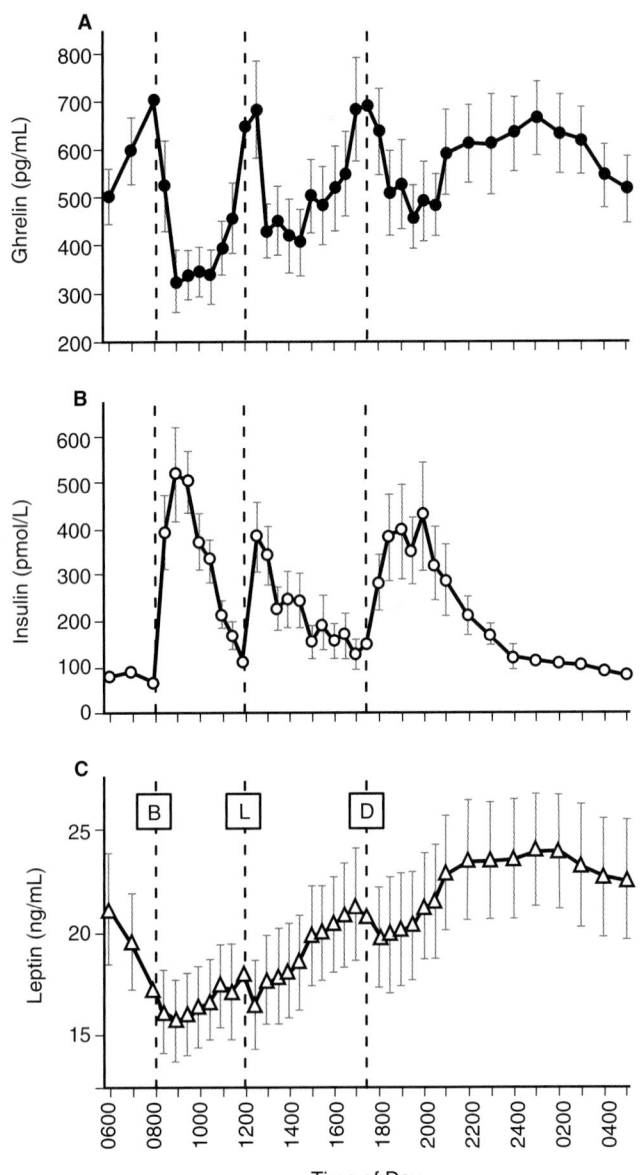

Figure 19-18 Twenty-four-hour profiles (mean ± standard error of the mean) of plasma ghrelin, insulin, and leptin levels in 10 healthy subjects 29 to 64 years old (body mass index 22–30 kg/m²) receiving breakfast, lunch, and dinner at 8:00 A.M., 12:00 P.M., and 5:30 P.M., respectively. (Adapted from Cummings DE, Purnell JQ, Frayo RS, et al: A preprandial rise in plasma ghrelin levels suggests a role in meal initiation in humans. Diabetes 50:1714–1719, 2001. Copyright © 2001 American Diabetes Association. Reprinted with permission from the American Diabetes Association.)

reported that human leptin levels are pulsatile,[333,353,356,360,361] including in subjects receiving continuous enteral nutrition rather than separate meals.[333]

Studies involving shifts of the meal schedule have shown that the timing of the daily maximum of plasma leptin levels is markedly dependent on the timing of meals.[362] However, the 24-hour rhythm of leptin concentrations is not simply a response to the feeding pattern. Indeed, the rhythm persists, albeit with a smaller amplitude, in subjects who receive continuous enteral nutrition.[333] After an abrupt shift of the sleep period, nocturnal leptin levels rise despite the absence of sleep and a second increase is observed after the onset of daytime recovery sleep,[333] indicating that both intrinsic circadian rhythmicity and sleep-wake homeostasis influence the release of leptin. Prolonged total sleep deprivation results in a

decrease in the amplitude of the leptin diurnal variation.[363] A recent study indicates that 1 week of sleep restriction (4 hours of bedtime per night), performed under controlled conditions of caloric intake and physical activity, is associated with a 20% to 30% reduction in mean leptin levels, acrophase, and amplitude of the diurnal variation (see Fig. 19-7).[116] The magnitude of this impact of sleep restriction on leptin levels is comparable with that observed in young adults under normal sleep conditions after 3 days of dietary restriction by approximately 900 kilocalories per day.[355] Morning leptin levels are elevated in patients with obstructive apnea.[131] In patients with narcolepsy, leptin levels are decreased and the nocturnal increase is abolished.[364]

The diurnal variations of leptin and cortisol levels are in an approximate mirror image. A possible relationship between the two rhythms has not been clearly identified.[356,361,365,366] Normal 24-hour leptin levels and diurnal leptin variations were found in patients with primary adrenal failure.[366] However, increased leptin levels,[367,368] caused by an equal amplification of basal and pulsatile secretion,[369] with a preservation of the diurnal pattern[367] have been reported in patients with Cushing's syndrome. A normal diurnal leptin pattern has also been reported in patients with GH deficiency[370] or with perinatal stalk-transection syndrome.[371]

Adiponectin

Adiponectin, a serum adipokine secreted exclusively from differentiated adipocytes, enhances insulin sensitivity.[372,373] In normal-weight men, adiponectin levels exhibit ultradian pulsatility as well as diurnal variation, with a significant nocturnal decrease, reaching minimal values in the early morning.[374] Interestingly, the 24-hour variations of the leptin-binding protein sOB-R are nearly identical to those of adiponectin but out-of-phase with the diurnal rhythm of plasma leptin.[374] Adiponectin levels are decreased in obesity and diabetes.[375] So far, possible relations between the adiponectin rhythm and sleep have not been reported.

Ghrelin

Ghrelin is a peptide—secreted primarily by the stomach and duodenum[218,376,377]—that is thought to have orexigenic properties. In addition, ghrelin stimulates GH secretion, displays ACTH- and prolactin-releasing activities,[218] and has been reported to promote SWS.[378] Daytime profiles of plasma ghrelin are primarily regulated by the schedule of food intake. Ghrelin levels rise sharply before each designated meal time and fall to trough levels within 1 hour after eating. A study examining spontaneous meal initiation in the absence of time- and food-related cues provided good evidence of a role for ghrelin in meal initiation.[379] This pattern seems to be exaggerated after the dinner meal because ghrelin levels peak around 1:00 A.M. and remain elevated until the later part of the night, when they tend to spontaneously decrease,[232,380,381] suggesting the existence of a robust diurnal rhythm (see Fig. 19-18).

The nocturnal ghrelin rise is slightly dampened during acute sleep deprivation.[382] A 2-day sleep restriction under controlled conditions of caloric intake and physical activity, was recently reported to be associated with a nearly 30% elevation in daytime ghrelin levels, concomitant with a nearly 20% reduction of leptin levels.[383] Thus, partial sleep curtailment simultaneously induced a decrease in anorexigenic leptin and an increase in orexigenic ghrelin levels. Moreover, sleep curtailment was also found to be associated with an increase in hunger. This increase in hunger was strongly correlated with the increase in ghrelin-to-leptin ratio,[383] suggesting that chronic sleep curtailment could be associated with excessive food intake and constitute a risk factor for obesity.

Ghrelin levels are decreased but the diurnal pattern remains largely unaltered in obese subjects.[232] A diet-induced weight loss was associated with increased 24-hour ghrelin levels.[232]

Acknowledgments

We thank Dr. K. Knutson and Dr. R. Leproult for assistance with manuscript preparation. This research was partially supported by grants RO1 DK-41814, RO1 HL-72694, and PO1 AG-11412 from the U.S. National Institutes of Health, and by a grant from the American Diabetes Association (E. Van Cauter).

REFERENCES

1. Turek FW: Circadian rhythms. Horm Res 49:103–113, 1998.
2. Borbely AA: Processes underlying sleep regulation. Horm Res 49:114–117, 1998.
3. Aschoff J: Circadian rhythms: General features and endocrinological aspects. In Krieger DT (ed): Endocrine Rhythms. New York, Raven Press, 1979, pp 1–61.
4. Wever RA: The Circadian System of Man: Results of Experiments under Temporal Isolation. New York, Springer-Verlag, 1979.
5. Lehman MN, Silver R, Bittman EL: Anatomy of suprachiasmatic nucleus grafts. In Klein DC, Moore RY, Reppert SM (eds): Suprachiasmatic Nucleus: The Mind's Clock. New York, Oxford University Press, 1991, pp 349–374.
6. Ralph M, Foster RG, Davis FC, et al: Transplanted suprachiasmatic nucleus determines circadian period. Science 247:975–978, 1990.
7. Earnest DJ, Sladek CD: Circadian vasopressin release from perifused rat suprachiasmatic explants in vitro: Effects of acute stimulation. Brain Res 422:398–402, 1987.
8. Gillette MU: SCN electrophysiology in vitro: Rhythmic activity and endogenous clock properties. In Klein DC, Moore RY, Reppert SM (eds): Suprachiasmatic Nucleus: The Mind's Clock. New York, Oxford University Press, 1991.
8a. Earnest DJ, Liang FQ, Ratcliff M, et al: Immortal time: Circadian clock properties of rat suprachias matic cell lines. Science 283:693–695, 1999.
9. Welsh DK, Logothetis DE, Meister M, et al: Individual neurons dissociated from rat suprachiasmatic nucleus express independently phased circadian firing rhythms. Neuron 14:697–706, 1995.
10. Reppert SM, Weaver DR: Coordination of circadian timing in mammals. Nature 418:935–941, 2002.
11. Yamazaki S, Numano R, Abe M, et al: Resetting central and peripheral circadian oscillators in transgenic rats Science 288:682–685, 2000.
12. Yoo SH, Yamazaki S, Lowrey PL, et al: PERIOD2::LUCIFERASE real-time reporting of circadian dynamics reveals persistent circadian oscillations in mouse peripheral tissues. Proc Natl Acad Sci U S A 101:5339–5346, 2004.
13. Davidson AJ, Yamazaki S, Menaker M: SCN: Ringmaster of the circadian circus or conductor of the circadian orchestra? Novartis Found Symp 253:110–125, 2003.
14. Dijk DJ, Czeisler CA: Contribution of the circadian pacemaker and the sleep homeostat to sleep propensity, sleep structure, electroencephalographic slow waves, and sleep spindle activity in humans. J Neurosci 15:3526–3538, 1995.
15. Czeisler CA, Duffy JF, Shanahan TL, et al: Stability, precision, and near-24-hour period of the human circadian pacemaker. Science 284:2177–2181, 1999.
16. Wright KP Jr, Hughes RJ, Kronauer RE, et al: Intrinsic near-24-h pacemaker period determines limits of circadian entrainment to a weak synchronizer in humans. Proc Natl Acad Sci U S A 98:14027–14032, 2001.
17. Card JP, Moore RY: The organization of visual circuits influencing the circadian activity of suprachiasmatic nucleus. In Klein DC, Moore RY, Reppert SM (eds): Suprachiasmatic Nucleus: The Mind's Clock. New York, Oxford University Press, 1991, pp 51–76.
18. Foster RG: Seeing the light . . . in a new way. J Neuroendocrinol 16:179–180, 2004.
19. Klein T, Martens H, Dijk DJ, et al: Circadian sleep regulation in the absence of light perception: Chronic non-24-hour circadian rhythm sleep disorder in a blind man with a regular 24-hour sleep-wake schedule. Sleep 16:333–343, 1993.
20. Turek FW: Pharmacological probes of the mammalian circadian clock: Use of the phase response curve approach. Trends Pharmacol Sci 8:212–217, 1987.
21. Lockley SW, Brainard GC, Czeisler CA: High sensitivity of the human circadian melatonin rhythm to resetting by short wavelength light. J Clin Endocrinol Metab 88:4502–4505, 2003.
22. Boivin DB, Duffy JF, Kronauer RE, et al: Dose-response relationships for resetting of human circadian clock by light. Nature 379:540–542, 1996.
23. Minors DS, Waterhouse JM, Wirz-Justice A: A human phase-response curve to light. Neurosci Lett 13:36–40, 1991.
24. Van Cauter E, Sturis J, Byrne MM, et al: Demonstration of rapid light-induced advances and delays of the human circadian clock using hormonal phase markers. Am J Physiol 266:E953–E963, 1994.
25. Khalsa SB, Jewett ME, Cajochen C, et al: A phase response curve to single bright light pulses in human subjects. J Physiol 549:945–952, 2003.
26. Czeisler CA, Kronauer RE, Allan JS, et al: Bright light induction of strong (type 0) resetting of the human circadian pacemaker. Science 244:1328–1333, 1989.
27. Jewett M, Kronauer RE, Czeisler CA: Light-induced suppression of endogenous circadian amplitude in humans. Nature 350:59–62, 1991.
28. Mendoza J, Dardente H, Escobar C, et al: Dark pulse resetting of the suprachiasmatic clock in Syrian hamsters: Behavioral phase-shifts and clock gene expression. Neuroscience 127:529–537, 2004.
29. Van Cauter E, Moreno-Reyes R, Akseki E, et al: Rapid phase advance of the 24-h melatonin profile in response to afternoon dark exposure. Am J Physiol 275:E48–E54, 1998.
30. Goichot B, Weibel L, Chapotot F, et al: Effect of the shift of the sleep-wake cycle on three robust endocrine markers of the circadian clock. Am J Physiol 275:E243–E248, 1998.
31. Buxton OM, L'Hermite-Balériaux M, Turek FW, et al: Daytime naps in darkness phase shift the human circadian rhythms of melatonin and thyrotropin secretion. Am J Physiol 278:R373–R382, 2000.
32. Mrosovsky N: Locomotor activity and non-photic influences on the circadian clock. Biol Rev 71:343–372, 1996.
33. Mrosovsky N: Phase response curves for social entrainment. J Comp Physiol A 162:35–46, 1988.
34. Turek FW: Effects of stimulated physical activity on the circadian pacemaker of vertebrates. J Biol Rhythms 4:135–148, 1989.
35. Turek FW, Smith R, Van Reeth O, et al: Disturbances of the activity rest cycle alter the circadian clock of mammals. In Inouye S, Krieger JM (eds): Endogenous Sleep Factors. The Hague, Netherlands, 1990, pp 277–283.
36. Zlomanczuk P, Schwartz WJ: Cellular and molecular mechanisms of circadian rhythms in mammals. In Turek FW, Zee PC (eds): Regulation of Sleep and Circadian Rhythms. New York, Marcel Dekker, 1999, pp 309–342.
37. Pickard GE, Rea MA: Serotonergic innervation of the hypothalamic suprachiasmatic nucleus and photic regulation of circadian rhythms. Biol Cell 89:513–523, 1997.
38. Van Reeth O, Sturis J, Byrne MM, et al: Nocturnal exercise phase delays circadian rhythms of melatonin and thyrotropin in normal men. Am J Physiol 266:E964–E974, 1994.
39. Buxton OM, Frank SA, L'Hermite-Balériaux M, et al: Roles of intensity and duration of nocturnal exercise in causing phase-shifts of human circadian rhythms. Am J Physiol 273:E536–E542, 1997.
40. Eastman CI, Hoese EK, Youngstedt SD, et al: Phase-shifting human circadian rhythms with exercise during the night shift. Physiol Behav 58:1287–1291, 1995.
41. Barger LK, Wright KP Jr, Hughes RJ, et al: Daily exercise facilitates phase delays of circadian melatonin rhythm in very dim light. Am J Physiol 286:R1077–R1084, 2004.
42. Baehr EK, Eastman CI, Revelle W, et al: Circadian phase-shifting effects of

nocturnal exercise in older compared with young adults. Am J Physiol 284:R1542–R1550, 2003.

43. Lewy AL, Ahmed S, Jackson JML, et al: Melatonin shifts human circadian rhythms according to a phase-response curve. Chronobiol Int 9:380–392, 1992.

44. Lewy AJ, Sack RL, Blood ML, et al: Melatonin marks circadian phase position and resets the endogenous circadian pacemaker in humans. In Chadwick DJ, Ackrill K (eds): Circadian Clocks and Their Adjustment (Ciba Foundation Symposium 183). New York, John Wiley & Sons, 1995, pp 303–321.

45. Geoffriau M, Brun J, Chazot G, et al: The physiology and pharmacology of melatonin in humans. Horm Res 49:136–141, 1998.

46. Rosenthal NE: Plasma melatonin as a measure of the human clock. J Clin Endocrinol Metab 73:225–226, 1991.

47. Shanahan TL, Czeisler CA: Light exposure induces equivalent phase shifts of the endogenous circadian rhythms of circulating plasma melatonin and core body temperature in men. J Clin Endocrinol Metab 73:227–235, 1991.

48. Lewy AJ, Bauer VK, Ahmed S, et al: The human phase response curve (PRC) to melatonin is about 12 hours out of phase with the PRC to light. Chronobiol Int 15:71–83, 1998.

49. Sack RL, Brandes RW, Kendall AR, et al: Entrainment of free-running circadian rhythms by melatonin in blind people. N Engl J Med 343:107–1077, 2000.

50. Challet E, Caldelas I, Graff C, et al: Synchronization of the molecular clockwork by light- and food-related cues in mammals. Biol Chem 384:711–719, 2003.

51. Davidson AJ, Poole AS, Yamazaki S, et al: Is the food-entrainable circadian oscillator in the digestive system? Genes Brain Behav 2:32–39, 2003.

52. Prosser RA, Bergeron HE: Leptin phase-advances the rat suprachiasmatic circadian clock in vitro. Neurosci Lett 336:139–142, 2003.

53. Rechtschaffen A, Kales A: A Manual of Standardized Terminology, Techniques and Scoring System for Sleep Stages of Human Subjects. Los Angeles, UCLA Brain Information Service/Brain Research Institute, Los Angeles, 1968.

54. Saper CB, Chou TC, Scammell TE: The sleep switch: Hypothalamic control of sleep and wakefulness. Trends Neurosci 24:726–731, 2001.

55. Sherin JE, Shiromani PJ, McCarley RW, et al: Activation of ventrolateral preoptic neurons during sleep. Science 271:216–219, 1996.

56. Gallopin T, Fort P, Eggermann E, et al: Identification of sleep-promoting neurons in vitro. Nature 404:992–995, 2000.

57. Gaus SE, Strecker RE, Tate BA, et al: Ventrolateral preoptic nucleus contains sleep-active, galaninergic neurons in multiple mammalian species. Neuroscience 115:285–294, 2002.

58. Lu J, Bjorkum AA, Xu M, et al: Selective activation of the extended ventrolateral preoptic nucleus during rapid eye movement sleep. J Neurosci 22:4568–4576, 2002.

59. Aschoff J: On the perception of time during prolonged temporal isolation. Hum Neurobiol 4:41–52, 1985.

60. Aschoff J, von Goetz C, Wildgruber C, et al: Meal timing in humans during isolation without time cues. J Biol Rhythms 1:151–162, 1986.

61. Aschoff J: On the dilatability of subjective time. Perspect Biol Med 35:276–280, 1992.

62. Czeisler CA, Weitzman E, Moore-Ede MC, et al: Human sleep: Its duration and organization depend on its circadian phase. Science 210:1264–1267, 1980.

63. Chou TC, Bjorkum AA, Gaus SE, et al: Afferents to the ventrolateral preoptic nucleus. J Neurosci 22:977–990, 2002.

64. Edgar DM, Dement WC, Fuller CA: Effect of SCN lesions on sleep in squirrel monkeys: Evidence for opponent processes in sleep-wake regulation. J Neurosci 13:1065–1079, 1993.

65. Mendelson WB, Bergmann BM, Tung A: Baseline and post-deprivation recovery sleep in SCN-lesioned rats. Brain Res 980:185–190, 2003.

66. Naylor E, Bergmann BM, Krauski K, et al: The circadian clock mutation alters sleep homeostasis in the mouse. J Neurosci 20:8138–8143, 2000.

67. Monk TH, Buysse DJ, Reynolds CF III, et al: Rhythmic versus homeostatic influences on mood, activation and performance in the elderly. J Gerontol 47:221–227, 1991.

68. Monk TH, Buysse DJ, Reynolds CF, et al: Circadian rhythms in human performance and mood under constant conditions. J Sleep Res 6:9–18, 1997.

69. Dijk DJ, Czeisler CA: Paradoxical timing of the circadian rhythm of sleep propensity serves to consolidate sleep and wakefulness in humans. Neurosci Lett 166:63–68, 1994.

70. Boivin DB, Czeisler CA, Dijk DJ, et al: Complex interaction of the sleep-wake cycle and circadian phase modulates mood in healthy subjects. Arch Gen Psychiatry 54:145–152, 1997.

71. Folkard S, Hume KI, Minors DS, et al: Independence of the circadian rhythm in alertness from the sleep-wake cycle. Nature 313:678–679, 1985.

72. Johnson MP, Duffy JF, Dijk DJ, et al: Short-term memory, alertness and performance: A reappraisal of their relationship to body temperature. J Sleep Res 1:24–29, 1992.

73. Akerstedt T, Folkard S: Validation of the S and C components of the three-process model of alertness regulation. Sleep 18:1–6, 1995.

74. Leproult R, Van Reeth O, Byrne MM, et al: Sleepiness, performance and neuroendocrine function during sleep deprivation: Effects of exposure to bright light or exercise. J Biol Rhythms 12:245–258, 1997.

75. Dijk DJ, Duffy JF: Circadian regulation of human sleep and age-related changes in its timing, consolidation and EEG characteristics. Ann Med 31:130–140, 1999.

76. Brandenberger G, Follenius M, Goichot B, et al: Twenty-four hour profiles of plasma renin activity in relation to the sleep-wake cycle. J Hypertens 12:277–283, 1994.

77. Van Cauter E, Polonsky KS, Scheen AJ: Roles of circadian rhythmicity and sleep in human glucose regulation. Endocr Rev 18:716–738, 1997.

78. Brandenberger G, Gronfier C, Weibel L, et al: Modulatory role of sleep on hormonal pulsatility. In Hayashi O, Inoue S (eds): Sleep and Sleep Disorders: From Molecule to Behavior. Tokyo, Academic Press, 1997, pp 195–198.

79. Van Cauter E, Spiegel K: Circadian and sleep control of endocrine secretion. In Turek FW, Zee PC (eds): Regulation of Sleep and Circadian Rhythms. New York, Marcel Dekker, 1999, pp 397–426.

80. Van Cauter E, Copinschi G: Interactions between growth hormone secretion and sleep. In Smith RG, Thorner MO (eds): Human Growth Hormone: Research and Clinical Practice. Totowa, NJ, Humana Press, 1999, pp 261–283.

81. van Coevorden A, Mockel J, Laurent E, et al: Neuroendocrine rhythms and sleep in aging men. Am J Physiol 260:E651–E661, 1991.

82. Czeisler CA, Dumont M, Duffy JF, et al: Association of sleep-wake habits in older people with changes in output of circadian pacemaker. Lancet 340:933–936, 1992.

83. Van Cauter E, Plat L, Leproult R, et al: Alterations of circadian rhythmicity and sleep in aging: endocrine consequences. Horm Res 49:147–152, 1998.

84. Van Cauter E, Leproult R, Plat L: Age-related changes in slow-wave sleep and REM sleep and relationship with growth hormone and cortisol levels in healthy men. JAMA 284:861–868, 2000.

85. Prinz PN: Sleep and sleep disorders in older adults. J Clin Neurophysiol 12:139–146, 1995.

86. Zee PC, Rosenberg RS, Turek FW: Effects of aging on entrainment and rate of resynchronization of the circadian locomotor activity. Am J Physiol 263:1099–1103, 1992.

87. Pittendrigh CS, Daan S: Circadian oscillations in rodents: A systematic increase of their frequency with age. Science 186:548–550, 1974.

88. Morin LP: Age-related changes in hamster circadian period, entrainment and rhythm splitting. J Biol Rhythms 3:237–248, 1988.

89. Yamazaki S, Straume M, Tei H, et al: Effects of aging on central and peripheral mammalian clocks. Proc Natl Acad Sci U S A 99:10801–10806, 2002.

90. Dijk DJ, Duffy JF, Riel E, et al: Ageing and the circadian and homeostatic regulation of human sleep during forced desynchrony of rest, melatonin and temperature rhythms. J Physiol 516:611–627, 1999.

91. Duffy JF, Czeisler CA: Age-related change in the relationship between circadian period, circadian phase, and diurnal preference in humans. Neurosci Lett 318:117–120, 2002.

92. Zhang Y, Kornhauser JM, Zee PC, et al: Effects of aging on light-induced phase-shifting of circadian behavioral rhythms, Fos expression, and Creb phosphorylation in the hamster suprachiasmatic nucleus. Neuroscience 70:951–961, 1996.

93. Van Reeth O, Zhang Y, Zee PC, et al: Aging alters feedback effects of the activity-rest cycle in the circadian clock. Am J Physiol 263:R981–R986, 1992.

94. Van Reeth O, Zhang Y, Reddy A, et al: Aging alters the entraining effects of an activity-inducing stimulus on the circadian clock. Brain Res 607:286–292, 1993.

95. Van Reeth O, Zhang Y, Zee PC, et al: Grafting fetal suprachiasmatic nuclei in the hypothalamus of old hamsters restores responsiveness of the circadian clock to a phase shifting stimulus. Brain Res 643:338–342, 1994.

96. Campbell SS, Kripke DF, Gillin JC, et al: Exposure to light in healthy elderly subjects and Alzheimer's patients. Physiol Behav 42:141–144, 1988.

97. Ehlers CL, Frank E, Kupfer DJ: Social zeitgebers and biological rhythms. Arch Gen Psychiatry 45:948–952, 1988.

98. Ancoli-Israel S, Kripke DF, Jones DW, et al: 24-hour sleep and light rhythms in nursing home patients. Sleep Res 20A:410, 1991.

99. Campbell SS, Dawson D, Anderson MW: Alleviation of sleep maintenance insomnia with timed exposure to bright light. J Am Geriatr Soc 41:829–836, 1993.

100. Mishima K, Okawa M, Shimizu T, et al: Diminished melatonin secretion in the elderly caused by insufficient environmental illumination. J Clin Endocrinol Metab 86:129–134, 2001.

101. Aschoff J, Hoffmann K, Pohl H, et al: Re-entrainment of circadian rhythms after phase-shifts of the zeitgeber. Chronobiologia 28:119–133, 1975.

102. Knutsson A, Akerstedt T, Orth-Gomer K, et al: Increased risk of ischaemic heart disease in shift workers. Lancet 89–92, 1986.

103. Czeisler CA, Johnson MP, Duffy JF, et al: Exposure to bright light and darkness to treat physiologic maladaptation to night work. N Engl J Med 322:1253–1259, 1990.

104. Rosa RR: Extended workshifts and excessive fatigue. J Sleep Res 4:51–56, 1995.

105. van Amelsvoort L, Schouten E, Kok F: Duration of shiftwork related to body mass index and waist to hip ratio. Int J Obes Relat Metab Disord 23:973–978, 1999.

106. Roden M, Koller M, Pirich K, et al: The circadian melatonin and cortisol secretion pattern in permanent night shift workers. Am J Physiol 265:R261–R267, 1993.

107. Weibel L, Spiegel K, Follenius M, et al: Internal dissociation of the circadian markers of the cortisol rhythm in night workers. Am J Physiol 270:E608–E613, 1996.

108. Weibel L, Spiegel K, Gronfier C, et al: Twenty-four-hour melatonin and core body temperature rhythms: Their adaptation in night workers. Am J Physiol 272:R948–R954, 1997.

109. Dawson D, Encel N, Lushington K: Improving adaptation to simulated night shift: Timed exposure to bright light versus daytime melatonin administration. Sleep 18:11–21, 1995.

110. Campbell SS, Dawson D: Enhancement of nighttime alertness and performance with bright ambient light. Physiol Behav 48:317–320, 1990.

111. Campbell SS: Effects of timed bright light exposure on shift work adaptation in middle-aged subjects. Sleep 18:408–416, 1995.

112. Eastman CI: High-intensity light for circadian adaptation to a 12-h shift of the sleep schedule. Am J Physiol 263:R428–R436, 1992.

113. Eastman CI, Steward KT, Mahoney MP, et al: Dark goggles and bright light improve circadian rhythm adaptation to night shift work. Sleep 17:535–543, 1994.

114. Eastman CI, Martin S: How to use light and dark to produce circadian adaptation to night shift work. Ann Med 31:87–98, 1999.

115. Spiegel K, Leproult R, Van Cauter E: Impact of sleep debt on metabolic and endocrine function. Lancet 354:1435–1439, 1999.

116. Spiegel K, Leproult R, L'Hermite-Balériaux M, et al: Leptin levels are dependent on sleep duration: Relationships with sympatho-vagal balance, carbohydrate regulation, cortisol and TSH. J Clin Endocrinol Metab 89:5762–5771, 2004.

117. Leproult R, Copinschi G, Buxton O, et al: Sleep loss results in an elevation of cortisol levels the next evening. Sleep 20:865–870, 1997.

118. Sherman B, Wysham C, Pfohl B: Age-related changes in the circadian rhythm of plasma cortisol in man. J Clin Endocrinol Metab 61:439–443, 1985.

119. Van Cauter E, Leproult R, Kupfer DJ: Effects of gender and age on the levels and circadian rhythmicity of plasma cortisol. J Clin Endocrinol Metab 81:2468–2473, 1996.

120. Plat L, Féry F, L'Hermite-Balériaux M, et al: Metabolic effects of short-term physiological elevations of plasma cortisol are more pronounced in the evening than in the morning. J Clin Endocrinol Metab 84:3082–3092, 1999.

121. McEwen BS: Stress, adaptation, and disease. Allostasis and allostatic load. Ann N Y Acad Sci 840:33–44, 1998.

122. Kripke DF, Garfinkel L, Wingard DL, et al: Mortality associated with sleep duration and insomnia. Arch Gen Psychiatry 59:131–136, 2002.

123. Vioque J, Torres A, Quiles J: Time spent watching television, sleep duration and obesity in adults living in Valencia, Spain. Int J Obes Relat Metab Disord 24:1683–1688, 2000.

124. Sekine M, Yamagami T, Hamanishi S, et al: Parental obesity, lifestyle factors and obesity in preschool children: Results of the Toyama Birth Cohort Study. J Epidemiol 12:33–39, 2002.

125. Ayas NT, White DP, Al-Delaimy WK, et al: A prospective study of self-reported sleep duration and incident diabetes in women. Diabetes Care 26:380–384, 2003.

126. Cooper BG, White JES, Ashworth LA, et al: Hormonal and metabolic profiles in subjects with obstructive sleep apnea syndrome and the effects of nasal continuous positive airway pressure (CPAP) treatment. Sleep 18:172–179, 1995.

127. Goldstein SJ, Wu RHK, Thorpy MJ, et al: Reversibility of deficient sleep entrained growth hormone secretion in a boy with achondroplasia and obstructive sleep apnea. Acta Endocrinol 116:95–101, 1987.

128. Saini J, Krieger J, Brandenberger G, et al: Continuous positive airway pressure treatment: Effects on growth hormone, insulin and glucose profiles in obstructive sleep apnea patients. Hormone Metab Res 25:375–381, 1993.

129. Spiegel K, Follenius M, Krieger J, et al: Prolactin secretion during sleep in obstructive sleep apnea patients. J Sleep Res 4:56–62, 1995.

130. Ozturk L, Unal M, Tamer L, et al: The association of the severity of obstructive sleep apnea with plasma leptin levels. Arch Otolaryngol Head Neck Surg 129:538–540, 2003.

131. Patel SR, Palmer LJ, Larkin EK, et al: Relationship between obstructive sleep apnea and diurnal leptin rhythms. Sleep 27:235–239, 2004.

132. Phillips BG, Kato M, Narkiewicz K, et al: Increases in leptin levels, sympathetic drive, and weight gain in obstructive sleep apnea. Am J Physiol 279:H234–H237, 2000.

133. Ip MS, Lam KS, Ho C, et al: Serum leptin and vascular risk factors in obstructive sleep apnea. Chest 118:580–586, 2000.

134. Manzella D, Parillo M, Razzino T, et al: Soluble leptin receptor and insulin resistance as determinant of sleep apnea. Int J Obes Relat Metab Disord 26:370–375, 2002.

135. Sanner BM, Kollhosser P, Buechner N, et al: Influence of treatment on leptin levels in patients with obstructive sleep apnoea. Eur Respir J 23:601–604, 2004.

136. Harsch IA, Konturek PC, Koebnick C, et al: Leptin and ghrelin levels in patients with obstructive sleep apnoea: Effect of CPAP treatment. Eur Respir J 22:251–257, 2003.

137. Shimizu K, Chin K, Nakamura T, et al: Plasma leptin levels and cardiac

sympathetic function in patients with obstructive sleep apnoea-hypopnoea syndrome. Thorax 57:429–434, 2002.

138. Chin K, Shimizu K, Nakamura T, et al: Changes in intra-abdominal visceral fat and serum leptin levels in patients with obstructive sleep apnea syndrome following nasal continuous positive airway pressure therapy. Circulation 100:706–712, 1999.

139. Harsch I, Schahin S, Bruckner K, et al: The effect of continuous positive airway pressure treatment on insulin sensitivity in patients with obstructive sleep apnoea syndrome and type 2 diabetes. Respiration 71:252–259, 2004.

140. Harsch IA, Schahin SP, Radespiel-Troger M, et al: Continuous positive airway pressure treatment rapidly improves insulin sensitivity in patients with obstructive sleep apnea syndrome. Am J Respir Crit Care Med 169:156–162, 2004.

141. Vgontzas AN, Bixler EO, Chrousos GP: Metabolic disturbances in obesity versus sleep apnoea: The importance of visceral obesity and insulin resistance. J Intern Med 254:32–44, 2003.

142. Punjabi NM, Sorkin JD, Katzel LI, et al: Sleep-disordered breathing and insulin resistance in middle-aged and overweight men. Am J Respir Crit Care Med 165:677–682, 2002.

143. Elmasry A, Lindberg E, Berne C, et al: Sleep-disordered breathing and glucose metabolism in hypertensive men: A population-based study. J Intern Med 249:153–161, 2001.

144. American Sleep Disorders Association: The International Classification of Sleep Disorders. Lawrence, KS, Allen Press, Inc., 1990.

145. Rosenthal RE, Vanderpool JRJ, Levendosky AA, et al: Phase-shifting effects of bright morning light as treatment for delayed sleep phase syndrome. Sleep 13:354–361, 1990.

146. Jones CR, Campbell SS, Zone SE, et al: Familial advance sleep phase syndrome: A short-period circadian rhythm variant in humans. Nat Med 5:1062–1065, 1999.

147. Kleitman N: Basic rest activity cycle: 22 years later. Sleep 5:311–317, 1982.

148. Chapotot F, Gronfier C, Jouny C, et al: Cortisol secretion is related to electroencephalographic alertness in human subjects during daytime wakefulness. J Clin Endocrinol Metab 83:4263–4268, 1998.

149. Lang DA, Matthews DR, Peto J, et al: Cyclic oscillations of basal plasma glucose and insulin concentrations in human beings. N Engl J Med 301:1023–1027, 1979.

150. O'Meara NM, Sturis J, Blackman JD, et al: Analytical problems in detecting rapid insulin secretory pulses in normal humans. J Clin Endocrinol Metab 27:231–238, 1993.

151. Goodner C, Walike B, Koerker D, et al: Insulin, glucagon, and glucose exhibit synchronous, sustained oscillations in fasting monkeys. Science 195:177–179, 1977.

152. Jaspan JB, Lever E, Polonsky KS, et al: In vivo pulsatility of pancreatic islet peptides. Am J Physiol 251:E215–E226, 1986.

153. Veldhuis JD, Iranmanesh A, Johnson ML, et al: Twenty-four-hour rhythms in plasma concentrations of adenohypophyseal hormones are generated by distinct amplitude and/or frequency modulation of underlying pituitary secretory bursts. J Clin Endocrinol Metab 71:1616–1623, 1990.

154. Veldhuis JD, Johnson ML, Lizarralde G, et al: Rhythmic and nonrhythmic modes of anterior pituitary gland secretion. Chronobiol Int 9:371–379, 1992.

155. Van Cauter E, van Coevorden A, Blackman JD: Modulation of neuroendocrine release by sleep and circadian rhythmicity. In Yen S, Vale W (eds): Advances in Neuroendocrine Regulation of Reproduction. Norwell, MA, Serono Symposis USA, 1990, pp 113–122.

156. Polonsky KS, Sturis J, Van Cauter E: Temporal profiles and clinical significance of pulsatile insulin secretion. Horm Res 49:178–184, 1998.

157. Simon C, Brandenberger G, Saini J, et al: Slow oscillations of plasma glucose and insulin secretion rate are amplified during sleep in humans under continuous enteral nutrition. Sleep 17:333–338, 1994.

158. Knobil E, Hotchkiss J: The menstrual cycle and its neuroendocrine control. In Knobil E, Neill JD (eds): The Physiology of Reproduction. New York, Raven Press, 1988, pp 1971–1994.

159. Conn PM, Crowley WF: Gonadotropin-releasing hormone and its analogues. N Engl J Med 324:93–103, 1991.

160. Sturis J, Scheen AJ, Leproult R, et al: 24-hour glucose profiles during continuous or oscillatory insulin infusion. J Clin Invest 95:1464–1471, 1995.

161. Halberg F, Tong YL, Johnson EA: Circadian system phase: An aspect of temporal morphology: Procedures and illustrative examples. In Mayersbach HV (ed): Cellular Aspects of Biorhythms. New York, Springer-Verlag, 1967, pp 20–48.

162. Cleveland WS: Robust locally weighted regression and smoothing scatterplots. J Am Stat Assoc 74:829–836, 1979.

163. Van Cauter E: Method for characterization of 24-h temporal variation of blood constituents. Am J Physiol 237:E255–E264, 1979.

164. Van Cauter E: Computer-assisted analysis of endocrine rhythms. In Rodbard D, Forti G (eds): Computers in Endocrinology. New York, Raven Press, 1990, pp 59–70.

165. Polonsky KS, Licinio-Paixao J, Given BD, et al: Use of biosynthetic human C-peptide in the measurement of insulin secretion rates in normal volunteers and type I diabetic patients. J Clin Invest 77:98–105, 1986.

166. De Nicolao G, Rocchetti M: Stable and efficient techniques for the deconvolution of hormone time series. In Guardabasso V, Rodbard D, Forti G (eds): Computers in Endocrinology: Recent Advances. New York, Raven Press, 1990, pp 83–91.

167. Veldhuis JD, Johnson ML: A review and appraisal of deconvolution methods to evaluate in vivo neuroendocrine secretory events. J Neuroendocrinol 2:755–771, 1990.

168. Sturis J, Polonsky KS, Shapiro ET, et al: Abnormalities in the ultradian oscillations of insulin secretion and glucose levels in type 2 (non-insulin-dependent) diabetic patients. Diabetologia 35:681–689, 1992.

169. Pincus SM, Keefe DL: Quantification of hormone pulsatility via an approximate entropy algorithm. Am J Physiol 262:E741–E754, 1992.

170. Urban RJ, Evans WS, Rogol AD, et al: Contemporary aspects of discrete peak-detection algorithms. I. The paradigm of the luteinizing hormone pulse signal in men. Endocr Rev 9:3–37, 1988.

171. Urban RJ, Kaiser DL, Van Cauter E, et al: Comparative assessment of objective pulse detection algorithms. II. Studies in men. Am J Physiol 254:E113–E119, 1988.

172. Veldhuis JD, Iranmanesh A, Johnson ML, et al: Amplitude, but not frequency, modulation of adrenocorticotropin secretory bursts gives rise to the nyctohemeral rhythm of the corticotropic axis in man. J Clin Endocrinol Metab 71:452–463, 1989.

173. Van Cauter E, Honinckx E: Pulsatility of pituitary hormones. Exp Brain Res 12(Suppl):41–60, 1985.

174. Lejeune-Lenain C, Van Cauter E, Desir D, et al: Control of circadian and episodic variations of adrenal androgens secretion in man. J Endocrinol Invest 10:267–276, 1987.

175. Weitzman ED, Zimmerman JC, Czeisler CA, et al: Cortisol secretion is inhibited during sleep in normal man. J Clin Endocrinol Metab 56:352–358, 1983.

176. Born J, Muth S, Fehm HL: The significance of sleep onset and slow wave sleep for nocturnal release of growth hormone (GH) and cortisol. Psychoneuroendocrinology 13:233–243, 1988.

177. Van Cauter E, Blackman JD, Roland D, et al: Modulation of glucose regulation and insulin secretion by circadian rhythmicity and sleep. J Clin Invest 88:934–942, 1991.

178. Weibel L, Follenius M, Spiegel K, et al: Comparative effect of night and daytime sleep on the 24-hour cortisol secretory profile. Sleep 18:549–556, 1995.

179. Follenius M, Brandenberger G, Bardasept J, et al: Nocturnal cortisol release in relation to sleep structure. Sleep 15:21–27, 1992.

180. Gronfier C, Luthringer R, Follenius M, et al: Temporal relationships between

pulsatile cortisol secretion and electroencephalographic activity during sleep in man. Electroencephalogr Clin Neurophysiol 103:405–408, 1997.

181. Bierwolf C, Struve K, Marshall L, et al: Slow wave sleep drives inhibition of pituitary-adrenal secretion in humans. J Neuroendocrinol 9:479–484, 1997.

182. Brabant G, Prank K, Ranft U, et al: Physiological regulation of circadian and pulsatile thyrotropin secretion in normal man and woman. J Clin Endocrinol Metab 70:403–409, 1990.

183. Spath-Schwalbe E, Gofferje M, Kern W, et al: Sleep disruption alters nocturnal ACTH and cortisol secretory patterns. Biol Psychiatry 29:575–584, 1991.

184. Pruessner JC, Wolf OT, Hellhammer DH, et al: Free cortisol levels after awakening: A reliable biological marker for the assessment of adrenocortical activity. Life Sci 61:2539–2549, 1997.

185. Caufriez A, Moreno-Reyes R, Leproult R, et al: Immediate effects of an 8-h advance shift of the rest-activity cycle on 24-h profiles of cortisol. Am J Physiol 282:E1147–E1153, 2002.

186. Scheer FA, Buijs RM: Light affects morning salivary cortisol in humans. J Clin Endocrinol Metab 84:3395–3398, 1999.

187. Leproult R, Colecchia EF, L'Hermite-Baleriaux M, et al: Transition from dim to bright light in the morning induces an immediate elevation of cortisol levels. J Clin Endocrinol Metab 86:151–157, 2001.

188. Linkowski P, Van Onderbergen A, Kerkhofs M, et al: Twin study of the 24-h cortisol profile: Evidence for genetic control of the human circadian clock. Am J Physiol 264:E173–E181, 1993.

189. Van Cauter E, Shapiro ET, Tillil H, et al: Circadian modulation of glucose and insulin responses to meals: Relationship to cortisol rhythm. Am J Physiol 262:E467–E475, 1992.

190. Born J, Hansen K, Marshall L, et al: Timing the end of nocturnal sleep. Nature 397:29–30, 1999.

191. Vgontzas AN, Bixler EO, Lin HM, et al: Chronic insomnia is associated with nyctohemeral activation of the hypothalamic-pituitary-adrenal axis: Clinical implications. J Clin Endocrinol Metab 86:3787–3794, 2001.

192. McEwen BS, Stellar E: Stress and the individual. Arch Intern Med 153:2093–2101, 1993.

193. McEwen B: Protective and damaging effects of stress mediators. N Engl J Med 338:171–179, 1998.

194. Dallman MF, Strack AL, Akana SF, et al: Feast and famine: Critical role of glucocorticoids with insulin in daily energy flow. Front Neuroendocrinol 14:303–347, 1993.

195. Dennison E, Hindmarsh P, Fall C, et al: Profiles of endogenous circulating cortisol and bone mineral density in healthy elderly men. J Clin Endocrinol Metab 84:3058–3063, 1999.

196. Nolten WE, Lindheimer MD, Rueckert PA, et al: Diurnal patterns and regulation of cortisol secretion in pregnancy. J Clin Endocrinol Metab 51:466–472, 1980.

197. Magiakou MA, Mastorakos G, Rabin D et al: The maternal hypothalamic-pituitary-adrenal axis in the third trimester of human pregnancy. Clin Endocrinol (Oxf) 44:419–428, 1996.

198. Rosman PM, Farag A, Benn R, et al: Modulation of pituitary-adrenal function: Decreased secretory episodes and blunted circadian rhythmicity in patients with alcoholic liver disease. J Clin Endocrinol Metab 55:709–717, 1981.

199. Boyar RM, Hellman LD, Roffwarg H, et al: Cortisol secretion and metabolism in anorexia nervosa. N Engl J Med 296:190–193, 1977.

200. Iranmanesh A, Lizarralde G, Johnson ML, et al: Dynamics of 24-hour endogenous cortisol secretion and clearance in primary hypothyroidism assessed before and after partial thyroid hormone replacement. J Clin Endocrinol Metab 70:155–161, 1990.

201. Gallagher TF, Hellman L, Finkelstein J, et al: Hyperthyroidism and cortisol secretion in man. J Clin Endocrinol Metab 34:919–927, 1972.

202. Refetoff S, Van Cauter E, Fang V, et al: The effect of dexamethasone on the 24-hour profiles of adrenocorticotropin and cortisol in Cushing's syndrome. J Clin Endocrinol Metab 60:527–535, 1985.

203. Van Cauter E, Refetoff S: Evidence for two subtypes of Cushing's disease based on the analysis of episodic cortisol secretion. N Engl J Med 312:1343–1344, 1985.

204. Roelfsema F, Pincus SM, Veldhuis JD: Patients with Cushing's disease secrete adrenocorticotropin and cortisol jointly more asynchronously than healthy subjects. J Clin Endocrinol Metab 83:688–692, 1998.

205. Linkowski P, Mendlewicz J, Leclercq R, et al: The 24-hour profile of adrenocorticotropin and cortisol in major depressive illness. J Clin Endocrinol Metab 61:429–438, 1985.

206. Rubin RT, Poland RE, Lesser IM, et al: Neuroendocrine aspects of primary endogenous depression: I. Cortisol secretory dynamics in patients and matched controls. Arch Gen Psychiatry 44:328–336, 1987.

207. Sachar ED (ed): Twenty-four-hour cortisol secretory patterns in depressed and manic patients. In Gispen WH, Van Wimersma Greidanus TB, Bohus B, De Wied D (eds): Hormones, Homeostasis and the Brain (Progress in Brain Research, vol. 42). Amsterdam, Elsevier, 1975, pp 81–91.

208. Linkowski P, Mendlewicz J, Kerkhofs M, et al: 24-hour profiles of adrenocorticotropin, cortisol, and growth hormone in major depressive illness: Effect of antidepressant treatment. J Clin Endocrinol Metab 65:141–152, 1987.

209. Yehuda R, Teicher MH, Trestman RL, et al: Cortisol regulation in posttraumatic stress disorder and major depression: A chronobiological analysis. Biol Psychiatry 15:79–88, 1996.

210. Yehuda R: Hypothalamic-pituitary-adrenal alterations in PTSD: Are they relevant to understanding cortisol alterations in cancer? Brain Behav Immunol 17:S73–S83, 2003.

211. Bremner JD, Vythilingam M, Anderson G, et al: Assessment of the hypothalamic-pituitary-adrenal axis over a 24-hour diurnal period and in response to neuroendocrine challenges in women with and without childhood sexual abuse and posttraumatic stress disorder. Biol Psychiatry 54:710–718, 2003.

212. MacHale SM, Cavanagh JT, Bennie J, et al: Diurnal variation of adrenocortical activity in chronic fatigue syndrome. Neuropsychobiology 38:213–217, 1998.

213. Wood B, Wessely S, Papadopoulos A, et al: Salivary cortisol profiles in chronic fatigue syndrome. Neuropsychobiology 37:1–4, 1998.

214. Crofford LJ, Young EA, Engleberg NC, et al: Basal circadian and pulsatile ACTH and cortisol secretion in patients with fibromyalgia and/or chronic fatigue syndrome. Brain Behav Immun 18:314–325, 2004.

215. Klerman EB, Goldenberg DL, Brown EN, et al: Circadian rhythms of women with fibromyalgia. J Clin Endocrinol Metab 86:1034–1039, 2001.

216. Pruessner JC, Hellhammer DH, Kirschbaum C: Burnout, perceived stress, and cortisol responses to awakening. Psychosom Med 61:197–204, 1999.

217. Muccioli G, Tschop M, Papotti M, et al: Neuroendocrine and peripheral activities of ghrelin: Implications in metabolism and obesity. Eur J Pharmacol 440:235–254, 2002.

218. van der Lely A, Tschop M, Heiman M, et al: Biological, physiological, pathophysiological, and pharmacological aspects of ghrelin. Endocr Rev 25:426–457, 2004.

219. Van Cauter E, Plat L, Copinschi G: Interrelations between sleep and the somatotropic axis. Sleep 21:553–566, 1998.

220. Mendlewicz J, Linkowski P, Kerkhofs M, et al: Genetic control of 24-hour growth hormone secretion in man: A twin study. J Clin Endocrinol Metab 84:856–862, 1999.

221. Ho KY, Evans WS, Blizzard RM, et al: Effects of sex and age on the 24-hour profile of growth hormone secretion in man: Importance of endogenous estradiol concentrations. J Clin Endocrinol Metab 64:51–58, 1987.

222. Shah N, Evans WS, Veldhuis JD: Actions of estrogen on pulsatile,

nyctohemeral, and entropic modes of growth hormone secretion. Am J Physiol R1351–R1358, 1999.

223. Caufriez A, Van Onderbergen A, L'Hermite-Balériaux M, et al: Daytime GH secretion is enhanced during luteal phase in normally cycling healthy women (in press).

224. Van Cauter E, Kerkhofs M, Caufriez A, et al: A quantitative estimation of GH secretion in normal man: Reproducibility and relation to sleep and time of day. J Clin Endocrinol Metab 74:1441–1450, 1992.

225. Holl RW, Hartmann ML, Veldhuis JD, et al: Thirty-second sampling of plasma growth hormone in man: Correlation with sleep stages. J Clin Endocrinol Metab 72:854–861, 1991.

226. Obal Jr F, Krueger JM: Biochemical regulation of non-rapid-eye-movement sleep. Front Biosci 8:520–550, 2003.

227. Ocampo-Lim B, Guo W, DeMott Friberg R, et al: Nocturnal growth hormone (GH) secretion is eliminated by infusion of GH-releasing hormone antagonist. J Clin Endocrinol Metab 81:4396–4399, 1996.

228. Van Cauter E, Plat L, Scharf M, et al: Simultaneous stimulation of slow-wave sleep and growth hormone secretion by gamma-hydroxybutyrate in normal young men. J Clin Invest 100:745–753, 1997.

229. Gronfier C, Luthringer R, Follenius M, et al: A quantitative evaluation of the relationships between growth hormone secretion and delta wave electroencephalographic activity during normal sleep and after enrichment in delta waves. Sleep 19:817–882, 1996.

230. Van Cauter E, Caufriez A, Kerkhofs M, et al: Sleep, awakenings and insulin-like growth factor I modulate the growth hormone secretory response to growth hormone-releasing hormone. J Clin Endocrinol Metab 74:1451–1459, 1992.

231. Jaffe C, Turgeon D, DeMott Friberg R, et al: Nocturnal augmentation of growth hormone (GH) secretion is preserved during repetitive bolus administration of GH-releasing hormone: Potential involvement of endogenous somatostatin—A clinical research center study. J Clin Endocrinol Metab 80:3321–3326, 1995.

232. Cummings DE, Weigle DS, Frayo RS, et al: Plasma ghrelin levels after diet-induced weight loss or gastric bypass surgery. N Engl J Med 346:1623–1630, 2002.

233. Dzaja A, Dalal M, Himmerich H, et al: Sleep enhances nocturnal plasma ghrelin levels in healthy subjects. Am J Physiol Endocrinol Metab 286:E963–E967, 2004.

234. Steiger A, Herth T, Holsboer F: Sleep-electroencephalography and the secretion of cortisol and growth hormone in normal controls. Acta Endocrinol 116:36–42, 1987.

235. Brandenberger G, Gronfier C, Chapotot F, et al: Effect of sleep deprivation on overall 24 h growth-hormone secretion. Lancet 356:1408, 2000.

236. Spiegel K, Leproult R, Colecchia EF, et al: Adaptation of the 24-h growth hormone profile to a state of sleep debt. Am J Physiol 279:R874–R883, 2000.

237. Vermeulen A: Nyctohemeral growth hormone profiles in young and aged men: Correlation with somatomedin-C levels. J Clin Endocrinol Metab 64:884–888, 1987.

238. Veldhuis J, Liem A, South S, et al: Differential impact of age, sex steroid hormones, and obesity on basal versus pulsatile growth hormone secretion in men as assessed in an ultrasensitive chemiluminescence assay. J Clin Endocrinol Metab 80:3209–3222, 1995.

239. Veldhuis JD, Iranmanesh A, Weltman A: Elements in the pathophysiology of diminished growth hormone (GH) secretion in aging humans. Endocrine 7:41–48, 1997.

240. Martin FC, Yeo AL, Sonksen PH: Growth hormone secretion in the elderly: Ageing and the somatopause. Baillieres Clin Endocrinol Metab 11:223–250, 1997.

241. Caufriez A, Frankenne F, Hennen G, et al: Regulation of maternal IGF-I by placental GH in normal and abnormal human pregnancies. Am J Physiol 265:E572–E577, 1993.

242. Eriksson L, Frankenne F, Eden S, et al: Growth hormone 24-h serum profiles during pregnancy—Lack of pulsatility for the secretion of the placental variant. Br J Obstet Gynaecol 96:949–953, 1989.

243. Veldhuis JD, Iranmanesh A, Ho KKY, et al: Dual defects in pulsatile growth hormone secretion and clearance subserve the hyposomatotropism of obesity in man. J Clin Endocrinol Metab 72:51–59, 1991.

244. Copinschi G, De Laet MH, Brion JP, et al: Simultaneous study of cortisol, GH and PRL circadian variations of hourly integrated concentrations in normal and obese subjects. Clin Endocrinol 9:15–26, 1978.

245. Ho KY, Veldhuis JD, Johnson ML, et al: Fasting enhances growth hormone secretion and amplifies the complex rhythms of growth hormone secretion in man. J Clin Invest 81:968–975, 1988.

246. Stoving RK, Veldhuis JD, Flyvbjerg A, et al: Jointly amplified basal and pulsatile growth hormone (GH) secretion and increased process irregularity in women with anorexia nervosa: Indirect evidence for disruption of feedback regulation within the GH-insulin-like growth factor I axis. J Clin Endocrinol Metab 84:2056–2063, 1999.

247. Edge JA, Dunger DB, Matthews DR, et al: Increased overnight growth hormone concentrations in diabetic compared with normal adolescents. J Clin Endocrinol Metab 71:1356–1362, 1990.

248. Laughlin GA, Dominguez CE, Yen SS: Nutritional and endocrine-metabolic aberrations in women with functional hypothalamic amenorrhea. J Clin Endocrinol Metab 83:25–32, 1998.

249. Morales AJ, Laughlin GA, Butzow T, et al: Insulin, somatotropic, and luteinizing hormone axes in lean and obese women with polycystic ovary syndrome: Common and distinct features. J Clin Endocrinol Metab 81:2854–2864, 1996.

250. Iranmanesh A, Lizarralde G, Johnson ML, et al: Nature of altered growth hormone secretion in hyperthyroidism. J Clin Endocrinol Metab 72:108–115, 1991.

251. Mendlewicz J, Linkowski P, Kerkhofs M, et al: Diurnal hypersecretion of growth hormone in depression. J Clin Endocrinol Metab 60:505–512, 1985.

252. Veldman RG, Frolich M, Pincus SM, et al: Growth hormone and prolactin are secreted more irregularly in patients with Cushing's disease. Clin Endocrinol 52:625–632, 2000.

253. Hartman ML, Veldhuis JD, Vance ML, et al: Somatotropin pulse frequency and basal concentrations are increased in acromegaly and are reduced by successful therapy. J Clin Endocrinol Metab 70:1375–1384, 1990.

254. Hartmann ML, Pincus SM, Johnson ML, et al: Enhanced basal and disorderly growth hormone secretion distinguish acromegalic from normal pulsatile growth hormone release. J Clin Invest 94:1277–1288, 1994.

255. van den Berg G, Pincus SM, Frolich M, et al: Reduced disorderliness of growth hormone release in biochemically inactive acromegaly after pituitary surgery. Eur J Endocrinol 138:164–169, 1998.

256. Sassin JF, Frantz AG, Weitzman ED, et al: Human prolactin: 24-hour pattern with increased release during sleep. Science 177:1205–1207, 1972.

257. Van Cauter E, L'Hermite M, Copinschi G, et al: Quantitative analysis of spontaneous variations of plasma prolactin in normal man. Am J Physiol 241:E355–E363, 1981.

258. Spiegel K, Follenius M, Simon C, et al: Prolactin secretion and sleep. Sleep 17:20–27, 1994.

259. Waldstreicher J, Duffy JF, Brown EN, et al: Gender differences in the temporal organization of prolactin (PRL) secretion: Evidence fort a sleep-independent circadian rhythm of circulating PRL levels—A clinical research center study. J Clin Endocrinol Metab 81:1483–1487, 1996.

260. Katznelson L, Riskind PN, Saxe VC, Klibanski A: Prolactin pulsatile characteristics in postmenopausal women. J Clin Endocrinol Metab 83:761–764, 1998.

261. Linkowski P, Spiegel K, Kerkhofs M, et al: Genetic and environmental influences on prolactin secretion during wake and during sleep. Am J Physiol 274:E909–E919, 1998.

262. Van Cauter E, Refetoff S: Multifactorial control of the 24-hour secretory profiles of pituitary hormones. J Endocrinol Invest 8:381–391, 1985.

263. Desir D, Van Cauter E, L'Hermite M, et al: Effects of "jet lag" on hormonal patterns. III. Demonstration of an intrinsic circadian rhythmicity in plasma prolactin. J Clin Endocrinol Metab 55:849–857, 1982.

264. Copinschi G, Van Onderbergen A, L'Hermite-Balériaux M, et al: Effects of the short-acting benzodiazepine triazolam, taken at bedtime, on circadian and sleep-related hormonal profiles in normal men. Sleep 13:232–244, 1990.

265. Copinschi G, Akseki E, Moreno-Reyes R, et al: Effects of bedtime administration of zolpidem on circadian and sleep-related hormonal profiles in normal women. Sleep 18:417–424, 1995.

266. Spiegel K, Luthringer R, Follenius M, et al: Temporal relationship between prolactin secretion and slow-wave electroencephalographic activity during sleep. Sleep 18:543–548, 1995.

267. Greenspan SL, Klibanski A, Rowe JW, et al: Age alters pulsatile prolactin release: Influence of dopaminergic inhibition. Am J Physiol 258:E799–E804, 1990.

268. Tay CC, Glasier AF, McNeilly AS: Twenty-four hour patterns of prolactin secretion during lactation and the relationship to suckling and the resumption of fertility in breast-feeding women. Hum Reprod 11:950–955, 1996.

269. Caufriez A, Désir D, Szyper M, et al: Prolactin secretion in Cushing's disease. J Clin Endocrinol Metab 53:843–846, 1981.

270. Iranmanesh A, Veldhuis JD, Carlsen EC, et al: Attenuated pulsatile release of prolactin in men with insulin-dependent diabetes mellitus. J Clin Endocrinol Metab 71:73–78, 1990.

271. Veldman RG, Frolich M, Pincus SM, et al: Basal, pulsatile, entropic, and 24-hour rhythmic features of secondary hyperprolactinemia due to functional pituitary stalk disconnection mimic tumoral (primary) hyperprolactinemia. J Clin Endocrinol Metab 86:1562–1567, 2001.

272. Groote Veldman R, van den Berg G, Pincus SM, et al: Increased episodic release and disorderliness of prolactin secretion in both micro- and macroprolactinomas. Eur J Endocrinol 140:192–200, 1999.

273. Boyar RM, Kapen S, Finkelstein JW, et al: Hypothalamic-pituitary function in diverse hyperprolactinemic states. J Clin Invest 53:1588–1598, 1974.

274. Spratt DI, O'Dea LL, Schoenfeld D, et al: Neuroendocrine-gonadal axis in men: Frequent sampling of LH, FSH and testosterone. Am J Physiol 254:E658–E666, 1988.

275. Fehm HL, Clausing J, Kern W, et al: Sleep-associated augmentation and synchronization of luteinizing hormone pulses in adult men. Neuroendocrinology 54:192–195, 1991.

276. Bremner WJ, Vitiello MV, Prinz PN: Loss of circadian rhythmicity in blood testosterone levels with aging in normal men. J Clin Endocrinol Metab 56:1278–1280, 1983.

277. Luboshitzky R, Herer P, Levi M, et al: Relationship between rapid eye movement sleep and testosterone secretion in normal men. J Androl 20:731–377, 1999.

278. Luboshitzky R, Zabari Z, Shen-Orr Z, et al: Disruption of the nocturnal testosterone rhythm by sleep fragmentation in normal men. J Clin Endocrinol Metab 86:1134–1139, 2001.

279. Carlsen E, Olsson C, Petersen JH, et al: Diurnal rhythm in serum levels of inhibin B in normal men: Relation to testicular steroids and gonadotropins. J Clin Endocrinol Metab 84:1664–1669, 1999.

280. Vermeulen A, Deslypere JP, Kaukman JM: Influence of antiopioids on luteinizing hormone pulsatility in aging men. J Clin Endocrinol Metab 68:68–72, 1989.

281. Veldhuis JD, Urban RJ, Lizarralde G, et al: Attenuation of luteinizing hormone secretory burst amplitude as a proximate basis for the hypoandrogenism of healthy aging in men. J Clin Endocrinol Metab 75:52–58, 1992.

282. Mulligan T, Iranmanesh A, Gheorghiu S, et al: Amplified nocturnal luteinizing hormone (LH) secretory burst frequency with selective attenuation of pulsatile (but not basal) testosterone secretion in healthy aged men: Possible Leydig cell desensitization to endogenous LH signaling—A clinical research center study. J Clin Endocrinol Metab 80:3025–3031, 1995.

283. Tenover JS, Matsumoto AM, Clifton DK, et al: Age-related alterations in the circadian rhythms of pulsatile luteinizing hormone and testosterone secretion in healthy. J Gerontol 43:M163–M169, 1988.

284. Veldhuis JD, Iranmanesh A, Demers LM, et al: Joint basal and pulsatile hypersecretory mechanisms drive the monotropic follicle-stimulating hormone (FSH) elevation in healthy older men: Concurrent preservation of the orderliness of the FSH release process: A general clinical research center study. J Clin Endocrinol Metab 84:3506–3514, 1999.

285. Penev P, Spiegel K, L'Hermite-Baleriaux M, et al: Relationship between REM sleep and testosterone secretion in older men. Ann Endocrinol 64:157, 2003.

286. Luboshitzky R, Shen-Orr Z, Herer P: Middle-aged men secrete less testosterone at night than young

287. Pincus SM, Mulligan T, Iranmanesh A, et al: Older males secrete luteinizing hormone and testosterone more irregularly, and jointly more asynchronously, than younger males. Proc Natl Acad Sci U S A 93:14100–14105, 1996.

288. Reame N, Sauder SE, Kelch RP, et al: Pulsatile gonadotropin secretion during the human menstrual cycle: Evidence for altered frequency of gonadotropin-releasing hormone secretion. J Clin Endocrinol Metab 59:328–337, 1984.

289. Filicori M, Santoro N, Merriam GR, et al: Characterization of the physiological pattern of episodic gonadotropin secretion throughout the menstrual cycle. J Clin Endocrinol Metab 62:1136–1144, 1986.

290. Hall JE, Schoenfeld DA, Martin KA, et al: Hypothalamic gonadotropin-releasing hormone secretion and follicle-stimulating hormone dynamics during the luteal-follicular transition. J Clin Endocrinol Metab 4:600–607, 1992.

291. Turek FW, Van Cauter E: Rhythms in reproduction. In Knobil E, Neill JD (eds): The Physiology of Reproduction. New York, Raven Press, 1993, pp 1789–1830.

292. Bergendahl M, Aloi JA, Iranmanesh A, et al: Fasting suppresses pulsatile luteinizing hormone (LH) secretion and enhances orderliness of LH release in young but not older men. J Clin Endocrinol Metab 83:1967–1975, 1998.

293. Sartorio A, Pizzocaro A, Liberati D, et al: Abnormal LH pulsatility in women with hyperprolactinaemic amenorrhoea normalizes after bromocriptine treatment: Deconvolution-based assessment. Clin Endocrinol 52:703–712, 2000.

294. Khoury SA, Reame NE, Kelch RP, et al: Diurnal patterns of pulsatile luteinizing hormone secretion in hypothalamic amenorrhea: Reproducibility and responses to opiate blockade and an alpha-adrenergic agonist. J Clin Endocrinol Metab 64:755–762, 1967.

295. Fumming DC, Vickovic MM, Fluker MR: Defects in pulsatile LH release in normally menstruating runners. J Clin Endocrinol Metab 60:810–812, 1985.

296. Zumoff B, Freeman R, Coupey S, et al: A chronobiologic abnormality in luteinizing secretion in teenage girls with the polycystic-ovary syndrome. N Engl J Med 309:1206–1209, 1983.

297. Porcu E, Venturoli S, Longhi M, et al: Chronobiologic evolution of luteinizing hormone secretion in adolescence: Developmental patterns and speculations on the onset of the polycystic ovary syndrome. Fertil Steril 67:842–848, 1997.

298. Venturoli S, Porcu E, Fabbri R, et al: Episodic pulsatile secretion of FSH, prolactin, oestradiol, oestrone, and LH circadian variations in polycystic ovary

syndrome. Clin Endocrinol 28:93–107, 1988.

299. Waldstreicher J, Santoro NF, Hall JE, et al: Hyperfunction of the hypothalamo-pituitary axis in women with polycystic ovarian disease: Indirect evidence for partial gonadotroph desensitization. J Clin Endocrinol Metab 66:165–172, 1998.

300. Blomquist CH, Holt JPJ: Chronobiology of the hypothalamo-pituitary-gonadal axis in men and women. In Touitou Y, Haus E (eds): Biological Rhythms in Clinical and Laboratory Medicine. New York, Springer-Verlag, 1992, pp 315–329.

301. Fachinetti F, Genazzani AD, Martignoni E, et al: Neuroendocrine correlates of premenstrual syndrome: Changes in the pulsatile pattern of plasma LH. Psychoneuroendocrinology 15:269–277, 1990.

302. Parry BL: Sleep, mood, and the menstrual cycle. Semin Reprod Med 8:81–88, 1990.

303. Spratt DI, Carr DB, Merriam GR, et al: The spectrum of abnormal patterns of gonadotropin-releasing hormone secretion in men with idiopathic hypogonadotropic hypogonadism: Clinical and laboratory correlations. J Clin Endocrinol Metab 64:283–291, 1987.

304. Luboshitzky R, Aviv A, Hefetz A, et al: Decreased pituitary-gonadal secretion in men with obstructive sleep apnea. J Clin Endocrinol Metab 87:3394–3398, 2002.

305. Luboshitzky R, Lavie L, Shen-Orr Z, et al: Pituitary-gonadal function in men with obstructive sleep apnea. The effect of continuous positive airways pressure treatment. Neuroendocrinol Lett 24:463–467, 2003.

306. Hangaard J, Andersen M, Grodum E, et al: Pulsatile luteinizing hormone secretion in patients with Addison's disease. Impact of glucocorticoid substitution. J Clin Endocrinol Metab 83:736–743, 1998.

307. Lopez-Alvarenga JC, Zarinan T, Olivares A, et al: Poorly controlled type I diabetes mellitus in young men selectively suppresses luteinizing hormone secretory burst mass. J Clin Endocrinol Metab 87:5507–5515, 2002.

308. Parker DC, Rossman LG, Pekary AE, et al: Effect of 64-hour sleep deprivation on the circadian waveform of thyrotropin (TSH): Further evidence of sleep-related inhibition of TSH release. J Clin Endocrinol Metab 64:157–161, 1987.

309. Goichot B, Brandenberger G, Saini J, et al: Nocturnal plasma thyrotropin variations are related to slow-wave sleep. J Sleep Res 1:186–190, 1992.

310. Gronfier C, Luthringer R, Follenius M, et al: Temporal link between plasma thyrotropin levels and electroencephalographic activity in man. Neurosci Lett 200:97–100, 1995.

311. Hirschfeld U, Moreno-Reyes R, Akseki E, et al: Progressive elevation of plasma thyrotropin during adaptation

to simulated jet lag: Effects of treatment with bright light or zolpidem. J Clin Endocrinol Metab 81:3270–3277, 1996.

312. Greenspan SL, Klibanski A, Schoenfeld D, et al: Pulsatile secretion of thyrotropin in man. J Clin Endocrinol Metab 63:661–668, 1986.

313. Brabant G, Brabant A, Ranft U, et al: Circadian and pulsatile thyrotropin secretion in euthyroid man under influence of thyroid hormone and glucocorticoid administration. J Clin Endocrinol Metab 65:83–88, 1987.

314. Kalsbeek A, Fliers, E, Franke AN, et al: Functional connections between the suprachiasmatic nucleus and the thyroid gland as revealed by lesioning and viral tracing techniques in the rat. Endocrinology 141:3832–3841, 2000.

315. Allan JS, Czeisler CA: Persistence of the circadian thyrotropin rhythm under constant conditions and after light-induced shifts of circadian phase. J Clin Endocrinol Metab 79:508–512, 1994.

316. Gary KA, Winokur A, Douglas SD, et al: Total sleep deprivation and the thyroid axis: Effects of sleep and waking activity. Aviat Space Environ Med 67:513–519, 1996.

317. Romijn JA, Wiersinga WM: Decreased nocturnal surge of thyrotropin in nonthyroidal illness. J Clin Endocrinol Metab 70:35–42, 1990.

318. Bartalena F, Martino E, Petrini L, et al: The nocturnal serum thyrotropin surge is abolished in patients with ACTH-dependent or ACTH-independent Cushing's syndrome. J Clin Endocrinol Metab 72:1195–1199, 1991.

319. Caron PJ, Nieman LK, Rose SR, et al: Deficient nocturnal surge of thyrotropin in central hypothyroidism. J Clin Endocrinol Metab 62:960–964, 1986.

320. Samuels MH, Lillehei K, Kleinschmidt-Demasters BK, et al: Patterns of pulsatile pituitary glycoprotein secretion in central hypothyroidism and hypogonadism. J Clin Endocrinol Metab 70:391–395, 1990.

321. Bartalena L, Cossu E, Grasso L, et al: Relationship between nocturnal serum thyrotropin peak and metabolic control in diabetic patients. J Clin Endocrinol Metab 76:983–987, 1993.

322. el-Hajj Fuleihan G, Klerman EB, Brown EN, et al: The parathyroid hormone circadian rhythm is truly endogenous—A general clinical research center study. J Clin Endocrinol Metab 82:281–286, 1997.

323. Kripke DF, Lavie P, Parker D, et al: Plasma parathyroid hormone and calcium are related to sleep stage cycles. J Clin Endocrinol Metab 47:1021–1027, 1978.

324. Logue FC, Fraser WD, O'Reilly DS, et al: Sleep shift dissociates the nocturnal peaks of parathyroid hormone (1-84), nephrogenous cyclic adenosine monophosphate, and

prolactin in normal men. J Clin Endocrinol Metab 75:25–29, 1992.

325. Fraser WD, Logue FC, Christie JP, et al: Alteration of the circadian rhythm of intact parathyroid hormone following a 96-hour fast. Clin Endocrinol 40:523–528, 1994.

326. Fraser WD, Logue FC, Christie JP, et al: Alteration of the circadian rhythm of intact parathyroid hormone and serum phosphate in women with established postmenopausal osteoporosis. Osteoporos Int 8:121–126, 1998.

327. Lobaugh B, Neelon FA, Oyama H, et al: Circadian rhythms for calcium, inorganic phosphorus, and parathyroid hormone in primary hyperparathyroidism: Functional and practical considerations. Surgery 106:1009–1017, 1989.

328. Luthringer R, Brandenberger G, Schaltenbrand N, et al: Slow wave electroencephalographic activity parallels renin oscillations during sleep in humans. Electroencephalogr Clin Neurophysiol 95:318–322, 1995.

329. Charloux A, Gronfier C, Lonsdorfer-Wolf E, et al: Aldosterone release during the sleep-wake cycle in humans. Am J Physiol 276:E43–E49, 1999.

330. Charloux A, Gronfier C, Chapotot F, et al: Sleep deprivation blunts the night time increase in aldosterone release in humans. J Sleep Res 10:27–33, 2001.

331. Brandenberger G, Charloux A, Grongier C, et al: Ultradian rhythms in hydromineral hormones. Horm Res 49:131–135, 1998.

332. Follenius M, Brandenberger G, Saini J: Lack of diurnal rhythm in plasma atrial natriuretic peptide. Life Sci 51:143–149, 1992.

333. Simon C, Gronfier C, Schlienger JL, et al: Circadian and ultradian variations of leptin in normal man under continuous enteral nutrition: Relationship to sleep and body temperature. J Clin Endocrinol Metab 83:1893–1899, 1998.

334. Plat L, Byrne MM, Sturis J, et al: Effects of morning cortisol elevation on insulin secretion and glucose regulation in humans. Am J Physiol 270:E36–E42, 1996.

335. Scheen AJ, Byrne MM, Plat L, et al: Relationships between sleep quality and glucose regulation in normal humans. Am J Physiol 271:E261–E270, 1996.

335a. Morgan L, Hampton S, Gibbs M, et al: Circadian aspects of postprandial metabolism. Chronobiol Int 29:795–808, 2003.

336. Simon C, Brandenberger G: Ultradian oscillations of insulin secretion in humans. Diabetes 51(Suppl 1):S258–S261, 2002.

337. Sturis J, Van Cauter E, Blackman JD, et al: Entrainment of pulsatile insulin secretion by oscillatory glucose infusion. J Clin Invest 87:439–445, 1991.

338. Sturis J: Possible Mechanisms Underlying Slow Oscillations of Human Insulin Secretion. Lingby, Denmark, The Technical University of Denmark, 1991.

338a. Song SH, Kjems L, Ritzel R, et al: Pulsatile insulin secretion by human pancreatic islets. J Clin Endocrinol Metab 87:213–221, 2002.

339. Porksen N, Hollingdal M, Juhl C, et al: Pulsatile insulin secretion: Detection, regulation, and role in diabetes. Diabetes 51(Suppl 1):S245–S254, 2002.

340. Courtney CH, Atkinson AB, Ennis CN, et al: Comparison of the priming effects of pulsatile and continuous insulin delivery on insulin action in man. Metab Clin Exp 52:1050–1055, 2003.

341. Meneilly GS, Veldhuis JD, Elahi D: Disruption of the pulsatile and entropic modes of insulin release during an unvarying glucose stimulus in elderly individuals. J Clin Endocrinol Metab 84:1938–1943, 1999.

342. Van Cauter E, Polonsky KS, Blackman JD, et al: Abnormal temporal patterns of glucose tolerance in obesity: Relationship to sleep-related growth hormone and circadian cortisol rhythmicity. J Clin Endocrinol Metab 79:1797–1805, 1994.

343. Bolli GB, Gerich JE: The "dawn phenomenon"—A common occurrence in both non-insulin-dependent and insulin-dependent diabetes mellitus. N Engl J Med 310:746–750, 1984.

344. Campbell PJ, Bolli GB, Cryer PE, et al: Pathogenesis of the dawn phenomenon in patients with insulin-dependent diabetes mellitus. N Engl J Med 312:1473–1479, 1985.

345. Davidson MB, Harris MD, Ziel FH, et al: Suppression of sleep-induced growth hormone secretion by anticholinergic agent abolishes dawn phenomenon. Diabetes 37:166–171, 1988.

346. Shapiro ET, Polonsky KS, Copinschi G, et al: Nocturnal elevation of glucose levels during fasting in noninsulin-dependent diabetes. J Clin Endocrinol Metab 72:444–454, 1991.

347. Banarer S, Cryer PE: Sleep-related hypoglycemia-associated autonomic failure in type 1 diabetes: Reduced awakening from sleep during hypoglycemia. Diabetes 52:1195–1203, 2003.

348. O'Meara NM, Sturis J, Van Cauter E, et al: Lack of control by glucose of ultradian insulin secretory oscillations in impaired glucose tolerance and in non-insulin-dependent diabetes mellitus. J Clin Invest 92:262–271, 1993.

349. Schmitz O, Juhl CB, Hollingdal M, et al: Irregular circulating insulin concentrations in type 2 diabetes mellitus: An inverse relationship between circulating free fatty acid and the disorderliness of an insulin time series in diabetic and healthy individuals. Metab Clin Exp 50:41–46, 2001.

350. Flier JS: Obesity wars: Molecular progress confronts an expanding epidemic. Cell 116:337–350, 2004.

351. Kershaw EE, Flier JS: Adipose tissue as an endocrine organ. J Clin Endocrinol Metab 89:2548–2556, 2004.

352. Sinha MK, Ohannesian JP, Heiman ML, et al: Nocturnal rise of leptin in lean, obese and non-insulin-dependent diabetes mellitus subjects. J Clin Invest 97:1344–1347, 1996.

353. Saad MF, Riad-Gabriel MG, Khan A, et al: Diurnal and ultradian rhythmicity of plasma leptin: Effects of gender and adiposity. J Clin Endocrinol Metab 83:453–459, 1998.

354. Kolaczynski JW, Considine RV, Ohannesian J, et al: Responses of leptin to short-term fasting and refeeding in humans: A link with ketogenesis but not ketones themselves. Diabetes 45:1511–1515, 1996.

355. Chin-Chance C, Polonsky KS, Schoeller D: Twenty-four hour leptin levels respond to cumulative short-term energy imbalance and predict subsequent intake. J Clin Endocrinol Metab 85:2685–2691, 2000.

356. Licino J, Negrao AB, Mantzoros C, et al: Sex differences in circulating human leptin pulse amplitude: Clinical implications. J Clin Endocrinol Metab 83:4140–4147, 1998.

357. Laughlin GA, Yen SS: Hypoleptinemia in women athletes: Absence of a diurnal rhythm with amenorrhea. J Clin Endocrinol Metab 82:318–321, 1997.

358. Balligand JL, Brichard SM, Brichard V, et al: Hypoleptinemia in patients with anorexia nervosa: Loss of circadian rhythm and unresponsiveness to short-term refeeding. Eur J Endocrinol 138:415–420, 1998.

359. Franceschini R, Corsini G, Cataldi A, et al: Twenty-four-hour variation in serum leptin in the elderly. Metabolism 48:1011–1014, 1999.

360. Sinha MK, Sturis J, Ohannesian J, et al: Ultradian oscillations of leptin secretion in humans. Biochem Biophys Res Commun 228:733–738, 1996.

361. Licino J, Mantzoros C, Negrao AB, et al: Human leptin levels are pulsatile and inversely related to pituitary-adrenal function. Nat Med 3:575–579, 1997.

362. Schoeller DA, Cella LK, Sinha MK, et al: Entrainment of the diurnal rhythm of plasma leptin to meal timing. J Clin Invest 100:1882–1887, 1997.

363. Mullington JM, Chan JL, Van Dongen HP, et al: Sleep loss reduces diurnal rhythm amplitude of leptin in healthy men. J Neuroendocrinol 15:851–854, 2003.

364. Kok SW, Meinders AE, Overeem S, et al: Reduction of plasma leptin levels and loss of its circadian rhythmicity in hypocretin (orexin)-deficient narcoleptic humans. J Clin Endocrinol Metab 87:805–809, 2002.

365. Eliman A, Knutsson U, Bronnegard M, et al: Variations in glucocorticoid levels within the physiological range affect plasma leptin levels. Eur J Endocrinol 139:615–620, 1998.

366. Purnell JQ, Samuels MH: Levels of leptin during hydrocortisone infusions that mimic normal and reversed diurnal cortisol levels in subjects with adrenal insufficiency. J Clin Endocrinol Metab 84:3125–3128, 1999.

367. Leal-Cerro A, Considine RV, Peino R, et al: Serum immunoreactive-leptin levels are increased in patients with Cushing's syndrome. Horm Metab Res 28:711–713, 1996.

368. Masuzaki H, Ogawa Y, Hosoda K, et al: Glucocorticoid regulation of leptin synthesis and secretion in humans: Elevated plasma leptin levels in Cushing's syndrome. J Clin Endocrinol Metab 82:2542–2547, 1997.

369. Veldman RG, Frolich M, Pincus SM, et al: Hyperleptinemia in women with Cushing's disease is driven by high-amplitude pulsatile, but orderly and eurhythmic, leptin secretion. Eur J Endocrinol 144:21–27, 2001.

370. Kousta E, Chrisoulidou A, Lawrence NJ, et al: The circadian rhythm of leptin is preserved in growth hormone deficient hypopituitary adults. Clin Endocrinol 48:685–690, 1998.

371. Pombo M, Herrera-Justiniano E, Considine RV, et al: Nocturnal rise of leptin in normal prepubertal and pubertal children and in patients with perinatal stalk-transection syndrome. J Clin Endocrinol Metab 82:2751–2754, 1997.

372. Yamauchi T, Kamon J, Waki H, et al: The fat-derived hormone adiponectin reverses insulin resistance associated with both lipoatrophy and obesity. Nat Med 7:941–946, 2001.

373. Kubota N, Terauchi Y, Yamauchi T, et al: Disruption of adiponectin causes insulin resistance and neointimal formation. J Biol Chem 277:25863–25866, 2002.

374. Gavrila A, Peng CK, Chan JL, et al: Diurnal and ultradian dynamics of serum adiponectin in healthy men: Comparison with leptin, circulating soluble leptin receptor, and cortisol patterns. J Clin Endocrinol Metab 88:2838–2843, 2003.

375. Weyer C, Funahashi T, Tanaka S, et al: Hypoadiponectinemia in obesity and type 2 diabetes: Close association with insulin resistance and hyperinsulinemia. J Clin Endocrinol Metab 86:1930–1935, 2001.

376. Date Y, Kojima M, Hosoda H, et al: Ghrelin, a novel growth hormone-releasing acylated peptide, is synthesized in a distinct endocrine cell type in the gastrointestinal tracts of rats and humans. Endocrinology 141:4255–4261, 2000.

377. Wren AM, Seal LJ, Cohen MA, et al: Ghrelin enhances appetite and

increases food intake in humans. J Clin Endocrinol Metab 86:5992–5995, 2001.

378. Weikel JC, Wichniak A, Ising M, et al: Ghrelin promotes slow-wave sleep in humans. Am J Physiol 284:E407–E415, 2003.

379. Cummings DE, Frayo RS, Marmonier C, et al: Plasma ghrelin levels and hunger scores in humans initiating meals voluntarily without time- and food-related cues.

Am J Physiol 287:E297–E304, 2004.

380. Cummings DE, Purnell JQ, Frayo RS, et al: A preprandial rise in plasma ghrelin levels suggests a role in meal initiation in humans. Diabetes 50:1714–1719, 2001.

381. Teff KL, Elliott SS, Tschop M, et al: Dietary fructose reduces circulating insulin and leptin, attenuates postprandial suppression of ghrelin, and increases triglycerides in women.

J Clin Endocrinol Metab 89:2963–2972, 2004.

382. Dzaja A, Dalal MA, Himmerich H, et al: Sleep enhances nocturnal plasma ghrelin levels in healthy subjects. Am J Physiol 286:E963–E967, 2004.

383. Spiegel K, Tasali E, Penev P, et al: Sleep curtailment in healthy young men is associated with decreased leptin levels, elevated ghrelin levels and increased hunger and appetite. Ann Intern Med 141:846–850, 2004.

Hypothalamic Syndromes

Glenn D. Braunstein

INTRODUCTION

The hypothalamus houses multiple nuclei along with afferent and efferent nerve fibers that connect the hypothalamus to the various portions of the brain and brain stem. It is divided into four regions: from anterior to posterior, the preoptic, supraoptic, tuberal, and mamillary regions; and three zones: laterally from the third ventricle, the periventricular, medial, and lateral[1-4] zones (Table 20-1, Figs. 20-1 and 20-2).

The hypothalamus is responsible for many of the body's homeostatic mechanisms, including water metabolism, temperature regulation, appetite control, the sleep-wake cycle, circadian rhythms, and control of the sympathetic and parasympathetic nervous systems. In addition, this area has activity in regard to emotional expression, behavior, and memory. Finally, the hypothalamus is essential to the neuroendocrine control of anterior pituitary function. Table 20-2 lists the various functions along with the hypothalamic nuclei or hypothalamic regions that have been identified as being responsible for these functions and the disorders that result from either destructive or stimulatory lesions in or around the nuclei or region.[1,4–24]

HYPOTHALAMIC DISORDERS: PATHOPHYSIOLOGIC PRINCIPLES

First, the small overall size of the hypothalamus and the close association of the nuclei and nerve tracts mean that a variety of different pathologic processes may give rise to the same signs and symptoms of neurologic and hypothalamic dysfunction.[4] The spectrum of disorders that can affect the hypothalamus is shown in Table 20-3. Tumors, infiltrative disorders, and infections, among other conditions, frequently give rise to headaches, neuro-ophthalmologic disorders, pyramidal tract or sensory nerve dysfunction, extrapyramidal cerebellar signs, and recurrent vomiting.[9,10] Other common manifestations include gonadal dysfunction, either hypogonadism or precocious puberty; diabetes insipidus; somnolence; dysthermia; and evidence of a caloric imbalance either with hyperphagia and obesity or with anorexia with emaciation.[9,10]

Second, although exceptions exist, most patients who have a systemic disorder, such as Langerhans' cell histiocytosis, sarcoidosis, tuberculosis, or leukemia, will exhibit manifestations of the disease outside of the hypothalamus and central nervous system.

Third, a lesion may disrupt a function that is subserved by a hypothalamic nucleus distant from the lesion. Because the afferent and efferent tracts to and from the hypothalamic nuclei traverse other areas of the hypothalamus and brain distant from the nuclei, lesions that affect those tracts may result in dysfunction of several hypothalamic nuclei.

Fourth, most lesions that result in chronic hypothalamic syndromes involve more than one nucleus. As can be seen in Table 20-2, most of the hypothalamic functions are controlled by more than one nucleus, and this redundancy allows some degree of compensation, should one nucleus be affected. In addition, most of the nuclei are paired, and destruction of a single nucleus may not be sufficient to result in a clinical syndrome. Thus, lesions that affect the basal tuberal region of the hypothalamus (pituitary adenomas with suprasellar extension, optic gliomas, and craniopharyngiomas), or are multiple (granulomatous disorders, metastatic tumors, infiltrative disease), or cause enlargement of the third ventricle (aqueductal stenosis, colloid cysts, pinealomas, germ cell tumors, midbrain gliomas) will more likely result in clinical hypothalamic dysfunction than will disorders affecting the more lateral portions of the hypothalamus.

Fifth, the rate of progression of the pathologic process affects the patient's clinical manifestations. Slowly progressive lesions may give few or no symptoms until they achieve a large size, at which time, altered endocrine function and deterioration of cognitive ability may be present, whereas small acute lesions may result in profound clinical manifestations such as alterations in consciousness, thermal dysregulation, and diabetes insipidus.

Sixth, the clinical syndrome due to involvement of a hypothalamic nucleus or tract may differ depending on whether the pathologic lesion is destructive or stimulatory. As an example, chronic, destructive lesions of the preoptic region may result in hypothermia and insomnia, whereas hyperthermia and lethargy may be seen with acute stimulatory lesions.

Finally, the clinical manifestations of the hypothalamic disease depend in part on the age of the patient. Thus, prepubertal gonadotropin deficiency results in sexual infantilism, whereas in the postpubertal state, regression, but not disappearance of, secondary sexual characteristics occurs. Similarly, prepubertal growth hormone deficiency because of a hypothalamic lesion disturbing growth hormone–releasing hormone (GHRH) function results in short stature, whereas a similar lesion occurring in an adult may be manifest only by the adult growth hormone deficiency syndrome.

Table 20-1 Major Hypothalamic Nuclei

	Zone		
Region	**Periventricular**	**Medial**	**Lateral**
Preoptic	Preoptic periventricular nucleus Anterior periventricular nucleus	Medial preoptic nucleus	Lateral preoptic nucleus
Supraoptic	Suprachiasmatic nucleus Paraventricular nucleus	Anterior hypothalamic nucleus Medial portion of supraoptic nucleus	Lateral portion of supraoptic nucleus
Tuberal	Arcuate (infundibular) nucleus	Dorsomedial hypothalamic nucleus Ventromedial hypothalamic nucleus	Lateral hypothalamic nucleus
Mamillary	Posterior hypothalamic nucleus	Premamillary nucleus Medial mamillary nucleus	Lateral mamillary nucleus Intercalatus nucleus

From Braunstein GD: The hypothalamus. In Melmed S (ed): The Pituitary, 2d ed. Cambridge, MA, Blackwell Scientific, 2002, pp 317–348, with permission.

MANIFESTATIONS OF HYPOTHALAMIC DISEASE (FIG. 20-3)

DISORDERS OF WATER METABOLISM

Central Diabetes Insipidus

Complete or partial central diabetes insipidus results from destruction of the antidiuretic hormone (ADH)-producing magnocellular neurons in the supraoptic and paraventricular

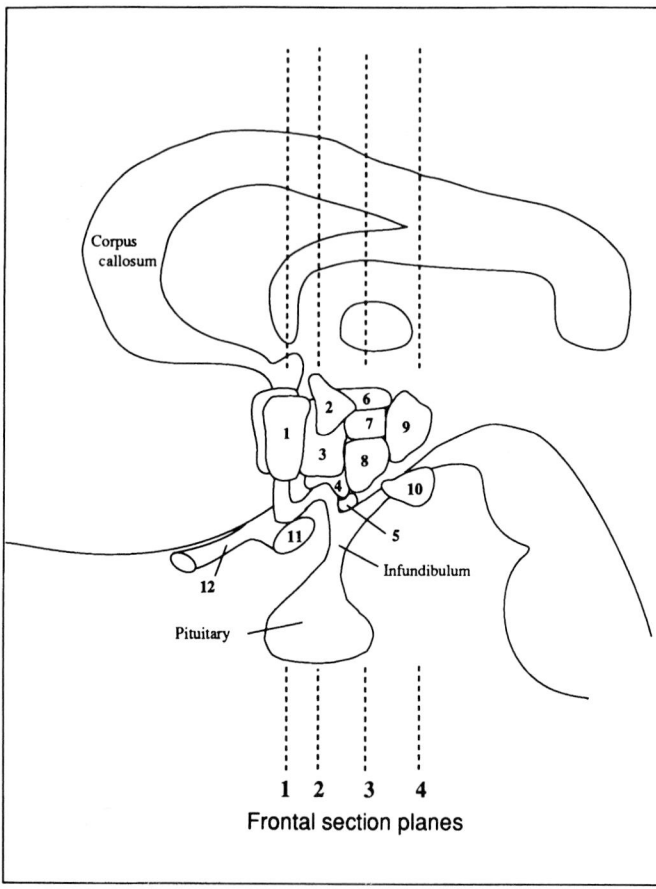

Figure 20-1 Schematic representation of lateral brain section demonstrating hypothalamic nuclei. *Dashed lines* represent the frontal (coronal) section planes illustrated in Figs. 20-2 and 20-3. *1,* preoptic nucleus; *2,* paraventricular nucleus; *3,* anterior hypothalamic areas; *4,* supraoptic nucleus; *5,* arcuate nucleus; *6,* dorsal hypothalamic area; *7,* dorsomedial nucleus; *8,* ventromedial nucleus; *9,* posterior hypothalamic area; *10,* mamillary body; *11,* optic chiasm; *12,* optic nerve. (From Braunstein GD: The hypothalamus. In Melmed S [ed]: The Pituitary, 2d ed. Cambridge, MA, Blackwell Scientific, 2002, pp 317–348, with permission.)

nuclei, or interruption of the transport of ADH through their axons, which terminate in the pituitary stalk and posterior pituitary. Diabetes insipidus is relatively common in patients with chronic hypothalamic disorders, being found in approximately 35% of such patients.[9,10] It also is frequently found in patients with acute insults to the hypothalamus or pituitary stalk, as is seen in vascular accidents and neurosurgical trauma. Obesity and hypogonadism frequently are present in patients with diabetes insipidus due to tumors or infiltrative disorders (see Fig. 20-3).

The majority of patients with diabetes insipidus have idiopathic or familial diabetes insipidus associated with gliosis of the supraoptic and paraventricular nuclei.[25] Approximately one third of patients with idiopathic diabetes insipidus have detectable anti-ADH producing cell antibodies, suggesting an autoimmune cause.[26] Autosomal-recessive, X-linked-recessive and autosomal-dominant forms of familial diabetes insipidus have been described. In the more common autosomal-dominant form, nucleotide deletions or substitutions in the *ADH* gene on chromosome 20 have been identified.[27] The DIDMOAD syndrome (Wolfram's syndrome) represents a rare autosomal-recessive form of central diabetes insipidus (DI) associated with type 1 diabetes mellitus (DM), optic atrophy (OA), bilateral sensorineural deafness (D), and, occasionally, ataxia and autonomic neurogenic bladder.[28] Diabetes insipidus is a frequent manifestation of suprasellar and pineal germinomas, sarcoidosis, lymphocytic infunidibuloneurohypophysitis, and the chronic disseminated form of Langerhans' cell histiocytosis.[29–36]

Adipsic or Essential Hypernatremia

Adipsic hypernatremia occurs when the osmoreceptors that are present in the anterior medial and anterior lateral preoptic regions are damaged. The affected patients have an impaired thirst mechanism, which results in insufficient fluid intake despite the hypernatremia. Although most of the affected patients have partial diabetes insipidus, their extracellular fluid volume remains normal, and they are not dehydrated. Therefore, they exhibit chronic elevations of serum sodium, but normal blood pressure, pulse rate, serum creatinine, and creatinine clearance, and can release ADH and concentrate their urine during fluid deprivation. When serum sodium concentrations are less than 160 mmol/L, few symptoms are present. However, between 160 and 180 mmol/L, patients may have fatigue, weakness, lethargy, muscle tenderness, cramps, anorexia, depression, and irritability, and 180 mmol/L stupor and coma may be present. Close to half of these patients have hypothalamic obesity and almost three fourths demonstrate some degree of anterior pituitary hormone deficiency.[6,9,10,13,37,38]

Essential hypernatremia has been described with a variety of lesions, including craniopharyngiomas, suprasellar germinomas, optic nerve gliomas, pineal tumors, Langerhans' cell his-

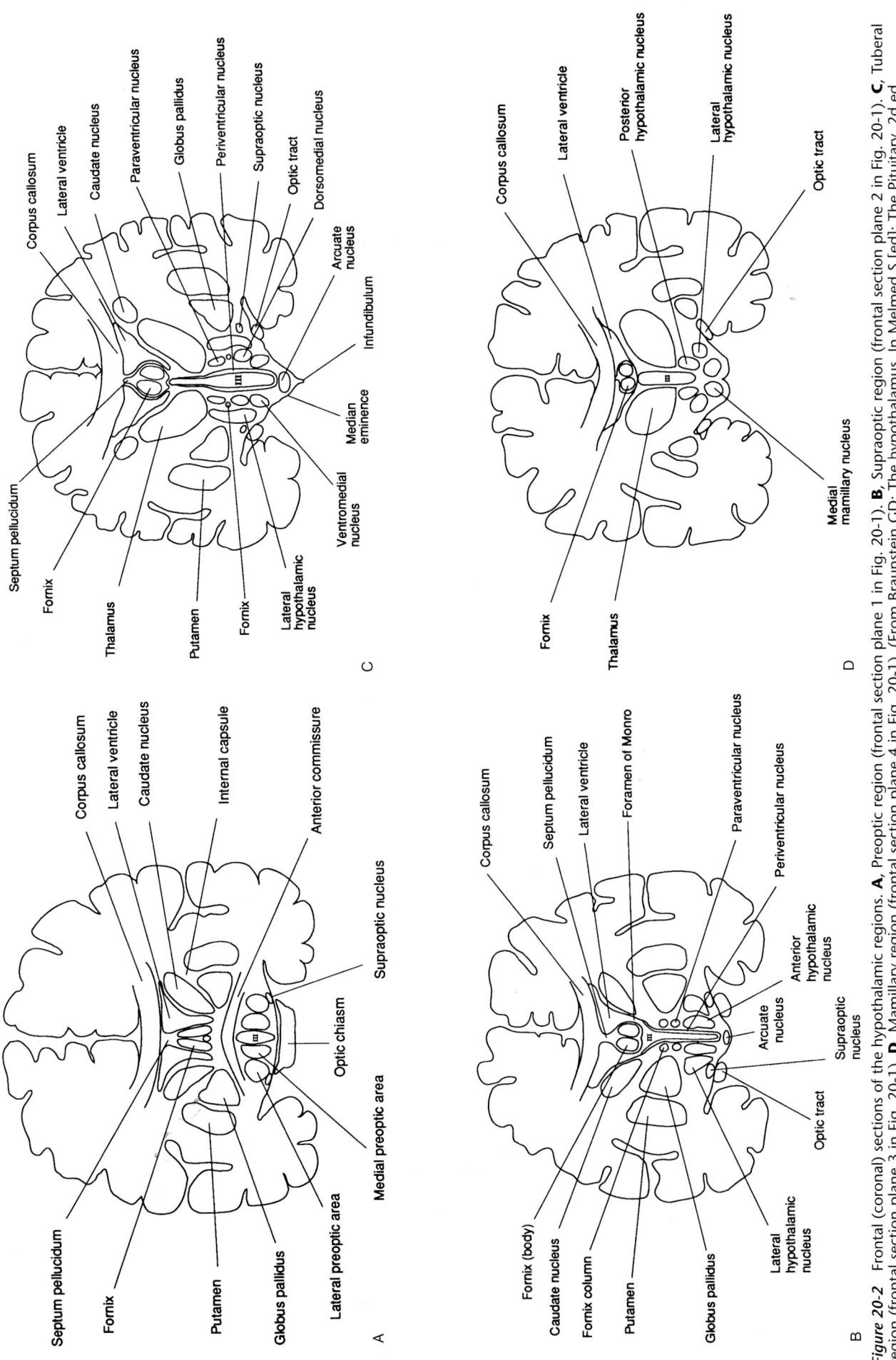

Figure 20-2 Frontal (coronal) sections of the hypothalamic regions. **A**, Preoptic region (frontal section plane 1 in Fig. 20-1). **B**, Supraoptic region (frontal section plane 2 in Fig. 20-1). **C**, Tuberal region (frontal section plane 3 in Fig. 20-1). **D**, Mamillary region (frontal section plane 4 in Fig. 20-1). (From Braunstein GD: The hypothalamus. In Melmed S [ed]: The Pituitary, 2d ed. Cambridge, MA, Blackwell Scientific, 2002, pp 317–348, with permission.)

tiocytosis, sarcoidosis, trauma, hydrocephalus, cysts, inflammatory conditions, ruptured aneurysms of the anterior communicating artery, and toluene exposure.[37-39] The Hayek-Peake syndrome is the association of essential hypernatremia with hypodipsia, obesity, lethargy, increased perspiration, central hypoventilation, hyperprolactinemia, hypothyroidism, and hyperlipidemia without an identifiable structural hypothalamic defect.[40,41]

Syndrome of Inappropriate Secretion of Antidiuretic Hormone

Syndrome of inappropriate secretion of antidiuretic hormone (SIADH) is characterized by serum hyponatremia and hypoosmolarity with an inappropriately elevated urine osmolarity in a patient with normal renal, adrenal, and thyroid function without evidence of intravascular or extracellular fluid volume expansion. The clinical symptoms depend on the rate of decrease of serum sodium, as well as the absolute serum sodium concentration. At serum sodium levels greater than 120 mmol/L, symptoms are generally mild and nonspecific and include anorexia, nausea, headache, weakness, and lethargy. At less than 120 mmol/L, these symptoms are accompanied by nausea, vomiting, and mental confusion, and, at very low levels, by seizure and coma. The syndrome is found with a variety of intracranial abnormalities, including head trauma, intracranial bleeding, meningitis, encephalitis, neurosurgery, hydrocephalus, acute intermittent porphyria, craniopharyngiomas, germinomas, and pinealomas.[6,13,29] An idiopathic form has been described in young women who exhibit menstrual irregularities, have enlarged lateral ventricles, and have SIADH cyclically. No structural defect has been described in these patients.[4]

DYSTHERMIA

Hyperthermia

The warm receptors present in the preoptic anterior hypothalamus are stimulated by an increase in the temperature of the blood. Together with signals from peripheral warm receptors that respond to an increase in external temperature, the afferent signals travel through the median forebrain bundle to the lateral portion of the posterior hypothalamus, which leads to vasodilation and sweating to dissipate heat. Conversely, stimulation of the preoptic anterior hypothalamic cold receptors through a decrease in temperature of the blood, or stimulation of the peripheral cold receptors through a decrease in ambient temperature, results in medial neurons in the posterior hypothalamus activating heat production through muscular shivering and heat conservation through vasoconstriction.[5,6]

Acute injury to the anterior hypothalamic and preoptic areas may result in a rapid temperature elevation as high as 41°C, associated with tachycardia and unconsciousness from failure of the heat-dissipating mechanisms to function while heat production continues. Chronic hyperthermia may be found with lesions in the tuberoinfundibular region, and in contrast to patients with elevated temperature from inflammation of infections, these patients generally do not experience malaise and paradoxically may have peripheral vasoconstriction.[1,5,6,9,11]

Wolff and colleagues[42] described a syndrome of hyperthermia associated with shaking chills, fever, hypertension, vomiting, and peripheral vasoconstriction that occurred cyclically at 3-week intervals, without a pathologic lesion in the hypothalamus being found. Similar paroxysms of hyperthermia have been noted in other patients without the cyclicity, and together these episodes may represent a variant of diencephalic epilepsy.[6,42,43]

In approximately 0.2% of patients receiving neuroleptic drugs, the neuroleptic malignant syndrome (NMS) develops, which is characterized by hyperthermia to 41°C or higher;

severe extrapyramidal signs, including "lead-pipe" muscle rigidity and tremor; signs of autonomic nervous system dysfunction such as pallor, tachycardia, arrhythmias, blood pressure lability, and diaphoresis; and changes in mental status, including mutism, delirium, and coma.[44] All antipsychotic medications have been reported to cause NMS, and most evidence suggests that disruption of the dopamine neurotransmission by neuroleptic-induced dopamine receptor blockade is the major pathophysiologic abnormality in susceptible individuals. Indeed, the greater the potency of the neuroleptic in regard to its dopamine D_2-receptor antagonism activity, the greater the frequency of NMS occurrence.[44] NMS is successfully treated with a variety of dopamine agonists. Injury to the preoptic medial and tuberal nuclei has been demonstrated at autopsy, as has a depletion of hypothalamic norepinephrine concentrations.[45] The syndrome generally begins within 2 weeks of initiating the neuroleptic and evolves over a 24- to 72-hour period. The most common complication is rhabdomyolysis, which may result in myoglobinuria and acute renal failure. The mortality of this syndrome is currently less than 10%, which reflects the increasing recognition and initiation of prompt therapy of the disorder.[44]

Hypothermia

Large destructive lesions of the anterior or posterior hypothalamus may result in inability to generate heat through vasoconstriction and muscular shivering. This occurs in 10% to 15% of patients with a variety of hypothalamic lesions, especially neoplasms, infiltrative disorders, and infections.[9,10,13] It also has been noted in patients with Parkinson's disease and Wernicke's encephalopathy, which are associated with lesions in the posterior hypothalamus and mamillary bodies, respectively.[46,47]

Diencephalic autonomic epilepsy refers to episodic or paroxysmal hypothermia, during which the body temperature decreases to 32°C or less over minutes to days, along with evidence of autonomic nervous system dysfunction, including flushing, sweating, hypotension, bradycardia, salivation, lacrimation, pupillary dilation, Cheyne-Stokes respiration, nausea, vomiting, asterixis, ataxia, and obtundation.[6,15,48-51] Electroencephalographic (EEG) abnormalities occur during the episodes. Autopsy studies have shown gliosis and loss of the arcuate nucleus and premamillary area in some patients, whereas others have been found to have tumors involving the floor and lower portion of the third ventricle.[15,48] The corpus callosum has been found to be absent in approximately half of the patients with episodic hypothermia, and these individuals also may exhibit diabetes insipidus, reset osmostat, growth hormone deficiency, hypogonadism, or precocious puberty (Shapiro's syndrome).[52-54]

Poikilothermia

When both the heat-loss and heat-conserving homeostatic mechanisms are impaired, wide fluctuations of body temperature might take place, without the patients experiencing thermal discomfort. This condition, known as poikilothermia, is found with both anterior and posterior hypothalamic destruction, as well as in patients with large lesions that may involve the posterior hypothalamus and rostal mesencephalon.[6,9,10] Rarely, patients with Wernicke's encephalopathy may experience poikilothermia.[6]

DISORDERS OF APPETITE CONTROL AND CALORIC BALANCE

Hypothalamic Obesity

Approximately 25% of patients with structural hypothalamic lesions exhibit hyperphagia and obesity.[9,10] Usually, the patients have lesions involving a large portion of the hypothalamus, although bilateral destruction of only the ventromedial nucleus may lead to hypothalamic obesity.[1,9,10,17,18,22,55] The majority of patients harbor a neoplasm, especially cranio-

Table 20-2 Hypothalamic Functions, the Nuclei or Regions Involved with the Specific Functions, and the Disorders Resulting from Stimulatory or Destructive Lesions in the Regions

Function	Nuclei [n] or Region Involved [r]	Disorders
Water metabolism	Supraoptic [n]; paraventricular [n]	Diabetes insipidus
	Circumventricular organs [r]	Essential hypernatremia
		SIADH
Temperature regulation	Preoptic anterior hypothalamic [r]	Hyperthermia
	Posterior hypothalamus [r]	Hypothermia
		Poikilothermia
Appetite control	Ventromedial [n] (satiety center)	Hypothalamic obesity
	Lateral hypothalamic [r] (feeding center)	Cachexia
		Anorexia nervosa
		Diencephalic syndrome
		Diencephalic glycosuria
Sleep-wake cycle and circadian rhythm	Ventrolateral preoptic anterior hypothalamic [r] (sleep center)	Somnolence
	Posterior hypothalamic [r] including tuberomamillary [n] (arousal center)	Reversal of sleep-wake cycle
		Alkinetic mutism
	Suprachiasmatic [n]	Coma
Visceral (autonomic) fraction	Posterior medial [r] (sympathetic region)	Sympathetic activation
	Preoptic anterior hypothalamus [r] (parasympathetic region)	Parasympathetic activation
Emotional expression and behavior	Ventromedial [n]	Sham rage
	Medial and posterior hypothalamus [r]	Fear or horror
	Caudal hypothalamic [r]	Apathy
		Hypersexual behavior
Memory	Ventromedial [n]	Short-term memory loss
	Mamillary bodies	
Control of anterior pituitary function	Arcuate [n]	Hyperfunction syndromes
	Preoptic [n]	
	Suprachiasmatic [n]	Hypofunction syndromes
	Paraventricular [n]	
	Neovascular zone (median eminence)	

SIADH, syndrome of inappropriate secretion of antidiuretic hormone.

pharyngioma, with a minority having inflammatory or granulomatous processes, a history of trauma, or infiltrative disorders.[55] Common clinical findings in these patients include headaches, visual abnormalities, hypogonadism, diabetes insipidus, and somnolence. Less commonly, behavioral abnormalities, such as antisocial behavior or sham rage, and seizures may be present.[55]

Diencephalic Syndrome of Infancy
Infants harboring a low-grade hypothalamic or optic nerve glioma, or rarely ependymomas, gangliogliomas, or dysgerminomas that destroy the ventromedial nuclei, may develop an unusual syndrome at approximately age 1 to 2 years, in which they begin to lose weight and subcutaneous fat, while maintaining an apparently good food intake and normal growth. They exhibit hyperactivity and a cheerful affect and often demonstrate nystagmus, pallor, vomiting, tremor, and optic atrophy. Endocrine evaluation is generally normal or may show nonspecific abnormalities including elevated growth hormone levels. If the patients live beyond age 2 years, they begin to gain weight and become obese. Their euphoria and cheerful affect disappear and are replaced by rage and irritability. Somnolence and precocious puberty also may be present.[5,56-58] A similar syndrome rarely has been described in adults with tumors involving the optic chiasm or anterior hypothalamic region.[59]

Hypothalamic Cachexia in Adults
In patients with destructive lesions of the lateral hypothalamus, rapid weight loss, decreased activity, hypophagia, muscle wasting, cachexia, and death may ensue, usually due to a neoplasm.[9,10,17,18,21] Malignant multiple sclerosis also may cause the lateral hypothalamic syndrome.[17,21]

Anorexia Nervosa
Anorexia nervosa is a common disorder, usually seen in young women beginning before the age of 25 years. Although it is not associated with a structural hypothalamic defect, functional hypothalamic abnormalities are present. These patients, with their distorted body image, exercise excessively, may induce vomiting, and have amenorrhea with a prepubertal pattern of gonadotropin release.[60] Elevations of basal serum growth hormone and ghrelin with reduction of insulin-like growth factor 1 (IGF-1) and leptin concentrations are found, and the patients may demonstrate abnormalities in hypothalamic-pituitary-adrenal activity with elevated plasma cortisol concentrations, decreased adrenocorticotropic hormone (ACTH) levels, and an attenuated ACTH response to corticotropin-releasing hormone (CRH). Low concentrations of thyroxine (T_4) and triiodothyronine (T_3) are found, with elevated reverse T_3 and a thyroid-stimulating hormone (TSH) response to thyrotropin-releasing hormone (TRH) that is either normal or demonstrates a delayed peak consistent with hypothalamic hypothyroidism.[61] Additionally, these patients may have hyperprolactinemia with galactorrhea, evidence of thermal dysregulation, and a partial diabetes insipidus.[62] The neuroendocrine and functional hypothalamic abnormalities remit when the patients regain their weight.

Diencephalic Glycosuria
Acute injuries to the tuberoinfundibular region from basal skull fractures, intracranial hemorrhage, or neurosurgical intervention around the third ventricle may lead to transient hyperglycemia and glycosuria.[1,63] Although many of the "stress hormones" with glucose contraregulatory activity are elevated in these patients, they do not appear to be responsible for the glucose abnormality.

SLEEP-WAKE CYCLE AND CIRCADIAN ABNORMALITIES
Approximately 10% of patients with hypothalamic disease will first be seen with somnolence, and this condition is found in 30% of such patients at some time during the course of their illness.[9,10] Somnolence is commonly seen in

Table 20-3	Causes of Hypothalamic Dysfunction

CONGENITAL
Acquired
  Developmental malformations
    Anencephaly
    Porencephaly
    Agenesis of the corpus callosum
    Septo-optic dysplasia
    Suprasellar arachnoid cyst
    Colloid cyst of the third ventricle
    Hamartoma
  Aqueductal stenosis
  Trauma
  Intraventricular hemorrhage
Genetic (familial or sporadic cases)
  Hypothalamic hypopituitarism
  Familial diabetes insipidus
  Prader-Willi syndrome
  Bardet-Biedl and associated syndromes
  DIDMOAD syndrome
  Pallister-Hall syndrome
  Leptin/leptin receptor mutations

TUMORS
Primary intracranial tumors
  Angioma of the third ventricle
  Craniopharyngioma
  Ependymoma
  Ganglioneuroma
  Germ cell tumors
  Glioblastoma multiforme
  Glioma
  Hamartoma
  Hemangioma
  Lipoma
  Lymphoma
  Medulloblastoma
  Meningioma
  Neuroblastoma
  Pinealomas
  Pituitary tumors
  Plasmacytoma
  Sarcoma
Metastatic tumors

INFILTRATIVE
Histiocytosis
Leukemia
Sarcoidosis

IMMUNOLOGIC
Idiopathic diabetes insipidus
Paraneoplastic syndrome

NUTRITIONAL, METABOLIC
Anorexia nervosa
Kernicterus
Wernicke-Korsakoff syndrome
Weight loss

DEGENERATIVE
Glial scarring
Parkinson's disease

INFECTIOUS
Bacterial
  Meningitis
Mycobacterial
  Tuberculosis
Spirochetal
  Syphilis
Viral
  Encephalitis
  Jakob-Creutzfeldt disease
  Kuru
  Poliomyelitis
  Varicella
  Cytomegalovirus infection

VASCULAR
Aneurysm
Arteriovenous malformation
Pituitary apoplexy
Subarachnoid hemorrhage

TRAUMA
Birth injury
Head injury
Postneurosurgical

FUNCTIONAL
Diencephalic epilepsy
Drugs
Hayek-Peake syndrome
Idiopathic syndrome of inappropriate secretion of antidiuretic hormone (SIADH)
Kleine-Levin syndrome
Periodic syndrome of Wolff
Psychosocial deprivation syndrome

OTHER
Radiation
Porphyria
Toluene exposure

DIDMOAD, diabetes insipidus, diabetes mellitus, optic atrophy, deafness.
Modified from Braunstein GD: The hypothalamus. In Melmed S (ed): The Pituitary, 2d ed. Cambridge, MA, Blackwell Scientific, 2002, pp. 317–348, with permission.

lesions involving the posterior hypothalamus, often in association with hypothermia.[1,6,64] Approximately 40% of patients with hypersomnolence also have hypothalamic obesity.[55] Most patients with these manifestations have neoplasms, especially craniopharyngiomas, epithelial pineal tumors, and suprasellar germinomas.[31,65] Encephalitis and Wernicke's nutritional encephalopathy are other causes of hypothalamic hypersomnia.[1,5,6] As previously noted, acute hypothalamic injury may lead to a transient coma. Narcolepsy, which is characterized by sudden episodes of sleep that last minutes to hours, may in some instances have a hypothalamic cause, as the syndrome has been found in patients with third ventricular tumors, with multiple sclerosis, after head injuries, and with encephalitis.[1] Deficiency of the hypothalamic orexin, hypocretin-1, have been found in the cerebrospinal fluid (CSF) of patients with narcolepsy, and

a loss of hypocretin neurons occurs in the lateral hypothalamus in affected patients.[66,67]

Patients with lesions of the anterior and preoptic hypothalamic nuclei may exhibit hyperactivity and insomnia or, more commonly, alterations in the sleep-wake cycle, with daytime sleepiness and nighttime hyperactivity.[6,23,68] This is characteristically seen in patients with cystic craniopharyngiomas. Anterior tuberal lesions also may lead to alterations in the sleep-wake cycle, as well as an akinetic mutism type of syndrome in which the patient appears awake but does not respond to verbal stimuli and demonstrates little spontaneous movement.[68]

The suprachiasmatic nuclei are responsible for the maintenance of many of our circadian rhythms, and lesions involving this region will alter the sleep-wake cycle, temperature control, and cognitive function.[66,69]

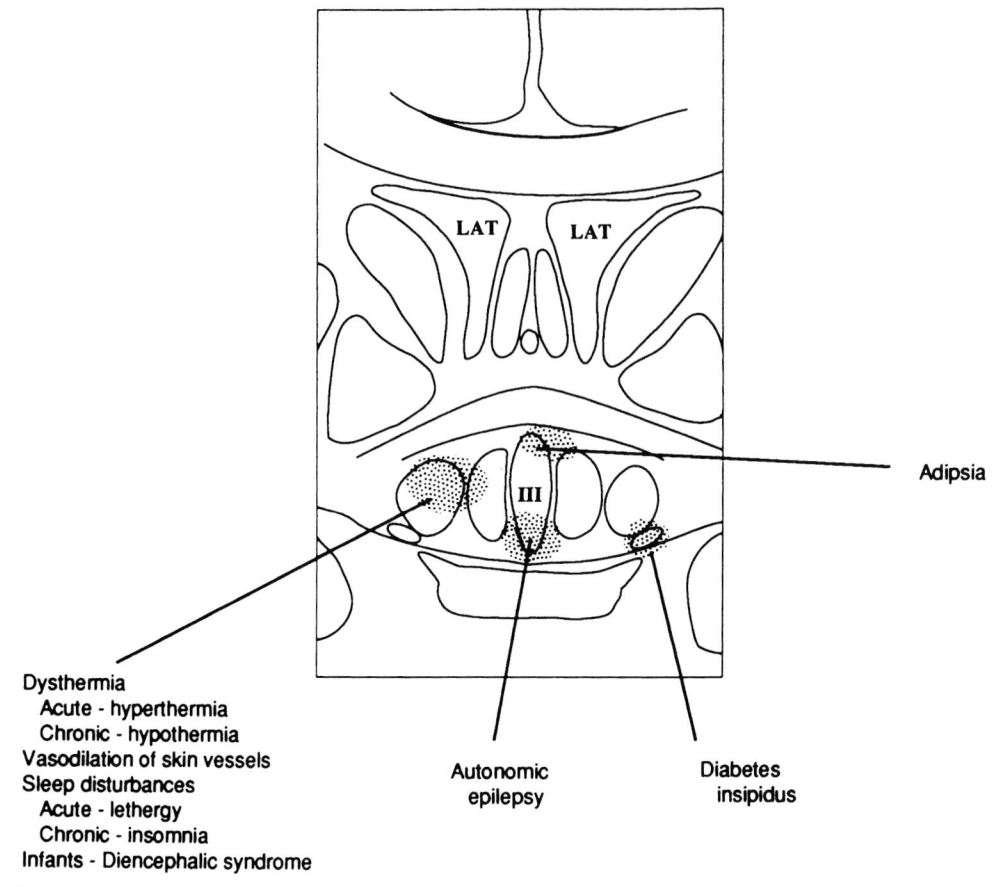

Adipsia

Dysthermia
   Acute - hyperthermia
   Chronic - hypothermia
Vasodilation of skin vessels
Sleep disturbances
   Acute - lethergy
   Chronic - insomnia
Infants - Diencephalic syndrome

Autonomic
epilepsy

Diabetes
insipidus

A

Diabetes insipidus

Acute-Hyperphagia
Chronic-Anorexia
    Wt. Loss
    Cachexia
    Apathy
    Decreased activity

Acute-polydipsia
Chronic-hypodipsia

Adipsia

Obesity
Hypogonadism
Hyperphagia
Finicky eating
Episodic rage

Paroxysmal
hyperthermia

Hypogonadism
Hypoadrenalism
Hypothyroidism
Diabetes insipidus

Hallucinations
Glycosuria

Figure 20-3 Clinical findings associated with hypothalamic lesions located at various anatomic sites. Clinicopathologic correlation based on multiple studies.[15–24] **A,** Corresponds to region depicted in Fig. 20-2A. **B,** Corresponds to region depicted in Fig. 20-2C.

B

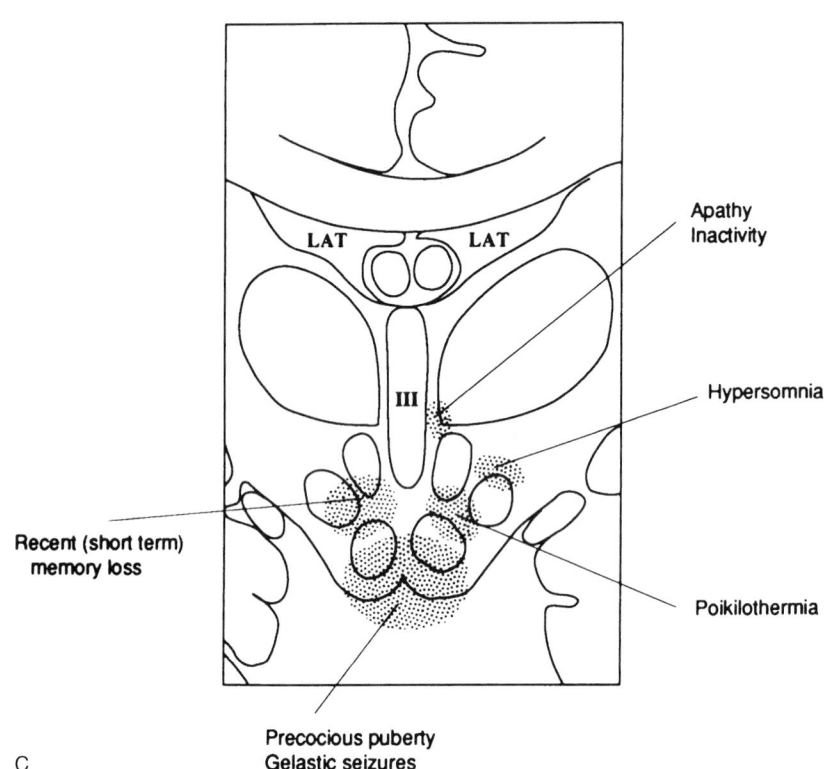

Apathy
Inactivity

Hypersomnia

Poikilothermia

Recent (short term)
memory loss

Precocious puberty
Gelastic seizures

Figure 20-3, cont'd **C,** Corresponds to section depicted in Fig. 20-2D. (From Braunstein GD: The hypothalamus. In Melmed S [ed]: The Pituitary, 2d ed. Cambridge, MA, Blackwell Scientific, 2002, pp 317–348, with permission.)

C

ABNORMALITIES OF EMOTIONAL EXPRESSION OR BEHAVIOR

Sham rage reactions with emotional lability, marked agitation, and aggressive, destructive behavior are found in patients with lesions involving the ventromedial nuclei.[6,23,64] Activation of the sympathetic nervous system is present during the episodes. In contrast, apathy, somnolence, and hypoactivity, as well as vocal and auditory unresponsiveness and akinetic mutism, have been found in patients with destruction of the mamillary bodies or lesions in the medial posterior hypothalamus.[1,6]

Hypersexual behavior is seen in individuals with lesions involving the caudal hypothalamus.[70] The Kleine-Levin syndrome is believed to represent a functional abnormality of the hypothalamus. It generally affects adolescent boys, who have recurrent episodes of somnolence, with periodic arousal that is associated with irritability, abnormal speech, forgetfulness, food gorging, and masturbation and other sexual activity. The episodes may occur at 3- to 6-month intervals and generally last 5 to 7 days. The disorder usually remits spontaneously in late adolescence or early adulthood.[71,72]

Gelastic or laughing seizures are a form of diencephalic epilepsy due to lesions involving the floor of the third ventricle and mamillary area, especially hamartomas of the tuber cinereum.[73] The affected child does not lose consciousness but stops his or her activity and begins to laugh or giggle or make bubbling noises, associated with a grimace from tightening of the facial muscles.[74,75] EEG abnormalities are present during the seizure.

DISORDERED CONTROL OF ANTERIOR PITUITARY FUNCTION

Hyperfunction Syndromes
Precocious Puberty
Isosexual pubertal development in girls younger than 8 years or boys younger than 9 years represents sexual precocity, which most often is due to premature activation of the hypothalamic-pituitary-gonadal axis. The majority of girls have no discernible lesion and are therefore classified as having idiopathic central precocious puberty, whereas only 10% of boys

have idiopathic precocious puberty.[76] In the latter, close to half have hypothalamic hamartomas, and a third have other benign or malignant neoplasms that are located in the posterior hypothalamus or near the mamillary bodies.[76] The spectrum of pathologic conditions that can cause central precocious puberty are listed in Table 20-4.[4,76–84] Some of these lesions may bring about early activation of the hypothalamic-pituitary-gonadal axis through increased intracranial pressure or irritation of the basal hypothalamus. Hypothalamic hamartomas involving the tuber cinereum are often associated with precocious puberty through premature activation of the normal hypothalamic gonadotropin-releasing hormone (GnRH) secretory mechanisms or through direct secretion of GnRH by the hamartoma, because GnRH has been located immunohistochemically within hamartomatous neurons.[85,86] In addition to pressure effects, germ cell tumors may result in precocious puberty through the secretion of human chorionic gonadotropin (hCG), which may stimulate the child's gonads to secrete sex steroid hormones, bringing about precocious sexual development. Finally, premature activation of the normal hypothalamic-pituitary-gonadal axis has been described in some patients who have had incomplete sexual precocity from congenital adrenal hyperplasia or polyostotic fibrous dysplasia (McCune-Albright) syndrome, in which the hypothalamus is exposed to elevated sex steroid hormone levels at an early age, and in patients with primary hypothyroidism, who also may exhibit galactorrhea with elevated prolactin levels (Van Wyk-Grumbach syndrome), in which the mechanism for the premature activation is unknown, but usually ceases with correction of the hypothyroidism.[84]

Acromegaly
Acromegaly due to the ectopic secretion of GHRH is rare, and in most instances, the source of the ectopic GHRH is a bronchial carcinoid, islet cell neoplasm, adrenal tumor, or lung carcinoma.[87,88] However, acromegaly also has been found in patients with hypothalamic hamartomas, gangliocytomas, gliomas, and choristomas.[87–90] Some of these tumors have been shown to contain GHRH, and they presumably

Table 20-4 Causes of Central Precocious Puberty

IDIOPATHIC

CONGENITAL ABNORMALITIES
Hypothalamic hamartoma
Arachnoid cyst
Myelomeningocele
Aqueductal stenosis with hydrocephalus
Tuberous sclerosis
Congenital optic nerve hypoplasia
Congenital adrenal hyperplasia
McCune-Albright syndrome
Septo-optic dysplasia

NEOPLASMS
Optic nerve glioma
Hypothalamic glioma
Neurofibroma
Astrocytoma
Ependymoma
Infundibuloma
Pinealoma
Neuroblastoma
Germinoma
Craniopharyngioma

INFLAMMATORY CONDITIONS
Tuberculosis
Sarcoidosis
Meningoencephalitis

SUBDURAL HEMATOMA

PRIMARY HYPOTHYROIDISM

From Braunstein GD: The hypothalamus. In Melmed S (ed): The Pituitary, 2d ed. Cambridge, MA, Blackwell Scientific, 2002, pp. 317–348, with permission.

secrete the releasing factor, which in turn stimulates the somatotrophs to hypersecrete growth hormone.

Cushing's Disease

Several lines of evidence suggest that Cushing's disease has a hypothalamic component to its pathophysiology.[91] First, it has been noted that the onset of the disease often follows an emotionally stressful event.[92] Because depression may be associated with pseudo-Cushing's syndrome with hypersecretion of glucocorticoids, it is conceivable that chronic corticotroph stimulation by hypothalamic CRH could lead to the development of a corticotroph adenoma and Cushing's disease and may account for the recurrence of Cushing's disease after apparently successful removal of an ACTH-secreting corticotroph adenoma.[93,94] Second, most patients with Cushing's disease, when given exogenous glucocorticoids in sufficient quantities, are able to suppress their ACTH secretion, a fact that has been known for some time and forms the basis for the high-dose portion of the dexamethasone suppression test.[91] Presumably, this phenomenon reflects an increased set point for negative feedback of glucocorticoids at the hypothalamic level. Third, some patients with Cushing's disease exhibit a reduction in ACTH and cortisol secretion and amelioration of symptoms after the administration of cyproheptadine, bromocriptine, or sodium valproate, which may work through the hypothalamus.[95–98] Nevertheless, most, if not all, corticotroph adenomas are of clonal origin rather than polyclonal, as would be anticipated if CRH hypersecretion were responsible for the pituitary abnormality.[99] Hypothalamic factors such as CRH may promote clonal expansion of corticotroph cells that have become intrinsically abnormal.[100] An unusual cause of pituitary-dependent Cushing's disease is the secretion of CRH by an intracranial neoplasm, as was demonstrated with an intrasellar gangliocytoma.[101]

Hyperprolactinemia

Because prolactin secretion by the lactotrophs is under hypothalamic dopamine inhibitory control, it is not surprising that patients with a variety of hypothalamic disorders may exhibit hyperprolactinemia. This is seen in 79% of patients with supersellar germinomas, 36% of patients with craniopharyngiomas, and 14% of patients with pineal germinomas.[31] Most patients have a prolactin concentration less than 70 ng/mL, and galactorrhea is infrequently seen, probably because of the coexistence of hypogonadism.[102] Nevertheless, amenorrhea and galactorrhea may be present in women, and impotence, in men.

Idiopathic hyperprolactinemia in patients without any demonstrable structural abnormality in the pituitary or hypothalamus is presumably due to a hypothalamic dopamine deficiency. The prolactin secretory dynamics of these patients in response to various stimulatory and inhibitory agents is similar to that seen in patients with prolactin-secreting pituitary adenomas. Indeed, some patients with idiopathic hyperprolactinemia when followed for a long period will eventually be found to have a prolactin-secreting pituitary microadenoma. Additional evidence supporting a hypothalamic cause for the pituitary adenoma is the finding of lactotroph hyperplasia in some patients who have had documented adenomas, as well as the recurrence of prolactin-secreting pituitary adenoma after successful removal of a microadenoma and an interval of normal prolactin-secretory dynamics.[103,104]

Hypofunction Syndromes

Hypothalamic Hypogonadism

Kallmann's syndrome (olfactory-genital dysplasia) is the most common form of congenital isolated gonadotropin deficiency and can occur sporadically or in a familial setting as an X-linked, autosomal-dominant, or -recessive trait with incomplete penetrance.[105] The X-linked disorder is due to a defect in the *KAL-1* gene whose product, anosmin-1, normally directs the migration of GnRH neurons from the olfactory placode to the hypothalamus. This results in a deficiency or absence of GnRH-secreting neurons in the hypothalamus, as well as agenesis or hypoplasia of the olfactory bulb, the latter defect being responsible for the hyposmia or anosmia seen in this syndrome. Boys are affected more commonly than are girls and often exhibit cryptorchidism and microphallus at birth, reflecting the lack of fetal gonadotropins, which stimulate testosterone secretion from the fetal testes. At the time of expected puberty, a failure of gonadotropins to increase, of testicular enlargement, or of development of secondary sexual characteristics to occur. After a single bolus injection of GnRH, little or no increase in gonadotropin levels is seen. However, if GnRH is given in a pulsatile fashion every 90 minutes, an increase in luteinizing hormone (LH) and follicle-stimulating hormone (FSH) will occur, reflecting the fact that the gonadotrophs are normal but understimulated in this syndrome. Pulsatile GnRH therapy may result in full virilization. Other components of this syndrome include color blindness, nerve deafness, cleft palate, exostosis, and renal abnormalities.[105]

Hypogonadotropic hypogonadism has been found with leptin and leptin-receptor gene mutations.[106] Congenital gonadotropin deficiency also is seen as a manifestation of panhypopituitarism, which may be on a hypothalamic basis, as well as with several complex hypothalamic disorders, including the Prader-Willi, Bardet-Biedl, and Laurence-Moon syndromes.

Hypogonadism is a relatively common manifestation of hypothalamic tumors and infiltrative disease, especially those that involve the floor of the third ventricle and median eminence. Obesity, diabetes insipidus, and neuroophthalmologic abnormalities often accompany the hypogonadism.[9,10]

Growth Hormone Deficiency

A variety of congenital structural defects involving the hypothalamus, such as anencephaly, holoprosencephaly, encephalocele, and septo-optic dysplasia, may result in growth hormone deficiency either alone or with other anterior pituitary hormone deficiencies.[4] Monotropic growth hormone deficiency may occur sporadically or on a familial basis because of a deficient production or secretion of GHRH. Such patients will demonstrate an increase in growth hormone secretion after multiple injections of GHRH. Growth hormone deficiency also occurs as a manifestation of panhypopituitarism and is the hormone that is most frequently absent in these patients. As in patients with isolated growth hormone deficiency, those with panhypopituitarism generally have a hypothalamic basis for the abnormality, with deficiencies of multiple hypothalamic-releasing hormones.[107]

At birth, patients with congenital growth hormone deficiency have a normal length and weight but may exhibit microphallus. During the first year, growth retardation is seen with a delay in both height and bone ages. Hypoglycemia may be found, because of the loss of the glucose contraregulation effect of growth hormone; during childhood, an increase in subcutaneous fat along with proportional short stature is noted. Even in the presence of normal gonadotrophs, puberty is often delayed in these patients. Treatment with growth hormone increases linear growth, reduces subcutaneous fat and glucose intolerance, and stimulates pubertal progression.[51]

Growth hormone deficiency is generally the earliest endocrine manifestation of a hypothalamic tumor or infiltrative process and results in growth retardation. Even in patients with structural hypothalamic disease who have no clinical evidence of growth retardation, provocative testing reveals a high frequency of inadequate growth hormone secretion.[105,108]

Hypothalamic Hypoadrenalism

Congenital or acquired isolated ACTH deficiency is quite rare. However, ACTH deficiency does occur commonly in association with deficiencies of other anterior pituitary hormones because of craniopharyngiomas, suprasellar germinomas, and septo-optic dysplasia.[30,77,78,105,108–111] Clinical manifestations include nausea, vomiting, hypotension, and hypoglycemia, without the hyperpigmentation and electrolyte abnormalities from aldosterone deficiency seen in primary adrenocortical insufficiency.

Hypothalamic Hypothyroidism

Isolated TSH deficiency also is quite rare. However, TSH deficiency is found in approximately one third of the patients with craniopharyngiomas, suprasellar germinomas, and in patients with septo-optic dysplasia.[29,30,77,78,105,108,110] Clinically, the patients may exhibit dry skin, puffiness, pallor, lethargy, bradycardia, hypothermia, and weight gain, with evidence of an atrophic thyroid gland. Serum-free T_4 levels are low, and the serum TSH may be low or slightly elevated, the latter reflecting abnormal glycoslyation of the TSH molecule, which results in decreased biologic activity.[112] After an injection of TRH, a delayed and prolonged increase in TSH is seen in patients with hypothalamic hypothyroidism.[29,30,71,72]

SPECIFIC HYPOTHALAMIC DISORDERS

PRADER-WILLI SYNDROME

Prader-Willi syndrome, first described in 1956, occurs in approximately 1 in 25,000 live births.[113,114] The major clinical manifestations include infantile hypotonia; feeding problems; failure to thrive; rapid weight gain occurring between ages 1 and 6 years; a characteristic dysmorphic facial appearance with a narrow bitemporal diameter, almond-shaped eyes, palpebral fissures, down-turned mouth; developmental delay and mental retardation; and hypogonadism, which

may be present at birth, with cryptorchidism, scrotal hypoplasia, and a small penis in boys, poor development of the labia minora and clitoris in girls, and delayed onset of puberty associated with low sex steroid hormones, low gonadotropins, and blunting of the gonadotropin response to GnRH. In addition, these patients have short stature, associated with growth hormone deficiency, and behavioral problems that appear during childhood and are characterized by temper tantrums, aggressive behavior, and obsessive-compulsiveness. One of the major characteristics of these patients is marked, indiscriminate hyperphagia and central obesity. These patients will exhibit abnormal food-seeking behavior, often eating discarded or spoiled food or pet food. Sleep disturbances and abnormalities in temperature control and heat generation also suggest a hypothalamic cause.[113–115] The only anatomic abnormality found in these patients is a decrease in the size of the paraventricular nuclei and oxytocin-producing neurons.[66]

Prader-Willi syndrome is a disorder of genetic (genomic) imprinting, in most cases due to a microdeletion of the paternally contributed chromosome 15q11-q13.[114,116] Thus, because only the paternal genes are normally expressed in this region, a mutation of the paternal gene results in absence of expression. A minority of patients have maternal uniparental disomy (both members of the chromosome pair inherited from the same parent). An even rarer cause is a translocation involving chromosome 15.[114,116]

BARDET-BIEDL AND RELATED SYNDROMES

The Bardet-Biedl syndrome represents an autosomal-recessive disorder characterized by retinal pigmentary dystrophy (retinitis pigmentosa), mental retardation, central obesity, polydactyly, a variety of renal abnormalities, and hypogonadotropic hypogonadism.[117] Those with the Laurence-Moon syndrome also exhibit retinal pigmentary dystrophy, mental retardation, and hypogonadotropic hypogonadism. These patients also have progressive spastic paraparesis and distal muscle weakness but do not exhibit polydactyly.[118] The Biemond syndrome is another autosomal-recessive condition with mental retardation, polydactyly or brachydactyly, obesity, and hypogonadotropic hypogonadism. Retinal pigmentary dystrophy does not occur in this condition; rather, these patients have iris coloboma. The autosomal-recessive Alström syndrome is associated with atypical retinal pigmentary dystrophy, obesity, nerve deafness, diabetes mellitus, and acanthosis nigricans. The affected patients have hypogonadism due to primary gonadal failure rather than hypothalamic dysfunction.[118,119] The overlapping features of these different syndromes raise the possibility that they are due to a similar genetic abnormality.

SEPTO-OPTIC PITUITARY DYSPLASIA

The anatomic features of septo-optic pituitary dysplasia, a midline developmental abnormality, are an absence of the septum pellucidum, agenesis of the corpus callosum, unilateral or bilateral hypoplasia of the optic nerves, and absence of the supraoptic and paraventricular nuclei with posterior pituitary hypoplasia.[77,78,109,110,120–122] The nonendocrine manifestations of this disease include visual abnormalities, mental retardation, nystagmus, seizures, and various forms of cerebral palsy.[77] Approximately two thirds of affected patients have short stature associated with growth hormone deficiency; approximately 40% have ACTH deficiency; 20%, TSH deficiency; and one fourth exhibit gonadotropin deficiency. Close to one fourth of the patients exhibit diabetes insipidus, and approximately 20% have hyperprolactinemia.[77,78,109,120–122] This disorder is caused by recessive mutation in the homeobox gene on chromosome 3, *HESX1*.[123]

HYPERPHAGIC SHORT STATURE (PSYCHOSOCIAL DWARFISM)

Hyperphagic short stature, a rare syndrome, which has its onset before age 2 years, occurs in some children exposed to a disturbed parent-child home environment. The clinical manifestations include short stature with delayed bone age associated with abnormal growth hormone response to provocative tests; low body weight despite an enormous appetite that is associated with gorging, pica, food hoarding, vomiting, and production of foul-smelling stools; polydipsia; bizarre behavior; emotional or mental retardation; and a protuberant abdomen. In addition to the abnormal growth hormone responses, these patients may have an inadequate ACTH response to provocative testing, although thyroid function and urine-concentrating ability are normal. The clinical findings are reversible and disappear when the children are placed in a nurturing environment.[124,125]

PSEUDOCYESIS

An extreme example of a functional hypothalamic disorder is seen in women in whom a conversion reaction develops, in which they think they are pregnant, but, in fact, are not. Amenorrhea, morning nausea, breast enlargement and engorgement, and abdominal distension due to retained colonic gas are present in these women. Hyperprolactinemia is found, and some women exhibit galactorrhea.[126,127] Elevated levels of LH may account for the persistent corpus luteum activity that is seen in this syndrome.[128] When these women are informed of the diagnosis, the clinical manifestations rapidly disappear.

HYPOTHALAMIC HAMARTOMA

These benign hyperplastic malformations contain ganglion cells, myelinated nerve fibers, and glial matrix, and are generally located between the tuber cinereum and mamillary bodies.[74,129] Most patients exhibit onset of clinical symptoms before age 2 years, with the major endocrine abnormality being isosexual precocious puberty. Other common manifestations include gelastic seizures, emotional lability, hyperactivity, and neurodevelopmental delay.[73,75,84,85,129–133] During late childhood or adolescence, obesity develops in many of these patients. The precocious puberty in these patients responds to long-acting GnRH agonists that downregulate GnRH receptors.[84] Neurosurgical removal of the hamartomas is indicated if signs of increased intracranial pressure, progressive growth, intractable seizures, or neurologic deterioration are present.[85]

The Pallister-Hall syndrome consists of hypothalamic hamartomas, panhypopituitarism, polydactyly, imperforate anus, and multiple craniofacial and limb abnormalities.[134–137] This may occur sporadically or be transmitted as an autosomal-dominant trait. An abnormality on chromosome 7 has been identified in some patients affected with the familial syndrome.[138]

SUPRASELLAR ARACHNOID CYST

Suprasellar arachnoid cyst, an uncommon developmental anomaly of the arachnoid membrane, leads to a CSF-filled cyst that obstructs CSF flow through the foramen of Monro, leading to hydrocephalus and increased intracranial pressure. Thus, headache, vomiting, lethargy, and increased head size are commonly found in these patients. The cysts also may compress the brain stem, optic nerve, and optic chiasm, leading to spasticity, ataxia, tremor, decreased visual acuity, and visual field defects. Endocrine abnormalities include growth hormone and ACTH deficiency, as well as precocious puberty.[139] Surgical decompression or percutaneous ventriculocystostomy is used to drain the cyst and reduce intracranial pressure.[140]

INFILTRATIVE DISORDERS

Sarcoidosis may involve the basal hypothalamus and floor of the third ventricle and lead to diminished visual acuity, visual field abnormalities, diabetes insipidus, thermal dysregulation, somnolence, personality changes, obesity, and hypothalamic hypopituitarism. Most patients with hypothalamic sarcoidosis also have involvement outside of the central nervous system.[33,34,36,141–143]

The chronic disseminated form of Langerhans' cell histiocytosis (Hand-Schüller-Christian disease) is classically composed of the triad of membranous bone lesions, exophthalmos, and diabetes insipidus. Growth retardation, hyperprolactinemia, hypogonadism, and hypodipsia or adipsia also may be found in these patients.[32,144]

HYPOTHALAMIC DYSFUNCTION AFTER BRAIN IRRADIATION

Both whole-brain irradiation and localized radiotherapy for brain or head or neck neoplasms are associated with a delayed onset of hypothalamic dysfunction most often manifest by progressive loss of growth hormone secretion and hyperprolactinemia. ACTH and gonadotropin deficiency also are found, as are changes in personality and abnormalities in thirst, sleep-wake cycle, and appetite regulation. Children are more susceptible to hypothalamic damage than are adults, and the incidence of hypothalamic abnormality increases with increasing radiation dose and decreasing intervals over which the radiation is administered.[145–148]

REFERENCES

1. Boshes B: Syndromes of the diencephalons: The hypothalamus and the hypophysis. In Vinken PJ, Bruyn GW (eds): Localization in Clinical Neurology: Handbook of Clinical Neurology, Vol 2. Amsterdam, North-Holland, 1969, pp 432–468.
2. Kirgis HD, Locke W: Anatomy and embryology. In Locke W, Schally AV (eds): The Hypothalamus and Pituitary in Health and Disease. Springfield, IL, Charles C Thomas, 1972, pp 3–21.
3. Bruesch SR: Anatomy of the human hypothalamus. In Givens JR, Kitabchi AE, Robertson JT (eds): The Hypothalamus. St. Louis, Mosby-Year Book, 1984, pp 1–16.
4. Braunstein GD: The hypothalamus. In Melmed S (ed): The Pituitary, 2d ed. Cambridge, MA, Blackwell Scientific, 2002, pp 317–348.
5. Carmel PW: Surgical syndromes of the hypothalamus. Clin Neurosurg 27:133–159, 1980.
6. Plum F, Van Uitert R: Nonendocrine diseases and disorders of the hypothalamus. In Reichlin S, Baldessarini RJ, Martin JB (eds): The Hypothalamus. New York, Raven Press, 1978, pp 415–473.
7. Sano K, Mayanagi Y, Sekino H, et al: Results of stimulation and destruction of the posterior hypothalamus in man. J Neurosurg 33:689–707, 1970.
8. Garnica AD, Netzloff ML, Rosenbloom AL: Clinical manifestations of hypothalamic tumors. Ann Clin Lab Sci 10:474–485, 1980.
9. Bauer HG: Endocrine and other clinical manifestations of hypothalamic disease: A survey of 60 cases, with autopsies. J Clin Endocrinol Metab 14:13–31, 1954.
10. Bauer HG: Endocrine and metabolic conditions related to pathology in the hypothalamus: A review. J Nerv Ment Dis 128:323–338, 1959.
11. Thompson HJ, Tkacs NC, Saatman KE, et al: Hypothermia following traumatic brain injury: A critical evaluation. Neurobiol Dis 12:163–173, 2003.

12. Dott NM: Surgical aspects of the hypothalamus. In Le Gros Clark WE, Beattie J, Riddoch G, et al (eds): The Hypothalamus: Morphological, Functional, Clinical and Surgical Aspects. London, Oliver & Boyd, 1938, pp 131–185.

13. Frohman LA: Clinical aspects of hypothalamic disease. In Motta M (ed): The Endocrine Functions of the Brain. New York, Raven Press, 1980, pp 419–446.

14. Riddoch G: Clinical aspects of hypothalamic derangement. In Le Gros Clark WE, Beattie J, Riddoch G, et al (eds): The Hypothalamus: Morphological, Functional, Clinical and Surgical Aspects. London, Oliver & Boyd, 1938, pp 101–130.

15. McLean AJ: Autonomic epilepsy. Arch Neurol 32:189–197, 1934.

16. Rothballer AB, Dugger GS: Hypothalamic tumor: Correlation between symptomatology, regional anatomy, and neurosecretion. Neurology 5:160–177, 1955.

17. White LE, Hain RF: Anorexia in association with a destructive lesion of the hypothalamus. Arch Pathol Lab Med 68:275–281, 1959.

18. Reeves AG, Plum F: Hyperphagia, rage, and dementia accompanying a ventromedial hypothalamic neoplasm. Arch Neurol 20:616–624, 1969.

19. Fox RH, Davies TW, Marsh FP, et al: Hypothermia in a young man with an anterior hypothalamic lesion. Lancet 2:185–188, 1970.

20. Lewin K, Mattingly D, Millis RR: Anorexia nervosa associated with hypothalamic tumour. Br Med J 2:629–630, 1972.

21. Kamalian N, Keesey RE, Zurhein GM: Lateral hypothalamic demyelination and cachexia in a case of "malignant" multiple sclerosis. Neurology 25:25–30, 1975.

22. Celesia GG, Archer CR, Chung HD: Hyperphagia and obesity: Relationship to medial hypothalamic lesions. JAMA 246:151–153, 1981.

23. Haugh RM, Markesbery WR: Hypothalamic astrocytomas: Syndrome of hyperphagia, obesity, and disturbances of behavior and endocrine and autonomic function. Arch Neurol 40:560–563, 1983.

24. Schwartz WJ, Busis NA, Hedley-Whyte ET: A discrete lesion of ventral hypothalamus and optic chiasm that disturbed the daily temperature rhythm. J Neurol 233:1–4, 1986.

25. Bergeron C, Kovacs K, Ezrin C, et al: Hereditary diabetes insipidus: An immunohistochemical study of the hypothalamus and pituitary gland. Acta Neuropathol 81:345–348, 1991.

26. Scherbaum WA: Autoimmune hypothalamic diabetes insipidus ("autoimmune hypothalamitis"). Prog Brain Res 93:283–293, 1992.

27. McLeod JF, Kouvacs L, Gaskill MB, et al: Familial neurohypophyseal diabetes insipidus associated with a signal peptide mutation. J Clin Endocrinol Metab 77:599A–599G, 1997.

28. Robertson GL: Antidiuretic hormone: Normal and disordered function. Neuroendocrinology 30:671–694, 2001.

29. Verbalis JG: Management of disorders of water metabolism in patients with pituitary tumors. Pituitary 22:119–132, 2002.

30. Buchfelder M, Fahlbusch R, Walther M, Mann K: Endocrine disturbances in suprasellar germinomas. Acta Endocrinol 120:337–342, 1989.

31. Jennings MT, Gelman R, Hochberg F: Intracranial germ-cell tumors: Natural history and pathogenesis. J Neurosurg 63:155–167, 1985.

32. Kaltsas GA, Powles TB, Evanson J, et al: Hypothalamo-pituitary abnormalities in adult patients with Langerhans cell histiocytosis: Clinical, endocrinological, and radiological features and response to treatment. J Clin Endocrinol Metab 85:1370–1376, 2000.

33. Delaney P: Neurologic manifestations in sarcoidosis: Review of the literature, with a report of 23 cases. Ann Intern Med 87:336–345, 1977.

34. Stuart CA, Neelon FA, Lebovitz HE: Hypothalamic insufficiency: The cause of hypopituitarism in sarcoidosis. Ann Intern Med 88:589–594, 1978.

35. Jawadi MH, Hanson TJ, Schemmel JE, et al: Hypothalamic sarcoidosis and hypopituitarism. Horm Res 12:1–9, 1980.

36. Vesely DL, Maldonado A, Levey GS: Partial hypopituitarism and possible hypothalamic involvement in sarcoidosis. Am J Med 62:425–431, 1977.

37. Ouma JR, Farrell VJR: Lymphocytic infundibulo-neurohypophysitis with hypothalamic and optic pathway involvement: Report of a case and review of the literature. Surg Neurol 57:49–54, 2002.

38. McKenna K, Thompson C: Osmoregulation in clinical disorders of thirst appreciation. Clin Endocrinol 49:139–152, 1998.

39. Teelucksingh S, Steer CR, Thompson CJ, et al: Hypothalamic syndrome and central sleep apnoea associated with toluene exposure. Q J Med 78:185–190, 1991.

40. Hayek A, Peake GT: Hypothalamic adipsia without demonstrable structural lesion. Pediatrics 70:275–278, 1982.

41. Du Rivage SK, Winter RJ, Brouillette RT, et al: Idiopathic hypothalamic dysfunction and impaired control of breathing. Pediatrics 75:896–898, 1985.

42. Wolff SM, Adler RC, Buskirk ER, et al: A syndrome of periodic hypothalamic discharge. Am J Med 36:956–967, 1964.

43. Martin JB, Reichlin S: Clinical Neuroendocrinology. Philadelphia, FA Davis, 1987, p 393.

44. Susman VL: Clinical management of neuroleptic malignant syndrome. Psychiatry Q 72:325–336, 2001.

45. Horn E, Lach B, Lapierre Y, et al: Hypothalamic pathology in the neuroleptic malignant syndrome. Am J Psychiatry 145:617–620, 1988.

46. Sandyk R, Iacono RP, Bamford CR: The hypothalamus in Parkinson disease. Ital J Neurol Sci 8:227–234, 1987.

47. Haak HR, van Hilten JJ, Roos RAC, et al: Functional hypothalamic derangement in a case of Wernicke's encephalopathy. Neth J Med 36:291–296, 1990.

48. Penfield W: Diencephalic autonomic epilepsy. Arch Neurol Psychiatry 22:358–369, 1929.

49. Fox RH, Wilkins DC, Bell JA, et al: Spontaneous periodic hypothermia: Diencephalic epilepsy. Br Med J 2:693–695, 1973.

50. Mooradian AD, Morley GK, McGeachie R, et al: Spontaneous periodic hypothermia. Neurology 34:79–82, 1984.

51. Flynn MD, Sandeman DD, Mawson DM, et al: Cyclical hypothermia: Successful treatment with ephedrine. J R Soc Med 84:752–753, 1991.

52. Shapiro WR, Williams GH, Plum F: Spontaneous recurrent hypothermia accompanying agenesis of the corpus callosum. Brain 92:423–436, 1969.

53. Bannister P, Sheridan P, Penney MD: Chronic reset osmoreceptor response, agenesis of the corpus callosum, and hypothalamic cyst. J Pediatr 104:97–99, 1984.

54. Page SR, Nussey SS, Jenkins JS, et al: Hypothalamic disease in association with dysgenesis of the corpus callosum. Postgrad Med J 65:163–167, 1989.

55. Bray GA, Gallagher TF Jr: Manifestations of hypothalamic obesity in man: A comprehensive investigation of eight patients and a review of the literature. Medicine (Baltimore) 54:301–330, 1975.

56. Russell A: A diencephalic syndrome of emaciation in infancy and childhood. Arch Dis Child 26:274, 1951.

57. Burr IM, Slonim AE, Danish RK, et al: Diencephalic syndrome revisited. J Pediatr 88:439–444, 1976.

58. Poussaint TY, Barnes PD, Nichols K, et al: Diencephalic syndrome: clinical features and imaging findings. Am J Neuroradiol 18:1499–1505, 1997.

59. Miyoshi Y, Yunoki M, Yano A, et al: Diencephalic syndrome of emaciation in an adult associated with a third ventricle intrinsic craniopharyngioma: Case report. Neurosurgery 52:224–227, 2003.

60. Rome ES: Eating disorders. Obstet Gynecol Clin North Am 30:353–377, 2003.

61. Muñoz MT, Argente J: Anorexia nervosa in female adolescents: Endocrine and bone mineral density disturbances. Eur J Endocrinol 147:275–286, 2002.

62. Mecklenberg RS, Loriaux DL, Thompson RH, et al: Hypothalamic dysfunction in patients with anorexia. Medicine (Baltimore) 53:147–159, 1974.

63. Clark LG: The hypothalamus in man. In Le Gros, Clark WE, Beattie J, et al (eds): The Hypothalamus: Morphological, Functional, Clinical and Surgical Aspects. London, Oliver & Boyd, 1938, pp 59–68.

64. Carpenter MB, Sutin J: Human Neuroanatomy. Baltimore, Williams & Wilkins, 1983, pp 552–578.

65. Locke W, Shally AV: The Hypothalamus and Pituitary in Health and Disease. Springfield, IL, Charles C Thomas, 1972, pp 427–432.

66. Overeem S, van Vliet JA, Lammers GJ, et al: The hypothalamus in episodic brain disorders. Lancet 1:437–444, 2002.

67. Thannickal TC, Moore RY, Nienhuis R, et al: Reduced number of hypocretin neurons in human narcolepsy. Neuron 27:469–474, 2000.

68. Martin JB, Reichlin S: Clinical Neuroendocrinology. Philadelphia, FA Davis, 1987, p 411.

69. Cohen RA, Albers HE: Disruption of human circadian and cognitive regulation following a discrete hypothalamic lesion: A case study. Neurology 41:726–729, 1991.

70. Fenzi F, Simonati A, Crosato F, et al: Clinical features of Kleine-Levin syndrome with localized encephalitis. Neuropediatrics 24:292–295, 1993.

71. Dauvilliers Y, Mayer G, Lecendreux M, et al: Kleine-Levin syndrome: An autoimmune hypothesis based on clinical and genetic analysis. Neurology 59:1739–1745, 2002.

72. Godoth N, Kesler A, Vainstein G, et al: Clinical and polysomnographic characteristics of 34 patients with Kleine-Levin syndrome. J Sleep Res 10:337–341, 2001.

73. Breningstall GN: Gelastic seizures, precocious puberty, and hypothalamic hamartoma. Neurology 35:1180–1183, 1985.

74. Sharma RR: Hamartoma of the hypothalamus and tuber cinereum: A brief review of the literature. J Postgrad Med 33:1–13, 1987.

75. Kuzniecky R, Guthrie B, Mountz J, et al: Intrinsic epileptogenesis of hypothalamic hamartomas in gelastic epilepsy. Ann Neurol 42:60–67, 1997.

76. Shankar RR, Pescovitz OH: Precocious puberty. Adv Endocrinol Metab 6:55–89, 1995.

77. Margalith D, Jan JE, McCormick AQ, et al: Clinical spectrum of congenital optic nerve hypoplasia: Review of 51 patients. Dev Med Child Neurol 26:311–322, 1984.

78. Margalith D, Tze WJ, Jan JE: Congenital optic nerve hypoplasia with hypothalamic-pituitary dysplasia. Am J Dis Child 139:361–366, 1985.

79. Gross RE: Neoplasms producing endocrine disturbances in childhood. Am J Dis Child 59:579–628, 1940.

80. Laue L, Comite F, Hench K, et al: Precocious puberty associated with neurofibromatosis and optic gliomas. Am J Dis Child 139:1097–1100, 1985.

81. Gillett GR, Symon L: Hypothalamic glioma. Surg Neurol 28:291–300, 1987.

82. Banna M: Pathology and clinical manifestations. In Hankinson J, Banna M (eds): Pituitary and Parapituitary Tumours. London, WB Saunders, 1976, pp 13–58.

83. Weinberger LM, Grant FC: Precocious puberty and tumors of the hypothalamus. Arch Intern Med 67:762–792, 1941.

84. Partsch C-J, Heger S, Sippell WG: Management and outcome of central precocious puberty. Clin Endocrinol 56:129–148, 2002.

85. Rosenfeld JV, Harvey AS, Wrennal J, et al: Transcallosal resection of hypothalamic hamartomas, with control of seizures, in children with gelastic epilepsy. Neurosurgery 48:108–118, 2001.

86. Judge DM, Kulin HE, Page R, et al: Hypothalamic hamartoma: A source of luteinizing hormone-releasing factor in precocious puberty. N Engl J Med 296:7–10, 1977.

87. Losa M, von Werder K: Pathophysiology and clinical aspects of the ectopic GH-releasing hormone syndrome. Clin Endocrinol 47:123–135, 1997.

88. Saeger W, Puchner MJA, Ludecke DK: Combined sellar gangliocytomas and pituitary adenoma in acromegaly or Cushing's disease. Virchows Arch 425:93–99, 1994.

89. Asa SL, Bilbao JM, Kovacks K, et al: Hypothalamic neuronal hamartoma associated with pituitary growth hormone cell adenoma and acromegaly. Acta Neuropathol 52:231–234, 1980.

90. Asa SL, Scheithauer BW, Bilbao JM, et al: A case for hypothalamic acromegaly: A clinicopathological study of six patients with hypothalamic gangliocytomas producing growth hormone releasing factor. J Clin Endocrinol Metab 58:796–803, 1984.

91. Biller BMK: Pathogenesis of pituitary Cushing's syndrome: Pituitary versus hypothalamic. Endocrinol Clin North Am 23:547–554, 1994.

92. Gifford S, Gunderson JG: Cushing's disease as a psychosomatic disorder: A selective review of the clinical and experimental literature and a report of ten cases. Perspect Biol Med 13:169–221, 1970.

93. Bigos ST, Somma M, Rasio E, et al: Cushing's disease: Management by transsphenoidal pituitary microsurgery. J Clin Endocrinol Metab 50:348–354, 1980.

94. Lamberts SW, Stefanko SZ, DeLang SE, et al: Failure of clinical remission after transsphenoidal removal of a microadenoma in a patient with Cushing's disease: Multiple hyperplastic and adenomatous cell nests in surrounding pituitary tissues. J Clin Endocrinol Metab 50:793–795, 1980.

95. Krieger DT, Amorosa L, Linick F: Cyproheptadine-induced remission of Cushing's disease. N Engl J Med 293:893–896, 1975.

96. Lankford HU, Tucker HS, Blackard WG: A cyproheptadine-reversible defect in ACTH control persisting after removal of the pituitary tumor in Cushing's disease. N Engl J Med 305:1244–1248, 1981.

97. Cavagnini F, Invitti C, Polli EE: Sodium valproate in Cushing's disease. Lancet 2:162–163, 1984.

98. Lamberts SWJ, Klijn JG, deQuijada M, et al: The mechanism of the suppressive action of bromocriptine on adrenocorticotropin secretion in patients with Cushing's disease and Nelson's syndrome. J Clin Endocrinol Metab 51:307–311, 1980.

99. Biller BMK, Alexander JM, Zervas NT, et al: Clonal origins of adrenocorticotropin-secreting pituitary tissue in Cushing's disease. J Clin Endocrinol Metab 75:1303–1309, 1992.

100. Faglia G, Spada A: The role of hypothalamus in pituitary neoplasia. Clin Endocrinol 9:225–242, 1995.

101. Asa SL, Kovacs K, Tindall GT, et al: Cushing's disease associated with an intrasellar gangliocytoma producing corticotrophin-releasing factor. Ann Intern Med 101:789–793, 1984.

102. Kapcala LP, Molitch ME, Post KD, et al: Galactorrhea, oligo/amenorrhea, and hyperprolactinemia in patients with craniopharyngiomas. J Clin Endocrinol Metab 51:798–800, 1980.

103. McKeel DW Jr, Fowler M, Jacobs LS: The high prevalence of prolactin cell hyperplasia in the human adenohypophysis. In Proceedings of the Endocrine Society 60th Annual Meeting, Miami Beach, 1978, abstract 353.

104. Feigenbaum SL, Downey DE, Wilson CB, et al: Transsphenoidal pituitary resection for preoperative diagnosis of prolactin-secreting pituitary adenoma in women: Long term follow-up. J Clin Endocrinol Metab 81:1711–1719, 1996.

105. Hardelin J-P: Kallmann syndrome: Towards molecular pathogenesis. Mol Cell Endocrinol 179:75–81, 2001.

106. Kalantaridou SN, Chrousos GP: Clinical review 148: Monogenic disorders of puberty. J Clin Endocrinol Metab 87:2481–2494, 2002.

107. Argente J, Abusrewil SA, Bona G, et al: Isolated growth hormone deficiency in children and adolescents. J Pediatr Endocrinol Metab 14(Suppl 2):1003–1008, 2001.

108. Fahlbusch R, Muller OA, Werder KV: Functional endocrinological disturbances in parasellar processes. Acta Neurochir 28(Suppl):456–460, 1979.

109. Arslanian SA, Rothfus WE, Foley TP Jr, et al: Hormonal, metabolic, and neuroradiologic abnormalities associated with septo-optic dysplasia. Acta Endocrinol 107:282–288, 1984.

110. Willnow S, Kiess W, Butenandt O, et al: Endocrine disorders in septo-optic dysplasia (De Morsier syndrome): Evaluation and follow up of 18 patients. Eur J Pediatr 155:179–184, 1996.

111. Korsgaard O, Lindholm J, Rasmussen P: Endocrine function in patients with suprasellar and hypothalamic tumours. Acta Endocrinol 83:1–8, 1976.

112. Beck-Peccoz P, Amr S, Menezes-Ferreira M, et al: Decreased receptor binding of biologically inactive thyrotropin in central hypothyroidism. N Engl J Med 312:1085–1090, 1985.

113. State MW, Dykens EM: Genetics of childhood disorders: XV. Prader-Willi syndrome: genes, brain, and behavior. J Am Acad Child Adolesc Psychiatry 39:797–800, 2000.

114. Cassidy SB: Prader-Willi syndrome. J Med Genet 34:917–923, 1997.

115. Hoybye C, Hilding A, Jacobsson H, et al: Metabolic profile and body composition in adults with Prader-Willi syndrome and severe obesity. J Clin Endocrinol Metab 87:3590–3597, 2002.

116. Cassidy SB, Schwartz S: Prader-Willi and Angelman syndromes: Disorders of genomic imprinting. Medicine (Baltimore) 77:140–151, 1998.

117. Beales PL, Elcioglu N, Woolf AS, et al: New criteria for improved diagnosis of Bardet-Biedl syndrome: Results of a population survey. J Med Genet 36:437–446, 1999.

118. Beales PL, Warner AM, Hitman GA, et al: Bardet-Biedl syndrome: A molecular and phenotypic study of 18 families. J Med Gent 34:922–928, 1997.

119. Charles SJ, Moore AT, Yates JAW, et al: Alstrom's syndrome: Further evidence of autosomal recessive inheritance and endocrinological dysfunction. J Med Genet 27:590–592, 1990.

120. Birkebaek NH, Patel L, Wright NB, et al: Endocrine status in patients with optic nerve hypoplasia: Relationship to midline central nervous system abnormalities and appearance of the hypothalamic-pituitary axis on magnetic resonance imaging. J Clin Endocrinol Metab 88:5281–5286, 2003.

121. Roessmann U, Velasco ME, Small EJ, et al: Neuropathology of "septo-optic dysplasia" (de Morsier syndrome) with immunohistochemical studies of the hypothalamus and pituitary gland. J Neuropathol Exp Neurol 46:597–608, 1987.

122. Yukizane S, Kimura Y, Yamashita Y, et al: Growth hormone deficiency of hypothalamic origin in septo-optic dysplasia. Eur J Pediatr 150:30–33, 1990.

123. Dattani MT, Martinez-Barbera JP, Thomas PQ, et al: Mutations in the homeobox gene HESX1/Hesx1 associated with septo-optic dysplasia in human and mouse. Nat Genet 19:125–133, 1998.

124. Skuse D, Albanese A, Stanhope R, et al: A new stress-related syndrome of growth failure and hyperphagia in children, associated with reversibility of growth-hormone insufficiency. Lancet 348:353–358, 1996.

125. Gilmour J, Skuse D, Pembrey M: Hyperphagic short stature and Prader-Willi syndrome: A comparison of behavioural phenotypes, genotypes and indices of stress. Br J Psychiatry 179:129–137, 2001.

126. Zuber T, Kelly J: Pseudocyesis. Am Fam Physician 30:131–134, 1984.

127. Bray MA, Muneyyirci-Delale A, Kofinas GD, et al: Circadian, ultradian, and episodic gonadotropin and prolactin secretion in human pseudocyesis. Acta Endocrinol 124:501–509, 1991.

128. Yen SSC, Rebar RW, Quesenberry W: Pituitary function in pseudocyesis. J Clin Endocrinol Metab 43:132–136, 1976.

129. List CF, Dowman CE, Bagchi BS, et al: Posterior hypothalamic hamartomas and gangliogliomas causing precocious puberty. Neurology 8:164–174, 1958.

130. Diebler C, Ponsot G: Hamartomas of the tuber cinereum. Neuroradiology 25:93–101, 1983.

131. Comite F, Psescovitz OH, Rieth KG: Luteinizing hormone-releasing hormone analog treatment of boys with hypothalamic hamartoma and true precocious puberty. J Clin Endocrinol Metab 59:888–892, 1984.

132. Sato M, Ushio Y, Arita N, et al: Hypothalamic hamartoma: Report of two cases. Neurosurgery 16:198–206, 1985.

133. Valdueza JM, Cristante L, Dammann O, et al: Hypothalamic hamartomas: With special reference to gelastic epilepsy and surgery. Neurosurgery 34:949–958, 1994.

134. Hall JG, Pallister PD, Clarren SK, et al: Congenital hypothalamic hamartoblastoma, hypopituitarism, imperforate anus, and postaxial polydactyly: A new syndrome? Part I: Clinical, causal, and pathogenetic considerations. Am J Med Genet 7:47–74, 1980.

135. Clarren SK, Alvord EC Jr, Hall JG: Congenital hypothalamic hamartoblastoma, hypopituitarism, imperforate anus, and postaxial polydactyly: A new syndrome? Part II: Neuropathological considerations. Am J Med Genet 7:75–83, 1980.

136. Biesecker LG, Abbott M, Allen J, et al: Report from the Workshop on Pallister-Hall Syndrome and Related Phenotypes. Am J Med Genet 65:76–81, 1996.

137. Biesecker LG, Graham JM Jr: Pallister-Hall syndrome. J Med Genet 33:585–589, 1996.

138. Kang S, Allen J, Graham JM Jr, et al: Linkage mapping and phenotypic analysis of autosomal dominant Pallister-Hall syndrome. J Med Genet 34:441–446, 1997.

139. Pierre-Kahn A, Capelle L, Brauner R, et al: Presentation and management of suprasellar arachnoid cysts: Review of 20 cases. J Neurosurg 73:355–359, 1990.

140. Rappaport ZH: Suprasellar arachnoid cysts: Options in operative management. Acta Neurochir 122:71–75, 1993.

141. Winnacker JL, Becker KL, Katz S: Endocrine aspects of sarcoidosis. N Engl J Med 278:427–434, 1968.

142. Winnacker JL, Becker KL, Katz S: Endocrine aspects of sarcoidosis (concluded). N Engl J Med 278:483–492, 1968.

143. Bell NH: Endocrine complications of sarcoidosis. Endocrinol Metab Clin North Am 20:645–654, 1991.

144. Kilborn TN, The J, Goodman TR: Paediatric manifestations of Langerhans cell histiocytosis: A review of the clinical and radiological findings. Clin Radiol 58:269–278, 2003.

145. Samaaan NA, Schultz PN, Yang K-PP, et al: Endocrine complications after radiotherapy for tumors of the head and neck. J Lab Clin Med 109:364–372, 1987.

146. Littley MD, Shalet SM, Beardwell CG: Radiation and hypothalamic-pituitary function. Baillieres Clin Endocrinol Metab 4:147–175, 1990.

147. Constine LS, Woolf PD, Cann D, et al: Hypothalamic-pituitary dysfunction after radiation for brain tumors. N Engl J Med 328:87–94, 1993.

148. Gleeson HK, Shalet SM: Endocrine complications of neoplastic diseases in children and adolescents. Curr Opin Pediatr 13:346–351, 2001.

Evaluation of Pituitary Masses

Shlomo Melmed

Both neoplastic and nonneoplastic sellar masses may arise from regions within and adjacent to the hypothalamus and pituitary. They manifest either as a result of their local pressure effects on surrounding vital structures or as a result of distant metabolic or hormonal derangements. Rarely, sellar masses may be the initial feature of a previously undiagnosed systemic disorder.

This chapter outlines the natural history and local and metabolic sequelae of mass lesions arising in the parasellar region; the characteristics of the specific lesions causing these sequelae are described. Although the functional anatomy of the hypothalamic regions has been well demarcated, the relatively close contiguity of these vital centers results in manifestations of distant metabolic derangements that do not necessarily depend on the nature or the exact localization of the parasellar mass lesion. In fact, similar hypothalamic "syndromes" may be caused by a large number of different pathologic processes, all of which arise in the general parasellar region.[1-3] Consequently, the natural history and long-term prognosis of a hypothalamic mass are important in managing the specific lesion, whose exact microanatomic localization in and of itself might not necessarily be clinically precise.

NATURAL HISTORY OF A PITUITARY OR PARASELLAR MASS

Before the advent of sensitive pituitary imaging techniques, a wide spectrum of clinical sequelae were evident from the effects of an enlarging mass arising from within the pituitary or its adjacent structures (Table 21-1). Although it is relatively uncommon today for such a mass to be invasive at the time of clinical diagnosis, the relative subtlety of clinical features can delay the anatomic imaging of such a mass by magnetic resonance imaging (MRI).

Most pituitary and hypothalamic masses are benign neoplasms, with the very rare occurrence of a true primary malignancy with proven distant metastases. Nevertheless, these benign lesions may be aggressively invasive locally into contiguous structures and can result in clinical features that depend on the anatomic location of the impinging mass. Hemorrhage and infarction, which can often be coincidental, may occur in these masses, especially during pregnancy, when the normal pituitary and its surrounding soft tissue structures are edematous and swollen. Diabetes mellitus and hypertension have also been associated with pituitary infarction. Hemorrhage and infarction of the pituitary and hypothalamus are true endocrine emergencies, leading to acute pituitary failure with hypoglycemia, hypothermia, hypotension, apoplexy, and death.

Sellar mass lesions may lead to clinically evident hormonal derangements caused by hormone hypersecretion or, more commonly, by failure of pituitary trophic hormone reserve. Many pituitary masses undergo silent infarction as evidenced by histologic proof of old infarct tissue in patients with otherwise normal pituitary function. Large infarcts may lead to the development of a partial or totally empty pituitary sella. Most of these patients have intact pituitary reserve, which implies that the surrounding rim of pituitary tissue is fully functional. Large cysts associated with the hypothalamic-pituitary unit may also give the radiologic appearance of an empty sella. Rarely, functional pituitary adenomas may arise within the remnant pituitary tissue, and these tumors, although their presence is indicated by classic endocrine hyperactivity, may not be visible by sensitive MRI (i.e., <2 mm in diameter). Acute or chronic infection with abscess formation may be an extremely rare occurrence in the pituitary or hypothalamic mass.

Pituitary hormone hyposecretion may be due to direct pressure effects of the expanding mass on anterior pituitary hormone-secreting cells. Alternatively, parasellar pressure effects

Table 21-1   Complications of a Pituitary or Parasellar Mass

Malignant transformation
Hormonal derangement
Local invasion
Malignant transformation
Hemorrhage
Infarction
Empty sella
Infection (abscess)
Hormonal derangement

may directly attenuate the synthesis or secretion of hypothalamic hormones, with resultant pituitary failure. In contrast, a not uncommon association of hypothalamic masses is overproduction of a specific hypothalamic hormone with resultant hyperfunctioning of a specific hypothalamic-pituitary-target hormone axis.

The important diagnostic dilemma facing the clinician is to effectively distinguish an adenoma arising from the anterior pituitary gland from other parasellar masses. The compelling reason for this diagnosis is the fact that the management and prognosis of true anterior pituitary neoplasms differ so markedly from those of other nonpituitary masses. Most masses arising from within the sella are benign, hormonally functional or nonfunctional adenomas, with relatively good prognosis after appropriate therapy. Their invasiveness is relatively limited, and only rarely will local vital structures be compromised. In contrast, parasellar masses arising from structures contiguous with the pituitary are often malignant or invasive and usually portend a less favorable prognosis.

MAGNETIC RESONANCE IMAGING

Safe and sensitive pituitary visualization is obtained by high-resolution MRI. The anterior pituitary is isodense with white matter, and the posterior pituitary exhibits a characteristic bright spot caused by neurosecretory phospholipid signals. Microadenomas can be detected by T1-weighted coronal spin echo MRI before and after gadolinium administration in approximately 90% of patients, when the mass does not enhance. Most clinically nonfunctioning pituitary masses are, however, macroadenomas at the time of clinical diagnosis and are readily detectable by imaging. MRI is invaluable in visualizing the optic tracts and evaluating the degree of soft tissue changes caused by the tumor. MRI cannot readily distinguish a pituitary adenoma from other intrasellar masses unless other characteristic signs (e.g., invasiveness, hemorrhage, suprasellar involvement) are considered. MRI may also be useful in the preoperative differential diagnosis of carotid artery aneurysms.

COMPUTED TOMOGRAPHY

Pituitary computed tomography (CT) offers the advantage of visualizing invasion of bony structures, including the sellar floor and clinoid bones. CT can also detect small calcifications characteristic of craniopharyngiomas, meningiomas, chordomas, and, rarely, aneurysms that would otherwise remain undiagnosed by MRI.

SOMATOSTATIN RECEPTOR SCINTIGRAPHY

The radiolabeled somatostatin analogue ^{111}In-pentetreotide may be used for in vivo imaging of pituitary tumors expressing somatostatin receptors. Although growth hormone cell adenomas are the most abundant expressors of SRIF (somatostatin) receptors, other pituitary tumor types also express the SRIF receptor to a varying degree. Single-photon emission

CT detects lesions approximately 1 cm in diameter. SRIF receptors that bind to the labeled analogue with high affinity have also been demonstrated in some nonfunctioning pituitary tumors, and variable positive scan imaging of nonfunctioning tumors has been reported. Scintigraphy has been proposed as an imaging technique to predict the response of these tumors to octreotide therapy, but this approach has proved disappointing.[3]

DOPAMINE RECEPTOR SCINTIGRAPHY

Prolactinomas may be imaged with a labeled D_2 receptor antagonist via ^{123}I-iodobenzamine single-photon emission CT. Nonfunctioning pituitary tumors have not been successfully identified with this imaging technique despite the fact that they possess membrane-bound dopamine receptors. This failure to image nonfunctioning tumors is probably due to the lower density of dopamine receptors found in these tumors in comparison to prolactinomas.[4]

LOCAL MASS EFFECTS OF AN ENLARGING SELLAR MASS

The anatomic location of the pituitary sella results in several possible local functional derangements caused by a mass in the midline region of the base of the brain (Table 21-2). The intrasellar mass may invade either soft tissue or surrounding bony structures. Because of its anatomic location, the dorsal roof of the sella presents the least resistance to expansion from within the confines of the bony sella. Nevertheless, both suprasellar and parasellar invasion inexorably occurs with an enlarging mass, with resultant clinical manifestations.

GENERAL EFFECTS

Headaches are common features of intrasellar tumors, even without demonstrable suprasellar extension. Because of the confined nature of the pituitary gland within the sella, even small changes in intrasellar pressure caused by a microadenoma are sufficient to increase pressure and stretching of the dural plate with resultant headache. Complaints of headache do not correlate with the size of the adenoma or the presence of suprasellar extension.[5] In fact, relatively minor distortions of the sellar diaphragm or dural impingement are accompanied by persistent headache. Importantly, medical management of small functional pituitary tumors with bromocriptine or octreotide is often accompanied by a remarkable disappearance of headache.

Table 21-2   Local Neurologic Effects of an Impinging Pituitary or Hypothalamic Mass

Affected Structure	Clinical Effect
Optic tract	Loss of red perception, bitemporal hemianopia, superior or bitemporal field defect, scotoma, blindness
Hypothalamus	Temperature dysregulation, appetite disorders, obesity, thirst disorders, diabetes insipidus, sleep disorders, behavioral dysfunction, autonomic nervous system dysfunction
Cavernous sinus	Ptosis, diplopia, ophthalmoplegia, facial numbness
Temporal lobe	Uncinate seizures
Frontal lobe	Personality disorder, anosmia
Central	Headache, hydrocephalus, psychosis, dementia, laughing seizures

OPTIC TRACT

Pressure on the optic chiasm as a result of dorsally expanding compression may result in visual defects ranging from small field defects to blindness.[5] The refinement of sensitive pituitary imaging techniques has resulted in earlier diagnosis of parasellar lesions than was previously feasible. Consequently, the incidence of presenting optic tract compression by a large mass is diminishing. Nevertheless, through 1972, 40% of 1000 patients with pituitary tumors had either bitemporal hemianopia or superior bitemporal defects.[5] One third of patients had evidence of blindness, scotomas, or other visual disturbances.[6]

Reproducible assessment of visual fields with perimetry techniques should be performed on all patients with an intrapituitary or extrapituitary mass lesion. Loss of red perception is an early sign of optic tract pressure, and red-colored visual signals should preferably be used.[6] Anterior frontal mass lesions may cause unilateral visual loss, whereas chiasmic or posterior pressure will usually result in bilateral defects. Classically, elevation and distortion of the optic chiasm result in bitemporal hemianopia, whereas dorsal chiasmic compression also results in field cuts. Homonymous hemianopia may result from tumor or vascular pressure on optic tract regions lying anterior to the chiasm. Transient visual disorders, asymmetric deficits, or enlargement of the blind spot may all indicate the presence of a parasellar mass. If the mass causes an internal hydrocephalus by obstructing the flow of cerebrospinal fluid (CSF), secondary visual disturbances and papilledema may ensue.

PITUITARY STALK

Compression of the stalk by an expanding intrasellar or parasellar mass may result in pituitary failure caused by encroachment of the portal vessels that normally provide pituitary access to the hypothalamic hormones. Stalk compression usually leads to hyperprolactinemia and failure of other pituitary trophic hormones.

CAVERNOUS SINUS

Lateral invasion of pituitary lesions or ventrolateral encroachment by parasellar or hypothalamic masses may impinge on the cavernous sinus and its neural contents. This invasion may lead to lesions of the third, fourth, and sixth cranial nerves, as well as the ophthalmic and maxillary branches of the fifth cranial nerve. Varying degrees of diplopia, ptosis, ophthalmoplegia, and decreased facial sensation occur, depending on the extent of neural involvement by the cavernous sinus mass.

SPHENOID SINUS

Dorsal extension into the sphenoid sinus implies that the parasellar mass has already eroded the bony sellar floor. Although no vital structures are located in the sinus, aggressive tumors may invade the roof of the palate and cause severe nasopharyngeal obstruction, infection, and even CSF leakage.

BRAIN

Both the temporal and frontal brain lobes may be invaded by the expanding parasellar mass. Uncinate seizures, personality disorders, and anosmia may result from localized tumor involvement.

METABOLIC SEQUELAE OF HYPOTHALAMIC LESIONS

In addition to the anatomic lesions caused by the expanding mass above, direct hypothalamic involvement of the encroaching mass may lead to important nonendocrine sequelae[7,8] (Table 21-3). Clinical features associated with hypothalamic masses depend to a large extent on the site of the lesion rather than the nature of the pathologic process. The enlarging hypothalamic mass, regardless of its etiology, will usually result in local pressure effects, including headaches and recurrent vomiting with or without associated extrapyramidal or pyramidal tract involvement. Common metabolic clinical sequelae, which occur in about one third of these patients, include precocious puberty or hypogonadism, diabetes insipidus, sleep disturbances, dysthermia, and appetite disorders (see Table 21-3). Because of the very close microanatomic contiguity of several highly specialized hypothalamic cells, precise site-specific functional effects of an expanding mass are rarely documented. Most patients therefore exhibit a spectrum of metabolic sequelae that occur regardless of the etiology or site of the pathologic process.

Temperature dysregulation, appetite and thirst disorders, sleep disorders, and behavioral and autonomic dysfunction[9-16] caused by hypothalamic lesions are more fully considered in Chapter 20.

PARASELLAR MASSES

A list of pituitary and nonpituitary masses is delineated in Table 21-4.

RATHKE'S CYST

During early embryogenesis, the anterior and intermediate lobes of the pituitary gland arise from Rathke's pouch. If the pouch fails to obliterate, cystic remnants remain at the interface between the anterior and posterior pituitary lobes. These small cysts (<5 mm) are found in about 20% of pituitary glands at autopsy.[17] Occasionally, a pituitary adenoma may also contain small cleft cysts.[18] MRI of these cysts reveals hyperdense or hypodense masses using either T1- or T2-weighted images. CT scanning reveals the presence of homogeneous hypodense areas that may allow differentiation from pituitary adenomas.[19] Other sellar cysts include arachnoid, epidermoid, and dermoid cysts. Although these lesions

---

Table 21-3 Metabolic Sequelae of Hypothalamic Mass Lesions

Temperature dysregulation
Hyperthermia
Hypothermia
Appetite disorders
Obesity
Hyperphagia
Anorexia and emaciation
Aphagia
Thirst disorders
Adipsia
Compulsive drinking
Hypernatremia
Sleep disorders
Reversal of sleep-wake cycle
Akinetic mutism
Somnolence and coma
Behavioral dysfunction
Hyperkinesis
Rage
Autonomic dysfunction
Cardiac arrhythmias
Loss of sphincter control
Cardiac failure

Source: Adapted from Martin JB, Reichlin S: Clinical Neuroendocrinology. Copyright © 1987 by Oxford University Press, Inc. Used by permission of Oxford University Press, Inc.

Table 21-4	Pituitary and Nonpituitary Sellar Masses

Cysts
  Rathke's
  Arachnoid
  Epidermoid
  Dermoid
Tumors
  Hormone-secreting or nonfunctional pituitary adenoma
  Granular cell tumor
  Craniopharyngioma
  Chordoma
  Meningioma
  Sarcomas
  Glioma
  Schwannoma
  Germ cell tumor
  Vascular tumor
  Solid or hematologic metastases
Malformation and hamartomas
  Ectopic pituitary, neurohypophysial, or salivary tissue
  Hypothalamic hamartoma
  Gangliocytoma
Miscellaneous lesions
  Aneurysms
  Lymphocytic hypophysitis
  Infections
  Sarcoidosis
  Giant cell granuloma
  Langerhans' histiocytosis

develop mainly in the cerebellopontine angle, they may also arise in the suprasellar region. Clinical features of compression include internal hydrocephalus, visual disturbances, and, rarely, growth hormone or adrenocorticotropic hormone (ACTH) deficiency, hyperprolactinemia, and diabetes insipidus.[20-23] Rarely, a squamous cell carcinoma may develop in the cyst.[24]

GRANULAR CELL TUMORS

Pituitary choristomas, or schwannomas, usually occur only after the age of 20 and are probably acquired lesions.[25,26] Their abundant cytoplasmic granules do not contain known pituitary hormones, nor are these tumors associated with endocrine syndromes. However, several pituitary adenomas have been coincidentally associated with these tumors.

CHORDOMAS

These midline tumors arise from remnants of the notochord, are slowly growing and locally invasive, and may metastasize.[27,28] Most arise from the vertebrae, but about one third involve the clivus region. Characteristically, they contain a mucin-rich matrix that allows for histologic diagnosis by fine-needle aspiration. On imaging, the tissue mass is associated with osteolytic bony erosion and calcification. MRI may allow visualization of the normal pituitary gland distinct from the very heterogeneous and often flocculent tumor mass. Nasopharyngeal obstruction may rarely occur, in addition to the more commonly encountered headaches and asymmetric visual disturbances. At surgery, these tumors appear rough and have a heterogeneous lobular appearance. Histologically, they exhibit markers for epithelial cells, including cytokeratin and vimentin. After surgical excision, local invasion and recurrence commonly occur, with mean patient survival of about 5 years. Rarely, chordomas become sarcomatous, with an aggressive natural history.

CRANIOPHARYNGIOMAS

These common parasellar tumors constitute about 3% of all intracranial tumors and up to 10% of childhood brain tumors.[12]

Although the tumor may occur at any age, it is commonly diagnosed during childhood and adolescence. The mass may arise from embryonic squamous remnants of Rathke's pouch extending dorsally toward the diencephalon. These tumors may be large (>10 cm in diameter) and invade the third ventricle and associated brain structures. About two thirds arise from within the sella, whereas remaining tumors arise from cell rests situated in the parasellar region.[29] The cystic mass is usually filled with cholesterol-rich viscous fluid, and calcification may be present. Histologic analysis shows these tumors to consist of two cell populations: squamous epithelium containing islands characterized by columnar cells lines the cyst; a mixed inflammatory reaction may also occur with calcification. Although craniopharyngiomas may be quite large and obstruct CSF flow, they rarely undergo malignant transformation.[30] Interestingly, cyst fluid contains immunoreactive human chorionic gonadotropin, which may actually leak into the CSF.[31] Features of increased intracranial pressure, including headache, projectile vomiting, papilledema, and somnolence, are usually encountered in children. Only about one third of patients are older than 40 years, and they commonly have asymmetric visual disturbances, including papilledema, optic atrophy, and field deficits. Other cranial nerves may also be involved, especially those situated within the cavernous sinus.

On CT imaging, most children and about half of all adults have a characteristic flocculent or convex calcification pattern of the tumor. Rarely, however, calcifications may also be observed in pituitary adenomas, other parasellar tumors, and even vascular sellar lesions.

Endocrine manifestations of craniopharyngioma usually result from partial or complete pituitary deficiency. Growth hormone deficiency, with resultant short stature and diabetes insipidus, and gonadal failure are common. Compression of the pituitary stalk or damage to the dopaminergic neurons in the hypothalamus results in hyperprolactinemia. This latter feature is especially important in the differential diagnosis of prolactinoma. Management of these common latter adenomas differs markedly from that of a craniopharyngioma, and careful imaging techniques might not easily distinguish the two lesions.[32] Certainly, a highly asymmetric mass (especially with preferential posterior or dorsal extension) that does not shrink after bromocriptine therapy should arouse suspicion of craniopharyngioma. The hyperprolactinemia associated with a craniopharyngioma will also respond quite effectively to dopamine agonists. This favorable biochemical response to treatment does not exclude the presence of a craniopharyngioma. Thus, craniopharyngioma may mimic a prolactinoma in terms of intrapituitary imaging, presence of hyperprolactinemia, and biochemical response to cabergoline.

Treatment options for these lesions include radical surgery, radiotherapy, or a combination of these modalities.[33,34] In selected centers, stereotactic irradiation of the mass has been performed with some success. Nevertheless, regardless of which form of therapy is chosen, ablation of the mass invariably results in anterior and/or posterior pituitary hormone deficits. Postoperative recurrence may occur in about a fifth of patients who undergo radical surgical excision,[35] whereas no appreciable difference is noted in the outcome of those who undergo subtotal surgical excision followed by radiotherapy. The presence of pure papillary squamous cellular elements may portend a higher surgical recurrence rate.[36] The long-term effects of childhood irradiation for these tumors are considered elsewhere (Chapter 22).

MENINGIOMAS

Meningiomas account for about one quarter of all intracranial tumors.[37] These tumors arise from arachnoid and meningioendothelial cells, and those occurring in the sellar and parasellar region account for about one fifth of all meningiomas.[38] They are usually more circumscribed and do not achieve the size of craniopharyngiomas. Suprasellar meningiomas may invade the pituitary ventrally, whereas an intrasellar tumor origin is extremely rare. Several patients with functional pituitary adenomas have also been described who harbored coincidental parasellar meningiomas.[39] These tumors are not hormonally active, although secondary hyperprolactinemia has been reported in up to 50% of patients. They usually cause local mass effects, including headache and progressive visual disturbances accompanied by optic atrophy. Imaging diagnosis by imaging is difficult because the differential radiologic diagnosis of a suprasellar meningioma with ventral extension from a pituitary adenoma with dorsal extension may be difficult. Improved MRI techniques have been used in attempts to distinguish the borders of meningiomas from adenomas, but the radiologic diagnosis remains difficult.[40] Typically, meningiomas are isodense on both T1- and T2-weighted imaging, in contrast to other parasellar lesions, which are usually hyperdense on T2-weighted imaging. Dural calcification may occasionally be discerned on CT scanning. Because of their rich vascularization, these tumors pose an increased intraoperative risk with a higher surgical mortality rate than is usually encountered for pituitary tumor resection.[41]

GLIOMAS

Optic gliomas and low-grade astrocytomas may cause optic atrophy, papilledema, visual loss, and pituitary failure in children; in adults, they may be more aggressively invasive. Most arise from within the optic chiasm or optic tracts, and fewer than one third are intraorbital.[42,43] Von Recklinghausen's disease is present in about one third of all patients with these tumors. Occasionally, these tumors may accompany growth retardation and delayed or precocious puberty,[44] and some may be malignant.[45] Mass effects include visual field disturbances, diencephalic syndrome, diabetes insipidus, and hydrocephalus.[46] Gliomas arising within the pituitary sella are exceedingly rare but, if present, may be associated with hyperprolactinemia and should be considered an uncommon mimicker of a prolactin-secreting pituitary adenoma. Important distinguishing features include the young age of these patients (80% <10 years old), relatively intact pituitary function, gross visual disturbances, and imaging localization of the mass. The tumor usually involves the optic chiasm, and optic nerve infiltration is also characteristic. Gliomas usually enhance after contrast injection, unlike hamartomas, which remain isodense.

HYPOTHALAMIC MASSES

Hypothalamic hamartomas are benign tumors composed of a mixture of neurons, astrocytes, and oligodendrocytes. These cell types are organized with varying degrees of differentiation, and they may express peptides released from the hypothalamus. Most commonly, these tumors occur before the age of 2 years and have been shown to express gonadotropin-releasing hormone (GnRH) with associated precocious puberty.[47] In tumors in which GnRH immunoreactivity could not be demonstrated, hypothalamic dysfunction was postulated as causing precocious puberty because GnRH injection results in a pubertal gonadotropin response.[48] Most patients have psychomotor delay and seizures. Curiously, these tumors may also be associated with laughing seizures, emotional lability, and rage.[49–53] The Pallister-Hall syndrome consists of hypothalamic hamartoblastoma; abnormalities of the craniofacial area, heart, kidneys, and lungs; imperforate anus; and hypopituitarism.[53] Although surgical excision is usually advocated for hamartomas, administration of long-acting GnRH analogues have been effective to downregulate gonadotropin secretion and control precocious puberty. Hypothalamic hamartomas are slowly growing tumors and rarely invasive. In contrast, gangliocytomas arising in the hypothalamic or intrasellar area do grow progressively. These tumors may be associated with pituitary tumors, and ganglion cells that are present with the pituitary adenoma may stain positively for hormones released from the hypothalamus. Although MRI distinction may be difficult,[54] when these tumors occur in association with concurrent pituitary adenomas, it has been tempting to speculate that the hypothalamic hormone that is expressed by the tumor is implicated in the pathogenesis of the pituitary adenoma.

Besides GnRH, these tumors have been shown to express growth hormone-releasing hormone[55–61] and corticotropin-releasing hormone[62,63] and are associated with acromegaly and Cushing's syndrome, respectively.

Suprasellar germ cell tumors may be histologically indistinguishable from germinomas, teratomas, embryonal carcinomas, and choriocarcinomas.[64–68] Some tumors express immunoreactive β-human chorionic gonadotropin, human placental lactogen, or other placental peptides. These tumors may be manifested by precocious puberty in addition to diabetes insipidus and visual field abnormalities. Unexplained pituitary stalk thickening in the presence of diabetes insipidus may be reflective of occult intracranial germinoma. Thirst disorders, with associated hypernatremia, emaciation, or even obesity, may also occur. Suppressed growth hormone secretion with growth delay is found in over 95% of these patients. After biopsy diagnosis, high-dose radiotherapy has proved to be effective, with about a 70% long-term survival rate.

Hypothalamic astrocytomas (gliomas), often arising in the anterior hypothalamus and associated with hypophagia of infancy, are rare tumors that may be malignant.

SECONDARY METASTASES TO THE PITUITARY REGION

Pituitary metastases occur quite commonly and are found in up to 5% of all cancer patients (Table 21-5). The posterior pituitary is the preferred site for blood-borne metastatic spread. This site preference may be explained by the vascular supply to the posterior pituitary; blood flows into it directly from the systemic circulation via the internal carotid arteries. The predominant blood supply to the anterior pituitary, in contrast, is by way of the hypothalamic portal system. Common primary carcinomas that metastasize to the pituitary include those of the lung, gastrointestinal tract, and breast. Up to one quarter of patients with metastatic breast cancer have pituitary metastases at autopsy, and approximately 18% of cases have demonstrable pituitary metastases.[69] Interestingly,

Table 21-5	Neoplastic Source of Pituitary Metastases in 238 Patients*	
Primary Neoplasm	**Percentage of Patients**
Breast	47
Lung	19
Gastrointestinal tract	6
Prostate	6
Leukemia	3
Pancreas	3
Unknown origin	2
Nasopharynx	<2
Melanoma	<2
Thyroid	<2
Plasmacytoma	<2
Endometrium	<1
Renal	<1
Ovary	<1
Liver	<1
Penis	<1

*Included are data from Post et al.,[84] Komninos et al.,[69] Palladino and Andrioli,[85] Max et al.,[86] and Juneau et al.[87]

Unable to display

symptomatic pituitary metastases may be the initial sign of previously undiscovered malignancy and even of malignancy of unknown origin. Although anterior pituitary failure is rare, an isolated metastatic deposit in the pituitary stalk without involvement of the anterior lobe may also be seen as pituitary failure (Table 21-6). Posterior pituitary metastases are common causes of failure, and about 15% of patients with diabetes insipidus harbor metastases from extrapituitary sources. Unfortunately, imaging of the pituitary mass does not distinguish these deposits from a pituitary adenoma unless extensive bony erosion is present. In fact, metastatic pituitary lesions may masquerade as a pituitary adenoma. In several instances, the diagnosis of pituitary metastasis will be made only by histologic study of a specimen removed at transsphenoidal surgery.

MISCELLANEOUS PARASELLAR MASSES

Acute lymphoblastic leukemia may be associated with periglandular pituitary infiltrates with minimal pituitary dysfunction. Rarely, the syndrome of inappropriate antidiuretic hormone secretion has been reported in this condition. Primary lymphoma may also involve the hypothalamus and pituitary stalk, and these patients may have resultant hypopituitarism. Isolated patients with solitary pituitary plasmacytomas in whom classic multiple myeloma does not develop have been reported, as have patients with primary lymphomas.[70] Rarely, Langerhans' histiocytosis (histiocytosis X) lesions may be confined to the hypothalamic-pituitary axis. These patients usually have diabetes insipidus and occasionally hyperprolactinemia caused by destruction of the hypothalamic portal tract.

HISTIOCYTOSIS X

Histiocytosis X lesions are composed of eosinophilic proliferative infiltrates that may be local or generalized. Although the form of the disorder may depend on location of the granulomatous infiltrate, most patients exhibit disordered hypothalamic pituitary function, including diabetes insipidus and growth disorders. Exophthalmos and focally lytic bone lesions are also characteristic. On MRI, the suprasellar mass

may be associated with signs of pituitary stalk and posterior pituitary involvement.

LYMPHOCYTIC HYPOPHYSITIS

Although more extensively described in Chapter 22, lymphocytic hypophysitis is an important cause of a sellar mass. This diffuse inflammatory process occurs predominantly in postpartum women and is characterized by a pituitary mass, pituitary failure, hyperprolactinemia, headache, and visual disturbances.[71] The natural history of the disorder is benign, most intrasellar processes resolving with time. On MRI, the mass enhances after contrast injection, often rendering it indistinguishable from an adenoma.[72] Pituitary failure should be treated, and some patients demonstrate mass resolution after steroid therapy.[73]

MUCOCELE

Expanding fluid accumulation in the sphenoid sinus may result in mucocele formation, which may compress parasellar structures. Severe headaches, visual disturbances (usually unilateral), and exophthalmos are characteristic features.[74] On MRI, the homogeneous sphenoid mass may be quite prominent, but occasionally it can be distinguished from the pituitary gland dorsally.

ANEURYSM

Aneurysms arising from within or adjacent to the parasellar vasculature may mimic a pituitary adenoma. Preoperative or intraoperative rupture is a potentially catastrophic complication, thus underscoring the absolute need for early diagnosis. Differentiating features from other pituitary masses may be subtle, including eye pain, very intense headaches, and relatively sudden onset of cranial nerve palsies. Although CT and MRI techniques can distinguish blood and hemorrhage from solid tumor or tissue, a highly vascular meningioma may be confused with an aneurysm.[75]

OTHER MASSES

Other rare parasellar masses include granulomas, sarcoidosis, and tuberculosis. Although evidence for systemic tuberculosis is usually present, isolated *sellar tuberculoma* may be encountered,[76,77] as may isolated sarcoid lesions. Infiltrative *sarcoidosis* of the hypothalamic-pituitary unit occurs in most patients with central nervous system sarcoid involvement.[78] Pituitary stalk thickening is also encountered. Typically, these patients have varying degrees of anterior pituitary failure with or without diabetes insipidus.

ABSCESS

Primary pituitary abscesses[79] may arise in immunocompromised subjects and may be caused by fungi (*Aspergillus*, *Nocardia*, or *Candida albicans*) or *Pneumocystis carinii*. Usually, these conditions manifest as diabetes insipidus, with or without anterior pituitary dysfunction, and hyperprolactinemia. Gonadal dysfunction may be an early peripheral endocrine sign in adults with these sellar masses.

APPROACH TO THE PATIENT WITH A SELLAR MASS

The clinical approach to a patient harboring a pituitary mass is compounded by the high (up to 25%) incidence of incidental silent pituitary microadenomas discovered at autopsy. Clinically inapparent pituitary cysts, hemorrhage, and infarctions are also not uncommonly discovered at autopsy. With widespread sensitive imaging techniques, asymptomatic

Table 21-6 **Initial Clinical Findings in 190 Patients with Clinically Apparent Pituitary Metastases**

Symptom/Finding	%
Diabetes insipidus	45
Cranial nerve II deficit	28
Anterior pituitary insufficiency (partial or total)	24
Cranial nerve palsy	22
Headaches/general malaise	16
Fatigue/general malaise	8
Hyperprolactinemia	6
Pituitary apoplexy	5
Nausea/vomiting	4
Anorexia/weight loss	3
Altered consciousness	3
Cognitive/psychiatric deficit	3
SIADH	1.5
Cerebral hemorrhage	1.5
Seizures	1.0
Amernorrhea/galactorrhea	1.0
Decreased libido	1.0
Cushing's syndrome	1.0
Acromegaly	1.0
Orthostatic hypotension	0.5
Tumor increase on dopamine agonist	0.5

pituitary lesions are being identified with increasing frequency,[80] and pituitary abnormalities compatible with the diagnosis of pituitary microadenoma are detectable in about 10% of the normal adult population. In view of the differential diagnosis of the intrasellar mass and in recognition of the fact that most lesions observed represent pituitary adenomas, several issues should be considered in the management of these masses. Of particular concern is whether the mass is hormonally functional and whether local mass effects are apparent at the time of diagnosis or develop in the future.[80]

Evaluation of pituitary mass function is important because the onset of symptoms and signs related to disordered hormone secretion is often insidious and may remain unnoticed for years. Clinical evaluation for changes compatible with ACTH, growth hormone, or prolactin hypersecretion or hyposecretion may reveal long-term serious systematic complications, and each may require distinct therapeutic approaches.[81] In the absence of clinical features of a humoral hypersecretory syndrome, recommendations for cost-effective laboratory screening are debatable. The incidence of hormone-secreting tumors in asymptomatic subjects with incidental pituitary masses is low, and low-grade asymptomatic hormone hypersecretion (e.g., for prolactin or α subunits) carries questionable long-term risk.

In the absence of evidence of hormone oversecretion, the presence of, or the potential for, local compressive effects must be considered. The risk for microadenoma enlargement to a compressive macroadenoma is low, so a decision to operate may be confidently postponed. For hypothalamic or parasellar masses of uncertain origin, histologic tissue examination may be the only direct approach to yield an accurate diagnosis. Although distinguishing MRI or CT features may be helpful in the differential diagnosis of a nonpituitary sellar mass, the final diagnosis usually remains elusive until pathologic confirmation is obtained. Benefits of pituitary surgery must also be weighed carefully against potential side effects,[82] although endoscopic approaches may facilitate safer access to sellar tissue for histologic diagnosis or resection.[83] If surgery is not indicated, subsequent imaging studies can determine the lesion's slow growth rate, if any. In the absence of tumor growth, the interval between scans may be prolonged, and surgery should not be recommended in these asymptomatic cases. When an incidentally asymptomatic macroadenoma is diagnosed, visual field and pituitary function should be comprehensively evaluated. If the findings are normal, imaging follow-up should be conducted, with the awareness that evidence of progressive enlargement or impingement of vital structures indicate a need for surgical intervention.

REFERENCES

1. Freda PU: Differential diagnosis of sellar masses. Endocrinol Metab Clin North Am 28:81–117, 1999.
2. Saeger W: Tumor-like lesions of the pituitary and sellar region. The Endocrinologist 12:300–314, 2002.
3. Maroldo TV, Dillon WP, Wilson CB: Advances in diagnostic techniques of pituitary tumors and prolactinomas. Oncology 4:105–115, 1992.
4. de Herder WW, Reijst AEM, Kwekkeboom DJ, et al: In vivo imaging of pituitary tumours using a radiolabelled dopamine D2 receptor radioligand. Clin Endocrinol 45:755–767, 1996.
5. Hollenhorst RW, Younge BR: Ocular manifestations produced by adenomas of the pituitary gland: Analysis of 1000 cases. In Kohler PO, Ross GT (eds): Diagnosis and Treatment of Pituitary Tumors. Amsterdam, Excerpta Medica, 1973, pp 53–64.
6. Melan O: Neuro-ophthalmologic features of pituitary tumors. Endocrinol Metab Clin North Am 16:585–608, 1987.
7. Marques PR, Illner P, Williams DD: Hypothalamic control of endocrine thermogenesis. Am J Physiol 241:E420, 1981.
8. Bauer HG: Endocrine and other clinical manifestations of hypothalamic disease. J Clin Endocrinol Metab 14:13–31, 1954.
9. Mooradian AD, Morley GK, McGeachie R, et al: Spontaneous periodic hypothermia. Neurology 34:79–82, 1984.
10. Newman MM, Halmi KA: The endocrinology of anorexia nervosa and bulimia nervosa. Neurol Clin 6:195–212, 1988.
11. Bray GA, Gallagher TJ Jr: Manifestations of hypothalamic obesity in man: A comprehensive investigation of eight patients and a review of the literature. Medicine (Baltimore) 54:301–330, 1975.
12. Burr IM, Slonim AE, Danish RK, et al: Diencephalic syndrome revisited. J Pediatr 88:439–444, 1976.
13. Scherbaum WA, Wass KAJ, Besser GM, et al: Autoimmune cranial diabetes insipidus: Its association with other endocrine diseases and with histiocytosis X. Clin Endocrinol 25:411–420, 1986.
14. DeRubertis FR, Michelis ME, Davis BB: "Essential" hypernatremia: Report of three cases and review of the literature. Arch Intern Med 134:889–895, 1974.
15. Hayek A, Peake GT: Hypothalamic adipsia without demonstrable structural lesion. Pediatrics 70:275–278, 1982.
16. Imura H, Kato Y, Nakai Y: Endocrine aspects of tumors arising from suprasellar, third ventricular regions. Prog Exp Tumor Res 30:313–324, 1987.
17. El-Mahdy W, Powell M: Transsphenoidal management of 28 symptomatic Rathke's cleft cysts, with special reference to visual and hormonal recovery. Neurosurgery 42:7–17, 1998.
18. Nishio S, Mizuno J, Barrow DL, et al: Pituitary tumors composed of adenohypophysial adenoma and Rathke's cleft cyst elements: A clinicopathological study. Neurosurgery 21:371–377, 1987.
19. Mukherjee JJ, Islam N, Kaltsas G, et al: Clinical, radiological and pathological features of patients with Rathke's cleft cysts: Tumors that may recur. J Clin Endocrinol Metab 82:2357, 1997.
20. Shin JL, Asa SL, Woodhouse LJ, et al: Cystic lesions of the pituitary clinicopathological features distinguishing craniopharyngioma, Rathke's cleft cyst, and arachnoid cyst. J Clin Endocrinol Metab 84:3972–3982, 1999.
21. Yamakawa K, Shitara N, Genka S, et al: Clinical course and surgical prognosis of 33 cases of intracranial epidermoid tumors. Neurosurgery 24:568–573, 1989.
22. Lewis AJ, Cooper PW, Kassel EE, Schwartz ML: Squamous cell carcinoma arising in a suprasellar epidermoid cyst: Case report. J Neurosurg 59:538–541, 1983.
23. Voelker JL, Campbell RL, Muller J: Clinical radiographic and pathological features of symptomatic Rathke's cleft cysts. J Neurosurg 74:535, 1991.
24. Schlachter LB, Tindall GT, Pearl GS: Granular cell tumor of the pituitary gland associated with diabetes insipidus. Neurosurgery 6:418–421, 1980.
25. Morrison JG, Gray GF, Dao AH, Adkins RB: Granular cell tumors. Am Surg 53:156–160, 1987.
26. Perzin KH, Pushparaj N: Nonepithelial tumors of the nasal cavity, paranasal sinuses, and nasopharynx: A clinicopathological study. XIV: Chordomas. Cancer 57:784–796, 1986.
27. Meyer JE, Oot RF, Lindfors KK: CT appearance of clival chordomas. J Comput Assist Tomogr 10:34–36, 1986.
28. Volpe R, Mazabraud A: A clinicopathologic review of 25 cases of chordoma (a pleomorphic and metastasizing neoplasm). Am J Surg Pathol 7:161–170, 1983.
29. Ogilvy-Stuart AL, Shalet SM: Tumour of the endocrine glands in children. Endocr Relat Cancer 1:27–41, 1994.
30. Petito CK, DeGirolami U, Earle KM: Craniopharyngiomas: A clinical and pathological review. Cancer 37:1944–1952, 1976.
31. Harris PE, Perry L, Chard T, et al: Immunoreactive human chorionic gonadotrophin from the cyst fluid and CSF of patients with craniopharyngioma. Clin Endocrinol 29:503–508, 1988.

32. Pigeau I, Sigal R, Halimi P, et al: MRI features of craniopharyngiomas at 1.5 tesla. J Neuroradiol 15:276–287, 1988.

33. Yasargil MG, Curcic M, Kis M, et al: Total removal of craniopharyngiomas: Approaches and long term-results in 144 patients. J Neurosurg 73:3–11, 1990.

34. Wen BC, Hussey DH, Staples J, et al: A comparison of the roles of surgery and radiation therapy in the management of craniopharyngiomas. Int J Radiat Oncol Biol Phys 16:17–24, 1989.

35. Adamson TE, Wiestler OD, Kleihues P, Yasargil MG: Correlation of clinical and pathological features in surgically treated craniopharyngiomas. J Neurosurg 73:12–17, 1990.

36. Honegger J, Buchfelder M, Fahlbusch R: Surgical treatment of craniopharyngiomas: Endocrinological results. J Neurosurg 90:251–257, 1999.

37. Rohringer M, Sutherland GR, Louw DE, Sima AAF: Incidence and clinicopathological features of meningioma. J Neurosurg 71:665–672, 1989.

38. Grisoli F, Vincentelli F, Raybaud C, et al: Intrasellar meningioma. Surg Neurol 20:36–41, 1983.

39. Yamada K, Hatayama T, Ohta M, et al: Coincidental pituitary adenoma and parasellar meningioma: Case report. Neurosurgery 19:267–270, 1986.

40. Donovan JL, Nesbit GM: Distinction of masses involving the sella and suprasellar space: Specificity of imaging features. Am J Roentgenol 167:597–603, 1996.

41. Andrews BT, Wilson CB: Suprasellar meningiomas: The effect of tumor location on postoperative visual outcome. J Neurosurg 69:523–528, 1988.

42. Alvord EC, Lofton S: Gliomas of the optic nerve or chiasm: Outcome by patient's age, tumor site, and treatment. J Neurosurg 68:85–98, 1988.

43. Rush JA, Younge BR, Campbell RJ, MacCarty CS: Optic glioma: Long term follow-up of 85 histopathologically verified cases. Ophthalmology 89:1213–1219, 1982.

44. Flickinger JC, Torres C, Deutsch M: Management of low-grade gliomas of optic nerve and chiasm. Cancer 61:635–642, 1988.

45. Rudd A, Rees JE, Kennedy P, et al: Malignant optic nerve gliomas in adults. J Clin Neuroophthalmol 5:238–243, 1985.

46. Albers GW, Hoyt WF, Forno LS, Shratter LA: Treatment response in malignant optic glioma of adulthood. Neurology 38:1071–1074, 1988.

47. Judge DM, Kulin HE, Page R, et al: Hypothalamic hamartoma: A source of luteinizing-hormone releasing factor in precocious puberty. N Engl J Med 296:7–10, 1977.

48. Hirsch-Pescovitz O, Comite F, Hench K, et al: The NIH experience with precocious puberty: Diagnostic subgroups and response to short term luteinizing hormone releasing hormone

analogue therapy. J Pediatr 108:47–54, 1986.

49. Curatolo P, Clismai R, Fitiocchi G, Boscherini B: Gelactic epilepsy and true precocious puberty, due to hypothalamic hamartoma. Dev Med Child Neurol 26:509–514, 1984.

50. Nishio S, Fujiwara S, Aiko N, et al: Hypothalamic hamartoma: Report of two cases. J Neurosurg 70:640–645, 1989.

51. Berkovic SF, Andermanii F, Melanson D, et al: Hypothalamic hamartomas and ictal laughter: Evolution of a characteristic epileptic syndrome and diagnostic value of magnetic resonance imaging. Ann Neurol 23:429–239, 1989.

52. Breningstall GN: Gelactic seizures, precocious puberty and hypothalamic hamartoma. Neurology 35:1180–1183, 1985.

53. Iafolla K, Fratkin JD, Spiegel PK, et al: Case report and delineation of the congenital hypothalamic hamartoblastoma syndrome (Pallister-Hall syndrome). Am J Med Genet 33:489–499, 1989.

54. Hubbard AM, Egelhoff JC: MR imaging of large hypothalamic hamartomas in two infants. Am J Neuroradiol 10:1277, 1989.

55. Bevan JS, Asa SL, Rossi ML, et al: Intrasellar gangliocytoma containing gastrin and growth hormone-releasing hormone associated with a growth hormone-secreting pituitary adenoma. Clin Endocrinol 30:213–224, 1989.

56. Markin RS, Leibrock LG, Huseman CA, McComb RD: Hypothalamic hamartoma: A report of two cases. Pediatr Neurosci 13:19–26, 1987.

57. Asa SL, Scheithauer BW, Bilbao JM, et al: A case for hypothalamic acromegaly: A clinicopathological study of six patients with hypothalamic gangliocytomas producing growth hormone-releasing factor. J Clin Endocrinol Metab 58:796–803, 1984.

58. Puchner MJ, Ludecke DK, Saeger W: Gangliocytomas of the sellar region: A review. Exper Clin Endocrinol 103:129–149, 1995.

59. Li JY, Racadot O, Kujas M, et al: Immunocytochemistry of four mixed pituitary adenomas and intrasellar gangliocytomas associated with different clinical syndromes: Acromegaly, amenorrhea-galactorrhea, Cushing's disease and isolated tumoral syndrome. Acta Neuropathol 77:320–328, 1989.

60. Yamada S, Stefaneanu I, Kovacs K, et al: Intrasellar gangliocytoma with multiple immunoreactivities. Endocr Pathol 1:58–63, 1990.

61. Freda PU, Wardlaw SL, Post KD: Unusual causes of sellar/parasellar masses in a large transsphenoidal surgery series. J Clin Endocrinol Metab 81:3455–3459, 1996.

62. Pelletier G, Desy L, Cote J, et al: Light microscope immunohistochemical localization of growth hormone-releasing factor (GRF) in the human

hypothalamus. Cell Tissue Res 245:461–464, 1986.

63. Asa SL, Kovacs K, Tindall GT, et al: Cushing's disease associated with an intrasellar gangliocytoma producing corticotrophin-releasing factor. Ann Intern Med 101:789–793, 1984.

64. Janmohamed S, Grossman AB, Metcalfe K, et al: Suprasellar germ cell ltumours: Specific problems and the evolution of optimal management with a combined chemoradiotherapy regimen. Clin Endocrinol 57:487–500, 2002.

65. Marsden HB, Birch IM, Swindell R: Germ cell tumours of childhood: A review of 137 cases. J Clin Pathol 34:879–883, 1981.

66. Furukawa F, Haebara H, Hamashima Y: Primary intracranial choriocarcinoma arising from the pituitary fossa: Report of an autopsy case with literature review. Acta Pathol 36:773–781, 1986.

67. Poon W, Ng HK, Wong K, South JR: Primary intrasellar germinoma presenting with cavernous sinus syndrome. Surg Neurol 30:402–405, 1988.

68. Mootha SL, Barkovich AJ, Grumbach MM: Idiopathic hypothalamic diabetes insipidus, pituitary stalk thickening, and the occult intracranial germinoma in children and adolescents. J Clin Endocrinol Metab 82:1362–1367, 1997.

69. Komninos J, Vlassopoulou V, Protopapa D, et al: Tumors metastatic to the pituitary gland: Case report and literature review. J Clin Endocrinol Metab 89:574–580, 2004.

70. Giustina A, Gola M, Doga M, Rosei EG: Clinical Review 136: Primary lymphoma of the pituitary: An emerging clinical entity. J Clin Endocrinol Metab 86:4567–4575, 2001.

71. Honeggar J, Fahlbusch R, Bonnerman A, et al: Lymphocytic and granulomatous hypophysitis: Experience with nine cases. Neurosurgery 40:713, 1997.

72. Ahmadi J, Meyers GS, Segall HD, et al: Lymphocytic adenohypophysitis: Contrast-enhanced MR imaging in five cases. Radiology 195:30, 1995.

73. Cheung CC, Ezzat S, Smyth HS, Asa SL: The spectrum and significance of primary hypophysitis. J Clin Endocrinol Metab 86:1048–1053, 2001.

74. Lanzieri CF, Shah M, Krauss D, et al: Use of gadolinium-enhanced MR imaging for differentiating mucoceles from neoplasms in the paranasal sinuses. Radiology 178:425, 1991.

75. Sharma MC, Arora R, Mahapatra AK: Intrasellar tuberculoma: An enigmatic pituitary infection: A series of 18 cases. Clin Neurol Neurosurg 102:72–77, 2000.

76. Ashkan K, Papadopoulos MC, Casey AT, et al: Sellar tuberculoma: Report of two cases. Acta Neurochir 139:523, 1997.

77. Taylor SL, Barakos JA, Harsh GR, et al: Magnetic resonance imaging of tuberculum sellae meningiomas: Preventing preoperative misdiagnosis as

pituitary macroadenoma. Neurosurgery 31:621, 1992.

78. Cannavo S, Romano C, Buffa R, Faglia G: Granulomatous sarcoidotic lesion of hypothalamic-pituitary region associated with Rathke's cleft cyst. J Endocrinol Invest 20:77–81, 1997.

79. Jain KC, Varma A, Mahapatra AK: Pituitary abscess: A series of six cases. Br J Neurosurg Psychiatry 41:972, 1978.

80. Greenman Y, Melmed S: Diagnosis and management of nonfunctioning pituitary tumors. Annu Rev Med 47:95–106, 1996.

81. Shimon I, Melmed S: Management of pituitary tumors. Ann Intern Med 129:472–483, 1998.

82. Ciric I, Ragin A, Baumgartner C, Pierce D: Complications of transsphenoidal surgery: Results of a national survey, review of the literature, and personal experience. Neurosurgery 40:225–237, 1997.

83. Jho HD, Carrau RL: Endoscopic endonasal transsphenoidal surgery: Experience with 50 patients. J Neurosurg 87:44–51, 1997.

84. Post KD, McCormick PC, Kandji AD, Hays AP: Metastatic carcinoma to pituitary adenoma: Report of two cases. Surg Neurol 30:286–292, 1988.

85. Palladino AR, Andrioli GC: Pituitary metastases as presenting lesions of malignancy. J Neurosurg Sci 36:51–54, 1992.

86. Max MB, Deck MDF, Rottenberg DA: Pituitary metastasis: Incidence in cancer patients and clinical differentiation from pituitary adenoma. Neurology 31:998–1002, 1981.

87. Juneau P, Schoene WC, Black P: Malignant tumors in the pituitary gland. Arch Neurol 49:555–558, 1992.

Hypopituitarism

Andreas Jöstel, Catherine Ann Lissett, and Stephen Michael Shalet

INTRODUCTION

Hypopituitarism is the deficiency of one or more pituitary hormones. It is relatively rare, with a prevalence of 45 per million and an annual incidence of about 4 per 100,000.[1] It is, however, seen commonly in endocrine practice and, importantly, is associated with increased morbidity and mortality. Clinical manifestations are influenced by the etiology, severity, and rate of onset of pituitary hormone deficiency.

MORTALITY IN HYPOPITUITARISM

Hypopituitarism is associated with excess mortality compared with that of the normal population. Six major epidemiologic studies of mortality rates in patients with hypopituitarism were published between 1990 and 2001.[2–7] These studies had certain features in common. Patients with acromegaly and Cushing's disease were excluded because of their known excess mortality. The median age of the patients was between 46 and 52 years, and 51% to 62% of patients were men. The duration of follow-up was between 10 and 13 years. Major differences between the studies were the relative frequencies of pituitary adenomas, the use of radiotherapy, and the degree of documented hypopituitarism.

In all studies, an excess mortality was recorded with standardized mortality rates (SMRs) of 1.2 to 2.2. Most of the increase in mortality was attributed to a higher incidence of cardiovascular and cerebrovascular disease; risk ratios for malignancies and respiratory disease varied. Common independent factors carrying a worse prognosis included craniopharyngioma as the primary pathology (SMR, 5 to 9) and female gender.

The exact contribution of hormonal deficiencies or suboptimal hormone replacement or both to the excess mortality is unresolved. Many believe that growth hormone (GH) defi-

ciency plays an important role: It is the hormone deficiency with the highest prevalence in pituitary hypofunction, and the negative effects on the cardiovascular risk profile in patients with untreated GH deficiency have been well documented (alterations in lipid fractions, blood vessel wall composition, nitric oxide availability, and inflammatory mediators). As a very high prevalence of GH deficiency is found in hypopituitary patients, documenting its contribution as an independent mortality risk factor is inherently difficult. Long-term controlled studies of GH replacement therapy could potentially provide such information, but so far, these studies have not been performed. Equally, other hormone deficiencies or their replacement had no consistent effect on mortality (i.e., untreated male gonadotropin deficiency was associated with reduced mortality in one study,[3] but with excess mortality in another[7]).

CAUSES

The causes of hypopituitarism are varied (Table 22-1). In adulthood, however, the most common cause is a pituitary adenoma or treatment with pituitary surgery or radiotherapy.

PITUITARY AND HYPOTHALAMIC MASS LESIONS

Pituitary adenomas account for the vast majority of pituitary mass lesions, although secondary tumors do occur, with metastases to the pituitary gland reported from carcinomas of the breast, lung, colon, and prostate. Pituitary microadenomas are surprisingly common, being found in between 1.5% and 27% of patients at autopsy[8]; these tumors are very rarely, if at all, associated with hypopituitarism and tend to run a benign course. Macroadenomas are less common but are more frequently associated with pituitary hormone deficiencies; some 30% of patients with pituitary macroadenomas

Table 22-1   Causes of Hypopituitarism

Neoplastic: Tumors involving the hypothalamic-pituitary (HP) axis
    Pituitary adenoma
    Craniopharyngioma
    Glioma (hypothalamus, third ventricle, optic nerve)
Surgery: for HP axis tumors
Radiotherapy
    HP axis tumors
    Brain tumors
    Head and neck cancer
    Acute lymphoblastic leukemia
Autoimmune
    Lymphocytic hypophysitis
Vascular
    Sheehan's syndrome
    Pituitary apoplexy
    Intrasellar carotid artery aneurysm
    Subarachnoid hemorrhage
Granulomatous diseases
    Sarcoidosis
    Tuberculosis
    Histiocytosis X
    Wegener's granulomatosis
Genetic (see Table 22-2)
    Combined pituitary hormone deficiencies
    Isolated pituitary hormone deficiencies
Developmental
    Midline cerebral and cranial malformations
Traumatic
    Head injury
    Perinatal trauma
Infection
    Encephalitis
    Pituitary abscess
Iron-overload states
    Hemochromatosis
    Hemosiderosis (thalassemia)
Idiopathic

have one or more anterior pituitary hormone deficiencies. Evidence suggests that the causative mechanism of hypopituitarism in these patients is compression of the portal vessels in the pituitary stalk, either secondary to the expanding tumor mass directly or to increased intrasellar pressure,[9] which explains the potential reversibility of pituitary dysfunction after surgery in some patients.

Craniopharyngiomas are the third most common intracranial tumor and account for the majority of parapituitary tumors. They are thought to arise from Rathke's pouch and may be cystic or solid, commonly showing calcification. Fifty percent occur in children younger than 15 years. Patients commonly are first seen with GH deficiency and diabetes insipidus, with or without a visual field defect.

Derangement of central endocrine regulation also occurs with other parapituitary space-occupying lesions such as chondromas, chordomas, suprasellar meningiomas, astrocytomas of the optic nerve, and primary tumors of the third ventricle.

PITUITARY SURGERY

Hypopituitarism is a common consequence of pituitary surgery. The incidence and degree of hypopituitarism depend on a number of factors, including the size of the original tumor, the degree of infiltration, and the experience of the surgeon. The patient should be warned of a possible deterioration of postoperative pituitary function, and assessment of pituitary function should be performed promptly after surgery. However, a postoperative decline in pituitary function is not universal. Surgery for pituitary adenomas may be associated with a significant recovery of pituitary function. About half of the patients recover at least one pituitary insufficiency after transsphenoidal

surgery. Postoperative improvement is more likely if no tumor is found on postoperative imaging and no neurosurgic or pathologic evidence that the tumor is of an invasive nature.[10] The most likely pituitary hormone to recover is thyroid-stimulating hormone (TSH), followed in order by adrenocorticotropic hormone (ACTH), gonadotropins, and GH.[11] Evidence exists that in those patients in whom recovery of pituitary function occurs, the process begins immediately after surgery.[12]

RADIOTHERAPY

Deficiency of one or more anterior pituitary hormones may follow treatment with external radiation when the hypothalamic-pituitary axis lies within the fields of radiation. Hypopituitarism has been described in patients who received radiation therapy for nasopharyngeal carcinomas, tumors of the pituitary gland or nearby structures, and primary brain tumors, as well as in children who underwent prophylactic cranial irradiation for acute lymphoblastic leukemia or total body irradiation (TBI) for a variety of tumors and other diseases.[13]

The radiobiologic impact of an irradiation schedule is dependent on the total dose, the number of fractions, and the duration. The same total dose given in fewer fractions over a shorter time is likely to cause a greater incidence of pituitary hormone deficiency than if the schedule is spread over a longer interval with a greater number of fractions. Equally, higher radiation doses tend to cause more severe pituitary hypofunction. Thus, after lower radiation doses, isolated GH deficiency ensues, whereas higher doses may produce panhypopituitarism (Fig. 22-1). Radiation dose also determines the speed of onset of hormonal deficiency. The greater the dose, the earlier GH deficiency will occur after treatment, so that between 2 and 5 years after irradiation, 100% of children receiving more than 30 Gy (over a 3-week period) to the hypothalamic-pituitary axis showed subnormal GH responses to an insulin tolerance test (ITT), whereas 35% of those receiving less than 30 Gy (over a 3-week period) still showed a

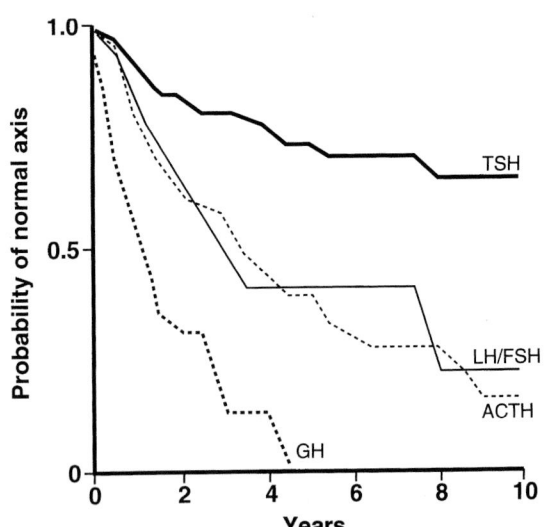

Figure 22-1   Life-table analysis indicating probabilities of initially normal hypothalamic-pituitary-target gland axes remaining normal after radiotherapy (3750 to 4250 cGy). Growth hormone (GH) secretion is the most sensitive of the anterior pituitary hormones to the effects of external radiotherapy, and thyroid-stimulating hormone (TSH) secretion is the most resistant. In two thirds of patients, gonadotropin deficiency develops before adrenocorticotropic hormone (ACTH) deficiency. LH, luteinizing hormone; FSH, follicle-stimulating hormone. (From Littley MD, Shalet SM, Beardwell CG, et al: Hypopituitarism following external radiotherapy for pituitary tumors in adults. Q J Med 70:145–160, 1989, with permission.)

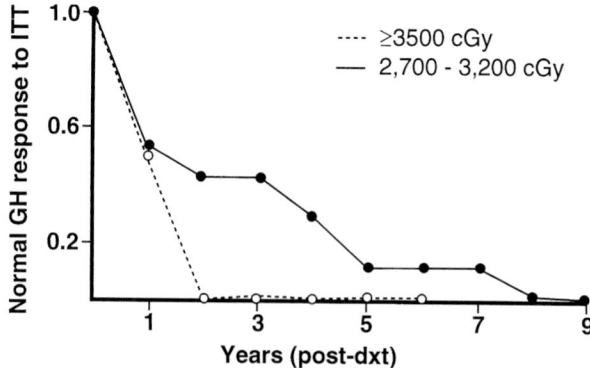

Figure 22-2   The incidence of growth hormone (GH) deficiency in children receiving 27 to 32 Gy or ≥35 Gy of cranial irradiation for a brain tumor in relation to time from irradiation (dxt). This illustrates that the speed at which individual pituitary hormone deficits develop is dose dependent; the higher the radiation dose, the earlier GH deficiency occurs. (Courtesy of the Department of Medical Illustrations, Withington Hospital, Manchester, England.)

normal GH response[14] (Fig. 22-2). Interpretation of the impact of radiation-induced damage to the hypothalamic-pituitary axis on GH status is, however, complicated in the early years after irradiation, when discordant results may be seen to different GH-provocative agents.[15]

Paradoxically, whereas high doses of cranial irradiation may render a child gonadotropin-deficient, lesser doses of irradiation may be associated with early puberty. The mechanism for early puberty after irradiation is likely to be related to disinhibition of cortical influences on the hypothalamus.

With increased survival, follow-up evaluation of patients irradiated for tumors of the brain and surrounding structures must focus less on the possibility of tumor recurrence and more on the delayed effects of therapy, including the endocrine effects.

GENETIC CAUSES

Our knowledge of genetic causes responsible for hypopituitarism has grown rapidly over recent years and has elucidated the pathophysiology of previously described "idiopathic" pituitary hormone deficiencies (Table 22-2). Gene mutations can (1) interfere with the development of different pituitary cell lineages (e.g., pituitary transcription factor defects), (2) cause alterations in hypothalamic releasing factors or their pituitary receptors (e.g., Kallmann syndrome), or (3) impair the production of pituitary hormones (e.g., isolated GH deficiency).

Table 22-2	Genetic Causes of Hypopituitarism	
	Gene Defect	**Hormone Deficiencies**
Combined	*Pit-1 (POU1F1, GHF1)*	GH, TSH, PRL
	PROP-1	GH, LH/FSH, TSH, ACTH, PRL
	HESX1 (Rpx)	GH, LH/FSH, TSH, ACTH, ADH
	LHX3/LHX4	GH, LH/FSH, TSH, PRL
	PITX2	GH, PRL
Isolated	*hGH*	GH
	GHRH receptor gene	GH
	KAL	FSH/LH
	GnRH receptor gene	FSH/LH
	DAX1/AHC	FSH/LH
	TBX19 (Tpit)	ACTH
	TSH-β gene	TSH
	TRH receptor gene	TSH

COMBINED PITUITARY HORMONE DEFICITS DUE TO TRANSCRIPTION FACTOR DEFECTS

A cascade of pituitary transcription factors regulates the differentiation of cells of Rathke's pouch into somatotrophs, lactotrophs, thyrotrophs, gonadotrophs, and corticotrophs. Mutations in early-appearing transcription factors tend to cause more extensive hormone deficiencies (e.g., multiple pituitary hormone deficiencies in mutations of *HESX1*, *PROP1*, *Pit-1*, and *LHX3/4*), whereas others can cause isolated deficiencies (e.g., ACTH deficiency due to *TBX19* mutations, GH deficiency in Rieger syndrome due to *PITX2* mutations).[16]

Pit-1

Pit-1 (pituitary-specific transcription factor-1), also termed GH factor-1 (*GHF-1*) or *POU1F1*, is a pituitary-specific transcription factor responsible for pituitary development and hormone expression in mammals. *Pit-1* contains two protein domains, termed *POU-specific* and *POU-homeo*, which are both necessary for high-affinity DNA binding of the GH and prolactin genes. *Pit-1* also is important for hormonal regulation of the prolactin and thyrotropin beta-subunit genes by thyrotropin-releasing hormone (TRH) and cyclic adenosine monophosphate (cAMP). Mutations of the *Pit-1* gene have been found in dwarf mice strains (Snell mouse) displaying hypoplasia of GH-, prolactin-, and TSH-secreting cells of the anterior pituitary, demonstrating the importance of *Pit-1* for the development of certain anterior pituitary cells. Humans with *Pit-1* deficiency resemble Snell mice in that they lack GH and prolactin, have variable degrees of TSH deficiency, and often exhibit pituitary hypoplasia. At a clinical level, *Pit-1* abnormalities account for only a small minority of the total number of worldwide cases of hypopituitarism. *Pit-1* gene mutations also have been discovered in patients with idiopathic GH deficiency associated with preserved basal prolactin and TSH secretion. This illustrates the variability of phenotypic presentation among these patients.

PROP1

A further, more recent discovery is a novel pituitary paired-like homeodomain factor, which seems to be an important prerequisite of the expression of *Pit-1*. This has been named *PROP1* (*Prophet of Pit-1*). Several multicenter studies of patients with otherwise unexplained multiple pituitary hormone deficiencies found underlying *PROP1* mutations in 40% to 50% of such patients. In individuals with a mutation of the *PROP1* gene, which causes reduced DNA-binding and transcriptional activation activity, progressive hypopituitarism develops, with GH, TSH, and gonadotropin deficiency typically present by the end of the second decade.[17] They also may have pituitary hyperplasia followed by degeneration and late appearance of partial ACTH deficiency.

HESX1

HESX1 ("homeobox gene expression in embryonic stem cells"), also called *Rpx* ("Rathke's pouch homeobox"), is a member of the pairedlike class of homeobox genes and is first expressed during mouse embryogenesis in a small patch of cells in the anterior midline visceral ectoderm, which are destined to give rise to the ventral prosencephalon. Mice lacking *HESX1* have variable anterior central nervous system (CNS) defects and pituitary dysplasia. A comparable and equally variable phenotype in humans is septo-optic dysplasia (SOD), which is associated with hypopituitarism, the latter possibly related to the interaction between *HESX1* and *PROP1*. Several human *HESX1* missense mutations have been described with phenotypes variably dominated by severe SOD, or relatively mild combined pituitary hormone deficiency, or isolated GH deficiency. Both homozygous and sporadic heterozygous mutations have been identified, the latter typically associated with milder phenotypes.[18]

LHX3/LHX4

LHX3 and *LHX4* belong to the Lhx ("LIM homeodomain transcription factor") family of transcription factors. *LHX3* is expressed in the pituitary, can bind to *Pit-1*, and can enhance *Pit-1* activity. It also contributes to the development of the alpha-subunit of the glycoprotein hormones. Netchine and coworkers[19] identified homozygous *LHX3* defects leading to panhypopituitarism (with the exception of ACTH deficiency) and rigidity of the cervical spine. *LHX4* has recently been implicated in familial hypopituitarism. An *LHX4* germline splice-site mutation has been found in one family with multiple pituitary deficits, short stature, and abnormalities of the pituitary gland, cerebellum, and skull base.[20]

PITX2

PITX2 is another pituitary homeodomain transcription factor, defects of which are seen in Rieger syndrome because of mutations in the *RIEG* gene. Some of those patients have been found to have GH deficiency and possibly impaired prolactin secretion.

ISOLATED GROWTH HORMONE DEFICIENCY

Two types of genetic defects that cause isolated GH deficiency have been identified.[21] These are mutations of the *GH* gene and of the GH-releasing hormone (GHRH) receptor gene. The human GH (*hGH*) gene is located on chromosome 17 in a cluster of five genes: *hGH-N* encodes the gene for pituitary GH, *hGH-V* encodes the gene for placental GH, and three genes encode for human chorionic somatotropin (hCS). Children with gene mutations or deletions of *hGH-N* have severe short stature and, in boys, microgenitalia. They have the characteristic phenotypic features of GH deficiency. Four types of mendelian disorders of the *GH* gene have been described: IGHD IA and IB are both inherited in an autosomal-recessive manner, resulting in absent or low GH levels. In patients with absent GH (IGHD IA), anti-GH antibodies often develop when they are treated with GH. IGHD II has an autosomal-dominant mode of inheritance with variable clinical severity. IGHD III is an X-linked disorder often associated with hypogammaglobulinemia.

Mutations of the gene encoding the GHRH receptor can result in a severely truncated receptor lacking the seven membrane-spanning domains. Such mutations have been identified in a number of kindreds with severe GH deficiency ("dwarfism of Sindh").[22] The GHRH receptor itself belongs to the family of G protein–coupled receptors. Heterozygous inactivating mutations in the Gs alpha gene, which are present in pseudohypoparathyroidism type Ia, can cause GHRH resistance (in addition to the well-documented hormone resistance to parathyroid hormone [PTH], TSH, gonadotropins, and glucagon), thereby causing GH deficiency.[23]

ISOLATED GONADOTROPIN DEFICIENCY

To date, several gene mutations have been identified as causes of idiopathic hypogonadotropic hypogonadism (IHH) in humans,[24] although the genetic basis of the condition is still unknown in the majority of patients. Inheritance is usually autosomal recessive, except for X-linked *KAL* and *DAX1* mutations.

Kallmann syndrome is the combination of IHH and anosmia or hyposmia, usually caused by defective GnRH secretion. Although the hypogonadotropic state can be explained by a failure of migration of GnRH neurons from their origin in the olfactory placode to the hypothalamus, anosmia is often, but not invariably, associated with agenesis of the olfactory bulbs. An X-linked form of Kallmann syndrome is caused by mutations in the *KAL* gene and is frequently associated with additional clinical features such as upper-limb mirror movements (bimanual synkinesia) and renal agenesis.

Mutations of the GnRH receptor gene can result in GnRH resistance at pituitary level, thereby causing gonadotropin deficiency. The *DAX1*-orphan nuclear receptor is expressed at multiple levels throughout the reproductive axis, and mutations in the *DAX-1/AHC* gene underlie the combined phenotype of adrenocortical failure and gonadotropin deficiency.

Other genes implicated in IHH are *PC1* (prohormone convertase, associated with defects in prohormone processing), *OB*, and *DB* (leptin and leptin receptor, associated with obesity), whereas inactivating mutations of luteinizing hormone *(LH)-beta* and follicle-stimulating hormone *(FSH)-beta* genes can cause isolated deficiencies of LH and FSH, respectively.

ISOLATED ACTH AND TSH DEFICIENCIES

Isolated deficiencies of TSH or ACTH are very rare; however, in a number of cases, a genetic abnormality has been described or proposed. Mutations of the coding region of the TSH-beta subunit gene[25] and TRH-receptor gene[26] have been found in a number of families as a cause of hereditary isolated TSH deficiency.

Recently, a pituitary transcription factor causing isolated ACTH deficiency was identified. *TBX19* (the human T-box pituitary transcription factor, analogous to *Tpit* in the mouse), has an essential role in differentiation of proopiomelanocortin (POMC) cells in the pituitary. At least two *TBX19* gene mutations causing isolated ACTH deficiency have been described.[27]

OTHER CAUSES

Posttraumatic

Pituitary dysfunction after severe head injuries tends to become apparent within 1 year after the trauma for the majority of patients, although in a significant proportion, it can remain undetected. A systematic evaluation of patients recovering from severe traumatic brain injuries revealed completely intact pituitary function in only 31 percent.[28] Another review[29] identified certain characteristics in patients in whom posttraumatic hypopituitarism develops: The majority had been unconscious for at least several days, and about half had associated skull fractures, whereas diabetes insipidus was present in only a third. The predominant autopsy findings in traumatic hypopituitarism are hypothalamic hemorrhage, anterior pituitary infarction, and posterior pituitary hemorrhage (each accounting for about 25% of the cases), whereas pituitary stalk lesions are seen in only a small minority. The reported predominance of hypogonadism in the majority of patients has not been uniformly confirmed.

Lymphocytic Hypophysitis

Lymphocytic hypophysitis, an immune-mediated diffuse infiltration of the anterior pituitary with lymphocytes and plasma cells, occurs predominantly in women and is often first evident in pregnancy or after delivery. The classic presentation is peripartum hypopituitarism, often with a pituitary mass and visual failure. ACTH deficiency is an almost universal feature that, when undiagnosed, has proved fatal. At an early stage, the pituitary gland is enlarged and cannot be distinguished from a pituitary tumor by computed tomography (CT) or magnetic resonance imaging (MRI), whereas in the later stages, the gland may atrophy, leaving an empty sella. Lymphocytic hypophysitis is more common in patients with other autoimmune endocrine diseases. Cytosolic autoantigens against the pituitary can be demonstrated in some cases but also are present in normal patients, and thus the definitive diagnosis of this condition remains difficult without pituitary biopsy. Spontaneous resolution of both the mass and the hypopituitarism has been reported, and, in some cases, neurosurgical intervention has led to irreversible pituitary failure. Therefore, conservative management is appropriate in the majority of patients.

Pituitary Apoplexy

Pituitary apoplexy is the abrupt destruction of pituitary tissue resulting from infarction or hemorrhage into the pituitary, usually into an underlying pituitary tumor. Severe headache accompanies a variable degree of visual loss or cranial nerve palsies. The consequent pituitary hormone deficiencies may develop rapidly. In Sheehan's syndrome, pituitary infarction occurs secondary to severe postpartum hemorrhage and ensuing circulatory failure. Once common, this complication is now confined mainly to areas where obstetric services are less well developed.

Granulomatous Diseases

Granulomatous diseases, including sarcoidosis, tuberculosis, and Langerhans' cell histiocytosis, can affect the hypothalamic-pituitary axis and cause hypopituitarism, including diabetes insipidus. Diabetes insipidus complicates sarcoidosis rarely (1%). It is more common, however, in Langerhans' cell histiocytosis, with diabetes insipidus developing in 15% of childhood cases, but it also may occur in patients first seen in adulthood.

Iron-overload States

Iron-overload states, that is, hemochromatosis and β-thalassemia treated with frequent blood transfusions, are associated with pituitary hyposecretion secondary to siderosis and a reduction of pituitary cell number. The gonadotrophs are particularly vulnerable to this mode of damage; however, as affected patients live longer owing to improved medical care, other pituitary hormone deficits, including deficits of GH and ACTH, are seen more frequently.

Hyperparathyroidism

Primary hyperparathyroidism due to a solitary adenoma can be associated with significantly impaired basal and stimulated GH secretion.[30] The pathogenetic mechanism is still speculative, but normality is restored after surgical removal of the adenoma.

CLINICAL FEATURES

The clinical features of hypopituitarism are affected principally by the degree, type, and speed of onset of the pituitary hormone deficiency. Local pressure effects or hormonal hypersecretion, however, can complicate the clinical picture.

In many forms of hypopituitarism, for example, secondary to a pituitary adenoma and after irradiation, a characteristic evolution of pituitary failure is apparent. Secretion of GH fails first, followed by LH, FSH, and finally by failure of ACTH and TSH secretion. Prolactin deficiency is rare except as a component of Sheehan's syndrome. Hyperprolactinemia is much more common, secondary to either interference with the secretion or delivery of dopamine to the pituitary, releasing the normal lactotrophs from tonic inhibition, or because of hypersecretion from a prolactinoma. Diabetes insipidus is not generally a feature of pituitary disease, and the presence of diabetes insipidus usually denotes a hypothalamic or stalk disorder, except when occurring after hypothalamic or pituitary surgery. The symptoms and signs of individual hormone deficiencies are listed in Table 22-3.

GROWTH HORMONE DEFICIENCY

GH secretion is a continuous variable, and a spectrum therefore exists from severe GH deficiency to mild GH insufficiency. Typically, the GH-deficient child has increased subcutaneous fat, especially around the trunk. The face is immature, with a prominent forehead and depressed midfacial development; this is related to the lack of GH effect on endochondral growth at the base of the skull, occiput, and

Table 22-3	Symptoms and Signs of Hormone Deficiencies
Hormone Deficiency	**Symptoms and Signs**
Growth hormone	Short stature in children, abnormal body composition, increased fracture rate, reduced well-being and performance
Gonadotropins	In men: poor libido/impotence, infertility, small soft testes, reduced facial/body hair
	In women: amenorrhea/oligomenorrhea dyspareunia, infertility, breast atrophy
Thyroid-stimulating hormone	Growth retardation in children, decrease in energy, constipation, sensitivity to cold, dry skin, weight gain
Adrenocorticotropic hormone	Weakness, tiredness, dizziness on standing, pallor, hypoglycemia
Prolactin	Failure of lactation
Antidiuretic hormone	Polyuria, polydipsia, nocturia, hypotension

the sphenoid bone. Dentition is delayed. In boys, the phallus may be small, and the average age of pubertal onset is delayed in both boys and girls (Fig. 22-3).

GH continues to have significant functions in adult life. Severe GH deficiency in adults is associated with impaired quality of life and adverse changes in body composition, bone mineral density (BMD), lipid profile, insulin sensitivity, endothelial integrity, cardiac function, and exercise capacity.[31] Adults with GH deficiency have a higher proportion of body fat than matched controls and a high waist-to-hip ratio, reflecting the predominantly central distribution of fat. On average, BMD in adults, particularly young adults, with GH deficiency is about 1 to 2 SD below the age-matched normal mean.[32] Correspondingly, a questionnaire-based study has estimated that the fracture rate in GH-deficient patients is increased twofold compared with that of an age-matched

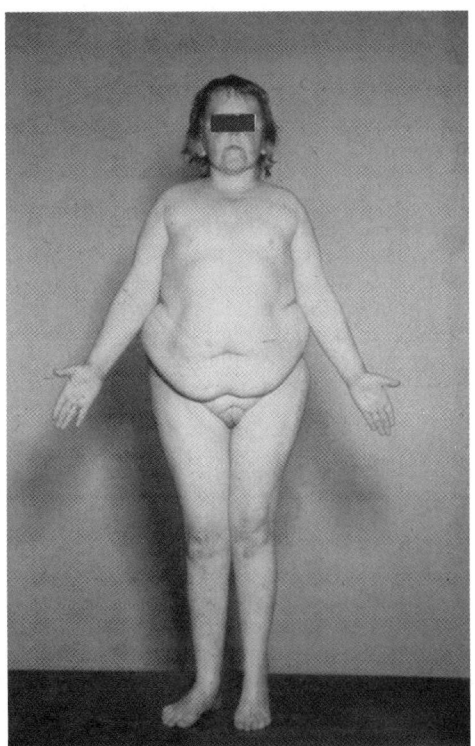

Figure 22-3 A 27-year-old man with combined congenital growth hormone (GH) and gonadotropin deficiency, first seen in adult life with extremely short stature (3 ft 9 in.), obesity with particular excess of truncal fat, immature face with depressed midfacial development, and microgenitalia.

group.[33] Studies in adults with varying degrees of hypopituitarism indicate that GH deficiency per se, rather than associated gonadotropin deficiency or overtreatment with glucocorticoid or thyroxine replacement, is responsible for the osteopenia. GH-deficient adults report more perceived health problems and a lower quality of life than controls. The conclusions from studies of the lipid profiles in GH-deficient adult patients are not in complete agreement. Nonetheless, a significant number of authors have reported a modest increase in total plasma cholesterol and an increase in the ratio of low-density (LDL) to high-density lipoprotein (HDL). In contrast to the pediatric experience, adults with hypopituitarism show elevated fasting and postprandial plasma insulin levels in comparison with controls, and data from euglycemic-hyperinsulinemic clamp studies confirm that these patients are insulin resistant.[34]

These adverse changes in the overall vascular risk profile underlie the suggestion that GH deficiency is responsible for the increased cardiovascular mortality in hypopituitarism.

GONADOTROPIN DEFICIENCY

Gonadotropin deficiency may result from deficient secretion of pituitary gonadotropins, faulty secretion of GnRH, and hyperprolactinemia, which impairs the pulsatile release of GnRH and thus causes secondary hypogonadism. Gonadotropin secretion also can be reduced in some functional disorders, most commonly in women, for example, with excessive weight loss or exercise. The clinical features of secondary or hypogonadotropic hypogonadism are similar to those of primary gonadal failure.

In male patients, the clinical features of gonadotropin deficiency differ according to whether the deficiency was acquired before or after pubertal age. If acquired before pubertal age, clinical examination reveals a small penis, small testes, and eunuchoid proportions (span exceeds height by >5 cm; Fig. 22-4). Hypogonadism acquired postpubertally is associated with a reduction in testicular size, loss of facial and body hair, and thinning of the skin, leading to the characteristic finely wrinkled facial skin of the "aging youth." Other effects include a decrease in skeletal muscle mass, BMD, sexual function, libido, and general well-being. Azoospermia is an almost inevitable consequence of hypogonadotropic hypogonadism, but exceptions exist. In the "fertile eunuch" variant, partial LH deficiency may result in low circulating testosterone levels and gynecomastia but preserved testicular size and fertility; presumably, intratesticular testosterone levels remain high enough to maintain spermatogenesis.

In a teenage girl, hypogonadotropic hypogonadism is associated with primary amenorrhea and absent breast development. In the adult woman, amenorrhea or oligomenorrhea, infertility, breast atrophy, vaginal dryness, and dyspareunia occur; pubic and axillary hair remain unless ACTH deficiency also is present.

ADRENOCORTICOTROPIC HORMONE DEFICIENCY

ACTH deficiency is the most life-threatening component of hypopituitarism. In addition to the other causes of pituitary failure discussed earlier, functional ACTH deficiency may occur after discontinuation of exogenous glucocorticoids or ACTH, even when these agents have been administered for only a few weeks. Isolated acquired ACTH deficiency also has been well documented, although its occurrence is rare.[35] The features of glucocorticoid deficiency due to ACTH deficiency are similar to those of Addison's disease. Weakness, tiredness, nausea, vomiting, and orthostatic hypotension are common. Weight loss and anorexia may mimic anorexia nervosa or a malignancy. Examination may reveal pallor of the skin, in contrast to the hyperpigmentation of Addison's disease, and in female patients particularly, loss of secondary sexual hair

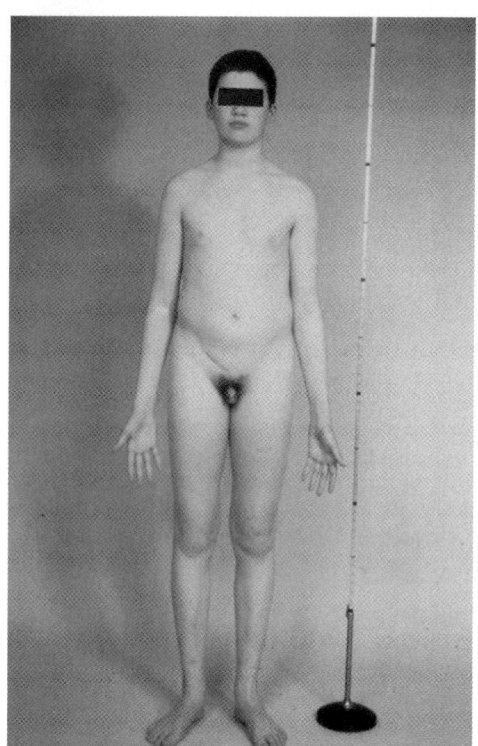

Figure 22-4 An 18-year-old man with Kallmann's syndrome initially seen in adult life. Note tall stature, eunuchoid proportions, lack of body hair, poor virilization, and an orchiopexy scar consistent with severe gonadotropin deficiency of very early onset.

occurs. In severe ACTH deficiency, particularly in childhood, hypoglycemia can occur: Cortisol deficiency results in increased insulin sensitivity and a decrease in hepatic glycogen reserves. Hyponatremia, although less commonly seen than in Addison's disease because of preservation of aldosterone secretion, may be the presenting feature of ACTH deficiency, particularly in the elderly. Acute cortisol insufficiency should be considered in the differential diagnosis of a patient with a history of anorexia and weight loss, increasing fatigue and weakness, and nausea and vomiting. The clinical features may include hypovolemic shock, fever, and an acute abdomen. A history of an acute headache, pituitary surgery, or irradiation may provide important pointers to the diagnosis.

THYROID-STIMULATING HORMONE DEFICIENCY

Thyroid-stimulating hormone (TSH) deficiency occurs late in most pituitary disorders. Symptoms include fatigue, weakness, inability to lose weight, constipation, and cold intolerance, in keeping with the symptoms of primary hypothyroidism. Symptoms are, however, generally milder than in primary hypothyroidism, because some residual TSH secretion is often preserved.

ANTIDIURETIC HORMONE DEFICIENCY

Polydipsia and polyuria with nocturia are the classic features of diabetes insipidus resulting from ADH deficiency. If the patient is unable to keep up with the fluid loss, hypotension and hypovolemia ensue. The features of diabetes insipidus may be masked in the presence of ACTH deficiency, because of the consequent hypovolemia and reduced glomerular filtration rate. Only when cortisol replacement therapy is commenced may the polyuria and polydipsia of diabetes insipidus be revealed.

PROLACTIN DEFICIENCY

Although prolactin deficiency per se is not known to have distinct clinical features, it almost always signifies more severe degrees of hypopituitarism, and GH deficiency is inevitable.[36]

DIAGNOSIS AND ENDOCRINE ASSESSMENT

Clinical examination can provide important clues to the cause and duration of hypopituitarism, and the physician must not neglect an assessment of height, weight, and pubertal status. Examination of the visual fields is essential and should be supported by either Goldmann or computer-assisted perimetry. The latter is more sensitive in detecting visual field defects that other techniques are unable to demonstrate.

IMAGING OF THE PITUITARY FOSSA

Imaging of the pituitary fossa is indicated when clinical evidence of a visual field defect or biochemical evidence of hypopituitarism is noted. CT and MRI have superseded the plain radiograph. MRI is the scanning technique of choice, as it offers higher resolution than CT scanning and is able to demonstrate microadenomas as small as 3 mm in diameter. If a pituitary adenoma is demonstrated, careful note should be taken of any extension of the tumor outside the pituitary fossa. In diabetes insipidus, the normal high-intensity posterior pituitary signal may be absent, and other causes of hypopituitarism may show classic CT or MRI findings (for example, craniopharyngioma).

An empty sella is not an uncommon finding. It refers to an enlarged or normal-sized pituitary fossa filled with cerebrospinal fluid. An empty sella may be caused by a congenital sellar diaphragmatic defect (primary) or may develop after lymphocytic hypophysitis, infarction of a pituitary tumor, Sheehan's syndrome, pituitary surgery, or radiation (secondary). The pituitary gland is usually flattened against the floor of the sella, and the pituitary stalk may be laterally deviated. The majority of patients with primary empty sella have normal pituitary function, but 15% have mild hyperprolactinemia, and it has been described in association with headache, endocrine dysfunction (particularly GH deficiency in children), and visual disturbances. The majority of patients with secondary empty sella have endocrine disturbances[37]; the severity is related to the underlying pathogenesis of the condition.

ENDOCRINE TESTING

The endocrine assessment of a patient with suspected hypopituitarism usually involves measurement of both baseline and stimulated hormone levels. Basal hormone levels yield much useful information, and therefore serum concentrations of prolactin, TSH, T_4, cortisol, LH, FSH, and testosterone in men, and estradiol in women, should be measured. As a general rule, suspected anterior pituitary hormone deficiency should be confirmed and corrected before possible ADH deficiency is investigated, as ACTH deficiency can mask the presence of ADH deficiency. Another important principle is that of retesting. This is important in two broad clinical contexts. The first is in young adults who received GH replacement in childhood. Over the last 10-year period, a number of studies reassessed the status of children who received GH replacement during childhood, after completion of growth and puberty. At reassessment, GH status was considered normal in 20% to 87%[31] of patients, most of whom had originally been classified as having isolated idiopathic GH deficiency. Those young adults with organic GH deficiency in childhood as a consequence of either a mass lesion, pituitary surgery, or irradiation to the hypothalamic-pituitary axis rarely reverted to normal GH secretory status. Hence, the etiology of the childhood diagnosis of GH deficiency should affect the strategy of retesting. Patients with isolated GH deficiency should undergo two tests of GH secretory status, whereas those with additional anterior pituitary hormone deficits require only one test at reassessment. The second cohort in whom retesting is indicated are those patients in whom progression of the hypopituitarism may be expected. This includes patients who were subject to irradiation of the hypothalamic-pituitary axis, patients after surgery, and in patients with an evolving pituitary or hypothalamic lesion. After irradiation, endocrine testing should be performed on a yearly basis for at least 10 years and again at 15 years. This is of particular importance because, although the classic sequence of pituitary hormone deficits (GH, gonadotropins, ACTH, and TSH) occurs in the majority of patients, other patterns may occur, most notably ACTH deficiency before gonadotropin deficiency.[38]

GROWTH HORMONE DEFICIENCY

GH replacement therapy has been offered to GH-deficient children for more than 30 years, but it became a licensed indication for GH-deficient adults in the United States, in a number of European countries, and in New Zealand only in 1996. Thus, in contrast to the long-standing pediatric literature and interest in the biochemical diagnosis of GH deficiency, the concerns of the endocrinologist treating adults have been addressed only recently.

GH secretion forms a spectrum between normality and abnormality, and therefore with rare exceptions, the diagnosis of GH deficiency must be made on arbitrary grounds. The more severe the GH deficiency, the less arbitrary the diagnosis, whereas the "lesser degrees of GH deficiency" merge into normality. Today, in many countries, children with all forms of GH insufficiency from mild to severe are considered for GH replacement, whereas in other countries, only those with severe GH deficiency receive GH replacement. In adulthood, however, only severe GH deficiency has been proved to be associated with any benefit from GH replacement, and thus in adulthood, the purpose of investigation is to diagnose severe GH deficiency.

GH secretion is pulsatile, and serum levels are low during many hours of the day. Therefore, a single basal GH estimation provides little useful information about GH secretory status. Twenty-four-hour GH profiles with 20-minute sampling are time consuming, expensive, and controversy exists as to their scientific and practical value; thus, in reality, a 24-hour GH profile remains a research investigation. Provocative tests are the most popular method of determining GH secretory status.[31]

At present the ITT is the "gold standard" for the biochemical diagnosis of severe GH deficiency. The ITT provokes a pronounced GH response in normal subjects, it allows the pituitary adrenal axis to be tested at the same time, and the morbidity associated with the performance of the test is low in experienced units.[39] For the diagnosis of severe GH deficiency in adults, a diagnostic cutoff of either 3 or 5 ng/mL has been evaluated by pooling the ITT data available from the literature, albeit with the necessary assumptions required when GH values from different centers are considered together. Nonetheless, based on a cutoff of 5 ng/mL, the ITT provides a specificity of 97%, a sensitivity of 100%, a positive predictive value of 99%, and a negative predictive value of 100%.[40] Nevertheless, each laboratory must establish its own diagnostic threshold values because of lack of standardization of GH assays rather than simply accepting the recommended cutoff level of 3 or 5 ng/mL.

A number of other GH provocative tests are available, including the arginine stimulation test and glucagon stimulation test. Each has advantages and disadvantages, either as an alternative to the ITT in patients in whom this test is contraindicated or as an adjunct in patients requiring a second provocative test. Clonidine is, however, unsuitable in adulthood, and the GHRH-pyridostigmine test fails to identify hypothalamic defects. It remains crucial that the results of each provocative test be interpreted in the context of normative values and local assays, as the cutoff used for the ITT is not broadly applicable to all other provocative tests, which may be more or less potent stimuli for GH secretion. The interpretation of stimulation tests should take into account the underlying pathology (e.g., radiation-induced GH deficiency might be evident only by using an ITT, whereas arginine-stimulated peak GH levels appear to be a less-sensitive indicator of GH deficiency under those circumstances).[41]

The pathophysiologic state of obesity is difficult to distinguish from organic GH deficiency in an adult. Substantial evidence indicates that morbid obesity is accompanied by suppression of GH release and that substantial weight loss may restore spontaneous and stimulated GH secretion. Even in clinically nonobese healthy adults, relative adiposity, in the abdominal region in particular, is a major negative determinant of stimulated GH secretion.[42] A study of age- and sex-matched subjects, however, suggested a much more profound reduction in total GH secretion in a group of individuals with organic GH deficiency compared with obese subjects.[43] Nonetheless, in the obese individual with pituitary disease and no other pituitary deficit, a reduced GH response to any of the standard provocative tests may reflect organic GH deficiency or obesity itself, and distinction between the two is now not easy.

GH secretion in healthy elderly adults is reduced compared with that in young adults. GH secretion declines by approximately 14% per decade from young adult life. Normal aging is associated with changes in body composition similar to those seen in patients with GH deficiency. In the clinical setting, this raises the question: Can the GH status of elderly patients with organic pituitary disease be distinguished from that of the normal elderly? Toogood and colleagues[44] established that GH secretion is significantly reduced in the elderly with pituitary disease compared with normal controls of similar age. This work suggested that the arginine stimulation test is a reasonable choice to assess GH status in elderly patients with two or three additional pituitary hormone deficits, particularly in an age group in which an ITT carries an increased theoretical risk of morbidity or mortality.

Serum insulin-like growth factor 1 (IGF-1) levels are stable throughout the day, mainly because of complexing of IGF-1 with IGF-binding proteins. Thus, assessing GH status with a single estimation of the circulating IGF-1 level, which is known to be GH dependent, was an attractive proposition and led to the hope that dynamic GH provocation tests would prove unnecessary. However, IGF-1 levels are affected by a number of other variables, including nutritional status, hepatic function, hypothyroidism, age, and pubertal status. Even in otherwise matched individuals, considerable overlap is found between values in GH-deficient and GH-sufficient individuals, particularly in those patients in whom GH deficiency developed in adulthood or who were rendered GH deficient by irradiation. Thus, an IGF-1 estimation is extremely useful for retesting young adults with a diagnosis of childhood-onset GH deficiency, moderately helpful (positive predictive value, ~30% to 50%) in middle-aged adults (age 25 to 55 years), and rarely helpful in the elderly (older than 60 years).

Within the limitations of the tests, we suggest that it is reasonable to perform only one provocative test of GH release in adult patients with two or three additional pituitary hormone deficiencies, as these patients are almost inevitably severely GH deficient. In the patient with a possible diagnosis of adult-onset isolated GH deficiency or GH deficiency plus one additional pituitary hormone deficit, two provocative tests of GH

release would be appropriate. The same strategy can be applied to reassessing the GH secretory status of young adults who received GH replacement for childhood GH deficiency. However, IGF-1 estimation itself should be considered adequate in those in whom multiple pituitary hormone deficits exist and could serve as one of the two tests of GH status in the much larger cohort of patients with a putative diagnosis of isolated GH deficiency, in whom retesting is required.

GONADOTROPIN DEFICIENCY

Adult gonadotropin deficiency is relatively easy to diagnose: In women of postmenopausal age, gonadotropin levels are clearly low or undetectable, whereas in premenopausal women, amenorrhea (or less commonly, oligomenorrhea), in addition to low estradiol levels and low or normal gonadotropin levels, provides sufficient evidence of the diagnosis. In adult men, a similar picture of low testosterone levels and low or inappropriately normal gonadotropin levels is seen.

A more difficult diagnostic situation lies in the distinction between isolated gonadotropin deficiency and constitutional delay of puberty in boys. Clinically, delayed puberty is defined by failure to develop signs of puberty by age 14 years (2 SD above the mean of chronologic age for the onset of puberty). More than 90% of boys age 14 years or older with delayed puberty have no endocrine abnormality and will go through puberty spontaneously at a later date. No biochemical tests reliably improve this epidemiologic prediction. The key clinical response is to deal with the pubertal needs of the child and return to the diagnosis later. If testicular volumes increase during androgen therapy, the diagnosis of constitutional delay in growth and puberty rather than gonadotropin deficiency is supported further.

ADRENOCORTICOTROPIC HORMONE DEFICIENCY

In normal people, the highest plasma cortisol levels are found between 6:00 A.M. and 8:00 A.M., and the lowest before midnight. Plasma cortisol and ACTH concentrations are elevated during physical and emotional stress, including acute illness, trauma, surgery, infection, and starvation.

If a 9:00 A.M. cortisol level is less than 100 nmol/L, particularly in an unwell patient, cortisol deficiency is highly likely, whereas a baseline level greater than 500 nmol/L indicates normality; many authors suggest that dynamic assessment of the hypothalamic-pituitary-adrenal (HPA) axis is not necessary under these circumstances.[45] Unless the patient is known to have pituitary disease, a paired plasma ACTH level will help distinguish between primary and secondary glucocorticoid deficiency: In primary cortisol deficiency (Addison's disease), the ACTH level will be high, whereas in secondary glucocorticoid deficiency, the ACTH level will be low or inappropriately normal.

If cortisol deficiency is suspected in an unwell patient, baseline cortisol and ACTH samples should be taken, and replacement therapy should be commenced immediately. Provocative testing can be performed at a later date.

The ITT is the gold standard for the assessment of the HPA axis and pituitary GH reserve. Neuroglycopenia occurs when the blood glucose is less than 2.2 mmol/L, resulting in the release of ACTH, cortisol, and GH. A serum cortisol response of more than 500 to 550 nmol/L is considered to indicate normality. The ITT is not without risk, however, and loss of consciousness and seizures are recognized, albeit rare, complications. Thus, it is contraindicated in those with known ischemic heart disease or a history of seizures; extreme age is a relative contraindication. When performed in an experienced endocrine unit, the ITT is associated with a low risk of complications.[39]

Other provocative tests useful for assessment of the HPA axis include the short Synacthen test and the intramuscular glucagon stimulation test. Each test has advantages and disadvantages, with some groups favoring the ITT, and others, the short Synacthen test. Of principal importance, however, is that the peak cortisol level achieved must be interpreted in light of the provocative test used. A typical cortisol cutoff level for the standard short Synacthen test is 550 nmol/L at 30 minutes. However, different cutoffs have been applied by various authors (460 to 600 nmol/L), depending on whether greater emphasis is placed on achieving a higher sensitivity or specificity and on the type of cortisol assay.[46-50] When glucagon is used as the provocative agent, the peak cortisol response occurs later (the test should be continued for 180 minutes), and it is smaller in magnitude than that seen in response to an ITT, and in a number (≤20%) of normal persons, a response is not seen.

As a consequence, although some patients can be classified as having "barn door" ACTH deficiency requiring glucocorticoid replacement therapy (i.e., cortisol response of <450 nmol/L to an ITT), a proportion belong in a gray zone where the results of testing must be interpreted in the light of clinical features (for example, patients with a cortisol response of between 450 and 500 nmol/L to an ITT may be advised to take glucocorticoid replacement only during an intercurrent illness or surgery). Last, tests of the HPA axis are not infallible, and consideration should be given to repeating a test if the results are at odds with the clinical picture.

THYROID-STIMULATING HORMONE DEFICIENCY

In secondary hypothyroidism, one might expect to find reduced concentrations of free or total T_4 in association with a serum TSH concentration below the normal range, analogous to the biochemical findings in secondary hypogonadism. This picture, however, is found only in a minority of patients, the majority having normal or occasionally elevated TSH levels. The mechanism behind this apparent contradiction is poorly understood, and a number of different explanations have been explored. One such is that in some cases of hypothalamic hypothyroidism, TSH may have reduced bioactivity,[51] suggesting that TRH regulates not only the secretion of TSH but also its specific molecular and conformational features.

The TSH response to TRH (TRH test) has been proposed as a tool to help differentiate between hypothalamic and pituitary hypothyroidism. Classically, in hypothyroidism secondary to a hypothalamic lesion and hence TRH deficiency, the TSH response is delayed (the 60-minute response is greater than the 20-minute response), whereas in hypothyroidism of pituitary origin, damage to the thyrotrophs results in an absent or impaired TSH response. Studies have revealed no clear-cut differences in biologic end points, however, between patients with hypothyroidism of pituitary and hypothalamic origin. Furthermore, the information gained has no therapeutic implications.

ANTIDIURETIC HORMONE DEFICIENCY

The diagnosis of ADH deficiency first requires confirmation of excess urine output. Polyuria is defined as the excretion of more than 3 L of urine per 24 hours (40 mL/kg/24 hours). Any patient with normal serum sodium and plasma osmolality who has a fluid output of less than 2 L/24 hours is likely to be normal and does not warrant further investigation.

Once excess urine output is confirmed, the usual first-line investigation is an 8-hour fluid-deprivation test. The basis for this test is the increase in plasma osmolality resulting from a lack of fluid intake for several hours, stimulating ADH secretion. The test should be performed under strict observation, because severe fluid and electrolyte depletion can occur. Plasma osmolality, urine volume, and osmolarity are measured hourly for 8 hours, after which a synthetic analogue of ADH (desmopressin) is given intramuscularly (IM). The urine osmolality is then remeasured. In a normal subject, ADH is secreted throughout the test, water is normally absorbed, and a subsequent elevation of urine osmolality occurs. In diabetes insipidus, the urine fails to concentrate (normal subjects achieve a urine osmolality at least twice the plasma osmolality) because of a lack of ADH; hence, plasma osmolality increases. Urine concentrates adequately only after administration of desmopressin. Sometimes in cases with long-standing polyuria, failure of urine concentration in response to desmopressin occurs not because of nephrogenic diabetes insipidus but because of a washout of interstitial solutes, including urea. This may lead to diagnostic difficulties. In cases in which the results of a water-deprivation test are inconclusive, the introduction of specific and sensitive radioimmunoassays for ADH has provided a further diagnostic avenue. A definitive diagnosis of ADH deficiency can be established by infusing hypertonic saline for 2 hours to increase plasma osmolality to more than 300 mOsm/kg, with regular 20- to 30-minute blood sampling to estimate plasma osmolality and ADH.

The ADH level after a period of fluid restriction reflects the two types of diabetes insipidus: In nephrogenic diabetes insipidus, ADH values are above the normal reference range, whereas in cranial diabetes insipidus, values are at the lower end of or below the normal reference range.

TREATMENT OF HYPOPITUITARISM

The treatment of hypopituitarism can be separated into those therapies directed at the underlying disease process and endocrine replacement therapy (Table 22-4). Endocrine replacement therapy should aim to mimic the normal

Table 22-4	Endocrine Replacement Therapy for Hormone Deficiencies
Hormone Deficiency	Replacement Hormones and Typical Daily Dose Range (Oral, if Not Stated Otherwise)
Growth hormone	Growth hormone: Subcutaneous: 0.3–0.7 mg (at night)
Gonadotropins (female)	Estrogen: Estradiol valerate: 1–2 mg, transdermal: 25–100 µg or conjugated equine estrogens: 0.625–1.25 mg PLUS Progesterone (examples): Norethisterone, 0.7–1 mg, transdermal: 170–250 µg or Levonorgestrel, 250 µg, transdermal: 7 µg or Medroxyprogesterone acetate, 5 mg
Gonadotropins (male)	Testosterone: Intramuscular (as testosterone esters): 250 mg every 2–3 wk or Transdermal: 5–7.5 mg or Implant: 600–800 mg every 4–6 mo
Thyroid-stimulating hormone	Thyroxine, 75–200 µg/day
Adrenocorticotropic hormone	Glucocorticoid (preferred schedule): Hydrocortisone, 10 mg morning, 5 mg noon, 5 mg evening, to 10 mg t.i.d.
Prolactin	Nil
Antidiuretic hormone	Desmopressin (DDAVP), 300–600 µg (in divided doses); intranasal, 10–40 µg (in divided doses)

hormonal milieu as far as possible, thus improving symptoms while avoiding overtreatment. It remains to be seen whether present regimens normalize the excess mortality in hypopituitary patients.

GROWTH HORMONE DEFICIENCY

Until 1989, the sole indication for GH therapy was in children with GH deficiency. With the availability of recombinant DNA-derived GH, the situation has gradually changed as the biologic consequences of GH deficiency in adult life have been appreciated.

GH-replacement therapy in adulthood induces favorable changes in body composition, with studies demonstrating a 15.5% reduction in fat mass and a 6% increase in lean body mass after 12 months of therapy. Correspondingly, an improvement is seen in indices of physical performance and maximal oxygen uptake. In response to GH therapy, the initial change in BMD over the first 3- to 6-month period is a decrease, believed to be due to increased bone remodeling activity. Markers of bone formation and resorption are increased early and remain elevated for at least 1 year. The subsequent response of bone differs between childhood-onset and adult-onset GH deficiency. By 6 months of treatment, the BMD is significantly increased in childhood-onset GH deficiency and continues to increase over an 18-month period of GH replacement. In adult-onset GH deficiency, BMD is not increased at 12 months, although a significant increase is noted at 24 months in those with lower baseline BMD scores. Evidence from placebo-controlled randomized studies suggests that significant improvement occurs in vitality, well-being, and overall quality of life in GH-deficient adults in response to GH replacement. The exact mechanism for the improved sense of well-being remains controversial: Possible explanations include increased exercise capacity, improved hydration status with normalization of extracellular volume, and a direct CNS effect.

The majority of GH-replacement studies show favorable changes in the lipid profile.[52] The most frequent finding has been a reduction in total cholesterol, LDL cholesterol, LDL/HDL cholesterol ratio, and apolipoprotein-B concentrations, with no significant change in either HDL cholesterol or triglyceride concentrations. Some studies suggested that GH-replacement therapy increases lipoprotein(a) levels, although poor assay standardization to date limit its use as a reliable predictor of cardiovascular risk.

GH replacement at higher doses can cause an increase in insulin resistance, with higher fasting glucose, fasting insulin, and glycated hemoglobin levels within 6 months after treatment. Most of those abnormalities improve over subsequent years, probably reflecting changes in body composition. However, patients receiving GH treatment will have to be monitored for alterations in glucose homeostasis; insulin resistance does not appear to be normalized on long-term GH therapy.[53] Several studies to date also documented favorable effects of GH treatment on impaired endothelial function, cardiac structure, and systemic vascular resistance but no change in fibrinogen levels.

GH-replacement therapy in the transition period from teenage years to adulthood deserves special consideration. Bone mass accrual continues for a number of years beyond achievement of final height and is greatly influenced by GH status. Therefore, continuation of GH-replacement therapy in severely GH-deficient young adults should be strongly recommended as an important preventive measure to avoid the complications of osteoporosis in later life.[54]

The majority of modern regimens use a low starting dose, that is, 0.3 mg/day as a single subcutaneous injection. This should then be increased every 4 to 6 weeks, based on clinical response and IGF-1 levels, until a steady replacement dose is reached. Because improvements in physiologic well-being and quality of life do not occur in all GH-deficient patients receiving replacement therapy, it is suggested that patients started on GH primarily for a quality-of-life indication should have an initial trial period of therapy; only those with definite improvement should continue treatment thereafter. Improvements in quality of life and body composition often occur only after several months of maintenance therapy, and therefore a trial of 6 months of GH at the correct maintenance dose is necessary to determine whether treatment is beneficial. At the end of this trial, patients should be reassessed by using a disease-specific questionnaire and with measurements of body composition and lipids. In patients started on GH for osteoporosis or osteopenia, therapy is reassessed after BMD estimation at 2 years. Such selection criteria are not being applied universally. In some countries, GH replacement is regarded simply as hormone substitution for an established deficiency, and therefore treatment is lifelong without the need for any qualifying criteria. The low-dose regimen is rarely associated with the side effects, such as peripheral edema, arthralgia, and myalgia, described when higher doses of GH replacement, particularly weight-based dosing regimens, were used. Monitoring of GH replacement should include regular measurement of weight, blood pressure, hemoglobin A_{1c}, lipid profile, IGF-1, fat distribution (waist/hip ratio), and assessment of quality of life by disease-specific questionnaire and patient interview.

GONADOTROPIN DEFICIENCY

In both sexes, sex steroid–replacement therapy is important for the maintenance of normal body composition, skeletal health, and sexual function, and it is the most appropriate form of replacement therapy in patients not desirous of fertility.

Estrogen Replacement

In women, this can be provided by many standard hormone-replacement therapy preparations. Progesterone must be given (cyclically or continuously) in all women with an intact uterus to prevent the possible effect of unopposed estrogen on the endometrium, that is, dysfunctional bleeding or endometrial cancer. The dose of estrogen should not be supraphysiologic (as in the oral contraceptive pill) unless a clear indication exists, such as strong patient preference, or in a patient with partial gonadotropin deficiency still having occasional menstrual cycles, with a desire for contraception. Estrogen can be delivered as a tablet, patch, gel, or implant. Although estrogen-replacement therapy can minimize the risk of osteoporosis, its long-term effects on the cardiovascular system in young hypopituitary women remain unknown. Estrogen-replacement therapy would typically be continued until age 50 years. Continuation after this time should be based on a discussion of the risks and benefits between the patient and physician, supported by BMD measurement.

Androgen Replacement

Androgen-replacement therapy for men is available in many modalities. The choice of preparation depends on local availability and the wishes of the patient. IM injection of testosterone 17α-hydroxyl esters every 2 to 3 weeks is a commonly used regimen of testosterone replacement. In some men, however, this mode of administration is associated with disturbing fluctuations in sexual function, energy level, and mood, mirroring the changes in testosterone concentrations. Changing to smaller doses on a more frequent basis or to another preparation can be helpful. Transdermal testosterone systems are an alternative, available as either patch systems (nonscrotal or scrotal) or the recently introduced testosterone gel. Both are able to maintain physiologic testosterone profiles in the majority of patients, but skin irritation, the need for scrotal shaving, or a drying time after gel application are some of the potential drawbacks of either transdermal system.

Less commonly used ways of administering testosterone are testosterone implants and oral androgen-replacement therapy. Subcutaneous implants consist of three to six 200-mg pellets, which can maintain normal testosterone levels for up to 6 months. The implantation of the pellets requires minor surgery and may be complicated in a minority of patients by local infection, extrusion, and scarring. Oral androgen-replacement therapy is available by using testosterone undecenoate, a 17α-hydroxyl ester of testosterone. However, this requires frequent dosing (2 to 4 times daily), and often subnormal testosterone levels are achieved because of variable absorption.

Androgen-replacement therapy should always be monitored to ensure physiologic mean testosterone levels. Suboptimal replacement doses result in low trough levels, whereas supraphysiologic doses can promote secondary polycythemia and progression of prostate cancer; therefore, regular monitoring of hemoglobin and prostate-specific antigen is recommended.

An area of debate now is the therapeutic use of testosterone in women. In postmenopausal women, particularly those who have undergone bilateral oophorectomy, evidence exists that combined estrogen and testosterone replacement results in substantial benefits in those who complain of loss of libido and impaired sexual function despite adequate estrogen replacement. The rationale behind such therapy is that after bilateral oophorectomy, circulating testosterone levels decrease by 50%. This reduction tends to be even greater in women with hypogonadotropic hypogonadism, who are likely to be ACTH as well as gonadotropin deficient; thus, symptomatic patients may benefit from low-dose testosterone-replacement therapy. Regimens with a 50-mg testosterone implant every 6 months have been used. This practice is, however, not universal, and insufficient research has been performed in the hypogonadotropic hypogonadal woman. Testosterone-replacement regimens are not approved for the latter indication by most regulatory authorities.

Gonadotropin and Gonadotropin-Releasing Hormone Therapy

In the hypogonadotropic hypogonadal patient fertility can be achieved with gonadotropin therapy. In men, excellent success rates can be achieved, provided primary testicular dysfunction does not coexist. Testosterone replacement should be discontinued before initiating therapy. The choice of therapy lies between gonadotropin replacement and GnRH. The former is the traditional therapeutic approach; initially, LH "activity" is provided by human chorionic gonadotropin (hCG) administered subcutaneously (SC) or IM at a dose of between 1000 and 2000 IU, 2 to 3 times weekly. Spermatogenesis is unlikely within the first 3 months of therapy. Treatment with hCG alone is continued for 6 months, with regular sperm counts to monitor progress. If adequate spermatogenesis is not achieved, then FSH in the form of human menopausal gonadotropin (hMG), or a more purified preparation of FSH, is added. The dose of FSH is increased if adequate spermatogenesis is not achieved after 6 months of combination therapy. The alternative regimen in patients with idiopathic hypogonadotropic hypogonadism and Kallmann's syndrome is pulsatile GnRH therapy. GnRH is administered SC via a catheter attached to a minipump. Its use implies a hypothalamic defect with essentially normal pituitary gonadotrophs. This regimen appears to have few advantages over gonadotropin therapy in men but may cause less gynecomastia. Both regimens may take up to 2 years to achieve adequate spermatogenesis, and thus once effective, consideration should be given to storing several samples of frozen sperm for any future attempts at pregnancy.

In women with hypogonadotropic hypogonadism, pregnancy rates of 83% after therapy with either pulsatile GnRH or gonadotropins are reported. These are better than rates achieved in women undergoing ovulation induction for other pathologic conditions. Again, the choice of therapy lies between gonadotropin therapy and pulsatile GnRH, but obvious advantages accrue to GnRH therapy if the patient has enough residual gonadotroph function.

Pulsatile GnRH therapy is more likely than hMG to result in development and ovulation of a single follicle, thereby reducing the risks of ovarian hyperstimulation and multiple gestation. However, in practice, GnRH therapy may not be practicable, and in more than 50% of women with organic pituitary disease, residual gonadotroph function is not sufficient to support this method.

ADRENOCORTICOTROPIC HORMONE DEFICIENCY

Any patient identified as having ACTH deficiency should be repeatedly educated about its clinical implications. It is crucial for the patient to understand the need to increase the replacement dose two- to threefold in case of an intercurrent illness or when undergoing surgery. Every patient with ACTH deficiency should wear an appropriate Medic-alert bracelet or necklace. Many patients also benefit from being issued with an IM hydrocortisone pack and taught how to self-administer IM hydrocortisone in the event of protracted vomiting.

As mentioned earlier, the decision to begin cortisol-replacement therapy should be based not only on the results of dynamic testing but also on clinical assessment. The next decision is the choice of glucocorticoid. Hydrocortisone is the logical choice, as it directly replaces the missing hormone. Alternatives include cortisone acetate, which is metabolized to cortisol, and therefore can be monitored in the same way as hydrocortisone. Its onset of action is slower, and its biologic activity is slightly longer, providing relative disadvantages and advantages over hydrocortisone, respectively. Other synthetic glucocorticoids, that is, prednisolone and dexamethasone, have significant disadvantages; monitoring is difficult, and, in the case of dexamethasone, the limited number of pharmaceutical preparations available makes small dose adjustments impossible.

Growing evidence now indicates that the traditional hydrocortisone regimen of 20 mg in the morning and 10 mg in the evening is far from ideal. First, this regimen is not physiologic, as the plasma half-life of cortisol is less than 2 hours. Thus, twice-daily dosing regimens are associated with very low cortisol levels in the late afternoon, and studies of a twice-daily regimen have demonstrated that quality-of-life scores are lower at this time. Thus, dosing 3 times daily is recommended. Second, the total daily dose of 30 mg hydrocortisone also is supraphysiologic, as production rates in the normal individual are significantly lower than previously believed.[55] Thus, a hydrocortisone regimen of 10 mg in the morning, 5 mg at noon, and 5 mg in the evening is likely to be a better starting schedule. Monitoring of therapy usually involves the use of an 8-hour day hydrocortisone curve, aiming to achieve normal cortisol levels. Such monitoring allows the detection of minor degrees of over- or under-replacement, which are unlikely to be clinically obvious. Minor over-replacement is associated with reduced BMD,[55] and it is likely that other factors, including blood pressure, insulin sensitivity, and body composition, also may be adversely affected.

THYROID-STIMULATING HORMONE DEFICIENCY

Secondary hypothyroidism is treated with thyroxine (T_4)-replacement therapy in the same way as is primary hypothyroidism. The normal starting dose in a young patient without evidence of cardiac disease is 100 μg/day. In the elderly or in a patient with evidence of ischemic heart disease, therapy should be started at lower doses, that is, 25 to 50 μg/day.

A complicating factor in secondary hypothyroidism, however, is that measurement of serum TSH is obviously unhelpful in the monitoring of T_4-replacement therapy. Thus, the biochemical objective should be to restore the serum-free T$_4$ concentration to the normal range.

Treatment of TSH deficiency always must be considered in the context of other pituitary hormone deficiencies. In a patient with suspected hypopituitarism, thyroxine therapy should be delayed until ACTH deficiency has been excluded or treated, as a risk of worsening the features of cortisol deficiency is present. Over-replacement with T$_4$ over long periods may be associated with reduced BMD, an increased risk of osteoporotic fracture, and an increase in the rate of development of atrial fibrillation; thus, excessive doses of T$_4$ should be avoided.

ANTIDIURETIC HORMONE DEFICIENCY

Desmopressin is the drug of choice for the treatment of ADH deficiency. It is a synthetic analogue of arginine vasopressin with two minor alterations in its molecular structure: a switch of arginine from the L- to the D-form in position 8, and deamination of cysteine in position 1. This results in a two- to fourfold increase in antidiuretic activity, prolongation of the biologic half-life to 6 to 8 hours, and absence of pressor activity, the latter eliminating side effects noted with arginine vasopressin, including hypertension, renal colic, coronary artery spasm, and abdominal colic.

Desmopressin is available in a number of preparations, including oral, intranasal, and parenteral. Dosages vary as much as 10-fold between individuals, with no apparent relation to age, sex, weight, or degree of polyuria. The drug should be started at low dose and increased gradually until urine output is controlled. Overdosage carries a risk of hyponatremia, and sodium levels should be checked after commencing or changing therapy.

STRATEGIES TO PREVENT HYPOPITUITARISM

Hypopituitarism increases morbidity and mortality in affected patients, requires therapy with complex drug regimens, and incurs significant cost by the health-care provider. The introduction of GH-replacement therapy has exacerbated the problem, with a yearly cost in U.S. dollars of $4500 to $6000 per patient. Thus, attention has turned to strategies that might reduce the incidence of hypopituitarism.

One area worthy of consideration is the routine use of radiotherapy after surgery for nonsecreting pituitary adenomas. Data suggest that recurrence rates after transcranial pituitary surgery are as high as 25% to 75%,[56] whereas recurrence after transsphenoidal surgery are reported to be between 12% and 22%. Data from Bradley and colleagues[57] indicate that in the subgroup of patients with complete tumor removal, as judged by the surgeon, without radiologic and surgical evidence of spread into the parapituitary structures or evidence of rapid tumor growth, a 90% recurrence-free survival occurs at 5 years. It should be pointed out, however, that surgical results are highly operator dependent in terms of tumor recurrence and that regular clinical and radiologic surveillance is mandatory. Nonetheless, by avoiding radiotherapy as a routine procedure, the incidence of long-term hypopituitarism will be significantly reduced.

Medical therapy offers an alternative to radiotherapy or surgery in patients with prolactinomas and now in patients with acromegaly. Dopamine-agonist drug therapy can shrink prolactinomas and restore normoprolactinemia in many patients, 70% of macroadenomas shrinking by 25% or more, and restoration of normoprolactinemia and normal gonadal function occurs in at least 75% of patients. Whether these agents also are associated with a restoration of other aspects of pituitary function is less clear. Variable recovery from both ACTH and TSH deficiency has been described, but the data regarding GH status, particularly in adults, are scanty. Furthermore, the advent of greater use of medical therapy for acromegaly with somatostatin analogues and a GH-receptor antagonist and the less frequent use of conventional radiotherapy should mean fewer hypopituitary patients in the future; the same advantage also may hold up for stereotactic surgery versus conventional radiotherapy.

REFERENCES

1. Regal M, Páramo C, Sierra SM, Garcia-Mayor RV: Prevalence and incidence of hypopituitarism in an adult Caucasian population in northwestern Spain. Clin Endocrinol (Oxf) 55:735–740, 2001.
2. Rosén T, Bengtsson BA: Premature mortality due to cardiovascular disease in hypopituitarism. Lancet 336:285–288, 1990.
3. Bates AS, Van't Hoff W, Jones PJ, Clayton RN: The effect of hypopituitarism on life expectancy. J Clin Endocrinol Metab 81:1169–1172, 1996.
4. Bülow B, Hagmar L, Mikoczy Z, et al: Increased cerebrovascular mortality in patients with hypopituitarism. Clin Endocrinol (Oxf) 46:75–81, 1997.
5. Bates AS, Bullivant B, Sheppard MC, Stewart PM: Life expectancy following surgery for pituitary tumours. Clin Endocrinol (Oxf) 50:315–319, 1999.
6. Nilsson B, Gustavasson-Kadaka E, Bengtsson BA, Jonsson B: Pituitary adenomas in Sweden between 1958 and 1991: Incidence, survival, and mortality. J Clin Endocrinol Metab 85:1420–1425, 2000.
7. Tomlinson JW, Holden N, Hills RK, et al: Association between premature mortality and hypopituitarism: West Midlands Prospective Hypopituitary Study Group. Lancet 357:425–431, 2001.
8. Molitch ME, Russell EJ: The pituitary "incidentaloma." Ann Intern Med 112:925–931, 1990.
9. Arafah BM, Prunty D, Ybarra J, et al: The dominant role of increased intrasellar pressure in the pathogenesis of hypopituitarism, hyperprolactinemia, and headaches in patients with pituitary adenomas. J Clin Endocrinol Metab 85:1789–1793, 2000.
10. Webb SM, Rigla M, Wägner A, et al: Recovery of hypopituitarism after neurosurgical treatment of pituitary adenomas. J Clin Endocrinol Metab 84:3696–3700, 1999.
11. Arafah BM: Reversible hypopituitarism in patients with large nonfunctioning pituitary adenomas. J Clin Endocrinol Metab 62:1173–1179, 1986.
12. Arafah BM, Kailani SH, Nekl KE, et al: Immediate recovery of pituitary function after transsphenoidal resection of pituitary macroadenomas.
J Clin Endocrinol Metab 79:348–354, 1994.
13. Littley MD, Shalet SM, Beardwell CG: Radiation and hypothalamic-pituitary function. Baillieres Clin Endocrinol Metab 4:147–175, 1990.
14. Shalet SM, Beardwell CG, Pearson D, Jones PH: The effect of varying doses of cerebral irradiation on growth hormone production in childhood. Clin Endocrinol (Oxf) 5:287–290, 1976.
15. Darzy KH, Shalet SM: Radiation-induced growth hormone deficiency. Horm Res 59(Suppl 1):1–11, 2003.
16. Cohen LE, Radovick S: Molecular basis of combined pituitary hormone deficiencies. Endocr Rev 23:431–442, 2002.
17. Deladoëy J, Flück C, Büyükgebiz A, et al: "Hot spot" in the PROP1 gene responsible for combined pituitary hormone deficiency. J Clin Endocrinol Metab 84:1645–1650, 1999.
18. Thomas PQ, Dattani MT, Brickman JM, et al: Heterozygous HESX1 mutations associated with isolated congenital pituitary hypoplasia and septo-optic dysplasia. Hum Mol Genet 10:39–45, 2001.

19. Netchine I, Sobrier ML, Krude H, et al: Mutations in LHX3 result in a new syndrome revealed by combined pituitary hormone deficiency. Nat Genet 25:182–186, 2000.
21. Binder G: Isolated growth hormone deficiency and the GH-1 gene: Update 2002. Horm Res 58(Suppl 3):2–6, 2002.
20. Machinis K, Pantel J, Netchine I, et al: Syndromic short stature in patients with a germline mutation in the LIM homeobox LHX4. Am J Hum Genet 69:961–968, 2001.
22. Netchine I, Talon P, Dastot F, et al: Extensive phenotypic analysis of a family with growth hormone (GH) deficiency caused by a mutation in the GH-releasing hormone receptor gene. J Clin Endocrinol Metab 83:432–436, 1998.
23. Mantovani G, Maghnie M, Weber G, et al: Growth hormone-releasing hormone resistance in pseudohypoparathyroidism type ia: New evidence for imprinting of the Gs alpha gene. J Clin Endocrinol Metab 88:4070–4074, 2003.
24. Quinton R, Duke VM, Robertson A, et al: Idiopathic gonadotrophin deficiency: Genetic questions addressed through phenotypic characterization. Clin Endocrinol (Oxf) 55:163–174, 2001.
25. Doeker BM, Pfäffle RW, Pohlenz J, Andler W: Congenital central hypothyroidism due to a homozygous mutation in the thyrotropin beta-subunit gene follows an autosomal recessive inheritance. J Clin Endocrinol Metab 83:1762–1765, 1998.
26. Collu R, Tang J, Castagné J, et al: A novel mechanism for isolated central hypothyroidism: Inactivating mutations in the thyrotropin-releasing hormone receptor gene. J Clin Endocrinol Metab 82:1561–1565, 1997.
27. Asteria C: T-box and isolated ACTH deficiency. Eur J Endocrinol 146:463–465, 2002.
28. Lieberman SA, Oberoi AL, Gilkison CR, et al: Prevalence of neuroendocrine dysfunction in patients recovering from traumatic brain injury. J Clin Endocrinol Metab 86:2752–2756, 2001.
29. Benvenga S, Campenní A, Ruggeri RM, Trimarchi F: Clinical review 113: Hypopituitarism secondary to head trauma. J Clin Endocrinol Metab 85:1353–1361, 2000.
30. Gasperi M, Cecconi E, Grasso L, et al: GH secretion is impaired in patients with primary hyperparathyroidism. J Clin Endocrinol Metab 87:1961–1964, 2002.
31. Shalet SM, Toogood A, Rahim A, Brennan BM: The diagnosis of growth hormone deficiency in children and adults. Endocr Rev 19:203–223, 1998.
32. Holmes SJ, Economou G, Whitehouse RW, et al: Reduced bone mineral density in patients with adult onset growth hormone deficiency. J Clin Endocrinol Metab 78:669–574, 1994.
33. Rosén T, Wilhelmsen L, Landin-Wilhelmsen K, et al: Increased fracture frequency in adult patients with hypopituitarism and GH deficiency. Eur J Endocrinol 137:240–245, 1997.
34. Beshyah SA, Gelding SV, Andres C, et al: Beta-cell function in hypopituitary adults before and during growth hormone treatment. Clin Sci (Lond) 89:321–328, 1995.
35. de Luis DA, Aller R, Romero E: Isolated ACTH deficiency. Horm Res 49:247–249, 1998.
36. Mukherjee A, Murray RD, Columb B, et al: Acquired prolactin deficiency indicates severe hypopituitarism in patients with disease of the hypothalamic-pituitary axis. Clin Endocrinol (Oxf) 59:743–748, 2003.
37. Cannavò S, Curtò L, Venturino M, et al: Abnormalities of hypothalamic-pituitary-thyroid axis in patients with primary empty sella. J Endocrinol Invest 25:236–239, 2002.
38. Littley MD, Shalet SM, Beardwell CG, et al: Hypopituitarism following external radiotherapy for pituitary tumours in adults. Q J Med 70:145–160, 1989.
39. Jones SL, Trainer PJ, Perry L, et al: An audit of the insulin tolerance test in adult subjects in an acute investigation unit over one year. Clin Endocrinol (Oxf) 41:123–128, 1994.
40. Hoffman DM, Ho KKY: Diagnosis of GH deficiency in adults. In Juul A, Jorgenson JOL (eds): Growth Hormone in Adults. Cambridge, UK, Cambridge University Press, 1996, pp 168–185.
41. Lissett CA, Saleem S, Rahim A, et al: The impact of irradiation on growth hormone responsiveness to provocative agents is stimulus dependent: Results in 161 individuals with radiation damage to the somatotropic axis. J Clin Endocrinol Metab 86:663–668, 2001.
42. Björntorp P: Endocrine abnormalities of obesity. Metabolism 44:21–23, 1995.
43. Salomon F, Cuneo RC, Umpleby AM, Sönksen PH: Interactions of body fat and muscle mass with substrate concentrations and fasting insulin levels in adults with growth hormone deficiency. Clin Sci (Lond) 87:201–206, 1994.
44. Toogood AA, O'Neill PA, Shalet SM: Beyond the somatopause: Growth hormone deficiency in adults over the age of 60 years. J Clin Endocrinol Metab 81:460–465, 1996.
45. Le Roux CW, Meeran K, Alaghband-Zadeh J: Is a 0900-h serum cortisol useful prior to a short Synacthen test in outpatient assessment? Ann Clin Biochem 39:148–150, 2002.
46. Hurel SJ, Thompson CJ, Watson MJ, et al: The short Synacthen and insulin stress tests in the assessment of the hypothalamic-pituitary-adrenal axis. Clin Endocrinol (Oxf) 44:141–146, 1996.
47. Clark PM, Neylon I, Raggatt PR, et al: Defining the normal cortisol response to the short Synacthen test: Implications for the investigation of hypothalamic-pituitary disorders. Clin Endocrinol (Oxf) 49:287–292, 1998.
48. Abdu TA, Elhadd TA, Neary R, Clayton RN: Comparison of the low dose short Synacthen test (1 microg), the conventional dose short Synacthen test (250 microg), and the insulin tolerance test for assessment of the hypothalamo-pituitary-adrenal axis in patients with pituitary disease. J Clin Endocrinol Metab 84:838–843, 1999.
49. Gonzálbez J, Villabona C, Ramón J, et al: Establishment of reference values for standard dose short Synacthen test (250 microgram), low dose short Synacthen test (1 microgram) and insulin tolerance test for assessment of the hypothalamo-pituitary-adrenal axis in normal subjects. Clin Endocrinol (Oxf) 53:199–204, 2000.
50. Gleeson HK, Walker BR, Seckl JR, Padfield PL: Ten years on: Safety of short Synacthen tests in assessing adrenocorticotropin deficiency in clinical practice. J Clin Endocrinol Metab 88:2106–2111, 2003.
51. Beck-Peccoz P, Amr S, Menezes-Ferreira MM, et al: Decreased receptor binding of biologically inactive thyrotropin in central hypothyroidism: Effect of treatment with thyrotropin-releasing hormone. N Engl J Med 312:1085–1090, 1985.
52. Murray RD, Wieringa GE, Lissett CA, et al: Low-dose GH replacement improves the adverse lipid profile associated with the adult GH deficiency syndrome. Clin Endocrinol (Oxf) 56:525–532, 2002.
53. Svensson J, Bengtsson BA: Growth hormone replacement therapy and insulin sensitivity. J Clin Endocrinol Metab 88:1453–1454, 2003.
54. Shalet SM, Shavrikova E, Cromer M, et al: Effect of growth hormone (GH) treatment on bone in postpubertal GH-deficient patients: A 2-year randomized, controlled, dose-ranging study. J Clin Endocrinol Metab 88:4124–4129, 2003.
55. Peacey SR, Guo CY, Robinson AM, et al: Glucocorticoid replacement therapy: Are patients overtreated and does it matter? Clin Endocrinol (Oxf) 46:255–261, 1997.
56. Shalet SM, Peacey SR: Treatment strategies in the prevention of growth hormone deficiency. In Lamberts SWJ (ed): The Diagnosis and Treatment of Pituitary Insufficiency. Bristol, UK, BioScientifica, 1997, pp 263–277.
57. Bradley KM, Adams CB, Potter CP, et al: An audit of selected patients with non-functioning pituitary adenoma treated by transsphenoidal surgery without irradiation. Clin Endocrinol (Oxf) 41:655–659, 1994.

Acromegaly

Shlomo Melmed

INTRODUCTION

Acromegaly is a disease of spectacular growth and metabolic disorders that has fascinated physicians for centuries. The natural history of the disorder, if left untreated, results in gross acral and facial disfigurement, musculoskeletal disability, cardiac failure, respiratory dysfunction, diabetes, and accelerated mortality.[1–3] If the disease occurs before epiphyseal closure, gigantism results.[1] After the first modern description of the disease in 1886 by Marie,[4] it was subsequently recognized that the disorder is associated with a growth hormone (GH)-secreting adenohypophyseal adenoma resulting in both a central mass lesion and the protean peripheral effects of sustained tissue exposure to high GH levels.[1,5–7]

PATHOGENESIS

The pathogenetic events that underlie the etiology of pituitary acromegaly include excessive pituitary somatotroph cell proliferation and unrestrained GH hypersecretion. GH is secreted by somatotroph cells, the largest differentiated compartment of the anterior pituitary. GH secretion is under dual hypothalamic inhibitory control: somatotropin release–inhibiting factor (SRIF) inhibits secretion and GH-releasing hormone (GHRH) stimulates both GH synthesis and secretion.[8,9] Ghrelin, a gut-derived peptide, binds to the GHS receptor and acts primarily at the hypothalamus to induce GH. Insulin-like growth factor 1 (IGF-1), the peripheral target molecule for GH action, participates in negative GH feedback inhibition by acting both at the hypothalamus to induce SRIF and directly at the pituitary to inhibit GH gene transcription.[10–12] Peripheral sex and adrenal steroids also regulate GH secretion.[8,13] GH itself binds to peripheral GH receptors that elicit signaling by JAK/STAT (Janus kinase/signal transducer and activator of transcription) intracellular phosphorylation cascades.[14] GH acts directly to attenuate insulin action and induce lipolysis.[15] The growth-promoting actions of GH are indirectly mediated by IGF-1, which is synthesized in the liver, kidney, pituitary, gastrointestinal tract, muscle, and cartilage.[12,16,17] GH actions mediated by IGF-1 include protein synthesis; amino acid transportation; muscle, cartilage, and bone growth; DNA and RNA synthesis; and cell proliferation.[18,19] Local production of IGF-1 may be under autocrine and paracrine regulation,[3,20,21] acting in concert with circulating IGF-1 and GH to elicit a final tissue impact.

EXCESS GROWTH HORMONE SECRETION

Tumors may arise from clonal expansion of one or more of the anterior pituitary differentiated cell types[22,23] and thereby result in specific hormone hypersecretory syndromes. The most common cause of acromegaly is a somatotroph (GH-secreting) adenoma of the anterior pituitary, which accounts for 30% of all hormone-secreting pituitary adenomas[1] (Table 23-1).

GH-secreting adenomas arise from differentiated cells secreting GH gene products[1,23,24] (Table 23-2). These cells include somatotrophs, mixed mammosomatotrophs (secreting both GH and prolactin [PRL]), or more primitive acidophilic stem cells. Regardless of their cellular origin, transformation and subsequent replication of these cells result in adenoma formation, as well as unrestrained GH secretion.[1] Most patients harbor densely granulated GH-cell adenomas, which are commonly encountered in older patients with indolent disease progression. Sparsely granulated GH-cell adenomas occur in younger patients with more aggressive disease onset and higher GH levels.[1,2] Mammosomatotroph cell tumors, or discrete mammotroph and somatotroph tumors, reflect the common stem cell origin of the somatotroph cell lineage.[2,24–26] Although acidophil stem cell adenomas secrete GH, their predominant product is PRL, thus accounting for the high incidence of hyperprolactinemic symptoms (galactorrhea, amenorrhea, infertility) initially seen in these patients.[27] Patients with McCune-Albright syndrome also may have acromegaly, although the presence of a discrete GH cell adenoma has been inconsistently reported in these cases.[28] Rarely, acromegaly may occur in patients with a partially empty sella.[29] The rim of pituitary tissue surrounding the empty sella may harbor a small endocrinologically active GH-secreting adenoma not visible on magnetic resonance imaging (MRI) (i.e., <2 mm in diameter). Because embryonic pituitary tissue originates from the nasopharyngeal Rathke's pouch, ectopic

Table 23-1 Causes of Acromegaly

Cause	Prevalence (%)
Excess GH secretion	
Pituitary	98
Densely or sparsely granulated GH cell adenoma	60
Mixed GH cell and PRL cell adenoma	25
Mammosomatotroph cell adenoma	10
Plurihormonal adenoma	
GH cell carcinoma or metastases	
Multiple endocrine neoplasia-1 (GH cell adenoma)	
McCune-Albright syndrome (rarely adenoma)	
Ectopic sphenoid or parapharyngeal sinus pituitary adenoma	
Extrapituitary tumor	
Pancreatic islet cell tumor	<1
Excess GH-releasing hormone secretion	
Central	<1
Hypothalamic hamartoma, choristoma, ganglioneuroma	<1
Peripheral	1
Bronchial carcinoid, pancreatic islet cell tumor, small cell lung cancer, adrenal adenoma, medullary thyroid carcinoma, pheochromocytoma	
Excess growth factor activity	
Acromegaloidism	<1

GH, growth hormone; PRL, prolactin.
Adapted from Melmed S: Acromegaly. N Engl J Med 322:966–977, 1990, with permission.

pituitary adenomas may arise in remnant nasopharyngeal tissue along the line of primitive adenohypophysial migration. These adenomas may not be detected on pituitary MRI fields, and more extensive skull base imaging may be required. Very rarely, ectopic GH production by pancreatic,[30] lung,[31] ovarian,[32] or lymphocytic neoplasms may result in acromegaly.[1]

EXCESS GROWTH HORMONE–RELEASING HORMONE SECRETION

Excessive circulating levels of GHRH may overstimulate the pituitary and cause somatotroph hyperplasia, GH hypersecretion, and acromegaly.[33] Central overproduction of GHRH may occur in patients harboring hypothalamic hamartomas or gangliocytomas.[33] These rare tumors are usually diagnosed by pathologic examination of a surgically resected sellar mass causing GH hypersecretion and acromegaly.[34] Ectopic GHRH production by carcinoid tumors, although rare, accounts for most cases of acromegaly.[35] The clinical association of acromegaly with carcinoid disease had long been recognized, and the pathogenesis of ectopic GHRH production is now elucidated. Subclinical GHRH immunoreactivity has been demonstrated in about 40% of lung, abdominal, and bony carcinoid tissue specimens.

Pituitary somatotroph hyperplasia plus acromegaly associated with ectopic GHRH production has been reported in more than 100 patients, and the original isolation of GHRH was accomplished from a pancreatic carcinoid tumor.[36] Because the peripheral features of hypersomatotropism are quite similar in all forms of pituitary and nonpituitary acromegaly, diagnosis of the etiology of the disease may be clinically challenging.[1]

Acromegaloidism is a very rare syndrome characterized by acromegalic features with no discernible pituitary tumor and normal serum GH and IGF-1 concentrations. It has been presumed that this disorder is due to excess secretion of a putative, as yet unidentified growth factor.[37]

ROLE OF THE HYPOTHALAMUS IN THE ETIOLOGY OF ACROMEGALY

Hypothalamic GHRH and SRIF selectively regulate GH gene expression and secretion.[8] These hypothalamic peptide hormones are expressed both within the anterior pituitary gland itself and within GH-secreting pituitary tumors.[38,39] GHRH, in addition to its hormonal regulation of GH production, induces somatotroph DNA synthesis.[40] Mice bearing an overexpressing GHRH transgene are subject to somatotroph hyperplasia and ultimately to pituitary adenomas.[41,42] In patients with carcinoid tumors and ectopic GHRH production, somatotroph hyperplasia and occasionally adenomas also may develop, which suggests that disordered endocrine or paracrine GHRH or SRIF action may be permissive for pituitary tumor growth.[43] GHRH signaling defects also have been identified in acromegaly. Constitutive activation of the GHRH receptor G protein signaling unit facilitates ligand-independent induction of GH gene expression. This *gsp* mutation results in guanosine triphosphatase (GTPase) inactivation with subsequent elevated cyclic adenosine monophosphate (cAMP) levels and GH hypersecretion.[44,45] Excessive CREB (cAMP

Table 23-2 Clinical and Pathologic Characteristics of GH-Secreting Pituitary Tumors

Cell Type	Hormonal Products	Clinical Features	Histologic Features
Densely granulated somatotroph	GH	Slow growing	Numerous somatotrophs with large secretory granules
Sparsely granulated somatotroph	GH	Rapidly growing Often invasive	Cellular pleomorphism
Mixed cell (somatotroph/lactotrope)	GH and PRL	Variable	Densely and sparsely granulated somatotrophs and lactotrophs
Mammosomatotroph	GH and PRL	Commonly in children Gigantism Mild hyperprolactinemia	Both GH and PRL in same cell, often same secretory granule
Acidophil stem cell	PRL and GH	Rapidly growing/invasive Hyperprolactinemia dominant	Distinctive ultrastructure Giant mitochondria
Plurihormonal cell	GH (PRL) with α-GSU, FSH/LH, TSH, or ACTH	Often, secondary hormonal products are clinically silent Rarely hyperthyroidism or Cushing's disease	Variable: either monomorphous or plurimorphous
Somatotroph carcinoma	GH	Aggressive and invasive	Rigorously documented extracranial metastasis

ACTH, adrenocorticotropic hormone; GH, growth hormone; GSU, α-glycoprotein subunit; LH, luteinizing hormone; PRL, prolactin; TSH, thyroid-stimulating hormone.
Adapted from Melmed S: Pathogenesis of pituitary tumors. Endocrinol Metab Clin North Am 21:553–574, 1992, with permission.

response element binding protein) serine phosphorylation also may account for activation of the CREB–Pit-1 (pituitary-specific transcription factor-1) signaling unit in a subset of GH cell adenomas.[46]

Pituitary tumor–derived paracrine GHRH or SRIF or both also may regulate tumor growth or function, although no consistent activating hormone receptor structural mutations have been identified. A truncated alternatively spliced GHRH receptor transcript has been described, but its functional significance is unclear.[47] In light of compelling evidence favoring intrinsic genetic defects occurring in GH-secreting pituitary tumors, as discussed later, it is apparent that hypothalamic influences may be permissive of tumor growth rather than being proximally involved in the initiation of somatotroph tumorigenesis.[43,48]

INTRINSIC PITUITARY LESIONS

Virtually all GH cell adenomas arise as discrete clonal expansions of a transformed cell[22] (Table 23-3). This monoclonal origin implies that intrinsic genetic alterations account for tumorigenic initiating events and supports abundant earlier clinical observations that resection of small well-circumscribed adenomas usually results in surgical cure of GH-secreting adenomas.[24,43,49] Because adenohypophyseal tissue surrounding the pituitary adenoma is histologically normal, it is unlikely that multiple independent cellular growth events (e.g., generalized hyperplasia) precede adenoma formation. Increasing evidence points to complex molecular cascades accounting for the cellular progression resulting in pituitary cell transformation and, ultimately, tumor formation. Multistep development of pituitary acromegaly involves a spectrum of genetic alterations associated with dysregulation of cell proliferation, differentiation, and GH production.[43] Activation of oncogene function or inactivation of tumor-suppressor genes or both may account for these changes[43,50,51] (see Table 23-3).

CANDIDATE GENES IN THE ETIOLOGY OF ACROMEGALY

Inactivating Mutations

Several transgenic animal models have shown that disruption of tumor-suppressor genes (including RB [retinoblastoma] and p27) results in a high incidence of pituitary tumor formation in afflicted mice.[52–54] Because a variety of chromosomal loss of heterogeneity (LOH) patterns are observed in human adenomas, loss of tumor-suppressor gene activity was similarly postulated for human tumors (Table 23-4).

Several chromosomal lesions occur in pituitary tumor tissue derived from patients with sporadic nonfamilial acromegaly. LOH involving chromosomes 11q13, 13, and 9 occurs in up to 20% of sporadic[50,55,56] pituitary tumors. Despite the multiple

---

Table 23-3 Evidence for an Intrinsic Pituitary Defect in the Pathogenesis of Acromegaly

GH-secreting adenomas are monoclonal
Absence of somatotroph hyperplasia in normal pituitary tissue surrounding pituitary adenomas
Successful surgical cure of well-circumscribed GH cell adenomas is achieved in >75% of patients
Adenoma transformation is rarely associated with generalized somatotroph hyperplasia
Unrestrained GH hypersecretion occurs independent of physiologic hypothalamic feedback control
Normalization of GH pulsatility often occurs after complete adenoma resection

GH, growth hormone.
Adapted from Drange MR, Melmed S: IGFs in the evaluation of acromegaly. In Rosenfeld RG, Roberts CT (eds): Contemporary Endocrinology. The IGF System: Molecular Biology, Physiology, and Clinical Applications. Totowa, NJ, Humana, 1999, pp 699–720, with permission.

---

endocrine neoplasia type 1 (MEN1) gene location on chromosome 11, non–MEN1 patients with sporadic pituitary tumors and 11q LOH harbor intact coding and intronic sequences, with appropriately expressed MEN1 messenger RNA (mRNA).[56] Lesions in chromosomes 13 and 9 also are more prevalent in invasive or larger adenomas.[51] Chromosome 13q LOH occurs in proximity to the RB locus and was found in 13 aggressive pituitary tumors, whereas small circumscribed tumors exhibit intact RB alleles.[57] These results suggest the presence of putative tumor-suppressor genes located on chromosomes 11 and 13 that may be involved in controlling the propensity for pituitary tumor proliferation. Despite these heterogeneous chromosomal LOH patterns, consistent loss of tumor-suppressor gene activity has not been identified for acromegaly. Although tumor invasiveness or size correlates with an increased propensity for chromosomal LOH,[51] identification of a specific molecular lesion leading to loss of antiproliferative activity in GH-secreting tumors remains elusive[43] (see Table 23-3).

Activating Mutations

GTPase acts to inactivate stimulatory G (G_s) proteins that induce adenyl cyclase and intracellular cAMP accumulation.[58] Missense mutations replacing residue 201 (Arg $\rightarrow$ Cys or His) or 227 (Gln $\rightarrow$ Arg or Leu), termed *gsp*, result in persistently elevated ligand-independent G_s activity and constitutively elevated cAMP and GH hypersecretion.[44] *Gsp* mutations occur in a subset of GH adenomas, with a prevalence ranging from 30% to 40% in whites[58–63] to only 10% in Japanese[64] patients with acromegaly. Clinical or biochemical correlations have not been associated with *gsp* mutations.[44,65] Thus, although these mutational events suggest a compelling mechanism for explaining GH cell hypersecretion, their clinical significance has not been apparent (see Table 23-4), as the natural course of the disease does not differ in *gsp* +ve or -ve patients.

Rarely, *ras* mutations have been observed in highly invasive pituitary tumors or their extrapituitary metastases.[66–68] Development of true GH cell carcinoma with documented extracranial metastases, however, is exceedingly rare[67] (see Table 23-4). A pituitary tumor-transforming gene (PTTG) was isolated from rat GH-secreting pituitary tumor cells,[69] and is functionally homologous to yeast securing, which regulates sister chromatid separation during mitosis.[70] PTTG overexpression results in cell transformation in vitro and experimental tumor formation in vivo. The PTTG gene is located on chromosome 5q33, a region with a known propensity for development of several malignancies.[43] PTTG mRNA is abundant in GH-producing tumors, with more than 10-fold increases evident in larger tumors.[71] The strong transforming potential of PTTG, as well as its widespread and abundant expression in pituitary tumors, indicates a key role in early induction of GH cell transformation, possibly by regulating the pituitary cell cycle[70] (see Table 23-4).

Familial Syndromes

Acromegaly may occur as a component of MEN syndromes, including the Carney complex or MEN1. The Carney complex consists of myxomas; spotty skin pigmentation; and testicular, adrenal, and pituitary tumors.[72–75] About 20% of patients with this autosomal-dominant syndrome associated with chromosome 2p16 harbor GH-secreting pituitary tumors.[50,72]

The MEN1 gene is located on chromosome 11q13, and LOH of chromosome 11q13 occurs in pancreatic, parathyroid, and pituitary tumors of patients with MEN1.[56,76] Inactivation of the MEN1 tumor-suppressor gene likely accounts for the syndrome, in accordance with Knudson's "two hit" theory whereby both inherited allelic germ-line mutations and a somatic deletion are required for inactivation of both specific alleles and subsequent tumor formation.[77] MEN1, an

Table 23-4 Tumor-Suppressor Genes and Oncogenes Associated with GH Cell Adenomas

$G_{s\alpha}$	Protein	Defect	Function
Tumor-suppressor genes			
MEN1	Menin	Mutation or deletion	Nuclear; function unknown
P16INK4a	p16	Methylation	CDK4 inhibitor; loss of cell-cycle regulation
Oncogenes			
gsp (GNAS1)	$G_{s\alpha}$ subunit of G protein	Missense mutation at codon 201 or 227	Inactivates intrinsic GTPase; constitutive activation of adenyl cyclase
H-ras	Ras	Missense mutation at codon 12, 13, or 61	Constitutive activation; associated with metastases
Pttg	PTTG	Overexpression	Promotes transformation

GH, growth hormone; GTPase, guanosine triphosphatase; PTTG, pituitary tumor–transforming gene.
Adapted from Drange M, Melmed S: Etiopatogenia de la acromegalia. In Webb S (ed): Libro De La Acromegalia. Accion Medica, Barcelona, Spain, 1998, with permission.

autosomal-dominant syndrome, consists of hyperplastic or adenomatous parathyroid glands, endocrine pancreas, and anterior pituitary.[76] Pituitary adenomas develop in almost half these patients, with GH cell adenomas reported in about 10% of afflicted subjects.

Isolated familial acromegaly or gigantism not associated with MEN has rarely been reported.[50,78,79] Chromosome 11q13 LOH with no discernible MEN 1 mutation was detected in the pituitary adenomas of two brothers with gigantism.[80]

EPIDEMIOLOGY OF ACROMEGALY

Acromegaly is a rare disease, and accurate assessment of its prevalence in the community has been difficult to ascertain. In Newcastle, England, an annual incidence of 2.8 new patients per million adult population was reported, with an approximate point prevalence of 38 cases per million adult population.[81] A higher incidence was reported in Sweden, where the average prevalence of the disease was reported to be 69 cases per million.[2,82] If these data are projected to the population of the United States, 750 to 900 new cases would be expected annually, and GH-secreting pituitary adenomas would be present, but undiagnosed, in another 10,000 to 20,000 persons. The mean age at diagnosis is 40 to 45 years, and its insidious onset may cause the disease to not be diagnosed until 10 to 12 years after symptom onset.[82–84] This long delay in diagnosis is often due to the subtle and slow onset of common symptoms, including headache, joint pains, jaw malocclusion, or mild type 2 diabetes. Furthermore, this relatively long time delay allows prolonged exposure of peripheral tissues to unacceptably elevated GH and IGF-1 levels.

DIAGNOSIS

Persistent GH hypersecretion is the hallmark of acromegaly. Excess GH stimulates hepatic production of IGF-1, which is responsible for most of the clinical manifestations of acromegaly.[85–87] The diagnosis is often delayed for up to 12 years because of slow clinical progression over many years. Although serum GH and IGF-1 concentrations are both increased in virtually all patients with acromegaly, serum IGF-1 levels may be discordant with GH increases. When a patient is suspected to have acromegaly, biochemical testing is required to confirm the clinical diagnosis, and imaging techniques are used to localize the cause of excess GH secretion (Table 23-5).

DOCUMENTING GROWTH HORMONE HYPERSECRETION

The diagnosis of acromegaly is confirmed by measurement of serum GH after a glucose load and by assessing levels of GH-dependent circulating molecules such as IGF-1 and IGF-binding protein-3 (IGFBP-3).[29] IGF-1 levels reflect the integrated bioeffects of GH hypersecretion, and age- and gender-matched elevated IGF-1 levels are pathognomonic of acromegaly.[88]

Measurement of the serum IGF-1 concentration is the most precise screening test for acromegaly. Unlike those of GH, serum IGF-1 concentrations do not fluctuate hourly according to food intake, exercise, or sleep, but rather reflect integrated GH secretion during the preceding day or longer. Serum IGF-1 concentrations, which are gender and age dependent, are elevated in virtually all patients with acromegaly, thus providing excellent discrimination from subjects without acromegaly.[2,85] In normal subjects, serum IGF-1 concentrations are highest during puberty and decline gradually thereafter; values are significantly lower in adults older than 60 years than in younger subjects. Females have higher levels than do males, and pregnancy may also be associated with elevated IGF-1 levels. Thus, an inappropriately controlled "normal" IGF-1 value in an elderly male patient may in fact be truly elevated and indicative of acromegaly. Serum GH should be measured in patients with equivocal or elevated age- and sex-adjusted serum IGF-1 values.

Although all patients with acromegaly have increased GH secretion, it may be difficult to distinguish elevated random GH levels from normal. As GH levels fluctuate widely throughout the day and night, measuring random GH levels rarely provides useful information for diagnosis of the disorder.[2] Short-term fasting, exercise, stress, and sleep are associated with elevated GH, and the availability of ultrasensitive GH assays has indicated that this pulsatile GH rhythm may occur at levels below the detectable sensitivity of previously available assays. Serum GH concentrations fluctuate widely, from less than 0.5 ng/mL (with ultrasensitive assays) during most of the day, to as high as 20 or 30 ng/mL at night or after vigorous exercise. As random serum GH concentrations may be elevated in patients with uncontrolled diabetes mellitus, liver disease, and malnutrition, dynamic tests have been proposed to confirm pituitary GH hypersecretion. The mean GH concentration obtained from 6-hourly samplings will generally provide an integrated summation of net GH secretion,

Table 23-5 Diagnosis of Acromegaly

Biochemical testing
    GH nadir >1 ng/mL during oral glucose load
    Elevated age- and gender-matched IGF-1 level
MRI
    Visualization of pituitary adenoma

GH, growth hormone; IGF-1, insulin-like growth factor 1; MRI, magnetic resonance imaging.

and averaged pooled levels greater than 5 ng/mL are usually encountered in acromegaly.[2]

The diagnostic hallmark of excess GH hypersecretion is failure to suppress GH levels to 0.4 ng/mL or less (chemiluminescent; immunoradiometric assay) during a 2-hour period after a 75-g oral glucose load.[29] Stringent ultrasensitive GH assays should have a nadir cut-off of <0.4 ng/mL. Invariably, patients who fail to suppress GH after glucose exhibit elevated total IGF-1 levels with a strong log-linear association between the 24-hour mean GH output and IGF-1 levels.[2,89] About 10% or fewer of patients may have apparently "normal" GH or IGF-1 levels or both at the time of diagnosis. Repeating the assays in a reputable laboratory may often resolve an apparent clinical-biochemical discordance. Alternatively, reinterpretation of a glucose suppression test or use of a rigorous GH assay may confirm the diagnosis.

About 60% of patients with acromegaly also exhibit an evoked GH response (>50%) to thyrotropin-releasing hormone (TRH; 500 μg given intravenously) or, less commonly, to gonadotropin-releasing hormone administration. These discordant responses are seen only in patients with tumorous GH hypersecretion and not in normal subjects. Conversely, levodopa (500 mg orally) reduces serum GH concentrations by 50% or more in about half of patients with acromegaly, whereas the drug increases GH levels in normal subjects.[2]

Because IGFBP-3 secretion is GH dependent, concentrations may be elevated in patients with acromegaly, thus suggesting that IGFBP-3 measurement may prove useful in diagnosis.[90] However, in contrast to the tight correlation of integrated mean 24-hour serum GH with total and free IGF-1 levels, IGFBP-3 levels do not correlate as tightly with disease activity.[91,92] Thirty-two percent of subjects with active acromegaly had normal IGFBP-3 levels, and in patients who failed to suppress GH, no consistent elevation of IGFBP-3 was observed.[91] Thus, the utility of IGFBP-3 measurements for acromegaly diagnosis or follow-up is limited.

LOCALIZING THE SOURCE OF EXCESS GROWTH HORMONE

Once a biochemical diagnosis of GH hypersecretion is confirmed, MRI of the pituitary to localize the source of hormone excess is indicated. MRI effectively delineates soft tissue pituitary masses, and gadolinium-enhanced MRI may detect adenomas 2 mm in diameter. In about 75% of patients, the tumor is a macroadenoma (tumor diameter of ≥10 mm) and may extend to parasellar or suprasellar regions or invade the cavernous sinus. More than 90% of patients exhibit a discrete

pituitary adenoma on MRI, whereas about 10% of patients may harbor a partial or even apparently total empty sella. Functional GH-secreting adenomas may arise in the remnant rim of pituitary tissue surrounding the empty sella and may not be visible on MRI. Rarely, other nonpituitary causes of acromegaly (see earlier) will require abdominal or chest imaging to localize the source of ectopic GHRH or, more rarely, GH production. Lateral skull radiographs with sellar coned-down tomography or pituitary computed tomographic scans are not usually indicated because they expose patients to unnecessary ionizing radiation and, when compared with MRI techniques, are insensitive, especially in delineating soft tissue changes.

Nonpituitary Acromegaly

Rare nonpituitary causes of acromegaly include a hypothalamic tumor secreting GHRH,[33,93] a nonendocrine tumor secreting GHRH,[36,94] or ectopic GH secretion by a nonendocrine tumor.[1,31,32] MRI of the head and pituitary should identify some of these tumors. If pituitary MRI findings are normal, abdominal and chest imaging should be performed, followed by catheterization studies in an attempt to demonstrate an arteriovenous GHRH gradient over the suspected tumor bed. In patients with ectopic GHRH secretion, serum GHRH and GH concentrations are both elevated, and pituitary MRI reveals a normal-sized or enlarged hyperplastic gland.[95]

An algorithm for the diagnostic evaluation of patients suspected of having acromegaly is shown in Figure 23-1. A normal age- and gender-controlled serum IGF-1 concentration is strong evidence excluding the diagnosis of acromegaly. If the serum IGF-1 concentration is high (or equivocal), serum GH should be measured within 2 hours after oral glucose administration. If pituitary MRI fails to reveal the presence of a discrete adenoma in the presence of clear-cut biochemical evidence of hypersomatotropism, studies to identify the rarely encountered GHRH- or GH-secreting tumors should be undertaken.

CLINICAL MANIFESTATIONS

The somatotroph adenoma itself, especially if a macroadenoma, may cause local symptoms such as headache, visual field defects (classically bitemporal hemianopia), and cranial nerve palsies. These compressive features are not unique to acromegaly and may occur with any enlarging sellar mass. Nevertheless, the headache associated with acromegaly is uniquely debilitating and may not be exclusively caused by pressure effects.

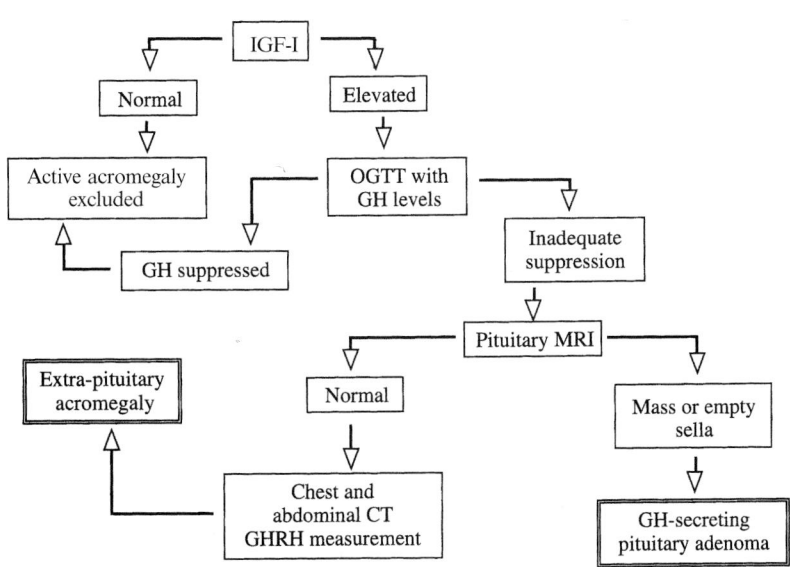

Figure 23-1 Diagnosis of acromegaly. CT, computed tomography; GH, growth hormone; GHRH, growth hormone–releasing hormone; IGF-1, insulin-like growth factor 1; MRI, magnetic resonance imaging; OGTT, oral glucose tolerance test. (Adapted from Melmed S, Kleinberg DL: Anterior pituitary. In Larsen R, Kronenberg H, Melmed S, Polonsky K [eds]: Williams Textbook of Endocrinology, 10th ed., Philadelphia, Saunders, 2003, pp. 177–280, with permission.)

The systemic clinical features of acromegaly occur as a consequence of the deleterious impact of elevated serum concentrations of both GH and IFG-1 on peripheral tissues (Table 23-6). The somatic impact of elevated GH includes growth stimulation of a variety of tissues, such as skin, connective tissue, cartilage, bone, and many epithelial tissues, including mucosal surfaces. The metabolic effects of excess GH include nitrogen retention, insulin antagonism, and enhanced lipogenesis.

The onset of acromegaly is insidious, and disease progression usually slow. At diagnosis, about 75% of patients are shown to harbor macroadenomas (tumor diameter of ≥10 mm), and some tumors extend to the parasellar or suprasellar regions.[15] Headaches are the initial symptoms in approximately 60% of patients, and 10% have visual symptoms.

Acral Overgrowth

Acral and soft-tissue overgrowth is invariably a feature of acromegaly. Characteristic findings include an enlarged protruding jaw (macrognathia) with associated mandibular overbite and enlarged, swollen hands and feet, resulting in increasing shoe and glove size and the need to enlarge rings. Facial features are coarse, with enlargement of the nose and frontal bones, as well as the jaw; the upper incisors are consequently spread apart. Despite the prominence of these findings, the rate of change is so slow that few patients seek care because their appearance has changed (e.g., only 13% of 256 patients in one series[5]).

Table 23-6	Risks of Long-Term Exposure to Elevated Growth Hormone Levels

Arthropathy
  Unrelated to age at onset or to GH levels
  Usually occurs with acromegaly of long duration
  Reversibility
    Rapid symptomatic improvement with treatment
    Irreversibility of bone and cartilage lesions
Neuropathy
  Peripheral nerves affected
    Intermittent anesthesias, paresthesias
    Sensorimotor polyneuropathy
    Impaired sensation
  Reversibility
    Onion bulbs (whorls) do not regress with lowered GH levels
Cardiovascular disease
  Cardiomyopathy
    Left ventricular diastolic function decreased
    Left ventricular mass increased; arrhythmias
    Fibrous hyperplasia of connective tissue
  Hypertension
    Exacerbates cardiomyopathic changes
  Reversibility
    May progress even with normalized GH levels
Respiratory disease
  Upper airway obstruction
    Caused by soft-tissue overgrowth and decreased pharyngeal
      muscle tone
  Reversibility
    Improved with reduction of GH levels
Malignancy
  Increased risk of malignancy
  Increased soft-tissue polyps
  Reversibility
    Effect of therapy on risk of malignancy unknown
Carbohydrate intolerance
  Occurs in one fourth of acromegalics, more often with family
    history of diabetes mellitus
  Reversibility
    Improves with reduced GH levels

GH, growth hormone.
From Melmed S, Dowling RH, Frohman L, et al: Acromegaly: Consensus for cure. Am J Med 97:468, 1994, with permission.

Rheumatologic Features

Musculoskeletal symptoms are leading causes of morbidity and serious functional disability in patients with acromegaly.[96,97] In several studies encompassing large series, at least half of all patients exhibited minor arthralgias, and severe, debilitating arthritic features ultimately developed in more than one third of patients.[97,98] The pathogenesis of joint disease in acromegaly generally begins with a noninflammatory osteoarthritic disorder and culminates in severe secondary joint and cartilage degeneration.[97] Excess GH and IGF-1 exposure leads to uneven cartilage proliferation that results in a mechanically unstable joint surface. Joint spaces then narrow as weight-bearing surfaces erode cartilage and cause excess intra-articular new fibrocartilage deposits. Subchondral cysts and osteophytes then develop in an irreversible self-perpetuating process. Severe physical deformity and functional disability result from these inexorable pathologic and mechanical stresses. Although symptomatic and functional relief of arthritic disorders is observed in most patients after reducing GH levels, structural changes are unfortunately not reversible.[98,99]

Joint arthralgias are a common initial feature of the disease, and back pain and kyphosis are common.[5] Synovial tissue and cartilage enlarge and cause hypertrophic arthropathy of the knees, ankles, hips, spine, and other joints.[97] Back pain also may occur because of osteoporosis caused either by GH excess itself or concurrent gonadal insufficiency from the enlarging pituitary tumor. Spine and hip bone density may be increased in women with acromegaly, but not if estrogen deficiency is present.[100] When excess GH secretion begins before epiphyseal fusion, linear growth increases and causes pituitary gigantism.

Skin and Soft Tissues

The skin thickens, and multiple recurrent skin tags may appear.[3,101] Hyperhidrosis at rest is common (present in 50% of patients)[2,3,5] and often malodorous. Hair growth increases, and some women have hirsutism.[2,5,102] Other manifestations of soft tissue overgrowth include macroglossia, deepening of the voice, and paresthesias of the hands (carpal tunnel syndrome) from nerve entrapment.[2,5–7,15,98] Other patients have a symmetric sensorimotor peripheral (rarely hypertrophic) neuropathy unrelated to entrapment.[96]

Thyroid

Thyroid enlargement may be diffuse or multinodular. In a study of 37 patients with acromegaly, 92% had an enlarged thyroid gland when assessed with ultrasound; mean thyroid size was increased more than 5 times normal.[103] Thyroid function is, however, usually normal.

Cardiovascular

Impaired cardiovascular function in acromegaly is an important determinant of morbidity and mortality.[3,104] The deleterious direct impact of excess GH and IGF-1, as well as the effect of hypertension, which is present in 30% of patients, contributes to the disorder.[5,105,106] Cardiac enlargement is disproportionate to the increased size of internal body organs,[107–109] and the severity of cardiomyopathy correlates significantly with the duration of exposure to hypersomatotropism.[104,108,110] Mean left ventricular mass may be significantly increased to more than 200 g, as opposed to a normal mean weight of 140 g, and end-systolic and diastolic volumes are attenuated. Concentric ventricular hypertrophy is associated with interstitial fibrosis, lymphocytic infiltration, and necrosis.[108] Resting diastolic blood pressure and left and right ventricular peak filling rates are elevated. Postexercise systolic and diastolic blood pressure may also be elevated, and the left ventricular ejection fraction is attenuated.[111] Because physiologic doses of replacement GH also may actually improve cardiac function in patients with adult GH deficiency, a fine equilibrium may exist for the respective impacts of GH excess and GH deficiency on maintaining healthy myocardial function.[108]

Sleep Apnea

Peripheral airway obstruction caused by macroglossia, mandible deformation, mucosal hypertrophy, and inspirational laryngeal collapse has long been recognized as causing airway obstruction,[5] snoring, and sleep apnea in up to two thirds of patients.[3] Macroglossia and enlargement of the soft tissues of the pharynx and larynx lead to obstructive sleep apnea in about 50% of patients; others have central sleep apnea, possibly resulting from altered central respiratory control.[112] Sleep apnea may be an important cause of mortality in these patients. Recently, a central form of sleep apnea was recognized in acromegaly.[112–114] This disorder appears to correlate more closely with elevated GH and IGF-1 levels and may reflect central respiratory suppression caused by the dysregulated hypothalamic-GH axis. Clearly, the strong association of sleep apnea with hypertension, coronary artery disease, and cardiac arrest also reflects the clinical phenotype of patients with acromegaly. Attenuation of GH levels, especially with octreotide, improves or abrogates sleep apnea.[112,115] After 6 months of treatment of 14 apneic acromegalic patients with octreotide, a 40% decrease in the number of apneic events per hour was seen, as well as a decrease in total apneic time from 28% to 15%. Maximum O_2 saturation rose from 76% to 84%, accompanied by a decline in daytime sleepiness, as well as improvement in central and obstructive apneic parameters.[112]

Diabetes

GH is a potent antagonist of insulin action, and glucose intolerance is encountered in up to 60% of patients. About 25% of patients may require insulin, and thus diabetes is an important systemic complication of hypersomatotropism. Diabetes is a major determinant of mortality, and only 30% of patients with diabetes at the time that acromegaly is diagnosed appear to survive 20 years.[83,116]

Gonadal Function

Women with acromegaly may have amenorrhea, with or without galactorrhea,[3,15,117] and some have hot flashes and vaginal atrophy. Men may have impotence, loss of libido, decreased facial hair growth, and testicular atrophy.[3,7,117] Hypogonadism is caused either by hyperprolactinemia (present in about 30% of patients)[102,117] or by impairment of gonadotropin secretion as the expanding pituitary tumor compresses normal pituitary gonadotroph cells. Asymptomatic reversible prostatic enlargement also is common, even in men with hypogonadism.[118,119]

Neoplasms

Acromegaly is associated with an enhanced risk for development of colonic polyps and [120–122] Prospective studies have reported premalignant adenomatous colonic polyps in up to 30% of patients, a prevalence not different from that in the general U.S. population.[122–124] Patients with acromegaly are more likely to have multiple adenomatous polyps, as well as polyps proximal to the splenic flexure, underscoring the need for full-length colonoscopy.[121,125] No difference in the duration or degree of acromegaly is evident in patients with or without adenomatous polyps. A multicenter retrospective study of 1362 patients with acromegaly found a lower cancer rate than in the general population (standardized incidence ratio of 0.76) but an increased colon cancer mortality rate.[126,127] The enhanced mortality correlated with persistently elevated serum GH concentrations but was not observed in patients with posttreatment serum GH levels less than 2.5 ng/mL.[128,129] Colonoscopy is therefore recommended at diagnosis for all patients and periodically thereafter. From the published literature, it appears that elevated GH/IGF-1 levels do not appreciably induce malignancies in patients with acromegaly. However, uncontrolled GH levels may act permissively to enhance morbidity and mortality from colon cancer. These findings underscore the requirement for tight GH control in these patients.

LABORATORY FINDINGS

Patients with acromegaly exhibit increased serum GH and IGF-1 concentrations and may have hyperglycemia, with frank diabetes occurring in 25% of patients. Some patients have hypertriglyceridemia. Hypercalciuria and hyperphosphatemia (not >5.5 mg/dL) occur in approximately 70% of patients as a result of direct stimulation of renal tubular phosphate reabsorption by IGF-1.[102]

Hyperprolactinemia occurs in about 30% of patients and is due to cosecretion of PRL and GH by the tumor or to stalk interference with hypothalamic-pituitary portal delivery of dopamine. Secretion of other pituitary hormones, especially gonadotropins, also may be decreased. Elevated plasma fibrinogen concentrations revert to normal with therapy, which suggests that effective treatment of acromegaly may prevent cardiovascular morbidity.[130]

MORTALITY

The overall mortality rate in acromegaly is about 2 to 4 times that of the general population.[126,129,131,132] Up to 50% of patients die before age 50 years, and up to 89% die before age 60 years.[2,133] In a series of 151 patients, survival was reduced an average of 10 years in comparison to age-matched controls.[83]

Although mortality and morbidity in acromegaly are significantly correlated with cardiovascular, pulmonary, and neoplastic disorders, the single most significant determinant of survival is the level of posttreatment GH[83] (Table 23-7). Several retrospective studies now indicate that survival in acromegaly may be normalized to a control age-matched rate by controlling GH levels[128,129]; in particular, life-table analysis showed that GH levels less than 2.5 ng/mL were associated with survival rates equal to those of the general population.[126,132,134] A recent postoperative follow-up of 53 patients for a mean of 12.7 years indicated that a normal IGF-1 level and GH nadir cutoff of less than 0.25 µg/L are associated with improved blood pressure control and glucose tolerance.[84] Thus, tight control of GH through aggressive multimodal therapy appears to reduce mortality risk to that expected for nonacromegalic subjects.[84,128,129] Less clarity exists on the predictive value of IGF-1 levels as mortality determinants,[126,131,132] and further prospective studies are awaited. In particular, the role of radiotherapy in adversely skewing mortality outcomes will have to be excluded from these evaluations.

Table 23-7 Outcome Determinants of Acromegaly

Causes of Death	%	Survival Determinants	P Value
Cardiovascular	38–62	Last known GH	0.0001
Respiratory	0–25	Hypertension	0.02
Malignancy	9–25	Cardiac disease	0.03
		Diabetes	0.03
		Symptom duration	0.04

Elevated mortality is reversed by suppressing growth hormone (GH). Data from Wright, 1969; Alexander et al., 1980; Nabarro, 1987; Bengtsson et al., 1988; Rajasoorya, 1994; Bates, 1994; Swearingen et al., 1998; Abosch et al., 1998; and Freda et al., 1998, with permission.

MANAGEMENT

TREATMENT GOALS FOR ACROMEGALY

Treatment goals for acromegaly embody principles that apply to treating hormonal hypersecretory tumors (Table 23-8). Treatment should be both safe and efficacious. GH and IGF-1 levels should be normalized, especially because elevated GH levels have been associated with mortality in these patients. Thus, tight GH control is an important therapeutic end point.[84] Tumor mass effects, especially central compression of visual tracts, should be alleviated. Importantly, the integrity of pituitary function should be preserved, and if hypopituitarism develops, patients require life-long pituitary replacement. Clinical features of the disease that lead to the characteristic morbidity and ultimately to mortality should be ameliorated. Several treatment options are available for acromegaly. Transsphenoidal surgical resection of the adenoma, pharmacologic therapy with somatostatin analogues (Table 23-9), dopamine agonists and a GH-receptor antagonist, and various modes of radiation therapy are used to treat GH-secreting adenomas. The challenge of tight GH control in acromegaly can now be met with greater stringency by using single or multimodal forms of therapy. Effective disease control should thus include sustained hormone suppression, a contained adenoma mass, improved systemic morbidity, and ultimately, normalized mortality (Tables 23-8 through 23-10).

SURGERY

Surgery for the treatment of GH-secreting pituitary tumors was pioneered in the early part of the century by Dr. Harvey Cushing, who demonstrated successful resection of such tumors by a transsphenoidal approach. This technique is standard, and only very rarely do large masses that extend far beyond the sella turcica require a transfrontal approach. The most important determinant of a successful surgical outcome is the experience of the surgeon. Recently, endoscopic approaches to pituitary adenoma resection have proved to be efficacious.[135,136]

Surgery rapidly alleviates acromegaly symptoms, removes the tumor mass, relieves optic tract pressure effects, and relieves headache. Tumor debulking, even if partial, also may be helpful in enhancing the effectiveness of subsequent therapy. Surgical control also is inversely correlated with initial tumor size and GH levels.[137,138] Not all patients are appropriate surgical candidates, usually because of coexisting cardiovascular and pulmonary disease, which may be a contraindication to anesthesia. If the tumor is sufficiently large or invasive and portends intraoperative damage to vital structures, the benefits of the procedure should be weighed against surgical risks.

Results of surgical resection of GH-secreting adenomas have only recently included more stringent biochemical criteria. Short-term remission (GH, 5 µg/L) was achieved in 76% of 254 patients, with most of 129 patients remaining in

Table 23-8 Treatment Goals for Acromegaly

Reduce IGF-1 level to age- and gender-matched normal
Control GH hypersecretion
   Serum GH should be <1 ng/mL during OGTT
Relieve symptoms and signs of acromegaly and prevent comorbidities and early death
Remove, reduce, or control tumor mass
Preserve pituitary function

IGF, insulin-like growth factor; GH, growth hormone, OGTT, oral glucose tolerance test.

Table 23-9 Long-acting Somatostatin Analogues

Drug	Frequency of Administration	Route of Administration	Needle Size
Oct LAR*	4 wks	IM	19 gauge
LAN 30 SR	7, 10, or 14 days	IM	Thin-walled 18 gauge
LAN 60 SR	21 or 28 days	IM	Thin-walled 18 gauge
Autogel 60, 90, 120 mg	28 days or longer	Deep SC	12-gauge trocar

LAR, long-acting release; LAN, lanreotide.
*Available in the United States.

long-term remission.[129] Although the biochemical parameter of "basal" GH less than 5 µg/L used in this study does not reflect normalization of GH hypersecretion, even with this less stringent criterion, the postsurgical mortality outcome was equivalent to that of age- and sex-matched controls, in contrast to the 2.4- to 4.8-fold enhanced mortality observed in patients with persistent disease (GH, >5 µg/L). Using more stringent criteria (normalized IGF-1 levels or GH suppression to ≥2 µg/L after glucose loading), more than 90% of patients with microadenomas successfully achieved control.[128,139,140] Unfortunately, most tumors encountered at diagnosis are large macroadenomas, and fewer than 50% of patients with macroadenomas are biochemically controlled.[128,138,139] In these invasive tumors, surgical resection is invariably followed by persistent GH and or IGF-1 hypersecretion. Visible residual tumor mass is often contiguous with or involves the cavernous sinus, internal carotid arteries, or suprasellar regions. Mortality risk in patients cured at surgery does not differ from that of controls, whereas in patients with persistent disease, even after adjuvant irradiation or medical therapy, mortality remains significantly increased (almost twofold). Thus, the level of GH attained postsurgically is the most important determinant of mortality outcome.[83] However, regardless of the treatment mode, normalization of GH restores mortality risk to that of age-matched population controls, and postoperative disease persistence is associated with a 3.5-fold relative mortality risk.[126,128,132]

Transnasal endoscopy[135,136] appears to offer a more facile tumor access and lower complication rates. Long-term outcomes are awaited to assess the efficacy of this approach.

Side Effects

The most important adverse surgical event is failure to resect invasive tumor totally and, consequently, persistent hormonal hypersecretion. Postoperative complications occur in approximately 10% of patients, and their incidence is largely dependent on the experience of the operating surgeon.[138,141] Complications include permanent diabetes insipidus, cerebrospinal fluid leaks requiring repair, meningitis, severe sinusitis, and hypopituitarism.[82,133,139–141] Perioperative morbidity and residual pituitary failure remain of concern in patients with invasive tumors, especially when operated on by less experienced surgeons.

In summary, surgical success is based largely on skill and experience and on tumor size or invasiveness. Surgery is useful for prompt reduction of GH levels, and tumor debulking may enhance the effectiveness of medical therapy. After apparent successful resection, however, up to 8% of tumors recur within 10 years. GH levels should be measured in the immediate postoperative period, and evidence of GH hypersecretion at this time portends either disease persistence or long-term recurrence. Overall, by immunoradiometric GH assay, postglucose GH values less than 1.0 µg/L are found in 50% of patients after surgery, and in 39% of patients

Table 23-10 Treatment Options for Acromegaly

Surgery	Somatostatin Analogue	Radiotherapy	Dopamine Agonists (High Dose)	GH-receptor Antagonist
EFFICACY				
Microsurgery GH controlled in 80%	GH controlled in ~65% of patients within weeks	GH <5 ng/mL in 90% of patients in 18 yr	GH <5 ng/mL in 15%	IGF-1 normalized in >95% GH elevated (inactive)
Macrosurgery GH controlled in <50%				
Normal IGF-1 in ~50%	Normal IGF-1 in ~70%	Normal IGF-1 in <5%	Normal IGF-1 in <10%	
ADVANTAGES				
Rapid onset	No hypopituitarism	Permanent	Oral administration	No hypopituitarism
One-time cost	Rapid onset	One-time cost	Low cost	Rapid onset
May be permanent	Continued efficacy	Good patient compliance	No hypopituitarism	Continued efficacy
DISADVANTAGES				
New hypopituitarism (10%)	Cost of drug and monitoring	Ineffective and slow onset	Relatively ineffective	Cost of drug and monitoring
	Asymptomatic gallstones (25%)	Hypopituitarism (50%)	Adverse events (~30%)	Daily injections
Diabetes insipidus (2–3%)	Monthy injections required	Visual/CNS dysfunction (~2%)	High dose required	Tumor growth not controlled
Local complications (~6%)	Gastrointestinal side effects	Cost of interim medical therapy		
				Elevated liver function tests (rare)
Cranial nerve/CNS damage (~1%)				GH deficiency (if overtreated)
Tumor persistence				

CNS, central nervous system; GH, growth hormone; IGF-1, insulin-like growth factor.
Adapted from Melmed S, Jackson I, Kleinberg D, et al: Current treatment guidelines for acromegaly. J Clin Endocrinol Metab 83:2646–2652, 1998, with permission.

with normalized IGF-1 levels, GH levels still fail to be suppressed.[142]

PITUITARY IRRADIATION

Techniques for pituitary radiotherapy include external radiation with either a cyclotron or a cobalt-60 source, and the radiotherapy is administered as a total dose of 4500 to 5000 rad. Higher doses are associated with a high incidence of side effects, whereas lower doses, although safer, appear to be less clinically effective. The total dose is given as 25 daily 180- to 200-rad fractions administered over a 6-week period.[143] Maximal tumor irradiation with minimal damage to nontumorous surrounding tissue has been achieved by advances in stereotactic MRI-directed tumor localization, focused beam direction, field size simulation, head immobilization, and isocentral rotational techniques.[144]

Proton-beam therapy also decreases GH secretion but is not widely available. Stereotactic ablation of GH-secreting adenomas by gamma knife radiosurgery is a promising new technique for which long-term results are not yet available. In 16 postsurgical patients monitored for up to 2.6 years, GH levels of less than 5 ng/mL and normalized IGF-1 concentrations were observed within 16 months of stereotactic radiosurgery.[145] However, the short follow-up precludes an assessment of complication outcome.

Tumor growth is invariably arrested after fractionated radiotherapy, but GH decline is slow, decreasing by approximately 20% per year. Within 18 years, 90% of patients have random serum GH concentrations lower than 5 ng/mL.[143] The degree and rapidity of GH attenuation are highly dependent on pretreatment GH levels.[143] However, few patients achieve the currently accepted rigorous goal of therapy, that is, a glucose-suppressed serum GH concentration less than 1 ng/mL. In one series, only 5 of 30 patients monitored for 10 or more years achieved this goal. After radiotherapy in 38 patients,

20 of whom had preradiotherapy IGF-1 data available, GH levels decreased by about 60% 3.5 years after irradiation and by about 80% 7 years after radiotherapy. However, plasma levels of IGF-1 remained almost unchanged and did not decrease to less than 80% of the initial value, even 7 years after radiotherapy. Only two patients ultimately exhibited normalized IGF levels.[146] The failure of irradiation to normalize IGF-1 levels effectively in the long term implies persistent, albeit low levels of GH hypersecretion in these patients. Subsequent studies have demonstrated improved efficacy, and longer-term outcomes are awaited.[146]

Side Effects

Pituitary failure develops in 50% of patients undergoing deep x-ray therapy by 10 years and require thyroid, gonadal, or adrenal steroid replacement or a combination of these.[1,29] Rarely, optic tract damage results in visual deficits. Ten years after radiotherapy, patients have a small but significant risk of a secondary brain malignancy, including glioma, in up to 1.7% of patients (relative risk of 16 vs. expected).[147–149] Radiation also may rarely induce brain parenchymal changes[149–151] and brain dysfunction manifested as depression, decreased memory, decreased general quality of life, loss of vision, and cranial nerve palsies.[141,152] Long-term controlled results and side effect profiles for gamma knife radiosurgery are not yet available, but a recent follow-up has been promising, indicating fewer local side effects, with no visual deficits reported in 30 patients for up to 4 years.[145]

Thus, radiotherapy is effective in acromegaly, although its benefits are dose and time dependent, and GH reduction is delayed by 10 to 15 years. Even with the most accurate techniques, GH levels less than 2.0 ng/mL and normalization of IGF-1 levels are infrequently achieved.[146,153] Therefore, radiation therapy may be useful for patients with growing pituitary tumors whose condition is not controlled by surgery or who are resistant to medical therapy.

MEDICAL MANAGEMENT

Octreotide

Octreotide is a synthetic octapeptide analogue of native naturally occurring somatostatin. This 8-amino acid analogue (molecular weight of 1019) binds selectively to the SSTR2 somatostatin receptor subtype.[154] After subcutaneous injection, octreotide is rapidly absorbed, and peak drug concentrations (5.5 ng/mL) are achieved within 24 minutes of a 100-μg injection. The plasma distribution is about 12 minutes, and the elimination half-life is 1.5 hours, as compared with 2 minutes for natural SRIF.[154,155] The drug inhibits pituitary GH secretion, also directly suppresses hepatic IGF-1 production,[156] controls tumor growth, and relieves soft tissue symptoms.

Octreotide inhibits GH, glucagon, and insulin release, but the analogue exhibits greater selectivity in suppressing GH and glucagon than does somatostatin.[154] In normal subjects, octreotide attenuates GH stimulation evoked by arginine,[156] exercise, and insulin-induced hypoglycemia.[157,158] The drug also may abrogate the postprandial release of gastrointestinal and pancreatic peptides.[158] Because native somatostatin suppresses thyroid-stimulating hormone (TSH) secretion, it is not surprising that octreotide also blocks the TRH-induced release of TSH.[156,158,159] In acromegaly, octreotide reduces GH levels (by >50%) in more than 95% of all patients.

In the long term, about 70% of patients will have integrated GH levels suppressed to less than 5 ng/mL, and about 55% of patients have GH levels suppressed to less than 2 ng/mL. Seventy percent or more of patients will have their IGF-1 levels normalized after long-term treatment with octreotide (Fig. 23-2). Hypopituitarism will not develop while the patient is taking octreotide because octreotide binds selectively to the somatostatin-receptor subtype that regulates GH secretion.[160] In addition to its effects on suppressing GH and IGF-1 levels, headache, fatigue, perspiration, joint pains, carpal tunnel syndrome, and paresthesias improve in most patients treated over the long term.

The starting dose of subcutaneous octreotide is 50 μg given subcutaneously in 8-hourly doses, and after 2 weeks, the dose can be increased to 100 μg 3 times daily. Thereafter, dose titrations to a maximum of 1500 μg/day may be made, depending on the nadir 2-hour postinjection GH level. The efficacy of octreotide also can be improved by increasing the dose frequency, although not necessarily increasing the total daily drug dose, or by administering the drug in a continuous-infusion minipump. Interestingly, long-term (>3 years) use of the drug is associated with enhanced sensitivity and improved biochemical control. Tachyphylaxis does not occur, and downregulation of receptor responses does not appear to be manifested clinically.[159] About half of all patients will exhibit tumor shrinkage (30% average tumor volume change).

Growth Hormone Response to Long-term Depot Preparations

Long-term depot somatostatin preparations include octreotide LAR (long-acting release) (approved in the United States) and, in Europe, lanreotide and autogel.[155,159,161,162] Octreotide LAR incorporates octreotide into microspheres of a biodegradable poly-D,L-lactide-co-glycolide glucose polymer. After 3-monthly injections of the depot preparation, sustained octreotide concentrations are maintained. Autogel is a water-soluble compound, allowing deep subcutaneous slow release of lanreotide.

Figure 23-3 depicts the pharmacokinetic response to octreotide LAR in acromegaly. After a single injection of octreotide LAR, drug levels peak at about 28 days after injection and decrease slowly thereafter. GH levels decline after the injection and, by day 14, are suppressed to less than 2 μg/L. GH suppression (as determined by measurement of integrated secretion over a 4-hour period) is sustained through day 49 and starts increasing thereafter. From the pharmacokinetic curve, it is apparent that a single injection administered every 30 days will allow GH levels to be persistently suppressed throughout the month. Figure 23-4 depicts the effects of a single, monthly injection of octreotide LAR in a group of patients with acromegaly whose average GH levels were suppressed for the duration of the study (≤54 months).

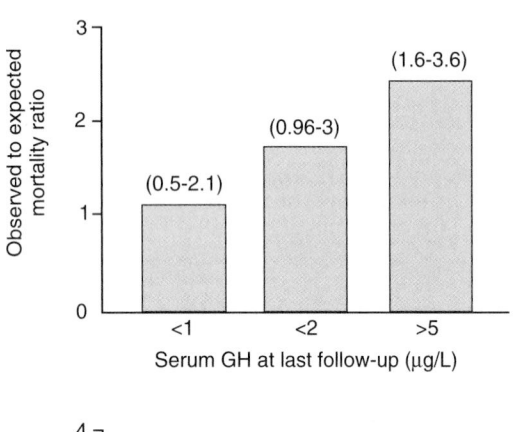

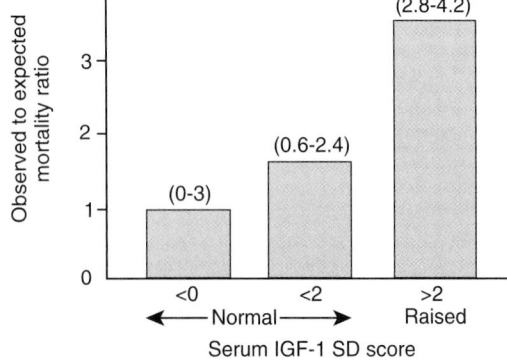

Figure 23-2 Growth hormone and insulin-like growth hormone-1 levels as mortality determinants. (From Holdaway IM, Rajasoorja RC, Gamble GD: Factors influencing mortality in acromegaly. J Clin Endcrinol Metab 89:667–674, 2004, with permission.)

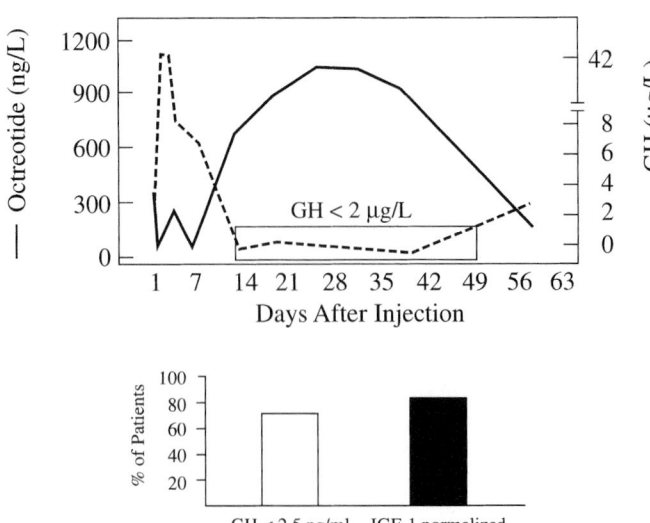

Figure 23-3 Pharmacokinetics of octreotide, long-acting release (LAR). GH, growth hormone; IGF-1, insulin-like growth factor 1.

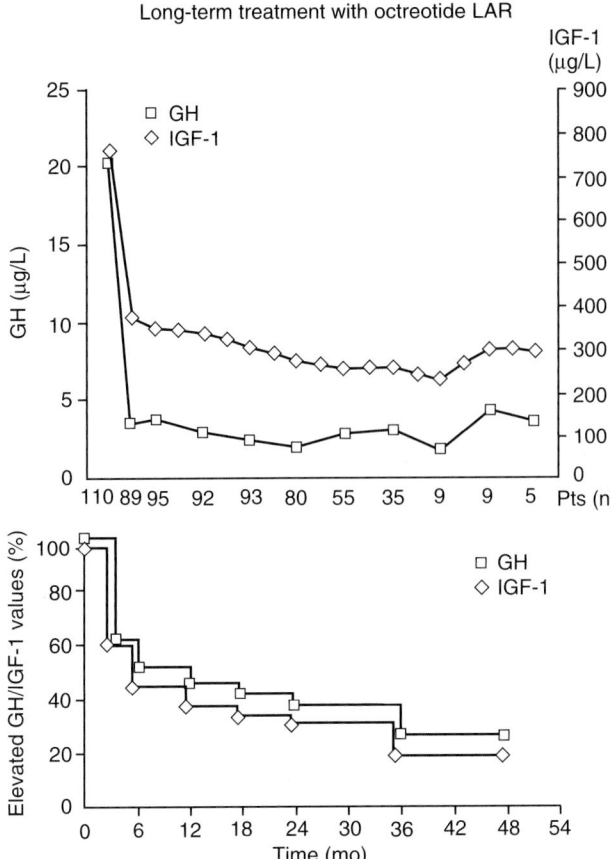

Figure 23-4 Long-term treatment with octreotide, long-acting release. (From Cozzi R, Attanasio R, Montini M, et al: Four-year treatment with octreotide-long-acting repeatable in 110 acromegalic patients: predictive value of short-term results? J Clin Endocrinol Metab 88:3090–3098, 2003, with permission.)

GH suppression appears to be sustained as long as patients receive monthly injections of octreotide LAR. About 80% of a total of 110 patients had IGF-1 levels normalized and GH suppressed to less than 2.5 ng/mL within 36 months.[155]

Clinical improvement is sustained, with little systemic or local intolerance. Thus, administration of octreotide LAR results in persistent therapeutic serum drug concentrations and sustained suppression of both GH and IGF-1 values. The incidence of gallstones, microlithiasis, biliary sediment, or biliary sludge does not differ from that after subcutaneous octreotide (see later).

Side Effects
Although octreotide is relatively safe in the long term, several important adverse events are reported. Asymptomatic echogenic gallbladder lesions develop in about 25% of patients.[29] These lesions include both sludge and gallstones, which are usually diagnosed within the first 2 years of treatment, with few if any new echogenic events encountered thereafter. The prevalence of gallstones during octreotide therapy appears to vary geographically. In China, gallstones will ultimately develop in most patients taking octreotide[163]; conversely, patients in southern Europe exhibit a far lower incidence. Clearly, dietary and/or other environmental factors play a role in their pathogenesis. Transient gastrointestinal symptoms, including anorexia, nausea, vomiting, flatulence, and loose stools, may occur, especially during the first 2 weeks of therapy; these symptoms may be ameliorated by injecting the medication between meals or at night. Rarely, fat malabsorption and bradycardia have been reported.

In summary, long-acting somatostatin analogues are effective and safe in managing GH hypersecretion in patients in whom surgical resection has failed to achieve a stringent biochemical remission. Somatostatin analogues also may be offered as primary therapy for patients who refuse surgery, have medical risk factors that contraindicate surgery, or have undergone irradiation, in whom GH levels may remain unacceptably elevated.[29,164] Most patients with macroadenomas have persistent postsurgical GH hypersecretion, and the use of SRIF analogues should be weighed against radiotherapy for these patients. Long-acting injectable depot analogues administered once every 14 to 30 days provide enhanced patient convenience and compliance while retaining drug sensitivity.[84,165,166] Prior surgery appears not to alter the long-term efficacy of somatostatin analogues in attaining biochemical control. However, drug cost and patient compliance must be factored in when deciding on therapeutic options.

DOPAMINE AGONISTS

High doses of dopamine agonists have been used for several years in the management of these patients, and bromocriptine is associated with GH normalization in fewer than 15% of patients.[167] A large meta-analysis revealed that only 20% of patients will achieve GH levels less than 5 ng/mL, which is not a maximal criterion for control. Only 10% or fewer of all patients will actually have IGF-1 levels normalized. However, bromocriptine does not carry with it a risk for hypopituitarism, and because it is an orally available medication, it is extremely convenient and cost effective for the patient.[168] Cabergoline, a long-acting dopamine agonist, has been used in acromegaly, but the long-term results are not yet compelling.[168–170]

Adverse Events
Because high doses (>20 mg/day) are required to achieve even moderate efficacy, the incidence of adverse events is far higher than usually seen when treating patients with prolactinomas. Patients receiving high doses of dopamine agonists complain of gastrointestinal symptoms, including nausea, vomiting, and abdominal cramps. Rarely, arrhythmias have been reported. Nasal stuffiness and sleep disturbances are common complaints.[167,171,172]

GROWTH HORMONE RECEPTOR ANTAGONIST

The growth hormone receptor antagonist (GHRA), pegvisomant, directly inhibits GH action in the periphery.[173] Unlike somatostatin and dopamine agonists that act centrally to inhibit GH secretion through somatotroph-cell somatostatin and dopamine receptors, pegvisomant interferes with the functional dimerization of two GH receptor subunits suppressing peripheral IGF-1 generation in almost all patients with GH-secreting pituitary tumors treated for up to 36 months. Pegvisomant binds one GHR unit on site 1, but cannot bind the mutated site 2.[173] The site 2 mutation in pegvisomant involves replacement of glycine by lysine at position 120 (G120), preventing functional GHR dimerization, blocking initiation of subsequent GH signal transduction.

Daily doses of pegvisomant (10, 15, or 20 mg), given for 12 weeks, normalized IGF-1 levels in 38%, 75%, and 82% of patients with acromegaly, respectively.[174,175] A concomitant dose-dependent reduction in serum IGF-1 levels is accompanied by a dose-dependent regression of soft-tissue swelling, excessive perspiration, and fatigue, with no significant improvement in arthralgia or headache. Pegvisomant also improves insulin sensitivity and glucose tolerance in patients with acromegaly, reducing fasting serum insulin levels and fasting serum glucose levels, without observed decreased glycated hemoglobin.

Short-term (≤3 months of treatment) side effects encountered in pegvisomant-treated patients (vs. placebo) included reversible injection-site reactions (11%), diarrhea, and nausea (14% vs. 3%) in an 18-month study.[174] GH levels are reversibly increased approximately twofold, mirroring the IGF-1 decrease. Despite detection of anti-GH antibodies in 17% of patients, no evidence of tachyphylaxis was found. Serum cholesterol elevation also was reported. Long-term side effects are yet unknown and require prospective surveillance.

A concern with prolonged pegvisomant therapy is tumor growth reminiscent of changes seen with Nelson's syndrome. Currently, 2 of 160 patients reported in the literature exhibit progression of tumor size while receiving pegvisomant; both patients had macroadenomas at baseline, and the exact cause of tumor growth is unclear. Therefore, regular pituitary MRI assessment is recommended. Two patients demonstrated reversible elevation of transaminases. Elevation monitoring of liver function tests (LFTs) is recommended during treatment.

The availability of pegvisomant allows a new approach for monitoring biochemical control of acromegaly. As GH levels are elevated in patients receiving pegvisomant therapy, IGF-1 levels must be used to monitor efficacy, emphasizing the need to standardize commercial IGF-1 assays and development of age- and gender-specific reference ranges. Possible overtreatment with pegvisomant may create GH deficiency, as pegvisomant may suppress IGF-1 levels below the lower limit of normal in patients with acromegaly. It seems reasonable to titrate IGF-1 levels to midnormal ranges in these patients. Although pegvisomant normalizes IGF-1 levels in somatostatin-resistant patients,[176] experience with pegvisomant and somatostatin analogue cotreatment is limited. Pegvisomant is approved for patients who are intolerant or partially or nonresponsive to conventional treatment. Pegvisomant effectively normalizes IGF-1 in patients with acromegaly with a low incidence of adverse events. However, experience is yet too short for adequate assessment of its proper place in life-long treatment of acromegaly.

INTEGRATED APPROACH TO THE MANAGEMENT OF ACROMEGALY

TREATMENT APPROACH FOR ACROMEGALY: PATIENTS WITH LIKELIHOOD OF GOOD SURGICAL OUTCOME

Once acromegaly is diagnosed, the likelihood of surgical cure is assessed (Fig. 23-5). For small, well-circumscribed tumors, surgical excision by an experienced pituitary surgeon is the treatment of choice. Surgical cure rates are maximal for noninvasive, well-encapsulated smaller tumors. If a good surgical outcome is predicted, that is, a 60% chance or better that the disease will be controlled by tumor excision, surgery is indicated. After surgery, patients are monitored to ensure that GH responses to a glucose load are less than 1 ng/mL and that IGF-1 levels are normalized (Fig. 23-6). If, however, after surgery, hormone levels are not controlled, indicative of disease persistence or recurrence, either short- or long-acting somatostatin analogues are indicated.[29] Pegvisomant is indicated after failure of other therapy. Careful assessment of pituitary tumor size by using MRI is recommended every 6 to 12 months, depending on baseline tumor size and location (Fig. 23-7). Patients should be followed up by measuring age- and gender-matched IGF-1 levels, aiming for the midnormal range levels. Pegvisomant treatment should be avoided in patients who have LFT abnormalities until further data are available, and LFTs should be evaluated monthly during the first 6 months of therapy. If the patient is still not biochemically controlled, a dopamine agonist is added, or reoperation or irradiation is considered.

Patients with a Poor Likelihood of Successful Surgical Outcome

Patients with large adenomas are likely to have a poor surgical outcome, and fewer than half of them will be biochemically controlled. Most patients in whom acromegaly is newly diagnosed have large macroadenomas, which portend a poor surgical outcome. These patients can be offered primary

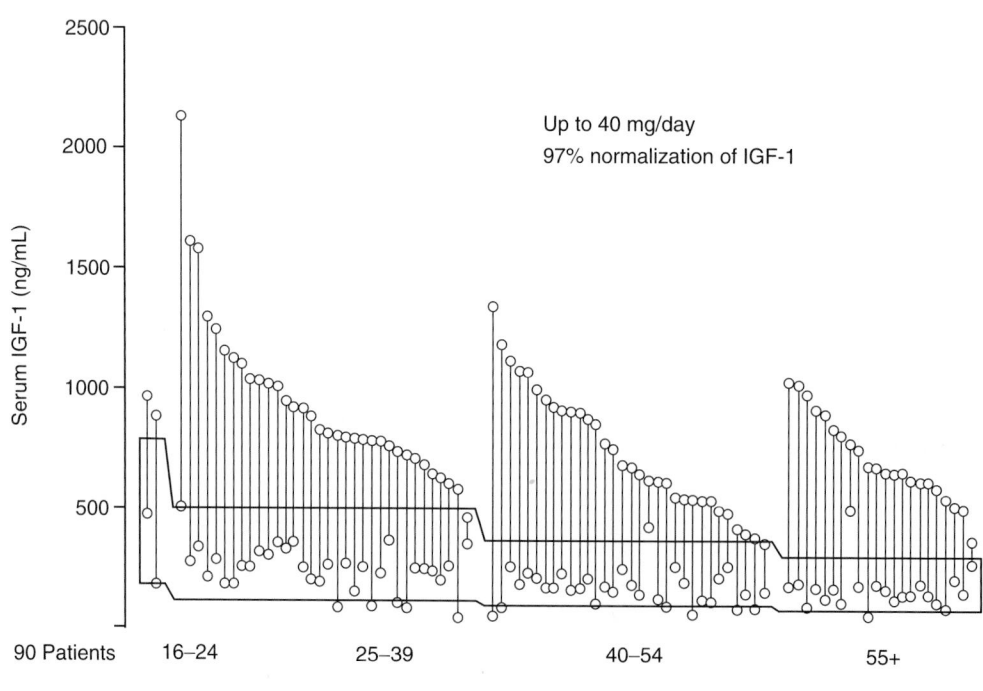

Figure 23-5 Insulin-like growth factor 1 levels at baseline and after 12 months of pegvisomant therapy. (From van der Lely AJ, Hutson RK, Trainer PJ, et al: Long-term treatment of acromegaly with pegvisomant, a growth hormone receptor antagonist. Lancet 358:1754–1759, 2001, with permission.)

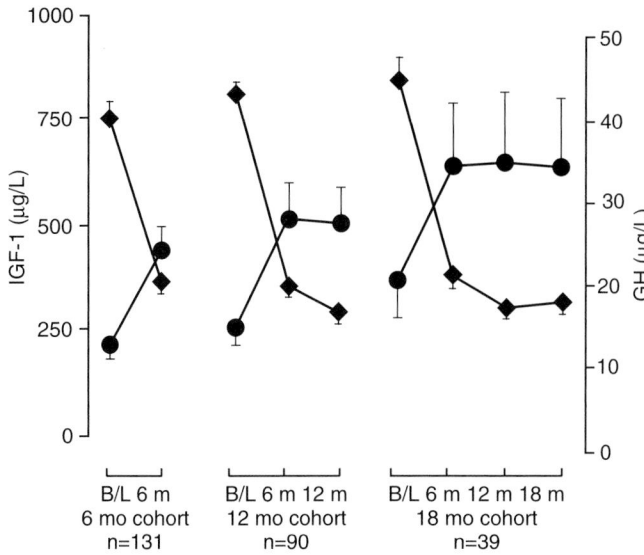

Dynamics of GH and IGF-1 during pegvisomant treatment

Figure 23-6 Dynamics of growth hormone and insulin-like growth factor 1 during pegvisomant treatment. (From van der Lely AJ, Hutson RK, Trainer PJ, et al: Long-term treatment of acromegaly with pegvisomant, a growth hormone receptor antagonist. Lancet 358:1754–1759, 2001, with permission.)

treatment with somatostatin analogues, as would patients in whom surgery is contraindicated or who decline surgery.[176] Because the drug reduces tumor bulk by approximately 50%,[161,176] subsequent surgery may be rendered easier, although no prospective data yet support this principle. If biochemical control is not achieved, drug efficacy may be improved by dose increases and the addition of a dopamine agonist, and these patients should be offered a GHRA.[29] If patients are resistant to medical treatment, second surgery or irradiation is indicated, depending on the size and location of the tumor remnant and the skill of the neurosurgeon.

FOLLOW-UP

Laboratory follow-up of patients includes performance of an oral glucose load and measurement of GH levels during the subsequent 2 hours. Stringent responses include GH less than 1 ng/mL, accompanied by a normalized IGF-1 level. If these goals are not achieved, medical treatment should be initiated, and if it is already being administered, efficacy may be improved by increasing medication dose frequency, adding a dopamine agonist or starting a GHRA. Reoperation and radiation therapy are further adjuvant options. Pituitary MRI should be repeated after 6 to 12 months in patients with macroadenomas, depending on the degree of local pressure signs. In patients with tumors that have been effectively excised, serial MRI is warranted only once every 2 years after surgery. Invasive residual tumors require more frequent MRI evaluation. Although tumor mass may not invariably shrink with somatostatin analogue therapy, further progressive tumor growth rarely occurs while patients are taking the medication.

GENERAL

Patients with acromegaly require management of multiple associated medical disorders. Colonoscopy should be performed at the time of diagnosis. The presence of more than three skin tags, a family history, age older than 50 years, or the presence of previous polyps requires more aggressive colonoscopic monitoring. Because cardiovascular morbidity is so high in patients with acromegaly, aggressive management of hypertension, left ventricular hypertrophy, cardiac failure, and arrhythmias should be pursued. Pulmonary function and sleep evaluation should be undertaken in all patients early in the course of the disorder, and debilitating arthritis requires aggressive rheumatologic management. Screening and therapy for insulin resistance and diabetes are important, and somatostatin analogues usually improve diabetes control dramatically. Insulin requirements may immediately decrease to 90% of pretreatment needs as GH is effectively suppressed. Headache is an extremely common symptom and usually improves with somatostatin

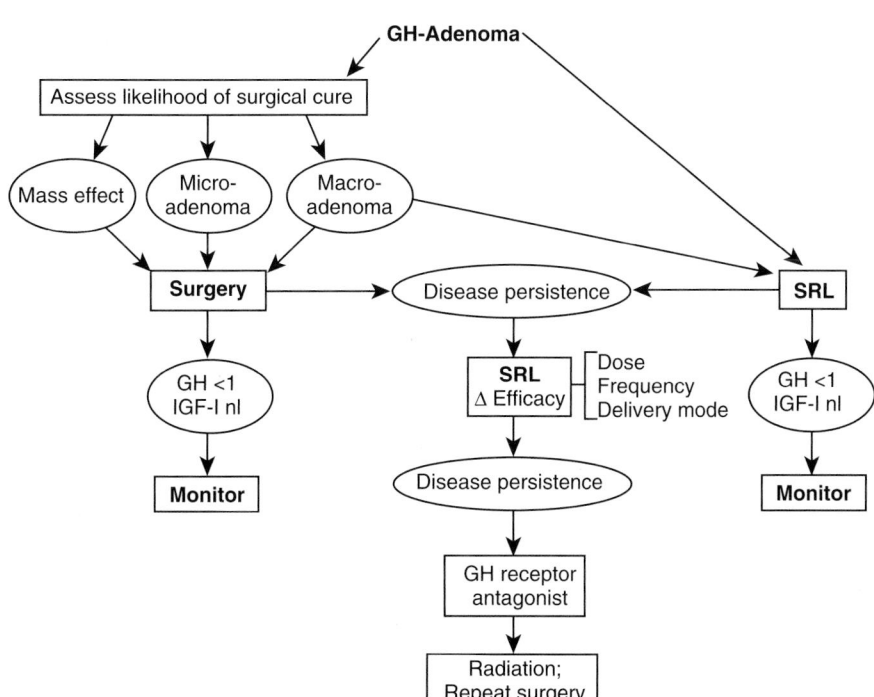

Figure 23-7 Management of acromegaly. GH, growth hormone; GHRA, GH receptor antagonist; IGF-1, insulin-like growth factor 1; SRL, somatostatin receptor ligand.

analogues; if not, potent analgesics may be indicated. Maxillofacial disorders may require dental, maxillary, and facial cosmetic surgery. Fertility is commonly of concern to patients, and several recent reports of successful pregnancies in women treated with octreotide provide optimistic guidelines for pregnancy management.[111,177] Nevertheless, octreotide is not approved by the Food and Drug Administration for use during pregnancy. Patients with acromegaly may be depressed and have low self-esteem and other psychosocial sensitivity.[174,178] Thus, careful individual or group counseling may be indicated to assist patients with these issues. Finally, because all the available treatment modes for acromegaly are associated with therapy-specific complications, they should be carefully watched for and, if they occur, promptly treated.

The availability of long-acting depot preparations of somatostatin analogues[179] and the GHRA have changed the approach to management, inasmuch as patient compliance and medication acceptance are expected to improve markedly. Slow-release somatostatin formulations require single injections once every 2 to 4 weeks and control acromegaly in about 70% of patients; their side effect profile appears quite similar. Availability of daily injectable GH receptor antagonists and oral formulations of SSR ligands[160,180] provide promising new therapeutic avenues for patients manifesting GH hypersecretory syndromes.

REFERENCES

1. Melmed S: Acromegaly. N Engl J Med 322:966–977, 1990.
2. Barkan AL: Acromegaly: Diagnosis and therapy. Endocrinol Metab Clin North Am 18:277–310, 1989.
3. Molitch ME: Clinical manifestations of acromegaly. Endocrinol Metab Clin North Am 21:597–614, 1992.
4. Marie P: Sur deux cas d'acromegalie: Hypertrophie singuliere non congenitale des extremities superieures et cephalique. Rev Med 6:297–333, 1886.
5. Nabarro JDN: Acromegaly. Clin Endocrinol (Oxf) 26:481–512, 1987.
6. Colao A, Ferone D, Marzullo P, Lombardi G: Systemic complications of acromegaly: Epidemiology, pathogenesis, and management. Endocr Rev 25:102–152, 2004.
7. Jadresic A, Banks LM, Child DF, et al: The acromegaly syndrome: Relation between clinical features, growth hormone values and radiological characteristics of the pituitary tumours. Q J Med 51:189–204, 1982.
8. Frohman LA, Jansson JO: Growth hormone-releasing hormone. Endocr Rev 7:223–253, 1986.
9. Thorner MO, Vance ML: Growth hormone. J Clin Invest 82:745–747, 1988.
10. Yamashita S, Melmed S: Insulin-like growth factor I regulation of growth hormone gene transcription in primary rat pituitary cells. J Clin Invest 79:449–452, 1987.
11. Berelowitz M, Szabo M, Frohman LA, et al: Somatomedin-C mediates growth hormone negative feedback by effects on both the hypothalamus and the pituitary. Science 212:1279–1281, 1981.
12. Melmed S, Yamashita S, Yamasaki H, et al: IGF-I receptor signaling: Lessons from the somatotroph. Recent Prog Horm Res 51:189–215, 1996.
13. Veldhuis JD, Liem AY, South S, et al: Differential impact of age, sex steroid hormones, and obesity on basal versus pulsatile growth hormone secretion in men as assessed in an ultrasensitive chemiluminescence assay. J Clin Endocrinol Metab 80:3209–3222, 1995.
14. Carter-Su C, Schwartz J, Smit LS: Molecular mechanism of growth hormone action. Annu Rev Physiol 58:187–207, 1996.
15. Melmed S, Jameson JL: Disorders of the anterior pituitary and hypothalamus. In Kasper DL, Fauci AS, Hauser SL, et al (eds): Harrison's Principles of Internal Medicine, 16th ed. New York, McGraw-Hill, 2005, pp 2076–2097.
16. D'Ercole AJ, Stiles AD, Underwood LE: Tissue concentrations of somatomedin C: Further evidence for multiple sites of synthesis and paracrine or autocrine mechanisms of action. Proc Natl Acad Sci U S A 81:935–939, 1984.
17. Drange MR, Melmed S: IGFs in the evaluation of acromegaly. In Rosenfeld RG, Roberts CT (eds): Contemporary Endocrinology: The IGF System: Molecular Biology, Physiology, and Clinical Applications. Clifton, NJ, Humana, 1999, pp 699–720.
18. Jones JI, Clemmons DR: Insulin-like growth factors and their binding proteins: Biological actions. Endocr Rev 16:3–34, 1995.
19. Van Wyk JJ: The somatomedins: Biological and physiologic control mechanisms. In Growth Factors. Orlando, FL, Academic Press, 1984, pp 81–125.
20. Isaksson OG, Lindahl A, Nilsson A, et al: Mechanism of the stimulatory effect of growth hormone on longitudinal bone growth. Endocr Rev 8:426–438, 1987.
21. Spencer GS, Hodgkinson SC, Bass JJ: Passive immunization against insulin-like growth factor-I does not inhibit growth hormone-stimulated growth of dwarf rats. Endocrinology 128:2103–2109, 1991.
22. Herman V, Fagin J, Gonsky R, et al: Clonal origin of pituitary adenomas. J Clin Endocrinol Metab 71:1427–1433, 1990.
23. Melmed S, Braunstein GD, Horvath E, et al: Pathophysiology of acromegaly. Endocr Rev 4:271–290, 1983.
24. Drange MR, Melmed S: Molecular pathogenesis of acromegaly. Pituitary 2:43–50, 1999.
25. Frawley LS, Boockfor FR: Mammosomatotropes: Presence and functions in normal and neoplastic pituitary tissue. Endocr Rev 12:337–355, 1991.
26. Asa SL, Kovacs K, Horvath E, et al: Human fetal adenohypophysis: Electron microscopic and ultrastructural immunocytochemical analysis. Neuroendocrinology 48:423–431, 1988.
27. Horvath E, Kovacs K, Singer W, et al: Acidophil stem cell adenoma of the human pituitary: Clinicopathologic analysis of 15 cases. Cancer 47:761–771, 1981.
28. Weinstein LS, Shenker A, Gejman PV, et al: Activating mutations of the stimulatory G protein in the McCune-Albright syndrome. N Engl J Med 325:1688–1695, 1991.
29. Melmed S, Casanueva F, Cavagnini F, et al: Guidelines for acromegaly management: A consensus statement. J Clin Endocrinol Metab 87:4054–4058, 2002.
30. Melmed S, Ezrin C, Kovacs K, et al: Acromegaly due to secretion of growth hormone by an ectopic pancreatic islet-cell tumor. N Engl J Med 312:9–17, 1985.
31. Sparagana M, Phillips G, Hoffman C, et al: Ectopic growth hormone syndrome associated with lung cancer. Metabolism 20:730–736, 1971.
32. Kaganowicz A, Farkouh NH, Frantz AG, et al: Ectopic human growth hormone in ovaries and breast cancer. J Clin Endocrinol Metab 48:5–8, 1979.
33. Sano T, Asa SL, Kovacs K: Growth hormone-releasing hormone-producing tumors: Clinical, biochemical, and morphological manifestations. Endocr Rev 9:357–373, 1988.
34. Asa SL, Scheithauer BW, Bilbao JM, et al: A case for hypothalamic acromegaly: A clinicopathological study of six patients with hypothalamic gangliocytomas producing growth hormone-releasing factor. J Clin Endocrinol Metab 58:796–803, 1984.
35. Oberg K, Norheim I, Wide L: Serum growth hormone in patients with carcinoid tumours: Basal levels and response to glucose and thyrotrophin releasing hormone. Acta Endocrinol (Copenh) 109:13–18, 1985.
36. Thorner MO, Perryman RL, Cronin MJ, et al: Somatotroph hyperplasia: Successful treatment of acromegaly by removal of a pancreatic islet tumor secreting a growth hormone-releasing factor. J Clin Invest 70:965–977, 1982.
37. Ashcraft MW, Hartzband PI, Van Herle AJ, et al: A unique growth factor in patients with acromegaloidism.

J Clin Endocrinol Metab 57:272–276, 1983.

38. Levy A, Lightman SL: Growth hormone-releasing hormone transcripts in human pituitary adenomas. J Clin Endocrinol Metab 74:1474–1476, 1992.

39. Levy L, Bourdais J, Mouhieddine B, et al: Presence and characterization of the somatostatin precursor in normal human pituitaries and in growth hormone secreting adenomas. J Clin Endocrinol Metab 76:85–90, 1993.

40. Billestrup N, Swanson LW, Vale W: Growth hormone-releasing factor stimulates proliferation of somatotrophs in vitro. Proc Natl Acad Sci U S A 83:6854–6857, 1986.

41. Mayo KE, Hammer RE, Swanson LW, et al: Dramatic pituitary hyperplasia in transgenic mice expressing a human growth hormone-releasing factor gene. Mol Endocrinol 2:606–612, 1988.

42. Kovacs M, Kineman RD, Schally AV, et al: Effects of antagonists of growth hormone-releasing hormone (GHRH) on GH and insulin-like growth factor I levels in transgenic mice overexpressing the human GHRH gene, an animal model of acromegaly. Endocrinology 138:4536–4542, 1997.

43. Shimon I, Melmed S: Genetic basis of endocrine disease: Pituitary tumor pathogenesis. J Clin Endocrinol Metab 82:1675–1681, 1997.

44. Spada A, Arosio M, Bochicchio D, et al: Clinical, biochemical, and morphological correlates in patients bearing growth hormone-secreting pituitary tumors with or without constitutively active adenylyl cyclase. J Clin Endocrinol Metab 71:1421–1426, 1990.

45. Vallar L, Spada A, Giannattasio G: Altered Gs and adenylate cyclase activity in human GH-secreting pituitary adenomas. Nature 330:566–568, 1987.

46. Bertherat J, Chanson P, Montminy M: The cyclic adenosine 3′,5′-monophosphate-responsive factor CREB is constitutively activated in human somatotroph adenomas. Mol Endocrinol 9:777–783, 1995.

47. Hashimoto K, Koga M, Motomura T, et al: Identification of alternatively spliced messenger ribonucleic acid encoding truncated growth hormone-releasing hormone receptor in human pituitary adenomas. J Clin Endocrinol Metab 80:2933–2939, 1995.

48. Molitch ME: Prolactinoma. In Melmed S (ed): The Pituitary. Cambridge, Blackwell, 1995, pp 443–477.

49. Melmed S, Ho K, Klibanski A, et al: Clinical review 75: Recent advances in pathogenesis, diagnosis, and management of acromegaly. J Clin Endocrinol Metab 80:3395–3402, 1995.

50. Gadelha MR, Prezant TR, Une KN, et al: Loss of heterozygosity on chromosome 11q13 in two families with acromegaly/gigantism is independent of mutations of the multiple endocrine neoplasia type I gene. J Clin Endocrinol Metab 84:249–256, 1999.

51. Bates AS, Farrell WE, Bicknell EJ, et al: Allelic deletion in pituitary adenomas reflects aggressive biological activity and has potential value as a prognostic marker. J Clin Endocrinol Metab 82:818–824, 1997.

52. Fero ML, Rivkin M, Tasch M, et al: A syndrome of multiorgan hyperplasia with features of gigantism, tumorigenesis, and female sterility in p27(Kip1)-deficient mice. Cell 85:733–744, 1996.

53. Jacks T, Fazeli A, Schmitt EM, et al: Effects of an Rb mutation in the mouse. Nature 359:295–300, 1992.

54. Nakayama K, Ishida N, Shirane M, et al: Mice lacking p27(Kip1) display increased body size, multiple organ hyperplasia, retinal dysplasia, and pituitary tumors. Cell 85:707–720, 1996.

55. Herman V, Drazin NZ, Gonsky R, et al: Molecular screening of pituitary adenomas for gene mutations and rearrangements. J Clin Endocrinol Metab 77:50–55, 1993.

56. Prezant TR, Levine J, Melmed S: Molecular characterization of the MEN-1 tumor suppressor gene in sporadic pituitary tumors. J Clin Endocrinol Metab 83:1388–1391, 1998.

57. Pei L, Melmed S, Scheithauer B, et al: Frequent loss of heterozygosity at the retinoblastoma susceptibility gene (RB) locus in aggressive pituitary tumors: Evidence for a chromosome 13 tumor suppressor gene other than RB. Cancer Res 55:1613–1616, 1995.

58. Spada A, Lania A, Ballare E: G protein abnormalities in pituitary adenomas. Mol Cell Endocrinol 142:1–14, 1998.

59. Barlier A, Gunz G, Zamora AJ, et al: Prognostic and therapeutic consequences of Gs alpha mutations in somatotroph adenomas. J Clin Endocrinol Metab 83:1604–1610, 1998.

60. Landis CA, Masters SB, Spada A, et al: GTPase inhibiting mutations activate the alpha chain of Gs and stimulate adenylyl cyclase in human pituitary tumours. Nature 340:692–696, 1989.

61. Clementi E, Malgaretti N, Meldolesi J, et al: A new constitutively activating mutation of the Gs protein alpha subunit-gsp oncogene is found in human pituitary tumours. Oncogene 5:1059–1061, 1990.

62. Lyons J, Landis CA, Harsh G, et al: Two G protein oncogenes in human endocrine tumors. Science 249:655–659, 1990.

63. Boggild MD, Jenkinson S, Pistorello M, et al: Molecular genetic studies of sporadic pituitary tumors. J Clin Endocrinol Metab 78:387–392, 1994.

64. Hosoi E, Yokogoshi Y, Horie H, et al: Analysis of the Gs alpha gene in growth hormone-secreting pituitary adenomas by the polymerase chain reaction-direct sequencing method using paraffin-embedded tissues. Acta Endocrinol (Copenh) 129:301–306, 1993.

65. Adams EF, Brockmeier S, Friedmann E, et al: Clinical and biochemical characteristics of acromegalic patients harboring gsp-positive and gsp-negative pituitary tumors. Neurosurgery 33:198–203, 1993.

66. Cai WY, Alexander JM, Hedley-Whyte ET, et al: Ras mutations in human prolactinomas and pituitary carcinomas. J Clin Endocrinol Metab 78:89–93, 1994.

67. Pei L, Melmed S, Scheithauer B, et al: H-ras mutations in human pituitary carcinoma metastases. J Clin Endocrinol Metab 78:842–846, 1994.

68. Karga HJ, Alexander JM, Hedley-Whyte ET, et al: Ras mutations in human pituitary tumors. J Clin Endocrinol Metab 74:914–919, 1992.

69. Pei L, Melmed S: Isolation and characterization of a pituitary tumor-transforming gene (PTTG). Mol Endocrinol 11:433–441, 1997.

70. Melmed S: Mechanisms for pituitary tumorigenesis: The plastic pituitary. J Clin Invest 112:1603–1618, 2003.

71. Zhang X, Horwitz GA, Heaney AP, et al: Pituitary tumor transforming gene (PTTG) expression in pituitary adenomas. J Clin Endocrinol Metab 84:761–767, 1999.

72. Stratakis CA, Carney JA, Lin JP, et al: Carney complex, a familial multiple neoplasia and lentiginosis syndrome: Analysis of 11 kindreds and linkage to the short arm of chromosome 2. J Clin Invest 97:699–705, 1996.

73. Stratakis CA, Jenkins RB, Pras E, et al: Cytogenetic and microsatellite alterations in tumors from patients with the syndrome of myxomas, spotty skin pigmentation, and endocrine overactivity (Carney complex). J Clin Endocrinol Metab 81:3607–3614, 1996.

74. Carney JA, Hruska LS, Beauchamp GD, et al: Dominant inheritance of the complex of myxomas, spotty pigmentation, and endocrine overactivity. Mayo Clin Proc 61:165–172, 1986.

75. Carney JA, Gordon H, Carpenter PC, et al: The complex of myxomas, spotty pigmentation, and endocrine overactivity. Medicine (Baltimore) 64:270–283, 1985.

76. Teh BT, Kytola S, Farnebo F, et al: Mutation analysis of the MEN1 gene in multiple endocrine neoplasia type 1, familial acromegaly and familial isolated hyperparathyroidism. J Clin Endocrinol Metab 83:2621–2626, 1998.

77. Knudson AGJ: Mutation and cancer: Statistical study of retinoblastoma. Proc Natl Acad Sci U S A 68:820–823, 1971.

78. Benlian P, Giraud S, Lahlou N, et al: Familial acromegaly: A specific clinical entity: Further evidence from the genetic study of a three-generation family. Eur J Endocrinol 133:451–456, 1995.

79. Ackermann F, Krohn K, Windgassen M, et al: Acromegaly in a family without a mutation in the menin gene. Exp Clin Endocrinol Diabetes 107:93–96, 1999.

80. Gadelha MR, Rhode K, Kineman RD, Frohman LA: Author's response: Isolated familial somatotropinomas: Does the disease map to 11q13 or to 2p16? J Clin Endocrinol Metab 85:4921, 2000.

81. Alexander L, Appleton D, Hall R, et al: Epidemiology of acromegaly in the Newcastle region. Clin Endocrinol (Oxf) 12:71–79, 1980.

82. Bengtsson BA, Eden S, Ernest I, et al: Epidemiology and long-term survival in acromegaly. Acta Med Scand 223:327–335, 1988.

83. Holdaway IM, Rajasoorya CR, Gamble GD, Stewart AW: Long-term treatment outcome in acromegaly. Growth Horm IGF-1 Res 13:185–192, 2003.

84. Serri O, Beauregard C, Hardy J: Long-term biochemical status and disease-related morbidity in 53 postoperative patients with acromegaly. J Clin Endocrinol Metab 89:658–661, 2004.

85. Clemmons DR, Van Wyk JJ, Ridgway EC, et al: Evaluation of acromegaly by radioimmunoassay of somatomedin-C. N Engl J Med 301:1138–1142, 1979.

86. Rieu M, Kuhn JM, Bricaire H, et al: Evaluation of treated acromegalic patients with normal growth hormone levels during oral glucose load. Acta Endocrinol 107:1–8, 1984.

87. Lee PD, Durham SK, Martinez V, et al: Kinetics of insulin-like growth factor (IGF) and IGF-binding protein responses to a single dose of growth hormone. J Clin Endocrinol Metab 82:2266–2274, 1997.

88. Melmed S: Confusion in clinical laboratory GH and IGF-1 reports. Pituitary 2:171–172, 1999.

89. Barkan AL, Beitins IZ, Kelch RP: Plasma insulin-like growth factor-I/somatomedin-C in acromegaly: Correlation with the degree of growth hormone hypersecretion. J Clin Endocrinol Metab 67:69–73, 1988.

90. Grinspoon S, Clemmons D, Swearingen B, et al: Serum insulin-like growth factor-binding protein-3 levels in the diagnosis of acromegaly. J Clin Endocrinol Metab 80:927–932, 1995.

91. de Herder WW, van der Lely AJ, Janssen JA, et al: IGFBP-3 is a poor parameter for assessment of clinical activity in acromegaly. Clin Endocrinol (Oxf) 43:501–505, 1995.

92. van der Lely AJ, de Herder WW, Janssen JA, et al: Acromegaly: The significance of serum total and free IGF-I and IGF-binding protein-3 in diagnosis. J Endocrinol 155(Suppl):9–16, 1997.

93. Shibasaki T, Kiyosawa Y, Masuda A, et al: Distribution of growth hormone-releasing hormone-like immunoreactivity in human tissue extracts. J Clin Endocrinol Metab 59:263–268, 1984.

94. Guillemin R, Brazeau P, Bohlen P, et al: Growth hormone-releasing factor from a human pancreatic tumor that caused acromegaly. Science 218:585–587, 1982.

95. Melmed S, Ziel FH, Braunstein GD, et al: Medical management of acromegaly due to ectopic production of growth hormone-releasing hormone by a carcinoid tumor. J Clin Endocrinol Metab 67:395–399, 1988.

96. Lieberman SA, Bjorkengren AG, Hoffman AR: Rheumatologic and skeletal changes in acromegaly. Endocrinol Metab Clin North Am 21:615–631, 1992.

97. Scarpa R, De Brasi D, Pivonello R, et al: Acromegalic axial arthropathy: A clinical case-control study. J Clin Endrocrinol Metab 89:598–603, 2004.

98. Bluestone R, Bywaters EG, Hartog M, et al: Acromegalic arthropathy. Ann Rheum Dis 30:243–258, 1971.

99. Dons RF, Rosselet P, Pastakia B, et al: Arthropathy in acromegalic patients before and after treatment: A long-term follow-up study. Clin Endocrinol (Oxf) 28:515–524, 1988.

100. Lesse GP, Fraser WD, Farquharson R, et al: Gonadal status is an important determinant of bone density in acromegaly. Clin Endocrinol (Oxf) 48:59–65, 1998.

101. Melmed S: Acromegaly. In Melmed S (ed): The Pituitary. Cambridge, MA, Blackwell, 2002.

102. Wass J: Acromegaly and gigantism. In Besser GM, Thorner MO (eds): Comprehensive Clinical Endocrinology, 3rd ed. St. Louis, Mosby, 2002, pp 57–71.

103. Cheung NW, Boyages SC: The thyroid gland in acromegaly: An ultrasonographic study. Clin Endocrinol (Oxf) 46:545–549, 1997.

104. Pereira AM, van Thiel SW, Lindner JR, et al: Increased prevalence of regurgitant valvular heart disease in acromegaly. J Clin Encrinol Metab 89:71–75, 2004.

105. Chanson P, Megnien JL, del Pino M, et al: Decreased regional blood flow in patients with acromegaly. Clin Endocrinol (Oxf) 49:725–731, 1998.

106. Lieberman SA, Hoffman AR: Sequelae to acromegaly: Reversibility with treatment of the primary disease. Horm Metab Res 22:313–318, 1990.

107. Colao A, Cuocolo A, Marzullo P, et al: Effects of 1-year treatment with octreotide on cardiac performance in patients with acromegaly. J Clin Endocrinol Metab 84:17–23, 1999.

108. Lombardi G, Colao A, Marzullo P, et al: Is growth hormone bad for your heart? Cardiovascular impact of GH deficiency and of acromegaly. J Endocrinol 155(Suppl):33–39, 1997.

109. Sacca L, Cittadini A, Fazio S: Growth hormone and the heart. Endocr Rev 15:555–573, 1994.

110. Colao A, Cuocolo A, Marzullo P, et al: Impact of patient's age and disease duration on cardiac performance in acromegaly: A radionuclide angiography study. J Clin Endocrinol Metab 84:1518–1523, 1999.

111. Colao A, Merola B, Ferone D, et al: Acromegaly. J Clin Endocrinol Metab 82:2777–2781, 1997.

112. Grunstein RR, Ho KK, Sullivan CE: Effect of octreotide, a somatostatin analog, on sleep apnea in patients with acromegaly. Ann Intern Med 121:478–483, 1994.

113. Grunstein RR, Ho KY, Sullivan CE: Sleep apnea in acromegaly. Ann Intern Med 115:527–532, 1991.

114. Grunstein RR, Ho KY, Berthon-Jones M, et al: Central sleep apnea is associated with increased ventilatory response to carbon dioxide and hypersecretion of growth hormone in patients with acromegaly. Am J Respir Crit Care Med 150:496–502, 1994.

115. Chanson P, Timsit J, Benoit O, et al: Rapid improvement in sleep apnea of acromegaly after short-term treatment with somatostatin analogue SMS 201-995 [Letter]. Lancet 1:1270–1271, 1986.

116. Melmed S: Unwanted effects of growth hormone excess in the adult. J Pediatr Endocrinol Metab 9:369–374, 1996.

117. Duncan E, Wass JAH: Investigation protocol: Acromegaly and its investigation. Clin Endocrinol (Oxf) 50:285–293, 1999.

118. Colao A, Marzullo P, Spiezia S, et al: Effect of growth hormone (GH) and insulin-like growth factor I on prostate diseases: An ultrasonographic and endocrine study in acromegaly, GH deficiency, and healthy subjects. J Clin Endocrinol Metab 84:1986–1991, 1999.

119. Colao A, Marzullo P, Ferone D, et al: Prostatic hyperplasia: An unknown feature of acromegaly. J Clin Endocrinol Metab 83:775–779, 1998.

120. Melmed S: Acromegaly and cancer: Not a problem? J Clin Endocrinol Metab 86:2929–2934, 2001.

121. Renehan AG, Pudhupalayan B, Painter JE, et al: The prevalence and characteristics of colorectal neoplasia in acromegaly. J Clin Endocrinol Metab 85:3417–3424, 2000.

122. Jenkins PJ, Besser M: Clinical Perspective: Acromegaly and cancer: A problem. J Clin Endocrinol Metab 86:2935–2941, 2001.

123. Ezzat S, Strom C, Melmed S: Colon polyps in acromegaly. Ann Intern Med 114:754–755, 1991.

124. Leiberman DA, Weiss DG: One-time screening for colorectal cancer with combined fecal occult-blood testing and examination of the distal colon. N Engl J Med 345:555–560, 2001.

125. Jenkins PJ, Fairclough PD, Richards T, et al: Acromegaly, colonic polyps and carcinoma. Clin Endocrinol (Oxf) 47:17–22, 1997.

126. Holdaway IM, Rajasoorja RC, Gamble GD: Factors influencing mortality in acromegaly. J Clin Endcrinol Metab 89:667–674, 2004.

127. Orme SM, McNally RJ, Cartwright RA, et al: Mortality and cancer incidence in acromegaly: A retrospective cohort study: United Kingdom Acromegaly Study Group. J Clin Endocrinol Metab 83:2730–2734, 1998.

128. Swearingen B, Barker FG, Katznelson L, et al: Long-term mortality after transsphenoidal surgery and adjunctive therapy for acromegaly. J Clin Endocrinol Metab 83:3419–3426, 1998.

129. Abosch A, Tyrrell JB, Lamborn KR, et al: Transsphenoidal microsurgery for growth hormone-secreting pituitary adenomas: Initial outcome and long-term results. J Clin Endocrinol Metab 83:3411–3418, 1998.

130. Landin-Wilhelmsen K, Tengborn L, Wilhelmsen L, et al: Elevated fibrinogen levels decrease following treatment of acromegaly. Clin Endocrinol (Oxf) 46:69–74, 1997.

131. Biermasz NR, Dekker FW, Pereira AM, et al: Determinants of survival in treated acromegaly in a single center: predictive value of serial insulin-like growth factor I measurements. J Clin Endocrinol Metab 89:2789–2796, 2004.

132. Ayuk J, Clayton RN, Holder G, et al: Growth hormone and pituitary radiotherapy, but not serum insulin-like growth factor-I concentrations, predict excess mortality in patients with acromegaly. J Clin Endocrinol Metab 89:1613–1617, 2004.

133. Krieger MD, Couldwell WT, Weiss MH: Assessment of long-term remission of acromegaly following surgery. J Neurosurg 98:719–724, 2003.

134. Bates AS, Van't Hoff W, Jones JM, et al: Does treatment of acromegaly affect life expectancy? Metabolism 44(Suppl 1):1–5, 1995.

135. Jho HD, Carrau RL: Endoscopic endonasal transsphenoidal surgery: Experience with 50 patients. J Neurosurg 87:44–51, 1997.

136. Cappabianca P, Cavallo LM, Colao A, de Divitiis E: Surgical complications associated with the endoscopic endonasal transsphenoidal approach for pituitary adenomas. J Neurosurg 97:293–298, 2002.

137. Biermasz NR, van Dulken H, Roelfsema F: Ten-year follow-up results of transsphenoidal microsurgery in acromegaly. J Clin Encrinol Metab 85:4596–4602, 2000.

138. Ahmed S, Elsheikh M, Stratton IM, et al: Outcome of transsphenoidal surgery for acromegaly and its relationship to surgical experience. Clin Endocrinol (Oxf) 50:561–567, 1999.

139. Kreutzer J, Vance ML, Lopes MB, Laws ER Jr: Surgical management of GH-secreting pituitary adenomas: An outcome study using modern remission criteria. J Clin Endocrinol Metab 86:4072–4077, 2001.

140. Shimon RL, Cohen ZR, Ram Z, Hadani M: Transsphenoidal surgery for acromegaly: Endocrinological follow-up of 98 patients. Neurosurgery 48:1239–1243, 2001.

141. Ciric I, Ragin A, Baumgartner C, et al: Complications of transsphenoidal surgery: Results of a national survey, review of the literature, and personal experience. Neurosurgery 40:225–236, 1997.

142. Freda PU, Post KD, Powell JS, et al: Evaluation of disease status with sensitive measures of growth hormone secretion in 60 postoperative patients with acromegaly. J Clin Endocrinol Metab 83:3808–3816, 1998.

143. Eastman RC, Gorden P, Glatstein E, et al: Radiation therapy of acromegaly. Endocrinol Metab Clin North Am 21:693–712, 1992.

144. Laws JE, Vance ML: Radiosurgery for pituitary tumors and craniopharyngiomas. Neurosurg Clin North Am 10:327–336, 1999.

145. Attanasio R, Epaminonda P, Motti E, et al: Gamma-knife radiosurgery in acromegaly: A 4-year follow-up study. J Clin Endocrinol Metab 88:3105–3112, 2003.

146. Barkan AL, Halasz I, Dornfeld KJ, et al: Pituitary irradiation is ineffective in normalizing plasma insulin-like growth factor I in patients with acromegaly. J Clin Endocrinol Metab 82:3187–3191, 1997.

147. Tsang RW, Laperriere NJ, Simpson WJ, et al: Glioma arising after radiation therapy for pituitary adenoma: A report of four patients and estimation of risk [published erratum appears in Cancer 73:492, 1994]. Cancer 72:2227–2233, 1993.

148. Ahmed M, Kanaan I, Rifai A, et al: An unusual treatment-related complication in a patient with growth hormone-secreting pituitary tumor. J Clin Endocrinol Metab 82:2816–2820, 1997.

149. Brada M, Ford D, Ashley S, et al: Risk of second brain tumour after conservative surgery and radiotherapy for pituitary adenoma. Br Med J 304:1343–1346, 1992.

150. Al-Mefty O, Kersh JE, Routh A, et al: The long-term side effects of radiation therapy for benign brain tumors in adults. J Neurosurg 73:502–512, 1990.

151. Alexander MJ, DeSalles AA, Tomiyasu U: Multiple radiation-induced intracranial lesions after treatment for pituitary adenoma: Case report. J Neurosurg 88:111–115, 1998.

152. Crossen JR, Garwood D, Glatstein E, et al: Neurobehavioral sequelae of cranial irradiation in adults: A review of radiation-induced encephalopathy. J Clin Oncol 12:627–642, 1994.

153. Jaffe CA: Reevaluation of conventional pituitary irradiation in the therapy of acromegaly. Pituitary 2:55–62, 1999.

154. Lamberts SWJ, van der Lely AJ, de Herder WW, et al: Octreotide. N Engl J Med 334:246–254, 1996.

155. Cozzi R, Attanasio R, Montini M, et al: Four-year treatment with octreotide-long-acting repeatable in 110 acromegalic patients: Predictive value of short-term results? J Clin Endocrinol Metab 88:3090–3098, 2003.

156. Murray RD, Kim K, Ren S-G, et al: Central and peripheral actions of somatostatin on the growth hormone-insulin-like growth factor-I axis. J Clin Invest 114:349–356, 2004.

157. Lightman SL, Fox P, Dunne MJ: The effect of SMS 201-995, a long-acting somatostatin analogue, on anterior pituitary function in healthy male volunteers. Scand J Gastroenterol Suppl 119:84–95, 1986.

158. Battershill PE, Clissold SP: Octreotide: A review of its pharmacodynamic and pharmacokinetic properties, and therapeutic potential in conditions associated with excessive peptide secretion. Drugs 38:658–702, 1989.

159. Gillis JC, Noble S, Goa KL: Octreotide long-acting release (LAR): A review of its pharmacological properties and therapeutic use in the management of acromegaly. Drugs 53:618–699, 1997.

160. Shimon I, Yan X, Taylor JE, et al: Somatostatin receptor (SSTR) subtype-selective analogues differentially suppress in vitro growth hormone and prolactin in human pituitary adenomas: Novel potential therapy for functional pituitary tumors. J Clin Invest 100:2386–2392, 1997.

161. Colao A, Ferone D, Marzullo P, et al: Long-term effects of depot long-acting somatostatin analog octreotide on hormone levels and tumor mass in acromegaly. J Clin Endocrinol Metab 86:2779–2786, 2001.

162. Attanasio R, Baldelli R, Pivonello R, et al: Lanreotide 60 mg, a new long-acting formulation: Effectiveness in the chronic treatment of acromegaly. J Clin Endocrinol Metab 88:5258–5265, 2003.

163. Shi YF, Zhu XF, Harris AG, et al: Prospective study of the long-term effects of somatostatin analog (octreotide) on gallbladder function and gallstone formation in Chinese acromegalic patients. J Clin Endocrinol Metab 76:32–37, 1993.

164. Ayuk J, Stewart SE, Stewart PM, Sheppard MC: Long-term safety and efficacy of depot long-acting somatostatin analogs for the treatment of acromegaly. J Clin Endocrinol Metab. 87:4142–4146, 2002.

165. Newman CB, Melmed S, Snyder PJ, et al: Safety and efficacy of long-term octreotide therapy of acromegaly: Results of a multicenter trial in 103 patients: A clinical research center study. J Clin Endocrinol Metab 80:2768–2775, 1995.

166. Caron P, Cogne M, Gusthiot-Joudet B, et al: Intramuscular injections of slow-release lanreotide (BIM 23014) in acromegalic patients previously treated with continuous subcutaneous infusion of octreotide (SMS 201-995). Eur J Endocrinol 132:320–325, 1995.

167. Jaffe CA, Barkan AL: Treatment of acromegaly with dopamine agonists. Endocrinol Metab Clin North Am 21:713–735, 1992.

168. Jackson SN, Fowler J, Howlett TA: Cabergoline treatment of acromegaly: A preliminary dose finding study. Clin Endocrinol (Oxf) 46:745–749, 1997.

169. Abs R, Verhelst J, Maiter D, et al: Cabergoline in the treatment of acromegaly: A study in 64 patients. J Clin Endocrinol Metab 83:374–378, 1998.

170. Muratori M, Arosio M, Gambino G, et al: Use of cabergoline in the long-term treatment of hyperprolactinemic and acromegalic patients. J Endocrinol Invest 20:537–546, 1997.

171. Colao A, Ferone D, Marzullo P, et al: Effect of different dopaminergic agents in the treatment of acromegaly. J Clin Endocrinol Metab 82:518–523, 1997.

172. Vance ML, Evans WS, Thorner MO: Drugs five years later: Bromocriptine. Ann Intern Med 100:78–91, 1984.

173. Kopchick JJ, Parkinson C, Stevens EC, Trainer PJ: Growth hormone receptor antagonists: Discovery, development and use in patients with acromegaly. Endocr Rev 23:623–646, 2002.

174. van der Lely AJ, Hutson RK, Trainer PJ, et al: Long-term treatment of acromegaly with pegvisomant, a growth hormone receptor antagonist. Lancet 358:1754–1759, 2001.

175. Trainer PJ, Drake WM, Katznelson L, et al: Treatment of acromegaly with the growth hormone-receptor antagonist pegvisomant. N Engl J Med 342:1171–1177, 2000.

176. Bonert VH, Zib K, Scarlett JA, Melmed S: Growth hormone receptor antagonist therapy in acromegalic patients resistant to somatostatin analogs. J Clin Endocrinol Metab 85:2958–2961, 2000.

177. Herman-Bonert V, Seliverstov M, Melmed S: Pregnancy in acromegaly: Successful therapeutic outcome. J Clin Endocrinol Metab 83:727–731, 1998.

178. Furman K, Ezzat S: Psychological features of acromegaly. Psychother Psychosom 67:147–153, 1998.

179. van der Hoek J, de Herder WW, Feelders RA, van der Lely: A single-dose comparison of the acute effects between the new somatostatin analog SOM230 and octreotide in acromegalic patients. J Clin Endocrinol Metab 89:638–645, 2004.

180. Bevan JS, Atkin SL, Atkinson AB, et al: Primary medical therapy for acromegaly: An open, prospective, multicenter study of the effects of subcutaneous and intramuscular slow-release octreotide on growth hormone, insulin-like growth factor-I, and tumor size. J Clin Endocrinol Metab 87:4554–4563, 2002.

Cushing's Syndrome

Damian G. Morris, Ashley B. Grossman, and Lynnette K. Nieman

INTRODUCTION

Harvey Cushing[1,2] was the first to codify the symptom complex of obesity, diabetes, hirsutism, and adrenal hyperplasia and to postulate that the basophilic adenomas found at autopsy in six of eight patients caused the disease that now bears his name. Shortly thereafter, Walters and colleagues[3] identified the etiologic contribution of adrenal tumors and the therapeutic role of adrenalectomy. Over the ensuing century, understanding of the pathogenesis of Cushing's syndrome has expanded to include ectopic production of adrenocorticotropic hormone (ACTH)[4] and corticotropin-releasing hormone (CRH)[5] and recognition of bilateral adrenal stimulation by factors other than ACTH.[6-9] The treatment options for Cushing's syndrome have increased to include medical agents that decrease the secretion or block the activity of circulating cortisol and surgical resection of eutopic and ectopic ACTH-producing tumors. Because florid Cushing's syndrome is ultimately fatal, early diagnosis and treatment have always been important. The variety of causes and the specific therapies now available dictate that correct diagnosis is also crucial. This chapter reviews the manifestations, etiologies, approaches to diagnosis, and treatment of this complicated and multifaceted syndrome.

DEFINITION

Cushing's syndrome is a symptom complex that reflects chronic excessive tissue exposure to glucocorticoids. The diagnosis cannot be made unless both clinical features and biochemical abnormalities are present.

ETIOLOGY AND PATHOPHYSIOLOGY

CUSHING'S SYNDROME

The causes of Cushing's syndrome can be divided into those that are ACTH dependent and ACTH independent (Table 24-1). The ACTH-dependent forms are characterized by excessive ACTH production from a corticotroph adenoma (known as pituitary-dependent Cushing's syndrome or Cushing's disease), from an ectopic tumoral source (ectopic ACTH syndrome), or from normal corticotrophs under the influence of excessive CRH production (ectopic CRH secretion). ACTH stimulates all three layers of the adrenal cortex to grow and secrete steroids. When excessive, this results in histologic hyperplasia and increased adrenal weight. Micronodules and macronodules (>1 cm) may be seen. Circulating glucocorticoids are increased, often associated with some increase in adrenal androgens.

ACTH-independent forms, apart from exogenous administration of glucocorticoids, represent adrenal activation by mechanisms other than trophic ACTH support. This enlarging group includes unilateral disease (adenoma and carcinoma), bilateral disease (primary pigmented nodular adrenal disease, McCune-Albright syndrome, and macronodular adrenal disease of unknown cause or caused by ectopic expression of receptors for ligands such as gastric inhibitory polypeptide [GIP], β-adrenergic agents, and vasopressin), and hyperfunction of adrenal rest tissue.

Adrenal adenomas, composed of zona fasciculata cells, produce only glucocorticoids, in contrast to activation of the entire adrenal cortex seen in other causes of Cushing's syndrome. ACTH levels are suppressed by hypercortisolism and the nonadenomatous tissue atrophies because of lack of this trophic factor. As a result, androgenic signs, such as pustular acne and hirsutism, are somewhat uncommon, and dehydroepiandrosterone sulfate levels are typically low.

Cushing's Disease

Cushing's disease is almost always caused by a solitary (probably monoclonal) corticotroph adenoma.[10] Although nodular corticotroph hyperplasia without evidence of a CRH-producing neoplasm does occur, it represents 2% or less of large surgical series.[11,12] The majority of tumors are intrasellar microadenomas (<1 cm in diameter), although macroadenomas account for approximately 10% of tumors, and extrasellar extension or invasion may occur. The cause(s) of Cushing's disease remains unknown, despite much work on the molecular characterization of these tumors. There has traditionally been debate as to whether the development of pituitary adenomas is due to abnormal hypothalamic hormonal stimulation

Table 24-1 Etiology of Cushing's Syndrome

ACTH dependent
Pituitary-dependent Cushing's syndrome (Cushing's disease)
Ectopic ACTH syndrome
Ectopic CRH secretion
Exogenous ACTH administration
ACTH independent
Adrenal adenoma
Adrenal carcinoma
Primary pigmented nodular adrenal disease (PPNAD), sporadic or
  associated with the Carney complex
AIMAH
AIMAH secondary to abnormal hormone receptor expression/
  function
McCune-Albright syndrome
Exogenous glucocorticoid administration

ACTH, adrenocorticotropic hormone; AIMAH, ACTH-independent bilateral macronodular adrenal hyperplasia; CRH, corticotropin-releasing hormone.

or feedback regulation or an intrinsic pituitary defect. More recently, a model has been proposed that encompasses both theories. Here tumors can arise either as a clonal expansion from a primary intrinsic pituitary defect or excessive hormonal stimulation/abnormal feedback leading to hyperplasia, which in turn predisposes the cells to mutate, with subsequent clonal expansion.[13] Analysis of the primary corticotroph stimulatory and negative feedback pathways have not revealed a common defect.[14,15] Similarly, the common oncogenes and tumor suppressor genes implicated in other cancers do not seem to be commonly involved in the pathogenesis of corticotropinomas. Studies of knockout mice and analysis of human pituitary tumor samples have implicated the cyclin-dependent kinase inhibitor p27(Kip1) in corticotroph tumorigenesis. Overall, reduced p27 protein levels in corticotropinomas and a high phosphorylated p27/p27 ratio suggest increased inactivation of this negative cell-cycle regulator, although the cause of this change remains to be elucidated.[16] Cytogenetic studies have revealed a surprising number of gross chromosomal changes in benign pituitary adenomas, and although the number of corticotroph tumors studied has been small, gain of chromosome 6p and loss of chromosomes 2, 15q, and 22 seem to be the most common abnormalities.[17-19] Perhaps improvement in molecular biologic techniques, particularly microarray analysis, will lead to the implication of new genes in the pathogenesis of these tumors that will require further study.[20]

Ectopic Adrenocorticotropic Hormone Syndrome

The syndrome of ectopic hormone secretion was first codified by Liddle and colleagues,[4] who defined it as "any hormone produced by a neoplasm which is derived from tissue not normally engaged in the production of the hormone in question." ACTH and other pro-opiomelanocortin (POMC) products were subsequently identified in many noncorticotroph tumors, although not all were associated with increased circulating levels or the development of Cushing's syndrome.[4,21]

Although small cell lung cancer is probably the most common cause of ectopic ACTH syndrome, it is not the most common seen in later larger series, and this probably represents differences in referral patterns as discussed later (Table 24-2). An intrathoracic neoplasm (carcinoma of the lung or carcinoid of the bronchus or thymus) accounts for approximately 60% of ectopic ACTH secretion, followed by pancreatic tumors (islet cell or carcinoid) and phaeochromocytoma (~5%–10%), and medullary carcinoma of the thyroid (<5%).

The mechanism whereby the POMC gene becomes derepressed in noncorticotroph tumors is not understood. One hypothesis is that these cells are derived from a common multipotential progenitor cell capable of producing peptide hormones, such that ACTH production is a reversion to a less differentiated state.[22] The observation that many ACTH-producing tumors are derived from neural crest amine precursor uptake and decarboxylation (APUD) cells may support this view.[23] However, because endodermally derived tumors also produce ACTH, the acquisition of amine precursor uptake and decarboxylation characteristics may be but one manifestation of dedifferentiation and may not represent the cause of ectopic ACTH production.

Although the mechanism of gene derepression is not understood, the regulation of POMC production and processing has been investigated. POMC, corticotropin-like intermediate lobe protein, and larger forms of ACTH ("big" or pro-ACTH) that are not usually secreted may circulate, and the intracellular ratio of the POMC products may be abnormal.[24,25] Investigation of cell lines of small cell carcinoma of the lung that synthesize POMC and pro-ACTH showed that only ACTH precursors were secreted, suggesting that processing to ACTH is defective.[26] The pattern of POMC mRNA species in ACTH-producing tumors has been characterized. A 1200-bp transcript similar to that of a corticotroph adenoma,[27] a shorter than normal 800-bp mRNA lacking a signal sequence for secretion,[27,28] and a larger 1400- to 1500-bp POMC transcript have been identified. The larger species appears to originate upstream of the usual pituitary promoter, with preservation of the normal translation start site.[29,30] It is possible that the promoters that initiate this transcription are not regulated by glucocorticoids, and this may explain in part the lack of responsiveness to glucocorticoid suppression noted clinically in these patients. In vitro investigation of human small cell cancer cell lines and pancreatic islet cell tumors with normal glucocorticoid receptor binding has

Table 24-2 Percentage Incidence of Tumor Types Causing Ectopic Adrenocorticotropic Hormone Syndrome in Four Large Series from 1969 to 2003

Tumor Type	Liddle et al., 1969[4] (N = 104)	Jex et al., 1985[452] (N = 21)	Torpy et al., 2002[453] (N = 58)	Morris and Grossman, 2003[454] (N = 32)
Lung carcinoma	50	20	2	19
Bronchial carcinoid	5	28	40	41
Thymic carcinoid	10	8	10	3
Pancreatic tumors	10	20	7	12
Pheochromocytoma, paraganglioma, neuroblastoma	5	12	5	3
Medullary thyroid carcinoma	2		3	9
Miscellaneous*	17	8	2	12

*Other tumors reported to uncommonly secrete adrenocorticotropic hormone include the appendix, breast, cloacogenic carcinoma of the anal canal, colon, esophagus, gallbladder, gastric carcinoid, kidney, melanoma, mesothelioma, myeloblastic leukaemia, ovary, prostate, salivary glands, and testes.

found, for the most part, no regulation of POMC, tyrosine aminotransferase, or the glucocorticoid receptor mRNA at doses of hydrocortisone that would normally suppress pituitary production.[31-33] However, clinical observation of suppression of ACTH production by some bronchial carcinoids during glucocorticoid administration suggests retention of a functional glucocorticoid response element that regulates POMC production, at least in some ectopic tumors.[34]

Ectopic Corticotropin-Releasing Hormone Secretion

Tumor secretion of CRH with or without ACTH secretion is a rare cause of Cushing's syndrome. Although many tumors immunostain for CRH, its secretion is less common, and most patients do not develop cushingoid features.[35] Thus, the diagnosis primarily rests on the demonstration of elevated plasma CRH levels. The literature includes fewer than 20 patients who fit this criterion. Tumors may have negative immunostaining for ACTH, but this may be related to reduced storage and rapid secretion. In cases such as these, a CRH and ACTH gradient across the tumor bed can be suggestive that, in fact, the tumor secretes both peptides.[36] Tumors include bronchial and thymic carcinoids, small cell lung cancer, medullary thyroid carcinoma, phaeochromocytoma, gangliocytoma, prostate carcinoma, and ganglioneuroblastoma.[37,38] The biochemical responses to diagnostic tests can be similar to those seen in ectopic ACTH secretion or pituitary ACTH-dependent disease.[38] It is important to note that many, if not all, ectopic secretors of CRH causing Cushing's syndrome are also ectopic ACTH secretors.

Primary Adrenal Disease

The primary adrenal forms of Cushing's syndrome do not share a common cause. Although the cause of adrenocortical neoplasia is not known, some events important in the development of adrenal cancer have been identified. Paternal isodisomy at 11p15.5 with overexpression of *IGF2* and reduced expression of *CDKN1C* (a G1 cyclin-dependent kinase inhibitor) and *H19* (a putative growth suppressor) seems to be a key event. Mutations of *p53* may be involved in a small subset of carcinomas. Other genes important in pathogenesis remain to be elucidated, although potential loci have been identified at chromosomes 17p, 1p, 2p16, and 11q13 for tumor suppressor genes, and chromosomes 4, 5, and 12 for oncogenes.[39] Adenomas and carcinomas tend to be monoclonal, although the nodular hyperplasias are often polyclonal.[40] Adrenal adenomas are encapsulated benign tumors, usually less than 40 g in weight. Adrenal carcinomas are usually encapsulated, generally weigh more than 100 g, and may lack classic histologic features of malignancy, although nuclear pleomorphism, necrosis, mitotic figures, and vascular or lymphatic invasion suggest the diagnosis.[41] The adjacent adrenal tissue is atrophic in both conditions.

Primary pigmented nodular adrenal disease (PPNAD), also known as micronodular adrenal disease, is a rare form of Cushing's syndrome characterized histologically by small to normal-size glands (combined weight <12 g) with cortical micronodules (average 2–3 mm) that may be dark or black in color. The intervening cortex is usually atrophic.[42] Approximately one half of the cases of PPNAD are apparently sporadic. The remainder occur as part of the Carney complex in association with a variety of other abnormalities, including myxomatous masses of the heart, skin, or breast; blue nevi or lentigines, and other endocrine disorders (sexual precocity; Sertoli cell, Leydig cell, or adrenal rest tumor; and acromegaly). The Carney complex is inherited as an autosomal-dominant condition, and Cushing's syndrome occurs in approximately 30% of cases.[43] The genes responsible have been mapped to chromosomes 2p16[43] and 17q22-24.[44] Recently, at the 17q22-24 locus, the tumor suppressor gene *PRKAR1A*, coding for the type 1a regulatory subunit of protein kinase A, has been shown to be mutated in approxi-

mately one half of patients with Carney complex, both familial and sporadic.[45] It may well be that more careful ascertainment will demonstrate that the majority of patients presenting with PPNAD will be shown to have Carney syndrome.

Cushing's syndrome resulting from bilateral nodular adrenal disease is an uncommon feature of the McCune-Albright syndrome,[46] which is characterized by fibrous dysplasia of bone, café-au-lait skin pigmentation, and endocrine dysfunction (usually precocious puberty). In this disease, an activating mutation at codon 201 of the α subunit of the G protein that stimulates cyclic adenosine monophosphate formation occurs in a mosaic pattern in early embryogenesis.[47] If this affects some adrenal cells, constitutive activation of adenylate cyclase and the steroidogenic cascade leads to nodule formation and glucocorticoid excess. The internodular adrenal cortex, where the mutation is not present, becomes atrophic.[48]

A missense mutation of the ACTH receptor resulting in its constitutive activation and ACTH-independent Cushing's syndrome has also been reported.[49]

ACTH-independent bilateral macronodular adrenal hyperplasia (AIMAH) is a rare form (<1%) of Cushing's syndrome that involves huge adrenal glands, causing confusion with Cushing's disease and biochemical tests that are consistent with a nonpituitary form of the disorder. Most cases are sporadic, but a few familial cases have been reported.[50] Although the cause remains unclear in most cases, some nodules express increased numbers of receptors normally found on the adrenal gland, or ectopic receptors for circulating ligands that then can stimulate cortisol production. Perhaps the best known example of this phenomenon is food-dependent Cushing's syndrome: The normal postprandial increase in gastric inhibitory peptide (GIP) appeared to cause Cushing's syndrome in two middle-aged women with bilateral multinodular adrenal enlargement, mildly elevated urinary free cortisol (UFC) values, and undetectable plasma ACTH values. Fasting morning serum cortisol values were low or normal. Cortisol values increased dramatically after meals and after in vivo or in vitro exposure to GIP.[7,8] In one patient, curative bilateral adrenalectomy revealed multinodular adrenal glands weighing 20 and 35 g.[8] In the other, treatment with octreotide ameliorated the syndrome.[7] Ectopic expression of GIP receptors was found in these patients, although in others eutopic increased expression of vasopressin receptors or ectopic expression of β-adrenergic receptors or luteinizing hormone/human chorionic gonadotropin receptors appeared to stimulate cortisol production.[51] However, it is possible that this apparent ectopic induction of receptors on the adrenal is a response to the adrenal hyperplasia rather than its cause.

Adrenal rest tissue in the liver, in the adrenal beds, or in association with the gonads may rarely cause Cushing's syndrome, usually in the setting of ACTH-dependent disease after adrenalectomy.[52-55] Ectopic cortisol production by an ovarian carcinoma has been reported.[56]

PSEUDO-CUSHING'S STATES

A pseudo-Cushing's state may be defined as one in which some or all of the clinical features that resemble true Cushing's syndrome and some evidence of hypercortisolism are present, but disappear after resolution of the underlying condition.[57] The pathophysiology of these states has not been established. One hypothesis is that these stressful conditions increase the activity of the CRH neuron, resulting in excessive ACTH secretion, adrenal hyperplasia, and increased cortisol production.[58] The model predicts only intermittent and modest hypercortisolism because of appropriate corticotroph reduction in ACTH secretion in response to negative feedback by cortisol (Figure 24-1). This construct presumes also that the hypertrophied adrenal glands produce excessive glucocorticoids in response to normal ACTH levels, an assumption that

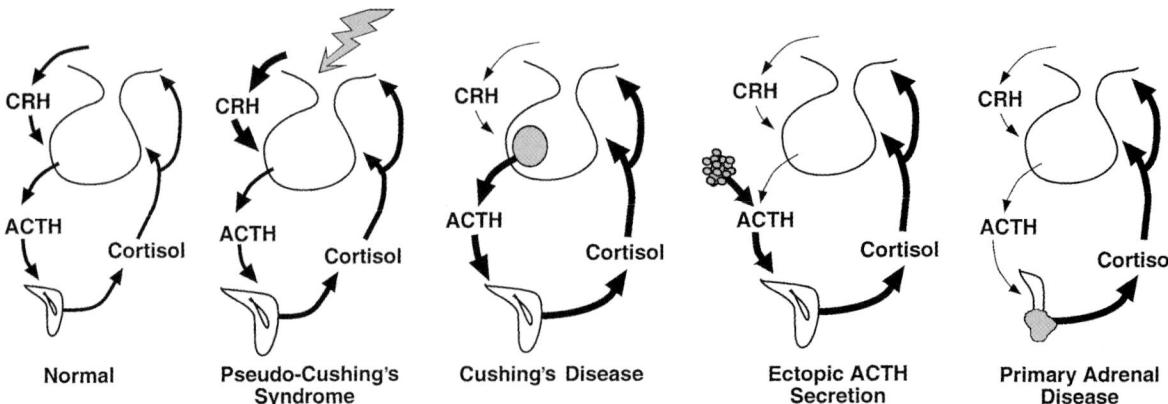

Figure 24-1   Physiology of the hypothalamic-pituitary-adrenal axis in normal individuals and hypercortisolemic states. Corticotropin-releasing hormone (CRH) secretion from the hypothalamus normally stimulates adrenocorticotropic hormone (ACTH) secretion from the pituitary gland. This in turn results in increased cortisol production from the adrenal glands. The system is modulated by negative feedback inhibition by cortisol of both CRH and ACTH secretion. In pseudo-Cushing's syndrome, the CRH neuron is activated by central input *(large shaded arrow)* resulting in increased CRH output that eventuates in hypercortisolism. Increased cortisol production restrains corticotroph activation but does not completely reverse the activation of the CRH neuron, so that mild to moderate hypercortisolism may persist. In Cushing's disease, a corticotroph adenoma secretes ACTH in excess and is only partially inhibited by rising cortisol levels. In this setting and that of ectopic ACTH secretion and primary adrenal disease, the CRH neuron is suppressed by hypercortisolism. In ectopic ACTH secretion, excessive secretion of ACTH from a nonpituitary tumor is not inhibited by glucocorticoid feedback. In this setting and that of autonomous production of cortisol by the adrenal gland, ACTH secretion by normal corticotrophs is suppressed by hypercortisolism.

is supported by the blunted ACTH, but not cortisol, response to exogenous CRH in anorexia nervosa,[59] depression,[60] and obligate athleticism.[61]

EPIDEMIOLOGY

Iatrogenic causes account for the majority of cases of Cushing's syndrome because of the common therapeutic use of high-dose glucocorticoids. Large series have reported the distribution of endogenous cases as follows: Cushing's disease (68%), adrenal adenomas (8%–19%), adrenal carcinoma (6%–7%), ectopic ACTH syndrome (6%–15%), and nodular adrenal hyperplasia (2%).[57,62] There is, however, a paucity of information on the true incidence of these causes. Perhaps the best data come from a population-based study covering the whole of Denmark (population of 5.3 million), which used stringent methods of data collection, aided by the small number of centers treating the disorder.[63] The incidence of Cushing's disease, adrenal adenoma, and adrenal carcinoma were 1.2 per million per year, 0.6 per million per year, and 0.2 per million per year, respectively. The reported incidence of ectopic ACTH syndrome was extremely low (0.1 per million per year). This is probably due (as the authors concede) to many cases never being recognized, but may partly be explained by a group of patients with ACTH-dependent Cushing's syndrome (0.5 per million per year) with presumed but unproven pituitary disease. Some of these may well have had ectopic ACTH syndrome. The incidence of ectopic ACTH syndrome is most certainly underestimated in the endocrine literature because most cases reaching endocrinologists are those caused by occult tumors as opposed to those caused by overt malignancy. However, given that Cushing's syndrome will be present in 3% to 12% of cases of small cell lung cancer[64,65] and the recent incidence of small cell lung cancer in Europe is approximately 120 per million per year in men, and 40 per million per year in women,[66] this is by far the most common cause. Other epidemiologic studies have looked at just the incidence of Cushing's disease and found rates between 0.7 per million per year in northern Italy[67] and 2.4 per million per year in northern Spain.[68]

Gender and age distribution varies with the cause of Cushing's syndrome. Adrenal adenomas and Cushing's disease present much more commonly in women than in men, and adrenal carcinoma is approximately 1.5 times as common as in men.[57,62] Nodular adrenal hyperplasia has an approximately equal gender ratio.

Ectopic ACTH syndrome is the only cause of the syndrome that is more common in men, although this may change as more women are developing small cell lung cancer. Lung cancer is more common after age 40, and this accounts for the increased mean age of patients with ectopic ACTH syndrome compared with Cushing's disease, which occurs between 25 and 40 years of age.[69] The other major cause of ectopic ACTH secretion, intrathoracic carcinoids, has a peak incidence around 40 years and only a slightly increased male-to-female ratio.[70] The age distribution of adrenal cancer is bimodal, with peaks in childhood and adolescence and late in life, although adrenal adenoma occurs most often around 35 years of age.

CLINICAL FEATURES

Excessive cortisol production has widespread systemic effects,[69,71–74] (Table 24-3). Although the full-blown cushingoid phenotype is unmistakable, the clinical diagnosis may be equivocal for patients with few of the typical characteristics (Fig. 24-2). Some nonspecific features consistent with the diagnosis of Cushing's syndrome, such as obesity, hypertension, and menstrual irregularity, are common in the general population and may provoke unwarranted and costly screening tests for patients not likely to be affected.

One useful strategy when considering the diagnosis of Cushing's syndrome is to look for evidence of progressive physical changes by examination of serial photographs, especially of individuals photographed at annual events such as holidays, birthdays, or school milestones (Fig. 24-3). Another approach relies on identification of signs and symptoms that correctly classify patients suspected of having the disorder. Truncal obesity, ecchymoses, plethora, proximal muscle weakness, osteopenia, and hypertension are discriminant indices for Cushing's syndrome, with ecchymoses and muscle weakness being the most reliable.[71,75]

Table 24-3 Percentage Frequency of Clinical Signs and Symptoms of Cushing's Syndrome as Described in Six Large Studies from 1952 to 2003

Signs and Symptoms (Men/Women)	Plotz et al., 1952[69] (N = 33)	Sprague et al., 1956[74] (N = 100)	Soffer et al., 1961[73] (N = 50)	Urbanic and George, 1981[72] (N = 31)	Ross and Linch, 1982[71] (N = 70)	Pecori Giraldi et al., 2003[127] (N = 280)
Obesity or weight gain	97	84	86	79	97	85/86
Hypertension	84	90	88	77	74	68/67
Weakness/muscle atrophy	83		58	90	56	64/46
Plethora	89	81	78		94	89/81
Round face	89	92	92		88	
Striae	60	64	50	51	56	72/51
Thin skin				84		
Ecchymoses	60	62	68	77	62	21/32
Hirsutism	73	74	84	64	81	
Acne	82	64		35	21	19/28
Female balding			51		13	
Dorsocervical fat pad		67	34		54	51/54
Edema	60		66	48	50	
Menstrual changes	86	35	72	69	84	
Decreased libido	86		100/33	55	100/	
Headache	58				47	
Backache	83			39	43	
Psychiatric disturbance	67		40	48	62	26/34
Recurrent infections		14		25		
Poor wound healing/severe infection	42					
Abdominal pain					21	
Renal calculi					15	21/6
Osteoporosis/fracture	83		56	48	50	47/32
Abnormal glucose tolerance	94		84	39	50	43/45

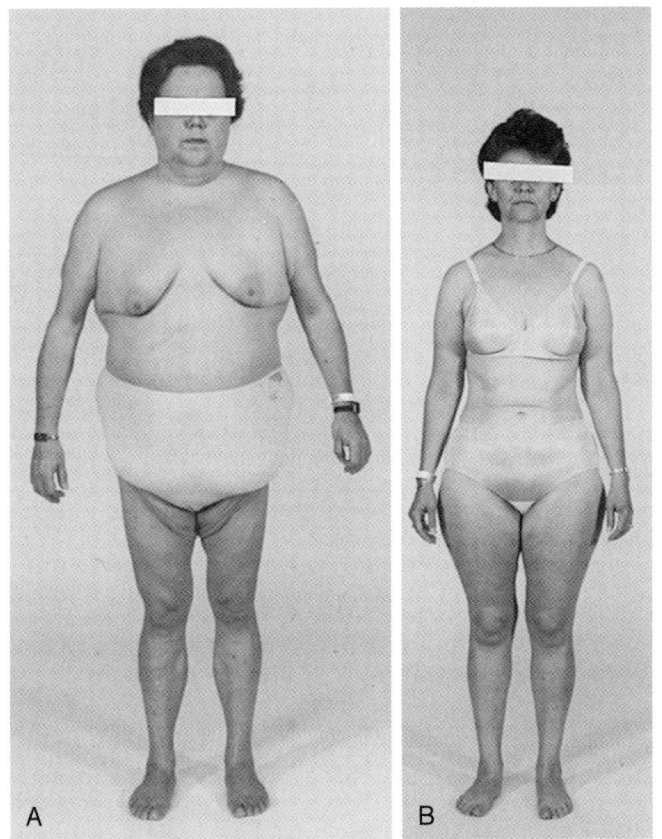

Figure 24-2 Body habitus of two patients with proven Cushing's syndrome. Features typical of the syndrome, central obesity, round face, and supraclavicular fat pads, are present in the patient in **A** but not in the patient in **B**, illustrating that the diagnosis is not always apparent from the initial physical examination.

Increased deposition of fat, one of the earliest signs, occurs in almost all patients and is reported as increasing weight or difficulty in maintaining weight. The distribution of fat is altered also in both men and women, with increased amounts in the visceral compartments[76] and subcutaneous sites on the face and neck. Increased intra-abdominal fat results in the truncal obesity described by Cushing in approximately 50% of patients. Increased fat in the face (moon facies), supraclavicular or temporal fossae, and the dorsocervical area ("buffalo hump") is uncommon in normal people. When extreme, the supraclavicular fat may present as a "collar" rising above the clavicles (Fig. 24-4); filling of the temporal fossae may prevent eyeglass frames from seating properly.

Abnormal fat deposition may occur in the epidural space. Spinal epidural lipomatosis causing neurologic deficit, a rare complication of long-term exogenous steroid use, has been reported in a few patients with endogenous Cushing's syndrome.[77,78] Lumbosacral findings were seen in both men and women, whereas thoracic obstruction was restricted to men. The condition can be diagnosed by magnetic resonance imaging (MRI).[79]

Loss of subcutaneous tissue results in a variety of skin abnormalities that are unusual in the general population and suggest hypercortisolism. Ecchymoses, often after minimal trauma, and cutaneous atrophy, seen as a fine "cigarette paper" wrinkling or tenting over the dorsum of the hand and elbows, are typical. Cutaneous atrophy is influenced by gender and age, with men and the young having greater skin thickness. Two maxims follow: First, it is useful to compare the patient's skin with that of a near age- and gender-matched healthy person, and second, skin thickness is relatively preserved in cushingoid women with increased androgen production or preservation of ovarian function (Fig. 24-5).

Facial plethora, especially over the cheeks, also reflects loss of subcutaneous tissue. Although plethora is more obvious in pale whites, it may be present and should be sought in darker skinned persons. Because erythema may be induced in

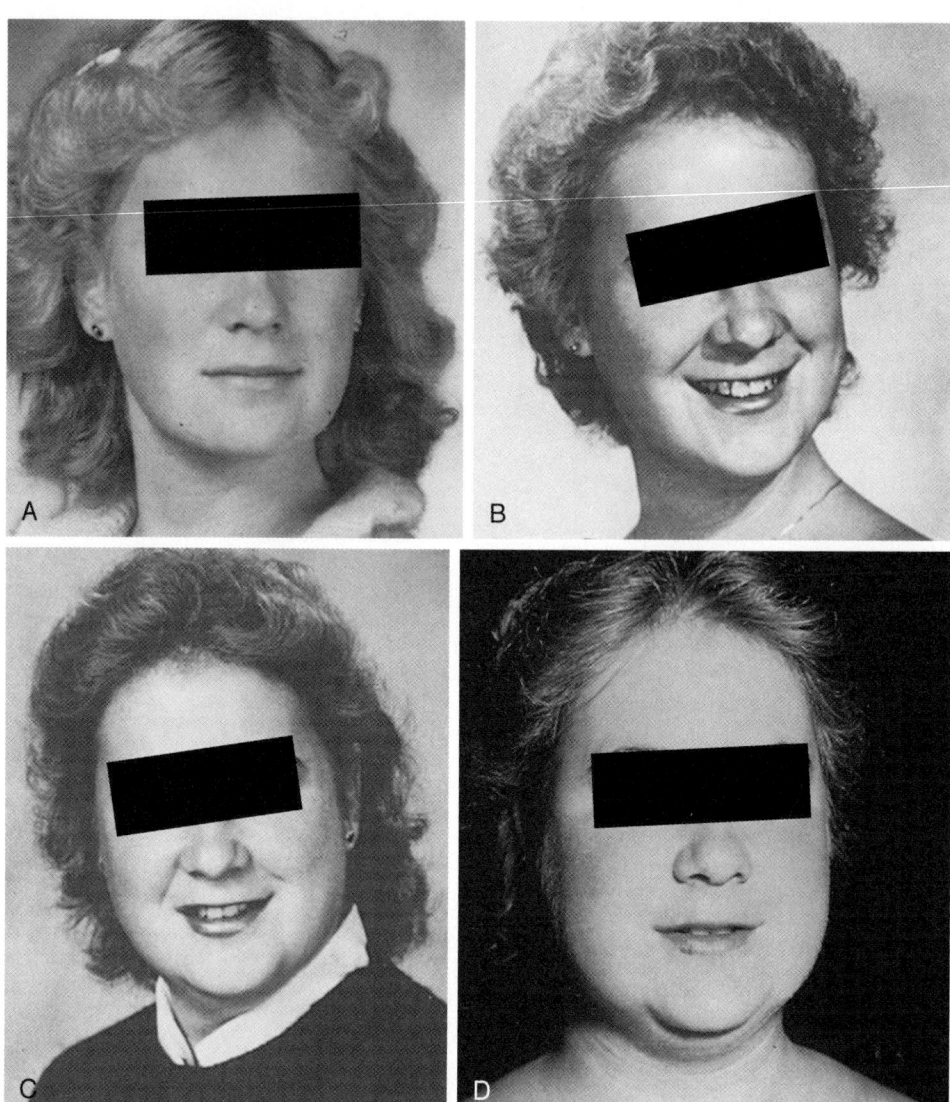

Figure 24-3 Progression of cushingoid features as shown in photographs taken at 1-year intervals (**A–D,** progress from earliest to latest).

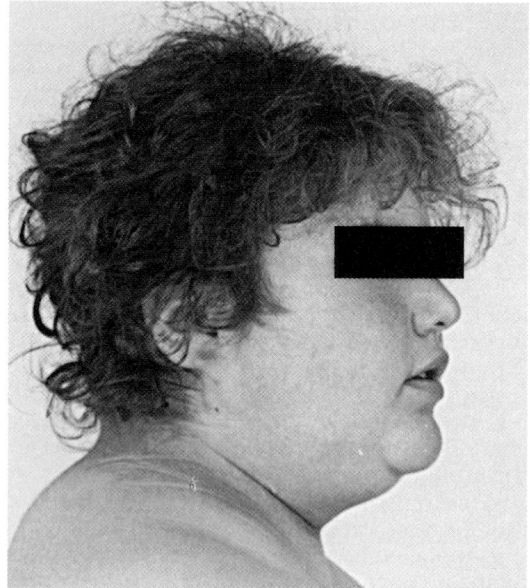

Figure 24-4 Fat may fill or, in this case, rise above the supraclavicular fossa of patients with Cushing's syndrome.

normal persons by ultraviolet radiation from lamps or sunlight, wind, or medications (including topical drying agents, glucocorticoids, and antipsoriatic treatments), exposure to these agents should be ascertained before plethora is ascribed to endogenous hypercortisolism. A demarcation line, representing collar, sleeve, or shoulder straps, may differentiate exogenous from endogenous causes. Flushing caused by other conditions (e.g., mastocytosis, thyrotoxicosis, vasomotor instability or estrogen insufficiency in women, carcinoid syndrome) should be considered.

Purple striae more than 1 cm in diameter are virtually pathognomonic for Cushing's syndrome (Fig. 24-6). Although the silvery, healed striae that are typical post partum are not caused by active Cushing's syndrome, other pink, less pigmented, and thinner striae are seen. Although most common over the abdomen, striae occur also over the hips, buttocks, thighs, breasts, and upper arms. The tear in the subcutaneous tissue may be best appreciated by indirect (side) lighting, which throws the striae into relief, or by light stroking of the skin. The violaceous hue is not dependent on ACTH-dependent pigmentation and may be seen in Cushing's syndrome secondary to primary adrenal causes.

Proximal muscle weakness with preservation of distal strength is a hallmark of Cushing's syndrome. Histologically, this is reflected in profound atrophy of fibers without necrosis.[80–82] Weakness is best assessed historically by questions

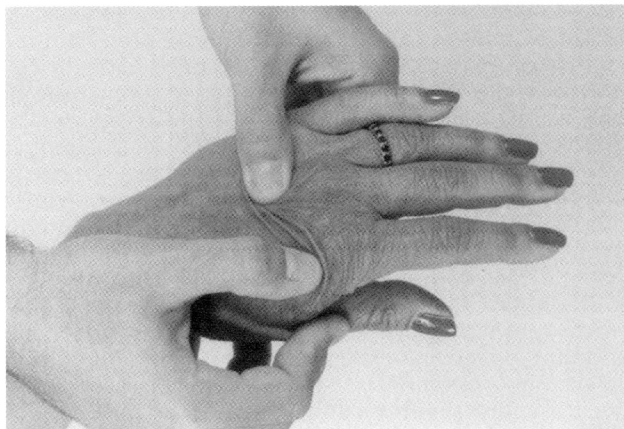

Figure 24-5 Thinning of the skin may be demonstrated by twisting the skin on the dorsum of the hand.

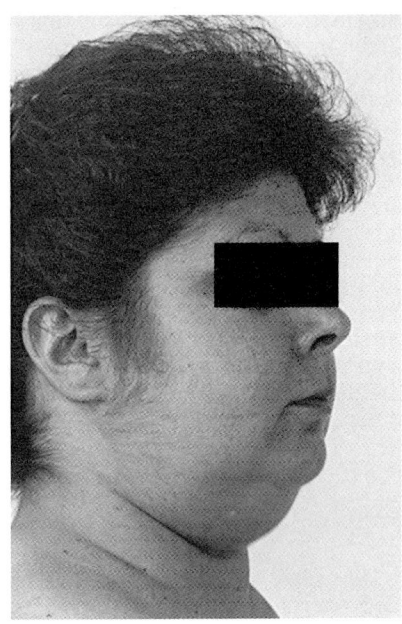

Figure 24-7 Vellus hirsutism, especially on the cheeks, is often present in women with Cushing's syndrome.

related to use of these muscles: Is there difficulty or weakness in climbing stairs, getting up from a chair or bed without using hand propulsion, or performing activities using the shoulders (e.g., brushing hair, reaching objects in overhead cabinets, changing ceiling light bulbs)? Formal muscle testing is useful. Assess the strength of the hip flexors by asking the patient to get out of a chair without using his or her arms. If this can be done, the patient is asked to rise from a squat. Inability to perform either task, in the absence of hip or lower extremity arthropathy or other myopathic processes, is suggestive of Cushing's syndrome. Leg extension while seated is a quantifiable test of proximal muscle strength. The number of seconds for which this position is held can be used to judge deterioration or progress after treatment.

Osteopenia is common. A history of fractures, typically of the feet, ribs, or vertebrae, may be one of the only signs of Cushing's syndrome, especially in men.[72,73,83] Avascular necrosis of bone, a rare complication of endogenous hypercortisolism, is more common in iatrogenic hypercortisolism.[84,85]

Vellus hypertrichosis of the forehead or upper cheeks distinguishes Cushing's syndrome from the more common causes of hirsutism and may be appreciated only by careful visual and tactile inspection (Fig. 24-7). Excessive terminal hair on the face and body, and acne, either pustular, reflecting increased androgens, or papular, reflecting pure gluco-

corticoid excess, may be present.[86] Severe hirsutism and virilization are uncommon and suggest adrenal carcinoma.

Most patients experience emotional and cognitive changes (including increased fatigue, irritability, crying, and restlessness), depressed mood; decreased libido; insomnia; anxiety; impaired memory, concentration, and verbal communication; and changes in appetite. These changes correlate with the degree of hypercortisolism.[87] Irritability, characterized as a decreased threshold for uncontrollable verbal outbursts, may be one of the earliest symptoms. The global impairment in neuropsychological function correlates well with performance of serial 7 subtractions and recall of the names of three cities, bedside tests that can be used by the clinician to quantify this symptom complex.[88]

Approximately 80% of patients meet strict criteria for a major affective disorder, 50% with unipolar depression and 30% with bipolar illness.[89,90] Although the quality of the depressed mood ranges from suicide attempts to sadness, the time course is characteristically intermittent, rarely lasting more than 3 days, in contrast to the constant dysphoria reported by depressed patients without Cushing's syndrome.[87] A minority of patients are manic. The improvement in neuropsychiatric findings after treatment of Cushing's syndrome, coupled with similar features in patients treated with exogenous steroids, and the association of hypercortisolism with poor cognitive performance in depressed patients both suggest glucocorticoid excess as a cause.[91,92]

Hypertension is present in approximately 80% of patients, and although hypertension is also common in the general population, its presence in patients younger than 40 years of age, especially if difficult to control, may alert one to the syndrome. In children with Cushing's syndrome, hypertension is present in approximately 50%.[93] Hypertension usually resolves with treatment of the Cushing's syndrome but may persist, possibly due to microvessel remodeling and/or underlying essential hypertension.[94]

The association of hypercortisolism and fungal infections of the skin, such as mucocutaneous candidiasis, tinea versicolor, and pityriasis, and poor wound healing are common features. Wound dehiscence occurs less often but is an important consideration in patients being treated surgically without medical pretreatment.

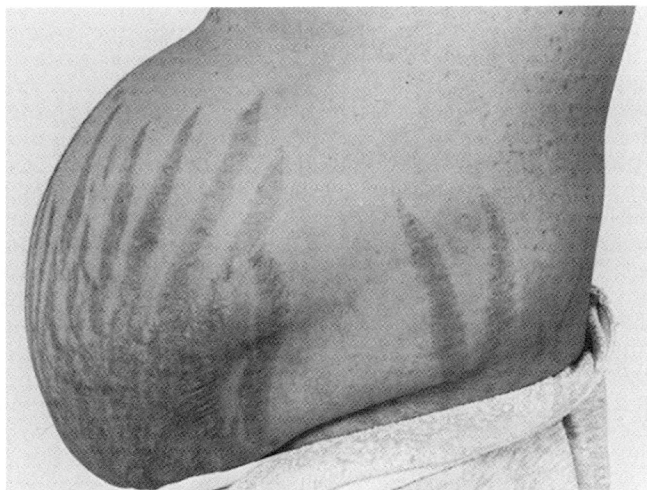

Figure 24-6 Typical abdominal striae of a patient with hypercortisolism. These are greater than 1 cm in width and violaceous.

Patients with marked hypercortisolism (plasma cortisol > 43 µg/dL [1200 nmol/L], UFC > 2000 µg/day [5520 nmol/day]) are at risk of two potentially catastrophic events: perforation of the viscera and severe infections, either bacterial or opportunistic such as *Pneumocystis carinii*, aspergillosis, nocardiosis, cryptococcosis, histoplasmosis, and *Candida*.[95-97] Classic clinical signs, such as loss of bowel sounds and fever, may be absent, and the typical leukocytosis of hypercortisolism may not increase further. Thus, the threshold of suspicion for opportunistic infections and a surgical abdomen must be low in patients with severe hypercortisolism.

Libido is decreased uniformly in men and to a lesser extent (44%) in women,[72] in whom increased libido may indicate excess androgen production by an adrenocortical carcinoma. Menstrual irregularities, amenorrhea, and infertility are common and may be the presenting complaints.[98] Impotence is common.

PATHOLOGY

The cardinal laboratory findings in endogenous Cushing's syndrome reflect overproduction of glucocorticoids. Although morning plasma cortisol values may be normal, an increased nighttime nadir blunts or obliterates the normal diurnal rhythm.[99-101] This increase in mean 24-hour plasma values is reflected in increased levels of free, or unbound, cortisol in urine[102] and saliva.[103] The capacity of corticosteroid-binding globulin for cortisol is exceeded at a serum cortisol value of approximately 20 µg/dL (~600 nmol/L). At this point, the excretion of free cortisol increases dramatically in direct proportion to the increased unbound circulating cortisol values.

Hypokalemic metabolic alkalosis is usually observed when daily urine cortisol excretion is greater than 1500 µg (4100 nmol), and thus mainly in cases of ectopic ACTH syndrome.[104] This probably represents a mineralocorticoid action of cortisol at the renal tubule due to saturation of the enzyme 11β-hydroxysteroid dehydrogenase type 2, which inactivates cortisol to cortisone.[105] However, although a common feature of ectopic ACTH secretion, it may also occur in approximately 10% of patients with Cushing's disease.

Serum albumin is inversely correlated with cortisol levels, but this is only of clinical significance at very high cortisol levels, and reverses with treatment of the Cushing's syndrome.[106] Drastic reductions in serum albumin should alert the physician to the possibility of concomitant pathology such as infection.

Circulating elevated glucocorticoids increase clotting factors including factor VIII, fibrinogen, and von Willebrand factor and reduce fibrinolytic activity, resulting in a fourfold risk of thrombotic events.[107-109]

Lipid abnormalities show increases in very low density lipoprotein, low-density lipoprotein, high-density lipoprotein, and consequently total cholesterol and triglycerides. The changes are probably caused by a direct cortisol effect of increased hepatic synthesis of very low density lipoprotein without altered clearance.[110,111]

Cushing's syndrome is characterized by insulin resistance and hyperinsulinemia,[112] with frank diabetes mellitus occurring in 30% to 40% of patients, and glucose intolerance in a further 20% to 30%.[113,114] A recent study has suggested that as many as 2% of overweight, poorly controlled patients with diabetes may have occult Cushing's syndrome if fully investigated.[115]

Patients with Cushing's disease show accelerated cardiovascular disease, including increased carotid artery intima-media thickness and atherosclerotic plaques on Doppler ultrasonography.[116] This increased risk is maintained even as long as 5 years after cure of the hypercortisolemia.[117]

Hypercortisolism suppresses the thyroidal, gonadal, and growth hormone axes. Thyrotropin-releasing hormone and thyroid-stimulating hormone release is disturbed and particularly the nocturnal surge of thyroid-stimulating hormone is lost, resulting in reduced total thyroxine, total triiodothyronine, and free triiodothyronine levels compared with controls.[118] Others have found no differences in free thyroxine or free triiodothyronine levels but have shown that there is a significantly increased prevalence of autoimmune thyroid disease in patients treated for Cushing's syndrome.[119,120] In both men and women, low levels of luteinizing hormone, follicle-stimulating hormone, and gonadal steroids consistent with hypogonadotrophic hypogonadism are common and correlate with the degree of hypercortisolemia.[121,122] In addition, the coexistence of polycystic ovarian syndrome in Cushing's syndrome may be more common than previously thought.[98] Hypercortisolemia causes reduced GH secretion during sleep and blunted GH responses to stimulation tests.[123]

The prevalence of osteoporosis as assessed by dual energy x-ray absorptiometry is approximately 50% in adult Cushing's syndrome.[124] It appears more common in adrenal Cushing's syndrome than Cushing's disease, and this may relate to increased adrenal androgens in the latter having a protective effect.[125]

The accentuated visceral fat distribution characteristic of Cushing's syndrome can be quite marked when visualized by computed tomography (CT),[76] and the liver is frequently (20%) steatotic on imaging.[126]

CLINICAL SPECTRUM

The typical patient with Cushing's disease presents at midlife complaining of the gradual development of symptoms, although males tend to present at an earlier age and with more severe clinical consequences.[127] Hypokalemia, virilization, and extremely high cortisol excretion (>10-fold normal) are distinctly uncommon and should alert the physician to an alternative cause. The clinical presentation of pituitary corticotroph macroadenomas, apart from visual field changes caused by suprasellar expansion, is not unique. By contrast, invasive pituitary adenomas present at a slightly younger age; cavernous sinus and dural involvement may result in cranial neuropathies and facial neuralgia.[128,129] Only a few case reports attest to cerebrospinal or extracranial metastasis of ACTH-producing pituitary tumors.[130]

Nelson's syndrome is characterized by the development of hyperpigmentation and high ACTH levels after bilateral adrenalectomy for Cushing's disease. The tumor growth after adrenalectomy has been attributed to the relative resistance of these tumors to physiologic glucocorticoid suppression.

An abrupt onset of severe Cushing's syndrome should prompt an evaluation for ectopic ACTH secretion. This variant of ectopic ACTH secretion classically presents as a paraneoplastic syndrome in the context of a known malignancy. The features were captured in the initial formulation of Liddle and colleagues[4]: weight loss, hypokalemia, weakness, and diabetes. However, Cushing's syndrome caused by occult ectopic ACTH secretion often present in the more classic way with weight gain and striae and can be difficult to differentiate clinically from Cushing's disease. It is patients with this syndrome who most often present a diagnostic dilemma. They tend to have UFC excretion in the range seen in pituitary disease and may not show hypokalemia, hyperpigmentation, or the other findings typical of severe ectopic ACTH secretion.

Adrenocortical carcinomas are inefficient producers of cortisol and tend to evince Cushing's syndrome when the tumor is large (>6 cm), if at all. Abdominal pain or a palpable mass suggests this cause. Feminization in a man or virilization and increased libido in a woman, indicating involvement of the zona reticularis, suggest adrenal cancer or the more rare macronodular adrenal disease. The typical patient with PPNAD is a child or young adult who may present with an intermittent course or a family history of associated signs: Lentigines may be the initial clue to this cause. By contrast, patients with the massive macronodular variant of ACTH-independent Cushing's syndrome tend to be older than 40 years of age.

DIAGNOSIS AND DIFFERENTIAL DIAGNOSIS

The diagnosis of Cushing's syndrome rests on the demonstration of both physical and biochemical features of glucocorticoid excess. Thus, the diagnosis is unequivocal in a typical patient with many of the physical features discussed earlier in the setting of UFC levels more than fourfold above normal.[131] However, many of the signs of hypercortisolism, such as obesity, hypertension, mood changes, menstrual irregularity, and hirsutism, are common in the general population. Similarly, mild glucocorticoid excess is seen in affective disorders,[132] strenuous exercise,[61] alcoholism and alcohol withdrawal states,[133] renal failure,[134] and hypoglycemia. Diagnostic strategies for distinguishing between these pseudo-Cushing's states and true Cushing's syndrome are discussed.

Glucocorticoid resistance is characterized by an abnormal glucocorticoid receptor number or binding, causing compensatory increases in ACTH and excessive glucocorticoid production to maintain normal glucocorticoid-mediated effects at the target tissues. The diagnosis should be considered in the hypokalemic, hypertensive, hypercortisolemic patient *without* typical glucocorticoid-mediated signs of Cushing's syndrome.[135]

ESTABLISHING THE DIAGNOSIS OF CUSHING'S SYNDROME

Biochemical confirmation of the diagnosis of Cushing's syndrome is needed when a careful history and physical examination reveal clinical features that could be consistent with the syndrome (Table 24-4). It is important to remember that the urgency for diagnosis and treatment of Cushing's syndrome is greatest when the symptoms are severe. In milder cases, the patient may be best served by waiting until the diagnosis is clear. Periodic reevaluation with urine screening tests and documentation of body habitus with photographs may reveal progression.

Initial Screening Tests

Hypercortisolemia demonstrated by the loss of the normal circadian rhythm of cortisol secretion and disturbed feedback of the hypothalamic-pituitary-adrenal (HPA) axis are the cardinal biochemical features of Cushing's syndrome. Tests to confirm the diagnosis are based on these principles. To screen for Cushing's syndrome, tests of high sensitivity should be used initially to avoid missing milder cases.

Urinary-Free Cortisol

Under normal conditions, 10% of plasma cortisol is free or unbound and physiologically active. Unbound cortisol is filtered by the kidney, with the majority being reabsorbed in the tubules and the remainder excreted unchanged. Thus, 24-hour UFC collection produces an integrated measure of serum cortisol, smoothing out the variations in cortisol during the day. UFC determinations first became clinically available in 1968[136] and have superseded the historical measurement of urinary metabolites of glucocorticoids and androgens (17-hydroxycorticosteroids [17-OHCS], 17-ketosteroids,

Table 24-4 Evaluation of Suspected Cushing's Syndrome

History
Increased weight
Growth retardation in children
Weakness
Easy bruising
Stretch marks
Poor wound healing
Fractures
Change in libido
Impotence/irregular or no menses
Emotional, cognitive, mood changes (fatigue, irritability, anxiety, insomnia, depression, impaired memory and concentration)

Examination
Fat distribution (centripetal obesity; rounded face; dorsocervical, supraclavicular, temporal fat pads)
Hypertension
Proximal muscle weakness and atrophy
Thin skin and ecchymoses
Purple striae
Hirsutism
Acne
Facial plethora
Edema
Impaired serial 7s/recall of 3 cities

Laboratory findings
Abnormal glucose tolerance/frank diabetes mellitus, hypokalemia

First-line screening tests
Elevated 24-hour urinary free cortisol (3 collections)
Lack of suppression to low-dose dexamethasone (LDDST)
Elevated late night salivary cortisol*

Additional screening tests (if required)
Cortisol circadian rhythm
Insulin tolerance test
Combined LDDST + CRH test*
Loperamide test*

*These tests require further evaluation.
CRH, corticotropin-releasing hormone; LDDST, low-dose dexamethasone suppression test.

and 17-ketogenic steroids). There are four major problems associated with the measurement of such steroid metabolites for the detection of Cushing's syndrome. First, a significant proportion of the material in a 24-hour sample does not represent cortisol metabolites. Second, the colorimetric and fluorometric assay methods are often affected by medications and other substances so that the assay cannot be performed or the result is not accurate. Third, 17-OHCS measurement is affected by hepatic and renal disease and is increased in many obese individuals relative to normal-weight subjects. Last, 17-ketosteroids and 17-ketogenic steroids represent both glucocorticoid and androgenic pathways and thus are not a good choice for discrimination of glucocorticoid excess.

The major drawback of the test is the potential for an inadequate 24-hour urine collection, and written instructions must be given to the patient. In addition, creatinine excretion in the collection should be measured to assess completeness and should equal approximately 1 g per 24 hours in a 70-kg patient (variations depend on muscle mass). This should not vary by more than 10% between collections in the same individual.[137] It cannot be used to correct for incomplete collection, however, because the rates of cortisol and creatinine excretion are not parallel over the 24-hour period. Various groups have tried to overcome the collection issue by proposing shorter collection periods, usually at night, when the loss of circadian rhythm differs most from normal controls,[138,139] but these have not been widely accepted. In children, UFC should be corrected for body surface area ($\times 1.72\ m^2$).[140]

When measuring UFC using conventional radioimmunoassay in cases of factitious Cushing's syndrome, there may be cross-reactivity of some exogenous glucocorticoids.[141] If such cases are suspected, UFC should be assayed by high-performance liquid chromatography, which specifically measures unbound urine cortisol.[142] Similarly, other usually structurally similar steroids may cross-react in an immunoassay, depending on the antibody used, which accounts for the twofold difference in the upper limit of normal urine cortisol of the antibody-based assays compared with high-performance liquid chromatography. These differences are important to note because they change the normal reference range. Occasionally, substances such as carbamazepine and digoxin can coelute with cortisol during high-performance liquid chromatography and cause falsely elevated results.[143]

If the previous caveats have been satisfied, the UFC measurement can be interpreted. In large series, measurement of an elevated UFC above the normal range has a high sensitivity for the diagnosis Cushing's syndrome (~95%–100%).[102,144] However, it should be noted that in the later study, 11% of 146 patients with proven Cushing's syndrome had at least one of four UFC collections within the normal range, which confirms the need for multiple collections. Values greater than fourfold normal (~400 µg/day [1100 nmol/day] in most radioimmunoassays) are rare except in Cushing's syndrome. Values between this and down to the upper limit of normal are compatible with either Cushing's syndrome or pseudo-Cushing's states, so that one must exclude the latter diagnosis. In summary, UFC measurements have a high sensitivity if collected correctly, and several completely normal collections make the diagnosis of Cushing's syndrome very unlikely. However, when biochemical evidence of Cushing's syndrome is not obtained in the setting of clinical features that suggest the diagnosis, repeated measurement of urine cortisol may demonstrate cyclicity or progression. The specificity is somewhat lower, and thus patients with marginally elevated levels require further investigation.[57]

Late-Night Salivary Cortisol

Salivary cortisol measurement offers an excellent reflection of the plasma-free cortisol concentration in normality and disease because it circumvents the changes in total cortisol due to corticosteroid-binding globulin alterations.[145,146] Due to the simple noninvasive collection procedure, which can conveniently be performed at home, it offers a number of attractive advantages over blood collection, particularly in children. Salivary cortisol is stable for some days at room temperature,[147] and the sample is obtained using a standard saliva collection kit. Analysis is performed using a modification of the plasma cortisol radioimmunoassay or enzyme-linked immunosorbent assay. Nighttime salivary cortisol estimation has been studied at a number of centers as a screening test for Cushing's syndrome in both adults[148–150] and children.[151,152] At the National Institutes of Health, 122 patients with Cushing's syndrome, 21 patients with pseudo-Cushing's states, 23 noncushingoid controls, and 34 healthy volunteers had nighttime salivary cortisol measurements made, mostly as inpatients (78%). A threshold of 0.55 µg/dL (15.2 nmol/L) for an inpatient midnight or outpatient bedtime salivary cortisol identified 93% of subjects with Cushing's syndrome and excluded all subjects without the disorder (100% specificity).[149] In a study of 300 patients (41 Cushing's syndrome, 33 pseudo-Cushing's states, 199 obese, and 27 healthy individuals), a midnight salivary cortisol cut-off of 9.7 nmol/L or more gave a sensitivity and specificity of 93% for the diagnosis of Cushing's syndrome.[150] Therefore, despite different criteria, the sensitivity of the late-night salivary cortisol appears the same in both of these large studies. However, the lower specificity of the latter study is probably attributable to the higher number of individuals without Cushing's syndrome being included, whereas in the former study, the diagnostic criteria were chosen with 100% specificity in mind. Several other diagnostic cut-off points for late-night

(11:00 P.M.–12:00 A.M.) salivary cortisol have also been proposed from smaller studies ranging from 0.13 µg/dL (3.6 nmol/L)[148] to 0.28 µg/dL (7.7 nmol/L)[153] in adults and 0.27 µg/dL (7.5 nmol/L)[151] to 0.28 µg/dL (7.7 nmol/L)[152] in children. From these studies, the sensitivity and specificity of this test appears to be relatively consistent at different centers, ranging from 92% to 100% and 93% to 100%, respectively. In summary, therefore, although late-night salivary cortisol appears to be a useful and convenient additional screening test for Cushing's syndrome, particularly in the outpatient setting, further large studies of its diagnostic accuracy are needed. In addition, validated commercial assays are not yet widely available.

Low-Dose Dexamethasone Suppression Tests

In normal individuals, administration of the potent synthetic glucocorticoid dexamethasone results in suppression of the HPA axis, whereas patients with Cushing's syndrome are resistant, at least partially, to this negative feedback. The original low-dose dexamethasone test (LDDST), described by Liddle in 1960, measured urinary 17-OHCS before and during 48 hours of 0.5 mg dexamethasone every 6 hours, and an excretion of greater than 4 mg/day on the second day of dexamethasone treatment was considered to indicate Cushing's syndrome.[154] Dexamethasone does not cross-react with modern cortisol immunoassays, and the simpler measurement of a single plasma cortisol post-dexamethasone has been validated in various series and gives the test a sensitivity of between 97% and 100% for the diagnosis of Cushing's syndrome.[155–158] The simpler overnight LDDST was proposed by Nugent and colleagues[159] in 1965; this measured a 9:00 A.M. plasma cortisol after a single dose of 1 mg dexamethasone taken at midnight. Since then, various other doses, between 0.5 and 2 mg, have been proposed for the overnight test, and various diagnostic cut-offs have been applied.[160–162] There appears to be no difference in discrimination between single doses of 1, 1.5, or 2 mg.[163] Higher doses significantly decrease the sensitivity of the test.[164] In a comprehensive review of the LDDST, both the original 2-day test and the 1-mg overnight protocol appear to have comparably high sensitivities (98%–100%), provided a conservative postdexamethasone serum cortisol cut-off of 1.8 µg/dL (50 nmol/L) is applied. However, the specificity of the overnight test (88%) is lower compared with the 2-day test, particularly if serum cortisol is measured at both 24 and 48 hours (97%–100%), with potential misclassification of patients with pseudo-Cushing's states and acute or chronic illnesses.[165,166] Many endocrinologists use the overnight test due to its greater simplicity and lower cost, although some centers still advocate the 48-hour test due to its high sensitivity and specificity, provided written instructions are given to the patient.[158] More recently, the LDDST has been used to measure salivary rather than serum cortisol and may be of potential benefit in terms of convenience but requires further evaluation.[152,153]

Factors such as variable absorption and increased or decreased dexamethasone metabolism due to other compounds (Table 24-5) can influence any oral dexamethasone test.[167] Therefore, a history of symptoms of malabsorption and a careful drug history should be taken before using the test in a patient. One solution to overcome demonstrated malabsorption is to use one of the published intravenous dexamethasone suppression tests.[168,169] Pregnancy and other causes of increased corticosteroid-binding globulin (such as exogenous estrogens) should also be excluded because these are likely to result in false-positive tests.

Second-Line Tests
Cortisol Circadian Rhythm
The normal diurnal rhythm of plasma cortisol is blunted or absent in Cushing's syndrome,[99–101] with normal or increased morning values and an increase in the nighttime nadir. Meal-

Table 24-5	Spurious Causes of Abnormal Dexamethasone Suppression test results

False positive
  Increased metabolism: barbiturates, phenytoin, carbamazepine, primidone, rifampicin, aminoglutethimide[167]
  Increased cortisol-binding globulin: pregnancy, oral estrogens, tamoxifen[455]
  Malabsorption
  Pseudo-Cushing's states
False negative
  Reduced metabolism: high-dose benzodiazepines, indomethacin,[456] liver disease[457]

related and stress-related increases in plasma cortisol may result in apparently elevated values in normal persons. As a result, plasma levels of cortisol discriminate patients with Cushing's syndrome best when obtained around midnight, either through an indwelling line for awake patients[170] or by direct venepuncture within 5 to 10 minutes of waking of sleeping patients.[157] In one study, 20 normal sleeping subjects had values less than 1.8 µg/dL (50 nmol/L), whereas all 150 patients with Cushing's syndrome had midnight plasma cortisol concentrations greater than this.[157] However, the best cut-off value to discriminate between *awake* patients with pseudo-Cushing's states and Cushing's syndrome was 7.5 µg/dL (207 nmol/L), with a 94% sensitivity and 100% specificity.[170] Similarly, patients with severe medical illness, depression, and mania may have cortisol values one to three times normal.[132,163] Therefore, a sleeping midnight cortisol value less than 1.8 µg/dL (50 nmol/L) effectively excludes active Cushing's syndrome, but higher values, unless very high, are less specific for Cushing's syndrome.

Other Second-Line Tests

The insulin tolerance test may be a useful adjunct to distinguish Cushing's syndrome from pseudo-Cushing's states. Serum cortisol values increase in normal people after acute hypoglycemia, presumably because of central stimulation of CRH and vasopressin. The sustained hypercortisolism of Cushing's syndrome suppresses CRH and vasopressin secretion and so blunts this response. The CRH/vasopressin neurons are presumed to be overactive in pseudo-Cushing's states, particularly depression associated, so a normal response to hypoglycemia (<40 mg/dL, <2.2 nmol/L) is usually maintained. Unfortunately, approximately 18% of patients with Cushing's syndrome, especially those with minimal hypercortisolism, show a normal response to adequate hypoglycemia.[163] If used, a dose of insulin of 0.3 U/kg should be used to overcome the insulin resistance in these patients.[132]

The opiate agonist loperamide (16 mg orally) has been shown to inhibit CRH and thus ACTH and cortisol levels in most normal individuals but not in patients with Cushing's syndrome. This has not been used by many groups but has been evaluated in one center in 151 patients referred with the putative diagnosis of Cushing's syndrome, in whom 41 were subsequently confirmed to have that diagnosis. Here the test had a sensitivity of 100% and specificity of 95%.[171,172] However, it is unclear as to how well this test may be at excluding pseudo-Cushing's states because a significant proportion of patients with depression also fail to suppress the HPA axis.[173] It does not appear to be affected by drugs that affect the metabolism of dexamethasone and could potentially be useful in assessing patients on such treatment.[172]

More recently, a combined dexamethasone-CRH test has been evaluated for the difficult scenario of the differentiation of pseudo-Cushing's states from true Cushing's syndrome in patients with only mild hypercortisolemia and equivocal physical findings.[174] Dexamethasone 0.5 mg every 6 hours was given for eight doses, ending 2 hours before administration of

ovine CRH (1 µg/kg intravenously) to 58 adults with UFC less than 360 µg/day (<1000 nmol/day). Subsequent evaluation proved 39 to have Cushing's syndrome and 19 to have a pseudo-Cushing's state. The plasma cortisol value 15 minutes after CRH was less than 1.4 µg/dL (38 nmol/L) in all patients with pseudo-Cushing's states and greater in all patients with Cushing's syndrome. A prospective follow-up study in 98 patients showed a reduction in the sensitivity and specificity to 99% and 96%, respectively.[175] Thus, this test may prove to be a major advance in the ability to distinguish between Cushing's syndrome and pseudo-Cushing's states but does require further evaluation. In particular, any advantage over the 2-mg, 2-day conventional low-dose dexamethasone test requires confirmation.

DIFFERENTIAL DIAGNOSIS OF CUSHING'S SYNDROME

Once the diagnosis of Cushing's syndrome is made, its cause must be determined. The strategy for the differential diagnosis of Cushing's syndrome (Fig. 24-8) begins with measurement of plasma ACTH to distinguish between ACTH-dependent and ACTH-independent causes. Modern two-site immunoradiometric assays are more sensitive than the older radioimmunoassays and therefore provide the best discrimination. Only assays that can reliably detect values to below 10 pg/mL should be used, and appropriate collection and processing of the sample are essential because ACTH is susceptible to degradation by peptidases so that the sample must be kept in an ice water bath and centrifuged, aliquoted, and frozen within a few hours to avoid a spuriously low result. Repeated measurements are usually necessary because patients with ACTH-dependent Cushing's disease have been shown to have on occasion ACTH levels less than 10 pg/mL (2 pmol/L) on conventional radioimmunoassay,[176] but consistent ACTH measurements of less than 10 pg/mL (2 pmol/L) at 9:00 A.M. with concomitant hypercortisolemia essentially confirm ACTH-independent Cushing's syndrome. When the basal ACTH level is indeterminate (10–20 pg/mL [2–4 pmol/L]), the response to CRH may be useful in this setting. Patients with primary adrenal disease rarely show maximal ACTH values greater than 20 pg/mL (4 pmol/L), although patients with Cushing's disease usually exceed this value.

Investigating Adrenocorticotropic Hormone–Independent Cushing's Syndrome

Radiologic tests are the mainstay in differentiating between the various types of ACTH-independent Cushing's syndrome. High-resolution CT scanning of the adrenal glands has excellent diagnostic accuracy for masses greater than 1 cm and allows evaluation of the contralateral gland.[177] MRI may be useful for the differential diagnosis of adrenal masses; the T_2-weighted signal is progressively darker in phaeochromocytoma, carcinoma, adenoma, and finally normal tissue.[178] MRI is at least as useful as CT in pediatric cases.[179] With this approach, adrenal tumors appear as a unilateral mass with an atrophic or less commonly normal-size contralateral gland.[180] If the lesion is greater than 5 cm in diameter, it should be considered to be malignant until proven otherwise, and imaging characteristics should not be relied on. Very rarely, bilateral adenomas can be present.[177,180,181] The adrenal glands in PPNAD appear normal or slightly lumpy from multiple small nodules but are not generally enlarged.[182] AIMAH is characterized by bilaterally huge (>5 cm) nodular or hyperplastic glands.[183,184] Exogenous administration of glucocorticoids results in adrenal atrophy; very small glands may be a clue as to this entity.

In some clinical settings, the adrenal glands in ACTH-independent and ACTH-dependent causes of Cushing's may have similar appearances on imaging. The CT appearance of the adrenals in AIMAH may be similar to the appearance seen in ACTH-dependent forms of Cushing's syndrome, in which

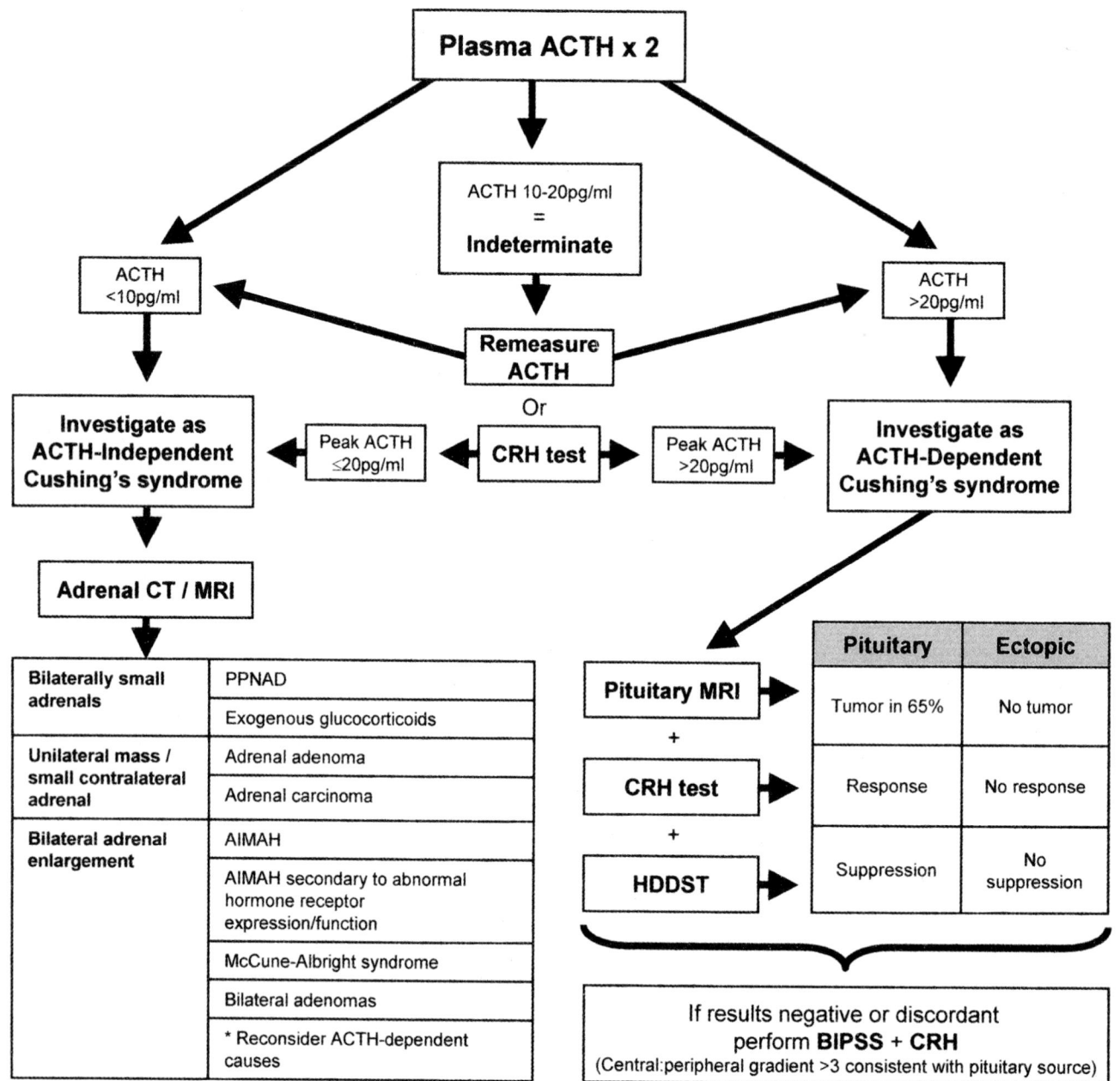

Figure 24-8 Suggested strategy for the differential diagnosis of Cushing's syndrome. ACTH, adrenocorticotropic hormone; AIMAH, ACTH-independent bilateral macronodular adrenal hyperplasia; BIPSS, bilateral inferior petrosal sinus sampling; CRH, corticotropin-releasing hormone; CT, computed tomography; HDDST, high-dose dexamethasone suppression test; MRI, magnetic resonance imaging; PPNAD, primary pigmented nodular adrenal disease.

adrenal enlargement is present in 70% of cases,[185] but the two can usually be distinguished by the ACTH level and the degree of adrenal enlargement. Some patients with the macronodular subset of Cushing's disease can develop a degree of adrenal autonomy that can cause biochemical confusion.[186,187] Occasionally, confusion can also arise with apparent unilateral adrenal lesions, when the biochemistry is consistent with an ACTH-dependent cause; we would generally rely on the biochemistry in this situation and would examine the contralateral gland to see whether it is hyperplastic. Iodocholesterol scintigraphy may be useful. In this technique, functional adrenal tissue takes up a radioactively tagged cholesterol analogue; Cushing's disease is the usual diagnosis if the contralateral gland is of normal size or enlarged and has some uptake with iodocholesterol scanning.[188,189] The converse pertains to patients with adrenal adenoma; the contralateral gland is atrophic, without iodocholesterol uptake.[177]

Differentiating between Adrenocorticotropic Hormone–Dependent Causes of Cushing's Syndrome

Although some patients with ectopic ACTH secretion, usually those with overt tumors, have extremely elevated values of plasma ACTH (>100 pg/mL [>20 pmol/L]), there is complete overlap between values in occult ectopic ACTH secretion and Cushing's disease.[190] Therefore, ACTH values alone cannot differentiate reliably the ACTH-dependent forms of Cushing's syndrome.

The ACTH-dependent forms of Cushing's syndrome present the greatest diagnostic challenge. Cushing's disease accounts for by far the majority of cases of ACTH-dependent Cushing's syndrome, overall approximately 80% to 90% in most series. This percentage is gender dependent, being higher in women than men,[191] although in childhood, there is an anomalous male preponderance. Therefore, even before one starts further investigation, the pretest probability that the patient has Cushing's disease is very high, and any investigation must improve on this. The specificity of any test should be as close to 100% for the diagnosis of Cushing's disease to avoid inappropriate pituitary surgery in patients with ectopic ACTH production. A variety of functional tests of the HPA axis has been developed to take advantage of the differences in pathophysiology between the ACTH-dependent causes of Cushing's syndrome. Some of these investigations have evolved and others have fallen by the wayside.

Bilateral Inferior Petrosal Sinus Sampling

Bilateral inferior petrosal sinus sampling is the best test for distinguishing ACTH-dependent forms of Cushing's syndrome as long as the patient has active hypercortisolemia, which should be confirmed at the time of the procedure.[192,193] The test exploits the normal venous drainage of each half of the pituitary gland via the cavernous sinus into the corresponding petrosal sinus. Each petrosal sinus is catheterized separately via a femoral approach, and blood for measurement of ACTH is obtained simultaneously from each sinus and a peripheral vein at two timepoints before and at 3 to 5 minutes and possibly also 10 minutes after the administration of ovine or human CRH (1 µg/kg or 100 µg intravenously, respectively)[194] (Fig. 24-9).

ACTH concentrations are greater in the central samples in Cushing's disease and increase after CRH administration, reflecting ACTH secretion by the corticotroph adenoma. In contrast, ACTH values in the central and peripheral specimens are similar in ectopic ACTH secretion and do not increase after CRH. A ratio of the central (i.e., petrosal) to peripheral ACTH values is calculated. In most large series, pre-CRH gradients greater than 2 are 100% specific for Cushing's disease,[195,196] but a single patient with ectopic ACTH secretion has been reported as having a ratio just over this value.[62]

Similarly, most post-CRH ratios in ectopic ACTH-secreting tumors are less than 2, but ratios of as high as 2.3 have been reported.[195] Hence, a conservative cut-off ratio of more than 3 seems rational to maintain a 100% specificity for the diagnosis of Cushing's disease. A number of patients with Cushing's disease (5%–20%) also have a basal gradient less than 2, but the sensitivity of the test is improved after CRH, and so we advocate its use in all cases. It should be remembered that the technique is highly specialized, and in experienced single centers with only a small number of radiologists doing the catheterization procedure, the test is able to achieve a sensitivity of 95% to 99% for correctly diagnosing Cushing's disease.[195,196] Allied with this are a number of important points. First, both petrosal sinuses must be adequately cannulated and catheter placement confirmed before and after sampling.[197] Second, the radiologist must confirm the venous anatomy because anomalous venous drainage can give false-negative results. Third, the procedure carries a small risk of complications. Transient ear discomfort or pain can occur, as can local groin hematomas. More serious transient and permanent neurologic sequelae have been reported, including brain stem infarction, although these are rare (<1%), and most have been related to a particular type of catheter used[198,199]; if there are any early warning signs of such events, the procedure should be immediately halted. Patients should be given heparin during sampling to prevent thrombotic events.[131] CRH itself is generally tolerated well, although patients may experience brief facial flushing and a metallic taste in the mouth. One case of CRH inducing pituitary apoplexy in a patient with Cushing's disease has been reported.[200]

Another potential advantage of bilateral inferior petrosal sinus sampling is to lateralize microadenomas within the pituitary using the inferior petrosal sinus ACTH gradient, with a basal or post-CRH intersinus ratio of at least 1.4 being the criterion for lateralization used in all large studies.[195,196,201,202] In these studies, the diagnostic accuracy of localization as assessed by operative outcome varied between 59% and 83%. This is improved if venous drainage is assessed to be symmetric.[203] The accuracy of lateralization appears to be higher in children (90%), a situation in which imaging is often negative.[204] There is some discrepancy between studies as to whether CRH improves the predictive value of the test.[205] If a reversal of lateralization is seen pre- and post-CRH, the test cannot be relied on.[206]

Some have advocated sampling of the cavernous sinus[207] or jugular venous sampling,[208] but overall neither procedure appears as sensitive as bilateral inferior petrosal sinus sampling for the determination of a pituitary ACTH source, although a recent small report using a complicated protocol of sampling from multiple cavernous sinuses sites and the inferior petrosal sinus have suggested this to be highly sensitive in lateralizing the tumor.[209]

High-Dose Dexamethasone Suppression Test

The original high-dose dexamethasone suppression test (HDDST) was described in the same paper as the 48-hour LDDST; 2 mg dexamethasone is used in place of 0.5 mg, with a 50% reduction in urinary 17-OHCS shown to differentiate 96% of patients with Cushing's disease from adrenal tumors.[154] The HDDST's role in the differential diagnosis of ACTH-dependent Cushing's syndrome is based on the same premise: that most pituitary corticotroph tumors retain some responsiveness (albeit reduced) to negative glucocorticoid feedback on ACTH secretion, whereas ectopic ACTH-secreting tumors, like adrenal tumors, typically do not. However, the main problem with applying the same suppression criteria is the high number of false positives (~10%–30%) seen in ectopic Cushing's syndrome.[190] In addition, in most centers, the measurement of UFC or plasma/serum cortisol has superseded that of urinary 17-OHCS. Shifting the criteria to a more

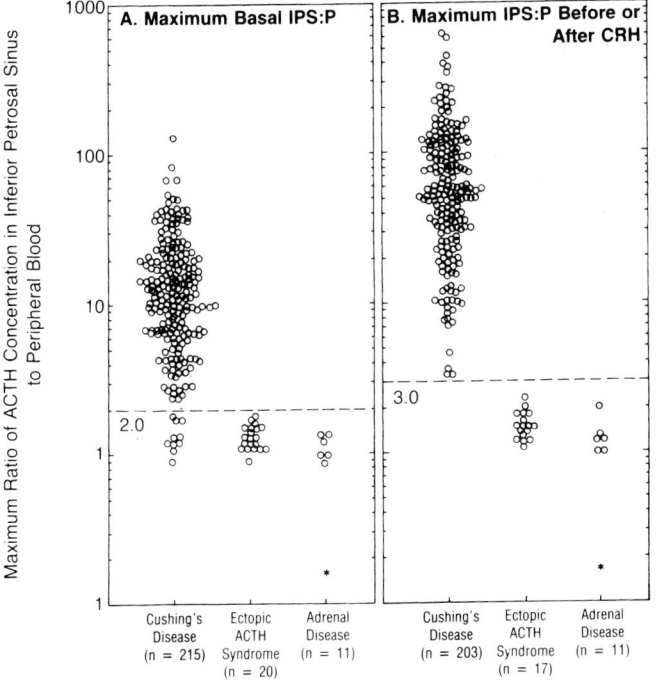

Figure 24-9 Maximal ratio of adrenocorticotropic hormone (ACTH) concentration in the inferior petrosal sinus to peripheral blood in patients with confirmed Cushing's disease, ectopic ACTH syndrome, or adrenal disease before corticotropin-releasing hormone (CRH) **(A)** or at any time before or after CRH administration **(B)**. A ratio of 3.0 had 100% sensitivity and specificity. (Data from Oldfield EH, Doppman JL, Nieman LK, et al: Petrosal sinus sampling with and without corticotropin-releasing hormone for the differential diagnosis of Cushing's syndrome. N Engl J Med 325:897–905, 1991.)

than 90% suppression of UFC initially resulted in improving the specificity to 100% but with a loss of sensitivity (65%–70%)[210,211] (Fig. 24-10); however, applying the same criteria to a larger cohort ($N = 185$) reduced the sensitivity to 59% and the specificity also decreased to 73%.[212] In this study, combining the criteria of suppression of UFC (>90%) or 17-OHCS (>69%), as previously suggested, only served only to increase the sensitivity marginally (72%) at the expense of specificity (67%). Using the criteria of a greater than 60% suppression in serum cortisol at 9:00 A.M. after the last dose of dexamethasone in a large series of 220 cases of ACTH-dependent Cushing's syndrome, the sensitivity and specificity of the HDDST were 91% and 80%, respectively.[158] Data from this study also showed that suppression to HDDST can be inferred by a greater than 30% suppression of serum cortisol to the 2-day LDDST (Fig. 24-11), and therefore the former may be an unnecessary extra investigation.

An overnight test has also been studied, using a single dose of 8 mg dexamethasone at 11:00 P.M., with a 50% reduction in plasma cortisol levels taken on the morning after administration giving 92% sensitivity and 100% specificity.[213] However, others have not found it to give such good discrimination, and even by adjusting the criteria, it probably only has discrimination equal to that of the original test.[211,214] Two multicenter reports have looked at the combined results of using either the 2-day or the overnight HDDST using the standard criteria of a more than 50% suppression of UFC or plasma cortisol.[62,215] When the HDDST is used in this way, its sensitivity (81%–86%) and specificity (67%–69%) are remarkably similar in both studies and comparable with those of single-center series. Therefore, although the sensitivity and specificity of the test are not high, dexamethasone is widely available and inexpensive, and the test is relatively convenient so that it is still widely used. However, it should not be forgotten that the patients are receiving large doses of glucocorticoids in addition to their high endogenous cortisol production, and one should be alert for the precipitation of psychosis and/or worsening of glycemic control or other complications.

Metyrapone Stimulation Test

This test is mentioned largely for historical reasons because it is rarely used in today's clinical practice. The original protocol was also originally devised for the differentiation of pituitary from adrenal tumors.[216] Metyrapone principally inhibits 11β-hydroxylase activity in the adrenal steroidogenic pathway. In Cushing's disease, lowering cortisol production results in a reduction in the negative feedback on ACTH production; increased ACTH causes an accumulation of products before the 11β-hydroxylase block (11-deoxycortisol, 17-OHCS, and 17-ketogenic steroids), and these can be measured in the urine and plasma. This does not occur in ACTH-independent Cushing's syndrome and only very rarely in ACTH syndrome in which the production of ACTH is relatively fixed. In the largest series to date looking specifically at its use in the differential diagnosis of ACTH-dependent Cushing's syndrome, a greater than 400-fold increase in plasma 11-deoxycortisol or a 70% increase in urinary 17-OHCS gave a 71% sensitivity and 100% specificity for Cushing's disease (169 patients) versus ectopic ACTH syndrome (15 patients).[212] Because it is complicated to perform and because of its poor performance, it can only be recommended in centers that are unable to perform CRH testing and bilateral inferior petrosal sinus sampling, and here it should be done in combination with the HDDST because this has been shown to increase the sensitivity to 88%.[212]

Corticotropin-Releasing Hormone Stimulation Test

The use of CRH stimulation for the differential diagnosis of ACTH-dependent Cushing's syndrome is based on two assumptions: (1) that corticotropinomas retain responsivity to CRH, although noncorticotroph tumors lack CRH receptors and cannot respond to the agent and (2) that hypercortisolism has been sufficient to inhibit the normal corticotroph response. Indeed, most patients with Cushing's disease respond to CRH, either 1 μg/kg or 100 μg intravenous synthetic ovine or human sequence CRH, with increases in plasma ACTH or cortisol, although patients with ectopic ACTH secretion typically do not.[217,218] Human sequence CRH has qualitatively similar properties to ovine CRH, although it is shorter acting with a slightly smaller increase in plasma cortisol and ACTH in normal and obese patients and in those with Cushing's disease[219]; this may be related to the more rapid clearance of the human sequence by endogenous CRH-binding protein.[220] The availability differs worldwide, with ovine CRH predominant in North America but human CRH elsewhere.

Because different centers have used differing protocols, including type of CRH and sampling timepoints, there is little consensus on a universal criterion for interpreting the test. However, where the test has been validated in experienced

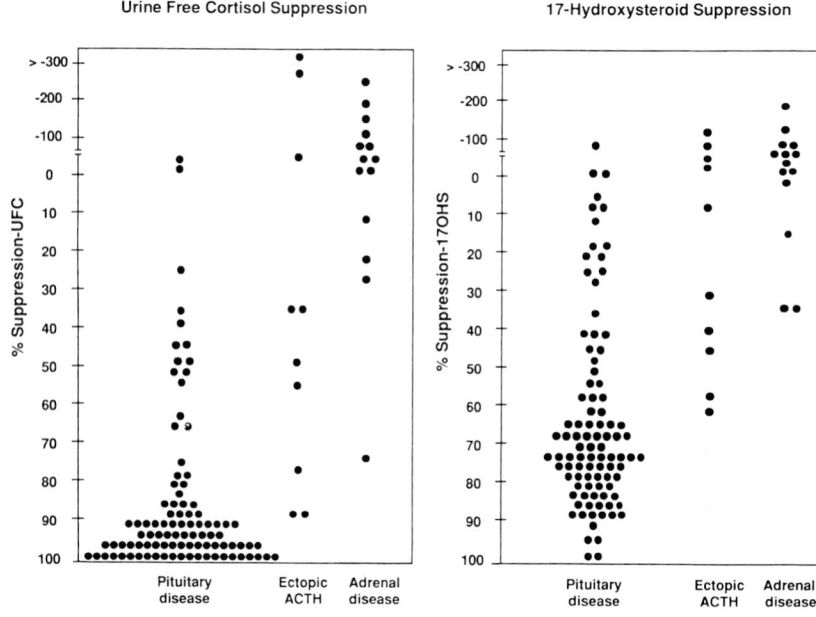

Figure 24-10 Suppression of urine free cortisol (UFC) and 17-hydroxycorticosteroid (17-OHCS) excretion during a standard high-dose dexamethasone suppression test in 118 patients with surgically confirmed Cushing's syndrome. The percentage of suppression represents the ratio of urine excretion on the second day of dexamethasone, 2 mg every 6 hours, divided by the mean of urine excretion on 2 baseline days, expressed as a percentage. The criterion of UFC greater than 90% suppression or 17-OHCS greater than 64% suppression for the diagnosis of Cushing's disease yielded 86% sensitivity and 100% specificity. The criterion of 64% suppression was later increased to 69% suppression to maintain 100% sensitivity. (Data from Flack MR, Oldfield EH, Cutler GB Jr, et al: Urine free cortisol in the high-dose dexamethasone suppression test for the differential diagnosis of the Cushing syndrome. Ann Intern Med 116:211–217, 1992; and Dichek HL, Nieman LK, Oldfield EH, et al: A comparison of the standard high-dose dexamethasone suppression test and the overnight 8-mg dexamethasone suppression test for the differential diagnosis of Cushing's syndrome. J Clin Endocrinol Metab 78:418–422, 1994.)

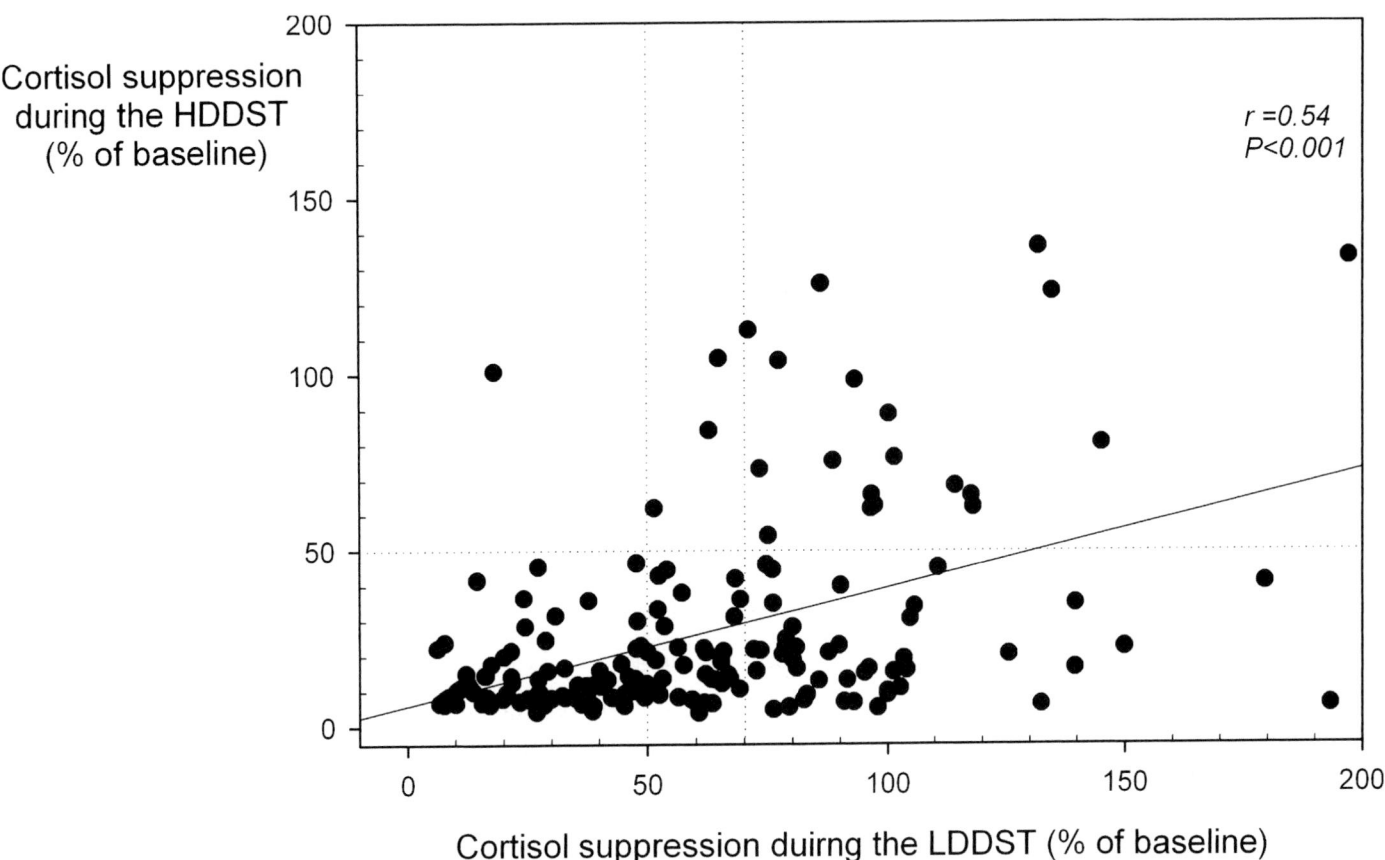

Figure 24-11   Correlation between the degree of suppression during the low-dose dexamethasone suppression test (LDDST) and the high-dose dexamethasone suppression test (HDDST) in 185 patients with Cushing's disease. (Reproduced with permission from Isidori AM, Kaltsas GA, Mohammed S, et al: Discriminatory value of the low-dose dexamethasone suppression test in establishing the diagnosis and differential diagnosis of Cushing's syndrome. J Clin Endocrinol Metab 88:5299–5306, 2003. Copyright © 2003, The Endocrine Society.)

centers, then the diagnostic utility appears similar. For instance, in the largest published series of the use of ovine CRH in ACTH-dependent Cushing's syndrome, an increase in ACTH by at least 35% from a mean basal (−5 and −1 minutes) to a mean of 15 and 30 minutes after ovine CRH in 100 patients with Cushing's disease and 16 patients with ectopic ACTH syndrome (Fig. 24-12) gave the test a sensitivity of 93% for diagnosing Cushing's disease and 100% specificity. The best cortisol criterion was an increase of at least 20% at a mean of 30 and 45 minutes, giving a sensitivity of 91% and a specificity of 88%.[221] Similarly, in the largest series of the use human CRH test in 101 patients with Cushing's disease and 14 with ectopic ACTH syndrome, the best criterion to differentiate Cushing's disease from ectopic ACTH syndrome was an increase in cortisol of at least 14% from a mean basal (−15 and 0 minutes) to a mean of 15 and 30 minutes, giving a sensitivity of 85% and a specificity of 100% (Fig. 24-13). In contrast, the best ACTH response was a maximal increase of at least 105%, giving 70% sensitivity and 100% specificity.[191] Thus, the CRH test is a useful discriminator between causes of ACTH-dependent Cushing's syndrome, but which cut-off to use must be evaluated at individual centers, and caution should be exercised because there will undoubtedly be patients with ectopic ACTH syndrome who respond outside these cut-offs. However, an increase in cortisol outside the normal range can also differentiate Cushing's disease from normality, albeit in only approximately 50% of cases, and, as noted previously, the measurement of plasma ACTH in the test can help discriminate ACTH-dependent and ACTH-independent causes of Cushing's syndrome when basal levels of ACTH are equivocal. We therefore believe that it plays a useful role in the investigation of patients with Cushing's syndrome.

Other Stimulation Tests

Vasopressin and desmopressin (a synthetic long-acting vasopressin analogue without the V1-mediated pressor effects) are thought to stimulate ACTH release in Cushing's disease through the corticotroph-specific V3 (or V1b) receptor. Hexarelin (a growth hormone secretagogue) also stimulates ACTH release sevenfold greater than human CRH; although the mechanism has not been entirely elucidated, this probably occurs through stimulation of vasopressin release in normal subjects[222] but by stimulation of aberrant growth hormone secretagogue receptors in patients with corticotroph tumors.[223] These peptides have all been used in a similar manner to CRH to try to improve the differentiation of ACTH-dependent Cushing's syndrome but have proved inferior.[224–226] A combined desmopressin (10 μg) and human CRH (100 μg) test initially looked extremely promising.[227] However, a recent study of this combined test in 26 patients with Cushing's disease and 5 patients with ectopic ACTH syndrome showed significant overlap in the responses.[228] The disappointing discriminatory outcome of these stimulants is undoubtedly due to the expression of both vasopressin and growth hormone secretagogue receptors by some ectopic ACTH-secreting tumors.[131,229]

Combined Test Strategies

Because none of the noninvasive tests have 100% diagnostic accuracy, a number of investigators have evaluated the utility of combined test strategies. The CRH and HDDST have been paired in this way, and combined have a diagnostic accuracy greater than that of either test alone, yielding 98% to 100% sensitivity and 88% to 100% specificity.[230–232] A similar high accuracy has been obtained by combining the results of the LDDST and the CRH test.[158]

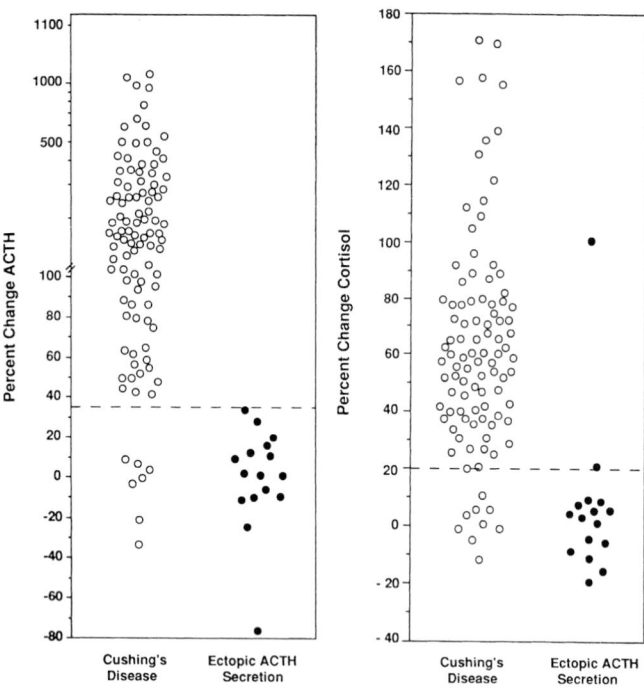

Figure 24-12 Response of adrenocorticotropic hormone (ACTH) and cortisol to ovine corticotropin-releasing hormone in patients with Cushing's disease and ectopic ACTH secretion. ACTH responses are expressed as the percentage of change in mean concentration 15 and 30 minutes after ovine corticotropin-releasing hormone from the mean basal value 1 and 5 minutes before the injection. The *dashed line* indicates a response of 35%, representing a diagnostic criterion with 100% specificity and 93% sensitivity. Cortisol responses are expressed as the percentage of change in mean cortisol concentration 30 and 45 minutes after ovine corticotropin-releasing hormone from the mean basal value 1 and 5 minutes before the injection. The *dashed line* indicates a response of 20%, representing a diagnostic criterion with 88% specificity and 91% sensitivity. (Data from Nieman LK, Oldfield EH, Wesley R, et al: A simplified morning ovine corticotropin-releasing hormone stimulation test for the differential diagnosis of ACTH-dependent Cushing syndrome. J Clin Endocrinol Metab 77:1308–1312, 1993.)

Imaging of the Adrenocorticotropin Hormone Source
Pituitary MRI imaging pre– and post–gadolinium enhancement should be performed in all patients with ACTH-dependent Cushing's syndrome and will identify an adenoma in approximately two thirds of patients with Cushing's disease[62,233] but also in approximately 10% of normal individuals.[234] The majority of these (95%) will exhibit a hypointense signal with no post–gadolinium enhancement, with the remaining 5% showing an isointense signal post–gadolinium enhancement.[235] CT imaging typically shows a hypodense lesion that fails to enhance postcontrast but is less sensitive than MRI in detecting small (<5 mm) adenomas.[62,236]

Imaging is the most helpful way to identify the source of ectopic ACTH production. Given the likely sites of tumors, CT and/or MRI of the neck, chest, and abdomen should be obtained. The most common source is bronchial carcinoid tumors, and small (<1 cm) lesions can often prove difficult to locate. Fine-cut high-resolution CT scanning with both supine and prone images can help differentiate between tumors and vascular shadows.[57] MRI can identify chest lesions that are not evident on CT scanning and characteristically show a high signal on T_2-weighted and short-inversion time inversion recovery (STIR) images.[237] CT-guided aspiration of masses for measurement of ACTH may provide useful functional information.[238]

In addition, measurement of marker peptides, such as calcitonin, gastrin, 5-hydroxyindoleacetic acid, serotonin, and catecholamine, may help to identify a neuroendocrine tumor.

Because the majority of ectopic ACTH-secreting tumors are of neuroendocrine origin and therefore may express somatostatin receptor subtypes, radiolabeled somatostatin analogue (^{111}In-pentetreotide) scintigraphy may be useful to show functionality of identified tumors, and there have been sporadic reports that it identifies lesions not apparent using conventional imaging.[239–241] However, in the majority of patients, including a recent series of 35 patients with ectopic ACTH secretion,[111] In-pentetreotide scintigraphy was not able to detect tumors when the MRI or CT scan was negative, and there are significant numbers of false-positive scans.[242] Thus, CT and MRI represent the best initial screening examinations, but scintigraphy may be a useful adjunctive imaging modality in selected cases. The role of positron-emission tomography remains unclear.

Strategy for Diagnosis and Differential Diagnosis of Cushing's Syndrome
After an international workshop in 2002, a consensus statement was published for the diagnosis and differential diagnosis of Cushing's syndrome. It is recommended that three 24-hour UFC and/or the LDDST be used as the first-line screening. Late-night salivary cortisol requires further evaluation but looks promising. False-positive results will be common, and second-line tests should be used as necessary for confirmation. Once the diagnosis of Cushing's syndrome is unequivocal, ACTH levels, the CRH test, and possibly the HDDST, together with appropriate imaging, are the most useful noninvasive investigations to determine the etiology, if both indicate Cushing's disease. Bilateral inferior petrosal sinus sampling is recommended in cases of ACTH-dependent Cushing's syndrome in which the clinical, biochemical, or radiologic results are discordant or equivocal.[131]

SPECIAL CLINICAL PRESENTATIONS AND PROBLEMS

Cyclical Cushing's Syndrome
Most patients with Cushing's syndrome demonstrate consistently elevated glucocorticoid values. A small subset show significant variability in glucocorticoid secretion, alternating normal and elevated values on a regular or irregular basis.[243] The few cases of spontaneous remission of Cushing's syndrome, including Cushing's first patient, may fit into this category.[2,244,245] The clinical course of patients with this type of intermittent, cyclic, or periodic Cushing's syndrome may be invariant, usually with mild signs and cushingoid symptoms, or it may parallel the biochemical abnormalities, with exacerbation of cushingoid features that parallel increased glucocorticoid production.

The etiologic distribution is altered; in one report, Cushing's disease, ectopic ACTH secretion, and primary adrenal causes accounted for 50%, 40%, and 10%, respectively, of 30 cases.[243] Carcinoid tumors of the thymus, lung, stomach, and kidney accounted for all but one case of ectopic ACTH secretion.

Patients with periodic Cushing's syndrome often show conflicting or "inappropriate" responses to standard diagnostic tests, particularly dexamethasone suppression.[246] Since as many as 50% of carcinoid tumors may suppress ACTH and thus glucocorticoid secretion during dexamethasone administration,[183,247] it is possible that increasing ACTH and cortisol levels in turn may inhibit POMC production in these tumors and in pituitary corticotrophs. Some patients with Cushing's disease show suppressed glucocorticoid production with hydrocortisone but not with dexamethasone.[248] In others, the response may reflect increasing or decreasing endogenous activity, without relationship to the action of the agent administered.[249,250] This may be deduced if a patient has conflicting patterns of response to multiple administrations of the test agent. Discrepant urine tests have been reported in these patients, with elevated 17-OHCS and normal UFC excre-

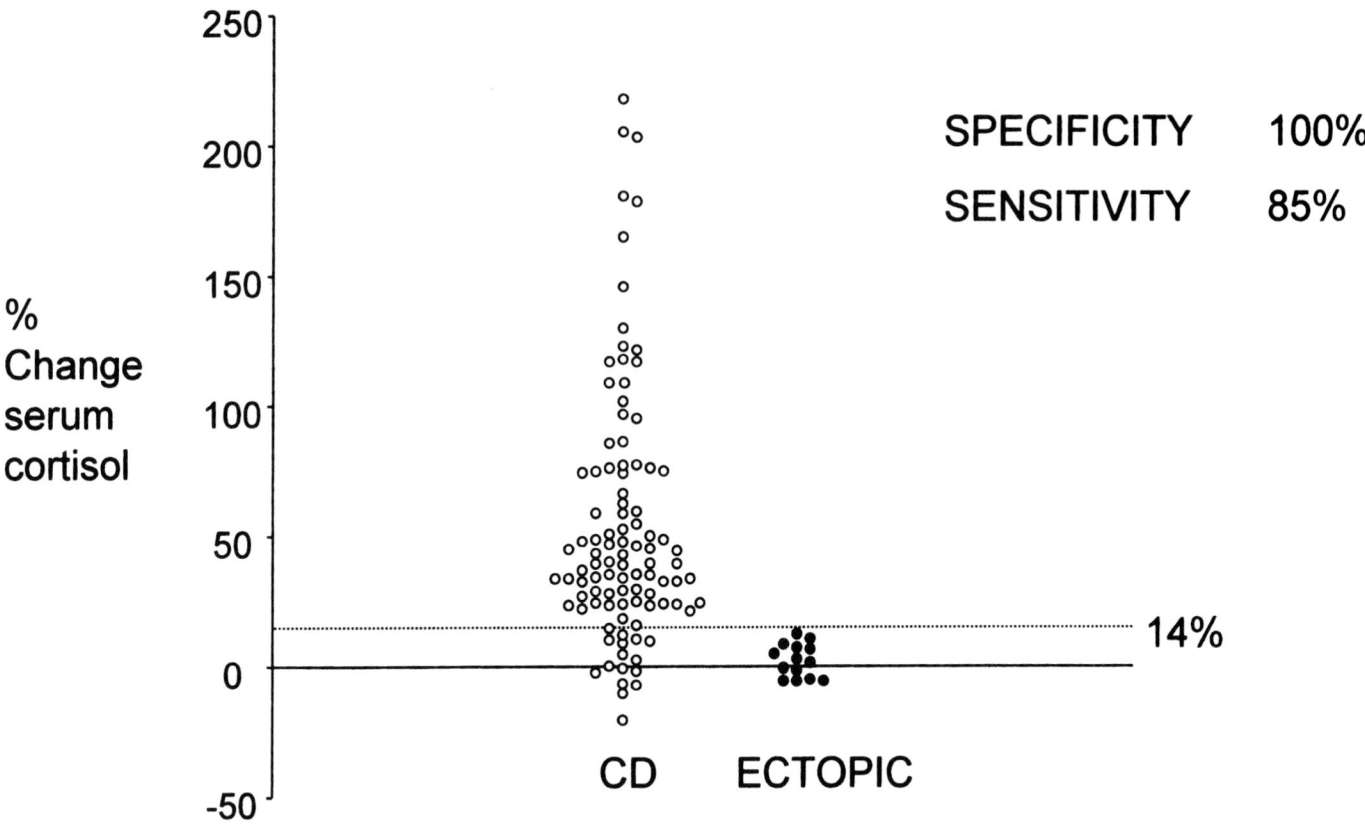

Figure 24-13 Percentage change in serum cortisol from a mean basal at –15 and 0 minutes to a mean value calculated from the levels at 15 and 30 minutes after the administration of human corticotropin-releasing hormone (100 mg intravenously) in 100 patients with Cushing's disease (CD) and 14 patients with ectopic adrenocorticotropic hormone syndrome. (Reproduced with permission from: Newll-Price J, Morris DG, Drake WM, et al: Optimal response criteria for the human CRH test in the differential diagnosis of ACTH-dependent Cushing's syndrome. J Clin Endocrinol Metab 87:1640–1645, 2002.)

tion.[251] If studied during a quiescent period, patients with nonpituitary disease may be misclassified as having Cushing's disease, and those with "normal" responses to the LDDST may be incorrectly diagnosed as not having Cushing's syndrome.[252] Dynamic testing should only be performed during a sustained period of hypercortisolism, as documented by failure to suppress on an LDDST, concurrent increased evening salivary or plasma cortisol, and/or elevated UFC excretion.

Iatrogenic and Factitious Cushing's Syndrome

Appropriate therapeutic but supraphysiologic doses of glucocorticoids given for a medical condition cause most cases of iatrogenic Cushing's syndrome, which is usually an expected, unavoidable adverse effect of therapy. Exogenous hypercortisolism may result also when a prescribed dose of glucocorticoid is increased inappropriately by the patient.[253] Although most common with oral agents, Cushing's syndrome may result from glucocorticoids administered to the nasal or rectal mucosa, tracheobronchial tree, or the skin.[254–256] The use of all prescription, over-the-counter medications, and herbal remedies,[257] including nasal drops, inhalants, and topical agents, should be assessed in all cushingoid patients. Agents not given for their glucocorticoid activity, such as fludrocortisone acetate and megestrol,[258] also may produce cushingoid features on occasion.

Factitious Cushing's syndrome, which may be a form of Münchausen's syndrome, is rare. The typical suppression of plasma ACTH and dehydroepiandrosterone sulfate may lead to a mistaken diagnosis of primary adrenal disease.[142] Plasma and urine cortisol values vary, depending on the route, schedule, and type of glucocorticoid ingested. For example, intravenous injection of hydrocortisone may suppress ACTH values and increase UFC levels without increasing

single random plasma cortisol values.[259] If basal urine or plasma cortisol values are low, it may be useful to screen the urine for synthetic glucocorticoids.[142]

Chronic Renal Failure

Plasma levels of cortisol are normal in chronic renal failure when assessed with radioimmunoassays using an organic extraction procedure[260,261] but may be increased if other assay techniques are used[262]; ACTH levels are increased.[260] Glomerular filtration rates of less than 30 mL/min result in decreased cortisol excretion, and the UFC may be normal despite excessive cortisol production.[263] The ACTH and cortisol responses to ovine CRH may be suppressed in patient with renal failure except for those undergoing continuous ambulatory peritoneal dialysis.[261] The metabolism of dexamethasone is normal in chronic renal failure, but the oral absorption can be altered in some patients and may necessitate measuring plasma dexamethasone levels.[264,265] The reduced degree of suppression of cortisol by dexamethasone suggests a prolonged half-life of cortisol. Normal suppression to the overnight 1-mg LDDST is uncommon, and the 2-day 2-mg/day protocol does better in this regard.[134,265,266] The cortisol response to insulin-induced hypoglycemia is normal or absent.[264,267] Cushing's syndrome has been described in the setting of chronic renal failure only rarely.[268–270]

Pediatric Cushing's Syndrome

The most common presentation of Cushing's syndrome in children is growth retardation, often with a decrease in height percentile over time as the weight percentile increases.[271–273] However, hypercortisolemic patients with virilizing adrenal tumors may show growth acceleration; thus, the absence of growth failure does not exclude the diagnosis of Cushing's syndrome.[274] Other virilizing signs such as acne and hirsutism are seen in approximately 50% of patients regardless of etiology.[273] Hypertension and striae are seen in approximately 50% of cases.[275] Muscle weakness may be less common in the pediatric patient.[72] This may reflect the effect of exercise rather than age because older patients who follow an exercise program tend to maintain strength. In addition to the spectrum of psychiatric and cognitive changes seen in adults, which can affect school performance, children may show "compulsive diligence" and actually do quite well academically.[271] Depression is less common in children than in adults. Headaches and fatigue are common.[273]

Cushing's disease accounts for the between 75% and 85% of Cushing's syndrome in children and adolescents, but before the age of 10 years, this proportion decreases to only 50%.[272,273] In prepubertal children, Cushing's disease has a male predominance.[276] ACTH-independent causes of Cushing's syndrome are more common in younger patients. Signs of virilization or feminization in the very young (<2 years) suggest adrenal carcinoma.[277] Two primary adrenal causes of Cushing's syndrome, McCune-Albright syndrome and PPNAD, are typically diseases of childhood or young adults. Ectopic secretion of ACTH occurs less frequently than in adults. Sources of ectopic ACTH production in children include Wilms' tumor,[278] neuroblastoma,[279] paraganglioma,[280] pancreatic islet cell tumor,[281] bronchial carcinoid,[273] and carcinoid tumor of the kidney.[282]

Cushing's Syndrome in Pregnancy

The pregnant woman with possible Cushing's syndrome presents a diagnostic challenge to the physician because of the physical and biochemical changes that are common to both conditions, including weight gain, fatigue, striae, hypertension, and glucose intolerance.[283] Total serum cortisol levels increase in pregnancy, beginning in the first trimester and peaking at 6 months, with a decrease only after delivery,[284] probably reflecting increased induction of hepatic corticosteroid-binding globulin production by estrogen. The diurnal pattern of serum cortisol is preserved, albeit at a higher level, so that nadir values range between 5 and 10 μg/dL (140–280 nmol/L) and peak levels between 32 and 56 μg/dL (880–1550 nmol/L).[285] Free cortisol levels in blood and urine increase to overlap those seen in Cushing's syndrome.[285] The set point for dexamethasone suppression of cortisol increases progressively throughout gestation.[286] Since no normative values are available for interpretation of the LDDST, UFC is most commonly used as a screening test, with allowance for a higher upper limit of normal.

TREATMENT

Optimal treatment for Cushing's syndrome renders the patient eucortisolemic with minimal morbidity and mortality. With the advent of synthetic glucocorticoid therapy, adrenalectomy became the treatment of choice because it conferred rapid and, in most cases, permanent resolution of Cushing's syndrome.[287] Improvements in neurosurgical techniques and appreciation of the sources of ectopic ACTH secretion have changed the therapeutic approach to Cushing's syndrome, so that surgery now is directed toward resection of abnormal tissue, whether ACTH or cortisol producing. This optimal approach cannot be realized if the patient is unable to safely undergo surgery or if the tumor is occult or metastatic. Other second-line therapies that are less specific and may have greater morbidity must be chosen in these settings.

MEDICAL TREATMENT

The medical treatments for hypercortisolism have two broad mechanisms of action. One class of compounds modulates ACTH release and is restricted to the treatment of ACTH-dependent Cushing's syndrome, principally Cushing's disease. The second class of agents reduces cortisol levels through inhibition of adrenal steroidogenesis or cortisol action by antagonism at the level of the receptor. These compounds are used in the treatment of all forms of Cushing's syndrome. The major current role of medical therapy is in the preoperative control of hypercortisolemia or as adjunctive treatment after failed surgical management, while other therapies such as radiotherapy are instituted.

Agents That Modulate Adrenocorticotropin Hormone Release

Neuromodulatory compounds that affect CRH or ACTH synthesis or release, including serotonin antagonists, dopamine agonists, somatostatin analogues, and sodium valproate, have been examined as therapeutic agents principally for Cushing's disease, but no large-scale, placebo-controlled trials have been reported.

Serotonin Antagonists

The nonselective serotonin antagonist cyproheptadine inhibits ACTH secretion in normal subjects.[288] There are reports of successful lowering of plasma ACTH in small numbers of patients with Cushing's disease, including Nelson's syndrome, using doses of as high as 24 mg/day,[289] and prolonged response as long as 11 years has been recorded.[290] Ritanserin and ketanserin, selective serotonin type 2 receptor antagonists, have also been shown to have a therapeutic response on ACTH production.[291,292] However, the percentage of responders and duration of response are limited for both compounds. Cyproheptadine increases appetite and may cause considerable weight gain. These agents are rarely used today.

Dopamine Agonists

The dopamine agonist bromocriptine normalizes cortisol levels in only a small percentage of patients with Cushing's disease, and the response may not be sustained.[293] High doses of bromocriptine (as high as 55 mg/day) may be required,[294] and the postural hypotension and nausea at these doses may limit this approach. There is, however, recent experience that suggests that cabergoline may have an important role in medical therapy: Further studies in this area are awaited with interest.[295] The ACTH response to acute challenge with bromocriptine, the response to dexamethasone, or the basal prolactin levels do not predict the long-term response to therapy.[296] It has been suggested that bromocriptine responsiveness is indicative of Cushing's disease of intermediate lobe origin.[297] However, bromocriptine responsiveness has also been demonstrated in Cushing's disease due to corticotroph hyperplasia and in an apparently normal pituitary.[298]

Sodium Valproate

Sodium valproate, a γ-aminobutyric acid reuptake inhibitor, decreases ACTH levels in patients receiving the agent for its antiseizure effects,[299] an action probably mediated by inhibition of hypothalamic CRH release.[300] Despite sporadic reports of ACTH inhibition and treatment with valproate in Cushing's disease,[301,302] two larger studies have produced very disappointing results with long-term treatment (600 mg/day).[296,303]

Somatostatin Analogues

Long-acting somatostatin analogues such as octreotide and lanreotide are widely used in the therapy of various neuroendocrine tumors, and somatostatin receptors have been demonstrated on corticotroph adenomas in addition to ectopic sources of ACTH.[304] Octreotide appears to inhibit ACTH release in Nelson's syndrome but rarely in patients with Cushing's disease, and this has been postulated to be due to somatostatin receptor downregulation from the circulating hypercortisolemia.[305] In ectopic ACTH-secreting tumors, octreotide has produced a prolonged (>3 months) reduction in ACTH and hypercortisolemia in approximately 70% of published cases. Preoperative assessment with pentetreotide scintigraphy may help predict which tumors might respond to treatment. Octreotide treatment produces a temporary response in GIP-dependent Cushing's syndrome but is unhelpful in other causes of ACTH-independent Cushing's syndrome.[306] There is so far little experience of the sustained release preparations in Cushing's syndrome. It is possible that the introduction of somatostatin analogues with a broader spectrum of activity for somatostatin receptor subtypes, such as SOM230 (Novartis, Basel, Switzerland) will increase the therapeutic role of these agents.

Agents Inhibiting Steroidogenesis

The oral inhibitors of adrenal steroidogenesis are the most commonly used medical agents in the treatment of Cushing's syndrome; these include metyrapone, ketoconazole, aminoglutethimide, mitotane, and trilostane. Etomidate is the only available agent that can be given parenterally. We would usually recommend partial inhibition of cortisol production (adjusted adrenal blockade) with frequent monitoring to identify a dosing regimen that maintains eucortisolism while avoiding adrenal insufficiency or excess. However, in some patients, particularly those with variable cortisol production, it can be difficult to achieve this. In cases of full adrenal blockade with glucocorticoid replacement to avoid symptoms of adrenal insufficiency (a block-and-replace regimen) may be advocated. In all forms of treatment, patients and their physicians must be alert to the signs and symptoms of adrenal insufficiency.

Mitotane

Mitotane, or o,p'-DDD, is derived from the family of insecticides that includes DDT. It inhibits adrenal steroidogenesis catalyzed by cholesterol desmolase,[307] 11- and 18-hydroxylase, and 3β-hydroxysteroid dehydrogenase.[308] It also has marked direct cytotoxic effects on the zona fasciculata and zona reticulosa, which led to its original use in high doses (5–20 g/day) as treatment for inoperable adrenocortical carcinoma.[309,310] In this condition, it is now more commonly used as adjunctive treatment to surgery, in which it controls hormonal hypersecretion in the majority of patients and induces tumor regression in some patients.[311] Its effect on lengthening survival in this aggressive condition remains controversial, but there is some evidence that it is beneficial.[312] Although high serum levels (> 14 µg/mL) were reported to be positively associated with tumor regression and survival in one study,[313] good results have also been obtained with low doses (1–2.5 g/day).[314,315] Where possible, monitoring of serum levels should be undertaken. Combined treatment of mitotane with standard chemotherapeutic agents such as cisplatin, etoposide, and doxorubicin have also been used in a number of small studies in advanced adrenal carcinoma with variable benefit.[316-318]

In Cushing's disease, mitotane alone in high doses (4–12 g/day) can achieve remission in as many as 83% of patients, but more commonly, mitotane is used in lower doses (0.5–4 g/day), sometimes in combination with radiation therapy, with clinical and biochemical remission achieved in approximately 80%.[319,320] Using low doses, the onset of effect can take approximately 6 to 8 weeks, and additional adjunctive medical treatment may be needed in this interim. Similarly, the agent has a long half-life (18–159 days), due in part to its lipophilic properties, and it effects can last for weeks or months after discontinuation of therapy. Mitotane has also proved useful in the treatment of hypercortisolism associated with ectopic secretion of ACTH, alone or in combination with metyrapone or aminoglutethimide.[321]

The utility of mitotane is limited by its gastrointestinal and neurologic toxicity. Nausea and anorexia are common at doses as high as 4 g/day and is ubiquitous at more than 4 g/day.[322] These side effects may be avoided by beginning at a dose of 0.5 to 1.0 g/day and increasing gradually, by 0.5 to 1.0 g every 1 to 4 weeks. Doses should be taken with meals or at bedtime with food. If significant adverse effects do occur, the drug should be discontinued for 3 to 5 days and then restarted at a lower dose.[320] At the higher doses, neurologic side effects occur in approximately 50% of patients and include drowsiness, gait disturbances, dizziness or vertigo, confusion, and problems with language. Other adverse effects include fatigue (perhaps due to decreased cortisol levels), gynecomastia, skin rash, hypouricemia, elevated liver enzymes, and abnormal platelet function.[310,311,323] The hypercholesterolemia, which is common even at low doses, can be reversed with 3-hydroxy-3-methylglutaryl coenzyme A reductase inhibitors such as simvastatin.[324] Mitotane is relatively contraindicated in women desiring fertility within 2 to 5 years. It may induce spontaneous abortion and act as a teratogen, effects that may persist for a number of years after discontinuation due to deposition in fat.[325]

Mitotane increases hormone-binding proteins (cortisol-binding globulin, sex hormone binding–globulin, and thyroxine-binding globulin).[326] Therefore, total serum cortisol cannot be relied on to monitor therapy, and UFC and/or plasma ACTH should be used instead. In addition, mitotane increases the metabolic clearance of exogenously administered steroids,[327] and replacement doses of glucocortiod must be increased by approximately one third.

Metyrapone

Metyrapone acts primarily to inhibit the enzyme 11β-hydroxylase,[328] and the subsequent elevation of 11-deoxycortisol can be monitored in the serum of patients treated with metyrapone. The decrease in cortisol is rapid, with trough levels at 2 hours postdose, and a test dose of 750 mg with hourly cortisol estimation for 4 hours can be used to predict response: A rapid and sustained decrease in cortisol to less than approximately 7 µg/dL (~200 nmol/L), as is often seen with ectopic ACTH and adrenal tumors, suggests that a smaller dose of metyrapone may be appropriate, whereas a decrease 10 to 12 µg/dL (~300 nmol/L), as often seen in Cushing's disease, would indicate a higher dose requirement.[329] Maintenance therapy is started at 0.75 to 1.5 g/day in three to four divided doses daily. The usual requirement is approximately 2 g/day, although higher doses (as high as 6 g/day) may be needed in ectopic ACTH syndrome.[329] Metyrapone is useful in treating patients with Cushing's syndrome from adrenal tumors, ectopic ACTH syndrome, and Cushing's disease.[329,330] The principal side effects are hirsutism and acne (as predicted by the increase in adrenal androgens), dizziness, and gastrointestinal upset. The androgenic effects can be particularly problematic and may preclude its use in some younger female patients. Hypokalemia, edema, and hypertension due to increased mineralocorticoids are infrequent[329] but may require cessation of therapy.[331] Our experience would suggest that the only major problems are associated with the increase in adrenal androgens; careful monitoring of treatment to avoid hypoadrenalism and education of the patient are required. Although not previously reported, we have seen a case of hemolysis in a patient with glucose 6-phosphate dehydrogenase deficiency.

Aminoglutethimide

Aminoglutethimide was introduced as an anticonvulsant in the late 1950s; it was noted to induce hypothyroidism and adrenal insufficiency and subsequently shown to inhibit the side-chain cleavage of cholesterol to pregnenolone.[332,333] It thus inhibits not only cortisol but also estrogen and aldosterone production. In addition, it also inhibits the enzymes

11β-hydroxylase, 18-hydroxylase, and aromatase.[334] Aminoglutethimide is begun at a dose of 500 mg/day in four divided doses and can be increased by 250 to 500 mg every 3 to 4 days to a total dose of 2 g/day.

The largest series of patients treated with aminoglutethimide consisted of 66 patients with Cushing's syndrome: 14 of 33 with Cushing's disease, all 6 with adrenal adenomas, 4 of 6 with ectopic ACTH syndrome, and 13 of 21 with adrenal carcinoma showed a favorable response to aminoglutethimide.[335] Overall, this drug seems to be less efficient in treating Cushing's disease compared with the other causes of Cushing's syndrome, which may be due to an increase in ACTH overcoming the enzymatic blockade.[336] The common side effects are a morbilliform rash, fever, dizziness, lethargy, and blurred vision. The incidence of adverse reactions is high, in as high as 58% of patients, particularly at doses of more than 1 g/day,[335] and they generally limit its use. Combination treatment with metyrapone has been used to try to reduce the dose (≤750 mg/day), and thus the toxicity of aminoglutethimide, and appears to be better tolerated.[337] However, we rarely use this treatment today.

Ketoconazole

Ketoconazole is an imidazole derivative whose primary indication is as an oral antifungal agent. However, reports of gynecomastia in some ketoconazole-treated patients led to the realization that it is an inhibitor of cytochrome P-450 enzymes, including side-chain cleavage, C17,20-lyase, 11β-hydroxylase, and 17β-hydroxylase.[338,339] It has also been reported to have a direct effect on ectopic ACTH secretion from a thymic carcinoid tumor.[340] Treatment for Cushing's syndrome is usually started at a dose of 200 mg twice daily, and its onset of action is slower than metyrapone. It has been used successfully to lower cortisol levels in patients with Cushing's syndrome of various etiologies including adrenal carcinoma, ectopic ACTH syndrome, and invasive ACTH-producing pituitary carcinoma, with doses required between 200 and 1200 mg/day in as many as four divided daily doses.[341-344]

The principal side effect of ketoconazole is hepatotoxicity. Reversible elevation of hepatic serum transaminases occurs in approximately 5% to 10% of patients and need not result in discontinuation of the agent if levels remain below two- to threefold the upper normal range. The incidence of serious hepatic injury is approximately 1 in 15,000 patients,[345] and it can be fatal or require liver transplantation.[346,347] The hepatotoxicity appears to be idiosyncratic and has been reported within 7 days of the start of treatment in a patient with Cushing's syndrome.[348] Other adverse reactions of ketoconazole include skin rashes and gastrointestinal upset, but these occur in less than 15%,[342] and one must always be wary of causing adrenal insufficiency.[349] Due to its C17-20 lyase inhibition and consequent antiandrogenic properties, ketoconazole is particularly useful in female patients in whom hirsutism is an issue, which may be worsened with metyrapone. Conversely, gynecomastia and reduced libido in male patients may be unacceptable and require alternative agents. One further advantage of ketoconazole is its inhibition of cholesterol synthesis, particularly low-density lipoprotein cholesterol.[342,350] We have found it to be particularly useful in combination with low doses of metyrapone.

Trilostane

Trilostane is a relatively weak inhibitor of steroidogenesis: Even at maximal daily doses of 980 mg, only a minority of patients achieve remission.[351,352] Although its use in combination therapy has not been reported, trilostane may prove to be a useful addition to such a therapeutic strategy. Side effects include abdominal discomfort, diarrhea, and paresthesia. Trilostane is detected in fluorometric assays for 11-hydroxycorticoids, including cortisol, and in radioimmunoassays for estrogen and testosterone, probably because of structural similarities to the steroids of interest. Radioimmunoassay cortisol or UFC should be used to monitor treatment.

Etomidate

Etomidate, an imidazole-derived anesthetic agent, was reported to have adrenolytic effects in 1983.[353] Compared with the other imidazole derivative ketoconazole, etomidate more potently inhibits adrenocortical 11β-hydroxylase, has a similar inhibition of 17-hydroxylase, but has less of an effect on C17-20 lyase.[354] At higher concentrations, it also appears to have an effect on cholesterol side-chain cleavage.[355] Etomidate has been used successfully to control severe hypercortisolemia in patients with Cushing's syndrome of various etiologies at doses of as high as 0.3 mg/kg/hr,[356] although such high doses tend to be sedative.[357] Most case reports have therefore reported the use of lower nonhypnotic total doses of between 1.2 and 8.3 mg/hr to good effect.[358-360] It may be more difficult to normalize cortisol levels in patients with Cushing's disease, which probably reflects the increased ACTH drive from the pituitary, as opposed to relatively fixed production from an ectopic source.[359] Clearly, etomidate is an effective adrenolytic agent that acts rapidly but is limited in its use by the fact it has to be given parenterally. However, in this situation, it may be lifesaving. It is important to recognize that the etomidate preparations available in Europe are dissolved in an alcohol-based vehicle, although the currently available preparation in the United States uses propylene glycol, which may have potential side effects such as nephrotoxicity.[360]

Glucocorticoid Receptor Antagonists

Mifepristone (RU 486) is a potent competitive antagonist of glucocorticoid and progesterone receptors.[361] It was developed primarily as an abortifacient agent. The major drawback is the lack of biochemical markers to monitor overtreatment, and its long half-life and minimal agonist activity leaves the patient open to hypoadrenalism. In 1985, Nieman and colleagues[362] reported clinical improvement in a patient with ectopic ACTH syndrome treated with mifepristone at doses of as high as 20 mg/kg/day for 9 weeks. The increase in plasma ACTH values after RU 486 administration in normal individuals[363] and patients with Cushing's disease[364] would probably limit its use in the latter condition. Thus, although it may be useful, the drug needs to be used with great caution in Cushing's syndrome.[365]

Potential Novel Medical Agents

In the rare cases of Cushing's syndrome due to AIMAH and aberrant receptor expression of GIP, β-adrenergic, and luteinizing hormone/human chorionic gonadotropin receptors, specific receptor antagonists may prove to be useful in such patients in the future.[366]

Retinoic acid has been found to inhibit ACTH secretion and cell proliferation both in vitro in ACTH-producing tumor cell lines and cultured human corticotroph adenomas and in vivo in nude mice.[367] These potential antisecretory and antiproliferative activities of this agent in Cushing's syndrome need to be investigated further.

The thiazolidinedione rosiglitazone, a peroxisome-proliferator-activated receptor γ (PPAR-γ) agonist, has been shown in suprapharmacologic doses to induce G_0/G_1 cell-cycle arrest and apoptosis and suppress ACTH secretion in human and murine corticotroph tumor cells. In addition, the development of murine corticotroph tumors, generated by subcutaneous injection of ACTH-secreting AtT20 cells, was prevented.[368] It appears that this is not specific to corticotroph adenomas but also applies to other forms of pituitary tumor.[369] We and others have only attempted this novel treatment strategy in a few selected cases of Cushing's disease and Nelson's syndrome, with limited success. Formal trials are awaited.

SURGERY

Preoperative Evaluation and Treatment

Many centers use routine preoperative medical adrenal blockade to attain a period of eucortisolemia for 4 to 6 weeks before surgery. The aim is to allow reversal of some of the metabolic and catabolic effects of the hypercortisolemia that may inhibit wound healing and cause other complications in the perioperative period. The disadvantage of this strategy is that the normal corticotrope may be disinhibited by the time of surgery so that the expected hypocortisolism after successful tumor resection does not occur, and this index of remission is not reliable. This rationale is only empirical, and a randomized trial to see whether this approach improves outcome would be welcomed.[370]

Because Cushing's syndrome is a prothrombotic state, anticoagulant prophylaxis should be considered perioperatively.[371] The lipid abnormalities, hypertension, and diabetes common in Cushing's syndrome predispose these patients to atherosclerotic cardiac disease and should be treated by conventional approaches.

Transsphenoidal Resection of Corticotropinoma

Transsphenoidal resection is regarded as the treatment of choice in Cushing's disease.[370,372] The procedure is usually performed using a gingival approach, as originally devised by Kanavel and Halsted and later popularized by Cushing.[373] The development of the operating microscope led to the introduction of transsphenoidal resection of pituitary microadenomas by Hardy in 1968. Further advancements have been made in the past decade by the use of rigid endoscopes and more recently flexible endoscopes.[374,375] The goal of surgery is a selective adenomectomy and thus preservation of as much normal pituitary tissue as possible, and the procedure should be performed by a neurosurgeon experienced in transsphenoidal surgery. If a tumor cannot be identified, hemihypophysectomy on the side of the gland with an ACTH gradient on petrosal sinus sampling is usually the best way to proceed, perhaps achieving cure without hypopituitarism. What defines apparent cure or remission after transsphenoidal surgery still causes much debate. Most large series report immediate remission rates of approximately 70% to 80%,[11,62,376,377] with lower rates for macroadenomas,[378] using variable remission criteria that include normal postoperative cortisol levels, normal UFC levels, and/or a normal response to an LDDST, associated with resolution of the disease clinically. However, what is clear is that long-term recurrence rates in these cohorts are significant at as high as 25% by 10 years after surgery. This is perhaps not surprising because ACTH production from normal corticotrophs surrounding a corticotroph adenoma should be suppressed, and after complete removal of that adenoma, circulating ACTH and cortisol levels should become very low or undetectable and may remain so for some time. Indeed, postoperative hypercortisolemia (<1.8 μg/dL [<50 nmol/L] at 9:00 A.M.) and the need for glucocorticoid replacement have been shown to be the best reflection of long-term cure,[379,380] but there is no guarantee.[381,382] Cortisol measurements should be made within 2 weeks of surgery and at least 24 hours after the last dose of hydrocortisone.[383] Thus, in reality, transsphenoidal surgery achieves long-term cure even in the best hands in only approximately 50% to 60% of adult patients and is therefore somewhat disappointing,[382,384] and the data emphasize the need for long-term endocrinologic follow-up of these patients. Similar results are seen in children with Cushing's disease.[385,386] The chance of successful remission is also reduced with macroadenomas and tumors that invade the cavernous sinus.[11,378] The success of surgery also depends on the correct diagnosis; retrospective analysis from a number of centers revealed that incorrect diagnosis accounts for as many as 12% of patients with surgical failure.[387]

The mortality of transsphenoidal surgery is approximately 1% to 2%.[11,376] Transient diabetes insipidus is probably the most common complication, being reported in as many as 28% of patients.[382] Other perioperative complications, including cerebrospinal fluid leak, meningitis, and profuse bleeding, occur in less than 10% of patients. Permanent complications such as persistent diabetes insipidus and injury to the optic nerve or nerves of the cavernous sinus (causing ptosis or diplopia) occur less frequently.[11,376] However, hypopituitarism, particularly growth hormone deficiency, is common (53%–59%), with other anterior hormone deficits occurring in approximately 35% to 45% of patients.[382,388] Such complications are more common after resection of larger tumors or larger amounts of normal pituitary tissue (or stalk) or after repeat surgery.

Postoperative Evaluation and Management

Patients typically receive supraphysiologic doses of glucocorticoids to cover transsphenoidal surgery at initial daily doses of as high as 400 mg hydrocortisone (4 mg dexamethasone), tapering off within 1 to 3 days. Morning (9:00 A.M.) serum cortisol measurements are then obtained for 3 days starting 24 hours after the last glucocorticoid administration, during which time the patient should be observed for development of signs of adrenal insufficiency. This approach allows prompt classification of likely cure, normocortisolemia, or persistent hypercortisolism. As discussed previously, postoperative hypercortisolemia (<1.8 μg/dL [50 nmol/L] at 9:00 A.M.) is probably the best indicator of the likelihood of long-term remission; however, one should be aware that early detectable serum cortisol levels may still be compatible with cure and may decrease within 2 weeks, reflecting either gradual infarction or remnant tumor or some degree of adrenal semiautonomy.[383,389] Dynamic tests have also been used to predict long-term remission. The cortisol and ACTH response to CRH in the early postoperative period may provide a useful index of the risk of recurrence of Cushing's disease, the rationale being that responsiveness may indicate residual tumor.[62,390] A study of postoperative responses to CRH in 221 patients suggested that a cortisol response greater than 5 μg/dL (138 nmol/L) at 60 minutes had a positive predictive value of 42% and a negative predictive value of 94% for recurrence of disease.[391] Because patients with partial recovery of the axis would be expected to have a normal response, regardless of the risk of recurrence, the CRH test cannot be interpreted and should not be used in this setting. There is also some evidence that persistence of the ACTH response to desmopressin postoperatively is probably linked to a higher rate of relapse.[392,393]

Patients who are hypocortisolemic should be started on glucocorticoid replacement, and 15 to 30 mg hydrocortisone (12–15 mg/m²) in two to three divided doses is the preferred choice. The first dose (usually half to two thirds of the total dose) should be taken before getting out of bed, and the last dose should be taken no later than 6:00 P.M. because later administration of glucocorticoids may result in disordered sleep.

All patients receiving chronic glucocorticoid replacement therapy should be instructed that they are "dependent" on taking glucocorticoids as prescribed, and that failure to take or absorb the medication will lead to adrenal crisis and possibly death. They should be prescribed a 100-mg hydrocortisone intramuscular injection pack for emergency use. They should also obtain a medical information bracelet or necklace that identifies this requirement (Medic Alert Foundation). Education should stress the effects of glucocorticoid withdrawal[394]; the need for compliance with the daily dose of glucocorticoid; the need to double the oral dose for nausea, diarrhea, and fever; and the need for parenteral administration and medical evaluation during emesis, trauma, or severe medical stress.

The patient should be told to expect desquamation of the skin, and flulike symptoms (malaise, joint aching, anorexia, and nausea) during the postoperative months and that these are signs that indicate remission. Most patients tolerate these symptoms of glucocorticoid withdrawal much better if they are forewarned and alerted to their positive nature. Physicians should not increase the glucocorticoid dose in the absence of intercurrent illness based on these symptoms alone but should seek signs of adrenal insufficiency, such as vomiting, electrolyte abnormalities, and postural hypotension.[395] The affective and cognitive changes associated with Cushing's syndrome are particularly slow to resolve. Postoperatively, assessment for deficiencies of other pituitary hormones should also be sought, and the appropriate replacement regimen initiated as necessary.

Diuresis is common after transsphenoidal surgery and may result from intraoperative or glucocorticoid-induced fluid overload or may be due to diabetes insipidus. For these reasons, assessment of paired serum and urine osmolality and the serum sodium concentration is essential. It is advisable to withhold specific therapy unless the serum osmolality is greater than 295 mOsm/kg, the serum sodium is greater than 145 mmol/L, and the urine output is greater than 200 mL/hour with an inappropriately low urine osmolality. Desmopressin (DDAVP, Ferring) 1 µg given subcutaneously will provide adequate vasopressin replacement for 12 hours or more. Hyponatremia may occur in as many as 20% of patients within 10 days of surgery. This may be due to injudicious fluid replacement or inappropriate antidiuretic hormone secretion as is frequently seen after extensive gland exploration, and fluid intake should be restricted.[396]

A small minority of patients proceed to (apparently) permanent diabetes insipidus, requiring long-term treatment with a vasopressin analogue. A dose and schedule of administration should be chosen to provide unbroken sleep but allow a period of "breakthrough" urination each day. This goal is often achieved using 10 to 20 µg desmopressin intranasally (or an equivalent oral dose) in the evening.

Some glucocorticoid-induced abnormalities, including hypokalemia, hypertension, and glucose intolerance, may be normalized during the postoperative period so that preoperative treatments for these need to reassessed. There is some evidence that deficits in bone mass may be partially reversed after treatment of hypercortisolemia.[397,398] Bisphosphonate treatment may induce a more rapid improvement in bone mineral density[399] and should be considered in patients with osteoporosis on bone density scanning, which is either especially severe or appears not be improving after treatment of Cushing's syndrome.

Persistent hypercortisolemia after transsphenoidal exploration should prompt reevaluation of the diagnosis of Cushing's disease, especially if previous diagnostic test results were indeterminate or conflicting or if no tumor was found on pathologic examination. Petrosal sinus sampling after transsphenoidal surgery can confirm a pituitary source of ACTH, but the rate of correct lateralization decreases, probably because of alterations in venous anatomy caused by the prior surgery; therefore, the procedure cannot be used to direct a second operative search or decision for hemihypophysectomy.

The treatment options for patients with persistent Cushing's disease include repeat surgery, radiation therapy, and adrenalectomy. If immediate surgical remission is not achieved at the first exploration, early repeat transsphenoidal surgery may be worthwhile in a significant proportion of patients, at the expense of increased likelihood of hypopituitarism.[400] The likelihood of remission after repeat surgery is greatest when some or all of the following outcome parameters are present: the diagnosis is correct, as evidenced by previous curative surgery with pathologic confirmation of an ACTH-staining adenoma; the initial exposure or resection was incomplete; or residual tumor is seen on CT or MRI scan without evidence of cavernous sinus invasion. Repeat sellar exploration is less likely to be helpful in patients with empty sella syndrome or very little pituitary tissue on CT or MRI scans. Patients with cavernous sinus or dural invasion identified at the initial procedure are not candidates for repeat surgery to treat hypercortisolism and should receive radiation therapy.

Recovery of the HPA axis can be monitored by measurement of 9:00 A.M. serum cortisol after omission of hydrocortisone replacement. Because recovery after transsphenoidal surgery rarely occurs before 3 to 6 months and is common at 1 year, initial testing at 6 to 9 months is cost effective.[401] If the cortisol is undetectable on 2 consecutive days, then recovery of the axis has not occurred and glucocorticoid replacement can be restarted. If the cortisol is measurable, adequate reserve of the HPA axis can be assessed using the insulin tolerance test,[402] with a peak cortisol value of >18 µg/dL (500 nmol/L), indicating adequate reserve on modern assays.[403] Many centers use the cortisol response to 250 µg synthetic (1-24) ACTH as an alternative means of assessing HPA reserve,[404,405] but there is some controversy as to its reliability in this situation.[406,407] If it is used instead of the insulin tolerance test, a 30-minute cortisol of 22 µg/dL (600 nmol/L) is probably more reliable than the traditional cut-off of 18 µg/dL (500 nmol).[403] Glucocorticoid replacement can be discontinued abruptly if the cortisol response is shown to be normal. Where recovery of the HPA axis is only partial on dynamic testing, but the 9:00 A.M. cortisol levels are above the lower limit of the normal range (7 µg/dL [200 nmol/L]), it is reasonable to reduce the hydrocortisone unless symptoms of adrenal insufficiency occur. Patients need to continue to be aware of the continuing need for additional glucocorticoids at times of stress or illness and should be given a supply of oral hydrocortisone and an intramuscular injection pack. For patients with detectable but low 9:00 A.M. cortisol levels, the hydrocortisone replacement dose can usually be adjusted down, and, if necessary, adequate replacement can be assessed by measuring serum cortisol at various points throughout the day, ensuring that levels are always sufficient (>1.8 µg/dL, 50 nmol/L) before each dose; this may mean that the peak levels after each dose appear to be unphysiologic, but there is a tradeoff between mirroring a normal physiologic rhythm as far as possible and the inconvenience of multiple dosing. Two late but unrelated conundrums may arise: the questions of recurrence and permanent lack of recovery of the axis. Patients who articulate that the Cushing's syndrome has returned are often correct, even before physical and biochemical evidence are unequivocal. Assessment is warranted in a patient with these complaints or with recurrent physical signs characteristic of the hypercortisolemic phase. If this is to be done as an outpatient, UFC can be measured initially on dexamethasone 0.5 mg/day, if not yet weaned from glucocorticoids. However, ideally assessment of a cortisol circadian rhythm can be done as an inpatient having stopped the hydrocortisone. If the UFC result is increased, evaluation of hypercortisolism should proceed. If the result is subnormal or low, the patient should be questioned about the actual dose of glucocorticoid that has been taken. Often, patients take additional hydrocortisone, either because they discover that this decreases the symptoms of glucocorticoid withdrawal or because they have increased the dose "for stress," often without following strict guidelines. These patients have a suppressed axis and very slow regression of cushingoid features because of exogenous hypercortisolism. They require education and support along with reduction in the daily dose of hydrocortisone to recommended levels. The patient who has a subnormal cortisol response to ACTH 2 years after transsphenoidal surgery (in the absence of overreplacement) may proceed to life-long ACTH deficiency. If recurrent Cushing's disease is diagnosed, the therapeutic options are the same as for persistent disease. Repeat transsphenoidal surgery performed as long as 10 years after the initial operation can achieve a success rate of approximately 70%.[408]

Adrenalectomy

Resection of the affected adrenal gland(s) is the treatment of choice only for non-ACTH-dependent hypercortisolism of adrenal origin or when a specific surgical approach to the ACTH-dependent causes is not feasible. In adrenal adenomas, the cure rate is 100% when performed by experienced adrenal surgeons.[409] Surgery is the mainstay of treatment of adrenal cancer; more aggressive surgical approaches probably account for the increase in life span reported in this disease.[86,410] This approach may require multiple operations to resect primary lesions, local recurrences, and hepatic, thoracic, and, occasionally, intracranial metastases. Adjuvant medical treatment with mitotane and other chemotherapeutic agents has been discussed already.

Bilateral adrenalectomy as a second line of treatment has the advantage of providing rapid resolution of hypercortisolism and has no risk of hypopituitarism, in contrast to radiation therapy. Adrenalectomy may be chosen over radiation therapy by young patients desiring fertility who have concerns about radiation-induced hypopituitarism and loss of reproductive function. Its disadvantages include perioperative morbidity and mortality and the life-long requirement of glucocorticoid and mineralocorticoid replacement therapy. In addition, in patients with Cushing's disease, there is the risk of developing Nelson's syndrome, which occurs more frequently if adrenalectomy is performed at a younger age and if a pituitary adenoma is confirmed at previous pituitary surgery.[377,411] Prophylactic pituitary radiotherapy appears to reduce the risk of developing Nelson's syndrome from 50% to 25%.[412]

The mortality and morbidity of traditional open adrenalectomy via an anterior or posterior incision range from 1% to 20% in various series, probably reflecting differences in the severity of Cushing's syndrome and the presence of associated conditions, such as cardiovascular disease.[178,287] Apart from resection of suspected carcinoma, these approaches have been supplanted by laparoscopic resection, which has a low mortality and morbidity when done by an experienced surgeon.[413] Glands as large as 7.5 cm may be removed using this approach.[414]

Plasma cortisol levels become undetectable after successful adrenalectomy. Early failure to achieve hypocortisolism usually is related to incomplete resection of the gland(s). Recurrence, especially in the ACTH-dependent forms of Cushing's syndrome, may be related to regrowth of adrenal cells in the surgical bed or to growth of adrenal rest tissue.

In the postoperative period after bilateral adrenalectomy, the hydrocortisone dose is maintained at approximately twice the replacement dose, and saline 0.9% is given intravenously until the patient can take oral medications. This provides sodium and sufficient mineralocorticoid activity until fludrocortisone 100 µg/day can be given by mouth. Serum cortisol measurement done to confirm adequacy of resection is then assessed while the patient receives dexamethasone 0.5 mg/day and fludrocortisone. The patient is then switched back to hydrocortisone and fludrocortisone and must be advised regarding adrenal insufficiency as previously discussed. The dose of fludrocortisone is adjusted according to the patient's blood pressure, exposure to heat, and salt intake; the usual dose is 100 µg/day but ranges from 50 to 400 µg. A normal plasma renin activity measurement provides evidence of adequate mineralocorticoid replacement and can be used to gauge therapy. After unilateral adrenalectomy, the components of the HPA axis gradually recover after surgical cure of Cushing's syndrome. The time to recovery may be as short as 3 months and as long as 2 years.[390,401] The duration of recovery may be shorter in patients with mild hypercortisolism and those with recurrence and longer after resection of an adrenal adenoma.

Surgery for Ectopic Adrenocorticotropic Hormone Syndrome

If an ectopic ACTH-secreting tumor is localized and amenable to surgical excision, such as in a lobectomy for a bronchial carcinoid tumor, the chance of cure of Cushing's syndrome is high. However, if significant metastatic disease is present, surgery is unlikely to be of benefit. If the source of ACTH cannot be localized or if metastatic disease precludes surgery, alternative treatment of hypercortisolism must be chosen. For the patient with occult disease, medical therapy allows interval tumor surveillance with the goal of eventual tumor resection. Because some tumors remain occult for as long as 20 years, this may not prove practical for all patients, and adrenalectomy is appropriate when the patient cannot tolerate the cost, medical side effects, or psychological effects of long-term medical therapy and monitoring. Long-term medical therapy also may be the treatment of choice for the patient with widely disseminated disease who is not a good surgical candidate for adrenalectomy.

Bilateral adrenalectomy is the treatment of choice for any patient requiring rapid correction of hypercortisolism or when hypercortisolism cannot be controlled with medical therapy, when previously effective medical therapy must be discontinued because of significant medical side effects or intolerance, or when a severely hypercortisolemic patient is unable to take oral medications or etomidate.

RADIOTHERAPY

Pituitary

The role of radiation therapy to the pituitary gland in Cushing's disease is usually as adjunctive treatment in those who have failed transsphenoidal surgery but is also a good primary option for patients who cannot undergo surgery and for those having a bilateral adrenalectomy in whom the risk of Nelson's syndrome is deemed great.

Conventional Radiotherapy

Conventional pituitary radiotherapy is delivered at a total dose of 4500 to 5000 cGy (rad) in 25 fractional doses over 35 days using a three-field (opposed lateral fields and vertex field) technique. This approach ensures that the daily dose to neural tissue does not exceed 180 cGy and avoids the complications of optic neuritis and cortical necrosis associated with larger total and fractional doses.[415] The latent onset of action of radiotherapy means that adjunctive medical therapy is usually instituted before or at the time of treatment. The therapeutic response is assessed at least with annual monitoring, with weaning of medical treatment if possible. When conventional radiotherapy is used as primary treatment of Cushing's disease, remission is only achieved in 40% to 60% of adult patients.[377,416-418] The response is even worse if a lower dose of radiation (2000 cGy) is used.[419] By contrast, similar regimens achieve remission in 80% of children treated before the age of 18 years, often within 12 months.[420] More usually, conventional radiotherapy is used in the setting of failure to cure after transsphenoidal surgery. In this regard, it performs rather better with reported remission rates of as high as 83% in adults,[417,421] and 100% in children.[422] After conventional radiotherapy, remission usually starts by 9 months after treatment, and most patients are in remission within 2 years, although it can take much longer.[423]

Hypopituitarism is the most common side effect of pituitary radiotherapy, with growth hormone deficiency occurring in 36% to 68% of treated adults.[388,421] The incidence is probably higher in children,[424] but prompt diagnosis and treatment with human growth hormone ensure acceptable growth acceleration and catch-up growth.[425] Gonadotropin and thyroid-stimulating hormone deficiency are seen less commonly. The risk of optic neuropathy is low and probably less than 1% as long as low-dose fractions are used (≤200 cGy).[426] Similarly, the occurrence of brain necrosis is exceedingly rare.[427] The issue of secondary tumors remains contentious: Although meningiomas and gliomas have been reported after pituitary radiotherapy, it is not clear whether the incidence is significantly greater than the background risk of developing such tumors in patients who already have one intracranial tumor.[426]

Stereotactic Radiosurgery

In stereotactic radiosurgery, concentrated beams of high doses of radiation are precisely aimed at the mapped discrete lesion, delivering very high doses to the tumor and relatively low doses to normal surrounding tissue. There are a number of techniques to do this: using narrow beams from multiple gamma cobalt sources (gamma knife), a single beam from a linear accelerator that is arced around the target (X-knife, SMART), or using heavy charged particles (proton or helium beams). The advent of high-resolution MRI for mapping has facilitated this therapy. Usually, only a single therapy dose is required, and this is biologically more effective than delivering the same dose in fractions.[428] Probably the most widely used technique currently for Cushing's syndrome is the gamma knife, and this has been used both as primary therapy and adjunctive treatment. In a pre-MRI era study that included long-term follow-up (mean 17 years) of 18 patients, in which the gamma knife was used as the primary treatment in 15, the overall remission rate was 83%. Other studies that have included MRI-mapped patients have shown similar success rates.[429,430] In 43 patients treated after failed transsphenoidal surgery, 27 (63%) achieved remission at a mean of 12 months, although three of these later relapsed. Tumor shrinkage was seen in 24 of 33 patients as evidenced by MRI.[431] Linear accelerator radiotherapy for Cushing's disease is less well described, and follow-up data are often scanty, but there are reports of some success in small numbers of patients, either as a single radiosurgical dose[432–434] or as fractionated therapy.[433,435] Radiosurgery of the pituitary gland using heavy charged particles from proton or helium beams has been available since the 1950s but has not been widely available. Published results for Cushing's disease have been good with remission seen in more than 90% of patients.[436,437] As with conventional forms of radiation therapy, it appears that younger patients have a better response.

Therefore, at least in the medium term, radiosurgery appears to be effective treatment. As with conventional radiotherapy, the main side effect is hypopituitarism, and although the perceived risk of damage to adjacent structures such as the optic chiasm is less, more studies and longer follow-up are needed.[438] Some centers use it mainly for salvage of difficult recurrent tumors, for example, in the cavernous sinus or Nelson's syndrome,[434,439] whereas others have suggested it as an alternative to conventional radiotherapy in adenomas smaller than 30 mm with a minimal distance from the optic chiasm of 2 to 3 mm.[427] In general, it is only really applicable where there is a clear and unambiguous target that is clear of the optic pathways.

Interstitial Radiotherapy

Two centers have used interstitial irradiation (yttrium-90 or gold-198 implants) as primary therapy for Cushing's disease.[440,441] Remission rates in these cohorts were high (75%–77%), although some required a second implant. The principal side effect was hypopituitarism.

Other Tumors

There is no significant evidence that radiotherapy improves overall survival in adrenocortical carcinoma, although there are sporadic reports that it may be helpful adjuvant treatment to radical surgery in selected cases.[442,443] Local radiotherapy after surgical resection of an ectopic ACTH-secreting source may also be beneficial, particularly in nonmetastatic thoracic carcinoid tumors.[444,445]

SPECIAL THERAPEUTIC PROBLEMS

Pregnancy

Maternal hypercortisolism is associated with a poor pregnancy outcome, including an increased rate of premature delivery and stillbirth.[283] It is unclear whether this is a toxic effect of hypercortisolism on the fetus or placenta or is related to associated medical conditions such as hypertension and diabetes. However, pregnancy outcome has been slightly better in women with adrenal causes of Cushing's syndrome who received surgical treatment while pregnant. An additional reason for early resection of adrenal masses is the significant incidence of adrenal carcinoma in pregnancy. Although anesthesia increases the risk of premature labor, both maternal and fetal outcome are improved by resolution of hypercortisolism, and surgery should not be delayed because of this concern.[446] Many patients with Cushing's disease have not been treated during pregnancy; although metyrapone, cyproheptadine, radiation therapy, and transsphenoidal surgery[447] have all been used in a few cases.[283] Because ketoconazole is teratogenic in animals and blocks steroidogenesis, its use is contraindicated.[448]

Exogenous Cushing's Syndrome

The treatment of exogenous Cushing's syndrome is to discontinue glucocorticoid ingestion. If this is possible, a weaning schedule should be followed until a replacement dose of hydrocortisone is reached, at which point the patient may be weaned very gradually, as discussed earlier for postoperative treatment. If the degree of suppression of the axis cannot be estimated from the medication and dose received, the response to synthetic ACTH can be used as a rough gauge of adrenal suppression.

For the patient in whom glucocorticoids cannot be discontinued, a change in dose or schedule may ameliorate symptoms of Cushing's syndrome. Patients requiring supraphysiologic glucocorticoid therapy should undergo measurement of bone density and be counseled to maintain adequate calcium intake, exercise, and receive bisphosphonate therapy when appropriate.

PROGNOSIS

The life expectancy of patients with nonmalignant causes of Cushing's syndrome, at one time a uniformly fatal illness, has improved dramatically with effective surgical and medical treatments and the availability of antibiotics, antihypertensive agents, and glucocorticoids. In a 1952 review, Plotz and colleagues[69] reported a 5-year mortality rate of 50% in actively hypercortisolemic patients, with 46% caused by bacterial infection and 40% due to cardiovascular complications (cardiac failure, cardiovascular accidents, or renal insufficiency). In 1961, the mortality rate was similar, but the causes had changed: two thirds were due to postoperative adrenal crisis before cortisone was available or from metastatic adrenal cancer. Cardiovascular events related to hypertension (stroke, heart failure, renal failure, myocardial infarction) led to death in approximately 20%; infectious causes had decreased to approximately 15%.[73] Ten years later, in 1971, 30% of patients with benign causes of Cushing's syndrome died within 5 years of diagnosis, most from cardiovascular disease or infection, despite decreased postoperative mortality.[449] In 1979, a lower incidence of death (6%) was noted within 2 to 10 years of radiation therapy, mitotane, or combination treatment of Cushing's disease.[319] The improvement may reflect earlier detection of Cushing's syndrome, better treatment of hypercortisolism, and the associated medical complications, such as hypertension, or lower perioperative mortality. Three recent studies on the long-term survival in Cushing's disease treated in the era of transsphenoidal surgery were reported. Two were epidemiologic studies from northern

Spain[68] and Denmark,[63] and the third was a series from a single neurosurgical center where all patients had undergone transsphenoidal surgery.[450] They report quite varying standardized mortality ratios of 3.8, 1.7, and 0.98, respectively. The discrepancy in the findings between the three series is not completely clear, but it is difficult to make absolute comparisons, not least because the study by Swearingen and colleagues[450] undoubtedly is affected by selection bias. However, what the latter two studies do appear to show is that after curative transsphenoidal surgery, long-term mortality is not significantly different from that in the general population. This is perhaps surprising because increased cardiovascular risk markers and evidence of atherosclerotic disease persist when measured 5 years after remission of Cushing's disease.[117] The outcome of pediatric Cushing's disease is excellent if treated at centers with appropriate experience.[275]

The prognosis of the potentially malignant causes of Cushing's syndrome is variable. Adrenal cancer, as reviewed earlier, has an extremely poor prognosis. Tumors that produce ACTH ectopically tend to have a poor prognosis, particularly when compared with tumors from the same tissue that do not produce ACTH. Small cell lung cancer, islet cell tumors, and thymic carcinoids[451] illustrate this phenomenon. As many as 82% of patients with small cell lung cancer and Cushing's syndrome die within 2 weeks from the start of chemotherapy.[65] Among the causes of ectopic ACTH syndrome, phaeochromocytoma and bronchial carcinoid appear to offer the best prognosis after tumor resection, but this is not universal.

REFERENCES

1. Cushing HW: The pituitary body and its disorders. Philadelphia, JB Lippincott, 1912.
2. Cushing HW: The basophil adenomas of the pituitary body and their clinical manifestations (pituitary basophilism). Bull Johns Hopkins Hosp 1:137–195, 1932.
3. Walters W, Wilder RM, Kepler EJ: The suprarenal cortical syndrome with presentation of ten cases. Ann Surg 100:670–688, 1934.
4. Liddle GW, Nicholson WE, Island DP, et al: Clinical and laboratory studies of ectopic humoral syndromes. Recent Prog Horm Res 25:283–314, 1969.
5. Howlett TA, Rees LH, Besser GM: Cushing's syndrome. Clin Endocrinol Metab 14:911–945, 1985.
6. Bertagna X: New causes of Cushing's syndrome. N Engl J Med 327:1024–1025, 1992.
7. Reznik Y, Allali-Zerah V, Chayvialle JA, et al: Food-dependent Cushing's syndrome mediated by aberrant adrenal sensitivity to gastric inhibitory polypeptide. N Engl J Med 327:981–986, 1992.
8. Lacroix A, Bolte E, Tremblay J, et al: Gastric inhibitory polypeptide-dependent cortisol hypersecretion— A new cause of Cushing's syndrome. N Engl J Med 327:974–980, 1992.
9. Malchoff CD, Orth DN, Abboud C, et al: Ectopic ACTH syndrome caused by a bronchial carcinoid tumor responsive to dexamethasone, metyrapone, and corticotropin-releasing factor. Am J Med 84:760–764, 1988.
10. Biller BM, Alexander JM, Zervas NT, et al: Clonal origins of adrenocorticotropin-secreting pituitary tissue in Cushing's disease. J Clin Endocrinol Metab 75:1303–1309, 1992.
11. Mampalam TJ, Tyrrell JB, Wilson CB: Transsphenoidal microsurgery for Cushing disease. A report of 216 cases. Ann Intern Med 109:487–493, 1988.
12. Young WF Jr, Scheithauer BW, Gharib H, et al: Cushing's syndrome due to primary multinodular corticotrope hyperplasia. Mayo Clin Proc 63:256–262, 1988.

13. Asa SL, Ezzat S: The cytogenesis and pathogenesis of pituitary adenomas. Endocr Rev 19:798–827, 1998.
14. Dahia PL, Grossman AB: The molecular pathogenesis of corticotroph tumors. Endocr Rev 20:136–155, 1999.
15. Rabbitt EH, Ayuk J, Boelaert K, et al: Abnormal expression of 11 beta-hydroxysteroid dehydrogenase type 2 in human pituitary adenomas: A prereceptor determinant of pituitary cell proliferation. Oncogene 22:1663–1667, 2003.
16. Korbonits M, Chahal HS, Kaltsas G, et al: Expression of phosphorylated p27(Kip1) protein and Jun activation domain-binding protein 1 in human pituitary tumors. J Clin Endocrinol Metab 87:2635–2643, 2002.
17. Trautmann K, Thakker RV, Ellison DW, et al: Chromosomal aberrations in sporadic pituitary tumors. Int J Cancer 91:809–814, 2001.
18. Metzger AK, Mohapatra G, Minn YA, et al: Multiple genetic aberrations including evidence of chromosome 11q13 rearrangement detected in pituitary adenomas by comparative genomic hybridization. J Neurosurg 90:306–314, 1999.
19. Fan X, Paetau A, Aalto Y, et al: Gain of chromosome 3 and loss of 13q are frequent alterations in pituitary adenomas. Cancer Genet Cytogenet 128:97–103, 2001.
20. Evans CO, Young AN, Brown MR, et al: Novel patterns of gene expression in pituitary adenomas identified by complementary deoxyribonucleic acid microarrays and quantitative reverse transcription-polymerase chain reaction. J Clin Endocrinol Metab 86:3097–3107, 2001.
21. Imura H: Ectopic hormone syndromes. Clin Endocrinol Metab 9:235–260, 1980.
22. de Bustros A, Baylin SB: Hormone production by tumours: Biological and clinical aspects. Clin Endocrinol Metab 14:221–256, 1985.
23. Pearse AG: Common cytochemical and ultrastructural characteristics of cells producing polypeptide hormones (the APUD series) and their relevance to thyroid and ultimobranchial C cells and calcitonin.

Proc R Soc Lond B Biol Sci 170:71–80, 1968.
24. Pullan PT, Clement-Jones V, Corder R, et al: ACTH LPH and related peptides in the ectopic ACTH syndrome. Clin Endocrinol (Oxf) 13:437–445, 1980.
25. Rees LH, Bloomfield GA, Gilkes JJ, et al: ACTH as a tumor marker. Ann N Y Acad Sci 297:603–620, 1977.
26. Stewart MF, Crosby SR, Gibson S, et al: Small cell lung cancer cell lines secrete predominantly ACTH precursor peptides not ACTH. Br J Cancer 60:20–24, 1989.
27. White A, Clark AJ, Stewart MF: The synthesis of ACTH and related peptides by tumours. Baillieres Clin Endocrinol Metab 4:1–27, 1990.
28. DeBold CR, Menefee JK, Nicholson WE, Orth DN: Proopiomelanocortin gene is expressed in many normal human tissues and in tumors not associated with ectopic adrenocorticotropin syndrome. Mol Endocrinol 2:862–870, 1988.
29. de Keyzer Y, Bertagna X, Luton JP, Kahn A: Variable modes of proopiomelanocortin gene transcription in human tumors. Mol Endocrinol 3:215–223, 1989.
30. Clark AJ, Lavender PM, Besser GM, Rees LH: Pro-opiomelanocortin mRNA size heterogeneity in ACTH-dependent Cushing's syndrome. J Mol Endocrinol 2:3–9, 1989.
31. Clark AJ, Stewart MF, Lavender PM, et al: Defective glucocorticoid regulation of proopiomelanocortin gene expression and peptide secretion in a small cell lung cancer cell line. J Clin Endocrinol Metab 70:485–490, 1990.
32. Roth KA, Newell DC, Dorin RI, et al: Aberrant production and regulation of proopiomelanocortin-derived peptides in ectopic Cushing's syndrome. Horm Metab Res 20:225–229, 1988.
33. Melmed S, Yamashita S, Kovacs K, et al: Cushing's syndrome due to ectopic proopiomelanocortin gene expression by islet cell carcinoma of the pancreas. Cancer 59:772–778, 1987.
34. Limper AH, Carpenter PC, Scheithauer B, Staats BA: The Cushing syndrome induced by bronchial

carcinoid tumors. Ann Intern Med 117:209–214, 1992.

35. Asa SL, Kovacs K, Vale W, et al: Immunohistologic localization of corticotrophin-releasing hormone in human tumors. Am J Clin Pathol 87:327–333, 1987.

36. Jessop DS, Cunnah D, Millar JG, et al: A phaeochromocytoma presenting with Cushing's syndrome associated with increased concentrations of circulating corticotrophin-releasing factor. J Endocrinol 113:133–138, 1987.

37. Zangeneh F, Young WF Jr, Lloyd RV, et al: Cushing's syndrome due to ectopic production of corticotropin-releasing hormone in an infant with ganglioneuroblastoma. Endocr Pract 9:394–399, 2003.

38. Wajchenberg BL, Mendonca BB, Liberman B, et al: Ectopic adrenocorticotropic hormone syndrome. Endocr Rev 15:752–787, 1994.

39. Sidhu S, Gicquel C, Bambach CP, et al: Clinical and molecular aspects of adrenocortical tumourigenesis. ANZ J Surg 73:727–738, 2003.

40. Beuschlein F, Reincke M, Karl M, et al: Clonal composition of human adrenocortical neoplasms. Cancer Res 54:4927–4932, 1994.

41. Weiss LM, Medeiros LJ, Vickery AL Jr: Pathologic features of prognostic significance in adrenocortical carcinoma. Am J Surg Pathol 13:202–206, 1989.

42. Travis WD, Tsokos M, Doppman JL, et al: Primary pigmented nodular adrenocortical disease. A light and electron microscopic study of eight cases. Am J Surg Pathol 13:921–930, 1989.

43. Stratakis CA, Carney JA, Lin JP, et al: Carney complex, a familial multiple neoplasia and lentiginosis syndrome. Analysis of 11 kindreds and linkage to the short arm of chromosome 2. J Clin Invest 97:699–705, 1996.

44. Casey M, Mah C, Merliss AD, et al: Identification of a novel genetic locus for familial cardiac myxomas and Carney complex. Circulation 98:2560–2566, 1998.

45. Kirschner LS, Sandrini F, Monbo J, et al: Genetic heterogeneity and spectrum of mutations of the PRKAR1A gene in patients with the Carney complex. Hum Mol Genet 9:3037–3046, 2000.

46. Kirk JM, Brain CE, Carson DJ, et al: Cushing's syndrome caused by nodular adrenal hyperplasia in children with McCune-Albright syndrome. J Pediatr 134:789–792, 1999.

47. Weinstein LS, Shenker A, Gejman PV, et al: Activating mutations of the stimulatory G protein in the McCune-Albright syndrome. N Engl J Med 325:1688–1695, 1991.

48. Boston BA, Mandel S, LaFranchi S, Bliziotes M: Activating mutation in the stimulatory guanine nucleotide-binding protein in an infant with Cushing's syndrome and nodular adrenal

hyperplasia. J Clin Endocrinol Metab 79:890–893, 1994.

49. Swords FM, Baig A, Malchoff DM, et al: Impaired desensitization of a mutant adrenocorticotropin receptor associated with apparent constitutive activity. Mol Endocrinol 16:2746–2753, 2002.

50. Findlay JC, Sheeler LR, Engeland WC, Aron DC: Familial adrenocorticotropin-independent Cushing's syndrome with bilateral macronodular adrenal hyperplasia. J Clin Endocrinol Metab 76:189–191, 1993.

51. Lacroix A, Ndiaye N, Tremblay J, Hamet P: Ectopic and abnormal hormone receptors in adrenal Cushing's syndrome. Endocr Rev 22:75–110, 2001.

52. Maschler I, Rosenmann E, Ehrenfeld EN: Ectopic functioning adrenocortico-myelolipoma in longstanding Nelson's syndrome. Clin Endocrinol (Oxf) 10:493–497, 1979.

53. Lalau JD, Vieau D, Tenenbaum F, et al: A case of pseudo-Nelson's syndrome: Cure of ACTH hypersecretion by removal of a bronchial carcinoid tumor responsible for Cushing's syndrome. J Endocrinol Invest 13:531–537, 1990.

54. Adeyemi SD, Grange AO, Giwa-Osagie OF, Elesha SO: Adrenal rest tumour of the ovary associated with isosexual precocious pseudopuberty and cushingoid features. Eur J Pediatr 145:236–238, 1986.

55. Contreras P, Altieri E, Liberman C, et al: Adrenal rest tumor of the liver causing Cushing's syndrome: Treatment with ketoconazole preceding an apparent surgical cure. J Clin Endocrinol Metab 60:21–28, 1985.

56. Marieb NJ, Spangler S, Kashgarian M, et al: Cushing's syndrome secondary to ectopic cortisol production by an ovarian carcinoma. J Clin Endocrinol Metab 57:737–740, 1983.

57. Newell-Price J, Trainer P, Besser M, Grossman A: The diagnosis and differential diagnosis of Cushing's syndrome and pseudo-Cushing's states. Endocr Rev 19:647–672, 1998.

58. Chrousos GP, Schuermeyer TH, Doppman J, et al: NIH conference. Clinical applications of corticotropin-releasing factor. Ann Intern Med 102:344–358, 1985.

59. Gold PW, Gwirtsman H, Avgerinos PC, et al: Abnormal hypothalamic-pituitary-adrenal function in anorexia nervosa. Pathophysiologic mechanisms in underweight and weight-corrected patients. N Engl J Med 314:1335–1342, 1986.

60. Gold PW, Loriaux DL, Roy A, et al: Responses to corticotropin-releasing hormone in the hypercortisolism of depression and Cushing's disease. Pathophysiologic and diagnostic implications. N Engl J Med 314:1329–1335, 1986.

61. Luger A, Deuster PA, Kyle SB, et al: Acute hypothalamic-pituitary-adrenal responses to the stress of treadmill exercise. Physiologic adaptations to physical training. N Engl J Med 316:1309–1315, 1987.

62. Invitti C, Giraldi FP, de Martin M, Cavagnini F: Diagnosis and management of Cushing's syndrome: Results of an Italian multicentre study. Study Group of the Italian Society of Endocrinology on the Pathophysiology of the Hypothalamic-Pituitary-Adrenal Axis. J Clin Endocrinol Metab 84:440–448, 1999.

63. Lindholm J, Juul S, Jorgensen JO, et al: Incidence and late prognosis of Cushing's syndrome: A population-based study. J Clin Endocrinol Metab 86:117–123, 2001.

64. Abeloff MD, Trump DL, Baylin SB: Ectopic adrenocorticotrophic (ACTH) syndrome and small cell carcinoma of the lung-assessment of clinical implications in patients on combination chemotherapy. Cancer 48:1082–1087, 1981.

65. Dimopoulos MA, Fernandez JF, Samaan NA, et al: Paraneoplastic Cushing's syndrome as an adverse prognostic factor in patients who die early with small cell lung cancer. Cancer 69:66–71, 1992.

66. Janssen-Heijnen ML, Coebergh JW: The changing epidemiology of lung cancer in Europe. Lung Cancer 41:245–258, 2003.

67. Ambrosi B, Faglia G: Epidemiology of pituitary tumours. In Faglia G, Beck-Peccoz P, Ambrosi B (eds): Pituitary Adenomas: New Trends in Basic and Clinical Research. Amsterdam, Excerpta Medica, 1991, pp 159–168.

68. Etxabe J, Vazquez JA: Morbidity and mortality in Cushing's disease: An epidemiological approach. Clin Endocrinol (Oxf) 40:479–484, 1994.

69. Plotz CM, Knowlton AI, Ragan C: The natural history of Cushing's syndrome. Am J Med 13:597–614, 1952.

70. Leinung MC, Young WF Jr, Whitaker MD, et al: Diagnosis of corticotropin-producing bronchial carcinoid tumors causing Cushing's syndrome. Mayo Clin Proc 65:1314–1321, 1990.

71. Ross EJ, Linch DC: Cushing's syndrome—Killing disease: Discriminatory value of signs and symptoms aiding early diagnosis. Lancet 2:646–649, 1982.

72. Urbanic RC, George JM: Cushing's disease—18 years' experience. Medicine (Baltimore) 60:14–24, 1981.

73. Soffer LJ, Iannaccone A, Gabrilove JL: Cushing's syndrome: A study of fifty patients. Am J Med 30:129–146, 1961.

74. Sprague RG, Randall RV, Salassa RM: Cushing's syndrome: Review of 100 cases. Arch Intern Med 98:389–398, 1956.

75. Nugent CA, Warner HR, Dunn JT, Tyler FH: Probability theory in the diagnosis of Cushing's syndrome. J Clin Endocrinol Metab 24:621–627, 1964.

76. Rockall AG, Sohaib SA, Evans D, et al: Computed tomography assessment of fat distribution in male and female patients with Cushing's syndrome. Eur J Endocrinol 149:561–567, 2003.

77. Roy-Camille R, Mazel C, Husson JL, Saillant G: Symptomatic spinal epidural

lipomatosis induced by a long-term steroid treatment. Review of the literature and report of two additional cases. Spine 16:1365–1371, 1991.

78. Noel P, Pepersack T, Vanbinst A, Alle JL: Spinal epidural lipomatosis in Cushing's syndrome secondary to an adrenal tumor. Neurology 42:1250–1251, 1992.

79. Healy ME, Hesselink JR, Ostrup RC, Alksne JF: Demonstration by magnetic resonance of symptomatic spinal epidural lipomatosis. Neurosurgery 21:414–415, 1987.

80. Pleasure DE, Walsh GO, Engel WK: Atrophy of skeletal muscle in patients with Cushing's syndrome. Arch Neurol 22:118–125, 1970.

81. Muller R, Kugelberg E: Myopathy in Cushing's syndrome. J Neurol Neurosurg Psychiatry 22:314–319, 1959.

82. Afifi AK, Bergman RA, Harvey JC: Steroid myopathy. Clinical, histologic and cytologic observations. Johns Hopkins Med J 123:158–173, 1968.

83. Vertebral compression fractures with accelerated bone turnover in a patient with Cushing's disease. Am J Med 68:932–940, 1980.

84. Kingsley GH, Hickling P: Polyarthropathy associated with Cushing's disease. Br Med J 292:1363, 1986.

85. Phillips KA, Nance EP Jr, Rodriguez RM, Kaye JJ: Avascular necrosis of bone: A manifestation of Cushing's disease. South Med J 79:825–829, 1986.

86. Bertagna C, Orth DN: Clinical and laboratory findings and results of therapy in 58 patients with adrenocortical tumors admitted to a single medical center (1951 to 1978). Am J Med 71:855–875, 1981.

87. Starkman MN, Schteingart DE: Neuropsychiatric manifestations of patients with Cushing's syndrome. Relationship to cortisol and adrenocorticotropic hormone levels. Arch Intern Med 141:215–219, 1981.

88. Starkman MN, Schteingart DE, Schork MA: Correlation of bedside cognitive and neuropsychological tests in patients with Cushing's syndrome. Psychosomatics 27:508–511, 1986.

89. Haskett RF: Diagnostic categorization of psychiatric disturbance in Cushing's syndrome. Am J Psychiatry 142:911–916, 1985.

90. Hudson JI, Hudson MS, Griffing GT, et al: Phenomenology and family history of affective disorder in Cushing's disease. Am J Psychiatry 144:951–953, 1987.

91. Rubinow DR, Post RM, Savard R, Gold PW: Cortisol hypersecretion and cognitive impairment in depression. Arch Gen Psychiatry 41:279–283, 1984.

92. Kathol RG: Etiologic implications of corticosteroid changes in affective disorder. Psychiatr Med 3:135–162, 1985.

93. Magiakou MA, Mastorakos G, Zachman K, Chrousos GP: Blood pressure in children and adolescents with Cushing's syndrome before and after surgical care. J Clin Endocrinol Metab 82:1734–1738, 1997.

94. Fallo F, Sonino N, Barzon L, et al: Effect of surgical treatment on hypertension in Cushing's syndrome. Am J Hypertens 9:77–80, 1996.

95. Bakker RC, Gallas PR, Romijn JA, Wiersinga WM: Cushing's syndrome complicated by multiple opportunistic infections. J Endocrinol Invest 21:329–333, 1998.

96. Graham BS, Tucker WS Jr: Opportunistic infections in endogenous Cushing's syndrome. Ann Intern Med 101:334–338, 1984.

97. Sarlis NJ, Chanock SJ, Nieman LK: Cortisolemic indices predict severe infections in Cushing syndrome due to ectopic production of adrenocorticotropin. J Clin Endocrinol Metab 85:42–47, 2000.

98. Kaltsas GA, Korbonits M, Isidori AM, et al: How common are polycystic ovaries and the polycystic ovarian syndrome in women with Cushing's syndrome? Clin Endocrinol (Oxf) 53:493–500, 2000.

99. Halbreich U, Zumoff B, Kream J, Fukushima DK: The mean 1300-1600 h plasma cortisol concentration as a diagnostic test for hypercortisolism. J Clin Endocrinol Metab 54:1262–1264, 1982.

100. Liu JH, Kazer RR, Rasmussen DD: Characterization of the twenty-four hour secretion patterns of adrenocorticotropin and cortisol in normal women and patients with Cushing's disease. J Clin Endocrinol Metab 64:1027–1035, 1987.

101. Refetoff S, Van Cauter E, Fang VS, et al: The effect of dexamethasone on the 24-hour profiles of adrenocorticotropin and cortisol in Cushing's syndrome. J Clin Endocrinol Metab 60:527–535, 1985.

102. Mengden T, Hubmann P, Muller J, et al: Urinary free cortisol versus 17-hydroxycorticosteroids: A comparative study of their diagnostic value in Cushing's syndrome. Clin Investig 70:545–548, 1992.

103. Evans PJ, Peters JR, Dyas J, et al: Salivary cortisol levels in true and apparent hypercortisolism. Clin Endocrinol (Oxf) 20:709–715, 1984.

104. Christy NP, Laragh JH: Pathogenesis of hypokalemic alkalosis in Cushing's syndrome. Nord Hyg Tidskr 265:1083–1088, 1961.

105. Stewart PM, Krozowski ZS: 11 beta-Hydroxysteroid dehydrogenase. Vitam Horm 57:249–324, 1999.

106. Putignano P, Kaltsas GA, Korbonits M, et al: Alterations in serum protein levels in patients with Cushing's syndrome before and after successful treatment. J Clin Endocrinol Metab 85:3309–3312, 2000.

107. Ambrosi B, Sartorio A, Pizzocaro A, et al: Evaluation of haemostatic and fibrinolytic markers in patients with Cushing's syndrome and in patients with adrenal incidentaloma. Exp Clin Endocrinol Diabetes 108:294–298, 2000.

108. Casonato A, Pontara E, Boscaro M, et al: Abnormalities of von Willebrand factor are also part of the prothrombotic state of Cushing's syndrome. Blood Coagul Fibrinolysis 10:145–151, 1999.

109. Patrassi GM, Dal Bo ZR, Boscaro M, et al: Further studies on the hypercoagulable state of patients with Cushing's syndrome. Thromb Haemost 54:518–520, 1985.

110. Taskinen MR, Nikkila EA, Pelkonen R, Sane T: Plasma lipoproteins, lipolytic enzymes, and very low density lipoprotein triglyceride turnover in Cushing's syndrome. J Clin Endocrinol Metab 57:619–626, 1983.

111. Friedman TC, Mastorakos G, Newman TD, et al: Carbohydrate and lipid metabolism in endogenous hypercortisolism: Shared features with metabolic syndrome X and NIDDM. Endocr J 43:645–655, 1996.

112. Page R, Boolell M, Kalfas A, et al: Insulin secretion, insulin sensitivity and glucose-mediated glucose disposal in Cushing's disease: A minimal model analysis. Clin Endocrinol (Oxf) 35:509–517, 1991.

113. Biering H, Knappe G, Gerl H, Lochs H: [Prevalence of diabetes in acromegaly and Cushing syndrome]. Acta Med Austriaca 27:27–31, 2000.

114. Krassowski J, Godziejewska M, Kurta J, Kasperlik-Zaluska A: [Glucose tolerance in adrenocortical hyperfunction. Analysis of 100 cases]. Pol Arch Med Wewn 92:70–75, 1994.

115. Catargi B, Rigalleau V, Poussin A, et al: Occult Cushing's syndrome in type-2 diabetes. J Clin Endocrinol Metab 88:5808–5813, 2003.

116. Faggiano A, Pivonello R, Spiezia S, et al: Cardiovascular risk factors and common carotid artery caliber and stiffness in patients with Cushing's disease during active disease and 1 year after disease remission. J Clin Endocrinol Metab 88:2527–2533, 2003.

117. Colao A, Pivonello R, Spiezia S, et al: Persistence of increased cardiovascular risk in patients with Cushing's disease after five years of successful cure. J Clin Endocrinol Metab 84:2664–2672, 1999.

118. Bartalena L, Martino E, Petrini L, et al: The nocturnal serum thyrotropin surge is abolished in patients with adrenocorticotropin (ACTH)-dependent or ACTH-independent Cushing's syndrome. J Clin Endocrinol Metab 72:1195–1199, 1991.

119. Colao A, Pivonello R, Faggiano A, et al: Increased prevalence of thyroid autoimmunity in patients successfully treated for Cushing's disease. Clin Endocrinol (Oxf) 53:13–19, 2000.

120. Niepomniszcze H, Pitoia F, Katz SB, et al: Primary thyroid disorders in endogenous Cushing's syndrome. Eur J Endocrinol 147:305–311, 2002.

121. Luton JP, Thieblot P, Valcke JC, et al: Reversible gonadotropin deficiency in male Cushing's disease. J Clin Endocrinol Metab 45:488–495, 1977.

122. Lado-Abeal J, Rodriguez-Arnao J, Newell-Price JD, et al: Menstrual abnormalities in women with Cushing's disease are correlated with hypercortisolemia rather than raised circulating androgen levels. J Clin Endocrinol Metab 83:3083–3088, 1998.

123. Giustina A, Bossoni S, Bussi AR, et al: Effect of galanin on the growth hormone (GH) response to GH-releasing hormone in patients with Cushing's disease. Endocr Res 19:47–56, 1993.

124. Kaltsas G, Manetti L, Grossman AB: Osteoporosis in Cushing's syndrome. Front Horm Res 30:60–72, 2002.

125. Ohmori N, Nomura K, Ohmori K, et al: Osteoporosis is more prevalent in adrenal than in pituitary Cushing's syndrome. Endocr J 50:1–7, 2003.

126. Rockall AG, Sohaib SA, Evans D, et al: Hepatic steatosis in Cushing's syndrome: A radiological assessment using computed tomography. Eur J Endocrinol 149:543–548, 2003.

127. Giraldi FP, Moro M, Cavagnini F: Gender-related differences in the presentation and course of Cushing's disease. J Clin Endocrinol Metab 88:1554–1558, 2003.

128. King AB: The diagnosis of carcinoma of the pituitary gland. Bull Johns Hopkins Hosp 89:339–353, 1951.

129. Martins AN, Hayes GJ, Kempe LG: Invasive pituitary adenomas. J Neurosurg 22:268–276, 1965.

130. Della CS, Corsello SM, Satta MA, et al: Intracranial and spinal dissemination of an ACTH secreting pituitary neoplasia. Case report and review of the literature. Ann Endocrinol (Paris) 58:503–509, 1997.

131. Arnaldi G, Angeli A, Atkinson AB, et al: Diagnosis and complications of Cushing's syndrome: A consensus statement. J Clin Endocrinol Metab 88:5593–5602, 2003.

132. Besser GM, Edwards CRW: Cushing's syndrome. Clin Endocrinol Metab 1:451–490, 1972.

133. Lamberts SW, Klijn JG, de Jong FH, Birkenhager JC: Hormone secretion in alcohol-induced pseudo-Cushing's syndrome. Differential diagnosis with Cushing disease. JAMA 242:1640–1643, 1979.

134. Wallace EZ, Rosman P, Toshav N, et al: Pituitary-adrenocortical function in chronic renal failure: Studies of episodic secretion of cortisol and dexamethasone suppressibility. J Clin Endocrinol Metab 50:46–51, 1980.

135. Werner S, Thoren M, Gustafsson JA, Bronnegard M: Glucocorticoid receptor abnormalities in fibroblasts from patients with idiopathic resistance to dexamethasone diagnosed when evaluated for adrenocortical disorders. J Clin Endocrinol Metab 75:1005–1009, 1992.

136. Murphy BE: Clinical evaluation of urinary cortisol determinations by competitive protein-binding radioassay. J Clin Endocrinol Metab 28:343–348, 1968.

137. Orth DN: Cushing's syndrome. N Engl J Med 332:791–803, 1995.

138. Contreras LN, Hane S, Tyrrell JB: Urinary cortisol in the assessment of pituitary-adrenal function: Utility of 24-hour and spot determinations. J Clin Endocrinol Metab 62:965–969, 1986.

139. Laudat MH, Billaud L, Thomopoulos P, et al: Evening urinary free corticoids: A screening test in Cushing's syndrome and incidentally discovered adrenal tumours. Acta Endocrinol (Copenh) 119:459–464, 1988.

140. Carpenter PC: Diagnostic evaluation of Cushing's syndrome. Endocrinol Metab Clin North Am 17:445–472, 1988.

141. Lin CL, Wu TJ, Machacek DA, et al: Urinary free cortisol and cortisone determined by high performance liquid chromatography in the diagnosis of Cushing's syndrome. J Clin Endocrinol Metab 82:151–155, 1997.

142. Cizza G, Nieman LK, Doppman JL, et al: Factitious Cushing syndrome. J Clin Endocrinol Metab 81:3573–3577, 1996.

143. Turpeinen U, Markkanen H, Valimaki M, Stenman UH: Determination of urinary free cortisol by HPLC. Clin Chem 43:1386–1391, 1997.

144. Nieman LK, Cutler GB Jr: The sensitivity of the urine free cortisol measurement as a screening test for Cushing's syndrome (abstract P-822). Program of the 72nd Annual Meeting of The Endocrine Society, Atlanta, GA, 1990.

145. Laudat MH, Cerdas S, Fournier C, et al: Salivary cortisol measurement: A practical approach to assess pituitary-adrenal function. J Clin Endocrinol Metab 66:343–348, 1988.

146. Putignano P, Dubini A, Toja P, et al: Salivary cortisol measurement in normal-weight, obese and anorexic women: Comparison with plasma cortisol. Eur J Endocrinol 145:165–171, 2001.

147. Chen YM, Cintron NM, Whitson PA: Long-term storage of salivary cortisol samples at room temperature. Clin Chem 38:304, 1992.

148. Raff H, Raff JL, Findling JW: Late-night salivary cortisol as a screening test for Cushing's syndrome. J Clin Endocrinol Metab 83:2681–2686, 1998.

149. Papanicolaou DA, Mullen N, Kyrou I, Nieman LK: Nighttime salivary cortisol: A useful test for the diagnosis of Cushing's syndrome. J Clin Endocrinol Metab 87:4515–4521, 2002.

150. Putignano P, Toja P, Dubini A, et al: Midnight salivary cortisol versus urinary free and midnight serum cortisol as screening tests for Cushing's syndrome. J Clin Endocrinol Metab 88:4153–4157, 2003.

151. Gafni RI, Papanicolaou DA, Nieman LK: Nighttime salivary cortisol measurement as a simple, noninvasive, outpatient screening test for Cushing's syndrome in children and adolescents. J Pediatr 137:30–35, 2000.

152. Martinelli CE Jr, Sader SL, Oliveira E, et al: Salivary cortisol for screening of Cushing's syndrome in children. Clin Endocrinol (Oxf) 51:67–71, 1999.

153. Castro M, Elias PC, Quidute AR, et al: Out-patient screening for Cushing's syndrome: The sensitivity of the combination of circadian rhythm and overnight dexamethasone suppression salivary cortisol tests. J Clin Endocrinol Metab 84:878–882, 1999.

154. Liddle GW: Tests of pituitary-adrenal suppressability in the diagnosis of Cushing's syndrome. J Clin Endocrinol Metab 20:1539–1560, 1960.

155. Kennedy L, Atkinson AB, Johnston H, et al: Serum cortisol concentrations during low dose dexamethasone suppression test to screen for Cushing's syndrome. Br Med J 289:1188–1191, 1984.

156. Hankin ME, Theile HM, Steinbeck AW: An evaluation of laboratory tests for the detection and differential diagnosis of Cushing's syndrome. Clin Endocrinol (Oxf) 6:185–196, 1977.

157. Newell-Price J, Trainer P, Perry L, et al: A single sleeping midnight cortisol has 100% sensitivity for the diagnosis of Cushing's syndrome. Clin Endocrinol (Oxf) 43:545–550, 1995.

158. Isidori AM, Kaltsas GA, Mohammed S, et al: Discriminatory value of the low-dose dexamethasone suppression test in establishing the diagnosis and differential diagnosis of Cushing's syndrome. J Clin Endocrinol Metab 88:5299–5306, 2003.

159. Nugent CA, Nichols T, Tyler FH: Diagnosis of Cushing's syndrome-single dose dexamethasone suppression test. Arch Intern Med 116:172–176, 1965.

160. Shimizu N, Yoshida H: Studies on the "low dose" suppressible Cushing's disease. Endocrinol Jpn 23:479–484, 1976.

161. McHardy-Young S, Harris PW, Lessof MH, Lyne C: Single dose dexamethasone suppression test for Cushing's syndrome. Br Med J 2:740–744, 1967.

162. Seidensticker JF, Folk RL, Wieland RG, Hamwi GJ: Screening test for Cushing's syndrome with plasma 11-hydroxycorticosteroids. JAMA 202:87–90, 1967.

163. Crapo L: Cushing's syndrome: A review of diagnostic tests. Metabolism 28:955–977, 1979.

164. Odagiri E, Demura R, Demura H, et al: The changes in plasma cortisol and urinary free cortisol by an overnight dexamethasone suppression test in patients with Cushing's disease. Endocrinol Jpn 35:795–802, 1988.

165. Lampe TH, Fariss BL, Risse SC, et al: Laboratory evaluation for Cushing's

syndrome in psychiatric patients with cortisol nonsuppression following the overnight dexamethasone suppression test. Biol Psychiatry 22:1264–1270, 1987.

166. Wood PJ, Barth JH, Freedman DB, et al: Evidence for the low dose dexamethasone suppression test to screen for Cushing's syndrome— Recommendations for a protocol for biochemistry laboratories. Ann Clin Biochem 34:222–229, 1997.

167. Putignano P, Kaltsas GA, Satta MA, Grossman AB: The effects of anti-convulsant drugs on adrenal function. Horm Metab Res 30:389–397, 1998.

168. Abou Samra AB, Dechaud H, Estour B, et al: Beta-lipotropin and cortisol responses to an intravenous infusion dexamethasone suppression test in Cushing's syndrome and obesity. J Clin Endocrinol Metab 61:116–119, 1985.

169. Atkinson AB, McAteer EJ, Hadden DR, et al: A weight-related intravenous dexamethasone suppression test distinguishes obese controls from patients with Cushing's syndrome. Acta Endocrinol (Copenh) 120:753–759, 1989.

170. Papanicolaou DA, Yanovski JA, Cutler GB Jr, et al: A single midnight serum cortisol measurement distinguishes Cushing's syndrome from pseudo-Cushing states. J Clin Endocrinol Metab 83:1163–1167, 1998.

171. Ambrosi B, Bochicchio D, Ferrario R, et al: Effects of the opiate agonist loperamide on pituitary-adrenal function in patients with suspected hypercortisolism. J Endocrinol Invest 12:31–35, 1989.

172. Ambrosi B, Bochicchio D, Colombo P, et al: Loperamide to diagnose Cushing's syndrome. JAMA 270:2301–2302, 1993.

173. Bernini GP, Argenio GF, Cerri F, Franchi F: Comparison between the suppressive effects of dexamethasone and loperamide on cortisol and ACTH secretion in some pathological conditions. J Endocrinol Invest 17:799–804, 1994.

174. Yanovski JA, Cutler GB Jr, Chrousos GP, Nieman LK: Corticotropin-releasing hormone stimulation following low-dose dexamethasone administration. A new test to distinguish Cushing's syndrome from pseudo-Cushing's states. JAMA 269:2232–2238, 1993.

175. Yanovski JA, Cutler GB Jr, Chrousos GP, Nieman LK: Prospective evaluation of the dexamethasone-suppressed corticotrophin-releasing hormone test in the differential diagnosis of Cushing's syndrome and pseudo-Cushing's states (abstract). Program of the 77th Annual Meeting of the Endocrine Society, Washington, DC, 1995, p 99.

176. Lytras N, Grossman A, Perry L, et al: Corticotrophin releasing factor: Responses in normal subjects and patients with disorders of the hypothalamus and pituitary. Clin Endocrinol (Oxf) 20:71–84, 1984.

177. Fig LM, Gross MD, Shapiro B, et al: Adrenal localization in the adrenocorticotropic hormone-independent Cushing syndrome. Ann Intern Med 109:547–553, 1988.

178. Perry RR, Nieman LK, Cutler GB Jr, et al: Primary adrenal causes of Cushing's syndrome. Diagnosis and surgical management. Ann Surg 210:59–68, 1989.

179. Hanson JA, Weber A, Reznek RH, et al: Magnetic resonance imaging of adrenocortical adenomas in childhood: Correlation with computed tomography and ultrasound. Pediatr Radiol 26:794–799, 1996.

180. Doppman JL, Miller DL, Dwyer AJ, et al: Macronodular adrenal hyperplasia in Cushing disease. Radiology 166:347–352, 1988.

181. Mimou N, Sakato S, Nakabayashi H, et al: Cushing's syndrome associated with bilateral adrenal adenomas. Acta Endocrinol (Copenh) 108:245–254, 1985.

182. Doppman JL, Travis WD, Nieman L, et al: Cushing syndrome due to primary pigmented nodular adrenocortical disease: Findings at CT and MR imaging. Radiology 172:415–420, 1989.

183. Malchoff CD, Rosa J, DeBold CR, et al: Adrenocorticotropin-independent bilateral macronodular adrenal hyperplasia: An unusual cause of Cushing's syndrome. J Clin Endocrinol Metab 68:855–860, 1989.

184. Doppman JL, Nieman LK, Travis WD, et al: CT and MR imaging of massive macronodular adrenocortical disease: A rare cause of autonomous primary adrenal hypercortisolism. J Comput Assist Tomogr 15:773–779, 1991.

185. Sohaib SA, Hanson JA, Newell-Price JD, et al: CT appearance of the adrenal glands in adrenocorticotrophic hormone-dependent Cushing's syndrome. Am J Roentgenol 172:997–1002, 1999.

186. Aron DC, Findling JW, Fitzgerald PA, et al: Pituitary ACTH dependency of nodular adrenal hyperplasia in Cushing's syndrome. Report of two cases and review of the literature. Am J Med 71:302–306, 1981.

187. Smals AG, Pieters GF, van Haelst UJ, Kloppenborg PW: Macronodular adrenocortical hyperplasia in long-standing Cushing's disease. J Clin Endocrinol Metab 58:25–31, 1984.

188. Leiba S, Shindel B, Weinberger I, et al: Cushing's disease coexisting with a single macronodule simulating adenoma of the adrenal cortex. Acta Endocrinol (Copenh) 112:323–328, 1986.

189. Schteingart DE, Tsao HS: Coexistence of pituitary adrenocorticotropin-dependent Cushing's syndrome with a solitary adrenal adenoma. J Clin Endocrinol Metab 50:961–966, 1980.

190. Howlett TA, Drury PL, Perry L, et al: Diagnosis and management of ACTH-dependent Cushing's syndrome: Comparison of the features in ectopic and pituitary ACTH production. Clin Endocrinol (Oxf) 24:699–713, 1986.

191. Newell-Price J, Morris DG, Drake WM, et al: Optimal response criteria for the human CRH test in the differential diagnosis of ACTH-dependent Cushing's syndrome. J Clin Endocrinol Metab 87:1640–1645, 2002.

192. Yamamoto Y, Davis DH, Nippoldt TB, et al: False-positive inferior petrosal sinus sampling in the diagnosis of Cushing's disease. Report of two cases. J Neurosurg 83:1087–1091, 1995.

193. Yanovski JA, Cutler GB Jr, Doppman JL, et al: The limited ability of inferior petrosal sinus sampling with corticotropin-releasing hormone to distinguish Cushing's disease from pseudo-Cushing states or normal physiology. J Clin Endocrinol Metab 77:503–509, 1993.

194. Miller DL, Doppman JL: Petrosal sinus sampling: Technique and rationale. Radiology 178:37–47, 1991.

195. Oldfield EH, Doppman JL, Nieman LK, et al: Petrosal sinus sampling with and without corticotropin-releasing hormone for the differential diagnosis of Cushing's syndrome. N Engl J Med 325:897–905, 1991.

196. Kaltsas GA, Giannulis MG, Newell-Price JD, et al: A critical analysis of the value of simultaneous inferior petrosal sinus sampling in Cushing's disease and the occult ectopic adrenocorticotropin syndrome. J Clin Endocrinol Metab 84:487–492, 1999.

197. McCance DR, McIlrath E, McNeill A, et al: Bilateral inferior petrosal sinus sampling as a routine procedure in ACTH-dependent Cushing's syndrome. Clin Endocrinol (Oxf) 30:157–166, 1989.

198. Miller DL: Neurologic complications of petrosal sinus sampling. Radiology 183:878, 1992.

199. Lefournier V, Gatta B, Martinie M, et al: One transient neurological complication (sixth nerve palsy) in 166 consecutive inferior petrosal sinus samplings for the etiological diagnosis of Cushing's syndrome. J Clin Endocrinol Metab 84:3401–3402, 1999.

200. Rotman-Pikielny P, Patronas N, Papanicolaou DA: Pituitary apoplexy induced by corticotrophin-releasing hormone in a patient with Cushing's disease. Clin Endocrinol (Oxf) 58:545–549, 2003.

201. Tabarin A, Greselle JF, San Galli F, et al: Usefulness of the corticotropin-releasing hormone test during bilateral inferior petrosal sinus sampling for the diagnosis of Cushing's disease. J Clin Endocrinol Metab 73:53–59, 1991.

202. Landolt AM, Schubiger O, Maurer R, Girard J: The value of inferior petrosal sinus sampling in diagnosis and treatment of Cushing's disease. Clin Endocrinol (Oxf) 40:485–492, 1994.

203. Lefournier V, Martinie M, Vasdev A, et al: Accuracy of bilateral inferior petrosal or cavernous sinuses sampling

in predicting the lateralization of
Cushing's disease pituitary
microadenoma: Influence of catheter
position and anatomy of venous
drainage. J Clin Endocrinol Metab
88:196–203, 2003.
204. Lienhardt A, Grossman AB, Dacie JE,
et al: Relative contributions of inferior
petrosal sinus sampling and pituitary
imaging in the investigation of
children and adolescents with ACTH-
dependent Cushing's syndrome. J Clin
Endocrinol Metab 86:5711–5714,
2001.
205. Morris DG, Grossman AB: Dynamic
tests in the diagnosis and differential
diagnosis of Cushing's syndrome.
J Endocrinol Invest 26:64–73, 2003.
206. Miller DL, Doppman JL, Nieman LK,
et al: Petrosal sinus sampling:
Discordant lateralization of ACTH-
secreting pituitary microadenomas
before and after stimulation with
corticotropin-releasing hormone.
Radiology 176:429–431, 1990.
207. Doppman JL, Nieman LK, Chang R,
et al: Selective venous sampling from
the cavernous sinuses is not a more
reliable technique than sampling from
the inferior petrosal sinuses in
Cushing's syndrome. J Clin Endocrinol
Metab 80:2485–2489, 1995.
208. Doppman JL, Oldfield EH, Nieman LK:
Bilateral sampling of the internal
jugular vein to distinguish between
mechanisms of adrenocorticotropic
hormone-dependent Cushing
syndrome. Ann Intern Med 128:33–36,
1998.
209. Kai Y, Hamada J, Nishi T, et al:
Usefulness of multiple-site venous
sampling in the treatment of
adrenocorticotropic hormone-
producing pituitary adenomas. Surg
Neurol 59:292–298, 2003.
210. Flack MR, Oldfield EH, Cutler GB Jr,
et al: Urine free cortisol in the
high-dose dexamethasone suppression
test for the differential diagnosis of the
Cushing syndrome. Ann Intern Med
116:211–217, 1992.
211. Dichek HL, Nieman LK, Oldfield EH,
et al: A comparison of the standard
high dose dexamethasone suppression
test and the overnight 8-mg
dexamethasone suppression test for
the differential diagnosis of
adrenocorticotropin-dependent
Cushing's syndrome. J Clin Endocrinol
Metab 78:418–422, 1994.
212. Avgerinos PC, Yanovski JA,
Oldfield EH, et al: The metyrapone and
dexamethasone suppression tests for
the differential diagnosis of the
adrenocorticotropin-dependent
Cushing syndrome: A comparison.
Ann Intern Med 121:318–327, 1994.
213. Tyrrell JB, Findling JW, Aron DC, et al:
An overnight high-dose
dexamethasone suppression test for
rapid differential diagnosis of
Cushing's syndrome. Ann Intern Med
104:180–186, 1986.
214. Bruno OD, Rossi MA, Contreras LN,
et al: Nocturnal high-dose

dexamethasone suppression test in the
aetiological diagnosis of Cushing's
syndrome. Acta Endocrinol (Copenh)
109:158–162, 1985.
215. Aron DC, Raff H, Findling JW:
Effectiveness versus efficacy: The
limited value in clinical practice of
high dose dexamethasone suppression
testing in the differential diagnosis of
adrenocorticotropin-dependent
Cushing's syndrome. J Clin Endocrinol
Metab 82:1780–1785, 1997.
216. Liddle GW, Estep Hl, Kendall JWJ,
et al: Clinical application of a new test
of pituitary reserve. J Clin Endocrinol
Metab 19:875–894, 1959.
217. Kaye TB, Crapo L: The Cushing
syndrome: An update on diagnostic
tests. Ann Intern Med 112:434–444,
1990.
218. Giraldi FP, Invitti C, Cavagnini F: The
corticotropin-releasing hormone test in
the diagnosis of ACTH-dependent
Cushing's syndrome: A reappraisal.
Clin Endocrinol (Oxf) 54:601–607,
2001.
219. Trainer PJ, Faria M, Newell-Price J,
et al: A comparison of the effects of
human and ovine corticotropin-
releasing hormone on the pituitary-
adrenal axis. J Clin Endocrinol Metab
80:412–417, 1995.
220. Trainer PJ, Woods RJ, Korbonits M,
et al: The pathophysiology of
circulating corticotropin-releasing
hormone-binding protein levels in the
human. J Clin Endocrinol Metab
83:1611–1614, 1998.
221. Nieman LK, Oldfield EH, Wesley R,
et al: A simplified morning ovine
corticotropin-releasing hormone
stimulation test for the differential
diagnosis of adrenocorticotropin-
dependent Cushing's syndrome. J Clin
Endocrinol Metab 77:1308–1312, 1993.
222. Korbonits M, Kaltsas G, Perry LA, et al:
The growth hormone secretagogue
hexarelin stimulates the hypothalamo-
pituitary-adrenal axis via arginine
vasopressin. J Clin Endocrinol Metab
84:2489–2495, 1999.
223. Korbonits M, Bustin SA, Kojima M,
et al: The expression of the growth
hormone secretagogue receptor ligand
ghrelin in normal and abnormal
human pituitary and other
neuroendocrine tumors. J Clin
Endocrinol Metab 86:881–887, 2001.
224. Tabarin A, San Galli F, Dezou S, et al:
The corticotropin-releasing factor test
in the differential diagnosis of
Cushing's syndrome: A comparison
with the lysine-vasopressin test. Acta
Endocrinol (Copenh) 123:331–338,
1990.
225. Malerbi DA, Mendonca BB,
Liberman B, et al: The desmopressin
stimulation test in the differential
diagnosis of Cushing's syndrome. Clin
Endocrinol (Oxf) 38:463–472, 1993.
226. Ghigo E, Arvat E, Ramunni J, et al:
Adrenocorticotropin- and
cortisol-releasing effect of hexarelin, a
synthetic growth hormone-releasing
peptide, in normal subjects and

patients with Cushing's syndrome.
J Clin Endocrinol Metab
82:2439–2444, 1997.
227. Newell-Price J, Perry L, Medbak S, et al:
A combined test using desmopressin
and corticotropin-releasing hormone
in the differential diagnosis of
Cushing's syndrome. J Clin Endocrinol
Metab 82:176–181, 1997.
228. Tsagarakis S, Tsigos C, Vasiliou V, et al:
The desmopressin and combined
CRH-desmopressin tests in the
differential diagnosis of ACTH-
dependent Cushing's syndrome:
Constraints imposed by the
expression of V2 vasopressin receptors
in tumors with ectopic ACTH
secretion. J Clin Endocrinol Metab
87:1646–1653, 2002.
229. Korbonits M, Jacobs RA, Aylwin SJ,
et al: Expression of the growth
hormone secretagogue receptor in
pituitary adenomas and other
neuroendocrine tumors. J Clin
Endocrinol Metab 83:3624–3630, 1998.
230. Nieman LK, Chrousos GP, Oldfield EH,
et al: The ovine corticotropin-releasing
hormone stimulation test and the
dexamethasone suppression test in the
differential diagnosis of Cushing's
syndrome. Ann Intern Med
105:862–867, 1986.
231. Hermus AR, Pieters GF, Pesman GJ,
et al: The corticotropin-
releasing-hormone test versus the
high-dose dexamethasone test in the
differential diagnosis of Cushing's
syndrome. Lancet 2:540–544, 1986.
232. Grossman AB, Howlett TA, Perry L,
et al: CRF in the differential diagnosis
of Cushing's syndrome: A comparison
with the dexamethasone suppression
test. Clin Endocrinol (Oxf)
29:167–178, 1988.
233. Doppman JL, Frank JA, Dwyer AJ, et al:
Gadolinium DTPA enhanced MR
imaging of ACTH-secreting
microadenomas of the pituitary gland.
J Comput Assist Tomogr 12:728–735,
1988.
234. Hall WA, Luciano MG, Doppman JL,
et al: Pituitary magnetic resonance
imaging in normal human volunteers:
Occult adenomas in the general
population. Ann Intern Med
120:817–820, 1994.
235. Findling JW, Doppman JL: Biochemical
and radiologic diagnosis of Cushing's
syndrome. Endocrinol Metab Clin
North Am 23:511–537, 1994.
236. Escourolle H, Abecassis JP, Bertagna X,
et al: Comparison of computerized
tomography and magnetic resonance
imaging for the examination of the
pituitary gland in patients with
Cushing's disease. Clin Endocrinol
(Oxf) 39:307–313, 1993.
237. Doppman JL, Pass HI, Nieman LK,
et al: Detection of ACTH-producing
bronchial carcinoid tumors: MR
imaging vs CT. Am J Roentgenol
156:39–43, 1991.
238. Doppman JL, Nieman L, Miller DL
et al: Ectopic adrenocorticotropic
hormone syndrome: Localization

studies in 28 patients. Radiology 172:115–124, 1989.

239. de Herder WW, Lamberts SW: Octapeptide somatostatin-analogue therapy of Cushing's syndrome. Postgrad Med J 75:65–66, 1999.

240. Tabarin A, Valli N, Chanson P, et al: Usefulness of somatostatin receptor scintigraphy in patients with occult ectopic adrenocorticotropin syndrome. J Clin Endocrinol Metab 84:1193–1202, 1999.

241. Tsagarakis S, Christoforaki M, Giannopoulou H, et al: A reappraisal of the utility of somatostatin receptor scintigraphy in patients with ectopic adrenocorticotropin Cushing's syndrome. J Clin Endocrinol Metab 88:4754–4758, 2003.

242. Torpy DJ, Chen CC, Mullen N, et al: Lack of utility (of111n)-pentetreotide scintigraphy in localizing ectopic ACTH producing tumors: Follow-up of 18 patients. J Clin Endocrinol Metab 84:1186–1192, 1999.

243. Shapiro MS, Shenkman L: Variable hormonogenesis in Cushing's syndrome. Q J Med 79:351–363, 1991.

244. Kammer H, Barter M: Spontaneous remission of Cushing's disease. A case report and review of the literature. Am J Med 67:519–523, 1979.

245. Hayslett JP, Cohn GL: Spontaneous remission of Cushing's disease. Report of a case. N Engl J Med 276:96–97, 1967.

246. Brown RD, Van Loon GR, Orth DN, Liddle GW: Cushing's disease with periodic hormonogenesis: One explanation for paradoxical response to dexamethasone. J Clin Endocrinol Metab 36:445–451, 1973.

247. Strott CA, Nugent CA, Tyler FH: Cushing's syndrome caused by bronchial adenomas. Am J Med 44:97–104, 1968.

248. Schweikert HU, Fehm HL, Fahlbusch R, et al: Cyclic Cushing's syndrome combined with cortisol suppressible, dexamethasone non-suppressible ACTH secretion: A new variant of Cushing's syndrome. Acta Endocrinol (Copenh) 110:289–295, 1985.

249. Kendall JW, Sloop PR Jr: Dexamethasone-suppressible adrenocortical tumor. N Engl J Med 279:532–535, 1968.

250. Braverman LE, Woeber KA, Ingbar SH: An unusual case of Cushing's syndrome. N Engl J Med 273:1018–1020, 1965.

251. Vagnucci AH, Evans E: Cushing's disease with intermittent hypercortisolism. Am J Med 80:83–88, 1986.

252. Kreze A, Veleminsky J, Spirova E: A follow-up of the "low dose suppressible" hypercortisolism. Endocrinol Exp 17:119–123, 1983.

253. Dixon RB, Christy NP: On the various forms of corticosteroid withdrawal syndrome. Am J Med 68:224–230, 1980.

254. Tsuruoka S, Sugimoto K, Fujimura A: Drug-induced Cushing syndrome in a patient with ulcerative colitis after betamethasone enema: Evaluation of plasma drug concentration. Ther Drug Monit 20:387–389, 1998.

255. Findlay CA, Macdonald JF, Wallace AM, et al: Childhood Cushing's syndrome induced by betamethasone nose drops, and repeat prescriptions. Br Med J 317:739–740, 1998.

256. Quddusi S, Browne P, Toivola B, Hirsch IB: Cushing syndrome due to surreptitious glucocorticoid administration. Arch Intern Med 158:294–296, 1998.

257. McConkey B: Adrenal corticosteroids in Chinese herbal remedies. Q J Med 96:81–82, 2003.

258. Mann M, Koller E, Murgo A, et al: Glucocorticoidlike activity of megestrol. A summary of Food and Drug Administration experience and a review of the literature. Arch Intern Med 157:1651–1656, 1997.

259. O'Hare JP, Vale JA, Wood S, Corrall RJ: Factitious Cushing's syndrome. Acta Endocrinol (Copenh) 111:165–167, 1986.

260. Luger A, Lang I, Kovarik J, et al: Abnormalities in the hypothalamic-pituitary-adrenocortical axis in patients with chronic renal failure. Am J Kidney Dis 9:51–54, 1987.

261. Siamopoulos KC, Dardamanis M, Kyriaki D, et al: Pituitary adrenal responsiveness to corticotropin-releasing hormone in chronic uremic patients. Perit Dial Int 10:153–156, 1990.

262. Nolan GE, Smith JB, Chavre VJ, Jubiz W: Spurious overestimation of plasma cortisol in patients with chronic renal failure. J Clin Endocrinol Metab 52:1242–1245, 1981.

263. Sederberg-Olsen P, Binder C, Kehlet H: Urinary excretion of free cortisol in impaired renal function. Acta Endocrinol (Copenh) 78:86–90, 1975.

264. Ramirez G, Gomez-Sanchez C, Meikle WA, Jubiz W: Evaluation of the hypothalamic hypophyseal adrenal axis in patients receiving long-term hemodialysis. Arch Intern Med 142:1448–1452, 1982.

265. Workman RJ, Vaughn WK, Stone WJ: Dexamethasone suppression testing in chronic renal failure: Pharmacokinetics of dexamethasone and demonstration of a normal hypothalamic-pituitary-adrenal axis. J Clin Endocrinol Metab 63:741–746, 1986.

266. Rosman PM, Farag A, Peckham R, et al: Pituitary-adrenocortical function in chronic renal failure: Blunted suppression and early escape of plasma cortisol levels after intravenous dexamethasone. J Clin Endocrinol Metab 54:528–533, 1982.

267. Rodger RS, Dewar JH, Turner SJ, et al: Anterior pituitary dysfunction in patients with chronic renal failure treated by hemodialysis or continuous ambulatory peritoneal dialysis. Nephron 43:169–172, 1986.

268. Sharp NA, Devlin JT, Rimmer JM: Renal failure obfuscates the diagnosis of Cushing's disease. JAMA 256:2564–2565, 1986.

269. Otokida K, Fujiwara T, Oriso S, Kato M: Cortisol and its metabolites in the plasma and urine in Cushing's syndrome with chronic renal failure (CRF), compared to Cushing's syndrome without CRF. Nippon Jinzo Gakkai Shi 31:651–656, 1989.

270. Jain S, Sakhuja V, Bhansali A, et al: Corticotropin-dependent Cushing's syndrome in a patient with chronic renal failure—A rare association. Ren Fail 15:563–566, 1993.

271. Streeten DH, Faas FH, Elders MJ, et al: Hypercortisolism in childhood: Shortcomings of conventional diagnostic criteria. Pediatrics 56:797–803, 1975.

272. Magiakou MA, Mastorakos G, Oldfield EH, et al: Cushing's syndrome in children and adolescents. Presentation, diagnosis, and therapy. N Engl J Med 331:629–636, 1994.

273. Weber A, Trainer PJ, Grossman AB, et al: Investigation, management and therapeutic outcome in 12 cases of childhood and adolescent Cushing's syndrome. Clin Endocrinol (Oxf) 43:19–28, 1995.

274. Lee PD, Winter RJ, Green OC: Virilizing adrenocortical tumors in childhood: Eight cases and a review of the literature. Pediatrics 76:437–444, 1985.

275. Savage MO, Lienhardt A, Lebrethon MC, et al: Cushing's disease in childhood: Presentation, investigation, treatment and long-term outcome. Horm Res 55(Suppl 1):24–30, 2001.

276. McArthur RG, Hayles AB, Salassa RM: Childhood Cushing disease: Results of bilateral adrenalectomy. J Pediatr 95:214–219, 1979.

277. Jones GS, Shah KJ, Mann JR: Adreno-cortical carcinoma in infancy and childhood: A radiological report of ten cases. Clin Radiol 36:257–262, 1985.

278. Pombo M, Alvez F, Varela-Cives R, et al: Ectopic production of ACTH by Wilms' tumor. Horm Res 16:160–163, 1982.

279. Normann T, Havnen J, Mjolnerod O: Cushing's syndrome in an infant associated with neuroblastoma in two ectopic adrenal glands. J Pediatr Surg 6:169–175, 1971.

280. Kitahara M, Mori T, Seki H, et al: Malignant paraganglioma presenting as Cushing syndrome with virilism in childhood. Production of cortisol, androgens, and adrenocorticotrophic hormone by the tumor. Cancer 72:3340–3345, 1993.

281. Styne DM, Isaac R, Miller WL, et al: Endocrine, histological, and biochemical studies of adrenocorticotropin-producing islet cell carcinoma of the pancreas in childhood with characterization of proopiomelanocortin. J Clin Endocrinol Metab 57:723–731, 1983.

282. Hannah J, Lippe B, Lai-Goldman M, Bhuta S: Oncocytic carcinoid of the kidney associated with periodic Cushing's syndrome. Cancer 61:2136–2140, 1988.

283. Sheeler LR: Cushing's syndrome and pregnancy. Endocrinol Metab Clin North Am 23:619–627, 1994.

284. Brien TG: Human corticosteroid binding globulin. Clin Endocrinol (Oxf) 14:193–212, 1981.

285. Nolten WE, Lindheimer MD, Rueckert PA, et al: Diurnal patterns and regulation of cortisol secretion in pregnancy. J Clin Endocrinol Metab 51:466–472, 1980.

286. Odagiri E, Ishiwatari N, Abe Y, et al: Hypercortisolism and the resistance to dexamethasone suppression during gestation. Endocrinol Jpn 35:685–690, 1988.

287. Sarkar R, Thompson NW, McLeod MK: The role of adrenalectomy in Cushing's syndrome. Surgery 108:1079–1084, 1990.

288. Cavagnini F, Panerai AE, Valentini F, et al: Inhibition of ACTH response to oral and intravenous metyrapone by antiserotoninergic treatment in man. J Clin Endocrinol Metab 41:143–148, 1975.

289. Whitehead HM, Beacom R, Sheridan B, Atkinson AB: The effect of cyproheptadine and/or bromocriptine on plasma ACTH levels in patients cured of Cushing's disease by bilateral adrenalectomy. Clin Endocrinol (Oxf) 32:193–201, 1990.

290. Tanakol R, Alagol F, Azizlerli H, et al: Cyproheptadine treatment in Cushing's disease. J Endocrinol Invest 19:242–247, 1996.

291. Sonino N, Boscaro M, Fallo F, Fava GA: Potential therapeutic effects of ritanserin in Cushing's disease. JAMA 267:1073, 1992.

292. Sonino N, Fava GA, Fallo F, et al: Effect of the serotonin antagonists ritanserin and ketanserin in Cushing's disease. Pituitary 3:55–59, 2000.

293. Boscaro M, Benato M, Mantero F: Effect of bromocriptine in pituitary-dependent Cushing's syndrome. Clin Endocrinol (Oxf) 19:485–491, 1983.

294. Mercado-Asis LB, Yasuda K, Murayama M, et al: Beneficial effects of high daily dose bromocriptine treatment in Cushing's disease. Endocrinol Jpn 39:385–395, 1992.

295. Pivonello R, Ferone D, de Herder WW, et al: Dopamine receptor expression and function in corticotroph pituitary tumors. J Clin Endocrinol Metab 89:2452–2462, 2004.

296. Koppeschaar HP, Croughs RJ, Thijssen JH, Schwarz F: Response to neurotransmitter modulating drugs in patients with Cushing's disease. Clin Endocrinol (Oxf) 25:661–667, 1986.

297. Lamberts SW, de Lange SA, Stefanko SZ: Adrenocorticotropin-secreting pituitary adenomas originate from the anterior or the intermediate lobe in Cushing's disease: Differences in the regulation of hormone secretion. J Clin Endocrinol Metab 54:286–291, 1982.

298. Croughs RJ, Koppeschaar HP, van't Verlaat JW, McNicol AM: Bromocriptine-responsive Cushing's disease associated with anterior pituitary corticotroph hyperplasia or normal pituitary gland. J Clin Endocrinol Metab 68:495–498, 1989.

299. Kritzler RK, Vining EP, Plotnick LP: Sodium valproate and corticotropin suppression in the child treated for seizures. J Pediatr 102:142–143, 1983.

300. Gomi M, Iida S, Itoh Y, et al: Unaltered stimulation of pituitary adrenocorticotrophin secretion by corticotrophin-releasing factor following sodium valproate administration in a patient with Nelson's syndrome. Clin Endocrinol (Oxf) 23:123–127, 1985.

301. Jones MT, Gillham B, Altaher AR, et al: Clinical and experimental studies on the role of GABA in the regulation of ACTH secretion: A review. Psychoneuroendocrinology 9:107–123, 1984.

302. Beckers A, Stevenaert A, Pirens G, et al: Cyclical Cushing's disease and its successful control under sodium valproate. J Endocrinol Invest 13:923–929, 1990.

303. Colao A, Pivonello R, Tripodi FS, et al: Failure of long-term therapy with sodium valproate in Cushing's disease. J Endocrinol Invest 20:387–392, 1997.

304. Greenman Y, Melmed S: Heterogeneous expression of two somatostatin receptor subtypes in pituitary tumors. J Clin Endocrinol Metab 78:398–403, 1994.

305. Lamberts SW, de Herder WW, Krenning EP, Reubi JC: A role of (labeled) somatostatin analogs in the differential diagnosis and treatment of Cushing's syndrome. J Clin Endocrinol Metab 78:17–19, 1994.

306. de Herder WW, Lamberts SW: Is there a role for somatostatin and its analogs in Cushing's syndrome? Metabolism 45:83–85, 1996.

307. Hart MM, Swackhamer ES, Straw JA: Studies on the site of action of o,p'-DDD in the dog adrenal cortex. II. Steroids 17:575–586, 1971.

308. Ojima M, Saitoh M, Itoh N, et al: [The effects of o,p'-DDD on adrenal steroidogenesis and hepatic steroid metabolism]. Nippon Naibunpi Gakkai Zasshi 61:168–178, 1985.

309. Bergenstal DM, Hertz R, Lipsett MB, Moy RH: Chemotherapy of adrenocortical cancer with O,p'DDD. Ann Intern Med 53:672–682, 1960.

310. Gutierrez ML, Crooke ST: Mitotane (o,p'-DDD). Cancer Treat Rev 7:49–55, 1980.

311. Luton JP, Cerdas S, Billaud L, et al: Clinical features of adrenocortical carcinoma, prognostic factors, and the effect of mitotane therapy. N Engl J Med 322:1195–1201, 1990.

312. Kasperlik-Zaluska AA: Clinical results of the use of mitotane for adrenocortical carcinoma. Braz J Med Biol Res 33:1191–1196, 2000.

313. van Slooten H, Moolenaar AJ, van Seters AP, Smeenk D: The treatment of adrenocortical carcinoma with o,p'-DDD: Prognostic implications of serum level monitoring. Eur J Cancer Clin Oncol 20:47–53, 1984.

314. Dickstein G, Shechner C, Arad E, et al: Is there a role for low doses of mitotane (o,p'-DDD) as adjuvant therapy in adrenocortical carcinoma? J Clin Endocrinol Metab 83:3100–3103, 1998.

315. Ilias I, Alevizaki M, Philippou G, et al: Sustained remission of metastatic adrenal carcinoma during long-term administration of low-dose mitotane. J Endocrinol Invest 24:532–535, 2001.

316. Bukowski RM, Wolfe M, Levine HS, et al: Phase II trial of mitotane and cisplatin in patients with adrenal carcinoma: A Southwest Oncology Group study. J Clin Oncol 11:161–165, 1993.

317. Berruti A, Terzolo M, Pia A, et al: Mitotane associated with etoposide, doxorubicin, and cisplatin in the treatment of advanced adrenocortical carcinoma. Italian Group for the Study of Adrenal Cancer. Cancer 83:2194–2200, 1998.

318. Williamson SK, Lew D, Miller GJ, et al: Phase II evaluation of cisplatin and etoposide followed by mitotane at disease progression in patients with locally advanced or metastatic adrenocortical carcinoma: A Southwest Oncology Group Study. Cancer 88:1159–1165, 2000.

319. Luton JP, Mahoudeau JA, Bouchard P, et al: Treatment of Cushing's disease by O,p'DDD. Survey of 62 cases. N Engl J Med 300:459–464, 1979.

320. Schteingart DE, Tsao HS, Taylor CI, et al: Sustained remission of Cushing's disease with mitotane and pituitary irradiation. Ann Intern Med 92:613–619, 1980.

321. Carey RM, Orth DN, Hartmann WH: Malignant melanoma with ectopic production of adrenocorticotropic hormone. Palliative treatment with inhibitors of adrenal steroid biosynthesis. J Clin Endocrinol Metab 36:482–487, 1973.

322. Hutter AM Jr, Kayhoe DE: Adrenal cortical carcinoma. Results of treatment with o,p'DDD in 138 patients. Am J Med 41:581–592, 1966.

323. Haak HR, Caekebeke-Peerlinck KM, van Seters AP, Briet E: Prolonged bleeding time due to mitotane therapy. Eur J Cancer 27:638–641, 1991.

324. Maher VM, Trainer PJ, Scoppola A, et al: Possible mechanism and treatment of o,p'DDD-induced hypercholesterolaemia. Q J Med 84:671–679, 1992.

325. Leiba S, Weinstein R, Shindel B, et al: The protracted effect of o,p'-DDD in Cushing's disease and its impact on adrenal morphogenesis of young

human embryo. Ann Endocrinol (Paris) 50:49–53, 1989.

326. van Seters AP, Moolenaar AJ: Mitotane increases the blood levels of hormone-binding proteins. Acta Endocrinol (Copenh) 124:526–533, 1991.

327. Hague RV, May W, Cullen DR: Hepatic microsomal enzyme induction and adrenal crisis due to o,p'DDD therapy for metastatic adrenocortical carcinoma. Clin Endocrinol (Oxf) 31:51–57, 1989.

328. Carballeira A, Fishman LM, Jacobi JD: Dual sites of inhibition by metyrapone of human adrenal steroidogenesis: Correlation of in vivo and in vitro studies. J Clin Endocrinol Metab 42:687–695, 1976.

329. Verhelst JA, Trainer PJ, Howlett TA, et al: Short and long-term responses to metyrapone in the medical management of 91 patients with Cushing's syndrome. Clin Endocrinol (Oxf) 35:169–178, 1991.

330. Jeffcoate WJ, Rees LH, Tomlin S, et al: Metyrapone in long-term management of Cushing's disease. Br Med J 2:215–217, 1977.

331. Connell JM, Cordiner J, Davies DL, et al: Pregnancy complicated by Cushing's syndrome: Potential hazard of metyrapone therapy. Case report. Br J Obstet Gynaecol 92:1192–1195, 1985.

332. Dexter RN, Fishman LM, Ney RL, Liddle GW: Inhibition of adrenal corticosteroid synthesis by aminoglutethimide: Studies of the mechanism of action. J Clin Endocrinol Metab 27:473–480, 1967.

333. Cash R, Brough AJ, Cohen MN, Satoh PS: Aminoglutethimide (Elipten-Ciba) as an inhibitor of adrenal steroidogenesis: Mechanism of action and therapeutic trial. J Clin Endocrinol Metab 27:1239–1248, 1967.

334. Shaw MA, Nicholls PJ, Smith HJ: Aminoglutethimide and ketoconazole: Historical perspectives and future prospects. J Steroid Biochem 31:–146, 1988.

335. Misbin RI, Canary J, Willard D: Aminoglutethimide in the treatment of Cushing's syndrome. J Clin Pharmacol 16:645–651, 1976.

336. Zachmann M, Gitzelmann RP, Zagalak M, Prader A: Effect of aminoglutethimide on urinary cortisol and cortisol metabolites in adolescents with Cushing's syndrome. Clin Endocrinol (Oxf) 7:63–71, 1977.

337. Child DF, Burke CW, Burley DM, et al: Drug controlled of Cushing's syndrome. Combined aminoglutethimide and metyrapone therapy. Acta Endocrinol (Copenh) 82:330–341, 1976.

338. Feldman D: Ketoconazole and other imidazole derivatives as inhibitors of steroidogenesis. Endocr Rev 7:409–420, 1986.

339. Engelhardt D, Weber MM, Miksch T, et al: The influence of ketoconazole on human adrenal steroidogenesis: Incubation studies with tissue slices.

Clin Endocrinol (Oxf) 35:163–168, 1991.

340. Steen RE, Kapelrud H, Haug E, Frey H: In vivo and in vitro inhibition by ketoconazole of ACTH secretion from a human thymic carcinoid tumour. Acta Endocrinol (Copenh) 125:331–334, 1991.

341. Mortimer RH, Cannell GR, Thew CM, Galligan JP: Ketoconazole and plasma and urine steroid levels in Cushing's disease. Clin Exp Pharmacol Physiol 18:563–569, 1991.

342. Sonino N, Boscaro M, Paoletta A, et al: Ketoconazole treatment in Cushing's syndrome: Experience in 34 patients. Clin Endocrinol (Oxf) 35:347–352, 1991.

343. Tabarin A, Navarranne A, Guerin J, et al: Use of ketoconazole in the treatment of Cushing's disease and ectopic ACTH syndrome. Clin Endocrinol (Oxf) 34:63–69, 1991.

344. Ahmed M, Kanaan I, Alarifi A, et al: ACTH-producing pituitary cancer: Experience at the King Faisal Specialist Hospital & Research Centre. Pituitary 3:105–112, 2000.

345. Lewis JH, Zimmerman HJ, Benson GD, Ishak KG: Hepatic injury associated with ketoconazole therapy. Analysis of 33 cases. Gastroenterology 86:503–513, 1984.

346. Duarte PA, Chow CC, Simmons F, Ruskin J: Fatal hepatitis associated with ketoconazole therapy. Arch Intern Med 144:1069–1070, 1984.

347. Knight TE, Shikuma CY, Knight J: Ketoconazole-induced fulminant hepatitis necessitating liver transplantation. J Am Acad Dermatol 25:398–400, 1991.

348. McCance DR, Ritchie CM, Sheridan B, Atkinson AB: Acute hypoadrenalism and hepatotoxicity after treatment with ketoconazole. Lancet 1:573, 1987.

349. Tucker WS Jr, Snell BB, Island DP, Gregg CR: Reversible adrenal insufficiency induced by ketoconazole. JAMA 253:2413–2414, 1985.

350. Miettinen TA: Cholesterol metabolism during ketoconazole treatment in man. J Lipid Res 29:43–51, 1988.

351. Dewis P, Anderson DC, Bu'lock DE, et al: Experience with trilostane in the treatment of Cushing's syndrome. Clin Endocrinol (Oxf) 18:533–540, 1983.

352. Semple CG, Beastall GH, Gray CE, Thomson JA: Trilostane in the management of Cushing's syndrome. Acta Endocrinol (Copenh) 102:107–110, 1983.

353. Ledingham IM, Watt I: Influence of sedation on mortality in critically ill multiple trauma patients. Lancet 1:1270, 1983.

354. Weber MM, Lang J, Abedinpour F, et al: Different inhibitory effect of etomidate and ketoconazole on the human adrenal steroid biosynthesis. Clin Investig 71:933–938, 1993.

355. Lamberts SW, Bons EG, Bruining HA, de Jong FH: Differential effects of the imidazole derivatives etomidate, ketoconazole and miconazole and of

metyrapone on the secretion of cortisol and its precursors by human adrenocortical cells. J Pharmacol Exp Ther 240:259–264, 1987.

356. Schulte HM, Benker G, Reinwein D, et al: Infusion of low dose etomidate: Correction of hypercortisolemia in patients with Cushing's syndrome and dose-response relationship in normal subjects. J Clin Endocrinol Metab 70:1426–1430, 1990.

357. Allolio B, Schulte HM, Kaulen D, et al: Nonhypnotic low-dose etomidate for rapid correction of hypercortisolaemia in Cushing's syndrome. Klin Wochenschr 66:361–364, 1988.

358. Herrmann BL, Mitchell A, Saller B, et al: [Transsphenoidal hypophysectomy of a patient with an ACTH-producing pituitary adenoma and an "empty sella" after pretreatment with etomidate]. Dtsch Med Wochenschr 126:232–234, 2001.

359. Drake WM, Perry LA, Hinds CJ, et al: Emergency and prolonged use of intravenous etomidate to control hypercortisolemia in a patient with Cushing's syndrome and peritonitis. J Clin Endocrinol Metab 83:3542–3544, 1998.

360. Krakoff J, Koch CA, Calis KA, et al: Use of a parenteral propylene glycol-containing etomidate preparation for the long-term management of ectopic Cushing's syndrome. J Clin Endocrinol Metab 86:4104–4108, 2001.

361. Baulieu EE: The steroid hormone antagonist RU486. Mechanism at the cellular level and clinical applications. Endocrinol Metab Clin North Am 20:873–891, 1991.

362. Nieman LK, Chrousos GP, Kellner C, et al: Successful treatment of Cushing's syndrome with the glucocorticoid antagonist RU 486. J Clin Endocrinol Metab 61:536–540, 1985.

363. Healy DL, Chrousos GP, Schulte HM, et al: Increased adrenocorticotropin, cortisol, and arginine vasopressin secretion in primates after the antiglucocorticoid steroid RU 486: Dose response relationships. J Clin Endocrinol Metab 60:1–4, 1985.

364. Bertagna X, Bertagna C, Laudat MH, et al: Pituitary-adrenal response to the antiglucocorticoid action of RU 486 in Cushing's syndrome. J Clin Endocrinol Metab 63:639–643, 1986.

365. Sartor O, Cutler GB Jr: Mifepristone: Treatment of Cushing's syndrome. Clin Obstet Gynecol 39:506–510, 1996.

366. Lacroix A, N'Diaye N, Mircescu H, et al: The diversity of abnormal hormone receptors in adrenal Cushing's syndrome allows novel pharmacological therapies. Braz J Med Biol Res 33:1201–1209, 2000.

367. Paez-Pereda M, Kovalovsky D, Hopfner U, et al: Retinoic acid prevents experimental Cushing syndrome. J Clin Invest 108:1123–1131, 2001.

368. Heaney AP, Fernando M, Yong WH, Melmed S: Functional PPAR-gamma

receptor is a novel therapeutic target for ACTH-secreting pituitary adenomas. Nat Med 8:1281–1287, 2002.

369. Heaney AP, Fernando M, Melmed S: PPAR-gamma receptor ligands: Novel therapy for pituitary adenomas. J Clin Invest 111:1381–1388, 2003.

370. Lamberts SW, van der Lely AJ, de Herder WW: Transsphenoidal selective adenomectomy is the treatment of choice in patients with Cushing's disease. Considerations concerning preoperative medical treatment and the long-term follow-up. J Clin Endocrinol Metab 80:3111–3113, 1995.

371. Boscaro M, Sonino N, Scarda A, et al: Anticoagulant prophylaxis markedly reduces thromboembolic complications in Cushing's syndrome. J Clin Endocrinol Metab 87:3662–3666, 2002.

372. Melby JC: Therapy of Cushing disease: A consensus for pituitary microsurgery. Ann Intern Med 109:445–446, 1988.

373. Welbourn RB: The evolution of transsphenoidal pituitary microsurgery. Surgery 100:1185–1190, 1986.

374. Jho HD, Carrau RL: Endoscopic endonasal transsphenoidal surgery: Experience with 50 patients. J Neurosurg 87:44–51, 1997.

375. Kawamata T, Kamikawa S, Iseki H, Hori T: Flexible endoscope-assisted endonasal transsphenoidal surgery for pituitary tumors. Minim Invasive Neurosurg 45:208–210, 2002.

376. Bochicchio D, Losa M, Buchfelder M: Factors influencing the immediate and late outcome of Cushing's disease treated by transsphenoidal surgery: A retrospective study by the European Cushing's Disease Survey Group. J Clin Endocrinol Metab 80:3114–3120, 1995.

377. Sonino N, Zielezny M, Fava GA, et al: Risk factors and long-term outcome in pituitary-dependent Cushing's disease. J Clin Endocrinol Metab 81:2647–2652, 1996.

378. Blevins LS Jr, Christy JH, Khajavi M, Tindall GT: Outcomes of therapy for Cushing's disease due to adrenocorticotropin-secreting pituitary macroadenomas. J Clin Endocrinol Metab 83:63–67, 1998.

379. Trainer PJ, Lawrie HS, Verhelst J, et al: Transsphenoidal resection in Cushing's disease: Undetectable serum cortisol as the definition of successful treatment. Clin Endocrinol (Oxf) 38:73–78, 1993.

380. McCance DR, Gordon DS, Fannin TF, et al: Assessment of endocrine function after transsphenoidal surgery for Cushing's disease. Clin Endocrinol (Oxf) 38:79–86, 1993.

381. Yap LB, Turner HE, Adams CB, Wass JA: Undetectable postoperative cortisol does not always predict long-term remission in Cushing's disease: A single centre audit. Clin Endocrinol (Oxf) 56:25–31, 2002.

382. Rees DA, Hanna FW, Davies JS, et al: Long-term follow-up results of transsphenoidal surgery for Cushing's disease in a single centre using strict criteria for remission. Clin Endocrinol (Oxf) 56:541–551, 2002.

383. McCance DR, Besser M, Atkinson AB: Assessment of cure after transsphenoidal surgery for Cushing's disease. Clin Endocrinol (Oxf) 44:1–6, 1996.

384. Newell-Price JDC, Norris J, Afshar F, et al: Transsphenoidal hypophysectomy in Cushing's disease—Results and follow-up in 103 patients. Abstract presented at the 16th Joint Meeting of the British Endocrine Societies, Harrogate, UK. J Endocrinol 152(Suppl):72, 1997.

385. Leinung MC, Kane LA, Scheithauer BW, et al: Long term follow-up of transsphenoidal surgery for the treatment of Cushing's disease in childhood. J Clin Endocrinol Metab 80:2475–2479, 1995.

386. Devoe DJ, Miller WL, Conte FA, et al: Long-term outcome in children and adolescents after transsphenoidal surgery for Cushing's disease. J Clin Endocrinol Metab 82:3196–3202, 1997.

387. Chandler WF, Schteingart DE, Lloyd RV, et al: Surgical treatment of Cushing's disease. J Neurosurg 66:204–212, 1987.

388. Hughes NR, Lissett CA, Shalet SM: Growth hormone status following treatment for Cushing's syndrome. Clin Endocrinol (Oxf) 51:61–66, 1999.

389. Rollin GAFS, Ferreira NP, Junges M, et al: Dynamics of serum cortisol levels after transsphenoidal surgery in a cohort of patients with Cushing's disease. J Clin Endocrinol Metab 89:1131–1139, 2004.

390. Avgerinos PC, Chrousos GP, Nieman LK, et al: The corticotropin-releasing hormone test in the postoperative evaluation of patients with Cushing's syndrome. J Clin Endocrinol Metab 65:906–913, 1987.

391. Nieman LK, Gumowski J, DeVroom H, et al: Prediction of long-term remission of Cushing's disease after successful transsphenoidal resection of ACTH-secreting tumor. Paper presented at the 80th Annual Meeting of the Endocrine Society, New Orleans, LA, 1998, P345.

392. Colombo P, Dall'Asta C, Barbetta L, et al: Usefulness of the desmopressin test in the postoperative evaluation of patients with Cushing's disease. Eur J Endocrinol 143:227–234, 2000.

393. Losa M, Mortini P, Dylgjeri S, et al: Desmopressin stimulation test before and after pituitary surgery in patients with Cushing's disease. Clin Endocrinol (Oxf) 55:61–68, 2001.

394. Byyny RL: Withdrawal from glucocorticoid therapy. N Engl J Med 295:30–32, 1976.

395. Leshin M: Acute adrenal insufficiency: Recognition, management, and prevention. Urol Clin North Am 9:229–235, 1982.

396. Olson BR, Rubino D, Gumowski J, Oldfield EH: Isolated hyponatremia after transsphenoidal pituitary surgery. J Clin Endocrinol Metab 80:85–91, 1995.

397. Manning PJ, Evans MC, Reid IR: Normal bone mineral density following cure of Cushing's syndrome. Clin Endocrinol (Oxf) 36:229–234, 1992.

398. Di Somma C, Pivonello R, Loche S, et al: Effect of 2 years of cortisol normalization on the impaired bone mass and turnover in adolescent and adult patients with Cushing's disease: A prospective study. Clin Endocrinol (Oxf) 58:302–308, 2003.

399. Di Somma C, Colao A, Pivonello R, et al: Effectiveness of chronic treatment with alendronate in the osteoporosis of Cushing's disease. Clin Endocrinol (Oxf) 48:655–662, 1998.

400. Ram Z, Nieman LK, Cutler GB Jr, et al: Early repeat surgery for persistent Cushing's disease. J Neurosurg 80:37–45, 1994.

401. Doherty GM, Nieman LK, Cutler GB Jr, et al: Time to recovery of the hypothalamic-pituitary-adrenal axis after curative resection of adrenal tumors in patients with Cushing's syndrome. Surgery 108:1085–1090, 1990.

402. Plumpton FS, Besser GM: The adrenocortical response to surgery and insulin-induced hypoglycemia incorticosteroid-treated and normal subjects. Br J Surg 55:857, 1968.

403. Bangar V, Clayton RN: How reliable is the short synacthen test for the investigation of the hypothalamic-pituitary-adrenal axis? Eur J Endocrinol 139:580–583, 1998.

404. Kehlet H, Lindholm J, Bjerre P: Value of the 30 min ACTH-test in assessing hypothalamic-pituitary-adrenocortical function after pituitary surgery in Cushing's disease. Clin Endocrinol (Oxf) 20:349–353, 1984.

405. Stewart PM, Corrie J, Seckl JR, et al: A rational approach for assessing the hypothalamo-pituitary-adrenal axis. Lancet 1:1208–1210, 1988.

406. Orme SM, Peacey SR, Barth JH, Belchetz PE: Comparison of tests of stress-released cortisol secretion in pituitary disease. Clin Endocrinol (Oxf) 45:135–140, 1996.

407. Ammari F, Issa BG, Millward E, Scanion MF: A comparison between short ACTH and insulin stress tests for assessing hypothalamo-pituitary-adrenal function. Clin Endocrinol (Oxf) 44:473–476, 1996.

408. Friedman RB, Oldfield EH, Nieman LK, et al: Repeat transsphenoidal surgery for Cushing's disease. J Neurosurg 71:520–527, 1989.

409. Valimaki M, Pelkonen R, Porkka L, et al: Long-term results of adrenal surgery in patients with Cushing's syndrome due to adrenocortical

adenoma. Clin Endocrinol (Oxf) 20:229–236, 1984.

410. Bellantone R, Ferrante A, Boscherini M, et al: Role of reoperation in recurrence of adrenal cortical carcinoma: Results from 188 cases collected in the Italian National Registry for Adrenal Cortical Carcinoma. Surgery 122:1212–1218, 1997.

411. Kemink L, Pieters G, Hermus A, et al: Patient's age is a simple predictive factor for the development of Nelson's syndrome after total adrenalectomy for Cushing's disease. J Clin Endocrinol Metab 79:887–889, 1994.

412. Jenkins PJ, Trainer PJ, Plowman PN, et al: The long-term outcome after adrenalectomy and prophylactic pituitary radiotherapy in adrenocorticotropin-dependent Cushing's syndrome. J Clin Endocrinol Metab 80:165–171, 1995.

413. McCallum RW, Connell JM: Laparoscopic adrenalectomy. Clin Endocrinol (Oxf) 55:435–436, 2001.

414. Wells SA, Merke DP, Cutler GB Jr, et al: Therapeutic controversy: The role of laparoscopic surgery in adrenal disease. J Clin Endocrinol Metab 83:3041–3049, 1998.

415. Sheline GE, Wara WM, Smith V: Therapeutic irradiation and brain injury. Int J Radiat Oncol Biol Phys 6:1215–1228, 1980.

416. Orth DN, Liddle GW: Results of treatment in 108 patients with Cushing's syndrome. N Engl J Med 285:243–247, 1971.

417. Howlett TA, Plowman PN, Wass JA, et al: Megavoltage pituitary irradiation in the management of Cushing's disease and Nelson's syndrome: Long-term follow-up. Clin Endocrinol (Oxf) 31:309–323, 1989.

418. Murayama M, Yasuda K, Minamori Y, et al: Long term follow-up of Cushing's disease treated with reserpine and pituitary irradiation. J Clin Endocrinol Metab 75:935–942, 1992.

419. Littley MD, Shalet SM, Beardwell CG, et al: Long-term follow-up of low-dose external pituitary irradiation for Cushing's disease. Clin Endocrinol (Oxf) 33:445–455, 1990.

420. Jennings AS, Liddle GW, Orth DN: Results of treating childhood Cushing's disease with pituitary irradiation. N Engl J Med 297:957–962, 1977.

421. Estrada J, Boronat M, Mielgo M, et al: The long-term outcome of pituitary irradiation after unsuccessful transsphenoidal surgery in Cushing's disease. N Engl J Med 336:172–177, 1997.

422. Storr HL, Plowman PN, Carroll PV, et al: Clinical and endocrine responses to pituitary radiotherapy in pediatric Cushing's disease: An effective second-line treatment. J Clin Endocrinol Metab 88:34–37, 2003.

423. Mahmoud-Ahmed AS, Suh JH: Radiation therapy for Cushing's disease: A review. Pituitary 5:175–180, 2002.

424. Carroll PV, Monson JP, Grossman AB, et al: Successful treatment of childhood-onset Cushing's disease is associated with persistent reduction in growth hormone secretion. Clin Endocrinol (Oxf) 60:169–174, 2004.

425. Lebrethon MC, Grossman AB, Afshar F, et al: Linear growth and final height after treatment for Cushing's disease in childhood. J Clin Endocrinol Metab 85:3262–3265, 2000.

426. Plowman PN: Pituitary adenoma radiotherapy—When, who and how? Clin Endocrinol (Oxf) 51:265–271, 1999.

427. Becker G, Kocher M, Kortmann RD, et al: Radiation therapy in the multimodal treatment approach of pituitary adenoma. Strahlenther Onkol 178:173–186, 2002.

428. Marks LB: Conventional fractionated radiation therapy vs. radiosurgery for selected benign intracranial lesions (arteriovenous malformations, pituitary adenomas, and acoustic neuromas). J Neurooncol 17:223–230, 1993.

429. Zhang N, Pan L, Dai J, et al: Gamma knife radiosurgery as a primary surgical treatment for hypersecreting pituitary adenomas. Stereotact Funct Neurosurg 75:123–128, 2000.

430. Vladyka V, Liscak R, Simonova G, et al: [Radiosurgical treatment of hypophyseal adenomas with the gamma knife: Results in a group of 163 patients during a 5-year period]. Cas Lek Cesk 139:757–766, 2000.

431. Sheehan JM, Vance ML, Sheehan JP, et al: Radiosurgery for Cushing's disease after failed transsphenoidal surgery. J Neurosurg 93:738–742, 2000.

432. Yoon SC, Suh TS, Jang HS, et al: Clinical results of 24 pituitary macroadenomas with linac-based stereotactic radiosurgery. Int J Radiat Oncol Biol Phys 41:849–853, 1998.

433. Mitsumori M, Shrieve DC, Alexander E III, et al: Initial clinical results of LINAC-based stereotactic radiosurgery and stereotactic radiotherapy for pituitary adenomas. Int J Radiat Oncol Biol Phys 42:573–580, 1998.

434. Swords FM, Allan CA, Plowman PN, et al: Stereotactic radiosurgery XVI: A treatment for previously irradiated pituitary adenomas. J Clin Endocrinol Metab 88:5334–5340, 2003.

435. Colin P, Delemer B, Nakib I, et al: [Unsuccessful surgery of Cushing's disease. Role and efficacy of fractionated stereotactic radiotherapy]. Neurochirurgie 48:285–293, 2002.

436. Linfoot JA, Nakagawa JS, Wiedemann E, et al: Heavy particle therapy: Pituitary tumors. Bull Los Angeles Neurol Soc 42:175–189, 1977.

437. Marova EI, Starkova NT, Kirpatovskaia LE, et al: [Results of treatment of Itsenko-Cushing disease using proton irradiation of the hypophysis]. Med Radiol (Mosk) 32:42–49, 1987.

438. Marcou Y, Plowman PN: Stereotactic radiosurgery for pituitary adenomas. Trends Endocrinol Metab 11:132–137, 2000.

439. Wolffenbuttel BH, Kitz K, Beuls EM: Beneficial gamma-knife radiosurgery in a patient with Nelson's syndrome. Clin Neurol Neurosurg 100:60–63, 1998.

440. Sandler LM, Richards NT, Carr DH, et al: Long term follow-up of patients with Cushing's disease treated by interstitial irradiation. J Clin Endocrinol Metab 65:441–447, 1987.

441. Molinatti GM, Limone P, Porta M: Treatment of Cushing's disease by interstitial pituitary irradiation: Short- and long-term follow-up. Panminerva Med 37:1–7, 1995.

442. Magee BJ, Gattamaneni HR, Pearson D: Adrenal cortical carcinoma: Survival after radiotherapy. Clin Radiol 38:587–588, 1987.

443. de Castro F, Isa W, Aguera L, et al: [Primary adrenal carcinoma]. Actas Urol Esp 17:30–34, 1993.

444. He J, Zhou J, Lu Z: Radiotherapy of ectopic ACTH syndrome due to thoracic carcinoids. Chin Med J (Engl) 108:338–341, 1995.

445. Andres R, Mayordomo JI, Cajal S, Tres A: Paraneoplastic Cushing's syndrome associated to locally advanced thymic carcinoid tumor. Tumori 88:65–67, 2002.

446. Bevan JS, Gough MH, Gillmer MD, Burke CW: Cushing's syndrome in pregnancy: The timing of definitive treatment. Clin Endocrinol (Oxf) 27:225–233, 1987.

447. Casson IF, Davis JC, Jeffreys RV, et al: Successful management of Cushing's disease during pregnancy by transsphenoidal adenectomy. Clin Endocrinol (Oxf) 27:423–428, 1987.

448. Sonino N: The use of ketoconazole as an inhibitor of steroid production. N Engl J Med 317:812–818, 1987.

449. Welbourn RB, Montgomery DA, Kennedy TL: The natural history of treated Cushing's syndrome. Br J Surg 58:1–16, 1971.

450. Swearingen B, Biller BM, Barker FG, et al: Long-term mortality after transsphenoidal surgery for Cushing disease. Ann Intern Med 130:821–824, 1999.

451. Wick MR, Rosai J: Neuroendocrine neoplasms of the thymus. Pathol Res Pract 183:188–199, 1988.

452. Jex RK, van Heerden JA, Carpenter PC, Grant CS: Ectopic ACTH syndrome. Diagnostic and therapeutic aspects. Am J Surg 149:276–282, 1985.

453. Torpy DJ, Mullen N, Ilias I, Nieman LK: Association of hypertension and hypokalemia with Cushing's syndrome caused by ectopic ACTH secretion: A series of 58 cases. Ann N Y Acad Sci 970:134–144, 2002.

454. Morris DG, Grossman AB: Cushing's syndrome—The diagnosis and differential diagnosis. In Gaillard RC

(ed): The ACTH Axis: Pathogenesis, Diagnosis and Treatment. Kluwer, 2003, p 229–257.

455. Aron DC, Tyrrell JB, Fitzgerald PA, et al: Cushing's syndrome: problems in diagnosis. Medicine (Baltimore) 60:25–35, 1981.

456. iebl R: Factors interfering with the dexamethasone suppression test. Klin Wochenschr 64:535–539, 1986.

457. Kapcala LP, Hamilton SM, Meikle AW: Cushing's disease with 'normal suppression' due to decreased dexamethasone clearance. Arch Intern Med 144:636–637, 1984.

Gonadotroph and Other Clinically Nonfunctioning Pituitary Adenomas

Peter J. Snyder

INTRODUCTION

Gonadotroph adenomas are pituitary adenomas that arise from gonadotroph cells of the pituitary gland. They are among the most common pituitary adenomas, comprising 40% to 50% of all macroadenomas and approximately 80% of clinically nonfunctioning adenomas. They are often not recognized as of gonadotroph cell origin, probably for two reasons. First, they secrete inefficiently. Second, what they do secrete—intact gonadotropins and their subunits—usually do not produce a recognizable clinical syndrome, that is, they are clinically nonfunctioning. Consequently, these adenomas are usually not recognized until they become so large that they cause neurologic symptoms. Other kinds of pituitary adenomas—corticotroph, somatotroph, lactotroph, and thyrotroph—usually cause clinical syndromes, but uncommonly they may also be clinically nonfunctioning.

HISTORY

Pituitary macroadenomas that are not associated with syndromes of hormonal excess have long been recognized. By the late nineteenth and early twentieth centuries, surgeons were attempting to excise macroadenomas that were causing visual impairment.[1] Also in the early twentieth century, Cushing described numerous patients whose pituitary macroadenomas were associated with hypopituitarism as well as bitemporal hemianopsia.[2] Because pituitary adenomas not associated with syndromes of hormone excess showed no staining with hematoxylin or eosin, in contrast to basophilic staining of adenomas associated with Cushing's syndrome and acidophilic staining of adenomas associated with acromegaly, they were called "chromophobe" adenomas. The first reports of pituitary adenomas associated with supranormal serum concentrations of intact gonadotropins appeared in the mid-1970s,[3,4] and the first report of adenomas associated with gonadotropin subunits within the next few years.[5,6] Only later was it appreciated that the majority of clinically nonfunctioning adenomas associated with nonelevated serum concentrations of intact gonadotropins and their subunits were also of gonadotroph origin. The origin of these adenomas, however, could be recognized only in vitro (e.g., by secretion by dispersed cells in culture[7]), by immunocytochemical staining,[8] or by expression of gonadotropin subunit mRNAs.[9] The term *gonadotroph cell adenomas*, later shortened to *gonadotroph adenomas*, was first used to refer to the full spectrum of these adenomas in 1985.[10]

PATHOGENESIS

ETIOLOGY

Gonadotroph adenomas appear to be true neoplasms, arising from a somatic mutation of a single progenitor cell that divides repetitively. The evidence for this view comes from studies that show that virtually all pituitary adenomas, including gonadotroph adenomas, are monoclonal; that is, they arise from a somatic mutation of a single cell. In one study of five women whose pituitary macroadenomas expressed some combination of follicle-stimulating hormone-β (FSH-β), luteinizing hormone-β (LH-β), and α subunit and whose peripheral leukocytes were heterozygous for hypoxanthine phosphoribosyltransferase (HPRT), the adenomas had predominantly one allele or the other, but not both (Fig. 25-1).[11] This study suggests that gonadotroph adenomas arise from a somatic mutation of a single progenitor cell that then proliferates, but what mutation and what causes the transformation remain unknown.

Specific mutations are known that are associated with the development of about 40% of somatotroph adenomas,[12] and the MEN-I mutation results in pituitary adenomas associated in patients with multiple endocrine neoplasia type I,[13] but the mutations that cause other pituitary adenomas, including gonadotroph adenomas, are not known. Investigators have searched for many other mutations that might be causally related to the development of other pituitary adenomas, but none of these has been clearly associated with the pathogenesis of any pituitary adenomas. Two genes have recently been identified that might be related to the pathogenesis of pituitary adenomas. One is the pituitary tumor transforming gene (PTTG), which was cloned from GH4 cells, a rat pituitary tumor cell line.[14] It is overexpressed in the majority of human pituitary adenomas of all cell types compared with nonadenomatous pituitary tissue.[15] The other is a truncated form of the fibroblast growth factor receptor-4, which has been identified in all types of human pituitary adenomas. Transgenic

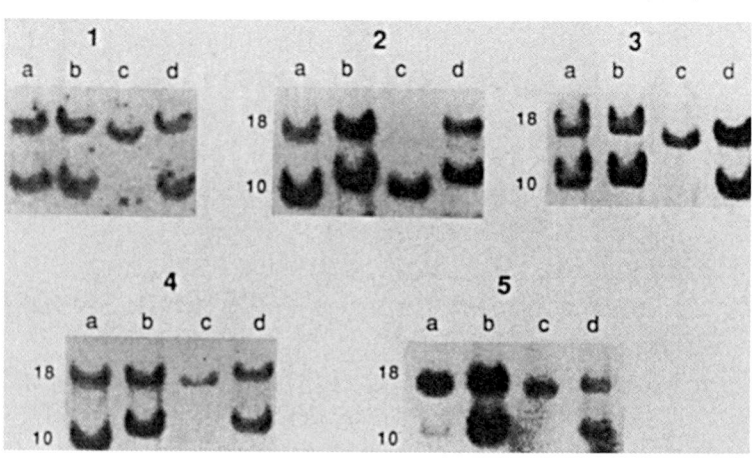

Figure 25-1 Demonstration of the apparent monoclonality of five pituitary adenomas. The bands represent DNA fragments of the hypoxanthine phosphoribosyltransferase gene from the peripheral leukocytes *(lanes a and b)* and pituitary adenoma cells *(lanes c and d)* of five women. The leukocytes of each patient show both alleles *(lane a)*, but the adenoma cells show only one allele *(lane c)*, supporting the hypothesis that these adenomas arose from clonal expansion of a single cell. (From Alexander JM, Biller BMK, Bikkal H, et al: Clinically nonfunctioning pituitary tumors are monoclonal in origin. J Clin Invest 86:336–340, 1990.)

mice that have been constructed to express this mutation in their lactotroph cells have developed lactotroph adenomas.[16]

External hormonal stimulation from the hypothalamus now seems unlikely to be a primary cause of gonadotroph adenomas, but it might have a secondary effect on adenoma growth and probably has an effect on adenoma secretion, since administration of the gonadotropin-releasing hormone (GnRH) antagonist Nal-Glu GnRH to patients who have gonadotroph adenomas and supranormal serum FSH concentrations lowers the FSH to normal.[17]

PATHOPHYSIOLOGY

Secretion by gonadotroph adenomas can be characterized as inefficient, incomplete, and inconsistent. Secretion is inefficient compared to other pituitary adenomas; whereas a lactotroph adenoma 2 cm in diameter usually produces a serum prolactin concentration 100 to 1000 times normal, a gonadotroph adenoma of that size produces a serum FSH concentration no more than 10 times normal and sometimes not supranormal at all.[10] Secretion is incomplete in that secretion of both intact FSH and LH is unusual; instead, secretion is usually of some combination of intact FSH and α, FSH-β, and LH-β subunit.[10–20] Secretion is inconsistent among adenomas in the relative amounts of intact FSH and LH and their subunits each secretes. These characteristics can be recognized

both in vivo and in vitro, and both basally and in response to stimulation.

Basal Secretion

Gonadotroph adenomas more often produce supranormal serum concentrations of intact FSH than of intact LH. In a series of 38 men who had clinically nonfunctioning pituitary adenomas, most of which had in vitro evidence of gonadotroph origin, 10 had supranormal serum FSH concentrations (Fig. 25-2).[20] The degree of FSH elevation may range from minimal to 10 times the upper limit of normal. The intact FSH secreted by gonadotroph adenomas appears to be normal or nearly normal in size,[18] charge,[21] and biologic activity in vitro.[22] Gonadotroph adenomas uncommonly produce supranormal serum concentrations of intact LH, rarely of sufficient degree to cause a supranormal serum testosterone concentration.[3,23,24] About 15% of men who have gonadotroph adenomas have supranormal basal serum concentrations of α, or FSH-β, or LH-β subunits, sometimes in combination with supranormal concentrations of intact FSH or LH.[20]

Stimulated Secretion

Administration of thyrotropin-releasing hormone (TRH) to patients who have gonadotroph adenomas often produces an increase in the serum concentrations of intact gonadotropins and their subunits, especially of the LH-β subunit.[19,20] These

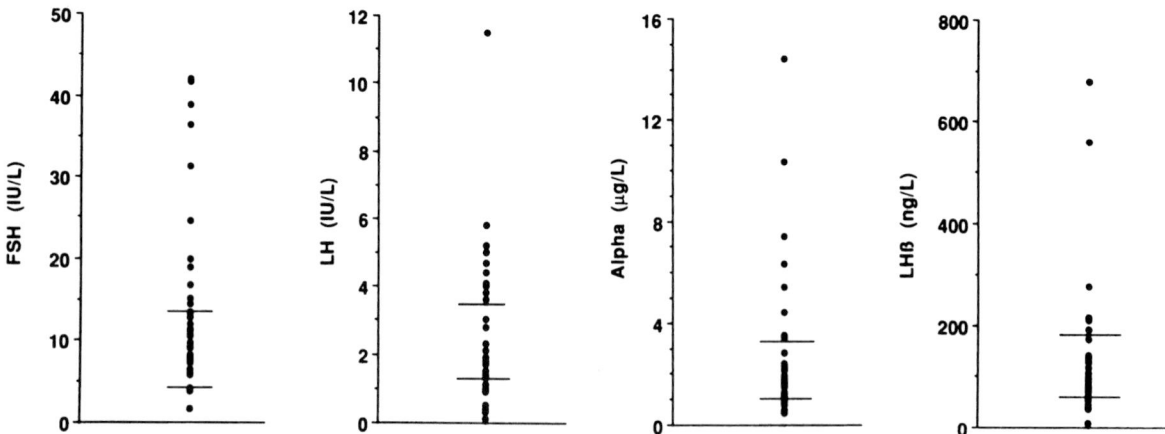

Figure 25-2 Basal serum concentrations of intact follicle-stimulating hormone (FSH) and luteinizing hormone (LH) and α and LH-β subunits in 38 men with pituitary macroadenomas that were considered "clinically nonfunctioning." Eleven had elevations of FSH, 10 of LH, 8 of α subunit, and 6 of LH-β subunit. Of the 38 adenomas, 36 were studied in cell culture and 29 could be identified as gonadotroph adenomas by their secretion in culture. (From Daneshdoost L, Gennarelli TA, Bashey HM, et al: Identification of gonadotroph adenomas in men with clinically nonfunctioning adenomas by the LH-β subunit response to TRH. J Clin Endocrinol Metab 77:1352–1355.)

responses are interpretable as characteristic of gonadotroph adenomas because healthy men and women show no response of intact gonadotropins and their subunits to TRH, or, in the case of intact LH and LH-β, no more than a 33% increase. In a study of 16 women with pituitary macroadenomas that were clinically nonfunctioning, 11 could be identified as being of gonadotroph origin by their LH-β subunit responses to TRH; 4 had responses of LH and 3 of FSH (Fig. 25-3).[19] Of 38 men who had pituitary macroadenomas that were clinically nonfunctioning, 14 had responses of LH-β, 5 of intact LH, and 4 of intact FSH.[20]

Administration of GnRH to patients who have gonadotroph adenomas results in greatly variable FSH and LH responses, from subnormal to normal,[25] but the responses cannot be interpreted because either normal or adenomatous gonadotroph cells could be the source of the FSH or LH.

Secretion In Vitro

Gonadotroph adenomas that are recognized in vivo by supranormal basal or stimulated serum concentrations of intact gonadotropins and/or subunits usually secrete in culture relatively large amounts of the same intact hormones and subunits they secreted in vivo. Of 11 women whose clinically nonfunctioning adenomas could be recognized as of gonadotroph origin by their LH-β responses to TRH, 9 were established in dispersed cell culture, and all 9 secreted readily detectable amounts of LH-β.[19] In addition, gonadotroph adenomas often secrete relatively large amounts of other gonadotroph cell products in culture.[19] Gonadotroph adenomas in culture respond to both TRH and GnRH by secreting both FSH and LH.[25] They respond to somatostatin[26] and bromocriptine[27] by decreased secretion of gonadotropins and their subunits. Gonadotroph adenomas express the somatostatin receptor, principally subtypes 1 and 5.[28]

CLINICAL FEATURES

Gonadotroph and other clinically nonfunctioning adenomas usually come to clinical attention when they become so large that they cause neurologic symptoms (Table 25-1). The large size is illustrated by a series of 100 patients whose gonadotroph adenomas, documented immunocytochemically, averaged 2.5 ± 0.7 cm in diameter and ranged from 1.1 to 4.5 cm.[29] These adenomas may also be detected as an incidental finding when an imaging procedure of the head is performed for an unrelated reason. Uncommonly, but with increasing frequency, they may come to medical attention because of hormonal hypersecretion. The large size of gonadotroph and other clinically nonfunctioning adenomas commonly causes hormonal hyposecretion from the nonadenomatous pituitary, but these deficiencies usually do not impel the patient to seek medical attention. Gonadotroph adenomas are probably not recognized when they are microadenomas because they are so inefficient at that size they probably do not result in supranormal serum concentrations of intact gonadotropins or their subunits.

Impaired vision is the neurologic symptom that most commonly leads a patient with a gonadotroph or other clinically nonfunctioning adenoma to seek medical attention because suprasellar extension of the adenoma elevates and compresses the optic chiasm. Although a bitemporal visual field defect is considered the most typical abnormality, asymmetric defects are also common. When compression becomes more severe, central visual acuity may also be impaired. The onset of the deficit is usually so gradual that patients often do not seek ophthalmologic consultation for months or even years. Other neurologic symptoms that may cause a patient with a gonadotroph adenoma to seek medical attention are headaches, caused presumably by expansion of the sella; diplopia, caused by oculomotor nerve compression due to lateral extension of the adenoma; cerebrospinal fluid (CSF) rhinorrhea, caused by inferior extension of the adenoma; and the excruciating headache and diplopia, caused by pituitary apoplexy.

Detection of a clinically nonfunctioning adenoma as an incidental finding when an imaging procedure of the head is performed for an unrelated reason, such as a motor vehicle accident or other trauma, is the next most common presentation.

The least common presentation is as a consequence of hormonal hypersecretion by the adenoma, although clinical

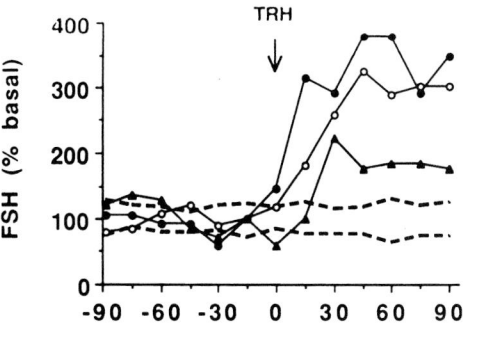

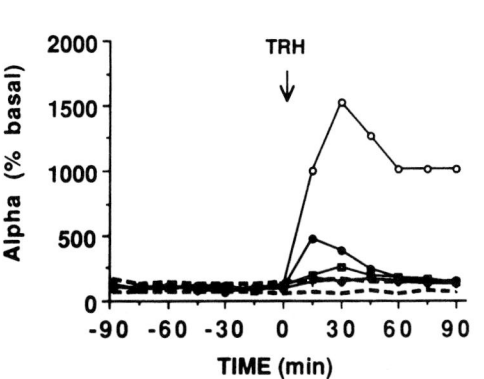

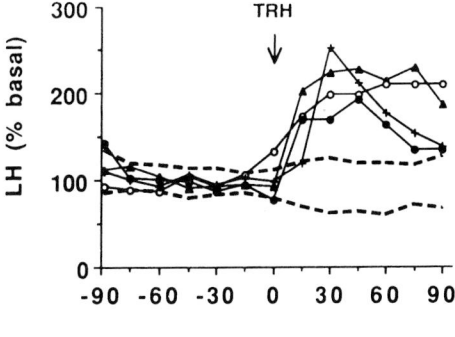

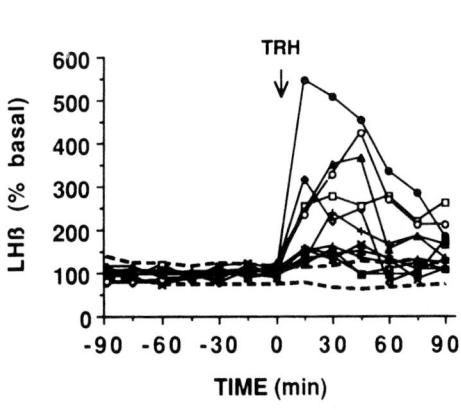

Figure 25-3 Increases in the serum concentrations of intact follicle-stimulating hormone (FSH), luteinizing hormone (LH), α subunit, and, mostly, LH-β subunit to thyrotropin-releasing hormone (TRH) in 16 women with adenomas that had been thought to be "nonsecreting" on the basis of basal hormone concentrations. The dashed lines show the ranges of serum concentrations in 16 age-matched healthy women. Eleven women with "nonsecreting" adenomas exhibited significant responses to TRH of LH-α subunit, four of intact LH and α subunit, and three of FSH. (From Daneshdoost L, Gennarelli TA, Bashey HM, et al: Recognition of gonadotroph adenomas in women. N Engl J Med 324:589–594, 1991.)

Table 25-1 Clinical Presentations of Gonadotroph Adenomas

NEUROLOGIC SYMPTOMS (MOST COMMON)
Visual impairment
Headache
Other (diplopia, seizures, cerebrospinal fluid rhinorrhea)

INCIDENTAL FINDING
(of a sellar mass when an imaging procedure is performed because of an unrelated symptom)

HORMONAL SYMPTOMS
Ovarian hyperstimulation in a premenopausal woman
Premature puberty in a prepubertal boy
Symptoms of hormonal deficiencies

syndromes are being recognized with increasing frequency. The most common of these is ovarian hyperstimulation syndrome caused by constant, and usually excessive, FSH secretion in a premenopausal woman.[30-37] These women usually present with oligo- or amenorrhea, and by pelvic ultrasound have multiple, large ovarian cysts and a thickened endometrial stripe. The serum concentration of estradiol is usually markedly elevated, often more than 500 pg/mL and as high as 2000 pg/mL. Concentrations of intact gonadotropins and their subunits basally and in response to TRH are similar to those in other gonadotroph adenomas, as described previously. Normal ovarian function can be restored if the adenoma is excised.[37] Ovarian hyperstimulation has also been reported in a prepubertal girl.[38] Another clinical syndrome is premature puberty in a prepubertal boy due to an adenoma secreting intact LH.[39,40]

At the time of initial presentation due to a neurologic symptom, many patients with gonadotroph and other clinically nonfunctioning adenomas, when questioned, admit to symptoms of hormonal deficiencies. Ironically, the most common pituitary hormonal deficiency is of LH, the result of compression of the normal gonadotroph cells by the adenoma and lack of secretion of a substantial amount of intact LH by the adenomatous gonadotroph cells. The result in men is a subnormal serum testosterone concentration, which produces decreased energy and libido. The result in premenopausal women is amenorrhea. Deficiencies of thyroid-stimulating hormone (TSH) and adrenocorticotropic hormone (ACTH), which lead to thyroxine and cortisol deficiencies, may also occur.

PATHOLOGY

Most tumors that arise from the gonadotroph cells, like tumors that arise from other pituitary cell types, are adenomas but are rarely carcinomas. Gonadotroph adenomas differ little, if any, from other pituitary macroadenomas in gross pathologic appearance or by light or electron microscopy. Gonadotroph adenomas can be reliably distinguished pathologically from other pituitary adenomas only by detecting the expression of the FSH-β, LH-β, or α subunit genes by immunospecific staining for the subunits in adenoma tissue, by extracting their mRNAs from adenoma tissue, or by secretion of intact gonadotropins or the subunits by cultured adenoma cells. Similarly, clinically nonfunctioning adenomas of other cell types can sometimes be identified only by in vitro techniques.

Gonadotroph adenomas do not differ in their gross pathologic characteristics from other pituitary adenomas of similar size. They may extend outside of the sella turcica in any direction—superiorly to elevate and compress the optic chiasm, laterally into the cavernous sinuses to compress the oculomotor

nerves, and inferiorly into the sphenoid sinus to cause CSF rhinorrhea. Gonadotroph carcinomas are recognized by distant metastases, mostly intracranial.[41-45]

By light microscopy, gonadotroph adenoma cells are not arranged in the normal pituitary glandular pattern but instead are in cords or sheets,[46,47] sometimes interspersed with varying amounts of fibrous tissue. In any one adenoma the cells are usually very similar in size, often monotonously so, but vary considerably among adenomas. The gonadotrophic nature of the adenomas can often be recognized by immunospecific staining for gonadotropin subunits. Not only do adenomas associated with elevated serum gonadotropin concentrations stain for gonadotropin subunits (Fig. 14-7),[46,47] but so do more than 70% of adenomas that are associated with no supranormal serum concentration of any pituitary hormone.[8,48,49] The percentage of cells that stain immunospecifically for gonadotropin subunits, however, is smaller than the percentage of somatotroph or lactotroph adenoma cells that stain for growth hormone of prolactin, and the intensity of staining is also less. Some gonadotroph adenomas, however, cannot be recognized at all by immunospecific staining. Many adenomas that do not stain immunospecifically for any pituitary hormone and are called "null cell" or "oncocytic" (because of densely packed mitochondria) secrete intact gonadotropins and/or their subunits in cell culture.[49]

The electron microscopic appearance is variable. Some adenomatous gonadotroph cells have numerous secretory granules of varying sizes and cytoplasmic organelles, and others have sparse secretory granules and few organelles.[46,50] Yet others have numerous mitochondria ("oncocytes") and few secretory granules.[31]

DIAGNOSIS

The process of making the diagnosis of a gonadotroph adenoma or other clinically nonfunctioning adenoma usually proceeds from recognizing that a patient's visual abnormality or other neurologic symptom could represent an intrasellar lesion, to confirming the presence of a sellar lesion by an imaging procedure, to attempting to characterize the lesion by its hormonal features.

TESTS OF VISION AND IMAGING OF THE PITUITARY

Neuroophthalmologic evaluation should include a computerized test of visual fields and of assessment of visual acuity. The sellar region should be imaged by magnetic resonance (Fig. 25-4), which will show the size, shape, and location of the lesion but will not distinguish a pituitary adenoma from other intrasellar lesions, a pituitary adenoma from the nonadenomatous pituitary, or one kind of pituitary adenoma from another.

HORMONAL TESTS

Intrasellar mass lesions detected by MRI should be evaluated further by measurement of serum concentrations of pituitary hormones to determine if the lesion is of pituitary or nonpituitary origin, and, if pituitary, the cell of origin. A prolactin concentration higher than 100 ng/mL, and especially above 200 ng/mL, suggests a lactotroph adenoma; an elevated IGF-1 concentration suggests a somatotroph adenoma even if the patient does not appear to be acromegalic; an elevated 24-hour urine cortisol suggests a corticotroph adenoma even if the patient does not appear to be cushingoid; and an elevated serum T4 and TSH that is not suppressed suggest a thyrotroph adenoma. Suspicion that the lesion is a gonadotroph adenoma depends on the absence of findings suggestive of another kind of adenoma plus the presence of specific combinations of basal and stimulated concentrations of intact

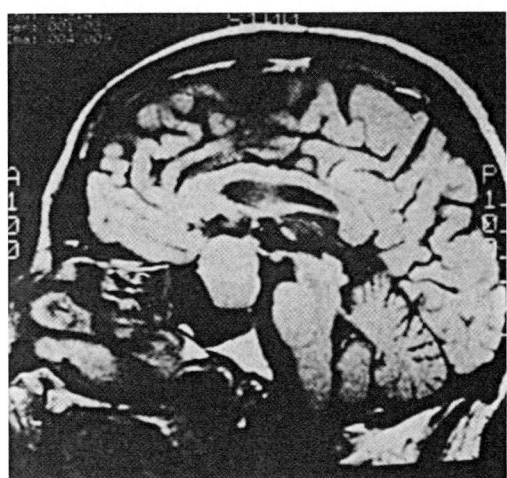

Figure 25-4   Magnetic resonance imaging showing a sagittal view of the head a large gonadotroph adenoma extending superiorly to elevate the optic chiasm. Gonadotroph adenomas are often not recognized until they become this large.

gonadotropins and their subunits (Table 25-2). The combinations differ somewhat in men and women.

In a man who has a pituitary macroadenoma, elevated basal serum concentrations of intact gonadotropins and/or their subunits alone or in combination with responses of any of these to TRH is strong evidence that the adenoma is of gonadotroph origin. An elevated basal FSH concentration is common, as are elevated basal α, FSH-β, and LH-β subunit concentrations. Patients who have elevated basal intact hormone and subunit secretion often exhibit responses of any of them to TRH.

In a woman of postmenopausal age, elevated basal serum concentrations of intact FSH or gonadotropin subunits are usually of little diagnostic value because either the adenoma or the nonadenomatous postmenopausal gonadotroph cells could be the source. In a few situations, however, basal concentrations can point to a gonadotroph adenoma as the source, such as when intact FSH is markedly elevated but LH is not elevated at all, or when one of the gonadotropin subunits is distinctly elevated but intact FSH and LH are not elevated.[19] More commonly, however, in vivo diagnosis usually depends on finding a response to TRH of intact FSH or LH

or, most commonly, of LH-β subunit. In a woman of premenopausal age, ovarian hyperstimulation, including elevated serum estradiol concentration, as discussed previously, elevated FSH out of proportion to LH, or elevated basal α subunit concentration basally all point to the gonadotroph nature of the sellar mass. The response to TRH, as in other circumstances, is most often useful.

DIFFERENTIAL DIAGNOSIS

Gonadotroph adenomas need to be distinguished from other kinds of clinically nonfunctioning pituitary adenomas, nonpituitary lesions arising within and around the sella, and long-standing primary hypogonadism. Although adenomas arising from other pituitary cells usually are recognized readily by the clinical syndromes they produce and by their secretory products, some somatotroph,[51,52] corticotroph,[53] and even lactotroph adenomas are clinically silent. Some of them do not produce the usual clinical syndrome but can be recognized by the usual hormonal abnormalities, such as elevated serum concentration of IGF-1 in the case of a somatotroph adenoma or an elevated 24-hour urine cortisol in the case of a corticotroph adenoma. Others appear to be nonsecreting in vivo and are recognized only when studied in vitro, such as by immunospecific staining. Magnetic resonance characteristics sometimes suggest that a lesion is more or less likely to be a pituitary adenoma rather than a nonpituitary lesion, but there is no characteristic that is pathognomic of a pituitary adenoma or any parasellar lesion. Long-standing primary hypogonadism can lead to gonadotroph cell hypertrophy and thus to pituitary enlargement, and in this way is similar to gonadotroph adenomas, as well as in elevated serum gonadotropin concentrations. The pituitary enlargement seen with primary hypogonadism, however, is not nearly so great as that with gonadotroph adenomas at the time of presentation. In primary hypogonadism, LH as well as FSH is elevated, and neither intact gonadotropins nor their subunits respond to TRH.[54]

CLINICAL UTILITY OF DIAGNOSIS

Making the diagnosis of a gonadotroph or other clinically nonfunctioning adenoma in vivo is valuable in distinguishing a lesion as of pituitary rather than nonpituitary origin and in providing a marker by which to monitor the response to treatment. Distinguishing an intrasellar lesion as of pituitary rather than nonpituitary origin is valuable because it can influence treatment. If surgery is needed, for example, a pituitary lesion, no matter how large, is almost always approached transsphenoidally because it is infradural, but a meningioma should be approached transcranially if it arises above the dura. Finding tumor markers characteristic of a gonadotroph adenoma, such as elevated basal FSH or α or LH-β subunit concentrations, or characteristic of a somatotroph adenoma, such as an elevated IGF-1, not only identifies the lesion as of gonadotroph or somatotroph origin, but it also provides a means by which to follow the response to treatment. When the basal serum FSH concentration is elevated prior to surgery, for example, the decrease after surgery correlates with reduction in adenoma mass seen by imaging.[55]

Table 25-2	Hormonal Criteria for the Diagnosis of Gonadotroph Adenomas*	
Men	**Women**
SUPRANORMAL BASAL SERUM CONCENTRATIONS OF	
FSH[†]	FSH but not LH
α, LH-β, or FSH-β subunits	Any subunit relative to intact FSH and LH
LH and testosterone	FSH and estradiol
SUPRANORMAL RESPONSE TO TRH OF	
FSH	FSH
LH	LH
LH-β (most common)	LH-β (most common)

*Assuming the patient has a pituitary macroadenoma. Approximately 50% to 75% of patients with gonadotroph adenomas have one or more of these abnormalities.

†Assuming the patient does not have a history of primary hypogonadism. FSH, follicle-stimulating hormone; LH, luteinizing hormone; TRH, thyrotropin-releasing hormone.

TREATMENT

Because gonadotroph and other clinically nonfunctioning adenomas are usually not detected until they become so large that they cause significant visual impairment, treatment usually must be directed at reducing adenoma mass and restoring vision as soon as possible. Surgery, usually transsphenoidal, is the only treatment that meets this criterion (Table 25-3). Pituitary adenomas are usually sensitive to radiation, which

Table 25-3 Comparison of Treatments for Gonadotroph Adenomas

Treatment	Indications	Complications
Transsphenoidal surgery	Intrasellar mass with suprasellar extension and severe visual impairment	Worsening of vision, oculomotor palsy, hematoma, cerebrospinal fluid rhinorrhea, meningitis, seizures, diabetes insipidus, hypopituitarism
Transcranial surgery	Large, residual symptomatic extrasellar tissue following transsphenoidal surgery	Same as above, but more likely
Supervoltage radiation	Primary treatment: intrasellar mass with only mild suprasellar extension. Adjuvant treatment: substantial residual adenoma tissue after surgery	Transient: fatigue, nausea, hair loss, loss of taste and smell. Permanent: hypopituitarism
Observation	Adenoma confined to sella; patient elderly or infirm	Visual impairment
Medications (dopamine agonists, somatostatin analogues, gonadotropin-releasing hormone antagonists	Experimental protocol; generally ineffective	

may be used to prevent regrowth if substantial adenoma tissue remains after surgery or to treat primarily if an adenoma is detected before it becomes so large as to cause neurologic symptoms. Several pharmacologic treatments have been tried, but none of them so far reduce adenoma size reliably.

SURGERY

Surgical Approaches
Transsphenoidal surgery is usually the preferred treatment for gonadotroph and other clinically nonfunctioning adenomas that impair vision significantly or cause severe headaches, diplopia, or other neurologic abnormalities or that elevate the optic chiasm without causing visual impairment. The transsphenoidal approach using an operating microscope is usually preferred over the transcranial as the initial procedure, no matter how great the suprasellar extension, because pituitary adenomas are infradural and the risk of serious side effects is lower. During the past decade some surgeons have employed an endoscopic approach to sellar masses.[56–58] No direct comparison has been made of the efficacy and risks of the two procedures. Other surgeons have used the more conventional operating microscope to remove as much adenoma tissue as possible and then used an endoscope, with its angled lenses, to determine if any adenoma tissue remains. Transcranial surgery may be performed when suprasellar adenoma tissue that remains after transsphenoidal surgery continues to cause clinically significant neurologic impairment. Neurologic side effects are somewhat more likely by this approach than by the transsphenoidal.

Efficacy
Seventy percent to 80% of patients who have abnormal visual fields due to a gonadotroph adenoma in one series experienced improvement following transsphenoidal surgery. This improvement is similar to that of macroadenomas generally. In one series of 230 patients whose visual fields were abnormal before transsphenoidal surgery, the fields improved in 73%, remained the same in 23%, and worsened in 4%.[59] In another series of 113 patients with pituitary adenomas that extended beyond the sella, 81% of those with visual field defects before surgery experienced improvement in fields after surgery, 19% remained the same, and none worsened.[60] The improvement in vision is paralleled by a decrease in hormonal hypersecretion.[55]

Complications
Serious complications of transsphenoidal surgery are uncommon but appear to be greater when the adenoma is very large and the surgeon has performed fewer transsphenoidal procedures. In a survey in which neurosurgeons were asked to

report their experience, complications reported by the 958 respondents included some that were serious, including carotid artery injury (1.1%), central nervous system injury (1.3%), loss of vision (1.8%), ophthalmoplegia (1.4%), hemorrhage or swelling of the residual tumor (2.9%), cerebrospinal fluid leak (3.9%), meningitis (1.5%), and death (0.9%).[61] The chances of anterior pituitary insufficiencies (19.4%) and diabetes insipidus (17.8%) were higher. The incidence of each complication was higher among neurosurgeons who were less experienced. Among neurosurgeons who reported performing fewer than 200 transsphenoidal procedures, 1.2% of procedures resulted in death; but among neurosurgeons who reported performing more than 500 procedures, only 0.2% resulted in death. Although these results are based on retrospective self-reporting via questionnaire, they provide a broader assessment of complications of transsphenoidal surgery than that provided by individual pituitary surgeons,[60,62] whose complication rates are closer to those of the most experienced group above.[61]

Complication rates are also greater in patients who have had prior pituitary surgery than in those who never had and even greater in those whose prior surgery was via craniotomy than in those whose prior surgery was transsphenoidal.[63]

Evaluation of the Results
The results of surgery should initially be evaluated 4 to 6 weeks afterwards by measurement of whatever hormones or subunits that had been elevated before surgery and by assessment of the functions of the nonadenomatous anterior pituitary and vasopressin secretion. Neuroophthalmologic function should likewise be reevaluated. Residual adenoma tissue should be evaluated by MRI, generally about 6 months after surgery, which allows time for blood and edema from surgery to resolve.

RADIATION

Techniques
Radiation therapy has been used to treat pituitary adenomas for decades. The standard technique during this period has employed a supervoltage source to deliver a total of 45 to 50 Gy in daily 2 Gy doses via three external portals. Other techniques have recently been used that employ various radiation sources delivered stereotactically, to attempt to minimize the amount of radiation to which the brain is exposed. One group of techniques, collectively called stereotactic radiosurgery, involves stereotactic administration of a large single dose of radiation from one of several possible sources, including protons from a cyclotron, high-energy x-rays from a linear accelerator, and gamma radiation from a ^{60}Co source

("gamma knife"). Another technique, called "conformal radiation," involves administration of supervoltage radiation in fractionated doses, as in conventional radiotherapy, but from multiple portals and guided by a computer-generated model so that the radiation conforms to boundaries of the lesion.

Efficacy
When conventional radiation is administered following surgery for a pituitary macroadenoma, it is usually effective in preventing regrowth of the adenoma.[64–66] In one study of men who had conventional radiation therapy following surgery for clinically nonfunctioning pituitary macroadenomas, only 7% of the 63 patients developed new visual impairment requiring additional treatment during the subsequent 15 years, but 66% of the 63 who did not receive radiation developed new visual impairment.[66] The efficacy of stereotactic methods of radiation delivery in preventing recurrence of pituitary adenomas and other sellar tumors remains to be determined.

Complications and Side Effects
There are both short-term and long-term side effects of conventional radiation. The short-term side effects include nausea, lethargy, loss of taste and smell, and loss of hair at the radiation portals. The first two remit within 2 months and the latter two usually remit within 6 months but may be permanent. The long-term side effects include hypopituitarism and neurologic complications. Hypopituitarism may begin as soon as 1 month after completion of radiation but usually not until a year or more. By 10 years afterwards, about 50% of patients have a deficiency of ACTH, TSH, or LH.[67–69]

Neurologic side effects are less common. Blindness due to optic neuritis,[70] brain tumors, and cerebrovascular accidents attributed to accelerated local atherosclerosis have been reported as case reports in some series,[71,72] but other series that have evaluated possible neurologic sequellae have found none.[73] Because the various stereotactic techniques for administering radiation to the sella area are designed to expose the structures surrounding the sella and the brain to less radiation than does the conventional technique, it is possible that these techniques reduce the risk of neurologic sequellae, but it is too soon to know if this hope will be realized. The larger amount of radiation given per dose during stereotactic radiosurgery, however, poses a greater risk of optic neuritis than does conventional radiation. In fact, radiation-induced optic neuritis has already been reported following this procedure.[74]

Management of Patients after Radiation
Hormonal evaluation, both for excessive secretion of whichever intact gonadotropins and their subunits were secreted excessively by the adenoma prior to treatment and for deficient secretion by the nonadenomatous pituitary, should be performed 6 and 12 months after radiation and once a year thereafter. Evaluation of size by MRI should be performed 1 year after radiation and, if the mass is smaller, less frequently thereafter. Neuroophthalmologic evaluation should be repeated after radiation if it was abnormal before.

PHARMACOLOGIC TREATMENT
Several drugs have been administered in attempts to treat gonadotroph adenomas, but so far none has been found that reduces their size consistently and substantially. Although dopamine does not decrease gonadotropin secretion to an appreciable degree in normal subjects, bromocriptine has been reported to reduce the secretion of intact gonadotropins and α subunit in a few patients and even to improve vision in one, but not to reduce adenoma size.[75] CV 205-504 has been reported to reduce secretion and adenoma size in occasional patients.[76] Cabergoline has been reported to reduce α subunit concentration in a single patient with a gonadotroph adenoma[77] and to decrease adenoma volume by 10% to 18% in 7 of 13 other patients with gonadotroph adenomas.[78]

The somatostatin analogue octreotide has been used to treat gonadotroph adenomas because gonadotroph adenomas express somatostatin receptors and because of the demonstration that somatostatin itself may decrease secretion by gonadotroph adenomas in vitro. Although there have been occasional reports of dramatic decreases in size of gonadotroph adenomas associated with octreotide administration[79,80] and some improvement in vision, the majority of patients have little if any reduction of adenoma or improvement of vision.[79–81]

Several agonist analogues of GnRH have been administered to patients with gonadotroph adenomas, based on the rationale that chronic administration of these agonists causes downregulation of GnRH receptors on, and decreased secretion of FSH and LH from, normal gonadotroph cells. Administration of GnRH agonist analogues to patients with gonadotroph adenomas, however, generally produces either an agonist effect or no effect on secretion and no effect on adenoma size.[82,83] Administration for 1 week of the GnRH antagonist, Nal-Glu GnRH, to men with gonadotroph adenomas reduced their elevated FSH concentrations to normal.[17] However, when Nal-Glu administration was continued for 6 months, although FSH remained suppressed, adenoma size did not decrease.[84]

The demonstration that many pituitary adenomas, including gonadotroph and other nonfunctioning adenomas, overexpress the nuclear hormone receptor PPAR-γ[85] suggests that administration of ligands for this receptor, such as thiazolidinediones, might be used to treat these adenomas.

REFERENCES

1. Fahlbusch R, Buchfelder M, Nomikos P: Pituitary Surgery. Malden, MA, Blackwell, 2002.
2. Cushing H: The Pituitary Body and Its Disorders. Philadelphia, Lippincott, 1912.
3. Snyder PJ, Sterling FH: Hypersecretion of LH and FSH by a pituitary adenoma. J Clin Endocrinol Metab 42:544–550, 1976.
4. Cunningham GR, Huckins C: An FSH and prolactin-secreting pituitary tumor: Pituitary dynamics and testicular histology. J Clin Endocrinol Metab 44:248–253, 1977.
5. Ridgway EC, Klibanski A, Ladenson PW, et al: Pure alpha-secreting pituitary adenomas. N Engl J Med 304:1254–1259, 1981.
6. Snyder PJ, Johnson J, Muzyka R: Abnormal secretion of glycoprotein α-subunit and follicle-stimulating hormone (FSH) β-subunit in men with pituitary adenomas and FSH hypersecretion. J Clin Endocrinol Metab 51:579–584, 1980.
7. Snyder PJ, Bashey H, Phillips JL, et al: Comparison of hormonal behavior of gonadotroph cells adenomas in vivo and in culture. J Clin Endocrinol Metab 61:1061–1065, 1985.
8. Black PM, Hsu DW, Klibanski A, et al: Hormone production in clinically nonfunctioning pituitary adenoma. J Neurosurg 66:244–250, 1987.
9. Jameson JL, Klibanski A, Black PM, et al: Glycoprotein hormone genes are expressed in clinically nonfunctioning pituitary adenomas. J Clin Invest 80:1472–1478, 1987.
10. Snyder PJ: Gonadotroph cell adenomas of the pituitary. Endocr Rev 6:552–563, 1985.
11. Alexander JM, Biller BMK, Bikkal H, et al: Clinically nonfunctioning pituitary tumors are monoclonal in origin. J Clin Invest 86:336–340, 1990.
12. Spada A, Arosio M, Bochicchio D, et al: Clinical, biochemical, and morphological correlates in patients bearing growth hormone-secreting pituitary tumors with or without constitutively active adenylyl cyclase. J Clin Endocrinol Metab 71:1421–1426, 1990.

13. Chandrasekhapappa SC, Guru SC, Manickam P, et al: Positional cloning of the gene for multiple endocrine neoplasia-type 1. Science 276:404–407, 1997.

14. Pei L, Melmed S: Isolation and characterization of a pituitary tumor-transforming gene (PTTG). Mol Endocrinol 11:433–441, 1997.

15. Zhang X, Horwitz GA, Heaney AP, et al: Pituitary tumor transforming gene (PTTG) expression in pituitary adenomas. J Clin Endocrinol Metab 84:761–767, 1999.

16. Ezzat S, Zheng L, Zhu XF, et al: Targeted expression of a human pituitary tumor-derived isoform of FGF receptor-4 recapitulates pituitary tumorigenesis. J Clin Invest 109:69–78, 2002.

17. Daneshdoost L, Pavlou S, Molitch ME: Inhibition of follicle-stimulating hormone secretion from gonadotroph adenomas by repetitive administration of a gonadotropin-releasing hormone antagonist. J Clin Endocrinol Metab 71:92–97, 1990.

18. Snyder PJ, Bashey HM, Kim SU, et al: Secretion of uncombined subunits of luteinizing hormone by gonadotroph cell adenomas. J Clin Endocrinol Metab 59:1169–1175, 1984.

19. Daneshdoost L, Gennarelli TA, Bashey HM, et al: Recognition of gonadotroph adenomas in women. N Engl J Med 324:589–594, 1991.

20. Daneshdoost L, Gennarelli TA, Bashey HM, et al: Identification of gonadotroph adenomas in men with clinically nonfunctioning adenomas by the LHa subunit response to TRH. J Clin Endocrinol Metab 77:1352–1355, 1993.

21. Chappel SC, Bashey HM, Snyder PJ: Similar isoelectric profiles of FSH from gonadotroph cell adenomas and non-adenomatous pituitaries. Acta Endocrinol 113:311–316, 1986.

22. Galway AB, Hsueh JW, Daneshdoost L, et al: Gonadotroph adenomas in men produce biologically active follicle-stimulating hormone. J Clin Endocrinol Metab 71:907–912, 1990.

23. Peterson RD, Kourides IA, Horwith M, et al: Luteinizing hormone and α-subunit-secreting pituitary tumor: Positive feedback of estrogen. J Clin Endocrinol Metab 51:692–698, 1981.

24. Klibanski A, Deutsch PJ, Jameson JL, et al: Luteinizing hormone-secreting pituitary tumor: Biosynthetic characterization and clinical studies. J Clin Endocrinol Metab 64:536–542, 1987.

25. Snyder PJ, Bigdeli H, Gardner DF, et al: Gonadal function in fifty men with untreated pituitary adenomas. J Clin Endocrinol Metab 48:309–314, 1979.

26. Klibanski A, Alexander JM, Bikkal HA, et al: Somatostatin regulation of glycoprotein hormone and free subunit secretion in clinically nonfunctioning and somatotroph adenomas in vitro. J Clin Endocrinol Metab 1248:1255, 1991.

27. Lamberts SWJ, Verleun T, Oosterom R: The effects of bromocriptine, thyrotropin-releasing hormone, and gonadotropin-releasing hormone on hormone secretion by gonadotropin-secreting pituitary adenomas in vivo and in vitro. J Clin Endocrinol Metab 64:524–530, 1987.

28. Pawlikowski M, Pisarek H, Kunert-Radek J, et al: Immunohistochemical detection of somatostatin receptor subtypes in "clinically nonfunctioning" pituitary adenomas. Endocr Pathol 14:231–238, 2003.

29. Young WF, Scheithauer BW, Kovacs KT, et al: Gonadotroph adenoma of the pituitary gland: A clinicopathologic analysis of 100 cases. Mayo Clin Proc 71:649–656, 1996.

30. Catargi B, Felicie-Dellan E, Tabarin A: Comment on gonadotroph adenoma causing ovarian hyperstimulation. J Clin Endocrinol Metab 84:3404, 1999.

31. Christin-Maitre S, Rongieres-Bertrand C, Kottler ML, et al: A spontaneous and severe hyperstimulation of the ovaries revealing a gonadotroph adenoma. J Clin Endocrinol Metab 83:3450–3453, 1998.

32. Djerassi A, Coutifaris C, West VA, et al: Gonadotroph adenoma in a premenopausal woman secreting follicle-stimulating hormone and causing ovarian hyperstimulation. J Clin Endocrinol Metab 80:591–594, 1995.

33. Murata Y, Ando H, Nagasaka T, et al: Successful pregnancy after bromocriptine therapy in an anovulatory woman complicated with ovarian hyperstimulation caused by follicle-stimulating hormone-producing plurihormonal pituitary microadenoma. J Clin Endocrinol Metab 88:1988–1993, 2003.

34. Pentz-Vidovic I, Skoric T, Grubisic G, et al: Evolution of clinical symptoms in a young woman with a recurrent gonadotroph adenoma causing ovarian hyperstimulation. Eur J Endocrinol 143:607–614, 2000.

35. Shimon I, Rubinek T, Bar-Hava I, et al: Ovarian hyperstimulation without elevated serum estradiol associated with pure follicle-stimulating hormone-secreting pituitary adenoma. J Clin Endocrinol Metab 86:3635–3640, 2001.

36. Valimaki MJ, Tiitinen A, Alfthan H, et al: Ovarian hyperstimulation caused by gonadotroph adenoma secreting follicle-stimulating hormone in 28-year-old woman. J Clin Endocrinol Metab 84:4204–4208, 1999.

37. Castelbaum AJ, Bigdeli H, Post KD, et al: Exacerbation of ovarian hyperstimulation by leuprolide reveals a gonadotroph adenoma. Fertil Steril 78:1311–1313, 2002.

38. Tashiro H, Katabuchi H, Ohtake H, et al: A follicle-stimulating hormone-secreting gonadotroph adenoma with ovarian enlargement in a 10-year-old girl. Fertil Steril 72:158–160, 1999.

39. Faggiano M, Criscuolo T, Perrone I, et al: Sexual precocity in a boy due to hypersecretion of LH and prolactin by a pituitary adenoma. Acta Endocrinol 102:167–172, 1983.

40. Ambrosi B, Basstti M, Ferrario R, et al: Precocious puberty in a boy with a PRL, LH- and FSH-secreting pituitary tumour: Hormonal and immunocytochemical studies. Acta Endocrinol 122:569–576, 1990.

41. Beauchesne P, Trouillas J, Barral F, et al: Gonadotropic pituitary carcinoma: Case report. Neurosurgery 37:810–815; discussion 815–816, 1995.

42. McCutcheon IE, Pieper DR, Fuller GN, et al: Pituitary carcinoma containing gonadotropins: Treatment by radical excision and cytotoxic chemotherapy: Case report. Neurosurgery 46:1233–1239; discussion 1239–1240, 2000.

43. O'Brien DP, Phillips JP, Rawluk DR, et al: Intracranial metastases from pituitary adenoma. Br J Neurosurg 9:211–218, 1995.

44. Pichard C, Gerber S, Laloi M, et al: Pituitary carcinoma: Report of an exceptional case and review of the literature. J Endocrinol Invest 25:65–72, 2002.

45. Roncaroli F, Nose V, Scheithauer BW, et al: Gonadotropic pituitary carcinoma: HER-2/neu expression and gene amplification. Report of two cases. J Neurosurg 99:402–408, 2003.

46. Trouillas J, Girod C, Sassolas G, et al: The human gonadotropic adenoma pathologic diagnosis and hormonal correlations in 26 tumors. Semin Diagn Pathol 3:42–57, 1986.

47. Horvath E, Kovacs K: Gonadotroph adenomas of the human pituitary sex-related fine-structural dichotomy. Am J Pathol 117:429–440, 1984.

48. Mashiter K, Adams E, Van Noorden S: Secretion of LH, FSH and PRL shown by cell culture and immunocytochemistry of human functionless pituitary adenomas. Clin Endocrinol 15:103–112, 1981.

49. Asa SL, Gerne BM, Singer W, et al: Gonadotropin secretion in vitro by human pituitary null cell adenomas and oncocytomas. J Clin Endocrinol Metab 62:1011–1019, 1986.

50. Kovacs K: Tumors of the pituitary gland. Atlas of Tumor Pathology. Washington, Armed Forces Institute of Pathology, 1986.

51. Klibanski A, Zervas NT, Kovacs K, et al: Clinically silent hypersecretion of growth hormone in patients with pituitary tumors. J Neurosurg 66:806–811, 1987.

52. Yamada S, Sano T, Stefaneanu L, et al: Endocrine and morphological study of a clinically silent somatotroph adenoma of the human pituitary. J Clin Endocrinol Metab 76:352–356, 1993.

53. Asa SL, Ezzat S: The cytogenesis and pathogenesis of pituitary adenomas. Endocr Rev 19:798–827, 1998.

54. Snyder PJ, Muzyka R, Johnson J, et al: Thyrotropin-releasing hormone provokes abnormal follicle-stimulating hormone (FSH) and luteinizing hormone responses in men who have pituitary adenomas and FSH hypersecretion. J Clin Endocrinol Metab 51:744–748, 1980.

55. Harris RI, Schatz NJ, Gennarelli T, et al: Follicle-stimulating hormone-secreting pituitary adenomas: Correlation of reduction of adenoma size with reduction of adenoma size with reduction of hormone hypersecretion after transsphenoidal surgery. J Clin Endocrinol Metab 56:1288–1293, 1983.

56. Cappabianca P, Cavallo LM, Colao A, et al: Endoscopic endonasal transsphenoidal approach: Outcome analysis of 100 consecutive procedures. Minim Invasive Neurosurg 45:193–200, 2002.

57. Jho HD: Endoscopic transsphenoidal surgery. J Neurooncol 54:187–195, 2001.

58. Kawamata T, Iseki H, Ishizaki R, et al: Minimally invasive endoscope-assisted endonasal trans-sphenoidal microsurgery for pituitary tumors: Experience with 215 cases comparing with sublabial trans-sphenoidal approach. Neurol Res 24:259–265, 2002.

59. Trautmann JC, Laws ER: Visual status after transsphenoidal surgery at the Mayo Clinic, 1971–1982. Am J Ophthalmol 96:200–208, 1983.

60. Black PM, Zervas NT, Candia GL: Incidence and management of complications of transsphenoidal operations for pituitary adenomas. Neurosurg 20:920–924, 1987.

61. Ciric I, Ragin A, Baumgartner C, et al: Complications of transsphenoidal surgery: Results of a national survey, review of the literature, and personal experience. Neurosurg 40:225–237, 1997.

62. Wilson CB: A decade of pituitary microsurgery. J Neurosurg 61:814–833, 1984.

63. Laws ER Jr, Fode NC, Redmond MJ: Transsphenoidal surgery following unsuccessful prior therapy. J Neurosurg 63:823–829, 1985.

64. Zaugg M, Adamman O, Pescia R, et al: External irradiation of macroinvasive pituitary adenomas with telecobalt: A retrospective study with long-term follow-up in patients irradiated with doses mostly of between 4045 Gy. Int J Radiat Oncol Biol Phys 32:671–680, 1995.

65. McCord MW, Buatti JM, Fennel EM, et al: Radiotherapy for pituitary adenoma: Long-tem outcome and sequellae. Int J Radiat Oncol 39:437–444, 1997.

66. Gittoes NJL, Bates AS, Tse W, et al: Radiotherapy for non-functioning pituitary adenomas. Clin Endocrinol 48:331–337, 1998.

67. Snyder PJ, Fowble B, Schatz NJ, et al: Hypopituitarism following radiation therapy of pituitary adenomas. Am J Med 81:457–462, 1986.

68. Littley MD, Shalet SM, Beardwell CG, et al: Hypopituitarism following external radiotherapy for pituitary tumours in adults. Q J Med 145:160, 1970.

69. Nelson P, Goodman M, Flickenger J, et al: Endocrine function in patients with large pituitary tumors treated with operative decompression and radiation therapy. Neurosurg 24:398–400, 1989.

70. Millar JL, Spry NA, Lamb DS, et al: Blindness in patients after external beam irradiation for pituitary adenoma: Two cases occurring after small daily fractional doses. Clin Oncol 3:291–294, 1991.

71. Brada M, Ford D, Ashley S, et al: Risk of second brain tumour after conservative surgery and radiotherapy for pituitary adenoma. Br Med J 304:1343–1346, 1993.

72. Fisher BJ, Gaspar LE, Noone B: Radiation therapy of pituitary adenoma: Delayed sequelae. Radiology 187:843–846, 1993.

73. Dowsett RJ, Fowble B, Sergott RC, et al: Results of radiotherapy in the treatment of acromegaly: Lack of ophthalmologic complications. Int J Radiat Oncol Biol Phys 19:453–459, 1990.

74. Girkin CA, Comey CH, Lunsford LD, et al: Radiation optic neuropathy after stereotactic radiosurgery. Ophthalmopathy 104:1634–1643, 1997.

75. Stewart PM, Kane KF, Stewart SE, et al: Depot long-acting somatostatin analog (Sandostatin-LAR) is an effective treatment for acromegaly. J Clin Endocrinol Metab 80:3267–3272, 1995.

76. Connor SE, Penney CC: MRI in the differential diagnosis of a sellar mass. Clin Radiol 58:20–31, 2003.

77. Giusti M, Bocca L, Florio T, et al: Cabergoline modulation of alpha-subunits and FSH secretion in a gonadotroph adenoma. J Endocrinol Invest 23:463–466, 2000.

78. Lohmann T, Trantakis C, Biesold M, et al: Minor tumour shrinkage in nonfunctioning pituitary adenomas by long-term treatment with the dopamine agonist cabergoline. Pituitary 4:173–178, 2001.

79. Warnet A, Harris AG, Renard E, et al: A prospective multicenter trial of octreotide in 24 patients with visual defects caused by nonfunctioning and gonadotropin-secreting pituitary adenomas. French Multicenter Octreotide Study Group. Neurosurgery 41:786–795; discussion 796–787, 1997.

80. Sy RAG, Bernstein R, Chynn KY, et al: Reduction in size of a thyrotropin- and gonadotropin-secreting pituitary adenoma treated with octreotide acetate (somatostatin analog). J Clin Endocrinol Metab 74:690–694, 1992.

81. Katznelson L, Oppenheim DS, Coughlin F, et al: Chronic somatostatin analog administration in patients with alpha subunit-secreting pituitary adenomas. J Clin Endocrinol Metab 75:1318–1325, 1992.

82. Roman SH, Goldstein M, Kourides IA, et al: The luteinizing hormone-releasing hormone (LHRH)agonist d-[TRT6PRO9NEt]LHRH increased rather than lowered LH and alpha subunit levels in a patient with an LH-secreting pituitary tumor. J Clin Endocrinol Metab 58:313–319, 1984.

83. Klibanski A, Jameson JL, Biller BMK, et al: Gonadotropin and alpha subunit responses to chronic gonadotropin-releasing hormone analog administration in patients with glycoprotein hormone-secreting pituitary tumors. J Clin Endocrinol Metab 68:81–86, 1989.

84. McGrath GA, Goncalves RJ, Udupa JK, et al: New technique for quantitation of pituitary adenoma size: Use in evaluating treatment of gonadotroph adenomas with gonadotropin-releasing hormone antagonist. J Clin Endocrinol Metab 76:1363–1368, 1993.

85. Heaney AP, Fernando M, Melmed S: PPAR-gamma receptor ligands: Novel therapy for pituitary adenomas. J Clin Invest 111:1381–1388, 2003.

TSH-Producing Adenomas

Paolo Beck-Peccoz and Luca Persani

INTRODUCTION

Pituitary thyrotropin-producing adenomas (TSH-omas) are rare tumors that cause hyperthyroidism by chronically stimulating an intrinsically normal thyroid gland.[1-4] The first case of hyperthyroidism secondary to TSH-oma (central hyperthyroidism) was reported in 1960 by measuring serum TSH levels with a bioassay.[5] In 1970, Hamilton and coworkers[6] documented the first case of TSH-oma that was indisputably proved by modern radioimmunoassay techniques. Since then, about 300 patients have been reported in the literature. Although early reports describe these tumors as invasive macroadenomas that cause high morbidity and, in general, are difficult to be removed surgically, some cases are now more easily cured owing to earlier diagnosis. In fact, with the advent of ultrasensitive immunometric assays for TSH measurement, which are routinely performed in association with direct measurement of circulating free thyroid hormones (free thyroxine [FT_4] and free triiodothyronine [FT_3]), it is expected that patients with TSH-oma at the stage of microadenoma will be recognized with increasing frequency, thus permitting an improved clinical outcome.

Classically, TSH-omas, together with resistance to thyroid hormone,[7-9] were defined as syndromes of "inappropriate secretion of TSH," based on the common hormonal profile characterized by high levels of FT_4 and FT_3 in the presence of measurable TSH concentrations, a finding that contrasted with that observed in primary hyperthyroidism in which TSH is always undetectable. Nonetheless, the term *central hyperthyroidism* seems to be more pertinent for these disorders. However, clinically and biochemically, euthyroid patients with pituitary adenomas that secrete TSH molecules, possibly with reduced bioactivity, have been described but not clearly documented.[10,11] Moreover, pituitary hyperplasia and, in rare instances, true adenoma[12-14] secondary to long-standing primary hypothyroidism are well-known clinical conditions, recently reviewed by us and others.[4] In the majority of these so-called feedback tumors, resolution of the pituitary lesion and normalization of TSH levels occur after levothyroxine replacement therapy, thus bringing into question the actual functional autonomy of such tumors (see Chapter 105).

The clinical importance of these rare entities is based on the diagnostic and therapeutic challenges they present. Failure to recognize these different diseases may result in dramatic consequences, such as improper thyroid ablation in patients with central hyperthyroidism or unnecessary pituitary surgery in patients with resistance to thyroid hormone. In contrast, early diagnosis and correct treatment of pituitary tumors prevent the occurrence of complications (visual defects by compression of the optic chiasm, hypopituitarism) and should improve the rate of cure.

EPIDEMIOLOGY

TSH-producing adenoma is a rare disorder, accounting for about 0.5% to 1% of all pituitary adenomas in both clinical and surgical or pathologic series.[15-17] The prevalence in the general population is 1 to 2 cases per million. However, it is worth considering that these data were calculated many years ago, when probably only a minority of these tumors was diagnosed. Indeed, the number of reported cases of TSH-omas has tripled since the late 1980s (Fig. 26-1). A recent report confirms this trend in a large surgical series, indicating that the occurrence of TSH-omas increased from fewer than 1% to 2.8% from 1989 to 1991.[18] This increased number of recorded cases results from the introduction of ultrasensitive immunoradiometric assays for TSH as a first-line test for the evaluation of thyroid function. On the basis of the finding of measurable serum TSH levels in the presence of elevated thyroid hormone concentrations, many patients who were previously thought to have Graves' disease can be correctly diagnosed as having a TSH-secreting pituitary adenoma or, alternatively, resistance to thyroid hormone. Moreover, an increased awareness by the endocrinologist and general practitioner regarding the existence of central hyperthyroidism has greatly contributed to the disclosure of a higher number of patients with such a rare disorder.

PATHOLOGY AND ETIOPATHOGENESIS

The thyrotroph is the cell type of origin in TSH-omas. These tumors are nearly always benign; at present, transformation of a TSH-oma into a carcinoma with multiple metastases has been reported in only one patient.[19] The majority of them (72%) secrete TSH alone, although this is often accompanied by unbalanced hypersecretion of the α subunit. About one fourth of TSH-omas are mixed adenomas, characterized by concomitant hypersecretion of other anterior pituitary hormones, mainly growth hormone (GH), prolactin (PRL), or both, which are known to share with TSH the common

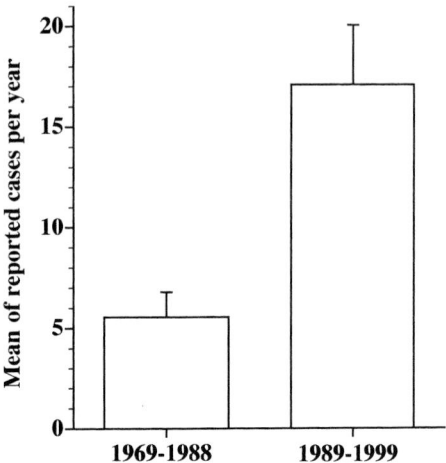

Figure 26-1 The significant increase of reported cases of TSH-producing adenoma in the last decade, when ultrasensitive TSH assay and direct methods for free thyroid hormone measurement became available as first-line tests of thyroid function.

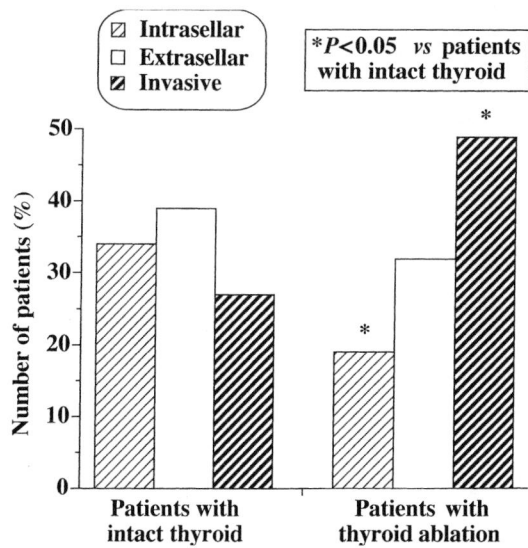

Figure 26-3 Effects of previous thyroid ablation on the size of TSH-producing adenomas. *Intrasellar* refers to both microadenomas and intrasellar macroadenomas, *extrasellar* to macroadenomas with suprasellar extension, and *invasive* to invasive macroadenomas. Data were calculated from 253 reported patients (163 with intact thyroid and 90 with thyroid ablation). Statistical analysis was carried out by Fisher's exact test.

transcription factor Pit-1. Indeed, hypersecretion of TSH and GH is the most frequent association (16%), followed by hypersecretion of TSH and PRL (10.4%) and occasionally TSH and gonadotropins (1.4%) (Fig. 26-2). No association with adrenocorticotropic hormone (ACTH) hypersecretion has been documented to date. Two ectopic TSH-producing adenomas have been documented in the pharyngeal hypophysis.[20,21]

At morphologic and histopathologic analysis, most TSH-omas are macroadenomas (87%), frequently with fibrous consistency, even in the absence of prior surgery or radiotherapy, and high local invasiveness.[22] However, previous thyroid ablation by surgery or radioiodine has deleterious effects on the size and invasiveness of the tumor (Fig. 26-3).[4,23] In fact, invasive macroadenomas were found in 49% of patients who had undergone thyroid ablation versus 27% in those who were untreated, whereas the figure was reversed in patients with microadenomas (diameter <1 cm) or intrasellar macroadenomas. Therefore, previous thyroid ablation may induce an aggressive transformation of the tumor, as is observed in Nelson's syndrome after adrenalectomy for Cushing's disease.

Light microscopy shows that adenoma cells are chromophobic, although they occasionally stain with either basic or acid dyes. Ultrastructurally, adenomatous cells frequently appear monomorphous, even if they hypersecrete TSH, α subunit, and other pituitary tropins.[24-26] Cells with abnormal morphologic features or mitoses,[27] which may be misinterpreted as pituitary malignancy or metastases from distant carcinomas, are present in poorly differentiated adenomas that are characterized by the presence of fusiform cells with sparse and small secretory granules (80 to 200 nm). Indeed, there are no clear criteria of malignancy for TSH-omas except for the presence of metastases. It is worth noting that the only carcinoma that has been reported so far exhibited a progressive malignant transformation accompanied by a decline of TSH and α subunit secretion.[19]

Immunostaining studies show the presence of TSH-β, either free or combined with the α subunit. By using double immunostaining, the existence of mixed TSH-α subunit adenomas composed of one cell type secreting α subunit alone and another cosecreting α subunit and TSH has been documented.[28] In addition to α subunit, TSH frequently colocalizes with other pituitary hormones in the same tumoral cell[29] or even in the same secretory granule.[24,28,30,31] Nonetheless, a positive immunohistochemistry panels for one or more pituitary hormones does not necessarily correlate with hypersecretion in vivo.[32] Indeed, positive immunostaining for ACTH and gonadotropins without evidence of in vivo hypersecretion has been reported.[33-37]

TSH-omas have been shown to be monoclonal in origin,[38] and several studies have screened a substantial number of adenomas for proto-oncogene activation[32,33,39-41] or loss of antioncogenes,[40,42] yielding negative results.[4] A highly variable expression of thyrotropin-releasing hormone (TRH) and dopamine receptors was documented in several adenomas,[43-45] whereas functional somatostatin receptors were constantly detected in TSH-omas,[46-49] thus providing the rationale for their medical treatment with somatostatin analogues.

Recently, somatic mutations[50] and aberrant alternative splicing[51] of thyroid hormone receptor b have been reported, along with dysregulation of iodothyronine deiodinase enzyme expression and function.[52,53] These findings may at

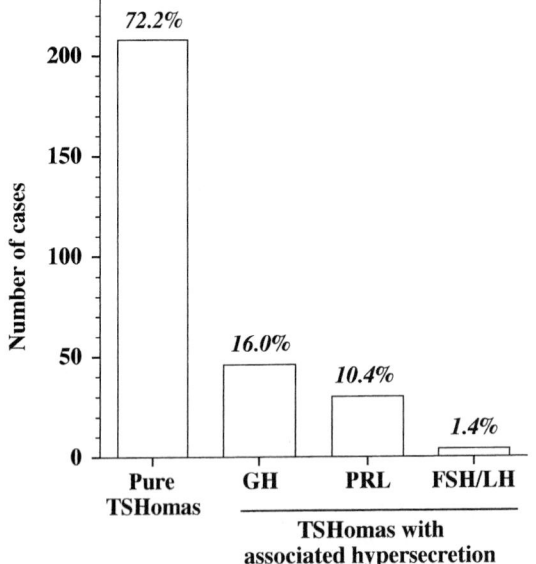

Figure 26-2 Classification of TSH-producing adenomas based on hormone secretion into circulation.

least in part explain the defects in negative regulation of TSH by thyroid hormones in some tumors.

CLINICAL FEATURES

Patients with TSH-oma present with the signs and symptoms of either hyperthyroidism or the mass effect of an expanding intracranial tumor (Table 26-1). TSH-omas may occur at any age (range, 11 to 84 years), although most patients are in the third to sixth decade of life. Unlike the female predominance seen in the other common thyroid disorders, TSH-omas occur with equal frequency in males and females. Goiter and clinical thyrotoxicosis are the most common presenting symptoms. Most patients presented with a long history of thyroid dysfunction, often mistakenly diagnosed as Graves' disease, and one third had inappropriate thyroidectomy, radioiodine thyroid ablation, or both. Thus, patients with TSH-omas may present to the specialist with hyperthyroidism that has been refractory to prior therapeutic attempts. In general, clinical features of hyperthyroidism are sometimes milder than expected on the basis of serum thyroid hormone levels. Moreover, individual patients with untreated TSH-oma were reported to be clinically euthyroid.[10,54–56] This emphasizes the importance of systematic measurement of TSH and FT_4 in all patients with pituitary tumor to disclose those with central hyperthyroidism or hypothyroidism. In some acromegalic patients, signs or symptoms of hyperthyroidism are missed, as they are overshadowed by those of acromegaly.[24,57] Severe thyrotoxic features clinically, such as atrial fibrillation, cardiac failure, and episodes of periodic paralysis,[58–60] are observed in one fourth of cases.

The presence of a goiter is the rule (93%), even in patients who have undergone previous partial thyroidectomy. As the thyroid is intrinsically normal in this disorder, it may regrow even after near total resection as a consequence of TSH hyperstimulation. Occurrence of multinodular goiter has been reported in several patients,[61] and differentiated thyroid carcinoma has been reported in some patients.[62–65] Progression toward functional autonomy seems to be infrequent.[66,67] In contrast to Graves' disease, the occurrence of circulating antithyroid autoantibodies is similar to that found in the general population. Unilateral exophthalmos due to orbital invasion by pituitary tumor was reported in only three patients with TSH-omas, whereas Graves'-associated bilateral ophthalmopathy was reported in five patients.[4]

Most patients bearing a TSH-producing macroadenoma seek medical attention with signs and symptoms of an expanding intracranial tumor. Indeed, as a consequence of tumor suprasellar extension or invasiveness, signs and symptoms of tumor mass prevail over those of thyroid hyperfunction in many patients. Visual field defects are present in about two thirds of patients and headache in one fifth. Moreover, partial hypopituitarism is common, and loss of gonadal function is present in about one third of patients.[22,68] Galactorrhea was recorded in almost all patients with mixed TSH- and PRL-secreting tumors.[69,70]

Finally, TSH-omas may occur in families with multiple endocrine neoplasia type 1[71–73] and in McCune-Albright syndrome.[74]

BIOCHEMICAL FINDINGS

TSH AND THYROID HORMONE LEVELS

High concentrations of thyroid hormones in the presence of detectable TSH levels are typically present in patients with hyperthyroidism due to a TSH-oma or with resistance to thyroid hormone. In the case of replacement therapy for prior thyroidectomy or thyroid ablation, it is crucial to assess patients in steady state, as TSH levels need 4 to 6 weeks to adjust to a change in levothyroxine dose. Thus, the diagnosis of TSH-producing adenoma may be difficult to establish in any patient who has had a dramatic change in thyroid hormone replacement therapy resulting from either physician instruction or poor compliance. Conversely, the finding of elevated TSH levels in patients who have undergone thyroid ablation and have been overtreated with levothyroxine should be regarded as a possible sign of previously undiagnosed TSH-oma.[75]

Various abnormalities in the pituitary-thyroid axis, as well as laboratory artifacts, may cause a biochemical profile similar to that characterizing central hyperthyroidism. These different conditions are more common than are TSH-omas and resistance to thyroid hormone and should be excluded before performing the extensive clinical assessment of the possible presence of central hyperthyroidism. Either familial or drug- or estrogen-induced increases of circulating thyroxine binding globulin (TBG) or variants of albumin or transthyretin lead to increases in the levels of total serum thyroid hormone, particularly T_4, thus producing a biochemical profile that may be confused with TSH-omas. Therefore, the measurement of free thyroid hormones is mandatory in these conditions and should be performed by means of direct "two-step" methods, that is, methods that are able to avoid contact between serum proteins and tracer at the time of assay.[76,77] Indeed, normal levels of total T_4 were recorded in several patients with TSH-oma, and only the measurement of FT_4 allowed the right diagnosis of central hyperthyroidism. Furthermore, inhibition of T_4 to T_3 conversion induced by iodine-containing drugs or nonthyroidal illness may cause hyperthyroxinemia and nonsuppressed TSH that are, however, associated with normal or low-normal T_3. In clinically ambiguous situations, the differential diagnosis rests on the recognition of the underlying disorder as well as documenting normalization of thyroid function test results at a later stage or after recovery of drug withdrawal.

Several laboratory artifacts may cause falsely high serum levels of either TSH or thyroid hormones (Table 26-2). The more common factors that interfere in TSH measurement are heterophilic antibodies directed against mouse gamma globulins[78] or anti-TSH antibodies. However, preventing the formation of the "sandwich," anti-TSH antibodies usually leads to an underestimation of the actual levels of TSH and rarely to an overestimation. The presence of anti-T_4, anti-T_3 autoantibodies, or both may cause FT_4, FT_3, or both to be overestimated, particularly when "one-step" analogue methods are employed.[77] Finally, because patients with a TSH-oma may have T_3 toxicosis as in other forms of hyperthyroidism, there is a need to measure T_3, in particular, free T_3 when T_4 levels are normal.

Table 26-1	**Clinical Characteristics of Patients with TSH-oma**
	Patients with TSH-oma % (n/total)[a]
Age (years)	41.1 ± 14.6 (199)[b]
Sex (female)	55 (152/276)
Previous thyroid ablation	33 (95/290)
Severe thyrotoxicosis	25 (46/184)
Goiter	93 (177/190)
Thyroid nodule(s)	72 (46/64)
Macroadenomas	86 (224/261)
Visual field defect	40 (56/141)
Headache	20 (23/117)
Menstrual disorders[c]	33 (25/75)

Source: Data from reports published up to December 2003.
[a]n/total refers to the number of patients for whom the information was available.
[b]Mean ± SD (n).
[c]Data include women with or without associated PRL hypersecretion.

Table 26-2   **Circulating Factors That May Interfere with the Measurement of TSH or Total and Free Thyroid Hormones Giving Overestimation of the Actual Serum Levels of These Hormones and Thus Simulating the Presence of a TSH-Producing Adenoma**

Heterophilic antibodies directed against mouse γ-globulins leading to interference with monoclonal antibodies used in the immunometric assay[a]
Anti-TSH autoantibodies or antibodies cross-reacting with TSH[b]
Anti-iodothyronine autoantibodies (anti-T4 and/or anti-T3)[c]
Abnormal forms of albumin or transthyretin (e.g., familial dysalbuminemic hyperthyroxinemia)[c]

[a]This interference is commonly prevented by the addition of a few milliliters of mouse serum to the assay buffer.
[b]Overestimation of TSH is very rare in the presence of such antibodies. The interference cannot be prevented, but it can be documented by performing dilution and recovery tests in the immunoassay.
[c]To prevent misdiagnosis, measure free T_4 and free T_3 by direct "two-step" methods (refs. 64, 65).

In TSH-omas, extremely variable levels of serum TSH and thyroid hormones have been reported (Table 26-3). Interestingly, in patients who were previously treated with thyroid ablation, TSH levels are dramatically higher than in untreated patients, although free thyroid hormone levels were still in the hyperthyroid range and the reduction of total thyroid hormone levels was minimal. The conserved sensitivity of tumoral thyrotroph cells to even small reductions of circulating free thyroid hormone levels is confirmed by the rapidly increased rate of TSH secretion during antithyroid drug administration.[57]

Although patients with TSH-oma have a TSH-dependent hyperstimulation of the thyroid gland, any significant correlation between immunoreactive TSH and free thyroid hormone levels is lacking, even though only untreated patients are taken into account. Moreover, in one third of these patients, high levels of free thyroid hormones are associated with immunoreactive TSH levels within the normal range. Variations of the biologic activity of secreted TSH molecules most likely account for these findings.[79] The first demonstration that circulating TSH in patients with TSH-oma may possess an enhanced bioactivity was made in one patient with a mixed GH-TSH-secreting pituitary adenoma in whom a ratio between biologic and immunologic activities of TSH significantly higher than that of controls was documented.[24] Other studies indicate that the circulating TSH biologic/immunologic activity ratio may be normal, reduced, or increased in patients with TSH-oma,[22,79,80] probably because of altered glycosylation of circulating TSH molecules. In fact, both intrapituitary and circulating TSH exist as multiple isoforms characterized by heterogeneity of oligosaccharide chains,

which has a great impact on hormone biologic properties, such as biologic activity and metabolic clearance rate. Tumoral transformation may be accompanied by variable alterations of the posttranslational processing within thyrotrophs, leading to the secretion of TSH molecules with peculiar glycosylation and biologic properties.[79,81,82]

GLYCOPROTEIN HORMONE α SUBUNIT

TSH-omas commonly secrete excessive quantities of the free α subunit, resulting in high levels of circulating free α subunit in two thirds of patients (see Table 26-3). This is another expression of the altered synthetic process within tumoral thyrotrophs and represents a helpful diagnostic clue to the presence of a TSH-oma. Secretion of the α subunit in these tumors is in excess not only of the TSH-β subunit, but also of the intact TSH molecule. This results in a molar ratio of α subunit to TSH, which is generally higher than 1. Although previous studies have suggested that a ratio greater than 1.0 is indicative of the presence of TSH-producing adenoma,[1,83] similar values have been observed in normal controls, particularly in postmenopausal women, indicating the need for appropriate control groups matched for TSH and gonadotropin levels.[4,61,84] Interestingly, microadenomas that frequently have α subunit levels within the normal range may show a high α subunit/TSH molar ratio. Furthermore, it has been suggested that extremely high levels of free α subunit might portend future malignant behavior and that a spontaneous and marked decrease of both TSH and α subunit might indicate that the tumor is becoming less differentiated and correlate with invasive and metastatic behavior.[19]

Table 26-3   **Biochemical Data of Patients with TSH-oma**

Parameter	Patients with Intact Thyroid	Patients with Thyroid Ablation	P
TSH mU/L[a]	9.6 ± 1.1 (120)	57.8 ± 10.2 (81)	<0.0002
α subunit μg/L[a]	17.8 ± 5.8 (68)	14.54 ± 2.7 (46)	NS
α subunit/TSH m.r.[a,b]	43.6 ± 15.4 (68)	3.7 ± 0.7 (46)	<0.03
TT4 nmol/L[a]	243.5 ± 19.9 (30)	177.1 ± 9.8 (45)	<0.002
FT4 pmol/L[a]	44.3 ± 2.6 (68)	28.7 ± 2.5 (30)	<0.0006
TT3 nmol/L[a]	5.0 ± 0.7 (29)	4.1 ± 0.3 (42)	NS
FT3 pmol/L[a]	16.6 ± 0.9 (52)	10.5 ± 0.9 (20)	<0.0005
Normal TSH levels[c]	34% (56/164)	11% (9/79)	<0.0005
High α subunit levels[c]	66% (65/99)	73% (35/48)	NS
High α subunit/TSH m.r.[c]	88% (84/96)	77% (37/48)	NS
High SHBG levels[c]	90% (19/21)	67% (6/9)	NS
Abnormal TSH response to TRH test[c,d]	80% (110/138)	83% (58/70)	NS
Abnormal TSH response to T3 suppression test[c,e]	100% (47/47)	100% (33/33)	NS

Source: Data from reports published up to December 2003.
[a]Mean ± SE (n).
[b]To calculate α subunit/TSH molar ratio divide α subunit (μg/liter) by TSH (mU/liter) and multiply by 10, provided that TSH IRP 80/558 is used in the immunometric assay.
[c]% (n/total).
[d]Net TSH increment <4.0 mU/L.
[e]Lack of complete TSH inhibition after 8 to 10 days of L-T3 administration (80 to 100 μg/day).

PARAMETERS EVALUATING PERIPHERAL THYROID HORMONE ACTION

The measurements of several parameters of peripheral thyroid hormone action both in vivo (basal metabolic rate, cardiac systolic time intervals, Achilles' reflex time) and in vitro (sex hormone–binding globulin [SHBG], cholesterol, angiotensin-converting enzyme, osteocalcin, blood red cell sodium content, carboxyterminal cross-linked telopeptide of type I collagen [ICTP], and so on)[85] may help in quantifying the degree of peripheral hyperthyroidism, particularly in patients with mild clinical signs and symptoms[34,57,61,86–90] (see Table 26-3). In particular, evaluations of SHBG and ICTP may help to differentiate hyperthyroid patients with TSH-oma, in whom these parameters are elevated, from those with resistance to thyroid hormone, in whom they are in the range of those of euthyroid subjects.

DYNAMIC TESTING

Several stimulatory and inhibitory tests have been employed to evaluate TSH secretory dynamics in patients with TSH-oma. None of these tests is of clear-cut diagnostic value, and the combination of some of them may increase their accuracy in disclosing the pituitary adenoma. Among the stimulatory tests, TRH-induced TSH secretion is absent or blunted in 83% of patients (see Table 26-3). Although the α subunit response to the preceding stimulatory agents usually paralleled that of TSH, discrepancy between α subunit and TSH response to TRH has been recorded in some cases. Such a discrepancy may be due to the presence of mixed adenomas, composed of distinct cell types that possess different receptor expression.[24,28] Most TSH-omas are unable to increase TSH secretion after administration of dopamine antagonists such as domperidone or sulpiride. Chronic treatment with antithyroid drugs induces an increase in serum TSH levels in most patients because of both the high sensitivity of adenomatous cells to the reduction of circulating levels of FT_4 and FT_3[57] and the recovered TSH secretion by normal thyrotrophs surrounding the adenoma in response to the activated feedback mechanism.[4,91] In keeping with this are the observations of significantly higher TSH levels in patients who have undergone thyroid ablation, as well as the more active proliferation of tumoral cells in treated patients.

Among inhibitory tests, a complete inhibition of both basal and TRH-stimulated TSH secretion after a T_3 suppression test (Werner test: 80 to 100 µg/day of levothyronine for 8 to 10 days) has never been recorded in a patient with a TSH-oma (see Table 26-3), although a slight TSH reduction may occur in a minority of patients. In patients who have undergone previous thyroid ablation, this test is the most sensitive and specific in documenting the possible presence of a TSH-oma. However, high doses of T_3 are contraindicated in elderly patients or in those with coronary heart disease. Dopamine (1 to 4 µg/kg body weight/min intravenously) or dopamine agonists, such as bromocriptine (2.5 mg orally), are generally ineffective in inhibiting TSH secretion, whereas native somatostatin or its analogues reduce TSH levels in the majority of cases and may be predictive of the efficacy of long-term treatment in the majority of patients.[61,92,93]

IMAGING STUDIES AND LOCALIZATION

In considering the diagnosis of a TSH-oma, full imaging studies, particularly high-resolution computed tomography (CT) or nuclear magnetic resonance imaging (MRI), are necessary. However, since most TSH-omas are macroadenomas, alterations of the sella profile on plain radiographs are present in many cases. Curiously, in two patients, pituitary stones have

been described.[94] Various degrees of suprasellar extension or sphenoidal sinus invasion are present in two thirds of cases.

Microadenomas are now reported with increasing frequency, accounting for about 13% of all recorded cases. In contrast to other secreting pituitary tumors,[95] no correlation between serum TSH levels and tumor size was found in untreated patients with TSH-oma. Pituitary scintigraphy with radiolabeled Tyr^3-substituted octreotide has been shown to successfully image TSH-omas.[96] Moreover, in vivo evidence for both somatostatin and dopamine D_2-receptors was obtained by using single-photon emission tomography with ^{111}In-pentetreotide and ^{123}I-iodobenzamide.[93,97] The presence of these receptors correlates with the sensitivity of the tumor to chronic medical treatment. ^{111}In-pentetreotide scintigraphy may also be useful in localizing possible ectopic TSH-producing adenomas. Finally, bilateral petrosal sinus sampling has been used in difficult cases, allowing the identification and lateralization of a microadenoma not seen on radiographic scans.[98] However, one should expect a certain number of false lateralizations, as has already been observed for ACTH-secreting pituitary tumors.

DIFFERENTIAL DIAGNOSIS

The presence of detectable TSH levels in a hyperthyroid patient rules out primary hyperthyroidism, whereas in patients receiving levothyroxine replacement for primary hypothyroidism, poor compliance is by far the most common cause of apparent inappropriate secretion of TSH, with TSH still too high for the levels of the thyroid hormones. This underscores the importance of studying patients in steady state. The first step in the case of hyperthyroxinemia and detectable TSH is to measure free thyroid hormone levels and repeat TSH measurement by ultrasensitive assays. The finding of normal TSH, FT_4, and FT_3 levels suggests euthyroid hyperthyroxinemia, whereas high FT_4 and FT_3 concentrations and suppressed TSH definitively indicate the presence of primary hyperthyroidism due to Graves' disease and other forms of thyrotoxicosis. If FT_4 and FT_3 concentrations are elevated in the presence of measurable TSH levels, it is important to exclude methodologic interference. When the existence of central hyperthyroidism is eventually confirmed, several diagnostic steps have to be carried out to differentiate a TSH-oma from resistance to thyroid hormone. This is particularly true for the variant of resistance to thyroid hormone with predominant pituitary resistance where there are clear clinical signs of hyperthyroidism.[7–9] Indeed, alterations of pituitary content on CT or MRI, as well as the possible presence of neurologic signs and symptoms (visual defects, headache) or clinical features of concomitant hypersecretion of other pituitary hormones (acromegaly, galactorrhea, amenorrhea) definitely point to the presence of a TSH-oma. Nevertheless, the differential diagnosis may be difficult when the pituitary adenoma is undetectable by CT or MRI or in the case of confusing (empty sella) or incidental pituitary lesions.[99,100] No significant differences in age, sex, previous thyroid ablation, TSH levels, or free thyroid hormone concentrations occur between patients with TSH-oma and those with resistance to thyroid hormone (Table 26-4). However, in contrast with resistance to thyroid hormone patients, familial cases of TSH-oma have never been documented. The finding of measurable TSH levels and high concentrations of FT_4 and FT_3 in one relative definitely points to the diagnosis of resistance to thyroid hormone. Serum TSH levels within the normal range are more frequently found in resistance to thyroid hormone, whereas elevated α subunit concentrations or a high α subunit/TSH molar ratio is typically present in patients with TSH-omas. Moreover, absent or impaired TSH responses to TRH administration and to the T_3 suppression test favor the presence of a TSH-oma. Circulating SHBG levels are in the hyperthyroid range in patients with

Table 26-4 Differential Diagnosis between TSH-Producing Adenomas (TSH-omas) and Resistance to Thyroid Hormones (RTH)

Parameter	TSH-omas	RTH	P
Age (years)	9-84	0.1 to 80	NS
Sex (F/M ratio)	1.4	1.3	NS
TSH mU/L[a]	2.8 ± 0.6	2.0 ± 0.3	NS
FT4 pmol/L[a]	42.0 ± 4.5	28.5 ± 2.7	NS
FT3 pmol/L[a]	14.2 ± 1.5	11.9 ± 1.0	NS
SHBG nmol/L[a]	117.0 ± 17.6	60.0 ± 4.1	<0.0001
Familial cases	0%	84%	<0.0001
Lesions at CT scan or MRI	98%	2%	<0.0001
High α subunit levels	68%	2%	<0.0001
High α subunit/TSH m.r.	84%	2%	<0.0001
Abnormal TSH response to TRH test[b]	85%	5%	<0.0001
Abnormal TSH response to T3 suppression test[c]	100%	100%[d]	NS

[a]Only patients with intact thyroid were taken into account. Data are obtained from patients followed at our institution (18 TSH-omas and 68 RTH) and are expressed as mean ± SE (n).
[b]Net TSH increment <4.0 mU/L.
[c]Werner's test (80 to 100 μg T3 for 8 to 10 days). Quantitatively normal responses to T3, i.e., complete inhibition of both basal and TRH-stimulated TSH levels, have never been recorded in either group of patients.
[d]Although abnormal in quantitative terms, TSH response to T3 suppression test is qualitatively normal in the majority of RTH patients.[7-9]

TSH-oma, the only patients with low SHBG being those with concomitant hypersecretion of GH, which potently inhibits SHBG secretion. The few patients with thyroid hormone resistance and high SHBG levels were those who were treated with estrogens or those showing profound hypogonadism.[88] Other parameters that may be useful in the differential diagnosis are the markers of bone turnover, such as ICTP (altered in TSH-omas, normal in resistance to thyroid hormone), or total cholesterol (rarely high in TSH-omas).[9,89] In difficult cases, particularly after thyroidectomy, genetic investigations on the thyroid hormone receptor-β_1 mutations may be the only diagnostic test. Finally, an apparent association between TSH-oma and resistance to thyroid hormone has been reported in a few patients.[86,101] Although genetic studies and familial investigations were not carried out in the Japanese patient, the occurrence of TSH-omas in patients with resistance to thyroid hormone is theoretically possible and therefore should be carefully considered.

TREATMENT AND OUTCOME

PITUITARY SURGERY AND RADIATION THERAPY

The primary goal in the treatment of TSH-omas is to remove the pituitary tumor and restore euthyroidism. Therefore, the first therapeutic approach to TSH-producing adenomas should be to surgically remove or debulk the tumor by transsphenoidal or subfrontal adenomectomy, the choice of route depending on the tumor volume and its suprasellar extension.[17,102,103] This may be particularly difficult because of the marked fibrosis of these tumors and the local invasion involving the cavernous sinus, internal carotid artery, or optic chiasm. To restore euthyroidism before surgery, antithyroid drugs or octreotide along with propranolol can be administered. If surgery is contraindicated or declined, pituitary radiotherapy (no less than 45 Gy fractionated at 2 Gy/day or 10 to 25 Gy in a single dose if a stereotactic gamma unit is available) and subsequent somatostatin analogue administration should be considered.

Surgery alone or combined with radiotherapy induces normalization of thyroid hormone levels and apparent complete removal of tumor mass in about one third of patients, whereas the normalization of thyroid hormones without a complete removal of the adenoma occurs in an another third of patients (Table 26-5). Collectively, about two thirds of TSH-omas are under control with surgery, irradiation, or both. In the remaining patients, the large size and the invasiveness of the tumor prevent successful removal of the tumor. Elevation

of α subunit or cosecretion of other pituitary hormones does not seem to be an unfavorable prognostic factor. Postsurgical deaths were reported in five cases. Partial or complete hypopituitarism may be the result of surgery. Evaluation of other pituitary functions, particularly ACTH secretion, should be carefully undertaken soon after surgery and checked again every year, especially in patients who are treated by radiotherapy. In addition, in the case of surgical cure, postoperative TSH is undetectable and may remain low for many weeks or months, causing central hypothyroidism. The time necessary for the recovery of normal thyrotrophs is variable, and permanent central hypothyroidism may occasionally occur because of damage to the normal thyrotroph by the tumor or during surgery. Thus, temporary or permanent levothyroxine replacement therapy may be necessary. In a few cases, total thyroidectomy was performed after pituitary surgery failed because the patients were at risk of thyroid storm.

MEDICAL TREATMENT

In terms of pharmacologic therapy of TSH-omas, antithyroid drugs must not be used as medical treatment of TSH-omas because they may cause more rapid growth and invasiveness of the tumors, and their use is recommended only as preparation of the patient for neurosurgery. For alleviating the symptoms of hyperthyroidism, β-blockers such as propranolol may be used. Glucocorticoids are effective in reducing TSH secretion, but they induce deleterious side effects in long-term treatment. Dopamine agonists, particularly bromocriptine, have been employed in some TSH-omas with variable results, the positive effects that are observed in some patients with mixed TSH- and PRL-secreting adenoma diminishing with time.[104,105] Currently, the medical treatment of TSH-omas rests on somatostatin analogues such as octreotide[48,92,93,106–108] or the new slow-release formulation of lanreotide.[109,110] Octreotide leads to a reduction of TSH and α subunit secretion in almost all cases, with restoration of the euthyroid state in the majority of them (see Table 26-5). Moreover, modifications of the TSH glycoisomer distribution pattern during octreotide treatment have been documented in one patient,[111] suggesting that restoration of euthyroidism in some patients who show no reduction in immunoreactive levels of TSH during octreotide therapy may be due to a reduction of the bioactivity of secreted molecules.[92,112] During octreotide therapy, tumor shrinkage occurs in about half of patients (see Table 26-5), and vision improvement is seen in 75%.

Tachyphylaxis occurred in 22% of patients and responded to increasing octreotide doses, whereas long-term studies

Table 26-5 Results of Pituitary Surgery Alone, Surgery Plus Irradiation (Rx), and Injection of Somatostatin Analogues in the Treatment of TSH-Producing Adenomas

	Surgery (n = 125)	Surgery + Rx (n = 57)	Somatostatin Analogues (n = 84)
REDUCTION OF TUMOR MASS			
Complete	34%	29%	0%
Partial	34%	40%	51%
Absent	32%	31%	49%
RESOLUTION OF CLINICAL SYMPTOMS			
Yes	57%	62%	95%
No	43%	38%	5%

demonstrated true escape from the inhibitory effects in few cases. In only 5% of cases was a true resistance to octreotide treatment documented. Octreotide treatment was effective in restoring euthyroidism in one pregnant woman with central hyperthyroidism and had no side effects on fetal development and thyroid function.[113,114] Patients taking octreotide have to be carefully monitored because untoward side effects, such as cholelithiasis and carbohydrate intolerance, may become manifested. The dose that is administered should be tailored for each patient, depending on therapeutic response and tolerance (including gastrointestinal side effects). The marked octreotide-induced suppression of TSH secretion and consequent biochemical hypothyroidism seen in some patients may require levothyroxine substitution. Whether somatostatin analogue treatment may be an alternative to surgery and irradiation in patients with TSH-oma remains to be established. However, the slow-release preparation of somatostatin, lanreotide-SR, and octreotide-LAR, may represent a useful tool for long-term treatment of such a rare pituitary adenoma.

CRITERIA OF CURE AND FOLLOW-UP

Evidence has accumulated about the criteria of cure and follow-up of patients undergoing operation or irradiation for TSH-omas.[4,57,61] In untreated hyperthyroid patients, it is reasonable to assume that cured patients have clinical and biochemical reversal of thyroid hyperfunction. However, normal free thyroid hormone concentrations or indices of peripheral thyroid hormone action in the euthyroid range may be associated with a partial removal or destruction of tumoral cells, since transient clinical remission and euthyroidism are frequently observed.[57,61] As it occurs for other pituitary tumors, disappearance of neurologic signs and symptoms only partially reflects the radicality of tumor removal, since it may occur even in the presence of an incomplete debulking of the tumor. Pituitary imaging performed after surgery has a low predictivity because of the high frequency of false-negative imaging results. The criteria of normalization of circulating TSH are not applicable to previously thyroidectomized patients or to those with normal basal values of TSH. In our experience, undetectable TSH levels 1 week after surgery are likely to indicate complete adenomectomy, provided that the patient was hyperthyroid and presurgical treatments were stopped at least 10 days before surgery.[48] Similarly, although normalization of α subunit or α subunit/TSH molar ratio is in general a good index for the evaluation of therapy efficacy, both parameters are normal in a remarkable number of patients with TSH-oma. The most sensitive and specific test to document the complete removal of the adenoma remains the T_3 suppression test (in the absence of clinical contraindication). In fact, regardless of the restoration of euthyroidism,

only patients in whom T_3 administration completely inhibits basal and TRH-stimulated TSH secretion appear to be truly cured (Fig. 26-4).

Data on the recurrence rate of TSH-oma in patients who are judged to be cured after surgery or radiotherapy are still lacking. However, the recurrence of the adenoma does not appear to be frequent, at least in the first years after successful surgery. In general, the patient should be evaluated clinically and biochemically two or three times the first year postoperatively and then every year. Pituitary imaging should be performed every 2 or 3 years but should be performed promptly whenever an increase in TSH and thyroid hormone levels or clinical symptoms occur. In the case of persistent macroadenoma, a close visual field follow-up is required, as the visual function is threatened.

CONCLUSIONS

Central hyperthyroidism due to TSH-secreting pituitary adenomas is a rare cause of thyrotoxicosis. The diagnosis is now facilitated by the recent introduction of ultrasensitive TSH immunoassays as well as direct free thyroid hormone measurement, which are not obscured by abnormal serum transport proteins. Increased awareness and early recognition of these tumors will prevent inappropriate treatment, such as thyroid ablation or long-term antithyroid drug administration, which undoubtedly increases TSH secretion, tumor size, and invasiveness. Although no single diagnostic test is pathognomonic in establishing the diagnosis, the elevation of α subunit levels and serum SHBG concentrations, as well as the frequently absent or impaired TSH responses to TRH and T_3 suppression tests, are the most useful markers to distinguish patients with TSH-omas from those with thyroid hormone resistance. Furthermore, high-resolution CT and MRI may help in detecting tumors as small as 3 mm in diameter. Surgery still remains the first therapeutic approach to the disease, followed by radiotherapy in the case of failure. The finding of measurable TSH levels after a simple T_3 suppression test definitely indicates that the removal of the tumor cells was incomplete, thus requiring a closer follow-up of the patient

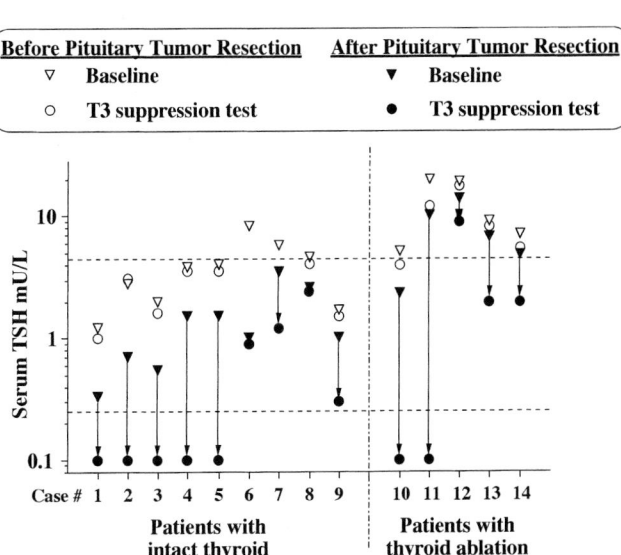

Figure 26-4 Results of T_3 suppression test carried out before and after pituitary surgery in patients with TSH-producing adenoma. *Horizontal dashed lines* indicate the normal range of serum TSH. Note the lack of TSH suppression in all patients before neurosurgery. Complete suppression of serum TSH levels (i.e., complete removal of the adenoma) was seen in about half of patients after neurosurgery, independent of previous thyroid ablation.

or additional therapies, or both. If needed, treatment with somatostatin analogues is worthwhile, allowing restoration of euthyroidism and even tumor shrinkage in many cases.

Acknowledgment

The authors thank Dr. Anna Spada for the critical reading of the manuscript.

REFERENCES

1. Smallridge RC: Thyrotropin-secreting tumors. In Mazzaferri EL, Samaan NA (eds): Endocrine Tumors. Boston, Blackwell, 1993, p 136.
2. Samuels MH, Ridgway EC: Glycoprotein-secreting pituitary adenomas. Baillieres Clin Endocrinol 9:337, 1995.
3. Greenman Y, Melmed S: Thyrotropin-secreting pituitary tumors. In Melmed S (ed): The Pituitary. Boston, Blackwell Science, 1995, p 546.
4. Beck-Peccoz P, Brucker-Davis F, Persani L, et al: Thyrotropin-secreting pituitary tumors. Endocr Rev 17:610, 1996.
5. Jailer JW, Holub DA: Remission of Graves' disease following radiotherapy of a pituitary neoplasm. Am J Med 28:497, 1960.
6. Hamilton C, Adams LC, Maloof F: Hyperthyroidism due to thyrotropin-producing pituitary chromophobe adenoma. N Engl J Med 283:1077, 1970.
7. Refetoff S, Weiss RE, Usala SJ: The syndromes of resistance to thyroid hormone. Endocr Rev 14:348, 1993.
8. Beck-Peccoz P, Asteria C, Mannavola D: Resistance to thyroid hormone. In Braverman LE (ed): Contemporary Endocrinology: Diseases of the Thyroid. Totowa, NJ, Humana Press, 1997, p 199.
9. Chatterjee VKK, Clifton-Bright RJ, Gurnell M: Thyroid hormone resistance. In Jameson JL (ed): Contemporary Endocrinology: Hormone Resistance Syndromes. Totowa, NJ, Humana Press, 1999, p 145.
10. Felix I, Asa SL, Kovacs K, et al: Recurrent plurihormonal bimorphous pituitary adenoma producing growth hormone, thyrotropin, and prolactin. Arch Pathol Lab Med 118:66, 1994.
11. Bertholon-Gregoire M, Trouillas J, Guigard MP, et al: Mono and plurihormonal thyrotropic pituitary adenomas: Pathological, hormonal and clinical studies in twelve patients. Eur J Endocrinol 140:519, 1999.
12. Katz MS, Gregerman RI, Horvath E, et al: Thyrotroph cell adenoma of the human pituitary gland associated with primary hypothyroidism: Clinical and morphological features. Acta Endocrinol 95:41, 1980.
13. Pioro EP, Scheithauer BW, Laws ER Jr, et al: Combined thyrotroph and lactotroph cell hyperplasia simulating prolactin-secreting pituitary adenoma in long-standing primary hypothyroidism. Surg Neurol 29:218, 1980.
14. Ghannam NN, Hammami MM, Muttair Z, et al: Primary hypothyroidism-associated TSH-secreting pituitary adenoma/hyperplasia presenting as a bleeding nasal mass and extremely elevated TSH level. J Endocrinol Invest. 22:419, 1999.

15. Saeger W, Ludecke DK: Pituitary adenomas with hyperfunction of TSH. Virchows Arch Am Pathol Anat Histol 394:255, 1982.
16. Wilson CB: A decade of pituitary microsurgery: The Herbert Olivecrona lecture. J Neurosurg 61:814, 1984.
17. Socin HV, Chanson P, Delemer B, et al: The changing spectrum of TSH-secreting pituitary adenomas: Diagnosis and management in 43 patients. Eur J Endocrinol 148:433, 2003.
18. Mindermann T, Wilson CB: Thyrotropin-producing pituitary adenomas. J Neurosurg 79:521, 1993.
19. Mixson AJ, Friedman TC, David AK, et al: Thyrotropin-secreting pituitary carcinoma. J Clin Endocrinol Metab 76:529, 1993.
20. Cooper DS, Wenig BM: Hyperthyroidism caused by an ectopic TSH-secreting pituitary tumor. Thyroid 6:337, 1996.
21. Pasquini E, Faustini-Fustini M, Sciarretta V, et al: Ectopic TSH-secreting pituitary adenoma of the vomerosphenoidal junction. Eur J Endocrinol 148:253, 2003
22. Gesundheit N, Petrick P, Nissim M, et al: Thyrotropin-secreting pituitary adenomas: Clinical and biochemical heterogeneity. Ann Intern Med 111:827, 1989.
23. Weintraub BD, Petrick PA, Gesundheit N, et al: TSH-secreting pituitary tumors. In Medeiros-Neto G, Gaitan S (eds): Frontiers in Thyroidology. New York, Plenum, 1986, p 71.
24. Beck-Peccoz P, Piscitelli G, Amr S, et al: Endocrine, biochemical, and morphological studies of a pituitary adenoma secreting growth hormone, thyrotropin (TSH), and α-subunit: Evidence for secretion of TSH with increased bioactivity. J Clin Endocrinol Metab 62:704, 1986.
25. Ozawa Y, Kameya T, Kasuga A, et al: A functional thyrotropin- and growth hormone-secreting pituitary adenoma with ultrastructurally monomorphic feature: A case study. Endocr J 45:211, 1998.
26. Ikeda H, Ogawa Y, Yoshimoto T: Ultrastructural characteristics of TSH-producing adenomas with special reference to its close similarity to BFA-treated pituitary adenoma cells. Pituitary 1:221,1999
27. Trouillas J, Girod C, Loras B, et al: The TSH secretion in the human pituitary adenomas. Pathol Res Pract 183:596, 1988.
28. Terzolo M, Orlandi F, Bassetti M, et al: Hyperthyroidism due to a pituitary adenoma composed of two different cell types, one secreting alpha-subunit alone and another cosecreting alpha-subunit and thyrotropin. J Clin Endocrinol Metab 72:415, 1991.

29. Jaquet P, Hassoun J, Delori P, et al: A human pituitary adenoma secreting thyrotropin and prolactin: Immunohistochemical, biochemical and cell culture study. J Clin Endocrinol Metab 59:817, 1984.
30. Kuzuya N, Inoue K, Ishibashi M, et al: Endocrine and immunohistochemical studies on thyrotropin (TSH)-secreting pituitary adenomas: Responses of TSH, alpha-subunit and growth hormone to hypothalamic releasing hormones and their distribution in adenoma cells. J Clin Endocrinol Metab 71:1103, 1990.
31. Malarkey WB, Kovacs K, O'Dorisio T: Response of GH- and TSH-secreting pituitary adenoma to a somatostatin analogue (SMS 201-995): Evidence that GH and TSH coexist in the same cell and secretory granules. Neuroendocrinology 49:267, 1989.
32. Sanno N, Teramoto A, Matsuno A, et al: Clinical and immunohistochemical studies on TSH-secreting pituitary adenoma: Its multihormonality and expression of Pit-1. Modern Pathol 7:893, 1994.
33. Dong Q, Brucker-Davis F, Weintraub BD, et al: Screening of candidate oncogenes in human thyrotroph tumors: Absence of activating mutations of the $G\alpha_q$, $G\alpha_{11}$, $G\alpha_s$, or thyrotropin-releasing hormone receptor genes. J Clin Endocrinol Metab 81:1134, 1996.
34. Lind P, Langsteger W, Koltringer P, et al: Transient prealbumin-associated hyperthyroxinemia in a TSH-producing pituitary adenoma. Nuklearmedizin 29:40, 1990.
35. Waldhausl W, Brautsch-Marrain P, Nowotony P, et al: Secondary hyperthyroidism due to thyrotropin hypersecretion: Study of pituitary tumor morphology and thyrotropin chemistry and release. J Clin Endocrinol Metab 49:879, 1979.
36. Stanley JM, Najjar SS: Hyperthyroidism secondary to a TSH-secreting pituitary adenoma in a 15-year-old-male. Clin Pediatr 30:109, 1991.
37. Patrick AW, Atkin SL, MacKenzie J, et al: Hyperthyroidism secondary to a pituitary adenoma secreting TSH, FSH, alpha-subunit and GH. Clin Endocrinol (Oxf) 40:275, 1994.
38. Ma W, Ikeda H, Watabe N, et al: A plurihormonal TSH-producing pituitary tumor of monoclonal origin in a patient with hypothyroidism. Horm Res 59:257, 2003
39. Pellegrini I, Barlier A, Gunz G, et al: Pit-1 gene expression in the human pituitary and pituitary adenomas. J Clin Endocrinol Metab 79:189, 1994.
40. Boggild MD, Jenkinson S, Pistorello M, et al: Molecular genetics studies of sporadic pituitary tumors. J Clin Endocrinol Metab 78:387, 1994.

41. Bamberger CM, Fehn M, Bamberger AM, et al: Reduced expression levels of the cell-cycle inhibitor p27Kip1 in human pituitary adenomas. Eur J Endocrinol 140:250, 1999.

42. Sumi T, Stefaneanu L, Kovacs K, et al: Immunohistochemical study of p53 protein in human and animal pituitary tumors. Endocr Pathol 4:95, 1993.

43. Chanson P, Li JY, LeDafniet M, et al: Absence of receptors for thyrotropin (TSH)-releasing hormone in human TSH-secreting pituitary adenomas associated with hyperthyroidism. J Clin Endocrinol Metab 66:447, 1988.

44. LeDafniet M, Brandi A-M, Kujas M, et al: Thyrotropin-releasing hormone (TRH) binding sites and thyrotropin response to TRH are regulated by thyroid hormones in human thyrotropic adenomas. Eur J Endocrinol 130:559, 1994.

45. Kim K, Arai K, Sanno N, et al: The expression of thyrotrophin-releasing hormone receptor 1 messenger ribonucleic acid in human pituitary adenomas. Clin Endocrinol (Oxf) 54:309, 2001.

46. Polak M, Bertherat J, Li JY, et al: A human TSH-secreting adenoma: Endocrine, biochemical and morphological studies: Evidence of somatostatin receptors by using quantitative autoradiography. Clinical and biological improvement by SMS 201-995 treatment. Acta Endocrinol 124:479, 1991.

47. Takano K, Ajima M, Teramoto A, et al: Mechanism of action of somatostatin on human TSH-secreting adenoma cells. Am J Physiol 268:E558, 1995.

48. Bertherat J, Brue T, Enjalbert A, et al: Somatostatin receptors on thyrotropin-secreting pituitary adenomas: Comparison with the inhibitory effects of octreotide upon in vivo and in vitro hormonal secretions. J Clin Endocrinol Metab 75:540, 1992.

49. Levy A, Eckland DJA, Gurney AM, et al: Somatostatin and thyrotropin-releasing hormone response and receptor status of a thyrotropin-secreting pituitary adenoma: Clinical and "in vitro" studies. J Neuroendocrinol 1:321, 1989.

50. Ando S, Sarlis NJ, Oldfield EH, Yen PM: Somatic mutation of TRbeta can cause a defect in negative regulation of TSH in a TSH-secreting pituitary tumor. J Clin Endocrinol Metab 86:5572, 2001.

51. Ando S, Sarlis NJ, Krishnan J, et al: Aberrant alternative splicing of thyroid hormone receptor in a TSH-secreting pituitary tumor is a mechanism for hormone resistance. Mol Endocrinol 15:1529, 2001.

52. Tannahill LA, Visser TJ, McCabe CJ, et al: Dysregulation of iodothyronine deiodinase enzyme expression and function in human pituitary tumours. Clin Endocrinol (Oxf) 56:735, 2002.

53. Baur A, Buchfelder M, Kohrle J: Expression of 5'-deiodinase enzymes in normal pituitaries and in various human pituitary adenomas. Eur J Endocrinol 147:263, 2002.

54. Yamakita N, Ikeda T, Murai T, et al: Thyrotropin-producing pituitary adenoma discovered as a pituitary incidentaloma. Intern Med 34:1055, 1995.

55. Koide Y, Kugai N, Kimura S, et al: A case of pituitary adenoma with possible simultaneous secretion of thyrotropin and follicle-stimulating hormone. J Clin Endocrinol Metab 54:397, 1982.

56. Scanlon MF, Howells S, Peters JR, et al: Hyperprolactinaemia, amenorrhoea and galactorrhoea due a pituitary thyrotroph adenoma. Clin Endocrinol 23:35, 1985.

57. Losa M, Giovanelli M, Persani L, et al: Criteria of cure and follow-up of central hyperthyroidism due to thyrotropin-secreting pituitary adenomas. J Clin Endocrinol Metab 81:3084, 1996.

58. Kiso Y, Yoshida K, Kaise K, et al: A case of thyrotropin (TSH)-secreting tumor complicated by periodic paralysis. Jpn J Med 29:399, 1990.

59. Alings AM, Fliers E, de Herder WW, et al: A thyrotropin-secreting pituitary adenoma as a cause of thyrotoxic periodic paralysis. J Endocrinol Invest 21:703, 1998.

60. Hsu FS, Tsai WS, Chau T, et al: Thyrotropin-secreting pituitary adenoma presenting as hypokalemic periodic paralysis. Am J Med Sci 325:48, 2003.

61. Brucker-Davis F, Oldfield EH, Skarulis MC, et al: Thyrotropin-secreting pituitary tumors: Diagnostic criteria, thyroid hormone sensitivity, and treatment outcome in 25 patients followed at the National Institutes of Health. J Clin Endocrinol Metab 84:476, 1999.

62. Calle-Pascual AL, Yuste E, Martin P, et al: Association of a thyrotropin-secreting pituitary adenoma and a thyroid follicular carcinoma. J Endocrinol Invest 14:499, 1991.

63. Gasparoni P, Rubello D, Persani L, et al: Unusual association between a thyrotropin-secreting pituitary adenoma and a papillary thyroid carcinoma. Thyroid 8:181, 1998.

64. Kishida M, Otsuka F, Kataoka H, et al: Hyperthyroidism in a patient with TSH-producing pituitary adenoma coexisting with thyroid papillary adenocarcinoma. Endocr J 47:731, 2000.

65. Ohta S, Nishizawa S, Oki Y, et al: Coexistence of thyrotropin-producing pituitary adenoma with papillary adenocarcinoma of the thyroid: A case report and surgical strategy. Pituitary 4:271, 2001

66. Beckers A, Abs R, Mahler C, et al: Thyrotropin-secreting pituitary adenomas: Report of seven cases. J Clin Endocrinol Metab 72:477, 1991.

67. Abs R, Stevenaert A, Beckers A: Autonomously functioning thyroid nodules in a patient with a thyrotropin-secreting pituitary adenoma: Possible cause-effect relationship. Eur J Endocrinol 131:355, 1994.

68. Sy ARG, Bernstein R, Chynn KI, et al: Reduction in size of a thyrotropin- and gonadotropin-secreting pituitary adenoma treated with octreotide acetate (somatostatin analogue). J Clin Endocrinol Metab 74:690, 1992.

69. Horn K, Erhardt F, Fahlbusch R, et al: Recurrent goiter, hyperthyroidism, galactorrhoea and amenorrhoea due to a thyrotropin and prolactin-producing pituitary tumor. J Clin Endocrinol Metab 43:137, 1976.

70. Adriaanse R, Brabant G, Endert E, et al: Pulsatile thyrotropin and prolactin secretion in a patient with a mixed thyrotropin- and prolactin-secreting pituitary adenoma. Eur J Endocrinol 130:113, 1994.

71. Burgess JR, Shepherd JJ, Greenaway TM: Thyrotropinomas in multiple endocrine neoplasia type 1 (MEN-1). Aust N Z J Med 24:740, 1994.

72. Wynne AG, Gharib H, Scheithauer BW, et al: Hyperthyroidism due to inappropriate secretion of thyrotropin in 10 patients. Am J Med 92:15, 1992.

73. Taylor TJ, Donlon SS, Bale AE, et al: Treatment of a thyrotropinoma with octreotide-LAR in a patient with multiple endocrine neoplasia-1. Thyroid 10:1001, 2000.

74. Gessl A, Freissmuth M, Czech T, et al: Growth hormone-prolactin-thyrotropin-secreting pituitary adenoma in atypical McCune-Albright syndrome with functionally normal Gsα protein. J Clin Endocrinol Metab 79:1128, 1994.

75. Langlois M-F, Lamarche JB, Bellabarba D: Long-standing goiter and hypothyroidism: An unusual presentation of a TSH-secreting adenoma. Thyroid 6:329, 1996.

76. Ekins R: Measurement of free hormones in blood. Endocr Rev 11:5, 1990.

77. Beck-Peccoz P, Piscitelli G, Cattaneo MG, et al: Evaluation of free thyroxine methods in the presence of iodothyronine binding autoantibodies. J Clin Endocrinol Metab 58:736, 1984.

78. Zweig MH, Csako G, Spero M: Escape from blockade of interfering heterophile antibodies in a two-site immunoradiometric assay for thyrotropin. Clin Chem 34:2589, 1988.

79. Beck-Peccoz P, Persani L: Variable biological activity of thyroid-stimulating hormone. Eur J Endocrinol 131:331, 1994.

80. Bevan JS, Burke CW, Esiri MM, et al: Studies of two thyrotropin-secreting pituitary adenomas: Evidence for dopamine receptor deficiency. Clin Endocrinol 31:59, 1989.

81. Magner JA, Kane J: Binding of thyrotropin to lentil lectin is unchanged by thyrotropin-releasing hormone administration in three patients with thyrotropin-producing pituitary adenomas. Endocr Res 8:163, 1992.

82. Magner JA, Klibanski A, Fein H, et al: Ricin and lentil lectin affinity chromatography reveals oligosaccharide heterogeneity of thyrotropin secreted by 12 human pituitary tumors. Metabolism 41:1009, 1992.

83. Kourides IA, Ridgway EC, Weintraub BD, et al: Thyrotropin-induced hyperthyroidism: Use of alpha and beta subunit levels to identify patients with primary tumors. J Clin Endocrinol Metab 45:534, 1977.

84. Beck-Peccoz P, Persani L, Faglia G: Glycoprotein hormone α-subunit in pituitary adenomas. Trends Endocrinol Metab 3:41, 1992.

85. Smallridge RC: Metabolic, physiologic, and clinical indexes of thyroid function. In Braverman LE, Utiger RD (eds): Werner and Ingbar's The Thyroid, 7th ed. Philadelphia, JB Lippincott, 1996, p 397.

86. Watanabe K, Kameya T, Yamauchi A, et al: Thyrotropin-producing adenoma associated with pituitary resistance to thyroid hormone. J Clin Endocrinol Metab 76:1025, 1993.

87. Azarnivar A, Chopra IJ: Tension pneumoencephalus after transsphenoidal resection of a thyrotropin (TSH)-secreting pituitary adenoma. Endocrinologist 5:308, 1995.

88. Beck-Peccoz P, Roncoroni R, Mariotti S, et al: Sex hormone-binding globulin measurement in patients with inappropriate secretion of thyrotropin (IST): Evidence against selective pituitary thyroid hormone resistance in nonneoplastic IST. J Clin Endocrinol Metab 71:19, 1990.

89. Persani L, Preziati D, Matthews CH, et al: Serum levels of carboxyterminal cross-linked telopeptide of type I collagen (ICTP) in the differential diagnosis of the syndromes of inappropriate secretion of TSH. Clin Endocrinol 47:207, 1997.

90. Morpurgo PS, Beck-Peccoz P, Reschini E, et al: Serum activin A levels in different thyroid disorders. Thyroid 12:1113, 2002.

91. Rubello D, Busnardo B, Girelli ME, et al: Severe hyperthyroidism due to neoplastic TSH hypersecretion in an old man. J Endocrinol Invest 12:571, 1989.

92. Chanson P, Weintraub BD, Harris AG: Octreotide therapy for thyroid stimulating hormone-secreting pituitary adenomas: A follow-up of 52 patients. Ann Intern Med 119:236, 1993.

93. Losa M, Magnani P, Mortini P, et al: Indium-111 pentetreotide single-photon emission tomography in patients with TSH-secreting pituitary adenomas: Correlation with the effect of a single administration of octreotide on serum TSH levels. Eur J Nucl Med 24:728, 1997.

94. Webster J, Peters JR, John R, et al: Pituitary stone: Two cases of densely calcified thyrotropin-secreting pituitary adenomas. Clin Endocrinol 40:137, 1994.

95. Nabarro JDN: Acromegaly. Clin Endocrinol (Oxf) 26:481, 1987.

96. Lamberts SWJ, Krenning EP, Reubi J-C: The role of somatostatin and its analogs in the diagnosis and treatment of tumors. Endocr Rev 12:450, 1991.

97. Verhoeff NPLG, Bemelman FJ, Wiersinga WM, et al: Imaging of dopamine D2 and somatostatin receptors in vivo using single-photon emission tomography in a patient with a TSH/PRL-producing pituitary macroadenoma. Eur J Nucl Med 20:555, 1993.

98. Frank SJ, Gesundheit N, Doppman JL, et al: Preoperative lateralization of pituitary microadenomas by petrosal sinus sampling: Utility in two patients with non-ACTH-secreting tumors. Am J Med 87:679, 1989.

99. Mariotti S, Anelli S, Bartalena L, et al: Familial hyperthyroidism due to nonneoplastic inappropriate TSH secretion associated with sellar abnormalities [Abstract]. J Endocrinol Invest 10(Suppl 1):20, 1987.

100. Hall WA, Luciano MG, Doppman JL, et al: Pituitary magnetic resonance imaging in normal human volunteers: Occult adenomas in the general population. Ann Intern Med 120:817, 1994.

101. Safer JD, Colan SD, Fraser LM, et al: A pituitary tumor in a patient with thyroid hormone resistance: A diagnostic dilemma. Thyroid 11:281, 2001.

102. McCutcheon IE, Weintraub BD, Oldfield EH: Surgical treatment of thyrotropin-secreting pituitary adenomas. J Neurosurg 73:674, 1990.

103. Losa M, Mortini P, Franzin A, et al: Surgical management of thyrotropin-secreting pituitary adenomas. Pituitary 2:127, 1999.

104. Carlson H, Linfoot J, Braunstein G, et al: Hyperthyroidism and acromegaly due to a thyrotropin- and growth hormone-secreting pituitary tumor: Lack of hormonal response to bromocriptine. Am J Med 74:915, 1983.

105. Zuniga S, Mendoza V, Espinoza IF, et al: A plurihormonal TSH-secreting pituitary microadenoma: Report of a case with an atypical clinical presentation and transient response to bromocriptine therapy. Endocr Pathol 8:81, 1997.

106. Comi R, Gesundheit N, Murray L, et al: Response of thyrotropin-secreting pituitary adenomas to a long-acting somatostatin analogue. N Engl J Med 317:12, 1987.

107. Gourgiotis L, Skarulis MC, Brucker-Davis F, et al: Effectiveness of long-acting octreotide in suppressing hormonogenesis and tumor growth in thyrotropin-secreting pituitary adenomas: report of two cases. Pituitary 4:135, 2001.

108. Caron P, Arlot S, Bauters C, et al: Efficacy of the long-acting octreotide formulation (octreotide-LAR) in patients with thyrotropin-secreting pituitary adenomas. J Clin Endocrinol Metab 86:2849, 2001.

109. Gancel A, Vuillermet P, Legrand A, et al: Effects of a slow-release formulation of the new somatostatin analogue lanreotide in TSH-secreting pituitary adenomas. Clin Endocrinol 40:421, 1994.

110. Kuhn JM, Arlot S, Lefebvre H, et al: Evaluation of the treatment of thyrotropin-secreting pituitary adenomas with a slow release formulation of the somatostatin analog lanreotide. J Clin Endocrinol Metab 85:1487, 2000.

111. Francis TB, Smallridge RC, Kane J, et al: Octreotide changes serum thyrotropin (TSH) glycoisomer distribution as assessed by lectin chromatography in a TSH macroadenoma patient. J Clin Endocrinol Metab 77:183, 1993.

112. Hill S, Falko J, Wilson C, et al: Thyrotropin-producing pituitary adenomas. J Neurosurg 57:515, 1982.

113. Caron P, Gerbaud C, Pradayrol L, et al: Successful pregnancy in an infertile woman with a thyrotropin-secreting macroadenoma treated with somatostatin analog (octreotide). J Clin Endocrinol Metab 81:1164, 1996.

114. Blackhurst G, Strachan MW, Collie D, et al: The treatment of a thyrotropin-secreting pituitary macroadenoma with octreotide in twin pregnancy. Clin Endocrinol (Oxf) 57:401, 2002.

CHAPTER 27

Disorders of Prolactin Secretion and Prolactinomas

Marcello D. Bronstein

Nongestational/puerperal prolactin (PRL) hypersecretion is the most prevalent hypothalamic-pituitary dysfunction, and its main cause is PRL-secreting pituitary adenomas (prolactinomas). Prolactinomas are the most common pituitary tumors, with an estimated prevalence of 500 cases/1 million inhabitants.[1] These tumors are classified either as microadenomas (diameter <10 mm) or macroadenomas (>10 mm) and can be enclosed, expansive, or invasive.[2] Prolactinomas are more common in women, especially microprolactinomas; macroprolactinomas have roughly the same prevalence in both genders. PRL-secreting pituitary carcinomas are exceedingly rare.[3,4] Because hyperprolactinemia usually is associated with menstrual disturbances, anovulation, and sexual impairment in both genders, and prolactinomas have a greater incidence in people in their 20s and 30s, these tumors are an important cause of infertility. To make the correct diagnosis of prolactinoma, other causes of hyperprolactinemia—physiologic, drug-induced, or pathologic—must be ruled out. It also is important to be aware of laboratory and imaging pitfalls that can mislead the diagnosis and treatment.[5] This chapter addresses the causes, clinical findings, diagnosis, and therapeutic options for prolactinomas and other causes of hyperprolactinemia.

HISTORY

"If a woman is neither pregnant nor has given birth, and produces milk, her menstruation has stopped." This sentence, attributed to Hippocrates (Aforisms, section 5, #39), shows that the association between menstrual disturbances and inappropriate milk secretion has been known since ancient times. It was only in the twentieth century, however, that such disturbances were associated with hypersecretion of a pituitary hormone. In 1928, Striker and Grueter[6] identified a pituitary factor that was able to induce milk secretion in rabbits. Early in the eighteenth century, Hunter discovered that "pigeon's milk," a substance secreted by male and female parents to feed the young pigeon, is secreted by the crop, and according to Hunter, "the crop behaves like the udder of mammalian females regarding uterine gestation." In 1933, Riddle and colleagues[7] identified the stimulatory effect of a pituitary hormone on pigeons' crop growth and differentiation, which also controlled milk secretion in mammals, and called it *prolactin*. The pigeon's crop model later was used for the PRL bioassay. Coincidentally, the association of amenorrhea, infertility, and galactorrhea were described better around the 1930s.

Afterward, this clinical picture was characterized in three different contexts: (1) postpartum without sellar enlargement (Chiari-Frommel syndrome),[8] (2) nonpuerperal period, also without sellar augmentation (Ahumada-Argonz-del Castillo syndrome),[9] and (3) associated with a pituitary tumor (Forbes-Albright syndrome).[10] The existence of a human PRL, distinct from the growth hormone (GH), remained controversial, however, until the development of a specific radioimmunoassay for PRL in the early 1970s,[11] when it was shown that all the above-mentioned syndromes were linked to elevated serum PRL levels. The development of pituitary microsurgery and, later on, of high-resolution imaging techniques showed that most of the cases with normal sella on plain x-rays, described as nontumoral, were small pituitary tumors (microadenomas). When PRL-secreting pituitary adenomas (prolactinomas) were proved as being the main cause of pathologic hyperprolactinemia, linked or not to a previous pregnancy, the division borne by the three eponymic amenorrhea-galactorrhea syndromes became obsolete. There are many other causes of hyperprolactinemia that must be differentiated from prolactinomas so that a correct therapeutic approach can be instituted.

EPIDEMIOLOGY

Hyperprolactinemia is the most prevalent hypothalamic-pituitary dysfunction, with prolactinomas being the main cause. These tumors represent roughly 25% of surgically removed pituitary adenomas and nearly 50% of adenohypophyseal tumors in autopsy series.[12,13] This apparent discrepancy may be due to the excellent results of medical treatment of prolactinomas with dopaminergic agonists. Their prevalence is estimated at 500 cases/1 million inhabitants, with an incidence of 27 cases/1 million/year.[1] Microprolactinomas (diameter <10 mm) represent about 60% of PRL-secreting adenomas and are more common in women than in men (20:1), whereas macroadenomas have roughly the same prevalence on both genders.[14,15] There are no sex-related differences in autopsy series.[12,16] Prolactinomas occur in all ages, with the diagnosis made predominantly in the 20s and 30s in both sexes.[14,15] They are the most frequent pituitary adenomas encountered in childhood and adolescence.[17] Prolactinomas represent the minority of pituitary tumors diagnosed after age 70, however. Prolactinomas are the most prevalent pituitary adenoma in the multiple endocrine neoplasia type 1 (MEN1) syndrome.[18,19] Isolated familial prolactinomas (not related to MEN1) have been described.[20] PRL-secreting pituitary carcinomas are exceedingly rare, with about 100 documented cases in the literature.[21]

PATHOGENESIS

Similar to other pituitary adenomas, prolactinomas are monoclonal in origin.[22] To date, the exact mechanisms leading to the development of lactotroph adenomas are not well established. Among the candidates are the pituitary tumor transforming gene (PTTG)[23,24] and the heparin-binding secretory transforming gene (*hst*),[25] both of which induce angiogenesis through fibroblast growth factors (FGF-2 and FGF-4). Estrogens seem to play a pivotal role in these mechanisms because estrogen modulator drugs, such as tamoxifen and raloxifene, and the antiestrogen ICI-182780 inhibit PTTG expression in prolactinomas in vitro and their growth in vivo (Fig. 27-1).[26] Reduction in the expression of the cytokine leukemia inhibitory factor[27] and nerve growth factor[28] and

the overexpression of bone morphogenetic protein 4[29] and the high mobility group A2 gene (*HMGA2*)[30] are among other events that potentially might be involved in prolactinoma tumorigenesis.

Studies on the microvascular density of prolactinomas show conflicting results: One study by electronic microscopy did not disclose differences between vascular density of the normal pituitary and microprolactinomas, but macroprolactinomas exhibited a much lower degree of vascularization. A more recent study using immunohistochemistry with antibodies for different endothelial markers observed that microprolactinomas are less vascular than macroprolactinomas. Additionally, microvascular density was related to tumor invasiveness and malignancy.[31]

The decrease of dopaminergic inhibition seems to play a role, at least a permissive one, in prolactinoma development. Lesions in the tuberoinfundibular dopaminergic neurons in female rats bearing prolactinomas were described.[32] Several studies have shown the development of prolactinomas in mice with D2 receptor knockout, with this phenotype being more severe and presenting a faster evolution in females and in animals treated with estrogens.[33–35] To date, no "natural" mutations were found in the D2 receptor gene.[36] PRLr(–/–) mice exhibited more intense hyperprolactinemia and larger tumors than did age-matched Drd2(–/–) mice, and there were cumulative effects in compound homozygous mutant male mice. This fact suggests that PRL inhibits lactotrophs not only by the activation of hypothalamic dopamine neurons, but also directly within the pituitary in a dopamine-independent fashion.

Prolactinomas associated with MEN1 present inactivating mutations characterized by loss of heterozygosity in locus 11q13 and mutations in the menin-codifying gene. They tend to be larger and more aggressive than their sporadic counterparts.[37,38] Sporadic prolactinomas may exhibit loss of heterozygosity, but without mutations in the menin gene detected to date, suggesting the presence of a tumor suppressor gene located within chromosome 11q13 yet distinct from MEN1.[39,40] Finally, mutations in the proto-oncogene *ras* and in the tumor suppressor gene p53 can be linked to the development of the rare PRL-secreting carcinomas.[21]

PATHOLOGY

The terms *microadenoma* and *macroadenoma*, coined by Hardy,[41] represent pituitary adenomas measuring less or more than 1 cm. Microprolactinomas are found mainly in young women, usually located in the lateral portions of the pituitary. They are generally enclosed within a pseudocapsule, but also can be invasive.[42] Macroprolactinomas also can be enclosed, but usually expand to the optic chiasmal region or invade local structures, such as the cavernous sinus or the sellar floor and sphenoid sinus.[42] Histologically, there are no differences between microprolactinomas and macroprolactinomas, which are usually "chromophobic" on hematoxylin-eosin staining. For this reason, many pituitary adenomas previously classified as "functionless" before the development of a radioimmunoassay for PRL were prolactinomas. This fact is explained by the use of electronic microscopy, which characterized most prolactinomas as sparsely granulated: oval and slight irregular nuclei, complex rough endoplasmic reticulum, large Golgi complexes, and sparse spherical or pleomorphic secretory granules, measuring 130 to 500 nm (Fig. 27-2).[43–45] The hallmark of these tumors is the so-called misplaced exocytosis, the extrusion of secretory granules along the lateral cell border.[46] This phenomenon diagnoses PRL secretion, either by normal or by neoplastic lactotrophs. The rare, densely granulated lactotroph adenoma is strongly acidophilic with strong diffuse immunostaining for PRL in the cytoplasm. The rough endoplasmic reticulum is less prominent, and the secretory

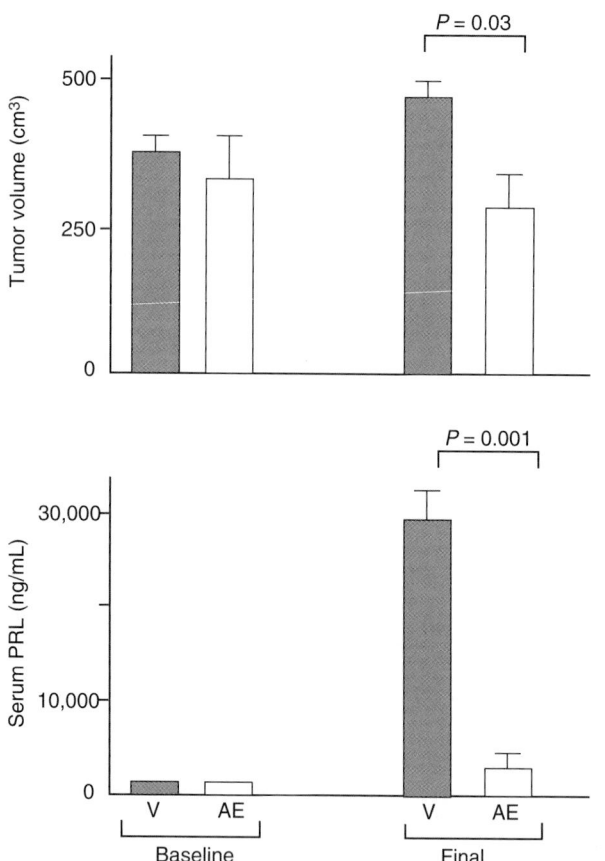

Figure 27-1 Selective antiestrogen treatment inhibits pituitary tumor growth in vivo. Pretreatment (baseline) and posttreatment tumor volumes and serum prolactin (PRL) levels after mini osmotic pumps infusion of vehicle or antiestrogen ICI-182780 (0.5 µg/day) was infused in 20 female Wistar-Furth rats harboring subcutaneous pituitary tumors. All animals developed tumors. Each bar represents mean ± SEM for 10 animals per group. *$P = 0.03$; **$P < 0.001$. (From Heaney AP, Fernando M, Melmed S: Functional role of estrogen in pituitary tumor pathogenesis. J Clin Invest 109:277–283, 2002.)

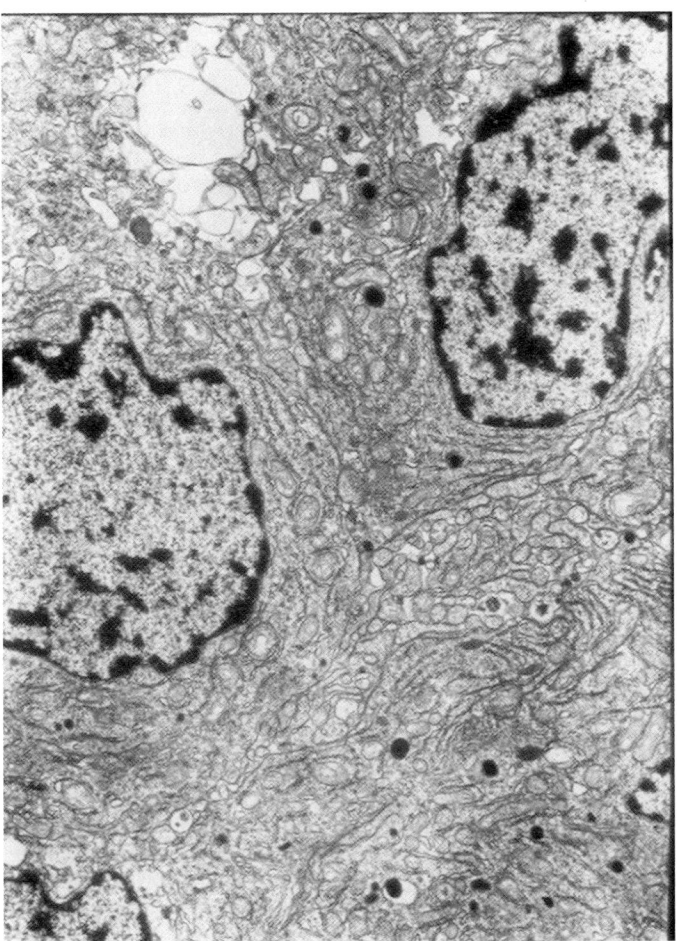

Figure 27-2 Electronic microscopy of a sparsely granulated prolactinoma, showing sparse secretory granules, well-developed rough endoplasmic reticulum, and prominent Golgi complexes.

granules are bigger (500 to 700 nm) and more numerous than in its sparsely granulated counterpart.[47]

Electron microscopy usually is not required for prolactinoma diagnosis since the immunohistochemical assessment of PRL production became routinely available. This technique directly characterizes PRL-secreting adenomas, ruling out "functionless" macroadenomas associated with hyperprolactinemia due to hypothalamus-pituitary disconnection, the so-called pseudoprolactinomas.[48] A study of 120 unselected necropsies showed that 27% of them harbored pituitary microadenomas without clinical expression, 40% of which immunostained for PRL.[49] These data indicate that there could be clinically and hormonally non–PRL-secreting pituitary adenomas that are immunohistochemically positive for this hormone. The significance of this finding for the natural history of prolactinomas is unknown.

ACIDOPHIL STEM CELL ADENOMA

Exceptionally hyperprolactinemic patients might exhibit mild or no clinical features of acromegaly associated with biochemical evidence of slight serum GH elevation. This situation is due to the presence of the rare and aggressive acidophil stem cell pituitary adenoma.[50] The acidophilia is attributable to mitochondrial accumulation called *oncocytic change*. Immunohistochemical analysis is positive for PRL, and occasionally there is a scant positivity for GH. The definitive diagnosis requires electron microscopy, which depicts enlarged mitochondria. Scattered cells containing juxtanuclear fibrous bodies are similar to cells of sparsely granulated somatotroph adenomas. Misplaced exocytosis is present. The secretory granules are sparse and small, measuring 150 to 200 nm.

NONTUMORAL LESIONS ASSOCIATED WITH HYPERPROLACTINEMIA

Many nontumoral conditions can be mistaken for prolactinomas. Thyrotroph hyperplasia is associated with primary hypothyroidism due to loss of feedback (Fig. 27-3).[51,52] It generally occurs in severe long-standing thyroid hypofunction, but has been described even in short-term hypothyroidism.[53] The correct diagnosis is important because this condition regresses with thyroid hormone replacement.[54] Idiopathic lactotroph hyperplasia is a rare cause of hyperprolactinemia that mistakenly can be taken for an expanding macroprolactinoma. The pituitary mass shape can help in the differential diagnosis. Inflammatory lesions, such as lymphocytic hypophysitis (occurring mainly during pregnancy and puerperium), and sarcoidosis can be misdiagnosed as lactotroph adenoma.[55–58]

PITUITARY PROLACTIN-SECRETING CARCINOMAS

Pituitary PRL-secreting carcinomas are exceedingly rare tumors that exhibit morphologic features indistinguishable from those of PRL-secreting adenomas. In addition to local invasiveness, distant intracranial and extracranial metastases in the nervous system and visceral metastases are the clues for the diagnosis of malignancy. Regarding intracranial lesions, sometimes it is difficult to distinguish between contiguity of

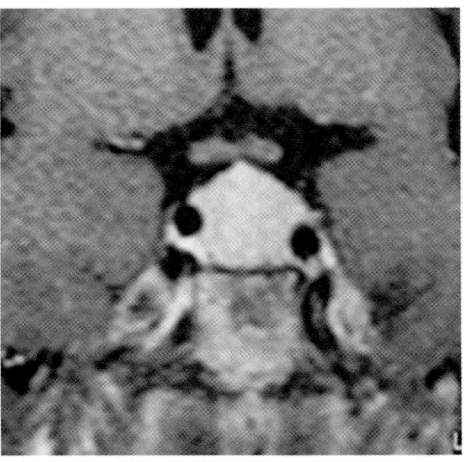
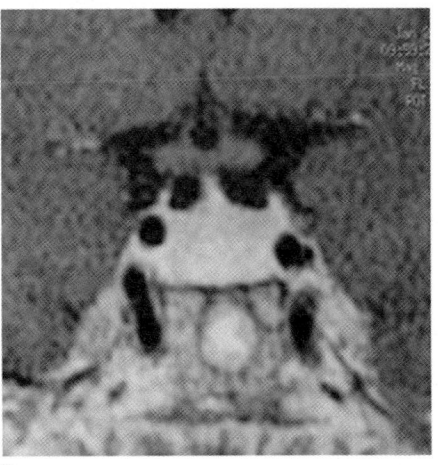

A   B

Figure 27-3 Magnetic resonance imaging (gadolinium-enhanced T1-weighted coronal views) of a 41-year-old woman with primary hypothyroidism before **(A)** and after 1 month on levothyroxine replacement therapy **(B)**. (From Bronstein MD: Problems in the differential diagnosis of the hyperprolactinemic patient. Clinical Endocrinology Update 2003, syllabus pp 241–247; with permission of the Endocrine Society.)

an invasive prolactinoma and true metastasis from a PRL-secreting carcinoma.[3,4]

DIFFERENTIAL DIAGNOSIS OF HYPERPROLACTINEMIA

The main causes of hyperprolactinemia are listed in Table 27-1.

PHYSIOLOGIC HYPERPROLACTINEMIA

Throughout pregnancy, the size of a normal pituitary increases up to 136%, according to magnetic resonance imaging (MRI) studies.[59] This extensive growth is due to estrogen-induced hypertrophy and hyperplasia of lactotrophs, leading to progressive increase in PRL production and its hypersecretion during pregnancy.[60,61] Placental estrogen production stimulates lactotroph mitosis, PRL mRNA levels, and PRL synthesis, leading to a stepwise increase in serum PRL levels, achieving mean levels of 200 ng/mL at the end of pregnancy and up to 450 ng/mL in some cases. Serum PRL levels decline quickly after delivery but are maintained slightly increased in

Table 27-1 Causes of Hyperprolactinemia

PHYSIOLOGIC
Pregnancy and puerperium
Neonatal period
Physical activity
"Stress"

DRUG-INDUCED
Dopamine receptor blockers
  Sulpiride
  Chlorpromazine
  Haloperidol
  Risperidone
  Metoclopramide
  Domperidone
Serotonin reuptake inhibitors
Cimetidine
Tricyclic antidepressants
Verapamil
Methyldopa
Protease inhibitors

PATHOLOGIC
Pituitary disease
  Prolactinomas
  Acromegaly
  Cushing's disease
  Nelson's syndrome
  Lymphocytic hypophysitis
  "Empty sella" syndrome
Hypothalamic disease and hypothalamus/pituitary disconnection
  Tumors
    Nonfunctioning pituitary adenomas
    Meningiomas
    Dysgerminomas
    Craniopharyngiomas
  Inflammatory/granulomatous
    Sarcoidosis
    Histiocytosis
  Stalk section
  Vascular
  Actinic
Neurogenic
  Chest wall lesions
  Spinal cord lesions
Miscellaneous
  Primary hypothyroidism
  Adrenal insufficiency
  Uremia
  Cirrhosis
  Paraneoplastic
  Idiopathic

nursing women several months, especially after breastfeeding. At birth, newborn serum PRL concentrations are elevated nearly 10-fold, probably as a result of the stimulatory effect of maternal estrogen levels.[62]

Because exercise and nonspecific stress are physiologic causes of hyperprolactinemia, there is a concern that the stress-induced PRL increase could lead to hormone elevation during venipuncture, and a period of rest before blood withdrawal is still recommended in many laboratories. A report by Vieira and coworkers,[63] which included a large population, provided evidence that rest before blood collection may be needed in only a few patients.

PHARMACOLOGIC HYPERPROLACTINEMIA

Among medications that increase serum PRL, dopamine receptor blockers are the most potent. Neuroleptics, such as sulpiride, haloperidol, chlorpromazine, and risperidone, and antiemetic drugs, such as metoclopramide and domperidone,[64–66] can elevate serum PRL to levels that usually are detected with prolactinomas. Serotoninergic and antihistaminergic drugs are less potent that antidopaminergic medications. The calcium channel blocker verapamil elevates serum PRL levels probably by decreasing central dopamine generation, possibly through N-type calcium channels.[67] It was shown that protease inhibitors used for treatment of acquired immunodeficiency syndrome can cause hyperprolactinemia, but the mechanism is unknown.[68] A detailed inquiry about drug use is mandatory for all hyperprolactinemic patients.

PATHOLOGIC HYPERPROLACTINEMIA

Hyperprolactinemia is present in about 40% of acromegalic patients as a result of GH/PRL cosecretion by the same or by different tumor cells or secondary to hypothalamus-pituitary disconnection.[69,70] Because of the characteristic features of acromegaly, the differential diagnosis is usually not a problem. As already mentioned, in patients harboring the rare acidophylic stem pituitary adenoma, serum GH is usually low compared with PRL levels, however, and acromegalic features are usually absent or minimally expressed.[50] In some cases, PRL resistance to dopamine agonists can be a clue for the differential diagnosis with prolactinomas.

Hyperprolactinemia secondary to impaired hypothalamic/tuberoinfundibular dopamine secretion or to stalk or even intrapituitary disconnection can be caused by tumors, inflammatory diseases, or trauma. In these cases, PRL is produced by normal lactotrophs and rarely exceeds 150 μg/L. The differential diagnosis of macroprolactinomas is mainly with the so-called clinically nonfunctioning pituitary adenomas (pseudoprolactinomas) and, to a lesser extent, with craniopharyngiomas.[48,70] Other tumoral lesions, such as meningiomas and chordomas, and nontumoral conditions, such as "empty sella" syndrome and even intrasellar aneurysms, can be associated with hyperprolactinemia, however (Fig. 27-4).[55] The differential diagnosis between macroprolactinomas and pseudoprolactinomas is crucial regarding their primary treatment—medical for macroprolactinomas and surgical for pseudoprolactinomas. Patients with nonfunctioning tumors treated with dopamine agonists were considered as having resistant macroprolactinomas due to the absence of tumor shrinkage, even with the (obvious) PRL decrease to very low or undetectable levels (Fig. 27-5).[71] A clue to differentiate pseudoprolactinomas from true prolactinomas is the dramatic early PRL decrease with bromocriptine doses of 1.25 mg/day.

Primary hypothyroidism can be associated with hyperprolactinemia, presumably due to high thyrotropin-releasing hormone levels that stimulate prolactin release, and presumably reduce prolactin metabolic clearance.[72,73] Thyrotroph hyperplasia may occur, leading to pituitary enlargement mimicking

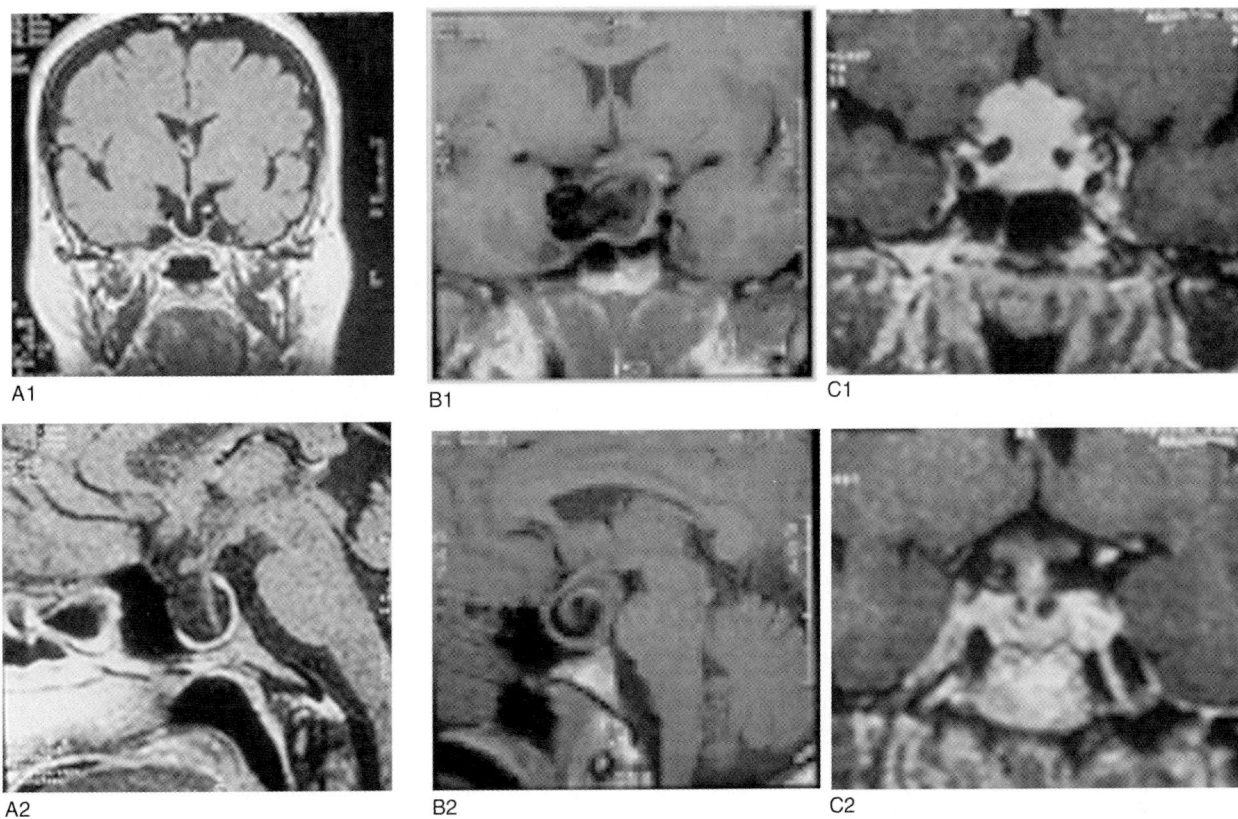

Figure 27-4 Magnetic resonance imaging of lesions (*1,* coronal views; *2,* sagittal views) associated with hyperprolactinemia: "empty sella" **(A1, A2)**, intrasellar aneurysm **(B1, B2)**, and meningioma **(C1, C2)**.

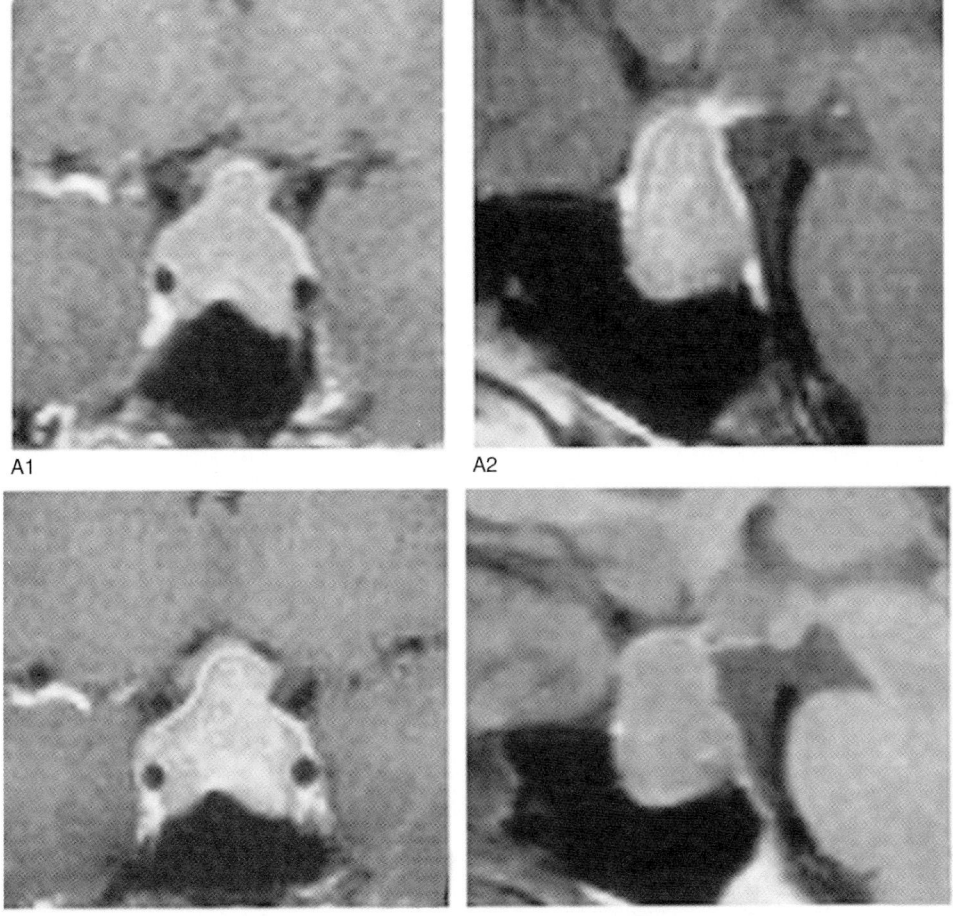

Figure 27-5 Magnetic resonance imaging of a 41-year-old woman with a nonfunctioning pituitary adenoma and serum prolactin level of 51 ng/mL before **(A1,** coronal views; **A2,** sagittal views) and during the 12th month of cabergoline "treatment" **(B1,** coronal views; **B2,** sagittal views). No tumor shrinkage was observed, despite serum prolactin decrease to 1.2 ng/mL. (From Bronstein MD: Problems in the differential diagnosis of the hyperprolactinemic patient. Clinical Endocrinology Update 2003, syllabus pp 241–247; with permission of the Endocrine Society.)

a pituitary adenoma (see Fig. 27-3).[51–53] Cushing's disease and adrenal insufficiency can be associated with hyperprolactinemia, which also can be present in Nelson's syndrome.[74,75] Polycystic ovary syndrome also may be associated with hyperprolactinemia.[76] Menstrual disturbances are prevalent in patients with polycystic ovary syndrome and in patients with prolactinomas, and sometimes the distinction between the two conditions may be difficult. The presence of mild hyperprolactinemia, negative pituitary imaging, high luteinizing hormone–to–follicle-stimulating hormone ratio, and clinical features suggestive of polycystic ovary syndrome can help in the differential diagnosis.

Uremia can be associated with hyperprolactinemia, mainly in patients with end-stage renal disease. The mechanism probably is related to reduced PRL clearance and to a presumably reduced dopaminergic tonus.[77] Serum PRL elevation is mild, but can be considerably increased in uremic patients taking drugs with a dopamine receptor–blocking effect.[78] Hyperprolactinemia is present in up to 20% of patients with liver cirrhosis, probably owing to an unbalanced estrogen-to-androgen ratio and to an altered dopaminergic tonus.[79] Nipple manipulation and chest wall lesions, such as herpes zoster and surgical scars, may increase serum PRL via stimulation of neuron pathways going through the spinal cord.[80–82] In contrast to paraneoplastic adrenocorticotropic hormone (ACTH) secretion, ectopic production of PRL has rarely been described.[83] Finally, when all the above-mentioned causes are ruled out, hyperprolactinemia is called *idiopathic* or *functional*. It is likely, however, that most patients with this condition harbor small microprolactinomas, which went undetected with less sensitive imaging tools used in the past, such as hypocycloidal polytomography and computed tomography (CT) and even with MRI. If there is no radiologic evidence of a prolactinoma at initial diagnosis of hyperprolactinemia, however, an identifiable adenoma is unlikely to develop in the long-term follow-up.[84]

DIAGNOSIS OF PROLACTINOMAS

CLINICAL FEATURES

Hyperprolactinemia and its impact on the gonadotropic axis is the hallmark of microprolactinomas and macroprolactinomas and their clinical manifestations. Macroprolactinomas also may cause neurologic and visual disturbances and impairment of other pituitary functions owing to the tumor mass effect (Table 27-2).[85] Loss of visual fields and impairment

of visual acuity are the main ophthalmologic manifestations.[86] Headache is the most common neurologic presentation, and it is attributed to dural stretch or cavernous sinus invasion and, less frequently, as part of the clinical symptoms of pituitary apoplexy.[87] There are few reports of special types of headache, such as the "SUNCT" syndrome secondary to prolactinomas, but the role of hyperprolactinemia as causative agent is obscure.[88] Other rare presentations of invasive macroprolactinomas are hydrocephalus,[89] neuropsychiatric manifestations, and otoneurologic manifestations.[90,91]

Women generally present with a correlation between the degree of serum PRL elevation and gonadal impairment, ranging from a short luteal phase to amenorrhea (Fig. 27-6).[92] Most PRL-secreting pituitary adenomas are associated with amenorrhea because hyperprolactinemia due to prolactinomas usually shows serum PRL levels greater than 100 ng/mL. Because hyperprolactinemia is present in about 20% of women with amenorrhea,[93] most patients with such menstrual disturbance and high serum PRL levels may harbor a prolactinoma. Because microprolactinomas can be associated with serum PRL levels between 40 and 100 ng/mL, and PRL biologic activity does not always correspond to routine laboratory assay levels,[94,95] however, some women with prolactinomas may exhibit milder forms of gonadotropic impairment, such as anovulatory cycles and oligomenorrhea.[96] In addition to menstrual disturbances, hyperprolactinemic women complain of loss of libido, vaginal dryness, dispareunia, and psychological distress.[97] Similar to other disorders associated with hypogonadism, osteoporosis is a frequent finding in women with hyperprolactinemia/prolactinomas, mainly in prolactinomas with long-standing hypogonadism.[98] The relative risk of developing osteoporosis in premenopausal women with prolactinomas can be 4.5.[99] Although a direct effect of PRL on bone has been considered, there is evidence that hyperprolactinemia is not a risk factor in itself for the development of osteoporosis, with the associated hypoestrogenism being the major determinant.[100,101]

Galactorrhea is a frequent finding in women with hyperprolactinemia, but it can be absent, mainly in patients with macroprolactinomas associated with severe hypogonadism. Breast examination, if not adequate, also may fail to disclose mild galactorrhea. These facts may explain the discrepancy among series, which show a prevalence of galactorrhea ranging from 30% to 84%.[93,102] Galactorrhea also may occur in normoprolactinemic women. A study including 235 patients with galactorrhea associated with diverse conditions showed that serum PRL was normal in 86% of women with idiopathic galactorrhea without amenorrhea.[103] The mechanism is unknown, being attributed to different causes, such as mammary hypersensitivity to PRL or "occult" transient hyperprolactinemia.

Table 27-2 Clinical Manifestations of Prolactinomas
RELATED TO HYPERPROLACTINEMIA
Gonadal impairment
Menstrual disturbances
Infertility
Sexual dysfunction
Osteoporosis
Galactorrhea
RELATED TO TUMOR MASS EFFECT
Visual disturbances
Visual field defects
Reduced visual acuity
Disturbances of ocular motility
Headache
Rare manifestations
Trigeminal neuralgia
Hydrocephalus
Otoneurologic
Neuropsychiatric
Impairment of other pituitary functions

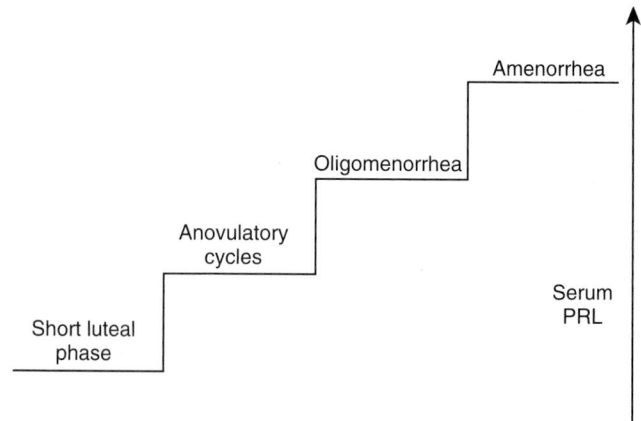

Figure 27-6 Serum prolactin (PRL) elevation and gonadal impairment.

Hyperprolactinemia in men is predominantly associated with macroprolactinomas. The main clinical manifestations are hypogonadism, which is usually severe, along with loss of libido and reduced body hair growth, visual impairment, and headache.[104,105] Only 22.5% of 80 patients with macroprolactinomas in our series sought medical assistance due to sexual complaints, whereas most patients requested appointments because of visual or neurologic disturbances. During the interview, 85% of the patients admitted, however, that loss of libido was of utmost importance.[106] In patients with microprolactinomas (n = 12), sexual dysfunction was the main complaint in 67% of the cases, but that number increased to 92% after the interview.[106] Although microadenomas are more frequent in women than in men, there are no sex-related differences in autopsy series, suggesting that the more objective clinical manifestations in women lead to more frequent and earlier searches for medical care. Testosterone replacement without serum PRL normalization seldom restores libido, an observation that points to a direct effect of PRL on sexual behavior, as previously suggested by animal models.[107,108] Galactorrhea is far less frequent in men than in women with prolactinomas.[109] It was disclosed in 15% and 25% of our patients with macroprolactinomas and microprolactinomas.[106] When present in men harboring pituitary tumors, however, it strongly suggests the presence of a prolactinoma (Fig. 27-7).[109] Osteoporosis also is present in hyperprolactinemic men.[110,111]

Although the prevalence of prolactinomas in both genders is higher in the 20s and 30s, prolactinomas can occur in elderly and in younger individuals. Data on 44 young patients (12 males and 32 females, aged 16.3 ± 1.9 years at diagnosis) with pituitary adenomas showed a predominance of macroadenomas (61%) over microadenomas (39%). Of those, prolactinomas were the most prevalent (68% of cases).[112] Other series on prolactinomas diagnosed in childhood or adolescence showed that the prevalence of macroadenomas was also higher (15 versus 11 cases)[113] or similar (24 versus 23 cases) compared with microadenomas.[114] The predominance of larger tumors in children and adolescents points to molecular mechanisms influencing proliferation rather than the time course of the disease influencing the progression of prolactinoma size and invasiveness.

LABORATORY EVALUATION

Basal serum PRL evaluation usually confirms the clinical suspicion of a prolactinoma. Serum PRL usually ranges from 50 to 300 ng/mL in the presence of microprolactinomas and from 200 to 5000 ng/mL in the presence of macroprolactinomas (normal values range from 2 to 15 ng/mL). Values of 30 ng/mL have been associated with microprolactinomas, however, and values of 35,000 ng/mL have been found in patients harboring large and invasive macroprolactinomas. Stimulation tests with thyrotropin-releasing hormone and metoclopramide or suppression tests using levodopa, previously popular mainly for the differential diagnosis of microprolactinomas and so-called idiopathic hyperprolactinemia,[115] give nonspecific results and have been largely abandoned.[116–118]

Hyperprolactinemia secondary to hypothalamus-pituitary disconnection rarely exceeds 150 ng/mL, and lesions that mimic macroprolactinomas, especially nonfunctioning pituitary adenomas, generally exhibit serum PRL less than this value (pseudoprolactinomas).[48,70] A laboratory artifact may lead to an erroneous differential diagnosis between macroprolactinomas and pseudoprolactinomas, however. When serum PRL is evaluated by two-site immunometric assays, large amounts of antigen—PRL in this case—saturate capture and signal antibodies, impairing their binding, causing serum PRL to be underestimated (the so-called high-dose hook effect). Patients bearing macroprolactinomas with extremely high serum PRL levels (generally >10,000 ng/mL, depending on the assay measuring range) may present with falsely lower levels, within the 30 to 150 ng/mL range, causing the patient to be misdiagnosed as harboring a nonfunctioning pituitary adenoma. To avoid unnecessary surgeries (treatment of choice for nonfunctioning tumors), PRL assays with serum dilution or using two-step incubation are recommended in patients with macroadenomas who may harbor a prolactinoma.[119–121] If such assays are not readily available, clinical clues pointing to prolactinomas are patient age younger than 50 years, presence of galactorrhea in male patients,[109] and tumor shrinkage under dopamine agonist drugs, as shown by fast visual improvement in cases with chiasmal compression or rapid tumor reduction evidenced by MRI.[119]

Another laboratory pitfall concerns the presence of high serum PRL levels in subjects with few or no symptoms related to PRL excess. Human PRL in circulation manifests as marked size heterogeneity, with three forms (23 kDa, 50 kDa, and 150 to 170 kDa) that are indistinguishable by routine assays.[122] The 23-kDa form (little PRL) is the most common form, but serum PRL can be elevated secondary to the presence of 150 to 170 kDa aggregates with low biologic activity (big-big PRL), leading to *macroprolactinemia*, a term coined by Jackson and colleagues[123] in the 1980s. Less frequently, the 50-kDa form

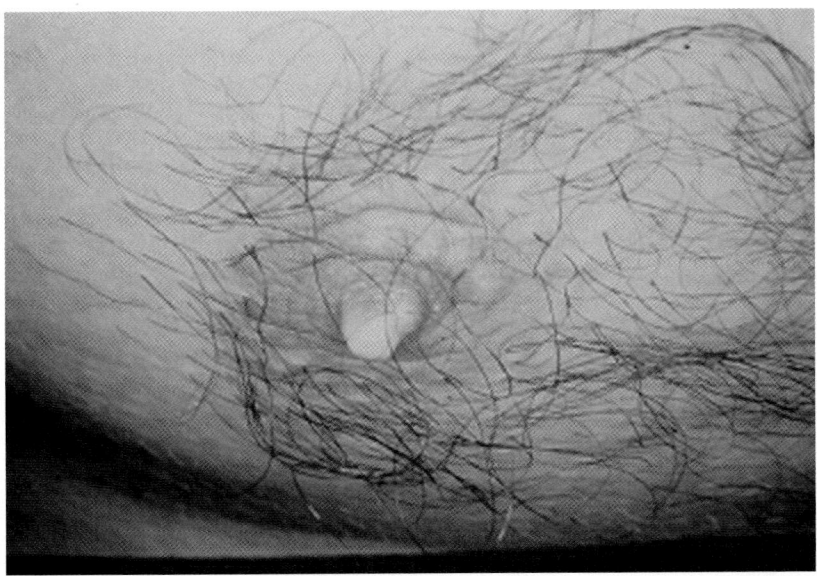

Figure 27-7 Galactorrhea in a man harboring a macroprolactinoma.

(big PRL) can be the prevalent circulating form.[124,125] The presence of molecular aggregates with low biologic activity, such as big-big PRL, should be suspected when high serum PRL levels are detected in patients without or with scarce signs and symptoms related to hyperprolactinemia.[5,126] Precipitation with polyethylene glycol is an excellent screening method.[127,128] The predominant molecular form recovered (i.e., assayed after the precipitation) is the highly biologically active little PRL. The gel filtration chromatography confirms the presence of big-big PRL (Fig. 27-8), but being a costly and time-consuming method, it is performed for practical clinical purposes only when polyethylene glycol precipitation results are inconclusive. Macroprolactinemia is a common finding, occurring in 8% to 42% of all cases of hyperprolactinemia.[5] The pathogenesis of macroprolactinemia is still unknown. It could be, in part, a complex of monomeric PRL with immunoglobulin G,[129] and anti-PRL autoantibodies were identified in some patients with idiopathic hyperprolactinemia.[130]

Big-big PRL biologic activity is still controversial in the literature. Studies in vitro with rat Nb2 cell bioassays show either the presence or the absence of biologic activity.[5] To explain the dissociation of presence of activity in vitro but not in vivo, we can speculate that, owing to its large molecular weight, macroprolactin does not cross the capillary barrier, and it is unable to reach target cells. Additionally, the PRL receptor forms of rat cells are different from those of humans, so a bioassay using human cells that addresses the biologic activity of macroprolactin is lacking. Despite these controversies in the literature concerning the biologic activity of PRL aggregates, most patients with macroprolactinemia do not manifest clinical features related to hyperprolactinemia and do not need any treatment. To avoid unnecessary medical or surgical procedures, macroprolactin screening is mandatory when clinical features and serum PRL assay results are conflicting.

Assessment of other pituitary functions is mandatory, mainly in the presence of macroprolactinomas. Insulin-like growth factor 1 must be followed either to verify GH deficiency or to disclose the rare cases of prolactinomas that progress with PRL/GH cosecretion.[131] Gonadotropin assessment may explain cases with persistent amenorrhea or sexual impairment despite PRL normalization. Although less frequently affected, thyrotropic and adrenocorticotropic axes also must be evaluated. Thyrotropin assessment also may disclose primary hypothyroidism as the cause of hyperprolactinemia.[72,73] Because restoration of pituitary function may occur after adenoma removal by surgery or tumor shrinkage attained by medical therapy,[91,132-134] these assessments have to be repeated after such procedures to avoid unnecessary hormone replacement.

IMAGING

The 1970s through 1990s witnessed the great advance in diagnosis by imaging, including neuroimaging of the hypothalamic-pituitary region, which evolved from polytomography (to disclose small masses)[135] and pneumocysternography (to assess suprasellar extension and "empty sella")[136] to MRI, passing through by CT. Concerning microadenomas, some studies point to a similar efficacy between CT and MRI. One study comparing the two methods in 33 patients with presumed microprolactinomas showed positive scans in 91% versus 64% of cases with MRI with gadolinium enhancement versus conventional CT scan. Respectively, when CT was performed with thin cuts and sequential imaging after iodinated contrast, however, the detection of microadenomas increased to 82%.[137] Another study of patients with surgically confirmed microadenomas showed similar sensitivity for the combination of conventional and dynamic serial CT scans compared with nonenhanced and gadolinium-enhanced MRI.[138] One report retrospectively correlating high-resolution coronal CT scans and surgical findings in 51 patients with a preoperative diagnosis of microprolactinomas showed, however, that only 39 of the patients had microadenomas at surgery. Twenty-three patients had identifiable lesions on CT scans. Of these, 21 had microadenomas, and 2 did not. Six patients with surgically proven microadenomas had normal CT scans.[139] This study shows a significant number of false-positive and false-negative cases of microprolactinomas in hyperprolactinemic patients evaluated by CT. Finally, many studies show better sensitivity of MRI compared with CT. One study disclosed only 3.2% of false-negativity with MRI versus 25.8% with CT.[140] Another study compared the two imaging modalities in 19 patients with suspected pituitary microadenomas who subsequently underwent transsphenoidal exploration of the pituitary fossa. CT correctly diagnosed microadenomas in 53% of the patients, whereas MRI was accurate in 89% of cases.[141] Although MRI is currently considered the gold standard imaging method for microprolactinomas, tumors measuring less than 2 mm may remain undetected by this technique. This fact is well known for the usually tiny ACTH-secreting adenomas leading to Cushing's disease, with about 50% of them not identified by MRI.[142] It is probable that many of the so-called idiopathic hyperprolactinemic patients harbor a small microprolactinoma. Procedures such as dynamic imaging with gadolinium enhancement may contribute to improve MRI sensitivity for such tiny adenomas (Fig. 27-9).

MRI is superior to CT for tumor boundary delineation, especially regarding its associations with the optic chiasm and cavernous sinus (Fig. 27-10). Additionally, tumor consistency, presence of hemorrhage, and presence of cystic lesions are

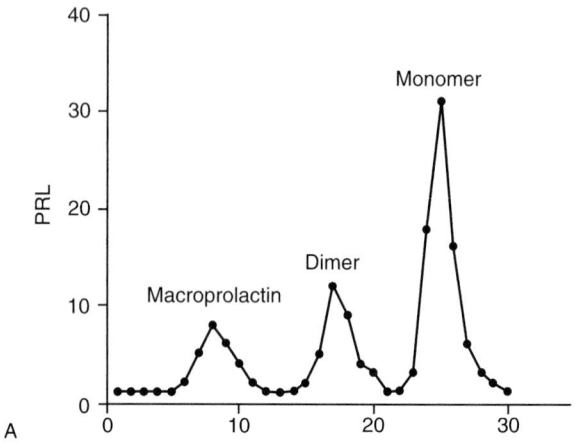

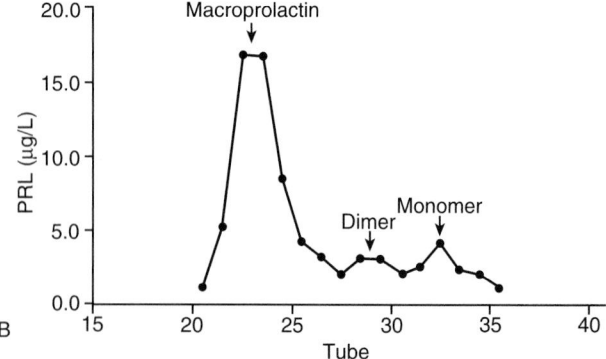

Figure 27-8 Gel filtration chromatography of a patient with symptomatic prolactinoma **(A)** and of an asymptomatic woman with macroprolactinemia **(B)**. PRL, prolactin.

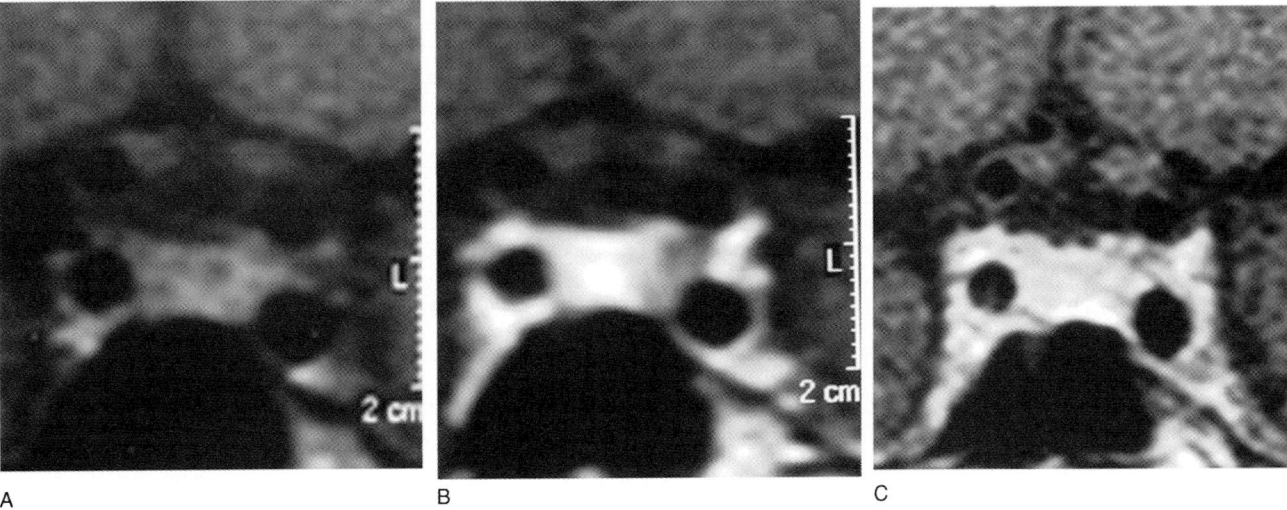

A   B   C

Figure 27-9 Magnetic resonance imaging (coronal views) of a microprolactinoma disclosed only during dynamic gadolinium-enhanced sequence. **A**, Before contrast injection. **B**, Lack of contrast enhancement on the left side of the pituitary gland suggestive of microadenoma. **C**, Whole gland contrasted.

better shown by MRI, especially comparing T1-weighted and T2-weighted images. CT has the advantage of showing bone erosion and calcifications[143,144]; however, this is dispensable if a plain skull x-ray, in addition to MRI, is available.

MRI can disclose the so-called *pituitary incidentaloma,* a term coined by Reincke in 1990 to describe incidentally discovered pituitary masses by imaging performed to evaluate conditions not linked to pituitary disease, including head trauma and sinusitis. Controversies exist in the literature concerning the definition of pituitary incidentalomas.[145] Molitch[146] included patients who presented with symptomatic pituitary disease and who were diagnosed only when a sellar mass was incidentally disclosed. In our opinion, the term *incidentaloma* should be reserved for cases with no endocrine or mass effects of a pituitary adenoma.[5] Incidental imaginig findings of pituitary adenomas, mainly microadenomas, are present in 26.7% of the autopsy findings in the general population.[12] Other imaging pitfalls include normal anatomic variations, such as asymmetric sphenoid septum with bulging of the sellar floor; displacement of the pituitary stalk[147]; artifacts, such as clips and prostheses; and global pituitary enlargement, either physiologic, as shown in puberty[148] and pregnancy,[149] or pathologic, as seen in primary hypothyroidism[53,54] and mental depression.[150]

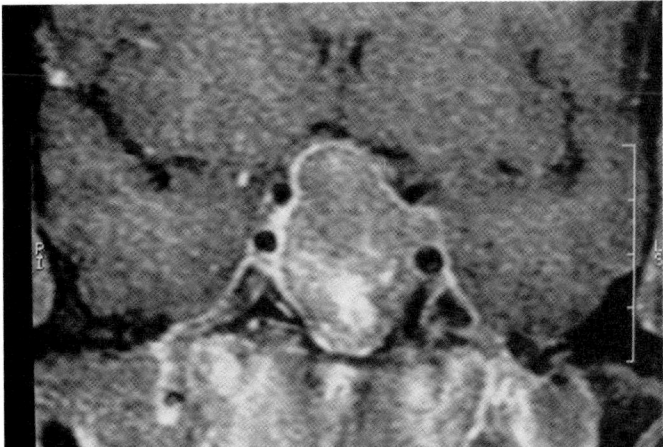

Figure 27-10 Magnetic resonance imaging (gadolinium-enhanced coronal view) showing optic chiasm compression and left cavernous sinus invasion by a macroadenoma.

Regarding the functional evaluation of prolactinomas by imaging, in vivo imaging by single-photon emission computed tomography using radiolabeled high-affinity benzamine derivatives to D2 receptors, such as iodine 123–methoxybenzamide or iodine 123–epipride, could serve as a response predictor to dopamine agonist treatment.[151,152] Positron emission tomography using 18-fluorodeoxyglucose, carbon 11–methionine, or dopamine D2 receptor ligands also has been used for in vivo assessment of the metabolic rate and D2 receptor density of macroprolactinomas and other pituitary tumors.[153] These methods are expensive and time consuming, however, and are better reserved for the study of tumors without a hormone marker, such as clinically nonfunctioning pituitary adenomas. Regarding prolactinomas, such techniques currently should be reserved for investigational purposes or for special cases, such as search for metastases in the rare malignant prolactinomas.[154] Figure 27-11 is a flow diagram for the diagnostic evaluation of hyperprolactinemia.

TREATMENT

The therapy of hyperprolactinemia/prolactinomas aims at reverting the symptoms dependent on hormone hypersecretion and the neurologic and visual manifestations due to tumor mass effect. The ideal treatment must spare or even improve other pituitary dysfunctions, if present. Good tolerance and low recurrence rates also are therapeutic goals.

Treatment of secundary hyperprolactinemia is intended to treat or remove the cause of the disorder. Levothyroxine usually corrects hyperprolactinemia associated with primary hypothyroidism. The surgical removal of a nonfunctioning pituitary adenoma with mass effect and withdrawal of drugs such as sulpiride and haloperidol, when possible, bring serum PRL down to normal levels.

As far as prolactinoma treatment is concerned, the 1970s brought, almost concomitantly, two powerful therapeutic advances: the improvement of pituitary microsurgery[2] and the development of ergot derivatives with potent dopaminergic agonistic activity.[155] Additionally, radiation therapy, including more recent stereotactic techniques, has a place, albeit restricted, in prolactinoma treatment (Table 27-3). Therapeutic strategy must consider several aspects, such as the patient's clinical presentation, the differences between microadenomas and macroadenomas concerning their natural history, the desire for pregnancy, and the patient's treatment preference, if applicable.

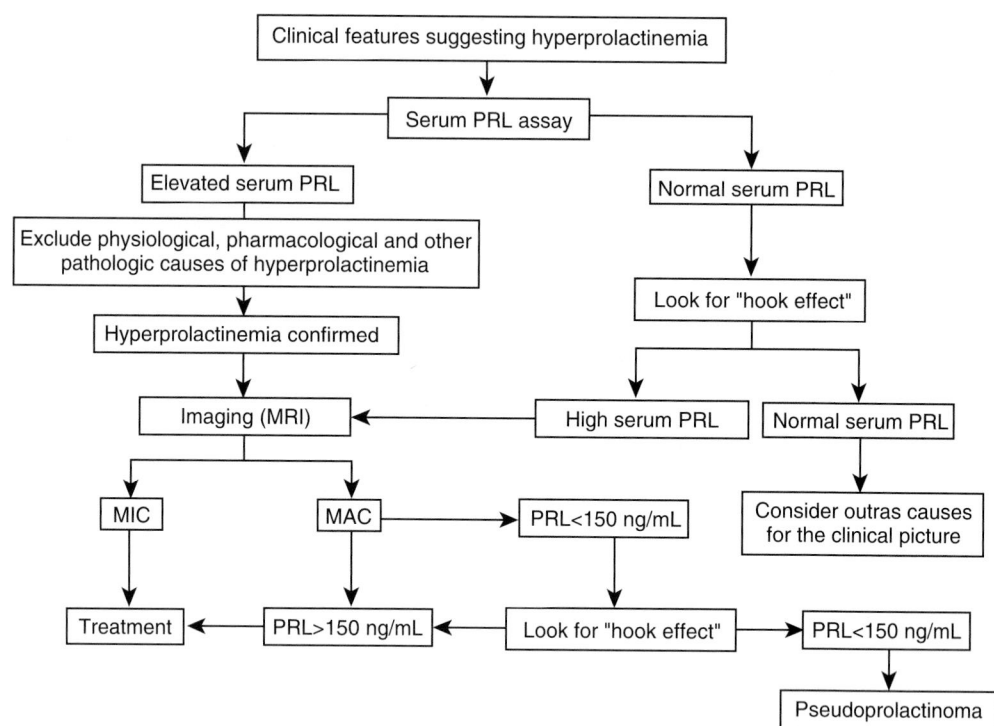

Figure 27-11 Flow diagram for the diagnostic evaluation of hyperprolactinemia. MAC, macroadenoma; MIC, microadenoma; PRL, prolactin.

SURGICAL THERAPY

Pituitary surgery by the transsphenoidal approach was used at the beginning of the twentieth century and was reintroduced in the early 1960s[156] and greatly improved when the surgical microscope was introduced.[2] More recently, endonasal endoscopic surgery has become available.[157] These developments made the selective removal of the pituitary adenoma possible, sparing the normal gland, along with low complication and mortality rates, mainly for surgeons with more than 500 operations.[158] Besides serum PRL normalization, this surgical modality aims at reducing or eliminating the mass effect of expanding macroadenomas, often leading to the resolution of neurologic and visual manifestations. The transcranial surgical approach is reserved solely for tumors with a predominance of extrasellar location, expanding out of the midline.[159]

The surgical success in normalizing serum PRL levels depends on the experience and ability of the surgeon and on the tumor size and invasiveness. Preoperative serum PRL levels, usually associated with tumor dimension and location, were found to be paramount in predicting surgical remission, being the only predictive factor in multivariate analysis in some reports.[160,161] Consequently, the best results were achieved in microprolactinomas with a preoperative serum PRL less than or equal to 100 ng/mL. In our own series, serum PRL was normalized in 62.5% of 64 patients with microprolactinomas (in 83% with preoperative PRL ≤100 ng/mL) and in 24% of 58 macroprolactinomas.[162] A study on the initial outcome of 219 women with prolactinomas operated on by transsphenoidal microsurgery showed a remission rate of 92% of cases with preoperative PRL less than or equal to 100 ng/mL and 91% with intrasellar microadenomas, but only 59% in women with microadenomas with cavernous sinus extension, leading to an overall remission rate of 82% for microadenomas. Of the women with macroprolactinomas, 88% with intrasellar adenomas, 86% with moderate suprasellar extension, and 80% with focal sphenoid sinus invasion achieved remission. Surgical remission in patients with diffuse sphenoid sinus invasion, cavernous sinus invasion, and major suprasellar extension was poor, however, ranging from 0% to 44%.[160] In another large series of 120 patients with prolactinomas (93 women and 27 men) who underwent pituitary surgery by the transsphenoidal route, PRL normalization occurred in 78% of patients with microadenomas, in 87.5% of patients with intrasellar macroadenomas, and in 27% of patients with extrasellar macroadenomas.[161]

A compilation of 34 published series showed that postsurgical serum PRL normalization was achieved in 73.7% of 1321 microprolactinomas and 32.4% of 1279 macroprolactinomas.[163] Comparison among the series is difficult, however, because many authors do not mention preoperative serum PRL levels, the tumor size, and degree of invasiveness. The grade of clinical improvement in cured patients is high, mainly in smaller tumors. Menses and fertility restoration is high, and pregnancy rates ranged from 75% to 90% in different series. Some patients can achieve menstrual regulation and even become pregnant without full PRL normalization.[161,164] Sexual improvement in men is less likely to occur, probably owing to irreversible gonadotropic damage caused by the higher frequency of extrasellar and invasive prolactinomas compared with women. Nonetheless, pituitary function generally is preserved in intrasellar adenomas, and is restored by the removal of suprasellar adenomas causing hypothalamus-pituitary disconnection.[161] In addition, neurologic and visual amelioration often is achieved after pituitary surgery.

Table 27-3	Treatment of Prolactinomas

MEDICAL
Dopamine agonist drugs
Sexual steroid replacement (for selective microprolactinomas)

SURGICAL
Transsphenoidal approach
    Sublabial
    Endonasal (with or without endoscope)

RADIOTHERAPY
Conventional
Stereotactic
    Cobalt-60 or linear acceleration (LINAC)
    Single shot ("radiosurgery") or multiple shots
Proton beam

Many patients bearing prolactinomas have undergone treatment with dopamine agonist drugs before surgery. The effect of previous medical therapy on surgical outcome is still a matter of debate. Some reports point to poorer results compared with nontreated patients[165,166]; others do not show significant differences.[161,162] There is also evidence, however, of improvement of surgical results in the medically pretreated group.[167] Because the issue of dopamine agonist–induced fibrosis remains unresolved, it is unclear whether the negative outcome was caused directly by the drug or whether it was biased by a tendency to treat medically large and invasive tumors, which present with the poorest surgical results.

An important caveat of surgical treatment is prolactinoma recurrence. This issue was raised in the early 1980s, when an article from the Montreal group reported recurrence rates in surgically "cured" patients to be 50% for microprolactinomas and 80% for macroprolactinomas.[168] Subsequently, several reports on this issue were published, but with less impressive figures. A literature compilation reported recurrence rates of 21% of 544 microprolactinomas and 19.8% of 253 macroprolactinomas.[163] In our series, the recurrence of hyperprolactinemia in surgically cured patients was 27% for microprolactinomas and 17% for macroprolactinomas.[164] Median time to recurrence varied among the different surgical series, from 1 to 7 years. Concerning recurrence predictors, many studies pointed to higher postoperative serum PRL levels in patients who recurred compared with patients without recurrence,[160,168–171] whereas others did not find serum PRL levels to be a predictor of late outcome.[172] Another marker of recurrence is the absence of PRL response to dynamic tests, especially to thyrotropin-releasing hormone.[161,170–172] These findings raise the question whether, in prolactinomas, serum PRL increase after surgical normalization represents true recurrence or important but incomplete tumor removal.

Although the occurrence of relapses contributes to the decrease of long-term surgical cure rate of prolactinomas, many patients with recurrent hyperprolactinemia remain asymptomatic and have no evidence of tumor regrowth.[160,171,173] Relapse can be transient. From a cohort of 44 patients with surgically cured microprolactinomas, 8 (18.2%) experienced recurrence and were followed up. Only two of the eight patients experienced permanent relapse.[174] Additional therapy is reserved only for patients with symptomatic recurrence.

Surgical treatment for prolactinomas is indicated for cases with persistent intolerance or hormonal or tumor resistance to dopamine agonists (see later); pituitary apoplexy[175,176]; tumor growth during medical therapy[177]; cerebrospinal fluid (CSF) leakage due to dopamine agonist–induced tumor shrinkage of invasive macroprolactinomas[178,179]; and, rarely, visual loss on medical therapy, secondary to optic chiasm herniation resulting from tumor retraction.[180] Additionally, surgery is an excellent alternative for patients harboring microprolactinomas, especially patients with serum PRL less than or equal to 100 ng/mL, with poor compliance to medical therapy.[160,162,181]

MEDICAL THERAPY

The knowledge that dopamine is a powerful inhibitor of PRL secretion has yielded insights regarding use of dopamine agonists in hyperprolactinemia treatment.

Bromocriptine

At the end of the 1960s, an ergot derivative, 2-bromo-α-ergocryptine (bromocriptine) was developed, and shortly thereafter its use in clinical trials was initiated.[155,182] Bromocriptine binds and stimulates the seven-membrane–spanning dopamine D2 receptors in normal and in adenomatous lactotrope cells, inducing activation of the G_i receptor (negatively coupled to adenylate cyclase) and, consequently, leading to postreceptor events that ultimately cause the inhibition of PRL synthesis and

secretion.[183] Although many other dopamine agonist drugs were developed thereafter, bromocriptine is still the one that presents the largest and longest worldwide experience (Table 27-4).

Pharmacokinetic studies with bromocriptine show that after a single oral dose of 2.5 mg, serum levels peak, and maximal suppressive action occurs between 1 and 3 hours. The drug has a relatively short mean elimination half-life (about 6.2 hours) and generally is administered twice a day.[184] Owing to a considerable interindividual variability in the PRL-lowering effects of a given dose of bromocriptine, however, some patients need to take the drug three times a day and others just once a day, mainly when higher doses are required or normoprolactinemia already has been achieved.[185]

Bromocriptine treatment results in serum PRL normalization and clinical improvement in most patients with hyperprolactinemia/prolactinomas. A compilation of 13 series from the literature encompassing 286 women treated with bromocriptine showed PRL normalization and return of menses from 64% to 100% and 57% to 100% of cases.[186] Our data showed evidence of normoprolactinemia in 55% of patients with microprolactinoma treated primarily or postsurgically with bromocriptine (mean dose 3.8 mg/day), with menses return in 98% of the patients. Of women without PRL normalization, 81% also recovered menses, making unnecessary the increase of bromocriptine dose, optimizing drug tolerance and reducing costs.[164] Although less frequent, microprolactinoma in men also can be treated successfully with dopamine agonists. Of 12 patients predominantly treated with bromocriptine, 83% achieved normal PRL level and clinical improvement.[187] Eleven men with microprolactinoma have been treated by us, with serum PRL and serum testosterone normalization in 73% and 86% of them.[106]

Because macroprolactinomas often present with mass effect, they were first surgically treated and, if not cured, then treated with bromocriptine. The observation by Corenblum and colleagues[188] in the mid-1970s that bromocriptine use reduces tumor size in addition to its PRL-lowering effect, consequently relieving neurologic and visual complaints, also allowed primary treatment for macroprolactinomas. In a prospective multicenter trial, normal PRL levels were achieved in 18 of 27 patients (67%) followed up for at least 12 months while receiving variable doses of bromocriptine.[189] All patients exhibited some degree of tumor shrinkage: 9, less than 25%; 5, between 25% and 50%; and 13, greater than 50% tumor size reduction. Another study with macroprolactinomas with extrasellar extension showed serum PRL normalization in all of the 10 men and 17 of 19 women, with mean bromocriptine doses of 13 mg/day and 8 mg/day. Tumor size was reduced by more than 50% in 18 of 29 patients (62%) with a secondary empty sella in 5 cases and by less than 50% in 11 patients. Visual field improved in most of the patients who initially presented with such abnormalities.[190] Patients with giant prolactinomas (diameter >4 cm) also achieved disease control with primary bromocriptine therapy.[191] In our series, serum PRL was normalized in 60% of women with macroprolactinomas (mean bromocriptine dose 7 mg/day); 72% of these women had menses recovery. Menses

Table 27-4	Main Dopamine Agonist Drugs
Drug	**Usual Dose**
Bromocriptine	2.5–10 mg/day
Pergolide	0.025–0.5 mg/day
Quinagolide*	0.075–0.6 mg/day
Cabergoline	0.5–2 mg/wk

*Not approved in the United States.

also were restored in 44% of patients who remained hyperprolactinemic.[164] The lower rate of menses normalization compared with women harboring microprolactinomas is probably due to the higher prevalence of gonadotropic impairment in the macroprolactinoma group. Regarding macroprolactinoma in men, serum PRL and testosterone levels normalized in 67% and 85% of 66 patients bearing macroprolactinomas, showing that also in men the gonadotropic axis may normalize even when PRL is not fully normalized.[106] Other series show different figures, with PRL returning to normal levels in 83% of patients, but with testosterone normalization in only 62% of them, probably reflecting different degrees of gonadotropic impairment. We obtained 80% of tumor reduction in primarily treated macroprolactinoma patients.

The mechanism of prolactinoma shrinkage by dopamine agonists is not yet fully understood. Some reports in the early 1980s suggested that tumor reduction was due to lactotrope cell size reduction.[192,193] Bromocriptine decreases mRNA and PRL synthesis within days and cell multiplication (antiproliferative and proapoptotic mechanisms have been suggested) and tumor growth.[194,195] These events are evidenced quickly microscopically by a decrease in the number of PRL secretory granules, involution of the rough endoplasmic reticulum and Golgi apparatus, and decrease of cytoplasmic volume. With longer periods of treatment (e.g., 6 months), there is evidence of cell vacuolization and fragmentation with collagen deposition.[196] These early and late morphologic changes of the tumor lactotropes may explain the rapid regrowth of macroprolactinomas when bromocriptine is discontinued after a short period of therapy,[197,198] whereas often no tumor expansion is observed when the drug is withdrawn after being used for a longer period.[199,200] Serum PRL levels may be suppressed in some patients without tumor shrinkage, although the converse does not occur.

The degree of macroprolactinoma reduction by bromocriptine and its time course have been carefully analyzed.[201] Data on 271 patients included from prospective series on primary therapy of true macroprolactinomas showed that 79% of patients presented with more than 25% shrinkage and that 89% of them had shrunk to some degree. Pretreatment serum PRL concentration and gender difference did not predict the degree of tumor reduction. Of 102 prolactinomas large enough to produce chiasmal compression, 85% showed tumor shrinkage of more than 25%. Another compilation, including eight series from the literature totaling 112 patients with macroprolactinomas,[202] showed that 40.2% had a greater than 50% reduction in tumor size; in 28.6%, the reduction was 25% to 50%; in 12.5%, the reduction was less than 25%; and 18.7% had no evidence of tumor size reduction (Table 27-5). The time course of macroprolactinoma shrinkage is highly variable. Some patients experience a dramatic improvement of visual acuity 12 hours after

bromocriptine has been introduced, with tumor shrinkage being documented within 1 week. In others, significant tumor reduction is observed only 1 year after medical therapy has been started. In the U.S. multicenter study cited previously,[189] 19 patients had tumor shrinkage in 6 weeks, but in 8 others, the reduction was not observed until the 6-month imaging reassessment was performed. General data from most series show that rapid shrinkage occurs during the first 6 months in most cases, with slower reduction thereafter, with additional decreases in tumor size observed after 1 year for several years in some cases. Visual improvement generally parallels and often precedes tumor shrinkage, unless the optic tract has been chronically and severely damaged. Figure 27-12 illustrates an unusual case of long-term macroprolactinoma shrinkage, showing that minor tumor reduction, even when not depicted by imaging, is sufficient for visual field improvement. In such situations, the clinical amelioration signified that the primary medical therapy was effective even without clear tumor shrinkage, and pituitary surgery could be postponed or, as it was in this case, needless.

Macroprolactinoma reexpansion during successful medical therapy, albeit uncommon, may occur and can lead to visual impairment recurrence.[177] Another rare situation is visual deterioration despite initial improvement, in parallel with tumor shrinkage during medical treatment, provoked by chiasm herniation, which may result from traction on the optic chiasm that is pulled down into the now partially empty sella. The two above-mentioned situations generally require surgical intervention, although drug reduction or discontinuation may repair the chiasm herniation.[180] In addition, pituitary surgery often is needed for a third rare situation, CSF leakage occurring in macroprolactinomas invading the sphenoid sinus, in cases treated with dopamine agonists (Fig. 27-13). In such cases, the tumor shrinkage behaves as the cork removed from a wine bottle, opening a pathway for CSF flow. CSF leakage, which brings a risk for meningitis, often

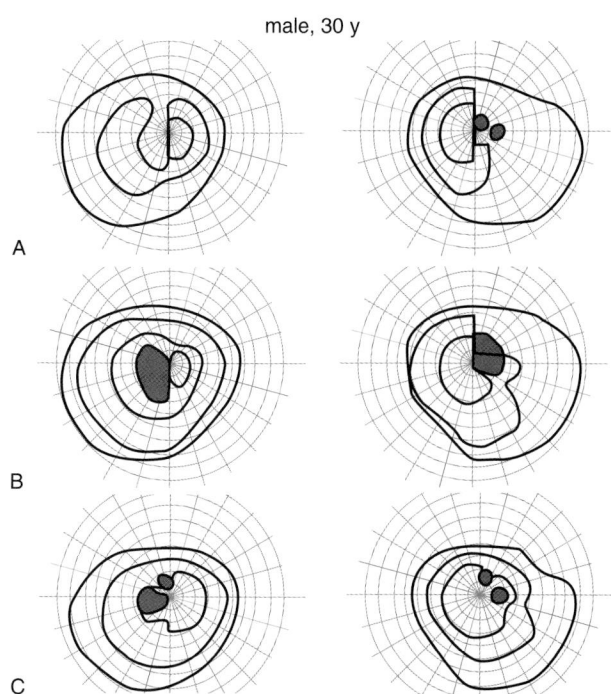

Figure 27-12 Visual fields (Goldman perimetry) of a 30-year-old man harboring a macroprolactinoma. Impaired visual fields before treatment (**A**) showed amelioration 3 days after the beginning of bromocriptine treatment (**B**) and almost normalized after 28 days (**C**) of drug therapy.

Table 27-5	Comparison of Efficacy of Dopamine Agonists in Effecting Tumor Size Reduction				
		Tumor Size Reduction (%)			
Dopamine Agonist	**No. Cases**	**>50**	**25–50**	**<25**	**No Change**
Bromocriptine	112	40.2	28.6	12.5	18.7
Pergolide	61	75.4	9.8	8.2	6.5
Quinagolide*	105	48.1	20.2	17.3	14.4*
Cabergoline	320	28.4	28.4	14.8	28.4

*Not approved in the United States.
From Molitch ME: Medical management of prolactin-secreting pituitary adenomas. Pituitary 5:55–65, 2002.

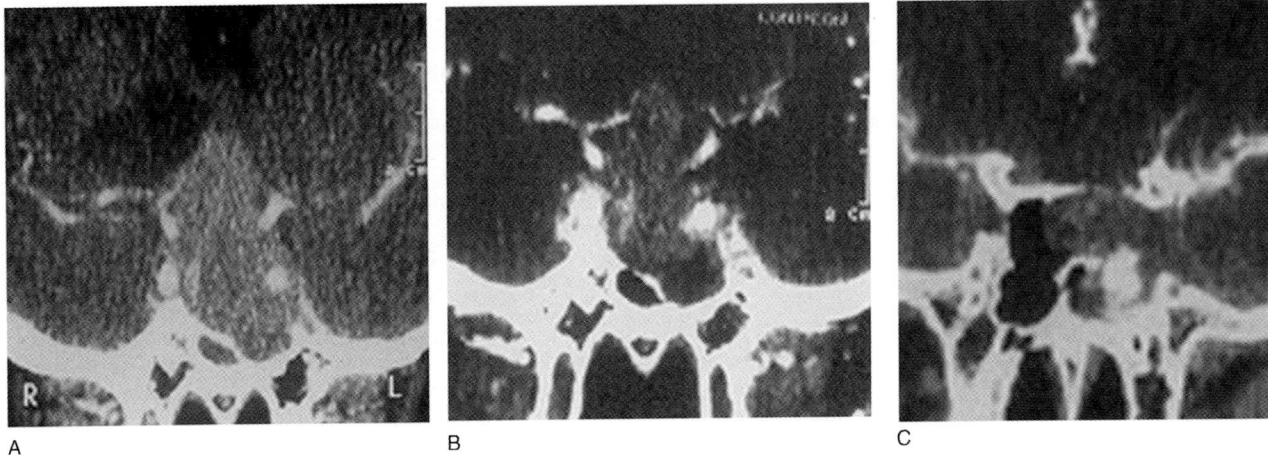

Figure 27-13 Computed tomography (coronal views) of a man harboring a macroprolactinoma invading the sphenoid sinus before **(A)** and 6 days after bromocriptine treatment showing shrinkage mainly of the sphenoid sinus mass **(B)** with cerebrospinal fluid leakage confirmed by metrizamide injection **(C)**.

occurs shortly after the beginning of medical therapy,[179] but may manifest several months later.[178]

Besides its effect on visual and neurologic symptoms, bromocriptine-induced shrinkage of macroprolactinomas can recover other impaired anterior pituitary functions as a result of the restoration of hypothalamus-pituitary connection, which has been compromised by the tumor mass effect.[91,132–134] To avoid the maintenance of unnecessary hormonal replacement, pituitary function must be reassessed in patients with macroprolactinoma and previous hypopituitarism successfully treated by dopamine agonists.

Despite the effectiveness of medical therapy for prolactinomas, one of the drawbacks is the need for long-term therapy. Treatment with bromocriptine and other dopamine agonist drugs generally is considered as "symptomatic" because bromocriptine discontinuation leads to recurrence of hyperprolactinemia in most patients and, as previously mentioned, to tumor regrowth, at least after short-term use. Concerning long-term therapy with bromocriptine, a retrospective study from our group showed that 25.8% of 62 patients with microprolactinomas and 15.9% of 69 patients with macroprolactinomas treated with bromocriptine for a median time of 47 months continued to be normoprolactinemic after a median time of 44 months of drug withdrawal.[203] There were no statistically significant differences regarding age, gender, bromocriptine initial dose and length of use, tumor size, pregnancy during treatment, and previous pituitary surgery or radiotherapy among patients who continued to be normoprolactinemic and patients who did not. Other reports from the literature point to a percentage of patients who remained normoprolactinemic after bromocriptine interruption ranging from 6.6% to 37.5% (Table 27-6).[203] The question regarding why long-term findings differ from short-term findings may be answered by the formerly described microscopic alterations of the lactotrope during bromocriptine administration, suggesting a cytostatic effect related to short-term therapy and a cytocidal effect related to long-term treatment, which could explain the maintenance of normoprolactinemia after drug withdrawal.[204]

Another factor that may influence remission of prolactinomas is their natural history. A study including 25 women with untreated hyperprolactinemia (18 microadenomas, 7 macroadenomas) for a mean period of 11.3 years (mean initial PRL levels 225 ng/mL) showed that 7 of 22 patients with amenorrhea resumed menses spontaneously. Galactorrhea resolved completely in 8 of 19 patients. Only one patient had a slight progression of sellar abnormality. At the reevaluation, mean PRL levels had decreased to 155 ng/mL.[205] Another report was concerned with 30 women with hyperprolactinemia (18 with normal pituitary imaging or empty sella) without treatment, followed for an average time of 5.2 years. Of the women, 35% showed improvement in clinical symptoms. Six of 30 women had increased PRL levels, 14 showed no changes, and 10 had a decrease with PRL normalization in 6.[206] A study of 41 patients with "idiopathic" hyperprolactinemia followed for 1 year found that 83% of patients had unchanged PRL levels or even showed a decrease, and 34% showed normalization of PRL levels.[84]

Table 27-6	Overview of Studies on Normoprolactinemia after Bromocriptine (BRC) Withdrawal				
Author	Year	No.	Normal Prolactin after BRC Withdrawal (%)	Mean Period of BRC Use (mo)	Period without BRC (mo)
Zarate et al.	1983	16	37.5	24	24 (mean)
Johnston et al.	1984	15	6.6	44	1.25–3.5
Rasmussen et al.	1987	75	44	24	≥6
Wang et al.	1987	24	21	24	12–48
Winkelmann et al.	1988	40	18.4	48	5–25
Van't Verlaat et al.	1991	12	8.3	58.8	12 (mean)
Passos et al.	2002	131	20.6	47	44 (mean)

From Passos VQ, Souza JJS, Musolino NRC, et al: Long-term follow-up of prolactininomas: Normoprolactinemia after bromocriptine withdrawal. J Clin Endocrinol Metab 87:3578–3582, 2002.

During a mean period of 31 months, 38 patients with microprolactinomas were followed without treatment. Nearly 55% of patients had normalization of PRL levels, and there was no evidence of tumor growth.[207] Finally, there is evidence that women with hyperprolactinemia who experience menopause have a significant chance of normalizing their PRL levels, pointing to estrogen influence.[208,209] These data on untreated patients indicate that natural history has an important role in the outcome of prolactinomas and PRL normalization. The mechanisms involved are yet to be clarified, however. Although bromocriptine use has been associated with pituitary apoplexy,[210] the evolution of one of our patients who became normoprolactinemic, shown in Figure 27-14, which shows a bright T1-weighted image without contrast on MRI highly indicative of hemorrhage before medical treatment, suggested that subclinical pituitary apoplexy may play a role in the natural history of prolactinomas and PRL normalization.

Whatever the mechanisms involved, there is a subset of patients with prolactinomas treated with bromocriptine who maintain normoprolactinemia after drug withdrawal without any predictive factor. We suggest that a gradual drug dose reduction should be attempted, along with PRL level monitoring in patients under dopamine agonist use who show normalization of PRL levels. To avoid unnecessary treatment, drug withdrawal can be attempted in this group of patients, with periodic reassessments.

Among the problems associated with medical treatment of prolactinomas, drug side effects are the most prevalent. Bromocriptine is generally well tolerated with doses between 2.5 and 20 mg/day. The most frequent side effects are nausea, vomiting, and orthostatic hypotension and, to a lesser extent, nasal congestion, headache, constipation, and psychotic events, such as auditory hallucinations, delusional ideas, and mood changes. The drug should be given carefully to psychiatric patients.[211] There are isolated reports of leukopenia, hepatitis, headaches, and cardiac arrhythmias. Higher doses (20 to 140 mg daily), used for patients with Parkinson's disease, may lead to pleural effusions, thickening and parenchymal lung changes, and retroperitoneal fibrosis.[212]

Bromocriptine side effects can be minimized by starting therapy at 1.25 mg at bedtime after food intake and progressively increasing it to include 1.25 mg a day after breakfast and at bedtime, according to individual tolerance, until the therapeutic dose is achieved. When normoprolactinemia is obtained, the dose can be reduced in many cases.[213] A subset of patients remain intolerant, however, even when all such recommendations are followed. Our data show persistent intolerance to bromocriptine in 24% and 12% of women harboring microprolactinomas and macroprolactinomas and in 5% of men with macroprolactinomas. Intolerance to bromocriptine may be overcome in some cases with a slow-releasing oral formulation (bromocriptine SRO), which also can be used as a once-a-day formulation.[214] We did not find better tolerance of this extended oral form, however, compared with the regular formulation. A single long-lasting injectable form (bromocriptine LA), with 50 mg of the drug, peaking after 2 hours and lasting for 28 days, which was developed for lactation inhibition, was efficacious for prolactinoma treatment, mainly in patients with intracranial hypertension and vomiting.[215] Thereafter an injectable repeatable form was developed (bromocriptine-LAR), with good local and systemic tolerance, even in patients who were previously intolerant to the oral formulation.[91,216] The injectable forms of bromocriptine are not commercially available, however. Additionally, the use of bromocriptine by the intravaginal route offered better tolerance for some patients, probably as a result of a slower drug absorption, but the absence of a local upper gastrointestinal effect of oral bromocriptine cannot be excluded.[217] The administration is bothersome, however, and there are local side effects, such as vaginal irritation. With the development of better-tolerated new oral drugs, the intravaginal administration of bromocriptine for prolactinoma treatment is now seldom employed.

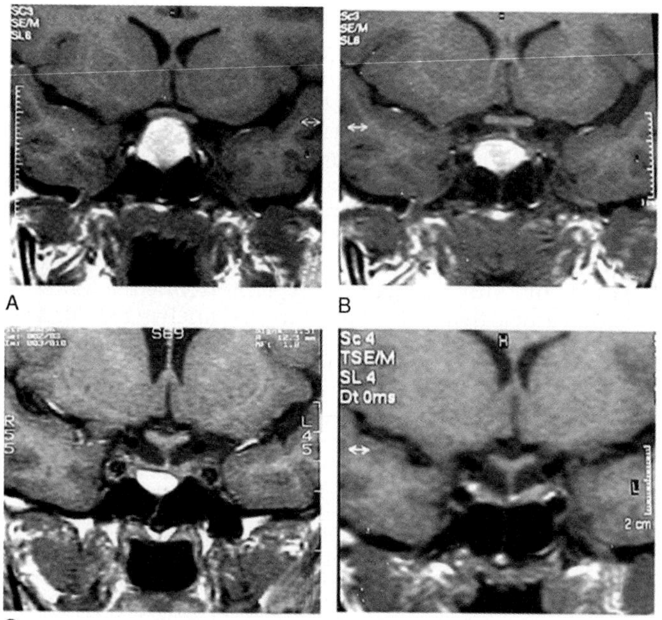

An even more vexing problem in the medical treatment of prolactinomas is their partial or complete lack of responsiveness to bromocriptine. The definition of bromocriptine resistance is arbitrary, with the failure of the drug in normalizing serum PRL levels or in reducing the tumor size using a dose equal to or greater than 15 mg/day for at least 3 months being the most currently accepted. According to this principle, about 10% of prolactinomas are resistant to bromocriptine.[218] This criterion has limitations regarding clinical practice, however. Patients who are intolerant to bromocriptine would not attain the dose established as limit, and although they are different conceptually, bromocriptine intolerance and resistance overlap. Patients harboring expanding tumors with visual impairment should not wait for 3 months without an improvement. As previously mentioned, clinical amelioration and tumor reduction may be achieved even if serum PRL is still above the normal range.[164] Pragmatically, bromocriptine resistance can be defined as the failure to obtain adequate clinical results in patients using the highest tolerable drug dose.

Mechanisms implicated for bromocriptine resistance of prolactinomas have not yet been fully elucidated. Studies in vivo and in vitro using radiolabeled dopamine antagonists as markers show that dopamine D2 receptor density is reduced in resistant prolactinomas compared with tumors that are responsive to bromocriptine.[219] When the D2 receptor density in lactotrope cell membranes is extremely low, the dopamine agonist drug paradoxically may lead to tumor growth.[219] The paucity of dopamine D2 receptors seems to be the main mechanism of bromocriptine resistance in prolactinomas. Additionally, postreceptor events have been described, includ-

Figure 27-14　Magnetic resonance imaging (T1-weighted coronal views without gadolinium enhancement) of a 14-year-old girl harboring a macroadenoma. A, Before treatment (prolactin, 108 ng/mL). B, 2 months on bromocriptine (2.5 mg/day). C, 8 months on bromocriptine (5 mg/day) (prolactin, 18 ng/mL). D, 16 months after bromocriptine withdrawal (prolactin, 13 ng/mL). (From Passos VQ, Souza JJ, Musolino NR, et al: Long-term follow-up of prolactinomas: Normoprolactinemia after bromocriptine withdrawal. J Clin Endocrinol Metab 87:3578–3582.)

ing decreased ratio between the short and long isoforms of the dopamine D2 receptor, derived from alternative splicing.[220] No mutations in the dopamine D2 receptor that could be ascribed to the bromocriptine resistance have been described to date.[36]

Some prolactinomas that are initially responsive to bromocriptine become resistant during therapy.[221] In such situations, especially in aggressive tumors, the diagnosis of the rare PRL-secreting carcinoma must be considered.[21,218]

Several other dopamine agonist drugs have been employed for the treatment of hyperprolactinemia/prolactinomas (see Table 27-3). Many show therapeutic efficacy, but three of them in particular merit detailed description, aiming mainly at overcoming intolerance and resistance to bromocriptine.

Pergolide
Pergolide is an ergot derivative, with an estimated potency 100 times that of bromocriptine, that has been approved by the U.S. Food and Drug Administration only for Parkinson's disease therapy. Considerable data concerning prolactinoma treatment have been collected, however, since the 1980s.[222–228] The drug can be given once daily in a dose ranging from 0.025 to 0.5 mg. Used in new patients or after a long period of other dopamine agonist drug withdrawal, pergolide has been effective in normalizing serum PRL levels in 31 of 47 patients with microprolactinomas and macroprolactinomas (with menses resumption in 76% of women and testosterone increase in 71% of men)[222] and in 68% of 44 patients with macroprolactinomas.[223,224] When pergolide is compared with bromocriptine, some studies point to similar efficacy and tolerance of both drugs,[225,226] whereas others favor pergolide.[227,228] Regarding tumor reduction, a compilation of 61 patients with macroprolactinoma shows 75.4% of cases with more than 50% shrinkage and 9.8% of patients with adenoma reduction between 25% and 50% (see Table 27-5).[202] A few cases of heart valvulopathy occurring in patients taking pergolide for Parkinson's disease have been reported.[229]

Quinagolide (CV 205-502)
Quinagolide is a nonergot dopamine agonist drug that has specific affinity to the dopamine D2 receptor. Its efficacy in normalizing serum PRL levels is similar to that of bromocriptine, ranging from 45% to 100%, with most studies with macroprolactinomas showing PRL normalization between 58% and 75%, paralleled by clinical improvement.[230–234] Quinagolide is administered once a day in doses ranging from 0.075 mg to 0.6 mg. Some studies point to better tolerance compared with bromocriptine.[233,234] Additionally, there is evidence that about 50% of patients with bromocriptine-resistant prolactinomas attained normoprolactinemia when switched to quinagolide.[235,236] Such tumors were partially responsive to bromocriptine, however, with the further decrease attributed to better patient tolerance and a higher affinity to the already reduced but still present dopamine D2 receptors. Prolactinoma patients who are severely resistant to bromocriptine are not expected to respond to quinagolide either. Tumor size reduction evaluated in 105 patients showed more than 50% shrinkage and reduction between 25% and 50% in 48.1% and 20.2% of cases (see Table 27-5).[202] Quinagolide is commercially available only in Europe.

Cabergoline
Cabergoline is a synthetic ergoline that shows high specificity and affinity for the dopamine D2 receptor. It is a potent and long-acting inhibitor of PRL secretion, with an elimination half-life ranging between 63 and 109 hours.[237] PRL-lowering effects occur rapidly within 3 hours and were evident after a single-dose administration at the end of follow up (21 days) in puerperal women and at 14 days in patients with hyperprolactinemia. This pharmacologic profile allows cabergoline to be administered once or twice a week in most patients,

usually at a weekly dose of 0.5 to 2 mg. In our experience, normoprolactinemia was maintained in some patients taking one tablet (0.5 mg) of cabergoline every 10 days and even every 2 weeks. Many studies have shown the efficacy of cabergoline in normalizing serum PRL levels and reducing tumor size, with consequent improvement of clinical and visual manifestations (Fig. 27-15). In 127 hyperprolactinemic patients (71 microprolactinomas, 19 macroprolactinomas, 37 idiopathic), cabergoline was administered at a dose between 0.25 and 3.5 mg/wk, given once or twice weekly in 114 patients and three times weekly or daily in 13 cases. Serum PRL levels were normalized in 114 patients (90%). Of 56 women with amenorrhea, 52 resumed menses; 17 women became pregnant; and sexual potency was restored in the three men. A total of 48 mild-to-moderate adverse events were reported by 29 patients (23%).[238]

In a study comprising 37 new patients, cabergoline normalized PRL levels in 88% of 26 microprolactinomas and in 100% of 11 macroprolactinomas. Regular menses were restored in 7 of 10 macroprolactinomas and in all oligomenorrheic patients with microadenoma; serum testosterone levels normalized in 2 of 3 hypogonadial men. Side effects developed in only three cases.[239] Another study with cabergoline (0.5 to 3 mg/wk) administered once per week was conducted in 15 patients (8 women) with macroprolactinomas. Normal PRL levels were attained in 73% of cases. Gonadal function was restored in all hypogonadial men and in 75% of premenopausal women with amenorrhea. Side effects were minimal.[240]

Many studies pointed to better efficacy and tolerance of cabergoline compared with bromocriptine (Table 27-7).[241–245] Of 37 bromocriptine-intolerant prolactinoma patients studied by our group, only 5 remained intolerant when switched to cabergoline.[244] In a large multicenter European comparative study encompassing 459 women with hyperprolactinemic amenorrhea, 0.5 to 1 mg of cabergoline twice weekly was more effective than 2.5 to 5 mg of bromocriptine twice daily in the treatment of hyperprolactinemic amenorrhea, restoring ovulatory cycles in 72% of women and normalizing plasma PRL levels in 83% compared with 52% and 59% for bromocriptine. Adverse effects were recorded in 68% of women taking cabergoline and 78% of women taking bromocriptine, but only 3% discontinued cabergoline, whereas 12% stopped taking bromocriptine due to drug intolerance.[241] Regarding cabergoline effect on macroprolactinoma size, in a compilation of 12 series including 320 patients, 28.4% had a greater than 50% tumor shrinkage, 28.4% had a reduction between 25% and 50%, and 43% had less than 25% or no reduction at all (see Table 27-5).[202] Because many of these patients had been previously intolerant or resistant to other dopamine agonists, the poorer cabergoline results for macroprolactinoma shrinkage compared with other drugs may have been biased. This bias can be illustrated by a study showing that the prevalence of macroprolactinoma shrinkage greater than 80% after cabergoline treatment was higher in naive patients (92.3%) than in patients who were previously intolerant (42.1%), resistant (30.3%), or responsive (38.4%) to bromocriptine or quinagolide.[246] As far as dopamine agonist resistance in prolactinomas is concerned, some studies indicate that cabergoline normalized serum PRL levels in patients who were resistant to bromocriptine and even to quinagolide. In two series dealing with bromocriptine-treated prolactinomas without full PRL normalization, normoprolactinemia was achieved in 70% and 85% of patients when they were switched to cabergoline.[243,247] As previously pointed out (see section on Quinagolide), such tumors did respond partially to bromocriptine, however, and the additional decrease brought up by cabergoline is probably related to its better tolerability and higher affinity to the reduced but still present dopamine D2 receptors. Consequently, severely resistant prolactinomas are not expected to respond to any

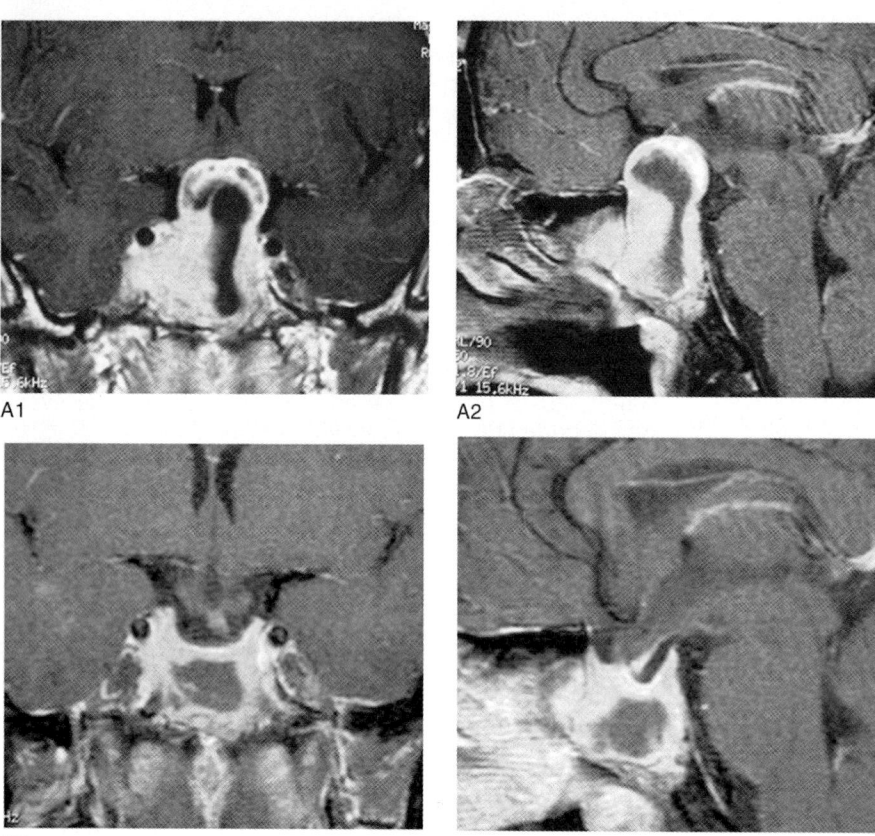

Figure 27-15 Magnetic resonance imaging (T1-weighted with gadolinium enhancement) of a man bearing a large macroprolactinoma. **A1** (coronal view) and **A2** (sagittal view), before treatment. **B1** (coronal view) and **B2** (sagittal view), after 1 month of cabergoline treatment, showing significant tumor shrinkage that was paralleled by visual improvement.

dopamine agonist drug and have to be treated by a different means.

Some studies pointed out maintenance of normoprolactinemia in 31% of patients after cabergoline withdrawal for 12 months, on average.[238,239,248] A long-term follow-up study including 200 hyperprolactinemic patients showed that after 2 to 5 years after cabergoline withdrawal, normoprolactinemia still persisted in 76% of patients with "nontumoral" hyperprolactinemia, in 70% of patients with microprolactinomas, and in 65% of patients with macroprolactinomas.[249]

These results suggest that cabergoline compares favorably with bromocriptine also in terms of maintenance of normal PRL levels after drug withdrawal.[203]

Medical therapy seems to be the first option for prolactinoma therapy, being more effective than surgery, especially for macroprolactinomas.[250] To date, cabergoline seems to be the first-choice drug for prolactinoma treatment in view of its remarkable tolerance, capacity to normalize serum PRL levels, reduce tumor size, and induce high rates of normoprolactinemia persistence after drug withdrawal.

RADIOTHERAPY

The efficacy of conventional radiation therapy for prolactinomas is lower than medical or surgical treatment. Our results of 19 patients submitted to radiotherapy after medical/surgical failure showed that only 3 (16%) achieved serum PRL normalization 5, 6, and 15 years after the procedure.[164] A study with 63 patients treated with radiation after noncurative surgery showed that only 30% had normal PRL levels by 10 years.[251] A compilation from the literature shows serum PRL normalization in less than one third of patients 5 to 15 years after conventional radiotherapy, with hypopituitarism occurring in 5.5% to 93.3% of cases.[252] This prevalence is probably greater because many series have underestimated GH deficiency in adults.

There are emerging data on gamma knife radiosurgery for prolactinomas. In one retrospective investigation, the authors examined the results of gamma knife radiosurgery for tumor remnants after unsuccessful open surgery and medical treatment in 20 patients with prolactinomas. Serum PRL levels decreased into the normal range in five cases (25%). Patients treated with dopamine agonists during gamma knife radiosurgery did significantly less well compared with the untreated group, suggesting a "radioprotective" effect of the drug.[253]

Table 27-7	Treatment of Hyperprolactinemia: Comparison between Bromocriptine (BRC) and Cabergoline (CAB) Efficacy and Tolerability		
Author (n)	**Treatment Characteristics**	**BRC**	**CAB**
Webster et al., 1994[241] (n = 459)	Prolactin normalization	58%	83%
	Ovulatory cycles	52%	72%
	Side effects	78%	68%
	Withdrawal	12%	3%
	Prevailing dose	2.5 mg 2×/day	0.5 mg 2×/wk
Sabuncu et al., 2001[245] (n = 34)	Prolactin normalization	59%	82%
	Side effects	53%	12%
Pascal-Vigneron et al., 1995[242] (n = 120)	Prolactin normalization	48%	93%
	Ovulatory cycles	48%	72%
	Side effects	65%	53%
	Digestive side effects	86%	37%

Another study including 128 patients estimated the efficacy of gamma knife radiosurgery as the primary therapy for prolactinomas. The mean follow-up time was 33.2 months (range, 6 to 72 months). Tumor control was observed in all but two patients who underwent surgery 18 and 36 months after gamma knife radiosurgery. Clinical cure was achieved in 67 cases (52%). Nine infertile women became pregnant 2 to 13 months after irradiation, and all gave birth to normal infants. There was no visual deterioration related to gamma knife radiosurgery. This study points to better results in terms of PRL normalization, but does not mention the impact of treatment on pituitary function, besides of mentioning five women who experienced "premature menopause."[254] More data and follow-up time are required to assess the superiority of gamma knife radiosurgery compared with conventional radiotherapy. To date, in the author's opinion, radiation therapy for prolactinomas is reserved for cases with medical and surgical failures, especially for invasive tumors.

THERAPEUTIC PERSPECTIVES

As a result of the efficacy of medical and surgical therapies, most patients with prolactinomas can be controlled adequately. A subset of patients resistant to dopamine agonists, especially patients harboring invasive macroadenomas, who are not expected to be surgically cured, pose an important therapeutic problem. Radiotherapy, as described earlier, is generally efficacious only in the long-term and usually leads to hypopituitarism.

Many studies did not find tumor enlargement in patients with "idiopathic" hyperprolactinemia or microprolactinomas, before or after menopause.[208,255,256] When pregnancy is not a concern, and galactorrhea is not disturbing, sexual steroid replacement can be considered for those patients, who must be followed carefully. Additionally, testosterone may be given to men harboring resistant microprolactinomas and even partially resistant macroprolactinomas, with monitoring of PRL levels and with imaging. The introduction of an aromatase inhibitor drug may be considered if there is evidence of tumor growth or serum PRL increase.[257]

Prolactinomas usually do not respond to somatostatin.[258] It has been shown, however, that a selective analogue of the somatostatin receptor subtype 5 inhibited PRL secretion in human prolactinoma cell culture.[259] Nevertheless, another in vitro study did not show better response of this selective analogue compared with quinagolide.[260] More recently, an analogue that acts in four of the five somatostatin receptor subtypes has been developed. Although some reports point to in vitro inhibition of PRL secretion,[261,262] more studies, mainly in vivo, are needed to verify the efficacy of this "universal" analogue and other somatostatin receptor subtype analogues for the treatment of resistant prolactinomas.

There is evidence that nerve growth factor expression is reduced in resistant prolactinomas[263] and that this growth factor restores p53 function in pituitary cell lines.[264] Nerve growth factor administration to athymic mice with transplanted human bromocriptine-resistant prolactinomas results in the expression of dopamine D2 receptors in the tumor and restores sensitivity to subsequent treatment with bromocriptine. This could be a promising therapy for patients who are refractory to dopamine-agonist treatment.[265]

Studies show that the human PTTG induces angiogenesis via basic fibroblast growth factor induction[266] and that estrogen is involved in paracrine regulation of pituitary tumorigenesis by PTTG. Selective estrogen receptor modulators, such as tamoxifen and raloxifene, and inhibitors, such as ICI 182780, abolished estrogen-induced pituitary PTTG expression in vivo, suppressed serum PRL concentrations by 88%, and attenuated PRL-secreting pituitary tumor growth by 41% in rats. Antiestrogen treatment of primary human pituitary tumor cultures reduced PTTG expression approximately 65%.[26] These findings may indicate a role for selective antiestrogens in prolactinoma treatment, including resistant ones. Figure 27-16 summarizes the current therapeutic approach to resistant prolactinomas.

PROLACTINOMAS AND PREGNANCY

The development of efficacious medical and surgical therapies for prolactinomas has made pregnancy possible for women bearing such tumors. Gestational risks due to the possibility of tumor growth during pregnancy, mainly in women with macroadenomas, raise a concern, however. The management of pregnancy in patients with prolactinomas submitted to different therapies is brought into focus here.

Regarding microprolactinomas, a study including 91 pregnancies mostly induced by bromocriptine, without previous surgery or radiotherapy, indicated symptomatic tumor growth in 5.5% of cases.[267] In a compilation of pregnancies in 246 women with microprolactinomas treated with bromocriptine only, tumor growth symptoms were reported in 1.6% of patients, although an asymptomatic increase of the tumor was shown in 4.5% of the cases. None of the patients needed surgical intervention during pregnancy.[268] We followed 71 term pregnancies, and the results were similar.[269] Of the 22 patients with previous surgery, none presented symptoms of tumor growth; of the 41 pregnant patients who underwent treatment with bromocriptine alone, only 1 (2.4%) presented with headaches in the third month of pregnancy, which regressed with drug reintroduction. Seven patients got pregnant without treatment and did not develop any complications. There was an asymptomatic increase of the tumor in one case with previous surgery and in two cases with bromocriptine alone, as assessed by scanning postpartum. Because of the low risk of tumor growth during pregnancy in patients with microprolactinomas, there is no need to perform periodic imaging or ophthalmologic examinations. These assessments should be reserved for cases with clinical complaints suggesting tumor growth, such as headache or visual field changes.

The risk of complications during pregnancy is much greater with macroprolactinomas. One study revealed symptomatic tumor growth in 41.3% of 56 pregnancies occurring in 46 patients who were medically treated only compared with 7.1% of 70 pregnancies that occurred in 67 women who previously had been submitted to surgery or radiotherapy.[267] A review from the literature pointed to symptoms related to

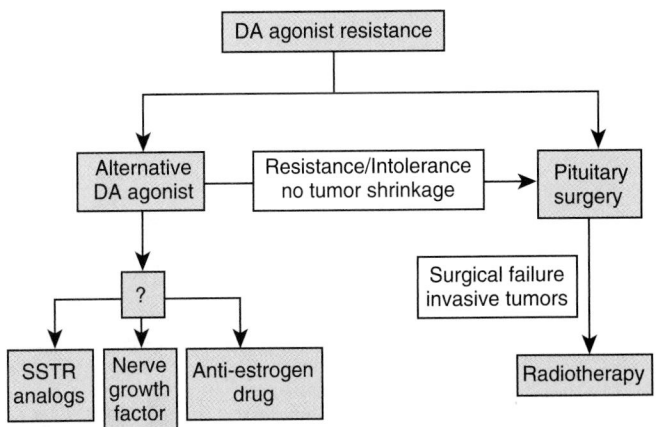

Figure 27-16 Algorithm of therapeutic strategies for resistant prolactinomas. DA, dopamine; SSTR analogues, somatostatin receptor subtype ligand specific analogues.

tumor growth in 15.5% of 45 patients with macroprolactinomas treated with bromocriptine only. The incidence of complications was only 4.3% in the 46 patients who underwent surgery or radiotherapy before pregnancy. Additionally, asymptomatic tumor growth was seen in 8.9% of the patients without prior surgery or radiotherapy.[268] We followed 51 term pregnancies in patients with macroprolactinomas.[269] Of those, 21 were in patients with previous surgery, and none of the patients presented with symptoms or signs of tumor growth. Of the 30 patients treated with pregestational bromocriptine only, 11 (37%) manifested complaints related to tumor growth: All of them presented with headaches, and seven had visual alterations (Fig. 27-17). Pituitary imaging after delivery was performed in 23 other patients, and an asymptomatic growth of the tumor was observed in 4 more cases.

These data show the higher risk of tumor growth in macroprolactinomas during pregnancy, necessitating a stricter follow-up (Fig. 27-18). The first recommendation should be the use of a nonhormonal contraceptive along with a dopamine agonist until tumor shrinkage has been shown within sellar boundaries. The duration of previous treatment with dopamine also might be important. A follow-up study of 37 pregnancies showed signs of tumor growth in 7, all of them treated with bromocriptine for less than 1 year. No tumor enlargement was found in the 14 macroprolactinoma patients treated for a longer time, suggesting that the duration of bromocriptine use before conception might be a good prognostic factor in pregnancy.[270]

After pregnancy has been confirmed, the dopamine agonist can be withdrawn, and the patient must be monitored closely for symptoms related to tumor growth. If there is a suspected tumor expansion, the confirmation can be made through MRI, after the fourth month of gestation, and by visual field testing (see Fig. 27-18). Monitoring serum PRL levels during pregnancy does not seem to be useful because they are not always related to tumor behavior during gestation. The reintroduction of bromocriptine in such cases often leads to clinical amelioration and tumor reduction.[271-274] In 9 of 11 patients who exhibited complications during pregnancy, bromocriptine reintroduction brought complete resolution of the symptoms related to tumor growth.[275] Surgery also can be employed as treatment for symptomatic tumor growth in pregnancy. Several authors have reported good results,[276,277] although the increased risk of spontaneous abortion in patients who undergo surgery is well known.[278]

The safety of bromocriptine reintroduction or even maintenance during pregnancy is supported by a large experience with this dopamine agonist reported in the literature. A large review[279] consisted of 2587 pregnancies and did not show an increase of maternal or fetal morbidity or mortality.

Since then, some authors have favored the maintenance of bromocriptine in pregnancy to prevent complications in patients with macroprolactinomas without previous surgery or radiotherapy.[280,281] It is our policy to indicate such an approach only when the patient gets pregnant after a short treatment period, mainly without confirmation of tumor shrinkage or when the tumor is outside sellar boundaries. Surgery is indicated before pregnancy in cases without tumor reduction during treatment with dopamine agonists or in patients who developed tumor growth in previous gestations.[275]

Pregnancy and Other Dopamine Agonist Drugs
In recent years, the use of new dopamine agonists, such as quinagolide, cabergoline, and pergolide, for the treatment of hyperprolactinemia has increased, and pregnancies have been described. Data were obtained on 176 pregnancies, in which quinagolide was used, on average, for 37 days. Miscarriages occurred in 14% of the cases, with one ectopic pregnancy. Fetal malformation was described in nine cases, although other drugs had been used in three patients.[282] Quinagolide was used successfully during pregnancy in two bromocriptine-resistant patients who presented symptoms of tumor growth.[236] Cabergoline has been the most used medication among the more recent dopamine agonist drugs, and reports on pregnancies during cabergoline therapy are emerging. We followed six full-term gestations in patients who withdrew cabergoline as soon as pregnancy was confirmed and did not observe malformations, but two premature births occurred.[275] The largest review to date was made in 1996, with 204 gestations, and they did not observe an increase of spontaneous abortion (12%) or malformations (four cases).[283] More recent publications regarding gestations induced by cabergoline have not reported complications either.[239,243] A patient who used cabergoline, 0.5 mg twice a week from 18 to 37 weeks' gestation, showed tumor reduction and delivered a healthy infant.[284] Nevertheless, the drug's long action, which persists 3 weeks after its withdrawal, associated with fewer data compared with bromocriptine (around 360 versus >6000 pregnancies) (Table 27-8), still limits its indication for patients who wish to conceive or its use during pregnancy. Regarding pergolide, animal data point to its safety in pregnancy.[285] No human data are available to date.

Follow-up after Delivery
Breastfeeding does not increase the risk of tumor growth in patients who progressed well during pregnancy.[270,275,286] Breastfeeding is contraindicated only when patients need to maintain the dopamine agonist after delivery, owing to tumor growth signs.

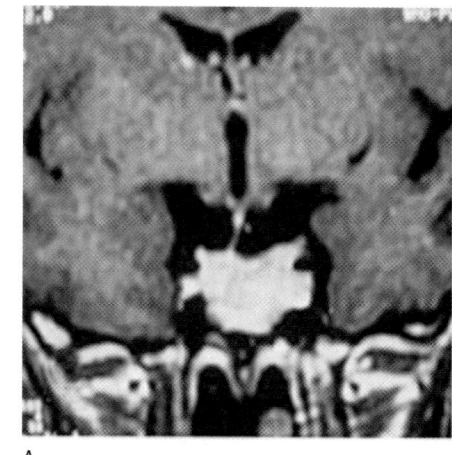
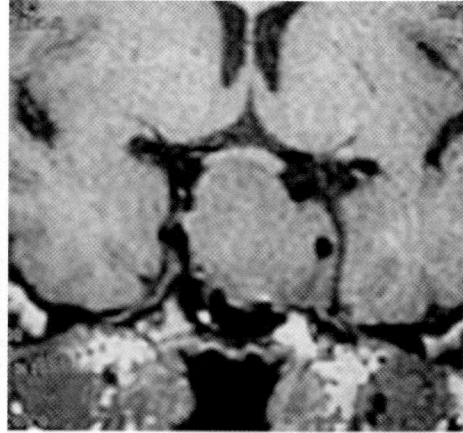

Figure 27-17 Magnetic resonance imaging (coronal views) of a patient with macroprolactinoma. **A,** Tumor is limited to sellar boundaries during bromocriptine treatment, before pregnancy. **B,** Tumor growth during the 4th month of pregnancy without bromocriptine use. (From Musolino NRC, Bronstein MD: Prolactinomas and pregnancy. In Bronstein MD [ed]: Pituitary Tumors in Pregnancy. Boston, Kluwer Academic Publishers, 2001, pp 91–108.)

A   B

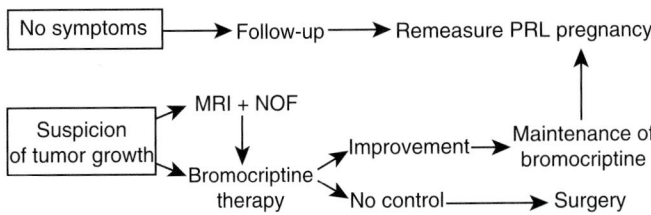

Figure 27-18 Suggested algorithm for the follow-up of patients with macroprolactinoma during pregnancy. NOF, neuroophthalmologic examination; PRL, prolactin. (From Musolino NRC, Bronstein MD: Prolactinomas and pregnancy. In Bronstein MD [ed]: Pituitary Tumors in Pregnancy. Boston, Kluwer Academic Publishers, 2001, pp 91–108.)

There have been several reports in the literature regarding reduction or normalization of serum PRL levels after delivery.[268,273,277,287] In our hands, 60% and 72% of patients with microprolactinomas and macroprolactinomas showed a decrease in PRL levels after delivery compared with pregestational levels. In 11% of all patients who conceived, PRL levels normalized after pregnancy, some with a new gestation without therapy. On average, PRL levels decreased from 336 ± 105 ng/mL to 133 ± 20 ng/mL in 62 patients who were available for comparison.[269] These results are similar to ones reported by other authors. A study observed a reduction in serum PRL in 19 of 38 patients and normalization in three other cases,[273] and another study[287] reported PRL normalization after pregnancy in 29% of women. Tumor reduction after preg-

nancy also has been described. A study with 16 patients harboring prolactinomas found 27% of tumor reduction or disappearance after delivery.[288] We also observed tumor reduction in 8 of 23 patients with macroprolactinomas, assessed by imaging before and after delivery. Two other patients developed asymptomatic apoplexy. The explanation for this "curative" effect of pregnancy is to be clarified. It may be related partly to modifications in the vasculature of the adenoma due to the estrogen stimulation, resulting in necrosis or microinfarctions of the adenomatous tissue. Hemorrhagic zones in prolactinoma patients receiving estrogen therapy already have been described.[289]

Another issue of concern is the outcome of the children whose mothers took dopamine agonist drugs during pregnancy. One study reported the follow-up spanning 4 months to 9 years in 546 children exposed to intrauterine bromocriptine.[279] The authors did not find any developmental impairment in the children. We followed 70 children born to mothers who conceived on bromocriptine.[269] At a mean follow-up of 67 months (range, 12 to 240 months), only two children presented with disorders of neuropsychomotor development: one case of idiopathic hydrocephaly and another of tuberous sclerosis. We did not find any similar reports in the literature. Fifteen of these children already had started puberty, one of them precociously.

TREATMENT PLANNING AND FOLLOW-UP

Based on the previously described evidence, to date, the gold-standard therapy for either microprolactinomas or macroprolactinomas is medical treatment with dopamine agonist drugs (Fig. 27-19). Physicians must motivate patients to embark on such long-term treatment based on the overall better results compared with surgery and, mainly based on more recent data,[203,249] the possibility of drug withdrawal for a substantial number of patients with maintenance of normoprolactinemia. Surgical treatment of prolactinomas is indicated for patients with persistent intolerance or hormonal or tumor resistance to more than one dopamine agonist drug—in particular if pregnancy is desired—or if the tumor has grown during medical treatment. In cases of resistance, rare conditions, such as acidophil stem cell adenoma or PRL-secreting carcinomas, must be considered. Malignant prolactinomas respond only temporarily, if they respond at all, when patients are switched to another dopamine agonist drug or undergo surgery. Chemotherapy also is usually ineffective. Surgical therapy also is indicated frequently in pituitary

Table 27-8 Effect of Bromocriptine on Pregnancies

	Bromocriptine		
	n	%	Normal Population (%)
Pregnancies	6239	100	100
Spontaneous abortion	620	9.9	10–15
Terminations	75	1.25	
Ectopic	31	0.5	0.5–1
Hydatidiform moles	11	0.2	0.05–0.7
Deliveries (known duration)	4139	100	100
At term (≥38 wk)	3620	87.5	85
Preterm (<38 wk)	519	12.5	15
Deliveries (known outcome)	5120	100	100
Single births	5031	9.3	8.7
Multiple births	89	1.7	1.3
Infants (known details)	5213	100	100
Normal	5030	96.5	95.0
With malformations	93	1.8	3–4
With perinatal disorders	90	1.7	≥2

Data from Krupp P, Monka C, Richter K: Program of the Second World Congress of Gynecology and Obstetrics, Rio de Janeiro, 1988, p 9.

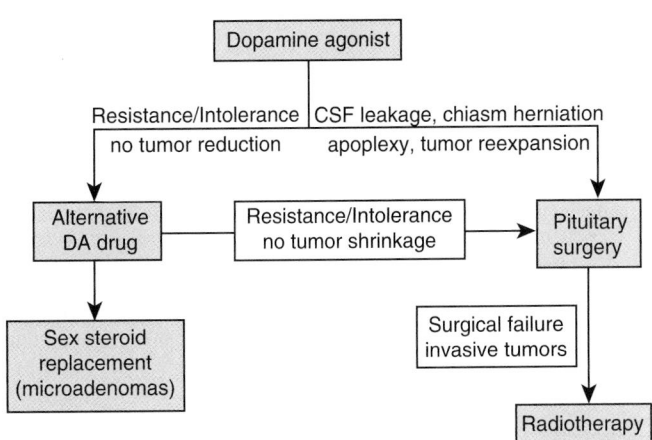

Figure 27-19 Suggested algorithm for treatment of prolactinomas. CSF, cerebrospinal fluid; DA, dopamine.

apoplexy, in dopamine agonist–induced CSF leakage occurring in invasive macroprolactinomas, and in the exceedingly rare occurrence of visual loss secondary to optic chiasm herniation during medical therapy. Additionally, surgery in skilled hands may be considered for patients not willing to be submitted to long-term medical therapy, especially patients harboring microprolactinomas and serum PRL levels less than 100 ng/mL. Radiotherapy, either conventional or stereotactic, is reserved for prolactinomas not responsive to medical or surgical treatment, particularly regarding the invasive ones.

There is evidence that, in general, estrogen replacement is not harmful for women harboring microprolactinomas. This approach may be used when fertility is not an issue for patients with intolerance or resistance to medical therapy and not cured by or not willing to undergo pituitary surgery. In addition, women successfully treated medically may use hormonal contraceptives if they have not adapted to barrier methods. Menopausal women bearing microprolactinomas can interrupt dopamine agonist drug use and are allowed to start hormone replacement therapy if it is indicated.[208] Although there is evidence of a PRL role in carcinogenesis in animal models, mainly carcinoma of the mammary gland, human data are still highly controversial.[290-293] It is now apparent that human mammary epithelial cells can synthesize PRL endogenously, permitting autocrine/paracrine actions within the mammary gland that are independent of pituitary PRL and probably not affected by dopamine agonist drugs. To date, the maintenance of high serum PRL levels in premenopausal and postmenopausal women is not a concern with regard to carcinogenesis. Finally, for macroprolactinomas that are not adequately controlled, the use of estrogens is generally discouraged, given their potential for inducing growth.

The follow-up planning for patients with prolactinomas depends on the tumor size and clinical, laboratory, and imaging response to therapy. Many patients are clinically controlled even if serum PRL levels are still above the normal range and do not need further drug dose increases. For microprolactinomas and especially for macroprolactinomas, significant tumor shrinkage or "disappearance" on MRI is a good prognostic marker, and in such cases, imaging reassessment can be performed sporadically. Medically or surgically controlled patients must be reassessed periodically clinically and hormonally to identify patients who may discontinue the dopamine agonist drug with maintenance of normoprolactinemia or patients with recurrence of hyperprolactinemia.

Acknowledgments
I would like to acknowledge Dr. Nina R. C. Musolino for her critical reading of the manuscript, for friendship, and for many years of collaborative scientific work.

REFERENCES

1. Miyai K, Ichibara K, Kondo L, et al: Asymptomatic hyperprolactinemia and prolactinoma in the general population mass screening by paired assays of serum prolactin. Clin Endocrinol (Oxf) 25:549–554, 1986.
2. Hardy J: Transsphenoidal microsurgery of the normal and pathological pituitary. Clin Neurosurg 16:185–217, 1969.
3. Saeger W, Bosse U, Pfingst E, et al: Prolactin producing hypophyseal carcinoma: Case report of an extremely rare metastatic tumor. Pathologe 16:354–358, 1995.
4. Gollard R, Kosty M, Cheney C, et al: Prolactin-secreting pituitary carcinoma with implants in the cheek pouch and metastases to the ovaries: A case report and literature review. Cancer 76:1814–1820, 1995.
5. Glezer A, D'Alva CB, Salgado LR, et al: Pitfalls in pituitary diagnosis: Peculiarities of three cases. Clin Endocrinol (Oxf) 57:135–139, 2002.
6. Striker P, Grueter F: Action du lobe antérieur de l'hypophyse sur la montée laiteuse. C R Soc Biol Paris 99:1978–1980, 1929.
7. Riddle O, Bartes RW, Dykshorn DW: The preparation, identification and assay of prolactin—a hormone of the anterior pituitary. Am J Physiol 105:191–216, 1933.
8. Mendel EB: Chiari-Frommel syndrome. Am J Obstet Gynecol 51:889–892, 1946.
9. Argonz J, del Castillo EB: A syndrome characterized by estrogenic insufficiency, galactorrhea and decreased urinary gonadotropin. J Clin Endocrinol Metab 13:79–87, 1953.
10. Forbes AP, Henneman PH, Griswold GC, et al: Syndrome characterized by galactorrhea, amenorrhea and low urinary FSH: Comparison with acromegaly and normal lactation. J Clin Endocrinol Metab 14:264–271, 1954.
11. Hwang P, Guyda H, Friesen H: A radioimmunoassay for human prolactin. Proc Natl Acad Sci U S A 68:1902–1906, 1971.
12. Burrow GN, Wortzman G, Rewcastle NB, et al: Microadenomas of the pituitary and abnormal sellar tomograms in an unselected autopsy series. N Engl J Med 304:156–158, 1981.
13. Mindermann T, Wilson CB: Age-related and gender-related occurrence of pituitary adenomas. Clin Endocrinol (Oxf) 41:359–364, 1994.
14. Faglia G: Epidemiology and pathogenesis of pituitary adenomas. Acta Endocrinol (Copenh) 129:1–5, 1993.
15. Drange MR, Fram NR, Herman-Bonert V, et al: Pituitary tumor registry: A novel clinical resource. J Clin Endocrinol Metab 85:168–174, 2000.
16. Molitch ME, Russell EJ: The pituitary "incidentaloma." Ann Intern Med 112:925–931, 1990.
17. De Menis E, Visentin A, Billeci D, et al: Pituitary adenomas in childhood and adolescence: Clinical analysis of 10 cases. J Endocrinol Invest 24:92–97, 2001.
18. Burgess JR, Shepherd JJ, Parameswaran V, et al: Spectrum of pituitary disease in multiple endocrine neoplasia type 1 (MEN 1): Clinical, biochemical, and radiological features of pituitary disease in a large MEN 1 kindred.
19. Corbetta S, Pizzocaro A, Peracchi M, et al: Multiple endocrine neoplasia type 1 in patients with recognized pituitary tumours of different types. Clin Endocrinol (Oxf) 47:507–512, 1997.
20. Berezin M, Karasik A: Familial prolactinoma. Clin Endocrinol (Oxf) 42:483–486, 1995.
21. Pernicone PJ, Scheithauer BW, Sebo TJ, et al: Pituitary carcinoma: A clinicopathologic study of 15 cases. Cancer 79:804–812, 1997.
22. Herman V, Fagin J, Gonsky R, et al: Clonal origin of pituitary adenomas. J Clin Endocrinol Metab 71:1427–1433, 1990.
23. Zhang X, Horwitz G, Prezant TR, et al: Structure, expression and function of human pituitary tumor transforming gene (PTTG). Mol Endocrinol 13:156–166, 1999.
24. Zhang X, Horwitz GA, Heaney AP, et al: Pituitary tumor transforming gene (PTTG) expression in pituitary adenomas. J Clin Endocrinol Metab 84:761–767, 1999.
25. Shimon I, Hinton DR, Weiss MH, et al: Prolactinomas express human heparin-binding secretory transforming gene (hst) protein product: Marker of tumour invasiveness. Clin Endocrinol (Oxf) 48:23–29, 1998.
26. Heaney AP, Fernando M, Melmed S: Functional role of estrogen in pituitary tumor pathogenesis. J Clin Invest 109:277–283, 2002.
27. Ben-Shlomo A, Miklovsky I, Ren SG, et al: Leukemia inhibitory factor regulates prolactin secretion in prolactinoma and lactotroph cells. J Clin Endocrinol Metab 88:858–863, 2003.
28. Fiorentini C, Guerra N, Facchetti M, et al: Nerve growth factor regulates dopamine D(2) receptor expression in prolactinoma cell lines via

p75(NGFR)-mediated activation of nuclear factor-kappaB. Mol Endocrinol 16:353–366, 2002.

29. Paez-Pereda M, Giacomini D, Refojo D, et al: Involvement of bone morphogenetic protein 4 (BMP-4) in pituitary prolactinoma pathogenesis through a Smad/estrogen receptor crosstalk. Proc Natl Acad Sci U S A 100:1034–1039, 2003.

30. Finelli P, Pierantoni GM, Giardino D, et al: The High Mobility Group A2 gene is amplified and overexpressed in human prolactinomas. Cancer Res 62:2398–2405, 2002.

31. Turner HE, Harris AL, Melmed S, et al: Angiogenesis in endocrine tumors. Endocr Rev 24:600–632, 2003.

32. Sarkar DK, Gottschall PE, Meites J: Damage to hypothalamic dopaminergic neurons is associated with development of prolactin-secreting pituitary tumors. Science 218:684–686, 1982.

33. Schuff KG, Hentges ST, Kelly MA, et al: Lack of prolactin receptor signaling in mice results in lactotroph proliferation and prolactinomas by dopamine-dependent and -independent mechanisms. J Clin Invest 110:973–981, 2002.

34. Cruz-Soto ME, Scheiber MD, Gregerson KA, et al: Pituitary tumorigenesis in prolactin gene-disrupted mice. Endocrinology 143:4429–4436, 2002.

35. Hentges ST, Low MJ: Pituitary tumorigenesis in prolactin gene-disrupted mice. Endocrinology 143:4429–4436, 2002.

36. Friedman E, Adams EF, Hoog A, et al: Normal structural dopamine type 2 receptor gene in prolactin-secreting and other pituitary tumors. J Clin Endocrinol Metab 78:568–574, 1994.

37. Marx SJ, Agarwal SK, Kester MB, et al: Multiple endocrine neoplasia type 1: Clinical and genetic features of the hereditary endocrine neoplasias. Recent Prog Horm Res 54:397–438, 1999.

38. Verges B, Boureille F, Goudet P, et al: Pituitary disease in MEN type 1 (MEN1): Data from the France-Belgium MEN1 multicenter study. J Clin Endocrinol Metab 87:457–465, 2002.

39. Prezant TR, Levine J, Melmed S: Molecular characterization of the men1 tumor suppressor gene in sporadic pituitary tumors. J Clin Endocrinol Metab 83:1388–1391, 1998.

40. Schmidt MC, Henke RT, Stangl AP, et al: Analysis of the MEN1 gene in sporadic pituitary adenomas. J Pathol 188:168–173, 1999.

41. Hardy J: Transsphenoidal surgery of hypersecreting pituitary tumors. In Kolhler G, Ross GT (eds): Diagnosis and Treatment of Pituitary Tumors. New York, Elsevier, 1973, pp 179–194.

42. Scheithauer BW, Kovacs KT, Laws ER Jr, et al: Pathology of invasive pituitary tumors with special reference to functional classification. J Neurosurg 65:733–744, 1986.

43. Kovacs K, Horvath E, Corenblum B, et al: Pituitary chromophobe adenomas consisting of prolactin cells:

A histologic, immunocytological and electron microscopic study. Virchows Arch 366:113–123, 1975.

44. Robert F, Hardy J: Prolactin secreting adenomas: A light and eletron microscopical study. Arch Pathol 99:625–633, 1975.

45. McComb DJ, Kovacs K: Ultrastructural morphometry of sparsely granulated prolactin cell adenomas of the human pituitary. Acta Endocrinol (Copenh) 89:21–29, 1978.

46. Kovacs K, Horvath E: Misplaced exocytosis: A distinct form of secretion in the anterior pituitary. Indian J Pathol Microbiol 19:85–89, 1976.

47. Horvath E, Kovacs K: Pathology of prolactin cell adenomas of the human pituitary. Semin Diagn Pathol 3:4–17, 1986.

48. Bevan JS, Burke CW, Esiri MM, et al: Misinterpretation of prolactin levels leading to management errors in patients with sellar enlargement. Am J Med 82:29–32, 1987.

49. Burrow GN, Wortzman G, Rewcastle NB, et al: Microadenomas of the pituitary and abnormal sellar tomograms in an unselected autopsy series. N Engl J Med 304:156–158, 1981.

50. Horvath E, Kovacs K, Singer W, et al: Acidophil stem cell adenoma of the human pituitary: Clinicopathologic analysis of 15 cases. Cancer 47:761–771, 1981.

51. Ozbey N, Sariyildiz E, Yilmaz L, et al: Primary hypothyroidism with hyperprolactinaemia and pituitary enlargement mimicking a pituitary macroadenoma. Int J Clin Pract 51:409–411, 1997.

52. Alkhani AM, Cusimano M, Kovacs K, et al: Cytology of pituitary thyrotroph hyperplasia in protracted primary hypothyroidism. Pituitary 1:291–295, 1999.

53. Himono T, Hatabu H, Kasagi K, et al: Rapid progression of pituitary hyperplasia in humans with primary hypothyroidism: Demonstration with MR imaging. Radiology 213:383–388, 1999.

54. Sarlis NJ, Brucker-Davis F, Doppman JL, et al: MRI-demonstrable regression of a pituitary mass in a case of primary hypothyroidism after a week of acute thyroid hormone therapy. J Clin Endocrinol Metab 82:808–811, 1997.

55. Saeger W: Space occupying processes of the sellar region with emphasis on tumor-like lesions. Pathologe 24:247–254, 2003.

56. Bellastella A, Bizzarro A, Coronella C, et al: Lymphocytic hypophysitis: A rare or underestimated disease? Eur J Endocrinol 149:363–376, 2003.

57. Nakao K, Noma K, Sato B, et al: Serum prolactin levels in eighty patients with sarcoidosis. Eur J Clin Invest 8:37–40, 1978.

58. Molina A, Mana J, Villabona C, et al: Hypothalamic-pituitary sarcoidosis with hypopituitarism: Long-term remission

with methylprednisolone pulse therapy. Pituitary 5:33–36, 2002.

59. Gonzalez JG, Elizondo G, Saldriar D, et al: Pituitary gland growth during normal pregnancy: An in vivo study using magnetic resonance imaging. Am J Med 85:217–220, 1988.

60. Scheithauer BW, Sano T, Kovacs KT, et al: The pituitary gland in pregnancy: A clinicpathologic and immunohistochemical study of 69 cases. Mayo Clin Proc 65:461–474, 1990.

61. Rigg LA, Lein A, Yen SSC: Pattern of increase in circulating prolactin levels during human gestation. Am J Obstet Gynecol 129:454–456, 1977.

62. Morris LF, Braunstein GD: Impact of pregnancy on normal pituitary function. In Bronstein MD (ed): Pituitary Tumors in Pregnancy. Boston, Kluwer Academic Publishers, 2001, pp 1–32.

63. Vieira JG, Tachibana T, Obara L, et al: Stress-related hyperprolactinemia: Evidence that rest before blood collection for serum prolactin measurement may be needed in only a minority of patients. EndoSociety 85th Annual Meeting, Philadelphia, 2003, PI-648, p 287.

64. Mielke DH, Gallatn DM, Kessler C: An evaluation of a unique new antipsychotic agent, sulpiride: Effects on serum prolactin and growth hormone levels. Am J Psychiatry 134:1371–1375, 1977.

65. Kleinberg DL, Davis JM, de Coster R, et al: Prolactin levels and adverse events in patients treated with risperidone. J Clin Psychopharmacol 19:57–61, 1999.

66. McCallum RW, Sowers JR, Hershman JM, et al: Metoclopramide stimulates prolactin secretion in man. J Clin Endocrinol Metab 42:148–152, 1976.

67. Kelley SR, Kamal TJ, Molitch ME: Mechanism of verapamil calcium channel blockade-induced hyperprolactinemia. Am J Physiol 270:96–100, 1996.

68. Hutchinson J, Murphy M, Harries R, et al: Galactorrhoea and hyperprolactinaemia associated with protease-inhibitors. Lancet 356:1003–1004, 2000.

69. Lloyd RV, Cano M, Chandler WF, et al: Human growth hormone and prolactin secreting pituitary adenomas analyzed by in situ hybridization. Am J Pathol 134:605–613, 1989.

70. Molitch ME, Reichlin S: Hypothalamic hyperprolactinemia: Neuroendocrine regulation of prolactin secretion in patients with lesions of the hypothalamus and pituitary stalk. In MacLeod RM, Thorner MO, Scapagnini U (eds): Prolactin: Basic and Clinical Correlates. Padova, Liviana Press, 1985, pp 709–719.

71. Grossman A, Ross R, Charlesworth M, et al: The effect of dopamine agonist therapy on large functionless pituitary tumours. Clin Endocrinol (Oxf) 22:679–686, 1985.

72. Honbo KS, Herle AJV, Kellet KA: Serum prolactin levels in untreated primary hypothyroidism. Am J Med 64:782–787, 1978.

73. Velardo A, Toschi E, Pantaleoni M, et al: Hyperprolactinemia in hypothyroidism: Effects of L-thyroxine therapy. Min Endocrinol 19:1–4, 1994.

74. Barbetta L, Dall'Asta C, Ambrosi B: Hyperprolactinemia preceding Cushing's disease. J Endocrinol Invest 23:491–492, 2000.

75. Stryker TD, Molitch ME: Reversible hyperthyrotropinemia, hyperthyroxinemia, and hyperprolactinemia due to adrenal insufficiency. Am J Med 79:271–276, 1985.

76. Estopinan Garcia V, Martinez Burgui JA, Ballester Ferrer A, et al: Prolactin and polycystic ovary síndrome. Med Clin (Barc) 116:759, 2001.

77. Veldhuis JD, Iranmanesh A, Wilkowski MJ, et al: Neuroendocrine alterations in the somatotropic and lactotropic axes in uremic men. Eur J Endocrinol 131:489–498, 1994.

78. Hou SH, Grossman S, Molitch ME: Hyperprolactinemia in patients with renal insufficiency and chronic renal failure requiring hemodialysis or chronic ambulatory peritoneal dialysis. Am J Kidney Dis 6:245–249, 1985.

79. Hasselbalch HC, Bech K, Eskildsen PC: Serum prolactin and thyrotropin responses to thyrotropin-releasing hormone in men with alcoholic cirrhosis. Acta Med Scand 209:37–40, 1981.

80. Boyd AE 3rd, Spare S, Bower B, et al: Neurogenic galactorrhea-amenorrhea. J Clin Endocrinol Metab 47:1374–1377, 1978.

81. Herman V, Kalk WJ, de Moor NG, et al: Serum prolactin after chest wall surgery: Elevated levels after mastectomy. J Clin Endocrinol Metab 52:148–151, 1981.

82. Modest GA, Fangman JJ: Nipple piercing and hyperprolactinemia. N Engl J Med 347:1626–1627, 2002.

83. Molitch ME, Schwartz S, Mukherji B: Is prolactin secreted ectopically? Am J Med 70:803–807, 1981.

84. Martin TL, Kim M, Malarkey WB: The natural history of idiopathic hyperprolactinemia. J Clin Endocrinol Metab 60:855–858, 1985.

85. Mah PM, Webster J: Hyperprolactinemia: Etiology, diagnosis, and management. Semin Reprod Med 20:365–374, 2002.

86. Poon A, McNeill P, Harper A: Patterns of visual loss associated with pituitary macroadenomas. Aust N Z J Ophthalmol 23:107–115, 1995.

87. Abe T, Matsumoto K, Kuwazawa J, et al: Headache associated with pituitary adenomas. Headache 38:782–786, 1998.

88. Matharu MS, Levy MJ, Merry RT, et al: SUNCT syndrome secondary to prolactinoma. J Neurol Neurosurg Psychiatry 74:1590–1592, 2003.

89. Zikel OM, Atkinson JL, Hurley DL: Prolactinoma manifesting with symptomatic hydrocephalus. Mayo Clin Proc 74:475–477, 1999.

90. Minniti G, Jaffrain-Rea ML, Santoro A, et al: Giant prolactinomas presenting as skull base tumors. Surg Neurol 57:99–103, 2002.

91. Bronstein MD, Musolino NR, Cardim CS, et al: Treatment of macroprolactinomas with a long-acting, parenteral and repeatable new form of bromocriptine. In Landolt AM, Heitz PU, Zapf J, et al (eds): Advances in Pituitary Adernoma Research. Oxford, Pergamon Press, 1988.

92. Del Pozo E, Schulz KD, Wyss H, et al: Effect of prolactin on the mechanisms of ovulation and on pregnancy: Some recent findings. In Robyn C, Harter M (eds): Progress in Prolactin Physiology and Pathology. Elsevier/North-Holland Biomedical Press, 1978.

93. Franks S, Murray MA, Jequier AM, et al: Incidence and significance of hyperprolactinaemia in women with amenorrhea. Clin Endocrinol (Oxf) 4:597–607, 1975.

94. Hattori N: Macroprolactinemia: A new cause of hyperprolactinemia. J Pharmacol Sci 92:171–177, 2003.

95. Amadori P, Dilberis C, Marcolla A: All the studies on hyperprolactinemia should not forget to consider the possible presence of macroprolactinemia. Eur J Endocrinol 150:93–94, 2004.

96. Serri O, Chik CL, Ur E, Ezzat S: Diagnosis and management of hyperprolactinemia. Can Med Assoc J 169:575–581, 2003.

97. Reavley A, Fisher AD, Owen D, et al: Psychological distress in patients with hyperprolactinaemia. Clin Endocrinol (Oxf) 47:343–348, 1997.

98. Kayath MJ, Lengyel AM, Vieira JG: Prevalence and magnitude of osteopenia in patients with prolactinoma. Braz J Med Biol Res 26:933–941, 1993.

99. Vartej P, Poiana C, Vartej I: Effects of hyperprolactinemia on osteoporotic fracture risk in premenopausal women. Gynecol Endocrinol 15:3–7, 2001.

100. Schlechte JA, Sherman B, Martin R: Bone density in amenorrheic women with and without hyperprolactinemia. J Clin Endocrinol Metab 56:1120–1123, 1983.

101. Ciccarelli E, Savino L, Carlevatto V, et al: Vertebral bone density in non-amenorrhoeic hyperprolactinaemic women. Clin Endocrinol (Oxf) 28:1–6, 1988.

102. Bronstein MD, Marino R Jr, Pereira DHM: Therapeutic alternatives for hyperprolactinemia: The role of bromoergocriptine. Rev Bras Ginecol Obstet 5:193, 1983.

103. Kleinberg DL, Noel GL, Frantz AG: Galactorrhea: A study of 235 cases, including 48 with pituitary tumors. N Engl J Med 296:589–600, 1977.

104. Berezin M, Shimon I, Hadani M: Prolactinoma in 53 men: Clinical characteristics and modes of treatment (male prolactinoma). J Endocrinol Invest 18:436–441, 1995.

105. Asano S, Ueki K, Suzuki I, et al: Clinical features and medical treatment of male prolactinomas. Acta Neurochir (Wien) 143:465–470, 2001.

106. Bronstein MD: Prolactinoma in men. Arq Bras Endocrinol Metab 43:338, 1999.

107. Carter JN, Tyson JE, Tolis G, et al: Prolactin-screening tumors and hypogonadismin 22 men. N Engl J Med 299:847–852, 1978.

108. Drago F, Scapagnini U: Side effects of drugs stimulating prolactin secretion on the behavior of male rats. Arch Int Pharmacodyn Ther 276:271–278, 1985.

109. Molitch ME, Thorner MO, Wilson C: Management of prolactinomas. J Clin Endocrinol Metab 82:996–1000, 1997.

110. Greenspan SL, Neer RM, Ridgway EC, et al: Osteoporosis in men with hyperprolactinemic hypogonadism. Ann Intern Med 104:777–782, 1986.

111. Di Somma C, Colao A, Di Sarno A, et al: Bone marker and bone density responses to dopamine agonist therapy in hyperprolactinemic males. J Clin Endocrinol Metab 83:807–813, 1998.

112. Cannavo S, Venturino M, Curto L, et al: Clinical presentation and outcome of pituitary adenomas in teenagers. Clin Endocrinol (Oxf) 58:519–527, 2003.

113. Colao A, Loche S, Cappa M, et al: Prolactinomas in children and adolescents: Clinical presentation and long-term follow-up. J Clin Endocrinol Metab 83:2777–2780, 1998.

114. Jallad RS, Goic MSZ, Musolino NR, et al: Prolactinomas in children and adolescents: Retrospective study on 47 patients. Arq Bras Endocrinol Metabol 44:300, 2000.

115. Cowden EA, Ratcliffe JG, Thomson JA, et al: Tests of prolactin secretion in diagnosis of prolactinomas. Lancet 1:1155–1158, 1979.

116. Prescott RW, Johnston DG, Taylor P, et al: The inability of dynamic tests of prolactin and TSH secretion to differentiate between tumorous and non-tumorous hyperprolactinemia. J Endocrinol Invest 8:49–54, 1985.

117. Le Moli R, Endert E, Fliers E, et al: Evaluation of endocrine tests: A. The TRH test in patients with hyperprolactinaemia. Neth J Med 61:44–48, 2003.

118. Di Sarno A, Rota F, Auriemma R, et al: An evaluation of patients with hyperprolactinemia: Have dynamic tests had their day? J Endocrinol Invest 26:39–47, 2003.

119. Cunha-Neto MB, Musolino NR, Batista MC, et al: Macroprolactinomas masquerading as pseudoprolactinomas: The high dose hook effect. Arq Bras Endocrinol Metab 41:98–101, 1997.

120. Barkan AL, Chandler WF: Giant pituitary prolactinoma with falsely low serum prolactin: The pitfall of the "high-dose hook effect": Case report. Neurosurgery 42:913–915, 1998.

121. Frieze TW, Mong DP, Koops MK: "Hook effect" in prolactinomas: Case

report and review of literature. Endocr Pract 8:296–303, 2003.

122. Sinha YN: Structural variants of prolactin: Occurrence and physiological significance. Endocr Rev 16:354–369, 1995.

123. Jackson RD, Wortsman J, Malarkey WB: Macroprolactinemia presenting like a pituitary tumor. Am J Med 78:346–350, 1985.

124. Tritos NA, Guay AT, Malarkey WB: Asymptomatic "big" hyperprolactinemia in two men with pituitary adenomas. Eur J Endocrinol 138:82–85, 1998.

125. Glezer A, Vieira JG, Giannella-Neto D, et al: Clinical asymptomatic hyperprolactinemia is not always linked to macroprolactinemia: Peculiarities of two cases. EndoSociety 85th Annual Meeting, Philadelphia, 2003, P3-649, p 630.

126. Vallette-Kasic S, Morange-Ramos I, Selim A, et al: Macroprolactinemia revisited: A study on 106 patients. J Clin Endocrinol Metab 87:581–588, 2002.

127. Vieira JG, Tachibana TT, Obara LH, et al: Extensive experience and validation of polyethylene glycol precipitation as a screening method for macroprolactinemia. Clin Chem 44:1758–1759, 1998.

128. Olukoga AO, Kane JW: Macroprolactinaemia: Validation and application of the polyethylene glycol precipitation test and clinical characterization of the condition. Clin Endocrinol 51:119–126, 1999.

129. Cavaco B, Leite V, Santos MA, et al: Some forms of big big prolactin behave as a complex of monomeric prolactin with an immunoglobulin G in patients with macroprolactinemia or prolactinoma. J Clin Endocrinol Metab 80:2342–2346, 1995.

130. Hattori N, Ikekubo K, Ishihara T, et al: A normal ovulatory woman with hyperprolactinemia: Presence of anti-prolactin autoantibody and the regulation of prolactin secretion. Acta Endocrinol (Copenh) 126:497–500, 1992.

131. Andersen M, Hagen C, Frystyk J, et al: Development of acromegaly in patients with prolactinomas. Eur J Endocrinol 149:17–22, 2003.

132. Warfield A, Finkel DM, Schatz NJ, et al: Bromocriptine treatment of prolactin-secreting pituitary adenomas may restore pituitary function. Ann Intern Med 101:783–785, 1984.

133. Sibal L, Ugwu P, Kendall-Taylor P, et al: Medical therapy of macroprolactinomas in males: I. Prevalence of hypopituitarism at diagnosis. II. Proportion of cases exhibiting recovery of pituitary function. Pituitary 5:243–246, 2002.

134. George LD, Nicolau N, Scanlon MF, et al: Recovery of growth hormone secretion following cabergoline treatment of macroprolactinomas. Clin Endocrinol (Oxf) 53:595–599, 2000.

135. Vezina JL, Sutton TJ: Prolactin-secreting pituitary microadenomas: Roentgenologic diagnosis. Am J Roentgenol Radium Ther Nucl Med 120:46–54, 1974.

136. Leclercq TA, Hardy J, Vezina JL, et al: Intrasellar arachnoidocele and the so-called empty sella syndrome. Surg Neurol 2:295–299, 1974.

137. Delecourt F, Leclerc X, Ardaens Y, et al: Searching for prolactin microadenoma: Scanner or MRI? Ann Endocrinol (Paris) 54:413–420, 1993.

138. Stadnik T, Spruyt D, van Binst A, et al: Pituitary microadenomas: Diagnosis with dynamic serial CT, conventional CT and T1-weighted MR imaging before and after injection of gadolinium. Eur J Radiol 18:191–198, 1994.

139. Davis PC, Hoffman JC Jr, Tindall GT, et al: Prolactin-secreting pituitary microadenomas: Inaccuracy of high-resolution CT imaging. Am J Roentgenol 144:151–156, 1985.

140. Juliani G, Avataneo T, Potenzoni F, et al: CT and MR compared in the study of hypophysis. Radiol Med (Torino) 77:51–64, 1989.

141. Johnson MR, Hoare RD, Cox T, et al: The evaluation of patients with a suspected pituitary microadenoma: Computed tomography compared to magnetic resonance imaging. Clin Endocrinol (Oxf) 36:335–338, 1992.

142. Buchfelder M, Nistor R, Fahlbusch R, et al: The accuracy of CT and MR evaluation of the sella turcica for detection of adrenocorticotropic hormone-secreting adenomas in Cushing disease. Am J Neuroradiol 14:1183–1190, 1993.

143. Davis PC, Hoffman JC Jr, Spencer T, et al: MR imaging of pituitary adenoma: CT, clinical, and surgical correlation. Am J Roentgenol 148:797–802, 1987.

144. Lundin P, Bergstrom K, Thuomas KA, et al: Comparison of MR imaging and CT in pituitary macroadenomas. Acta Radiol 32:189–196, 1991.

145. Aron DC, Howlett TA: Pituitary incidentalomas. Endocrinol Metab Clin North Am 29:205–221, 2000.

146. Molitch ME: Pituitary incidentalomas. Endocrinol Metab Clin North Am 26:725–740, 1997.

147. Hall WA, Luciano MG, Doppman JL, et al: Pituitary magnetic resonance imaging in normal human volunteers: Occult adenomas in the general population. Ann Intern Med 120:817–820, 1994.

148. Elster AD, Chen MYM, Williams DW 3rd, et al: Pituitary gland: MR imaging of physiologic hypertrophy in adolescence. Radiology 174:681–685, 1990.

149. Elster AD, Sanders TG, Vines FS, et al: Size and shape of the pituitary gland during pregnancy and post partum: Measurement with MR imaging. Radiology 181:531–535, 1991.

150. Krishnan KRR, Doraiswamy PM, Lurie SN, et al: Pituitary size in depression. J Clin Endocrinol Metab 72:256–259, 1991.

151. Scillitani A, Dicembrino F, Di Fazio P, et al: In vivo visualization of pituitary dopaminergic receptors by iodine-123 methoxybenzamide (IBZM) correlates with sensitivity to dopamine agonists in two patients with macroprolactinomas. J Clin Endocrinol Metab 80:2523–2525, 1995.

152. de Herder WW, Reijs AE, de Swart J, et al: Comparison of iodine-123 epidepride and iodine-123 IBZM for dopamine D2 receptor imaging in clinically non-functioning pituitary macroadenomas and macroprolactinomas. Eur J Nucl Med 26:46–50, 1999.

153. Bergstrom M, Muhr C, Lundberg PO, et al: PET as a tool in the clinical evaluation of pituitary adenomas. J Nucl Med 32:610–615, 1991.

154. Petrossians P, de Herder W, Kwekkeboom D, et al: Malignant prolactinoma discovered by D2 receptor imaging. J Clin Endocrinol Metab 85:398–401, 2000.

155. Fluckiger E, Wagner HR: 2-Br-alpha-ergokryptin: Influence on fertility and lactation in the rat. Experientia 24:1130–1131, 1968.

156. Guiot G, Bouche J, Hertzog E, et al: Hypophysectomy by trans-sphenoidal route. Ann Radiol (Paris) 6:187–192, 1963.

157. Cho DY, Liau WR: Comparison of endonasal endoscopic surgery and sublabial microsurgery for prolactinomas. Surg Neurol 58:371–375, 2002.

158. Ciric I, Ragin A, Baumgartner C, et al: Complications of transsphenoidal surgery: Results of a national survey, review of the literature, and personal experience. Neurosurgery 40:225–236, 1997.

159. Laws ER Jr, Thapar K: Pituitary surgery. Endocrinol Metab Clin North Am 28:119–131, 1999.

160. Tyrrell JB, Lamborn KR, Hannegan LT, et al: Transsphenoidal microsurgical therapy of prolactinomas: Initial outcomes and long-term results. Neurosurgery 44:254–261, 1999.

161. Losa M, Mortini P, Barzaghi R, et al: Surgical treatment of prolactin-secreting pituitary adenomas: Early results and long-term outcome. J Clin Endocrinol Metab 87:3180–3186, 2002.

162. Marino R Jr, Bronstein MD: The role of pituitary surgery in the treatment of prolactinomas. In Meirelles RMR, Machado A, Povoa LC (eds): Clinical Endocrinology. Amsterdam, Excepta Medica, 1988, pp 53–56.

163. Molitch ME: Disorders of prolactin secretion. Endocrinol Metab Clin North Am 30:585–610, 2001.

164. Bronstein M, Musolino N, Cunha-Neto M, et al: Hyperprolactinemia therapy: Lessons learned from long-term follow-up. Eur J Endocrinol 130:116, 1994.

165. Landolt AM, Keller PJ, Froesch ER, et al: Bromocriptine: Does it jeopardise the result of later surgery for prolactinomas? Lancet 2:657–658, 1982.

166. Soule SG, Farhi J, Conway GS, et al: The outcome of hypophysectomy for prolactinomas in the era of dopamine agonist therapy. Clin Endocrinol (Oxf) 44:711–716, 1996.

167. Perrin G, Treluyer C, Trouillas J, et al: Surgical outcome and pathological effects of bromocriptine preoperative treatment in prolactinomas. Pathol Res Pract 187:587–592, 1991.

168. Serri O, Rasio E, Beauregard H, et al: Recurrence of hyperprolactinemia after selective transsphenoidal adenomectomy in women with prolactinoma. N Engl J Med 309:280–283, 1983.

169. Amar AP, Couldwell WT, Chen JC, et al: Predictive value of serum prolactin levels measured immediately after transsphenoidal surgery. J Neurosurg 97:307–314, 2002.

170. Webster J, Page MD, Bevan JS, et al: Low recurrence rate after partial hypophysectomy for prolactinoma: The predictive value of dynamic prolactin function tests. Clin Endocrinol (Oxf) 36:35–44, 1992.

171. Schlechte JA, Sherman BM, Chapler FK, et al: Long term follow-up of women with surgically treated prolactin-secreting pituitary tumors. J Clin Endocrinol Metab 62:1296–1301, 1986.

172. Maira G, Anile C, De Marinis L, et al: Prolactin-secreting adenomas: Surgical results and long-term follow-up. Neurosurgery 24:736–743, 1989.

173. Massoud F, Serri O, Hardy J, et al: Transsphenoidal adenomectomy for microprolactinomas: 10 to 20 years of follow-up. Surg Neurol 45:341–346, 1996.

174. Thomson JA, Gray CE, Teasdale GM: Relapse of hyperprolactinemia after transsphenoidal surgery for microprolactinoma: Lessons from long-term follow-up. Neurosurgery 50:36–39, 2002.

175. Deb S: Clinical significance of pituitary apoplexy. J Indian Med Assoc 96:302–303, 1998.

176. da Motta LA, de Mello PA, de Lacerda CM, et al: Pituitary apoplexy: Clinical course, endocrine evaluations and treatment analysis. J Neurosurg Sci 43:25–36, 1999.

177. Kupersmith MJ, Kleinberg D, Warren FA, et al: Growth of prolactinoma despite lowering of serum prolactin by bromocriptine. Neurosurgery 24:417–423, 1989.

178. Bronstein MD, Musolino NR, Benabou S, et al: Cerebrospinal fluid rhinorrhea occurring in long-term bromocriptine treatment for macroprolactinomas. Surg Neurol 32:346–349, 1989.

179. Barlas O, Bayindir C, Hepgul K, et al: Bromocriptine-induced cerebrospinal fluid fistula in patients with macroprolactinomas: Report of three cases and a review of the literature. Surg Neurol 41:486–489, 1994.

180. Jones SE, James RA, Hall K, et al: Optic chiasmal herniation—an under recognized complication of dopamine agonist therapy for macroprolactinoma. Clin Endocrinol (Oxf) 53:529–534, 2000.

181. Turner HE, Adams CB, Wass JA: Trans-sphenoidal surgery for microprolactinoma: An acceptable alternative to dopamine agonists? Eur J Endocrinol 140:43–47, 1999.

182. Besser GM, Parke L, Edwards CR, et al: Galactorrhoea: Successful treatment with reduction of plasma prolactin levels by brom-ergocryptine. Br Med J 3:669–672, 1972.

183. Ben-Jonathan N: Regulation of prolactin secretion. In Imura H (ed): The Pituitary Gland. New York, Raven Press, 1994, p 261.

184. Shran HF, Bhuta SI, Schwarz HJ, Thorner MO: The pharmacokinetics of bromocriptine in man. In Goldstein M, Calne DB, Lieberman A, Thorner MO (eds): Ergot Compounds and Brain Function: Neuroendocrine and Neuropsychiatric Aspect. New York, Raven Press, 1980, p 125.

185. Ciccarelli E, Mazza E, Ghigo E, et al: Long term treatment with oral single administration of bromocriptine in patients with hyperprolactinemia. J Endocrinol Invest 10:51–53, 1987.

186. Vance ML, Evans WS, Thorner MO: Bromocriptine. Ann Intern Med 100:78–91, 1984.

187. Pinzone JJ, Katznelson L, Danila DC, et al: Primary medical therapy of micro- and macroprolactinomas in men. J Clin Endocrinol Metab 85:3053–3057, 2000.

188. Corenblum B, Webster BR, Mortimer CB, et al: Possible antitumour effect of 2 bromoergocryptine in 2 patients with large prolactin-secreting pituitary adenomas. Clin Res 23:614A, 1975.

189. Molitch ME, Elton RL, Blackwell RE, et al: Bromocriptine as primary therapy for prolactin-secreting macroadenomas: Results of a prospective multicenter study. J Clin Endocrinol Metab 60:698–705, 1985.

190. Essais O, Bouguerra R, Hamzaoui J, et al: Efficacy and safety of bromocriptine in the treatment of macroprolactinomas. Ann Endocrinol (Paris) 63:524–531, 2002.

191. Shrivastava RK, Arginteanu MS, King WA, et al: Giant prolactinomas: Clinical management and long-term follow up. J Neurosurg 97:299–306, 2002.

192. Rengachary SS, Tomita T, Jefferies BF, et al: Structural changes in human pituitary tumor after bromocriptine therapy. Neurosurgery 10:242–251, 1982.

193. Tindall GT, Kovacs K, Horvath E, et al: Human prolactin-producing adenomas and bromocriptine: A histological, immunocytochemical, ultrastructural, and morphometric study. J Clin Endocrinol Metab 55:178–183, 1982.

194. Lloyd HM, Jacobi JM, Willgoss DA: DNA synthesis by pituitary tumours, with reference to plasma hormone levels and to effects of bromocriptine. Clin Endocrinol (Oxf) 43:79–85, 1995.

195. Gruszka A, Pawlikowski M, Kunert-Radek J: Anti-tumoral action of octreotide and bromocriptine on the experimental rat prolactinoma: Anti-proliferative and pro-apoptotic effects. Neuroendocrinol Lett 22:343–348, 2001.

196. Kovacs K, Stefaneanu L, Horvath E, et al: Effect of dopamine agonist medication on prolactin producing pituitary adenomas: A morphological study including immunocytochemistry, electron microscopy and in situ hybridization. Virchows Arch 418:439–446, 1991.

197. Thorner MO, Perryman RL, Rogol AD, et al: Rapid changes of prolactinoma volume after withdrawal and reinstitution of bromocriptine. J Clin Endocrinol Metab 53:480–483, 1981.

198. Orrego JJ, Chandler WF, Barkan AL: Rapid re-expansion of a macroprolactinoma after early discontinuation of bromocriptine. Pituitary 3:189–192, 2000.

199. Johnston DG, Hall K, Kendall-Taylor P, et al: Effect of dopamine agonist withdrawal after long-term therapy in prolactinomas: Studies with high-definition computerised tomography. Lancet 2:187–192, 1984.

200. van't Verlaat JW, Croughs RJ: Withdrawal of bromocriptine after long-term therapy for macroprolactinomas: Effect on plasma prolactin and tumour size. Clin Endocrinol (Oxf) 34:175–178, 1991.

201. Bevan JS, Webster J, Burke CW, et al: Dopamine agonists and pituitary tumor shrinkage. Endocr Rev 13:220–240, 1992.

202. Molitch ME: Medical management of prolactin-secreting pituitary adenomas. Pituitary 5:55–65, 2002.

203. Passos VQ, Souza JJ, Musolino NR, et al: Long-term follow-up of prolactinomas: Normoprolactinemia after bromocriptine withdrawal. J Clin Endocrinol Metab 87:3578–3582, 2002.

204. Gen M, Uozumi T, Ohta M, et al: Necrotic changes in prolactinomas after long term administration of bromocriptine. J Clin Endocrinol Metab 59:463–470, 1984.

205. Koppelman MC, Jaffe MJ, Rieth KG, et al: Hyperprolactinemia, amenorrhea, and galactorrhea: A retrospective assessment of twenty-five cases. Ann Intern Med 100:115–121, 1984.

206. Schlechte J, Dolan K, Sherman B, et al: The natural history of untreated hyperprolactinemia: A prospective analysis. J Clin Endocrinol Metab 68:412–418, 1989.

207. Sisam DA, Sheehan JP, Sheeler LR: The natural history of untreated microprolactinomas. Fertil Steril 48:67–71, 1987.

208. Touraine P, Deneux C, Plu-Bureau G, et al: Hormonal replacement therapy in menopausal women with a history of hyperprolactinemia. J Endocrinol Invest 21:732–736, 1998.

209. Karunakaran S, Page RC, Wass JA: The effect of the menopause on prolactin levels in patients with hyperprolactinaemia. Clin Endocrinol (Oxf) 54:295–300, 2001.
210. Pinto G, Zerah M, Trivin C, et al: Pituitary apoplexy in an adolescent with prolactin-secreting adenoma. Horm Res 50:38–41, 1998.
211. Turner TH, Cookson JC, Wass JA, et al: Psychotic reactions during treatment of pituitary tumours with dopamine agonists. Br Med J 289:1101–1103, 1984.
212. Kains JP, Hardy JC, Chevalier C, et al: Retroperitoneal fibrosis in two patients with Parkinson's disease treated with bromocriptine. Acta Clin Belg 45:306–310, 1990.
213. Liuzzi A, Dallabonzana D, Oppizzi G, et al: Low doses of dopamine agonists in the long-term treatment of macroprolactinomas. N Engl J Med 313:656–659, 1985.
214. Merola B, Colao A, Caruso E, et al: Effectiveness and long-term tolerability of the slow release oral form of bromocriptine on tumoral and non-tumoral hyperprolactinemia. J Endocrinol Invest 15:173–176, 1992.
215. Bronstein MD, Cardim CS, Marino R Jr: Short-term management of macroprolactinomas with a new injectable form of bromocriptine. Surg Neurol 28:31–37, 1987.
216. Beckers A, Petrossians P, Abs R, et al: Treatment of macroprolactinomas with the long-acting and repeatable form of bromocriptine: a report on 29 cases. J Clin Endocrinol Metab 75:275–280, 1992.
217. Jasonni VM, Raffelli R, de March A, et al: Vaginal bromocriptine in hyperprolactinemic patients and puerperal women. Acta Obstet Gynecol Scand 70:493–495, 1991.
218. Brue T, Pellegrini I, Priou A, et al: Prolactinomas and resistance to dopamine agonists. Horm Res 38:84–89, 1992.
219. Pellegrini I, Rasolonjanahary R, Gunz G, et al: Resistance to bromocriptine in prolactinomas. J Clin Endocrinol Metab 69:500–509, 1989.
220. Caccavelli L, Feron F, Morange I, et al: Decreased expression of the two D2 dopamine receptor isoforms in bromocriptine-resistant prolactinomas. Neuroendocrinology 60:314–322, 1994.
221. Delgrange E, Crabbe J, Donckier J: Late development of resistance to bromocriptine in a patient with macroprolactinoma. Horm Res 49:250–253, 1998.
222. Kleinberg DL, Boyd AE 3rd, Wardlaw S, et al: Pergolide for the treatment of pituitary tumors secreting prolactin or growth hormone. N Engl J Med 309:704–709, 1983.
223. Blackwell RE, Bradley EL Jr, Kline LB, et al: Comparison of dopamine agonists in the treatment of hyperprolactinemic syndromes: A multicenter study. Fertil Steril 39:744–748, 1983.
224. Ahmed SR, Shalet SM: Discordant responses of prolactinoma to two different dopamine agonists. Clin Endocrinol (Oxf) 24:421–426, 1986.
225. Lamberts SW, Quik RF: A comparison of the efficacy and safety of pergolide and bromocriptine in the treatment of hyperprolactinemia. J Clin Endocrinol Metab 72:635, 1991.
226. Berezin M, Avidan D, Baron E: Long-term pergolide treatment of hyperprolactinemic patients previously unsuccessfully treated with dopaminergic drugs. Isr J Med Sci 27:375–379, 1991.
227. Freda PU, Andreadis CI, Khandji AG, et al: Long-term treatment of prolactin-secreting macroadenomas with pergolide. J Clin Endocrinol Metab 85:8–13, 2000.
228. Orrego JJ, Chandler WF, Barkan AL: Pergolide as primary therapy for macroprolactinomas. Pituitary 3:251–256, 2000.
229. Van Camp G, Flamez A, Cosyns B, et al: Heart valvular disease in patients with Parkinson's disease treated with high-dose pergolide. Neurology 61:859–861, 2003.
230. Vance ML, Lipper M, Klibanski A, et al: Treatment of prolactin-secreting pituitary macroadenomas with the long-acting non-ergot dopamine agonist CV 205-502. Ann Intern Med 112:668–673, 1990.
231. Serri O, Beauregard H, Lesage J, et al: Long term treatment with CV 205-502 in patients with prolactin-secreting pituitary macroadenomas. J Clin Endocrinol Metab 71:682–687, 1990.
232. van der Lely AJ, Brownell J, Lamberts SW: The efficacy and tolerability of CV 205-502 (a nonergot dopaminergic drug) in macroprolactinoma patients and in prolactinoma patients intolerant to bromocriptine. J Clin Endocrinol Metab 72:1136–1141, 1991.
233. Kvistborg A, Halse J, Bakke S, et al: Long-term treatment of macroprolactinomas with CV 205-502. Acta Endocrinol (Copenh) 128:301–307, 1993.
234. Glaser B, Nesher Y, Barziliai S: Long-term treatment of bromocriptine-intolerant prolactinoma patients with CV 205-502. J Reprod Med 39:449–454, 1994.
235. Brue T, Pellegrini I, Gunz G, et al: Effects of the dopamine agonist CV 205-502 in human prolactinomas resistant to bromocriptine. J Clin Endocrinol Metab 74:577–584, 1992.
236. Morange I, Barlier A, Pellegrini I, et al: Prolactinomas resistant to bromocriptine: Long-term efficacy of quinagolide and outcome of pregnancy. Eur J Endocrinol 135:413–420, 1996.
237. Del Dotto P, Bonuccelli U: Clinical pharmacokinetics of cabergoline. Clin Pharmacokinet 42:633–645, 2003.
238. Ferrari C, Paracchi A, Mattei AM, et al: Cabergoline in the long-term therapy of hyperprolactinemic disorders. Acta Endocrinol (Copenh) 126:489–494, 1992.
239. Cannavo S, Curto L, Squadrito S, et al: Cabergoline: A first-choice treatment in patients with previously untreated prolactin-secreting pituitary adenoma. J Endocrinol Invest 22:354–359, 1999.
240. Biller BM, Molitch ME, Vance ML, et al: Treatment of prolactin-secreting macroadenomas with the once-weekly dopamine agonist cabergoline. J Clin Endocrinol Metab 81:2338–2343, 1996.
241. Webster J, Piscitelli G, Polli A, et al: A comparison of cabergoline and bromocriptine in the treatment of hyperprolactinemic amenorrhea. Cabergoline Comparative Study Group. N Engl J Med 331:904–909, 1994.
242. Pascal-Vigneron V, Weryha G, Bosc M, et al: Hyperprolactinemic amenorrhea: Treatment with cabergoline versus bromocriptine: Results of a national multicenter randomized double-blind study. Presse Med 24:753–757, 1995.
243. Verhelst J, Abs R, Maiter D, et al: Cabergoline in the treatment of hyperprolactinemia: A study in 455 patients. J Clin Endocrinol Metab 84:2518–2522, 1999.
244. Musolino NR, Cunha Neto MB, Bronstein MD: Cabergoline as an alternative for the medical treatment of prolactinomas: Experience in bromocriptine intolerance/resistance. Arq Bras Endocrinol Metab 44:139–143, 2000.
245. Sabuncu T, Arikan E, Tasan E, et al: Comparison of the effects of cabergoline and bromocriptine on prolactin levels in hyperprolactinemic patients. Intern Med 40:857–861, 2001.
246. Colao A, Di Sarno A, Landi ML, et al: Macroprolactinoma shrinkage during cabergoline treatment is greater in naive patients than in patients pretreated with other dopamine agonists: A prospective study in 110 patients. J Clin Endocrinol Metab 85:2247–2252, 2000.
247. Colao A, Di Sarno A, Sarnacchiaro F, et al: Prolactinomas resistant to standard dopamine agonists respond to chronic cabergoline treatment. J Clin Endocrinol Metab 82:876–883, 1997.
248. Muratori M, Arosio M, Gambino G, et al: Use of cabergoline in the long-term treatment of hyperprolactinemic and acromegalic patients. J Endocrinol Invest 20:537–546, 1997.
249. Colao A, Di Sarno A, Cappabianca P, et al: Withdrawal of long-term cabergoline therapy for tumoral and nontumoral hyperprolactinemia. N Engl J Med 349:2023–2033, 2003.
250. Acquati S, Pizzocaro A, Tomei G, et al: A comparative evaluation of effectiveness of medical and surgical therapy in patients with macroprolactinoma. J Neurosurg Sci 45:65–69, 2001.

251. Tsang RW, Brierley JD, Panzarella T, et al: Role of radiation therapy in clinical hormonally-active pituitary adenomas. Radiother Oncol 41:45–53, 1996.

252. Molitch ME: Pathologic hyperprolactinemia. Endocrinol Metab Clin North Am 21:877–901, 1992.

253. Landolt AM, Lomax N: Gamma knife radiosurgery for prolactinomas. J Neurosurg 93:14–18, 2000.

254. Pan L, Zhang N, Wang EM, et al: Gamma knife radiosurgery as a primary treatment for prolactinomas. J Neurosurg 93:10–13, 2000.

255. Corenblum B, Donovan L: The safety of physiological estrogen plus progestin replacement therapy and with oral contraceptive therapy in women with pathological hyperprolactinemia. Fertil Steril 59:671–673, 1993.

256. Testa G, Vegetti W, Motta T, et al: Two-year treatment with oral contraceptives in hyperprolactinemic patients. Contraception 58:69–73, 1998.

257. Gillam MP, Middler S, Freed DJ, et al: The novel use of very high doses of cabergoline and a combination of testosterone and an aromatase inhibitor in the treatment of a giant prolactinoma. J Clin Endocrinol Metab 87:4447–4451, 2002.

258. Bronstein MD, Knoepfelmacher M, Liberman B, et al: Absence of suppressive effect of somatostatin on prolactin levels in patients with hyperprolactinemia. Horm Metab Res 19:271–274, 1987.

259. Shimon I, Yan X, Taylor JE, et al: Somatostatin receptor (SSTR) subtype-selective analogues differentially suppress in vitro growth hormone and prolactin in human pituitary adenomas: Novel potential therapy for functional pituitary tumors. J Clin Invest 100:2386–2392, 1997.

260. Jaquet P, Ouafik L, Saveanu A, et al: Quantitative and functional expression of somatostatin receptor subtypes in human prolactinomas. J Clin Endocrinol Metab 84:3268–3276, 1999.

261. Hofland LJ, Bruns C, Weckbecker G, et al: Differential desensitization of GH release after continuous exposure to octreotide and the novel somatostatin peptidomimetic SOM 230. The Endocrine Society's 84th annual meeting, San Francisco, 2002, P2-108.

262. Hofland LJ, van der Hoek J, van Koetsveld PM, et al: The novel somatostatin analog SOM230 has a broad spectrum of inhibitory action on hormone release by human somatotroph, corticotroph and PRL-secreting pituitarty adenomas in vitro. The Endocrine Society's 85th annual meeting, Philadelphia, 2003, P2-449, p 416.

263. Missale C, Boroni F, Losa M, et al: Nerve growth factor suppresses the transforming phenotype of human prolactinomas. Proc Natl Acad Sci U S A 90:7961–7965, 1993.

264. Facchetti M, Uberti D, Memo M, et al: Nerve growth factor restores p53 function in pituitary tumor cell lines via trkA-mediated activation of phosphatidylinositol 3-kinase. Mol Endocrinol 18:162–172, 2004.

265. Missale C, Losa M, Boroni F, et al: Nerve growth factor and bromocriptine: A sequential therapy for human bromocriptine-resistant prolactinomas. Br J Cancer 72:1397–1399, 1995.

266. Ishikawa H, Heaney AP, Yu R, et al: Human pituitary tumor-transforming gene induces angiogenesis. J Clin Endocrinol Metab 86:867–874, 2001.

267. Gemzell C, Wang CF: Outcome of pregnancy in women with pituitary adenoma. Fertil Steril 31:363–372, 1979.

268. Molitch ME: Pregnancy and the hyperprolactinemic woman. N Engl J Med 312:1364–1370, 1985.

269. Musolino NRC, Bronstein MD: Prolactinomas and pregnancy. In Bronstein MD (ed): Pituitary Tumors in Pregnancy. Boston, Kluwer Academic Publishers, 2001, pp 91–108.

270. Holmgren U, Bergstrand G, Hagenfeldt K, et al: Women with prolactinoma-effect of pregnancy and lactation on serum prolactin and on tumour growth. Acta Endocrinol (Copenh) 111:452–459, 1986.

271. van Roon E, van der Vijver JCM, Gerretsen G, et al: Rapid regression of a suprasellar extending prolactinoma after bromocriptine treatment during pregnancy. Fertil Steril 36:173–177, 1981.

272. Maeda T, Ushiroyama T, Okuda K, et al: Effective bromocriptine treatment of a pituitary macroadenoma during pregnancy. Obstet Gynecol 61:117–120, 1983.

273. Bergh T, Nillius SJ, Wide L: Clinical course and outcome of pregnancies in amenorrhoeic women with hyperprolactinaemia and pituitary tumours. Br Med J 1:875–880, 1978.

274. Tan SL, Jacobs HS: Rapid regression through bromocriptine therapy of a suprasellar extending prolactinoma during pregnancy. Int J Gynaecol Obstet 24:209–215, 1986.

275. Bronstein MD, Salgado LR, Musolino NR: Medical management of pituitary adenomas: The special case of the pregnant woman. Pituitary 5:99–107, 2002.

276. Chil DF, Gordoon H, Mashiter K, et al: Pregnancy, prolactin and pituitary tumours. Br Med J 4:87–89, 1975.

277. Crosignani PG, Ferrari C, Scarduelli C, et al: Spontaneous and induced pregnancies in hyperprolactinemic women. Obstet Gynecol 58:708–713, 1981.

278. Brodsky JB, Cohen EN, Brown BW Jr, et al: Surgery during pregnancy and fetal outcome. Am J Obstet Gynecol 138:1165–1167, 1980.

279. Krupp P, Monka C: Bromocriptine in pregnancy: Safety aspects. Klin Wochenschr 65:823–827, 1987.

280. Canales ES, Garcia IC, Ruiz JE, et al: Bromocriptine as prophylactic therapy in prolactinoma during pregnancy. Fertil Steril 36:524–526, 1981.

281. Konopka P, Raymond JP, Merceron RE, et al: Continuous administration of bromocriptine in the prevention of neurological complications in pregnant women with prolactinomas. Am J Obstet Gynecol 146:935–938, 1983.

282. Webster J: A comparative review of the tolerability profiles of dopamine agonists in treatment of hyperprolactinaemia and inhibition of lactation. Drug Saf 14:228–238, 1996.

283. Robert E, Musatti L, Piscitelli G, et al: Pregnancy outcome after treatment with the ergot derivative, cabergoline. Reprod Toxicol 10:333–337, 1996.

284. Liu C, Tyrrell JB: Successful treatment of a large macroprolactinoma with cabergoline during pregnancy. Pituitary 4:179–185, 2001.

285. Buelke-Sam J, Cohen IR, Tizzano JP, et al: Developmental toxicity of the dopamine agonist pergolide mesylate in CD-1 mice: II. Perinatal and postnatal exposure. Neurotoxicol Teratol 13:297–306, 1991.

286. Zarate A, Canales ES, Alger M, et al: The effect of pregnancy and lactation on pituitary prolactin-secreting tumours. Acta Endocrinol (Copenh) 92:407–412, 1979.

287. Crosignani PG, Mattei AM, Severini V, et al: Long-term effects of time, medical treatment and pregnancy in 176 hyperprolactinemic women. Eur J Obstet Gynaecol Reprod Biol 44:175–180, 1992.

288. Badawy SZ, Marziale JC, Rosenbaum AE, et al: The long-term effects of pregnancy and bromocriptine treatment on prolactinomas—the value of radiologic studies. Early Pregnancy 3:306–311, 1997.

289. Peillon F, Racadot J, Moussy D, et al: Prolactin-secreting adenomas: A correlative study of morphological and clinical data. In Fahlbuch R, von Werder K (eds): Treatment of Pituitary Adenomas. Stuttgart, Thieme, 1978, p 114.

290. Wang PS, Walker AM, Tsuang MT, et al: Dopamine antagonists and the development of breast cancer. Arch Gen Psychiatry 59:1147–1154, 2002.

291. Manjer J, Johansson R, Berglund G, et al: Postmenopausal breast cancer risk in relation to sex steroid hormones, prolactin and SHBG (Sweden). Cancer Causes Control 14:599–607, 2003.

292. Rose-Hellekant TA, Arendt LM, Schroeder MD, et al: Prolactin induces ERα-positive and ERα-negative mammary cancer in transgenic mice. Oncogene 22:4664–4674, 2003.

293. Liby K, Neltner B, Mohamet L, et al: Prolactin overexpression by MDA-MB-435 human breast cancer cells accelerates tumor growth. Breast Cancer Res Treat 79:241–252, 2003.

Pituitary Surgery

Paolo Cappabianca, Luigi Maria Cavallo, and Oreste de Divitiis

HISTORICAL BACKGROUND
SURGICAL ANATOMY

SURGERY
    Transsphenoidal Approaches
    Transcranial Approaches
    Radiosurgery
COMPLICATIONS

Pituitary surgery is a distinct subspecialty of neurosurgery that demands precise knowledge of basic neurosurgical techniques and associated skills, together with specific knowledge, interest, and appreciation of pituitary pathophysiology, allowing the surgeon to make the right choice at the right moment. It is currently possible to manage many of the different pituitary syndromes with more than one option, including medical, surgical, and radiotherapeutic, alone or in various combinations. Pituitary surgery yields the best outcomes when performed in centers where the entire range of pituitary specialties is offered in an environment of effective teamwork. Such teamwork demands a "teamwork attitude," which is not just the addition of the expertise of the single contributors, but rather a cultural and psychological attitude, with the single units working with a goal of true exchange and sincere collaboration, which allows cooperative effort for the benefit of the patient and positive feedback for physicians and surgeons. Pituitary surgery, perhaps more than other areas of neurosurgery, requires careful and specific postoperative management and long-term patient follow-up, which can make the difference between a satisfactory result and a poor result. A patient can be operated on successfully, but the outcome may not be as brilliant as the surgical procedure if mutual exchange between specialists such as the pathologist, the ophthalmologist, the neuroradiologist, and the endocrinologist is not established. If teamwork logic is established, each participant contributes to the final outcome of the patient while promoting growth of the other components, which calls for further work and better allocation of competencies and effectiveness: A virtuous circuit develops.

It is in such a context that pituitary surgery should exist today, where the neurosurgeon dealing with techniques, indications, and results is a member of an orchestra who is playing a refined instrument. The neurosurgeon must have keen perception, good instincts, steady hands, and the ability to perform an operation made to measure for the individual patient and not mass-produced. To realize these goals, the neurosurgeon must know detailed anatomy, learned in the laboratory before working in an operating room; he or she must be experienced in neuroimaging, must know pathophysiology and the natural history of pituitary disease, and must be familiar with the various therapeutic options. The neurosurgeon plays a crucial role, fully informed about current therapeutic possibilities in the interest of the patient and of the institution where the operation is done.

HISTORICAL BACKGROUND

Pituitary surgery has developed and advanced on the basis of repeated innovations and exchanges between Europe and the New World. The first operation on a pituitary tumor was performed by Horsley in 1889, who published in 1906[1] the results obtained on a series of 10 patients first by means of a frontal craniotomy and later a temporal approach.[2] The first surgeon reporting on an operation specifically for a pituitary tumor was a British general surgeon, Paul; in 1893, he performed a temporal decompression in an acromegalic patient without actually reaching the tumor.[3,4]

The next milestone was the first transsphenoidal approach achieved by the Viennese surgeon Schloffer in Innsbruck, Austria, in 1907.[5] The existence of a direct route through the nose toward the brain was not absolutely new: Many centuries ago, the Egyptians used to extract the cerebral tissue transnasally in the mummification process by means of special hooked instruments, without disfiguring the face. Based on the anatomic studies of the Italian physician Giordano, chief surgeon of the Hospital of Venice,[6,7] Schloffer performed a lateral rhinotomy, reflecting the nose to the right; removed the turbinates; and opened the maxillary, ethmoid, and sphenoid sinuses before reaching the sella. In the same year, von Eiselberg,[8] in Vienna, performed a similar, if even more extended, procedure. The next evolutionary step, approaching the modern transsphenoidal approach, was realized in 1909 by Kocher, professor of surgery in Berne, Switzerland, who was awarded the Nobel Prize for Medicine and Physiology in 1909 for his contributions concerning the thyroid; he performed a transseptal submucosal approach, by means of an external midline incision on the nasal bridge,[9,10] but without exenteration of frontal, ethmoidal, and maxillary sinuses. Another remarkable contribution was that of Kanavel,[11,12] who proposed an approach through an infranasal skin incision. The first totally endonasal procedure, without complete dislocation of the nose, was achieved in 1910 in five stages with the patient under local anesthesia by Hirsch, a Viennese rhinologist, who was the first to incorporate a nasal speculum.[13] He used the technique of his teacher Hajek,[14] previously employed for purulent infections of the sphenoid sinus, opening first the posterior ethmoid sinus, then enlarging the opening into the sphenoid sinus, after a submucosal resection of the septum, according to Kocher's and Kilian's techniques,[9,15] beginning with a hemitransfixion incision in the right nasal cavity. Hirsch moved to the United States in 1938, to escape the Nazis, and worked in Boston with the neurosurgeon Hamlin.[16]

In 1910, Halstead[17,18] was a pioneer of the sublabial approach, initially performed in a multistage operation in Chicago. Cushing performed his first transsphenoidal procedure in 1909,[19] but his classic sublabial, transseptal, transsphenoidal approach[20] was the evolution of his technique and a combination of different methods reported by other authors, such as Halstead, Hirsch, Kanavel, and Kocher (i.e., sublabial incision + submucosal paraseptal approach to the sphenoid sinus + use of the nasal speculum + use of an electric headlamp). Cushing later abandoned this procedure[10,21,22] likely because of better recovery of vision in patients operated transcranially owing to difficulty with hemostasis and completeness of tumor removal in large suprasellar tumors and owing to difficulty in preoperative differential diagnosis. His advocacy of the transcranial option prompted most neurosurgeons to follow his recommendations. Another leading American neurosurgeon, Dandy, stated, "the nasal route is impractical and can never be otherwise."[23] In 1918, at the Johns Hopkins Medical Society, Dandy had presented his experience in about 20 cases operated on by an intracranial intradural approach to the chiasm, according to a frontotemporal route to the pituitary along the sylvian fissure, originally conceived by Heuer in 1914.[24,25] The two main transcranial options, the subfrontal and the frontotemporal, are still used today together with more recent skull base approaches.

The late 1920s to the 1960s were a relatively dark period for transsphenoidal surgery, related to the absence of antibiotics and replacement therapy for adrenocortical hormones, to the lack of adequate illumination, and to the opinions of the most authoritative opinion leader, Cushing. The only pupil of Cushing who did not abandon the transsphenoidal method was Dott, neurosurgeon of the Royal Infirmary at Edinburgh.[10,26] He had learned the method from Cushing when he had been awarded a 1-year Rockefeller Fellowship at the Peter Bent Brigham Hospital in 1923. It is not clear why Dott did not publish his results, but he kept the procedure alive, improved the technique by adding two light bulbs to the speculum designed by Cushing, and taught the method to the French neurosurgeon Guiot during his visit at the Royal Infirmary in 1956. Guiot at the Hôpital Foch in Paris and Guiot's trainee Hardy in Montreal deserve the credit for the "transsphenoidal renaissance" in the late 1960s and 1970s. Modern transsphenoidal surgery takes advantage of the innovations of intraoperative image intensification and fluoroscopy, introduced by Guiot, and of the use of the operating microscope, according to Hardy,[27] who introduced the concept of microadenoma and selective microsurgical resection.

No new progress was made until the 1990s, when the latest innovation, the endoscope, was introduced. By analogy with the evolution of Picasso's painting, the "cubist evolution" of transsphenoidal surgery occurred, from the devastating transfacial approaches to the minimally invasive contemporary procedures[28]: using the endoscope as a visualizing instrument for pituitary surgery. Used for the first time by Guiot in 1963[29] as an adjunct to the microscope to expand the field of vision (endoscope-assisted microneurosurgery), then abandoned for many years because still technically insufficient, the endoscope has come into regular use as a stand-alone visualizing and operating tool (pure endoscopic transsphenoidal surgery) thanks primarily to the work of Jho in Pittsburgh[30,31] and of our group in Naples, Italy,[32,33] who have standardized a unilateral endonasal anterior sphenoidotomy approach to the sella, without the use of the operating microscope or of a transsphenoidal retractor. Further advancement and evolution of the technique is expected through intraoperative magnetic resonance imaging (MRI), robotics, and miniaturization, in addition to the rapidly emerging biomolecular frontiers, which are expected to change the world of pituitary surgery.

SURGICAL ANATOMY

The pituitary gland, or hypophysis cerebri, is situated within the hypophyseal fossa, a fibro-osseous compartment near the center of the cranial base (Fig. 28-1). This fossa is limited laterally and superiorly by reflections of dura mater and

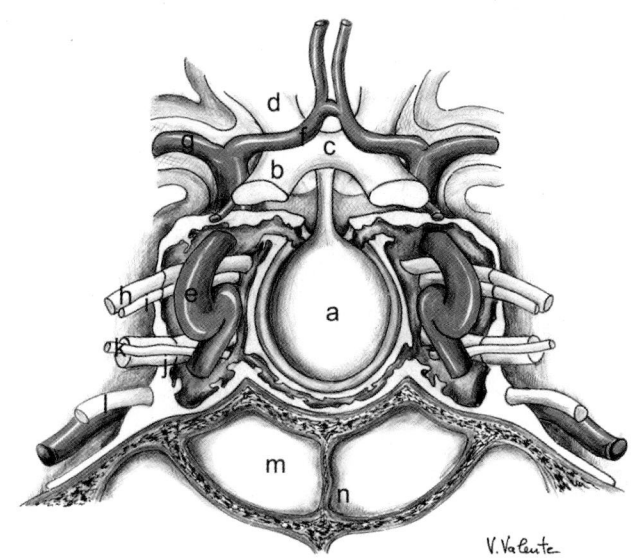

Figure 28-1 Frontal view: schematic drawing of the sellar region. *a,* pituitary gland; *b,* optic nerve; *c,* optic chiasm; *d,* optic tract; *e,* internal carotid artery; *f,* anterior cerebral artery; *g,* middle cerebral artery; *h,* oculomotor nerve; *i,* trochlear nerve; *j,* ophthalmic branch (V1) of the trigeminal nerve; *k,* abducent nerve; *l,* maxillary branch (V2) of the trigeminal nerve; *m,* sphenoid sinus; *n,* sphenoid septum. (Courtesy of V. Valente, MD.)

anteriorly, posteriorly, and inferiorly by the sella turcica, a depression in the body of the sphenoid bone. At the superior edge of the anterior wall of the sella turcica, there is a bony protrusion called tuberculum sellae, and its posterior wall is the dorsum sellae.

The degree of pneumatization of the sphenoid bone and the thickness of the bone separating the sphenoid sinus from the hypophyseal fossa are highly variable. Three sinus types are distinguished by their shape and size: In the *conchal type* (approximately 3%), the area below the sella is a solid block of bone without an air cavity; in the *presellar type* (approximately 17%), the air cavity does not penetrate beyond a vertical plane parallel to the anterior sellar wall; and in the *sellar type* (approximately 80%), the air cavity extends into the body of the sphenoid below the sella and as far posteriorly as the clivus. The conchal type is most common in children before the age of 12 years, at which time pneumatization progresses within the sphenoid sinus. The greater the degree of pneumatization of the sphenoid sinus, the easier is the access to the sellar region through the transsphenoidal approach.

The space within the sphenoid sinus is subdivided by one or more septa. Single septa are not always located in the midline, and in 20% of cases, the posterior attachment of the sphenoid septum to the sphenoid sinus is on the carotid protuberance, becoming an important landmark for preventing injury to the carotid artery.

The diaphragma sellae, a fold of dura with a central aperture, forms an incomplete roof above the sella turcica. The diaphragma separates the anterior lobe from the overlying optic chiasm. The central opening of the diaphragma is of variable size and transmits the pituitary stalk and its blood supply. The subarachnoid space of the chiasmatic cistern can extend through the aperture of the diaphragma and into the sella turcica for varying distances above the gland. When there is an incompetent diaphragma sellae (i.e., wide central aperture of the diaphragma), the chiasmatic cistern herniates to fill the sella turcica partially, leading to remodeling and enlargement of the hypophyseal fossa and flattening of the pituitary gland, a condition called *empty sella,*[34] which is found in 5% to 23% of cases at autopsy.[35] When this condition is associated with the presence of an adenoma, usually a microadenoma, the surgeon must be careful to avoid entering the subarachnoid space (i.e., the chiasmatic cistern herniated into the sella), to prevent an intraoperative cerebrospinal fluid (CSF) leak, which could increase the difficulty of resecting the lesion.

The folds of the dura mater form the lateral walls of the hypophyseal fossa and the medial wall of the so-called cavernous sinuses, these latter consisting of a series of compartmentalized venous channels separated by fibrous trabeculae and communicating with each other by means of the anterior and posterior intercavernous sinuses.[36–40] The oculomotor nerve, the trochlear nerve, and first two divisions of the trigeminal nerve are embedded in the lateral wall of the cavernous sinus, lying between the endothelial lining and the dura mater, whereas the abducens nerve is contained within the sinus itself. The cavernous sinus also envelops a portion of the internal carotid artery (ICA) and the sympathetic nerve plexus encircling it. The intracavernous segment of the ICA extends forward, adjacent to the superolateral surface of the body of the sphenoid bone, in a groove called the *carotid sulcus*. The carotid arteries and the bone layers overlying them in the sphenoid sinus form two protuberances, which represent important landmarks in the transsphenoidal approach, particularly at the level of the sellar floor, where they are considered the lateral margins of a correct opening of the sella.

The pituitary gland derives its blood supply from two groups of arteries. The superior hypophyseal artery primarily supplies the anterior lobe, the pituitary stalk, and the inferior surface of the optic nerve and chiasm, whereas the inferior hypophyseal artery is primarily related to the pars nervosa. The superior hypophyseal artery can arise from the supraclinoid portion of the ICA or from the posterior communicating artery, whereas the inferior hypophyseal artery arises from the meningohypophyseal trunk, a branch of the cavernous segment of the ICA.

The pituitary gland is overlaid by the visual pathways and the hypothalamus. The relationships between the pituitary gland, diaphragma sellae, sulcus chiasmatis, and optic apparatus are important determinants of the visual deficits produced by an expanding pituitary tumor.[41] In some cases, the anterior border of the optic chiasm is closely applied to the sulcus chiasmatis of the sphenoid bone; this leads to a lower position of the optic chiasm, which is much nearer to the diaphragma sellae. This condition, called *prefixed chiasm* and present in 5% to 10% of cases,[42,43] must be considered during the transcranial approaches and in the transsphenoidal opening of the upper portion of the sellar floor as in the extended approaches to the planum sphenoidale because of the possibility of producing iatrogenic damage to the optic chiasm. In other cases, the optic chiasm is located above the anterior part of the diaphragma sellae, making it extremely vulnerable to the suprasellar extension of a pituitary tumor. This pattern is found in about 12% of cases.[42,43] In most cases (75%), the optic chiasm is placed more posteriorly, lying over the posterior aspect of the diaphragma sellae, near the dorsum sellae,[42,43] which is the more favorable relationship for the removal of a sellar lesion because in such a circumstance the suprasellar region is free from the optic chiasm. The remaining pattern is that of an optic chiasm located on and behind the dorsum sellae, called *postfixed chiasm* (4% to 11% of cases).[42,43] In such cases, the intracranial course of the optic nerves is longer, and the medial aspects of the optic nerves are more vulnerable to the suprasellar extension of the pituitary tumor.

Anatomy should represent an uninterrupted line in the surgeon's mind. The surgeon must have a thorough knowledge of anatomy and refer to it before, during, and after the surgical procedure. Only in this way can the surgeon determine the correct surgical approach, the exact plan for each operation; perform the necessary intraoperative controls; and check the ultimate results of the intervention.

Progress in diagnostic imaging techniques (computed tomography [CT] and MRI) has given the neurosurgeon preoperative detailed knowledge of the anatomy of each patient and of the surgical route to follow, rendering the surgical procedure safer and more comfortable for the patient and surgeon. CT of the nasal and paranasal structures provides precise information on the surgical route to follow, particularly useful for the endoscopic transsphenoidal procedure, revealing the possible presence of turbinate hypertrophy; nasal septal deviation; concha bullosa; unusual sphenoid sinus type (sellar, presellar, or conchal type); single or multiple sphenoid septa; presence of an Onodi cell, representing a potential risk for the optic nerve; and any bone structure alteration caused by the sellar lesion, such as thinning or erosion or both of the sellar floor. MRI of the sellar area, before and after intravenous administration of a paramagnetic contrast medium (gadolinium-diethylene-triamine-pentaacetic acid), is fundamental. Imaging permits the precise localization of the lesion with its peculiar characteristics, localization of the anatomic endosellar and parasellar structures (cisterns, optic nerves, medial wall of the cavernous sinus with the ICA), and knowledge of their mutual relationships. In clinical practice, MRI is performed in the sagittal and coronal planes: The sagittal sections give good definition of the morphology and size of the lesion; of the pituitary gland and of the pituitary stalk, when recognizable; of the suprasellar cisterns; and of the optic chiasm. The coronal slices add an evaluation of symmetry, at the sellar and parasellar level. In the axial plane, the images are obtained as completion, to define better the anterosellar and retrosellar extensions of the lesion.

The need to define intraoperatively the exact location of a lesion and its relationships with surrounding vascular and nervous structures has led to the development of neuronavigation and intraoperative MRI, which provide continuous anatomic information. The neuronavigator is a computer-based system that offers the surgeon real-time information relating to the operating site. The basic function of the navigator is to obtain the location of a probe tip within the surgical field and to translate it into the CT/MRI coordinates. The patient's head is initially related to the CT/MRI coordinates; this relationship is established preoperatively using a set of fiducial markers on the patient's head. During transsphenoidal surgery, it can obviate the need for intraoperative fluoroscopy, avoiding the exposure of the operating room staff and the patient to radiation. Its employment is particularly useful in the presence of a conchal or presellar type of sphenoid sinus, in identifying the boundaries of the sella, and in some cases of recurrences in which prior surgery has altered the landmarks needed to reach the sella safely.[44–49]

Intraoperative MRI, using a magnetic resonance magnet positioned in a specially designed operating room with a movable operating table that allows the translation of the patient from the surgical equipment to the MRI imager, offers the opportunity of a "second look" during the same surgical procedure. In transsphenoidal surgery, intraoperative MRI allows documentation of the extent of surgical resection of the sellar lesion, and the removal of the suprasellar portion of the tumor can be reliably evaluated.[50–55]

SURGERY

Therapy for pituitary adenomas is targeted to achieve multiple goals, as follows:

1. Normalization of excess hormone secretion
2. Preservation or restoration of normal pituitary function
3. Elimination of mass effect
4. Preservation or restoration of normal neurologic function, usually visual acuity or visual field (or both) being more frequently affected

5. Prevention of tumor recurrence
6. Achievement of a complete histologic diagnosis
7. Obtaining tissue for scientific studies

Despite advances in the medical treatment of pituitary adenomas, most of these tumors are managed surgically. Indications for surgery of pituitary adenomas are as follows:

- Pituitary apoplexy, a relatively rare condition presenting with sudden headache, abrupt visual loss, ophthalmoplegia, altered level of consciousness, and collapse from acute adrenal insufficiency. It is caused by a hemorrhage into the tumor or its acute necrosis, with subsequent swelling and frequent spreading into the subarachnoid space, leading to other signs of meningeal irritation; the related acute and severe clinical syndrome demands glucocorticoid replacement and surgical decompression, usually transsphenoidal, if visual loss is severe and progressive.[56–59] If the patient has a mild form of apoplexy and is clinically stable, it is prudent to measure the serum prolactin because some patients with prolactinoma present in this fashion and can be treated successfully with medical therapy.
- Progressive mass effect, producing compression of the surrounding neurovascular structures and usually causing visual deficit (due to compression of the optic chiasm) or less frequently cranial nerve palsy (due to compression of cranial nerves inside the cavernous sinus). In cases of prolactin-secreting macroadenomas, dopamine agonist administration can be considered as the first treatment option because of the predictable dramatic shrinkage of the lesion, with rapid recovery of neurologic deficits. In such circumstances, frequent visual field and imaging controls are necessary to monitor the clinical evolution.

Because pituitary tumors are biologically, endocrinologically, and pathologically a heterogeneous group of lesions, the role of surgery differs for the different pituitary tumor subtypes. The primary role of surgery is established in the following conditions:

- Nonfunctioning pituitary tumors
- Cushing's disease because of the present inadequacy of pharmacologic agents
- Acromegaly, in combination with medical treatment (preoperative and postoperative, if necessary)
- Thyroid-stimulating hormone–secreting adenomas

The role of surgery in prolactinoma is secondary, but still necessary in selected conditions. Indications for surgery also include the following:

- Failure of or resistance to medical treatment or intolerable side effects of medical therapy
- Recurrences, in combination or in association with the other therapeutic options, medical or radiotherapeutic or both

Indications for surgery have changed over time and with the refinement of the surgical techniques and according to the evaluation of results and experiences, to the development of knowledge about the biology of pituitary tumors, and to the use of effective new pharmacologic agents[60–62] and radiation techniques. Large invasive pituitary tumors are difficult to cure regardless of the approach because the removal of every fragment of the tumor is often impossible. Extended transsphenoidal approaches sometimes can represent a valid alternative to transcranial options; excellent visual outcomes derive from the transsphenoidal method.[58,63] Visual impairment does not indicate the need for a transcranial operation, as Cushing believed at one time.[64]

The surgical approach, with respect to the basic principles for resecting pituitary adenomas, can be performed by two main approaches, each of them with several subcategories:

1. Transsphenoidal
  a. Microsurgical
    (1) Transnasal
    (2) Sublabial
    (3) Endonasal
  b. Endoscopic
2. Transcranial
  a. Subfrontal unilateral
  b. Frontolateral or pterional
  c. Subfrontal bilateral interhemispheric

After an initial flourishing of transsphenoidal surgery in the early 1900s, transcranial approaches obtained success and were popular in the first half of the twentieth century. This fundamental debate lasted for decades, until the introduction of intraoperative fluoroscopy and microscopy effectively put it to rest. With these new imaging techniques, adequate exposure and thorough exploration of the sella turcica became possible without the need for a craniotomy and associated brain retraction. As a result, the transseptal transsphenoidal approach came to be accepted as the procedure of choice for the surgical management of most pituitary lesions.[65,66]

The success of the transsphenoidal approach is based on solid foundations: It is the least traumatic route to the sella, it lacks visible scars, it provides excellent visualization of the pituitary gland and adjacent pathology, it offers a lower morbidity and mortality rate compared with transcranial procedures, and it requires only a brief hospital stay. Indications for transsphenoidal surgery today include more than 95% of the surgical indications in the sellar area and approximately 96% of all pituitary adenomas.[67] The well-established indications for this route are as follows:

- Almost all adenomatous lesions[68]
- Nonneoplastic intrasellar cysts[34,69–71]
- Craniopharyngiomas, preferably cystic, extra-arachnoidal,[72] and infradiaphragmatic,[73] with an enlarged sella[74–76]

Absolute indications were established in the 1970s and are still valid today; they include the following[77]:

- Elevated surgical risk of the transcranial route
  - In the elderly
  - In long-standing compression of the chiasm, not able to tolerate additional trauma
  - In case of acute endosellar hypertension
  - In most cases of pituitary apoplexy
  - In pan-invasive, not radically removable adenomas
- Adenomas with downward development
- Microadenomas

To these classic guidelines for the transsphenoidal option, in more recent decades the following can be added:

- The extended transsphenoidal approaches to the sphenoethmoid planum, for suprasellar craniopharyngiomas, Rathke's cleft cysts, some tuberculum sellae meningiomas, and anterior cranial base CSF leaks[78–88]; to the clival area, for chordomas[79,89–93]; and to the parasellar compartment,[37,79,91,94–99] for invasive adenomas and chordomas. The development of the extended transsphenoidal approaches has now provided transsphenoidal access to several lesions that previously would have been considered accessible by transcranial approaches only. The spectrum of lesions accessible to transsphenoidal surgery is widening. The extended approaches today represent standard procedures in selected centers and in experienced hands and are expected to experience further progress in the near future with additional technical and instrumental development.
- A sequential transsphenoidal approach, in intrasuprasellar adenomas, as an intentionally two-staged transsphenoidal operation. This operation is designed to encourage the descent of a suprasellar remnant of the adenoma

incompletely removed in the first step, to limit the risks of a brisk decompression of huge lesions, and to manage the lesions with a second surgery.[100]

The striking figure indicating that 19% of primary brain tumors treated in academic centers in the United States are operated transsphenoidally is testimony to what we have reported about the evolving modern and contemporary indications for the transsphenoidal approach. There are conditions that limit and sometimes contraindicate the choice of the transsphenoidal approach in favor of the transcranial, either related to the anatomy of the surgical pathway or to the morphology and consistency of the lesion. The size of the sella, its degree of mineralization, the size and the pneumatization of the sphenoid sinus, and the position and tortuosity of the carotid arteries can increase remarkably the difficulty of the transsphenoidal procedure and the final surgical result and may determine the opportunity or even the necessity for the transcranial alternative.

Indications for transcranial surgery include the following[68,73]:

1. Tumors with extensive intracranial invasion, into the anterior cranial fossa or lateral or posterior extension into the middle and posterior cranial fossae.[101]
2. Tumors with asymmetric suprasellar development, particularly if major vessel involvement is present.
3. Tumors with intracranial extension separated from the intrasellar portion by a narrow neck (dumbbell adenoma), showing an hourglass configuration.[102]
4. Suprasellar tumors not completely resectable through the transsphenoidal route.[103]
5. Recurrent or residual pituitary tumors in patients who already have had unsuccessful transsphenoidal surgery.
6. When preoperative MRI assessment, on the basis of long thyroid hormone receptor (TR) signal, suggests a firm consistency of the adenoma, preventing easy debulking with subsequent collapse and descent into the sella, when resected from below.[104–106] This may occur after radiotherapy[107]; increased fibrosis also has been reported after treatment with dopamine agonists[108] or somatostatin analogues,[109,110] but these reports do not reflect our experience.
7. When the sphenoid sinus is not pneumatized and the sella is small or does not make it easy to reach the suprasellar extension of the tumor.[111]
8. When coexisting vascular[96,112] and tumoral surgical pathology is evident and one-time surgical treatment of both conditions is chosen.

TRANSSPHENOIDAL APPROACHES

One or another variation of the transsphenoidal approach represents the most physiologic and minimally traumatic corridor of surgical access to the sella, providing direct and superior visualization of the pituitary gland and adjacent pathology.[92,113] The transsphenoidal approach represents a midline approach that has been performed since the 1960s by means of the *operating microscope* as visualizing tool, through transnasal transseptal, sublabial transseptal, or endonasal procedures (microsurgical transsphenoidal procedures). The transsphenoidal approach also can be performed by means of the *endoscope* as the sole visualizing tool during the entire surgical procedure, realizing a "pure" endoscopic endonasal transsphenoidal approach. The combined use of the microscope and the endoscope during the same approach defines the condition of *endoscope-assisted microsurgery*.

Microsurgical Transsphenoidal Approaches
Although many different transsphenoidal procedures and variations have been described, currently there are three basic microsurgical transsphenoidal approaches to pituitary tumors: the *transnasal* transseptal transsphenoidal approach,

the *sublabial* transseptal transsphenoidal approach, and the *endonasal* transsphenoidal approach. The patient can be positioned on the operating table supine, as originally proposed by Cushing, with the surgeon behind the patient's head, or in the semisitting position, as favored by Guiot, with the surgeon standing in front of the patient. The procedure is performed with an operating microscope for visualization, illumination, and magnification of the surgical field. Intermittent fluoroscopy is used for trajectory guidance, or, more recently, neuronavigational systems permit the surgeon to gather information about the current position of anatomic structures or instruments during the procedure itself.[44–49] Intraoperative MRI is capable of enhancing safety and providing additional knowledge about the completeness of lesion removal.[50,51,53–55] The three main transsphenoidal methods differ slightly one from each other primarily in the initial phase up to the exposure of the sphenoid sinus; they then follow the same surgical sphenoidal and sellar steps.

Microsurgical Transnasal Transseptal Transsphenoidal Approach
In a diffused version of the transnasal approach (Fig. 28-2), the operation starts in the right nostril, with the retraction of the columella to the patient's left to expose through incision in the nostril the anterior edge of the septal cartilage, 2 to 3 cm behind the mucosal-cutaneous junction. The nasal mucosa usually adheres tightly to the most anterior region of the septum: Its dense, fibrous strands are divided with a combination of sharp and blunt dissection. The submucosal dissection is extended posteriorly, elevating the nasal mucosa away from the septal cartilage up to its junction with the bony septum. The cartilaginous septum is dissected from the mucoperichondrium along its right side, then is laterally pushed on the left side, at the junction point, to free the cartilaginous septum from the bony septum. Posterior submucosal tunnels are created along both sides of the bony septum, which is partially removed to facilitate the introduction of a self-retaining transsphenoidal retractor, following the use of a nasal speculum in the dissection of the nasal septum. Care must be taken to avoid mucosal perforation during these maneuvers.

Microsurgical Sublabial Transseptal Transsphenoidal Approach
The upper lip is retracted, and an incision is made along the buccogingival junction, between the two canine fossae

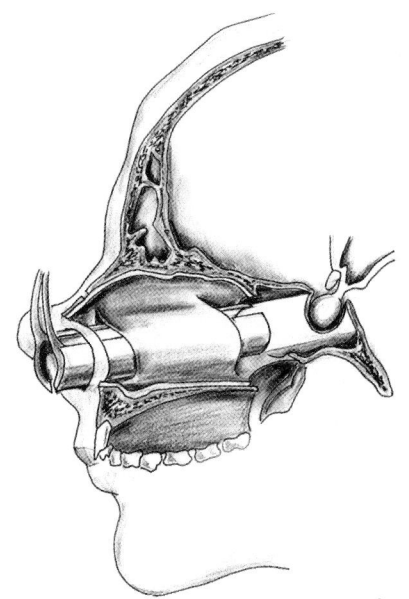

Figure 28-2 Sagittal view: schematic drawing of the microsurgical transnasal transseptal transsphenoidal approach. (Courtesy of V. Valente, MD.)

(Fig. 28-3). The upper lip and the periosteum are elevated to expose the anterior nasal spine and the inferior border of the pyriform aperture of the nasal cavities. The mucosa of the floor of the nose is elevated first on both sides with a small periosteal elevator, which is introduced along the nasal septum to detach the mucosa from the cartilage. The elevated mucosa is held in place by a nasal speculum, allowing further mucosal elevation from the bony nasal septum. The inferior and posterior portion of the cartilaginous septum is dissected from the bony nasal septum and is deflected laterally. The self-retaining nasal speculum is introduced and opened widely to hold the retracted mucosa out of the field. The sublabial approach permits a more anterior trajectory with respect to the transnasal option, which can be useful in lesions that extend in the suprasellar area or toward the planum sphenoidale.

Microsurgical Endonasal Transsphenoidal Approach

A hand-held speculum is inserted into the nostril along the middle turbinate, which reliably leads to the sphenoid sinus (Fig. 28-4). In the posterior nasal cavity, an elevator is used to make a vertical mucosal incision at the junction of the keel of the sphenoid bone and the posterior nasal septum. The septum, with its intact mucosa, is pushed off the midline by the medial blade of the hand-held speculum. Bilateral mucosal flaps over the keel of the sphenoid bone are elevated and reflected laterally, with the identification of the sphenoid ostia. The hand-held speculum is replaced by a thin nasal speculum, which is placed up to the face of the sphenoid bone. After lesion removal, the speculum is withdrawn, the nasal septum is returned to the midline, and the ipsilateral out-fractured middle turbinate may be moved toward the midline to prevent a maxillary sinus mucocele. Nasal packing is placed for 24 hours in selected cases, but is not routinely employed.[114,115]

When the anterior wall of the sphenoid sinus has been reached by one of the aforementioned three routes, bone punches are used to make a large opening of the anterior wall of the sphenoid sinus, which extends beyond the sphenoid ostia to provide adequate sellar floor exposure. After opening the anterior wall of the sphenoid sinus, one or more septa can be identified. The surgeon should review the anatomy of the

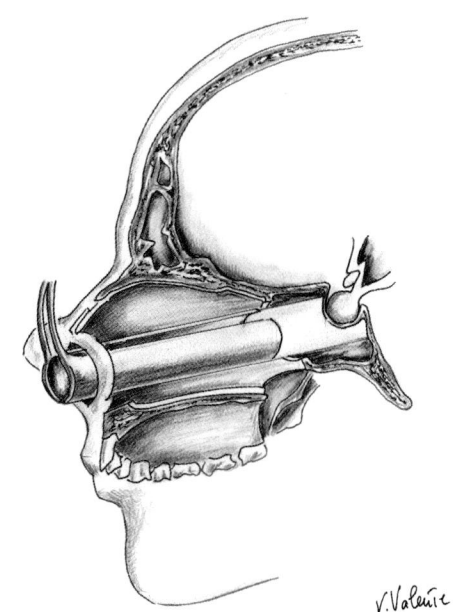

Figure 28-4   Sagittal view: schematic drawing of the microsurgical endonasal transsphenoidal approach. (Courtesy of V. Valente, MD.)

sphenoid sinus on the preoperative nasal and paranasal cavity CT scans and compare them with the intraoperative ones, particularly when the septa are implanted on one of the carotid prominences and the sphenoid sinus is of a presellar type. The insertion of the septum along the posterior wall of the sphenoid sinus may be a useful anatomic landmark to identify the sellar floor and to define the medial extent of the cavernous sinus. Even if in selected cases it is not necessary to remove all the sphenoid septa, their removal must allow exposure of all the crucial anatomic findings visible inside the sphenoid cavity.

Usually, the sphenoid mucosa is displaced laterally as much as necessary to open the sellar floor, unless adenomatous infiltration is evident or suspected, and the mucosa is resected in such cases. Its preservation is thought to ensure adequate mucociliary transport, with its associated function in maintaining the physiology of nasosinusal ventilation.

After completing the removal of the sphenoid septa, on the posterior wall of the sphenoid sinus the sella is recognizable; its anatomic boundaries, when not clearly visible, are confirmed by C-arm fluoroscopy or neuronavigation. An adequate bony exposure of the sellar floor is crucial to the success of the approach, particularly when dealing with large tumors.

With a presellar or a conchal type of sphenoid sinus, the sphenoidotomy calls for some precautions.[116] In these two variants of incomplete sphenoid sinus pneumatization, a microdrill is used to open the sellar floor. In these cases, fluoroscopy or neuronavigation is extremely useful, if not essential, for identification of the superior and inferior edges of the sella, even in experienced hands. The method of opening of the sellar floor depends on its consistency: If it is intact, opening is achieved by means of a microdrill or bone punches or both; if it is eroded or thinned, opening is achieved by means of a dissector, sometimes realizing an osteoplastic opening useful for sellar repair.[117]

The dura is incised in a midline position, in a linear or cross fashion, and a fragment of dura can be taken for histologic examination if it appears infiltrated.[118] When the dura is incised, the surgeon must keep in mind that the perisellar sinuses,[119] and particularly the superior and the inferior intercavernous sinuses, are compressed and usually obliterated by macroadenomas, making the dural incision bloodless. The situation is different with microadenomas, particularly in cases of Cushing's disease, in which it is not unusual to find the

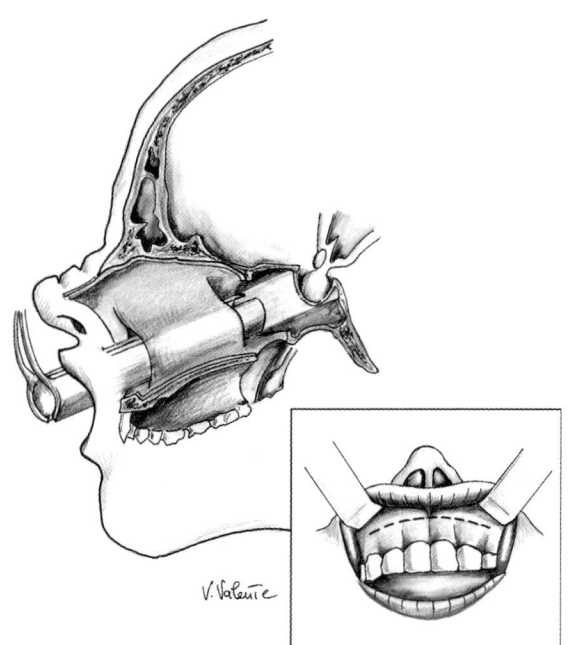

Figure 28-3   Sagittal view: schematic drawing of the microsurgical sublabial transseptal transsphenoidal approach. See detail of the sublabial incision on the right. (Courtesy of V. Valente, MD.)

entire sellar dura covered by one or two venous channels that can bleed during tumor resection. Caution is necessary when incising the dura in microadenomas to avoid damaging a possibly ectatic carotid artery, which may be located within the sella, especially in acromegalic patients.

Before removing an adenoma, the surgeon must keep in mind that the pituitary gland is an extra-arachnoid structure, situated below the diaphragma sellae. During the removal of a pituitary adenoma, the surgical maneuvers must respect these structures, to avoid postoperative CSF leaks and other major complications. Concerning the removal of a microadenoma, if it is visible on the surface of the gland, a cleavage plane between the microadenoma and the residual anterior pituitary should be found, with the aim of delimiting the lesion. When the microadenoma is not superficial, and there is no change in the appearance of the overlying anterior pituitary, such as discoloration or attenuated texture, a small incision can be made in the normal pituitary gland on the same side of the microadenoma, and the lesion can be removed with the help of small ring curettes. After the curettage of the adenoma, a small cottonoid is inserted inside the tumor cavity and with a forceps is turned in alternate directions to mobilize fragments of the lesion or of the neoplastic capsule. Concerning the removal of macroadenomas, the surgeon first must try to remove the tumor tissue from the interior of the sella and from any lateral extension, to avoid cumbersome obstruction of the surgical field by a down-hanging, inverted diaphragma sellae. If a gradual descent of the suprasellar portion of the lesion is not observed, it is useful to ask the anesthetist to perform the Valsalva maneuver, which may cause a protrusion into the sellar cavity of a part of the dura and arachnoid covering the suprasellar tumor extension (suprasellar cistern), or to inject air through a lumbar drain preoperatively positioned for the same purpose.[120]

After the intracapsular emptying of the adenoma, its capsule can be dissected from the suprasellar cistern, when possible. As the macroadenoma grows, it sometimes distends the residual normal anterior pituitary, which appears as a thin layer of tissue surrounding the adenoma capsule, sometimes seen on MRI, the removal of which could cause a postoperative hypopituitarism. It is also important to recognize the neurohypophysis, sometimes present in front of the dorsum sellae, where curettage or aspiration must be avoided, to prevent the development of postoperative diabetes insipidus.

After lesion removal, closure of the sellar floor is performed, especially when an intraoperative CSF leak has occurred, using a variety of techniques (intradural or extradural closure of the sella, packing of the sella with or without packing of the sphenoid sinus) and different autologous and synthetic materials.[121,122] Overpacking of the sella must be avoided to prevent compression of the optic system.

Similar to the removal of lesions that often originate or develop inside the intra-arachnoid compartment, such as craniopharyngiomas or Rathke's cleft cysts, further considerations are appropriate. These lesions develop primarily in the suprasellar region, with an intact or only slightly enlarged sellar cavity. In such cases, an extended approach is often necessary to manage the lesion. The anterior sellar wall, the tuberculum sellae, and the posterior portion of the planum sphenoidale are drilled away, according to the circumstances, with the use of a microdrill with a diamond bur. The superior intercavernous sinus is identified, coagulated, and divided in a midline position. When the lesion is exposed, it is removed, trying to respect as much as possible the arachnoid membrane to avoid intraoperative and postoperative complications, which seem to be higher than in conventional transsphenoidal surgery.[83]

Endoscopic Endonasal Transsphenoidal Approach

Endoscopic endonasal transsphenoidal surgery (Fig. 28-5) is a novel, minimally invasive transsphenoidal approach performed

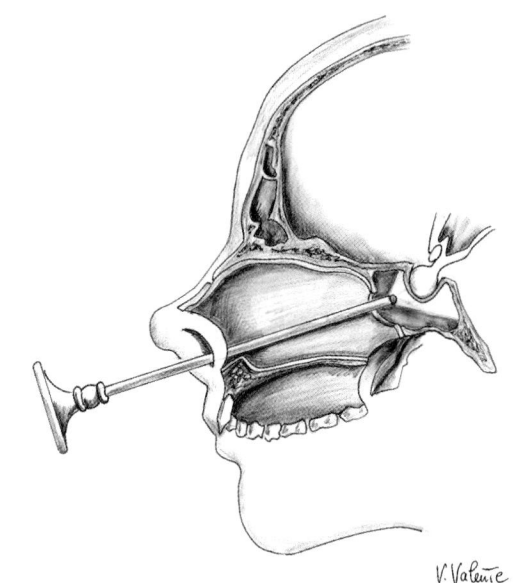

Figure 28-5 Sagittal view: schematic drawing of the endoscopic endonasal transsphenoidal approach. (Courtesy of V. Valente, MD.)

by means of the endoscope as a stand-alone visualizing and operating instrument, without the need of the transsphenoidal retractor. It has the same indications as the conventional microsurgical technique[33,123] and since the 1990s has enjoyed progressive acceptance among surgeons and patients for its minimal invasiveness and for the excellent surgical view it provides.[30–33,124–127] It requires specific endoscopic skills and is based on a different concept because the endoscopic view that the surgeon receives on the video monitor is not the transposition of the real image, as it would be looking through the eyepiece of a microscope, but is the result of a microprocessor's elaboration.

The patient is positioned supine with the trunk elevated 10 degrees and the head turned 10 degrees toward the surgeon, not fixed in a Mayfield headrest with pins, but just in a horseshoe-type headrest. The endoscopic equipment (monitor, light source, video camera, video recorder) is ergonomically positioned behind the head of the patient and in front of the operator, who is on the patient's right. The anesthetist with his or her equipment is positioned on the left of the patient at the level of the head, the assistant is positioned on the patient's left, and the nurse is positioned at the level of the patient's legs. The table-mounted endoscope holder, which holds the endoscope in the sphenoid and sellar phases of the operation, allowing the surgeon to work with two hands, is fixed next to the patient's shoulder and is tilted so as not to interfere with the maneuvers of the surgical instruments. Before beginning the surgical procedure, the anesthesiologist helps to ensure bloodless nasal cavities, sometimes by means of a slight controlled hypotension and always with excellent analgesia, to minimize mucosal bleeding, especially until the anterior sphenoidotomy has been performed.

The endoscope (4 mm in diameter, 0-degree angled lens, 18 cm in length) is introduced through the chosen nostril, tangential to the floor of the nasal cavity. The first structures to be identified are the inferior turbinate laterally and the nasal septum medially. Above the inferior turbinate, one can see the head of middle turbinate, usually close to the nasal septum. As the endoscope advances along the floor of the nasal cavity, it reaches the choana. Cottonoids soaked with diluted epinephrine (1:100,000) or with xylometazoline hydrochloride are positioned between the middle turbinate and the nasal septum to enlarge the space between them and to obtain the decongestion of the nasal mucosa (which has a rich innervation and vascularization). The head of the middle turbinate is delicately dislocated laterally to widen further the virtual space between the middle turbinate and the nasal septum and to create an adequate surgical pathway. After the creation of suitable space between the middle turbinate and the nasal septum, the endoscope is angled upward along the roof of the choana and the sphenoethmoid recess, until it reaches the sphenoid ostium, usually located about 1.5 cm above the roof of the choana. When the sphenoid cavity is reached, coagulation of the sphenoethmoid recess and of the area around the sphenoid ostium is performed, starting about 0.5 cm from the top of the choana up to the superior border of the nasal cavity to avoid arterial bleeding originating from septal branches of the sphenopalatine artery.

At this point, a microdrill with a cutting bur separates the nasal septum from the sphenoid rostrum. The whole anterior wall of the sphenoid sinus is now visible and is enlarged circumferentially, using bone punches or a microdrill; care must be taken in the inferolateral direction, where the sphenopalatine artery or its major branches lie. To avoid these vessels, it is sufficient to cut away the nasal mucosa slightly in an inferolateral direction and to coagulate it with the bipolar forceps to expose the sphenoid rostrum completely. The sphenoid rostrum is removed in fragments and not "en bloc" because this last maneuver could cause lacerations and bleeding in the nasal mucosa while passing through the nasal cavity. It is mandatory to remove widely the anterior wall of the sphenoid sinus, especially downward, before reaching the sella; otherwise, the instruments would not be able to reach all the areas visible by the endoscope. When the anterior sphenoidotomy is completed, small amounts of bleeding originating from the edges of the sphenoidotomy must be controlled to avoid occluding the lens of the endoscope during the next phases.

The sphenoid and the sellar phases of the endoscopic procedure are performed according to the same rules and principles of the microsurgical transsphenoidal approach. Nevertheless, because of the characteristics of the endoscopic approach and owing to intrinsic properties of the endoscope itself, some procedural considerations should be made, as follows:

- After the removal of the sphenoid septa, thanks to the wider view offered by the endoscope, the posterior and lateral walls of the sphenoid sinus are visible, with the sellar floor at the center, the sphenoethmoid planum above it, and the clival indentation below; lateral to the sellar floor, the bony prominences of the ICA and of the optic nerves can be seen and between them the optocarotid recess, molded by the pneumatization of the optic strut of the anterior clinoid process. These prominences and depressions, especially in a well-pneumatized sphenoid sinus, not invaded by a sellar lesion, define a sort of "fetal face," where the forehead corresponds to the sphenoid planum, the eyes to the two optocarotid recesses, the eyebrows to the two optic nerve protuberances, the nose to the sella, and the mouth to the clivus, laterally limited by the two paraclival carotid artery protuberances, representing the cheeks. Nevertheless, in most sellar-type sphenoid sinuses, all these landmarks may not be clearly recognizable because of the different degree of sphenoid sinus pneumatization or extension of the lesion, but the identification of the sphenoethmoid planum, of the clival indentation, and of the bony protuberances of the ICA can be considered enough to determine safely the edges of the sellar floor. Because of the paucity of anatomic landmarks, only in the presence of a presellar or a conchal sphenoid sinus or in some recurrences, a neuronavigation system or C-arm fluoroscopy is needed to avoid lateral misdirection, close to the parasellar and paraclival courses of the ICAs.
- Before opening the sellar floor, a longer endoscope (4 mm in diameter, 0-degree angled lens, 30 cm in length), fixed to

the holder, is positioned inside the upper portion of the nasal cavity to free both of the surgeon's hands and to allow comfortable introduction of two instruments under the endoscope, without coming into conflict with it.

- The opening of the sellar floor, dural incision, and lesion removal are performed following the already well-defined rules of the microsurgical transsphenoidal approach. If there is enough space in the sellar cavity, during or after lesion removal, angled endoscopes (30-degree and 45-degree) can be advanced to verify the presence of possible tumor remnants, often imprisoned in the recesses created by the descent of the suprasellar cistern. When the lesion extends toward the medial wall of the cavernous sinus, its removal can be accomplished under direct endoscopic vision, using curved instruments and suction cannulas.
- After removal of the tumor, if there is evidence or risk of a CSF leak, closure of the sella is performed according to common guidelines. Sellar reconstruction is performed also with the purpose of creating a barrier outward, of reducing the dead space, and of preventing the descent of the chiasm in the sellar cavity[122]; in certain other cases, no plugging is used.[121] Because of the minimal invasiveness of the endoscopic procedure, no autologous bone or cartilage from the nasal septum is usually available, and different synthetic or resorbable materials,[128] when necessary,[121] must be employed to obtain a safe and effective repair of the sella. Lumbar drainage is adopted in case of intraoperative CSF leaks, only when the closure is not judged absolutely watertight, in extended approaches, or when minimal unexpected postoperative CSF leak occurs.
- At the end of the procedure, hemostasis is obtained; final irrigation is performed; the endoscope is gradually removed; and the middle turbinate is gently restored in a medial direction, avoiding contact with the nasal septum, to prevent the formation of synechiae. Packing of the nasal cavity is not commonly considered necessary except in cases of diffuse intraoperative bleeding from the nasal mucosa, as can occur in some acromegalic patients or in poorly controlled hypertensive patients, where it is applied for a few hours.

Because transsphenoidal endoscopy is a more recent contribution to pituitary surgery, some advantages, pitfalls, and peculiar aspects related to this technique must be highlighted:

- The main advantages of the endoscopic procedure compared with the microsurgical procedures are related to the properties of the endoscope itself and to the absence of the nasal speculum.[33,125] Avoiding the use of the nasal speculum, which creates a "fixed tunnel" and an almost coaxial restriction of the microinstruments, the endoscope discloses its superior properties, permitting a wider vision of the surgical field, with a close-up "look" inside the anatomy. The angled lens endoscopes enable the surgeon to work on tumors located in suprasellar and parasellar regions under direct visual control.
- The whole procedure seems to be less traumatic, and the percentage of many complications is reduced compared with the traditional microsurgical approach.[129] Because the real operation starts from the natural ostium of the sphenoid sinus and the submucosal nasal phase is avoided, septal perforations, nasal scars, damage to the nasal spine, and orodental complications due to the incision in the buccogingival junction are prevented.
- In almost all cases, no nasal packing is employed, and postoperative breathing difficulties are reduced.
- The use of an endoscopic approach is particularly advantageous in the case of recurrent or residual tumors already treated with a transsphenoidal operation,[130] in which the surgeon usually finds distorted anatomy and may encounter nasal synechiae, septal perforations, mucoceles,

and intrasellar scarring. With the endoscopic procedure, thanks to the avoidance of the submucosal nasal phase of the microsurgical operation, the real beginning of the operation is at the sphenoid sinus, already enlarged by the former approach, rendering the procedure faster and more straightforward compared with the microsurgical transsphenoidal method. The wide anatomic view of the surgical field the endoscope offers in the sphenoid and sellar area minimizes the chance of a misdirected orientation, when the midline anatomic landmarks are not recognizable or absent, reducing the possibility of injury to the intrasellar and parasellar structures.

• The endoscopic endonasal approach can be employed in cases of intentionally two-staged transsphenoidal operations[100] because of its excellent ability in reaching the sellar region during the second operation.

Disadvantages of the endoscopic approach include requiring a steep learning curve to become confident with the unfamiliar anatomy of the nasal cavities and with the specific endoscopic dexterity. Nevertheless, after adequate experience, the operating time becomes the same or shorter than that required for transsphenoidal microsurgery, especially in case of recurrences. The endoscope offers only bidimensional vision on the video monitor. The sense of depth can be gained with the surgeon's experience, making the endoscope execute in and out movements, looking for many useful different anatomic landmarks and referring to the many protuberances and depressions in the sphenoid sinus, representing reflections and shadows corresponding to different structures. Dedicated microsurgical endoscopic instruments with secure grip, straight and not bayonet shaped, provided with different and variably angled tips are necessary to reach the surgical targets, particularly the targets that the angled endoscopes are able to show.[131,132]

TRANSCRANIAL APPROACHES

With the selected indications described previously, there are many different standard transcranial or alternative skull base approaches routinely used, depending on the direction of the extrasellar growth of the lesion. Most surgeons become familiar with one or two approaches and tend to use them in most cases. We describe just the major variations of the transcranial techniques that remain in popular use for the resection of pituitary tumors with extensive suprasellar and parasellar extension: the *unilateral subfrontal approach, pterional approach,* and *bilateral subfrontal interhemispheric approach.* Depending on the particular compartment where the tumor is located, the size of the opening must be commensurate with the best and the safest removal of the tumor, "as small as possible, as large as necessary, but cosmetically optimal."[133] With all of the variations, the operating microscope and dedicated microinstruments are employed, according to the general principles of central nervous system microneurosurgery, and in more recent times the condition of endoscope-assisted microsurgery is sometimes realized.

The unilateral subfrontal approach (Fig. 28-6), described for the first time with an extradural version by McArthur in 1912,[134] then by Frazier in 1913,[135] and by Krause in Berlin in 1914, with a right frontal osteoplastic flap,[136] was adopted by Cushing[21,64] and is still in current use. This approach is indicated mainly for large suprasellar adenomas with an asymmetric supraparasellar extension and when the tumor has expanded into the upper prepontine cistern. It gives excellent bilateral access to the optic nerves and the chiasm.[137]

The patient is placed on the surgical table in a supine position with the head slightly elevated, rotated to the contralateral side and extended 20 to 40 degrees to facilitate the spontaneous movement of the frontal lobes away from

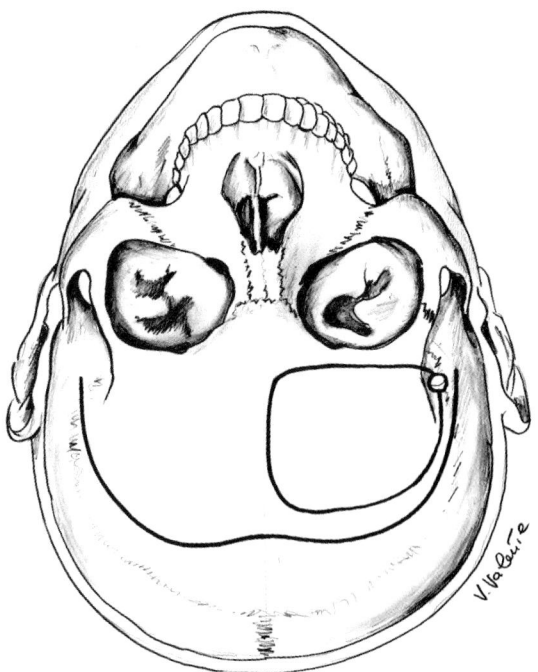

Figure 28-6 Schematic drawing of the unilateral subfrontal approach (seen from a surgical point of view). The bottom, curved line shows the skin incision, and the circular line shows the border of the craniotomy. (Courtesy of V. Valente, MD.)

the orbital roof. Different skin incisions fit the purpose, but usually a bicoronal skin incision is adopted that begins less than 1 cm anterior to the tragus and proceeds in a curvilinear fashion to the superior temporal line near the opposite tragus behind the hairline. The craniotomy usually is performed through a single keyhole, made on the right side, positioned in the anterosuperior margin of the right temporalis muscle, immediately below the superior orbital ridge, for cosmetic purposes. If a correct dissection of the dura cannot be accomplished from a single bur hole, a second bur hole is made, and dural separation from the bone is completed by means of a blunt dissector, minimizing injury to the subjacent brain. The craniotome is introduced, and a quadrangular craniotomy is performed, keeping the basal cut as low as possible. Preoperatively, the surgeon should have a clear idea of the size of the frontal sinuses to avoid entering them with the craniotome. If the frontal sinus is opened, before the dural opening, it should be stripped of mucosa—a procedure called *cranialization*—and packed, then covered in a layer of galea capitis, temporalis fascia, tensor fascia lata, or dural substitute, which then is fixed in position to prevent the leakage of CSF.

After the dural opening, the olfactory nerve is microscopically freed from its arachnoid attachments; care must be taken to avoid damage to the small vascular feeders. The frontal lobe is retracted gently so that the parachiasmatic cisterns can be opened carefully until the optic nerves, the chiasm, the A1 segments, and the anterior communicating artery are well exposed. The lesion is identified. After bipolar coagulation and incision of the capsule, between the optic nerves, the adenoma is debulked and can be removed gently, preserving the pituitary stalk. During retrochiasmatic removal, care must be taken to minimize the manipulations, avoiding damage to the optic pathways.

The frontolateral craniotomy, initially reported by Dandy in 1918,[23,138] subsequently modified and popularized by Yasargil[133] as the pterional approach (Fig. 28-7), is a versatile craniotomy that gives good exposure of the inferolateral portion of the frontal lobe and the anterior temporal lobe. The pterional approach provides a short distance to the suprasellar

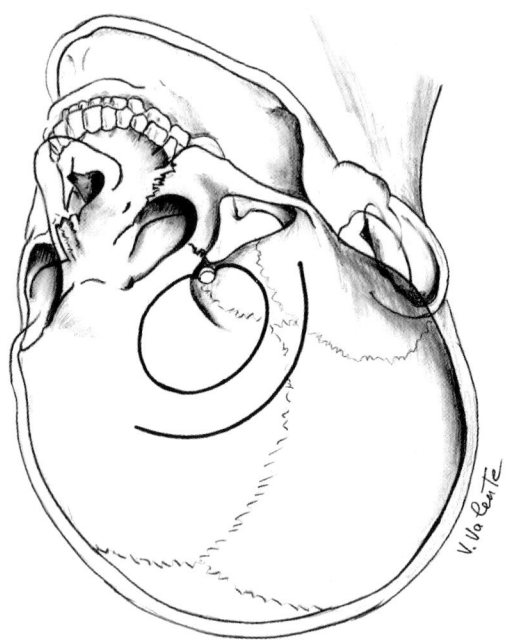

Figure 28-7 Schematic drawing of the pterional approach (seen from a surgical point of view). The curved line shows the skin incision, and the circle shows the border of the craniotomy. (Courtesy of V. Valente, MD.)

region and is the craniotomy of choice for adenomas with unilateral extrasellar parasellar extension, when there is the need to expose the compartment between the optic nerve and the ICA or the ICA and the third cranial nerve. It may be useful when cavernous sinus area invasion[39] or a significant retrochiasmatic component is present. The opening of the basal cisterns early in the approach is employed to minimize brain retraction; mannitol is used when further cerebral relaxation is necessary.

For a pterional scalp and bone flap, the patient is positioned supine on a standard operating table. The head is secured with a three-point pin fixation system, directed 20 degrees vertex down, and rotated 30 degrees toward the side where the craniotomy will be done. The incision starts posterior to the frontal branch of the facial nerve, just anterior to the tragus; swings forward with a large radius arc; and terminates at the midline, posterior to the hairline, high on the forehead. Bur holes in a pterional craniotomy usually are placed at the intersection of the zygomatic bone, the superior temporal line, and the supraorbital ridge (keyhole) and just superior to the zygoma 1 cm anterior to the tragus. The two craniotome cut segments when joined together create a relatively circular pterional craniotomy bone flap.

The laterobasal frontal and anteromedial temporal lobes lie within the perimeter of the craniotomy bone flap. The dura is opened in a curvilinear fashion, centered over the sphenoid wing, draped inferiorly, and fixed with dural stitches. The sylvian fissure should be opened on the frontal side of the sylvian vein to dissect free the M1 segment, by splitting the arachnoid spanning from the surface of the basal frontal to the temporal lobes; the frontal lobe must be mobilized, giving the surgeon access to the sellar and parasellar regions, in a basic of extracerebral approach (Yasargil's pterional-transsilvian approach).

At this time, the sequence of cisternal openings depends on the extension of the lesion: The carotid cistern is completely opened, revealing the carotid artery and its branches. The tumor can be found in the optochiasmatic cistern, the interpeduncular cistern (Lilliequist's membrane), and the cistern of lamina terminalis. In the case of intraventricular

extension, the adenoma can be reached through the translamina terminalis corridor (Fig. 28-8).[139–142]

The optimal technique is to decompress the tumor between the optic nerves and to mobilize it from the opticocarotid space to the interoptic space. The intracapsular debulking starts between the two optic nerves with suction, ring curettes, or ultrasonic aspirator, according to the consistency. Working within and without the tumor capsule, the adenoma is removed from the surrounding neurovascular structures.

When a large pituitary tumor invades the parasellar-cavernous sinus area and the adjacent central skull base regions, this approach can be modified following Dolenc's technique.[39] A transbasal approach is performed: It is extradural and consists of an osteoplastic frontotemporoparietal craniotomy; unroofing of the orbit; resecting the sphenoid wing and the anterior clinoid process; opening the optic canal; and exposing cranial nerves III, IV, and VI.

The bilateral interhemispheric subfrontal approach (Fig. 28-9), initially described by Killiani[143] in 1904 for the removal of chiasmatic lesions and variously used by many neurosurgeons for selected anterior cranial fossa lesions, such as large olfactory groove meningiomas, is not used today as frequently as the other two options we have described. It has been revised more recently[144–146] for the treatment of large craniopharyngiomas with retrochiasmatic extension. It offers a wide exposure of the anterior cranial base with a good overview of the sellar, suprasellar, and parasellar areas. It affords an excellent midline orientation and may be used for the treatment of huge pituitary adenomas with large bilateral suprasellar extension because occasionally a unilateral approach is insufficient for adequate bilateral management of the lesion. This technique requires patience and time, which can be fully rewarded by the technical advantages of excellent exposure of the surgical field.

The extracranial steps of the bilateral interhemispheric subfrontal approach are identical to the steps described earlier except that the craniotomy is extended on both sides. Two bur holes are made on each side with a high-speed drill. Through the use of a craniotome, an osteoplastic osteotomy or a free bone flap is performed, extending close to the orbital roof anteriorly and along the cranial convexity posteriorly. If the frontal sinus is entered, it must be treated before the dura is opened, as already described. The dura is opened fronto-basally; the sagittal sinus is ligated in its most anterior extremity and is divided with proper technique, and the falx is transected up to its insertion on the crista galli and retracted

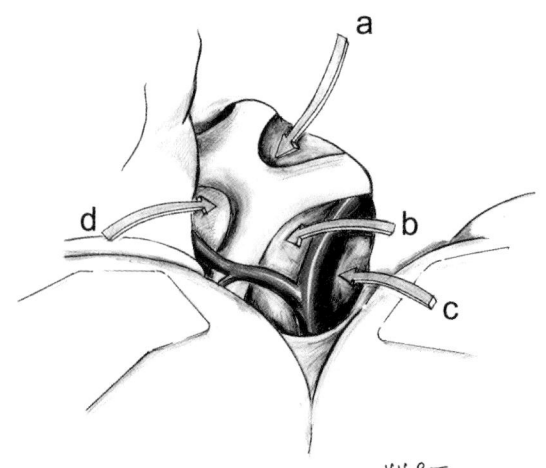

Figure 28-8 Schematic drawing of the different surgical corridors available by means of the pterional approach. *a*, interoptic corridor; *b*, optocarotid corridor; *c*, corridor lateral to the internal carotid artery; *d*, translamina terminalis corridor. (Courtesy of V. Valente, MD.)

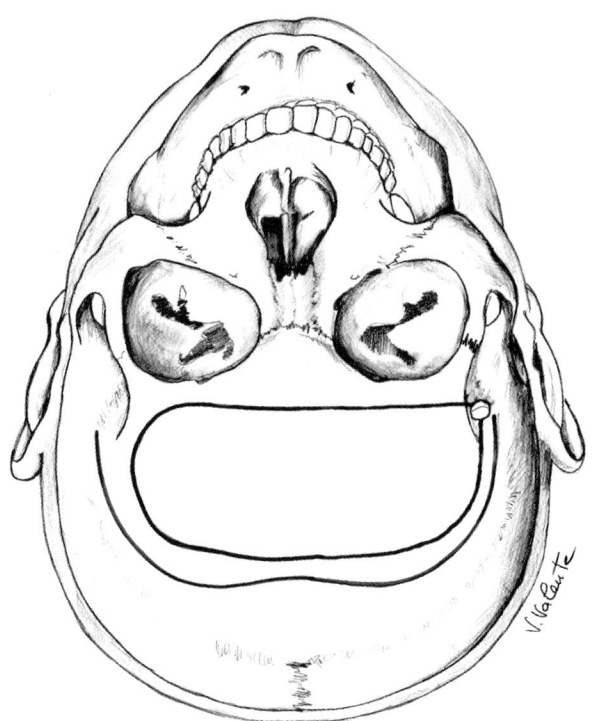

Figure 28-9 Schematic drawing of the bilateral subfrontal approach (seen from a surgical point of view). The bottom, curved line shows the skin incision, and the circular line shows the border of the craniotomy. (Courtesy of V. Valente, MD.)

with the frontal lobes. The interhemispheric and the bilateral olfactory cisternae are opened to drain CSF and to avoid excessive retraction. Both olfactory nerves should be dissected symmetrically, as performed in the unilateral subfrontal approach. After that, the surgical overview can visualize better both olfactory nerves and both optic nerves. The tumor capsule can be seen, and the dissection between the carotid artery and the capsule is performed on both sides. After this step, debulking of the tumor can be done, and the resection is performed. The tumor is removed with sharp and blunt dissection from beneath and around the optic nerves and chiasm and from surrounding brain and blood vessels.

These craniotomy approaches, which at first sight might seem traumatic, often provide excellent results for the patient, especially when the more modern technologic advances are employed (i.e., microscopic magnification, ultrasonic aspiration, bipolar coagulation, neuronavigation) by suitably trained neurosurgeons.

RADIOSURGERY

In addition to the traditional forms of pituitary surgery, either transsphenoidal or transcranial, a third kind of "surgery" should be considered—*radiosurgery*. It consists of a way of treating brain disorders with precise delivery of a single high dose of radiation usually in a 1-day session. Treatment involves the use of focused radiation beams delivered stereotactically to a specific area of the brain and has such a dramatic effect on the target zone that the changes are considered "surgical." Through the use of three-dimensional, computer-aided planning and the high degree of immobilization provided by stereotactic head fixation, the treatment can minimize the amount of radiation to healthy brain tissue. The patient's head is secured to a stereotactic frame and positioned so that the tumor is centered in the spot where all the beams intersect. In this way, the tumor receives a great deal of radiation, while the surrounding brain tissue receives very little radiation. Each low-energy radiation beam passes

harmlessly through scalp, skull, and overlying brain, but all beams focus on the tumor.

Radiosurgery usually is proposed as a second-line therapy after surgery, if the tumor volume is small and the distance of the adenoma surface to the optic pathways is broad enough to allow a safe procedure (5 mm). It is indicated in some patients with recurrent adenomas that are known to be locally invasive in the cavernous sinus, bone, or dura or when the recurrence is clearly manifested by a return of symptoms, and the tumor is considered unlikely to respond to additional resection.

There are three basic forms of radiosurgery, delivered by three different technologic instruments: the gamma knife, the linear accelerator (LINAC), and the cyclotron. Each instrument operates differently, with a different source of radiation—gamma rays or x-rays for the gamma knife, the LINAC and charged particles (protons or helium ions) for the cyclotron.

In the gamma knife, the radiation is produced from decay of Cobalt-60 radiation sources; there are 201 beams from fixed radiation sources, which intersect in the center of the unit. The Cobalt-60–based machines provide extremely accurate targeting and precise treatment for brain lesions. They are dedicated mainly to treating brain tumors and arteriovenous malformations in a 1-day treatment.

In the LINAC, the radiation beam is produced electronically by a linear accelerator, resulting in a similar type of energy. The beam is moving constantly around its isocenter in a spherical arc, but there is only one beam that intersects itself from many different directions. The LINAC-based machines can perform radiosurgery on larger tumors and can fractionate treatments over several days. Treatments that are given over time are referred to as *fractionated stereotactic radiotherapy*.

Because the main limitation of gamma knife or LINAC radiosurgery is the distance between the tumor margin and the optic chiasm, the appropriate candidates for these treatments[147] are patients with a small residual tumor or a tumor confined to the cavernous sinus, in whom the risk of damage to vision is minimized. The delay in reducing excessive hormone secretion to normal is shorter than with conventional radiotherapy.[148–150]

The particle beam or cyclotron is in limited use in the United States and, in addition to brain tumors, it treats other cancers in a fractionated manner. Dedicated neurosurgeons with specific expertise and close cooperation with physicists and radiation oncologists are involved in this special field, which is not yet fully developed.

COMPLICATIONS

Complications of pituitary surgery depend on the surgical route employed to reach the sella. We refer to *transsphenoidal* (microsurgical and endoscopic) and *transcranial* complications. Microsurgical transsphenoidal surgery, with its lack of visible scars and lower mortality and morbidity compared with the conventional transcranial approaches, is appealing to patients and physicians. Serious complications of transsphenoidal surgery are uncommon and seem to be related to the size of the tumor and the experience of the surgeon. Nevertheless, even if the mortality rate is low (usually <1%),[151–154] complications still occur.[155] Major morbidity (CSF leak, meningitis, stroke, intracranial hemorrage, and visual loss) occurs in 3.4% of cases, whereas minor complications (sinus disease, nasal septal perforations) are present in approximately 4.6% of procedures.[67] Microsurgical transsphenoidal approach complications can be divided into different groups, according to the anatomic structures and to the systems that may be involved. The following categories can be identified:

1. Nasofacial complications (approach complications)
2. Sphenoid sinus complications
3. Sella turcica complications
4. Suprasellar and parasellar complications
5. Endocrine complications

Nasofacial complications, including nasal septal perforations, bleeding from the mucosal branches of the sphenopalatine artery, injury or fracture of the cribriform plate with subsequent CSF leak, anesthesia of the upper lip and of the anterior maxillary teeth, saddle nose, anosmia caused by undue superior nasal septum dissection, diastasis of the maxilla, or fracture of the hard palate due to overspreading of the speculum, have been reported. *Sphenoid sinus complications* more frequently occurring are sinusitis and mucocele, a rare and usually late-onset disorder, caused by obstruction of the airflow at the osteomeatal complex. Fracture of the sphenoid body with injury to the optic nerves and the carotid arteries, sometimes due to thin or absent bone, is exceptional, but must be kept in mind. *Sella turcica complications* that may occur include CSF leak due to violation of the arachnoid membrane, subarachnoid hemorrhage, vasospasm, and tension pneumocephalus. A wide range of *suprasesllar and parasellar complications* have been reported: hypothalamic injury, as a result of direct surgical injury or from hemorrage or ischemia provoked by the procedure; visual damage, owing to direct surgical trauma, hemorrhage, or ischemia; vascular injury to one of the vessels of the circle of Willis, which represents one of the main sources of operative mortality[66,156]; meningitis, related to a CSF leak or to contamination; cavernous sinus injury (ICA; sixth, thirth, and fourth cranial nerve injury), owing to surgical maneuvers to remove the lesion extending into the parasellar area; and brain stem injury, owing to a misdirected approach toward the clivus. These complications occur infrequently. The *endocrine sequelae* are the most frequent complications after a transsphenoidal procedure. The loss of one or more anterior pituitary functional axes occurs in approximately 3% of microadenomas, whereas in macroadenomas it occurs in about 5% of cases.[67] Permanent diabetes insipidus occurs in 3% of cases.[67]

For the endoscopic transsphenoidal approach, differences in the type of complications are noted compared with complications described with the microsurgical transsphenoidal approach. These differences arise from the different type of approach and from the absence of the nasal speculum in the endoscopic procedure. The endoscopic approach is endonasal, whereas the microsurgical approach has a phase in which the oral mucosa or nasal septum or both are dissected, and this, even if rarely, can be the reason for anesthesia of the upper lip and of the anterior maxillary teeth, nasal septal perforations, saddle nose, and anosmia. The lack of the nasal speculum avoids the development of other rare complications, such as diastasis of the maxilla or fracture of the hard palate, due to overspreading of the speculum; fracture of the orbit; and injury or fracture of the cribriform plate and subsequent CSF leak. Bleeding from the mucosal branches of the sphenopalatine artery[157] also is possible with the endoscopic approach. Series of endoscopic operations[125,127,129] show an overall decreased incidence of complications compared with historical microsurgical transsphenoidal series.[152] There is not only a decrease in functional and esthetic nasofacial complications, but also there is a correlated decrease in all the other complications described in the literature. The explanation for the reduced complication rate might be found in the wider "overview inside the anatomy," facilitated by the endoscope, and in the decreased surgical trauma of the endoscopic approach itself.

The transcranial approaches are associated with a significantly higher morbidity and mortality compared with the transsphenoidal route; morbidity and mortality have decreased in the microsurgical era. A direct comparison of the complications between the two groups is not possible because the respective inclusion criteria have changed over the years. One aspect that should not be underestimated is that nowadays transcranial surgery usually is employed for giant and invasive pituitary adenomas[73,158,159] or adenomas invading the parasellar compartment or the central skull base,[160] representing a cohort of subjects with the most difficult surgical management and intricate surgical problems. Despite these considerations, a surprisingly high total tumor resection rate (63% to 96%) has been reported more recently.[160] In a similar subset of patients, the recurrence rate has been 15.2%.[73]

Specific complications, common to any supratentorial craniotomy, are related to traction on the frontal and temporal lobes, dissection of major or perforating vessels, and manipulation of the optic or oculomotor nerves.[161] The most feared complication is postoperative hematoma in the sellar and suprasellar region, leading to coma and autonomic deterioration. The most common postoperative complication is diabetes insipidus, immediate, delayed (4 to 5 days), or triphasic; transient (31.8%) or permanent (21.1%); followed by hemiparesis, transient (33.3%), or permanent (9.1%).[73] Loss of vision can occur, most commonly due to disruption of the blood supply to the chiasm or the optic nerves. Other complications, such as worsening of anterior pituitary function, epilepsy, infection, and CSF leak, also can occur. The strict operative mortality (5%) or mortality from disease-related complications (11.3%) is not negligible.[73]

Surgery, either transsphenoidal or transcranial, should accomplish the goal of a total removal of the lesion during the first operation, if possible, for the patient's best chance of "cure." Only a reasonable risk can be borne by the patient in terms of complications and postoperative deficits, however, because long-term benefits optimizing the results of surgery can be obtained by means of additional medical or radiotherapeutic treatment. The surgeon always must attempt a complete and radical result, but at the same time always must remember that a wide variety of different options—medical, surgical, and radiotherapeutic—are now available. What is crucial, regardless of the surgical option selected for a single case, whether transsphenoidal or transcranial, is to relate the goal of surgery to the patient's needs. Never is there a reason to take unnecessary risks. What is most important is the concept that one must be able to select the best option for the actual condition of the patient among all the options available, surgical or otherwise.

Another aspect has major importance in the general perspective, and that is the necessity of a long-term postoperative follow-up, together with the attitude of teamwork of the entire neuroendocrine unit. This is of equal value to the surgical technical aspects and indications we have discussed in this chapter.

Acknowledgments
We wish to thank our teacher, Professor Enrico de Divitiis, for his constant guidance; Professor Edward R. Laws, Jr., for his encouragement and support; all the colleagues of our team, especially the endocrinologists and AnnaMaria Colao, MD, PhD, for their extraordinary partnership; and Vinicio Valente, MD, for the artwork.

REFERENCES

1. Fahlbusch R, Buchfelder M, Nomikos P: Pituitary Surgery. In Melmed S (ed): The Pituitary. Malden, MA, Blackwell, 2002, pp 405–417.

2. Horsley V: Address in surgery on the technic of operation on the central nervous system. Br Med J 2:411–423, 1906.

3. Caton R, Paul FT: Notes on a case of acromegaly treated by operation. Br Med J 2:1421–1423, 1893.

4. Jane JA Jr, Thapar K, Laws ER Jr: A history of pituitary surgery. Oper Tech Neurosurg 5:200–209, 2002.

5. Schloffer H: Erfolgreiche Operationen eines Hypophysentumors auf Nasalem Wege. Wien Clin Wochenschr 20:621–624, 1907.

6. Artico M, Pastore FS, Fraioli B, et al: The contribution of Davide Giordano (1864–1954) to pituitary surgery: The transglabellar-nasal approach. Neurosurgery 42:909–912, 1998.

7. Giordano D: Compendio di Chirurgia Operativa Italiana. Torino, UTET, 1911, pp 100–103.

8. von Eiselsberg A, von Frankl-Hochwart L: Uber die operative Behandlung der Tumoren der Hypophysisgegend. Neurol Centralblatt 26:994–1001, 1907.

9. Kocher T: Ein Fall von Hypophysis-Tumor mit Operativer Heilung. Dtsch Zeitschrift Chir 100:13–37, 1909.

10. Lanzino G, Laws ER Jr: Pioneers in the development of transsphenoidal surgery: Theodor Kocher, Oskar Hirsch, and Norman Dott. J Neurosurg 95:1097–1103, 2001.

11. Kanavel AB: The removal of tumors of the pituitary body by an infranasal route: A proposed operation with a description of the technique. JAMA 53:1704–1707, 1909.

12. Kanavel AB, Grinker J: Removal of tumors of the pituitary body with a suggestion as to a two-step route, and a report of a case with a malignant tumor operated upon with primary recovery. Surg Gynecol Obstet 10:414–418, 1910.

13. Hirsch O: Uber Methoden der Behandlung von Hypophysistumoren auf endonasalem Wege. Arch Laryngol Rhinol 24:129–177, 1911.

14. Hajek M: Zur Diagnose und intranasalen chirurgischen Behandlung der Eiterungen der Keilbeinhöhle und des hinteren Siebbeinlabyrinthes. Arch Laryngol Rhinol 16:105–143, 1904.

15. Kilian G: Die submuköse Fensterresektion der Nasenscheidewand. Arch Laryngol Rhinol 16:362–387, 1904.

16. Hamlin H: Oskar Hirsch. Surg Neurol 16:391–393, 1981.

17. Halstead AE: The operative treatment of tumors of the hypophysis. Surg Gynecol Obstet 10:494, 1910.

18. Halstead AE: Remarks on the operative treatment of tumors of the hypophysis: With the report of two cases operated on by an oronasal method. Tran Am Surg Assoc 28:73–93, 1910.

19. Cushing H: Partial hypophysectomy for acromegaly: With remarks on the functions on the hypophysis. Ann Surg 30:1002–1017, 1909.

20. Cushing H: Surgical experiences with pituitary disorders. JAMA 63:1515–1525, 1914.

21. Cushing H: Intracranial Tumors: Notes upon a Series of Two Thousand Verified Cases with Surgical-Mortality Percentages Pertaining Thereto. Springfield, IL, Charles C Thomas, 1932, pp 69–79.

22. Rosegay H: Cushing's legacy to transsphenoidal surgery. J Neurosurg 54:448–454, 1981.

23. Dandy WE: The brain. In Lewis D (ed): Practice of Surgery. Hagerstown, MD, WF Prior, 1934, pp 556–605.

24. Heuer GJ: Surgical experiences with an intracranial approach to chiasmal lesions. Arch Surg 1:368–381, 1920.

25. Heuer GJ: The surgical approach and the treatment of tumors and other lesions about the optic chiasm. Surg Gynecol Obstet 53:489–518, 1931.

26. Liu JK, Das K, Weiss MH, et al: The history and evolution of transsphenoidal surgery. J Neurosurg 95:1083–1096, 2001.

27. Hardy J: Transsphenoidal microsurgery of the normal and pathological pituitary. Clin Neurosurg 16:185–217, 1969.

28. Cappabianca P, de Divitiis O, Maiuri F: Evolution of transsphenoidal surgery. In de Divitiis E, Cappabianca P (eds): Endoscopic Endonasal Transsphenoidal Surgery. New York, Springer, 2003, pp 1–7.

29. Guiot G, Rougerie J, Fourestier M, et al: Explorations endoscopiques intracraniennes. Presse Med 71:1225–1228, 1963.

30. Carrau R, Jho HD, Ko Y: Transnasal-transsphenoidal endoscopic surgery of the pituitary gland. Laryngoscope 106:914–918, 1996.

31. Jho HD, Carrau RL, Ko Y: Endoscopic pituitary surgery. In Wilkins H, Rengachary S (eds): Neurosurgical Operative Atlas. Park Ridge, IL, American Association of Neurological Surgeons, 1996, pp 1–12.

32. Cappabianca P, Alfieri A, de Divitiis E: Endoscopic endonasal transsphenoidal approach to the sella: Towards functional endoscopic pituitary surgery (FEPS). Minim Invasive Neurosurg 41:66–73, 1998.

33. de Divitiis E, Cappabianca P, Cavallo LM: Endoscopic endonasal transsphenoidal approach to the sellar region. In de Divitiis E, Cappabianca P (eds): Endoscopic Endonasal Transsphenoidal Surgery. New York, Springer, 2003, pp 91–130.

34. de Divitiis E, Spaziante R, Stella L: Empty sella and benign intrasellar cysts. In Krayenbühl H (ed): Advances and Technical Standards in Neurosurgery. New York, Springer-Verlag, 1981, pp 3–74.

35. Aron DC, Findling JW, Tyrell JB: Hypothalamus and pituitary. In Greenspan FS, Strewler GJ (eds): Basic and Clinical Endocrinology. Stanford, Appleton & Lange, 1997, pp 95–156.

36. Alfieri A, Jho HD: Endoscopic endonasal cavernous sinus surgery: An anatomical study. Neurosurgery 48:827–837, 2001.

37. Alfieri A, Jho HD: Endoscopic endonasal approaches to the cavernous sinus: Surgical approaches. Neurosurgery 49:354–362, 2001.

38. Cavallo LM, Cappabianca P, Galzio R, et al: Endoscopic transnasal approach to the laterosellar compartment (LSC) versus transcranial route: Anatomical study. Neurosurgery 2004, in press.

39. Dolenc VV: Transcranial epidural approach to pituitary tumors extending beyond the sella. Neurosurgery 41:542–550, 1997.

40. Partington M, Davis DH, Laws ER, et al: Pituitary adenomas in childhood and adolescence. J Neurosurg 80:209–216, 1994.

41. Amar AP, Weiss MH: Pituitary anatomy and physiology. Neurosurg Clin North Am 13:11–23, 2003.

42. Kirgis HD, Locke W: Anatomy and embriology. In Locke W, Schally AV (eds): The Hypothalamus and Pituitary in Health and Disease. Springfield, IL, Charles C Thomas, 1972, pp 3–65.

43. Schaeffer JP: Some points in the regional anatomy of the optic pathway, with special reference to tumors of the hypophysis cerebri and resulting ocular changes. Anat Rec 28:243–279, 1924.

44. Elias WJ, Chadduck JB, Alden TD, et al: Frameless stereotaxy for transsphenoidal surgery. Neurosurgery 45:271–277, 1999.

45. Jane JA Jr, Thapar K, Alden TD, et al: Fluoroscopic frameless stereotaxy for transsphenoidal surgery. Neurosurgery 48:1302–1308, 2001.

46. Kajiwara K, Nishikazi T, Ohmoto Y, et al: Image-guided transsphenoidal surgery for pituitary lesions using Mehrkoordinaten Manipulator (MKM) navigation system. Minim Invasive Neurosurg 46:78–81, 2003.

47. Lasio G, Ferroli P, Felisati G, et al: Image-guided endoscopic transnasal removal of recurrent pituitary adenomas. Neurosurgery 51:132–137, 2002.

48. Ohhashi G, Kamio M, Abe T, et al: Endoscopic transnasal approach to the pituitary lesions using a navigation system (Insta Trak system): Technical note. Minim Invasive Neurosurg 45:120–123, 2002.

49. Sandeman D, Moufid A: Interactive image-guided pituitary surgery: An experience of 101 procedures. Neurochirurgie 44:331–338, 1998.

50. Bohinski RJ, Warnick RE, Gaskill-Shipley MF, et al: Intraoperative magnetic resonance imaging to determine the extent of resection of pituitary macroadenomas during transsphenoidal microsurgery. Neurosurgery 49:1133–1144, 2001.

51. Fahlbusch R, Ganslandt O, Buchfelder M, et al: Intraoperative magnetic resonance imaging during transsphenoidal surgery. J Neurosurg 95:381–390, 2001.

52. Lewin JS, Metzger A, Selman WR: Intraoperative magnetic resonance image guidance in neurosurgery. J Magn Reson Imaging 12:512–524, 2000.

53. Martin CH, Schwartz R, Jolesz F, et al: Transsphenoidal resection of pituitary adenomas in an intraoperative MRI unit. Pituitary 2:155–162, 1999.

54. Nimsky C, Ganslandt O, Hofmann B, et al: Limited benefit of intraoperative low-field magnetic resonance imaging in craniopharyngioma surgery. Neurosurgery 53:72–81, 2003.

55. Steinmeier R, Fahlbusch R, Ganslandt O, et al: Intraoperative magnetic resonance imaging with the magnetom open scanner: Concepts, neurosurgical indications, and procedures: A preliminary report. Neurosurgery 43:739–748, 1998.

56. Bills D, Meyer F, Laws ER Jr, et al: A retrospective analysis of pituitary apoplexy. Neurosurgery 33:602–609, 1993.

57. Ebersold MJ, Laws ER Jr, Scheithauer BW, et al: Pituitary apoplexy treated by transsphenoidal surgery: A clinicopathological and immunocytochemical study. J Neurosurg 58:315–320, 1983.

58. Laws ER Jr, Trautmann JC, Hollenhorst RW Jr: Trans-sphenoidal decompression of the optic nerve and chiasm: Visual results in 62 patients. J Neurosurg 46:717–722, 1977.

59. Laws ER Jr: Surgical management of pituitary apoplexy. In Welch K, Caplan L, Reis D (eds): Primer on Cerebrovascular Diseases. New York, Academic Press, 1997, pp 508–510.

60. Colao A, Ferone D, Marzullo P, et al: Long-term effect of depot long-acting somatostatin analog octreotide on hormone levels and tumor mass in acromegaly. J Clin Endocrinol Metab 86:2779–2786, 2001.

61. Colao A, Di Sarno A, Cappabianca P, et al: Withdrawal of long-term cabergoline therapy for tumoral and nontumoral hyperprolactinemia. N Engl J Med 349:2023–2033, 2003.

62. Di Sarno A, Landi ML, Cappabianca P, et al: Resistance to cabergoline as compared with bromocriptine in hyperprolactinemia: Prevalence, clinical definition, and therapeutic strategy. J Clin Endocrinol Metab 86:5256–5261, 2001.

63. Cohen AR, Cooper PR, Kupersmith MJ, et al: Visual recovery after transsphenoidal removal of pituiatry adenomas. Neurosurgery 17:446–452, 1985.

64. Henderson WR: The pituitary adenomata: A follow-up study of the surgical results in 338 cases (Dr Harvey Cushing's series). Br J Surg 26:811–921, 1939.

65. Laws ER Jr: Pituitary surgery. Endocrinol Metab Clin North Am 16:647–665, 1987.

66. Laws ER Jr, Thapar K: Pituitary surgery. Endocrinol Metab Clin North Am 28:119–131, 1999.

67. Thapar K, Laws ER Jr: Pituitary tumors. In Kaye AW, Laws ER Jr (eds): Brain Tumors. London, Churchill Livingstone, 2001, pp 804–854.

68. Wilson CB: Role of surgery in the management of pituitary tumors. Neurosurg Clin North Am 1:139–159, 1990.

69. Baskin DS, Wilson CB: Transsphenoidal treatment of non-neoplastic intrasellar cysts: A report of 38 cases. J Neurosurg 60:8–13, 1984.

70. El-Mahdy W, Powell M: Transsphenoidal management of 28 symptomatic Rathke's cleft cysts, with special reference to visual and hormonal recovery. Neurosurgery 42:7–17, 1998.

71. Ross DA, Norman D, Wilson CB: Radiologic characteristics and results of surgical management of Rathke's cysts in 43 patients. Neurosurgery 30:173–179, 1992.

72. Ciric IS, Cozzens JW: Craniopharyngiomas: Transsphenoidal method of approach—for the virtuoso only? Clin Neurosurg 27:169–187, 1980.

73. Yasargil MG: Transcranial surgery for large pituitary adenomas. In Yasargil MG (ed): Microneurosurgery: Microneurosurgery of CNS Tumors. Stuttgart, Georg Thieme Verlag, 1996, pp 200–204, 207.

74. Abe T, Lüdecke DK: Transnasal surgery for infradiaphragmatic craniopharyngiomas in pediatric patients. Neurosurgery 44:957–966, 1999.

75. Laws ER Jr: Transsphenoidal microsurgery in the management of craniopharyngioma. J Neurosurg 52:661–666, 1980.

76. Spaziante R, de Divitiis E: Drainage techniques for cystic craniopharyngiomas. Neurosurg Quart 7:183–208, 1997.

77. Guiot G: Transsphenoidal approach in surgical treatment of pituitary adenomas: General principles and indications in non-functioning adenomas. In Kohler PO, Ross GT (eds): Diagnosis and Treatment of Pituitary Adenomas. Amsterdam, Excerpta Medica, 1973, pp 159–178.

78. Castelnuovo P, Locatelli D, Mauri S, et al: Extended endoscopic approaches to the skull base. Anterior cranial base CSF leaks. In de Divitiis E, Cappabianca P (eds): Endoscopic Endonasal Transsphenoidal Surgery. New York, Springer, 2003, pp 137–158.

79. de Divitiis E, Cappabianca P, Cavallo LM: Endoscopic transsphenoidal approach: Adaptability of the procedure to different sella lesions. Neurosurgery 51:699–707, 2002.

80. Jane JA Jr, Thapar K, Kaptain GJ, et al: Pituitary surgery: Transsphenoidal approach. Neurosurgery 51:435–444, 2002.

81. Jho HD: The expanding role of endoscopy in skull-base surgery: Indications and instruments. Clin Neurosurg 48:287–305, 2001.

82. Jho HD: Endoscopic endonasal approach to the optic nerve: A technical note. Minim Invasive Neurosurg 44:190–193, 2001.

83. Kaptain GJ, Vincent DA, Sheehan JP, et al: Transsphenoidal approaches for extracapsular resection of midline suprasellar and anterior cranial base lesions. Neurosurgery 49:94–101, 2001.

84. Kato T, Sawamura J, Abe H, et al: Transsphenoidal-transtuberculum sellae approach for supradiaphragmatic tumours: Technical note. Acta Neurochir 140:715–719, 1998.

85. Kim J, Choe I, Bak K, et al: Transsphenoidal supradiaphragmatic intradural approach: Technical note. Minim Invasive Neurosurg 43:33–37, 2000.

86. Kouri JG, Chen MY, Watson JC, et al: Resection of suprasellar tumors by using a modified transsphenoidal approach. J Neurosurg 92:1028–1035, 2000.

87. Mason RB, Nieman LK, Doppman JL, et al: Selective excision of adenomas originating in or extending into the pituitary stalk with preservation of pituitary function. J Neurosurg 87:343–351, 1997.

88. Weiss WH: The transnasal transsphenoidal approach. In Apuzzo MLJ (ed): Surgery of the Third Ventricle. Baltimore, Williams & Wilkins, 1987, pp 476–494.

89. Jho HD, Carrau RL, McLaughlin ML, et al: Endoscopic transsphenoidal resection of a large chordoma in the posterior fossa. Acta Neurochir 139:343–348, 1997.

90. Kelley TF, Stankiewicz JA, Chow JM, et al: Endoscopic closure of postsurgical anterior cranial fossa cerebrospinal fluid leaks. Neurosurgery 39:743–746, 1996.

91. Lalwani AK, Kaplan MJ, Gutin PH: The transsphenoethmoid approach to the sphenoid sinus and clivus. Neurosurgery 31:1008–1014, 1992.

92. Laws ER Jr: Transsphenoidal surgery. In Apuzzo MLJ (ed): Brain Surgery: Complications Avoidance and Management. New York, Churchill Livingstone, 1993, pp 357–362.

93. Maira G, Pallini R, Anile C, et al: Surgical treatment of clival chordomas: The transsphenoidal approach revisited. Neurosurgery 85:784–792, 1996.

94. Fraioli B, Esposito V, Santoro A, et al: Transmaxillosphenoidal approach to tumors invading the medial compartment of the cavernous sinus. J Neurosurg 82:63–69, 1995.

95. Frank G, Pasquini E: Extended endoscopic approaches to the skull base: Approach to the cavernous sinus. In de Divitiis E, Cappabianca P (eds): Endoscopic Endonasal Transsphenoidal Surgery. New York, Springer, 2003, pp 159–175.

96. Hermier M, Turjman F, Tournut P, et al: Intracranial aneurysm associated with pituitary adenoma shown by MR angiography: Case report. Neuroradiology 36:115–116, 1994.

97. Inoue T, Rhoton AL Jr, Theele D, et al: Surgical approaches to the cavernous sinus: A microsurgical study. Neurosurgery 26:903–932, 1990.

98. Kitano M, Taneda M: Extended transsphenoidal approach with submucosal posterior ethmoidectomy for parasellar tumors: Technical note. J Neurosurg 94:999–1004, 2001.

99. Sabit I, Schaefer SD, Couldwell T: Extradural extranasal combined transmaxillary transsphenoidal approach to the cavernous sinus: A minimally invasive microsurgical model. Laryngoscope 110:286–291, 2000.

100. Saito K, Kuwayama A, Yamamoto N, et al: The transsphenoidal removal of non functioning pituitary adenomas with suprasellar extension: The open sella method and intentionally staged operation. Neurosurgery 36:668–676, 1995.

101. Mortini P, Giovanelli M: Transcranial approaches to pituitary tumors. Oper Tech Neurosurg 5:1–13, 2002.

102. Van Alpen HA: Microsurgical fronto-temporal approach to pituitary adenomas with extrasellar extension. Clin Neurol Neurosurg 78:246–256, 1975.

103. Alleyne CH Jr, Barrow DL, Oyesiku NM: Combined transsphenoidal and pterional craniotomy approach to giant pituitary tumors. Surg Neurol 57:380–390, 2002.

104. Ishii K, Ikeda H, Takahashi S, et al: MR imaging of pituitary adenomas with sphenoid sinus invasion: Characteristic MR findings indicating fibrosis. Radiat Med 14:173–178, 1996.

105. Iuchi T, Saeki N, Tanaka M, et al: MRI prediction of fibrous pituitary adenomas. Acta Neurochir 140:779–786, 1998.

106. Snow RB, Johnson CE, Morgello S, et al: Is magnetic resonance imaging useful in guiding the operative approach to large pituitary tumors? Neurosurgery 26:801–803, 1990.

107. Patterson RH: The role of transcranial surgery in the management of pituitary adenoma. Acta Neurochir 65(Suppl):16–17, 1996.

108. Esiri M, Bevan JS, Burke CW, et al: Effect of bromocriptine treatment on the fibrous tissue content of prolactin-secreting and nonfunctioning macroadenomas of the pituitary gland. J Clin Endocrinol Metab 63:383–388, 1986.

109. Barkan AL, Lloyd RV, Chandler WF, et al: Preoperative treatment of acromegaly with long-acting somatostatin analog SMS 201-995: Shrinkage of invasive pituitary macroadenomas and improved surgical remission rate. J Clin Endocrinol Metab 67:1040–1048, 1988.

110. Ezzat S, Horvath E, Harris AG, et al: Morphological effects of octreotide on growth hormone-producing pituitary adenomas. J Clin Endocrinol Metab 79:113–118, 1994.

111. Rhoton AL Jr: Operative techniques and instrumentation for neurosurgery. Neurosurgery 53:907–934, 2003.

112. Revuelta R, Arriada-Mendicoa N, Ramirez-Alba J, et al: Simultaneous treatment of a pituitary adenoma and an internal carotid artery aneurysm through a supraorbital keyhole approach. Minim Invasive Neurosurg 45:109–111, 2002.

113. Elias WJ, Laws ER Jr: Transsphenoidal approach to lesions of the sella. In Schmidek HH (ed): Schmidek and Sweet Operative Neurosurgical Techniques. Philadelphia, WB Saunders, 2000, pp 373–384.

114. Rhoton AL Jr: The supratentorial cranial space: Microsurgical anatomy and surgical approaches. Neurosurgery 51(Suppl 1):335–374, 2002.

115. Zada G, Kelly DF, Cohan P, et al: The endonasal transsphenoidal approach for pituitary adenomas and other sellar lesions: An assessment of efficacy, safety and patient impressions. J Neurosurg 98:350–358, 2003.

116. Landolt AM, Schiller Z: Surgical technique: Transsphenoidal approach. In Landolt AM, Vanve ML, Reilly PR (eds): Pituitary Adenomas. New York, Churchill Livingstone, 1996, pp 315–331.

117. de Divitiis E, Spaziante R: Osteoplastic opening of the sellar floor in transsphenoidal surgery: Technical note. Neurosurgery 20:445–446, 1987.

118. Meij B, Lopes MB, Ellegala DB, et al: The long term significance of microscopic dural invasion in 354 patients with pituitary adenomas treated with transsphenoidal surgery. J Neurosurg 96:195–208, 2002.

119. de Divitiis E, Spaziante R, Iaccarino V, et al: Phlebography of the cavernous and intercavernous sinuses. Surg Neurol 15:306–312, 1981.

120. Spaziante R, de Divitiis E: Forced subarachnoid air in transsphenoidal excision of pituitary tumours (pumping technique). J Neurosurg 71:864–867, 1989.

121. Cappabianca P, Cavallo LM, Esposito F, et al: Sellar repair in endoscopic endonasal transsphenoidal surgery: Results of 170 cases. Neurosurgery 51:1365–1372, 2002.

122. Spaziante R, de Divitiis E, Cappabianca P: Repair of the sella after transsphenoidal surgery. In Schmideck HH (ed): Schmidek and Sweet Operative Neurosurgical Techniques. Philadelphia, WB Saunders, 2000, pp 398–416.

123. Jho HD: Endoscopic surgery of pituitary adenomas. In Krisht AF, Tindall GT (eds): Comprehensive Management of Pituitary Disorders. Hagerstown, MD, Lippincott Williams & Wilkins, 1999, pp 389–403.

124. Cappabianca P, Cavallo LM, Colao A, et al: Endoscopic endonasal transsphenoidal approach: Outcome analysis of 100 consecutive procedures. Minim Invasive Neurosurg 45:1–8, 2002.

125. de Divitiis E, Cappabianca P: Endoscopic endonasal transsphenoidal surgery. In Pickard JD (ed): Advances and Technical Standards in Neurosurgery. New York, Springer Verlag, 2002, pp 137–177.

126. Jho HD, Carrau RL: Endoscopic endonasal transsphenoidal surgery: Experience with 50 patients. J Neurosurg 87:44–51, 1997.

127. Jho HD: Endoscopic transsphenoidal surgery. In Schmidek HH (ed): Schmidek and Sweet Operative Neurosurgical Techniques. Philadelphia, WB Saunders, 2000, pp 385–397.

128. Cappabianca P, Cavallo LM, Mariniello G, et al: Easy sellar reconstruction in endoscopic transsphenoidal surgery with polyester-silicone dural substitute and fibrin glue: Technical note. Neurosurgery 49:473–476, 2001.

129. Cappabianca P, Cavallo LM, Colao A, et al: Surgical complications of the endoscopic endonasal transsphenoidal approach for pituitary adenomas. J Neurosurg 97:293–298, 2002.

130. Cappabianca P, Alfieri A, Colao A, et al: Endoscopic endonasal transsphenoidal surgery in recurrent and residual pituitary adenomas: Technical note. Minim Invasive Neurosurg 43:38–43, 2000.

131. Cappabianca P, Alfieri A, Thermes S, et al: Instruments for endoscopic endonasal transsphenoidal surgery. Neurosurgery 45:392–396, 1999.

132. Leonhard M, Cappabianca P, de Divitiis E: The endoscope, endoscopic equipment and instrumentation. In de Divitiis E, Cappabianca P (eds): Endoscopic Endonasal Transsphenoidal Surgery. New York, Springer, 2003, pp 9–19.

133. Yasargil MG: General operative techniques. In Yasargil MG (ed): Microneurosurgery: Microsurgical Anatomy of the Basal Cisterns and Vessels of the Brain, Diagnostic Studies, General Operative Techniques and Pathological Considerations of the Intracranial Aneurysms, vol I. New York, Georg Thieme Verlag, 1984, pp 215–233.

134. McArthur LL: An aseptic surgical access to the pituitary body and its neighbourhood. JAMA 58:2009–2011, 1912.

135. Frazier CH: Lesions of the hypophysis from the viewpoint of the surgeon. Surg Gynecol Obstet 17:724–736, 1913.

136. Krause F: Freilegung der Hypophyse. In Krause F (ed): Chirurgie der Gehirnkrankheiten. Stuttgart, Ferdinand Enke, 1914, pp 465–470.

137. Powell MP, Pollock JR: Transcranial surgery. In Powell MP, Lightman SL, Laws ER Jr (eds): Management of Pituitary Tumors. Totowa, NJ, Humana Press, 2003, pp 147–159.

138. Dandy WE: A new hypophysis operation. Bull Johns Hopkins Hosp 29:154–155, 1918.

139. Bhagwati SN, Deopujari CE, Parulekar GD: Lamina terminalis approach for retrochiasmal craniopharyngiomas. Childs Nerv Syst 6:425–429, 1990.

140. de Divitiis O, Angileri F, d'Avella D, et al: Microsurgical anatomic features of the lamina terminalis. Neurosurgery 50:563–570, 2002.

141. King TT: Removal of intraventricular craniopharyngiomas through the lamina terminalis. Acta Neurochir 45:277–286, 1979.

142. Maira G, Anile C, Colosimo C, et al: Craniopharyngiomas of the third ventricle: Trans-lamina terminalis approach. Neurosurgery 47:563–570, 2000.

143. Killiani OGT: Some remarks on tumors of the chiasm, with a proposal how to reach the same by operation. Ann Surg 40:35–43, 1904.

144. Fahlbusch R, Honegger J, Paulus W, et al: Surgical treatment of craniopharyngiomas: Experience with 168 patients. J Neurosurg 90:237–250, 1999.

145. Samii M, Tatagiba M: Craniopharyngioma. In Kaye AW, Laws ER Jr (eds): Brain Tumors. London, Churchill Livingstone, 1995, pp 873–894.

146. Suzuki J: The bifrontal anterior interhemispheric approach. In Apuzzo MLJ (ed): Surgery of the Third Ventricle. Baltimore, Williams & Wilkins, 1998, pp 489–515.

147. Ganz JC: Gamma knife treatment of pituitary adenomas. In Landolt A, Vance M, Reilly P (eds): Pituitary Adenomas. Edinburgh, Churchill Livingstone, 1996, pp 461–474.

148. Degerblad M, Rahn T, Bergstrand G, et al: Long-term results of stereotactic radiosurgery to the pituitary gland in Cushing's disease. Acta Endocrinol 112:310–314, 1986.

149. Landolt A, Haller D, Lomax N, et al: Stereotactic radiosurgery for recurrent surgically treated acromegaly: Comparison with fractionated radiotherapy. J Neurosurg 88:1002–1008, 1998.

150. Vance ML, Laws ER Jr: Gamma Knife radiosurgery for secretory pituitary adenomas. In Powell SL, Lightman SL, Laws ER Jr (eds): Management of Pituitary Tumors. Totowa, NJ, Humana Press, 2003, pp 221–229.

151. Black PMcL, Zervas NT, Candia GL: Incidence and management of complications of transsphenoidal operation for pituitary adenomas. Neurosurgery 20:920–924, 1987.

152. Ciric I, Ragin A, Baumgartner C, et al: Complications of transsphenoidal surgery: Results of a national survey, review of the literature, and personal experience. Neurosurgery 40:225–237, 1997.

153. Laws ER Jr, Kern EB: Complications of trans-sphenoidal surgery. Clin Neurosurg 23:401–416, 1976.

154. Zervas NT: Surgical results in pituitary adenomas: Results of an international survey. In Black PMcL, Zervas NT, Ridgway EC Jr, Martin JB (eds): Secretory Tumors of the Pituitary Gland. New York, Raven Press, 1984, pp 377–385.

155. Laws ER Jr, Kern EB: Complications of trans-sphenoidal surgery. In Laws ER Jr, Randall RV, Kern EB (eds): Management of Adenomas and Related Lesions. New York, Appleton-Century-Crofts, 1982, pp 329–346.

156. Laws ER Jr: Vascular complications of transsphenoidal surgery. Pituitary 2:163–170, 1999.

157. Cockroft KM, Carew JF, Trost D, et al: Delayed epistaxis resulting from external carotid artery injury requiring embolization: A rare complication of transsphenoidal surgery: Case report. Neurosurgery 47:236–239, 2000.

158. Guiot G, Derome P: Surgical problems of pituitary adenomas. In Krayenbühl H (ed): Advances and Technical Standards in Neurosurgery. New York, Springer Verlag, 1976, pp 3–33.

159. Mohr G, Hardy J, Comtois R, et al: Surgical management of giant adenomas. Can J Neurol Sci 17:62–66, 1990.

160. Dolenc VV: Pituitary tumors extending beyond the sella. In Microsurgical Anatomy and Surgery of the Central Skull Base. New York, Springer, 2003, pp 236–252.

161. Fahlbusch R, Buchfelder M: Surgical complications. In Landolt AM, Vance ML, Reilly PR (eds): Pituitary Adenomas. New York, Churchill Livingstone, 1996, pp 395–408.

Evaluation and Management of Childhood Hypothalamic and Pituitary Tumors

Cristina Traggiai and Richard Stanhope

Intracranial and spinal cord tumors are the most frequent type of childhood cancer after leukemia. Tumors in the pediatric age group differ from adults in the types and location of tumors; the value of extensive surgical resection of malignant tumors; the importance of chemotherapy; improved prognosis; and the delay in using radiotherapy. The relationship between tumor location and tumor type is close. Advances in the therapy of malignant brain tumors in children have led to a significant improvement in survival rates over the last few years. Radiation therapy still plays a major role in the management of intracranial malignancies, together with surgical resection and, more recently, chemotherapy and this has led to improvement in the outcomes of several tumor types. Endocrine symptoms are well-recognized as sequelae of the treatment of intracranial tumors; much less commonly hypothalamic tumors can result in children presenting with growth failure and/or endocrine dysfunction. Endocrinopathies are significant consequences of childhood intracranial tumors and their treatment. The risk of developing these adverse events is related to the underlying tumor, as well as surgery, chemotherapy, and irradiation therapy.

EPIDEMIOLOGY

Intracranial and spinal cord tumors are the second most frequent type of childhood malignancy after leukemia, accounting for approximately 20% of cases.[1] While much is known about the epidemiology of malignant intracranial tumors in childhood, there is a paucity of information about benign tumors. The incidence of brain tumors in childhood is of 3 per 100,000. The highest age-adjusted incidence, 31.4 per million, was observed in the Nordic countries, and rates between 24 and 27 per million were found in most other predominantly white populations. In the United States, the age-adjusted incidence rate was 36% higher in males and 68% higher in females than the rate based on malignant tumors alone. Black children had a significantly lower incidence than white children. Lower rates were seen in South America, Africa, and Asia; the lowest rates were for Chinese populations and for blacks in Africa, both below 15 per million. Among white populations, astrocytoma were the most common histologic type, often with an incidence of at least 10 per million, followed by medulloblastoma, 5 to 6 per million, and

ependymoma, 2 to 4 per million. In other regions with lower incidence rates, these three types accounted for similar proportions of the total. Black children in the United States had a higher incidence of craniopharyngioma than white children and there was an unusually high incidence of pineal tumors in Japan, 0.9 per million compared with 0.3 to 0.4 in many other countries. An incidence rate of 2.76 per 100,000 people younger than 18 years of age was found. Tumors in the suprasellar/hypothalamic region are unusual, the most common being craniopharyngiomas, which are approximately 9% of childhood intracranial tumors; other tumors are much rarer. The incidence of intracranial germinoma is only 0.26 cases per million children per year.[1,2] Considerable progress has been made toward improving survival for children with brain tumors, and yet there is still relatively little known regarding the molecular genetic events that contribute to tumor initiation or progression. Nonrandom patterns of chromosomal deletions in several types of childhood brain tumors suggest that the loss or inactivation of tumor suppressor genes is a critical event in tumorigenesis. Deletions of chromosomal regions 10q, 11, and 17p, for example, are frequent events in medulloblastoma, whereas loss of a region within 22q11.2, which contains the INI1 gene, is involved in the development of atypical teratoid and rhabdoid tumors.

CLASSIFICATION

Intracranial tumors are most commonly situated in the posterior fossa in 70% of cases, and in the supratentorial region in 30%, and can occur at any age although the most frequent age is between 2 and 5 years. The classification can be made either on the basis of histology or on the location of tumor site (Table 29-1). Many sellar and suprasellar tumors in childhood, such as craniopharyngiomas and Rathke's cysts do not originate from the central nervous system and are not "brain tumors." Hypothalamic tumors are usually hypothalamic hamartoma, low grade astrocytoma, Langerhans' cell histiocytosis (LCH), and dermoid and epidermoid tumors. Tumors such as craniopharyngiomas and germinomas tend to affect the hypothalamus indirectly, originating in the peripituitary or pituitary region, and extending upward. The pituitary stalk is typically affected from lesions such as germinomas, LCH, and craniopharyngiomas. LCH commonly affects the middle

Table 29-1 **Histologic Classification of Intracranial Tumors**

Supratentorial midline tumors:	Low-grade glioma Craniopharyngioma Germ cell tumor Pineal cell tumors (pineocytoma/pineoblastoma)
Supratentorial hemispheric tumors Infratentorial tumors	

of the pituitary stalk, in a similar appearance to tuberculosis and sarcoidosis, which may be related to LCH cells involving the cerebrospinal fluid. The anterior pituitary is frequently affected from benign pituitary adenoma, whereas the posterior pituitary is the common location of pilocytic astrocytoma and LCH. Malignant glioma, meningioma, Schwann cell, and pituitary tumors, as well as metastases which are the most common intracranial tumors in adults, are comparatively uncommon in children.[3] In contrast, benign glioma, primitive neuroectodermal tumors, and craniopharyngiomas account for a substantially higher percentage of intracranial tumors in children than in adults.[4,5] Classification of primitive neuroepithelial cells is based on appearance of the tumor as determined by light microscopy, immunocytochemical techniques, and ultrastructural features without consideration for site of origin.[6]

SYMPTOMS AND SIGNS

The mode of presentation depends on the age of the child as well as the location of the tumor. Symptoms and signs can be usefully divided into those from raised intracranial pressure, focal neurologic signs, and endocrinopathy. Nonspecific symptoms if raised intracranial pressure are the following: repeated and frequent headaches, especially if they are worsening and associated with nausea or vomiting, often occurring in the early morning; irritability; listlessness; vomiting; failure to thrive; macrocephaly; and loss of developmental milestones.[7] Epilepsy may be the initial presenting feature of an intracranial tumor. This may be due to the structural abnormality caused by the space-occupying lesion, but may be secondary to the associated endocrinopathies of hypoglycemia (secondary to growth hormone and/or cortisol insufficiency) or hyponatremia (from the syndrome of inappropriate antidiuretic hormone secretion). Although young children are more likely than infants to manifest localizing neurologic abnormalities, these are by no means uniformly present. In older children, a larger percentage of tumors manifest with localizing symptoms and signs that often suggest the location as well as the histologic identity of the tumor. Midline tumors often present in an insidious onset with various symptoms and signs: visual defects such as nystagmus, complete loss of vision, and diplopia because of paralysis of the lateral rectus muscles due to a sixth nerve palsy or due to raised intracranial pressure because of obstruction of the cerebrospinal fluid pathways; neuroendocrine dysfunction, behavioral and appetite disturbances, and regression of motor skills, or they may reflect their compression or infiltration of adjacent structures. Pineal region tumors typically manifest with eye movement abnormalities, such as Parinaud's syndrome or hydrocephalus and alteration of consciousness.[8]

ENDOCRINE DYSFUNCTION

For both benign and malignant tumors, presenting symptoms usually reflect the age of the child and the position of the tumor. Growth failure in children with occult intracranial tumors is characteristic. In idiopathic (congenital) growth hormone deficiency (GHD), birth length is relatively short but growth rate is normal until approximately 18 months of age, when a gradual deceleration occurs. Idiopathic GHD is usually easily distinguished from the growth failure associated with an occult intracranial tumor, in which growth is initially normal and height is appropriate for the parental percentiles, and followed by a marked growth deceleration. This is usually due to GHD but may exceptionally be due to the presence of the intracranial tumor with normal endocrine function. Absence of puberty, more than 2 standard deviation (SD), will require neuroradiologic imaging, but delayed puberty with growth deceleration is usually due to constitutional delay of growth and puberty. Even a child with suspected constitutional delay who does not respond to sex steroid therapy should be investigated endocrinologically and neuroradiologically. Craniopharyngiomas commonly present with failure to enter puberty or arrested puberty associated with an abnormal growth spurt; they usually demonstrate an absence of the normal consonance of puberty.[9]

The idiopathic form of central precocious puberty (CPP) occurs in 74% of the girls, and in 60% of the boys, who are more likely to have an occult intracranial tumor than girls.[10,11] Although it is commonly recognized that gonadotropin-dependent precocious puberty (or CPP) in boys is usually caused by an intracranial lesion, it used to be believed that girls had an idiopathic etiology and did not require neuroradiologic imaging. Recent large series of girls with gonadotropin-dependent precocious puberty have shown that girls, as well as boys, should have neuroradiologic imaging. Although in girls with CPP, hypothalamic hamartoma is the most common lesion, other tumors such as astrocytomas may present in this fashion; it is important not to miss the opportunity for an early diagnosis. Intracranial tumors causing CPP in girls are histologically specific, despite being in the same anatomic site involving the hypothalamus between the mamillary bodies and the median eminence, and it may be related to the secretion of specific local growth factors. CPP may be caused by hypothalamic hamartomas, astrocytomas, optic gliomas, pineal tumors, and arachnoid cysts. Interestingly, some other suprasellar tumors such as craniopharyngiomas, germinomas, and LCH are only rarely associated with the development of gonadotropin-dependent precocious puberty, despite the lesion being in the same anatomic site. High risk factors for the presence of an intracranial tumor in children with CPP are: a young age of onset (under age 3), high serum luteinizing hormone concentrations not associated with the development of a luteinizing hormone surge, and high serum leptin concentrations. However, it is impossible to exclude an intracranial lesion in a child with CPP without performing a magnetic resonance imaging (MRI) scan.[12,13] Diencephalic syndrome is a rare cause of failure-to-thrive in infancy and early childhood. The syndrome is characterized by profound emaciation despite normal or increased caloric intake, absence of cutaneous adipose tissue, locomotor hyperactivity, euphoria, and alertness. It commonly occurs in association with chiasmatic and hypothalamic gliomas. It has also been described in association with other lesions, such as midline cerebellar astrocytomas, suprasellar ependymomas, suprasellar spongioblastomas, and thalamic tumors.[14] Such children may even present to an eating disorder clinic and their growth failure attributed to an anorexic illness.[15]

The onset of diabetes insipidus (DI) with or without an evolving anterior pituitary endocrinopathy is suspicious of a space-occupying lesion. DI followed by an evolving anterior pituitary deficiency, including growth failure from GHD, is usually due to a sella/suprasellar tumor. Although DI is also common in midline cerebral malformations (such as septo-optic dysplasia), this usually follows or is contemporaneous with anterior pituitary failure.[16]

The term *Cushing's disease* describes the symptoms and signs of hypercortisolism due to a pituitary overproduction of adrenocorticotropic hormone, and has to be distinguished from *Cushing's syndrome*, which results from any etiology causing glucocorticoid excess. Symptoms and signs of Cushing's disease are similar to those of adults and often these have been present for many years prior to the diagnosis: obesity, hirsutism, acne, moon facies, hypertension, buffalo hump on the back of the neck, muscular weakness, psychiatric disturbance, depression, and osteoporosis. However, the initial and most characteristic symptom in childhood is growth arrest and this, combined with rapid weight gain, should point to the diagnosis. In young children, Cushing's syndrome is usually an adrenal etiology, including McCune-Albright syndrome. However, in older children and adolescents, it is more likely to be Cushing's disease with excessive adrenocorticotropic hormone production from a tumor of the anterior pituitary.

Pituitary gigantism is a rare disorder due to growth hormone (GH) hypersecretion, usually secondary to an adenoma of the anterior pituitary. Overproduction of GH secretion is responsible for gigantism in a patient with open epiphyses, and of acromegaly in a patient with closed epiphyses. The physical signs of GH excess are common to both disorders but the signs in pituitary gigantism are usually less obvious because of the shorter duration of the endocrinopathy. From what data are available, surprisingly such children appear to continue to grow for many years even after epiphyseal closure. GH-secreting tumors may occur in multiple endocrine neoplasia type 1 and McCune-Albright syndrome. Pituitary gigantism is a rare component of McCune-Albright syndrome, whereas the more usual manifestations are characteristic cutaneous pigmentation, polyostotic fibrous dysplasia, and gonadotropin-independent precocious puberty. Rarely, endocrine manifestations are adrenal dependent, Cushing's syndrome, thyrotoxicosis, and hyperparathyroidism.

The most common endocrine presentation of macroprolactinoma (in children and adolescents it is more common than microprolactinoma) is delayed/absent puberty due to prolactin (PRL) suppression of gonadotropins pulsatility, combined with gynecomastia in boys, and galactorrhea in girls. The presentation may be part of multiple endocrine neoplasia type 1. Macroprolactinoma usually extend upward and encroach on the visual pathway and are often accompanied by visual field defects. It is important to measure the serum PRL in every child with pituitary enlargement, particularly before any surgery is contemplated.[17]

Isolated adrenocorticotropic hormone insufficiency may occur in lymphocytic hypophysitis, although this condition is not a malignant tumor but presents as the differential diagnosis of a central pituitary mass. This tumor usually occurs in the puerperium and is extremely rare in childhood.[18]

Patients with arachnoid cyst tended to be older at initial diagnosis than craniopharyngioma or those with Rathke's cleft cyst. Patients with craniopharyngioma generally present with a long duration of symptoms, especially visual symptoms. Mass effects, such as visual problems and headaches, are common symptoms of all three cystic lesions, but psychiatric symptoms, eating disorders, and calcification of solid tumor components on neuroimaging are characteristic of craniopharyngioma. Children are more likely to present with neurologic symptoms than adults.

DIAGNOSIS

MRI scans have become the preferred diagnostic study for pediatric intracranial tumors. MRI is preferred under most circumstances, providing superior resolution and multiplanar imaging capabilities, and avoiding the "spray" artifact from the petrous ridge that may obscure computed tomographic images of the base of the brain, without a radiation burden to the child. The administration of gadolinium diethylenetriamine-pentaacetic acid appears to be a safe and effective contrast agent for MRI and provides a more accurate method of imaging in the follow-up of brain tumors in pediatric patients. Where clinical suspicion remains (normal neuroradiologic imaging in patients with DI) scans reported as normal should be sent for expert review and consideration of repeat imaging with time. The intervals for scanning should also be guided clinically as any set interval is empirical. MRI scan should be performed at a minimum of yearly intervals.[19] For lesions with a high frequency of cerebrospinal fluid dissemination, such as primitive neuroectodermal tumors and germ cell tumors, a neuraxis staging evaluation by spinal MRI, if not obtained preoperatively, should be performed approximately 2 weeks after surgery. In children with pineal region tumors, measurement of α-fetoprotein and β human chorionic gonadotropin in the blood is useful for the diagnosis of malignant germ cell tumors (pinealoblastomas); however, cerebrospinal fluid markers are of limited assistance. Placental alkaline phosphatase is a clinically useful tumor marker for primary intracranial germinoma.[20]

Thyroid function tests (as well as serum PRL concentration) are always required prior to surgery of a suspected pituitary tumor.[17] An elevated serum PRL concentration requires the distinction between stalk compression with moderate rise in PRL from the very high PRL concentrations associated with a PRL-secreting tumor. Macroprolactinomas usually have a very high PRL secretion and there is little ambiguity about the diagnosis. It is important to distinguish thyroid-stimulating hormone secreting adenomas, which are extremely rare, from the pituitary hyperplasia associated with long-standing primary hypothyroidism. After prolonged and severe primary hypothyroidism, with increased thyroid-stimulating hormone secretion, there is usually an increased size of the pituitary gland, which may attain a suprasellar extension and compression of the optic chiasm/nerves and may be accompanied by a gonadal form of premature sexual maturation, which is not true puberty (isolated breast development in girls and large testicular volumes with minimal virilization in boys).[21] These signs of premature maturation and pituitary enlargement decrease or resolve following the decrease in thyroid-stimulating hormone secretion within 6 months of commencing appropriate thyroxin replacement.

THERAPY

GENERAL PRINCIPLES OF TREATMENT

In general, the aim of therapy is to eradicate the tumor with minimal morbidity and mortality, since prognosis is correlated with the extent of resection. If no biopsy has been obtained, histology will be undertaken postoperatively. Because the details of treatment for many types have evolved over time and likely will continue to evolve, treatment decisions for individual patients are best made in the context of a multidisciplinary "team" approach (Table 29-2). The neurosurgeons estimate the extent of resection but it must be confirmed by computed tomography or MRI examination, preferably within the first 48 hours postoperatively. Postoperatively, computed tomography or MRI provides an objective assessment of the volume of residual tumor. These studies should be performed within 48 hours of surgery, if possible, to minimize the confounding effect of postsurgical enhancement around the operative bed. After diagnosis and initiation of treatment, follow-up imaging studies in children with malignant tumors are generally obtained every 3 months for 1 year, every 6 months for up to 5 years, and periodically thereafter. Imaging in benign tumors is typically obtained 3 to 6 months postoperatively and every 12 to 24 months thereafter for at least 5 years, the frequency largely depending on whether or not a complete resection has been confirmed on the initial postoperative scan. However, the optimal frequency of follow-up studies remains uncertain.

Table 29-2 Management Scheme for Pediatric Intracranial Tumors

Tumor Type	Surgery	Radiotherapy	Chemotherapy
Chiasmatic-hypothalamic glioma Craniopharyngioma	Exophytic lesions Gross total resection Subtotal resection Stereotaxic approaches	Progressive lesions (older children) Improves disease control after subtotal resection	Progressive lesions (young children) No proven benefit (except for local cyst control)
Germinoma	Biopsy to establish diagnosis to determine if results equal those of radiotherapy with less morbidity	Effective therapy	Studies ongoing
Malignant germ cell tumors	Biopsy Gross total resection	Craniospinal	Platinum-based appear beneficial
Pineal parenchymal tumors (pineoblastoma, pineocytoma)	Biopsy Gross total resection	Craniospinal for pineoblastoma	Probably beneficial for Local or stereotaxic therapy for nondisseminated pineocytoma

PERIOPERATIVE MANAGEMENT

Use of glucocorticoids to reduce peritumoral edema, cerebrospinal fluid diversion to treat hydrocephalus, anticonvulsants to prevent seizures, and hormonal replacement for patients with tumors in the hypothalamic-pituitary region are essential components of the perioperative management. Since edema commonly exacerbates the neurologic impairment produced by the tumor, glucocorticoids (e.g., dexamethasone 0.1 mg/kg/6 hr) are generally started preoperatively, continued intraoperatively, and then discontinued within 5 to 7 days postoperatively. In patients with pineal region tumors, a third ventriculostomy is a useful alternative to external ventricular drainage or shunt insertion. In patients with hypothalamic tumors, high doses of corticosteroids (e.g., hydrocortisone) are administered in the perioperative period unless dexamethasone is being used.

SURGICAL THERAPY

For the majority of pediatric brain tumors, direct open biopsy coupled with tumor resection is preferred. Although complete tumor removal is often feasible only for well-circumscribed benign tumors, a "near complete" resection can be achieved with many parenchymal tumors, affording substantial cytoreduction and relieving symptoms of mass effect. Transsphenoidal approach for hypothalamic-pituitary tumors is possible over the age of approximately 8 years. In younger children, this approach is not usually possible due to the small size of the nasal passages and the nonaeration of the sphenoid sinus.

CHEMOTHERAPY

A radiosensitizing effect of certain drugs is often postulated. Among patients with malignant brain tumors, infants and very young children have the worst prognosis and the most severe treatment-related neurotoxic effects. Chemotherapy appears to be an effective primary postoperative treatment for many malignant brain tumors in young children. Disease control for 1 or 2 years in a large minority of patients permits a delay in the delivery of radiation and, on the basis of preliminary results, a reduction in neurotoxicity. For patients who had undergone total surgical resection or who had a complete response to chemotherapy, the results are sufficiently encouraging to suggest that radiation therapy may not be needed in this subgroup of children after at least 1 year of chemotherapy.[22] Also, a significant proportion of children with malignant brain tumors can avoid radiotherapy and prolonged maintenance chemotherapy yet still achieve durable remission by administering myeloablative consolidation chemotherapy with autologous bone marrow reconstitution after maximal surgical resection and conventional induction chemotherapy.[23] No long-term side effects on height, bone mineral density, body composition, and bone maturation were found in patients with leukemia treated with chemotherapy alone. It causes growth retardation, but catch-up growth occurs after cessation of treatment.[24] Gonadal damage after cyclophosphamide (dose-related and it may be reversible) and busulphan (the association may cause permanent ovarian failure) is well-documented in adults; it seems that prepubertal and pubertal ovaries are more resistant than ovaries of adults. Ovaries are more resistant than testes; and seminiferous tubules are more sensitive.[25]

RADIOTHERAPY

The indications for radiotherapy of pediatric intracranial tumors and the parameters for radiation delivery have evolved in several ways during the last decade. Tumors have conventionally been treated with 5000 to 6000 cGy in 180 to 200 cGy/day fractions using multiple portals. Newer approaches, such as hyperfractionated irradiation and interstitial irradiation (stereotactic radiosurgery and interstitial brachytherapy) attempt to improve therapeutic efficacy while minimizing irradiation of surrounding brain and correspondingly reduce toxicity. Nevertheless, as more children are surviving brain tumors following surgery and radiation therapy, the price of the successful therapy is being increasingly realized in terms of adverse effects, particularly in the very young child. Chemotherapy is increasingly used to delay or avoid using irradiation in children younger than 3 years of age with high-grade and incompletely resected low-grade tumors. Because of improvements in imaging and dose delivery techniques, radiotherapy administration can be tailored to the geometry of the tumor. Hyperfractionated irradiation technique is based on the premise that normal cells are better able than tumor cells to repair sublethal damage between doses and that multiple fractions are more likely to irradiate proliferating cells in a sensitive part of the cell cycle.[26] Finally, novel approaches for focal irradiation, such as stereotactic radiosurgery and interstitial brachytherapy, are increasingly being employed in selected unresectable lesions to provide high doses of radiation to the tumor while minimizing irradiation of surrounding brain.[27,28] Radiosurgery is ideally suited to the treatment of small foci of unresectable disease and has led to long-term disease control in well-circumscribed benign lesions. In addition, ongoing studies in older children with selected lesions, such as "standard-risk" medulloblastoma and germinoma, use reduced doses of radiotherapy in conjunction with chemotherapy to minimize radiation-induced neurotoxicity. For many low-grade gliomas that have been extensively resected, adjuvant therapy often is deferred, because these tumors may remain quiescent for extended periods.

SEQUELAE OF TREATMENT

The small increase in incidence noted over the past two decades most likely represents advancements in diagnostic technology rather than true changes in disease frequency, though this is controversial. Survivors of childhood intracranial tumors are 13 times more likely to die than healthy age- and sex-matched peers.[29] Disease recurrence remains the single most common cause of late deaths. The sequelae of surgical treatment are evident soon after the operation but the sequelae of irradiation and chemotherapy become apparent over many decades. Neurologic, neurocognitive, and endocrine disturbances are the most prevalent disabilities observed among the long-term survivors of pediatric intracranial tumors. Maximum quality of life for the individual patient can only be achieved by long-term care and close cooperation of specialists in the different medical disciplines involved. It has been demonstrated that cranial irradiation has been implicated as the major cause for cognitive dysfunction. In that study, intellectual functioning was significantly lower in children whose treatment included cranial irradiation than in those treated without cranial irradiation, and this effect was more pronounced in nonverbal than in verbal intellectual abilities.[30] Some authors also showed that children younger than 7 years at diagnosis had a mean IQ loss of 27 points, while children over 7 years at diagnosis showed no significant decrease in IQ. They also demonstrated that decline in IQ occurred between baseline and year 2 of follow-up; none could be documented between years 2 and 4. All children younger than 7 years at diagnosis were receiving special education at follow-up; 50% of the children over 7 years at diagnosis were receiving supplemental educational services.[30] In Packer's study, children demonstrated a wide range of dysfunction including deficits in fine motor, visual-motor, and visual-spatial skills and memory difficulties; although not retarded, they had a multitude of neurocognitive deficits that detrimentally affected school performance after 2 years from treatment. The younger the child is at the time of treatment, the greater is the likelihood and severity of damage.[31] Reimers and colleagues tried to identify subgroups of children who are at increased risk for cognitive deficits; they showed that younger age at diagnosis, tumor site in the cerebral hemisphere, hydrocephalus treated with a shunt, and treatment with radiation therapy were found to be significant predictors of lower cognitive function. Radiation therapy was the most important risk factor for impaired intellectual outcome. The mean observed full scale IQ was 97 for the nonirradiated patients and 79 for the irradiated patients. Verbal IQ, but not performance and full scale IQ, had a significant negative correlation to biologic effective dose of irradiation to the tumor site.[32] Tumor involving the hypothalamic-pituitary area often produces a loss of endocrine function during a characteristic sequence in time, an evolving endocrinopathy. The risk of developing these adverse events is related to the underlying disease and its treatment with cytotoxic drugs and radiation therapy. The incidence and time course of disorders and the number of anterior pituitary hormones that are deficient depend on the sensitivity of the hormone itself to such therapy, on the dose, fractionation, and time elapsed since irradiation. Early detection and appropriate replacement therapy before clinical manifestations occur may carry important benefits in terms of normal pubertal and social development, growth, fertility, and bone mineralization.[33] The GH axis is the most sensitive and the adrenal axis the most resistant to the effects of direct irradiation to the hypothalamic-pituitary region. Patients who have received high doses (>30 Gy) of cranial, craniospinal irradiation, or total body irradiation are likely to develop GHD within 2 to 5 years from cessation of treatment.[34] Growth may be further impaired by spinal irradiation, which directly interferes with spinal growth, and is not due to an endocrinopathy.

In the rare syndrome of "growth without GH" normal or accelerated growth continues despite the patient having GHD and this occurs at the expense of hyperphagia and rapid weight gain. It is considered that the etiology of this condition is related to insulin and insulin-like peptides, which allow growth in the presence of GH insufficiency. This phenomenon usually occurs after craniopharyngioma surgery. Indeed, the first sign of a recurrence of a treated intracranial tumor while on GH therapy may be growth deceleration.[35] GHD newborns can have a length within the normal range, which suggests that other growth factors dominate longitudinal gain during gestation. Obese children grow at a normal rate despite their low serum GH levels and reduced response to pharmacologic stimulation tests. Children with hypopituitarism secondary to craniopharyngioma resection may continue to grow and may even show growth rate acceleration if their weight increases significantly. Several possible mechanisms might underlie the growth stimulation in obese children, such as elevated levels of insulin and reduced levels of insulin-like growth factor binding protein11. Recently, elevated sex hormone levels and elevated leptin levels in obese children were found to affect epiphyseal growth, and it may be that leptin also participates in the growth without GH observed in obesity, especially after craniopharyngioma removal. In the absence of GH, the sex hormones stimulate growth through a direct GH-independent effect on the epiphyses. Leptin, insulin, and sex hormones locally activate the insulin-like growth factor system in the epiphyseal growth plate.[36]

There is a correlation between the age at diagnosis (the immature hypothalamus may be more sensitive to irradiation), the dose of radiation given, different regimens, fractionation of irradiation, and pubertal development. Gonadal dysfunction can be induced both by a direct injury to the gonads (hypergonadotropic hypogonadism), and less frequently, by neuroendocrine injury to the hypothalamic-pituitary axis (hypogonadotropic hypogonadism).[37] Low doses of cranial irradiation (18–24 Gy) can cause precocious puberty especially in girls, with a compromised growth spurt leading to a loss in final height, whereas delayed puberty has been reported after high doses (>40 Gy) used to treat solid tumors adjacent to the hypothalamus. Either low-dose cranial irradiation given as prophylaxis in the treatment of acute lymphoblastic leukemia, or high-dose irradiation for tumors distant from the hypothalamic-pituitary axis can cause hypogonadism.[38] The irradiation to the gonads from the spinal irradiation could potentially cause oligo/azoospermia with total doses of 6 Gy; the Leydig cell damage is common after total doses greater than 20 Gy.[39,40] Early menopause has been reported as well.[41] The possibility of using gonadotropin-releasing hormone agonists to prevent ovarian damage has been proposed. A number of treatment options for preserving fertility are available for cancer survivors. Sperm banking should be offered even to young adolescent boys. Sperm are present in urine from the early teens onward and can be obtained and banked. Ovary banking will be a technique in the future as some centers develop the procedures. Concern that residual cancer cells are not also banked with the ovarian cells is an issue still to be addressed. Cryopreservation of embryos is part of current practice, and is useful in cases when couples desire it.[42] Further information on the ability of both ovary and uterus to sustain a pregnancy is crucial in deciding which treatment option to pursue. Pregnancy presents a cardiorespiratory stress; peripartum heart failure in women treated as children with anthracycline chemotherapy is a known complication.[43] Survivors who have been exposed to anthracycline therapy with or without radiation to the heart and those who received therapy known to induce pulmonary fibrosis or cardiopulmonary radiation therapy may benefit from a cardiac evaluation or pulmonary function test before pregnancy.[44] Delayed puberty development was reported in boys and girls after a total body irradiation (TBI) containing conditioning regimen, whereas patients given bone marrow transplantation for severe aplastic anemia (without total body irradiation) presented a normal puberty.[45] Other authors demonstrated that children who have been treated with a dose of 25 Gy for acute lymphoblastic leukemia at an early age (<7 years) had normal pubertal development. Girls, who had a late presentation of acute lymphoblastic leukemia, and a late treatment, had delayed puberty.[37] Deficiency of thyroid stimulating hormone, adrenocorticotropic hormone, and hyperprolactinemia can be seen following high-dose radiotherapy (>40 Gy) of the hypothalamic-pituitary axis, especially among young women.[46,47]

Patients in whom the pituitary stalk is injured during surgery often manifest a triphasic response of impaired fluid regulation characterized by an initial period of vasopressin insufficiency lasting 1 to 2 days; a subsequent period of inappropriate antidiuretic hormone release lasting several days; and final phase of persistent DI. In view of the rapid changes in vasopressin secretion in the perioperative period, careful attention to fluid replacement and cautious administration of synthetic vasopressin, if needed, are essential to avoid electrolyte and fluid imbalance. The presence of DI may be masked by cortisol insufficiency and not revealed until glucocorticoids have been administered. One of the most difficult hypothalamic diseases to treat during childhood is hypoadipsia combined with DI. This usually results in difficult management of DI and repeated episodes of hypernatremia or hyponatremia associated with intercurrent infections, especially with gastroenteritis. The condition is usually managed by training the child to take a fixed fluid intake by mouth every hour, and then titrate the dose of vasopressin that is required. Although relatively easy to achieve homoeostasis when the child is well, the predominant problems revolve around intercurrent illnesses, especially if the child has concurrent anterior pituitary failure and has seizures treated with carbamazepine and/or lamotrigine; both interfere with fluid secretion from the renal tubules. It is unusual for children with adipsia and DI to survive childhood.

The incidence of second malignancies ranges from 1% to more than 3%. The majority of second tumors are thyroid cancer, malignant gliomas, meningiomas, and sarcomas that occur within radiotherapy treatment fields 10 to 20 years after irradiation; an increased incidence of hematologic malignancies has been noted after chemotherapy.[48] Thyroid ultrasound scan should be performed once a year. Cranial radiation has also been associated with carotid occlusive disease, which often manifests as Moyamoya syndrome with progressive ischemic cerebrovascular symptoms. This syndrome is particularly common in patients irradiated for parasellar lesions, such as chiasmatic-hypothalamic gliomas.[49]

TREATMENT OF SPECIFIC TUMORS

The treatment of hypothalamic hamartoma is generally pharmacologic as surgical intervention is difficult and does not usually lead to resolution of the early puberty. The hamartoma usually remains the same size. Surgery would be very unlikely to be successful for the resolution of CPP. However, surgical resection, especially if the hamartoma is pedunculated, would be an option for frequent and inadequately controlled gelastic seizures.[50]

Lateralization, using petrosal sinus sampling, as well as transsphenoidal surgical approach, is difficult in young children with adrenocorticotropic hormone-secreting adenoma. Plasma cortisol measurements the day after surgery will confirm surgical cure.

The treatment of a macroprolactinoma is medical and does not usually require surgery. However, in the occasional child who presents with chiasmal compression from a large mass lesion, resection may be performed urgently. Treatment with dopamine agonists, such as bromocriptine and cabergoline, usually results in rapid tumor shrinkage and additional treatment of surgery and/or radiotherapy may not be necessary. In a child who is awake and alert, with a large mass lesion that is producing substantial mass effect, resection is performed on the next operating day.

OPTIC CHIASMATIC-HYPOTHALAMIC GLIOMAS

Optic chiasmatic-hypothalamic gliomas have been considered benign tumors and self-limiting in growth potential because of their histologic appearance. Chiasmatic and chiasmatic-hypothalamic tumors are different entities; most clinical series have reported significant morbidity and mortality especially with the more extensive, posteriorly positioned tumors. The biologic behavior of optic chiasmatic-hypothalamic gliomas is age-dependent with patients younger than 5 years and older than 20 years typically having tumors that exhibit aggressive growth. There are no specific pathologic features to help differentiate the clinical behavior of such tumors. The emergence of modern imaging techniques, including MRI, has facilitated the monitoring of the natural history of the disease and the determination of the effects of therapy. Most patients with optic chiasmatic-hypothalamic gliomas survive for many years. The management of optic chiasmatic gliomas is controversial, partly related to failure to separate out those tumors involving the optic chiasm only (chiasmatic tumors) from those also involving the hypothalamus (chiasmatic-hypothalamic tumors). Some authors suggested a conservative treatment for patients with optic chiasmatic-hypothalamic gliomas in the context of neurofibromatosis type 1 (NF-1) without visual failure, with cerebrospinal fluid shunting for hydrocephalus if present, and medical therapy for endocrine dysfunction.[51,52] For the chiasmatic-hypothalamic tumors, there was more morbidity and no prolongation of time to progression when radical resections were compared to more limited resections. However, over 90% of children with optic glioma without NF-1 will require some form of therapy.[53] Therefore, if surgery is performed, it may be appropriate to do a surgical procedure that strives only to provide a tissue diagnosis and to decompress the optic apparatus and/or ventricular system.[54] After tumor resection, patients whose vision is significantly compromised or who show progression of their disease on serial neuroimaging scans receive chemotherapy. A variety of regimens have been employed (e.g., carboplatinum, vincristine; and 6-thioguanine, procarbazine, dibromodulcitol), with response or stabilization rates of 75% to 100%.[55] Radiation therapy is effective in stabilization or improvement of vision and prevention of tumor progression in both optic pathway and chiasmatic-hypothalamic gliomas to children over 5 years old.[56] Optic chiasmatic-hypothalamic gliomas have an excellent long-term prognosis with a 10-year survival of over 85%.[57]

Chemotherapy is an increasing component of the management of diencephalic gliomas. It can result in tumor shrinkage and significant disease control in some patients. However, decisions concerning the initiation of treatment should be based on the goals of treatment. Factors include: age of the patient; whether the child has neurofibromatosis type 1; tumor size and location; the potential sequelae of radiotherapy; and the acute and long-term toxicity of the chemotherapeutic approach used. The erratic natural history of diencephalic tumors confounds evaluation of efficacy of the regimen chosen.

CYSTIC SELLA TUMORS

The distinction among craniopharyngioma, Rathke's cleft cyst, and intrasellar arachnoid cyst remains a difficult preoperative problem, although the presence of calcification makes the diagnosis of the former more likely. Accurate diagnosis of these rare pituitary lesions is important to determine the type of treatment and predict prognostic outcome. Only 10% of craniopharyngiomas are completely solid. The treatment of craniopharyngioma remains controversial. Although craniopharyngioma is a benign tumor, its location makes even advanced microsurgical techniques difficult to perform, because of adherence to the optic chiasm, hypothalamus, and vessels of the circle of Willis. Despite advances in microsurgical techniques, the complete removal of the tumor is possible in only 66% to 90% of patients.[58] Radiosurgery avoids the shortcoming of surgical resection near the hypothalamic-pituitary axis without the morbidity of open surgery.[59-61] In tumors with a large cystic component, stereotactic drainage or instillation of radioactive and/or chemotherapeutic agents have been used. Only several authors have reported the use of bleomycin for the treatment of recurrent cystic craniopharyngioma, although there is not an established protocol for using it. However, the risk of local complications after the administration of intratumoral bleomycin in these patients is around 10%, and some fatal toxic reactions have been recently reported.[62] Intracystic administration of bleomycin is a valid option as adjuvant therapy for craniopharyngioma in patients with recurrences that are not surgical candidates because of the high risk of complications. Other authors suggest that cystic lesions may be treated with intracavitary instillation of phosphorus-32 to deliver a cyst wall radiation dose of approximately 20,000 cGy.[63] If a treatment algorithm has been devised and followed that combines both surgery (radical and conservative) and radiotherapy (both external fractionated and intracyst instillations), long-term tumor control and minor disability are achieved. Endocrinologic deficits, had the worst prognosis after surgery, especially DI combined with absent thirst. Tumor recurrence occurred both radiographically and clinically, typically in the first 3 to 4 years after surgery; this suggests a need for close surveillance initially with neuroimaging, particularly in younger children, and also clinical examination. Lack of calcification at diagnosis is associated with a tendency to remain free of relapse. Predictors of high morbidity included severe hydrocephalus, intraoperative adverse events, and age younger than 5 years at presentation. Large tumor size, young age, and severe hydrocephalus were predictors of tumor recurrence, whereas complete tumor resection (as determined by postoperative neuroimaging) and radiotherapy given electively after subtotal excision were less likely to be associated with recurrent disease. However, patients treated with surgery alone have a significantly worse freedom from progression when compared to patients treated with surgery and radiation therapy or radiation therapy alone.[58] In the extensive experience of Yasargil and colleagues from the University of Zurich, using an aggressive surgical approach total resection was achieved in 90% of 144 patients

with an operative mortality rate of 16% and a good functional outcome in 67%.[59] In general, if total resection can be obtained, long-term control rate is between 50% and 80%; however, after subtotal resection, 50% to 100% of children experience local recurrence.[64,65] Since craniopharyngioma are potentially radioresponsive, external beam radiation therapy has long been used in the treatment of craniopharyngioma following incomplete surgical resection. Regine and Kramer reported a 60% 20-year survival rate in these patients.[66] In the series from the Royal Marsden Hospital, in 25 patients treated with salvage radiotherapy, the 15-year progression-free survival rate was 72%.[67] Recommended doses have ranged from 50 to 60 Gy in 180 to 200 cGy daily fractions.[68] Although the addition of fractionated postoperative radiation therapy has shown to reduce the recurrence rate, the incidence of hypothalamic and pituitary disorders is increased as seen with radical surgery.[58,69] Merchant and colleagues concluded that DI was the only endocrine deficiency that differed substantially in frequency between the groups treated with surgery and with radiotherapy, respectively.[70] Other complications of conventional radiation therapy include radiation necrosis, optic neuritis, and dementia. Obesity and the metabolic syndrome secondary to hypothalamic dysfunction seem to be important complications of craniopharyngioma treatment.[71]

PINEAL TUMORS

It is now recognized that the wide variety of tumor types found in the pineal region necessitates different modes of treatment; improved microsurgical and stereotactic surgical techniques have made mortality and morbidity rates acceptably low. The secondary deposits from pineal tumors, especially germinomas, are common in the suprasellar region. Benign teratomas, if resected totally, may require no further therapy; lesions that have been resected subtotally are treated with local radiotherapy. Nondisseminated germinomas are highly radiosensitive. Nongerminomatous germ cell tumors are treated with craniospinal radiation and chemotherapy; however, even with aggressive therapy, 5-year survival is less than 50%.[72-74] Pineoblastomas are considered to be primitive neuroectodermal tumors and their treatment and outcome are comparable to those of high-risk medulloblastomas; chemotherapy without radiotherapy appears to be ineffective therapy for young children, and for children more than 18 months of age at diagnosis treated with craniospinal radiation therapy and chemotherapy.[75,76] Some authors concluded that most pineal cysts are clinically benign, and they should be followed up for many years.[77] Pineocytomas, although benign histologically, show a propensity for local recurrence and cerebrospinal fluid dissemination; these lesions have been treated with local or craniospinal radiotherapy and, in some cases, chemotherapy.

REFERENCES

1. Stiller CA, Nectoux J: International incidence of childhood brain and spinal tumours. Int J Epidemiol 23:458–464, 1994.
2. Keene DL, Hsu E, Ventureyra E: Brain tumors in childhood and adolescence. Pediatr Neurol 20:198–203, 1999.
3. Reed UC, Rosemberg S, Gherpelli JL, et al: Brain tumors in the first two years of life: A review of forty cases. Pediatr Neurosurg 19:180–185, 1993.
4. Rickert CH, Probst-Cousin S, Gullotta F: Primary intracranial neoplasms of infancy and early childhood. Childs Nerv Syst 13:507–513, 1997.
5. Pollack IF: Brain tumors in children [Review]. N Engl J Med 331:1501–1507, 1994.

6. Rorke LB: The cerebellar medulloblastoma and its relationship to primitive neuroectodermal tumors. J Neuropathol Exp Neurol 42:1–15, 1983.
7. Albright AL: Pediatric brain tumors. CA Cancer J Clin 43:272–288, 1993.
8. Pollack IF: Pediatric brain tumors [Review]. Semin Surg Oncol 16:73–90, 1999.
9. Stanhope R, Adams J, Brook CG: Disturbances of puberty. Clin Obstet Gynaecol 12:557–577, 1985.
10. De Sanctis V, Corrias A, Rizzo V, et al: Etiology of central precocious puberty in males: The results of the Italian Study Group for Physiopathology of Puberty.

J Pediatr Endocrinol Metab 13:687–693, 2000.
11. Cisternino M, Arrigo T, Pasquino AM, et al: Etiology and age incidence of precocious puberty in girls: A multicentric study. J Pediatr Endocrinol Metab 13:695–701, 2000.
12. Chemaitilly W, Trivin C, Adan L, et al: Central precocious puberty: Clinical and laboratory features. Clin Endocrinol (Oxf) 54:289–294, 2001.
13. Stanhope R: Central precocious puberty and occult intracranial tumours. Clin Endocrinol (Oxf) 54:287–288, 2001.
14. Russell A: A diencephalic syndrome of emaciation in infancy and childhood. Arch Dis Child 26:274, 1951.

§

15. De Vile CJ, Sufraz R, Lask BD, Stanhope R: Occult intracranial tumours masquerading as early onset anorexia nervosa. Br Med J 311:1359–1360, 1995.

16. Mootha SL, Barkovich AJ, Grumbach MM, et al: Idiopathic hypothalamic diabetes insipidus, pituitary stalk thickening, and the occult intracranial germinoma in children and adolescents. J Clin Endocrinol Metab 82:1362–1367, 1997.

17. Torpiano J, Vanderpump M, Stanhope R: The management of sellar masses: Not all pituitary tumours require surgery for diagnosis and/or therapy. J Pediatr Endocrinol Metab 17:663–664, 2004.

18. Cemeroglu AP, Blaivas M, Muraszko KM, et al: Lymphocytic hypophysitis presenting with diabetes insipidus in a 14-year-old girl: Case report and review of the literature. Eur J Pediatr 156:684–688, 1997.

19. Sherwood MC, Stanhope R, Preece MA, Grant DB: Diabetes insipidus and occult intracranial tumours. Arch Dis Child 61:1222–1224, 1986.

20. Shinoda J, Yamada H, Sakai N, et al: Placental alkaline phosphatase as a tumor marker for primary intracranial germinoma. J Neurosurg 68:710–720, 1988.

21. Pringle PJ, Stanhope R, Hindmarsh P, Brook CG: Abnormal pubertal development in primary hypothyroidism. Clin Endocrinol (Oxf) 28:479–486, 1988.

22. Duffner PK, Horowitz ME, Krischer JP, et al: Postoperative chemotherapy and delayed radiation in children less than three years of age with malignant brain tumors. N Engl J Med 328:1725–1731, 1993.

23. Mason WP, Grovas A, Halpern S, et al: Intensive chemotherapy and bone marrow rescue for young children with newly diagnosed malignant brain tumors. J Clin Oncol 16:210–221, 1998.

24. Van der Sluis I, van der Heuvel-Eibrink MM, Hahlen K, et al: Bone mineral density, body composition, and height in long term survivors of acute lymphoblastic leukemia in childhood. Med Pediatr Oncol 35:415–420, 2000.

25. Kumar R, Biggart JD, McEvoy J, McGeown MG: Cyclophosphamide and reproductive function. Lancet 1:1212–1214, 1972.

26. Packer RJ, Boyett JM, Zimmerman RA, et al: Hyperfractionated radiotherapy (72 Gy) for children with brain stem gliomas. A Children's Cancer Group Phase I/II Trial. Cancer 72:1414–1421, 1993.

27. Grabb PA, Lunsford LD, Albright AL, et al: Stereotactic radiosurgery for glial neoplasms of childhood. Neurosurgery 38:696–702, 1996.

28. McDermott MW, Gutin PH, Larson DA, Sneed PK: Interstitial brachytherapy [Review]. Neurosurg Clin North Am 1:801–824, 1990.

29. Sklar CA: Childhood brain tumors. J Pediatr Endocrinol Metab 15(Suppl):669, 2002.

30. Radcliffe J, Packer RJ, Atkins TE, et al: Three- and four-year cognitive outcome in children with noncortical brain tumors treated with whole-brain radiotherapy. Ann Neurol 32:551–554, 1992.

31. Packer RJ, Sutton LN, Atkins TE, et al: A prospective study of cognitive function in children receiving whole-brain radiotherapy and chemotherapy: 2-year results. J Neurosurg 70:707–713, 1989.

32. Reimers TS, Ehrenfels S, Mortensen EL, et al: Cognitive deficits in long-term survivors of childhood brain tumors: Identification of predictive factors. Med Pediatr Oncol 40:26–34, 2003.

33. Cohen LE: Endocrine late effects of cancer treatment. Curr Opin Pediatr 15:3–9, 2003.

34. Livesey EA, Hindmarsh PC, Brook CG, et al: Endocrine disorders following treatment of childhood brain tumours. Br J Cancer 61:622–625, 1990.

35. Locatelli F, Giorgiani G, Pession A, Bozzola M: Late effects in children after bone marrow transplantation: A review. Haematol 78:319–328, 1993.

36. Phillip M, Moran O, Lazar L: Growth without growth hormone. J Pediatr Endocrinol Metab 15(Suppl):1267–1272, 2002.

37. Hughes IA, Napier A, Thompson EN: Pituitary-gonadal function in children treated for acute lymphoblastic leukaemia. Acta Paediatr Scand 69:691–692, 1980.

38. Rappaport R, Brauner R, Czernichow P, et al: Effect of hypothalamic and pituitary irradiation on pubertal development in children with cranial tumors. J Clin Endocrinol Metab 54:1164–1168, 1982.

39. Castillo LA, Craft AW, Kernahan J, et al: Gonadal function after 12-Gy testicular irradiation in childhood acute lymphoblastic leukaemia. Med Pediatr Oncol 18:185–189, 1990.

40. Leiper AD, Grant DB, Chessells JM: Gonadal function after testicular radiation for acute lymphoblastic leukaemia. Arch Dis Child 61:53–56, 1986.

41. Byrne J: Infertility and premature menopause in childhood cancer survivors. Med Pediatr Oncol 33:24–28, 1999.

42. Edwards RG, Morcos S, Macnamee M, et al: High fecundity of amenorrhoeic women in embryo-transfer programmes. Lancet 338:292–294, 1991.

43. Katz A, Goldenberg I, Maoz C, et al: Peripartum cardiomyopathy occurring in a patient previously treated with doxorubicin. Am J Med Sci 314:399–400, 1997.

44. Collis CH: Chemotherapy-related morbidity to the lungs. In Plowman PN, McElwain TJ, Meadows AT (eds): Complications of Cancer Management. Guildford, England, Butterworth Scientific Ltd, 1991, pp 250–271.

45. Sanders JE: The impact of marrow transplant preparative regimens on subsequent growth and development. The Seattle Marrow Transplant team. Semin Hematol 28:244–249, 1991.

46. Ogilvy-Stuart AL, Clark DJ, Wallace WH, et al: Endocrine deficit after fractionated total body irradiation. Arch Dis Child 67:1107–1110, 1992.

47. Wittert G, Donald RA, Espiner EA, et al: The hormonal effects of pituitary surgery and irradiation: A review of 59 cases. N Z Med J 98:93–97, 1985.

48. Hawkins MM, Draper GJ, Kingston JE: Incidence of second primary tumours among childhood cancer survivors. Br J Cancer 56:339–347, 1987.

49. Bitzer M, Topka H: Progressive cerebral occlusive disease after radiation therapy. Stroke 26:131–136, 1995.

50. de Brito VN, Latronico AC, Arnhold IJ, et al: Treatment of gonadotropin dependent precocious puberty due to hypothalamic hamartoma with gonadotropin releasing hormone agonist depot. Arch Dis Child 80:231–234, 1999.

51. Alshail E, Rutka JT, Becker LE, Hoffman HJ: Optic chiasmatic-hypothalamic glioma. Brain Pathol 7:799–806, 1997.

52. Wisoff JH, Abbott R, Epstein F: Surgical management of exophytic chiasmatic-hypothalamic tumors of childhood. J Neurosurg 73:661–667, 1990.

53. Jenkin D, Angyalfi S, Becker L, et al: Optic glioma in children: Surveillance, resection or irradiation? Int J Radiat Oncol Biol Phys 25:215–225, 1993.

54. Steinbok P, Hentschel S, Almqvist P, et al: Management of optic chiasmatic/hypothalamic astrocytomas in children. Can J Neurol Sci 29:132–138, 2002.

55. Gajjar A, Heideman RL, Kovnar EH, et al: Response of pediatric low grade gliomas to chemotherapy [Review]. Pediatr Neurosurg 19:113–120, 1993.

56. Erkal HS, Serin M, Cakmak A: Management of optic pathway and chiasmatic-hypothalamic gliomas in children with radiation therapy. Radiother Oncol 45:11–15, 1997.

57. Pollack IF, Claassen D, al-Shboul Q, et al: Low-grade gliomas of the cerebral hemispheres in children: An analysis of 71 cases. J Neurosurg 82:536–547, 1995.

58. De Vile CJ, Grant DB, Kendall BE, et al: Management of childhood craniopharyngioma: Can the morbidity of radical surgery be predicted? Neurosurg 85:73–81, 1996.

59. Yasargil MG, Curcic M, Kis M, et al: Total removal of craniopharyngiomas. Approaches and long-term results in 144 patients. J Neurosurg 73:3–11, 1990.

60. Carmel PW: Craniopharyngiomas. In Wilkins RH, Rengachary SS (eds): Neurosurgery. New York, McGraw-Hill, 1985, pp 905–916.

61. Pang D: Surgical management of craniopharyngioma. In Sekhar LN, Janecka IP (eds): Surgery of Cranial Base Tumors. New York, Raven Press, 1993, pp 787–807.

62. Hader WJ, Steinbok P, Hukin J, Fryer C: Intratumoral therapy with bleomycin

for cystic craniopharyngiomas in children. Pediatr Neurosurg 33:211–218, 2000.

63. Pollock BE, Lunsford LD, Kondziolka D, et al: Phosphorus-32 intracavitary irradiation of cystic craniopharyngiomas: Current technique and long-term results. Int J Radiat Oncol Biol Phys 33:437–446, 1995.

64. Kalapurakal JA, Goldman S, Hsieh YC, et al: Clinical outcome in children with craniopharyngioma treated with primary surgery and radiotherapy deferred until relapse. Med Pediatr Oncol 40:214–218, 2003.

65. Kalapurakal JA, Goldman S, Hsieh YC, et al: Clinical outcome in children with recurrent craniopharyngioma after primary surgery. Cancer J 6:388–393, 2000.

66. Regine WF, Kramer S: Pediatric craniopharyngiomas: Long term results of combined treatment with surgery and radiation. Int J Radiat Oncol Biol Phys 24:611–617, 1992.

67. Bloom HJG: Combined modality therapy for intracranial tumors. Cancer 35:111–120, 1975.

68. Tarbell N, Barnes P, Scott RM, et al: Advances in radiation therapy for craniopharyngiomas. Pediatr Neurosurg 21(Suppl):101–107, 1994.

69. Honegger J, Buchfelder M, Fahlbusch R: Surgical treatment of craniopharyngiomas: Endocrinological results. J Neurosurg 90:251–257, 1999.

70. Merchant TE, Kiehna EN, Sanford RA, et al: Craniopharyngioma: The St. Jude Children's Research Hospital experience 1984–2001. Int J Radiat Oncol Biol Phys 53:533–542, 2002.

71. Harz KJ, Muller HL, Waldeck E, et al: Obesity in patients with craniopharyngioma: Assessment of food intake and movement counts indicating physical activity. J Clin Endocrinol Metab 88:5227–5231, 2003.

72. Regis J, Bouillot P, Rouby-Volot F, et al: Pineal region tumors and the role of stereotactic biopsy: Review of the mortality, morbidity, and diagnostic rate in 370 cases. Neurosurgery 39:907–914, 1996.

73. Edwards MS, Hudgins RJ, Wilson CB, et al: Pineal region tumors in children. J Neurosurg 68:689–697, 1988.

74. Balmaceda C, Heller G, Rosenblum M, et al: Chemotherapy without irradiation—a novel approach for newly diagnosed CNS germ cell tumors: Results of an international cooperative trial. J Clin Oncol 14:2908–2915, 1996.

75. Jakacki RI, Zeltzer PM, Boyett JM, et al: Survival and prognostic factors following radiation and/or chemotherapy for primitive neuroectodermal tumors of the pineal region in infants and children: A report of the Children's Cancer Group. J Clin Oncol 13:1377–1383, 1995.

76. Dirks PB, Harris L, Hoffman HJ, et al: Supratentorial primitive neuroectodermal tumors in children. J Neurooncol 29:75–84, 1996.

77. Mandera M, Marcol W, Bierzynska-Macyszyn G, Kluczewska E: Pineal cysts in childhood. Childs Nerv Syst 19:750–775, 2003.

Vasopressin, Diabetes Insipidus, and Syndrome of Inappropriate Antidiuresis

Stephen G. Ball and Peter H. Baylis

INTRODUCTION

Vasopressin (VP), the antidiuretic hormone of most vertebrates, is the major determinant of renal solute-free water excretion and therefore plays a central role in the maintenance of water balance.

In 1895, Oliver and Schäfer[1] reported potent hypertensive effects of fresh pituitary gland extracts injected intravenously into mammals. The pressor activity was subsequently shown to reside solely in the neurohypophysis.[2] The renal effects of posterior pituitary extracts were described later, with the demonstration that they could reverse the polyuria caused by mechanical injury to the pituitary.[3] The efficacy of pituitary extract in the treatment of patients with diabetes insipidus was described independently by two sources in 1913.[4,5] Verney[6] in 1947 was the first to propose that secretion of the pituitary antidiuretic hormone was regulated by the osmolality of body water. He concluded that intracranial osmoreceptors, sensitive to changes in the concentration of sodium and other solutes, controlled production. However, it was not until 1954 that the chemical structure of arginine VP (AVP) was described and subsequently synthesized by du Vigneaud and associates.[7] The gene coding for AVP was cloned and characterized in 1982.[8]

ANATOMY AND NEUROPHYSIOLOGY OF THE NEUROHYPOPHYSIS

AVP is produced predominantly by neurosecretory neurons within specific regions of the hypothalamus and released from their nerve endings terminating in the posterior pituitary. AVP production is influenced by a series of sensory signals reflecting osmotic status, circulating volume, and blood pressure. The anatomic and functional relations of the hypothalamic nuclei and the sensory afferents involved in this process are the key to understanding the physiology and pathophysiology of the VP axis (Fig. 30-1).

The neurohypophysis is a structural and functional unit consisting of three parts: the supraoptic (SON) and paraventricular (PVN) nuclei of the hypothalamus, which contain the cell bodies of magnocellular neurosecretory neurons that synthesize VP and the related hormone oxytocin (OT); the supraoptico-hypophyseal tract, which carries the axons of these neurons; and the posterior pituitary, where the axons terminate on capillaries of the inferior hypohyseal artery. Small dendrites branch from the magnocellular neurons as they project toward the supraoptico-hypophyseal tract.

The SON is situated along the proximal portion of the optic tract and consists of the cell bodies of discrete vasopressinergic and oxytotic magnocellular neurons projecting to the posterior pituitary. The PVN contains a similar population, with similar projections. In humans, vasopressinergic neurons are found predominantly in the ventral SON but centrally within the PVN. Smaller parvocellular vasopressinergic neurons also are found in the suprachiasmatic nucleus and PVN.[9] A group of these PVN parvocellular neurons cosecrete AVP and corticotrophin-releasing factor (CRF) and project via the median eminence to the hypophyseal-portal vascular bed of the anterior pituitary. Functionally, they have a role in the regulation of adrenocorticotropic hormone (ACTH) release. These neurons act to integrate a number of stress inputs (neural and endocrine) to determine appropriate portal release of AVP and CRF. Interleukin-1 (IL-1) stimulates both AVP and CRF gene expression in parvocellular neurons and is thus implicated directly in immune-neuroendocrine integration.[10] Additional vasopressinergic neurons, predominantly from the PVN, project to extrahypothalamic sites in the forebrain, brain stem, and spinal cord.[11] In contrast to the anterior pituitary, the posterior pituitary gland is derived from the forebrain during development and is composed predominantly of

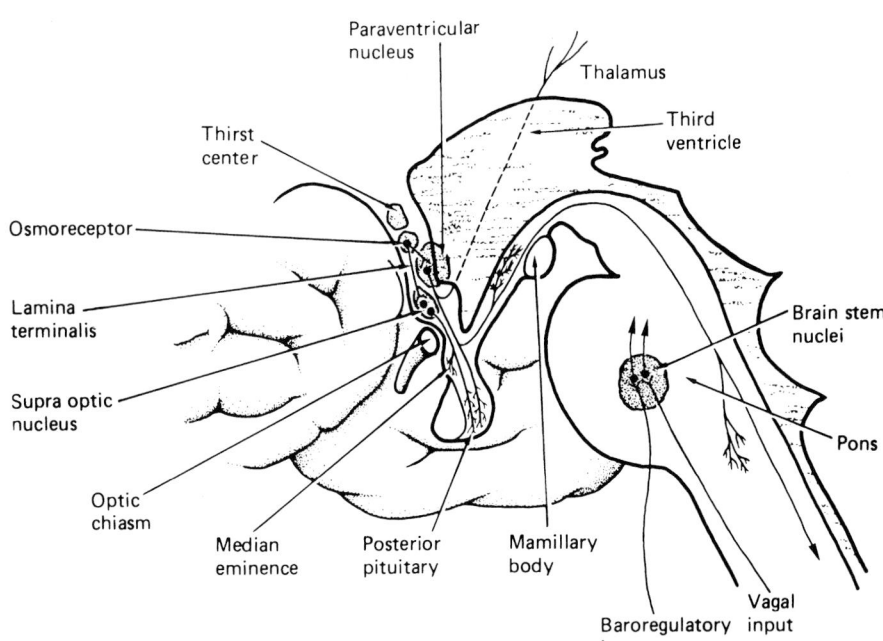

Figure 30-1 Schematic representation of the neurohypophysis and afferent connections. Sensory afferents from central osmoreceptors relay to the supraoptic (SON) and paraventricular nuclei (PVN), from where vasopressinergic magnocellular and parvocellular neurons project to the posterior pituitary and median eminence. Volume-sensitive afferents project to the SON and PVN via brain stem nuclei.

neural tissue. In the adult, the posterior pituitary constitutes some 20% of the total pituitary mass of about 600 mg.[12] It lies in a close anatomic relation with (immediately below) the hypothalamus.

The blood supply of the neurohypophysis is intimately linked with its function and pathophysiology. The posterior pituitary receives an arterial blood supply from the inferior hypophyseal artery and the artery of the trabecula (a branch of the superior hypophyseal artery), both of which are derived from the internal carotid and its branches. The SON and PVN receive an arterial supply from a number of branch arteries: the suprahypophyseal, anterior communicating, anterior cerebral, posterior communicating, and posterior cerebral arteries (all derived from the circle of Willis). Venous drainage of the neurohypophysis is through the dural, cavernous, and inferior petrosal sinuses.

SYNTHESIS AND METABOLISM OF VASOPRESSIN

VP is a strongly basic cyclical nonapeptide (isolectric point pH, 10.9) with a disulfide bridge between cysteine residues at positions 1 and 6 (Fig. 30-2).[13] Most mammals have the amino acid arginine at position 8 (AVP), giving a molecular mass of 1084 Da. Lysine vasopressin (LVP) is the antidiuretic hormone of the pig family, arginine at position 8 being substituted by lysine. Biologic activity is readily destroyed by oxidation or reduction of the disulfide bond.[14] The structure of OT differs from that of AVP by two amino acids: isoleucine at position 3 and leucine at position 8. Nonmammalian species have a variety of nonapeptides related closely to

VP and OT (Table 30-1), with amino acid substitutions occurring predominantly at positions 3, 4, and 8. This considerable structural conservation has led to the hypothesis that a single ancestral gene evolved along two evolutionary lines, one leading to vasotocin-vasopressin and the other to isotocin-mesotocin-OT.[15] However, additional data suggest that the numerous VP-like hormones are derived independently from multiple ancestral genes.[16]

MOLECULAR BIOLOGY OF VASOPRESSIN

The VP gene lies in tandem array (although in opposite transcriptional orientation) with the OT gene on chromosome 20, separated by some 8 Kb in humans.[17] The gene is composed of three exons and encodes a 145-amino acid polypeptide precursor with a modular structure: an amino-terminal signal peptide; the VP coding sequence; a VP-specific midmolecule peptide, neurophysin-II (NPII); and a carboxyl-terminal peptide that ultimately undergoes posttranslational glycosylation (Fig. 30-3). The OT gene also has three exons, and its product shares the same modular structure. Moreover, considerable homology exists between the NP sequences of the VP and OT genes. Positions 10 to 74 of NPII and NPI (the OT-specific neurophysin) are highly conserved at the amino acid level.

The VP gene is expressed in specific groups of hypothalamic neurons in addition to extrahypothalamic tissues such as adrenal gland, gonad, cerebellum, and the pituicytes of the posterior pituitary gland. A full description of the *cis*-acting elements mediating site-specific VP gene expression is not currently available. Sequences within the intergenic region

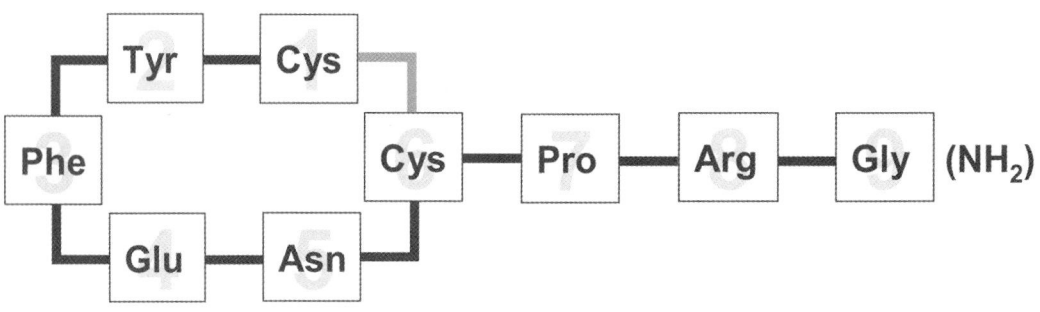

Figure 30-2 Schematic structure of arginine vasopressin. Arginine vasopressin (AVP) is a 9-amino acid, cyclic peptide with a disulfide bridge between cysteine residues at positions 1 and 6.

Table 30-1 Amino Acid Sequences of Arginine Vasopressin and Related Peptides

	Amino Acid Position									
Peptide	1	2	3	4	5	6	7	8	9	Distribution
Arginine vasopressin	Cys	Tyr	Phe	Glu	Asp	Cys	Pro	Arg	Gly	Most mammals
Lysine vasopressin			Phe	Glu				Lys		Pig family
Arginine vasotocin			Ile	Glu				Arg		Nonmammalian vertebrates
Oxytocin			Ile	Glu				Leu		Mammals, birds
Mesotocin			Ile	Glu				Ile		Reptiles
Isotocin			Ile	Ser				Ile		Fish
Glumitocin			Ile	Ser				Glu		Fish
Valitocin			Ile	Glu				Val		Fish
Aspartocin			Ile	Asp				Leu		Fish

(IGR) between the VP and OT genes are crucial for cell-specific expression.[18] A 178–base pair domain immediately downstream of exon 3 of the VP gene contains putative hypothalamus-specific enhancer motifs in common with sequences conferring hypothalamus-specific expression of the OT gene. It is postulated that these sites interact with hypothalamus-specific transcription factors to mediate, at least in part, tissue-limited expression.[19] However, whereas it is clear that the proximal 5′-promoter region of the VP gene is not sufficient to determine cell-specific expression, elements within the 3-Kb 5′-flanking sequence are important for this purpose. In addition, important roles may exist for neuron-specific repressors (e.g., neuron-restrictive silencer factor) in determining expression patterns.[10]

Regulation of VP gene expression in response to physiological stimuli is mediated through both positive and negative elements in the proximal promoter, which interact with several transcription factors. Of these *trans*-factors, adaptor protein 1 (AP1), AP2, and cyclic adenosine monophosphate (cAMP) response element binding protein (CREB) stimulate VP gene transcription, whereas the glucocorticoid receptor (GR) represses expression. VP magnocellular neurons do not express large amounts of GR under conditions of normal hydration. However, expression is stimulated in the hypo-osmolar state. This osmotic stimulation of GR expression may act further to suppress VP production in conditions such

as persistent hyponatremia.[10] Lactation triggers transcription of both OT and VP genes.[20] VP magnocellular neurons express estrogen receptor-β (ERβ), expression being inversely correlated with plasma osmolality. This impact on ERβ may modulate the inhibitory effects of gonadal steroids on VP release.[21] Salt loading causes a dramatic upregulation of VP gene transcription and accumulation of VP messenger RNA (mRNA) in the neurohypophysis.[22] In addition, water deprivation is associated with an increase in the length of the poly(A)-tail of AVP mRNA. This may affect mRNA stability and represent a rapid, transcription-independent mechanism for stimulating AVP synthesis.[23] VP mRNA contains a complex dendritic localization sequence (DLS) within part of the coding and 3′ untranslated region (3′UTR). The DLS interacts with a multifunctional poly(A)-binding protein (PABP), known to bind to the poly(A) tails of a number of mRNAs. DLS-PABP interactions play key roles in RNA stabilization, initiation of translation, and translational silencing.[24] Specifically, however, PABP interaction with the DLS can direct VP transcripts to be translated locally within dendrites of magnocellular neurons, generating a pool of locally synthesized hormone for dendritic release. Dendritic and axonal release of VP by magnocellular neurons is governed independently, and local control of translation within dendrites may be one of the mechanisms by which this is achieved.[25]

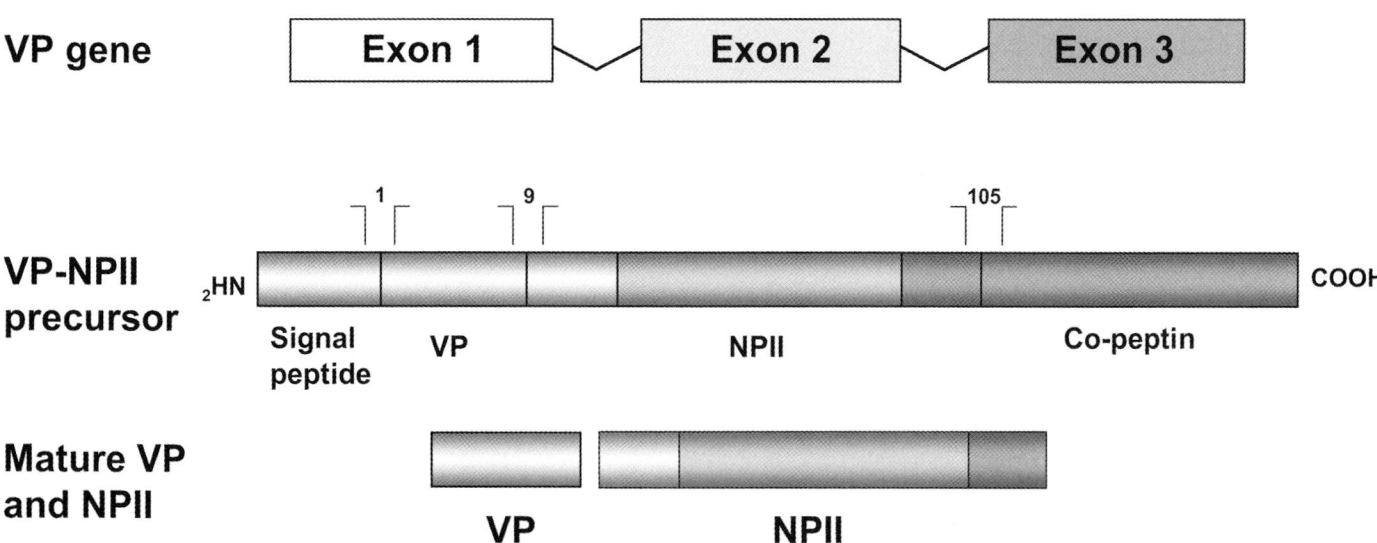

Figure 30-3 Schematic structure of the arginine vasopressin (AVP) gene and primary translation product. Numbers above the precursor relate to amino acid number with reference to the first amino acid of the AVP moiety.

BIOSYNTHESIS AND METABOLISM OF VASOPRESSIN

Synthesis of the VP precursor (VP-NPII preprohormone) occurs principally in the cell bodies of the hypothalamic neurons of the SON and PVN. Production of the mature hormone entails significant posttranslational processing. After translation, the carboxyl-terminal domain is glycosylated and packaged into vesicles of the regulated secretory pathway. As these migrate along the axons at some 2 mm per hour, the precursor undergoes successive cleavage by basic endopeptidases such as prohormone convertase (PC)1/3 and PC2, ultimately leaving the mature hormone, its associated NPII and a C-terminal glycopeptide, which are stored in secretory granules within nerve terminals.[26] Increased firing frequency of vasopressinergic neurons opens voltage-gated Ca^{2+} channels in nerve-terminal membranes, leading to transient Ca^{2+} influx, fusion of neurosecretory granules with the nerve terminal membrane, and release of VP and NPII in equimolar amounts.[27] Not all VP that is synthesized and processed is ultimately released. Some VP-containing neurosecretory granules migrate from the nerve endings as a result of an aging process, and their contents become unavailable.[28] Apart from acting as a carrier protein for VP during axonal migration, NPII appears to serve no other biologic function. Expression of a native AVP transgene in nonendocrine cells lacking the appropriate enzymes for posttranslational processing leads to the production of a nonprocessed AVP precursor, which is not biologically active. However, bioactive AVP can be produced by nonendocrine cells transfected with a bioengineered transgene encoding an AVP precursor in which the sequence between the AVP and NPII moieties has been mutated to encode amino acids recognized by the ubiquitous endopeptidase furin.[29]

As some VP mRNA is translated within the dendrites of magnocellular neurons, selective release of VP may occur from discrete intracellular pools within the same neuron, processed through different and discrete pathways, and subject to differential regulation.[30]

AVP has a short circulating half-life of about 5 to 15 minutes.[31] AVP circulates unbound to plasma proteins, although it does bind to specific receptors on platelets. AVP concentrations in platelet-rich plasma are fivefold higher than those of platelet-depleted plasma.[32] Several circulating and endothelial peptidases are responsible for AVP degradation, and at least four main sites of enzymatic cleavage have been identified on the AVP molecule.[31] During pregnancy and the immediate postpartum period, an extremely active cysteine aminopeptidase or vasopressinase (EC 3.4.11.3) of placental origin degrades AVP rapidly, further compromising circulating half-life.[31]

ACTIONS OF VASOPRESSIN

VASOPRESSIN RECEPTORS

The effects of VP are mediated by binding to receptors (V-Rs) on the plasma membranes of target cells.[33] Three V-R subtypes exist: V_1 to V_3 (Table 30-2). All have a seven–trans-membrane spanning domain modular structure typical of G protein–coupled receptors. They are encoded by different genes and differ in tissue distribution, signal transduction, and function. Rat and human V-Rs are 70% to 80% homologous at the amino acid level. The human V_2-R has been mapped to chromosome Xq28. The murine V_2-R maps to a syntenic X locus. The V_1-R is subject to both rapid homologous (VP-mediated) and heterologous desensitization through internalization. The V_2-R is subject to homologous desensitization.[34]

RENAL EFFECTS OF VASOPRESSIN

The principal physiologic action of AVP in humans is in the regulation of renal water resorption by the kidney, where the hairpin structure and electrolyte-transport processes of the nephron allow production of both concentrated and dilute urine in response to the prevailing AVP concentration. Active transport of solute out of the thick ascending limb of the loop of Henle generates an osmolar gradient in the renal interstitium that increases from cortex to inner medulla, a gradient through which distal parts of the nephron pass en route to the collecting duct. The presence of selective water channels (aquaporins) in the distal nephron allows resorption of water from the collecting-duct lumen along an osmotic gradient and excretion of concentrated urine.

Eleven different mammalian aquaporins (AQPs) have been identified to date, seven of which (AQP1–4, AQP6–8) are found in the kidney.[35] Targeted deletion studies suggest that a significant degree of functional redundancy is found in AQPs other than AQP1–3.[36] AQP1 is present in the apical and basolateral membranes of the proximal tubule and descending loop of Henle. It is a constitutively expressed water channel, facilitating isotonic fluid movement. Targeted deletion of AQP1 in the mouse significantly impairs renal concentrating ability, and loss-of-function mutations of AQP1 in humans

Table 30-2	Classification of Vasopressin Receptors		
	Receptor		
	V_1	**V_2**	**V_3**
Expression	Vascular smooth muscle Liver Platelets Central nervous system	Basolateral membrane of distal nephron	Pituitary corticotroph
Amino acid structure (human)	418 amino acids	370 amino acids	424 amino acids
Second messenger system	Gq/11-mediated phospholipase C activation: Ca^{2+}, inositol triphosphate, and diacyl glycerol mobilization	Gas–mediated adenylate cyclase activation: cAMP production and protein kinase A stimulation	As V_1
Physiologic effects	Smooth muscle contraction Stimulation of glycogenolysis Enhanced platelet adhesion Neurotransmitter and neuromodulatory function	Increased production and action of aquaporin-2	Enhanced ACTH release

ACTH, adrenocorticotropic hormone; cAMP, cyclic adenosine monophosphate.

lead to defective renal water conservation.[37,38] AQP3 and 4 are expressed constitutively in the basolateral membrane of the principal cells of the collecting duct. Targeted deletion of AQP3 in mouse leads to severe polyuria (although this could be attributed in part to the coincident reduction in AQP2 expression), whereas targeted deletion of AQP4 produces only a mild defect in concentrating ability. To date no phenotypes have been attributed to loss of function of either in humans. AQP6 is expressed in intracellular vesicles of acid-secreting cells of the collecting duct. AQP7 is found on the brush border of the proximal tubule, and AQP8 is present in low abundance intracellularly in proximal tubule and collecting duct cells. AQP2 is expressed on the luminal surface of collecting duct cells and is responsible for VP-dependent water transport from the lumen of the nephron into collecting duct cells. AVP partially modulates the expression of AQP3, but expression of AQP2 is AVP dependent. Binding of AVP to V_2-Rs on the interstitial surface of principal cells in the collecting duct produces a biphasic increase in expression of the water channel. V_2-R activation triggers an intracellular phosphorylation cascade, leading to enhanced AQP2 gene expression through a positive CRE site in the 5'-flanking promoter. Interestingly, an additional tonicity-responsive element is found in the 5'-flanking sequence, distal to and distinct from the CRE site.[39] AQP2 acts as a homotetramer. In addition to increasing AQP2 gene expression, V_2-R activation also accelerates the trafficking of presynthesized AQP2 protein to the luminal membrane and assembly of functional tetrameric water channels (Fig. 30-4).

A sigmoidal relation is found between plasma AVP concentration and urine osmolality (Fig. 30-5). At plasma concentrations of immunoreactive AVP of 0.5 pmol/L or less, maximum diuresis occurs. Maximum urine concentration is achieved at plasma AVP concentrations more than 3 to 4 pmol/L. Further elevation of plasma AVP above these values does not increase water resorption further.

After chronic elevation of VP secretion, antidiuresis may diminish, consistent with an apparent desensitization to the renal effects of the hormone. VP-independent downregulation of both V_2-R function and AQP2 expression are thought to play a role in this VP escape phenomenon.[39]

At sites other than the collecting duct, AVP has additional effects that contribute to its physiologic role. AVP decreases renal medullary blood flow and stimulates active urea transport from the distal collecting duct into the renal interstitium. In addition, AVP stimulates active sodium transport into the renal interstitium from the lumen of the thick ascending limb of the loop of Henle. These actions contribute to the generation and maintenance of a hypertonic medullary interstitium and augment AVP-dependent water resorption.[40-44]

CARDIOVASCULAR EFFECTS OF VASOPRESSIN

The cardiovascular effects of AVP are mediated by the V_1-R. AVP is a potent pressor agent, although marked effects on systemic blood pressure are apparent only at plasma concentrations many times higher than those observed under normal conditions.[45] Nevertheless, the use of specific V_1-R antagonists has highlighted the importance of AVP in maintaining blood pressure in mild volume depletion. The pressor effect of AVP varies according to vascular bed, and it can produce considerable constriction of regional arteries and arterioles (e.g., splanchnic, renal, hepatic) at near-physiologic concentrations (10 pmol/L).[46-48] Differential pressor effects on intrarenal vessels account for the shunting of blood from the medulla to the cortex under the influence of AVP.[49] Cardiac output and oxygen consumption are reduced by AVP through a variety of mechanisms.[50]

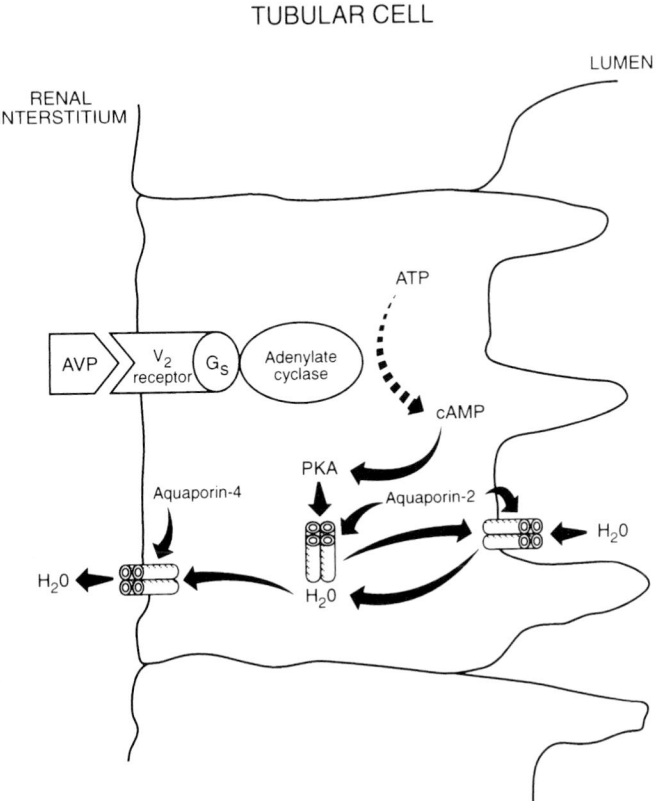

TUBULAR CELL

Figure 30-4 The action of arginine vasopressin (AVP) on renal collecting duct cells. Schematic representation of an AVP-sensitive collecting duct cell. The binding of AVP to the V_2-R on the basolateral membrane triggers G protein–mediated activation of a signal cascade via protein kinase A (PKA). This, in turn, leads to both increased aquaporin-2 (*AQP2*) gene expression and accelerates assembly of previously synthesized AQP2 monomers into functional tetrameric water channels in the luminal membrane. Aquaporin-4 is not AVP sensitive.

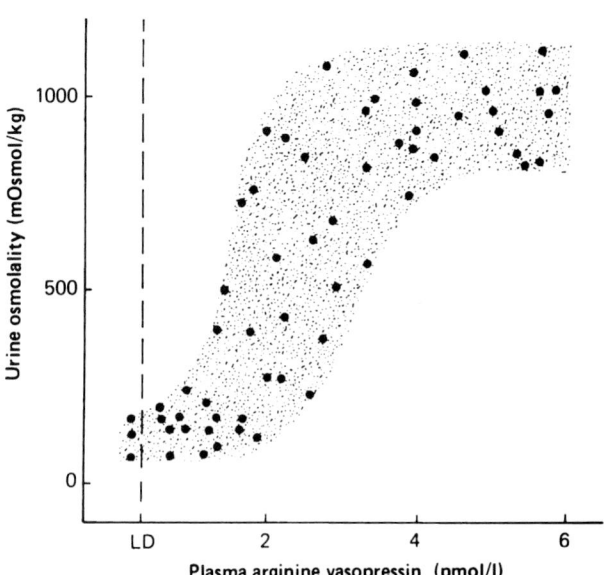

Figure 30-5 Relation between plasma AVP (pAVP) and urine osmolality. Data were obtained during water loading and fluid restriction in a group of healthy adults. Maximal urine concentration is achieved by pAVP values of 3–4 pmol/L. LD, Limit of detection of the AVP assay, 0.3 pmol/L.

EFFECTS OF VASOPRESSIN IN THE PITUITARY

AVP is an ACTH secretogogue. Although the effect is weak in isolation, AVP and CRF act synergistically. A group of PVN parvocellular neurons coexpressing AVP and CRF project via the median eminence and terminate on the hypohyseal-portal bed feeding the anterior pituitary. AVP and CRF expression by these parvocellular neurons is subject to negative feedback control by glucocorticoids. The effects of AVP on pituitary ACTH release are mediated by the corticotroph-specific V_3-R.[51-53] Regulation of corticotropin secretion by AVP is physiologically important. AVP does not influence the secretion of other anterior pituitary hormones.

CENTRAL NERVOUS SYSTEM AND MISCELLANEOUS EFFECTS OF VASOPRESSIN

Vasopressinergic nerve fibers and V-Rs are present in many areas of the central nervous system, including the cerebral cortex and the limbic system. These networks appear functionally and anatomically distinct from the neurohypophysis, and their physiologic role remains unclear. In rodent, central vasopressinergic systems have been shown to have important roles in mediating complex social behavior.[54,55] Additional miscellaneous effects of AVP are given in Table 30-3.[56-65]

REGULATION OF VASOPRESSIN RELEASE

OSMOREGULATION OF VASOPRESSIN RELEASE

An exquisitely sensitive relationship exists between plasma osmolality and plasma AVP concentrations.[66-68] In healthy adults, the infusion of hypertonic saline (855 mmol/L) to steadily increase plasma osmolality results in a progressive increase in peripheral plasma AVP concentrations. As the plasma AVP level increases, antidiuresis and urinary concentration increase. Although pulsatile release of AVP can be detected in the internal jugular vein, such pulses are not apparent as minute-to-minute fluctuation in AVP concentration in peripheral veins.[69] A direct correlation exists between plasma osmolality and plasma AVP concentration (Fig. 30-6), which is defined by the following function:

$$pAVP = 0.43 \, (pOs - 284), \quad r = +0.96, \quad P < 0.001$$

where pAVP indicates plasma AVP concentration, and pOs indicates plasma osmolality. This relationship defines two important physiologic characteristics: (1) the osmotic threshold for AVP release; and (2) the sensitivity of the osmoregulatory mechanism coupling plasma osmolality and AVP release.

The abscissal intercept of the regression line describing the change in plasma AVP concentration with changing plasma osmolality, 284 mOsm/kg, indicates the plasma osmolality at which plasma AVP starts to increase. This provides a measure of the set point of the osmoreceptor mechanism, or the osmotic threshold for AVP release.[70] Whether AVP secretion can be completely suppressed remains unclear. Data derived from very sensitive cytochemical methods for measurement

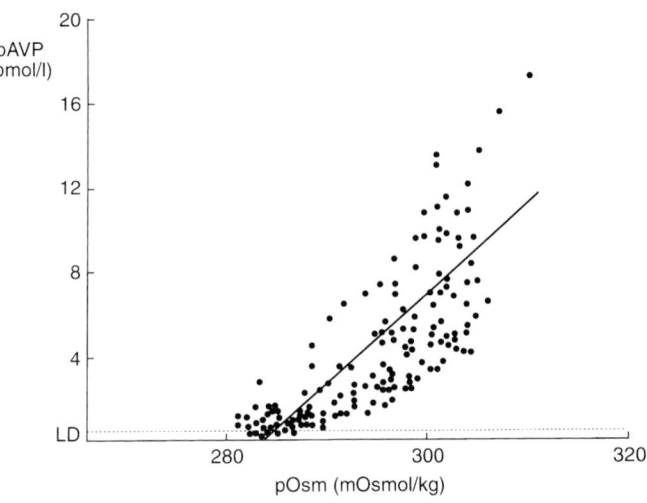

Figure 30-6 Relation between plasma osmolality (pOsm) and plasma AVP (pAVP). Increases in pAVP in response to hypertonicity induced by infusion of 855 mmol/L saline in a group of healthy adults. The mean regression line (*dashed line*) is defined by the equation: pAVP = 0.43 (pOsm − 284); r = +0.96; P < 0.001. LD, Limit of detection of the AVP assay, 0.3 pmol/L.

of plasma AVP suggest that secretion cannot be switched off by hypotonicity.[71] Nevertheless, the concept of an osmotic threshold for AVP release remains a pragmatic means to characterize osmoregulatory function and to analyze disorders of osmoregulation.[68] The slope of the regression line describing the change in plasma AVP concentration with changing plasma osmolality reflects the sensitivity of the osmoreceptor-AVP–releasing unit. Complete disconnection of AVP-secreting neurons from their osmoreceptors appears to cause persistent low-grade AVP release, resulting in plasma AVP values of about 1.0 pmol/L.[72] Thus, AVP secretion is increased from this "basal" rate by stimulation of facilitatory osmoreceptor cells but must be decreased to minimal values by activation of inhibitory cells.

Although considerable variation is found in both the osmotic threshold and sensitivity of AVP release between individuals, these parameters remain unchanged within an individual tested over a short period.[73] Studies have shown that they are similar in monozygotic twins, suggesting a genetic determinant for the set of the osmoregulatory system.[74] Further data suggest that a generational influence may affect osmoregulation, the osmolar threshold for AVP release being higher in the neonatal offspring of ewes exposed to hypertonic dehydration.[75]

In a number of physiologic situations, the conventional relationship between plasma osmolality and plasma AVP concentration is altered. Fast rates of hypertonic saline infusion result in exaggerated AVP responses,[66] thereby creating a curvilinear relation between plasma AVP and plasma osmolality. Pregnancy causes a lowering of the threshold for AVP secretion without alteration of the gain of the osmoreceptor in both rats[76] and humans,[77] which accounts for the hypo-osmolality of pregnancy. In the luteal phase of the normal human ovulatory menstrual cycle, a small but significant decrease in plasma osmolality occurs as a result of lowering of thresholds for thirst and AVP release.[78] Similar changes are found in patients with superovulation syndrome.[79] Drinking produces a rapid decline in plasma AVP concentration out of proportion to the change in plasma osmolality, reflecting additional nonosmotic sensory inputs, probably from oropharyngeal afferents. The aging process has a considerable effect on osmoregulation and fluid and electrolyte homeostasis.[80] Basal circulating AVP concentrations increase with age, and the response to osmotic stimulation is enhanced.[81,82] Thirst appreciation, however, is blunted, and fluid intake is reduced.[83] In

Table 30-3	Miscellaneous Effects of Vasopressin	
Action		**Receptor**
Clotting	Factor VII release from hepatocytes	V_2
	Von Willebrand factor release from vascular endothelium	V_2
Bone	Maintenance of bone mineral density	V_2
Liver	Glycogen phosphorylase activation	V_2

addition, both renal free water excretion and maximal concentrating ability are reduced, exposing the elderly to increased risk of both hyponatremia and hypernatremia.[84,85]

The response of the osmoreceptor to solutes other than sodium chloride is variable. In the presence of insulin, moderate hyperglycemia fails to stimulate AVP secretion,[86] but insulinopenic rats do release AVP after severe hyperglycemia.[87] Urea has about one third the stimulatory effect on AVP release of isosmolar sodium chloride.[86] Alcohol suppresses AVP secretion.[88]

BAROREGULATION OF VASOPRESSIN RELEASE

Both blood volume and pressure influence AVP secretion. Reduction in arterial blood pressure of 5% to 10% increases circulating immunoreactive AVP concentrations (Fig. 30-7).[89,90] In contrast to the simple linear correlation between plasma osmolality and plasma AVP, the relation between blood pressure and AVP is exponential.

Changes in circulating volume and blood pressure trigger an autonomic and endocrine cascade, of which AVP release is a part, resulting in a coordinated physiologic response. AVP responses can be modified by other neurohumoral influences that also are activated as part of the coordinated process. Atrial natriuretic peptides inhibit baroregulated AVP responses, whereas norepinephrine augments responses.[91] Furthermore, an interrelation exists between osmoregulatory and baroregulatory AVP secretion, such that the AVP osmoregulatory line is shifted to the left of normal as hypovolemia develops.[92,93] Thus, under conditions of moderate hypovolemia, osmoregulation is preserved around a lower set point of plasma osmolality (Fig. 30-8).[92] As hypovolemia becomes more severe, very high plasma AVP values are attained that override the osmoregulatory system such that nonosmoregulated AVP release can persist despite significant hyponatremia.

OTHER MECHANISMS REGULATING VASOPRESSIN RELEASE

In addition to osmotic and baro stimuli, AVP release is triggered in a number of physiologic and pathophysiologic situations. In primates, circulating AVP values in excess of 500 pmol/L have been recorded that are independent of

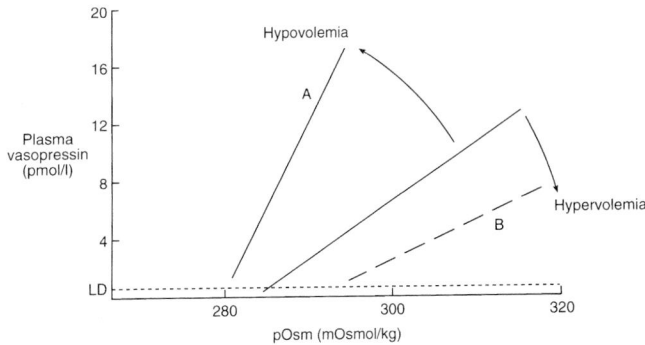

Figure 30-8 Diagrammatic representation of the effect of circulating volume on osmoregulated arginine vasopressin (AVP) release. Hypovolemia (*A*) reduces the osmolar threshold and increases the sensitivity of AVP release in response to osmotic stimulation. Hypervolemia (*B*) has the counter effect.

osmotic and hemodynamic input.[94,95] Nausea, emesis, neuroglycopenia, and manipulation of abdominal contents at surgery are all potent stimuli to AVP secretion.[96,97] Several factors may thus contribute to the high plasma AVP values observed after gastrointestinal surgery and predispose to hyponatremia if excess fluid is administered in the postoperative period. Posterior pituitary AVP production is increased by systemic immune stressors. Histamine and bacterial lipopolysaccharide stimulate AVP production through the local formation of prostaglandins, highlighting the role of these mediators in posterior pituitary hormone responses to immunochallenges.[98] Although AVP release is triggered during episodes of physiologic and pathophysiologic stress, its role as a true stress hormone remains controversial.

NEUROPHYSIOLOGIC REGULATION OF VASOPRESSIN RELEASE

Osmotic regulation of VP production is mediated by sensory afferents originating in the lamina terminalis, situated on the anterior wall of the third ventricle, anatomically distinct from the SON and PVN. The lamina terminalis is composed of the subfornical organ (SFO); the median preoptic nucleus (MnPO); and the organum vasculosum of the lamina terminalis (OVLT). The blood-brain barrier is incomplete in the region of the SFO and OVLT, and cells in these regions are thus exposed to the hormonal, ionic, and osmolar environment of the systemic circulation. Afferents sensitive to osmolality (osmoreceptors) are situated in the dorsal cap of the OVLT, and possibly also around the periphery of the SFO and MnPO. A non–N-methyl-D-aspartate (NMDA) receptor glutaminergic pathway relays osmotic inputs from OVLT to vasopressinergic magnocellular neurons in the SON. Inhibitory γ-aminobutyric acid (GABA)ergic neurons also project to the SON from the lamina terminalis. Atrial natriuretic peptide (ANP) may act presynaptically to inhibit glutaminergic signals from OVLT afferents.[99]

Baroregulatory influences on AVP production by the neurohypophysis derive from peripheral high- and low-pressure receptors located in the aortic arch, the carotid sinus, the cardiac atria, and the great veins within the thorax. Stretch-sensitive afferents (low-pressure receptors) at the junction of the cardiac atria and cava mediate the inhibitory effects of volume expansion on vasopressinergic magnocellular neurons. Afferents project via cranial nerves IX and X to the nucleus tractus solitarius (NTS) in the dorsomedial medulla oblongata and thence rostrally in the adrenergic cell group of the ventrolateral medulla, via the perinuclear zone of the SON, to the SON and PVN. Inhibitory afferents originating from arterial baroreceptors (high-pressure receptors) project via similar routes and converge on the perinuclear zone of

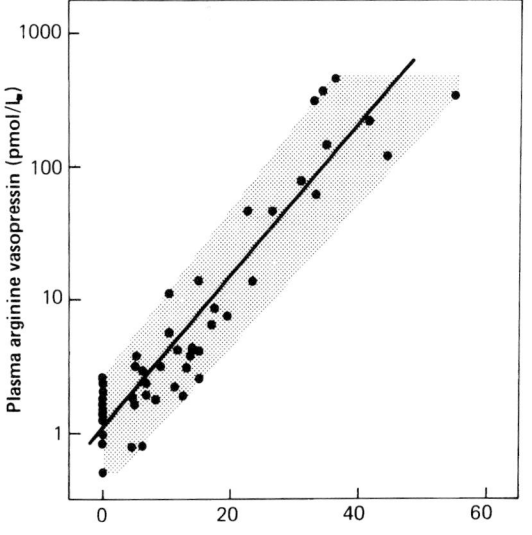

Figure 30-7 Relation of plasma AVP (pAVP) to the percentage decline in mean arterial blood pressure (MABP). Arterial blood pressure was reduced by infusing increasing doses of trimetaphan in healthy men. The regression line is defined by the equation: log (pAVP) = 0.06 (MABP + 0.67); r = +0.98; P < 0.001, N = 48.

the SON, which may thus act to integrate inputs reflecting volume status.[100] Interruption of the ascending baroregulatory pathway increases plasma AVP levels, consistent with a degree of tonic baroreceptor-dependent inhibition of AVP production.[101]

Vasopressinergic magnocellular neuronal dendrites also can release AVP. Indeed, axonal and dendritic VP release have different dynamics, suggestive of differential regulation. Dendritic OT released by oxytotic magnocellular neurons can act as a retrograde transmitter in the SON, inhibiting excitatory glutamate release from presynaptic terminals inputting to OT magnocellular neurons. As vasopressinergic magnocellular neurons express V-Rs in addition to synthesizing and releasing the hormone, it has been proposed that dendritic release of AVP may alter magnocellular AVP output either directly, through a short autofeedback loop, or indirectly, through affecting excitatory afferent input.[102,103] Dendritic VP release may thus play an important role in fine-tuning magnocellular neuron VP release into the general circulation.

INTER-RELATIONSHIP OF VASOPRESSIN AXIS AND THIRST

Both thirst and the drinking response are key components in the maintenance of fluid homeostasis. Thirst perception and the regulation of water ingestion involve complex, integrated neural and neurohumoral pathways. Current data suggest that central osmoreceptors involved in thirst perception are located in the OVLT and the AV3V region or the SFO of the anterior hypothalamus (or both) probably anatomically distinct from those mediating VP production.[104] The relative sensitivity of these regions to sodium or total osmolar load remain unclear.[105] Rostral projections remain largely unmapped, although lesions in the ventral nucleus medianus can produce both adipsia and hyperdipsia in rodents, suggesting that this may be one route through which afferents project to the cortex. Little doubt exists, however, that thirst is an extremely powerful sensation that drives the seeking and ingestion of water.

A linear relation exists between thirst, as determined by visual analogue scale, and plasma osmolalities in the physiologic range. In a similar manner to the relation of plasma osmolality and plasma AVP concentration, this can be defined by the function:

$$\text{Thirst} = 0.39 \text{ (plasma osmolality} - 285), r = +0.95, P < 0.001$$

The abscissal intercept of the regression line describing changes in thirst with changes in plasma osmolality, 285 mOsm/kg, represents the osmotic threshold for thirst perception (Fig. 30-9), effectively the same as the threshold for AVP release. Indeed, the functional characteristics of the osmoregulatory lines for AVP release and thirst are very similar. Despite wide individual variations in the value of the osmotic threshold for thirst, it remains remarkably consistent within individuals.[73] Drinking causes a dramatic fall in osmo-stimulated thirst analogue scores, identical to the rapid decline in circulating AVP concentrations that are seen on drinking.[106]

Thirst also can be stimulated by extracellular volume depletion. Underfill of the low-pressure thoracic circulation leads to drinking in animals, an effect probably mediated by the volume-sensitive left atrial receptors and vagal afferents.[107] The diagonal band of Broca is important in mediating thirst responses to volume depletion, although it does not seem to have a role in determining basal water intake.[108] Peripheral and central generation of the powerful dipsogen angiotensin II by volume-dependent activation of the renin-angiotensin system is a key component of the integrated behavioral and cardiovascular response to volume depletion.[109,110]

The osmoregulatory system for thirst and AVP secretion maintains plasma osmolality within the narrow limits of

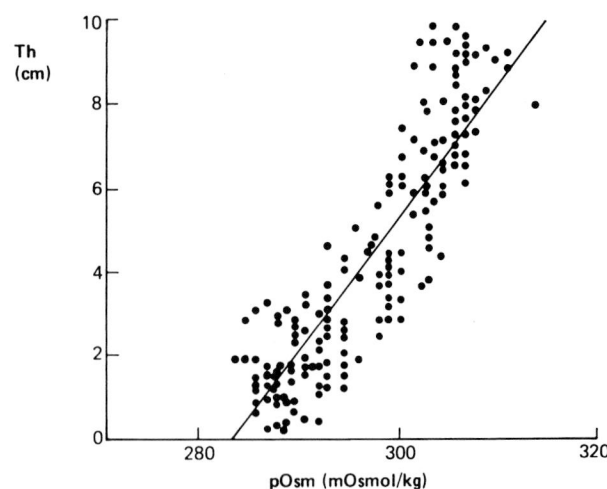

Figure 30-9   Relation between thirst (Th) and plasma osmolality (pOsm). Increases in thirst during hypertonic (855 mmol/L) saline infusion in a group of healthy adults. The mean regression line is defined by the equation: Th = 0.39 (pOsm − 285); r = +0.95; P < 0.001.

about 284 to 295 mOsm/kg. In response to increasing plasma osmolality from 284 mOsm/kg (osmotic threshold for AVP release), the plasma AVP concentration increases progressively, with parallel increases in urine osmolality. Plasma osmolalities in the region of 295 mOsm/kg and plasma AVP concentrations of 3 to 4 pmol/L produce a maximal antidiuresis. Although further increases in plasma osmolality result in more AVP release, they do not result in further conservation of renal water. Dehydration could ensue if fluid were not ingested. This is avoided in healthy individuals by the stimulation of thirst to promote drinking.[66,111] Intake should be sufficient to return plasma osmolality to levels at which renal water excretion can again be regulated by changes in AVP secretion (i.e., <295 mOsm/kg). In a healthy individual who has elevated plasma AVP concentration because of osmotic stimulation, the act of drinking causes a rapid decrease in plasma AVP concentration disproportionate to the change in plasma osmolality.[106] If fluid volumes greater than those demanded by thirst are consumed, AVP secretion is suppressed to very low levels (<0.3 pmol/L), at which the kidney is capable of excreting 15 to 20 L of urine in 24 hours. Ingestion of fluid volumes in excess of this results in further lowering of plasma osmolality in healthy adults.

DIABETES INSIPIDUS

The pathophysiology of AVP, disturbances in production or action of the hormone, manifest as clinical problems in sodium and water balance. This reflects the major role of AVP in body-fluid homeostasis. An additional related group of clinical problems reflect primary disturbances in thirst. Problems in both areas may coincide, highlighting the close functional and anatomic relation between the two processes of AVP production and thirst.

CLASSIFICATION OF DIABETES INSIPIDUS

Diabetes insipidus (DI), excess production of a dilute urine, is characterized by the excretion of urine in excess of 40 mL/kg per 24 hours in adults, or more than 100 mL/kg per 24 hours in infants. One of three pathogenetic mechanisms may be responsible (Table 30-4).[112–114]

- A deficiency, usually not absolute, of AVP: hypothalamic diabetes insipidus (HDI).

Table 30-4 Classification of Diabetes Insipidus

A. HYPOTHALAMIC DIABETES INSIPIDUS

Primary	Genetic	DIDMOAD (Wolfram) syndrome
		Autosomal dominant
		Autosomal recessive
	Developmental syndromes	Septo-optic dysplasia
		Lawrence-Moon-Biedl syndrome
	Idiopathic	
Secondary/acquired	Trauma	Head injury
		After surgery (transcranial, transphenoidal)
	Tumor	Craniopharyngioma, pinealoma, germinoma, metastases, pituitary macroadenoma
	Inflammatory	Granulomata
		Sarcoidosis, Histiocytosis
		Infection
		Meningitis, Encephalitis
		Infundibulo-neurohypophysitis
		Guillain-Barré syndrome
		Autoimmune (antivasopressin neuron antibodies)
	Vascular	Aneurysm
		Infarction
		Sheehan's syndrome
		Sickle-cell disease
	Pregnancy (associated with vasopressinase)	

B. NEPHROGENIC DIABETES INSIPIDUS

Primary	Genetic	X-linked recessive (*V2R* defect)
		Autosomal recessive (*AQP2* defect)
		Autosomal dominant (*AQP2* defect)
	Idiopathic	
Secondary	Chronic renal disease	Polycystic kidneys
		Obstructive uropathy
	Metabolic disease	Hypercalcemia
		Hypokalemia
	Drug induced	Lithium
		Demeclocycline
	Osmotic diuretics	Glucose
		Mannitol
	Systemic disorders	Amyloidosis
		Myelomatosis
	Pregnancy	

C. DIPSOGENIC DIABETES INSIPIDUS

Compulsive water drinking		
Associated with affective disorders		
Drug induced		
Structural/organic hypothalamic disease		Sarcoid
		Tumors involving hypothalamus
		Head injury
		Tuberculous meningitis

- Partial or total renal resistance to the antidiuretic action of AVP: nephrogenic diabetes insipidus (NDI).
- Excessive inappropriate drinking: dipsogenic diabetes insipidus (DDI) or primary polydipsia (PP).

HYPOTHALAMIC DIABETES INSIPIDUS

HDI (also known as neurogenic, central, or cranial DI) is a polyuric syndrome resulting from impaired osmoregulated AVP secretion. Most patients have detectable plasma AVP concentrations, but they are inappropriately low with respect to the concomitant plasma osmolalities. Although persistent polyuria can lead to hypertonic dehydration, most patients maintain water balance through an intact thirst mechanism. Presentation with HDI implies loss of function of more than 80% of AVP magnocellular neurons. HDI is a rare disorder, with an estimated prevalence of 1:25,000. An equal gender distribution is found.

The majority of HDI is acquired during adult life. Improved imaging, together with increased awareness of inflammatory and autoimmune etiologies, has reduced the number of cases designated as idiopathic.[115,116] Indeed, up to 30% of those patients previously classified as having idiopathic HDI may have a primary autoimmune etiology, characterized by the presence of circulating antibodies against AVP-secreting cells; age at onset younger than 30 years; and pituitary stalk thickening on magnetic resonance imaging (MRI).[117] However, the presence of circulating antibodies directed against AVP-secreting cells is not specific in isolation and can occur as an epiphenomenon in patients with HDI from other causes. The majority of children and young adults with HDI have abnormal brain or pituitary imaging or both, with tumors affecting the hypothalamus (craniopharyngioma, germinoma) and central nervous system (CNS) malformation being present in up to 50% of cases. More than 50% of cases in this age group have other anterior pituitary hormone deficiencies, or they may subsequently develop.[114,118]

Trauma to the hypothalamus, pituitary stalk, or posterior pituitary from open or closed head injury or surgery can lead to HDI. A triphasic disturbance in water balance can develop.[119] This is characterized by an immediate polyuric phase characteristic of HDI, followed within a few days by a more prolonged period (≤1 week) of antidiuresis. The second phase can be followed by either recovery or development of recurrent, persistent HDI. This characteristic "triple response" reflects initial magnocellular neuron damage; the subsequent release of large, unregulated amounts of preprocessed AVP; and finally either recovery or development of permanent HDI, as determined by the degree of initial neuropraxia or axonal shearing. Inhibitors of AVP action have been identified in the circulation during the second polyuric phase.[120] These may represent partly processed AVP precursors. All three phases may not be manifest in all cases.

Pituitary tumors that compress or invade the posterior lobe rarely cause HDI, although metastatic deposits in the hypothalamus, often from carcinoma of the breast or bronchus, result in HDI. Lymphocytic infiltration of the neurohypophysis (infundibulo-neurohypophysitis), recognized by a thickened pituitary stalk and inflammatory infiltrates of T lymphocytes and plasma cells with eosinophils, is a well-described cause of HDI.[121] HDI is present in up to 30% of adult patients with Langerhans' cell histiocytosis (LCH).[122]

Sheehan's syndrome remains an uncommon cause of HDI, but maximal urine-concentrating ability appears to be impaired in some patients, implying a minimal defect in osmoregulated AVP release without marked polyuria.[123] Selective vascular damage affecting the inferior hypophyseal arteries has been causally linked with a significant (≤20%) proportion of cases of idiopathic HDI.[124] Very rarely, HDI occurs in pregnancy. In some instances, this is due to increased activity of circulating vasopressinase, the aminopeptidase of placental origin.[125] After delivery, symptoms may resolve. Pregnancy can unmask partial HDI in patients with pituitary disease, in which case, the symptoms may recur, dependent on the natural history of the pituitary lesion. HDI in pregnancy must be differentiated from the transient NDI that is seen very occasionally.[126] Additional, unusual causes of HDI have been described. Cytomegalovirus infection of the hypothalamus leading to HDI was demonstrated in a patient with acquired immunodeficiency syndrome.[127] HDI as a consequence of carbon monoxide poisoning also was reported.[128]

Familial HDI constitutes 5% of total cases, in a number of different forms. Autosomal-dominant HDI (adHDI) is caused by loss-of-function mutations in the *AVP* gene, resulting in the production of a folding-incompetent peptide precursor that accumulates in the secretory pathway apparatus of magnocellular neurons.[129,130] The mutant precursor stimulates an autophagocytic process, resulting in neurotoxicity and a progressive loss of VP neurons.[131] The presence of a single mutant allele is sufficient for this process to occur. To date, mutations associated with adHDI have been described in the signal peptide, NPII, and VP moieties of the VP gene product. The majority affect exons 1 and 2 of the *AVP* gene (Fig. 30-10).[132,133] Although typically it is initially seen in childhood, the age at presentation can vary, reflecting differences in the rate of progressive loss of magnocellular neurons.[134] Intriguingly, the production of *AVP* by parvocellular neurons supplying *AVP* and corticotropin-releasing hormone to the median eminence appears normal in individuals with adHDI, suggesting neuron-specific differences in either mutant precursor processing, neurotoxicity, or AVP gene transcription.[135] A single nucleotide deletion in the VP gene also is the cause of HDI in the Brattleboro rat.[136]

Wolfram (WS) or DIDMOAD syndrome is a rare autosomal-recessive, progressive neurodegenerative disorder characterized by the association of H*D*I with *d*iabetes *m*ellitus, *o*ptic *a*trophy and bilateral sensorineural *d*eafness. Although expression is variable, presentation is generally with diabetes mellitus and optic atrophy in the first decade and HDI and deafness in the second decade. Patients may go on to develop the additional problems of renal outflow tract dilatation (secondary to reduced nerve fibers in the bladder wall) and progressive ataxia with brain stem atrophy. The syndrome is associated with premature death, often of respiratory failure. Gonadal atrophy also can occur.[137] WS is associated with loss-of-function mutations in the *WFSI* gene on Ch.4p16.1, which encodes an 890-amino acid glycoprotein (wolframin) found in the endoplasmic reticulum. Interestingly, noninactivating mutations in the same gene are associated with nonsyndromic autosomal-dominant sensorineural hearing loss.[138] An additional locus for WS has been identified recently at Ch.4q22-24, suggesting that the syndrome may be genetically heterogeneous.[139]

NEPHROGENIC DIABETES INSIPIDUS

NDI is due to renal resistance to the antidiuretic effects of VP. An outline of potential causes is given in Table 30-4. Most commonly, NDI is due to a variety of acquired metabolic or

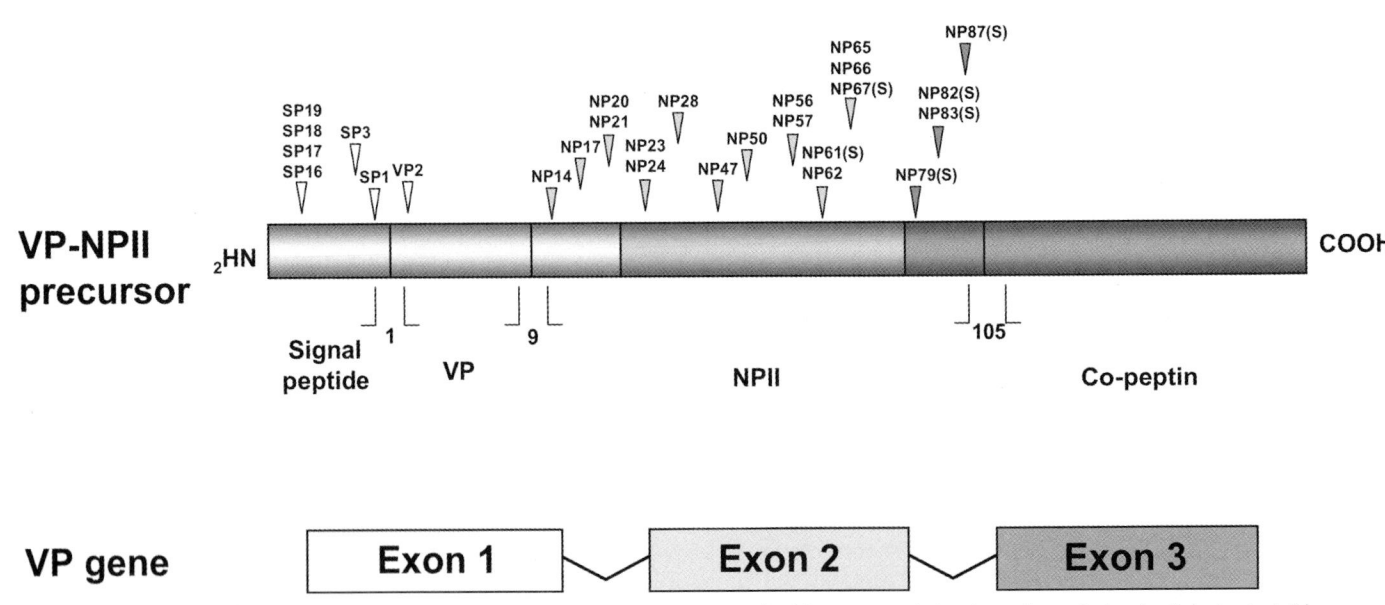

Figure 30-10 The spectrum of arginine vasopressin (AVP) mutations associated with autosomal-dominant hypothalamic diabetes insipidus (adHDI). Schematic representation of the AVP precursor depicting positions of known mutations associated with adHDI. The majority occur in exon 2 of the *VP* gene, and affect the NPII moiety. However, mutations affecting both the signal peptide and AVP sequence have been identified. Numbers reflect amino acid position in relation to first amino acid of VP. SP, signal peptide; VP, vasopressin; NP, neurophysin; (S), mutation resulting in premature translation termination (stop codon).

drug effects. Hypokalemia and hypercalcemia can produce acquired NDI, which is generally reversible with correction of the underlying cause. In contrast, NDI secondary to lithium toxicity can persist after drug discontinuation and may not always be reversible. Prolonged polyuria of any cause may itself cause NDI, due to dilution of the medullary interstitial solute concentration gradient, which is an obligate requirement for VP-dependent water resorption from the distal nephron.

A number of forms of familial NDI are found, all of which are rare. X-linked-recessive familial NDI (X-FNDI) is caused by inherited loss-of-function mutations in the V_2-R. More than 70 different mutations have been described, affecting all aspects of receptor physiology including expression, ligand binding, and G protein coupling. Most are associated with complete loss of function and lead to presentation in the first year of life. A few mutations have been described that are associated with a milder phenotype.[140] Approximately 10% of kindreds with FNDI have an autosomal-recessive form (AR-FNDI). Affected individuals harbor loss-of-function mutations of the gene encoding AQP2. The majority of mutations described to date occur in the region of the gene encoding the transmembrane domain of the water-channel protein. Rare kindreds have been described with an autosomal-dominant NDI (AD-NDI) due to loss-of-function mutations in *AQP2* affecting the carboxyl-terminal intracellular domain of the protein. NDI is expressed in these kindreds because the protein product of the mutant allele forms mixed oligomers with the product of the wild-type allele, resulting in sequestration within the Golgi or mistargeting to the basolateral rather than the apical membrane in a dominant negative manner.[141,142]

DIPSOGENIC DIABETES INSIPIDUS

DDI is a syndrome of polyuria that is a direct result of excessive fluid intake. Rarely, the problem may be associated with structural abnormalities affecting the neurohypophysis (such as hypothalamic sarcoidosis or craniopharyngioma). However, imaging is generally normal. DDI can be associated with a number of different abnormalities of thirst perception including a low osmotic threshold for thirst; an exaggerated thirst response to osmotic challenge; and an inability to suppress thirst at low osmolalities (see Fig. 30-9). However, the structural and functional basis of these abnormalities has not been determined. DDI is associated with affective disorders, and up to 20% of patients with chronic schizophrenia have DDI. Although DDI in these patients may reflect thought disorder, abnormalities in thirst and AVP production have been described.[143] Whether these abnormalities reflect primary defects in central processing or other factors (such as the effects of prior or concurrent drug treatment) remains to be determined.

MANAGEMENT OF DIABETES INSIPIDUS

Diagnosis of Diabetes Insipidus
No specific clinical features definitely identify the cause of polyuria in a particular patient. Diagnosis therefore rests on the results of investigations. Direct measurement of plasma AVP during osmotic stimulation establishes the diagnosis of HDI. However, because reliable methods to measure AVP have not always been readily available, indirect methods of assessing antidiuretic activity (a surrogate indicator of AVP production) during fluid deprivation have been developed.

Having established that the adult patient is polyuric (24-hour urine volume, >3 L), a fluid-deprivation test can be performed, with subsequent assessment of renal concentrating ability in response to exogenous VP (Table 30-5).[92] Patients with severe HDI have a low urine osmolality (<300 mOsm/kg) and high plasma osmolality (>295 mOsm/kg) after dehydration, and urine concentration to greater than

Table 30-5 Protocol for Water-Deprivation/Desmopressin Test	
Preparation phase	Free access to fluid overnight before test
	Avoid caffeine and smoking
Dehydration phase	0750 hr, weigh patient
	0800, Plasma and urine osmolality and urine volume
	Restrict fluids for 8 hr
	Weigh patient at 2-hr intervals
	Plasma and urine osmolality, and urine volume measurements every 2 hr
	Stop test if weight loss exceeds 5% of starting weight, or thirst is intolerable
	Supervise patient closely to avoid nondisclosed drinking
Desmopressin acetate (DDAVP) phase	Inject intramuscularly, 1 µg desmopressin
	Allow patient to eat and drink up to 1.5–2.0 times the volume of urine passed during dehydration phase
	Plasma and urine osmolality and urine volume measurements hourly to 2000 hr
	Plasma sodium and osmolality, 0900 hr next day

750 mOsm/kg after administration of exogenous desmopressin (1-desamino-8-D-arginine vasopressin, DDAVP, a synthetic analogue of VP). In contrast, severe NDI can be identified by failure to increase urine osmolality to greater than 300 mOsm/kg after dehydration and administration of DDAVP. Unfortunately, significant difficulties arise in establishing a diagnosis with fluid-deprivation tests. Many patients have partial defects, and mild forms of HDI, NDI, and DDI cannot always be differentiated with this type of test.[144] Furthermore, prolonged polyuria from any cause leads to partial resistance to the antidiuretic action of VP, because of dilution of the renal medullary interstitium.[145]

An accurate diagnosis of HDI can be made by direct measurement of plasma AVP concentration during graded osmotic stimulation, produced by infusion of hypertonic saline[145,146] (Fig. 30-11A). Patients with HDI are identified by undetectable or subnormal plasma AVP concentrations with respect to plasma osmolalities, with values to the right of the normal distribution. Patients with DDI and NDI have plasma AVP responses in the normal range. DDI and NDI can be distinguished by relating plasma AVP concentration to urine osmolality. NDI is characterized by inappropriately high plasma AVP values for the concomitant urine osmolality, whereas DDI patients show an appropriate relation (see Fig. 30-11B). Parallel assessment of thirst responses to graded osmotic stimulation (by using a visual analogue scale) is important, as concurrent problems in thirst perception may have a key bearing on management.

As accurate AVP assays may not be readily available, an alternative approach to diagnosis can be made by instituting a careful therapeutic trial of DDAVP while maintaining the patient under close observation. Administration of 10 µg of DDAVP intranasally once daily for 2 to 4 weeks causes progressive dilutional hyponatremia in DDI. Patients with NDI remain unaffected. Those with HDI experience an improvement in thirst and polyuria but remain normonatremic. As the concentrations of AVP in urine are higher than those in plasma, and thus detectable by a wider range of available assays, measurement of urinary AVP concentration during osmotic stress has been proposed as an additional alternative to the measurement of plasma AVP in the diagnosis of HDI.[147]

Figure 30-11 Dynamic tests of the arginine vasopressin (AVP) axis in patients with polyuria. **A,** Plasma AVP (pAVP) and osmolality (pOsm) responses to hypertonic (855 mmol/L) saline infusion. **B,** pAVP and urine osmolality (uOsm) responses to a period of fluid restriction in the same group of patients. *Shaded areas,* Range of the normal response. ○ and ●, Patients with hypothalamic diabetes insipidus (HDI); ■, patients with nephrogenic diabetes insipidus (NDI); ▲, patients with dipsogenic diabetes insipidus (DDI).

Imaging of the pituitary gland and the surrounding structures is mandatory in all patients with HDI. MRI is the method of choice. Imaging may demonstrate an associated structural lesion due to tumor or inflammation. Alternatively, evidence may be found of associated developmental anomaly. The posterior pituitary has as a characteristic bright signal on T_1-weighted MRI (T_1-MRI). The signal-intensity ratio of posterior lobe to pons correlates strongly with AVP content, and the majority of patients with HDI lose the normal signal seen on T_1-MRI (Fig. 30-12).[148] The posterior lobe signal also is diminished in the elderly, in patients with anorexia nervosa, in septic shock, in poorly controlled diabetes mellitus, and in those undergoing hemodialysis. It is thought that this may represent persistent hypersecretion and thus decreased VP-NPII complex content. Noninvasive dynamic MRI after contrast injection can identify abnormalities in posterior pituitary blood supply in patients with isolated HDI.[124] In the absence of other causal factors, this technique may have a role in diagnosing occult vasculopathy.

Other tests of pituitary function should be performed in patients diagnosed with HDI. Those diagnosed with NDI should have urine microscopy, renal tract ultrasound (to exclude obstruction), and tests of other aspects of tubular function. Debate is ongoing as to the merits of renal biopsy if creatinine clearance is normal. Genetic studies in cases of suspected familial disease remain research based, although the next 10 years is likely to see them move into the clinical service arena.

Treatment of Diabetes Insipidus

The polyuria of severe HDI is a great inconvenience and may lead to secondary renal tract problems of bladder distension, hydroureter, hydronephrosis, and secondary NDI. The treatment of choice for these patients is DDAVP, a synthetic, long-acting VP analogue that possesses minimal pressor activity and has twice the antidiuretic potency of AVP.[149] It can be administered as an intranasal spray (5 to 100 μg daily), parenterally (0.5 to 2.0 μg daily), or orally in the dose range from

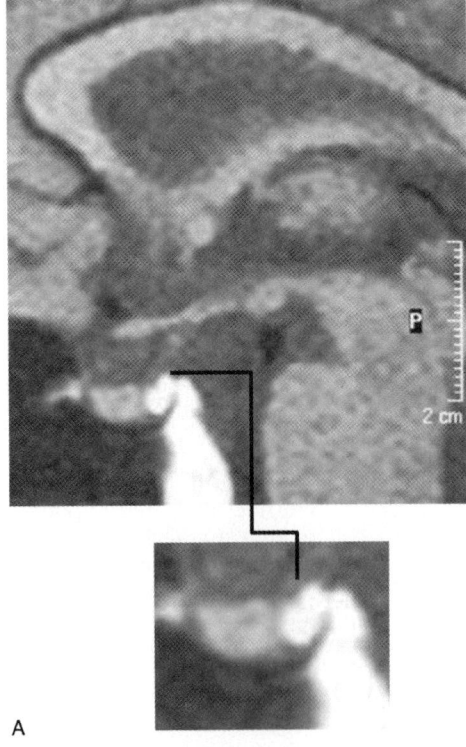
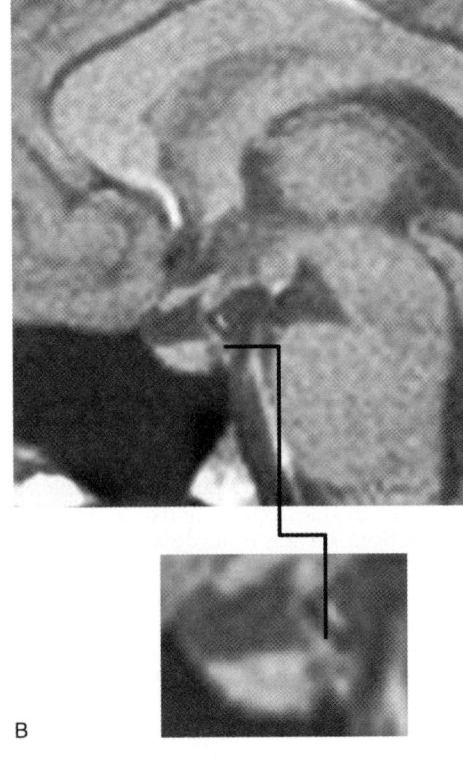

Figure 30-12 Magnetic resonance imaging (MRI) appearances of the posterior pituitary in hypothalamic diabetes insipidus (HDI). **A,** The normal posterior pituitary appears as a high-signal-intensity bright spot posterior in the pituitary fossa on T_1-weighted MRI. **B,** HDI is associated with loss of this high-signal-intensity bright spot.

100 to 1800 µg/day in divided doses. The individual variation in the dose required to control symptoms is considerable. To avoid the potential complication of dilutional hyponatremia, patients can be advised to omit DDAVP for a short period at regular intervals, perhaps once weekly, to allow breakthrough polyuria. If standard doses prove too potent, intranasal DDAVP spray can be diluted to 2.5 to 5.0 µg per activation. Patients with mild forms of HDI (urine volume, <4 L per 24 hours) can be managed with adequate fluids to quench thirst. It is important to monitor plasma electrolytes at regular intervals after the introduction of treatment. Any evidence of a decrease in plasma sodium concentration should trigger review of the patient and therapy.

NDI due to an acquired metabolic problem (hypokalemia or hypercalcemia, lithium toxicity) is best managed by addressing the underlying cause and maintaining adequate hydration while function recovers. For those patients with congenital NDI or in whom the acquired defect is irreversible, a number of additional measures can be introduced. However, these rarely reduce urine volumes by more than 50%. Nevertheless, this can lead to a significant improvement in quality of life. As many cases of acquired NDI are partial, with some nephrons retaining a degree of responsiveness to AVP, high-dose DDAVP (4 µg IM, b.i.d.) can reduce urine output. Further measures, which can be tried serially or in combination, include thiazide diuretics (hydrochlorothiazide, 25 mg/24 hours); nonsteroidal anti-inflammatories (ibuprofen, 200 mg/24 hours); and dietary salt restriction. All probably work through a combination of reducing glomerular filtration rate and interference with the diluting capacity of the distal nephron.

As with other causes of DI, the approach to DDI should try to address the underlying cause. This may be difficult. Switching treatment to alternative agents may help those patients with chronic schizophrenia and a history of hyponatremia. Individuals with persistent DDI are at risk of hyponatremia if treated with DDAVP. Reduction in fluid intake is the only rational treatment.

SYNDROME OF INAPPROPRIATE ANTIDIURESIS

HYPONATREMIA

Hyponatremia, defined as a serum sodium level less than 130 mmol/L, is a common electrolyte disorder, occurring in about 15% of hospitalized patients.[150] A pragmatic classification is given in Table 30-6. Clinical features of hyponatremia (Table 30-7) develop as serum sodium decreases slowly to less than 120 mmol/L or if a very rapid decrease occurs in serum sodium.[151–153] Values of serum sodium around 100 mmol/L are life threatening. However, many patients appear asymptomatic. This may reflect the chronicity of the condition together with appropriate physiologic adaptation or our inability to detect subtle alterations in higher function in this context. Hyponatremia is not associated invariably with reduced plasma osmolality. High concentrations of other osmolytes (commonly glucose) can result in hyponatremia but normal plasma osmolality. Hyponatremia from a reduction in the aqueous phase of plasma is rarely a problem with most up-to-date clinical biochemistry autoanalyzers.

DIAGNOSIS OF SYNDROME OF INAPPROPRIATE ANTIDIURESIS

The actions of AVP make inappropriate production of the hormone a prime candidate as a mediator of pathophysiologic hyponatremia. However, it is important to recognize that AVP production in the face of concurrent hyponatremia is not always inappropriate. During intravascular volume depletion, baroregulated AVP production may persist at plasma sodium levels significantly below the osmolar threshold. Hyponatremia

Table 30-6	Classification of Hyponatremia	
PSEUDOHYPONATREMIA		
Hyperglycemia		
Hyperlipidemia		
Nonphysiologic osmolyte		
SODIUM DEPLETION		
Renal loss (urine sodium > 20 mmol/L)		Diuretics
		Salt-wasting nephropathy
		Hypoadrenalism
		Central salt wasting
Extrarenal loss (urine sodium < 10 mmol/L)		Gut loss
		Burns
EXCESS WATER INTAKE		
Dipsogenic diabetes insipidus		
Sodium-free, hyposmolar irrigant solutions		
Dilute infant-feeding formula		
REDUCED RENAL FREE WATER CLEARANCE		
Hypovolemia		
Cardiac failure		
Nephrotic syndrome		
Hypothyroidism		
Hypoadrenalism		
Syndrome of inappropriate antidiuresis (urine sodium >20 mmol/L)		
Drugs		
Renal failure		
Portal hypertension and ascites		
Hypoalbuminaemia		
Sepsis and vascular leak syndromes		
Fluid sequestration		

may result, which can become chronic. However, the AVP production is not inappropriate. Although clinical assessment identifies the volume status of many patients, problems can arise in distinguishing mild forms of hypovolemia from euvolemia, and in assessing the relative size of the vascular component in clinical situations of extracellular volume expansion. Criteria for attributing hyponatremia to a syndrome of inappropriate antidiuresis (SIAD) secondary to inappropriate AVP production were defined by Bartter and Schwartz in 1967 (Table 30-8).[154] Most hyponatremic patients have detectable or elevated plasma AVP concentrations, and their urine osmolality tends to be higher than their plasma osmolality.[155,156] Neither is therefore diagnostic of SIAD. Measurement of urinary sodium concentration aids classification (see Table 30-6). Increased urinary excretion of AQP2 can be used as a surrogate marker of exaggerated AVP-dependent antidiuresis.[157]

ETIOLOGY OF SIAD

Many conditions are associated with SIAD. The mechanisms underlying the syndrome are not clear in all cases (Table 30-9). SIAD is a nonmetastatic manifestation of small cell cancer of

Table 30-7	Clinical Features of Hyponatremia Secondary to Syndrome of Antidiuresis
Anorexia	
Headache	
Nausea	
Vomiting	
Muscle cramps	
Lethargy	
Disorientation	
Ataxia	
Ileus	
Seizure	
Coma	
Osmotic demyelination	
Brain stem herniation	

Table 30-8 Diagnostic Criteria for Syndrome of Inappropriate Diuresis

Hyponatremia with appropriately low plasma osmolality
Urine osmolality greater than plasma osmolality
Renal sodium excretion, >20 mmol/L
Absence of hypotension, hypovolemia, and edema-forming states
Normal renal and adrenal function

the bronchus (SCC). AVP has been demonstrated in tumor extracts, and synthesis of AVP by SCC tissue has been demonstrated in vitro.[158] However, not all patients with SIAD associated with neoplastic disease have ectopic VP production. Inappropriate, excessive AVP secretion from the posterior pituitary has been demonstrated in this situation.[159] Interestingly, ectopic tumor production of VP does not always result in SIAD. Abnormal forms of AVP, with altered bioactivity, are secreted by some tumors, whereas others have been shown to synthesize AVP ectopically, but SIAD does not result.

PATHOPHYSIOLOGY OF SIAD

In most cases of SIAD, failure to suppress AVP secretion maximally occurs as plasma osmolality decreases below the theoretical osmotic threshold for AVP release. Thus, AVP continues to circulate at concentrations that are inappropriately high in relation to osmolar status, although the absolute AVP values may not be particularly elevated. For reasons not well understood, patients continue to drink. This, combined with the persistent antidiuresis due to circulating AVP, leads to dilutional hyponatremia.[160] Investigation of osmoregulated AVP secretion in a large group of patients fulfilling the SIAD criteria laid down by Bartter and Schwartz, and who had a variety of underlying disorders, revealed four distinct patterns of AVP release (Fig. 30-13).[159]

The first pattern (type A) is characterized by wide fluctuations in plasma AVP concentration that occur at random and bear no relation to changes in plasma osmolality. Such erratic release could be accounted for by ectopic secretion from neoplastic tissue. However, similar patterns occur in SIAD associated with nonneoplastic disease, suggesting a lesion in the posterior pituitary or the afferent pathways regulating VP release. The type A subtype accounts for about 35% of cases of SIAD.

A second group (type B), accounting for one third of cases, demonstrates resetting of the osmostat to the left of normal. In these patients, plasma AVP is responsive to changes in plasma osmolality, but the threshold for AVP release is subnormal. Such patients retain the ability to osmoregulate water excretion and to dilute and concentrate urine, but this occurs around a plasma osmolar set point that is lower than normal. Again, this pattern of AVP release is associated with both neoplastic and nonneoplastic disease. Because similar shifts to the left of normal are observed in hypovolemia and hypotension, one suspected cause is a lesion in the afferent baroregulatory pathways.

In type C SIAD, AVP secretion cannot be entirely suppressed, and constitutive low-level VP release at low plasma osmolality is present. However, in contrast to type B, increasing plasma osmolality results in a normal plasma VP response. Patients with type D SIAD, which accounts for fewer than 10% of cases, have entirely normal osmoregulated AVP secretion. Nevertheless, the patients fulfill the criteria of Bartter and Schwartz: They fail to excrete a water load and cannot maximally dilute urine. It is not known whether this subtype is due to an increase in renal sensitivity to low concentrations of AVP or to the action of another antidiuretic factor.

TREATMENT OF SIAD

Patients with chronic SIAD who have plasma sodium concentrations greater than 125 mmol/L rarely have significant symptoms from hyponatremia itself and may not require specific treatment. With more severe degrees of hyponatremia, some form of therapy may be required.

Table 30-9 Causes of Syndrome of Inappropriate Diuresis

NEOPLASTIC DISEASE	Empyema
Carcinoma (bronchus, duodenum, pancreas, bladder, ureter, prostate)	Cystic fibrosis
	Pneumothorax
	Aspergillosis
Thymoma	
Mesothelioma	**DRUGS**
Lymphoma, Leukemia	Sulphonylureas
Ewing's sarcoma	Opiates
Carcinoid	Alkylating agents and Vinca alkaloids
Bronchial adenoma	Thiazides and loop diuretics
NEUROLOGIC DISORDERS	Dopamine antagonists
Head injury, neurosurgery	Tricyclic antidepressants
Brain abscess or tumor	Monoamine oxidase inhibitors
Meningitis, encephalitis	Selective serotonin reuptake inhibitors
Guillain-Barré syndrome	
Cerebral hemorrhage	3,4-MDMA ("Ecstasy")
Cavernous sinus thrombosis	Anticonvulsants
Hydrocephalus	**MISCELLANEOUS**
Cerebellar and cerebral atrophy	Idiopathic
Shy-Drager syndrome	Psychosis
Peripheral neuropathy	Porphyria
Seizures	Abdominal surgery
Subdural hematoma	
Alcohol withdrawal	
CHEST DISORDERS	
Pneumonia	
Tuberculosis	

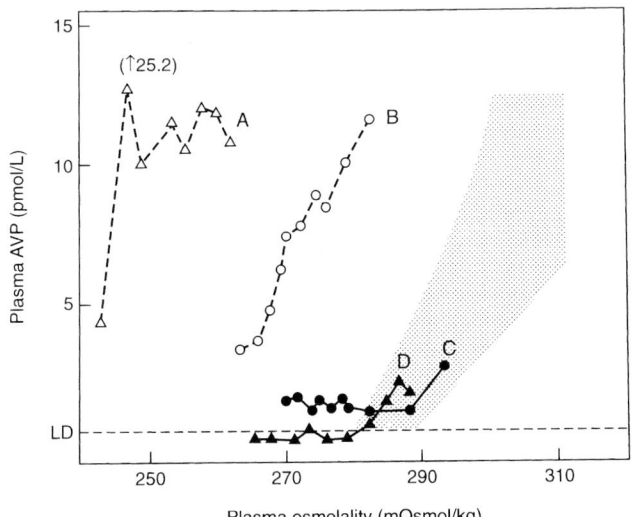

Figure 30-13 Plasma arginine vasopressin (AVP) response to infusion of hypertonic (855 mmol/L) saline in patients with syndrome of inappropriate antidiuresis (SIAD). *A,* SIAD type A, demonstrating erratic release of AVP independent of plasma osmolality. *B,* SIAD type B, demonstrating a reset osmolar threshold but normal sensitivity. *C,* SIAD type C, demonstrating inability to switch off AVP production at low plasma osmolalities. *D,* Normal individual.

Adequate treatment directed toward the underlying cause of SIAD is most appropriate, but if this fails, and the patient has mild to moderate symptoms, total fluid intake should be restricted to 500 mL per 24 hours, with the intention of increasing serum sodium levels slowly to no higher than 125 to 130 mmol/L.[153,161–163] Because fluid restriction can be distressing, particularly when it is prolonged, additional drug therapy may be required to manage chronic SIAD. The antidiuretic action of AVP can be blocked by demeclocycline (600 to 1200 mg daily) or the less reliable and more toxic lithium carbonate (600 to 1800 mg daily).[164] The NDI induced by these drugs may take up to 6 weeks to develop fully. An alternative therapeutic approach is the administration of oral furosemide (40 to 80 mg daily) together with salt supplementation (3 g daily).[165]

The development of specific peptide and nonpeptide V_2-R antagonists that act to increase renal solute-free water excretion without effects on renal salt excretion (aquaretics) constitutes an alternative approach to the management of SIAD. Although their efficacy has been confirmed in animals, peptide antagonists have failed to fulfill their potential in humans.[166] SIAD patients treated with a nonpeptide antagonist have shown substantial improvement in their degree of hyponatremia.[167,168] Nonpeptide aquaretics also may have an important role in the management of hyponatremia associated with chronic liver disease and congestive cardiac failure.[169]

The neurologic manifestations of hyponatremia are dependent on a number of factors: the degree of hyponatremia; the speed of onset and duration of the disturbance; and individual patient characteristics. When hyponatremia is chronic or has developed slowly or both, brain cell edema is limited by the efflux of organic solutes. This limited adaptive process is not apparent in acute hyponatremia. However, the adaptive processes limiting brain swelling in chronic hyponatremia can complicate corrective treatment. Rapid correction of hyponatremia when CNS adaptation has occurred can lead to changes in neuronal volume that trigger demyelination (osmotic demyelination).[170,171] This serious neurologic complication can occur within 1 to 4 days of correction of plasma sodium. Clinical manifestations are dominated by brain stem features and include quadriplegia, ophthalmoplegia, pseudobulbar palsy, and coma. Diagnosis is made in the context of an appropriate history and signs and confirmed by MRI. Risk factors for the development of osmotic demyelination include the rate and magnitude of increase in plasma sodium (although it can occur when hyponatremia is corrected more slowly), concurrent hypokalemia, poor nutritional status before the development of hyponatremia, and alcohol-related liver dysfunction.[172]

The management of both significant chronic hyponatremia (plasma sodium <110 mmol/L) and acute hyponatremia associated with life-threatening neurologic signs is thus a dilemma. Conservative management with fluid restriction may prolong the period of exposure to a dangerous internal environment. Aggressive management to correct the disturbance in electrolytes risks iatrogenic problems. No consensus exists on the optimal approach.[150] However, SIAD-induced hyponatremia associated with severe symptoms, especially if it has occurred rapidly (which is relatively unusual), may benefit from treatment with hypertonic fluids. A number of models exist for quantifying both the degree of water excess and the solute requirement for correction of hyponatremia in this clinical situation. However, all have flaws.[173] Moreover, given the potential complications of treatment, the preferred target should be a plasma sodium that reverses life-threatening complications of hyponatremia, rather than one that is normal. Plasma sodium should increase by no more than 1 to 2 mmol/hour, and by no more than 10 mmol/24 hours. Hypertonic fluids can be stopped when life-threatening complications of hyponatremia (e.g., seizures) are no longer apparent; non-life-threatening manifestations have been modified; or when plasma sodium concentration is greater than 125 mmol/L.

ADIPSIA AND HYPODIPSIA

Adipsic and hypodipsic syndromes are characterized by inadequate spontaneous fluid intake due to abnormalities in osmoregulated thirst. They are uncommon. Patients deny thirst and do not drink. If the defect is mild or partial, the resultant dehydration, hypernatremia, and volume depletion is well tolerated. More severe disorders can lead to profound hypernatremia, seizures, and coma. Because of the close functional and anatomic relation between the centers involved in both processes, abnormalities of thirst are commonly associated with disturbances in osmoregulated AVP release. Nonosmotic AVP production can be normal.[174]

ETIOLOGY OF ADIPSIA AND HYPODIPSIA

Thirst-deficiency syndromes develop as a result of a variety of pathologic processes involving the putative thirst osmoreceptor cells in the anterior circumventricular organs of the hypothalamus or their neuronal connections. Table 30-10 lists the specific diseases recognized to cause hypodipsic or adipsic hypernatremia.[153,175] The regions of the hypothalamus containing the osmoreceptors regulating both thirst and AVP release receive an arterial blood supply from perforating branches of the anterior cerebral artery (ACA). Rupture or repair or both of the ACA aneurysm can thus lead to combined adipsic HDI (ADI). Vascular causes account for some 15% of ADI.[176] Tumors and granulomatous disease make up the majority of other etiologies.

PATHOPHYSIOLOGY OF ADIPSIA AND HYPODIPSIA

Four patterns of adipsia/hypodipsia syndrome are recognized, differentiated by characteristic differences in thirst and associated AVP production.[143] Appropriate classification can be important, as important differences exist in natural history and management.

Patients with ADI type A (also known as essential hypernatremia) have a supranormal set point for both osmoregulated thirst and VP release. Sensitivities of both processes to changes in osmolar status are normal. Patients thus

Table 30-10 Causes of Adipsic and Hypodipsic Syndromes

NEOPLASTIC (50%)
Primary
  Craniopharyngioma
  Pinealoma
  Meningioma
Secondary
  Pituitary tumor
  Bronchial carcinoma
  Breast carcinoma

GRANULOMATOUS (20%)
Histiocytosis
Sarcoidosis

MISCELLANEOUS (15%)
Hydrocephalus
Ventricular cyst
Trauma
Toluene poisoning

VASCULAR (15%)
Internal carotid artery ligation
Anterior communicating artery aneurysm
Intrahypothalamic hemorrhage

osmoregulate around a higher set point but do not experience extreme hypernatremia. Nonosmotic AVP production is normal. Patients with ADI type B have normal osmotic thresholds for thirst and VP production, but the sensitivities of both processes are reduced. Nonosmotic AVP production is normal. As with the type A syndrome, patients are relatively protected from extreme hypernatremia. Patients with ADI type C have no thirst response to osmotic stimulation, and persistent constitutive low-level AVP release that is not responsive to osmotic stimuli. Nonosmotic AVP production can be normal. Patients generally are first seen with HDI, hypernatremia, and dehydration. However, patients with ADI type C are at risk of both severe hyper- and hyponatremia, as they can neither drink or produce AVP in response to an osmolar stimulus nor completely switch off AVP production in response to significant fluid loads. ADI type D is characterized by absent osmoregulated thirst but normal osmoregulated AVP production.[177]

MANAGEMENT OF ADIPSIA AND HYPODIPSIA

Hypodipsic patients, such as those with ADI type A and type B, rarely develop life-threatening hypernatremia because thirst develops when plasma osmolality levels increase sufficiently. Patients are thus recommended to maintain an obligate fluid intake of some 2 L/24 hours, adjusted for climate and season. Sometimes adequate fluid balance cannot be maintained during intercurrent illness, and patients may require supervised fluid therapy in a hospital setting.

Adipsia with absent osmoregulated AVP secretion (ADI type C) presents a major management problem, and these patients run the risk of profound hypernatremia. Management can be complicated by short-term memory impairment and deficits in functional task organization due to concurrent temporal lobe syndromes that are a consequence of the original lesion (such as ACA aneurysm and repair). One pragmatic approach is to determine a convenient antidiuresis with a fixed dose of DDAVP (1 to 2 L/24 hours) and to vary daily fluid intake as dictated by day-to-day fluctuation in body weight in relation to a target weight at which the patient is normonatremic and euvolemic. Frequent intermittent checks of plasma electrolytes are essential to avoid extreme fluctuations in serum sodium levels.[178] This approach can result in stable fluid balance and independent living, although wide swings from hypernatremia to hyponatremia can still occur.

REFERENCES

1. Oliver G, Schäfer EA: On the physiological actions of the pituitary body and certain other glands. J Physiol 18:277–279, 1895.
2. Howell TH: The physiological effects of extracts of the hypophysis cerebri and infundibular body. J Exp Med 3:245–248, 1898.
3. Schäfer EA: The functions of the pituitary body. Proc R Soc 81(series B):442–468, 1909.
4. Farini F: Diabete insipido ed opoterapia ipofisaria. Gazz Osp Clin 34:1135–1139, 1913.
5. von den Velden RL: Die Nierenwirkung von Hypophysenextrakten beim Menschen. Berl Klin Wochenschr 50:2083–2086, 1913.
6. Verney EB: The antidiuretic hormone and the factors which determine its release. Proc R Soc London 135(series B):25–105, 1947.
7. du Vigneaud V, Gish DT, Katsoyannis PG: A synthetic preparation possessing biological properties associated with arginine-vasopressin. J Am Chem Soc 76:4751–4752, 1954.
8. Land H, Schultz G, Schmale H, Richter D: Nucleotide sequence of cloned cDNA encoding for bovine arginine vasopressin-neurophysin II precursor. Nature 295:299–303, 1982.
9. Zimmerman EA, Nilaver G, Hou-yu A, Silverman AJ: Vasopressinergic and oxytocinergic pathways in the central nervous system. Fed Proc 43:91–96, 1984.
10. Itoi K, Jiang Y-Q, Iwasaki Y, et al: Regulatory mechanisms of corticotrophin-releasing hormone and vasopressin gene expression in the hypothalamus. J Neuroendocrinol 16:348–355, 2004.
11. Sofroniew MV: Projections from vasopressin, oxytocin and neurophysin neurons to neural targets in the rat and human. J Histochem Cytochem 28:475–478, 1980.
12. Rasmussen AT: The weight of the principal components of the normal male adult human hypophysis cerebri. Am J Anat 42:1–27, 1928.
13. Schally AV: Hormones of the neurohypophysis. In Lock W, Schally AV (eds): The Hypothalamus and Pituitary in Health and Disease. Springfield, IL, Charles C Thomas, 1972, pp 154–171.
14. Schally AV, Bowers CY, Kuroshima A, et al: Effect of lysine vasopressin dimers on blood pressure and some endocrine functions. Am J Physiol 207:378–384, 1964.
15. Acher R: Chemistry of the neurohypophysial hormones: An example of molecular evolution. In Knobil E, Sawyer WH (eds): Handbook of Physiology, section 7: Endocrinology, vol 4, pt 1. Washington, DC, American Physiological Society, 1974, pp 119–130.
16. Acher R, Chauvet J: Structure, processing and evolution of the neurohypophyseal, hormone-neurophysin precursors. Biochemie 70:1197–1207, 1988.
17. Mohr E, Schmitz E, Richter D: A single rat genomic cDNA fragment encodes both the oxytocin and vasopressin genes separated by 11 kilobases and orientated in opposite transcriptional directions. Biochemie 70:649–654, 1988.
18. Murphy D, Wells S: In vivo gene transfer studies on the regulation and function of the vasopressin and oxytocin genes. J Neuroendocrinol 15:109–125, 2003.
19. Fields RL, House SB, Gainer H: Regulatory domains in the intergenic region of the oxytocin and vasopressin genes that control their hypothalamus-specific expression in vitro. J Neurosci 23:7801–7809, 2003.
20. Zingg HH, Lefebvre DL: Oxytocin and vasopressin gene expression during gestation and lactation. Mol Brain Res 4:1–6, 1988.
21. Somponpun SJ, Sladek CD: Osmotic regulation of estrogen receptor-beta in rat vasopressin and oxytocin neurons. J Neurosci 23:4261–4269, 2003.
22. Murphy D, Levy A, Lightman S, Carter D: Vasopressin RNA in the neural lobe of the pituitary: Dramatic accumulation in response to salt loading. Proc Natl Acad Sci U S A 86:9002–9005, 1989.
23. Carter DA, Murphy D: Rapid changes in poly(A) tail length of vasopressin and oxytocin mRNAs from common early components of neurohypophyseal peptide gene activation following physiological stimulation. Neuroendocrinology 5:1–6, 1991.
24. Mohr E, Kachele I, Mullin C, et al: Rat vasopressin mRNA: A model system to characterize cis-acting elements and trans-acting factors in dendritic mRNA sorting. Prog Brain Res 139:211–224, 2002.
25. Mohr E, Richter D: Subcellular vasopressin mRNA trafficking and local translation in dendrites. J Neuroendocrinol 16:333–339, 2004.
26. Russell JT, Brownstein MJ, Gainer H: Biosynthesis of vasopressin, oxytocin and neurophysins: Isolation and characterization of two common precursors (propressophysin and prooxyphysin). Endocrinology 107:1880–1891, 1980.
27. Dutton A, Dyball REJ: Phasic firing enhances vasopressin release from the rat neurohypophysis. J Physiol 290:433–440, 1979.
28. Nordmann JJ, Labouesse J: Neurosecretory granules: Evidence for an aging process within the neurohypophysis. Science 211:595–597, 1981.
29. Yoshida M, Iwasaki Y, Asai M, et al: Gene therapy for central diabetes insipidus: Effective antidiuresis by

muscle-targeted gene transfer. Endocrinology 145:261–268, 2004.

30. Ludwig M, Sabatier N, Dayanilhi G, et al: The active role of dendrites in the regulation of magnocellular neurosecretory cell behavior. Prog Brain Res 139:247–256, 2002.

31. Lauson HD: Metabolism of neurohypophysial hormones. In Knobil E, Sawyer WH (eds): Handbook of Physiology, section 7: Endocrinology, vol 4, pt 1. Washington, DC, American Physiological Society, 1974, pp 287–393.

32. Bichet DG, Arthus M-F, Barjon JN, et al: Human platelet fraction arginine-vasopressin: Potential physiological role. J Clin Invest 79:881–887, 1987.

33. Zing HH: Vasopressin and oxytocin receptors. Baillieres Clin Endocrinol Metab 10:75–96, 1996.

34. Birnbaumer M: Vasopressin receptors. Trends Endocrinol Metab 11:406–410, 2000.

35. King LS, Yasui M: Aquaporins and disease: Lessons from mice to humans. Trends Endocrinol Metab 13:355–360, 2002.

36. Verkman AS: Physiological importance of aquaporin water channels. Ann Med 34:192–200, 2002.

37. Marples D: Water channels: Who needs them anyway? Lancet 355:1571–1572, 2000.

38. King LS, Choi M, Fernandez PC, et al: Defective urinary concentrating ability due to a complete deficiency of aquaporin-1. N Engl J Med 345:175–179, 2001.

39. Ishikawa S, Saito K, Kasono K: Pathological role of aquaporin-2 in impaired water excretion and hyponatraemia. J Neuroendocrinol 16:293–296, 2004.

40. Nielson S, Knepper MA: Vasopressin activates collecting duct urea transporters and water channels by distinct physical processes. Am J Physiol 265:F204–F213, 1993.

41. Knepper MA, Sands JM, Chou CL: Independence of water and urea transport in the rat inner medullary collecting duct. Am J Physiol 256:F610–F621, 1989.

42. Imbert-Teboul M, Chabardes D, Montegut M, et al: Vasopressin-dependent adenylate cyclase activities in the rat kidney medulla: Evidence for two separate sites of action. Endocrinology 102:1254–1261, 1978.

43. Wittner M, Di Stefano A, Wangemann P, et al: Differential effects of ADH on sodium, chloride, potassium, calcium and magnesium transport in cortical and medullary thick ascending limbs of mouse nephron. Pflugers Arch 412:516–523, 1988.

44. Hebert SC, Culpepper RM, Andreoli TE: NaCl transport in mouse medullary thick ascending limbs, I: Functional nephron heterogeneity and ADH-stimulated NaCl cotransport. Am J Physiol 241:412–431, 1981.

45. Montani JP, Liard JF, Schoun J, Mohring J: Hemodynamic effects of exogenous and endogenous vasopressin at low plasma concentrations in conscious dogs. Circ Res 47:346–355, 1980.

46. Altura BM, Altura BT: Actions of vasopressin, oxytocin, and synthetic analogs on vascular smooth muscle. Fed Proc 43:80–86, 1984.

47. Aisenbrey GA, Handelman WA, Arnold P, et al: Vascular effects of arginine vasopressin during fluid deprivation. J Clin Invest 67:961–968, 1981.

48. Liard J-F: Acute hemodynamic effects of antidiuretic agents. In Cowley AW, Liard J-F, Ausiello DA (eds): Vasopressin: Cellular and Integrative Functions. New York, Raven Press, 1988, pp 461–466.

49. Johnson MD, Park CS, Malvin RL: Antidiuretic hormone and the distribution of renal cortical blood flow. Am J Physiol 232:F111–F116, 1977.

50. Liard J-F: Vasopressin reduces oxygen uptake in intact dogs but not in sinoaortic denervated dogs. Am J Physiol 257:R1–R9, 1989.

51. Du Pasquier D, Loup F, Dubois-Dauphin M, et al: Binding sites for vasopressin in the human pituitary are associated with corticotrophs and may differ from other known vasopressin receptors. J Neuroendocrinol 3:237–247, 1991.

52. Sawchenko PE, Swanson LW, Vale WW: Co-expression of corticotrophin-releasing factor and vasopressin immunoreactivity in parvocellular neurosecretory neurons of the adrenalectomized rat. Proc Natl Acad Sci USA 81:1877–1883, 1984.

53. Baldino F, Davis LG: Glucocorticoid regulation of vasopressin messenger RNA. In Uhl GR (ed): In Situ Hybridization in the Brain. New York, Plenum Press, 1986, p 97.

54. Young LJ, Nilsen R, Waymire KG, et al: Increased affiliative response to vasopressin in mice expressing the V1a receptor from a monogamous vole. Nature 400:766–768, 1999.

55. Bielsky IF, Hu S-B, Szegda KL, et al: Profound impairment in social recognition and reduction in anxiety-like behaviour in vasopressin V1a receptor knockout mice. Neuropsychopharmacology 29:483–493, 2004.

56. Mannucci PM, Ruggeri ZM, Pareti FI, Capitanio A: DDAVP: A new pharmacological approach to the management of hemophilia and von Willebrand disease. Lancet 1:869–872, 1977.

57. Hashemi S, Tackaberry ES, Palmer DS, et al: DDAVP induced release of von Willebrand factor from endothelial cells in vitro: The effect of plasma and red cells. Biochim Biophys Acta 1052:63–70, 1990.

58. Mannucci PM, Federici AB: Release of factor VIII and von Willebrand factor by vasopressin and derivatives. In Jard S, Jamison R (eds): Vasopressin. Montrouge. France, John Libbey, 1991, pp 331–337.

59. Pivonello R, Colao A, di Somma C, et al: Impairment of bone status in patients with central diabetes insipidus. J Clin Endocrinol 83:2275–2280, 1998.

60. Hems DA, Rodrigues LM, Whitton PD: Rapid stimulation by vasopressin, oxytocin and angiotensin II of glycogen degradation in hepatocyte suspensions. Biochem J 172:311–312, 1978.

61. Spruce BA, McCulloch AJ, Burd J, et al: The effect of vasopressin infusion on glucose metabolism in man. Clin Endocrinol 22:463–468, 1985.

62. Pittman QJ, Landgraf R: Vasopressin in thermoregulation and blood pressure control. In Jard S, Jamison R (eds): Vasopressin. Montrouge. France, John Libbey, 1991, pp 177–184.

64. Ferris CF, Singer EA, Meenan DM, Albers HE: Inhibition of vasopressin-stimulated flank marking behaviour by V1-receptor antagonists. Eur J Pharmacol 154:153–159, 1988.

65. Sangal A, Keith AB, Wright C, Edwardson JA: Failure of vasopressin to enhance memory in a passive avoidance task in rats. Neurosci Lett 28:87–92, 1982.

66. Robertson GL, Shelton RL, Athar S: The osmoregulation of vasopressin. Kidney Int 10:25–37, 1976.

67. Hammer M, Ladefoged J, Olgaard K: Relationship between plasma osmolality and plasma vasopressin in human subjects. Am J Physiol 238:E313–E317, 1980.

68. Baylis PH, Thompson CJ: Osmoregulation of vasopressin secretion and thirst in health and disease. Clin Endocrinol 29:549–576, 1988.

69. Baylis PH, Gill GV: Investigation of polyuria. Clin Endocrinol Metab 13:295–310, 1984.

70. Moses AM, Miller M: Osmotic threshold for vasopressin release as determined by hypertonic saline infusion and dehydration. Neuroendocrinology 7:219–226, 1971.

71. Baylis PH, Pippard C, Gill GV, Burd J: Development of a cytochemical assay for plasma vasopressin: Application to studies on water loading normal man. Clin Endocrinol 24:383–392, 1986.

72. Robertson GL: Physiology of ADH secretion. Kidney Int 32(Suppl 21):S20–S26, 1987.

73. Thompson CJ, Selby P, Baylis PH: Reproducibility of osmotic and non-osmotic tests of vasopressin secretion in man. Am J Physiol 60:R533–R539, 1991.

74. Zerbe RL: Genetic factors in normal and abnormal regulation of vasopressin secretion. In Schrier RW (ed): Vasopressin. New York, Raven Press, 1985, pp 213–220.

75. Desai M, Guerra C, Wang S, Ross MG: Programming of hypertonicity in neonatal lambs: Resetting of the threshold for vasopressin secretion. Endocrinology 144:4332–4337, 2003.

76. Durr JA, Stamoutsos BA, Lindheimer MD: Osmoregulation during pregnancy in the rat: Evidence for resetting of the threshold for vasopressin secretion during gestation. J Clin Invest 68:337–346, 1981.

77. Davison JM, Gilmore EA, Durr J, et al: Altered threshold for vasopressin secretion and thirst in human pregnancy. Am J Physiol 246:F105–F109, 1984.

78. Spruce BA, Baylis PH, Burd J, Watson MJ: Variation in osmoregulation of arginine vasopressin during the human menstrual cycle. Clin Endocrinol 22:37–42, 1985.

79. Evbuomwan IO, Davison JM, Baylis PH, Murdoch A: Altered osmotic thresholds for arginine vasopressin secretion and thirst during superovulation and in the ovarian hyperstimulation syndrome (OHSS): Relevance to the pathophysiology of OHSS. Fertil Steril 75:933–941, 2001.

80. Miller M: Fluid and electrolyte homeostasis in the elderly: Physiological changes of ageing and clinical consequences. Baillieres Clin Endocrinol Metab 11:367–387, 1997.

81. Johnson AG, Crawford GA, Kelly D: Arginine vasopressin and osmolality in the elderly. J Am Geriatr Soc 42:399–404, 1994.

82. Helderman JH, Vestal RE, Rowe JW, et al: The response of arginine vasopressin to intravenous alcohol and hypertonic saline in man: The impact of ageing. J Gerontol 33:39–47, 1978.

83. Phillips PA, Rolls BJ, Ledingham JGG: Reduced thirst after water deprivation in healthy elderly men. N Engl J Med 311:753–759, 1984.

84. Crowe MJ, Forsling ML, Rolls BJ: Altered water excretion in healthy elderly men. Age Ageing 16:285–293, 1987.

85. Lewis WH, Alving AS: Changes with age in the renal function in adult men. Am J Physiol 123:500–515, 1938.

86. Zerbe RL, Robertson GL: Osmoregulation of thirst and vasopressin secretion in human subjects: Effect of various solutes. Am J Physiol 244:E607–E614, 1983.

87. Vokes TP, Aycinena PR, Robertson GL: Effect of insulin on osmoregulation of vasopressin. Am J Physiol 252:E538–E548, 1987.

88. Eisenhofer G, Johnson RH: Effect of ethanol ingestion on plasma vasopressin and water balance in humans. Am J Physiol 242:R522–R527, 1982.

89. Johnson JA, Zehr JE, Moore WW: Effects of separate and concurrent osmotic and volume stimuli on plasma ADH in sheep. Am J Physiol 218:1273–1280, 1970.

90. Baylis PH: Posterior pituitary function in health and disease. Clin Endocrinol Metab 12:747–770, 1983.

91. Goetz KL, Zhu JL, Leadley RJ, et al: Hemodynamic and hormonal influences on the secretion of vasopressin. In Jard S, Jamison R (eds): Vasopressin. Montrouge. France, John Libbey, 1991, pp 279–286.

92. Dunn FL, Brennan TJ, Nelson AE, Robertson GL: The role of blood osmolality and volume in regulating vasopressin secretion in the rat. J Clin Invest 52:3212–3219, 1973.

93. Goldsmith SR, Dodge D, Cowley AW: Nonosmotic influences on osmotic stimulation of vasopressin in humans. Am J Physiol 252:H85–H88, 1987.

94. Rowe JW, Shelton RL, Helderman JH, et al: Influence of the emetic reflex on vasopressin release in man. Kidney Int 16:729–735, 1979.

95. Verbalis JG, Richardson DW, Stricker EM: Vasopressin release in response to nausea-producing agents and cholecystokinin in monkeys. Am J Physiol 252:R749–R753, 1987.

96. Ukei M, Moran WH, Zimmerman B: The role of visceral afferent pathways on vasopressin secretion and urinary excretory patterns during surgical stress. Ann Surg 168:16–28, 1968.

97. Baylis PH, Robertson GL: Arginine vasopressin response to insulin-induced hypoglycemia in man. J Clin Endocrinol Metab 53:935–940, 1981.

98. Krigge U, Kjaer A, Kristofferson U, et al: Histamine and prostaglandin interaction in regulation of oxytocin and vasopressin secretion. J Neuroendocrinol 15:940–945, 2003.

99. McKinley MJ, Mathai M, McAllen RM et al: Vasopressin secretion: Osmotic and hormonal regulation by the lamina terminalis. J Neuroendocrinol 16:340–347, 2004.

100. Cunningham JT, Bruno SB, Grindstaff RR, et al: Cardiovascular regulation of supraoptic vasopressin neurons. Prog Brain Res 139:257–273, 2002.

101. Ishikawa S, Schrier RW: Pathophysiological roles of arginine vasopressin and aquaporin-2 in impaired water excretion. Clin Endocrinol 58:1–17, 2003.

102. Kombian SB, Hirasawa M, Mouginot D, et al: Modulation of synaptic transmission by oxytocin and vasopressin in the supraoptic nucleus. Prog Brain Res 139:235–246, 2002.

103. Ludwig M, Sabatier N, Dayanilhi G, et al: The active role of dendrites in the regulation of magnocellular neurosecretory cell behavior. Prog Brain Res 139:247–256, 2002.

104. Thrasher TN, Keil LC, Ramsay DJ: Lesions of the organum vasculosum of the lamina terminalis (OVLT) attenuate osmotically induced drinking and vasopressin secretion in the dog. Endocrinology 110:1837–1839, 1982.

105. McKinley MJ, Denton DA, Weisinger RW: Sensors for antidiuresis and thirst osmoreceptors or CSF sodium detectors? Brain Res 141:89–103, 1978.

106. Thompson CJ, Burd JM, Baylis PH: Acute suppression of plasma vasopressin and thirst after drinking in hypernatremic humans. Am J Physiol 252:R1138–R1142, 1987.

107. Andersson B, Rundgroen M: Thirst and its disorders. Annu Rev Med 33:231–239, 1982.

108. Sullivan MJ, Cunningham JT, Mazella D, et al: Lesions in the diagonal band

of Broca enhance drinking in the rat. J Neuroendocrinol 15:907–915, 2003.

109. Fitzsimons JT: The physiological basis of thirst. Kidney Int 10:3–11, 1976.

110. McKinley MJ, Denton DA, Park RG, Weisinger RS: Ablation of subforniceal organ does not prevent angiotensin-induced water drinking in sheep. Am J Physiol 250:R1052–R1059, 1986.

111. Thompson CJ, Bland J, Burd J, Baylis PH: The osmotic thresholds for thirst and vasopressin release are similar in healthy man. Clin Sci 71:651–656, 1986.

112. Thompson CJ: Polyuric states in man. In Baylis PH (ed): Water and Salt Homeostasis in Health and Disease. London, Bailliere Tindall, 1989, pp 473–497.

113. Robertson GL: Diabetes insipidus. Endocrinol Metab Clin North Am 24:549–572, 1995.

114. Baylis PH, Cheetham T: Diabetes insipidus. Arch Dis Child 79:84–89, 1998.

115. Blotner H: Primary or idiopathic diabetes insipidus: A system disease. Metabolism 7:191–206, 1958.

116. Baylis PH: Understanding the cause of idiopathic cranial diabetes insipidus: A step forward. Clin Endocrinol 40:171–172, 1994.

117. Pivoello R, De Bellis A, Faggiano A, et al: Central diabetes insipidus and autoimmunity: Relationship between the occurrence of antibodies to arginine vasopressin-secreting cells and clinical, immunological, and radiological features in a large cohort of patients with central diabetes insipidus of known and unknown etiology. J Clin Endocrinol Metab 88:1629–1636, 2003.

118. Maghnie M, Cosi G, Genovese R, et al: Central diabetes insipidus in children and young adults. N Engl J Med 343:998–1007, 2000.

119. Hollinshead WH: The interphase of diabetes insipidus. Proc Mayo Clin 39:95–100, 1964.

120. Seckl JR, Dunger DB, Bevan JS, et al. Vasopressin antagonist in early postoperative diabetes insipidus. Lancet 355:1353–1356, 1990.

121. Imura H, Nakao K, Shimatsu A, et al: Lymphocytic infundibuloneurohypophysitis as a cause of central diabetes insipidus. N Engl J Med 329:683–689, 1993.

122. Arico M, Girschikofsky M, Genereau T, et al: Langerhans cell histiocytosis in adults: Report from the International Registry of the Histiocyte Society. Eur J Cancer 39:2341–2348, 2003.

123. Jialal I, Desai K, Rajput MC: An assessment of posterior pituitary function in patients with Sheehan's syndrome. Clin Endocrinol 27:91–95, 1987.

124. Maghnie M, Altobelli M, Iorgin N-D, et al: Idiopathic central diabetes insipidus is associated with abnormal blood supply to the posterior pituitary gland caused by vascular impairment of the inferior hypophyseal artery

system. J Clin Endocrinol Metab 89:1891–1896, 2004.

125. Baylis PH, Thompson CJ, Burd JM, et al: Recurrent pregnancy-induced polyuria and thirst due to hypothalamic diabetes insipidus: An investigation into possible mechanisms responsible for polyuria. Clin Endocrinol 24:459–466, 1986.

126. Barron WM, Cohen LH, Ulland LA, et al: Transient vasopressin-resistant diabetes insipidus of pregnancy. N Engl J Med 310:442–444, 1984.

127. Moses AM, Thomas DG, Canfield MC, Collins G: Central diabetes insipidus due to cytomegalovirus infection of the hypothalamus in a patient with acquired immunodeficiency syndrome: A clinical, pathological, and immunohistochemical case study. J Clin Endocrinol Metab 88:51–54, 2003.

128. Chang M-Y, Lin J-L: Central diabetes insipidus following carbon monoxide poisoning. Am J Nephrol 21:145–149, 2001.

129. Ito M, Jameson JL, Ito M: Molecular basis of autosomal dominant neurohypophyseal diabetes insipidus: Cellular toxicity caused by the accumulation of mutant vasopressin precursors within the endoplasmic reticulum. J Clin Invest 99:2897–2905, 1997.

130. Eubank S, Nguyen TL, Deeb R, et al: Effects of diabetes insipidus mutations on neurophysin folding and function. J Biol Chem 276:29671–29680, 2001.

131. Davies J, Murphy D: Autophagy in hypothalamic neurones of rats expressing a familial neurohypophyseal diabetes insipidus transgene. J Neuroendocrinol 14:629–637, 2002.

132. Rittig S, Sigaard C, Ozata M, et al: Autosomal dominant neurohypophyseal diabetes insipidus due to substitution of histidine for tyrosine-2 in the vasopressin moiety of the hormone precursor. J Clin Endocrinol Metab 87:3351–3355, 2002.

133. Christenson JH, Sigaard C, Corydon TJ, et al: Impaired trafficking of mutated AVP prohormone in cells expressing rare disease genes causing autosomal dominant familial neurohypophyseal diabetes insipidus. Clin Endocrinol 60:125–136, 2004.

134. Elias PCL, Ellias LLK, Torres N, et al: Progressive decline of vasopressin secretion in familial autosomal dominant neurohypophyseal diabetes insipidus presenting a novel mutation in the vasopressin-neurophysin II gene. Clin Endocrinol 59:511–518, 2003.

135. Mahoney CP, Weinberger E, Bryant C, et al: Effects of aging on vasopressin production in a kindred with autosomal dominant neurohypophyseal diabetes insipidus due to a ΔE47 neurophysin mutation. J Clin Endocrinol Metab 87:870–876, 2002.

136. Schmale H, Richter D: Single base deletion in the vasopressin gene is the cause of diabetes insipidus in the Brattleboro rat. Nature 308:705–709, 1984.

137. Barrett TG, Bundey SE: Wolfram (DIDMOAD) syndrome. J Med Genet 34:838–841, 1997.

138. Cryns K, Sivakumaran TA, Van den Ouweland JMW, et al: Mutational spectrum of the WFS1 gene in Wolfram syndrome, non-syndromic hearing impairment, diabetes mellitus and psychiatric disease. Hum Mutat 22:275–287, 2003.

139. Domenecch E, Gomez-Zaera M, Nunes V: WFS1 mutations in Spanish patients with diabetes mellitus and deafness. Eur J Hum Genet 10:421–426, 2002.

140. Barbieris C, Mouillac B, Durroux T: Structural basis of vasopressin/oxytocin receptor function. J Endocrinol 156:223–229, 1998.

141. Mulders SM, Bichet DG, Rijss JPL, et al: An aquaporin-2 water channel mutant which causes autosomal dominant nephrogenic diabetes insipidus is retained in the Golgi complex. J Clin Invest 102:57–66, 1998.

142. Asai T, Kuwahara M, Kurihara H, et al: Pathogenesis of nephrogenic diabetes insipidus by aquaporin-2 C-terminus mutations. Kidney Int 64:2–10, 2003.

143. McKenna K, Thompson C: Osmoregulation in clinical disorders of thirst and thirst appreciation. Clin Endocrinol 49:139–152, 1998.

144. Zerbe RL, Robertson GL: A comparison of plasma vasopressin measurements with a standard indirect test in the differential diagnosis of polyuria. N Engl J Med 305:1539–1546, 1981.

145. Robertson GL: Diagnosis of diabetes insipidus. In Czernichow P, Robinson AG (eds): Diabetes Insipidus in Man: Frontiers of Hormone Research, vol 13. Basel, S. Karger, 1985, pp 176–189.

146. Baylis PH, Robertson GL: Vasopressin response to hypertonic saline infusion to assess posterior pituitary function. J R Soc Med 73:255–260, 1980.

147. Diedrich S, Eckmanns T, Exner P, et al: Differential diagnosis of polyuric/polydipsic syndromes with the aid of urinary vasopressin measurement in adults. Clin Endocrinol 54:665–671, 2001.

148. Fujisawa I: Magnetic resonance imaging of hypothalamic-neurohypophyseal system. J Neuroendocrinol 16:297–302, 2004.

149. Cobb WE, Spare S, Reichlin S: Neurogenic diabetes insipidus: Management with DDAVP (1-desamino-8-D-arginine vasopressin). Ann Intern Med 88:183–188, 1978.

150. Adrogue HJ, Madias NE: Hyponatremia. N Engl J Med 342:1581–1589, 2000.

151. Berl T, Anderson RJ, McDonald KM, Schrier RW: Clinical disorders of water metabolism. Kidney Int 10:117–132, 1976.

152. Arieff AL, Flach F, Massry SG: Neurological manifestations and morbidity of hyponatremia: Correlation with brain, water and electrolytes. Medicine 55:121–129, 1976.

153. Fried LF, Palevsky PM: Hyponatremia and hypernatremia. Med Clin North Am 81:585–609, 1997.

154. Bartter FC, Schwartz WB: The syndrome of inappropriate secretion of antidiuretic hormone. Am J Med 42:790–806, 1967.

155. Anderson RJ, Chung H-M, Kluge R, Schrier RW: Hyponatremia: A prospective analysis of its epidemiology and the pathogenetic role of vasopressin. Ann Intern Med 102:164–168, 1985.

156. Gross PA, Pehrisch H, Rascher W, et al: Pathogenesis of clinical hyponatremia: Observations of vasopressin and fluid intake in 100 hyponatremic medical patients. Eur J Clin Invest 17:123–129, 1987.

157. Ishikawa S-E, Saito T, Fugagawa A, et al: Close association of urinary excretion of aquaporin-2 with appropriate and inappropriate arginine vasopressin dependent antidiuresis in hyponatraemia in elderly subjects. J Clin Endocrinol Metab 86:1665–1671, 2001.

158. Carney DN, Gazdar AF, Oie HK, et al: The in vitro growth and characterization of small cell lung cancer. In Greco FA (ed): Biology and Management of Lung Cancer. Boston, Martinus Nijhoff, 1983, pp 1–24.

159. Zerbe R, Stropes L, Robertson GL: Vasopressin function in the syndrome of inappropriate antidiuresis. Annu Rev Med 31:315–327, 1980.

160. Rolls B: Thirst in human hypo- and hypernatremic states. In Jard S, Jamison R (eds): Vasopressin. Montrouge, France, John Libbey, 1991, pp 549–556.

161. Kovacs L, Robertson GL: Disorders of water balance: Hyponatremia and hypernatremia. Clin Endocrinol Metab 6:107–127, 1992.

162. Arieff AI: Management of hyponatremia. Br Med J 307:305–308, 1993.

163. Ellis SJ: Severe hyponatremia: Complications and treatment. Q J Med 88:905–909, 1995.

164. Forrest JN Jr, Cox M, Hong C, et al: Superiority of demeclocycline over lithium in the treatment of chronic syndrome of inappropriate secretion of antidiuretic hormone. N Engl J Med 298:173–177, 1978.

165. Decaux G, Waterlot Y, Gennette F, et al: Inappropriate secretion of antidiuretic hormone treated with furosemide. Br Med J 285:89–90, 1982.

166. Kinter LB, Ilson BE, Caltabianol S, et al: Antidiuretic hormone antagonism in humans: Are there predictors? In Jard S, Jamison R (eds): Vasopressin. Montrouge, France, John Libbey, 1991, pp 321–329.

167. Ohnishi A, Orita Y, Okahara R, et al: Potent aquaretic agent: A novel non-peptide selective vasopressin 2 antagonist (OPC-31260) in men. J Clin Invest 92:2653–2659, 1993.

168. Saito T, Ishikawa S, Abe K, et al: Acute aquaresis by the non-peptide arginine vasopressin (AVP) antagonist OPC-31260 improves hyponatremia in patients with syndrome of inappropriate secretion of antidiuretic hormone. J Clin Endocrinol Metab 82:1054–1057, 1997.

169. Ferguson JW, Therapondus G, Newby DE, Hayes PC: Therapeutic role of vasopressin receptor antagonism in patients with liver cirrhosis. Clin Sci 105:1–8, 2003.

170. Sterns RH, Riggs J, Schochet SS: Osmotic demyelination syndrome following correction of hyponatremia. N Engl J Med 314:1535–1542, 1986.

171. Verbalis JG: Adaptation to acute and chronic hyponatremia: Implications for symptomatology, diagnosis and treatment. Semin Nephrol 18:3–19, 1998.

172. Verbalis JG, Martinez AJ: Determinants of brain myelinolysis following correction of chronic hyponatremia in rats. In Jard S, Jamison R (eds): Vasopressin. Montrouge, France, John Libbey, 1991, pp 539–547.

173. Nguyen MK, Kurtz I: A new quantitative approach to the treatment of the dysnatraemias. Clin Exp Nephrol 7:125–137, 2003.

174. Smith D, McKenna K, Moore K, et al: Baroregulation of vasopressin release in adipsic diabetes insipidus. J Clin Endocrinol Metab 87:4564–4568, 2002.

175. Robertson GL, Aycinena P, Zerbe RL: Neurogenic disorders of osmoregulation. Am J Med 72:339–353, 1982.

176. Nguyen BN, Yablon SA, Chen SY: Hypodipsic hypernatraemia and diabetes insipidus following anterior communicating artery aneurysm clipping: Diagnostic and therapeutic challenges in the amnestic rehabilitation patient. Brain Inj 15:975–980, 2001.

177. Hammond DN, Moll GW, Robertson GL, Chelmicka-Schorr E: Hypodipsic hypernatremia with normal osmoregulation of vasopressin. N Engl J Med 315:433–436, 1986.

178. Ball SG, Vaidja B, Baylis PH: Hypothalamic adipsic syndrome: Diagnosis and management. Clin Endocrinol 47:405–409, 1997.

The Pineal Gland: Basic Physiology and Clinical Implications

Josephine Arendt

STRUCTURE AND BIOCHEMISTRY OF THE PINEAL GLAND

STRUCTURE

The pineal gland (epiphysis cerebri) is a small, unpaired central structure, essentially an appendage of the brain. Great variation in size and position is seen even within species.[1] In humans, the pineal gland weighs around 100 to 150 mg. It assumes a shape resembling a pine cone (hence *pineal*) and, again owing to its shape, has been referred to as the "penis of the brain."

The mammalian pineal gland is a secretory organ, whereas in fish and amphibians, it is directly photoreceptive, and in reptiles and birds, it has a mixed photoreceptor and secretory function.[2] The extracranial parietal (parapineal, frontal) organ found in some lower vertebrates has been referred to as the "third eye."[1,2] The principal cellular component is the pinealocyte, and elements of its photoreceptive evolutionary history remain in both structure and function.[1-3] In some species, including humans, calcified lumps are frequently present in pineal tissue after puberty, although this calcification does not appear to be associated with a decline in metabolic activity except in the sense that activity declines in general with aging.[4-6] The gland is richly vascularized. Its principal innervation is sympathetic and arises from the superior cervical ganglion.[7] In addition, good evidence has been presented for parasympathetic, commissural, and peptidergic innervation.[8] Its primary function in all species that have been studied to date is to transduce information concerning light-dark cycles to body physiology, particularly for the organization of body rhythms.[9] This information is encoded

in the secretion patterns of the major pineal hormone melatonin (5-methoxy-*N*-acetyltryptamine).[10]

SYNTHESIS AND METABOLISM OF MELATONIN

Melatonin is synthesized within pinealocytes—cell types derived from photoreceptors—from tryptophan via the pathway shown in Figure 31-1.[11,12] Most synthetic activity occurs during the dark phase, with a major increase (7- to 150-fold) in the activity of the rate-limiting enzyme serotonin-*N*-acetyltransferase (arylalkylamine *N*-acetyltransferase [AA-NAT]). The rhythm of production is endogenous in that it is generated in the suprachiasmatic nucleus (SCN), the major central rhythm-generating system or "clock" in mammals[12] (the pineal gland itself is a self-sustaining "clock" in some, if not all, lower vertebrates[13]). The melatonin rhythm is generated by a closed loop negative feedback of clock gene expression in the SCN, *Clock* and *Bmal* being positive stimulatory elements, *Per* and *Cry* being negative elements, subsequently influencing clock-controlled genes. *Per* and *NAT mRNA* oscillate in the pineal gland, although posttranscription control is evident in some species.[12] The elucidation of the molecular machinery underlying circadian rhythm generation has been a major scientific endeavor over the last few years. The subject has been extensively reviewed (see Ref. 14, for example).

The rhythm is synchronized to 24 hours primarily by the light-dark cycle acting via the retina and the retinohypothalamic projection to the SCN. The cDNAs encoding both AA-NAT and the *O*-methylating enzyme hydroxyindole-*O*-methyltransferase (see Fig. 31-1) have been cloned, and studies of molecular regulation of melatonin production show some species differences.[12] It is likely that the human

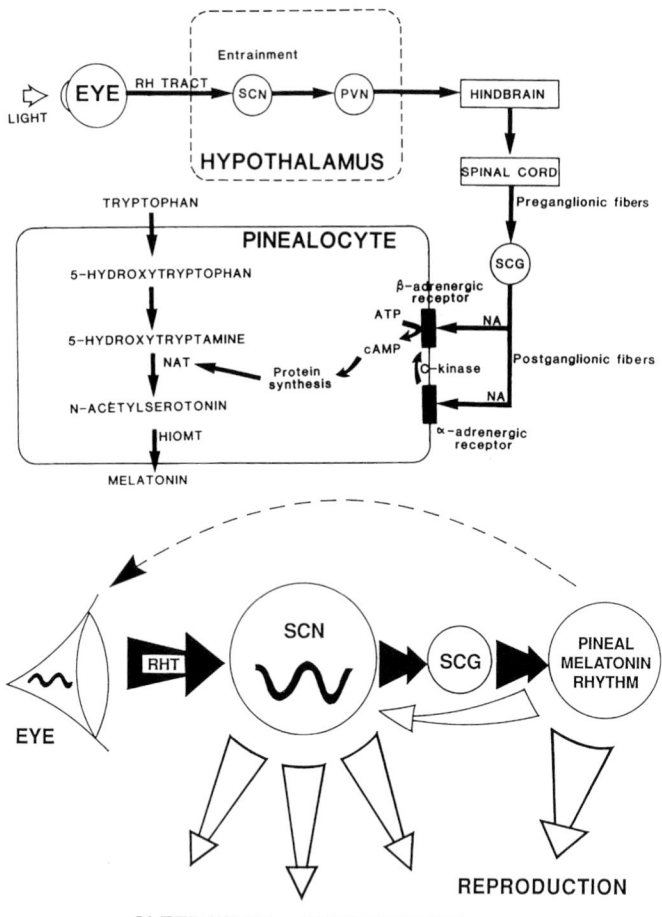

Figure 31-1 **A,** Control of melatonin synthesis in the pineal gland. The rhythm of secretion is generated in the suprachiasmatic nucleus (SCN) and entrained by the light-dark cycle. HIOMT, hydroxyindole-O-methyltransferase; NA, norepinephrine; NAT, 5-hydroxytryptamine (serotonin)-N-acetyltransferase; PVN, paraventricular nucleus; RH, retinohypothalamic; SCG, superior cervical ganglion. **B,** A model for closed loop feedback of melatonin within the circadian system. Functional melatonin receptors are found in both the suprachiasmatic nucleus (SCN) and the retina. Rhythm generation in the SCN can be modulated in phase and amplitude by melatonin. The mammalian retina generates rhythmic melatonin production in vitro, which together with pineal-derived melatonin may serve to influence retinal processes.

enzyme is regulated primarily at a posttranscriptional level, whereas in rodents, the key event appears to be cyclic adenosine monophosphate (cAMP)-dependent phosphorylation of a transcription factor that binds to the AA-NAT promoter. Rapid decline in activity with light treatment at night appears to depend on proteasomal proteolysis.[15] The role of 14-3-3 proteins in the control of melatonin synthesis has recently been described. These proteins form a complex with AA-NAT, triggered by cAMP-dependent phosphorylation of the enzyme, which is then activated and protected against proteolysis (usually at night). The enzyme is dephosphorylated during light exposure, dissociates from 14-3-3 protein, and is then destroyed by proteolysis.[16] Phosphorylation of the transcription factor CREB (cAMP-response element binding protein) is an important step in the signal transduction cascade that activates melatonin biosynthesis in the mammalian pineal organ.[17] According to distribution studies of AA-NAT mRNA, this enzyme is expressed in the pineal gland, retina, and, to a much lesser extent, some other brain areas, the pituitary, and the testis,[12] but apart from the pineal gland, these structures contribute little to circulating concentrations in

mammals.[9] Within the rodent retina, a self-sustaining "clock" maintains rhythmic production of melatonin in vitro as it does in many lower vertebrates.[18] Whether this pattern is true in humans remains to be seen.

Melatonin is metabolized primarily within the liver by 6-hydroxylation, followed by sulfate and/or glucuronide conjugation. A number of minor metabolites are also formed through ring splitting, cyclization of the side chain, or demethylation (see Arendt[9] for a bibliography). In humans and rodents, exogenous oral or intravenous melatonin has a short metabolic half-life (20 to 60 minutes, depending on the author and species), with a large hepatic first-pass effect and a biphasic elimination pattern. In ruminants, longer half-lives are seen after oral administration.[9,19]

OTHER PINEAL FACTORS

Although the pineal gland contains and synthesizes a multitude of other indoles together with biologically active peptides (for reviews, see Refs. 20 and 21), they have not yet been attributed important physiologic functions. Most effects of pinealectomy can be reversed by melatonin in physiologic concentrations; hence, it is difficult to consider other compounds major pineal hormones.

NEURAL CONTROL OF MELATONIN SYNTHESIS

In mammals, pineal denervation, or ganglionectomy, abolishes the rhythmic synthesis of melatonin and the light-dark control of its production. Norepinephrine is clearly the major transmitter and acts via β_1-adrenoceptors with potentiation by α_1-stimulation, but the role of neural serotonin is probably not negligible. A day-night variation is seen in pineal norepinephrine, with the highest values at night, approximately 180 degrees out of phase with the pineal serotonin rhythm. cAMP acts as a second messenger and stimulates AA-NAT activity. β-Adrenergic receptor-binding sites in the rat pineal vary over a 24-hour period, the lowest number being found toward the end of the dark phase and increasing shortly after lights go on.[11,12]

OTHER CONTROL MECHANISMS

The pineal gland contains very large numbers of other neuroreceptors and hormone receptors, but evaluation of their physiologic importance has not led to major insights into pineal function as yet. There is evidence for modulation of the noradrenergic stimulation of melatonin secretion by various peptides such as vasoactive intestinal peptide (VIP), neuropeptide Y, pituitary adenylate cyclase-activating peptide (PACAP), and opioids together with gamma-aminobutyric acid (GABA), dopamine, and glutamate.

PHYSIOLOGY OF THE PINEAL GLAND

LIGHT-DARK CONTROL OF MELATONIN SYNTHESIS

A Darkness Hormone

In virtually all species that have been studied to date, whether nocturnal or diurnal, melatonin is synthesized and secreted during the dark phase of the day.[9] Remarkably, even the unicellular alga *Gonyaulax* appears to produce melatonin during the dark phase, and it appears to be present in higher plants.[22,23] Melatonin production is clearly a highly evolutionarily conserved phenomenon. In most vertebrates, the rhythm is endogenous, that is, internally generated. It persists in the absence of time cues (*free-running*), in general assuming a period that deviates slightly from 24 hours, and is thus a true circadian rhythm.[24–27] Lesions of the SCN lead to loss of the vast majority of circadian rhythms, such as locomotor activity, sleep, behavior,[28] hormones including melatonin, and urinary constituents. Circadian rhythms are entrained (synchronized) to the 24-hour day primarily by light-dark cycles. Many blind people with no light perception at all (conscious or unconscious) show free-running melatonin and other rhythms (e.g., sleep, cortisol, core temperature) in a normal environment.[29,30] In addition to entraining the rhythm, day length (photoperiod) determines the duration of nighttime secretion both by direct suppression of melatonin and by determining the length of the signal emitted by the SCN.[31]

Factors (zeitgebers) other than light-dark cycles that are involved in entrainment include behavioral imposition such as forced activity and rest (particularly in darkness), social and nutritional (rhythmic feeding) cues, temperature variations, knowledge of clock time, certain drugs, and melatonin itself.[32]

Melatonin Secretion in Relation to Day Length
In most species, melatonin secretion is related to the length of the night: The longer the night, the longer the duration of secretion.[9] This phenomenon has been particularly well demonstrated in sheep, in which melatonin levels rise within a few minutes of lights off and, in photoperiods of more than around 14 hours of light, do not decline until lights on. In such photoperiods, light serves to entrain the rhythm and suppress secretion at the beginning and/or the end of the dark phase (Fig. 31-2).

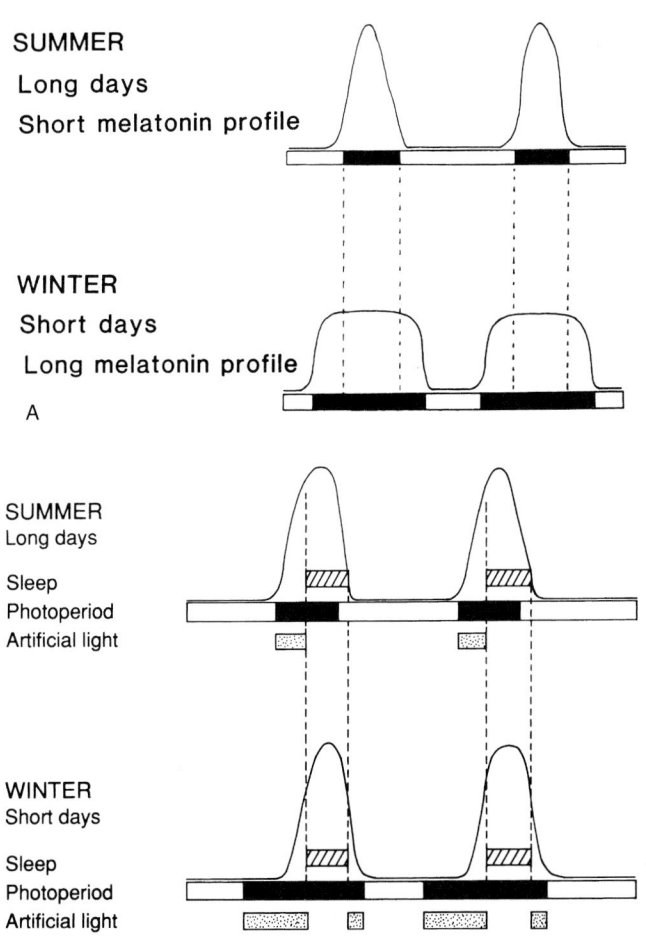

SUMMER
Long days
Short melatonin profile

WINTER
Short days
Long melatonin profile
A

SUMMER
Long days

Sleep
Photoperiod
Artificial light

WINTER
Short days

Sleep
Photoperiod
Artificial light
B

Figure 31-2 Diagrammatic representation of melatonin secretion in relation to day length. **A,** The change in duration, with length of the natural dark phase acts as a seasonal time cue in photoperiodic species. **B,** Social behavior and artificial lighting in humans lead to minimal change in duration but phase advances in summer. If a long or short dark phase is imposed, the pattern reverts to that shown in **A.**

The most consistent observation in humans is that melatonin profiles show a phase change from winter to summer, with earlier secretion in summer than in winter (see Arendt[9] for references). However, if humans are kept strictly in darkness for 14 hours per day for a period of 2 months, the melatonin secretion pattern expands to cover almost the entire dark period, and concomitantly, in extended periods of 16 hours of light, the rhythm contracts to less than 9 hours, with accompanying changes in body temperature and sleep.[33] Small changes in duration of the profile have been seen between winter and summer in high latitudes. Short-term imposition of artificial short days leads to a change in phase of endogenous melatonin.[34] Many clinical studies have not controlled sufficiently for exposure to natural or artificial light, making interpretation of data difficult.

Light Suppression of Melatonin Secretion
Even brief exposure to light of suitable intensity, duration, and spectral quality suppresses melatonin production at night.[35,36] Short wavelengths (~465 nm) are most effective in mice and humans.[37,38] Since the action spectrum derived from irradiance response curves does not correspond to either scotopic or photopic action spectra, a new photoreceptor system has been invoked.[39]

The amount of light that is required to suppress melatonin secretion during the night varies from species to species, with the time of night, and with previous light exposure.[35] In humans, Lewy and colleagues originally observed that 2500-lux broad-spectrum white light (domestic light is around 300 to 500 lux) is required to completely suppress melatonin at night.[36] However, much lower intensities will partially suppress and shift the rhythm in humans.[40,41]

This observation has been of very considerable importance for a general appreciation of the role of light in human physiology, in particular, its importance in the control of human rhythms and in the treatment of winter depression (seasonal affective disorder[42]).

Entrainment of the Melatonin Rhythm
A single daily light pulse of suitable intensity and duration in otherwise constant darkness is sufficient to phase-shift and synchronize the melatonin rhythm to 24 hours in animals.[43] Phase shifting and entrainment have been demonstrated in humans with suitable intensity and duration of light treatment.[9,44,45] It is likely that short wavelengths are also most effective for entrainment of the rhythm to 24 hours.[46,47] However, the relative contribution of light to the entrainment of melatonin in a normal environment remains to be fully determined. If subjects are maintained for 2 weeks exclusively in domestic intensity broad spectrum white light (12 hours of 200 lux and 12 hours of near darkness [<5 lux] daily) with no structured activity or rest periods, the circadian timing system drifts to later and later times.[48] Studies in Antarctica suggest that a structured social routine in a dim light environment suffices to synchronize melatonin to 24 hours.[9] However, as many blind people with no conscious or unconscious light perception living in a normal social environment show desynchronized melatonin and other circadian rhythms, it is clear that at least some perception of light is of primary importance.[49–51]

ROLE IN PHOTOPERIODIC SEASONAL FUNCTIONS

Photoperiodism
Most species, even humans, show seasonal variations in their physiology and behavior. The reproductive cycle is timed so that environmental conditions are propitious for growth of the young, and variations in behavior, pelage (coat growth and color), appetite, body weight, and fat are such that survival in ambient temperature conditions is optimized and camouflage protects against predators. When seasonal

functions are timed primarily by day length, species are referred to as photoperiodic.[52] Photoperiod is often critical for the timing of pubertal development.[53] In general, puberty is reached only during the adult mating season. It is clear that in photoperiodic mammals and marsupials, an intact inner-vated pineal gland is essential for the perception of photope-riodic change.[54,55] Most information is derived from studies on reproductive function in hamsters and sheep.

Role of Melatonin

Pinealectomy removes the vast majority of circulating mela-tonin in rodents, primates, and ungulates.[54] It was therefore the first pineal hormone to be investigated as a pineal pho-toneuroendocrine transducer. It is possible to administer melatonin by daily infusion or feeding to generate at will circulating profiles with a duration that is characteristic of particular photoperiods in an intact or pinealectomized animal.[54,55] In this way, it has become clear that a particular melatonin duration is a necessary and sufficient condition for induction of a given seasonal response and is equipotent with a particular photoperiod. Long-duration melatonin is equiva-lent to short days, and short-duration melatonin is equivalent to long days (see Fig. 31-2). Interpretation of the signal, as with day length, depends on the physiology (for example, long- or short-day breeder) of the species in question. In sheep, the evidence is good that long days or short-duration melatonin can time the whole seasonal cycle, at least of repro-duction, and act as a seasonal zeitgeber for a presumed endogenous annual rhythm.[55] Animals become refractory to a specific duration of melatonin, as they do to a particular pho-toperiod. For example, a period of long days (or a long-day melatonin signal) is required before a short-day melatonin signal advances the reproductive cycle in sheep.[54,55]

Puberty

The photoperiod via melatonin secretion determines the tim-ing of puberty in some species, provided that a sufficient degree of physical maturity has been reached.[53] Interestingly, photoperiod perception by the fetus is present before birth in rodents and ungulates and ensures a rate of development that is appropriate to environmental conditions.[56] Melatonin crosses the placenta in a number of species, and mela-tonin injection in the mother can dictate the timing of postnatal reproductive development.

The laboratory rat is only marginally photoperiodic. Nevertheless, injections of melatonin during the late light phase, during a small window in the late dark phase, or even via continuous-release implants, specifically during the period of pubertal development, delay reproductive matu-rity in both males and females.[9,56,57] Full sexual maturity is eventually achieved; thus, the system is not perma-nently compromised. Moreover, in vitro melatonin inhibits gonadotropin-releasing hormone (GnRH)-induced luteinizing hormone (LH) release by cultured rat pituitary glands from prepubertal animals, and there is recent evidence for an influence of melatonin on neuronal GnRH gene expression.[58]

Nonreproductive Seasonal Functions

The pineal gland via melatonin secretion probably plays a role in all photoperiod-dependent functions in mammals. Evidence exists to substantiate this statement with respect to behavior, body weight, coat constitution and color (for exam-ple, the white winter coat of some polar species), prolactin variations, antler growth, thyroid activity, appetite, ther-moregulation, delayed implantation, embryonic diapause, and hibernation.[9,54,55,59] Partly because the ability to control reproduction is of applied interest in commercially important domestic species such as sheep, this aspect has received more attention than others. The winter coat of animals such as mink, arctic foxes, and cashmere goats also has commercial significance and can be manipulated by photoperiod and

melatonin administration. Implanted melatonin induces short-day effects, and a number of commercial preparations of melatonin have been developed to this end.

ROLE OF THE PINEAL GLAND AND MELATONIN IN CIRCADIAN RHYTHMS

An extensive literature has described the importance of the pineal gland (and also the retina) in the control of circadian rhythms in lower vertebrates. Melatonin is produced rhyth-mically by both the pineal gland and the retina in many lower vertebrates and probably serves as the common humoral signal for circadian organization.[9,32]

ROLE OF THE PINEAL GLAND IN MAMMALIAN CIRCADIAN RHYTHMS

Until quite recently, opinion was that the pineal gland did not have a role in the mammalian circadian system. However, in rats, pinealectomy increases the rate of reentrainment to forced phase shifts of the light-dark cycle, and pinealectomy of hamsters in constant light leads to major disruption of the circadian system.[60,61] In humans, it is likely that the phase-shifting effects of light do not depend on melatonin suppres-sion[62] but that the presence of endogenous or exogenous melatonin can in some circumstances modulate the effects of light on the circadian system.[63] Further insights into the cir-cadian role of melatonin in humans are considered in subse-quent sections. A substantial body of work implicates melatonin in circadian thermoregulation (see Badia et al.[59] for a review). Many such effects may involve the thyroid gland.[64] Melatonin has also been implicated in rhythmic and other aspects of cardiovascular function. Pinealectomy of rodents leads to hypertension, and there is a body of evidence indicating an influence of melatonin on blood pressure.[9]

EFFECTS OF TIMED ADMINISTRATION OF MELATONIN

Behavior, Hormones, and Temperature

In rats, daily melatonin injections synchronize free-running activity and temperature rhythms in constant darkness and are reported to partially or completely synchronize disrupted activity rhythms in constant light, although the latter obser-vation is somewhat controversial.[32,61,65] A phase-response curve to single injections of melatonin can be demonstrated with small phase advances of at most 1 hour during the late subjective day.[65] Timed administration hastens adaptation of activity and melatonin production to forced phase shift and can change the direction of reentrainment.[65–67] Some strains of adult hamster can be synchronized by melatonin adminis-tration,[68,69] and fetal hamsters can be entrained by mater-nal injections of melatonin at 24-hour intervals in specific circadian phases.[56]

Gestation

In the rat, gestation length depends on the ambient light-dark cycle. Small advances or delays in parturition can be induced by day lengths that are shorter or longer than 24 hours, and the effect can partially be mimicked by timed melatonin administration.[70]

Estrous Cycle

Because the pineal gland is involved in circadian timing, the presumption must be that it is concerned with timing of the LH surge and, indeed, with general estrous timing. In rats, timed melatonin administration has been demonstrated to mimic the effects of extending the light-dark cycle on timing of the LH surge. Observations of the melatonin rhythm itself show a decreased amplitude during proestrus in rodents but with conflicting reports in other species (see elsewhere[9,71] for reviews).

Aging

A fairly consistent observation in pineal research is the decline in amplitude of the melatonin rhythm in old age (see Arendt[9] for references). Pinealectomy accelerates the aging process, and the possible antiaging effects of melatonin have generated considerable publicity.[72] Several hypotheses have been put forward to explain these often flawed,[73,74] insubstantial, but interesting observations. One proposes that melatonin enhances immune responses via an opiatergic mechanism. Another considers that appropriately timed daily melatonin administration optimizes circadian relationships, especially of phase, and increases circadian amplitude (see Armstrong and Redman[75] for references). The most widely published explanation is that melatonin acts as a free radical scavenger and antioxidant.[76–78] Being an easily oxidized molecule, melatonin does indeed have some antioxidant activity. Whether this property is physiologically relevant in mammals remains an open question. It has been suggested that this activity was its primary evolutionary function in primitive species.[77] Certainly, much publicity has attended this property of the molecule; numerous subsequent publications describe the potential applications of melatonin as an antioxidant, and most recently, evidence has been presented to suggest that the antioxidant capacity in vivo is related to plasma melatonin levels. However, the quantities of exogenous melatonin that are required to generate significant antioxidant activity in vivo remain to be specified.

In Vitro Phase Shifts

The metabolic activity of the rodent SCN in vivo and the electrical activity of various in vitro SCN preparations can be modified by melatonin; it inhibits 2-deoxyglucose uptake into the nuclei in the late subjective day with no effect at other times and inhibits electrical activity, also during the late subjective day.[32] By far the most convincing evidence is the phase-advancing effect of melatonin on the circadian rhythm of electrical activity in cultured SCN.[79] The effect was large, acute, and time dependent, shifts of up to several hours being observed. Thus, melatonin acts directly on a central biologic clock to change its phase.

Retinal Rhythms

Melatonin appears to function as a paracrine signal within the retina. It enhances retinal function in low-intensity light by inducing photomechanical changes and regulating turnover rates of the photoreceptive apparatuses of rods, cones, and the surrounding pigment epithelium.[80]

Summary

The pineal gland, the retina, and the SCN together form the basic structures that perceive and transduce the nonvisual effects of light. Melatonin provides a closed loop to this system (see Fig. 31-1; Fig. 31-3). It is reasonable to conclude that in adult mammals, melatonin serves to modulate circadian phase and strengthen coupling. In fetal and neonatal mammals, it helps to program the circadian system and determine the timing of developmental stages, especially puberty.

THE PINEAL GLAND IN HUMAN PHYSIOLOGY AND PATHOLOGY

Clearly, the importance of the pineal gland in humans depends on the importance of light in human physiology. It is reasonable to assume that the pineal gland conveys information concerning light-dark cycles for the organization of seasonal and circadian rhythms in humans as in animals. Pinealectomy in humans removes virtually all plasma melatonin.[81] Other consequences of the operation consist of diffuse neurologic problems that do not add up to a consistent functional effect as yet and may be more related to

nonspecific effects of the operation. Recent work suggests that melatonin is absent or very low in treated or untreated pineal germinomas, but the consequences remain to be defined.[82]

HUMAN MELATONIN PRODUCTION

Basic Characteristics

Mechanisms

Early work demonstrated the presence of hydroxyindole-O-methyltransferase activity in tissue from postmortem pineal glands. The melatonin content of human pineal glands is related to the time of death, with higher values at night, as expected. Pathologic or traumatic denervation of the pineal gland abolishes the plasma melatonin rhythm. β-Adrenergic antagonists suppress melatonin production, and increased availability of norepinephrine and serotonin is stimulatory (see Ref. 9 for a bibliography). Good evidence has thus been presented that the neural and biochemical pathways that are known to control pineal function in rats are similar in humans.

Melatonin and 6-Sulfatoxymelatonin Production

In a "normal" environment, melatonin is secreted during the night in healthy humans, as in all other species. The average maximum levels attained in plasma in adults are of the order of 60 to 70 pg/mL when measured with high-specificity assays. Mean maximum concentrations of 6-sulfatoxymelatonin attain 80 to 100 pg/mL (different mammalian species have a relatively narrow range of circulating concentrations, although birds have more). Minimum concentrations of both compounds are usually below 10 pg/mL. Peak concentrations of melatonin in plasma normally occur between 2:00 and 4:00 A.M. The onset of secretion is usually around 9:00 to 10:00 P.M., and the offset is usually at 7:00 to 9:00 A.M. in adults in temperate zones. The appearance and peak levels of 6-sulfatoxymelatonin in plasma are delayed by 1 to 2 hours, and the morning decline is delayed by 3 to 4 hours[9] (Fig. 31-4). In urine, 50% to 80% of 6-sulfatoxymelatonin appears in the overnight sample (midnight to 8:00 A.M.), and it is low but rarely undetectable in the afternoon and early evening.

The rhythm is endogenous, with a period that is usually greater than 24 hours.[26,27,83] Possibly the most striking characteristic of the normal human melatonin rhythm is its reproducibility from day to day and from week to week in normal individuals, rather like a hormonal fingerprint.[84] This stability leads to the extensive use of melatonin in plasma or saliva and aMT6s in urine as marker rhythms for circadian phase, for example, in the investigation of sleep disorders, and evaluating adaptation to abrupt phase shifts as in shift work and jet lag. The large interindividual variations have been ascribed to the size of the pineal gland rather than to variations in enzymic activity.[85] A small number of apparently normal individuals have no detectable melatonin in plasma at all times of day.[86]

Association with Temperature

Many associations of melatonin with temperature exist in humans. The most striking is the reciprocal relationship in circadian profiles, in which the temperature nadir correlates closely with the peak of melatonin.[87] The increase in core temperature that is induced by light at night and is associated with melatonin suppression could be at least partially opposed by replacement melatonin.[88] Possibly half of the nighttime decline in core temperature might be ascribed to the hypothermic effects of endogenous melatonin.[89] A causal relationship is also indicated, as exogenous melatonin during the "biologic daytime," that is, during the period of low melatonin secretion, can acutely depress body temperature in humans.[89,90] This effect is posture dependent.[91] The ovulatory rise in temperature during the menstrual cycle is associated

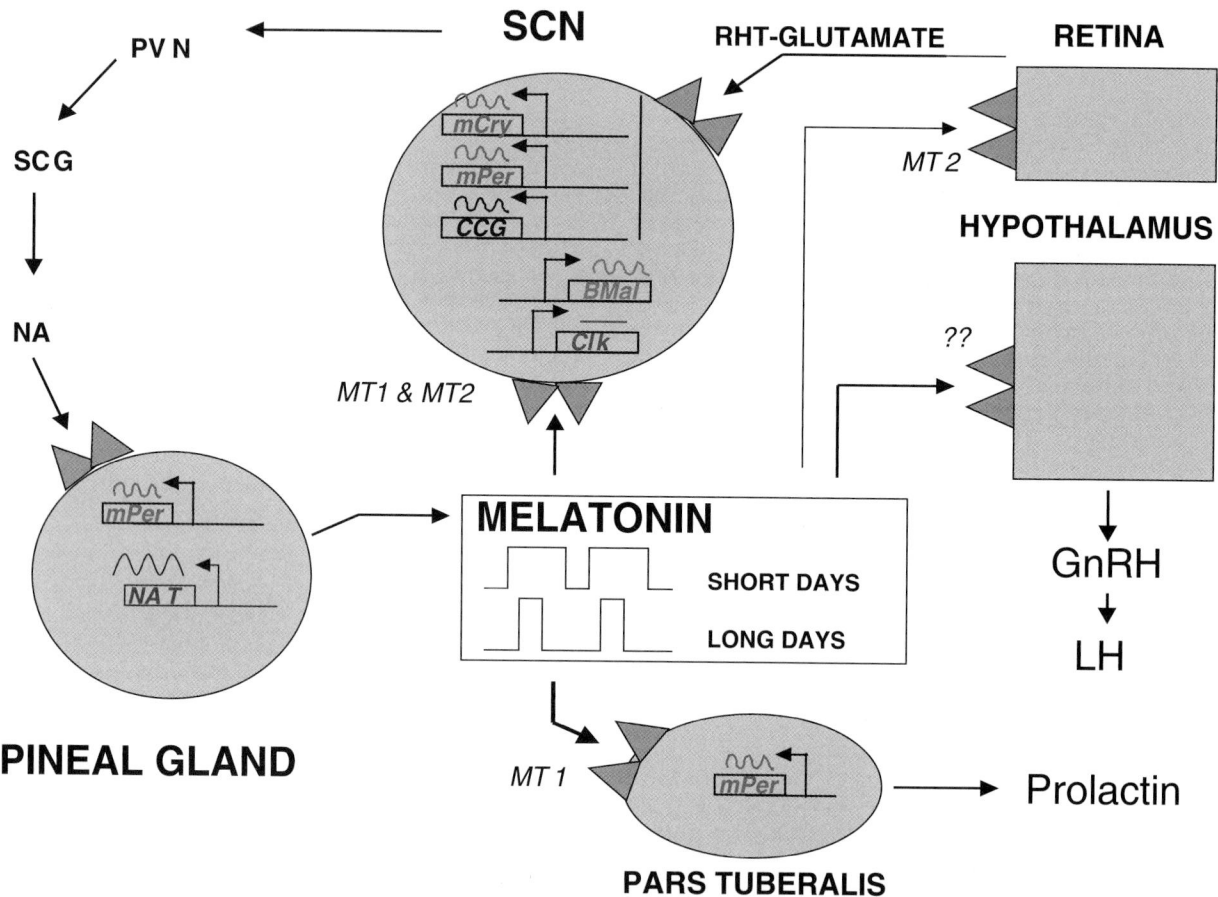

Figure 31-3 Diagrammatic representation of the control of production and the functions of melatonin, with regard to seasonal and circadian timing mechanisms. RHT, retinohypothalamic tract; NA, noradrenalin; SCN, suprachiasmatic nucleus; PVN, paraventricular nucleus; SCG, superior cervical ganglion; MT1 and MT2, melatonin receptor subtypes. The melatonin rhythm is generated by a closed loop negative feedback of clock gene expression in the SCN; *Clock* and *Bmal,* positive stimulatory elements; *Per, Cry,* negative elements; *CCG,* clock-controlled genes. *Per* and *NAT* mRNA oscillate in the pineal gland, although posttranscription control is evident in some species. Melatonin influences SCN activity via two or more receptors. MT2 appears to be the phase-shifting receptor in rodents, whereas MT1 is associated with suppression of SCN electrical activity. The MT2 receptor was first characterized in the retina and influences dopamine release. Melatonin conveys photoperiodic information influencing the pattern of *per* expression in the pars tuberalis for the control of seasonal prolactin variations via an MT1 receptor. Melatonin target sites in the hypothalamus that influence seasonal variations in reproductive hormones have yet to be fully defined. (Source: Based, with permission, on an original diagram by Dr Elisabeth Maywood, MRC Laboratory of Molecular Biology, Neurobiology Division, Hills Road, Cambridge, CB2 2QH, UK.)

with a reported decline in the amplitude of melatonin, but the decline in melatonin is not a consistent observation.

Association with Sleep
Obvious correlations are noted between melatonin production at night and sleep. However, sleep deprivation does not abolish the melatonin rhythm and in very dim light does not affect secretion.[87] During sleep deprivation, self-rated fatigue exhibits a circadian rhythm that is closely correlated with plasma melatonin levels.[87] The association between the evening rise of circulating melatonin and the evening increase in sleep propensity suggests a causal relationship.[92] The timing of sleep spindles and certain other electroencephalographic (EEG) characteristics also relates to the circadian phase of melatonin.[93] Careful observations in constant routine conditions of the profiles of melatonin, core body temperature, sleep propensity, sleepiness, cortisol, rapid eye movement (REM), and so on have led to a definition of biologic night in

humans.[92,94] This corresponds to the period during which melatonin is secreted, with an apparent switch process at "dusk" and "dawn" that is common to melatonin onset and offset, core temperature rise and decline, and increasing and decreasing sleep propensity. The so-called forbidden zone for sleep or wake maintenance zone occurs just prior to the onset of melatonin secretion and can be overcome by melatonin administration to advance the evening rise.[95,96]

The peak of melatonin secretion is associated with the nadirs of alertness and performance, together with increased blood lipid levels at night (Fig. 31-5).[97]

Patients suffering from non-24-hour sleep-wake disorder (largely blind subjects with no perception of light) intermittently secrete melatonin during the daytime. This is strongly associated with the presence of naps during the day.[98] Daytime melatonin production is seen in Smith-Magenis syndrome (caused by a deletion in chromosome 17p11.2); these patients have excessive daytime sleepiness, poor nighttime

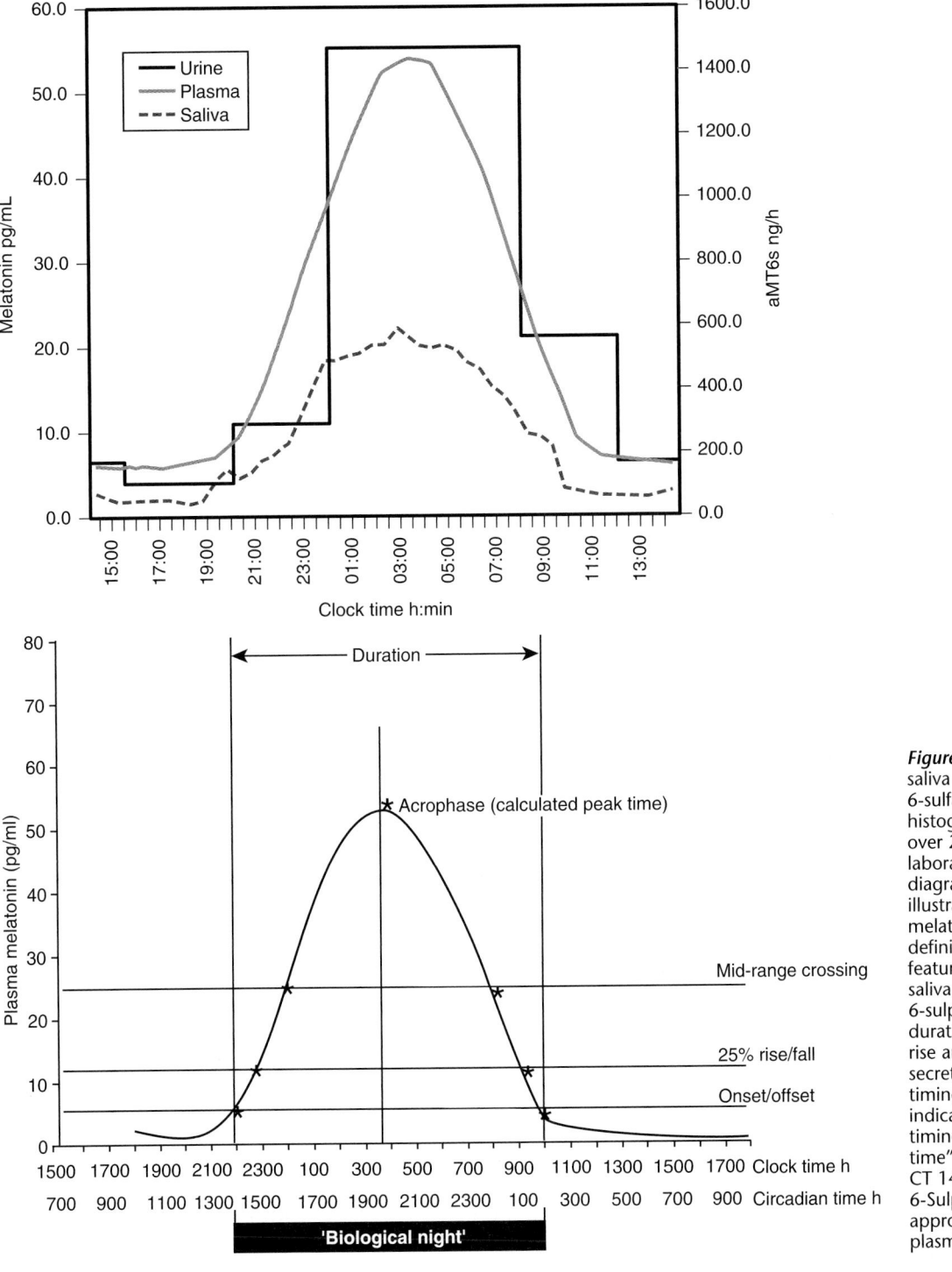

Figure 31-4 **A,** Plasma melatonin, saliva melatonin, and urinary 6-sulfatoxymelatonin (aMT6s, histogram). Mean normal values over 24 hours from the author's laboratory are represented diagrammatically. **B,** Diagram to illustrate the normal profile of melatonin secretion (plasma) defining "biologic night." The features of this profile and that of salivary melatonin and urinary 6-sulphatoxymelatonin (acrophase, duration, midrange crossing, 25% rise and fall, onset and offset of secretion), used to characterize the timing of the circadian clock are indicated. Melatonin treatment timing is often based on "circadian time" (CT), where, by convention, CT 14 is melatonin onset. 6-Sulphatoxymelatonin acrophase is approximately 2 hours after the plasma melatonin acrophase.

Continued

sleep, but normal cortisol rhythms. Treatment of these patients with atenolol to suppress daytime melatonin successfully reduces daytime sleepiness.[99] These various observations support a role for melatonin in reinforcing human sleepiness or sleep.

Other Associations
Obviously, any variable with a marked circadian rhythm shows correlations with melatonin, if necessary, displaced in time. Examples include cortisol, prolactin, thyroid-stimulating hormone, aspects of the immune system, and many others.[9] The relationships of stress, exercise,[100] and some other nonpharmacologic interventions in modification of melatonin

production are somewhat unclear and do not appear to play a major role in humans.

Development, Puberty, and Aging
Shortly after birth, very little melatonin or 6-sulfatoxymelatonin is detectable in body fluids. A robust melatonin rhythm appears around 6 to 8 weeks of life.[101] Whether in specific individuals this rhythm corresponds to the organization and synchronization of other circadian variables such as sleep remains a question of very considerable interest. The plasma concentration of melatonin increases rapidly thereafter and reaches a lifetime peak on average at 3 to 5 years of age.[102] The increment is much greater at night. Subsequently, a steady

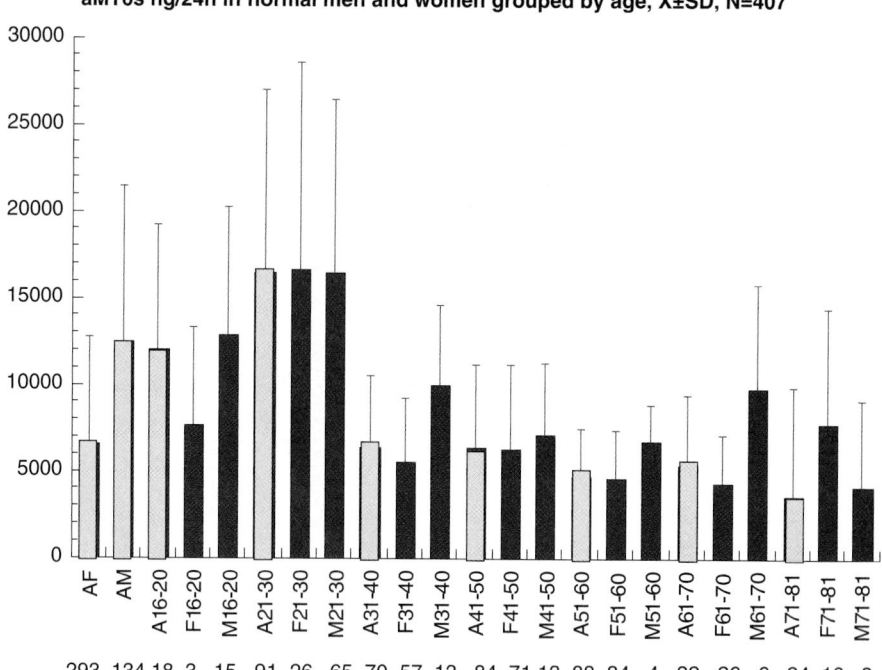

Figure 31-4, cont'd **C,** Production of 6-sulphatoxymelatonin (ng/24 hours) at different ages in men and women (A = all, M = male, F = female), normal values from the author's laboratory. Note the decline with age.

decrease is seen, with mean adult concentrations attained in the mid to late teens and the major decline occurring before puberty. Values remain relatively unchanged until 35 to 40 years of age, and a final decline in amplitude then takes place until (on average) low levels are seen in old age, with the exception of one study using very healthy elderly subjects[103] (see Arendt[9] for references). Reports of association of differences in secretion in adults with gender, height, or body weight are not consistent. The decline in plasma melatonin in early life in no way proves that it is involved in human pubertal development. Although a lower melatonin concentration has been reported in children with precocious puberty and higher concentrations in those with delayed puberty and hypothalamic amenorrhea than in age-matched controls,[104-106] these associations remain correlative and not causal. Ovarian suppression with a GnRH analogue in precocious girls is not accompanied by changes in melatonin secretion.[107] However, in some case reports, induction of sexual development was associated with a decline in melatonin production.[108,109]

Menstrual Cycle

Some of the very earliest reports on human melatonin described low preovulatory concentrations the morning before ovulation and suggested that low melatonin was facilitatory to the preovulatory LH peak.[9] This observation is inconsistent, however, and more recent work indicates that neither the amplitude nor the phase of melatonin is altered in the course of the normal cycle.[9,71] The effects of melatonin on core body temperature are reported to vary in the course of the cycle, and herein may lie a physiologic function.[110] LH pulses are amplified in the early follicular phase by oral melatonin at 8:00 A.M.[111] Attempts to develop melatonin as a contraceptive pill in combination with a synthetic progestin minipill have not been successful.[112]

Very large doses (100 mg daily) potentiate testosterone-induced LH suppression.[113] A series of studies in males with and without hypogonadism has reinforced the perception that melatonin is essentially inhibitory to human reproductive function (e.g., Luboshitzky et al.[114,115]). Because humans appear to conceive more readily in long photoperiods, an explanation may reside in residual human photoperiodism.[116] The results of these studies partially support the contention

that melatonin, suitably administered, can inhibit human reproductive activity. Other, more recent data, however, indicate that over periods of 8 days to several weeks, daily melatonin administration (low pharmacologic doses) has no effect on a number of pituitary/gonadal hormones.[96,117,118]

In the author's opinion, low, timed doses of melatonin used to reinforce circadian organization are likely to increase fertility in humans.

PATHOLOGY

Pineal Hyperplasia and Hypoplasia

A number of reports of variations in postmortem pineal weight as a function of the cause of death have been summarized by Tapp.[5] Of the most interesting, hypoplasia of the pineal gland in association with retinal disease may be causally interrelated. Tapp has reported that pineal glands in patients dying of carcinoma of the breast or melanoma are heavier than those from patients with other cancers. Very large pineal glands (1 g) have been described in a rare genetic syndrome with insulin resistance.[119] Sudden infant death syndrome is associated with small pineal glands and decreased melatonin production.[120,121] Such deaths usually occur at night and may be associated with abnormalities of sleep. If melatonin helps to coordinate circadian organization in the developing infant, its underproduction may contribute to the disorder.

Pineal Tumors

Tumors of the pineal region in children are frequently associated with abnormal pubertal development.[122] The original hypothesis to explain precocious puberty in boys with pineal tumors was that the tumors destroyed the capacity of the pineal gland to inhibit sexual development. In fact, much evidence suggests that precocity is due to production of the β subunit of human chorionic gonadotropin (β-hCG) by germ cell tumors of the pineal gland.[123,124] This relationship has nevertheless stimulated much work on the possible role of the pineal gland through the secretion of melatonin as a means of timing human puberty.

Pineal tumors are heterogeneous and may arise from germ cells (teratomas, germinomas, choriocarcinomas, endodermal

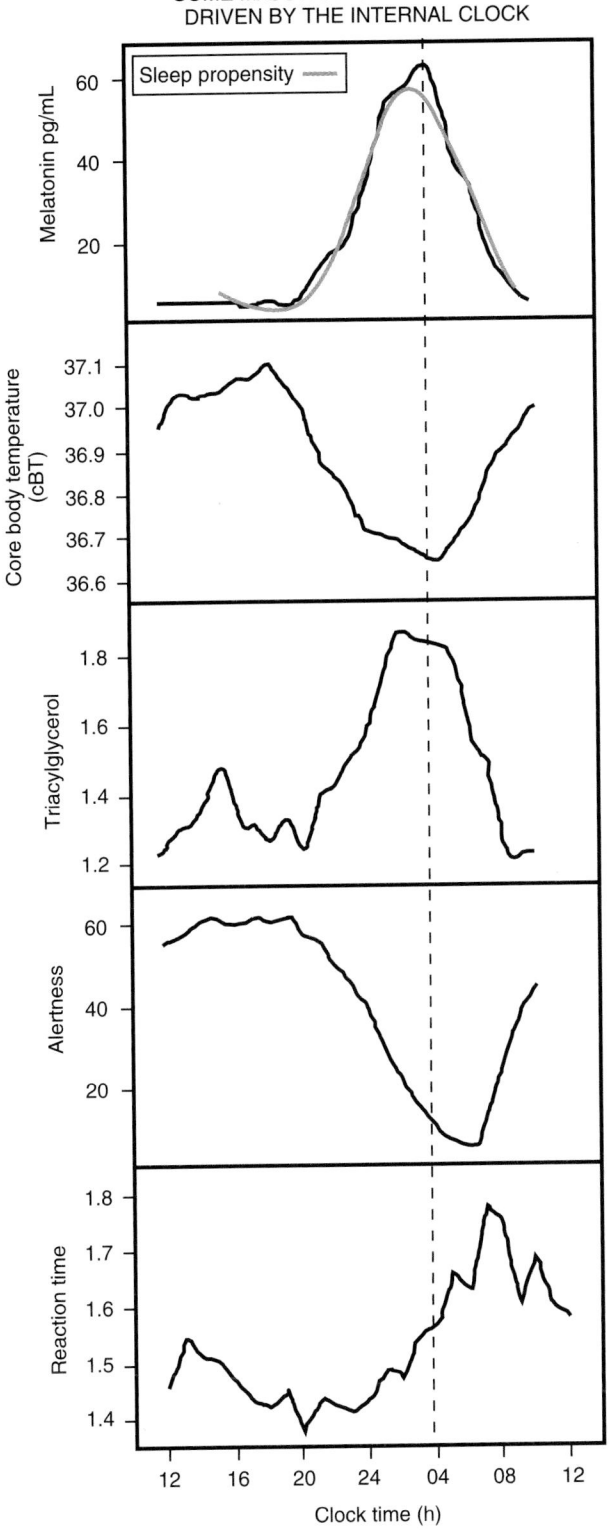

SOME MAJOR CIRCADIAN RHYTHMS
DRIVEN BY THE INTERNAL CLOCK

Figure 31-5 Relationship of plasma melatonin to other major circadian rhythms. Note the close correspondence between the core temperature nadir and the melatonin peak. (Source: Reproduced from Rajaratnam SMW and Arendt J. Lancet 358:999–1005, 2001, by permission.)

sinus tumors, mixed germ cell tumors), pineal parenchymal cells (pineoblastoma and pineocytoma), and the supporting stroma (gliomas).[125,126] All are rare (fewer than 1% of intracranial space-occupying lesions) and tend to occur in individuals younger than 20 years, with the exception of parenchymal cell tumors, which occur equally in adults and children. Germinomas respond well to radiation therapy, whereas primary surgery is more frequently the treatment of choice in other types. Tumor markers in cerebrospinal fluid (CSF), such as α-fetoprotein and β-hCG, together with CSF cytology and imaging (computed tomography or magnetic resonance imaging) aid in the differential diagnosis. The most common symptoms are secondary to hydrocephalus (headache, vomiting, and drowsiness), together with the triad of visual problems, diabetes insipidus, and reproductive abnormalities.[125] Germinomas and teratomas occur predominantly in males. Both precocious puberty and delayed puberty have been associated with pineal tumors. Precocious puberty is more commonly associated with teratoma. Cohen and coworkers[124] have reviewed the occurrence of precocious puberty in parallel with β-hCG-secreting pineal tumors. Because β-hCG is identical to β-LH, they conclude that pubertal development can be directly attributed to ectopic β-hCG production in many cases. Moreover, the predominance in boys may be explained on the basis that LH alone can stimulate testosterone production, whereas in girls, both LH and follicle-stimulating hormone (FSH) are required for ovarian follicular development and estrogen production

No information is consistent on overproduction or underproduction of melatonin with specific types of tumor. Recent work suggests that melatonin is absent or very low in treated or untreated pineal germinomas, but the consequences remain to be defined.[82]

However, pinealectomy removes circulating melatonin,[9,81] and radiation therapy appears to greatly suppress melatonin. At present, long-term evaluation of patients after surgery indicates that headache, disturbance of vision, afternoon sleepiness, mood disorders, visual and auditory hallucinations, and convulsive seizures are among the sequelae that have been reported following pineal ablation, although to what extent any of these relates to absence of the pineal gland is debatable.[127]

Other Solid Tumors

The relationship of the pineal gland and melatonin to cancer is a subject that has aroused much interest after early work suggesting that the pineal gland contains oncostatic activity. Cohen and coworkers proposed in 1978 that human breast cancer is a melatonin-deficient disease.[128] Since that time, many clinical studies have been performed to assess melatonin secretion in cancer patients. Low levels may be associated at least with (stage-dependent) breast and prostatic cancer[129,130]; however, not all studies are consistent. A number of broad studies that have included various oncologic conditions report significant differences, both increases and decreases, in plasma melatonin between types of cancer and control populations. At present, these studies are difficult to interpret. Some data suggest that the growth of human benign prostate epithelial cells depends on both steroids and melatonin.[131]

Considerable prominence has been given to the hypothesis that an increased risk of breast cancer in night shift workers is due to suppression of melatonin by light at night.[132] A causal connection has not been established, and many other factors (such as continual disruption of the circadian system in general) may be involved. Moreover, the association of childhood leukemia with environmental exposure to electromagnetic fields (EMF) has also been attributed to melatonin suppression by EMF. There is little convincing evidence for this association, and most recent data deny any acute suppression of melatonin in humans by EMF.[133]

General Pathology

Many clinical attempts have been made to relate circulating melatonin to endocrine and other pathology. The common finding (if sampling is suitable for rhythm detection) is usually that abnormal timing or amplitude of the rhythm is seen in disease. The results are often difficult to interpret. Liver disease such as cirrhosis, which impairs metabolic function, leads to higher than normal plasma concentrations of melatonin. Drugs that stimulate or suppress hydroxylation and conjugation mechanisms, that compete for metabolic pathways, or that modify pineal neural input mechanisms can be expected to affect circulating melatonin. Drugs that modify light sensitivity may well also affect melatonin.

Low melatonin is reported to associate (inter alia) with cardiovascular disease and diabetic autonomic neuropathy.[134,135] Studies of intensive care unit patients have shown very abnormal rhythms, but the data are confounded by the concomitant medication. Surprisingly, little evidence exists for a disturbance in melatonin secretion in major sleep disorders such as narcolepsy and Kleine-Levin syndrome.[9] In delayed sleep-phase insomnia, a small delay in the rhythm is usually found.[9,136]

Many clinical studies have not adequately controlled for factors unrelated to disease that influence melatonin (e.g., ambient light, posture, hospitalized patients versus outpatient control population). If all of these are taken into account, it would not be surprising if a patient, recumbent, in hospital lighting, with hospital hours of waking up, meals, and so on, and subjected to invasive procedures, has an abnormal melatonin rhythm compared to free-living humans.

Psychiatry

Abnormalities in circadian function have been postulated in depression and mania. Melatonin is arguably the best index of biologic clock function; only bright light and, to a smaller extent, posture "mask" expression of the endogenous rhythm,[25,137] and it has been extensively used in psychiatry and other fields to assess biologic clock status. Studies have shown a decline in amplitude of the melatonin rhythm in patients with depression, together with an increase in cortisol and possibly an increase in mania, although not all studies are consistent.[138]

Little evidence for abnormal timing of melatonin has been found, although Lewy and coworkers have reported exceptionally delayed melatonin rhythms in winter in patients with seasonal affective disorder as compared with the small delay seen in normal individuals,[139] and Parry and coworkers have observed abnormal melatonin patterns and response to light in patients with premenstrual dysphoric disorder.[140] At present, no consensus has been reached regarding what causes seasonal affective disorder. The treatment that was originally proposed for patients with this disorder was the creation of an artificial summer day length by using 3 hours of bright full-spectrum light (Vitalite, 2500 lux) in the morning and evening.[42] The melatonin hypothesis predicted that such light treatment would shorten the duration of melatonin secretion, thus generating a summer day length signal by analogy with animal work. The light treatment appears to be efficient (albeit with a large placebo effect), but it does not appear to work through suppression of melatonin. However, there is good evidence that morning light is somewhat more effective than evening light, which supports the phase-delay hypothesis.

Many pharmacologic antidepressant treatments stimulate melatonin secretion by acting through increased availability of the precursors tryptophan and serotonin and the major pineal neurotransmitter norepinephrine or by direct action on serotonin and catecholamine receptors.[138] A link between an increase in melatonin production and the efficacy of treatment may be possible, and this prospect merits exploration.

EFFECTS OF MELATONIN IN HUMANS

THERAPEUTIC POTENTIAL AND SIGNIFICANCE TO HEALTH

A very large number of people would benefit from the ability to manipulate rhythms at will. Circadian rhythm disturbance is associated with shift work, jet lag, blindness, insomnia, and old age (among other things). A search for a general chronobiotic—a compound that is able to rapidly shift the biologic clock in all its manifestations—occupies much scientific time and effort. Bright light in suitable intensity, timing, spectral composition, and duration is able to shift the biologic clock. A number of pharmaceutical products and steroid hormones have been shown to shift aspects of the circadian system in animals, usually the activity-rest cycle. Importantly, the use of melatonin and its analogues in this area has become evident. Many claims have been made for therapeutic actions other than adjustment of rhythms, and indeed melatonin does have effects on numerous systems. However, human data are rather sparse, and to the author's knowledge, no clinical consensus has emerged other than for its actions on sleep and the circadian system. Moreover, confusion reigns as to whether the apparently nonchronobiotic effects of melatonin nevertheless relate to biologic rhythmicity via, for example, optimization of internal phase relationships.

EARLY WORK

Enormous doses of up to 6.6 g (the daily production of about 200,000 people!) in the daytime had no beneficial effects on parkinsonism, Huntington's chorea, depression (which was worsened), and schizophrenia. Skin pigmentation was not affected; human pigment cells do not resemble amphibian melanophores in pigment migration phenomena. Small decreases in plasma LH and FSH were observed (see Arendt[9] for references). Large amounts of melatonin such as these may produce headache, abdominal cramps, and somnolence.

Much lower (2 mg intranasally, 0.3 to 240 mg orally or intravenously) doses of melatonin during the "biologic day," that is, when endogenous melatonin levels are low, can induce transient sleepiness or sleep and lower core body temperature in suitably controlled circumstances (posture is important, the greatest effects being seen with recumbent subjects in very dim light).[96,136,141,142] The first evidence dates from 40 years ago when Aaron Lerner, who first isolated the substance, took 100 mg and described sleepiness after the dose.[143] Early investigations used EEG characteristics to delimit an acute mild sedative and "hypnotic" effect in both animals (cats, rats, chickens) and humans.[9,141,142] Subsequently, a substantial body of literature, generally using much lower doses, has described advance shifts in the timing of sleep after early evening administration, transient sleepiness at several different times of day within 2 to 4 hours of the dose, time-dependent increases in sleep propensity, effects on the waking EEG comparable to but not identical with those of benzodiazepines, a lengthening of the first rapid eye movement episode after early evening administration, increases in the fast EEG frequencies after evening naps or nighttime sleep, and "beneficial effects" when taken at bedtime. The subject has been extensively reviewed recently.[141,142,144] A brief decline in performance, but with no effect on memory, has been reported after daytime melatonin administration.[145] Acute oral doses of melatonin stimulate prolactin secretion.[146] This enhanced prolactin secretion may relate to the ability of melatonin in pharmacologic amounts to inhibit some dopaminergic functions. Acute effects on other pituitary hormones are somewhat inconsistent, although a relationship between melatonin and vasopressin secretion has recently been established.[147]

ACUTE PHARMACOLOGY

The acute pharmacologic properties of melatonin in animals include sedation, hypothermia, anxiolysis, muscle hypotonia, decrease in locomotor activity with a rebound increase on increasing the dose, slight analgesia, slight protection against electroconvulsive shock, constriction of cerebral arteries, potentiation of noradrenalin-induced vasoconstriction, and very low toxicity.[148–150]

A large number of publications now address the "neuroprotective" effects of melatonin (as antioxidant and free-radical scavenger) in animal models, with as yet little human data. The interactions of melatonin with peripheral and central membrane receptors, nuclear receptors and intracellular proteins, such as calmodulin- or tubulin-associated proteins, as well as its direct or indirect antioxidant effects open the way to possible effects on multiple systems. However, the most convincing and largest body of data supports its effects as a chronobiotic: a substance that changes the timing of the biologic clock. In this respect, the timing of treatment is critical.

TIMED ADMINISTRATION

In early work, daily feeding of low-dose (2 to 5 mg) melatonin in the late afternoon advanced the timing of evening self-rated fatigue, the endogenous melatonin rhythm, and the morning decline in prolactin when compared with placebo. No significant effects were seen on self-rated mood or on LH, FSH, testosterone, cortisol, growth hormone, or thyroxine. No deleterious effects were reported by the subjects.[9] Thus, in low doses, melatonin has some chronobiotic effects in humans. Melatonin has rapid, transient, mild sleep-inducing effects and lowers alertness and body temperature during the 3 to 4 hours after low doses (0.5 to 5 mg) during the daytime, these effects being opposite to the acute effects of bright light given at night.[89,151] In the same dose range, melatonin is able to shift timing of the internal clock to both later and earlier times when administration is appropriately timed.[96,151–154] As for light, the appropriate timing can be predicted from a phase-response curve in subjects whose body clock phase is known. The phase-response curve to melatonin is essentially the reverse of that to light.[153] Melatonin given approximately 8 to 13 hours before core temperature minimum will produce phase advances and when given around 1 to 4 hours after core temperature minimum will produce phase delays (Fig. 31-6). A recent carefully controlled study showed convincingly that daily administration of a "surge-sustained" release preparation (1.5 mg) of melatonin at 1600h followed by recumbency and very dim light for 16 hours led to substantial phase advances of a number of circadian marker rhythms and an advanced timing and redistribution of sleep during the dark phase.[96] No increase in total sleep time was seen, reinforcing the view that melatonin acts on the timing mechanisms of sleep rather than being a hypnotic. There were no deleterious effects on pituitary/gonadal hormones or daytime alertness. In this dose, reinforced by recumbency and dim light, melatonin is clearly very effective at shifting the circadian clock and sleep timing.[96]

Most important, perhaps, recent data (Fig. 31-7) have shown that timed melatonin administration (0.5 to 5 mg at 24-hour intervals, usually at desired bedtime) can fully entrain (or synchronize) the free-running circadian rhythms of most blind subjects exhibiting this phenomenon, with a consequent improvement in sleep and daytime alertness.[155,156] These observations, from two competing laboratories, indicate that melatonin can be as effective as light for circadian rhythm management and is the treatment of choice for non-24-hour sleep-wake disorder of the blind.

JET LAG AND SHIFT WORK

Melatonin treatment that is timed to induce phase advances and delays has been used in the alleviation of jet lag in at least 14 real-life and simulation conditions, 11 of which reported beneficial effects. Field studies show that self-rated jet lag both westward and eastward can be reduced on average by 50% with appropriately timed treatment (reviewed in Refs. 157 and 158). The improvement appears to be greater with larger numbers of time zones. The subjective impressions are reinforced by improved latency and quality of sleep, greater daytime alertness, and slightly more rapid resynchronization of melatonin and cortisol rhythms. Comparable simulation studies have shown a significant increase in the rate of reentrainment of both hormonal and electrolyte rhythms and an immediate effect of lowering body temperature that persists as more rapid reentrainment.[158] Neither the dose nor the timing of melatonin administration has been fully optimized, although one study reported, with respect to alleviating sleep problems, that 5 mg was more effective than 0.5 mg and a slow-release preparation taken at bedtime after flight.[158] Three studies have shown no effect; a common factor in two was that the subjects were not adapted to local time before departure, with consequent problems for timing the treatment. The third also appeared to use inappropriate timing of treatment. Unpredictable exposure to bright light can theoretically act in opposition to the desired result. A Cochrane review recently concluded that timed melatonin was effective as a jet lag treatment.[159]

Exposure to bright light sufficient to suppress melatonin secretion during the night is clearly beneficial to night-shift workers in terms of alertness and reduced sleepiness. Preliminary work suggested improved sleep and increased daytime alertness in night-shift workers receiving melatonin at the desired bedtime during a night-shift week as compared with placebo and baseline conditions.[157] A number of recent studies have successfully used melatonin to adapt to simulated or real shift work (reviewed in Ref. 160), although it has to be said that several reports in the literature have shown no beneficial effects. Questions of posture, light environment, and timing need to be resolved in field studies.

BLINDNESS

Only a small number of subjects have been studied to date, but undoubtedly, most blind or visually impaired subjects who report sleep problems derive benefit from melatonin ingestion at the desired bedtime or specifically timed according to the circadian phase (see Fig. 31-7).[144,157,161–164] Melatonin was strikingly effective at improving sleep and behavior in multiply handicapped children with or without visual impairment.[165]

SLEEP PROBLEMS OF OLD AGE

Increasing numbers of positive reports now indicate that some subjects will derive benefit from melatonin administration. It is possible that very low doses are more useful than 2 to 5 mg and that improvement is seen when an underlying rhythm disorder is present rather than nonspecific insomnia. Dose timing and formulation remain to be optimized.[141,166]

DELAYED SLEEP-PHASE INSOMNIA

Patients with delayed sleep-phase insomnia cannot sleep at the socially acceptable time of night; they delay sleep onset until the early hours of the morning and sleep through much of the day. This condition has been successfully treated with bright light in the early morning to induce phase advances of the clock. In others, evening melatonin (5 mg at 10:00 P.M.

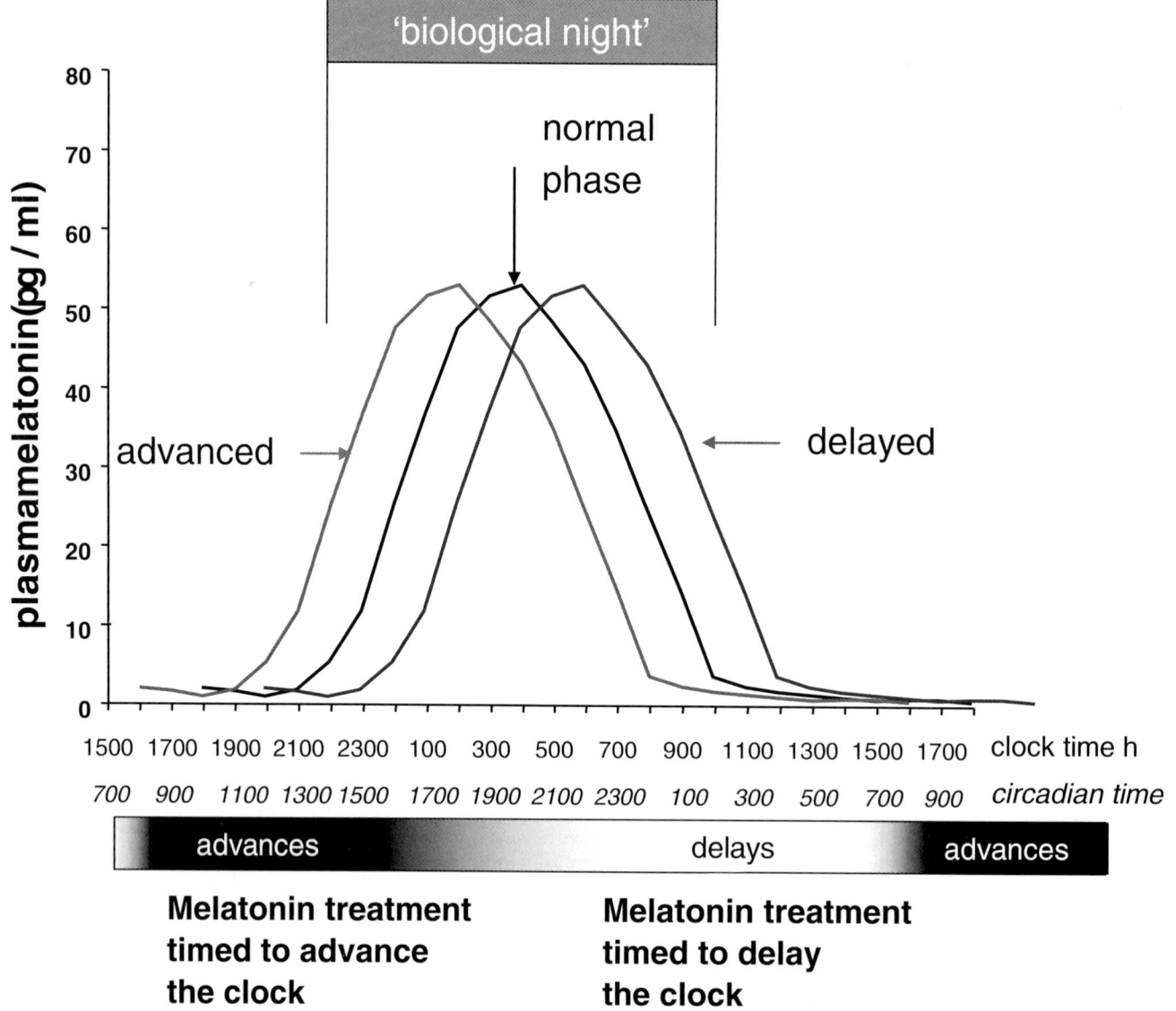

Figure 31-6 Diagram to illustrate the timing of melatonin treatment, relative to the endogenous melatonin rhythm, to induce phase advances or phase delays, based on published phase response curves[152,153,154] reproduced from Ref. 144 by permission. The probability of obtaining advances or delays is maximum in the totally dark or the totally light sections of the bar; in gray areas, individual differences are apparent.

or 5 hours ahead of endogenous melatonin onset[144]) also advances sleep time significantly. Judicious, timed application of both melatonin and bright light as time cues may well be the treatment of choice for such rhythm disturbances.

CANCER

Animal studies have provided good evidence for photoperiod dependency and/or melatonin responsiveness of the initiation and evolution of certain cancers, particularly hormone-dependent cancers. Oncostatic effects are reported in some human cell lines, and in general, the pineal gland and melatonin appear to have antitumor activity.[9,167–170] In dimethylbenzanthracene-induced mammary tumors in rats, pinealectomy greatly increased the incidence of induced tumor growth, and daily melatonin administration in the late light phase greatly decreased its incidence.[167] Not all reports show positive results, however. Positive effects of combination therapy-melatonin and tamoxifen, melatonin, and interleukin have been reported; most recently, survival time and quality of life were significantly enhanced by adjunct

melatonin therapy in small cell carcinoma of the lung.[170] Melatonin, when appropriately administered, may have stimulatory effects on aspects of the immune system, and positive effects on cancer may be a consequence. The evidence that melatonin may also act as a free-radical scavenger has been discussed previously. A recent review[170] addresses the general question of the circadian system in relation to cancer.

SITES AND MECHANISM OF ACTION OF MELATONIN

TARGET SITES

The actions of melatonin are multiple, and many must derive essentially from modification of events in the central nervous system. However, peripheral actions are of considerable interest. The molecule is highly lipophilic, with widely distributed potential sites of action. Obvious potential target sites in mammals, from the foregoing discussion, are the retina, the SCN and other central neuroendocrine control systems, and the pituitary gland. Concentrations of melatonin in the CSF

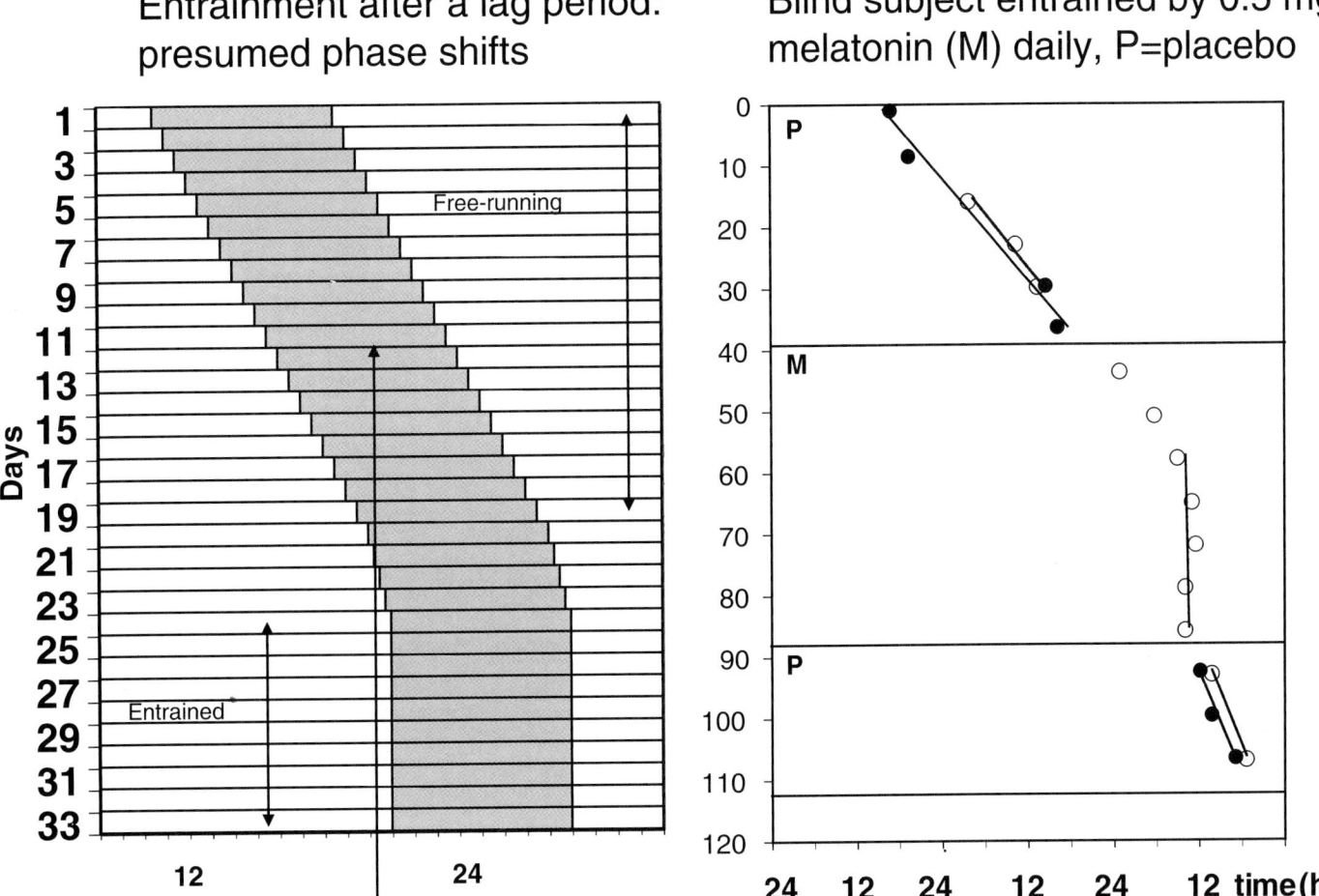

Entrainment after a lag period: presumed phase shifts

Blind subject entrained by 0.5 mg melatonin (M) daily, P=placebo

Melatonin daily at the same clock time

Period of melatonin secretion: biological night

Figure 31-7 Use of melatonin to entrain free running subjects to 24 hours. **Left panel,** Theoretical diagram; the gray bars show the period of melatonin secretion ("biologic night") free-running with placebo or no treatment, with presumed phase shifts due to melatonin treatment (2130h). Melatonin (daily from day 12 of free run) is initially timed such that the daily circadian delay due to free run moves the treatment time into a phase advance position. Small phase advances (shortening the period) and eventual entrainment occur. **Right panel,** Actual data from a totally blind subject treated with melatonin (M, 0.5 mg fast release) or placebo (P, lactose-gelatin) daily at bedtime, initially in a phase delay window, entrainment after a lag (3 to 4 weeks) occurs when the treatment falls within a phase advance window. Urinary cortisol (*open circles*) and 6-sulphatoxymelatonin (*solid circles*) acrophases are derived at weekly intervals. Free-running rhythms are evident during placebo treatment followed by entrainment with melatonin. Most subjects treated with 0.5 mg fast-release melatonin have been entrained. (Source: From Refs. 144 and 163 by permission.)

of ungulates are reported to be much higher than those in plasma.

Lesions of the SCN and the anterior hypothalamic area can block the photoperiodic and/or circadian effects of melatonin in some rodents, but with a degree of disparity between laboratories.[171] Implants or infusion of melatonin in the hypothalamus mimics or blocks photoperiodic responses in several species.[171-174] In prepubertal rats, melatonin inhibits GnRH-induced LH release in pituitary cultures at concentrations comparable to those circulating in the blood.[58] Melatonin clearly influences GnRH secretion from the hypothalamus (for example, in cocultures of the median eminence and pars tuberalis).[175] Good evidence indicates that melatonin controls the seasonal variations in prolactin secretion in ungulates via receptors in the pars tuberalis. It also appears that a circannual rhythm in prolactin is generated within the pars tuberalis itself.[176]

EFFECTS ON CLOCK GENES

Probably the most interesting development in the mechanistic aspects of the effects of melatonin concerns its influence on gene expression in the pars tuberalis. Many clock genes are expressed in the pars tuberalis (*Bmal1, Clock, Per1, Per2, Cry1, Cry2*) with a 24-hour rhythmicity that is different from their expression in the SCN. *Per1* is activated at the beginning of the light phase, and *Cry1* at the beginning of the dark phase. Long or short photoperiod information is encoded within the SCN. Melatonin synthesis, driven by the SCN, conveys this photoperiodic information to the pars tuberalis by virtue of its pattern of secretion. This in turn influences the pattern of expression of the clock genes *Per1* and *Cry1* within the pars tuberalis providing a means of translating the melatonin signal for the control of seasonal prolactin variations. Melatonin target sites in the hypothalamus influencing seasonal variations in reproductive hormones have yet to be fully defined, and so far, melatonin does not appear to influence clock gene expression in the SCN. However, it has been proposed that other "calendar" cells will be identified in the CNS that regulate seasonal changes other than prolactin and may use the relative phasing of clock gene expression for translating the photoperiodic (melatonin) signal.[177]

In rodent pars tuberalis cells, rhythmic expression of *Per1* appears to be dependent on sensitization of adenosine A2b receptors, which in turn depends on melatonin activation of MT1 receptors.[178,179] Clearly, it is possible that the melatonin signal is a widespread humoral mechanism related to biologic timing, acting through modification of clock gene expression. It appears not to be of major importance to SCN oscillations, but it is within the peripheral pars tuberalis system. The effects of melatonin on peripheral, as well as central, clock gene expression is likely to be a rich field of inquiry.

UPTAKE AND BINDING STUDIES

The development of 2-^{125}I-iodomelatonin as a high-specific-activity ligand has permitted the identification of high-affinity (K_d of 25 to 175 pM), saturable, specific, and reversible melatonin binding to cell membranes in the central nervous system, initially in the SCN[180] and the pars tuberalis of the pituitary[181] and subsequently in many brain and other areas, including cells of the immune system, a number of cancer cell lines, the gonads, the kidney, and, importantly, the cardiovascular system. The SCN shows clear binding in human postmortem tissue.[182,183] Species variation of melatonin-binding sites in the brain is of course apparent. The most consistent (but not universal) binding site between mammalian species is the pars tuberalis, primarily implicated in transduction of the effects of photoperiod, via melatonin, on seasonal variations in prolactin secretion in ruminants.[184]

Changes in detectable binding are seen with age; for example, in fetal rats, the first appearance of binding is in the pituitary: pars distalis and pars tuberalis, with SCN labeling appearing in later gestation. Pars distalis binding is absent in adult rats but persists after birth in the neonate.[185] This finding suggests that binding may indeed underlie function, inasmuch as melatonin inhibits GnRH-induced pituitary LH release in prepuberty but not in adulthood. Changes are also seen with the time of day, with season, and as a function of exposure to melatonin.[186-189]

Krause and Dubocovich have demonstrated a functional melatonin receptor initially in rabbit and chicken retina (inhibition of calcium-dependent dopamine release) that is localized in rabbit dopamine-containing amacrine cells in the inner plexiform, in the outer and inner segments in mice, and possibly in the pigmented layer in some mammals.[189]

The interaction of melatonin with nuclear receptors and intracellular proteins, such as calmodulin or tubulin-associated proteins, has also been reported.[182]

MELATONIN RECEPTOR PHARMACOLOGY

White and coworkers initially demonstrated that melatonin-induced pigment aggregation in amphibian melanophores is a pertussis toxin-sensitive system and that melatonin inhibits forskolin-activated cAMP formation.[190] Inhibition of cAMP production may be a general feature of melatonin receptors. Intensive investigation of the properties of the pars tuberalis–binding site has revealed that physiologic doses of melatonin inhibit forskolin-activated cAMP production in vitro in a time- and dose-related manner.[181,191] Other studies have provided good evidence that most binding sites are coupled to G proteins. Guanosine triphosphate analogues, which interfere with the regeneration of G_i-coupled receptors, decrease the affinity and sometimes the capacity of ^{125}I-melatonin binding in reptiles, birds, and mammals.

Melatonin receptors have been cloned, and three subtypes were initially named Mel-1a, Mel-1b, and Mel-1c.[191] The Mel 1a receptor gene has been mapped to human chromosome 4q35.1. Its primary expression is in the pars tuberalis of the pituitary and the SCN. Mel 1b has been mapped to chromosome 11q21-22, and its main expression is in the retina and the brain. Mel 1c is not found in mammals. Two cloned mammalian receptors (Mel 1a, Mel 1b) have now been renamed MT1 and MT2.[192] They are a new family of G protein–coupled receptors, have high affinity (K_d 20 to 160 picomolar), and inhibit forskolin-stimulated cAMP formation. Using gene knockout technology and pharmacologic manipulations, the results to date suggest that the phase shifting receptor is MT2, while MT1 is associated with acute suppression of SCN electrical activity in addition to its important actions within the pars tuberalis. Several other physiologic responses have been ascribed to MT1 and MT2 receptors, including (MT1) melatonin-mediated potentiation of adreneregic vasoconstriction and (MT2) modulation of dopamine release in the retina.[193-195] Genetic polymorphism has been identified within melatonin receptors, and further investigation of these polymorphisms in relation to photoperioidism, human disease, sensitivity to melatonin, and so on is ongoing.[196]

MELATONIN ANTAGONISTS AND AGONISTS

Large numbers of putative and actual melatonin agonists together with some antagonists have now been described. It is anticipated that much new information in this area will be available shortly; however, to the author's knowledge, none are available as yet as a registered medication.[197]

SUMMARY

The pineal gland, the retina, and the SCN together form the basic structures that perceive and transduce the nonvisual effects of light. Melatonin forms a closed loop to this system. The primary physiologic role of melatonin is to serve as a humoral signal of day length information for the timing of seasonal events in photoperiodic species, whether nocturnal or diurnal, long or short day breeders. Evidence of residual human seasonality and photoperiodic responses suggests that in the right conditions, it has the potential to act as a seasonal time cue in humans. However, the almost universal presence of artificial lighting and the imposed artificial work and sleep times in temperate zones are likely to be responsible for the minor seasonal changes that are evident in urban humans. Although changes in melatonin are associated with human puberty (normal and pathologic), a role in human puberty remains elusive. In diurnal humans, nighttime melatonin secretion reinforces events that occur at night (sleep, for example). It does not appear to be essential for normal circadian function but modulates response to changing time cues as an adjunct to light and possibly, in some circumstances, in conflict with light. Its ability to facilitate sleep and to shift the timing of the circadian clock has led to substantial therapeutic applications in circadian rhythm disorders (Fig. 31-8). In particular, it is the treatment of choice for non-24-hour sleep-wake disorder of the blind. It has generally been found to have anticancer effects, but the mechanisms that are involved remain to be clarified. Its actions as a free-radical scavenger and possible immunostimulant may well be of therapeutic interest, as well as numerous other effects. SCN receptors mediate the central circadian effects of melatonin, those in the mediobasal hypothalamus and pars tuberalis influence photoperiodic seasonal reproduction with regard to gonadotropin secretion and prolactin, respectively, and those in the retina mediate the retinal processes influenced by melatonin. Melatonin receptors are widespread in

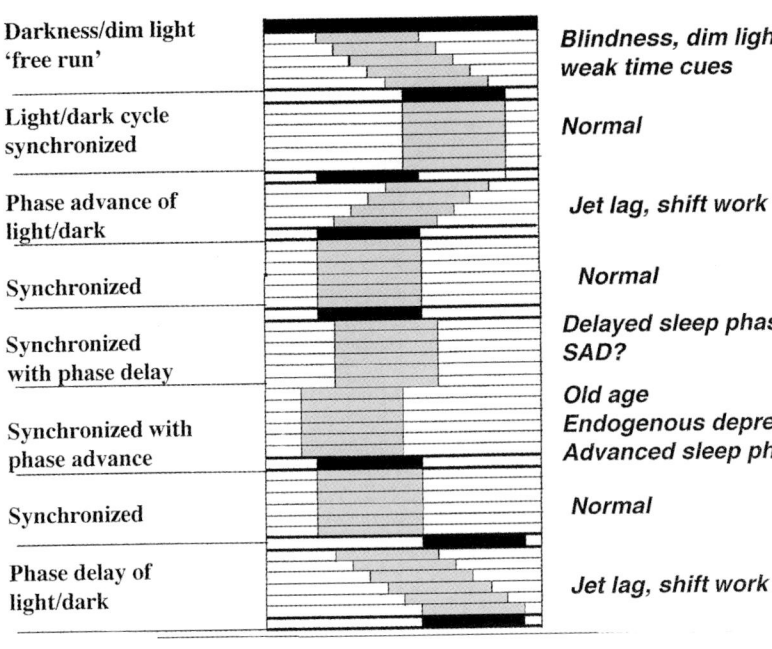

Darkness/dim light 'free run'

Light/dark cycle synchronized

Phase advance of light/dark

Synchronized

Synchronized with phase delay

Synchronized with phase advance

Synchronized

Phase delay of light/dark

Blindness, dim light weak time cues

Normal

Jet lag, shift work

Normal

Delayed sleep phase SAD?

Old age Endogenous depression Advanced sleep phase

Normal

Jet lag, shift work

Figure 31-8 Circadian rhythm disorders. *White and black filled bars* represent the light-dark cycle. *Gray filled bars* represent the timing of an endogenous circadian rhythm. In constant darkness or dim light with weak time cues, circadian rhythms free run, usually by delay, and show endogenous periodicity (*top panel*). In a normal environment, rhythms are synchronized to 24 hours (*second panel*). After an abrupt advance shift (eastward) of time cues, endogenous rhythms adapt via "transients"; during this time of desynchrony, sleep, alertness, performance, gastrointestinal function, metabolism, and other systems are disturbed (*third panel*). In the *fourth panel*, rhythms are synchronized to the new time cues. The *fifth panel* shows synchronized rhythms but with a phase delay relative to the environment. In the *sixth panel*, rhythms are synchronized but with a phase advance relative to the environment. The *seventh panel* shows normally synchronized rhythms. In the *eighth panel* is an abrupt phase delay (westward) of the light-dark cycle and adaptation by transients. Westward adaptation is usually faster than eastward. All these conditions are susceptible to timed treatment by substances (such as melatonin) that shift rhythms or by manipulating rhythms with light of suitable intensity and duration. (Source: Adapted from Arendt J: Melatonin and the Mammalian Pineal Gland. London, Chapman & Hall, 1995, p 71. With kind permission of Kluwer Academic Publishers.)

peripheral as well as central tissues, and the potential for modification of peripheral gene expression (as well as the demonstrable influence on gene expression in the pars tuberalis) is of interest. It is reasonable to conclude that in humans, melatonin serves to modulate circadian phase and strengthen coupling. It is likely that disturbed circadian rhythms are associated with many conditions other than the commonly cited jet lag and shift work—hence the importance of this "hormone of darkness."

Acknowledgments

This review was written during the tenure of grants from the Health and Safety Executive (UK), the Institute of Petroleum (UK), the National Grid (UK), and the Antarctic funding Initiative (UK). The author is grateful to these bodies as well as to the numerous funding agencies and commercial organizations that have supported her work on the pineal gland, melatonin, and biologic rhythms for many years.

REFERENCES

1. Vollrath L: The Pineal Organ. Heidelberg, Germany, Springer-Verlag, 1981.
2. Collin JP: Differentiation and regression of the cells of the sensory line in the epiphysis cerebri. In Wolstenholme GEW, Knight J (eds): The Pineal Gland. Edinburgh, Churchill Livingstone, 1972, pp 79–125.
3. Korf H-W, Moller M, Gery I, et al: Immunocytochemical demonstration of retinal S antigen in the pineal organ of four mammalian species. Cell Tissue Res 239:81–85, 1985.
4. Welsh MG: Pineal calcification: Structural and functional aspects. Pineal Res Rev 3:41–68, 1985.
5. Tapp E: The histology and pathology of the human pineal gland. Prog Brain Res 52:481–500, 1979.
6. Bojkowski C, Arendt J: Factors influencing urinary 6-sulphatoxymelatonin, a major melatonin metabolite, in normal human subjects. Clin Endocrinol 33:435–444, 1990.
7. Kappers JA: Innervation of the epiphysis cerebri in the albino rat. Anat Rec 136:220–221, 1960.
8. Moller M, Baeres FMM. The anatomy and innervation of the mammalian pineal gland. Cell Tissue Res 309:139–150, 2002.
9. Arendt J: Melatonin and the Mammalian Pineal Gland. London, Chapman & Hall, 1995.
10. Lerner AB, Case JD, Takahashi Y, et al: Isolation of melatonin, pineal factor that lightens melanocytes. J Am Chem Soc 80:2587, 1958.
11. Axelrod J: The pineal gland: A neurochemical transducer. Science 184:1341–1348, 1974.
12. Klein DC, Coon SL, Roseboom PH, et al: The melatonin rhythm generating enzyme: Molecular regulation of serotonin-N-acetyl transferase in the pineal gland. Rec Prog Horm Res 52:307–358, 1997.
13. Cassone VM, Natesan AK: Time and time again: The phylogeny of melatonin as a transducer of biological time. J Biol Rhythms 12:489–497, 1997.
14. Reppert SM, Weaver DR: Molecular analysis of mammalian circadian rhythms. Annu Rev Physiol 63:647–676, 2001.
15. Gastel J, Roseboom PH, Rinaldi PA, et al: Melatonin production: Proteasomal proteolysis in serotonin N-acetyltransferase regulation. Science 279:1358–1360, 1998.
16. Klein DC, Ganguly S, Coon S, et al: 14-3-3 Proteins and photoneuroendocrine transduction: Role in controlling the daily rhythm in melatonin. Biochem Soc Trans 30:365–373, 2002.
17. Maronde E, Schomerus C, Stehle JH, Korf HW: Control of CREB phosphorylation and its role for induction of melatonin synthesis in rat pinealocytes. Biol Cell 89:505–511, 1998.
18. Tosini G, Menaker M: Circadian rhythms in cultured mammalian retina. Science 272:419–421, 1996.
19. Cavallo A, Ritschel WA: Pharmacokinetics of melatonin in human sexual maturation. J Clin Endocrinol Metab 81:1882–1886, 1996.
20. Pevet P: Physiological role of neuropeptides in the mammalian pineal gland. Adv Pineal Res 6:275–282, 1991.
21. Simonneaux V, Ribelayga C: Generation of the melatonin endocrine message in mammals: a review of the complex regulation of melatonin synthesis by norepinephrine, peptides, and other pineal transmitters. Pharmacol Rev 55(2):325–395, 2003.
22. Poggeler B, Balzer I, Hardeland R, Lerchl A: Pineal hormone melatonin oscillates also in the dinoflagellate Gonyaulax polyedra. Naturwissenschaften 78:268–269, 1991.

23. Murch SJ, Simmons CB, Saxena PK: Melatonin in feverfew and other medicinal plants. Lancet 350:1598–1599, 1997.
24. Evered D, Clark S (eds): Photoperiodism, Melatonin and the Pineal. Ciba Foundation Symposium 117. London, Pitman, 1985.
25. Wever RA: Light effects on human circadian rhythms: A review of recent Andechs experiments. J Biol Rhythms 4:161–185, 1989.
26. Middleton B, Arendt J, Stone B. Human circadian rhythms in constant dim light (<8 lux) with knowledge of clock time. J Sleep Res 5:69–76, 1996.
27. Czeisler CA, Duffy JF, Shanahan TL, et al: Stability, precision, and near-24-hour period of the human circadian pacemaker. Science 284:5423 2177–2181, 1999.
28. Rusak B, Zucker I: Neural regulation of circadian rhythms. Physiol Rev 59:449–526, 1979.
29. Lewy AJ, Newsome DA: Different types of melatonin circadian secretory rhythms in some blind subjects. J Clin Endocrinol Metab 56:1103–1107, 1983.
30. Lockley SW, Skene DJ, Arendt J, et al: Relationship between melatonin rhythms and visual loss in the blind. J Clin Endocrinol Metab 82:3763–3770, 1997.
31. Sumova A, Jac M, Sladek M, Sauman I, Illnerova H: Clock gene daily profiles and their phase relationship in the rat suprachiasmatic nucleus are affected by photoperiod. J Biol Rhythms 18(2):134–144, 2003.
32. Cassone VM: Effects of melatonin on vertebrate circadian systems. Trends Neurosci 13:457–463, 1990.
33. Wehr TA: The durations of human melatonin secretion and sleep respond to changes in daylength (photoperiod). J Clin Endocrinol Metab 73:1276–1280, 1991.
34. Vondrasova-Jelinkova D, Hajek I, Illnerova H: Adjustment of the human melatonin and cortisol rhythms to shortening of the natural summer photoperiod. Brain Res 816:249–253, 1999.
35. Reiter RJ: Action spectra, dose-response relationships and temporal aspects of light's effects on the pineal gland. Ann N Y Acad Sci 453:215–230, 1985.
36. Lewy AJ, Wehr TA, Goodwin FK, et al: Light suppresses melatonin secretion in humans. Science 210:1267–1269, 1980.
37. Thapan K, Arendt J, Skene D: An action spectrum for melatonin suppression: Evidence for a novel non-rod, non-cone photoreceptor system in humans. J Physiol 535:261–267, 2001.
38. Brainard GC, Hanifin JP, Greeson JM, et al: Action spectrum for melatonin regulation in humans: evidence for a novel circadian photoreceptor. J Neurosci 21:6405–6412, 2001.
39. Foster RG, Hankins MW: Non-rod, non-cone photoreception in the vertebrates. Prog Retin Eye Res 21:507–527, 2002.
40. Bojkowski CJ, Aldhous M, English J, et al: Suppression of nocturnal plasma melatonin and 6-sulphatoxymelatonin by bright and dim light in man. Horm Metab Res 19:437–440, 1987.
41. Boivin DB, Czeisler CA: Resetting of circadian melatonin and cortisol rhythms in humans by ordinary room light. Neuroreport 9:779–782, 1998.
42. Rosenthal NE, Sack DA, Gillin JC, et al: Seasonal affective disorder. A description of the syndrome and preliminary findings with light therapy. Arch Gen Psychiatry 41:72–79, 1984.
43. Lincoln GA, Ebling FJP, Almeida OFX: Generation of melatonin rhythms. In Evered D, Clark S (eds): Photoperiodism, Melatonin and the Pineal. Ciba Foundation Symposium 117. London, Pitman, 1985, pp 129–141.
44. Broadway J, Arendt J, Folkard S: Bright light phase shifts the human melatonin rhythm during the Antarctic winter, Neurosci Lett 79:185–189, 1987.
45. Shanahan TL, Czeisler CA: Light exposure induces equivalent phase shifts of the endogenous circadian rhythms of circulating plasma melatonin and core body temperature in man. J Clin Endocrinol Metab 73:227–235, 1991.
46. Warman VL, Dijk D-J, Warman GR, et al: Phase advancing human circadian rhythms with short wavelength light. Neurosci Lett 342:37–40, 2003.
47. Lockley SW, Brainard GC, Czeisler CA: High sensitivity of the human circadian melatonin rhythm to resetting by short wavelength light. J Clin Endocrinol Metab 88:4502–4505, 2003.
48. Middleton B, Stone BM, Arendt J: Human circadian phase in 12:12h, 200:<8 lux and 1000:<8 lux light-dark cycles, without scheduled sleep or activity. Neurosci Lett 329:41–44, 2002.
49. Lockley SW, Skene DJ, Tabandeh H, et al: Relationship between napping and melatonin in the blind. J Biol Rhythms 12:16–25, 1997.
50. Sack R L, Lewy A J, Blood ML, et al: Melatonin administration to blind people: Phase advances and entrainment. J Biol Rhythms 6:249–261, 1991.
51. Czeisler CA, Shanahan TL, Klerman EB, et al: Suppression of melatonin secretion in some blind patients by exposure to bright light. N Engl J Med 332:6–11, 1995.
52. Hoffman K: Photoperiodism in vertebrates. In Aschoff J (ed): Handbook of Behavioural Neurobiology, vol 4. New York, Plenum, 1981, pp 449–473.
53. Ebling FJP, Foster DL: Pineal melatonin rhythms and the timing of puberty in mammals. Experientia 45:946–955, 1989.
54. Arendt J: Role of the pineal gland and melatonin in seasonal reproductive function in mammals. Oxf Rev Reprod Biol 8:266–320, 1986.
55. Malpaux B, Migaud M, Tricoire H, Chemineau P: Biology of mammalian photoperiodism and the critical role of the pineal gland and melatonin. J Biol Rhythms 16:336–347, 2001.
56. Davis F: Melatonin: Role in development. J Biol Rhythms 12:498–508, 1997.
57. Sizonenko PC, Lang U, Rivest RW, et al: The pineal and pubertal development. In Evered D, Clark S (eds): Photoperiodism, Melatonin and the Pineal. Ciba Foundation Symposium 117. London, Pitman, 1985, pp 208–230.
58. Vanecek J: Inhibitory effect of melatonin on GnRH-induced LH release. Rev Reprod 4:67–72, 1999.
59. Badia P, Myers B, Murphy P: Melatonin and thermoregulation. In Reiter RJ, Yu HS (eds): Melatonin: Biosynthesis, Physiological Effects, and Clinical Applications. Boca Raton, FL, CRC Press, 1992.
60. Quay WB: Precocious entrainment and associated characteristics of activity patterns following pinealectomy and reversal of photoperiod. Physiol Behav 5:1281–1290, 1970.
61. Cassone V: The pineal gland influences rat circadian activity rhythms in constant light. J Biol Rhythms 7:27–40, 1992.
62. Krauchi K, Cajochen C, Danilenko KV, Wirz-Justice A: The hypothermic effect of late evening melatonin does not block the phase delay induced by concurrent bright light in human subjects. Neurosci Lett 232:57–61, 1997.
63. Deacon S, English J, Tate J, Arendt J: Atenolol facilitates light induced phase shifts. Neurosci Lett 242:53–56, 1997.
64. Vriend J: Evidence for pineal gland modulation of the neuroendocrine-thyroid axis. Neuroendocrinology 36:68–78, 1983.
65. Armstrong SM: Melatonin and circadian control in mammals. Experientia 45:932–939, 1989.
66. Chesworth MJ, Cassone VM, Armstrong SM: Effects of daily melatonin injections on activity rhythms of rats in constant light. Am J Physiol 253:R101–R107, 1987.
67. Illnerova H: In Klein DC, Moore RY, Reppert SM (eds): Suprachiasmatic Nucleus, The Mind's Clock. Oxford, England, Oxford University Press, 1991, pp 197–219.
68. Schuhler S, Pitrosky B, Kirsch R, Pevet P: Entrainment of locomotor activity rhythm in pinealectomized adult Syrian hamsters by daily melatonin infusion. Behav Brain Res 133:343–350, 2002.
69. Hastings MH, Duffield GE, Ebling FJ, et al: Non-photic signalling in the suprachiasmatic nucleus. Biol Cell 89:495–503, 1998.
70. Bosc MJ: Time of parturition in rats after melatonin administration or change of photoperiod. J Reprod Fertil 80:563–568, 1987.
71. Reiter RJ: Melatonin and human reproduction. Ann Med 1:103–108, 1998.
72. Pierpaoli W, Regelson W: The Melatonin Miracle. New York, Simon & Schuster, 1995.

73. Reppert SM, Weaver DR: Melatonin madness. Cell 83:1059–1062, 1995.

74. Arendt J: Melatonin. Br Med J 312:1242–1243, 1996.

75. Armstrong SM, Redman J: Melatonin: A chronobiotic with anti-aging properties. Med Hypotheses 34:300–309, 1991.

76. Tan DX, Reiter RJ, Manchester LC, et al: Chemical and physical properties and potential mechanisms: Melatonin as a broad spectrum antioxidant and free radical scavenger. Curr Top Med Chem 2:181–197, 2002.

77. Hardeland R, Behrmann G, Fuhrberg B, et al: Evolutionary aspects of indoleamines as radical scavengers: Presence and photocatalytic turnover of indoleamines in a unicell, Gonyaulax polyedra. Adv Exp Med Biol 398:279–284, 1996.

78. Marshall KA, Reiter RJ, Poeggeler B, et al: Evaluation of the antioxidant activity of melatonin in vitro. Free Radic Biol Med 21:307–315, 1996.

79. Gillette MU, McArthur AJ: Circadian actions of melatonin at the suprachiasmatic nucleus. Behav Brain Res 73:135–139, 1996.

80. Iuvone M: In Djamgoz MBA, Archer S, Vallerga S (eds): Neurobiology and Clinical Aspects of the Outer Retina. London, Chapman & Hall, 1995, pp 25–55.

81. Neuwelt EA, Mickey B, Lewy AJ: The importance of melatonin and tumour markers in pineal tumours. J Neural Transm Suppl 21:397–413, 1986.

82. Murata J, Sawamura Y, Ikeda J, et al: Twenty-four hour rhythm of melatonin in patients with a history of pineal and/or hypothalamo-neurohypophyseal germinoma. J Pineal Res 25:159–166, 1998.

83. Czeisler CA: The effect of light on the human circadian pacemaker. In Circadian Clocks and their Adjustment. Ciba Foundation Symposium 183. Chichester, England, Wiley, 1995, pp 254–302.

84. Arendt J: Melatonin. Clin Endocrinol 29:205–229, 1988.

85. Coon SL, Zarazaga LA, Malpaux B, et al: Genetic variability in plasma melatonin in sheep is due to pineal weight, not to variations in enzyme activities. Am J Physiol 277:E792–E797, 1999.

86. Arendt J: Mammalian pineal rhythms. Pineal Res Rev 3:161–213, 1985.

87. Akerstedt T, Froberg JE, Friberg W, Wetterberg L: Melatonin excretion, body temperature and subjective arousal during 64 hours of sleep deprivation. Psychoneuroendocrinology 4:219, 1979.

88. Strassman RJ, Qualls CR, Lisansky EJ, Peake GT: Elevated rectal temperature produced by all-night bright light is reversed by melatonin infusion in men. J Appl Physiol 71:2178–2182, 1991.

89. Cagnacci A, Elliot JA, Yen SS: Melatonin: A major regulator of the circadian rhythm of core body temperature in humans. J Clin Endocrinol Metab 75:447–452, 1992.

90. Deacon S, English J, Arendt J: Acute phase-shifting effects of melatonin associated with suppression of core body temperature in humans. Neurosci Lett 178:32–34, 1994.

91. Krauchi K, Cajochen C, Wirz-Justice A. A relationship between heat loss and sleepiness: effects of postural change and melatonin administration. J Appl Physiol 83:134–139, 1997.

92. Wehr TA, Moul DE, Barbato G, et al: Conservation of photoperiod-responsive mechanisms in humans. Amer J Physiol (Regulatory, Integrative and Comparative Physiology) 265:R846–R857, 1993.

93. Dijk DJ, Shanahan TL, Duffy JF, et al: Variation of electroencephalographic activity during non-rapid eye movement and rapid eye movement sleep with phase of circadian melatonin rhythm in humans. J Physiol (Lond) 505:851–858, 1997.

94. Wehr TA, Aeschbach D, Duncan WC Jr: Evidence for a biological dawn and dusk in the human circadian timing system. J Physiol 535:937–951, 2001.

95. Shochat T, Haimov I, Lavie P: Melatonin: The key to the gate of sleep. Ann Med 30:109–114, 1998.

96. Rajaratnam SM, Dijk DJ, Middleton B, et al: Melatonin phase-shifts human circadian rhythms with no evidence of changes in the duration of endogenous melatonin secretion or the 24-hour production of reproductive hormones. J Clin Endocrinol Metab 88:4303–4309, 2003.

97. Rajaratnam SMW, Arendt J: Health in the 24-hour society. Lancet 358:999–1005, 2001.

98. Lockley SW, Skene DJ, Tabandeh H, et al: Relationship between napping and melatonin in the blind. J Biol Rhythms 12:16–25, 1997.

99. De Leersnyder H, de Blois MC, Bresson JL, et al: Inversion of the circadian melatonin rhythm in Smith-Magenis syndrome. Rev Neurol (Paris) 159(Suppl 6):S21–S26, 2003.

100. Strassman RJ, Appenzeller O, Lewy AJ, et al: Increase in plasma melatonin, beta-endorphin, and cortisol after a 28.5-mile mountain race: Relationship to performance and lack of effect of naltrexone. J Clin Endocrinol Metab 69:540–545, 1989.

101. Kennaway D, Stamp G, Goble F: Development of melatonin production in infants and the impact of prematurity. J Clin Endocrinol Metab 75:367–369, 1992.

102. Waldhauser F, Frisch H, Waldhauser M, et al: Fall in nocturnal serum melatonin during prepuberty and pubescence. Lancet 1:362–365, 1984.

103. Zeitzer JM, Daniels JE, Duffy JF, et al: Do plasma melatonin concentrations decline with age? Am J Med 107:432–436, 1999.

104. Attanasio A, Borrelli P, Marini R, et al: Serum melatonin in children with early and delayed puberty. Neuroendocrinol Lett 5:387, 1983.

105. Waldhauser F, Boepple P, Schemper M, Crowley WF: Serum melatonin in central precocious puberty is lower than in age matched pre-pubertal children. J Clin Endocrinol Metab 73:793–796, 1991.

106. Berga SL, Mortola JF, Yen SSC: Amplification of nocturnal melatonin secretion in women with functional hypothalamic amenorrhea. J Clin Endocrinol Metab 66:242–244, 1988.

107. Berga SL, Jones KL, Kaufmann S, Yen SSC: Nocturnal melatonin levels are unaltered by ovarian suppression in girls with central precocious puberty. Fertil Steril 52:937–941, 1989.

108. Arendt J, Labib MH, Bojkowski C, et al: Rapid decrease in melatonin production during treatment of delayed puberty with oestradiol in a case of craniopharyngioma. Lancet 1:1326, 1989.

109. Luboshitzky R, Shen-Orr Z, Ishai A, et al: Melatonin hypersecretion in male patients with adult-onset idiopathic hypogonadotropic hypogonadism. Exp Clin Endocrinol Diabetes 108:142–145, 2000.

110. Cagnacci A, Krauchi K, Wirz-Justice A, Volpe A: Homeostatic versus circadian effects of melatonin on core body temperature in humans. J Biol Rhythms 12:509–517, 1997.

111. Cagnacci A, Elliot JA, Yen SSC: Amplification of pulsatile LH secretion by exogenous melatonin in women. J Clin Endocrinol Metab 73:210–212, 1991.

112. Voordow BCG, Euser R, Verdonk RER, et al: Melatonin and melatonin-progestin combinations alter pituitary-ovarian function in women and can inhibit ovulation. J Clin Endocrinol Metab 74:108–117, 1992.

113. Anderson RA, Lincoln GA, Wu FCW: Melatonin potentiates testosterone-induced suppression of luteinising hormone secretion in normal men. Hum Reprod 8:1819–1822, 1993.

114. Luboshitzky R, Wagner O, Lavi S: Abnormal melatonin secretion in male patients with hypogonadism. J Mol Neurosci 7:91–98, 1996.

115. Luboshitzky R, Wagner O, Lavi S, et al: Abnormal melatonin secretion in hypogonadal men: The effect of testosterone treatment. Clin Endocrinol 47:463–469, 1997.

116. Roenneberg T, Aschoff J: Annual rhythms in human reproduction: I. Biology, sociology or both? J Biol Rhythms 5:195–216, 1990.

117. Luboshitzky R, Levi M, Shen-Orr Z, et al: Long–term melatonin administration does not alter pituitary-gonadal hormone secretion in normal men. Hum Reprod 15:60–65, 2000.

118. Wright J, Aldhous M, Franey C, English J, Arendt J: The effects of exogenous melatonin on endocrine function in man. Clin Endocr 24:375–382, 1986.

119. West RJ, Leonard JV: Familial insulin resistance with pineal hyperplasia: Metabolic studies and effect of hypophysectomy. Arch Dis Child 55:619–621, 1980.

120. Sparks DL, Hunsaker JC III: The pineal gland in sudden infant death syndrome: Preliminary observations. J Pineal Res 5:111–118, 1988.

121. Sturner WQ, Lynch HJ, Deng MH, Wurtman RJ: Melatonin levels in the sudden infant death syndrome. Forensic Sci Int 45:171–180, 1990.

122. Axelrod L: Endocrine dysfunction in patients with tumours of the pineal region. In Schmidek HH (ed): Pineal Tumours. New York, Masson, 1977, pp 61–77.

123. Wass JAL, Jones AE, Rees LH, Besser GM: hCGb producing pineal choriocarcinoma. Clin Endocrinol 17:423–431, 1982.

124. Cohen AR, Wilson JA, Sadeghi-Nejad A: Gonadotrophin-secreting pineal teratoma causing precocious puberty. Neurosurgery 28:597–602, 1991.

125. Horowitz MB: Central nervous system germinomas: A review. Arch Neurol 48:652–657, 1991.

126. Drummond KJ, Rosenfeld JV: Pineal region tumours in childhood: A 30-year experience. Childs Nerv Syst 15:119–126, 1999.

127. Chazot G, Claustrat B, Broussolle E, Lapras C: Headache and depression: Recurrent symptoms in adult pinealectomized patients. In Nappi G (ed): Headache and Depression: Serotonin Pathways as a Common Clue. New York, Raven Press, 1991, pp 299–303.

128. Sánchez-Barceló EJ, Cos S, Fernández R, Mediavilla MD: Melatonin and mammary cancer: A short review. Endocr Relat Cancer 10:153–159, 2003.

129. Tamarkin L, Danforth D, Lichter A, et al: Decreased nocturnal plasma melatonin peak in patients with estrogen receptor positive breast cancer. Science 216:1003–1005, 1982.

130. Bartsch C, Bartsch H: Melatonin in cancer patients and in tumor-bearing animals. Adv Exp Med Biol 467:247–264, 1999.

131. Gilad E, Matzkin H, Zisapel N: Interplay between sex steroids and melatonin in regulation of human benign prostate epithelial cell growth. J Clin Endocrinol Metab 82:2535–2541, 1997.

132. Schernhammer ES, Schulmeister K: Melatonin and cancer risk: Does light at night compromise physiologic cancer protection by lowering serum melatonin levels? Br J Cancer 90:941–943, 2004.

133. Warman GR, Tripp H, Warman VL, Arendt J: Acute exposure to circularly polarized 50-Hz magnetic fields of 200–300 micro T does not affect the pattern of melatonin secretion in young men. J Clin Endocrinol Metab 88:5668–5673, 2003.

134. Sewerynek E: Melatonin and the cardiovascular system. Neuroendocrinol Lett 23(Suppl 1):79–83, 2002.

135. O'Brien IAD, Lewin IG, O'Hare JP, et al: Abnormal circadian rhythm of melatonin in diabetic autonomic neuropathy. Clin Endocrinol 24:359–364, 1986.

136. Nagtegaal JE, Kerkhof GA, Smits MG, et al: Delayed sleep phase syndrome: A placebo-controlled cross-over study on the effects of melatonin administered five hours before the individual dim light melatonin onset. J Sleep Res 7:135–143, 1998.

137. Deacon S, Arendt J: Posture influences melatonin concentrations in plasma and saliva in humans. Neurosci Lett 167:191–194, 1994.

138. Arendt J: Melatonin: A new probe in psychiatric investigation? Br J Psychiatry 155:585–590, 1989.

139. Lewy AJ, Sack RL, Miller LS, Hoban TM: Anti-depressant and circadian phase-shifting effects of light. Science 235:352–354, 1987.

140. Parry BL, Berga SL, Mostofi N, et al: Plasma melatonin circadian rhythms during the menstrual cycle and after light therapy in premenstrual dysphoric disorder and normal control subjects. J Biol Rhythms 12:47–64, 1997.

141. Zhadnova IV, Wurtman RJ: Efficacy of melatonin as a sleep promoting agent. J Biol Rhythms 12:644–650, 1997.

142. Arendt J: Sleep science: Integrating basic research and clinical practice. In Schwartz W (ed): Melatonin. Karger Monographs in Clinical Neuroscience. Basel, Karger, 1997, pp 196–228.

143. Lerner AB, Nordlund JJ: Melatonin: Clinical pharmacology. J Neural Transm Suppl 13:339–347, 1978.

144. Arendt J, Skene DJ: Melatonin as a chronobiotic [and other articles in the same volume]. Sleep Med Rev 2004, in press.

145. Graw P, Werth E, Krauchi K, et al: Early morning melatonin administration impairs psychomotor vigilance. Behav Brain Res 121:167–172, 2001.

146. Waldhauser F, Steger H, Vorkapic P: Melatonin secretion in man and the influence of exogenous melatonin on some physiological and behavioural variables. Adv Pineal Res 2:207–223, 1987.

147. Forsling ML: Diurnal rhythms in neurohypophysial function. Exp Physiol 85:179S–186S, 2000.

148. Sugden D: Psychopharmacological effects of melatonin in mouse and rat. J Pharmacol Exp Ther 227:587–591, 1983.

149. Guardiola-Lemaitre B: Toxicology of melatonin. J Biol Rhythms 12:697–706, 1997.

150. Mahle CD, Coggins GD, Agarwal P, et al: Melatonin modulates vascular smooth muscle tone. J Biol Rhythms 12:690–696, 1997.

151. Deacon S, Arendt J: Melatonin-induced temperature suppression and its acute phase-shifting effects correlate in a dose-dependent manner in humans. Brain Res 688:77–85, 1995.

152. Lewy AJ, Ahmed S, Jackson JML, Sack RL: Melatonin shifts human circadian rhythms according to a phase-response curve. Chronobiol Int 9:380–392, 1993.

153. Lewy AJ, Bauer VK, Ahmed S, et al: The human phase response curve (PRC) to melatonin is about 12 hours out of phase with the PRC to light. Chronobiol Int 15:71–83, 1998.

154. Middleton B, Arendt J, Stone B: Complex effects of melatonin on human circadian rhythms in constant dim light. J Biol Rhythms 12:467–475, 1997.

155. Lockley SW, Skene DJ, James K, et al: Melatonin administration can entrain the free-running circadian system of blind subjects. J Endocrinol 164:R1–R6, 2000.

156. Sack RL, Brandes RW, Kendall AR, Lewy AJ: Entrainment of free-running circadian rhythms by melatonin in blind people. N Engl J Med 343:1070–1077, 2000.

157. Arendt J, Skene DJ, Middleton B, et al: Efficacy of melatonin treatment in jet lag, shift work, and blindness. J Biol Rhythms 12:604–617, 1997.

158. Arendt J, Stone B, Skene DJ: Sleep disruption in jet lag and other circadian rhythm disorders. In Turek F (section ed): Principles and Practice of Sleep Medicine, 4th ed. New York, Elsevier, 2004, in press.

159. Herxheimer A, Petrie KJ: Melatonin for the prevention and treatment of jet lag. Cochrane Database Syst Rev, CD001520. London, UK Cochrane Centre, 2002.

160. Burgess HJ, Sharkey KM, Eastman CI: Bright light, dark and melatonin can promote circadian adaptation in night shift workers. Sleep Med Rev 6:407–420, 2002.

161. Arendt J: Safety of melatonin in long term use. J Biol Rhythms 12:673–681, 1997.

162. Lewy AJ, Bauer VK, Hasler BP, et al: Capturing the circadian rhythms of free-running blind people with 0.5 mg melatonin. Brain Res 918:96–100, 2001.

163. Hack LM, Lockley SW, Arendt J, et al: The effects of low-dose 0.5-mg melatonin on the free-running circadian rhythms of blind subjects. J Biol Rhythms 18:420–429, 2003.

164. Arendt J: Melatonin, sleep and circadian rhythms [Editorial]. New Engl J Med 343:1114–1116, 2000.

165. Palm L, Blennow G, Wetterberg L: Long-term melatonin treatment in blind children and young adults with circadian sleep-wake disturbances. Dev Med Child Neurol 39:319–325, 1997.

166. Hughes RJ, Sack RL, Lewy AJ: The role of melatonin and circadian phase in age-related sleep-maintenance insomnia: Assessment in a clinical trial of melatonin replacement. Sleep 21:52–68, 1998.

167. Tamarkin L, Cohen M, Roselle D, et al: Melatonin inhibition and pinealectomy enhancement of 7,12-dimethylbenz(a)anthracene-induced mammary tumours in the rat. Cancer Res 41:4432–4436, 1981.

168. Conti A, Maestroni GJM: The clinical neuroimmunotherapeutic role of melatonin in oncology. J Pineal Res 19:103–110, 1995.

169. Lissoni P, Chilelli M, Villa S, et al: Five years survival in metastatic non-small cell lung cancer patients treated with chemotherapy alone or chemotherapy and melatonin: A randomized trial. J Pineal Res 35:12–15, 2003.

170. Fu L, Lee CC: The circadian clock: Pacemaker and tumour suppressor. Nature Rev Cancer 3:350–361, 2003.

171. Hastings MH, Maywood ES, Ebling FJP, et al: Sites and mechanism of action of melatonin in the photoperiodic control of reproduction. Adv Pineal Res 5:147–157, 1991.

172. Maywood ES, Hastings MH: Lesions of the iodomelatonin-binding sites of the mediobasal hypothalamus spare the lactotropic, but block the gonadotropic response of male Syrian hamsters to short photoperiod and to melatonin. Endocrinology 136:144–149, 1995.

173. Lincoln GA: Administration of melatonin into the mediobasal hypothalamus as a continuous or intermittent signal affects the secretion of follicle-stimulating hormone and prolactin in the ram. J Pineal Res 12:135–144, 1992.

174. Lincoln G, Maeda K: Effects of placing micro-implants of melatonin in the mediobasal hypothalamus and preoptic area on the secretion of prolactin and β-endorphin in rams. J Endocrinol 134:437–448, 1992.

175. Nakazawa K, Marubayashi U, McCann SM: Mediation of the short-loop feedback of luteinising hormone (LH) on LH-releasing hormone release by melatonin-induced inhibition of LH release from the pars tuberalis. Proc Natl Acad Sci U S A 88:7576–7579, 1991.

176. Lincoln GA, Andersson H, Hazlerigg D: Clock genes and the long term regulation of prolactin secretion: Evidence for a photoperiod/cirannual timer in the pars tuberalis. J Neuroendocrinol 15:390–397, 2003.

177. Lincoln GA, Andersson H, Loudon A: Clock genes in calendar cells as the basis of annual timekeeping in mammals: A unifying hypothesis. J Endocrinol 179:1–13, 2003.

178. Stehle JH, von Gall C, Korf HW: Melatonin: A clock output, a clock input. J Neuroendocrinol 15:383–389, 2003.

179. Von Gall C, Garabette ML, Kell CA, et al: Rhythmic gene expression in pituitary depends on heterologous sensitization by the neurohormone melatonin. Nat Neurosci 5:234–238, 2002.

180. Vanecek J, Pavlik A, Illnerova H: Hypothalamic melatonin receptor sites revealed by autoradiography. Brain Res 453:359–362, 1987.

181. Morgan PJ, Williams LM: Central melatonin receptors: Implications for a mode of action. Experientia 45:955–965, 1989.

182. Masana MI, Dubocovich ML: Melatonin receptor signaling: Finding the path through the dark. Science 107:1–5, 2002.

183. Reppert SM, Weaver DR, Godson C: Melatonin receptors step into the light: Cloning and classification of subtypes. Trends Pharmacol Sci 17:100–102, 1996.

184. Lincoln GA, Clarke IJ: Photoperiodically induced cycles in the secretion of prolactin in hypothalamo-pituitary disconnected rams: Evidence for translation of the melatonin signal in the pituitary gland. J Neuroendocrinol 6:251–260, 1994.

185. Williams LM, Martinoli MG, Titchener LT, Pelletier G: The ontogeny of central melatonin binding sites in the rat. Endocrinology 128:2083–2090, 1991.

186. Skene DJ, Masson-Pevet M, Pevet P: Seasonal changes in melatonin binding sites in the pars tuberalis of male European hamsters and the effect of testosterone manipulation. Endocrinology 132:1682–1686, 1993.

187. Dardente H, Klosen P, Pevet P, et al: MT1 melatonin receptor mRNA expressing cells in the pars tuberalis of the European hamster: Effect of photoperiod. J Neuroendocrinol 15:778–786, 2003.

188. Hazlerigg DG, Morgan PJ, Messager S: Decoding photoperiodic time and melatonin in mammals: What can we learn from the pars tuberalis? J Biol Rhythms 16:326–335, 2001.

189. Krause DN, Dubocovich ML: Regulatory sites in the melatonin system of mammals. Trends Neurosci 13:464–470, 1990.

190. White BH, Sekura RD, Rollag MD: Pertussis toxin blocks melatonin-induced aggregation in Xenopus dermal melanophores. J Comp Physiol [B] 157:153–159, 1987.

191. Reppert SM: Melatonin receptors: Molecular biology of a new family of G-protein-coupled receptors. J Biol Rhythms 12:528–531, 1997.

192. Dubocovich ML, Cardinali DP, Guardiola-Lemaitre B, et al: Melatonin receptors. In The IUPHAR Compendium of Receptor Characterization and Classification. London, IUPHAR Media, 1998, pp 187–193.

193. Reppert SM: Nature's knockout: The Mel1b receptor is not necessary for reproductive and circadian responses to melatonin in Siberian hamsters. Mol Endocrinol 10:1478–1487, 1996.

194. Dubocovich ML, Rivera-Bermudez MA, Gerdin MJ, et al: Molecular pharmacology, regulation and function of mammalian melatonin receptors. Front Biosci 8:1093–1108, 2003.

195. von Gall C, Stehle JH, Weaver DR. Mammalian melatonin receptors: Molecular biology and signal transduction. Cell Tissue Res 309:151–162, 2002.

196. Ebisawa T, Uchiyama M, Kajimura N, et al: Genetic polymorphisms of human melatonin 1b receptor gene in circadian rhythm sleep disorders and controls. Neurosci Lett 280:29–32, 2000.

197. Delagrange P, Atkinson J, Boutin JA, et al: Therapeutic perspectives for melatonin agonists and antagonists. J Neuroendocrinol 15:442–448, 2003.

GROWTH AND MATURATION

Growth Hormone

John J. Kopchick

GROWTH HORMONE

OVERVIEW

A growth-promoting principle of the pituitary gland was discovered in 1921.[1] In 1944, bovine growth hormone (GH) was isolated.[2] In the early 1960s, human growth hormone (hGH) was first used in GH-deficient children. In 1979, the cDNA encoding hGH was cloned,[3] and in 1985, recombinant hGH was approved for clinical use. During this time, a major scientific goal has been the correlation of GH structure with its biologic activities. Toward this end, a combination of in vitro and in vivo assays for GH's activities have been used. Throughout this review, the predominant theme will be the structure of the GH molecule as it relates to its function. I will then attempt to summarize the molecular events at the cellular level that lead to GH-induced biologic activities. Many findings concerning the structure and activity of GH and its interaction with GH receptors (GHRs) have been published since the last writing of this review. Unfortunately, I cannot cite all of these results. However, three important items have surfaced since the publication of that review: (1) the approval of a GH antagonist, Pegvisomant (Somavert®), for use in acromegalic individuals; (2) the findings that GH antagonists do not inhibit GHR dimerization but impede proper or functional GHR dimerization; and (3) the establishment that GHRs exist as dimers independent of GH binding. These three pivotal findings as well as others will be described in this review.

GENERAL BACKGROUND

GH, chorionic somatomammotropin (CS, placental lactogen), and prolactin (Prl) belong to a family of hormones that are thought to have evolved from a common precursor.[4,5] The GH family members are encoded by genes that span approximately 2.0 kilobases (kb) and contain five exons and four intervening sequences. The translation start and stop codons are located in exons 1 and 5 of the genes, respectively.[4]

The GH family of proteins contain approximately 200 amino acids with two (GH) or three (Prl) disulfide bonds.[6] The proteins' molecular masses are approximately 22,000, with similar sedimentation and diffusion coefficients.[6,7] The amino acid composition and sequence of the molecules are comparable, ranging from approximately 60% to 90% in amino acid sequence identity. The molecules are synthesized as precursor proteins; that is, they contain amino-terminal secretory signal peptides.[4] A comprehensive list of the amino acid sequences of GH molecules from various species has been presented,[8] and a pictorial representation of the percent identity between the amino acid sequences has been compiled.[9]

The hGH gene family consists of the 191-amino-acid hGH molecule, a GH variant termed *hGH-V, hCS*, and *hPrl*. Unlike hGH, which is expressed primarily in the pituitary and is not glycosylated, hGH-V is glycosylated, is expressed in the placenta, and is found in the serum during pregnancy.[10–12] It differs from pituitary hGH in 13 of 191 amino acid residues,[4] and like hGH, it promotes growth.[13] Another variant of hGH, termed *20 kDa* (20K), has been found in the pituitary and blood. It is produced by alternative splicing of the hGH precursor mRNA and lacks amino acids 32 to 46.[14] Two forms of hCS have been found, hCS-A and hCS-B, that differ by only one amino acid residue located in the secretory signal peptide. hCS is expressed by the placenta and, despite possessing 161 amino acid residues in common with hGH, retains minimal growth-promoting activity.[15] hPrl is expressed by the pituitary gland and contains 199 amino acids, though only 30 are identical to hGH in amino acid alignment.[4] hPrl has been reported to be phosphorylated and glycosylated and is the subject of Chapter 17.

The hGH gene family members are located on the long arm of chromosome 17. The 5' to 3' order of these genes are GH, a CS pseudogene, CS-A, GH-V, and CS-B.[16]

GH ACTIVITIES

During the late 1950s and early 1960s, a great deal of work was performed on GH and GH isoforms. Several heterogeneous types of GHs have been reported.[6,17–22] The heterogeneity of GH genes, isohormones, and variants has been reviewed and will not be described here.[23]

As the name implies, GH's major function is growth promotion. In vertebrates, hyposecretion of GH during childhood development leads to a growth hormone–deficient state that results in dwarfism (covered in Chapter 37), whereas hypersecretion of GH before puberty leads to gigantism. In adults, hypersecretion of GH from pituitary adenomas results in a clinical condition known as acromegaly, characterized by enlarged bones of the face, hands, and feet; enlarged heart, liver, and kidney tissue; fatigue; and weight gain. Approximately 25% of individuals with acromegaly develop type 2 diabetes, which results from chronically elevated circulating insulin levels and subsequent insulin resistance.[24] The subject of acromegaly has been nicely reviewed[25–30] and is covered in Chapter 23.

In healthy adults, GH exerts several metabolic effects, including those on protein, fat, and carbohydrate. Among the many metabolic activities of GH, two contradictory actions have been described. They are acute or early insulin-like activities and the chronic or late anti-insulin effects. This chronic effect is also described as GH's diabetogenic activity. Acute insulin-like activities include hypoglycemia,[31,32] increased glucose and amino acid transport and metabolism,[33–36] increased protein synthesis,[34] increased glycogenesis,[37,38] and increased lipogenesis.[39,40] These insulin-like activities are seen primarily in vitro or under special circumstances such as following hypophysectomy. GH's anti-insulin activities include hyperglycemia,[41] hyperinsulinemia,[42] increased lipolysis,[43,44] decreased glucose transport,[45] increased serum levels of nonesterified fatty acids,[46] decreased glucose metabolism,[47] and insulin resistance.[48–50] These anti-insulin activities have been found after relatively long periods of GH treatment, that is, after chronic exposure both in cultured cells and in vivo, and are thought to represent a major physiologic effect of GH.

To explain these two related but opposite activities, as well as other multiple GH activities, three hypotheses have been presented: (1) the existence of multiple GH receptors (R),[51,52] (2) the presence of multiple "active centers" in the GH molecule,[53] and (3) the presence of small, active GH fragments that result in multiple activities.[54–58] Work continues to test these three hypotheses.

In addition to the insulin-like and anti-insulin-like activities of the molecule, other in vivo assays for GH activity include an influence on rat tibia size,[59] metabolic and growth effects in hypophysectomized animals,[60] and the enhancement of growth rates in transgenic mice.[61–68] Additionally, in vitro or cultured cell–based assays include those in which the GHR gene is either endogenously expressed or expressed via transfection of cells. Assays that use these types of cells include GH-stimulated transcription of cotransfected reporter genes or GH's ability to stimulate cell differentiation and/or cell division.

Many of the functional effects of GH actually result from the action of insulin-like growth factor one (IGF-I), which is produced in liver, bone, and other tissues in response to GH.[69] In 1985, Green put forth the dual-effector theory of GH action.[70] In this theory, he postulated that GH acts directly on cells to promote differentiation, while IGF-I promotes cell multiplication. Now, an important experimental task is to determine which of the GH-associated effects are the direct outcome of GH and which are caused indirectly through IGF-I. Results of these important experiments will either support or reject the dual-effector theory of GH action.[70] Related to this issue, the IGF-1 gene has been conditionally disrupted in the liver of mice.[71,72] Although serum IGF-1 levels are significantly reduced in these animals, their rates of growth were not affected. Thus, the levels of serum IGF-1 do not coincide with growth rates, implying that the paracrine and/or autocrine actions of IGF-1 are important. The subject of IGF-1 is covered in Chapter 34.

A great deal of work describing the structure of the GH molecule as it relates to GH's biologic activities has been performed, and several excellent reviews concerning this subject have been presented.[4,6,8,23,40,73–79]

GH FRAGMENTS

Considerable work has proceeded attempting to determine the biologic activity of GH and various GH fragments. For example, Li and Graf[80] showed that cleavage of hGH by plasmin resulted in two fragments, that is, residues 1 to 134 and 141 to 191, each of which possessed reduced biologic activity. These two fragments were shown to react noncovalently, resulting in an hGH molecule that possessed full biologic activity[81] when evaluated using the pigeon crop-sac assay[82] and the rat tibia assay.[59] Additionally, Li and Bewley in 1976 presented the first structural representation of GH that included 191 amino acids and two disulfide bonds.[81]

Sonenberg and his colleagues found that a tryptic peptide of bGH (fragment A-2) that included amino acid residues 96 to 133 had low but significant levels of activity in the rat tibia width and weight gain assays[83,84] and stimulated hGH-like effects in humans.[85] However, the remaining fragment, termed A-1 (bGH 1 to 95, 134 to 191), possessed little activity.[85] On analyses of the fragments using far ultraviolet circular dichroism and intrinsic fluorescence emission spectroscopy and employing Chou-Fasman protein structure predictions,[86,87] a two-dimensional representation of the three-dimensional structure of GH was presented[88] (Fig. 32-1). Three α-helical regions were predicted in this model. Note that the fragment containing residues 96 to 133 included a α-helix. Thus, the first predicted secondary structure of GH was presented in 1978, complete with α-helical regions, β-sheets, and disulfide bonds (see Fig. 32-1).

Several lines of research suggested that endogenous GH fragments do in fact exist. Though most of these GH fragments were found to be artifacts of experimental manipulation,[23] several studies were performed on such GH fragments. For example, hGH 1 to 15 was found to possess insulin-like activity,[54–57] while hGH 177 to 191 had anti-insulin activity.[58,89] Also, the hGH variant (20K), which is generated by alternative GH precursor mRNA splicing and lacks amino acid residues 32 to 46, also lacked the insulin-like activity but possessed growth-promoting, lactogenic, and diabetogenic activities.[19,51,90,91] Salem in 1988 showed that an hGH amino terminal peptide (1–43) was an insulin potentiator that increased insulin-stimulated glucose clearance and glucose metabolism without affecting insulin secretion.[92] Also, Towns and colleagues have found that the N-terminus of hGH is involved in the growth-promoting, diabetogenic, and insulin-like activities of the molecule.[93]

Additionally, the ability of the 22-kDa, 20K, and 5-kDa amino terminal peptide forms of hGH to promote growth in transgenic mice has been evaluated.[94] Both the 22-kDa and 20K forms of hGH stimulated linear mouse growth, while the 5-kDa form did not.

A wide variety of experiments have been performed on other GH fragments. The reader is referred to a list of approximately 90 GH fragments with their corresponding biologic activities.[95]

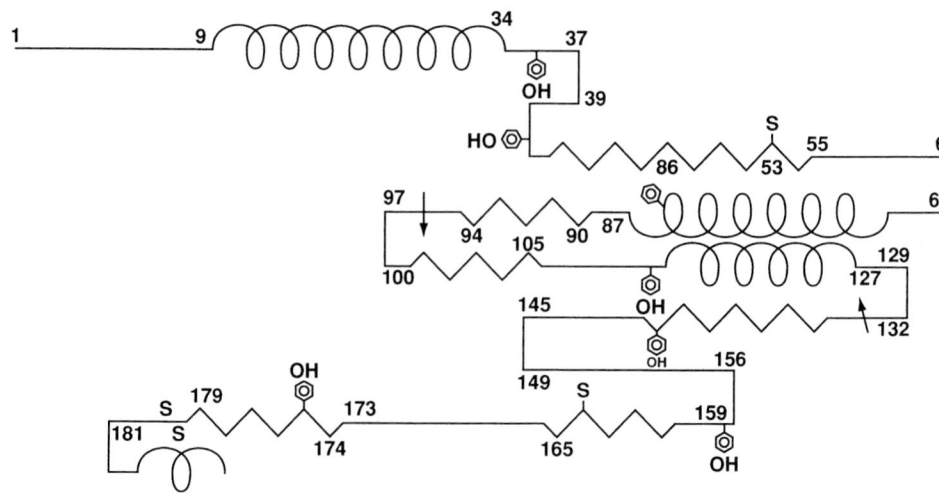

Figure 32-1 Schematic representation of bGH. Arrows indicate the trypsin cleavage sites located between amino acids 96 to 97 and 132 to 133. Also shown are three α-helical regions. This figure was adapted from Hara and colleagues.[88]

CRYSTAL STRUCTURE OF GH

The crystal structure of the GH molecule, in particular porcine (p) GH, was solved by Abdel-Meguid and coworkers in 1987[96] (Fig. 32-2). This momentous disclosure came 11 years after the first graphic representation of the GH molecule[81] and 66 years after the discovery of the growth-promoting principle of the pituitary gland.[1] GH was found to be an elongated molecule with approximate dimensions of 55 angstroms by 35 angstroms by 35 angstroms. The molecule contains four α-helices, which are tightly packed as antiparallel bundles aligned in an *up-up-down-down* orientation; 54% of GH's 191 amino acids are contained in these four α-helices. The molecule also contains a "large loop" between residues 33 and 75, a "smaller loop" between residues 129 and 154, and a "small loop" located at the carboxyl terminus.[96] This model has been used to generate and test many hypotheses in the GH field and represents the prototypic model for the GH family members.

DISULFIDE BONDS IN GH

Members of the GH family possess either two (GH) or three (Prl) disulfide bonds. Bovine (b) GH has four Cys residues located at positions 53, 164, 181, and 189. When aligned to optimize amino acid similarity, the four Cys residues were found to be conserved among all GH, Prl, and placental lac-

togen (PL) molecules.[6,75] This conservation may indicate that these residues are important for the structural integrity and biologic activity of the molecules. The four Cys residues form two disulfide bridges that are located between Cys 53 and Cys 164, which results in a large loop, and between Cys 181 and Cys 189, which forms a small C-terminal loop. The integrity of the small loop has been found to be nonessential for the biologic activity of GH[68,97] or ovine (o) Prl.[98]

When both disulfide bonds of hGH were split and the sulfur atoms were carbamidomethylated, total hGH potency was retained when analyzed in the rat tibia and pigeon crops-sac GH-dependent bioassays.[99] In a similar manner, Campbell and colleagues. have found that the two disulfide bridges of hGH are not required for lipolytic or antilipolytic activities in chicken adipose tissue.[100] However, when hGH was reduced and alkylated, substantial loss of biologic activity was found.[101] Loss of biologic activity was also found when both of the disulfide bonds of pGH were reduced and aminoethylated.[102] These contrasting results suggest that the biologic significance of the disulfide bonds' integrity may be species-specific.

Using site-directed mutagenesis techniques, Cys residue conversion experiments have been performed. When Cys 165 of hGH (equivalent to Cys 164 of bGH) was changed to Ala, this hGH analogue retained full biologic activity with respect to native hGH.[103] However, when the disulfide bonds in bGH were disrupted by amino acid substitution of Cys for Ser residues and assayed for their ability to enhance growth in transgenic mice, only those animals that expressed bGH analogues with the large loop intact demonstrated a growth-enhanced phenotype. These results suggested that the integrity of the large loop, but not that of the small loop, is essential for GH's growth-enhancing activity.[68]

HOMOLOGUE AND ALANINE SCANNING OF GH

The information about functional domains of GH obtained through fragment experiments is limited, since the overall conformation of the protein has been altered. In the early 1990s, a novel approach toward the understanding of the structure of GH was employed using recombinant DNA techniques. Cloned DNA sequences encoding hPrl, which possess minimal GHR binding affinity, were substituted for the corresponding regions of hGH. Since Prl and GH are somewhat homologous, the term *homologue scanning* was used to describe these experiments. The Prl/GH chimeric molecules were assayed for their ability to bind Prl or GH receptors. This approach was very effective in defining the receptor-binding domains of hGH.[104] It was found that the receptor-binding domains of hGH are mainly located in the NH₂-terminal portion of α-helix I, a loop region between amino acid residues 54 to 74, and the COOH-terminal portion of α-helix IV.[104]

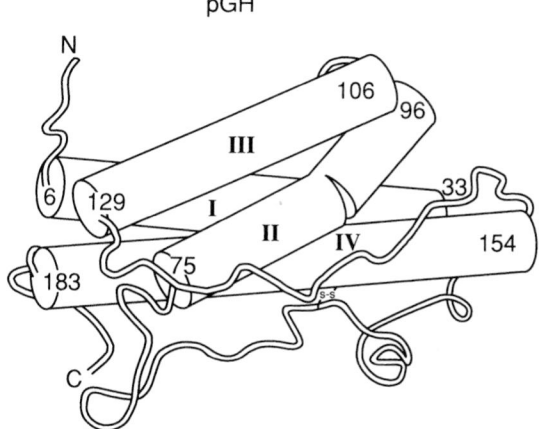

pGH

Figure 32-2 Crystal representation of the pGH at the 2.8-angstrom resolution level. Four α-helices are depicted (cylindric rods). The nonhelical region is shown as a thin tube. Also, one of the two disulfide bonds is shown; the other is hidden behind helix IV. The amino and carboxyl termini are located in the upper-left and lower-left corners, respectively. This figure was modified from Abdel-Meguid and colleagues.[96]

Systematic replacement of fragments of hGH with sequences derived from nonbinding GH homologues has generated information regarding GH/GHR-binding parameters. However, these experiments could not identify the specific residues involved in the ligand/receptor interaction.

Following the GH homologue-scanning studies, a more refined approach was applied to the structure/binding relationships of GH and GHR. In this approach, alanine codons were systematically substituted for many codons in the GH gene including those encoding residues found in α-helix I, the large loop, and α-helix IV. This "alanine-scanning" approach was used to define specific amino acid residues that are important for GHR binding.[105] It was reported that amino acid residues 10, 54, 56, 58, 64, 68 (loop region), and 171, 172, 175, 178, 182, and 185 (C-terminus) were involved in GHR binding.[104–106] The scanning mutagenesis studies largely ignored the third α-helix of GH because amino acid substitutions in the 3(rd) α-helix of GH resulted in little change in receptor-binding affinity.

THE THIRD α-HELIX OF GH

As was stated above, search for a growth-related domain in GH was pioneered by Sonenberg's group in late 1960s and early 1970s.[83,88,107,108] Their main finding was that a short sequence, generated by tryptic digestion of bGH, containing residues 96 to 133 (see Fig. 32-1) retained low but significant rat tibia bone growth-stimulating activity whereas the segments 1 to 95 and 134 to 191 had much less activity. The tryptic peptide, 96 to 133, contains the third α-helix of GH. Subsequently, it was reported that an hGH fragment (1 to 134) was fully active in the IM-9 human lymphocyte assay[109] and had lower but significant bioactivity in the rat tibia test.[80] Recently, recombinant hormones possessing different portions of GH, Prl, or PL have been generated and analyzed. hGH 1 to 134 was linked to hPL 141 to 191, and hPL 1 to 134 was linked to hGH 141 to 191 through a Cys53 to Cys165 disulfide bond.[22] These recombinant hormones were then tested for their immunoreactivities as well as receptor-binding properties. It was found that the recombinant hGH (1 to 134)–hPL (141 to 191) retains hGH immunoreactivity and full somatogenic receptor-binding ability but had little hPL activity. On the other hand, the recombinant hPL (1 to 134)–hGH (141 to 191) possessed a large amount of hPL immunoreactivity and lactogenic receptor-binding characteristics, with

negligible hGH activity. These results showed that immunoreactivity and biologic activity of the hormones were determined primarily by the NH2-terminal fragment (residues 1 to 134). The COOH-terminus appears to have little effect in determining specificity of biologic activity. Together, these results suggested that GH activity could be ascribed to different regions of the GH molecule and the 96 to 133 segment might be an "active core" required for growth promotion. These two lines of evidence lay the foundation for the structure/function studies of the third α-helix of GH.

MUTAGENESIS OF THE GH GENE ENCODING α-HELIX III

By combining site-specific mutagenesis of the GH gene with the ability of the resulting bGH analogues to enhance growth of transgenic mice, we have reported a growth-promoting region of GH localized in the third α-helix.[62–67] This α-helix possesses amphiphilic characteristics, that is, the hydrophobic residues are geographically separated from the hydrophilic residues (Fig. 32-3A). The third α-helix is imperfect in that Glu 117 (a hydrophilic residue) is found in the hydrophobic half of the α-helix while Ala 122 (a hydrophobic residue) and Gly 119 are positioned in the hydrophilic portion of the α-helix.

IMPORTANCE OF AMPHIPHILIC α-HELICES

Amphiphilic secondary structures have been proposed to be important functional domains for many peptide hormones.[110–118] It has been demonstrated that a GH-releasing hormone (GHRH) analogue with an optimized amphiphilic α-helix had enhanced biologic activity compared to native GHRH.[117] In addition, a calcitonin analogue was designed such that it had no amino acid sequence similarity to native calcitonin but maintained an identical length and amphiphilic properties. This analogue was nearly as potent as native calcitonin in mobilizing calcium.[114,115] Also, a yeast transcriptional activator, GCN4, contains an activation domain composed of 19 amino acids that is located outside its DNA-binding region. This short stretch of amino acids forms an amphiphilic α-helix that is sufficient for transcriptional activation.[116] It was suggested that this 19-amino-acid region in GCN4 might serve as a recognition signal for one or more components of the transcriptional apparatus.[116]

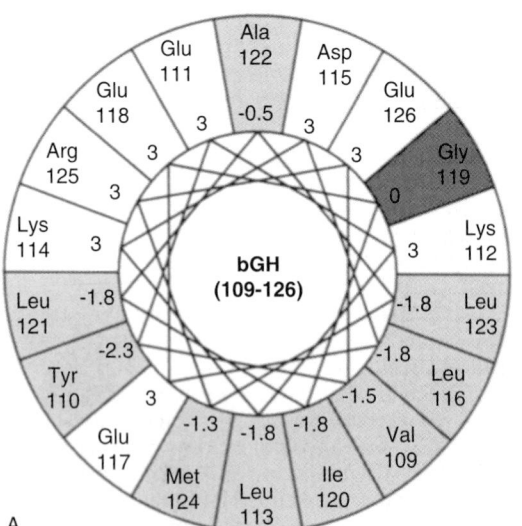

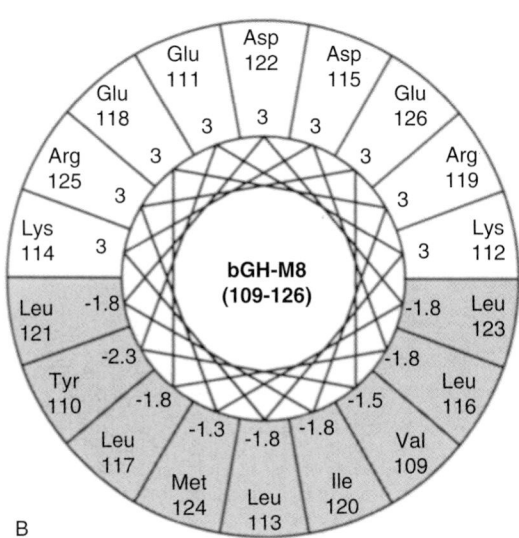

Figure 32-3 Axial projection of the third α-helix[109–126] of native bGH **(A)** and amino acid–substituted bGH **(B)**. Amino acid residues and corresponding hydrophilicity values are given. Amino acids in the open boxes are hydrophilic (top half of the wheel); those in the shaded boxes are hydrophobic (bottom half). The Gly residue[119] is depicted with darker shading. The figure is from Chen and colleagues.[62]

DESIGNING A GH ANALOGUE WITH A PERFECT AMPHIPHILIC α-HELIX

To convert GH's imperfect third amphiphilic α-helix to a "perfect" α-helix, we substituted Glu 117, Gly 119, and Ala 122 for Leu, Arg, and Asp, respectively[62] (Fig. 32-3B). When these amino acid substitutions were performed and the resulting GH analogue was purified and assayed, we found that it bound to GHRs with the same affinity as native GH. However, when the Glu117Leu, Gly119Arg, Ala122Asp GH analogue (termed *M8*) was assayed for its ability to enhance growth in transgenic mice, this GH analogue did not enhance growth, as does expression of wild-type GH transgenes,[61] but actually suppressed growth. Surprisingly, these animals possessed a dwarf phenotype[62] (Fig. 32-4). This was the first report of a GH antagonist.[62]

Thus, three amino acid substitutions (Glu117Leu, Gly119Arg, and Ala122Asp) in the third α-helix of bGH altered the activities of GH from those of a growth enhancer to those of a growth suppressor or antagonist.[62] In a subsequent study, we extended this observation by individually substituting Glu 117, Gly 119, and Ala 122 for Leu, Arg, and Asp, respectively. When assayed for their ability to bind to GHRs and to enhance growth in transgenic mice, the substitution of Leu 117 for Glu resulted in a GH analogue that behaved identically to native GH,[63] that is a giant mouse (see Fig. 32-4). Glu 117 is conserved in GHs from mammals to chickens.[6] Since the substitution mutation at this position (bGH-Glu117Leu) showed no effect on bGH growth-promoting activity, we conclude that residue 117 of bGH is not likely to be involved in growth-promoting activity. Again, this analogue retains the same activities as native bGH.

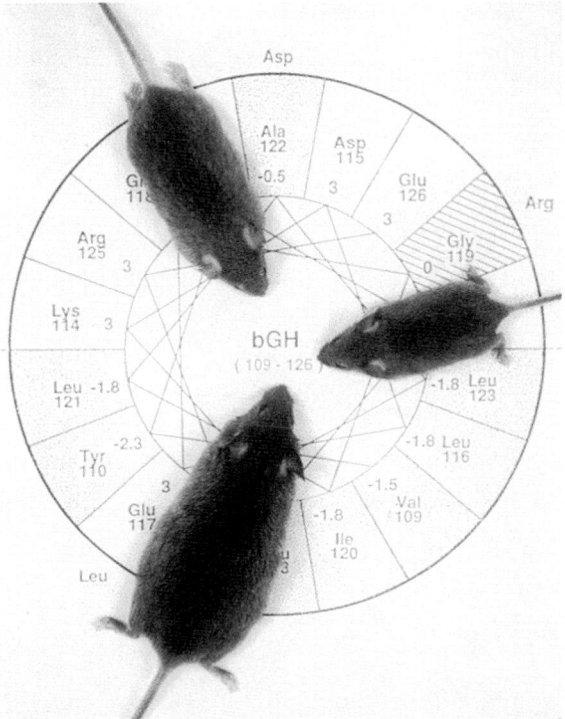

Figure 32-4 Representative transgenic mice that express different bGH analogues superimposed on the Edmonson wheel projection of the third α-helix of bGH. The mouse at the lower left expresses bGH-Glu-117 Leu and possesses an enhanced growth phenotype similar to animals that express wild-type bGH. The animal at the top expresses bGH-Ala122Asp and, despite having elevated serum levels of this GH analogue, possesses a normal growth phenotype. The mouse on the far right expresses bGH-Gly 119 Arg (the second reported GH antagonist) and possesses a dwarf phenotype. This figure is from Chen and colleagues.[63]

However, the bGH analogue, Gly119Arg, was found to bind to GHRs with the same affinity as native GH, but surprisingly, transgenic mice that expressed this analogue were about one half the size of their nontransgenic littermates[63] (see Fig. 32-4). This was the second report of a GH antagonist. We further confirmed this observation by generating hGH-Gly120Arg dwarf transgenic mice.[66] Additionally, several other amino acids were substituted for bGH Gly119. The following substitutions at amino acid position 119 (bGH-Gly119X, X = Arg, Lys, Leu, Pro, Trp) resulted in GH analogues in which the ability to bind to GHRs was uncoupled from the ability to enhance growth in transgenic mice. When these analogues were present at relatively high levels in the serum of transgenic mice, a dwarf phenotype resulted.[63] Thus, several GH antagonists were reported by our group; however, all were a result of the glycine in the third α-helix being replaced by another amino acid.

Finally, substitution of Asp for Ala at residue 122 results in a bGH analogue that binds to GH receptor but does not enhance (or suppress) growth in transgenic mice (see Fig. 32-4). However, unlike bGH-Gly119X analogues, the ability to retard mouse growth at relatively high serum levels was diminished. Thus, it appears that amino acid substitutions at position 119 (bGH) or 120 (hGH) are more effective than those at position 122 in growth suppression when the analogues are expressed at similar levels in transgenic mice. bGH-Ala122Asp may be acting as a partial agonist. Regardless, the salient feature of bGH-Ala122Asp and bGH-Gly119X is the apparent uncoupling of the ability to bind GHR with that of enhancing growth in transgenic mice.[62,63,66] Together, these studies were the first to document the discovery of GH antagonists.

GH ANTAGONISTS

Gly 119 is conserved among all members of the GH family including Prl and PL.[6] Gly is unique among amino acids in that it possesses a single hydrogen atom as a side chain. This small side chain has been suggested to increase molecule flexibility.[86] Consequently, it is the least favored residue for the formation of a stable α-helical structure.[86] The absolute conservation of this α-helix-destabilizing amino acid within a strong α-helical-forming region of GH's helix III implies a crucial role for this residue. As was stated above, when bGH Gly 119 or hGH Gly 120 was replaced with a variety of amino acids and the mutated genes were expressed in transgenic mice, dwarf animals resulted[62,63,66] (see Fig. 32-4). We also tested for the ability of the GH-substituted molecules to inhibit GH-dependent conversion of mouse preadipocytes to adipocytes. The bGH Gly119Arg or hGH Gly120Arg analogues were found to inhibit this reaction by 50% at equal molar concentrations of GH and analogues.[119,120] Thus, these GH molecules, in which α-helix III Glys were replaced by a variety of amino acids, acted as GH antagonists both in vitro and in vivo.[62-67,119-121] A confirmatory report on the generation of a GH antagonist by substituting arginine for glycine at position 120 in hGH was subsequently reported.[122]

Another hGH gene mutation has resulted in a "natural" GH antagonist.[123,124] In this case, the codon for Arg 77 was found to be mutated so as to encode Cys. The child in which this mutation was discovered possessed a dwarf phenotype. The molecule was shown to inhibit GH-stimulated Janus kinase 2 (JAK2) phosphorylation in vitro.[124] Expression of this GH analogue, hGHarg77cys, in transgenic mice resulted in giant animals and not dwarfs individuals (Stevens and Kopchick, unpublished results). Thus, the molecular mechanism by which this molecule act as a GH antagonist is not known.

GH ANTAGONISTS AS THERAPEUTIC AGENTS

In vitro and in vivo studies of hGH antagonists (GHAs)[62-67,119,121,122,125] have demonstrated that they possess a great potential to counteract the pathologic conditions of excess hGH in clinical settings. These pathologic situations include acromegaly, diabetic nephropathy,[121,126,127] diabetic retinopathy,[128,129] and certain cancers. For example, transgenic mice that express GH antagonists do not develop GH-induced glomerulosclerosis[126] (Fig. 32-5). Also, these animals are resistant to diabetes-induced kidney end organ damage.[121,130] Similarly, GHA mice have reduced levels of ischemia-induced retinal neovascularization compared to that seen in nontransgenic mice.[129] Additionally, when GH (giant) and GHA (dwarf) mice are crossed, the resulting offspring are intermediate in size, suggesting that GHAs may overcome the growth-enhancing properties of GH.[131] Thus, the use of transgenic animals that express GHAs have yielded data supporting the concept that this type of molecule may be used as a new class of therapeutic agent.

However, to elicit a sufficient pharmacologic effect, GHA should be present in the plasma long enough to antagonize the endogenous effects of GH. Studies on a GHA (hGH-Gly120Lys) have shown that this molecule has a serum half-life of less than 1 hour when injected intraperitoneally in mice.[132] This short half-life may render an hGH antagonist not practical for routine clinical use. There are several ways to improve the half-life of a therapeutic reagent. One is to conjugate the therapeutic molecules with polyethylene glycol (PEG), which prolongs the half-life of the molecules.[133–137] Clark and colleagues have shown that PEG of GH will significantly increase the serum half-life of the molecule.[138]

hGH antagonists have been pegylated[139] and used in vivo. We have found that hGH-Gly120Lys, when pegylated with four to six PEGs, has a half-life of approximately 18 hours after single intravenous, intraperitoneal, or subcutaneous injection.[132] When mice received a daily subcutaneous single injection of various doses (0.25 to 4 mg/kg) of Gly120Lys-PEG or vehicle for 5 days, a significant, dose-dependent suppression of IGF-I became obvious starting at day 3. The maximum suppression (up to 70%) of IGF-I production was achieved by 1 mg/kg dosing at day 6 after the first injection. Also, hepatic GHRs were significantly increased on day 8, also in a dose-dependent manner (Chen et al., unpublished data). These results suggest that exogenous administration of Gly120Lys-PEG can dramatically decrease serum IGF-I levels and may lead to the use of GHAs as therapeutic agents. In this regard, it has been shown that injection of a pegylated GHA (hGH-Gly120Lys) into mice results in an inhibition of diabetes-induced kidney damage.[140]

A GH receptor antagonist, Pegvisomant (Somavert), represents a new class of drugs that has been recently approved for use in acromegalic individuals. The data describing the results of Pegvisomant in acromegalic individuals have been described[141–145] and are discussed in Chapter 23. The antagonistic properties of Pegvisomant are derived from a substitution of Lys for Gly at position 120 of hGH identical to what has been described above. Additionally, eight amino acid substitutions in GH binding site 1 have been incorporated into the molecules that were originally thought to enhance binding of GH to GHRs. This form of the molecule was termed *B2036*. Additionally, four to five PEG moieties have been covalently linked to the protein backbone to prolong the circulating half-life and lower immunogenic potential.[139]

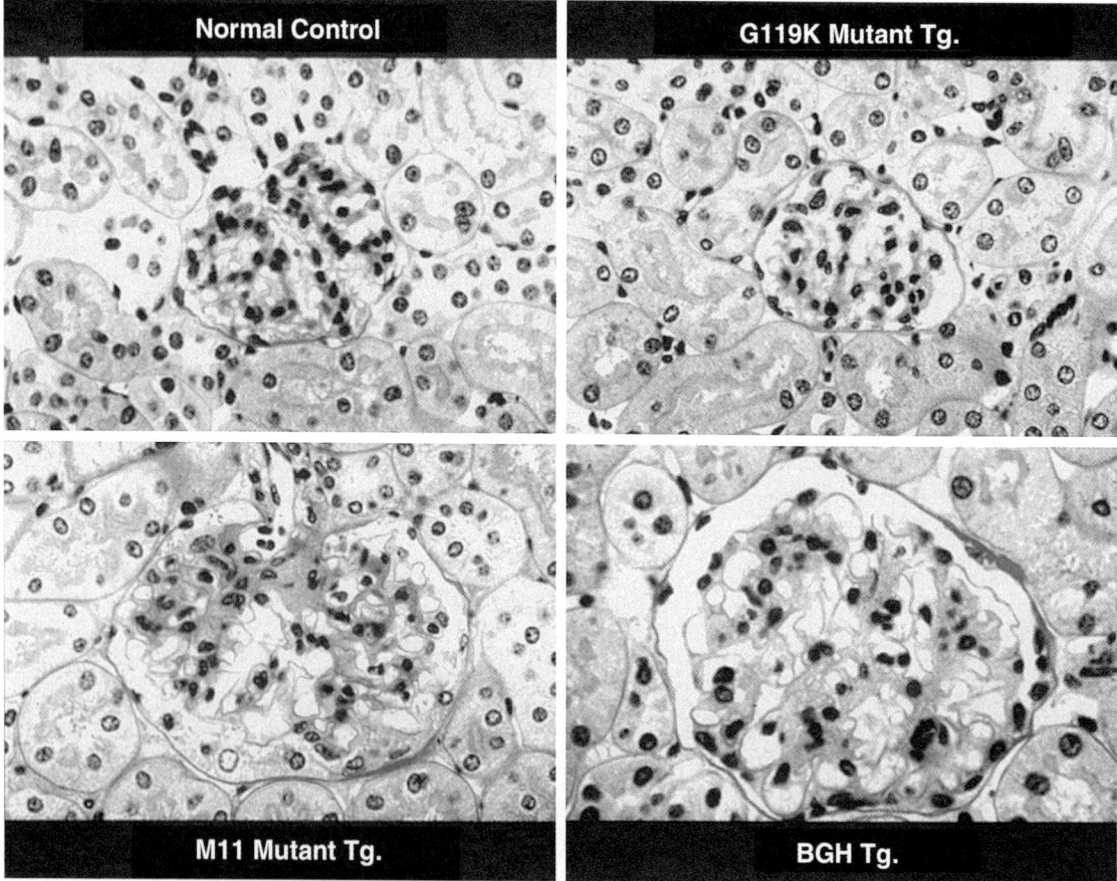

Figure 32-5 Kidney histopathologies of 9-month-old transgenic and control mice. A glomerulus of a control (Normal Control) and that of a GH antagonist (G119K) mouse are shown in the upper-right and upper-left portions of the figure, respectively. Glomeruli of bGH M11 (M11 Mutant Tg) and that of a bGH (BGH TG) transgenic mouse are shown in the lower-left and lower-right sectors of the figure, respectively. Kidneys from normal control and antagonists animals show no abnormal pathology. However, severe glomerulosclerosis is seen in kidneys from M11 and bGH transgenic mice.[126,127,288] This figure was modified from Yang and colleagues.[127]

When hGH Gly120Lys was compared to B2036 and to PEG-B2036 (Pegvisomant), unexpected binding properties were found.[146] B2036 was found to possess a greater affinity for GHBP than hGHGly120Lys; however, it retains the same affinity for full-length, membrane-bound GHRs.[146] Thus, the eight site 1 amino acid substitutions in B2036 do not increase affinity of the molecule to GHR, as was originally thought. However, Pegvisomant does have a greater affinity to GHRs than Peg hGH Gly120Lys does. This has been explained by the fact that ala and arg replaced the two native lysines in binding site 1, namely, hGH Lys168 and Lys172. Since conjugation of PEG to proteins occurs at primary amines, pegylation of these two residues in hGH Gly120Lys would interfere with binding site 1 of the GH molecule and thus decrease the affinity for full-length membrane-bound GHRs. In B2036 PEG, one would not observe this interference with binding site 1, since the Lys and Arg residues in this site have been substituted with other amino acids.[146] In summary, Pegvisomant has an approximately fourfold decrease in binding affinity to the GHBP and an approximately 30-fold decreased binding affinity to membrane-bound GHR relative to B2036.[146]

Pegvisomant could be used in clinical situations in which elevated levels of GH are present or where the action of GH warrants downregulation. As was stated above, results of Pegvisomant treatment in acromegalic individuals have been described[141-145] and are discussed in Chapter 23. Other potential uses of GHA include diabetes-induced end-organ damage and several types of cancers. Animal data in the areas of diabetes-induced end-organ damage[121,129,147-149] and in cancer[150-152] have shown promising results. Also, the possibility of the use of a GH antagonist to lower insulin and glucose levels has been suggested.[143,153]

OTHER AMINO ACID SUBSTITUTIONS IN THE HYDROPHILIC REGION OF GH'S THIRD α-HELIX

We further generated a series of bGH analogues with single or double amino acid substitutions in the hydrophilic region of the α-helix.[67] Corresponding transgenic mice lines were generated and analyzed. On the basis of results of growth rates of these transgenic mice, the analogues were categorized as full growth-promoting analogues (Glu111Ala, Lys112Leu-Lys114Trp, Leu116Ala, Glu117Leu, Glu111Ala-Glu118Ala, Arg125Leu, Glu126Gly); partial growth-promoting analogues or partial agonists (Asp115Ala, Leu123Ile); growth inhibitory

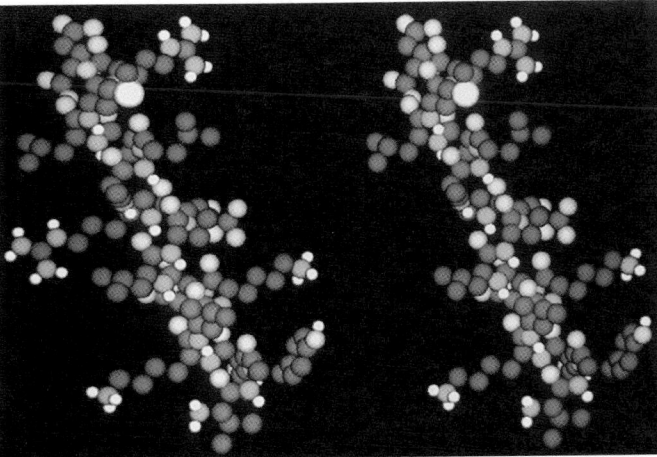

Figure 32-6 A space-filling model of the third α-helix of GH *(right)* and a GH antagonist *(left)*. The amino-terminal of the helices is located on the top of the figure, and the COOH end at the bottom. Note the cleft that is located in the middle of the wild-type helix *(right)* and the occupancy of this cleft with the side chain of Arg *(left)*. This figure is taken from Chen and colleagues.[63]

analogues (Gly119Xs); or non-growth-promoting analogues (deletion of residue 119, Δ-119).

It is important to note that analogues with amino acid substitutions that resulted in changes in growth-promoting activity are located within a region of nine amino acids, that is, between Asp 115 and Leu 123. These amino acids form two turns of the α-helix. By viewing the side chains of these potentially important amino acids, it appears that Gly 119 and Ala 122, two amino acids with relatively small side chains, form a hingelike or "cleft" structure, which we had predicted[63] (Fig. 32-6) and which has been shown to exist in the crystal structure of hGH.[154] The "cleft" is located near the center of this α-helix due primarily to Gly 119. Ala 122 is at the same phase of the α-helix, which extends the cleft owing to its relatively small side chain. We postulated that this cleft is important for the growth-promoting activity of the GH molecule.[63] If this cleft is important for growth-related biologic activity of the molecule, then Gly may be the only residue that is tolerable at this position. Extension of this model would yield the prediction that any other amino acid substitution at this position would decrease the flexibility of the molecule and/or "fill" the cleft, which would ultimately result in decreased biologic activity.

The amino acid residues that were chosen to substitute for Gly 119 in our study were representative of various amino acid groups, including Leu (hydrophobic, 2.8), Lys (hydrophilic and positively charged, 2.8), Trp (bulky hydrophobic, 3.8), and Pro (helix breaker with bulky side chain, 2.2). The number in parenthesis indicates the relative volume increase of the amino acid side chain as compared to Gly after the substitution mutation at position 119.

Finally, Asp 115 and Leu 123, amino acids with negatively charged (Asp) and long (Leu) side chains, respectively, flank the cleft and may be involved in the interaction with GH targets such as GHR or cellular targets.

To further substantiate the importance of the cleft in the third α-helix, we designed a bGH-analogue with a deletion at Gly 119 (△119). Transgenic mice that expressed this analogue demonstrated a phenotype similar to that of their littermates.[67] This data provide supportive evidence for the importance of the cleft structure in the third α-helix. It is interesting to point out that all bGH analogues tested in this study were able to bind to the GHR with an affinity similar to bGH including △119 (deletion mutation, inactive analogue), SAP (scrambled helix, weak antagonist), and Gly119Arg (potent antagonist).

To accommodate all of the data concerning the amino acid substitutions in GH, including those derived from the alanine-scanning studies[105] and those directed at the third α-helix of GH,[62] we proposed the second target hypothesis for GH action.[62] In this model, residues in α-helices I and IV and the large loop region interact with the GHR as reported by Cunningham and Wells.[105] Additionally, we postulated that the cleft region in the third α-helix interacts with an unidentified target and that the tripartite complex is the functional unit that is responsible for induction of GH action.[62]

COCRYSTALLIZATION OF GH WITH THE GHR

The second target hypothesis for GH action predicted that the cleft region in the third α-helix of GH would interact with an unidentified target, forming a GH/GHR/second target complex.[62] In 1992, the crystal structure of hGH along with the GH-binding protein (BP) was solved[154] (Fig. 32-7). Again, four GH α-helices were detected: α-helix I (residues 9 to 34), α-helix II (residues 72 to 92), α-helix III (residues 106 to 128), and α-helix IV (residues 155 to 184). Two small minihelices, residues 38 to 47 and 64 to 79, were also found in the large loop between α-helices I and II. Importantly, in the cocrystal, two identical GHBP molecules were found to interact with one GH molecule. Two sites on the GH molecule were found

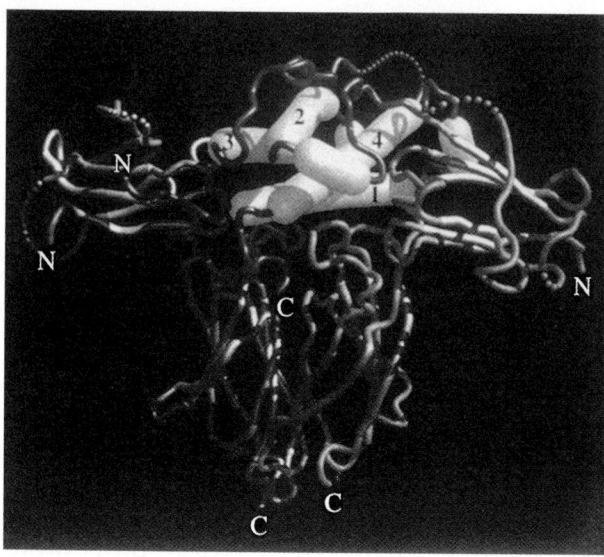

Figure 32-7   A representation of the GH/GHR cocrystal structure. The GH α-helices are indicated as cylinders and labeled 1, 2, 3, and 4. α-helices 1 and 4 (Site 1) are shown interacting with one GHBP; α-helix 3 (Site 2) is shown interacting with a second GHBP. This figure is taken from the cover of Science 1992 by de Vos and colleagues.[154]

to make contact with two identical GHRs. Amino acids, predicted from the alanine-scanning data,[105] were found to form the first contact site with the GHBP (Site 1), while the cleft region in the third α-helix, in particular Gly 120, and several amino acids at the amino terminus of the molecule were found to make contact with a second GHBP (Site 2). This observation was a substantial finding in the general fields of molecular endocrinology and in the area of growth factor and cytokine molecular and cellular biology. Significantly, it is one of the most fundamental findings in the GH field. Details concerning the interaction are described below. Thus, the cocrystallization of one GH molecule with two GHBPs supported the GH second target hypothesis of GH action, that is, the "second target" was another GHR. It should be pointed out that reagents used in these cocrystallization studies include nonglycosylated, bacterially synthesized GHBP and not a membrane-associated full-length GHR. Also, GH has not been found in a GHBP dimer in vivo.

GHR

BACKGROUND

Somatotropic cells of the anterior pituitary are the major site of GH synthesis and secretion. Production is regulated by the opposing actions of two hypothalamic neuropeptides: growth hormone–releasing hormone (GHRH), which stimulates synthesis and secretion of GH, and somatostatin (SST), which inhibits secretion of GH[69,155] (see Chapter 33). GH's essential role in growth promotion was once thought to be accomplished indirectly by the GH-induced synthesis of IGF-I (see Chapter 33). However, this point is still controversial, since the growth phenotype may be a combination of GH's direct tissue effects and the indirect effect of inducing synthesis of IGF-I. In contrast, GH's effect on energy metabolism in the nongrowing adult probably results from direct interaction with GHRs on target tissues.[156]

GHRs have been found on the cell surface of many tissues throughout the body, including liver, muscle, adipose, and kidney[157] and in early embryo and fetal tissue,[158–163] including an effect on embryonic tooth development.[164] Evidence linking

the importance of the GHR to the "growth" phenotype has come from the admirable studies on dwarf individuals who are GH-resistant. In these individuals, expression of different mutations located throughout the GHR gene result in the dwarf phenotype and a growth hormone–insensitive state that has been termed *Laron syndrome*.[165–170] GHR gene mutations have also been found in certain strains of sex-linked dwarf chickens.[171,172] The ultimate proof of the importance of the GHR was shown with the disruption of the GHR- and GH-binding protein (BP) genes in mice.[173] The knockout of these genes resulted in dwarf mice (Fig. 32-8). These mice are approximately half the size of wild-type mice. It was found that these mice have very low levels of IGF-1 and insulin, high levels of GH, and an extended life span.[174–176]

GHR AND GH-BINDING PROTEIN

The GHR is a member of the class 1 hematopoietic cytokine family.[177] The human GHR gene encompasses 10 exons and approximately 90 kb and encodes an extracellular domain, a small transmembrane domain, and an intracellular domain. The protein-coding region of the receptor gene is encoded by exons 2 to 10.[178] Exon 2 of the GHR gene encodes the secretory signal peptide and first six amino acids of the mature form of the protein; exons 3 to 7 encode the extracellular domain; exon 8 encodes the transmembrane domain; and exon 9 and 10 encode the intracellular domain.

The structure of the extracellular portion of the GHR consists of two domains, each containing seven β strands arranged to form a sandwich of two antiparallel β sheets.[154] This arrangement is also found in immunoglobins, CD4, and fibronectin. Stabilizing the GHR structure is a salt bridge between Arg 39 and Asp 132 and hydrogen bonds between Arg 43 and Glu 169.[154] Also, three disulfide bonds exist between Cys 38-48, Cys 83-94, and Cys 108-122[154,179] and are thought to be important in the overall structure integrity of the GHR.

A soluble portion of the GHR extracellular domain is termed the *GH-binding protein* (BP). In mice and rats, it is encoded by an additional exon, Exon 8A[180–182] and is produced by alternative splicing of the GHR precursor mRNA.[183,184] In other vertebrates, it is believed to be generated by proteolytic cleavage of the extracellular domain of the GHR. The function of the GHBP is unknown, but it might increase the activity of GH by enhancing its half-life or reduce the activity of GH by sequestering the molecule from the GHR. Until the GHBP gene alone has been disrupted, the ultimate function of the molecule remains unknown. The reader is referred to several GHBP reviews and papers.[23,73,183–189]

GH/GHR DIMERIZATION

Examination of the 2.8-angstrom crystal structure of the complex between the hormone and the extracellular domain of the GHR produced by *Escherichia coli* (hGHBP) demonstrated that the complex consisted of one molecule of GH and two molecules of receptor.[154] Furthermore, the crystal structure reveals how a nonsymmetric molecule, that is, GH, binds to two copies of the GHR (see Fig. 32-7).

Amino acid residues in the hGHR (actually hGH BP) involved in contact with hGH have been determined from the cocrystallization analyses of the GH/GHR complex.[154,190,191] The major binding determinants in the GH molecule (Site 1) are located in the two minihelices between α-helices 1 and 2 and between the center and carboxyl terminus of helix 4. GHR Site 1 residues are amino acids 40 to 45 and 101 to 106, which interact with GH amino acids 168 to 176 in α-helix 4 and residues 60 to 63 in the second minihelix. GHR Trp 169 interacts with hGH residues 171 to 179 in α-helix 4. The Site 2 binding determinants in the GHR are the same residues

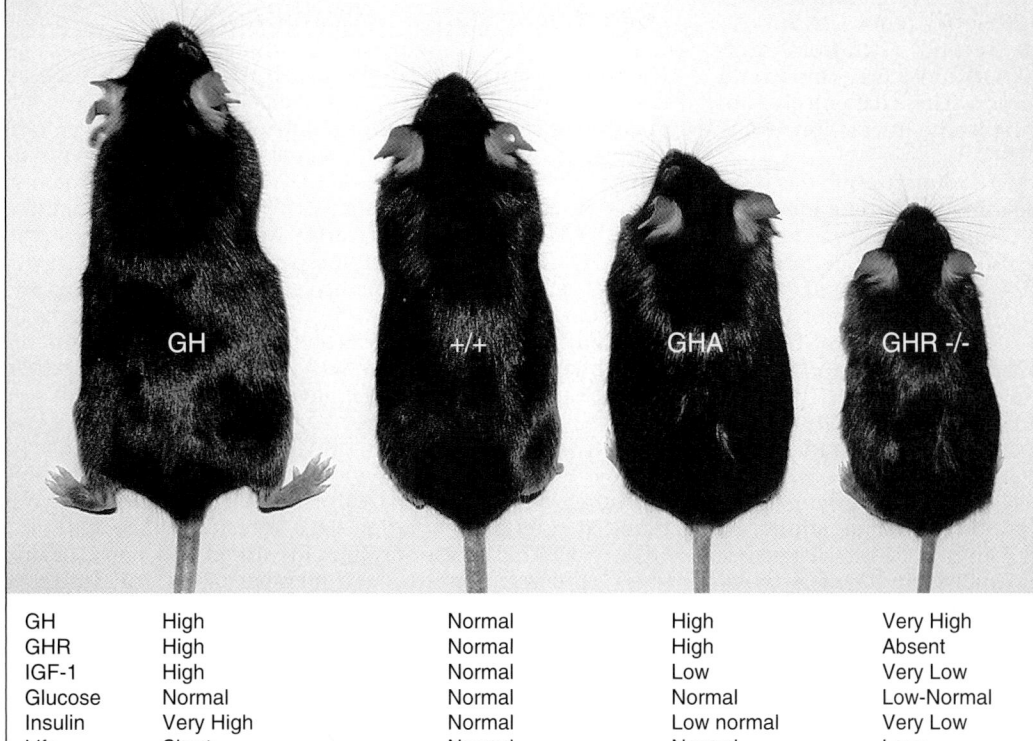

GH	High	Normal	High	Very High
GHR	High	Normal	High	Absent
IGF-1	High	Normal	Low	Very Low
Glucose	Normal	Normal	Normal	Low-Normal
Insulin	Very High	Normal	Low normal	Very Low
Life	Short	Normal	Normal	Long

Figure 32-8 GH transgenic, wild–type (+/+), GH antagonist (GHA) transgenic, and GHR/BP gene-disrupted (GHR –/–) mice. A wild-type mouse is shown second from the left (+/+). The GHR/BP (–/–) mouse is approximately half the size of the normal, wild-type (+/+) mouse and slightly smaller than the GHA transgenic mice. General endocrine values and life spans are noted.

(except for Asn 218) as for GHR Site I, especially Trp 104 and Trp 109. In terms of GH Site 2 residues that are important for contact and dimerization, only Phe 1, Ile 4, and Asp 116 in the third α-helix are significant.[192] Of particular interest is the close encounter with GH Gly 120 and GHR Trp 104 in this Site 2 interaction. Recently, the energetics governing the regulation of GH-induced receptor homodimerization has been presented.[193] In this study using *E. coli*–produced GHBP, two extracellular domains in the GHR were found to be important for GH binding. The authors found that most amino acid residues in the two binding interfaces act in an additive fashion, and six residues that are found in both domains contribute differently to GHR homodimerization depending on which extracellular domain they reside in.[193]

It must be pointed out that most if not all of these GH/GHBP interactive studies use a nonglycosylated, bacterially expressed GHBP and not the membrane-bound GHR. Reviews of the contact points between GH and the GHR have been presented.[194,195]

Attempts to generate a more potent GH agonist by altering Site 1 have been successful. For example, monovalent phage display techniques have yielded GH analogues with increased binding affinity to the GHR.[196] Also, GH analogues in which residues have been altered in the C-terminus of the first helix have resulted in GH agonists with increased GHR-binding affinity.[197,198]

In the GHR, a GH-induced dimerization domain exists. A Cys residue, Cys 241, has been reported to undergo GH-induced intermolecular disulfide bonding, thus bridging together two GHR.[199] Also, eight hGHR amino acid residues are involved in the salt bridge and the hydrogen bond interactions across the extracellular dimerization domain.[154] For hGHR1, the residues are Ser 145, Leu 146, Thr 147, His 150, Asp 152, and Ser 201; for hGHR2, they are Asp 152, Ser 201, Asn 143, and Tyr 200. Of these eight residues, five are important for GH/GHR-mediated signal transduction, Ser 145, His 150, Asp 152, Try 200, and Ser 201 but not Leu 146 or Thr 147.[200] This study as well as others,[201] including those using monoclonal antibodies to induce a GH response,[202] suggest

that a GH-induced conformational change in the GHR is required for a full biologic response. Additionally, the subtle but significant differences between the 1hGH/2GHR[154] and 1 hGH/1GHR[203] cocrystal structures suggest that a conformational change does occur in the one ligand–two receptor complex.

Members of the cytokine receptor family possess disulfide bonds and a WSXWS "box" in their extracellular domain. The GHR, unlike the other members of the cytokine receptor family, does not possess a WSXWS box, but an equivalent YGEFS sequence has been noted.[204] A similar sequence has been found in the extracellular domain of the PrlR.[205] This sequence has been reported to be important for binding GHR accessory molecules[206] or provides a stabilizing effect on the receptor's structure.[204,207]

I have touched on only a few of the structural characteristics of the GHR. For a more exhaustive review of this subject, the reader is referred to an excellent review by Waters.[195]

GH/GHR INTERACTION: A MODEL

The cocrystallization of GH with GHBP[154] was, and is, a remarkable scientific finding (see Fig. 32-7). However, one must remember that in this crystal structure, GHBP, not the full-length GHR, was used. Also, since the GHBP was produced by *E. coli*, it was not glycosylated, as is the native GHBP and GHR. Nonetheless, the interaction of one GH with two GHBP has been extrapolated to the in vivo interaction of GH with the GHR. This finding has led to the theory of a sequential binding mechanism in which hGH binds to two GHRs.[192] In this model, hGH must first binds to one GHR using as high-affinity receptor-binding site that subsequently allows binding of the second receptor. Binding site 1 of hGH is located at residues identified by Ala scanning mutagenesis studies,[105] that is, α-helix one, the loop between amino acids 54 and 74, and α-helix four. Binding site 2 is located at the N-terminal (Ile 4) and the third α-helix, namely, Gly 120. The model predicts that a Typ 104 residue of the GHR "fits" into the "cleft" of the third α-helix of GH. The authors also proposed that the reason that hGH-Gly120Arg acted as a GH antagonist is because the substitution of Arg for Gly at position 120 blocked or inhibited the "second" GHR from interacting with binding site 2 on the GH molecule. This would inhibit GH-induced GHR dimerization. These data nicely supported the "cleft" theory pertaining to the interaction of GH Gly 120 with a second target.[62–67,119–121]

The importance of GH-induced GHR dimerization has been shown recently in humans. An adenine-to-guanine mutation was found in the hGH gene that results in the conversion of Asp112 to Gly. In the heterozygous state, the mutation is believed to be the cause of dwarfism in a female child.[208] This hGH analogue binds to hGHR in vitro but does not induce GHR dimerization and does not activate JAK2 and STAT5,[208] thus stressing the importance of GHR dimerization for biologic activity.

Recently, studies with GH antagonists (bGH Gly119Arg, hGH Gly120Lys, B2036, and Pegvisomant) have dramatically changed the GH-induced dimerization theory. The initial GH antagonists (bGH Gly119Arg and hGH Gly120Lys) were shown to bind to membrane-bound GHR with the same affinity as wild-type GH.[62,66] They were also found to be internalized at the same rate as wild-type GH. Finally, by chemical cross-linking studies, they were found to exist in a complex with 2 GHR.[209] Similar findings have recently been presented.[210] Thus, these data showed that GH antagonists do not prevent GHR dimerization but inhibit proper or functional GHR dimerization. This idea of GHR dimerization was further advanced by studies comparing binding and internalization rates of several GH antagonists, including hGH Gly120Lys, B2036, Peg-hGH Gly120 Lys, and Pegvisomant.[146] Again, these results showed that GH antagonists do not inhibit GHR dimerization or internalization but interfere with proper GHR dimerization. Finally, the elegant work of Gent and colleagues using coimmunoprecipitation and epitope-tagged truncated GHRs have now conclusively shown that ligand-independent GHR dimerization occurs in the endoplasmic reticulum and on cell membranes independent of GH binding.[211] A model of the interaction of GH with a preformed GHR dimer and of the GH antagonist (GHA) with a preformed GHR dimer is shown in Figure 32-9.

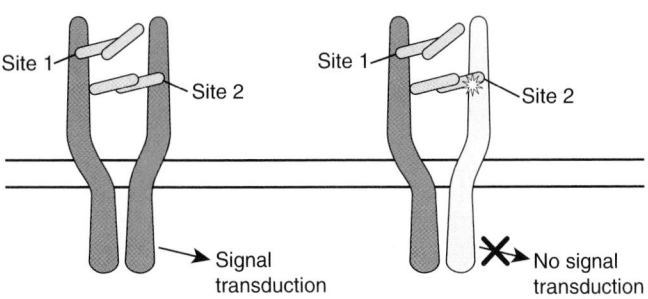

A   GH/GHR interaction   B   GHA/GHR interaction

Figure 32-9 **A,** The one-GH/two-GHR model of GH action. The GH molecule and its four α-helices are represented by the horizontal cylinders. The preformed GHR is shown as crossing the cellular membrane *(dark horizontal lines)*. The interaction of GH with the preformed GHR at Site 1 and Site 2 is indicated. Not shown are the several N-linked glycosylation sites on the GHR. **B,** The interaction of a GH antagonist with the preformed GHR dimer. The GH antagonist (GHA) and its four α-helices are represented by horizontal cylinders. The gly to lys change in the third α-helix is depicted by a star. The interaction of GHA with the preformed GHR at Site 1 and Site 2 is indicated. An improper or nonfunctional GHA/GHR dimer is indicated by the light shade of gray in the second GHR molecules found in the preformed dimer. Not shown are the several N-linked glycosylation sites on the GHR.

GH-INDUCED SIGNAL TRANSDUCTION

The molecular mechanisms by which GH transmits its signals via its receptor have been largely elucidated by experiments in cultured cells or hypophysectomized rats.[212] However, GH-induced, in vivo, tissue-specific signal transduction systems are still largely unknown and the subject of continued research in our own lab[213] as well as others.[214,215] Below are summarized several GH-mediated intracellular signal transduction pathways (Fig. 32-10). Some of these pathways may overlap with signal transduction intermediates induced by insulin and other hormones, thus providing opportunities of "biologic cross-talk" between these molecules. Several reviews on the subject have been recently presented.[79,212,216–221] Also, excellent reviews on the GHR and PRLR have been published.[195,219]

JAK ACTIVATION

In the early 1990s, GH treatment of responsive cells was found to induce association of a tyrosine kinase with the GHR.[222–224] This kinase was later identified as a 121-kDA protein[225] and was found to be a member of the JAK family of proteins, in particular JAK2.[226,227] Activation of JAKs appears to be an initial step in one of the GH-induced signal transduction systems (see Fig. 32-10). Although three JAK molecules are involved in the GH/GHR signal transduction, JAK2 exhibits the greatest degree of activation.[226,228–230] GH-dependent JAK2 activation requires interaction between JAK2 and the membrane-proximal, proline-rich motif (termed *box 1*) located in the intracellular region of GHR.[231–234] Since GHR itself has no intrinsic kinase activity, it is thought that the colocalization of two JAK2 molecules by the dimerized GHR results in transphosphorylation of one JAK2 by the other, resulting in JAK2 activation.[212,218] Activated JAK2, in turn, is thought to phosphorylate GHR on multiple tyrosine residues, possibly providing docking sites for STAT5.[235,236]

SIGNAL TRANSDUCERS AND ACTIVATORS OF TRANSCRIPTION (STAT) SIGNALING PATHWAY

Many of the physiologic effects of GH result from transcriptional regulation of a variety of genes. Several different signaling pathways contribute to this regulation (see Fig. 32-10), but the pathway that was discovered in the mid-1990s and perhaps the most universal pathway implicated in GH action involves the signal transducers and activators of transcription (STAT) proteins. On phosphorylation, cytoplasmic STAT proteins form either homodimers or heterodimers, translocate into the nucleus, bind DNA, and activate transcription.[218,237]

GH-dependent tyrosyl phosphorylation requiring JAK2 activation has been demonstrated for STAT1, STAT3, and STAT5.[228,234,238–243] In addition, STAT5 activation requires regions of GHR that are not involved in JAK2 activation, suggesting that STAT5 also interacts directly with GHR.[228,234,235,244] The docking of STAT5 with the GHR requires phosphorylated tyrosine residues that are presumably mediated by JAK2. The tyrosine residues that were found to be phosphorylated and important in the STAT5 docking and subsequent activation reaction have been reported.[235,243,245,246] While STAT5 has been found to directly associate with the GHR,[243] STAT1 and STAT3 probably do not but interact with the GHR but interact with JAK2 instead.[228,234,244] A model of this interaction has been presented.[235]

STAT1, STAT3, STAT5, and possibly STAT4 have also been identified in GH-induced DNA-binding complexes of several genes. For example, STAT1, STAT3, and in some cells STAT4 have been shown to bind to the *cis*-inducible element (SIE) of the c-*fos* promoter/enhancer.[239–241,247] Similarly, STAT5 has been shown to bind to the interferon-γ-activated sequence (GAS)-like response element in the serine protease inhibitor

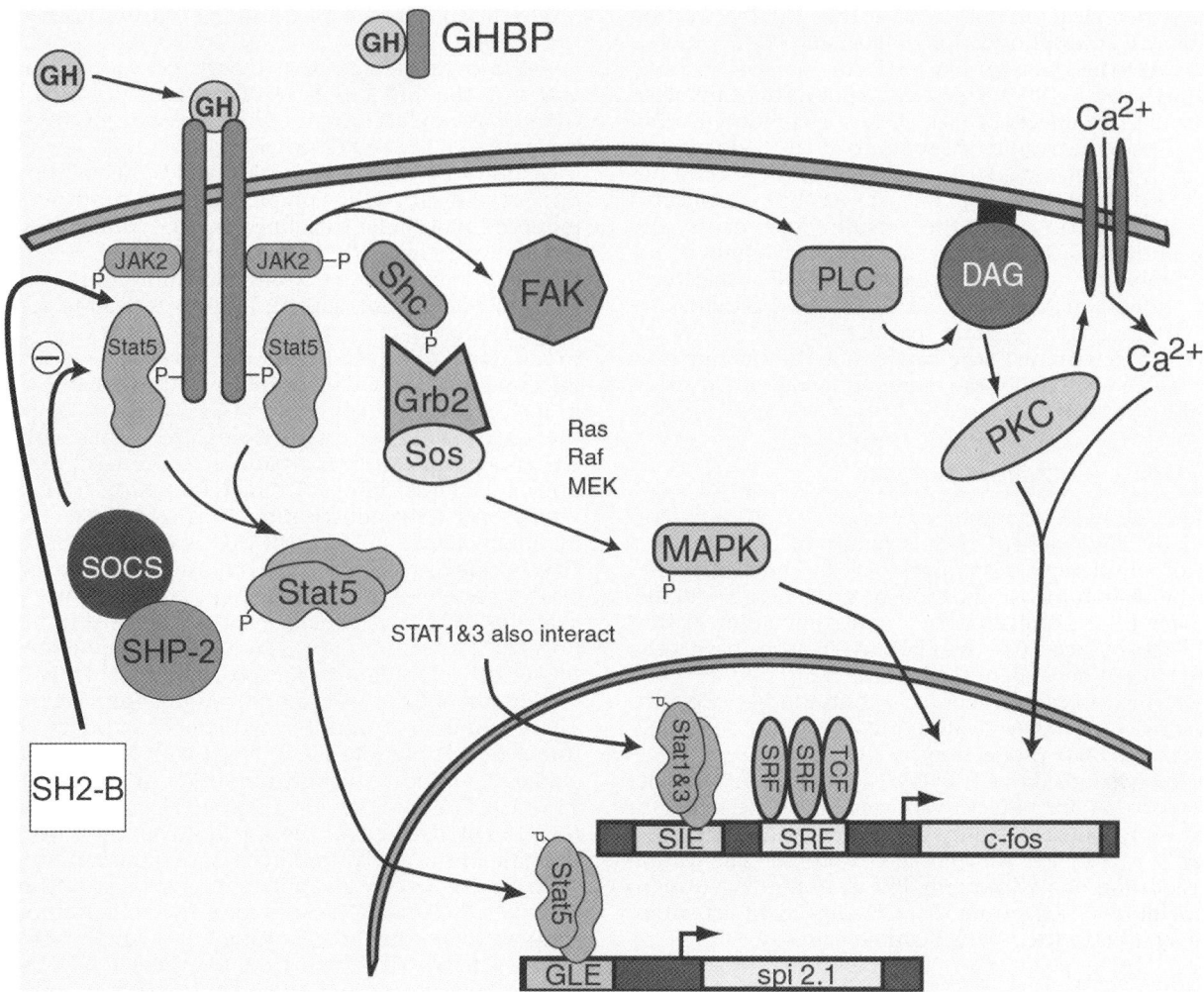

Figure 32-10 A model depicting intracellular signaling intermediates induced by binding of GH with the GHR. This figure is taken has been modified from Kopchick and Andry.[79]

(*spi*) 2.1 gene.[248] Their presence is required for maximum transcriptional gene activation.[249,250]

MITOGEN-ACTIVATED PROTEIN KINASE (MAPK) SIGNALING PATHWAY

Another GH-inducible pathway that ultimately culminates in transcriptional regulation of a number of genes involves activation of two mitogen-activated protein kinases (MAPKs), termed *extracellular signal regulated kinase (ERK) 1 and ERK2*.[251–254] (see Fig. 32-10). This pathway was first described for insulin-mediated signal transduction. The pathway most likely begins with GH-stimulated binding of SHC family members to phosphorylated residues in both GHR and JAK2 followed by phosphorylation of the SHCs by JAK2.[255] Subsequently, the tyrosyl phosphorylated SHC proteins interact with growth factor receptor bound 2 (GRB2), which, in turn, interacts with *son of sevenless* (SOS).[255,256] Finally, GH activates RAS, RAF, and MAP-ERK kinase (MEK).[256] These studies, as well as those by Winston and Hunter,[257] implicate GH as the inducer of the SHC-GRB2-SOS-RAS-RAF-MEK pathway for activation of MAPK. GH has also been shown to activate insulin receptor substrates (IRS)-1[258,259] and IRS-2,[260] which can also lead to activation of the RAS-MEK-signaling pathway (see below).

GH has been shown to activate the S6 kinase, p90(RSK), most likely via MAPK.[251] p90(RSK), in turn, can phosphorylate a transcription factor, termed *serum response factor* (SRF), that binds to the GH-responsive serum response element

(SRE) of the c-*fos* promoter/enhancer.[247,261] GH may activate another protein, the ternary complex factor p62(TCF)/ELK1, which interacts with SRF to bind SRE but is directly activated by ERKs 1 and 2.[262,263] Further evidence that MAPKs are involved in the GH-dependent transcriptional regulation of c-*fos* comes from the observation that the same regions of GHR required for activation of MAPK are also required for c-*fos* gene induction.[264] As was mentioned above, STAT proteins are also involved in c-*fos* gene regulation, demonstrating a convergence of at least two divergent GH-signaling pathways in the regulation of a single gene. MAPK activation, also inducible by a number of growth factors, may represent a common signal transduction system, whereas activation of STAT proteins (in particular STAT5) may be more specific to GH.[265]

The MAPK-signaling pathway may also contribute to the insulin-like activity of GH, that is, stimulation of glucose uptake.[264] An inhibitor that blocks GH-induced tyrosyl phosphorylation of ERKs 1 and 2 but not JAK2 also partially inhibits GH-stimulated glucose uptake, implicating involvement of inhibitor-sensitive kinases downstream of JAK2 but upstream of ERKs 1 and 2 in this activity.[264]

INSULIN RECEPTOR SUBSTRATE SIGNALING PATHWAY

In addition to the MAPK pathway intermediates, GH also activates members of an additional insulin-signaling pathway, IRS-1, and IRS-2[258,260] (see Fig. 32-10). Although the nature of the interaction between the IRS molecules and the GHR/JAK2 complex is not clear, it does appear that JAK2 activation results in tyrosyl phosphorylation of IRS-1 and IRS-2, which is involved in the insulin-like effects of GH.[259,260,266] Phosphatidylinositol (PI) 3′-kinase also appears to be involved in the insulin-like effects of GH, since a GH-induced interaction between the regulatory subunit of PI 3′-kinase and tyrosyl phosphorylated IRS-1 and -2 has been demonstrated.[259,260,267,268] PI 3′-kinase, in turn, has been implicated in the translocation of the insulin-dependent glucose transporter GLUT4 from low-density microsomes to the plasma membrane, nuclear translocation of ERK1, and regulation of protein kinase C (PKC). Whether these activities are directly GH inducible remains speculative.[260,269–271] Also, it has not been determined whether or not the IRS-signaling pathway is also involved in the more physiologically relevant anti-insulin effects of GH.

PROTEIN KINASE C SIGNALING PATHWAY

Experiments designed to inhibit or deplete PKC activity have suggested the involvement of this family of enzymes in a number of physiologic responses to GH. These responses include the insulin-like stimulation of lipogenesis,[272] induction of c-fos gene expression,[273,274] and stimulation of Ca^{2+} uptake.[275] GH-induced Ca^{2+} oscillations, in turn, have been implicated in GH-dependent spi 2.1 gene transcription[276] and the refractoriness of certain cells to GH's insulin-like effects.[277]

One pathway for PKC activation involves GH-induced 1,2-diacylglycerol (DAG) production by phospholipase C (PLC) that is possibly coupled to GHR via a G protein.[278,279] Another proposed pathway for PKC activation involves the IRS/PI 3′-kinase pathway, but its inability to act independently on GH is unclear.[212,271] We have shown that GH promotes activation and translocation of a PK isoform, PKC-ε, from the cytosol to plasma membrane, suggesting that GH-dependent activation of PKC may involve the IRS/PI 3′-kinase pathway.[280]

SUPPRESSORS OF CYTOKINE-SIGNALING AND PROTEIN TYROSINE PHOSPHATASES

Recently, several molecules have been implicated in inhibiting GH-induced intracellular signaling. Suppressors of cytokine-signaling (SOCS) proteins are important in the regulation of GHR/JAK2 signaling (see Fig. 32-10). There are eight members of the SOCS family, and GH induces SOCS 1, 2, and 3. SOCS proteins are thought to downregulate GH signaling by inhibiting the kinase activity of JAK2.[221] In addition to SOCS proteins, several protein tyrosine phosphatases have been found to be involved in termination of GH-activated STAT signaling. Two candidate phosphatases are the SH2 domain containing phosphatases, SHP1 and SHP2, and have been implicated in dephosphorylation of JAK-2 and GHR tyrosines (see Fig. 32-10).[220,221]

As was mentioned earlier, the GH-responsive pathways described above have been elucidated primarily by experiments performed in cell culture or under special in vivo circumstances. An important challenge that is just beginning to be addressed is the verification of these pathways in normal animals.[214,215] The ultimate challenge, however, will be the correlation of physiologic GH functions with a particular tissue-specific signal transduction pathway.

THE MECHANISM OF GH ACTION: PROBLEMS AND OPPORTUNITIES

PROBLEMS WITH THE 1GH/2GHR DIMERIZATION MODEL

Dimerization of the GHR appears to be essential for GH action and has become the model when describing the molecular interaction of GH with the GHR.[122,154] However, several

results, listed below, should lead to more exhaustive testing of the model.

One must remember that in this crystal structure, GHBP, and not the full-length GHR, was used. Also, since the GHBP was produced by E. coli, it was not glycosylated, as is the native GHBP and GHR.

GH-induced GHR dimerization and subsequent internalization of the GH/GHR complex are not sufficient for GH-induced intracellular signaling, since GH antagonists do form dimers with the GHR and are internalized.[209] Also, experiments with monoclonal antibodies indicate that binding of GH, but not GH antagonists, appears to lead to a conformational change in the extracellular domain of GHR, giving rise to an active dimer configuration necessary for signal transduction.[201,202] These data fit nicely with the subtle differences in the cocrystal structures of the GH/GHR 2:1 complex versus the 1:1 GH antagonist/GHR complex.[203] Thus, although the GH antagonist can bind to and promote GHR dimer formation, apparently "proper" dimer formation is not induced. This proper GHR dimerization apparently leads to a conformational change in the GHR that is required for subsequent GH specific intracellular signal transduction (see Fig. 32-9).

Data presented in studies using transgenic mice as in vivo assay for various GH analogues have resulted in mouse phenotypes that cannot be explained simply by employing the one-GH/two-GHR model for GH action.[67,281] Different mouse growth phenotypes were found, ranging from dwarf to giants. These results that cannot be explained simply by the altered interaction at binding site 2 of GH with its receptor. In these studies,[67] amino acid substitutions in bGH at positions Asp 115 (Asp 116 of hGH), Ala 122 (Thr 123 of hGH), or Leu 123 (Leu 124 of hGH) have been shown to have less than a sixfold decrease in the ability to induce GHR dimerization in vitro[122] yet have a significant and different effect on growth-promoting activities.[66] Thus, GH-induced GHR dimerization cannot simply explain the different mouse growth phenotypes.

One alternative explanation for these results is that the third α-helical region of GH interacts with an unknown second target(s) that participates in the regulation growth. The second target postulation is substantiated by the finding that hGH 108–129, a sequence encompassing the third α-helix of hGH, binds to a site other than the GHR and evokes a mitogenic response.[282]

hGH Ile 4 has been shown to be an important residue in the site 2 interaction between GH and the GHR. Replacement of Ile 4 with alanine greatly diminishes the ability of GH-induced GHR dimerization,[192] yet expression of this GH analogue (hGH-Ile4Ala) in transgenic mice results in large animals or full GH activity.[66] Thus, if the hGH analogue (Ile-4-Ala) is decreasing proper GHR dimerization, then it is not affecting the ability of GH to promote growth in transgenic mice.

In the cocrystal structure of hGH with the hGHBP, Trp 104 of the GHR closely aligns with hGH Gly 120.[154] Transgenic mice that express hGH Gly120Lys possess a dwarf phenotype.[66] However, if hGH Gly 120 is replace by Ala, one would predict that GHR Trp 104 would be somewhat displaced from the hGH molecule, since it can not "fit" into the cleft of the third α-helix. This molecule would be predictive to inhibit or destabilize GHR dimerization. However, this molecule acts as a full agonist in its ability to promote growth in transgenic mice.[66]

Thus, is GH-induced GHR dimerization the universal mechanism by which GH elicits its many activities? Perhaps not.

ARE THERE OTHER GHRs?

As was stated above, although the cocrystal structure of GH and the GH/GHBP has been solved,[154] one should not become dogmatic in terms of the one-ligand/two-receptor hypothesis when attempting to explain all of GH's in vivo activities.

Continuing on the possibility of other GHRs, it has been reported that hGH fragment 44–191 binds with low affinity to the GHR and at high, nonphysiologic levels stimulates proliferation of a myeloid cell transfected with the hGHR. Also, the 44–191 fragment can antagonize GH action, presumably by blocking proper GHR dimerization. In contrast, hGH fragment 44–191 has been shown to have an order of magnitude higher diabetogenic activity than hGH.[283] Could another GHR be responsible for these activities?

Also, when one compares the ability of GH to induce differentiation with its ability to stimulate glucose uptake (GH's insulin-like activity) in 3T3-L1 cells (preadipocytes), one finds a difference in ED50 values for these two activities.[284,285] The ED50 for GH promotion of differentiation is approximately 0.1 nM,[284] while that of its insulin-like activity is 1.0 nM.[285] If GH were acting via the same GHR and intracellular signaling system, then the same ED50 values may be predicted for each activity. However, this is clearly not the case.

Cunningham and coworkers have reported that hGH analogues with amino acid substitutions at site I resulted in GH analogues with affinities for the GHR that are similar to or greater than those of wild-type GH; however, they have markedly decreased bioactivity.[104,105,192]

Staten and colleagues[286] have shown that bovine PL forms a 1:1 complex with bGHR, however, bGH will induce a 1:2 complex under similar conditions. Surprisingly, both are able to induce and increase in circulating IGF-1 and nitrogen retention in cattle.

Additionally, the first described GH antagonist (bGH Gly 119-Arg) represses growth in transgenic mice[62] and inhibits GH-induced preadipocyte differentiation.[119,120] Surprisingly, this molecule antagonizes the lipolytic effect but retains full insulin-like activity of GH in a chicken adipose tissue.[287]

Thus, is GH interacting with the same GHR to induce these activities?

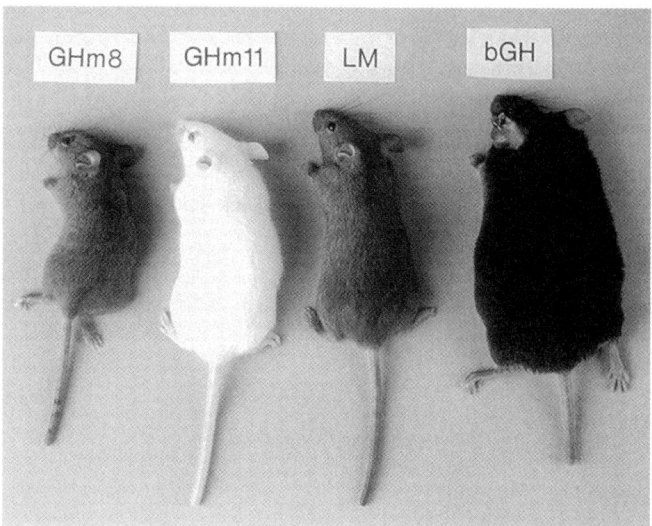

Figure 32-11 Growth phenotypes of mice that express different GH analogues. The animal shown are 6-month-old males.
A nontransgenic control animal is indicated as the littermate (LM). A mouse that expresses wild-type bGH is shown on the right and is labeled bGH. A mouse that expressed the bGH antagonist, bGH-Gly119Arg, is shown on the left and is labeled GHm8. A mouse that express a bGH analogue in which the third α-helix is destabilized by substitution of proline residues at selected sites[127] and is labeled GHm11. Note that the LM and GHm11 mice are approximately the same size, the bGH animal is approximately twice the size of LM, and GHm8 is approximately half the size of LM. The LM and GHm8 mice live to approximately 3 years of age, bGH animal dies at 9 to 12 months of age, and GHm11 dies at 12 to 15 months of age. This figure was taken from Yang and colleagues.[127]

GH ASSAYS

One of the most important issues concerning discoveries in the GH area, or perhaps the most important issue, is the types of assays used to quantify GH and to identify the activity of the molecule. Further work is needed to standardize quantification of GH. One cannot screen for the ability of GH analogues to bind to GHRs in vitro and expect to predict the activity of the molecule in vivo. If this were the only assay used, then GH antagonists would not have been discovered.[62] Additional assays involving the in vivo action of GH are needed.

At times somewhat unexpected, yet important, results are derived from in vivo studies, For example, in a structure/function approach to the activities of GH in which mutated GH genes are expressed in transgenic mice and the growth of the animals is monitored, our group has shown that one can uncouple the ability of GH to enhance IGF-1 production and promote growth from a deleterious effect, that is, GH-induced glomerulosclerosis (Fig. 32-11; see also Fig. 32-6). Expression of wild-type GH gene in transgenic mice results in animals with elevated serum IGF-1 levels and a corresponding enhanced growth phenotype (see Fig. 32-8).[61,62] These "giant" GH transgenic mice have been found to die prematurely, with glomerulosclerosis as one of the primary causes of death phenotype[149] (see Fig. 32-5). Importantly, transgenic IGF-1 mice do not develop glomerulosclerosis.[149] Thus, GH appears to be acting directly on the kidney independent of IGF-1. Support for this concept of GH direct action on peripheral tissue comes from studies on another strain of transgenic mice. When the third α-helix of GH was destabilized by the substitution of proline residues as selected sites and these mutated GH genes (termed *M11*) were subsequently expressed in transgenic mice, animals with normal growth phenotypes and normal serum IGF-1 levels resulted (see Fig. 32-11). However, severe glomerulosclerosis was observed in these animals[126,127] (see Fig. 32-5). Thus, the ability of GH to promote growth and

enhance IGF-1 production was uncoupled from the ability to induce glomerulosclerosis. Therefore, it appears that GH is acting directly on the kidney, independently of IGF-1. This is an important observation, since it is the first to report that GH may indeed act independently of IGF-1.

The data from in vitro binding studies, cell-based assays, or in vivo assays must be carefully interpreted to precisely define the function of novel GH analogues. For example, the ability of GH analogues to act as mitogenic agents might not be the proper cell-based assay to uncover GH's mechanism of action, since some believe that GH is not a mitogenic agent.[54] While a variety of cell-based and several in vivo assays abound, none sufficiently depict the action of the molecule as it acts in "normal" conditions. Thus, an important future challenge is to develop assays which reflect the action of GH. Since the in vivo molecule actions of GH are not known, the opportunity exists for the discovery and development of these assays.

CONCLUDING REMARKS

The study of the mechanism by which GH elicits its many and varied responses has proceeded vigorously for nearly seven decades. The recent advances in obtaining the crystal structure of GH[96] (see Fig. 32-2), the discovery of GHAs[62] (see Figs. 32-3 and 32-4), cocrystallization of GH with GHBP[154] (see Fig. 32-7), elucidation of the GHR as a preexisting dimer,[211] and disruption of the mouse GHR/BP gene[173] (see Fig. 32-8) have resulted in new ideas and research directions in the GH area. With this new information and the proteomics and genomics age upon us, the future for testing hypotheses based on the action of GH remains fertile. Important areas for new discovery include elucidation of in vivo, tissue-specific GH/GHR-induced signal transduction pathways, the possibility of other GHRs, and breakthroughs concerning therapeutic molecules that might influence the activity of GH.

Several important questions arise related to the above discussion:

1. Do all of GH biologic activities arise via proper or functional GH-induced dimerization of the GHR?
2. Do other GHRs exist?
3. Does GH act directly on tissue, independent of the action of IGF-1?

These as well as other unanswered questions will be solved in the future; however, inspection of the preliminary data would suggest the following respective answers: No, yes, yes.

Acknowledgments

My work on GH is currently supported by grants from DiAthegen LLC, Ohio University's Edison Biotechnology Institute, the College of Osteopathic Medicine, and Eminent Scholar's Program, which include a grant form Milton and Lawrence Goll. Previously, the GH work was supported by the above, with additional funding derived from the USDA, NIH, Merck & Co., the Juvenile Diabetes International Foundation, the Central Ohio Diabetes Association, and Sensus Corp.

I would like to thank all of my current and former graduate students, postdoctoral fellows, technicians, undergraduate students, visiting scientists, and collaborators who participated in many of the studies reported in this review and whose scientific and personal friendships I cherish.

REFERENCES

1. Evans HM, Long JA: The effect of the anterior lobe administered intraperitoneally upon growth, maturity and oestrus cycles of the rat. Anat Rec 21:62–63, 1921.
2. Li CH, Evans HM: The isolation of pituitary growth hormone. Science 99:183–184, 1944.
3. Martial JA, Hallewell RA, Baxter JD, et al: Human growth hormone: Complementary DNA cloning and expression in bacteria. Science 205:602–607, 1979.
4. Miller WL, Eberhardt NL: Structure and evolution of the growth hormone gene family. Endocr Rev 4:97–130, 1983.
5. Niall HD, Hogan ML, Sauer R, et al: Sequences of pituitary and placental lactogenic and growth hormones: Evolution from a primordial peptide by gene reduplication. Proc Natl Acad Sci U S A 68:866–870, 1971.
6. Watahiki M, Yamamoto M, Yamakawa M, et al: Conserved and unique amino acid residues in the domains of the growth hormones. Flounder growth hormone deduced from the cDNA sequence has the minimal size in the growth hormone prolactin gene family. J Biol Chem 264:312–316, 1989.
7. Li CH: The chemistry of human pituitary growth hormone: 1967–1973. In Li CH (ed): Hormonal Proteins and Peptides, vol 3. New York, Academic Press, 1975, pp 1–33.
8. Scanes CG, Campbell RM: Growth hormone: Chemistry. In Harvey S, Scanes CG, Daughaday WH (eds): Growth Hormone. Boca Raton, CRC Press, 1995, pp 1–24.
9. Kopchick JJ, Chen WY: Structure function relationships of growth hormone (GH) and other members of the GH gene family. Handbook Physiol 2000, pp 325–360.
10. Hennen G, Frankenne F, Closset J, et al: A human placental GH: Increasing levels during second half of pregnancy with pituitary GH suppression as revealed by monoclonal antibody radioimmunoassays. Int J Fertil 30:27–33, 1985.
11. Daughaday WH, Trivedi B, Winn HN, et al: Hypersomatotropism in pregnant women, as measured by a human liver radioreceptor assay. J Clin Endocrinol Metab 70:215–221, 1990.
12. Frankenne F, Rentier-Delrue F, Scippo ML, et al: Expression of the growth hormone variant gene in human placenta. J Clin Endocrinol Metab 64:635–637, 1987.
13. Selden RF, Wagner TE, Blethen S, et al: Expression of the human growth hormone variant gene in cultured fibroblasts and transgenic mice. Proc Natl Acad Sci U S A 85:8241–8245, 1988.
14. Lewis UJ: Variants of growth hormone and prolactin and their posttranslational modifications. Annu Rev Physiol 46:33–42, 1984.
15. Wallis M: The molecular evolution of pituitary growth hormone prolactin and placental lactogen: A protein family showing variable rates of evolution. J Mol Evol 17:10, 1981.
16. Chen EY, Liao YC, Smith DH, et al: The human growth hormone locus: Nucleotide sequence, biology, and evolution. Genomics 4:479–497, 1989.
17. Kaplan SL, Grumbach MM: Electrophoretic and immunological characteristics of native and purified human growth hormone. Nature 196:336–338, 1962.
18. Lewis UJ, Brink NC: Crystalline human growth hormone. J Am Chem Soc 80:4429–4430, 1958.
19. Lewis UJ, Dunn JT, Bonewald LF, et al: A naturally occurring structural variant of human growth hormone. J Biol Chem 253:2679–2687, 1978.
20. Li CH, Liu WK, Dixon JS: Human pituitary growth hormone. VI: Modified procedure of isolation and NH$_2$-terminal amino acid sequence. Arch Biochem Biophys (Suppl I):327–332, 1962.
21. Roos P, Fevold HR, Gemzell CA: Preparation of human growth hormone by gel filtration. Biochim Biophys Acta 74:525–531, 1965.
22. Russell J, Sherwood LM, Kowalski K, et al: Recombinant hormones from fragments of human growth hormone and human placental lactogen. J Biol Chem 256:296–300, 1981.
23. Baumann G: Growth hormone heterogeneity: Genes, isohormones, variants, and binding proteins. Endocr Rev 12:424–449, 1991.
24. Sonksen PH, Salomon F, Cuneo R: Metabolic effects of hypopituitarism and acromegaly. Horm Res 36:27–31, 1991.
25. Daughaday WH: Growth hormone, insulin-like growth factors, and acromegaly. In DeGrout LJ (ed): Endocrinology, vol 3. Philadelphia, WB Saunders, 1995, pp 303–329.
26. Melmed S, Braunstein GD, Horvath E, et al: Pathophysiology of acromegaly. Endocr Rev 4:271–290, 1983.
27. Melmed S, Ho K, Klibanski A, et al: Clinical review 75: Recent advances in pathogenesis, diagnosis, and management of acromegaly. J Clin Endocrinol Metab 80:3395–3402, 1995.
28. Melmed S: Acromegaly. Metabolism 45:51–52, 1996.
29. Melmed S: Unwanted effects of growth hormone excess in the adult. J Pediatr Endocrinol Metab 9(Suppl 3):369–374, 1996.
30. Melmed S: Medical management of acromegaly: What and when? Acta Endocrinol (Copenh) 129(Suppl 1):13–17, 1993.
31. Milman AE, Russell JA: Some aspects of purified pituitary growth hormone on carbohydrate metabolism in the rat. Endocrinology 47:114–119, 1950.
32. Swislocki NL: Effects of nutritional status and the pituitary on the acute plasma free fatty acid and glucose responses of rats to growth hormone administration. Metabolism 17:174–180, 1968.
33. Hjalmarson A, Ahren K: Sensitivity of the rat diaphragm to growth hormone. II: Early and late effects of growth hormone on amino acid and pentose uptake. Acta Endocrinol (Copenh) 56:347–358, 1967.
34. Kostyo JL, Nutting DF: Acute in vivo effects of growth hormone on protein synthesis in various tissues of hypophysectomized rats and their relationship to the levels of thymidine factor and insulin in the plasma. Horm Metab Res 5:167–172, 1973.
35. Batchelor BR, Mahler RJ: Growth hormone-induced enhancement of insulin sensitivity in adipose tissue. Horm Metab Res 4:87–92, 1972.
36. Goodman HM: The effects of growth hormone on the utilization of L-leucine in adipose tissue. Endocrinology 102:210–217, 1978.

37. Newman JD, Armstrong JM, Bornstein J: Effects of part sequences of human growth hormone on in vivo hepatic glycogen metabolism in the rat. Biochim Biophys Acta 544:234–244, 1978.

38. Porterfield SP: The effects of growth hormone, thyroxine and insulin on the activities of reduced nicotinamide adenine dinucleotide phosphate dehydrogenase, glucose-6-phosphatase and glycogen phosphorylase in fetal rat liver. Horm Metab Res 11:444–448, 1979.

39. Goodman HM, Schwartz J: Growth hormone and lipid metabolism. In Knobil E, Sawyer WH (eds): Handbook of Physiology, vol 4. Washington, DC, American Physiological Society, 1974, pp 211–232.

40. Pandian MR, Gupta SL, Talwar GP: Studies on the early interactions of growth hormone: Effect in vitro on lipogenesis in adipose tissue. Endocrinology 88:928–936, 1971.

41. de Bodo R, Altszuler N: The metabolic effects of growth hormone and their physiological significance. Vitam Horm 15:206–211, 1957.

42. Altszuler N, Steele R, Rathgeb I, et al: Influence of growth hormone on glucose metabolism and plasma insulin levels in the dog. In Pecile A, Muller EE (eds): Growth Hormone: Proceedings of the First International Symposium, Amsterdam. Excerpta Medica Int. Congress Ser. 158, 1968, pp 309–315.

43. Fain JN, Kovacev VP, Scow RO: Effect of growth hormone and dexamethasone on lipolysis and metabolism in isolated fat cells of the rat. J Biol Chem 240:3522–3529, 1965.

44. Goodman HM, Grichting G: Growth hormone and lipolysis: A reevaluation. Endocrinology 113:1697–1702, 1983.

45. Goodman HM, Grichting G: Growth hormone action on adipocytes. In Raiti S, Tolman RH (eds): Human Growth Hormone. New York, Plenum Press, 1986, pp 499–512.

46. Hollobaugh SL, Tzagournis M, Folk RL, et al: The diabetogenic action of human growth hormone: Glucose–fatty acid interrelationships. Metabolism 17:485–491, 1968.

47. Altszuler N, Steele R, Rathgeb I, et al: Glucose metabolism and plasma insulin level during epinephrine infusion in the dog. Am J Physiol 212:677–682, 1967.

48. Fraser R, Joplin JF, Opie M, et al: The augmented insulin tolerance test for detecting insulin resistance. J Endocrinol 25:299–303, 1962.

49. MacGorman LR, Rizza RA, Gerich JE: Physiological concentrations of growth hormone exert insulin–like and insulin antagonistic effects on both hepatic and extrahepatic tissues in man. J Clin Endocrinol Metab 53:556–559, 1981.

50. Maloff BL, Levine JH, Lockwood DH: Direct effects of growth hormone on insulin action in rat adipose tissue maintained in vitro. Endocrinology 107:538–544, 1980.

51. Smal J, Closset J, Hennen G, et al: The receptor binding properties of the 20K variant of human growth hormone explain its discrepant insulin-like and growth promoting activities. Biochem Biophys Res Commun 134:159–165, 1986.

52. Sigel MB, Thorpe NA, Kobrin MS, et al: Binding characteristics of a biologically active variant of human growth hormone (20K) to growth hormone and lactogen receptors. Endocrinology 108:1600–1603, 1981.

53. Kostyo JL: The multivalent nature of growth hormone. In Raiti S, Tolman RH (eds): Human Growth Hormone, New York, Plenum Press, 1986, pp 449–454.

54. Armstrong JM, Bornstein J, Bromley JO, et al: Parallel insulin-like actions of human growth hormone and its part sequence hGH 7-13. Acta Endocrinol (Copenh) 102:492–498, 1983.

55. Ng FM, Bornstein J, Welker C, et al: Insulin potentiating action of synthetic peptides relating to the amino terminal sequence of human growth hormone. Diabetes 23:943–949, 1974.

56. Ng FM, Bornstein J: Insulin-potentiating action of a synthetic amino-terminal fragment of human growth hormone (hGH 1–15) in streptozotocin-diabetic rats. Diabetes 28:1126–1130, 1979.

57. Ng FM, Harcourt JA: Stimulation of 2-deoxyglucose uptake in rat adipocytes by a human growth hormone fragment (hGH 4-15). Diabetologia 29:882–887, 1986.

58. Wade JD, Ng FM, Bornstein J, et al: Effect of C-terminal chain shortening on the insulin-antagonistic activity of human growth hormone 177–191. Acta Endocrinol (Copenh) 101:10–14, 1982.

59. Greenspan FS, Li CH, Simpson ME, et al: Bioassay of hypophyseal growth hormone: The tibia test. Endocrinology 45:455–463, 1949.

60. Davidson MB: Effect of growth hormone on carbohydrate and lipid metabolism. Endocr Rev 8:115–131, 1987.

61. Palmiter RD, Brinster RL, Hammer RE, et al: Dramatic growth of mice that develop from eggs microinjected with metallothionein-growth hormone fusion genes. Nature 300:611–615, 1982.

62. Chen WY, Wight DC, Wagner TE, et al: Expression of a mutated bovine growth hormone gene suppresses growth of transgenic mice. Proc Natl Acad Sci U S A 87:5061–5065, 1990.

63. Chen WY, Wight DC, Mehta BV, et al: Glycine 119 of bovine growth hormone is critical for growth-promoting activity. Mol Endocrinol 5:1845–1852, 1991.

64. Chen WY, White ME, Wagner TE, et al: Functional antagonism between endogenous mouse growth hormone (GH) and a GH analog results in dwarf transgenic mice. Endocrinology 129:1402–1408, 1991.

65. Chen WY, Wight DC, Chen NY, et al: Mutations in the third alpha-helix of bovine growth hormone dramatically affect its intracellular distribution in vitro and growth enhancement in transgenic mice. J Biol Chem 266:2252–2258, 1991.

66. Chen WY, Chen N, Yun J, et al: In vitro and in vivo studies of the antagonistic effects of human growth hormone analogs. J Biol Chem 269:15892–15897, 1994.

67. Chen WY, Chen NY, Yun J, et al: Amino acid residues in the third alpha-helix of growth hormone involved in growth promoting activity. Mol Endocrinol 9:292–302, 1995.

68. Chen XZ, Shafer AW, Yun JS, et al: Conversion of bovine growth hormone cysteine residues to serine affects secretion by cultured cells and growth rates in transgenic mice. Mol Endocrinol 6:598–606, 1992.

69. Strobl JS, Thomas MJ: Human growth hormone. Pharmacol Rev 46:1–34, 1994.

70. Green H, Morikawa M, Nixon T: A dual effector theory of growth-hormone action. Differentiation 29:195–198, 1985.

71. Sjögren K, Liu JL, Blad K, et al: Liver-derived insulin-like growth factor I (IGF-I) is the principal source of IGF-I in blood but is not required for postnatal body growth in mice. Proc Natl Acad Sci U S A 96:7088–7092, 1999.

72. Yakar S, Liu JL, Stannard B, et al: Normal growth and development in the absence of hepatic insulin-like growth factor I. Proc Natl Acad Sci U S A 96:7324–7329, 1999.

73. Baumann G: Growth hormone binding proteins and various forms of growth hormone: Implications for measurements. Acta Paediatr Scand Suppl 370:72–80, 1990.

74. Kostyo JL: The search for the active core of pituitary growth hormone. Metabolism 23:885–899, 1974.

75. Nicoll CS, Mayer GL, Russell SM: Structural features of prolactins and growth hormones that can be related to their biological properties [published erratum appears in Endocr Rev 1987 Feb;8(1):43]. Endocr Rev 7:169–203, 1986.

76. Goffin V, Martial JA, Summers NL: Use of a model to understand prolactin and growth hormone specificities. Protein Eng 8:1215–1231, 1995.

77. Goffin V, Shiverick KT, Kelly PA, et al: Sequence-function relationships within the expanding family of prolactin, growth hormone, placental lactogen, and related proteins in mammals. Endocr Rev 17:385–410, 1996.

78. Kopchick JJ, Bellush LL, Coschigano KT: Transgenic models of growth hormone action. Ann Rev Nutr 19:437–461, 1999.

79. Kopchick JJ, Andry JM: Growth hormone (GH), GH receptor, and signal transduction. Mol Genet Metab 71:293–314, 2000.

80. Li CH, Graf L: Human pituitary growth hormone: Isolation and properties of two biologically active fragments from plasmin digests. Proc Natl Acad Sci U S A 71:1197–1201, 1974.

81. Li CH, Bewley TA: Human pituitary growth hormone: Restoration of full biological activity by noncovalent interaction of two fragments of the hormone. Proc Natl Acad Sci U S A 73:1476–1479, 1976.

82. Nicoll CS: Bio-assay of prolactin: Analysis of the pigeon crop-sac response to local prolactin injection by an objective and quantitative method. Endocrinology 80:641–655, 1967.

83. Sonenberg M, Kikutani M, Free CA, et al: Chemical and biological characterization of clinically active tryptic digests of bovine growth hormone. Ann N Y Acad Sci 148:532–558, 1968.

84. Yamasaki N, Shimanaka J, Sonenberg M: Studies on the common active site of growth hormone: Revision of the amino acid sequence of an active fragment of bovine growth hormone. J Biol Chem 250:2510–2514, 1975.

85. Levine LS, Sonenberg M, New MI: Metabolic effects in children of a 37 amino acid fragment of bovine growth hormone. J Clin Endocrinol Metab 37:607–615, 1973.

86. Chou PY, Fasman GD: Prediction of protein conformation. Biochemistry 13:222–245, 1974.

87. Garnier J, Osguthorpe DJ, Robson B: Analysis of the accuracy and implications of simple methods for predicting the secondary structure of globular proteins. J Mol Biol 120:97–120, 1978.

88. Hara K, Hsu Chen CJ, Sonenberg M: Recombination of the biologically active peptides from a tryptic digest of bovine growth hormone. Biochemistry 17:550–556, 1978.

89. Wade JD, Pullin CO, Ng FM, et al: The synthesis and hyperglycaemic activity of the amino acid sequence 172–191 of human growth hormone. Biochem Biophys Res Commun 78:827–832, 1977.

90. Frigeri LG, Peterson SM, Lewis UJ: The 20,000-dalton structural variant of human growth hormone: Lack of some early insulin-like effects. Biochem Biophys Res Commun 91:778–782, 1979.

91. Shaar CJ, Grinnan EL, Short WG, et al: Hyperglycemic activity in dogs of recombinant DNA-derived 20,000 dalton variant of methionyl human growth hormone. Endocr Res 12:21–35, 1986.

92. Salem MA: Effects of the amino-terminal portion of human growth hormone on glucose clearance and metabolism in normal, diabetic, hypophysectomized, and diabetic-hypophysectomized rats. Endocrinology 123:1565–1576, 1988.

93. Towns R, Kostyo JL, Vogel T, et al: Evidence that the N-terminus of human growth hormone is involved in expression of its growth promoting, diabetogenic, and insulin-like activities. Endocrinology 130:1225–1230, 1992.

94. Stewart TA, Clift S, Pitts-Meek S, et al: An evaluation of the functions of the 22-kilodalton (kDa), the 20-kDa, and the N-terminal polypeptide forms of human growth hormone using transgenic mice. Endocrinology 130:405–414, 1992.

95. Paladini AC, Pena C, Parks E: Molecular biology of growth hormone. CRC Crit Rev Biochem 15:25–56, 1983.

96. Abdel-Meguid SS, Shieh HS, Smith WW, et al: Three-dimensional structure of a genetically engineered variant of porcine growth hormone. Proc Natl Acad Sci U S A 84:6434–6437, 1987.

97. Graf L, Li CH, Bewley TA: Selective reduction and alkylation of the COOH-terminal disulfide bridge in bovine growth hormone. Int J Pept Protein Res 7:467–473, 1975.

98. Doneen BA, Bewley TA, Li CH: Studies on prolactin: Selective reduction of the disulfide bonds of the ovine hormone. Biochemistry 18:4851–4860, 1979.

99. Dixon JS, Li CH: Retention of the biological potency of human pituitary growth hormone after reduction and carbamidomethylation. Science 154:785–786, 1966.

100. Campbell RM, Kostyo JL, Scanes CG: Lipolytic and antilipolytic effects of human growth hormone, its 20-kilodalton variant, a reduced and carboxymethylated derivative, and human placental lactogen on chicken adipose tissue in vitro. Proc Soc Exp Biol Med 193:269–273, 1990.

101. Necessary PC, Andersen TT, Ebner KE: Activity of alkylated prolactin and human growth hormone in receptor and cell assays. Mol Cell Endocrinol 39:247–254, 1985.

102. Nutting DF, Kostyo JL, Mills JB, et al: A cyanogen bromide fragment of reduced and S-aminoethylated porcine growth hormone with anabolic activity. Biochim Biophys Acta 200:601–604, 1970.

103. Tokunaga T, Tanaka T, Ikehara M, et al: Synthesis and expression of a human growth hormone (somatotropin) gene mutated to change cysteine-165 to alanine. Eur J Biochem 153:445–449, 1985.

104. Cunningham BC, Jhurani P, Ng P, et al: Receptor and antibody epitopes in human growth hormone identified by homolog-scanning mutagenesis. Science 243:1330–1336, 1989.

105. Cunningham BC, Wells JA: High-resolution epitope mapping of hGH-receptor interactions by alanine-scanning mutagenesis. Science 244:1081–1085, 1989.

106. Cunningham BC, Bass S, Fuh G, et al: Zinc mediation of the binding of human growth hormone to the human prolactin receptor. Science 250:1709–1712, 1990.

107. Hara K, Sonenberg M: Polyalanylation of bovine somatotropin peptide 96-133. Biochim Biophys Acta 492:95–101, 1977.

108. Yamasaki N, Kangawa K, Kobayashi S, et al: Amino acid sequence of a biologically active fragment of bovine growth hormone. J Biol Chem 247:3874–3880, 1972.

109. Aston R, Ivanyi J: Antigenic, receptor-binding and mitogenic activity of proteolytic fragments of human growth hormone. EMBO J 2:493–497, 1983.

110. Blanc JP, Taylor JW, Miller RJ, et al: Examination of the requirement for an amphiphilic helical structure in beta-endorphin through the design, synthesis, and study of model peptides. J Biol Chem 258:8277–8284, 1983.

111. Blanc JP, Kaiser ET: Biological and physical properties of a beta-endorphin analog containing only D-amino acids in the amphiphilic helical segment 13-31. J Biol Chem 259:9549–9556, 1984.

112. Edmunson AB: Amino–acid sequence of sperm whale myoglobin. Nature 205:883–887, 1965.

113. Kaiser ET, Kezdy FJ: Amphiphilic secondary structure: Design of peptide hormones. Science 223:249–255, 1984.

114. Moe GR, Kaiser ET: Design, synthesis, and characterization of a model peptide having potent calcitonin-like biological activity: Implications for calcitonin structure/activity. Biochemistry 24:1971–1976, 1985.

115. Moe GR, Miller RJ, Kaiser ET: Design of a peptide hormone: Synthesis and characterization of a model peptide with calcitonin-like activity. J Am Chem Soc 105:4100–4102, 1983.

116. Stanojevic D, Verdine GL: Deconstruction of GCN4/GCRE into a monomeric peptide-DNA complex. Nat Struct Biol 2:450–457, 1995.

117. Tou JS, Kaempfe LA, Vineyard BD, et al: Amphiphilic growth hormone releasing factor (GRF) analogs: Peptide design and biological activity in vivo. Biochem Biophys Res Commun 139:763–770, 1986.

118. Xing H, Shapiro DJ: An estrogen receptor mutant exhibiting hormone-independent transactivation and enhanced affinity for the estrogen response element. J Biol Chem 268:23227–23233, 1993.

119. Okada S, Chen WY, Wiehl P, et al: A growth hormone (GH) analog can antagonize the ability of native GH to promote differentiation of 3T3-F442A preadipocytes and stimulate insulin-like and lipolytic activities in primary rat adipocytes. Endocrinology 130:2284–2290, 1992.

120. Okada S, Kopchick JJ: Effects of growth hormone antagonist (hGH-G120R) on 3T3-F442A adipocytes. Diabetes 44:135A, 1995.

121. Chen NY, Chen WY, Bellush L, et al: Effects of streptozotocin treatment in growth hormone (GH) and GH antagonist transgenic mice. Endocrinology 136:660–667, 1995.

122. Fuh G, Cunningham BC, Fukunaga R, et al: Rational design of potent antagonists to the human growth hormone receptor. Science 256:1677–1680, 1992.

123. Takahashi Y, Kaji H, Okimura Y, et al: Brief report: Short stature caused by a mutant growth hormone [see comments] [published erratum appears in N Engl J Med 1996 May 2;334(18):1207]. N Engl J Med 334:432–436, 1996.

124. Chihara K, Takahashi Y, Kaji H, et al: Short stature caused by a natural growth hormone antagonist. Horm Res 49:41–45, 1998.

125. Dattani MT, Hindmarsh PC, Brook CG, et al: G120R, a human growth hormone antagonist, shows zinc-dependent agonist and antagonist activity on Nb2 cells. J Biol Chem 270:9222–9226, 1995.

126. Yang CW, Striker LJ, Kopchick JJ, et al: Glomerulosclerosis in mice transgenic for native or mutated bovine growth hormone gene. Kidney Int Suppl 39:S90–S94, 1993.

127. Yang CW, Striker LJ, Pesce C, et al: Glomerulosclerosis and body growth are mediated by different portions of bovine growth hormone. Studies in transgenic mice. Lab Invest 68:62–70, 1993.

128. Foley ED, Aiello LP, Pierce EA, et al: The effect of growth hormone on a mouse model of proliferative retinopathy [abstract]. Investigative Ophthalmology & Visual Science Meeting 36:S1047, 1995.

129. Smith LE, Kopchick JJ, Chen W, et al: Essential role of growth hormone in ischemia-induced retinal neovascularization. Science 276:1706–1709, 1997.

130. Chen NY, Chen WY, Kopchick JJ: Liver and kidney growth hormone (GH) receptors are regulated differently in diabetic GH and GH antagonist transgenic mice. Endocrinology 138:1988–1994, 1997.

131. Chen NY, Chen WY, Striker LJ, et al: Co-expression of bovine growth hormone (GH) and human GH antagonist genes in transgenic mice. Endocrinology 138:851–854, 1997.

132. Chen WY, Zhao GH, Gu Y, et al: Pharmacokinetic & Pharmacodynamic Studies of Human Growth Hormone Antagonist G120K-PEG in Mice, vol 10. International Congress of Endocrinology, 1996, p 275.

133. Allen TM, Hansen C, Martin F, et al: Liposomes containing synthetic lipid derivatives of poly(ethylene glycol) show prolonged circulation half-lives in vivo. Biochim Biophys Acta 1066:29–36, 1991.

134. Inoue H, Kadoya T, Kabaya K, et al: A highly enhanced thrombopoietic activity by monomethoxy polyethylene glycol-modified recombinant human interleukin-6. J Lab Clin Med 124:529–536, 1994.

135. Klibanov AL, Maruyama K, Beckerleg AM, et al: Activity of amphipathic poly(ethylene glycol) 5000 to prolong the circulation time of liposomes depends on the liposome size and is unfavorable for immunoliposome binding to target. Biochim Biophys Acta 1062:142–148, 1991.

136. Tsutsumi Y, Kihira T, Tsunoda S, et al: Intravenous administration of polyethylene glycol-modified tumor necrosis factor-alpha completely regressed solid tumor in Meth-A murine sarcoma model. Jpn J Cancer Res 85:1185–1188, 1994.

137. Yamaoka T, Tabata Y, Ikada Y: Distribution and tissue uptake of poly(ethylene glycol) with different molecular weights after intravenous administration to mice. J Pharm Sci 83:601–606, 1994.

138. Clark R, Olson K, Fuh G, et al: Long-acting growth hormones produced by conjugation with polyethylene glycol. J Biol Chem 271:21969–21977, 1996.

139. Olson K, Gehant R, Mukku V, et al: Preparation and characterization of poly(ethylene gycol)ylated human growth hormone antagonist. In Harris JM, Zalipsky S (eds): Poly(ethylene glycol) Chemistry and Biological Applications, Washington, DC, American Chemical Society, 1997, pp 170–181.

140. Flyvbjerg A, Bennett WF, Rasch R, et al: Inhibitory effect of a growth hormone receptor antagonist (G120K-PEG) on renal enlargement, glomerular hypertrophy and urinary albumin excretion in experimental diabetes in mice. Diabetes 48:377–382, 1999.

141. Kopchick JJ, Parkinson C, Stevens EC, et al: Growth hormone receptor antagonists: Discovery, development, and use in patients with acromegaly. Endocr Rev 23:623–646, 2002.

142. Trainer PJ, Drake WM, Katznelson L, et al: Treatment of acromegaly with the growth hormone-receptor antagonist pegvisomant. N Engl J Med 342:1171–1177, 2000.

143. van der Lely AJ, Hutson RK, Trainer PJ, et al: Long-term treatment of acromegaly with pegvisomant, a growth hormone receptor antagonist. Lancet 358:1754–1759, 2001.

144. Thorner MO, Strasburger CJ, Wu Z, et al: Growth hormone (GH) receptor blockade with a PEG-modified GH (B2036-PEG) lowers serum insulin-like growth factor-I but does not acutely stimulate serum GH. J Clin Endocrinol Metab 84:2098–2103, 1999.

145. Drake WM, Parkinson C, Besser GM, et al: Clinical use of a growth hormone receptor antagonist in the treatment of acromegaly. Trends Endocrinol Metab 12:408–413, 2001.

146. Ross RJ, Leung KC, Maamra M, et al: Binding and functional studies with the growth hormone receptor antagonist, B2036-PEG (pegvisomant), reveal effects of pegylation and evidence that it binds to a receptor dimer. J Clin Endocrinol Metab 86:1716–1723, 2001.

147. Flyvbjerg A, Bennet WF, Rasch R, et al: Inhibitory effect of a growth hormone receptor antagonist (G120K-PEG) on renal enlargement, glomerular hypertrophy and urinary albumin excretion in experimental diabetes in mice. Diabetes 48:377–382, 1999.

148. Chen NY, Chen WY, Kopchick JJ: A growth hormone antagonist protects mice against streptozotocin induced glomerulosclerosis even in the presence of elevated levels of glucose and glycated hemoglobin. Endocrinology 137:5163–5165, 1996.

149. Doi T, Striker LJ, Quaife C, et al: Progressive glomerulosclerosis develops in transgenic mice chronically expressing growth hormone and growth hormone releasing factor but not in those expressing insulinlike growth factor-1. Am J Pathol 131:398–403, 1988.

150. Friend KE: Cancer and the potential place for growth hormone receptor antagonist therapy. Growth Horm IGF Res 11(Suppl A):S121–S123, 2001.

151. Friend KE, Khandwala HM, Flyvbjerg A, et al: Growth hormone and insulin-like growth factor. I: Effects on the growth of glioma cell lines. Growth Horm IGF Res 11:84–91, 2001.

152. Pollak M, Blouin MJ, Zhang JC, et al: Reduced mammary gland carcinogenesis in transgenic mice expressing a growth hormone antagonist. Br J Cancer 85:428–430, 2001.

153. Yakar S, Setser J, Zhao H, et al: Inhibition of growth hormone action improves insulin sensitivity in liver IGF-1-deficient mice. J Clin Invest 113:96–105, 2004.

154. de Vos AM, Ultsch M, Kossiakoff AA: Human growth hormone and extracellular domain of its receptor: Crystal structure of the complex. Science 255:306–312, 1992.

155. Kopchick JJ, Woodley FW: Regulation of Growth Hormone Gene Expression: Advances in Molecular and Cellular Endocrinology, vol 1, JAI Press, 1997, pp 51–82.

156. Goodman HM: Growth hormone and metabolism. In Schreibman MP, Scanes CG, Pang PKT (eds): The Endocrinology of Growth, Development, and Metabolism in Vertebrates. San Diego, Academic Press, 1993, pp 93–115.

157. Roupas P, Herington AC: Cellular mechanisms in the processing of growth hormone and its receptor. Mol Cell Endocrinol 61:1–12, 1989.

158. Garcia-Aragon J, Lobie PE, Muscat GE, et al: Prenatal expression of the growth hormone (GH) receptor/binding protein in the rat: A role for GH in embryonic and fetal development? Development 114:869–876, 1992.

159. Klempt M, Bingham B, Breier BH, et al: Tissue distribution and ontogeny of growth hormone receptor messenger ribonucleic acid and ligand binding to hepatic tissue in the midgestation sheep fetus. Endocrinology 132:1071–1077, 1993.

160. Barnard R, Thordarson G, Lopez MF, et al: Expression of growth hormone-binding protein with a hydrophilic carboxyl terminus by the mouse placenta: Studies in vivo and in vitro. J Endocrinol 140:125–135, 1994.

161. Hill DJ, Riley SC, Bassett NS, et al: Localization of the growth hormone receptor, identified by immunocytochemistry, in second trimester human fetal tissues and in placenta throughout gestation. J Clin Endocrinol Metab 75:646–650, 1992.

162. Werther GA, Haynes K, Waters MJ: Growth hormone (GH) receptors are expressed on human fetal mesenchymal tissues: Identification of messenger ribonucleic acid and GH-binding protein. J Clin Endocrinol Metab 76:1638–1646, 1993.

163. Ohlsson C, Lovstedt K, Holmes PV, et al: Embryonic stem cells express growth hormone receptors: Regulation by retinoic acid. Endocrinology 133:2897–2903, 1993.

164. Zhang CZ, Li H, Young WG, et al: Evidence for a local action of growth hormone in embryonic tooth development in the rat. Growth Factors 14:131–143, 1997.

165. Laron Z, Pertzelan A, Mannheimer S: Genetic pituitary dwarfism with high serum concentration of growth hormone: A new inborn error of metabolism? Isr J Med Sci 2:152–155, 1966.

166. Laron Z, Klinger B, Erster B, et al: Serum GH binding protein activities identifies the heterozygous carriers for Laron type dwarfism. Acta Endocrinol (Copenh) 121:603–608, 1989.

167. Laron Z, Lilos P, Klinger B: Growth curves for Laron syndrome. Arch Dis Child 68:768–770, 1993.

168. Laron Z: Laron syndrome: From description to therapy. Endocrinologist 3:21–28, 1993.

169. Savage MO, Blum WF, Ranke MB, et al: Clinical features and endocrine status in patients with growth hormone insensitivity (Laron syndrome). J Clin Endocrinol Metab 77:1465–1471, 1993.

170. Rosenfeld RG, Rosenbloom AL, Guevara-Aguirre J: Growth hormone (GH) insensitivity due to primary GH receptor deficiency. Endocrin Rev 15:369–390, 1994.

171. Duriez B, Sobrier ML, Duquesnoy P, et al: A naturally occurring growth hormone receptor mutation: In vivo and in vitro evidence for the functional importance of the WS motif common to all members of the cytokine receptor superfamily. Mol Endocrinol 7:806–814, 1993.

172. Huang N, Cogburn LA, Agarwal SK, et al: Overexpression of a truncated growth hormone receptor in the sex-linked dwarf chicken: Evidence for a splice mutation. Mol Endocrinol 7:1391–1398, 1993.

173. Zhou Y, Xu BC, Maheshwari HG, et al: A mammalian model for Laron syndrome produced by targeted disruption of the mouse growth hormone receptor/binding protein gene (the Laron mouse). Proc Natl Acad Sci U S A 94:13215–13220, 1997.

174. Coschigano KT, Holland AN, Riders ME, et al: Deletion, but not antagonism, of the mouse growth hormone receptor results in severely decreased body weights, insulin and IGF-1 levels and increased lifespan. Endocrinology 144:3799–3810, 2003.

175. Coschigano KT, Bellush LL, Kopchick JJ: Analysis of a mouse model for Laron syndrome. The Endocrine

Society's 80th Annual Meeting, New Orleans, LA, 1998, p 302.

176. Coschigano KT, Clemmons D, Bellush LL, et al: Assessment of growth parameters and life span of GHR/BP gene-disrupted mice. Endocrinology 141:2608–2613, 2000.

177. Bazan JF: Haemopoietic receptors and helical cytokines. Immunol Today 11:350–354, 1990.

178. Godowski PJ, Leung DW, Meacham LR, et al: Characterization of the human growth hormone receptor gene and demonstration of a partial gene deletion in two patients with Laron-type dwarfism. Proc Natl Acad Sci U S A 86:8083–8087, 1989.

179. Fuh G, Mulkerrin MG, Bass S, et al: The human growth hormone receptor: Secretion from Escherichia coli and disulfide bonding pattern of the extracellular binding domain. J Biol Chem 265:3111–3115, 1990.

180. Zhou Y, He L, Kopchick JJ: An exon encoding the mouse growth hormone binding protein (mGHBP) carboxy terminus is located between exon 7 and 8 of the mouse growth hormone receptor gene. Receptor 4:223–227, 1994.

181. Zhou Y, He L, Kopchick JJ: Structural comparison of a portion of the rat and mouse growth hormone receptor/binding protein genes. Gene 177:257–259, 1996.

182. Edens A, Southard JN, Talamantes F: Mouse growth hormone-binding protein and growth hormone receptor transcripts are produced from a single gene by alternative splicing. Endocrinology 135:2802–2805, 1994.

183. Sadeghi H, Wang BS, Lumanglas AL, et al: Identification of the origin of the growth hormone-binding protein in rat serum. Mol Endocrinol 4:1799–1805, 1990.

184. Baumbach WR, Horner DL, Logan JS: The growth hormone-binding protein in rat serum is an alternatively spliced form of the rat growth hormone receptor. Genes Dev 3:1199–1205, 1989.

185. Talamantes F: The structure and regulation of expression of the mouse growth hormone receptor and binding protein. Proc Soc Exp Biol Med 206:254–256, 1994.

186. Frick GP, Tai LR, Baumbach WR, et al: Tissue distribution, turnover, and glycosylation of the long and short growth hormone receptor isoforms in rat tissues. Endocrinology 139:2824–2830, 1998.

187. Bingham B, Oldham ER, Baumbach WR: Regulation of growth hormone receptor and binding protein expression in domestic species. Proc Soc Exp Biol Med 206:195–199, 1994.

188. Oldham ER, Bingham B, Baumbach WR: A functional polyadenylation signal is embedded in the coding region of chicken growth hormone receptor RNA. Mol Endocrinol 7:1379–1390, 1993.

189. Baumann G: Growth hormone binding proteins. In Melmed ES (ed): Endocrine Update Book Series. Norwell, MA, Kluwer Academic Publishers, 1999.

190. Clackson T, Wells JA: A hot spot of binding energy in a hormone-receptor interface. Science 267:383–386, 1995.

191. Clackson T, Ultsch MH, Wells JA, et al: Structural and functional analysis of the 1:1 growth hormone:receptor complex reveals the molecular basis for receptor affinity. J Mol Biol 277:1111–1128, 1998.

192. Cunningham BC, Ultsch M, De Vos AM, et al: Dimerization of the extracellular domain of the human growth hormone receptor by a single hormone molecule. Science 254:821–825, 1991.

193. Bernat B, Pal G, Sun M, et al: Determination of the energetics governing the regulatory step in growth hormone-induced receptor homodimerization. Proc Natl Acad Sci U S A 27:27, 2003.

194. Waters MJ, Barnard RT, Lobie PE, et al: Growth hormone receptors: Their structure, location and role. Acta Paediatr Scand Suppl 366:60–72, 1990.

195. Waters MJ: The growth hormone receptor. In Kostyo JL (ed): Handbook of physiology. Section 7: The endocrine system. Vol V: Hormonal control of growth. Oxford, England, Oxford University Press, 1999, pp 397–444.

196. Lowman HB, Wells JA: Affinity maturation of human growth hormone by monovalent phage display. J Mol Biol 234:564–578, 1993.

197. Rowlinson SW, Barnard R, Bastiras S, et al: Evidence for involvement of the carboxy terminus of helix 1 of growth hormone in receptor binding: Use of charge reversal mutagenesis to account for calcium dependence of binding and for design of higher affinity analogues. Biochemistry 33:11724–11733, 1994.

198. Rowlinson SW, Barnard R, Bastiras S, et al: A growth hormone agonist produced by targeted mutagenesis at binding site 1: Evidence that site 1 regulates bioactivity. J Biol Chem 270:16833–16839, 1995.

199. Frank SJ, Gilliland G, Van Epps C: Treatment of IM-9 cells with human growth hormone (GH) promotes rapid disulfide linkage of the GH receptor. Endocrinology 135:148–156, 1994.

200. Chen C, Brinkworth R, Waters MJ: The role of receptor dimerization domain residues in growth hormone signaling. J Biol Chem 272:5133–5140, 1997.

201. Mellado M, Rodriguez-Frade JM, Kremer L, et al: Conformational changes required in the human growth hormone receptor for growth hormone signaling. J Biol Chem 272:9189–9196, 1997.

202. Rowlinson SW, Behncken SN, Rowland JE, et al: Activation of chimeric and full-length growth hormone receptors by growth hormone receptor monoclonal antibodies: A specific

conformational change may be required for full-length receptor signaling. J Biol Chem 273:5307–5314, 1998.

203. Ultsch MH, Somers W, Kossiakoff AA, et al: The crystal structure of affinity-matured human growth hormone at 2 A resolution. J Mol Biol 236:286–299, 1994.

204. Baumgartner JW, Wells CA, Chen CM, et al: The role of the WSXWS equivalent motif in growth hormone receptor function. J Biol Chem 269:29094–29101, 1994.

205. Somers W, Ultsch M, De Vos AM, et al: The X-ray structure of a growth hormone-prolactin receptor complex [see comments]. Nature 372:478–481, 1994.

206. Kossiakoff AA, Somers W, Ultsch M, et al: Comparison of the intermediate complexes of human growth hormone bound to the human growth hormone and prolactin receptors. Protein Sci 3:1697–1705, 1994.

207. Rozakis–Adcock M, Kelly PA: Identification of ligand binding determinants of the prolactin receptor. J Biol Chem 267:7428–7433, 1992.

208. Takahashi Y, Shirono H, Arisaka O, et al: Biologically inactive growth hormone caused by an amino acid substitution. J Clin Invest 100:1159–1165, 1997.

209. Harding PA, Wang X, Okada S, et al: Growth hormone (GH) and a GH antagonist promote GH receptor dimerization and internalization. J Biol Chem 271:6708–6712, 1996.

210. van Kerkhof P, Govers R, Alves dos Santos CM, et al: Endocytosis and degradation of the growth hormone receptor are proteasome-dependent. J Biol Chem 275:1575–1580, 2000.

211. Gent J, van Kerkhof P, Roza M, et al: Ligand-independent growth hormone receptor dimerization occurs in the endoplasmic reticulum and is required for ubiquitin system-dependent endocytosis. Proc Natl Acad Sci U S A 99:9858–9863, 2002.

212. Argetsinger LS, Carter-Su C: Mechanism of signaling by growth hormone receptor. Physiol Rev 76:1089–1107, 1996.

213. Cataldo LA, Kopchick JJ: Characterization of Growth Hormone Mediated Signal Transduction in Mouse Liver vol 80. Chevy Chase, MD, The Endocrine Society, 1998, p 143.

214. Chow JC, Ling PR, Qu Z, et al: Growth hormone stimulates tyrosine phosphorylation of JAK2 and STAT5, but not insulin receptor substrate-1 or SHC proteins in liver and skeletal muscle of normal rats in vivo. Endocrinology 137:2880–2886, 1996.

215. Thirone ACP, Carvalho CRO, Saad MJA: Growth hormone stimulates the tyrosine kinase activity of JAK2 and induces tyrosine phosphorylation of insulin receptor substrates and shc in rat tissues. Endocrinology 140:55–62, 1999.

216. Carter-Su C, Schwartz J, Smit LS: Molecular mechanism of growth hormone action. Annu Rev Physiol 58:187–207, 1996.

217. Carter-Su C, Smit LS: Signaling via JAK tyrosine kinases: Growth hormone receptor as a model system. Recent Prog Horm Res 53:61–82, 1998.

218. Ihle JN, Witthuhn BA, Quelle FW, et al: Signaling by the cytokine receptor superfamily: JAKs and STATs. Trends Biochem Sci 19:222–227, 1994.

219. Kelly PA, Ali S, Rozakis M, et al: The growth hormone/prolactin receptor family. Recent Prog Horm Res 48:123–164, 1993.

220. Piwien-Pilipuk G, Huo JS, Schwartz J: Growth hormone signal transduction. J Pediatr Endocrinol Metab 15:771–786, 2002.

221. Herrington J, Carter-Su C: Signaling pathways activated by the growth hormone receptor. Trends Endocrinol Metab 12:252–257, 2001.

222. Carter-Su C, Stubbart JR, Wang XY, et al: Phosphorylation of highly purified growth hormone receptors by a growth hormone receptor-associated tyrosine kinase. J Biol Chem 264:18654–18661, 1989.

223. Campbell GS, Christian LJ, Carter-Su C: Evidence for involvement of the growth hormone receptor-associated tyrosine kinase in actions of growth hormone. J Biol Chem 268:7427–7434, 1993.

224. Wang X, Uhler MD, Billestrup N, et al: Evidence for association of the cloned liver growth hormone receptor with a tyrosine kinase. J Biol Chem 267:17390–17396, 1992.

225. Wang X, Moller C, Norstedt G, et al: Growth hormone-promoted tyrosyl phosphorylation of a 121-kDa growth hormone receptor-associated protein. J Biol Chem 268:3573–3579, 1993.

226. Argetsinger LS, Campbell GS, Yang X, et al: Identification of JAK2 as a growth hormone receptor-associated tyrosine kinase. Cell 74:237–244, 1993.

227. Carter-Su C, Argetsinger LS, Campbell GS, et al: The identification of JAK2 tyrosine kinase as a signaling molecule for growth hormone. Proc Soc Exp Biol Med 206:210–215, 1994.

228. Smit LS, Meyer DJ, Billestrup N, et al: The role of the growth hormone (GH) receptor and JAK1 and JAK2 kinases in the activation of Stats 1, 3, and 5 by GH. Mol Endocrinol 10:519–533, 1996.

229. Johnston JA, Kawamura M, Kirken RA, et al: Phosphorylation and activation of the Jak-3 Janus kinase in response to interleukin-2. Nature 370:151–153, 1994.

230. Argetsinger LS, Carter-Su C: Growth hormone signalling mechanisms: Involvement of the tyrosine kinase JAK2. Horm Res 45:22–24, 1996.

231. VanderKuur JA, Wang X, Zhang L, et al: Domains of the growth hormone receptor required for association and activation of JAK2 tyrosine kinase. J Biol Chem 269:21709–21717, 1994.

232. Frank SJ, Gilliland G, Kraft AS, et al: Interaction of the growth hormone receptor cytoplasmic domain with the JAK2 tyrosine kinase. Endocrinology 135:2228–2239, 1994.

233. Dinerstein H, Lago F, Goujon L, et al: The proline-rich region of the GH receptor is essential for JAK2 phosphorylation, activation of cell proliferation, and gene transcription. Mol Endocrinol 9:1701–1707, 1995.

234. Wang YD, Wood WI: Amino acids of the human growth hormone receptor that are required for proliferation and Jak-STAT signaling. Mol Endocrinol 9:303–311, 1995.

235. Wang X, Darus CJ, Xu BC, et al: Identification of growth hormone receptor (GHR) tyrosine residues required for GHR phosphorylation and JAK2 and STAT5 activation. Mol Endocrinol 10:1249–1260, 1996.

236. VanderKuur JA, Wang X, Zhang L, et al: Growth hormone-dependent phosphorylation of tyrosine 333 and/or 338 of the growth hormone receptor. J Biol Chem 270:21738–21744, 1995.

237. Schindler C, Darnell JE Jr: Transcriptional responses to polypeptide ligands: The JAK-STAT pathway. Annu Rev Biochem 64:621–651, 1995.

238. Gronowski AM, Rotwein P: Rapid changes in nuclear protein tyrosine phosphorylation after growth hormone treatment in vivo: Identification of phosphorylated mitogen-activated protein kinase and STAT91. J Biol Chem 269:7874–7878, 1994.

239. Meyer DJ, Campbell GS, Cochran BH, et al: Growth hormone induces a DNA binding factor related to the interferon-stimulated 91-kDa transcription factor. J Biol Chem 269:4701–4704, 1994.

240. Campbell GS, Meyer DJ, Raz R, et al: Activation of acute phase response factor (APRF)/Stat3 transcription factor by growth hormone. J Biol Chem 270:3974–3979, 1995.

241. Gronowski AM, Zhong Z, Wen Z, et al: In vivo growth hormone treatment rapidly stimulates the tyrosine phosphorylation and activation of Stat3. Mol Endocrinol 9:171–177, 1995.

242. Gouilleux F, Pallard C, Dusanter-Fourt I, et al: Prolactin, growth hormone, erythropoietin and granulocyte-macrophage colony stimulating factor induce MGF-Stat5 DNA binding activity. EMBO J 14:2005–2013, 1995.

243. Xu BC, Wang X, Darus CJ, et al: Growth hormone promotes the association of transcription factor STAT5 with the growth hormone receptor. J Biol Chem 271:19768–19773, 1996.

244. Sotiropoulos A, Moutoussamy S, Renaudie F, et al: Differential activation of Stat3 and Stat5 by distinct regions of the growth hormone receptor. Mol Endocrinol 10:998–1009, 1996.

245. Hansen LH, Wang X, Kopchick JJ, et al: Identification of tyrosine residues in the intracellular domain of the growth hormone receptor required for transcriptional signaling and Stat5 activation. J Biol Chem 271:12669–12673, 1996.

246. Hansen JA, Hansen LH, Wang X, et al: The role of GH receptor tyrosine phosphorylation in Stat5 activation. J Mol Endocrinol 18:213–221, 1997.

247. Meyer DJ, Stephenson EW, Johnson L, et al: The serum response element can mediate induction of c-fos by growth hormone. Proc Natl Acad Sci U S A 90:6721–6725, 1993.

248. Wood TJ, Sliva D, Lobie PE, et al: Mediation of growth hormone-dependent transcriptional activation by mammary gland factor/Stat 5. J Biol Chem 270:9448–9453, 1995.

249. Chen C, Clarkson RW, Xie Y, et al: Growth hormone and colony-stimulating factor 1 share multiple response elements in the c-fos promoter. Endocrinology 136:4505–4516, 1995.

250. Bergad PL, Shih HM, Towle HC, et al: Growth hormone induction of hepatic serine protease inhibitor 2.1 transcription is mediated by a Stat5-related factor binding synergistically to two gamma-activated sites. J Biol Chem 270:24903–24910, 1995.

251. Anderson NG: Growth hormone activates mitogen-activated protein kinase and S6 kinase and promotes intracellular tyrosine phosphorylation in 3T3-F442A preadipocytes. Biochem J 284:649–652, 1992.

252. Campbell GS, Pang L, Miyasaka T, et al: Stimulation by growth hormone of MAP kinase activity in 3T3-F442A fibroblasts. J Biol Chem 267:6074–6080, 1992.

253. Winston LA, Bertics PJ: Growth hormone stimulates the tyrosine phosphorylation of 42- and 45-kDa ERK-related proteins. J Biol Chem 267:4747–4751, 1992.

254. Moller C, Hansson A, Enberg B, et al: Growth hormone (GH) induction of tyrosine phosphorylation and activation of mitogen-activated protein kinases in cells transfected with rat GH receptor cDNA. J Biol Chem 267:23403–23408, 1992.

255. VanderKuur J, Allevato G, Billestrup N, et al: Growth hormone-promoted tyrosyl phosphorylation of SHC proteins and SHC association with Grb2. J Biol Chem 270:7587–7593, 1995.

256. VanderKuur JA, Butch ER, Waters SB, et al: Signaling molecules involved in coupling growth hormone receptor to mitogen-activated protein kinase activation. Endocrinology 138:4301–4307, 1997.

257. Winston LA, Hunter T: JAK2, Ras, and Raf are required for activation of extracellular signal-regulated kinase/mitogen-activated protein kinase by growth hormone. J Biol Chem 270:30837–30840, 1995.

258. Souza SC, Frick GP, Yip R, et al: Growth hormone stimulates tyrosine phosphorylation of insulin receptor substrate-1. J Biol Chem 269:30085–30088, 1994.

259. Argetsinger LS, Hsu GW, Myers MG, Jr, et al: Growth hormone, interferon-gamma, and leukemia inhibitory factor promoted tyrosyl phosphorylation of insulin receptor substrate-1. J Biol Chem 270:14685–14692, 1995.

260. Argetsinger LS, Norstedt G, Billestrup N, et al: Growth hormone, interferon-gamma, and leukemia inhibitory factor utilize insulin receptor substrate-2 in intracellular signaling. J Biol Chem 271:29415–29421, 1996.

261. Rivera VM, Miranti CK, Misra RP, et al: A growth factor-induced kinase phosphorylates the serum response factor at a site that regulates its DNA-binding activity. Mol Cell Biol 13:6260–6273, 1993.

262. Gille H, Kortenjann M, Thomae O, et al: ERK phosphorylation potentiates Elk-1-mediated ternary complex formation and transactivation. EMBO J 14:951–962, 1995.

263. Hill CS, Treisman R: Transcriptional regulation by extracellular signals: Mechanisms and specificity. Cell 80:199–211, 1995.

264. Gong TW, Meyer DJ, Liao J, et al: Regulation of glucose transport and c-fos and egr-1 expression in cells with mutated or endogenous growth hormone receptors. Endocrinology 139:1863–1871, 1998.

265. Harding PA, Wang XZ, Kopchick JJ: Growth hormone (GH)-induced tyrosine-phosphorylated proteins in cells that express GH receptors. Receptor 5:81–92, 1995.

266. Eriksson H, Ridderstrale M, Tornqvist H: Tyrosine phosphorylation of the growth hormone (GH) receptor and Janus tyrosine kinase-2 is involved in the insulin-like actions of GH in primary rat adipocytes. Endocrinology 136:5093–5101, 1995.

267. Ridderstrale M, Tornqvist H: PI-3-kinase inhibitor Wortmannin blocks the insulin-like effects of growth hormone in isolated rat adipocytes. Biochem Biophys Res Commun 203:306–310, 1994.

268. Ridderstrale M, Degerman E, Tornqvist H: Growth hormone stimulates the tyrosine phosphorylation of the insulin receptor substrate-1 and its association with phosphatidylinositol 3-kinase in primary adipocytes. J Biol Chem 270:3471–3474, 1995.

269. Cheatham B, Vlahos CJ, Cheatham L, et al: Phosphatidylinositol 3-kinase activation is required for insulin stimulation of pp70 S6 kinase, DNA synthesis, and glucose transporter translocation. Mol Cell Biol 14:4902–4911, 1994.

270. Urich M, el Shemerly MY, Besser D, et al: Activation and nuclear translocation of mitogen-activated protein kinases by polyomavirus middle-T or serum depend on phosphatidylinositol 3-kinase. J Biol Chem 270:29286–29292, 1995.

271. Toker A, Meyer M, Reddy KK, et al: Activation of protein kinase C family members by the novel polyphosphoinositides PtdIns-3,4-P2 and PtdIns-3,4,5-P3. J Biol Chem 269:32358–32367, 1994.

272. Smal J, De Meyts P: Role of kinase C in the insulin-like effects of human growth hormone in rat adipocytes. Biochem Biophys Res Commun 147:1232–1240, 1987.

273. Gurland G, Ashcom G, Cochran BH, et al: Rapid events in growth hormone action. Induction of c-fos and c-jun transcription in 3T3-F442A preadipocytes. Endocrinology 127:3187–3195, 1990.

274. Slootweg MC, de Groot RP, Herrmann-Erlee MP, et al: Growth hormone induces expression of c-jun and jun B oncogenes and employs a protein kinase C signal transduction pathway for the induction of c-fos oncogene expression. J Mol Endocrinol 6:179–188, 1991.

275. Gaur S, Yamaguchi H, Goodman HM: Growth hormone increases calcium uptake in rat fat cells by a mechanism dependent on protein kinase C. Am J Physiol 270:C1485–C1492, 1996.

276. Billestrup N, Bouchelouche P, Allevato G, et al: Growth hormone receptor C-terminal domains required for growth hormone-induced intracellular free Ca2+ oscillations and gene transcription. Proc Natl Acad Sci U S A 92:2725–2729, 1995.

277. Schwartz Y, Yamaguchi H, Goodman HM: Growth hormone increases intracellular free calcium in rat adipocytes: Correlation with actions on carbohydrate metabolism. Endocrinology 131:772–778, 1992.

278. Rogers SA, Hammerman MR: Growth hormone activates phospholipase C in proximal tubular basolateral membranes from canine kidney. Proc Natl Acad Sci U S A 86:6363–6366, 1989.

279. Catalioto RM, Ailhaud G, Negrel R: Diacylglycerol production induced by growth hormone in Ob1771 preadipocytes arises from phosphatidylcholine breakdown. Biochem Biophys Res Commun 173:840–848, 1990.

280. Okada S, Kopchick JJ: Growth Hormone Inhibits Translocation of Protein Kinase C-a and -g Stimulated by Insulin in 3T3-F422A Cells, vol 78. Chevy Chase, MD, The Endocrine Society, 1996, p 275.

281. Kopchick J, Chen XZ, Li Y, et al: Differential in vivo activities of bovine growth hormone analogues. Transgenic Res 7:61–71, 1998.

282. Jeoung DI, Allen DL, Guller S, et al: Mitogenic and receptor activities of human growth hormone 108-129 [published erratum appears in J Biol Chem 1995 Nov 3;270 (44):26721]. J Biol Chem 268:22520–22524, 1993.

283. Lewis UJ, Lewis LJ, Salem MA, et al: A recombinant-DNA-derived modification of human growth hormone (hGH44-191) with enhanced diabetogenic activity. Mol Cell Endocrinol 78:45–54, 1991.

284. Nixon T, Green H: Contribution of growth hormone to the adipogenic activity of serum. Endocrinology 114:527–532, 1984.

285. Silverman MS, Mynarcik DC, Corin RE, et al: Antagonism by growth hormone of insulin-sensitive hexose transport in 3T3-F442A adipocytes. Endocrinology 125:2600–2604, 1989.

286. Staten NR, Byatt JC, Krivi GG: Ligand-specific dimerization of the extracellular domain of the bovine growth hormone receptor. J Biol Chem 268:18467–18473, 1993.

287. Campbell RM, Chen WY, Wiehl P, et al: A growth hormone (GH) analog that antagonizes the lipolytic effect but retains full insulin-like (antilipolytic) activity of GH. Proc Soc Exp Biol Med 203:311–316, 1993.

288. Yang CW, Striker GE, Chen WY, et al: Differential expression of glomerular extracellular matrix and growth factor mRNA in rapid and slowly progressive glomerulosclerosis: Studies in mice transgenic for native or mutated growth hormone. Lab Invest 76:467–476, 1997.

Growth Hormone–Releasing Hormone, Ghrelin, and Growth Hormone Secretagogues

Márta Korbonits, Bruce D. Gaylinn, Ralf Nass, and Michael O. Thorner

BASIC PHYSIOLOGY
   Growth Hormone–Releasing Hormone
   Ghrelin and Growth Hormone Secretagogues
CLINICAL IMPLICATIONS
   Growth Hormone–Releasing Hormone
   GHRH Therapy in GH-Deficient Children

GHRH Treatment in Adults
Growth Hormone Secretagogues
Ghrelin and Growth Hormone Secretagogues
Ghrelin Levels in Pathologic Conditions
SUMMARY

BASIC PHYSIOLOGY

GROWTH HORMONE–RELEASING HORMONE

History

Growth hormone–releasing hormone (GHRH), the last of the originally proposed hypophysiotropic factors, was identified structurally in 1982. A generation earlier, Reichlin proposed the existence of a GHRH because selective hypothalamic lesions yielded a growth hormone (GH) deficiency state and growth failure.[1,2] Although many groups attempted to isolate GHRH, success was achieved first by isolation of GHRH from GHRH-producing abdominal tumors rather than from the traditional physiologic source, the hypothalamus. In 1973, it was first reported that extracts of various human tumors enhance GH release.[3] Eight cases of presumed ectopic GHRH-secreting tumors were described,[4–13] and a partial purification of GHRH from an extrapituitary tumor was reported in 1980.[14] In October 1980, we studied in Charlottesville, Virginia, a patient with acromegaly and Turner's syndrome. Her acromegaly was due to somatotroph hyperplasia rather than a pituitary adenoma,[15] a diagnosis that became evident after her acromegaly persisted despite transsphenoidal surgery. Therefore, we sought a source for ectopic GHRH secretion and found a 5-cm tumor in the tail of the pancreas. It was from this tumor that two different teams isolated a 40-amino acid peptide, GHRH(1–40)-OH, then designated growth hormone–releasing factor (GH-RF).[16–18] Simultaneously, the Guillemin laboratory sequenced three GHRH peptides from a tumor obtained in Lyon, France: GHRH(1–44)-NH$_2$, GHRH(1–40)-OH, and GHRH(1–37)-OH.[19,20] The amino acid sequences were identical for all three peptides, with varying C-terminal extensions indicating the possibility of processing prior to release. The full biologic activity resided in residues 1 to 29,[21] and the sequence demonstrated that this was a member of the glucagon-secretin family of peptides. There were no disulfide bonds and no evidence of glycosylation of this peptide factor. These GHRHs eventually fulfilled the requirements of a hypophysiotropic GHRH. This chapter provides a limited summary of basic and clinical GHRH research.

Molecular and Cellular Biology

GHRH is a peptide hormone produced predominantly by neurons in the arcuate nucleus of the hypothalamus. These neurons send processes to the median eminence where GHRH is released into the pituitary portal circulation. GHRH then acts to stimulate the pulsatile release of GH from soma-

totrophs of the anterior pituitary.[22] Both GHRH(1–44)-NH$_2$ and GHRH(1–40)-OH can be found in the human hypothalamus[23–25] and in pituitary tumors of acromegalic patients.[26] GHRH is also produced in other tissues, where it may serve autocrine or paracrine roles. GHRH can be made synthetically[17,27] and recombinantly in *Escherichia coli.*[28] Human GHRH has also been introduced into transgenic mice.[29]

GHRH Peptide

GHRH is a member of a family of homologous peptides that includes secretin, glucagon, glucagon-like peptides (GLP-1, GLP-2), vasoactive intestinal peptide (VIP), pituitary adenylate cyclase–activating peptide (PACAP), PACAP-related peptide, peptide histidine-methionine (PHM, known as PHI in other species where the C-terminal residue is isoleucine), and glucose-dependent insulinotrophic polypeptide (also called gastric inhibitory peptide).[30–32] These peptides are thought to have arisen from a common ancestor through a series of gene duplications.[32] They retain sequence and structural similarities and can, to varying extents, interact at each other's receptors.[30]

The GHRH peptide sequence is known for several mammals, and GHRH-like sequences have been found in birds, fish, and even protochordate invertebrates.[33–35] GHRH sequences shown in Table 33-1 demonstrate that the N-terminal (1–29) residues that are required for receptor binding in the human[21] are 62% identical in the mouse (the most divergent known mammal) and less conserved in more distant species. This is in contrast to related peptides like PACAP, VIP, and glucagon, which are 100% identical in many mammals and more than 90% identical in more distant species.[32,35]

It has been proposed that the active tertiary structure of the GHRH peptide is an amphiphilic α helix that runs from residue 4 onward.[36,37] This helical structure, with polar and hydrophobic faces, is presumably stabilized when the peptide is bound to its receptor but is not stable in aqueous solution.[38] Circulating GHRH is rapidly inactivated in vivo by dipeptidylaminopeptidase IV (DPP-IV) acting at alanine 2[39] and is also partially inactivated by oxidation at methionine 27.[21] Medicinal chemists have used the GHRH scaffold to develop peptidic GHRH analogues with increased stability and potency. These efforts have used combinations of strategies that include increasing the stability of the α helix with helix-forming residues or ring structures; introducing unnatural amino acids or polyethylene glycol residues to decrease dipeptidylaminopeptidase, tryptic, and chymotryptic protease susceptibility and thereby prolong the half-life of the peptide in the circulation and subcutaneous tissues; and replacing the oxidizable methionine.[21,40–44] Substituting the alanine at position 2 with D-arginine was found to produce GHRH antagonists.[45,46] More stable, higher-affinity versions of this type of antagonist have recently been developed[47,48] and may prove useful to block the mitogenic affects of GHRH.[49] While GHRH acts as a low-affinity agonist at the VIP receptor, GHRH analogues such as N-Ac-Tyr[1], D-Phe[2]GHRH(1–29)-NH$_2$ have been developed as VIP antagonists.[50]

Gene and mRNA

Messenger RNA extracted from human tumors allowed complementary DNA (cDNA) probes to be constructed and the single-copy GHRH gene to be identified on human chromosome 20.[51] The human,[52] rat,[53] and mouse[54] genes span about 10 kb of DNA and include five exons. The third exon encodes the 1–31 sequence, which is sufficient for the known biologic activities of GHRH. The human mRNA encodes a 108-amino acid precursor protein, the middle region of which is processed to form the mature GHRH peptide. Brain-, placental-, and gonadal-specific forms of GHRH mRNA are known.[53,55,56] These tissue-specific messages initiate at different gene promotors and result in mRNAs of different sizes, but the encoded precursor protein remains identical. Immunologic evidence shows that the C-terminal fragment of the precursor protein is processed into an additional peptide known as GHRH-related peptide (GHRH-RP; see Table 33-1). GHRH-RP is expressed in the human hypothalamus,[57] where its role is not known, and in rat testis, where it is reported to regulate Sertoli cell function.[58] An additional alternatively spliced mRNA found in rat placenta but not hypothalamus encodes the normal GHRH but includes an altered GHRH-RP.[59]

Tissue Distribution

In the human and a number of species, GHRH immunoreactivity is present in the basal hypothalamus, appropriate anatomically for release into the pituitary portal vessels.[25,60–64] GHRH cell bodies directing processes to the median eminence originate from both the perifornical nucleus[63] and the arcuate (rat) or infundibular (human) nucleus.[25,60,61,63] GHRH perikarya are also found in the ventromedial nucleus,[62,63,65] a region that can induce increased GH release upon electrical stimulation.[9] There is a reciprocal innervation between GHRH and somatostatin neurons in the rat hypothalamus,[66] providing the potential for direct communication between the major stimulatory and inhibitory neurons governing GH release. This relationship may participate in the ultradian oscillation of hypothalamic GHRH and somatostatin mRNAs.[67] GHRH neurons also directly express somatostatin receptors.[68] A number of other brain regions outside of the hypothalamus contain immunoreactive GHRH.[61–63] The ontogeny of GHRH neurons suggests that they appear in the human fetus between 18 and 29 weeks of gestation[60,69] and in the rat on embryonic day 18, reaching adult levels by postnatal day 30.[70]

There is much evidence for GHRH outside the central nervous system in a number of cell types and tissues in humans and in rodents, but its function outside the GH axis remains to be established. Messenger RNA for GHRH, immunoactive GHRH, or bioactive GHRH content is reported in the anterior pituitary,[71] ovary,[72] testis,[56,73] placenta,[55,56,74–76] leukocytes,[77–79] adrenal medulla,[80] pancreas,[81,82] gastrointestinal tract,[82,83] and in tumors associated with the GH axis[26,71,84,85] as well as many other tumor types including human breast, endometrium, and ovary.[86] Ultrasensitive reverse transcription-polymerase chain reaction (RT-PCR) techniques can detect trace amounts of GHRH mRNA in most rat tissues examined.[87] Studies in the somatotrope found immunoreactive GHRH in secretory granules and the cell nuclei.[88] Additional data demonstrate somatotrope uptake of labeled GHRH into secretory granules, lysosomes, and the nuclear membrane.[89,90]

GHRH Signaling

GHRH Receptor

GHRH acts through a high-affinity G protein–coupled receptor (GHRHR) found in the anterior pituitary and coupled to cyclic adenosine monophosphate (cAMP).[91] Upon the molecular cloning of the receptor from human pituitary tumor and rat and mouse pituitary,[92–94] it was found to be a member of the G protein–coupled receptor family B, also called the secretin family. The GHRHR protein has 47%, 42%, 35%, and 28% sequence identity with receptors for VIP, secretin, calcitonin, and parathyroid hormone, respectively.[92,93] The isolated cDNAs encoded a 423-amino acid protein that has seven putative transmembrane domains, and a 108-residue N-terminal extracellular domain (after signal peptide cleavage) containing one glycosylation site (Fig. 33-1). The rat and human protein sequences are 82% identical.[92] The GHRHR sequence predicts

Table 33-1 Growth Hormone–Releasing Hormone Sequences

	1 29	44	% Identity*
Human	YADAIFTNSYRKVLGQLSARKLLQDIMSR	QQGESNQERGARARL	100
Porcine	YADAIFTNSYRKVLGQLSARKLLQDIMSR	QQGERNQEQGARVRL	100
Bovine†	YADAIFTNSYRKVLGQLSARKLLQDIM**N**R	QQGERNQEQGAKVRL	97
Ovine	YADAIFTNSYRK**I**LGQLSARKLLQDIM**N**R	QQGERNQEQGAKVRL	93
Hamster	YADAIFT**S**SYRKVLGQLSARKLLQDIMSR	QQGERNQEQGPRVRL	97
Rat	**H**ADAIFT**SS**YR**RI**LGQLY**A**RKLL**HE**IMSR	QQGERNQEQRSRFN	72
Murine	**HV**DAIFT**TT**NYRKLL**S**QLYARK**VI**QDIM**NK**	Q·GERIQEQRARLS	62
Chicken	**H**AD**GIFSK**AYRKLLGQLSARNYL**HSLMAK**	RVGGASSGLGDEAEPLS	55
Carp	**H**AD**GMFNK**AYRKAL**GQLSARKYLHTLMAK**	RVGGG·SMIEDDNEPLS	55
Catfish	**H**AD**GLLDRALRDILVQLSARKYLHSLTAV**	RVGEE·EEDEEDSEPLS	38
Tunicate	**HSDGIFTKDYRKYLGQLRAQKFLQWLMKR**		59
Related human peptides:			
hVIP	**HSDAVFTDNYTRLRKQMAVKKYLNSILN**		31
hPACAP	**HSDGIFTDSYSRYRKQMAVKKYLAAVLGK**	RYKQRVKNK	31
hPHM	**HADGVFTSDFSKLLGQLSAKKYLESLM**		48
hGHRH-RP	**QVDSMWAE·····QKQMELESILVALL···QKHSRNSQG**		10

Residues that differ from the human in the 1–29 region are shown in bold.
*Identity calculated for residues 1–29 that are required for activity at the GHRH receptor.
†Bovine and caprine sequences are identical.
. Indicates gap in alignment.
hGHRH-RP: hGHRH-related peptide, see text.

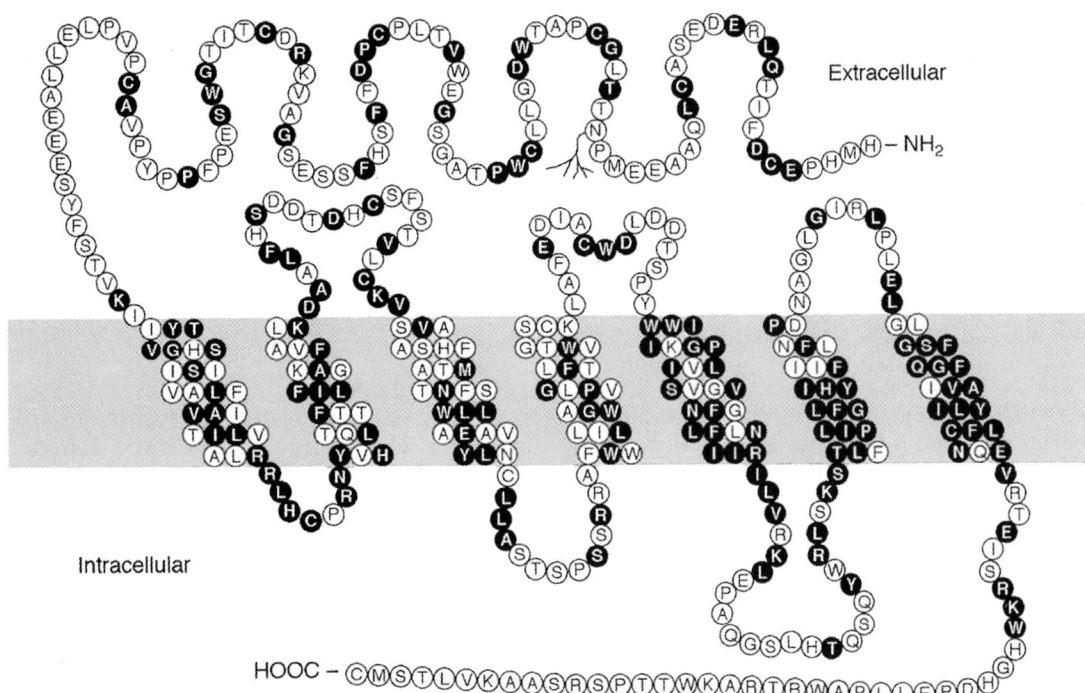

Figure 33-1 Cartoon representation of the deduced sequence of the human pituitary growth hormone–releasing hormone receptor. Shaded amino acids are conserved in closely related receptors. (Reprinted with permission from Gaylinn BD, Harrison JK, Zysk JR, et al: Molecular cloning and expression of a human anterior pituitary receptor for GHRH. Mol Endocrinol 7:77–84, 1993.)

10 extracellular cysteine residues that are also found in secretin, VIP, and PACAP receptors. Eight of these 10 are conserved in nearly all reported members of this receptor family. These cysteine residues are proposed to form sulfhydral crosslinks that stabilize an extracellular domain involved in hormone binding.[95]

The cloned pituitary GHRHR expressed in cell lines demonstrated saturable, high-affinity, GHRH-specific binding and also stimulated the accumulation of intracellular cAMP in response to physiologic concentrations of GHRH.[92–94] Unlike some related receptors that could signal through both cAMP:PKA and phospholipase C:IP$_3$:PKC pathways, only cAMP activation could be detected. Though GHRH was not seen to activate the phospholipase C pathway in somatotrope cells, it does stimulate phospholipid turnover. A specific GHRH antagonist blocked both binding and second messenger responses.

Data from the cloned receptor were consistent with photoaffinity crosslinking studies of GHRHR in sheep pituitary membranes that revealed high-affinity binding sites with an apparent molecular weight of 55 kilodaltons and one glycosylation site. After deglycosylation and taking into account the mass of the coupled GHRH-analogue, the molecular weight of the native ovine receptor protein was estimated at 42 kilodaltons,[96] in agreement with the prediction from the human cDNA sequence of 45 kilodaltons, assuming cleavage of a signal peptide.[93] Further, the binding characteristics of the natural sheep receptor and the cloned human receptor are largely in agreement with a single high-affinity site with a K_d of approximately 0.2 nM.

Various radiolabeled forms of GHRH bind to membranes of the pituitary, thymus, and spleen. The dissociation constants estimated in these studies vary wildly from 41 pM[97] to 590 nM.[98] No binding was measurable in three nonfunctional pituitary adenomas, while there was consistent GHRH binding to five acromegalic adenomas, with dissociation constants averaging 0.3 nM.[99]

Studies attempting to delineate the receptor's GHRH-binding domains using chimeric receptor constructs[95] or GHRH crosslinking[100] suggest that while the large N-terminal extracellular domain plays a major role in GHRH binding, other domains are also essential for ligand selectivity and binding.

GHRH Receptor mRNA and Gene

Two GHRHR mRNA transcripts of approximately 2.5 and 4 kilobases were identified in rat pituitary, 2.0 and 2.1 kilobases in mouse, and 3.5 kilobases in ovine pituitary.[92–94] Further, in the mouse it has been shown that the receptor is expressed in a spatial and temporal pattern corresponding to GH gene expression.[94] In the mouse, the first evidence of a pituitary-specific transcription factor (Pit-1) expression occurred at embryonic day 14.5, while transcripts encoding the cloned receptor first appeared on embryonic day 16.5.[94] Mutations that cause a loss of Pit-1 expression, such as in dw/dw mice, lead to a lack of GHRHR gene expression and somatotrope hypoplasia.[94]

The human GHRHR gene is divided into 13 exons separated by variably sized introns that spread its length to over 15 kb, the complete sequence of which is known.[101] Fluorescent in situ hybridization localized the gene to human chromosome 7p14–15.[102,103] Studies of the receptor gene's promotor region found no traditional initiator motifs such as a TATA box.[104,105] Putative binding sites for several transcription factors including Pit-1, Oct-1, Brn-2, NF-1, cAMP response element, and estrogen receptor response elements were identified. An in vitro reporter system demonstrated that expression was enhanced by Pit-1 and glucocorticoids and inhibited by estrogen.[104] Pit-1 stimulation is consistent with previous studies in Snell and Jackson dwarf mice showing Pit-1 dependence of receptor expression.[94] The glucocorticoid effect on the promotor may be the mechanism for glucocorticoid upregulation of GHRH-binding sites[106] and receptor mRNA[107,108] in rats. The estrogen inhibition of promotor transcription is consistent with the observed sexual dimorphism in receptor mRNA expression.[109] Studies have suggested that GHRHR expression is upregulated by GHRH itself.[110–112] While a putative cAMP response element that could explain this effect was found in the receptor gene promoter, in vitro regulation of the promoter by forskolin could not be demonstrated.

The structure of the rat GHRHR gene[113] closely matches that of the human, but includes an additional exon that would predict an alternatively spliced receptor message. This alternative long form encodes 41 additional amino acids in the third intracellular loop. Rat and mouse GHRHR cDNA clones demonstrate this alternative long form.[92,94] However, analysis of rat pituitary mRNA by polymerase chain reaction (PCR) revealed only evidence of the shorter form.[92] Alternative splicing at the homologous site in the PACAP receptor results in functional receptors that differ in their relative signaling through cAMP and phospholipase C second messenger pathways.[114] When the long form of the rat GHRHR is stably expressed in cell lines, it binds GHRH, but no intracellular signaling through any pathway, cAMP, or phospholipase C could be detected.[113]

In the mouse, there is evidence of alternative splicing encoding a receptor devoid of the first transmembrane domain.[94] Alternatively spliced GHRH mRNA encoding a receptor lacking the last two transmembrane domains has been reported in human pituitary tumors and in normal pituitary.[115] In the rat, an alternative splice replacing the last 5 amino acid residues at the C-terminus with a new 17-residue sequence has been found by PCR.[116] This receptor variant appears to signal cAMP normally. No functional role for any of these alternatively spliced GHRHR messages has been established, though it is proposed that a truncated receptor variant expressed in tumors can act as a dominant negative in inhibiting GHRH signaling.[117]

Several studies have shown that synthetic GHRH antagonists can inhibit the growth and proliferation of a variety of human tumors and tumor cell lines.[118–122] This antiproliferative effect of antagonists is consistent with the hypothesis that GHRH can act as a local autocrine/paracrine factor in the stimulation of cell growth[123] and with the mitogenic actions of GHRH at the somatotroph.[124] The mechanism for this action has been unclear because full-length GHRH receptor could not be detected in these cell lines responsive to GHRH antagonist.[122] Recently, it has been found that many tumor cells, and also normal human prostate, express low levels of alternatively spliced forms of GHRH receptor messages not found in the pituitary.[122,125] Recent studies suggest that a receptor splice variant with an alternative N-terminal domain (SV1) may be the site of action for the antiproliferative effects of GHRH antagonists[126–128] and for ligand-independent stimulation of tumor growth.[129]

GHRHR mutations resulting in dwarfism have recently been identified in mouse and humans. The first such mutation was found in the *little* mouse. This dwarf strain has an inherited autosomal defect resulting in low levels of GH and pituitary hypoplasia, but is still responsive to exogenous GH. The mutation was mapped by linkage analysis to mouse chromosome 6.[130] Pituitary cells from these mice would not respond to GHRH but could release GH in response to other activators of cAMP, suggesting a receptor defect.[131] After the cloning of the GHRHR cDNA, two groups localized the mouse gene to the midregion of chromosome 6 and went on to sequence the receptor from the *little* mouse.[132,133] They found an Asp-to-Gly point mutation at residue 60 of the receptor's extracellular domain. This residue is highly conserved in related receptors and its mutation resulted in a complete loss of cAMP signaling. Further studies demonstrated that the mutant *little* mouse receptor protein was expressed and localized in the cell membrane, but was unable to bind GHRH.[132,133]

A variety of loss of function GHRHR mutations have been identified in studies of human GH deficiency. Two such mutations are found in large kindreds. One GHRHR mutation has been identified in three distantly related kindreds from India,[134] Pakistan,[135] and Sri Lanka.[136] These patients all share a recessive mutation mapping to chromosome 7p14. A single-base-pair change encodes a premature stop codon at residue 72, resulting in a severe receptor truncation and loss of all

function. Another receptor mutation has been identified in a large Brazilian kindred.[137] In this case, the mutation interferes with a splice donor site resulting in the retention of intron 1. The translational reading frame is disrupted at residue 20 within the signal peptide and no part of the mature receptor protein can be made. It is likely that other receptor mutations will be identified in GH-deficient patients, and it is possible that activating mutations may be associated with some cases of acromegaly. It is now suggested that 10% of all human familial isolated GH deficiency type 1 is caused by GHRHR defects.[138] Screening of pituitary tumors for activating mutations of GHRHRs have yielded ambiguous[139] or negative results.[140,141]

Intracellular Signaling

At the somatotrope, GHRH activates many of the classical signaling systems including cAMP, calmodulin, calcium mobilization, and phospholipid pathways, indicating a significant commitment of the somatotrope to respond to GHRH. As with many secretory cells, GHRH-accelerated GH release requires both calcium,[142–146] and calmodulin.[143,147] Intracellular calcium is elevated within seconds of a GHRH stimulus, in both pituitary cells[148–150] and thymocytes.[151] This calcium response is dependent on influx of extracellular calcium and is not due to the release of intracellular stores.[152] cAMP also signals to the cell nucleus regulating multiple transcription factors to affect gene expression.[153]

cAMP Metabolism cAMP analogues and calcium stimulate GHRH release from cultured hypothalamus, while protein kinase C modulates these effectors.[154] At the somatotrope, GHRH stimulates cAMP accumulation and GH release, and these responses are blocked by somatostatin.[142–144,155–165] Glucocorticoid pretreatment enhances both the potency and efficacy of GHRH in driving cAMP accumulation and GH release[166]; this steroid is necessary for GHRH-induced cAMP accumulation after several days in culture. Adenylate cyclase activity in membranes of normal rat pituitary or human acromegalic tumors[167] is enhanced by GHRH in a guanine nucleotide-[147,168] and calmodulin-sensitive[147] manner. Pertussis toxin enhances GHRH-initiated cAMP accumulation and GH release.[155,158,162] The spontaneous reduction in GHRH-stimulated cAMP levels that occurs over time can be blocked by cycloheximide,[155] while the stimulatory ability of GHRH is potentiated by protein kinase C activation.[161,162,165,169] This indicates that another receptor system, which stimulates C kinase, may directly enhance the productivity of the GHRHR-coupling protein-adenylate cyclase complex[170,171]; a candidate for which is growth hormone secretagogue receptor.[169]

Phospholipids GHRH increases phosphatidylinositol labelling[172] as well as free arachidonate levels[173] in the pituitary. Although in most systems no effect of GHRH on polyphosphoinositide hydrolysis is detectable,[174] a report shows that in a specific subclass of porcine somatotropes (low-density somatotropes) GHRH stimulates both cAMP and inositol phosphate-dependent second messenger pathways.[175] Other metabolic pathways involving phospholipid metabolism may be activated by or modulate GHRH activity.[149,160] cAMP metabolism can be dissociated from GH release after GHRH with some phospholipid metabolic enzyme inhibitors, indicating they can act distal to the cAMP system to evoke exocytosis.[160]

Mitogenic Signaling In vivo, insufficient GHRH signaling during development through a GHRHR defect[133] or as a result of GHRH antisera administration[176] results in somatotrope hypoplasia. Excess GHRH signaling through tumor expression,[15] Gs mutation,[177] or transgenic overexpression[178] stimulates somatotrope hyperplasia. In vitro, GHRH is a mitogenic signal for somatotrope proliferation.[179] The mitogen-activated protein kinase (MAPK) pathway is a potential mechanism for this action. Recent evidence demonstrates a dose-dependent GHRH stimulation of the tyrosine phosphorylation of MAPK.[180–182] The pathways through which GHRH activates MAPK are not established.

GH mRNA and Release Dynamics in Culture

GHRH stimulates the level or transcription rate of GH mRNA,[180,181] the release of newly synthesized GH,[182] and total GH (stored plus released),[183] as well as the proliferation of somatotropes in vitro.[179] The GHRH effect on the somatotrope varies according to the anatomic location of the somatotrope within the pituitary[184] and the GH releasing effect is further enhanced by acute administration of glucocorticoids,[27,166,185] possibly through increased GHRH binding.[97] Like glucocorticoids, triiodothyronine[185] and GH-releasing peptide[169] can amplify GHRH-stimulated GH secretion. In contrast, insulin-like growth factor 1 (IGF-I)[27] and somatostatin[163,185] are noncompetitive inhibitors of GHRH-accelerated GH release in vitro.

Accelerated GH release occurs immediately after exposure to GHRH[155,157,186–189] and remains elevated for the duration of the GHRH pulse,[155,157,186,188,189] albeit at declining rates of release after about 10 minutes.[8,157,183,186,189–191] This spontaneous decline could occur without GH content depletion[8] and could be blocked by cycloheximide, suggesting the participation of a rapidly turning over inhibitory protein.[155] The reciprocal interaction of GHRH and somatostatin, suggested neuroanatomically,[66] and in pituitary portal blood measurements[192,193] results in a greater mass of GH release per GHRH pulse. This has been demonstrated in perifusion culture.[194]

Picomolar to nanomolar concentrations of GHRH that likely are present in pituitary portal blood[192,193] regulate a graded GH response from the somatotrope.[17,20,27,156] GHRH also stimulates modest prolactin release at low GHRH concentrations in vitro[195,196] and the secretion of a protein known as peptide 23 (identical to pancreatitis-associated protein and a member of the C-type lectin supergene family).[197,198] As GHRH can interact with VIP receptors (VIP is a prolactin secretagogue) in intestinal epithelium[199] and GH_3 cells,[200] it is possible that pharmacologic or pathologic levels of GHRH can activate this and other receptor types.

Animal Studies

GHRH Release

The pulsatile release of GH is influenced by numerous factors including nutrition, body composition, metabolism, age, sex steroids, adrenal corticoids, thyroid hormones, and renal and hepatic functions.[201] A major common pathway for these factors is through their effects on GHRH release from the hypothalamus through direct actions on GHRH neurons and also through interplay with somatostatin neurons. These effects may be mediated through other factors such as growth hormone secretagogues,[202] catecholamines,[203] interleukin-1,[204] somatostatin,[204] opioids,[203] leptin,[205–207] inhibin,[208] and neuropeptide Y (NPY).[209]

GHRH Effects on the GH Axis

GHRH was first demonstrated to stimulate GH release in vivo using anesthetized rats.[210,211] These GH responses to GHRH could be enhanced by passive immunization against somatostatin[212–214] or blocked by passive immunization against rat GHRH.[212,213] It was soon found that GHRH could enhance GH secretion in every vertebrate species tested, including monkey,[215] bovine,[216–219] swine,[220] chicken,[221] and carp.[34]

GHRH is necessary for endogenous pulsatile GH secretion as anti-GHRH antisera treatment eliminated these pulses in rats and sheep.[222,223] However, recent data[224] suggest that rhythmic GH secretion persists in an amplitude-miniaturized version in the absence of a GHRHR signal, at least in men. This observation is supported by Jessup and colleagues,[225] who found a gender-specific difference after administration of a GHRH antagonist, with no change in basal secretion in men but a significant decrease in women. Antisera to GHRH also decreased statural growth[226] and GHRHR mRNA expression[111] in the rat. Conversely, GHRH administered over several days to weeks, enhances body or organ growth and function in experimental animals.[219,227–229] The effect is particularly striking in mice transgenic for GHRH.[230,231] Pulses of GHRH are measured in pituitary portal plasma of unanesthetized sheep, with peak values of 25 to 40 pg/mL and a period of 71 minutes.[193] Temporal analysis of GH pulses in these sheep suggested a complex regulation that can be only partially explained by GHRH and somatostatin pulses and suggest the involvement of other factors such as an endogenous ligand corresponding to the synthetic GH secretagogues.[169]

During development, basal GH responses to exogenous GHRH decrease from postnatal day 1 to 28 in the rhesus monkey.[232] Passive immunization against GHRH shows that endogenous GHRH is an active secretagogue up to day 9.[233] In the rat, GHRH injections do not increase GH levels at postnatal day 2,[234] whereas stimulatory responses of similar magnitude are measured at postnatal days 10, 30, and 75, as well as at 14 months.[235] Likewise, 5 days of GHRH injections elevate GH biosynthesis in rat pituitaries at postnatal day 10.[236] Rat pituitary GHRHR mRNA expression was highest in early gestation, declined to a nadir at 12 days of age, increased at the onset of sexual maturation, and then declined with aging.[237]

There are significant changes in GHRH status during aging. In the hypothalamus there is a reduction in GHRH gene expression and content,[238] as well as a decrease in GHRH binding to pituitary in 18-month-old rats.[239] GHRHR mRNA is correspondingly decreased in 18-month-old rats, but can be brought back toward levels observed in younger animals by treatment with GHRH.[240] Decreased GHRHR expression may contribute to the diminished pituitary response to GHRH in aged male rats[241–243] and humans.[83,244]

The GHRH system is also strongly influenced by gender (or gonadal steroids). Hypothalamic GHRH mRNA levels are greater in male than female rats[245,246] and are reduced by orchidectomy and increased by testosterone treatment in intact[247] or castrated[248] male rats. Estradiol has no effect on hypothalamic GHRH mRNA.[247,249] The ability of GHRH to elicit a GH response in vivo varies during the rat estrous cycle,[250] is of greater magnitude in the male than female,[235,251] and is strongly sex steroid dependent.[251] Somatotropes from male rats, likewise, have a greater cAMP and GH response to GHRH than those from female rats when studied in static[159] or perifusion[251] cultures. Furthermore, the intact and castrated male rat treated with testosterone yields the most GHRH responsive somatotropes,[251] as does direct testosterone treatment of cultured somatotropes.[252] Gender differences can be measured at the level of the single somatotrope using the hemolytic plaque assay[253]; testosterone (administered in vivo) increases secretory capacity and recruits a subpopulation of somatotropes, while estradiol has the opposite effects.[254] GHRH receptor message levels are dramatically lower in female than in male rats,[109] and estrogen acts at the receptor gene to inhibit GHRHR mRNA expression.[104]

In addition to sex steroid effects, free fatty acids[255] and GH itself[256] reduce the in vivo release of GH in response to GHRH. GH treatment decreases hypothalamic GHRH content in intact rats[246] and after hypophysectomy GHRH levels in the hypothalamus rise,[257] suggesting feedback regulation of GHRH by GH. Thyroxine replacement can restore hypothalamic immunoreactive GHRH levels reduced by thyroidectomy in rats,[258] and both triiodothyronine and cortisol can protect against the reduction in GHRH-stimulated GH release in hypothyroid,[259] or adrenalectomized rats,[260,261] respectively. Indeed, chronic glucocorticoids in vivo decrease GHRH expression in GHRH neurons of the arcuate nucleus.[262,263]

Months of excess GHRH exposure in transgenic mice is associated with increased pituitary mass and mammosomatotrope hyperplasia[230,231] that eventually results in adenoma formation after 12 months.[264,265] This is reminiscent of the clinical findings in patients with ectopic GHRH secretion. What was surprising was the rapidity of this effect; GHRH infusions were capable of inducing enlargement of the anterior pituitary within days in intact, normal rats.[266] The dose range of this acute effect has yet to be defined, and this observation does not address the potential risks of replacement of GHRH in deficiency states. In pituitary allograph studies, in orchidectomized hamsters, exogenous GHRH maintains somatotrope size without affecting the percent of GH cells.[267]

GHRH Effects on Functions Outside of the GH Axis

GHRH stimulates gastrin release and epithelial cell proliferation in the digestive tract.[268] It also stimulates insulin, glucagon, and somatostatin secretion from the pancreas.[269-271] In the brain, GHRH coexists with tyrosine hydroxylase[272] and can enhance its activity,[273] as well as that of choline acetyltransferase,[274] while inhibiting thyrotropin-releasing hormone secretion from the rat hypothalamus.[275] GHRH influences eating behavior,[276-279] and circulating GHRH is increased by feeding in humans.[280] The latter effect is due to release of GHRH from extra central nervous system sites. GHRH enhances non–rapid eye movement sleep in rats.[281] GHRH antisera[282] or GHRH antagonists[283] inhibit sleep, and sleep deprivation enhances hypothalamic GHRH mRNA levels.[284,285] GHRH-Ab treatment of female rats results in osteopenic effects,[286] and plasmid-mediated GHRH expression in an animal model of cancer cachexia was able to prevent weight loss.[287] Most of these activities, including the control of GH status, suggest that GHRH predominantly acts as a nutrient-partitioning hormone to regulate body composition.

GHRELIN AND GROWTH HORMONE SECRETAGOGUES

History

Opiates have been recognized to stimulate GH secretion. The GH secretagogue (GHS) story evolved from the seminal observation by Bowers and colleagues that met-enkephalin analogs, which lacked analgesic activity, preserved their GH-releasing activity.[288] Bowers and colleagues developed these GH-releasing peptides, and the most promising of the initial compounds that they developed was GHRP-6, a hexapeptide with two D-amino acids.[289] This compound did not interact with the GHRHR and in vivo synergized with GHRH.[290,291] A characteristic of GHSs is that they have rather weak effects on GH stimulation from the pituitary in vitro while they are very efficacious when administered in vivo. This observation, together with the simple structure of the GHRPs, made them attractive molecules to be developed to enhance GH secretion. Thus, the pharmaceutical industry became interested and expended major resources to developing peptide and non-peptide compounds. A remarkable achievement by the

Merck group was that they took one of their synthetic compounds, MK-0677, as a tool and succeeded in the expression cloning of the GHS-receptor (GHS-R).[292] Thus, the structure of the GHS-R was known prior to the isolation and characterization of any natural ligand for the receptor.[293] A natural ligand for the receptor, ghrelin,[294] was identified in 1999 as a result of a "reverse pharmacology" process. Although the highest concentration of the receptor is in the hypothalamus and pituitary, ghrelin was surprisingly identified from the stomach. Ghrelin has been detected in a number of tissues,[294-296] suggesting that it represents a new member of the brain-gut peptide family, though there remains some controversy as to whether it is present in significant amounts in the hypothalamus.[297-299] Following earlier reports on positive effects on appetite of some GHSs, the profound GH-independent orexigenic effects of ghrelin were recognized.[300]

An endogenous ligand of the GHS-R type 1a was named ghrelin from the Proto-Indo-European word "*ghre,*" which means grow, and "*relin*" as it had GH-releasing activities.[294] Ghrelin is a 28-amino acid peptide with a fatty acid chain modification on the N-terminal third amino acid (Fig. 33-2). At the same time, a stomach-derived mRNA sequence was identified by another group, coding for a protein with sequence similarities to motilin and named motilin-related peptide m46.[301] This peptide later turned out to be identical to ghrelin, although the fatty acid modification was not recognized as a result of being identified from its mRNA rather than peptide sequence.

The 117-amino acid long preproghrelin is coded by the ghrelin gene situated on chromosome 3 (3p25–26).[294] Preproghrelin contains a 23-amino acid signal peptide, the 28 amino acid ghrelin and a 66 amino acid tail. There are several physiologically occurring variants of ghrelin with similar biologic activity to the originally described molecule.[302,303] The acylation of the hydroxyl group of Ser[3] is necessary for the activities mediated by the GHS-1a receptor (calcium mobilization, GH release, and appetite effect),[294,304,305] but not for others (proliferative and anti-apoptotic effects).[306-309] In initial reports, the majority (90% to 95%) of circulating 28-amino acid ghrelin was in desoctanoyl form, while C-terminal proghrelin concentration was found to be 1.5 times higher than ghrelin.[310] However, more recent reports using samples collected under acid conditions in the presence of esterase inhibitors suggest that 15% to 40% of circulating ghrelin is in the acyl form, with the higher levels of the active form seen when ghrelin levels (and presumable secretion rates) are higher.[311,312]

Ghrelin has been identified in a wide variety of species, and its receptor GHS-R has been conserved for over 400 million years as it has been identified in puffer fish.[313] Ghrelin was originally isolated from the stomach. There are a number of different types of endocrine cells in the stomach. About 20% of the chromogranin A–immunoreactive endocrine cells contain ghrelin mRNA.[314] Ghrelin cells are equivalent to those known as A cells or X/A-like cells, whose hormonal product was

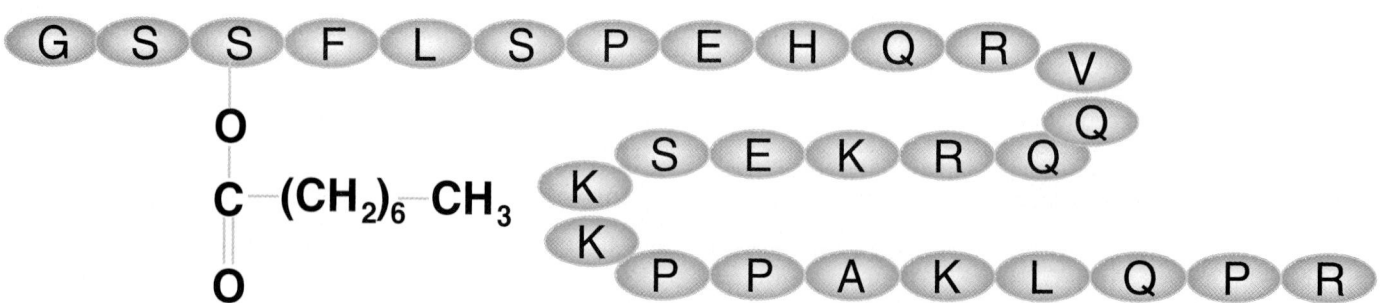

Figure 33-2 The structure of the mature human ghrelin peptide.

previously unidentified. A smaller number of immunopositive cells are found in the small and large intestine. The concentration of ghrelin found in the circulation of rats decreases by 80% following surgical removal of the acid-producing part of the stomach, suggesting that the oxyntic mucosa is the major source of circulating ghrelin.[315] A similar reduction of ghrelin levels was found in humans following gastrectomy.[316]

Outside the intestinal tract, ghrelin expression has been identified in a number of tissues at the mRNA or protein level or both. Whether significant levels of ghrelin are expressed in the hypothalamus remains controversial. Ghrelin peptide has been detected by immunostaining in the hypothalamus[294–296,317,318] and was localized in the internuclear space between the hypothalamic nuclei and the ependymal layer of the third ventricle. Ghrelin was also seen in the axon terminals and these axons innervated the arcuate, ventromedial, paraventricular, and dorsomedial nucleus and the lateral hypothalamus, as well as outside the hypothalamus in the bed nucleus of the stria terminalis, amygdala, thalamus, and habenula.[296] But other studies could not detect significant levels of ghrelin message or protein product, suggesting a role for circulating ghrelin.[297,298]

Ghrelin mRNA expression has been described in all the normal human tissues studied,[319] as well as in different tumors including pituitary adenomas, neuroendocrine tumors, thyroid and medullary thyroid carcinomas, and endocrine tumors of the pancreas and lung.[295,320–325] Ghrelin peptide has been shown to be expressed in pituitary,[295] immune cells,[326,327] ß and α cells of the pancreas,[328,329] as well as a new islet cell type, ε cell, which contains ghrelin and no other known hormones,[330,331] lung,[332] placenta,[333] testis,[334,335] kidney[336] and cyclical expression in the ovary.[337,338] Within the pituitary, ghrelin immunostaining colocalized to prolactin, growth hormone, and thyroid-stimulating hormone–secreting cells but not to adrenocorticotropic hormone (ACTH) or gonadotroph cells.[339] Circulating ghrelin might reach the hypothalamic nuclei directly from the bloodstream (arcuate nucleus) or via crossing the blood-brain barrier,[305] but peripheral (vagal) connections to the brain stem may also play an important role in the effect of ghrelin (see Fig. 33-5).

Assays for Ghrelin

Most studies in the literature to date have examined total ghrelin using commercially available radioimmunoassay (RIA) or enzyme-linked immunosorbent assay kits. These assays are directed to the C-terminal end of the peptide and do not distinguish if the acylation on serine 3 is present. Newer assays to measure active ghrelin are now available. Most of these assays are directed to the N-terminal region of ghrelin and are specific for the acylated form. These assays also cross-react with short N-terminal fragments of ghrelin that have negligible biological activity and whose abundance in the blood is unknown. Sandwich assays that are specific for full-length acylated ghrelin have just become commercially available. Each of these types of assays report somewhat different information about the forms of ghrelin that are present and so must be interpreted appropriately.

Due to an endogenous esterase activity, acylated "active" ghrelin in blood samples is unstable. Thus, measured ghrelin levels can be a function of sample collection, handling, and storage methods. Current techniques collect blood samples into chilled tubes containing esterase/protease inhibitors, centrifuge promptly to separate the plasma, and then acidify the plasma to inactivate enzymatic activities.

Regulation of Ghrelin

Factors shown to be important in ghrelin regulation are listed in Table 33-2. In the human, ghrelin levels are high in the fasting state and fall immediately after food intake. Higher levels are observed during the night.[340,341] After prolonged fasting (>3 days), ghrelin levels are not elevated.[312,342] Chronic

Table 33-2 Regulation of Ghrelin Secretion

Increased with	Decreased with
Fasting (short term), low BMI	Food intake, high BMI
GHRH	Glucose
Thyroid hormones	Insulin
Testosterone	Somatostatin
Parasympathetic activity	GH (short term)
	GHS, ghrelin
	PYY$_{3-36}$

regulation is influenced by body weight, with high levels in subjects with low body mass index (BMI) and low levels in obese subjects.[343–345] Insulin appears to be the most important regulator of ghrelin levels as both insulin resistance and hyperinsulinemia predicts low ghrelin levels in a population consisting of insulin-resistant and insulin-sensitive subjects who have equal body mass index.[346] Most studies suggest that ghrelin levels are similar in males and females, but some data showed higher ghrelin levels in females.[347,348]

Physiology and Molecular Biology

Properties of Synthetic Peptide and Peptidomimetic GHS Compounds

The first GHS developed by Bowers and colleagues was GHRP (Table 33-3), a synthetic peptide derived from met-enkephalin that retained the ability to release GH from somatotrophs in vitro, but had little opioid activity.[288,359] This compound showed no in vivo activity. Refinement of GHRP resulted in GHRP-6 which has significantly improved stability and potency.[289] GHRP-6 is active both in vitro and in vivo, and has served as the model GHS from which many new compounds have been developed. GHRP-2 (KP 102)[360] is an improved structure with sixfold greater potency in rats. In an effort to extend the in vivo half-life of GHRP-6, the first tryptophan was stabilized by the addition of a methyl group.[361] The resulting compound, known as hexarelin appears equivalent to GHRP-2 in human studies.[362] GHRP-6, GHRP-2, and hexarelin are generally administered IV or SC. These peptides can stimulate GH following administration intranasally[363] or orally, although much higher doses are required.

In a pioneering effort to develop an orally active GHS that would be better absorbed, a group at Merck Research Laboratories engineered a non-peptide benzolactam compound that closely mimicked the structure of GHRP-6.[364] This compound, referred to as MK-0751 (L-692,429), was active and well tolerated in humans,[365,366] but had low oral bioavailability. An alternative spiroindane structure was developed and modified to produce MK-0677 (L-163,191) which had significantly improved oral potency and duration of action (>60% oral bioavailability in dogs with 5- to 6- hr half-life).[352] These non-peptide GHSs were shown to act specifically and through the same mechanism as GHRP-6, being synergistic with GHRH, not blocked by GHRH antagonists, ineffective after saturating GHRP-6 and competing at the cloned GHS-R.[367]

A large number of pharmaceutical companies and research groups are actively developing GHSs, and many new peptide and non-peptide compounds have been identified. The GHSs discussed here are difficult to compare as they differ in their pharmacokinetics and pharmacodynamics, potency in different assays and species specificity. Though some compounds are reported to elevate prolactin, ACTH, and cortisol,[362] others may have greater specificity.[368,369] GHSs are also reported to have specific effects on appetite,[370,371] sleep,[372] and cardiac function.[373,374] Different GHSs seem to differ in their relative potencies for these effects, suggesting differing cross-reactivities at unknown receptor subtypes and raising hopes for new compounds tailored specifically for these sites.

Table 33-3 Some Peptide and Peptidomimetic Growth Hormone Secretagogue (GHS) Compounds

Name	Structure	Orally Active	ED$_{50}$ (nM)*
GHRP	Tyr-D-Trp-Gly-Phe-Met-NH$_2$ aka (D-Trp)^2)-metenkephalin	No[288]	
GHRP-6	His-D-Trp-Ala-Trp-D-Phe-Lys-NH$_2$	Yes	2.2–6.2[349–351]
GHRP-2	D-Ala-D-βNal-Ala-Trp-D-Phe-Lys-NH$_2$ aka Pralmorelin, KP-102,	Yes	1.8[350, 351]
Hexarelin	His-D-Mrp-Ala-Trp-D-Phe-Lys-NH$_2$	Yes	1.8[350, 351]
MK-751	L-692,429 Benzolactam peptidomimetic	Yes	60[352]
MK-0677	L-163,191 Spiroindoline peptidomimetic	Yes	0.4–1.3[350–352]
G7039	Modified pentapeptide	No	0.18[349]
EP-51389	Modified tripeptide	Yes[353]	
Ipamorelin	Modified pentapeptide	No	1.3[350, 351]
NN-703	Modified tripeptide	Yes	2.7[350, 351]
CP-424,391	Pyrazolinone-piperidine aka Capromorelin	Yes	3[354]
SM-130686	Oxindole derivative, nonpeptide	Yes	6.3[355]
EP-1572	Peptidomimetic, similar to MK-0677 in oral potency for GH release	Yes[353]	
Ghrelin	Stimulates both GH release and appetite	No	2.1[294, 356]
EP-40737	Stimulates GH release but not appetite[357]		
EP-40904	Stimulates appetite but not GH release[357]		
BIM-28163	Antagonist for GH secretion, agonist for appetite and weight gain[358]		

*ED$_{50}$ in rat pituitary cell growth hormone release assay. ED$_{50}$, median effective dose; GHRP, growth hormone–releasing peptide; D-Mrp, 2-methyl-D-tryptophan; D-βNal, β-(2-naphthyl)D-alanine.

GHSs: Sites of Action

Considerable evidence suggests that GHSs act at the level of the hypothalamus, as well as at the pituitary.[349,375–378] The major site of GHSs action, however, seems to be at the hypothalamus.[290,378–380] This hypothalamic action is thought to explain why GHSs are much more effective in vivo than in vitro and also the marked synergy that is seen when GHS and GHRH are given together in vivo. The dominant role of this hypothalamic action is demonstrated by the fact that GHSs are unable to release GH in children and adults with pituitary stalk transsection.[381,382] An alternative explanation is that GHRH is required for GH synthesis and in its absence GHSs are largely ineffective. This is supported by studies in pigs where exogenous GHRH overcomes the effect of stalk transection and allow GHS responses.[383]

GHS Receptor

Ghrelin and the GHSs act on somatotrophs through a phospholipase C inositol triphosphate-PKC signaling pathway distinct from the cAMP-PKA pathway activated by GHRH.[294,384,385] Studies demonstrated a high-affinity, low-abundance (^{35}S)MK-0677 binding site in the anterior pituitary and hypothalamus that has the Mg^{2+} and guanosine triphosphate–dependence characteristic of a G protein–coupled receptor.[386] This allowed MK-0677-induced calcium-activated chloride currents in *Xenopus* oocytes to be used as a method for the expression cloning of a GHS-R from swine pituitary mRNA.[292] When this cDNA was used as a probe, two types (Ia and Ib) of receptor cDNA were identified in both swine and human pituitary libraries. The human type Ia cDNA encodes a 366-amino acid seven-transmembrane receptor of the rhodopsin family. This cDNA conferred high-affinity (K_d = 0.4 nM), saturable, and specific binding of MK-0677 that was competed by both peptide and nonpeptide GHSs. The type Ib GHS-R cDNA represented an alternatively spliced message from the same gene, but encoded only 289 amino acids representing the first five transmembrane domains and appeared to be nonfunctional.[292] Athough the mRNA of the type Ib form is widely detectable in tissues, it is unclear whether the type Ib receptor is expressed as a protein.[319]

At the time it was cloned, the GHS-R represented a new branch in the rhodopsin family of the G protein–coupled receptors, with only 35% and 29% identity with the closest known sequences, which were for neurotensin and thyrotropin-releasing hormone receptors. More recently, several orphan receptors more closely related to the GHS-R have been cloned,[387,388] and the one most similar to GHS-R (52% identity) has been identified as a receptor for the gut peptide motilin.[389] This suggested that the endogenous ligand for the GHS-R is a peptide with homology to motilin—this prediction proved correct in that ghrelin has approximately 30% amino acid homology to motilin and no significant homology to other known sequences.[301]

Ribonuclease protection assays demonstrated that GHS-R mRNA was a rare message present in low abundance in human pituitary and hippocampus.[292] In the rat brain, in situ hybridization showed GHS-R in the arcuate and ventromedial nuclei of the hypothalamus,[292] two sites thought to be involved in the regulation of GH secretion. Other brain regions not traditionally associated with GH secretion express GHS-R including the choroid plexus and the hippocampus.[376,390,391] This finding suggests a wider role for GHSs in the brain, for example, in the control of feeding behavior.[370,371,392] In peripheral tissues, very low but detectable levels of GHS-R mRNA are reported in the pancreas and renal pelvis.[391,393]

GHS-R mRNA has also been demonstrated in human pituitary adenomas.[394–396] The highest abundance has been demonstrated in GH-secreting pituitary adenomas, of which 100% expressed the receptor message, some at 200-fold the levels of normal pituitary.[394,395,397] GHS-R message was also present in some thyroid-stimulating hormone–secreting, ACTH-secreting, and gonadotroph adenomas, as well as in prolactinomas.

Ligand binding to the GHS-R activates phospholipase C to hydrolyze phosphatidyl-inositol-4,5-biphosphate, stored in the plasma membrane, to give both diacylglycerol and inositol-triphosphate (IP$_3$). A rapid transient elevation of calcium levels is a result of release of calcium from intracellular stores in response to IP$_3$, while diacylglycerol activates protein kinase C in the plasma membrane. Protein kinase C through tyrosine phosphorylation inhibits the potassium channel, causing depolarization: This depolarization causes the opening of voltage-dependent L-type calcium channels. Data suggest that cAMP levels are elevated when coadministered with GHRH, but the exact mechanism of this synergism is not known.[398,399] The GHS-R, as other G protein–coupled receptors, shows desensitization in its calcium and GH effects, although a long-term human study showed sustained elevation of IGF-1 levels over 1 year.[400–402]

The GHS-R was found to be highly constitutively active in a ligand-independent manner in transfected COS-7 and HEK293 cells. While ghrelin and GHSs further increased inositol phosphate turnover, a low-potency antagonist (substance P antagonist) was found to be a high-affinity inverse agonist.[403] These data might open the possibility for development of inverse agonist compounds to oppose the effect of activation of the receptor.

Regulation of GHS Receptor

Studies using the dw/dw rat model or normal rats to investigate the effects of GH on hypothalamic and pituitary GHS-R expression suggested that GHS-Rs are involved in feedback regulation of GH.[380,404] Whether these effects occur directly at the pituitary level or are mediated indirectly through the hypothalamus has yet to be determined. In addition, the expression of the pituitary GHS-R mRNA seems to be sex dependent, whereas the hypothalamic expression of this receptor showed no significant sex difference.[405] GHRH appears to positively regulate the pituitary GHS-R in rats.[406] The regulation of GHS-R is summarized in Table 33-4.

Evidence for alternative ligands for the GHS-R receptor have been presented: Adenosine seems to act as a partial ligand to the GHS-R.[407,408] It elevated intracellular Ca^{2+} levels but did not cause GH release from pituitary cultures. Cortistatin, a 14-amino acid neuropeptide with similarity to somatostatin, has also been shown to bind to GHS-R in the pituitary.[409,410]

Alternative binding sites for ghrelin and some GHSs have been identified in the pituitary, thyroid gland, heart, and other tissues,[411] and ghrelin has been found to be associated with a high-density lipoprotein in plasma.[412] Hexarelin-like peptidyl GHSs but not ghrelin can affect heart function through actions at macrophage scavenger receptor CD36.[413,414]

Evidence for GHS Receptor Subtypes

GHSs are synthetic compounds developed for their ability to stimulate GH release. We now know that this is due to their ability to signal at the GHS-R. To date, only one type of GHS-R is well characterized. In examining the range of GHS effects, it is difficult to distinguish possible coincidental effects at unrelated receptors from specific actions at related receptor subtypes. Data suggesting GHS-R subtypes are beginning to accumulate. Binding studies at pituitary and hypothalamic membranes have shown GHS-binding sites with different relative affinity for peptidyl and non-peptidyl GHS. Whereas the non-peptidyl GHS MK-0677 binds specifically to the high-affinity site, GHRP-6 binds preferentially to medium- and low-affinity sites.[386,415,416] Characterization of high-affinity hexarelin-binding and -crosslinking sites in the pituitary and brain has suggested the existence of different GHS-R subtypes. In these studies, the relative affinities for different GHSs and the molecular size of the crosslinked binding site do not seem to match the properties of the cloned GHS-R.[390,417] While hexarelin stimulates both GH release and feeding behavior, new hexarelin analogues appear specific for one effect or the other, suggesting that they act at different brain receptors.[371] Hexarelin is also reported to have GH-independent beneficial cardiac effects that persist after hypophysectomy and have been attributed to specific hexarelin-binding sites in the heart.[373,374,418] This hexarelin-binding site has now been identified as CD36, a class B

scavenger receptor that recognizes a variety of hydrophobic ligands.[419] While ghrelin and desoctanoyl ghrelin also bind to cardiovascular tissue, their binding sites appear to be different from the one related to hexarelin and they do not share the same cardiovascular effects as hexarelin.[414]

Regulation of GH Release

At the pituitary, GHSs can directly stimulate the release of GH.[169,349,364,384,400,420,421] GHSs cause somatotroph depolarization and raise intracellular Ca^{2+} but use a different receptor and signaling mechanism from GHRH.[422-426] At the level of individual pituitary cells examined with the reverse hemolytic plaque assay, GHSs increased the number of GH-secreting cells without altering the amount of GH released per cell. In contrast, GHRH increased both the amount of GH secreted per cell and the number of GH-secreting cells, while somatostatin predominantly acted to decrease the number of secreting cells; this is the opposite of the effect of GHSs and supports the view that GHSs act as functional antagonists of somatostatin.[422]

It is widely accepted that the synthesis of GH in the pituitary is under the control of GHRH.[181] In the absence of GHRH, GHSs can also stimulate GH synthesis. In rat pups treated with GHRH antiserum from birth, 5-day treatment with hexarelin results in a restoration of pituitary GH mRNA levels to that of controls.[379,427] Similar findings were made in GHRH-deficient young adult male rats.[427]

At the level of the hypothalamus, the mechanisms underlying GHS stimulation of pituitary GH release are not yet defined. Many data explain GHS actions through indirect effects on the hypothalamus and the involvement of GHRH[428-431] and somatostatin.[424] Other evidence suggests that GHS increases GH secretion independently of GHRH or somatostatin.[379,430,432]

In the hypothalamus a subset of GHRH neurons express GHS-R[433] and GHSs have been shown to enhance the expression of c-fos in some GHRH and NPY neurons.[434] Some but not all data suggest a direct GHRH-releasing effect of GHSs or ghrelin from the hypothalamus.[428,435,436] GHS treatment does decrease hypothalamic somatostatin mRNA levels in the aged rat to levels seen in young controls.[437] The direct actions of GHSs, together with interactions with GHRH and somatostatin, are proposed by some to be insufficient to explain the observed synergism with GHRH and GHS responses when GHRH action is blocked.[202,290] This suggests the alternative hypothesis that in addition to the known mechanisms, GHSs can also act to release an unknown hypothalamic factor (U factor), which acts as a potent stimulator of GH release from the pituitary.[290] Such a U factor could explain why the major actions of GHS require an intact hypophyseal stalk, but also points out that there is much we do not know about the actions of GHRH and ghrelin.

CLINICAL IMPLICATIONS

GROWTH HORMONE–RELEASING HORMONE

Measurement of GHRH Levels

Following the synthesis of GHRH, RIAs to measure the peptide were developed rapidly and have been used to document concentrations of the releasing hormone in tissues and body fluids. Initially, it was hoped that GHRH in the peripheral circulation would be principally of hypothalamic origin and its measurement would thus serve as an index of hypothalamic secretion. However, it is clear that most circulating GHRH is not of hypothalamic origin but instead comes from the gut.[438-441] Further, an RIA would ideally measure intact biologically active hormone. However, GHRH(1–44)-NH_2 has a very short half-life in the circulation of 6.8 minutes, and the metabolite GHRH(3–44)NH_2 appears within 1 minute of an

Table 33-4	Regulation of GHS-R Expression
Upregulation	**Downregulation**
GH deficiency	GH treatment
GHRH agonist	GHS treatment (or upregulation or no effect)
Glucocorticoids	
Estrogen	
Thyroid hormones	

intravenous injection of GHRH(1–44)NH$_2$.[442] GHRH is cleaved by a dipeptidylaminopeptidase IV in the circulation. The biologic activity of GHRH(3–44)NH$_2$ is less than 10^{-3} that of GHRH(1–44)NH$_2$.[39] Unfortunately, most RIAs measure GHRH(1–44)-NH$_2$ and GHRH(3–44)-NH$_2$ with equal efficiency and therefore do not reflect biologic activity in the circulation. Most assays are directed to the midportion of the GHRH molecule and therefore do not distinguish between different circulating forms. Besides the RIA, more sensitive enzyme immunoassays for GHRH measurement have been developed.[443] One of the few indications for measuring serum GHRH is GHRH-producing tumors.

GHRH Levels in Acromegaly
There has been intense interest in the frequency of ectopic GHRH as a cause of acromegaly. Two extensive studies have addressed this issue. In a study of 80 patients with acromegaly, 76 had GHRH levels in the normal range.[439] Of the four with elevated levels, one was known to harbor a GHRH-secreting tumor. Extensive evaluation of the other three failed to determine a source for the GHRH. In a second study, three of 177 patients with acromegaly exhibited elevated serum levels of GHRH.[444] In all cases, the GHRH levels were markedly elevated (i.e., in the ng/mL range), and the patients were previously known to have GHRH-secreting tumors. Thus, although apparently rare, ectopic secretion of GHRH must be considered as a possible cause of acromegaly, and measurement of peripheral GHRH seems prudent as a part of the evaluation. Since it is known that the release of ectopic hormones may be intermittent, and since only 300 pg/mL of GHRH is necessary to stimulate GH release in normal subjects, a single normal or modestly elevated GHRH determination may not exclude ectopic GHRH-associated acromegaly.

The subject of GHRH-producing tumors has been previously reviewed.[445,446] GHRH-producing tumors associated with acromegaly are rare. Unique features of patients with acromegaly harboring tumors secreting GHRH were young age, female preponderance, foregut derivation of the tumors, benign biologic behavior, small secretory granules in the tumor, and frequent association with multiple endocrine neoplasia type 1 (MEN1) syndrome. The pancreas and lung are common primary sites. GHRH-containing tumors unassociated with acromegaly include those of gut and thymus, small cell carcinoma of lung, and medullary carcinoma of thyroid. Several tumors are plurihormonal. In contrast to somatotroph adenoma seen in patients with classic acromegaly, the hypophyseal lesion represents somatotroph hyperplasia in acromegalic patients with GHRH-producing tumor. This finding indicates that GHRH not only increases somatotroph secretory activity but causes somatotroph proliferation. Studies of GHRH-producing tumors are of fundamental importance to obtain insight into endocrine activity of pituitary somatotrophs and the pathogenesis of GH-secreting pituitary adenomas associated with acromegaly; the importance of GHRH in the etiology of acromegaly is still unresolved. Preliminary evidence suggests that the amount of GHRH mRNA expression in somatotroph adenomas is associated with the progression and aggressiveness of these tumors.[85] The GHRH receptor mRNA is specifically expressed in GH-producing adenomas and somatotrophs.[84] To address whether GHRH can produce tumors, transgenic mice expressing the human GHRH gene have been developed. These animals, exposed to excessive quantities of GHRH throughout development and life, developed mammosomatotrope or somatotrope adenomas.[262,265] The significance of these observations to the human disease is unclear and further studies are needed. Early studies have investigated the beneficial effects of GHRH antagonists in animal and human studies. Interestingly, in one single reported clinical case, ectopic GHRH secretion was associated with empty sella syndrome.[447]

Treatment of transgenic mice overexpressing the human GHRH gene with GHRH antagonists resulted in suppression of GH and IGF-I secretion.[448] The relationship between GHRH-secreting tumors and MEN1 syndrome is controversial; further studies are required to elucidate whether they represent two distinct entities or whether GHRH-producing tumors accompanied by acromegaly are only *forme fruste* manifestations of MEN1 syndrome. Several cases of acromegaly due to ectopic GHRH secretion associated with MEN1 syndrome have been described.[449-453]

Eutopic GHRH Secretion
Occasionally, hypothalamic gangliocytomas may be associated with acromegaly. Immunocytochemical staining of such tumors for GHRH has been described. It has been suggested that these tumors should be considered as an unusual cause of acromegaly.[454] On occasion these tumors are intrasellar; in such cases, the observation that somatotrophs are in close anatomic association with neurons suggests that GHRH not only stimulates GH secretion but may also cause adenoma formation. An intrasellar gangliocytoma with somatotroph adenoma has been described. The gangliocytoma was strongly positive for gastrin and weakly positive for GHRH. Since gastrin administered intracerebroventricularly increases GH secretion, it has been suggested that gastrin release may act in a paracrine fashion on gangliocytoma to enhance GHRH secretion and thus cause somatotrope adenoma.[455-457]

GHRH Levels in GH-Deficient Children
Many reports concerning serum and cerebrospinal fluid concentrations of GHRH in children with various forms of growth deficiency have appeared. Of 22 children with the diagnosis of constitutional short stature (defined as 2 to 3 SD below the predicted mean height for age, peak levels of GH in excess of 10 µg/L during at least one provocation test, and bone age approximating chronologic age), basal GHRH levels (8 to 148 pg/mL) were no different from those noted in normal children.[458] In addition, in five of nine children, GHRH levels rose twofold 15 minutes after administration of levodopa (500 mg PO). In another study of 16 children with idiopathic delayed puberty, the peak serum GHRH concentration following levodopa was 41 ± 10 pg/mL and this compared with 96 ± 25 pg/mL in children with constitutional short stature.[459] Similarly, in patients with hypothalamic hypopituitarism, there was no increase in circulating GHRH levels after levodopa, which contrasts with responses in normal subjects.[460,461] These patients with hypothalamic hypopituitarism do respond to exogenous GHRH administration. Insulin-induced hypoglycemia increased circulating GHRH levels in normal subjects, but not in six patients with isolated GH deficiency.[462] In 10 children with short stature, GHRH levels increased at 15 minutes after hypoglycemia from 10 ± 0.5 to 17.1 ± 3.1 pg/mL.[463] There was no increase in GHRH after arginine, even though hypoglycemia alone or arginine alone increased GH concentrations.

However, in contrast to children with constitutional short stature, five children with GH deficiency associated with hypothalamic germinomas were reported to have undetectable concentrations of GHRH in the cerebrospinal fluid.[464] In addition, children with idiopathic GH deficiency have GHRH present in the cerebrospinal fluid but at concentrations lower than those in normal children (15.1 ± 1.0 vs. 29.3 ± 2.0 pg/mL; mean ± SEM).

GHRH as a Diagnostic Agent
Until 1985, the use of cadaveric GH was strictly controlled and limited to use in children with short stature due to severe GH deficiency. Dynamic tests of GH reserve were, therefore, of clinical significance in pediatric endocrinology and were performed primarily for academic interest in adults with hypothalamic-pituitary disease. With the advent of recombinant

human GH, now available in unrestricted quantities, and its approval for use in adults with GH deficiency resulting from hypothalamic pituitary disease in the United States, Europe, and Australia, the need to diagnose GH deficiency safely and effectively has become an important issue in adult endocrinology.[465]

Many of the tests used to determine GH status are either hazardous under certain circumstances (the insulin tolerance test [ITT] is contraindicated in the elderly, and in patients with ischemic heart disease or a history of seizures) or associated with unpleasant side effects (glucagon causes nausea and delayed hypoglycemia, clonidine is associated with drowsiness and hypotension, and arginine causes dizziness and phlebitis). Tests that are effective in children, such as those using arginine or clonidine as the stimulus, are less effective at releasing GH in adults.[466] The ITT is frequently quoted as the gold standard investigation for diagnosing GH deficiency in children and adults, but many endocrinologists shy away from this procedure because of concerns about the effects of hypoglycemia in their patients and because the test has to be supervised for its duration by a physician.

GHRH and the GH-releasing substances (e.g., GHRP-6, GHRP-1, GHRP-2, hexarelin, MK-0677) are powerful GHSs that are safe and well tolerated in both adults and children. These agents have attracted increasing attention as stimuli used to determine GH status in both adults and children.

Typically, tests of GH reserve in both children and adults have used procedures that depend on effects mediated by the hypothalamus. For example, agents such as arginine, glucagon, clonidine, or levodopa and insulin-induced hypoglycemia are assumed to elicit a hypothalamic signal that acts upon the somatotrophs to stimulate the release of GH. A lesion of the hypothalamus or the pituitary may produce an abnormal GH response to these stimuli. The use of GHRH to stimulate GH release directly from the somatotrophs allows a theoretical distinction to be made between patients with a pituitary abnormality, who will have an abnormal response to GHRH, and those with hypothalamic lesions who may respond normally to GHRH. This may be important when determining the therapeutic strategy for an individual patient.

Administration of GHRH to Normal Subjects
The effects of GHRH and its analogues given as a bolus have been studied in healthy men, women, and children.[467-477] Following an intravenous injection of GHRH, GH levels begin to rise within 5 minutes and reach a peak between 30 and 60 minutes. The ability of GHRH to release GH is dose-dependent,[476] the maximal response being observed following a dose of 1 µg/kg or higher.[471] In adults, the GH response to GHRH is similar in men and women, although women are more sensitive to GHRH than men; the dose of GHRH required for half-maximal GH secretion is 0.4 µg/kg in men and 0.2 µg/kg in women. The GH response to GHRH in women is not altered by the changes in sex steroid hormones that occur during the menstrual cycle.[475]

The effect of pubertal development on the GH response to GHRH is slight.[478,479] When 68 prepubertal children were compared with 66 children at various stages of puberty, no overall difference in GH response to GHRH was observed.[478] In a more detailed study that examined children at each stage of puberty, a slight decrease in GH response to GHRH was seen in boys during midpuberty. Although a similar decrease was not observed in girls, the GH response to GHRH did not differ significantly between the sexes during puberty.[479] In prepubertal children being evaluated for poor growth, priming the hypothalamic-pituitary-GH axis with sex steroids can normalize a suboptimal GH response to some stimuli. The GH response to GHRH is not affected by priming with estrogen,[480] suggesting that sex steroids assert their effects at the hypothalamus, either reducing somatostatin tone or increasing GHRH release, not at the pituitary.

The ability of GHRH to release GH is similar in prepubertal and pubertal children and in young adults. Over the course of the adult life span, however, the magnitude of the GH peak following GHRH declines with increasing age.[243,467,481,482] The likely mechanism for the age-related decline of the response to GHRH is an increase in somatostatin tone.[483] Support for this is found in studies that use GHRH in combination with pyridostigmine or arginine.[484,485] These agents have both been used alone as diagnostic tests for GH deficiency, producing a GH pulse by reducing somatostatin tone.[486,487] Arginine and pyridostigmine act synergistically with GHRH, producing large GH pulses similar to those seen in younger adults.

The GHRH Test: Which Analogue to Use? The potencies of the two naturally occurring analogues of GHRH, GHRH(1–40) and GHRH(1–44), have been compared and found to be equal. These two compounds have also been compared with the synthetic analogue GHRH(1–29)-NH_2 and have been found to be equipotent in terms of stimulating GH release.[488] At present, GHRH(1–29)-NH_2 is the analogue commercially available in the United States and Europe for use in clinical practice as a diagnostic agent, and in the United States for the treatment of children with GH deficiency.

Test Procedure The GHRH test is typically performed in the morning after an overnight fast. GHRH is administered as an intravenous bolus through a cannula inserted into a forearm vein. The dose of GHRH is determined by the weight of the patient; 1 µg/kg is used in both adults and children. Blood is drawn for estimation of GH levels 15 minutes and immediately before the injection of GHRH is given, then at 15, 30, 45, and 60 minutes following the administration of GHRH.

Side Effects Overall, side effects are uncommon following the administration of GHRH, and when they occur they are usually mild. The most frequently reported side effect is transient warmth and flushing of the face that passes within 5 minutes of administration. Other side effects reported are pain and redness at the injection site, nausea, vomiting, headache, a strange taste in the mouth, and tightness in the chest. These symptoms are transient and resolve rapidly.

What Constitutes a Normal GH Response to GHRH? With any test used in clinical practice, it is important to determine what constitutes a normal response. Accordingly, several studies have addressed this question for the GHRH test. Ranke and colleagues[489] defined the normal range of GH responses to GHRH in 86 children with a normal GH axis as 11.8 to 172.4 µg/L, by determining the mean response ±2 SD. This study also concluded that a GH response of less than 10 µg/L should be used as the diagnostic threshold for GH deficiency in children.

The diagnostic threshold of 10 µg/L has been used in other studies using the GHRH test[490-492] and is now generally accepted in pediatric practice. This peak is similar to that used to define GH deficiency when using the majority of stimuli in children despite its being recognized that the different stimuli are not equal in their ability to release GH.[478] Such thresholds are defined arbitrarily despite attempts to rationalize them.[493] This may reflect the fact that the diagnosis of GH deficiency in a child depends primarily on the clinical finding of poor growth, and that the stimulation test is used to confirm the presence of GH deficiency.

In adults, the diagnostic threshold used to identify patients with GH deficiency is lower than that used in pediatric practice. For example, a GH peak of less than 3 µg/L during an ITT is considered to be indicative of severe GH deficiency that warrants therapy with exogenous GH. If arginine were to be used as the stimulus, the diagnostic cutoff would be even lower than this.[493,494] In adults, the GHRH test is generally a more potent stimulus of GH secretion, resulting in higher pulses than those seen following the ITT, arginine, or glucagon.[495] This would suggest that the diagnostic cutoff for severe GH deficiency might be higher than 3 µg/L using the GHRH test in adults, but this has not been determined.

The GHRH Test in Children with Short Stature Normal Hypothalamic-Pituitary-GH Axis
The GH response elicited by GHRH in children with short stature due to a variety of etiologies has been well-characterized.[489–491,496–505] Children who have constitutional short stature, with no underlying pathology, have a normal GH peak following GHRH administration,[489,498,500,501,503,505] but the timing of that peak may be delayed.[496,499] Children that are short as a result of intrauterine growth retardation also have a normal GH response to GHRH.

GH Deficiency
GHRH is a powerful secretagogue and generally elicits a greater GH response than many of the traditional tests of GH status. Children with GH deficiency defined using conventional tests frequently have a greater response to GHRH than to other tests of GH status.[496] In a study of prepubertal children undergoing investigation of abnormal growth, subjects were divided into groups according to their response to conventional tests. GH status was considered normal if the peak GH response to a conventional test was greater than 10 µg/L; partial and severe GH deficiency were defined as a peak GH response between 5 and 10 µg/L and less than 5 µg/L, respectively.

Assuming a diagnostic cutoff of 10 µg/L for the GHRH test, 76% of the children with partial, and 39% with severe, GH deficiency had a GH peak greater than 10 µg/L during the GHRH test. Conversely, 10% of the children considered to have a normal GH axis had a peak GH response less than 10 µg/L, a figure consistent with the findings of other studies. This study demonstrated a considerable discordance between conventional tests of GH status and the GHRH test. It also indicated that, in a significant proportion of children with GH deficiency diagnosed clinically and confirmed using conventional tests, somatotroph function may be preserved, the cause of their impaired GH status being hypothalamic rather than pituitary dysfunction.

Patients who develop GH deficiency following cranial irradiation also exhibit discordance between the GHRH test and conventional tests of GH status. Typically, such patients have received radiotherapy for a tumor distant from the hypothalamic-pituitary axis, but this region was included in the radiation field, or cranial irradiation was given prophylactically during the treatment of acute lymphoblastic leukemia. The GH response to GHRH in such patients was greater than the response to the ITT and the arginine test in 80% of patients in one study.[506] This response suggests that radiation primarily affects the hypothalamic mechanisms that regulate GH secretion from the anterior pituitary. The magnitude of the GH peak during the GHRH test decreases as the time from radiation increases, suggesting that the effects of radiation do, ultimately, impinge upon somatotroph function. This may be a direct effect of radiation on the somatotrophs or the indirect effect of long-standing GHRH deficiency depleting the available GH pool within the somatotroph. The latter is supported by the observation that priming with GHRH for several days prior to the GHRH test can increase the GH response to GHRH significantly.[507]

GHRH and the Diagnosis of GH Deficiency in Adults
There are surprisingly few data on the use of GHRH alone as a diagnostic test in adults. Much of the work was carried out before the advent of recombinant human GH when the diagnosis of GH deficiency in adults was not an issue. The few studies in the literature were performed on small numbers of patients, the majority of whom had childhood-onset GH deficiency. More recently, studies that have investigated GHRH as a diagnostic agent in adults have used it in combination with other agents, the aim being to normalize the GH response across the adult life span (see later discussion).

Limitations of the GHRH Test
The use of GHRH alone as a diagnostic test for GH deficiency is limited by several factors. The discordance observed between the results of the GHRH test and the results of other stimulation tests such as the ITT can lead to difficulties interpreting the results of the GHRH test. There is considerable interindividual and intraindividual variation in the results of the GHRH test. The coefficient of variation for the GHRH test has been reported to be 60% for children[508] and 45% for adults,[495] although the variability diminishes with increasing age in adults.[509] The sensitivity of the GHRH test is relatively poor in children with short stature and varies with the severity of the GH deficiency as determined by other tests of GH status. In one study, the sensitivity of the GHRH test was 24% in patients with GH insufficiency (GH peak 5.0 to 10.0 µg/L to conventional tests) and 61% in patients with severe GH deficiency (GH peak <5.0 µg/L).[496] The specificity of the GHRH test has been reported to be 85% to 90%.[478,496]

The ability to interpret the GHRH test is confounded further by the inhibition of the GH response in obese subjects.[510–512] This may be particularly important when assessing patients with GH deficiency who have abnormal body composition with a propensity to abdominal obesity. The GH response to GHRH in obese patients with pituitary tumors is reduced, making it difficult to define their GH status accurately, particularly if the GH deficiency is isolated.[513]

The GHRH test is safe, associated with few side effects, and requires minimal medical supervision, making it an attractive test for use in the outpatient setting. However, the problems previously outlined make it difficult to interpret the results of the GHRH test in clinical practice and it must, therefore, be used with caution. A GH peak greater than 10 µg/L does not exclude GH deficiency in a child with poor growth, and further evaluation of the hypothalamic-pituitary axis should be undertaken. A positive result (i.e., a GH peak <10 µg/L) will be indicative of GH deficiency, but, because 10% to 15% of normal children fall into this group, further evaluation to confirm the diagnosis of GH deficiency will be necessary. The relatively good specificity of the GHRH test suggests that a positive result is significant and the child should be evaluated further with additional investigations and monitoring. At the present time, the primary role of the GHRH test is to determine which children are candidates for GHRH therapy.

Tests Using GHRH in Combination with Other Agents
The observation that GHRH acts synergistically with agents that reduce somatostatin tone has led to the development of tests that combine GHRH with arginine, pyridostigmine, and clonidine. GHRH acts synergistically with these agents, producing large GH pulses, the magnitude of which frequently exceeds 50 µg/L in healthy subjects.[478,484,495,514–516] The addition of these agents to GHRH increases the reproducibility of the test and improves diagnostic accuracy.

GHRH in combination with pyridostigmine or arginine causes profound release of GH. In one study of normal children and adolescents, the normal range for GHRH plus pyridostigmine was 22.6 to 90.0 µg/L (n = 94), and that of GHRH plus arginine, 22.4 to 108 µg/L (n = 81).[478] The results of these tests were not influenced by pubertal stage in either girls or boys.[478,517] However, a study of Maghnie and colleagues[518] concludes that in patients with acquired childhood-onset GH deficiency the number of pituitary hormone deficits and the patient's age affect the GH response to the combined GHRH and arginine test. The data of Groisne and colleagues suggest that BMI and age do have an impact in the GHRH-arginine test in children with idiopathic GH deficiency.[519] Both studies were conducted with a small number of patients.

In children with GH deficiency, in the GHRH-pyridostigmine test, used with the diagnostic threshold of 20 µg/L, the diagnosis was confirmed in 100% of patients with organic GH deficiency (caused by craniopharyngioma) and 80% of patients with idiopathic GH deficiency.[515] GHRH in combination with arginine has been extensively evaluated in adults with pituitary disease in the hope that it will provide a safer alternative to the ITT, which is currently considered to be the gold standard investigation of GH status in adults. There is no difference in sensitivity and specificity in young adults among the ARG + GHRH test, the PD + GHRH test, and the ITT in assessing GH secretion.[520] The combination of GHRH with arginine was chosen over pyridostigmine because the side effects with pyridostigmine were unpleasant and the GH response to GHRH plus arginine is not affected by age.[521] In adults, the GH response to GHRH and arginine is not affected by gender or age; similar results are achieved in male and female subjects and young and old adults.[516,521,522] Across the adult life span, the third percentile limit of GH response to GHRH plus arginine is 16.5 µg/L and the first percentile limit is 9 µg/L.

Adults with GH deficiency all had a peak GH response to GHRH plus arginine that fell below 16.5 µg/L, and 92% of patients had a peak below 9 µg/L. The GH peaks achieved during the GHRH-arginine test correlate well with those during the ITT, although the absolute GH response to GHRH plus arginine is considerably greater than that to the ITT. Of the seven patients that had achieved a peak GH greater than 9 µg/L during the GHRH-arginine test, six had achieved a GH peak higher than the diagnostic threshold for the ITT (3 µg/L). It was suggested by the authors that the diagnostic cutoff for the GHRH-arginine test should be 9 µg/L for severe GH deficiency in adults and 16.5 µg/L for GH insufficiency. The comparison of sensitivity and specificity of six different tests: ITT, arginine (ARG), levodopa (L-dopa), ARG plus L-dopa, and ARG + GHRH in the diagnosis of GH deficiency found the greatest diagnostic accuracy with the ARG + GHRH test and the ITT. The first was preferred over the latter due to fewer side effects.[523] In the clinical situation of radiation-induced GH deficiency, ITT should be used instead of the GHRH-arginine test.[524]

GHRH THERAPY IN GH-DEFICIENT CHILDREN

The potential of GHRH as a therapeutic agent for GH-deficient children has been examined in several studies. The majority of GH-deficient children with short stature and growth failure have a disorder of hypothalamic regulation of the pituitary rather than a defect of the somatotroph. In these children, injections of GHRH, as well as other GHSs, might be a useful treatment option. One of the first studies published in 1985 reported the use of GHRH (1–40)-OH administered SC with a peristaltic pump every 3 hours to two children with organic hypopituitarism (posttraumatic, hydrocephalus).[525] The children received 3 hourly doses of 1 or 3 µg/kg GHRH for 6 months. Both children increased their growth rate by about 1.5- to 6-fold compared to the growth rate before administration of GHRH(1–40)-OH. The rationale for using this dose regimen was based on the observation that, in growing children, five to nine pulses of GH are detected every 24 hours.

Since then, several studies have been performed to evaluate the benefits of GHRH therapy in GH-deficient children with different GHRH injection regimens and different doses. However, the groups of children who were treated were not homogeneous; their diagnoses varied from GH deficiency and short stature to normal variant short stature without GH deficiency. The GHRH preparations used included GHRH(1–40)-OH, GHRH(1–44)-NH$_2$, and GHRH(1–29)-NH$_2$.

GHRH Given by Pump

Table 33-5 shows the results of GHRH treatment by pump.[526-528] The response with this kind of treatment varied from 71% to 100%. The growth rate on GHRH therapy varied from 6.2 to 10 cm per year over the first 6 months and was maintained in patients for up to 5 years. The growth velocity appears to be related to the total daily dosage, which ranged from 10 to 2150 µg per day. So far no studies have evaluated whether it is the frequency of administration or the total daily dose that has the greatest impact on the therapeutic outcome. The first study, which looked at administration by pump or single injections of GHRH, was published in 1988.[526] It described the effects of different routes of GHRH administration in 24 GH-deficient children. GHRH(1–40) was given either by pump every 3 hours SC or every 3 hours SC overnight only. Alternatively, GHRH was given twice daily in a dose of 1 to 4 µg/kg per dose for 6 months. In all three circumstances, the growth velocity increased between 1.8-fold and 2.9-fold, with the greatest effects seen during the pump therapy with injections every 3 hours.

Unfortunately, there are no long-term comparative studies examining the growth-promoting effects of GHRH with GH. Two short-term studies (6 months' treatment) provided conflicting results: One suggested a comparable growth response with GHRH similar to GH treatment,[529] whereas the other suggested that GHRH was less effective.[530]

Table 33-5 Children Treated with Subcutaneous Growth Hormone–Releasing Hormone (GHRH) by Pump

References	n	Diagnosis* (Peak GH µg/L)	GHRH	Dose (µg/kg)	Total Dose (µg/day)†	Growth Velocity (cm/yr) (Mean ± SEM)		Responders	Comments
						Pre	During		
Thorner et al.[526]	10	GHD (<10)	1–40	1–3 q 3 hr	200–600	3.5 ± 1.4 (±SD)	10.0 ± 2.2 (6 mo)	100%	Ab-11/20
	10	GHD (<10)	1–40	1–2 q 3 hr overnight only	100–200	3.4 ± 1.0	6.2 ± 2.1 (6 mo)	80%	
Low[527]	7	GHD (<2)	1–44	1–2 q 3 hr	200–400	2.7 ± 0.2	8.4 ± 2.5 (2 mo) 5.4 ± 0.7 (12 mo)	71%	Ab-none
Brain et al.[528]	5 (12 mo)	Partial GHD (<10)	1–29	Continuous	2150	4.6 ± 0.3 (±SD)	7.0 ± 1.4 (12 mo)	100%	Ab-all
	3 (3–6 mo)						(similar GV in 3 at 3–6 mo)		

*Peak GH response to standard pharmacologic tests.
†Assumes 25-kg child.
Ab, antibodies; GH, growth hormone; GHD, growth hormone deficiency; GV, growth velocity.

GHRH Given SC Twice a Day
The most impressive results with GHRH injections given twice daily were achieved in a multicenter study using GHRH(1–44)-NH₂ in 20 GH-deficient children (Table 33-6).[526,531–538] All of the children responded with accelerated growth velocity. The growth velocity increased from 3.6 cm per year before treatment to 8.6 after 6 months, and 8.1 after 12 months. Ogilvy-Stuart and colleagues[538] reported a significant beneficial effect of GHRH(1–29) given in a dose of 30 μg/kg/day over 1 year, which resulted in a 1.8-fold increase of growth velocity per year in nine children with radiation-induced GH deficiency.

The effects of GHRH(1–29) therapy in growth retardation caused by chronic renal failure were examined in nine children by Pasqualini and coworkers.[537] They either were treated conservatively or with dialysis or had renal transplantation. GHRH(1–29) 52 μg/kg/day was administered for 3 to 6 months. The growth velocity increased from 3.8 to 8 cm per year.

GHRH Given SC Once a Day
Several groups have investigated the effects of GHRH given SC by once-daily injections, and the results are summarized in Table 33-7.[507,539–543] A study investigating 110 GH-deficient children treated with a dose of 30 μg/kg/day of GHRH (1–29)[544] showed a significant increase in linear growth velocity with 4.1 cm per year before treatment and 7.2 cm per year after 1 year of treatment (Fig. 33-3). The largest number of children was investigated in the GHRH European Multicenter Study,[541] which reported the treatment of 111 GH-deficient children.

Height velocity increased from 3.8 cm per year before, to 6 cm per year during 6 months of treatment. The group of Bozzola[540] reported an increase of growth velocity from 3.5 cm per year to 7.3 cm per year after 6 months of treatment in 10 GH-deficient children with GHRH(1–44). The optimal growth velocity was observed in the first 9 months of therapy in most of the studies.[539] Lanes and Carrillo[543] reported that therapy with GHRH(1–29) in 16 prepubertal GH-deficient children given once daily SC over 12 to 24 months resulted in a significant increase in growth velocity.

Which Children Should Be Considered for GHRH Therapy?
The use of GHRH(1–29)-NH₂ treatment of idiopathic GH deficiency in children with growth failure has now been

Table 33-6 Children Treated with Subcutaneous Growth Hormone–Releasing Hormone (GHRH) by Twice-Daily Injections

References	n	Diagnosis* (μg/L)	GHRH	Dose (μg/kg)	Total Dose (μg/day)†	Growth Velocity (cm/yr) (Mean ± SD) Pre	Growth Velocity (cm/yr) (Mean ± SD) During	Responders	Comments
Ross et al.[531]	18	GHD (<3.5) (including 10 IGHD, 4 MPHD, 3 cranial irradiation, 1 septo-optic dysplasia)	1–29	≤25‡	500–1000	1.7 ±1.2 (after 3 mo 3.4 ± 1.6)	7.2 ± 2.5 (6 mo) 3.0 ±1.2 (6 mo)	44%	Ab 14/17
Takano et al.[532]	4	2 IGHD (<7), 2 germinoma	1–44	50–100 μg/dose	100–200	#1 3.5 #2 3.1 #3 2.0 #4 1.0	8.2 (6 mo) 3.8 (# 1 & 3) 9.8 0.8	50%	Ab 2/4
Thorner et al.[526]	4	GHD (<10)	1–40	4	200	3.2 ±1.8	7.9 ±2.4 (6 mo)	100%	Ab 1/4
Smith and Brook[533]	8	GHD (8.5), some MPHD	1–29	4–8	200–400		5.1 ±0.3 (4 μg) 5.9 ±0.4 (8 μg) (mean—9 mo)	63%	Ab not done
Butenandt and Staudt[534]	7	GHD (<3)	1–29	4–6	200–300	3.0 (1.9–3.8) (6–15 mo)	4.0 (0.5–8.2)	29%	7/7 respond to subsequent GH Ab not done
Duck et al.[535]	20	GHD (<10)	1–44	10–20§	500–1000	3.6 ± 1.1	8.6 ± 2.5 (6 mo) 8.1 ± 1.5 (12 mo)	100%	Ab—none
Kirk et al.[536]	18	Height < third percentile	1–29	20	1000	4.8	7.2		
Pasqualini et al.[537]	9	Growth retardation because of CRF:3 treated conservatively, 3 on dialysis, 3 after renal transplantation	1–29	26	1300	3.8	8.0		
Ogilvy-Stuart et al.[538]	9	GHD, radiation-induced (<20 mU/L)	1–29	15	750	3.3	6.0		

*Peak GH to standard pharmacologic tests.
†Assumes 25-kg child.
‡Dose 250 μg if weight <20 kg (n = 8) or 500 μg dose if weight >20 kg (n = 10).
§Sixteen subjects, 10-μg dose for 1 year; 4 subjects, 10 μg for 6 months, and 20 μg for second 6 months.
Ab, antibodies; CRF, chronic renal failure; GHD, growth hormone deficiency; IGHD, isolated GHD; MPHD, multiple pituitary hormone deficiency.

Table 33-7 Children Treated with Subcutaneous Growth Hormone Releasing Hormone (GHRH) by Once Daily Injection

References	n	Diagnosis* (μg/L)	GHRH	Dose (μg/kg)	Total Dose (μg/day)†	Growth Velocity (cm/yr) (Mean ± SD) Pre	During	Responders	Comments
Rochiccioli et al.[539]	6	Partial GHD (<11)	1–44	10	250	4.2 ± 1.1 (±SD)	10 ±3.3 (6 mo) 8.6 ±1.8 (12 mo)	83% (at 12 mo)	Reduced GV at 9–12 mo; Ab 1/6
Bozzola et al.[540]	25	10 GHD (<5)	1–44	1.6–1.8	40–450	3.5 ±0.2 3.7 ±0.2	7.3 ±0.4 (6 mo)‡ 4.1 ±0.3	40% (at 6 mo) 32% (at 12 mo)	Responders Nonresponders Ab 6/25
		15 partial GHD (<10)							
Romer et al.[507]	11 9	GHD (<5) GHD (<3)	1–44 1–44	10 10 (3 ×/wk)	250	3.3 (n=20)	2.6 (6 mo) 3.0 (for all 20)	0%	Older children 19/21 pretreated with GH; 2/20 > 2 cm/yr
Lievre et al.[541]	111	GHD (<10)	1–44	1.3–23.1	30–300	≤ – 2 SD 6 ±0.2	> 2 cm/yr (6 mo)	50% increased GV	Ab 13.5%; 42% had catch-up growth
Wit et al.§[542]	5	GHD (<10)	1–44	7.5	190	2.5	4.6 (3 mo)	40% >2 cm/yr	"Insufficient response;" 10 pretreated with GH; Ab—none
	6			15	380	2.7	7.0 (3 mo)	50%	
Lanes et al.[543]	16	GHD (<10)	1–29	30	750	3.4 ±0.7	6.8 ±0.1 (6 mo) 6.2 ±0.9 (12 mo) 6.6 ±1.0 (18 mo) 6.5 ±0.7 (24 mo)	68% > 2 cm/yr over baseline	GHRH Ab were detected in 4/11 and 6/11 responders at 6 and 12 mo and in 2/5 responders at 6 mo
Thorner et al.[526]	110	GHD (<10)	1–29	30	750	4.1 ±0.9	8.0 ±1.5 (6 mo) 7.2 ±1.3 (12 mo)	74% > 2 cm/yr	Overall 62% had at least 1 positive Ab result at some point during treatment

*Peak GH to standard pharmacologic tests.
†Assumes 25 kg child.
‡After withdrawal of GHRH, responders' growth velocity decreased from 7.3 ± 0.4 to 5.1 ± 1.7; treated with GH (0.6 IU/kg for 6 mo).
§Three-month study of 10/12 pretreated with GH.
See Table 33-5 for abbreviations.
Subsequent methionyl-GH treatment (8 IU/wk): at 3 months average growth velocity similar for those on higher dose of GHRH; three had better response on GHRH.

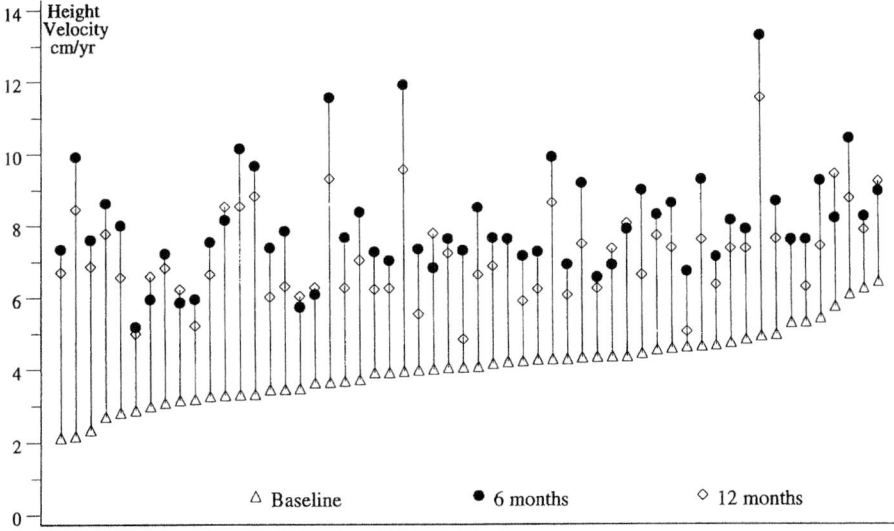

Figure 33-3 The effect of 6 and 12 months' growth hormone–releasing hormone (1–29) treatment in growth hormone–deficient children. The height velocities at baseline *(triangle)* and after 6 months *(circle)* and 12 months *(diamond)* of treatment are plotted by increasing baseline values. (Reprinted with permission from Thorner MO, Rochiccioli P, Colle M, et al: Once daily subcutaneous growth hormone–releasing hormone therapy accelerates growth in growth hormone–deficient children during the first year of therapy. J Clin Endocrinol Metab 81:1189–1196, 1996.)

approved by the Food and Drug Administration. The recommended daily dose is 30 µg/kg/day given SC at bedtime. The patients should be selected according to the following criteria: All children should be prepubertal, with a bone age of less than 7.5 years for females and less than 8 years for males. Children who do not adequately respond (i.e., peak GH level of ≤2 µg/L) to a GH stimulation test with GHRH prior to the study should not be treated with GHRH.

Adverse Effects

Development of antibodies during GHRH treatment has been described.[526,528–532,539,541,543,544] Treatment-related adverse events have been reported including local injection reactions characterized by pain, swelling, or redness, as well as headache, flushing, dysphagia, dizziness, hyperactivity, and urticaria. There are few reported data on thyroid function in children with GH deficiency. One study reported an increase in thyroid replacement requirements in one of seven patients.[545] Another study reported a 5% incidence of hypothyroidism.[526] The mechanism underlying the change in thyroid function is unclear, but it has been hypothesized that an increase in GH levels results in an increase in somatostatin tone with subsequent inhibition of thyroid-stimulating hormone secretion.[546]

GHRH TREATMENT IN ADULTS

Optimal GHRH therapy requires the functional integrity of somatotroph cells.[547] While in GH-deficient adults this is no longer the case, older adults, in whom the somatotroph hyposecretion is thought to be caused by the decreased activity of GHRH-secreting neurons,[548] still have an intact hypothalamic-pituitary axis. In addition, the pituitary GH-releasable pool in the elderly is comparable to that in young adults.

In fact, the few available studies dealing with the administration of GHRH in adults have been performed in the elderly to investigate whether GHRH treatment could counteract the age-dependent decline of GH. Twice-daily injections of GHRH(1–29) for 2 weeks,[549] as well as continuous GHRH(1–44) infusions for 2 weeks in healthy older men,[550] partially reversed the age-related decrease of GH, as well as IGF-1 levels. Another study, performed over 6 weeks,[551] suggested that GHRH administration to the elderly might attenuate some effects of aging on muscle strength. The results of further long-term studies on the effects of GHRH treatment in the elderly are awaited.

GROWTH HORMONE SECRETAGOGUES

Since the first studies reporting the GH-releasing capabilities of GHSs in humans, there has been interest in their potential as diagnostic agents. Peptide and non-peptide GHSs are powerful stimulators of GH release, effective when administered IV, SC, intranasally,[552] or PO.[366] These agents typically cause GH release in excess of that observed following GHRH or during the ITT.

GHS Action in Healthy Subjects

The GHSs cause the release of GH in a dose-dependent fashion.[553] They are more potent than GHRH: 1 µg/kg of GHRP-6 peptide results in significantly greater GH release than the same dose of GHRH. The effect of GHSs on GH release is more reproducible than the effect of GHRH. The peptide GHSs (e.g., GHRP-6, GHRP-1, GHRP-2, and hexarelin) and the non-peptide GHSs (e.g., MK-0677) differ in terms of their pharmacokinetics. MK-0677 has been developed specifically as an orally active agent. The peptidyl GHSs are active PO, but only at doses several hundred times higher than that required when administered IV.

An intact hypothalamic-pituitary axis is vital to facilitate the maximal effect of GHSs on GH release. GHRH and somatostatin both influence the action of GHSs, augmenting and diminishing the magnitude of the GH pulse, respectively. When GHRH is administered in combination with GHSs, the effect is synergistic, the magnitude of the GH pulse being greater than that obtained from the sum of the two agents administered separately.[291,554–559] The presence of GHRH is required for GHSs to exert their effects on GH secretion. In a family from the remote Valley of Sind in Pakistan, a missense mutation in the GHRH receptor that changes the glycine at residue 72 in the extracellular domain to a stop results in a phenotype analogous to the *little* mouse.[560] When members of the family who were homozygous for the mutation were challenged with hexarelin, there was no detectable GH response. In addition, studies performed in children who are GH-deficient as a result of pituitary stalk transection are unresponsive to GHSs.[561] Thus, somatotroph exposure to GHRH is necessary for GHSs to exert their action.

Manipulation of somatostatin tone also affects the GH response to GHSs. When hexarelin was given to subjects in combination with somatostatin, the amount of GH released was significantly reduced.[562] When arginine was administered to the elderly, a group proposed to have increased somatostatin tone, GH levels following the administration of GHRP-6 increased significantly, to levels seen in younger subjects.[563]

GHSs demonstrate GH-releasing activity during the neonatal period at a level which persists during prepubertal life.[564] During puberty there is an increased GH response to GHSs, which persists into adult life.[565–567] Subsequently, over the course of the adult life span, the GH response to GHSs declines, in line with the reduction in spontaneous GH secretion.[555,563,568]

The response to GHSs does not vary with sex apart from during puberty, when girls exhibit a greater response to GHSs than do boys.[566] The response in adult women is similar to that observed in men. Over the course of the adult life span, as with other stimuli, the magnitude of the GH response to GHSs diminishes, in line with the fall in spontaneous GH secretion observed with aging.[547] Women who received GHSs at various times during the menstrual cycle achieved similar peaks whether studied during the early-follicular, late-follicular, or luteal phase.[569]

GHSs and the Diagnosis of GH Deficiency

Although the effects of acute administration of GHSs have been extensively studied in healthy adults and children, few studies have evaluated their potential as diagnostic agents in patients with GH deficiency. The primary reason for this is the age-dependent decline in secretagogue-stimulated GH release, making it necessary to determine age-specific normative data. Instead of undertaking this considerable task, efforts have concentrated on finding ways of overcoming the effects of age by administering a GHS in combination with arginine or GHRH.

The combination of GHRH and GHS is the most potent stimulus of GH release known to endocrinologists and provides a promising alternative to the ITT. In normal subjects, the lower limit of the normal range (third percentile) of responses to GHRH and hexarelin was 55.5 µg/L, which was considerably higher than the lower limit of normal following GHRH and arginine (third percentile = 17.5 µg/L). The response to GHS plus GHRH is reproducible within an individual; the GH levels attained are similar among individuals and do not appear to decline with age.[557,570] Perhaps the most important feature of the GHS-GHRH test is its ability to discriminate GH-deficient patients from normal subjects. In two studies the combination of GHS and GHRH had a specificity and sensitivity of 100%.[571,572] The combination of GHS and GHRH is safe and well tolerated; side effects are similar to those seen when the two agents are administered separately.

The GHRH and GHS Test in Difficult Diagnostic Situations

The power of the combined stimulus of GHRH and GHS has resulted in its application to difficult diagnostic situations in which GH release, both spontaneous and stimulated, is reduced by a coexisting process. The problem of aging has already been discussed, but other situations, particularly obesity and syndromes of glucocorticoid excess, may confound the diagnosis of GH deficiency.

Obesity

Spontaneous and stimulated GH secretion is reduced in obese subjects.[511] The exact cause of the hyposomatotropism is uncertain, but a variety of mechanisms have been suggested. Among the hypotheses put forward are increased somatostatin tone, a reduction in the secretion of GHRH or of the natural ligand for the GHS receptor, or any combination of these.[573] What is known for certain is that the GH response to a number of stimuli, including GHRH,[510] GHRP-6,[556] and hexarelin,[574] is inversely correlated with body fat mass, specifically abdominal fat mass. The diminished GH response can make it difficult to accurately define the GH status of an obese patient with hypothalamic-pituitary disease, particularly those in whom GH deficiency may be the only hormone abnormality.

The combination of GHRH with either arginine[512] or GHS[556] administered to an obese subject causes a GH response far greater than any other stimulus, although the GH level does not quite reach that seen in normal controls. These tests are useful tools in the differentiation of true GH deficiency from hyposomatotropism caused by obesity.

Syndromes of Glucocorticoid Excess

In rats, glucocorticoids potentiate GHRH action and enhance spontaneous GH secretion. In normal humans, there is a biphasic effect of pharmacologic doses of glucocorticoids. When normal men were treated with a single IV bolus of dexamethasone 4 mg and 3 hours later were challenged with a bolus injection of GHRH, the peak GH response to GHRH increased from 9.9 ± 2.0 μg/L to 29.2 ± 5.7 μg/L. When the dexamethasone dose was increased to 8 mg IV 12 hours prior to a GHRH bolus, the peak GH response to GHRH was attenuated to 3 ± 1.1 μg/L. These results suggest an acute stimulatory response followed by a later inhibitory effect.[575] The pretreatment with pyridostigmine before administering GHRH partially reversed the effects of 48 hours of dexamethasone therapy, suggesting that somatostatin tone may be increased by glucocorticoids.[576] Patients with glucocorticoid excess caused by Cushing's syndrome or by exogenous steroids have markedly impaired GH secretion.[577] This may result from the combined effects of chronic exposure to glucocorticoids and the changes in body composition associated with Cushing's syndrome, particularly the central adiposity. The suppression of GH in these patients may persist for up to 1 year after resolution of the glucocorticoid excess,[578] which may give rise to misinterpretation of a patient's GH status. GHRH and GHRP-6 have been administered to patients with Cushing's syndrome separately and in combination. The effect of GHRH in these patients was almost abolished, and the response to GHRP-6 was considerably reduced compared to controls. The combination of GHRH and GHRP-6 was considerably more potent than either GHRH or GHRP-6 used alone, but the GH peaks were only 20% of those seen in normal subjects.[579] An earlier study had shown that the response to GHRH and pyridostigmine increased threefold following 7 days' priming with GHRH.[580] These data suggest that the effects of chronic glucocorticoid excess are primarily caused by reduced GH secretion. Whether the combination of GHRH and GHS will be able to predict which patients with Cushing's disease will recover normal GH secretion is a matter for further study.

The combination of GHS and GHRH provides a promising alternative to the ITT as the gold standard investigation to determine GH deficiency in adults and possibly children. Once GHSs are freely available, this test can be evaluated in everyday clinical practice by endocrinologists and may replace the ITT as the first-line investigation when diagnosing GH deficiency. Until then, the use of GHSs in the diagnosis of GH deficiency will be limited to a handful of academic centers around the world.

Therapeutic Potential of GHSs

Since the discovery of GHRPs in 1976, 5 years before the discovery of GHRH,[581] several different types of GHSs have been developed, including a series of non-peptidyl GHSs.[349,352,424,582] The concept that these agents amplify the pulsatile GH secretory pathway, instead of overriding normal physiology, has made this group of drugs the target of intensive research. The initial enthusiasm which accompanied the concept of orally available peptidergic and non-peptidergic GHSs, however, has been mitigated by the controversial results of several studies suggesting that there are no benefits in terms of changes in body composition, as well as a report of tolerance.[583] Others could not find development of tolerance and described beneficial effects on body composition.[584]

Therefore, the area of GHSs as therapeutic agents remains controversial. Some areas are discussed later where a GHS might be a useful agent, especially under the assumption that new compounds with higher efficacy and better oral availability will be developed. It is essential for the reader to recognize that each GHS is unique in terms of its bioavailability profile, its metabolism, and its specificity of action. Thus, no two GHSs may be compared except on a superficial level. It is not sound to extrapolate from one GHS to another.

Therapeutic Potential of GHSs in Children

The use of GHSs in children with growth retardation has been thought to have therapeutic potential. Several studies have proved the GH-releasing effects of these compounds, peptidergic as well as non-peptidergic, in short-term infusion studies in children. As a GH stimulus, they are as potent or even more potent than GHRH. Loche and coworkers[585] demonstrated that IV bolus infusions of hexarelin, 2 μg/kg of body weight, can increase GH release in short-statured children (familial short stature and constitutional delay of growth).

In a trial performed by Mericq et al.,[586] GHRP-2 was administered SC to six prepubertal children of short stature with GH deficiency, defined as a GH response of less than 7 μg/L to at least two standard provocative tests and a growth velocity of 4 cm per year or less. The agents were administered for 6 months at increasing doses (0.3–1.0 to 3.0 μg/kg/day). At months 7 and 8, the children received GHRP-2 3 μg/kg/day together with GHRH 3 μg/kg/day. The maximal overnight GH and GH peak amplitude showed a progressive increase at the higher doses. Growth velocities were increased when compared to baseline (5.3 ± 0.8 vs. 3.0 ± 0.5 cm/year, $P <.05$). During the long treatment period, the GHRP-2 injections were well tolerated. However, the study was not placebo controlled.

To date, only two studies report the effects of non-peptidergic GHSs in children.[587,588] In a short-term pilot study of 8 days, MK-0677 increased GH, IGF-1, and IGFBP-3 in some children with GH deficiency. In the following long-term double-blind placebo-controlled study by Yu and coworkers[587] with the GHS MK-0677 with 94 previously untreated, prepubertal GH-deficient children (height < fifth percentile, growth velocity < 25th percentile, peak GH < 10 ng/mL on two tests), the GHS was well tolerated. The children were treated for 6 months with either 0.4 mg/kg/day or 0.8 mg/kg/day. Mean growth velocity increased by more than 3 cm per year at 6 months.[587]

Similar results have been reported[589] in a group of prepubertal non-GH-deficient children. In this study, eight prepubertal children with constitutional short stature were treated with hexarelin administered three times daily intranasally. After treatment for up to 8 months, the growth velocity increased significantly (mean ± SD) from 5.3 ± 0.8 to 8.3 ± 1.7 cm per year in this group. Whether these changes would translate into increased adult height in these children after a longer therapy period is unclear to date.

Altogether, in preliminary studies, the growth response to GHS in GH-deficient children has been lower than that seen with GH treatment. Whether this is explained by the type of GH-deficient children selected for the trials or a suboptimal dosing regimen has yet to be determined. The development of new compounds with improved pharmacodynamic properties might bring improved results.

The use of GHSs in children with non-GH-deficient short stature has to be evaluated very carefully in the future.

Therapeutic Potential of GHSs in Adults
GH therapy has been approved in adults with organic GH deficiency[465] caused by hypothalamic-pituitary disease and for the acquired immunodeficiency syndrome–related wasting syndrome[590] in the United States. As adults with GH deficiency very often do not have an intact hypothalamic-pituitary axis, only some of these patients would probably benefit from the use of GHSs.[591] Currently, no data exist investigating the potential positive effects of GHS treatment in the acquired immunodeficiency syndrome–related wasting syndrome. Another potential field of research is the catabolic state of severe illness.

It seems that in the prolonged catabolic state of critical severe illness, a relative hyposomatotropism occurs, which seems to be partly of hypothalamic origin.[592] Infusion studies with GHRP-2 showed that given alone or together with GHRH, the somatotrophs can respond in this condition. In addition, there seems to occur a significant responsiveness to GH under GHRP infusion to these patients.[593-595] A 5-day infusion of GHRP-2 and thryotropin-releasing hormone in protracted critical illness not only reactivated the blunted GH and thyroid-stimulating hormone secretion but also showed metabolic effectiveness in this condition.[596] A double-blind placebo-controlled study[597] showed in a small number of healthy volunteers that diet-induced nitrogen wasting can be reduced after 7 days of treatment with an oral GH secretagogue (MK-0677). Studies by Neary and coworkers[598] suggest that ghrelin is able to increase energy intake in cancer patients. Similar data in animal cancer models support the anticachectic effect of ghrelin.[599] These findings support the concept of GHS use in the catabolic state. Further evaluation of the merits of the use of GHSs in adult patients on maintenance hemodialysis is warranted.[600]

The use of GHSs for treatment of critically ill patients has to be evaluated carefully. A previous study[601] showed that treatment with high doses of GH (0.07–0.13 mg/kg/day) leads to an increase in morbidity and mortality in these patients.

Another potential field of application for GHSs is in the normal older population, as there is an age-dependent decrease in GH secretion.[483] Some of the changes in body composition seen in the elderly resemble the changes seen in the GH-deficient adults.[483] Studies investigating the effects of GH treatment in the elderly have shown that GH treatment in the elderly might have beneficial effects on lean body mass, adipose tissue, and bone mineral density.[602] In addition, the releasable GH pool of the pituitary is preserved in the elderly.

The few existing studies investigating the effects of GHSs in the elderly have shown conflicting results. One study, using the peptidergic GHS hexarelin, could not show a beneficial effect on body composition after 16 weeks of SC treatment. The same investigators reported a partial and reversible

attenuation of the GH response to hexarelin, measured 4 weeks after cessation of hexarelin therapy. IGF-1 did not change significantly.[583]

Studies performed with an oral non-peptidergic GHS (MK-0677) resulted in a significant increase in IGF-1 concentration compared to that of young adults after 4 weeks of treatment with 25 mg given once a day. This increase was accompanied by an increase in the mean 24-hour GH concentration, GH pulse height, and interpulse nadir concentrations of these volunteers. There were no significant changes in the pulse number observed. No desensitization of the hypothalamic-pituitary GH axis occurred. Despite the fact that GHSs have been shown to have ACTH and prolactin (PRL)-releasing activity,[564] no change in cortisol secretion was found in this study.[603] The PRL levels rose slightly but remained within the normal range. Fasting insulin levels, as well as glucose levels, have been reported to increase under MK-0677 treatment.[604] First results of a double-blind placebo-controlled trial show that MK-0677 is able to significantly increase IGF-1 levels in healthy older men for 2 years.[605] In a randomized placebo-controlled study with 292 postmenopausal women, the effects of a GHS (MK-0677) on bone mineral density alone and in combination with an antiresorptive agent (alendronate) resulted in an increased bone mineral density (BMD) at the femoral neck when given together.[606] In a 6-month study in healthy older adults recovering from hip fracture, treatment with MK-0677 resulted in a greater improvement relative to placebo in some lower extremity measures. The overall performance measures did not show a significant change.[607] However, to date, the interpretation of such functional data is difficult as meaningful end points are hard to define. These divergent results underline once again that each GHS is unique in terms of its bioavailability and specificity profiles. Long-term studies are needed to further investigate the potential benefits of GHSs in the older population, that is, an increase in muscle mass and strength, as well as positive changes in body composition such as reduction in visceral fat.

Whether the use of GHSs in obesity will be of any benefit is questionable and requires further careful evaluation. The GH-releasing effects in obesity are decreased when compared with a normal population.[510,608] Eight weeks of treatment with the GHS MK-0677 at a dose of 25 mg per day in 24 obese men showed no change in total or visceral fat.[584] Of interest, the fat-free mass increased significantly and IGF-1 levels increased approximately 40% in this study.

Another potential therapeutic use for GHSs might be their use to improve cardiac function in certain stages of heart failure.[374] This is most likely caused by a direct effect of the GHSs at the heart, where cardiac-specific GHS binding sites have been identified.[609]

GHRELIN AND GROWTH HORMONE SECRETAGOGUES

Ghrelin stimulates GH, ACTH, and PRL release, feeding, gastric acid secretion, gastric motility, and cell proliferation (Table 33-8). However, data from the recently described ghrelin knockout mice suggest that alternative pathways can compensate for all the known effects of ghrelin (see following section)[610]; however, in one study of ghrelin knockout mice, endogenous ghrelin seemed important in determining the type of metabolic substrate (i.e., fat vs. carbohydrate) that is used for maintenance of energy balance, particularly under conditions of high fat intake.[297]

GH-Related Effects
The GH release, the first recognized effect of ghrelin, acts via a dual mechanism involving the hypothalamus and the pituitary. In in vitro studies, with rat pituitary cultures, ghrelin has been shown to specifically activate the GHS-R and stimulate GH release.[294] The effect of GHSs in vivo is much stronger than the in vitro effect; IV administration of ghrelin to freely

Table 33-8 Effects of Ghrelin/GHSs

Growth hormone release
ACTH and cortisol release
Prolactin release
Orexigenesis
Carbohydrate metabolism
Gastric motility
Immune
Sleep
Bone
Heart (inotropic)
Vasodilatation
Proliferative
Autonomous nervous system
Thermoregulation

moving rats caused a dose-dependent increase in GH release,[611–613] but the effect depends on the presence of GHRH. Although hypothalamic activation can be seen in the GHRH receptor–mutated *lit/lit* mouse, no GH release is observed.[614] Interestingly, in humans with GHRHR mutations, a very small but significant GH response can be observed with sensitive GH assays,[615] while the ACTH and PRL-releasing effects of GHSs are intact.[616] The efficacy of GHSs or ghrelin is greatly attenuated following administration of anti-GHRH serum in rats[429,617–619] or a GHRH antagonist in humans.[620] Pituitary stalk lesions cause attenuation of GHS or ghrelin effects but less so if the lesion occurred recently and the pituitary somatotrophs are not atrophic due to long-term GHRH deficiency.[621–625] Coadministration of GHS with GHRH causes a synergistic GH release,[579] and this effect can be used for diagnostic purposes to diagnose adult GH deficiency.[626] Continuous ghrelin administration leads to attenuation of the effect, while intermittent administration causes long-lasting effects.[627]

GHSs do not stimulate GH synthesis in adult somatotroph cells, although a positive effect on GH synthesis was shown in infant rat pituitary.[628–630]

In humans, the GH rise after an equivalent dose (1 µg/kg) of IV bolus GHRH, hexarelin, and ghrelin shows significantly different responses, with ghrelin being the most effective (peak mean GH ± SEM: 26.7 ± 8.7 µg/L, 68.4 ± 14.7 µg/L and 92.1 ± 16.7 µg/L, respectively). Ghrelin's GH-releasing effect decreases with age, similar to the effects of GHSs, while there is no age or sex dependence in the ACTH, cortisol, and prolactin effects and in the glucose (increase) and insulin (decrease) effects.[631] A reduced GH release is observed in obese subjects compared to normal subjects in response to ghrelin or to GHSs.[632] Food intake decreases the effect of ghrelin on GH release in both animal and human studies.[633,634]

Both peripherally or centrally administered GHSs and ghrelin stimulate the hypothalamic arcuate nucleus GHS-R, as well as directly acting at the pituitary GHS-R to release GH. However, recent data suggest that blockade of the afferent fibers of the vagus nerve abolished peripheral ghrelin-induced GH release.[635] Therefore, the exact mechanism of GH release elucidated by peripheral ghrelin remains to be clarified.

Despite the powerful GH-releasing effects of externally administered ghrelin or GHSs, it is uncertain whether ghrelin has a role in physiologic GH regulation. There is no difference in ghrelin levels during GH peak and trough periods.[636] No change was observed in GH levels after the administration of a GHS antagonist or after immunoneutralization of ghrelin.[637] A GHRH antagonist inhibited GH release but did not change plasma ghrelin levels in humans.[348] GH secretion is normal in patients with gastric bypass operation where there are very low ghrelin levels.[341] In a patient with ghrelin-secreting pancreatic tumor and 50 times higher ghrelin levels, GH and IGF levels were in the normal range, although desensitization and downregulation of the GHS-R is possible in this situation.[638] Ghrelin-deficient mice have normal growth hormone levels and growth characteristics.[610] However, acute GH injection inhibited ghrelin levels in GH-deficient patients,[639] while there are controversial data on long-term GH treatment. A study using a new ghrelin inhibitor, which directly binds to the active form of ghrelin, showed inhibition of ghrelin-induced GH release in rats.[637] After 1 year of GH replacement therapy, no change was observed in ghrelin levels in one study, while another treating subjects for 9 months found a significant 29% drop in ghrelin levels, although this could be also influenced by the increased insulin levels observed.[640] In a transgenic mouse model using antisense GHS-R mRNA expression under the control of tyrosine hydroxylase promoter, lower GH and IGF-1 levels were found in female animals,[641] and lower IGF-1 levels were reported in the GHS-R knockout animals.[642] A possible negative-feedback regulation of ghrelin by GH (GH administration or acromegaly) might suggest that ghrelin is part of the GH regulatory axis[640,643,644] even though such a potential feedback loop between GH and ghrelin has not been found consistently[298,348,518–520,645] It is possible that ghrelin plays a role in the diurnal rhythm of GH secretion, allowing higher GH levels during the night.[646] Whether the role of ghrelin as a GH secretion modulator is important in normal physiologic conditions or only becomes more prominent during states of negative energy balance remains to be clarified.[619]

Other Hormone-Related Effects

When treated in vitro, pituitary cells do not respond to GHSs or ghrelin with ACTH secretion, but in vivo administration results in a significant rise in ACTH levels with a consequent rise in cortisol levels.[647,648] The stimulatory effect on the hypothalamic-pituitary-adrenal axis is independent of GHRH and probably depends on hypothalamic vasopressin and corticotropin-releasing hormone stimulation,[318,435,436] while no direct effect has been shown on the adrenal gland. Both GHSs and ghrelin show exaggerated ACTH and cortisol response in patients with Cushing's disease,[649–651] which could be at least partly explained by the increased expression of GHS-R1a in corticotroph adenomas.[295,396] The stimulation of the hypothalamic-pituitary-adrenal axis attenuates during prolonged treatment with long-acting GHSs.[603,652,653] Ghrelin and GHSs release prolactin by activation of the somato-mammotroph cells in the pituitary.[367,654]

Feeding Effect

Ghrelin stimulates feeding in both animal and human studies.[300,659–662] Similar effects were actually shown earlier for GHSs.[392,623,663,664] Ghrelin specifically stimulates fat accumulation and has been shown to have direct stimulatory effects on adipocyte proliferation and on PPAR-γ synthesis.[300,662,665]

Acute peripheral administration of ghrelin to rats or mice briefly stimulates food intake and increases respiratory quotient (increases carbohydrate use). Because the rodent diet used is rich in carbohydrate, and because a momentary increase in food intake of such a diet is associated with a more sustained increased respiratory quotient, it is difficult to separate the acute effects of ghrelin on carbohydrate use from its ability to stimulate appetite. However, if no food is available, ghrelin administration does not stimulate respiratory quotient, suggesting that the substrate usage changes observed may be mediated by stimulated feeding (personal communication, Mark Heiman, 9/2004).

Ghrelin acts via stimulating NPY/AGRP cells and orexin cells and indirectly inhibiting pro-opiomelanocortin cells in the hypothalamus (Fig 33-4).[296,666,667] The vagus also seems to play an important role in the feeding effects as vagotomy inhibits the feeding effect of peripheral ghrelin.[635] Therefore,

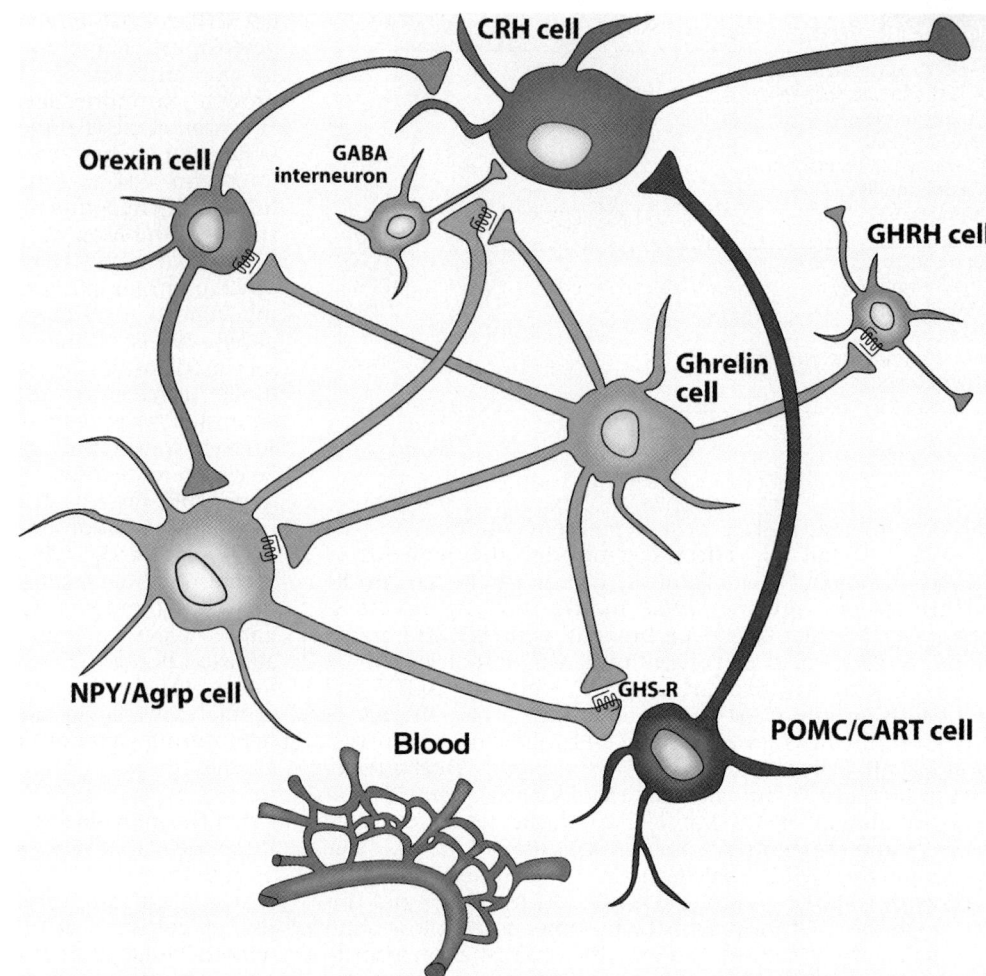

Figure 33-4 Possible ghrelin effects in the hypothalamus.[655] Ghrelin (either via the bloodstream or via hypothetical local ghrelin cells) stimulates presynaptic GHS-R located on NPY cell axons connecting to POMC cells in the arcuate nucleus and stimulates the release of the inhibitory neurotransmitter GABA to inhibit the anorexigenic POMC neurons. The effect of ghrelin in the PVN on CRH cells is more complex. Here, presynaptic GHS-R receptors stimulate NPY release, which, in turn, inhibit GABA release from GABA interneurons,[656] resulting in disinhibition, that is, stimulation of CRH neurons leading to ACTH and cortisol release.[318,647] Ghrelin cells may also connect to orexigenic orexin neurons in the lateral hypothalamus and stimulate their activity.[317] GHS-R is expressed on GHRH neurons, and these cells could be stimulated by GHSs.[657,658]

the feeding effect of ghrelin could occur via three possible mechanisms (Fig 33-5): (1) via peripheral ghrelin reaching the arcuate nucleus and stimuling orexigenic cells; (2) via GHS-R in the peripheral vagal afferents and the nucleus tractus solitarius; or (3) via locally produced ghrelin-stimulating arcuate and lateral hypothalamus orexigenic cells and/or inhibiting anorectic cells, although it has to be emphasized that some studies were not able to detect ghrelin and/or ghrelin cells in the hypothalamus.[297-299]

Effects on Carbohydrate Metabolism
Most human studies observed that ghrelin inhibits insulin levels, while it stimulates glucose levels.[668] Ghrelin has been shown to be present in the islet cells of the pancreas; α cells, ß cells, or a new cell type, ε cells, have been suggested as potential sources for ghrelin synthesis in the islet.[328-331] Ghrelin has a direct effect on insulin signaling in hepatoma cells.[669]

Adipose Tissue Effects
Chronic ghrelin administration has been shown to increase body fat content in rodents.[300,662] Interestingly, ghrelin-treated animals pair-fed to saline treated animals do not increase their weight but increase their fat tissue content as assessed by magnetic resonance imaging,[670] suggesting a specific effect independent of food intake and weight gain. The level of GHS-R mRNA increased by up to fourfold in adipose tissue from epididymal and parametrial regions as the rat aged from 4 to 20 weeks and was significantly elevated during the differentiation of preadipocytes in vitro.[665] Ghrelin (10^{-8} M) for 10 days stimulated the activity of glycerol-3-phosphate dehydrogenase and the differentiation of rat parametrial preadipocytes in vitro. Ghrelin treatment also significantly

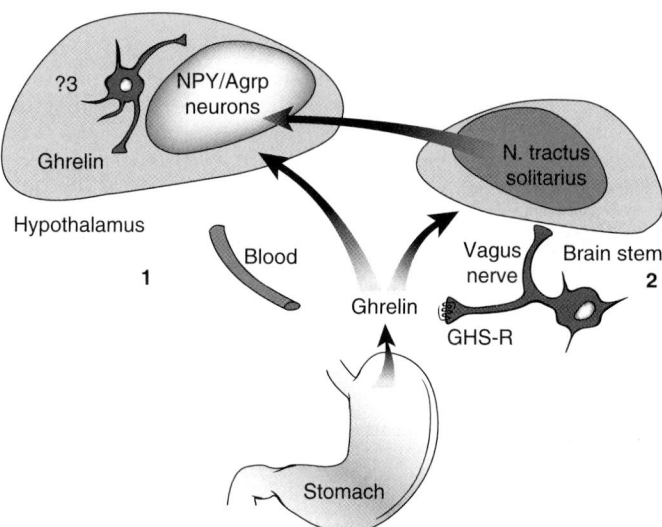

Figure 33-5 Ghrelin exerts its effects in the hypothalamus via three different pathways.[655] **1,** Ghrelin synthesized in the stomach reaches the arcuate nucleus via the bloodstream and possibly other brain areas via an active transport through the blood-brain barrier.[294,305] **2,** Ghrelin synthesized in the periphery stimulates vagal afferents, which have been shown to express GHS-R, and vagal connections reach the nucleus tractus solitarius in the brain stem, which then communicate with the hypothalamus.[635] **3,** There is controversy whether ghrelin cells are present in the hypothalamus,[297-299] but some data suggest that ghrelin is synthesized locally in the hypothalamus and has direct connections with NPY/AGRP and other hypothalamic cells.[296]

increased the levels of PPAR-γ mRNA in primary cultured rat differentiated adipocytes. However, this effect of ghrelin on PPAR-γ mRNA has not been found consistently.[671] In addition, isoproterenol-stimulated lipolysis was significantly reduced by simultaneous ghrelin treatment in a dose-dependent manner in vitro. Ghrelin (as well as desoctanoyl ghrelin) infused to the bone marrow specifically stimulates bone marrow fat cell proliferation.[307]

Cardiovascular Effects

GHSs and ghrelin have GH-independent effects on the cardiovascular system. Acute administration of peptide GHSs and ghrelin causes an elevation in the left ventricular ejection fraction in healthy subjects or in patients with ischemic cardiomyopathy, but not in patients with dilated cardiomyopathy.[373,672–674] Ghrelin is also effective in improving cardiac performance in chronic heart failure.[675,676] Ghrelin has vasodilator effects, and the density of ghrelin binding is increased in atherosclerosis.[677] Ghrelin inhibits apoptosis via an MAPK and Akt-dependent pathway in cardiomyocytes. Desoctanoyl ghrelin has also been shown to produce similar effects, and also showed binding in H9c2 cells that do not express the GHS-R1a mRNA.[308] It seems that at least some of the cardiovascular effects of ghrelin and hexarelin on cardiac function are different; this is apparently due to hexarelin's specific actions at the CD36 receptor.[413]

Reproductive Axis

Ghrelin is synthesized in the endometrium, placenta, ovaries, and testes, and direct effects have been shown in these tissues. Taking into account the fact that the reproductive axis is highly dependent on nutritional status, ghrelin, acting at central and peripheral levels, could be one of the signal mechanisms linking nutritional status to the hypothalamic-pituitary gonadal axis.[337]

Cell Proliferation

In some cell types (thyroid, breast), ghrelin has inhibitory effects, while in others (prostate, hepatoma, adrenal, pancreatic, cardiac, adipose cells, and pituitary) stimulatory effects on cell proliferation have been reported. The proliferative effect occurs via the MAPK pathway and desoctanoyl ghrelin also seems to have the same effect, suggesting that these do not occur via the GHS-R1a receptor.[306]

Other Effects

Ghrelin has inhibitory effect on cardiovascular sympathetic activity,[306] a stimulatory effect on gastrointestinal parasympathetic activity (gastric acid secretion and gastric motility)[678] and has inhibitory effect on vagal afferent discharge.[679] Ghrelin stimulates gastric motility, similar to motilin, and also stimulates gastric acid secretion.

Both GHSs and ghrelin have been shown to promote sleep in humans, although GHRP-2 showed an increase of stage 2 sleep, while MK-0677 and ghrelin increase slow wave sleep.[372,680–682] Interestingly, in lit/lit mice with a nonfunctional GHRH receptor, ghrelin increased food intake but had no effect on sleep, suggesting that GHRH is involved in the sleep effect of ghrelin.[683]

GHS-R has been identified in the hippocampus, and ghrelin administration increases anxiety.[680,684] These findings suggest that ghrelin may have a role in mediating neuroendocrine and behavioral responses to stressors and that the stomach might play an important role in the regulation of anxiety.

GHRELIN LEVELS IN PATHOLOGIC CONDITIONS

Abnormal Body Weight

Ghrelin is negatively correlated with weight, and higher ghrelin levels were found in patients on a low-calorie diet,[341,685] in patients suffering from anorexia due to cancer,[686,687] and in patients with cardiac disease[688] or anorexia nervosa.[689–692] Fasting increases circulating ghrelin levels, and it has been suggested that the fasting-related elevation of circulating GH could be a consequence of increased ghrelin levels.[693] However, on more prolonged fasting (3 day), ghrelin levels are no longer elevated.[342] Patients with anorexia nervosa have high ghrelin levels, and weight gain decreases ghrelin concentrations.[343,689,692,694,695]

Neonates with intrauterine growth retardation have higher ghrelin levels than normal neonates, and the increased orexigenic drive could contribute to postnatal catch-up growth.[696–698]

Obese subjects have lower ghrelin levels than lean subjects.[344] Weight loss through dieting increases circulating ghrelin levels.[341,685] Data suggest that ghrelin is regulated by insulin and does not depend directly on fat mass or fat distribution.[346,347]

The most effective treatment for morbid obesity is gastric surgery with Roux-en-Y gastric bypass or adjustable gastric banding. It has long been observed that Roux-en-Y gastric bypass has effects beyond the restriction of the capacity of the stomach, and long-term reduction in appetite is achieved. It has been suggested that decreased ghrelin levels, probably due to the loss of stomach tissue involved in food processing, could be the cause of loss of appetite after gastric bypass surgery.[699] However, a recent study involving 66 obese subjects investigated before and after surgery suggested that ghrelin levels increased in line with the weight loss.[700]

Diabetes Mellitus and Insulin Resistance

Patients with insulin resistance (type 2 diabetes, polycystic ovary syndrome) have lower ghrelin levels than BMI-matched controls.[701–705] The causality between higher insulin concentration (and/or the pathologic process of insulin resistance) and lower ghrelin levels cannot be determined by these data. Low ghrelin levels appeared to be associated with high blood pressure independent of BMI in a population-based study, as well as in pregnant women.[701,706]

Prader-Willi Syndrome

While all forms of human obesity, including simple obesity, congenital leptin deficiency, leptin receptor or melanocortin-4 receptor mutations, or hypothalamic obesity from craniopharyngioma, show low ghrelin levels, patients with Prader-Willi syndrome have inappropriately high ghrelin levels in the range of patients with anorexia nervosa.[707–710] Prader-Willi syndrome is the most common syndromal cause of genetic obesity, caused by loss of expression of imprinted genes on the paternally inherited chromosome 15q11-q13, and characterized by life-threatening childhood-onset hyperphagia and obesity, as well as GH deficiency and hypogonadism, thought to be due to hypothalamic abnormalities.[711] Hyperghrelinemia, three to four times higher than BMI-matched controls, could contribute to the severe hyperphagia observed in these patients. It remains to be determined whether ghrelin is directly involved in the pathogenesis of the different symptoms in Prader-Willi syndrome.

Acromegaly

Ghrelin levels increase after surgery in acromegalic subjects in inverse correlation with GH, IGF-1, and insulin levels, suggesting that one or a combination of these hormones result in suppressed ghrelin levels in active acromegaly.[643,644]

Hyperthyroidism

Ghrelin levels are reduced in hyperthyroidism, suggesting that ghrelin is not involved in the hyperphagia of hyperthyroidism.[712] As the known factors suppressing ghrelin levels (high BMI, high insulin or somatostatin) cannot play a role here, and the decreased body weight of hyperthyroidism should rather stimulate ghrelin levels, it is assumed that thyroid hormones have a direct inhibitory effect on ghrelin.

Knockout Animal Models

Ghrelin knockout animals are indistinguishable from their wild-type littermates in terms of body size, food intake, GH and IGF-1 levels, reproduction, bone density, activity or behavior, blood chemistry, organ weight or tissue pathology, and response to ghrelin injection.[610] However, under high-fat diet, ghrelin knockout animals use more fat, suggesting that ghrelin influences the type of metabolic substrate used for the maintenance of energy balance.[297]

A selective hypothalamic knockout model using antisense GHS-R mRNA expression under the tyrosine hydroxylase control showed lower GH and IGF-1 levels in female animals.[641] Recent data suggest that the complete GHS-R knockout mice are smaller and have a 20% decrease in their IGF level.[642]

A number of single-nucleotide polymorphisms have been identified in the human ghrelin and GHS-R genes, but further studies are necessary to investigate if any of these have biologic relevance.

SUMMARY

Ghrelin is a peptide hormone secreted into the circulation from the stomach but also synthesized in a number of tissues, suggesting both endocrine and paracrine effects. The acyl group of the peptide is necessary for GH release and orexigenisis, but not for some other effects, including cell proliferation in various cell types. GHSs and ghrelin were originally considered as potent secretagogues of GH, but the role of peripheral ghrelin in the regulation of normal GH is unclear at the present time. The appetite-inducing and lipogenic effects of ghrelin seem to be important but the controversial knockout animal data suggest that further studies are needed. The concept that ghrelin is lipogenic independent of its orexigenic effect has not been substantiated. Little is known of the importance of circulating ghrelin and desoctanoyl ghrelin in regulation of physiologic processes as ghrelin knockout animals are apparently completely normal, but the well-known redundancy in other appetite-inducing agents could mask relevant effects of this peptide. Further studies are necessary to reveal the exact mechanism involved in ghrelin physiology and pathophysiology, and possible phenotypic roles for changes in ghrelin levels, such as those seen with insulin-resistant states (type 2 diabetes mellitus, obesity, polycystic ovarian syndrome) and the unexpected hyperghrelinemia in patients with Prader-Willi syndrome. Further studies exploring potential clinical applications for ghrelin, as well as orally available ghrelin mimetics, are necessary. Similarly, further clinical treatment applications for GHRH have still to be determined, and further research will be necessary in this field as well.

REFERENCES

1. Reichlin S: Growth and the hypothalamus. Endocrinology 67:760–773, 1960.
2. Reichlin S: Growth hormone content of pituitaries from rats with hypothalamic lesions. Endocrinology 69:225–230, 1961.
3. Beck C, Larkins RG, Martin TJ, et al: Stimulation of growth hormone release from superfused rat pituitary by extracts of hypothalamus and of human lung tumours. J Endocrinol 59(2):325–333, 1973.
4. Dabek FT: Bronchial carcinoid tumour with acromegaly in two patients. J Clin Endocrinol Metab 38(2):329–333, 1974.
5. Sonksen PH, Ayres AB, Braimbridge M, et al: Acromegaly caused by pulmonary carcinoid tumours. Clin Endocrinol 5(5):503–513, 1976.
6. Caplan RH, Koob L, Abellera RM, et al: Cure of acromegaly by operative removal of an islet cell tumor of the pancreas. Am J Med 64(5):874–882, 1978.
7. Shalet SM, Beardwell CG, MacFarlane IA, et al: Acromegaly due to production of a growth hormone releasing factor by a bronchial carcinoid tumor. Clin Endocrinol 10(1):61–67, 1979.
8. Zafar MS, Mellinger RC, Fine G, et al: Acromegaly associated with a bronchial carcinoid tumor: Evidence for ectopic production of growth hormone-releasing activity. J Clin Endocrinol Metab 48:66–71, 1979.
9. Leveston SA, McKeel DW Jr, Buckley PJ, et al: Acromegaly and Cushing's syndrome associated with a foregut carcinoid tumor. J Clin Endocrinol Metab 53(4):682–689, 1981.
10. Southern AL: Functioning metastatic bronchial carcinoid with elevated levels of serum and cerebrospinal fluid serotonin and pituitary adenoma. J Clin Endocrinol Metab 20:298–305, 1960.
11. Weiss L, Ingram M: Adenomatoid bronchial tumors: A consideration of the carcinoid tumors and the salivary tumors of the bronchial tree. Cancer 14:161–178, 1961.
12. Buse J, Buse MG, Roberts WJ: Eosinophilic adenoma of the pituitary and carcinoid tumors of the rectosigmoid area. J Clin Endocrinol Metab 21:735–738, 1961.
13. Ballard HS, Frame B, Hartsock RJ: Familial multiple endocrine adenoma-peptic ulcer complex. Medicine 43:481–516, 1964.
14. Frohman LA, Szabo M, Berelowitz M, et al: Partial purification and characterization of a peptide with growth hormone-releasing activity from extrapituitary tumors in patients with acromegaly. J Clin Invest 65(1):43–54, 1980.
15. Thorner MO, Perryman RL, Cronin MJ, et al: Somatotroph hyperplasia: Ssuccessful treatment of acromegaly by removal of a pancreatic islet tumor secreting a growth hormone-releasing factor. Transact Assoc Am Phys 95:177–187, 1982.
16. Spiess J, Rivier J, Thorner M, et al: Sequence analysis of a growth hormone releasing factor from a human pancreatic islet tumor. Biochemistry 21(24):6037–6040, 1982.
17. Rivier J, Spiess J, Thorner M, et al: Characterization of a growth hormone-releasing factor from a human pancreatic islet tumour. Nature 300(5889):276–278, 1982.
18. Esch FS, Bohlen P, Ling NC, et al: Characterization of a 40 residue peptide from a human pancreatic tumor with growth hormone releasing activity. Biochem Biophys Res Comm 109(1):152–158, 1982.
19. Sassolas G, Chayvialle JA, Partensky C, et al: Acromegaly, clinical expression of the production of growth hormone releasing factor in pancreatic tumors. Ann Endocrinol 44(6):347–354, 1983.
20. Guillemin R, Brazeau P, Bohlen P, et al: Growth hormone-releasing factor from a human pancreatic tumor that caused acromegaly. Science 218(4572):585–587, 1982.
21. Campbell RM, Lee Y, Rivier J, et al: GRF analogs and fragments: Correlation between receptor binding, activity and structure. Peptides 12(3):569–574, 1991.
22. Frohman LA, Jansson JO: Growth hormone-releasing hormone. Endocr Rev 7(3): 223–253, 1986.
23. Bohlen P, Brazeau P, Bloch B, et al: Human hypothalamic growth hormone releasing factor (GRF): Evidence for two forms identical to tumor derived GRF-44-NH2 and GRF-40. Biochem Biophys Res Comm 114(3):930–936, 1983.
24. Ling N, Esch F, Bohlen P, et al: Isolation, primary structure, and synthesis of human hypothalamic somatocrinin: Growth hormone-releasing factor. Proc Natl Acad Sci U S A 81(14):4302–4306, 1984.
25. Lin HD, Bollinger J, Ling N, et al: Immunoreactive growth hormone-releasing factor in human stalk median eminence. J Clin Endocrinol Metab 58(6):1197–1199, 1984.
26. Asa SL, Kovacs K, Thorner MO, et al: Immunohistological localization of

growth hormone-releasing hormone in human tumors. J Clin Endocrinol Metab 60(3):423–427, 1985.

27. Brazeau P, Ling N, Bohlen P, et al: Growth hormone releasing factor, somatocrinin, releases pituitary growth hormone in vitro. Proc Natl Acad Sci U S A 79:7909–7913, 1982.

28. Engels JW, Glauder J, Mullner H, et al: Enzymatic amidation of recombinant (Leu27) growth hormone releasing hormone-Gly45. Protein Eng 1:195–199, 1987.

29. Brar AK, Downs TR, Heimer EP, et al: Biosynthesis of human growth hormone-releasing hormone (hGRH) in the pituitary of hGRH transgenic mice. Endocrinology 129(6):3274–3280, 1991.

30. Christophe J, Svoboda M, Dehaye J-P, et al: The VIP/PHI/secretin/helodermin/helospectin/GRF family: Structure-function relationships of the natural peptides, their precursors and synthetic analogues as tested in vitro on receptors and adenylate cyclase in a panel of tissue membranes. In Martinez J (ed): Peptide Hormones as Prohormones: Processing, Biological Activity, Pharmacology. E. Horwood Chichester, England, Halstead Press, 1989, pp 211–243.

31. Bell GI: The glucagon superfamily: Precursor structure and gene organization. Peptides 7(Suppl 1):27–36, 1986.

32. Campbell RM, Scanes CG: Evolution of the growth hormone-releasing factor (GRF) family of peptides. Growth Regulation 2(4):175–191, 1992.

33. McRory JE, Parker RL, Sherwood NM: Expression and alternative processing of a chicken gene encoding both growth hormone-releasing hormone and pituitary adenylate cyclase-activating polypeptide. DNA Cell Biol 16(1):95–102, 1997.

34. Vaughan JM, Rivier J, Spiess J, et al: Isolation and characterization of hypothalamic growth-hormone releasing factor from common carp, Cyprinus carpio. Neuroendocrinology 56(4):539–549, 1992.

35. McRory J, Sherwood NM: Two protochordate genes encode pituitary adenylate cyclase-activating polypeptide and related family members. Endocrinology 38(6):2380–2390, 1997.

36. Kaiser ET, Kezdy FJ: Amphiphilic secondary structure: Design of peptide hormones. Science 223(4633):249–255, 1984.

37. Campbell RM, Bongers J, Felix AM: Rational design, synthesis, and biological evaluation of novel growth hormone releasing factor analogues. Biopolymers 37(2):67–88, 1995.

38. Clore GM, Martin SR, Gronenborn AM: Solution structure of human growth hormone releasing factor. Combined use of circular dichroism and nuclear magnetic resonance spectroscopy. J Mol Biol 191(3):55–61, 1986.

39. Frohman LA, Downs TR, Heimer EP, et al: Dipeptidylpeptidase IV and trypsin-like enzymatic degradation of

human growth hormone-releasing hormone in plasma. J Clin Invest 83(5):1533–1540, 1989.

40. Kovacs M, Gulyas J, Bajusz S, et al: An evaluation of intravenous, subcutaneous, and in vitro activity of new agmatine analogs of growth hormone-releasing hormone hGH-RH (1-29)NH2. Life Sci 42(1):27–35, 1988.

41. Coy DH, Hocart SJ, Murphy WA: Human growth hormone-releasing hormone analogues with much improved in vitro growth hormone-releasing potencies in rat pituitary cells. Eur J Pharmacol 204(2):179–185, 1991.

42. Zarandi M, Serfozo P, Zsigo J, et al: Potent agonists of growth hormone-releasing hormone. Part I. Int J Peptide Protein Res 39(3):211–217, 1992.

43. Campbel RM, Heimer EP, Ahmad M, et al: Pegylated peptides. V. Carboxy-terminal PEGylated analogs of growth hormone-releasing factor (GRF) display enhanced duration of biological activity in vivo. J Peptide Res 49(6):527–537, 1997.

44. Cervini LA, Donaldson CJ, Koerber SC, et al: Human growth hormone-releasing hormone hGHRH(1-29)-NH2: Systematic structure-activity relationship studies. J Med Chem 41(5):717–727, 1998.

45. Coy DH, Murphy WA, Sueiras-Diaz J, et al: Structure-activity studies on the N-terminal region of growth hormone releasing factor. J Med Chem 28(2):181–185, 1985.

46. Robberecht P, Coy DH, Waelbroeck M, et al: Structural requirements for the activation of rat anterior pituitary adenylate cyclase by growth hormone-releasing factor (GRF): Discovery of (N-Ac-Tyr1, D-Arg2)-GRF(1-29)-NH2 as a GRF antagonist on membranes. Endocrinology 117(5):1759–1764, 1985.

47. Zarandi M, Horvath JE, Halmos G, et al: Synthesis and biological activities of highly potent antagonists of growth hormone-releasing hormone. Proc Natl Acad Sci U S A 91(25):12298–12302, 1994.

48. Toth K, Kovacs M, Zarandi M, et al: New analogs of human growth hormone-releasing hormone (1-29) with high and prolonged antagonistic activity. J Peptide Res 51(2):134–141, 1998.

49. Jungwirth A, Schally AV, Pinski J, et al: Growth hormone-releasing hormone antagonist MZ-4-71 inhibits in vivo proliferation of Caki-I renal adenocarcinoma. Proc Natl Acad Sci U S A 94(11):5810–5813, 1997.

50. Waelbroeck M, Robberecht P, Coy DH, et al: Interaction of growth hormone-releasing factor (GRF) and 14 GRF analogs with vasoactive intestinal peptide (VIP) receptors of rat pancreas. Discovery of (N-Ac-Tyr1,D-Phe2)-GRF(1-29)-NH2 as a VIP antagonist. Endocrinology 116(6):2643–2649, 1985.

51. Gubler U, Monahan JJ, Lomedico PT, et al: Cloning and sequence analysis of

cDNA for the precursor of human growth hormone-releasing factor, somatocrinin. Proc Natl Acad Sci U S A 80(14):4311–4314, 1983.

52. Mayo KE, Cerelli GM, Lebo RV, et al: Gene encoding human growth hormone-releasing factor precursor: Structure, sequence, and chromosomal assignment. Proc Natl Acad Sci U S A 82(1):63–67, 1985.

53. Mayo KE, Cerelli GM, Rosenfeld MG, et al: Characterization of cDNA and genomic clones encoding the precursor to rat hypothalamic growth hormone-releasing factor. Nature 314(6010):464–467, 1985.

54. Frohman MA, Downs TR, Chomczynski P, et al: Cloning and characterization of mouse growth hormone-releasing hormone (GRH) complementary DNA: Increased GRH messenger RNA levels in the growth hormone-deficient lit/lit mouse. Mol Endocrinol 3(10):1529–1536, 1989.

55. Gonzalez-Crespo S, Boronat A: Expression of the rat growth hormone-releasing hormone gene in placenta is directed by an alternative promoter. Proc Natl Acad Sci U S A 88(19):8749–8753, 1991.

56. Berry SA, Srivastava CH, Rubin LR, et al: Growth hormone-releasing hormone-like messenger ribonucleic acid and immunoreactive peptide are present in human testis and placenta. J Clin Endocrinol Metab 75(1):281–284, 1992.

57. Bloch B, Baird A, Ling N, et al: Immunohistochemical evidence that growth hormone-releasing factor (GRF) neurons contain an amidated peptide derived from cleavage of the carboxyl-terminal end of the GRF precursor. Endocrinology 118(1):156–162, 1986.

58. Breyer PR, Rothrock JK, Beaudry N, et al: A novel peptide from the growth hormone releasing hormone gene stimulates Sertoli cell activity. Endocrinology 137(5):2159–2162, 1996.

59. Perez-Riba M, Gonzalez-Crespo S, Boronat A: Differential splicing of the growth hormone-releasing hormone gene in rat placenta generates a novel pre-proGHRH mRNA that encodes a different C-terminal flanking peptide. FEBS Lett 402(2-3):273–276, 1997.

60. Bloch B, Gaillard RC, Brazeau P, et al: Topographical and ontogenetic study of the neurons producing growth hormone-releasing factor in human hypothalamus. Regul Pept 8(1):21–31, 1984.

61. Bugnon C, Gouget A, Fellmann D, et al: Immunocytochemical demonstration of a novel peptidergic neurone system in the cat brain with an anti-growth hormone-releasing factor serum. Neurosci Lett 38(2):131–137, 1983.

62. Jacobowitz DM, Schulte H, Chrousos GP, et al: Localization of GRF-like immunoreactive neurons in the rat brain. Peptides 4(4):521–524, 1983.

63. Merchenthaler I, Vigh S, Schally AV, et al: Immunocytochemical localization of growth hormone-releasing factor in

the rat hypothalamus. Endocrinology 114(4):1082–1085, 1984.

64. Sawchenko PE, Swanson LW, Rivier J, et al: The distribution of growth-hormone-releasing factor (GRF) immunoreactivity in the central nervous system of the rat: An immunohistochemical study using antisera directed against rat hypothalamic GRF. J Comp Neurol 237(1):100–115, 1985.

65. Bloch B, Brazeau P, Bloom F, et al: Topographical study of the neurons containing hpGRF immunoreactivity in monkey hypothalamus. Neurosci Lett 37(1):23–28, 1983.

66. Horvath S, Palkovits M, Gorcs T, et al: Electron microscopic immunocytochemical evidence for the existence of bidirectional synaptic connections between growth hormone-releasing hormone- and somatostatin-containing neurons in the hypothalamus of the rat. Brain Res 481(1):8–15, 1989.

67. Zeitler P, Tannenbaum GS, Clifton DK, et al: Ultradian oscillations in somatostatin and growth hormone-releasing hormone mRNAs in the brains of adult male rats. Proc Natl Acad Sci U S A 88:8920–8924, 1991.

68. Tannenbaum GS, Zhang WH, Lapointe M, et al: Growth hormone-releasing hormone neurons in the arcuate nucleus express both Sst1 and Sst2 somatostatin receptor genes. Endocrinology 139(3):1450–1453, 1998.

69. Bresson JL, Clavequin MC, Fellmann D, et al: Ontogeny of the neuroglandular system revealed with HPGRF 44 antibodies in human hypothalamus. Neuroendocrinology 39(1):68–73, 1984.

70. Ishikawa K, Katakami H, Jansson JO, et al: Ontogenesis of growth hormone-releasing hormone neurons in the rat hypothalamus. Neuroendocrinology 43(5):537–542, 1986.

71. Joubert D, Benlot C, Lagoguey A, et al: Normal and growth hormone (GH)-secreting adenomatous human pituitaries release somatostatin and GH-releasing hormone. J Clin Endocrinol Metab 68:572–577, 1989.

72. Bagnato A, Moretti C, Ohnishi J, et al: Expression of the growth hormone-releasing hormone gene and its peptide product in the rat ovary. Endocrinology 130(3):1097–1102, 1992.

73. Tsagarakis S, Ge F, Besser GM, et al: Similar high molecular weight forms of growth hormone-releasing hormone are found in rat brain and testis. Life Sci 49(22):1627–1634, 1991.

74. Suhr ST, Rahal JO, Mayo KE: Mouse growth-hormone-releasing hormone: Precursor structure and expression in brain and placenta. Mol Endocrinol 3(11):1693–1700, 1989.

75. Margioris AN, Brockmann G, Bohler HC Jr, et al: Expression and localization of growth hormone-releasing hormone messenger ribonucleic acid in rat placenta: In vitro secretion and regulation of its peptide product. Endocrinology 126(1):151–158, 1990.

76. Meigan G, Sasaki A, Yoshinaga K: Immunoreactive growth hormone-releasing hormone in rat placenta. Endocrinology 123(2):1098–1102, 1988.

77. Weigent DA, Blalock JE: Immunoreactive growth hormone-releasing hormone in rat leukocytes. J Neuroimmunol 29(1–3):1–13, 1990.

78. Stephanou A, Knight RA, Lightman SL: Production of a growth hormone-releasing hormone-like peptide and its mRNA by human lymphocytes. Neuroendocrinology 53(6):628–633, 1991.

79. Weigent DA, Riley JE, Galin FS, et al: Detection of growth hormone and growth hormone-releasing hormone-related messenger RNA in rat leukocytes by the polymerase chain reaction. Proc Soc Exper Biol Med 198:643–648, 1991.

80. Nicholson WE, DeCherney GS, Jackson RV, et al: Pituitary and hypothalamic hormones in normal and neoplastic adrenal medullae: Biologically active corticotropin-releasing hormone and corticotropin. Regul Pept 18:173–188, 1987.

81. Shibasaki T, Kiyosawa Y, Masuda A, et al: Distribution of growth hormone-releasing hormone-like immunoreactivity in human tissue extracts. J Clin Endocrinol Metab 59(2):263–268, 1984.

82. Bosman FT, Van Assche C, Nieuwenhuyzen Kruseman AC, et al: Growth hormone releasing factor (GRF) immunoreactivity in human and rat gastrointestinal tract and pancreas. J Histochem Cytochem 32(11):1139–1144, 1984.

83. Christofides ND, Stephanou A, Suzuki H, et al: Distribution of immunoreactive growth hormone-releasing hormone in the human brain and intestine and its production by tumors. J Clin Endocrinol Metab 59(4):747–751, 1984.

84. Lopes MB, Gaylinn BD, Thorner MO, et al: Growth hormone-releasing hormone receptor mRNA in acromegalic pituitary tumors. Am J Pathol 150(6):1885–1891, 1997.

85. Thapar K, Kovacs K, Stefaneanu L, et al: Overexpression of the growth-hormone-releasing hormone gene in acromegaly-associated pituitary tumors. An event associated with neoplastic progression and aggressive behavior. Am J Pathol 151(3):769–784, 1997.

86. Kahan Z, Arencibia JM, Csernus VJ, et al: Expression of growth hormone-releasing hormone (GHRH) messenger ribonucleic acid and the presence of biologically active GHRH in human breast, endometrial, and ovarian cancers. J Clin Endocrinol Metab 84(2):582–589, 1999.

87. Matsubara S, Sato M, Mizobuchi M, et al: Differential gene expression of growth hormone (GH)-releasing hormone (GRH) and GRH receptor in various rat tissues. Endocrinology 136(9):4147–4150, 1995.

88. Morel G, Mesguich P, Dubois MP, et al: Ultrastructural evidence for endogenous growth hormone-releasing factor-like immunoreactivity in the monkey pituitary gland. Neuroendocrinology 38:123–133, 1984.

89. Mentlein R, Buchholz C, Krisch B: Binding and internalization of gold-conjugated somatostatin and growth hormone-releasing hormone in cultured rat somatotropes. Cell Tissue Res 258:309–317, 1989.

90. Morel G: Uptake and ultrastructural localization of a [125I] growth hormone releasing factor agonist in male rat pituitary gland: Evidence for internalization. Endocrinology 129(3):1497–1504, 1991.

91. Mayo KE, Miller TL, DeAlmeida V, et al: The growth-hormone-releasing hormone receptor: Signal transduction, gene expression, and physiological function in growth regulation. Ann N Y Acad Sci 805: 184–203, 1996.

92. Mayo KE: Molecular cloning and expression of a pituitary-specific receptor for growth hormone-releasing hormone. Mol Endocrinol 6(10):1734–1744, 1992.

93. Gaylinn BD, Harrison JK, Zysk JR, et al: Molecular cloning and expression of a human anterior pituitary receptor for growth hormone-releasing hormone. Mol Endocrinol 7(1):77–84, 1993.

94. Lin C, Lin SC, Chang CP, et al: Pit-1-dependent expression of the receptor for growth hormone releasing factor mediates pituitary cell growth. Nature 360(6406):765–768, 1992.

95. DeAlmeida VI, Mayo KE: Identification of binding domains of the growth hormone-releasing hormone receptor by analysis of mutant and chimeric receptor proteins. Mol Endocrinol 12(5): 750–765, 1998.

96. Gaylinn BD, Lyons CE, Zysk JR, et al: Photoaffinity cross-linking to the pituitary receptor for growth hormone-releasing factor. Endocrinology 135(3):950–955, 1994.

97. Seifert H, Perrin M, Rivier J, et al: Binding sites for growth hormone releasing factor on rat anterior pituitary cells. Nature 313:487–489, 1985.

98. Abribat T, Boulanger L, Gaudreau P: Characterization of [125I-Tyr10]human growth hormone-releasing factor (1-44) amide binding to rat pituitary: Evidence for high and low affinity classes of sites. Brain Res 528(2):291–299, 1990.

99. Ikuyama S, Natori S, Nawata H, et al: Characterization of growth hormone-releasing hormone receptors in pituitary adenomas from patients with acromegaly. J Clin Endocrinol Metab 66(6):1265–1271, 1988.

100. Gaylinn BD, Lyons CE, Thorner MO: Mapping of the GHRH receptor binding site by photoaffinity crosslinking from different residues of

GHRH. in 79th Annual Meeting of the Endocrine Society, Minneapolis, 1997.

101. Andrews S, Dubbelde C, Ryan E: The sequence of Homo sapiens PAC clone DJ0877J02. 1998, US National Center for Biotechnology Information, National Library of Medicine: GenBank accession AC005155 http://www.ncbi.nlm.gov/.

102. Gaylinn BD, von Kap-Herr C, Golden WL, et al: Assignment of the human growth hormone-releasing hormone receptor gene (GHRHR) to 7p14 by in situ hybridization. Genomics 19(1):193–195, 1994.

103. Wajnrajch MP, Chua SC, Green ED, et al: Human growth hormone-releasing hormone receptor (GHRHR) maps to a YAC at chromosome 7p15. Mamm Genome 5(9):595, 1994.

104. Petersenn S, Rasch AC, Heyens M, et al: Structure and regulation of the human growth hormone-releasing hormone receptor gene. Mol Endocrinol 12(2):233–247, 1998.

105. Iguchi G, Okimura Y, Takahashi T, et al: Cloning and characterization of the 5'-flanking region of the human growth hormone-releasing hormone receptor gene. J Biol Chem 274(17):12108–12114, 1999.

106. Seifert H, Perrin M, Rivier J, et al: Growth hormone-releasing factor binding sites in rat anterior pituitary membrane homogenates: Modulation by glucocorticoids. Endocrinology 117(1):424–426, 1985.

107. Tamaki M, Sato M, Matsubara S, et al: Dexamethasone increases growth hormone (GH)-releasing hormone (GRH) receptor mRNA levels in cultured rat anterior pituitary cells. J Neuroendocrinol 8(6):475–480, 1996.

108. Mille TL, Mayo KE: Glucocorticoids regulate pituitary growth hormone-releasing hormone receptor messenger ribonucleic acid expression. Endocrinology 138(6):2458–2465, 1997.

109. Ono M, Miki N, Murata Y, et al: Sexually dimorphic expression of pituitary growth hormone-releasing factor receptor in the rat. Biochem Biophys Res Comm 216(3):1060–1066, 1995.

110. Bilezikjian LM, Seifert H, Vale W: Desensitization to growth hormone-releasing factor (GRF) is associated with down-regulation of GRF-binding sites. Endocrinology 118(5):2045–2052, 1986.

111. Horikawa R, Hellmann P, Cella SG, et al: Growth hormone-releasing factor (GRF) regulates expression of its own receptor. Endocrinology 137(6):2642–2645, 1996.

112. Aleppo G, Moskal SF II, De Grandis PA, et al: Homologous down-regulation of growth hormone-releasing hormone receptor messenger ribonucleic acid levels. Endocrinology 138(3):1058–1065, 1997.

113. Miller TL, Godfrey PA, Dealmeida VI, et al: The rat growth hormone-releasing hormone receptor gene: Structure, regulation, and generation of receptor isoforms with different signaling properties. Endocrinology 140(9):4152–4165, 1999.

114. Journot L, Waeber C, Pantaloni C, et al: Differential signal transduction by six splice variants of the pituitary adenylate cyclase-activating peptide (PACAP) receptor. Biochem Soc Transact 23(1):133–137, 1995.

115. Tang J, Lagace G, Castagne J, et al: Identification of human growth hormone-releasing hormone receptor splicing variants. J Clin Endocrinol Metab 80(8):2381–2387, 1995.

116. Zeitler P, Stevens P, Siriwardana G: Functional GHRH receptor carboxyl terminal isoforms in normal and dwarf (dw) rats. J Mol Endocrinol 21(3):363–371, 1998.

117. Motomura T, Hashimoto K, Koga M, et al: Inhibition of signal transduction by a splice variant of the growth hormone-releasing hormone receptor expressed in human pituitary adenomas. Metabolism 47(7):804–808, 1998.

118. Halmos G, Schally AV, Varga JL, et al: Human renal cell carcinoma expresses distinct binding sites for growth hormone-releasing hormone. Proc Natl Acad Sci U S A 97(19):10555–10560, 2000.

119. Kiaris H, Schally AV, Varga JL, et al: Growth hormone-releasing hormone: An autocrine growth factor for small cell lung carcinoma. Proc Natl Acad Sci U S A 96(26):14894–14898, 1999.

120. Kiaris H, Schally AV, Varga JL: Suppression of tumor growth by growth hormone-releasing hormone antagonist JV-1-36 does not involve the inhibition of autocrine production of insulin-like growth factor II in H-69 small cell lung carcinoma. Canc Lett 161(2):149–155, 2000.

121. Kiaris H, Schally AV, Armatis P: Direct action of growth hormone-releasing hormone agonist JI-38 on normal human fibroblasts: Evidence from studies on cell proliferation and c-myc proto-oncogene expression. Regul Pept 96(3):119–124, 2001.

122. Rekasi Z, Czompoly T, Schally AV, et al: Isolation and sequencing of cDNAs for splice variants of growth hormone-releasing hormone receptors from human cancers. Proc Natl Acad Sci U S A 97(19):10561–10566, 2000.

123. Kineman RD: Antitumorigenic actions of growth hormone-releasing hormone antagonists. Proc Natl Acad Sci U S A 97(2):532–534, 2000.

124. Billestrup N, Swanson LW, Vale W: Growth hormone-releasing factor stimulates proliferation of somatotrophs in vitro. Proc Natl Acad Sci U S A 83(18):6854–6857, 1986.

125. Chopin LK: A potential autocrine pathway for growth hormone releasing hormone (GHRH) and its receptor in human prostate cancer cell lines. Prostate 49(2):116–121, 2001.

126. Kiaris H, Schally AV, Busto R, et al: Expression of a splice variant of the receptor for GHRH in 3T3 fibroblasts activates cell proliferation responses to GHRH analogs. Proc Natl Acad Sci U S A 99(1):196–200, 2002.

127. Halmos G, Schally AV, Czompoly T, et al: Expression of growth hormone-releasing hormone and its receptor splice variants in human prostate cancer. J Clin Endocrinol Metab 87(10):4707–4714, 2002.

128. Garcia-Fernandez MO, Schally AV, Varga JL, et al: The expression of growth hormone-releasing hormone (GHRH) and its receptor splice variants in human breast cancer lines; the evaluation of signaling mechanisms in the stimulation of cell proliferation. Breast Cancer Res Treat 77(1):15–26, 2003.

129. Kiaris H, Chatzistamou I, Schally AV, et al: Ligand-dependent and -independent effects of splice variant 1 of growth hormone-releasing hormone receptor. Proc Natl Acad Sci U S A 100(16):9512–9517, 2003.

130. Eicher EM, Beamer WG: Inherited ateliotic dwarfism in mice. Characteristics of the mutation, little, on chromosome 6. J Hered 67(2):87–91, 1976.

131. Jansson JO, Downs TR, Beamer WG, et al: Receptor-associated resistance to growth hormone-releasing factor in dwarf "little" mice. Science 232(4749):511–512, 1986.

132. Godfrey P, Rahal JO, Beamer WG, et al: GHRH receptor of little mice contains a missense mutation in the extracellular domain that disrupts receptor function. Nat Genet 4(3):227–232, 1993.

133. Lin SC, Lin CR, Gukovsky I, et al: Molecular basis of the little mouse phenotype and implications for cell type-specific growth. Nature 364(6434):208–213, 1993.

134. Wajnrajch MP, Gertner JM, Harbison MD, et al: Nonsense mutation in the human growth hormone-releasing hormone receptor causes growth failure analogous to the little (lit) mouse. Nat Genet 12(1):88–90, 1996.

135. Baumann G, Maheshwari H: The dwarfs of Sindh: Severe growth hormone (GH) deficiency caused by a mutation in the GH-releasing hormone receptor gene. Acta Paediatrica (Suppl) 423:33–38, 1997.

136. Netchine I, Talon P, Dastot F, et al: Extensive phenotypic analysis of a family with growth hormone (GH) deficiency caused by a mutation in the GH-releasing hormone receptor gene. J Clin Endocrinol Metab 83(2):432–436, 1998.

137. Salvatori R, Hayashida CY, Aguiar-Oliveira MH, et al: Familial dwarfism due to a novel mutation of the growth hormone-releasing hormone receptor gene. J Clin Endocrinol Metab 84(3):917–923, 1999.

138. Salvatori R: Isolated growth hormone (GH) deficiency due to compound heterozygosity for two new mutations in the GH-releasing hormone receptor gene. Clin Endocrinol 54(5): 681–687, 2001.

139. Adams EF, Symowski H, Buchfelder M, et al: A polymorphism in the growth hormone (GH)-releasing hormone (GHRH) receptor gene is associated with elevated response to GHRH by human pituitary somatotrophinomas in vitro. Biochem Biophys Res Comm 275(1):33–36, 2000.

140. Lee EJ, Kotlar TJ, Ciric I, et al: Absence of constitutively activating mutations in the GHRH receptor in GH-producing pituitary tumors. J Clin Endocrinol Metab 86(8):3989–3995, 2001.

141. Salvatori R: Absence of mutations in the growth hormone (GH)-releasing hormone receptor gene in GH-secreting pituitary adenomas. Clin Endocrinol 54(3):301–307, 2001.

142. Bilezikjian LM, Vale WW: Stimulation of adenosine 3′,5′-monophosphate production by growth hormone-releasing factor and its inhibition by somatostatin in anterior pituitary cells in vitro. Endocrinology 113(5):1726–1731, 1983.

143. Mougin C, Brazeau P, Ling N, et al: Roles of cyclic AMP and calcium in the mechanism of the release of growth hormone by somatocrinin. Comptes Rendus De L Academie Des Sciences 299:83–88, 1984.

144. Brazeau P, Ling N, Esch F, et al: Somatocrinin (growth hormone releasing factor) in vitro bioactivity; Ca++ involvement, cAMP mediated action and additivity of effect with PGE2. Biochem Biophys Res Comm 109:588–594, 1982.

145. Beck-Peccoz P, Volpi A, Maggioni AP, et al: Evidence for an inhibition of thyroid hormone effects during chronic treatment with amiodarone. Horm Metab Res 18(6):411–414, 1986.

146. Hart GR, Ray KP, Wallis M: Mechanisms involved in the effects of TRH on GHRH-stimulated growth hormone release from ovine and bovine pituitary cells. Mol Cell Endocrinol 56:53–61, 1988.

147. Schettini G, Cronin MJ, Hewlett EL, et al: Human pancreatic tumor growth hormone-releasing factor stimulates anterior pituitary adenylate cyclase activity, adenosine 3′,5′-monophosphate accumulation, and growth hormone release in a calmodulin-dependent manner. Endocrinology 115(4):1308–1314, 1984.

148. Holl RW, Thorner MO, Leong DA: Intracellular calcium concentration and growth hormone secretion in individual somatotropes: Effects of growth hormone-releasing factor and somatostatin. Endocrinology 122(6):2927–2932, 1988.

149. Snyder GD, Yadagiri P, Falck JR: Effect of epoxyeicosatrienoic acids on growth hormone release from somatotrophs. Am J Physiol 256:E221–E226, 1989.

150. Rawlings SR, Hoyland J, Mason WT: Calcium homeostasis in bovine somatotrophs: Calcium oscillations and calcium regulation by growth hormone-releasing hormone and somatostatin. Cell Calcium12:403–414, 1991.

151. Guarcello V, Weigent DA, Blalock JE: Growth hormone releasing hormone receptors on thymocytes and splenocytes from rats. Cell Immunol 136:291–302, 1991.

152. Thorner MO, Holl RW, Leong DA: The somatotrope: An endocrine cell with functional calcium transients. J Exper Biol 139:169–179, 1988.

153. Bertherat J: Nuclear effects of the cAMP pathway activation in somatotrophs. Horm Res 47(4–6):245–250, 1997.

154. Cugini CD, Millard WJ, Leidy JW: Signal transduction systems in growth hormone-releasing hormone and somatostatin release from perifused rat hypothalamic fragments. Endocrinology 129:1355–1362, 1991.

155. Cronin MJ, Hewlett EL, Evans WS, et al: Human pancreatic tumor growth hormone (GH)-releasing factor and cyclic adenosine 3′,5′-monophosphate evoke GH release from anterior pituitary cells: The effects of pertussis toxin, cholera toxin, forskolin, and cycloheximide. Endocrinology 114(3):904–913, 1984.

156. Cronin MJ, Rogol AD, Dabney LG, et al: Selective growth hormone and cyclic AMP stimulating activity is present in human pancreatic islet cell tumor. J Clin Endocrinol Metab 55(2):381–383, 1982.

157. Cronin MJ, Rogol AD, MacLeod RM, et al: Biological activity of a growth hormone-releasing factor secreted by a human tumor. Am J Physiol 244(4):E346–353, 1983.

158. Cronin MJ, Rogol AD: Sex differences in the cyclic adenosine 3′:5′-monophosphate and growth hormone response to growth hormone-releasing factor in vitro. Biol Reprod 31:984–988, 1984.

159. Cronin MJ, Rogol AD, Myers GA, et al: Pertussis toxin blocks the somatostatin-induced inhibition of growth hormone release and adenosine 3′,5′-monophosphate accumulation. Endocrinology 113:209–215, 1983.

160. Cronin MJ, MacLeod RM, Canonico PL: Modification of basal and GRF-stimulated cyclic AMP levels and growth hormone release by phospholipid metabolic enzyme inhibitors. Neuroendocrinology 40:332–338, 1985.

161. Cronin MJ, Canonico PL: Tumor promoters enhance basal and growth hormone releasing factor stimulated cyclic AMP levels in anterior pituitary cells. Biochem Biophys Res Comm 129:404–410, 1985.

162. Cronin MJ, Summers ST, Sortino MA, et al: Protein kinase C enhances growth hormone releasing factor (1-40)-stimulated cyclic AMP levels in anterior pituitary. Actions of somatostatin and pertussis toxin. J Biol Chem 261:13932–13935, 1986.

163. Arimura A, Culler MD, Turkelson CM, et al: In vitro pituitary hormone releasing activity of 40 residue human pancreatic tumor growth hormone releasing factor. Peptides 4(1):107–110, 1983.

164. Culler MD, Kenjo T, Obara N, et al: Stimulation of pituitary cAMP accumulation by human pancreatic GH-releasing factor-(1-44). Am J Physiol 247(5 Pt 1):E609–E615, 1984.

165. Ray KP, Wallis M: Regulation of growth hormone secretion and cyclic AMP metabolism in ovine pituitary cells: Interactions involved in activation induced by growth hormone-releasing hormone and phorbol esters. Mol Cell Endocrinol 58:243–252, 1988.

166. Michel D, Lefevre G,Labrie F: Dexamethasone is a potent stimulator of growth hormone-releasing factor-induced cyclic AMP accumulation in the adenohypophysis. Life Sci 35: 597–602, 1984.

167. Spada A, Vallar L, Giannattasio G: Presence of an adenylate cyclase dually regulated by somatostatin and human pancreatic growth hormone (GH)-releasing factor in GH-secreting cells. Endocrinology 115:1203–1209, 1984.

168. Labrie F, Gagne B, Lefevre G: Growth hormone-releasing factor stimulates adenylate cyclase activity in the anterior pituitary gland. Life Sci 33(22):2229–2233, 1983.

169. Cheng K, Chan WW, Barreto A Jr, et al: The synergistic effects of His-D-Trp-Ala-Trp-D-Phe-Lys-NH2 on growth hormone (GH)-releasing factor-stimulated GH release and intracellular adenosine 3′,5′-monophosphate accumulation in rat primary pituitary cell culture. Endocrinology 124(6):2791–2798, 1989.

170. Summers ST, Cronin MJ: Phorbol esters induce two distinct changes in GH3 pituitary cell adenylate cyclase activity. Arch Biochem Biophys 262:12–18, 1988.

171. Summers ST, Cronin MJ: Phorbol esters enhance basal and stimulated adenylate cyclase activity in a pituitary cell line. Biochem Biophys Res Comm 135:276–281, 1986.

172. Canonico PL, Cronin MJ, Thorner MO, et al: Human pancreatic GRF stimulates phosphatidylinositol labeling in cultured anterior pituitary cells. Am J Physiol 245(6):E587–E590, 1983.

173. Canonico PL, Speciale C, Sortino MA, et al: Growth hormone releasing factor (GRF) increases free arachidonate levels in the pituitary: A role for lipoxygenase products. Life Sci 38:267–272, 1986.

174. Dobson PRM, Merritt JE, Baird JG, et al: The effect of growth hormone releasing factor on cyclic AMP accumulation and

phosphatidylinositol breakdown. In 5th International Conference on Cyclic Nucleotides Protein Phosphorylation,1983.

175. Ramirez JL, Torronteras R, Malagon MM, et al: Growth hormone-releasing factor mobilizes cytosolic free calcium through different mechanisms in two somatotrope subpopulations from porcine pituitary. Cell Calcium 23(4):207–217, 1998.

176. Cella SG, Locatelli V, Broccia ML, et al: Long-term changes of somatotrophic function induced by deprivation of growth hormone-releasing hormone during the fetal life of the rat. J Endocrinol 140(1):111–117, 1994.

177. Landis CA, Masters SB, Spada A, et al: GTPase inhibiting mutations activate the alpha chain of Gs and stimulate adenylyl cyclase in human pituitary tumours. Nature 340(6236):692–696, 1989.

178. Lloyd RV, Jin L, Chang A, et al: Morphologic effects of hGRH gene expression on the pituitary, liver, and pancreas of MT-hGRH transgenic mice. An in situ hybridization analysis. Am J Pathol 141(4):895–906, 1992.

179. Billestrup N, Swanson LW, Vale W: Growth hormone-releasing factor stimulates proliferation of somatotrophs in vitro. Proc Natl Acad Sci U S A 83:6854–6857, 1986.

180. Barinaga M, Yamonoto G, Rivier C, et al: Transcriptional regulation of growth hormone gene expression by growth hormone-releasing factor. Nature 306(5938):84–85, 1983.

181. Barinaga M, Bilezikjian M, Vale WW, et al: Independent effects of growth hormone releasing factor on growth hormone release and gene transcription. Nature 314(6008):279–281, 1985.

182. Stachura ME, Tyler JM, Farmer PK: Fractional reduction of somatostatin concentration interacted with rat growth hormone releasing hormone to titrate the magnitude of pulsatile growth hormone and prolactin release in perifusion. Neuroendocrinology 48:500–506, 1988.

183. Dieguez C, Foord SM, Shewring G, et al: The effects of long term growth hormone releasing factor (GRF 1-40) administration on growth hormone secretion and synthesis in vitro. Biochem Biophys Res Comm 121:111–117, 1984.

184. Perez FM, Hymer WC: A new tissue-slicing method for the study of function and position of somatotrophs contained within the male rat pituitary gland. Endocrinology 127:1877–1886, 1990.

185. Vale W, Vaughan J, Yamamoto G, et al: Effects of synthetic human pancreatic (tumor) GH releasing factor and somatostatin, triiodothyronine and dexamethasone on GH secretion in vitro. Endocrinology 112:1553–1555, 1983.

186. Borges JL, Uskavitch DR, Kaiser DL, et al: Human pancreatic growth hormone-releasing factor-40 (hpGRF-40) allows stimulation of GH release by TRH. Endocrinology 113(4):1519–1521, 1983.

187. Almeida OF, Schulte HM, Rittmaster RS, et al: Potency and specificity of a growth hormone-releasing factor in a primate and in vitro. J Clin Endocrinol Metab 58(2):309–312, 1984.

188. Vigh S, Schally AV: Interaction between hypothalamic peptides in a superfused pituitary cell system. Peptides 5(Suppl 1):241–247, 1984.

189. Badger TM, Millard WJ, McCormick GF, et al: The effects of growth hormone (GH)-releasing peptides on GH secretion in perifused pituitary cells of adult male rats. Endocrinology 115(4):1432–1438, 1984.

190. Ceda GP, Hoffman AR: Growth hormone-releasing factor desensitization in rat anterior pituitary cells in vitro. Endocrinology 116:1334–1340, 1985.

191. Gelato MC, Rittmaster RS, Pescovitz OH, et al: Growth hormone responses to continuous infusions of growth hormone-releasing hormone. J Clin Endocrinol Metab 61:223–228, 1985.

192. Plotsky PM, Vale W: Patterns of growth hormone-releasing factor and somatostatin secretion into the hypophysial-portal circulation of the rat. Science 230(4724):461–463, 1985.

193. Frohman LA, Downs TR, Clarke IJ, et al: Measurement of growth hormone-releasing hormone and somatostatin in hypothalamic-portal plasma of unanesthetized sheep. Spontaneous secretion and response to insulin-induced hypoglycemia. J Clin Invest 86(1):17–24, 1990.

194. Weiss J, Cronin MJ, Thorner MO: Periodic interactions of GH-releasing factor and somatostatin can augment GH release in vitro. Am J Physiol 253(5 Pt 1):E508–E514, 1987.

195. Law GJ, Ray KP, Wallis M: Effects of growth hormone-releasing factor, somatostatin and dopamine on growth hormone and prolactin secretion from cultured ovine pituitary cells. FEBS Lett 166:189–193, 1984.

196. Stachura ME, Tyler JM, Farmer PK: Human pancreatic growth hormone-releasing factor-44 differentially stimulates release of stored and newly synthesized rat growth hormone in vitro. Endocrinology 116:698–706, 1985.

197. Tachibana K, Marquardt H, Yokoya S, et al: Growth hormone-releasing hormone stimulates and somatostatin inhibits the release of a novel protein by cultured rat pituitary cells. Mol Endocrinol 2:973–978, 1988.

198. Katsumata N, Chakraborty C, Myal Y, et al: Molecular cloning and expression of peptide 23, a growth hormone-releasing hormone-inducible pituitary protein. Endocrinology 136(4):1332–1339, 1995.

199. Bergstrom RW, Hansen KL, Clare CN, et al: Hypogonadotropic hypogonadism and anosmia (Kallmann's syndrome) associated with a marker chromosome. J Androl 8(1):55–60, 1987.

200. Zeytin F, Brazeau P: GRF (somatocrinin) stimulates release of neurotensin, calcitonin and cAMP by a rat C cell line. Biochem Biophys Res Comm 123:497–506, 1984.

201. Muller EE, Locatelli V, Cocchi D: Neuroendocrine control of growth hormone secretion. Physiol Rev 79(2):511–607, 1999.

202. Casanueva FF, Dieguez C: Growth hormone secretagogues: Physiological role and clinical utility. Trends Endocrinol Metab 10(1):30–38, 1999.

203. Miki N, Ono M, Shizume K: Evidence that opiatergic and alpha-adrenergic mechanisms stimulate rat growth hormone release via growth hormone-releasing factor (GRF). Endocrinology 114:1950–1952, 1984.

204. Honegger J, Spagnoli A, D'Urso R, et al: Interleukin-1 beta modulates the acute release of growth hormone-releasing hormone and somatostatin from rat hypothalamus in vitro, whereas tumor necrosis factor and interleukin-6 have no effect. Endocrinology 129:1275–1282, 1991.

205. Tannenbaum GS, Gurd W, Lapointe M: Leptin is a potent stimulator of spontaneous pulsatile growth hormone (GH) secretion and the GH response to GH-releasing hormone. Endocrinology 139(9):3871–3875, 1998.

206. Cocchi D, De Gennaro Colonna V, Bagnasco M, et al: Leptin regulates GH secretion in the rat by acting on GHRH and somatostatinergic functions. J Endocrinol 162(1):95–99, 1999.

207. Carro E, Senaris RM, Seoane LM, et al: Role of growth hormone (GH)-releasing hormone and somatostatin on leptin-induced GH secretion. Neuroendocrinology 69(1): 3–10, 1999.

208. Carro E, Senaris RM, Mallo F, et al: Regulation of hypothalamic somatostatin and growth hormone releasing hormone mRNA levels by inhibin. Brain Res 66(1-2): 91–94, 1999.

209. Carro E, Seoane LM, Senaris R, et al: Interaction between leptin and neuropeptide Y on in vivo growth hormone secretion. Neuroendocrinology 68(3):187–191, 1998.

210. Wehrenberg WB, Ling N, Bohlen P, et al: Physiological roles of somatocrinin and somatostatin in the regulation of growth hormone secretion. Biochem Biophys Res Comm 109:562–567, 1982.

211. Wehrenberg WB, Ling N, Brazeau P, et al: Somatocrinin, growth hormone releasing factor, stimulates secretion of

growth hormone in anesthetized rats. Biochem Biophys Res Comm 109:382–387, 1982.

212. Wehrenberg WB, Bloch B, Phillips BJ: Antibodies to growth hormone-releasing factor inhibit somatic growth. Endocrinology 115:1218–1220, 1984.

213. Wehrenberg WB, Brazeau P, Luben R, et al: Inhibition of the pulsatile secretion of growth hormone by monoclonal antibodies to the hypothalamic growth hormone releasing factor (GRF). Endocrinology 111(6):2147–2148, 1982.

214. Tannenbaum GS, Ling N: The interrelationship of growth hormone (GH)-releasing factor and somatostatin in generation of the ultradian rhythm of GH secretion. Endocrinology 115(5):1952–1957, 1984.

215. Koritnik DR, Cronin MJ, Orth DN, et al: Pituitary response to intravenous hypothalamic releasing peptides in cynomolgus monkeys treated with contraceptive steroids. J Clin Endocrinol Metab 65:37–45, 1987.

216. Johke T, Hodate K, Ohashi S, et al: Growth hormone response to human pancreatic growth hormone releasing factor in cattle. Endocrinologia Japonica 31:55–61, 1984.

217. Moseley WM, Krabill LF, Friedman AR, et al: Administration of synthetic human pancreatic growth hormone-releasing factor for five days sustains raised serum concentrations of growth hormone in steers. J Endocrinol 104:433–439, 1985.

218. Moseley WM, Krabill LF, Friedman AR, et al: Growth hormone response of steers injected with synthetic human pancreatic growth hormone-releasing factors. J Anim Sci 58:430–435, 1984.

219. Enright WJ, Chapin LT, Moseley WM, et al: Growth hormone-releasing factor stimulates milk production and sustains growth hormone release in Holstein cows. J Dairy Sci 69:344–351, 1986.

220. Peticlerc D, Pelletier G, Lapierre H, et al: Dose response of two synthetic human growth hormone-releasing factors on growth hormone release in heifers and pigs. J Anim Sci 65:996–1005, 1987.

221. Leung FC, Taylor JE: In vivo and in vitro stimulation of growth hormone release in chickens by synthetic human pancreatic growth hormone releasing factor (hpGRFs). Endocrinology 113:1913–1915, 1983.

222. Ono M, Miki N, Demura H: Effect of antiserum to rat growth hormone (GH)-releasing factor on physiological GH secretion in the female rat. Endocrinology 129(4):1791–1796, 1991.

223. Magnan E, Mazzocchi L, Cataldi M, et al: Effect of actively immunizing sheep against growth hormone-releasing hormone or somatostatin on spontaneous pulsatile and neostigmine-induced growth hormone secretion. J Endocrinol 144(1):83–90, 1995.

224. Maheshwari HG, Pezzoli SS, Rahim A, et al: Pulsatile growth hormone secretion persists in genetic growth hormone-releasing hormone resistance. Am J Physiol Endocrinol Metab 282(4):E943–E951, 2002.

225. Jessup SK, Dimaraki EV, Symons KV, et al: Sexual dimorphism of growth hormone (GH) regulation in humans: Endogenous GH-releasing hormone maintains basal GH in women but not in men [see comment]. J Clin Endocrinol Metab 88(10):4776–4780, 2003.

226. Cella SG, Locatelli V, Mennini T, et al: Deprivation of growth hormone-releasing hormone early in the rat's neonatal life permanently affects somatotropic function. Endocrinology 127:1625–1634, 1990.

227. Thorner MO, Cronin MJ: Growth hormone-releasing factor: Clinical and basic studies. In Mueller EE, MacLeod RM, Frohman LA (eds): Neuroendocrine Perspectives. Amsterdam, Elsevier, 1985, pp 95–144.

228. Ling N, Zeytin F, Bohlen P, et al: Growth hormone releasing factors. Ann Rev Biochem 54: 403–423, 1985.

229. Clark RG, Robinson IC: Growth induced by pulsatile infusion of an amidated fragment of human growth hormone releasing factor in normal and GHRF-deficient rats. Nature 314:281–283, 1985.

230. Mayo KE, Hammer RE, Swanson LW, et al: Dramatic pituitary hyperplasia in transgenic mice expressing a human growth hormone-releasing factor gene. Mol Endocrinol 2: 606–612, 1988.

231. Stefaneanu L, Kovacs K, Horvath E, et al: Adenohypophysial changes in mice transgenic for human growth hormone-releasing factor: A histological, immunocytochemical, and electron microscopic investigation. Endocrinology 125(5):2710–2718, 1989.

232. Wheeler MD, Wehrenberg WW, Styne DM: Growth hormone regulation by growth hormone-releasing hormone in infant rhesus monkeys. Biol Neonate 60:19–28, 1991.

233. Wheeler MD, Styne DM: Longitudinal changes in growth hormone response to growth hormone-releasing hormone in neonatal rhesus monkeys. Pediatr Res 28:15–18, 1990.

234. Acs Z, Lonart G, Makara GB: Role of hypothalamic factors (growth-hormone-releasing hormone and gamma-aminobutyric acid) in the regulation of growth hormone secretion in the neonatal and adult rat. Neuroendocrinology 52(2):156–160, 1990.

235. Ge F, Tsagarakis S, Rees LH, et al: Relationship between growth hormone-releasing hormone and somatostatin in the rat: Effects of age and sex on content and in-vitro release from hypothalamic explants. J Endocrinol 123(1):53–58, 1989.

236. Cozzi MG, Zanini A, Locatelli V, et al: Growth hormone-releasing hormone

and clonidine stimulate biosynthesis of growth hormone in neonatal pituitaries. Biochem Biophys Res Comm 138:1223–1230, 1986.

237. Korytko AI, Zeitler P, Cuttler L: Developmental regulation of pituitary growth hormone-releasing hormone receptor gene expression in the rat. Endocrinology 137(4):1326–1331, 1996.

238. De Gennaro Colonna VD, Zoli M, Cocchi D, et al: Reduced growth hormone releasing factor (GHRF)-like immunoreactivity and GHRF gene expression in the hypothalamus of aged rats. Peptides 10:705–708, 1989.

239. Abribat T, Deslauriers N, Brazeau P, et al: Alterations of pituitary growth hormone-releasing factor binding sites in aging rats. Endocrinology 128(1):633–635, 1991.

240. Girard N, Boulanger L, Denis S, et al: Differential in vivo regulation of the pituitary growth hormone-releasing hormone (GHRH) receptor by GHRH in young and aged rats. Endocrinology 140(6):2836–2842, 1999.

241. Sonntag WE, Gough MA: Growth hormone releasing hormone induced release of growth hormone in aging male rats: Dependence on pharmacological manipulation and endogenous somatostatin release. Neuroendocrinology 47:482–488, 1988.

242. Ceda GP, Valenti G, Butturini U, et al: Diminished pituitary responsiveness to growth hormone-releasing factor in aging male rats. Endocrinology 118(5):2109–2114, 1986.

243. Lang I, Kurz R, Geyer G, et al: The influence of age on human pancreatic growth hormone releasing hormone stimulated growth hormone secretion. Horm Metab Res 20(9):574–578, 1988.

244. Pavlov EP, Harman SM, Merriam GR, et al: Responses of growth hormone (GH) and somatomedin-C to GH-releasing hormone in healthy aging men. J Clin Endocrinol Metabol 62(3):595–600, 1986.

245. Argente J, Chowen JA, Zeitler P, et al: Sexual dimorphism of growth hormone-releasing hormone and somatostatin gene expression in the hypothalamus of the rat during development. Endocrinology 128(5):2369–2375, 1991.

246. Maiter DM, Gabriel SM, Koenig JI, et al: Sexual differentiation of growth hormone feedback effects on hypothalamic growth hormone-releasing hormone and somatostatin. Neuroendocrinology 51:174–180, 1990.

247. Zeitler P, Argente J, Chowen-Breed JA, et al: Growth hormone-releasing hormone messenger ribonucleic acid in the hypothalamus of the adult male rat is increased by testosterone. Endocrinology 127(3):1362–1368, 1990.

248. Zeitler P, Vician L, Chowen-Breed JA, et al: Regulation of somatostatin and

growth hormone-releasing hormone gene expression in the rat brain. Metabol Clin Experiment 39:46–49, 1990.

249. Maiter D, Koenig JI, Kaplan LM: Sexually dimorphic expression of the growth hormone-releasing hormone gene is not mediated by circulating gonadal hormones in the adult rat. Endocrinology 128:1709–1716, 1991.

250. Aguilar E, Pinilla L: Ovarian role in the modulation of pituitary responsiveness to growth hormone-releasing hormone in rats. Neuroendocrinology 54(3):286–290, 1991.

251. Evans WS, Krieg RJ, Limber ER, et al: Effects of in vivo gonadal hormone environment on in vitro hGRF-40-stimulated GH release. Am J Physiol 249(3 Pt 1):E276–E280, 1985.

252. Hertz P, Silbermann M, Even L, et al: Effects of sex steroids on the response of cultured rat pituitary cells to growth hormone-releasing hormone and somatostatin. Endocrinology 125:581–585, 1989.

253. Leong DA, Lau SK, Sinha YN, et al: Enumeration of lactotropes and somatotropes among male and female pituitary cells in culture: Evidence in favor of a mammosomatotrope subpopulation in the rat. Endocrinology 116(4):1371–1378, 1985.

254. Ho KY, Thorner MO, Krieg RJ, et al: Effects of gonadal steroids on somatotroph function in the rat: Analysis by the reverse hemolytic plaque assay. Endocrinology 123(3):1405–1411, 1988.

255. Alvarez CV, Mallo F, Burguera B, et al: Evidence for a direct pituitary inhibition by free fatty acids of in vivo growth hormone responses to growth hormone-releasing hormone in the rat. Neuroendocrinology 53(2):185–189, 1991.

256. Grings EE, Scarborough R, Schally A, et al: Response to a growth hormone-releasing hormone analog in heifers treated with recombinant growth hormone. Domest Anim Endocrinol 5:47–53, 1988.

257. Levy A, Matovelle MC, Lightman SL, et al: The effects of pituitary stalk transection, hypophysectomy and thyroid hormone status on insulin-like growth factor 2-, growth hormone releasing hormone-, and somatostatin mRNA prevalence in rat brain. Brain Res 579(1):1–7, 1992.

258. Katakami H, Downs TR, Frohman LA: Decreased hypothalamic growth hormone-releasing hormone content and pituitary responsiveness in hypothyroidism. J Clin Invest 77:1704–1711, 1986.

259. Edwards CA, Dieguez C, Scanlon MF: Effects of hypothyroidism, tri-iodothyronine and glucocorticoids on growth hormone responses to growth hormone-releasing hormone and His-D-Trp-Ala-Trp-D-Phe-Lys-NH2. J Endocrinol 121:31–36, 1989.

260. Wehrenberg WB, Baird A, Ling N: Potent interaction between glucocorticoids and growth hormone-releasing factor in vivo. Science 221:556–558, 1983.

261. Wehrenberg WB, Baird A, Klepper R, et al: Interactions between growth hormone-releasing hormone and glucocorticoids in male rats. Regul Pept 25:147–155, 1989.

262. Miell J, Corder R, Miell PJ, et al: Effects of glucocorticoid treatment and acute passive immunization with growth hormone-releasing hormone and somatostatin antibodies on endogenous and stimulated growth hormone secretion in the male rat. J Endocrinol 131:75–86, 1991.

263. Senaris RM, Lago F, Coya R, et al: Regulation of hypothalamic somatostatin, growth hormone-releasing hormone, and growth hormone receptor messenger ribonucleic acid by glucocorticoids. Endocrinology 137(12):5236–5241, 1996.

264. Asa SL, Kovacs K, Stefaneanu L, et al: Pituitary mammosomatotroph adenomas develop in old mice transgenic for growth hormone-releasing hormone. Proc Soc Exper Biol Med 193(3):232–235, 1990.

265. Asa SL: The role of hypothalamic hormones in the pathogenesis of pituitary adenomas. Pathol Res Pract 187:581–583, 1991.

266. Cronin MJ, Burnier J, Clarke RG: Growth hormone releasing hormone infusion in normal rats enlarges the pituitary within days. J Endocrinol Invest 14(1):34, 1991.

267. Horacek MJ, Campbell GT, Blake CA: Effects of growth hormone-releasing hormone on somatotrophs in anterior pituitary gland allografts in hypophysectomized, orchidectomized hamsters. Cell Tissue Res 253:287–290, 1988.

268. Lehy T, Accary JP, Dubrasquet M, et al: Growth hormone-releasing factor (somatocrinin) stimulates epithelial cell proliferation in the rat digestive tract. Gastroenterology 90(3):646–653, 1986.

269. Hermansen K, Kappelgaard AM: Characterization of growth hormone-releasing hormone stimulation of the endocrine pancreas: Studies with alpha- and beta-adrenergic and cholinergic antagonists. Acta Endocrinologica 114(4):589–594, 1987.

270. Bailey CJ, Wilkes LC, Flatt PR, et al: Effects of growth hormone-releasing hormone on the secretion of islet hormones and on glucose homeostasis in lean and genetically obese-diabetic (ob/ob) mice and normal rats. J Endocrinol 123(1):19–24, 1989.

271. Green IC, Southern C, Ray K: Mechanism of action of growth-hormone-releasing hormone in stimulating insulin secretion in vitro from isolated rat islets and dispersed islet cells. Horm Res 33(5):199–204, 1990.

272. Horvath S, Mezey E, Palkovits M: Partial coexistence of growth hormone-releasing hormone and tyrosine hydroxylase in paraventricular neurons in rats. Peptides 10:791–795, 1989.

273. Kentroti S, Vernadakis A: Growth hormone-releasing hormone influences neuronal expression in the developing chick brain. I. Catecholaminergic neurons. Brain Res 49:275–280, 1989.

274. Kentroti S, Vernadakis A: Growth hormone-releasing hormone and somatostatin influence neuronal expression in developing chick brain. II. Cholinergic neurons. Brain Res 512:297–303, 1990.

275. Mitsuma T, Nogimori T, Hirooka Y: Effects of growth hormone-releasing hormone and corticotropin-releasing hormone on the release of thyrotropin-releasing hormone from the rat hypothalamus in vitro. Exper Clin Endocrinol 90:365–368, 1987.

276. Imaki T, Shibasaki T, Hotta M, et al: The satiety effect of growth hormone-releasing factor in rats. Brain Res 340:186–188, 1985.

277. Dickson PR, Vaccarino FJ: Characterization of feeding behavior induced by central injection of GRF. Am J Physiol 259(3 Pt 2):R651–R657, 1990.

278. Vaccarino FJ, Bloom FE, Rivier J, et al: Stimulation of food intake in rats by centrally administered hypothalamic growth hormone-releasing factor. Nature 314:167–168, 1985.

279. Ruckebusch Y, Malbert CH: Stimulation and inhibition of food intake in sheep by centrally-administered hypothalamic releasing factors. Life Sci 38:929–934, 1986.

280. Penny ES, Sopwith AM, Patience RL, et al: Characterization by high-performance liquid chromatography of circulating growth hormone-releasing factors in normal subjects. J Endocrinol 111:507–511, 1986.

281. Wehrenberg WB, Ehlers CL: Effects of growth hormone-releasing factor in the brain. Science 232(4755):1271–1273, 1986.

282. Obal F Jr, Payne L, Opp M, et al: Growth hormone-releasing hormone antibodies suppress sleep and prevent enhancement of sleep after sleep deprivation. Am J Physiol 263(5 Pt 2):R1078–R1085, 1992.

283. Zhang J, Obal F Jr, Zheng T, et al: Intrapreoptic microinjection of GHRH or its antagonist alters sleep in rats. J Neurosci 19(6):2187–2194, 1990.

284. Toppila J, Alanko L, Asikainen M, et al: Sleep deprivation increases somatostatin and growth hormone-releasing hormone messenger RNA in the rat hypothalamus. J Sleep Res 6(3):171–178, 1997.

285. Zhang J, Chen Z, Taishi P, et al: Sleep deprivation increases rat hypothalamic growth hormone-releasing hormone mRNA. Am J Physiol 275(6 Pt 2):R1755–R1761, 1998.

286. Sibilia V, Rigamonti AE, Pagani F, et al: Long-term effects on bone of postnatal

immunization against GHRH in female and male rats. J Endocrinol 177(1):93–100, 2003.

287. Draghia-Akli R, Cummings KK, Khan AS, et al: Effects of plasmid-mediated growth hormone-releasing hormone in severely debilitated dogs with cancer. Mol Ther 6(6):830–836, 2002.

288. Bowers CY, Momany F, Reynolds GA, et al: Structure-activity relationships of a synthetic pentapeptide that specifically releases growth hormone in vitro. Endocrinology 106(3):663–667, 1980.

289. Bowers CY, Momany FA, Reynolds GA, et al: On the in vitro and in vivo activity of a new synthetic hexapeptide that acts on the pituitary to specifically release growth hormone. Endocrinology 114(5):1537–1545, 1984.

290. Bowers CY, Sartor AO, Reynolds GA, et al: On the actions of the growth hormone-releasing hexapeptide, GHRP. Endocrinology 128(4):2027–2035, 1991.

291. Bowers CY, Reynolds GA, Durham D, et al: Growth hormone (GH)-releasing peptide stimulates GH release in normal men and acts synergistically with GH-releasing hormone. J Clin Endocrinol Metab 70(4):975–982, 1990.

292. Howard AD, Feighner SD, Cully DF, et al: A receptor in pituitary and hypothalamus that functions in growth hormone release. Science 273(5277):974–977, 1996.

293. Conn PM, Bowers CY: A new receptor for growth hormone-release peptide. Science 273(5277):923, 1996.

294. Kojima M, Hosada H, Date Y, et al: Ghrelin is a growth-hormone-releasing acylated peptide from stomach. Nature 402:656–660, 1999.

295. Korbonits M, Bustin SA, Kojima M, et al: The expression of the growth hormone secretagogue receptor ligand ghrelin in normal and abnormal human pituitary and other neuroendocrine tumors. J Clin Endocrinol Metab 86:881–887, 2001.

296. Cowley MA, Smith RG, Diano S, et al: The distribution and mechanism of action of ghrelin in the CNS demonstrates a novel hypothalamic circuit regulating energy homeostasis. Neuron 37:649–661, 2003.

297. Wortley KE, Anderson KD, Garcia K, et al: Genetic deletion of ghrelin does not decrease food intake but influences metabolic fuel preference. Proc Natl Acad Sci U S A 101(21):8227–8232, 2004.

298. Nass R, Liu J, Hellman P, et al: Chronic changes in peripheral growth hormone levels do not affect ghrelin stomach mRNA expression and serum ghrelin levels in three transgenic mouse models. J Neuroendocrinol 16(8):669–675, 2004.

299. Katakami H, Shimizu K, Kimura N, et al: Cloning and characterization of ghrelin and GHRH in the rhesus monkey, Macaca mulatto. 86th Annual Meeting of the Endocrine Society, New Orleans., 2004. Abstr. OR47-2.

300. Tschöp M, Smiley DL, Heiman ML: Ghrelin induces adiposity in rodents. Nature 407:908–913, 2000.

301. Tomasetto C, Karam SM, Ribieras S, et al: Identification and characterization of a novel gastric peptide hormone: The motilin-related peptide. Gastroenterology 119:395–405, 2000.

302. Hosoda H, Kojima M, Matsuo H, et al: Purification and characterization of rat des-Gln14-Ghrelin, a second endogenous ligand for the growth hormone secretagogue receptor. J Biol Chem 275:21995–22000, 2000.

303. Hosoda H, Kojima M, Mizushima T, et al: Structural divergence of human ghrelin. Identification of multiple ghrelin-derived molecules produced by post-translational processing. J Biol Chem 278:64–70, 2003.

304. Broglio F, Benso A, Gottero C, et al: Non-acylated ghrelin does not possess the pituitaric and pancreatic endocrine activity of acylated ghrelin in humans. J Endocrinol Invest 26:192–196, 2003.

305. Banks WA, Tschöp M, Robinson SM, et al: Extent and direction of ghrelin transport across the blood-brain barrier is determined by its unique primary structure. J Pharmacol Exp Ther 302:822–827, 2002.

306. Nanzer AM, Khalaf S, Mozid AM, et al: Ghrelin exerts a proliferative effect on a rat pituitary somatotroph cell line via the mitogen-activated protein kinase (MAPK) pathway. Eur J Endocrinol 151:233–240, 2004.

307. Thompson NM, Gill DA, Davies R, et al: Ghrelin and des-octanoyl ghrelin promote adipogenesis directly in vivo by a mechanism independent of GHS-R1a. Endocrinology 145:232–242, 2004.

308. Baldanzi G, Filigheddu N, Cutrupi S, et al: Ghrelin and des-acyl ghrelin inhibit cell death in cardiomyocytes and endothelial cells through ERK1/2 and PI 3-kinase/AKT. J Cell Biol 159:1029–1037, 2002.

309. Cassoni P, Papotti M, Ghe C, et al: Identification, characterization, and biological activity of specific receptors for natural (ghrelin) and synthetic growth hormone secretagogues and analogs in human breast carcinomas and cell lines. J Clin Endocrinol Metab 86:1738–1745, 2001.

310. Pemberton C, Wimalasena P, Yandle T, et al: C-terminal pro-ghrelin peptides are present in the human circulation. Biochem Biophys Res Commun. 310:567–573, 2003.

311. Sloan JH, Green NK, Mistry JS, et al: Developement of radioimmunoassays to measure different molecular forms of ghrelin. Proceedings of the 85th Meeting of the Endocrine Society, 3–88, 496, 2003.

312. Liu J, Gaylinn BD, Nass RM, et al: Effects of prolonged fasting on circulating ghrelin levels in healthy young men. Proceedings of the 86th Meeting of the Endocrine Society, 1–49, 166, 2004.

313. Palyha OC, Feighner SD, Tan CP, et al: Ligand activation domain of human orphan growth hormone (GH) secretagogue receptor (GHS-R) conserved from pufferfish to humans. Mol Endocrinol 14:160–169, 2000.

314. Date Y, Kojima M, Hosoda H, et al: Ghrelin, a novel growth hormone-releasing acylated peptide, is synthesized in a distinct endocrine cell type in the gastrointestinal tracts of rats and humans. Endocrinology 141: 4255–4261, 2000.

315. Dornonville dlC, Bjorkqvist M, Sandvik AK, et al: A-like cells in the rat stomach contain ghrelin and do not operate under gastrin control. Regul Pept 99:141–150, 2001.

316. Leonetti F, Silecchia G, Iacobellis G, et al: Different plasma ghrelin levels after laparoscopic gastric bypass and adjustable gastric banding in morbid obese subjects. J Clin Endocrinol Metab 88:4227–4231, 2003.

317. Toshinai K, Date Y, Murakami N, et al: Ghrelin-induced food intake is mediated via the orexin pathway. Endocrinology 144:1506–1512, 2003.

318. Mozid AM, Tringali G, Forsling ML, et al: Ghrelin is released from rat hypothalamic explants and stimulates corticotrophin-releasing hormone and arginine-vasopressin. Horm Metab Res 35:455–459, 2003.

319. Gnanapavan S, Kola B, Bustin SA, et al: The tissue distribution of the mRNA of ghrelin and subtypes of its receptor, GHS-R, in humans. J Clin Endocrinol Metab 87:2988–2991, 2002.

320. Korbonits M, Kojima M, Kangawa K, et al: Presence of ghrelin in normal and adenomatous human pituitary. Endocrine 14:101–104, 2001.

321. Kanamoto N, Akamizu T, Hosoda H, et al: Substantial production of ghrelin by a human medullary thyroid carcinoma cell line. J Clin Endocrinol Metab 86:4984–4990, 2001.

322. Papotti M, Cassoni P, Volante M, et al: Ghrelin-producing endocrine tumors of the stomach and intestine. J Clin Endocrinol Metab 86:5052–5059, 2001.

323. Volante M, Allia E, Fulcheri E, et al: Ghrelin in fetal thyroid and follicular tumors and cell lines: Expression and effects on tumor growth. Am J Pathol 162:645–654, 2003.

324. Iwakura H, Hosoda K, Doi R, et al: Ghrelin expression in islet cell tumors: Augmented expression of ghrelin in a case of glucagonoma with multiple endocrine neoplasm type I. J Clin Endocrinol Metab 87:4885–4888, 2002.

325. Rindi G, Savio A, Torsello A, et al: Ghrelin expression in gut endocrine growths. Histochem Cell Biol 117:521–525, 2002.

326. Hattori N, Saito T, Yagyu T, et al: GH, GH receptor, GH secretagogue receptor, and ghrelin expression in human T cells, B cells, and neutrophils. J Clin Endocrinol Metab 86:4284–4291, 2001.

327. Dixit VM, Schaffer EM, Taub DD: Ghrelin is expressed and secreted from human T lymphocytes and inhibits activation and leptin induced inflammatory cytokine expression via functional, lipid raft-associated growth hormone secretagogue receptors (GHS-R). Proceedings of the 85th Annual Meeting of the Endocrine Society, 2003. OR51-3.

328. Volante M, Allia E, Gugliotta P, et al: Expression of ghrelin and of the GH secretagogue receptor by pancreatic islet cells and related endocrine tumors. J Clin Endocrinol Metab 87:1300–1308, 2002.

329. Date Y, Nakazato M, Hashiguchi S, et al: Ghrelin is present in pancreatic alpha-cells of humans and rats and stimulates insulin secretion. Diabetes 51:124–129, 2002.

330. Wierup N, Svensson H, Mulder H, et al: The ghrelin cell: A novel developmentally regulated islet cell in the human pancreas. Regul Pept 107:63–69, 2002.

331. Prado CL, Pugh-Bernard AE, Elghazi L, et al: Ghrelin cells replace insulin-producing {beta} cells in two mouse models of pancreas development. Proc Natl Acad Sci U S A 101:2924–2929, 2004.

332. Volante M, Fulcheri E, Allia E, et al: Ghrelin expression in fetal, infant, and adult human lung. J Histochem Cytochem 50:1013–1021, 2002.

333. Gualillo O, Caminos J, Blanco M, et al: Ghrelin, a novel placental-derived hormone. Endocrinology 142:788–794, 2001.

334. Barreiro ML, Gaytan F, Caminas JE, et al: Cellular location and hormonal regulation of ghrelin expression in rat testis. Biol Reprod 67:1768–1776, 2002.

335. Tena-Sempere M, Barreiro ML, Gonzalez LC, et al: Novel expression and functional role of ghrelin in rat testis. Endocrinology 143:717–725, 2002.

336. Mori K, Yoshimoto A, Takaya K, et al: Kidney produces a novel acylated peptide, ghrelin. FEBS Lett 486:213–216, 2000.

337. Caminos JE, Tena-Sempere M, Gaytan F, et al: Expression of ghrelin in the cyclic and pregnant rat ovary. Endocrinology 144:1594–1602, 2003.

338. Gaytan F, Barreiro ML, Chopin LK, et al: Immunolocalization of ghrelin and its functional receptor, the type 1a growth hormone secretagogue receptor, in the cyclic human ovary. J Clin Endocrinol Metab 88:879–887, 2003.

339. Caminos JE, Nogueiras R, Blanco M, et al: Cellular distribution and regulation of ghrelin mRNA in the rat pituitary gland. Endocrinology 144:5089–5097, 2003.

340. Cummings DE, Purnell JQ, Frayo RS, et al: A preprandial rise in plasma ghrelin levels suggests a role in meal initiation in humans. Diabetes 50:1714–1719, 2001.

341. Cummings DE, Weigle DS, Frayo RS, et al: Plasma ghrelin levels after diet-induced weight loss or gastric bypass surgery. N Engl J Med 346:1623–1630, 2002.

342. Chan JL, Bullen J, Lee JH, et al: Ghrelin levels are not regulated by recombinant leptin administration and/or three days of fasting in healthy subjects. J Clin Endocrinol Metab 89(1):335–343, 2004.

343. Ariyasu H, Takaya K, Tagami T, et al: Stomach is a major source of circulating ghrelin, and feeding state determines plasma ghrelin-like immunoreactivity levels in humans. J Clin Endocrinol Metab 86:4753–4758, 2001.

344. Tschöp M, Weyer C, Tataranni P, et al: Circulating ghrelin levels are decreased in human obesity. Diabetes 50:707–709, 2001.

345. Shiiya T, Nakazato M, Mizuta M, et al: Plasma ghrelin levels in lean and obese humans and the effect of glucose on ghrelin secretion. J Clin Endocrinol Metab 87:240–244, 2002.

346. McLaughlin T, Abbasi F, Lamendola C, et al: Plasma ghrelin concentrations are decreased in insulin-resistant obese adults relative to equally obese insulin-sensitive controls. J Clin Endocrinol Metab 89(4):1630–1635, 2004.

347. Purnell JQ, Weigle DS, Breen P, et al: Ghrelin levels correlate with insulin levels, insulin resistance, and high-density lipoprotein cholesterol, but not with gender, menopausal status, or cortisol levels in humans. J Clin Endocrinol Metab 88:5747–5752, 2003.

348. Barkan AL, Dimaraki EV, Jessup SK, et al: Ghrelin secretion in humans is sexually dimorphic, suppressed by somatostatin, and not affected by the ambient growth hormone levels. J Clin Endocrinol Metab 88:2180–2184, 2003.

349. Elias KA, Ingle GS, Burnier JP, et al: In vitro characterization of four novel classes of growth hormone-releasing peptide. Endocrinology 136(12):5694–5699, 1995.

350. Hansen BS, Raun K, Nielsen KK, et al: Pharmacological characterisation of a new oral GH secretagogue, NN703. Eur J Endocrinol 141(2):180–189, 1990.

351. Hansen BS, Ankersen M, Hansen TK, et al: Pharmakokinetics of NN703. Eur J Endocrinol 141:180–189, 1999.

352. Patchett AA, Nargund RP, Tata JR, et al: Design and biological activities of L-163,191 (MK-0677): A potent, orally active growth hormone secretagogue. Proc Natl Acad Sci U S A 92(15):7001–7005, 1995.

353. Guerlavais V, Boeglin D, Mousseaux D, et al: New active series of growth hormone secretagogues. J Med Chem 46(7):1191–1203, 2003.

354. Pan LC, Carpino PA, Lefker BA, et al: Preclinical pharmacology of CP-424,391, an orally active pyrazolinone-piperidine [correction of pyrazolidinone-piperidine] growth hormone secretagogue [erratum appears in Endocrine 2001 Apr;14(3):437]. Endocrine 14(1):121–132, 2001.

355. Nagamine J, Nagata R, Seki H, et al: Pharmacological profile of a new orally active growth hormone secretagogue, SM-130686. J Endocrinol 171(3):481–489, 2001.

356. Kojima M, Hosoda H, Locatelli V, et al: Ghrelin is a growth-hormone-releasing acylated peptide from stomach. Nature 402(6762):656–660, 1999.

357. Torsello A, Locatelli V, Melis MR, et al: Differential orexigenic effects of hexarelin and its analogs in the rat hypothalamus: Indication for multiple growth hormone secretagogue receptor subtypes. Neuroendocrinology 72(6):327–332, 2000.

358. Halem HA, Taylor JE, Dong JZ, et al: Novel analogs of ghrelin: Physiological and clinical implications. Eur J Endocrinol 151(Suppl 2):S071–S075, 2004.

359. Momany FA, Bowers CY, Reynolds GA, et al: Design, synthesis, and biological activity of peptides which release growth hormone in vitro. Endocrinology 108(1):31–39, 1981.

360. Bowers CY: GH releasing peptides-structure and kinetics. J Pediatr Endocrinol 6:21–31, 1993.

361. Deghenghi R, Cananzi MM, Torsello A, et al: GH-releasing activity of Hexarelin, a new growth hormone releasing peptide, in infant and adult rats. Life Sci 54(18):1321–1328, 1994.

362. Arvat E, di Vito L, Maccagno B, et al: Effects of GHRP-2 and hexarelin, two synthetic GH-releasing peptides, on GH, prolactin, ACTH and cortisol levels in man. Comparison with the effects of GHRH, TRH and hCRH. Peptides 18(6):885–891, 1997.

363. Ghigo E, Arvat E, Camanni F: Orally active growth hormone secretagogues: State of the art and clinical perspectives. Ann Med 30(2):159–168, 1998.

364. Cheng K, Chan WW, Butler B, et al: Stimulation of growth hormone release from rat primary pituitary cells by L-692,429, a novel non-peptidyl GH secretagogue. Endocrinology 132(6):2729–2731, 1993.

365. Gertz BJ, Barrett JS, Eisenhandler R, et al: Growth hormone response in man to L-692,429, a novel nonpeptide mimic of growth hormone-releasing peptide-6. J Clin Endocrinol Metab 77(5):393–397, 1993.

366. Aloi JA, Gertz BJ, Hartman ML, et al: Neuroendocrine responses to a novel growth hormone secretagogue, L-692,429, in healthy older subjects. J Clin Endocrinol Metab 79(4):943–949, 1994.

367. Smith RG, Van der Ploeg LH, Howard AD, et al: Peptidomimetic regulation of growth hormone secretion. Endocrine Rev 18(5):621–645, 1997.

368. Chapman IM, Hartman ML, Pezzoli SS, et al: Enhancement of pulsatile growth hormone secretion by continuous infusion of a growth

hormone-releasing peptide mimetic, L-692,429, in older adults—a clinical research center study. J Clin Endocrinol Metab 81(8):2874–2880, 1996.

369. Raun K, Hansen BS, Johansen NL, et al: Ipamorelin, the first selective growth hormone secretagogue. Eur J Endocrinol 139(5):552–561, 1998.

370. Locke W, Kirgis HD, Bowers CY, et al: Intracerebroventricular growth-hormone-releasing peptide-6 stimulates eating without affecting plasma growth hormone responses in rats. Life Sci 56(16):1347–1352, 1995.

371. Torsello A, Luoni M, Schweiger F, et al: Novel hexarelin analogs stimulate feeding in the rat through a mechanism not involving growth hormone release. Eur J Pharmacol 360(2–3):123–129, 1998.

372. Frieboes RM, Murck H, Maier P, et al: Growth hormone-releasing peptide-6 stimulates sleep, growth hormone, ACTH and cortisol release in normal man. Neuroendocrinology 61(5):584–589, 1995.

373. Bisi G, Podio V, Valetto MR, et al: Acute cardiovascular and hormonal effects of GH and hexarelin, a synthetic GH-releasing peptide, in humans. J Endocrinol Invest 22(4):266–272, 1999.

374. Broglio F, vM, Podio V, et al: The acute administration of hexarelin, a synthetic GHRP, but not of growth hormone increases left ventricular ejection fraction in normal man. 80th Endocrine Society Meeting, 1998. Abstr. OR 15-3.

375. Locatelli V, Torsello A: Growth hormone secretagogues: Focus on the growth hormone-releasing peptides. Pharmacol Res 36(6):415–423, 1997.

376. Dickson SL, Leng G, Dyball RE, et al: Central actions of peptide and non-peptide growth hormone secretagogues in the rat. Neuroendocrinology 61(1):36–43, 1995.

377. Sirinathsinghji DJ, Chen HY, Hopkins R, et al: Induction of c-fos mRNA in the arcuate nucleus of normal and mutant growth hormone-deficient mice by a synthetic non-peptidyl growth hormone secretagogue. Neuroreport 6(15):1989–1992, 1995.

378. Torsello A, Grilli R, Luoni M, et al: Mechanism of action of Hexarelin. I. Growth hormone-releasing activity in the rat. Eur J Endocrinol 135(4):481–488, 1996.

379. Locatelli V, Grilli R, Torsello A, et al: Growth hormone-releasing hexapeptide is a potent stimulator of growth hormone gene expression and release in the growth hormone-releasing hormone-deprived infant rat. Pediatr Res 36(2):169–174, 1994.

380. Bennett PA, Thomas GB, Howard AD, et al: Hypothalamic growth hormone secretagogue-receptor (GHS-R) expression is regulated by growth hormone in the rat. Endocrinology 138(11):4552–4557, 1997.

381. Loche S, Cambiaso P, Merola B, et al: The effect of hexarelin on growth hormone (GH) secretion in patients with GH deficiency. J Clin Endocrinol Metab 80(9):2692–2696, 1995.

382. Popovic V, Damjanovic S, Micic D, et al: Blocked growth hormone-releasing peptide (GHRP-6)-induced GH secretion and absence of the synergic action of GHRP-6 plus GH-releasing hormone in patients with hypothalamopituitary disconnection: Evidence that GHRP-6 main action is exerted at the hypothalamic level. J Clin Endocrinol Metab 80(3):942–947, 1995.

383. Hickey GJ, Drisko J, Faidley T, et al: Mediation by the central nervous system is critical to the in vivo activity of the GH secretagogue L-692,585. J Endocrinol 148(2):371–380, 1996.

384. Cheng K, Chan WW, Butler B, et al: Evidence for a role of protein kinase-C in His-D-Trp-Ala-Trp-D-Phe-Lys-NH2-induced growth hormone release from rat primary pituitary cells. Endocrinology 129(6):3337–3342, 1991.

385. Akman MS, Girard M, O'Brien LF, et al: Mechanisms of action of a second generation growth hormone-releasing peptide (Ala-His-D-beta Nal-Ala-Trp-D-Phe-Lys-NH2) in rat anterior pituitary cells. Endocrinology 132(3):1286–1291, 1993.

386. Pong SS, Chaung LY, Dean DC, et al: Identification of a new G-protein-linked receptor for growth hormone secretagogues. Mol Endocrinol 10(1):57–61, 1996.

387. McKee KK, Tan CP, Palyha OC, et al: Cloning and characterization of two human G protein-coupled receptor genes (GPR38 and GPR39) related to the growth hormone secretagogue and neurotensin receptors. Genomics 46(3):426–434, 1997.

388. Tan CP, McKee KK, Liu Q, et al: Cloning and characterization of a human and murine T-cell orphan G-protein-coupled receptor similar to the growth hormone secretagogue and neurotensin receptors. Genomics 52(2):223–229, 1998.

389. Feighner SD, Tan CP, McKee KK, et al: Receptor for motilin identified in the human gastrointestinal system. Science 284(5423):2184–2188, 1999.

390. Muccioli G, Ghe C, Ghigo MC, et al: Specific receptors for synthetic GH secretagogues in the human brain and pituitary gland. J Endocrinol 157(1):99–106, 1998.

391. Guan XM, Yu H, Palyha OC, et al: Distribution of mRNA encoding the growth hormone secretagogue receptor in brain and peripheral tissues. Brain Res 48(1):23–29, 1997.

392. Okada K, Ishii S, Minami S, et al: Intracerebroventricular administration of the growth hormone-releasing peptide KP-102 increases food intake in free-feeding rats. Endocrinology 137(11):5155–5158, 1996.

393. Yokote R, Sato M, Matsubara S, et al: Molecular cloning and gene expression of growth hormone-releasing peptide receptor in rat tissues. Peptides 19(1):15–20, 1998.

394. Adams EF, Huang B, Buchfelder M, et al: Presence of growth hormone secretagogue receptor messenger ribonucleic acid in human pituitary tumors and rat GH3 cells. J Clin Endocrinol Metab 83(2):638–642, 1998.

395. Skinner MM, Nass R, Lopes B, et al: Growth hormone secretagogue receptor expression in human pituitary tumors. J Clin Endocrinol Metab 83(12):4314–4320, 1998.

396. Korbonits M, Jacobs RA, Aylwin SJ, et al: Expression of the growth hormone secretagogue receptor in pituitary adenomas and other neuroendocrine tumors. J Clin Endocrinol Metab 83(10):3624–3630, 1998.

397. Renner U, Brockmeier S, Strasburger CJ, et al: Growth hormone (GH)-releasing peptide stimulation of GH release from human somatotroph adenoma cells: Interaction with GH-releasing hormone, thyrotropin-releasing hormone, and octreotide. J Clin Endocrinol Metab 78(5):1090–1096, 1994.

398. Cheng K, Chan WW, Barreto A Jr, et al: The synergistic effects of His-D-Trp-Ala-Trp-D-Phe-Lys-NH2 on growth hormone(GH)-releasing factor-stimulated GH release and intracellular adenosin 3′,5′-monophosphate accumulation in rat pituitary cell culture. Endocrinology 124:2791–2798, 1989.

399. Cunha SR, Mayo KE: Ghrelin and growth hormone (GH) secretagogues potentiate GH-releasing hormone (GHRH)-induced cyclic adenosine 3′,5′-monophosphate production in cells expressing transfected GHRH and GH secretagogue receptors. Endocrinology 143:4570–4582, 2002.

400. Cheng J, Wu TJ, Butler B, et al: Growth hormone releasing peptides: A comparison of the growth hormone releasing activities of GHRP-2 and GHRP-6 in rat primary pituitary cells. Life Sci 60(16):1385–1392, 1997.

401. Orkin RD, New DI, Norman D, et al: Rapid desensitisation of the growth hormone secretagogue (ghrelin) receptor to hexarelin in vitro. J Endocrinol Invest 26:743–747, 2003.

402. Murphy MG, Weiss S, McClung M, et al: Effect of alendronate and MK-677 (a growth hormone secretagogue), individually and in combination, on markers of bone turnover and bone mineral density in postmenopausal osteoporotic women. J Clin Endocrinol Metab 86:1116–1125, 2001.

403. Holst B, Cygankiewicz A, Jensen TH, et al: High constitutive signaling of the ghrelin receptor-identification of a potent inverse agonist. Mol Endocrinol 17:2201–2210, 2003.

404. Kamegai J, Wakabayashi I, Miyamoto K, et al: Growth hormone-

dependent regulation of pituitary GH secretagogue receptor (GHS-R) mRNA levels in the spontaneous dwarf Rat. Neuroendocrinology 68(5):312–318, 1998.

405. Kamegai J, Wakabayashi I, Kineman RD, et al: Growth hormone-releasing hormone receptor (GHRHR) and growth hormone secretagogue receptor (GHS-R) mRNA levels during postnatal development in male and female rats. J Neuroendocrinology 11(4):299–306, 1999.

406. Kineman RD, Kamegai J, Frohman LA: Growth hormone (GH)-releasing hormone (GHRH) and the GH secretagogue (GHS), L692,585, differentially modulate rat pituitary GHS receptor and GHRH receptor messenger ribonucleic acid levels. Endocrinology 140(8):3581–3586, 1999.

407. Smith RG, Griffin PR, Xu Y, et al: Adenosine: A partial agonist of the growth hormone secretagogue receptor. Biochem Biophys Res Commun 276:1306–1313, 2000.

408. Tullin S, Hansen BS, Ankersen M, et al: Adenosine is an agonist of the growth hormone secretagogue receptor. Endocrinology 141:3397–3402, 2000.

409. Deghenghi R, Papotti M, Ghigo E, et al: Cortistatin, but not somatostatin, binds to growth hormone secretagogue (GHS) receptors of human pituitary gland. J Endocrinol Invest 24:RC1–RC3, 2001.

410. Muccioli G, Papotti M, Locatelli V, et al: Binding of 125I-labelled ghrelin to membranes from human hypothalamus and pituitary gland. J Endocrinol Invest 24(3):RC7–RC9, 2001.

411. Papotti M, Ghe C, Cassoni P, et al: Growth hormone secretagogue binding sites in peripheral human tissues. J Clin Endocrinol Metab 85:3803–3807, 2000.

412. Beaumont NJ, Skinner VO, Tan TM, et al: Ghrelin can bind to a species of high-density lipoprotein associated with paraoxonase. J Biol Chem 278(11):8877–8880, 2003.

413. Bodart V, Febbraio M, Demers A, et al: CD36 mediates the cardiovascular action of growth hormone-releasing peptides in the heart. Circ Res 90:844–849, 2002.

414. Torsello A, Bresciani E, Rossoni G, et al: Ghrelin plays a minor role in the physiological control of cardiac function in the rat. Endocrinology 144(5):1787–1792, 2003.

415. Sethumadhavan K, Veeraragavan K, Bowers CY: Demonstration and characterization of the specific binding of growth hormone-releasing peptide to rat anterior pituitary and hypothalamic membranes. Biochem Biophys Res Comm 178(1):31–37, 1991.

416. Codd EE, Shu AY, Walker RF: Binding of a growth hormone releasing hexapeptide to specific hypothalamic and pituitary binding sites.

Neuropharmacology 28(10):1139–1144, 1989.

417. Ong H, McNicoll N, Escher E, et al: Identification of a pituitary growth hormone-releasing peptide (GHRP) receptor subtype by photoaffinity labeling. Endocrinology 139(1):432–435, 1998.

418. De Gennaro Colonna V, Rossoni G, et al: Cardiac ischemia and impairment of vascular endothelium function in hearts from growth hormone-deficient rats: Protection by hexarelin. Eur J Pharmacol 334(2–3):201–217, 1997.

419. Bodart V, Febbraio M, Demers A, et al: CD36 mediates the cardiovascular action of growth hormone-releasing peptides in the heart. Circ Res 90(8):844–849, 2002.

420. Lei T, Buchfelder M, Fahlbusch R, et al: Growth hormone releasing peptide (GHRP-6) stimulates phosphatidylinositol (PI) turnover in human pituitary somatotroph cells. J Mol Endocrinol 14(1):135–138, 1995.

421. Mitani M, Kaji H, Abe H, et al: Growth hormone (GH)-releasing peptide and GH releasing hormone stimulate GH release from subpopulations of somatotrophs in rats. J Neuroendocrinol 8(11):825–830, 1996.

422. Goth MI, Lyons CE, Canny BJ, et al: Pituitary adenylate cyclase activating polypeptide, growth hormone (GH)-releasing peptide and GH-releasing hormone stimulate GH release through distinct pituitary receptors. Endocrinology 130(2):939–944, 1992.

423. Soliman EB, Hashizume T, Kanematsu S: Effect of growth hormone (GH)-releasing peptide (GHRP) on the release of GH from cultured anterior pituitary cells in cattle. Endocrine J 41(5):585–591, 1994.

424. Smith RG, Pong SS, Hickey G, et al: Modulation of pulsatile GH release through a novel receptor in hypothalamus and pituitary gland. Rec Prog Horm Res 51:261–285; discussion 285–286, 1996.

425. Chen C, Wu D, Clarke IJ: Signal transduction systems employed by synthetic GH-releasing peptides in somatotrophs. J Endocrinology 148(3):381–386, 1996.

426. Giustina A, Bonfanti C, Licini M, et al: Hexarelin, a novel GHRP-6 analog, stimulates growth hormone (GH) release in a GH-secreting rat cell line (GH1) insensitive to GH-releasing hormone. Regul Pept 70(1):49–54, 1997.

427. Torsello A, Luoni M, Grilli R, et al: Hexarelin stimulation of growth hormone release and mRNA levels in an infant and adult rat model of impaired GHRH function. Neuroendocrinology 65(2):91–97, 1997.

428. Guillaume V, Magnan E, Cataldi M, et al: Growth hormone (GH)-releasing hormone secretion is stimulated by a

new GH-releasing hexapeptide in sheep. Endocrinology 135(3):1073–1076, 1994.

429. Bercu BB, Yang SW, Masuda R, et al: Role of selected endogenous peptides in growth hormone-releasing hexapeptide activity: Analysis of growth hormone-releasing hormone, thyroid hormone-releasing hormone, and gonadotropin-releasing hormone. Endocrinology 130(5):2579–2586, 1992.

430. Conley LK, Teik JA, Deghenghi R, et al: Mechanism of action of hexarelin and GHRP-6: Analysis of the involvement of GHRH and somatostatin in the rat. Neuroendocrinology 61(1):44–50, 1995.

431. Jansson J-O, Downs TR, Beamer WG, Frohman LA: The dwarf 'little' (lit/lit) mouse is resistant to growth hormone (GH)-releasing peptide (GH-RP-6) as well as to GH releasing hormone (GRH). In 68th Annual Meeting of the Endocrine Society. Anaheim, California, 1986.

432. Fletcher TP, Thomas GB, Willoughby JO, et al: Constitutive growth hormone secretion in sheep after hypothalamopituitary disconnection and the direct in vivo pituitary effect of growth hormone releasing peptide 6. Neuroendocrinology 60(1):76–86, 1994.

433. Tannenbaum GS, Lapointe M, Beaudet A, et al: Expression of growth hormone secretagogue-receptors by growth hormone-releasing hormone neurons in the mediobasal hypothalamus. Endocrinology 139(10):4420–4423, 1998.

434. Dickson SL, Luckman SM: Induction of c-fos messenger ribonucleic acid in neuropeptide Y and growth hormone (GH)-releasing factor neurons in the rat arcuate nucleus following systemic injection of the GH secretagogue, GH-releasing peptide-6. Endocrinology 138(2):771–777, 1997.

435. Korbonits M, Little JA, Forsling ML, et al: The effect of growth hormone secretagogues and neuropeptide Y on hypothalamic hormone release from acute rat hypothalamic explants. J Neuroendocrinology 11(7):521–528, 1999.

436. Wren AM, Small CJ, Fribbens CV, et al: The hypothalamic mechanisms of the hypophysiotropic action of ghrelin. Neuroendocrinol 76:316–324, 2002.

437. Cattaneo L, Luoni M, Settembrini B, et al: Effect of long-term administration of Hexarelin on the somatotrophic axis in aged rats. Pharmacol Res 36(1):49–54, 1997.

438. Rosskamp R, Becker M, Haverkamp F, et al: Plasma levels of growth hormone-releasing hormone and somatostatin in response to a mixed meal and during sleep in children. Acta Endocrinologica 116:549–554, 1987.

439. Penny ES, Penman E, Price J, et al: Circulating growth hormone releasing

factor concentrations in normal subjects and patients with acromegaly. Br Med J 289(6443):453–455, 1984.

440. Inoue S, Katakami H, Hidaka H, et al: Peripheral plasma levels of human growth hormone releasing hormone (GHRH) during the sleep test in short children. Endocrine J 45(Suppl):S71–S75, 1998.

441. Sopwith AM, Penny ES, Lytras N, et al: Dissociation between circulating concentrations of immunoreactive growth hormone releasing factor and growth hormone in normal human subjects. Clin Sci 72(2):181–185, 1987.

442. Frohman LA, Downs TR, Williams TC, et al: Rapid enzymatic degradation of growth hormone-releasing hormone by plasma in vitro and in vivo to a biologically inactive product cleaved at the NH2 terminus. J Clin Invest 78:906–913, 1986.

443. Katakami H, Hashida S, Hidaka H, et al: Development and clinical application of a highly sensitive enzyme immunoassay (EIA) for human growth hormone-releasing hormone (hGHRH) in plasma. Endocrine J 45(Suppl):S67–S70, 1998.

444. Thorner MO, Frohman LA, Leong DA, et al: Extrahypothalamic growth-hormone-releasing factor (GRF) secretion is a rare cause of acromegaly: Plasma GRF levels in 177 acromegalic patients. J Clin Endocrinol Metab 59(5):846–849, 1984.

445. Sano T, Asa SL, Kovacs K: Growth hormone-releasing hormone-producing tumors: Clinical, biochemical, and morphological manifestations. Endocrine Rev 9(3):357–573, 1988.

446. Faglia G, Arosio M, Bazzoni N: Ectopic acromegaly. Endocrinol Metab Clin North Am 21(3):575–595, 1992.

447. Osella G, Orlandi F, Caraci P, et al: Acromegaly due to ectopic secretion of GHRH by bronchial carcinoid in a patient with empty sella [see comment]. J Endocrinol Invest 26(2):163–169, 2003.

448. Kovacs M, Kineman RD, Schally AV, et al: Effects of antagonists of growth hormone-releasing hormone (GHRH) on GH and insulin-like growth factor I levels in transgenic mice overexpressing the human GHRH gene, an animal model of acromegaly. Endocrinology 138(11):4536–4542, 1997.

449. Sano T, Yamasaki R, Saito H, et al: Growth hormone-releasing hormone (GHRH)-secreting pancreatic tumor in a patient with multiple endocrine neoplasia type I. Am J Surg Pathol 11(10):810–819, 1987.

450. Asa SL, Singer W, Kovacs K, et al: Pancreatic endocrine tumour producing growth hormone-releasing hormone associated with multiple endocrine neoplasia type I syndrome. Acta Endocrinologica 115(3):331–337, 1987.

451. Ramsay JA, Kovacs K, Asa SL, et al: Reversible sellar enlargement due to growth hormone-releasing hormone production by pancreatic endocrine tumors in a acromegalic patient with multiple endocrine neoplasia type I syndrome. Cancer 62(2):445–450, 1988.

452. Yamasaki R, Saito H, Sano T, et al: Ectopic growth hormone-releasing hormone (GHRH) syndrome in a case with multiple endocrine neoplasia type I. Endocrinologia Japonica 35(1): 97–109, 1988.

453. Liu SW, van de Velde CJ, Heslinga JM, et al: Acromegaly caused by growth hormone-relating hormone in a patient with multiple endocrine neoplasia type I. Jap J Clin Oncol 26(1):49–52, 1996.

454. Asa SL, Scheithauer BW, Bilbao JM, et al: A case for hypothalamic acromegaly: A clinicopathological study of six patients with hypothalamic gangliocytomas producing growth hormone-releasing factor. J Clin Endocrinol Metab 58(5):796–803, 1984.

455. Bevan JS, Asa SL, Rossi ML, et al: Intrasellar gangliocytoma containing gastrin and growth hormone-releasing hormone associated with a growth hormone-secreting pituitary adenoma. Clin Endocrinol 30:213–224, 1989.

456. Kojima K, Miyake M, Nakagawa H, et al: Multiple gastric carcinoids and pituitary adenoma in type A gastritis. Int Med 36(11):787–789, 1997.

457. Garcia-Rojas JF, Mangas A, Barba A, et al: Role of growth hormone-releasing hormone on pentagastrin-induced growth hormone release in normal subjects. J Endocrinol Invest 14(3):241–244, 1991.

458. Donnadieu M, Evain-Brion D, Tonon MC, et al: Variations of plasma growth hormone (GH)-releasing factor levels during GH stimulation tests in children. J Clin Endocrinol Metab 60:1132–1134, 1985.

459. Argente J, Evain Brion D, Donnadieu M, et al: Impaired response of growth hormone-releasing hormone (GHRH) measured in plasma after L-dopa stimulation in patients with idiopathic delayed puberty. Acta Paediatr 76(2):266–270, 1987.

460. Mitsuhashi S, Yamasaki R, Miyazaki S, et al: Effect of oral administration of L-dopa on the plasma levels of growth hormone-releasing hormone (GHRH) in normal subjects and patients with various endocrine and metabolic diseases. Nippon Naibunpi Gakkai Zasshi—Folia Endocrinologica Japonica 63:934–946, 1987.

461. Chihara K, Kashio Y, Kita T, et al: L-dopa stimulates release of hypothalamic growth hormone-releasing hormone in humans. J Clin Endocrinol Metab 62: 466–473, 1986.

462. Kashio Y, Chihara K, Kita T, et al: Effect of oral glucose administration on plasma growth hormone-releasing hormone (GHRH)-like immunoreactivity levels in normal subjects and patients with idiopathic

GH deficiency: Evidence that GHRH is released not only from the hypothalamus but also from extrahypothalamic tissue. J Clin Endocrinol Metab 64:92–97, 1987.

463. Rosskamp R, Becker M, Tegeler A, et al: Effect of insulin-induced hypoglycemia on circulating levels of plasma growth hormone-releasing hormone and somatostatin in children. Horm Res 27:121-125, 1987.

464. Kashio Y, Chihara K, Kaji H, et al: Presence of growth hormone-releasing factor-like immunoreactivity in human cerebrospinal fluid. J Clin Endocrinol Metab 60:396–398, 1985.

465. Growth Hormone Research Society: Consensus guidelines for the diagnosis and treatment of adults with growth hormone deficiency: Summary statement of the Growth Hormone Research Society Workshop on Adult Growth Hormone Deficiency. J Clin Endocrinol Metab 83:379–381, 1998.

466. Rahim A, Toogood AA, Shalet SM: The assessment of growth hormone status in normal young adult males using a variety of provocative tests. Clin Endocrinol 45:557–562, 1996.

467. Shibasaki T, Shizume K, Nakahara M, et al: Age-related changes in plasma growth hormone response to growth hormone-releasing factor in man. J Clin Endocrinol Metab 58(1):212–214, 1984.

468. Thorner MO, Rivier J, Spiess J, et al: Human pancreatic growth-hormone-releasing factor selectively stimulates growth-hormone secretion in man. Lancet 1(8314-5):24–28, 1983.

469. Wood SM, Ch'ng JL, Adams EF, et al: Abnormalities of growth hormone release in response to human pancreatic growth hormone releasing factor (GRF (1-44)) in acromegaly and hypopituitarism. Br Med J 286:1687–1691, 1983.

470. Rosenthal SM, Schriock EA, Kaplan SL, et al: Synthetic human pancreas growth hormone-releasing factor (hpGRF1-44-NH2) stimulates growth hormone secretion in normal men. J Clin Endocrinol Metab 57:677–679, 1983.

471. Gelato MC, Pescovitz OH, Cassorla F, et al: Dose-response relationships for the effects of growth hormone-releasing factor-(1-44)-NH2 in young adult men and women. J Clin Endocrinol Metab 59:197–201, 1984.

472. Sassolas G, Chatelain P, Cohen R, et al: Effects of human pancreatic tumor growth hormone-releasing hormone (hpGRH1-44-NH2) on immunoreactive and bioactive plasma growth hormone in normal young men. J Clin Endocrinol Metab 59: 705–709, 1984.

473. Lang I, Schernthaner G, Pietschmann P, et al: Effects of sex and age on growth hormone response to growth hormone-releasing hormone in healthy individuals. J Clin Endocrinol Metab 65:535–540, 1987.

474. Chihara K, Kashio Y, Abe H, et al: Idiopathic growth hormone (GH)

deficiency, and GH deficiency secondary to hypothalamic germinoma: Effect of single and repeated administration of human GH-releasing factor (hGRF) on plasma GH level and endogenous hGRF-like immunoreactivity level in cerebrospinal fluid. J Clin Endocrinol Metab 60:269–278, 1985.

475. Evans WS, Borges JL, Vance ML, et al: Effects of human pancreatic growth hormone-releasing factor-40 on serum growth hormone, prolactin, luteinizing hormone, follicle-stimulating hormone, and somatomedin-C concentrations in normal women throughout the menstrual cycle. J Clin Endocrinol Metab 59(5):1006–1010, 1984.

476. Vance ML, Borges JL, Kaiser DL, et al: Human pancreatic tumor growth hormone-releasing factor: Dose-response relationships in normal man. J Clin Endocrinol Metab 58(5):838–844, 1984.

477. Gelato M, Malozowski S, Nicoletti M: Responses to growth hormone releasing hormone during development and puberty in normal boys and girls. In Symposium on Recent Developments in the Study of Growth Factors: GRF and Somatomedin, Paris, 1985.

478. Ghigo E, Bellone J, Aimaretti G, et al: Reliability of provocative tests to assess growth hormone secretory status. Study in 472 normally growing children. J Clin Endocrinol Metab 81(9):3323–3327, 1996.

479. Gelato MC, Malozowski S, Caruso-Nicoletti M, et al: Growth hormone (GH) responses to GH-releasing hormone during pubertal development in normal boys and girls: Comparison to idiopathic short stature and GH deficiency. J Clin Endocrinol Metab 63:174–179, 1986.

480. Ross RJ, Grossman A, Davies PS, et al: Stilboestrol pretreatment of children with short stature does not affect the growth hormone response to growth hormone-releasing hormone. Clin Endocrinol 27:155–161, 1987.

481. Iovino M, Monteleone P, Steardo L: Repetitive growth hormone-releasing hormone administration restores the attenuated growth hormone (GH) response to GH-releasing hormone testing in normal aging. J Clin Endocrinol Metab 69(4):910–913, 1989.

482. Coiro V, Volpi R, Cavazzini U, et al: Restoration of normal growth hormone responsiveness to GHRH in normal aged men by infusion of low amounts of theophylline. J Gerontol 46(5):M155–M158, 1991.

483. Corpas E, Harman SM, Blackman MR: Human growth hormone and human aging. Endocrine Rev 14:20–39, 1993.

484. Ghigo E, Goffi S, Nicolosi M, et al: Growth hormone (GH) responsiveness to combined administration of arginine and GH-releasing hormone

does not vary with age in man. J Clin Endocrinol Metab 71(6):1481–1485, 1990.

485. Ghigo E, Goffi S, Arvat E, et al: Pyridostigmine partially restores the GH responsiveness to GHRH in normal aging. Acta Endocrinologica 123(2):169–173, 1990.

486. Alba-Roth J, Muller OA, Schopohl J, et al: Arginine stimulates growth hormone secretion by suppressing endogenous somatostatin secretion. J Clin Endocrinol Metab 67(6):1186–1189, 1988.

487. Ross RJ, Tsagarakis S, Grossman A, et al: GH feedback occurs through modulation of hypothalamic somatostatin under cholinergic control: Studies with pyridostigmine and GHRH. Clin Endocrinol 27(6):727–733, 1987.

488. Grossman A, Savage MO, Besser GM: Growth hormone releasing hormone. Clin Endocrinol Metab 15(3):607–627, 1986.

489. Ranke MB, Gruhler M, Rosskamp R, et al: Testing with growth hormone-releasing factor (GRF(1-29)NH2) and somatomedin C measurements for the evaluation of growth hormone deficiency. Eur J Pediatr 145(6):485–492, 1986.

490. Bozzola M, Tato L, Cisternino M, et al: Synthetic growth hormone-releasing hormone (GHRH 1-44) in the differential diagnosis between hypothalamic and pituitary GH deficiency. J Endocrinol Invest 9:503–506, 1986.

491. Takano K, Hizuka N, Shizume K, et al: Plasma growth hormone (GH) response to GH-releasing factor in normal children with short stature and patients with pituitary dwarfism. J Clin Endocrinol Metab 58:236–241, 1984.

492. Schonberg D: Diagnosis of growth hormone deficiency. Baillieres Clin Endocrinol Metab 6(3):527–546, 1992.

493. Shalet SM, Toogood A, Rahim A, et al: The diagnosis of growth hormone deficiency in children and adults. Endocrine Rev 19:203–223, 1998.

494. Toogood AA, Jones J, O'Neill PA, et al: The diagnosis of severe growth hormone deficiency in elderly patients with hypothalamic-pituitary disease. Clin Endocrinol 48:569–576, 1998.

495. Hoeck HC, Jakobsen PE, Vestergaard P, et al: Differences in reproducibility and peak growth hormone responses to repeated testing with various stimulators in healthy adults. Growth Horm IGF Res 9(1):18–24, 1999.

496. Chatelain P, Alamercery Y, Blanchard J, et al: Growth hormone (GH) response to a single intravenous injection of synthetic GH-releasing hormone in prepubertal children with growth failure. J Clin Endocrinol Metab 65(3):387–394, 1987.

497. Schriock EA, Lustig RH, Rosenthal SM, et al: Effect of growth hormone (GH)-releasing hormone (GRH) on plasma GH in relation to magnitude and duration of GH deficiency in

26 children and adults with isolated GH deficiency or multiple pituitary hormone deficiencies: Evidence for hypothalamic GRH deficiency. J Clin Endocrinol Metab 58:1043–1049, 1984.

498. Laron Z, Keret R, Bauman B, et al: Differential diagnosis between hypothalamic and pituitary hGH deficiency with the aid of synthetic GH-RH 1-44. Clin Endocrinol 21:9–12, 1984.

499. Pintor C, Puggioni R, Fanni V, et al: Growth-hormone releasing factor and clonidine in children with constitutional growth delay. Evidence for defective pituitary growth hormone reserve. J Endocrinol Invest 7:253–256, 1984.

500. Reiter JC, Craen M, van Vliet G: Decreased growth hormone response to growth hormone-releasing hormone in Turner's syndrome: Relation to body weight and adiposity. Acta Endocrinologica 125:38–42, 1991.

501. Sartorio A, Spada A, Conti A, et al: Effect of two consecutive administrations of GHRH in children with constitutional growth delay. Eur J Pediatr 149:678–679, 1990.

502. Lannering B, Albertsson-Wikland K: Growth hormone release in children after cranial irradiation. Horm Res 27(1):13–22, 1987.

503. Takano K, Shizume K, Imura H, et al: Plasma growth hormone (GH) response to GH-releasing factor (SM-8144) in children of short stature and patients with GH deficiency. Endocrinologia Japonica 34(1):117–128, 1987.

504. Cappa M, Loche S, Borrelli P, et al: Growth hormone response to growth hormone releasing hormone 1-40 in Turner's syndrome. Horm Res 27(1):1–6, 1987.

505. Rogol AD, Blizzard RM, Johanson AJ, et al: Growth hormone release in response to human pancreatic tumor growth hormone-releasing hormone 1-40 in children with short stature. J Clin Endocrinol Metab 59(4):580–586, 1984.

506. Ahmed SR, Shalet SM: Hypothalamic growth hormone releasing factor deficiency following cranial irradiation. Clin Endocrinol 21:483–488, 1984.

507. Romer TE, Rymkiewicz-Kluczynska B, Olivier M, et al: Growth hormone-releasing hormone reverses secondary somatotroph unresponsiveness. J Clin Endocrinol Metab 72:503–506, 1991.

508. Hindmarsh PC, Swift PG: An assessment of growth hormone provocation tests. Arch Dis Child 72(4):362–367; discussion 367–368, 1995.

509. Dysken MW, Skare SS, Burke MS, et al: Intrasubject reproducibility of growth hormone-releasing hormone-stimulated growth hormone in older women, older men, and younger men. Biol Psychiatry 33(8–9):610–617, 1993.

510. Williams T, Berelowitz M, Joffe SN, et al: Impaired growth hormone responses to growth hormone-releasing

factor in obesity. A pituitary defect reversed with weight reduction. N Engl J Med 311(22):1403–1407, 1984.

511. Scacchi M, Pincelli AI, Cavagnini F: Growth hormone in obesity. Int J Obes Relat Metab Disord 23(3):260–271, 1999.

512. Ghigo E, Procopio M, Boffano GM, et al: Arginine potentiates but does not restore the blunted growth hormone response to growth hormone-releasing hormone in obesity. Metabolism 41(5):560–563, 1992.

513. Bing-You RG, Bigos ST, Oppenheim DS: Serum growth hormone response to growth hormone-releasing hormone in non-obese and obese adults with hypopituitarism. Metabolism 42(6):790–794, 1993.

514. Cordido F, Casanueva FF, Dieguez C: Cholinergic receptor activation by pyridostigmine restores growth hormone (GH) responsiveness to GH-releasing hormone administration in obese subjects: Evidence for hypothalamic somatostatinergic participation in the blunted GH release of obesity. J Clin Endocrinol Metab 68(2):290–293, 1989.

515. Ghigo E, Imperiale E, Boffano GM, et al: A new test for the diagnosis of growth hormone deficiency due to primary pituitary impairment: Combined administration of pyridostigmine and growth hormone-releasing hormone. J Endocrinol Invest 13(4):307–316, 1990.

516. Valetto MR, Bellone J, Baffoni C, et al: Reproducibility of the growth hormone response to stimulation with growth hormone-releasing hormone plus arginine during lifespan. Eur J Endocrinol 135(5):568–572, 1996.

517. Cappa M, Loche S, Salvatori R, et al: The growth hormone response to pyridostigmine plus growth hormone releasing hormone is not influenced by pubertal maturation. J Endocrinol Invest 14(1):41–45, 1991.

518. Maghnie M, Cavigioli F, Tinelli C, et al: GHRH plus arginine in the diagnosis of acquired GH deficiency of childhood-onset. J Clin Endocrinol Metab 87(6):2740–2744, 2002.

519. Groisne C, Trivin C, Souberbielle JC, et al: Factors influencing the growth hormone response to growth hormone-releasing hormone in children with idiopathic growth hormone deficiency. Horm Res 58(2):94–98, 2002.

520. Donaubauer J, Kiess W, Kratzsch J, et al: Re-assessment of growth hormone secretion in young adult patients with childhood-onset growth hormone deficiency. Clin Endocrinol 58(4):456–463, 2003.

521. Ghigo E, Aimaretti G, Gianotti L, et al: New approach to the diagnosis of growth hormone deficiency in adults. Eur J Endocrinol 134(3):352–356, 1996.

522. Aimaretti G, Corneli G, Razzore P, et al: Comparison between insulin-induced hypoglycemia and growth hormone (GH)-releasing hormone + arginine as provocative tests for the diagnosis of GH deficiency in adults. J Clin Endocrinol Metab 83(5):1615–1618, 1998.

523. Biller BM, Samuels MH, Zagar A, et al: Sensitivity and specificity of six tests for the diagnosis of adult GH deficiency. J Clin Endocrinol Metab 87(5):2067–2079, 2002.

524. Darzy KH, Aimaretti G, Wieringa G, et al: The usefulness of the combined growth hormone (GH)-releasing hormone and arginine stimulation test in the diagnosis of radiation-induced GH deficiency is dependent on the post-irradiation time interval. J Clin Endocrinol Metab 88(1):95–102, 2003.

525. Thorner MO, Reschke J, Chitwood J, et al: Acceleration of growth in two children treated with human growth hormone-releasing factor. N Engl J Med 312(1):4–9, 1985.

526. Thorner MO, Rogol AD, Blizzard RM, et al: Acceleration of growth rate in growth hormone-deficient children treated with human growth hormone-releasing hormone. Pediatr Res 24(2):145–151, 1988.

527. Low LC: The therapeutic use of growth-hormone-releasing hormone. J Pediatr Endocrinol 6(1):15–20, 1993.

528. Brain CE, Hindmarsh PC, Brook CG: Continuous subcutaneous GHRH(1-29)NH2 promotes growth over 1 year in short, slowly growing children. Clin Endocrinol 32(2):153–163, 1990.

529. Neyzi O, Yordam N, Ocal G, et al: Growth response to growth hormone-releasing hormone(1-29)-NH2 compared with growth hormone. Acta Paediatrica 388(suppl):16–21; discussion 22, 1993.

530. Chen RG, Shen YN, Yei J, et al: A comparative study of growth hormone (GH) and GH-releasing hormone(1-29)-NH2 for stimulation of growth in children with GH deficiency. Acta Paediatrica 388(Suppl):32–35; discussion 36, 1993.

531. Ross RJ, Rodda C, Tsagarakis S, et al: Treatment of growth-hormone deficiency with growth-hormone-releasing hormone. Lancet 1(8523):5–8, 1987.

532. Takano K, Hizuka N, Asakawa K, et al: Human growth hormone-releasing hormone (hGH-RH; hGRF) treatment of four patients with GH deficiency. Endocrinologia Japonica 35:775–781, 1988.

533. Smith PJ, Brook CG: Growth hormone releasing hormone or growth hormone treatment in growth hormone insufficiency? Arch Dis Child 63(6):629–634, 1988.

534. Butenandt O, Staudt B: Comparison of growth hormone releasing hormone therapy and growth hormone therapy in growth hormone deficiency. Eur J Pediatr 148(5):393–395, 1989.

535. Duck SC, Schwarz HP, Costin G, et al: Subcutaneous growth hormone-releasing hormone therapy in growth hormone-deficient children: First year of therapy. J Clin Endocrinol Metab 75(4):1115–1120, 1992.

536. Kirk JM, Trainer PJ, Majrowski WH, et al: Treatment with GHRH(1-29)NH2 in children with idiopathic short stature induces a sustained increase in growth velocity. Clin Endocrinol 41(4):487–493, 1994.

537. Pasqualini T, Ferraris J, Fainstein-Day P, et al: Growth acceleration in children with chronic renal failure treated with growth-hormone-releasing hormone (GHRH). Medicina 56(3):241–246, 1996.

538. Ogilvy-Stuart AL, Stirling CJH, Kelnar MO, et al: Treatment of radiation-induced growth hormone deficiency with growth hormone-releasing hormone. Clin Endocrinol 46(5):571–578, 1997.

539. Rochiccioli PE, Tauber MT, Coude FX, et al: Results of 1-year growth hormone (GH)-releasing hormone-(1-44) treatment on growth, somatomedin-C, and 24-hour GH secretion in six children with partial GH deficiency. J Clin Endocrinol Metab 65:268–274, 1987.

540. Bozzola M, Biscaldi I, Cisternino M, et al: Long term growth hormone (GH)-releasing hormone and biosynthetic GH therapy in GH-deficient children: comparison of therapeutic effectiveness. J Endocrinol Invest 13(3):235–239, 1990.

541. Lievre M, Chatelain P, Van Vliet G, et al: Treatment with growth hormone-releasing hormone (GHRH) 1-44 in children with idiopathic growth hormone deficiency: A randomized double-blind dose-effect study. The GHRH European Multicenter Study (GEMS) Group. Fundam Clin Pharmacol 6(8–9):359–366, 1992.

542. Wit JM, Otten BJ, Waelkens JJ, et al: Short-term effect on growth of two doses of GRF 1-44 in children with growth hormone deficiency: Comparison with growth induced by methionyl-GH administration. Horm Res 27:181–189, 1987.

543. Lanes R, Carrillo E: Long-term therapy with a single daily subcutaneous dose of growth hormone releasing hormone (1-29) in prepubertal growth hormone deficient children. Venezuelan Collaborative Study Group. J Pediatr Endocrinol 7(4):303–308, 1994.

544. Thorner M, Rochiccioli P, Colle M, et al: Once daily subcutaneous growth hormone-releasing hormone therapy accelerates growth in growth hormone-deficient children during the first year of therapy. Geref International Study Group. J Clin Endocrinol Metab 81(3):1189–1196, 1996.

545. Low LC, Wang C, Cheung PT, et al: Long term pulsatile growth hormone (GH)-releasing hormone therapy in children with GH deficiency. J Clin Endocrinol Metab 66(3):611–617, 1988.

546. Lippe BM, Van Herle AJ, LaFranchi SH, et al: Reversible hypothyroidism in

growth hormone-deficient children treated with human growth hormone. J Clin Endocrinol Metab 40(4):612–618, 1975.

547. Ghigo E, Arvat E, Aimaretti G, et al: Diagnostic and therapeutic uses of growth hormone-releasing substances in adult and elderly subjects. Baillieres Clin Endocrinol Metab 12(2):341–358, 1998.

548. Nakamura S, Mizuno M, Katakami H, et al: Aging-related changes in in vivo release of growth hormone-releasing hormone and somatostatin from the stalk-median eminence in female rhesus monkeys (Macaca mulatta). J Clin Endocrinol Metab 88(2):827–833, 2003.

549. Corpas E, Harman SM, Pinegro MA, et al: Growth hormone (GH)-releasing hormone-(1-29) twice daily reverses the decreased GH and insulin-like growth factor-I levels in old men. J Clin Endocrinol Metab 75(2):530–535, 1992.

550. Corpas E, Harman SM, Pinegro MA, et al: Continuous subcutaneous infusions of growth hormone (GH) releasing hormone 1-44 for 14 days increase GH and insulin-like growth factor-I levels in old men. J Clin Endocrinol Metab 76(1):134–138, 1993.

551. Vittone J, Blackman M, Busby-Whitehead J, et al: Effects of single nightly injections of growth hormone-releasing hormone (GHRH 1-29) in healthy elderly men. Metabolism 46(1):89–96, 1997.

552. Laron Z, Frenkel J, Gil-Ad I, et al: Growth hormone releasing activity by intranasal administration of a synthetic hexapeptide (hexarelin). Clin Endocrinol 41(4):539–541, 1994.

553. Imbimbo BP, Mant T, Edwards M, et al: Growth hormone-releasing activity of hexarelin in humans. A dose-response study. Eur J Clin Pharmacol 46(5):421–425, 1994.

554. Casanueva FF, Micic D, Pombo M, et al: Role of the new growth hormone-releasing secretagogues in the diagnosis of some hypothalamopituitary pathologies. Metabolism 45(8 Suppl 1):123–126, 1996.

555. Arvat E, Gianotti L, Grottoli S, et al: Arginine and growth hormone-releasing hormone restore the blunted growth hormone-releasing activity of hexarelin in elderly subjects. J Clin Endocrinol Metab 79(5):1440–1443, 1994.

556. Cordido F, Penalva A, Dieguez C, et al: Massive growth hormone (GH) discharge in obese subjects after the combined administration of GH-releasing hormone and GHRP-6: Evidence for a marked somatotroph secretory capability in obesity. J Clin Endocrinol Metab 76(4):819–823, 1993.

557. Micic D, Popovic V, Doknic M, et al: Preserved growth hormone (GH) secretion in aged and very old subjects after testing with the combined stimulus GH-releasing hormone plus GH-releasing hexapeptide-6. J Clin Endocrinol Metab 83(7):2569–2572, 1998.

558. Penalva A, Carballo A, Pombo M, et al: Effect of growth hormone (GH)-releasing hormone (GHRH), atropine, pyridostigmine, or hypoglycemia on GHRP-6-induced GH secretion in man. J Clin Endocrinol Metab 76(1):168–171, 1993.

559. Micic D, Mallo F, Peino R, et al: Regulation of growth hormone secretion by the growth hormone releasing hexapeptide (GHRP-6). J Pediatr Endocrinol 6(3–4):283–289, 1993.

560. Maheshwari HG, Rahim A, Shalet SM, et al: Selective lack of growth hormone (GH) response to the GH-releasing peptide hexarelin in patients with GH-releasing hormone receptor deficiency. J Clin Endocrinol Metab 84(3):956–959, 1999.

561. Maghnie M, Spica-Russotto V, Cappa M, et al: The growth hormone response to hexarelin in patients with different hypothalamic-pituitary abnormalities. J Clin Endocrinol Metab 83(11):3886–3889, 1998.

562. Arvat E, Gianotti L, Di Vito L, et al: Modulation of growth hormone-releasing activity of hexarelin in man. Neuroendocrinology 61(1):51–56, 1995.

563. Ghigo E, Arvat E, Rizzi G, et al: Arginine enhances the growth hormone-releasing activity of a synthetic hexapeptide (GHRP-6) in elderly but not in young subjects after oral administration. J Endocrinol Invest 17(3):157–162, 1994.

564. Ghigo E, Arvat E, Muccioli G, et al: Growth hormone-releasing peptides. Eur J Endocrinol 136(5):445–460, 1997.

565. Laron Z, Bowers CY, Hirsch D, et al: Growth hormone-releasing activity of growth hormone-releasing peptide-1 (a synthetic heptapeptide) in children and adolescents. Acta Endocrinologica 129(5):424–426, 1993.

566. Bellone J, Aimaretti G, Bartolotta E, et al: Growth hormone-releasing activity of hexarelin, a new synthetic hexapeptide, before and during puberty. J Clin Endocrinol Metab 80(4):1090–1094, 1995.

567. Loche S, Bizzarri C, Maghnie M, et al: The growth hormone-releasing activity of hexarelin, a new synthetic hexapeptide, in short normal and obese children and in hypopituitary subjects. J Clin Endocrinol Metab 80(2):674–678, 1995.

568. Ghigo E, Arvat E, Rizzi G, et al: Growth hormone-releasing activity of growth hormone-releasing peptide-6 is maintained after short-term oral pretreatment with the hexapeptide in normal aging. Eur J Endocrinol 131(5):499–503, 1994.

569. Penalva A, Pombo M, Carballo A, et al: Influence of sex, age and adrenergic pathways on the growth hormone response to GHRP-6. Clin Endocrinol 38(1):87–91, 1993.

570. Micic D, Popovic V, Kendereski A, et al: The sequential administration of growth hormone-releasing hormone followed 120 minutes later by hexarelin, as an effective test to assess the pituitary GH reserve in man. Clin Endocrinol 45(5):543–551, 1996.

571. Gasperi M, Aimaretti G, Scarcello G, et al: Low dose hexarelin and growth hormone (GH)-releasing hormone as a diagnostic tool for the diagnosis of GH deficiency in adults: Comparison with insulin-induced hypoglycemia test. J Clin Endocrinol Metab 84(8):2633–2637, 1999.

572. Peino R, Leal A, Garcia-Mayor RV, et al: The use of growth hormone (GH) secretagogues in the diagnosis of GH deficiency in humans. Growth Horm IGF Res 9(Suppl A):101–105, 1999.

573. Casanueva FF, Dieguez C: Interaction between body composition, leptin and growth hormone status. Baillieres Clin Endocrinol Metab 12(2):297–314, 1998.

574. Rahim A, O'Neill PA, Shalet SM: The effect of body composition on hexarelin-induced growth hormone release in normal elderly subjects. Clin Endocrinol 49(5):659–664, 1998.

575. Casanueva FF, Burguera B, Tome MA, et al: Depending on the time of administration, dexamethasone potentiates or blocks growth hormone releasing hormone-induced growth hormone release in man. Neuroendocrinology 47:46–49, 1988.

576. Trainer PJ, Kirk JM, Savage MO, et al: Pyridostigmine partially reverses dexamethasone-induced inhibition of the growth hormone response to growth hormone-releasing hormone. J Endocrinol 134(3):513–517, 1992.

577. Frantz AG, Rabkin MT: Human growth hormone: Clinical measurement, response to hypoglycaemia and suppression by corticosteroids. N Engl J Med 271:1375–1381, 1964.

578. Magiakou MA, Mastorakos G, Gomez MT, et al: Suppressed spontaneous and stimulated growth hormone secretion in patients with Cushing's disease before and after surgical cure. J Clin Endocrinol Metab 78(1):131–137, 1994.

579. Leal-Cerro A, Pumar A, Garcia E, et al: Inhibition of growth hormone release after the combined administration of GHRH and GHRP-6 in patients with Cushing's syndrome. Clin Endocrinol 41(5):649–654, 1994.

580. Leal-Cerro A, Pumar A, Villamil F, et al: Growth hormone releasing hormone priming increases growth hormone secretion in patients with Cushing's syndrome. Clin Endocrinol 38(4):399–403, 1993.

581. Momany FA, Bowers CY, Reynolds GA, et al: Conformational energy studies and in vitro and in vivo activity data on growth hormone-releasing

peptides. Endocrinology 114(5):1531–1536, 1984.

582. McDowell RS, Elias KA, Stanley MS, et al: Growth hormone secretagogues: Characterization, efficacy, and minimal bioactive conformation. Proc Natl Acad Sci U S A 92(24):11165–11169, 1995.

583. Rahim A, O'Neill PA, Shalet SM: Growth hormone status during long-term hexarelin therapy. J Clin Endocrinol Metab 83(5):1644–1649, 1998.

584. Svensson J, Lonn L, Jansson JO, et al: Two-month treatment of obese subjects with the oral growth hormone (GH) secretagogue MK-677 increases GH secretion, fat-free mass, and energy expenditure. J Clin Endocrinol Metab 83(2):362–369, 1998.

585. Loche S, Colao A, Cappa M, et al: The growth hormone response to hexarelin in children: reproducibility and effect of sex steroids. J Clin Endocrinol Metab 82(3):861–864, 1997.

586. Mericq V, Cassorla F, SalazarT, et al: Effects of eight months treatment with graded doses of a growth hormone (GH)-releasing peptide in GH-deficient children. J Clin Endocrinol Metab 83(7): 2355–2360, 1998.

587. Yu H, Cassorla F, Tiulpakov A, Si Y-F, et al: A double blind placebo-controlled efficacy trial of an oral growth hormone (GH) secretagogue (MK-0677) in GH deficient (GHD) children. In 80th Annual Meeting US Endocrine Society, New Orleans, 1998.

588. Codner E, Cassorla F, Tiulpakov AN, et al: Effects of oral administration of ibutamoren mesylate, a nonpeptide growth hormone secretagogue, on the growth hormone-insulin-like growth factor I axis in growth hormone-deficient children. Clin Pharmacol Ther 70(1):91–98, 2001.

589. Laron Z, Frenkel J, Deghenghi R, et al: Intranasal administration of the GHRP hexarelin accelerates growth in short children. Clin Endocrinol 43(5):631–635, 1995.

590. Schambelan M, Mulligan K, Grunfeld C, et al: Recombinant human growth hormone in patients with HIV-associated wasting. A randomized, placebo-controlled trial. Serostim Study Group. Ann Intern Med 125(11):873–882, 1996.

591. Chapman IM, Pescovitz OH, Murphy G, et al: Oral administration of growth hormone (GH) releasing peptide-mimetic MK-677 stimulates the GH/insulin-like growth factor-I axis in selected GH-deficient adults. J Clin Endocrinol Metab 82(10):3455–3463, 1997.

592. Van den Berghe G, deZegher F, Bouillon R: The somatotrophic axis in critical illness: Effects of growth hormone secretagogues. Growth Horm IGF Res 8:153–155, 1998.

593. Van den Berghe G, de Zegher F, Bowers CY, et al: Pituitary responsiveness to GH-releasing hormone, GH-releasing peptide-2 and thyrotrophin-releasing hormone in critical illness. Clin Endocrinol 45(3):341–351, 1996.

594. Van den Berghe G, de Zegher F, Veldhuis JD, et al: The somatotropic axis in critical illness: effect of continuous growth hormone (GH)-releasing hormone and GH-releasing peptide-2 infusion. J Clin Endocrinol Metab 82(2):590–599, 1997.

595. Van den Berghe G, de Zegher F, Baxter RC, et al: Neuroendocrinology of prolonged critical illness: Effects of exogenous thyrotropin-releasing hormone and its combination with growth hormone secretagogues. J Clin Endocrinol Metab 83(2):309–319, 1998.

596. Van den Berghe G, Wouters P, Weekers F, et al: Reactivation of pituitary hormone release and metabolic improvement by infusion of growth hormone-releasing peptide and thyrotropin-releasing hormone in patients with protracted critical illness. J Clin Endocrinol Metab 84(4):1311–1323, 1999.

597. Murphy MG, Plunkett LM, Gertz BJ, et al: MK-677, an orally active growth hormone secretagogue, reverses diet-induced catabolism. J Clin Endocrinol Metab 83(2):320–325, 1998.

598. Neary NM, Small CJ, Wren AM, et al: Ghrelin increases energy intake in cancer patients with impaired appetite: Acute, randomized, placebo-controlled trial. J Clin Endocrinol Metabol 89(6):2832–2836, 2004.

599. Hanada T, Toshinai K, Kajimura N, et al: Anti-cachectic effect of ghrelin in nude mice bearing human melanoma cells. Biochem Biophys Res Comm 301(2):275–279, 2003.

600. Jenkins RC, El Nahas AM, Wikie ME, et al: The effect of dose, nutrition, and age on hexarelin-induced anterior pituitary hormone secretion in adult patients on maintenance hemodialysis. J Clin Endocrinol Metab 84(4):1220–1225, 1999.

601. Takala J, Ruokonen E, Webster NR, et al: Increased mortality associated with growth hormone treatment in critically ill adults. N Engl J Med 341:785–792, 1999.

602. Rudman D, Feller AG, Nagraj HS, et al: Effects of human growth hormone in men over 60 years old. N Engl J Med 323(1):1–6, 1990.

603. Chapman IM, Bach MA, Van Cauter E, et al: Stimulation of the growth hormone (GH)-insulin-like growth factor I axis by daily oral administration of a GH secretogogue (MK-677) in healthy elderly subjects. J Clin Endocrinol Metab 81(12):4249–4257, 1996.

604. Copinschi G, Van Onderbergen A, L'Hermite-Baleriaux M, et al: Effects of a 7-day treatment with a novel, orally active, growth hormone (GH) secretagogue, MK-677, on 24-hour GH profiles, insulin-like growth factor I, and adrenocortical function in normal young men. J Clin Endocrinol Metab 81(8):2776–2782, 1996.

605. Nass R, Pezzoli SS, Clasey JL, et al: Effects of 1-year treatment with MK-677 on 24-h mean GH levels and body composition in healthy older men: A double-blind, placebo-controlled, crossover study of an orally active GH secretagogue. 86th Annual Meeting of the Endocrine Society, New Orleans, 2004. Abstr. P1-427.

606. Murphy MG, Weiss S, McClung M, et al: Effect of alendronate and MK-677 (a growth hormone secretagogue), individually and in combination, on markers of bone turnover and bone mineral density in postmenopausal osteoporotic women. J Clin Endocrinol Metab 86(3):1116–1125, 2001.

607. Bach MA, Rockwood K, Zetterberg C, et al: The effects of MK-0677, an oral growth hormone secretagogue, in patients with hip fracture. J Am Geriatr Soc 52(4):516–523, 2004.

608. Kirk SE, Gertz BJ, Schneider SH, et al: Effect of obesity and feeding on the growth hormone (GH) response to the GH secretagogue L-692,429 in young men. J Clin Endocrinol Metab 82(4):1154–1159, 1997.

609. Locatelli V, Rossoni G, Schweiger F, et al: Growth hormone-independent cardioprotective effects of hexarelin in the rat. Endocrinology 140(9):4024–4031, 1999.

610. Sun Y, Ahmed S, Smith RG: Deletion of ghrelin impairs neither growth nor appetite. Mol Cell Biol 23:7973–7981, 2003.

611. Seoane LM, Tovar S, Baldelli R, et al: Ghrelin elicits a marked stimulatory effect on GH secretion in freely-moving rats. Eur J Endocrinol 143:R7–R9, 2000.

612. Tolle V, Zizzari P, Tomasetto C, et al: In vivo and in vitro effects of ghrelin/motilin-related peptide on growth hormone secretion in the rat. Neuroendocrinol 73:54–61, 2001.

613. Date Y, Murakami N, Kojima M, et al: Central effects of a novel acylated peptide, ghrelin, on growth hormone release in rats. Biochem Biophys Res Commun 275:477–480, 2000.

614. Dickson SL, Doutrelantviltart O, Leng G: GH-deficient dw/dw rats and lit/lit mice show increased fos expression in the hypothalamic arcuate nucleus following systemic injection of GH-releasing peptide-6. J Endocrinol 146:519–526, 1995.

615. Gondo RG, Aguiar-Oliveira MH, Hayashida CY, et al: Growth hormone-releasing peptide-2 stimulates GH secretion in GH-deficient patients with mutated GH-releasing hormone receptor. J Clin Endocrinol Metab 86:3279–3283, 2001.

616. Maheshwari HG, Rahim A, Shalet SM, et al: Selective lack of growth hormone (GH) response to the GH-releasing peptide hexarelin in patients with GH-releasing hormone receptor deficiency. J Clin Endocrinol Metab 84(3):956–959, 1999.

617. Clark RG, Carlsson L, Trojnar J, Robinson ICAF: The effect of growth hormone-releasing peptide and growth hormone-releasing factor on conscious and anaesthetized rats. J Neuroendocrinol 1:249–255, 1989.

618. Conley LK, Teik JA, Deghenghi R, et al: Mechanism of action of hexarelin and GHRP-6—analysis of the involvement of GHRH and somatostatin in the rat. Neuroendocrinology 61:44–50, 1995.

619. Tannenbaum GS, Epelbaum J, Bowers CY: Interrelationship between the novel peptide ghrelin and somatostatin/growth hormone-releasing hormone in regulation of pulsatile growth hormone secretion. Endocrinology 144:967–974, 2003.

620. Pandya N, De Mott-Friberg R, Bowers CY, et al: Growth hormone (GH) releasing peptide-6 requires endogenous hypothalamic GH-releasing hormone for maximal GH stimulation. J Clin Endocrinol Metab 83:1186–1189, 1998.

621. Hayashi S, Kaji H, Ohashi S, et al: Effect of intravenous administration of growth hormone-releasing peptide on plasma growth hormone in patients with short stature. Clin Paediatr Endocrinol 2(Suppl 2):69–74, 1993.

622. Hickey GJ, Drisko J, Faidley T, et al: Mediation by the central nervous system is critical to the in vivo activity of the GH secretagogue L-692,585. J Endocrinol 148:371–380, 1996.

623. Locke W, Kirgis HD, Bowers CY, et al: Intracerebroventricular growth-hormone-releasing peptide-6 stimulates eating without affecting plasma growth-hormone responses in rats. Life Sci 56:1347–1352, 1995.

624. Popovic V, Damjanovic S, Micic D, et al: Blocked growth hormone-releasing peptide (GHRP-6)-induced growth hormone secretion and absence of the synergic action of GHRP-6 plus growth hormone-releasing hormone in patients with hypothalamopituitary disconnection—evidence that GHRP-6 main action is exerted at the hypothalamic level. J Clin Endocrinol Metab 80:942–947, 1995.

625. Popovic V, Miljic D, Micic D, et al: Ghrelin main action on the regulation of growth hormone release is exerted at hypothalamic level. J Clin Endocrinol Metab 88:3450–3453, 2003.

626. Popovic V, Leal A, Micic D, et al: GH-releasing hormone and GH-releasing peptide-6 for diagnostic testing in GH-deficient adults. Lancet 356:1137–1142, 2000.

627. Thompson NM, Davies JS, Mode A, et al: Pattern-dependent suppression of growth hormone (GH) pulsatility by ghrelin and GHRP-6 in moderately GH deficient rats. Endocrinology 144:4859–4867, 2003.

628. Soto JL, Castrillo JL, Dominguez F, et al: Regulation of the pituitary-specific transcription factor GHF-1/PIT-1 messenger-ribonucleic-acid levels by growth-hormone-secretagogues in rat anterior-pituitary-cells in monolayer-culture. Endocrinology 136:3863–3870, 1995.

629. Locatelli V, Grilli R, Torsello A, et al: Growth hormone-releasing hexapeptide is a potent stimulator of growth hormone gene expression and release in the growth hormone-releasing hormone-deprived infant rat. Pediatr Res 36:169–174, 1994.

630. Garcia A, Alvarez CV, Smith RG, et al: Regulation of pit-1 expression by ghrelin and GHRP-6 through the GH secretagogue receptor. Mol Endocrinol 15:1484–1495, 2001.

631. Broglio F, Benso A, Castiglioni C, et al: The endocrine response to ghrelin as a function of gender in humans in young and elderly subjects. J Clin Endocrinol Metab 88:1537–1542, 2003.

632. Tassone F, Broglio F, Destefanis S, et al: Neuroendocrine and metabolic effects of acute ghrelin administration in human obesity. J Clin Endocrinol Metab 88:5478–5483, 2003.

633. Hewson AK, Tung LY, Connell DW, et al: The rat arcuate nucleus integrates peripheral signals provided by leptin, insulin, and a ghrelin mimetic. Diabetes 51:3412–3419, 2002.

634. DeMarinis L, Mancini A, Valle D, et al: Role of food intake in the modulation of hexarelin-induced growth hormone release in normal human subjects. Horm Metab Res 32:152–156, 2000.

635. Date Y, Murakami N, Toshinai K, et al: The role of the gastric afferent vagal nerve in ghrelin-induced feeding and growth hormone secretion in rats. Gastroenterology 123:1120–1128, 2002.

636. Okimura Y, Ukai K, Hosoda H, et al: The role of circulating ghrelin in growth hormone (GH) secretion in freely moving male rats. Life Sci 72:2517–2524, 2003.

637. Helmling S, Maasch C, Eulberg D, et al: Inhibition of ghrelin action in vitro and in vivo by an RNA-Spiegelmer. Proc Natl Acad Sci U S A 101(36):13174–13179, 2004.

638. Corbetta S, Peracchi M, Cappiello V, et al: Circulating ghrelin levels in patients with pancreatic and gastrointestinal neuroendocrine tumors: Identification of one pancreatic ghrelinoma. J Clin Endocrinol Metab 88:3117–3120, 2003.

639. Dall R, Kanaley J, Hansen TK, et al: Plasma ghrelin levels during exercise in healthy subjects and in growth hormone-deficient patients. Eur J Endocrinol 147:65–70, 2002.

640. Eden-Engstrom B, Burman P, Holdstock C, et al: Effects of growth hormone (GH) on ghrelin, leptin, and adiponectin in GH-deficient patients. J Clin Endocrinol Metab 88:5193–5198, 2003.

641. Shuto Y, Shibasaki T, Otagiri A, et al: Hypothalamic growth hormone secretagogue receptor regulates growth hormone secretion, feeding, and adiposity. J Clin Invest 109:1429–1436, 2002.

642. Sun Y, Wang P, Zheng H, Smith RG: Generation and characterization of growth hormone secretagogue receptor knockout mice. Proceedingsof the 85th Annual Meeting of the Endocrine Society, 2003. P1–P216.

643. Freda PU, Reyes CM, Conwell IM, et al: Serum ghrelin levels in acromegaly: Effects of surgical and long-acting octreotide therapy. J Clin Endocrinol Metab 88:2037–2044, 2003.

644. Cappiello V, Ronchi C, Morpurgo PS, et al: Circulating ghrelin levels in basal conditions and during glucose tolerance test in acromegalic patients. Eur J Endocrinol 147:189–194, 2002.

645. Murdolo G, Lucidi P, Di Loreto C, et al: Circulating ghrelin levels of visceral obese men are not modified by a short-term treatment with very low doses of GH replacement. J Endocrinol Invest 26(3):244-249, 2003.

646. Dimaraki EV, Jaffe CA, Bowers CY, et al: Pulsatile and nocturnal growth hormone secretions in men do not require periodic declines of somatostatin. Am J Physiol Endocrinol Metab 285:E163–E170, 2003.

647. Arvat E, Maccario M, Di Vito L, et al: Endocrine activities of ghrelin, a natural GH secretagogue, in humans: Comparison and interactions with hexarelin, a non natural peptidyl GHS, and GH-releasing hormone. J Clin Endocrinol Metab 86:1169–1174, 2001.

648. Korbonits M, Trainer PJ, Besser GM: The effect of an opiate antagonist on the hormonal changes induced by hexarelin. Clin Endocrinol (Oxf) 43:365–371, 1995.

649. Arvat E, Giordano R, Ramunni J, et al: Adrenocorticotropin and cortisol hyperresponsiveness to hexarelin in patients with Cushing's disease bearing a pituitary microadenoma, but not in those with macroadenoma. J Clin Endocrinol Metab 83:4207–4211, 1998.

650. Ghigo E, Arvat E, Ramunni J, et al: Adrenocorticotropin- and cortisol-releasing effect of hexarelin, a synthetic growth hormone-releasing peptide, in normal subjects and patients with Cushing's syndrome. J Clin Endocrinol Metab 82:2439–2444, 1997.

651. Leal-Cerro A, Torres E, Soto A, et al: Ghrelin is no longer able to stimulate growth hormone secretion in patients with Cushing's syndrome but instead induces exaggerated corticotropin and cortisol responses. Neuroendocrinology 76:390–396, 2002.

652. Copinschi G, Van Onderbergen A, L'Hermite-Baleriaux M, et al: Effects of a 7-day treatment with a novel, orally active, growth hormone (GH) secretagogue, MK-677, on 24-hour GH profiles, insulin-like growth factor I, and adrenocortical function in normal young men. J Clin Endocrinol Metab 81:2776–2782, 1996.

653. Rahim A, O'Neill PA, Shalet SM: The effect of chronic hexarelin

administration on the pituitary-adrenal axis and prolactin. J Endocrinol 156:P200, 1998.

654. Cheng K, Chan WW, Butler B, et al: A novel non-peptidyl growth hormone secretagogue. Horm Res 40:109–115, 1993.

655. Korbonits M, Goldstone AP, Gueorguiev M, Grossman AB: Ghrelin—A hormone with multiple functions. Front Neuroendocrinol 25:27–68, 2004.

656. Cowley MA, Pronchuk N, Fan W, et al: Integration of NPY, AGRP, and melanocortin signals in the hypothalamic paraventricular nucleus: Evidence of a cellular basis for the adipostat. Neuron 24:155–163, 1999.

657. Tannenbaum GS, Lapointe M, Beaudet A, et al: Expression of growth hormone secretagogue receptors by growth hormone-releasing hormone neurons in the mediobasal hypothalamus. Endocrinology 139:4420–4423, 1998.

658. Dickson SL, Luckman SM: Induction of c-fos messenger ribonucleic acid in neuropeptide Y and growth hormone (GH)-releasing factor neurones in the rat arcuate nucleus following systemic injection of the GH secretagogue, GH-releasing peptide-6. Endocrinology 138:771–777, 1997.

659. Nakazato M, Murakami N, Date Y, et al: A role for ghrelin in the central regulation of feeding. Nature 409:194–198, 2001.

660. Shintani M, Ogawa Y, Ebihara K, et al: Ghrelin, an endogenous growth hormone secretagogue, is a novel orexigenic peptide that antagonizes leptin action through the activation of hypothalamic neuropeptide Y/Y1 receptor pathway. Diabetes 50:227–232, 2001.

661. Asakawa A, Inui A, Kaga T, et al: Antagonism of ghrelin receptor reduces food intake and body weight gain in mice. Gut 52:947–952, 2003.

662. Lall S, Tung LY, Ohlsson C, et al: Growth hormone (GH)-independent stimulation of adiposity by GH secretagogues. Biochem Biophys Res Commun 280:132–138, 2001.

663. Shibasaki T, Yamauchi N, Takeuchi K, et al: The growth hormone secretagogue KP-102-induced stimulation of food intake is modified by fasting, restraint stress, and somatostatin in rats. Neurosci Lett 255:9–12, 1998.

664. Torsello A, Luoni M, Schweiger F, et al: Novel hexarelin analogs stimulate feeding in the rat through a mechanism not involving growth hormone release. Eur J Pharmacol 360:123–129, 1998.

665. Choi K, Roh SG, Hong YH, et al: The role of ghrelin and growth hormone secretagogues receptor on rat adipogenesis. Endocrinology 144:754–759, 2003.

666. Lawrence CB, Snape AC, Baudoin FM, et al: Acute central ghrelin and GH secretagogues induce feeding and activate brain appetite centers. Endocrinology 143:155–162, 2002.

667. Yamanaka A, Beuckmann CT, Willie JT, et al: Hypothalamic orexin neurons regulate arousal according to energy balance in mice. Neuron 38:701–713, 2003.

668. Broglio F, Arvat E, Benso A, et al: Ghrelin, a natural GH secretagogue produced by the stomach, induces hyperglycemia and reduces insulin secretion in humans. J Clin Endocrinol Metab 86:5083–5086, 2001.

669. Murata M, Okimura Y, Iida K, et al: Ghrelin modulates the downstream of insulin signaling in hepatoma cells. J Biol Chem 277:5667–5674, 2002.

670. Wren AM, Small CJ, Thomas EL, et al: Continuous subcutaneous administration of ghrelin results in accumulation of adipose tissue, independent of hyperphagia or body weight gain. 23rd Joint Meeting of the British Endocrine Societies with the European Federation of Endocrine Societies, Brighton, UK, 2004. 7 OC35.

671. Zhang W, Zhao L, Lin TR, et al: Inhibition of Adipogenesis by Ghrelin. Mol Biol Cell 5(5):2484–2491, 2004.

672. Muccioli G, Broglio F, Valetto MR, et al: Growth hormone-releasing peptides and the cardiovascular system. Ann Endocrinol 61:27–31, 2000.

673. Enomoto M, Nagaya N, Uematsu M, et al: Cardiovascular and hormonal effects of subcutaneous administration of ghrelin, a novel growth hormone-releasing peptide, in healthy humans. Clin Sci 105:431–435, 2003.

674. Imazio M, Bobbio M, Broglio F, et al: GH-independent cardiotropic activities of hexarelin in patients with severe left ventricular dysfunction due to dilated and ischemic cardiomyopathy. Eur J Heart Fail 4:185–191, 2002.

675. Nagaya N, Kangawa K: Ghrelin improves left ventricular dysfunction and cardiac cachexia in heart failure. Curr Opin Pharmacol 3:146–151, 2003.

676. Nagaya N, Kangawa K: Ghrelin, a novel growth hormone-releasing peptide, in the treatment of chronic heart failure. Regul Pept 114:71–77, 2003.

677. Katugampola SD, Pallikaros Z, Davenport AP: [125I-His(9)]-ghrelin, a novel radioligand for localizing GHS orphan receptors in human and rat tissue: Up-regulation of receptors with atherosclerosis. Br J Pharmacol 134:143–149, 2001.

678. Matsumura K, Tsuchihashi T, Fuji K, et al: Neural regulation of blood pressure by leptin and the related peptides. Regul Pept 114:79-86, 2003.

679. Masuda Y, Tanaka T, Inomata N, et al: Ghrelin stimulates gastric acid secretion and motility in rats. Biochem Biophys Res Commun 276:905-908, 2000.

680. Asakawa A, Inui A, Kaga T, et al: A role of ghrelin in neuroendocrine and behavioral responses to stress in mice. Neuroendocrinol 74:143–147, 2001.

681. Weikel JC, Wichniak A, Ising M, et al: Ghrelin promotes slow-wave sleep in man. Am J Physiol Endocrinol Metab 284:E407–E415, 2002.

682. Copinschi G, Leproult R, Van Onderbergen A, et al: Prolonged oral treatment with MK-677, a novel growth hormone secretagogue, improves sleep quality in man. Neuroendocrinol 66:278–286, 1997.

683. Obal JF, Alt J, Taishi P, et al: Sleep in mice with non-functional growth hormone releasing hormone receptors. Am J Physiol Regul Integr Comp Physiol 284:R131–R139, 2003.

684. Carlini VP, Monzon ME, Varas MM, et al: Ghrelin increases anxiety-like behavior and memory retention in rats. Biochem Biophys Res Commun 299:739–743, 2002.

685. Hansen TK, Dall R, Hosoda H, et al: Weight loss increases circulating levels of ghrelin in human obesity. Clin Endocrinol (Oxf) 56:203–206, 2002.

686. Wisse BE, Frayo RS, Schwartz MW, et al: Reversal of cancer anorexia by blockade of central melanocortin receptors in rats. Endocrinology 142:3292–3301, 2001.

687. Shimizu Y, Nagaya N, Isobe T, et al: Increased plasma ghrelin level in lung cancer cachexia. Clin Cancer Res 9:774–778, 2003.

688. Nagaya N, Uematsu M, Kojima M, et al: Elevated circulating level of ghrelin in cachexia associated with chronic heart failure: Relationships between ghrelin and anabolic/catabolic factors. Circulation 104:2034–2038, 2001.

689. Otto B, Cuntz U, Fruehauf E, et al: Weight gain decreases elevated plasma ghrelin concentrations of patients with anorexia nervosa. Eur J Endocrinol 145:669–673, 2001.

690. Nakai Y, Hosoda H, Nin K, et al: Plasma levels of active form of ghrelin during oral glucose tolerance test in patients with anorexia nervosa. Eur J Endocrinol 149:R001–R003, 2003.

691. Nedvidkova J, Krykorkova I, Bartak V, et al: Loss of meal-induced decrease in plasma ghrelin levels in patients with anorexia nervosa. J Clin Endocrinol Metab 88:1678–1682, 2003.

692. Tolle V, Kadem M, Bluet-Pajot MT, et al: Balance in ghrelin and leptin plasma levels in anorexia nervosa patients and constitutionally thin women. J Clin Endocrinol Metab 88:109–116, 2003.

693. Muller AF, Lamberts SW, Janssen JA, et al: Ghrelin drives GH secretion during fasting in man. Eur J Endocrinol 146:203–207, 2002.

694. Tanaka M, Naruo T, Yasuhara D, et al: Fasting plasma ghrelin levels in subtypes of anorexia nervosa. Psychoneuroendocrinology 28:829–835, 2003.

695. Krsek M, Rosicka M, Papezova H, et al: Plasma ghrelin levels and malnutrition: A comparison of two etiologies. Eat Weight Disord 8:207–211, 2003.

696. Iniguez G, Ong K, Pena V, et al: Fasting and post-glucose ghrelin levels in SGA infants: Relationships with size and weight gain at one year of age. J Clin Endocrinol Metab 87:5830–5833, 2002.

697. Cortelazzi D, Cappiello V, Morpurgo PS, et al: Circulating levels of ghrelin in human fetuses. Eur J Endocrinol 149:111–116, 2003.

698. Farquhar J, Heiman M, Wong AC, et al: Elevated umbilical cord ghrelin concentrations in small for gestational age neonates. J Clin Endocrinol Metab 88:4324–4327, 2003.

699. Geloneze B, Tambascia MA, Pilla VF, et al: Ghrelin: A gut-brain hormone: Effect of gastric bypass surgery. Obes Surg 13:17–22, 2003.

700. Holdstock C, Engstrom BE, Ohrvall M, et al: Ghrelin and adipose tissue regulatory peptides: Effect of gastric bypass surgery in obese humans. J Clin Endocrinol Metab 88:3177–3183, 2003.

701. Pöykkö SM, Kellokoski E, Horkko S, et al: Low plasma ghrelin is associated with insulin resistance, hypertension, and the prevalence of type 2 diabetes. Diabetes 52:2546–2553, 2003.

702. Ostergard T, Hansen TK, Nyholm B, et al: Circulating ghrelin concentrations are reduced in healthy offspring of Type 2 diabetic subjects, and are increased in women independent of a family history of Type 2 diabetes. Diabetologia 46:134–136, 2003.

703. Anderwald C, Brabant G, Bernroider E, et al: Insulin-dependent modulation of plasma ghrelin and leptin concentrations is less pronounced in type 2 diabetic patients. Diabetes 52:1792–1798, 2003.

704. Pagotto U, Gambineri A, Vicennati V, et al: Plasma ghrelin, obesity, and the polycystic ovary syndrome: Correlation with insulin resistance and androgen levels. J Clin Endocrinol Metab 87:5625–5629, 2002.

705. Schöfl C, Horn R, Schill T, et al: Circulating ghrelin levels in patients with polycystic ovary syndrome. J Clin Endocrinol Metab 87:4607–4610, 2002.

706. Makino Y, Hosoda H, Shibata K, et al: Alteration of plasma ghrelin levels associated with the blood pressure in pregnancy. Hypertension 39:781–784, 2002.

707. Haqq AM, Farooqi IS, O'Rahilly S, et al: Serum ghrelin levels are inversely correlated with body mass index, age, and insulin concentrations in normal children and are markedly increased in Prader-Willi syndrome. J Clin Endocrinol Metab 88:174–178, 2003.

708. Cummings DE, Clement K, Purnell JQ, et al: Elevated plasma ghrelin levels in Prader-Willi syndrome. Nat Med 8:643–644, 2002.

709. DelParigi A, Tschop M, Heiman ML, et al: High circulating ghrelin: A potential cause for hyperphagia and obesity in Prader-Willi syndrome. J Clin Endocrinol Metab 87:5461–5464, 2002.

710. Goldstone AP, Thomas EL, Brynes AE, et al: Elevated fasting plasma ghrelin in Prader-Willi syndrome adults is not solely explained by their reduced visceral adiposity and insulin resistance. J Clin Endocrinol Metab 89:1718–1726, 2004.

711. Goldstone AP: Prader-Willi syndrome: Advances in genetics, pathophysiology and treatment. Trends Endocrinol Metab 15:12–20, 2004.

712. Riis AL, Hansen TK, Moller N, et al: Hyperthyroidism is associated with suppressed circulating ghrelin levels. J Clin Endocrinol Metab 88:853–857, 2003.

Insulin-like Growth Factor 1 and Its Binding Proteins

David R. Clemmons

INTRODUCTION

The family of insulin-like growth factors (IGFs) is unusual when considered in the context of traditional hormones. Although like classically defined hormones, these substances are secreted into extracellular fluids and act on cells within tissues of distal target sites, they also act on cells that are adjacent to the cell of origin and on the cells of origin themselves, such as fibroblasts, a process that has been termed *autocrine* or *paracrine growth stimulation*. Therefore, these substances can be viewed as either traditional hormones or as locally produced growth factors. The ability to manipulate animals genetically has resulted in a greater understanding of the role of locally produced IGF-1 in regulating growth in vivo. Although knowledge is still evolving in this area, it is clear that the full understanding of the mechanism of action of polypeptide growth factors, such as IGF-1, cannot be elucidated without an appreciation for both their systemic endocrine effects, which can be demonstrated in classic in vivo infusion experiments or these local actions that require tissue-specific gene knockout experiments, wherein local production can be attenuated. Clearly, both of these sources of peptide (i.e., autocrine produced and endocrine transported) are important for regulation of growth in vivo. Likewise, attempts in clinical medicine to manipulate growth factors, such as in treating cancers that are growth factor dependent, will have to consider ablation of systemically produced circulating growth factors and ablation of local tissue production. Thus, a true understanding of the physiologic mechanisms that regulate both types of production is necessary.

The IGFs belong to a family of polypeptides that evolved from a common ancestral precursor into IGF-1, IGF-2, and proinsulin. All three members of the family probably evolved before the emergence of a pituitary gland, although growth hormone (GH) control of IGF-1 appeared near the time that IGF-1 and insulin diverged. Unlike insulin, both IGF-1 and IGF-2 circulate bound to high-affinity binding proteins. This results in a very different plasma half-life and differences in their target cell actions as compared with those of insulin. Similarly, the IGFs have distinct cellular receptors that bind IGF-1 and -2 with much higher affinity than insulin. The insulin receptor has similar selectivity. Because they are ubiquitously secreted in all tissues, and the IGF-1 receptor is present on all cell types, the IGFs represent important systemic regulators of growth. This ubiquitous tissue production and receptor distribution is a major determinant of balanced organ and tissue growth.

IGF-1 was originally discovered because of its property of stimulating sulfation of proteoglycans that are present in cartilage.[1] It was later determined that it was an important stimulant of cartilage DNA synthesis.[2] This effect of IGF-1 was discovered while trying to develop in vitro assays for GH activity. When GH was added to cartilage in vitro, it was a poor stimulant of cartilage sulfation. However, the administration of GH to hypophysectomized animals resulted in induction of a substance in serum that was a potent stimulant of cartilage sulfation. This suggested that a separate growth factor was induced in the serum of these animals. Purification of this substance led to determination of its primary amino acid sequence and to studies that showed that it could stimulate the growth of whole animals.[3,4]

Molecular technology has made it possible to determine the structure of the receptors for the IGFs and for GH. These

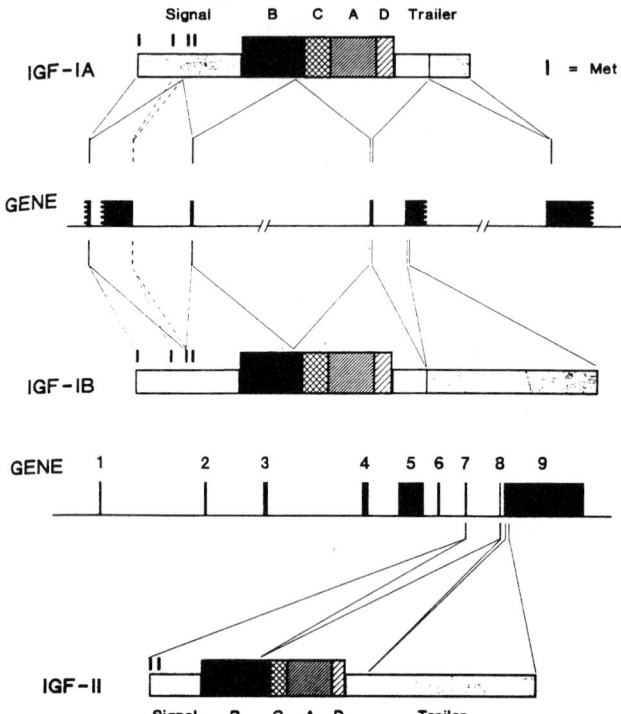

Figure 34-1 Structure of the human insulin-like growth factor 1 (IGF-1) gene and the precursor proteins it encodes. The *black* boxes that are shown represent exons. The portions of each exon that encode parts of the precursor protein are shown by *lines*. The IGF-1A and -1B precursor forms are represented by *boxes*. The B, C, A, and D domains of the mature peptides are noted.

studies also led to the identification of signal-transduction pathways that are linked to each receptor. All three peptides can induce activation of similar signaling molecules, although in several cases, activation of the IGF-1 receptor clearly induces a subset of signaling molecules that are distinct. A more complete description of the relative roles of IGF-1, insulin, and GH in growth and metabolic regulation ultimately awaits the elucidation of all of the proteins that are induced by activa-

tion of each receptor. This should lead to a better definition of their respective target cell roles, as well as their relative hierarchic importance in growth regulation.

IGF-1 GENE AND PROTEIN STRUCTURES

The IGF-1 gene is a complex, multicomponent gene, with six exons.[5] The gene structure is shown in Figure 34-1. The first and second exons encode the 5'-untranslated and pre-propeptide regions of IGF-1. Exon 3 encodes the distal propeptide sequence and the regions of the mature peptide that are homologous to the B chain of insulin, and the region homologous to the C peptide and to the A chain region. Exon 4 encodes a D-extension peptide. The fifth and sixth exons are shuffled and can encode one of two sequences termed *IGF-1A* and *IGF-1B*.[6] This alternative splicing occurs in multiple tissues, and both IGF-1A and IGF-1B have been found as gene products of specific cell types in culture.[7,8]

Several forms of IGF-1 messenger RNA (mRNA) are transcribed, and at least four specific transcripts are often detected in tissues.[9] The most abundant transcript detected is the 6-kB IGF-1 transcript, which includes multiple polyadenylation sites and a long 3'-untranslated sequence. The abundance of this transcript is regulated by GH.[10] GH increases transcription of IGF-1 by inducing STAT5B, which binds to an intronic region between exons 2 and 3 and initiates transcription. Several different fetal and tissue-specific promoters of IGF-1 have been identified, and they account for distinct transcript patterns in various tissues and the appearance of various forms at specific periods in development.[11] Other abundant transcripts include a 3.2-kB transcript, a 2.7-kB transcript, and a 0.9-kB transcript. Stimuli other than GH have been shown to influence the abundance of these transcripts in various tissues.[12,13] The small, 0.9-kB transcript is one source of the mature 70-amino acid IGF-1 peptide. This transcript is present in the liver, and this is believed to be an important source of the peptide that is present in the systemic circulation. Alternative processing of IGF-1 mRNA after its transcription has been shown to occur in multiple tissues and may be physiologically relevant in specific situations. Variable polyadenylation sites and regulation of processing of the 3'-untranslated RNA extensions have been shown to occur and can result in different-length transcripts.[14]

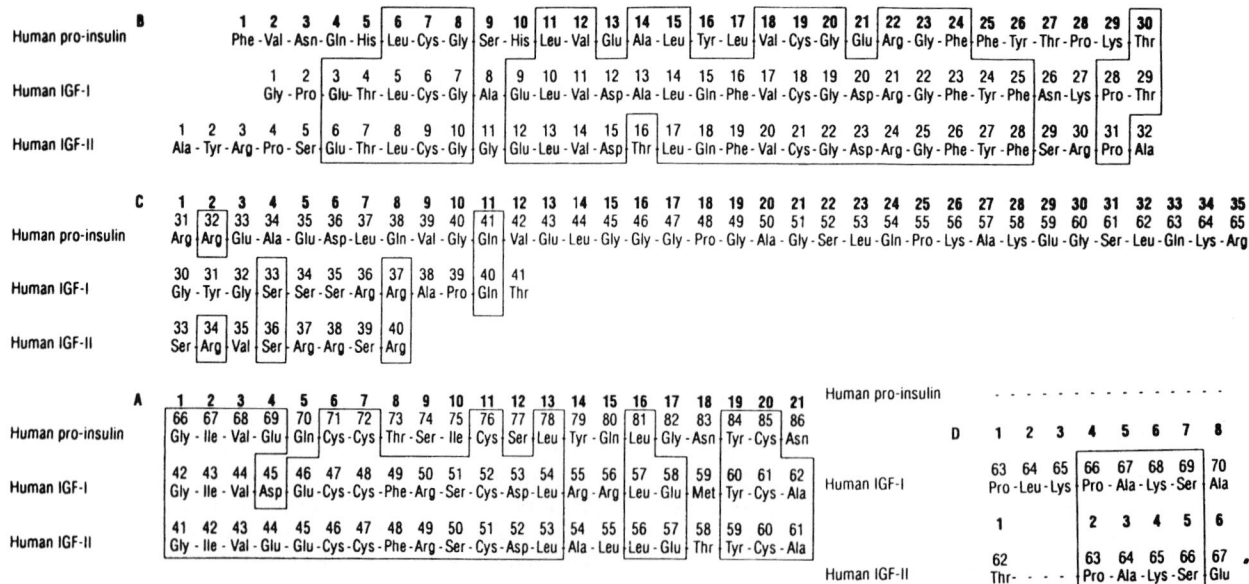

Figure 34-2 The sequences of proinsulin, insulin-like growth factor (IGF)-1, and IGF-2. The sequences are divided into the B, C, A, and D domains.

The polypeptide structures of three members of the IGF gene family are shown in Figure 34-2. Mature IGF-1 and IGF-2 contain 70 and 67 amino acids, respectively.[15] Proinsulin has a longer C-peptide region compared with the C-peptide region in IGF-1 or IGF-2. The sequence in this region is not conserved. The A chain and B chain peptide regions are of similar length. The sequences in this region are 41% and 43% homologous with proinsulin. IGF-1 and -2 contain D-domain extensions of eight and six amino acids, respectively. Unlike proinsulin, IGF-1 and -2 are not cleaved into two-chain polypeptides during intracellular processing, but rather they are secreted as intact single-chain proteins. Forms of IGF-1 have been isolated from serum and from cell culture supernatants that contain the E-peptide extensions (e.g., both A and B), but the relative abundance of these forms in most tissues has not been determined.[7,8] The frequency of processing of the E-peptide domains is unclear, because longer forms of IGF-1A or IGF-1B have been shown to be secreted by cells in culture. However, some cells do not secrete IGF-1 with the E-peptide extension, so the physiologic role of this sequence in regulating IGF-1 and -2 actions is not well defined.

Specific amino acids within the IGF-1 molecule have been shown by site-directed mutagenesis to account for receptor or binding protein association or both (Table 34-1). Specifically, tyrosine 24, tyrosine 60, and, to some extent, tyrosine 31 are required for IGF-1-receptor recognition.[16,17] The tyrosines at positions 24 and 60 are conserved within IGF-2, but tyrosine 31 is not present. The residue within the proinsulin sequence that is homologous to Tyr24 (e.g., Phe25) is important for insulin binding to its receptor. Tyr60 appears to be necessary for IGF-1 to maintain a stable conformation. Studies using mutant forms of IGF-1 with large deletions indicate that the region between residues 24 and 37 contains the primary receptor-binding site.[18] Mutations in this region have very little effect on binding protein affinity. More recent crystallographic[19,20] and nuclear magnetic resonance (NMR) studies[21,22] confirmed the importance of these residues. These studies highlighted the importance of Phe16 and Leu54 for ligand-induced activation and suggest that they are required by full activation of the receptor kinase.

IGF-1 and -2 contain four amino acids that account for most of the binding protein activity. These include the amino acids at positions 3, 4, 15, and 16 of the B chain region of IGF-1 and the homologous residues 6, 7, 18, and 19 in IGF-2.[23] These residues are critical for recognition by all six forms of IGF-binding proteins (IGFBPs). Mutant forms of IGF-1 that contain substitutions of proinsulin residues in these four positions have a nearly total loss of binding protein activity.[24] In addition, residues at amino acids 49, 50, and 51 in the A chain are important for recognition by four of the six high-affinity-binding proteins.[25] The major exception is IGFBP-3, wherein only the B chain residues appear to be important. Recent x-ray crystallographic studies of the IGF-1/IGFBP-5 complex confirmed the importance of these residues and

showed that they are the primary sites within IGF-1 that interact with IGFBP-5.[21] Studies of the tertiary structures of IGF-1 and IGF-2 have predicted that these residues are surface exposed and therefore should be available for binding to binding proteins. A recent NMR study showed that two of three helices that are present in IGF-1 form a surface exposed hydrophobic patch that contains these A and B chain residues. A peptide that bound to this patch inhibited IGF-1/IGFBP binding.[22] The C-peptide regions in each of the three proteins are divergent, and this accounts for the most of the heterogeneity of sequence between IGF-1 and IGF-2. The three disulfide linkages are conserved in all three peptides.

The structure of IGF-1 is highly conserved across species. Bovine IGF-1 is identical to that of the human, and that of rat differs by only three amino acids.[26] IGF-1-like molecules have been detected in all vertebrates that have been analyzed, and even in species as low on the phylogenetic tree as *Caenorhabditis elegans* contain IGF-1-like molecules. Computer modeling studies have indicated that the three-dimensional structure of IGF-1 is probably similar to that of insulin, which has been analyzed by x-ray crystallography.[19,20,27] Different forms of IGF-1 have been found to be present in human serum and tissues. The most extensively studied form is des-1-3 IGF-1, which occurs in brain and in serum.[28,29] This molecule is believed to be important because it has much lower affinity for binding proteins and therefore, if generated in vivo, can provide a more biologically active form of IGF-1.

IGF-1 RECEPTOR

The IGF-1 receptor is ubiquitously present and has been shown to be present in cell types derived from all three embryonic lineages. When animal tissues have been analyzed, this receptor can be detected uniformly. This probably accounts for the ability of IGF-1 to stimulate growth of all tissues. The receptor number appears to be very tightly controlled, because receptor number per cell varies within the range of 20,000 to 35,000. This may be an important, protective regulatory function, because cellular transformation in response to IGF-1 usually requires more than 1 million receptors per cell.[30] This hypothesis is supported by the fact that, when cells are genetically engineered to contain more than a million IGF-1 receptors per cell, they become tumorigenic, whereas cells that have fewer than 100,000 receptors per cell do not induce tumors. Thus, the variables that regulate IGF-1 receptor number could be important in terms of the genesis of neoplasia.

The hormonal regulation of receptor number has been analyzed in great detail. Hormones such as GH, follicle-stimulating hormone (FSH), luteinizing hormone (LH), progesterone, estradiol, and thyroxine have been shown to increase receptor expression.[31,32] Similarly, platelet-derived growth factor (PDGF), epidermal growth factor (EGF), fibroblast growth factor (FGF), and angiotensin II upregulate receptor expression in specific cell types.[33,34] After hormone binding, downregulation of the receptor number occurs with internalization of receptors. However, possibly due to IGFBPs, the rate of internalization of IGF-1 receptors is substantially slower than that of other growth factors, such as EGF or insulin.

The biochemical structure of the receptor is similar to that of other polypeptide growth factor receptors (Fig. 34-3). The receptor is a heterotetrameric glycoprotein composed of two ligand-binding subunits, termed *alpha subunits*, which contain 706 amino acids, and two *beta subunits*, which contain 627 amino acids. Only the beta subunits have a transmembrane domain (see Fig. 34-3). In humans, the protein is translated from a single mRNA transcript derived from a gene that contains 21 exons located on chromosome 15, Q25-Q26.[35] The prepropeptide is 1367 amino acids, and the signal peptide is removed cotranslationally. The precursor is cleaved between Lys708/Arg709 to generate the alpha and beta subunits.

Table 34-1	Specific Amino Acids in Insulin-Like Growth Factor 1 (IGF-1) That Mediate Binding Protein and Receptor Association	
Region of IGF-1	**Ligand Interaction**	
B chain		
Glu3, Thr4, Gln15, Phe16	Required for binding to IGF-binding proteins (IGFBPs) 1–6	
A chain		
Phe49, Arg50, Ser51	Required for optimal binding to IGFBP-1, -2, -4, -5	
Tyr24, Tyr31, Tyr60	IGF-1 receptor	
Tyr24-Arg37	Contains the primary receptor binding site	
Tyr60	Necessary for a stable conformation	

Ligand Affinities: Ins >> IGF-I > IGF-II   IGF-I > IGF-II >> Ins   IGF-I > IGF-II > Ins

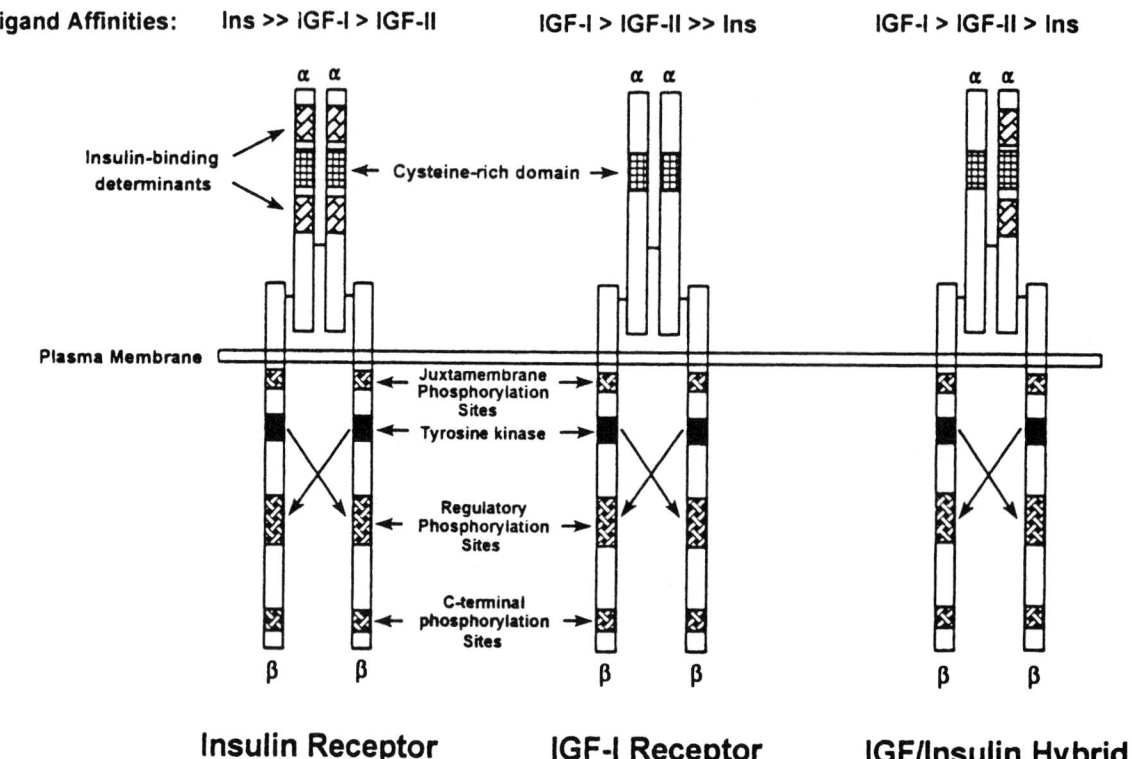

Figure 34-3 Structural characteristics of the insulin, insulin-like growth factor (IGF)-1, and hybrid receptors.

These are linked together by disulfide bonds to form the heterotetrameric receptor. Amino acid–sequence comparison with the insulin receptor reveals 46% amino acid identity.[35]

The alpha subunit contains three domains that are essential for ligand binding. The ligand-binding domain of the alpha subunit binds IGF-1 with an association constant of approximately 10^{-9} mol/L. IGF-2 binds with sixfold lower affinity, and insulin, with a 200- to 300-fold lower affinity.[5,36] The structure of the a subunit has been analyzed by crystallography, which shows that two L domains flank a central cysteine-rich region.[37] Mutagenesis studies have shown that the residues within the L_1 domain (1–50) are important for binding. The cysteine-rich region (290–300) contains four residues that are essential to maintain high affinity. A short C-terminal region (692–702) also is very important because changes in 7 of these 10 residues reduced binding affinity from 10- to 30-fold.[38]

The beta subunit of the receptor is composed of a transmembrane domain between positions 906 and 929, followed by a long, intracytoplasmic domain. This region contains intrinsic tyrosine kinase (TK) activity and critical sites of tyrosine and serine phosphorylation. The TK domain is 84% homologous with the insulin-receptor TK domain.[39] The catalytic domain contains an adenosine triphosphate (ATP)-binding motif and a catalytic lysine at position 1003. Substitution for this lysine abolishes IGF-1-stimulated biologic actions.[40] Ligand binding to the alpha subunit triggers a conformational change and dimerization that leads to autoactivation.[41,42] This, in turn, leads to transreceptor phosphorylation, wherein specific tyrosines located on one beta subunit are transphosphorylated by the TK activity located on the paired beta subunit. This mode of TK activation that results in tyrosine autophosphorylation is similar to that which occurs in the insulin receptor.[42–44]

At least six important tyrosines are contained within the cytoplasmic domain and are phosphorylated by the intrinsic TK. The most important is a triple tyrosine motif at positions 1149, 1150, and 1151. Substitutions for these tyrosines abolish IGF-1 signaling.[40,45] Recent crystal structure analysis of the beta subunit showed that phosphorylation of all three tyrosines is required to obtain the optimal conformation.[46] Phosphorylation of two or three tyrosines yields a structure in which the central domain is trapped in a half-closed loop, whereas after phosphorylation of all three residues, the loop is opened, facilitating catalysis.[47] After phosphorylation of these residues in response to activation of intrinsic TK activity by hormone binding to the receptor, the TK is further activated to phosphorylate intracellular substrates, such as insulin receptor substrate-1 and -2 (IRS-1 and -2) (see later). After receptor autophosphorylation, tyrosine 950 is phosphorylated, and this is the principal IRS-1-binding site. Substitution for this residue attenuates IRS-1 phosphorylation and biologic signaling.[48] IRS-1 affinity for the phosphorylated receptor is increased ninefold.[49] After adherence of IRS-1 to the receptor, the intrinsic TK activity is further activated, and it phosphorylates additional sites on IRS-1. This provides binding sites for adaptor proteins, such as Grb-2, which in turn leads to Ras activation. Other kinases, such as phosphotidylinositol-3 (PI 3)-kinase are activated by binding to phosphorylated IRS-1. Mutation of tyrosine 1316 abrogates the ability to activate PI 3-kinase, and alteration of tyrosines 1250 and 1251, not found in the insulin receptor, results in only a slight effect on autophosphorylation but induces a major reduction in the cellular proliferation response.[50] The receptor also can phosphorylate other substrates directly, including Shc, Crk, and Grb-10.[51,52] Phosphorylation of residues 1280 and 1283 is necessary for binding to 14-3-3, an additional signaling intermediate, and for maintaining IGF-1 antiapoptotic activity. The NPXY motif, which is located near the transmembrane domain, is required for internalization.[53,54]

Chimeric receptors that contain heterodimers of the IGF-1 and insulin receptor have been described.[55] These dimers are disulfide linked. Receptor hybrids have been detected in several tissues and cell types. It is possible that they exist in all cells in which both IGF-1 and insulin receptors are expressed. The ligand specificity and affinity properties of hybrid receptors are much closer to those of the IGF-1 receptor than with the insulin receptor. Hybrid receptor activation has been shown to lead to stimulation of signal transduction and IGF-1 biologic actions in vitro[56,57]; however, the biologic significance of hybrid receptor formation has not been determined.

The IGF-1 receptor has been overexpressed in several types of cells in culture. Overexpression can lead to the ability of cells to grow in soft agar and to form tumors in nude mice.[30] This suggests that tight regulation of receptor number is responsible for controlling the ability of IGF-1 to transform cells. Recent studies using antisense oligonucleotides to reduce the IGF-1 receptor number confirmed its importance for growth and transforming activity of human tumor cells.[58] Importantly, deletion of specific tyrosines, mainly substitution for tyrosine 1250 or 1251, results in a marked diminution in the transforming property of the IGF-1 receptor, although mitogenesis in vitro is still preserved.[59,60] In addition to its ability to transform cells, the receptor appears to be extremely important for IGF-1 to modulate the effects of other growth factors. Mouse fibroblasts containing deficient numbers of IGF-1 receptors do not undergo DNA synthesis in response to the addition of EGF. Similarly, overexpression of the EGF and PDGF receptors does not lead to proliferation of fibroblasts in soft agar in the absence of IGF-1 receptors.[61,62] Reexpression of the IGF-1 receptor allows proliferation to occur. Large T-antigen induction by the cellular transforming virus, SV40, requires expression of the IGF-1 receptor, and wild-type Ras activation has a lesser effect on cellular transformation if the IGF-1 receptor is absent.[63] Likewise, Src oncogene expression results in transforming activity only in the presence of an IGF-1 receptor.

The IGF-1 receptor has an important role in normal development and normal fetal growth. Animals that have had the IGF-1 receptor deleted by homologous recombination are born approximately 40% of normal size.[64] These animals are not viable at birth because of hypoplasia of the diaphragmatic muscle. Defects in the development of the nervous system, skin, and bones have been noted. These developmental abnormalities apparently occur relatively late in gestation. Fibroblasts obtained from these embryos have a markedly attenuated growth response compared with fibroblasts from normal embryos.[65]

The receptor also is important for prevention of apoptosis. IGF-1 and its receptor support the viability of nonproliferating cells in culture, such as neurons. The extent of apoptosis that can be induced in neurons by osmotic hyperglycemia,

ischemia, or potassium shock is dependent on normal IGF-1-receptor expression, suggesting that it is neuroprotective.[66] Hematopoietic cells that are dependent on interleukin-3 (IL-3) for proliferation and undergo apoptosis if IL-3 is withdrawn are protected by IGF-1 exposure if IGF-1 receptors are present. Plating tumor cells on a surface that does not allow ligand binding to integrins results in susceptibility to apoptosis, and this susceptibility can be reversed by incubation with IGF-1.[67] Mutation of tyrosine 1251, Lys1294, or His1293 eliminates the capacity of the receptor to protect against apoptosis, whereas mutations of Tyr1250, 1316, and 950 have no effect.[68]

In contrast to that of the IGF-1 receptor, overexpression of the insulin receptor is nontransforming. Likewise, overexpression of a chimeric receptor bearing the beta subunit of the insulin receptor is nontransforming, but if the IGF-1-receptor beta subunit is expressed with the insulin-receptor alpha subunit, then mitogenic activity of insulin is detected at much lower ligand concentrations, and this receptor construct allows transformation to occur.[69]

RECEPTOR-MEDIATED SIGNAL TRANSDUCTION

After activation of the intrinsic TK activity and phosphorylation of the triple tyrosine domain of the receptor, the docking protein, IRS-1, binds directly to the receptor (Fig. 34-4). A functionally similar protein termed *IRS-2* has been shown to bind by a similar mechanism.[70] After binding, IRS-1 is then tyrosine phosphorylated by the receptor at multiple sites, creating docking motifs that are critical for binding of intracellular proteins that contain *Src* homology-2 (SH-2) domains. These domains contain approximately 100 amino acids that share sequence similarity cellular oncogene, *Src*. Six of the tyrosines in IRS-1 occur within YXXM sequences, a recognition motif within SH-2 domains.[71] IRS-1 gene deletion in mice results in a major decrease in body weight with proportionate reduction in liver, heart, and spleen.[72] Activation of signaling pathways that lead to enhanced IRS-1 degradation results in attenuation of IGF-1 signaling.[73,74]

Signaling proteins that bind directly to the phosphorylated tyrosines on IRS-1 include the adaptor proteins Nck and Grb-2.[75] Grb-2 forms a complex with the Ras activating protein

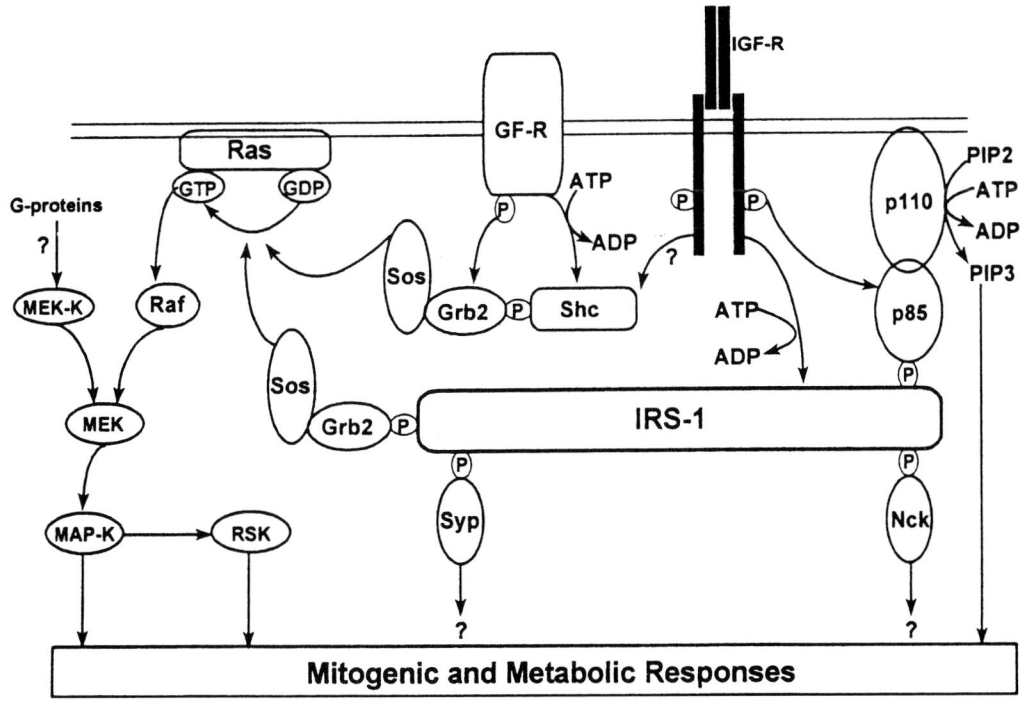

Figure 34-4 Major signaling pathways that are used by the insulin-like growth factor (IGF)-1 receptor. Shown for comparison are the pathways used by other growth factors, such as epidermal growth factor and platelet-derived growth factor. P-110 and P-85 represent the major subunits of phosphatidylinositol-3'-kinase.

(son of sevenless [SOS]), and this complex leads to subsequent P-21 Ras activation, which activates Raf and downstream components of the mitogen-activated protein kinase (MAPK) pathway. Activation of this pathway is important for the mitogenic function of IGF-1.[51,76] The IGF-1 receptor can directly phosphorylate Shc, and this leads to association of activated of Grb-2 and Shc independent of IRS-1. Shc/Grb-2 activation by IGF-1R leads directly to MAPK activation. An additional signaling molecule that is activated by the receptor is Crk, a Grb-2-like protein, with SH-2 and SH-3 domains. Crk then activates Grb-2 and SOS after it is phosphorylated by the IGF-1 receptor.[52] Other signaling pathways that have been shown to be activated include protein kinase-C, phospholipase-C, and direct stimulation of calcium-permeable ion channels.[77–79] Additional signaling molecules that have been shown to interact with the IGF-1 receptor include RACK-1[80] and Grb-10.[81] Activation of these proteins leads to activation of downstream signaling cascades including G protein activation.

IRS-1 activation induces the two subunits of PI-3 kinase to associate. This results in catalytic activation, the generation of inositol triphosphate, and activation of protein tyrosine kinase B.[82,83] This kinase activates P70 S6 kinase and GSK-3, a kinase that is involved in glucose transport. This pathway also is important for IGF-1-induced increases in protein synthesis, cell motility, and for inhibition of apoptosis.[84]

Because specificity exists between insulin and IGF-1 in terms of their metabolic and growth-promoting actions,[85,86] it was presumed that major differences would be detected in the signal-transduction pathways that each hormone used. However, IGF-1 and insulin-receptor kinase domains are 84% identical, and similar residues are autophosphorylated. Presumably, either distinct domains are activated in the IRS-1 and -2 or separate combinations of signaling pathways are activated. Although the degree of phosphorylation of IRS-1, IRS-2, and Shc appears to be nondistinguishable between insulin and IGF-1 receptors, activation of Crk-2 is specific for the IGF-1 receptor.[52] Because Crk-2 has transforming activity, its activation may partially account for the ability of overexpression of IGF-1 receptors to be transforming. Likewise, insulin-receptor activation results in dephosphorylation of tyrosine residues on focal adhesion kinase, whereas IGF-1 receptor does not have this effect.[87] Similarly, insulin and IGF-1 receptors have been shown to use different G protein--signaling components.[88] Activation of Src kinase results in phosphorylation of the IGF-1 receptor, but not of the insulin receptor.[89] One example of a molecular explanation that could account for some differences is the observation that activation of IRS-1 by the respective receptors results in binding to phosphorylated tyrosines in different domains.[90] The insulin receptor binds preferentially to tyrosines 987 and 727, whereas the IGF-1 receptor binds preferentially to tyrosine 895. Gene-targeting experiments have confirmed that the IGF-1 receptor has effects that are different from those of the insulin receptor, but how these effects are mediated in vivo beyond ligand-binding selectivity remains undetermined.[91]

Blocking specific functions of intracellular signaling pathways has been shown to attenuate specific IGF-1 actions. The PI-3 kinase pathway appears important for glucose transport and for cell migration.[82,83] Specific inhibitors of PI-3 kinase result in attenuation of these IGF-1-stimulated actions. Similarly, the MAPK pathway appears to be the predominant pathway for mitogenesis and rescue from apoptosis, and specific blockade of these phosphorylation reactions results in a preferential effect on these IGF-1-stimulated actions.[68] However, the requirement for either pathway is not absolute, because high concentrations of specific inhibitors of these pathways result in inhibition of overlapping functions. For example, 1.0 μmol/L PD98059 inhibits MAPK effectively, and it is a potent inhibitor of IGF-1-stimulated DNA synthesis, but it has no effect on cell migration. However, a 50 μmol/L concentration of this compound will inhibit cell migration significantly, even though it has a weak effect on PI-3 kinase activity. This suggests that overlapping contributions may exist of these pathways to multiple cellular functions. Protein kinase C also appears to be essential for IGF-1-stimulated migration and stimulation of the transcription of specific genes.

IGF-2 MANNOSE-6 PHOSPHATE RECEPTOR

The IGF-2/cation-independent mannose-6 phosphate receptor is a single-chain membrane-spanning glycoprotein that contains 2451 amino acids. It binds mannose-6 phosphate residues on lysosomal enzymes, as well as IGF-2. A large extracellular domain is present, a 23-amino acid transmembrane domain, and a 164-residue carboxy-terminal intracytoplasmic domain. The extracellular domain is composed of 15 repeating motifs.[92] Motifs 7 to 9 bind mannose-6 phosphate, and motif 11 contains the IGF-2-binding region.[93] Intracellularly, this receptor functions to translocate newly synthesized lysosomal enzymes into endosomes. On the cell surface, it binds to mannose-6 phosphate–containing extracellular glycoproteins, which are endocytosed into endosomes. The receptors are then recycled back to the cell surface. Proteins other than lysosomal enzymes that have been described as binding to this receptor include proliferin, thyroglobulin, and latent transforming growth factor β (TGF-β). Binding of latent TGF-β has been shown to result in cleavage of the inactive form into active TGF-β.[94] In adipocytes, it has been shown that insulin is a potent stimulant of redistribution of mannose-6 phosphate receptors from intracellular locations to the plasma membrane.[95] The receptor binds IGF-2 with an affinity in the range of kDa 1 to 3 nM. The affinity for IGF-1 is 80-fold lower, and the receptor does not bind insulin.[96] Mannose-6 phosphate–containing proteins bind to a site that is distinct from IGF-1 or IGF-2, and the receptor can bind both ligands simultaneously. Once IGF-2 is bound, it is internalized and degraded. The extracellular portion of the receptor can be proteolytically cleaved in certain cell types, and the cleavage product is released. This soluble form has been detected in plasma; however, the physiologic significance of its release into plasma has not been determined.[97]

The role of this receptor in IGF physiology is incompletely understood. Deletion of the receptor or mutations that result in loss of IGF-2 binding result in death of fetal mice at approximately 15 days of gestation.[98] The receptor is subject to parental imprinting, such that only the maternal allele of the IGF-2 receptor and the paternal allele of IGF-2 are expressed. Therefore, mice that inherit a receptor allele containing a mutation from the mother have functionally altered IGF-2 receptors. These mice develop severe edema in utero before death.[99] They are also larger than fetuses of comparable developmental age. If IGF-2 is concomitantly deleted, approximately 50% of the fetuses survive birth; however, postnatal survival is poor. The hypothesis has been that these mice lack the putative scavenging function of the IGF-2 receptor and accumulate toxic levels of IGF-2. Although the scavenging function of the receptor is well accepted, it is less clear whether this receptor mediates important actions mediated by the IGF-1 receptor, such as growth stimulation. The receptor does not contain a TK domain. Whether it stimulates intracellular signaling mechanisms in vivo is unknown. In certain cell types in culture, mutant forms of IGF-2 that bind poorly to the IGF-1 receptor stimulate some cellular events, such as cell migration.[100] Increases in calcium flux have been shown to occur after stimulation of 3T3 cells by IGF-2 binding to this receptor. Additionally, the receptor has been shown to activate guanosine triphosphate (GTP)-binding proteins, but the exact functional significance of these effects is undetermined.[101] The cytoplasmic portion of the receptor encodes regions that are necessary for specific subcellular localization and endocytosis, as well as binding to GTP-binding proteins.[100] In addition, it contains residues that are phosphorylated by intracellular kinases, but the role of this phosphorylation is unknown. Partitioning of the receptor after internalization can be hormonally regulated. Treatment with insulin was found to cause an increase in the fraction of surface receptors, without a change in total number. Mannose-6 phosphate stimulates a similar increase, and this can be blocked by pretreatment with pertussis toxin, implying both stimulatory and inhibitory GTP-binding protein regulation.[102] However, a specific antibody that blocks IGF-1-receptor action can completely inhibit IGF-2-mediated cellular growth responses in some cell types. This suggests that many of the growth-promoting effects of IGF-2 are mediated through the IGF-1 receptor.

IGF-BINDING PROTEINS

A characteristic of IGF-1 and IGF-2 that distinguishes them from proinsulin is the ability to bind to high-affinity IGF-binding proteins (IGFBPs). The IGFBPs are a family of six proteins that each have high affinity for IGF-1 and IGF-2.[103] In each case, this affinity is greater than the affinity of the type 1 IGF receptor for IGF-1. One or more members of this family is present in all extracellular fluids. Therefore, they control the ability of IGF-1 and -2 to bind to receptors. In addition to this property, the major functions of the IGFBPs include (1) transporting the IGFs in the vasculature, (2) controlling their access to the extravascular space, (3) controlling tissue localization and distribution, and (4) controlling access to receptors and thereby modulating the biologic responses of cells to IGF-1.

The gene structure of the IGFBPs has been presented in several reviews. All of the six forms of IGFBPs contain four exons.[104] The mRNA species range in size from 1.4 Kb (IGFBP-2) to 6 Kb (IGFBP-5). When their protein structures are examined, a great deal of similarity is seen between the IGFBPs. Of the 18 cysteines, all are conserved in five of the six binding proteins. IGFBP-4 has two additional cysteines, and IGFBP-6 has only 16 cysteines. If the cysteine structure is disrupted, IGF-1 binding is markedly attenuated. All are secreted proteins and contain a hydrophobic leader sequence. The affinity of each protein for IGF-1 and -2 is shown in Table 34-2. As can be seen from the table, the greatest difference is in IGFBP-6, which has a 40-fold higher affinity for IGF-2.

An important general property of the IGF-binding proteins is their conservation of sequence in the N-terminal and C-terminal thirds of each protein. A high degree of sequence homology is seen in these two modules among each protein.[104] Similarly, the sequences in these regions are highly conserved across species. In contrast, the middle third sequence diverges completely. This may be important, functionally, because this is the major site of proteolytic cleavage for IGFBPs and suggests that distinct proteases cleave specific forms. Two of the proteins are N-glycosylated, and glycosylation sites occur in the middle third of the sequence, therefore providing specificity for this property among the different proteins.

SPECIFIC PROPERTIES OF EACH FORM OF IGF-BINDING PROTEIN

IGFBP-1 has an estimated mass of approximately 25,271 Daltons. It is not glycosylated, but it contains an Arg-Gly-Asp near its carboxyl terminus.[105] This sequence has been shown to bind to the $\alpha5B_1$ integrin.[106] IGFBP-1 is unique in that it appears intact in multiple types of extracellular fluids and is, of the six, the most resistant to proteolytic cleavage. The affinity of IGFBP-1 for IGF-1 and -2 is nearly equal.

IGFBP-2 contains 289 amino acids and has a mass estimate of 32,444 Daltons. Its sequence is highly conserved across species, especially in the C terminus.[107] IGFBP-2 is not glycosylated. It also has an Arg-Gly-Asp sequence near its carboxyl terminus, but it has not been shown to bind to the $\alpha5B_1$ integrin. The protein is cleaved in many types of physiologic fluids, and the fragments that are generated have reduced affinity for IGF-1 and -2.[108]

IGFBP-3 contains 266 amino acids and is variably N-glycosylated.[109] This accounts for varying molecular weight estimates between 43 and 56 kDa. Three potential N-linked glycosylation sites are present, all of which are used. Digestion with N-glycanase reduces the estimated molecular mass to 34 kDa. Glycosylation does not alter the affinity of this protein. No Arg-Gly-Asp sequence is present. IGFBP-3 contains a highly basic region between residues 216 and 244, in which 10 of 18 amino acids are basic. This region accounts for its heparin-binding activity and its ability to adhere to glycosaminoglycans.[110,111]

IGFBP-4 is a 24,532-Dalton protein containing 237 amino acids. It is N-glycosylated and therefore migrates with molecular masses of 28 kDa in the glycosylated form and 24 kDa in the nonglycosylated form.[112] Glycosylation does not affect the affinity for IGF-1 or -2. Two extra cysteines are present in the central core region of IGFBP-4, but their functional significance is undefined. IGFBP-4 is cleaved in most physiologic fluids to 16- and 14-kDa fragments that have very low affinity for IGF-1 and -2.[113]

IGFBP-5 has a molecular mass of 31,393 Daltons, and human IGFBP-5 contains 252 amino acids. IGFBP-5 is the most highly conserved form of IGF-binding protein, with 97% homology in sequence between the mouse and human forms.[114] It is most closely related in sequence to IGFBP-3, with approximately 50% homology in the amino- and carboxy-terminal ends. IGFBP-5 contains the same heparin-binding domain as IGFBP-3, located between amino acids 201 and 218.[111] Seventeen of 18 residues in this sequence are identical to those in IGFBP-3. Mutagenesis of these residues results in loss of heparin binding.[115] In addition, this sequence mediates binding to the extracellular matrix (ECM), and some of the proteins in the ECM that bind IGFBP-5 are not proteoglycans.[116,117] IGFBP-5 is O-glycosylated and has size estimates between 31 and 34 kDa. This protein has a high affinity for IGF-1 and -2. It is proteolytically cleaved into a 22-kDa fragment in physiologic fluids that has a much lower affinity for these ligands.[118]

IGFBP-6 has a molecular mass estimate of 31,413 Daltons. Its cysteine content differs among species, with 14 cysteines in the rat and 16 cysteines in the human.[119] No Arg-Gly-Asp sequence is present. The protein is O-glycosylated but not N-glycosylated.[120] It has a high affinity for IGF-2 compared with IGF-1, but the physiologic significance of this difference has not been ascertained.[121] IGFBP-6 is proteolytically cleaved in physiologic fluids.

CONTROL OF IGF-1 CONCENTRATIONS IN SERUM

Before the advent of molecular biologic techniques that made it possible to obtain sufficient highly purified IGF-1 to administer to humans, the primary means of assessing the effects of IGF-1 on anabolism was to make inferences from changes

Table 34-2	Affinities of Insulin-Like-Binding Proteins (IGFBPs) for Insulin-Like Growth Factor (IGF)-1 and -2	
	Affinity ($K_a \times 10^9$) L/M	
IGFBPs	IGF-1	IGF-2
IGFBP-1	1.1	1.2
IGFBP-2	3.4	10.9
IGFBP-3	8.9	22.1
IGFBP-4	2.6	6.0
IGFBP-5	38	41
IGFBP-6	0.1	4.4

in plasma or tissue IGF-1 concentrations.[122] Correlations between IGF-1 levels and parameters of anabolism, such as growth rate, rates of total body protein synthesis, and nitrogen balance were undertaken, and inferences were drawn based on changes in IGF-1 serum levels in response to variables such as GH administration.[122,123] These studies formed the basis of several principles of IGF-1 physiology that have been confirmed directly by manipulation of IGF-1 expression in transgenic animals or by infusion of IGF-1 into animals and humans and indirectly by measurements of changes in IGF-1 concentrations in states of GH deficiency or excess.

Age is an important determinant of the normal serum IGF-1 concentrations. Plasma concentrations increase from very low levels, 20 to 60 ng/mL, at birth to a peak values between 600 and 1100 ng/mL at puberty.[124] The concentrations then decrease rapidly in the second decade, reaching mean values of 350 ng/mL by age 20 years and then decline more slowly over each decade. They are 50% of the 20-year-old values by age 60 years.[125] A portion of this change is due to age-dependent changes in GH secretion. Although this may account for much of the decline that occurs during adulthood, it clearly does not account for all of the major increase that occurs during childhood.

Important genetic determinants are found of plasma IGF-1 concentrations. Studies in twins have shown that approximately 40% of each individual's IGF-1 variability can be accounted for on the basis of undefined genetic factors, which are linked to height.[126] A very close correlation exists between IGF-1 concentrations and height in many different types of populations that have been studied, and these appear to be due, at least in part, to this genetic factor. This genetic determinant is independent of intrinsic GH secretion. Recently, a polymorphism in the IGF-1 gene that occurs in 12% of whites has been shown to be associated with a lower mean serum IGF-1 concentration (~30% reduction) and a decreased final adult height (e.g., ~2 cm). The presence of this polymorphism in individuals older than 60 years was associated with a twofold increase in the prevalence of type 2 diabetes and an increased incidence of heart attacks and strokes.[127,128]

The major hormonal determinant of plasma IGF-1 concentrations is GH. Children with definitive evidence of GH deficiency (GHD) usually have IGF-1 values that are below the 95% confidence interval.[129,130] Because values vary so much throughout childhood, however, age-adjusted normative data are required to interpret low plasma IGF-1 values (Fig. 34-5). Consideration of developmental stage (skeletal age) also is important for interpreting low values.[131] A normal IGF-1 value is strong evidence that GHD is not present. Conversely, a low value does not definitively prove that GHD is present.[123,132] Other causes of growth retardation can be associated with a low IGF-1, although causes such as constitutional growth delay are usually associated with normal levels. However, values less than the 95% confidence interval can occur in such children, usually when nutritional intake is suboptimal. Administration of GH to patients with GHD results in a substantial increase in IGF-1, and this occurs in the first 4 to 6 hours after an injection.[133] The values peak at 24 hours and then begin to attenuate. Because GH also increases the plasma concentrations of IGFBP-3 and a third protein, termed *acid labile subunit* (ALS), the formation of the ternary complex accounts for the extended duration of this change in serum IGF-1. The IGF-1 response of a short child to GH administration has not proven to be a useful diagnostic test.[134,135] In spite of these problems in interpreting low values, basal IGF-1 measurements are very useful as a screening test for selecting individuals who should undergo stimulation testing to assess their GH secretory response.[123,129,130,132]

In states of GH excess, IGF-1 values are invariably increased. The mean IGF-1 for patients with acromegaly is approximately 7 times the normal age-adjusted control value.[136]

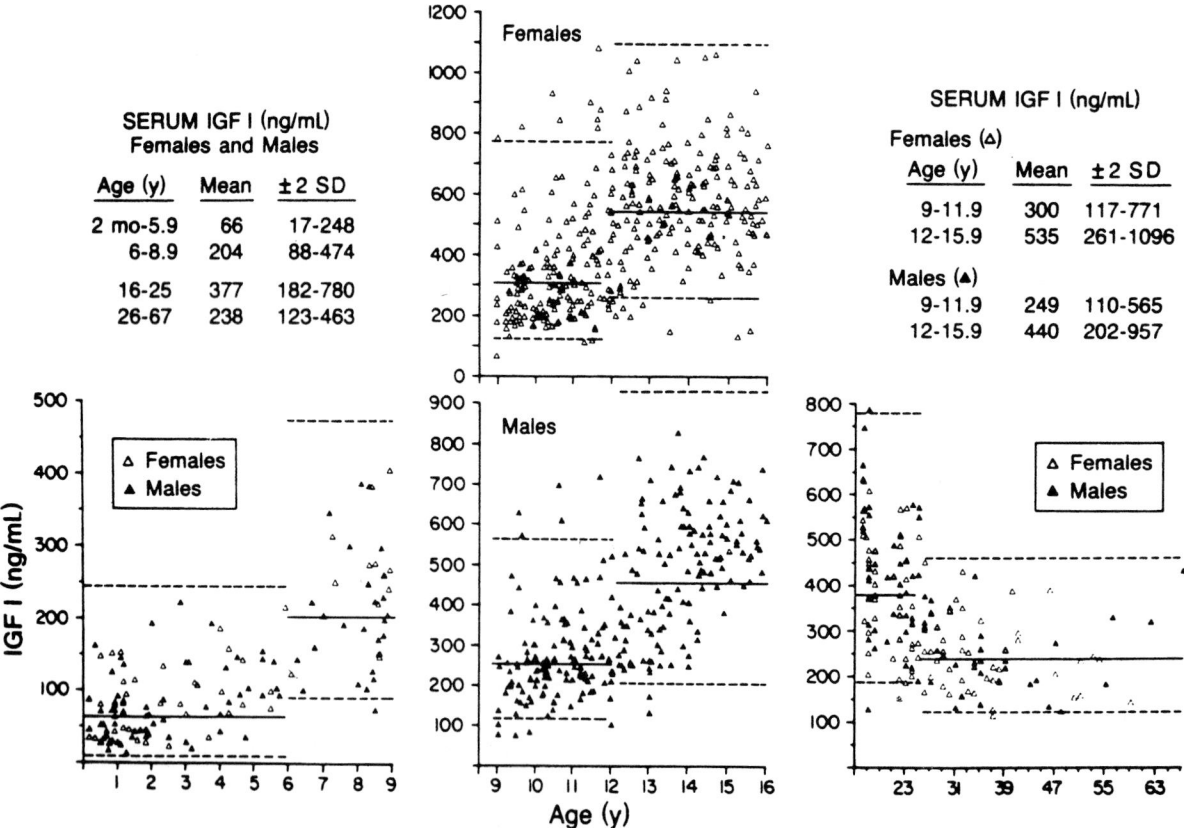

SERUM IGF I (ng/mL) Females and Males		
Age (y)	Mean	±2 SD
2 mo-5.9	66	17-248
6-8.9	204	88-474
16-25	377	182-780
26-67	238	123-463

SERUM IGF I (ng/mL)		
Females (△)		
Age (y)	Mean	±2 SD
9-11.9	300	117-771
12-15.9	535	261-1096
Males (▲)		
9-11.9	249	110-565
12-15.9	440	202-957

Figure 34-5 Serum concentrations of insulin-like growth factor (IGF)-1 in healthy subjects, age 2 months to 68 years. The 95% confidence intervals are shown as *dashed lines*.

The sensitivity and specificity of a single IGF-1 measurement for accurately diagnosing acromegaly in patients older than 20 years is more than 97%.[137] The severity of the IGF-1 abnormality appears to correlate with disease activity, and values correlate with measurement of soft tissue growth, such as heel-pad thickness.[136] IGF-1 measurements are useful in monitoring the response to therapy and correlate well with residual GH secretion in these patients.[138] Generally, if 24-hour mean GH values are less than 1.6 ng/mL, then IGF-1 will be within the age-adjusted 95% confidence interval. IGF-1 values also are elevated during the last trimester of pregnancy, presumably because of increases in placental GH secretion.[139]

Another hormonal variable that controls IGF-1 concentrations is thyroxine. Plasma IGF-1 concentrations are low in severe thyroxine deficiency and increase with thyroid hormone replacement.[140] Values are not suppressed in Turner's syndrome, and estrogen replacement results in little change. Prolactin has a weak, stimulatory effect on plasma IGF-1. In subjects who are severely GHD, prolactin concentrations of 200 ng/mL or greater can maintain IGF-1 in the normal range.

Nutritional status is an important determinant of plasma IGF-1 concentrations. Adequate caloric and protein intake have to be maintained to maintain an adequate serum IGF-1, in both children and adults.[141,142] Fasting for 3 days results in substantial reduction in total serum IGF-1 and a blunted response to the administration of GH.[143] Ten days of fasting results in a 70% decrease in plasma IGF-1. After a 5-day fast, values decline by 53%, and subjects must be refed for at least 8 days for values to return to normal. During fasting and refeeding, the change in IGF-1 correlates with the change in nitrogen balance.[144] The change is due to both energy and protein deficiency. An energy intake of 20 Kcal/kg is required to maintain a normal IGF-1, whereas an intake of 0.6 g/kg of protein is required. The energy must be supplied as at least 100 g of carbohydrate. Similarly, the quality of the protein intake (e.g., the amount of essential amino acids) is an important determinant of IGF-1 at protein intakes less than 0.5 g/kg/day. Children with severe protein-calorie malnutrition have low IGF-1 values that respond to treatment.[141] Other catabolic conditions, such as hepatic failure, inflammatory bowel diseases, or renal failure are associated with low serum IGF-1 concentrations.[145,146] Insulin is an important determinant of IGF-1 concentrations. Although it is difficult to differentiate between nutritional regulation and insulin action, insulin perfusion of the liver in diabetic animals results in a substantial increase in plasma IGF-1.[147] Patients with poorly controlled type 1 diabetes mellitus have low normal IGF-1 values that increase into the normal range with adequate insulin treatment.[148] Furthermore, in poorly controlled type 1 diabetes, a correlation exists between hemoglobin A_1C values and IGF-1.[149] Similarly, patients with severe insulin resistance have low IGF-1 values.[150]

CONTROL OF IGFBP CONCENTRATIONS IN BLOOD AND EXTRACELLULAR FLUIDS

Four forms of IGFBPs are easily detected in plasma: IGFBP-1, -2, -3, and -4. IGFBP-3 not only is the most abundant, but also has the highest affinity for IGF-1 and -2.[151] The IGFBPs in serum perform three functions. The first is to act as transport proteins for the IGFs. The second is to regulate their half-lives, and the third is to provide a specific means for transcapillary transport into extravascular fluid compartments.

The plasma concentrations of IGFBP-3 are regulated by GH. IGFBP-3 concentrations are low in patients with GHD and increase after GH treatment.[152] This increase is partially due to a direct effect of GH on IGFBP-3 synthesis; however, it also is due to the fact that the half-life of IGFBP-3 is prolonged by binding to the two other proteins to form a ternary complex

(consisting of IGF-1 or IGF-2, IGFBP-3, and ALS). ALS is an 88-kDa glycoprotein containing several leucine-rich domains that are known to facilitate protein-protein interaction, and it is this domain structure that accounts for its binding to IGFBP-3.[153] Because IGF-1 and ALS synthesis also are increased by GH, all three components are increased, and this acts to prolong the half-life of each component. The binding of IGF-1 to this complex in plasma functions to prolong its half-life from 6 minutes in the free form, which is similar to that of insulin, to 16 hours.[154] The prolongation of the half-life of ALS-associated IGF-1/IGFBP-3 complexes also is due to the fact that this macromolecular complex (150 kDa) cannot freely cross capillary barriers, and therefore it is not excreted by the kidney. If sufficient IGF-1 and IGFBP-3 are infused to exceed the binding capacity of ALS, then their half-lives are shortened substantially, indicating that it is the ternary complex that maintains the stability and prolongs their half-lives. The molar concentration of IGFBP-3 in serum is generally equal to the sum of those of IGF-1 and -2, and therefore it is usually saturated. The affinity of IGFBP-3 for IGF-1 and -2 is not reduced by binding to ALS, and its high affinity and its long half-life account for the fact that 75% of the IGF-1 and -2 in plasma is carried in this complex.[155] The exact function of this large storage pool of IGF-1 and -2 in serum is unknown. However, it is clear that changes in the IGF-1 concentrations within this large complex correlate with the anabolic response to GH administration. Plasma IGFBP-3 levels are elevated in patients with acromegaly and low in patients with GH deficiency, as are ALS levels.[156,157] Age is an important determinant of IGFBP-3 concentrations, and they vary with age in a manner that is similar to those of IGF-1.[131]

Hormones other than GH can influence the synthesis of IGFBP-3, and, therefore, its plasma concentration. This protein is low in prepubertal boys and increases after testosterone administration. It decreases 40% after menopause and can be increased in postmenopausal women with physiologic estrogen replacement.[158] IGFBP-3 concentrations are low in patients with hypothyroidism and increase 55% after administration of thyroxine.[159]

Insulin enhances the IGFBP-3-synthesis response to GH, but it does not appear to have a direct effect. Insulin also stimulates ALS, and severe diabetes results in reduced ALS levels and reduced ternary complex formation. Although GH directly stimulates IGFBP-3 and ALS synthesis, infusion of IGF-1, although increasing serum IGFBP-3 transiently, acts to suppress its concentrations over time by suppressing GH release from the pituitary and thereby reducing ALS synthesis.[160] Because the ALS concentration is rate limiting for complex formation, the total complex levels decrease after infusion of high doses of IGF-1 for several days.

IGFBP-3 abundance in serum also is regulated by protease activity.[161,162] Several proteases that degrade IGFBP-3 have been described, including prostate-specific antigen (PSA) and plasmin, but the exact identity of the serum protease has not been determined.[163] Protease concentrations are abundant in human pregnancy serum[161,162] and also are present in GH-resistant states.[164] Proteolytic cleavage reduces the affinity of IGFBP-3 greatly, and the IGF-1 that is released binds to unsaturated IGFBP-1, -2, and -4, wherein it can equilibrate much more readily with the interstitial fluids.[165] Therefore, an important function of proteases that cleave IGFBP-3 may be to liberate IGF-1 from the IGFBP-3/ALS complex and allow them to bind to lower-affinity forms of IGFBPs that can cross capillary barriers, thus facilitating a more favorable equilibrium with the extravascular space.

The next most abundant IGFBP in plasma is IGFBP-2.[166] The affinity of IGFBP-2 for IGF-1 is less than that of IGFBP-3, and its plasma concentrations are substantially lower. IGFBP-2 concentrations are inversely regulated by GH; that is, they are high in GH deficiency, suppressed with administration of GH, and are low in acromegaly.[167] Unlike IGFBP-3, IGFBP-2 does not bind to ALS, and no ternary complex is found in plasma; therefore, its half-life when bound to IGF-1 is approximately 90 minutes. It is not saturated, and excess binding capacity exists. Intact IGFBP-2 crosses the capillary barriers.[168] IGFBP-2 also is degraded by a protease, and fragments with reduced affinity have been detected in plasma. Hepatocytes appear to be the major source of serum IGFBP-2, and the abundance of its mRNA in liver is regulated in parallel with its plasma concentrations.[169] Hypophysectomy in experimental animals results in a major increase in IGFBP-2 mRNA expression in liver. GH administration to GHD humans results in substantial reduction of plasma IGFBP-2. One of the major stimuli of IGFBP-2 concentrations in serum is IGF-1. After IGF-1 administration to GHD humans or patients with diabetes, a threefold to fourfold increase in IGFBP-2 occurs.[170] Plasma IGFBP-2 concentrations also are increased by IGF-2, and they are elevated in patients with retroperitoneal tumors that produce IGF-2.[171] Hepatic IGFBP-2 mRNA expression is significantly increased in diabetic rats and suppressed with insulin administration.[172] Severely limiting nutrient intake in humans results in increases in plasma IGFBP-2, as does poorly controlled type 1 diabetes.[173] Prolonged nutrient deprivation results in an approximately twofold increase in plasma IGFBP-2 concentrations. This appears to be dependent on protein intake, because it can be mimicked with low-protein diets that contain a normal caloric content, and IGFBP-2 expression in animals is increased during protein restriction.[174,175] Because the half-life of the IGF-1 bound to IGFBP-2 is considerably less than that of IGF-1 bound to IGFBP-3, it has been assumed that IGF-1 that is bound to IGFBP-2 is in more rapid equilibrium with IGF-1 in the extravascular space.

The third most abundant protein in serum is IGFBP-1. IGFBP-1 also circulates in binary complexes with IGF-1 and -2. Its affinity for the two growth factors is coequal (see Table 34-2). IGFBP-1 is acutely regulated by insulin.[176,177] Insulin-deficient states, such as fasting or type 1 diabetes, are associated with very high concentrations of IGFBP-1, whereas administration of insulin or ingestion of a meal results in marked suppression (fivefold to sixfold) of serum IGFBP-1 concentrations.[173,177] Major sites of synthesis of IGFBP-1 are highly restricted, and the liver is the principal site of synthesis, although kidney, maternal placenta, and uterus are other sources of this peptide. Plasma concentrations are controlled primarily by hepatic synthesis and release. Hepatic synthesis is primarily under the control of insulin,[176] although other hormones, such as GH and cortisol, also have effects.[178] IGFBP-1 in blood is unsaturated, and therefore IGFBP-1 is proposed to be a major modulator of free IGF-1 levels, particularly in response to food intake. Postprandially, changes in serum insulin result in a fourfold to fivefold decrease in IGFBP-1. This change is due to direct suppression of synthesis in the liver. IGFBP-1 mRNA expression is decreased in experimental animals after insulin administration to diabetic animals.[176] This is due to a direct effect of insulin on IGFBP-1 gene transcription, and there is an insulin response element in the 5′-flanking region of the IGFBP-1 gene.[179] IGFBP-1 crosses intact capillary beds, and the amount that crosses in a fixed period is dependent on ambient insulin concentrations.[180]

Because IGFBP-1 can bind free IGF-1, it has been proposed to have a glucoregulatory function, that is, because IGF-1 enhances insulin sensitivity, factors that lead to excessive IGFBP-1 may lead to reduced insulin sensitivity. In states of significant insulin resistance, enhanced phosphorylation of IGFBP-1 occurs, which increases its affinity for IGF-1 and therefore results in further attenuation of its ability to enhance insulin sensitivity.[181] Both fasting and diabetes have been shown to cause disproportionate increases in serum IGFBP-1 concentrations.[173,177] In addition, administration of glucocorticoid increases IGFBP-1, presumably by a direct effect on IGFBP-1 gene transcription. Administration of large

concentrations of IGFBP-1 to hypophysectomized rats have resulted in slight increases in glucose concentrations, suggesting that IGFBP-1 may have some role in regulating the insulin-like actions of IGF-1.[182] Because IGF-1 increases insulin sensitivity, the high concentrations of IGFBP-1 that occur in diabetes may contribute to insulin resistance.[183]

The exact roles of IGFBP-1 and IGFBP-2 in controlling the distribution of the IGFs has not been determined. In catabolic states, such as nutritional deprivation, GH deficiency, or renal failure, IGFBP-1 and IGFBP-2 levels are increased, and they may become the major binding component.[184–186] Similarly, in these conditions, the amount of IGF-1 that is bound to IGFBP-3 is decreased.

IGFBP-4 concentrations in serum have been shown to correlate with changes in bone physiology. Specifically, in states of low bone turnover and low parathyroid hormone concentrations, serum IGFBP-4 concentrations are increased. A correlation exists between sunlight exposure and IGFBP-4, suggesting that vitamin D, or one of its active metabolites, regulates IGFBP-4.[187]

IGFBP-5 exists in serum mostly as proteolytic fragments, and intact IGFBP-5 is present at very low concentrations. The fragments that are present have very low affinity for IGF-1 and -2, and therefore their plasma concentrations are unlikely to be major regulators of IGF-1 action. IGFBP-5 in plasma binds to ALS, and its concentrations are regulated by GH and IGF-1. Both intact IGFBP-5 and its major fragment increase substantially when GH is administered to GHD patients.[188]

IGF-binding proteins are synthesized by several cell types. Table 34-3 lists the various forms of IGFBPs in tissues, their cell type of origin and the major variables that have been shown to regulate their concentrations.

CONTROL OF IGF-1 SYNTHESIS IN TISSUES

Although it is beyond the scope of this chapter to discuss the expression of IGF-1 in all tissues that have been studied, some general principles are important for a fundamental understanding of the autocrine/paracrine–mediated actions of this growth factor. Connective tissue cells within a given tissue or organ are often the origin of IGF-1 transcripts.[189] In situ hybridization studies have shown that fibroblasts and other cells of mesenchymal origin are the primary extrahepatic source of IGF-1 in vivo.[190] Importantly, the abundance of this transcript in connective tissue cells is increased in response to GH.[191] Fibroblast synthesis also is regulated by growth factors such as PDGF.[192]

In cartilage, both GH and FGF have been shown to be potent stimuli of IGF-1 synthesis by prechondrocytes.[193] Its synthesis is most abundant in those cells that are actively differentiating, and, when chondrocytes reach the hypertrophic state, IGF-1 synthesis is diminished. Fetal chondrocytes, during development, have been shown to be an abundant source of IGF-1 mRNA.

Similar to cartilage, bone osteoblasts are a source of IGF-1 peptide, and it is synthesized in fetal calvarial tissue.[194] GH also increases IGF-1 synthesis by osteoblasts. IGF-1 synthesis rates correlate with changes in osteoblast DNA synthesis, type I collagen synthesis, and synthesis of other components of bone ECM.[195] Several bone trophic factors, such as bone morphogenic proteins (BMPs), stimulate the synthesis of IGF-1 mRNA by these cells. Both BMP-2 and BMP-3 stimulate IGF-1 synthesis.[196,197] In bone, IGF-1 mRNA expression is downregulated by glucocorticoids. In contrast, estrogen stimulates the expression of IGF-1.[198] Prostaglandins also are potent inducers of IGF-1 gene transcription by osteoblasts, and PTH is a potent stimulator of IGF-1 gene transcription.[189,199] PTH mediates its effect through cyclic adenosine monophosphate (cAMP) induction, which enhances IGF-1 gene transcription.[200] In contrast, the bone growth factors, FGF, PDGF, and TGF-β, downregulate IGF-1 expression. IGF-1 appears to be an important factor for erythropoiesis. Red cell

Table 34-3 The Various Forms of Insulin-Like Growth Factor–Binding Proteins (IGFBPs)

Tissue	Primary Cell Type of Origin or Area	Form of IGFBP Secreted	Variables That Control Synthesis or Secretion
Uterus, decidua	Stroma and epithelium	IGFBP-1	Estrogen, progesterone
	Stroma	IGFBP-2, -4, -5, -6	
	Endothelium	IGFBP-3	
	Myometrium	IGFBP-2, -3, -5	
Placenta	Epithelium	IGFBP-1	Hypoxia, dexamethasone
		IGFBP-2, -3, -4	Fetal development
Brain	Choroid plexus, meninges	IGFBP-2	
	Capillaries	IGFBP-3	
	Olfactory bulb, Schwann cells	IGFBP-2, -6	
	White matter, nerves	IGFBP-5	
	Glial cells	IGFBP-2, -3	Hypoxic injury
	Focal neuronal concentrations	IGFBP-4	
Kidney	Collecting ducts	IGFBP-1	
	Distal tubules	IGFBP-2	Work induction by furosemide
	Mesangial cells	IGFBP-5	
Lung	Mesenchymal cells (fetus)	IGFBP-2	
	Epithelium (fetus)	IGFBP-2	
	Pneumatocytes	IGFBP-4	
	Interstitial cells	IGFBP-5	
Breast	Epithelium	IGFBP-2, -3	Increased IGFBP-5 during lactation
	Stroma	IGFBP-3, -4, -5	Increased IGFBP-5 during lactation withdrawal
Cartilage	Prechondrocytes	IGFBP-3, -4, -5	
	Hypertrophic chondrocytes	IGFBP-3, -5	
Bone	Osteoblasts	IGFBP-5	Age-related decrease
		IGFBP-4	Vitamin D
	Capillaries	IGFBP-3	
Gut	Epithelium	IGFBP-2, -4	
		IGFBP-3	Nutrient deprivation
	Lamina propria	IGFBP-3, -5	Increase in response to injury
Bladder	Smooth muscle	IGFBP-2, -4, -5	Hypertrophy increases IGFBP-2
Prostate	Stroma	IGFBP-2, -3	
Liver	Hepatocytes	IGFBP-1, -2, -4, -6	Fasting increases IGFBP-1, -2; insulin deprivation increases IGFBP-1, -2
	Sinusoids, stroma	IGFBP-3, -5	GH increases IGFBP-3
Ovary	Theca	IGFBP-2, -4	LH increases IGFBP-2; involution increases IGFBP-4
	Stroma	IGFBP-5	
	Stroma, capillaries	IGFBP-3	
	Corpus luteum	IGFBP-3	
Connective tissue	Fibroblasts	IGFBP-3, -4, -5	IGF-1, IGF-2, RA increase IGFBP-3; TNF-α, IL-1 increase IGFBP-4; dexamethasone increases IGFBP-4 and decreases IGFBP-5; IGF-1 increases IGFBP-5
Skeletal muscle	Myoblasts, myocytes	IGFBP-2, -4, -5	Differentiation increases IGFBP-2 and -5
Blood vessels	Endothelium	IGFBP-2, -3, -4, -6	
	Smooth muscle	IGFBP-2, -4, -5	Injury increases IGFBP-5

GH, growth hormone; LH, luteinizing hormone; RA, retinoic acid; TNF-α, tumor necrosis factor-α; IL-1, interleukin-1.

mass is decreased in GHD animals, and it is restored to normal with IGF-1 administration.[201] Erythroid precursor cells have been shown to synthesize IGF-1, and its synthesis can be stimulated in these cells both by GH and erythropoietin. Similarly, granulocyte precursor cells synthesize IGF-1 mRNA, and this is stimulated by granulocyte-macrophage colony-stimulating factor.[202]

Reproductive Tract
IGF-1 expression is decreased in the ovary of the hypophysectomized rat, and ovarian expression increases in response to GH. Estrogen can increase ovarian IGF-1 expression, and this has been localized primarily to the thecal cells of the early follicle.[203] IGF-1 receptors also are present in these follicles, indicating the possibility for an autocrine loop. Follicular fluid contains IGF-1 and -2 peptides, and their concentrations are increased after FSH administration.[204] Several studies suggest that the effects of IGF-2 predominate over time of IGF-1 in the ovary, and much more IGF-2 is produced in that organ. In the oviduct, IGF-1 and -2 have been shown to be present in oviductal fluid, and oviductal cells express the encoding by mRNA of both IGF-1 and -2, as well as IGF-1 receptors. Endometrium normally expresses IGF-1 mRNA, and, in rats, a 20-fold increase can be induced with estradiol administration.[9] Estrogen induces IGF-1 expression primarily in the epithelium, whereas progesterone induces it in the endometrial stroma. In the late proliferative phase, IGF-1 mRNA is present almost exclusively in the stroma. Similarly, IGF-1-receptor mRNA is upregulated during the secretory phase of the menstrual cycle. The testes express IGF-1 mRNA, and the source of origin is the Leydig cell.[205] IGF-1 expression by Leydig cells is downregulated by IL-1 and stimulated by LH.

Neural Tissue
Circulating plasma IGF-1 crosses the blood-brain barrier. However, much of the IGF-1 that is present in cerebrospinal fluid (CSF) is believed to arise from IGF-1 synthesis within the central nervous system (CNS). The major sites of IGF-1 mRNA are the Purkinje cells of the cerebellum, the olfactory bulb, and the hippocampus.[206] The retina also is a site of postnatal

expression. Astroglial cells in the cerebellum also are an important site of IGF-1 synthesis. Immunohistochemical staining has shown that IGF-1 is transported along axons and dendrites, and that IGF-1 peptide is present in the choroid plexus. Factors that regulate IGF-1 synthesis in peripheral tissues such as nutrition,[207] thyroid hormone,[208] and estrogen,[209] also regulate CNS IGF-1 expression. TNF-α downregulates IGF-1 expression.[210]

Muscle

IGF-1 mRNA is expressed in the satellite cells and myoblasts of skeletal muscle.[211,212] After an ischemic or toxic injury, a major increase is found in IGF-1 mRNA expression.[211] The wave of increase of expression after skeletal muscle injury coincides with the appearance of regenerating tissue and rapid cell division. Work-induced hypertrophy in muscle also can lead to an increase in expression of IGF-1 and -2, indicating that this change is GH independent.[213] The IGF-1B transcript is selectively increased.[214] Cardiac muscle also is a site of IGF-1 synthesis, and it is increased in models of cardiac hypertrophy that have been induced either by pressure or by volume overload.[215,216] Blood vessels also are an important site of IGF-1 synthesis. Both endothelial and smooth muscle cells contain IGF-1 mRNA. Pressure overload results in increased IGF-1 expression.[217] After blood vessel injury, an increase in IGF-1 expression by smooth muscle cells is found.[218]

Liver

IGF-1 expression in liver correlates extremely well with changes in plasma GH concentrations. Expression in hepatic tissue is low in hypophysectomized animals and increases after administration of GH.[219] The effect of GH has been shown to be mediated through the transcription factor STAT5B.[220] Likewise, nutritional deprivation results in a major decrease in IGF-1 mRNA abundance, and this can be restored with refeeding.[221] A part of this change is due to a change in transcription, and part is due to a change in mRNA stability.

The liver is a major site of insulin action, and insulin regulates IGF-1 mRNA expression.[222] Similarly, the effect of thyroxine on serum IGF-1 is mediated through its effect on hepatic IGF-1 expression.[223]

Development

IGF-1 transcripts are easily detected in developing rats, in intestine, liver, lung, and brain. Expression is present in as early as 11-day embryos, and IGF-1 mRNA abundance increases 8.6-fold by day 13.[224] In early embryos, IGF-1 is detected in yolk sac, hepatic bud, dermal myotomes, sclerotomes, as well as brachial arch mesoderm. In late fetal development, IGF-1 content is increased in muscle, precartilaginous mesenchymal condensations, perichondrium, and the immature chondrocyte periosteum, as well as in ossification centers.[225] In human fetal embryos, IGF-1 mRNA levels are relatively low at 16 weeks, and the highest levels are found in placenta and stomach. At 20 weeks, fetal kidney, placenta, lung, brain, cartilage, as well as liver, have detectible transcripts. The perisinusoidal cells of the liver and the perichondrium appear to be foci of intense expression in 20-week fetuses, and the cells of origin appear to be fibroblast-like. Postnatally, IGF-1 expression increases markedly in skin, nerve, and muscle.

IGF-1 Expression in Kidney

IGF-1 is expressed at low levels in the fetal kidney; however, in the adult kidney in rats, IGF-1 mRNA is abundant.[226] Immunohistochemical staining shows moderate amounts of IGF-1 in both the proximal and distal tubules of human fetuses. In adult rats, IGF-1 is localized primarily over the collecting ducts. Overexpression of IGF-1 in transgenic animal kidneys has been shown to result in renal growth, and GH

administration to GHD rats results in increased expression of IGF-1 in the kidney. Unilateral nephrectomy in rats results in compensatory growth of the contralateral kidney and in increased mRNA expression 24 hours after nephrectomy.[227] This increase in compensatory synthesis is partly dependent on GH, because it is less intense in hypophysectomized animals. After ischemic injury, increased IGF-1 immunoreactivity is noted in the regenerating cells of the proximal tubules.

Control of IGFBP Concentrations in Tissues

Because IGF-1 and -2 function not only as endocrine hormones, but also as paracrine regulators of growth and differentiation in tissues, the primary role of the IGFBPs in tissues may be to control the amount of locally produced IGF that is accessible to receptors. The exact regulation of the six binding proteins in each tissue in which they are expressed is beyond the scope of this chapter. As shown in Table 34-3, each tissue appears to express different combinations of binding proteins differentially.

THE ACTIONS OF THE IGFs: IGF-1 ACTIONS IN VITRO

IGF-1 receptors are present in almost all cell types and mediate most of the effects of IGF-1 and IGF-2 in vitro, as well as the growth-promoting effects of insulin, when it is present in sufficiently high concentrations to activate this receptor (e.g., concentrations greater than 10^{-7} mol/L). Several biologic actions of IGF-1 have been studied by using cells in culture, including anabolic effects such as increases in protein synthesis and cell size; effects on carbohydrate metabolism, such as glucose transport, glucose oxidation, and lipid synthesis; and the effects on cell growth, including stimulation of DNA synthesis, mitogenesis, and inhibition of cell death. Other generalized processes that have been analyzed include cell-cycle progression, cell differentiation, and cellular migration. Specific events, such as synthesis of individual proteins, have been analyzed, as well as the ability of IGF-1 to augment specific functions of differentiated cells that are stimulated by other hormones or growth factors.

CELL-CYCLE PROGRESSION

One of the most commonly studied effects of IGF-1 in vitro is its ability to stimulate DNA synthesis. IGF-1 appears to act principally by stimulating entry into DNA synthesis from the latter part of the G_1 phase of the cell cycle.[228] In some systems, its presence is required for progression through all 12 hours of G_1. IGF-1 is not as potent in stimulating quiescent cells to enter G_1 compared with other growth factors, such as PDGF or FGF, but once cells have entered the cycle, it is often sufficient to stimulate progression through to S phase.[229] In some cell types, it is possible to alter this requirement by overexpressing EGF, the c-myb proto-oncogene, or SV40 T antigen.[230] Generally, these manipulations cause cells to secrete more autocrine-produced IGF-1 and thereby stimulate the IGF-1 receptor. Support for the hypothesis that constitutively synthesized IGF-1 is still required in such systems derives from studies in which antibodies that inhibit IGF-1 binding to its receptor block DNA synthesis, and cells that have had the IGF-1 receptor deleted do not grow in response to stimulation by other growth factors.[231] Similarly, in some systems, enhanced expression of the IGF-1 receptor will abrogate the need for PDGF or FGF.[232]

Other growth factors have been shown to work cooperatively with IGF system components. PDGF and FGF increase the number of IGF-1-binding sites, and FGF increases constitutive tyrosine phosphorylation of the IGF-1 receptor kinase.[233] IGF-1 is a mitogen for essentially every type of cell that possesses IGF-1 receptors. These include all mesenchymal cell types, many types of epithelial cells, including neuronal epithelium, and multiple endodermally derived cell types. Cell lines in culture that have been shown to have an increased number of IGF-1 receptors are more sensitive to the growth-promoting actions of IGF-1. A factor complicating the interpretation of all of the studies that analyze IGF-1 effects on growth in vitro is the autocrine secretion of IGF-1. This autocrine-synthesized IGF-1 is capable of binding to receptors and potentiating IGF-1 action through the IGF-1 receptor.[234] Therefore, analysis of the effects of IGF-1 added to cells in culture often must take into account this confounding variable. In many of the studies in which synergism between IGF-1 and other growth factors has been observed, their effects are partially due to autocrine-secreted IGF-1. Hormones, such as TSH and FSH, and growth factors, such as PDGF and EGF, may exert part of their proliferative effects by stimulating autocrine secretion of IGF-1.[235]

EFFECTS OF IGF-1 ON THE PROLIFERATION OF DIFFERENT TYPES OF CELLS

Cartilage

Many of the growth-promoting actions of GH on skeletal growth are believed to be due to the local production of IGF-1 by prechondrocytes or early differentiating chondrocytes within the epiphyseal growth plate.[236] In vitro, IGF-1 stimulates cartilage cell division and size, as well as proteoglycan synthesis, which contributes to enhanced extracellular matrix synthesis.[237] IGF-1 also inhibits apoptosis in these cells.[238] Transplantation of articular chondrocytes that had been transfected with IGF-1 complementary DNA (cDNA) showed increased cell growth and matrix synthesis.[239]

Bone

IGF-1 stimulates several anabolic effects on bone cells in culture. Exposure of preosteoblast cells to IGF-1 results in stimulation of type I collagen synthesis, DNA and RNA synthesis, as well as total protein synthesis.[240] In addition, skeletal tissue is a rich source of stored IGF-1. Osteoblasts themselves can synthesize IGF-1, and several of the IGF-binding proteins that bind to bone extracellular matrix can act as a storage reservoir.[112] IGF-1 expression has been shown to be stimulated by a number of hormones and cytokines that are potent trophic growth factors for bone, implying that many of their effects may be mediated locally through IGF-1 production. Genetic models in which components of the IGF system have been altered have verified the importance of locally synthesized IGF-1.[241] Targeted overexpression of IGF-1 in bone is associated with increased bone mineral density,[242] and targeted deletion of the IGF-1 receptor is associated with poor responsiveness to parathyroid hormone.[243] Targeted deletion of hepatic IGF-1 gene expression that reduces serum IGF-1 results in decreased cortical bone thickness.[244]

Skin

Proliferation of primary human keratinocytes in culture has been shown to be stimulated by IGF-1, and IGF-1 is produced by dermal fibroblasts, but not by skin epithelial cells, which suggests that paracrine stimulation of skin epithelium by IGF-1 derived from dermal fibroblasts may be the primary mechanism by which this growth factor contributes to epithelial proliferation.[245]

Skeletal Muscle

Several types of myoblasts in culture have been shown to respond to IGF-1 addition. Both IGF-1 and -2 stimulate muscle cell protein synthesis, as well as DNA synthesis.[246] Their effects are complex, because they are linked to the differentiation program of these cells (see later). IGF-1 is synthesized by the satellite cells that are premyoblast precursors and synthesis in satellite cells is controlled by the need to maximize the proliferative pool. After stimulation of myoblast proliferation, prolonged exposure to higher concentrations of IGF-1 results in terminal differentiation.[247] This effect is linked to the ability of IGF-1 to enhance the expression of the myogenic differentiation protein, myogenin. Muscle-specific deletion of the IGF-1 receptor results in muscle hypoplasia at birth,[214] and IGF-1 overexpression enhances DNA synthesis during regeneration after injury.[248] Increased expression also increases muscle DNA synthesis and cell number in normal animals.[249,250] Cardiac muscle IGF-1 overexpression has been shown to reduce ventricular dilatation in models of cardiomyopathy.[251]

Smooth Muscle

Targeted overexpression of IGF-1 results in enhanced smooth muscle cell growth in response to balloon injury.[252] The expression of contractile proteins such as myosin heavy chain is increased in these animals, leading to enhanced contractility.[253] Similarly, IGF-1 overexpression in intestinal smooth muscle leads to increased growth of the muscularis.[254]

Nervous System

The major cell types that grow in response to IGF-1 are astrocytes and glial cell precursors.[255] In end-terminally differentiated neurons, IGF-1 has been shown to stimulate neurite outgrowth and myelin synthesis.[256] Cells derived from the sympathetic nervous system, such as adrenal chromaffin cells, are stimulated to divide by IGF-1.[257] IGF-1 is a stimulant of neurite outgrowth in axons damaged by denervation.[258,259] In animals, IGF-1 is required for normal growth of the olfactory bulb.[260] Deletion of IGF-1 or IGF-1R results in brain growth retardation, and localized increase in cerebellar expression increased cerebellar size.[261] Detailed analysis has shown that some of these changes are due to changes in cell number.[262] Similarly, after injury, animals that had had IGF-1-receptor expression deleted in brain showed decreased changes in oligodendrocytes and reduced myelin synthesis.[263]

Other Cell Types

Other cell types that have been shown to be IGF-1 responsive include mammary epithelial cells, vascular smooth muscle cells, endothelial cells, mesangial cells, erythroid progenitor cells, oocytes, adrenal fasciculata cells, granulosa cells, promyelocytic cells, granulocyte colony-forming cells, fetal hepatocytes, pancreatic islet cells, oligodendrocytes, Sertoli cells, and spermatogonia.[225]

EFFECTS ON CELL DEATH

In many systems, IGF-1 has been shown to be a potent inhibitor of programmed cell death. The systems that have been the best characterized are hematopoietic and neuronal cell precursors. In hematopoietic cells, erythroid progenitor cells can be induced to undergo apoptosis with serum or erythropoietin deprivation, and this effect is suppressed by IGF-1.[264] IGF-1 inhibits apoptosis in myeloid precursors that occurs after the discontinuation of stimulatory cytokines, such as IL-3.[265] In many tumor cell types, transfection with a dominant negative form of the IGF-1 receptor (a form of IGF receptor that has a TK-defective subunit) results in enhancement of the apoptotic effect that is induced by cytotoxic agents.[266] During ovarian follicle development, IGF-1 stimulation by gonadotropins may prevent apoptosis of the developing follicular cells.[267] IGF-1 has been shown to inhibit the apoptosis that occurs during development in myoblasts, neurons, and oligodendrocytes.[93]

EFFECTS ON CELLULAR DIFFERENTIATION

In cultured myoblasts, IGF-1 induces the expression of myogenin, a specific myoblast differentiation factor, and myogenin induction can be blocked with antisense oligonu-cleotides that inhibit the synthesis of autocrine-stimulated IGF-1.[268] Autocrine-produced IGF-2 may have similar effects. The programmed events that occur during differentiation in response to IGF-1 are time specific because, in L-6 myoblasts, cellular exposure to high concentrations of IGF-1 early in the differentiation program acts to inhibit differentiation, but at later times, it is accelerated.[247,268] IGF-2 also may inhibit apoptosis that occurs during transition from proliferation to differentiation in myoblastic cell lines. Differentiation markers also have been shown to be preferentially stimulated in response to IGF-1 or -2 in osteoclasts, chondrocytes, and neural cells.[269–271] The addition of IGF-1 to different types of cultured neurons has been shown to enhance neuronal differentiation. Maintenance of neuroepithelial cultures in several model systems has been shown to be enhanced by IGF-1, probably by inhibiting apoptosis.

EFFECTS ON SPECIFIC CELLULAR FUNCTIONS

Production of steroids by ovarian granulosa cells and thecal cells has been shown to be stimulated by IGF-1 and -2, and their effects are synergistic with FSH.[204] IGF-1 also stimulates steroid hormone secretion by adrenocorticotropic hormone (ACTH)-responsive, adrenal cortical cells.[272] IGF-1 stimulates testosterone secretion from Leydig cells and acts synergistically with LH to increase the response.[273] Similarly, thyroglobulin production by thyroid follicular cells is synergistically enhanced with TSH plus IGF-1.[274] Thymulin is a specific secretory product of thymic epithelium that is stimulated by IGF-1. GH secretion by pituitary cells is inhibited by IGF-1.[275] Histamine release from beta cells in response to immunoglobulin E is potentiated by IGF-1. IGF-1 inhibits glutamate-stimulated release of γ-aminobutyric acid (GABA) from Purkinje cells. IGF-1 is a specific stimulant of IGFBP-5 synthesis by muscle cells and fibroblasts.[276] Other specific proteins whose synthesis is stimulated by IGF-1 include elastin by smooth muscle cells,[277] crystallin by lens epithelial cells,[278] and cholesterol side-cleavage enzyme by adrenal cortical cells.[279] Some proteins whose expression is increased after IGF-1 have been shown to result in specific functional changes in that cell type (e.g., the increased α-actin in skeletal muscle[280] and the increased myelin in neuronal cells[281]). Microarray studies have shown that IGF-1 selectively upregulates the expression of several genes and some, such as heparin-binding EGF and twist, may have important implications for cellular growth.[282,283]

Several generalized metabolic processes that are stimulated by IGF-1 in a variety of cell types have been analyzed. These include glucose uptake, glycolysis, glycogen synthesis, and glucose oxidation in fat cells and skeletal muscle cells.[284] These metabolic effects can be mediated by the insulin receptor if sufficient IGF-1 is added in vitro (e.g., concentrations $>10^{-8}$ mol/L); however, antibody-blocking studies have indicated that IGF-1 can have direct effects on this process through its own receptor in some cell types. Similarly, the hybrid IGF-1/insulin receptor may play a role in mediating these effects in some cell types. Total protein synthesis, ECM protein synthesis and cell migration, and the synthesis of proteoglycans and collagen, in particular, have been analyzed extensively in connective tissue cells. IGF-1 often acts in concert with other growth factors to stimulate connective tissue cell protein synthesis. IGF-1 is a potent stimulant of cell migration and stimulates this process by both chemotaxis and chemokinesis.[285] IGF-1 is not directly angiogenic, but it can stimulate the synthesis of angiogenic peptides, such as vascular endothelial cell growth factor.

ROLE OF IGF-1 IN MALIGNANT TUMORS

Because IGF-1 is a potent inhibitor of apoptosis, it has been proposed that it may function to enhance tumor formation in

several experimental animal models. The presence of an intact IGF-1 receptor is required for tumor propagation.[19,286] In the absence of IGF-1 receptors, C6 glioma cells do not form tumors, and they undergo apoptosis.[266] Often, the presence of a normal IGF-1-receptor number is inadequate for tumor formation, and the IGF-1 receptors must be overexpressed.[30] However, several processes that are necessary for tumor formation can be facilitated by IGF-1, even in the absence of enhanced receptor number, such as prevention of cell death. Deletion of the receptor results in inability of cells that would normally be tumorigenic in nude mice to form tumors, and mutation of specific tyrosine residues on the receptor and expression of these mutated receptors results in lack of tumor formation.[59,287] In human tumors, a direct causal role for the receptor in pathogenesis has been difficult to prove. All of the data that exist are correlative. In Wilms' tumor, small cell lung carcinoma, and uterine cancer, IGF-1-receptor number is increased.[288] No mutations of the receptor have been identified as a cause of human tumors.

Several cell types that form tumors in animals have been shown to overproduce IGF-1 or IGF-2. However, in these systems, antisense IGF-1 often does not inhibit tumor formation or induce apoptosis, in contrast to the effects that are induced by blocking receptor synthesis. Transgenic mice that overexpress IGF-2 have a higher rate of hepatic tumor formation.[289] Precancerous liver nodules that occur in virally induced models of hepatic cancers overexpress IGF-2. Pancreatic tumor cells that have been transformed with SV40 T antigen require IGF-2 for continued growth.[290] Certain fetal tumors, such as Wilms' tumor and neuroblastoma, are accompanied by loss of imprinting of the IGF-2 gene, and overproduction of IGF-2 accompanies tumor formation.[291] The IGF-2 receptor also has been implicated as a tumor suppressor in hepatocellular carcinomas, possibly through its role in the clearance and degradation of IGF-2.[292] The only paraneoplastic syndrome that is known to be definitively linked to IGF-2 overproduction occurs with retroperitoneal sarcomas. Overproduction of IGF-2 by the tumor results in hypoglycemia.[293] The mechanism that has been proposed is that IGF-2 binds to lower-molecular-weight forms of IGFBPs in plasma (such as IGFBP-2), and this allows accelerated equilibration of IGF-1 and -2 with extravascular fluids, thus leading to increase the IGF-1 in interstitial fluids and to hypoglycemia. Studies in mice have shown that IGF-1 overexpression is associated with mammary intraepithelial neoplasia; conversely, expression of dominant/negative forms of the IGF-1 receptor is associated with decreased tumor progression.[294,295] Similarly, animals with low serum IGF-1 due to gene targeting of hepatic IGF-1 have delayed onset and reduced severity of many tumors. Transgenic overexpression of IGF-1 in mouse prostate also leads to a higher prevalence of tumors at younger ages compared with control animals.[296]

CONTROL OF IGF-1 ACTIONS IN CELLS AND TISSUES BY IGFBPs

Because the IGFBPs are ubiquitously present in all tissues and have a high affinity for IGF-1, they function in regulate IGF-1 actions by controlling access to receptors. The most important determinant of this capacity to modulate IGF-1 action is their affinity, although other variables, such as binding to their own receptors, which leads to IGF-1-independent actions, may play a role.

VARIABLES THAT REGULATE IGFBP AFFINITY

The affinity of each binding protein is shown in Table 34-3. The estimates vary, but they range between twofold and 50-fold greater than the affinity of the type 1 IGF receptor for IGF-1.

The biologic consequence of this high-affinity binding is the inhibition of IGF-1 or IGF-2 binding to cell-surface receptors. Variables that reduce IGFBP affinity to levels that are less than the IGF-1 receptor, such as proteolysis, function to allow an increase in the amount of receptor-associated IGF. In contrast, variables that reduce IGFBP affinity into a range where it approximates that of the receptor but leaves the form of IGFBP intact may result in prolonged but enhanced diffusion of IGF-1 and -2 onto receptors. Either process may result in enhancement of IGF-1 actions, but the type of effect that is enhanced may differ. Additionally, IGFBPs may function to alter the clearance rate of IGF-1 and -2 in tissues and thereby provide a more stable reservoir of peptides. At present, three variables have been identified that significantly alter the affinity of one or more of the IGFBPs. These include proteolysis, phosphorylation, and adherence to cell surfaces or ECM.

PROTEOLYSIS

Proteolysis of IGFBP-3 by serum proteases has been shown to result in marked reduction in affinity for IGF-1 and a significant, but less-intense change in affinity for IGF-2. The principal fragment that is retained, the 32-kDa fragment, has at least a 20-fold reduction in affinity for IGF-1.[297] This protease is present in high concentrations in pregnancy serum and after nutritional deprivation. It also is detectable in states of GHD and in poorly controlled diabetes.[298] The nature of the protease is unknown, although a significant amount of data supports the hypothesis that it is a cation-dependent, serine protease. Matrix metalloproteases (MMPs), such as MMP-1, MMP-2, and MMP-9, degrade several forms of IGFBPs, including IGFBP-3, and constitute part of the IGFBP-3 serum protease activity that is noted during pregnancy.[299] Several well-defined proteases have been shown to degrade IGFBP-3, including plasmin, cathepsin-D, and prostate-specific antigen.[300-302] IGFBP-3 proteolytic activity has been noted in lymph, follicular fluid, peritoneal fluid, and amniotic fluid. The IGFBP-2 protease also is a cation-dependent serine protease and cleaves IGFBP-2 into fragments that have very low affinity for IGF-1 and -2. To cleave IGFBP-2 optimally, this protease requires that IGF-1 or -2 be bound to IGFBP-2.[303] IGFBP-5 has been shown to be cleaved by proteases in a variety of physiologic fluids, including serum, and by the complement C1s that is present in cell-culture supernatants from fibroblasts, osteoblasts, and smooth muscle cells.[304] IGFBP-5, like IGFBP-3, also is cleaved by MMP-2 and -9.[305] The fragments of IGFBP-5 that are generated have very low affinity. Blocking proteolytic cleavage by incubating IGF-1 with a mutated, protease-resistant form of IGFBP-5 was shown to inhibit IGF-1-stimulated cell growth. IGFBP-4 proteases also are present in several physiologic fluids. Like IGFBP-2, IGFBP-4 proteolytic activity is enhanced by IGF binding to IGFBP-4.[306] Correlative data suggest that degradation of IGFBP-4 results in relief of inhibition of IGF-1 actions.[307] Plasma associated pregnancy protein-A (PPAP-A), a metalloprotease, has been shown to cleave IGFBP-4.[308]

IGFBP PHOSPHORYLATION

Three of the six forms of IGFBP have been shown to be phosphorylated: IGFBP-1, -3, and -5. IGFBP-1 is phosphorylated on serine residues at positions 101, 119, and 169. Caseine kinase-2 is one of two kinases that can actively phosphorylate IGFBP-1.[309] Phosphorylation increases the affinity of IGFBP-1 for IGF-1 by sixfold. Different degrees of phosphorylated IGFBP-1 have been found in different physiologic fluids, and during poorly controlled diabetes, a very highly phosphorylated form of IGFBP-1 predominates.[152] IGFBP-3 is phosphorylated at positions 111 and 113,[310] and IGF-1 stimulates its phosphorylation. Caseine kinase-2 phosphorylates IGFBP-3.

ADHERENCE TO CELL SURFACE, EXTRACELLULAR MATRIX, AND GLYCOSAMINOGLYCANS

Both IGFBP-3 and IGFBP-5 have been shown to adhere to cell surfaces. Proteoglycans may be important cell surface–binding components for both proteins. Specific receptors have been postulated to exist for IGFBP-3. The type V TGF-β receptor is an important cell-surface moeity that binds IGFBP-3.[311] IGF-1 that is bound to ECM or cell-associated IGFBP-3 is in more favorable equilibrium with receptors, because IGFBP-3 binding to cells reduces its affinity by approximately 10-fold.[312] IGFBP-5 binding to ECM or to proteoglycans causes an eightfold reduction in its affinity.[116] However, proteoglycans are not the only type of ECM protein that can bind to IGFBP-5. Plasminogen activator inhibitor-1,[313] osteopontin, and thrombospondin[314] have been shown to bind to IGFBP-5 with high affinity. Localization of IGFBP-5 within the ECM may provide an important means for focally concentrating IGF-1 or -2 in the pericellular environment.[315-318]

EFFECTS OF SPECIFIC FORMS OF IGFBP ON IGF-1 ACTIONS

IGFBP-1

Detailed analysis of IGFBP-1 actions in vitro has shown that this protein, when added in excess over IGF-1, is generally inhibitory. That is, if highly phosphorylated, high-affinity forms of IGFBP-1 are added in a 4:1 molar excess over IGF-1, they inhibit DNA synthesis, as well as glucose incorporation and glucose transport.[319,320] IGFBP-1 has been shown to block IGF-1 binding to receptors on human endometrial membranes, and it inhibits differentiated functions such as steroidogenic response of human granulosa cells to IGF-1. IGFBP-1 also can enhance the cellular response to IGF-1. If the dephosphorylated form of IGFBP-1 is used and added in an equimolar ratio or less with IGF-1, IGFBP-1 can potentiate the in vitro response of smooth muscle cells, keratinocytes, and fibroblasts to IGF-1.[321,322] IGFBP-1 has been shown to stimulate migration of CHO cells, fibroblasts, and trophoblasts directly by binding to the α5β1 integrin receptor through its RGD sequence.[106,323] This effect does not require IGF-1 binding to IGFBP-1.

IGFBP-2

IGFBP-2 also has been shown to be inhibitory in most in vitro experiments. By using purified IGFBP-2, it was shown to inhibit IGF-1-stimulated thymidine incorporation into chick embryo fibroblasts and rat astroglial cells, as well as into a human lung carcinoma cell line. IGFBP-2 inhibited IGF-1- or IGF-2-stimulated protein synthesis in Madin-Darby bovine kidney (MDBK) cells, and des-IGF-1, which did not bind to IGFBP-2, was fully stimulatory.[324] Overexpression in renal epithelial cells in vitro resulted in inhibition of IGF-1 actions.[325] IGFBP-2 was shown to mediate the inhibitory effect of TGF-β on lung epithelial cell growth.[326] IGFBP-2 has been shown to stimulate IGF-1-stimulated glucose incorporation and aminoisobutyric acid (AIB) transport in microvascular endothelial cells and DNA synthesis in smooth muscle cells.[327,328] IGFBP-2 was shown to enhance glioblastoma invasion[329] and to stimulate the growth of prostate cancer cells.[330]

IGFBP-3

IGFBP-3, if added in molar excess, inhibits glucose incorporation into fat cells, as well as IGF-1-stimulated DNA synthesis in human fibroblasts. Maximal inhibition was noted at a 5:1

molar ratio. IGFBP-3 inhibits IGF-1-stimulated glucose incorporation.[331] If IGFBP-3 is preincubated with muscle cells and then removed from the medium, it can potentiate their AIB transport response to IGF-1.[332] With this experimental paradigm, IGFBP-3 also was shown to enhance the IGF-1-stimulated DNA-synthesis response of human fibroblasts, but coincubation with IGFBP-3 was inhibitory.[333] IGFBP-3 inhibited IGF-1-stimulated cAMP generation by rat granulosa cells and inhibited IGF-1-stimulated collagen synthesis by osteoblasts.[334] Addition of IGFBP-3 to breast epithelial cells results in growth inhibition.[335] In addition, it inhibits the growth of breast cancer cells in part by stimulating the activity of a phosphatase that downregulates IGF-1 signaling.[336]

IGF-INDEPENDENT EFFECTS

IGFBP-3 has been shown to bind to the type V TGF-β receptor. Direct addition of IGFBP-3 has been shown to attenuate the effects of several growth factors, including FGF, on cell growth.[337] TGF-β is believed to cause part of its growth inhibitory effect in breast carcinoma cells through induction of IGFBP-3.[338] Increasing the expression of IGFBP-3 has been shown to inhibit the antiproliferative actions of several factors.[339-341] Antibodies to IGFBP-3 block the stimulation of apoptosis by TGF-β in prostate carcinoma cells. IGFBP-3 can inhibit growth of fibroblasts that do not possess IGF-1 receptors. These findings indicate that IGFBP-3 clearly has some growth-suppressive effects, at least in vitro, that are independent of IGF-1. IGFBP-3 also has been shown to stimulate apoptosis in certain cell lines, including cells that do not possess IGF-1 receptors. In addition to its ability to bind to the type V TGF-β receptor, IGFBP-3 has been shown to bind the retinoid X receptor α (RXRα) receptor and to inhibit retinoic acid signaling.[342] This response requires nuclear translocation of IGFBP-3, which has been demonstrated to occur.[343]

Modulation of IGF Actions by IGFBP-4

IGFBP-4 has been consistently shown in some in vitro experiments to inhibit the actions of IGF-1 on cartilage and bone growth.[344] IGFBP-4 that is synthesized constitutively by intestinal carcinoma cells inhibits this growth.[345] Several differentiated functions of IGF-1 have been shown to be inhibited by IGFBP-4, including the generation of cAMP by osteoblasts, protein synthesis by prostatic cells, and glycogen synthesis by osteosarcoma cells, as well as the steroidogenic response of granulosa cells to FSH. IGFBP-4 potently inhibits smooth muscle cell replication, as well as AIB transport.[346] A protease-resistant mutant of IGFBP-4 inhibited osteoblast proliferation.[347] Cultured myoblasts overexpressing IGFBP-4 showed impaired proliferation and differentiation.[348]

IGFBP-5

IGFBP-5 has been shown to potentiate the effects of IGF-1 in stimulating protein synthesis and DNA synthesis in skeletal tissue, including myoblasts, smooth muscle cells, fibroblasts, osteoblasts, and chondrocytes.[304,349] The potentiation of IGF-1-stimulated fibroblast and smooth muscle cell growth is believed to occur by association of IGFBP-5 with ECM.[116] ECM binding requires a specific region of basic amino acids that are located between positions 201 and 218, and mutation of specific basic residues within this motif results in the loss of ECM association and an inability of IGFBP-5 to potentiate the effects of IGF.[350] IGFBP-5 also can potentiate the effect of IGF-2 on mouse osteoblast, DNA, and protein synthesis. IGFBP-5 has been shown to have effects that are independent of IGF-1. A fragment of IGFBP-5 that does not bind IGF-1 has been shown to potentiate the effect of IGF-1 on osteoblast DNA synthesis[351] and to stimulate mesangial cell migration.[352] Overexpression of IGFBP-5 has been shown to activate MAPK independent of IGF-1.[353] In contrast, some studies have demonstrated that IGFBP-5 overexpression results in growth inhibition.[354-356] Schwann cell differentiation that is stimulated by IGF-1 has been shown to be potentiated by IGFBP-5.[357]

IGFBP-6 appears preferentially to inhibit the effects of IGF-2 in bone, and the response of neuroblastoma cells in culture to IGF-1 is inhibited by IGFBP-6.[358,359] Addition of IGFBP-6 inhibited cartilage growth,[360] and its overexpression in rhadomyosarcoma or bronchial epithelial cells resulted in growth inhibition.[361,362]

In summary, IGF-binding proteins are important modulators of IGF action. They function to control the half-life of IGF in blood and its distribution among tissues and extracellular fluids. In extracellular fluids, they clearly control the ability of IGF-1 and -2 to associate with receptors. Factors that alter the affinity of IGFBPs for IGF-1 and -2 can result in enhancement of IGF-1 actions. The exact role of each of these binding proteins in particular tissues in vivo is currently a major focus of research.

ACTIONS OF IGF-1 IN VIVO

IGF-1 was termed *somatomedin* initially because it mediated the growth-promoting actions of GH, and it was presumed to be a growth stimulant for all tissues. Several correlative types of experiments were conducted to support this hypothesis. These included hypophysectomy of animals, resulting in low serum GH and IGF-1 concentrations and a balanced reduction in growth.[363] Likewise, states of GH excess induced by implanting GH-producing tumors into animals resulted in generalized tissue overgrowth and high circulating IGF-1 concentrations. Serum IGF-1 concentrations were shown to correlate with changes in GH secretion and growth rates that occurred during postnatal life.[152] Based on these observations, it was presumed that GH acted primarily by stimulating IGF-1 synthesis in the liver, with concomitant increases in plasma IGF-1, and that IGF-1 was transported to skeletal tissues where it acted to stimulate growth. The development of cDNA probes for IGF-1 allowed new types of experiments that led to refinement of this hypothesis. Hepatic IGF-1 expression was shown to be decreased after hypophysectomy, and it was increased after GH administration.[221] Subsequently, it was shown that IGF-1 was synthesized in multiple extrahepatic tissues and that paracrine-synthesized IGF-1 could stimulate growth.[235,364] This raised the question as to what percentage of the generalized growth-promoting actions of IGF-1 was mediated by autocrine/paracrine secretion and what percentage was mediated by endocrine effects.

Administration of IGF-1 to whole animals results in balanced growth.[4] If the animal has been hypophysectomized, the effect is enhanced. A rate-limiting factor is the amount of IGF-1 that can be infused, because very high concentrations will induce hypoglycemia.[365] IGF-1 also feeds back on the pituitary and suppresses GH. This results in a reduction in total serum IGF-1 concentrations due to suppression of ALS and IGFBP-3. If animals are made catabolic, either by nutritional deprivation[366] or by administration of glucocorticoids,[367,368] administration of IGF-1 results in a partial reversal of this catabolic effect. Likewise, systemic administration of IGF-1 has been shown to improve wound healing, recovery of renal function after kidney injury,[369] and whole-body protein accretion.[370] When IGF-1 is given to nutritionally compromised animal models, the increase in the weight of organs such as spleen and kidney appears to be enhanced preferentially as compared with changes in skeletal growth.[370,371] In contrast, in well-nourished, hypophysectomized rats and mice, proportionate body growth occurs in response to IGF-1, with skeletal tissue being stimulated in a manner nearly identical to that in nonskeletal tissue.[371] IGF-1 stimulates an increase in glomerular filtration rate and has a direct, trophic effect on gut epithelial proliferation.[372] Infusion of IGF-1 tends to reduce IGFBP-3 and increase IGFBP-2, changes similar to those that occur in GHD. Infusion of IGF-1 to insulin-deficient, diabetic rats results in improved growth and more normal utilization of glucose.[373] Similarly, peripheral glucose uptake and glycerol synthesis are stimulated. Infusion of IGF-1 into the insulin-deficient BB rat results in suppression of hepatic glucose output, possibly due to suppressive effect on glucagon and GH, and these actions lead to enhanced sensitivity to insulin.[374] Diabetic animals that receive IGF-1 have less increase in body fat compared with animals treated with insulin.

MODULATION OF IN VIVO ACTIONS BY IGFBPs

In vivo studies have been performed wherein specific forms of IGFBPs have been administered with IGF-1. Administration of an equimolar amount of IGFBP-1 with IGF-1 to animals reduces the growth response of hypophysectomized rats compared with IGF-1 alone.[375] Administration of a large, single dose of IGFBP-1 without IGF-1 resulted in a modest increase (6%) in plasma glucose concentrations.[182] Acute increases in plasma IGFBP-1 result in decreased protein synthesis basally and in response to IGF-1.[376] In contrast, administration of IGFBP-1 with IGF-1 (1:4 molar ratio) to wounds results in enhanced wound healing, including increases in reepithelialization and formation of granulation tissue.[377] Similarly targeted deletion of IGFBP-1 in liver decreases hepatic regeneration after injury[378] and overexpression in placenta results in increased placental mass.[379] In addition, overexpression of IGFBP-1 in pancreas in vivo was shown to have a trophic effect on islet cells.[380] These findings indicate that in some specialized circumstances, increased tissue expression of IGFBP-1 may enhance IGF-1 actions as compared with the global inhibition that occurs when IGFBP-1 is infused into blood. Subcutaneous administration of IGFBP-2 together with IGF-2 has been shown to stimulate bone formation and to inhibit the development of mouse osteoporosis.[381] Administration of a complex of IGFBP-2 and IGF-2 stimulated osteoblast differentiation.[382]

IGFBP-3

Because of its role in carrying IGFs in serum, animal studies in which IGF-1 and IGFBP-3 are infused together have been important for defining the endocrine actions of IGF-1. In vivo administration of a combination of IGF-1 and IGFBP-3 has consistently been shown to enhance the trophic effects of IGF-1.[383] Administration of an equimolar concentration of IGF-1/IGFBP-3 to hypophysectomized rats showed increased bone mineralization and increased growth rates compared with IGF-1 alone. Administration of equimolar concentrations of IGF-1/IGFBP-3 to estrogen-deficient rats resulted in approximately 30% improvement in bone mineral density.[383] Muscle mass also was increased in these animals. A polyclonal anti-IGF-1 antibody that functions like an IGFBP also enhances the effects of IGF-1 when administered concomitant with IGF-1 to experimental animals.[384]

TRANSGENIC ANIMAL AND GENE-TARGETING STUDIES

Several transgenic animal models of IGF-1 action have been used, in which IGF-1 has been overexpressed. One particularly interesting model was used in which GH secretion was attenuated by cytotoxic destruction of somatotrophs, and then IGF-1 replacement therapy was performed by expressing IGF-1 mRNA in several tissues.[385] These animals grew normally, although some disproportionate growth of the kidneys, liver, pancreas, and spleen were noted.[386] Additionally,

small bowel length and mass are greater as is villus height and crypt depth.[387] Likewise, brain size appeared to be particularly sensitive to IGF-1 transgene overexpression. If IGF-1 is overexpressed on a background of no GHD, then more modest increases in somatic growth compared with control animals are noted; however, total body size can be increased by 30%.[386] Brain size is increased disproportionately by 50%. The effect is due in part to inhibition of apoptosis.[388] Whether suppression of GH results in the inability to attain greater growth rates after IGF-1 overexpression is unknown. Interestingly, the GHD mice have a somewhat hypoplastic liver, and this effect is not totally reversed by IGF-1 transgene overexpression.[385] The major conclusion from these studies was that the majority of the growth-promoting effects of GH were mediated by IGF-1 by using both autocrine/paracrine and endocrine mechanisms and that local expression of IGF-1 in tissues such as brain results in disproportionate increases in growth.

Attempts to determine the effects of IGFBPs also used transgenic animals. IGFBP-1 transgenic animals show variable phenotypes, depending on which organs express the transgene. Mice who had expression predominantly in pancreas, kidney, and brain had normal organ sizes, except brain, which was decreased in size.[389] Because IGFBP-1 is not constitutively expressed in brain, it presumably bound to IGF-1 or IGF-2, and the animals had a reduction in brain growth. In contrast, in mice with abundant hepatic expression, a slight growth retardation occurred at birth and a 10% to 15% reduction in postnatal growth.[390] Similarly, moderate glucose intolerance was found.[391] Abundant expression of IGFBP-1 in the liver has been shown to result in more severe growth retardation and delayed skeletal maturation.[392] Overexpression of IGFBP-2 results in fetal and postnatal growth maturation.[393] This effect is present even in the face of GH and IGF-1 excess.[394]

In IGFBP-3 transgenic animals, an increase in liver, spleen, and kidney size is seen, although total body weight and length are not significantly greater than control.[395]

Analysis of bone has shown that resorption is increased, and formation is decreased.[396] Overexpression that resulted in 4.9-fold to 7.7-fold increase in plasma IGFBP-3 resulted in modest growth retardation, even though IGF-1 levels were increased by 1.9-fold to 2.8-fold.[397] Targeted overexpression of IGFBP-4 in smooth muscle or in bone has been shown to attenuate IGF-1 actions. Cancellous bone formation is reduced, and this is associated with impaired growth.[398] In organs with a high smooth muscle content (e.g., bladder and uterus), disproportionate growth impairment is noted.[399] IGFBP-5 administration to IGF-1-deficit mice resulted in increase mouse bone cell proliferation and alkaline phosphatase activity.[400] In contrast, forced overexpression in bone resulted in osteopenia.[401] Similar overexpression in mammary gland resulted in apoptosis.[356]

A great deal of information regarding the skeletal and postnatal growth-promoting effects of IGF-1 has been obtained by homologous recombination experiments. In experiments in which the IGF-1 gene was deleted, the fetuses were born alive and were 60% of normal birth length and weight.[402] Homozygous animals had extremely high juvenile mortality rates, and only approximately 10% to 20% of these animals survived to adulthood. This appears to be due somewhat to the gene-dosage effects, because animals (created by one group that had a leaky promoter that resulted in a partial reduction in IGF-1 expression but not total attenuation) were larger at birth, but, more important, nearly 100% of the animals survived into adulthood.[403] This suggests that some threshold lower limit of IGF-1 concentration accounts for the excessive mortality. The animals that do survive to adulthood are disproportionately short and have an abnormally slow growth rate during the juvenile period.[402,403] They reach 30% of normal adult size. They also have poor Leydig cell development and small brains. Skeletal abnormalities also were noted.

The cause for the increased premature death is unknown. No apparent abnormalities of differentiation have been noted. Fetal growth retardation begins at day 13.5 in utero, and body size is reduced progressively at each stage up to birth.

Deletion of the IGF-1 receptor results in a much more severe phenotype. The animals are 45% of the normal size at birth.[64,402] None survives birth. All have a hypoplastic diaphragm and fail to take a normal first breath. Likewise, multiple skeletal and skin defects are seen, indicating that the receptor is necessary for normal muscle, skin, and bone development in utero. Haploinsufficiency of the IGF-1 receptor results in survival and modest growth retardation (e.g., 8% reduction in adult size).[404] These animals tolerate oxidative stress better than controls and have a 16% to 33% increase in life span.[405] Deletion of IGF-1-receptor expression in endothelium resulted in some protection against the development of neovascularization.[406]

IGF-2 gene deletion gives a very different phenotype. The animals are approximately 60% of normal size at birth, but, unlike the IGF-1 mice, they grow normally postnatally and do not die in excessive numbers.[407] No differentiation defects or structural tissue defects are noted. Deletion of both IGF-1 and -2 resulted in extremely small mice that are approximately 30% of normal size. This manipulation is lethal, because the mice cannot generate a normal inspiration. They are phenotypically similar to the mice lacking the IGF-1 receptor.

IGFBP-2

Deletion of the IGFBP-2 gene resulted in animals with large spleens, but no other change in organ growth was noted.[408] Body size was unchanged at birth and remains normal through juvenile development. This implicates a role for IGFBP-2 in fetal splenic development. Analysis of organ size in adult animals showed a reduction in spleen size, but liver weight was increased.[409]

IGFBP-4

Although IGFBP-4 has consistently been shown to inhibit IGF action in vitro, deletion of this gene in vivo resulted in a slight enhancement of fetal growth (e.g., a 15% increase in size at birth).[410] These differences persisted postnatally, but no further acceleration in growth rate occurred. This suggests that the in vitro actions of IGFBP-4 may not always mimic the in vivo activity.

AUTOCRINE/PARACRINE REGULATION OF IGF-1-MEDIATED GROWTH

Experimental animal models have been useful in readdressing the question of autocrine/paracrine effects of IGF-1. Because multiple animal studies showed that IGF-1 mRNA transcripts were expressed in connective tissue cells, principally fibroblasts, and in the equivalent cell types in some organs, such as the intestine, wherein the cells in the lamina propria express abundant IGF-1 transcripts, a major question was whether this material was regulated in a way similar to that of IGF-1 that was expressed in the liver and secreted into blood. Administration of GH to hypophysectomized rats showed that IGF-1 transcripts were increased in skeletal tissue, such as cartilage, bone, muscle, skin, and other organs, such as the brain, indicating that this autocrine/paracrine-produced IGF-1, much of which was presumed not to enter the circulation, could be regulated locally. This raised the important question of the extent to which autocrine/ paracrine-produced IGF-1 contributed to growth, as opposed to IGF-1 produced in the liver.

Cell-culture experiments reinforced the hypothesis that IGF-1 production is widespread and regulated by many factors. PDGF was shown to stimulate IGF-1 synthesis by fibro-blast cells, suggesting that autocrine/paracrine IGF-1 might be regulated by factors other than GH. An outstanding example of local control of IGF-1 is the response to injury that occurs after several types of injury models, such as freezing ear cartilage or thermal burns.[411] Fibroblast or chondrocyte precursor cells surrounding the damaged area immediately begin to synthesize IGF-1, and the peak of synthesis usually occurs between 3 and 7 days after injury. Balloon denudation of blood vessels is another example of such injury. The wave of IGF-1 synthesis usually coincides with an increase in the number of precursor cells that are entering the proliferative pool.[412,413] This continues for several days and then begins to subside. Therefore, it has been assumed that local regulation of growth, particularly in response to injury, but also in response to other stimuli, such as unilateral nephrectomy, wherein the contralateral kidney makes more IGF-1 and enlarges, may be more responsive to local IGF-1 regulation.

Another method for analyzing this problem has been to use hypophysectomized or GHD animal models, in which the IGF-1 gene is expressed in tissues other than liver. In this setting, if IGF-1 expression is ubiquitous and can be maintained at high enough levels, the animals develop reasonably normal IGF-1 plasma concentrations and grow normally. Another model of regulation has been analysis of brain growth. The blood-brain barrier provides some partitioning between blood IGF-1 and locally produced IGF-1. Transgenic animals in which there is intense expression of IGF-1 within the CNS show larger brains than do animals without this intense expression, indicating a paracrine stimulation of growth that is probably partially independent of blood IGF-1 concentrations.[218,385,386] However, the excellent correlation between changes in blood concentrations of IGF-1 after GH administration to hypophysectomized animals and growth rates suggests that excellent correlation also exists between endocrine-produced IGF-1 and growth.

A recent experimental animal model helped to understand further the relative components of autocrine/paracrine-produced IGF-1 as compared with blood-transported IGF-1. By using the Cre Lox expression system, investigators selectively targeted IGF-1 expression in the liver.[414,415] No IGF-1 expression occurred in the liver, and plasma IGF-1 concentrations were reduced by 80%. In contrast to IGF-1 knockout animals, in which the expression of IGF-1 in peripheral tissues as well as in liver is destroyed, all other tissues in these animals synthesized IGF-1 normally. Deletion of IGF-1 expression from the liver was not associated with growth inhibition. These animals were normal size at birth and grew normally postnatally. This indicates that deletion of IGF-1 expression in the liver results in a major reduction in endocrine-produced IGF-1 and that autocrine/paracrine IGF-1 in these experimental mice is adequate to allow normal statural growth. Because peripheral tissue IGF-1 expression also is under the control of GH, this type of experiment does not distinguish between how much of the locally produced IGF-1 is regulated by factors other than GH and how much is under GH control. It does eliminate the possibility that, to grow normally, one must have a completely normal blood IGF-1 concentration and proves definitively that the major source of blood IGF-1 is the liver. Although it might not be surprising that fetal growth was normal in these animals, because IGF-2 is an important fetal growth factor, it is striking that no juvenile growth retardation was found, in spite of these low plasma IGF-1 concentrations. These studies have been extended by simultaneously deleting liver ALS expression. This dual inhibition results in a 30% reduction in growth and a more severe decrease in serum IGF-1.[416] These animals also have reduced bone mineral density. In contrast, deletion of ALS alone resulted in mild growth retardation.[417] This model also allowed a better analysis of the role of plasma IGF-1 in glucose metabolism. Animals with the liver-specific IGF-1 gene deletion have a fourfold increase in serum GH, which results in insulin resistance.[418] Blocking the hepatic action of this increase in GH restores insulin sensitivity to normal.[419] However, animals with *IGF-1* and *ALS* deletions had elevated free IGF-1, and although they also had increased GH, they had normal insulin sensitivity, suggesting a direct insulin-sensitizing role for free IGF-1 in plasma.[420]

EFFECTS OF IGF-1 IN HUMANS

The data regarding IGF-1 infusion into humans as compared with administration of GH must be reevaluated in light of recent findings regarding autocrine/paracrine actions of IGF-1. As noted previously, when GH is administered, IGF-1 mRNA is induced in multiple tissues in experimental animals that have been made GHD, and an increase in serum IGF-1 is found. This indicates that both autocrine/paracrine mechanisms, as well as endocrine ones, are activated by GH. In contrast, administration of IGF-1 alone intravenously to GHD animals or humans does not result in autocrine/paracrine activation of *IGF-1* gene expression. Similarly, other unknown but important growth-regulatory molecules that are synthesized in response to GH may not be increased by IGF-1; therefore, IGF-1 administration may not always induce the same anabolic changes as does GH.

Administration of IGF-1 to normal humans results in changes that are comparable to those noted previously in animal studies. A large bolus of rapidly administered IGF-1 (e.g., 100 μg/kg) results in hypoglycemia.[421] When analyzed on a molar basis, IGF-1 is one twelfth as potent as insulin in reducing glucose and free fatty acid levels. A continuous infusion of 24 μg/kg/hr of IGF-1 to normal humans results in a 50% reduction in C peptide but maintenance of euglycemia. Peripheral glucose uptake is increased at these infusion rates of IGF-1, and hepatic glucose production and free fatty acid levels are suppressed. Protein breakdown also is decreased.[422] However, with lower infusion rates (5 μg/kg/hr), which do not necessitate supplemental glucose to avoid hypoglycemia, no effect on protein breakdown is seen.[423] Insulin sensitivity also is enhanced, as assessed by insulin-to-glucose ratios measured during the IGF-1 infusion. IGF-1 has consistently suppressed insulin levels and resulted in more efficient glucose responsiveness to insulin.[424] Because GH also is suppressed, inhibition of several of the known insulin-antagonist actions of GH may contribute to this change. IGF-1 also suppresses glucagon, and such suppression probably contributes to the enhanced insulin sensitivity that is observed during IGF-1 infusions.[422,424]

Administration of exogenous IGF-1 to catabolic subjects results in improvement in nitrogen balance at an infusion rate of 12 μg/kg/hr. The degree of improvement is comparable to that achieved with GH administration.[425] A second study that used the same design (i.e., 6 days of a 50% caloric restriction) showed that concomitant administration of GH with 12-μg/kg/hr infusion of IGF-1 resulted in further enhancement of nitrogen retention compared with either treatment alone. GH inhibited the development of symptomatic hypoglycemia. Infusion of IGF-1 alone resulted in suppression of IGFBP-3 concentrations and suppression of the acid-labile subunit, but administration of concomitant GH resulted in maintenance of normal levels of this complex in plasma.[160] This high level of the IGF-1/IGFBP-3 complex may have contributed to improved nitrogen balance. Several other studies suggested that maintenance of complex activity results in a better anabolic response. Administration of the complex to patients with severe burns resulted in increased protein-synthesis rates.[426] Similarly, administration of both proteins to osteoporotic patients after hip fracture showed that it was anabolic and improved bone density.[427]

IGF-1 alone also caused a threefold increase in IGFBP-2 concentrations, suggesting that a larger fraction of the IGF-1 would be bound to IGFBP-2 under these conditions and thus have a shorter half-life. A reduced anabolic response to IGF-1

alone may occur as a consequence of these changes in IGFBP profiles. Cholesterol also is reduced in response to IGF-1 infusion, as is potassium. Renal function improves, with an approximately 25% increase in glomerular filtration rate and renal blood flow.[428] The fractional excretion of phosphate is decreased, which probably contributes to the antiphosphaturic effect noted in acromegaly.

GH selectively stimulates whole-body protein synthesis and has a lesser effect on inhibiting proteolysis. IGF-1 infusions at relatively high concentrations inhibit proteolysis but have no effect on protein synthesis. With prolonged administration of IGF-1 (e.g., 5 to 7 days given as a subcutaneous injection), no effect on proteolysis, but a marked increase in protein synthesis is found, and the effects are indistinguishable from those of GH.[429] Therefore, the mode of administration and the actual dose of IGF-1 that is given are important determinants of whether IGF-1 has an short-term insulin-like effect on protein synthesis (e.g., inhibiting proteolysis) or a long-term GH-like effect in preferentially stimulating protein synthesis. The combination of GH plus IGF-1 has a greater effect on decreasing protein oxidation in GHD subjects compared with either substance given alone.[430] Others were not able to demonstrate a greater protein anabolic effect in normal, healthy, fed subjects when the GH and IGF-1 were given simultaneously compared with GH alone.[431] When catabolism is induced by administering high doses of glucocorticoids, IGF-1 has a significant effect on attenuating proteolysis and a small effect on increasing protein synthesis.[432] These effects are less dramatic than those with GH. The effect of IGF-1 in enhancing insulin sensitivity appears to be preserved even in dexamethasone-treated patients.

BONE METABOLISM

Short-term IGF-1 administration to normal subjects results in increased bone turnover, with a preferential effect on bone formation.[433] Young women with anorexia nervosa and severe osteopenia also respond by increasing bone turnover, and a short-term anabolic effect is noted.[434] IGF-1 also is an effective stimulant of bone formation in men with osteoporosis.[435] Patients with GHD also respond to IGF-1 with increased bone turnover.[436] The peptide has been given to elderly subjects with osteoporosis and results in improved markers of bone formation, such as pyridiniline cross-links in the urine. However, increases in markers of bone resorption indicate that bone turnover is stimulated.[437] The net effect of long-term administration of IGF-1 alone on bone mineral content is unknown. Studies in rats have shown that administration of IGF-1, in combination with IGFBP-3, may be a potent stimulant of cortical bone formation, and a 4-month treatment in humans with osteoporosis supported this conclusion.[427] These enhanced effects of IGF-1/IGFBP-3 compared with IGF-1 alone may be due to the inability of IGF-1 administration alone to sustain high plasma IGF-1 concentrations over prolonged periods.

OTHER EFFECTS OF IGF-1

In addition to its effects in suppressing free fatty acids, ketones bodies, and triglycerides in the short term, IGF-1 suppresses apolipoprotein B-100 levels. IGF-1 administration also suppresses plasminogen activator inhibitor-I levels, and this has the potential to reduce the risk of thrombosis in patients with atherosclerosis. IGF-1 has been shown to be neurotrophic in humans, and trials in amyotropic lateral sclerosis have shown some improvement in nerve regeneration and a slight prolongation of survival, indicating improved muscle function.

IGF-1 in Diabetes

When insulin sensitivity is assessed formally with a euglycemic hyperinsulinemic clamp method, IGF-1 administration results in a substantial improvement in sensitivity to insulin.[126] This occurs in normal subjects, insulin-deficient diabetics, and patients with extreme insulin-resistance syndromes, including those involving mutations of the insulin receptor. Preliminary studies have indicated that administration of IGF-1 to patients with severe insulin resistance results in long-term reduction of glucose and improved insulin sensitivity.[438] Adolescents with type 1 diabetes who were treated for 4 weeks with subcutaneously administered IGF-1 had reduced insulin requirements and improved their metabolic control. These effects were attributed to suppression of the Dawn phenomenon.[439] Administration of IGF-1 to patients with type A extreme insulin resistance has resulted in improved metabolic control. Some studies, however, have not seen the same degree of improvement in patients with type A insulin resistance. Administration of IGF-1 to subjects with type 2 diabetes shows that it results in a 3.4-fold improvement in insulin resistance, as assessed by direct measurement.[440] More important, IGF-1 reduces hemoglobin A1C by approximately 1.7% and results in improved glucose tolerance. Insulin concentrations are reduced in these patients, suggesting that a change in insulin sensitivity is the primary mechanism accounting for this improvement. Similarly, the requirement for exogenous insulin can be reduced in type 1 diabetics by IGF-1, while maintaining good glycemic control.[441] In a large ($N = 208$) group of type 2 diabetics who were treated with four different doses of IGF-1 for 3 months, the groups that received the two highest doses had a 1.6% reduction in hemoglobin A1C, indicating that long-term improvement in diabetic control is achievable with IGF-1.

Side effects have been noted both in normal subjects and in diabetics who have received high concentrations of IGF-1 for several weeks. These include parotid gland tenderness, subcutaneous edema, and a 10% increase in heart rate. In rare subjects, edema of the retina occurs, and, occasionally, pseudotumor cerebri has been noted. Other unusual side effects include Bell's palsy and severe myalgias. All of these side effects have been noted to be reversible and remit after stopping IGF-1.[440,441] Administration of the combination of IGFBP-3 and IGF-1 to those with type 1 diabetes for 2 weeks resulted in a 48% reduction in insulin dosage and a 23% reduction in blood glucose, indicating improvement in insulin sensitivity. This combination was associated with a reduction in side effects.[442]

Growth Hormone Insensitivity Syndrome

Short-term administration of IGF-1 to patients with GH insensitivity syndrome in which mutations of the GH receptor and very low serum IGF-1 concentrations are found results in improvement in nitrogen and phosphate retention and decreases in glucose and insulin.[443] Analysis of growth rates in nine such subjects who were treated for 1 year showed that they grew approximately 7.5 cm in the first year, as compared with pretreatment growth rates of approximately 4 cm/yr. Longer-term follow-up, administering IGF-1 at 50 µg/kg twice a day, subcutaneously, to patients with GH insensitivity syndrome, has shown that the first-year growth velocity cannot be maintained in the second year, and the growth rates are reduced to 6 cm per year.[444–447] This growth rate has been maintained for periods as long as 4 years in subjects who received IGF-1, and therefore the growth benefit, if projected to adulthood, would result in significant improvement in final adult stature. However, the growth rates during the second through fifth years are not so robust as those in GHD subjects who received GH during a similar interval. Hypoglycemia occurs occasionally in these patients but is usually avoidable with a dosage adjustment. Other side effects that have been noted with short-term, high-dose administration of IGF-1 to adults have not been observed in these children. One child with a GH insensitivity syndrome did develop pseudotumor cerebri, which resolved while treatment was continued. Another troublesome feature that has been noted, however, is a coarsening of the facial features, particularly in those subjects who are receiving the treatment during initiation of adolescence. This effect appears to be more significant than that noted with GH administration during puberty. Evaluation of these patients 1 to 2 years after stopping IGF-1 shows that their coarse facial features resolve. Whether the suboptimal growth rates and coarsening of facial features are due to stimulation by IGF-1 in the absence of the direct actions of GH that are mediated through the GH receptor is unknown.

A single patient has been described in whom a mutation resulted in deletion of a major portion of the *IGF-1* gene.[448] This resulted in severe growth retardation at birth that persisted into adulthood. Head circumference also was reduced. Administration of IGF-1 before epiphyseal fusion resulted in growth acceleration. It also resulted in improvement in insulin sensitivity.[448] Four patients have been described with either a single allele or point mutation in the IGF-1 receptor.[449–451] All cases resulted in growth retardation. One child with two point mutations responded to high doses of GH with an increase in growth.[451]

REFERENCES

1. Salmon WD Jr, Daughaday WH: A hormonally controlled serum factor which stimulates sulfate incorporation by cartilage in vitro. J Lab Clin Med 49:825, 1957.
2. Daughaday WH, Reeder C: Synchronous activation of DNA synthesis in hypophysectomized rat cartilage by growth hormone. J Lab Clin Med 68:357, 1966.
3. Rinderknecht E, Humbel RE: The amino acid sequence of human insulin-like growth factor I and its structural homology with proinsulin. J Biol Chem 253:2769, 1978.
4. Schoenle E, Zapf J, Humbel RE, et al: Insulin-like growth factor I stimulates growth in hypophysectomized rats. Nature 296:252, 1982.
5. Ullrich A, Gray A, Tam AW, et al: Insulin-like growth factor-I receptor primary structure: Comparison with insulin receptor suggests structural determinants that define functional specificity. EMBO J 5:2503, 1986.
6. Rotwein P, Pollack KM, Didier DK, et al: Organization and sequence of the human insulin-like growth factor I gene. J Biol Chem 261:4828, 1986.
7. Conover CA, Baker BK, Hintz RL: Cultured fibroblasts secrete insulin-like growth factor-I A. J Clin Endocrinol Metab 69:25, 1989.
8. Clemmons DR, Shaw DS: Purification and biologic properties of fibroblast somatomedin. J Biol Chem 263:2841, 1986.
9. Murphy LJ, Freisen HG: Differential effects of estrogen and growth hormone on uterine and hepatic insulin like growth factor-I gene expression in ovariectomized and hypophysectomized rat. Endocrinology 122:325, 1988.
10. Murphy LJ, Bell GI, Duckworth ML, et al: Identification, characterization, and regulation of complementary dexoxyribonucleic acid which evokes insulin-like growth factor I. Endocrinology 121:684, 1987.
11. Holt EC, Van Wyk JJ, Lund PK: Tissue and development specific regulation of a complex family of insulin-like growth factor I messenger ribonucleic acids. Mol Endocrinol 2:1077, 1988.
12. Carlsson B, Carlsson L, Billig H: Estrus cycle dependent covariation of the insulin-like growth factor I (IGF-I) messenger ribonucleic acid and protein in rat ovary. Mol Cell Endocrinol 64:271, 1989.
13. McCarthy TL, Centrella M, Canalis E: Cortisol inhibits the synthesis of insulin-like growth factor-I in skeletal cells. Endocrinology 126:1569, 1990.
14. Hepler JE, VanWyk JJ, Lund PK: Different half lives of insulin-like growth factor-I mRNA that differ in length of 3'-untranslated sequence. Endocrinology 127:155, 1990.
15. Rinderknecht E, Humbel RE: Primary structure of human insulin-like growth factor II. FEBS Lett 89:283, 1978.
16. Cascieri MA, Chicchi GC, Applebaum J, et al: Mutants of human insulin like

growth factor I with reduced affinity for the type I insulin like growth factor receptor. Biochemistry 27:3229, 1988.

17. Bayne ML, Applebaum J, Chicchi GG, et al: The roles of tyrosines 24, 31, and 60 in the high affinity binding of insulin-like growth factor-I to the type 1 insulin-like growth factor receptor. J Biol Chem 265:15648, 1990.

18. Bayne ML, Applebaum J, Underwood D, et al: The C region of human insulin-like growth factor (IGF) I is required for high affinity binding to the type I IGF receptor. J Biol Chem 264:11004, 1989.

19. Vajdos FF, Ultsch M, Schaffer ML, et al: Crystal structure of human insulin-like growth factor-1: Detergent binding inhibits binding protein interactions. Biochemistry 40:11022, 2001.

20. Brzozowski AM, Dodson EJ, Dodson GG, et al: Structural origins of the functional divergence of human insulin-like growth factor-I and insulin. Biochemistry 41:9389, 2002.

21. Zeslawski W, Beisel HG, Kamionka M, et al: The interaction of insulin-like growth factor-I with the N-terminal domain of IGFBP-5. EMBO J 20:3638, 2001.

22. Schaffer ML, Deshayes K, Nakamura G, et al: Complex with a phage display-derived peptide provides insight into the function of insulin-like growth factor I. Biochemistry 42:9324, 2003.

23. Clemmons DR, Dehoff MH, Busby WH, et al: Competition for binding to insulin-like growth factor (IGF) binding protein-2, 3, 4, and 5 by the IGFs and IGF analogs. Endocrinology 131:890, 1992.

24. Bayne ML, Applebaum J, Chicchi GG, et al: Structural analogues of human insulin-like growth factor-I with reduced affinity for serum binding protein and the type II insulin-like growth factor receptor. J Biol Chem 263:6233, 1988.

25. Clemmons DR, Cascieri MA, Camacho-Hubner C, et al: Discrete alterations of the IGF-I molecule that alter its affinity for IGF binding proteins result in changes in bioactivity. J Biol Chem 265:12210, 1990.

26. Tamura K, Kobayashi M, Ishii Y, et al: Primary structure of rat insulin-like growth factor I. Endocrinology 112:2215, 1983.

27. Blundell TL, Bedarkar S, Rinderknecht E, et al: Insulin-like growth factor: A model for tertiary structure accounting for immunoreactivity and receptor binding. Proc Natl Acad Sci U S A 75:180, 1978.

28. Sara V, Carlsson-Skwirut C, Anderson C, et al: Characterization of somatomedin from fetal brain: Identification of a variant form of insulin-like growth factor-I. Proc Natl Acad Sci U S A 83:4904, 1986.

29. Yamamoto H, Murphy LJ: Generation of des 1-3 insulin-like growth factor-I in serum by acid protease. Endocrinology 135:2432, 1994.

30. Kaleko M, Rutter WJ, Miller D: Overexpression of the human insulin-like growth factor-I receptor promotes ligand dependent neoplastic transformation. Mol Cell Biol 10:464, 1990.

31. Hernandez ER: Regulation of the genes for insulin-like growth factor (IGF) I and II and their receptors by steroids and gonadotrophins in the ovary. J Steroid Biochem Mol Biol 53:219, 1995.

32. Moreno B, Rodriguez MJ, Perez CA, et al: Thyroid hormone controls expression of insulin-like growth factor-I receptor gene at different levels in lung and heart in developing and adult rats. Endocrinology 138:1194, 1997.

33. Hernandez-Sanchez C, Werner H, Roberts CT, et al: Differential regulation of insulin-like growth factor-I receptor gene expression by IGF-I and basic fibroblast growth factor. J Biol Chem 272:4663, 1997.

34. Du J, Meng XP, Delafontaine P: Transcriptional regulation of the insulin-like growth factor-I receptor gene: Evidence for protein kinase C dependent and independent pathways. Endocrinology 138:1378, 1996.

35. Abbott AM, Bueno R, Pedrin MT, et al: Insulin-like growth factor-I receptor gene structure. J Biol Chem 267:10759, 1992.

36. LeRoith D, Werner H, Beitner-Johnson D, et al: Molecular and cellular aspects of the insulin-like growth factor-I receptor. Endocr Rev 16:143, 1995.

37. Garrett TP, McKern NM, Lou M, et al: Crystal structure of the first three domains of the type-1 insulin like growth factor receptor. Nature 394:395, 1998.

38. Whittaker J, Groth AV, Mynarcik DC, et al: Alanine scanning mutagenesis of a type I insulin-like growth factor receptor ligand binding site. J Biol Chem 276:43980, 2001.

39. Sepp-Lorczino L: Structure and function of the insulin-like growth factor-I receptor. Breast Cancer Res Treat 47:235, 1998.

40. Kato H, Faria TN, Stannard B, et al: Role of tyrosine kinase activity in signal transduction by the insulin-like growth factor receptor. J Biol Chem 268:2655, 1992.

41. Gual P, Baron U, Adengian F, et al: A conformational change in the beta subunit of the insulin-like growth factor-I receptor identified by anti-peptide antibodies. Endocrinology 136:5298, 1995.

42. Iterie N, Yoshino H, Moses AC, et al: Evidence that receptor aggregation may play a role in transmembrane signaling through the insulin-like growth factor-I receptor. Mol Endocrinol 2:83, 1998.

43. Treadway JL, Frattali AL, Pessin JE: Intramolecular subunit interactions between insulin and insulin-like growth factor-I alpha beta half receptors induced by ligand and Mn/Mg ATP binding. Biochemistry 31:11801, 1992.

44. Longolis WJ, Sasaroka T, Yip CL, et al: Functional characterization of hybrid receptors composed of a truncated insulin receptor and wild type insulin-like growth factor-I or insulin receptors. Endocrinology 136:1978, 1995.

45. Gronberg M, Wulff BS, Rasmussen JS, et al: Structure-function relationship of the insulin-like growth factor receptor tyrosine kinase. J Biol Chem 268:23435, 1990.

46. Pautsch A, Zoephel A, Ahorn H, et al: Crystal structure of bisphosphorylated IGF-1 receptor kinase: Insight into domain movements upon kinase activation. Structure 9:955, 2001.

47. Favelyukis S, Till JH, Hubbard SR, et al: Structure and autoregulation of the insulin-like growth factor I receptor kinase. Nat Struct Biol 8:1058, 2001.

48. Yamasaki H, Pager D, Gebremedhin S, et al: Human insulin-like growth factor-I receptor 950 tyrosine is required for somatotroph growth factor signal transduction. J Biol Chem 267:20953, 1992.

49. Huang M, Lai WP, Wong MS, et al: Effect of receptor phosphorylation on the binding between IRS-1 and IGF-1R as revealed by surface plasmon resonance biosensor. FEBS Lett 505:31, 2001.

50. Blakesley VA, Scrimgeour A, Esposito D, et al: Signaling via the insulin-like growth factor-I receptor: Does it differ from insulin receptor signaling? Cytokine Growth Factor Rev 7:153, 1996.

51. Giorgetti S, Pelicci PG, Pelicci G, et al: Involvement of Src-homology/collagen SHC proteins in signaling through the insulin and IGF-I receptors. Eur J Biochem 233:195, 1994.

52. Beitner-Johnson D, LeRoith D: Insulin-like growth factor-I stimulates tyrosine phosphorylation of endogenous c-crk. J Biol Chem 270:5187, 1995.

53. Prager D, Li HL, Yamasaki H, et al: Human insulin-like growth factor-I receptor internalization: Role for juxtamembrane domain. J Biol Chem 269:11934, 1994.

54. Hsu D, Knudson PE, Zapf J, et al: NPXY motif in the insulin-like growth factor-I receptor is required for efficient ligand mediated receptor internalization and biologic signaling. Endocrinology 134:744, 1994.

55. Soos MA, Field CE, Siddle K: Purified hybrid insulin/insulin-like growth factor-I receptors bind insulin-like growth factor-I but not insulin with high affinity. Biochem J 290:419, 1993.

56. Pandini G, Frasca F, Mineo R, et al: Insulin/insulin-like growth factor I hybrid receptors have different biological characteristics depending on the insulin receptor isoform involved. J Biol Chem 277:39684, 2002.

57. Sakai K, Clemmons DR: Glucosamine induces resistance to insulin-like growth factor I (IGF-I) and insulin Hep G2 cell cultures: biological significance of IGF-I/insulin hybrid receptors. Endocrinology 144:2388, 2003.

58. Bohula EA, Salibury, AJ, Sohail M, et al: The efficacy of small interfering RNAs targeted to the type 1 insulin-like

growth factor receptor (IGF1R) is influenced by secondary structure in the IGF1R transcript. J Biol Chem 278:15991, 2003.

59. Esposito D, Blakesley VA, Koval AP, et al: Tyrosine residues in the C-terminal domain of the insulin-like growth factor I (IGF-I) receptors mediate mitogenic and tumorogenic signals. Endocrinology 138:2979, 1997.

60. Li S, Resnicoff M, Boneya R: Effect of mutations at serines 1280-1281 on the mitogenic and transforming activities of the IGF-I receptor. J Biol Chem 271:12254, 1996.

61. Coppola D, Ferber A, Miura M, et al: A functional IGF-I receptor is a requirement for mitogenic and transforming activities of the epidermal growth factor receptor. Mol Cell Biol 14:4588, 1994.

62. DeAngelis T, Ferber A, Baserga R: The insulin-like growth factor I receptor is a requirement for the mitogenic and transforming activities of the platelet derived growth factor receptor. J Cell Physiol 164:214, 1995.

63. Sell C, Rubini R, Rubin R, et al: Simian virus 40 large tumor antigen is unable to transform mouse embryo fibroblasts lacking type I insulin like growth factor receptor. Proc Natl Acad Sci U S A 90:11217, 1993.

64. Liu JP, Baker J, Perkins AS, et al: Mice carrying null mutations of the genes encoding insulin like growth factor I (IGF-I) and type 1 IGF receptor (IGF/r). Cell 75:73, 1993.

65. Sell C, Dumenil G, Deneaud C, et al: Effect of a null mutation of the insulin-like growth factor I receptor gene on growth and transformation of mouse embryo fibroblasts. Mol Cell Biol 14:3604, 1994.

66. D'Mello SR, Galli C, Ciott T, et al: Induction of apoptosis in cerebellar granule neurons by low potassium: Inhibition of death by insulin-like growth factor-I and cAMP. Proc Natl Acad Sci U S A 90:10989, 1993.

67. Rubin R, Baserga R: Biology of disease: Insulin-like growth factor-I receptor: Its role in cell proliferation, apoptosis, and tumorigenicity. Lab Invest 13:311, 1995.

68. O'Connor R, Kauffman ZA, Liu Y, et al: Identification of domains of the insulin-like growth factor-I receptor that are required for protection from apoptosis. Mol Cell Biol 17:427, 1997.

69. Faria TN, Blakesley VA, Kato H, et al: Role of the carboxy-terminal domain of the insulin and insulin-like growth factor-I receptors in receptor function. J Biol Chem 269:13922, 1994.

70. Sun XJ, Wang LM, Zhang Y, et al: Role of IRS-2 in insulin and cytokine signaling. Nature 377:173, 1995.

71. Sun XJ, Rothenberg P, Kahn CR, et al: Structure of the insulin receptor substrate IRS-1 defines a unique signal transduction protein. Nature 351:73, 1991.

72. Pete G, Fuller CR, Oldham JM, et al: Postnatal growth responses to insulin-like growth factor I in insulin receptor substrate-1-deficient mice. Endocrinology 140:5478, 1999.

73. Morelli C, Garofalo C, Bartucci M, et al: Estrogen receptor-alpha regulates the degradation of insulin receptor substrates 1 and 2 in breast cancer cells. Oncogene 22:4007, 2003.

74. Zhang H, Hoff H, Sell C: Downregulation of IRS-1 protein in thapsigargin-treated human prostate epithelial cells. Exp Cell Res 289:352, 2003.

75. Myers MJ, White MF: The IRS-1 signaling system. Trends Biol Sci 19:289, 1994.

76. Skolnik EY, Batzer A, Li N, et al: The function of Grb-2 in linking the insulin receptor to ras signaling pathways. Science 260:1953, 1993.

77. Takasu W, Takasu M, Komiya I, et al: Insulin-like growth factor-I stimulates inositol phosphate accumulation: A rise in cytosol free calcium, and proliferation in cultured thyroid cells. J Biol Chem 264:18485, 1989.

78. Kojima I, Mogami H, Ogata E: Oscillation of cytoplasmic free calcium concentration induced by insulin-like growth factor-I. Am J Physiol 262:E307, 1992.

79. Neri LM, Billi AM, Monzoli L, et al: Selective nuclear translocation of protein kinase C alpha in Swiss 3T3 cells treated with IGF-I. FEBS Lett 347:63, 1991.

80. Kiely PA, Sant A, O'Connor R: RACK1 is an insulin-like growth factor 1 (IGF-1) receptor-interacting protein that can regulate IGF-I mediated Akt activation and protection from cell death. J Biol Chem 277:22581, 2002.

81. Giovannone B, Lee E, Laviola L, et al: Two novel proteins that are linked to insulin-like growth factor (IGF-I) receptors by the Grb10 adapter and modulate IGF-I signaling. J Biol Chem 278:31564, 2003.

82. Myers MJ, White MF: Insulin signal transduction and the IRS proteins. Annu Rev Pharmacol 36:615, 1996.

83. Myers MG, Sun XJ, Cheatham B, et al: IRS-I is a common element in insulin and insulin-like growth factor I signalling to the phosphatidylinositol 5'-kinase. Endocrinology 132:1421, 1993.

84. Baserga R: The insulin like growth factor receptor: A key to tumor growth? Cancer Res 55:249, 1995.

85. Kim JJ, Park BC, Kido Y, et al: Mitogenic and metabolic effects of type I IGF receptor overexpression in insulin receptor-deficient hepatocytes. Endocrinology 142:3354, 2001.

86. Kim JJ, Accili D: Signalling through IGF-I and insulin receptors: Where is the specificity? Growth Horm IGF Res 12:81, 2002.

87. Pillay TS, Sasoka T, Olefsky JM: Insulin stimulates tyrosine dephosphorylation of pp125 focal adhesion kinase. J Biol Chem 270:991, 1995.

88. Dalle S, Ricketts W, Imamura T, et al: Insulin and insulin-like growth factor I receptors utilize different G protein signaling components. J Biol Chem 276:15688, 2001.

89. Peterson JE, Jelinik T, Kaleko M, et al: C phosphorylation and activation of the IGF-I receptor in Src-transformed cells. J Biol Chem 269:27315, 1994.

90. Xu B, Bird VG, Miller WT: Substrate specificity of the insulin and insulin like growth factor I receptor tyrosine kinase catalytic domains. J Biol Chem 270:29825, 1995.

91. Nakae J, Kido Y, Accili D: Distinct and overlapping functions of insulin and IGF-I receptors. Endocr Rev 22:818, 2001.

92. Kornfeld S: Structure and function of the mannose 6 phosphate insulin-like growth factor II receptors. Am Rev Biochem 61:307, 1992.

93. Stewart CS, Rotwein P: Growth, differentiation, and survival: Multiple physiologic functions for insulin-like growth factors. Physiol Rev 76:1005, 1966.

94. Flaument RS, Kojima S, Abe M, et al: Activation of latent transforming growth factor beta. Adv Pharmacol 24:51, 1993.

95. Appell KC, Simpson IA, Cushman SW: Characterization of the stimulatory action of insulin and insulin-like growth factor II binding in rat adipose cells: Differences in the mechanism of insulin action on insulin like growth factor II receptors and glucose transporters. J Biol Chem 263:10824, 1998.

96. Nielsen FC: The molecular and cellular biology of insulin like growth factor II. Prog Growth Factor Res 4:257, 1992.

97. Keiss W, Greenstein LA, White RM, et al: Type II insulin like growth factor receptor is present in rat serum. Proc Natl Acad Sci U S A 84:7720, 1987.

98. Lau MM, Stewart CHE, Liu Z, et al: Loss of imprinted IGF-II cation independent mannose 6 phosphate receptor results in fetal overgrowth and perinatal lethality. Gene Dev 8:2953, 1994.

99. Filson AJ, Louvi A, Efstratiadis A, et al: Rescue of T-associated maternal effect in mice carrying null mutations in IGF-II and IGF-IIr, two reciprocally imprinted genes. Development 118:731, 1993

100. Minniti C, Kohn EC, Grubb JH, et al: The insulin-like growth factor II (IGF-II)/mannose 6-phosphate receptor mediates IGF-II-induced motility in human rhabdomyosarcoma cells. J Biol Chem 267:9000, 1992.

101. McKinnon T, Chakraborty C, Gleeson L, et al: Stimulation of human extravillous trophoblast migration by IGF-II is mediated by IGF type 2 receptor involving inhibitory G protein(s) and phosphorylation. J Clin Endocrinol Metab 86:3665, 2001.

102. Okomoto T, Katada T, Murayama Y, et al: A simple structure encodes G protein activity function of the IGF-I/mannose 6 phosphate receptor. Cell 62:709, 1990.

103. Jones JI, Clemmons DR: Insulin like growth factor and their binding

proteins: Biologic actions. Endocr Rev 16:3, 1995.

104. Clemmons DR: Insulin like growth factor binding proteins. In Kostyo JL (ed): Handbook of Physiology: Hormonal Control of Growth, vol 5. New York, Oxford University Press, 1999, p 1901.

105. Brewer MT, Stetler GL, Squires CH, et al: Cloning, characterization and expression of a human insulin-like growth factor binding protein. Biochem Biophys Res Commun 152:1289, 1988.

106. Jones JI, Gockerman A, Busby WH Jr, et al: Insulin-like growth factor binding protein 1 stimulates cell migration and binds to the α5β1 integrin by means of its Arg-Gly-Asp sequence. Proc Natl Acad Sci U S A 90:10553, 1993.

107. Rechler MM: Insulin like growth factor binding proteins. Vitam Horm 47:1, 1993.

108. Pucilowska JB, Davenport ML, Kabir I, et al: The effect of dietary protein supplementation on insulin like growth factors (IGFs) and IGF binding proteins in children with shigellosis. J Clin Endocrinol Metab 77:1516, 1993.

109. Hossenlopp P, Seurin D, Segovia-Quinson B, et al: Analysis of serum insulin-like growth factor binding proteins using Western blotting: Use of the method for titration of the binding proteins and competitive binding studies. Anal Biochem 154:138, 1986.

110. Booth BA, Boes M, Dake BL, et al: Structure function relationships in the heparin binding C-terminal region of insulin-like growth factor binding protein-3. Growth Regul 6:206, 1996.

111. Baxter RC: Glycosaminoglycans inhibit formation of the 140-kDa insulin like growth factor binding protein complex. Biochem J 271:773, 1990.

112. Bautista CM, Baylink DJ, Mohan S: Isolation of a novel insulin-like growth factor (IGF) binding protein from human bone: A potential candidate for fixing IGF-II in human bone. Biochem Biophys Res Commun 176:756, 1991.

113. Durham SK, Keifer MR, Riggs BL, et al: Regulation of insulin like growth factor binding protein-4 by a specific insulin like growth factor binding protein-4 protease in normal human osteoblast like cells: Implications on human cell physiology. J Bone Miner Res 9:111, 1994.

114. James PL, Jones SB, Busby WH, et al: IGF binding protein-5 is expressed in myoblast differentiation and is highly conserved. J Biol Chem 268:22305, 1993.

115. Arai T, Clarke JB, Parker A, et al: Substitution of specific amino acids in insulin-like growth factor-binding protein-5 alters heparin binding and its change in affinity for IGF-I in response to heparin. J Biol Chem 271:6099, 1996.

116. Jones JI, Gockerman A, Busby WH, et al: Extracellular matrix contains insulin-like growth factor binding protein-5: Potentiation of the effects of IGF-I. J Cell Biol 121:679, 1993.

117. Nam TJ, Busby WH, Clemmons DR: Insulin-like growth factor binding protein-5 binds to plasminogen activator inhibitor-I. Endocrinology 138:2972, 1997.

118. Camacho-Hubner C, Busby WH, McCusker RH, et al: Identification of the forms of insulin-like growth factor binding proteins produced by human fibroblasts and the mechanisms that regulate their secretion. J Biol Chem 267:11949, 1992.

119. Keifer MD, Masiarz FR, Bauer D, et al: Identification and molecular cloning of two new 30 kDa insulin-like growth factor binding proteins isolated from adult human serum. J Biol Chem 266:9043, 1991.

120. Bach LA, Thotakura NR, Rechler MM: Human IGFBP-6 is O-glycosylated. Biochem Biophys Res Commun 186:301, 1992.

121. Martin JL, Willetts KE, Baxter RC: Purification and properties of a novel insulin-like growth factor-II binding protein from transformed human fibroblasts. J Biol Chem 265:4124, 1990.

122. Clemmons DR, Van Wyk JJ: Factors controlling blood concentrations in somatomedin-C. Clin Endocrinol Metab 13:113, 1984.

123. Underwood LE, D'Ercole AJ, Van Wyk JJ: Somatomedin-C and the assessment of growth. Pediatr Clin North Am 27:771, 1980.

124. Underwood LE, VanWyk JJ: Normal and aberrant growth. In Williams Textbook of Endocrinology, 8th ed. Philadelphia, WB Saunders, pp 1079–1104.

125. Rudman DG, Kutner MH, Rogers CM: Impaired growth hormone secretion in the adult population: Relation to age and adiposity. J Clin Invest 67:1361, 1981.

126. Hong Y, Pedesen NL, Brismar K, et al: Quantitative genetic analyses of insulin like growth factor I (IGF-I), IGF binding protein-1 and insulin levels in middle-aged and elderly twins. J Clin Endocrinol Metab 81:1791, 1996.

127. Vaessen N, Heutink P, Janssen JA, et al: A polymorphism in the gene for IGF-I: Functional properties and risk for type 2 diabetes and myocardial infarction. Diabetes 50:637, 2001.

128. Schut AF, Janssen JA, Deinum J, et al: Polymorphism in the promoter region of the insulin-like growth factor I gene is related to carotid intima-media thickness and aortic pulse wave velocity in subjects with hypertension. Stroke 34:1623, 2003.

129. Zapf J, Walter H, Froesch ER: Radioimmunological determinations of IGF-I and IGF-II in normal subjects and in patients with growth disorders and extrapancreatic tumor hypoglycemia. J Clin Invest 68:1321, 1981.

130. Nunez SB, Municchi G, Barnes KM, et al: Insulin-like growth factor I (IGF-I) and IGF binding protein-3 concentrations compared to stimulated and night growth hormone in the evaluation of short children: A clinical research center study. J Clin Endocrinol Metab 81:1927, 1996.

131. Juul A, Dalgaard P, Blum WF, et al: Serum levels of insulin-like growth factor (IGF) binding protein-3 (IGFBP-3) in healthy infants, children, and adolescents: The relation to IGF-I, IGF-II, IGFBP-1, IGFBP-2, age, sex, body mass index, and pubertal maturation. J Clin Endocrinol Metab 80:2534, 1995.

132. Hasegawa Y, Hasegawa T, Aso T, et al: Comparison between insulin-like growth factor-I (IGF-I) and IGF binding protein-3 (IGFBP-3) measurement in the diagnosis of growth hormone deficiency. Endocrine J 40:185, 1996.

133. Copeland KC, Johnson DM, Kuehl RJ, et al: Estrogen stimulates growth hormone and somatomedin-C in castrate and intact female baboons. J Clin Endocrinol Metab 58:698, 1984.

134. Dean HJ, Kellet JG, Bala RM: The effect of growth hormone treatment on somatomedin levels in growth hormone deficient children. J Clin Endocrinol Metab 55:1167, 1982.

135. Moore DC, Rogelio HA, Smith EK, et al: Plasma somatomedin-C as a screening test for growth hormone deficiency in children and adolescents. Horm Res 16:49, 1982.

136. Clemmons DR, Underwood LE, Ridgway EC: Evaluation of acromegaly by radioimmunoassay of somatomedin-C. N Engl J Med 301:1138, 1979.

137. Melmed S: Acromegaly. N Engl J Med 322:966, 1990.

138. Juul A, Main K, Blum WF, et al: The ratio between serum levels of insulin-like growth factor-I (IGF-I) and the IGF binding proteins (IGFBP-1, 2 and 3) decreases with age in healthy adults and is increased in acromegalic patients. Clin Endocrinol 41:85, 1994.

139. Furlanetto RW, Underwood LE, Van Wyk JJ, et al: Serum immunoreactive somatomedin-C is elevated in late pregnancy. J Clin Endocrinol Metab 47:695, 1979.

140. Chernausek SD, Underwood LE, Utiger RD, et al: Growth hormone secretion and plasma somatomedin-C in primary hypothyroidism. Clin Endocrinol 19:337, 1983.

141. Phillips LS, Unterman TG: Somatomedin activity in disorders of nutrition and metabolism. Clin Endocrinol Metab 13:145, 1984.

142. Clemmons DR, Klibanski A, Underwood LE, et al: Reduction of plasma immunoreactive somatomedin-C during fasting in humans. J Clin Endocrinol Metab 53:1247, 1981.

143. Merimee TJ, Zapf J, Froesch ER: Insulin-like growth factors in fed and fasted states. J Clin Endocrinol Metab 55:999, 1982.

144. Isley WL, Underwood LE, Clemmons DR: Dietary components that regulate

serum somatomedin-C in humans. J Clin Invest 71:175, 1983.

145. Tonshoff B, Blum WF, Wingen A, et al: Serum insulin-like growth factors (IGFs) and IGF binding proteins 1, 2, and 3 in children with chronic renal failure: Relationship to height and glomerular filtration rate. J Clin Endocrinol Metab 80:2684, 1995.

146. Mock DM: Growth retardation in chronic inflammatory bowel disease. Gastroenterology 11:1019, 1986.

147. Goldstein S, Sertich GJ, Levan KR, et al: Nutrition and somatomedin XIX molecular regulation of insulin-like growth factor I in streptozotocin-diabetic rats. Mol Endocrinol 2:1093, 1988.

148. Bereket A, Lang CH, Blethen SL, et al: Insulin-like growth factor binding protein-2 and insulin: Studies in children with type I diabetes mellitus and maturity-onset diabetes of the young. J Clin Endocrinol Metab 80:3647, 1995.

149. Dills DG, Allen C, Palta M, et al: Insulin-like growth factor-I is related to glycemic control in children and adolescents with newly diagnosed insulin-dependent diabetes. J Clin Endocrinol Metab 80:2139, 1995.

150. Morrow LA, O'Brien MB, Moller DE, et al: Recombinant human insulin-like growth factor-I therapy improves glycemic control and insulin action in the type A syndrome of severe insulin resistance. J Clin Endocrinol Metab 79:205, 1994.

151. Baxter RC, Martin JL: Radioimmunoassay of growth hormone dependent insulin-like growth factor binding protein in human plasma. J Clin Invest 78:1504, 1986.

152. Blum WF, Albertsson-Wikland K, Rosberg S, et al: Serum levels of insulin-like growth factor I (IGF-I) and IGF binding protein 3 reflect spontaneous growth hormone secretion. J Clin Endocrinol Metab 76:1610, 1993.

153. Leogney SR, Baxter RC, Carrerato T, et al: Structure and functional expression of acid labile subunit of the insulin-like growth factor binding protein complex. Mol Endocrinol 6:870, 1992.

154. Guler H-P, Zapf J, Schmid C, et al: Insulin-like growth factors I and II in healthy man: Estimations of half-lives and production rates. Acta Endocrinol 121:753, 1989.

155. Baxter RC, Martin JL: Structure of the Mr 140,000 growth hormone-dependent insulin-like growth factor binding protein complex: Determination by reconstitution and affinity labeling. Proc Natl Acad Sci U S A 86:6898, 1989.

156. De Boer H, Blok GJ, Popp-Snijders C, et al: Monitoring of growth hormone replacement therapy in adults, based on measurements of serum markers. J Clin Endocrinol Metab 81:1371, 1996.

157. Grinspoon S, Clemmons DR, Swearingen B, et al: Serum insulin-like growth factor-binding protein-3 levels in the diagnosis of acromegaly. J Clin Endocrinol Metab 80:927, 1995.

158. Pfeilschifter J, Scheidt-Nave C, Leidig-Bruckner G, et al: Relationship between circulating insulin-like growth factor components and sex hormones in a population based sample of 50- to 80-year-old men and women. J Clin Endocrinol Metab 81:2534, 1996.

159. Miell JP, Taylor AM, Zini M, et al: Effects of hypothyroidism and hyperthyroidism on insulin-like growth factors (IGFs) and growth hormone- and IGF binding proteins. J Clin Endocrinol Metab 76:950, 1993.

160. Kupfer SR, Underwood LE, Baxter RC, et al: Enhancement of the anabolic effects of growth hormone and insulin like growth factor-I by the use of both agents simultaneously. J Clin Invest 91:391, 1993.

161. Guidice LC, Farrell EM, Pham H, et al: Insulin like growth factor binding proteins in maternal serum throughout gestation and in the puerperium. J Clin Endocrinol Metab 71:806, 1990.

162. Hossenlopp P, Segovia B, Lassare C, et al: Enzymatic evidence of degradation of insulin-like growth factor binding protein in 150 k complex during pregnancy. J Clin Endocrinol Metab 71:797, 1990.

163. Bang P: Serum proteolysis of IGFBP-3. Prog Growth Fact Res 6:285, 1995.

164. Walker JL, Baxter RC, Young S, et al: Effects of recombinant insulin-like growth factor I on IGF binding proteins and the acid-labile subunit in growth hormone insensitivity syndrome. Growth Regul 3:109, 1993.

165. Lassare C, Binoux M: Insulin-like growth factor binding protein-3 is functionally altered in pregnancy plasma. Endocrinology 134:1254, 1994.

166. Blum WF, Brier BH: Radioimmunoassays for IGFs and IGFBPs. Growth Regul 4:11, 1994.

167. Clemmons DR, Busby WH, Snyder DK: Variables controlling the secretion of insulin-like growth factor binding protein-2 in normal human subjects. J Clin Endocrinol Metab 73:727, 1991.

168. Bar RS, Clemmons DR, Boes M, et al: Transcapillary permeability and subendothelial distribution of endothelial and amniotic fluid IGF-binding proteins in rat heart. Endocrinology 127:1078, 1990.

169. Ooi GT, Orlowski CC, Brown AL, et al: Different tissue distribution and hormonal regulation of messenger RNAs encoding rat insulin-like growth factor binding proteins-1 and 2. Mol Endocrinol 4:321, 1990.

170. Young SCJ, Smith-Banks A, Underwood LE, et al: Effects of recombinant IGF-I and GH treatment upon serum IGF binding proteins in calorically restricted adults. J Clin Endocrinol Metab 75:603, 1992.

171. Daughaday WH, Trivedi B, Baxter RC: Serum "big" insulin-like growth factor-II from patients with tumor hypoglycemia lacks normal E-domain O-linked glycosylation: A possible determinant of normal propeptide processing. Proc Natl Acad Sci U S A 90:5283, 1993.

172. Schmid C, Schlapfer I, Waldvogel M, et al: Differential regulation of insulin-like growth factor binding protein (IGFBP)-2 mRNA in liver and bone cells by insulin and retinoic acid in vitro. FEBS Lett 303:205, 1992.

173. Smith WJ, Underwood LE, Clemmons DR: Effects of caloric or protein restriction on insulin-like growth factor-I (IGF-I) and IGF-binding proteins in children and adults. J Clin Endocrinol Metab 80:443, 1995.

174. Straus DS, Takemoto CD: Effect of dietary protein deprivation insulin-like growth factor IGF-I and II, IGF binding protein-2 and serum albumin gene expression in the rat. Endocrinology 127:1849, 1990.

175. Ooi GT, Tseng LY, Tran MQ, et al: Insulin rapidly decreases insulin-like growth factor-binding protein-1 gene transcription in streptozotocin-diabetic rats. Mol Endocrinol 6:2219, 1992.

176. Suikkari A-M, Koivisto VA, Koistinen R, et al: Dose-response characteristics for suppression of low molecular weight plasma insulin-like growth factor binding protein by insulin. J Clin Endocrinol Metab 68:135, 1989.

177. Busby WH, Snyder DK, Clemmons DR: Radioimmunoassay of a 26,000 dalton plasma insulin like growth factor binding protein: Control by nutritional variables. J Clin Endocrinol Metab 67:1225, 1988.

178. Powell DR, Lee PDK, DePaolis LA, et al: Dexamethasone stimulates expression of insulin-like growth factor-binding protein-1 gene expression in human hepatoma cells. Growth Regul 3:11, 1993.

179. Unterman T, Oehler DT, Ngyuen H, et al: A novel DNA/protein complex interacts with the insulin-like growth factor binding protein-1 (IGFBP-1) insulin response sequence and is required for maximal effects of insulin and glucocorticoids on promoter function. Prog Growth Fact Res 6:119, 1995.

180. Bar RS, Boes M, Clemmons DR, et al: Insulin differentially alters transcapillary movement of intravascular IGFBP-1, IGFBP-2 and endothelial cell IGF binding proteins in rat heart. Endocrinology 127:497, 1990.

181. Westwood M, Gibson JM, Williams AC, et al: Hormonal regulation of circulating insulin-like growth factor-binding protein-1 phosphorylation status. J Clin Endocrinol Metab 80:3520, 1995.

182. Lewitt MS, Denyer GS, Cooney GJ, et al: Insulin-like growth factor binding protein-1 modulates blood glucose levels. Endocrinology 129:2254, 1991.

183. Bereket A, Lang CH, Blethen SL, et al: Effect of insulin on the insulin-like growth factor system in children with new onset insulin-dependent diabetes mellitus. J Clin Endocrinol Metab 80:1312, 1995.

184. Davies SC, Wass JAH, Ross RJM, et al: Induction of a specific protease for insulin-like growth factor binding protein-3 in the circulation during severe illness. J Endocrinol 130:469, 1991.

185. Davenport ML, Isley WL, Pucilowska J, et al: Insulin-like growth factor binding protein-3 proteolysis is induced following elective surgery. J Clin Endocrinol Metab 130:2505, 1992.

186. Holt RI, Jones JS, Stone NM, et al: Sequential changes in insulin like growth factor I and IGF-binding proteins in children with end stage liver disease before and after orthotopic liver transplantation. J Clin Endocrinol Metab 81:160, 1996.

187. Scharla SH, Strong DD, Mohan S, et al: 1,25 Dihydroxyvitamin D_3 differentially regulates the production of insulin-like growth factor I (IGF-I) and IGF-binding protein-4 in mouse osteoblasts. Endocrinology 129:3139, 1991.

188. Ono T, Kanzaki S, Seino Y, et al: Growth hormone (GH) treatment of GH-deficient children increases serum levels of insulin-like growth factors (IGFs), IGF-binding protein-3 and -5, and bone alkaline phosphatase isoenzyme. J Clin Endocrinol Metab 81:2111, 1996.

189. Roberts CT, Lasky SR, Lowe WL, et al: Molecular coding of rat insulin-like growth factor-I complementary DNA: Differential messenger RNA processing of regulation by growth hormone in extrahepatic tissue. Mol Endocrinol 1:243, 1987.

190. Han VKM, D'Ercole AJ, Lund PK: Cellular location of somatomedin (insulin-like growth factor) messenger RNA in the human fetus. Science 236:193, 1987.

191. Hynes MA, Van Wyk JJ, Brooks PJ, et al: Growth hormone dependence of somatomedin-C/insulin-like growth factor I and insulin-like growth factor II messenger ribonucleic acids. Mol Endocrinol 1:233, 1987.

192. Clemmons DR, Underwood LE, Van Wyk JJ: Hormonal control of immunoreactive somatomedin production by cultured human fibroblasts. J Clin Invest 67:10, 1981.

193. Isgaard J, Nilsson A, Vikma A, et al: Growth hormone regulates the level of IGF-I mRNA in rat growth plate. Endocrinology 122:1515, 1988.

194. McCarthy TL, Centrella M, Canalis E: Parathyroid hormone enhances transcript and polypeptide levels of insulin-like growth factor-I in osteoblast enriched cultures from fetal rat bone. Endocrinology 124:1247, 1989.

195. Silver DM, Fudo H, Halperin D, et al: Differential expression of insulin like growth factor I (IGF-I) and IGF-II messenger ribonucleic acid in growing rat bone. Endocrinology 132:1158, 1993.

196. McCarthy TL, Ji C, Centrella M, et al: Links among growth factors: Hormones, and nuclear factors with essential roles in bone formation. Crit Rev Oral Biol Med 11:409, 2000.

197. Rosen V, Wozney JM: Bone morphogenetic proteins. In Bilezikian JP, Raisz LG, Rodan GA (eds): Principles of Bone Biology, 2d ed. San Diego, Academic Press, 2002, p 919.

198. Earnst M, Heath JK, Rodan GA: Estradiol effects on proliferation messenger ribonucleic acid for collagen and insulin like growth factor I and parathyroid hormone stimulation of adenylate cyclase activity in osteoblast cells from calvaric and long bones. Endocrinology 125:825, 1989.

199. Bichell DP, Rotwein P, McCarthy TL: Prostaglandin E_2 avidly stimulates insulin like growth factor I gene expression in primary osteoblast cultures: Evidence for transcriptional control. Endocrinology 133:1020, 1993.

200. Billiard J, Grewal SS, Lukaesko L, et al: Hormonal control of insulin-like growth factor I gene transcription in human osteoblasts: Dual actions of cAMP-dependent protein kinase on CCAAT/enhancer-binding protein delta. J Biol Chem 276:31238, 2001.

201. Phillips AF, Persson B, Hall K, et al: The effects of biosynthetic insulin like growth factor I supplementation on somatic growth, maturation and erythropoiesis on the neonatal rat. Pediatr Res 23:298, 1988.

202. Adamo ML: Regulation of insulin like growth factor I gene expression. Diabetes Rev 3:2, 1995.

203. Hernandez ER, Horowitz A, Vera A, et al: Expression of genes encoding the insulin like growth factors and their receptors in the human ovary. J Clin Endocrinol Metab 74:419, 1992.

204. Guidice LC: Insulin like growth factors and ovarian follicular development. Endocrine Rev 13:641, 1992.

205. Smith EP, Dickson BA, Chernausek SD: Insulin like growth factor binding protein-3 secretion from cultured rat Sertoli cells: Dual regulation by follicle stimulating hormone and IGF-I. Endocrinology 127:27441, 1990.

206. Bondy CA, Lee WH: Patterns of insulin-like growth factor gene expression in brain: Functional implications. Ann N Y Acad Sci 692:33, 1993.

207. Ye P, Lee KH, D'Ercole AJ: Insulin-like growth factor-I (IGF-I) protects myelination from undernutritional insult: Studies of transgenic mice overexpressing IGF-I in brain. J Neurosci Res 62:700, 2000.

208. Elder DA, Karayal AF, D'Ercole AJ, et al: Effects of hypothyroidism on insulin-like growth factor-I expression during brain development in mice. Neurosci Lett 293:99, 2000.

209. Cheng CM, Cohen M, Wang J, et al: Estrogen augments glucose transporter and IGF-1 expression in primate cerebral cortex. FASEB J 15:907, 2001.

210. Ye P, Price W, Kassiotics G, et al: Tumor necrosis factor-alpha regulation of insulin-like growth factor-I, type 1 IGF receptor, and IGF binding protein expression in cerebellum of transgenic mice. J Neurosci Res 71:721, 2003.

211. Edwall D, Schalling M, Jennische E, et al: Induction of insulin-like growth factor I messenger ribonucleic acid during regeneration of rat skeletal muscle. Endocrinology 124:820, 1989.

212. Tollefsen SE, Lajara R, McCusker RH, et al: Insulin-like growth factors (IGF) in muscle development. J Biol Chem 264:13810, 1989.

213. Paul AC, Rosenthal N: Different modes of hypertrophy in skeletal muscle fibers. J Cell Biol 156:751, 2002.

214. Fernandez AM, Dupont J, Farrar RP, et al: Muscle-specific inactivation of the IGF-I receptor induces compensatory hyperplasia in skeletal muscle. J Clin Invest 109:347, 2002.

215. Donohue TJ, Lance DD, Largo MN, et al: Induction of myocardial insulin-like growth factor I gene expression in left ventricular hypertrophy. Circulation 89:799, 1994.

216. Hanson MC, Kenneth AF, Alexander RW, et al: Induction of cardiac insulin-like growth factor-I gene expression in pressure overload hypertrophy. Am J Med Sci 306:69, 1993.

217. Fath KA, Alexander RW, Delafontaine P: Abdominal coarctation increases insulin-like growth factor I mRNA levels in rat aorta. Circ Res 72:271, 1993.

218. Cercek B, Fishbein MC, Forrester JS, et al: Induction of insulin-like growth factor I messenger RNA in rat aorta after balloon denudation. Circ Res 66:1755, 1990.

219. Adamo ML, Bach MA, Roberts CT, LeRoith D: Regulation of insulin, IGF-I, and IGF-II gene expression. In LeRoith D (ed): Insulin-Like Growth Factors: Molecular and Cellular Aspects. Boca Raton, FL, CRC Press, 1990, p 271.

220. Woelfle J, Billiard J, Rotwein P: Acute control of insulin-like growth factor-I gene transcription by growth hormone through Stat5b. J Biol Chem 278:22696, 2003.

221. Lowe WL, Adam OM, Werner H, et al: Regulation by fasting of insulin-like growth factor I and its receptor: Effects on gene expression and binding. J Clin Invest 84:619, 1989.

222. Butler ST, Marr AL, Pelton SH, et al: Insulin restores GH responsiveness during lactation-induced negative energy balance in dairy cattle: Effects on expression of IGF-I and GH receptor 1A. J Endocrinol 176:205, 2003.

223. Ramos S, Goya L, Alvarez C, et al: Effect of thyroxine administration on

the IGF/IGF binding protein system in neonatal and adult thyroidectomized rats. J Endocrinol 169:111, 2001.

224. Rotwein P, Pollack KM, Watson M, et al: Insulin-like growth factor gene expression during rat embryonic development. Endocrinology 121:2141, 1987.

225. DePaulo F, Scott LA, Roth J: Insulin and insulin-like growth factor I in early development: peptides, receptors, and biological events. Endocr Rev 4:558, 1990.

226. Hirschberg R: The physiology and pathophysiology of IGF-I in the kidney. Adv Exp Med Biol 343:345, 1993.

227. Fagin JA, Melmed S: Relative increase in insulin-like growth factor-I messenger ribonucleic acid levels in compensatory renal hypertrophy. Endocrinology 120:718, 1987.

228. Stiles CD, Capone GT, Scher CD, et al: Dual control of cell growth by somatomedin and platelet-derived growth factor. Proc Natl Acad Sci U S A 76:1279, 1979.

229. Leof EB, Wharton W, Van Wyk JJ, et al: Epidermal growth factor and somatomedin-C regulate G_1 progression in competent BALB/c 3T3 cell. Exp Cell Res 141:107, 1982.

230. Travali S, Reiss K, Ferber A, et al: Constitutively expressed c-*myb* abrogates the requirement for insulin-like growth factor-I in 3T3 fibroblasts. Mol Cell Biol 11:731, 1991.

231. Coppola D, Ferber A, Miura A, et al: A functional insulin-like growth factor I receptor is required for the mitogenic and transforming activities of the epidermal growth factor receptor. Mol Cell Biol 14:4588, 1994.

232. Pietrzkowski Z, Lammers R, Carpenter G, et al: Constitutive expression of insulin-like growth factor-I and insulin-like growth factor-I receptor abrogates all requirements for exogenous growth factors. Cell Growth Differ 3:199, 1992.

233. Pfeifle B, Boeder H, Ditschuneit H: Interaction of receptors for insulin-like growth factor I, platelet-derived growth factor, and fibroblast growth factor in rat aortic cells. Endocrinology 120:2251, 1987.

234. Clemmons DR, Van Wyk JJ: Evidence for a functional role of endogenously produced somatomedin-like peptides in the regulation of DNA synthesis in cultured human fibroblasts and porcine smooth muscle cells. J Clin Invest 75:1914, 1985.

235. Lowe WL: Biologic actions of the insulin-like growth factors. In LeRoith D (ed): Insulin-like Growth Factors: Molecular and Cellular Aspects. Boca Raton, FL, CRC Press, 1991, p 49.

236. Vetter U, Zapf J, Heit W, et al: Human fetal and adult chondrocytes: Effect of insulin-like growth factors I and II, insulin, and growth hormone on clonal growth. J Clin Invest 77:1903, 1986.

237. Kemp SF, Kearns GL, Smith WG, et al: Effects of IGF-I on the synthesis and processing of glycosaminoglycans in cultured chick chondrocytes. Acta Endocrinol 119:245, 1988.

238. Loeser RF, Shanker G: Autocrine stimulation by insulin-like growth factor 1 and insulin like growth factor 2 mediates chrondocyte survival in vitro. Arthritis Rheum 43:1552, 2000.

239. Madry H, Zurakowski D, Trippel SB: Overexpression of human insulin-like growth factor-I promotes new tissue formation in an ex vivo model of articular chrondrocyte transplantation. Gene Ther 8:1443, 2001.

240. Hock JM, Centrella M, Canalis E: Insulin-like growth factor-I has independent effects on bone matrix formation and cell replication. Endocrinology 122:254, 1988.

241. Yakar S, Rosen C: From mouse to man: Redefining the role of insulin-like growth factor-I in the acquisition of bone mass. Proc Soc Exp Biol Med 228:245, 1998.

242. Zhao G, Monier-Faugere MC, Langub MC, et al: Targeted overexpression of insulin-like growth factor I to osteoblasts of transgenic mice: Increased trabecular bone volume without increased osteoblast proliferation. Endocrinology 141:2674, 2000.

243. Zhang M, Xuan S, Bouxsein ML, et al: Conditional mutagenesis of the IGF1 receptor gene in osteoblasts reduces cancellous bone volume and increases turnover. J Biol Chem 277:44005, 2002.

244. Sjogren K, Sheng M, Moverare S, et al: Effects of liver-derived insulin-like growth factor I on bone metabolism in mice. J Bone Miner Res 17:1977, 2002.

245. Barreca A, Delena P, Del Monte S, et al: *In vitro* paracrine regulation of human growth by fibroblast derived growth factors. J Cell Physiol 151:262, 1992.

246. Dodson MV, Allen RE, Hossner KL: Ovine somatomedin, multiplication stimulating activity, and insulin promote skeletal muscle satellite cell proliferation *in vitro*. Endocrinology 117:2357, 1985.

247. Florini JR, Ewton DZ, Root SL: IGF-I stimulates terminal myogenic differentiation by induction of myogenin gene expression. Mol Endocrinol 5:718, 1991.

248. Takahashi T, Ishida K, Itoh K, et al: IGF-I gene transfer by electroporation promotes regeneration in a muscle injury model. Gene Ther 10:612, 2003.

249. Fiorotto ML, Schwartz RJ, Delaughter MC: Persistent IGF-I overexpression in skeletal muscle in transiently enhances DNA accretion and growth. FASEB J 17:59, 2003.

250. Banu J, Wang L, Kalu DN: Effects of increased muscle mass on bone in male mice overexpressing IGF-I in skeletal muscles. Calcif Tissue Int 73:196, 2003.

251. Welsh S, Plank D, Witt S, et al: Cardiac-specific IGF-1 expression

attenuates dilated cardiomyopathy in tropomodulin-overexpressing transgenic mice. Circ Res 90:641, 2002.

252. Zhu B, Zhao G, Witte DP, et al: Targeted overexpression of IGF-I in smooth muscle cells of transgenic mice enhances neointimal formation through increased proliferation and cell migration after intraarterial injury. Endocrinology 142:3598, 2001.

253. Zhao G, Sutliff RL, Weber CS, et al: Smooth muscle-targeted overexpression of insulin-like growth factor I results in enhanced vascular contractility. Endocrinology 142:623, 2001.

254. Williams KL, Fuller CR, Fagin J, et al: Mesenchymal IGF-I overexpression: paracrine effects in the intestine, distinct from endocrine actions. Am J Physiol Gastrointest Liver Physiol 283:875, 2002.

255. Cao Y, Gunn AJ, Bennet L, et al: Insulin-like growth factor (IGF)-1 suppresses oligodendrocyte caspase-3 activation and increases glial proliferation after ischemia in near-term fetal sheep. J Cereb Blood Flow Metab 23:739, 2003.

256. Caroni P, Grandes P: Nerve sprouting in innervated adult skeletal muscle induced by exposure to high levels of insulin-like growth factor-I. J Cell Biol 110:1307, 1990.

257. Frondin M, Gammeltoft S: Insulin-like growth factors act synergistically with fibroblast growth factor and nerve growth factor to promote chromaffin cell proliferation. Proc Natl Acad Sci U S A 91:1771, 1994.

258. Caroni P, Schneider C: Signalling by insulin-like growth factors in paralyzed skeletal muscle: Rapid induction of IGF-I expression in muscle fiber and prevention of interstitial cell proliferation by IGFBP-5 and IGFBP-4. J Neurosci 14:3378, 1994.

259. Hansson HA, Dahlin LB, Danielsen N, et al: Evidence indicating trophic importance of IGF-I in regenerating peripheral nerves. Acta Physiol Scand 126:609, 1986.

260. Vicario-Abejon C, Yusta-Boyo MJ, Fernandez-Moreno C, et al: Locally born olfactory bulb stem cells proliferate in response to insulin-related factors and require endogenous insulin-like growth factor-I for differentiation into neurons and glia. J Neurosci 23:895, 2003.

261. Ye P, Xing YZ, Dai ZH, et al: In vivo actions of insulin-like growth factor-I (IGF-I) on cerebellum development in transgenic mice: Evidence that IGF-I increases proliferation of granule cell progenitors. Brain Res 95:44, 1996.

262. D'Ercole AJ, Ye P, O'Kusky JR: Mutant mouse models of insulin-like growth factor actions in the central nervous system. Neuropeptides 36:209, 2002.

263. Mason J, Xuan S, Dragatsis I, et al: Insulin-like growth factor (IGF) signaling through type 1 IGF receptor plays an important role in

remyelination. J Neurosci 23:7710, 2003.

264. Muta K, Krontes B: Apoptosis of human erythroid colony forming cells is decreased by stem cell factor and insulin-like growth factor-I as well as erythropoietin. J Cell Physiol 156:264, 1993.

265. Rodriguez-Tarduchy G, Collins MKL, Garcia I, et al: Insulin-like growth factor I inhibits apoptosis in IL-3 dependent hematopoietic cells. J Immunol 149:535, 1992.

266. Resnicoff MD, Abraham W, Yutaboonchai HL, et al: The insulin-like growth factor-I receptor protects tumor cells from apoptosis *in vitro*. Cancer Res 55:2463, 1995.

267. Claun SY, Billig H, Tilly JL, et al: Gonadotrophin suppression of apoptosis in cultured preovulatory follicles: Mediatory role of endogenous insulin-like growth factor-I. Endocrinology 135:1845, 1994.

268. Florini JR, Ewton DZ, Root SL: Insulin-like growth factors, muscle growth and myogenesis. Diabetes Rev 3:73, 1995.

269. Mochizuki H, Hakeda Y, Watatsuki N, et al: Insulin-like growth factor I supports formation and activation of osteoblasts. Endocrinology 131:1075, 1992.

270. Geduspen JS, Solursh M: Effects of the mesonephros and insulin-like growth factor-I on chondrogenesis. Dev Biol 156:500, 1993.

271. Palmer S, Myerson G, Lindgren E, et al: Insulin-like growth factor-I shifts from promoting cell division to potentiating maturation during normal differentiation. Proc Natl Acad Sci U S A 88:9994, 1991.

272. Penhoat A, Naville D, Jaillard L, et al: Hormonal regulation of insulin-like growth factor-I secretion by bovine adrenal cells. J Biol Chem 264:6858, 1989.

273. Kasson BC, Hseuh AJ: Insulin-like growth factor-I augments androgen biosynthesis by rat testicular cells. Mol Cell Endocrinol 52:27, 1987.

274. Satisteban P, Kohn DL, DiLauro R: Thyroglobulin gene expression is regulated by insulin and insulin-like growth factor I as well as thyrotropin in FRTL 5 cells. J Biol Chem 262:4068, 1987.

275. Yamasaki H, Prager D, Gebremedhin S, et al: Insulin-like growth factor-I (IGF-I) attenuation of growth hormone is enhanced by overexpression of pituitary IGF-I receptors. Mol Endocrinol 5:890, 1991.

276. Duan C, Hawes S, Prevette T, et al: Insulin like growth factor-I (IGF-I) stimulates IGF binding protein-5 synthesis through transcriptional activation of the gene in aortic smooth muscle cells. J Biol Chem 271:4280, 1996.

277. Wolfe BL, Rich CB, Goud HD, et al: Insulin-like growth factor-I regulates transcription of the elastin gene. J Biol Chem 268:124418, 1993.

278. Alemany J, Borras T, dePablo F: Transcriptional stimulation of the delta 1-crystallin gene by insulin-like growth factor I and insulin requires DNA cis elements in chicken. Proc Natl Acad Sci U S A 87:3353, 1990.

279. Urban RJ, Shupnik MA, Bodenburg YH: Insulin-like growth factor-I increases expression of the porcine P-450 cholesterol side chain cleavage gene through a GC-rich domain. J Biol Chem 269:25761, 1994.

280. Spangenburg EE, Bowles DK, Booth FW: IGF-I induced transcriptional activity of the skeletal {alpha} action gene is regulated by signaling mechanisms linked to voltage-gated calcium channels during myoblast differentiation. Endocrinol 2003, epub.

281. Carson MJ, Behringer RR, Brinster RI, et al: Insulin-like growth factor I increases brain growth and central nervous system myelination in transgenic mice. J Neurosci 10:779, 1993.

282. Dupont J, Fernandez AM, Glackin CA, et al: Insulin-like growth factor I (IGF-I) induced twist expression is involved in the anti-apoptotic effects of the IGF-I receptor. J Biol Chem 276:26699, 2001.

283. Mulligan C, Rochford J, Denyer G, et al: Microarray analysis of insulin and insulin-like growth factor-I (IGF-I) receptor signaling reveals the selective up-regulation of the mitogen heparin-binding EGF-like growth factor by IGF-1. J Biol Chem 277:42480, 2002.

284. Dimitridas G, Billings M, Bevan S, et al: Effects of insulin-like growth factor-I on the rates of glucose transport and utilization in rat skeletal muscle *in vitro*. Biochem J 285:269, 1992.

285. Zheng B, Clemmons DR: Blocking ligand occupancy of the αVβ3 integrin inhibits IGF-I signaling in vascular smooth muscle cells. Proc Natl Acad Sci U S A 95:11217, 1998.

286. Morrione A, DeAngelis T, Baserga R: Evidence of the bovine papilloma virus to transform mouse embryo fibroblasts with targeted gene disruption of the insulin-like growth factor-I receptor gene. J Virol 169:5260, 1995

287. Li S, Resnicoff MD, Baserga R: Effect of substituting tyrosines 1280-1281 on the mitogenic and transforming actions of the insulin like growth factor-I receptor. J Biol Chem 271:12254, 1996.

288. LeRoith D, Werner H, Beitner-Johnson D, et al: Molecular and cellular aspects of the insulin like growth factor I receptor. Endocr Rev 16:143, 1995.

289. Schiramacher P, Held WA, Yang D, et al: Reactivation of insulin-like growth factor II during hepatocarcinogenesis in transgenic mice suggests a role in malignant growth. Cancer Res 5:2549, 1992.

290. Christofori G, Naiki P, Hanahan D: A second signal supplied by insulin like growth factor II in oncogene induced tumorigenesis. Nature 369:414, 1994.

291. Ogawa O, Eccles MA, Szeto J, et al: Relation of insulin like growth factor II gene imprinting implicated in Wilms' tumor. Nature 362:749, 1993

292. De Sousa AT, Hinbrirs GR, Washington MK, et al: Frequent loss of heterozygote on 69 at the mannose 6 phosphate/insulin like growth factor II receptor locus in human hepatocellular tumors. Oncogene 10:1725, 1995

293. Baxter RC, Daughaday WH: Impaired function of the ternary insulin like growth factor binding complex in patients with hypoglycemia due to non-islet cell tumors. J Clin Endocrinol Metab 73:696, 1991.

294. Hadsell DL, Murphy KL, Bonnette SG, et al: Cooperative interaction between mutant p53 and des$^{1-3}$ IGF-I accelerates mammary tumorigenesis. Oncogene 19:889, 2000.

295. Sachdev D, Hartell JS, Lee AV, et al: A dominant negative type I insulin-like growth factor receptor inhibits metastasis of human cancer cells. J Biol Chem 2003, epub.

296. DiGiovanni J, Kiguchi K, Frijhoff A, et al: Deregulated expression of insulin-like growth factor 1 in prostate epithelium leads to neoplasia in transgenic mice. Proc Natl Acad Sci U S A 97:3455, 2000.

297. Davenport ML, D'Ercole AJ, Underwood LE: Effects of maternal fasting on fetal growth serum insulin like growth factors (IGFs) and tissue IGF messenger ribonucleic acids. Endocrinology 126:2062, 1990.

298. Bang P, Brismar K, Rosenfeld RG: Increased proteolysis of insulin-like growth factor-binding protein-3 (IGFBP-3) in noninsulin-dependent diabetes mellitus serum, with elevation of a 20-kildalton (kDa) glycosylated IGFBP-3 fragment contained in the approximately 130-150 kDa ternary complex. J Clin Endocrinol Metab 78:1119, 1994.

299. Fowlkes J, Enghild JJ, Suzukik N, et al: Matrix metalloproteases degrade insulin like growth factor binding protein-3 in dermal fibroblast cultures. J Biol Chem 269:25742, 1994.

300. Cohen P, Graves HC, Peehl D, et al: Prostate specific antigen PSA is an insulin-like growth factor binding protein-3 protease found in seminal plasma 2. Clin Endocrinol Metab 75:1046, 1992.

301. Nunn SE, Peehl DM, Cohen P: Acid-activated insulin-like growth factor binding protein protease activity of cathepsin D in normal and malignant prostatic epithelial cells and seminal plasma. J Cell Physiol 171:196, 1997.

302. Bunn RC, Fowlkes JL: Insulin-like growth factor binding protein proteolysis. Trends Endocrinol Metab 14:176, 2003.

303. Gockerman A, Clemmons DR: Porcine aortic smooth muscle cells secrete a

serine protease for insulin like growth factor binding protein-2. Circ Res 76:514, 1995.

304. Clemmons DR: Insulin-like growth factor binding proteins and their role in controlling IGF actions. Cytokine Growth Factor Rev 8:45, 1997.

305. Thrailkill KM, Quarles P, Nagase H, et al: Characterization of insulin like growth factor binding protein 5 degrading proteases produced throughout murine osteoblast differentiation. Endocrinology 136:3527, 1995.

306. Conover CA: A unique receptor independent mechanism by which insulin like growth factor I regulates the availability of insulin like growth factor binding protein in normal and transformed fibroblasts. J Clin Invest 88:1354, 1991.

307. Rees C, Clemmons DR, Horvitz GD, et al: A protease-resistant form of insulin-like growth factor binding protein-4 (IGFBP-4) inhibits IGF-I actions. Endocrinology 139:4182, 1998.

308. Lawrence JB, Oxvig C, Overgaard MT, et al: The insulin-like growth factor (IGF-I)-dependent IGF binding protein-4 protease secreted by human fibroblasts is pregnancy-associated plasma protein-A. Proc Natl Acad Sci U S A 196:3149, 1999.

309. Ankrapp DP, Jones JI, Clemmons DR: Characterization of insulin like growth factor binding protein-1 kinases from human hepatoma cells. J Cell Biochem 60:387, 1996.

310. Coverley JA, Baxter RC: Regulation of insulin-like growth factor (IGF) binding protein-3 phosphorylation by IGF-I. Endocrinology 136:5778, 1995.

311. Leal SM, Liu Q, Huang GS, et al: The type V transforming growth factor beta receptor is a putative insulin like growth factor binding protein 3 receptor. J Biol Chem 272:20572, 1997.

312. McCusker RH, Camacho-Hubner C, Bayne ML, et al: Insulin-like growth factor (IGF) binding to human fibroblast and glioblastoma cells: The modulating effect of cell released IGF binding proteins (IGFBPs). J Cell Physiol 144:244, 1990.

313. Nam TJ, Busby WH Jr, Clemmons DR: Insulin-like growth factor binding protein-5 binds to plasminogen activator inhibitor-I. Endocrinology 138:2972, 1997.

314. Nam TJ, Busby WH Jr, Rees C, et al: Thrombospondin and osteopontin bind to insulin-like growth factor (IGF)-binding protein-5 leading to an alteration in IGF-I stimulated cell growth. Endocrinology 141:1100, 2000.

315. Wirtz MK, Xu H, Rust K, et al: Insulin-like growth factor binding protein-5 expression by human trabecular meshwork. Invest Ophthalmol Vis Sci 39:45, 1998.

316. Kiepe D, Andress DL, Mohan S, et al: Intact IGF-I binding protein-4 and -5 and their respective fragments isolated from chronic renal failure serum differentially modulate IGF-I actions in culture growth plate chrondrocytes. J Am Soc Nephrol 12:2400, 2001.

317. Campbell PG, Andress DL: Insulin-like growth factor (IGF)-binding protein-5-(201-218) region regulates hydroxyapatite and IGF-I binding. Am J Physiol 273:E1005, 1997.

318. Parker A, Clarke JB, Busby WH Jr, et al: Identification of the extracellular matrix binding sites for insulin like growth factor-binding protein 5. J Biol Chem 271:13523, 1996.

319. Burch WW, Correa J, Shaveley JE, et al: The 25 kDa insulin-like growth factor (IGF) binding protein inhibits both basal and IGF mediated growth in chick embryonic pelvic cartilage in vitro. J Clin Endocrinol Metab 70:173, 1990.

320. Okajimina T, Iwashita M, Takeda Y, et al: Inhibitory effects insulin-like growth factor binding proteins 1 and 3 on IGF activated glucose consumption in mouse BALB/c3T3 fibroblasts. J Endocrinol 133:457, 1993.

321. Elgin RG, Busby WH, Clemmons DR: An insulin-like growth factor binding protein enhances the biologic response to IGF-I. Proc Natl Acad Sci U S A 84:3254, 1987.

322. Kratz G, Lake M, Ljungstrom K, et al: Effect of recombinant IGF binding protein-1 on primary cultures of human keratinocytes and fibroblasts: Selective enhancement of IGF-I but not IGF-II induced cell proliferation. Exp Cell Res 202:381, 1992.

323. Gleeson LM, Charkraborty C, McKinnon T, et al: Insulin-like growth factor-binding protein 1 stimulates human trophoblast migration by signaling through alpha 5 beta 1 integrin via mitogen-activated protein kinase pathway. J Clin Endocrinol Metab 86:2484, 2001.

324. Ross M, Francis GL, Szabo L, et al: Insulin-like growth factor (IGF)-binding proteins inhibit the biological activities of IGF-1 and IGF-2 but not des-(1-3)-IGF-1. Biochemistry J 258:267, 1989.

325. Wolf E, Lahm H, Wu M, et al: Effects of IGFBP-2 overexpression in vitro and in vivo. Pediatr Nephrol 14:572, 2000.

326. Dong F, Wu HB, Hong J, et al: Insulin-like growth factor binding protein-2 mediates the inhibition of DNA synthesis by transforming growth factor-beta in mink lung epithelial cells. J Cell Physiol 190:63, 2002.

327. Bar RS, Booth BA, Bowes M, et al: Insulin-like growth factor binding proteins from cultured endothelial cells: Purification, characterization, and intrinsic biologic activities. Endocrinology 125:1910, 1989.

328. Bourner MJ, Busby WH, Siegel NR, et al: Cloning and sequence determination of bovine insulin-like growth factor binding protein-2 (IGFBP-2): Comparison of its structural and functional properties with IGFBP-1. J Cell Biochem 48:215, 1992.

329. Wang H, Wang H, Shen W, et al: Insulin-like growth factor binding protein 2 enhances glioblastoma invasion by activating invasion-enhancing genes. Cancer Res 63:4315, 2003.

330. Moore MG, Wetterau LA, Francis MJ, et al: Novel stimulatory role for insulin-like growth factor binding protein-2 in prostate cancer cells. Int J Cancer 105:14, 2003.

331. Zapf J, Schoenle E, Jagars G, et al: Inhibition of the action of nonsuppressible insulin-like activity on isolated fat cells by binding to its carrier protein. J Clin Invest 63:1077, 1979.

332. Conover CA: Potentiation of insulin-like growth factor (IGF) action by IGF-binding protein-3: Studies of underlying mechanism. Endocrinology 130:3191, 1992.

333. DeMellow JSM, Baxter RC: Growth hormone dependent insulin-like growth factor binding protein both inhibits and potentiates IGF-I stimulated DNA synthesis in skin fibroblasts. Biochem Biophys Res Commun 156:199, 1988.

334. Schmid C, Rutishauser J, Schlapfer I, et al: Intact but not truncated insulin-like growth factor binding protein-3 blocks IGF-I induced stimulation of osteoblasts: Control of IGF signalling to bone cells by IGFBP-3 specific proteolysis. Biochem Biophys Res Commun 179:579, 1991.

335. Strange, KS, Wilkinson D, Emerman JT: Mitogenic properties of insulin-like growth factors I and II, insulin-like growth factor binding protein-3 and epidermal growth factor for on human breast carcinoma cells. Breast Cancer Res Treat 75:203, 2002.

336. Ricort JM, Binoux M: Insulin-like growth factor-binding protein-3 activates a phosphotyrosine phosphatase: Effects on the insulin-like growth factor signaling pathway. J Biol Chem 277:19448, 2002.

337. Blat C, Delbe J, Villaudy J, et al: Inhibitory diffusible factor-45 bifunctional activity as a cell growth inhibitor and as an insulin-like growth factor I-binding protein. J Biol Chem 264:12449, 1989.

338. Oh Y, Muller HL, Ng L, et al: Transforming growth factor-beta-induced cell growth inhibition in human breast cancer cells is mediated through insulin-like growth factor-binding protein-3 action. J Biol Chem 270:13589, 1995.

339. Gucev ZS, Oh Y, Kelley KM, et al: Insulin-like growth factor binding protein 3 mediates retinoic acid and transforming growth factor β2-induced growth inhibition in human breast cancer cells. Cancer Res 56:1545, 1996.

340. Huynh H, Yang XF, Pollak M: Estradiol and antiestrogens regulate a growth inhibitory insulin like growth factor binding protein 3 autocrine loop in human breast cancer cells. J Biol Chem 271:1016, 1996.

341. Boyle BJ, Zhao XY, Cohen P, et al: Insulin-like growth factor binding protein-3 mediates 1α25-dihydroxyvitamin D₃ growth inhibition in the LNCaP prostate cancer cell lines through p21/WAF1. J Urol 165:1319, 2001.

342. Liu B, Lee HY, Weinzimer SA, et al: Direct functional interactions between insulin-like growth factor-binding protein-3 and retinoid X receptor-a regulate transcriptional signaling and apoptosis. J Biol Chem 275:33607, 2000.

343. Schedlich LJ, Young TF, Fifth SM, et al: Insulin-like growth factor-binding protein (IGFBP)-3 and IGFBP-5 share a common nuclear transport pathway in T47D human breast carcinoma cells. J Biol Chem 273:18347, 1998.

344. Mohan S, Bautista CM, Wergedal J, et al: Isolation of inhibitory insulin-like growth factor (IGF) binding protein from bone cell conditioned medium: A potential local regulator of IGF action. Proc Natl Acad Sci U S A 86:8338, 1989.

345. Coulouscou JM, Shoyab M: Purification of a colon cancer cell growth inhibitor and its identification as insulin-like growth factor binding protein-4. Cancer Res 51:2813, 1991.

346. Conover CA, Durham SK, Zapf J, et al: Cleavage analysis of insulin-like growth factor (IGF)-dependent IGF-binding protein-4 proteolysis and expression of protease-resistant IGF-binding protein-4 mutants. J Biol Chem 270:4395, 1995.

347. Qin X, Byun D, Strong DD, et al: Studies on the role of human insulin-like growth factor-II (IGF-II) dependent IGF binding protein (hIGFBP)-4 protease in human osteoblasts using protease-resistant IGFBP-4 analogs. J Bone Miner Res 15:2079, 1999.

348. Damon SE, Haugk KL, Birnbaum RS, et al: Retrovirally mediated overexpression of insulin-like growth factor binding protein 4: Evidence that insulin-like growth factor is required for skeletal muscle differentiation. J Cell Physiol 175:109, 1998.

349. Duan C, Clemmons DR: Differential expression and biological effects of insulin-like growth factor binding protein-4 and -5 in vascular smooth muscle cells. J Biol Chem 273:16836, 1998.

350. Parker A, Rees C, Clarke JB, et al: Binding of insulin-like growth factor binding protein-5 to smooth muscle cell extracellular matrix is a major determinant of the cellular response to IGF-I. Mol Biol Cell 9:2383, 1998.

351. Andress DL, Birnbaum RS: A novel human insulin-like growth factor binding protein secreted by osteoblast cells. Biochem Biophys Res Commun 176:213, 1991.

352. Abrass CK, Berfield AK, Andress DL: Heparin binding domain of insulin-like growth factor binding protein-5 stimulates mesangial cell migration. Am J Physiol 273:899, 1997.

353. Kuemmerle JF, Zhou H: Insulin-like growth factor-binding protein-5 (IGFBP-5) stimulates growth and IGF-I secretion in human intestinal smooth muscle by Ras-dependent activation of p38 MAP kinase and Erk1/2 pathways. J Biol Chem 277:20563, 2002.

354. Butt AJ, Dickson KA, McDougall F, et al: Insulin-like growth factor-binding protein-5 inhibits the growth of human breast cancer cells in vitro and in vivo. J Biol Chem 278:29676, 2003.

355. Schneider MR, Zhou R, Hoeflich A, et al: Insulin-like growth factor binding protein-5 inhibits growth and induces differentiation of mouse osteosarcoma cells. Biochem Biophys Res Commun 288:435, 2001.

356. Marshman E, Green KA, Flint DJ, et al: Insulin-like growth factor binding protein-5 and apoptosis in mammary epithelial cells. J Cell Sci 116:675, 2003.

357. Cheng HL, Feldman EL: Insulin-like growth factor-I (IGF-I) and IGF binding protein-5 in Schwann cell differentiation. J Cell Physiol 171:161, 1997.

358. Gabbitas B, Canalis E: Cortisol enhances the transcription of insulin-like growth factor-binding protein-6 in cultured osteoblasts. Endocrinology 137:1687, 1996.

359. Babajko S, Leneuve P, Loret C, et al: IGF-binding protein-6 is involved in growth inhibition in SH-SY5Y human neuroblastoma cells: Its production is both IGF- and cell density-dependent. J Endocrinol 152:221, 1997.

360. Kiepe D, Ulinski T, Powell DR, et al: Differential effects of insulin-like growth factor binding proteins-1, -2, -3 and -6 on cultured growth plate chondrocytes. Kidney Int 62:1591, 2002.

361. Gallicchio MA, Kneen M, Hall C, et al: Overexpression of insulin-like growth factor binding protein-6 inhibits rhabdomyosarcoma growth in vivo. Int J Cancer 94:645, 2001.

362. Sueoka N, Lee HY, Walsh GL, et al: Insulin-like growth factor binding protein-6 inhibits the growth of human bronchial epithelial cells and increases in abundance with all-trans-retinoic acid treatment. Am J Respir Cell Mol Biol 23:297, 2000.

363. Van Wyk JJ, Underwood LE, Hintz RL, et al: The somatomedins: A family of insulin-like hormones under growth hormone control. Recent Prog Horm Res 30:259, 1974.

364. D'Ercole AJ, Stiles AD, Underwood LE: Tissue concentrations of somatomedin-C: Further evidence for multiple sites of synthesis and paracrine or autocrine mechanisms of action. Proc Natl Acad Sci U S A 81:935, 1984.

365. Jacob RJ, Barrett E, Plewe G, et al: Acute effects of insulin-like growth factor-I on glucose and amino acid metabolism in the awake fasted rat. J Clin Invest 83:1717, 1989.

366. Douglas RG, Gluckman PD, Ball B, et al: The effects of infusion of insulin-like growth factor I (IGF-I), IGF-II and insulin on glucose and protein metabolism in fasted lambs. J Clin Invest 88:614, 1991.

367. Tomas FM, Knowles SE, Owens PC, et al: Insulin-like growth factor-I (IGF-I) and especially IGF-I variants are anabolic in dexamethasone-treated rats. Biochem J 282:91, 1992.

368. Chrysis D, Zhang J, Underwood LE: Divergent regulation of proteasomes by insulin-like growth factor I and growth hormone in skeletal muscle of rats made catabolic with dexamethasone. Growth Horm IGF Res 12:434, 2002.

369. Miller SB, Martin DR, Kissone J, et al: Insulin-like growth factor I accelerates recovery from ischemic acute tubular necrosis in the rat. Proc Natl Acad Sci U S A 89:11876, 1992.

370. Lang CH, Frost RA: Role of growth hormone, insulin-like growth factor-I and insulin-like growth factor binding proteins in the catabolic response to injury and infection. Curr Opin Nutr Metab Care 5:271, 2002.

371. Thissen JP, Underwood LE, Maiter DM, et al: Failure of IGF-I infusion to promote growth in protein-restricted rats despite normalization of serum IGF-I concentrations. Endocrinology 128:885, 1991.

372. Olanrewaju H, Patel L, Seidel ER: Trophic action of local intraileal infusion of insulin like growth factor I: polyamine dependence. Am J Physiol 263:E282, 1992.

373. Schweiller E, Guler H-P, Merryweather J: Growth restoration of insulin deficit diabetic rats by recombinant human insulin-like growth factor I. Nature 323:169, 1986.

374. Jacob RJ, Sherwin RS, Bowen L, et al: Metabolic effects of IGF-I and insulin in spontaneously diabetic BB/w rats. Am J Physiol 260:E262, 1991.

375. Cox GN, McDermott MJ, Merkel E, et al: Recombinant human insulin-like growth factor binding protein-1 inhibits growth stimulated by IGF-I and growth hormone in hypophysectomized rats. Endocrinology 35:1913, 1994.

376. Lang CH, Vary TC, Frost RA: Acute in vivo election of insulin-like growth factor (IGF) binding protein-1 decreases plasma free IGF-I and muscle protein synthesis. Endocrinology 144:3922, 2003.

377. Galiano RD, Zhao L, Clemmons DR, et al: Interaction between the insulin-like growth factor family and the integrin receptor family in tissue repair processes. J Clin Invest 98:2462, 1996.

378. Leu JI, Crissey MA, Taub R: Massive hepatic apoptosis associated with TGF-beta1 activation after Fas ligand treatment of IGF binding protein-1-deficient mice. J Clin Invest 111:129, 2003.

379. Crossey PA, Pillai CC, Miell JP: Altered placental development and intrauterine growth restriction in IGF

binding protein-1 transgenic mice. J Clin Invest 110:411, 2002.

380. Dheen ST, Rajkumar K, Murphy LJ: Islet cell proliferation and apoptosis in insulin-like growth factor binding protein-1 in transgenic mice. J Endocrinol 155:551, 1997.

381. Conover CA, Johnstone EW, Turner RT, et al: Subcutaneous administration of insulin-like growth factor IGF-II/IGF binding protein-2 complex stimulates bone formation and prevents loss of bone mineral density in a rat model of disuse osteoporosis. Growth Horm IGF Res 12:178, 2002.

382. Palermo C, Manduca P, Gazzerro E, et al: Potentiating role of insulin-like growth factor binding protein (IGFBP)-2 on IGF-II-stimulated alkaline phosphatase activity in differentiating osteoblasts. Am J Physiol Endocrinol Metab 2003; epub.

383. Bagi CM, Brommage R, Adams SO, et al: Benefit of systemically administered rh IGF-I and rh IGF-I/IGBP-3 on cancellous bone in oophorectomized rats. J Bone Miner Res 9:1301, 1994.

384. Stewart CH, Bates DC, Calder TA, et al: Potentiation of insulin like growth factor (IGF-I) activity by an antibody: Supportive evidence for enhancement of IGF-I bioavailability in vivo by IGF binding proteins. Endocrinology 133:1462, 1993.

385. Behringer RR, Lewin TM, Quaife CJ, et al: Expression of insulin-like growth factor I stimulates normal somatic growth in growth hormone deficient transgenic mice. Endocrinology 127:1033, 1990.

386. Matthews LS, Hammer RE, Beheringer R, et al: Growth enhancement of transgenic mice expressing human insulin-like growth factor-I. Endocrinology 123:2827, 1988.

387. Ohneda K, Ulshen MH, Fuller CR, et al: Enhanced growth of small bowl in transgenic mice expressing human insulin-like growth factor I. Gastroenterology 112:444, 1997.

388. Chrysis D, Calikoglu AS, Ye P, et al: Insulin-like growth factor-I overexpression attenuates cerebellar apoptosis by altering the expression of Bcl family proteins in a developmentally specific manner. J Neurosci 21:1481, 2001.

389. Dai A, Xing Y, Boney CM, et al: Human insulin-like growth factor binding protein-1 (hIGFBP-1) transgenic mice: Characterization and insights into the regulation of IGFBP-1 expression. Endocrinology 135:1316, 1994.

390. Rajkumar K, Barron D, Lewitt M, et al: Growth retardation and hyperglycemia in insulin-like growth factor binding protein-1 transgenic mice. Endocrinology 136:4029, 1995.

391. Crossey PA, Jones JS, Miell JP: Dysregulation of the insulin/IGF binding protein-1 axis in transgenic mice is associated with hyperinsulinemia and glucose intolerance. Diabetes 49:457, 2000.

392. Ben Lagha N, Menuelle P, Seurin P, et al: Bone formation in the context of growth retardation induced by hIGFBP-1 overexpression in transgenic mice. Connect Tissue Res 43:515, 2002.

393. Eckstein F, Pavicic T, Nedbal S, et al: Insulin-like growth factor binding protein-2 (IGFBP-2) overexpression negatively regulates bone size and mass, but not density, in the absence and presence of growth hormone/IGF-I excess in transgenic mice. Anat Embryol (Berl) 206:139, 2003.

394. Hoeflich A, Nedbal S, Blum WF, et al: Growth inhibition in giant growth hormone transgenic mice by overexpression of insulin-like growth factor-binding protein-2. Endocrinology 142:1889, 2001.

395. Murphy LJ, Molnar P, Lu X, et al: Expression of human insulin-like growth factor-binding protein-3 in transgenic mice. J Mol Endocrinol 15:293, 1995.

396. Silha JV, Mishra S, Rosen CJ, et al: Perturbations in bone formation and resorption in insulin-like growth factor binding protein-3 transgenic mice. J Bone Miner Res 18:1834, 2003.

397. Modric T, Silha JV, Shi Z, et al: Phenotypic manifestations of insulin-like growth factor-binding protein-3 overexpression in transgenic mice. Endocrinology 142:1958, 2001.

398. Zhang M, Faugere MC, Malluche H, et al: Paracrine overexpression of IGFBP-4 in osteoblasts of transgenic mice decreases bone turnover and causes global growth retardation. J Bone Miner Res 18:836, 2003.

399. Wang J, Niu W, Witte DP, et al: Overexpression of insulin-like growth factor binding protein-4 (IGFBP-4) in smooth muscle cells of transgenic mice through a smooth muscle alpha-actin-IGFBP-4 fusion gene induces smooth muscle hypoplasia. Endocrinology 139:2605, 1998.

400. Miyakoshi N, Richman C, Kasukawa Y, et al: Evidence that IGF-binding protein-5 functions as a growth factor. J Clin Invest 107:73, 2001.

401. Devlin RD, Du Z, Buccilli V, et al: Transgenic mice overexpressing insulin-like growth factor binding protein-5 display transiently decreased osteoblastic function and osteopenia. Endocrinology 143:3955, 2002.

402. Baker J, Liu JP, Robertson EJ, et al: Role of insulin like growth factors in embryonic and postnatal growth. Cell 75:83, 1993.

403. Powell-Braxton L, Hollingshead P, Warburton C, et al: IGF-I is required for normal embryonic development in mice. Genes Dev 7:2609, 1993.

404. Holzenberger M, Leneuve P, Hamard G, et al: A targeted partial invalidation of the insulin-like growth factor receptor gene in mice causes a postnatal growth deficit. Endocrinology 141:2557, 2000.

405. Holzenberger M, Dupont J, Ducos B, et al: IGF-I receptor regulates lifespan and resistance to oxidative stress in mice. Nature 421:182, 2003.

406. Kondo T, Vicent D, Suzuma K, et al: Knockout of insulin and IGF-I receptors on vascular endothelial cells protects against retinal neovascularization. J Clin Invest 111:1835, 2003.

407. DeChiara RM, Efstratiadis A, Robertson EJ: A growth deficiency phenotype in heterozygous mice carrying an insulin-like growth factor II gene disruption. Nature 345:78, 1990.

408. Pintar JE, Schuller A, Cerro JA, et al: Genetic ablation of IGFBP-2 suggests functional redundancy in the IGFBP family. Prog Growth Fact Res 6:437, 1995.

409. Wood TL, Rogler LE, Czick ME, et al: Selective alterations in organ sizes in mice with a targeted disruption of the insulin-like growth factor binding protein-2 gene. Mol Endocrinol 14:1472, 2000.

410. Shuller AGP, Pintar JE: Embryonic growth deficit in IGFBP-4 deficient mice: Presented to the 80th Endocrine Society Meeting, New Orleans, LA, June 14–18, 1998; R6-1[Abstract].

411. Jennische E, Skottner A, Hansson HA: Dynamic changes in insulin-like growth factor I immunoreactivity correlate with repair events in rat ear after freeze-thaw injury. Exp Mol Pathol 47:193, 1987.

412. Hansson HA, Jennische E, Skottner A: Regenerating endothelial cells express insulin-like growth factor-I immunoreactivity after arterial injury. Cell Tissue Res 250:499, 1987.

413. Khorsondi MJ, Fagin JA, Ginnella-Neto, et al: Regulation of insulin-like growth factor I and its receptor in rat aorta after balloon degradation: Evidence for local bioactivity. J Clin Invest 90:1926, 1992.

414. Yakar S, Liu JU, Stannard B, et al: Normal growth and development in the absence of insulin-like growth factor-I. Proc Natl Acad Sci U S A 96:7324, 1999.

415. Sjogren K, Liu JL, Blad K, et al: Liver-derived insulin-like growth factor I (IGF-I) is the principal source of IGF-I in blood but is not required for postnatal body growth in mice. Proc Natl Acad Sci U S A 96:7088, 1999.

416. Yakar S, Rosen CJ, Beamer WG, et al: Circulating levels of IGF-I directly regulate bone growth and density. J Clin Invest 110:771, 2002.

417. Ueki I, Ooi GT, Tremblay ML, et al: Inactivation of the acid labile subunit gene in the mice results in mild retardation of postnatal growth despite profound disruptions in the circulating insulin-like growth factor system. Proc Natl Acad Sci U S A 97:6868, 2000.

418. Yakar S, Liu JL, Fernandez AM, et al: Liver-specific IGF-1 gene deletion leads

to muscle insulin insensitivity. Diabetes 50:1110, 2001.

419. Yakar S, Setser J, Zhao H, et al: Inhibition of growth hormone action improves insulin sensitivity in liver IGF-1 deficient mice. J Clin Invest 113:96, 2004.

420. Haluzik M, Yakar S, Gavirilova O, et al: Insulin resistance in the liver specific IGF-1 gene-deleted mouse is abrogated by deletion of the acid-labile subunit of the IGF-binding protein-3 complex: Relative roles of growth hormone and IGF-I in insulin resistance. Diabetes 52:2483, 2003.

421. Guler H-P, Zapf J, Froesch ER: Short-term metabolic effects of recombinant human insulin-like growth factor-I in healthy adults. N Engl J Med 317:137, 1987.

422. Boulware S, Tamborlane W, Sherwin R: Diverse effects of insulin like growth factor I on glucose lipid-I amino acid metabolism. Am J Physiol 262:130, 1992.

423. Mauras N, Horber FF, Haymond MW: Low dose recombinant human insulin like growth factor-I fails to affect protein anabolism but alters islet cell secretion in humans. J Clin Endocrinol Metab 75:1192, 1992.

424. Kerr D, Tamborlane V, Rife F, et al: Effect of insulin-like growth factor-I on the responses to and recognition of hypoglycemia in humans: A comparison with insulin. J Clin Invest 91:141, 1993.

425. Clemmons DR, Smith-Banks A, Celniker AC, et al: Reversal of diet-induced catabolism by infusion of recombinant insulin-like growth factor-I (IGF-I) in humans. J Clin Endocrinol Metab 75:234, 1992.

426. Herndon DN, Ramzy PI, DebRoy MA, et al: Muscle protein catabolism after severe burn: Effects of IGF-1/IGFBP-3 treatment. Ann Surg 229:713, 1999.

427. Boonen S, Rosen C, Bouillon R, et al: Musculoskeletal effects of the recombinant human IGF-I/IGF binding protein-3 complex in osteoporotic patients with proximal femoral fracture: A double-blind, placebo-controlled pilot study. J Clin Endocrinol Metab 87:1593, 2002.

428. Guler H-P, Schmid C, Zapf J, et al: Effects of recombinant insulin-like growth factor-I on insulin secretion and renal function in normal human subjects. Proc Natl Acad Sci U S A 86:2868, 1989.

429. Mauras N: Combined recombinant human growth hormone and recombinant human insulin-like growth factor I: Lack of synergy on whole body protein anabolism in normally fed subjects. J Clin Endocrinol Metab 80:2633, 1995.

430. Hussain MA, Schmitz O, Mengel A, et al: Insulin-like growth factor I stimulate lipid oxidation, reduces protein oxidation, and enhances insulin sensitivity in humans. J Clin Invest 92:2249, 1993.

431. Berneis K, Nianis R, Girard J, et al: Effects of insulin-like growth factor I combined with growth hormone on glucocorticoid induced whole body protein catabolism. J Clin Endocrinol Metab 82:2528, 1997.

432. Mauras N, Beaufree B: Recombinant human insulin like growth factor I enhances whole body protein anabolism and significantly diminishes the protein catabolic effects of prednisone in humans without a diabetogenic effect. J Clin Endocrinol Metab 80:869, 1995.

433. Ebling PR, Jones JD, O'Fallon WM, et al: Short term effects of recombinant human insulin like growth factor I on bone turnover in normal women. J Clin Endocrinol Metab 77:1384, 1993.

434. Grinspoon S, Baum HBA, Lee K, et al: Effects of short term rhIGF-I on bone turnover in osteopenic women with anorexia nervosa. J Clin Endocrinol Metab 81:3364, 1996.

435. Johansson AG, Lindh E, Blum WF, et al: Effects of growth hormone and insulin-like growth factor-I in men with osteoporosis. J Clin Endocrinol Metab 81:44, 1996.

436. Biandi T, Glatz Y, Bouillon R, et al: Effects of short term insulin-like growth factor-I (IGF-I) or growth hormone treatment on bone metabolism and on production of 1,25 dihyroxycholecalciferol in GH deficient adults. J Clin Endocrinol Metab 83:81, 1998.

437. Ghiron L, Thompson JL, Holloway L: Effects of recombinant insulin like growth factor I and growth hormone on bone turnover in elderly women. J Bone Miner Res 10:1844, 1995.

438. Kuzuya H, Matsuura N, Sakamoto M, et al: Trial of insulin-like growth factor-I therapy for patients with extreme insulin resistance syndromes. Diabetes 42:696, 1993.

439. Cheetham TD, Jones J, Taylor AM, et al: The effects of recombinant insulin-like growth factor I administration or growth hormone levels and insulin requirements in adolescents with type 1 insulin-dependent diabetes mellitus. Diabetologia 36:678, 1993.

440. Moses AC, Young SCJ, Morrow LA, et al: Recombinant human insulin-like growth factor I increases insulin sensitivity and improves glycemic control in type II diabetes. Diabetes 45:95, 1996.

441. Quattrin T, Thrailkill K, Baler L, et al: Dual hormonal replacement with insulin and recombinant insulin like growth factor I in insulin dependent diabetes mellitus: Effects on glycemic control, IGF-I levels, and safety profiles. Diabetes Care 20:374, 1997.

442. Clemmons DR, Moses AC, McKay MJ, et al: The combination of insulin-like growth factor I and insulin-like growth factor-binding protein-3 reduces insulin requirements in insulin-dependent type 1 diabetes: Evidence for in vivo biological activity. J Clin Endocrinol Metab 85:1518, 2000.

443. Walker JL, Ginalska-Malinowska M, Romer TC, et al: Effects of infusion of insulin-like growth factor-I in a child with growth hormone insensitivity syndrome. N Engl J Med 324:1483, 1991.

444. Walker JL, VanWyk JJ, Underwood LE: Stimulation of statural growth by recombinant insulin-like growth factor-I in a child with growth hormone insensitivity syndrome (Laron-type). J Pediatr 121:641, 1992.

445. Rosenfeld RG, Rosenbloom AL, Guevara-Aguirre J: Growth hormone (GH) insensitivity due to primary GH receptor deficiency. Endocrine Rev 15:369, 1994.

446. Guevara-Aguirre J, Vasconez O, Martinez V, et al: A randomized double blind placebo controlled trial of safety and efficacy of recombinant human insulin like growth factor I in children with growth hormone receptor deficiency. J Clin Endocrinol Metab 80:1393, 1995.

447. Backeljaw PF, Underwood LE: Prolonged treatment with recombinant insulin like growth factor I in children with growth hormone insensitivity syndrome: A clinical research center study. J Clin Endocrinol Metab 81:3312, 1996.

448. Camacho-Hubner C, Woods KA, Miraki-Moud F, et al: Effects of recombinant human insulin-like growth factor I (IGF-I) therapy on the growth hormone IGF system of a patient with partial IGF-I gene deletion. J Clin Endocrinol Metab 84:1611, 1999.

449. de Lacerda L, Carvalho JA, Stannard B, et al: In vitro and in vivo responses to short-term recombinant human insulin-like growth factor-1 (IGF-I) in a severely growth-retarded girl with ring chromosome 15 and deletion of a single allele for the type 1 IGF receptor gene. Clin Endocrinol 51:541, 1999.

450. Okubo Y, Siddle K, Firth H, et al: Cell proliferation activities on skin fibroblasts from a short child with absence of one copy of the type 1 insulin-like growth factor receptor (IGF1R) gene and a tall child with three copies of the IGF1R gene. J Clin Endocrinol Metab 88:5981, 2003.

451. Abuzzahab MJ, Schneider A, Goddard A, et al: IGF-I receptor mutations resulting in intrauterine and postnatal growth retardation. N Engl J Med 349:2211, 2003.

Peptide Growth Factors Other than Insulin-like Growth Factors or Cytokines

Peter Rotwein

INTRODUCTION

Growth factors are secreted proteins that exert diverse effects on cell growth, metabolism, differentiation, and on the growth and development of organisms as distinct as fish, worms, flies, frogs, and humans.[1] Although the term *growth factor* was used initially to describe secreted substances that enhanced cell division, the phrase now includes proteins that stimulate or inhibit progression through the cell cycle, that control cell viability or death, or that act principally to regulate cellular differentiation.[1,2] To accomplish these and other biologic actions, growth factors activate specific cellular receptors. Receptors are modular transmembrane proteins that can bind growth factors at their extracellular domains with high affinity and specificity and can transmit the information generated by binding into changes in cellular economy.[3] Growth factors also may interact with other cell-associated or secreted binding proteins. In general, binding proteins do not mediate biologic effects directly, but they modulate growth factor availability or stability.

The last few decades have seen an explosive increase in knowledge about growth factors and their actions. This has included the characterization of many growth factors, their receptors, and binding proteins. The structural information derived from the determination of the amino acid sequences of these proteins and results of studies of biologic function have led to the classification of growth factors into several discrete families. The information explosion has been enhanced

by the advent of molecular cloning in the early 1980s and by the ability to produce pure recombinant growth factors through molecular biologic techniques. Table 35-1 lists the major growth factor families.

GENERAL PRINCIPLES OF GROWTH FACTOR ACTION

DISTINGUISHING AMONG HORMONES, GROWTH FACTORS, AND CYTOKINES

As discussed throughout this textbook, hormones also regulate the growth and development of cells and tissues and thus could be classified as growth factors. In general, hormones are substances that are produced in endocrine glands, are secreted into the bloodstream, and act at locations distant from their sites of synthesis. Although this *endocrine* mode of action is shared by some growth factors (e.g., see Chapter 34 on the insulin-like growth factor [IGF] family), fundamental differences exist between these two classes of molecules. Unlike hormones, growth factors are produced by many tissues in the body and thus are not exclusively synthesized by specific glands. Growth factors are proteins, whereas hormones may be proteins, small peptides, or lipid derivatives. Growth factors also use modes of action that distinguish them from hormones, termed *paracrine, autocrine,* and *juxtacrine* modes. A *paracrine* mode of action occurs when a growth factor that is secreted by one cell has an effect on adjacent cells. A *juxtacrine*

Table 35-1 Major Growth Factor Families

Name	Abbreviation	No. of Members
Epidermal growth factor	EGF	11
Fibroblast growth factor	FGF	~22
Insulin-like growth factor	IGF	2
Nerve growth factor	NGF	4
Platelet-derived growth factor	PDGF	4
Transforming growth factor-β	TGF-β	~29

mode is similar, although the growth factor is bound to the cell membrane or extracellular matrix. *Autocrine* actions are mediated by a growth factor on its cell of origin after its secretion into the extracellular environment. A variation on this theme has been termed *intracrine* and was first described for an oncogenic variant of platelet-derived growth factor (PDGF) termed *v-sis*.[4,5] *Intracrine* actions occur inside the cell of origin and are thus independent of growth factor secretion. These modes of action are outlined in Figure 35-1.

Cytokines are secreted proteins produced principally by lymphocytes, macrophages, and precursors of blood cells. These proteins act to regulate the function of the immune and hematopoietic systems. Cytokines are thus similar to traditional growth factors in their modes of action. They are described in detail in other chapters of this text.

GROWTH FACTOR RECEPTORS AND SIGNALING PATHWAYS

As noted earlier, the effects of growth factors are mediated by activation of specific receptors. Growth factor receptors are transmembrane proteins that consist of at least three domains: an extracellular region that binds the growth factor with high affinity and specificity, a membrane-spanning segment, and one or more intracellular domains that interact with signaling molecules inside the cell.[6-8] Despite the diversity of growth factors and receptors characterized to date, all receptors share these structural features. All growth

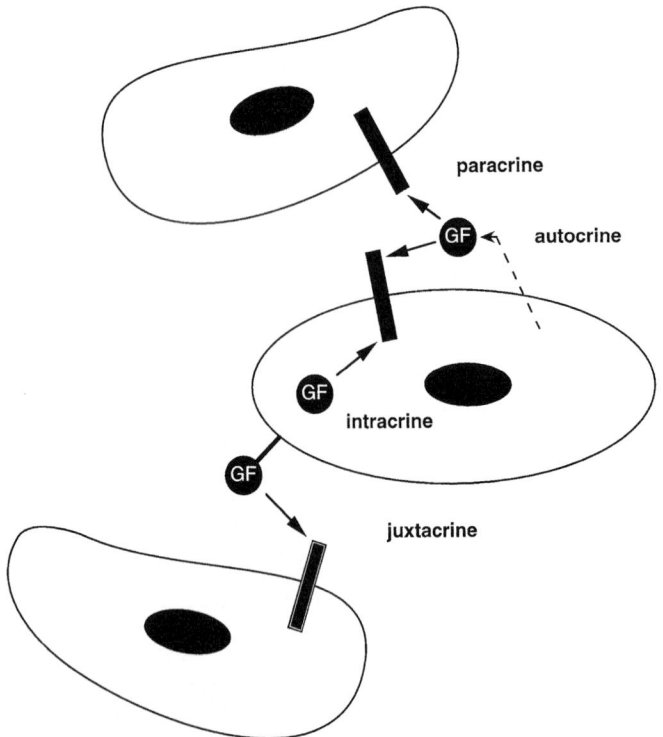

Figure 35-1 Modes of growth factor action: autocrine, paracrine, intracrine, and juxtacrine.

factor receptors also function as ligand-activated intracellular enzymes. With the exception of receptors for the transforming growth factor-β (TGF-β) family, all growth factor receptors studied to date show tyrosine kinase activity. Receptors for TGF-β and related molecules phosphorylate substrates on serine and threonine residues rather than tyrosines.[9,10]

Several general principles govern the steps by which growth factors activate their receptors, although the specific details differ for each growth factor–receptor combination. Binding of a growth factor to the extracellular domain of its receptor first leads to receptor dimerization or oligomerization. Dimerization of the receptor occurs either because the growth factor exists as a dimer and binds to two receptors (e.g., PDGF, TGF-β, nerve growth factor [NGF]), because a growth factor monomer has two binding sites for its receptor (e.g., epidermal growth factor [EGF]), or because the receptor is a preformed dimer (e.g., IGF-1).[7,8] The conformational changes induced by ligand binding then activate the intracellular kinase domain of the receptor, leading sequentially to phosphorylation of the receptor itself (usually on multiple amino acids) by a transphosphorylation mechanism, and then to the phosphorylation of other substrates.[6-8] Autophosphorylation, particularly on tyrosine residues, creates a series of docking sites for other intracellular proteins that contain modules termed *SH2 domains*, for their similarity to a region of approximately 100 amino acids first identified in the cellular oncogene, *c-src*.[11-13] Different proteins containing SH2 domains bind to distinct docking sites on the receptor, based on the context of each phosphorylated tyrosine, which is defined by the sequence of amino acids adjacent to this modified residue.[6] More recently, another class of phosphotyrosine binding sites termed the *PTB domain* was identified.[14] Although structurally distinct from the SH2 domain, it appears to be functionally equivalent in mediating interactions between a phosphorylated tyrosine residue and a signaling protein. Thus, activated growth factor receptors with multiple phosphorylated tyrosines in different amino acid contexts become the focal point for the transient intracellular aggregation of many SH2- or PTB-containing proteins (Fig. 35-2). These proteins include a variety of intermediates in signal-transduction pathways, with the ultimate effects being amplification and diversification of the initial signal induced on growth factor binding to its receptor. As an example, the activated PDGF receptor binds a series of adapter molecules (Shc, Nck, Grb2), enzymes (PI 3-kinase regulatory subunit, phospholipase Cγ [PLCγ], protein tyrosine phosphatase 1D [PTP1D], c-src), and other proteins, which together participate in the pleiotropic biologic effects of PDGF.[15] Analogous pathways are stimulated by other growth factor receptors. See other chapters for more detailed discussions of signal-transduction pathways.

NUCLEAR ACTIONS OF GROWTH FACTORS

The long-term changes within cells induced by growth factors are secondary to alterations in gene expression. These changes are but several outcomes of the multiple signaling pathways induced after the assembly of proteins on the activated growth factor receptor. For example, the binding of the adapter molecule Grb2 to a phosphorylated tyrosine of an activated receptor brings this protein and its partner, termed *Son of Sevenless* (SOS), a guanine nucleotide exchange protein, to the cell membrane. SOS can then physically associate with the membrane-bound signaling intermediate, c-ras, leading to ras activation through stimulation of its guanoxine triphosphate (GTP)-bound form.[16,17] This sets into motion a series of enzymatic reactions, which lead to the phosphorylation and activation of a pair of serine-threonine protein kinases, the mitogen-activated protein kinase (MAPK) or extracellular signal–regulated kinase (ERK) 1 and 2.[16,17] MAPKs in turn phosphorylate and activate several cytoplasmic and nuclear

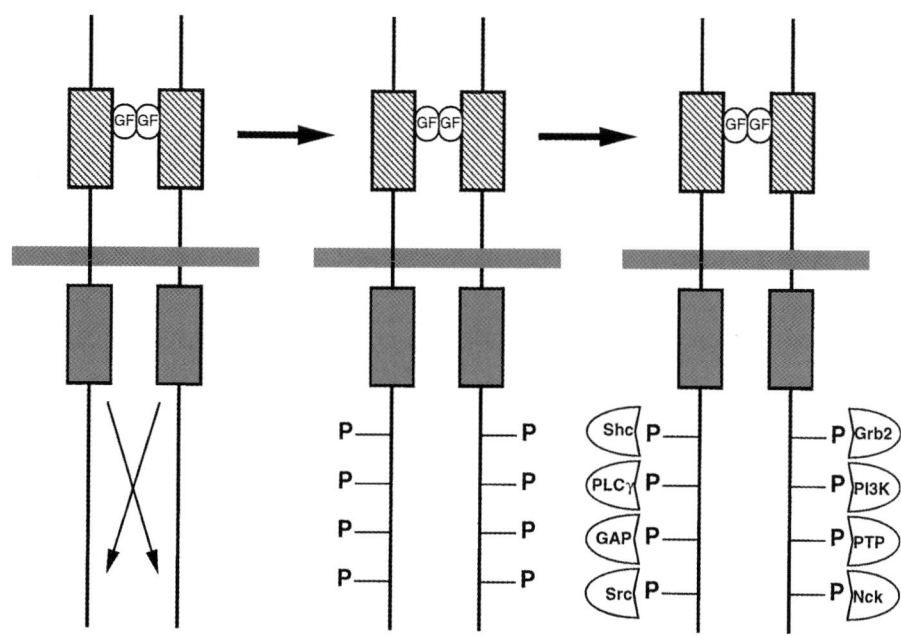

Figure 35-2 An overview of signal transduction by tyrosine kinase receptors. **Left,** Binding of a growth factor to the extracellular part of its receptor leads to receptor dimerization and activates the receptor kinase. **Center,** Tyrosine phosphorylation of the receptor occurs by transphosphorylation. **Right,** Intracellular substrates with SH2 (src homology 2) domains bind to phosphorylated tyrosine residues of the activated receptor. The ligand-binding domain of the receptor and the tyrosine kinase domain are indicated by *boxes*. The growth factor (GF) is shown as a dimer. Shc, Nck, Grb2, adaptor molecules; PLC, phospholipase; GAP, guanosine (GTP)ase-activating protein; PI 3-K, PI 3-kinase regulatory subunit; PTP, protein tyrosine phosphatase.

proteins, including the transcriptional activator, ternary complex factor, which stimulates expression of the gene encoding c-*fos*.[18–20] This pathway reflects a primary response to growth factors, because it is dependent on a series of protein-protein interactions and enzymatic steps that do not require new synthesis of cellular proteins. The protein c-*fos* combines with c-*jun* as components of the transcription factor, adaptor protein 1 (AP1), which in turn regulates the activity of a variety of genes.[18,20,21] Thus, gene expression and protein biosynthesis are altered after growth factor signaling is stimulated.

A related pathway mediated by activated growth factor receptors leads to the stimulation of another member of the MAPK family termed c-*Jun N-terminal kinase* (JNK, also known as stress-activated protein kinase or SAPK). JNK/SAPK phosphorylates c-*jun* on two serine residues that are critical for its activation as a transcription factor.[20] Thus, both c-*jun* and c-*fos* may be induced through growth factor–stimulated signaling pathways. Other MAPK cascades with different nuclear effects also are activated by growth factor receptors.[21]

SUMMARY

Peptide growth factors are multifunctional proteins that regulate diverse biologic processes through interactions with cellular receptors that function as ligand-activated intracellular enzymes. The enzymatic pathways that are initiated by the binding of a growth factor to its receptor lead to long-term changes in gene expression and protein synthesis that alter the phenotypes of individual cells and tissues and have profound effects on growth and development in the whole animal. Table 35-2 summarizes some of the salient features of growth factor

biology. Specific details pertinent to individual growth factor families are described in the following sections.

EPIDERMAL GROWTH FACTOR AND RELATED MOLECULES

INTRODUCTION

EGF was one of the first peptide growth factors to be identified.[22] The EGF family now consists of seven structurally similar proteins that are capable of binding to and activating the EGF receptor (also known as ErbB1), and four groups of neuregulins, related proteins that bind to and activate other receptors of the ErbB family.[23–25] The four ErbBs are receptor tyrosine kinases that function as homo- and heterodimers to activate a variety of intracellular signaling processes.[25,26] Both the EGF ligands and their ErbB receptors are widely expressed and are active in embryonic development and adult life.

STRUCTURE OF EGF AND RELATED MOLECULES

The 11 members of the EGF and neuregulin families and three related proteins are listed in Table 35-3. A common feature of this family is that the proteins are synthesized as large transmembrane precursors that are proteolytically cleaved to release the soluble form of the mature growth factor. The larger, membrane-anchored protein precursors also appear to be biologically active and to exert their actions through a juxtacrine mechanism.[23,24] All members of the EGF family share a region of amino acid similarity of 45 to 55 residues known as the EGF-like domain that is necessary and sufficient for

Table 35-2	**Principles of Growth Factor Biology**

1. Growth factors are secreted peptides that exert major effects on cell growth, differentiation, and metabolism, and on the growth and development of the whole organism
2. Growth factors may be grouped into families that share structural and functional properties
3. Growth factor action is mediated by interactions with cellular receptors and with cell-associated or secreted binding proteins
4. Growth factor receptors are transmembrane proteins that function as ligand-activated protein kinases. Changes in phosphorylation of intracellular substrates regulate signaling pathways that ultimately transmit the biologic effects of growth factors, resulting in changes in cell motility, survival, proliferation, differentiation, or metabolism
5. Abnormalities in growth factors or their receptors may contribute to disorders of growth, development, and differentiation, and to cancer

Table 35-3 Epidermal Growth Factor Family

Epidermal growth factor
Transforming growth factor-α
Amphiregulin
Heparin-binding epidermal growth factor
Betacellulin
Epiregulin
Epigen

NEUREGULIN SUBFAMILY
Heregulin/neu-differentiation factor
Glial growth factor
Acetylcholine receptor–inducing activity
Sensory and motor neuron–derived factor

NEUREGULIN-2 SUBFAMILY

NEUREGULIN-3 SUBFAMILY

NEUREGULIN-4 SUBFAMILY

DISTANTLY RELATED PROTEINS
Cripto
Cryptic-1
Vaccinia virus growth factor

binding to ErbB receptors.[27] This protein segment contains six characteristically spaced cysteine residues that form three intramolecular disulfide bonds and define a characteristic three-loop secondary structure that is required for binding to ErbB receptors.[27]

EGF is a conserved 53-amino acid single-chain protein that is synthesized from a 1217-amino acid membrane-bound precursor.[28] The precursor protein contains eight additional segments with structural homology to EGF, as well as a transmembrane domain and a short intracellular carboxyl-terminal tail. TGF-α, the second member of the EGF family to be characterized, is a 50-residue peptide derived from a 160-amino acid precursor.[29] The EGF-like domain is 44% identical to EGF. Amphiregulin consists of either a 78- or an 84-residue mature protein and is derived from a 252-amino acid precursor.[30] It was isolated initially from the MCF7 breast cancer cell line.[30] Heparin-binding EGF-like growth factor (HB-EGF) was first identified in the conditioned culture medium derived from the U937 macrophage cell line.[31] The 184- to 206-amino acid transmembrane precursor is processed into a series of biologically active mature proteins of 72 to 87 residues that differ at their amino termini.[31,32] HB-EGF is distinguished from other members of the EGF family by being heavily O-glycosylated and by containing amino acid motifs that allow the protein to interact strongly with heparan sulfate proteoglycans.[32,33] The membrane-based precursor of HB-EGF also has been identified as the cell-surface receptor for diphtheria toxin and has been shown to be required for toxin entry into susceptible cells.[34] Betacellulin, an 80-residue protein derived from a larger precursor, was characterized from pancreatic B-cell tumors derived from transgenic mice expressing SV40 T-antigen in their insulin-producing cells.[35] Epiregulin, a 46–amino acid peptide derived from a larger precursor, was purified from a subclone of the mouse NIH3T3 cell line.[36] Epigen was initially characterized as an expressed DNA sequence tag from a keratinocyte complementary DNA (cDNA) library and was found to encode a 51-residue active peptide that could bind to and activate ErbB1.[37]

The neuregulins comprise a discrete subclass of the EGF family that do not bind to the EGF receptor, ErbB1, but interact with other ErbBs. The neuregulins, including glial growth factor, acetylcholine receptor–inducing activity, sensory and motor-neuron-derived factor, and others, are protein products of a very large single gene of more than 1.4 million nucleotide pairs on human chromosome 8 that is alternatively processed into multiple messenger RNA (mRNA) species.[24] Neuregulins

contain a shared EGF-like domain of either 77 amino acids (α) or 62 residues (β) in addition to other isoform-specific protein sequences. In general, β neuregulins have been shown to exert more potent biologic effects than α-containing proteins. Related molecules termed *neuregulins-2, -3,* and *-4* also have been characterized, and have motif structures similar to neuregulins.[24,38–40]

Three additional proteins share structural similarity with EGF family members. Cripto, a gene cloned serendipitously from a human embryonal cancer cell line,[41,42] and cryptic-1, a gene characterized in differentiating mouse embryonic stem cells,[43] each contain an EGF-like motif with six cysteine residues. Because the spacing of the cysteines differs from that of other members of the EGF family, with the first disulfide loop being absent, these proteins appear not to bind to ErbB receptors.[44] Pox viruses, such as vaccinia, encode a gene product termed *vaccinia virus growth factor* that is 37% identical to EGF.[45] This 77–amino acid protein, secreted when cells are infected with vaccinia, can bind to and activate the EGF receptor.[45]

ErbB RECEPTORS AND SIGNALING MECHANISMS

The four ErbB receptors are structurally related transmembrane proteins consisting of an extracellular domain with two cysteine-rich segments, a single membrane-spanning region, and a large intracellular segment composed of a tyrosine kinase domain and several tyrosines that become phosphorylated upon receptor activation (Fig. 35-3). The human receptors also are known as HER1 to HER4, and ErbB2/HER2 is also called Neu.[25] As described earlier for receptor tyrosine kinases, binding of EGF family members to ErbB molecules induces receptor dimerization, which triggers kinase activation and autophosphorylation of tyrosine residues in the intracytoplasmic region of the receptors, leading to creation of docking sites for intracellular signaling intermediates and effector proteins.[25,26]

Despite overall sequence and structural similarities, the four ErbB receptors mediate signal diversification and discrimination through at least three different mechanisms.[25–27] First,

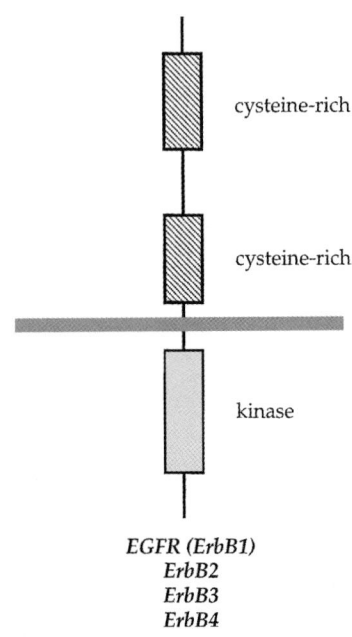

Figure 35-3 Epidermal growth factor receptor (EGFR) and related receptors. The two cysteine-rich segments in the extracellular region and the intracellular tyrosine kinase domain are depicted by *boxes*.

individual receptors are able to bind distinct subsets of EGF family members. EGF, TGF-α, amphiregulin, HB-EGF, betacellulin, epiregulin, and epigen can bind to the EGF receptor, ErbB1. Neuregulin, neuregulin-2, neuregulin-3, neuregulin-4, HB-EGF, betacellulin, and epiregulin are able to bind to ErbB4. Neuregulin or neuregulin-2 can bind to ErbB3. ErbB2 has no known ligand and thus appears to be an orphan receptor.[25]

Second, ligand binding may lead to either receptor homodimerization or to heterodimerization, with the dimerization pattern being defined through both ligand specificity and receptor availability. For example, EGF binding to ErbB1 may lead to the formation of ErbB1 homodimers or to heterodimers of ErbB1 with ErbB2, ErbB3, or ErbB4.[25,27] Because each ErbB family member has a distinct but overlapping profile of preferred interactions with intracellular signaling intermediates, each combination of receptor dimers has the potential to induce a unique pattern of biologic effects depending on the signaling molecules activated.

Third, ErbB3 does not contain any functional kinase but rather is a substrate for other ErbB kinases.[25–27] This effectively limits the range of signaling intermediates activated by receptor heterodimers containing ErbB3.

In addition to the mechanisms described earlier, several other types of molecular interactions have the potential to extend or modify the range of biologic actions of ErbB receptors. Decorin is a proteoglycan that plays a structural role in modulating assembly of the extracellular matrix.[46] It also may bind to and inhibit some of the actions of TGF-β.[46] Decorin is able to activate the EGF receptor, ErbB1, by directly binding to its extracellular domain, leading to stimulation of receptor kinase activity and to sustained activation of the MAPK signal-transduction pathway.[46] The growth hormone receptor (GHR) also uses ErbB1 as a signaling component, but in a mechanistically different way than does decorin. The GHR is a member of the cytokine receptor family. Members of this family lack intrinsic protein kinase activity but associate with and activate nonreceptor tyrosine kinases of the JAK family (see other chapters for details). In liver cells, stimulation of the GHR by its ligand GH leads to induction of MAPKs through tyrosine phosphorylation of ErbB1 by JAK2.[25,47] Similar results have been observed for the prolactin receptor after binding of its ligand, prolactin.[25] The tyrosine kinase activity of ErbB1 appears to be dispensable for this effect, implying that ErbB1 acts as a substrate for JAK2 and as an intermediate in the signal-transduction pathway leading to activation of MAPKs by the GHR or the prolactin receptor. An analogous pattern of receptor cross-talk has been observed between another member of the cytokine receptor family, the gp130 subunit of the interleukin-6 receptor, and ErbB2, which also leads to activation of MAPKs.[25,48] The physiologic and clinical significance of these signaling interactions between cytokine receptors and ErbB receptors and between decorin and ErbB1 remain to be evaluated.

Cross-talk also occurs between ErbB receptors and G protein–coupled receptors.[25,49–51] Several ligands that activate different G protein–coupled receptors, including thrombin, lysophosphatidic acid, and endothelin-1, also stimulate tyrosine phosphorylation of ErbB1 and ErbB2 in cultured fibroblasts, leading to induction of MAPKs.[49,50] In other cultured cells, ErbB1 appears able to activate G proteins through phosphorylation of Gsα, leading to stimulation of adenylyl cyclase activity.[50,51] As with cytokine receptors, the biologic significance of such cross-talk remains to be defined.

BIOLOGIC EFFECTS

As revealed by targeted gene-disruption experiments in mice, EGF family members play key roles in the differentiation of tissues composed principally of epithelial cells, in mesenchymal-epithelial interactions, and in development of components of the central and peripheral nervous systems. Targeted

deficiency of ErbB1 caused defective or delayed epithelial development.[52–54] These abnormalities were manifested by reduced placental size, by immature and poorly inflated lungs, by progressive cystic dilatation of renal collecting ducts, by diminished thickness of epidermis of the skin, by decreased hair growth secondary to abnormalities of hair follicles, and by diminished development of the eyelids and cornea.[52–54] Depending on strain-specific modifiers, these defects and others led to a host of phenotypic alterations ranging from death at the peri-implantation period to the birth of live mice with multiorgan abnormalities.[52–54] Because lack of one of the ligands for ErbB1, TGF-α, caused only a subset of defects seen in the ErbB1 knockout mice,[55] these results indicate that the multiple ligands for ErbB1 are required to regulate receptor actions appropriately during development.

Targeted disruption of the genes encoding ErbB2, ErbB4, and neuregulin-1 also showed an overlapping spectrum of developmental abnormalities.[56–59] These mice all died before embryonic day 11 secondary to cardiac malfunction caused by defects in the trabecular extensions of the ventricular myocardium.[56–58] Because ErbB2 and ErbB4 are expressed in myocardial cells, and neuregulin-1 is produced by the adjacent endocardium, these results define a paracrine signaling network in which activation of ErbB2 and ErbB4 by neuregulin-1 is required for proper myocardial differentiation and function. As these mice had distinct but overlapping defects in their nervous systems, it seems likely that other ligands that activate the two receptors in different combinations play important roles in differentiation and maturation in regions of the brain, spinal code, and peripheral nervous system.[56–58]

A mutation in *cripto*, one of the divergent members of the EGF family, also was a lethal abnormality.[60] Mice engineered to lack this protein died before embryonic day 11 and had major defects in mesoderm and endoderm formation and in organization of the anterior-posterior body axis.[60] Membrane-bound *cripto* may act in part by functioning both as a co-receptor for TGF-β family members, *nodal* and related proteins, and as an inhibitor of the actions of another TGF-β family member, activin.[61]

ErbB signaling pathways also are involved in postnatal development. Treatment of developing mammary glands with EGF, TGF-α, or neuregulin-1 enhanced terminal alveolar differentiation.[62–64] At least three ErbB receptors (ErbB1, 3, and 4) are expressed during mammary development and mediate these biologic effects.[25,65,66]

ErbB proteins appear to play a role in viral pathogenesis. ErbB1 was identified as a key component of the cellular receptor for human cytomegalovirus, an important pathogen for individuals with compromised immune systems.[67] Human cytomegalovirus gains entry into susceptible cells through binding to ErbB1 or to ErbB1-ErbB3 heterodimers and activates receptor-mediated signaling pathways.[67]

ErbB receptors also play roles in epithelial carcinogenesis. Amplification and overexpression of ErbB2 in breast cancer correlates with both cancer recurrence and poor survival.[68] Other ErbB receptors also are overexpressed or mutated in breast, colon, ovarian, lung, and other cancers, and have been implicated in disease progression.[69,70] In non–small cell lung carcinomas, overexpression of ErbB1 has been correlated with high metastatic rate and diminished patient survival.[71,72] In a small subset of these patients, potential gain-of-function mutations of ErbB1 additionally have been identified.[71,72]

THERAPEUTIC USES

EGF treatment induces the shedding of wool and is used as an alternative to shearing sheep. Antibodies to ErbB2 have provided diagnostic information for clinical staging of breast cancer.[69,70] A humanized antibody to ErbB2 (trastuzumab or Herceptin) has been proven to be an effective therapeutic agent in metastatic breast cancer,[25] whereas a small-molecule inhibitor (gefitinib or Iressa) has been shown to be effective in preliminary studies in patients with non–small cell lung cancer who have gain-of-function mutations in ErbB1.[71,72] A role for ErbB inhibitors also may be anticipated in counteracting infections with cytomegalovirus in immunocompromised individuals.

FIBROBLAST GROWTH FACTOR FAMILY

INTRODUCTION

Fibroblast growth factors (FGFs) comprise a family of heparin-binding growth factors with diverse effects on wound healing, development, angiogenesis, and other biologic processes. The term *FGF* was initially applied to two proteins, acidic FGF (now FGF-1) and basic FGF (FGF-2), which were isolated from brain and pituitary gland extracts based on their ability to stimulate DNA synthesis in fibroblasts.[73,74] The FGF family now contains at least 22 members (FGF-1 through FGF-23; there is no FGF-19).[74] FGF action is mediated by interactions with transmembrane FGF receptors and with heparin sulfate proteoglycans (HSPGs). FGF receptors (FGFRs) also comprise a family that consists of four related genes termed FGFR1 through 4.[75-78] Several different receptor isoforms are the products of alternative RNA splicing.[76-78]

STRUCTURE OF FIBROBLAST GROWTH FACTORS

The 22 known FGFs show structural and amino acid sequence similarities in a core region that is required for binding to FGF receptors and to HSPGs. FGF-1 and -2 are both highly conserved 155–amino acid proteins that are 55% identical to each other.[73,74] Both proteins lack classic amino-terminal signal sequences for directing protein secretion. Despite considerable investigation, how these proteins reach the extracellular environment remains an unsolved problem. FGF-2 mRNA also can be translated beginning with upstream CUG codons, leading to variants with extended amino termini. The FGF-3 precursor also exhibits alternative translation initiation, although this protein contains a signal peptide, as do FGF-4 through -8, -10, -15, -17, -18, and FGF-21 through -23. Like FGF-1 and -2, FGF-9, FGF-16, and FGF-20 lack a signal peptide, and their mechanisms of secretion are unknown.[73,74] FGF-11 through -14 also do not contain a signal sequence but are not secreted and remain intracellular.[74]

FIBROBLAST GROWTH FACTOR RECEPTORS AND BINDING PROTEINS

FGFRs are the protein products of four highly related genes and share between 60% and 95% amino acid similarity.[74,75,77] They function as ligand-activated tyrosine protein kinases with different specificities for the different FGF ligands.[74,75,77] FGFRs are composed of an extracellular, ligand-binding domain, a single transmembrane segment, and an intracellular region consisting of a tyrosine kinase domain that is split into two parts by a kinase insert region and a COOH-terminal tail of 55 to 66 residues (Fig. 35-4A). This latter segment is divergent in sequence among FGFRs and may be responsible for interactions with cellular substrates that are distinct for each receptor.[73,75,77]

The extracellular domains of FGFRs are composed of two or three immunoglobulin (Ig)-like motifs (Fig. 35-4B) that result from different combinations of alternative RNA splicing of each primary gene transcript.[74,75,77] A short unique segment, known as the acidic box domain (because of the high concentration of glutamic and aspartic acid residues), is found between Ig1 and Ig2.[75]

FGFRs exist in both transmembrane and secreted forms (Fig. 35-4B). Transmembrane versions of FGFR1 contain three Ig domains or lack domain 1. The absence of the first Ig region does not alter binding to FGF-1 or -2.[74,75,77] Binding affinity may be modified, depending on which of three alternatively spliced exons is used to code for the carboxyl-terminal half of the third Ig domain. Receptors using segment IIIb bind FGF-1 with higher affinity than FGF-2, whereas receptors containing region IIIc bind both growth factors equally, and also bind FGF-4 equivalently.[79] Binding of FGF-3, and FGF-5 through -9 is more variable.[79] Receptors containing segment IIIa are secreted and potentially function as FGF-binding proteins (Fig. 35-4B). Additional minor receptor variants have been characterized that do not affect ligand binding.

Expression of different FGFRs and splicing variants is controlled in both tissue-specific and developmental-specific ways.[75] In addition, it has been shown that several receptor isoforms are coexpressed in the same tissues.[75] This receptor diversity provides one mechanism for regulating FGF action in different tissues and at different developmental stages.

In addition to the FGFRs, FGFs also bind with lower affinity to several HSPGs, including syndecans 1 to 4, glypican, and perlecan.[80,81] Interactions with HSPGs are essential for high-affinity binding to FGFRs.[80,81] HSPGs in the extracellular

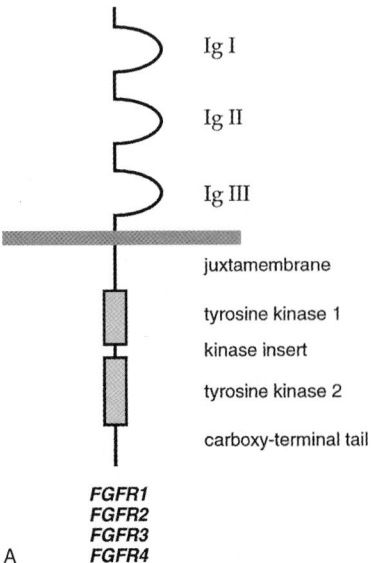

Figure 35-4 **A,** Diagram of fibroblast growth factor (FGF) receptors. The different domains are labeled. Ig indicates immunoglobulin-like domains. **B,** Alternative RNA splicing of the *FGFR1* gene regulates synthesis of multiple receptor isoforms. Receptors with two or three Ig domains and with different exons encoding the carboxy-terminal part of Ig domain III are illustrated. Additional receptor subtypes with minor variations on these patterns have been described.

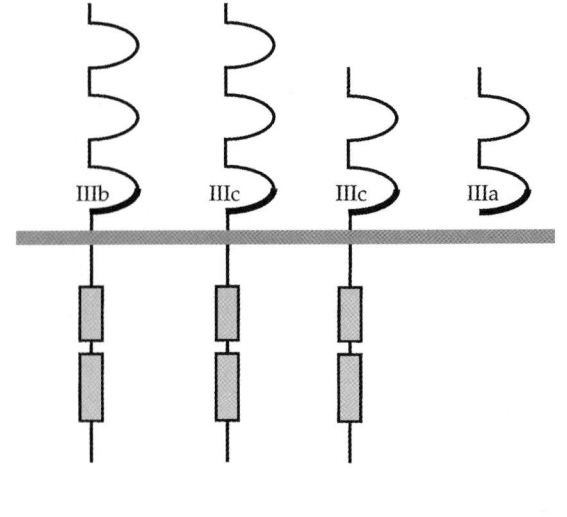

matrix also serve as storage pools for FGFs, providing mechanisms for modulating biologic effects by enhancing local growth factor concentrations, limiting degradation, and regulating access to receptors.[82]

Other ligands besides FGFs also bind to FGFRs. Human FGFR1 functions as a coreceptor with HSPGs for adeno-associated virus 2.[83] Cells that express only one of these components fail to bind virus and are thus resistant to infection. In addition, FGF-1 antagonizes viral infection by competing for binding to FGFR-1.[83] Because adeno-associated virus 2–based vectors are being tested for application to human gene therapy, these observations have potential clinical implications.

Binding of FGFs to FGFRs leads to rapid receptor dimerization and to autophosphorylation by a transphosphorylation mechanism. Because FGFs do not form dimers and are not bivalent ligands, the mechanism of receptor dimerization has been unclear. One potential role for cell-surface HSPGs is to provide the equivalent of a dimerization interface for FGFs by binding several growth factor molecules simultaneously.[84] This would allow the FGF-HSPG complex to interact with several receptor molecules at the same time and thus stimulate receptor oligomerization. Experimental evidence for this idea has been demonstrated.[81]

BIOLOGIC AND CLINICAL EFFECTS

A variety of studies have underscored the critical roles of different members of the FGF family in growth, development, and morphogenesis in many different species. Experiments using dominant-negative FGFRs and other approaches have demonstrated a requirement for FGF signaling in the induction and patterning of mesoderm that occurs early in the development of the frog, *Xenopus laevis*.[85] FGF action is needed for induction of a subset of mesodermal cell types, particularly skeletal muscle. FGFs also may collaborate with activins (members of the TGF-β family) in induction of the notochord.[85] Similar collaborative interactions may be required for induction of other tissue types.

Several FGFs and their receptors have been shown to play critical roles in mouse development, as assessed by targeted gene disruptions and overexpression strategies. A knockout of the *FGFR1* or *FGFR2* genes in mice led to early embryonic death. Nullizygous embryos died before midgestation, soon after the onset of gastrulation, and had multiple defects in mesodermal derivatives.[78,86,87] In contrast, loss of *FGFR4* had no developmental consequences.[78] FGF-3 deficiency caused abnormalities in formation of the tail and inner ear.[88] The absence of FGF-5 led to mice with abnormally long hair, implying a key role for this growth factor in regulation of the hair growth cycle.[89] A homozygous knockout of the *FGF-4*

gene was a lethal abnormality.[90] Embryos developed minimally after implantation into the uterus. FGF-10-deficient embryos failed to form lung buds.[91] Mice with diminished expression of FGF-8 developed abnormalities in the left to right axis during early gestation, with failure to establish normal patterning on the left side.[92] This contrasts with the situation in the chick embryo, where FGF-8 appears to function as a determinant of right-sided identity.[92] FGF-22, along with FGF-7 and FGF-10, was shown recently to act in the central nervous system (CNS) in the local differentiation of axons to form nerve terminals at their target sites.[93]

A key role for FGF action in limb development has been defined in the chicken, mouse, and human. Implantation of beads soaked in FGF-1, FGF-2, FGF-4, FGF-6, or FGF-10 into the flank of an early chick embryo caused the appearance of an extra limb bud and led to the formation of supernumerary limbs.[94] It is likely that this concentrated source of FGF mimics the normal situation by enhancing local cell proliferation and also by modulating the expression of several other factors that control limb patterning and morphogenesis.[94]

Regulated FGF action also is required for normal bone growth during embryonic development. In mice, targeted deficiency of FGFR3 caused larger than normal bone length and enhanced expression of proliferating and hypertrophic chondrocytes within the growth plate.[95] In humans, a variety of heterozygous gain-of-function mutations of FGFRs causes craniosynostosis syndromes and chondrodysplasias[78] (Table 35-4).

Craniosynostosis is the premature fusion of skull bone sutures. Different syndromes have been defined based on the association of craniosynostosis with other malformations.[78,95] Pfeiffer syndrome consists of craniosynostosis plus flattening of the midface, abnormalities in the great toes and thumbs, and occasionally syndactyly (cutaneous and bony fusion of the digits) affecting other fingers and toes. Crouzon syndrome includes craniosynostosis with ptosis (bulging of eyes). In Apert syndrome, craniosynostosis is associated with severe syndactyly of the hands and feet. In Jackson-Weiss syndrome, craniosynostosis is accompanied by variable other malformations, and in Beare-Stevenson syndrome, craniosynostosis occurs with furrowed skin and acanthosis nigricans (thickening and darkening of the skin). Achondroplasia is the most common form of dwarfism associated with shortened limbs. Thanatophoric dysplasia is a severe form of achondroplasia, in which the ribs also are shortened. Hypochondroplasia is a milder form of achondroplasia.

Some of the known causes for each of these syndromes are heterozygous activating mutations of *FGFR1*, *FGFR2*, or *FGFR3* (see Table 35-4). To date, more than 60 distinct mutations have been identified.[78] One general class of lesions leads to an unpaired cysteine residue within the extracellular

Table 35-4 Human FGF Receptor Mutations			
Syndrome	**Phenotype**	**Receptor**	**Mutation**
Pfeiffer	Craniosynostosis; flattening of midface abnl great toes and thumbs; syndactyly	FGFR1 FGFR2	Pro252Arg Multiple residues
Crouzon	Craniosynostosis; ptosis	FGFR2 FGFR3	Multiple residues Ala391Glu
Apert	Craniosynostosis; severe syndactyly	FGFR2	Ser252Trp Pro253Arg
Jackson-Weiss	Craniosynostosis; syndactyly; other abnormalities	FGFR2	Cys342Arg Ala344Gly
Beare-Stevenson	Craniosynostosis; furrowed skin; acanthosis nigricans	FGFR2	Ser372Cys Tyr375Cys
Achondroplasia	Shortening of limbs	FGFR3	Transmembrane domain
Hypochondroplasia	Shortening of limbs	FGFR3	Asn540Lys
Thanatophoric dysplasia	Severe shortening of limbs; abnormalities in vertebrae, ribs, skull	FGFR3	Linker between Ig II and III; carboxy-terminal tail (type I); Lys650Glu (type II)

region of the affected FGFR. It has been hypothesized that these mutations alter patterns of disulfide bonding within a given receptor, leading to an activating conformational change.[78,95] Other classes of mutations represent substitutions of highly conserved amino acids in conserved segments of the receptors. These mutations also may lead to activating conformational alterations.[78,95] The amino acid substitutions that cause the different craniosynostosis syndromes tend to be located in the extracellular domains of *FGFR1* through *FGFR3*, whereas the mutations responsible for achondroplasias and related abnormalities have been found mostly in the transmembrane and intracellular regions of *FGFR3* (see Table 35-4). Surprisingly, mutations in *FGFR4* have not been identified to date in these disorders.

POTENTIAL DIAGNOSTIC AND THERAPEUTIC USES

DNA-based diagnostic tests are potentially available for craniosynostosis and achondroplasia syndromes, although not all cases of these disorders have been linked to *FGFR* genes. If gene therapy with vectors based on adeno-associated viruses becomes a clinical reality, then manipulation of expression of *FGFR1* will have important implications.

NERVE GROWTH FACTOR FAMILY AND OTHER NEUROTROPHIC FACTORS

INTRODUCTION

NGF was the first growth factor characterized[96] and was the first trophic agent shown to be critical for survival of sympathetic neurons.[97] Currently, four members are known of the NGF or neurotrophin family (Table 35-5). These proteins exert diverse effects on the survival and differentiation of different components of the nervous system by activating three related neurotrophic receptors, TrkA, TrkB, and TrkC, and by binding to a low-affinity NGF receptor (NGFR).

STRUCTURE OF NEUROTROPHINS

Human NGF is a 120–amino acid protein with three intrachain disulfide bonds. It is synthesized as a precursor with an amino-terminal extension.[98] Brain-derived neurotrophic factor (BDNF), and neurotrophins 3 and 4 (NT3, NT4) are secreted proteins of 118 to 130 residues with three intrachain disulfide bonds.[98] The four neurotrophic factors are approximately 50% to 60% identical in amino acid sequence, and their structures are similar. All four proteins bind to their receptors as homodimers.[98]

NEUROTROPHIN RECEPTORS AND SIGNALING

The high-affinity neurotrophin receptors or Trk family of tyrosine protein kinases were identified initially through studies of an oncogene found in colon cancer. A gene rearrangement resulted in the fusion of a then-novel tyrosine kinase with tropomyosin.[99] Analysis of the cellular proto-oncogene led to the characterization of a receptor-like molecule, TrkA, whose tissue distribution corresponded with that of NGF-responsive neurons.[100] Later studies identified two additional members of this family, TrkB and TrkC. The Trks

are conserved structurally (Fig. 35-5). They share approximately 80% amino acid identity in their intracellular tyrosine kinase domains but diverge in the extracellular ligand-binding regions.[101] Like other growth factor receptors, Trks are activated by ligand binding to their extracellular domain, which leads to receptor dimerization, kinase activation, and transphosphorylation of sites within the intracytoplasmic region. The phosphorylated tyrosines then serve as docking sites for intracellular proteins with SH2 domains. Distinct specificities exist for ligand binding. TrkA binds NGF; TrkB binds BDNF, NT3, and NT4; and TrkC binds NT3.[101,102]

In addition to the Trks, a structurally distinct lower-affinity NGFR termed *p75* also has been described.[101,103] It is related to Fas/ApoA1 and to the receptors for tumor necrosis factor and lymphotoxin B.[104] These proteins have typical cysteine-rich motifs in their extracellular domains, a single transmembrane segment, and a characteristic short region, termed the *death domain*, in their intracellular portions.[101,103] Binding of NGF to p75 triggers activation of at least two signaling pathways, one leading to stimulation of the transcription factor, nuclear factor κB (NFκβ), and the other, enhancing conversion of sphingomyelin to ceramide.[103,104] Although other neurotrophins also bind to p75, they are not able to trigger sustained signaling responses.[104,105]

BIOLOGIC EFFECTS

The key role of NGF was first shown when injected neutralizing antibodies led to the disappearance of the peripheral sympathetic nervous system in newborn rats.[97] Subsequent studies indicated that target tissues synthesized neurotrophic peptides that maintained neuronal survival and promoted innervation. These observations led to the concept of "target-derived neurotrophic factors."[105] Gene-disruption studies in mice have validated this hypothesis and have defined specific and essential functions for neurotrophins and their receptors. Homozygous mutation of *TrkA* resulted in loss of peripheral sympathetic neurons and disappearance of distinct populations of pain- and temperature-sensitive neurons.[106] This lethal mutation caused alterations that were similar to those seen after treatment of newborn rodents with NGF antibodies. *TrkB*-deficient mice exhibited defects in cranial and spinal

Table 35-5	Nerve Growth Factor Family
Nerve growth factor
Brain-derived neurotrophic factor
Neurotrophin 3
Neurotrophin 4

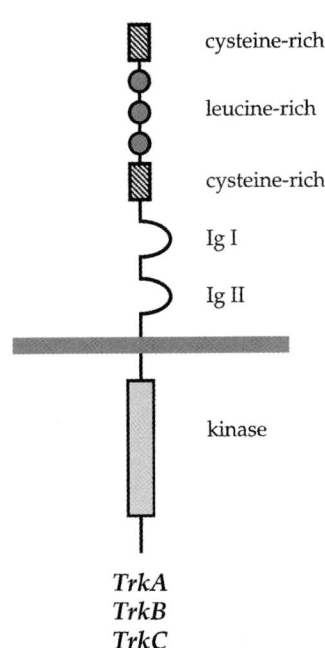

Figure 35-5 Trks A, B, and C encode high-affinity receptors for neurotrophins. Different domains are labeled. Ig indicates an immunoglobulin-like domain.

sensory neurons and loss of some cranial and spinal motor neurons.[107] The sensory deficits were more severe than those seen with homozygous deficiency of either BDNF or NT4, a result consistent with the observation that both neurotrophins are ligands of *TrkB*.[108,109] *TrkB* deficiency also was lethal, as was *TrkC* deficiency. In these latter mice, loss of proprioceptive neurons in the spinal chord and the muscle spindle was seen.[110] Proprioceptive neurons mediate awareness of limb position. Spinal proprioceptive neurons also were diminished in NT3-deficient mice.[111]

Ablation of p75 led to defects in a portion of the peripheral sensory nervous system responsible for sensing changes in skin temperature. The mice were otherwise viable, and the sympathetic nervous system was normal.[112]

Although marked abnormalities were observed throughout the spinal chord and peripheral nervous system in Trk-deficient and neurotrophin-deficient mice, minimal changes were seen in the CNS, despite the widespread distribution of TrkB and TrkC in the CNS. This may reflect functional redundancy of neurotrophin signaling in the CNS or the collaborative effects of other neurotrophic molecules. It has been reported that NGF induces cell death of retinal neurons during early development in the chick.[113] These results and other observations have implicated p75 as a NGF-activated death receptor under certain circumstances.[103]

OTHER NEUROTROPHIC FACTORS

Glial-derived neurotrophic factor (GDNF) is a 134–amino acid protein first characterized by its ability to promote survival of midbrain dopaminergic neurons.[114] It is the founding member of a new family of putative neurotrophic agents that includes neurturin (NTN), artemin, and persephin.[102,115–117] These four proteins are approximately 40% identical in primary amino acid sequence.[118] Members of the GDNF family are unrelated in structure or sequence to the NGF family but show distant kinship with the TGF-β superfamily[9] (Table 35-6). GDNF signaling is initiated by its binding to a heterodimeric receptor composed of α and β subunits that are products of separate genes.[118] The α subunit, termed *GFRα*, is a glycoprotein that is linked to the extracellular face of the cell membrane by a glycophosphatidylinositol anchor. To date, four GFRα proteins have been characterized.[119–123] GFRα1 preferentially binds GDNF, GFRα2 binds NTN, whereas GFRα3 binds artemin, and GFRα4 binds persephin.[116,120–122,124] The β subunit is the protooncogene, *ret*, a transmembrane, ligand-activated tyrosine protein kinase.[118] Activating mutants in *ret* cause multiple endocrine neoplasia, type 2, and familial medullary thyroid carcinoma.[118] whereas inactivating mutations are found in Hirschsprung's disease, a congenital disorder characterized by absence of parasympathetic ganglia from the enteric nervous system.[118]

In cell types lacking *ret*, GDNF can bind to a transmembrane isoform of the neural cell adhesion molecule, NCAM, and in association with GFRα1, can activate several signaling pathways.[125] GFRα1 also can interact with NCAM in the absence of GDNF and, under these circumstances, can impair NCAM-mediated cell-cell adhesion.[125,126]

Gene-disruption experiments have revealed identical phenotypes for mice lacking *ret* or GDNF. In both cases, renal agenesis, neuronal loss in peripheral ganglia, and profound deficits in the enteric nervous system were found, with nearly all neurons distal to the stomach being absent, and in males, defective spermatogenesis.[126–129] Similar abnormalities in development of the kidney and the enteric nervous system were seen in mice engineered to lack GFRα1.[130] Mice deficient in NTN or GFRα2 showed defects in enteric and parasympathetic innervation, whereas mice lacking GFRα4 were normal.[118,126] The absence of GFRα2 also led to postweaning growth impairment.[118] Lack of artemin or GFRα3 caused few abnormalities, although the mice developed ptosis (drooping

Table 35-6 Transforming Growth Factor-β Family

TGF-B SUBFAMILY
TGF-β1
TGF-β2
TGF-β3

ACTIVIN SUBFAMILY
Activin AA
Activin AB
Activin BB

BMP2 SUBFAMILY
BMP2
BMP4

BMP3 SUBFAMILY
BMP3
GDF10

BMP5 SUBFAMILY
BMP5
BMP6/Vgr1
BMP7
BMP8

VG1 SUBFAMILY
GDF1/Vg1
GDF3/Vgr2

GDF5 SUBFAMILY
GDF5
GDF6
GDF7

INTERMEDIATE MEMBERS
Nodal
Dorsalin
GDF8
GDF9

DISTANTLY RELATED MEMBERS
MIS
Inhibins
GDNF
Artemin
Neurturin
Persephin

eyelids), secondary to loss of sympathetic innervation to the lid elevator muscle.[118]

THERAPEUTIC USES

Little information is available linking primary abnormalities in neurotrophic factors or their receptors with any disorders, except for the connection between mutations in *ret* and both Hirschsprung's disease and multiple endocrine neoplasia type 2, as noted earlier. However, in Huntington's disease, diminished delivery of BDNF to striatal neurons occurs in the cerebral cortex, where it normally plays a role in their survival.[131] Because of this and other considerations, pharmacologic treatment with neurotrophic agents, either alone or in concert with other growth factors, may prove beneficial in treating several neurodegenerative disorders. In addition, because of its physiologic role in spermatogenesis, GDNF may be a potential pharmacologic target for development of a male contraceptive.

PLATELET-DERIVED GROWTH FACTOR FAMILY

INTRODUCTION

PDGF was discovered as a protein released from the α granules of platelets that was responsible for much of the effect of serum on the proliferation of cells in culture. It was purified from platelets as a highly basic 30-kilodalton dimeric protein.[132,133] Purified PDGF was found to consist of two related chains, PDGF-A and PDGF-B, products of separate genes.[133] PDGF binds to two cell-surface receptors, PDGFR-α and PDGFR-β, which also are related in structure and sequence but are distinct gene products.[134] Both growth factors and their receptors are expressed in a wide variety of cell and tissue types.[133,135]

STRUCTURE OF PLATELET-DERIVED GROWTH FACTOR

Mature PDGF-A and -B chains are 109 amino acids in length and are 60% identical.[133,134] Eight cysteine residues are completely conserved between the two proteins. Both PDGF chains are synthesized as precursor proteins that undergo processing to yield mature glycoproteins. The B chain is homologous to *v-cis*, the transforming protein of simian sarcoma virus.[135] All three combinations of growth factor dimers have been isolated from tissues: AA, AB, BB. In addition to platelet α granules, PDGF has been isolated from several cell types including macrophages and from aortic smooth muscle cells.[133] Recently, two divergent members of the PDGF family were identified and termed *PDGF-C* and *-D*.[136–138] These proteins are 43% identical to one another, are nearly three times larger than PDGF-A or -B, and are secreted as latent factors requiring limited proteolysis for activation.[139] The proteases involved in cleavage have not been characterized. PDGF-C and -D appear able to form only homodimers.[139]

PLATELET-DERIVED GROWTH FACTOR RECEPTORS AND SIGNALING

The two PDGFRs are ligand-activated tyrosine protein kinases.[134] The receptors are composed of an extracellular region that contains five Ig-like domains, a transmembrane segment, and an intracellular region with a tyrosine kinase domain that is split by a kinase insert of approximately 100 amino acids (Fig. 35-6). The binding of PDGF to the extracellular region of the receptor induces receptor dimerization. Both homo- and heterodimers can form, depending on the ligand and the relative receptor abundance. PDGFR-β homodimers bind only PDGF BB and DD; PDGFR-α homodimers bind PDGF AA, AB, BB, and CC; whereas PDGFR-αβ heterodimers bind PDGF BB, AB, CC, and DD.[133,139] As indicated for other GFRs, ligand binding triggers the receptor kinase, leading to autophosphorylation by a transphosphorylation mechanism. Tyrosine phosphorylation creates docking sites for signal-transduction molecules that contain SH2 domains. At least 10 different SH2-containing proteins have been shown to bind to different sites on the two PDGFRs, including adaptors (Grb2, Grb7, Nck, Crk), enzymes (PI 3-kinase, Src kinases, phospholipase Cγ, the tyrosine phosphatase, SHP-2/PTP-1D, and GTPase activating protein for Ras), and transcription factors (Stats 1, 3, and 5).[140]

BIOLOGIC EFFECTS

PDGF action is essential for normal development.[141] A mutation in PDGF-A or -B, or either receptor, is associated with lethal developmental anomalies in mice. Absence of the *PDGFR-α* gene caused death by midgestation, with major defects in formation of bones of the skull and face, spina bifida, and fusions of cervical vertebrae and ribs.[142] A targeted homozygous mutation in the *PDGFR-β* gene also was lethal,[143] with death during late gestation secondary to hemorrhage. *PDGFR-β*-deficient mice also showed maldevelopment of the kidneys, with absence of mesangial cells.[143] A similar phenotype is seen in mice with a homozygous null mutation in the PDGF B-chain gene, as predicted because it is the sole ligand for the β receptor.[144] The cause of hemorrhage in these mice appears to be secondary to absence of microvascular pericytes,

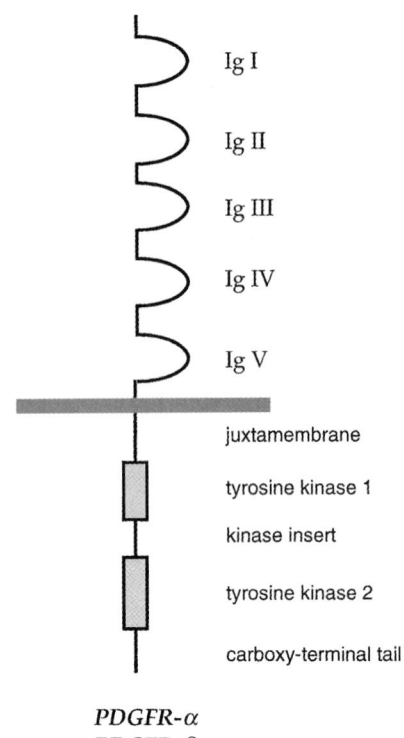

Figure 35-6 Structure of the two platelet-derived growth factor (PDGF) receptors. Different regions are labeled. Ig indicates an immunoglobulin-like domain.

which normally contribute to the mechanical stability of the capillary wall.[144] A defect in PDGF A-chain expression also led to a lethal phenotype.[145] In some populations of mice, death occurred before midgestation by unknown mechanisms.[145] Other mice lived for up to several weeks after birth but died secondary to emphysema because of loss of alveolar myofibroblasts in the lung. These latter cells are responsible for production of elastin during the phase of lung maturation that occurs normally during the first 2 postnatal weeks.[145] The outcome of engineered deficiencies of PDGF-C or -D has not been reported.

One of the major actions of PDGF in the adult is in wound healing.[146] Tissue injury leads to the rapid release of abundant PDGF AB by degranulating platelets. Other short-term sources of growth factor include activated macrophages and endothelial cells. Later in the history of a wound, keratinocytes also are induced to produce PDGF. PDGF has several actions during wound healing. It is chemotactic for smooth muscle cells, fibroblasts, neutrophils, and monocytes and stimulates macrophage activation. It acts as a vasoconstrictor to assist in closure of damaged blood vessels. It is a potent mitogen for fibroblasts and smooth muscle cells and stimulates their proliferation in collaboration with other growth factors.[146] PDGF induces expression of fibronectin, of collagenase, and of some types of collagen, and these proteins participate in the tissue remodeling that occurs during wound healing.[146]

The actions of PDGF that follow injury to the intima of blood vessels are similar to those occurring after a wound and contribute to the pathophysiology of atherosclerosis.[134] Release of PDGF by aggregating platelets will trigger the same effects seen in a peripheral wound, leading to the proliferative changes that are associated with atherosclerotic plaques.[134,146] Activation of *PDGFR-β* also may be enhanced in vascular smooth muscle cells through downregulation of expression of the low-density lipoprotein (LDL) receptor-related protein, which is able to modulate responsiveness to PDGF-BB.[147]

PDGF and PDGFR abnormalities have been associated with different human cancers.[148] Amplification of the gene for *PDGFR-α* has been seen in a subset of patients with malignant gliomas.[148] Activating gene fusions of *PDGFR-β* with other proteins have been described in individuals with chronic myelomonocytic leukemia,[149] and mutations of *PDGFR-α* have been detected in patients with gastrointestinal stromal tumors.[150] Some individuals with dermatofibrosarcoma protuberans have been found to have activating translocations of the PDGF-B gene, leading to enhanced production of PDGF-B and stimulation of *PDGFR-β*.[148] The tumors in some of these individuals have responded favorably to treatment with the tyrosine kinase inhibitor STI571 or Gleevac, indicating a role for signaling through the *PDGFR-β* in tumor progression.[148] Signaling through *PDGFR-β* also may contribute to the abnormal angiogenesis seen in cancer.[151]

THERAPEUTIC USES

Exogenous PDGF accelerates the healing of incisional wounds in experimental animals[146] and has been shown to enhance closure of chronic pressure ulcers in human studies.[152] In several models of wound healing, PDGF is most active when used in combination with other growth factors. As noted earlier, therapy directed against PDGFRs may be effective in certain types of cancers.

TRANSFORMING GROWTH FACTOR-β FAMILY

INTRODUCTION

TGF-β is a dimer of 25 kilodaltons composed of two identical disulfide-linked 12.5-kilodalton proteins. In mammals, three isoforms have been described, TGF-β1, TGF-β2, and TGF-β3.[153] These proteins are prototypical members of a large family of growth factors with diverse biologic effects in many different species.[153-156] TGF-β and related proteins control aspects of development, differentiation, and determination; regulate immune function and the response to inflammation; and play pivotal roles in reproduction.[154-157] TGF-β action is controlled by interactions with several classes of receptors and with cell-associated and extracellular-binding proteins. Two classes of high-affinity TGF-β receptors have been defined. Type I and type II receptors are ligand-activated serine-threonine protein kinases.[9,154,155,158] A type III receptor modulates binding of TGF-β to type I and type II receptors but lacks its own signaling capability.[9]

TRANSFORMING GROWTH FACTOR-β AND RELATED PROTEINS

The TGF-β superfamily contains nearly 30 members in vertebrates (see Table 35-6); multiple homologues exist in invertebrates as well.[153,155] Many of these proteins are synthesized as larger precursors with amino-terminal extensions. Amino acid sequence similarity among family members is confined to the mature 110- to 140-residue growth factor.[153,155] Proteolytic cleavage releases the mature protein, which in biologically active form is a dimer.[154,155] Members of the TGF-β family share seven cysteine residues that are nearly invariant. Six cysteines are involved in the formation of intrachain disulfide bonds that link the protein into a rigid structure termed a *cysteine knot*, as initially defined in the crystal structure of TGF-β2.[153] The seventh cysteine forms the interchain disulfide bridge, which joins two monomers into a TGF-β dimer.

Transforming Growth Factor-β
Three structurally related TGF-β molecules have been characterized in mammals, TGF-β1, TGF-β2, and TGF-β3, and two others have been identified in nonmammalian vertebrates.[153]

The mature proteins are 64% to 82% identical. Mammalian TGF-β monomers are 112 amino acids in length and contain nine cysteines. They are synthesized as precursors of approximately 350 to 400 residues and are secreted as latent complexes of approximately 100 kilodaltons.[153,159] Latent complexes consist of the mature TGF-β dimer noncovalently associated with a dimer of the remainder of the precursor protein, which is termed *latency-associated peptide* (LAP). This small latent complex is unable to bind to TGF-β receptors. A larger latent complex also exists. It consists additionally of a 125- to 160-kilodalton cysteine-rich glycoprotein known as latent TGF-β binding protein (LTBP). Activation of latent complexes provides one potential mechanism for regulating growth factor availability.[159] Although the precise pathway of activation has not been elucidated, it appears to involve proteolysis at the cell surface.

Inhibins and Activins
Inhibins were identified as proteins found in ovarian follicular fluid that inhibited pituitary secretion of follicle-stimulating hormone (FSH). The two inhibins are heterodimers between a distinct α subunit and one of two β subunits, βA and βB. Activins were characterized as stimulators of FSH secretion and are composed of dimers of inhibin β chains. Three isoforms have been isolated: AA, AB, and BB. Inhibins and activins are functional antagonists.[160] The biologic properties of these proteins are described in detail in Chapter 141.

Bone Morphogenetic Proteins
Seven bone morphogenetic proteins (BMPs) have been characterized, termed *BMP2 through 8*.[153-155] These proteins are composed of dimers of molecular mass 26 to 31 kilodaltons. BMPs were identified initially by their ability to induce cartilage and bone.[161,162] BMP2 and BMP4 are closely related in sequence to each other and to the *Drosophila* protein decapentaplegic (dpp). Dpp plays essential roles in morphogenesis and in bodily patterning in the fly.[153] BMP5 through 8 are 74% to 91% identical to one another.[163] BMP6 also is known as vegetal-related 1 (Vgr1).[9] Additional proteins that are closely related to the BMPs include vegetal 1 (Vg1), also termed *growth-differentiation factor* 1 (GDF1), and GDF3, also known as Vgr2.[9] Other more distant relatives include *nodal*, dorsalin, and GDF5 to 10.[9,153] The biologic actions of some of the BMPs and related proteins are described later. A more comprehensive review of BMPs may be found elsewhere.[162,164]

Müllerian Inhibitory Substance
Müllerian inhibitory substance (MIS) was characterized as a factor secreted by male mammalian embryos that caused regression of the müllerian duct, which otherwise would develop into the oviducts, uterus, and upper one third of the vagina.[165] It is a disulfide-linked dimer that is secreted as a dimeric precursor of approximately 140 kilodaltons. MIS is distantly related in sequence to TGF-β (~30% amino acid similarity). Its biologic actions are described elsewhere in this textbook.

Glial-derived Neurotrophic Growth Factor
Glial-derived neurotrophic growth factor (GDNF) was isolated through its ability to promote survival and differentiation of dopaminergic neurons and binds to its own heterodimeric receptor, which is unrelated to TGF-β family receptors.[118,126] GDNF and related proteins are less than 25% identical to other members of the TGF-β family. The biologic actions of GDNF were described earlier in this chapter.

TRANSFORMING GROWTH FACTOR-β RECEPTORS

Type I and Type II Receptors
TGF-β binds to three major cell-surface proteins that were initially termed *type I*, *type II*, and *type III*, based on approximate molecular masses of 53, 70, and more than 200

kilodaltons.[154,155,158] Several cDNAs encoding each class of receptor were subsequently cloned. Type I and type II receptors are structurally related glycoproteins (Fig. 35-7). Both are composed of extracellular ligand-binding domains of 102 to 196 amino acids containing a short cysteine-rich box, a single transmembrane region, and an intracytoplasmic portion of approximately 400 to 500 residues. The intracellular portion contains a kinase domain that will phosphorylate itself and exogenous substrates on serine and threonine residues.[154,155,158] Related receptors bind activins and BMPs. Type I and type II proteins interact to create functional signaling receptors.

Type III Receptors and Transforming Growth Factor-β-Binding Proteins

The type III receptor acts as an accessory molecule in TGF-β action. Type III receptors do not have an intrinsic signaling function but regulate access to signaling receptors.[9] Two related molecules compose the type III TGF-β receptors.[166] Betaglycan is a transmembrane proteoglycan with a protein core molecular mass of 130 kilodaltons. It can bind TGF-β1, β2, β3, or inhibin with high affinity. Betaglycan is structurally related to endoglin, the other type III receptor protein, a transmembrane glycoprotein composed of two disulfide-linked 95-kilodalton subunits.[155] Endoglin has been shown to bind TGF-β1 and TGF-β3.[155] Betaglycan and endoglin both consist of large extracellular domains, a single transmembrane segment, and a short intracytoplasmic region. In addition to presenting TGF-β to signaling receptors, type III receptors also may function in the storage and clearance of TGF-β.[9]

Other TGF-β-binding proteins include LTBP, described earlier, and follistatin, a widely distributed, secreted glycoprotein that binds activin and BMPs and inhibits their actions.[160] The developmental regulators, noggin, chordin, and Cerberus, all bind to BMPs and modulate their interactions with receptors.[155] Cripto, a member of the EGF family described earlier in this chapter, may facilitate binding of nodal and Vg1 to activin receptors.[155] In addition, α_2-macroglobulin, a serum protein, binds both mature TGF-β and activin and may play a role in growth-factor clearance from the circulation.[9]

RECEPTOR ACTIVATION AND SIGNAL-TRANSDUCTION PATHWAYS

Ligand binding induces formation of a heteromeric complex of type I and type II receptors.[154,155] Current evidence indicates that this complex contains two or more type I receptor molecules and two or more type II molecules per TGF-β dimer (Fig. 35-8). Complex formation leads to phosphorylation of type I receptors on serine and threonine residues by the type II receptor kinase.[154,155,158] Type I receptors then phosphorylate and activate their major substrates, Smad proteins, which are then transduced to the nucleus.[154,155,158] (see Fig. 35-8). Smads are intracellular proteins composed of two conserved regions, an amino-terminal MH1 domain of approximately 130 residues and a carboxyl-terminal MH2 domain of approximately 200 amino acids, separated by a central linker segment of variable length.[154,155,158] Three classes of Smads are based on both functional and structural considerations. Receptor-regulated Smads are direct substrates of type I receptors. Smads 2 and 3 are phosphorylated by the type I TGF-β receptor, and Smads 1, 5, and 8, by type I BMP receptors.[154,155] A second class of Smads participates in signaling through association with receptor-activated Smads. Smad 4 is the only such co-Smad identified to date. Smad 4 binds to a receptor-activated Smad when the latter becomes phosphorylated by the type I receptor kinase.[154,155] The oligomer is then translocated to the nucleus (see Fig. 35-8). Antagonistic Smads, including Smads 6 and 7, block the signaling functions of receptor-activated Smads. Smad 7 inhibits signaling induced by TGF-β and BMPs, whereas Smad 6 preferentially blocks BMP signaling.[154,155,158]

Once in the nucleus, the Smad complex functions to stimulate gene transcription. The primary mechanisms of gene regulation involve physical interactions with other sequence-specific transcription factors and transcriptional coactivators.[154,155,158] The Smad pathway is diagrammed in Figure 35-8.

Other signaling pathways also may modulate the actions of TGF-β. A novel MAPK/extracellular signal-regulated kinase

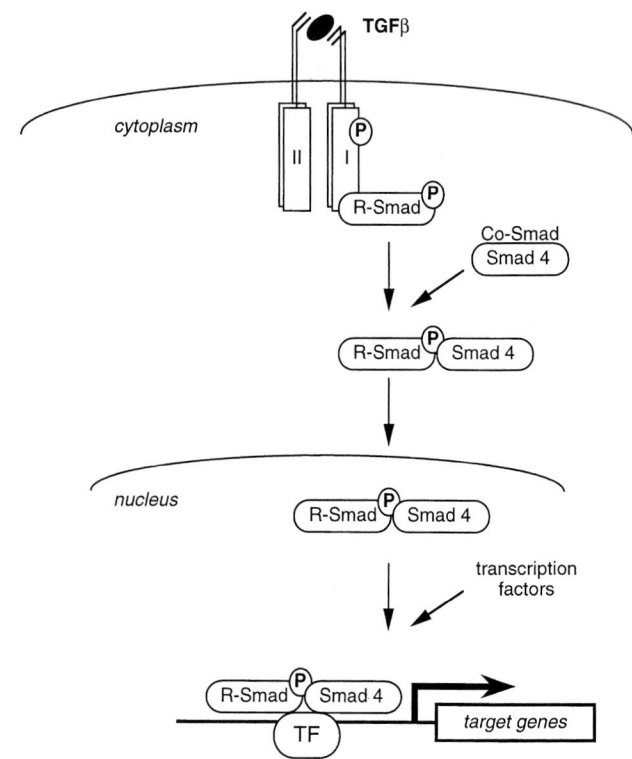

Figure 35-8   The transforming growth factor-β receptor-Smad pathway. Receptor-regulated Smads (R-Smads) are phosphorylated by the activated receptor complex, leading to binding of the Co-Smad, Smad4. The Smad complex is then transduced to the nucleus, where in association with distinct transcription factors (TFs), it binds to sites on target genes to regulate their transcription.

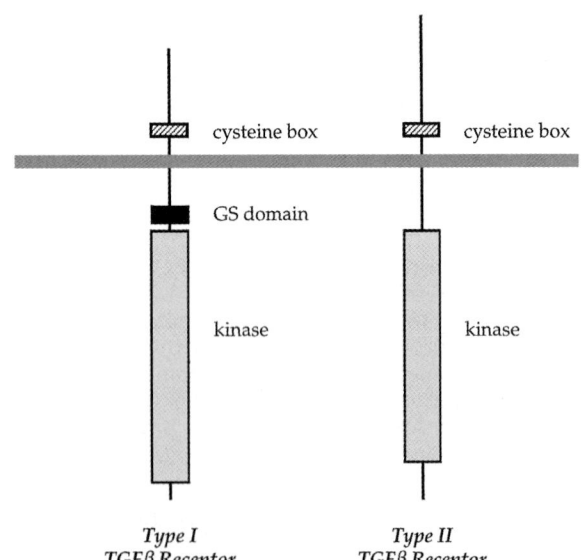

Figure 35-7   Structure of type I and type II transforming growth factor-β (TGF-β) receptors. Different regions are labeled. The GS domain is unique to type I receptors.

(MEK kinase) termed *TAK1* (for TGF-β-activated kinase) was characterized based on its complementation of a MAPK pathway in yeast.[167] Other MAPKs also may play roles in TGF-β-regulated gene expression.[158]

BIOLOGIC EFFECTS

As noted earlier, members of the TGF-β family exert diverse biologic effects. The actions of activins, inhibins, and MIS are described in other chapters. This section outlines some of the functions of other members of this growth-factor family.

Development

Genetic studies indicate major roles for several TGF-β-related proteins in early development. The *Drosophila* protein *dpp* is essential for normal dorsoventral patterning, for development of the gastrointestinal tract, and for other aspects of cell-lineage determination.[153] In the nematode *Caenorhabditis elegans*, homologues of type I and type II receptors (daf-1 and daf-4, respectively) control a signal-transduction pathway that is required for formation of a special larval stage (dauer larva) when population density exceeds food supply.[153] During the early development of the frog, *Xenopus laevis*, Vg1, activins, and BMPs exert striking effects on the formation and patterning of mesoderm. Similarly, in mice, mutations in *nodal* disrupt normal mesoderm formation.[153] GDF8, also termed *myostatin*, is an inhibitor of skeletal muscle growth and is mutated in a naturally occurring double-muscling syndrome in cattle.[168]

Mutations in the BMP genes also cause marked developmental abnormalities. Deletion of *BMP2* or *BMP5* genes in mice causes embryonic lethality.[164] A null mutation in *BMP5* leads to alterations in the size, shape, and number of skeletal components and a diminution in the size of the external ear.[164] Mutation of *BMP7* causes death in the perinatal period secondary to malformations of kidneys and eyes.[164]

TGF-β1 also is important in mouse development. A targeted disruption of the TGF-β1 gene leads to neonatal death secondary to cardiac abnormalities.[169] This phenotype is seen only in progeny of TGF-β1-deficient mothers, because transplacental passage of TGF-β1 and absorption of TGF-β1 in mother's milk normally compensates for the lack of growth-factor production by the nullizygous fetus and infant.[169] TGF-β2 deficiency leads to alterations in the size and shape of limb rudiments.[170]

Control of Inflammation and the Response to Tissue Injury

Mice born from heterozygous mothers with a homozygous null mutation for TGF-β1 have no morphologic abnormalities at birth but die soon after weaning of multiple organ failure secondary to massive infiltration of inflammatory cells.[171,172] This result potentially reflects the bivalent actions of TGF-β in inflammation and repair of tissue injury. Normally after an injury, TGF-β1 is released by platelets and functions as a strong chemotactic agent for neutrophils, monocytes, lymphocytes, and fibroblasts.[157] Monocytes and lymphocytes are then induced to produce other growth factors and cytokines, whereas fibroblasts are stimulated to synthesize extracellular matrix proteins. More TGF-β also is synthesized by these cells; it then downregulates the inflammatory process by inhibiting the functions of activated inflammatory cells. The normal result is cessation of inflammation as the wound heals. This last step does not occur in TGF-β1-deficient mice once the source of maternal TGF-β has dissipated, and massive inflammation persists.[169]

Excessive production of TGF-β may enhance tissue fibrosis and may contribute to the pathogenesis of fibrotic disorders, including glomerulopathies, liver cirrhosis, rheumatoid arthritis, and others.[173] In experimental glomerulonephritis and diabetic glomerulosclerosis, neutralizing antibodies to TGF-β1 are able to prevent accumulation of extracellular matrix proteins and minimize fibrosis and kidney damage.[174]

MUTATIONS AND DISEASE

One of the major actions of TGF-β is to inhibit cell proliferation.[9] It was thus postulated that mutations in TGF-β signaling pathways might be found in cancer, because enhanced proliferation contributes to tumorigenesis. This prediction was demonstrated in analysis of human colon cancers with microsatellite instability, in which inactivating mutations of the type II TGF-β receptor were identified.[175] Microsatellite instability is a common feature of hereditary nonpolyposis colorectal cancer and also has been found in nonhereditary gastrointestinal cancers.[175] Other mutations in the type II receptor have been detected in squamous carcinomas of the head and neck, gastric cancers, and others.[9,156]

Smad mutations also have been found in human cancers. *Smad 4* was initially characterized as a candidate tumor-suppressor gene that was mutated or deleted in nearly half of human pancreatic carcinomas.[176] Inactivating mutations were subsequently found in colorectal tumors and in a small population of other cancers.[9] *Smad 2* mutations also have been identified in colon cancer.[156,177]

Mutations in other components of TGF-β signaling pathways are found several inherited disorders in humans. The type III receptor, endoglin, and the type I receptor, Alk1, are expressed at high levels in the vascular endothelium. Inactivating mutations in each of these genes have been linked to hereditary hemorrhagic telangiectasia, a disorder characterized by a tendency toward bleeding in the gastrointestinal tract and nasal mucosa secondary to vascular epithelial dysplasia at these sites.[156,178–180] Primary pulmonary hypertension is a rare and potentially fatal disorder characterized by the ablation of small arteries and arterioles in the lungs, leading to pulmonary vascular hypertension and right-sided heart failure. Loss-of-function mutations in the gene encoding a BMP type II receptor have been found in up to 50% of affected individuals with the familial form of the disease and in approximately 25% of patients with the sporadic form.[156] Inactivating mutations in the genes for a BMP type I receptor and for *Smad4* have been identified in families with juvenile polyposis syndrome.[156] This disorder is characterized by gastrointestinal hamartomatous polyps that have the potential to cause systemic symptoms, including bowel obstruction and bleeding, and place affected individuals at increased risk for colorectal cancer.[156] Potentially inactivating mutations in the *GDF5* gene have been found in Hunter-Thompson and Grebe-type acromesomelic chondrodysplasias, recessive disorders with skeletal abnormalities limited to the distal bones.[181] A phenotypically similar disorder has been observed in mice with mutations in the same gene.[182] Camurati-Engelmann disease is an uncommon autosomal-dominant disorder characterized by progressive hyperosteosis and sclerosis of the diaphysis of long bones.[183] Missense mutations within the coding region of the *TGF-β1* gene have been found in several affected families.[183]

THERAPEUTIC USES

One use of TGF-β is in wound healing. A single local treatment accelerates wound repair in experimental animals.[157,173] Topical TGF-β2 has clinical application in repair of retinal tears. Antagonists of TGF-β action also have potential as antifibrotic agents.[173,174] BMPs have potential use in repair of bone and joint defects.[162,184]

OTHER GROWTH FACTOR FAMILIES

Many growth factors have been identified that do not fit into the framework of the families described in previous sections. Several of these proteins have not been characterized completely, or their biologic effects have not been examined fully.

They are not reviewed here. For several others, specific actions have been defined. Two examples whose properties are summarized below are hepatocyte growth factor (HGF), and vascular endothelial growth factor (VEGF).

HEPATOCYTE GROWTH FACTOR

HGF is a disulfide-linked heterodimer consisting of a 69-kilodalton α chain and a 34-kilodalton β chain that was identified as a potent serum-derived stimulator of liver cell growth in tissue culture[185] and as an effector of enhanced cell motility ("scatter factor"[186]). HGF binds to and activates a heterodimeric tyrosine kinase receptor that is the cellular homologue of the *v-met* oncogene (c-*met*).[187] This receptor has a wide tissue distribution, and HGF has been shown to exert diverse effects on multiple cell types.[188–191]

HGF is synthesized as a 728–amino acid single-chain protein.[192,193] The secreted inactive precursor is cleaved between arginine 494 and valine 495 to generate the biologically active two-chain molecule.[193,194] The HGF precursor is a substrate for several proteases found in serum, including urokinase-type and tissue-type plasminogen, blood coagulation factor XII, and another serine protease structurally similar to factor XII.[194]

HGF is related in amino acid sequence and overall structure to macrophage-stimulating protein (MSP), which was originally characterized as an activator of peritoneal macrophages,[195] and to plasminogen.[194] All three proteins contain a series of amino-terminal "kringle" domains in the α chain,[188,194] followed by a serine protease domain in the carboxyl-terminal segment of the β chain (Fig. 35-9). Kringles are segments of approximately 80 amino acids in length that form a double-looped structure that resembles a pretzel.[188,194] Alterations of critical amino acids at the putative catalytic site in the β chain have rendered HGF and MSP devoid of protease activity.[188,192]

As noted earlier, the receptor for HGF is a ligand-activated tyrosine kinase encoded by the cellular homologue of the c-*met* oncogene. The receptor is synthesized as a glycosylated single-chain precursor that undergoes posttranslational cleavage to generate the mature disulfide-linked αβ heterodimer (Fig. 35-10). The 50-kilodalton α chain is extracellular; the transmembrane 145-kilodalton β chain contains an extracellular ligand-binding region, a single membrane-spanning segment, and an intracellular region with a tyrosine kinase domain and two tyrosine residues near the carboxyl terminus that bind signal-transduction molecules when phosphorylated.[189,190,193] Ligand binding activates the receptor kinase, leading to autophosphorylation and recruitment and activation of signaling intermediates, including MAPK and PI 3-kinase pathways, src kinases, and others.[189,191] Several of these signaling outcomes are enhanced by the interaction of c-*met* with distinct cell-surface proteins, including the α6β5 integrin, Plexin B1, and CD44.[189]

The HGF receptor is closely related to two other tyrosine kinases, termed *Ron* and *Sea* (an acronym for sarcoma, erythroblastosis, and anemia).[196,197] Both glycoproteins are proto-oncogenes. Ron is the receptor for MSP, whereas Sea is the chicken homologue of Ron.[190,191]

Activation of Met by HGF initiates a diverse series of biologic actions. Mice with a targeted disruption of the HGF gene die in midstation secondary to abnormal development of

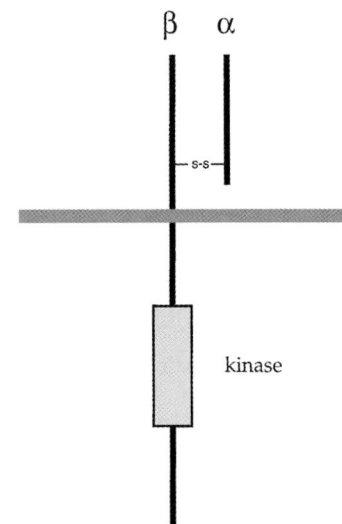

Figure 35-10   Structure of the hepatocyte growth factor (HGF) receptor. The two chains are indicated, as is the disulfide bond that joins them. The kinase domain in the intracellular portion of the β chain is depicted as a *box*.

the placenta and liver.[198,199] Inactivation of Met also is a lethal mutation.[200] These mice also die during midstation with placental and hepatic abnormalities and additionally show severe defects in limb musculature,[200] indicating the importance of Met in promoting the normal migration of skeletal myoblasts.

HGF expression is potently induced in the kidney in rats during experimentally stimulated compensatory renal hypertrophy.[194] Because of its strong mitogenic and morphogenic effects on renal tubular cells, HGF is considered to be a potentially therapeutically important renotropic factor[194] and may prove to be useful in counteracting the tissue fibrosis that occurs during the development of chronic renal disease.[201] It also is a potent locally produced mitogen and motility factor for gastric epithelial cells[202] and thus may be of therapeutic benefit in peptic ulcer disease.[202] A similar role for *HGF* has been postulated in response to liver injury,[188] and protective effects of *HGF* gene therapy have been demonstrated in experimental liver cirrhosis in rats.[203] Recent studies also implicate activation of c-*met* by HGF in the liver as critical for initial infection of hepatocytes by *Plasmodium* sporozoites, the causative agents in malaria.[204] This observation suggests that local inhibition of HGF or c-*met* could become a useful antimalarial therapy.

VASCULAR ENDOTHELIAL GROWTH FACTOR

Development of the vasculature and delivery of blood to tissues are essential for organogenesis during embryonic development and for normal wound healing and tissue maintenance in the adult. Conversely, abnormal angiogenesis plays a central role in the pathogenesis of a diverse array of diseases, including the growth and metastasis of malignant neoplasms, development of proliferative retinopathies, and other disorders.[205,206] Although several different growth factors and cytokines have been implicated as potential regulators of normal and pathologic angiogenesis, recent studies have established a critical role for VEGF and its receptors in development of the vasculature and in mediating abnormal vasculogenesis in disease.[206–208]

VEGF is a disulfide-linked dimeric glycoprotein of approximately 36 to 56 kilodaltons that is distantly related to PDGF. Human VEGF consists of four isoforms of 121, 165, 186, and 206 amino acids that are the protein products of alternatively

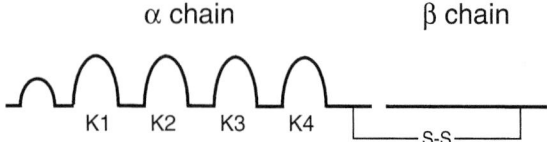

Figure 35-9   Structure of hepatocyte growth factor (HGF). The four kringle domains in the α chain, K1 to K4, are indicated, as is the disulfide bond joining the α and β chains.

spliced transcripts of the *VEGF* gene. VEGF$_{165}$, the major isoform, is a 45-kilodalton heparin-binding glycoprotein.[206]

VEGF was the first member characterized of a gene family that currently contains at least five distinct proteins in mammals. Placental growth factor (PlGF) is a dimeric glycoprotein whose amino acid sequence is approximately 40% identical to that of VEGF.[209,210] VEGF-B is a 188-residue protein with approximately 43% identity to VEGF.[211–213] Several isoforms of both proteins have been characterized. VEGF-C is a 399-residue protein that is 32% identical to VEGF in its amino-terminal domain,[213,214] whereas VEGF-D is 60% identical to VEGF-C.[215] In addition to these proteins, a related molecule is encoded by a parapoxvirus, sheep Orf virus.[206]

VEGF binds with high affinity to two related transmembrane tyrosine kinase receptors, VEGFR-1 (also called flt-1 for fms-like tyrosine kinase), and VEGFR-2 (also known as flk-1/KDR for fetal liver kinase-1/kinase domain region).[206,216] PlGF and VEGF-B also bind to VEGFR-1.[206,216] VEGFR-1 and -2 have seven immunoglobulin (Ig)-like segments in their extracellular region, a single membrane-spanning domain, and a tyrosine kinase region that is interrupted by a kinase-insert domain (Fig. 35-11). The second Ig-like domain contains the binding site for VEGF.[206] A related protein, flt-4/VEGFR-3, is the critical receptor for VEGF-C and VEGF-D, although these proteins also are able to bind to VEGFR-2.[206,216] All three receptors are structurally related to the two PDGF receptors.[205] VEGFR-1 and VEGFR-2 are expressed predominantly in vascular endothelium,[217,218] thus accounting for the specific actions of VEGF in the vasculature, whereas VEGFR-3 is expressed during early development throughout the vasculature but becomes progressively restricted to lymphatic endothelial cells in the adult.[216] Recent work has shown that VEGFR-1 is a negative regulator of VEGF, at least in the vasculature, and that VEGFR-2 and VEGFR-3 are signaling receptors.[206] On ligand binding, both VEGFR-2 and VEGFR-3 are able to activate signaling molecules containing SH2 domains, which appear to interact with phosphorylated tyrosine residues located within their intracellular segments.[206,216] The signaling properties of VEGF ligands are enhanced by coreceptors termed *neuropilins*.[206,216]

As demonstrated by results of targeted gene-disruption experiments, all three VEGFRs are essential for vasculogenesis in the embryo.[219–221] Mice lacking VEGFR-1 died in utero before embryonic day 10 and failed to organize normal vascular channels.[219] In contrast, mice expressing a mutant VEGFR-1 lacking its kinase domain, but retaining normal binding capacity for VEGF, developed normally and had normal vasculature, supporting the idea that VEGFR-1 is a negative modulator of the actions of VEGF.[222] Mice homozygous for disruption of the VEGFR-2 gene also died before embryonic day 10. These mice lacked blood vessels and additionally had marked deficits in precursors of blood cells.[220] Mice deficient in VEGFR-3 died before embryonic day 10 secondary to defective vascular remodeling.[221] Mice heterozygous for a targeted mutation in VEGF died before embryonic day 12 and had severe abnormalities in the developing forebrain, heart, and aorta, had major defects in the vasculature of many organs and tissues, and showed deficient blood cell formation.[223,224] In contrast, mice with complete deficiencies of either PlGF or VEGF-B developed normally.[225,226]

VEGF and its receptors also play key roles in the vascular repair that accompanies wound healing.[206,216] VEGF has been shown to be a potent mitogen for endothelial cells[227] and has been found to stimulate angiogenesis in both in vitro and in vivo model systems.[228,229] VEGF also stimulates microvascular leakage and was identified during its initial characterization as a vascular permeability factor.[230,231] Enhanced microvascular permeability has been hypothesized to be a key step in angiogenesis, by giving rise to a extravascular fibrin gel that can serve as a substrate for endothelial cell growth.[232]

VEGF is a central component of the pathologic angiogenesis that accompanies tumor growth and metastasis and other disorders.[207] *VEGF* gene expression is enhanced in the majority of human cancers.[205] Inhibition of VEGF function with neutralizing antibodies or by blocking receptor function has been shown to abrogate growth of human tumor cell lines in mice.[233–235] Initial clinical trials involving several different approaches toward inhibiting VEGF function in patients with cancer have been encouraging and are continuing.[236–238] The neovascularization that characterizes advanced diabetic retinopathy and other eye disorders is a consequence of retinal ischemia, which leads to increased local production of VEGF and subsequent pathologic angiogenesis.[208] Neovascularization also is a major contributor to visual loss in age-related macular degeneration, a leading cause of blindness in adults, and is thought to be secondary to local production of VEGF in the eye. Anti-VEGF therapy also has been promising in initial trials.[239]

OTHER VASCULAR ENDOTHELIAL GROWTH FACTORS

A novel family of tissue-restricted angiogenic growth factors has been characterized recently.[240,241] Endocrine gland–derived VEGF proteins (EG-VEGF) are expressed primarily in steroid-producing tissues, including the adrenal glands, ovary, and testes.[241] They are unrelated in amino acid sequence or structure to the VEGF family and stimulate their effects through novel G protein–coupled receptors found on the vascular endothelium of steroid hormone–producing glands.[241] The biologic actions of EG-VEGF are described in other chapters of this text.

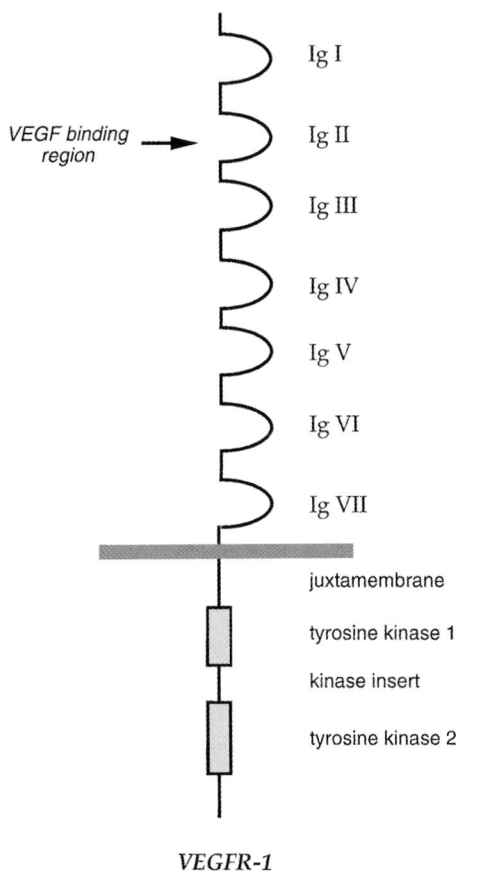

VEGF binding region →

Ig I
Ig II
Ig III
Ig IV
Ig V
Ig VI
Ig VII

juxtamembrane
tyrosine kinase 1
kinase insert
tyrosine kinase 2

VEGFR-1
VEGFR-2

Figure 35-11 Structure of vegetative endothelial growth factor (VEGF) receptors. Different regions are depicted. Ig indicates an immunoglobulin-like domain. The region binding VEGF in Ig II is labeled.

SUMMARY AND PERSPECTIVE

Growth factors are multifunctional proteins that exert their diverse biologic effects by activating specific transmembrane receptors, which are ligand-regulated protein kinases. The actions of growth factors lead to short-term alterations in cellular function and to long-term changes in the whole organism. As described in this chapter, growth factors play critical roles in many aspects of development, regulate somatic growth of a variety of tissues and organs, and modulate tissue maturation and repair. Although as emphasized in this chapter, each growth factor is able to mediate a unique spectrum of biologic effects, in the whole organism, different growth factors collaboratively regulate different functions. Only recently has the potential of growth factors for therapeutic use been recognized. Studies in the coming decade should lead to further understanding of the roles of growth factors in many areas of biology and medicine.

REFERENCES

1. Sporn MB, Roberts AB: Peptide growth factors are multifunctional. Nature 332:217–218, 1998.
2. Raff MC: Size control: The regulation of cell numbers in animal development. Cell 85:173–175, 1996.
3. Pazin MJ, Williams LT: Triggering signaling cascades by receptor tyrosine kinases. Trends Biochem Sci 17:374–378, 1992.
4. Keating MT, Williams LT: Autocrine stimulation of intracellular PDGF receptors in v-sis-transformed cells. Science 239:914–916, 1988.
5. Bejcek BE, Li DY, Deuel TF: Transformation by v-sis occurs by an internal autoactivation mechanism. Science 245:1496–1499, 1989.
6. Fantl WJ, Johnson DE, Williams LT: Signaling by receptor tyrosine kinases. Annu Rev Biochem 63:453–481, 1993.
7. Lemmon MA, Schlessinger J: Regulation of signal transduction and signal diversity by receptor oligomerization. Trends Biochem Sci 19:459–463, 1994.
8. Heldin C-H: Dimerization of cell surface receptors in signal transduction. Cell 80:213–223, 1995.
9. Massague J: TGF-β signal transduction. Annu Rev Biochem 67:853–891, 1998.
10. Attisano L, Wrana JL: Mads and Smads in TGFβ signalling. Curr Opinion Cell Biol 10:188–194, 1998.
11. Koch CA, Anderson D, Moran MF, et al: SH2 and SH3 domains: Elements that control interactions of cytoplasmic signaling proteins. Science 252:668–674, 1991.
12. Anderson D, Koch CA, Grey L, et al: Binding of SH2 domains of phospholipase C gamma 1, GAP, and Src to activated growth factor receptors. Science 250:979–982, 1990.
13. Matsuda M, Mayer BJ, Fukui Y, et al: Binding of transforming protein, P47gag-crk, to a broad range of phosphotyrosine-containing proteins. Science 248:1537–1539, 1990.
14. Kavanaugh WM, Williams LT: An alternative to SH2 domains for binding tyrosine-phosphorylated proteins. Science 266:1862–1865, 1994.
15. Claesson-Welsh L: Platelet-derived growth factor receptor signals. J Biol Chem 269:32023–32026, 1994.
16. Egan SE, Weinberg RA: The pathway to signal achievement. Nature 365:781–783, 1993.
17. Roberts TM: A signal chain of events. Nature 360:534–565, 1992.
18. Karin M: Signal transduction from the cell surface to the nucleus through the phosphorylation of transcription factors. Curr Opin Cell Biol 6:415–424, 1994.
19. Whitmarsh AJ, Shore P, Sharrocks AD, et al: Integration of MAP kinase signal transduction pathways at the serum response element. Science 269:403–407, 1995.
20. Karin M: The regulation of AP-1 activity by mitogen-activated protein kinases. J Biol Chem 270:16483–16486, 1995.
21. Hill CS, Treisman R: Transcriptional regulation by extracellular signals: Mechanisms and specificity. Cell 80:199–211, 1995.
22. Cohen S: Isolation of a mouse submaxilliary gland protein accelerating incisor eruption and eyelid opening in the new-born animal. J Biol Chem 237:1555–1562, 1962.
23. Harris RC, Chung E, Coffey RJ: EGF receptor ligands. Exp Cell Res 284:2–13, 2003.
24. Falls DL: Neuregulins: Functions, forms, and signaling strategies. Exp Cell Res 284:14–30, 2003.
25. Holbro T, Hynes NE: ErbB receptors: Directing key signaling networks throughout life. Annu Rev Pharmacol Toxicol 44:195–217, 2004.
26. Burgess AW, Cho HS, Eigenbrot C, et al: An open-and-shut case? Recent insights into the activation of EGF/ErbB receptors. Mol Cell 12:541–552, 2003.
27. Riese DJII, Stern DF: Specificity within the EGF family/ErbB receptor family signaling network. Bioessays 20:41–48, 1998.
28. Bell G, Fong NM, Stempien MM, et al: Human epidermal growth factor precursor: cDNA sequence, expression in vitro and gene organization. Nucleic Acids Res 14:8427–8433, 1986.
29. Derynck R, Roberts AB, Winkler ME, et al: Human transforming growth factor-alpha: Precursor structure and expression in E. coli. Cell 38:287–297, 1984.
30. Shoyab M, Plowman GD, McDonald VL, et al: Structure and function of human amphiregulin: A member of the epidermal growth factor family. Science 243:1074–1076, 1989.
31. Higashiyama S, Abraham JA, Miller J, et al: A heparin-binding growth factor secreted by macrophage-like cells that is related to EGF. Science 251:936–939, 1991.
32. Raab G, Klagsbrun M: Heparin-binding EGF-like growth factor. Biochim Biophys Acta 1333:F179–F199, 1997.
33. Thompson SA, Higashiyama S, Wood K, et al: Characterization of sequences within heparin-binding EGF-like growth factor that mediate interaction with heparin. J Biol Chem 269:2541–2549, 1994.
34. Naglieh JG, Metherall JE, Russell DW, et al: EGF-like growth factor precursor. Cell 69:1051–1061, 1992.
35. Shing Y, Christofori G, Hanahan D, et al: Betacellulin: A mitogen from pancreatic β cell tumors. Science 259:1604–1607, 1993.
36. Toyoda H, Komurasaki T, Uchida D, et al: Epiregulin: A novel epidermal growth factor with mitogenic activity for rat primary hepatocytes. J Biol Chem 270:7495–7500, 1995.
37. Strachan L, Murison JG, Prestidge RL, et al: Cloning and biological activity of epigen, a novel member of the epidermal growth factor superfamily. J Biol Chem 276:18265–18271, 2001.
38. Carraway KLIII, Weber JL, Unger MJ, et al: Neuregulin-2, a new ligand of ErbB3/ErbB4-receptor tyrosine kinases. Nature 387:512–516, 1997.
39. Chang H, Riese DJ II, Gilbert W, et al: Ligands for ErbB-family receptors encoded by a neuregulin-like gene. Nature 387:509–512, 1997.
40. Harari D, Tzahar E, Romano J, et al: Neuregulin-4: A novel growth factor that acts through the ErbB-4 receptor tyrosine kinase. Oncogene 18:2681–2689, 1999.
41. Ciccodicola A, Dono R, Obici S, et al: Molecular characterization of a gene of the "EGF family" expressed in undifferentiated human NTERA2 teratocarcinoma cells. EMBO J 8:1987–1997, 1989.
42. Brandt R, Normanno N, Gullick WJ, et al: Identification and biological characterization of an epidermal growth factor-related protein: Cripto-1. J Biol Chem 269:17320–17328, 1994.
43. Shen MM, Wang H, Leder P: A differential display strategy identifies Cryptic, a novel EGF-related gene expressed in the axial and lateral mesoderm during mouse gastrulation. Development 124:429–442, 1997.
44. Kannan S, DeSantis M, Lohmeyer M, et al: Cripto enhances the tyrosine phosphorylation of Shc and activates mitogen-activated protein kinase (MAPK) in mammary epithelial cells. J Biol Chem 272:3330–3335, 1997.
45. Stroobant P, Rice AP, Gullick WJ, et al: Purification and characterization of vaccinia virus growth factor. Cell 42:383, 393, 1985.

46. Iozzo RV, Moscatello DK, McQuillan DJ, et al: Decorin is a biological ligand for the epidermal growth factor receptor. J Biol Chem 274:4489–4492, 1999.

47. Yamauchi T, Ueki K, Tobe K, et al: Tyrosine phosphorylation of the EGF receptor by the kinase Jak2 is induced by growth hormone. Nature 390:91–96, 1997.

48. Qiu Y, Ravi L, Kung HJ: Requirement of ErbB2 for signaling by interleukin-6 in prostate carcinoma cells. Nature 393:83–85, 1998.

49. Daub H, Weiss FU, Wallasch C, et al: Role of transactivation of the EGF receptor in signalling by G-protein-coupled receptors. Nature 379:557–560, 1996.

50. Nair BG, Parikh B, Miligan G, et al: Gsα mediates epidermal growth factor-elicited stimulation of rat cardiac adenylate cyclase. J Biol Chem 265:23117–23122, 1990.

51. Poppleton H, Sun H, Fulgham D, et al: Activation of Gsα by the epidermal growth factor receptor involves phosphorylation. J Biol Chem 271:6947–6951, 1996.

52. Miettinen PJ, Berger JE, Meneses J, et al: Epithelial immaturity and multiorgan failure in mice lacking epidermal growth factor receptor. Nature 376:337–341, 1995.

53. Threadgill DW, Dlugosz AA, Hansen LA, et al: Targeted disruption of mouse EGF receptor effect of genetic background on mutant phenotype. Science 269:230–233, 1995.

54. Sibilia M, Wagner EF: Strain-dependent epithelial defects in mice lacking the EGF receptor. Science 269:234–237, 1995.

55. Luetteke NC, Qiu TH, Peiffer RL, et al: TGFα deficiency results in hair follicle and eye abnormalities in targeted and waved-1 mice. Cell 73:263–278, 1993.

56. Meyer D, Birchmeier C: Multiple essential functions of neuregulin in development. Nature 378:386–398, 1995.

57. Gasman M, Casagranda F, Orioll D, et al: Aberrant neural and cardiac development in mice lacking the ErbB4 neuregulin receptor. Nature 378:390–394, 1995.

58. Lee K-F, Simon H, Chen H, et al: Requirement for neuregulin receptor erbB2 in neural and cardiac development. Nature 378:394–398, 1995.

59. Kramer R, Bucay N, Kane DJ, et al: Neuregulins with an Ig-like domain are essential for mouse myocardial and neuronal development. Proc Natl Acad Sci U S A 93:4833–4838, 1996.

60. Ding J, Yang L, Yan Y-T, et al: Cripto is required for correct orientation of the anterior-posterior axis in the mouse embryo. Nature 395:702–707, 1998.

61. Shen MM: Decrypting the role of Cripto in tumorigenesis. J Clin Invest 112:500–502, 2003.

62. Halter SA, Dempsey P, Matsui Y, et al: Distinctive patterns of hyperplasia in transgenic mice with mammary tumor virus transforming growth factor-alpha: Characterization of mammary gland and skin proliferations. Am J Pathol 140:1131–1146, 1992.

63. Spitzer E, Zschiesche W, Binas B, et al: EGF and TGF alpha modulate structural and functional differentiation of the mammary gland from pregnant mice in vitro: Possible role of the arachidonic acid pathway. J Cell Biochem 57:495–508, 1995.

64. Yang Y, Spitzer E, Meyer D, et al: Sequential requirement of hepatocyte growth factor and neuregulin in the morphogenesis and differentiation of the mammary gland. J Cell Biol 131:215–226, 1995.

65. Jones FE, Jerry DJ, Guarino BC, et al: Heregulin induces in vivo proliferation and differentiation of mammary epithelium into secretory lobuloalveoli. Cell Growth Differ 7:1031–1038, 1996.

66. Alroy I, Yarden Y: The ErbB signaling network in embryogenesis and oncogenesis: Signal diversification through combination ligand-receptor interactions. FEBS Lett 410:83–86, 1997.

67. Wang X, Huong SM, Chiu ML, et al: Epidermal growth factor receptor is a cellular receptor for human cytomegalovirus. Nature 424:456–461, 2003.

68. Slamon DJ, Godolphin W, Jones LA, et al: Studies of the HER-2/neu proto-oncogene in human breast and ovarian cancer. Science 244:707–712, 1989.

69. Bacus SS, Zelnick CR, Plowman G, et al: Expression of the erbB-2 family of growth factor receptors and their ligands in breast cancers. Am J Clin Pathol 102:S13–S24, 1994.

70. Plowman GD, Culousco JM, Whitney GS, et al: Ligand-specific activation of HER4/p180erbB4, a fourth member of the epidermal growth factor receptor family. Proc Natl Acad Sci U S A 90:1746–1750, 1993.

71. Paez JG, Janne PA, Lee JC, et al: EGFR mutations in lung cancer: Correlation with clinical response to gefitinib therapy. Science 304:1497–1500, 2004.

72. Lynch TJ, Bell DW, Sordella R, et al: Activating mutations in the epidermal growth factor receptor underlying responsiveness of non-small-cell lung cancer to gefitinib. N Engl J Med 350:2129–2139, 2004.

73. Galzie Z, Kinsella AR, Smith JA: Fibroblast growth factors and their receptors. Biochem Cell Biol 75:669–685, 1997.

74. Dono R: Fibroblast growth factors as regulators of central nervous system development and function. Am J Physiol Regul Integr Comp Physiol 284:R867–R881, 2003.

75. McKeehan WL, Wang F, Kan M: The heparan sulfate-fibroblast growth factor family: Diversity of structure and function. Prog Nucleic Acid Res Mol Biol 59:135–176, 1998.

76. Gorlin RJ: Fibroblast growth factors, their receptors and receptor disorders. J Craniomaxilofac Surg 25:69–79, 1997.

77. Johnson DE, Williams LT: Structural and functional diversity in the FGF receptor multigene family. Adv Cancer Res 60:1–41, 1993.

78. Coumoul X, Deng CX: Roles of FGF receptors in mammalian development and congenital diseases. Birth Defects Res Part C Embryo Today 69:286–304, 2003.

79. Ornitz DM, Xu J, Colvin JS, et al: Receptor specificity of the fibroblast growth factor family. J Biol Chem 271:15292–15297, 1996.

80. Ornitz DM, Yayon A, Flanagan JG, et al: Heparin is required for cell free binding of basic fibroblast growth factor to a soluble receptor and for mitogenesis. Mol Cell Biol 12:240–247, 1992.

81. Yayor A, Klagsbrun M, Esko JD, et al: Cell surface, heparin like molecules are required for binding of basic fibroblast growth factor to its high affinity receptor. Cell 64:841–848, 1991.

82. Vlodavsky I, Bar-Shavit R, Ishai-Michaeli R, et al: Extracellular sequestration and release of fibroblast growth factor: A regulatory mechanism? Trends Biochem Sci 16:268–271, 1991.

83. Qing K, Mah C, Hansen J, et al: Human fibroblast growth factor receptor 1 is a co-receptor for infection by adeno-associated virus 2. Nat Med 5:71–75, 1999.

84. Spivak-Kroizman T, Lemmon MA, Dikic I, et al: Heparin-induced oligomerization of FGF molecules is responsible for FGF receptor dimerization, activation and cell proliferation. Cell 79:1015–1024, 1994.

85. Isaacs HV: New perspectives on the role of the fibroblast growth factor family in amphibian development. Cell Mol Life Sci 53:350–361, 1997.

86. Deng C-X, Wynshaw-Boris A, Shen MM, et al: Murine FGFR-1 is required for early postimplantation growth and axial organization. Genes Dev 8:3045–3057, 1994.

87. Yamaguchi TP, Harpal K, Henkemeyer M, et al: FGFR-1 is required for embryonic growth and mesodermal patterning during mouse gastrulation. Genes Dev 8:3032–3044, 1994.

88. Mansour SL: Targeted disruption of int-2 (fgf-3) causes developmental defects in the tail and inner ear. Mol Reprod Dev 39:62–68, 1994.

89. Hebert JM, Rosenquist T, Gotz J, et al: FGF5 as a regulator of the hair growth cycle: evidence from targeted and spontaneous mutations. Cell 78:1017–1025, 1994.

90. Feldman B, Poueymirou W, Papaioannou VE, et al: Requirement of FGF-4 for postimplantation mouse development. Science 267:246–249, 1995.

91. Min H, Danilenko DM, Scully SA, et al: Fgf-10 is required for both limb and lung development and exhibits striking functional similarity to *Drosophilia* branchless. Genes Dev 12:3156–3161, 1998.

92. Meyers EN, Martin GR: Differences in left-right axis pathways in mouse and chick: functions of FGF8 and SHH. Science 285:403–406, 1999.

93. Umemori H, Linhoff MW, Ornitz DM, et al: FGF22 and its close relatives are presynaptic organizing molecules in the mammalian brain. Cell 118:257–270, 2004.

94. Szebenyi G, Fallon JF: Fibroblast growth factors as multifunctional signaling factors. Int Rev Cytol 185:45–106, 1999.

95. Deng C, Wynshaw-Boris A, Zhou F, et al: Fibroblast growth factor receptor 3 is a negative regulator of bone growth. Cell 84:911–921, 1996.

96. Cohen S: Purification of a nerve-growth promoting protein from the mouse salivary gland and its neuro-cytotoxic antiserum. Proc Natl Acad Sci U S A 46:302–311, 1960.

97. Levi-Montalcini R, Booker B: Destruction of the sympathetic ganglia in mammals by an antiserum to a nerve growth protein. Proc Natl Acad Sci U S A 46:384–391, 1960.

98. Lindsay RM: Neutrophins and receptors. Prog Brain Res 103:3–14, 1994.

99. Pulciani S, Santos E, Lauver AV, et al: Oncogenes in solid human tumors. Nature 300:539–542, 1982.

100. Martin-Zanca D, Barbacid M, Parada LF: Expression of the trk proto-oncogene is restricted to the sensory cranial and spinal ganglia of neural crest origin in mouse development. Genes Dev 4:683–694, 1990.

101. Huang EJ, Reichardt LF: Trk receptors: Roles in neuronal signal transduction. Annu Rev Biochem 72:609–642, 2003.

102. Ibanez CF: Emerging themes in structural biology of neurotropic factors. Trends Neurosci 21:438–444, 1998.

103. Chao M, Casaccia-Bonnefil P, Carter B, et al: Neurotrophin receptors: Mediators of life and death. Brain Res Rev 26:295–301, 1998.

104. Bothwell M: p75ntr: A receptor after all. Science 272:506–507, 1996.

105. Frade JM, Barde Y: Nerve growth factor: Two receptors, multiple functions. Bioessays 20:137–145, 1998.

106. Smeyne RJ, Klein R, Schnapp A, et al: Severe sensory and sympathetic neuropathies in mice carrying a disrupted trk/NGF receptor gene. Nature 368:246–249, 1994.

107. Klein R, Smeyne RJ, Wurst W, et al: Targeted disruption of the trkB neurotrophin receptor gene results in nervous system lesions and neonatal death. Cell 75:113–122, 1993.

108. Ernfors P, Lee KF, Jaenisch R: Mice lacking brain-derived neurotrophic factor develop sensory deficits. Nature 368:147–150, 1994.

109. Conover JC, Erickson JT, Katz DM, et al: Neuronal deficits, not involving motor neurons, in mice lacking BDNF and/or NT4. Nature 375:235–238, 1995.

110. Klein R, Silos-Santiago I, Smeyne RJ, et al: Disruption of the neutrophin 3 receptor gene trkC eliminates Ia muscle afferents and results in abnormal movements. Nature 368:249–251, 1994.

111. Ernfors P, Lee KF, Kucera J, et al: Lack of neurotrophin 3 leads to deficiencies in the peripheral nervous system and loss of limb proprioceptive afferents. Cell 77:503–512, 1994.

112. Lee K-F, Davies AM, Jaenisch R: p75-deficient embryonic dorsal root sensory and neonatal sympathetic neurons display a decreased sensitivity to NGF. Development 120:1027–1033, 1994.

113. Frade J-M, Rodriguez-Tebar A, Barde Y-A: Induction of cell death by endogenous nerve growth factor through its p75 receptor. Nature 383:166–168, 1996.

114. Lin L-FH, Doherty DH, Lile JD, et al: GDNF: A glial cell line-derived neurotrophic factor for midbrain dopaminergic neurons. Science 260:1130–1132, 1993.

115. Kotzbauer PT, Lampe PA, Heuckeroth RO, et al: Neurturin, a relative of glial-cell-line-derived neurotropic factor. Nature 384:467–470, 1996.

116. Milbrandt J, deSauvage FJ, Fahrner TJ, et al: Persephin, a novel neurotrophic factor related to GDNF and neurturin. Neuron 20:245–253, 1998.

117. Baloh RH, Enomoto H, Johnson EMJ, et al: The GDNF family ligands and receptors: Implications for neural development. Curr Opin Neurobiol 10:103–110, 2000.

118. Airaksinen MS, Saarma M: The GDNF family: signaling, biological functions and therapeutic value. Nat Rev Neurosci 3:383–394, 2002.

119. Baloh RH, Gorodinsky A, Golden JP, et al: GFRα3 is an orphan member of the GDNF/neurturin/perephin receptor family. Proc Natl Acad Sci U S A 95:5801–5806, 1998.

120. Jing S, Wen D, Yu Y, et al: GDNF-induced activation of the ret protein tyrosine kinase is mediated by GDNFR-alpha, a novel receptor for GDNF. Cell 85:1113–1124, 1996.

121. Treanor JJ, Goodman L, de Sauvage F, et al: Characterization of a multicomponent receptor for GDNF. Nature 382:80–83, 1996.

122. Baloh RH, Tansey MG, Golden JP, et al: TrnR2, a novel receptor that mediates neurturin and GDNF signaling through Ret. Neuron 18:793–802, 1997.

123. Sanicola M, Hession C, Worley D, et al: Glial cell line-derived neurotrophic factor-dependent RET activation can be mediated by two different cell-surface accessory proteins. Proc Natl Acad Sci U S A 94:6238–6243, 1997.

124. Lindahl M, Poteryaev D, Yu L, et al: Human glial cell line-derived neurotrophic factor receptor alpha 4 is the receptor for persephin and is predominantly expressed in normal and malignant thyroid medullary cells. J Biol Chem 276:9344–9351, 2001.

125. Paratcha G, Ledda F, Ibanez CF: The neural cell adhesion molecule NCAM is an alternative signaling receptor for GDNF family ligands. Cell 113:867–879, 2003.

126. Sariola H, Saarma M: Novel functions and signaling pathways for GDNF. J Cell Sci 116:3855–3862, 2003.

127. Pichel JG, Shen L, Hui SZ, et al: Defects in enteric innervation and kidney development in mice lacking GDNF. Nature 382:73–76, 1996.

128. Sanchez MP, Silos-Santiago I, Frisen J, et al: Renal agenesis and the absence of enteric neurons in mice lacking GDNF. Nature 382:70–73, 1996.

129. Schuchardt A, D'Agati V, Larsson-Blomberg L, et al: Defects in the kidney and enteric nervous system of mice lacking the tyrosine kinase receptor Ret. Nature 367:380–383, 1994.

130. Enomoto H, Araki T, Jackman A, et al: GFRα1-deficient mice have deficits in the enteric nervous system and kidneys. Neuron 21:317–324, 1998.

131. Gauthier LR, Charrin BC, Borrell-Pages M, et al: Huntingtin controls neurotrophic support and survival of neurons by enhancing BDNF vesicular transport along microtubules. Cell 118:127–138, 2004.

132. Ross R, Glomset J, Kariya B, et al: A platelet-dependent serum factor that stimulates the proliferation of arterial smooth muscle cells in vitro. Proc Natl Acad Sci U S A 71:1207–1210, 1974.

133. Heldin C-H, Westermark B: Platelet-derived growth factor: Mechanism of action and possible in vivo function. Cell Regul 1:555–566, 1990.

134. Heldin CH, Ostman A, Ronnstrand L: Signal transduction via platelet-derived growth factor receptors. Biochim Biophys Acta 1378:F79–F113, 1998.

135. Westermark B, Heldin C-H: Platelet-derived growth factor: Structure, function and implications in normal and malignant cell growth. Acta Oncol 32:101–105, 1993.

136. Li X, Ponten A, Aase K, et al: PDGF-C is a new protease-activated ligand for the PDGF alpha-receptor. Nat Cell Biol 2:302–309, 2000.

137. Bergsten E, Uutela M, Li X, et al: PDGF-D is a specific, protease-activated ligand for the PDGF beta-receptor. Nat Cell Biol 3:512–516, 2001.

138. LaRochelle WJ, Jeffers M, McDonald WF, et al: PDGF-D, a new protease-activated growth factor. Nat Cell Biol 3:517–521, 2001.

139. Li X, Eriksson U: Novel PDGF family members: PDGF-C and PDGF-D. Cytokine Growth Factor Rev 14:91–98, 2003.

140. Heldin CH: Simultaneous induction of stimulatory and inhibitory signals by PDGF. FEBS Lett 410:17–21, 1997.

141. Hoch RV, Soriano P: Roles of PDGF in animal development. Development 130:4769–4784, 2003.

142. Soriano P: The PDGFα receptor is required for neural crest cell development and for normal patterning of the somites. Development 124:2691–2700, 1997.

143. Soriano P: Abnormal kidney development and hematological disorders in PDGF β-receptor mutant mice. Genes Dev 8:1888–1896, 1994.

144. Lindahl P, Johansson BR, Leveen P, et al: Pericyte loss and microaneurysm formation in PDGF-β-deficient mice. Science 277:242–244, 1997.

145. Bostrom H, Willetts K, Pekny M, et al: PDGF-A signaling is a critical event in lung alveolar myofibroblast development and alveogenesis. Cell 85:863–873, 1996.

146. Betsholtz C, Raines EW: Platelet-derived growth factor: A key regulator of connective tissue cells in embryogenesis and pathogenesis. Kidney Int 51:1361–1369, 1987.

147. Herz J: LRP: A bright beacon at the blood-brain barrier. J Clin Invest 112:1483–1485, 2003.

148. Pietras K, Sjoblom T, Rubin K, et al: PDGF receptors as cancer drug targets. Cancer Cell 3:439–443, 2003.

149. Magnusson MK, Meade KE, Brown KE, et al: Rabaptin-5 is a novel fusion partner to platelet-derived growth factor beta receptor in chronic myelomonocytic leukemia. Blood 98:2518–2525, 2001.

150. Heinrich MC, Corless CL, Duensing A, et al: PDGFRA activating mutations in gastrointestinal stromal tumors. Science 299:708–710, 2003.

151. Jain RK, Booth MF: What brings pericytes to tumor vessels? J Clin Invest 112:1134–1136, 2003.

152. Robson MC, Phillips LG, Thomason A, et al: Platelet-derived growth factor BB for the treatment of chronic pressure ulcers. Lancet 339:23–25, 1992.

153. Kingsley DM: The TGF-β superfamily: New members, new receptors, and new genetic tests of function in different organisms. Genes Dev 8:133–146, 1994.

154. Derynck R, Zhang YE: Smad-dependent and Smad-independent pathways in TGF-beta family signaling. Nature 425:577–584, 2003.

155. Shi Y, Massague J: Mechanisms of TGF-beta signaling from cell membrane to the nucleus. Cell 113:685–700, 2003.

156. Waite KA, Eng C: From developmental disorder to heritable cancer: It's all in the BMP/TGF-beta family. Nat Rev Genet 4:763–773, 2003.

157. Letterio JJ, Roberts AB: Regulation of immune responses by TGF-β. Annu Rev Immunol 16:137–161, 1998.

158. ten Dijke P, Hill CS: New insights into TGF-beta-Smad signaling. Trends Biochem Sci 29:265–273, 2004.

159. Flaumenhaft R, Kojima S, Abe M, et al: Activation of latent transforming growth factor β. Adv Pharmacol 24:51–76, 1993.

160. Ying SY: Inhibins, activins and follistatins. J Steroid Biochem 33:705–713, 1989.

161. Wozney JM: The bone morphogenetic protein family and osteogenesis. Mol Reprod Dev 32:160–167, 1992.

162. Sakou T: Bone morphogenetic proteins: From basic studies to clinical approaches. Bone 22:591–603, 1998.

163. Shibuya H, Yamagichi K, Shirakabe K, et al: TAB1: An activator of the TAK1 MAPKKK in TGF-β signal transduction. Science 272:1179–1182, 1996.

164. Wozney JM: The bone morphogenetic protein family: Multifunctional cellular regulators in the embryo and adult. Eur J Oral Sci 106:160–166, 1998.

165. Josso N, Cate RL, Picard JY, et al: Anti-mullerian hormone: The Jost factor. Recent Prog Horm Res 48:1–59, 1993.

166. Cheifetz S, Weatherbee JA, Tsang ML, et al: The transforming growth factor-beta system, a complex pattern of cross-reactive ligands and receptors. Cell 48:409–415, 1987.

167. Yamaguchi K, Shirakabe K, Shibuya H, et al: Identification of a member of the MAPKKK family as a potential mediator of TGF-beta signal transduction. Science 270:2008–2011, 1995.

168. McPherron AC, Lee SJ: Double muscling in cattle due to mutations in the myostatin gene. Proc Natl Acad Sci U S A 94:12457–12461, 1997.

169. Letterio JJ, Geiser AG, Kulkarni AB, et al: Maternal rescue of transforming growth factor-β1 null mice. Science 264:1936–1938, 1994.

170. Sanford LP, Ormsby I, Gittenberger-de Groot AC, et al: TGFbeta2 knockout mice have multiple developmental defects that are non-overlapping with other TGFbeta knockout phenotypes. Development 124:2659–2670, 1997.

171. Shull MM, Ormsby I, Kier AB, et al: Targeted disruption of the mouse transforming growth factor-beta 1 gene results in multifocal inflammatory disease. Nature 359:639–644, 1992.

172. Kulkarni AB, Huh CG, Becker D, et al: Transforming growth factor beta 1 null mutation in mice causes excessive inflammatory response and early death. Proc Natl Acad Sci U S A 90:770–774, 1993.

173. Border WA, Nobel NA: Transforming growth factor β in tissue fibrosis. N Engl J Med 331:1286–1292, 1994.

174. Ziyadeh FN: Mediators of diabetic renal disease: The case for TGF-β as the major mediator. J Am Soc Nephrol 15(Suppl 1):S55–S57, 2004.

175. Markowitz S, Wang J, Myeroff L, et al: Inactivation of the type II TGF-β receptor in colon cancer cells with microsatellite instability. Science 268:1336–1338, 1995.

176. Hahn SA, Schutte M, Hoque AT, et al: DPC4, a candidate tumor suppressor gene at human chromosome 18q21.1. Science 271:350–353, 1996.

177. Eppert K, Scherer SW, Ozcelik H, et al: MADR2 maps to 18q21 and encodes a TGFbeta-regulated MAD-related protein that is functionally mutated in colorectal carcinoma. Cell 86:543–552, 1996.

178. McAllister KA, Grogg KM, Johnson DW, et al: Endoglin, a TGF-beta binding protein of endothelial cells, is the gene for hereditary haemorrhagic telangiectasia type 1. Nat Genet 8:345–351, 1994.

179. McAllister KA, Baldwin MA, Thukkani AK, et al: Six novel mutations in the endoglin gene in hereditary hemorrhagic telangiectasia type 1 suggest a dominant-negative effect of receptor function. Hum Mol Genet 4:1983–1985, 1995.

180. Johnson DW, Berg JN, Baldwin MA, et al: Mutations in the activin receptor-like kinase 1 gene in hereditary haemorrhagic telangiectasia type 2. Nat Genet 13:189–185, 1996.

181. Polinkovsky A, Robin NH, Thomas JT, et al: Mutations in CDMP1 cause autosomal dominant brachdactyly type C. Nat Genet 17:18–19, 1997.

182. Storm EE, Huynh TV, Copeland NG, et al: Limb alterations in brachypodism mice due to mutations in a new member of the TGF beta-superfamily. Nature 368:639–643, 1994.

183. Kinoshita A, Saito T, Tomita H, et al: Domain-specific mutations in TGFB1 result in Camurati-Engelmann disease. Nat Genet 26:19–20, 2000.

184. Serra R, Chang C: TGF-beta signaling in human skeletal and patterning disorders. Birth Defects Res Part C Embryo Today 69:333–351, 2003.

185. Nakamura T, Teramoto H, Ichihara A: Purification and characterization of a growth factor from rat platelets for mature parenchymal hepatocytes in primary cultures. Proc Natl Acad Sci U S A 83:6489–6493, 1986.

186. Stoker M, Gherardi E, Perryman M, et al: Scatter factor is a fibroblast-derived modulator of epithelial cell motility. Nature 327:239–242, 1987.

187. Bottaro DP, Rubin JS, Faletto DL, et al: Identification of the hepatocyte growth factor receptor as the c-met proto-oncogene product. Science 251:802–804, 1991.

188. Trusolino L, Pugliese L, Comoglio PM: Interactions between scatter factors and the receptors: Hints for therapeutic applications. FASEB J 12:1267–1280, 1998.

189. Bertotti A, Comoglio PM: Tyrosine kinase signal specificity: lessons from the HGF receptor. Trends Biochem Sci 28:527–533, 2003.

190. Rosario M, Birchmeier W: How to make tubes: Signaling by the Met receptor tyrosine kinase. Trends Cell Biol 13:328–335, 2003.

191. Danilkovitch-Miagkova A, Zbar B: Dysregulation of Met receptor tyrosine kinase activity in invasive tumors. J Clin Invest 109:863–867, 2002.

192. Chirgadze DY, Hepple J, Byrd RA, et al: Insights into the structure of hepatocyte growth factor/scatter factor (HGF/SF) and implications for receptor activation. FEBS Lett 430:126–129, 1998.

193. Maggiora P, Gambarotta G, Olivero M, et al: Control of invasive growth by the HGF receptor family. J Cell Physiol 173:183–186, 1997.

194. Balkovetz DF, Lipschutz JH: Hepatocyte growth factor and the kidney: It is not just for the liver. Int Rev Cytol 186:225–260, 1999.

195. Skeel A, Yoshimura T, Showalter SD, et al: Macrophage stimulating protein: Purification, partial amino acid sequence, and cellular activity. J Exp Med 173:1227–1234, 1991.

196. Gaudino G, Follenzi A, Naldini L, et al: RON is a heterodimeric tyrosine kinase receptor activated by the HGF homologue MSP. EMBO J 13:3524–3532, 1994.

197. Hayman MJ, Kitchener G, Vogt PK, et al: The putative transforming protein of S13 avian erythroblastosis virus is a transmembrane glycoprotein with an associated protein kinase activity. Proc Natl Acad Sci U S A 82:8237–8241, 1985.

198. Schmidt C, Bladt F, Goedecke E, et al: Scatter factor/hepatocyte growth factor is essential for liver development. Nature 373:699–702, 1995.

199. Uehara Y, Minowa O, Mori C, et al: Placental defect and embryonal lethality in mice lacking hepatocyte growth factor/scatter factor. Nature 373:702–705, 1995.

200. Bladt F, Riethmacher D, Isenmann S, et al: Essential role for the c-met receptor in the migration of myogenic precursor cells into the limb bud. Nature 376:768–771, 1995.

201. Liu Y: Hepatocyte growth factor in kidney fibrosis: Therapeutic potential and mechanisms of action. Am J Physiol Renal Physiol 287:F7–F16, 2004.

202. Takahashi M, Ota S, Shimda T, et al: Hepatocyte growth factor is the most potent endogenous stimulant of rabbit gastric epithelial cell proliferation and migration in primary culture. J Clin Invest 95:1994–2003, 1995.

203. Ueki T, Kaneda Y, Tsustui H, et al: Hepatocyte growth factor gene therapy of liver cirrhosis in rats. Nat Med 5:226–230, 1999.

204. Carrolo M, Giordano S, Cabrita-Santos L, et al: Hepatocyte growth factor and its receptor are required for malaria infection. Nat Med 9:1363–1369, 2003.

205. Ferrara N, Davis-Smyth T: The biology of vascular endothelial growth factor. Endocr Rev 18:4–25, 1997.

206. Ferrara N, Gerber HP, LeCouter J: The biology of VEGF and its receptors. Nat Med 9:669–676, 2003.

207. Luttun A, Autiero M, Tjwa M, et al: Genetic dissection of tumor angiogenesis: Are PlGF and VEGFR-1 novel anti-cancer targets? Biochim Biophys Acta 1654:79–94, 2004.

208. Frank RN: Diabetic retinopathy. N Engl J Med 350:48–58, 2004.

209. Maglione D, Guerrerio V, Viglietto G, et al: Isolation of a human placenta cDNA coding for a protein related to the vascular permeability factor. Proc Natl Acad Sci U S A 88:9267–9271, 1991.

210. Hauser S, Weich HA: A heparin-binding form of placenta growth factor (PlGF-2) is expressed in human umbilical vein endothelial cells and in placenta. Growth Factors 9:259–268, 1993.

211. Olofsson B, Pajusola K, Kaipainen A, et al: Vascular endothelial growth factor B, a novel growth factor for endothelial cells. Proc Natl Acad Sci U S A 93:2576–2581, 1996.

212. Grimmond S, Lagencrantz J, Drinkwater C, et al: Cloning and characterization of a human gene related to vascular endothelial growth factor. Genome Res 6:124–131, 1996.

213. Joukov V, Kaipainen A, Jeltsch M, et al: Vascular endothelial growth factors VEGF-B and VEGF-C. J Cell Physiol 173:211–215, 1997.

214. Joukov V, Pajusola K, Kaipainen A, et al: A novel vascular endothelial growth factor, VEGF-C, is a ligand for the FLT (VEGFR-3) and KDR (VEGFR-2) receptor tyrosine kinases. EMBO J 15:290–298, 1996.

215. Achen MG, Jeltsch M, Kukk E, et al: Vascular endothelial growth factor D (VEGF-D) is a ligand for the tyrosine kinases VEGF receptor 2 (Flk1) and VEGF receptor 3 (Flt4). Proc Natl Acad Sci U S A 95:548–553, 1998.

216. Cross MJ, Dixelius J, Matsumoto T, et al: VEGF-receptor signal transduction. Trends Biochem Sci 28:488–494, 2003.

217. Jakeman LB, Winer J, Bennett GL, et al: Binding sites for vascular endothelial growth factor are localized on endothelial cells in adult rat tissues. J Clin Invest 89:244–253, 1992.

218. Jakeman LB, Armanini M, Phillips HS, et al: Developmental expression of binding sites and mRNA for vascular endothelial growth factor suggests a role for this protein in vasculogenesis and angiogenesis. Endocrinology 133:848–859, 1993.

219. Fong G-H, Rossant J, Gertenstein M, et al: Role of Flt-1 receptor tyrosine kinase in regulation of assembly of vascular endothelium. Nature 376:66–67, 1995.

220. Shalabi F, Rossant J, Yamaguchi TP, et al: Failure of blood island formation and vasculogenesis in Flk-1 deficient mice. Nature 376:62–66, 1995.

221. Dumont DJ, Jussila L, Taipale J, et al: Cardiovascular failure in mouse embryos deficient in VEGF receptor-3. Science 282:946–949, 1998.

222. Hiratsuka S, Minowa O, Kuno J, et al: Flt-1 lacking the tyrosine kinase domain is sufficient for normal development and angiogenesis in mice. Proc Natl Acad Sci U S A 95:9349–9354, 1998.

223. Carmeliat P, Ferreira V, Breier G, et al: Abnormal blood vessel development and lethality in embryos lacking a single VEGF allele. Nature 380:435–439, 1996.

224. Ferrara N, Carvermoore K, Chen H, et al: Heterozygous embryonic lethality induced by targeted inactivation of the VEGF gene. Nature 380:439–442, 1996.

225. Carmeliet P, Moons L, Luttun A, et al: Synergism between vascular endothelial growth factor and placental growth factor contributes to angiogenesis and plasma extravasation in pathological conditions. Nat Med 7:575–583, 2001.

226. Bellomo D, Headrick JP, Silins GU, et al: Mice lacking the vascular endothelial growth factor-B gene (vegfb) have smaller hearts, dysfunctional coronary vasculature, and impaired recovery from cardiac ischemia. Circ Res 86:E29–E35, 2000.

227. Leung DW, Cachianes G, Kuang W-J, et al: Vascular endothelial growth factor is secreted angiogenic mitogen. Science 246:1306–1309, 1989.

228. Wilting J, Christ B, Weich HA: The effects of growth factors on the day 13 chorioallantoic membrane (CAM): A study of VEGF165 and PDGF-BB. Anat Embryol 186:251–257, 1992.

229. Takeshita S, Zheng LP, Brogi E, et al: Therapeutic angiogenesis. J Clin Invest 59:662–670, 1994.

230. Senger DR, Galli SJ, Dvorak AM, et al: Tumor cells secrete a vascular permeability factor that promotes accumulation of ascites fluid. Science 219:983–985, 1983.

231. Connolly DT, Olander JV, Heuvelman D, et al: Human vascular permeability factor. Isolation from U937 cells. J Biol Chem 254:20017–20024, 1989.

232. Dvorak HF, Harvey VS, Estrella P, et al: Fibrin containing gels induce angiogenesis: Implications for tumor stroma generation and wound healing. Lab Invest 57:673–686, 1987.

233. Kim KJ, Li B, Winer J, et al: Inhibition of vascular endothelial growth factor-induced angiogenesis suppresses tumor growth in vivo. Nature 362:841–844, 1993.

234. Millauer B, Shawver LK, Plate KH, et al: Glioblastoma growth is inhibited in vivo by a negative dominant Flk-1 mutant. Nature 367:576–579, 1994.

235. Millauer B, Longhi MP, Plate KH, et al: Dominant-negative inhibition of Flk-1 suppresses the growth of many tumor types in vivo. Cancer Res 56:1615–1162, 1996.

236. Holash J, Davis S, Papadopoulos N, et al: VEGF-Trap: A VEGF blocker with potent antitumor effects. Proc Natl Acad Sci U S A 99:11393–11398, 2002.

237. Kabbinavar F, Hurwitz HI, Fehrenbacher L, et al: Phase II, randomized trial comparing bevacizumab plus fluorouracil (FU)/leucovorin (LV) with FU/LV alone

in patients with metastatic colorectal cancer. J Clin Oncol 21:60–65, 2003.

238. Yang JC, Haworth L, Sherry RM, et al: A randomized trial of bevacizumab, an anti-vascular endothelial growth factor antibody, for metastatic renal cancer. N Engl J Med 349:427–434, 2003.

239. Krzystolik MG, Afshari MA, Adamis AP, et al: Prevention of experimental choroidal neovascularization with intravitreal anti-vascular endothelial growth factor antibody fragment. Arch Ophthalmol 120:338–346, 2002.

240. LeCouter J, Kowalski J, Foster J, et al: Identification of an angiogenic mitogen selective for endocrine gland endothelium. Nature 412:877–884, 2001.

241. Ferrara N, LeCouter J, Lin R, et al: EG-VEGF and Bv8: A novel family of tissue-restricted angiogenic factors. Biochim Biophys Acta 1654:69–78, 2004.

Somatic Growth and Maturation

Leona Cuttler and Robert L. Rosenfield

Growth is an inherent property of life. Normal somatic growth requires the integrated function of many of the hormonal, metabolic, and other growth factors discussed in preceding chapters. This chapter first briefly reviews the determinants of growth. Then it deals in detail with the overall result of these processes—normal patterns of linear growth. Finally, the differential diagnosis and management of disorders of growth are discussed.

DETERMINANTS OF NORMAL GROWTH

CELLULAR GROWTH

Normal growth requires an intrinsically normal cell that is nourished by an optimal milieu (with respect to pH, trace minerals, and substrates for structural and energy purposes) and exposed to the necessary growth factors. It is regulated by the same molecular mechanisms that determine physiologic responses in the mature cell.

The body grows primarily through proliferation of cells by mitosis.[1,2] Increase in cell size generally plays more of a role in organ growth as development approaches completion. Growth factors and other environmental signals affect cell division by modulating passage through the first phase of the mitotic cell cycle (G_1).[3,4] The first subphase of G_1 requires "competence factors," such as fibroblast growth factor, which induce cells to become competent to synthesize DNA. Cells then require essential amino acids to progress to a critical point in the cycle at which "progression factors" can induce completion of G_1. Progression factors are exemplified by insulin-like growth factors (IGFs), insulin, thyroxine, and hydrocortisone. Growth factors modulate the internal regulatory pathways governed by cyclins and cyclin-dependent kinases (CDKs), which are *proto-oncogenes*, and CDK inhibitors (CDKI), which are *tumor suppressors*. The balance between cyclin, CDK, and CDKI activity determines the start of DNA synthesis (S phase of the cell cycle). From this point onward, cell-cycle processes depend entirely on intracellularly triggered controls involving cyclins. After completing DNA synthesis, the cell finishes doubling its entire contents (G_2 phase) and then undergoes the M phase of the cycle during which cell division is completed.

The cell cycle is to a great extent regulated by nuclear factor-κB (NF-κB).[5] This transcription factor is held inactive in the cytoplasm when bound to its inhibitory partner Iκβ. When Iκβ undergoes regulated serine phosphorylation, it is polyubiquinated, which targets it for degradation with the proteosome. This releases NF-κB to move to the nucleus, where it promotes cell-cycle progression and inhibits programmed cell death (apoptosis).

During each mitotic cycle, a portion of the terminal end (the telomere) of each chromosome is lost, which eventually shortens the chromosome to the point where cell proliferation becomes impossible and the cell dies.[6] The enzyme telomerase supports the synthesis of telomeric DNA, which maintains telomere length and proliferative potential. Telomerase is present in somatic cells of the fetus, permitting continued growth. With maturation of the fetus, however, telomerase levels begin to fall and decline progressively with aging, limiting mortality.

SOMATIC GROWTH

Prenatal Growth

Prenatal and postnatal requirements for growth differ in several respects. Embryonic growth is primarily determined by genetic programming of local sequential inductions.[7] Coordination of cell differentiation and morphogenesis requires a class of developmental genes belonging to the homeobox family.[8–10] Homeobox genes encode transcription factors that bind DNA, thereby controlling gene expression, cell differentiation, and organ development. Abnormalities of several homeobox genes are known to cause organ malformations and to affect linear growth (see Chapter 16). Fetal growth depends heavily on the delivery of nutrients, metabolic substrates, and oxygen from the mother. The placenta regulates these as well as contributes to the fetal nutritional and hormonal milieu.[11–13] Placental size is a determinant of fetal growth, and placental growth is itself influenced by genomic factors,[13,14] maternal nutrition (perhaps via leptin),[15,16] and uterine blood flow. Placental regulation of fetal blood flow is, in turn, a determinant of growth; the discordance in size of monozygous twins has been attributed to the unequal distribution of blood flow that results from placental arteriovenous anastomoses.[17]

Both placental growth and function involve hormones. Specific deletion of placental IGF-2, which is an imprinted gene expressed from the paternal allele, sequentially reduces placental growth, decreases nutrient delivery, and restricts fetal growth.[13] The placenta also influences fetal growth through its elaboration of hormones. For example, human placental lactogen seems to influence regulation of fetal IGF-1.[18] There is evidence that leptin, produced by the placenta or fetal tissues, regulates fetal growth.[16] Umbilical cord leptin appears to be an index of fetal nutrition in humans, and correlates with birth size independent of IGF-1.[16,19] Familial and environmental variables that correlate with birth size independent of gestational age include maternal weight, sibling birth weight, parity, altitude, and, inversely, uterine constraints, such as the number of fetuses carried.[20-25]

Some of the hormonal requirements for fetal growth differ from those regulating postnatal growth. Prenatal growth is less dependent on GH and thyroxine. Individuals with congenital GH deficiency or resistance often have normal birth length, although in large population studies average birth length is reduced by 1 standard deviation (SD).[11,26] Similarly, newborns with congenital hypothyroidism typically have normal birth size, although their bone maturation lags during the last trimester.[27]

The IGF system affects prenatal as well as postnatal growth, although specific influences and regulatory components differ according to stage of development. Immunoreactive IGF is present in most fetal tissues. Rodent models lacking IGF-1, IGF-2, or the IGF-1 receptor have reduced birth weights, suggesting a role for both IGF-1 and IGF-2 in prenatal growth.[28-31] Such models also indicate that IGF-2 is equal in importance to IGF-1 for fetal growth, each contributing about 33%.[31,32] The IGF-1 receptor mediates all of the IGF-1 effect and 90% of the IGF-2 effect, the insulin receptor about 10%. Whereas animals lacking IGF-2 that survive may have relatively normal postnatal growth, those with IGF-1 deficiency remain stunted, indicating another distinction between prenatal and postnatal regulation of growth. There is evidence that, during fetal life, IGF-1 is relatively independent of GH and regulated greatly by nutritional status (particularly glucose availability and the consequent fetal insulin secretion) and placental lactogen.[7,11,18,26] Although the serum IGF level is even lower prenatally than in infancy, it rises during gestation and correlates with size at birth.[11] IGF-2 blood levels are higher than those of IGF-1 in utero, in contrast to postnatal life. Human correlates, substantiating the role of IGFs in prenatal growth, are the identification of a patient with homozygous partial deletion of the gene encoding IGF-1 and identification of patients with IGF-1 receptor mutations with severe intrauterine growth retardation as well as postnatal growth failure.[33]

In addition to IGFs, insulin influences fetal growth. Infants of diabetic mothers and children with Beckwith-Weidemann syndrome (with hyperinsulinism) have excessive fetal growth, while those with pancreatic agenesis have poor fetal growth.

Sex hormones may also play a subtle role in normal fetal growth: Plasma levels of testosterone, estradiol, and dehydroepiandrosterone are at or above pubertal levels by midgestation; estrogen promotes fetal bone development[34]; and androgen action seems to account for the greater birth weight of boys compared to girls.[7,26]

The embryologic development of the pituitary gland and placental physiology are discussed further in Chapters 16 and 181.

Understanding the regulation of fetal growth has assumed particular importance because of potential links between prenatal growth and later disease. There is strong experimental evidence in animal models to indicate that an adverse fetal environment, as reflected in birth size, can lead to a poor health outcome in adults.[35] Mechanisms as diverse in origin as undernutrion or glucocorticoid exposure have similar deleterious effects on such cardiovascular risk factors as blood pressure and glucose tolerance. Considerable human data support such a "fetal origins of adult disease" model.[36] Animal and human data are compatible with a model that proposes that diverse prenatal insults cause a significant defect in placental inactivation of maternal cortisol due to decreased 11β-hydroxysteroid dehydrogenase activity, leading to elevated fetal cortisol, which, in turn, is responsible for intrauterine growth retardation (IUGR) and reprogramming of the hypothalamic-pituitary-adrenal axis for hyperresponsiveness to stress.[37] Cortisol excess, in turn, has been proposed to

predispose to features of the metabolic (insulin-resistance) syndrome.[37-41] Some data suggest that catch-up growth by mid-childhood, particularly excess weight gain, seems to worsen the outcome with respect to glucose intolerance.[38-40,42] On the other hand, the fetal origins model has been hotly disputed.[36,43-45] Alternatively, polymorphisms in the IGF-1 gene and the vitamin D receptor have been claimed to account for some of the associations between fetal size and various adverse adult outcomes.[46,47]

Postnatal Growth

Genetic determinants exist for both prenatal and postnatal growth.[48] Some of the determinants for bone growth reside on the sex chromosomes. Genes on the Y chromosome seem to enhance stature commencing in antenatal life.[48,49] The X chromosome clearly carries genetic determinants that promote linear growth and regulate body proportions.[48,50] Recently, several clusters of autosomal genes were found to be involved in growth because they behave differently when they come from the mother than when from the father. This is because of the epigenetic process of genomic imprinting, which, like X-inactivation, is due to genes being methylated to silence them.[14] Although the exact nature of most imprinted genes is unknown, the IGF-2 and IGF-2 receptor genes on chromosome 15 are known to be imprinted. The IGF-2 gene is silenced in eggs and, thus, in the maternal contribution to the embryo's genome ("maternal imprinting"). The IGF-2 receptor is imprinted the opposite way; it is paternally imprinted, that is, only the gene derived from the mother's egg is expressed.

The axial and appendicular skeleton account for the vast majority of postnatal linear growth. These bones are formed by endochondral ossification, which commences with chondrocytes of the epiphyses laying down an orderly cartilage template, which osteoblasts then convert to bone.[51-53] The cranium and some of the clavicle are formed by direct intramembranous ossification. The cycle of bone cell remodeling for structural purposes is closely linked to the overall metabolic needs for calcium and phosphorus homeostasis, primarily by the actions of parathormone and calciferol. Chondrocyte proliferation is inhibited by parathyroid hormone–related protein (PTHrP) and fibroblast growth factor (FGF) paracrine signaling mediated through the PTH receptor and FGF receptor 3 (FGFR3). This effect is opposed by Indian hedgehog signaling, which operates in a negative feedback loop with PTHrP. The natriuretic factor system, particularly involving the C type, similarly appears to play a local role in endochondral ossification, in this case as positive regulators.[54,55]

Nutrition and metabolism must be adequate for normal growth. Adult height has been used as a marker for the nutritional status of populations during childhood and has been shown to relate to cognitive function.[56,57] Calories seem particularly critical for cell multiplication. Two percent to 13% of normal energy consumption goes into promoting growth.[1,58] Protein intake is particularly important for normal growth in cellular size. It must be adequate with respect to both amount and provision of essential amino acids or their ketoanalogues.[59-61] Essential fatty acids are necessary for normal growth in lower animals, but this may not hold true for primates.[62] Vitamins A and D are important for normal growth.[1,63] Trace metals, such as zinc and copper, are probably essential for normal growth and sexual maturation[64-67] because of their role as cofactors for enzyme function. The pH must be maintained at optimal levels to conserve mineral homeostasis.[68]

The general level of *activity* seems to promote overall body growth, just as normal muscular activity is necessary for limb growth. The mechanism is unclear; it may be related to neural trophic factors or blood flow. The efficiency of nitrogen accretion and growth are decreased in inactive rats.[69]

Hormones are essential "catalysts" of growth. Under normal circumstances, the growth hormone (GH)-IGF system, thyroid hormone, and sex steroids are fundamental regulators of linear growth.

Growth hormone (GH) ontogeny, biology, and secretion are reviewed in detail Chapter 32. A complex interplay of extracellular peptides and intracellular transcription factors and signaling systems governs the development of the hypothalamic and pituitary GH secretory system.[70,71] Pituitary secretion of GH is normally under the immediate control of hypothalamic hormones: somatostatin, which inhibits its release; and growth hormone releasing hormone (GHRH). GHRH stimulates GH synthesis as well as secretion. Defects in GHRH synthesis or action stunt growth in mouse models, and humans with a defect in the GHRH receptor similarly show growth failure,[72] attesting to the fundamental importance of GHRH in GH secretion and growth.

The balance between GHRH and somatostatin is determined by a complex flux of input from higher cerebral centers, which mediate nutritional, metabolic, and endocrine signals (Fig. 36-1).[73–81] Diverse neurotransmitters are involved; they include acetylcholine, galanin, and neuropeptide Y. Dopamine is inhibitory to GH release in the newborn period.[82]

Endocrine input includes the recently discovered endogenous GH secretagogue (GHS) ghrelin, an orexigenic peptide originating in the stomach and hypothalamus. Ghrelin stimulates GH release, primarily through promoting GHRH release, but also by acting directly on the pituitary, through specific receptors (GHSR). In addition, there is negative feedback on GH secretion by circulating IGF-1, which is primarily of hepatic origin, and glucose levels.[83,84]

GH secretion is also influenced by androgens and estrogen (which appear responsible for the rise in GH secretion during normal puberty), as well as by thyroxine and glucocorticoids (hypothyroidism and cortisol excess reduce GH secretion).

After secretion, GH is approximately 50% bound to GH-binding protein (GHBP). GHBP rises through childhood.[85] It is the extracellular domain of the GH receptor (GHR), its underlying alternate splicing may be differentially regulated from the intact GHR.[86] GHR is a member of the cytokine family. One molecule of GH binds to two GHR molecules, indicating receptor dimerization, which is critical for GH action. (This leads to activation of a receptor-associated Janus tyrosine kinase [JAK-2] and, in turn, transduction through a number of pathways, including the MAPK [mitogen-activated protein kinase] and STAT [signal transducers and activators of transcription] pathways.) These paths result in activation of genes (including IGF-1) that mediate GH's biologic effects. Abnormalities of the GHR and its signaling system result in GH insensitivity and growth failure (see discussion to follow). GH-activated intracellular signaling is illustrated in Figure 36-2.[87]

GH appears to stimulate growth by a combination of direct effects and effects mediated by IGFs.[88] It stimulates the production of endocrine IGF-1 and its major binding protein (IGFBP-3). It also directly induces the clonal expansion and differentiation of target stem cells (such as prechondrocytes), and these differentiating cells (chondrocytes) then respond to GH by forming IGF-1 and IGF-1 receptors, which makes them responsive to the growth-promoting effect of both endocrine IGF-1 and IGFs secreted locally (autocrine and paracrine IGFs).[89,90]

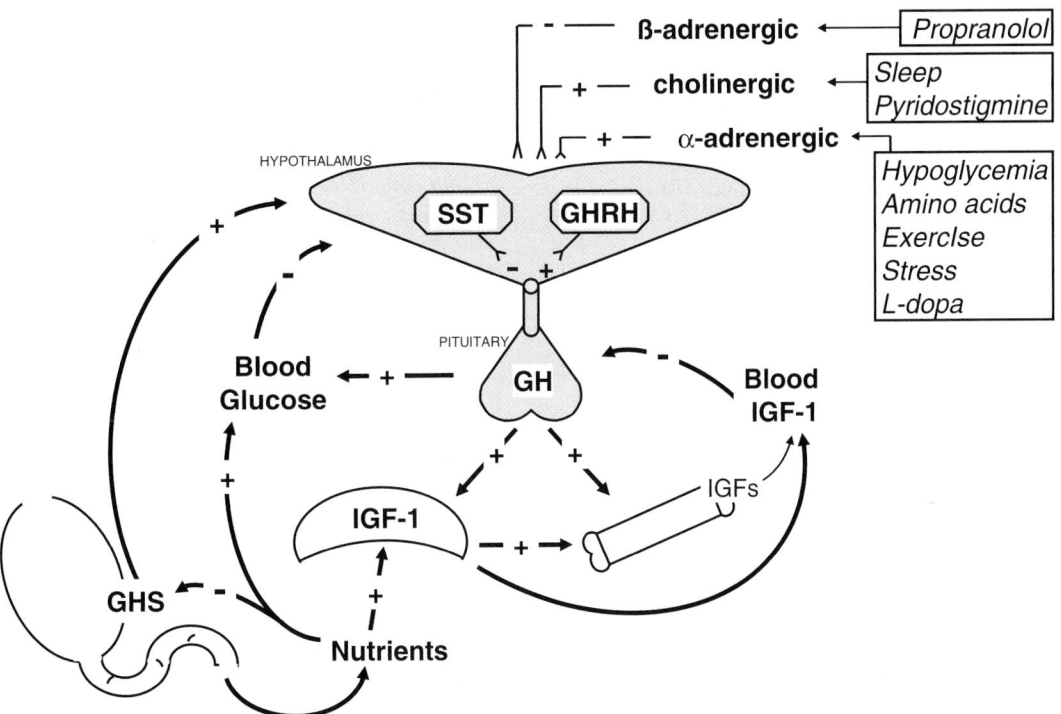

Figure 36-1 GH regulatory axis: Major factors regulating growth hormone (GH) release. GH is secreted after the integration of diverse hypothalamic stimuli. It stimulates insulin-like growth factor 1 (IGF-1) production by the liver, bone, and other tissues, as well as gluconeogenesis. GH release from the pituitary gland is under tonic inhibition by hypothalamic somatostatin, and GH-releasing hormone (GHRH) stimulates GH release when somatostatin (SST) tone wanes due to fluctuations in input from higher neural centers. Ghrelin is an endogenous GH secretagogue (GHS) and orexogenic peptide mainly secreted by the stomach in response to fasting. Its major effect on GH is indirectly to antagonize SST release at the level of the hypothalamus. Small amounts of GHS are formed in the hypothalamus, however, and weakly stimulate GHRH release directly; neonatally, GHS pituitary expression is high. SST tone is inhibited by cholinergic, dopaminergic, and α-adrenergic neuronal inputs to the hypothalamus and stimulated by β-adrenergic ones. Negative feedback effects are exerted primarily by the long-loop actions of blood glucose and IGF-1, but also by short-loop signals between the various signal peptides of the axis. IGF-1 and blood glucose also exert negative feedback effects on GH release. Pharmacologic stimuli to GH release are shown in boxes. *Solid lines* indicate major regulatory pathways, *dotted lines* minor ones. +, stimulator of GH, GHS, or IGF-1 release; −, inhibitor of GH, GHS, or IGF-1 release.

IGF-1, produced by the liver and other tissues, is a critical regulator of postnatal growth and represents a major mechanism by which GH promotes growth. Circulating IGF-binding proteins (IGFBPs) sequester IGFs, whereas at the cell surface they can promote IGF action and exert novel actions.[91] The IGFs and IGF-binding proteins are discussed in detail in Chapter 34. Defects in IGF-1 synthesis or action lead to growth failure in humans as well as laboratory animals. The effects of IGF-1 may depend on the tissue of origin. Local production of IGF-1 in peripheral tissues appears to mediate GH-induced somatic growth, whereas circulating IGF-1, originating primarily in the liver, may not be essential for growth, but provides negative feedback for the GH axis.[90] The free (unbound) IGF-1 is thought to be the biologically active fraction of circulating IGF-1, but the validity of current assays for this moiety is in question.[92,93] IGF-1 production is primarily regulated by GH when nutrition is normal. IGF-2 is produced by cells independently of GH, and seems to be normally important only for local growth regulation.[94] IGF-2 levels seem to be modulated locally by the activity of a metabolizing receptor complex consisting of the IGF-2 receptor and glypican-3.[95]

There is more to the regulation of plasma IGF-1 concentrations and bioactivity than GH. Hepatic IGF-1, the major source of blood IGF-1, is fundamentally under broad regulation by nutrition. Undernutrition decreases plasma IGF-1 levels despite normal or elevated GH concentrations. Overnutrition (i.e., obesity) has the opposite effect.[73] Studies in rats suggest that insulin plays a role in mediating nutritional effects on hepatic IGF-1 formation through its stimulation of amino acid uptake.[96,97] The increased plasma-free IGF-1 concentration in obese patients has been attributed to the suppressive effect of their insulin excess on IGFBP-1.[98] Thyroid hormone and cortisol are necessary for hepatic IGF-1 production, and prolactin has a slight effect on it.[99]

Factors other than GH and nutrition—including age—determine IGF production, and these are poorly understood. Plasma IGF-1, IGFBP-3 levels,[100] and somatomedin activity[101] rise slowly during the prepubertal years without any change in GH production (Fig. 36-2).[102] As a result, IGF-1 levels in normal children younger than 5 years of age overlap with those of GH-deficient children, making use of these tests in diagnosing GH deficiency difficult in young children. During puberty, IGF-1 levels rise further, and since IGFBP-3 levels rise to a lesser degree, free-plasma IGF-1 rises even more markedly.[100] The pubertal increase in IGF-1 is mediated by sex hormone stimulation of GH secretion,[103–105] although a separate direct effect on IGF-1 has been suggested.[106] IGF-1 levels during adolescence, therefore, correlate more with pubertal development and bone age than with chronologic age.

The relationship of plasma IGF-1 levels to normal linear growth is not a simple one. Plasma IGF-1 levels do not correlate with growth rate in childhood except during the pubertal growth spurt.[107] IGFBPs in plasma determine the unbound concentration of IGF-1, transport the IGFs to target cells, and influence the interaction of IGFs with their receptors; a tissue IGFBP-protease system modulates IGF-1 bioavailability to target cells.[89,91,108,109] IGFBPs also appear to be bioactive molecules that have IGF-independent functions.[91,109] IGF bioactivity may also be influenced by circulating somatomedin inhibitory activity, which is attributable to both glucocorticoids and incompletely characterized peptides.[110,111] The cytokines interleukin-6 and tumor necrosis factor-α have direct inhibitory effects on chondrocytes.[112]

Growth may be normal with subnormal GH production in the poorly understood "growth without growth hormone syndrome."[113] Most often, this syndrome has been identified after treatment for pituitary tumors, but the syndrome has occasionally been recognized in benign forms of hypopituitarism.[114] IGF-1 levels may be low, but bioactivity normal. Most such patients are obese, so insulin excess or sensitivity has been suspected to be the underlying growth factor. Individual variation in local aromatase activity and thus availability of estrogen has also been suggested.[115] Hyperprolactinemia is seldom found.

Thyroid hormone is necessary for postnatal bone growth because of both indirect effects on the GH-IGF axis and direct effects on bone growth.[116] Thyroid hormone is required for normal GH secretion in response to GHRH and for normal GH action as indexed by GHBP, IGF, and IGFBP levels. Hypothyroidism (and, to a lesser degree, mutations of the thyroid receptor-β) produces short stature and delays bone maturation.

Glucocorticoids in above-normal amounts are inhibitors of linear growth.[111,117] The mechanism is both indirect and direct. Glucocorticoid excess inhibits spontaneous GH secretion by stimulating somatostatin tone. The bioactivity of plasma IGF-1 falls during glucocorticoid therapy; this may reflect an increase in IGF-binding protein.[118,119] Glucocorticoids themselves directly hinder cartilage growth,[120] perhaps in part by inhibiting GH and IGF-1 induction of their respective receptors.[121]

Increased secretion of *sex hormones* clearly initiates the pubertal growth spurt. The growth-promoting actions of sex hormones require adequate GH; GH-deficient children will not undergo a normal pubertal growth spurt unless GH is

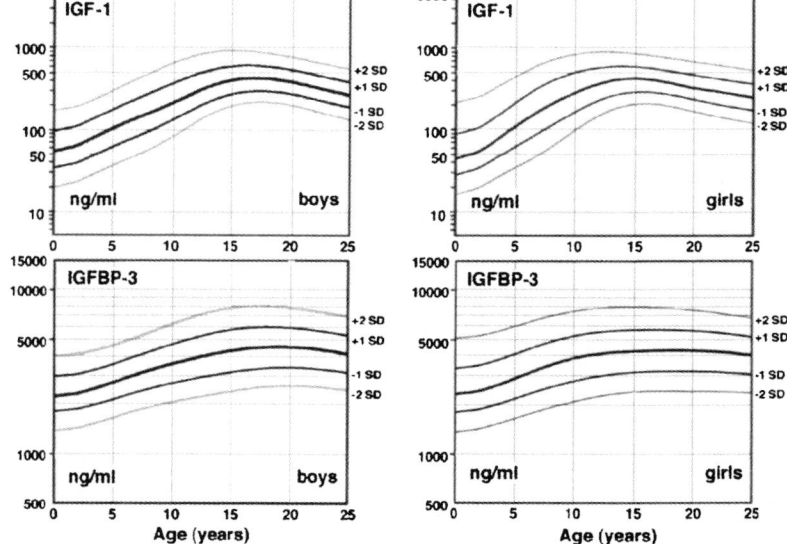

Figure 36-2 Plasma insulin-like growth factor 1 (IGF-1) and IGF-binding protein-3 (IGFBP-3) normal ranges from infancy to adulthood. The increases after 10 years of age are related to pubertal stage rather than age. IGF-1 values are given in terms of the World Health Organization reference preparation 87/518, which is of low (44%) purity with respect to authentic recombinant human IGF-1, so the values shown are in excess of the true IGF-1 concentration.[41] (Data from Diagnostic Systems Laboratories, 1997.)

replaced. About half of the contribution of sex hormones to the pubertal growth spurt is due to their stimulation of the GH-IGF axis, which appears to be primarily mediated by estrogen.[75,103,104,122] The remainder of the effects of sex steroids on growth is direct or mediated by a direct effect on IGF.[106,123–125]

Estrogen and androgen both stimulate bone growth, bone turnover, and epiphyseal growth.[106,126,127] Androgen appears to stimulate and estrogen to inhibit periosteal bone formation, while estrogen promotes greater cortical thickening. Estrogen is particularly effective in reducing bone turnover, however, and estrogens are responsible for epiphyseal closure.[128] To some extent, these effects may be exerted prenatally, since maternal estrogen can have permanent effects on fetal bone development.[129] Differences between these actions of sex hormones account for women's bones being shorter and narrower than men's.

Early pubertal amounts of estradiol (about 0.25 mg/month) stimulate growth in girls, in contrast to inhibition of growth on high doses of estrogen.[130] Peak growth velocity of boys occurs at a testosterone production rate of about 50 to 100 mg/month.[131] Whether other sex steroids play an independent role in growth is unknown; it has been reported that dehydroepiandrosterone sulfate promotes calcification of cartilage and subandrogenic doses of androstenedione promote growth.[34]

PATTERNS OF NORMAL SOMATIC GROWTH

INTRAUTERINE GROWTH

During the first trimester, tissue patterns and organ systems develop. In the second trimester, there is major cellular hyperplasia in the fetus and its growth velocity is maximal. During the third trimester, organ systems mature and weight gain is maximal.

Standards for intrauterine growth are shown in Figure 36-3.[132] Race, altitude, and gender cause subtle differences from these norms.[133] Fetal growth is more rapid than postnatal growth. The first fetal epiphyseal center to ossify is the calcaneous (at an average gestational age of 24 weeks), followed by the talus (28 weeks), distal femoral epiphysis (36 weeks), proximal tibial epiphysis (38 weeks), and cuboid (42 weeks).[134] Weight increases relatively more than length during the third trimester due to the accumulation of fat and muscle.

Healthy infants born prematurely have weights appropriate for gestational age and continue to grow at the same rate they would have grown in utero.[135] When corrected for postconceptional age, length and weight follow postnatal standards. Consequently, the lengths of children born prematurely remain slightly less through infancy than those of children born at term, but the differences become negligible with time. Very premature infants, however, require intensive care to survive and uniformly lose weight during the first weeks of life; it takes several years for the great majority to catch up to the weight and length of term infants, and females achieve more catch-up growth than males.[136,137] In contrast to premature infants, 10% to 15% of those born small for gestational age prove to have persistent short stature beyond 4 years of age[138] (see discussion to follow).

POSTNATAL GROWTH

Postnatal growth patterns of normal children are well characterized, resulting in several clinical parameters for assessment of growth.

1. *Linear growth* is assessed as supine *length* until 2 to 3 years of age (using a firm box with inflexible head board

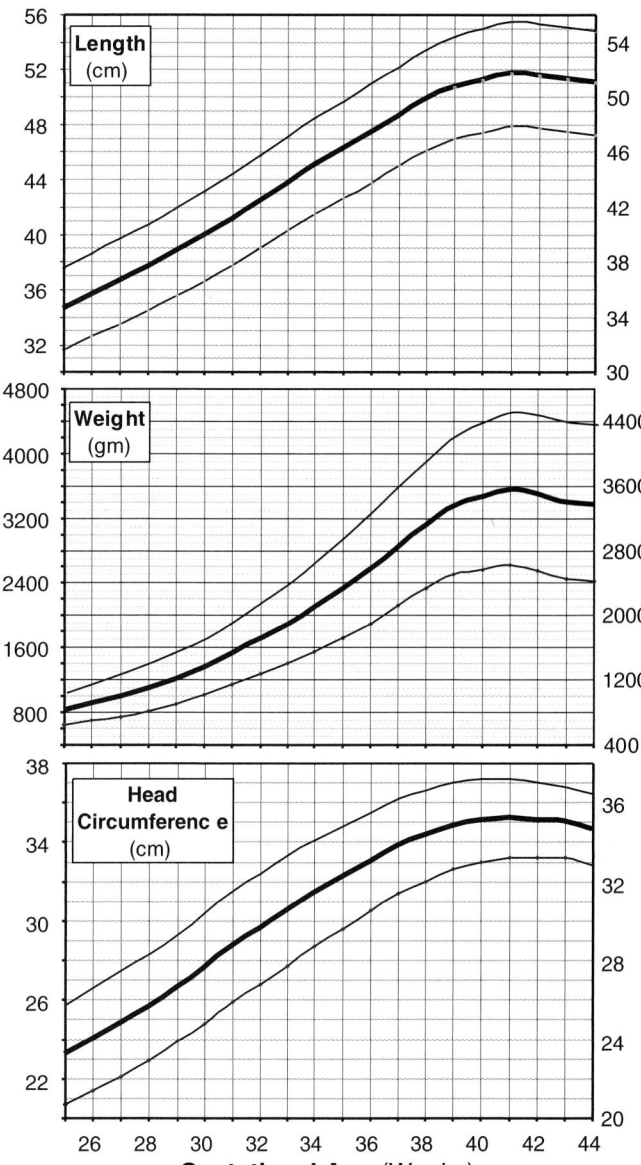

Figure 36-3 Intrauterine growth charts. Data represent birth weights according to gestational age of live-born Caucasian infants at sea level. Infants with major congenital malformations were excluded. (From Usher R, McLean F: Intrauterine growth of live-born Caucasian infants at sea level: Standards obtained from measurements in seven dimensions of infants born between 25 and 44 weeks of gestation. J Pediatr 74(6):901–910, 1969.)

and movable foot board) and, thereafter, as erect *height* measured using calibrated stadiometers. Stature is then plotted on growth charts. Traditionally, these linear growth standards have been derived from cross-sectional data as shown in Figure 36-4.[139] Since differences in the timing of puberty can influence normal growth rates, longitudinal growth charts are useful in sequential assessment of individual children.[140,141] Height SDs in relation to the mean for age and gender can be determined from the Centers for Disease Control and Prevention website.[139] Syndrome-specific growth charts have been developed for Turner's syndrome, Down syndrome, and achondroplasia.[142–144] There is a "secular trend" toward increasing height of populations with time in association with improvements in nutrition and health,[145] although the most recent U.S. data suggest little change in the past 25 years.

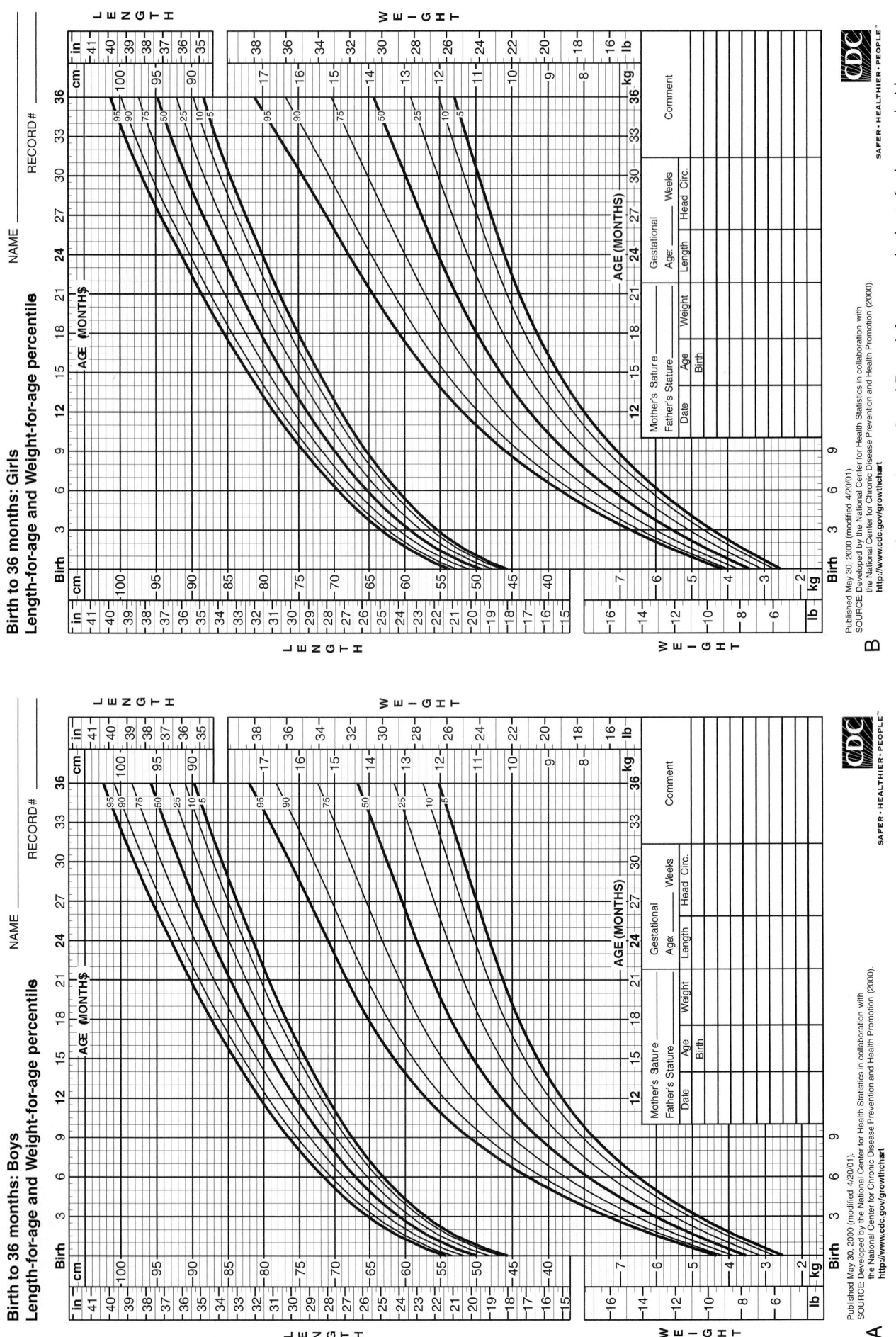

Birth to 36 months: Boys
Length-for-age and Weight-for-age percentile

NAME _____

RECORD # _____

Published May 30, 2000 (modified 4/20/01).
SOURCE: Developed by the National Center for Health Statistics in collaboration with
the National Center for Chronic Disease Prevention and Health Promotion (2000).
http://www.cdc.gov/growthchart

A

Birth to 36 months: Girls
Length-for-age and Weight-for-age percentile

NAME _____

RECORD # _____

Published May 30, 2000 (modified 4/20/01).
SOURCE: Developed by the National Center for Health Statistics in collaboration with
the National Center for Chronic Disease Prevention and Health Promotion (2000).
http://www.cdc.gov/growthchart

B

Figure 36-4 Postnatal growth standards. Current standards for height and weight of normal children in the United States. Figures **A** and **B** are infant growth charts for boys and girls, respectively.

702

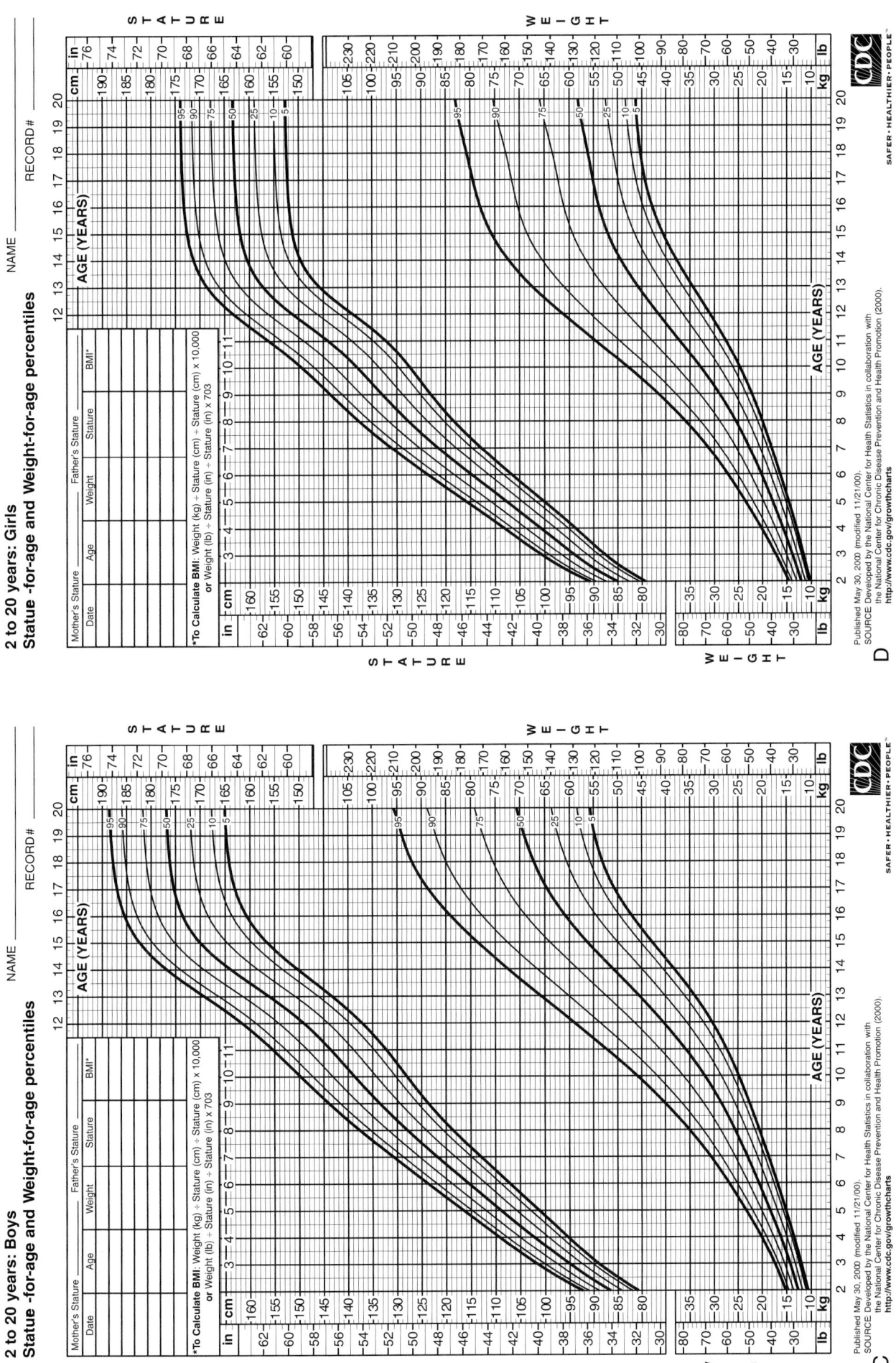

2 to 20 years: Boys
Statue -for-age and Weight-for-age percentiles

2 to 20 years: Girls
Statue -for-age and Weight-for-age percentiles

Figure 36-4, cont'd Figures **C** and **D** are for older boys and girls, respectively. (From Centers for Disease Control and Prevention. CDC growth charts: United States. National Center for Health Statistics. Available at: *http://www.cdc.gov/growthcharts/.* Accessed May 30, 2000; see Color Plate xx.)

2. *Weight and body mass index* (BMI; weight[kg]/height[cm]^2) are measured and plotted on appropriate growth charts.[139] Weight is a labile parameter relative to height, being sensitive to acute illnesses and short-term changes in feeding and activity patterns, as well as muscle mass. Whether nutrition is appropriate can be estimated by comparing a child's percentile position for weight with respect to height age or by calculating the BMI. During puberty, fat stores tend to increase slightly in girls and decrease in boys. The waist/hip ratio decreases during adolescence in girls due to a relatively great increase in hip circumference.[146]

3. *Growth velocity* is assessed from sequential height measurements, and can be plotted on growth velocity charts (Fig 36-5).[140,141] A minimum of 6 months' interval is needed for meaningful assessments of growth velocity. Growth occurs in three phases—infantile, childhood, and pubertal—which each have distinct characteristics.[147] Linear growth velocity is most rapid in infancy, averaging 15 cm/year in the first 2 years of life. Two thirds of infants cross percentile channels on the linear growth curves.[148] The growth of infants seems to result from an initial steep vector, which is generated by the GH- and thyroxine-independent cell proliferation that uniquely drives intrauterine growth, superimposed on a shallow vector, which is dependent on the endocrine factors that determine subsequent growth during childhood.

4. *Growth patterns*: In childhood, after infancy until puberty begins, growth normally proceeds along a channel that closely corresponds to a given height-attained percentile on cross-sectional growth standards. A child normally establishes this channel by 2 to 3 years of age,[148] although, on rare occasions, a gradual drift by as many as 40 percentile positions in height attained may occur over a period of several years in normal children.[149] These channels have a slightly decelerating velocity that averages about 6 cm per year in mid-childhood (see Fig. 36-5).[141] However, normal children cross height-velocity percentiles to maintain their height-attained channel (Fig. 36-6).[140,150,151] Growth consistently along the third percentile for height velocity will lead to a subnormal height.

The growth channel seems to be genetically determined. Children grow as if to reach a genetically predetermined

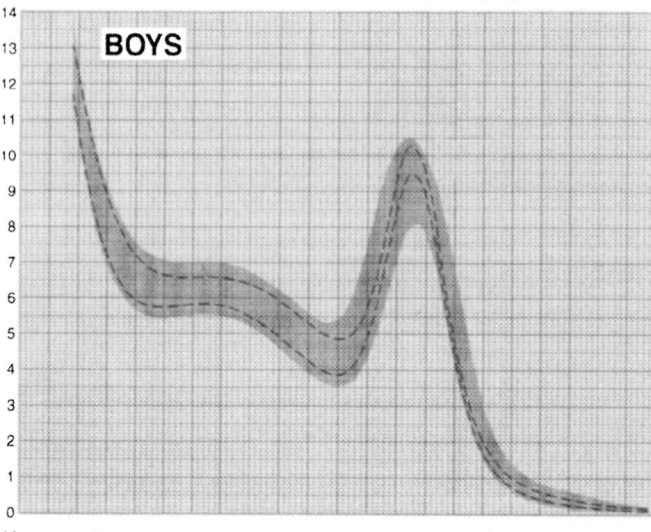

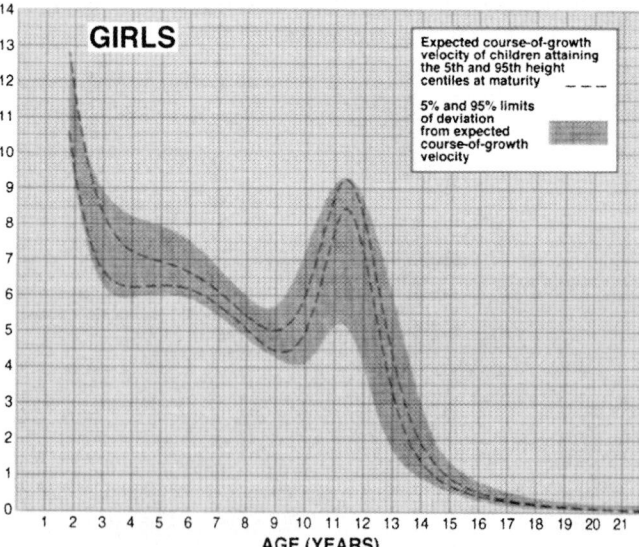

HEIGHT VELOCITY (cm/yr)

Figure 36-5 Longitudinal height velocity standards derived from the Fels, Berkely, and Denver growth studies.[141] (Courtesy of RD Bock.)

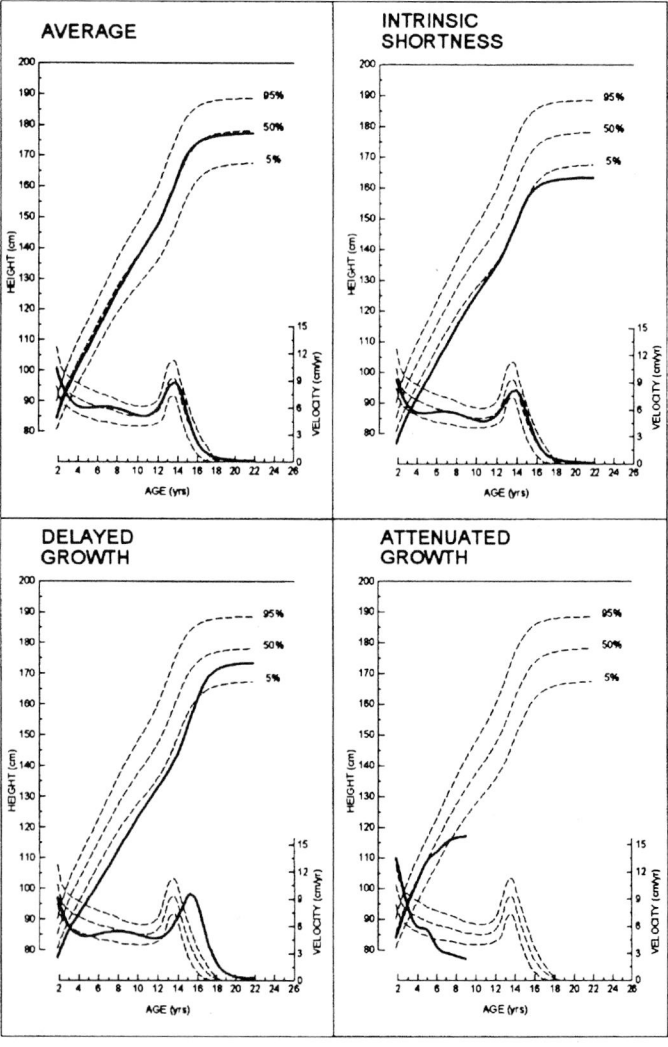

Figure 36-6 Linear growth curves in children with various types of growth patterns. Note that three prepubertal children of similar short stature at 9 years of age have different prognoses for growth. The growth curve of an average-size child is shown for comparison. On each chart, the upper scale shows the height attained, and the lower scale shows the height velocity. Normal percentiles are from the National Center for Health Statistics. Growth curves were generated by the TRI-FOUR program of Bock et al. (Bock RD, du Toit SHC, Thissen D: A.U.X.A.L: Auxological Analysis of Longitudinal Data. Chicago, Scientific Software, 1993. Courtesy of RD Bock.)

height. This *target height*, representing the child's genetic potential, can be approximated by calculating the mid-parental height (the average of the parents' heights) and adding 6.5 cm for boys or subtracting 6.5 cm for girls (to adjust for the average differences between men and women). Alternative functions have been proposed for children with short parents. However, all such predictions are only accurate within a range of 7 to 10 cm.[152]

Deflections from this channel are firmly resisted, as if growth is being developmentally canalized.[153] The mechanisms by which the growth channel is maintained are unknown. They may involve recognition of cell density, which is a determinant of the cell population in culture systems.[154] In the course of a year, healthy children maintain their percentile position with respect to height attained by means of short-term fluctuations in growth velocity, termed stasis and saltation.[155] These oscillations may be marked, growth sometimes seeming nil over 3-month periods, and are a potential source of error in growth diagnosis. GH variability has been reported to increase during periods of short-term growth.[156] The variations tend to be seasonal, a "blooming" trend most often occurring in the spring.

During puberty, children may again cross height-attained percentiles, because the pubertal growth spurts of individuals occur out of phase. The magnitude of this pubertal growth spurt is only apparent from growth-velocity standards based on age of menarche or longitudinal data. Peak growth velocity occurs approximately 1 year prior to menarche[157] in girls, and at a bone age of approximately 12 years in girls and 13 years in boys.[158] Girls on average achieve only 7 cm further growth after menarche.[159] During the course of sexual maturation, the epiphyseal cartilage plates become progressively obliterated, and growth ceases when the process is complete. Only about 1 cm of growth occurs after fusion is complete in the femur and tibia.

Some of the greater ultimate height of boys than of girls results from their later puberty and consequent longer period of prepubertal growth[151]; boys additionally have a slightly greater peak linear growth velocity than girls.[140] Early maturers have more brisk pubertal growth than late maturers.[140] This tendency occurs at comparable levels of bone maturation (Table 36-1).[160] The growth patterns of nonwhite American children differ from that of whites in some particulars.[161] Immigrant children go into a phase of catch-up growth in an optimum nutritional environment.[162]

5. *Body proportions* (arm span and upper-to-lower segment ratio) change in concert with growth. The limbs are relatively short in infancy. By about 11 years of age, adult proportions are reached (Figs. 36-7 and 36-8).[163,164] Occasional marked changes in segmental proportions appear during puberty.[165] Many growth disorders are characterized by abnormal body proportions (see later discussion).

6. *Head circumference* increases most rapidly during early infancy (Fig. 36-9).[166] It is related to both skeletal and brain growth, and about half the variation is familial.[167-169]

CATCH-UP GROWTH AND COMPENSATORY GROWTH

Catch-up growth occurs upon relief from any disorder that has caused a deviation from a child's genetic growth channel and restores the child to his or her original channel.[153,170-172] In classic ("type 1") catch-up growth, the rate of growth is supranormal and exceeds that expected for the age at which growth had been arrested. During adolescence, it may resemble the pubertal growth spurt. This type of catch-up growth has been further subclassifed.[173] A different kind of catch-up growth ("type 2") occurs following adequate therapy of sexual precocity.[174] In this situation, restoration of height potential occurs because restitutional linear growth proceeds without bone maturation advancement, that is, height age catches up to bone age (Table 36-2). Complete compensation for growth failure can occur upon correction of the disorder. Catch-up may be incomplete, however, if the growth disorder is of many years' duration and extends into the age at which puberty normally occurs. The mechanism of catch-up growth is unclear: GH is permissive and possible roles of IGF-1 and leptin have been suggested,[175] but the intrinsic epiphyseal factors determining developmental canalization of growth seem to be key.

Compensatory growth is the term used for the local organ regeneration that occurs after the mass of an organ has

---

Table 36-1 Percentage of Adult Height Achieved at Successive Bone Ages, Variation in Height Prediction from Bone Age, and Variation in Bone Age in Relation to Chronologic Age

	Bone Age (yr)												
	6.0	7.0	8.0	9.0	10.0	11.0	12.0	13.0	14.0	15.0	16.0	17.0	18.0
Percentage of mature height													
Boys													
Average*		69.5	72.3	75.2	78.4	80.4	83.4	87.6	92.7	96.8	98.2	99.1	99.6
Accelerated*		67.0	69.6	72.0	74.7	76.7	80.9	85.0	90.5	95.8	98.0	99.0	
Retarded*	68.0	71.8	75.6	78.6	81.2	82.3	84.5	88.0					
Girls													
Average	72.0	75.7	79.0	82.7	86.2	90.6	92.2	95.8	98.0	99.0	99.6	99.9	100.0
Accelerated		71.2	75.0	79.0	82.8	88.3	90.1	94.5	97.2	98.6	99.3	99.8	
Retarded	73.3	77.0	80.4	84.1	87.4	91.8	93.2	96.4	98.3	99.4	99.8	100.0	
	Chronologic Age (yr)												
	6.0	7.0	8.0	9.0	10.0	11.0	12.0	13.0	14.0	15.0	16.0	17.0	18.0
Height prediction standard deviation (inches)													
Boys		1.47	1.27	1.33	1.14	1.09	1.21	1.21	0.88	0.49	0.41		
Girls		1.73	1.46	1.37	1.15	1.06	0.6	0.42	0.38	0.26	0.20		
Bone age standard deviation (mo)													
Boys	9.3	10.1	10.8	11.0	11.4	10.5	10.4	11.1	12.0	14.2	15.1	15.4	
Girls	9.0	8.3	8.8	9.3	10.8	12.3	14.0	14.6	12.6	11.2			

*With respect to whether bone age is within 1 year of chronologic age.

From Gruelich WW, Pyle SI: Radiographic Atlas of Skeletal Development of the Hand and Wrist. Palo Alto, CA, Stanford University Press, 1959.

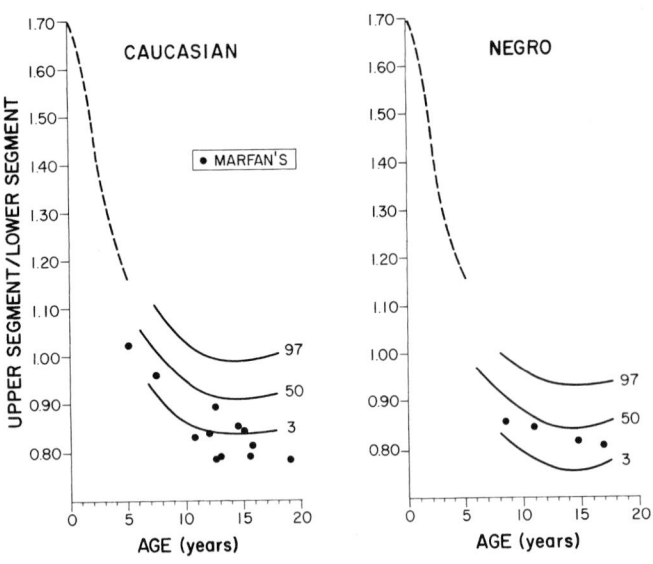

Figure 36-7 Normal standards for the ratio of the upper segment to the lower segment of the body. The lower segment is the measurement from the top of the symphysis pubis to the heel; the upper segment is computed by subtracting the lower segment from height. The *dotted line* shows the average for young children in 1932. (Percentile and Marfan data from McKusick VA: Heritable Disorders of Connective Tissue, ed 4. St Louis, Mosby, 1972.)

been reduced, as by removal or destruction of a portion of that organ.[153] Examples include the compensatory growth that occurs after partial hepatectomy or loss of a kidney. Local IGF-1 and IGF-2 are involved in this type of growth.[94]

BONE AGE IN PREDICTION OF ADULT HEIGHT AND PUBERTAL MILESTONES

Bone growth is accompanied by a predictable pattern of bone maturation. After epiphyseal ossification centers first appear, they undergo modeling in shape and then fuse with the shaft. Bone maturation is assessed as bone age (BA, skeletal age) (see Table 36-2). Figures 36-10 and 36-11 schematically show the Gruelich and Pyle BA standards.[176,177] The normal range for BA is indicated in Table 36-1. The evaluation is most reliable if the maturation of each center is assessed for calculation of the average,[178] to circumvent the normal variations in the epiphyseal ossification pattern.[179] Other atlas methods are available for assessing bone maturation.[180] Skeletal development of young black children is about 0.67 SD advanced over whites of comparable economic status.[181] Other ethnic differences exist that are, to an unknown extent, nutritional.[180]

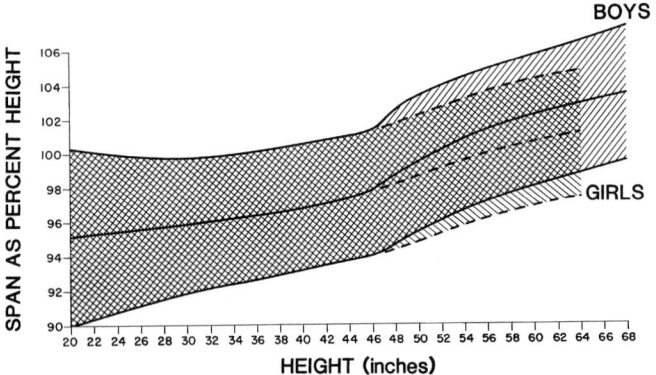

Figure 36-8 Standards for arm span as a percentage of height. The *shaded area* represents the normal range, smoothed. (Data from Engelbach W: Endocrine Medicine, vol 1. Springfield, IL, Charles C Thomas, 1932, p 261.)

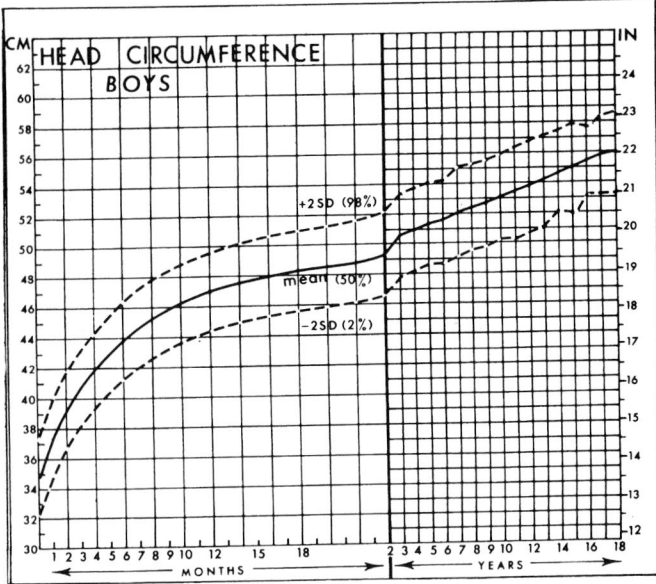

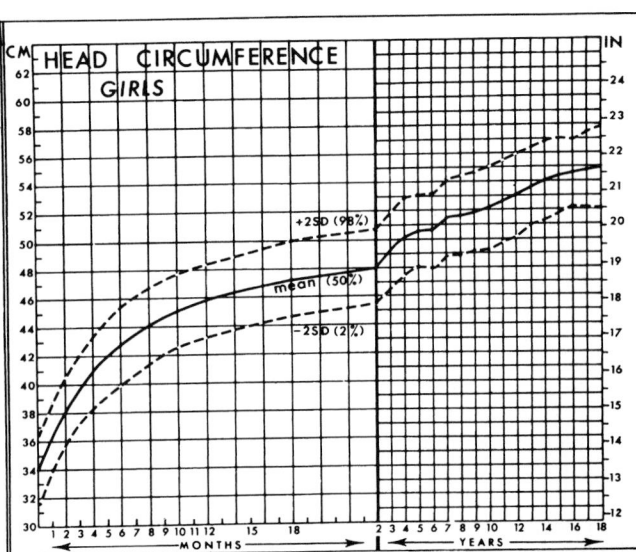

Figure 36-9 Interracial standards for maximal fronto-occipital head circumference. Boys' measurements are about 1 cm greater than those of girls at all ages. (From Nellhaus G: Head circumference from birth to eighteen years. Pediatrics 41:106, 1968. Copyright American Academy of Pediatrics, 1968.)

BA is a better predictor of pubertal milestones than chronologic age. It is as if bone and neuroendocrine maturation have common genetic, nutritional, and endocrine determinants.[182] A BA of 11 to 12 years corresponds better to the onset of puberty in girls and boys, respectively, than these chronologic ages. Peak height-velocity phase differences are 25% less when plotted against BA instead of chronologic age.[150] In girls, menarche has been demonstrated to occur at a mean skeletal age of approximately 13 years.[176,183]

Table 36-2	Definitions of Growth Parameters
Parameter	**Definition**
Bone age	Age for which bone maturation is average
Chronologic age	Calendar age
Height age	Age for which height is average
Weight age	Age for which weight is average

MALE

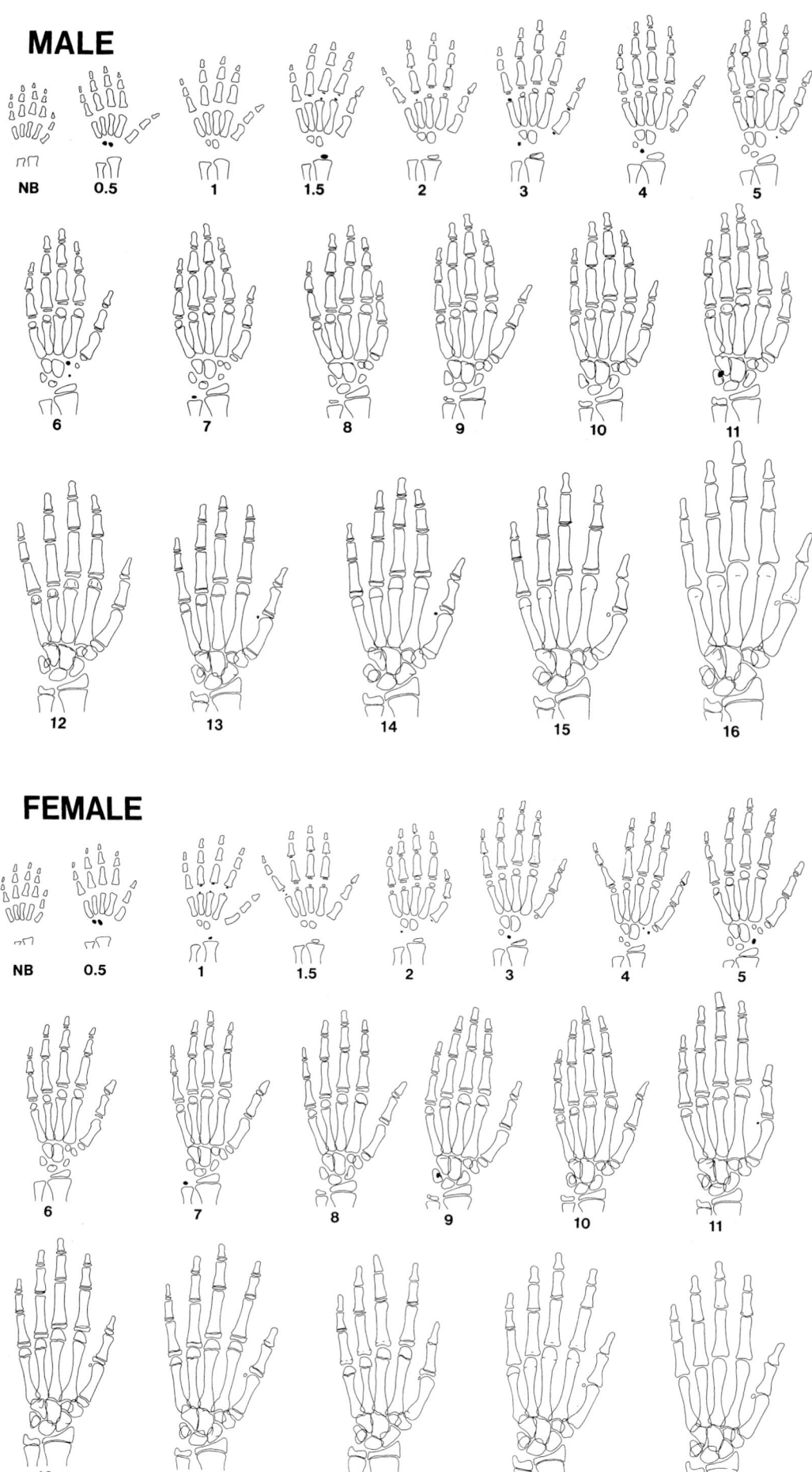

Figure 36-10 Progression of ossification of the hand and wrist in boys. Tracings are modified from the standards of Gruelich and Pyle[105] according to the manner of Wilkins.[106] Newly apparent ossification centers are shown in *black*. Late prefusion is depicted as a *single line* at the junction of the epiphysis and shaft. Bony projections, which appear as a *double contour* within the outlines of a center, are not illustrated after their appearance has matured.

FEMALE

Figure 36-11 Progression of ossification of the hand and wrist in girls. See legend for Figure 35-10.

Table 36-3 Factors Causing Short Stature, with Representative Clinical Conditions

Factors Affecting Height	Representative Conditions	Clinical and Laboratory Features
GENETIC		
Normal Variants	Familial intrinsic shortness	Family history of shortness, normal bone age; no clinical or laboratory abnormalities
	Constitutional delay in growth	Family history of delayed growth, delayed bone age; no other clinical or laboratory abnormalities
Chromosomal aneuploidy	Turner's syndrome	Short, gonadal dysgenesis, otherwise variable phenotype, karyotype necessary to exclude, X deletion
	Trisomy 13–15	Mental retardation, congenital heart disease, bilateral cleft palate and lip, microphthalmia, colobomata, holoprosencephaly, IUGR
	Trisomy 16–18	Mental retardation, congenital heart disease, foot/hand deformities, IUGR
	Down syndrome (trisomy 21)	"Mongoloid" facies, hypotonia, mental retardation
Skeletal dysplasias	See Table 36-4	
Dysmorphic syndromes	Noonan's syndrome	Similar to Turner's (see Table 36-5), normal karyotype, and present in both sexes, PPN11 mutation in half
	Russell-Silver syndrome	IUGR, relative macrocephaly, small triangular face, asymmetry, UPD7 in 10%
	Prader-Willi syndrome	Obesity, hypogonadism, hypotonia, intellectual and behavioral deficits, chromosome 15 abnormalities
	Williams syndrome	"Elfin facies," supravalvular aortic stenosis, ± infantile hypercalcemia, IUGR,[442] 7q11.23 deletion[198]
	Leprechaunism	Congenital lipodystrophy, "puckish" facies, IUGR, insulin resistance and receptor mutation[199]
	Bloom syndrome	Photosensitive dermatitis with telangiectactic erythema, malar hypoplasia, small nose, DNA helicase mutation[206]
	Smith-Lemli-Opitz sydrome	Male pseudohermaphroditism, microcephaly, syndactyly, characteristic facies, cholesterol biosynthetic defect[200]
	Fanconi's syndrome	Radial aplasia, GH deficiency,[201] DNA instability mutations[202]
	Rubinstein-Taybi syndrome	Broad thumbs, antimongoloid eyes, hypoplastic maxilla, mental retardation,[443] subset with CBP mutations[203]
	Cockayne's syndrome	Onset in early childhood, lipodystrophy, retinitis pigmentosa, photosensitivity, mental retardation, microcephaly, DNA repair defect[204]
	Progeria (Hutchinson-Gilford syndrome)	Onset in infancy, characteristic facies, arteriosclerosis, lipodystrophy, mental retardation, lamin A/C mutation[205]
	Werner's syndrome	Onset in late childhood, characteristic facies, atherosclerosis, cataract, lamin A/C[205] or DNA helicase mutation[206]
	Rothmund-Thomson syndrome	"Marbled" pigmentation ± photosensitivity (poikiloderma congenital), cataract, ± ectodermal dysplasia, DNA helicase mutation[206]

INTRAUTERINE	Growth Retardation	Small for gestational age	Ongoing growth failure in a minority of nonsyndromic cases; diverse maternal, placental and fetal disorders, most unexplained
		Fetal alcohol syndrome	Characteristic facies (short palpebral fissure length, thin upper lip, indistinct philtrum),[444] microcephaly, mental retardation
		Fetal hydantoin syndrome	Hypertelorism, terminal digit hypoplasia, mental retardation, seizures
		Congenital rubella syndrome	Hepatosplenomegaly, pancytopenia, patent ductus arteriosus, cataract, deafness
NUTRITIONAL	Inadequate Intake	Starvation	Weight generally depressed more than height
		Psychosocial feeding problems	
		Anorexia due to chronic disease	
	Vitamin/Mineral Deficiency	Rickets	Nutritional deficiency in vitamin D is most common cause, but there are diverse other acquired and genetic causes; alkaline phosphatase elevated in most types
		Zinc deficiency	
	Nutrient Loss	Malabsorption	Symptoms of gastrointestinal, liver, or pancreatic disease; respiratory problems if due to cystic fibrosis
		Chronic vomiting	Obstruction to gastrointestinal tract, achalasia of esophagus, electrolyte disturbances, increased intracranial pressure
	Metabolic Wastage	Uncontrolled diabetes mellitus	High glycohemoglobin, hepatomegaly (Mauriac syndrome); exclude other causes of poor growth; fetal diabetes causes IUGR
		Hyperthyroidism	Goiter, eye signs, abnormal thyroid function tests
PSYCHOSOCIAL	Psychosocial dwarfism	See description under GH/IGF-1	
HORMONAL	GH/IGF-1 Deficiency	Congenital	May have neonatal hypoglycemia, midline defects; may have only short stature
		Acquired	May have history of trauma, CNS insult, or abnormal CNS exam
		Psychosocial deprivation	May show abnormal behavior, hyperphagia; may mimic panhypopituitarism; growth improves with better environment
		GH/IGF-1 resistance	
	Hypothyroidism		Growth failure may be only symptom
	Glucocorticoid	Excess	Supraphysiologic levels attenuate growth. Often associated with obesity
	Sex Steroids	Deficiency	Deficiency after 10-11 years of age impairs growth
CHRONIC ILLNESS			May have history or symptoms of chronic condition or short stature may be presenting feature; weight often impaired more than height

CBP, CREB-binding protein; GH, growth hormone; IGF-1, insulin-like growth factor 1; IUGR, intrauterine growth retardation.

The bone age can be used to predict ultimate height potential, since the degree of bone maturation is inversely proportional to the amount of epiphyseal cartilage growth remaining. It follows that if a child's BA and height age (HA; see Table 36-2) are equal, he or she has the potential to reach an average adult height. The fraction of final height achieved at each BA is known (see Table 36-1). Therefore, *predicted adult height* can be calculated by dividing a child's current height by this fraction (method of Bayley and Pinneau).[160] The error inherent in this method is less than 1.5 inches in normal children (see Table 36-1). However, spontaneous shifts by as much as 5 inches in predicted height may occur in 3% of the population for reasons that are unclear.[184] The error is not reduced by serial readings.[178] The error is greater in children who are very short[185] or have bone dysplasias.

In order to reduce the error in height prediction, elaborate tables have been devised that take into consideration not only a child's BA and height but also the genetic target height and weight.[186] Genetic influences on height predicted from bone age can be roughly accounted for by adding one third the amount that the midparental height differs from the average.[159]

Three methods for assessing height predictions based, in part, on bone age have been developed.[160,186,187] All are based on data from normal children. The Bayley-Pinneau method can be simply applied to young children with abnormal bone ages, so it is used most frequently in children with growth disorders; however, its accuracy has not been verified in many of these.

GROWTH DISORDERS

Children presenting for inadequate or excessive linear growth generally have either a genetically based, normal variant growth pattern or a disorder of the factors that control growth, as discussed previously. In some children, no etiology for abnormal growth can be identified (idiopathic short stature). The following section first categorizes the disorders that cause short stature according to the factors that influence growth. Endocrinopathies are discussed here only insofar as they affect growth; detailed discussion of these disorders can be found in other chapters. Then we present an approach to the differential diagnosis of these disorders according to the clinical assessment of growth pattern with which the patient presents, along with those clinical features and laboratory tests that discriminate among these disorders. Discussion of treatment of short stature follows. Tall stature is discussed in a parallel manner in the final section.

SHORT STATURE

Causes of Short Stature (Table 36-3)
Genetic and Familial Conditions
Familial Normal Variants　Conditions traditionally considered to be normal variants dominate as the most frequent causes of short stature. Two major nonpathologic familial patterns of growth cause the great majority of short stature. One is *familial intrinsic short stature* (sometimes termed *familial* or *genetic short stature*), in which normal children's growth approximates that of their short parents. The other is *constitutional delay in growth and pubertal development*, in which healthy children who are short (delayed puberty may be the most prominent symptom) spontaneously achieve their normal growth potential at a later-than-average age. Characteristically, a parent or close relative has a similar growth pattern. In both of these growth patterns that are traditionally considered normal variants, the typical patient is of normal birth size, and length progressively crosses growth channels to fall below the fifth percentile by 2 to 3 years of age. Height age and bone age then characteristically advance at a normal rate, so that height

is below but closely parallel to the fifth percentile through the prepubertal years. These two normal variants differ, however, because in the former the bone age is normal and puberty occurs at a normal age, whereas in the latter the bone age is delayed and there is a corresponding delay of puberty until the child reaches a pubertal bone age, at which time a growth spurt results in an adult height that is generally normal for the family target height. These diagnoses rest on the family history, growth pattern, bone age, and exclusion of other abnormalities. Predictions of adult heights are particularly prone to overestimation of growth potential in some very short children.[185] As the molecular controls of growth are elucidated, it is likely that some subgroup(s) of these children will be found to have specific diseases.

Skeletal Dysplasias　*Osteochondrodysplasias* are a large group of developmental disorders of chondro-osseous tissue, characterized by disproportionate growth, deformation of the skeleton or of individual bones or groups of bones, and genetic transmission; they are often associated with short stature. They include over 150 mostly rare conditions, the number expanding as underlying molecular defects are characterized (Table 36-4).[188,189] Abnormal body proportions, such as upper body segment abnormally longer than lower body segment (see Fig. 36-7),[163] or arm span disproportionate to height (see Fig. 36-8)[164] are diagnosed by these features together with specific radiologic bone abnormalities.

The most common is achondroplasia, an autosomal-dominant condition, which has a frequency of about 1 in approximately 20,000, with about 90% of cases representing fresh mutations.[190] It causes short stature (often apparent at birth and with deceleration of growth rate in infancy), short limbs, macrocephaly, a low nasal bridge, caudal narrowing of the spinal canal, and, occasionally, hydrocephalus (Fig. 36-12).[190] The average adult height is about 125 cm in females and 131 cm in males.[190] Achondroplasia is generally caused by a gain of function mutation in the FGFR3 gene.[191,192] Inactivating mutation of Indian hedgehog leads to a similar phenotype.[193]

Hypochondroplasia is an allelic variant of achondroplasia.[191,192] It manifests with short stature and dysmorphic features that are often more mild than achondroplasia. Newborns may be slightly small, but short stature generally becomes evident by 3 years of age. There are few craniofacial abnormalities in hypochondroplasia. These children are minimally short limbed. The hands and feet are usually stubby, and genu varum may occur. The most objective radiologic finding is narrowing of the lower lumbosacral interpedicular distances.

Osteochondrodysplasias may cause specific patterns of disproportion. In spondoepiphyseal dysplasia, the spine is disproportionately affected and growth slows in mid-childhood, causing an attenuated growth pattern. On the other hand, some bone dysplasias cause proportionate dwarfism. Tubular stenosis is a proportionate form of bone dysplasia associated with congenital hypoparathyroidism.[194] Activating mutation of the PTH/PTHrP receptor has been discovered to cause Jansen's metaphyseal dysplasia, which is associated with asymptomatic hypercalcemia.[195] Various atlases are available to distinguish among the known types of bone dysplasias.[153,190,196,197] In recent years, it has become possible to make a specific genetic diagnosis in many cases.[191]

Chromosomal Abnormalities, Monogenic Disorders, and Syndromes　Several syndromes are associated with short stature (see Table 36-3).[190,198-206] Those in which short stature or endocrine problems are prominent are discussed here.

Turner's Syndrome　Turner's syndrome (gonadal dysgenesis), caused by deletion of X-chromosomal material, is the most common pathologic cause of short stature in girls. Haploinsufficiency for the SHOX (short stature homeobox-

Table 36-4 Representative Types of Skeletal Dysplasia of Known Genetic Basis

Dysplasia Group	Inheritance	IUGR	Genetic Basis
ACHONDROPLASIA GROUP			
Achondroplasia	AD	+	FGF R3 activating mutation
Hypochondroplasia	AD	–	FGFR3 activating mutation
TYPE II COLLAGENOPATHIES			
Spondyloepiphyseal dysplasia (SED) congenital	AD	+	COL2A1
TYPE IX COLLAGENOPATHIES			
Stickler dysplasia	AD	+	COL11A1
OTHER SPONDYLOEPIPHYSEAL DYSPLASIAS			
X-linked SED tarda	XLD		Xp22.2-p22.1
PSEUDOACHONDROPLASIA AND MULTIPLE EPIPHYSEAL DYSPLASIAS (MED)			
Pseudoachondroplasia and MED (Fairbanks type)	AD	–	COMP/cartilage oligomeric matrix protein
MED (other types)	?	–	COL9A2
CHONDRODYSPLASIA PUNCTATA			
Zellweger syndrome	AR	+	PEX1,2,5,6/peroxins
Brachytelephalangic type	XLR	+	ARSE/arylsulfatase E
METAPHYSEAL DYSPLASIA			
Jansen type	AD	+	PTHR
Schmid type	AD	–	COL10A1/COL10 α-chain
Adenosine deaminase deficiency	AD	–	ADA/adenosine deaminase
ACROMELIC AND ACROMESOMELIC DYSPLASIAS			
Trichorhinophalangeal syndrome types	AD	+	TRPS1±EXT1
Grebe and Hunter-Thompson dysplasias	AR	+	CDMP1/cartilage-derived morphogenic protein
Albright hereditary osteodystrophy		–	GNAS1/guanine nucleotide α subunit, inactive
DYSPLASIAS WITH PROMINENT MEMBRANOUS BONE INVOLVEMENT			
Cleidocranial dysplasia	AD	+	CBFA1/core-binding factor α subunit
BENT BONE DYSPLASIAS			
Campomelic dysplasia	AD	+	SOX9/SRY box-9
DYSOSTOSIS MULTIPLEX			
Mucopolysaccharidosis II	XLR	–	IDS/iduronate-2-sulfatase
Mucopolysaccharidosis, others	AR	–	Diverse
DYSPLASIAS WITH DECREASED BONE DENSITY			
Osteogenesis imperfecta (diverse)	AD/AR	±	COLA1 or 2/α(1 or 2) I procollagen
DYSPLASIAS WITH DEFECTIVE MINERALIZATION			
Hypophosphatasia, infantile type	AR	+	ALPL/alkaline phosphatase
Hypophosphatemic rickets	XLD	–	PHEX
INCREASED BONE DENSITY WITHOUT MODIFICATION OF BONE SHAPE			
Osteopetrosis/renal tubular acidosis	AR	+	CA2/carbonic anhydrase II
Pyknodysostosis	AR	+	CTSK/cathepsin K
DISORGANIZED DEVELOPMENT OF CARTILAGINOUS AND FIBROUS COMPONENTS OF SKELETON			
Fibrous dysplasia (McCune-Albright syndrome)	Spmos	–	GNAS1, activating
Fibrodysplasia ossificans progressiva	AD	+	BMP4/bone morphogenetic protein 4

AD, autosomal dominant; AR, autosomal recessive; SPmos, sporadic mosaic; XLD, X-linked dominant; XLR, X-linked recessive.
From International Working Group on Constitutional Diseases of Bone: International nomenclature and classification of the osteochondrodysplasias (1997). Am J Med Genet 79(5):376–382, 1998; and Superti-Furga A, Bonafe L, Rimoin DL: Molecular-pathogenetic classification of genetic disorders of the skeleton. Am J Med Genet 106(4):282–293, 2001.

containing) gene has been found to contribute to short stature in Turner's syndrome.[207,208] The SHOX gene is located on the pseudoautosomal region of the distal short arm of the X and Y chromosomes.[207,209] Abnormalities of the SHOX gene were also found responsible for Leri-Weill dyschondrosteosis, and Langer mesomelic dysplasia (associated with severe dwarfism) was found due to SHOX nullizygosity.[210]

The incidence of Turner's syndrome is 1 in 2500 newborn girls. The average birth size of these children is at the lower end of the normal range. Although there are significant variations among affected individuals, typically height drops below the third percentile by 2 to 3 years of age and this is followed by gradual and progressive deviation from the normal growth channels.[211] Growth may become further attenuated in the teenage years and epiphyseal closure is delayed, in part because of hypogonadism.[212] The most characteristic features

of Turner's syndrome are short stature and gonadal dysgenesis. The presence of pubertal development should not deter consideration of the diagnosis because about 10% of patients have some residual ovarian tissue rather than streak gonads. Thus, these patients may have spontaneous menarche, although few sustain regular menses.[213] Additional manifestations of Turner's syndrome include lymphedema, particularly in the newborn period, and the dysmorphic features and congenital anomalies listed in Table 36-5. Variation in the physical manifestations of Turner's syndrome are illustrated in Figure 36-13.[190] Aortic root dilatation and renal anomalies are infrequent but important.[214] There is an increased incidence of autoimmune thyroiditis and diabetes mellitus. Karyotype analysis is essential in the investigation of any girl with unexplained short stature. Without growth-promoting therapy, adult height averages 56.5 inches.[211]

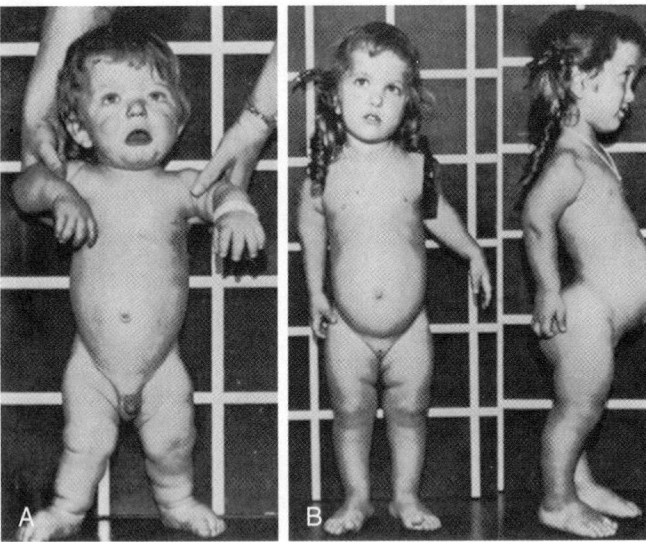

Figure 36-12 Achondroplasia. *A*, One-year-old boy with a height age of 4 months. *B*, Four-year-old girl with a height age of 20 month (From Jones KL [ed]: Smith's Recognizable Patterns of Human Malformation, 4th ed. Philadelphia, WB Saunders, 1988.)

Table 36-5 Approximate Incidence of Somatic Abnormalities in Turner's and Noonan's Syndromes*

Abnormality	Turner's Syndrome[93,118,119] (%)	Noonan's Syndrome[93,120–124] (%)
Short stature (<10%)	100/80[†]	90/90
Gonadal failure	99/85?	≤10/≤10[‡]
Cryptorchidism	NA/33	NA/75
Hypertelorism	<25	100
High palate	80	75
Neck webbed	50	10
Neck short	68	100
Cubitus valgus	68	30
Chest deformity[§]	50	50
Coarctation of aorta	20	<1
Pulmonic stenosis	10	50[¶]
Mental retardation	10**	25
Pigmented moles, multiple	50	<10

*Defined on the basis of the presence (Turner) or absence (Noonan) of a sex chromosome abnormality. Turner's syndrome in females results from deletion of genetic material on the X chromosome. Various sex chromosomal abnormalities have been reported in Turner's syndrome in males—for example, XO, XXY, XO/XY, XO/XY/XYY, XX/XXY.
[†]Female/male.
[‡]The distinction between delayed puberty and hypogonadism has seldom been made.
[§]Pectus or an apparent increase in intermipple distance.
[¶]The high incidence of congenital heart disease in Noonan's syndrome may be due to ascertainment bias, Dr. Noonan being a cardiologist. A variety of other congenital heart defects have been reported in both syndromes.
**Males seem to have a greater incidence of mental retardation, although finding this may be a matter of ascertainment.
NA, not applicable.

Although Turner's syndrome does not involve GH deficiency as a cause of the growth impairment, GH treatment (particularly in doses higher than those used for GH deficiency) appears to improve growth. Results suggest that long-term GH treatment increases adult height in many recipients by about 2 cm for each year of treatment, although reports vary in the degree of height gained with no discernable gain in some.[211,215–217] GH treatment is currently recommended when the height of a girl with Turner's syndrome drops below the fifth percentile on the normal female growth curve. The side effects of GH treatment are discussed later. To induce pubertal development in girls with ovarian failure due to Turner's syndrome, very low dose exogenous estrogen therapy (and, eventually, cycling with progesterone) is needed in adolescence and beyond.[130]

Noonan's Syndrome Noonan's syndrome, originally called "male Turner's syndrome," is now diagnosed in patients of either sex with normal external genitalia who have a Turner-like phenotype but normal sex chromosomes.[218–222] It may be transmitted as an autosomal-dominant disorder. Mutations in

PTPN11, the gene encoding the nonreceptor-type protein tyrosine phosphatase SHP-2, account for about half the cases.[223–225] Although the anomalies in an individual may resemble those in Turner's syndrome, the overall incidence of malformations is different, with predominantly right-sided cardiac lesions in Noonan's and left-sided lesions in Turner's syndrome (see Table 36-5). Patients with Noonan's syndrome have a better prognosis for gonadal function (delayed puberty rather than gonadal failure) and become somewhat taller than patients with Turner's syndrome, having adult heights that average 162.5 cm in males and 152.7 cm in females.[226] Some studies have noted an improvement in growth with GH

Figure 36-13 Variable phenotypes of Turner's syndrome: five girls with 45,X syndrome illustrating the variability of features such as webbed neck and broad chest. (From Jones KL [ed]: Smith's Recognizable Patterns of Human Malformation, 4th ed. Philadelphia, WB Saunders, 1988.)

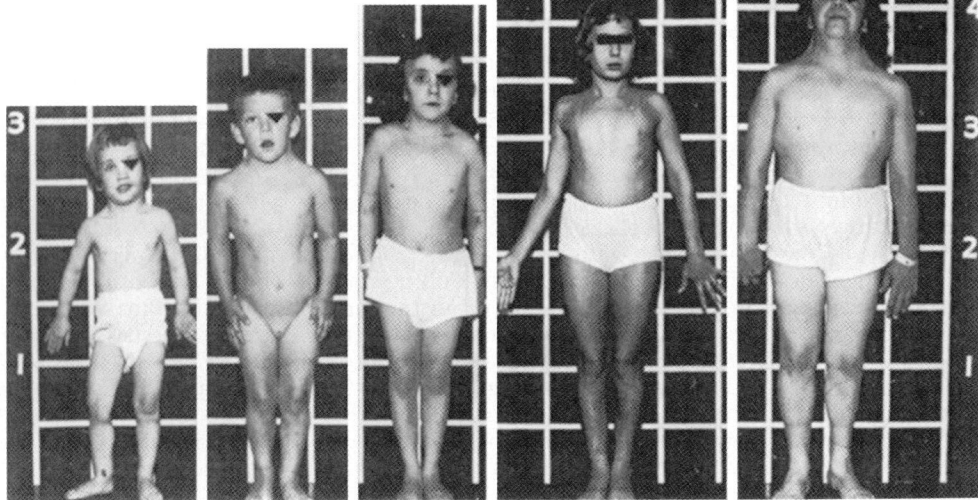

treatment,[227] but further large and well-controlled studies are needed.

Prader-Willi Syndrome In Prader-Willi syndrome, short stature is associated with neonatal failure to thrive and hypotonicity, obesity of onset at about 2 years of age due to development of a voracious appetite, intellectual impairment, and hypogonadism. It is associated with deletion of a critical region of the proximal part of the long arm of chromosome 15 in 70% of cases and unimaternal disomy of this region in the others (Fig. 36-14).[228,229] Some may have GH deficiency. GH therapy may improve growth and weight.[230–232]

18q Deletions Deletions of 18q occur in about 1 of 40,000 children. Approximately two thirds of affected children have heights more than 2 SDs below the mean, and most have abnormal growth velocities.[233] These patients may be at increased risk for GH deficiency.[233]

Down Syndrome Stunting of growth and cerebral dysfunction are virtually uniform features of autosomal aneuploidy. Down syndrome (trisomy 21 and variants thereof) is the most common multiple malformation syndrome in humans. Adult height averages 155 cm in affected males, 145 cm in females.[144]

Intrauterine Growth Retardation and Small for Gestational Age
Intrauterine growth retardation (IUGR) is a term generally used to designate individuals with persistent short stature due to the presence of an intrinsic growth disorder of prenatal onset. It may be diagnosed before birth because of poor growth prenatally (IUGR) or diagnosed retrospectively because of persistent growth failure in children born small for gestational age (SGA). SGA has been variously defined as weight or length below the third to tenth percentile.[132,234,235] IUGR is a common condition that affects approximately 10% of infants born SGA.

The etiology of IUGR is mutifactorial and includes genetic alterations, congenital malformations, placental factors, and maternal factors (see Tables 36-3 and 36-4). Genetic causes of IUGR include chromosome abnormalities, single gene defects, and uniparental disomy (UPD).[236,237] Congenital diabetes mellitus and insulin receptor mutations are uniformly associated with IUGR.[11,97] Congenital IGF-1 deficiency and IGF-1 receptor mutations in humans, as well as IGF disruption in animal models, cause IUGR.[29,33,238] However, the exact etiology in any given child remains unknown in up to 60% of cases.[239]

Russell-Silver syndrome is a term applied to some children with IUGR in association with dysmorphic features such as pseudohydrocephalus (a relatively large head with a small face), clinodactyly, and subtle body asymmetry. It is a heterogeneous condition with unclear diagnostic features: About half of patients with the syndrome have delayed puberty and reach a normal adult height,[240] but the remainder may be quite short.[241] It is clearly not a single entity. It has been suggested that approximately 10% have uniparental disomy of maternal chromosome 7.[236]

Other cases of IUGR with ongoing growth failure postnatally are nonsyndromic and occur as the seemingly nonspecific result of such dissimilar disorders as maternal heroin addiction,[242] intrauterine infections,[243] placental insufficiency,[244] fetal malnutrition,[245,246] or hypoxia-related congenital anomalies.[247] A common thread to these may be a decreased endowment in total body cell number.[248] Another mechanism may be via fetal hypercortisolism.[37] Unexplained IUGR may also have genomic roots in view of the fact that maternal uniparental disomy for chromosome 6 has been reported to be associated with IUGR only because it unmasked congenital adrenal hyperplasia, an autosomal-recessive trait.[237]

The clinical management of children with short stature attributed to IUGR requires attempts to ascertain and manage the underlying cause of the condition.[234] For those SGA

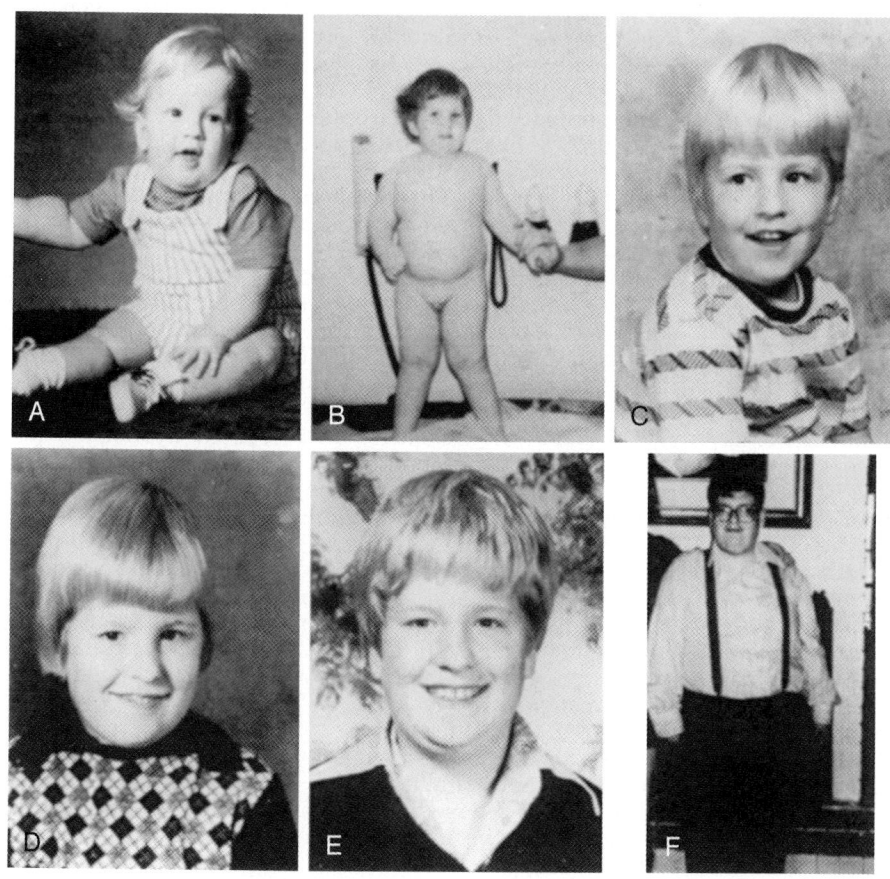

Figure 36-14 Evolution of the phenotype in Prader-Willi syndrome in a patient with a 15q deletion. *A*, 11 months; *B*, 2.5 years; *C*, 3.5 years; *D*, 7 years; *E*, 13 years; *F*, 27 years. (From Cassidy SB: Prader-Willi syndrome. J Med Genet 34:917–923, 1997.)

children who fail to manifest catch-up growth in height by 2 to 3 years of age, the U.S. Food and Drug Administration has approved GH therapy.[249,250] GH has been found to increase growth rate in these children in a dose-dependent manner.[234,251–253] One study has reported reduction in insulin sensitivity in short SGA children treated with GH.[254]

Undernutrition

Undernutrition sufficient to reduce calorie intake below 82% to 91% of the recommended level will arrest growth.[255,256] This degree of undernutrition is suggested by weight for height, BMI, or body fat below the tenth percentile.[257] Undernutrition may result from inadequate nutrient intake (due to psychosocial feeding or eating disorders, or poor appetite due to chronic disease), excessive nutrient output (chronic vomiting or malabsorption as in inflammatory bowel disease, celiac disease, cystic fibrosis, or hepatic disease), or metabolic wastage (e.g., as in poorly controlled diabetes mellitus).[258,259] A unique cause of malnutrition in infants is the diencephalic syndrome. This is characterized by a paucity of body fat resembling lipodystrophy in a hyperalert, otherwise healthy child. Radiosensitive brain tumors in the anterior hypothalamic area are the usual cause. Disturbance of the regulation of appetite, the secretion of pituitary lipolytic hormones such as GH, or increased energy expenditure have been postulated as the mechanism.[260,261] Deficiency of trace metals such as zinc and copper by itself causes growth failure.[66,67]

Chronic Nonendocrine Diseases

Chronic nonendocrine disorders of virtually any organ system may attenuate growth.[262] Generally, weight is suppressed more than height, in contrast to primary endocrine disorders. The mechanisms of growth impairment vary according to the disease and often include undernutrition, medication effects (e.g., supraphysiologic doses of glucocorticoids), chronic acidosis, and/or secondary endocrine dysfunction. Examples include celiac disease, inflammatory bowel disease, chronic renal failure, cardiovascular disease, hematologic disorders, poorly controlled diabetes mellitus, chronic acidosis, cystic fibrosis, and chronic infections. Although the primary disorder is evident in many cases of short stature due to chronic illness, short stature is sometimes the primary presenting feature. This occurs notably in inflammatory bowel disease, celiac disease, and renal dysfunction.

Celiac disease and Crohn's disease are notorious for presenting as short stature without gastrointestinal complaints. Measurement of transglutamidase (endomysial) antibodies is a sensitive screening test for celiac disease,[263] and sometimes referral to a gastroenterologist is needed. Poor growth in Crohn's disease reflects poor food intake, malabsorption, and direct effects of the inflammatory process on the growth axis.[264–266] Growth can also be adversely affected by glucocorticoid therapy and may improve with nutritional interventions or surgery.[266,267]

Renal disease suppresses growth; this probably reflects chronic acidosis, poor intake, anemia, subnormal formation of 1,25-dihydroxycholecalciferol, and, at times, the medications required. In addition, serum IGF-1 is generally normal, but IGF bioactivity and free IGF-1 have been reported to be low,[268,269] probably because of excessive circulating IGF-binding proteins.[270] The Food and Drug Administration has approved GH for the treatment of short stature due to renal failure before transplantation. GH has also been used in some studies after transplantation, with promising results.[271]

Metabolic disorders may affect growth. Either chronic acidosis[68] or chronic alkalosis[272] cause growth failure. Chronic anemia[273] and rickets cause a delayed growth pattern.[274,275] A defect in zinc action has resulted in growth failure.[276] Diabetes mellitus, when poorly controlled, can lead to Mauriac syndrome, involving growth failure and hepatomegaly due to excessive glycogen deposition. In thalassemia, growth impairment may reflect not only chronic anemia, but also endocrine dysfunction due to hemosiderosis.[277]

Endocrine Disorders

GH Deficiency   GH deficiency is the most difficult to diagnose of the endocrine disorders causing short stature since it may cause no phenotypic abnormalities other than slow linear growth, and diagnostic tests are controversial. If untreated, GH deficiency can result in adults with proportionate extreme short stature (formerly termed *midgets*). Recent advances in our understanding of molecular loci influencing GH synthesis and secretion have elucidated specific etiologies of previously unexplained GH-related growth failure.

GH deficiency can be congenital or acquired, and may be isolated or coexist with other pituitary hormone deficiencies (panhypopituitarism). Congenital forms of GH deficiency may be due to primary hypothalamic and/or pituitary defects.

Congenital hypothalamic-pituitary disorders may be associated with midline defects such as septo-optic dysplasia (involving varying degrees of hypoplasia of the optic nerves, chiasm, and infundibular region of the hypothalamus), holoprosencephaly, cleft palate, or a single central incisor.[278–281] Mutations in HESX1, a homeodomain transcription factor, can cause a broad spectrum of phenotypes—including septo-optic dysplasia, interruption of the pituitary stalk (ectopic posterior pituitary), and isolated GH deficiency—which can present in infancy or evolve over years.[282] Diverse patterns of pituitary hormone deficiency can result from mutations of other homeodomain transcription factors, such as POU1F1 (Pit-1), Prop-1, LHX3, LHX4, and PTX2, that are essential for pituitary development.[10,283–296] Combined pituitary hormone deficiency (CPHD) of GH, prolactin, and thyroid-stimulating hormone (TSH) is the typical outcome of inactivating mutations of both POU1F1 and PROP1, while PROP1 defects also sometimes cause follicle-stimulating hormone (FSH), luteinizing hormone (LH), and adrenocorticotropic hormone (ACTH) deficiencies, often with pituitary enlargement. POU1F1 defects can be transmitted as autosomal dominant or recessive. In one study, 35 of 73 subjects with CPHD, belonging to 18 unrelated families, had PROP1 gene defects.[288] Other congenital primary pituitary disorders include defects in the GH gene,[297–300] bioinactive GH,[301] and mutations in the GHRH-receptor gene.[302,303] Surprisingly, primary genetic defects of the GHRH gene have not yet been identified. Genetic disorders of pituitary development leading to hypopituitarism are discussed in detail in Chapters 16 and 22.

Most isolated, and presumably congenital, GH deficiency is currently considered idiopathic, and this occurs in 1 in 3500 children.[304] Magnetic resonance imaging shows abnormalities, including a small anterior pituitary, an attenuated pituitary stalk, and/or ectopic posterior pituitary, in over 70% of GH-deficient children.[305–307]

Congenital GH deficiency may lead to neonatal hypoglycemia. The combination of neonatal hypoglycemia, prolonged neonatal jaundice, and, in males, micropenis suggests panhypopituitarism.[308] Congenital GH deficiency may also present with short stature in early infancy or childhood. In addition to shortness, GH deficiency typically causes relative adiposity, reduced musculature, a cherubic appearance, and a high-pitched voice. These manifestations are not present in all children with the disorder, however. The diagnosis of GH deficiency should be considered in all children with subnormal growth velocity.

Acquired GH deficiency may result from head trauma, tumors such as craniopharyngioma, Rathke's pouch cyst, histiocytosis, cranial irradiation, or chemotherapy.[309–314] These children show attenuation of growth after an initial period of normal growth. Acquired, isolated, permanent idiopathic GH deficiency is considered rare.

Functional hypopituitarism is another form of acquired GH deficiency. The prototypic cause of this is the psychosocial deprivation syndrome. This "deprivation dwarfism" may be seen in children who are not malnourished or overtly disturbed, but who show abnormal behavior patterns, including hyperphagia, hoarding food, drinking from toilets, or sleepwalking.[315–317] GH deficiency in this condition rapidly resolves in a nurturing environment. In one study, initial catch-up growth did not correlate with final height, and the mean final height attained was significantly lower than the midparental target height.[318] Anorexia nervosa may also occasionally cause functional GH deficiency.[319]

The diagnosis of GH deficiency has classically rested on demonstration of a subnormal GH response to two or more provocative pharmacologic tests of GH reserve (i.e., a GH peak less than 5 ng/mL indicative of complete deficiency and 5–10 ng/dL indicative of partial deficiency using a polyclonal GH assay[320]; some use 7 ng/mL as the cutoff point between complete and partial GH deficiency) in a child with slow growth velocity, a delayed bone age, and no other disorder that accounts for slow growth. Monoclonal antibodies yield GH values that are about half the values of assays using polyclonal antisera.[321] Provocative tests include arginine, L-dopa, clonidine, glucagon, and insulin-induced hypoglycemia.[322,323] Two pharmacologic tests are traditionally used because approximately 15% to 20% of apparently normal children have a poor response to a given single test of GH reserve. Untreated hypothyroidism, obesity, and glucocorticoid treatment may falsely lower GH levels. Sex steroid priming with estrogen or androgen for 1 to 7 days before the GH provocative test is sometimes utilized to distinguish GH deficiency from constitutional delay in growth and development.[324–326] Although this classic definition continues to have support, concern has been raised because of potential false-positive and false-negative diagnoses using this approach and because of inconsistencies in GH assays.[324,327–329] Some have considered the false-positive rate related to evolving cutoff points in the diagnosis of GH deficiency and to inconsistencies in how GH tests have been used.[330] Alternative approaches have been proposed to diagnose forms of GH deficiency, such as neurosecretory defects and bioactive GH. These include 12- to 24-hour measurement of spontaneous GH secretion. Measurement of IGF-1 and/or IGFBP-3 have been widely suggested for the diagnosis; however, IGF-1 and IGFBP-3 levels are affected by undernutrition, chronic systemic diseases, and delayed puberty, and they must be interpreted in terms of age and pubertal stage (see Fig. 36-2).[331,332] Combination testing with GHRH and a somatostatin suppressor such as arginine has been introduced[74] as an alternative diagnostic procedure, this is a synergistic stimulus that can induce normal GH release in children with congenital hypopituitarism who meet all classic criteria for isolated GH deficiency.[333] Because GH levels are higher in newborns than infants and children, the diagnosis of GH deficiency has been made in neonates by demonstrating a random GH level of less than 20 ng/mL in the appropriate clinical situation (e.g., microphallus or hypoglycemia). Therapeutic trials of GH have also been suggested as a means to assess GH deficiency by examining the growth response to GH, but their interpretation is difficult (see later discussion). Overall, no single method has yet emerged as a gold standard alternative to the classical definition. Following the diagnosis of GH deficiency, magnetic resonance imaging is indicated to determine whether the hypopituitarism is due to structural lesions or tumors.

Recombinant GH therapy (usually in a dose of 0.3 mg/kg/week subcutaneously, divided daily or 6 days/week) is the standard treatment for GH deficiency, and is remarkably successful for this condition (Fig. 36-15). In GH-deficient children treated with GH daily, the growth rate during the first year of treatment is, on average, 11.5 cm[334]; although it declines somewhat thereafter, it remains markedly above

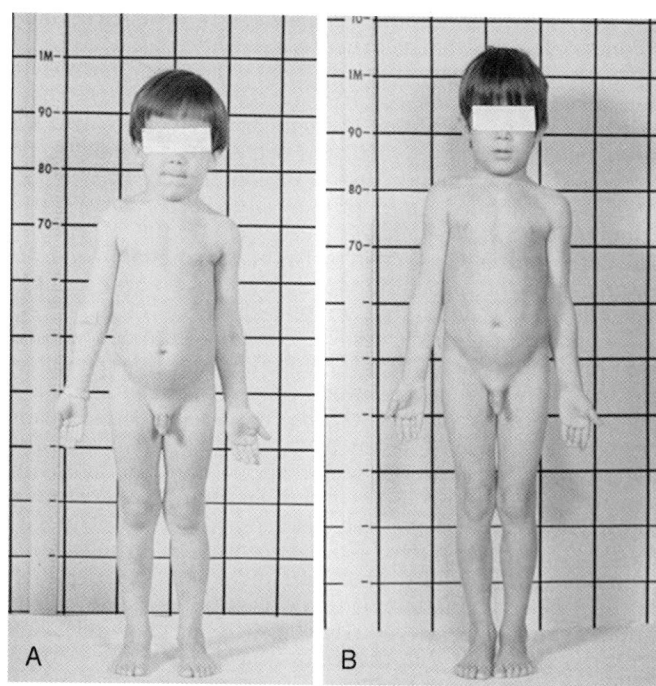

Figure 36-15 Growth hormone (GH)-deficient patient before **(A)** and after **(B)** treatment with GH for 1 year. Note that the growth spurt is accompanied by normal maturation of body proportions.

pretreatment growth velocity. Recombinant GH therapy is effective in bringing adult height into the normal range when it is begun early.[335] GH treatment also increases bone mass and lean tissue mass in children with GH deficiency.[336]

Potential adverse effects of recombinant GH include fluid retention (sometimes with cerebral edema), pancreatitis, glucose intolerance and/or insulin resistance, transient gynecomastia, slipped capital femoral epiphysis, and growth of nevi.[337–340] Concerns about leukemia and second tumors have not been confirmed among children who do not have other predisposing factors, although ongoing surveillance continues.[341–345] Growth deceleration associated with high-affinity, high-capacity antibodies to GH has been reported but appears very rare. Retinopathy has been described in patients with renal failure receiving GH to improve growth.[346] Some children with Prader-Willi syndrome treated with GH have died of respiratory causes.[347] The long-term risk of cancer from childhood GH therapy appears low, but exact risk is not known.[348,349] A systematic review, however, found that circulating concentrations of IGF-1 and IGFBP-3 are associated with an increased risk of common cancers, although associations are modest.[350] In addition to GH treatment, those children with GH deficiency associated with other pituitary hormone deficiencies (i.e., panhypopituitarism) require adequate replacement of these hormones. A review of the Canadian experience suggests that adrenal insufficiency represents a potentially avoidable cause of death in children with panhypopituitarism.[351]

Traditionally, GH therapy for GH-deficient children has been stopped after adult height is reached and epiphyses have fused. It is important not to discontinue GH therapy before secondary sex characteristics are advanced since GH potentiates sex hormone effects.[125,352,353] A major emerging issue in GH deficiency is GH treatment beyond the end of linear growth, as studies suggest that low doses of GH may somewhat improve metabolic status, body composition, and well-being in adults with GH deficiency.[324] The use of GH in adults is discussed further in Chapter 38. Alternatives to standard GH therapy, including oral GH secretagogues, IGF-1, inhaled GH, and GH-releasing factor, are under study or under development.[354–358]

GH Insensitivity Syndromes Whereas GH deficiency causes secondary IGF-1 deficiency, there is a growing class of disorders know to cause primary IGF-1 deficiency. These are termed *GH insensitivity (GHI) syndromes*. In these conditions, patients tend to have clinical manifestations similar to children with GH deficiency; however, in GHI, GH secretion is adequate, but peripheral tissues are incapable of responding normally to GH. GHI is subdivided into primary and secondary forms. Primary GHI includes hereditary defects in (1) the GH receptor (the defects initially described by Laron and often termed *Laron dwarfism*), (2) GH signal transduction system (i.e., postreceptor defects), (3) defects in the synthesis or action of IGF-1, and (4) bioinactive GH molecules.[301,359-364] Large kindreds with GH receptor defects have been described in the Mediterranean region as well as Equador. Several different point mutations of the GH receptor have been described in such patients. A postreceptor defect in STAT5b has been reported and likely other postreceptor defects will be identified.[87,363] Growth failure due to primary defects of IGF-1 synthesis and to primary defects of the IGF-1 receptor have also been reported.[33,238,365] In general, the clinical phenotype associated with GHI includes severe postnatal growth failure, small face and frontal bossing, high-pitched voice, premature aging, delayed bone age, and other features common to severe GH deficiency.[362,364] Blue sclera and limited extensibility at the elbow have also been variably described. The patient with the IGF-1 synthetic defect had, in addition to postnatal growth failure, intrauterine growth failure, mental retardation, sensorineural deafness, and insulin resistance. It has been suggested that the manifestations of GHI are heterogeneous and that mild forms of GHI may exist.[33,364,366] It has also been suggested that some children with idiopathic short stature will be found to have forms of GHI.[367]

The diagnosis of GHI is suggested by extreme short stature, decreased serum concentrations of IGF-1, IGF-2, and IGFBP-3, and increased serum concentrations of GH. Decreased serum concentrations of GHBP are highly suggestive of a GH-receptor defect, but are not necessarily present.[368] Inability to adequately generate IGF-1 in response to GH administration is an important aspect of demonstrating GHI, although diagnostic criteria that distinguish mild GHI from normal are currently imprecise.[367,369,370] Diagnostic criteria for GH-receptor defects have been proposed.[371,372] Treatment with recombinant IGF-1 seems to be effective in some of these conditions.[359,360,373-375]

GH resistance may also be secondary to a variety of illnesses. This GH resistance may be due to malnutrition or inhibitors of GH action, among which are glucocorticoids. Antibodies to exogenous GH on rare occasions impair the response to GH therapy.[376]

Hypothyroidism *Hypothyroidism* in childhood is characterized by slow linear growth velocity and, if chronic, causes short stature and retards bone age. Acquired hypothyroidism, most commonly due to autoimmune thyroiditis, may have few clear clinical features aside from growth impairment. Congenital hypothyroidism, if untreated, can also stunt growth and, additionally, will often cause profound mental retardation if not treated within the first few months of life. Fortunately, neonatal screening programs in many countries enable early detection and treatment of most cases. Hypothyroidism is diagnosed by measurement of free thyroxine (T_4) and TSH using age-related norms; additional studies such as measurement of thyroid antibodies can help to establish the etiology of hypothyroidism. It has been suggested that mild central hypothyroidism may contribute to 10% of idiopathic short stature.[377] The replacement dose of thyroid hormone in children averages 100 μm/m²/day.[378] Catch-up growth is expected after treatment of juvenile hypothyroidism if the diagnosis is made early.[153] However, once treatment is begun, skeletal maturation may accelerate unduly, resulting in patients not reaching their expected adult heights.[379]

Glucocorticoid Excess *Glucocorticoid excess*, whether endogenous or exogenous, profoundly slows growth. Doses of cortisol greater than about 12 to 15 mg/m²/day (prednisone 3–5 mg/m²/day) impair growth in normal prepubertal children.[111] Growth failure may be the only clear clinical sign of glucocorticoid excess in children.[380,381] Cushing's syndrome is usually iatrogenic, resulting from supraphysiologic doses of glucocorticoid treatment by any route, including topical. Endogenous glucocorticoid excess may be due to adrenal tumors (particularly in infants), primary pigmented nodular adrenocortical disease, bilateral adrenal hyperplasia secondary to ACTH-producing pituitary adenoma (Cushing's disease), or ectopic ACTH production. The growth attenuation with Cushing's syndrome of any cause contrasts with exogenous obesity, in which height velocity is normal. Significant virilization also occurs with adrenal tumors that secrete androgen as well as glucocorticoids, and growth inhibition may be counteracted by androgen.[382] The diagnosis of endogenous glucocorticoid excess is based on clinical evidence, assessment of suppressibility of endogenous glucocorticoids by exogenous glucocorticoid (dexamethasone suppression test), and radiologic studies to attempt localization of the lesion. Treatment of endogenous glucocorticoid excess focuses on removal or ablation of the underlying lesion (transsphenoidal removal of pituitary microadenoma in the case of Cushing's disease).[383-386] Early and effective treatment of glucocorticoid excess enables catch-up growth.[153]

In cases in which growth inhibition is attributable to glucocorticoid treatment of nonendocrine disease, there are four possible alternatives: (1) Use another form of therapy; (2) lower the daily steroid dose if the underlying disease can be so controlled; (3) switch the patient to alternate-morning glucocorticoid therapy[387]; or (4) switch the patient to topical (e.g., inhaled) steroid therapy.[388] Alternate day "pulses" of prednisone or topical administration often results in preservation of the desired therapeutic effect while avoiding the unwanted cushingoid changes, but neither are certain solutions to the dilemma. GH therapy may partially counterbalance growth suppression due to moderate doses of glucocorticoid, with considerable variability of response.[117]

Idiopathic Short Stature

The term *idiopathic short stature* (short stature of unknown cause) is generally used to include children who appear to have none of the previously described conditions. However, it is sometimes applied to children with familial intrinsic short stature, constitutional delay, or intrauterine growth retardation. It is likely that some subgroups of children now considered to have idiopathic short stature will be found to have specific molecular defects in GH, IGF-1, or new genes that influence growth. Some have advocated therapeutic trials of GH in individual children with idiopathic short stature to discern whether individuals should have continuing GH treatment; however, the robust growth response of many children with idiopathic short stature to short-term GH therapy suggests that short-term trials may not be particularly useful.[389] Long-term data suggest that GH can increase adult height by 4 to 7 cm in children with idiopathic short stature, and the Food and Drug Administration recently approved GH for the "long-term treatment of idiopathic short stature, also called non-growth hormone deficient short stature, defined by height SDs ≤ 2.25, and associated with growth rates unlikely to permit attainment of adult height in the normal range, in patients whose epiphyses are not closed and for whom diagnostic evaluation excludes other causes associated with short stature that should be observed or treated by other means."[389,390] Thus, depending on how this criterion is applied, 1.2% of U.S. children are potentially eligible for GH treatment, with resulting policy and practice implications.[391-394]

Differential Diagnosis of Short Stature by Growth Pattern

To individualize the workup of short stature, it is useful to classify patients according to the relationships among *chronologic age* (CA), *height age* (HA), *weight age* (WA), *bone age* (BA), and *growth rate*. These terms are defined in Table 36-2.

Diagnostic decisions can be simplified by first categorizing the disorder of growth with regard to whether it is a primary disturbance of weight (undernutrition) or height by the relationship between HA and WA. If the child's WA is depressed out of proportion to the HA (e.g., weight below the tenth percentile for height), primary nutritional disorders or chronic disease should be the principal diagnostic considerations. If the height and weight are proportionately depressed (or height is depressed out of proportion to weight), genetic, endocrinologic, or metabolic disorders are more likely to be responsible.

Primary linear growth disturbances result from inherent aberrations of bone growth or of systemic factors extrinsic to bone that affect its rate of growth. Disturbances of linear growth can be understood on the basis of three general principles: (1) Normal linear growth during childhood proceeds toward a genetically determined target height by following a predictable channel that is achieved by the end of infancy; (2) normal bone growth is accompanied by a predictable rate of advance of BA; and (3) children normally enter puberty at a pubertal BA. Based on these principles, linear growth disturbances can be categorized into three growth patterns: *intrinsic* shortness, *delayed* growth, or *attenuated* growth (see Fig. 36-6; Table 36-6).[395]

Intrinsic shortness is characterized by inherent limitation of bone growth that destines affected children to be short adults. The growth curves typically fall below normal by 3 years of age and then approximately parallel the normal curves in those children destined to be modestly short. The growth rates of these children are within or slightly below the normal range. In the more severe disorders of bone growth, such as Turner's syndrome and achondroplasia, however, the poor growth rates lead to the growth curve deviating progressively further below normal with time. The BA typically approximates the CA. Puberty occurs at a normal age (barring associated hypogonadism, as in Turner's syndrome). For example, a 9-year-old child with an HA of 6.5 years and a BA of 9 years will be small as an adult. Examples of this growth pattern include normal variant familial intrinsic short stature, Turner's syndrome and bone dysplasias, primary dysmorphic syndromes such as

Prader-Willi syndrome and Russell-Silver syndrome, severe intrauterine growth retardation–related short stature, and impaired spinal growth secondary to irradiation.

Children with a *delayed* growth pattern have delayed puberty and continue to grow for longer than their peers, thus potentially reaching normal adult heights. By 3 years of age, the growth curves of these children closely parallel the normal growth channels, with growth rates within or close to the normal range. In contrast to children with intrinsic shortness, the bone age is significantly delayed, typically to approximately the same extent as the height age. For example, a 9-year-old child with a height age of 6.5 and a bone age of 6.5 ordinarily has normal growth potential. Constitutional delay in growth and pubertal development is by far the most common cause of a delayed growth pattern. Other examples of conditions that may be associated with a delayed growth pattern are mild undernutrition and indolent chronic disease, such as anemia and persistent poorly controlled asthma. Because familial intrinsic short stature and constitutional delay are each so common, they occur together about as often as they occur alone. When they coexist, the growth rate is likely to be slightly subnormal and resemble the attenuated pattern.

Children with an *attenuated* growth pattern have low growth rates, resulting in their progressive deviation from the normal growth channels. BA is approximately equal to HA (or even less in hypothyroidism). The delayed BA indicates that adult height potential is normal, *if* the underlying disorder is treated effectively. Beyond 3 years of age, this pattern virtually always indicates underlying pathology. The underlying disorders, unless optimally treated, preclude normal achievement of the height potential. Thus, a 9-year-old child with an HA and BA of 6.5 and subnormal growth velocity has an attenuated growth pattern; this child has an endocrine, metabolic, or systemic disease until proven otherwise. Examples of conditions causing this growth pattern are GH deficiency, hypothyroidism, glucocorticoid excess, severe chronic illness, and malnutrition.

Diagnostic Evaluation

Given the many potential causes of short stature, establishing a diagnosis depends on eliciting several features on history, physical examination, and laboratory studies. Documentation of the growth rate and bone age are key, as discussed in the previous section on growth patterns. If the child has a normal bone age, suggesting an intrinsically short

Table 36-6 Differential Diagnosis of Short Stature by Growth Pattern

Type of Growth Pattern	Bone Age Approximates	Growth Rate	Differential Diagnostic Categories
Intrinsic shortness	Chronologic age (BA = CA > HA)	Approximates normal Normal/subnormal	Familial normal variant Genetic syndromes • Chromosomal anomalies • Bone dysplasia • Dysmorphic syndromes • Intrauterine growth retardation, nonspecific • Spinal irradiation
Delayed growth	Height age (BA = HA < CA)	Approximates normal	"Constitutional" normal variant Chronic disease Undernutrition
Attenuated growth	Height age (BA = HA < CA)	Subnormal	Endocrinopathies • GH deficiency • GH insensitivity • Hypothyroidism • Cushing's syndrome • Hypogonadism after 10–12 years of age • Acid-base disturbances • Chronic disease, severe (e.g., Crohn's disease) • Malnutrition

BA, bone age; CA, chronologic age; HA, height age.

growth pattern, it is important to seek a history of IUGR, presence/absence of neonatal lymphedema (suggestive of Turner's syndrome), a history of tetany or seizures (compatible with pseudohypoparathyroidism), and a family history of short stature. Physical examination in this group of patients should be directed toward a search for body disproportion and dysmorphisms as well as pubertal status. When the clinical assessment strongly suggests a particular diagnosis, appropriate and specific diagnostic tests, such as karyotype, gonadotropin and calcium levels, and a skeletal survey, can proceed.

In the child with a significantly delayed bone age, indicating a delayed or attenuated growth pattern, review of systems should be comprehensive. It should focus on weight changes, appetite, food intolerance, vomiting, abdominal cramping, and stool characteristics; genitourinary symptoms, particularly polyuria and enuresis; headache and visual disturbances (suggestive of CNS lesion); lethargy or cold intolerance (suggestive but not necessarily present in hypothyroidism); and pubertal development. The past medical history and history of the use of medications, particularly glucocorticoids in any form, may be important. A classic triad for congenital hypopituitarism is perinatal hypoglycemia, prolonged jaundice, and, in boys, micropenis. The clinician should seek a family history of delay of puberty or extreme short stature. The clinician should perform a careful general physical examination. Specific features on physical examination include the weight/height ratio, a search for finger clubbing or perianal sores (regarding inflammatory bowel disease), fundoscopy and examination of visual fields (to assess perichiasmatic central nervous system lesions such as craniopharyngiomas), assessment for goiter, and pubertal staging.

Constitutional delay in growth and development is principally a diagnosis of exclusion and, in extreme cases, is difficult to distinguish from isolated defects of gonadotropin or GH production. While puberty is delayed, the growth rate may fall to subnormal levels. Testing shows a delayed bone age, and the IGF-1 level remains at a prepubertal level, compatible with the bone age. Gonadotropin secretion may remain in the prepubertal range until the bone age has reached 11 to 12 years. The distinction between hypogonadism and delayed puberty can sometimes be made by determination of gonadotropin levels during sleep or in response to a gonadotropin-releasing hormone agonist test by 14 years of age.[396] GH tests may be compatible with GH deficiency unless performed after sex steroid priming.[324-326] Indeed, transient GH deficiency is sometimes associated with delayed puberty.

When the clinical assessment strongly suggests a particular diagnosis, appropriate and specific diagnostic tests can proceed. If the weight is below the tenth percentile for height, it may be difficult to distinguish undernutrition from constitutional underweight. Calorie counting, sweat test, and screening tests for occult chronic disease may be helpful. These include complete blood count, urinalysis, chemistry profile, erythrocyte sedimentation rate, and antiendomyseal antibodies.

If the cause of poor growth is still not clear, but the child's growth rate is subnormal (i.e., leading to an attenuated growth pattern) or the child's height is markedly below age-appropriate standards or the family target height, additional tests to assess possible hypothyroidism (free thyroxine, thyrotropin) and GH deficiency (IGF-1, IGFBP-3, provocative tests of GH reserve such as clonidine, arginine, insulin), and, in girls, karyotype for assessment for Turner's syndrome are indicated. Controversies in the diagnostic tests for GH deficiency are described at the beginning of this section. Less common tests are generally based on clinical suspicion of the underlying condition (e.g., methylation analysis to diagnose Prader-Willi syndrome, SHOX protein, GH-binding protein, and so forth).

Not uncommonly, previous measurements are unavailable and the child's pattern of growth is not clear, although the child seems healthy overall. In this situation, it would be reasonable to follow the child's height at regular intervals to establish a pattern of growth that dictates whether further tests are indicated.

Management

When at all possible, treatment should be directed at the primary cause of pathologic short stature. Examples include nutritional counseling for undernutrition, gluten-free diet for celiac disease, psychotherapy for eating disorders, thyroid hormone for hypothyroidism, and growth hormone for GH deficiency. Many of these disorders are hereditary; genetic counseling should not be overlooked.

For conditions considered normal variants (familial short stature, constitutional delay), reassurance and explanation of the wide range of normal are often very helpful. In discussing therapeutic options, the clinician must advise child and family about the unknown factors (for example, errors are inherent in height predictions). Many children often choose to forego medical intervention at this point.

Low-dose sex steroid therapy is indicated for the treatment of hypogonadism if puberty is delayed beyond 13 (girls) or 14 (boys) years of age.[397,398] In extreme cases of constitutional delay, this modality is useful for a limited period of time in order to boost self-image by advancing secondary sex characteristics gently with a mild corresponding growth spurt. In order to minimize the possibility of loss of growth potential, we recommend that the initial course of therapy for the induction of sexual development consists of six monthly injections of 50 mg/m^2 repository testosterone in boys and 0.2 mg depot estradiol in girls.[130,398] A reasonable alternative regimen for girls begins with 5 μg ethinyl estradiol by mouth daily.[399] Such a course of therapy has no deleterious effect on height potential and has positive effects on self-image. The patient's growth, development, and predicted height should be carefully reevaluated immediately on completion of the therapeutic regimen and again 6 months later before undertaking a second course of therapy. Depot testosterone, 100 mg/m^2/ month, and depot estradiol, 1.0 mg/month, closely approximate midpubertal sex hormone production in boys and girls, respectively. We prefer administering injections of repository forms of sex hormones to avoid the occasional side effects of 17-alkylated steroid analogues. However, the anabolic steroid oxandrolone 0.1 mg/kg/day for 3 to 6 months has been used without compromising final height.[400] Premature use of adult replacement doses of androgen or estrogen (about twofold greater than the midpubertal doses) will cause a disproportionate advance of BA relative to linear growth and compromise height potential. Children with delayed puberty should be followed closely from 10 years of age onward because, particularly in the most severely delayed cases with the most immature body proportions, puberty inexplicably occurs at an earlier than expected bone age, leading to the children falling well short of predicted height.[185,397]

GH therapy is currently approved by the Food and Drug Administration for the treatment of short stature due to GH deficiency (0.18–0.3 mg/kg/week, divided into daily subcutaneous doses), Turner's syndrome (up to 0.375 mg/kg/week), chronic renal failure prior to transplantation (up to 0.35 mg/kg/week),[230] persistent short stature after SGA status (i.e., IUGR) (0.48 mg/kg/week), Prader-Willi syndrome (0.24 mg/kg/week), and selected children with idiopathic short stature (up to 0.37 mg/kg/week) as described in previous sections.[249] A higher dose for GH-deficient adolescents in puberty has also been approved. Varying lines of data suggest that long-term GH therapy may promote growth in a variety of other conditions, although there have been inconsistencies in the findings. (See Refs. 230, 340, 391, and 401–413 for a review of medical, ethical, and policy issues concerning GH therapy for nontraditional indications.) It has been recommended that children on GH therapy have routine monitoring of IGF-1 and IGFBP-3 (and perhaps IGFBP-2).[414,415]

Since long-term gonadotropin releasing hormone (GnRH) agonist therapy is successful in improving adult height of children with idiopathic sexual precocity by delaying epiphyseal fusion, as discussed at the end of this chapter, attempts have been made to use this as a nonstandard method to promote growth in children with idiopathic short stature. The height prognosis in isolated GH deficiency seems to be improved by adding GnRH agonist to GH therapy.[416] Although significant improvement in adult height of normal short children has been achieved by years of GnRH agonist therapy, to the extent of about 1 cm for each year of therapy, this has been accompanied by significantly less accretion of bone mineral density; accordingly, long-term GnRH agonist treatment is not recommended for this condition.[417,418] Adding GH to GnRH therapy is reported to yield approximately twice as much increase in final height; the possibility that this combination will counteract the deleterious effect of GnRH agonist alone on bone mineral density is unknown.[419]

TALL STATURE

Causes of Tall Stature

Genetic normal variants cause most tall stature (Table 36-7). Two distinct familial variants, which lead to different outcomes in tall children, can be identified. One is *familial intrinsic tall stature* (sometimes called genetic tallness); children are typically normal size at birth and a high-normal growth rate is established by 3 years of age. Thus, the child typically crosses height percentile during the first 3 years of life and thereafter maintains a height-attained channel above and closely parallel to the 95th percentile. Children with *constitutionally advanced growth and pubertal development* grow similarly during childhood, but they have an advanced BA and go into puberty early, so they stop growing at a normal height. Both these groups of children have a family history of a similar growth pattern, and the child does not show clinical or biochemical features of the disorders described as follows.

Genetic and chromosomal disorders are known causes of tall stature. Hyperploidy of sex chromosomes predisposes to tall stature.[48] The most common of these disorders is Klinefelter's syndrome (47,XXY). It is characterized by decreased upper to lower segment ratio dating from the prepubertal years, hypogonadism, and gynecomastia; it is often associated with mild mental retardation. The prototypic genetic syndrome associated with tall stature is Marfan syndrome, which usually segregates with mutations in the fibrillin gene.[48,420] It is classically characterized by musculoskeletal signs (such as arachnodactyly and hyperextensibility), cardiovascular findings (such as aortic aneurysm), ocular signs (such as lens subluxation), decreased upper to lower body ratio, and autosomal-dominant heredity. Arachnodactyly can be quantitated from either the body proportions or the metacarpal index (ratio of length to midshaft breadth of metacarpals II–V; normal: male < 8.0:1, female < 8.7:1) on a BA. Congenital contractural arachnodactyly is a genetically closely related syndrome. Homocystinuria has marfanoid features but also may involve mental retardation, joint contractures, and a tendency to thromboembolism. Sipple's syndrome (type 2 polyendocrine syndrome) may also have marfanoid features; the presence of mucosal neuromas may be a specific clue to its presence.

Sotos' syndrome ("cerebral gigantism") is characterized by the presence of overgrowth during early childhood, a moderately advanced BA, macrocephaly, developmental retardation, and dysmorphisms, particularly acromegaloid facial feature.[421–423] Most are long and slender at birth; they reach an above average, occasionally excessive, adult height. The great majority of cases are due to mutation of nuclear receptor binding SET-domain 1 (NSD1),[423,424] sometimes in association with a chromosome *5q35* microdeletion. Weaver syndrome, which has somewhat different facial dysmorphisms, is sometimes an allelic variant. Sotos' syndrome can be mimicked by fragile X syndrome. Disproportionate bone age advancement characterizes some other congenital overgrowth disorders, such as Marshall-Smith syndrome, characterized by poor weight gain.[190]

The prototypic congenital macrosomia syndrome is Beckwith-Weidemann syndrome. The most consistent features

---

Table 36-7 Factors Causing Tall Stature, with Representative Clinical Conditions

Factors Affecting Height	Representative Conditions		Clinical and Laboratory Features
Genetic	Normal variants	Familial intrinsic tallness	Growth parallels 95th percentile; family history of tall stature; normal physical exam, puberty, and BA
		Constitutionally advanced	Growth parallels 95th percentile; puberty and BA slightly advanced
	Chromosomal abnormalities	Klinefelter's syndrome	Hypogenitalism and hypogonadism, eunuchoid; 47,XXY
		Fragile X syndrome	Mental retardation; macroorchidism in males
	Dysmorphic syndromes	Marfan syndrome	Arachnodactyly, hyperextensibility, lens subluxation, aortic dilation
		Beckwith-Wiedemann syndrome	Infant gigantism, macroglossia, umbilical defects, neonatal syndrome hypoglycemia due to pancreatic β-cell hyperplasia, may develop embryonal tumors
		Sotos' syndrome	Cerebral gigantism: dolichocephalic large head, coarse facies, cerebral dysfunction
Nutrition	Primary obesity		IGF-1 blood level nutrition-driven, "growth without GH"
Hormones	GH excess		Accelerated growth, acromegaloid signs with advancing age, occasional hyperprolactinemia; may be associated with McCune-Albright syndrome
	Hyperthyroidism		Hypermetabolic features, goiter, eye abnormalities
	Sex steroid	Excess	Precocious puberty: premature secondary sexual characteristics and epiphyseal fusion, leading to compromise of adult height
		Deficiency	Deficiency beyond teenage years permits prolonged growth and may lead to eunuchoid habitus

BA, bone age; GH, growth hormone; IGF-1, insulin-like growth factor 1.

are overgrowth, macroglossia, umbilical defects ranging from hernia to omphalocele, and earlobe pits. Hyperplasia of various visceral (especially kidney) and endocrine organs (especially pancreatic β cells) is the rule. Birth size is above average, growth velocity is high until midchildhood, and adult height is 2.5 SD above normal. Children with this syndrome are predisposed to develop embryonal intra-abdominal tumors in early childhood, most commonly Wilms' tumor and adrenocortical carcinoma. The disorder is associated with loss of heterozygosity at chromosomal locus *11p15.5* due to duplications, translocation/inversion, unipaternal disomy, or mutation of the CDKI *p57*[KIP2], which cause imbalance between the function of growth-promoting genes such as IGF-2 and tumor suppressor genes on this imprinted region.[425] The Simpson-Golabi-Behmal syndrome is similar in having macrosomia, macroglossia, omphalocele, and Wilms' tumor, but has a different pattern of associated features, such as "bulldog facies," polydactyly, fingernail hypoplasia, and even greater adult height.[95] It is caused by an X-linked mutation of glypican-3, a receptor that modulates IGF-2 action.

Lipodystrophy, particularly the total forms, whether congenital or acquired, is associated with tall stature.[426] Insulin resistance is frequently so severe as to cause pseudoacromegaly and hyperlipidemia is prominent.

Overnutrition (exogenous obesity) during childhood typically accelerates growth slightly and advances BA comparably to HA. IGF-1 levels are normal in the presence of low GH levels.[73]

Hormonal disorders of GH, sex steroids, and thyroid hormone can cause tall stature. *GH excess is* a rare but important cause of accelerated growth. This condition, termed *gigantism* during childhood, may be associated with acromegaloid features in older children (Fig. 36-16).[427,428] It is usually due to

a pituitary somatotroph adenoma or to somatotroph hyperplasia. Activating mutations of G_{sa} have been described in isolated pituitary adenomas and in patients with McCune-Albright syndrome associated with hypersecretion of hormones such as GH.[429,430] Hyperprolactinemia may coexist.

Hyperthyroidism accelerates bone growth and maturation.[426] Affected infants may have premature cranial synostosis.[431]

Sexual precocity accelerates height. Classically, BA is stimulated disproportionately, which leads to premature epiphyseal fusion. Thus, these children become tall, but stop growing prematurely, so their adult height is stunted. Slowly progressive forms of precocious puberty do not necessarily deleteriously affect adult height, however.[432]

Sex hormone deficiency, conversely, prolongs the growing period because the epiphyses do not close. This leads to increased height and eunuchoid proportions in hypogonadal individuals.[433] Through the discovery of patients deficient in aromatase or with inactivating mutation of the estrogen receptor, estradiol has been found to be the critical hormone that brings about epiphyseal fusion.[106]

Differential Diagnosis of Tall Stature by Growth Pattern

Since supranormal height occurs either because of inherent endowment or an excessive stimulation of the rate of bone growth, the diagnostic approach based on the relationships of CA, HA, BA, and growth velocity is analogous to that described for short stature. Four patterns of growth causing tall stature can be distinguished: intrinsic tallness, advanced growth, accelerated growth, and prolonged growth (Table 36-8, Fig. 36-17).[395,434]

Intrinsic tallness is the term applied to literally long-boned individuals. They come to grow above, but approximately parallel, to the 95th percentile on height-attained curves.

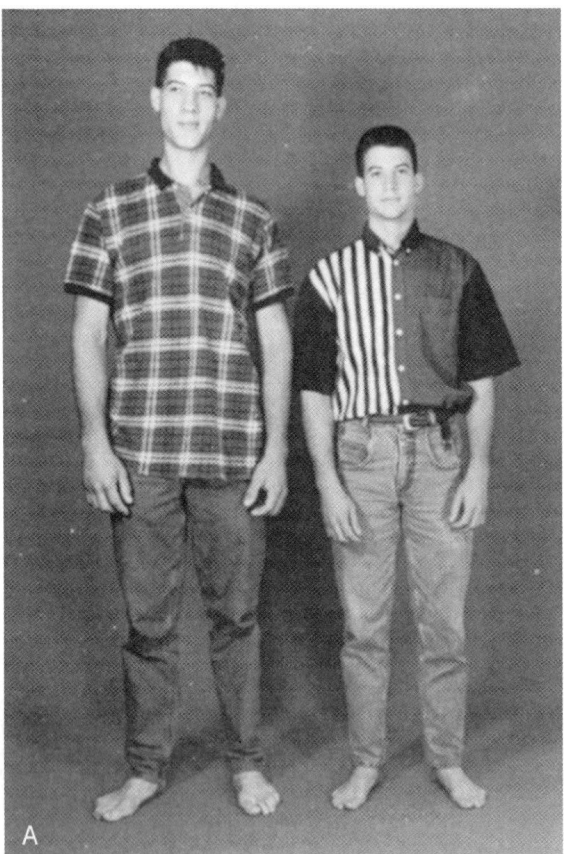
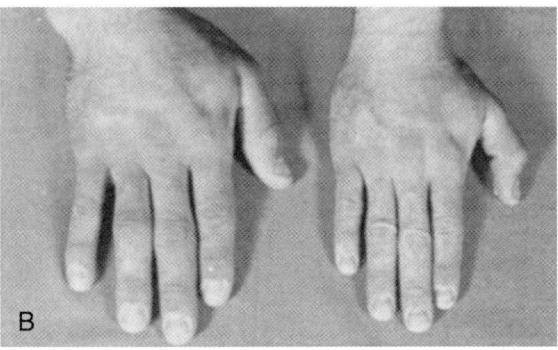
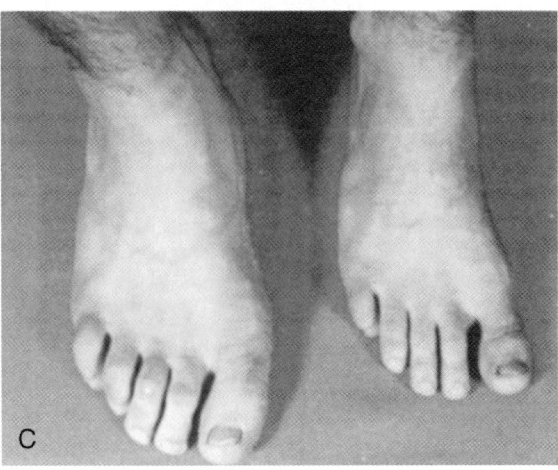

Figure 36-16 Pituitary gigantism. A 22-year-old-man with gigantism caused by excess growth hormone is shown to the left of his identical twin. The increased height (**A**) and enlarged hand (**B**) and foot (**C**) of the affected twin are apparent. Their height and features began to diverge at approximately 13 years of age. (From Gagel RF, McCutcheon IE: Images in clinical medicine. Pituitary gigantism. N Engl J Med 340:524, 1999).

Table 36-8 Differential Diagnosis of Tall Stature by Growth Pattern

Type of Growth Pattern	Bone Age Relationships	Growth Rate	Differential Diagnostic Categories
Intrinsic tallness	BA ≈ CA < HA	Approximates normal	Familial tallness Chromosomal disorders • XXY, fragile X, XXX • XYY • *8p* trisomy Genetic disorders • Marfanoid syndromes • Cerebral gigantism syndromes • Congenital macrosomia syndromes
Advanced growth	BA ≈ HA > CA	Approximates normal	"Constitutional" normal variant Obesity Lipodystrophy Hyperthyroidism
Accelerated growth	BA > HA > CA BA ≤ HA > CA	Supranormal Supranormal	Sexual precocity GH or IGF excess
Prolonged growth	BA < HA > CA	Normal	Hypogonadism Estrogen deficiency

BA, bone age; CA, chronologic age; HA, height age.

Their BA and age of puberty are normal. This is usually a normal variant (familial intrinsic tallness), but rarely is due to genetic disorders such as Marfan syndrome or homocystinuria.

Advanced growth is a pattern with similar growth in childhood, with a growth velocity that maintains them approximately parallel to the 95th percentile on height-attained curves, but they go into puberty early so stop growing at a normal size. This pattern is indicated by a BA advanced in proportion to HA. Examples include normal variant (constitutionally advanced), obesity, and hyperthyroidism. Mild forms of sexual precocity also cause this growth pattern.

Accelerated growth refers to that pattern in which growth rate is excessive. Adult height is abnormal unless the underlying disorder is corrected. Adult height is subnormal in rapidly progressive sexual precocity, and is excessive in GH excess.

Prolonged growth results from deficiency of sex hormones, particularly estrogen. Such patients continue growing into adulthood.

Diagnostic Evaluation

The tall child whose height parallels the 95th percentile and has tall parents, no dysmorphic features, normal pace of puberty, and a normal bone age is likely to have *intrinsic tallness* on a familial origin without a pathologic basis. Further investigations are often not needed. However, chromosomal disorders, Marfan syndrome, homocystinuria, and occasionally excessive GH can simulate the clinical picture. The presence of dysmorphic features, macroorchidism, or intellectual impairment in a tall child suggests the need for chromosome analysis, plasma amino acid assay, or genetics consultation to evaluate these possibilities. An increase in the concentration of IGF-2 and the IGF-2/IGFBP-3 ratio have been noted in some children with constitutional tall stature, and suggested as a mechanism for increased growth.[435]

The tall child with an *advanced growth pattern* (i.e., BA advanced in proportion to HA) is likely to have "constitutional" normal variant tallness, particularly if the height

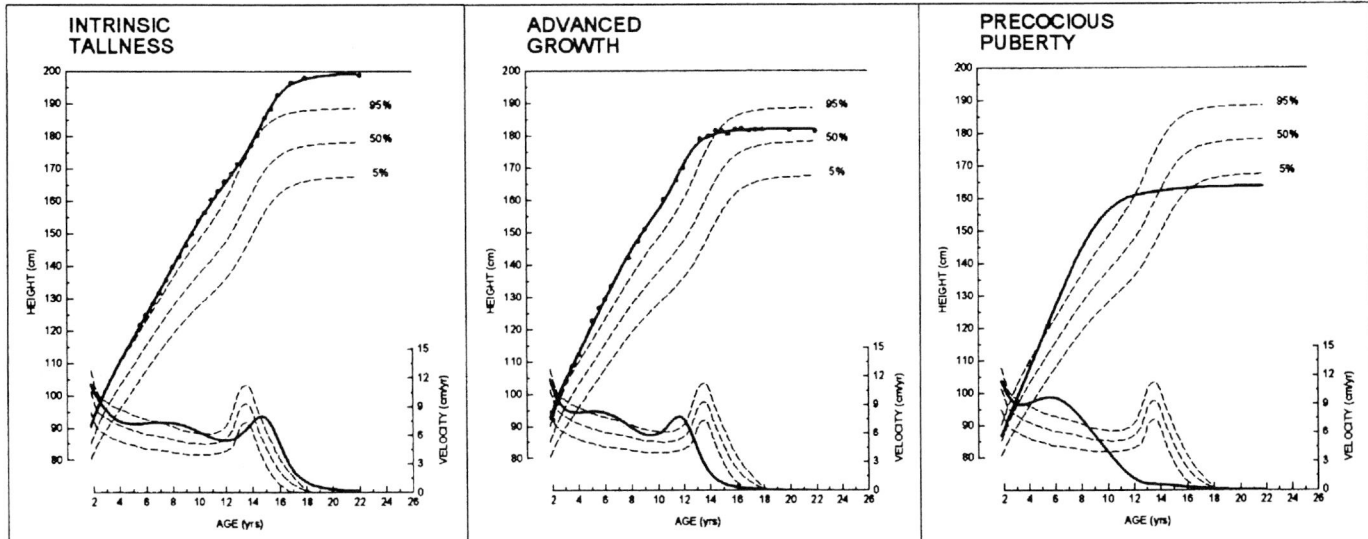

Figure 36-17 Growth patterns of three boys of similar prepubertal tall stature. Growth data on the two boys on the left are from the Fels Institute files. One became a tall adult (intrinsic tall stature); the other grew to be of normal adult height after undergoing an early pubertal growth spurt (advanced height). Growth data on the boy with precocious puberty are derived from the data of Thamdrup.[284] (Courtesy of RD Bock.)

parallels the 95th percentile, there is a compatible family history, and the clinical examination is otherwise normal. Since hyperthyroidism may mimic this presentation, the clinical examination includes evaluation for goiter, ophthalmologic abnormalities, and hypermetabolism; thyroid function studies will provide confirmation. Exogenous obesity, in the absence of dysmorphic features or intellectual impairment, may present this pattern of tall stature. In the absence of puberty or symptoms or signs suggestive of a hypothalamic disturbance or hypoglycemia, the tall stature virtually excludes an endocrine basis for obesity.

An *accelerated growth pattern* (involving progressive deviation of height above the 95th percentile and an advanced bone age) requires assessment for sexual precocity. This includes clinical assessment of primary and secondary sexual characteristics, as well as evaluation for the possibility of central nervous system disorders or abdominal masses and a search for nevi and bone deformities. If the BA is significantly advanced, screening should commence with determination of blood levels of estradiol, testosterone, dehydroepiandrosterone sulfate, gonadotropins (preferably in a third-generation assay), and possibly serum hCG. Screening for excessive GH secretion should be initiated with random GH, IGF-1, and IGFBP-3 blood levels. The definitive test for the diagnosis of GH excess is the failure of serum GH to suppress below 2 ng/mL after an oral glucose load (1.75 g/kg, maximum 100 g), although some false-positive tests have been reported.[427] Hyperprolactinemia often exists together with GH excess. The most reliable confirmatory test is one of suppressibility of serum GH after a glucose load. If there is evidence of GH excess, serum GHRH may be measured (to assess the rare possibility of ectopic GHRH production) and appropriate imaging studies performed. The clinician should also consider the possibilities of McCune-Albright syndrome, multiple endocrine adenomatosis type I, and carcinoid syndrome in children and adolescents with GH excess.

A *prolonged growth pattern* suggests sex hormone deficiency or resistance. Evaluation of pubertal development, sense of smell (to evaluate Kallmann's syndrome), and body proportions (eunuchoid habitus with long legs and low upper/lower body segment ratio is characteristic of sex hormone deficiency) are needed. Laboratory studies include ascertainment of circulating sex hormone and gonadotropin levels, chromosome analysis, and, when indicated, imaging studies.

Management

Since familial intrinsic tall stature represents a variant of the normal, reassurance and support are needed. In certain cases (e.g., predicted adult height in excess of 183 cm for girls), familial tall stature may be particularly distressing, and treatment to curtail growth by accelerating epiphyseal fusion can be undertaken. Estrogen in large amounts (e.g., 0.3 mg/day of ethinyl estradiol) can be begun just before or early in puberty, given daily without interruption, and continued until epiphyseal fusion has occurred. A progestin (e.g., 100 mg of progesterone) taken orally daily for 10 days for the first 10 days of each month is also given to yield regular menses. Potential risks of estrogen therapy include thrombosis, hyperlipidemia, glucose intolerance, nausea, mild hypertension, and weight gain. Although there is evidence that estrogen therapy can reduce adult height as much as 3.5 to 7.3 cm below that predicted, the results cannot be assured.[436,437] Because of the potential adverse effects, relatively few endocrinologists offer high-dose estrogen for growth suppression.[438] Somatostatin analogue may be an alternative treatment to reduce adult height in selected cases; some authors have reported comparable treatment with estrogen for girls with Marfan syndrome, androgen insensitivity, and other overgrowth problems.[436] Depot testosterone in highly virilizing doses (about 400 mg every 2 weeks) has been used to reduce predicted adult height in selected tall boys, but experience is limited.[436]

Hypersecretion of GH due to pituitary adenomas is generally treated by surgery and/or a somatostatin analogue. Pituitary radiation has also been utilized. Pituitary hyperplasia causing GH excess (as in McCune-Albright syndrome) can be treated with somatostatin analogue. In ectopic GHRH-producing tumors, surgical removal is the treatment of choice.

The compromised height potential resulting from gonadotropin-dependent sexual precocity is treated by suppressing gonadotropins with long-acting gonadotropin-releasing hormone agonists. The most widely used agent in the United States is depot leuprolide (ordinarily given as a monthly depot intramuscular injection). The treatment is effective when started at an early age, with an average height gain above pretreatment height prediction of about 1.4 cm for each year of therapy.[439] Coincident GH deficiency must be treated for optimal growth.[440] Furthermore, GH-sufficient patients with central precocity who are started on treatment relatively late and whose height velocity falls below the prepubertal normal range after 2 to 3 years gain an average of 2 cm per year when GH therapy is added.[441] Otherwise, premature puberty is treated by specific therapy where possible, for example, using cortisol replacement for congenital adrenal hyperplasia or inhibitors of steroidogenesis for McCune-Albright syndrome. Conversely, sex hormone deficiency can be replaced.

REFERENCES

1. Cheek DB: Human Growth. Philadelphia, Lea & Febiger, 1968.
2. Winick M, Noble A: Quantitative changes in DNA, RNA, and protein during prenatal and postnatal growth in the rat. Dev Biol 12(3):451–466, 1965.
3. Orlowski CC, Furlanetto RW: The mammalian cell cycle in normal and abnormal growth. Endocrinol Metab Clin North Am 25:491–502, 1996.
4. Meredith JE Jr, Winitz S, Lewis JM, et al: The regulation of growth and intracellular signaling by integrins. Endocr Rev 17(3):207–220, 1996.
5. Mitchell BS: The proteasome: An emerging therapeutic target in cancer. N Engl J Med 348(26):2597–2598, 2003.
6. Zipursky A: Telomerase, immortality, and cancer. Pediatr Res 47(2):174, 2000.
7. Styne DM: Fetal growth. Clin Perinatol 25:917–938, 1998.
8. Zhao Y, Westphal H: Homeobox genes and human genetic disorders. Curr Mol Med 2(1):13–23, 2002.
9. Markakis EA: Development of the neuroendocrine hypothalamus. Front Neuroendocrinol 23(3):257–291, 2002.
10. Cushman LJ, Showalter AD, Rhodes SJ: Genetic defects in the development and function of the anterior pituitary gland. Ann Med 34(3):179–191, 2002.
11. Gluckman PD: The endocrine regulation of fetal growth in late gestation: The role of insulin-like growth factors. J Clin Endocrinol Metab 80:1047–1050, 1994.
12. Brooks AA, Johnson MR, Steer PJ, et al: Birth weight: nature or nurture? Early Hum Dev 42(1):29–35, 1995.
13. Constancia M, Hemberger M, Hughes J, et al: Placental-specific IGF-II is a major modulator of placental and fetal growth. Nature 417(6892):945–948, 2002.
14. Lindgren V: Genomic imprinting in disorders of growth. Endocrinol Metab Clin North Am 25(3):503–521, 1996.
15. Coutant R, Boux de Casson F, Douay O, et al: Relationships between placental GH concentration and maternal smoking, newborn gender, and maternal leptin: Possible implications for birth weight. J Clin Endocrinol Metab 86(10):4854–4859, 2001.
16. Christou H, Serdy S, Mantzoros CS: Leptin in relation to growth and developmental processes in the fetus. Semin Reprod Med 20(2):123–130, 2002.

17. Schinzel AA, Smith DW, Miller JR: Monozygotic twinning and structural defects. J Pediatr 95(6):921–930, 1979.
18. Handwerger S, Freemark M: The roles of placental growth hormone and placental lactogen in the regulation of human fetal growth and development. J Pediatr Endocrinol Metab 13(4):343–356, 2000.
19. Vatten LJ, Nilsen ST, Odegard RA, et al: Insulin-like growth factor I and leptin in umbilical cord plasma and infant birth size at term. Pediatrics 109(6):1131–1135, 2002.
20. Lubchenco LO, Hansman C, Dressler M, Boyd E: Intrauterine growth as estimated from liveborn birth-weight data at 24 to 42 weeks gestation. Pediatrics 32:793–800, 1963.
21. Thomson AM, Billewicz WZ, Hytten FE: The assessment of fetal growth. J Obstet Gynecol Br Commonw 75:90, 1968.
22. Wingerd J, Schoen EJ: Factors influencing length at birth and height at five years. Pediatrics 53(5):737–741, 1974.
23. Beck GJ, van der Berg BJ: The relationship of the rate of intrauterine growth of low-birth-weight infants to later growth. J Pediatr 86:504, 1975.
24. Gardoni J, Chang A, Kalyan B, et al: Customized antenatal growth charts. Lancet 339:283–287, 1991.
25. Yip R, Binkin NJ, Trowbridge FL: Altitude and childhood growth. J Pediatr 113:486–489, 1988.
26. de Zegher F, Francois I, van Helvoirt M, Van den Berghe G: Small as fetus and short as child: From endogenous to exogenous growth hormone. J Clin Endocrinol Metab 82:2021–2026, 1997.
27. Smith DW, Popick C: Large fontanels in congenital hypothyroidism: A potential clue toward earlier recognition. J Pediatr 80:753, 1972.
28. DeChiara TM, Efstratiadis A, Robertson EJ: A growth-deficiency phenotype in heterozygous mice carrying an insulin-like growth factor II gene disrupted by targeting. Nature 345(6270):78–80, 1990.
29. Liu JP, Baker J, Perkins AS, et al: Mice carrying null mutations of the genes encoding insulin-like growth factor I (Igf-1) and type 1 IGF receptor (Igf1r). Cell 75(1):59–72, 1993.
30. Baker J, Liu JP, Robertson EJ, Efstratiadis A: Role of insulin-like growth factors in embryonic and postnatal growth. Cell 75(1):73–82, 1993.
31. Louvi A, Accili D, Efstratiadis A: Growth-promoting interaction of IGF-II with the insulin receptor during mouse embryonic development. Dev Biol 189(1):33–48, 1997.
32. Lassarre C, Hardouin S, Daffos F, et al: Serum insulin-like growth factors and insulin-like growth factor binding proteins in the human fetus: Relationships with growth in normal subjects and in subjects with intrauterine growth retardation. Pediatr Res 29(3):219–225, 1991.

33. Woods KA, Camacho-Hubner C, Savage MO, Clark AJ: Intrauterine growth retardation and postnatal growth failure associated with deletion of the insulin-like growth factor I gene. N Engl J Med 335(18):1363–1367, 1996.
34. Rosenfield RL: Role of androgens in growth and development of the fetus, child, and adolescent. Adv Pediatr 19:171, 1972.
35. Gluckman PD: Editorial: nutrition, glucocorticoids, birth size, and adult disease. Endocrinology 142(5):1689–1691, 2001.
36. Barker DJ, Eriksson JG, Forsen T, Osmond C: Fetal origins of adult disease: Strength of effects and biological basis. Int J Epidemiol 31(6):1235–1239, 2002.
37. Houang M, Morineau G, le Bouc Y, et al: The cortisol-cortisone shuttle in children born with intrauterine growth retardation. Pediatr Res 46(2):189–193, 1999.
38. Cianfarani S, Geremia C, Scott CD, Germani D: Growth, IGF system, and cortisol in children with intrauterine growth retardation: Is catch-up growth affected by reprogramming of the hypothalamic-pituitary-adrenal axis? Pediatr Res 51(1):94–99, 2002.
39. Hofman PL, Cutfield WS, Robinson EM, et al: Insulin resistance in short children with intrauterine growth retardation. J Clin Endocrinol Metab 82(2):402–406, 1997.
40. Soto N, Bazaes RA, Pena V, et al: Insulin sensitivity and secretion are related to catch-up growth in small-for-gestational-age infants at age 1 year: Results from a prospective cohort. J Clin Endocrinol Metab 88(8):3645–3650, 2003.
41. Ibañez L, Ferrer A, Ong K, et al: Insulin sensitization early after menarche prevents progression from precocious pubarche to polycystic ovary syndrome. J Pediatr 144(1):23–29, 2004.
42. Bhargava SK, Sachdev HS, Fall CH, et al: Relation of serial changes in childhood body-mass index to impaired glucose tolerance in young adulthood. N Engl J Med 350(9):865–875, 2004.
43. McCance DR, Pettitt DJ, Hanson RL, et al: Birth weight and non–insulin dependent diabetes: Thrifty genotype, thrifty phenotype, or surviving small baby genotype? Br Med J 308(6934):942–945, 1994.
44. Morley R, Dwyer T: Fetal origins of adult disease? Clin Exp Pharmacol Physiol 28(11):962–966, 2001.
45. Huxley R, Neil A, Collins R: Unraveling the fetal origins hypothesis: Is there really an inverse association between birthweight and subsequent blood pressure? Lancet 360(9334):659–665, 2002.
46. Vaessen N, Janssen JA, Heutink P, et al: Association between genetic variation in the gene for insulin-like growth factor-I and low birthweight. Lancet 359(9311):1036–1037, 2002.

47. Lorentzon M, Lorentzon R, Nordstrom P: Vitamin D receptor gene polymorphism is associated with birth height, growth to adolescence, and adult stature in healthy Caucasian men: A cross-sectional and longitudinal study. J Clin Endocrinol Metab 85(4):1666–1670, 2000.
48. Sotos JF: Overgrowth. Section IV. Genetic disorders associated with overgrowth. Clin Pediatr (Phila) 36(1):39–49, 1997.
49. Kirsch S, Weiss B, Schon K, Rappold GA: The definition of the Y chromosome growth-control gene (GCY) critical region: Relevance of terminal and interstitial deletions. J Pediatr Endocrinol Metab 15(Suppl 5):1295–1300, 2002.
50. Zinn A: Growing interest in Turner syndrome. Nature Genet 16:3–4, 1997.
51. Baron R: General principles of bone biology. In Favus M (ed): Primer on the Metabolic Bone Disorders and Disorders of Mineral Metabolism, 5th ed. Philadelphia, Lippincott Williams & Wilkins, 2003.
52. Robson H, Siebler T, Shalet SM, Williams GR: Interactions between GH, IGF-I, glucocorticoids, and thyroid hormones during skeletal growth. Pediatr Res 52(2):137–147, 2002.
53. Horton WA: Skeletal development: Insights from targeting the mouse genome. Lancet 362(9383):560–569, 2003.
54. Matsukawa N, Grzesik WJ, Takahashi N, et al: The natriuretic peptide clearance receptor locally modulates the physiological effects of the natriuretic peptide system. Proc Natl Acad Sci U S A 96(13):7403–7408, 1999.
55. Miyazawa T, Ogawa Y, Chusho H, et al: Cyclic GMP-dependent protein kinase II plays a critical role in C-type natriuretic peptide-mediated endochondral ossification. Endocrinology 143(9):3604–3610, s2002.
56. Tanner JM: Growth at Adolescence. London, Blackwell, 1962.
57. Abbott RD, White LR, Ross GW, et al: Height as a marker of childhood development and late-life congnitive function: The Honolulu-Asia aging study. Pediatrics 102:602–603, 1998.
58. Hommes FA, Drost YM, Geraets WXM, Reijenga MAA: The energy requirement for growth: An application of Atkinson's metabolic price system. Pediatr Res 9:51, 1975.
59. Holt LE Jr: Some problems in dietary amino acid requirements. Am J Clin Nutr 21:367, 1968.
60. Fisch RO, Gravem HJ, Feinberg SB: Growth and bone characteristics of phenylketonurics: Comparative analysis of treated and untreated phenylketonuric children. Am J Dis Child 112(1):3–10, 1966.
61. Cahill GF Jr: Editorial: Nitrogen versatility in bats, bears and man. N Engl J Med 290(12):686–687, 1974.
62. Holman RT: Essential fatty acid deficiency. Prog Chem Fats Lipids 9:275, 1968.

63. Chesney RW: Requirements and upper limits of vitamin D intake in the term neonate, infant, and older child [see comments]. J Pediatr 116(2):159–166, 1990.

64. Clement DH, Fomon SJ, Forbes GB, et al: Trace elements in infant nutrition. Pediatrics 26:715, 1960.

65. Ulmer DD: Trace elements. N Engl J Med 297(6):318–321, 1977.

66. Nakamura T, Nishiyama S, Futagoishi-Suginohara Y, et al: Mild to moderate zinc deficiency in short children: Effect of zinc supplementation on linear growth velocity [see comments]. J Pediatr 123(1):65–69, 1993.

67. Danks DM, Campbell PE, Walker-Smith J, et al: Menkes kinky-hair syndrome. Lancet 1:1100, 1972.

68. Cooke RE, Boyden DG, Haller E: The relationship of acidosis and growth retardation. J Pediatr 57:326, 1960.

69. Viteri FE: The effect of inactivity on the growth of rats fed diets adequate or restricted with respect to normal caloric intake. New Concepts about Old Aspects of Malnutrition. Academia Mexicana de Pediatria, 1973.

70. Rosenfeld MG, Briata P, Dasen J, et al: Multistep signaling and transcriptional requirements for pituitary organogenesis in vivo. Recent Prog Horm Res 55:1–13, discussion 13–14, 2000.

71. Treier M, Gleiberman AS, O'Connell SM, et al: Multistep signaling requirements for pituitary organogenesis in vivo. Genes Dev 12(11):1691–1704, 1998.

72. Mayo KE, Miller T, DeAlmeida V, et al: Regulation of the pituitary somatotroph cell by GHRH and its receptor. Recent Prog Horm Res 55:237–266, discussion 266–237, 2000.

73. Giustina A, Veldhuis JD: Pathophysiology of the neuroregulation of growth hormone secretion in experimental animals and the human. Endocr Rev 6:717–797, 1998.

74. Ghigo E, Aimaretti G, Arvat E, Camanni F: Growth hormone–releasing hormone combined with arginine or growth hormone secretagogues for the diagnosis of growth hormone deficiency in adults. Endocrine 15(1):29–38, 2001.

75. Veldhuis J, Bowers C: Three-peptide control of pulsatile and entropic feedback-sensitive modes of growth hormone secretion: Modulation by estrogen and aromatizable androgen. J Pediatr Endocrinol Metab 16 (Suppl 3):587–605, 2003.

76. Tannenbaum GS, Epelbaum J, Bowers CY: Interrelationship between the novel peptide ghrelin and somatostatin/growth hormone–releasing hormone in regulation of pulsatile growth hormone secretion. Endocrinology 144(3):967–974, 2003.

77. Torsello A, Scibona B, Leo G, et al: Ontogeny and tissue-specific regulation of ghrelin mRNA expression suggest that ghrelin is primarily involved in the control of extraendocrine functions in the rat. Neuroendocrinology 77(2):91–99, 2003.

78. Wang G, Lee HM, Englander E, Greeley GH Jr: Ghrelin—not just another stomach hormone. Regul Pept 105(2):75–81, 2002.

79. Le Roith D, Bondy C, Yakar S, et al: The somatomedin hypothesis: 2001. Endocr Rev 22(1):53–74, s2001.

80. Wallenius K, Sjogren K, Peng XD, et al: Liver-derived IGF-I regulates GH secretion at the pituitary level in mice. Endocrinology 142(11):4762–4770, 2001.

81. Gasperi M, Cecconi E, Grasso L, et al: GH secretion is impaired in patients with primary hyperparathyroidism. J Clin Endocrinol Metab 87(5):1961–1964, 2002.

82. De Zegher F, Van Den Berghe G, Devlieger H, et al: Dopamine inhibits growth hormone and prolactin secretion in the human newborn. Pediatr Res 34(5):642–645, 1993.

83. Melmed S, Yamashita S, Yamasaki H, et al: IGF-I receptor signaling: Lessons from the somatotroph. Recent Prog Horm Res 51:189–215, discussion 215–186, 1996.

84. Korytko AI, Cuttler L: Regulation of GHRH receptor gene expression in the neonatal and adult rat pituitary. Growth Horm IGF Res 11(5):282–288, 2001.

85. Wallis M: Growth hormone–binding proteins. Clin Endocrinol 35:291–293, 1991.

86. Walker JL, Moats-Staaats BM, Stiles AD, Underwood LE: Tissue-specific developmental regulation of the messenger ribonucleic acids encoding the growth hormone receptor and the growth hormone binding protein in rat fetal and postnatal tissues. Pediatr Res 31:335–339, 1992.

87. Eugster E: New revelations about the role of STATs in stature. N Engl J Med 349(12):1110–1112, 2003.

88. Lupu F, Terwilliger JD, Lee K, et al: Roles of growth hormone and insulin-like growth factor 1 in mouse postnatal growth. Dev Biol 229(1):141–162, 2001.

89. Spagnoli A, Rosenfeld RG: The mechanisms by which growth hormone brings about growth: The relative contributions of growth hormone and insulin-like growth factors. Endocrinol Metab Clin North Am 25:615–632, 1996.

90. Le Roith D, Scavo L, Butler A: What is the role of circulating IGF-I? Trends Endocrinol Metab 12(2):48–52, 2001.

91. Firth SM, Baxter RC: Cellular actions of the insulin-like growth factor binding proteins. Endocr Rev 23(6):824–854, 2002.

92. Daughaday WH: Free insulin-like growth factor (IGF) in disorders of IGF binding protein 3 complex formation. J Clin Endocrinol Metab 89(1):3–5, 2004.

93. Domene HM, Bengolea SV, Martinez AS, et al: Deficiency of the circulating insulin-like growth factor system associated with inactivation of the acid-labile subunit gene. N Engl J Med 350(6):570–577, 2004.

94. D'Ercole AJ: Insulin-like growth factors and their receptors in growth. Endocrinol Metab Clin North Am 25:573–590, 1996.

95. Weksberg R, Squire JA, Templeton DM: Glypicans: A growing trend [news, comment]. Nat Genet 12:225–227, 1996.

96. Pao C-I, Farmer PK, Begovic S, et al: Regulation of insulin-like growth factor-I (IGF-I) and IGF-binding protein 1 gene transcription by hormones and provision of amino acids in rat hepatocytes. Mol Endocrinol 7:1561–1568, 1993.

97. Menon RK, Sperling MA: Insulin as a growth factor. Endocrinol Metab Clin North Am 25:633–648, 1996.

98. Argente J, Caballo N, Barrios V, et al: Multiple endocrine abnormalities of the growth hormone and insulin-like growth factor axis in prepubertal children with exogenous obesity: Effect of short- and long-term weight reduction. J Clin Endocrinol Metab 82:2076–2083, 1997.

99. Schalch DS, Heinrich UE, Draznin B, et al: Role of the liver in regulating somatomedin activity: Hormonal effects on the synthesis and release of insulin-like growth factor and its carrier protein by the isolated perifused rat liver. Endocrinol 104:1044, 1979.

100. Juul A, Holm K, Kastrup KW, et al: Free insulin-like growth factor I serum levels in 1430 healthy children and adults, and its diagnostic value in patients suspected of growth hormone deficiency. J Clin Endocrinol Metab 82:2497–2502, 1997.

101. Van den Brande JL, DeCaju MVL: Plasma somatomedin activity in children with growth disturbances. In: Raiti S (ed): Advances in Human Growth Hormone Research. Washington, DC, US Government Printing Office, 1974, p 98.

102. Quarmby V, Quan C, Ling V, et al: How much insulin-like growth factor I (IGF-I) circulates? Impact of standardization on IGF-I assay accuracy. J Clin Endocrinol Metab 83:1211–1216, 1998.

103. Clark PA, Rogol AD: Growth hormones and sex steroid interactions at puberty. Endocrinol Metab Clin North Am 25:665–682, 1996.

104. Roemmich JN, Clark PA, Mai V, et al: Alterations in growth and body composition during puberty: III. Influence of maturation, gender, body composition, fat distribution, aerobic fitness, and energy expenditure on nocturnal growth hormone release. J Clin Endocrinol Metab 83:1440–1447, 1998.

105. Rosenfield RL, Furlanetto R: Physiologic testosterone or estradiol induction of puberty increases plasma somatomedin-C. J Pediatr 107(3):415–417, 1985.

106. Bachrach BE, Smith EP: The role of sex steroids in bone growth and development: Evolving new concepts. Endocrinol 6:362–368, 1996.

107. Schaff-Blass E, Burstein S, Rosenfield RL: Advances in diagnosis and treatment of short stature, with special reference to the role of growth hormone. J Pediatr 104(6):801–813, 1984.

108. Collett-Solberg PF, Cohen P: The role of the insulin-like growth factor binding proteins and the IGFBP proteases in modulating IGF action. Endocrinol Metab Clin North Am 25:591–614, 1996.

109. Mohan S, Baylink DJ: IGF-binding proteins are multifunctional and act via IGF-dependent and -independent mechanisms. J Endocrinol 175(1):19–31, 2002.

110. Phillips LS, Fusco AC, Unterman TC, del Greco F: Somatomedin inhibitor in uremia. J Clin Endocrinol Metab 59:764, 1984.

111. Allen DB: Growth suppression by glucocorticoid therapy. Endocrinol Metab Clin North Am 25:699–718, 1996.

112. Ballinger A: Fundamental mechanisms of growth failure in inflammatory bowel disease. Horm Res 58(Suppl 1):7–10, 2002.

113. Geffner ME: The growth without growth hormone syndrome. Endocrinol Metab Clin North Am 25:649–664, 1996.

114. Den Ouden DT, Kroon M, Hoogland PH, et al: A 43-year-old male with untreated panhypopituitarism due to absence of the pituitary stalk: From dwarf to giant. J Clin Endocrinol Metab 87(12):5430–5434, 2002.

115. Faustini-Fustini M, Balestrieri A, Rochira V, Carani C: The apparent paradox of tall stature with hypopituitarism: New insights from an old story. J Clin Endocrinol Metab 88(8):4002–4003, author reply 4003, 2003.

116. Weiss RE, Refetoff S: Effect of thyroid hormone on growth: Lessons from the syndrome of resistance to thyroid hormone. Endocrinol Metab Clin North Am 25:719–730, 1996.

117. Allen DB, Julius JR, Breen TJ, Attie KM: Treatment of glucocorticoid-induced growth suppression with growth hormone. J Clin Endocrinol Metab 83:2824–2829, 1998.

118. Mehls O, Himmele R, Homme M, et al: The interaction of glucocorticoids with the growth hormone–insulin-like growth factor axis and its effects on growth plate chondrocytes and bone cells. J Pediatr Endocrinol Metab 14(Suppl 6):1475–1482, 2001.

119. Hochberg Z: Mechanisms of steroid impairment of growth. Horm Res 58(Suppl 1):33–38, 2002.

120. Baron J, Klein KO, Colli MJ, et al: Catch-up growth after glucocorticoid excess: A mechanism intrinsic to the growth plate. Endocrinol 135:1367–1371, 1994.

121. Canalis E: Inhibitory actions of glucocorticoids on skeletal growth: Is local insulin-like growth factor I to blame? [editorial; comment]. Endocrinology 139(7):3041–3042, 1998.

122. Daughaday WH, Rotwein P: Insulin-like growth factors I and II: Peptide, messenger ribonucleic acid and gene structures, serum, and tissue concentrations. Endocr Rev 10(1):68–91, 1989.

123. Rosenfeld RG, Rosenbloom AL, Guevara-Aguirre J: Growth hormone (GH) insensitivity due to primary GH receptor deficiency. Endocr Rev 15(3):369–390, 1994.

124. Abu AO, Horner A, Kusec V, et al: The localization of androgen receptors in human bone. J Clin Endocrinol Metab 82:3493–3497, 1997.

125. Zachmann M, Prader A, Sobel E, et al: Pubertal growth in patients with androgen insensitivity: Indirect evidence for the importance of estrogens in pubertal growth of girls. J Pediatr 108:694–697, 1986.

126. Kousteni S, Bellido T, Plotkin LI, et al: Nongenotropic, sex-nonspecific signaling through the estrogen or androgen receptors: Dissociation from transcriptional activity. Cell 104(5):719–730, 2001.

127. Seeman E: The structural and biomechanical basis of the gain and loss of bone strength in women and men. Endocrinol Metab Clin North Am 32(1):25–38, 2003.

128. Smith EP, Boyd J, Frank GR, et al: Estrogen resistance caused by a mutation in the estrogen-receptor gene in a man. N Engl J Med 331(16):1056–1061, 1994.

129. Migliaccio S, Newbold RR, Bullock BC, et al: Alterations of maternal estrogen levels during gestation affect the skeleton of female offspring. Endocrinology 137(5):2118–2125, 1996.

130. Rosenfield RL, Perovic N, Devine N, et al: Optimizing estrogen replacement treatment in Turner syndrome. Pediatrics 102:486–488, 1998.

131. Rosenfield R: Low-dose testosterone effect on somatic growth. Pediatrics 77:853–857, 1986.

132. Usher R, McLean F: Intrauterine growth of live-born Caucasian infants at sea level: Standards obtained from measurements in seven dimensions of infants born between 25 and 44 weeks of gestation. J Pediatr 74(6):901–910, 1969.

133. Thomas P, Peabody J, Turnier V, Clark RH: A new look at intrauterine growth and the impact of race, altitude, and gender. Pediatrics 106(2):e21, 2000.

134. Pryse-Davies J, Smitham JH, Napier KA: Factors influencing development of secondary ossification centres in the fetus and newborn: A postmortem radiological study. Arch Dis Child 49(6):425–431, 1974.

135. Shaffer SG, Quimiro CL, Anderson JV, Hall R: Postnatal weight changes in low birth weight babies. 602–603 79:702, 1983.

136. Niklasson A, Engstrom E, Hard AL, et al: Growth in very preterm children: A longitudinal study. Pediatr Res 54(6):899–905, 2003.

137. Hack M, Schluchter M, Cartar L, et al: Growth of very low birth weight infants to age 20 years. Pediatrics 112(1 Pt 1):e30–e38, 2003.

138. Sas T, de Waal W, Mulder P, et al: Growth hormone treatment in children with short stature born small for gestational age: 5-year results of a randomized, double-blind, dose-response trial. J Clin Endocrinol Metab 84(9):3064–3070, 1999.

139. Centers for Disease Control and Prevention: CDC growth charts: United States. National Center for Health Statistics. Available at: http://www.cdc.gov/growthcharts/. Accessed May 30, 2000.

140. Tanner JM, Davies PS: Clinical longitudinal standards for height and height velocity for North American children. J Pediatr 107(3):317–329, 1985.

141. Bock RD, Rosenfield RL: Course-of-growth norms for longitudinal height velocity. Hummanbiol (Budapest) 25:575–586, 1994.

142. Lyon AJ, Preece MA, Grant DB: Growth curve for girls with Turner syndrome. Arch Dis Child 60(10):932–935, 1985.

143. Horton WA, Rotter JI, Kaitila I, et al: Growth curves in achondroplasia. Birth Defects Orig Artic Ser 13(3C):101–107, 1977.

144. Cronk C, Crocker AC, Pueschel SM, et al: Growth charts for children with Down syndrome: 1 month to 18 years of age. Pediatrics 81(1):102–110, 1988.

145. Fredriks AM, van Buuren S, Burgmeijer RJ, et al: Continuing positive secular growth change in the Netherlands 1955–1997. Pediatr Res 47(3):316–323, 2000.

146. Hammer LD, Wilson DM, Litt IF, et al: Impact of pubertal development on body fat distribution among white, Hispanic, and Asian female adolescents. J Pediatr 118(6):975–980, 1991.

147. Karlberg J: On the construction of the infancy-childhood-puberty growth standard [see comments]. Acta Paediatr Scand Suppl 356:26–37, 1989.

148. Smith DW, Truog W, Rogers JE, et al: Shifting linear growth during infancy: Illustration of genetic factors in growth from fetal life through infancy. J Pediatr 89(2):225–230, 1976.

149. Reed RB, Stuart HC: Patterns of growth in height and weight from birth to 18 years of age. Pediatrics 29:904–921, 1959.

150. Tanner JM, Whitehouse RH, Takaishi M: Standards from birth to maturity for height, weight, height velocity, and weight velocity: British children, 1960. Arch Dis Child 41:454, 1966.

151. Bock RD, Thissen D: Statistical problems of fitting individual growth curves. In Johnson F, Roche A, C S (eds): Human Physical Growth and Maturation. New York, Plenum, 1980, p 265.

152. Tanner JM, Goldstein H, Whitehouse RH: Standards for children's height at ages 2–9 years allowing for heights of parents. Arch Dis Child 45(244):755–762, 1970.

153. Boersma B, Wit JM: Catch-up growth. Endocr Rev 18(5):646–661, 1997.

154. Glinos AD: Density dependent regulation of growth and differentiated function in suspension cultures of mouse fibroblasts. In Kulonen E, Pikkarainen J (eds): Biology of Fibroblast. New York, Academic, 1973, p 155.

155. Tillmann V, Thalange NK, Foster PJ, et al: The relationship between stature, growth, and short-term changes in height and weight in normal prepubertal children. Pediatr Res 44(6):882–886, 1998.

156. Gill MS, Tillmann V, Veldhuis JD, Clayton PE: Patterns of GH output and their synchrony with short-term height increments influence stature and growth performance in normal children. J Clin Endocrinol Metab 86(12):5860–5863, 2001.

157. Shuttleworth FK: Sexual maturation and physical growth of girls age 6 to 19. Monogr Soc Res Child Dev 2:5, 1937.

158. Cara JF, Rosenfield RL, Furlanetto RW: A longitudinal study of the relationship of plasma somatomedin-C concentration to the pubertal growth spurt. Am J Dis Child 41:562–564, 1987.

159. Tanner JM, Whitehouse RH, Marshall WA, Carter BS: Prediction of adult height from height, bone age, and occurrence of menarche, at ages 4 to 16 with allowance for midparent height. Arch Dis Child 50(1):14–26, 1975.

160. Bayley N, Pinneau S: Tables for predicting adult height from skeletal age: Revised for use with the Gruelich-Pyle hand standards. J Pediatr 40:432–441, 1952.

161. Russell DL, Keil MF, Bonat SH, et al: The relation between skeletal maturation and adiposity in African American and Caucasian children. J Pediatr 139(6):844–848, 2001.

162. Barr GD, Allen CM, Shinefield HR: Height and weight of 7500 children of three skin colors. Am J Dis Child 124:866, 1972.

163. McKusick VA: Heritable Disorders of Connective Tissue, 4th ed. St. Louis, Mosby, 1972.

164. Engelbach W: Endocrine Medicine, Vol 1. Springfield, IL, Thomas, 1932.

165. Maresh MM: Linear growth of long bones of extremities from infancy through adolescence. Am J Dis Child 89:725, 1955.

166. Nellhaus G: Head circumference from birth to 18 years: Practical composite international and interracial graphs. Pediatrics 41(1):106–114, 1968.

167. Weaver DD, Christian JC: Familial variation of head size and adjustment for parental head circumference. J Pediatr 96:990–994, 1980.

168. Krieger I: Head circumference, mental retardation and growth failure. Pediatrics 37:384, 1966.

169. Cloutier MD, Stickler GB: Head circumference in children with idiopathic hypopituitarism. Pediatrics 42(1):209–210, 1968.

170. Prader A: Catch-up growth. Postgrad Med J 54(Suppl 1):133–146, 1978.

171. Ranke MB: Catch-up growth: New lessons for the clinician. J Pediatr Endocrinol Metab 15(Suppl 5):1257–1266, 2002.

172. Wit JM, Boersma B: Catch-up growth: definition, mechanisms, and models. J Pediatr Endocrinol Metab 15(Suppl 5):1229–1241, 2002.

173. Boersma B, Houwen RH, Blum WF, et al. Catch-up growth and endocrine changes in childhood celiac disease: Endocrine changes during catch-up growth. Horm Res 58(Suppl 1):57–65, 2002.

174. Bongiovanni AM: Letter: Maturational deceleration following treatment with testosterone. J Pediatr 83(6):1095, 1973.

175. Ranke MB, Cutfield WS, Lindberg A, et al: A growth prediction model for short children born small for gestational age. J Pediatr Endocrinol Metab 15(Suppl 5):1273, 2002.

176. Gruelich WW, Pyle SI: Radiographic Atlas of Skeletal Development of the Hand and Wrist. Palo Alto, CA, Stanford University Press, 1959.

177. Wilkins L: The Diagnosis and Treatment of Endocrine Disorders in Childhood and Adolescence, 3d ed. Springfield, IL, 1965.

178. Roche AF, Eyman SL, Davila GH: Skeletal age prediction. J Pediatr 78:997, 1971.

179. Baer MJ, Durkatz J: Bilateral asymmetry in skeletal maturation of the hand and wrist. Am J Phys Anthropol 15:180, 1957.

180. Tanner J, Oshman D, Bahhage F, Healy M: Tanner-Whitehouse bone age reference values for North American children [see comments]. J Pediatr 131(1 Pt 1):34–40, 1997.

181. Garn SM, Sandusky ST, Nagy JM, McCann MB: Advanced skeletal development in low-income Negro children. J Pediatr 80(6):965–969, 1972.

182. Flor-Cisneros A, Leschek EW, Merke DP, et al: In boys with abnormal developmental tempo, maturation of the skeleton and the hypothalamic-pituitary-gonadal axis remains synchronous. J Clin Endocrinol Metab 89(1):236–241, 2004.

183. Frisancho AR, Garn SM, Rohmann CG: Age at menarche: A new method of prediction and retrospective assessment based on hand x-rays. Hum Biol 41:42, 1969.

184. Bayer LM, Bayley N: Growth pattern shifts in healthy children spontaneous and induced. J Pediatr 62:631, 1963.

185. Hintz RL, Attie KM, Baptista J, Roche A: Effect of growth hormone treatment on adult height of children with idiopathic short stature. N Engl J Med 340:502–507, 1999.

186. Roche AF, Wainer H, Thissen D: The RWT method for the prediction of adult stature. Pediatrics 56(6):1027–1033, 1975.

187. Tanner JM, Healy MJR, Goldstein H, Cameron N: Assessment of Skeletal Maturity and Prediction of Adult Height (TW3 Method), 3d ed. London, WB Saunders, 2001.

188. International Working Group on Constitutional Diseases of Bone: International nomenclature and classification of the osteochondrodysplasias (1997). Am J Med Genet 79(5):376–382, 1998.

189. Superti-Furga A, Bonafe L, Rimoin DL: Molecular-pathogenetic classification of genetic disorders of the skeleton. Am J Med Genet 106(4):282–293, 2001.

190. Jones K: Smith's Recognizable Patterns of Human Malformation, Vol 4, 4th ed. Philadelphia, WB Saunders, 1988.

191. Horton WA: Molecular genetic basis of the human chondrodysplasias. Endocrinol Metab Clin North Am 25:683–698, 1996.

192. Horton WA: Fibroblast growth factor receptor 3 and the human chondrodysplasias. Curr Opin Pediatr 9:437–442, 1997.

193. Hellemans J, Coucke PJ, Giedion A, et al: Homozygous mutations in IHH cause acrocapitofemoral dysplasia, an autosomal recessive disorder with cone-shaped epiphyses in hands and hips. Am J Hum Genet 72(4):1040–1046, 2003.

194. Fanconi S, Fischer JA, Wielandd P, et al: Kenny syndrome: Evidence for idiopathic hypoparathyroidism in two patients and for abnormal parathyroid hormone in one. J Pediatr 109:469, 1986.

195. Schipani E, Langman CB, Parfitt AM, et al: Constitutively activated receptors for parathyroid hormone and parathyroid hormone-related peptide in Jansen's metaphyseal chondrodysplasia [see comments]. N Engl J Med 335(10):708–714, 1996.

196. Silverman RN: Caffey's Pediatric X-Ray Diagnosis, Vol 1, 8th ed. Chicago, Year Book Medical Publications, 1985.

197. Shapiro F: Epiphyseal disorders. New Engl J Med 317:1702–1710, 1987.

198. Morris CA, Mervis CB, Hobart HH, et al: GTF2I hemizygosity implicated in mental retardation in Williams syndrome: Genotype-phenotype analysis of five families with deletions in the Williams syndrome region. Am J Med Genet 123A(1):45–59, 2003.

199. Maassen JA, Tobias ES, Kayserilli H, et al: Identification and functional assessment of novel and known insulin receptor mutations in five patients with syndromes of severe insulin resistance. J Clin Endocrinol Metab 88(9):4251–4257, 2003.

200. Moebius FF, Fitzky BU, Glossmann H: Genetic defects in postsqualene cholesterol biosynthesis. Trends Endocrinol Metab 11(3):106–114, 2000.

201. Dupuis-Girod S, Gluckman E, Souberbielle JC, Brauner R: Growth hormone deficiency caused by pituitary stalk interruption in Fanconi's anemia. J Pediatr 138(1):129–133, 2001.

202. Tischkowitz MD, Morgan NV, Grimwade D, et al: Deletion and reduced expression of the Fanconi anemia FANCA gene in sporadic acute myeloid leukemia. Leukemia 18(3):420–425, 2004.

203. Bartsch O, Wagner A, Hinkel GK, et al: FISH studies in 45 patients with Rubinstein-Taybi syndrome: Deletions associated with polysplenia, hypoplastic left heart and death in infancy. Eur J Hum Genet 7(7):748–756, 1999.

204. Lehmann AR: DNA repair-deficient diseases, xeroderma pigmentosum, Cockayne syndrome and trichothiodystrophy. Biochimie 85(11):1101–1111, 2003.

205. Hegele RA: Drawing the line in progeria syndromes. Lancet 362(9382):416–417, 2003.

206. Hickson ID: RecQ helicases: Caretakers of the genome. Nat Rev Cancer 3(3):169–178, 2003.

207. Rao E, Weiss B, Fukami M, et al: Pseudoautosomal deletions encompassing a novel homeobox gene cause growth failure in idiopathic short stature and Turner syndrome. Nat Genet 16(1):54–63, 1997.

208. Ross JL, Scott C Jr, Marttila P, et al: Phenotypes Associated with SHOX Deficiency. J Clin Endocrinol Metab 86(12):5674–5680, 2001.

209. Ogata T, Matsuo N: Sex chromosome aberrations and stature: Deduction of the principal factors involved in the determination of adult height. Hum Genet 91(6):551–562, 1993.

210. Zinn AR, Wei F, Zhang L, et al: Complete SHOX deficiency causes Langer mesomelic dysplasia. Am J Med Genet 110(2):158–163, 2002.

211. Rosenfeld RG, Attie KM, Frane J, et al: Growth hormone therapy of Turner's syndrome: Beneficial effect on adult height. J Pediatr 132:319–324, 1998.

212. Saenger P: Turner syndrome. Curr Ther Endocrinol Metab 6:239–243, 1997.

213. Pasquino AM, Passeri F, Pucarelli I, et al: Spontaneous pubertal development in Turner syndrome. J Clin Endocrinol Metab 82:1810–1813, 1997.

214. Committee on Genetics, American Academy of Pediatrics: Health supervision for children with Turner syndrome. Pediatrics 96(6):1166–1173, 1995.

215. van Pareren YK, de Muinck Keizer-Schrama SM, Stijnen T, et al: Final height in girls with turner syndrome after long-term growth hormone treatment in three dosages and low dose estrogens. J Clin Endocrinol Metab 88(3):1119–1125, 2003.

216. Cave CB, Bryant J, Milne R: Recombinant growth hormone in children and adolescents with Turner syndrome. Cochrane Database Syst Rev 3:CD003887, 2003.

217. Quigley CA, Crowe BJ, Anglin DG, Chipman JJ: Growth hormone and low dose estrogen in Turner syndrome: Results of a United States multi-center trial to near-final height. J Clin Endocrinol Metab 87(5):2033–2041, 2002.

218. Summitt RL: Turner syndrome and Noonan's syndrome. J Pediatr 75(4):730–731, 1969.

219. Carballo EC: Turner syndrome and Noonan's syndrome. J Pediatr 75(4):729–730, 1969.

220. Curts FL, Pucci E, Scappaaticci S, et al: XO and male phenotype. Am J Dis Child 128:90, 1974.

221. Heller RH: The Turner phenotype in the male. J Pediatr 66:48,1965.

222. Anonymous: Noonan's syndrome. Lancet 340:22, 1992.

223. Tartaglia M, Kalidas K, Shaw A, et al: PTPN11 mutations in Noonan syndrome: Molecular spectrum, genotype-phenotype correlation, and phenotypic heterogeneity. Am J Hum Genet 70(6):1555–1563, 2002.

224. Kosaki K, Suzuki T, Muroya K, et al: PTPN11 (protein-tyrosine phosphatase, nonreceptor-type 11) mutations in seven Japanese patients with Noonan syndrome. J Clin Endocrinol Metab 87(8):3529–3533, 2002.

225. Saenger P: Editorial: Noonan syndrome—certitude replaces conjecture. J Clin Endocrinol Metab 87(8):3527–3528, 2002.

226. Ranke MB, Heidemann P, Knupfer C, et al: Noonan syndrome: Growth and clinical manifestations in 144 cases. Eur J Pediatr 148:220–227, 1988.

227. Kelnar CJ: Growth hormone therapy in noonan syndrome. Horm Res 53(Suppl 1):77–81, 2000.

228. Holm VA, Cassidy SB, Butler MG, et al: Prader-Willi syndrome: Consensus diagnostic criteria. Pediatrics 91:398–402, 1993.

229. Cassidy SB: Prader-Willi syndrome. J Med Genet 34:917–923, 1997.

230. Furlanetto RW, Allen D, Gertner J, et al: Guidelines for the use of growth hormone in children with short stature: A report by the Drug and Therapeutics Committee of the Lawson Wilkins Pediatric Endocrine Society. J Pediatr 127:857–867, 1995.

231. Carrel AL, Myers SE, Whitman BY, Allen DB: Growth hormone improves body composition, fat utilization, physical strength and agility, and growth in Prader-Willi syndrome: A controlled study. J Pediatr 134(2):215–221, 1999.

232. Lindgren AC, Hagenaas L, Muller J, et al: Growth hormone treatment of children with Prader-Willi syndrome affects linear growth and body composition favorably. Acta Paediatr 87:28–31, 1998.

233. Hale DE, Cody JD, Baillargeon J, et al: The spectrum of growth abnormalities in children with 18q deletions. J Clin Endocrinol Metab 85(12):4450–4454, 2000.

234. Lee PA, Chernausek SD, Hokken-Koelega AC, Czernichow P: International Small for Gestational Age Advisory Board consensus development conference statement: Management of short children born small for gestational age, April 24–October 1, 2001. Pediatrics 111(6 Pt 1):1253–1261, 2003.

235. Robertson C: Catch-up growth among very-low-birth-weight preterm infants: A historical perspective. J Pediatr 143(2):145–146, 2003.

236. Eggermann T, Wollmann HA, Kuner R, et al: Molecular studies in 37 Silver-Russell syndrome patients: Frequency and etiology of uniparental disomy. Hum Genet 100:415–419, 1997.

237. Spiro RP, Christian SL, Ledbetter D, et al: Intrauterine growth retardation associated with maternal uniparental disomy for chromosome 6 unmasked by congenital adrenal hyperplasia. Pediatr Res 43(Part 2)(4):128A (Abst 736), 1998.

238. Abuzzahab MJ, Schneider A, Goddard A, et al: IGF-I receptor mutations resulting in intrauterine and postnatal growth retardation. N Engl J Med 349(23):2211–2222, 2003.

239. Lin CC, Santolaya-Forgas J: Current concepts of fetal growth restriction: Part I. Causes, classification, and pathophysiology. Obstet Gynecol 92(6):1044–1055, 1998.

240. Saal HM, Pagon RA, Pepin MG: Reevaluation of Russell-Silver syndrome. J Pediatr 107(5):733–737, 1985.

241. Davies PS, Valley R, Preece MA: Adolescent growth and pubertal progression in the Silver-Russell syndrome. Arch Dis Child 63(2):130–135, 1988.

242. Kandall SR, Albin S, Lowinson J, et al: Differential effects of maternal heroin and methadone use on birthweight. Pediatrics 58(5):681–685, 1976.

243. Chiriboga-Klein S, Oberfield SE, Casullo AM, et al: Growth in congenital rubella syndrome and correlation with clinical manifestations [see comments]. J Pediatr 115(2):251–255, 1989.

244. Soothill P, Nicolaides KH, Bilardo CM, Campbell S: Relation of fetal hypoxia in growth retardation to mean blood velocity in the fetal aorta. Lancet 2:1118, 1986.

245. Bergner L, Susser MW: Low birth weight and prenatal nutrition: An interpretative review. Pediatrics 46(6):946–966, 1970.

246. Naeye RL, Blanc W, Paul C: Effects of maternal nutrition on the human fetus. Pediatrics 52(4):494–503, 1973.

247. Naeye R: Organ abnormalities in a human parabiotic syndrome. Am J Pathol 46:299, 1965.

248. Medovy H: New parameters in neonatal growth: Cell number and cell size. J Pediatr 711:459, 1967.

249. Physician's Desk Reference, 57th ed. Montvale, NJ, Thompson PDR, 2003.

250. Saenger P: US experience in evaluation and diagnosis of GH therapy of intrauterine growth retardation/small-for-gestational-age children. Horm Res 58(Suppl 3):27–29, 2002.

251. Ranke MB, Lindberg A, Cowell CT, et al: Prediction of response to growth hormone treatment in short children born small for gestational age: analysis of data from KIGS (Pharmacia International Growth Database). J Clin Endocrinol Metab 88(1):125–131, 2003.

252. Pomerance JJ: Management of short children born small for gestational age. Pediatrics 112(1 Pt 1):180–182, 2003.

253. Lee PA, Kendig JW, Kerrigan JR: Persistent short stature, other potential outcomes, and the effect of growth hormone treatment in children who are born small for gestational age. Pediatrics 112(1 Pt 1):150–162, 2003.

254. Cutfield WS, Jackson WE, Jefferies C, et al: Reduced insulin sensitivity during growth hormone therapy for short children born small for gestational age. J Pediatr 142(2):113–116, 2003.

255. Sandberg DE, Smith MM, Fornari V, et al: Nutritional dwarfing: Is it a consequence of disturbed psychosocial functioning? Pediatrics 88(5):926–933, 1991.

256. Pugliese MT, Lifshitz F, Grad G, et al: Fear of obesity: A cause of short stature and delayed puberty. N Engl J Med 309(9):513–518, 1983.

257. Frisch RE, McArthur JW: Menstrual cycles: Fatness as a determinant of minimum weight for height necessary for their maintenance or onset. Science 185(4155):949–951, 1974.

258. Winter RJ, Phillips LS, Green OC, Traisman HS: Somatomedin activity in the Mauriac syndrome. J Pediatr 97(4):598–600, 1980.

259. Taylor AM, Sharma AK, Avasthy N, et al: Inhibition of somatomedin-like activity by serum from streptozotocin-diabetic rats: Prevention by insulin treatment and correlation with skeletal growth. Endocrinology 121(4):1360–1365, 1987.

260. Addy DP, Hudson FP: Diencephalic syndrome of infantile emaciation: Analysis of literature and report of further three cases. Arch Dis Child 47(253):338–343, 1972.

261. Vlachopapadopoulou E, Tracey KJ, Capella M, et al: Increased energy expenditure in a patient with diencephalic syndrome. J Pediatr 122:922, 1993.

262. Zeitler PS, Travers S, Kappy MS: Advances in the recognition and treatment of endocrine complications in children with chronic illness. Adv Pediatr 46:101–149, 1999.

263. Maki M, Mustalahti K, Kokkonen J, et al: Prevalence of celiac disease among children in Finland. N Engl J Med 348(25):2517–2524, 2003.

264. Sawczenko A, Ballinger AB, Croft NM, et al: Adult height in patients with early onset of Crohn's disease. Gut 52(3):454–455; author reply 455, 2003.

265. Alemzadeh N, Rekers-Mombarg LT, Mearin ML, et al: Adult height in patients with early onset of Crohn's disease. Gut 51(1):26–29, 2002.

266. Ballinger A: Management of growth retardation in the young patient with Crohn's disease. Expert Opin Pharmacother 3(1):1–7, 2002.

267. Sentongo TA, Stettler N, Christian A, et al: Growth after intestinal resection for Crohn's disease in children, adolescents, and young adults. Inflamm Bowel Dis 6(4):265–269, 2000.

268. Kapila P, Jones J, Rees L: Effect of chronic renal failure and prednisolone on the growth hormone–insulin-like growth factor axis. Pediatr Nephrol 16(12):1099–1104, 2001.

269. Frystyk J, Ivarsen P, Skjaerbaek C, et al: Serum-free insulin-like growth factor I correlates with clearance in patients with chronic renal failure. Kidney Int 56(6):2076–2084, 1999.

270. Tonshoff B, Blum WF, Wingen AM, Mehls O: Serum insulin-like growth factors (IGFs) and IGF binding proteins 1, 2, and 3 in children with chronic renal failure: Relationship to height and glomerular filtration rate. The European Study Group for Nutritional Treatment of Chronic Renal Failure in Childhood. J Clin Endocrinol Metab 80(9):2684–2691, 1995.

271. Fine RN, Stablein D, Cohen AH, et al: Recombinant human growth hormone post–renal transplantation in children: A randomized controlled study of the NAPRTCS. Kidney Int 62(2):688–696, 2002.

272. Simopoulos AP, Bartter FC: Growth characteristics and factors influencing growth in Bartter's syndrome. J Pediatr 81:56, 1972.

273. Platt OS, Rosenstock W, Espeland MA: Influence of sickle hemoglobinopathies on growth and development. N Engl J Med 311:7, 1984.

274. Glorieux FH: Rickets, the continuing challenge [editorial; comment]. N Engl J Med 325(26):1875–1877, 1991.

275. Alon U, Donaldson DL, Hellerstein S, et al: Metabolic and histologic investigation of the nature of nephrocalcinosis in children with hypophosphatemic rickets and in the Hyp mouse. J Pediatr 120:899–905, 1991.

276. Sampson B, Kovar IZ, Rauscher A, et al: A case of hyperzincemia with functional zinc depletion: A new disorder? Pediatr Res 42(2):219–225, 1997.

277. Italian Working Group on Endocrine Complications in Non-endocrine Diseases: Multicentre study on prevalence of endocrine complications in thalassaemia major. Clin Endocrinol (Oxf) 42(6):581–586, 1995.

278. Ellenberger C, Runyan TE: Holoprosencephaly with hypoplasia of the optic nerve, dwarfish and agenesis of the septum pellucidum. Am J Opthal 70:960, 1970.

279. Rudman D, Davis T, Priest JH, et al: Prevalence of growth hormone deficiency in children with cleft lip or palate. J Pediatr 93(3):378–382, 1978.

280. Roessler E, Belloni E, Gaudenz L, et al: Mutations in the human sonic hedgehog gene cause holoprosencephaly. Nat Genet 14:357–360, 1996.

281. Berry SA, Pierpont ME, Gorlin RJ: Solitary maxillary central incisor and short stature. J Pediatr 104:877, 1984.

282. Carvalho LR, Woods KS, Mendonca BB, et al: A homozygous mutation in HESX1 is associated with evolving hypopituitarism due to impaired repressor-corepressor interaction. J Clin Invest 112(8):1192–1201, 2003.

283. Cohen LE, Wondisford FE, Radovick S: Role of Pit-1 in the gene expression of growth hormone, prolactin, and thyrotropin. Endocrinol Metab Clin North Am 25:523–540, 1996.

284. Mendonca BB, Osorio MGF, Laatronico AC, et al: Longitudinal hormonal and pituitary imaging changes in two females with combined pituitary hormone deficiency due to deletion of A301,G302 in the PROP1 gene. J Clin Endocrinol Metab 84:942–945, 1999.

285. Dattani ML, Martinez-Barbera J, Thomas PQ, et al: Molecular genetics of septo-optic dysplasia. Horm Res 53(Suppl 1):26–33, 2000.

286. Parks JS, Brown MR, Hurley DL, et al: Heritable disorders of pituitary development. J Clin Endocrinol Metab 84(12):4362–4370, 1999.

287. Brickman JM, Clements M, Tyrell R, et al: Molecular effects of novel mutations in Hesx1/HESX1 associated with human pituitary disorders. Development 128(24):5189–5199, 2001.

288. Deladoey J, Fluck C, Buyukgebiz A, et al: "Hot spot" in the PROP1 gene responsible for combined pituitary hormone deficiency. J Clin Endocrinol Metab 84(5):1645–1650, 1999.

289. Paracchini R, Giordano M, Corrias A, et al: Two new PROP1 gene mutations responsible for compound pituitary hormone deficiency. Clin Genet 64(2):142–147, 2003.

290. Vieira TC, Dias da Silva MR, Cerutti JM, et al: Familial combined pituitary hormone deficiency due to a novel mutation R99Q in the hot spot

region of Prophet of Pit-1 presenting as constitutional growth delay. J Clin Endocrinol Metab 88(1):38–44, 2003.

291. Netchine I, Sobrier ML, Krude H, et al: Mutations in LHX3 result in a new syndrome revealed by combined pituitary hormone deficiency. Nat Genet 25(2):182–186, 2000.

292. Sloop KW, Parker GE, Hanna KR, et al: LHX3 transcription factor mutations associated with combined pituitary hormone deficiency impair the activation of pituitary target genes. Gene 265(1–2):61–69, 2001.

293. Raetzman LT, Ward R, Camper SA: Lhx4 and Prop1 are required for cell survival and expansion of the pituitary primordia. Development 129(18):4229–4239, 2002.

294. Dattani MT: DNA testing in patients with GH deficiency at the time of transition. Growth Horm IGF Res 13(Suppl):S122–S129, 2003.

295. Baumann G: Genetic characterization of growth hormone deficiency and resistance: Implications for treatment with recombinant growth hormone. Am J Pharmacogenomics 2(2):93–111, 2002.

296. Drouin J, Lamolet B, Lamonerie T, et al: The PTX family of homeodomain transcription factors during pituitary developments. Mol Cell Endocrinol 140(1–2):31–36, 1998.

297. Wagner JK, Eble A, Hindmarsh PC, Mullis PE: Prevalence of human GH-1 gene alterations in patients with isolated growth hormone deficiency. Pediatr Res 43:105–110, 1998.

298. Phillips JA III: Mutations of the GH gene. J Pediatr Endocrinol Metab 15(Suppl 5):1435–1436, 2002.

299. Millar DS, Lewis MD, Horan M, et al: Novel mutations of the growth hormone 1 (GH1) gene disclosed by modulation of the clinical selection criteria for individuals with short stature. Hum Mutat 21(4):424–440, 2003.

300. Moseley CT, Phillips JA III: Pituitary gene mutations and the growth hormone pathway. Semin Reprod Med 18(1):21–29, 2000.

301. Takahashi Y, Kaji H, Okimura Y, et al: Brief report: Short stature caused by a mutant growth hormone [see comments] [published erratum appears in N Engl J Med 334(18):1207, 1996]. N Engl J Med 334(7):432–436, 1996.

302. Gertner JM, Wajnrajch MP, Leibel RL: Genetic defects in the control of growth hormone secretion. Horm Res 49:S9–S14, 1998.

303. Carakushansky M, Whatmore AJ, Clayton PE, et al: A new missense mutation in the growth hormone–releasing hormone receptor gene in familial isolated GH deficiency. Eur J Endocrinol 148(1):25–30, 2003.

304. Lindsay R, Feldkam M, Harris D, et al: Utah growth study: Growth standards and the prevalence of growth hormone deficiency. J Pediatr 125:29–35, 1994.

305. Hamilton J, Blaser S, Daneman D: MR imaging in idiopathic growth hormone deficiency. Am J Neuroradiol 19(9):1609–1615, 1998.

306. Kornreich L, Horev G, Lazar L, et al: MR findings in growth hormone deficiency: Correlation with severity of hypopituitarism. Am J Neuroradiol 19(8):1495–1499, 1998.

307. Meszaros F, Vergesslich K, Riedl S, et al: Posterior pituitary ectopy in children with idiopathic growth hormone deficiency. J Pediatr Endocrinol Metab 13(6):629–635, 2000.

308. Choo-Kang LR, Sun CC, Counts DR: Cholestasis and hypoglycemia: Manifestations of congenital anterior hypopituitarism. J Clin Endocrinol Metab 81(8):2786–2789, 1996.

309. Newman CB, Levine LS, New MI: Endocrine function in children with intrasellar and suprasellar neoplasms. Am J Dis Child 135:259, 1981.

310. Thomsett MJ, Conte FA, Kaplan SL, et al: Endocrine and neurologic outcome in childhood craniopharyngioma: Review of effect of treatment in 42 patients. J Pediatr 97:728, 1980.

311. Sklar CA, Grumbach MM, Kaplan SL, Conte FA: Hormonal and metabolic abnormalities associated with central nervous system germinoma in children and adolescents and the effect of therapy: Report of 10 patients. J Clin Endocrinol Metab 52(1):9–16, 1981.

312. Román J, Villaizdán CJ, Garcia-Foncillas J, et al: Growth and growth hormone secretion in children with cancer treated with chemotherapy. J Pediatr 131:105–112, 1997.

313. Adan L, Trivin C, Sainte-Rose C, et al: GH deficiency caused by cranial irradiation during childhood: Factors and markers in young adults. J Clin Endocrinol Metab 86(11):5245–5251, 2001.

314. Matsuno A, Nagashima T, Teramoto A, Kirino T: Endocrinologic aspects of 23 patients with Rathke's cleft cyst. Endocrinologist 11:245–246, 2001.

315. Silver HK, Finkelstein M: Deprivation dwarfism. J Pediatr 70:317, 1967.

316. Powell GF, Brasel JA, Blizzard RM: Emotional deprivation and growth retardation simulating idiopathic hypopituitarism. I. Clinical evaluation of the syndrome. N Engl J Med 276(23):1271–1278, 1967.

317. Skuse D, Albanese A, Stanhope R, et al: A new stress-related syndrome of growth failure and hyperphagia in children, associated with reversibility of growth-hormone insufficiency [see comments]. Lancet 348(9024):353–358, 1996.

318. Gohlke BC, Stanhope R: Final height in psychosocial short stature: Is there complete catch-up? Acta Paediatr 91(9):961–965, 2002.

319. Huseman C, Johanson A: Growth hormone deficiency in anorexia nervosa. J Pediatr 87(6 Pt 1):946–948, 1975.

320. Porter BA, Rosenfield RL, Lawrence AM: The levodopa test of growth hormone reserve in children. Am J Dis Child 126(5):589–592, 1973.

321. Blethen SL, Chasalow FI: Use of a two-site immunoreadiometric assay for growth hormone (GH) in identifying children with GH-dependent growth failure. J Clin Endocrinol Metab 57:1031, 1983.

322. Frasier SD: A review of growth hormone stimulation tests in children. Pediatrics 53:979, 1974.

323. Cara JF, Johanson AJ: Growth hormone for short stature not due to classic growth hormone deficiency. Pediatr Clin North Am 37:1229–1254, 1990.

324. Shalet SM, Toogood A, Rahim A, Brennan BMDI: The diagnosis of growth hormone deficiency in children and adults. Endocr Rev 19:203–223, 1998.

325. Moll GW Jr, Rosenfield RL, Fang VS: Administration of low-dose estrogen rapidly and directly stimulates growth hormone production. Am J Dis Child 140(2):124–127, 1986.

326. Marin G, Domene HM, Barnes KM, et al: The effects of estrogen priming and puberty on the growth hormone response to standardized treadmill exercise and arginine-insulin in normal girls and boys [see comments]. J Clin Endocrinol Metab 79(2):537–541, 1994.

327. Rosenfeld RG, Albertsson-Wiklund K, Cassorla F, et al: Diagnostic controversy: The diagnosis of childhood growth hormone deficiency revisited. J Clin Endocrinol Metab 80:1532–1540, 1995.

328. Ghigo E, Bellone J, Aimaretti G, et al: Reliability of provocative tests to assess growth hormone secretory status: Study in 472 normally growing children. Endocrinol Metab 81:3323–3327, 1996.

329. Carel JC, Tresca J-P, Letrait M, et al: Growth hormone testing for the diagnosis of growth hormone deficiency in childhood: A population register-based study. J Clin Endocrinol Metab 82:2117–2121, 1997.

330. Guyda HJ: Growth hormone testing and the short child. Pediatr Res 48(5):579–580, 2000.

331. Juul A, Dalgaard P, Blum WF, et al: Serum levels of insulin-like growth factor (IGF)-binding protein-3 (IGFBP-3) in healthy infants, children, and adolescents: The relation to IGF-I, IGF-II, IGFBP-1, IGFBP-2, age, sex, body mass index, and pubertal maturation. J Clin Endocrinol Metab 80(8):2534–2542, 1995.

332. Andrade Olivie MA, Garcia-Mayor RV, Gonzalez Leston D, et al: Serum insulin-like growth factor (IGF) binding protein-3 and IGF-I levels during childhood and adolescence: A cross-sectional study. Pediatr Res 38(2):149–155, 1995.

333. Maghnie M, Salati B, Bianchi S, et al: Relationship between the morphological evaluation of the pituitary and the growth hormone (GH) response to GH-releasing hormone plus arginine in children and adults with congenital hypopituitarism. J Clin Endocrinol Metab 86(4):1574–1579, 2001.

334. MacGillivray MH, Baptista J, Johanson A: Outcome of a four-year randomized study of daily versus three times weekly somatropin treatment in prepubertal naive growth hormone–deficient children. Genentech Study Group. J Clin Endocrinol Metab 81(5):1806–1809, 1996.

335. Blethen SL, Baptista J, Kuntze J, et al: Adult height in growth hormone (GH) deficient children treated with biosynthetic GH. Genentech Growth Study Group. J Clin Endocrinol Metab 82:418–420, 1997.

336. Boot AM, Engels MA, Boerma GJ, et al: Changes in bone mineral density, body composition, and lipid metabolism during growth hormone (GH) treatment in children with GH deficiency. J Clin Endocrinol Metab 82:2423–2428, 1997.

337. Blethen SL, Allen DB, Graves D, et al: Safety of recombinant deoxyribonucleic acid–derived growth hormone: The National Cooperative Growth Study experience. J Clin Endocrinol Metab 80:1704–1710, 1996.

338. Malozowski S, Tanner LA, Wysowski D, Fleming GA: Growth hormone, insulin-like growth factor I, and benign intracranial hypertension [letter]. N Engl J Med 329(9):665–666, 1993.

339. Bramnert M, Segerlantz M, Laurila E, et al: Growth hormone replacement therapy induces insulin resistance by activating the glucose–fatty acid cycle. J Clin Endocrinol Metab 88(4):1455–1463, 2003.

340. Wilson TA, Rose SR, Cohen P, et al: Update of guidelines for the use of growth hormone in children: The Lawson Wilkins Pediatric Endocrinology Society Drug and Therapeutics Committee. J Pediatr 143(4):415–421, 2003.

341. Fradkin J, Mills J, Schonberger L, et al: Risk of leukemia after treatment with pituitary growth hormone. JAMA 270(23):2829–2832, 1993.

342. Leukemia in patients treated with growth hormone. Lancet 1:1159–1160, 1988.

343. Shalet SM, Brennan BM, Reddingius RE: Growth hormone therapy and malignancy. Horm Res 48(Suppl):29–32, 1997.

344. Moshang T Jr, Rundle AC, Graves DA, et al: Brain tumor recurrence in children treated with growth hormone: The National Cooperative Growth Study experience. J Pediatr 128:S4–S7, 1996.

345. Moshang T Jr, Grimberg A: The effects of irradiation and chemotherapy on growth. Endocrinol Metab Clin North Am 25:731–742, 1996.

346. Koller DA, Green L, Gertner JM, et al: Retinal changes mimicking diabetic retinopathy in two nondiabetic, growth hormone–treated patients. J Clin Endocrinol Metab 83:2380–2383, 1998.

347. Vliet GV, Deal CL, Crock PA, et al: Sudden death in growth hormone–treated children with Prader-Willi syndrome. J Pediatr 144(1):129–131, 2004.

348. Swerdlow AJ, Higgins CD, Adlard P, Preece MA: Risk of cancer in patients treated with human pituitary growth hormone in the UK, 1959–85: A cohort study. Lancet 360(9329):273–277, 2002.

349. Sperling MA, Saenger PH, Ray H, et al: Growth hormone treatment and neoplasia: Coincidence or consequence? J Clin Endocrinol Metab 87(12):5351–5352, 2002.

350. Renehan A, Zwahlen M, Minder C, et al: Insulin-like growth factor (IGF)-I, IGF binding protein-3, and cancer risk: Systematic review and meta-regression analysis. Lancet 363(9418):1346–1353, 2004.

351. Taback SP, Dean HJ: Mortality in Canadian children with growth hormone (GH) deficiency receiving GH therapy 1967–1992. J Clin Endocrinol Metab 81:1693–1696, 1996.

352. Zachman MM, Prader A: Anabolic and androgenic effect of testosterone on sexually immature boys and its dependency on growth hormone. J Clin Endocrinol Metab 40:85, 1970.

353. Rilemma JA: Development of the mammary gland and lactation. Trends Endocrinol Metab 5:149, 1994.

354. Johnson OL, Cleland JL, Lee HJ, et al: A month-long effect from a single injection of microencapsulated human growth hormone. Nat Med 2(7):795–799, 1996.

355. Smith RG, Van der Ploeg LH, Howard AD, et al: Peptidomimetic regulation of growth hormone secretion. Endocr Rev 18:621–645, 1997.

356. Pihoker C, Badger TM, Reynolds GA, Bowers CY: Treatment effects of intranasal growth hormone releasing peptide-1 in children with short stature. J Endocrinol 155:79–86, 1997.

357. Thorner M, Rochiccoli P, Collee M, et al: Once daily subcutaneous growth hormone–releasing hormone therapy accelerates growth in growth hormone deficient children during the first year of therapy. J Clin Endocrinol Metab 81:1189–1196, 1996.

358. Silverman BL, Blethen SL, Reiter EO, et al: A long-acting human growth hormone (Nutropin Depot): Efficacy and safety following 2 years of treatment in children with growth hormone deficiency. J Pediatr Endocrinol Metab 15(Suppl 2):715–722, 2002.

359. Rosenbloom AL, Rosenfeld RG, Guevara-Aguirre J: Growth hormone insensitivity. Pediatr Clin North Am 44:423–442, 1997.

360. Sobrier ML, Dastot F, Duquesnoy, et al: Nine novel growth receptor gene mutations in patients with Laron syndrome. J Clin Endocrinol Metab 82:432–437, 1997.

361. Heath-Monnig E, Wohltmann HJ, Mills-Dunlap B, Daughaday WH: Measurement of insulin-like growth factor I (IGF-I) responsiveness of fibroblasts of children with short stature: Identification of a patient with IGF-I resistance. J Clin Endocrinol Metab 64(3):501–507, 1987.

362. Laron Z: Growth hormone insensitivity (Laron syndrome). Rev Endocr Metab Disord 3(4):347–355, 2002.

363. Kofoed B: Growth hormone insensitivity associated with a STAT5b mutation. N Engl J Med 349(12):1139–1147, 2003.

364. Burren CP, Woods KA, Rose SJ, et al: Clinical and endocrine characteristics in atypical and classical growth hormone insensitivity syndrome. Horm Res 55(3):125–130, 2001.

365. Woods KA, Camacho-Hubner C, Bergman RN, et al: Effects of insulin-like growth factor I (IGF-I) therapy on body composition and insulin resistance in IGF-I gene deletion. J Clin Endocrinol Metab 85(4):1407–1411, 2000.

366. Woods KA, Dastot F, Preece MA, et al: Phenotype: Genotype relationships in growth hormone insensitivity syndrome. J Clin Endocrinol Metab 82(11):3529–3535, 1997.

367. Blair JC, Savage MO: The GH–IGF-I axis in children with idiopathic short stature. Trends Endocrinol Metab 13(8):325–330, 2002.

368. Attie KM, Carlsson LM, Rundle AC, Sherman BM: Evidence for partial growth hormone insensitivity among patients with idiopathic short stature. The National Cooperative Growth Study. J Pediatr 127(2):244–250, 1995.

369. Buckway CK, Selva KA, Burren CP, et al: IGF generation in short stature. J Pediatr Endocrinol Metab 15(Suppl 5):1453–1454, 2002.

370. Buckway CK, Selva KA, Pratt KL, et al: Insulin-like growth factor binding protein-3 generation as a measure of GH sensitivity. J Clin Endocrinol Metab 87(10):4754–4765, 2002.

371. Savage MO, Rosenfeld RG: Growth hormone insensitivity: A proposed revised classification. Acta Paediatr Suppl 428:147, 1999.

372. Blum WF, Ranke MB, Savage MO, Hall K: Insulin-like growth factors and their binding proteins in patients with growth hormone receptor deficiency: Suggestions for new diagnostic criteria. The Kabi Pharmacia Study Group on Insulin-like Growth Factor I Treatment in Growth Hormone Insensitivity Syndromes. Acta Paediatr Suppl 383:125–126, 1992.

373. Guevara-Aguirre J, Rosenbloom AL, Vasconez O, et al: Two-year treatment of growth hormone (GH) receptor deficiency with recombinant insulin-

like growth factor I in 22 children: Comparison of two dosage levels and to GH-treated GH deficiency. J Clin Endocrinol Metab 82(2):629–633, 1997.

374. Backeljauw PF, Underwood LE: Prolonged treatment with recombinant insulin-like growth factor I in children with growth hormone insensitivity syndrome: A clinical research center study. J Clin Endocrinol Metab 81:3312–3317, 1996.

375. Backeljauw PF, Underwood LE: Therapy for 6.5–7.5 years with recombinant insulin-like growth factor I in children with growth hormone insensitivity syndrome: A clinical research center study. J Clin Endocrinol Metab 86(4):1504–1510, 2001.

376. Kaplan SL, Savage DCL, Suter S, et al: Antibodies to human growth hormone arising in patients treated with human growth hormone: Incidence, characteristics, and effects on growth. In: Raiti S (ed): Advances in Human Growth Hormone Research. Washington, DC, US Government Printing Office, 1974, p 725.

377. Pitukcheewanont P, Rose SR: Nocturnal TSH surge: A sensitive diagnostic test for central hypothyroidism in children. Endocrinologist 7:226–232, 1997.

378. Rezvani I, DiGeorge AM: Reassessment of the daily dose of oral thyroxine for replacement therapy in hypothyroid children. J Pediatr 90(2):291–297, 1977.

379. Rivkees SA, Bode HH, Crawford JD: Long-term growth in juvenile acquired hypothyroidism: The failure to achieve normal adult stature. N Engl J Med 318(10):599–602, 1988.

380. Lee PA, Weldon W, Migeon CV: Short stature as the only clinical sign of Cushing's syndrome. J Pediatr 86:89, 1975.

381. McArthur RG, Hayles AB, Salassa RM: Growth retardation in Cushing disease. J Pediatr 96:783, 1979.

382. Shahidi NT, Crigler JF Jr: Evaluation of growth and/or endocrine systems in testosterone-corticosteroid-treated patients with aplastic anemia. J Pediatr 70:233, 1967.

383. Leinung MC, Zimmerman D: Cushing's disease in children. Endocrinol Clin North Am 23:629–639, 1994.

384. Leinung MC, Kane LA, Scheithauer BW, et al: Long-term follow-up for transsphenoidal surgery for the treatment of Cushing's disease in childhood. J Clin Endocrinol Metab 80:2475–2479, 1995.

385. Styne DM, Grumbach MM, Kaplan SL: Treatment of Cushing's disease in childhood and adolescence by transsphenoidal microadenomectomy. N Engl J Med 310:889, 1984.

386. Lebrethon MC, Grossman AB, Afshar F, et al: Linear growth and final height after treatment for Cushing's disease in childhood. J Clin Endocrinol Metab 85(9):3262–3265, 2000.

387. Soyka LF: Alternate-day corticosteroid therapy. Adv Pediatr 19:47, 1972.

388. Hollman GA, Allen DB: Overt glucocorticoid excess due to inhaled corticosteroid therapy. Pediatrics 81:452–455, 1988.

389. Finkelstein BS, Imperiale TF, Speroff T, et al: Effect of growth hormone therapy on height in children with idiopathic short stature: A meta-analysis. Arch Pediatr Adolesc Med 156(3):230–240, 2002.

390. FDA talk paper: FDA approves Humatrope for short stature. Available at: http://www.fda.gov/bbs/topics/ANSWERS/2003/ANS01242.html. Accessed August 26, 2003.

391. Cuttler L, Silvers JB: Growth hormone treatment for idiopathic short stature: Implications for practice and policy. Arch Pediatr Adolesc Med 158(2):108–110, 2004.

392. Angier N: Ideas and Trends: Short Men, Short Shrift. Are Drugs the Answer? New York Times, June 22, 2003: 12.

393. Kaufman M: FDA approves wider use of growth hormone. Washington Post, July 26, 2003: A12.

394. Que V, Prakash S: Human Growth Hormone: FDA approves drug for use in healthy, short children. National Public Radio. Available at: http://discover.npr.org/features/feature.jhtml?wfId=1392897. Accessed August 14, 2003, 2003.

395. Rosenfield RL: Essentials of growth diagnosis. Endocrinol Metab Clin North Am 25:743–758, 1996.

396. Ghai K, Cara JF, Rosenfield RL: Gonadotropin releasing hormone agonist (nafarelin) test to differentiate gonadotropin deficiency from constitutionally delayed puberty in teen-age boys: A clinical research center study. J Clin Endocrinol Metab 80(10):2980–2986, 1995.

397. Albanese A, Stanhope R: Predictive factors in the determination of final height in boys with constitutional delay of growth and puberty. J Pediatr 126(4):545–550, 1995.

398. Rosenfield RL: Diagnosis and management of delayed puberty. J Clin Endocrinol Metab 70:559–562, 1990.

399. Ross JL, Long LM, Skerda M, et al: The effect of low dose ethinyl estradiol on 6 month growth rates and predicted height in patients with Turner syndrome. J Pediatr 109:950, 1986.

400. Tse W-Y, Buyukgebiz A, Hindmarsh PC, et al: Long-term outcome of oxandrolone treatment in boys with constitutional delay of growth and puberty. J Pediatr 117:588, 1990.

401. Lantos J, Siegler M, Cuttler L: Ethical issues in growth hormone therapy. JAMA 261:1020–1024, 1989.

402. Underwood LE: Growth hormone therapy for short stature: Yes or no? Hosp Pract 27:192–198, 1992.

403. Sandberg DE: Should short children who are not deficient in growth

hormone be treated? West J Med 172(3):186–189, 2000.

404. Finkelstein BS, Silvers JB, Marrero U, et al: Insurance coverage, physician recommendations, and access to emerging treatments: Growth hormone therapy for childhood short stature. JAMA 279:663–668, 1998.

405. Zimet G, Oweens RP, Dahms WT, et al: Psychosocial outcome of children evaluated for short stature. Arch Pediatr Adolesc Med 151:1017–1023, 1997.

406. Zimet GD, Cutler M, Litvene M, et al: Psychological adjustment of children with non–growth hormone deficient short stature. J Ped Adolesc Psychol 16:264–170, 1995.

407. Kodish E, Cuttler L: Ethical issues in emerging new treatments such as growth hormone therapy for children with Down syndrome and Prader-Willi syndrome. Curr Opin Pediatr 8:401–405, 1996.

408. Downie AB, Mulligan J, McCaughey ES, et al: Psychological response to growth hormone treatment in short normal children. Arch Dis Child 75:32–35, 1996.

409. Lippe BM, Nakamoto JM: Conventional and nonconventional uses of growth hormone. Recent Prog Horm Res 48:179–235, 1993.

410. Allen DB, Fost NC: Growth hormone therapy for short stature: Panacea or Pandora's box? [see comments]. J Pediatr 117(1 Pt 1):16–21, 1990.

411. Voss LD: Growth hormone therapy for the short normal child: Who needs it and who wants it? The case against growth hormone therapy. J Pediatr 136(1):103–106, 2000.

412. Saenger P: The case in support of Gh therapy. J Pediatr 136(1):106–109, discussion 109–110, 2000.

413. Cuttler L, Silvers JB, Singh J, et al: Short stature and growth hormone therapy: A national study of physician recommendation patterns. JAMA 276(7):531–537, 1996.

414. Das U, Whatmore AJ, Khosravi J, et al: IGF-I and IGF-binding protein-3 measurements on filter paper blood spots in children and adolescents on GH treatment: Use in monitoring and as markers of growth performance. Eur J Endocrinol 149(3):179–185, 2003.

415. Ranke MB, Schweizer R, Elmlinger MW, et al: Relevance of IGF-I, IGFBP-3, and IGFBP-2 measurements during GH treatment of GH-deficient and non-GH-deficient children and adolescents. Horm Res 55(3):115–124, 2001.

416. Mul D, Wit JM, Oostdijk W, Van den Broeck J: The effect of pubertal delay by GnRH agonist in GH-deficient children on final height. J Clin Endocrinol Metab 86(10):4655–4656, 2001.

417. Lee MM: Is treatment with a luteinizing hormone-releasing hormone agonist justified in short adolescents? N Engl J Med 348(10):942–945, 2003.

418. Yanovski JA, Rose SR, Municchi G, et al: Treatment with a luteinizing hormone-releasing hormone agonist in adolescents with short stature. N Engl J Med 348(10):908–917, 2003.

419. Pasquino AM, Pucarelli I, Roggini M, Segni M: Adult height in short normal girls treated with gonadotropin-releasing hormone analogs and growth hormone. J Clin Endocrinol Metab 85(2):619–622, 2000.

420. Pereira L, Levran O, Ramirez F, et al: A molecular approach to the stratification of cardiovascular risk in families with Marfan's syndrome [see comments]. N Engl J Med 331(3):148–153, 1994.

421. Sotos JF: Overgrowth. Section V. Syndromes and other disorders associated with overgrowth. Clin Pediatr (Phila) 36(2):89–103, 1997.

422. Douglas J, Hanks S, Temple IK, et al: NSD1 mutations are the major cause of Sotos syndrome and occur in some cases of Weaver syndrome but are rare in other overgrowth phenotypes. Am J Hum Genet 72(1):132–143, 2003.

423. Visser R, Matsumoto N: Genetics of Sotos syndrome. Curr Opin Pediatr 15(6):598–606, 2003.

424. Kurotaki N, Imaizumi K, Harada N, et al: Haploinsufficiency of NSD1 causes Sotos syndrome. Nat Genet 30(4):365–366, 2002.

425. Li M, Squire JA, Weksberg R: Molecular genetics of Wiedemann-Beckwith syndrome [in process citation]. Am J Med Genet 79(4):253–259, 1998.

426. Sotos JF: Overgrowth. Section III. Other hormonal causes. Clin Pediatr (Phila) 35(12):637–648, 1996.

427. Sotos JF: Overgrowth. Section II. Hormonal causes. Clin Pediatr (Phila) 35(11):579–590, 1996.

428. Gagel RF, McCutcheon IE: Images in clinical medicine: Pituitary gigantism. N Engl J Med 340(7):524, 1999.

429. Cuttler L: The regulation of growth hormone secretion. Endocrinol Metab Clin North Am 25:541–572, 1996.

430. Dotsch J, Kiess W, Hanze J, et al: Gs alpha mutation at codon 201 in pituitary adenoma causing gigantism in a 6-year-old boy with McCune-Albright syndrome. J Clin Endocrinol Metab 81(11):3839–3842, 1996.

431. Wilroy RS Jr, Etteldorf JN: Familial hyperthyroidism including two siblings with neonatal Graves disease. J Pediatr 78:625, 1971.

432. Brauner R, Adan L, Malandry A, Zantleifer D: Adult height in girls with idiopathic true precocious puberty. J Clin Endocrinol Metab 79:415–420, 1994.

433. Uriarte MM, Baron J, Garcia HB, et al: The effect of pubertal delay on adult height in men with isolated hypogonadotropic hypogonadism [published erratum appears in J Clin Endocrinol Metab 75(4):1009, 1992]. J Clin Endocrinol Metab 74(2):436–440, 1992.

434. Thamdrup E: Precocious Sexual Development. Springfield, IL, Thomas, 1961.

435. Garrone S, Radetti G, Sidoti M, et al: Increased insulin-like growth factor (IGF)-II and IGF/IGF-binding protein ratio in prepubertal constitutionally tall children. J Clin Endocrinol Metab 87(12):5455–5460, 2002.

436. Sotos JF: Overgrowth. Section I. Overgrowth disorders. Clin Pediatr (Phila) 35(10):517–529, 1996.

437. Drop SLS, de Waal WJ, Keizer-Schrama SM: Sex steroid treatment of constitutionally tall stature. Endocr Rev 19:540–558, 1998.

438. Barnard ND, Scialli AR, Bobela S: The current use of estrogens for growth-suppressant therapy in adolescent girls. J Pediatr Adolesc Gynecol 15(1):23–26, 2002.

439. Paul D, Conte FA, Grumbach MM, Kaplan SL: Long-term effect of gonadotropin-releasing hormone agonist therapy on final and near-final height in 26 children with true precocious puberty treated at a median age of less than 5 years. J Clin Endocrinol Metab 80(2):546–551, 1995.

440. Adan L, Souberbielle JC, Zucker JM: Adult height in 24 patients treated for growth hormone deficiency and early puberty. J Clin Endocrinol Metab 82:229–233, 1997.

441. Pasquino AM, Pucarelli I, Segni M, et al: Adult height in girls with central precocious puberty treated with gonadotropin-releasing hormone analogues and growth hormone. J Clin Endocrinol Metab 84:449–452, 1999.

442. Partsch C-J, Dreyer G, Gosch A, et al: Longitudinal evaluation of growth, puberty, and bone maturation in children with Williams syndrome. J Pediatr 134:82–89, 1999.

443. Petrij F, Giles RH, Dauwerse HG, et al: Rubinstein-Taybi syndrome caused by mutations in the transcriptional co-activator CBP [see comments]. Nature 376(6538):348–351, 1995.

444. Astley SJ, Clarren SK: A case definition and photographic screening tool for the facial phenotype of fetal alcohol syndrome. J Pediatr 129(1):33–41, 1996.

Growth Hormone Deficiency in Children

Mehul T. Dattani and Peter C. Hindmarsh

INTRODUCTION

The height of an individual is the culmination of a complex process that results from an interaction between genes, nutritional status, hormonal milieu, and environmental factors. In terms of adult height, fetal growth is critical and has major implications for the ultimate stature of an individual. Birth length is approximately 30% of final height and, with a crown-rump length velocity of 50 to 60 cm/year, this period represents the fastest rate of growth achieved by an individual. This growth is mediated by maternal nutrition and a number of growth factors such as insulin-like growth factor 1 (IGF-1), IGF-2, fibroblast growth factor, epidermal growth factor, transforming growth factors α and β, and insulin. Any compromise in maternal nutrition or in the production of these growth factors is associated with intrauterine growth restriction.

Postnatal growth is best described by the ICP (infancy-childhood-pubertal) model of growth.[1] These three phases are regulated by different components of the endocrine system. During the infancy phase, growth is rapid but at a sharply decelerating rate. Growth at this stage is principally dependent on nutrition, although endocrine factors in the form of the growth hormone (GH)–IGF axis play an increasingly important role during the first year of life. Over the first 2-year period, "catch-up" or "catch-down" growth commonly occurs while the infant establishes his or her own growth trajectory with a marked increase in the correlation between current height and final height ($r = 0.8$) by age 3 years. As a result, growth along a predictable channel is a hallmark of the healthy child. Poor growth may be a manifestation of any underlying illness, reflecting a wide variety of genetic, constitutional, and pathologic conditions, of which GH deficiency (GHD) is but one cause.

By age 4 years, average height velocity has declined to 7 cm/year, with a further decline to a rate of 5 to 5.5 cm/year at age 8 years (Fig. 37-1). The onset of the childhood phase of growth is apparent from age 6 months, when overlap occurs between the childhood and infancy phases of growth. This childhood growth is dependent mainly on endocrine factors such as GH and thyroxine.[2] The third phase of postnatal growth, the pubertal phase, is dependent on the normal secretion of GH and sex steroids. It is extremely variable in terms of timing, with marked sexual dimorphism that gives rise to the average difference of 12.5 cm in adult height between the sexes.

GH is the main mediator of postnatal growth,[2] and virtually any chronic childhood illness will modify secretion. Care must be exercised in the evaluation of GH secretion in these situations. Although GHD may be considered a form of IGF deficiency,[3] this approach may be limited, and as GH receptor and postreceptor issues (Chapter 32) and GHD in adults (Chapter 38) are considered elsewhere, this chapter focuses primarily on GHD, as related to disorders of the hypothalamopituitary axis in children.

HISTORY

The history of GHD starts with the pursuit of therapeutic interventions that antedate attempts to measure serum concentrations of GH. In 1932, a treatment to promote growth with a crude anterior pituitary extract was reported,[4] but it was not until Raben's observations of 1958[5] and the general availability of methods of GH extraction that large studies could be conducted. These larger studies showed a beneficial effect of human GH in promoting growth in children with clear physical signs suggestive of GH deficiency.[6-9]

GH immunoassays postdated the initial therapeutic studies of GH.[10] The advent of radioimmunoassay allowed the measurement of the concentration of GH in blood in response to a variety of pharmacologic stimuli, thereby paving the way to a better understanding of which children might benefit from the then limited supplies of GH. This limitation in supply largely dictated clinical research until the advent of unlimited supplies of biosynthetic human GH (r-hGH) resulting from bioengineering technology in the late 1970s and early 1980s.

Our understanding of the physiology of GH secretion stemmed from the pioneering work of Geoffrey Harris and his group in Oxford, who suggested that release of GH from the pituitary was under the control of a releasing factor secreted from the hypothalamus. The demonstration by Brazeau and colleagues.[11] of a GH release–inhibiting factor (somatostatin) led to a radical change in the thinking around the control of GH secretion. The final demonstration of a GH stimulating factor came in 1982 when GH-releasing hormone was isolated

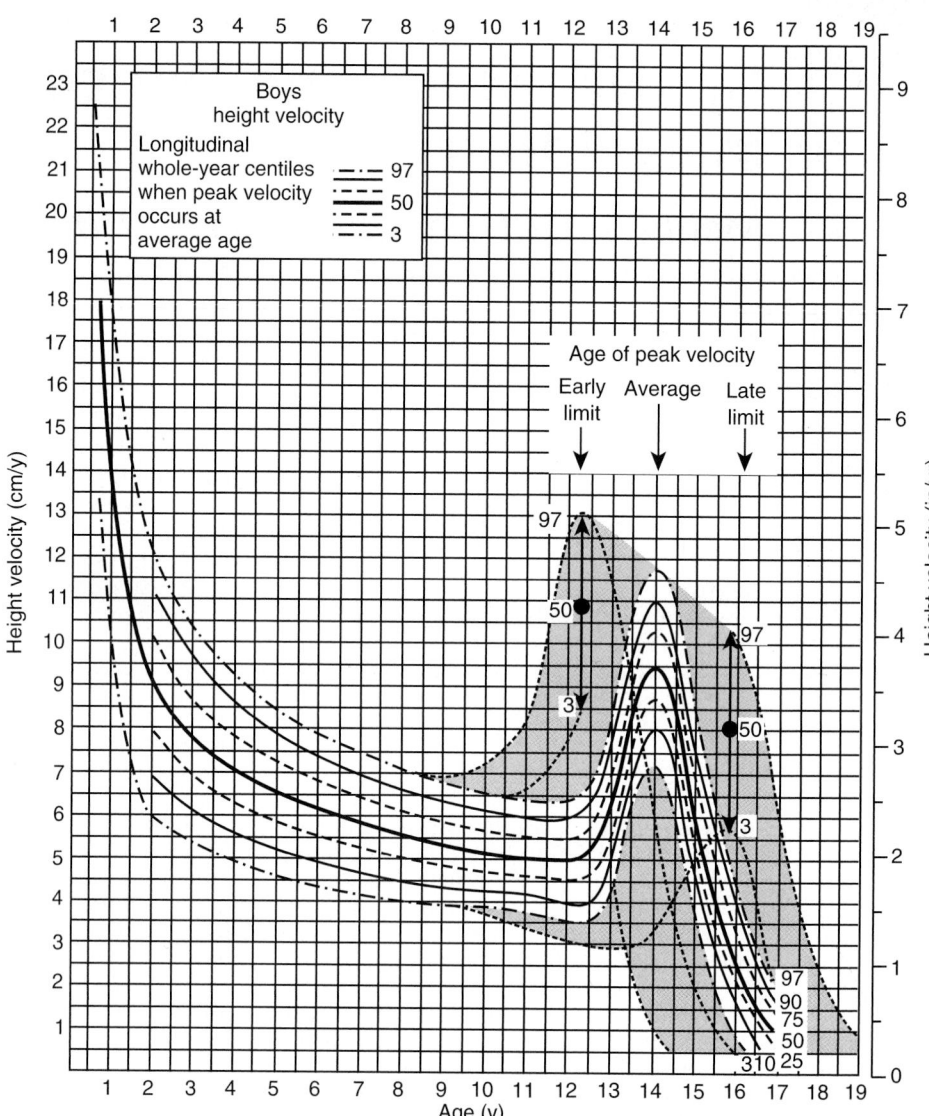

Figure 37-1 Height velocity chart for boys aged 0 to 19 years. Centiles 3 to 97 illustrated with 50th centile in *bold.* *Shaded zone,* Variation in timing of pubertal growth spurt. Visually, the chart depicts the rapid but rapidly decelerating growth during the first 4 years of life followed by a much slower declination until the onset of the pubertal growth spurt. (Copyright Castlemead Publications.)

and characterized from two pancreatic tumors.[12,13] During the search for the releasing factor, little was made of a further stimulating factor described by Bowers and colleagues,[14] which, although synthetic in nature, formed the basis from which GH-releasing substances and their receptors were identified. Finally, the natural ligand, ghrelin, was isolated from the stomach.

For a considerable period, GH was believed to act via the generation of a further endocrine factor from the liver, somatomedin-C or IGF-1.[15] Further work led to the realization that liver was not the only source of IGF-1, and in a series of classic experiments, Green[16] and Isaksson[17] demonstrated in adipose tissue and cartilage, respectively, that IGF-1 was generated locally and acted in a paracrine manner to promote clonal expansion of the cell population.

EPIDEMIOLOGY

The reported incidence of GHD is, to a large extent, dependent on the criteria used to establish the diagnosis and reflects the wide variation in the stringency of diagnostic testing. In one United Kingdom study, an incidence of 1 in 60,000 live births was reported,[18] although a survey of Scottish schoolchildren led to a calculated prevalence of 1 per 4000 live births,[19] a value similar to that of the Utah Growth Study (1 in 3480 live births).[20]

Several large surveys have indicated that approximately 25% of children diagnosed with GHD have an underlying "organic" cause for their condition, such as trauma, central nervous system (CNS) tumors, inflammation, irradiation, or anatomic abnormalities of the hypothalamus or pituitary.[21,22] The remainder are labeled "idiopathic" GHD. Such surveys are likely to overestimate the number of true cases of idiopathic GHD because of variation in the diagnosis of GHD. Recent advances in developmental endocrinology suggest that many patients labeled previously as having idiopathic GHD have genetic abnormalities or subtle anatomic abnormalities affecting the hypothalamus or pituitary, or both.

PATHOGENESIS

A list of causes of GHD is provided in Table 37-1. As mentioned already, idiopathic GHD constitutes by far the largest group of patients, although advances in developmental biology are forcing a rethink in this area.

GENETIC AND STRUCTURAL ABNORMALITIES

Pituitary Development
The pituitary gland, which consists of anterior, intermediate, and posterior lobes, is a central regulator of growth, metabolism, and development. Its complex functions are mediated

Table 37-1 Causes of Growth Hormone Deficiency

CONGENITAL

GENETIC
See Table 37-2

ASSOCIATED WITH STRUCTURAL DEFECTS OF THE BRAIN
Agenesis of the corpus callosum
Septo-optic dysplasia
Holoprosencephaly
Encephalocele
Hydrocephalus

ASSOCIATED WITH MIDLINE FACIAL DEFECTS
Cleft lip/palate
Single central incisor

IDIOPATHIC

ACQUIRED

TRAUMA
Perinatal trauma
Postnatal trauma

INFECTION
Meningitis/encephalitis

CNS TUMORS
Craniopharyngioma
Pituitary germinoma
Histiocytosis

AFTER CRANIAL IRRADIATION

AFTER CHEMOTHERAPY

PITUITARY INFARCTION

NEUROSECRETORY DYSFUNCTION

TRANSIENT
Peripubertal
Psychosocial deprivation
Hypothyroidism

via hormone-signaling pathways that act to regulate the finely balanced homeostatic control in vertebrates by coordinating signals from the hypothalamus to peripheral endocrine organs (thyroid, adrenals, and gonads) (Table 37-2). The mature anterior pituitary gland is populated by five neuroendocrine cell types, defined by the hormone produced: corticotrophs (adrenocorticotropic hormone [ACTH]), thyrotrophs (thyroid-stimulating hormone [TSH]), gonadotrophs (luteinizing hormone [LH]; follicle-stimulating hormone [FSH]), somatotrophs (GH), and lactotrophs (prolactin [PRL]).[23] The posterior gland secretes vasopressin and oxytocin. The origins of the anterior and posterior lobes of the pituitary gland are embryologically distinct. Rathke's pouch, the primordium of the anterior pituitary, arises from the oral ectoderm, whereas the posterior pituitary derives from neural ectoderm. Development of the anterior gland follows a similar pattern in a number of different species, but has been best studied in rodents.

In the mouse, anterior pituitary development occurs in four distinct stages: pituitary placode formation; the development of a rudimentary Rathke's pouch; the formation of a definitive pouch; and, finally, the terminal differentiation of the various cell types in a temporally and spatially regulated manner (Fig. 37-2). The apposition of Rathke's pouch and the diencephalon, which later develops into the hypothalamus, is maintained throughout the early stages of pituitary organogenesis[24] and appears to be critical for normal anterior pituitary development. A number of signaling molecules—fibroblast growth factor-8 (Fgf8),[24–26] bone morphogenetic protein 4 (Bmp4),[24,25] and Nkx2.1[26]—that are expressed in the neural ectoderm and not in Rathke's pouch are thought to play a significant role in normal anterior pituitary development, as illustrated by the phenotype of mouse mutants that are either null or hypomorphic for these alleles. These signaling molecules activate or repress key regulatory genes encoding transcription factors such as *Hesx1*, *LIM homeobox 3* (*Lhx3*), and *LIM homeobox 4* (*Lhx4*) within the developing

Table 37-2 Genes Implicated in Isolated Growth Hormone Deficiency and Combined Pituitary Hormone Deficiencies

Gene (Murine/Human)	Protein (Murine/Human)	Murine Loss of Function Phenotype	Human Phenotype	Inheritance Murine/Human
Hesx1/HESX1	Hesx1/HESX1	Anophthalmia or microphthalmia, agenesis of corpus callosum, absence of septum pellucidum, pituitary dysgenesis or aplasia	Variable: SOD, CPHD, IGHD with EPP/dominant or recessive	Dominant or recessive in both
Sox3/SOX3	Sox3/SOX3	Unknown	Isolated GHD with mental retardation	Unknown in mouse; X-linked in humans
Lhx3/LHX3	Lhx3/LHX3	Hypoplasia of Rathke's pouch	GH, TSH, gonadotropin deficiency with pituitary hypoplasia. Corticotrophs spared. Short, rigid cervical spine with limited rotation	Recessive in both
Lhx4/LHX4	Lhx4/LHX4	Mild hypoplasia of anterior pituitary	GH, TSH, cortisol deficiency, persistent craniopharyngeal canal and abnormal cerebellar tonsils	Recessive in mouse, dominant in humans
Prop1/PROP1	Prop1/PROP1	Hypoplasia of anterior pituitary with reduced somatotrophs, lactotrophs, thyrotrophs, and gonadotrophs	GH, TSH, prolactin, and gonadotropin deficiency. Evolving ACTH deficiency. Enlarged pituitary with later involution	Recessive in both
Pit1/POU1F1 (PIT1)	Pou1f1/POU1F1	Anterior pituitary hypoplasia with reduced somatotrophs, lactotrophs, and thyrotrophs	Variable anterior pituitary hypoplasia with GH, TSH, and prolactin deficiencies	Recessive in mouse, dominant/recessive in humans
Ghrhr/GHRHR	Ghrhr/GHRHR	Reduced somatotrophs with anterior pituitary hypoplasia	GH deficiency with anterior pituitary hypoplasia	Recessive
Gh-1/GH-1	Growth hormone (GH)		GH deficiency	Recessive, dominant, or X-linked in humans

SOD, superoxide dismutase; IGHD, isolated GH deficiency; CPHD, combined pituitary hormone deficiency; EPP, eye pigment transporter; GHD, growth hormone deficiency; TSH, thyroid-stimulating hormone; ACTH, adrenocorticotropic hormone.

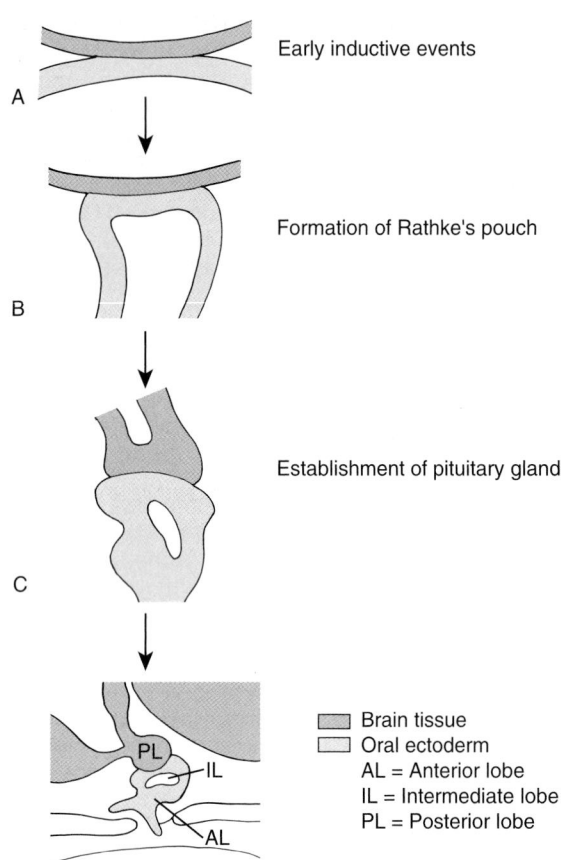

Figure 37-2 Formation of the pituitary gland. Four-stage process commencing with early inductive events as the infundibulum of the diencephalon abuts the roof of the oral cavity. Pituitary established with signaling gradients generating spatial defined patterns of gene expression and specific cell lineages in the definitive gland. (Reproduced from Valette-Kasic and Enjalbert, *Topical Endocrinology*, February 2003.)

Rathke's pouch that are essential for subsequent development of the pituitary[23,24] (Fig. 37-3).

The final stage of pituitary gland development entails the terminal differentiation of the progenitor cells into the distinct cell types found within the mature pituitary gland. This process is tightly regulated by extrinsic factors (*Fgf8*, *Bmp2*, *Bmp4*, and *Bmp7*) that emanate from the surrounding infundibulum and the juxtapituitary mesenchyme. These then establish gradients of transcription factors (*Lhx3*, *Six3*, *Prophet of Pit1 [Prop1]*, *Pit1*, *Nkx3.1*, *Islet-1 [Isl1]*, *Lhx4*, *Six1*, *Brain-4 [Brn4]*, and *Pituitary-forkhead [P-frk]*).[25–28] These genetic gradients lead to a wave of cell differentiation. Each of the five anterior pituitary cell types differentiates in a temporally and spatially regulated manner (Fig. 37-4),[29–32] and this process is dependent on a number of transcription factors such as Pit1 and steroidogenic factor 1 (Sf1).[33,34]

Less is known about pituitary development in humans, but it appears to mirror that in the rodent. Spontaneous or artificially induced mutations in the mouse have led to significant insights into human pituitary disease, and identification of mutations associated with human pituitary disease have in turn been invaluable in defining the genetic cascade responsible for the development of this complex structure.

Disorders of Pituitary and Extrapituitary Development in Humans

A number of genetic abnormalities have been identified in children who were previously thought to have idiopathic GHD or combined pituitary hormone deficiency (CPHD)[35–37] (see Table 37-2). In some cases, extrapituitary manifestations may be associated. Mutations within the *paired-like* homeobox gene *HESX1* are associated with the phenotypes of GHD, CPHD, and septo-optic dysplasia, a condition characterized by forebrain, pituitary, and eye abnormalities such as optic nerve hypoplasia.[38–40] The inheritance and phenotypes are variable, with both dominant and recessive modes of inheritance described. Intriguingly, *HESX1* mutations are classically associated with anterior pituitary hypoplasia with an undescended posterior pituitary and an absent or thin infundibulum. An example is shown in Figure 37-5.

Mutations within the LIM-domain genes *LHX3* and *LHX4* are associated with CPHD with extrapituitary manifestations

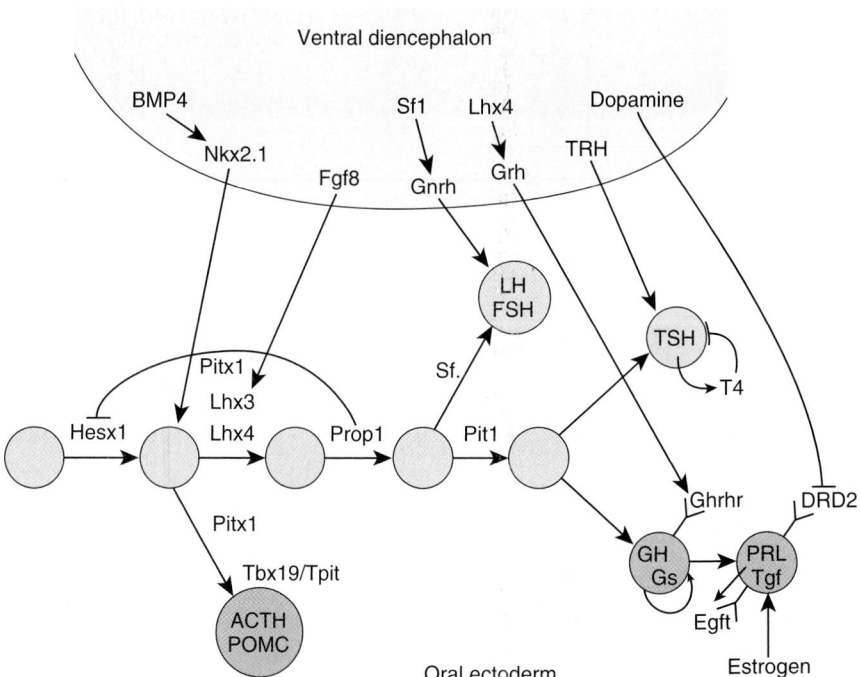

Figure 37-3 Sequence cascade of factors involved in pituitary development. Apposition factors as well as gradient factors are involved in determination and situation of pituitary cell types. See text for full description of interactions.

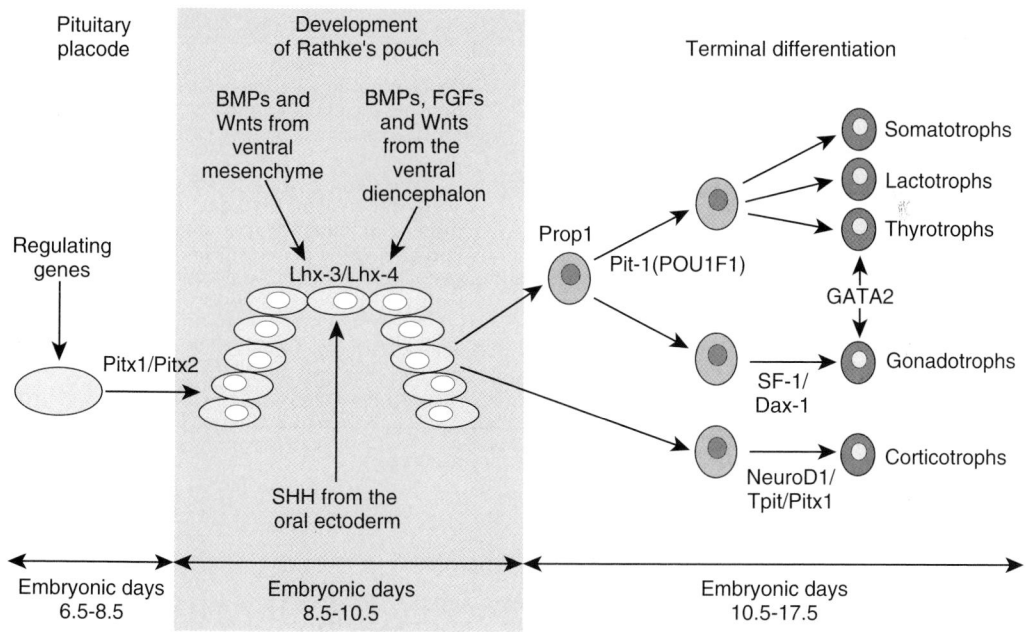

Figure 37-4 Temporal sequence of events of pituitary development in the mouse. (Reproduced from Valette-Kasic and Enjalbert, Topical Endocrinology, February 2003.)

such as a short neck and steep cervical spine in the case of *LHX3*[41] and an abnormal cerebellum in the case of *LHX4*.[42] The inheritance of *LHX3* mutations is recessive, whereas that associated with *LHX4* mutations is dominant, unlike the murine phenotype.

Recent studies with *SOX3* suggest a possible explanation for the predominance of males in many series of GHD. *SOX3* is sited on the X chromosome (Xq26-27) and appears to be important not only in pituitary development but also is associated with mental retardation.[43] These observations of GHD and brain developmental abnormalities are particularly important, as neurodevelopmental handicap has often been ascribed to untreated neonatal hypoglycemia, whereas structural developmental problems may be a more pertinent explanation.

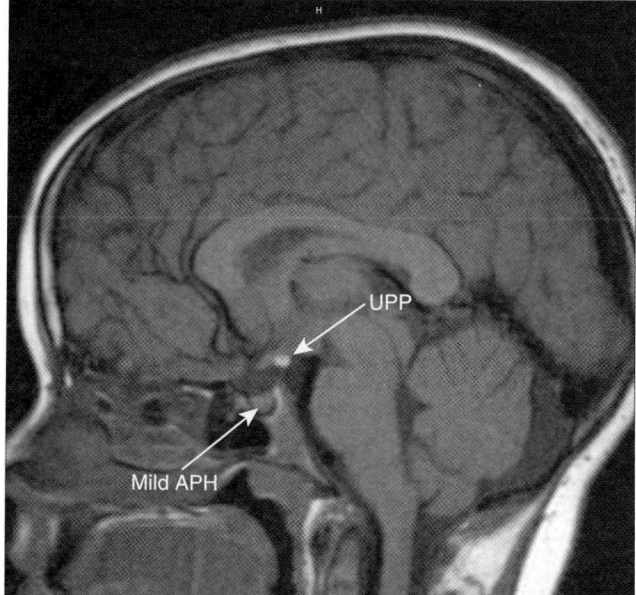

Figure 37-5 Sagittal magnetic resonance scan of a patient with isolated growth hormone deficiency showing undescended posterior pituitary (UPP) as a bright spot at base of hypothalamus and mild anterior pituitary hypoplasia (APH).

It is clear that our understanding of the etiology of hypopituitarism is rudimentary, and that the mechanisms whereby mutations in the genes that have been identified to date lead to a particular phenotype are largely unknown. Additionally, many cases of hypopituitarism may be due to changes in regulatory regions of known genes, or perhaps within novel genes that have yet to be identified.

Growth Hormone–Releasing Hormone and Growth Hormone–Releasing Hormone Receptor (GHD Type IB)

As growth hormone–releasing hormone (GHRH) and its receptor are critical to somatotroph population expansion, abnormalities in either are likely to be associated with severe GHD. Although no mutations of the human GHRH gene have been identified, mutations in GHRH receptor (GHRHR) have been identified in a number of pedigrees.[44] Two large pedigrees have been identified in Pakistan (Glu72Stop mutation)[45] and in northeastern Brazil.[46] All patients reported to date have been homozygous for mutations of the GHRHR gene. Serum GH concentrations fail to increase after standard provocative testing, as well as after GHRH administration. The patients resemble the *little* mouse (lit/lit), which has a mutation of the GHRHR gene affecting the ligand-binding domain.[47]

Somatotroph Development

A number of mouse models exist in which somatotroph development has been impaired. These include the Ames, the Jackson, and the Snell dwarf mice. A missense point mutation within the Prophet of Pit1 or Prop1 gene (S83P) has been shown to be responsible for the Ames dwarf mouse.[48] The phenotype results from a failure of initial determination of the Pit-1 lineage required for production of GH, PRL, and TSH. The Ames pituitary gland contains less than 1% of the normal complement of somatotrophs and decreased numbers of lactotrophs and thyrotrophs. In humans, mutations within the transcription factor *PROP1* are associated with CPHD in the form of GH, PRL, TSH, and gonadotropin deficiency.[49,50] In a proportion of individuals with *PROP1* mutations, cortisol deficiency will develop.[51] Additionally, a number of individuals with mutations within *PROP1* have transient pituitary masses with subsequent involution[52] (Fig. 37-6). The exact mechanism underlying this phenomenon remains unclear, but it is clearly important to exclude mutations within *PROP1* in patients with pituitary "tumors,"

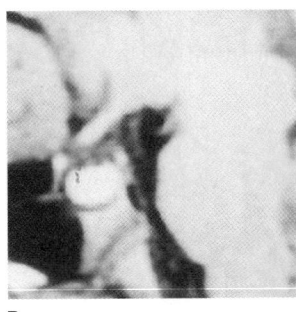

A   B

Figure 37-6 Radiologic features in a patient with *PROP-1* mutation. **A,** Plain skull radiograph, showing large sella turcica. **B,** Magnetic resonance image of pituitary, showing large mass occupying the sella turcica. (Reproduced from Mendonca BB, Osorio MG, Latronico AC, et al: Longitudinal hormonal and pituitary imaging changes in two females with combined pituitary hormone deficiency due to deletion of A301,G302 in the *PROP1* gene. J Clin Endocrinol Metab 84:942–945, 1999.)

Table 37-3	**Genetic Abnormalities in GH-1**
A. Type 1	Type 1A Autosomal-recessive GHD due to total absence of GH synthesis Type 1B Autosomal-recessive GHD due to splicing defects in *GH-1* or defects in *GHRHR* gene
B. Type 2	Autosomal-dominant GHD due to splice site and missense mutations in the *GH-1* gene resulting in dominant negative expression of the *GH-1* gene. Abnormal folding of mutant interferes with storage and secretion
C. Type 3	X-linked GHD. Xq21-q22 with X-linked agamma-globulinemia and Xq22-q27 with X-linked mental retardation

GHD, growth hormone deficiency.

especially the nonfunctional variety. Considerable variability exists in the timing of the endocrinopathy, and a number of patients will actually commence puberty, but then arrest halfway through. Recently, a mutation within *PROP1* was identified in a patient who actually achieved a normal final height without receiving any GH treatment. *PROP1* mutations are thought to be the most common cause of familial CPHD and are usually recessive.

Pit-1[53,54] is a member of the POU family of homeodomain proteins and contains a highly conserved bipartite DNA-binding domain, consisting of the POU homeodomain, required for low-affinity DNA binding, and a POU-specific domain, responsible for the specificity of DNA binding and potential interactions with other proteins. The Snell dwarf mouse, characterized by pituitary hypoplasia and GH, PRL, and TSH deficiencies, has a point mutation (W261C) within the Pit-1 gene, affecting the third helix of the POU homeodomain. This abrogates binding of Pit-1 to its target promoter sequences. Several mutations and deletions of the PIT1 gene have been identified in humans with CPHD, characterized by the combination of GH, PRL, and TSH deficiency.[55–57] Mutations have been described that separately affect the DNA-binding capacity of POU1F-1 or its transactivation properties. Autosomal-dominant transmission, resulting from a dominant negative effect, has been observed in mutations affecting dimerization of POU1F1, transactivation (P24L), or in the relatively common R271W mutation, which results in increased binding to promoter elements and disruption of transcriptional activation.[58] Autosomal-recessive transmission is found in other mutations, such as A172stop, E250stop, R143G, A158P, and P239S.[59] Variability in phenotype has been reported, although most patients exhibit growth retardation during the first year of life. GH and PRL deficiency is complete; TSH secretion may be observed during infancy but declines progressively during the early months of life. Magnetic resonance imaging (MRI) scanning revealed a marked variability in the size of the anterior pituitary, with some patients demonstrating a normal pituitary, whereas others have a hypoplastic pituitary. After appropriate GH and thyroxine replacement, patients appear to enter puberty normally and have normal fertility. Lactation may be impaired.

GH1 Gene

The *GH1* gene is located on chromosome 17 and is part of a cluster of five structurally related genes (*GH1, CSHP* [chorionic somatomammotropin pseudogene], *CSH* [chorionic somatomammotropin], *GH2* [or placental variant], and *CSH2*). Mutations within the *GH-1* gene are associated with isolated GH deficiency (Table 37-3). Large recessive inherited

deletions are associated with absence of GH protein (type 1A GHD). Complete loss of pituitary GH secretion occurs, secondary to deletions resulting from nonhomologous crossing over at different sites in the GH and chorionic somatomammotropin (CS) gene cluster. The most common deletion is 6.7 kb, but deletions of 7.0, 7.6, and greater than 45 kb also have been observed.[60] Wagner and colleagues[61] described the GHD IA phenotype in a patient with a point mutation in the GH signal peptide, E23X, resulting in premature termination of translation. Patients typically have an excellent initial response to GH therapy, but because of the absence of a normal GH molecule in fetal life, an attenuation of the growth response to exogenous GH may result from the development of anti-GH antibodies,[62] although this event has been described less frequently with newer GH preparations.

Type IB GHD is due to homozygous splice-site mutations within the GH1 gene or homozygous mutations within the GHRHR. It is associated with an excellent response to GH treatment with no formation of antibodies.

Type II GHD is autosomal dominant and associated with splice-site mutations.[63,64] These mutations lead to the production of two alternatively spliced GH molecules, 20- and 17.5-kilodalton hGH. Mutations in an exon splice enhancer within exon 3 of the *GH-1* gene also have been associated with autosomal-dominant GHD.[65] The generation of the 17.5-kilodalton form of hGH has a dominant negative effect and prevents the secretion of the normal wild-type 22-kilodalton hGH, with a consequent deleterious effect on pituitary somatotrophs. In a murine model of this dominant negative mutation, loss of somatotroph number[66] occurs and progressive damage to adjacent pituitary cells (with later failure of prolactin, TSH, and gonadotropin secretion).[67]

Seven different splice-site mutations have been reported to date. In addition, three missense mutations (R183H, P89L, and V110F) were recently implicated in isolated growth hormone deficiency (IGHD) type II. These patients have a normal GH1 allele but are unable to secrete the normal form of GH in appropriate concentrations. The mutant protein therefore exerts a dominant negative effect.

GHD type III, an X-linked form of IGHD, has been reported in patients with hypogammaglobulinemia. To date, no alteration in the *GH1* gene has been identified in this condition, and the genetic mechanisms remain unknown. Recently, a polyalanine expansion within the transcription factor SOX3, which lies at Xq26-27, has been associated with X-linked GHD and mental retardation.[43] Intriguingly, duplications of this region of the X chromosome have been associated with X-linked panhypopituitarism, although the exact mechanism remains unclear.

Bioinactive Growth Hormone Molecule

Because the GH molecule exists in multiple molecular forms, resulting from alternative splicing or posttranslational processing, some cases of short stature have been hypothesized to be the consequence of abnormal ratios of the various GH forms.[68,69] The first report with detailed biochemistry and molecular genetics was described by Takahashi and associates.[70,71] of two individuals heterozygous for point mutations in the GH gene. The mutant GH molecules (R77C and D112G) were capable of binding to the GHR, perhaps even with increased affinity, but were unable to stimulate tyrosine phosphorylation of GH-activated intracellular signaling intermediates in a normal manner. The ability of the R77C mutant to behave in a dominant negative manner was demonstrated by its ability to inhibit the in vitro actions of wild-type GH.

Structural Abnormalities

In addition to the structural abnormalities associated with the genetic problems described earlier, GHD can occur in the setting of other cranial or midline abnormalities such as holoprosencephaly, nasal encephalocele, single central incisor, and cleft lip and palate.

As methods of radiologic evaluation of the CNS have improved, an increasing percentage of patients with idiopathic GHD have been identified to have structural abnormalities.[72–80] Many of these are associated with some of the genetic abnormalities described earlier, but the findings are worthy of separate consideration. In particular, the finding on MRI of an undescended (erroneously called *ectopic*) posterior pituitary (UPP) was more common in male than in female patients (3:1 when UPP present vs. 1:1 if normal anatomy), in patients with CPHD as compared with IGHD (49% vs. 12%), breech delivery (32% vs. 7%), and associated congenital brain anomalies (12% vs. 7%).

These findings appear to be best explained by a defect in induction of the mediobasal structure of the brain in the early embryo, rather than the product of birth trauma, as previously suggested.[76] Whether pituitary insufficiency is the result of hypothalamic or pituitary dysgenesis, or the product of hypoplasia or sectioning of the pituitary stalk, is not always clear. Perinatal problems, however, including breech presentation, may prove to be the consequence, rather than the cause, of underlying CNS abnormality. The concept that UPP, stalk section or hypoplasia, and pituitary hypoplasia may represent abnormal embryonic development, rather than the consequences of birth trauma, is supported by the finding of similar anatomic abnormalities in patients with septo-optic dysplasia, type I Arnold-Chiari syndrome, holoprosencephaly, and increasingly in patients with mutations in the genes controlling pituitary development.

In the empty sella syndrome, abnormalities of the sellar diaphragm allow herniation of the suprasellar subarachnoid space into the region of the sella turcica.[81] This may result in damage to the sella, including the pituitary. Empty sella syndrome may be the consequence of surgery or irradiation or may be idiopathic. It is often found in patients with mutations in *PROP-1*, when it may have been preceded by a pituitary mass.

ACQUIRED DEFECTS

Destructive Lesions of the Hypothalamus and Pituitary

A wide range of destructive lesions involving the hypothalamus or pituitary may appear with isolated GHD or CPHD. Birth trauma, associated with abrupt delivery, prolonged labor, or extensive use of forceps, has been associated frequently with subsequent hypothalamic or pituitary dysfunction.[82,83] An increased incidence of GHD has been reported in breech deliveries, although it is still unclear whether such deliveries lead to acquisition of pituitary dysfunction, or,

conversely, whether preexisting CNS abnormalities result in higher rates of abnormal birth presentations.

Tumors

CNS tumors are an important cause of isolated GHD and CPHD and must be excluded in every child with GHD who does not have an obvious alternative explanation for growth failure. Midline brain tumors include germinomas, meningiomas, gliomas, colloid cysts of the third ventricle, ependymomas, and optic nerve gliomas. GHD or CPHD also may occur from local extension of tumors affecting the head or neck, such as craniopharyngeal carcinomas and lymphomas.

The major pediatric tumor involving the pituitary is craniopharyngioma, which is probably an evolving congenital malformation that develops from remnants of Rathke's pouch.[84] Arising from rests of squamous cells at the embryonic junction of the adenohypophysis and neurohypophysis, it forms an enlarging cyst filled with degenerating cells, leading to cyst fluid or calcifications, but never to malignant degeneration. These calcifications may be seen, at times, on skull films and constitute an important diagnostic sign. Although craniopharyngiomas represent the consequences of a congenital malformation, they may appear clinically at any age. Although significant growth failure may be observed at the time of diagnosis, patients most commonly are first seen with complaints of increased intracranial pressure, such as headaches, vomiting, and oculomotor disturbances; visual field defects are frequently noted at the time of diagnosis.[84] From 50% to 80% of patients have deficiency of at least one pituitary hormone, most commonly GH or gonadotropins; diabetes insipidus is reported in 25% to 50% of patients at diagnosis.[84,85]

Langerhans' cell histiocytosis also may appear at any age. Depending on the sites and extent of histiocytic infiltration, these disorders may manifest with isolated GHD or CPHD with or without diabetes insipidus.[86] The pituitary stalk is usually thickened on MRI scanning.

Irradiation of the Central Nervous System

Cranial irradiation used for the therapy of solid brain tumors and as prophylaxis for leukemia can lead to abnormal hypothalamopituitary (HP) function. The sensitivity of the HP axis to radiation depends on the dose, fractionation, tissue location, and the age of the patient.[87] Such damage is, typically, difficult to assess precisely, because the hypothalamus and pituitary may differ in the extent of involvement, and the loss of function may evolve with time. Sensitivity to CNS radiation may differ among patients, although the majority of children will experience some degree of hypothalamic or pituitary dysfunction within 5 years of receiving 30 Gy.[88,89] GHD also occurs with doses of 18 to 24 Gy,[90] and subtle dysfunction may be observed at even lower doses. GH secretion, generally, appears to be the most sensitive to irradiation, followed by TSH, gonadotropins, and, finally, ACTH. This may relate to the unique position of the GHRH neurons on the surface of the hypothalamus and not deep within the structure, as previously thought.[91]

As pituitary dysfunction evolves over several years after irradiation, such children should be monitored for growth deceleration. Whereas provocative GH testing may be within normal limits, measures of spontaneous GH secretion frequently demonstrate abnormalities.[92] Serum concentrations of IGF-1 or IGF-binding protein-3 (IGFBP-3) may not be reduced in the early years after cranial irradiation.[93,94]

Cranial irradiation also may result in precocious puberty, leading to an early pubertal growth spurt, advanced skeletal maturation, and, ultimately, reduced stature. This may be superimposed on any growth restriction that results from the spinal irradiation for the primary problem.[95–97] Low-dose irradiation is frequently associated with a precocious onset of puberty; higher doses may result in gonadotropin deficiency and pubertal delay. In the irradiated child with early puberty, therapy with gonadotropin-releasing hormone (GnRH) analogues should be considered, with or without GH treatment, to delay epiphyseal fusion.

Lower doses of radiation (24 Gy) also are associated with GHD in approximately 30% to 60% of cases. Craniospinal irradiation used in the treatment of posterior fossa tumors and total body irradiation used in conditioning regimens for bone marrow transplant also are associated with damage to the epiphyses, with subsequent disproportionate short stature.

Infiltrative and Inflammatory Disorders

Infiltrative diseases are uncommon causes of GHD in the pediatric population, but pituitary insufficiency may be observed secondary to CNS involvement in tuberculosis,[98] sarcoidosis,[99] or toxoplasmosis. Inflammation associated with bacterial, viral, fungal, or parasitic disease may also result in hypothalamic-pituitary dysfunction. Lymphadenoid hypophysitis also has been reported.

Vascular Lesions

Aneurysms may behave as space-occupying lesions and cause hypothalamic or pituitary destruction.

Psychosocial Dwarfism

Psychosocial dwarfism is a form of poor growth associated with bizarre eating and drinking behavior, social withdrawal, delayed speech, and, on occasion, other evidence of developmental delay.[100] Periodic hyperphagia is associated with decreased GH responsiveness to standard provocative stimuli, but also with subnormal responses to exogenous GH therapy.[101] Removal from the stressful environment, which usually involves removal from the home, is accompanied by a restoration of normal GH secretion, typically within weeks, and a period of catch-up growth.[102,103] The mechanisms for this reversible form of GHD are unclear, but it is of note that a variety of psychiatric conditions in adults may be associated with decreased spontaneous and provocative GH secretion. Establishment of the diagnosis of psychosocial dwarfism requires documentation of catch-up growth and restoration of normal GH secretion after correction of the environmental situation.

PHYSIOLOGY OF THE HYPOTHALAMO-PITUITARY-SOMATOTROPH AXIS

Growth hormone (GH) is secreted by somatotrophs in the anterior pituitary gland. The secretory pattern is pulsatile, with discrete pulses of GH every 3 to 4 hours and virtually undetectable GH concentrations in between. GH secretion varies considerably with age[104,105] and shows a sexually dimorphic pattern,[106] with a greater average daily GH output in women. This pattern is the result of an interaction between the hypothalamic peptides GHRH and somatostatin (SS). The amplitude of the GH peak is determined by GHRH that stimulates the pituitary somatotrophs to increase both the secretion of stored GH and GH gene transcription. SS determines trough levels of GH by inhibition of GHRH release from the hypothalamus and GH release from the pituitary. Withdrawal of SS conversely determines the timing of a GH pulse.

More recently, the use of synthetic GH-releasing peptides (GHRPs) has led to the identification of a GH secretagogue (GHS) receptor (GHSR type 1a). The receptor is strongly expressed in the hypothalamus, but specific binding sites for GHRP also have been identified in other regions of the CNS and peripheral endocrine and nonendocrine tissues in both humans and other organisms.[107–109] The endogenous ligand for the GHS receptor, ghrelin, was isolated from the stomach and is an octynylated peptide consisting of 28 amino acids.[110] It is expressed predominantly in the stomach, but lower

amounts are present within the bowel, pancreas, kidney, immune system, placenta, pituitary, testis, ovary, and hypothalamus.[111,112] Ghrelin leads not only to the secretion of GH, but also stimulates PRL and ACTH secretion. Additionally, it influences endocrine pancreatic function and glucose metabolism, gonadal function, appetite, and behavior. It also can control gastric motility and acid secretion and has cardiovascular and antiproliferative effects. The role of endogenous ghrelin in normal growth during childhood remains unclear. Both ghrelin and GHRPs release GH synergistically with GHRH.

The expression of the human GH gene, located on chromosome 17, is regulated not only by a proximal promoter, but also by a locus control region (LCR) 15 to 32 kB upstream of the hGH-1 gene. The LCR confers pituitary-specific, high-level expression of hGH.[113,114] The full-length transcript from the GH1 gene encodes a 191-amino acid 22-kilodalton protein that accounts for 85% to 90% of circulating GH. Alternative splicing of the messenger RNA (mRNA) transcript generates a 20-kilodalton form of GH that accounts for the remaining 10% to 15%. Within both the proximal promoter and the LCR are located binding sites for the pituitary-specific transcription factor Pit1. Additional binding sites for the transcription factor Zn15 also are located within the proximal promoter.

In the circulation, GH binds to two binding proteins, high-affinity GHBP and low-affinity GHBP.[115,116] Little is known about the low-affinity GHBP, which accounts for approximately 10% to 15% of GH binding, with a preference for binding to 20-kilodalton hGH. The high-affinity GHBP is a 61-kilodalton glycosylated protein that represents a soluble form of the extracellular domain of the GH receptor that can bind to both 20- and 22-kilodalton hGH, and thereby prolong the half-life of GH. In vivo studies that have coadministered GH and GHBP to hypophysectomized and GHD rats have demonstrated a potentiation of weight gain and bone growth, although similar studies have not as yet been performed in humans.[117]

The GH receptor (GHR) is present in a number of tissues. The hormone sequentially dimerizes its receptor, activating a receptor-associated tyrosine kinase JAK2 that in turn is autophosphorylated and also phosphorylates the GHR. This then leads to signal transduction by using the mitogen-activated protein kinase (MAPK), signal transduction and activators of transcription (STAT), and phosphatidylinositol kinase (PI 3-kinase) pathways. The result is activation of a number of genes that mediate the effects of GH. These include early-response genes encoding transcription factors such as c-jun, c-fos, and c-myc implicated in cell growth, proliferation, and differentiation, and IGF-1, which mediates the growth-promoting effects of GH.[118,119]

IGF-1 and IGF-2 are single-chain polypeptide hormones that are widely expressed, and, together with a family of specific binding proteins, they are believed to mediate most of the actions of GH. Extensive and authoritative reviews cover this aspect of the GH axis[120] (Chapter 32).

CLINICAL FEATURES

NEONATAL PRESENTATION

Recent studies in humans and in animal models have demonstrated marked similarities, but also critical differences, between the clinical features of GHD and various forms of IGF deficiency.[121–123] In GHD, prenatal growth is near normal, although mild reductions in birth length and weight have been observed. GHD does not cause severe intrauterine growth restriction (IUGR), whereas loss of placental GH does.[124] However, loss of IGF-1 in utero results in severe IUGR in both humans and mice,[125,126] suggesting that IGF-1 and the IGF-1 receptor are critically involved in intrauterine growth. IGF-1 synthesis and secretion in utero are not regulated primarily by pituitary GH.

IGF-1 production comes under GH regulation either in the last few months of fetal life or shortly after birth and is well established by age 6 months. Growth failure is greater for skeletal growth than for body weight, so infants and young children have an appearance of relative adiposity. Neonates may have hypoglycemia, and this suggests the possibility of other pituitary hormone deficiencies, especially ACTH. Normoglycemia is maintained only when cortisol replacement therapy is commenced, suggesting that ACTH and, consequently, cortisol secretion is critical for glucose homeostasis. However, the GH–IGF-1 axis also plays a role in maintaining glucose homeostasis, although IGHD is rarely associated with neonatal hypoglycemia. A diagnostic fast may be required to dissect CPHD from other causes of hypoglycemia, although the distinguishing feature from hyperinsulinism is the absence of ketone body formation in the latter.[127]

The presence of concomitant gonadotropin deficiency is suggested by the presence of microphallus, cryptorchidism, and scrotal hypoplasia. Genital ambiguity would not be expected because of placental production of human chorionic gonadotropin (hCG). Prolonged jaundice with conjugated hyperbilirubinemia and cholestasis also may be observed, typically in patients with CPHD. The relative contributions of GH, ACTH, and TSH deficiency to this presentation are unclear. It is imperative that the diagnosis of pituitary insufficiency be considered in any infant (especially term) with hypoglycemia, cryptorchidisim, and microphallus, or conjugated hyperbilirubinemia. Associated features that might indicate more widespread problems (midline defects of the face, a single central incisor, nystagmus or optic nerve hypoplasia or both) should be looked for and MRI undertaken.

INFANT AND CHILDHOOD YEARS

After the perinatal period, the defining feature of GHD is growth failure. Reduced skeletal growth may be observed during the first 6 months of life in congenital GHD, but by age 6 to 12 months, early growth failure is almost inevitable.[128–131] Height velocity is usually between −2 and −5 standard deviations (SDs) from the mean leading to progressive height centile crossing. In patients with acquired GHD, the critical feature is a change in growth rate. Between age 2 years and the onset of puberty, children maintain their height percentile with remarkable integrity. Deviation from this channel (either acceleration or deceleration) needs investigation. Thus, a child who has been growing along the 75th percentile, but moves across to the 25th percentile, warrants evaluation, even though his or her height may still be within the normal range.

Bone age is often delayed in patients with GHD. This may not be so in acquired GHD because of the close proximity of time to the growth failure or when acquired GHD is accompanied by accelerated puberty, as occasionally seen in patients with intracranial tumors, when bone age may be accelerated.[96,97] Delayed dentition may be observed, but in the absence of midline craniofacial abnormalities, is otherwise normal. Other skeletal appearances include hypoplasia of facial bones, hypoplastic nasal bridge, frontal bossing, and delayed closure of sutures. Head circumference is usually at the lower limits of normal, indicating normal brain growth.

An increase in adiposity, particularly central adiposity, can be detected by careful measurement of skin-fold thicknesses. Genital growth, before the onset of puberty, is usually proportional to body size. Puberty may be delayed, but, in the absence of other endocrine deficiencies, is otherwise normal.

Limited data are available on the adult height of untreated GHD patients. These results are often difficult to interpret because of (1) heterogeneity in the timing of GHD; (2) het-

erogeneity in the severity of GHD; (3) the presence or absence of other pituitary deficiencies; and (4) delay in puberty, resulting in late epiphyseal fusion. Wit and colleagues[132] summarized the results from studies of 22 untreated men and 14 untreated women[133–135] with severe isolated GHD and reported a mean adult height of −4.7 SD. In patients with untreated autosomal-recessive GHD, Rimoin and associates[133] reported mean adult heights of −7.4 SD. In patients with CPHD, adult height is often not as severely affected as in IGHD, presumably reflecting pubertal delay and late epiphyseal fusion.[135]

DIAGNOSIS OF GROWTH HORMONE DEFICIENCY IN CHILDHOOD

The diagnostic evaluation of children with growth failure is complex, as multiple causes exist for short stature (Table 37-4). In the pursuit of the diagnosis of GHD, other causes for short stature need to be considered and excluded. This is because the diagnosis of GHD is one of exclusion[136] and as GH is the final common pathway for postnatal growth many causes of poor growth may secondarily affect GH secretion.[137] A number of tests are available for assessing GH status. Considerable attention has been paid to the underlying mechanisms assessed by the tests, how the samples should be collected, and what type of measurement should be performed. Less attention has been paid to the statistical assumptions underlying the performance

Table 37-4 Causes of Short Stature

NONPATHOGENIC
Constitutional delay of growth and puberty
Familial short stature
Nutritional

LOW BIRTH WEIGHT

SYSTEMIC DISORDERS
Cardiovascular disease (e.g., congenital heart disease)
Renal (e.g., chronic renal failure, renal tubular disease)
Respiratory (e.g., cystic fibrosis, asthma)
Gastrointestinal disease (e.g., Crohn's disease)
Neurologic (e.g., brain tumor)
Psychological (e.g., anorexia nervosa, child abuse)

ENDOCRINE CAUSES
GH-RELATED CAUSES
Growth hormone (GH) deficiency: isolated or combined with other hormone deficiencies
Resistance to GH due to defects in the GH receptor
Defects in post–GH receptor signaling: mutation in *STAT5b*
IGF-1 deficiency
Abnormality of ALS (acid labile subunit)
IGF type 1 receptor mutation

HYPOTHYROIDISM

PSEUDOHYPOPARATHYROIDISM

GLUCOCORTICOID EXCESS
Cushing's syndrome
Congenital adrenal hyperplasia
Exogenous administration

GENETIC CAUSES
Turner's syndrome
Noonan's syndrome
Down syndrome
Skeletal dysplasias: hypochondroplasia, achondroplasia, spondyloepiphyseal dysplasia
Russell-Silver syndrome
Seckl's syndrome
Prader-Willi syndrome
Miscellaneous: other syndromes (e.g., Rothmund-Thompson, Leri-Weill syndrome, progeria, mucopolysaccharidoses)

IGF-1, insulin-like growth factor type 1.

of diagnostic tests. The statistical theory behind many tests is complex because the results do not follow an all-or-none law. Rather than being left with a clear-cut answer to the initial diagnostic question, the clinician is more likely to be left with a series of probabilities as to whether the patient is likely to have GHD.

GUIDANCE DERIVED FROM CLINICAL ASSESSMENT

Neonatal Period
Several pointers to the diagnosis of GHD were considered earlier. In the neonatal period, GHD may be isolated or associated with other pituitary hormone deficiencies. Small genitalia may point to associated gonadotropin deficiency. Hypoglycemia in the newborn period is often a feature of ACTH deficiency, although, on an arbitrary basis, a serum GH of less than 10 ng/mL is considered consistent with a diagnosis of GHD under these circumstances.[138] This is not universal, however, and caution must be exercised in interpreting the GH response to hypoglycemia under different circumstances.[139] Prolonged neonatal jaundice raises the question of thyroxine (unconjugated) or cortisol (conjugated hyperbilirubinemia) deficiency. Given these features, it might be possible on the basis of pattern recognition to ascribe the diagnosis of GHD to a patient with a high degree of certainty. MRI of the brain should be obtained to look for an undescended posterior pituitary, anterior pituitary hypoplasia, hypoplasia or absence of the pituitary stalk, hypoplasia of the optic chiasm, and absence or hypoplasia of the corpus callosum and septum pellucidum.[72-81]

Infancy and Childhood
Diagnostic evaluation in children must be based on auxology. Although a number of clinical features of GHD are said to be classic, none is specific. For example, obesity is listed as a clinical feature of GHD, but if we simply restricted biochemical evaluation to patients with obesity as the main feature, testing the GH axis would yield a large number of individuals with a poor GH response, because obesity per se is associated with blunted GH responses to various stimuli.[140,141] Individuals who are GHD are often obese, but the converse is clearly not the case.

Little is known of the sensitivity and specificity of many of the clinical observations, either alone or in combination. The prevalence of many of the clinical features within the general population is unknown, which heightens the problem. Even the presence of specific features or combinations of features will increase only slightly the likelihood of disease if they are relatively insensitive.

The manifestation of GHD as a result of a GH gene deletion is early and poor growth can be detected as early as the sixth month of postnatal life. With advancing age, more GH has to be secreted to maintain concentrations of GH sufficient for growth, so idiopathic isolated pituitary GHD may appear at any time. It is the degree of deficiency that dictates when the individual comes to medical attention. Table 37-5 provides general clinical rules that are a useful aid when selecting patients for further study of the GH axis.

PRINCIPLES OF TESTING

The aim of any diagnostic test is to take the clinical history and examination to the point at which the care of the patient is altered. A vast and bewildering literature exists on GH testing, but the clinician can be guided by asking the questions detailed in Table 37-6.

Two points deserve special mention. First, it is unusual in endocrinology for there to be a diagnostic gold standard. The anterior pituitary is not accessible, and molecular biology is not sufficiently advanced to give definitive answers. Second, care must be taken in ascribing the role of a gold standard. It

Table 37-5 Clinical Indicators for Further Evaluation of the GH Axis

1. Height, at any age, below the 0.4th centile on the UK Reference Charts.[142] The 0.4 level is chosen to improve diagnostic return from evaluation. The previous cut-off (3rd or 5th centile) lacks sensitivity and specificity.
2. Crossing of one or more height centiles on the UK Reference Charts over a period of ≥1 years. Centiles are equispaced (0.7 SD) allowing general rules to be applied at all ages
3. A height that is inappropriately low for the heights of the parents
4. Predisposing condition (tumor, radiation, etc.) or features suggestive of an underlying syndrome
5. Neonatal signs consistent with pituitary hormone deficiencies

GH, growth hormone.

may change with time, and the test must be well validated by application to large numbers of individuals with and without the condition. The temptation is to use the extremes, but this may lead to a considerable overestimate of sensitivity and specificity[143] that may not be borne out in field studies.[144,145]

Two principles operate when using diagnostic tests[146]: The first probability is a useful marker of diagnostic uncertainty. This is when the sensitivity (ability to detect a target disorder when present, or true-positive rate) and specificity (ability to identify correctly the absence of the disorder or true-negative rate) become important. If both were 85%, 15% of patients with disease would have a negative result (false negative), and 15% without disease would have a positive result (false positive). Abnormal results would occur in patients with and without disease. Whatever the result, new information has been generated that may or may not influence decision making. Second, diagnostic tests should be obtained only when they can alter the management of the case, that is, if the test result alters the probability of the disease.

Pre- and Posttest Probability
The relation between the probability of disease after the results of diagnostic tests are known (the posttest probability) and pretest probability test of disease depends on the sensitivity and specificity of the test, as shown in Figure 37-7. Two important points exist: The first is that the more certain the clinician is of the diagnosis before the test is performed, the less effect the confirmatory test has on the probability of disease. The obverse also is true. The second point is that tests will have major effects on probability of disease in the intermediate zone. Testing is not likely to be beneficial if the pretest probability is very high or low. This is one reason that screening for GH problems in short children on the basis of biochemical tests is unhelpful, as the pretest probability is 1 in 3000 or 0.003%.

Clinicians are often faced with the situation in which they are really sure the patient has the condition, but the test does not confirm this. Table 37-7 analyses this concept. Here, specificity and sensitivity have been fixed, and the effects on posttest probability are considered. In the situation in which

Table 37-6 Underlying Principles of Assessing Tests

1. Has there been an independent blind comparison with the diagnostic "gold standard"?
2. Was the test conducted in a wide range of patients with and without the condition?
3. Is the test reproducible?
4. What was the definition of normal in the test situation?
5. How might the test interact with others in a diagnostic sequence?
6. Does the test entail risk or reduce risk for the patient?

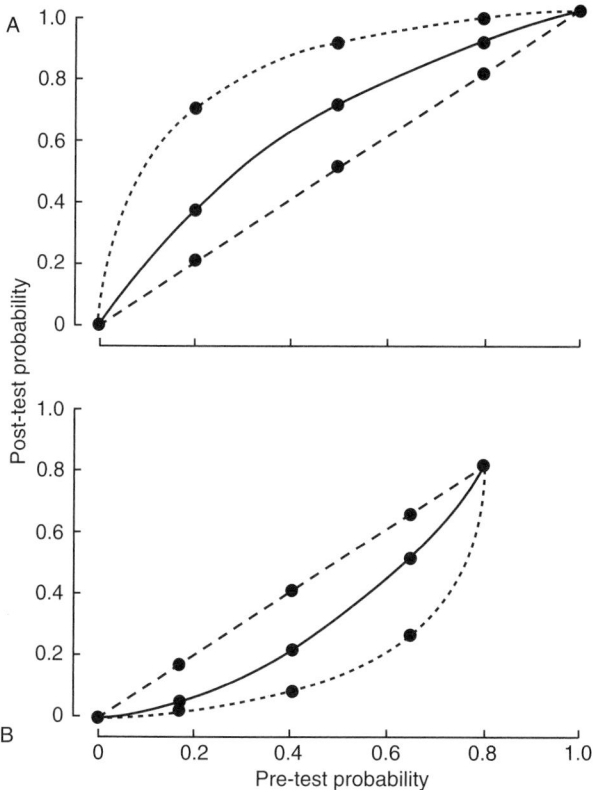

Figure 37-7 The relation between pretest and posttest probability of disease. The data were constructed by using Bayes' theorem with a test sensitivity and specificity of either 70% (*solid line*) or 90% (*dashed line*). **A,** The posttest probability if the test were positive; **(B)** the posttest probability if the test were negative. If the posttest probability were the same as the pretest probability, then the relation would be given by the line of identity. (Reproduced from Brok CGD, Hindmarsh PC, Jacobs HS [eds]: Clinical Pediatric Endocrinology, 4th ed. London, Blackwell Publishers, 2001.)

a 90% pretest probability exists that the patient is GHD, then, even if the test is negative in the individual, still a 67% probability (reduced by 23%) remains that the patient has the condition, so treatment would still be justified. When the pretest probability was 5% (very certain that the patient does not have GHD) and the test is positive, all the result says is that the patient has a 1 in 4 chance of having the condition, so we would probably not treat. In the middle, certainty in either direction is dramatically improved.

Multiple Tests
Table 37-7 could have been made much larger by introducing any number of pretreatment probabilities. There comes a point, however, when posttest probability changes to a level where a decision has to be made to stop and either accept or reject the proposal that the condition is present. The decision to stop investigation and to treat or not depends on how convinced the clinician is of the diagnosis, the benefits and risks of the therapy, and the potential yield and risks of further tests. Two ways exist to assist this situation: Conduct another test, or use a more sophisticated analysis rather than a simple positive or negative.

This is problematic in the GH field because the methodology assumes that the results of the two tests are independent. In normal individuals, undergoing repeated GHRH tests, dependence cannot be assumed.[147] Where repeated tests have been performed in children, concordance was observed 50% of the time, a value close to that calculated for independent events by using a test with 70% to 85% efficiency. Another important issue is whether the test might change in individuals as they age. Some evidence indicates that the clonidine test is less effective in releasing GH in young adults compared with children.[148] Whether the magnitude of the response to other stimuli can be assumed to remain unchanged is unknown.

Assuming that the two tests are performed (on different days) and that they are dependent, then if both tests must be positive for diagnosis, this maximizes specificity and avoids falsely labeling normal children, but it misses many treatable individuals. Insisting that both tests be negative maximizes sensitivity, minimizes misdiagnoses, but falsely labels many more normal children.

One special area of two tests is the question of retesting after completion of GH therapy. Several recent publications suggested that individuals who were originally diagnosed with GHD do not appear to have the biochemical abnormality when the test is repeated later.[149,150] This has led to statements being made that these individuals are no longer GHD. Two issues are worth considering: the first is that the population studied during the second test is not the same as that during the first. Those thought unlikely to have the condition have been excluded. The second point also relates to some extent to the original diagnosis. It is worth rehearsing the scenario that has led to the second test. The child was initially evaluated because of concerns over short stature and poor growth. At that point, a test was conducted because the clinician required an answer with which to rule in or rule out the diagnosis, and the result was sufficient in terms of posttest probability for therapy to be offered. If the posttest probability of the child having the condition was 87%, then this value now forms the pretest probability for the second test, not the 50:50 situation the clinician faced before the original investigation. Information has been collected that influences the probability of the disease process being present.

DIAGNOSIS OF GROWTH HORMONE DEFICIENCY

Assessment of GH secretion is problematic, in part because of the pulsatile nature of GH secretion.[151] The most consistent GH surges accompany slow-wave electroencephalographic rhythms during phases 3 and 4 of sleep. Although this rhythmicity is characteristic of GH secretion at all ages, the size of the amplitudes and the total integrated GH secretion varies with sex, age, pubertal status, and nutrition.[152,153] Between pulses, serum GH concentrations are extremely low, often less than 0.1 ng/mL. Consequently, measurement of random serum GH concentrations is of no value in the diagnosis of GHD. Measurement of spontaneous GH secretion requires multiple sampling, typically every 15 minutes over a 12- to 24-hour period.[151-155] Such methods are inconvenient and expensive, and although they allow identification of the patient with severe GHD, it is not clear that they can discriminate between partial GHD and normal secretory variation.[156] However, even the reproducibility of GH secretory patterns in children from day to day is uncertain. Rose and colleagues[156] reported that measurement of spontaneous GH

Table 37-7	Effect on Posttest Probability of Differing Pretest Certainty Assuming Constant Sensitivity and Specificity		
		Posttest Probability	
Pretest Probability (%)		Test Positive	Test Negative
90		98 (+8)	67 (−23)
50		87 (+37)	19 (−32)
5		25 (+20)	1 (−4)

Change from pretest probability in parentheses.

secretion identified only 57% of children diagnosed as GHD by provocative testing. Lanes[157] reported that approximately 25% of normally growing children have low overnight GH concentrations. A longitudinal study of GH secretion in normal boys during puberty indicated wide intersubject variation,[152,153] and day-to-day variation has been noted among normal subjects.[158]

An alternative approach has been the measurement of urinary GH concentrations.[159-163] This method requires a timed urinary collection and a GH assay of high sensitivity, as urinary GH concentrations are low. The theoretic advantages of this approach include its relative ease of performance and noninvasive nature, as well as the requirement for only a single GH measurement. This must be balanced, however, by the need to assess the effects of renal function, the wide interindividual variation, and the lack of adequate age- and sex-related reference ranges.

As a result of these difficulties, the standard for the diagnosis of GHD has been provocative testing of GH "secretory reserve"[138] (Table 37-8). Physiologic stimuli for such tests have included sleep[164] and exercise,[165,166] and pharmacologic stimuli have included a wide variety of agents.[167-175] None of these tests truly mimics normal GH secretory physiology, and none has been evaluated adequately in normal children and normal short children. The limitations of provocative GH testing in the diagnosis of GHD are described later and should be considered in light of statistical theory (see earlier):

1. Provocative testing, by its nature, is nonphysiologic. None of the commonly used stimuli truly mimics normal regulation of GH secretion.
2. The definition of a "normal" response to stimulation is arbitrary. Normal values are difficult to obtain in pediatric practice, and reference ranges would be needed for tall, normal, and short children because their GH secretion differs.[176] In addition, both age and pubertal stage influence GH secretion,[152,153,176] as does body composition.[140,141] Values for these would also have to be included.

   The classic approach of defining normal data in terms of a gaussian distribution does not come without hazard. Endocrine testing rarely fits this distribution, and even if it did, it would imply that the lowest and highest 2.5% of values are abnormal and that all diseases have the same frequency—clearly unlikely. Creating upper and lower limits does not help either. It is more appropriate to identify a range of diagnostic test results beyond which the disorder of GHD is likely.

Most decisions on placing the value have been empirical rather than statistical. In practice, cut-off values could be chosen at an absolute extreme. If 100 short children were studied and GH sufficiency or deficiency were defined by a peak response of less than 3 ng/mL, only 3% to 5% might have a response at this level. When testing the next 100 children, we might find that one or two normal individuals might have such a response. They will be outliers, but they are important because the more patients studied, the greater the chance of finding outliers.

Moving the cut-off to more extreme values to exclude these patients restricts the population of treatable individuals. Relaxing the criteria interposes normal individuals into the diagnosis zone. Placing the cut-off is based partly on clinical judgment. As no disadvantage exists, apart from financial cost, in falsely labeling someone with GHD and treating them, a relaxed cut-off would be acceptable.

3. The dependence of GH secretion on other factors must be taken into account. Marin and colleagues[177] demonstrated that when exercise and arginine stimulation tests were performed on normal-stature children without sex steroid priming, the lower limits of normal (–2 SD) peak serum GH concentration for prepubertal children was as low as 1.9 ng/mL and increased to 7.2 ng/mL on estrogen priming. Thyroxine and cortisol, which directly alter gene transcription, influence the results obtained, and these must be controlled before undertaking a diagnostic study.[178] Similarly, the presence of high levels of glucose or free fatty acids may influence the response obtained.[179]
4. GH assays may measure a variety of immunoreactive molecular forms of GH.[180] These GH variants do not necessarily possess equivalent growth-promoting actions. Furthermore, considerable interassay variability exists in the measurement of these GH molecular variants.[181-183] Individual standards must be established for each laboratory.[184] It is not likely that these problems will be resolved by immunofunctional GH assays, which may face many of the same issues.[185]
5. Most endocrine tests are conducted over short periods, and results are extrapolated to longer time frames. GH provocation tests take 2 hours to perform, and the results are then compared with height velocity measurements obtained over a longer period, often 1 year. That a relation exists is perhaps surprising; that there are high false-positive and -negative rates probably is not.

Table 37-8	Growth Hormone Stimulation Tests		
Stimulus	**Dose**	**Sampling Protocol (min)**	**Notes**
Exercise	Cycle for 10–15 min	15 min for 90 min	Variable response, highly dependent on degree of exercise
Levodopa	<15 kg, 125 mg 15–30 kg, 250 mg >30 kg, 500 mg	15 min for 90 min	Nausea
Clonidine	0.15 mg/m^2	30 min for 90 min	Tiredness; postural hypotension
Arginine HCl	0.5 g/kg (max, 30 g) IV, given as 10% arginine HCl in 0.9% NaCl over 30 min	15 min for 90 min	May cause insulin release
Insulin	0.05–0.1 U/kg IV	15 min for 120 min	Hypoglycemia; requires supervision. Can also measure cortisol reliably
Glucagon	0.1 mg/kg IM (max, 1 mg)	30 min for 180 min	Nausea
GHRH	1 μg/kg IV	15 min for 120 min	Flushing. Only assesses pituitary reserve not whole H-P axis
GHRH-Arginine			Needs further work to assess value in pediatrics

Tests should be performed after an overnight fast. Patients should be documented to be euthyroid. Prepubertal children should be primed with gonadal steroids.
IV, intravenous; IM, intramuscular; GHRH, GH-releasing hormone.

6. Hormone pulsatility also may influence diagnostic tests if the test itself (e.g., the stimulus applied) is influenced by oscillations within the system under study. The GH response at any time is going to be heavily dependent on the interplay between the hypothalamic regulatory peptides involved in GH release (GHRH and somatostatin).[186] Somatostatin, in particular, is a key determinant of the amount of GH released as a result of GHRH stimulation. Attempts have been made to take control of this variable[187] by pretreatment with somatostatin. GHRH combined with arginine is an alternative approach.[188] It was hoped that the ghrelin-like agents would be an advance in this area because of their potent GH-releasing qualities, but they appear to have the same problems of reproducibility.[189]

7. Endocrine systems also are subject to feedback from target tissues, and this is an issue not only in the interpretation of single provocation tests but also where second tests are performed in rapid succession to the first. A diminished response to GHRH can be observed if the second stimulus is applied 1, 2, or 3 hours after the first.[147] The implication of doing two tests on the same day, often following each other, are immense, because the cut-off that might be implied to determine normality or not may not be the same for the second test as for the first, especially if the second stimulus is different from the first.

8. Provocative testing fails to give any consideration to the effect of negative feedback by serum IGF-1.[190-193] It probably makes more sense to interpret serum GH concentrations in light of serum IGF concentrations, much as TSH concentrations are best assessed with a knowledge of circulating thyroxine concentrations.

9. In assessing the results of endocrine evaluations, it is generally assumed that the single or multiple samples measured are relatively stable, at least over short periods. When important changes are postulated to be taking place, for example, in a disease process, some knowledge of the inherent variability within the measurement system is required. In the short term, a number of studies have demonstrated variability within and between individuals in terms of GH tests.[158,194] Group data are usually reproducible, but problems can arise if it is assumed that individual oscillatory profiles are consistent from day to day. Table 37-9 summarizes data relating to intraindividual coefficients of variation in 24-hour GH and IGF-1 profiles measured over the course of 1 year.[194] These observations add an additional dimension to the comparison of studies obtained under one series of circumstances with a set obtained under another series of circumstances, particularly if they are separated by long periods.

10. In considering provocative tests, the situation may arise in which no response is observed: A possible explanation is that the strength of the stimulus was insufficient to provoke hormone release. In such a situation, it is valuable to have an independent marker of stimulus application. In the insulin-induced hypoglycemia test, this marker is glucose and the attainment of adequate hypoglycemia. In the glucagon test, it may be the release of glucose. In other tests, no independent markers may be present, so that doubt may be cast on the reliability of the nonresponse.

11. Provocative GH testing is expensive, uncomfortable, and has risk. Insulin-induced hypoglycemia should be performed only in a supervised setting. Deaths have been documented in patients rendered hypoglycemic and corrected in an overly vigorous manner.

Of the provocative tests listed in Table 37-8, it should be noted that stimulation with GHRH is not designed to document whether a patient has GHD, but rather whether GHD, established by other methods, is the result of pituitary or hypothalamic dysfunction.[195] Failure to respond to GHRH suggests that the abnormality is at the pituitary level. This test may be enhanced by the addition of arginine or pyridostigmine.[196]

PRACTICAL APPROACH TO DIAGNOSTIC EVALUATION

A practical approach to the diagnosis of a child with GHD is grounded on clinical assessment with allocation of pretest probability of disease presence. In the prepubertal child with abnormal growth, serum concentrations of IGF-1, IGFBP-3, amyotrophic lateral sclerosis (ALS), or a combination of these provides a means for excluding a diagnosis of GHD. Provocative GH testing with appropriate sex steroid priming will provide information on GH secretory capability, and GHRH stimulation, with or without arginine or pyridostigmine, will allow determination of whether the defect is at the hypothalamic or pituitary level. All data must be interpreted together with known test performances and integrated with the pretest probability to generate a posttest probability, which would then lead to a decision as to whether intervention is required. The interpretation of second tests of GH secretion is problematic from both the physiological and statistical standpoints and should be analyzed with extreme caution

Documentation of GHD also requires that other pituitary functions be assessed periodically, including TSH, ACTH, and gonadotropin status. Other pituitary deficiencies may not be evident on initial assessment but may develop over time. MRI of the hypothalamus and pituitary should be performed initially, to determine whether evidence exists of intracranial tumors, pituitary hypoplasia, or midline defects. Even if the baseline MRI is normal, in the absence of an alternative explanation for GHD or CPHD, the possibility of tumors or structural defects should not be dismissed permanently. With increasing knowledge of the genetics of pituitary disorders, these should be looked for, as they affect the likelihood of other pituitary hormone deficiencies evolving with time and allow genetic counseling to be undertaken.

TREATMENT

GROWTH HORMONE

The first successful treatment of human GHD with human pituitary-derived GH (HGH) was in the 1950s, and this was followed by a series of publications that documented the efficacy of GH in patients with GHD.[6-9,136] Treatment used human cadaver pituitary–derived HGH, which brought with it a series of problems surrounding supply. Limited supplies mandated the use of suboptimal dosages, interrupted treatment periods, and frequent cessation of therapy before maximal height had been attained. The use of human pituitary–derived HGH was halted in 1985 after the discovery of several cases of Creutzfeldt-Jakob disease associated with its

Table 37-9	Within-individual Coefficients of Variation for GH and IGF-1 with Testosterone as Comparison	
	Mean Coefficient of Variation [%] (Range)
Mean 24-hr serum GH concentration	35 (9–58)
Serum IGF-1 concentration	21 (14–34)
Serum testosterone concentration	13 (8–19)

GH, growth hormone; IGF, insulin-like growth factor.

use. Pituitary-derived HGH was replaced with recombinant DNA–derived r-hGH, which allowed potentially unlimited supplies, obviating the need for low-dose use and interrupted therapeutic regimens. The initial r-hGH preparation was an N-terminal methionine (met-r-hGH), which was fully active biologically but was ultimately replaced by the mature 191-amino acid protein. The biopotency of current preparations of r-hGH, expressed as International Units per milligram of the new World Health Organization (WHO) r-hGH reference reagent for somatropin (88/624), is 3 International Units/mg.

Dose Studies
Investigations of optimal dosing of r-hGH have been complicated by the use of heterogeneous study populations, so that studies frequently include patients with unequivocal and complete GHD, together with patients with partial GHD. Several studies have demonstrated a dose-response relation for HGH, but the slope of the response is relatively shallow.[197] MacGillivray and colleagues[198] compared the growth responses of 99 children treated with pituitary HGH at a mean dosage of 0.1 mg/kg/week, with those of 77 children treated with r-hGH at a dosage of 0.3 mg/kg/week. The mean time required to reach normal height (greater than –2 SD) was 48 months for the low-dose group and 27 months for the high-dose group. Fifty-one percent of the low-dose group never reached this point compared with 23% in the high-dose group. Cohen and colleagues[199] compared the growth responses of prepubertal, naive patients randomized to r-hGH at a dosage of 0.175, 0.35, or 0.7 mg/kg/week for the first 2 years of treatment. Significantly greater height velocities and gains in height SD resulted from the 0.35 mg/kg/week versus 0.175 mg/kg/week, but no further significant improvement was observed with the 0.7-mg/kg/week dosage. Ultimately, the issues that should determine dosage in the child with GHD are (1) how best to return the GHD child to the normal growth curve; (2) how best to ensure that the child attains his or her genetic height potential; (3) risks; and (4) cost. For the child with severe GHD, weekly dosages of 0.175 mg/kg, administered in seven daily doses, either by a subcutaneous or an intramuscular route, are usually sufficient to increase growth rates from 3 to 4 cm/year to more than 10 cm/year.

Frequency of Administration
Several studies have compared the short-term effects of administering HGH either daily or thrice weekly.[200,201] Generally, daily injections are more effective, but increasing the frequency more than this makes little difference.[202] Sustained-release r-hGH preparations, which may be administered as infrequently as every 2 to 4 weeks[203] are unlikely to be effective and have potentially greater side effects because of the pulsatile nature of GH physiology.

Prediction Models
A series of models have been derived[8,204] that describe factors that might influence response but none has gone on to test these in formal randomized control trials. It has been reported that in children with GHD, auxologic parameters, such as chronologic age (the younger the patient, the better the response), and the difference between target height and actual height (the smaller the patient, the better the response) are better predictors of growth response than the cumulative weekly GH dosage. Several problems are found with these types of models:

1. Although prediction models are useful to give an average effect, they are not individualizable.
2. They often only focus on one outcome, usually short-term growth, whereas interest may be more centered on final height. The two need not necessarily be related, and the factors that influence response in the first year

of treatment may differ totally from those that lead to prediction of the individual's final height.
3. Very few prediction models have been constructed from an a priori hypothesis, and care must be taken that no interference has occurred from other factors accompanying the disease that might affect prognosis. The problem is that importance can be ascribed to factors that are merely "markers" for other factors of real importance. Examples of this can be seen in models that demonstrate that individuals who are extremely short, growing very poorly, and whose heights are subsequently further away from their genetic height respond best to treatment. All these factors are simply a marker of "how bad the disease is" and could perhaps be more easily summarized by a similar single factor that actually describes the severity of the condition.
4. Specific issues associated with growth-response models are summarized in Table 37-10.
   a) The first problem relates to the method by which response to GH is defined. In several studies, acceleration in growth rate or the difference between the pretreatment growth rate and that observed during the year of treatment is used. Using either, however, leads potentially to the generation of artefact. This is because if difference (e.g., change in height velocity) is plotted against pretreatment states (e.g., pretreatment height velocity), then a good relation will always be demonstrated, purely and simply because pretreatment height velocity is contributing to both variables.[205,206] Examination of the association between change in a variable, and its initial value is complicated. It is possible, for example, if high values are recorded at one stage, and the same measure is performed at a later date, low values may be recorded even in the absence of treatment. This effect, "regression to the mean," will be most marked in those with highest or lowest initial recorded values and will induce a spurious association between change and initial value. Several methods are available to overcome this problem.[207,208]
   b) The prediction gives the average effect, and the confidence interval of the response is smallest at the average value of the independent variable. The difficulty comes in applying this information to the individual. Simply stating the average expected improvement is not much help. To convey this information, consideration must be given to the patient's perception of what the treatment can do. If the patient wishes a growth response that will put him or her into the upper half of the normal height distribution, then disappointment might ensue. It is far better to provide the individual with an understanding of the chance of a successful outcome, and the concept "Number Needed to Treat" is useful.[209]
   c) If the treatment effect varies among individuals with the same true initial height value, then spurious trends may emerge in the overall model prediction. Even though it is clear that most treatments will not affect all individuals equally, this is not well

Table 37-10 Specific Issues with Prediction Models of Response to Growth Hormone Treatment Development

1. Regression to the mean
2. Prediction gives average effect. How to apply to individuals for prognosis
3. Predictors may not be independent of each other. Assumptions made in linear and multiple regression modeling
4. Assumptions about uniformity of response
5. Spurious correlations involving time

understood. Whether a child with GHD with a tall or a short parent will have a better or worse response than a child with average-height parents is difficult to determine, as at present no easy markers of GH sensitivity are available.

d) Inherent problems exist with making predictions from previous data (e.g., how does year 1 influence year 2) or from the original data set. If we are looking at serial effects on height, it is important to recognize that the data going into such analyses are highly correlated. A person that is taller than average after 1 year also will tend to be taller than average after 2 years of follow-up. It is important to realize that any two quantities changing over time will show a statistical association. Methods are available to assist in this area, but of necessity, the time component must be removed.[210]

Height Outcomes and the Influence of Puberty

Early initiation of therapy, combined with careful attention to dosage adjustments and compliance, is the best predictor of cumulative growth response in patients with GHD. Final height correlates with height at the initiation of puberty, so it is important to maximize growth during the prepubertal period, within the limits of safety and economy.[211–220] Analysis of data on final heights of r-hGH-treated GHD is complicated by the heterogeneity of patient groups and dosage, but the most common observation is a general failure of children to reach their full genetic height potential, especially in the case of IGHD, and particularly in female patients. Price and Ranke[221] reported final heights of −1.26 SD and −1.45 SD from the mean in boys and girls, respectively, with IGHD, and −0.22 SD and −0.52 SD from the mean in boys and girls, respectively, with CPHD. In patients with longer durations of treatment and higher dosages of r-hGH, adult heights tended to be greater, although still failing to achieve full genetic height potential.

It is clear that the timing of puberty has a significant impact on adult height of the r-hGH-treated GHD child.[219,220,222,223] The duration of r-hGH treatment and the height gained prepubertally are, typically, greater when puberty is induced rather than spontaneous. In the study by Ranke and colleagues,[222] final height was attained at 17.8 and 19.2 years in boys and at 16.0 and 17.0 years in girls after spontaneous and induced puberty, respectively. Final heights were greater after induced puberty compared with spontaneous puberty in boys (171.3 vs. 166.0 cm) and in girls (157.0 vs. 155.0 cm). Therapy designed to delay the onset of puberty (both normal and precocious) may augment the cumulative growth response to r-hGH.

Burns and colleagues[219] reported that final height in GHD patients who enter puberty spontaneously is less than in patients in whom puberty must be induced because of gonadotropin deficiency. Final height gain can be particularly variable in children who have had treatment for malignancies. The GHD is often complicated by skeletal damage after traumatic brain injury (TBI) or craniospinal irradiation, early puberty, hypothyroidism, gonadotropin deficiency, malnutrition, and concomitant chemotherapy. Gonadotropin-releasing hormone analogue (GnRHa) therapy to arrest early puberty has been used in conjunction with GH treatment in this group of patients, with encouraging results.[224] The use of the GnRHa reduces the concentration of sex steroid, with a consequent delay in epiphyseal fusion. However, the use of GH and GnRHa combination therapy in children with GHD[225] is not widely used at present. It may be beneficial under certain circumstances, for example, where the diagnosis of GHD has been delayed. The effects of GnRHa in the long term are unknown, and, additionally, the cost of this combination therapy would have to be weighed against the benefits.

Although considerable attention has been paid to growth, it is important to realize that GH treatment in childhood also can normalize body composition, with a reduction in body fat, although effects on lean body mass are less evident. It also is associated with reversible insulin insensitivity and an increase in the ratio of high-density lipoprotein (HDL) to total cholesterol. Glomerular filtration rate (GFR) is increased, and bone remodeling accelerated, with a marked increase in bone mineral mass.[226]

Adverse Effects of Human Growth Hormone

r-hGH has had an excellent safety record.[227,228] Reports of anti-GH antibodies in patients receiving r-hGH have been few, with no untoward effect on the growth response. Fluid retention and carpal tunnel syndrome are observed in adults but are seldom significant in children. Whereas the incidence of type 1 diabetes mellitus is not higher in patients with idiopathic GHD than in the general population, the incidence of type 2 diabetes mellitus is greater in those patients treated with GH, although this tends to be in those predisposed to developing this condition.[229] Idiopathic intracranial hypertension (pseudotumor cerebri) has been observed occasionally but resolves with cessation of treatment and then a gradual reintroduction of r-hGH, but commencing at a lower dose.[228] Slipped capital femoral epiphysis has been reported, but it is not clear that the incidence is greater than that observed in normal children during rapid periods of growth. Other possible rare and still unproven complications include acute pancreatitis, increased growth of pigmented nevi, and prepubertal gynecomastia.

The most important theoretical risk with r-hGH therapy has been malignancy.[227,228,230–236] Epidemiologic assessment has been complicated by the fact that many r-hGH recipients are at increased risk of malignancy because of chromosomal abnormalities, prior malignancies, or prior histories of chemotherapy or irradiation. Additionally, it has been suggested that, in some cases, GH deficiency itself may predispose to development of malignancy.[228] Although a number of early reports suggested a link between HGH treatment and leukemia, Blethen and colleagues[227] reported that an analysis of 47,000 patient-years of treatment in more than 19,000 children indicated that in children without known risk factors, r-hGH therapy was not associated with an increased occurrence of tumors or recurrence rate of leukemia or CNS tumors. Despite these assurances, it is customary to delay r-hGH treatment in children with treated brain tumors until they have been shown to be tumor free for at least 1 to 2 years.

More recently, the long-term follow-up of these patients has revealed a higher than expected incidence and mortality of colonic cancer and Hodgkin's disease.[237] However, these data must be put in context. The affected patients had been treated with high GH doses given 2 to 3 times/week. Hence, one could speculate that the IGF-1 concentrations generated by this mode of GH therapy may be excessive. IGF-1 concentrations at the upper end of the normal range (top quartile for colon and prostate, and top tertile for breast) have been associated with colon, breast, and prostatic cancer.[238–242] Because lower doses of GH are given on a daily basis, it would be incorrect, at this stage at least, to extrapolate the data from the earlier studies to the present treatment regimens.

End Points of Therapy

Given the discussion outlined earlier in terms of efficacy, safety, and clinical governance, Table 37-11 illustrates some suggested outcomes that can be monitored and used as a basis of short- and long-term audit, as well as safety monitoring.

GROWTH HORMONE–RELEASING HORMONE

In children whose GHD is due to a hypothalamic abnormality, treatment with GHRH would appear to be an appropriate therapeutic option.[243–245] Both GHRH (1-44) and (1-29) are biologically active in humans. Unfortunately, although it can

Table 37-11   Short-, Medium-, and Long-term End Points of Growth Hormone Therapy in GHD Children

	End Point	Rationale	Measure
Short term	1. Growth acceleration	1. Assess response	1. Minimum response of >2 cm/yr
	2. Reduction in adipose mass	2. Assess response	2. Skinfold thickness
	3. Correct dose	3. Optimize therapy	3. IGF-1 and growth
	4. Vision and headaches	4. Increased intracranial pressure	4. Fundoscopy
	5. Assessment of limp	5. Slipped femoral epiphysis	5. X-ray
Medium term	1. Bone maturation	1. Rate of skeletal maturation	1. Yearly bone age
	2. Pubertal status	2. Early puberty or rapid progression	2. 6-month Tanner staging
	3. Correct dose	3. Optimize therapy	3. IGF-1 and growth response. Return to target height within 6 years of therapy
	4. Thyroid status	4. Altered status or evolving endocrinopathy	4. Yearly thyroid function tests
	5. Other hormones	5. Evolving endocrinopathy	5. Gonadotroph and corticotroph function
	6. Metabolic status	6. Insulin insensitivity	6. Fasting glucose and insulin
Long term	1. Growth	1. Outcome	1. Final height within target height of parents
	2. Bone mineralization	2. GH effect on bone	2. DEXA scan
	3. Malignancy risk	3. ? GH cancer link	3. Cancer registry
	4. Cardiovascular risk	4. Hyperinsulinism or GH effect (? long-term GHD)	4. Fasting glucose and insulin, blood pressure, fasting lipids

GHD, growth hormone deficiency; DEXA, dual-energy x-ray absorptiometry; IGF, insulin-like growth factor.

be absorbed nasally, this route of administration has not proved to be effective,[246] and treatment must be via subcutaneous or intramuscular injection, as is the case with r-hGH. Direct comparisons of r-hGH and GHRH have not been performed, but a number of studies indicate that GHRH, administered once or twice daily, can increase the growth rates of children with GHD. No specific therapeutic advantage of GHRH over r-hGH has been demonstrated to date, although further studies are warranted to investigate optimization of dosage and frequency of administration.

GROWTH HORMONE–RELEASING PEPTIDES AND NONPEPTIDYL GROWTH HORMONE SECRETAGOGUES

Since the discovery of growth hormone–releasing peptides (GHRPs) by Bowers and coworkers in the 1980s,[14] a variety of small GHRPs and nonpeptidyl small-molecule GH secretagogues have been manufactured.[247] These molecules are potent stimulators of GH release, especially when administered together with GHRH, and may be active when administered by intravenous, intramuscular, subcutaneous, nasal, and oral routes. These potential advantages must be balanced by the likelihood that normal GHRH production is required to see maximal benefit from such agents.[248,249] Clinical trials have proven disappointing, however.

TRANSITION TO ADULT CARE

It has been suggested that, at the end of statural growth, GH secretion should be reassessed in all patients after a washout period of at least 1 to 3 months.[250–252] The investigation of choice is an insulin tolerance test (ITT),[253] although the arginine + GHRH test has recently been proposed as a safer alternative, particularly in patients who have a contraindication to an ITT.[254] In between 25% and 75% of patients, the GH response to provocation is in the normal range, as would be expected from the earlier discussion on testing, and probability theory should be used to determine whether therapy should be continued.[255] In the remainder, continuation of GH therapy should be considered in those with a peak GH less than 3 µg/L, who can be described as having severe GHD. Patients with a peak GH between 3 and 7 µg/L have moderate GHD and should be followed up by an adult endocrinologist. In these individuals, adverse changes in body composition, quality of life, and bone mineral density may be an indication to recommence GH treatment,[256] although it is less likely that these individuals will develop adult GHD syndrome.[255] In those patients with multiple pituitary hormone deficiency, GHD due to a congenital lesion and GHD secondary to radiotherapy, surgery, or a mass lesion, the GHD is highly unlikely to reverse.[257]

REFERENCES

1. Karlberg J: On the modelling of human growth. Stat Med 6:185–192, 1987.
2. Hindmarsh PC, Smith PJ, Brook CGD, Matthews DR: The relationship between growth velocity and growth hormone secretion in short prepubertal children. Clin Endocrinol 27:581–591, 1987.
3. Rosenfeld RG: Disorders of growth hormone/IGF secretion and action. In Sperling M (ed): Pediatric Endocrinology. Philadelphia, WB Saunders, 1996, pp 117–169.
4. White P: Diabetes in Childhood and Adolescence. Philadelphia, Lea & Febiger, 1932.
5. Raben MS: Treatment of a pituitary dwarf with human growth hormone. J Clin Endocrinol Metab 18:901–903, 1958.
6. Soyka ZF, Ziskind A, Crawford JD: Treatment of short stature in children and adolescents with human pituitary growth hormone (Raben): Experience with 35 cases. N Engl J Med 271:754–764, 1964.
7. Prader A, Zachmann M, Poley JR, et al: Long term treatment with human growth hormone (Raben) in small doses: Evaluation of 18 hypopituitary patients. Helv Paediatr Acta 22:423–439, 1967.
8. Tanner JM, Whitehouse RH, Hughes PCR, Vince FP: Effect of human growth hormone treatment for 1 to 7 years on growth of 100 children with growth hormone deficiency, low birth weight, inherited smallness, Turner syndrome and other complaints. Arch Dis Child 45:745–779, 1971.
9. Aceto T, Frasier SD, Hayles AB, et al: Collaborative study of the effects of human growth hormone in growth hormone deficiency, 1.:First year of therapy. J Clin Endocrinol Metab 35:483–496, 1972.
10. Hunter WM, Greenwood FC: Preparation of iodine-131 labelled human growth hormone of high specific activity. Nature 194:495–496, 1962.
11. Brazeau P, Vale W, Burgus R, et al: Hypothalamic polypeptide that inhibits the secretion of immunoreactive pituitary growth hormone. Science 178:77–79, 1973.
12. Guillemin R, Brazeau P, Bohien P, et al: Growth hormone releasing factor from a human pancreatic tumour that caused acromegaly. Science 218:585–587, 1982.

13. Rivier J, Spiess J, Thorner MO, Vale W: Characterisation of a growth hormone-releasing factor from a human pancreatic islet tumour. Nature 300:276–278, 1982.

14. Bowers CY, Momany F, Reynolds GA, et al: Structure-activity relationships of a synthetic pentapeptide that specifically releases growth hormone in vitro. Endocrinology 106:663–667, 1980.

15. Salmon WD, Daughaday WH: A hormonally controlled serum factor which stimulates sulphate incorporation by cartilage in vivo. J Lab Clin Med 49:825–836, 1957.

16. Zezulak KM, Green H: The generation of insulin-like growth factor 1 sensitive cells by growth hormone action. Science 233:551–553, 1986.

17. Isgaard J, Nilsson A, Lindahl A, et al: Effects of local administration of GH and IGF-1 on longitudinal bone growth in rats. Am J Physiol 250:E367–E372, 1986.

18. Parkin JM: Incidence of growth hormone deficiency. Arch Dis Child 49:904–905, 1974.

19. Vimpani GV, Vimpani AF, Lidgard GP, et al: Prevalence of severe growth hormone deficiency. Br Med J 2:427–430, 1977.

20. Lindsay R, Feldkamp M, Harris D, et al: Utah Growth Study: Growth standards and the prevalence of growth hormone deficiency. J Pediatr 125:29–35, 1994.

21. Wilton P: Progress in Growth Hormone Therapy: 5 Years of KIGS. Mannheim, Germany, JJ Verlag, 1994, pp 62–66.

22. Genentech National Cooperative Growth Study Summary Report 18. San Francisco, Genentech, 1994, pp 6–13.

23. Dasen JS, Rosenfeld MG: Signaling and transcriptional mechanisms in pituitary development. Annu Rev Neurosci 24:327–355, 2000.

24. Takuma N, Sheng HZ, Furuta Y, et al. Formation of Rathke's pouch requires dual induction from the diencephalon. Development 125:4835–4840, 1998.

25. Ericson J, Norlin S, Jessell TM, Edlund T: Integrated FGF and BMP signaling controls the progression of progenitor cell differentiation and the emergence of pattern in the embryonic anterior pituitary. Development 125:1005–1015, 1998.

26. Lazzaro D, Price M, De Felice M, Di Lauro R: The transcription factor TTF-1 is expressed at the onset of thyroid and lung morphogenesis and in restricted regions of the foetal brain. Development 113:1093–1104, 1991.

27. Sheng HZ, Moriyama K, Yamashita T, et al: Multistep control of pituitary organogenesis. Science 278:1809–1812, 1997.

28. Treier M, Gleiberman AS, O'Connell SM, et al: Multistep signaling requirements for pituitary organogenesis in vivo. Genes Dev 12:1691–1704, 1998.

29. Rosenfeld MG, Briata P, Dasen J, et al: Multistep signaling and transcriptional requirements for pituitary organogenesis in vivo. Recent Prog Horm Res 55:1–13, 2000.

30. Sheng HZ, Westphal H: Early steps in pituitary organogenesis. Trends Genet 15:236–40, 1999.

31. Simmons DM, Voss JW, Ingraham HA, et al: Pituitary cell phenotypes involve cell-specific Pit-1 mRNA translation and synergistic interactions with other classes of transcription factors. Genes Dev 4:695–711, 1990.

32. Japon MA, Rubinstein M, Low MJ: In situ hybridization analysis of anterior pituitary hormone gene expression during fetal mouse development. J Histochem Cytochem 42:1117–1125, 1994.

33. Li S, Crenshaw EB III, Rawson EJ, et al: Dwarf locus mutants lacking three pituitary cell types result from mutations in the POU-domain gene pit-1. Nature 347:528–533, 1990.

34. Ingraham HA, Lala DS, Ikeda Y, et al: The nuclear receptor steroidogenic factor 1 acts at multiple levels of the reproductive axis. Genes Dev 8:2302–2312, 1994.

35. Dattani MT, Robinson ICAF: The molecular basis for developmental disorders of the pituitary gland in man. Clin Genet 57:337–346, 2000.

36. Cohen LE, Wondisford FE, Salvatoni A, et al: A "hot spot" in the Pit-1 gene responsible for combined pituitary hormone deficiency: Clinical and molecular correlates. J Clin Endocrinol Metab 80:679–684, 1995.

37. Cohen LE, Radovick S: Molecular basis of combined pituitary hormone deficiencies. Endocr Rev 23:431–442, 2002.

38. Dattani MT, Martinez-Barbera JP, Thomas PQ, et al: Mutations in the homeobox gene HESX1/Hesx1 associated with septo-optic dysplasia in human and mouse. Nat Genet 19:125–133, 1998.

39. Thomas PQ, Dattani MT, Brickman JM, et al: Heterozygous HESX1 mutations associated with isolated congenital pituitary hypoplasia and septo-optic dysplasia. Hum Mol Genet 10:39–45, 2001.

40. Brickman JM, Clements M, Tyrell R, et al: Molecular effects of novel mutations in Hesx1/HESX1 associated with human pituitary disorders. Development 128:5189–5199, 2001.

41. Netchine I, Sobrier ML, Krude H, et al: Mutations in LHX3 result in a new syndrome revealed by combined pituitary hormone deficiency. Nat Genet 25:182–186, 2001.

42. Machinis K, Pantel J, Netchine I, et al: Syndromic short stature in patients with a germline mutation in the LIM homeobox LHX4. Am J Hum Genet 69:961–968, 2001.

43. Laumonnier F, Ronce N, Hamel BC, et al: Transcription factor SOX3 is involved in X-linked mental retardation with growth hormone deficiency. Am J Hum Genet 71:1450–1455, 2002.

44. Wajnrajch MP, Gertner JM, Harbison MD, et al: Nonsense mutations of the human growth hormone releasing hormone receptor (GHRHR) causes growth failure analogous to that of the little (lit) mouse. Nat Genet 12:88–90, 1996.

45. Baumann G, Maheshwari H: Severe growth hormone (GH) deficiency caused by a mutation in the GH-releasing hormone receptor gene. Acta Paediatr Suppl 423:33–38, 1997.

46. Salvatori R, Hagashida CY, Aguiar-Olivera MH, et al: Familial dwarfism due to a novel mutation of the growth hormone-releasing hormone receptor gene. J Clin Endocrinol Metab 84:917–923, 1999.

47. Godfrey P, Rahal JO, Beamer WG, et al: GHRH receptor of little mouse contains missense mutation in the extracellular domain that disrupts receptor function. Nat Genet 4:227–232, 1993.

48. Sornson MW, Wu W, Daser JS, et al: Pituitary lineage determination by the Prophet of Pit-1 homeodomain factor defective in Ames dwarfism. Nature 384:327–333, 1996.

49. Wu W, Cogan JD, Pfaffle RW, et al: Mutations in PROP1 cause familial combined pituitary hormone deficiency. Nat Genet 18:147–149, 1998.

50. Deladoey J, Fluck C, Buyukgebiz A, et al: "Hot spot" in the PROP1 gene responsible for combined pituitary hormone deficiency. J Clin Endocrinol Metab 84:1645–1650, 1999.

51. Pernasetti F, Toledo SP, Vasilyev VV, et al: Impaired adrenocorticotropin-adrenal axis in combined pituitary hormone deficiency caused by a two-base pair deletion (301-302delAG) in the prophet of Pit-1 gene. J Clin Endocrinol Metab 85:390–397, 2000.

52. Mendonca BB, Osorio MG, Latronico AC, et al: Longitudinal hormonal and pituitary imaging changes in two females with combined pituitary hormone deficiency due to deletion of A301,G302 in the PROP1 gene. J Clin Endocrinol Metab 84:942–945, 1999.

53. Bodner M, Castrillo J-L, Theill LE, et al: The pituitary-specific transcription factor GHF-1 is a homeobox-containing protein. Cell 55:505–518, 1988.

54. Mangalam HJ, Albert VR, Ingraham HA, et al: A pituitary POU domain protein, pit-1, activates both growth hormone and prolactin promoters transcriptionally. Genes Dev 3:946–958, 1989.

55. Li S, Crenshaw EB, Rawson EJ, et al: Dwarf locus mutants lacking three pituitary cell types result from mutations in the POU-domain gene. Nature 347:528–533, 1990.

56. Tatsumi K, Miyai K, Notomi T, et al: Cretinism with combined hormone deficiency caused by a mutation in the PIT1 gene. Nat Genet 1:56–58, 1992.

57. Radovick S, Nations M, Du Y, et al: A mutation in the POV-homeodomain of Pit-1 responsible for combined pituitary hormone deficiency. Science 257:1115–1118, 1992.

58. Pfaffle R, Kim C, Otten B, et al: Pit-1: Clinical aspects. Horm Res 45(Suppl 1):25–28, 1996.

59. Pernasetti F, Milner RDG, Al Ashwal AAL, et al: Pro239Ser: A novel recessive mutation of the *Pit-1* gene in seven Middle Eastern children with growth hormone, prolactin, and thyrotropin deficiency. J Clin Endocrinol Metab 83:2079–2083, 1998.

60. Procter A, Phillips JA III, Cogan J: The molecular genetics of growth hormone deficiency. Hum Genet 103:255–272, 1998.

61. Wagner JK, Eble A, Hindmarsh PC, et al: Prevalence of human GH-1 gene alterations in patients with isolated growth hormone deficiency. Pediatr Res 43:105–110, 1998.

62. Illig R, Prader A, Ferrandez A, et al: Hereditary prenatal growth hormone deficiency with increased tendency to growth hormone antibody formation ("A-type" of isolated growth hormone deficiency). Acta Paediatr Scand 60:607, 1971.

63. Phillips JA III, Cogan J: Genetic basis of endocrine disease, 6: Molecular basis of familial human growth hormone deficiency. J Clin Endocrinol Metab 78:11–16, 1994.

64. Binder G, Ranke M: Screening for growth hormone (GH) gene splice-site mutations in sporadic cases with severe isolated GH deficiency using ectopic transcript analysis. J Clin Endocrinol Metab 80:1247–1252, 1995.

65. Moseley C, Mullis P, Prince M, Phillips JA III: An exon splice enhancer mutation causes autosomal dominant GH deficiency. J Clin Endocrinol Metab 87:847–852, 2002.

66. McGuiness L, Magoulas C, Mathers K, et al: Autosomal dominant growth hormone deficiency disrupts secretory vesicles: In vitro and in vivo studies in transgenic mice. Endocrinology 144:720–731, 2003.

67. Ryther RCC, McGuiness LM, Phillips JA III, et al: Disruption of exon definition produces a dominant-negative growth hormone isoform that causes somatotroph death and IGHD II. Hum Genet 113:140–148, 2003.

68. Valenta LJ, Sigtel MB, Lesniak MA, et al: Pituitary dwarfism in a patient with circulating abnormal growth hormone polymers. N Engl J Med 312:214–217, 1985.

69. Kowarski AA, Schneider J, Ben-Galim E, et al: Growth failure with normal serum RIA-GH and low somatomedin activity: Somatomedin restoration and growth acceleration after exogenous GH. J Clin Endocrinol Metab 47:461–464, 1978.

70. Takahashi Y, Kaji H, Okimura Y, et al: Short stature caused by a mutant growth hormone. N Engl J Med 334:432–436, 1996.

71. Takahashi Y, Shirono H, Arisaka O, et al: Biologically inactive growth hormone caused by an amino acid substitution. J Clin Invest 100:1159–1165, 1997.

72. Fujisawa I, Kikuchi K, Nishimura K, et al: Transection of the pituitary stalk: Development of an ectopic posterior lobe assessed with MR imaging. Radiology 165:487–489, 1987.

73. Abrahams JJ, Trefelner E, Boulware SD: Idiopathic growth hormone deficiency MR findings in 35 patients. Am J Neuroradiol 12:155–160, 1991.

74. Kuroiwa T, Okabe Y, Hasuo K, et al: MR imaging of pituitary dwarfism. Am J Neuroradiol 12:161–164, 1991.

75. Cacciari E, Zucchini S, Carla G, et al: Endocrine function and morphological findings in patients with disorders of the hypothalamo-pitutitary area: A study with magnetic resonance. Arch Dis Child 65:1199–1202, 1990.

76. Maghnie M, Larizza D, Triulzi F, et al. Hypopituitarism and stalk agenesis: A congenital syndrome worsened by breech delivery? Horm Res 35:104–108, 1991.

77. Brown RS, Bhatia V, Hayes E: An apparent cluster of congenital hypopituitarism in central Massachusetts: Magnetic resonance imaging and hormonal studies. J Clin Endocrinol Metab 72:12–18, 1991.

78. Root AW, Martinez CR: Magnetic resonance imaging in patients with hypopituitarism. Trends Endocrinol Metab 3:283–287, 1992.

79. Argyopoulou M, Perignon F, Brauner R, et al: Magnetic resonance imaging in the diagnosis of growth hormone deficiency. J Pediatr 120:886–891, 1992.

80. Triulzi F, Scotti G, diNatale B, et al: Evidence of a congenital midline brain anomaly in pituitary dwarfs: A magnetic resonance imaging study in 101 patients. Pediatrics 93:409–416, 1994.

81. Wilkinson IA, Duck SC, Gager WE, et al: Empty sella syndrome: Occurrence in childhood. Am J Dis Child 136:245–248, 1992.

82. Albertsson-Wikland K, Niklasson A, Karlberg P: Birth data for patients who later develop growth hormone deficiency: Preliminary analysis of a national register. Acta Paediatr Suppl 370:115–120, 1990.

83. Craft WH, Underwood LE, Van Wyk JJ: High incidence of perinatal insult in children with idiopathic hypopituitarism. J Pediatr 96:397–402, 1980.

84. DeVile CJ, Grant DB, Hayward RD, Stanhope R: Growth and endocrine sequelae of craniopharyngioma. Arch Dis Child 75:108–114, 1996.

85. Tiulpakov AN, Mazerkina NA, Brook CG, et al: Growth in children with craniopharyngioma following surgery. Clin Endocrinol (Oxf) 49:733–738, 1998.

86. Nanduri VR, Bareille P, Pritchard J, Stanhope R: Growth and endocrine disorders in multisystem Langerhans' cell histiocytosis. Clin Endocrinol (Oxf) 53:509–515, 2000.

87. Ogilvy-Stuart AL, Clark DJ, Wallace WH, et al: Endocrine deficit after fractionated total body irradiation. Arch Dis Child 67:1107–1110, 1992.

88. Clayton PE, Shalet SM: Dose dependency of time of onset of radiation-induced growth hormone deficiency. J Pediatr 118:226–228, 1991.

89. Rappaport R, Brauner R: Growth and endocrine disorders secondary to cranial irradiation. Pediatr Res 25:561–567, 1989.

90. Sklar C, Mertens A, Walter A, et al: Final height after treatment for childhood acute lymphoblastic leukemia: Comparison of no cranial irradiation with 1800 and 2400 centigrays of cranial irradiation. J Pediatr 123:56–64, 1993.

91. Balthasar N, Mery PF, Magoulas CB, et al: Growth hormone-releasing hormone (GHRH) neurons in GHRH-enhanced green fluorescent protein transgenic mice: A ventral hypothalamic network. Endocrinology 144:2728–2740, 2003.

92. Blatt J, Bercu BB, Gillin JC, et al: Reduced pulsatile growth hormone secretion in children after therapy for acute lymphoblastic leukemia. J Pediatr 104:182–186, 1984.

93. Sklar CA, Sarafoglou K, Whittam E: Effects of insulin-like growth factor binding protein 3 in predicting the growth hormone response to provocative testing in children treated with cranial irradiation. Acta Endocrinol 129:511–515, 1993.

94. Nivot S, Benelli C, Clot JP, et al: Nonparallel changes of growth hormone (GH) and insulin-like growth factor binding protein-3, and GH-binding protein, after craniospinal irradiation and chemotherapy. J Clin Endocrinol Metab 78:597–601, 1995.

95. Leiper AD, Stanhope R, Kitching P, et al: Precocious and premature puberty associated with treatment of acute lymphoblastic leukemia. Arch Dis Child 72:1107–1112, 1992.

96. Ogilvy-Stuart AL, Shalet SM: Growth and puberty after growth hormone treatment after irradiation for brain tumors. Arch Dis Child 73:141–146, 1995.

97. Quigley C, Cowell C, Jimenez M, et al: Normal or early development of puberty despite gonadal damage in children treated for acute lymphoblastic leukemia. N Engl J Med 321:143–151, 1989.

98. Bartsocas CS, Pantelakis SN: Human growth hormone therapy in hypopituitarism due to tuberculous meningitis. Acta Paediatr Scand 62:304–306, 1973.

99. Stuart CA, Neelon FA, Lebovitz HE: Hypothalamic insufficiency: The cause of hypopituitarism in sarcoidosis. Ann Intern Med 88:589–594, 1978.

100. Powell GF, Brasel JA, Blizzard RM: Emotional deprivation and growth retardation simulating idiopathic hypopituitarism. N Engl J Med 276:1271–1278, 1967.

101. Stanhope R, Adlard P, Hamill G, et al: Physiological growth hormone (GH) secretion during the recovery from psychosocial dwarfism: A case report.

Clin Endocrinol (Oxf) 28:335–339, 1988.

102. Skuse D, Albanese A, Stanhope R: A new stress-related syndrome of growth failure and hyperphagia in children, associated with reversibility of growth-hormone insufficiency. Lancet 348:353–358, 1996.

103. Albanese A, Hamill G, Jones J, et al: Reversibility of physiological growth hormone secretion in children with psychosocial dwarfism. Clin Endocrinol 40:687–692, 1994.

104. Gluckman PD: Maturation of hypothalamic-pituitary function in the ovine fetus and neonate. Ciba Found Symp 86:5–42, 1981.

105. Hindmarsh PC, Matthews DR, Brook CGD: Growth hormone secretion in children determined by time series analysis. Clin Endocrinol (Oxf) 29:35–44, 1988.

106. Jaffe CA, Ocampo-Lim B, Guo W, et al: Regulatory mechanisms of growth hormone secretion are sexually dimorphic. J Clin Invest 102:153–164, 1998.

107. Papotti M, Ghe C, Cassoni P, et al: Growth hormone secretagogue binding sites in peripheral human tissues. J Clin Endocrinol Metab 85:3803–3807, 2000.

108. Muccioli G, Broglio F, Valetto MR, et al: Growth hormone-releasing peptides and the cardiovascular system. Ann Endocrinol (Paris) 61:27–31, 2000.

109. Gnanapavan S, Kola B, Bustin SA, et al: The tissue distribution of the mRNA of ghrelin and subtypes of its receptor, GHS-R, in humans. J Clin Endocrinol Metab 87:2988, 2002.

110. Kojima M, Hosoda H, Date Y, et al: Ghrelin is a growth-hormone-releasing acylated peptide from stomach. Nature 402:656–660, 1999.

111. Date Y, Kojima M, Hosoda H, et al: Ghrelin, a novel growth hormone-releasing acylated peptide, is synthesized in a distinct endocrine cell type in the gastrointestinal tracts of rats and humans. Endocrinology 141:4255–4261, 2000.

112. Smith RG, Palyha OC, Feighner SD, et al: Growth hormone releasing substances: Types and their receptors. Horm Res 51(Suppl 3):1–8, 1999.

113. Bennani-Baiti IM, Asa SL, Song D, et al: DNase I-hypersensitive sites I and II of the human growth hormone locus control region are a major developmental activator of somatotrope gene expression. Proc Natl Acad Sci U S A 95:10655–10660, 1998.

114. Shewchuk BM, Asa SL, Cooke NE, Liebhaber SA: Pit-1 binding sites at the somatotrope-specific DNase I hypersensitive sites I, II of the human growth hormone locus control region are essential for in vivo hGH-N gene activation. J Biol Chem 274:35725–35733, 1999.

115. Baumann G: Growth hormone heterogeneity: Genes, isohormones, variants, and binding proteins. Endocr Rev 12:424–449, 1991.

116. Baumann G: Genetic characterization of growth hormone deficiency and resistance: Implications for treatment with recombinant growth hormone. Am J Pharmacogenomics 2:93–111, 2002.

117. Clark RG, Mortensen DL, Carlsson LM, et al: Recombinant human growth hormone (GH)-binding protein enhances the growth-promoting activity of human GH in the rat. Endocrinology 137:4308–4315, 1990.

118. Carter-Su C, Schwartz J, Smit LS: Molecular mechanism of growth hormone action. Annu Rev Physiol 58:187–207, 1996.

119. Smit LS, Meyer DJ, Billestrup N, et al: The role of the growth hormone (GH) receptor and JAK1 and JAK2 kinases in the activation of Stats 1, 3, and 5 by GH. Mol Endocrinol 10:519–533, 1996.

120. Rosenfeld RG: An endocrinologist's approach to the growth hormone–insulin-like growth factor axis. Acta Paediatr Suppl 423:17–19, 1997.

121. Rosenfeld RG, Rosenbloom AL, Guevara-Aguirre J: Growth hormone (GH) insensitivity due to primary GH receptor deficiency. Endocr Rev 15:369–390, 1994.

122. Rosenfeld RG, Rosenbloom AL, Guevara-Aguirre J: Abnormalities of growth hormone action. In Kelnar CJH, Savage MO, Stirling HF, et al (eds): Growth Disorders. Pathophysiology and Treatment. London, Chapman & Hall, 1998, pp 549–564.

123. Woods KA, Dastot F, Preece MA, et al: Phenotype:genotype relationships in growth hormone insensitivity syndrome. J Clin Endocrinol Metab 82:3529–3535, 1997.

124. Rygaard K, Revol A, Esquivel-Escobedo D, et al: Absence of human placental lactogen and placental growth hormone (hGH-V) during pregnancy: PCR analysis of the deletion. Hum Genet 102:87–92, 1998.

125. DeChiara TM, Efstratiadis A, Robertson EJ: A growth-deficiency phenotype in heterozygous mice carrying an insulin-like growth factor II gene disrupted by targeting. Nature 345:78–80, 1990.

126. Woods KA, Camacho-Hubner C, Savage MD, Clark AJ: Intrauterine growth retardation and postnatal growth failure associated with deletion of the insulin-like growth factor I gene. N Engl J Med 335:1363–1367, 1996.

127. Hussain K, Aynsley-Green A: Management of hyperinsulinism in infancy and childhood. Ann Med 32:544–551, 2000.

128. Goossens M, Brauner R, Czernichow P, et al: Isolated growth hormone deficiency type 1A associated with a double deletion in the human growth hormone gene cluster. J Clin Endocrinol Metab 62:712–716, 1986.

129. Wit JM, Van Unen H: Growth of infants with neonatal growth hormone deficiency. Arch Dis Child 67:920–924, 1982.

130. Herber SM, Milner RDG: Growth hormone deficiency presenting under age 2 years. Arch Dis Child 59:557–560, 1984.

131. Gluckman PD, Gunn A-J, Wray A: Congenital idiopathic growth hormone deficiency associated with early postnatal growth failure. J Pediatr 121:920–923, 1992.

132. Wit JM, Kamp G, Rikken B: Spontaneous growth and response to growth hormone treatment in children with growth hormone deficiency and idiopathic short stature. Pediatr Res 39:295–302, 1996.

133. Rimoin DL, Merimee TJ, Rabinowitz D, et al: Genetic aspects of clinical endocrinology. Recent Prog Horm Res 24:365–437, 1968.

134. Ranke MB: A note on adults with growth hormone deficiency. Acta Paediatr Suppl 331:80–82, 1987.

135. van der Werff ten Bosch JJ, Bot A: Growth of males with idiopathic hypopituitarism without growth hormone treatment. Clin Endocrinol (Oxf) 32:707–717, 1990.

136. Milner RDG, Russell-Fraser T, Brook CGD, et al: Experience with human growth hormone in Great Britain: The report of the MRC Working Party. Clin Endocrinol 11:15–38, 1979.

137. Vanderschuren-Lodeweyckx M, Wolter R, Mulla A, et al: Plasma growth hormone in coeliac disease. Acta Pediatr (Helv) 28:349–357, 1973.

138. Rosenfeld RG, Albertsson-Wikland K, Cassorla F, et al: The diagnosis of childhood growth hormone deficiency revisited. J Clin Endocrinol Metab 80:1532–1540, 1995.

139. Hussain K, Hindmarsh P, Aynsley-Green A: Spontaneous hypoglycemia in childhood is accompanied by paradoxically low serum growth hormone and appropriate cortisol counterregulatory hormonal responses. J Clin Endocrinol Metab 88:3715–3723, 2003.

140. Rahim A, O'Niell P, Shalet SM: The effect of body composition on hexerelin-induced growth hormone release in normal elderly subjects. Clin Endocrinol 49:659–664, 1988.

141. Iranmanesh A, Lizaralde G, Veldhuis JD: Age and relative adiposity are specific negative determinants of the pregnancy and amplitude of growth hormone (GH) secretory bursts and the half-life of endogenous GH in healthy men. J Clin Endocrinol Metab 73:1081–1088, 1991.

142. Freeman JV, Cole TJ, Chinn S, et al: Cross sectional stature and weight reference curves for the UK, 1990. Arch Dis Child 73:17–24, 1995.

143. Blum WF, Ranke MB, Kietzmann K, et al: A specific radioimmunoassay for the growth hormone (GH)-dependent somatomedin-binding protein: Its use for diagnosis of GH deficiency. J Clin Endocrinol Metab 70:1292–1298, 1990.

144. Tillman V, Buckler JM, Kibirge MS, et al: Biochemical tests in the diagnosis of childhood growth hormone deficiency. J Clin Endocrinol Metab 82:531–535, 1997.

145. Mitchell H, Dattani MT, Nanduri V, et al: Failure of IGF-1 and IGFBP-3 to diagnose growth hormone insufficiency. Arch Dis Child 80:443–447, 1999.

146. Sox HC Jr: Probability theory in the use of diagnostic tests. Ann Intern Med 104:60–66, 1986.

147. Suri D, Hindmarsh PC, Matthews DR, et al: The pituitary gland is capable of responding to two successive doses of growth hormone releasing hormone (GHRH). Clin Endocrinol 34:13–17, 1991.

148. Rahim A, Toogood A, Shalet SM: The assessment of growth hormone status in normal young adult males using a variety of provocative tests. Clin Endocrinol 45:557–562, 1996.

149. Wacharasindhu S, Cotterill AM, Comacho-Hubner C, et al: Normal growth hormone secretion in growth hormone insufficient children re-tested after completion of linear growth. Clin Endocrinol 45:553–556, 1996.

150. Tauber M, Houlin P, Pienkowski C, et al: Growth Hormone (GH) retesting and auxological data in 131 GH-deficient patients after completion of treatment. J Clin Endocrinol Metab 82:352–356, 1997.

151. Thomas GB, Robinson ICAF: Central regulation of growth hormone secretion. In Kelnar CJH, Savage MO, Stirling HF, et al (eds): Growth Disorders. Pathophysiology and Treatment. London, Chapman & Hall, 1998, pp 99–125.

152. Martha PM Jr, Rogol AD, Veldhuis JD, et al: Alterations in the pulsatile properties of circulating growth hormone concentrations during puberty in boys. J Clin Endocrinol Metab 69:563–570, 1989.

153. Martha PM, Gorman KM, Blizzard RM, et al: Endogenous growth hormone secretion and clearance rates in normal boys as determined by deconvolution analysis: Relationship to age, pubertal status and body mass. J Clin Endocrinol Metab 74:336–344, 1992.

154. Spiliotis BE, August GP, Hung W, et al: Growth hormone neurosecretory dysfunction: A treatable cause of short stature. JAMA 252:2223–2230, 1984.

155. Bercu BB, Shulman D, Root AW, et al: Growth hormone (GH) provocative testing frequently does not reflect endogenous GH secretion. J Clin Endocrinol Metab 86:709–716, 1986.

156. Rose SR, Ross JL, Uriarte M, et al: The advantage of measuring stimulated as compared with spontaneous growth hormone levels in the diagnosis of growth hormone deficiency. N Engl J Med 319:201–207, 1988.

157. Lanes R: Diagnostic limitations of spontaneous growth hormone measurements in normally growing prepubertal children. Am J Dis Child 143:1284–1286, 1989.

158. Donaldson DL, Hollowell JG, Pan F, et al: Growth hormone secretory profiles: Variation on consecutive nights. J Pediatr 115:51–56, 1989.

159. Hourd P, Edwards R: Current methods for the measurement of growth hormone in urine. Clin Endocrinol (Oxf) 40:155–170, 1994.

160. Albini CH, Quattrin T, Vandlen RL, et al: Quantitation of urinary growth hormone in children with normal and subnormal growth. Pediatr Res 23:89–92, 1988.

161. Granada ML, Sanmarti ALA, et al: Clinical usefulness of urinary growth hormone measurements in normal and short children according to different expressions of urinary growth hormone data. Pediatr Res 32:73–76, 1992.

162. Phillip M, Chalew SA, Stene MA, et al: The value of urinary growth hormone determination for assessment of growth hormone deficiency and compliance with growth hormone therapy. Am J Dis Child 147:553–557, 1993.

163. Skinner AM, Clayton PE, Price DA, et al: Urinary growth hormone excretion in the assessment of children with disorders of growth. Clin Endocrinol (Oxf) 39:201–206, 1993.

164. Underwood LE, Azumi K, Voina SJ, et al: Growth hormone levels during sleep in normal and growth hormone deficient children. Pediatrics 48:946–954, 1971.

165. Buckler JMH: Plasma growth hormone response to exercise as a diagnostic aid. Arch Dis Child 48:565–567, 1973.

166. Lacey KA, Hewison A, Parkin JM: Exercise as a screening test for growth hormone deficiency in children. Arch Dis Child 48:508–512, 1973.

167. Coller R, Leboeuf G, Letarte J: Stimulation of growth hormone secretion by levodopa propranolol in children and adolescents. Pediatrics 56:262–266, 1975.

168. Youlton R, Kaplan SL, Grumbach MM: Growth and growth hormone, IV: Limitations of the growth hormone response to insulin and arginine in the assessment of growth hormone deficiency in children. Pediatrics 43:989–1004, 1969.

169. Lanes R, Hurtado E: Oral clonidine: An effective growth hormone-releasing agent in prepubertal subjects. J Pediatr 100:710–714, 1982.

170. Mitchell ML, Bryne MJ, Sanchez Y, et al: Detection of growth deficiency: The glucagon stimulation test. N Engl J Med 282:539–541, 1970.

171. Merimee TJ, Rabinowitz D, Fineberg SE: Arginine-initiated release of human growth hormone. N Engl J Med 280:1434–1438, 1969.

172. Fass B, Lippe BM, Kaplan SA: Relative usefulness of three growth hormone stimulation screening tests. Am J Dis Child 133:931–933, 1979.

173. Weldon VV, Gupta SK, Klingensmith G: Evaluation of growth hormone release in children using arginine and L-dopa in combination. J Pediatr 87:540–544, 1975.

174. Reiter EO, Martha PM Jr: Pharmacological testing of growth hormone secretion. Horm Res 33:121–127, 1990.

175. Raiti S, Davis WT, Blizzard RM: A comparison of the effects of insulin hypoglycemia and arginine infusion on release of human growth hormone. Lancet 2:1182–1183, 1967.

176. Albertsson-Wikland K, Rosberg S: Analysis of 24-hour growth hormone profiles in children: Relation to growth. J Clin Endocrinol Metab 67:493–500, 1988.

177. Marin G, Domene HM, Barnes KM, et al: The effects of estrogen priming and puberty on the growth hormone response to standardized treadmill exercise and arginine-insulin in normal girls and boys. J Clin Endocrinol Metab 79:537–541, 1994.

178. Pringle PJ, Stanhope R, Hindmarsh P, Brook CGD: Abnormal pubertal development in primary hypothyroidism. Clin Endocrinol 28:479–486, 1988.

179. Cordido F, Fernandez T, Martinez T, et al: Effect of acute pharmacological reduction of plasma free fatty acids on growth hormone (GH) releasing hormone-induced GH secretion in obese adults with and without hypopituitarism. J Clin Endocrinol Metab 83:4350–4354, 1998.

180. Lewis UJ, Singh RNP, Tutwiler GH, et al: Human growth hormone: A complex of proteins. Recent Prog Horm Res 36:477–508, 1980.

181. Reiter EO, Morris AH, MacGillivray MH, et al: Variable estimates of serum growth hormone concentrations by difference radioassay systems. J Clin Endocrinol Metab 66:68–71, 1988.

182. Celniker AC, Chem AB, Wert RM Jr, et al: Variability in the quantitation of circulating growth hormone using commercial immunoassays. J Clin Endocrinol Metab 68:469–476, 1989.

183. Barth JH, Smith JH, Clarkson P: Wide diversity in measurements of growth hormone after stimulation tests in short children are due to assay variability. Ann Clin Biochem 32:369–372, 1995.

184. Dattani MT, Pringle PJ, Hindmarsh PC, Brook CGD: What is a normal stimulated growth hormone concentration? J Endocrinol 133:447–450, 1992.

185. Strasburger CJ, Wu Z, Pflaum C-D, et al: Immunofunctional assay of human growth hormone (hGH) in serum: A possible consensus for quantitative hGH measurement. J Clin Endocrinol Metab 81:2613–2620, 1996.

186. Devesa J, Lima L Lois N, et al: Reasons for the variability in growth hormone (GH) responses to GHRH challenge: The endogenous

hypothalamic-somatotroph rhythm (HSR). Clin Endocrinol 30:367–377, 1989.

187. Tzanela M, Guyada H, Van Vliet G, Tannenbaum GS: Somatostatin pretreatment enhances growth hormone responsiveness to GH-releasing hormone: A potential new diagnostic approach to GH deficiency. J Clin Endocrinol Metab 81:2487–2494, 1996.

188. Bernasconi S, Volta C, Cozzini A, et al: GH response to GHRH, insulin, clonidine and arginine after GHRH pretreatment in children. Acta Endocrinol 126:105–108, 1992.

189. Massoud AF, Hindmarsh PC, Matthews DR, Brook CGD: The effect of repeated administration of hexarelin, a growth hormone releasing peptide, and growth hormone releasing hormone (GHRH) on growth hormone (GH) responsivity. Clin Endocrinol 44:555–562, 1996.

190. Berelowitz M, Szabo M, Frohman LA, et al: Somatomedin-C mediates growth hormone negative feedback by effects on both the hypothalamus and pituitary. Science 212:1279–1281, 1981.

191. Yamashita S, Melmed S: Insulin-like growth factor I action on rat anterior pituitary cells: Suppression of growth hormone secretion and messenger ribonucleic acid levels. Endocrinology 118:176–182, 1986.

192. Abe H, Molitch M, Van Wyk JJ, et al: Human growth hormone and somatomedin-C suppress the spontaneous release of growth hormone in unanesthetized rats. Endocrinology 113:1319–1324, 1983.

193. Ceda GP, Davis WT, Rosenfeld RG, et al: The growth hormone (GH) releasing hormone (GHRH)-GH-somatomedin axis: Evidence for rapid inhibition of GHRH-elicited GH release by insulin-like growth factors I and II. Endocrinology 120:1658–1662, 1987.

194. Saini S, Hindmarsh PC, Matthews DR, et al: Reproducibility of 24-hour serum growth hormone profiles in man. Clin Endocrinol 34:455–462, 1991.

195. Shriock EA, Hulse JA, Harris DA, et al: Evaluation of hypothalamic dysfunction in growth hormone (GH)-deficient patients using single versus multiple doses of growth hormone-releasing hormone (GHRH-44) and evidence for diurnal variation in somatotroph responsiveness to GHRH in GH deficient patients. J Clin Endocrinol Metab 65:1177–1182, 1987.

196. Ghigo E, Bellone J, Aimasetti G, et al: Reliability of provocative tests to assess growth hormone secretory status: Study in 472 normally growing children. J Clin Endocrinol Metab 81:3323–3327, 1996.

197. Frasier SD: Human pituitary growth hormone (hGH) therapy in growth hormone deficiency. Endocr Rev 4:155–170, 1983.

198. MacGillivray MH, Baptista J, Johanson A, et al: Outcome of a four year randomized study of daily versus three times weekly somatotropin treatment in prepubertal naive growth hormone deficient children. J Clin Endocrinol Metab 81:1806–1809, 1996.

199. Cohen P, Bright GM, Rogol AD, et al: Effects of dose and gender on the growth and growth factor response to GH in GH-deficient children: Implications for efficacy and safety. J Clin Endocrinol Metab 87:90–98, 2002.

200. Smith PJ, Hindmarsh PC, Brook CGD: Contribution of dose and frequency of administration to the therapeutic effect of growth hormone. Arch Dis Child 63:491–494, 1998.

201. Albertsson-Wikland K: The effect of human growth hormone injection frequency on linear growth rate. Acta Paediatr Scand Suppl 337:110–116, 1987.

202. Hakeem V, Hindmarsh PC, Brook CGD: Intermittent versus continuous administration of growth hormone treatment. Arch Dis Child 68:783–784, 1993.

203. Johnson OL, Cleleand TL, Lee HJ, et al: A month-long effect from a single injection of microencapsulated human growth hormone. Nat Med 2:795–799, 1969.

204. Ranke MB, Lindberg A, Guilbaud O: Prediction of growth in response to treatment with growth hormone. In Ranke MB, Gunnarsson R (eds): Progress in Growth Hormone Therapy: 5 Years of KIGS. Mannheim, Germany, JJ Verlag, 1994, pp 97–111.

205. Bland JM, Altman DG: Statistical methods for assessing agreement between two methods of clinical measurement. Lancet i:307–310, 1986.

206. Blomqvist N: On the bias caused by regression to the mean in studying the relation between change and initial value. J Clin Periodontol 13:34–37, 1986.

207. Hayes RJ: Methods for assessing whether change depends on initial value. Stat Med 7:915–927, 1988.

208. Gardner MJ, Heady JA: Some effects of within-person variability in epidemiological studies. J Chron Dis 26:781–795, 1973.

209. Taback SP, Van Vliet G: Managing the short stature of Turner syndrome: An evidence based approval to the suggestion of growth hormone supplementation. In Hindmarsh PC (ed): Current Indications for Growth Hormone Therapy. Basel, Karger, 1999, pp 102–117.

210. Matthews JNS, Altman DG, Campbell MJ, Royston P: Analysis of serial measurements in medical research. Br Med J 300:230–235, 1990.

211. Bundak R, Hindmarsh PC, Brook CGD: Long-term auxologic effects of human growth hormone. J Pediatr 112:875–879, 1990.

212. Libber SM, Plotnick LP, Johanson AJ, et al: Long-term follow-up of hypopituitary patients treated with human growth hormone. Medicine 69:46–55, 1990.

213. Bramswig JH, Schlosser H, Kiese K: Final height in children with growth hormone deficiency. Horm Res 43:126–128, 1995.

214. Chipman JJ, Hicks JR, Holcombe JH, et al: Approaching final height in children treated for growth hormone deficiency. Horm Res 43:129–131, 1995.

215. Frisch H, Birnbacher R: Final height and pubertal development in children with growth hormone deficiency after long-term treatment. Horm Res 43:132–134, 1995.

216. Severi F: Final height in children with growth hormone deficiency. Horm Res 43:138–140, 1995.

217. Blethen SL, Compton P, Lippe BM, et al: Factors predicting the response to growth hormone (GH) therapy in prepubertal children with GH deficiency. J Clin Endocrinol Metab 74:574–579, 1993.

218. Arrigo T, DeLuca F, Bernasconi S, et al: Catch-up growth and height prognosis in early treated children with congenital hypopituitarism. Horm Res 44(Suppl):26–31, 1996.

219. Burns EC, Tanner JM, Preece MA, et al: Final height and pubertal development in 55 children with idiopathic growth hormone deficiency, treated for between 2 and 15 years with human growth hormone. Eur J Pediatr 137:155–164, 1981.

220. Bourguignon JP, Vandeweghe M, Vanderschuren-Lodeweyckx M, et al: Pubertal growth and final height in hypopituitary boys: A minor role of bone age at onset of puberty. J Clin Endocrinol Metab 63:376–382, 1986.

221. Price DA, Ranke MB: Final height following growth hormone treatment. In Ranke MB, Gunnarsson R (eds): Progress in Growth Hormone Therapy: 5 Years of KIGS. Mannheim, Germany, JJ Verlag, 1994, pp 574–579.

222. Ranke MB, Price DA, Albertsson-Wikland K, et al: Factors determining pubertal growth and final height in growth hormone treatment of idiopathic growth hormone deficiency. Horm Res 48:62–71, 1997.

223. Blethen SL, Baptista J, Kuntze J, et al: Adult height in growth hormone (GH)-deficient children treated with biosynthetic GH. J Clin Endocrinol Metab 82:418–420, 1997.

224. Adan L, Souberbielle JC, Zucker JM, et al: Adult height in 24 patients treated for growth hormone deficiency and early puberty. J Clin Endocrinol Metab 82:229–233, 1997.

225. Tanaka T, Satoh M, Yasunaga T, et al: GH and GnRH analog treatment in children who enter puberty at short stature. J Pediatr Endocrinol Metab 10:623–628, 1987.

226. Saggese G, Baroncelli GI, Bertelloni S, Barsanti S: The effect of long-term growth hormone (GH) treatment on bone mineral density in children with GH deficiency: Role of GH in the

attainment of peak bone mass. J Clin Endocrinol Metab 81:3077–3083, 1996.

227. Blethen SL, Alster DK, Graves D, et al: Safety of recombinant DNA-derived growth hormone (rhGH): The National Cooperative Growth Study experience. J Clin Endocrinol Metab 81:1704–1710, 1996.

228. Wilton P: Adverse events during growth hormone treatment: 5 years' experience. In Ranke B, Gunnarsson R (eds): Progress in Growth Hormone Therapy: 5 Years of KIGS. Mannheim, Germany, JJ Verlag, 1994, pp 291–307.

229. Cutfield WS, Wilton P, Bennmarker H, et al: Incidence of diabetes mellitus and impaired glucose tolerance in children and adolescents receiving growth-hormone treatment. Lancet 355:610–613, 2000.

230. Watanabe S, Yamagucki N, Tsunematsu Y, et al: Risk factors for leukemia occurrence among growth hormone users. Jpn J Cancer 80:822–825, 1989.

231. Fisher DA, Job J, Preece M, et al: Leukemia in patients treated with growth hormone. Lancet 1:1159–1160, 1988.

232. Fradkin JE, Mills JL, Schonberger LB, et al: Risk of leukemia after treatment with pituitary growth hormone. JAMA 270:2829–2832, 1993.

233. Oglivy-Stuart AL, Ryder WD, Gattamaneni HR, et al: Growth hormone and tumor recurrence. Br Med J 304:1601–1605, 1992.

234. Tuffli GA, Johanson A, Rundle AC, et al: Lack of increased risk for extracranial, nonleukemic neoplasms in recipients of recombinant deoxyribonucleic acid growth hormone. J Clin Endocrinol Metab 80:1416–1422, 1995.

235. Moshang T, Rundle AC, Graves DA, et al: Brain tumor recurrence in children treated with growth hormone: The National Cooperative Growth Study experience. J Pediatr 128:S4–S7, 1996.

236. Swerdlow AJ, Reddingius RE, Higgins CD, et al: Growth hormone treatment of children with brain tumors and risk of tumor recurrence. J Clin Endocrinol Metab 85:4444–4449, 2000.

237. Swerdlow AJ, Higgins CD, Adlard P, Preece MA: Risk of cancer in patients treated with human pituitary growth hormone in the UK, 1959-85: A cohort study. Lancet 360:273–277, 2002.

238. Ma J, Pollak MN, Giovannucci E, et al: Prospective study of colorectal cancer risk in men and plasma levels of insulin-like growth factor (IGF)-I and IGF-binding protein-3. J Natl Cancer Inst 91:620–625, 1999.

239. Hankinson SE, Willett WC, Colditz GA, et al: Circulating concentrations of insulin-like growth factor-I and risk of breast cancer. Lancet 351:1393–1396, 1998.

240. Chan JM, Stampfer MJ, Giovannucci E, et al: Plasma insulin-like growth factor-I and prostate cancer risk: A prospective study. Science 279:563–566, 1998.

241. Palmqvist R, Hallmans G, Rinaldi S, et al: Plasma insulin-like growth factor 1, insulin-like growth factor binding protein 3, and risk of colorectal cancer: A prospective study in northern Sweden. Gut 50:642–646, 2002.

242. Furstenberger G, Senn HJ: Insulin-like growth factors and cancer. Lancet Oncol 5:298–302, 2002.

243. Thorner MO, Rogol AD, Blizzard RM, et al: Acceleration of growth rate in growth hormone-deficient children treated with human growth hormone-releasing hormone. Pediatr Res 24:145–151, 1988.

244. Thorner MO, Rochiccioli P, Colle M, et al: Once daily subcutaneous growth hormone-releasing hormone therapy accelerates growth in growth hormone-deficient children during the first year of therapy: Geraf International Study Group. J Clin Endocrinol Metab 81:1189–1196, 1996.

245. Huerta MG, Rogol AD: Growth hormone-releasing hormone and other growth hormone secretagogues. In Kelnar CJH, Savage MO, Stirling HF, et al (eds): Growth Disorders. Pathophysiology and Treatment. London, Chapman & Hall, 1998, pp 701–720.

246. Hummelink R, Sippell WG, Benoit KG: Intranasal administration of growth hormone-releasing hormone (1-29)-NH$_2$ in children with growth hormone deficiency: Effects on growth hormone secretion and growth. Acta Paediatr Suppl 388:23–26, 1993.

247. Bowers CY, Alster DK, Frentz JM: The growth hormone-releasing activity of a synthetic hexapeptide in normal men and short stature children after oral administration. J Clin Endocrinol Metab 74:292–298, 1992.

248. Bowers CY: On a peptidomimetic growth hormone-releasing peptide. J Clin Endocrinol Metab 79:940–942, 1994.

249. Smith RG, van der Ploey LHT, Howard AD, et al: Peptidomimetic regulation of growth hormone secretion. Endocr Rev 18:621–645, 1997.

250. Allen DB: Issues in the transition from childhood to adult growth hormone therapy. Pediatrics 104:1004–1010, 1999.

251. Monson JP, Hindmarsh P: The assessment of growth hormone deficiency in children and adults with particular reference to the transitional period. Clin Endocrinol (Oxf) 53:545–547, 2000.

252. Rosenfeld RG: Transitioning patients with childhood-onset growth hormone deficiency to treatment in adulthood. J Pediatr Endocrinol Metab 15:1361–1365, 2002.

253. GH Research Society: Consensus guidelines for the diagnosis and treatment of growth hormone (GH) deficiency in childhood and adolescence: Summary statement of the GH Research Society. J Clin Endocrinol Metab 85:3990–3993, 2000.

254. Donaubauer J, Kiess W, Kratzsch J, et al: Re-assessment of growth hormone secretion in young adult patients with childhood-onset growth hormone deficiency. Clin Endocrinol (Oxf) 58:456–463, 2003.

255. de Boer H, van der Veen EA: Why retest young adults with childhood-onset growth hormone deficiency? J Clin Endocrinol Metab 82:2032–2036, 1997.

256. Saggese G, Ranke MB, Saenger P, et al: Diagnosis and treatment of growth hormone deficiency in children and adolescents: Towards a consensus: Ten years after the availability of recombinant human growth hormone workshop held in Pisa, Italy, 27–28 March, 1998. Horm Res 50:320–340, 1998.

257. Shalet SM, Toogood A, Rahim A, Brennan BM: The diagnosis of growth hormone deficiency in children and adults. Endocr Rev 19:203–223, 1998.

Growth Hormone Deficiency in Adults

Ken K. Y. Ho

INTRODUCTION

Adult patients with organic hypopituitarism receive substitutive hormone treatment for secondary glucocorticoid, sex steroid, and thyroid hormone deficiency. Until recently, growth hormone (GH) deficiency in these patients was not regarded as a clinical problem, as it was assumed that GH had no physiological relevance after cessation of childhood growth.

The critical role of GH in stimulating childhood growth is well recognized, and its use in treating dwarfism due to GH deficiency is an unchallenged indication world-wide. Body growth represents the result of the stimulation by GH of a complex and integrated series of metabolic processes that are readily demonstrable in adults, even after cessation of body growth. Growth stops at the end of puberty as a result of fusion of the growth plates in long bones. However, GH continues to be produced throughout adult life and is the most abundant hormone in the adult pituitary gland. Hormones exert their actions by binding to specific receptors on tissues. All body tissues examined to date contain receptors for GH. This observation suggests that effects of GH are widespread and that the hormone plays a general role in maintaining the metabolic process and the integrity of many tissues.

Raben[1] first reported nearly four decades ago of improved vigor and well being in an adult women with hypopituitarism treated with GH. A major reason for past neglect of treating hypopituitary adult patients with GH was the very limited availability of pituitary-derived GH outside the pediatric setting. The advent of genetic engineering resulting in abundant supplies of recombinant GH has led to a major reappraisal of its physiologic role in adult life Many countries including the United States, United Kingdom, member countries of the European Union, and Australia have approved the use of GH for replacement therapy in adults with GH deficiency.

EPIDEMIOLOGY

Limited information is available on the epidemiology of hypopituitarism. A Swedish survey estimates the prevalence of hypopituitarism to be 175 cases per million.[2] A Spanish study has reported a prevalence of hypopituitarism of 290 and 450 cases per million from two cross-sectional surveys in 1992 and 1999, respectively. in a regional center, and a corresponding incidence of 60 per million per year.[3] Sixty percent of the patients were GH deficient, giving a prevalence of GH deficiency of 114 to 270 cases per million and an incidence of 24 per million per year. In patients with pituitary tumors evaluated before surgery, about 50% of patients already had evidence of GH, gonadotropin, or cortisol deficiency.[4] After surgery, about 80% had evidence of GH or gonadotropin deficiency. In patients who received postoperative radiotherapy, evaluation after 5 years revealed that all patients were GH deficient.[4]

The etiology of adult GH deficiency from four series totaling 1798 patients is shown in Table 38-1.[5-8] Approximately 50% arise from pituitary tumors, 18% from extrapituitary tumors, 5% from inflammatory or infiltrative lesion, and up to 15% are idiopathic. The treatment of pituitary and extrapituitary tumors is the most common cause of deficiency, accounting for nearly two thirds of cases. The frequency of causes differs between patients with childhood-onset and adult-onset GH deficiency.[6] Idiopathic causes, representing the largest group in childhood disease, are likely to represent a heterogeneous collection of congenital developmental abnormalities including mutations of *pit-1* and *PROP* genes, causing multiple pituitary hormone deficiencies.

CONSEQUENCES OF GROWTH HORMONE DEFICIENCY

One of the first indications of the deleterious effects of GH deficiency in adults came from an epidemiologic study in 1990,[5] which reported a twofold increase in cardiovascular mortality in hypopituitary patients receiving conventional hormone replacement (Fig. 38-1). Three more recent studies provide further evidence that adults with hypopituitarism have reduced life expectancy from cardiovascular and cerebrovascular mortality.[9-11] Radiotherapy and craniopharyngioma were independent predictors of mortality.[11] The recent observation of reduced life expectancy in patients with congenital isolated GH deficiency[12] suggests that GH deficiency rather than suboptimal hormone-replacement regimens account for the increased mortality rate in hypopituitarism.

Table 38-1	Causes of Growth Hormone Deficiency in 1798 Patients		
		Number	%
Pituitary		991	55.1
Extra pituitary			
	Cerebral*	83	4.6
	Extracerebral†	233	13.0
Non tumoral			
	Inflammatory	66	3.7
	Trauma	40	2.2
	Infiltrative	21	1.2
	Other‡	20	6.7
Idiopathic		244	13.6
Total		**1798**	**100**

Data are derived from four studies (Refs. 5–8).
*Includes gliomas, pinealomas, dysgerminomas.
†Includes craniopharyngiomas, meningiomas, epidermoid cysts, Rathke's cysts.
‡Includes developmental malformations, irradiation other than for pituitary treatment, empty sella.

Table 38-2	Syndrome of Adult Growth Hormone Deficiency

SYMPTOMS
Increased body fat
Reduced muscle bulk
Reduced strength and physical fitness
Reduced sweating
Impaired psychological well-being
  Depressed mood
  Anxiety
  Reduced physical stamina
  Reduced vitality and energy
  Increased social isolation

SIGNS
Overweight
Increased adiposity, especially abdominal
Poor muscular development
Reduced exercise performance
Thin, dry skin
Depressed affect

INVESTIGATIONS
Peak GH response to hypoglycemia <3 μg/L (all patients)
Low IGF-1 (60% of patients)
Hyperlipidemia: high LDL cholesterol, low HDL cholesterol
Elevated fasting insulin
Reduced bone mineral density

GH, growth hormone; IGF, insulin-like growth factor; LDL, low-density lipoprotein; HDL, high-density lipoprotein.

In addition to having a reduced life expectancy, adults with GH deficiency, whether dating from childhood or acquired in later adult life, have a range of metabolic, body compositional, and functional abnormalities. These patients have a recognizable clinical syndrome, associated with a characteristic history, symptoms, signs, and investigative findings (Table 38-2).

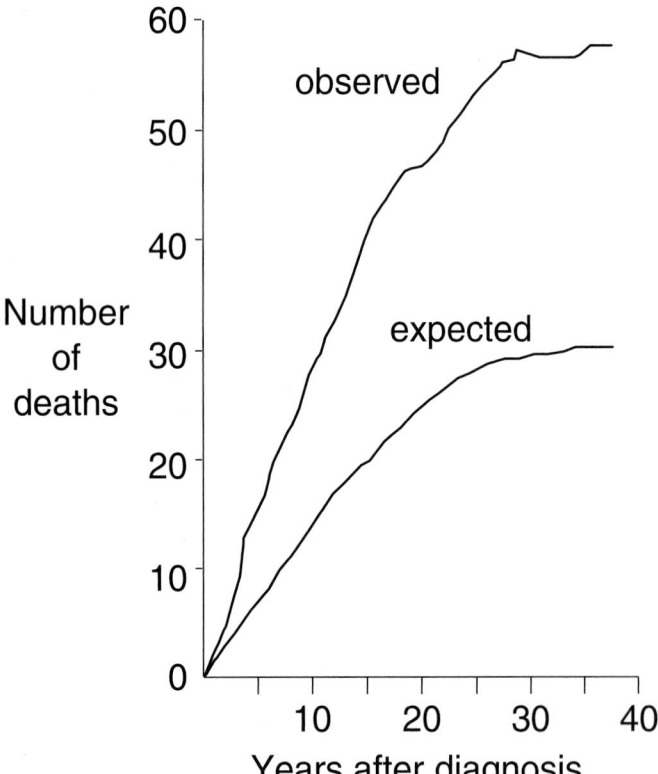

Figure 38-1 Mortality rate in adult patients with hypopituitarism receiving conventional hormone-replacement therapy. (Reproduced from Rosen A, Rosen T, Bengtsson B-A: Premature mortality due to cardiovascular disease in hypopituitarism. Lancet 336:285–288, 1990, with permission.)

METABOLISM

Hypopituitary patients unreplaced with GH display biochemical abnormalities that are strongly linked to the development of vascular disease. These patients have higher concentrations of total and low-density lipoprotein (LDL) cholesterol as well as apolipoprotein B.[12–14] Evidence exists from ultrasonographic studies of intima and media thickening and premature atherosclerosis of large vessels.[15,16] These patients also have a higher level of plasminogen inhibitory activity and higher concentration of fibrinogen,[17] both markers of increased atherothrombotic propensity. Fibrinogen also is a risk factor for stroke and myocardial infarction. Circulating levels of proinflammatory factors linked to the development of vascular disease, such as C-reactive protein (CRP) also are increased.[18]

BODY COMPOSITION

Marked abnormality of body composition is characterized by increased proportion of body fat and reduced lean mass.[19,20] These changes are a consequence of the loss of the lipolytic and anabolic actions of GH. The effects of GH on body fat and muscle can be seen in Figure 38-2, which shows the striking changes in body physique in a man before and 5 years after acquiring GH deficiency after surgery for a pituitary tumor.

These patients not only are more obese but also display a disproportionate increase in central abdominal fat.[20] The tendency for central fat deposition is important because visceral obesity is linked to the development of insulin resistance, diabetes, and cardiovascular disease.[21] Adults with GH deficiency have evidence of insulin resistance[22] and a higher prevalence of impaired glucose tolerance.[23]

The reduction of lean body mass in adult GH deficiency arises from combined reduction of bone, muscle and visceral mass, and extracellular fluid volume. Bone mass at different skeletal sites is reduced in patients with childhood-onset and adult-onset GH deficiency.[24,25] The risk of fractures is increased between two- to threefold.[26,27]

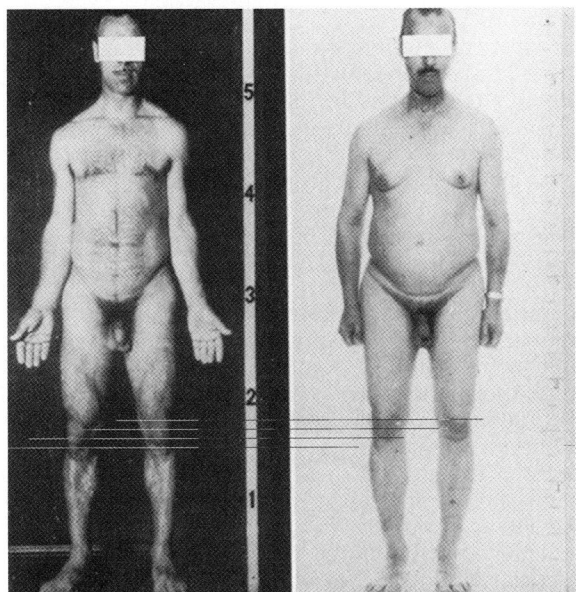

Figure 38-2 Body physique in a normal man before and 5 years after acquiring growth hormone deficiency as a result of pituitary surgery for a macroadenoma. Note the striking change in body composition with an accumulation of body fat, particularly in the abdomen, and marked loss of musculature. (Courtesy of Professor Peter Sonksen.)

PHYSICAL PERFORMANCE

The abnormalities of body composition are accompanied by a significant impairment of physical performance and muscle strength.[28,29] Physical fitness, as determined by cycle ergometry, has consistently been shown to be reduced in adult GH deficiency, with rates of maximal oxygen uptake reduced on average by about 30%.[30] Exercise performance is a complex parameter dependent on a number of factors including cardiorespiratory and neuromuscular muscle function. These patients have impaired cardiac function with reduced ventricular muscle mass, reduced ejection fraction, impaired ventricular filling,[31-33] and reduced lung size, all of which contribute to reduced exercise capacity. As the skin is a target tissue of GH action, another likely contributing factor to reduced exercise endurance is impairment of sweating, which arises from hypoplasia of the eccrine sweat glands. The skin of GH-deficient subjects is atrophic and dry.[14] Reduced sweating increases the susceptibility to hyperthermia during exercise and may limit exercise performance.[34]

QUALITY OF LIFE

The metabolic, body compositional, and functional abnormities in adult GH deficiency are accompanied by significant impairment of psychological well-being and reduced quality of life. Fatigue, easy exhaustion, and lack of vitality are common symptoms. Early studies using generic questionnaires revealed lower self-perception of quality of life with patients regarding themselves as having reduced health, self-control, vitality, and experiencing more anxiety.[35,36] A Dutch survey of social integration reported that GH-deficient adults had impaired social status.[37] These patients were on a lower professional scale, had lower income, and were generally without partners and living at home with their parents. Recent studies based on disease-specific questionnaires evaluating life satisfaction revealed marked impairment in quality of life regardless of country and cultural background.[38] On average, scores from GH-deficient patients were approximately half those of the normal population.[39]

Thus, the collective evidence indicate that adults who lack GH are not normal but suffer from metabolic abnormalities, disordered body composition, reduced physical fitness, impaired psychological well being and reduced quality of life.

DIAGNOSIS OF ADULT GROWTH HORMONE DEFICIENCY

Although the features of GH deficiency are recognizable, they are not particularly distinct and mimic body compositional and biochemical changes of the aging process.[40] GH secretion itself decreases progressively with aging, associated with a progressive increase in adiposity, which itself reduces GH secretion.[41,42] Thus, clinical suspicion must be confirmed by accurate biochemical diagnosis to ensure that GH-deficient patients are accurately identified and treated.

WHO TO TEST

GH deficiency should be defined biochemically within an appropriate clinical context. Biochemical testing for GH deficiency should be considered in patients with a high probability of hypothalamus-pituitary disease and manifest clinical features of the syndrome.[43] This includes patients with a history of organic hypothalamic-pituitary dysfunction, cranial irradiation, or known childhood onset of GH deficiency. Patients with childhood-onset GH deficiency should be retested as adults before committing them to long-term GH replacement.

BIOCHEMICAL DIAGNOSIS

Three widely accepted approaches for assessing GH secretory status include measuring (1) the peak GH response to a provocative test, (2) spontaneous GH secretion, and (3) serum concentrations of GH-regulated proteins such as insulin-like growth factor 1(IGF-1) and IGF-binding protein-3 (IGFBP-3).

Provocative Tests

The diagnosis of adult GH deficiency is established by provocative testing of GH secretion. Patients should be receiving adequate and stable hormone replacement for other hormonal deficits before testing. A number of provocative tests include insulin tolerance test (ITT), arginine, glucagon, clonidine, and growth hormone–releasing hormone (GHRH) alone or in combination with arginine or pyridostigmine. However, the GH-releasing potency differs between these agents, with the ITT being a better stimulator of GH release than arginine or clonidine.

The Growth Hormone Research Society has recommended the ITT as the diagnostic test of choice.[43] It is superior to measuring integrated 24-hour GH concentration or IGF-1[44] (Fig. 38-3). Provided adequate hypoglycemia (<2.2 mmol/L or 40 mg/dL) is achieved, the ITT distinguishes GH deficiency from the reduced GH secretion that accompanies normal aging and obesity. The ITT should be performed in experienced endocrine units under supervision. The test is contraindicated in patients with electrocardiographic evidence or history of ischemic heart disease or in patients with seizure disorders. Given these precautions, the ITT is safe, with a risk of adverse event of less than 1 in 450.[45] Normal subjects respond to insulin-induced hypoglycemia with a peak GH concentration of more than 5 μg/L.[45] Severe GH deficiency is defined by a peak GH response to hypoglycemia of less than 3 μg/L. These cut-off values were defined in GH assays using polyclonal competitive radioimmunoassays. However, GH immunoassay results vary between different methods, and therefore the cut-off value may require appropriate adjustment.

In patients in whom the ITT is contraindicated, alternative provocative tests of GH secretion must be used with appropriate cut-offs because of their varying ability to stimulate GH release. At present, alternatives to the ITT that have been

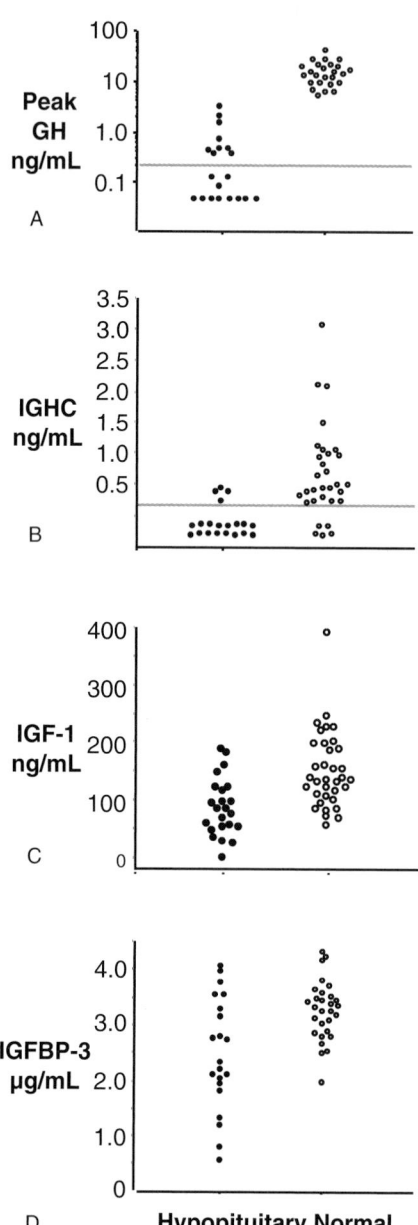

Figure 38-3 Comparison of peak growth hormone (GH) concentration obtained during an insulin tolerance test **(A)**, integrated GH concentration (IGHC) obtained from blood withdrawal every 20 minutes for 24 hours **(B)**, insulin-like growth factor (IGF)-1 **(C)** and IGF-binding protein (IGFBP)-3 concentrations **(D)** in patients with organic hypopituitarism and age- and sex-matched normal subjects. *Dotted line,* Limit of reading. (Reproduced from Hoffman DM, O'Sullivan AJ, Baxter RC, Ho KKY: Diagnosis of growth hormone deficiency in adults. Lancet 343:1064–1068, 1994, with permission.)

validate include (1) combined arginine and GHRH test,[46] and (2) combined GHRH with GHRP-2 or GHRP-6 test.[47,48] Some patients with idiopathic GH deficiency identified by a failed GH response to the ITT show a robust GH response to combined administration of GHRH and growth hormone–releasing peptide (GHRP)-6.[49] It is possible that these secretagogues restored GH secretion by acting directly on the pituitary of patients in whom GH deficiency arose from hypothalamic disease. Caution should be exercised in the selection of patients for diagnostic testing with combined GHRH and GHRP administration. Thus, the combined test may be best used to assess patients with organic pituitary disease causing GH deficiency.[50]

Spontaneous Secretion

This is most commonly estimated by measuring GH from frequent samples obtained over a 24-hour period. Integrated GH measurements obtained in this way do not readily discriminate GH-deficient patients from normal subjects, even with the use of highly sensitive assays.[51] Together with the labor-intensive nature of the procedure, this procedure is more suitable as a research tool and cannot be recommended as a practical or reliable diagnostic test for GH deficiency (see Fig. 38-3).[44]

Biochemical Markers of Growth Hormone Action

These markers include IGF-1, IGFBP-3, and the acid-labile subunit of the IGF-1-BP complex. Of the three biochemical markers, the merit of IGF-1 has been the most intensively studied. Serum IGF-1 concentrations are useful only when age-adjusted normal ranges are used. Although IGF-1 levels are reduced in adult GH deficiency, a normal concentration does not exclude the diagnosis (see Fig. 38-3). A subnormal IGF-1 level in an adult patient with coexisting pituitary hormone deficits is strongly suggestive of GH deficiency, particularly in the absence of conditions known to reduce IGF-1 levels, such as malnutrition, liver disease, poorly controlled diabetes mellitus, and hypothyroidism. The separation of IGF-1 values between GH-deficient and normal subjects is greatest in the young. As IGF-1 levels decline in normal subjects with aging, IGF-1 becomes less reliable as a biochemical marker of GH deficiency in patients older than 50 years when the values merge with those of normal subjects.[46] Measurement of IGFBP-3 or the acid-labile subunit does not offer any advantage over IGF-1.[52]

Thus, the biochemical diagnosis of adult GH deficiency is normally established by the ITT in patients with a history of pituitary disease. A low IGF-1 level in such patients signifies hyposomatotropism, although a normal level dose not exclude the diagnosis.

Which Patients Do Not Require a Stimulation Test?

In patients with organic hypothalamic-pituitary disease, the prevalence of GH deficiency is strongly linked to the number of pituitary hormone deficits, ranging from approximately 25% to 40% with no deficit to virtually 95% to 100% when more than three pituitary hormone deficiencies are present[53] (Fig. 38-4). A recent study reported that the positive predictive value is 95% for GH deficiency in patients with more than three additional pituitary hormone deficiencies and a low IGF-1 level (<88 ng/mL).[54] Thus, patients with these criteria need not proceed to a stimulation test to establish GH deficiency.

GROWTH HORMONE REPLACEMENT THERAPY

The beneficial effects of GH replacement in hypopituitary adults were first reported in 1989.[20,55] Since then, the impact of GH replacement has been extensively studied, and long-term experience of up to 10 years indicates sustained benefits.[56]

METABOLISM

GH treatment induces profound effects on protein and fat metabolism, which result in significant changes in body composition. The anabolic effects arise from direct stimulation of protein synthesis and reduction of protein oxidation. GH stimulates lipolysis and fat oxidation, enhancing the utilization of fat for energy metabolism. The marked effects of GH on substrate metabolism are accompanied by a significant stimulation of resting energy expenditure.[20]

In addition to exerting effects on the oxidative metabolism of fat, GH also reduces a significant shift of lipoprotein metabolism to a less atherogenic profile.

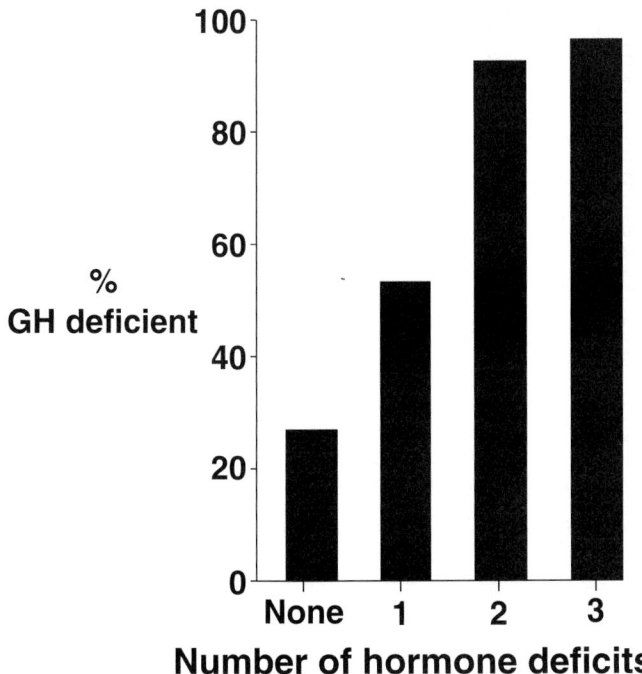

Figure 38-4   Relation between the number of anterior pituitary hormone deficits and the prevalence of growth hormone deficiency in 190 patients with known pituitary disease. (Reproduced from Toogood AA, Beardwell C, Shalet SM: The severity of growth hormone deficiency in adults with pituitary disease is related to the degree of hypopituitarism. Clin Endocrinol 41:511–516, 1994, with permission.)

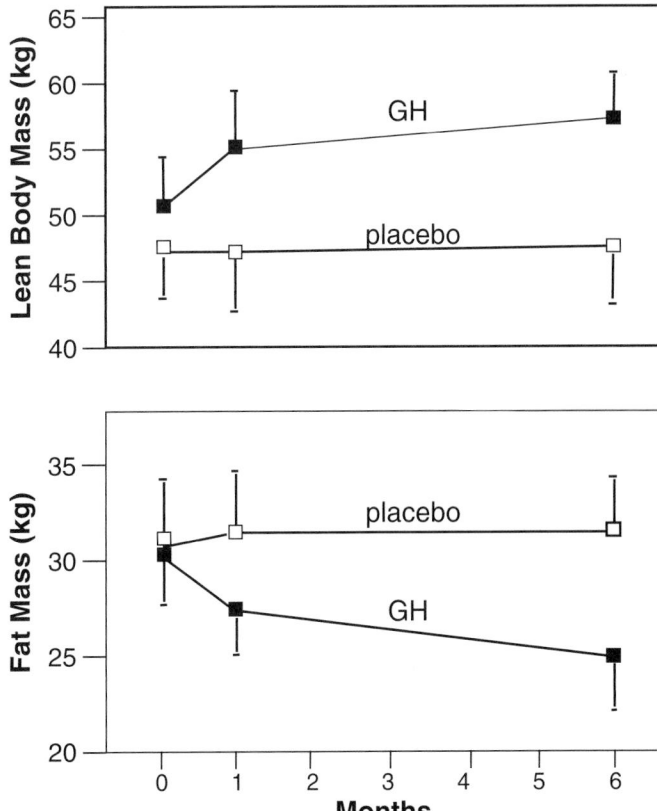

Figure 38-5   Body composition in growth hormone (GH)-deficient adult during treatment with either GH or placebo for 6 months. **A,** Body fat and **(B)** lean body mass. (Reproduced from Salomon F, Cuneo RC, Hesp R, Sonksen PH: The effects of treatment with recombinant human growth hormone on body composition and metabolism in adults with growth hormone deficiency. N Engl J Med 321:1797–1803, 1989, with permission.)

Most studies report a decrease in total cholesterol.[14] Less consistently reported are effects on increasing high-density lipoprotein (HDL) cholesterol and reducing levels of LDL cholesterol and apolipoprotein.[57-59] The favorable effects of improving the lipoprotein profile are more evident after treatment for more than a year.[59,60] Most studies report little effect on triglyceride levels.[14] Mechanisms accounting for a less-atherogenic profile include GH induction of hepatic LDL receptors and reduction in central adiposity, accompanied by an improvement in insulin sensitivity.

GH treatment reduces intima-media thickness of the carotid arteries and improves flow-mediated endothelium-dependent dilatation.[16,61] The mean intima-media thickness of the carotid vessels was significantly less after 10 years of GH treatment when compared with that of an untreated GH-deficient group.[56] The changes are not correlated to the reductions in plasma lipids. Proinflammatory factors such as CRP and interleukin (IL)-6, strongly implicated in the pathogenesis of vascular disease, decrease significantly with GH treatment.[62] It is yet to be established that the improvement in these risk markers translates to a reduction of cardiovascular mortality.

BODY COMPOSITION

GH replacement induces striking changes in body composition.[6,14,20,55,58] One of the first studies of adult replacement reported a significant reduction of 18% body fat and a corresponding increase of lean body mass of 10% over a 6-month treatment period (Fig. 38-5). These changes in body composition occurred without a significant change in body weight. Regional studies of body composition show that the greatest reduction of body fat occurs in abdominal and visceral fat.[63] The restoration of body composition is largely completed by the first 12 months of treatment, although a small reduction

in body fat and increase in lean and muscle mass may continue for longer.[60]

The increase in lean body mass arises from combined increase in skeletal muscle mass, visceral mass, and bone mass, as well as in extracellular fluid volume. Studies using computed tomography (CT) scanning show that the cross-sectional area of thigh muscle increases by 5% to 8% after 6 months of treatment, with values becoming normal after 3 years of continuous treatment.[29,64] Significant increases in extracellular water also occur. These changes occur as a consequence of the antinatriuretic properties of GH, which are dose dependent and involve activation of the renin-angiotensin system, as well as a direct renal tubular effect.[65] Renal plasma flow and glomerular filtration rate are increased.

Bone remodeling is activated by GH. Markers of bone formation such as osteocalcin, alkaline phosphatase, and bone Gla protein, along with markers of resorption such as urinary hydroxyproline, are increased by GH treatment.[14] Initial studies reporting changes in bone mineral density (BMD) over 6 to 12 months of treatment gave conflicting results. However, more recent studies reporting long-term data show a progressive increase in BMD beyond 12 to 18 months of treatment[66-68] (Fig. 38-6). The gain is more marked in those with low densities before starting GH treatment.[66] The collective findings indicated that GH induces a biphasic effect, with initial predominance of bone resorption followed by net accretion after 12 months, reaching a plateau after 3 years.[60,69] Markers of bone turnover increase in the first 12 months but return to baseline after 3 to 4 years.[70]

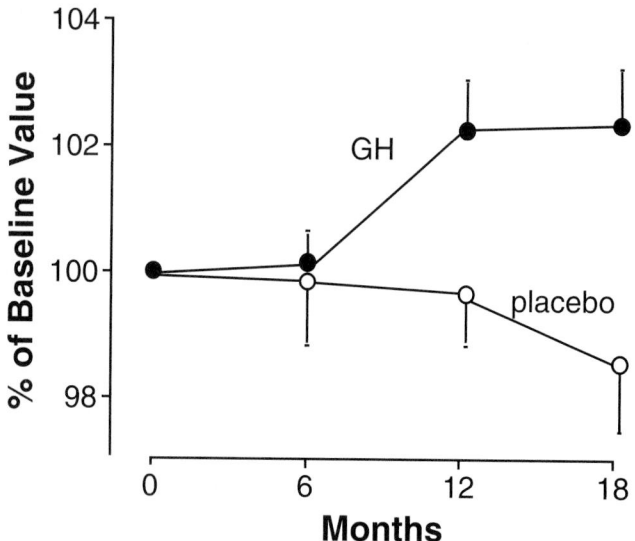

Figure 38-6   Bone mineral density of the lumbar spine in growth hormone (GH)-deficient adults during treatment with either GH or placebo for 18 months. (Reproduced from Baum HB, Biller BM, Finkelstein JS, Klibanski A: Effect of physiologic growth hormone therapy on bone density and body composition in patients with adult onset growth hormone deficiency: A randomised, placebo-controlled trial. Ann Intern Med 125:883–890, 1996, with permission.)

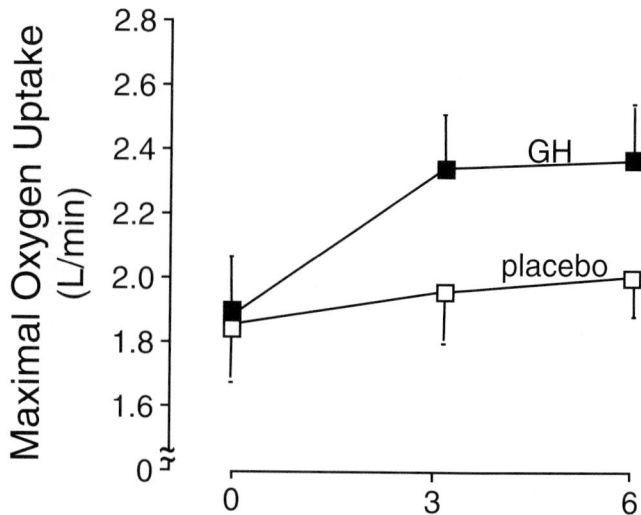

Figure 38-7   Maximal exercise capacity in growth hormone (GH)-deficient adults during treatment with either GH or placebo for 6 months. Exercise capacity was measured as maximal oxygen uptake during incremental cycle ergometry. (Reproduced from Cuneo RC, Salomon F, Wiles CM, et al: Growth hormone treatment of growth hormone deficient adults, II. Effects on exercise performance. J Appl Physiol 70:695–700, 1991, with permission.)

GH replacement causes progressive thickening of skin, restoration of eccrine function, and hair growth. The venous vasculature is more prominent and renders cannulation easier. The general anabolic effects are seen in various tissues and organs. Heart size and ventricular mass increase along with an expansion of plasma volume and red cell mass.[71]

GH treatment of the GH-deficient child is normally terminated when final height and epiphyseal closure are reached. Strong evidence indicates that biologic maturity is attained after the postpubertal period in the early years of adulthood. Muscle mass and strength continue to increase in normal subjects after puberty, and this does not occur in GH-deficient subjects.[72,73] The bone mineral content of GH-treated subjects doubled that of unreplaced GH-deficient subjects after 2 years in the postpubertal period.[74] Thus, compelling reasons exist for GH-deficient children to continue GH treatment after puberty to allow complete physical maturation.

PHYSICAL PERFORMANCE

Several studies reported that the increase in lean body and muscle mass during GH treatment is accompanied by an improvement in muscle strength. Quadriceps or hip muscle strength improves significantly after 6 months of treatment.[29,64] Muscle strength normalized after 2 years, without further significant change at 5 years.[75,76]

Many studies reported improvement in exercise capacity and performance in parallel with an increase in maximal oxygen uptake[30,77] (Fig. 38-7). Exercise training alone significantly improves aerobic capacity of GH-deficient adults and are not additive to the effects of GH treatment alone.[78]

In patients with GH deficiency, submaximal exercise performance, estimated as anaerobic threshold, increases significantly during GH treatment, suggesting that physical activities of daily living may be accomplished by less metabolic stress and subjective perception of effort.[79] Maximal workload and oxygen consumption increased progressively over a 5-year period of GH treatment.[69] In addition to increases in muscle strength, many other factors may contribute to an improvement in exercise performance. These include enhanced cardiac function and improved heat dissipation through increased sweating. The data supporting a

positive effect of GH on cardiac function are strong. Stroke volume, cardiac output, and diastolic function improve during GH treatment.[30,80,81]

QUALITY OF LIFE

The psychological well-being and quality of life of GH-deficient patients receiving replacement have been assessed by using self-administered questionnaires that address general health and well-being. Although these tools are not disease specific, several double-blind, placebo-controlled studies have reported improvement in mood, energy, sleep, and vitality scores with GH treatment,[35,58,63] with continued improvement in these domains during the open phase. In general, GH replacement improved perceived health status and subjective well-being in the domains of health-related quality of life within 6 months. These findings were confirmed in a large randomized placebo-controlled blinded trial based on partner evaluation by questionnaire. According to the partner, the patients were more alert, active, and industrious, and had greater vitality and endurance during GH treatment.[82] Disease-specific tools have reported unequivocal improvement in measures of life satisfaction after GH treatment.[39] A large survey in 304 patients showed not only an improvement in quality of life, but also significant reduction in the numbers of sick leave and doctor visits during 12 months of GH therapy[83] (Fig. 38-8).

Significant differences are noted in clinical and biochemical presentation and responses to GH therapy between patients with childhood-onset and those with adult-onset GH deficiency.[6,76] Height, body weight, and lean body mass are lower in those with childhood-onset GH deficiency. The quality of life appears to be less disrupted in childhood-onset disease. During GH treatment, this group display greater changes in body composition, greater increases in BMDs and in muscle strength, but lesser improvement in lipid profiles and quality-of-life measures than do their adult-onset counterparts. The interesting differences at baseline and in responses to GH are likely to reflect the biologic roles of GH at difference phases of life as well as the psychological impact of GH injections in the developing child. A patient with adult-onset disease is likely to recognize the restoration of a quality of life to a level once experienced before acquiring GH deficiency. In contrast,

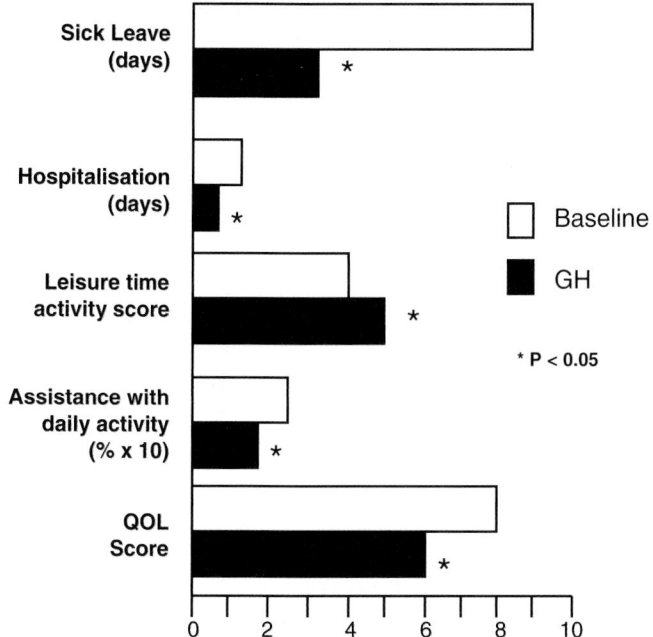

Figure 38-8 Changes in health care utilization and quality of life (QOL) measured at baseline and after 12 months of growth hormone replacement. The number of days of sick leave and hospitalization in the previous 6 months were taken as the baseline measures. QOL was assessed by a disease-specific questionnaire. (Reproduced from Hernberg-Stahl E, Luger A, Abs R, et al: Healthcare consumption decreases in parallel with improvements in quality of life during GH replacement in hypopituitary adults with GH deficiency. J Clin Endocrinol Metab 86:5277–5281, 2001, with permission.)

TREATMENT

DOSAGE

The Growth Hormone Research Society recommended that GH be commenced at a low dose (0.15 to 0.3 mg/day; 0.45 to 0.9 International Units/day), and that the dose gradually be increased in accordance with clinical and biochemical responses.[43] The maintenance dosage may vary considerably, is influenced by gender and age, but rarely exceeds 1 mg/day (3 International Units/day). Women appear to require higher doses than men, whereas the elderly require lower doses. A recent study of dose optimization designed to achieve normal IGF-1 levels reported the average daily maintenance dose to be 1.2 International Units in women and 0.8 International Units in men.[84] GH should be administered subcutaneously each day in the evening. Over a 5-year treatment period, the average weight-adjusted dose for women was 30% higher than that for men whose IGF-1 was one standard deviation higher than that in women[60] (Fig. 38-9). Thus, women require a larger dose of GH than do men.

What clinical end points should be monitored? A physical examination and careful history, with particular attention to quality-of-life questions, are of great value in monitoring treatment, and where possible, the partner's input should be sought. Serum IGF-1 is the most useful biochemical marker of GH response, the level of which should be maintained within an age-adjusted normal range. Clinical monitoring should include assessment of body composition (e.g., waist circumference, skin folds, or dual x-ray absorptiometry) and lipid measurements.

INTERACTIONS

GH may influence the metabolism of many substances including hormones and medications. GH stimulates the activity of the hepatic cytochrome P-450 system, a major pathway of the oxidative metabolism of several drugs including anticonvulsants and theophylline. It is likely that dosage adjustments may be necessary in patients commencing GH treatment. Cortisol also is metabolized by the hepatic cytochrome P-450 system. Biochemical evidence indicates that GH increases the metabolic disposition of cortisol and may increase the risk of adrenal insufficiency,[85] which has been reported in some studies.[58] Although a causal relation remains unproven, GH-deficient patients receiving GH therapy should be strongly

adults who received GH as a developing child have grown up with and adapted to the condition and are likely to harbor negative recollections of enforced daily injections. As GH therapy is terminated on epiphysial closure, which occurs before somatic maturation, conventionally GH-treated children may not reach their physical and developmental potential on termination of GH treatment for dwarfism.[72] The data suggest the existence of two clinical entities, developmental and metabolic, reflecting the function of GH at different stages of life.[6]

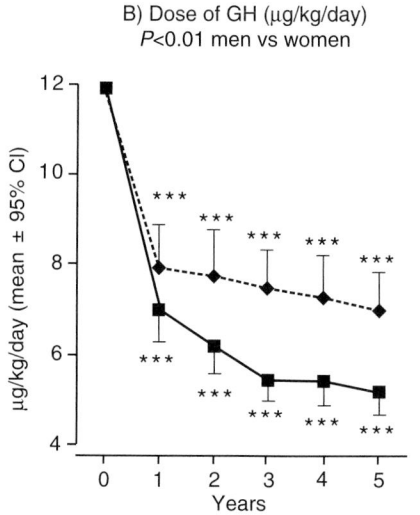

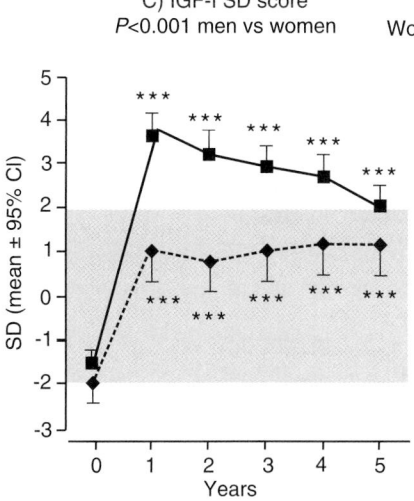

Figure 38-9 Growth hormone (GH) dose (µg/kg/day) and insulin-like growth factor (IGF)-1 standard deviation score in a group of 70 men and 48 women with GH deficiency treated for 5 years. The mean GH dose was lower, yet men attained higher IGF-1 responses than did women. (Reproduced from Gotherstrom G, Svensson J, Koranyi J, et al: A prospective study of 5 years of GH replacement therapy in GH-deficient adults: Sustained effects on body composition, bone mass and metabolic indices. J Clin Endocrinol Metab 86:4657–4665, 2001, with permission.)

advised to increase the dosage of glucocorticoids when unwell, as is generally recommended.

GH stimulates the peripheral conversion of T_4 to T_3. This effect may be frequently seen as a decrease in circulating T_4 levels, particularly in patients taking thyroid hormone replacement for hypopituitarism.[86] If T_3 is not monitored during GH replacement, a decrease in T_4 may be misinterpreted as inadequate substitution and may lead to unnecessary increase in the dosage of thyroid hormone replacement.

Sex steroids exert significant modulatory effects on GH action. Estrogen exerts significant effects on hepatic function that are dependent on the route of administration. When compared with the transdermal route, oral estrogen reduces IGF-1 and fat oxidation, effects that are opposite to those of GH.[87] GH-deficient women who are also hypogonadal should receive estrogen by a nonoral route during GH replacement. This is because oral but not transdermal estrogen attenuates the biologic effects of GH.[88] Fifty percent more GH was required during oral estrogen treatment to maintain an equivalent IGF-1 level than that during transdermal administration (see Fig. 38-8). In contrast, androgens enhance the metabolic effects of GH. The divergent effects of estrogens and androgens on GH action are a likely explanation for the observation that women are less responsive than men to GH[60,89] (Fig. 38-10).

SAFETY

The principle of hormone-replacement therapy predicates that hormone replacement restores the untreated, morbid hormone-deficient state to normal. Side effects may be encountered as a consequence of inappropriate dosage or the failure of the mode of hormone replacement to induce a pharmacokinetic profile that mimics normal physiology. The same issues apply to GH-replacement therapy. The experience from several large multicenter clinical trials indicates that GH treatment is safe and well tolerated.[58,90,91]

The most common side effects arise from the antinatriuretic action of GH, which causes fluid retention (Table 38-3). These manifest as dependent edema, paresthesia, and carpal tunnel syndrome and occur with greater frequency in older patients. However, these symptoms are mild, dose related, and resolve in the majority of patients either spontaneously or with dosage reduction.[92] The early trials used somewhat supraphysiologic doses of GH and encountered these side effects in up to 50% of patients. More recent trials using a dosage regimen designed to maintain IGF-1 levels in the normal range have encountered virtually no untoward effects.[67] GH-replacement dosage must be individualized, as is the case for other types of hormone-replacement therapies.

Although GH antagonizes insulin action, the risk of developing hyperglycemia is very low. Only two case of reversible diabetes were reported from two European multicenter trials with a combined total of 400 patients,[90,91] whereas diabetes developed in none of 166 patients in an Australian study.[58] Insulin sensitivity improves and may normalize after some months of treatment.[93] This paradoxical effect arises from the reduction in central abdominal fat, which ameliorates insulin resistance. No deterioration in insulin sensitivity was observed after 7 years of GH treatment.[94]

As GH promotes the growth of tissues, concern has been expressed that GH therapy may increase the risk of pituitary tumor recurrence or the development of neoplasia. Analysis of the extensive pediatric experience shows no convincing evidence for a causal link between GH treatment and tumor recurrence or the development of neoplasia,[95] including leukemia.[96] It was recently reported that mean IGF-1 levels are higher in patients with prostate and breast cancers than in controls.[97,98] One interpretation of these observations is that elevating IGF-1, which occurs with GH treatment, may increase the risk of developing prostate and breast cancers. If this is true, patients with acromegaly who have sustained elevated IGF-1 levels should have a higher incidence of these malignancies. Conflicting reports exist about whether cancer incidence is increased in this disease, and many have lacked statistical power. The best study to date, involving more than 1000 acromegalic patients, found overall cancer incidence rates to be lower than those in the general population.[99] No significant increase was found in site-specific cancer rates, including breast cancer. These data in acromegaly provide the strongest evidence against a causal association between IGF-1 and malignancy. Nevertheless, it is important for future

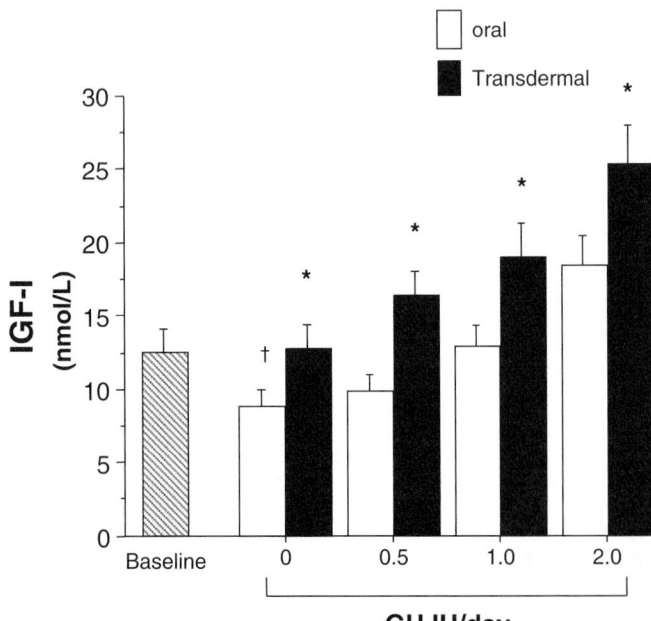

Figure 38-10 Mean insulin-like growth factor (IGF)-1 levels before and during incremental doses of growth hormone (GH; 0.5, 1.0, and 2.0 Units/day) during oral and transdermal estrogen therapy in eight GH-deficient adult women. (Reproduced from Wolthers T, Hoffman DM, Nugent AG, et al: Oral estrogen therapy impairs the metabolic effects of growth hormone [GH] in GH deficient women. Am J Physiol 281:E1191-E1196, 2001, with permission.)

Table 38-3	Treatment Guidelines for Growth Hormone (GH) Replacement in Adult GH Deficiency
Pretherapy	Adequate replacement of other hormone deficiencies
	Pituitary imaging
	Body composition
	IGF-1, BSL, lipids
Starting dose	0.15–0.3 mg/day (0.5–1.0 International Units)
Adjustments	Small monthly increment, 0.01–0.15 mg/day
Monitor	IGF-1 (dose titration)
	BSL, lipids
	Weight, body composition, quality-of-life measures
Side effects	Edema, arthralgia, myalgia, paresthesia
Dosage considerations	Avoid weight-based regimens
	Women require more GH than men
	Elderly require less GH than the young
	Requirements greater with oral than with transdermal estrogen therapy in women
Contraindications	Malignancy, intracranial hypertension, proliferative retinopathy

IGF-1, insulin-like growth factor 1; BSL, blood sugar level.

studies to establish whether the incidence of cancer or tumor recurrence in GH-replaced hypopituitary patients is different from that in untreated patients.

A workshop convened by the Growth Hormone Research Society concluded that GH replacement is safe. No evidence indicates that GH or IGF-1 induces tumor formation,[100] although GH and IGF-1 can stimulate growth of established tumors. Therefore, current recommendations for cancer prevention and early detection should be practiced in the adult with hypopituitarism treated with GH. Good clinical practice requires regular imaging of residual pituitary tumor. A baseline scan should be done before starting treatment. GH replacement does not impose a need for intensifying follow-up.

CONTRAINDICATIONS

Contraindications to GH replacement include active malignancy, benign intracranial hypertension, and proliferative retinopathy. Pregnancy is not a contraindication, although treatment should be discontinued in the second trimester, as GH is produced by the placenta.[43]

CONCLUSION

Adult patients with GH deficiency have impaired health characterized by abnormalities of fuel metabolism, body composition, physical performance, and psychological function, which adversely affect quality of life. Most, if not all, of these abnormalities improve or normalize with GH replacement. Side effects are minor, mostly relate to fluid retention, and can be minimized by individualizing dosage requirement. Because GH remains expensive, it is important that its use in adults be restricted to patients with proven GH deficiency. Based on the global evidence of efficacy and safety, adults with GH deficiency should have replacement with GH, a principle consistent with the tenet of hormone replacement for hormone deficiency in the practice of endocrinology.

REFERENCES

1. Raben MS: Growth hormone, 2: Clinical uses of human growth hormone. N Engl J Med 266:82–86, 1992.
2. Rosen T, Bengtsson BA: Epidemiology of adult onset hypopituitarism in Goteborg, Sweden during 1956-1987. Presented at the International Symposium on Growth Hormone and Growth Factors, Gothenburg, 1994, pp A3–A60 [Abstract].
3. Regal M, Paramo C, Sierra SM, Garcia-Mayor RV: Prevalence and incidence of hypopituitarism in an adult Caucasian population in northwestern Spain. Clin Endocrinol (Oxf) 55:735–740, 2001.
4. Littley MD, Shalet SM, Beardwell CG, et al: Hypopituitarism following external radiotherapy for pituitary tumours in adults. Q J Med 70:145–160, 1989.
5. Rosen T, Bengtsson B-A: Premature mortality due to cardiovascular disease in hypopituitarism. Lancet 336:285–288, 1990.
6. Attanasio AF, Lamberts SWJ, Matranga AMC: Adult growth hormone deficient patients demonstrate heterogeneity between childhood-onset and adult-onset before and during human GH treatment. J Clin Endocrinol Metab 82:82–88, 1997.
7. Abs R, Verhelst J, Maiter D, et al: Cabergoline in the treatment of acromegaly: A study in 64 patients. J Clin Endocrinol Metab 83:374–378, 1998.
8. Christ ER, Carroll PV, Sonksen PH: The etiology of growth hormone deficiency in human adult. In Bengtsson B-A (ed): Growth Hormone. Boston, Kluwer Academic Publishers, 1999, pp 97–108.
9. Bulow B, Hagmart L, Mikoczy Z, et al: Increased cerebrovascular mortality in patients with hypopituitarism. Clin Endocrinol 46:75–81, 1997.
10. Bates AS, Van't Hoff W, Jones JP, Clayton RN: The effect of hypopituitarism on life expectancy. J Clin Endocrinol Metab 81:1169–1172, 1996.
11. Tomlinson JW, Holden N, Hills RK, et al: Association between premature mortality and hypopituitarism: West Midlands Prospective Hypopituitary Study Group. Lancet 357:425–431, 2001.
12. Besson A, Salemi S, Gallati S, et al: Reduced longevity in untreated patients with isolated growth hormone deficiency. J Clin Endocrinol Metab 88:3664–3667, 2003.
13. De Boer H, Blok GJ, Voerman HJ, et al: Serum lipid levels in growth hormone deficient men. Metabolism 43:199–203, 1994.
14. Carroll PV, Christ ER, Bengtsson BA, et al: Growth hormone deficiency in adulthood and the effects of growth hormone replacement: A review. J Clin Endocrinol Metab 83:382–395, 1998.
15. Markussis V, Beyshah SA, Fisher C, et al: Detection of premature atherosclerosis by high resolution ultrasonography in symptom-free hypopituitary adults. Lancet 340:1188–1192, 1992.
16. Pfeiffer M, Verhovec R, Zizek B, et al: Growth hormone (GH) treatment reverses early atherosclerotic changes in GH-deficient adults. J Clin Endocrinol Metab 84:453–457, 1991.
17. Johansson JO, Landin K, Tengborn L, et al: High fibrinogen and plasminogen activator inhibitory activity in growth hormone-deficiency adults. Arterioscler Thromb 14:434–437, 1994.
18. Sesmilo G, Miller KK, Hayden D, Klibanski A: Inflammatory cardiovascular risk markers in women with hypopituitarism. J Clin Endocrinol Metab 86:5774–5781, 2001.
19. Hoffman DM, O'Sullivan AJ, Freund J, Ho KKY: Adults with growth hormone deficiency have abnormal body composition but normal energy metabolism. J Clin Endocrinol Metab 80:72–77, 1995.
20. Salomon F, Cuneo RC, Hesp R, Sonksen PH: The effects of treatment with recombinant human growth hormone on body composition and metabolism in adults with growth hormone deficiency. N Engl J Med 321:1797–1803, 1989.
21. Reaven G: Banting Lecture 1988: Role of insulin resistance in human disease. Diabetes 37:1595–1607, 1988.
22. Hew FL, Koschmann M, Christopher M, Alford K: Insulin resistance in growth hormone deficient adults: Defects in glucose utilisation and glycogen synthetase activity. J Clin Endocrinol Metab 81:555–564, 1996.
23. Beshyah SA, Henderseon A, Nithayanathan R, et al: Metabolic abnormalities in growth hormone deficient adults: Carbohydrate tolerance and lipid metabolism. Endocrinol Metab 1:173–180, 1994.
24. Kaufman J, Taelman P, Vermelen A, Vandeweghe M: Bone mineral status in growth hormone deficient males with isolated and multiple pituitary deficiencies. J Clin Endocrinol Metab 74:118–123, 1932.
25. Holmes SJ, Economou G, Whitehouse RW, et al: Reduced bone mineral densities in patients with adult onset growth hormone deficiency. J Clin Endocrinol Metab 78:669–674, 1994.
26. Wuster C, Abs R, Bengtsson BA, Bennmarker H, et al: The influence of growth hormone deficiency, growth hormone replacement therapy, and other aspects of hypopituitarism on fracture rate and bone mineral density. J Bone Miner Res 16:398–405, 2001.
27. Rosen T, Wilhelmsen L, Landin-Wilhelmsen K, et al: Increased fracture frequency in adults with hypopituitarism and growth hormone deficiency. Eur J Endocrinol 137:240–245, 1998.
28. Rutherford OM, Beshyah SA, Johnston DG: Quadriceps strength before and after growth hormone replacement in growth hormone deficient adults. Endocrinol Metab 1:44–47, 1994.
29. Cuneo RC, Salomon F, Wiles CM, et al: Growth hormone treatment of growth hormone deficient adults, I: Effects on muscle mass and strength. J Appl Physiol 70:688–694, 1991.

30. Cuneo RC, Salomon F, Wiles CM, et al: Growth hormone treatment of growth hormone deficient adults, II. Effects on exercise performance. J Appl Physiol 70:695–700, 1991.

31. Amato G, Carella C, Fazio S, et al: Body composition, bone metabolism, and heart structure and function in growth hormone (GH) deficient adults before and after GH replacement therapy. J Clin Endocrinol Metab 77:1671–1676, 1993.

32. Merola B, Cittadini A, Coloa A, et al: Cardiac structural and functional abnormalities in adult patients with growth hormone deficiency. J Clin Endocrinol Metab 77:1658–1661, 1993.

33. Shahi M, Beshyah SA, Hackett D, et al: Myocardial dysfunction in treated adult hypopituitarism: A possible explanation for increased cardiovascular mortality. Br Heart J 67:92–96, 1002.

34. Juul A, Behrenscheer A, Tims T, et al: Impaired thermoregulation in adults with growth hormone deficiency during heat exposure and exercise. Clin Endocrinol 38:237–244, 1993.

35. McGauley GA, Cuneo RC, Salomon FC, Sonksen PH: Psychological well-being before and after growth hormone treatment in adults with growth hormone deficiency. Horm Res 33(Suppl):52–54, 1990.

36. Rosen T, Wiren L, Wilhemsen L, et al: Decreased psychological well-being in adult patients with growth hormone deficiency. Clin Endocrinol 40:111–116, 1994.

37. Rikken B, Van Busschbach J, Le Cessie S, et al: Impaired social status of growth hormone deficient adults as compared to controls with short or normal stature. Clin Endocrinol 43:205–211, 1995.

38. Blum WF, Shavrikova EP, Edwards DJ, et al: Decreased quality of life in adult patients with growth hormone deficiency compared with general populations using the new, validated, self-weighted questionnaire, questions on life satisfaction hypopituitarism module. J Clin Endocrinol Metab 88:4158–4167, 2003.

39. Rosilio M, Blum WF, Edwards DJ, et al: Long-term improvement of quality of life during growth hormone (GH) replacement therapy in adults with GH deficiency, as measured by questions on life satisfaction-hypopituitarism (QLS-H). J Clin Endocrinol Metab 89:1684–1693, 2004.

40. Rudman D: Growth hormone, body composition and aging. J Am Geriatr Soc 33:800–807, 1985.

41. Ho KY, Evans WS, Blizzard RM, et al: Effects of sex and age on the 24 hour secretory profile of GH secretion in man: Importance of endogenous estradiol concentrations. J Clin Endocrinol Metab 64:51–58, 1987.

42. Iranmanesh A, Lizarralde G, Veldhuis JD: Age and relative adiposity are specific negative determinants of the frequency and amplitude of growth hormone (GH) secretory bursts and the half-life of endogenous GH in healthy men. J Clin Endocrinol Metab 73:1081–1088, 1991.

43. Growth Hormone Research Society: Consensus guidelines for the diagnosis and treatment of adults with growth hormone deficiency: Summary statement of the Growth Hormone Research Society Workshop on Adult Growth Hormone Deficiency. J Clin Endocrinol Metab 83:379–381, 1998.

44. Hoffman DM, O'Sullivan AJ, Baxter RC, Ho KKY: Diagnosis of growth hormone deficiency in adults. Lancet 343:1064–1068, 1994.

45. Hoffman DM, Ho KKY: Diagnosis of GH deficiency in adults. In Juul A, Jorgensen JOL (eds): Growth hormone in adults. Cambridge, Cambridge University Press, 1996, pp 168–185.

46. Ghigo E, Aimaretti G, Gianotti L, et al: New approach to the diagnosis of growth hormone deficiency in adults. Eur J Endocrinol 134:352–356, 1996.

47. Popovic V, Leal A, Micic D, et al: Combined administration of growth (GH) releasing hormone and GH-releasing peptide-6 as an effective diagnostic test of GH deficiency in adult. Lancet 356:1137–1142, 2000.

48. Mahajan T, Lightman SL: A simple test for growth hormone deficiency in adults. J Clin Endocrinol Metab 85:1473–1476, 2000.

49. Leal-Cerro A, Garcia E, Astorga R, et al: Growth hormone (GH) responses to the combined administration of GH-releasing peptide 6 in adults with GH deficiency. Eur J Endocrinol 132:712–715, 1995.

50. Ho KKY: Diagnosis of GH deficiency in adults [Editorial]. Lancet 356:1125–1126, 2000.

51. Reutens AT, Hoffman DM, Leung KC, Ho KKY: Evaluation and application of a highly sensitive assay for serum growth hormone (GH) in the study of adult GH deficiency. J Clin Endocrinol Metab 80:480–485, 1995.

52. Arosio M, Garrone S, Bruzzi P, et al: Diagnostic value of the acid-labile subunit in acromegaly: Evaluation in comparison with insulin-like growth factor (IGF) I, and IGF binding protein-1, –2, –3. J Clin Endocrinol Metab 86:1091–1098, 2001.

53. Toogood AA, Beardwell C, Shalet SM: The severity of growth hormone deficiency in adults with pituitary disease is related to the degree of hypopituitarism. Clin Endocrinol 41:511–516, 1994.

54. Hartman ML, Crowe BJ, Biller BM, et al: Which patients do not require a GH stimulation test for the diagnosis of adult GH deficiency? J Clin Endocrinol Metab 87:477–485, 2002.

55. Jorgensen JOL, Theusen L, Ingemann-Hansen T, et al: Beneficial effects of growth hormone treatment in GH-deficient adults. Lancet 1:1221–1225, 1989.

56. Gibney J, Wallace JD, Spinks T, et al: The effect of 10 years of recombinant human growth hormone (GH) in adult GH-deficient patients. J Clin Endocrinol Metab 184:2596–2602, 1999.

57. Weaver JU, Monson JP, Noonan K, et al: The effect of low dose recombinant human growth hormone replacement on regional fat distribution, insulin sensitivity and cardiovascular risk factors in hypopituitary patients. J Clin Endocrinol Metab 80:153–159, 1995.

58. Cuneo RC, Judd S, Wallace JD, et al: The Australian multicentre trial of growth hormone treatment in GH-deficient adults. J Clin Endocrinol Metab 83:107–116, 1998.

59. Beshyah SA, Henderson A, Niththyananthan R, et al: The effects of short and long term growth hormone replacement in hypopituitary adults on lipid metabolism and carbohydrate tolerance. J Clin Endocrinol Metab 80:356–363, 1995.

60. Gotherstrom G, Svensson J, Koranyi J, et al: A prospective study of 5 years of GH replacement therapy in GH-deficient adults: Sustained effects on body composition, bone mass and metabolic indices. J Clin Endocrinol Metab 86:4657–4665, 2001.

61. Borson-Chazot F, Serusclat A, Kalfallah Y, et al: Decrease in carotid intima-media thickness after one year growth hormone (GH) treatment in adults with GH deficiency. J Clin Endocrinol Metab 84:1329–1333, 1999.

62. Sesmilo G, Biller BM, Llevadot J, et al: Effects of growth hormone administration on inflammatory and other cardiovascular risk markers in men with growth hormone deficiency. A randomized, controlled clinical trial. Ann Intern Med 133:111–122, 2000.

63. Bengtsson B-A, Eden S, Lonn L, et al: Treatment of adults with growth hormone (GH) deficiency with recombinant human GH. J Clin Endocrinol Metab 76:309–317, 1993.

64. Jorgensen JOL, Theusen L, Muller J, et al: Three years of growth hormone treatment in growth-hormone deficient adults: Near normalisation of body composition and physical performance. Acta Endocrinol 130:224–228, 1994.

65. Hoffman DM, Crampton L, Sernia C, et al: Short term growth hormone (GH) treatment of GH deficient adults increases body sodium and extracellular water but not blood pressure. J Clin Endocrinol Metab 81:1123–1128, 1996.

66. Johannsson G, Rosen T, Bosaues I, et al: Two years of growth hormone treatment increases bone mineral content and density in hypopituitary patients with adult-onset growth hormone deficiency. J Clin Endocrinol Metab 81:2865–2873, 1996.

67. Baum HB, Biller BM, Finkelstein JS, Klibanski A: Effect of physiologic growth hormone therapy on bone density and body composition in patients with adult onset growth hormone deficiency: A randomised, placebo-controlled trial. Ann Intern Med 125:883–890, 1996.

68. Vandeweghe M, Taelman P, Kaufman J-M: Short and long term

effects of growth hormone treatment on bone turnover and bone mineral content in adult growth hormone-deficient males. Clin Endocrinol 39:409–415, 1993.

69. Ter Maaten JC, Be Boer H, Kamp O, et al: Long-term effects of growth hormone (GH) replacement in men with childhood-onset GH deficiency. J Clin Endocrinol Metab 84:2373–2380, 1999.

70. Valimaki MJ, Salmela PI, Salmi J, et al: Effects of 42 months of GH treatment on bone mineral density and bone turnover in GH-deficient adults. Eur J Endocrinol 140:545–554, 1999.

71. Christ ER, Cummins MH, Westwood NB, et al: The importance of growth hormone in the regulation of erythropoiesis, red cell mass, and plasma volume in adults with growth hormone deficiency. J Clin Endocrinol Metab 82:2985–2990, 1997.

72. Rutherford OM, Jones DA, Round JM, et al: Changes in skeletal muscle and body composition after discontinuation of growth hormone treatment in growth hormone deficient young adults. Clin Endocrinol 34:469–475, 1991.

73. Hulthen L, Bengtsson BA, Sunnerhagen KS, et al: GH is needed for the maturation of muscle mass and strength in adolescents. J Clin Endocrinol Metab 86:4765–4770, 2001.

74. Shalet SM, Shavrikova E, Cromer M, et al: Effect of growth hormone (GH) treatment on bone in postpubertal GH-deficient patients: A 2-year randomized, controlled, dose-ranging study. J Clin Endocrinol Metab 88:4124–4129, 2003.

75. Johannsson G, Grimby G, Sunnerhagen KS, Bengtsson BA: Two years of growth hormone (GH) treatment increase isometric and isokinetic muscle strength in GH-deficient adults. J Clin Endocrinol Metab 82:2877–2884, 1997.

76. Koranyi J, Svensson J, Gotherstrom G, et al: Baseline characteristics and the effects of five years of GH replacement therapy in adults with GH deficiency of childhood or adulthood onset: A comparative, prospective study. J Clin Endocrinol Metab 86:4693–4699, 2001.

77. Nass R, Huber RM, Klauss V, et al: effect of growth hormone (hGH) replacement therapy on physical work capacity and cardiac and pulmonary function in patients with hGH deficiency acquired in adulthood. J Clin Endocrinol Metab 80:552–557, 1995.

78. Thomas SG, Esposito JG, Ezzat S: Exercise training benefits growth hormone (GH)-deficient adults in the absence or presence of GH treatment. J Clin Endocrinol Metab 88:5734–5738, 2003.

79. Woodhouse LJ, Asa SL, Thomas SG, Ezzat S: Measures of submaximal aerobic performance evaluate and predict functional response to growth hormone (GH) treatment in GH-deficient adults. J Clin Endocrinol Metab 84:4570–4577, 1999.

80. Caidahl K, Eden S, Bengtsson BA: Cardiovascular and renal effects of growth hormone. Clin Endocrinol 40:393–400, 1994.

81. Valcavi R, Gaddi O, Zini M, et al: Cardiac performance and mass in adults with hypopituitarism: Effect of one year of growth hormone treatment. J Clin Endocrinol Metab 80:659–666, 1995.

82. Burman P, Broman JE, Hetta J, et al: Quality of life in adults with growth hormone (GH) deficiency: Response to treatment with recombinant GH in a placebo-controlled 21 month trial. J Clin Endocrinol Metab 80:3585–3590, 1995.

83. Hernberg-Stahl E, Luger A, Abs R, et al: Healthcare consumption decreases in parallel with improvements in quality of life during GH replacement in hypopituitary adults with GH deficiency. J Clin Endocrinol Metab 86:5277–5281, 2001.

84. Drake WM, Coyte D, Camacho-Hubner C, et al: Optimizing growth hormone replacement therapy by dose titration in hypopituitary adults. J Clin Endocrinol Metab 83:3913–3919, 1998.

85. Weaver JU, Thaventhiran L, Noonan K, et al: The effect of growth hormone replacement on cortisol metabolism and glucocorticoid sensitivity in hypopituitary adults. Clin Endocrinol 41:639–648, 1994.

86. Jorgensen JOL, Pedersen SA, Lauberg P, et al: Effects of growth hormone therapy on thyroid function of growth hormone-deficient adults with and without concomitant thyroxine-substituted central hypothyroidism. J Clin Endocrinol Metab 69:1127–1132, 1989.

87. O'Sullivan AJ, Crampton L, Freund J, Ho KKY: Route of estrogen replacement confers divergent effects on energy metabolism and body composition in postmenopausal women. J Clin Invest 102:1035–1040, 1998.

88. Wolthers T, Hoffman DM, Nugent AG, et al: Oral estrogen therapy impairs the metabolic effects of growth hormone (GH) in GH deficient women. Am J Physiol 281:E1191–E1196, 2001.

89. Burman P, Johansson AG, Siegbahn A, et al: Growth hormone (GH)-deficient men are more responsive to GH replacement therapy than women. J Clin Endocrinol Metab 82:550–555, 1997.

90. Mardh G, Lundin K, Borg G, et al: Growth hormone replacement therapy in adult hypopituitary patients with growth hormone deficiency: Combined data from 12 European placebo-controlled trials. Endocrinol Metab 1(Suppl A):43–49, 1994.

91. Chipman JJ, Attanasio AF, Birkett MA, et al: The safety profile of growth hormone replacement therapy in adults. Clin Endocrinol 46:473–481, 1997.

92. De Boer H, Blok GJ, Popp-Snijders C, et al: Monitoring of growth hormone replacement therapy in adult based on measurement of serum markers. J Clin Endocrinol Metab 80:2069–2076, 1996.

93. Hwu CM, Kwok CF, Lai TY, et al: Growth hormone replacement reduces total body fat and normalises insulin sensitivity in GH-deficient adults: A report of one-year clinical experience. J Clin Endocrinol Metab 82:3285–3292, 1997.

94. Svensson J, Fowelin J, Landin K, et al: Effects of seven years of GH-replacement therapy on insulin sensitivity in GH-deficient adults. J Clin Endocrinol Metab 87:2121–2127, 2002.

95. Allen D: National Cooperative Growth Study Safety Symposium: Safety of human growth hormone therapy. J Pediatr 128:S8–S13, 1996.

96. Nishi Y, Tanaka T, Takano K, et al: Recent status in the occurrence of leukemia in growth hormone-treated patients in Japan. J Clin Endocrinol Metab 84:1961–1965, 1999.

97. Chan JM, Stampfe MJ, Giovannucci E, et al: Plasma insulin-like growth factor 1 and prostate cancer risk: A prospective study. Science 279:563–566, 1998.

98. Hankinson SE, Willett WC, Colditz GA, et al: Circulating concentrations of insulin-like growth factor-I and risk of breast cancer. Lancet 351:1393–1396, 1998.

99. Orme SM, McNally RI, Cartwright RA, et al: Mortality and cancer incidence in acromegaly: A retrospective cohort study. J Clin Endocrinol Metab 83:2730–2734, 1998.

100. Growth Hormone Research Society: Consensus: Critical evaluation of the safety of recombinant human growth hormone administration: Statement from the Growth Hormone Research Society. J Clin Endocrinol Metab 86:1868–1870, 2001.

IMMUNOLOGY AND ENDOCRINOLOGY

CHAPTER 39

Immunologic Mechanisms Causing Autoimmune Endocrine Disease

Monica Girotra, Jeffrey A. Bluestone, and Kevan C. Herold

It has been shown that many endocrine disorders are mediated by autoimmune mechanisms. These autoimmune attacks can target almost any of the endocrine glands, leading to diverse clinical manifestations ranging from the destruction of the organ (e.g., Hashimoto's disease or type 1 diabetes mellitus) to overstimulation of the endocrine gland and hypersecretion of hormones (e.g., Graves' disease) (Table 39-1). Studies point to common pathways that lead to these diseases involving the dysregulation of immune T and B lymphocytes. This chapter provides an overview of the basic processes that control the immune response and relates these mechanisms to the pathogenesis of autoimmune endocrine diseases. The identification and improved understanding of these pathways may represent targets for immune therapy.

STRUCTURAL AND FUNCTIONAL BIOLOGY OF T LYMPHOCYTES

In most experimental models of autoimmune endocrine diseases, T cells play a central role in the pathogenesis of the disease. In an animal model of spontaneous thyroiditis, the OS chicken, the disease is mediated by T cells. T-cell depletion, within a day of hatching, prevents later development of thyroiditis.[1] In all animal models of type 1 diabetes mellitus, T-cell depletion prevents disease, and diabetes can be adoptively transferred by T cells or splenocytes.[2–4] T-cell clones that proliferate in response to autoantigens have been isolated from animal models of and patients with type 1 diabetes mellitus.[5] These T cells are thought to play an important role in the immune-mediated destruction of β cells in type 1 diabetes mellitus.

The precise prevalence of cellular responses to endocrine tissues in the general population is unknown. It is likely, however, that cell-mediated responses are more frequent than initially suspected. Focal thyroiditis can be found at autopsy in 6% of men and 22% of women without known thyroid disease.[6] Low levels of cellular autoimmunity are tolerated in many normal individuals without progression to autoimmune disease. Identifying the factors that modulate progression

from tolerable levels to autoimmune disease is key to understanding disease pathogenesis and designing interventions to prevent disease.

STRUCTURE AND ACTIVATION PATHWAYS OF THE T-CELL RECEPTOR

T cells express a receptor complex consisting of unique antigen-specific receptors (T-cell receptors [TCRs]) associated with a multimolecular complex of molecules, CD3ε, CD3δ, CD3γ, and CD3ζ. These associated monomorphic proteins are responsible for signal transduction (Fig. 39-1).[7–10] The part of the TCR complex that binds to antigen includes a heterodimer consisting of α/β or γ/δ chains. In humans, 95% of circulating T cells are α/β (TCR αβ), and the remainder express γ/δ chains (TCR γδ). α/β T cells can be differentiated further by expression of CD4 or CD8 molecules on their cell surfaces. These molecules are members of the immunoglobulin family of cell surface molecules. CD4 or CD8 molecules bind to class II or class I major histocompatibility complex (MHC) molecules on antigen-presenting cells (APCs) (discussed later), playing a crucial role in T-cell development and subsequent antigen recognition.[10,11]

The signaling through the TCR/CD3 complex has been shown to depend on a cascade of biochemical events dependent on tyrosine phosphorylation and subsequent downstream kinase activation (Fig. 39-2).[12] Ligation of the TCR leads to the immediate activation of the associated src kinases (p56lck and p59fyn). This activation results in the phosphorylation of tyrosines localized within intracellular domains of the TCR/CD3 complex proteins, CD3γ, CD3δ, CD3ε, and CD3ζ. These tyrosines are part of a regulatory sequence of amino acids, termed the *immune receptor tyrosine activation motif (ITAM)*.[13] The phosphorylation of the ITAMs leads to a cascade of subsequent kinase activation, phosphorylation, and dephosphorylation of downstream proteins.[14] An important early event in T-cell activation is the phosphorylation of the membrane-anchored adapter protein, LAT (linker of activation of T cells), by the tyrosine kinase ZAP-70. Adapter proteins set in motion two major signaling cascades, one involving

Table 39-1   **Endocrine Diseases Most Likely Due to Autoimmune Mechanisms**

Chronic lymphocytic thyroiditis (Hashimoto's disease)
Graves' disease
Postpartum thyroiditis
Type 1 diabetes mellitus
Type B insulin resistance
Autoimmune hypoglycemia (insulin autoantibodies)
Autoimmune oophoritis
Autoimmune orchitis
Addison's disease
Autoimmune hypophysitis
Autoimmune hypoparathyroidism
Type 1 polyendocrine autoimmunity
   Chronic mucocutaneous candidiasis
   Hypoparathyroidism
   Addison's disease
Adrenal medullary autoantibodies
Primary (adrenal) pigmented and nodular forms of Cushing's syndrome

phospholipase Cγ1 (PLCγ-1) activation and the other involving activation of the cellular protein ras. These events result in additional biochemical signals ultimately leading to the activation of the mitogen-activated protein kinase (MAPK) pathway and the phosphatase calcineurin. Calcineurin promotes activation of the nuclear transcription factors, AP-1, NFAT, and NFκB, which leads to cytokine transcription. Protein phosphorylation, after receptor engagement, controls T-lymphocyte behavior.

Defects in TCR signaling have been postulated to play a role in the development of autoimmune endocrine disease. Rapoport and colleagues[15] described impaired TCR activation pathways in the nonobese diabetic (NOD) mouse, a model of spontaneous type 1 diabetes mellitus. They identified defective TCR-mediated signaling along the protein kinase C/Ras/MAPK pathway of T-cell activation. In addition, the FcR non-binding anti-CD3 monoclonal antibody (mAb) and altered peptide ligands (discussed later) proposed for treatment of autoimmune diseases are thought to alter the normal T-cell activation cascade.[16,17]

PHENOTYPICALLY AND FUNCTIONALLY DISTINCT T-CELL SUBSETS

Initial studies of TCR αβ T lymphocytes showed two distinct subsets based on the expression of CD4 or CD8 glyproteins.

These subsets differentially recognize peptides in the context of class II versus class I MHC molecules.[11] It has become increasingly clear, however, that CD4+ and CD8+ T cells can be subclassified further into functionally distinct subsets. Naive T cells activated by antigen/MHC complexes (a process called *T-cell priming*) can differentiate into mature effector phenotypes based on the production of different soluble mediators called *cytokines*. This paradigm, delineated initially in mice, also occurs in humans.[18,19] The most distinctive subsets of CD4+ or T-helper cells are designated *Th0, Th1,* and *Th2*. Th0 cells, the least differentiated subset, can be driven by stimulation with antigen and costimulatory signals to differentiate into Th1 cells, which secrete interleukin (IL)-2 and interferon (IFN)-γ, or Th2 cells, which secrete IL-4.[20] Th1 cells mediate classic delayed hypersensitivity reactions, whereas Th2 cells provide help for B cells as they differentiate into antibody-producing plasma cells. Even Th1 cells influence antibody production, however, by altering the immunoglobulin isotypes produced during an immune response. In humans, the IgG subclass IgG4 is associated with Th2 responses (IgG1 in mice), whereas IgG1 is associated with Th1 responses (IgG2a in mice).[21] Several families of T-cell transcription factors have been identified, including Ikaros, LKLF, GATA3, and c-maf, which control differentiation of T cells at the molecular level.[22] Studies in mice indicate that the affinity of the TCR for its ligand interactions between T cells and costimulatory molecules and cytokines themselves can alter T-cell differentiation into one or another phenotype.[23,24] This is most apparent in mouse models in which T cells from TCR transgenic mice can differentiate into either Th1 or Th2 cells depending on the inflammatory milieu in which they differentiate. IFN-γ and IL-12 promote differentiation of precursor cells into Th1 cells by preventing the outgrowth of Th2 cells and augmentation of Th1 differentiation.[25] The transcription factor, T-bet, regulates lineage commitment of T-helper lymphocytes partly by activating IFN-γ.[26] IL-15 also has been shown to stimulate human Th1-cell differentiation, whereas the transcription factors, GATA-3 and c-MAF, and the prototypic Th2 cytokine, IL-4, have the greatest influence in driving Th2 differentiation.[25,27–29]

Since at least the 1970s, there has been the notion that in addition to the above-noted T-cell subsets, which are essential to promote immunity, there are classes of regulatory/suppressor T cells that exist to control immunity. CD8+ T cells have been identified that suppress immune responses through their direct cytotoxicity on antigen-bearing cells or through the production of suppressive cytokines.[30] The modern view of CD4+ regulatory T cells began with the observation by

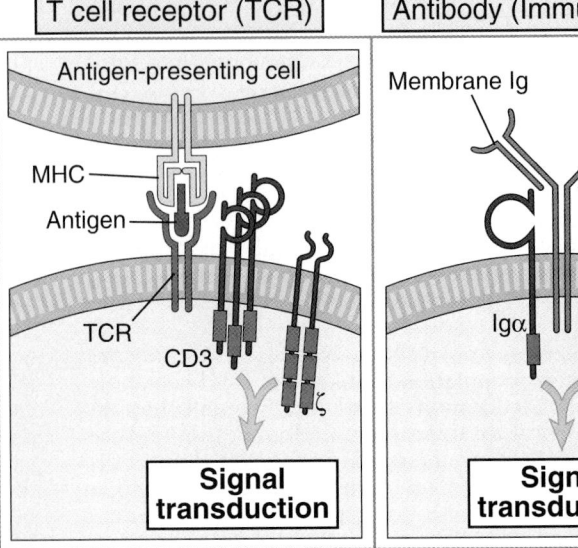

Figure 39-1   Antigen recognition and signaling of lymphocyte antigen receptors. **A,** The T-cell receptor (TCR) is the antigen receptor on the T lymphocyte that recognizes antigen presented by MHC molecules on antigen-presenting cells. The TCR is associated with CD3 proteins, which are responsible for signal transduction. **B,** The membrane immunoglobulin (mIg) is the antigen receptor on the B lymphocyte. The signal transduction component of the mIg comprises a disulfide-bonded heterodimer of the Igα and Igβ molecules. (From Abbas AK, Lichtman AH: Cellular and Molecular Immunology. Philadelphia, WB Saunders, 2003.)

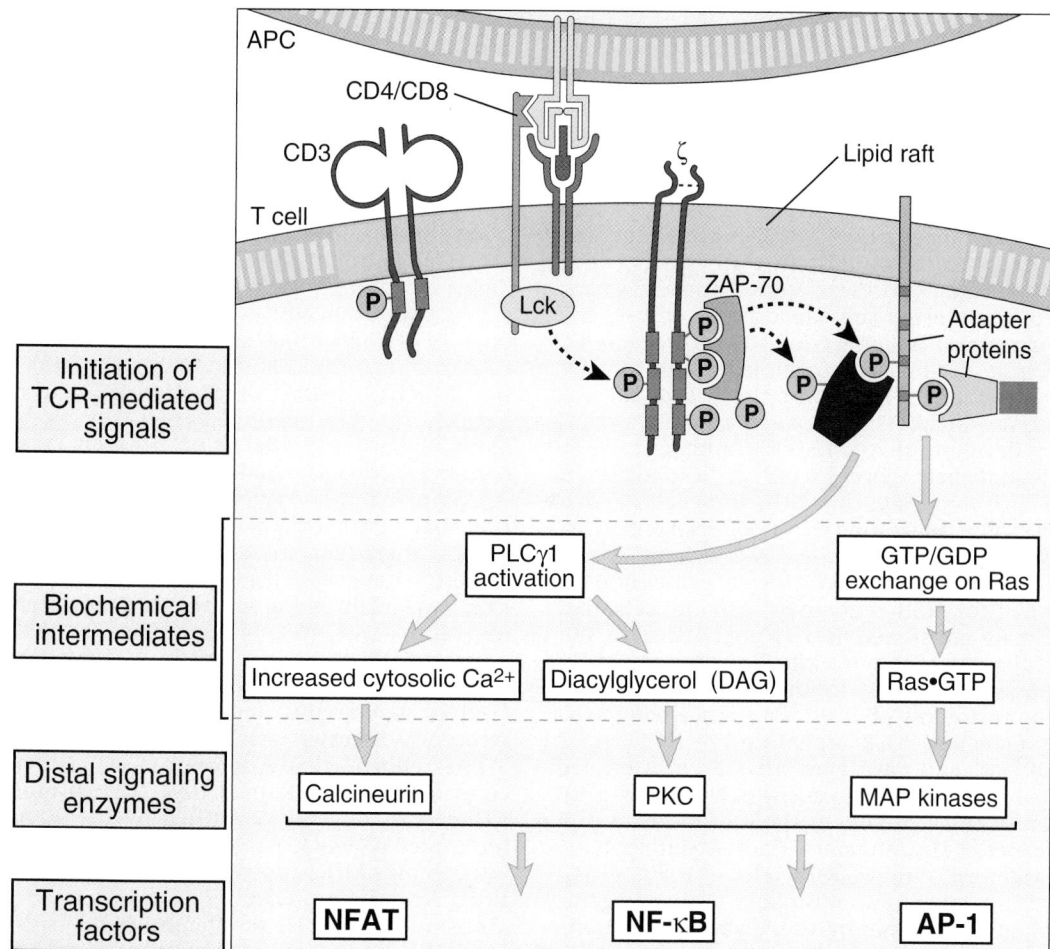

Figure 39-2   Intracellular signaling events during T-cell activation. Binding of the T-cell receptor (TCR) to the antigen-MHC complex on the antigen-presenting cell (APC) initiates proximal signaling events, which lead to the phosphorylation of the CD3ζ molecule, binding and activation of ZAP-70, phosphorylation of adapter proteins, and activation of various cellular enzymes. These enzymes ultimately activate transcription factors that lead to the expression of genes involved in T-cell responses. (From Abbas AK, Lichtman AH: *Cellular and Molecular Immunology.* Philadelphia, WB Saunders, 2003.)

Wood and Sakaguchi[31] that the adoptive transfer of T cells depleted of CD25+ cells induced multiorgan autoimmunity in the recipient animals. This observation was extended from studies carried out almost 40 years earlier, which showed that thymectomy of mice 3 days after birth leads to systemic autoimmunity.[32] Similar to Th1 and Th2 cells, regulatory T-cell (T_{reg}) development and function is controlled by a specific transcription factor, Foxp3 (forkhead box p3). Foxp3 controls expression of the suppressive phenotype and is the master control gene for these cells. Studies have shown that regulatory T cells that develop in the periphery under certain immune contexts can be characterized by the expression of Foxp3.[33]

T_{reg} cells can be delineated into two subsets: natural and adaptive regulatory T cells. Natural T_{reg} cells are characterized most commonly by the constitutive expression of CD25 and only represent a minor (5% to 10%) component of CD4+ T cells (but possess potent suppressive activity in vivo and in vitro[34]). Natural T_{reg} cells develop during the normal process of T-cell maturation in the thymus, resulting in an endogenous, or "natural," population of antigen-specific T_{reg} cells that survives as a long-lived population in the periphery poised to prevent potentially pathologic autoimmune reactions. The second subset of "adaptive" T_{reg} cells develops as a consequence of activation of mature T cells under particular conditions of suboptimal antigen exposure or costimulation or both.[34] The adaptive subset of T_{reg} cells functions mainly

as a homeostatic control over various adaptive immune responses by producing immunosuppressive cytokines, such as transforming growth factor (TGF)-β and IL-10.[35]

Several variables associated with T-cell activation affect the development of the final phenotype.[21] The antigen dose and the antigen itself may affect differentiation. Weak TCR signals also have been found to promote differentiation into Th2 cells, whereas strong signals can cause differentiation into Th1 cells.[36] Likewise, ligands that provide an altered signal to the TCR, such as altered peptide ligands and the FcR nonbinding anti-CD3 antibody, have been shown to skew differentiation toward a Th2 response.[16,17,37] In addition to the TCR signal, costimulatory signals and cytokines (discussed later) are important variables contributing to T-cell activation and the resulting cell phenotype. The involvement of particular costimulatory ligands and cytokines depends on several other factors, such as the tissue involved and other associated cells. Regulatory T cells also are influenced greatly by antigen context and concentration during thymic development and in the periphery. Low doses of continual antigenic exposure or altered signaling, as in the case of altered peptide ligands or dimeric anti-CD3 therapy, leads to a profound increase in regulatory T-cell activity.[33,38]

The final phenotype of a cell has important implications for the cell's ability to mediate autoimmune disease. In most instances, cell-mediated immune responses associated with autoimmune endocrine diseases have been associated with Th1 cytokines (IFN-γ and IL-2), and protection from autoimmune endocrine disease has been associated with Th2 cytokines (IL-4). In all models of type 1 diabetes mellitus, IFN-γ can be found in the islets of Langerhans, and the blockade of IFN-γ with anti-IFN-γ antibody prevents the disease in a mouse model of type 1 diabetes mellitus.[39,40]

The relationships between T-cell phenotype and autoimmune endocrine disease have been studied extensively in a murine model of spontaneous type 1 diabetes mellitus, the NOD mouse. In these mice, insulitis first appears between 2 and 4 weeks of age, and diabetes is detected beginning after 15 weeks of age. As discussed subsequently, T cells are the mediators of the disease, although B lymphocytes are required for initiation of insulitis. In NOD mice, expression of Th1 cytokines can be detected by 1 to 2 months of age. There is an increase in expression of Th1 cytokines in female mice, in which diabetes develops in 70% to 90%, but a decrease in male mice, in which diabetes develops only in 10% to 20%.[41] Genetic absence of IFN-γ delays, but does not prevent, diabetes in the NOD mouse, suggesting that IFN-γ is an enhancer, rather than a requirement, for disease.[42] Monoclonal T cells expressing a TCR reactive with islet antigen cause autoimmune diabetes when they differentiate in vitro into cells that produce IFN-γ and are transferred into young NOD mice, but not when they differentiate in vitro into IL-4 producers.[43] In addition, differentiation of cells toward a Th1 phenotype, enhanced by administration of IL-12, can exacerbate NOD diabetes.[44] The defective TCR signaling in NOD mice described by Rapoport and colleagues[45] has been associated with impaired IL-4 production. Treatment of NOD mice with IL-4 or expression of this cytokine in the islets leads to protection from diabetes.[46] The situation is not as simple, however, as progression of disease with Th1 cytokines and protection with Th2 cytokines. Although TCR transgenic T cells of a Th2 phenotype do not transfer diabetes into young NOD mice, they do so into NOD/scid animals, which have defective T-cell and B-cell development secondary to the scid mutation.[47] Finally, the role of regulatory cytokines produced in part by suppressor CD4+ and CD8+ T cells remains complex. Although treatment of NOD mice with IL-10 protected against diabetes,[48] Wogensen and colleagues[49] found that in NOD mice producing IL-10 in islets as a transgene developed accelerated diabetes, even though the islet infiltrating cells were of a Th2 phenotype. In addition, IL-10 knockout NOD mice also develop diabetes.[50,51] The basis for this difference is unclear, but perhaps under certain circumstances IL-10 controls TGF-β production. TGF-β may control diabetes in certain conditions, whereas in others, IL-10 may precipitate disease.[51]

This and other observations, discussed subsequently, suggest that an interaction between the cytokine milieu at the time of antigen recognition and a diverse population of cells present at that site ultimately determines the pathogenicity of the response. Another example is that NOD mice expressing IL-4 as a transgene in the islets of Langerhans do not develop diabetes. When the T-cell repertoire of the IL-4 transgenic animal is restricted to a single subtype reactive toward a specific antigen, however, the protection with IL-4 is lost, and the mice develop disease. These studies have been interpreted to indicate that cytokines, including IL-4 and IL-10, are important in preventing the progression of pathogenic antigen-specific responses, but the targets of their action are not the primary effector T cells.[52]

REQUIREMENT FOR COSTIMULATION FOR T-CELL ACTIVATION

Engagement of the TCR alone is insufficient to cause conventional activation of T cells and differentiation into effector cells. Delivery of the TCR signal alone, in the absence of a costimulatory signal, may result in T-cell unresponsiveness (or anergy) or even apoptosis (programmed cell death).[53,54] A second costimulatory signal is required for the development of

fully competent T cells and B cells. Costimulation regulates expansion of antigen-reactive populations of T cells, migration of cells to sites of inflammation, production of soluble mediators of inflammation, and differentiation of T cells into the subsets discussed earlier. It is expected that these interactions can control autoimmune endocrine disease.

Costimulatory signals are generated through the interaction between receptors on the surfaces of T cells and ligands on the surfaces of APCs. The interactions between these molecules are not antigen-specific. The combination of signals delivered through the TCR and costimulatory molecules are synergistic for T-cell activation. Activation leads to the production of IL-2 with other cytokines and chemokines, rescues cells from apoptosis, and leads to expansion of mature effector T cells capable of mediating a sustained immune response.[55,56] Most peripheral tissues do not express costimulatory signals, and interaction between T cells reactive with peripheral antigens would not normally be expected to result in competent T-cell activation. This control of T-cell activation may be important in regulating tolerance to peripheral tissues, including endocrine organs. Several costimulatory receptors have now been described. These can be separated into two main groups: the immunoglobulin superfamily, including CD28, CTLA-4 (cytotoxic T lymphocyte–associated antigen 4), PD-1 (programmed cell death-1), ICOS (inducible T-cell costimulator), and the tumor necrosis factor receptor (TNFR) superfamily, including CD40, OX-40, and 4-1BB receptors (discussed later) (Table 39-2).

The cell surface glycoprotein, CD28, interacts with molecules on the APC termed *B7-1* (CD80) and *B7-2* (CD86).[57] CD28 originally was identified by the ability of anti-CD28 molecules to block T-cell anergy after their encounter with antigen plus MHC complexes. B7-1 (CD80) was the first identified ligand for CD28. B7-1 transfectants can costimulate antigen-driven T-cell proliferation and IL-2 production and block the induction of anergy of T-cell clones.[58-61] There is considerable evidence for the relevance of CD28 and B7-1/B7-2 costimulatory signals in endocrine disease.[62] As noted earlier, most peripheral tissues do not express costimulatory signals. B7-1 expression has been found, however, on thyroid follicular cells in patients with Hashimoto's thyroiditis.[63,64] It has been postulated that this expression may lead preferentially to a Th1 cytokine pattern resulting in thyroid cell destruction.[64,65] In a mouse model of type 1 diabetes mellitus, Lenschow and coworkers[66] found that a soluble CD28 antagonist, human CTLA-4 (hCTLA-4Ig), can prevent diabetes. The blockade of CD28 costimulation by this agent resulted in skewing of the T-cell responses toward a Th2 phenotype. In this regard, treatment of mice with anti-CD28 antibodies also blocked disease progression, highlighting the crucial role of costimulation in the pathogenesis of type 1 diabetes mellitus

Table 39-2	Costimulatory Receptors and Ligands	
Costimulatory Molecule	Ligand(s)	Reference
STIMULATORY MOLECULES		
CD28	B7-1 (CD80), B7-2 (CD86)	57
?	B7-H3	409, 410
ICOS	B7-H1	97, 409, 411
CD40L (CD154)	CD40	107, 118, 121
OX40	OX40R	
4-1BB (CD137)	4-1BBL	117
ICAM-1	LFA-1, LFA-3	412
INHIBITORY MOLECULES		
CTLA-4 (CD152)	CD80, CD86	78, 267
CD30	CD30L	117
PD-1	PD-L1, PD-L2	84, 86, 88

in this model.[67] Transgenic expression of B7-1 on islet cells in the NOD mouse leads to accelerated diabetes, and its expression on islets of normal mice leads to susceptibilty to autoimmune diabetes induced with multiple low doses of streptozotocin.[68–70] β-cell B7-1 expression in transgenic mice also disrupts the natural resistance of the pancreas to T cell–mediated autoimmune destruction, resulting in severe insulitis and diabetes after exposure to autoantigen.[71] These studies indicated that provision of a CD28 costimulatory signal subsequent to antigen recognition is sufficient to activate islet antigen-reactive cells. Antibodies against B7-1 do not block T-cell stimulation completely, however, and cells from mice deficient in B7-1 still can stimulate antigen-specific T-cell responses.[58] NOD mice deficient in B7-1 develop accelerated diabetes, suggesting an important role in immune regulation.[58]

A second CD28 ligand, B7-2, was subsequently identified and cloned.[72,73] A combination of antibodies against B7-1 and B7-2 completely inhibits antigen-specific T-cell responses in vitro. In contrast to B7-1, NOD mice deficient in B7-2 are completely protected from diabetes, but develop a peripheral neuropathy at a later age.[74] The cells from the B7-2 knockout NOD mouse are capable of immune responsiveness, but either are not receiving signals needed for a destructive islet response or are controlled by immune regulatory cells (discussed later). The role of B7-1 and B7-2 in the differentiation of immune regulatory cells in diabetes was shown by Salomon and associates.[75] This group found that mice lacking CD28 or B7-1 and B7-2 developed diabetes because they failed to develop CD4+/CD25+ regulatory T cells.[75] In murine autoimmune thyroiditis, blockade of B7-2 inhibited priming and in vitro activation of effector T cells.[76] By virtue of their ability to induce cytokine production, costimulatory signals can affect autoimmune responses in positive and negative ways. Arreaza and coworkers[77] found that the treatment of young NOD mice with an agonistic anti-CD28 mAb restored deficient IL-4 production and prevented autoimmune diabetes. These results contrast with the results of Lenschow and colleagues, in which treatment with the CD28 antagonist, human CTLA-4Ig, promoted Th2 function.[58] These conflicting studies exemplify the complex role of costimulation in the regulation of autoimmunity due to its effects on T-cell differentiation, survival, and regulatory pathways. CD28/B7 costimulation can affect characteristics of the immune response, which ultimately may determine its ability to induce disease.

Rather than an activation signal, the second B7 ligand, CTLA-4, imparts a negative signal to T cells. CTLA-4 inhibits TCR signal transduction by binding to the TCR and inhibiting tyrosine phosphorylation after T-cell activation.[78] This important interaction can regulate T-cell activation and differentiation.[79] Similar to CD28, CTLA-4 binds ligands B7-1 and B7-2, but does so with much higher affinity; this is believed to play a role in the modulation of immune responses after activation because CTLA-4 expression is increased after T-cell activation.[80,81] Its importance in control of autoimmune responses has been shown in many animal models, with mice deficient in CTLA-4 dying of autoimmune disease involving the heart, pancreas, and other organs at a young age (discussed later).[82]

The tryptophan-degrading enzyme indoleamine 2,3-dioxygenase (IDO) seems to be involved in regulating antigen activation and proliferation of T cells and is linked closely to the CD28/CTLA-4 costimulatory pathway. Human monocyte-derived dendritic cells (DCs) express IDO and are able to suppress antigen-driven T-cell proliferation. The enhanced expression of IDO on DCs requires ligation of B7 on DCs by CTLA-4 or CD28 expressed on T cells. IDO activation via engagement of B7-1/B7-2 molecules on DCs may regulate T-cell responses and help limit autoimmunity.[83]

Another negative regulatory molecule has been described, named *programmed death-1* (PD-1).[84–86] This molecule is found on activated T cells and binds to two known ligands, PD-L1 (also named *B7-H1*) and PD-L2 (also named *B7-DC*), found on APCs and on diverse parenchymal cell types.[86–88] Ligation of the PD-1 receptor inhibits cell proliferation and IL-2 production and induces cell cycle arrest.[89] The development of an autoimmunity in the absence of PD-1 is analogous to the phenotype of CTLA-4–deficient animals.[90] This situation has led to the hypothesis that PD-1 may play a central role in the maintenance of peripheral tolerance toward autoantigens.[91] In animal models, this molecule has been implicated in the pathogenesis of type 1 diabetes mellitus, autoimmune cardiomyopathy, and a lupus-like syndrome (discussed later).

ICOS, also a member of the immunoglobulin superfamily of receptors, is expressed on activated T cells. The ligand for ICOS, B7H, is constitutively expressed on B cells and non-lymphoid tissues, including the lung, brain, and heart.[95] ICOS plays an important role in T-cell activation and proliferation and may help regulate Th2 cell differentiation.[96–98] In addition, ICOS has been shown to have a crucial role in humoral responses, with ICOS-deficient mice having defects in T cell–dependent antibody isotype switching and germinal center formation.[99] Homozygous mutation of ICOS in humans leads to an immunodeficiency syndrome characterized by the severe reduction in all immunoglobulin subclasses.[100] With respect to autoimmune disease, ICOS knockout mice develop more severe experimental allergic encephalomyelitis, a mouse model of multiple sclerosis.[101] It has been suggested that ICOS may be an important signaling molecule for regulatory T cells that control autoimmune diabetes in the NOD model.[102]

CD40, a member of the TNFR superfamily, was first identified as the receptor on T cells for the costimulatory ligand CD40L (CD154) on B lymphocytes.[103] Humans with a genetic mutation of CD40L are immunodeficient and develop the hyper-IgM syndrome. This disease is characterized by elevated levels of IgM; low levels of IgA, IgG, and IgE; and the absence of lymph node germinal centers. This observation and other murine studies indicate a primary role of CD40/CD154 interactions in the regulation of B-cell proliferation and function.[104] CD40/CD154 interactions can regulate APC function of B cells and DCs through induction of other costimulatory ligands, especially B7 molecules. Initial studies suggested that CD40/CD40L interactions may be important primarily as an inducer of B7 expression on APCs. Full reconstitution of cellular and humoral immunity was achieved in CD40L-deficient mice by administration of an activating antibody to CD40 that increased expression of B7-2.[105] CD40/CD40L interactions also provide additional functional effects in addition to B7-1 and B7-2 interactions and can costimulate T cells independently.[106] CD40L/CD40 interactions are thought to be important early in the immune response, but less important after initiation. Blockade of CD40/CD40L interactions can prevent diabetes in the NOD mouse only if administered early in life and cannot block recurrent insulitis.[107,108] In the setting of allograft rejection of pancreatic islets, blockade of CD40L with anti-CD154 mAb was effective in preventing graft loss in nonhuman primates. Long-term follow-up of these animals suggested that treatment with anti-CD154 mAb may have induced tolerance to the islet grafts.[109,110] A combination of anti-CD154 mAb with donor spleen cells has been shown to induce immunologic tolerance in a rodent model of diabetes and islet transplantation.[111,112] It was a great disappointment when human trials with anti-CD154 mAb were halted because of the development of thromboses secondary to the expression of CD154 on activated platelets.[113] Efforts are under way, however, to develop anti-CD40 mAbs to block the CD40 receptor, which, it is hoped, may limit toxicity. With respect to thyroid disease, human thyroid follicular cells have been shown to express CD40.[114,115] CD40 expressed by these nonimmune cells may interact with CD40L on T cells and contribute to the progression in autoimmune thyroid disease.[64] In the NOD mouse model of diabetes, regulation of DCs by CD4+ regulatory T cells has been shown to be controlled by CD40/CD40L interactions.[116]

Other costimulatory interactions also have been found to be important in autoimmune responses, particularly in the absence of costimulation by CD28, CD40L, or the cytokines IL-2 or IL-4. The OX-40 (OX-40R) and 4-1BB (CD137) receptors are additional members of the TNFR superfamily and are present on activated T cells.[117] When engaged by an agonist, such as anti-OX-40 antibody or the OX-40 ligand (OX-40L) during antigen presentation to T-cell lines, the OX-40R generates a costimulatory signal that is as potent as CD28 costimulation.[118] These signals help regulate the accumulation of antigen-reactive T cells during immune responses.[119] Engagement of OX-40R enhances effector and memory-effector T-cell function by upregulating IL-2 production and increasing the life span of effector T cells. Blocking OX-40/OX-40R interactions has been found to decrease experimental allergic encephalomyelitis, a model of multiple sclerosis.[120-122] 4-1BB receptor signaling also promotes effector and memory T-cell function and is thought to perform similar functions as OX-40R.[117,123,124] Transgenic NOD mice overexpressing a 4-1BB agonist in pancreatic β cells develop more severe diabetes than nontransgenic NOD mice. These mice overexpressing the 4-1BB agonist had earlier diabetes onset, more severe insulitis, and higher mortality.[125]

FUNCTIONAL BIOLOGY OF B LYMPHOCYTES

The hallmark of autoimmune endocrine diseases is the presence of autoantibodies directed against organ-specific antigens. Autoantibodies to endocrine antigens are common in the general population. In one cross-sectional study, 10.3% of women and 2.7% of men without thyroid dysfunction were found to have thyroid autoantibodies.[126] Likewise, 3.1% of first-degree relatives of patients with type 1 diabetes have islet cell antibodies. Only 1% of relatives progress to diabetes over a 7-year period, however.[127] These clinical observations suggest that autoreactive B cells do not always result in clinical disease and are tolerated by the host. These observations also indicate that autoantibodies alone are not sufficient to cause autoimmune endocrine disease.

The antigen-specific–binding receptor on B cells is membrane immunoglobulin (mIg), which is a tetrameric complex of immunoglobulin heavy (H) and light (L) chains.[128] Similar to T cells, B-cell function also depends on signal transduction pathways.[129] The signal transduction component of the mIg comprises a disulfide-bonded heterodimer of the Igα and Igβ molecules (see Fig. 39-1). Within the Igα and Igβ subunits of the mIg is an ITAM that induces protein tyrosine kinase activation and calcium mobilization. The signaling function of the ITAM depends on two conserved tyrosine residues, which are sites of phosphorylation after B-cell receptor (BCR) engagement. Two distinct signals are delivered through the BCR: an activation signal that leads to cell entry into the cell cycle and upregulation of costimulatory molecules and a persistence signal, which is needed for normal B-cell development. The membrane immunoglobulin is associated with a protein complex that is homologous to the CD3 complex associated with the TCR. The components of this disulfide-linked heterodimeric complex binds to cytoplasmic effectors, including src-family tyrosine kinases. The receptor-associated src-family kinases activate numerous downstream signaling pathways leading to transcription factor activation. These transcription factors induce the expression of genes whose products stimulate the growth and differentiation of B cells. A unique feature of B cells is their ability to respond to antigen in different structural contexts with different biologic responses.[128,130] The encounter of a B cell with antigen may lead to clonal deletion and receptor editing (discussed later),

which represent inhibited responses. If the antigen is encountered in multimeric form complexed with carbohydrate, however, the B cell is induced to proliferate. In the latter situation, anergy can result if T-cell help is not provided.

In contrast to T cells, B lymphocytes cannot be unequivocally grouped into subsets on the basis of unique surface markers alone. All B cells make and secrete antibodies, although two major subpopulations of B cells display sufficient functional diversity to justify their classification as distinct subsets.[131] CD5+ B cells (B1) differentiate in the omentum and constitute the predominant B-cell type during fetal life.[132,133] They tend to produce IgM antibodies with broad specificity for bacterial antigens and self-antigens. Although rheumatoid factor activity and anti-DNA antibodies are produced most frequently by B1 cells, they are not responsible for autoantibodies against endocrine cells. The responses of B1 cells are thymus independent and provide a first line of defense against common bacterial antigens. The B1 responses do not lead to immunologic memory.

B2 cells represent the conventional B cells that secrete all immunoglobulin classes and represent the subset most relevant to autoimmune endocrine diseases.[134] These cells are thymus dependent and require physical interaction with T cells specific for the same antigen (cognate help). These cells are the likely sources of autoantibodies, such as antithyroglobulin, antimicrosomal, anti-GAD, and anti-IA-2/ICA512 antibodies.

The B2 cell relies on its surface immunoglobulin clonal receptors to bind and internalize antigen, which is processed and presented on class II MHC molecules to helper T cells.[135] After engagement of the TCRs with the MHC plus peptide complex, many pairs of cell adhesion molecules participate actively in the T-cell–B-cell interaction. Several of these pairs deliver costimulatory signals to the B cell to promote its clonal expansion and differentiation. In addition, the activated T cells secrete cytokines, such as IL-4, IL-5, and others, which stimulate B-cell differentiation. The process of T cell–dependent B-cell differentiation is complex and highly regulated resulting in several possible outcomes, including generation of memory cells and highly differentiated effector cells that secrete immunoglobulins.[136]

ROLE OF IMMUNOGLOBULINS IN AUTOIMMUNE ENDOCRINE DISEASES

In a few examples, including Graves' disease (antibodies against the thyroid-stimulating hormone [TSH] receptor), autoimmune hypoglycemia (antibodies against insulin), and type B insulin resistance (antibodies against the insulin receptor), autoantibodies are direct mediators of disease. In other autoimmune endocrine disease, autoantibodies are markers of the autoimmune process and have helped to elucidate the disease pathogenesis, but are not the direct mediators of disease.[137-140] Autoantibodies have identified islet antigens, such as ICA512 (IA-2), GAD65, and insulin in type 1 diabetes mellitus, that may be the target of pathogenic T cells. The absolute dependence on T cells as mediators of type 1 diabetes mellitus has been supported by the finding that T-cell clones can transfer diabetes to immune-deficient NOD mice in the absence of B cells and, more recently, by the identification of a patient with X-linked agammaglobulinemia who developed type 1 diabetes mellitus.[141,142] In this patient, T-cell responses to islet antigens could be detected. Other experimental data indicate an important role, however, for either B cells or immunoglobulins in experimental autoimmune diabetes. In the NOD mouse, diabetes does not occur in the absence of B cells.[143,144] Greeley and associates[145] found that the offspring of B cell–deficient NOD mothers were protected from spontaneous diabetes, whereas the offspring of B cell–deficient fathers were not protected. This study points to the maternal transmission of β cell–reactive antibodies as an important step influencing the development of immune-mediated β-cell destruction in NOD mice. B cells also may serve as APCs and provide necessary costimulatory signals for early T-cell activation. This idea is supported by the observation that later in the disease process, B lymphocytes seem to be dispensable because diabetes can be adoptively transferred by B cell–depleted spleen cells from diabetic mice.[146]

Regardless of the pathogenic role of autoantibodies in disease progression, autoantibodies have facilitated studies on the natural history of autoimmune endocrine diseases. In type 1 diabetes, studies of discordant twins and triplets who later developed diabetes showed that autoimmunity may be present for years before disease is clinically apparent and at a time when only subtle abnormalities of insulin secretion can be detected. The antigens recognized by the autoantibodies seem to identify a natural progression of disease. The three most predictive antibodies, anti-insulin, anti-GAD65, and anti-ICA512, appear sequentially, suggesting an evolution of the disease process.[140,147,148] Studies of autoantibodies in type 1 diabetes mellitus support the notion that the disease develops over a period of about 3 years. The presence of autoantibodies to multiple autoantigens in relatives of patients with type 1 diabetes mellitus is the strongest predictor of development of type 1 diabetes mellitus. In addition, autoantibodies have led to the identification of antigens that are targets of autoreactive T cells and involved in the pathogenesis of disease (Table 39-3). The antigen glutamic acid decarboxylase (GAD65) originally was found through the search for the antigen recognized by antibodies reactive with a 64-kDa islet cell membrane protein in found in type 1 diabetics and BB/W rats, a rat model of type 1 diabetes mellitus.[149–153]

ANTIGEN PRESENTATION TO LYMPHOCYTES

The immune responses that cause autoimmune endocrine diseases are antigen specific. That is, they are focused toward certain target peptides, rather than involving generalized immune dysregulation. The specificity of this response is conferred by the ability of immune cells to respond exclusively to organ-specific antigens. Antigen recognition by T and B lymphocytes differs, however. The antigen receptors on T cells recognize protein sequences of 8 to 20 amino acids in length presented by the MHC molecule (discussed later). Immunoglobulins, which are the antigen receptors on B cells, recognize three-dimensional structures present on unprocessed antigens.[154–160] The processing of proteins and the presentation of their peptide components to T cells require a complex series of interrelated events that take place in specialized APCs, such as macrophages, DCs, and, in certain situations, B cells. APCs perform two essential functions required for the initiation of immune responses: (1) They

display antigenic fragments associated with specialized antigen-presenting molecules, and (2) they deliver costimulatory signals required for lymphocyte activation and differentiation.

The specialized antigen-presenting molecules are the cell surface glycoproteins encoded in the highly polymorphic MHC genes called *MHC class I* and *class II*. In humans, these genes are called *human leukocyte antigen (HLA) genes*. There are three class I genes—HLA-A, HLA-B, and HLA-C. There are also three regions of class II genes—HLA-DR, HLA-DP, and HLA-DQ. MHC genes are codominantly expressed, with individuals expressing MHC alleles inherited from each parent. An individual's MHC haplotype consists of the set of MHC alleles on each chromosome. HLA alleles are named numerically with heterozygous individuals having two HLA haplotypes (i.e., HLA-DR3/DR4, HLA-DP2/DP3, and HLA-DQ3/DQ4). Studies of human MHC genes have revealed extensive polymorphism. More than 250 alleles have been found for some HLA loci.[161] An example of the HLA genes constructing an HLA-DR3 and HLA-DR4 haplotype is shown in Figure 39-3.

MHC molecules are peptide-binding molecules that present antigen for recognition by T cells (see Fig. 39-1). Conventional (CD4$^+$ and CD8$^+$) T cells recognize only the complex of MHC plus peptide. T-cell recognition is said to be MHC restricted. In this manner, only peptides that can bind to MHC molecules can be "seen" by T cells. MHC molecules sample the contents of the cellular compartments and bring representative peptides to the cell surface for T-cell scrutiny. Class I MHC molecules are found on all cells, although the relative level of expression may differ considerably among organs, cell types, and individual cells.[156] MHC class I molecules specialize in the binding of *intracellular* peptides in the endoplasmic reticulum and in their subsequent transport to the cell surface for recognition by T cells expressing the MHC class I–binding molecules, CD8 (CD8$^+$ T cells). MHC class I–associated peptides are formed through the proteolysis of cytosolic proteins. These peptides are transported to the endoplasmic reticulum, where they form stable complexes with MHC class I molecules. These MHC class I–antigen complexes travel through the Golgi apparatus and are transported to the cell surface by exocytic vesicles. In contrast, MHC class II molecules (also referred to as *Ia*) bind peptides generated by proteolysis of extracellular material in the endosomal compartment and present them on the surface for recognition by T cells expressing the MHC class II–binding molecule CD4 (CD4$^+$ T cells).[157,159] The expression of class II MHC molecules is more restricted than that of class I. They are found on APCs such as macrophages and DCs, B lymphocytes, thymic epithelial cells, and, in humans, activated T lymphocytes. APCs first bind and internalize native antigen from the extracellular compartment. These proteins are then degraded and transported to vesicles, where they associate with MHC class II molecules synthesized in the endoplasmic reticulum. The MHC II molecule from the endoplasmic reticulum is bound to a peptide known as *CLIP* (class II–associated invariant chain peptide), which prevents the class II molecule from binding other peptides before encounter with antigen. CLIP is removed from the class II–binding pocket by proteolytic enzymes and the HLA-DM molecule. HLA-DM is similar in structure to the class II molecule and serves as a peptide exchanger by aiding in the removal of CLIP and the binding of processed peptides to the class II molecule. This stable MHC class II–peptide complex is transported and expressed on the cell surface for recognition by CD8$^+$ T cells.[161]

The structures of MHC class I and II molecules reflect their specialized functions. Class I and II molecules contain NH$_2$ terminal peptide–binding baskets sitting on a structural platform composed of two immunoglobulin domains. MHC class I consists of a chain with three extracellular domains associated noncovalently with the non-MHC peptide β$_2$-microglobulin. The MHC class I basket is composed of the α$_1$ and β$_2$ domains

---

Table 39-3 Autoantigens Identified in Type 1 Diabetes Mellitus

Antigen	Reference
Proinsulin	221
Insulin B chain*	208
IA-2/ICA512*	209
IA-2β/phogrin	210
GAD65*	211
ICA69	212
Imogen	213
Heat shock protein	214
IGRP†	216

*Autoantibodies against these antigens are most predictive of type 1 diabetes mellitus
†Islet-specific glucose-6-phosphatase catalytic subunit–related protein

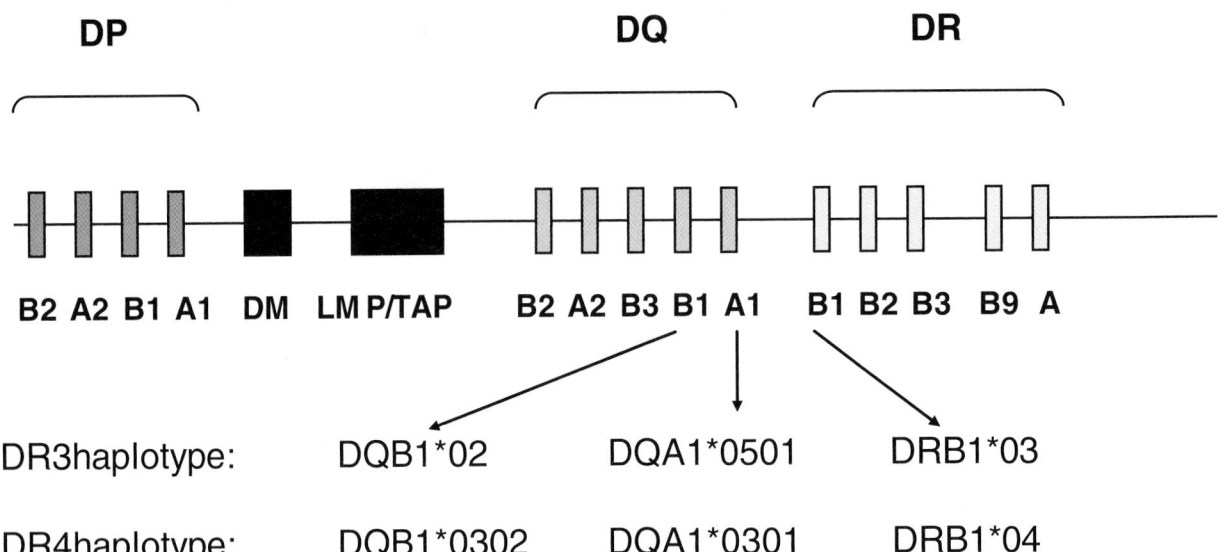

Figure 39-3 HLA MHC II region and construction of HLA-DR3 and HLA-DR4 haplotypes. This is a simplified representation of the human MHC II genes omitting genes with unknown function. The HLA alleles DP, DQ, and DR are shown. The DM, LMP, and TAP regions are involved in antigen processing. DM region encodes for the DM molecule, which catalyzes peptide binding to MHC class II molecules. LMP region encodes subunits of proteasomes, which degrade cytoplasmic proteins. TAP (transporter associated with antigen processing) region encodes the TAP transporter, which transports peptides in antigen processing. An example of a HLA-DR3 and HLA-DR4 haplotype is shown. This DR3 haplotype is found in several autoimmune endocrine diseases, including type 1 diabetes mellitus, Graves' disease, autoimmune hypothyroidism, Addison's disease, and primary ovarian failure. The DR4 haplotype is associated with type 1 diabetes mellitus with the greatest susceptibility to disease in HLA-DR3/DR4 heterozygote individuals. (Adapted from Tait KF, Gough SC: The genetics of autoimmune endocrine disease. Clin Endocrinol [Oxf] 59:1–11, 2003; and Abbas AK, Lichtman AH: Cellular and Molecular Immunology. Philadelphia, WB Saunders, 2003.)

supported by the immunoglobulin α_3 and β_2-microglobulin domains.[154] MHC class II is a heterodimer of α and β chains, both of which are integral membrane proteins with two extracellular domains. The α_1 and β_1 domains create the MHC class II basket that sits on top of the immunoglobulin α_2 and β_2 domains.[157] For both classes of MHC molecules, the peptide-binding basket is composed of two domains, each contributing four β-pleated sheets and one α helix. The β sheets form the bottom of the basket and the α helix the sides. Most of the polymorphic residues in MHC molecules reside in the sites involved in peptide binding.

MHC class I molecules have been shown to be important in the pathogenesis of type 1 diabetes mellitus through the development of MHC class I–deficient NOD mice using targeted disruption of the β_2-microglobulin gene. β_2-microglobulin is a non–MHC-encoded protein that is needed for MHC class I antigen expression. β_2-microglobulin-deficient NOD mice do not develop type 1 diabetes mellitus spontaneously.[162] Restoring β-cell MHC class I expression in these mice allows for the development of a nondestructive insulitis but not full diabetes, illustrating the complex of role of MHC class I molecules during disease progression.[163] The postulated significance of these observations is that class I–restricted T cells, CD8+ cells, are required for initiation of insulitis in the NOD model. In addition, T cell–predominant infiltration to islets (insulitis) and hyperexpression of MHC class I antigens on islet cells have been found in pancreatic biopsy specimens of patients with recent-onset type 1 diabetes mellitus.[164-166]

There has been much debate concerning the hypothesis that aberrant expression of MHC molecules on endocrine cells may lead to the presentation of antigens and activation of autoreactive T cells. MHC II molecules are aberrantly expressed on thyroid follicular cells in Graves' disease and Hashimoto's thyroiditis along with increased numbers of MHC class I molecules.[167,168] In autoimmune thyroid disease, there are many cells expressing MHC II molecules potentially capable of presenting autoantigens. These include "professional" APCs, such as DCs, and "nonprofessional" APCs, such as MHC II–expressing thyroid follicular cells.[64,169]

Thyroid follicular cells aberrantly express MHC II antigens and upregulate their MHC I expression in Graves' disease and Hashimoto's thyroiditis.[167,168] A potential function of this increased MHC II expression has been illustrated given that thyroid follicular cells expressing MHC II can present viral peptide antigens to cloned T cells.[170] Together with the data on the expression of the costimulatory molecules CD40 and B7-1 on Hashimoto's thyroid follicular cells, these thyroid follicular cells may function as efficient APCs capable of initiating and propagating the autoimmune response in Hashimoto's thyroiditis. The absence of B7-1 on thyroid follicular cells in Graves' disease may limit their role in autoantigen presentation because it has been shown that autoantigen presentation in this disorder is primarily by professional B7-positive APCs.[171] Nonetheless, the aforementioned findings indicate mechanisms through which thyrocytes may crosstalk with immune cells. A similar hypothesis concerning the expression of MHC class II molecules by endocrine cells in the islets of Langerhans has been suggested.[172-175] Careful analysis of the MHC class II–expressing cells in islets of the NOD mouse has suggested, however, that the class II–positive cells are also CD45+, indicating a lymphoid origin.[176] The etiology of MHC II–expressing cells in the islets of humans with type 1 diabetes mellitus is still unclear.

It follows from the previous discussion that the ability of a T cell to respond to any given antigen depends not only on the binding characteristics of antigenic peptides, but also on the physical properties of the MHC molecules. It is not surprising that genes of the MHC have been associated most strongly with autoimmune endocrine diseases. Multiple associations with Graves' disease and class I and class II HLA alleles have been reported (see Fig. 39-3). HLA B8 was among the first associations with the disease.[177,178] The strongest association in whites is found with the HLA DR3 haplotype.[178,179] HLA-DQA1*0501 has been found to be independently associated in some studies.[180,181] In other studies, this apparent association of HLA-DQA1*0501 and Graves' disease has been found to be the result of linkage dysequilibrium with DR3. Linkage dysequilibrium signifies that these two alleles may be in close proximity on the DNA strand and that the true association may be with DR3 and Graves' disease.[181] In addition, HLA-DR3 has been associated with autoimmune hypothyroidism and primary ovarian failure in smaller studies.[178,182] With respect to Hashimoto's thyroiditis, the HLA DRB1*04-DQB1*0301 haplotype also has been shown to confer an increased susceptibility to disease in an Italian population.[183] Addison's disease is a complex genetic disorder that has been associated with a specific HLA-DR and HLA-DQ genotype.[184-187] The highest susceptibility to Addison's disease is in patients with a heterozygous HLA-DR4-DQ8/HLA-DR3-DQ2 genotype.[184,188,189] Addison's disease also has been strongly linked with a mutated allele (5.1) of a nonclassic HLA molecule, MHC class I chain–related A (MIC-A).[184,190,191]

The MHC locus is the strongest genetic determinant of susceptibility to type 1 diabetes mellitus, contributing approximately 50% to familial clustering.[192,193] Mean logarithm of odds (lod) scores, a statistical estimate of whether two gene loci are likely to lie near each other on a chromosome and to be inherited together, have been shown to be greater than 10 in several studies.[194] This lod score reflects an extremely high likelihood that type 1 diabetes mellitus is associated with certain MHC genes. Among whites, HLA-DR3 and HLA-DR4 alleles (see Fig. 39-3) confer increased susceptibility to type 1 diabetes mellitus, and 94% of white type 1 diabetes patients carry these alleles.[195-197] The greatest genetic risk for type 1 diabetes mellitus is the DR3/DR4 heterozygous state. The strength of the association with the MHC is reflected by comparing the risk of type 1 diabetes mellitus in HLA-nonidentical siblings (1.2%) with the age-corrected empirical risk in HLA identical siblings (15.5%). Studies of North American white patients with these alleles showed that the association is closer to the DQ region of the MHC. Todd and coworkers[198] found that the absence of an aspartic acid at position 57 of the DQ β chain best explained susceptibility to type 1 diabetes mellitus. An analogous finding exists in the unique I-A^{g7} class II allele of the NOD mouse.[199] DQ haplotypes lacking aspartic acid, such as DQ*0201 and DQ*0302, are associated with increased risk, whereas alleles with aspartic acid, such as DQ*0602 and DQ*0102, are protective. The phenotype of protective alleles is dominant.[197]

The fact that specific sequences of the DQ β chain increases type 1 diabetes mellitus susceptibility suggested that the antigen-binding properties conferred by DQ's protein sequence might affect T-cell activation and tolerance or other functional immune responses regulating islet reactive T cells. Transgenic expression of another amino acid residue at position 57 of the DQ β chain inhibited diabetes development in the NOD mouse.[200-202] The unique diabetes-susceptible class II MHC molecules have unique peptide-binding properties. Peptides eluted from I-A^{g7} of the NOD mouse have sequences that implicate an acidic residue in the C terminus of the peptide as important for binding. Reich and colleagues[203] showed the role of this residue in binding by direct peptide-binding analysis. Other than the C-terminal amino acid, however, the I-A^{g7} class II–binding peptides lack other identifiable binding motifs, but rather interact via general hydrophobic amino acid residues.

More recently, another molecular basis of the MHC linkage is beginning to be elucidated based on the unusual physical properties of the DQ and I-A^{g7} molecules. First, these MHC class II molecules fail to form stable αβ dimers in association with binding peptides. In contrast to murine MHC alleles, such as I-A^d, I-A^b, and I-A^k, there are few stable αβ dimers on the surfaces of NOD APCs. The dimers are short lived and present antigenic peptides to T cells poorly[204,205]; this may preclude negative selection of autoreactive T cells in the thymus (discussed later) or affect activation of diabetogenic T cells in the periphery.

The human cluster of differentiation 1 (CD1) family of cell surface molecules has been characterized as non-MHC antigen presenting molecules.[160] In contrast to class I and II MHC molecules, the antigen-binding groove of CD1 is made up of hydrophobic residues suggesting that CD1 binds hydrophobic ligands such as lipids. Antigens presented by CD1 are lipid and glycoprotein in nature instead of peptides. CD1 molecules are recognized by natural killer (NK)–like T cells.[206] These cells can be activated in vivo by α-galactosylceramide (α-GalCer), an NK T-cell ligand. These cells are thought to be a source of IL-4 in the early stages of an immune response. As discussed earlier, the local cytokine environment at the time of T-cell activation affects differentiation of T cells. In humans, T cells expressing the Vα24JαQ TCR, a characteristic of NK T cells, reduced production of IL-4 in relatives of patients who progressed to diabetes compared with relatives of patients who did not progress to diabetes.[207] These investigators suggest the reduced IL-4 production by this subset of cells leads to immune responses skewed toward IFN-γ production, which is needed for autoimmune diabetes.

ANTIGENIC TARGETS OF THE ENDOCRINE AUTOIMMUNE RESPONSE

Work in recent years has identified antigenic targets of the immune responses in autoimmune endocrine diseases.[208-221] These targets are listed in Tables 39-3 and 39-4. In general, the antigens represent intracellular proteins without structural anomalies. The fact that these proteins have a vital role in normal human physiology and that they are expressed at high levels in the organism highlights the importance of the various control mechanisms discussed previously in regulating responses to them.

Alternatively, several lines of evidence support the notion that mimicry between foreign peptides and autoantigens may result in autoreactivity. Glutamic acid decarboxylase (GAD), which has been shown to be the target of autoantibodies in human type 1 diabetes mellitus and pathogenic T cells in the NOD mouse, has molecular homology with the coxsackie viral protein P2-C.[222] The similarities between these two epitopes may lead to autoreactivity in genetically predisposed persons. A similar mechanism also may account for the high rate of development of type 1 diabetes mellitus in offspring of women who have had congenital rubella. Karjalainen and associates[223] reported that patients with type 1 diabetes mellitus have antibodies that react with a discrete segment of bovine serum albumin (BSA, ABBOS), suggesting the possibility that mimicry between the BSA antigen and an islet antigen may trigger an anti-islet immune response. Although these mechanisms of molecular mimicry are suggested by epidemiologic data, there is little direct evidence to support their role in human disease. Other factors are needed for activation of antigen-reactive T cells highlighted in the subsequent discussion of clonal ignorance.

Table 39-4	Autoantigens Identified in Human Autoimmune Thyroid Diseases
Antigen	**Reference**
Heat shock protein	413
Flavoprotein subunit of mitochondrial succinate dehydrogenase*	217
Na/I transporter	218
TG	219
TPO†	220
TSH receptor	220

*Formerly unidentified 64-kDa protein.
†Formerly microsomal antigen.
Na/I, sodium/iodide; TG, thyroglobulin; TPO, thyroid peroxidase; TSH, thyroid-stimulating hormone.

An important concept, elucidated primarily from studies of autoreactive T cells from animal models, is the spreading and diversification of the antigenic targets of autoimmune responses, or epitope spreading, during disease pathogenesis.[224] Although the initial immune response may be to a particular peptide sequence of an antigen, with time, other peptides of the same antigen become targets of the autoimmune response (intramolecular spreading), and even additional antigens are involved (intermolecular spreading). This involvement has been shown in the NOD mouse for T-cell responses to GAD and insulin.[225,226] The extent to which the response to the primary antigen or to the spread antigens account for tissue destruction is not clearly understood. An implication of this understanding is that it may be difficult to identify inciting antigens by studying the autoimmune response late in its course. Immune interventions with specific antigens must be early in the evolving response because with time, the proportion of T cells reactive with the inciting antigen diminishes.

MECHANISMS OF TOLERANCE

The development of endocrine disease by immunologic mechanisms represents a failure to develop or maintain tolerance to self-antigens. In this setting, *tolerance* refers to the absence of immunologic destruction of a tissue and does not imply the absence of autoreactive cells or antibodies. In most instances, the initiators of the immune response that results in disease have not been identified. Among the antigens that have been described as targets of autoimmunity, most are cellular components that are constitutively expressed (e.g., thyroid peroxidase, GAD, insulin). More recent interest has focused on understanding how tolerance toward self-proteins is established and maintained by the immune system and the failures of this system that result in endocrine diseases (Fig. 39-4).

The random rearrangement of individual variable components of the TCR and BCR genes is designed to maximize diversity, anticipating all possible MHC/antigenic structures.[227] An important implication of the random nature of TCR and BCR gene arrangement is that every individual, even monozygotic twins, has a unique immune cell repertoire. This fact has been invoked to explain the discordance of autoimmune endocrine diseases, such as type 1 diabetes mellitus, among identical twins, although environment also likely plays an important role.

The chance rearrangement of TCR and BCR genes that leads to the diverse reactivity implies that self-reactive receptors will be present in the repertoire. Mechanisms to eliminate, control, or restrict responses to self are paramount to avoid autoimmune disease (see Fig. 39-4).

CLONAL DELETION

The most important and efficacious mechanism for tolerance is clonal deletion. Clonal deletion of T cells occurs predominantly in the thymus, and deletion of B cells occurs in the bone marrow through the elimination of immature lymphocytes.[228] In the thymus, several developmental steps occur that ultimately lead to export of T cells reactive with antigens in the context of self-MHC molecules (see Fig. 39-4A). First, to ensure that only cells that are capable of responding to antigens presented by self-MHC molecules constitute the final repertoire, cells that respond to antigen in the context of self-MHC undergo a process termed *positive selection*, whereas cells not restricted by self-MHC molecules do not mature further and die by apoptosis. Clonal deletion occurs predominantly in immature lymphocytes. Apoptosis is developmentally regulated in lymphocytes to ensure their timely death after encounters with self-antigens. The success of clonal deletion depends on the availability of self-antigens at toleragenic concentrations and the correct functioning of the lymphocyte's apoptotic machinery. In general, self-reactive clones with high-affinity receptors are more likely to be clonally deleted than clones expressing low affinity for self. Studies with intrathymically transplanted islet cells and in transgenic mice expressing TCR specific for the male antigen (H-Y), selective class II or class I MHC molecules, and specific peptides have been used to show that clonal deletion occurs between migration from the thymic cortex to medulla. This process is responsible for the elimination of potentially autoreactive T cells from the repertoire of mature peripheral T cells.[228-233]

The ability of clonal deletion to eliminate autoreactive T cells depends on the following: (1) the ability of the MHC molecules to bind and present autoantigens, (2) the expression of the antigen in the thymus at the time of development, and (3) the function of the activation pathways needed for negative selection. As discussed earlier, a failure to delete autoreactive lymphocytes may be tightly linked to the MHC genes through the MHC molecules' unique binding characteristics. These binding characteristics may be poor in the case of DQ or IA^{g7} molecules associated with type 1 diabetes. Expression of known islet antigens in the thymus at the time of T-cell development has been shown to result in loss of susceptibility to autoimmune diabetes induced with multiple low doses of streptozotocin in the BB/W rat and NOD mouse.[232-234] Transplantation of islets into the thymus of younger patients has been suggested as one approach to induce tolerance to islets to prevent either type 1 diabetes mellitus or the rejection of transplanted islet allografts.

Clonal deletion affects only antigens expressed or that traffic into the thymus, and cells reactive with antigens expressed outside the thymus are not deleted from the repertoire. It has been shown that medullary thymic epithelial cells express a diverse range of tissue-specific antigens, including disease-associated autoantigens. This may help induce tolerance to self-antigens that otherwise would be temporally or spatially isolated from the immune system.[235] Many antigens previously considered to be expressed exclusively in the periphery are expressed in the thymus. Insulin, the 69-kDa islet cell autoantigen (ICA69), and GAD, thought to be important autoantigens in type 1 diabetes mellitus, are expressed by specialized APCs in the thymus.[236,237] It has been postulated that the association between polymorphisms of the insulin gene and type 1 diabetes mellitus may be accounted for by the effects of these polymorphisms on expression of insulin in the thymus, perhaps by affecting negative selection of autoreactive T cells.[238] In the NOD mouse model of disease, it has been shown that mice deficient in insulin-2, but not insulin-1, develop accelerated diabetes. Insulin-2 is the isoform of insulin that is expressed in the mouse thymus, suggesting that its absence leads to accelerated diabetes by failure to remove autoantigen (i.e., insulin) reactive T cells.[239] Conversely, knockout of the insulin-1 gene, which is expressed predominantly in the islets with little thymic expression, protects mice from disease. It is suggested that the absence of insulin-1 may prevent autoantigen-stimulated destruction of islet cells and does not compromise the removal of insulin-reactive T cells in the thymus.[240] Finally, data have suggested that the costimulatory molecule, CTLA-4, may be associated with clonal deletion of potentially autoreactive T cells in the thymus. Intrathymic CTLA-4 blockade dramatically inhibits anti-CD3-mediated depletion of CD4$^+$/CD8$^+$ double positive immature thymocytes.[241] This finding suggests the possibility that the genetic associations between autoimmune endocrine diseases and CTLA-4 genotypes may have a functional correlate related to the acquisition of central tolerance (see later).[242-244]

An example of thymic expression of peripheral endocrine cell antigens as a determinant of autoimmunity is the autoimmune polyendocrine syndrome type 1 (APS-1). This syndrome includes candidiasis, hypoparathyroidism, Addison's disease, and often type 1A diabetes and is associated with hypothyroidism, pernicious anemia, alopecia, vitiligo, hepatitis, ovarian atrophy, and keratitis. The syndrome is due to mutations in the autoimmune-suppressor gene (AIRE, autoimmune regulator).[245–249] The AIRE gene encodes a transcription factor that has been shown to promote the ectopic expression of peripheral tissue–restricted antigens in medullary epithelial cells of the thymus. AIRE-deficient thymic medullary cells show a specific reduction in ectopic expression of genes encoding peripheral antigens. It is thought that the absence of thymic expression of these peripheral antigens results in autoimmunity and the onset of this polyglandular syndrome. Humans expressing a defective form of the AIRE gene develop autoimmunity, which is modeled by mice expressing a mutant form of this gene.[245] These mutant mice display a partial defect in promiscuous gene expression by thymic medullary epithelial cells (mTECs) resulting in a defined profile of autoimmune diseases dependent on the absence of AIRE in the thymus. AIRE-deficient mTECs show a specific reduction in ectopic transcription of genes encoding peripheral antigens. These findings emphasize the importance of thymically imposed "central" tolerance in the prevention of autoimmunity. Although promiscuous gene expression by mTECs and its role in self-tolerance in mice are currently undisputed, it has been unclear until more recently whether this tolerance mechanism has been conserved across species barriers during evolution, including humans. Gotter and colleagues[235] showed that the promiscuous expression of tissue-specific self-antigens in the thymus is preserved between mice and humans; this strengthens the validity of analogies drawn between human autoimmune diseases and corresponding animal models, particularly with respect to APS-1.

Clonal deletion is also a mechanism for removal of self-reactive B cells from the peripheral lymphoid compartment. Immature B cells that encounter self-antigen are eliminated from the immune repertoire by negative selection.[250,251] Lysozyme-binding B cells in the spleen and lymph nodes are deleted in double-transgenic mice expressing antilysozyme immunoglobulin and a membrane bound form of lysozyme. Negative selection has been proposed to take place by two distinct mechanisms: (1) deletion by apoptosis and (2) alteration of the antigen receptor specificity by receptor editing. *Receptor editing* refers to a process by which selection occurs at the level of the BCR so that self-reactive receptors that encounter autoantigen in the bone marrow are altered through secondary rearrangement.[252] Whether receptor editing is effective for preventing autoreactivity to organ-specific B cells has not been shown.

Studies of B-cell tolerance to endocrine organs suggest that clonal deletion does not occur for cells reactive with organ-specific antigens. Systemic expression of membrane-bound hen-egg lysozyme (mHEL) results in elimination or inactivation of circulating HEL-reactive B cells. When mHEL is expressed exclusively on thyroid cells, however, elimination or inactivation of circulating HEL-reactive B cells does not occur.[253] Other mechanisms must be operational to avoid autoreactivity. One possibility is that antigens are sequestered from circulating preimmune B cells similar to clonal ignorance discussed subsequently.

CLONAL IGNORANCE

In general, naive T cells do not circulate into the peripheral tissues. *Clonal ignorance* refers to a situation in which self-reactive lymphocytes with the functional capacity to respond to their target antigens coexist with that antigen.[254–257] In one example, expression of the alloantigen IA^d on the β cells of H-2^b mice failed to induce an inflammatory response and subsequent development of diabetes, even though cells reactive with the alloantigen were present in the animal and responded

to the alloantigen in vitro.[258] This is a precarious state because self-reactive lymphocyte clones operationally ignore self-antigens only as long as local conditions permit. The condition may be reversed by the presence of inflammatory mediators, antigen mimicry, or other mechanisms that can induce T-cell migration to sites of antigen and expression of activation molecules.[259] Mice expressing a transgene encoding a glycoprotein from the lymphocytic choriomeningitis virus in the pancreatic β cells and a TCR that recognized the glycoprotein plus MHC are functionally tolerant of the glycoprotein.[260] The tolerance is broken if the mouse is infected with live lymphocytic choriomeningitis virus (LCMV). If a third gene, termed *adenovirus E3*, which among other things, inhibits expression of class I molecules on β cells, is also present, tolerance is not broken by LCMV infection. This occurs even though LCMV reactive cells are found in the spleen.[261] This example illustrates that functional tolerance may be local.

Control of T-cell migration also may be related to induction of tolerance to peripheral antigens induced in neonates. In mouse bone marrow chimeras generated at different ages, recent thymic emigrants were tolerized to a skin-expressed MHC class I antigen during the neonatal period, but not during adulthood.[262] Blockade of T-cell migration neonatally prevented tolerance induction. T-cell trafficking through nonlymphoid tissues in the neonate is crucial for the establishment of self-tolerance to sessile, skin-expressed antigens.

CLONAL ANERGY

Clonal anergy refers to a state of functional nonresponsiveness of lymphocytes. Bretcher and Cohn[263] suggested that B cells required two signals for effective activation, the first provided by the antigen-specific receptor, the second by another noncognate costimulatory receptor. The notion was that the autoreactive response could be controlled, at least in part, by alterations of activation involving the TCR/BCR or costimulatory signals. Mueller and colleagues[55] and Lenschow and coworkers[57] hypothesized that these types of interventions would lead to the development of anergy. There is now ample evidence that this form of peripheral regulation occurs in vivo.[55,57,264] Under certain circumstances of signal 1 or signal 2 blockade, the T cells not only fail to respond to antigen, but also do not respond when rechallenged with the antigen even when appropriate activating signals are delivered.

Clonal anergy can be induced in T cells by providing an altered "signal 1"/signal via the TCR or by providing signal 1 in the absence of "signal 2"/costimulatory signal. Allen and colleagues[265] found that "altered peptide ligands" that bind TCR can induce nonresponsiveness of antigen-reactive T cells, and Smith and associates[16] reported that FcR nonbinding anti-CD3 mAb can induce anergy of Th1 cells by delivering an altered signal to activated T cells. The molecular mechanisms that are thought to underlie this induced nonresponsiveness involve qualitative changes in the phosphorylation of TCR components. The basis for the selective effects on phenotypic subsets is not clear because similar changes in TCR signaling have been observed in Th1 and Th2 cells. Nonetheless, these studies make the point that the TCR is not exclusively an "on" or "off" switch—*quantitatively* different TCR signals can result in *qualitatively* different outcomes. The selective effects make this approach attractive for immune therapies. These observations also are consistent with the notion of tolerance induction as an active process that involves delivery of "altered" activation signals.[264]

Tolerance of B cells involves changes in antigen receptor signaling.[266] B cells in transgenic mice expressing a BCR for HEL and circulating HEL populate the peripheral lymphoid organs, but do not respond to HEL.[266] These same cells proliferate in response to the bacterial antigen, lipopolysaccharide, and retain responsiveness to stimulation via CD40 and IL-4. This clonal anergy to the HEL antigen is analogous to the

CENTRAL T CELL TOLERANCE

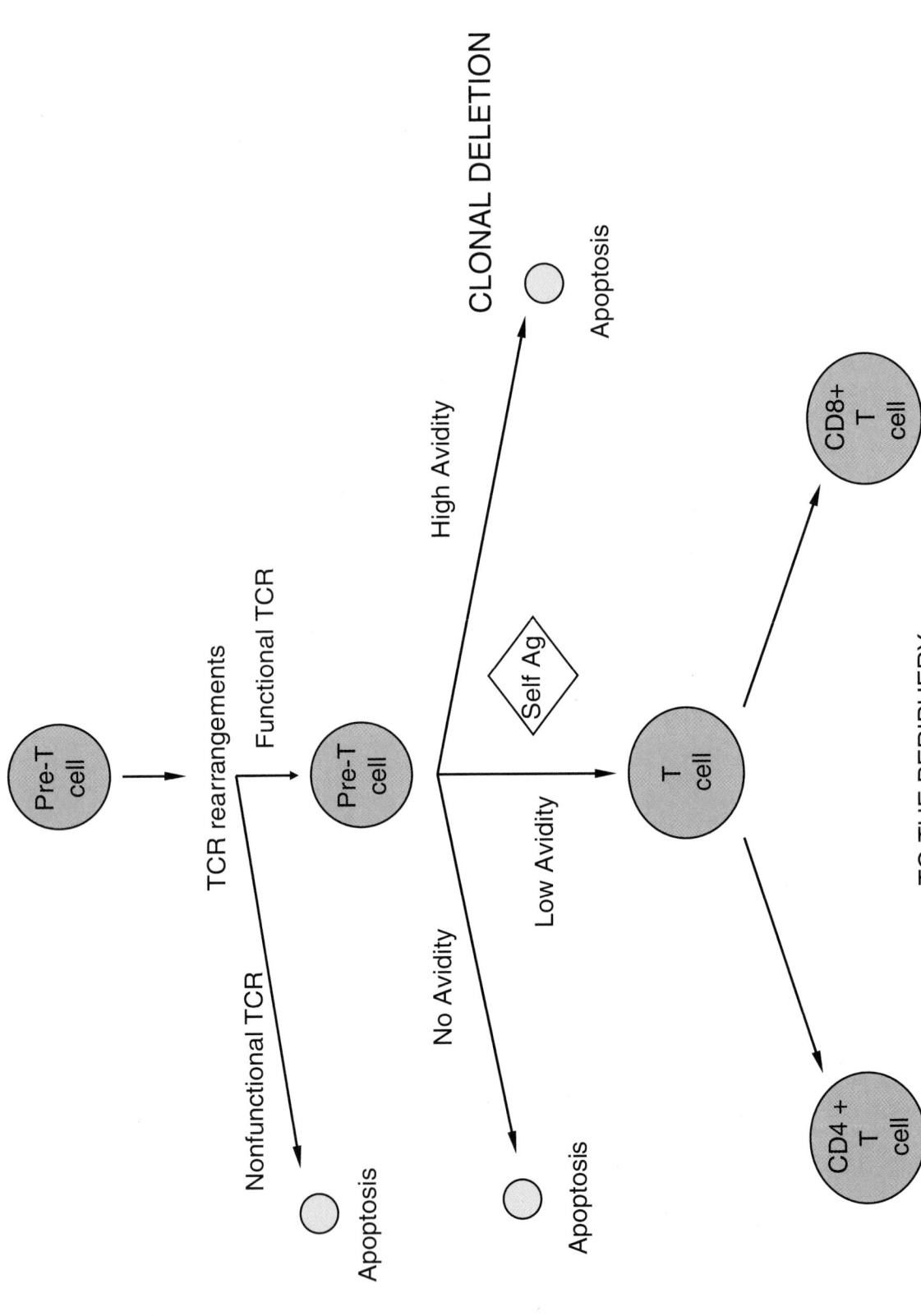

Figure 39-4 Mechanisms of tolerance. **A,** Central tolerance (at the level of the thymus). First, immature T cells rearrange their T-cell receptors (TCRs) to have a functional TCR with αβ chains. Cells with nonfunctional TCRs die via apoptosis. Subsequently, pre–T cells with no affinity for self-antigen also are destroyed through apoptosis. Self-reactive T-cell clones with high-affinity receptors are more likely to be clonally deleted than clones expressing low affinity for self. Successful clonal deletion depends on the availability of self-antigens at toleragenic concentrations and the intact functioning of the apoptotic machinery. T cells with low avidity for self migrate to the periphery.

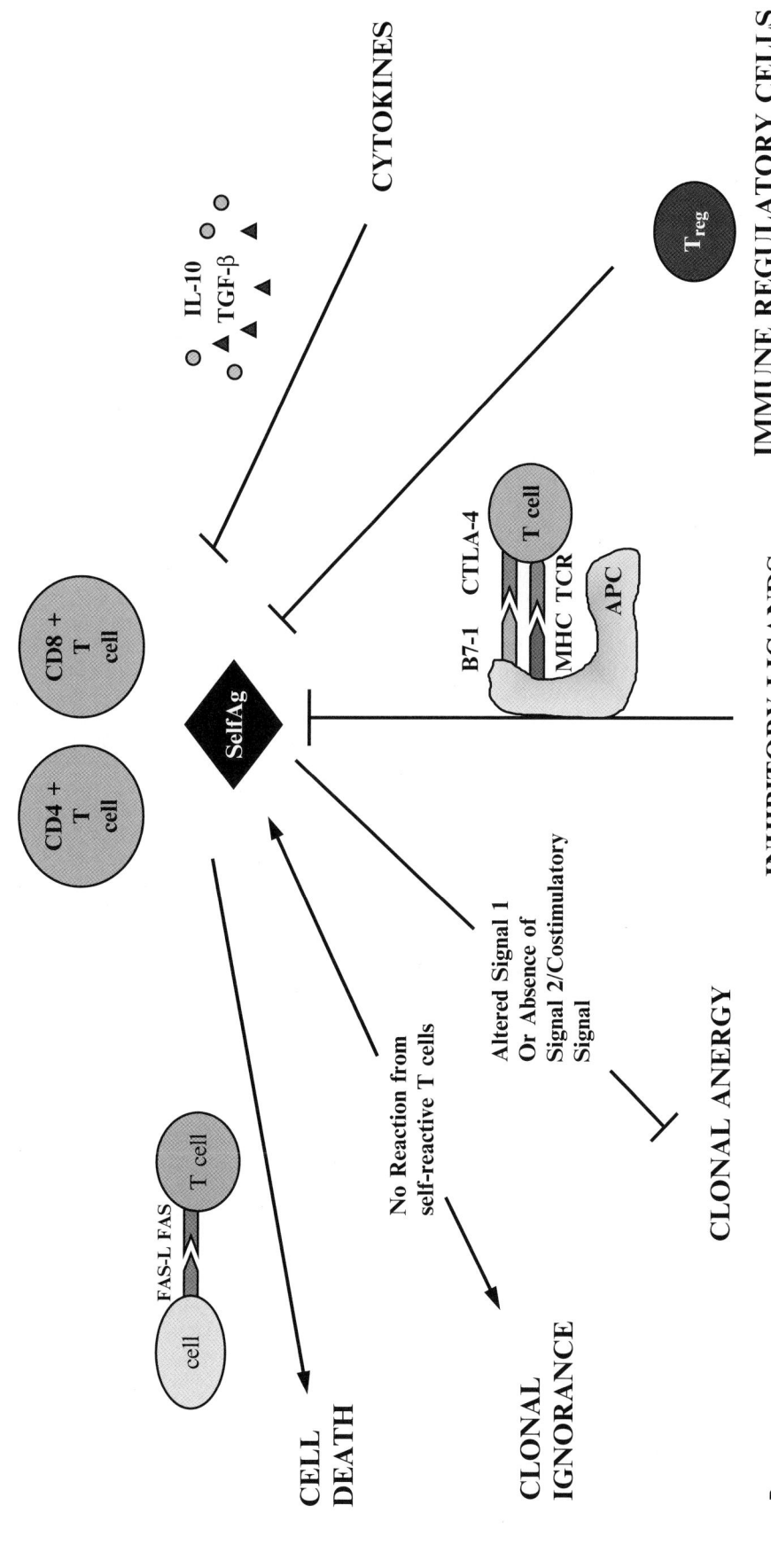

PERIPHERAL T CELL TOLERANCE

CYTOKINES

IL-10

TGF-β

IMMUNE REGULATORY CELLS

T_reg

INHIBITORY LIGANDS

B7-1   CTLA-4

T cell

MHC TCR

APC

CD4 + T cell

CD8 + T cell

SelfAg

Altered Signal 1 Or Absence of Signal 2/Costimulatory Signal

CLONAL ANERGY

No Reaction from self-reactive T cells

CLONAL IGNORANCE

FAS-L FAS

T cell

cell

CELL DEATH

Figure 39-4, cont'd **B,** Peripheral tolerance. Tolerance in the periphery may be accomplished by the following mechanisms to limit autoimmune responses (described in detail in the text): (1) clonal ignorance, (2) clonal anergy, (3) inhibitory ligands action, (4) cell death of autoreactive cells, (5) immune regulatory cell action, and (6) cytokine action. (Adapted from Greenspan FS, Gardner DG: Basic and Clinical Endocrinology. New York, Lange, 2001.)

B

effects of TCR activation in the absence of costimulatory signals. Silencing of autoreactive B cells involves changes in antigen receptor function and changes in the cells' potential to differentiate.

INHIBITORY T-CELL LIGANDS

Costimulatory molecules, as discussed earlier, also can send inhibitory signals to regulate immune responses. CTLA-4 originally was identified as a homologue of CD28 and was thought to be a costimulatory molecule, but instead CTLA-4 inhibits T-cell responses and has been shown, in several animal models of autoimmune disease, to play a key role in the unfolding of the autoimmune diathesis.[82,267–273] These studies emphasize the role of CTLA-4 in maintenance of tolerance in the periphery with the engagement of CTLA-4 potently downregulating immune responses. In a transgenic mouse model of autoimmune diabetes, CTLA-4 interactions regulate pancreatic islet-reactive T cells, supported by the finding that mAb blockade of CTLA-4 rapidly induces diabetes in animals that would not normally develop disease until many months later.[274] This effect is observed only early in the course of disease. More recent studies have indicated that it is during the reencounter of previously activated T cells with their target antigen that CTLA-4 engagement is most critical, rather than during initial T-cell priming.[275] Likewise, in mice, engagement of CTLA-4 can prevent autoimmune thyroiditis and experimental allergic encephalomyelitis.[276,277] The inhibitory effect of CTLA-4 seems most important for responses of peripheral blood cells because the T-cell repertoire of CTLA-4-deficient mice seems to be normal.[278] Other studies have suggested a role of CTLA-4 in central tolerance regulated in the thymus. Mice with defective CTLA-4 function or expression may possess a skewing toward increased affinities for self-MHC antigen complexes. In CTLA-4-deficient mice with a bias toward self-reactivity could contribute, jointly with impaired peripheral control of T cells, to the autoimmunity observed in these animals.[279]

It has been shown that splice variant of CTLA-4, named ligand-independent CTLA-4 (liCTLA-4), strongly inhibits T-cell responses by binding and dephosphorylating the TCR ζ-chain independent of ligand activation. This form of CTLA-4 was found to be higher in memory T cells from diabetes-resistant NOD mice compared with normal NOD mice, suggesting that this increased expression and negative signaling delivered by liCTLA-4 may regulate development of T cell–mediated autoimmune responses.[280] Because of the central role of this molecule in regulating immune responses, the identified genetic associations between CTLA-4 with autoimmune thyroid disease and type 1 diabetes mellitus are of immunologic interest.[279,281–286]

Yanagawa and colleagues[279] found an association between polymorphisms in the CTLA-4 gene and Graves' disease. Similarly, Ueda and associates[244] identified polymorphisms of the CTLA-4 gene associated with Graves' disease, autoimmune hypothyroidism, and type 1 diabetes mellitus. Although the relationship of the CTLA-4 gene with type 1 diabetes mellitus and autoimmune hypothyroidism has not been as reproducible compared with studies in patients with Graves' disease.[284–286] In the NOD mouse, a diabetes susceptibility locus also has been found on chromosome 1 within a region that encompasses CTLA-4 and CD28.[281–283] Colucci and coworkers[283] found that there is defective expression of CD28 and CTLA-4 in these mice. The role of CTLA-4 in controlling T-cell responsiveness makes this locus an interesting candidate gene for disease susceptibility. It has been suggested that failure to deliver T-cell inhibitory signals in the periphery or even during thymic development because of functional differences in CTLA-4 alleles may result in unchecked T-cell responses or failure to delete autoreactive cells during T-cell ontogeny.

PD-1, another negative regulatory molecule discussed previously, has been shown to play an important role in the maintenance of peripheral tolerance to autoantigens in animal models.[91] PD-1-deficient animals develop diverse autoimmune conditions, including an autoimmune dilated cardiomyopathy and a lupus-like syndrome with arthritis and nephritis depending on the genetic background of the animal.[92,93] PD-1 has been shown to contribute to the pathogenesis of type 1 diabetes mellitus and experimental autoimmune encephalomyelitis in murine models. Blockade of PD-1 or its ligand, PD-L1, rapidly precipitates diabetes in prediabetic NOD mice.[94] Similarly, blockade of PD-1 or its other known ligand, PD-L2, has been shown to accelerate the murine model of multiple sclerosis, experimental autoimmune encephalomyelitis.[287] Taken together, these results indicate a role for this receptor-ligand interaction in the prevention of autoimmune responses.

CD30, a member of the TNFR superfamily, is another T-cell ligand that may deliver inhibitory signals, particularly for cells that have not been deleted through the Fas pathway of activation-induced cell death (discussed later). In a transplantation model, Kurts and associates[288] found that CD8+/CD30− cells were 6000 times more aggressive for pancreatic islets than wild-type CD8+ T cells.

Stimulatory and inhibitory mechanisms are controlled by costimulatory signals. Manipulation of costimulatory signals would be an attractive target for immune therapy because it specifically would target autoantigen reactive T cells and spare naive cells. Because inhibitory and activation signals are delivered to T cells through costimulatory ligands, however, a clearer understanding of the role of these ligands is needed before considering clinical studies with agonists or antagonists of these molecules.

PERIPHERAL TOLERANCE VIA CELL DEATH

After activation of T cells in the periphery, T-lymphocyte death occurs through two mechanisms: (1) passive cell death, which occurs via growth factor withdrawal or after antigen clearance and subsequent cessation of TCR signals, or (2) activation-induced cell death.[289] In activation-induced cell death, death of activated cells is mediated by cytokines such as TNF-α and IL-2, and interactions between the Fas Ligand (FasL) and it receptor Fas, which deliver apoptotic signals to activated T cells.[290,291] Elimination of activated cells by death signals is one means of preventing autoreactivity. One of the unique characteristics of "immune privileged" sites is the expression of FasL. The expression of FasL causes the death of activated T cells that express Fas and prevents T-cell responses against the FasL-expressing organ. IL-2 is also a key promoter of this process.[292,293] In contrast, IL-15 protects activated T cells from passive cell death.[292] Data support a primary role for activation-induced cell death and growth factor withdrawal in allotransplantation. Turka, Strom, and others showed that apoptosis of activated, alloreactive T cells is essential for the induction of tolerance.[294–296] The use of an IL-2 agonist with an antagonist to IL-15 has been shown to enable long-term engraftment/tolerance in allotransplantation models, including transplantation of allogeneic islets into overtly diabetic NOD mice.[295] This tolerance to the allograft occurs in part by promoting the death of activated T cells, which could destroy the graft while preserving CD4+/CD25+ T cell–dependent immunoregulatory cells.[296] In sharp contrast, global immunosuppression, such as with cyclosporine, blocks T-cell activation and apoptosis, but precludes the induction of tolerance possibly by destroying activated T effector cells and regulatory T cells.[264,297,298]

MECHANISMS OF CELL DEATH IN AUTOIMMUNE DISEASE

Conversely, Fas/FasL interactions, leading to apoptosis of target cells,[299] also have been incriminated in autoimmune endocrine diseases. Chervonsky and associates[300] found that the ability to upregulate Fas is acquired by β cells during the natural course of diabetes in NOD mice. Their studies, using Fas-deficient, NOD[lpr/lpr] mice, which are resistant to spontaneous diabetes, support a crucial role for this pathway in causing β-cell destruction. In addition, immunohistochemical analysis of pancreas biopsy specimens of patients with recent-onset type 1 diabetes mellitus and insulitis on biopsy has shown Fas expression in β cells and infiltrating cells. In patients with insulitis, FasL was expressed exclusively in islet-infiltrating cells, including CD8[+] cells, macrophages, and CD4[+] cells. The authors concluded that the interaction between Fas on β cells and FasL on infiltrating cells may trigger selective apoptotic β-cell death in inflamed islets, leading to type 1 diabetes mellitus.[301] The importance of Fas/FasL interactions also has taken an interesting turn, however, in studies of thyroid glands from patients with Hashimoto's thyroiditis.[302] These studies suggest that fratricide rather than homicide may account for cell death. Giordano and colleagues[302] found that thyrocytes from glands with Hashimoto's thyroiditis, but not normal thyroids, express Fas. FasL was shown to be constitutively expressed in normal and diseased glands. They postulated that expression of Fas, induced in glands with Hashimoto's disease, ligated FasL expressed by the same or a neighboring cell leading to cell death; this was consistent with their finding that exposure to IL-1β induced thyrocyte apoptosis, which was prevented by antibodies that block Fas. IL-1β-induced (or other inflammatory cytokine) Fas expression could lead to death by suicide or fratricide. In addition to the upregulation of Fas in Hashimoto's thyroiditis, it has been shown that the anti-apoptotic molecule Bcl-2 is reduced in these glands, which together may lead to thyrocyte death and hypothyroidism. In contrast, the same researchers showed reduced levels of Fas/FasL and increased levels of Bcl-2 in thyrocytes of Graves' disease. This finding could favor thyrocyte survival and the hypertrophy associated with TSH receptor antibodies.[303]

Studies of sequential involvement of T-cell subsets in the NOD mouse have begun to shed light on mechanisms of cell death in this model of type 1 diabetes mellitus. Studies involving adoptive transfer of splenocytes from NOD mice into immune-deficient NOD/scid mice have suggested that CD8[+] cells are needed early in the disease and CD4[+] cells are involved in later stages of islet destruction.[304] This suggestion is consistent with the observation that in the absence of class I MHC molecules (to which CD8 molecules bind), insulitis is not seen in the NOD mouse.[305,306] The mechanism of cell death is not clear, however, and may partly involve perforin, an enzyme from cytotoxic granules in CD8[+] T cells that mediates cell lysis. NOD mice deficient in perforin have delayed onset of diabetes.[307] Diabetogenic CD8[+] T-cell clones can destroy islet cells in a Fas-dependent, perforin-independent manner, however.[308–310]

The cytokine milieu, created by activated T cells, can be directly toxic to the insulin-producing β cells. TNF-α and IFN-γ are perhaps the most important cytokines that mediate islet destruction.[311] Using transgenic and knockout NOD mice, Pakala and associates[312] showed the role of these molecules in tissue destruction. Islets deficient in Fas, IFN-γ receptor, or inducible nitric oxide synthase had normal diabetes development. The specific lack of TNF-α receptor 1 caused protection from diabetes, however, by altering the ability of islet reactive CD4[+] T cells to establish insulitis and destroy β cells

REGULATORY T CELLS AND TOLERANCE

Regulatory T cells are likely to be an important contributor to tolerance. There are numerous examples of T$_{reg}$ cells influencing natural and induced disease states in a variety of mouse models of autoimmunity.[313,314] Seddon and Mason[315]

identified a potential regulatory population of CD4[+] peripheral T cells or CD4[+] thymocytes that can prevent induction of autoimmune thyroiditis. Development of these cells is antigen specific, and their activity depends on endogenously produced IL-4 and TGF-β. Generation of "regulatory" T cells from thymic emigrant precursors is driven by peripheral autoantigen. In another illustration, BB/W rats have been shown to be lymphopenic and spontaneously develop autoimmune diabetes.[316] These rats fail to develop T cells expressing RT6[+], which have been shown to inhibit diabetes. Depletion of RT6[+] T cells in diabetes-resistant (DR) BB rats precipitates disease.[317] In the NOD mouse, a population of CD28-dependent CD4[+]/CD25[+]/L-selectin-positive T cells are able to inhibit transfer of diabetes by T cells from diabetic mice.[318] These cells can be shown to be antigen specific.[319] Similar CD4[+] regulatory T cells have been identified in numerous systems, including bone marrow transplantation and oral tolerance induction.[320,321] In most cases, these other cell subsets, termed Th3 or Tr1 cells, mediate immune suppression through IL-10 or TGF-β or both, although it is not clear how related these different T-cell subsets are.

Emerging data in humans suggest that animal models of T$_{reg}$ cells are relevant to human disease. Genetic disruption of the FoxP3 gene leads to profound multiorgan autoimmunity.[322–325] The syndrome of X-linked polyendocrinopathy, immune dysfunction, and diarrhea (known as XPID) is a rare disorder resulting in widespread, aggressive autoimmunity and early death.[184] Mutations in the FoxP3 gene have been identified in patients with this disorder. Research in the mouse model of this disease suggests that autoimmunity may stem from a lack of functioning regulatory T cells.[326] The importance of T$_{reg}$ cells was again highlighted in findings from patients with patients with another multiorgan autoimmune disease, the autoimmune polyglandular syndrome type 2 (APS-2). The common phentotype in this disorder consists of Addison's disease, type 1A diabetes, and autoimmune thyroid disease, although many other autoimmune disorders have been reported.[187] Regulatory T cells isolated from APS-2 patients were shown to be defective in their suppressive capacity.[327] This finding is consistent with results in several murine models in which depletion of T$_{reg}$ cells causes a similar syndrome.[328] Regulatory T cells have been identified to be deficient in patients with type 1 diabetes mellitus and other immunologic diseases.[329–331] These observations in human disease suggest that in addition to autoimmune effector cells, cells with a regulatory role develop in the thymus and may play an important role in controlling activation of the disease-causing cells.

Several groups have described regulatory CD8[+] T cells as well. In some systems, these cells react directly with activated CD4[+] T cells and may limit CD4[+] responses involved in autoimmunity.[332,333] In other settings, the CD8[+] cells interact with APCs, which stimulate the production of CD4[+]/CD25[+] regulatory T cells.[334] As in the case of regulatory CD4[+] cells, the role of CD8[+] cells during the induction or development of autoimmune diseases is still under investigation.

PERIPHERAL TOLERANCE VIA ACTIVE REGULATION

Many investigators have shown the enormous potential of T$_{reg}$ cells to suppress pathologic immune responses in autoimmune diseases, transplantation, and graft-versus-host disease.[313] Some of the earliest studies of tolerance induction using mAbs directed at CD4 or CD8 showed that tolerance to skin grafts in mice could be induced in a robust and long-lasting manner.[335] This tolerance developed over 4 weeks, but when established, the tolerance could affect naive cells transferred into the mice (dominant tolerance). Tolerance depended on the presence of host CD4[+] T cells, which were focused to the site of antigen. Further studies with a third-party graft indicated that regulation operated in a local microenvironment where antigen acts to focus naive antigen-specific T cells into the vicinity of regulatory CD4+ T cells. Even naive T cells would acquire tolerance, however, by cohabitation with the tolerant cells. This phenomenon, termed *infectious tolerance,*[336] suggested that active immune regulation was a fundamental mechanism of immune tolerance. Since the late 1990s, it has been clear that immune regulation in many of these antibody therapeutic systems was due to a novel subset of CD4+ T cells that coexpressed CD25 and a variety of other cell surface/intracellular markers.[337] The relevance of T$_{reg}$ cells to disease was obvious from the first descriptions of these cells, based on their ability to regulate autoimmunity.[338]

As discussed earlier, autoimmune endocrine diseases have been associated with a Th1-type cytokine response, whereas Th2 and T$_{reg}$ cells cytokines are protective. By modifying the cytokine milieu, cytokines can prevent or exacerbate autoimmune disease, most likely by modifying the differentiation or function of other cells in the local environment. The cytokine environment at the time of T-cell activation and the cells' ability to produce cytokines is likely to be an important determinant of progression of disease. A finding suggestive of this concept is that in HLA-matched control subjects without diabetes, T cells secreted increased levels of IL-10 in response to islet peptides, whereas patients with type 1 diabetes mellitus secreted IFN-γ and IL-10.[339] It is not surprising that one of the essential roles of T$_{reg}$ cells is to produce cytokines that can alter the activation milieu of potentially pathogenic T cells. The timing of T$_{reg}$ cell migration into the site may be critical for it effects. In this regard, in the NOD mouse, treatment with IL-10 can prevent diabetes when given at a later stage of the disease, but exacerbates diabetes when expressed as a transgene in the β cells.[340,341] At this point, it is not clear whether these differences in responses are the cause or effect of the disease, but they suggest a mechanism for maintenance of tolerance to autoantigens in normal individuals by production of nonpathogenic and even immune regulatory cytokines.[342]

Perhaps the most important cytokine postulated to be produced during tolerogenic responses is TGF-β. It has been shown that a transient pulse of TGF-β in the islets during an early phase of diabetes in NOD mice is sufficient to inhibit disease onset by promoting the expansion of intraislet CD4+/CD25+ T cells. These T cells exhibit characteristics of regulatory T cells, including small size, high level of intracellular CTLA-4, expression of Foxp3, and transfer of protection against diabetes to mice prone to develop type 1 diabetes mellitus.[343] TGF-β also was shown to induce the proliferation of these CD4+/CD25+ regulatory T cells in vivo. The induction of TGF-β-producing T$_{reg}$ cells may require an IL-10-producing precursor.[344] These findings suggested a critical interrelationship between regulatory T cells, IL-10, and TGF-β by which TGF-β inhibits autoimmune diseases via regulation of the number of CD4+/CD25+ regulatory T cells, which produce essential regulatory cytokines or promote tolerance through antigen-specific cell-cell contact.[345] In this regard, TGF-β is produced in an inactive form that is often found bound to the cell surface via a TGF-latency associated peptide. The apparently conflicting notion that regulatory T cells act locally and with some bystander effects may be reconciled by this novel activity. Finally, TGF-β also is thought to be involved in tolerance induced to ingested antigens (oral tolerance).[346] It has been postulated that this mechanism may be invoked to prevent autoimmune disease.[347] In the NOD mouse, it has been possible to prevent diabetes by feeding insulin to animals.[348] This observation forms the basis for the ongoing "oral tolerization" arm of the Diabetes Prevention Trial–1, in which insulin is administrated orally to patients at high risk for developing type 1 diabetes mellitus in hopes to prevent or delay disease onset (discussed later).

ROLE OF CYTOKINES AND OTHER SOLUBLE FACTORS IN THE AUTOIMMUNE RESPONSE

As discussed earlier, activated T cells produce soluble products that also affect the differentiation of an immune response and may affect its pathogenicity directly. One of the important early mediators of differentiation of autoimmune cells is IFN-α. Its presence has been detected in the pancreas in early lesions of autoimmune diabetes, and transgenic expression of IFN-α in islet cells causes diabetes.[349,350]

In addition, rather than a clear distinction between progression of disease with Th1 cytokines and prevention with Th2 cytokines, most studies have suggested an evolving process that can exhibit a varying phenotype. In NOD mice, expression of Th1 cytokines can be detected by 1 to 2 months of age, and there is an increase in expression of Th1 cytokines in male mice, in which diabetes develops in 70% to 90% of mice, but a decrease in female mice, in which diabetes occurs only in 10% to 20%.[41] Shimada and coworkers[351] reported that the expression of IFN-γ in islets from NOD mice occurs as a relatively late process, shortly before clinical appearance of hyperglycemia. Andre-Schmutz and associates[310] found in TCR transgenic NOD mice that treatment with cyclophosphamide precipitates diabetes, and the coordinate expression of IL-18, IL-12, and TNF-α was required for the onset of islet destruction. There was no cellular or molecular evidence of cell contact–mediated mechanisms of β cell death in their studies. In autoimmune thyroid disease, the response may vary with the phenotype and stage of the disease. Th1 and Th2 phenotypes can be found in glands from patients with Graves' disease and Hashimoto's thyroiditis. The difference between diseases may be the effect of a functionally dominant population at a given time.[352]

The precise mechanism whereby cytokines affect the autoimmune response may involve maintenance/loss of tolerance, direct toxic effects on target tissues, and effects on the differentiation of T effector cells. TNF-α and IFN-γ are perhaps the most important cytokines that mediate islet destruction.[311] Using transgenic and knockout NOD mice, Pakala and associates[312] showed the role of these molecules in tissue destruction. Islets deficient in Fas, IFN-γ receptor, or inducible nitric oxide synthase had normal diabetes development. The specific lack of TNF-α receptor 1 caused protection from diabetes, however, by altering the ability of islet reactive CD4+ T cells to establish insulitis and destroy β cells. Cytokines produced by Th1 cells, including IFN-γ together with IFN-α, can inhibit glucose-stimulated insulin release from islets in vitro.[353] It is postulated that these cytokines can cause production of free radicals that may injure β cells directly. Sarvetnick and colleagues[354] showed that the transgenic expression of IFN-γ and class II MHC molecules in β cells resulted in insulitis, loss of tolerance to islet antigens, and diabetes. IFN-γ may not be a prerequisite, however, for the development of diabetes, given that the genetic absence of IFN-γ in NOD mice does not prevent either insulitis or diabetes, but only delays the time to onset of disease. The same is true of NOD mice deficient in IL-4 and IL-10. It has been suggested that Th1/Th2 cytokine shifts may be an outcome rather than a cause of immune stimulation in this mouse model.[355] Other studies using IFN-γ receptor mutant mice suggest that the important effect of this cytokine is on APCs causing class I MHC upregulation on pancreatic β cells, but not the induction of diabetes.[356] In the case of IL-2-induced hypothyroidism, IL-2 may activate primed intrathyroidal lymphocytes, which then destroy thyroid tissue.[357]

The previous discussion has highlighted the fact that the T cells' microenvironment may affect cell activation and differentiation into mature phenotypes. Consistent with this role of soluble factors is the observation that subclinical thyroiditis may become exacerbated by treatment of patients with IL-2.[358] Hypothyroidism may evolve from subclinical thyroiditis after treatment of patients with interferon-α. Soluble factors produced by T cells and other cells may affect the access of T cells to sites of antigen and sites of antigen presentation.[359,360] Picarella and associates[361] found that transgenic expression of TNF-α leads to invasive insulitis and TNF-β peri-insulitis. Chemokines are produced by activated T cells and may cause recruitment of lymphocytes and other activated cells into the pancreas.[362,363] Another example of chemokine effects was seen studying the prevention of type 1 diabetes mellitus in mouse models by LCMV. A cure of diabetes through LCMV infection was found to involve the recruitment of T lymphocytes along a cytokine (IP-10) gradient into pancreatic lymph nodes.[364] Memory CD4[+] T cells expressing the chemokine receptor CCR4 also are found in the insulitis of NOD mice, which appear to be recruited in response to macrophage-derived chemokines.[365]

SPECIAL CASE OF POLYENDOCRINOPATHIES

Frequently, more than one autoimmune endocrinopathy occurs in the same individual. These syndromes include the autoimmune polyendocrine syndrome type 1 (common phenotype: candidiasis, hypoparathyroidism, Addison's disease); autoimmune polyendocrine syndrome type 2 (common phenotype: Addison's disease, autoimmune thyroid disease, type 1A diabetes); and X-linked polyendocrinopathy, immune dysfunction, and diarrhea as noted previously. More common associations include type 1 diabetes mellitus and autoimmune thyroid disease or type 1 diabetes mellitus with celiac sprue.[366,367] The mechanistic basis for APS-1 and X-linked polyendocrinopathy has been identified involving mutations of the AIRE (autoimmune regulator) and FoxP3 genes that affect antigen presentation in the thymus and the generation of regulatory T cells as described earlier.[184] In most cases, the basis for the coexistence of more than one disease is not clear. In certain cases, shared HLA genes are involved (i.e., HLA-DR3 in type 1 diabetes mellitus and autoimmune thyroid disease), which may work in concert with genes that regulate tolerance and recurrent tissue inflammation resulting in these disease entities.

TREATMENT OF AUTOIMMUNE ENDOCRINE DISEASES BY IMMUNE MODULATION

As an understanding of the mechanisms of autoimmune endocrine diseases has developed, novel immunotherapies have evolved to prevent or treat these diseases. Most clinical trials have involved treatment of new-onset type 1 diabetes mellitus (Fig. 39-5). Initial trials used conventional, broad-spectrum, immune-suppressive agents, including cyclosporine and azathioprine with prednisone.[368-375] Treatment with these agents altered the natural history of the disease over the first year from diagnosis. In an analysis of responders to cyclosporine, investigators found that the most important predictor of response to the drug was the metabolic status (C peptide levels in the plasma) at entry into the trial. None of these drugs was able to induce a lasting clinical remission of the disease. Three years after treatment with cyclosporine, none of the patients remained independent from insulin.[371] Other broad-spectrum, immune-suppressive agents that have been tried without sustained success include azathioprine with prednisone, antithymocyte globulin and prednisone, and methotrexate.[376-378] The toxicity of these broad-spectrum, immune-suppressive agents has led most investigators to abandon their use in this setting.

The aforementioned immune-suppressive agents prevent T-cell responses through depletion or inactivation of T cells. Agents such as glucocorticoids and cyclosporine block cytokine gene transcription, preventing the production of T-cell growth factors.[372,373] A more specific approach was tested using a ricin-conjugated anti-CD5 mAb, which targets the CD5[+] cell antigen and ricin A chain, a ribosomal inhibitor protein. This therapy improved the rate of preservation of C peptide in patients with new-onset type 1 diabetes mellitus in this pilot study.[379] These tested approaches do not induce immunologic tolerance, however—disease recurs after the drug is discontinued. An exception is treatment with the mAb against the CD3 molecule on the TCR.[380-385] Chatenoud and others[381,384,385] reported that an anti-CD3 monoclonal antibody can prevent or reverse diabetes in mouse models of type 1 diabetes mellitus. In a randomized trial, a humanized non-FcR-binding anti-CD3 mAb, hOKT3γ1(Ala-Ala), was given over a 14-day course in patients with newly diagnosed type 1 diabetes mellitus. This single 14-day course of anti-CD3 mAb treatment decreased the rate of loss of insulin production over 1 year and improved glycemic control with reduction in insulin use.[383] This outcome was achieved without the need for continuous immune suppression and persisted at a time when T cells were quantitatively normal. At the conclusion of drug treatment, a subpopulation of CD4[+] T cells that were producing IL-10 but not IFN-γ were identified in drug-treated patients. These cells were proposed potentially to impart a regulatory function and be protective against the development of type 1 diabetes mellitus.[386] Studies that followed, from NOD mice treated with anti-CD3 mAb, suggested that the antibody induced a subpopulation of CD4[+]/CD25[+] regulatory T cells that produced TGF-β, which was required for the regulation of autoimmune diabetes in this model.[35] Non-FcR-binding anti-CD3 molecules originally were designed to reduce the "cytokine release" syndrome induced with the FcR-binding anti-CD3 mAb (i.e., OKT3) when this antibody cross-links with the receptor for immunoglobulin Fc regions.[387] Studies in vitro indicated that these mAbs induced a quantitatively reduced signal to T cells compared with the FcR-binding form.[16,388] These findings support the concept discussed earlier that *quantitative* differences in TCR stimulation result in *qualitative* different responses.

The identification of antigens in type 1 diabetes mellitus has led to the design of antigen-specific approaches to immunotherapy.[389] The 60-kDa heat shock protein (hsp60) is another potential target self-antigen in the pathogenesis of type 1 diabetes[390,391] and has served as the basis of clinical diabetes trials. An immunomodulatory peptide from hsp60, DiaPep277, has been shown to arrest β-cell destruction and maintain insulin production in newly diabetic NOD mice.[392-395] Based on this observation, Raz and colleagues[396] initiated a randomized, double-blind, phase II study of treatment with this peptide in patients with newly diagnosed (<6 months) type 1 diabetes mellitus. Thirty-five patients with type 1 diabetes mellitus and basal C peptide concentrations greater than 0.1 nmol/L were randomized to receive either subcutaneous injections of DiaPep277 or placebo injections. At 10 months, mean C peptide concentrations had decreased in the placebo group but were maintained in the DiaPep277 group. The requirement for exogenous insulin was higher in the placebo group than in the DiaPep277 group. T-cell reactivity to hsp60 and to DiaPep277 in the treatment arm showed an enhanced Th2 cytokine phenotype. Although a small study, the treatment of newly diagnosed type 1 diabetes mellitus with DiaPep277 may preserve endogenous insulin production by inducing a shift from Th1 to Th2 cytokine production.

Keller and coworkers[397] reported that type 1 diabetes mellitus could be prevented in nondiabetic relatives at high risk for developing the disease by treatment with subcutaneous insulin at a time when their tolerance to oral glucose was normal. The preliminary clinical observation was supported by studies in the NOD mouse and BB/W rat models of type 1 diabetes mellitus, although the mechanisms involved were not understood.[398] Possible mechanisms included the induc-

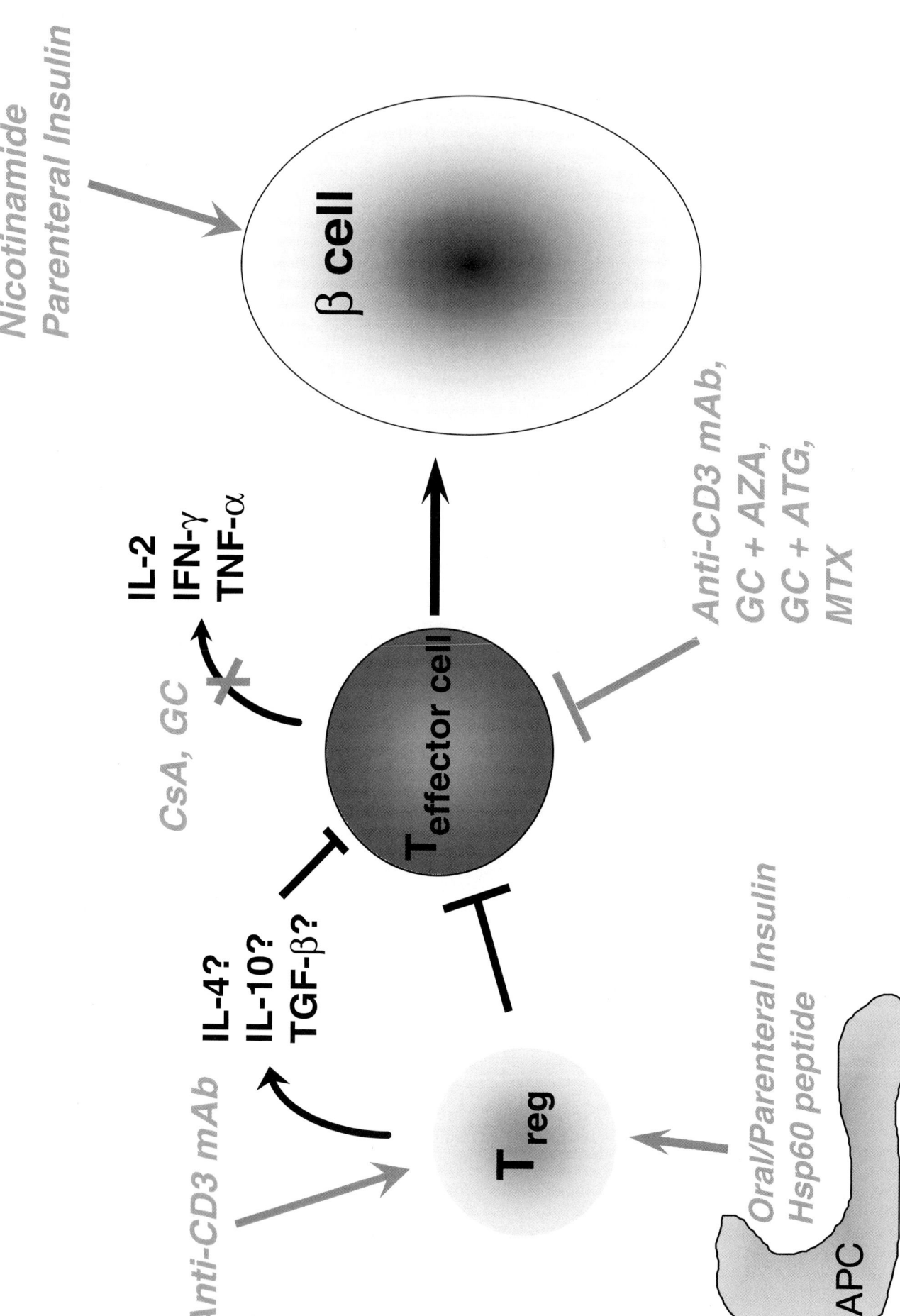

Figure 39-5 Postulated sites of action of agents in recent and past type 1 diabetes mellitus treatment or prevention trials. Animal models have suggested a dynamic interaction between effector and regulatory T cells, which may be affected by many treatment strategies (*italicized*) as outlined in the text. APC, antigen-presenting cells; ATG, antithymocyte globulin; AZA, azathioprine; CsA, cyclosporine; GC, glucocorticoids; IFN, interferon; IL, interleukin; TGF, transforming growth factor. (Modified from Herold KC: Treatment of type 1 diabetes mellitus to preserve insulin secretion. Endocrinol Metab Clin North Am 33:93–111, 2004.)

tion of tolerance to a diabetes-specific antigen and metabolic rest of the β cell, which may limit the presentation of antigens required for immune-mediated islet destruction. This initial clinical observation has led to a large multicenter trial, the Diabetes Prevention Trial–Type 1 Diabetes (DPT-1), to test the ability of treatment with insulin to prevent or modify the onset of diabetes in relatives of patients who are at risk for the disease—either parenteral insulin in high-risk patients or oral insulin in moderate-risk patients.[399] The parenteral trial had negative results; there was no beneficial effect of subcutaneous insulin injections. Although with an intention-to-treat analysis, the oral insulin trial also was negative, more recent examination of the data has raised the question about efficacy in a subgroup of individuals with high levels of anti-insulin antibodies, a population at potentially greater risk for type 1 diabetes mellitus.[400] In a European trial of oral insulin, however, there was no clinically beneficial effect.[401] Finally, other investigators have taken a different approach—to prevent islet damage and the presentation of islet antigens to immune cells by administering nicotinamide to individuals at high risk of disease. Although successful in rodent models of the disease, this clinical trial also was negative with no difference in the development of diabetes between treatment and control groups after the administration of oral nicotinamide for 5 years.[402] A similar approach is the basis for combination trial with vitamin E in hopes that this antioxidant could contribute to the potential protection of islets with nicotinamide. This trial showed that the use of nicotinamide alone or in combination with vitamin E, along with intensive insulin therapy, preserved baseline C peptide secretion for 2 years after diagnosis in patients with recent-onset type 1 diabetes mellitus.[403] The disagreement between the outcomes of the large clinical trials and preclinical results in the most widely studied models of type 1 diabetes mellitus has led some investigators to question the value of the murine models of the disease. Many have cited the clear differences between murine and human immune responses. In addition, the comparison between spontaneous type 1 diabetes mellitus that develops in highly inbred murine strains in germ-free environments with human disease that occurs in an outbred population exposed to many different environmental agents has been questioned, given that these environmental conditions have been incriminated as causative of disease.[404–406] Although the resolution of this dilemma requires further comparisons, the studies of rodent models have been irreplaceable for understanding the mechanisms of autoimmunity.

The experience with clinical trials to treat autoimmune thyroiditis is more limited. Investigators have examined the effects of immune suppression on the exacerbation of ophthalmopathy, which occurs after radioiodine therapy for hyperthyroidism.[407] This manifestation is thought to be related to an increase in levels of circulating thyroid autoantibodies related to leakage of antigens after radioactive iodine therapy. Bartalena and colleagues[408] reported that exacerbation of this manifestation may be ameliorated by treatment of patients with corticosteroids at the time of radioiodine therapy.

One clinical observation has been the *appearance* of autoimmune thyroiditis after administration of cytokines for other conditions. Hypothyroidism and hyperthyroidism have been reported after treatment with IFN-α.[359,360] The mean incidence of IFN-α-induced thyroid dysfunction has been reported to be 6%, but at least one antithyroid antibody has been found in 17% of patients. Spontaneous resolution occurs in more than half of affected individuals with discontinuation of IFN-α treatment. The presence of thyroid autoantibodies before therapy was a predictor for thyroid dysfunction. Hypothyroidism also is a frequent occurrence after lymphokine-activated killer cell therapy.[358] The hypothyroidism seems to be due to activation of intrathyroidal lymphocytes by IL-2 and induction of IFN-γ, a potent inhibitory cytokine for thyroid cells. These studies suggest a mechanism of thyroid dysfunction in which primed cells are activated by administration of high doses of cytokines and support the models of pathogenesis suggested earlier.

CONCLUSION

Experimental data, primarily based on animal models of human diseases, suggest that autoimmune endocrine diseases result from dysregulated immune responses directed against normal constituents of the endocrine glands. The fact that these diseases often follow a progressive course resulting in complete cellular destruction may reflect the activation of the response by the continued presence of the antigen, the impact of local inflammation, epitope spreading, and genetically predetermined sensitivity to the target tissue. Ongoing studies of genetic predisposition of these diseases have suggested new testable hypotheses about pathologic mechanisms. These include failure to remove autoreactive cells from the repertoire resulting from unusual binding properties of certain class II MHC molecules; low, nontoleragenic levels of autoantigen expression in the thymus; and defective costimulatory and negative regulatory signals.

In the periphery, other events are needed for activation of the autoimmune response, such as costimulatory signals and chemokine and cytokine activity, which also may be awry in the autoimmune setting. Little is known about how these events are initiated and regulated in human disease—the possibility of an infectious event resulting in cross-reactivity between antigens of that agent and the islet cells remains. Under these circumstances, normal mechanisms of immune tolerance, such as clonal anergy, deletion, or immune regulation via cytokines or regulatory T cells, may fail, leading to unwanted pathogenic autoreactivity.

The new developments in understanding mechanisms of autoimmune endocrine disease have suggested novel approaches to immunotherapy, in particular, targeting lymphocyte activation pathways and induction of lymphocyte anergy. The new developments also have indicated that previous attempts to induce sustained reversal of disease by broad immune suppression are not likely to be successful and may counteract the new toleragenic protocols. These newer strategies will attempt to target "antigen-specific" immune pathways, pathogenic and regulatory, so that lasting tolerance can be achieved.

REFERENCES

1. Pointes de Carvallio LP, Templeman J, Wick G, Roitt IM: The role of self-antigen in the development of autoimmunity in obese strain chickens with spontaneous autoallergic thyroiditis. J Exp Med 155:1255–1266, 1982.
2. Miller BH, Appel MC, O'Neil JJ, Wicker LS: Both the Lyt2+ and L3T4+ T cell subsets are required for the transfer of diabetes in non-obese diabetic (NOD) mice. J Immunol 140:52–62, 1988.
3. Koevary S, Rossini AA, Stoller W, et al: Passive transfer of diabetes in the BB/W rat. Science 220:727–729, 1983.
4. Herold KC, Montag AG, Fitch FW: Treatment with anti-T lymphocyte antibodies prevents induction of insulitis in mice given multiple low doses of streptozotocin. Diabetes 36:796–801, 1987.
5. Roep BO, Arden SD, deVries RRP, Hutton JC: T cell clones from a type 1 diabetes patient respond to insulin secretory granule proteins. Nature 345:632–634, 1990.
6. Williams ED, Donaich I: The post-mortem incidence of focal thyroiditis. J Pathol 83:255–264, 1962.

7. Davis M: T cell receptor gene diversity and selection. Annu Rev Biochem 59:475–496, 1990.

8. Jorgensen JL, Reay PA, Ehrich EW, Davis M: Molecular components of T cell recognition. Annu Rev Immunol 10:835–873, 1992.

9. Alberola-Ila J, Takaki S, Kerner JD, Permutter R: Differential signaling by lymphocyte antigen receptors. Annu Rev Immunol 15:125–154, 1997.

10. Janeway CA Jr: The T cell receptor as a multicomponent signaling machine: CD4/CD8 coreceptors and CD45 in T cell activation. Annu Rev Immunol 10:645–674, 1992.

11. Fleury SG, Crouteau G, Sekaly R-P: CD4 and CD8 recognition of class II and class I molecules of the major histocompatibility complex. Semin Immunol 3:177–186, 1991.

12. Qian D, Griswold-Prenner I, Rosner RM, Fitch FW: Multiple components of the T cell antigen receptor complex become tyrosine-phosphorylated upon activation. J Biol Chem 268:4488–4494, 1993.

13. Weiss A, Littman DR: Signal transduction by lymphocyte antigen receptors. Cell 76:263–278, 1994.

14. Perlmutter RM, Levine SD, Appleby MW, et al: Regulation of lymphocyte function by protein phosphorylation. Annu Rev Immunol 11:451–499, 1993.

15. Rapoport MJ, Lazarus AH, Jaramillo A, et al: Thymic T cell anergy in autoimmune nonobese diabetic mice is mediated by defective T cell receptor regulation of the pathway of p21ras activation. J Exp Med 177:1221–1232, 1993.

16. Smith JA, Tang Q, Bluestone JA: Partial TCR signals delivered by FcR-nonbinding anti-CD3 monoclonal antibodies differentially regulate individual Th subsets. J Immunol 160:4841–4849, 1998.

17. Pfeiffer C, Stein K, Southwood SHK, et al: Altered peptide ligands can control CD4 T lymphocyte differentiation in vivo. J Exp Med 181:1569–1574, 1995.

18. Kelso A, Troutt AB, Maraskovsky E, et al: Heterogeneity in lymphokine profiles of CD4+ and CD8+ T cells and clones activated in vivo and in vitro. Immunol Rev 123:85–114, 1991.

19. Rogmani S: Lymphokine production by human T cells in disease states. Annu Rev Immunol 12:227–258, 1994.

20. Constant SL, Bottomly K: Induction of the Th1 and Th2 CD4+ T cell responses: Alternative approaches. Annu Rev Immunol 15:297–322, 1997.

21. Coffman RL, Seymour BWP, Lebman DA, et al: The role of helper T cell products in mouse B cell differentiation and isotype regulation. Immunol Rev 102:5–28, 1988.

22. Kuo CT, Leiden JM: Transcriptional regulation of T lymphocyte development and function. Annu Rev Immunol 17:149–188, 1999.

23. Lenschow DJ, Herold KC, Rhee L, et al: CD28/B7 regulation of Th1 and Th2 subsets in the development of autoimmune diabetes. Immunity 5:285–293, 1996.

24. Nakamura T, Kamogawa Y, Bottomly K, Flavell RA: Polarization of IL-4- and IFN-gamma-producing CD4+ T cells following activation of naive CD4+ T cells. J Immunol 158:1085–1094, 1997.

25. Murphy KM, Ouyang W, Farrar JD, et al: Signaling and transcription in T helper development. Annu Rev Immunol 18:451–494, 2000.

26. Szabo SJ, Sullivan BM, Stemmann C, et al: Distinct effects of T-beta in TH1 lineage commitment and IFN-gamma production in CD4 and CD8 T cells. Science 295:338–342, 2002.

27. Swain SL, Weinberg AD, English M, Huston G: IL-4 and IFNγ direct the development of distinct subsets of helper T cells. Fed Proc 4:2020, 1990.

28. Lodolce JP, Burkett P, Koka RM, et al: Regulation of lymphoid homeostasis by interleukin-15. Cytokine Growth Factor Rev 13:429–439, 2002.

29. Seder RA, Gazzinelli R, Sher A, Paul WE: IL-12 acts directly on CD4+ T cells to enhance priming for IFNγ production and diminishes IL-4 inhibition of such priming. Proc Natl Acad Sci U S A 90:10188–10192, 1993.

30. Chess L, Jiang H: Resurrecting CD8+ suppressor T cells. Nat Immunol 5:469–471, 2004.

31. Wood KJ, Sakaguchi S: Regulatory T cells in transplantation tolerance. Nat Rev Immunol 3:199–210, 2003.

32. Saoudi A, Seddon B, Fowell D, Mason D: The thymus contains a high frequency of cells that prevent autoimmune diabetes on transfer into prediabetic recipients. J Exp Med 184:2393–2398, 1996.

33. Walker MR, Kasprowicz DJ, Gersuk VH, et al: Induction of FoxP3 and acquisition of T regulatory activity by stimulated human CD4+CD25− T cells. J Clin Invest 112:1437–1443, 2003.

34. Bluestone JA, Abbas AK: Natural versus adaptive regulatory T cells. Nat Rev Immunol 3:253–257, 2003.

35. Belghith M, Bluestone JA, Barriot S, et al: TGF-beta-dependent mechanisms mediate restoration of self-tolerance induced by antibodies to CD3 in overt autoimmune diabetes. Nat Med 9:1202–1208, 2003.

36. Evavold BD, Sloan-Lancaster J, Allen PM: Tickling the TCR: Selective T-cell functions stimulated by altered peptide ligands. Immunol Today 14:602–609, 1993.

37. Smith JA, Tso JY, Clark MR, et al: Nonmitogenic anti-CD3 monoclonal antibodies deliver a partial T cell receptor signal and induce clonal anergy. J Exp Med 185:1413–1422, 1997.

38. Apostolou I, Von Boehmer H: In vivo instruction of suppressor commitment in naive T cells. J Exp Med 199:1401–1408, 2004.

39. Herold KC, Vezys V, Sun Q, et al: Regulation of cytokine production during development of autoimmune diabetes induced with multiple low-doses of streptozotocin. J Immunol 156:3521–3527, 1996.

40. Zipris D, Greiner DL, Malkani S, et al: Cytokine gene expression in islets and thyroids of BB rats: IFN-gamma and IL-12p40 mRNA increase with age in both diabetic and insulin-treated nondiabetic BB rats. J Immunol 156:1315–1321, 1996.

41. Fox CJ, Danska JS: IL-4 expression at the onset of islet inflammation predicts nondestructive insulitis in nonobese diabetic mice. J Immunol 158:2414–2424, 1997.

42. Hultgren B, Huang X, Dybdal N, Stewart TA: Genetic absence of gamma-interferon delays but does not prevent diabetes in NOD mice. Diabetes 45:812–817, 1996.

43. Katz JD, Benoist C, Mathis D: T helper cell subsets in insulin dependent diabetes. Science 268:1185–1188, 1995.

44. Tremblau S, Penna G, Bosi E, et al: Interleukin 12 administration induces T helper type 1 cells and accelerates autoimmune diabetes in NOD mice. J Exp Med 181:817–821, 1995.

45. Rapoport M, Jaramillo A, Zipris D, et al: Interleukin 4 reverses T cell proliferative unresponsiveness and prevents the onset of diabetes in nonobese diabetic mice. J Exp Med 178:87–98, 1993.

46. Gallichan WS, Balasa B, Davies JD, Sarvetnick N: Pancreatic IL-4 expression results in islet-reactive Th2 cells that inhibit diabetogenic lymphocytes in the nonobese diabetic mouse. J Immunol 163:1696–1703, 1999.

47. Pakala SV, Kurrer MO, Katz JD: T helper 2 (Th2) T cells induce acute pancreatitis and diabetes in immune-compromised nonobese diabetic (NOD) mice. J Exp Med 186:299–306, 1997.

48. Pennline KH, Roque-Gaffrey E, Monahan M: Recombinant human IL-10 prevents the onset of diabetes in the nonobese diabetic mouse. Clin Immunol Immunopathol 71:169–175, 1994.

49. Wogensen L, Lee MS, Sarvetnick N: Production of interleukin 10 by islet cells accelerates immune-mediated destruction of beta cells in nonobese diabetic mice. J Exp Med 179:1379–1384, 1994.

50. Balasa B, Van Gunst K, Jung N, et al: IL-10 deficiency does not inhibit insulitis and accelerates cyclophosphamide-induced diabetes in the nonobese diabetic mouse. Cell Immunol 202:97–102, 2000.

51. Balasa B, Sarvetnick N: The paradoxical effects of interleukin 10 in the immunoregulation of autoimmune diabetes. J Autoimmun 9:283–286, 1996.

52. Mueller R, Bradley LM, Krahl T, Sarvetnick N: Mechanism underlying counterregulation of autoimmune diabetes by IL-4. Immunity 7:411–418, 1997.

53. Jenkins MK: The ups and downs of T cell costimulation. Immunity 1:442–446, 1994.

54. Jenkins MK, Schwartz RH: Antigen presentation by chemically modified splenocytes induces antigen-specific T cell unresponsiveness in vitro and in vivo. J Exp Med 165:302–319, 1987.

55. Mueller DL, Jenkins MK, Schwartz RH: Clonal expansion versus functional clonal inactivation: A costimulatory pathway determines the outcome of T cell receptor occupancy. Annu Rev Immunol 7:4545–4580, 1989.

56. Herold KC, Lu J, Rulifson I, et al: Regulation of chemokine production by CD28/B7 costimulation. J Immunol 159:4150–4153, 1997.

57. Lenschow DJ, Walunas TL, Bluestone JA: CD28/B7 system of T cell costimulation. Annu Rev Immunol 14:233–258, 1996.

58. Linsley PS, Ledbetter JA: The role of the CD28 coreceptor during T cell responses to antigen. Annu Rev Immunol 11:191–212, 1993.

59. June CH, Ledbetter JA, Linsley PS, THompson CB: Role of the CD28 receptor in T cell activation. Immunol Today 11:211–216, 1990.

60. Harding RA, McArthur JG, Gross JA, et al: CD28-mediated signalling costimulates murine T cells and prevents induction of anergy in T cell clones. Nature 356:607–609, 1992.

61. Linsley PS, Brady W, Grosmaire L, et al: Binding of the B cell activation antigen B7 to CD28 costimulates T cell proliferation and interleukin 2 mRNA accumulation. J Exp Med 173:721–730, 1991.

62. Lenschow DJ, Herold KC, Rhee L, et al: CD28/B7 regulation of Th1 and Th2 subsets in the development of autoimmune diabetes. Immunity 5:285–293, 1996.

63. Battifora M, Pesce G, Paolieri F, et al: B7.1 costimulatory molecule is expressed in thyroid follicular cells in Hashimoto's thyroiditis, but not in Graves' disease. J Clin Endocrinol Metab 83:4130–4139, 1998.

64. Salmaso C, Olive D, Pesce G: Costimulatory molecules and autoimmune thyroid diseases. Autoimmunity 35:159–167, 2002.

65. Kuchroo VK, Das MP, Brown JA: B7.1 and B7.2 costimulatory molecules differentially activate the Th1/Th2 developmental pathways: Application for autoimmune disease therapy. Cell 80:707–718, 1995.

66. Lenschow DJ, Ho SC, Sattar H, et al: Differential effects of B7-1 and B7-2 mAb treatment on the development of diabetes in the NOD mouse. J Exp Med 181:1145–1155, 1995.

67. Zhang J, Salojin KV, Delovitch TL: CD28 co-stimulation restores T cell responsiveness in NOD mice by overcoming deficiencies in Rac-1/p38 mitogen-activated protein kinase signaling and IL-2 and IL-4 gene transcription. Int Immunol 13:377–384, 2001.

68. Wong S, Guerder S, Visintin I, et al: Expression of the costimulatory molecule B7-1 in pancreatic beta cells accelerates diabetes in the NOD mouse. Diabetes 44:326–329, 1995.

69. Harlan DM, Barnett MA, Abe R, et al: Very-low dose streptozotocin induces diabetes in insulin promoter mB7-1 transgenic mice. Diabetes 44:816–823, 1995.

70. Herold KC, Vezys V, Koons A, et al: CD28/B7 co-stimulation regulates autoimmune diabetes induced with multiple low doses of streptozotocin. J Immunol 158:984–991, 1997.

71. Pechhold K, Karges W, Blum C, et al: Beta cell-specific CD80 (B7-1) expression disrupts tissue protection from autoantigen-specific CTL-mediated diabetes. J Autoimmun 20:1–13, 2003.

72. Freeman GH, Gribben JG, Boussiotis VA, et al: Cloning of B7-2: A CTLA-4 counter-receptor that costimulates human T cell proliferation. Science 262:909–911, 1993.

73. Lenschow DJ, Su GH, Zuckerman LA, et al: Expression and functional significance of an additional ligand for CTLA-4. Proc Natl Acad Sci U S A 90:11054–11063, 1993.

74. Salomon B, Rhee L, Bour-Jordan H, et al: Development of spontaneous autoimmune peripheral polyneuropathy in B7-2-deficient NOD mice [erratum in J Exp Med 2001 Nov 5;194(9):1393]. J Exp Med 194:677–684, 2001.

75. Salomon B, Lenschow DJ, Rhee L, et al: B7/CD28 costimulation is essential for the homeostasis of the CD4+CD25+ immunoregulatory T cells that control autoimmune diabetes. Immunity 12:431–440, 2000.

76. Peterson KE, Sharp GC, Tang H, Braley-Mullen H: B7.2 has opposing roles during the activation versus effector stages of experimental autoimmune thyroiditis. J Immunol 162:1859–1867, 1999.

77. Arreaza GA, Cameron MJ, Jaramillo A, et al: Neonatal activation of CD28 signaling overcomes T cell anergy and prevents autoimmune diabetes by an IL-4-dependent mechanism. J Clin Invest 100:2243–2255, 1997.

78. Lee KM, Chuang E, Griffin M, et al: Molecular basis of T cellinactivation by CTLA-4. Science 282:2263–2266, 1998.

79. Chambers CA, Kuhns MS, Egen JG, Allison JP: CTLA-4-mediated inhibition in regulation of T cell responses: Mechanisms and manipulation in tumor immunotherapy. Annu Rev Immunol 19:565–594, 2001.

80. Krummel MF, Allison JP: CD28 and CTLA-4 have opposing effects on the response of T cells to stimulation. J Exp Med 182:459–465, 1995.

81. Chambers CA, Allison JP: Co-stimulation in T cell responses. Curr Opin Immunol 9:396–404, 1997.

82. Tivol EA, Borriello F, Schweitzer AN, et al: Loss of CTLA-4 leads to massive lymphoproliferation and fatal multiorgan tissue destruction, revealing a critical negative regulatory role of CTLA-4. Immunity 5:541–547, 1995.

83. Munn DH, Sharma MD, Mellor AL: Ligation of B7-1/B7-2 by human CD4(+) T cells triggers indoleamine 2,3-dioxygenase activity in dendritic cells. J Immunol 172:4100–4110, 2004.

84. Ishida Y, Agata Y, Shibahara K, Honjo T: Induced expression of PD-1, a novel member of the immunoglobulin gene superfamily, upon programmed cell death [abstract]. EMBO J 11:3887–3895, 1992.

85. Agata Y, Kawasaki A, Nishimura H, et al: Expression of the PD-1 antigen on the surface of stimulated mouse T and B lymphocytes. Int Immunol 8:765–772, 1996.

86. Freeman GJ, Long AJ, Iwai Y, et al: Engagement of the PD-1 immunoinhibitory receptor by a novel B7 family member leads to negative regulation of lymphocyte activation. J Exp Med 192:1027–1034, 2000.

87. Dong H, Zhu G, Tamada K, Chen L: B7-H1, a third member of the B7 family, co-stimulates T-cell proliferation and interleukin-10 secretion. Nat Med 5:1365–1369, 1999.

88. Latchman Y, Wood CR, Chernova T, et al: PD-L2 is a second ligand for PD-1 and inhibits T cell activation. Nat Immunol 2:261–268, 2001.

89. Carter L, Fouser LA, Jussif J, et al: PD-1:PD-L inhibitory pathway affects both CD4(+) and CD8(+) T cells and is overcome by IL-2. Eur J Immunol 32:634–643, 2002.

90. Tivol EA, Borriello F, Schweitzer AN, et al: Loss of CTLA-4 leads to massive lymphoproliferation and fatal multiorgan tissue destruction, revealing a critical negative regulatory role of CTLA-4. Immunity 3:541–547, 1995.

91. Nishimura H, Honjo T: PD-1: An inhibitory immunoreceptor involved in peripheral tolerance. Trends Immunol 22:265–268, 2001.

92. Nishimura H, Nose M, Hiai H, et al: Development of lupus-like autoimmune diseases by disruption of the PD-1 gene encoding an ITIM motif-carrying immunoreceptor. Immunity 11:141–151, 1999.

93. Nishimura H, Okazaki T, Tanaka Y, et al: Autoimmune dilated cardiomyopathy in PD-1 receptor-deficient mice. Science 291:319–322, 2001.

94. Ansari MJ, Salama AD, Chitnis T, et al: The programmed death-1 (PD-1) pathway regulates autoimmune diabetes in nonobese diabetic (NOD) mice. J Exp Med 198:63–69, 2003.

95. Swallow MM, Wallin JJ, Sha WC: B7h, a novek costimulatory homolog of B7.1 and B7.2, is induced by TNF-alpha. Immunity 11:423–432, 1999.

96. Coyle AJ, Lehar S, Lloyd C, et al: The CD28-related molecule ICOS is required for effective T cell-dependent immune responses. Immunity 13:95–105, 2000.

97. Tafuri A, Shahinian A, Bladt F, et al: ICOS is essential for effective T-helper-cell responses. Nature 409:105–109, 2001.

98. Dong C, Nurieva RI, Prasad DVR: Immune regulation by novel costimulatory molecules. Immunol Res 28:39–48, 2003.

99. McAdam AJ, Greenwald RF, Levin MA, et al: ICOS is critical for CD40-mediated antibody class switching. Nature 409:102–105, 2001.

100. Grimbacher B, Warnatz K, Peter HH: The immunological synapse for B-cell memory: The role of the ICOS and its ligand for the longevity of humoral immunity. Curr Opin Allergy Clin Immunol 3:409–419, 2003.

101. Rottman JB, Smith T, Tonra JR, et al: The costimulatory molecule ICOS plays an important role in the immunopathogenesis of EAE. Nat Immunol 2:605–611, 2001.

102. Herman AE, Freeman GJ, Mathis D, Benoist C: T regulatory cells dependent on ICOS promote regulation of effector cells in the prediabetic lesion. J Exp Med 199:1479–1489, 2004.

103. Noelle RJ, Ledbetter JA, Aruffo A: CD40 and its ligand, an essential ligand-receptor pair for thymus-dependent B-cell activation. Immunol Today 13:431–433, 1992.

104. Foy TM, Aruffo A, Bajorath J, et al: Immune regulation by CD40 and its ligand GP39. Annu Rev Immunol 14:591–617, 1996.

105. Yang Y, Wilson JM: CD40 ligand-dependent T cell activation: Requirement of B7-CD28 signaling through CD40. Science 273:1862–1864, 1996.

106. Judge TA, Wu Z, Zheng XG, et al: The role of CD80, CD86, and CTLA4 in alloimmune responses and the induction of long-term allograft survival. J Immunol 162:1947–1951, 1999.

107. Balasa B, Krahl T, Patstone G, et al: CD40 ligand-CD40 interactions are necessary for the initiation of insulitis and diabetes in nonobese diabetic mice. J Immunol 159:4620–4627, 1997.

108. Markees TG, Serreze DV, Phillips NE, et al: NOD mice have a generalized defect in their response to transplantation tolerance induction. Diabetes 48:967–974, 1999.

109. Kenyon NS, Chatzipetrou M, Masetti M, et al: Long-term survival and function of intrahepatic islet allografts in rhesus monkeys treated with humanized anti-CD154. Proc Natl Acad Sci U S A 96:8132–8137, 1999.

110. Kenyon NS, Fernandez LA, Lehmann R, et al: Long-term survival and function of intrahepatic islet allografts in baboons treated with humanized anti-CD154. Diabetes 48:1473–1481, 1999.

111. Gordon EJ, Woda BA, Shultz LD, et al: Rat xenograft survival in mice treated with donor-specific transfusion and anti-CD154 antibody is enhanced by elimination of host CD4+ cells. Transplantation 71:319–327, 2001.

112. Gordon EJ, Markees TG, Phillips NE, et al: Prolonged survival of rat islet and skin xenografts in mice treated with donor splenocytes and anti-CD154 monoclonal antibody. Diabetes 47:1199–1206, 1998.

113. Henn V, Slupsky JR, Grafe M, et al: CD40 ligand on activated platelets triggers an inflammatory reaction of endothelial cells. Nature 391:591–594, 1998.

114. Metcalfe RA, McIntosh RS, Marelli-Berg F, et al: Detection of CD40 on human thyroid follicular cells: Analysis of expression and function. J Clin Endocrinol Metab 83:1268–1274, 1998.

115. Smith TJ, Sciaky D, Phipps RP, Jennings TA: CD40 expression in human thyroid tissue: Evidence for involvement of multiple cell types in autoimmune and neoplastic diseases. Thyroid 9:749–755, 1999.

116. Serra P, Amrani A, Yamanouchi J, et al: CD40 ligation releases immature dendritic cells from the control of regulatory CD4+CD25+ T cells. Immunity 19:877–889, 2003.

117. Croft M: Co-stimulatory members of the TNFR family: Keys to effective T-cell immunity? Nat Rev Immunol 3:609–620, 2003.

118. Akiba H, Miyahira Y, Atsuta M, et al: Critical contribution of OX40 ligand to T helper cell type 2 differentiation in experimental leishmaniasis. J Exp Med 191:275–380, 2000.

119. Bansal-Pakala P, Halteman BS, Cheng MH, Croft M: Costimulation of CD8 T cell responses by OX40. J Immunol 172:4821–4825, 2004.

120. Ndhlovu LC, Ishii N, Murata K, et al: Critical involvement of OX40 ligand signals in the T cell priming events during experimental autoimmune encephalomyelitis. J Immunol 167:2991–2999, 2001.

121. Weinberg AD, Wegmann KW, Funatake C, Whitham RH: Blocking OX-40/OX-40 ligand interaction in vitro and in vivo leads to decreased T cell function and amelioration of experimental allergic encephalomyelitis. J Immunol 162:1818–1826, 1999.

122. Nohara C, Akiba H, Nakajima A, et al: Amelioration of experimental autoimmune encephalomyelitis with anti-OX40 ligand monoclonal antibody: A critical role for OX40 ligand in migration, but not development, of pathogenic T cells. J Immunol 166:2108–2115, 2001.

123. Kienzle G, von Kempis J: CD137 (ILA/4-1BB), expressed by primary human monocytes, induces monocyte activation and apoptosis of B lymphocytes. Int Immunol 12:73–82, 2000.

124. Mittler RS, Bailey TS, Klussman K, et al: Anti-4-1BB monoclonal antibodies abrogate T cell-dependent humoral immune responses in vivo through the induction of helper T cell anergy. J Exp Med 190:1535–1540, 1999.

125. Sytwu HK, Lin WD, Roffler SR, et al: Anti-4-1BB-based immunotherapy for autoimmune diabetes: Lessons from a transgenic non-obese diabetic (NOD) model. J Autoimmun 21:247–254, 2003.

126. Turnbridge WMG, Evered DC, Hall R, et al: The spectrum of thyroid disease in the community: The Whickham survey. Clin Endocrinol 7:481–492, 1977.

127. Riley WJ, Maclaren NK, Krisher J, et al: A prospective study of the development of diabetes in relatives of patients with insulin-dependent diabetes. N Engl J Med 323:1167–1172, 1990.

128. Pleiman CM, Clark MR: Signal transduction by the B cell antigen receptor and its coreceptors. Annu Rev Immunol 12:457–486, 1994.

129. Kurosaki T: Genetic analysis of B cell antigen receptor signaling. Annu Rev Immunol 17:555–592, 1999.

130. Reth M, Hombach J, Weinands J, et al: The B-cell antigen receptor complex. Immunol Today 12:196–201, 1991.

131. Casali P, Notkins AL: CD5+ B lymphocytes, polyreactive antibodies and the human B cell repertoire. Immunol Today 10:364–369, 1989.

132. Solvason N, Kearney JF: The human fetal omentum: A site of B cell generation. J Exp Med 175:397–404, 1992.

133. Hardy RR: Variable gene usage, physiology ad development of Ly-1+ (CD5+) B cells. Curr Opin Immunol 4:181–185, 1992.

134. Tarlinton DM, McLean M, Nossal GJ: B1 and B2 cells differ in their potential to switch immunoglobulin isotype. Eur J Immunol 25:3388–3393, 1995.

135. Finkelman FD, Lees A, Morris SC: Antigen presentation by B lymphocytes to CD4+ T lymphocytes in vivo: Importance for B lymphocytes and T lymphocyte activation. Semin Immunol 4:247–256, 1992.

136. Williams AF, Barclay AN: The immunoglobulin superfamily: Domains for cell surface recognition. Annu Rev Immunol 6:381–405, 1988.

137. Kriss JP, Pleshakow V, Chien JR: Isolation and idenfication of the long-acting tyroid stimulator and its relation to hyperthyroidism and circumscribed pretibial myxedema. J Clin Endocrinol Metab 24:1005–1028, 1964.

138. Goldman J, Baldwin D, Rubenstein AH, et al: Characterization of circulating insulin and proinsulin binding antibodies in autoimmune hypoglycemia. J Clin Invest 63:1050–1059, 1979.

139. Moller DE, Flier JS: Insulin resistance: Mechanisms, syndromes, and implications. N Engl J Med 325:938–948, 1991.

140. Eisenbarth G: Type 1 diabetes mellitus: a chronic autoimmune disease. N Engl J Med 314:1360, 1986.

141. Martin S, Wolf-Eichbaum D, Duinkerken G, et al: Development of

type 1 diabetes despite severe hereditary B-lymphocyte deficiency. N Engl J Med 345:1036–1040, 2001.

142. Miller BJ, Appel MC, O'Neil JJ, Wicker LS: Both the Lyt-2+ and L3T4+ T cell subsets are required for the transfer of diabetes in nonobese diabetic mice. J Immunol 140:52–58, 1988.

143. Noorchashm H, Noorchashm N, Kern J, et al: B-cells are required for the initiation of insulitis and sialitis in nonobese diabetic mice. Diabetes 46:941, 1997.

144. Serreze DV, Chapman HD, Varnum DS, et al: B lymphocytes are essential for the initiation of T cell-mediated autoimmune diabetes: Analysis of a new "speed congenic" stock of NOD.Igμ^{null} mice. J Exp Med 184:2049, 1996.

145. Greeley SA, Katsumata M, Yu L, et al: Elimination of maternally transmitted autoantibodies prevents diabetes in nonobese diabetic mice. Nat Med 8:399–402, 2002.

146. Miller BJ, Appel MC, O'Neil JJ, et al: Both the Lyt-2^{+} and L3T4^{+} T cell subsets are required for the transfer of diabetes in nonobese diabetic mice. J Immunol 140:52, 1988.

147. Yu L, Robles DT, Abiru N, et al: Early expression of antiinsulin autoantibodies of humans and the NOD mouse: Evidence for early determination of subsequent diabetes. Proc Natl Acad Sci U S A 97:1701–1706, 2000.

148 Tisch R, Yang X, Singer SM, et al: Immune response to glutamic acid decarboxylase correlates with insulitis in non-obese diabetic mice. Nature 366:72, 1993.

149. Baekkeskov S, Aanstoot H-J, Christgau S, et al: Identification of the 64K autoantigen in insulin-dependent diabetes as the GABA-synthesizing enzyme glutamic acid decarboxylase. Nature 347:151, 1990.

150. Kaufman DL, Erlander MG, Clare-Salzler M, et al: Autoimmunity to two forms of glutamate decarboxylase in insulin-dependent diabetes mellitus. J Clin Invest 89:283, 1992.

151. Hagopian W, Michelsen B, Karlsen AE: Autoantibodies in IDDM primarily recognize the 65,000-Mr rather than the 67,000-Mr isoform of glutamic acid decarboxylase. Diabetes 42:631, 1993.

152. Hagopian W, Sanjeevi C, Kockum I, et al: Glutamate decarboxylase-, insulin-, and islet cell-autoantibodies and HLA typing to detect diabetes in a general population-based study of Swedish children. J Clin Invest 95:1505, 1995.

153. Hagopian W, Michelsen B, Karlsen AE: Autoantibodies in IDDM primarily recognize the 65,000-Mr rather than the 67,000-Mr isoform of glutamic acid decarboxylase. Diabetes 42:631, 1993.

154. Bjorkman PH, Saper MA, Samraoui B, et al: The foreign antigen binding site and T cell recognition regions of class I histocompatibility antigens. Nature 329:512–518, 1987.

155. Brown JH, Jardetzky T, Saper MA, et al: A hypothetical model of the foreign antigen binding site of class II histocompatibility molecules. Nature 332:845–850, 1988.

156. van Bleek GM, Nathensen SG: Presentation of antigenic peptides by MHC class I molecules. Trends Cell Biol 2:202–207, 1992.

157. Germain RN, Hendrix LR: MHC class II structure, occupancy and surface expression determined by post-endoplasmic reticulum antigen binding. Nature 353:134–139, 1991.

158. Rothbard JB, Gefter MC: Interactions between immunogenic peptides and MHC proteins. Annu Rev Immunol 9:527–565, 1991.

159. Watts C: Capture and processing of exogenous antigens for presentation on MHC molecules. Annu Rev Immunol 15:821–850, 1997.

160. Porcelli SA, Modlin RL: The CD1 system: Antigen-presenting molecules for T cell recognition and glycolipids. Annu Rev Immunol 17:297–330, 1999.

161. Abbas AK, Lichtman AH: Cellular and Molecular Immunology. Philadelphia, WB Saunders, 2003.

162. Serreze DV, Leiter EH, Christianson GJ, et al: Major histocompatibility complex class I-deficient NOD-B2 mnull mice are diabetes and insulitis resistant. Diabetes 43:505, 1994.

163. Kay TW, Parker JL, Stephens LA, et al: RIP-beta 2-microglobulin transgene expression restores insulitis, but not diabetes, in beta 2-microglobulin null nonobese diabetic mice. J Immunol 157:3688, 1996.

164. Imagawa A, Hanafusa T, Tamura S, et al: Pancreatic biopsy as a procedure for detecting in situ autoimmune phenomena in type 1 diabetes: Close correlation between serological markers and histological evidence of cellular autoimmunity. Diabetes 50:1269–1273, 2001.

165. Imagawa A, Hanafusa T, Miyagawa J, Matsuzawa Y: A proposal of three distinct subtypes of type 1 diabetes mellitus based on clinical and pathological evidence. Ann Med 32:539–543, 2000.

166. Imagawa A, Hanafusa T, Itoh N, et al: Immunological abnormalities in islets at diagnosis paralleled further deterioration of glycaemic control in patients with recent-onset Type 1 (insulin-dependent) diabetes mellitus. Diabetologia 42:574–578, 1999.

167. Hanafusa T, Pujol-Borrell R, Chiovato L, et al: Aberrant expression of HLA-DR antigen on thyrocytes in Graves' disease: Relevance for autoimmunity. Lancet 2:1111–1115, 1983.

168. Lucas-Martin A, Foz-Sala M, Todd I, et al: Occurrence of thyrocyte HLA class II expression in a wide variety of thyroid diseases: Relationship with lymphocytic infiltration and thyroid autoantibodies. J Clin Endocrinol Metab 66:367–375, 1988.

169. Kabel PJ, Voorbij HA, De Haan M, et al: Intrathyroidal dendritic cells. J Clin Endocrinol Metab 66:199–207, 1988.

170. Londei M, Lamb JR, Bottazzo GF, Feldmann M: Epithelial cells expressing aberrant MHC class II determinants can present antigen to cloned human T cells. Nature 312:639–641, 1984.

171. Matsuoka N, Eguchi K, Kawakami A, et al: Lack of B7-1/BB1 and B7-2/B70 expression on thyrocytes of patients with Graves'disease: Delivery of costimulatory signals from bystander professional antigen-presenting cells. J Clin Endocrinol Metab 81:4137–4143, 1996.

172. Bottazzo GF, Dean BM, McNally JM, et al: In situ characterization of autoimmune phenomena and expression of HLA molecules in the pancreas in diabetic insulitis. N Engl J Med 313:353–360, 1985.

173. Foulis AK, Farquharson MA: Aberrant expression of HLA-DR antigens by insulin-containing beta-cells in recent-onset type I diabetes mellitus. Diabetes 35:1215–1224, 1986.

174. Dean BM, Walker R, Bone AJ, et al: Pre-diabetes in the spontaneously diabetic BB/E rat: Lymphocyte subpopulations in the pancreatic infiltrate and expression of rat MHC class II molecules in endocrine cells. Diabetologia 28:464–466, 1985.

175. Hanafusa T, Fujino-Kurihara H, Miyazaki A, et al: Expression of class II major histocompatibility complex antigens on pancreatic B cells in the NOD mouse. Diabetologia 30:104–108, 1987.

176. McInerney MF, Rath S, Janeway CA Jr: Exclusive expression of MHC class II proteins on CD45+ cells in pancreatic islets of NOD mice. Diabetes 40:648–651, 1991.

177. Farid NR, Bear J: The human major histocompatibility complex and endocrine disease. Endocr Rev 2:50, 1981.

178. Baker JR: Autoimmune endocrine disease. JAMA 278:1931, 1997.

179. Brix TH, Kyvik KO, Hegedus L: What is the evidence of genetic factors in the etiology of Graves' disease? A brief review. Thyroid 8:627, 1998.

180. Badenhoop K, Walfish PG, Rau H, et al: Susceptibility and resistance alleles of human leukocyte antigen (HLA) DQA1 and HLA DQB1 are shared in endocrine autoimmune disease. J Clin Endocrinol Metab 80:2112, 1995.

181. Lavard L, Madsen HO, Perrild H, et al: HLA class II associations in juvenile Graves' disease: Indication of a strong protective role of the DRB1'0701,DQA1'0201 haplotype. Tissue Antigens 50:639, 1997.

182. Tait KF, Gough SC: The genetics of autoimmune endocrine disease. Clin Endocrinol (Oxf) 59:1–11, 2003.

183. Petrone A, Giorgi G, Mesturino CA, et al: Association of DRB1*04-DQB1*0301 haplotype and lack of association of two polymorphic sites at CTLA-4 gene with Hashimoto's thyroiditis in an Italian population. Thyroid 11:171–175, 2001.

184. Eisenbarth GS, Gottlieb PA: Autoimmune polyendocrine syndromes. N Engl J Med 350:2068–2079, 2004.

185. Maclaren N, Riley W: Inherited susceptibility to autoimmune Addison's disease is linked to human leukocyte antigens-DR3 and/or DR4, except when associated with type I autoimmune polyglandular syndrome. J Clin Endocrinol Metab 62:455, 1986.

186. Weetman AP, Zhang L, Tandon N, Edwards OM: HLA associations with autoimmune Addison's disease. Tissue Antigens 38:31–33, 1991.

187. Donner H, Braun J, Seidl C, et al: Codon 17 polymorphism of the cytotoxic T lymphocyte antigen 4 gene in Hashimoto's thyroiditis and Addison's disease. J Clin Endocrinol Metab 82:4130, 1997.

188. Yu L, Brewer KW, Gates S, et al: DRB1*04 and DQ alleles: Expression of 21-hydroxylase autoantibodies and risk of progression to Addison's disease. J Clin Endocrinol Metab 84:328–335, 1999.

189. Myhre AG, Undlien DE, Lovas K, et al: Autoimmune adrenocortical failure in Norway: Autoantibodies and human leukocyte antigen class II associations related to clinical features. J Clin Endocrinol Metab 87:618–623, 2002.

190. Park YS, Sanjeevi CB, Robles D, et al: Additional association of intra-MHC genes, MICA and D6S273, with Addison's disease. Tissue Antigens 60:155–163, 2002.

191. Gambelunghe G, Falorni A, Ghaderi M, et al: Microsatellite polymorphism of the MHC class I chain-related (MIC-A and MIC-B) genes marks the risk for autoimmune Addison's disease. J Clin Endocrinol Metab 84:3701–3707, 1999.

192. Redondo MJ, Eisenbarth GS: Genetic control of autoimmunity in Type I diabetes and associated disorders. Diabetologia 45:605–622, 2002.

193. Mein CA, Esposito L, Dunn MG, et al: A search for type 1 diabetes susceptibility genes in familes from the United Kingdom. Nat Genet 19:297–300, 1998.

194. Todd JA: Genetics of type 1 diabetes. Pathol Biol 45:219–227, 1997.

195. Nepom G: Immunogenetics of HLA-associated diseases. Concepts Immunopathol 5:80, 1988.

196. Bach FH, Rich SS, Barbosa R, et al: Insulin-dependent diabetes-associated HLA-D region encoded determinants. Hum Immunol 12:59, 1985.

197. Baisch JM, Weeks T, Giles R, et al: Analysis of HLA-DQ genotypes and susceptibility in insulin-dependent diabetes mellitus. N Engl J Med 322:1836, 1990.

198. Todd JA, Bell JI, McDevitt H: HLA-DQB gene contributes to susceptibility and resistance to insulin-dependent diabetes mellitus. Nature 329:599, 1987.

199. Davies J, Kawaguchi Y, Bennett S, et al: A genome-wide search for human type 1 diabetes susceptibility genes. Nature 371:130, 1994.

200. Lund T, O'Reilly L, Hutchings P, et al: Prevention of insulin-dependent diabetes mellitus in non-obese diabetic mice by transgenes encoding modified I-A beta-chain or normal I-E alpha-chain. Nature 345:727–729, 1990.

201. Miyazaki T, Uno M, Uehira M, et al: Direct evidence for the contribution of the unique I-ANOD to the development of insulitis in non-obese diabetic mice. Nature 345:722–724, 1990.

202. Slattery RM, Kjer-Nielsen L, Allison J, et al: Prevention of diabetes in non-obese diabetic I-Ak transgenic mice. Nature 345:724–726, 1990.

203. Reich EP, von Grafenstein H, Barlow A, et al: Self peptides isolated from MHC glycoproteins of non-obese diabetic mice. J Immunol 152:2279–2288, 1994.

204. Kanagawa O, Shimizu J, Unanue ER: The role of I-Ag7 beta chain in peptide binding and antigen recognition by T cells. Int Immunol 9:1523–1526, 1997.

205. Carrasco-Marin E, Shimizu J, Kanagawa O, Unanue ER: The class II MHC I-Ag7 molecules from non-obese diabetic mice are poor peptide binders. J Immunol 156:450–458, 1996.

206. Exley M, Garcia J, Balk SP, Porcelli S: Requirements for CD1d recognition by human invariant Vα2+CD4–CD8– T cells. J Exp Med 186:109–120, 1997.

207. Wilson SB, Kent SC, Patton KT, et al: Extreme Th1 bias of invariant Valpha24JalphaQ T cells in type 1 diabetes. Nature 391:177–181, 1998.

208. Palmer JP, Asplin C, Clemons P, et al: Insulin antibodies in insulin-dependent diabetics before insulin treatment. Science 222:1337, 1983.

209. Rabin D, Pleasic S, Shapiro H, et al: Islet cell antigen 512 is a diabetes-specific islet autoantigen related to protein tyrosine phosphatases. J Immunol 152:3183, 1994.

210. Hawkes K, Wasmeier C, Christie MR, et al: Identification of the 37k-antigen in insulin-dependent diabetes as a tyrosine phosphatase-like protein (phogrin) related to IA-2. Diabetes 45:1187, 1996.

211. Baekkeskov S, Aanstoot H-J, Christgau S: Identification of the 64K autoantigen in insulin-dependent diabetes as the GABA-synthesizing enzyme glutamic acid decarboxylase. Nature 347:151, 1990.

212. Pietropaolo M, Castaño L, Babu S, et al: Islet cell autoantigen 69 kD (ICA69): Molecular cloning and characterization of a novel diabetes-associated autoantigen. J Clin Invest 92:359, 1993.

213. Arden SD, Roep BO, Neophytou PI, et al: Imogen 38: A novel 38-kD islet mitochondrial autoantigen recognized by T cells from a newly diagnosed type 1 diabetic patient. J Clin Invest 97:551, 1996.

214. Abulafia-Lapid R, Gillis D, Yosef O, et al: T cells and autoantibodies to human HSP70 in type 1 diabetes in children. J Autoimmun 20:313–321, 2003.

215. Abulafia-Lapid D, Elias I, Raz Y, et al: T-cell proliferation responses of Type 1 diabetes patients and healthy individuals to human HSP60 and its peptides. J Autoimmun 12:121–129, 1999.

216. Lieberman SM, Evans AM, Han B, et al: Identification of the beta cell antigen targeted by a prevalent population of pathogenic CD8+ T cells in autoimmune diabetes. Proc Natl Acad Sci U S A 100:8384–8388, 2003.

217. Kubota S, Gunji K, Ackrell BAC, et al: The 64-kilodalton eye muscle protein is the flavoprotein subunit of mitochondrial succinate dehydrogenase: The corresponding serum antibodies are good markers of an immune-mediated damage to the eye muscle in patients with Graves' hyperthyroidism. J Clin Endocrinol Metab 83:443, 1998.

218. Morris JC, Bergert ER, Bryant WP: Binding of immunoglobulin G from patients with autoimmune thyroid disease to rat sodium-iodide symporter pepetides: Evidence for the iodide transporter as an autoantigen. Thyroid 7:527, 1997.

219. Tomer Y: Anti-thyroglobulin autoantibodies in autoimmune thyroid diseases: Cross-reactive or pathogenic? Clin Immunol Immunopathol 82:3, 1997.

220. McKenzie JM, Zakarija M: Antibodies in autoimmune thyroid disease. In Braverman L, Utiger R (eds): The Thyroid: A Fundamental and Clinical Text, 7th ed. Philadelphia, Lipincott, 1996, p 416.

221. French MB, Allison J, Cram DS, et al: Transgenic expression of mouse proinsulin II prevents diabetes in nonobese diabetic mice. Diabetes 46:34–39, 1997.

222. Endl J, Otto H, Jung G, et al: Identification of naturally processed T cell epitopes from glutamic acid decarboxylase presented in the context of HLA-DR alleles by T lymphocytes of recent onset IDDM patients. J Clin Invest 99:2405–2415, 1997.

223. Karjalainen J, Martin JM, Knip M, et al: A bovine albumin peptide as a possible trigger of insulin-dependent diabetes N Engl J Med 327:302–307, 1992.

224. Lehmann PV, Sercarz EE, Forsthuber T, et al: Determinant spreading and the dynamics of the autoimmune T-cellrepertoire. Immunol Today 14:203–208, 1993.

225. Wong FS, Karttunen J, Dumont C, et al: Identification of an MHC

class I-restricted autoantigen in type 1 diabetes by screening an organ-specific cDNA library. Nat Med 5:1026–1031, 1999.

226. Kaufman DL, Clare-Salzler M, Tian J, et al: Spontaneous loss of T-cell tolerance to glutamic acid decarboxylase in murine insulin-dependent diabetes. Nature 366:69, 1993.

227. Schatz DG, Oettinger MA, Schlissel MS: V(D)J recombination: Molecular biology and regulation. Annu Rev Immunol 10:359–384, 1992.

228. Von Boehmer H: The developmental biology of T lymphocytes. Annu Rev Immunol 6:309–326, 1988.

229. MacDonald HR, Hengartner H, Pedrazzini T: Intrathymic deletion of self reactive cells prevented by neonatal anti-CD4 antibody treatment. Nature 335:730–733, 1988.

230. Blackman M, Kappler J, Marrack P: The role of the T cell receptor in positive and negative selection of developing T cells. Science 248:1335–1337, 1990.

231. Posselt AM, Barker CF, Friedman AI, Naji A: Prevention of autoimmune diabetes in the BB rat by intrathymic islet transplantation at birth. Science 256:1321–1324, 1992.

232. Koevary SB, Blomberg M: Prevention of diabetes in BB/Wor rats by intrathymic islet injection. J Clin Invest 89:512–520, 1992.

233. Herold KC, Montag AG, Buckingham F: Induction of tolerance to autoimmune diabetes with islet antigens. J Exp Med 176:1107–1114, 1992.

234. Gerling IC, Atkinson MA, Leiter EH: The thymus as a site for evaluating the potency of candidate beta cell autoantigens in NOD mice. J Autoimmun 7:851–858, 1994.

235. Gotter J, Brors B, Hergenhahn M, Kyewski B: Medullary epithelial cells of the human thymus express a highly diverse selection of tissue-specific genes colocalized in chromosomal clusters. J Exp Med 199:155–166, 2004.

236. Jolicoeur C, Hanahan D, Smith KM: T-cell tolerance toward a transgenic beta-cell antigen and transcription of endogenous pancreatic genes in thymus. Proc Natl Acad Sci U S A 91:6707–6711, 1994.

237. Pugliese A: Central and peripheral autoantigen presentation in immune tolerance. Immunology 111:138–146, 2004.

238. Pugliese A, Zeller M, Fernandez A Jr: The insulin gene is transcribed in the human thymus and transcription levels correlated with allelic variation at the INS VNTR-IDDM2 susceptibility locus for type 1 diabetes. Nat Genet 15:293–297, 1997.

239. Chentoufi AA, Polychronakos C: Insulin expression levels in the thymus modulate insulin-specific autoreactive T-cell tolerance: the mechanism by which the IDDM2 locus may predispose to diabetes. Diabetes 51:1383–1390, 2002.

240. Moriyama H, Abiru N, Paronen J, et al: Evidence for a primary islet autoantigen (preproinsulin 1) for insulitis and diabetes in the nonobese diabetic mouse. Proc Natl Acad Sci U S A 100:10376–10381, 2003.

241. Cilio CM, Daws MR, Malashicheva A, et al: Cytotoxic T lymphocyte antigen 4 is induced in the thymus upon in vivo activation and its blockade prevents anti-CD3-mediated depletion of thymocytes. J Exp Med 188:1239–1246, 1998.

242. Takara M, Kouki T, DeGroot LJ: CTLA-4 AT-repeat polymorphism reduces the inhibitory function of CTLA-4 in Graves' disease. Thyroid 13:1083–1089, 2003.

243. Kouki T, Gardine CA, Yanagawa T, Degroot LJ: Relation of three polymorphisms of the CTLA-4 gene in patients with Graves' disease. J Endocrinol Invest 25:208–213, 2002.

244. Ueda H, Howson JM, Esposito L, et al: Association of the T-cell regulatory gene CTLA4 with susceptibility to autoimmune disease. Nature 423:506–511, 2003.

245. Anderson MS, Venanzi ES, Klein L, et al: Projection of an immunological self shadow within the thymus by the aire protein. Science 298:1395–1401, 2002.

246. The Finnish-German APECED (Autoimmune Polyendocrinopathy-Candidiasis-Ectodermal Dystrophy) Consortium: An autoimmune disease, APECED, caused by mutations in a novel gene featuring two PHD-type zinc-finger domains. Nat Genet 17:399–403, 1997.

247. Pearce SH, Cheetham T, Imrie H, et al: A common and recurrent 13-bp deletion in the autoimmune regulator gene in British kindreds with autoimmune polyendocrinopathy type 1. Am J Hum Genet 63:1675–1684, 1998.

248. Scott HS, Heino M, Peterson P, et al: Common mutations in autoimmune polyendocrinopathy-candidiasis-ectodermal dystrophy patients of different origins. Mol Endocrinol 12:1112–1119, 1998.

249. Kumar PG, Laloraya M, She JX: Population genetics and functions of the autoimmune regulator (AIRE). Endocrinol Metab Clin North Am 31:321–338, 2002.

250. Goodnow CC: Transgenic mice and analysis of B cell tolerance. Annu Rev Immunol 10:489–518, 1992.

251. Nemazee D, Russell D, Arnold B, et al: Clonal deletion of autospecific B lymphocytes. Immunol Rev 122:117–132, 1991.

252. Retter MW, Nemazee D: Receptor editing: Genetic reprogramming of autoreactive lymphocytes. Cell Biochem Biophys 31:81–88, 1999.

253. Akkaraju S, Canaan K, Goodnow C: Self-reactive B cells are not eliminated or inactivated by autoantigen expressed on thyroid epithelial cells. J Exp Med 186:2005–2012, 1997.

254. Miller JFAP, Morahan G: Peripheral T cell tolerance. Annu Rev Immunol 10:51–70, 1992.

255. Miller J, Daitch L, Rath P, Selsing E: Tissue specific expression of allogeneic calss II molecules induces neither islet rejection nor clonal inactivation of alloreactive T cell. J Immunol 144:334–341, 1990.

256. Hammerling G, Schonrich G, Momburg R, et al: Non-deletional mechanisms of peripheral and central tolerance: Studies with transgenic mice with tissue specific expression of a foreign MHC class I antigen. Immunol Rev 122:47–67, 1991.

257. Ransdell F, Fowlkes BJ: Maintenance of in vivo tolerance of persistence of antigen. Science 257:1130–1133, 1992.

258. Lo D, Burkly LC, Widera G, et al: Diabetes and tolerance in transgenic mice expressing class II MHC molecules in pancreatic beta cells. Cell 53:159–168, 1988.

259. Ohashi PS, Oehen S, Buerki K, et al: Ablation of "tolerance" and induction of diabetes by virus infection in viral antigen transgenic mice. Cell 65:305–317, 1991.

260. Oldstone MBA, Nerenberg M, Southern P, et al: Virus infection triggers insulin dependent diabetes mellitus in a transgenic model. Cell 65:319–331, 1991.

261. Von Herrath MG, Efrat S, Oldstone MBA, Horwitz MS: Expression of adenoviral E3 transgenes in β cells prevents autoimmune diabetes. Proc Natl Acad Sci U S A 94:9808–9813, 1997.

262. Alferink J, Aigner S, Reibke R, et al: Peripheral T-cell tolerance: The contribution of permissive T-cell migration into parenchymal tissues of the neonate. Immunol Rev 169:255–261, 1999.

263. Bretcher P, Cohn M: A theory of self-nonself discrimination. Science 169:1042–1046, 1970.

264. Li Y, Li XC, Zheng XX, et al: Blocking both signal 1 and signal 2 of T-cell activation prevents apoptosis of alloreactive T cells and induction of peripheral allograft tolerance. Nat Med 11:1298–1302, 1999.

265. Daniel C, Grakoui A, Allen PM: Inhibition of an in vitro CD4+ T cell alloresponse using altered peptide ligands. J Immunol 160:3244–3250, 1998.

266. Nossal GJV, Pike BL: Clonal anergy: Persistence in tolerant mice of antigen-binding B lymphocytes incapable of responding to antigens or mitogen. Proc Natl Acad Sci U S A 77:1602–1606, 1980.

267. Brunet JF, Denizot F, Luciani MF, et al: A new member of the immunoglobulin superfamily CTLA-4. Nature 328:267–270, 1987.

268. Walunas TL, Lenschow DJ, Balcker CY, et al: CTLA-4 can function as a negative regulator of T cell activation. Immunity 1:405–413, 1994.

269. Krummel MF, Allison JP: CTLA-4 engagement inhibits IL-2 accumulation and cell cycle progression upon activation of resting T cells. J Exp Med 183:2533–2540, 1996.

270. Walunas TL, Bakker CY, Bluestone JA: CTLA-4 ligation blocks CD28-dependent T cell activation. J Exp Med 183:2541–2550, 1996.

271. Karandiker NJ, Vanderglut CL, Walunas TL, et al: CTLA-4: A negative regulator of autoimmune disease. J Exp Med 184:783–788, 1996.

272. Alegre ML, Noel PJ, Eisfelder BJ, et al: Regulation of surface and intracellular expression of CTLA4 on mouse T cells. J Immunol 157:4762–4770, 1996.

273. Luhder F, Hoglund P, Allison JP, et al: Cytotoxic T lymphocyte-associated antigen 4 (CTLA-4) regulates the unfolding of autoimmune diabetes. J Exp Med 187:427–432, 1998.

274. Luhder F, Hoglund P, Allison JP, et al: Cytotoxic T lymphocyte-associated antigen4 (CTLA-4) regulates the unfolding of autoimmune diabetes. J Exp Med 187:427–432, 1998.

275. Luhder F, Chambers C, Allison JP, et al: Pinpointing when T cell costimulatory receptor CTLA-4 must be engaged to dampen diabetogenic T cells. Proc Natl Acad Sci U S A 97:12204–12209, 2000.

276. Karandikar NJ, Eagar TN, Vanderlugt CL, et al: CTLA-4 downregulates epitope spreading and mediates remission in relapsing experimental autoimmune encephalomyelitis. J Neuroimmunol 109:173–180, 2000.

277. Vasu C, Gorla SR, Prabhakar BS, Holterman MJ: Targeted engagement of CTLA-4 prevents autoimmune thyroiditis. Int Immunol 15:641–654, 2003.

278. Walunas TL, Sperling AI, Khattri R, et al: CD28 expression is not essential for positive and negative selection of thymocytes or peripheral T cell tolerance. J Immunol 156:1006–1013, 1996.

279. Yanagawa T, Hidaka Y, Guimaraes V, et al: CTLA-4 gene polymorphism associated with Graves' disease in a Caucasian population. J Clin Endocrinol Metab 80:41–45, 1995.

280. Vijayakrishnan L, Slavik JM, Illes Z, et al: An autoimmune disease-associated CTLA-4 splice variant lacking the B7 binding domain signals negatively in T cells. Immunity 20:563–575, 2004.

281. Hill NJ, Lyons PA, Armitage N, et al: NOD Idd5 locus controls insulitis and diabetes and overlaps the orthologous CTLA4/IDDM12 and NRAMP1 loci in humans. Diabetes 49:1744–1747, 2000.

282. Lamhamedi-Cherradi SE, Boulard O, Gonzalez C, et al: Further mapping of the Idd5.1 locus for autoimmune diabetes in NOD mice. Diabetes 50:2874–2878, 2001.

283. Colucci F, Bergman ML, Penha-Goncalves C, et al: Apoptosis resistance of nonobese diabetic peripheral lymphocytes linked to the Idd5 diabetes susceptibility region. Proc Natl Acad Sci U S A 94:8670–8674, 1997.

284. Nistico L, Buzzetti F, Pritchard LE, et al: The CTLA-4 gene region of chromosome 2q33 is linked to and associated with, type 1 diabetes. Belgian Diabetes Registry. Hum Mol Genet 5:1075–1080, 1996.

285. Chistiakov DA, Turakulov RI: CTLA-4 and its role in autoimmune thyroid disease. J Mol Endocrinol 31:21–36, 2003.

286. Djilali-Saiah I, Larger E, Harfouch-Hammoud E, et al: No major role for the CTLA-4 gene in the association of autoimmune thyroid disease with IDDM. Diabetes 47:125–127, 1998.

287. Salama AD, Chitnis T, Imitola J, et al: Critical role of the programmed death-1 (PD-1) pathway in regulation of experimental autoimmune encephalomyelitis [erratum in J Exp Med 2003 Aug 18;198(4):677]. J Exp Med 198:71–78, 2003.

288. Kurts S, Carbone FR, Krummel MF, et al: Signalling through CD30 protects against autoimmune diabetes mediated by CD8 T cells. Nature 398:341–344, 1999.

289. Rudin CM, Thompson CB: Apoptosis and disease: Regulation and clinical relevance of programmed cell death. Annu Rev Med 48:267–281, 1997.

290. Webb S, Morris C, Sprent J: Extrathymic tolerance of mature T cells: Clonal elimination as a consequence of immunity. Cell 63:1249–1256, 1990.

291. Ashkenazi A, Dixit VM: Death receptors: Signaling and modulation. Science 281:1305–1308, 1998.

292. Waldman TA, Dubois S, Tagaya Y: Contrasting roles of IL-2 and IL-15 in the life and death of lymphocytes: Implications for immunotherapy. Immunity 14:105–110, 2001.

293. Lenardo M, Chan KM, Hornung F, et al: Mature T lymphocyte apoptosis—immune regulation in a dynamic and unpredictable antigenic environment. Annu Rev Immunol 17:221–253, 1999.

294. Chiffokau E, Walsh PT, Turka L: Apoptosis and transplantation to tolerance. Immunol Rev 193:124–145, 2003.

295. Zheng XX, Sanchez-Fueyo A, Sho M, et al: Favorably tipping the balance between cytopathic and regulatory T cells to create transplant tolerance. Immunity 19:503–514, 2003.

296. Ricordi C, Strom TB: Clinical islet transplantation: Advances and immunological challenges. Nat Rev Immunol 4:259–268, 2004.

297. Jankins MK, Schwartz RH, Pardoll DH: Effects of cyclosporin A on T cell development and clonal deletion. Science 241:1655–1658, 1988.

298. Gao E-K, Lo D, Cheney R, et al: Abnormal differentiation of thymocytes in mice treated with cyclosporin A. Nature 336:176–179, 1988.

299. Kurrer MO, Pakala SV, Hanson HL, Katz JD: β cell apoptosis in T cell-mediated autoimmune diabetes. Proc Natl Acad Sci U S A 94:213–218, 1997.

300. Chervonsky AV, Wang Y, Wong FS, et al: The role of Fas in autoimmune diabetes. Cell 89:17–24, 1997.

301. Moriwaki M, Itoh N, Miyagawa J, et al: Fas and Fas ligand expression in inflamed islets in pancreas sections of patients with recent-onset Type I diabetes mellitus. Diabetologia 42:1332–1340, 1999.

302. Giordano C, Stassi G, De Maria R, et al: Potential involvement of Fas and its ligand in the pathogenesis of Hashimoto's. Science 275:960–963, 1997.

303. Salmaso C, Bagnasco M, Pesce G, et al: Regulation of apoptosis in endocrine autoimmunity: Insights from Hashimoto's thyroiditis and Graves' disease. Ann N Y Acad Sci 966:496–501, 2002.

304. Christianson SW, Shultz LD, Leiter EH: Adoptive transfer of diabetes into immunodeficient NOD-scid/scid mice: Relative contributions of CD4+ and CD8+ T-cells from diabetic versus prediabetic NOD.NON-Thy-1a donors. Diabetes 42:44–55, 1993.

305. Serreze DV, Chapman HD, Varnum DS, et al: Initiation of autoimmune diabetes in NOD/Lt mice is MHC class I-dependent. J Immunol 158:3978–3986, 1997.

306. Wicker LS, Leiter EH, Todd JA, et al: Beta 2-microglobulin-deficient NOD mice do not develop insulitis or diabetes. Diabetes 43:500–504, 1994.

307. Kagi D, Odermatt B, Seiler P, et al: Reduced incidence and delayed onset of diabetes in perforin-deficient nonobese diabetic mice. J Exp Med 186:989–997, 1997.

308. Amrani A, Verdaguer J, Anderson B, et al: Perforin-independent beta-cell destruction by diabetogenic CD8(+) T lymphocytes in transgenic nonobese diabetic mice. J Clin Invest 103:1201–1209, 1999.

309. Kagi D, Odermatt B, Seiler P, et al: Reduced incidence and delayed onset of diabetes in perforin-deficient nonobese diabetic mice. J Exp Med 7:989–997, 1997.

310. Andre-Schmutz I, Hindelang C, Benoist C, Mathis D: Cellular and molecular changes accompanying the progression from insulitis to diabetes. Eur J Immunol 29:245–255, 1999.

311. Haskins K, Wegmann D: Diabetogenic T-cell clones. Diabetes 45:1299–1305, 1996.

312. Pakala SV, Chivetta M, Kelly CB, Katz JD: In autoimmune diabetes the transition from benign to pernicious insulitis requires an islet cell response to tumor necrosis factor alpha. J Exp Med 189:1053–1062, 1999.

313. Chatenoud L, Salomon B, Bluestone JA: Suppressor T cells—they're back and critical for regulation of autoimmunity. Immunol Rev 182:149–163, 2001.

314. Sakaguchi S, Sakaguchi N, Shimizu J, et al: Immunologic tolerance maintained by CD25+ CD4+ regulatory T cells: Their common role in controlling autoimmunity, tumor immunity, and transplantation tolerance. Immunol Rev 182:18–32, 2001.

315. Seddon B, Mason D: Regulatory T cells in the control of autoimmunity: The essential role of transforming growth bactor beta and interleukin 4 in the prevention of autoimmune thyroiditis in rats by peripheral CD4(+)CD45FC– cells and CD4+CD8– thymocytes. J Exp Med 189:279–288, 1999.

316. Greiner DL, Mordes JP, Handler ES, et al: Depletion of RT6.1+ T lymphocytes induces diabetes in resistant biobreeding/Worcester (BB/W) rats. J Exp Med 166:461–475, 1987.

317. Greiner DL, Mordes JP, Handler ES, et al: Depletion of RT6.1+ T lymphocytes induces diabetes in resistant biobreeding/Worcester (BB/W) rats. J Exp Med 166:461–475, 1987.

318. Herbelin A, Gombert J-M, Lepault F, et al: Mature mainstream TCRαβ+ CD4+ thymocytes express L-selectin mediate "active tolerance" in the nonobese diabetic mouse. J Immunol 161:2620–2628, 1998.

319. Tang Q, Henriksen KJ, Bi M, et al: In vitro-expanded antigen-specific regulatory T cells suppress autoimmune diabetes. J Exp Med 199:1455–1465, 2004.

320. Weiner HL: Induction and mechanism of action of transforming growth factor-beta-secreting Th3 regulatory cells. Immunol Rev 182:207–214, 2001.

321. Chen ZM, O'Shaughnessy MJ, Gramaglia I, et al: IL-10 and TGF-beta induce alloreactive CD4+CD25– T cells to acquire regulatory cell function. Blood 101:5076–5083, 2003.

322. Wildin RS, Ramsdell F, Peake J, et al: X-linked neonatal diabetes mellitus, enteropathy and endocrinopathy syndrome is the human equivalent of mouse scurfy. Nat Genet 27:18–20, 2001.

323. Wildin RS, Smyk-Pearson S, Filipovich AH: Clinical and molecular features of the immunodysregulation, polyendocrinopathy, enteropathy, X linked (IPEX) syndrome. J Med Genet 39:537–545, 2002.

324. Schubert LA, Jeffery E, Zhang Y, et al: Scurfin (FOXP3) acts as a repressor of transcription and regulates T cell activation. J Biol Chem 276:37672–37679, 2001.

325. Fontenot JD, Gavin MA, Rudensky AY: Foxp3 programs the development and function of CD4+CD25+ regulatory T cells. Nat Immunol 4:330–336, 2003.

326. Hori S, Nomura T, Sakaguchi S: Control of regulatory T cell development by the transcription factor Foxp3. Science 299:1057–1061, 2003.

327. Kriegel MA, Lohmann T, Gabler C, et al: Defective suppressor function of human CD4+ CD25+ regulatory T cells in autoimmune polyglandular syndrome type II. J Exp Med 199:1285–1291, 2004.

328. Sakaguchi S, Sakaguchi N, Asano M, et al: Immunologic self-tolerance maintained by activated T cells expressing IL-2 receptor alpha-chains (CD25): Breakdown of a single mechanism of self-tolerance causes various autoimmune diseases. J Immunol 155:1151–1164, 1995.

329. Kukreja A, Cost G, Marker J, et al: Multiple immuno-regulatory defects in type-1 diabetes. J Clin Invest 109:131–140, 2002.

330. Sullivan KE, McDonald-McGinn D, Zackai EH: CD4(+) CD25(+) T-cell production in healthy humans and in patients with thymic hypoplasia. Clin Diagn Lab Immunol 9:1129–1131, 2002.

331. Viglietta V, Baecher-Allan C, Weiner HL, Hafler DA: Loss of functional suppression by CD4+CD25+ regulatory T cells in patients with multiple sclerosis. J Exp Med 199:971–979, 2004.

332. Jiang H, Kashleva H, Xu LX, et al: T cell vaccination induces T cell receptor Vbeta-specific Qa-1-restricted regulatory CD8(+) T cells. Proc Natl Acad Sci U S A 95:4533–4537, 1998.

333. Ware R, Jiang H, Braunstein N, et al: Human CD8+ T lymphocyte clones specific for T cell receptor V beta families expressed on autologous CD4+ T cells. Immunity 2:177–184, 1995.

334. Filaci G, Suciu-Foca N: CD8+ T suppressor cells are back to the game: Are they players in autoimmunity? Autoimmun Rev 1:279–283, 2002.

335. Waldmann H, Cobbold S: How do monoclonal antibodies induce tolerance? A role for infectious tolerance? Annu Rev Immunol 16:619–644, 1998.

336. Cobbold S, Waldmann H: Infectious tolerance. Curr Opin Immunol 10:518–524, 1998.

337. Cobbold SP, Nolan KF, Graca L, et al: Regulatory T cells and dendritic cells in transplantation tolerance: Molecular markers and mechanisms. Immunol Rev 196:109–124, 2003.

338. Hori S, Takahashi T, Sakaguchi S: Control of autoimmunity by naturally arising regulatory CD4+ T cells. Adv Immunol 81:331–371, 2003.

339. Arif S, Tree TI, Astill TP, et al: Autoreactive T cell responses show proinflammatory polarization in diabetes but a regulatory phenotype in health. J Clin Invest 113:451–463, 2004.

340. Groux H, Bigler M, de Vries JE, Roncarolo MG: Interleukin-10 induces a long-term antigen-specific anergic state in human CD4+ T cells. J Exp Med 184:19–29, 1996.

341. Pennline KJ, Roque-Gaffney E, Monahan M: Recombinant human IL-10 prevents the onset of diabetes in the nonobese diabetic mouse. Clin Immunol Immunopathol 71:169–175, 1994.

342. Herold KC: Achieving antigen-specific immune regulation. J Clin Invest 113:346–349, 2004.

343. Peng Y, Laouar Y, Li MO, et al: TGF-beta regulates in vivo expansion of Foxp3-expressing CD4+CD25+ regulatory T cells responsible for protection against diabetes. Proc Natl Acad Sci U S A 101:4572–4577, 2004.

344. Levings MK, Sangregorio R, Sartirana C, et al: Human CD25+CD4+ T suppressor cell clones produce transforming growth factor beta, but not interleukin 10, and are distinct from type 1 T regulatory cells. J Exp Med 196:1335–1346, 2002.

345. Horwitz DA, Zheng SG, Gray JD: The role of the combination of IL-2 and TGF-beta or IL-10 in the generation and function of CD4+ CD25+ and CD8+ regulatory T cell subsets. J Leukoc Biol 74:471–478, 2003.

346. Weiner HL, Freidman A, Miller A, et al: Oral tolerance: Immunologic mechanisms and treatment of animal and human organ specific autoimmune diseases by oral administration of autoantigens. Annu Rev Immunol 12:809–838, 1994.

347. Ma S-W, Zhao D-L, Yin Z-Q, et al: Transgenic plants expressing autoantigens fed to mice to induce oral immune tolerance. Nat Med 3:793–801, 1997.

348. Zhang ZJ, Davidson L, Eisenbarth G, et al: Suppression of diabetes in nonobese diabetic mice by oral administration of porcine insulin. Proc Natl Acad Sci U S A 88:10252–10261, 1991.

349. Stewart TA, Hultgren B, Huang X, et al: Induction of type I diabetes by interferon-alpha in transgenic mice. Science 260:1942–1946, 1993.

350. Huang X, Hultgren B, Dybdal N, Stewart TA: Islet expression of interferon-alpha precedes diabetes in both the BB rat and streptozotocin-treated mice. Immunity 1:469–478, 1994.

351. Shimada A, Charlton B, Taylor-Edwards C, Fathman CG: Beta-cell destruction may be a late consequence of the autoimmune process in nonobese diabetic mice. Diabetes 45:1063–1067, 1996.

352. Roura-Mir C, Catalfamo M, Sospedra M, et al: Single-cell analysis of intrathyroidal lymphocytes shows differential cytokine expression in Hashimoto's and Graves' disease. Eur J Immunol 27:3290–3302, 1997.

353. Rabinovitch A, Sumoski W, Rajotte RV, Warnock GL: Cytotoxic effects of cytokines on human pancreatic islet cells in monolayer culture. J Clin Endocrinol Metab 71:152–156, 1990.

354. Sarvetnick N, Shizuru J, Liggitt D, et al: Loss of pancreatic islet tolerance induced by β cell expression of interferon γ. Nature 346:844–847, 1990.

355. Serreze DV, Chapman HD, Post CM, et al: Th1 to Th2 cytokine shifts in

nonobese diabetic mice: Sometimes an outcome, rather than the cause, of diabetes resistance elicited by immunostimulation. J Immunol 166:1352–1359, 2001.

356. Thomas HE, Parker JL, Schreiber RD, Kay TW: IFN-gamma action on pancreatic beta cells causes class I MHC upregulation but not diabetes. J Clin Invest 102:1249–1257, 1998.

357. Meloni G, Trisolini SM, Capria S, et al: How long can we give interleukin-2? Clinical and immunological evaluation of AML patients after 10 or more years of IL2 administration. Leukemia 16:2016–2018, 2002.

358. Atkins MH, Mier JW, Parkinson DR, et al: Hypothyroidism after treatment with interleukin-2 and lymphokine-activated killer cells. N Engl J Med 318:1557–1563, 1988.

359. Vial T, Descotes J: Immune-mediated side-effects of cytokines in humans. Toxicology 105:31–57, 1995.

360. Conlon KC, Urba WJ, Smith JW 2d: Exacerbation of symptoms of autoimmune disease in patients receiving alpha-interferon therapy. Cancer 65:2237–2242, 1990.

361. Picarella DE, Kratz A, Li CB, et al: Transgenic tumor necrosis factor (TNF)-alpha production in pancreatic islets leads to insulitis, not diabetes: Distinct patterns of inflammation in TNF-alpha and TNF-beta transgenic mice. J Immunol 150:4136–4150, 1993.

362. Meagher C, Sharif S, Hussain S, et al: Cytokines and chemokines in the pathogenesis of murine type 1 diabetes. Adv Exp Med Biol 520:133–158, 2003.

363. Baggiolini M, Dewald B, Moser B: Human chemokines: An update. Annu Rev Immunol 15:675–705, 1997.

364. Christen U, Benke D, Wolfe T, et al: Cure of prediabetic mice by viral infections involves lymphocyte recruitment along an IP-10 gradient. J Clin Invest 113:74–84, 2004.

365. Kim SH, Cleary MM, Fox HS, et al: CCR4-bearing T cells participate in autoimmune diabetes. J Clin Invest 110:1675–1686, 2002.

366. Ide A, Eisenbarth GS: Genetic susceptibility in type 1 diabetes and its associated autoimmune disorders. Rev Endocr Metab Disord 4:243–253, 2003.

367. Liu E, Eisenbarth GS: Type 1A diabetes mellitus-associated autoimmunity. Endocrinol Metab Clin North Am 31:391–410, 2002.

368. The Canadian-European Randomized Control Trial Group: Cyclosporin-induced remission of IDDM after early intervention: Association of 1 yr of cyclosporin treatment with enhanced insulin secretion. Diabetes 37:1574–1582, 1988.

369. Stiller CF, Dupre J, Gent M: Effects of cyclosporine immunosuppression in insulin-dependent diabetes mellitus of recent onset. Science 223:1362–1367, 1984.

370. Bougneres FP, Carel JC, Castano L, et al: Factors assiacted with early remission of type 1 diabetes in children treated with cyclosporine. N Engl J Med 318:663–670, 1988.

371. Bougneres PF, Landais P, Boisson C: Limited duration of remission of insulin dependency in children with recent overt type 1 diabetes treated with low-dose cyclosporin. Diabetes 39:1264–1272, 1990.

372. Staruch MJ, Sigal NH, Dumont FJ: Differential effects of the immunosuppressive macrolides FK-506 and rapamycinon activation-induced T-cell apoptosis. Int J Immunopharmacol 13:677–685, 1991.

373. Sigal NH, Dumont FJ: Cyclosporin A, FK-506, and rapamycin: Pharmacologic probes of lymphocyte signal transduction. Annu Rev Immunol 10:519–560, 1992.

374. Cook JJ, Hudson I, Harrison LC, et al: Double-blind controlled trial of azathioprine in children with newly diagnosed type 1 diabetes. Diabetes 38:779–783, 1989.

375. Silverstein J, MacLaren N, Riley W, et al: Immunosuppression with azathioprine and prednisone in recent-onset insulin-dependent diabetes mellitus. N Engl J Med 319:599–604, 1988.

376. Silverstein J, Maclaren N, Riley W, et al: Immunosuppression with azathioprine and prednisone in recent-onset insulin-dependent diabetes mellitus. N Engl J Med 319:599–604, 1988.

377. Buckingham BA, Sandborg CI: A randomized trial of methotrexate in newly diagnosed patients with type 1 diabetes mellitus. Clin Immunol 96:86–90, 2000.

378. Eisenbarth GS, Srikanta S, Jackson R, et al: Anti-thymocyte globulin and prednisone immunotherapy of recent onset type 1 diabetes mellitus. Diabetes Res 2:271–276, 1985.

379. Skyler JS, Lorenz TJ, Schwartz S, et al: Effects of an anti-CD5 immunoconjugate (CD5-plus) in recent onset type I diabetes mellitus: A preliminary investigation. The CD5 Diabetes Project Team. J Diabetes Complications 7:224–232, 1993.

380. Chatenoud L, et al: Anti-CD3 antibody induces long-term remission of overt autoimmunity in nonobese diabetic mice. Proc Natl Acad Sci U S A 91:123–127, 1994.

381. Herold KC, Bluestone JA, Montag AG, et al: Prevention of autoimmune diabetes with nonactivating anti-CD3 monoclonal antibody. Diabetes 41:385–391, 1992.

382. Chatenoud L, Primo J, Bach JF: CD3 antibody-induced dominant self tolerance in overtly diabetic NOD mice. J Immunol 158:2947–2954, 1997.

383. Herold KC, Hagopian W, Auger JA, et al: Anti-CD3 monoclonal antibody in new-onset type 1 diabetes mellitus. N Engl J Med 346:1692–1698, 2002.

384. Chatenoud L, Thervet E, Primo J, et al: Anti-CD3 antibody induces long-term remission of overt autoimmunity in nonobese diabetic mice. Proc Natl Acad Sci U S A 91:123–127, 1994.

385. Chatenoud L, Primo J, Bach JF: CD3 antibody-induced dominant self tolerance in overtly diabetic NOD mice. J Immunol 158:2947–2954, 1997.

386. Herold KC, Burton JB, Francois F, et al: Activation of human T cells by FcR nonbinding anti-CD3 mAb, hOKT3gamma1(Ala-Ala). J Clin Invest 111:409–418, 2003.

387. Chatenoud L, Bach JF: Anti-CD3 antibodies. Immunol Ser 59:175–191, 1993.

388. Smith JA, Tso Jy, Clark MR, et al: Nonmitogenic anti-CD3 monoclonal antibodies deliver a partial T cell receptor signal and induce clonal anergy. J Exp Med 185:1413–1422, 1997.

389. Tian J, Clare-Salzler M, Herschenfeld A, et al: Modulating autoimmune responses to GAD inhibits disease progression and prolongs islet graft survival in diabetes-prone mice. Nat Med 2:1348–1354, 1996.

390. Elias D, Cohen IR: Treatment of autoimmune diabetes and insulitis in NOD mice with heat shock protein 60 peptide p277. Diabetes 44:1132–1138, 1995.

391. Elias D, Meilin A, Ablamunits V, et al: Hsp60 peptide therapy of NOD mouse diabetes induces a Th2 cytokine burst and downregulates autoimmunity to various β-cell antigens. Diabetes 46:758–764, 1997.

392. Muir A, Peck A, Clare-Salzler M, et al: Insulin immunization of nonobese diabetic mice induces a protective insulitis characterized by diminished intraislet interferon-gamma transcription. J Clin Invest 95:628–634, 1995.

393. Elias D, Markovits D, Reshef T, et al: Induction and therapy of autoimmune diabetes in the non-obese diabetic (NOD/LT) mouse by a 65-kDa heat shock protein. Proc Natl Acad Sci U S A 87:1576–1580, 1990.

394. Elias D, Cohen IR: Peptide therapy for diabetes in NOD mice. Lancet 343:704–706, 1994.

395. Elias D, Reshef T, Birk OS, et al: Vaccination against autoimmune mouse diabetes with a T-cell epitope of the human 65 kDa heat shock protein. Proc Natl Acad Sci U S A 88:3088–3091, 1991.

396. Raz I, Elias D, Avron A, et al: Beta-cell function in new-onset type 1 diabetes and immunomodulation with a heat-shock protein peptide (DiaPep277): A randomised, double-blind, phase II trial. Lancet 358:1749–1753, 2001.

397. Keller RJ, Eisenbarth GS, Jackson RA: Insulin prophylaxis in individuals at

high risk of type I diabetes. Lancet 341:927–928, 1993.

398. Atkinson MA, Maclaren NK, Luchetta R: Insulitis and diabetes in NOD mice reduced by prophylactic insulin therapy. Diabetes 39:933, 1990.

399. Diabetes Prevention Trial—Type 1 Diabetes Study Group: Effects of insulin in relatives of patients with type 1 diabetes mellitus. N Engl J Med 346:1685–1691, 2002.

400. Skyler J: Oral presentation. American Diabetes Association, Orlando, FL, June 4–8, 2004.

401. Pozzilli P, Pitocco D, Visalli N, et al: No effect of oral insulin on residual beta-cell function in recent-onset type I diabetes (the IMDIAB VII). IMDIAB Group. Diabetologia 43:1000–1004, 2000.

402. Gale EA, Bingley PJ, Emmett CL, Collier T, and the European Nicotinamide Diabetes Intervention Trial (ENDIT) Group: European Nicotinamide Diabetes Intervention Trial (ENDIT): A randomized controlled trial of intervention before the onset of type 1 diabetes. Lancet 363:925–931, 2004.

403. Crino A, Schiaffini R, Manfrini S, et al, on behalf of the IMDIAB group: A randomized trial of nicotinamide and vitamin E in children with recent onset type 1 diabetes (IMDIAB IX). Eur J Endocrinol 150:719–724, 2004.

404. Karjalainen J, Martin JM, Knip M, et al: A bovine albumin peptide as a possible trigger of insulin-dependent diabetes mellitus [erratum in N Engl J Med 1992 Oct 22;327(17):1252]. N Engl J Med 327:302–307, 1992.

405. Ziegler AG, Schmid S, Huber D, et al: Early infant feeding and risk of developing type 1 diabetes–associated autoantibodies. JAMA 290:1721–1728, 2003.

406. Norris JM, Barriga K, Klingensmith G, et al: Timing of initial cereal exposure in infancy and risk of islet autoimmunity. JAMA 290:1713–1720, 2003.

407. Tallstedt L, Lundell G, Torring O, et al: Occurrence of ophthalmopathy after treatment for Graves' hyperthyroidism. The Thyroid Study Group. N Engl J Med 326:1733–1738, 1992.

408. Bartalena L, Marcocci C, Bogazzi F, et al: Relation between therapy for hyperthyroidism and the course of Graves' ophthalmopathy. N Engl J Med 338:73–78, 1998.

409. Abbas AK, Sharpe AH: T cell stimulation: An abundance of B7s. Nat Med 5:1345–1346, 1999.

410. Swallow MM, Wallin JJ, Sha WC: B7h, a novel costimultory homolog of B7.1 and B7.2 is induced by TNF-alpha. Immunity 11:423–432, 1999.

411. Dong H, Zhy G, Tamada K, Chen L: B7-H1, a third member of the B7 family, co-stimulates T cell proliferation and interleukin-10 secretion. Nat Med 5:1365–1369, 1999.

412. Kim JJ, Tsai A, Nottingham LK, et al: Intracellular adhesion molecule-1 modulates beta-chemokines and directly costimulates T cells in vivo. J Clin Invest 103:869–877, 1999.

413. Appetecchia M, Castelli M, Delpino A: Anti-heat shock proteins autoantibodies in autoimmune thyroiditis: Preliminary study. J Exp Clin Cancer Res 16:395, 1997.

Interactions of the Endocrine and Immune Systems

George P. Chrousos and Ilia J. Elenkov

THERAPEUTIC PERSPECTIVES

The neuroendocrine and immune systems play major roles in adaptation. Any *stressor*, or threat to the stability of the internal milieu, is counteracted by responses of the organism, the *adaptive responses*. The effectors of these responses are the corticotropin-releasing hormone (CRH)/arginine-vasopressin (AVP) and locus caeruleus–noradrenaline (LC-NA)/autonomic (sympathetic) neurons of the hypothalamus and brain stem, which regulate the peripheral activities of the hypothalamic-pituitary-adrenal (HPA) axis and the systemic/adrenomedullary sympathetic nervous systems (SNS), respectively. Activation of the HPA axis and LC-NA/autonomic system result in systemic elevations of glucocorticoids and catecholamines (CAs), respectively, that act in concert to maintain the steady state or *homeostasis*.[1]

Since Selye's time, in the late 1930s, stress hormones, especially glucocorticoids, have been progressively known to shrink the thymus and lymph nodes; to inhibit lymphocyte proliferation, migration, and cytotoxicity; and to suppress the secretion of certain cytokines, such as interleukin-2 (IL-2) and interferon-γ (IFN-γ). These early observations and the broad use of glucocorticoids as potent anti-inflammatory/immunosuppressant agents in the last 50 years led to the initial conclusion that stress was, in general, immunosuppressive. Recently, however, there has been convincing evidence that glucocorticoids and CAs, at levels that can be achieved during stress, influence the immune response in a less monochromatic way. This new understanding helps to explain some well-known, but often contradictory, effects of stress on the immune system and on the onset and course of certain infectious, autoimmune/inflammatory, allergic, and neoplastic diseases. Here, we provide a brief up-to-date review of this understanding.

HISTORIC MILESTONES

Neuroendocrinology and immunology developed independently of each other for many years. Celsius defined four of the five cardinal signs of inflammation almost 2000 years ago, and Eustachius described the adrenal glands in 1563. The question, however, as to how the brain communicates with the immune system remained unknown or enigmatic until recently. Evidence that lymphoid organs are innervated dates back to the end of the nineteenth century when nerves, independently of blood vessels, were found to enter lymph nodes.[2] In 1898, von Fürth described a bioactive principle in extracts from animal adrenal glands, which he called "suprarenin." Three years later, Takamine and Aldrich independently isolated suprarenin in crystalline form (cf. Ref. 3) and named it *adrenaline*; their investigation determined the correct formula ($C_9H_{13}NO_3$) of this substance, which represents the first hormone to be isolated from animal tissues. During later experiments, in 1907, a "by-product" of the synthesis of adrenaline or epinephrine was identified; this substance became commercially available as "arterenol" in 1908. It was, in fact, noradrenaline or norepinephrine, which was formally discovered and isolated from tissues 40 years later.

At the end of the nineteenth century and the beginning of the twentieth century, Metchnicoff and Ehrlich, respectively, developed the concepts of cellular and humoral immunity (see Ref. 4). In 1904, Loeper and Crouzon[5] were the first to describe a pronounced leukocytosis after subcutaneous injection of epinephrine in humans. In the 1920s, Metal'nikov and Chorine[6] showed that immune reactions could be conditioned by classic Pavlovian means. In the 1930s, Selye described involution of the thymus in animals that were exposed to stressors and expanded on the concept of the stress response initially introduced by Cannon.[7] Cannon had called this response the *fight or flight* reaction and had linked it to stress and to CA secretion. Cannon had also emphasized the "generalized" sympathetic response or the "wisdom of the body" that occurs during stress, contrasting it with the more "discrete" functions of parasympathetic pathways.[8,9]

In the 1940s, von Euler[10] isolated norepinephrine (NE) from a lymphoid organ, the spleen, and later provided evidence that NE was the major neurotransmitter released from sympathetic nerves. Cortisone, the active principle of the adrenal glands, was isolated by Kendal and Reichstein in the late 1940s and shown to suppress immune functions. These scientists, along with Hench, received the Nobel Prize in Medicine and Physiology, after Hench showed that cortisone produced a spectacular amelioration of rheumatoid arthritis.[11,12] Interestingly, in the 1950s Dougherty and Frank[13] noticed a 400% increase of what they called "stress-lymphocytes" within 10 minutes after subcutaneous injection of epinephrine. These cells had the morphology of large granular lymphocytes or natural killer (NK) cells, whose function and characteristics were described in the late 1970s (see Ref. 3).

It was in the 1970s and 1980s, however, that Besedovsky and coworkers demonstrated that classic hormones and newly described cytokines were involved in a functionally relevant *cross-talk* between the brain and the immune system.[14–16] They showed that an immune response induced an increase of plasma glucocorticoid concentrations,[14,16,17] altered the activity of hypothalamic noradrenergic neurons,[18] and decreased the content of NE in the spleen.[15,19] At about the same time, the first comprehensive morphologic studies provided evidence that both primary and secondary lymphoid organs were innervated by sympathetic/noradrenergic nerve fibers. Furthermore, it was shown that classic behavioral conditioning,[20] stressful stimuli,[1,21,22] or lesions in specific regions of the brain[23] reproducibly altered immune function. Finally, evidence was obtained in experimental animals that the susceptibility to autoimmune diseases was determined to a great extent by the activity of the stress system[24–26] or that stress mediators exert both proinflammatory and anti-inflammatory effects.[1,27] Subsequently, we witnessed an explosive growth of a new interdisciplinary research area that studies the neuroimmune communication, and our understanding of the interactions between the neuroendocrine system and the immune and inflammatory reaction has expanded enormously.

ORGANIZATION OF THE STRESS SYSTEM

The HPA axis and the systemic sympathetic and adrenomedullary (sympathetic) system are the peripheral limbs of the stress system, whose main function is to maintain basal and stress-related homeostasis.[8,28] The central components of this system are located in the hypothalamus and the brain stem (Fig. 40-1). They include the parvocellular neurons of the paraventricular nuclei of the hypothalamus that release CRH and AVP, the CRH neurons of the paragigantocellular and parabrachial nuclei of the medulla, and the A1, A2, A3, and A6 (locus caeruleus) mostly noradrenergic cell groups of the medulla and pons.

Each of the paraventricular nuclei has three parvocellular divisions: a medial group, producing mostly CRH and projecting and secreting into the hypophysial portal system; an intermediate group producing mostly AVP and also projecting and secreting into the hypophysial portal system; and a lateral group, producing primarily CRH and projecting to and innervating noradrenergic and other neurons of the stress system in the brain stem (Fig. 40-2).[8,28,29] Some parvocellular neurons contain and secrete both CRH and AVP, and this neural population increases with stress.[30,31] Other paraventricular CRH neurons project to and innervate pro-opiomelanocortin-containing neurons of the central stress system in the arcuate nucleus of the hypothalamus, as well as neurons of pain control areas of the hindbrain and spinal cord (see Figs. 40-1 and 40-2). Activation of the stress system leads to CRH-induced secretion of pro-opiomelanocortin-derived and other opioid peptides,[32,33] which enhance analgesia.[8,28] These peptides also simultaneously inhibit the activity of the stress system by suppressing CRH and norepinephrine secretion.[8,28]

CRH stimulates the secretion of adrenocorticotropic hormone (ACTH) by the corticotrophs of the anterior pituitary.[34,35]

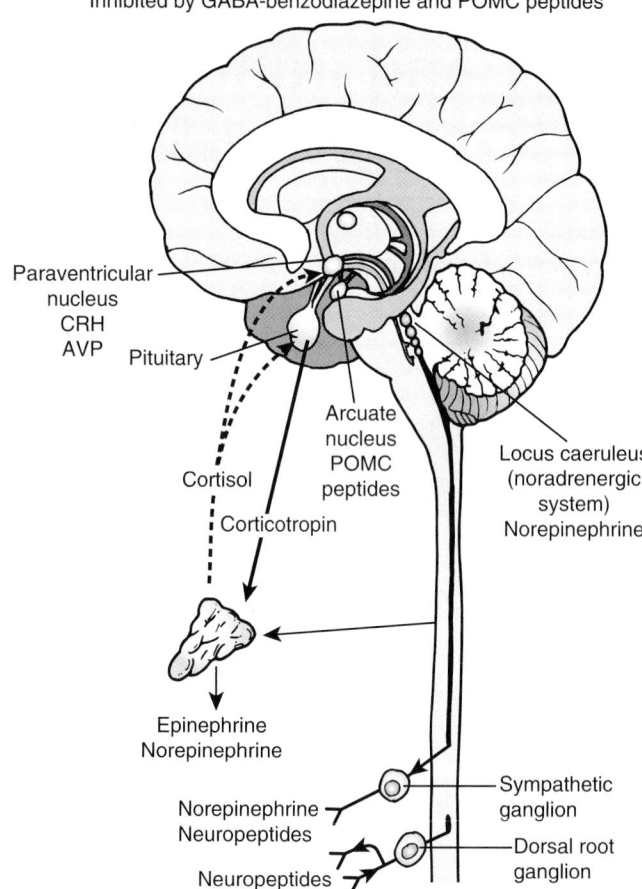

Figure 40-1 Major components of the central and peripheral stress system. The paraventricular nucleus and the locus caeruleus/noradrenergic system are shown, along with their peripheral limbs, the pituitary-adrenal axis, and the adrenomedullary and systemic sympathetic systems. The hypothalamic corticotropin-releasing hormone (CRH) and central noradrenergic neurons mutually innervate and activate each other, while they exert presynaptic autoinhibition through collateral fibers. Arginine vasopressin (AVP) from the paraventricular nucleus synergizes with CRH on stimulating corticotropin (ACTH) secretion. The cholinergic and serotonergic neurotransmitter systems stimulate both components of the central stress system, while the gamma aminobutyric acid/benzodiazepine (GABA/BZD) and arcuate nucleus pro-opiomelanocortin (POMC) peptide systems inhibit it. The latter is directly activated by the stress system and is important in the enhancement of analgesia that takes place during stress (Source: Chrousos GP: The hypothalamic-pituitary-adrenal axis and immune-mediated inflammation. N Engl J Med 332:1351–1362, 1995.)

Its effect on the pituitary is also permissive, because when CRH is absent, very little ACTH secretion takes place. AVP alone has very little ACTH secretagogue activity but is a potent synergistic factor with CRH. CRH and AVP may act synergistically on other target tissues with CRH and AVP receptors in the central nervous system (CNS) and perhaps the periphery.[36]

Every hour, the parvocellular neurons secrete two or three mostly synchronous pulses of CRH and AVP into the hypophysial portal system.[37–41] In early morning, the amplitudes of these pulses are highest, increasing the amplitude and apparent frequency of ACTH and cortisol secretory episodes. The frequency appears to increase, because previously undetectable pulses of ACTH and cortisol become measurable by standard assays. During acute stress, the amplitude

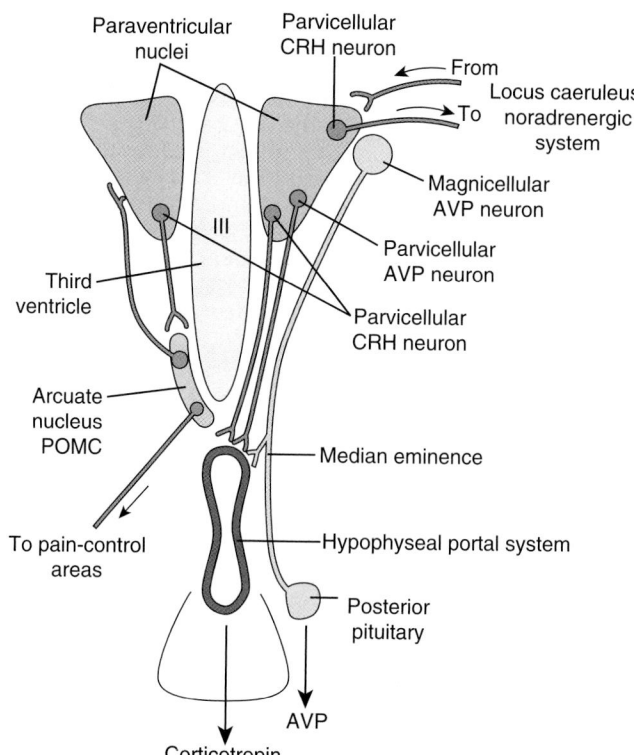

Figure 40-2 A close-up view of the paraventricular nuclei of the hypothalamus. Parvocellular CRH- and arginine vasopressin (AVP)–secreting neurons project to and secrete into the hypophysial portal system. Parvocellular CRH neurons also project to the brain stem to innervate neurons of the locus coeruleus/noradrenergic system. Magnocellular AVP-secreting neurons terminate at the posterior pituitary and secrete into the systemic circulation; they also have collateral terminals in the portal system. CRH is permissive for and stimulates pituitary corticotropin (ACTH) secretion, while AVP has a major synergistic role with CRH in the secretion of ACTH, however. The arcuate pro-opiomelanocortin (POMC) nucleus is shown, along with the mutual innervation between CRH and POMC-peptide-secreting neurons (Source: Chrousos GP: The hypothalamic-pituitary-adrenal axis and immune-mediated inflammation. N Engl J Med 332:1351–1362, 1995.)

of CRH and AVP pulses also increases, resulting in increases in the amplitude and apparent frequency of ACTH and cortisol pulses; in this case, the stress system recruits additional secretagogues of CRH, AVP, or ACTH, such as magnocellular AVP and angiotensin II.[8,28,42,43]

Circulating ACTH of pituitary origin is the key regulator of glucocorticoid secretion by the adrenal gland's *zona fasciculata*. Other hormones, including CAs, neuropeptide Y (NPY), from the adrenal medulla, and additional autonomic neural input to the adrenal cortex also take part in the regulation of glucocorticoid secretion.[41,44–47] ACTH participates in the control of aldosterone secretion by the *zona glomerulosa* and of adrenal androgen secretion by the *zona reticularis*.

The sympathetic system originates in nuclei within the brain stem and gives rise to preganglionic efferent fibers that leave the CNS through the thoracic and lumbar spinal nerves ("thoracolumbar system"). Most of the sympathetic preganglionic fibers terminate in ganglia located in the paravertebral chains that lie on either side of the spinal column. The remaining sympathetic ganglia are located in prevertebral ganglia, which lie in front of the vertebrae. From these ganglia, postganglionic sympathetic fibers run to the tissues that are innervated. Most postganglionic sympathetic fibers release NE; they are noradrenergic fibers, that is, they act by releasing NE. Adrenal medulla contains chromaffin cells,

embryologically and anatomically homologous to the sympathetic ganglia also derived from the neural crest. The adrenal medulla, unlike the postganglionic sympathetic nerve terminals, releases mainly epinephrine and, to a lesser extent, NE (the approximate ratio is 4:1); typical preganglionic sympathetic nerve terminals, whose main neurotransmitter is acetylcholine, innervate the chromaffin cells of the adrenal medulla.

CAs are synthesized from tyrosine that is transported into the noradrenergic endings or varicosities by a sodium-dependent carrier. Tyrosine is converted to dopamine (the rate-limiting step in the NE synthesis) by the enzyme tyrosine hydroxylase (TH) and a carrier that can be blocked by reserpine transports dopamine into the secretory vesicles. Dopamine is converted to NE within these vesicles by dopamine-β-hydroxylase. In the adrenal medulla, NE is further converted to epinephrine.

ROLE OF STRESS SYSTEM IN MAINTAINING BASAL AND STRESS-RELATED HOMEOSTASIS

Living organisms survive by maintaining an immensely complex dynamic steady state of the internal milieu or *homeostasis*, a term coined by Cannon. When homeostasis is disturbed or threatened, by internal or external challenges, both the HPA axis and the SNS become activated, resulting in increased peripheral levels of glucocorticoids and CAs that act in concert to maintain homeostasis. Selye defined this reaction in the 1930s as the "general adaptation or stress syndrome."[8]

The stress system has a baseline, circadian activity but also responds on demand to physical and emotional stressors. At rest, via glucocorticoids and CAs, it maintains basal *homeostasis*, as major regulators of fuel metabolism, heart rate, blood vessel tone, and thermogenesis, while during stress it adjusts these functions accordingly. This system integrates and responds to a great diversity of distinct circadian, neurosensory, blood-borne, and limbic signals. This includes humoral signals from the immune and inflammatory reaction. Indeed, any immune challenge that threatens the stability of the internal milieu can be regarded as a stressor, that is, a stimulus to the organism that activates the stress system to help reattain homeostasis.

The last 15 years have provided evidence that certain cytokines, particularly the pro-inflammatory ones, including tumor necrosis factor (TNF)-α and interleukin (IL)-1 and IL-6, activate both the HPA axis and the SNS.[1,48] Moreover, these cytokines, alone or in conjunction with components of the stress system, induce fever, sleepiness, fatigue, loss of appetite, and decreased libido and activate the hepatic synthesis of acute phase proteins, changes referred to as *sickness behavior* and *acute phase response*, respectively. Stress that is associated with an immune challenge has been called *immune* or *inflammatory stress*[1] and, like other forms of stress, is coordinated by the central stress system and its peripheral arms.

Functionally, the CRH and LC-NE/sympathetic systems seem to participate in a positive, reverberatory feedback loop so that activation of one system tends to activate the other as well.[8,28,49,50] This includes projections of CRH-secreting neurons from the lateral PVN to the central sympathetic systems in the hindbrain and, conversely, projections of catecholaminergic fibers from the LC-NE system via the ascending noradrenergic bundle to the PVN in the hypothalamus. Thus, CRH stimulates norepinephrine secretion through its specific receptors, while norepinephrine stimulates CRH secretion through primarily α1-noradrenergic receptors.[8,28,50] Autoregulatory, ultrashort negative feedback loops are also present in these neurons, with CRH and norepinephrine collateral fibers acting in an inhibitory fashion on presynaptic CRH and α2-noradrenergic receptors, respectively. The CRH, AVP, and noradrenergic neurons receive stimulatory input from the serotonergic, cholinergic, and histaminergic systems and inhibitory input from the gamma-aminobutyric acid (GABA)/benzodiazepine and opioid peptide neuronal systems of the brain.[8,28,49,50] Centrally secreted substance P has inhibitory actions on the hypothalamic CRH but not AVP neurons and stimulatory effects on the central noradrenergic system.[50-52]

Activation of the stress system leads to adaptive behavioral and physical changes.[8,28] Centrally, the behavioral changes include enhanced arousal and accelerated motor reflexes, better attention span and cognitive function, decreased feeding and sexual behavior, and increased ability to withstand pain. Peripherally, the activation of the stress system results in increased sympathetic output, that is, increase of the release of NE from the sympathetic nerve terminals and epinephrine/NE from the adrenal medulla, and in increased secretion of glucocorticoids by the adrenal cortex. These changes are related to the physical adaptation that includes changes in cardiovascular function, intermediary metabolism, and modulation of the immune and inflammatory reaction.

INNERVATION OF LYMPHOID ORGANS

Sympathetic/noradrenergic and sympathetic/NPY postganglionic nerve fibers innervate both the smooth muscle of the vasculature and the parenchyma of specific compartments of primary and secondary lymphoid organs.[53,54] These nerve fibers and their varicosites do travel in plexuses that run adjacent to and along the blood vessels in these organs; it is hence possible that both NE and NPY, released from these fibers, play a role in controlling blood flow to these organs and the traffic of leukocytes within their vessels. However, some noradrenergic fibers that are not associated with blood vessels are present in the parenchyma of lymphoid organ tissue.[53,54] NE released from their nerve fibers may exert immunomodulatory roles by altering the activity of local leukocytes. Noradrenergic innervation of lymphoid tissues appears to be regional and specific; generally, zones of T cells, macrophages and plasma cells are richly innervated, while nodular and follicular zones of developing or maturing B cells are poorly innervated.[53]

The main target cells of the noradrenergic innervation of lymphoid organs appear to be immature and mature thymocytes, thymic epithelial cells, T lymphocytes, macrophages, mast cells, plasma cells, and enterochromaffin cells. Noradrenergic nerve fibers in the thymus are closely associated with mast cells within both the perivascular and parenchymal zones, suggesting a possible humoral role for NE and histamine in the maturation of T cells. Noradrenergic innervation is present early in development, and the arrival of the fibers generally precedes the development of the cellular compartment of the immune system, suggesting a role for NE in the development of this system. For example, at the time of development and reorganization of the periarteriolar lymphatic sheath in the spleen (postnatal day 14 in the rat), the noradrenergic plexus around the central arterioles and its branches increases in density, displaying an adult pattern of both vascular and parenchymal innervation.[55]

In addition to the autonomic/sympathetic innervation, all lymphoid organs also receive sensory peptidergic innervation that is confined mostly to the parenchyma.[56] The most abundantly present neuropeptides are the tachykinins, substance P and neurokinin A, calcitonin gene-related peptide (CGRP), and vasoactive intestinal polypeptide/peptide histidine isoleucine. Double immunofluorescence reveals the coexistence of tachykinins with CGRP and of TH with NPY. This coexistence pattern conforms to the general scheme described for the peripheral innervation of nonimmune organs.

A close spatial relationship between peptidergic nerve fibers and mast cells, T cells, and macrophages is observed in immune organs.[56] Peptidergic nerves, however, are sparse in pure B-cell regions. Neuro-mast cell contacts are present in lymphoid organs, except the spleen.[56] Mast cells bear receptors for and respond to substance P (SP); the latter triggers the release of granules containing histamine, cytokines, and lipid mediators of inflammation, including leukotrienes. NE, on the other hand, through the stimulation of α_2- or β_2-adrenoreceptors, stimulates or inhibits the release of histamine from mast cells. Thus, apart from their direct immunomodulatory effects, SP antidromically released from sensory nerves, or NE released from postganglionic noradrenergic nerve terminals may exert indirect immunomodulatory effects via changes in mast cell degranulation within the parenchyma of lymphoid organs.

Neuro-mast cell connections and neuro-macrophage connections, as well as neuro-T-cell contacts, are not restricted to the preformed lymphoid organs and tissues, but are also regularly encountered in most nonimmune tissues.[56] Mast cells, T cells, and macrophages are regularly seen contacted by the terminals of peripheral nerves from the sympathetic and sensory ganglia. In the skin, postcapillary venules, macrophages, mast cells, and peptidergic nerves stained for tachykinins/CGRP form a typical quadrad, while in the outer wall of larger blood vessels, the quadrad is joined by TH/NPY fibers. Further, close interrelations but no coincidence of TH/NPY and SP/CGRP immunoreactive fibers are frequently observed in perivascular regions.[56]

THE IMMUNE RESPONSE AND THE INFLAMMATORY REACTION

Any immune response involves, first, recognition of a pathogen, and, second, mounting of a reaction against it. Broadly speaking, the different types of immune response fall into two categories: the *innate* (or nonspecific) and *adaptive* (or specific) immune responses.

Phagocytic cells, such as monocytes, macrophages, and polymorphonuclear neutrophils bind to microorganisms, internalize them, and kill them. Since they use primitive nonspecific recognition systems, which allow them to bind to a variety of microbial products, they mediate innate immune responses, acting as a first line of defense.[57] However, a subgroup of lymphocytes known as large granular lymphocytes (LGLs) also have the capacity to recognize surface changes that occur on a variety of tumor or virally infected cells and to destroy these cells using nonspecific recognition systems; this action is often called NK cell activity. Both monocytes/macrophages and LGLs may also recognize and destroy target cells (or pathogens) coated with specific antibody.

Lymphocytes, such as T lymphocytes (or T cells) and B lymphocytes (or B cells), are central components of the adaptive immune response, since they specifically recognize individual pathogens, whether they are inside host cells or outside in the tissue fluids or blood. B cells combat extracellular pathogens and their products by releasing antibodies, which specifically recognize and bind target molecules, the antigens. Antigens may be molecules on the surface of pathogens or soluble toxins produced by them. One group of lymphocytes, the T-helper (Th) cells, exert regulatory function, that is, they interact with B cells and help them divide, differentiate, and make antibody; this group also interacts with mononuclear lymphocytes and help them destroy intracellular pathogens. Another group of T cells, the T-cytotoxic (Tc), are responsible for the destruction of host cells, which have become infected by viruses or other intracellular pathogens. T cells use a specific receptor, the T-cell antigen receptor (TCR), to recognize antigens, but only in association with familiar markers on host cells. This receptor is related, both in structure and function to the surface antibody, which B cells use as their antigen receptors. T cells generate their effects either by releasing cytokines or by direct cell-cell interactions.[57]

The cells of the immune system are widely distributed throughout the body, but if an infection occurs, it is necessary to mobilize a large number of them at the site of infection. The process by which this occurs manifests itself as inflammation and includes[1] increased blood supply to the infected area by local vasodilatation,[2] increased capillary permeability to permit diapedesis of leukocytes, and exudation of plasma-containing soluble mediators of immunity. The migration of leukocytes is assisted by a process of chemical attraction known as chemotaxis (Fig. 40-3).

The cells that participate in the inflammatory reaction are monocytes, polymorphonuclear leukocytes (including neutrophils, basophils, and eosinophils), and lymphocytes, all attracted from the blood to the inflammatory site, and local immune accessory cells, such as endothelial cells, mast cells, tissue fibroblasts, and resident macrophages. In the earliest stages of inflammation, neutrophils are particularly prevalent, but in the later stages, monocytes and lymphocytes take on a primary role. Local generation of secretory products, including cytokines, lipid mediators of inflammation, and neuropeptides, is crucial for further chemoattraction of cells and for the coordinated activation of the effector cells.[58,59] Most of the time, these events are clinically undetectable. Occasionally, however, clinical inflammation occurs, generating high concentrations of local and circulating levels of cytokines and other mediators of inflammation associated with activation of the stress system and sickness behavior.

The sensory afferent fibers and postganglionic sympathetic neurons of the peripheral nervous system also influence inflammation (see Fig. 40-3).[60–64] The sensory fibers sense the local threat and not only send signals to the central nervous system, but also secrete proinflammatory or anti-inflammatory substances, such as the neuropeptides substance P or somatostatin, respectively, in the site of inflammation. The neurotransmitter NE that is released from the postganglionic sympathetic nerve fibers exerts mostly anti-inflammatory effects locally (see text below).

ROLE OF Th1 AND Th2 CELLS AND TYPE 1 AND TYPE 2 CYTOKINES IN THE REGULATION OF CELLULAR AND HUMORAL IMMUNITY

Immune responses are regulated by antigen-presenting cells (APCs), such as monocytes/macrophages, dendritic cells, and other phagocytic cells, which are components of *innate immunity* and by the recently described lymphocyte subclasses Th1 and Th2, which are components of *adaptive immunity*.[65,66] Th1 cells primarily secrete IFN-γ, IL-2, and TNF–β, which promote cellular immunity, whereas Th2 cells secrete a different set of cytokines, primarily IL-4, IL-10, and IL-13, which promote humoral immunity (Fig. 40-4).

Naive CD4[+] (antigen-inexperienced) Th0 cells are clearly bipotential and serve as precursors of Th1 and Th2 cells. Among the factors that are currently known to influence the differentiation of these cells toward Th1 or Th2, cytokines produced by cells of the innate immune system are the most important. Thus, IL-12, produced by activated monocytes/macrophages or other APCs, is a major inducer of Th1 differentiation and hence cellular immunity; this cytokine acts in concert with NK-derived IFN-γ to further promote Th1 responses.[67] APC-derived IL-12 and TNF-α in concert with NK cell- and Th1 cell-derived IFN-γ, stimulate the functional

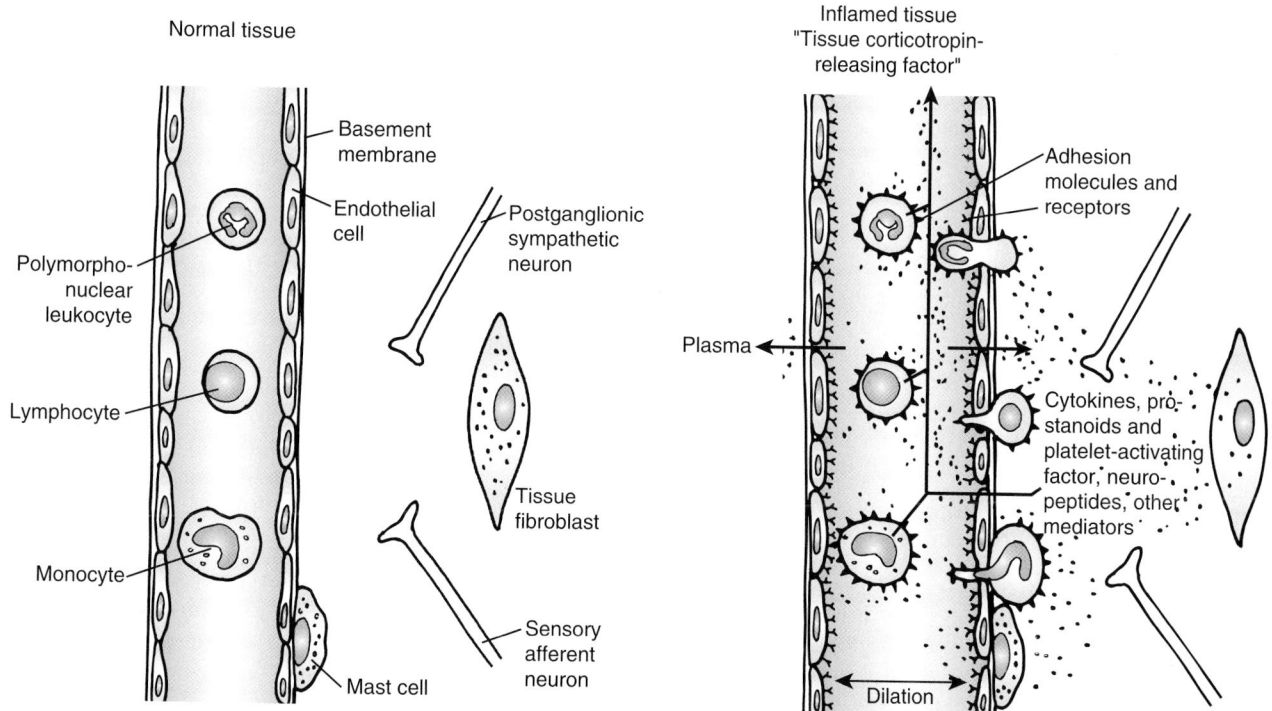

Figure 40-3 Major components and events of inflammation. Quiescent circulating leukocytes, local immune accessory cells, and the terminals of peripheral postganglionic sympathetic and sensory afferent neurons are shown (*left panel*). In inflamed tissue (*right panel*), there is vasodilation, increased permeability of the vessel, and exudation of plasma. Activated leukocytes and endothelial cells express adhesion molecules and adhesion-molecule receptors. Cells attach to the vessel wall, and diapedesis takes place, with chemotaxis toward a chemokine gradient at the focus of inflammation. Activated circulating cells, migrant cells, local immune accessory cells, and peripheral nerves secrete cytokines, prostanoids, platelet-activating factor, neuropeptides, and other mediators of inflammation. Some of these substances, such as interleukin-6, leukotrienes, complement component 5α, corticotropin-releasing hormone, and transforming growth factor-β, have chemokinetic activity. Some substances, such as the inflammatory cytokines tumor necrosis factor α, interleukin-1, and interleukin-6, escape in the systemic circulation, causing systemic symptoms and activating the hypothalamic-pituitary-adrenal axis. Because of such effects, these substances were historically referred to as "tissue corticotropin releasing factor (CRF)" (see text) (Source: Chrousos GP: The hypothalamic-pituitary-adrenal axis and immune-mediated inflammation. N Engl J Med 332:1351–1362, 1995.)

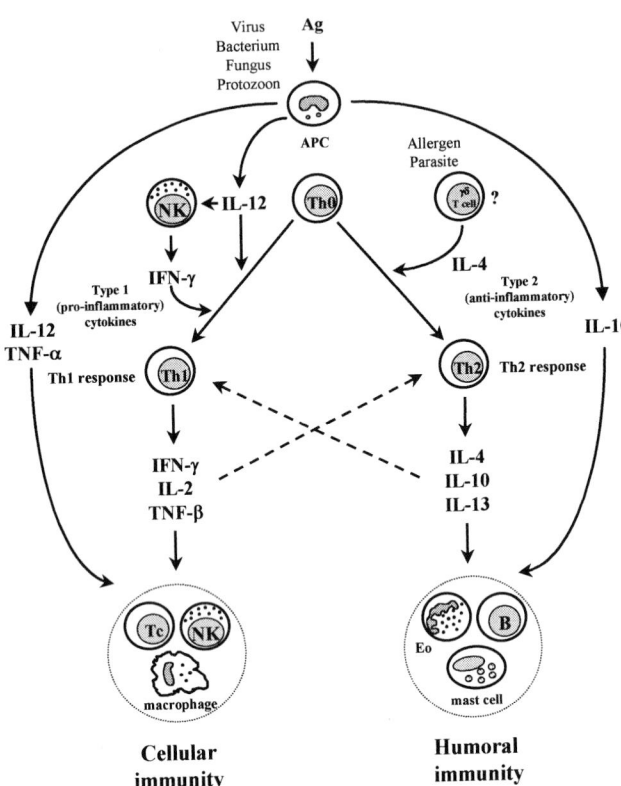

Figure 40-4   Role of Th1 and Th2 cells and type 1 and type 2 cytokines in the regulation of cellular and humoral immunity. Cellular immunity provides protection against intracellular bacteria, protozoa, fungi, and several viruses, while humoral immunity provides protection against multicellular parasites, extracellular bacteria, some viruses, soluble toxins, and allergens (see text). *Solid lines* represent stimulation; *dashed lines* represent inhibition. Ag, antigen; APC antigen-presenting cell; NK, natural killer cell; T, T cell; B, B cell; Th, T-helper cell; Tc, T-cytotoxic cell; Eo, eosinophil; IL, interleukin; TNF, tumor necrosis factor; IFN, interferon. (Source: Elenkov I, Chrousos G: Stress hormones, Th1/Th2 patterns, pro/anti-inflammatory cytokines and susceptibility to disease. Trends Endocrinol Metab 10(9):359–368, 1999.)

activity of Tc cells, NK cells, and activated macrophages, that is, the major components of cellular immunity. All three cytokines, IL-12, TNF-α, and IFN-γ, also stimulate the synthesis of nitric oxide and other inflammatory mediators that drive chronic delayed-type inflammatory responses. Because of these crucial and synergistic roles in inflammation, IL-12, TNF-α, and IFN-γ are considered the major proinflammatory cytokines.[65-67]

Th1 and Th2 responses are mutually inhibitory. Thus, IL-12 and IFN-γ inhibit Th2, and, conversely, IL-4 and IL-10 inhibit Th1 responses. IL-4 and IL-10 promote humoral immunity by stimulating the growth and activation of mast cells and eosinophils, the differentiation of B cells into antibody-secreting B cells, and B-cell immunoglobulin switching to IgE. Importantly, these cytokines inhibit macrophage activation, T-cell proliferation and the production of proinflammatory cytokines.[65,66] Thus, IL-4 and IL-10 are the major anti-inflammatory cytokines[65,66] (see Fig. 40-4).

EFFECTS OF THE HPA AXIS AND THE SNS ON THE IMMUNE AND INFLAMMATORY REACTION

ADRENOCORTICAL HORMONES

The anti-inflammatory and immunosuppressive properties of glucocorticoids, exerted via their ubiquitous intracellular

receptors, make them invaluable therapeutic agents in numerous diseases.[68] The glucocorticoid receptor is a 777-amino-acid cytoplasmic protein with three major functional domains and several subdomains. The carboxyterminal region binds glucocorticoid, and the middle portion domain binds to specific sequences of DNA in the regulatory regions of glucocorticoid-responsive genes (glucocorticoid-responsive elements).[68,69]

Glucocorticoids influence the traffic of circulating leukocytes and inhibit many functions of leukocytes and immune accessory cells.[8,28,68,69] They suppress the immune activation of these cells, inhibit the production of cytokines and other mediators of inflammation, and cause cytokine resistance. Subgroups of T lymphocytes are particularly affected by glucocorticoids. Thus, these hormones suppress T-helper 1 function and stimulate apoptosis of eosinophils and certain groups of T lymphocytes. Glucocorticoids also inhibit the expression of adhesion and adhesion receptor molecules on the surface of immune and other cell[70] and potentiate the acute-phase reaction.[71] All of these effects depend on altering the transcription rates of glucocorticoid-responsive genes or changing the stability of messenger RNAs of several proteins involved in inflammation.[72-74] For instance, glucocorticoids suppress production of IL-6 and IL-1 by decreasing both the transcription rate of the genes for these interleukins and the stability of their messenger RNA.

Among the many proteins that are regulated by glucocorticoids are the phospholipase A2, cyclooxygenase 2, and inducible nitric oxide synthetase 2 genes.[68,74-78] Suppression of these proteins decreases production of prostanoids, platelet-activating factor, and nitric oxide, three key molecules in the inflammatory response. The activated glucocorticoid receptor also inhibits the proinflammatory activity of many growth factors and cytokines by directly interacting with and blocking the third messenger systems for these hormones.[68,69] These include the transcription factors c-*jun*, NF-κB, and cyclic adenosine monophosphate (cAMP) response element binding protein (CREB). In a mutual fashion, elevated intracellular concentrations of these factors prevent the activated glucocorticoid receptor from exerting its effects on the genome.

Several circadian immune functions cause disease-associated diurnal changes that correspond to plasma glucocorticoid levels.[79,80] For example, the delayed hypersensitivity reaction, which is particularly sensitive to glucocorticoids, is greatest in the evening, when glucocorticoids are low, and least in the morning, when they are high.[79]

The secretion of adrenal androgens, which, like cortisol, follow the circadian pattern of ACTH, is associated with a distinct developmental pattern with highest levels in utero, during puberty, and in early adulthood.[81] Adrenal androgens with the Δ5 configuration in the A ring have been suggested as modulators of immune function.[82-85] An orphan receptor of the steroid-thyroid receptor superfamily specific for Δ5 adrenal androgens has been detected in T lymphocytes and presumably mediates the potentiation of T-helper 1 cells by these androgens, enhancing cellular immunity.[85]

CATECHOLAMINES

Lymphocyte traffic and circulation are under the influence of SNS and CAs. In the short term, acutely (<30 min) CAs mobilize NK cells from depots, while in the long term, chronically, CAs decrease the number of lymphocytes, particularly of NK cells in the peripheral blood.[3] CAs or β-adrenoreceptor (AR) agonists inhibit the T-cell proliferation that is induced by mitogens.[86,87] This is usually accompanied by an increase of cAMP in lymphocytes, and the amount of cAMP produced by T cells stimulated with isoproterenol, a β-AR agonist, is proportional to the degree of inhibition of the proliferation.[88,89] β-AR agonists exert similar inhibitory effect on the proliferative response of human highly purified T cells stimulated with immobilized anti-CD3 monoclonal antibody through the CD3/TCR complex.[89,90]

In vitro and in vivo studies reveal that CAs mediate, both acutely and chronically, an inhibition of NK cell activity.[91,92] Central administration of CRH that is known to increase the sympathetic autonomic outflow is accompanied by decreased NK activity in the periphery, an effect that is independent of adrenocortical activation.[93–95] This effect of central CRH is also rapid: Within 20 minutes of the infusion, lytic values of splenic NK cells decline by nearly 50%, while the cytotoxicity of peripheral NK cells is reduced within 1 hour.[93,95]

Moreover, several lines of evidence suggest that stress, which is accompanied by increased levels of peripheral CAs, inhibits several components of cellular immunity and particularly NK cell activity, an effect that is mediated mainly by the CRH-SNS axis.[93] Thus, in animals, the central application of anti-CRH antibodies completely blocks the inhibitory effect of footshock stress on NK activity.[93] It appears that NK cells are the most "sensitive" cells to the suppressive effect of stress, and not surprisingly, NK cell activity has become a bona fide index of stress-induced suppression of cellular immunity, employed in many studies (for a review, see Ref. 93). Apart from a direct and acute effect, chronically, during subacute or chronic stress, CAs may suppress NK activity indirectly, through their potent inhibition of the production of IL-12 and IFN-γ,[96] cytokines that are essential for NK activity (see text below).

CAs appear to mediate both inhibitory and stimulatory effects on macrophage activity. This process is influenced by several factors, such as availability of type 1/proinflammatory cytokines; the presence or absence of antigen; the presence in the microenvironment of proinflammatory mediators, such as SP, peripheral (immune) CRH, and histamine released from the sensory and postganglionic-sympathetic neurons or mast cells, respectively; and the state of activation or differentiation of macrophages, which may determine the β-ARs' responsiveness and the expression of α-ARs. CAs also exert enhancing effects on the initiation of Tc responses, in contrast to inhibition of effector Tc cell function. CAs inhibit both neutrophil phagocytosis and the release of lysosomal enzymes from neutrophils.[97] Furthermore, the superoxide generation and formation of oxygen radicals that play an important microbicidal role are suppressed at nanomolar concentrations of epinephrine, an effect that is mediated by β2-ARs.[98,99]

When B cells and Th cells are exposed to Th cell–dependent antigen, NE, through stimulation of β2 receptors, exerts an enhancing effect on B-cell antibody (Ab) production.[100,101] One mechanism for this enhancement may involve a β2-AR-induced increase in the frequency of B cells differentiating into Ab-secreting cells. Moreover, Th cells not only activate B cells via cell-to-cell interaction, but also provide the cytokines necessary for B-cell growth. Here again CAs may play an important modulatory role through their differential effect on type 1 and type 2 cytokine production (see text below). Thus, the β-AR agonists salbutamol and fenoterol potentiate IL-4-induced immunoglobulin E (IgE) production by human peripheral blood mononuclear cells (PBMCs), while they inhibit IFN-γ production by the same cells.[102] Furthermore, salbutamol induces an increase of the ex vivo *release* of IL-4, IL-6, and IL-10 by human PBMCs.[103]

STRESS HORMONES SUPPRESS CELLULAR AND POTENTIATE HUMORAL IMMUNITY

Effects of Glucocorticoids

Glucocorticoids suppress the production of TNF-α, IFN-γ, and IL-2 in vitro and in vivo in animals and humans.[1] As was recently shown, glucocorticoids also act through their classic cytoplasmic/nuclear receptors on APCs to suppress the production of the main inducer of Th1 responses IL-12 in vitro

and ex vivo.[96,104] Since IL-12 is extremely potent in enhancing IFN-γ and inhibiting IL-4 synthesis by T cells, the inhibition of IL-12 production may represent a major mechanism through which glucocorticoids affect the Th1/Th2 balance. Thus, glucocorticoid-treated monocytes/macrophages produce significantly less IL-12, leading to a decreased capacity of these cells to induce IFN-γ production by antigen-primed CD4+ T cells; the same treatment of monocytes/macrophages is also associated with an increased production of IL-4 by T cells, probably resulting from disinhibition from the suppressive effects of IL-12 on Th2 activity[105] (Fig. 40-5).

Furthermore, glucocorticoids potently downregulate the expression of IL-12 receptors on T and NK cells. This explains why human peripheral blood mononuclear cells stimulated with immobilized anti-CD3 lose their ability to produce IFN-γ in the presence of glucocorticoids.[106] Thus, although glucocorticoids may have a direct suppressive effect on Th1 cells, the overall inhibition of IFN-γ production by these cells appears to result mainly from the inhibition of IL-12 production by APCs and from the loss of IL-12 responsiveness of NK and Th1 cells.

It is particularly noteworthy that glucocorticoids have no effect on the production of the potent anti-inflammatory cytokine IL-10 by monocytes, yet lymphocyte-derived IL-10 production is upregulated by glucocorticoids.[96,107] Thus, rat CD4+ T cells that have been pretreated with dexamethasone

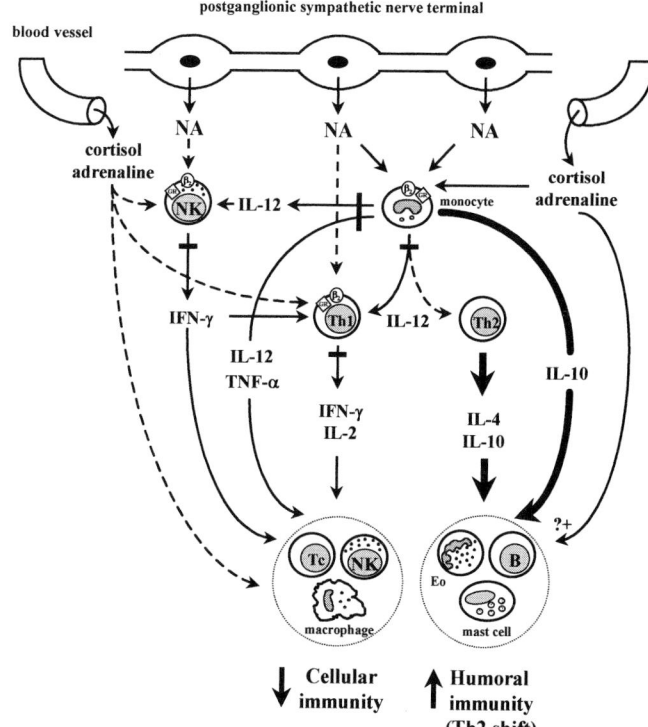

Figure 40-5 Effect of glucocorticoids and catecholamines on Th1/Th2 balance, cellular and humoral immunity. Stress influences immunity by stimulating cortisol and adrenaline secretion from the adrenal cortex and medulla, respectively, and the release of noradrenaline from the postganglionic sympathetic nerve terminals in blood vessels and lymphoid organs; systemic effects of glucocorticoids and catecholamines on the production of key regulatory type 1 and type 2 cytokines, Th1 and Th2 functions and, respectively, components of cellular and humoral immunity. NA, noradrenaline; NK, natural killer cell; GR, glucocorticoid receptor; T, T cell; B, B cell; Th, T-helper cell; Tc, T-cytotoxic cell; Eo, eosinophil; IL, interleukin; TNF, tumor necrosis factor; IFN, interferon. (Source: Elenkov I, Chrousos G: Stress hormones, Th1/Th2 patterns, pro/anti-inflammatory cytokines and susceptibility to disease. Trends Endocrinol Metab 10(9):359–368, 1999.)

exhibit increased levels of mRNA for IL-10.[108] Similarly, during experimental endotoxemia or cardiopulmonary bypass or in multiple sclerosis patients having an acute relapse, the treatment with glucocorticoids is associated with increased plasma IL-10 secretion.[107,109,110] This might have resulted from a direct stimulatory effect of glucocorticoids on T-cell IL-10 production and/or from the disinhibition of the restraining inputs of IL-12 and IFN-γ on monocyte/lymphocyte IL-10 production.

Effects of Catecholamines

CAs drive a Th2 shift, at the level of both APCs and Th1 cells (see Fig. 40-5). We recently demonstrated that NA and adrenaline potently inhibited or enhanced the production of IL-12 and IL-10, respectively, in human whole blood cultures that have been stimulated with LPS ex vivo.[96] These effects are mediated by stimulation of β-ARs, since they are completely prevented by propranolol, a β-AR antagonist. Our findings were subsequently extended by other laboratories showing that nonselective β- and selective $β_2$-AR agonists inhibited the production of IL-12 in vitro and in vivo.[111,112] In conjunction with their ability to suppress IL-12 production, $β_2$-AR agonists inhibited the development of Th1-type cells while promoting Th2 cell differentiation.[111]

$β_2$-ARs are expressed on Th1 cells but not on Th2 cells.[100] This may provide an additional mechanistic basis for a differential effect of CAs on Th1/Th2 functions. In fact, in both murine and human systems, $β_2$-AR agonists inhibit IFN-γ production by Th1 cells but do not affect IL-4 production by Th2 cells.[100,113] Importantly, the differential effect of CAs on Th1/Th2 cytokine production also operates in in vivo conditions. Thus, increasing sympathetic outflow in mice by selective $α_2$-AR antagonists or application of β-AR agonists results in inhibition of LPS-induced TNF-α and IL-12 production[112,114,115]; in humans, the administration of the $β_2$-AR agonist salbutamol results in inhibition of IL-12 production ex vivo[111] and acute brain trauma that is followed by massive release of CAs triggers secretion of substantial amounts of systemic IL-10.[116]

CAs exert inhibition on the production of proinflammatory cytokines in vivo. Application of propranolol, a β-AR antagonist that blocks their inhibitory effect on cytokine-producing cells, results in substantial increases of LPS-induced secretion of TNF-α and IL-12 in mice.[112,115] Thus, systemically, both glucocorticoids and CAs, through inhibition and stimulation, respectively, of Th1 and Th2 cytokine secretion, cause selective suppression of cellular immunity and a shift toward Th2-mediated humoral immunity. This is further substantiated by studies showing that stress hormones inhibit effector function of cellular immunity components, that is, the activity of NK, Tc, and activated macrophages.

The above general conclusion on the effects of stress hormones on Th1/Th2 balance might not pertain to certain conditions or local responses at specific compartments of the body. Thus, the synthesis of transforming growth factor beta (TGF-β), another type 2 cytokine with potent anti-inflammatory activities, is differentially regulated by glucocorticoids: It is enhanced in human T cells but suppressed in glial cells.[117] In addition, NA, via stimulation of $α_2$-ARs, can augment LPS-stimulated production of TNF-α from mouse peritoneal macrophages,[118] while hemorrhage, a condition associated with elevations of systemic CA concentrations, increases through stimulation of α-AR the expression of TNF-α and IL-1 by lung mononuclear cells.[119]

Since the response to β–AR agonist stimulation wanes during maturation of the human monocyte to macrophage,[120] it is possible that at certain compartments of the body, the α-AR-mediated effect of CAs becomes transiently dominant. Through this mechanism, CAs may actually boost local cellular immune responses in a transitory fashion. This is further substantiated by the finding that CAs potentiate the production of IL-8 from PBMCs and epithelial cells of the lung,[121]

thus probably promoting recruitment of polymorphonuclear leukocytes to this organ. The "paradoxic" stress-induced potentiation of inflammation in the lung might explain why the adult respiratory distress syndrome develops frequently in patients with major infections associated with profound activation of the stress system.[122] Thus, in summary, while stress hormones suppress Th1 responses and proinflammatory cytokine secretion and boost Th2 responses systemically, they may affect differently certain local responses. Further studies are needed to address this question.

THE CRH–MAST CELL–HISTAMINE AXIS

Central, hypothalamic CRH influences the immune system indirectly, through activation of the end products of the peripheral stress response, that is, glucocorticoids and CAs. CRH, however, is also secreted peripherally at inflammatory sites (peripheral or immune CRH) and influences the immune system directly, through local modulatory actions.[1,27] We first localized immunoreactive CRH in inflamed tissues of animals with experimental carrageenan-induced subcutaneous aseptic inflammation,[27] streptococcal cell wall– and adjuvant-induced arthritis, and retinol-binding protein (RBP)-induced uveitis and in human tissues from patients with various autoimmune/inflammatory diseases, including rheumatoid arthritis, autoimmune thyroid disease, and ulcerative colitis (cf. Ref. 123). The demonstration of CRH-like immunoreactivity in the dorsal horn of the spinal cord, dorsal root ganglia, and sympathetic ganglia support the hypothesis that the majority of immune CRH in early inflammation is of peripheral nerve rather than of immune cell origin (cf. Ref. 123).

Peripheral CRH has proinflammatory and vascular permeability-enhancing and vasodilatory actions. Thus, systemic administration of specific CRH antiserum blocks the inflammatory exudate volume and cell number in carrageenan-induced inflammation and RBP-induced uveitis and inhibits stress-induced intracranial mast cell degranulation.[27,124] In addition, CRH administration to humans or nonhuman primates causes major peripheral vasodilation that is manifested as flushing and increased blood flow and hypotension[125]; an intradermal CRH injection induces a marked increase of vascular permeability and mast cell degranulation.[126] Importantly, this effect is blocked by a CRH type 1 receptor antagonist and is stronger than the effect of an equimolar concentration of C48/80, a potent mast cell secretagogue.[126]

Thus, it appears that the mast cell is a major target of immune CRH. This has an anatomic prerequisite: In blood vessels, periarterial sympathetic plexuses are closely associated with mast cells lining the perivascular regions, and plexuses of nerve fibers (noradrenergic and peptidergic) within lymphoid parenchyma are also closely associated with clusters of mast cells. Histamine, a major product of mast cell degranulation, is a well-recognized mediator of acute inflammation and allergic reactions. These actions are mainly mediated by activation of H1 histamine receptors and include vasodilation, increased permeability of the vessel wall, edema, and in the lungs bronchoconstriction. Thus, it is conceivable that CRH activates mast cells via a CRH receptor type 1–dependent mechanism, leading to release of histamine and other contents of the mast cell granules that subsequently cause vasodilatation, increased vascular permeability, and other manifestations of inflammation (Fig. 40-6).

The last 10 to 15 years have provided strong evidence that histamine may have important immunoregulatory functions via H2 receptors expressed on immune cells (for a review, see Ref. 127). We have recently found that histamine, via stimulation of H2 receptors on peripheral monocytes and subsequent elevation of cAMP, inhibits the secretion of human IL-12 and stimulates the production of IL-10.[128] Our data are consistent with previous studies showing that histamine, via H2 receptors, also inhibits TNF-α production from monocytes

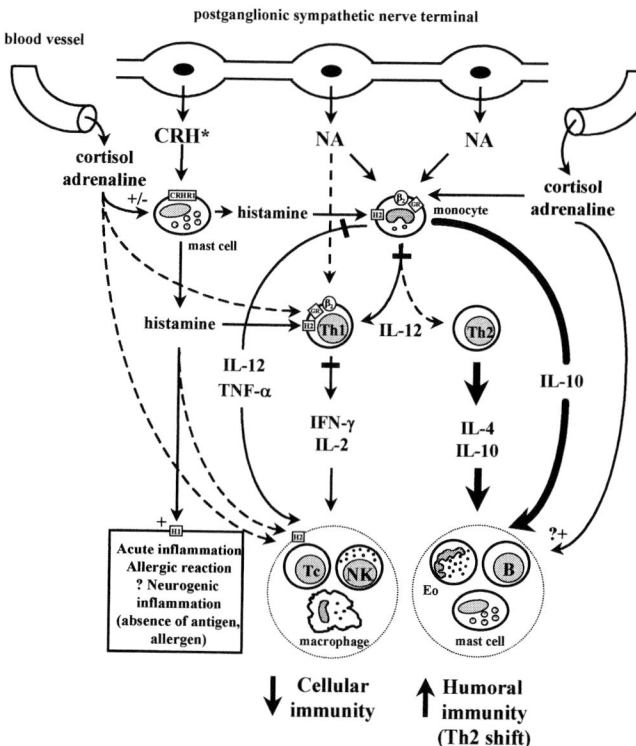

Figure 40-6 Effect of corticotropin releasing hormone–mast cell–histamine axis, glucocorticoid and catecholamines on Th1/Th2 balance, cellular and humoral immunity. Stress and CRH influence immune/inflammatory and allergic responses by stimulating glucocorticoid, catecholamines, and peripheral (immune) CRH secretion and by altering the production of key regulatory cytokines and histamine (see text). *CRH is also released from sensory nerves upon their activation. *Solid lines* represent stimulation, while *dashed lines* inhibition. CRH, peripheral (immune) corticotropin-releasing hormone; NA, noradrenaline; NK, natural killer cell; GR, glucocorticoid receptor; T, T cell; B, B cell; Th, T-helper cell; Tc, T-cytotoxic cell; Eo, eosinophil; IL, interleukin, TNF, tumor necrosis factor; IFN, interferon. (Source: Elenkov I, Chrousos G: Stress hormones, Th1/Th2 patterns, pro/anti-inflammatory cytokines and susceptibility to disease. Trends Endocrinol Metab 10(9):359–368, 1999.)

and IFN-γ production by Th1-like cells but has no effect on IL-4 production from Th2 clones.[129] Thus, histamine, similarly to CAs, appears to drive a Th2 shift both at the level of APCs and Th1 cells. Thus, the activation of CRH–mast cell–histamine axis through stimulation of H1 receptors may induce acute inflammation and allergic reactions, while through activation of H2 receptors, it may induce suppression of Th1 responses and a Th2 shift (see Fig. 40-6).

Stress-immune system interactions are undoubtedly complex. The evidence presented earlier, accumulated over the last decade, strongly suggests that stress hormones differentially regulate Th1/Th2 patterns and type1/type 2-cytokine secretion. Although interest in the Th2 response was initially directed at its protective role in helminthic infections and its pathogenic role in allergy, this response may have important regulatory functions in countering the tissue-damaging effects of macrophages and Th1 cells.[65] Thus, an excessive immune response, through activation of the stress system, and hence through glucocorticoids and CAs, suppresses the Th1 response and causes a Th2 shift. This may protect the organism from "overshooting" by type 1/proinflammatory cytokines and other products of activated macrophages with tissue-damaging potential.

Locally, as was stated previously, stress may exert proinflammatory or anti-inflammatory effects. This may be influ-

enced by several factors, such as presence or absence of antigen, the nature of antigen, and/or the presence and relative expression of particular receptor subtypes on the surface of immune cells (e.g., β_2- versus α_2-adrenergic or H1- versus H2-histaminergic receptors) or the organ involved. In addition, recent evidence indicates that stress is not a uniform, non-specific reaction[130]; different type of stressors with their own central neurochemical and peripheral neuroendocrine "signatures" might have different effects on the immune response.

EFFECTS OF THE IMMUNE AND INFLAMMATORY REACTION ON THE HPA AXIS AND THE SNS

The last two to three decades provided evidence that during an immune response, certain cytokines can signal the CNS, which, through a complex CRH-dependent pathway, triggers activation of both the HPA axis and the SNS.[16,18,131–136] Most of the HPA axis-stimulating activity in plasma comes from three cytokines, TNF-α, IL-1, and IL-6, which are produced at inflammatory sites and elsewhere in response to inflammation. In most situations, TNF-α appears first, followed by tandem secretion of IL-1 and IL-6.[137–139] All three cytokines stimulate their own secretion from the cells that produce them. In addition, TNF-α and IL-1 stimulate secretion of IL-6, whereas IL-6 inhibits secretion of TNF-α and IL-1. IL-6 acts synergistically with glucocorticoids in stimulating production of acute phase reactants.[68,71] Secretion of systemic IL-6 is also increased during stress of noninflammatory etiology, presumably stimulated by stress-induced CAs through a β_2-adrenergic receptor mechanism.[140,141]

All three inflammatory cytokines independently activate the HPA axis; in combination, their effects are synergistic.[132,134,142–144] Activation can be blocked with CRH-neutralizing antibodies, glucocorticoids, and prostanoid synthesis inhibitors. All three cytokines also directly stimulate CRH secretion in rat hypothalamic explants, and this effect can also be blocked by glucocorticoids and prostanoid synthesis inhibitors in vitro. The three inflammatory cytokines also mediate the stimulatory effect of bacterial lipopolysaccharide on the HPA axis. Antibodies to IL-6 almost completely inhibit this effect, suggesting a central role for IL-6 in axis stimulation.[145]

The elevations of ACTH and cortisol that are attained by IL-6 in human beings are well above those observed with maximal stimulating doses of CRH, suggesting that IL-6 in addition to CRH stimulates parvocellular AVP and other ACTH secretagogues.[146,147] ACTH levels are already maximal at doses of IL-6 that do not increase peripheral AVP levels. At higher doses, however, IL-6 causes peripheral elevations of AVP, indicating that this cytokine can also activate magnocellular AVP-secreting neurons. This suggests that elevations of IL-6 may be a common etiologic factor in the syndrome of inappropriate secretion of antidiuretic hormone observed in diverse states, such as infectious or inflammatory diseases or trauma.[147]

The HPA axis and the SNS are involved in a long feedback loop between the immune system and the CNS. The afferent limb of this loop seems to operate by blood-borne cytokines, which via circulation or through the afferents of the vagus nerve[148] activate the central components of the stress system. How inflammatory cytokines reach the hypothalamic CRH and AVP neurons is unclear, given that the blood-brain barrier protects the cellular bodies of both kinds of neurons.[142,149,150] The cytokines may cause the endothelial and glial cells to secrete prostanoids, IL-6, and other mediators of inflammation, which reach the CRH and AVP neurons in a cascade-like fashion.[145,151] Alternatively, a special transport system may be present for one or more of the inflammatory cytokines. Also, the inflammatory cytokines may directly activate the terminals of the CRH and AVP neurons in the median eminence, which is outside the blood-brain barrier. Because NE released in this region might exert tonic inhibitory control on CRH release through stimulation of α_2-ARs,[152,153] it was suggested that TNF-α by inhibiting NE release, that is, by disinhibition of this control, might trigger an increase of CRH release and subsequently an increase of ACTH from the anterior pituitary.[154]

Inflammation may also activate the HPA axis indirectly, by stimulation of the central noradrenergic stress system through cytokines and other mediators, which act first on stress system neurons of the area postrema that lie outside the blood-brain barrier or on neuron bodies inside the barrier through the endothelial-glial-neuronal cascade mentioned earlier. In addition, nociceptive, visceral, and somatosensory afferent neurons of the peripheral nervous system from inflammatory sites acutely stimulate the noradrenergic and CRH stress systems through an ascending neural spinal or cerebral nerve route.[155,156] In fact, several lines of evidence indicate that certain cytokines, such as IL-1 and IFN-α, stimulate both the central and peripheral components of the SNS. Thus, administration of IL-1 in the periphery increases the turnover of NE in the hypothalamus[133] and increases peripheral NE and epinephrine plasma levels.[157] Intracerebroventricular and peripheral injection of IFN-α or IL-1β produces a long-lasting increase of the sympathetic activity of the splenic nerve and an increased turnover of NE in the spleen.[158] As a result, the release of NE in the spleen is enhanced, as indicated by a recent in vivo microdialysis study.[159]

In addition to their acute effects on the hypothalamus, the inflammatory cytokines can apparently directly stimulate pituitary ACTH and adrenal cortisol secretion at high concentrations or given adequate time for interaction with these tissues.[134,142,160–164] Normally, the anterior pituitary and adrenal glands produce IL-1 and IL-6, which may influence local hormone production.[142,165,166] These cytokines might not always stimulate the pituitary gland or the adrenal cortex, however. IL-6, TNF-α, and IFN-γ inhibit the stimulatory effect of CRH on anterior pituitary cell cultures,[167,168] whereas TNF-α is a potent inhibitor of ACTH-induced cortisol production by cultured adrenocortical cells.[169]

Other inflammatory mediators and cytokines, including IFN-α, IL-2, epidermal growth factor, TGF-β, prostanoids, and platelet-activating factor, may also participate in the modulation of the HPA axis activity by inflammation (Table 40-1). The interferons and IL-2 may do so indirectly, by causing secretion of inflammatory cytokines. Prostanoids and platelet-activating factor, however, are autacoid amplifiers of hypothalamic CRH and AVP secretion. Receptors for these substances are present in the PVN, and CRH and AVP neurons respond to them.

Certain cytokines or combinations of cytokines have been shown to cause their target tissues to become resistant to glucocorticoids.[170,171] IL-2 and IL-4 together cause glucocorticoid resistance in T cells by markedly decreasing the affinity of the glucocorticoid receptor for its ligand by an as yet unclear mechanism.[171] In addition, changes in the intracellular metabolism of cortisol into less active or inactive metabolites in cells of the immune system alter the sensitivity of these cells to glucocorticoids.[172]

AMPHIDROMOUS INTERACTIONS BETWEEN THE STRESS AND IMMUNE SYSTEMS

SHORT- AND LONG-TERM ADAPTATIONS

Chronic activation of either the HPA axis or the immune and inflammatory reaction results in reciprocally protective adaptations. Thus, the immune suppression of patients with chronic endogenous Cushing syndrome is quite mild, suggesting that these patients become somewhat tolerant to glucocorticoids. Indeed, even though neutrophilia and eosinopenia persist, the lymphocyte phenotypes and function in these patients are similar to those of age- and gender-matched controls. Animals with chronic inflammatory disease, on the other hand, have mild rather than severe hypercortisolism, which is surprisingly associated with low CRH and high AVP messenger RNA expression and peptide secretion in the hypothalamus.[173–175]

Peripheral inflammation-induced hypothalamic elevation of substance P, an inhibitor of CRH secretion, has been considered the mechanism by which CRH neuron suppression occurs in certain painful inflammatory states.[50–52] In addition, elevated levels of inflammatory cytokines and interferon may participate in the restraint of the HPA axis by blocking the stimulatory effects of CRH and ACTH on the pituitary gland and adrenal cortex, respectively.[167–169] Human examples of this are certain patients with septic shock or acquired immunodeficiency syndrome (AIDS) and most patients with African trypanosomiasis, who have impaired adrenal responses to stress or exogenous stimuli like CRH and corticotropin.[176–179]

Chronic activation of the HPA axis is also associated with another adrenocortical adaptation, which leads to a relative decrease in the production of Δ^5 adrenal androgens.[180] This in turn may alter the T-helper phenotype of chronically affected patients toward predominance of T-helper 2.[82–84]

INFLUENCES OF REPRODUCTIVE HORMONES

In general, autoimmune diseases affect females more than males. In animal models, androgens usually suppress the immune response, whereas estrogens stimulate it.[181,182] The mechanisms of these effects are insufficiently characterized, although estrogens are known to stimulate adhesion molecules and adhesion molecule receptors in immune and immune accessory cells, while the CRH gene and hence immune CRH expression are responsive to estrogen.[70,183,184] Recent evidence indicates that estradiol (E2), similarly to glucocorticoids does not affect the production of IL-10 by monocytes; yet, lymphocyte-derived IL-10 production is upregulated by E2. In the presence of high doses of E2, the majority of the antigen-specific T-cell clones show enhancement of antigen- and anti-CD3-stimulated human IL-10 production.[185] This is relevant to the finding that E2 may polyclonally increase the production of IgG, including IgG anti-dsDNA, in systemic lupus erythematosus (SLE) patients' PBMCs by enhancing B-cell activity and by promoting IL-10 production, evidence that supports the involvement of E2 in the pathogenesis of SLE.[186] E2 also decreases LPS-induced TNF-α production by inhibition of the transcription factor NF-κB.[187] E2 might exert biphasic effects on secretion of TNF-α, with enhancement occurring at low doses of E2, and inhibition at high concentrations.[185] Interestingly, an estrogen deficiency has been linked to induction of bone loss by enhancing T-cell production of

Table 40-1	Cytokines and Other Mediators of Inflammation that Influence the Hypothalamic-Pituitary-Adrenal Axis

INFLAMMATORY CYTOKINES
Tumor necrosis factor-α
Interleukin-1α and interleukin-1β
Interleukin 6
Interleukin 8

OTHER CYTOKINES
Interferon-α
Interferon-γ
Interleukin-2

GROWTH FACTORS
Epidermal growth factor
Transforming growth factor-β

LIPID MEDIATORS
Prostanoids
Platelet-activating factor

TNF-α.[188] The differentiation of cells of the monocytes lineage into mature osteoclasts is specifically induced by TNF-related factor, RANKL (receptor activator of NF-κB ligand). T cells from ovariectomized mice produce increased amounts of TNF, which augments RANK-induced osteoclastogenesis.[189] This evidence indicates that the enhanced T-cell production of TNF resulting from increased bone marrow T-cell number might represent a key mechanism by which estrogen deficiency induces bone loss in vivo.[189,190]

Progesterone also favors the Th2 development, mainly through induction of IL-4 and IL-5 and through inhibition of TNF-α. Progesterone decreases steady-state levels of TNF-α mRNA and the production of intracellular and secreted TNF-α. Importantly, progesterone, at concentrations comparable to those present at the maternofetal interface, induces the development of Ag-specific CD4+ T-cell lines and clones that show enhanced ability to produce IL-4 and IL-5 without affecting the secretion of IL-10.[191] Moreover, progesterone also induces the expression of IL-4 mRNA and production in established human Th1 clones.[191] Estrogens and progesterone are most likely to drive a substantial Th2 shift only at concentrations (up to 35,000 pg/mL) associated with pregnancy. Prolactin appears to potentiate the immune and inflammatory reaction in vitro and in animals.[192] Inhibition of pituitary prolactin secretion in humans with autoimmune disease has not been effective therapeutically, perhaps because local, autacoid prolactin production might not respond to dopaminergic inhibition.[25]

INFLUENCE OF 1,25-DIHYDROXY VITAMIN D3

$1,25(OH)_2$ vitamin D3 preferentially targets Th1 activity by inhibiting the secretion of both IFN-γ and IL-2 and by suppressing the production of the pro-Th1 cytokine IL-12 by APCs.[193,194] The hormone inhibits IL-12 production by activated macrophages and DCs by downregulation of NF-κB activation and binding to the p40-kappaB sequence.[193] $1,25(OH)_2$ vitamin D3 has little or no effect on IL-4 production but enhances IL-10 secretion by DCs and IL-10 and IL-5 by PBMCs. Similarly to GCs $1,25(OH)_2$ vitamin D3 upregulates lymphocyte-derived IL-10 but does not affect the production of IL-10 by monocytes. Thus, $1,25(OH)2$ vitamin D3 may selectively inhibit Th1 functions and favor Th2 responses. Therefore, the development of less hypercalcemic analogues of $1,25(OH)_2$ vitamin D3 might open a new therapeutic area in autoimmunity and organ transplantation. In fact, it has recently been shown that by inhibiting IL-12 and Th1 development, administration of such analogues prevents or ameliorates chronic-relapsing experimental allergic encephalomyelitis (EAE) and autoimmune diabetes in mice.[195,196] In addition, the clinical improvement in psoriasis after application of calcipotriene, a synthetic analogue of $1,25(OH)_2$ vitamin D3, has been linked to the reduction of IL-8 and the increase of IL-10 production that are induced by this drug.[197]

DISTURBANCES IN THE INTERACTION BETWEEN THE STRESS AND IMMUNE SYSTEMS

DEFECTS OF THE HPA AXIS

Disturbances of the feedback relationship between the HPA axis and the immune and inflammatory reaction have been observed in animals and human states and can have two kinds of opposing effects (Table 40-2). An excessive HPA response to inflammation can mimic the stress or hypercortisolemic state and can increase susceptibility to infectious agents and tumors, and cause resistance to autoimmune or inflammatory disease. Conversely, a defective HPA axis response can mimic the glucocorticoid-deficient state and

Table 40-2	States Potentially Associated with Suppression or Activation of the Immune and Inflammatory Reaction Through Defects in the Hypothalamic-Pituitary-Adrenal (HPA) Axis or Its Target Tissues
Suppression of Immune and Inflammatory Reaction	**Activation of Immune and Inflammatory Reaction**

INCREASED HPA AXIS ACTIVITY
 Cushing's syndrome
 Melancholic depression
 Chronic active alcoholism
 Chronic stress
 Chronic excessive exercise
 Pregnancy (last trimester)
 Fischer rat
	DECREASED HPA AXIS ACTIVITY
	 Adrenal insufficiency
	 Rheumatoid arthritis
	 Atypical/seasonal depression
	 Chronic fatigue/fibromyalgia
	 Hypothyroidism
	 Posttraumatic stress disorder
	    Nicotine withdrawal
	 Post Cushing's syndrome cure
	 Post glucocorticoid therapy
	 Postpartum period
	 Post chronic stress
	 Lewis rat
	 Obese chicken (autoimmune
	    thyroiditis)

HYPERSENSITIVITY TO GLUCOCORTICOIDS HIV-1 infection (vpr)	**RESISTANCE TO GLUCOCORTICOIDS** Rheumatoid arthritis Steroid-resistant asthma AIDS and glucocorticoid resistance Degenerative osteoarthritis Systemic lupus erythematosus*

*Secondary to increased catabolism of cortisol in target tissues.
Source: Chrousos G: The hypothalamic-pituitary-adrenal axis and immune-mediated inflammation. N Engl J Med 332:1351–1362, 1995.

thus cause resistance to infections and neoplasms but increased susceptibility to autoimmune and inflammatory disease. Indeed, such properties were identified in Fischer and Lewis rats, two highly inbred strains that were selected for their resistance (Fischer) or susceptibility (Lewis) to inflammatory disease.[24,198] In the Lewis rat, the responsiveness of the HPA axis to inflammatory stimuli is decreased, whereas in the Fischer rat, HPA axis responsiveness to the same stimuli is increased.

Lewis rats are susceptible to a host of inflammatory diseases such as a rheumatoid arthritis–like syndrome in response to streptococcal cell-wall peptidoglycan, uveitis in response to immunization with retinol-binding protein, and encephalomyelitis in response to myelin basic protein. Fischer rats, by contrast, resist these experimentally induced diseases. The defect in the Lewis rat was localized to the hypothalamic CRH neuron, which was globally defective in its response to all stimulatory neurotransmitters.[199] The overall HPA axis response to stress was decreased in the Lewis rat; in addition, these animals exhibited chronic elevations of vasopressin as well as behaviors reminiscent of atypical depression in humans, a state characterized by low hypothalamic CRH secretion.[8,28,200,201]

Do the abnormalities in Lewis rats have parallels in humans? A subgroup of patients with active rheumatoid arthritis might qualify. These patients have low or normal circadian concentrations of ACTH and cortisol despite elevated plasma concentrations of IL-1β and IL-6.[202,203] Such patients have a poor response to the stress associated with that of major surgery, such as large joint replacement, despite dramatic postoperative elevations of IL-1β and IL-6.[203] Like Lewis rats, these patients also have consistently elevated levels of circulating AVP. Similarly to Lewis rats with streptococcal cell-wall peptidoglycan-induced arthritis, the inflamed joints of these patients have markedly elevated concentrations of immunoreactive CRH.[204,205] None of these abnormalities of the HPA axis were present in control patients with osteomyelitis (inflammatory disease) or degenerative osteoarthritis.

A key question about human rheumatoid arthritis is whether the hyporesponsiveness of the HPA axis is genetic constitutional or secondary to a particular type of chronic inflammation or both. To date, the data point to a genetic disturbance that defines increased susceptibility.[206] Prospective studies of families with autoimmune inflammatory disease should test this hypothesis, using a quantifiable benign inflammatory stimulus such as recombinant IL-6.[146,147]

Other examples suggest that a defective HPA axis increases susceptibility to autoimmune disease or increased immune reactivity[8,28,207,208] (see Table 40-2). Given the many behavioral effects of CRH, it is not surprising that fatigue, dysthymia, irritability, or even frank depression are frequent in many of these low CRH states.[8,28]

DEFECTS OF THE GLUCOCORTICOID TARGET TISSUES

Glucocorticoid hypersensitivity of the immune system can mimic the immunosuppression of hypercortisolism, while glucocorticoid resistance of the immune system may result in excessive immune system activity, and inflammatory activity may also arise from glucocorticoid resistance in target tissues[69,208-213] (see Table 40-2). Four diseases illustrate this mechanism. In rheumatoid arthritis, the concentration of glucocorticoid receptors in circulating leukocytes is reduced by approximately 50 percent.[208,209] This phenomenon cannot be attributed to hypercortisolism. Leukocyte resistance to glucocorticoids also occurs in steroid-resistant asthma.[210,211] Most patients with this disorder have marked but reversible decreases of affinity of glucocorticoid receptors in T-lymphocytes, suggesting an acquired problem, probably associated with elevations of transcription factors such as c-jun, NF-κB, and CREB, that interact with and neutralize activated glucocorticoid receptors; however, in a small subgroup of patients, glucocorticoid receptor concentrations are irreversibly decreased in all leukocyte subtypes, suggesting a congenital syndrome.[211] In some patients with AIDS, leukocytes also have a marked decrease in the affinity of glucocorticoid receptors for cortisol.[212] In these patients, the glucocorticoid resistance may be generalized, since there are signs of glucocorticoid deficiency, including postural hypotension and hyponatremia, despite elevated levels of corticotropin and cortisol. A fourth disease in which the reduced expression of glucocorticoid receptors and glucocorticoid resistance may have a role is degenerative osteoarthritis.[213] Osteoarthritic chondrocytes contain approximately half of the glucocorticoid receptors of normal chondrocytes and resist dexamethasone-induced suppression of metalloprotease synthesis. Metalloprotease participates in the limited inflammatory destruction of the cartilage in the joints of patients with osteoarthritis. Finally, glucocorticoid resistance has also been observed in patients with Crohn's disease.[214]

STRESS-INDUCED Th2 SHIFT: CLINICAL IMPLICATIONS

Infections

A major factor governing the outcome of infectious diseases is the selection of Th1 versus Th2-predominant adaptive responses during and after the initial invasion of the host. Thus, stress, and hence a stress-induced Th2 shift, may have a profound effect on the susceptibility of the organism to, and/or may influence the course of, an infection, the defense against which is primarily through cellular immunity mechanisms (Table 40-3).

Cellular immunity, and particularly IL-12 and IL-12-dependent IFN-γ secretion in humans, seems essential in the control of mycobacterial infections.[215] In the 1950s, Thomas Holmes (cf. Ref. 204) reported that individuals who had experienced stressful life events were more likely to develop tuberculosis and less likely to recover from it. Although it is still a matter of some speculation, stress hormone–induced inhibition of IL-12 and IFN-γ production and the consequent suppression of cellular immunity may amply explain the pathophysiologic mechanisms of these observations.

Helicobacter pylori infection is the most common cause of chronic gastritis that in some cases progresses to peptic ulcer

Table 40-3	Putative Pathophysiologic Roles of Stress Hormone-Induced Alterations of Th1/Th2 Balance in Certain Infections, Infectious Complications After Major Injury, Autoimmune/Inflammatory, Allergic or Neoplastic Diseases		
Condition	**Host Response**	**Pathogenic Response**	**Role of Stress**

Infections
  Mycobacterium tuberculosis
  Helicobacterium pylori
HIV
Common cold viruses
	Th1 protects	Suppressed cellular immunity, deficit of IL-12 and IFN-γ, Th2 shift with progression of infection	Stress-induced Th2 shift may contribute to increased susceptibility to or progression of these infections.

Major injury	Th2 protects?	Suppressed cellular immunity and IL-12, and IFN-γ production, overproduction of IL-10, Th2 shift	Increased levels of stress hormones may contribute to suppression of cellular immunity, resulting in infectious complications.

Autoimmunity
  RA, MS, ATD, type 1 diabetes
  mellitus
	Excessive Th1 response	Th1 shift, overproduction of IL-12 , TNF-α, IFN-γ; deficit of IL-10	A hypoactive stress system may facilitate/sustain the Th1 shift and flares of these autoimmune diseases.*

SLE	Excessive Th2 response	Th2 shift, deficit of IL-12 and TNF-α, overproduction of IL-10	Stress (Th2 shift) may induce/facilitate flares of SLE.
Allergy (Atopy)	Excessive Th2 response	Th2 shift, deficit of IL-12, overproduction of IL-4, IL-10	Stress hormone (and histamine)–induced Th2 shift may induce/facilitate/sustain allergic reactions.*
Tumors	Th1 protects	Suppressed cellular immunity, deficit of IL-12, TNF-α, overproduction of IL-10	Stress hormone (and histamine)–induced Th2 shift may contribute to increased susceptibility to or progression of certain tumors.

*The role of stress in autoimmunity and atopy is more complex; see text for details. Th, T helper; IL, interleukin; TNF, tumor necrosis factor; IFN, interferon; RA, rheumatoid arthritis; MS, multiple sclerosis; ATD, autoimmune thyroid disease; SLE, systemic lupus erythematosus.

Source: Elenkov I, Chrousos G: Stress hormones, Th1/Th2 patterns, pro/anti-inflammatory cytokines and susceptibility to disease. Trends Endocrinol Metab 10(9):359–368, 1999.

disease. The role of stress in promoting peptic ulcers has been recognized for many years. Thus, increased systemic stress hormone levels, in concert with an increased local concentration of histamine, induced by inflammatory or stress-related mediators, may skew the local responses toward Th2 and thus may allow the onset or progression of a *Helicobacter pylori* infection.

Human immunodeficiency virus (HIV)-positive patients have IL-12 deficiency, while disease progression has been correlated with a Th2 shift. The innervation (primarily sympathetic/noradrenergic) of lymphoid tissue may be particularly relevant to HIV infection, since lymphoid organs represent the primary site of HIV pathogenesis. In fact, as was recently shown, NA, the major sympathetic neurotransmitter that is released locally in lymphoid organs,[54,217] is able to directly accelerate HIV-1 replication by up to 11-fold in acutely infected human PBMCs.[218] The effect of NA on viral replication is transduced via the β-AR-adenylyl cyclase-cAMP-PKA signaling cascade.[218] The HIV-1 itself may contribute to the induction of intracellular cAMP through immunosuppressive, retroviral envelope peptide, which causes a shift in the cytokine balance and leads to suppression of cell-mediated immunity.[219]

Progression of HIV infection is also characterized by increased cortisol secretion in both the early and late stages of the disease. Thus, increased glucocorticoid production, triggered by the chronic infection, was recently proposed to contribute to HIV progression.[220] In another recent study, Kino and colleagues found that one of the HIV-1 accessory proteins, Vpr, acts as a potent coactivator of the host glucocorticoid receptor, rendering lymphoid cells hyperresponsive to glucocorticoids.[221] Thus, on one hand, stress hormones suppress cellular immunity and directly accelerate HIV replication, while, on the other hand, the virus itself may suppress cell-mediated immunity using the same pathways by which stress hormones, including CAs and glucocorticoids alter the Th1/Th2 balance.

In a recent study, an association was demonstrated between stress and the susceptibility to common cold among 394 people who had been intentionally exposed to five different upper respiratory viruses. Psychologic stress was associated in a dose-dependent manner with an increased risk of acute infectious respiratory illness, and this risk was attributed to increased rates of infection rather than to an increased frequency of symptoms after infection.[22] Thus, stress hormones, through their selective inhibition of cellular immunity, may play substantial roles in the increased risk of an individual to acute respiratory infections caused by common cold viruses.

Major Injury

Major injury (serious traumatic injury and major burns) or major surgical procedures often lead to severe immunosuppression that contributes to delayed wound healing and infectious complications and, in some cases, to sepsis, the most common cause of late death after trauma. A strong stimulation of the SNS and the HPA axis correlates with the severity of both cerebral and extracerebral injury and an unfavorable prognosis (cf. Ref. 116). In patients with traumatic major injury and in animal models of burn injury, the suppressed cellular immunity is associated with diminished production of IFN-γ and IL-12 and increased production of IL-10, that is, a Th2 shift.[222] A recent study indicated that systemic release of IL-10 triggered by SNS activation might be a key mechanism of immunosuppression after injury. Thus, high levels of systemic IL-10 documented in patients with "sympathetic storm" due to acute accidental or iatrogenic brain trauma were associated with high incidence of infection.[116] In a rat model, the increase of IL-10 was prevented by β-AR blockade,[116] while cellular immunity was improved in burned mice after H2 histamine receptor blockade.[127] Therefore, stress hor-

mones and histamine secretion triggered by major injury, via an induction of a Th2 shift may contribute to the severe immunosuppression observed in these conditions.

Autoimmunity

Several autoimmune diseases are characterized by common alterations of Th1 versus Th2 and IL-12/TNF-α versus IL-10 balance (see Table 40-3). In rheumatoid arthritis (RA), multiple sclerosis (MS), type 1 diabetes mellitus, autoimmune thyroid disease (ATD), and Crohn's disease (CD), the balance is skewed toward Th1 and an excess of IL-12 and TNF-α production, while Th2 activity and the production of IL-10 are deficient. This appears to be a critical factor that determines the proliferation and differentiation of Th1-related autoreactive cellular immune responses in these disorders.[223] On the other hand, SLE is associated with a Th2 shift and an excessive production of IL-10, while IL-12 and TNF-α production appear to be deficient.

The effect of stress on autoimmunity is extremely complex; often stress is related to both induction/exacerbation and amelioration of disease activity.[26,224] Animal studies and certain clinical observations suggest that a hyperactive or hypoactive stress system may be associated with decreased or increased vulnerability to different types of autoimmune diseases. Thus, Fischer rats, which have a hyperactive stress system, are extremely resistant to experimental induction of Th1-mediated autoimmune states, including arthritis, uveitis, and EAE.[26] Similarly, women in the third trimester of pregnancy, who have increased levels of cortisol, experience remission of Th1 type–mediated autoimmune diseases, such as RA, MS, type 1 diabetes mellitus, and ATD, possibly via suppression of proinflammatory (IL-12 and TNF-α) and potentiation of anti-inflammatory (IL-4 and IL-10) cytokine production.[26,225] In fact, we have recently shown that cortisol-, norepinephrine-, and 1,25-dihydroxyvitamin-induced inhibition and subsequent rebound of IL-12 and TNF-α production may represent a major mechanism via which pregnancy and postpartum alter the course of or susceptibility to Th1 type–mediated autoimmune disorders.[226] Through a reciprocal mechanism, Th2 type–mediated autoimmune disorders that are mainly driven by IL-10, such as SLE, may flare up in high cortisol and CA output states, that is, during stress or pregnancy.[26,225]

Conversely, Lewis rats, which possess a hypoactive HPA axis are extremely prone to develop experimentally induced Th1-mediated states, such as arthritis, uveitis, or EAE.[26] Similarly, clinical situations associated with decreased stress system activity are associated with increased expression or susceptibility to Th1 type–mediated autoimmune diseases such as RA, MS, and ATD. These are the postpartum period and the period that follows cure of endogenous Cushing's syndrome or discontinuation of glucocorticoid therapy.[1,26,96] This might also include the period that follows cessation of chronic stress or a rebound effect upon relief from stressors.

Epidemiologic studies suggest that severe stress, as reported by many patients, often precedes the development of certain Th1-mediated autoimmune states. Viral induction of autoimmunity is thought to occur by either bystander T-cell activation or molecular mimicry. Recent studies suggest that tissue-tropic Coxsackie B4 virus is associated by bystander damage with the development of type 1 diabetes mellitus, while human parvoviruses may be causative agents for rheumatoid arthritis.[227,228] If future studies confirm these hypotheses, severe stress, and hence severe suppression of cellular immunity may turn out to be a critical factor that facilitates the establishment of pathogenic and tissue-tropic viral infection followed by "autoimmune" tissue damage. At a later stage, severe stress, by skewing the balance toward Th2, may ameliorate disease activity, while acute stress and peripheral release of immune CRH, through its proinflammatory effects, may in some cases exacerbate disease activity.

Allergy/Atopy

Allergic reactions of type 1 hypersensitivity (atopy), such as asthma, eczema, hay fever, urticaria, and food allergy, are characterized by dominant Th2 responses, overproduction of histamine, and a shift to IgE production. As in the case of autoimmunity, the effects of stress on atopic reactions are complex, are at multiple levels, and can be at either direction. Stress hormones acting at the level of APCs and lymphocytes may induce a Th2 shift and thus facilitate or sustain atopic reactions; however, this can be antagonized by their effects on the mast cell (see Fig. 40-6). Glucocorticoids and CAs (through β_2-ARs) suppress the release of histamine by mast cells, thus abolishing its proinflammatory, allergic, and bronchoconstrictor effects. Thus, reduced levels of epinephrine and cortisol in the very early morning could contribute to nocturnal wheezing and have been linked to high circulating histamine levels in asthmatics.[229] This may also explain the beneficial effect of glucocorticoids and β_2-agonists in asthma. Infusion of high doses of adrenaline, however, causes a rise in circulating histamine levels that may be due to an α-adrenergic-mediated increase in mediator release (cf. Ref. 229). Thus, severe acute stress associated with high adrenaline concentrations and/or high local secretion of CRH could lead to mast cell degranulation. As a result, a substantial amount of histamine could be released, which consequently would not antagonize, but rather amplify, the Th2 shift through H2 receptors, while in parallel, by acting on H1 receptors, it could initiate a new episode or exacerbate a chronic allergic condition (see Fig. 40-6).

Glucocorticoids, alone or in combination with β_2-AR agonists, are broadly used in the treatment of atopic reactions, and particularly asthma. In vivo, ex vivo, and in vitro exposure to glucocorticoids and β_2-agonists result in a reduction of IL-12 production, which persists at least several days.[96,105,111] Thus, glucocorticoid and/or β_2-AR-agonist therapy is likely to reduce the capacity of APC to produce IL-12, to greatly suppress type 2 cytokine synthesis in activated but not resting T cells, and to abolish eosinophilia.[105] If, however, resting (cytokine-uncommitted) T cells are subsequently activated by APCs that have been preexposed to glucocorticoids and/or β_2-AR agonists, enhanced IL-4, production but limited IFN-γ synthesis could be induced.[105] Thus, while in the short term, the effect of glucocorticoids and β_2-AR agonists may be beneficial, their long-term effects might be to sustain the increased vulnerability of the patient to the allergic condition. This is further substantiated by the observations that both glucocorticoids and β_2-AR agonists potentiate the IgE production in vitro and in vivo.[230,231]

Tumor Growth

The amount of IL-12 that is available at the tumor site appears to be critical for tumor regression.[232] Thus, low levels of IL-12 have been associated with tumor growth, as opposed to tumor regression observed with administration of IL-12 delivered in situ or systemically. On the other hand, local overproduction of IL-10 and TGF-β, by inhibiting the production of IL-12 and TNF-α, and the cytotoxicity of NK and Tc cells, seems to play an inappropriate immunosuppressive role, allowing increased malignant tumor growth, as is seen, for example, in melanoma.[233] These and other studies suggest that Th1 function is locally downregulated during tumor growth.

Several lines of evidence suggest that stress can increase the susceptibility to tumors, tumor growth, and metastases. In animals, β-AR stimulation suppresses NK cell activity and compromises resistance to tumor metastases[234]; stress decreases the potential of spleen cells to turn into antitumor Tc against syngeneic B16 melanoma, and it significantly suppresses the ability of tumor-specific CD4$^+$ cells to produce IFN-γ and IL-2.[235] In humans, the augmentation of the rate of tumor progression and cancer-related death has been associated with stress (cf. Ref. 222), while treatment with cimetidine, an H2 histamine antagonist, correlated with increased survival in patients with gastric and colorectal cancer.[236] In fact, high concentrations of histamine have been measured within colorectal and breast cancer tissues, and large numbers of mast cells have been identified within certain tumor tissues (cf. Ref. 128). These data suggest that stress hormone/histamine-induced suppression of cellular immunity may contribute to increased growth of certain tumors.

THERAPEUTIC PERSPECTIVES

Glucocorticoids and agents that potentiate their actions are options for treatment of autoimmune inflammatory diseases.[237] By potentiating the secretion or the effects of hypothalamic CRH with CRH secretagogues, CRH agonists, or CRH-binding protein antagonists that cross the blood-brain barrier may prevent the development of inflammatory disease in susceptible people with a hypofunctional HPA axis and at the same time correct CNS symptoms of CRH deficiency. Such an action could be envisioned for nonpeptidic substance P antagonists, which would be expected to reverse the CRH suppression that occurs in chronic inflammatory states, and at the same time act as a local anti-inflammatory agent.

Antagonists of proinflammatory peptides may control inflammatory diseases or processes in which these peptides have a primary pathogenic role. Depending on their ability to cross the blood-brain barrier and the location of the therapeutic target, these antagonists could be used systemically or in a compartmentalized fashion.

Once the mechanisms of acquired glucocorticoid resistance in rheumatoid arthritis, steroid-resistant asthma, AIDS, and other inflammatory diseases are elucidated, therapy with the appropriate intracellular agents that will sensitize the cascade of glucocorticoid action in immune cells, or treatment with cytokines or their antagonists, or pharmacologic agents that influence their secretion and action may become available for the management of these disorders.

The potential immunopotentiating effects of Δ^5 adrenal androgens on T-helper 1 cells may be useful in the treatment of diseases such as SLE and the final stages of AIDS. A prospective, placebo-controlled study of dehydroepiandrosterone administration to patients with SLE was associated with marked clinical improvement and minimal adverse effects. A similar therapy might be beneficial in other such diseases.

Moreover, blocking the effect of stress by β_2-AR and/or H2 antagonists might result in boosting Th1 responses that might be useful in the management of certain infections or tumors, while the combined administration of β_2-AR agonists and glucocorticoids might help in the management of certain Th1-mediated autoimmune diseases. Finally, CRH antagonists might help to prevent stress-induced Th1-suppression and triggering of stress-induced allergic or vasokinetic phenomena. Such antagonists are at hand and show promise in preclinicals studies.[238]

REFERENCES

1. Chrousos GP: The hypothalamic-pituitary-adrenal axis and immune-mediated inflammation [see comments]. N Engl J Med 332:1351–1362, 1995.

2. Tonkoff W: Zur kenntnis der nerven der lymphdrüsen. Anat Anz 16:456–459, 1899.

3. Benschop RJ, Rodriguez-Feuerhahn M, Schedlowski M: Catecholamine-induced leukocytosis: Early observations, current research, and future directions. Brain Behav Immun 10:77–91, 1996.

4. Paul W (ed): Fundamental Immunology, 3rd ed. New York, Raven Press, 1993.

5. Loeper M, Crouzon O: L'action de l'adrenaline sur le sang. Arch Med Exp Anat Pathol 16:83–108, 1904.

6. Metal'nikov S, Chorine V: Rôle des réflexes conditionnels dans l'immunité. Ann Inst Pasteur Paris 40:893–900, 1926.

7. Selye H: Thymus and adrenals in the response of the organism to injuries and intoxications. Br J Exp Pathol 17:234–238, 1936.

8. Chrousos GP, Gold PW: The concepts of stress and stress system disorders. Overview of physical and behavioral homeostasis. JAMA 267:1244–1252, 1992. (Erratum appears in JAMA 268(2):200, 2000)

9. Janig W, McLachlan EM: Characteristics of function-specific pathways in the sympathetic nervous system. Trends Neurosci 15:475–481, 1992.

10. von Euler US: The presence of a substance with sympathin E properties in spleen extracts. Acta Physiol Scand 11:168–173, 1946.

11. Nobelstiftelsen: Les Prix Nobel. Stockholm, Sweden, Imprimerie Royal Norstedt and Soner, 1951.

12. Hench PS, Kendall EC, Slocumb CH, et al: The effect of a hormone of the adrenal cortex (17-hydroxy-11-dehydro-corticosterone: compound E) and of pituitary adrenocorticotropic hormone on rheumatoid athritis. Mayo Clin Proc 24:181–197, 1949.

13. Dougherty TF, Frank JA: The quantitative and qualitative responses of blood lymphocytes to stress stimuli. J Lab Clin Med 42:530–537, 1953.

14. Besedovsky HO, Sorkin E, Keller M, et al: Changes in blood hormone levels during the immune response. Proc Soc Exp Biol Med 150:466–470, 1975.

15. Besedovsky HO, Del Rey A, Sorkin E, et al: Immunoregulation mediated by the sympathetic nervous system. Cell Immunol 48:346–355, 1979.

16. Besedovsky H, del RA, Sorkin E, et al: Immunoregulatory feedback between interleukin-1 and glucocorticoid hormones. Science 233:652–654, 1986.

17. Besedovsky HO, del Rey AE, Sorkin E: Lymphokine-containing supernatants from Con A-stimulated cells increase corticosterone blood levels. J Immunology 126:385–389, 1981.

18. Besedovsky HO, del Rey AE, Sorkin E, et al: The immune response evokes changes in braion noradrenergic neurons. Science 221:564–566, 1983.

19. Del Rey A, Besedovsky HO, Sorkin E, et al: Sympathetic immunoregulation: Difference between high and low-responder animals. Am J Physiol 242:R30–R33, 1982.

20. Ader R, Cohen N: Behaviorally conditioned immunosuppression and murine systemic lupus erythematosus. Science 215:1534–1536, 1982.

21. Keller SE, Weiss JM, Schleifer SJ, et al: Stress-induced suppression of immunity in adrenalectomized rats. Science 221:1301–1304, 1983.

22. Cohen S, Tyrrell DA, Smith AP: Psychological stress and susceptibility to the common cold [see comments]. N Engl J Med 325:606–612, 1991.

23. Carlson SL, Felten DL: Involvement of hypothalamic and limbic structures in neural-immune communication. In Goetzl, EJ, Spector, NH (eds): Neuroimmune networks: Physiology and diseases, New York, Alan R. Liss, 1989.

24. Sternberg EM, Young WS, Bernardini R, et al: A central nervous system defect in biosynthesis of corticotropin-releasing hormone is associated with susceptibility to streptococcal cell wall-induced arthritis in Lewis rats. Proc Natl Acad Sci U S A 86:4771–4775, 1989.

25. Sternberg EM, Hill JM, Chrousos GP, et al: Inflammatory mediator-induced hypothalamic-pituitary-adrenal axis activation is defective in streptococcal cell wall arthritis-susceptible Lewis rats. Proc Natl Acad Sci U S A 86:2374–2378, 1989.

26. Wilder RL: Neuroendocrine-immune system interactions and autoimmunity. Annu Rev Immunol 13:307–338, 1995.

27. Karalis K, Sano H, Redwine J, et al: Autocrine or paracrine inflammatory actions of corticotropin-releasing hormone in vivo. Science 254:421–423, 1991.

28. Chrousos GP: Regulation and dysregulation of the hypothalamic-pituitary-adrenal axis: The corticotropin-releasing hormone perspective. Endocrinol Metab Clin North Am 21:833–858, 1992.

29. Saper CB, Loewy AD, Swanson LW, et al: Direct hypothalamo-autonomic connections. Brain Res 117:305–312, 1976.

30. Whitnall MH: Stress selectively activates the vasopressin-containing subset of corticotropin-releasing hormone neurons. Neuroendocrinology 50:702–707, 1989.

31. de Goeij DC, Kvetnansky R, Whitnall MH, et al: Repeated stress-induced activation of corticotropin-releasing factor neurons enhances vasopressin stores and colocalization with corticotropin-releasing factor in the median eminence of rats. Neuroendocrinology 53:150–159, 1991.

32. Nikolarakis KE, Almeida OF, Herz A: Stimulation of hypothalamic beta-endorphin and dynorphin release by corticotropin-releasing factor (in vitro). Brain Res 399:152–155, 1986.

33. Burns G, Almeida OF, Passarelli F, et al: A two-step mechanism by which corticotropin-releasing hormone releases hypothalamic beta-endorphin: The role of vasopressin and G-proteins. Endocrinology 125:1365–1372, 1989.

34. Lamberts SW, Verleun T, Oosterom R, et al: Corticotropin-releasing factor (ovine) and vasopressin exert a synergistic effect on adrenocorticotropin release in man. J Clin Endocrinol Metab 58:298–303, 1984.

35. Rittmaster RS, Cutler GBJ, Gold PW, et al: The relationship of saline-induced changes in vasopressin secretion to basal and corticotropin-releasing hormone-stimulated adrenocorticotropin and cortisol secretion in man. J Clin Endocrinol Metab 64:371–376, 1987.

36. Elkabir DR, Wyatt ME, Vellucci SV, et al: The effects of separate or combined infusions of corticotrophin-releasing factor and vasopressin either intraventricularly or into the amygdala on aggressive and investigative behaviour in the rat. Regul Pept 28:199–214, 1990.

37. Redekopp C, Irvine CH, Donald RA, et al: Spontaneous and stimulated adrenocorticotropin and vasopressin pulsatile secretion in the pituitary venous effluent of the horse. Endocrinology 118:1410–1416, 1986.

38. Ixart G, Barbanel G, Conte-Devolx B, et al: Evidence for basal and stress-induced release of corticotropin releasing factor in the push-pull cannulated median eminence of conscious free-moving rats. Neurosci Lett 74:85–89, 1987.

39. Engler D, Pham T, Fullerton MJ, et al: Studies of the secretion of corticotropin-releasing factor and arginine vasopressin into the hypophysial-portal circulation of the conscious sheep: I. Effect of an audiovisual stimulus and insulin-induced hypoglycemia. Neuroendocrinology 49:367–381, 1989.

40. Carnes M, Lent SJ, Goodman B, et al: Effects of immunoneutralization of corticotropin-releasing hormone on ultradian rhythms of plasma adrenocorticotropin. Endocrinology 126:1904–1913, 1990.

41. Calogero AE, Norton JA, Sheppard BC, et al: Pulsatile activation of the hypothalamic-pituitary-adrenal axis during major surgery. Metabolism 41:839–845, 1992.

42. Holmes MC, Antoni FA, Aguilera G, et al: Magnocellular axons in passage through the median eminence release vasopressin. Nature 319:326–329, 1986.

43. Phillips MI: Functions of angiotensin in the central nervous system. Annu Rev Physiol 49:413–435, 1987.

44. Hinson JP: Paracrine control of adrenocortical function: A new role for the medulla? J Endocrinol 124:7–9, 1990.

45. Andreis PG, Neri G, Mazzocchi G, et al: Direct secretagogue effect of corticotropin-releasing factor on the rat adrenal cortex: The involvement of the zona medullaris. Endocrinology 131:69–72, 1992.

46. Vinson GP, Whitehouse BJ, Henvill KL: The actions of alpha-MSh on the adrenal cortex, the melanotrophic peptides. In Hadley ME (ed): Biological Roles. Boca Raton, FL, CRC Press, 1988.

47. Ottenweller JE, Meier AH: Adrenal innervation may be an extrapituitary mechanism able to regulate adrenocortical rhythmicity in rats. Endocrinology 111:1334–1338, 1982.

48. Besedovsky HO, Del Rey A, Sorkin E, et al: Immunoregulatory feedback between interleukin-1 and glucocorticoid hormones. Science 233:652–654, 1986.

49. Sawchenko PE, Imaki T, Potter E, et al: The functional neuroanatomy of corticotrophin-releasing factor. In Chadwick DJ, Marsh J, Ackrill K (eds): Corticotrophin-Releasing Factor. Chichester, United Kingdom, John Wiley, 1993.

50. Larsen PJ, Jessop D, Patel H, et al: Substance P inhibits the release of anterior pituitary adrenocorticotrophin via a central mechanism involving corticotrophin-releasing factor-containing neurons in the hypothalamic paraventricular nucleus. J Neuroendocrinol 5:99–105, 1993.

51. Culman J, Tschope C, Jost N, et al: Substance P and neurokinin A induced desensitization to cardiovascular and behavioral effects: Evidence for the involvement of different tachykinin receptors. Brain Res 625:75–83, 1993.

52. Jessop DS, Chowdrey HS, Larsen PJ, et al: Substance P: Multifunctional peptide in the hypothalamo-pituitary system? J Endocrinol 132:331–337, 1992.

53. Felten DL, Felten SY, Carlson SL, et al: Noradrenergic and peptidergic innervation of lymphoid tissue. J Immunol 135:755s–765s, 1985.

54. Vizi ES, Orso E, Osipenko ON, et al: Neurochemical, electrophysiological and immunocytochemical evidence for a noradrenergic link between the sympathetic nervous system and thymocytes. Neuroscience 68:1263–1276, 1995.

55. Ackerman KD, Felten SY, Bellinger DL, et al: Noradrenergic sympathetic innervation of the spleen: III. Development of innervation in the rat spleen. J Neurosci Res 18:49–54, 1987.

56. Weihe E, Nohr D, Michel S, et al: Molecular anatomy of the neuro-immune connection. Int J Neurosci 59:1–23, 1991.

57. Roitt I, Brostoff J, Male D (eds): Immunology, 4th ed. London, Mosby, 1996.

58. Gallin JI, Goldstein IM, Snyderman R: Overview. In Gallin JI, Goldstein IM, Snyderman R (eds): Inflammation: Basic Principles and Clinical Correlates. New York, Raven Press, 1988.

59. Paul WE, Seder RA: Lymphocyte responses and cytokines. Cell 76:241–251, 1994.

60. Celander DR, Folkow B: The nature and distribution of afferent fibers provided with the axon reflex arrangements. Acta Physiol Scand 359–370, 1953.

61. Payan DG, Goetzl EJ: Modulation of lymphocyte function by sensory neuropeptides. J Immunol 135:783s–786s, 1985.

62. Engel D: The influence of the sympathetic nervous system on capillary permeability. Res Exp Med (Berl) 173:1–8, 1978.

63. Holzer P: Local effector functions of capsaicin-sensitive sensory nerve endings: Involvement of tachykinins, calcitonin gene-related peptide and other neuropeptides. Neuroscience 24:739–768, 1988.

64. Coderre TJ, Basbaum AI, Levine JD: Neural control of vascular permeability: Interactions between primary afferents, mast cells, and sympathetic efferents. J Neurophysiol 62:48–58, 1989.

65. Fearon DT, Locksley RM: The instructive role of innate immunity in the acquired immune response. Science 272:50–53, 1996.

66. Mosmann TR, Sad S: The expanding universe of T-cell subsets: Th1, Th2 and more [see comments]. Immunol Today 17:138–146, 1996.

67. Trinchieri G: Interleukin-12: A proinflammatory cytokine with immunoregulatory functions that bridge innate resistance and antigen-specific adaptive immunity. Annu Rev Immunol 13:251–276, 1995.

68. Boumpas DT, Chrousos GP, Wilder RL, et al: Glucocorticoid therapy for immune-mediated diseases: Basic and clinical correlates. Ann Intern Med 119:1198–1208, 1993.

69. Chrousos GP, Detera-Wadleigh SD, Karl M: Syndromes of glucocorticoid resistance [see comments]. Ann Intern Med 119:1113–1124, 1993.

70. Cronstein BN, Kimmel SC, Levin RI, et al: A mechanism for the antiinflammatory effects of corticosteroids: The glucocorticoid receptor regulates leukocyte adhesion to endothelial cells and expression of endothelial-leukocyte adhesion molecule 1 and intercellular adhesion molecule 1. Proc Natl Acad Sci U S A 89:9991–9995, 1992.

71. Hirano T, Akira S, Taga T, et al: Biological and clinical aspects of interleukin 6 [see comments]. Immunol Today 11:443–449, 1990.

72. Lee SW, Tsou AP, Chan H, et al: Glucocorticoids selectively inhibit the transcription of the interleukin 1 beta gene and decrease the stability of interleukin 1 beta mRNA. Proc Natl Acad Sci U S A 85:1204–1208, 1988.

73. Zanker B, Walz G, Wieder KJ, et al: Evidence that glucocorticosteroids block expression of the human interleukin-6 gene by accessory cells. Transplantation 49:183–185, 1990.

74. Nakano T, Ohara O, Teraoka H, et al: Glucocorticoids suppress group II phospholipase A2 production by blocking mRNA synthesis and post-transcriptional expression. J Biol Chem 265:12745–12748, 1990.

75. Vishwanath BS: Glucocorticoid deficiency increases phospholipase A2 activity in rats. J Clin Invest 92:1974–1980, 1993.

76. O'Banion MK, Winn VD, Young DA: cDNA cloning and functional activity of a glucocorticoid-regulated inflammatory cyclooxygenase. Proc Natl Acad Sci U S A 89:4888–4892, 1992.

77. Conrad DJ, Kuhn H, Mulkins M, et al: Specific inflammatory cytokines regulate the expression of human monocyte 15-lipoxygenase. Proc Natl Acad Sci U S A 89:217–221, 1992.

78. Moncada S, Higgs A: The L-arginine-nitric oxide pathway. N Engl J Med 329:2002–2012, 1993.

79. Cove-Smith JR, Kabler P, Pownall R, et al: Circadian variation in an immune response in man. Br Med J 2:253–254, 1978.

80. Harkness JA, Richter MB, Panayi GS, et al: Circadian variation in disease activity in rheumatoid arthritis. Br Med J (Clin Res Ed) 284:551–554, 1982.

81. Mastorakos G, Chrousos G: Adrenal hyperandrogenism. In Adashi E, Rock J, Rosenwaks Z (eds): Reproductive Endocrinology, Surgery, and Technology. New York, Raven Press, 1995.

82. Daynes RA, Dudley DJ, Araneo BA: Regulation of murine lymphokine production in vivo: II. Dehydroepiandrosterone is a natural enhancer of interleukin 2 synthesis by helper T cells. Eur J Immunol 20:793–802, 1990.

83. Blauer KL, Poth M, Rogers WM, et al: Dehydroepiandrosterone antagonizes the suppressive effects of dexamethasone on lymphocyte proliferation. Endocrinology 129:3174–3179, 1991.

84. Suzuki T: Dehydroepiandrosterone enhances IL2 production and cytotoxic effector function of human T cells. Clin Immunol Immunopathol 61:202–211, 1991.

85. Meikle AW: The presence of a dehydroepiandrosterone-specific receptor binding complex in murine T cells. J Steroid Biochem Mol Biol 42:293–304, 1992.

86. Hadden JW, Hadden EM, Middleton E Jr: Lymphocyte blast transformation: I. Demonstration of adrenergic receptors in human peripheral lymphocytes. Cell Immunol 1:583–595, 1970.

87. Chambers DA, Cohen RL, Perlman RL: Neuroimmune modulation: Signal transduction and catecholamines. Neurochem Int 22:95–110, 1993.

88. Carlson SL, Brooks WH, Roszman TL: Neurotransmitter-lymphocyte interactions: Dual receptor modulation of lymphocyte proliferation and cAMP production. J Neuroimmunol 24:155–162, 1989.

89. Bartik MM, Brooks WH, Roszman TL: Modulation of T cell proliferation by stimulation of the beta-adrenergic receptor: Lack of correlation between inhibition of T cell proliferation and cAMP accumulation. Cell Immunol 148:408–421, 1993.

90. Elliott L, Brooks W, Roszman T: Inhibition of anti-CD3 monoclonal antibody-induced T-cell proliferation by dexamethasone, isoproterenol, or prostaglandin E2 either alone or in combination. Cell Mol Neurobiol 12:411–427, 1992.

91. Whalen MM, Bankhurst AD: Effects of beta-adrenergic receptor activation, cholera toxin and forskolin on human natural killer cell function. Biochem J 272:327–331, 1990.

92. Hellstrand K, Hermodsson S: An immunopharmacological analysis of adrenaline-induced suppression of human natural killer cell cytotoxicity. Int Arch Allergy Appl Immunol 89:334–341, 1989.

93. Irwin M: Stress-induced immune suppression: Role of brain corticotropin releasing hormone and autonomic nervous system mechanisms. Adv Neuroimmunol 4:29–47, 1994.

94. Irwin M, Hauger R, Brown M: Central corticotropin-releasing hormone activates the sympathetic nervous system and reduces immune function: Increased responsivity of the aged rat. Endocrinology 131:1047–1053, 1992.

95. Strausbaugh H, Irwin M: Central corticotropin-releasing hormone reduces cellular immunity. Brain Behav Immun 6:11–17, 1992.

96. Elenkov IJ, Papanicolaou DA, Wilder RL, et al: Modulatory effects of glucocorticoids and catecholamines on human interleukin-12 and interleukin-10 production: Clinical implications. Proc Assoc Am Physicians 108:374–381, 1996.

97. Zurier RB, Weissmann G, Hoffstein S, et al: Mechanisms of lysosomal enzyme release from human leukocytes: II. Effects of cAMP and cGMP, autonomic agonists, and agents which affect microtubule function. J Clin Invest 53:297–309, 1974.

98. Weiss M, Schneider EM, Tarnow J, et al: Is inhibition of oxygen radical production of neutrophils by sympathomimetics mediated via beta-2 adrenoceptors? J Pharmacol Exp Ther 278:1105–1113, 1996.

99. Barnett CCJ, Moore EE, Partrick DA, et al: Beta-adrenergic stimulation down-regulates neutrophil priming for superoxide generation, but not elastase release. J Surg Res 70:166–170, 1997.

100. Sanders VM, Baker RA, Ramer-Quinn DS, et al: Differential expression of the beta2-adrenergic receptor by Th1 and Th2 clones: Implications for cytokine production and B cell help. J Immunol 158:4200–4210, 1997.

101. Sanders VM: The role of adrenoceptor-mediated signals in the modulation of lymphocyte function. Adv Neuroimmunol 5:283–298, 1995.

102. Coqueret O, Dugas B, Mencia-Huerta JM, et al: Regulation of IgE production from human mononuclear cells by beta 2-adrenoceptor agonists [see comments]. Clin Exp Allergy 25:304–311, 1995.

103. Coqueret O, Lagente V, Frere CP, et al: Regulation of IgE production by beta 2-adrenoceptor agonists. Ann N Y Acad Sci 725:44–49, 1994.

104. Blotta MH, DeKruyff RH, Umetsu DT: Corticosteroids inhibit IL-12 production in human monocytes and enhance their capacity to induce IL-4 synthesis in CD4+ lymphocytes. J Immunol 158:5589–5595, 1997.

105. DeKruyff RH, Fang Y, Umetsu DT: Corticosteroids enhance the capacity of macrophages to induce Th2 cytokine synthesis in CD4+ lymphocytes by inhibiting IL-12 production. J Immunol 160:2231–2237, 1998.

106. Wu CY, Wang K, McDyer JF, et al: Prostaglandin E2 and dexamethasone inhibit IL-12 receptor expression and IL-12 responsiveness. J Immunol 161:2723–2730, 1998.

107. van der Poll T, Barber AE, Coyle SM, et al: Hypercortisolemia increases plasma interleukin-10 concentrations during human endotoxemia: A clinical research center study. J Clin Endocrinol Metab 81:3604–3606, 1996.

108. Ramierz F, Fowell DJ, Puklavec M, et al: Glucocorticoids promote a TH2 cytokine response by CD4+ T cells in vitro. J Immunol 156:2406–2412, 1996.

109. Tabardel Y, Duchateau J, Schmartz D, et al: Corticosteroids increase blood interleukin-10 levels during cardiopulmonary bypass in men. Surgery 119:76–80, 1996.

110. Gayo A, Mozo L, Suarez A, et al: Glucocorticoids increase IL-10 expression in multiple sclerosis patients with acute relapse. J Neuroimmunol 85:122–130, 1998.

111. Panina-Bordignon P, Mazzeo D, Lucia PD, et al: Beta2-agonists prevent Th1 development by selective inhibition of interleukin 12. J Clin Invest 100:1513–1519, 1997.

112. Hasko G, Szabo C, Nemeth ZH, et al: Stimulation of beta-adrenoceptors inhibits endotoxin-induced IL-12 production in normal and IL-10 deficient mice. J Neuroimmunol 88:57–61, 1998.

113. Borger P, Hoekstra Y, Esselink MT, et al: Beta-adrenoceptor-mediated inhibition of IFN-gamma, IL-3, and GM-CSF mRNA accumulation in activated human T lymphocytes is solely mediated by the beta2-adrenoceptor subtype. Am J Respir Cell Mol Biol 19:400–407, 1998.

114. Hasko G, Elenkov IJ, Kvetan V, et al: Differential effect of selective block of alpha 2-adrenoreceptors on plasma levels of tumour necrosis factor-alpha, interleukin-6 and corticosterone induced by bacterial lipopolysaccharide in mice. J Endocrinol 144:457–462, 1995.

115. Elenkov IJ, Hasko G, Kovacs KJ, et al: Modulation of lipopolysaccharide-induced tumor necrosis factor-alpha production by selective alpha- and beta-adrenergic drugs in mice. J Neuroimmunol 61:123–131, 1995.

116. Woiciechowsky C, Asadullah K, Nestler D, et al: Sympathetic activation triggers systemic interleukin-10 release in immunodepression induced by brain injury. Nat Med 4:808–813, 1998.

117. Batuman OA, Ferrero A, Cupp C, et al: Differential regulation of transforming growth factor beta-1 gene expression by glucocorticoids in human T and glial cells. J Immunol 155:4397–4405, 1995.

118. Spengler RN, Allen RM, Remick DG, et al: Stimulation of alpha-adrenergic receptor augments the production of macrophage-derived tumor necrosis factor. J Immunol 145:1430–1434, 1990.

119. Le Tulzo Y, Shenkar R, Kaneko D, et al: Hemorrhage increases cytokine expression in lung mononuclear cells in mice: Involvement of catecholamines in nuclear factor-kappaB regulation and cytokine expression. J Clin Invest 99:1516–1524, 1997.

120. Baker AJ, Fuller RW: Loss of response to beta-adrenoceptor agonists during the maturation of human monocytes to macrophages in vitro. J Leukoc Biol 57:395–400, 1995.

121. Linden A: Increased interleukin-8 release by beta-adrenoceptor activation in human transformed bronchial epithelial cells. Br J Pharmacol 119:402–406, 1996.

122. Meduri GU, Chrousos GP: Duration of glucocorticoid treatment and outcome in sepsis: Is the right drug used the wrong way? [editorial; comment]. Chest 114:355–360, 1998.

123. Webster EL, Torpy DJ, Elenkov IJ, et al: Corticotropin-releasing hormone and inflammation. Ann N Y Acad Sci 840:21–32, 1998.

124. Theoharides TC, Spanos C, Pang X, et al: Stress-induced intracranial mast cell degranulation: A corticotropin-releasing hormone-mediated effect. Endocrinology 136:5745–5750, 1995.

125. Udelsman R, Gallucci WT, Bacher J, et al: Hemodynamic effects of corticotropin releasing hormone in the anesthetized cynomolgus monkey. Peptides 7:465–471, 1986.

126. Theoharides TC, Singh LK, Boucher W, et al: Corticotropin-releasing hormone induces skin mast cell degranulation and increased vascular permeability, a possible explanation for its proinflammatory effects. Endocrinology 139:403–413, 1998.

127. Rocklin RE (ed): Histamine and H2 antagonists in inflammation and immunodeficiency, New York, Marcel Dekker, 1990.

128. Elenkov IJ, Webster E, Papanicolaou DA, et al: Histamine potently suppresses human IL-12 and stimulates IL-10 production via H2 receptors. J Immunol 161:2586–2593, 1998.

129. Lagier B, Lebel B, Bousquet J, et al: Different modulation by histamine of IL-4 and interferon-gamma (IFN-gamma) release according to the phenotype of human Th0, Th1 and Th2 clones. Clin Exp Immunol 108:545–551, 1997.

130. Pacak K, Palkovits M, Yadid G, et al: Heterogeneous neurochemical responses to different stressors: A test of Selye's doctrine of nonspecificity. Am J Physiol 275:R1247–R1255, 1998.

131. Berkenbosch F, van OJ, del RA, et al: Corticotropin-releasing factor-producing neurons in the rat activated by interleukin-1. Science 238:524–526, 1987.

132. Sapolsky R, Rivier C, Yamamoto G, et al: Interleukin-1 stimulates the secretion of hypothalamic corticotropin-releasing factor. Science 238:522–524, 1987.

133. Dunn AJ: Systemic interleukin-1 administration stimulates hypothalamic norepinephrine metabolism parallelling the increased plasma corticosterone. Life Sci 43:429–435, 1988.

134. Bernardini R, Kamilaris TC, Calogero AE, et al: Interactions between tumor necrosis factor-a, hypothalamic corticotropin-releasing hormone, and adrenocorticotropin secretion in the rat. Endocrinology 126:2876–2881, 1990.

135. Elenkov IJ, Kovacs K, Kiss J, et al: Lipopolysaccharide is able to bypass corticotrophin-releasing factor in affecting plasma ACTH and corticosterone levels: Evidence from rats with lesions of the paraventricular nucleus. J Endocrinol 133:231–236, 1992.

136. Kovacs KJ, Elenkov IJ: Differential dependence of ACTH secretion induced by various cytokines on the integrity of the paraventricular nucleus. J Neuroendocrinol 7:15–23, 1995.

137. Akira S, Hirano T, Taga T, et al: Biology of multifunctional cytokines: IL 6 and related molecules (IL 1 and TNF). FASEB J 4:2860–2867, 1990.

138. Hesse DG, Tracey KJ, Fong Y, et al: Cytokine appearance in human endotoxemia and primate bacteremia. Surg Gynecol Obstet 166:147–153, 1988.

139. van Deventer SJ, Buller HR, ten Cate JW, et al: Experimental endotoxemia in humans: Analysis of cytokine release and coagulation, fibrinolytic, and complement pathways. Blood 76:2520–2526, 1990.

140. van Gool J, van Vugt H, Helle M, et al: The relation among stress, adrenalin, interleukin 6 and acute phase proteins in the rat. Clin Immunol Immunopathol 57:200–210, 1990.

141. Komaki G, Gottschall PE, Somogyvari-Vigh A, et al: Rapid increase in plasma IL-6 after hemorrhage, and posthemorrhage reduction of the IL-6 response to LPS, in conscious rats: Interrelation with plasma corticosterone levels. Neuroimmunomodulation 1:127–134, 1994.

142. Imura H, Fukata J, Mori T: Cytokines and endocrine function: An interaction between the immune and neuroendocrine systems. Clin Endocrinol (Oxf) 35:107–115, 1991.

143. Naitoh Y, Fukata J, Tominaga T, et al: Interleukin-6 stimulates the secretion of adrenocorticotropic hormone in conscious, freely-moving rats. Biochem Biophys Res Commun 155:1459–1463, 1988.

144. Perlstein RS, Mougey EH, Jackson WE, et al: Interleukin-1 and interleukin-6 act synergistically to stimulate the release of adrenocorticotropic hormone in vivo. Lymphokine Cytokine Res 10:141–146, 1991.

145. Perlstein RS, Whitnall MH, Abrams JS, et al: Synergistic roles of interleukin-6, interleukin-1, and tumor necrosis factor in the adrenocorticotropin response to bacterial lipopolysaccharide in vivo. Endocrinology 132:946–952, 1993.

146. Mastorakos G, Weber JS, Magiakou MA, et al: Hypothalamic-pituitary-adrenal axis activation and stimulation of systemic vasopressin secretion by recombinant interleukin-6 in humans: Potential implications for the syndrome of inappropriate vasopressin secretion [see comments]. J Clin Endocrinol Metab 79:934–939, 1994.

147. Mastorakos G, Chrousos GP, Weber JS: Recombinant interleukin-6 activates the hypothalamic-pituitary-adrenal axis in humans. J Clin Endocrinol Metab 77:1690–1694, 1993.

148. Maier SF, Goehler LE, Fleshner M, et al: The role of the vagus nerve in cytokine-to-brain communication. Ann N Y Acad Sci 840:289–300, 1998.

149. Tilders FJ, DeRijk RH, Van Dam AM, et al: Activation of the hypothalamus-pituitary-adrenal axis by bacterial endotoxins: Routes and intermediate signals. Psychoneuroendocrinology 19:209–232, 1994.

150. Reichlin S: Neuroendocrine-immune interactions. N Engl J Med 329:1246–1253, 1993.

151. De Simoni MG, Sironi M, De Luigi A, et al: Intracerebroventricular injection of interleukin 1 induces high circulating levels of interleukin 6. J Exp Med 171:1773–1778, 1990.

152. Vizi ES, Harsing LGJR, Zimanyi I, et al: Release and turnover of noradrenaline in isolated median eminence: Lack of negative feedback modulation. Neuroscience 16:907–916, 1985.

153. Plotsky PM, Cunningham ET Jr, Widmaier EP: Catecholaminergic modulation of corticotropin-releasing factor and adrenocorticotropin secretion. Endocr Rev 10:437–458, 1989.

154. Elenkov IJ, Kovacs K, Duda E, et al: Presynaptic inhibitory effect of TNF-alpha on the release of noradrenaline in isolated median eminence. J Neuroimmunol 41:117–120, 1992.

155. Gordon ML: An evaluation of affeent nervous impulses in the adrenal cortical responseto trauma. Endocrinology 47:347–350, 1950.

156. Chapman LF, Goodell H: The participation of the nervous system in the inflammatory reaction. Ann N Y Acad Sci 116:990–1017, 1963.

157. Berkenbosch F, de Goeij DEC, del Rey AE, et al: Neuroendocrine, sympathetic and metabolic responses induced by interleukin-1. Neuroendocrinology 50:570–576, 1989.

158. Katafuchi T, Hori T, Take S: Central administration of interferon-alpha enhances rat sympathetic nerve activity to the spleen. Neurosci Lett 125(1):37–40, 1991.

159. Shimizu N, Hori T, Nakane H: An interleukin-1 b-induced noradrenaline release in the spleen is mediated by brain corticotropin-releasing factor: An in vivo microdialysis study in conscious rats. Brain Behav Immun 7:14–23, 1994.

160. Spangelo BL, Judd AM, Isakson PC, et al: Interleukin-6 stimulates anterior pituitary hormone release in vitro. Endocrinology 125:575–577, 1989.

161. Roh MS: Direct stimulation of the adrenal cortex by interleukin-1. Surgery 102:140–146, 1987.

162. Salas MA, Evans SW, Levell MJ, et al: Interleukin-6 and ACTH act synergistically to stimulate the release of corticosterone from adrenal gland cells. Clin Exp Immunol 79:470–473, 1990.

163. Tominaga T, Fukata J, Naito Y, et al: Prostaglandin-dependent in vitro stimulation of adrenocortical steroidogenesis by interleukins. Endocrinology 128:526–531, 1991.

164. Vankelecom H, Carmeliet P, Van Damme J, et al: Production of interleukin-6 by folliculo-stellate cells of the anterior pituitary gland in a histiotypic cell aggregate culture system. Neuroendocrinology 49:102–106, 1989.

165. Schultzberg M, Andersson C, Unden A, et al: Interleukin-1 in adrenal chromaffin cells. Neuroscience 30:805–810, 1989.

166. Vankelecom H, Carmeliet P, Heremans H, et al: Interferon-gamma inhibits stimulated adrenocorticotropin, prolactin, and growth hormone secretion in normal rat anterior pituitary cell cultures. Endocrinology 126:2919–2926, 1990.

167. Gaillard RC, Turnill D, Sappino P, et al: Tumor necrosis factor alpha inhibits the hormonal response of the pituitary gland to hypothalamic releasing factors. Endocrinology 127:101–106, 1990.

168. Jaattela M, Ilvesmaki V, Voutilainen R, et al: Tumor necrosis factor as a potent inhibitor of adrenocorticotropin-induced cortisol production and steroidogenic P450 enzyme gene expression in cultured human fetal adrenal cells. Endocrinology 128:623–629, 1991.

169. Almawi WY, Lipman ML, Stevens AC, et al: Abrogation of glucocorticoid-mediated inhibition of T cell proliferation by the synergistic action of IL-1, IL-6, and IFN-gamma. J Immunol 146:3523–3527, 1991.

170. Kam JC, Szefler SJ, Surs W, et al: Combination IL-2 and IL-4 reduces glucocorticoid receptor-binding affinity and T cell response to glucocorticoids. J Immunol 151:3460–3466, 1993.

171. Klein A, Buskila D, Gladman D, et al: Cortisol catabolism by lymphocytes of patients with systemic lupus erythematosus and rheumatoid arthritis. J Rheumatol 17:30–33, 1990.

172. Harbuz MS, Lightman SL: Stress and the hypothalamo-pituitary-adrenal axis: Acute, chronic and immunological activation. J Endocrinol 134:327–339, 1992.

173. Dallman MF: Stress update: Adaptation of the hypothalamic-pituitary-adrenal axis to chronic stress. Trends Endocrinol Metabol 62–69, 1993.

174. Swain MG, Patchev V, Vergalla J, et al: Suppression of hypothalamic-pituitary-adrenal axis responsiveness to stress in a rat model of acute cholestasis. J Clin Invest 91:1903–1908, 1993.

175. Rothwell PM, Udwadia ZF, Lawler PG: Cortisol response to corticotropin and survival in septic shock [see comments]. Lancet 337:582–583, 1991.

176. Kidess AI, Caplan RH, Reynertson RH, et al: Transient corticotropin deficiency in critical illness. Mayo Clin Proc 68:435–441, 1993.

177. Dluhy RG: The growing spectrum of HIV-related endocrine abnormalities [editorial; comment]. J Clin Endocrinol Metab 70:563–565, 1990.

178. Reincke M, Heppner C, Petzke F, et al: Impairment of adrenocortical function associated with increased plasma tumor necrosis factor-alpha and interleukin-6 concentrations in African trypanosomiasis. Neuroimmunomodulation 1:14–22, 1994.

179. Parker LN, Levin ER, Lifrak ET: Evidence for adrenocortical adaptation to severe illness. J Clin Endocrinol Metab 60:947–952, 1985.

180. Berczi I: Gonadotrophins and sex hormones. In Berczi I (ed): Pituitary Function and Immunity. Boca Raton, FL, CRC Press, 1986.

181. Raveche ES, Steinberg AD: Sex hormones and autoimmunity. In Berczi I: Pituitary Function and Immunity. Boca Raton, FL, CRC Press, 1986.

182. Cid MC, Kleinman HK, Grant DS, et al: Estradiol enhances leukocyte binding to tumor necrosis factor (TNF)-stimulated endothelial cells via an increase in TNF-induced adhesion molecules E-selectin, intercellular adhesion molecule type 1, and vascular cell adhesion molecule type 1. J Clin Invest 93:17–25, 1994.

183. Vamvakopoulos NC, Chrousos GP: Evidence of direct estrogenic regulation of human corticotropin-releasing hormone gene expression: Potential implications for the sexual dimophism of the stress response and immune/inflammatory reaction. J Clin Invest 92:1896–1902, 1993.

184. Berczi I, Nagy E: Prolactin and other iactogenic hormones. In Berczi I (ed): Pituitary Function and Immunity. Boca Raton, FL, CRC Press, 1986.

185. Gilmore W, Weiner LP, Correale J: Effect of estradiol on cytokine secretion by proteolipid protein-specific T cell clones isolated from multiple sclerosis patients and normal control subjects. J Immunol 158:446–451, 1997.

186. Kanda N, Tsuchida T, Tamaki K: Estrogen enhancement of anti-double-stranded DNA antibody and immunoglobulin G production in peripheral blood mononuclear cells from patients with systemic lupus erythematosus. Arthritis Rheum 42:328–337, 1999.

187. Zang YC, Halder JB, Hong J, et al: Regulatory effects of estriol on T cell migration and cytokine profile: Inhibition of transcription factor NF-kappa B. J Neuroimmunol 124(1–2):106–114, 2002.

188. Cenci S, Weitzmann MN, Roggia C, et al: Estrogen deficiency induces bone loss by enhancing T-cell production of TNF-alpha. J Clin Invest 106(10):1229–1237, 2000.

189. Roggia C, Gao Y, Cenci S, et al: Up-regulation of TNF-producing T cells in the bone marrow: A key mechanism by which estrogen deficiency induces bone loss in vivo. Proc Natl Acad Sci U S A 98(24):13960–13965, 2001.

190. Srivastava S, Toraldo G, Weitzmann MN, et al: Estrogen decreases osteoclast formation by down-regulating receptor activator of NF-kappa B ligand (RANKL)-induced JNK activation. J Biol Chem 276(12):8836–8840, 2001.

191. Piccinni MP, Giudizi MG, Biagiotti R, et al: Progesterone favors the development of human T helper cells producing Th2-type cytokines and promotes both IL-4 production and membrane CD30 expression in established Th1 cell clones. J Immunol 155:128–133, 1995.

192. Gellersen B, Kempf R, Telgmann R, et al: Nonpituitary human prolactin gene transcription is independent of Pit-1 and differentially controlled in lymphocytes and in endometrial stroma. Mol Endocrinol 8:356–373, 1994.

193. D'Ambrosio D, Cippitelli M, Cocciolo MG, et al: Inhibition of IL-12 production by 1,25-dihydroxyvitamin D3: Involvement of NF-kappaB downregulation in transcriptional repression of the p40 gene. J Clin Invest 101:252–262, 1998.

194. Lemire JM, Archer DC, Beck L, Spiegelberg HL: Immunosuppressive actions of 1,25-dihydroxyvitamin D3: Preferential inhibition of Th1 functions. J Nutr 125:1704S–1708S, 1995.

195. Mattner F, Smiroldo S, Galbiati F, et al: Inhibition of Th1 development and treatment of chronic-relapsing experimental allergic encephalomyelitis by a non-hypercalcemic analogue of 1,25-dihydroxyvitamin D(3). Eur J Immunol 30(2):498–508, 2000.

196. Gregori S, Giarratana N, Smiroldo S, et al: A 1alpha, 25-dihydroxyvitamin D(3) analog enhances regulatory T-cells and arrests autoimmune diabetes in NOD mice. Diabetes 51(5):1367–1374, 2002.

197. Kang S, Yi S, Griffiths CE, et al: Calcipotriene-induced improvement in psoriasis is associated with reduced interleukin-8 and increased interleukin-10 levels within lesions. Br J Dermatol 138:77–83, 1998.

198. Calogero AE, Sternberg EM, Bagdy G, et al: Neurotransmitter-induced hypothalamic-pituitary-adrenal axis responsiveness is defective in inflammatory disease-susceptible Lewis rats: In vivo and in vitro studies suggesting globally defective hypothalamic secretion of corticotropin-releasing hormone. Neuroendocrinology 55:600–608, 1992.

199. Patchev VK, Kalogeras KT, Zelazowski P, et al: Increased plasma concentrations, hypothalamic content, and in vitro release of arginine vasopressin in inflammatory disease-prone, hypothalamic corticotropin-releasing hormone-deficient Lewis rats. Endocrinology 131:1453–1457, 1992.

200. Sternberg EM, Glowa JR, Smith MA, et al: Corticotropin releasing hormone related behavioral and neuroendocrine responses to stress in Lewis and Fischer rats. Brain Res 570:54–60, 1992.

201. Neeck G, Federlin K, Graef V, et al: Adrenal secretion of cortisol in patients with rheumatoid arthritis. J Rheumatol 17:24–29, 1990.

202. Chikanza IC, Petrou P, Kingsley G, et al: Defective hypothalamic response to immune and inflammatory stimuli in patients with rheumatoid arthritis [see comments]. Arthritis Rheum 35:1281–1288, 1992.

203. Masi AT, Josipovic DB, Jefferson WE: Low adrenal androgenic-anabolic steroids in women with rheumatoid arthritis (RA): Gas-liquid chromatographic studies of RA patients and matched normal control women indicating decreased 11-deoxy-17-ketosteroid excretion. Semin Arthritis Rheum 14:1–23, 1984.

204. Crofford LJ, Sano H, Karalis K, et al: Local expression of corticotropin-releasing hormone in inflammatory arthritis. Ann N Y Acad Sci 771:459–471, 1995.

205. Crofford LJ, Sano H, Karalis K, et al: Corticotropin-releasing hormone in synovial fluids and tissues of patients with rheumatoid arthritis and osteoarthritis. J Immunol 151:1587–1596, 1993.

206. Sternberg EM: Hyperimmune fatigue syndromes: Diseases of the stress response? [editorial; corrected; comment]. J Rheumatol 20:418–421, 1993. (Erratum appears in J Rheumatol 20(5):925, 1993.)

207. Dekaris D, Sabioncello A, Mazuran R, et al: Multiple changes of immunologic parameters in prisoners of war: Assessments after release from a camp in Manjaca, Bosnia. JAMA 270:595–599, 1993.

208. Schlaghecke R, Kornely E, Wollenhaupt J, et al: Glucocorticoid receptors in rheumatoid arthritis. Arthritis Rheum 35:740–744, 1992.

209. Kirkham BW, Corkill MM, Davison SC, et al: Response to glucocorticoid treatment in rheumatoid arthritis: In vitro cell mediated immune assay predicts in vivo responses. J Rheumatol 18:821–825, 1991.

210. Corrigan CJ, Brown PH, Barnes NC, et al: Glucocorticoid resistance in chronic asthma: Peripheral blood T lymphocyte activation and comparison of the T lymphocyte inhibitory effects of glucocorticoids and cyclosporin A. Am Rev Respir Dis 144:1026–1032, 1991.

211. Sher ER, Leung DY, Surs W, et al: Steroid-resistant asthma: Cellular mechanisms contributing to inadequate response to glucocorticoid therapy. J Clin Invest 93:33–39, 1994.

212. Norbiato G, Bevilacqua M, Vago T, et al: Cortisol resistance in acquired immunodeficiency syndrome. J Clin Endocrinol Metab 74:608–613, 1992.

213. DiBattista JA, Martel-Pelletier J, Antakly T, et al: Reduced expression of glucocorticoid receptor levels in human osteoarthritic chondrocytes: Role in the suppression of metalloprotease synthesis. J Clin Endocrinol Metab 76:1128–1134, 1993.

214. Franchimont D, Louis E, Dupont P, et al: Dig Dis Sci 44:1208–1215, 1999.

215. Altare F, Durandy A, Lammas D, et al: Impairment of mycobacterial immunity in human interleukin-12 receptor deficiency. Science 280:1432–1435, 1998.

216. Lerner BH: Can stress cause disease?: Revisiting the tuberculosis research of Thomas Holmes, 1949–1961. Ann Intern Med 124:673–680, 1996.

217. Elenkov IJ, Vizi ES: Presynaptic modulation of release of noradrenaline from the sympathetic nerve terminals in the rat spleen. Neuropharmacology 30:1319–1324, 1991.

218. Cole SW, Korin YD, Fahey JL, et al: Norepinephrine accelerates HIV replication via protein kinase A-dependent effects on cytokine production. J Immunol 161:610–616, 1998.

219. Haraguchi S, Good RA, James-Yarish M, et al: Induction of intracellular cAMP by a synthetic retroviral envelope peptide: A possible mechanism of immunopathogenesis in retroviral infections. Proc Natl Acad Sci U S A 92:5568–5571, 1995.

220. Clerici M, Bevilacqua M, Vago T, et al: An immunoendocrinological hypothesis of HIV infection [see comments]. Lancet 343:1552–1553, 1994.

221. Kino T, Gragerov A, Kopp JB, et al: The HIV-1 virion-associated protein vpr is a coactivator of the human glucocorticoid receptor. J Exp Med 189:51–62, 1999.

222. O'Sullivan ST, Lederer JA, Horgan AF, et al: Major injury leads to predominance of the T helper-2 lymphocyte phenotype and diminished interleukin-12 production associated with decreased resistance to infection [see comments]. Ann Surg 222:482–490, 1995.

223. Segal BM, Dwyer BK, Shevach EM: An interleukin (IL)-10/IL-12 immunoregulatory circuit controls susceptibility to autoimmune disease. J Exp Med 187:537–546, 1998.

224. Rogers MP, Fozdar M: Psychoneuroimmunology of autoimmune disorders. Adv Neuroimmunol 6:169–177, 1996.

225. Elenkov IJ, Hoffman J, Wilder RL: Does differential neuroendocrine control of cytokine production govern the expression of autoimmune diseases in pregnancy and the postpartum period? Mol Med Today 3:379–383, 1997.

226. Elenkov IJ, Wilder RL, Bakalov VK, et al: IL-12, TNF-alpha, and hormonal changes during late pregnancy and early postpartum: Implications for autoimmune disease activity during these times. J Clin Endocrinol Metab 86:4933–4938, 2001.

227. Horwitz MS, Bradley LM, Harbertson J, et al: Diabetes induced by Coxsackie virus: Initiation by bystander damage and not molecular mimicry. Nat Med 4:781–785, 1998.

228. Takahashi Y, Murai C, Shibata S, et al: Human parvovirus B19 as a causative agent for rheumatoid arthritis. Proc Natl Acad Sci U S A 95:8227–8232, 1998.

229. Barnes P, FitzGerald G, Brown M, et al: Nocturnal asthma and changes in circulating epinephrine, histamine, and cortisol. N Engl J Med 303:263–267, 1980.

230. Zieg G, Lack G, Harbeck RJ, et al: In vivo effects of glucocorticoids on IgE production [see comments]. J Allergy Clin Immunol 94:222–230, 1994.

231. Coqueret O, Lagente V, Frere CP, et al: Regulation of IgE production by beta 2-adrenoceptor agonists. Ann N Y Acad Sci 725:44–49, 1994.

232. Colombo MP, Vagliani M, Spreafico F, et al: Amount of interleukin 12 available at the tumor site is critical for tumor regression. Cancer Res 56:2531–2534, 1996.

230. Chouaib S, Asselin-Paturel C, Mami-Chouaib F, et al: The host-tumor immune conflict: From immunosuppression to resistance and destruction. Immunol Today 18:493–497, 1997.

234. Shakhar G, Ben–Eliyahu S: In vivo beta-adrenergic stimulation suppresses natural killer activity and compromises resistance to tumor metastasis in rats. J Immunol 160:3251–3258, 1998.

235. Li T, Harada M, Tamada K, et al: Repeated restraint stress impairs the antitumor T cell response through its suppressive effect on Th1-type CD4+ T cells. Anticancer Res 17:4259–4268, 1997.

236. Matsumoto S: Cimetidine and survival with colorectal cancer [letter; comment]. Lancet 346:115, 1995.

237. Franchimont D, Kino T, Galon T, et al: Glucocorticoids and inflammation revisited. Neuroimmunomodulation 10:247–260, 2003.

238. Grammatopoulos D, Chrousos G: Functional characteristics of CRH receptors and potential clinical applications of CRH-receptor antagonists. Trends Endocrinol Metab 13:436–444, 2002.

Autoimmune Polyglandular Syndromes

Noel K. Maclaren

Constellations of multiple endocrine gland autoimmunities often associated with immune-mediated diseases of nonendocrine organs, notably the skin, liver, and gastrointestinal tract, afflict both patients and their families. These constellations are well circumscribed and seldom encroach into the connective tissue or non-organ-specific autoimmune disease clusters. The study of such patients and their family members are revealing insights into their underlying immunodysregulation and thereby into the mechanisms involved in single-organ autoimmunities, such as type 1 diabetes.

Recognition of these autoimmune polyglandular syndromes (APSs) has greatly evolved over the last century, as summarized in Table 41-1. In 1849, Thomas Addison first described the clinical and pathologic features of adrenocortical failure in patients, some of whom also appeared to have pernicious anemia.[1] In his autopsy series, several patients were described (and drawn) with vitiligo in addition to adrenal atrophy with adrenalitis. In their 1908 review of polyglandular insufficiencies (islet, thyroid, gonad, adrenal, anterior pituitary), Claude and Gourgerot postulated that there might be a common pathogenesis for these conditions.[2] Mononuclear leukocyte infiltrates of goitrous thyroid glands were first noted by Hashimoto in 1912,[3] and a similar lesion of pancreatic islets, termed *insulitis*, was described by von Meyenburg in 1940.[4] It was Schmidt in 1926 who documented the association between adrenocortical failure and thyroiditis,[5] whereas Carpenter and colleagues in 1964 expanded Schmidt's syndrome to include type 1 diabetes.[6] A second association between mucocutaneous candidiasis and hypoparathyroidism was first suggested in 1929 by Thorpe and Handley.[7] Whitaker and colleagues expanded this latter association to a triad including adrenocortical insufficiency in 1956.[8] The autoimmune pathogenesis of these disorders began to emerge that same year when Roitt and coworkers discovered circulating precipitating autoantibodies to thyroglobulin in patients with Hashimoto's thyroiditis[9]; in 1963, Blizzard and Kyle identified antibodies to the adrenal gland in a proportion of patients with Addison's disease.[10] In 1980, Neufeld and colleagues distinguished two major APSs that contained Addison's disease (APS-1 and APS-2) and one APS that was like APS-2 but without the involvement of Addison's disease, which was classified as APS-3.[11] In retrospect, the latter two APSs are sufficiently related that APS-2a with Addison's disease and APS-2b without Addison's disease would seem more appropriate and have been used herein. Additional work is needed to characterize these latter groups and to identify their underlying genetics and pathogeneses (Table 41-2).

APS-1 is diagnosed when a patient manifests at least two of the following three key features: hypoparathyroidism, hypoadrenocorticism, and mucocutaneous candidiasis. This rare syndrome usually begins with persistent candidiasis during the first decade of life, most often presenting during infancy. It has been reported to affect males and females almost equally in a large American series,[12] but a modest female bias was observed in another collection of smaller reports.[13] The more common APS-2a is characterized by adrenocortical insufficiency in conjunction with thyroiditis and/or type 1 diabetes. Its prevalence has not been formally established, but it has been estimated to affect 14 to 20 persons per million population.[14] The diagnosis of APS-2 is frequently made during early adulthood through midlife, and it affects females three to four times more commonly than males. APS-2b revolves around thyrogastric autoimmunities, in association with vitiligo and type 1 diabetes. Should Addison's disease also develop in such patients, their condition would be reclassified as APS-2a. However, as emphasized herein, patients and their close relatives with any one autoimmune disease of the group are highly prone to develop others.

Immunogenetic studies suggest that human leukocyte antigen (HLA) class 2 genes are associated with APS-2a and b, whereas a recessively inherited gene that has been mapped to the long arm of chromosome 21 (q22.3) is now known to be responsible for APS-1. However, HLA class 2 genes may prove in part responsible for component diseases in APS-1. Multiple mutations were found in this APS-1 gene, named autoimmune regulator (*AIRE*), in patients with APS-1 (but not APS-2), thus justifying the clinical classification of APS-1 from APS-2. The test for *AIRE* gene mutations can now help distinguish APS-1 from APS-2, which can occasionally become blurred in individual patients, especially if their problems develop when they are adults. Furthermore, the findings of homozygous *AIRE* gene mutations in siblings of patients with APS-1 could be used to predict development of the component diseases in them. Functional studies of the *AIRE* gene product have been undertaken since the gene was discovered and are providing insights into normal versus pathologic immune tolerance mechanisms. The roles of the AIRE protein in the thymic deletion of autoreactive T cells and their downregulation when they escape into the periphery, have been emphasized in the recent literature. In addition, understanding of the cell-mediated immune responses involved in the pathophysiologic mechanism of APS is beginning to progress. Moreover, most of the more significant autoantigens for the component diseases of APS were identified in the 1990s. Autoantibodies to these autoantigens can be used as disease

Table 41-1 Emergence of the Polyglandular Syndromes

Event	Year	Reference
Description of adrenocortical atrophy in patients with pernicious anemia	1849	1
Hypothesis that polyglandular disease arises from a single process	1908	2
Description of mononuclear leukocyte infiltrate in goitrous thyroid glands	1912	3
Schmidt's syndrome described (thyroiditis and adrenalitis)	1926	5
Description of association between hypoparathyroidism and candidiasis	1929	7
Description of mononuclear leukocyte infiltrate in islets of Langerhans of diabetic patients	1940	4
Triad of hypoadrenocorticism, hypoparathyroidism, and candidiasis described	1956	8
Thyroid autoantibodies observed	1956	9
Thyroiditis induced in rabbits by immunizing with gland extract	1956	174
Indirect immunofluorescence labeling technique described	1959	175
Carpenter et al. expand Schmidt's syndrome to include insulin-dependent diabetes mellitus	1964	6
Clinical classification of distinct polyglandular autoimmune syndromes	1980	11, 12
AIRE gene responsible for APS-1 mapped to chromosome 21q22.3	1994	115
AIRE gene identified, thus confirming the clinical classification of APS	1997	119, 120

APS, autoimmune polyglandular syndrome.

markers to either facilitate diagnosis of the involved component diseases or to predict them. This chapter is designed to review the pathogenesis of the APSs, the current knowledge of their molecular immunogenetics, and the clinical translation of research findings into improved care of affected patients and their families.

PATHOPHYSIOLOGY

Evidence supporting the autoimmune nature of the component diseases of APS is compelling: (1) affected organs demonstrate a chronic inflammatory infiltrate composed mainly of lymphocytes, sometimes aggregating into follicle formation; (2) some of the component diseases are associated with immune response genes encoded by class II loci of the HLA complex and, more recently, the cytotoxic T lymphocyte antigen-4 (CTLA-4) locus; and (3) the syndromes are replete with autoantibodies reacting to target tissue–specific antigens, which are often targeted organ-specific enzymes. The initiating events and autoimmune pathogenic processes of APS remain largely undiscovered, but it is probable that both genetic and environmental factors are involved. In patients with APS-1 and the same *AIRE* gene mutations, different disease components develop in different orders with various ages of onset, which suggests the involvement of environmental factors and/or other background genetic factors such as HLA-D genotypes.

Autoantibodies may arise spontaneously through a breakdown in normal immunologic tolerogenesis or by immunization with an environmental agent that is a molecular mimic of a self-antigen (see later discussion). They could arise as part of a bystander immune response to self, after direct viral infection or damage to the target organ by a chemical agent. Other autoantibodies appear to arise as a secondary immune response, stimulating an immune response upon the release of normally sequestered intracellular antigens from damaged glands. The three main classes of organ-specific self-antigens to which autoantibodies are produced in APS (Table 41-3) are: organ-specific surface receptor molecules; intracellular enzymes, which have a central role in a vital and unique cellular function of the target cell; and secreted proteins such as hormones produced by the autoimmunity targeted organs. Examples of surface receptor molecules affected by autoimmunity include the thyrotropin receptor, which is involved in Graves' disease (stimulatory type) and atrophic thyroiditis (blocking type), and a component of the glucose transport system of the pancreatic β cell, which has been implicated as a target in immune-mediated type 1 diabetes. Important enzymes that act as autoantigens include thyroid peroxidase (previously called thyroid microsomal antigen) in Hashimoto's chronic lymphocytic thyroiditis and the P-450 steroidogenic enzyme 21-hydroxylase (21-OHase), essential to steroid hormone biosynthesis, in autoimmune Addison's disease. Thyroglobulin, as targeted in Hashimoto's thyroiditis, or insulin and pro-insulin, as involved in type 1 diabetes, are examples of autoantigenic endocrine cell products important to their respective autoimmune diseases.

It is perplexing why the component diseases of APS so coexist. One possibility is that sharing of target antigenic epitopes

Table 41-2 The Autoimmune Polyglandular Syndromes

APS-1	APS-2a	APS-2b	Frequency (%)
Hypoparathyroidism	Adrenocortical insufficiency	Thyroiditis, type 1 diabetes, pernicious anemia, vitiligo	>40
Mucocutaneous candidiasis	Thyroiditis		
Adrenocortical insufficiency	Insulin-dependent diabetes mellitus		
Ungual dystrophy, enamel hypoplasia, hypogonadism			
Malabsorption, alopecia (totalis or universalis) pernicious anemia (juvenile onset), thyroiditis chronic active hepatitis			10–40
Vitiligo	Hypogonadism	Hypogonadism	<10
Sjögren's syndrome	Vitiligo	Alopecia (adult onset)	
Anterior hypophysitis	Alopecia	Myasthenia gravis	
Type 1 diabetes	Pernicious anemia (adult onset)	Celiac disease	
Alopecia universalis	Myasthenia gravis	Rheumatoid arthritis	
	Celiac disease	Sjögren's syndrome	
	Rheumatoid arthritis		
	Sjögren's syndrome		

APS, autoimmune polyglandular syndrome.

Table 41-3 Types of Autoantigens in Autoimmune Polyglandular Syndromes

Target Organ	Enzymes	Receptors	Secreted Cell Products
Islet	Glutamic acid decarboxylase$_{65}$	Insulin receptor	Insulin
	Tyrosine phosphatase IA2/IA-2β	Glucose transporter (GLUT2)	Proinsulin
Thyroid	Thyroid peroxidase	Thyrotropin	Thyroglobulin
Parathyroid		Parathyroid	
Adrenal	21α-Hydroxylase	Calcium-sensing receptor	
	17α-Hydroxylase	ACTH	
Gonad	17α-Hydroxylase, side-chain cleavage enzyme	Gonadotropin	
Gastric intestine	H$^+$, K$^+$-ATPase, tryptophan hydroxylase, tissue transglutaminase		Intrinsic factor
Liver	P-450 IID6, 2C9, 1A2, AADC		
Melanocytes	Tyrosinase/binding protein		

AADC, amino acid decarboxylase; ACTH, adrenocorticotropic hormone.

between affected glands could be responsible. Whereas experimental evidence for this possibility is generally lacking, the P-450 17-OHase and side chain cleavage enzymes are present in all "steroidal cells" of the testes, ovary, placenta, and adrenal cortex. Thus, indirect immunofluorescent testing of all of these tissue substrates can be used to identify steroidal cell autoantibodies in patients of either gender. In addition, partial autoantibody cross-reactivity between the P-450 21-OHase and 17-OHase enzymes has been proposed in view of the amino acid sequence homology of the epitope region of these two molecules.[15] This theory is supported by evidence that absorption by recombinant 17-OHase could partially remove the reactivity of sera from patients with APS-1 against recombinant 21-OHase, and vice versa, thus suggesting both the presence of cross-reactive antibodies to 17-OHase and 21-OHase and a separate population of antibodies to 21-OHase and 17-OHase in the sera of patients with APS-1.[16] However, for the remaining component autoimmune diseases, no evidence of antigen cross-reactivity has been found. More likely is that the APSs have an underlying immunodeficiency affecting tolerance to self antigens as discussed later; however, the restricted list of autoimmune diseases found in an APS still remains to be explained.

HUMORAL AUTOIMMUNITY

One of the prominent features of APS is the presence of circulating autoantibodies to autoantigens normally present in the endocrine organs involved in the disease. Such autoantibodies can occur long before appearance of the respective clinical diseases. Patients with any APS may have autoantibodies against the same autoantigen, and many of the targeted autoantigens are enzymes as mentioned (see Table 41-3). Identification of circulating organ-specific autoantibodies provided the earliest and strongest evidence for an autoimmune pathogenesis of the APSs. Whereas patients with collagen vascular diseases synthesize immunoglobulins that recognize non-organ-specific cellular targets, such as nucleic acids or nucleoproteins, endocrine autoimmunities are associated with autoantibodies that react to organ-specific antigens. Although the pathogenicity of organ-specific autoantibodies remains unclear, their importance as diagnostic indicators and predictive markers of future disease is well established.[17-21] Indirect immunofluorescent assays continue to be a useful and convenient method to screen for autoantibodies to the autoantigens present in target organs. Procedures for procurement and processing of fresh frozen human substrate tissues for such testing must be meticulously followed to obtain consistent and reliable results.[22] Biochemical assays, such as immunoprecipitation assays using autoantigens labeled with radioisotopes are, however, increasingly used for measuring specific autoantibodies and have shown high

sensitivity and good reproducibility, and can be used to rapidly screen large numbers of serum samples.

Adrenocortical Autoantibodies

Adrenocortical autoantibodies (AAs) detected by indirect immunofluorescent labeling have been reported in most patients with non-tuberculous Addison's disease when tested at the time of their diagnoses.[23] All layers of the adrenal cortex bind AAs, with striking sparing of the adrenal medulla. Fluorescence of the zona glomerulosa, in particular, gives a distinctive pattern when viewed by ultraviolet microscopy. Some 15% of AA-positive patients with Addison's disease also have an autoantibody that cross-reacts with other steroid-producing cells, such as placental syncytiotrophoblasts, ovarian luteal cells, and/or testicular Leydig cells, and most of these patients have APS-1. These steroidal cell autoantibodies (SCAs) are distinguished from AAs by their ability to be adsorbed from serum by preincubation with adrenal, gonadal (ovarian or testicular), or placental homogenates, whereas AAs are exclusively removed from positive sera by prior exposure to adrenal homogenates. When detected, SCAs indicate a high risk for future gonadal failure, especially in females with high titers.[18,24] Patients with premature ovarian failure and a positive test for AAs have a higher risk for the development of Addison's disease than do those who do not test positive.[25]

The major steroid cell autoantigens involved in the reaction of AAs have now been identified, as mentioned previously; they include 21-OHase, 17α-OHase, and P-450 side chain cleavage (see Table 41-3). The major antigen for SCA is 17-OHase, a 55 kDa gonadal and adrenal steroid biosynthetic P-450 microsomal enzyme.[26] Most patients with non-tuberculous Addison's disease have antibodies to 21-OHase, although the reported frequencies may vary depending on the techniques used.[27-32] Antibodies to 21-OHase are generally found at higher frequency and titer in patients with Addison's disease in association with APS than in patients with isolated Addison's disease. The frequency of antibodies to 17-OHase and P-450 side-chain cleavage is also considerably higher in patients with APS than in patients with isolated Addison's disease.[31,33,34] The presence of antibodies to 17-OHase or P-450 side-chain cleavage in patients with isolated Addison's disease may, therefore, indicate progression toward hypogonadism in an APS. The dominant epitopes on 21-OHase commonly recognized by autoantibodies from patients with Addison's disease as an isolated disease or in association with APS are located in the C-terminal end and in a central region of 21-OH.[35,36] The epitopes on 21-OHase can be either conformational[37] or linear in nature.[38]

Autoantibodies to 21-OHase or AAs are useful markers indicating a risk for the development of Addison's disease. Occasionally, AA-positive individuals who do not have overt adrenocortical failure can be identified by screening patients with autoimmune diseases, especially autoimmune endocrine diseases, and their family members. About 20% of asymptomatic AA-positive relatives were reported to have elevated basal serum levels of adrenocorticotropic hormone (ACTH) and/or renin or blunted adrenocortical responses to an intravenous infusion of ACTH, features that are indicative of subclinical glandular dysfunction (Fig. 41-1). In two separate studies, autoantibodies to 21-OHase were found at frequencies of 2.3% (7/304)[16] and 1.7% (11/629)[39] in patients with type 1 diabetes. These results are similar to the frequencies of AA found a decade previously.[40] Furthermore, many of these patients had raised ACTH/renin levels indicative of impending Addison's disease.[19] It is reported that 25% of patients without clinical symptoms of hypoadrenalism but with a positive test for AAs were actually at a stage of subclinical hypoadrenalism.[41] In addition, Addison's disease may subsequently develop in up to 40% of such individuals over a follow-up period of 6 months to 10 years.[19,41] This risk was observed to be especially high if the autoantibodies fixed complement in vitro or were present at high titer. Thus, close attention should be paid to patients with positive tests for autoantibodies to 21-OHase and those with risk HLA alleles, such as DRB1*03/DQB1*0201, which is associated with both type 1 diabetes and Addison's disease.[42,43] In addition, all patients with features suggestive of APS-1 but without overt Addison's disease should be tested for AAs because at least 20% of APS-1 patients without symptoms of Addison's disease are positive for antibodies to 21-OHase.[44] Symptoms of adrenal deficiency may not be manifested until most of the adrenal cortex has been destroyed.[19] However, 21-OHase autoantibody positive patients with subclinical Addison's disease can be identified by increased levels of resting plasma renin activity and/or raised afternoon serum ACTH levels tested after patients have been recumbent for 1 hour. Giordano and coworkers has suggested that cortisol and dehydroepiandrosterone secretion in response to low doses of ACTH 1–24 may be impaired early in impending Addison's disease. As the disease progresses, depressed ACTH-stimulated cortisol responses and electrolyte disturbances can eventually be noted.[19] In patients with long-standing Addison's disease, the adrenal-specific autoantibodies can often be found years after the clinical onset, making identification of the autoimmune nature and, thus, risk of APS possible in hindsight.

Whereas cellular immune mechanisms are thought to cause the glandular destruction seen in autoimmune endocrinopathies, a pathogenic role for humoral autoreactivity in autoimmune oophoritis has been suggested by studies showing complement-mediated cytotoxicity of cultured granulosa cells in the presence of sera from affected patients but not in the presence of sera from control patients.[45] Binding of SCAs to granulosa cells by indirect immunofluorescence, however, can be demonstrated only when autoantibodies are present in high titer. Antibodies of patients with Addison's disease had been shown to have inhibitory effects on recombinant 21-OHase enzyme activity in vitro,[46] but such enzyme inhibitory effects are not so evident in vivo[47] and are conceptually unlikely to account for the resultant disease because such antibodies cannot penetrate adrenocortical cells to inhibit steroidogenesis.

Parathyroid Autoantibodies

Autoantibodies to the parathyroid gland were detected in 38% of 74 patients with idiopathic hypoparathyroidism by indirect immunofluorescent assay.[48] However, subsequent investigations have found that antiparathyroid serologic immunoreactivity is rare in patients with failed glands[49] and is not usually parathyroid specific.[50] Indeed, antibodies considered to be against parathyroid antigens in previous reports have, we believe, been confused with mitochondrial autoantibodies, and humoral sensitivity to parathyroid tissue may have delineated a tissue-specific response to antigens within the endothelial component of the gland.[51] In a recent study from our laboratory involving Western blotting, the calcium-sensing receptor was recognized in 32% (8/25) of patients with hypoparathyroidism associated with either APS-1 or hypothyroidism, with the major epitope located on the external domain of the receptor.[52] This finding suggests that such autoantibodies could have a pathogenic role involving down-regulation of parathyroid hormone secretion through signal transduction events in parathyroid cells. Such was actually demonstrated by Kifor and colleagues in two patients with autoimmune hypoparathyroidism.

Pancreatic β-Cell Autoantibodies

The intensive studies of humoral autoimmunities against antigens expressed by the pancreatic β cell (e.g., islet gangliosides, insulin, proinsulin, glutamic acid decarboxylase

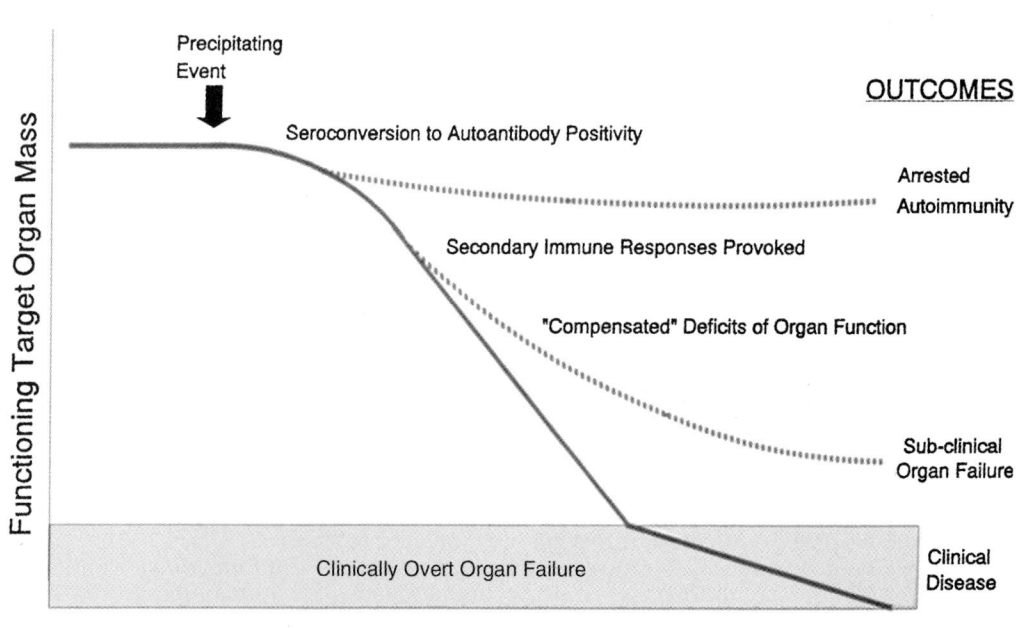

Figure 41-1 The proposed natural history of endocrine autoimmunity. Autoimmune attack of target organs often begins in people who have a genetic predisposition after an unknown precipitating event *(arrow)*. The early process manifests itself by provoking autoantibody production, and it may arrest at that stage *(top broken line)*. Progressive disease, associated with secondary responses against antigens released by damaged tissue, is initially detectable by minimal biochemical abnormalities, such as elevations of trophic hormones. Organ function loss may plateau before the critical organ mass threshold is reached *(lower broken line)*, or it may progress to clinically overt disease *(solid line)*. Hormone replacement therapy may decelerate the destruction of surviving tissue, but at this late stage, complete organ atrophy is inevitable.

[GAD$_{65}$], and tyrosine phosphatases [IA-2 and IA2-β]) highlight the complexity of disease-autoantibody relationships. The presence of islet cell autoantibodies detected by immunofluorescence, together with insulin autoantibody and/or anti-GAD or IA-2, has a high predictive value for the development of type 1 diabetes. However, islet cell autoantibodies, as well as GAD autoantibodies, also occur in many patients with APS-1,[53,54] a syndrome with only a low likelihood of progression to clinically overt diabetes,[12,53] at least in U.S. patients. Recent studies indicate that autoantibodies to islet cell autoantigens in patients with APS-1 have different reactive characteristics from those of patients with type 1 diabetes as in APS-2a and b. For example, GAD$_{65}$ autoantibodies are readily detectable by Western blotting in the sera of patients with APS-1,[53] similar to the GAD autoantibodies present in the sera of patients with stiff-man syndrome, an autoimmune neurologic disorder,[55] thus indicating that these autoantibodies recognize linear epitopes on denatured GAD$_{65}$. However, the GAD$_{65}$ autoantibodies present in patients with type 1 diabetes usually react with conformational epitopes of native or undenatured proteins,[56] which suggests that different immunoregulation mechanisms could have been involved in driving the production of these two sets of GAD$_{65}$ autoantibodies. It also suggests that the presence of islet cell autoimmunity in APS-1 is not necessarily an indicator of the destruction of islet cells, at least in APS-1 and stiff-man syndrome. It presumably lacks other components of the pathogenic process (e.g., antigen-specific cytotoxic T lymphocytes) that are necessary to produce β-cell damage and, thus, overt hyperglycemia. Alternatively, the islet cell nondestructive autoimmune response in patients with APS-1 may result from an impaired cellular immunoregulatory mechanism different from that in APS-2a; however, these speculations need to be systematically proved through specific studies. In the author's experience, some APS patients with high titers of GAD autoantibodies may exhibit neurologic symptoms, such as cognitive loss, muscular spasms, and partial epilepsy. Whereas these associations need to be confirmed, the possibility that loss of neuronal γ-amino butyric acid (or GABA) by action of GAD autoantibodies passing the blood-brain barrier needs to be explored.

Thyroid Autoantibodies

Autoantibodies in patients with APS react with thyroid gland proteins, including thyroid peroxidase, thyroglobulin, and thyrotropin receptors. Although immunoglobulins against the thyrotropin receptor may stimulate or inhibit both thyroid gland activity and the growth of thyrocytes, no consistently discernible effect on thyroid function has yet been attributed to autoantibodies that recognize thyroid peroxidase or thyroglobulin (see Table 41-3). Nevertheless, immunization of susceptible strains of mice with thyroglobulin in complete Freund's adjuvant induces a thyroid-specific immune infiltrate in experimental allergic thyroiditis.[57] Strangely, autoimmunity against the thyroid gland is distinctly unusual in APS-1.

Other Autoantibodies in APS

Primary hypogonadism, hypopituitarism, pernicious anemia, malabsorption, alopecia, chronic active hepatitis, and/or vitiligo may develop in patients with APS. Screening for marker autoantibodies for these associated diseases facilitates early diagnosis and treatment of the corresponding diseases. Weight loss and malabsorption are most often seen in patients with Addison's disease, especially those with APS-1,[58] which may indicate the underlying jejunal giardiasis, celiac disease, intestinal bacterial overgrowth, or autoimmune loss of intestinal endocrine cells. Thus, patients with APS should also be screened for associated endocrine and nonendocrine diseases by testing for the corresponding autoantibodies as available.

Interestingly, autoantibodies to tryptophan hydroxylase have recently been associated with malabsorption in patients with APS-1.[59] Also, celiac disease, which can occur in patients with APS-1 or APS-2, is characterized by damage to absorptive villi and flattening and hypoplasia of the crypts of the small intestine. Autoantibodies have been detected to tissue transglutaminase, in patients with celiac disease,[60] in line with the known evidence for its autoimmune nature.[61,62] In this disease, ingestion of gliadin in wheat appears to provoke a reversible autoimmunity with transglutaminase-associated symptoms. Thus, detection of autoantibodies to tissue transglutaminase in patients with Addison's disease, regardless of its association with APS, would help identify the existence of celiac disease in the patients tested. We do not advise testing for these autoantibodies in patients without possible symptoms of relevance since the finding of such autoantibodies in the absence of such symptoms, leads to therapeutic uncertainty about if and when to begin a rigorous wheat-free diet.

Achlorhydria and pernicious anemia occurring as part of the APSs are associated with the presence of circulating autoantibodies against gastric parietal cell autoantibodies (PCAs) and, less frequently, against intrinsic factor. Approximately 10% of patients with type 1 diabetes have coexisting circulating PCAs, and achlorhydria develops in many of these patients.[63] The pathogenic importance of these immunoglobulins is suggested by their toxic effects on the gastric mucosa of frogs and guinea pigs.[64,65] The parietal cell proton pump (H^+,K^+-ATPase) represents at least one target of PCA.[66] Thus, PCAs appear to be primarily associated with achlorhydria, whereas intrinsic factor may arise secondarily as a consequence of gastric cell damage and is associated with an increased likelihood of clinical pernicious anemia.

Vitiligo is often seen in patients with APS-1, and anti-melanocyte autoantibodies have been demonstrated in a small number of individuals with APS-1 and vitiligo.[67] The author has noted that chronic lymphocyte infiltrations in the margin of active vitiligo lesions are common when biopsies are performed. Furthermore, tyrosinase, the rate-limiting enzyme for melanin formation, is one target for autoantibodies in patients with vitiligo associated with endocrine diseases.[68] However, controversy on the frequency of autoantibodies to tyrosinase in patients with vitiligo has been reported.[69,70] It appears that patients with vitiligo in association with APS tend to have higher frequencies of antibodies to tyrosinase than do patients with vitiligo only. Tyrosinase-reactive T cells are present in the normal immune system and are responsible for the stimulation of peptides derived from tyrosinase.[71] Immunization by tyrosinase-related protein-1 has recently been shown to induce destruction of melanocytes in mice,[72] whereas the Smyth chicken model of vitiligo is characterized by autoantibodies to tyrosine-related protein-1.[73]

Antibodies detected by indirect immunofluorescent labeling of hypothalamic vasopressin-producing cells have also been reported in a small number of patients with central diabetes insipidus who had other autoimmune endocrinopathies.[22] In a report of 19 patients with a variety of endocrine autoimmunities, autoantibodies against anterior pituitary lactotrophs were detected,[74] and scattered reports of humoral responses against somatotrophs and, perhaps even gonadotrophs, have also been published but not independently confirmed. Rarely, if ever have these patients had symptomatic disease of their hypothalamic-pituitary axis, however. In contrast, among 30 reported patients with proven or presumed symptomatic lymphocytic hypophysitis, autoantibodies directed against the pituitary gland have been described.[75] With the use of transformed rodent pituitary cell lines as a substrate in an indirect immunofluorescence assay, immunoglobulins that specifically bound the hypophyseal cells in culture were observed in the serum of patients with the empty sella syndrome.[76] However, the empty sella syndrome has become increasingly explained by hypoplasia of the anterior hypophysis because of genetic lesions in one of the required differentiation factors. The author believes that pituitary autoimmunity is an area of potential research that needs more attention.

The antibodies previously described that react with cellular enzymes or hormones generally have unknown pathogenic significance. The functional role of autoantibodies that alter organ function by binding to their hormone receptors is, however, readily understandable. Whereas autoantibodies that bind thyrotropin and acetylcholine receptors have long been recognized to have pathogenic importance in Graves' disease and myasthenia gravis, respectively, a similar mechanism has only recently emerged as a potential pathogenic process in other endocrine autoimmunities. Thus, immunoglobulins that recognize receptors for gonadotropins, insulin, calcium-sensing receptors, or ACTH receptors may inhibit the action of their respective hormone ligands (see Table 41-3).[77]

In APS-1 patients with chronic active hepatitis, autoantibodies against mitochondrial, nuclear, or smooth muscle antigens are frequently found, although their clinical significance is unclear. Cytochrome P-450 proteins are often the common targets of autoantibodies from patients with APS and in patients with autoimmune liver diseases.[78] While abnormal B-lymphocyte functions have been variably described in patients with APS, deficiency of IgA is the most common feature, and high levels of IgG and IgE have also been observed in some patients.[79,80] Deficient secretion of IgA immunoglobulins by the intestine may result in small intestinal bacterial overgrowth and subsequent diarrhea.

CELLULAR AUTOIMMUNITY

Pathologic observations and experimental investigations of cellular immunity in multi-organ autoimmunity have yielded results similar to those found in the more intensive studies of isolated autoimmune thyroid and pancreatic islet diseases. In this section, therefore, information derived from research into APSs and other autoimmune disorders will be combined to review the principles of autoimmunity that are important to APS.

The gross and microscopic pathologic changes in APS-1 and APS-2 are similar to those of component-isolated endocrinopathies. Histologic examination of affected adrenal, thyroid, and parathyroid glands, ovaries, pancreatic islets, skin, and gastric mucosa has yielded similar results.[23,81–89] A mononuclear leukocyte infiltrate that is composed mainly of lymphocytes with some macrophages, natural killer cells, and plasma cells is typically seen. Neutrophils are characteristically absent. The infiltrating lymphocytes are of both B- and T-cell lineage, and the T-cell population includes both CD4+ and CD8+ subsets, often displaying activation markers.[81,85] Sparing of adjacent nontarget tissue is striking in all organs. As the disease approaches its final stages, scarring and atrophy predominate within the gland, mediated in part through target cell–induced apoptosis. Fibrosis eventually becomes a prominent finding in most affected glands and may highlight islands of surviving endocrine tissue that are both hyperplastic and hypertrophied, as illustrated by "regenerative nodules" in the adrenalitis lesions of Addison's disease. Such attempts at regeneration are invariably accompanied by continued inflammation.

Effector Functions

The presence of circulating tissue-specific autoreactive leukocytes in patients with APS was first demonstrated by the elaboration of migration inhibitory factors after the incubation of target organ homogenates with peripheral blood mononuclear cells (PBMCs) from affected individuals. Subsequently, increased levels of PBMCs expressing activation markers such

as HLA class II antigens have been observed in patients with early but not end-stage type 1 diabetes, Graves' disease, chronic lymphocytic thyroiditis, Addison's disease, and oophoritis.[81,90] Because surface antigen phenotyping does not reliably distinguish lymphocytes with different functions, cytokine production profiles of PBMCs are coming under scrutiny. Decreased production of interleukin-4 and increased production of interferon-γ in response to mitogen has been observed in patients with new-onset type 1 diabetes.[91,92] In contrast, autologous thyroid cells elicited interferon-γ production by PBMCs harvested from patients with autoimmune thyroid disease but not from those with nontoxic goiters or thyroid cancer.[93] Examination of affected end organs obtained early in the disease process will ultimately be more informative than examination of circulating lymphocytes. Unfortunately, tissue specimens obtained at or after the time that disease becomes clinically apparent contain infiltrates that represent a complex response against a multitude of antigens. Animal models of disease are now being used to observe the kinetics of leukocyte infiltration of autoimmune targets. In non-obese diabetic mice, reports of early insulitis have described initial infiltration by macrophages and CD8+ T lymphocytes, followed by CD4+ T lymphocytes and B lymphocytes.[94]

It appears unlikely that the action of a single T-lymphocyte clone can result in clinically important organ failure inasmuch as adoptive transfer of either type 1 diabetes or thyroiditis requires the transfusion of both CD4+ and CD8+ lymphocytes. Nonetheless, it is likely that autoimmunity against one of several discrete antigens can initiate disease. One recent report, however, in which insulin gene promotor-linked GAD antisense DNA was used to reduce islet cell expression of the antigen suggested that islet cell autoimmune diabetes was promptly abrogated.[95] Target organ invasion by restricted T-cell families, identified by their expression of T-cell receptor genes that contain uniquely rearranged variable (V) or complementarity-determining regions (e.g., CDR3) or by monoclonal expansion of B lymphocytes, has not been demonstrated convincingly in APSs. Preferential use of certain T-cell receptor families may occur, however, in an antigen-specific fashion during the inductive events.[96]

Despite the multitude of investigations, the sequence of effector events leading to eventual cell destruction has not been resolved with any certainty. It has been difficult to determine how the local effects of cytokines (released from either leukocytes, damaged endothelium, or possibly endocrine epithelium)[23,97] and the aberrant expression of major histocompatibility complex antigens (class I and/or class II)[81,86,98] and adhesion molecules (intercellular adhesion molecule-1)[99,100] on the endocrine epithelium surface contribute to the pathologic process. In diabetic rodents, β-cell expression of class I major histocompatibility complex is observed early in the pathogenic sequence, perhaps enhancing the ability of CD8+ T cells to lyse these cellular targets. Later, enhanced class II reactivity may occur as a result of the invasion of macrophages and perhaps some patchy aberrant expression of these antigens on pancreatic β cells.

Recurrent mucocutaneous candidal infections in APS-1, which are often resistant to treatment, most certainly reflect an abnormality in T-lymphocyte function. No specific T-cell defect to account for these findings has been consistently identified, although one must exist.[87] The possible role of the elusive transfer factor remains unclear.[101] Again, this area needs further investigation, especially regarding function of the newly identified *AIRE* gene.

IMMUNOREGULATORY FUNCTIONS

The classic concept of autoimmune disease arising from a "forbidden" lymphocyte clone that has escaped intrathymic deletion is incomplete inasmuch as some potentially autoreactive T lymphocytes are regularly found circulating in healthy individuals. Normal tolerance to self is achieved by the active induction of clonal deletion by the thymus, clone-specific anergy, or cytokine deviation by a peripheral regulatory process that remains poorly defined. Deficiencies in such immunoregulation may allow potentially autoreactive lymphocyte clones to become activated and thus pathogenic. The non-obese diabetic mouse has low levels of cytokine-rich natural killer T cells, and transfer of such cells to non-obese diabetic mice prevents the development of diabetes.[102] Wilson and colleagues found that natural killer T-cell clones derived from patients with type 1 diabetes often lacked interleukin-4 and had increased interferon-γ.[103] Kukeja found that natural killer T cells detectable in peripheral blood by antibodies to their restricted Vπja24/Vπjb11 T-cell receptor are reduced in type 1 diabetes, as well as in certain otherwise normal persons. However, this has proven to be a controversial finding in the hands of others. Recently, antigen-presenting cells have been shown to play important roles in autoimmune disease, particularly in type 1 diabetes. Antigen-presenting cells, which include dendritic cells, macrophages, and B lymphocytes, are the first cell types to appear in the pancreatic inflammatory process in non-obese diabetic mice.[104] Furthermore, dendritic cells are abundantly present in progressive human insulitis.[105] It has been indicated in one study that dendritic cells are both phenotypically and functionally impaired in humans at risk for type 1 diabetes.[106] It has been hypothesized that a defect in dendritic cell function in the thymus in type 1 diabetes–prone humans reduces the editing of self-reactive T cells or, in the periphery, impairs induction of regulatory T cells to prevent type 1 diabetes.[106]

Environmental Factors

If environmental precipitators of autoimmunity exist, and they probably do, their identification continues to be elusive. As an environmental factor, virus has long been suspected of being an agent that induces autoimmune disease. The pathogenic effects of virus on autoimmunity could result in a bystander attack on a particular target organ or in molecular mimicry, in which a viral peptide and a peptide of a host protein have immunologic cross-reactivity. Viral infection may also result in an immune response that accelerates an ongoing autoimmune response and eventually precipitates the clinical disease. An infectious trigger of polyglandular autoimmunity has not been reported in human epidemiologic studies. Reovirus type I infection in susceptible mice can cause type 1 diabetes and growth failure associated with antibodies to the anterior pituitary and pancreatic islets. However, a recent report on the expression of a human endogenous retrovirus (HERVK-10) as a cause of type 1 diabetes[107] has not been substantiated.[108–110]

Genetics

APS-1 is not associated with any class II HLA alleles,[111] but rather has been linked to a newly identified gene (*AIRE*) located on chromosome 21. APS-2a and APS-2b are associated with HLA class II genes with apparently distinctive HLA alleles for each of them. These two latter syndromes remain to be further defined genetically, especially with respect to their underlying non-HLA genes.

Genetic Studies in APS-1

APS-1 is an autosomal recessive disease with a pattern of inheritance initially derived from analysis of patients with idiopathic Addison's disease and hypoparathyroidism[112] and later reported by others in different racial groups.[11,58,113,114] By allelic association and linkage analysis, a candidate gene was initially mapped to the long arm of chromosome 21 (21q22.3) in 14 Finnish families of patients with APS-1.[115] This gene was later narrowed down to a range of less than 500 kb, around the gene encoding phosphofructokinase of the liver type (PFKL), by linkage analysis and physical mapping in relative homogeneous Finnish and European patients with APS-1,[116,117] and later in a heterogeneous group of U.S. patients with APS-1.[118] Ultimately, two individual groups identified the responsible gene, *AIRE* (autoimmune regulator), located proximal to the gene for *PFKL* on the long arm of chromosome 21.[119,120] The *AIRE* gene consists of 14 exons and encodes a protein with an estimated 545 amino acids that contains two plant homeodomain (PHD) zinc-finger motifs, three LXXLL motifs, and a proline-rich region, suggestive of its putative role as a nuclear transcriptional regulator (Fig. 41-2). Multiple mutations have been detected in patients with APS-1 and different racial backgrounds, thus indicating that this gene is the disease gene responsible for APS-1.

Characteristics of the *AIRE* Gene in Patients with APS-1

More than 30 separate mutations in the *AIRE* gene have been detected, either as homozygous or heterozygous forms with different frequencies in APS-1 patients of various ethnic backgrounds (see Fig. 41-2). The reader is referred to more updated reviews of the subject for minor mutational lesions in APS-1. The predicted outcomes for most of the *AIRE* mutations are

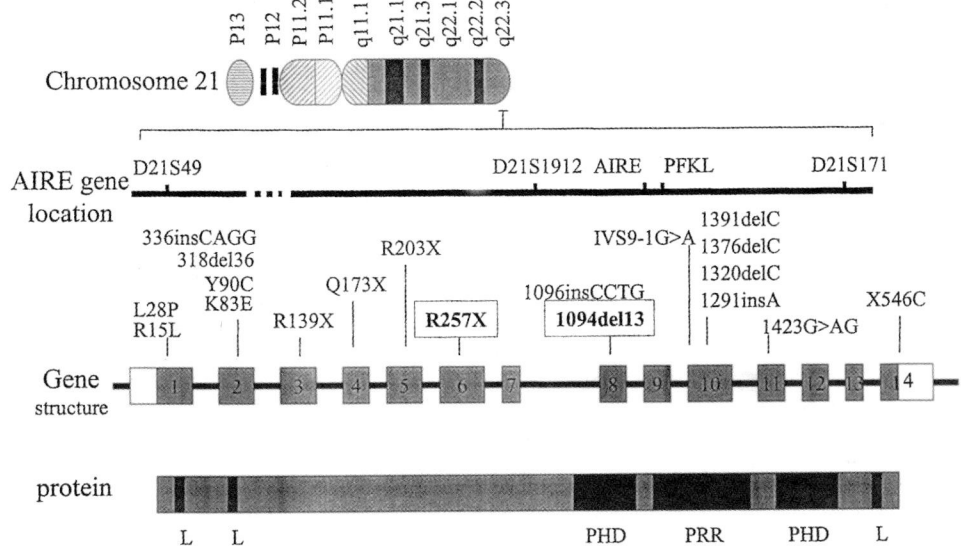

Figure 41-2 *AIRE* gene location, mutations, and characteristics of AIRE protein. The *AIRE* gene is located on chromosome 21q22.3, close to the gene encoding phosphofructokinase of the liver type (*PFKL*). R257X and 1094de113 are commonly present in patients with APS-1 syndrome among the total of more than 30 detected mutations. Two plant homeodomain (PHD) zinc-finger motifs, three LXXLL motifs (L), and aproline-rich region (PRR) are present in the AIRE protein. The nomenclature of the mutations was based on the AIREcDNA sequence (GenBank Accession # AB006682). More updated reviews of the genetic lesions of APS-1 can be found in the recent literature; however, no clear AIRE genotype/phenotype relationships have been identified.

truncated AIRE proteins in which one or two of its zinc finger motifs are disrupted. This effect is due to the introduction of either a stop codon or a frameshift in the coding gene. However, four missense mutations, R15L, L28P, Y90C, and K83E, result in the substitution of a single amino acid in exon 1 or 2. It remains to be confirmed how such missense mutations have a disrupting impact on the function of AIRE protein.

Of these separate mutations, two are most frequently detected in various racial groups. One is named R257X and is located at exon 6; the other one is 1094del13 and is located at exon 8 of the *AIRE* gene. The remaining mutations are much less frequent, and some of them have been detected only in a single allele. R257X is a substitution of C for T at amino acid position 257. This substitution results in change of an Arg codon (CCA) to a stop codon (TGA) and would produce a truncated protein with about 256 amino acids.[119] R257X is a dominant mutation in Finnish patients with APS-1 and is also frequently present in patients with other ethnic backgrounds, such as in northern Italians, Swiss, British, Germans, New Zealanders, and white Americans.[121,122] 1094del13, a 13-bp deletion at nucleotide positions 1094 to 1106, results in a frameshift to produce a truncated 372-amino acid residue. 1094del13 has been detected in APS-1 patients of various ethnic backgrounds.[120,121-124] In our group, Chen found this form of the *AIRE* gene mutation to be the most common in U.S. patients. In addition, 1094del13 is a dominant *AIRE* gene lesion in British patients with APS-1 inasmuch as 74% (17/23) of mutated *AIRE* gene alleles from British patients with APS-1 contain this deletion.[124]

Founder effects exist for some genetically isolated populations, as determined by analysis of mutations and haplotypes in patients with polymorphic markers closely associated with the *AIRE* gene locus. Recombination events are less common when two genomic markers are closer, and linkage disequilibrium is thus stronger with polymorphic markers of closely located genes. Therefore, individuals are likely to have common ancestors if they share the same haplotype for polymorphic markers that are in linkage disequilibrium, especially when they arise from genetically isolated populations. Haplotype analysis of polymorphic markers located close to the *AIRE* gene in Finnish patients has suggested that more than 85% of cases of APS-1 in Finnish patients are due to one major mutation that is commonly present in the ancestors of the Finnish population.[116] This result is in concordance with the finding that the mutation R257X is present in up to 82% of Finnish patients with APS-1 and is accompanied by one predominant haplotype of closely linked polymorphic markers, such as *D21S1912* and *PFKL*.[119,120] *D21S1912* is located approximately 130 kb upstream of the *AIRE* gene, and *PFKL* is located 1.5 kb downstream of the *AIRE* gene.[119,120] This evidence suggests that R257X occurred as a single mutation event in the relatively homologous Finnish population. Studies of 12 British families with APS-1 for *AIRE* gene mutations found that 17 of the 24 possible mutant *AIRE* alleles tested had 1094del13 with a common haplotype spanning the *AIRE* gene locus, which suggests the presence of a founder effect also for the British patients.[124] Similarly, a founder effect may be present in the Sardinian population, which has until recently been a genetically isolated population.[125] Mutation R139X has been found in 90% (18/20) of independent alleles with identical haplotypes for *D21S1912-PFKL* in that ethnic group.[123]

That patients with the same *AIRE* gene mutations often had different closely linked haplotypes suggests that either ancient mutational events or multiple independent events occurred to account for the *AIRE* mutations and haplotypes observed. For example, R257X is also a major mutation present in patients from European countries other than Finland. However, non-Finnish patients with R257X have more diversified haplotypes of *D21S1912-PFKL*.[121] Such is also the case

for the other major mutation, 1094del13, inasmuch as different haplotypes are present in patients with different ethnic origins. For example, 9 of 15 alleles of 1094del13 detected in 13 patients from a group of white, American patients with APS-1 had different *D21S1912-PFKL* haplotypes,[122] thus suggesting that multiple independent events led to the 1094del13 mutation. This result should be expected because the patients were of heterogeneous origins, typical of the North American population. Thus, the genetic data are now in hand for diagnosis and genetic counseling in families affected by APS-1.

Role of the *AIRE* Gene in the Pathogenesis of APS-1

An understanding of the biologic role of the AIRE protein should provide needed insight into the mechanism of tolerance and autoimmunity, particularly to APS-1, which displays T-cell abnormalities as well as multiple autoimmune endocrinopathies. The *AIRE* gene is particularly well-expressed as mRNA in the thymus, as well as in other tissues such as lymph nodes, pancreas, adrenal cortex, and PBMCs.[119,120] Attention has already been drawn to its nuclear localization and its probable role in transcriptional regulation of the encoded protein based on analysis of the predicted amino acid sequence.[119,120] The pattern of the two zinc-finger motifs in AIRE-1 is similar to the pattern seen in the Mi-2 and TIF1 autoantigens.[126] Mi-2 autoantigen is a 240-kilodalton human nuclear protein recognized by sera from patients with autoimmune dermatomyositis.[127] The Mi-2 autoantigen is actually a recently identified partial fragment of a chromohelicase DNA (CHD)-binding protein, CHD3.[128] The family of CHD proteins is known to play roles in gene expression and regulation.[129] Also, TIF1 is actively involved in transcriptional control of the estrogen receptor.[124,127] Accordingly, the *AIRE* gene most likely participates in transcriptional regulation of the expression of another gene(s).

No obvious correlations have been found between mutant genotypes of the *AIRE* gene and clinical phenotypes of APS-1, which suggests that the outcome of the syndrome may be influenced by environmental factors or non-*AIRE* genes. As mentioned previously, the core phenotype of APS-1 includes the three diseases: mucocutaneous candidiasis, hypoparathyroidism, and Addison's disease. Patients with APS-1 also frequently have one or more other autoimmune diseases, such as chronic active hepatitis, alopecia, vitiligo, or evidence of an immunodeficiency state, including chronic diarrhea/malabsorption, chronic mucocutaneous candidiasis, and oropharyngeal carcinomas. Not all patients with APS-1 express all three core component diseases or the frequently accompanied diseases. Even patients of the same ethnic origin with the same *AIRE* mutation may have different component diseases of APS-1 or a different order of appearance of the component diseases.[121,123,124] Different phenotype expressions are also present in affected siblings.

However, specific component diseases may develop in some ethnic groups of patients with APS-1, thus suggesting that the outcome of the syndrome is influenced by background genes within a population. For example, candidiasis is relatively rare in Iranian Jewish patients with APS-1.[114] Also, type 1 diabetes is rarely seen in patients with APS-1 in the United States; however, it does occur in some 15% of Finnish patients with APS-1, especially with increasing age. Finns, however, suffer the world's highest rates of type 1 diabetes and must have a high gene pool for the disease. Finnish patients with APS-1 often have ectodermal and enamel hypoplasia.[58] Calcium deficiency secondary to hypoparathyroidism should not be the primary cause for enamel dystrophy because in Finnish patients, ectodermal and enamel hypoplasia occurs in APS-1 patients with or without hypoparathyroidism.[58,130] In addition, those non-Finnish patients with APS-1 who had hypoparathyroidism are seldom seen with enamel hypoplasia.[114,118] Background genes or genes with epistatic effects may be responsible for variations in the expressed phenotype.[116] Alternatively, more than one gene may be responsible for the development of APS-1, although this possibility is becoming increasingly unlikely. Thus, studies on the function of the *AIRE* gene could shed more light on the pathogenic mechanism of APS-1.

Genetic Studies in APS-2a and APS-2b

APS-2a and APS-2b often affects individuals in many generations of the same family, which suggests that they are inherited as an autosomal-dominant trait with incomplete penetrance.[80,111,131] Addison's disease, either as a component disease of APS-2a or as an individual disease, is reported to be associated with HLA-DR3 and HLA-DR4,[132,133] however the HLA-DR4 haplotype, when seen in APS-2 might rather relate to coexisting β-cell autoimmunity.[42] However, thyroid autoimmunity in pedigrees with type 1 diabetes may segregate independently from the HLA complex.[63] DR3-DQB1*0201/DQB1*0302 is associated with APS-2 when type 1 diabetes is present.[134] Such HLA associations suggest that particular molecules of HLA are required for the development of component autoimmune diseases and that the expression of a particular autoimmune phenotype depends on the involvement of these plus other gene products, especially in a multi-component autoimmune syndrome such as APS-2. Unlike APS-1, the order of appearance of the component diseases of APS-2 varies greatly. Individual patients can initially have Addison's disease and, subsequently, type 1 diabetes and/or autoimmune thyroid disease or any other sequence. This variation could indicate the presence of different pathogenic pathways during the development of APS-2. Thus, it might be expected that non-HLA genes plus particular alleles of HLA genes could influence the susceptibility of individual patients to a constellation of diseases. For example, the association of DQB1*0302 with APS-2 was abolished in our study when patients with APS-2 and overt clinical type 1 diabetes or positive autoantibodies to islet antigens were excluded from analysis.[42] Also, development of the same disease with different susceptible HLA alleles has been observed in interracial studies of HLA susceptibility.[135] In addition, multigenetic involvement in development of the individual component diseases of APS-2a/b has been proved, such as linkage of type 1 diabetes to more than a dozen loci in non-HLA genomic regions,[136] and autoimmune thyroid disease appears to be polygenic as well.[137–139]

Patients with APS-2b lack Addison's disease and definitive genetic features except for their associations with its component diseases and their associated HLA alleles. For example, DQB1*0301 is increased when Hashimoto's thyroiditis is present; DRB1*03 and DRB3 are increased when Graves' disease, or type 1 diabetes, or both are present; and DRB1*13 is associated with vitiligo. Non-HLA genes are, however, expected to also be involved in the development of APS-2b, and attempts have been made to map for non-HLA genes responsible for the component disease of APS-2b. For example, Tomer and colleagues linked a susceptible locus for Graves' disease to within a 6 centimorgans at the chromosome 20q11.2.[140] Although this susceptible locus is waiting to be confirmed, the finding of a gene for the component disease of APS-2b would help in understanding the pathogenesis of the syndrome. The susceptible locus at chromosome 20q11.2 was linked to Graves' disease but not to Hashimoto's thyroiditis. This finding again suggests that the cause of pathogenic autoimmunity may involve different pathogenic processes and that alternative pathways exist for the breakdown in immune system self-tolerance. Thus, genetic studies of autoimmune endocrine syndromes should facilitate understanding of the pathogenic process of these diseases, which may be applicable to the component autoimmunities.

CLINICAL SPECTRUM OF AUTOIMMUNE POLYGLANDULAR SYNDROMES

An important responsibility for clinicians managing patients with endocrine gland deficiencies is to consider whether an individual with a single endocrine autoimmunity is at risk for the occurrence of a polyglandular disorder. Clues uncovered by a thorough history and physical examination plus laboratory findings of organ-specific autoantibodies may reveal the true polyglandular nature of a patient's condition. Subclinical or "compensated" deficiencies, identified by elevations in tropic hormone levels (e.g., normal thyroxine but elevated thyrotropin in Hashimoto's disease), reflect early gland destruction with initial compensation before overt gland failure with decreases in thyroxine are seen. Once an organ-specific autoantibody is found, the respective hormone deficiency should be monitored and treated with the same therapeutic replacement regimens as those used for patients who have isolated gland dysfunction. The authors urge the use of full diagnostic autoantibody panels, followed by monitoring of the function of any targeted organ in all probands with Addison's disease and their immediate relatives. We suggest screening all patients with type 1 diabetes for thyroid (thyroid peroxidase and thyroglobulin) and adrenal cortical (21-OHase) autoantibodies, the former because of its high frequency and the diagnostic difficulty of recognizing thyroid insufficiency in its early stages, and the latter because of its potential lethality if not recognized and treated. Older type 1 diabetic patients, especially females, should also be screened for gastric parietal cell and intrinsic factor autoantibodies and possibly vitamin B$_{12}$ and iron levels since pernicious anemia is common, especially when there is coexisting thyroid autoimmunity.

APS-1

APS-1 is diagnosed when two of the three defining diseases are present, that is, mucocutaneous candidiasis, hypoparathyroidism, and adrenocortical insufficiency. The first sign is invariably mucocutaneous candidiasis. Any young person afflicted by troublesome moniliasis should be assessed for a possible T-lymphocyte deficiency state and for type APS-1 as well. In one study, nearly 45% of pediatric patients with refractory monilial infections but no overt underlying T-cell defect had an autoimmune endocrinopathy.[141] Of patients with APS-1 in whom recurrent monilial infections develop, most have lesions that are restricted to the skin, nails, and oral and perianal mucosa. Although remissions of varying length occur, progressive or relapsing courses are common, and gastrointestinal involvement can become severe, especially when complicated by bacterial overgrowth, chronic diarrhea, or gastrointestinal hemorrhage. Hypoparathyroidism develops in more than 75% of patients with APS-1, usually before 10 years of age. Severe hypocalcemia manifested by carpopedal spasms, seizures, or laryngospasm can be the initial feature of APS-1, especially in young children. Adrenocortical failure typically develops after the onset of hypoparathyroidism between the ages of 3 and 30 years. Deficiencies of mineralocorticoids and glucocorticoids usually arise simultaneously, but their onset can be separated by 5 or more years.[58]

Females suffer from gonadal insufficiency more often than males do and usually have maturational arrest after the onset of pubarche or menarche. The author is unaware of female patients affected by APS-1 who have had a natural birth. Autoimmune oophoritis may also be manifested as failed pubertal development or as menstrual irregularities and polycystic ovaries.[142]

Fat malabsorption, which may be episodic, has been linked by some to hypoparathyroidism. More likely causes include

IgA deficiency, gluten sensitivity, and bacterial overgrowth of the upper portion of the small bowel. Malabsorption has been found to be linked to autoantibodies to tryptophan hydroxylase and to GAD, and to lack of serotonin secretion of intestinal endocrine cells.[59] Deficiencies of iron or vitamin B_{12} result from parietal cell autoimmunity, with the subsequent early appearance of achlorhydria followed by intrinsic factor deficiency and pernicious anemia. Typical atrophic gastritis arises in 15% of APS-1 patients, with a mean age at onset of 16 years.[58] Studies of Finnish patients have particularly emphasized manifestations of APS-1 in the teeth and integument. In decreasing order of frequency, enamel hypoplasia, ungual dystrophy (pitting), keratopathy, and tympanic membrane sclerosis have all been reported at rates from 33% to 77%.[58] Vitiligo may be missed if not specifically sought by ultraviolet light (Wood's lamp examination). Alopecia totalis or universalis is frequent, but all types of alopecia occur. It has been suggested that hair loss may diminish after treatment of hypoparathyroidism is started,[13] but such amelioration does not reflect the authors' experience. The appearance of hepatomegaly or jaundice with dark urine and clay-colored stool often heralds the onset of chronic active hepatitis. It occurs in up to 10% of patients and is not associated with persistent immunologic hypersensitivity to hepatitis viruses. Sjögren's syndrome (parotitis, arthritis, and sicca syndrome) is not infrequent, whereas type 1 diabetes, chronic thyroiditis, and hypophysitis are distinctly uncommon. We have now seen several patients in whom oropharyngeal and gastric carcinomas have developed, a situation sometimes seen in others with chronic defects in T-cell immunity or prolonged immunosuppressive therapy, albeit gastric atrophy is a known precursor of gastric neoplasias.

APS-2A AND APS-2B

APS-2a is far more common than APS-1 and is diagnosed when a patient has adrenocortical deficiency with combinations of type 1 diabetes, chronic lymphocytic thyroiditis, vitiligo, pernicious anemia, and Graves' disease. Unlike APS-1, this syndrome can be more difficult to recognize before the onset of clinically significant multiglandular disease. The disease is most commonly manifested in the third or fourth decade, but it is not uncommon before or after these ages. It is heralded by adrenocortical failure in almost half the cases, although this estimate may be skewed by a selection bias in the literature. As many as 20 years can elapse before the full extent of the polyglandular involvement becomes evident. Furthermore, although isolated thyroiditis and type 1 diabetes are common enough in these age groups, routine adrenal or 21-OHase autoantibody screening of such affected patients is difficult is justified in all owing to the serious consequences of missing adrenal failure when it becomes fully expressed as a clinical entity. The author also recommends routine thyroid autoantibody screening of all patients with type 1 diabetes since as many as one out of four female patients are found affected by thyroid autoimmunity as well as diabetes. Males have about half this rate. A family history of polyglandular failure is often present in past generations and can serve as a flag for patients who need extra monitoring. The presence of extra endocrinologic manifestations, such as alopecia or vitiligo, is less common than in APS-1, but when such manifestations are present, they are important clinical indicators of widespread autoimmunity, especially if they are profound. The risk of mortality from untreated adrenocortical failure in the 2% of patients with myasthenia gravis in whom associated endocrinopathies develop requires that all such patients younger than 40 years be assessed closely for endocrinologic disorders during their initial investigation.

APS-2b is more common than APS-2a and is most frequently seen in middle-aged women but it can occur at any age and in males. It is defined according to the accompanying autoimmune endocrinopathies, which include autoimmune thyroid diseases and/or type 1 diabetes, plus one of other autoimmune diseases such as pernicious anemia and vitiligo, but not Addison's disease. It is like APS-2a but without adrenocortical involvement. Once Addison's disease has appeared, such patients are reclassified as having APS-2a.

OTHER ASSOCIATIONS WITH APS

Rarer diagnoses have on occasion been reported in association with an APS. The authors and others have monitored patients with APS-1 in whom severe, idiopathic, noninflammatory myopathy with eventual respiratory failure developed. Hyposplenism may not be uncommon. Separate reports suggested that pure red cell hypoplasia and male infertility in patients with APS-1 responded well to glucocorticoid therapy.[142,143] In rare cases, neo-osseous porosis and sarcoidosis have been linked to APS-1 and type APS-2a, respectively.[144,145] Nephrocalcinosis develops in many patients with APS-1 and may be related to vitamin D therapy overdosage for hypoparathyroidism. It could also be related to antibodies to calcium-sensing receptors on the proximal renal tubules, although this association is speculative.

DIFFERENTIAL DIAGNOSIS

The differential diagnosis of APS during the initial assessment varies according to the disease manifested. When evidence of a second autoimmunity is present, consideration should be given to whether the patient has APS-1 or an APS-2 because future monitoring and the prognosis are different for these syndromes. Other diagnostic considerations are summarized in Table 41-4. Chromosomal disorders such as trisomy 21 and Turner's syndrome (45,XO and its genetic variants) are associated with an increased risk of endocrine autoimmunities, especially Hashimoto's thyroiditis (up to 30%) and immune-mediated type 1 diabetes (IMD) (approximately 5%).[146,147] The primary hypogonadism of Turner's syndrome, however, is not of autoimmune origin, and the apparent growth hormone deficiencies in some of these females may resolve after estrogen priming. DiGeorge's syndrome is a developmental disorder of the branchial arches that results in facial deformities, aortic arch anomalies such as truncus arteriosus, and thymic and parathyroid gland agenesis. Hypoparathyroidism and mucocutaneous candidiasis develop in these patients, with the diagnosis usually made in infancy, and they have few to no circulating T lymphocytes but produce no autoantibodies and Addison's disease never develops. Kearns-Sayre syndrome is a myopathic disease associated with hypoparathyroidism,

---

Table 41-4 Differential Diagnosis of Autoimmune Polyglandular Syndromes (APSs)

APS-1
APS-2a
APS-2b
Thyrogastric autoimmunity
Chromosomal disorder (45X,O; trisomy 21)
Kearns-Sayre syndrome
Congenital rubella
DiGeorge's syndrome
Wolfram's syndrome (DIDMOAD)
POEMS syndrome
Thymoma
Hemochromatosis
Myotonic dystrophy

APS, autoimmune polyglandular syndrome; DIDMOAD, diabetes insipidus, diabetes mellitus, optic atrophy, and neural deafness; POEMS, polyneuropathy, organomegaly, endocrinopathy, M protein, and skin changes.

primary hypogonadism, type 1 diabetes, and hypopitu-itarism. Cardiac conduction defects are common, and muscle biopsies are usually diagnostic. Wolfram's syndrome or DID-MOAD (diabetes insipidus, diabetes mellitus, optic atrophy, and nerve deafness) is an uncommon congenital condition that occurs in young children. Congenital hypoparathy-roidism has been reported to be caused by the biosynthetic effects of parathyroid hormone. Congenital rubella is associated with later onset of type 1 diabetes and hypothyroidism. The POEMS syndrome (plasma cell dyscrasia with polyneu-ropathy, organomegaly, endocrinopathy, M protein, and skin changes) occurs mainly in Japanese patients. It is associated with type 1 diabetes and primary hypogonadism. Thymomas (malignant more so than benign) are associated with myas-thenia gravis in up to 50% of cases. They arise most com-monly after 40 years of age in myasthenic patients and may be seen in association with Cushing's syndrome, Graves' dis-ease, or Addison's disease.[148] The author has an interesting African-American family in which all of three children (one to a different father) developed type 1 diabetes between 1 and 2 years of age associated with the usual autoantibodies. However, one of these children had also developed myasthe-nia gravis and was found to have septo-optic dysplasia with hypopituitarism. Hemochromatosis is usually manifested as lethargy, malaise, abdominal pain, and hypermelanotic skin lesions. The similarity to Addison's disease can become con-fusing in patients with either type 1 diabetes or secondary hypogonadism induced by pancreatic or hypophyseal iron deposition. Rarely, thyroid, parathyroid, or adrenocortical insufficiencies have been reported in hemochromatosis. Myotonic dystrophy is associated with primary testicular atro-phy, alopecia, and less frequently, diabetes mellitus (usually related to insulin resistance).

DIAGNOSTIC PROTOCOLS

Three major laboratory approaches are used to diagnose an APS, including serologic test for autoantibodies, function tests for the secretion of organ-specific hormones, and genetic tests for *AIRE* mutations and mutations in HLA-D genes. First, serum screening for autoantibodies are used to (1) verify the autoimmune nature of the disease in patients with polyglan-dular insufficiency; (2) identify patients affected by an iso-lated endocrinopathy in whom multi-organ autoimmunity is likely to develop; and (3) screen family members of patients with APS, even if those relatives are currently asymptomatic. A complete screening panel includes assessment of adrenal (21-OHase), steroidal cell (17-OH and P-450 ssc enzymes), thyroid (peroxidase and thyroglobulin), islet cell (GAD_{65} and IA-2/IA2-β), and parietal cell (H^+,K^+-ATPase) and intrinsic fac-tor autoantibodies (see Table 41-3). Thyroid-stimulating immunoglobulins may be useful in selected patients. A single negative examination does not rule out the possibility of future disease, and annual to biannual follow-up tests are pru-dent. The predictive value of a positive result has been presented above.

Second, in autoantibody-positive individuals, assessment of end-organ function is required. Serum levels of thyrotropin, calcium, phosphorus, and fasting glucose determined annu-ally can effectively assess thyroid, parathyroid, and pancreatic islet function of asymptomatic patients. Suspicion of subclin-ical gland dysfunction should prompt a complete functional evaluation of the suspect gland before determining a final diagnosis. Gonadal dysfunction is diagnosed when random serum gonadotropin (FSH) levels are elevated in the face of low sex steroid levels.

Although depression of early morning serum cortisol levels and electrolyte disturbances represent changes that occur at or just before the clinical onset of adrenocortical failure, it is best to monitor individuals at high risk for hypoadreno-corticism (those with AAs or SCAs) annually by seeking

inappropriate elevations of basal serum ACTH levels (mid-afternoon or later) and supine (>1 hr) plasma renin activity. To date, the author has determined no clinically relevant advantage to screening for adrenal gland dysfunction by for-mal ACTH stimulation testing or plasma renin activity assess-ment after salt deprivation. In our studies, raised serum ACTH levels beyond early morning indicated that the anterior hypophysis was responding to impending adrenocortical insufficiency and thus warranted follow-up with complete assessment of adrenocortical function.[19]

Annual hemoglobin or hematocrit determinations are essential, with accompanying examination of the blood film for erythrocyte and polymorphonuclear neutrophil morphology. When nutritional deficiencies are suspected, serum levels of ferritin and/or vitamin B_{12} and red cell folate determinations are indicated.

Fat malabsorption in APS may occur for many reasons, some of which are reversed with proper treatment. It is, there-fore, mandatory that fat malabsorption be completely inves-tigated. Stool examination for ova and parasites is helpful for diagnosing *Giardia lamblia* infection, but it may be necessary to obtain duodenal fluid or a jejunal biopsy for direct exami-nation and culture. Bacterial overgrowth can be diagnosed by duodenal aspirates, and a small bowel biopsy is required to diagnose villous atrophy morphologically. Serum IgA levels should also be assessed. Malabsorption/chronic diarrhea is unfortunately refractory to therapy. Antibodies to tryptophan hydroxylase, when present, may indicate absence of intestinal serotonin-containing cells.

Third, *AIRE* gene mutational analyses should be performed in patients with suspected APS-1 and in siblings of patients with APS-1, especially those in whom symptoms of compo-nent diseases of APS-1 have developed. For example, children or adolescents with suspected recurrent mucocutaneous can-didal infections that have been refractory to topical medica-tion should have the diagnosis confirmed at least initially by culturing scrapings from the periphery of an affected area. Such patients should be tested for *AIRE* gene mutation to con-firm the diagnosis of APS-1. The presence of homozygous *AIRE* gene mutations would indicate the diagnosis of APS-1 and may predict development of the component diseases of APS-1. However, failure to detect *AIRE* gene mutations should not exclude a diagnosis of APS-1 inasmuch as the known *AIRE* gene mutations are not detected in 10% to 30% of patients with an established diagnosis of APS-1, depending on their racial origin. This observation suggests that defects other than in the *AIRE* gene coding region may have similar effects as *AIRE* gene mutation on the development of APS-1, perhaps through defects in *AIRE* gene regulation. Obligate heterozy-gous carriers such as parents of a child with APS-1 may gen-erate APS-1 like autoantibodies, but they are infrequent, usually of low titer, and seldom associated with the respective autoimmune disease.

THERAPY

It has already been suggested that the key to successfully man-aging patients with an APS is to identify and treat their autoimmunities before they cause significant morbidity and mortality. Treatment of organ insufficiency is identical whether it occurs in isolation or as part of an APS. Replacement therapy remains the cornerstone. Patient educa-tion about the nature of the disease is often critical to early recognition of new autoimmunities, and as with any chronic disease, individualized needs for psychosocial support must be assessed. Genetic counseling is also warranted, and addi-tional affected family members should be sought by specific tests. Emergency identification should be worn at all times by APS patients, and the use of increased corticosteroid doses at times of acute stress usually averts adrenal crisis in those with Addison's disease. The authors believe that exogenous glucocorticoid supplements given at times of acute stress are well advised in asymptomatic individuals who have biochemical evidence of asymptomatic adrenocortical disease.

Of all the endocrine components of an APS, only type 1 diabetes does not carry a satisfactory prognosis when managed with well-monitored hormone replacement therapy. The long-term vascular complications have thus made type 1 diabetes a candidate for aggressive experimental approaches. Results of controlled trials using cyclosporine and azathioprine for treating newly diagnosed type 1 diabetes have indicated that some metabolic benefits are provided, although they are not often long lived, even with continued immunotherapy.[149,150] Anecdotal reports of improved orchitis,[151] oophoritis,[152] and hypophysitis[153] after immunosuppressive corticosteroid treatment are provocative but require systematic evaluation. For now, all immunomodulating therapies must be considered experimental and should be prescribed only in the setting of a controlled clinical trial. The author has had good experience with courses of intravenous immune globulin in APS-1 patients with chronic diarrhea, however, this experience could be fortuitous. As more autoantigens are identified and the disease pathogenesis becomes better understood, selective antigen-based therapies that do not cause generalized immunosuppression may be developed. Still further in the future lies the prospect of curative organ transplantation. Pancreatic and, to a lesser extent, islet transplants are currently used in kidney graft recipients with type 1 diabetes.[154] Adrenal gland transplants have been experimentally successful in rodents[155] and humans.[156] Whether thymic transplantation or gene therapy has any further roles in the treatment of APS-1 remains to be discovered.

The introduction of ketoconazole has greatly helped in the treatment of chronic mucocutaneous candidiasis, which is commonly resistant to topical antimicrobials.[157] The drug frequently causes gastrointestinal upset and can interfere with adrenal and glucocorticoid and sex steroid biosynthesis. Elevations of hepatic transaminases are usually transient, but fatal hepatic necrosis can rarely be caused by ketoconazole. In large doses, ketoconazole and its derivatives can induce adrenal suppression.

Management of fat malabsorption should first be aimed at diagnosing and treating reversible causes. Bacterial overgrowth often responds to broad-spectrum oral antibiotics. *G. lamblia* is best treated with quinacrine hydrochloride or metronidazole, and villous atrophy, seen especially in APS-2a, typically responds to dietary gluten withdrawal. If no specific cause of fat malabsorption is found, nutritional support with fat-soluble vitamin and medium-chain fatty acid supplements may be required. Such management is best done in consultation with a nutrition or gastroenterology specialist. Unfortunately, in our experience some patients remain refractory to all approaches.

Improved survival for patients with chronic active hepatitis has been achieved with new regimens of immunomodulating agents such as prednisone, cyclosporine, and azathioprine.[154] Tertiary hepatic care is indicated for patients in whom chronic active hepatitis develops.

PROGNOSIS

The impact of an APS on a given patient's lifestyle varies considerably because of differences in a host of disease-dependent, patient-dependent, family-dependent, and physician-dependent factors. All patients with either APS-1 or APS-2 are committed to a regimen of lifelong hormone, mineral, and/or vitamin replacement. Although it is usually best to counsel patients to continue participating in all their regular activities, health care providers must be mindful that an APS disease can dramatically alter a patient's life (e.g., an airline pilot in whom type 1 diabetes develops).

Systematic studies of the long-term prognosis in APS patients are lacking, but clinical impressions are that patients with APS-2a have rates of morbidity and mortality that are identical to those of the component diseases when they occur in isolation. Adrenal crises are still a significant cause of preventable mortality, and uncontrolled thyroid hormone imbalances can on rare occasion be emergencies, especially in the elderly. The complications of type 1 diabetes, both acute and chronic, are as important in the APS setting as in isolated pancreatic disease.

Although many patients in whom APS-1 is diagnosed lead a full and vigorous life,[58] poorer outcomes are common. In some, a course of recurrent illness initially develops in their second decade of life. Problems include asthenia, which is often of uncertain etiology; recurrent opportunistic infections, which presumably arise because of a T-lymphocyte deficiency; chronic active hepatitis, which continues to be one of the most common causes of mortality in APS-1; and oropharyngeal or gastric carcinoma, which can be fatal unless diagnosed early. Mortality near the end of the second or during the third decade is not uncommon.

CONCLUSION

Syndromes of multi-organ failure induced by autoimmunity occur in well-recognized patterns and can be detected at an asymptomatic stage by screening high-risk individuals for circulating autoantibodies. Such autoantibodies are also of diagnostic importance in symptomatic patients. Detection of *AIRE* gene mutations has become a useful indication for the diagnosis of APS-1. Optimal management includes close anticipatory monitoring so that early treatment of organ failure can be instituted, thereby preventing irreversible morbidity or even death, especially for untreated Addison's disease. Currently, treatment is limited to pharmacologic replacement and psychosocial support; however, increases in our understanding of the pathogenesis of these conditions should lead to treatments that will prevent progression to complete end-organ destruction. Over recent years, dramatic progress has been made in the identification of target antigens and epitopes involved in the autoimmune organ-specific diseases that are components of the APSs. Studies of the function of the *AIRE* gene product would promote understanding of the pathogenesis of APS-1 and immune tolerance in general. Gene therapies based on the disease genes identified are needed for the eventual cure and prevention of APS.

Whereas the number of *AIRE* gene mutations has grown since the last writing of this chapter (the reader is directed to reviews on the subject),[158-160] there has been novel genotype-phenotype relationships identified, albeit one report has indicated that individual component diseases in APS-1 have the same HLA-genotype associations as they do in APS-2.[160] The identification of the *AIRE* gene underlying APS-1 has provided an area of major stimulation to research into the pathogenesis of autoimmune disorders. The AIRE transcript has the highest expression in adult thymus and fetal liver.[161] AIRE protein is mostly expressed in thymic medullary epithelium but in a rare subset of cells in lymph nodes, spleen, and fetal liver.[162] AIRE transcripts were reported to be restrictively expressed in peripheral CD14-positive monocytes but not in polymorphonuclear neutrophils or T cells, while AIRE protein was also found in differentiated dendritic cells.[163] While *AIRE* gene knockout mice generally develop normally, they do develop multi-organ lymphocytic infiltrates, autoantibodies, and infertility and when antigenically challenged, show inhanced T-cell proliferation.[164] The absence of *AIRE* gene expression in knockout mice was associated with loss of expression of peripheral antigens in medullary cells of the thymus.[165] In transgenic *AIRE* gene knockout mice, where the transgene results in CD4+ T cells against a pancreatic antigen, the mice were deficient in eradicating these autoreactive T cells,[166] emphasizing the role of central tolerance associated with *AIRE* gene functioning. Others have reported that E3 ubiquitin ligase activity is mediated by the first plant homeodomain of the *AIRE* gene, suggesting a mechanism by which *AIRE* gene mutations mediate loss of central tolerance.[167] Murine *AIRE* gene transfectants have been shown to result in downregulation of IL-1 receptor antagonist (IL-1Ra) and class-11 molecules as mediated by competition of the transcriptional coactivator (CREB-binding protein or CBP), perhaps explaining the autoimmune and immunodeficient nature of APS-1.[168] In respect to APS-2, patients with single autoimmune endocrinopathies have been reported by Kukreja and Kreigel and coworkersl to have low peripheral levels of CD25+ T cells (T regulator cells). More importantly, these cells in patients with APS-2a were shown to be defective in their suppressor capacity.[169] Another locus of functional importance to diseases of APS-2 that has emerged through the work of the Oxford group of Todd and colleagues is CTLA-4, as reviewed recently.[170] Another report has indicated a high rate of APS-2 diseases in patients with sarcoidosis.[171] This calls to question whether such patients have sarcoidosis on an infectious basis because of their inherent immunodeficiency. The author has experience with the father of a patient with APS-2a who had chronic inflammatory bowel disease and then developed pulmonary sarcoidosis. Activating autoantibodies to the CaSR of parathyroid glands has been demonstrated in patients with hypoparathyroidism[171] while the clinical problem of infertility in women with APS-1 has been suggested to be addressed by in vitro fertilization.[171] However, the author knows of no report concerning experience with the latter.

REFERENCES

1. Addison T: Anaemia: Disease of the suprarenal capsules. Lond Med Gaz 8:517–518, 1849.
2. Claude H, Gourgerot H: Insuffisance pluriglandulaire endocrinienne. J Physiol Pathol Gen 10:469–480, 1908.
3. Hashimoto H: Zur kenntnis der lymphomatosen veranderung der schilddruse (struma lymphomatosa). Acta Klin Chir 97:219–248, 1912.
4. von Meyenburg H: Uber "Insulitis" bei diabetes. Schweiz Med Wochenschr 71:554–557, 1940.
5. Schmidt MB: Eine biglandulare Erkrankung (Nebennieren und Schilddrusse) bei Morbus Addisonii. Verh Dtsch Ges Pathol 21:212–221, 1926.
6. Carpenter CCJ, Solomon N, Silverberg SG, et al: Schmidt's syndrome (thyroid and adrenal insufficiency): A review of the literature and a report of fifteen new cases including ten instances of coexistent diabetes mellitus. Medicine (Baltimore) 43:153–180, 1964.
7. Thorpe ES, Handley HE: Chronic tetany and chronic mycelial stomatitis in a child aged four-and-one-half years. Am J Dis Child 38:328–338, 1929.
8. Whitaker J, Landing BH, Esselborn VM, Williams RR: The syndrome of familial juvenile hypoadrenocorticism, hypoparathyroidism and superficial moniliasis. J Clin Endocrinol 16:1374–1387, 1956.
9. Roitt IM, Doniach D, Campbell PN, Hudson RV: Autoantibodies in Hashimoto's disease (lymphadenoid goitre). Lancet 2:820–821, 1956.
10. Blizzard RM, Kyle MA: Studies of the adrenal antigens and antibodies in Addison's disease. J Clin Invest 42:1653–1660, 1963.
11. Neufeld M, Maclaren N, Blizzard R: Autoimmune polyglandular syndromes. Pediatr Ann 9:154–162, 1980.
12. Neufeld M, Maclaren NK, Blizzard RM: Two types of autoimmune Addison's disease associated with different polyglandular autoimmune (PGA) syndromes. Medicine (Baltimore) 60:355–362, 1981.
13. Brun JM: Juvenile autoimmune polyendocrinopathy. Horm Res 16:308–316, 1982.
14. Maclaren NK, Riley WJ: Autoimmune endocrinopathies. In Samter M, Talmage DW, Frank MM, et al (eds): Immunological Diseases of the Endocrine System. Boston, Little, Brown, 1988, pp 1737–1764.
15. Peterson P, Krohn KJ: Mapping of B cell epitopes on steroid 17 alpha-hydroxylase, an autoantigen in autoimmune polyglandular syndrome type I. Clin Exp Immunol 98:104–109, 1994.
16. Peterson P, Uibo R, Peranen J, Krohn K: Immunoprecipitation of steroidogenic enzyme autoantigens with autoimmune polyglandular syndrome type I (APS-1) sera; further evidence for independent humoral immunity to P450c17 and p450c21. Clin Exp Immunol 107:335–340, 1997.
17. Riley WJ, Maclaren NK, Krischer J, et al: A prospective study of the development of diabetes in relatives of patients with insulin-dependent diabetes. N Engl J Med 323:1167–1172, 1990.
18. Elder M, Maclaren N, Riley W: Gonadal autoantibodies in patients with hypogonadism and/or Addison's disease. J Clin Endocrinol Metab 52:1137–1142, 1981.
19. Ketchum CH, Riley WJ, Maclaren NK: Adrenal dysfunction in asymptomatic patients with adrenocortical autoantibodies. J Clin Endocrinol Metab 58:1166–1170, 1984.
20. Betterle C, Scalici C, Presotto F, et al: The natural history of adrenal function in autoimmune patients with adrenal autoantibodies. J Endocrinol 117:467–475, 1988.
21. Leisti S, Ahonen P, Perheentupa J: The diagnosis and staging of hypocortisolism in progressing autoimmune adrenalitis. Pediatr Res 17:861–867, 1983.
22. Scherbaum WA: Autoimmune hypothalamic diabetes insipidus. Prog Brain Res 93:283–292, 1992.
23. Bigazzi PE: Autoimmunity of the adrenals. In Volpe R (ed): Autoimmunity and Endocrine Disease. New York, Marcel Dekker, 1985, pp 345–373.
24. Ahonen P, Miettinen A, Perheentupa J: Adrenal and steroidal cell antibodies in patients with autoimmune polyglandular disease type I and risk of adrenocortical and ovarian failure. J Clin Endocrinol Metab 64:494–500, 1987.
25. Betterle C, Volpato M, Rees Smith B, et al: Adrenal cortex and steroid 21-hydroxylase autoantibodies in adult patients with organ-specific autoimmune diseases: Markers of low progression to clinical Addison's disease. J Clin Endocrinol Metab 82:932–938, 1997.
26. Krohn K, Uibo R, Aavik E, et al: Identification by molecular cloning of an autoantigen associated with Addison's disease as steroid 17α-hydroxylase. Lancet 339:770–773, 1992.
27. Winqvist O, Karlsson F, Kampe O: 21-Hydroxylase, a major autoantigen in idiopathic Addison's disease. Lancet 339:1559–1562, 1992.
28. Baumann-Antczak A, Wedlock N, Bednarek J, et al: Autoimmune Addison's disease and 21-hydroxylase. Lancet 340:429–430, 1992.
29. Bednarek J, Furmaniak J, Wedlock N, et al: Steroid 21-hydroxylase is a major autoantigen involved in adult onset autoimmune Addison's disease. FEBS Lett 309:51–55, 1992.
30. Falorni A, Nikoshkov A, Laureti S, et al: High diagnostic accuracy for idiopathic Addison's disease with a sensitive radiobinding assay for autoantibodies against recombinant human 21-hydroxylase. J Clin Endocrinol Metab 80:2752–2755, 1995.
31. Chen S, Sawicka J, Betterle C, et al: Autoantibodies to steroidogenic enzymes in autoimmune polyglandular syndrome, Addison's disease, and premature ovarian failure. J Clin Endocrinol Metab 81:1871–1876, 1996.
32. Tanaka H, Perez MS, Powell M, et al: Steroid 21-hydroxylase autoantibodies: Measurements with a new immunoprecipitation assay. J Clin Endocrinol Metab 82:1440–1446, 1997.
33. Winqvist O, Gustafsson J, Rorsman F, et al: Two different cytochrome P450 enzymes are the adrenal antigens in

autoimmune polyendocrine syndrome type I and Addison's disease. J Clin Invest 92:2377–2385, 1993.

34. Seissler J, Schott M, Steinbrenner H, et al: Autoantibodies to adrenal cytochrome P450 antigens in isolated Addison's disease and autoimmune polyendocrine syndrome type II. Exp Clin Endocrinol Diabetes 107:208–213, 1999.

35. Wedlock N, Asawa T, Baumann-Antczak A, et al: Autoimmune Addison's disease. Analysis of autoantibody binding sites on human steroid 21-hydroxylase. FEBS Lett 332:123–126, 1993.

36. Volpato M, Prentice L, Chen S, et al: A study of the epitopes on steroid 21-hydroxylase recognized by autoantibodies in patients with or without Addison's disease. Clin Exp Immunol 111:422–428, 1998.

37. Asawa T, Wedlock N, Baumann-Antczak A, et al: Naturally occurring mutations in human steroid 21-hydroxylase influence adrenal autoantibody binding. J Clin Endocrinol Metab 79:372–376, 1994.

38. Song YH, Connor E, Li Y, et al: The role of tyrosinase in autoimmune vitiligo. Lancet 344:1049–1052, 1994.

39. Brewer KW, Parziale VS, Eisenbarth GS: Screening patients with insulin-dependent diabetes mellitus for adrenal insufficiency. N Engl J Med 337:202, 1997.

40. Riley WJ, Maclaren NK, Neufeld M: Adrenal autoantibodies and Addison disease in insulin-dependent diabetes mellitus. J Pediatr 97:191–195, 1980.

41. Betterle C, Volpato M, Rees Smith B, et al: Adrenal cortex and steroid 21-hydroxylase autoantibodies in adult patients with organ-specific autoimmune diseases: Markers of low progression to clinical Addison's disease. J Clin Endocrinol Metab 82:932–938, 1997.

42. Huang W, Connor E, Rosa TD, et al: Although DR3-DQB1*0201 may be associated with multiple component diseases of the autoimmune polyglandular syndromes, the human leukocyte antigen DR4-DQB1*0302 haplotype is implicated only in beta-cell autoimmunity. J Clin Endocrinol Metab 81:2559–2563, 1996.

43. Peterson P, Salmi H, Hyoty H, et al: Steroid 21-hydroxylase autoantibodies in insulin-dependent diabetes mellitus. Childhood Diabetes in Finland (DiMe) Study Group. Clin Immunol Immunopathol 82:37–42, 1997.

44. Uibo R, Aavik E, Peterson P, et al: Autoantibodies to cytochrome P450scc, P450c17, and P450c21 in autoimmune polyglandular disease types I and II and in isolated Addison's disease. J Clin Endocrinol Metab 78:323–328, 1994.

45. McNatty KP, Short RV, Barnes EW, Irvine WJ: The cytotoxic effect of serum from patients with Addison's disease and autoimmune ovarian failure on human granulosa cells in culture. Clin Exp Immunol 22:378–384, 1975.

46. Furmaniak J, Talbot D, Reinwein D, et al: Immunoprecipitation of human adrenal microsomal antigen. FEBS Lett 231:25–28, 1988.

47. Boscaro M, Betterle C, Volpato M, et al: Hormonal responses during various phases of autoimmune adrenal failure: No evidence for 21-hydroxylase enzyme activity inhibition in vivo. J Clin Endocrinol Metab 81:2801–2804, 1996.

48. Blizzard RM, Chee D, Davis W: The incidence of parathyroid and other antibodies in the sera of patients with idiopathic hypoparathyroidism. Clin Exp Immunol 1:119–128, 1966.

49. Chapman CK, Bradwell AR, Dykks PW: Do parathyroid and adrenal autoantibodies coexist? J Clin Pathol 39:813–814, 1986.

50. Betterle C, Caretto A, Zeviani M, et al: Demonstration and characterization of anti-human mitochondria autoantibodies in idiopathic hypoparathyroidism and in other conditions. Clin Exp Immunol 62:353–360, 1985.

51. Fattorossi A, Aurbach GD, Sakaguchi K, et al: Anti-endothelial cell antibodies: Detection and characterization in sera from patients with autoimmune hypoparathyroidism. Proc Natl Acad Sci U S A 85:4015–4019, 1988.

52. Li Y, Song YH, Rais N, et al: Autoantibodies to the extracellular domain of the calcium sensing receptor in patients with acquired hypoparathyroidism. J Clin Invest 97:910–914, 1996.

53. Velloso LA, Winqvist O, Gustafsson J, et al: Autoantibodies against a novel 51 kDa islet antigen and glutamate decarboxylase isoforms in autoimmune polyendocrine syndrome type I. Diabetologia 37:61–69, 1994.

54. Tuomi T, Bjorses P, Falorni A, et al: Antibodies to glutamic acid decarboxylase in autoimmune polyendocrine syndrome type 1. J Clin Endocrinol Metab 82:147–150, 1997.

55. Solimena M, Folli F, Aparisi R, et al: Autoantibodies to GABA-ergic neurons and pancreatic beta cells in stiff-man syndrome. N Engl J Med 322:1555–1560, 1990.

56. Tuomi T, Rowley MJ, Knowles WJ, et al: Autoantigenic properties of native and denatured glutamic acid decarboxylase: Evidence for a conformational epitope. Clin Immunol Immunopathol 71:53–59, 1994.

57. Elrehewy M, Kong YM, Giraldo AA, Rose NR: Syngeneic thyroglobulin is immunogenic in good responder mice. Eur J Immunol 11:146–151, 1981.

58. Ahonen P, Myllarniemi S, Sipila I, et al: Clinical variation of autoimmune polyendocrinopathy-candidiasis-ectodermal dystrophy (APECED) in a series of 68 patients. N Engl J Med 322:1829–1836, 1990.

59. Ekwall O, Hedstrand H, Grimelius L, et al: Identification of tryptophan hydroxylase as an intestinal autoantigen. Lancet 352:279–283, 1998.

60. Dieterich W, Ehnis T, Bauer M, et al: Identification of tissue transglutaminase as the autoantigen of celiac disease. Nat Med 3:797–801, 1997.

61. Picarelli A, Maiuri L, Frate A, et al: Production of antiendomysial antibodies after in-vitro gliadin challenge of small intestine biopsy samples from patients with coeliac disease. Lancet 348:1065–1067, 1996.

62. Maki M: Coeliac disease and autoimmunity due to unmasking of cryptic epitopes? Lancet 348:1046–1047, 1996.

63. Maclaren NK, Riley WJ: Thyroid, gastric, and adrenal autoimmunities associated with insulin-dependent diabetes mellitus. Diabetes Care 8(suppl 1):34–38, 1985.

64. Loveridge N, Bitensky L, Chayen J, et al: Inhibition of parietal cell function by human gammaglobulin containing gastric parietal cell antibodies. Clin Exp Immunol 41:264–270, 1980.

65. Tanaka N, Glass GBJ: Effect of prolonged administration of parietal cell antibodies from patients with atrophic gastritis and pernicious anemia on the parietal cell mass and hydrochloric acid output in rats. Gastroenterology 58:482–494, 1970.

66. Burman P, Mardh S, Norberg L, Karlsson FA: Parietal cell antibodies in pernicious anemia inhibit H+, K+-adenosine triphosphatase, the proton pump of the stomach. Gastroenterology 96:1434–1438, 1989.

67. Betterle C, Mirakian R, Doniach D, et al: Antibodies to melanocytes in vitiligo. Lancet 1:159, 1984.

68. Song YH, Connor E, Li Y, et al: The role of tyrosinase in autoimmune vitiligo. Lancet 344:1049–1052, 1994.

69. Baharav E, Merimski O, Shoenfeld Y, et al: Tyrosinase as an autoantigen in patients with vitiligo. Clin Exp Immunol 105:84–88, 1996.

70. Xie Z, Chen D, Jiao D, Bystryn JC: Vitiligo antibodies are not directed to tyrosinase. Arch Dermatol 135:417–422, 1999.

71. Visseren MJ, van Elsas A, van der Voort EI, et al: CTL specific for the tyrosinase autoantigen can be induced from healthy donor blood to lyse melanoma cells. J Immunol 154:3991–3998, 1995.

72. Overwijk WW, Lee DS, Surman DR, et al: Vaccination with a recombinant vaccinia virus encoding a "self" antigen induces autoimmune vitiligo and tumor cell destruction in mice: Requirement for CD4(+) T lymphocytes. Proc Natl Acad Sci U S A 96:2982–2987, 1999.

73. Austin LM, Boissy RE: Mammalian tyrosinase-related protein-1 is recognized by autoantibodies from vitiliginous Smyth chickens. An avian model for human vitiligo. Am J Pathol 146:1529–1541, 1995.

74. Bottazzo GF, Pouplard A, Florin-Christensen A, Doniach D: Autoantibodies to prolactin-secreting

cells of human pituitary. Lancet 2:97–101, 1975.

75. Cosman F, Kalmon DP, Holub DA, Wardlaw SL: Lymphocytic hypophysitis: Report of 3 new cases and review of the literature. Medicine (Baltimore) 68:240–256, 1989.

76. Komatsu M, Kondo T, Yamauchi K, et al: Antipituitary antibodies in patients with the primary empty sella syndrome. J Clin Endocrinol Metab 67:633–638, 1988.

77. Wilkin TJ: Receptor autoimmunity in endocrine disorders. N Engl J Med 323:1318–1324, 1990.

78. Manns MP: Recent developments in autoimmune liver diseases. J Gastroenterol Hepatol 12(Suppl):256–271, 1997.

79. Arulanantham K, Dwyer JM, Genel M: Evidence for defective immunoregulation in the syndrome of familial candidiasis endocrinopathy. N Engl J Med 300:164–168, 1979.

80. Eisenbarth GS, Wilson PN, Ward F, et al: The polyglandular failure syndrome: Disease inheritance, HLA-type, and immune function studies in patients and families. Ann Intern Med 91:528–533, 1979.

81. Volpe R: Immunology of human thyroid disease. In Volpe R (ed): Autoimmune Diseases of the Endocrine System. Boca Raton, FL, CRC Press, 1990, pp 73–239.

82. Brenner O: Addison's disease with atrophy of the cortex of the suprarenals. Q J Med 22:121–144, 1928.

83. Gloor E, Hurlimann J: Autoimmune oophoritis. Am J Clin Pathol 81:105–109, 1984.

84. Sedmak DD, Hart WR, Tubbs RR: Autoimmune oophoritis: A histopathologic study of involved ovaries with immunologic characterization of the mononuclear cell infiltrate. Int J Gynecol Pathol 6:73–81, 1987.

85. Bottazzo GF, Dean BM, McNally JM, et al: In situ characterization of autoimmune phenomena and expression of HLA molecules in the pancreas in diabetic insulitis. N Engl J Med 313:353–360, 1985.

86. Foulis AK, Liddle CN, Farquharson MA, et al: The histopathology of the pancreas in type I (insulin-dependent) diabetes mellitus: A 25-year review of deaths in patients under 20 years of age in the United Kingdom. Diabetalogia 29:267–274, 1986.

87. Muir A, Schatz DA, Maclaren NK: Autoimmune Addison's disease. In Bach JF (ed): Immunoendocrinology: Seminars in Immunopathology, vol 14. New York, Springer-Verlag, 1993, pp 275–284.

88. Craig JM, Schiff LH, Boone JE: Chronic moniliasis associated with Addison's disease. Am J Dis Child 89:669–684, 1955.

89. Roitt IM, Doniach D: Gastric autoimmunity. In Miescher PA, Muller-Eberhard HJ (eds): Textbook of Immunopathology. New York, Grune & Stratton, 1976, pp 737–749.

90. Muir A, Maclaren NK: Autoimmune diseases of the adrenal glands, parathyroid glands, gonads, and hypothalamic-pituitary axis. Endocrinol Metab Clin North Am 20:619–644, 1991.

91. Berman MA, Sandborg CI, Wang Z, et al: Decreased IL-4 production in new onset type I insulin-dependent diabetes mellitus. J Immunol 157:4690–4696, 1996.

92. Kallmann BA, Huther M, Tubes M, et al: Systemic bias of cytokine production toward cell-mediated immune regulation in IDDM and toward humoral immunity in Graves' disease. Diabetes 46:237–243, 1997.

93. Aguayo J, Sakatsume Y, Jamieson C, et al: Nontoxic nodular goiter and papillary carcinoma of the thyroid gland are not associated with peripheral blood lymphocyte sensitization to thyroid cells. J Clin Endocrinol Metab 68:145–149, 1989.

94. Jarpe AJ, Hickman MR, Anderson JT, et al: Flow cytometric enumeration of mononuclear cell populations infiltrating the islets of Langerhans in prediabetic NOD mice: Development of a model of autoimmune insulitis for type I diabetes. Reg Immunol 3:305–307, 1991.

95. Yoon JW, Yoon CS, Lim HW, et al: Control of autoimmune diabetes in NOD mice by GAD expression or suppression in beta cells. Science 284:1183–1187, 1999.

96. Davies TF, Martin A, Concepcion ES, et al: Evidence of limited variability of antigen receptors on intrathyroidal T cells in autoimmune thyroid disease. N Engl J Med 325:238–244, 1991.

97. Campbell IL, Harrison LC: Molecular pathology of type I diabetes. Mol Biol Med 7:299–309, 1990.

98. Bottazzo GF, Todd I, Rirakian R, et al: Organ-specific autoimmunity: A 1986 overview. Immunol Rev 94:137–169, 1986.

99. Bagnasco M, Caretto A, Olive D, et al: Expression of intercellular adhesion molecule-1 (ICAM-1) on thyroid epithelial cells in Hashimoto's thyroiditis but not in Graves' disease or papillary thyroid cancer. Clin Exp Immunol 83:309–313, 1991.

100. Campbell IL, Cutri A, Wilkinson D, et al: Intercellular adhesion molecule-1 is induced on endocrine islet cells by cytokines but not by reovirus infection. Proc Natl Acad Sci U S A 86:4282–4286, 1989.

101. Kirkpatrick CH: Transfer factor. CRC Crit Rev Clin Lab Sci 12:87–122, 1980.

102. Baxter AG, Kinder SJ, Hammond KJ, et al: Association between $\alpha\beta TCR^+CD4^-CD8^-$ T-cell deficiency and IDDM in NOD/Lt mice. Diabetes 46:572–582, 1997.

103. Wilson SB, Kent SC, Patton KT, et al: Extreme Th1 bias of invariant $V\alpha 24 J\alpha Q$ T cells in type 1 diabetes. Nature 391:177–181, 1998.

104. Rosmalen JG, Leenen PJ, Katz JD, et al: Dendritic cells in the autoimmune insulitis in NOD mouse models of diabetes. Adv Exp Med Biol 417:291–294, 1997.

105. Jansen A, Voorbij HA, Jeucken PH, et al: An immunohistochemical study on organized lymphoid cell infiltrates in fetal and neonatal pancreases. A comparison with similar infiltrates found in the pancreas of a diabetic infant. Autoimmunity 15:31–38, 1993.

106. Takahashi K, Honeyman MC, Harrison LC: Impaired yield, phenotype, and function of monocyte-derived dendritic cells in humans at risk for insulin-dependent diabetes. J Immunol 161:2629–2635, 1998.

107. Conrad B, Weissmahr RN, Boni J, et al: A human endogenous retroviral superantigen as candidate autoimmune gene in type I diabetes. Cell 90:303–313, 1997.

108. Lan MS, Mason A, Coutant R, et al: HERV-K10s and immune-mediated (type 1) diabetes. Cell 95:14–16, 1998.

109. Lower R, Tonjes RR, Boller K, et al: Development of insulin-dependent diabetes mellitus does not depend on specific expression of the human endogenous retrovirus HERV-K. Cell 95:11–14, 1998.

110. Murphy VJ, Harrison LC, Rudert WA, et al: Retroviral superantigens and type 1 diabetes mellitus. Cell 95:9–11, 1998.

111. Maclaren NK, Riley WJ: Inherited susceptibility to autoimmune Addison's disease is linked to human leukocyte antigens-DR3 and/or DR4, except when associated with type I autoimmune polyglandular syndrome. J Clin Endocrinol Metab 62:455–459, 1986.

112. Spinner MW, Blizzard RM, Childs B: Clinical and genetic heterogeneity in idiopathic Addison's disease and hypoparathyroidism. J Clin Endocrinol Metab 28:795–804, 1968.

113. Ahonen P: Autoimmune polyendocrinopathy-candidosis-ectodermal dystrophy (APECED): Autosomal recessive inheritance. Clin Genet 27:535–542, 1985.

114. Zlotogora J, Shapiro MS: Polyglandular autoimmune syndrome type I among Iranian Jews. J Med Genet 29:824–826, 1992.

115. Aaltonen J, Bjorses P, Sandkuijl L, et al: An autosomal locus causing autoimmune disease: Autoimmune polyglandular disease type I assigned to chromosome 21. Nat Genet 8:83–87, 1994.

116. Bjorses P, Aaltonen J, Vikman A, et al: Genetic homogeneity of autoimmune polyglandular disease type I. Am J Hum Genet 59:879–886, 1996.

117. Aaltonen J, Horelli-Kuitunen N, Fan JB, et al: High-resolution physical and transcriptional mapping of the autoimmune polyendocrinopathy-candidiasis-ectodermal dystrophy locus on chromosome 21q22.3 by FISH. Genome Res 7:820–829, 1997.

118. Chen QY, Lan MS, She JX, Maclaren NK: The gene responsible for autoimmune polyglandular syndrome type 1 maps to chromosome 21q22.3 in US patients. J Autoimmun 11:177–183, 1998.

119. Nagamine K, Peterson P, Scott HS, et al: Positional cloning of the APECED gene. Nat Genet 17:393–398, 1997.

120. The Finnish-German APECED Consortium: An autoimmune disease, APECED, caused by mutations in a novel gene featuring two PHD-type zinc-finger domains. Nat Genet 17:399–403, 1997.

121. Scott HS, Heino M, Peterson P, et al: Common mutations in autoimmune polyendocrinopathy-candidiasis-ectodermal dystrophy patients of different origins. Mol Endocrinol 12:1112–1119, 1998.

122. Heino M, Scott HS, Chen Q, et al: Mutation analyses of North American APS-1 patients. Hum Mutat 13:69–74, 1999.

123. Rosatelli MC, Meloni A, Meloni A, et al: A common mutation in Sardinian autoimmune polyendocrinopathy-candidiasis-ectodermal dystrophy patients. Hum Genet 103:428–434, 1998.

124. Pearce SH, Cheetham T, Imrie H, et al: A common and recurrent 13-bp deletion in the autoimmune regulator gene in British kindreds with autoimmune polyendocrinopathy type 1. Am J Hum Genet 63:1675–1684, 1998.

125. Cavalli-Sforza LL, Menozzi P, Piazza A: The History and Geography of Human Genes. Princeton, NJ, Princeton University Press, 1994.

126. Thenot S, Henriquet C, Rochefort H, Cavailles V: Differential interaction of nuclear receptors with the putative human transcriptional coactivator hTIF1. J Biol Chem 272:12062–12068, 1997.

127. Ge Q, Nilasena DS, O'Brien CA, et al: Molecular analysis of a major antigenic region of the 240-kD protein of Mi-2 autoantigen. J Clin Invest 96:1730–1737, 1995.

128. Woodage T, Basrai MA, Baxevanis AD, et al: Characterization of the CHD family of proteins. Proc Natl Acad Sci U S A 94:11472–11477, 1997.

129. Le Douarin B, Zechel C, Garnier JM, et al: The N-terminal part of TIF1, a putative mediator of the ligand-dependent activation function (AF-2) of nuclear receptors, is fused to B-raf in the oncogenic protein T18. EMBO J 14:2020–2033, 1995.

130. Lukinmaa PL, Waltimo J, Pirinen S: Polyendocrinopathy-candidiasis-ectodermal dystrophy (APECED): Report of three cases. J Craniofac Genet Dev Biol 16:174–181, 1996.

131. Butler MG, Hodes ME, Conneally PM, et al: Linkage analysis in a large kindred with autosomal dominant transmission of polyglandular autoimmune disease type II (Schmidt syndrome). Am J Med Genet 18:61–65, 1984.

132. Santamaria P, Barbosa JJ, Lindstrom AL, et al: HLA-DQB1-associated susceptibility that distinguishes Hashimoto's thyroiditis from Graves' disease in type I diabetic patients. J Clin Endocrinol Metab 78:878–883, 1994.

133. Tamai H, Kimura A, Dong RP, et al: Resistance to autoimmune thyroid disease is associated with HLA-DQ. J Clin Endocrinol Metab 78:94–97, 1994.

134. Boehm BO, Manfras B, Seidl S, et al: The HLA-DQ beta non-Asp-57 allele: A predictor of future insulin-dependent diabetes mellitus in patients with autoimmune Addison's disease. Tissue Antigens 37:130–132, 1991.

135. She JX: Susceptibility to type I diabetes: HLA-DQ and DR revisited. Immunol Today 17:323–329, 1996.

136. Todd JA: Genetics of type 1 diabetes. Pathol Biol (Paris) 45:219–227, 1997.

137. Yanagawa T, Hidaka Y, Guimaraes V, et al: CTLA-4 gene polymorphism associated with Graves' disease in a Caucasian population. J Clin Endocrinol Metab 80:41–45, 1995.

138. Donner H, Rau H, Walfish PG, et al: CTLA4 alanine-17 confers genetic susceptibility to Graves' disease and to type 1 diabetes mellitus. J Clin Endocrinol Metab 82:143–146, 1997.

139. Sale MM, Akamizu T, Howard TD, et al: Association of autoimmune thyroid disease with a microsatellite marker for the thyrotropin receptor gene and CTLA-4 in a Japanese population. Proc Assoc Am Physicians 109:453–461, 1997.

140. Tomer Y, Barbesino G, Greenberg DA, et al: Linkage analysis of candidate genes in autoimmune thyroid disease. III. Detailed analysis of chromosome 14 localizes Graves' disease-1 (GD-1) close to multinodular goiter-1 (MNG-1). International Consortium for the Genetics of Autoimmune Thyroid Disease. J Clin Endocrinol Metab 83:432–4327, 1998.

141. Herrod HG: Chronic mucocutaneous candidiasis in childhood and complications of non-Candida infection: A report of the pediatric immunodeficiency collaborative study group. Pediatrics 116:377–382, 1990.

142. Mandel M, Etzioni A, Theodor R, Passwell JH: Pure red cell hypoplasia associated with polyglandular autoimmune syndrome type I. Isr J Med Sci 25:138–141, 1989.

143. Tsatsoulis A, Shalet SM: Antisperm autoantibodies in the polyglandular autoimmunity (PGA) syndrome type I: Response to cyclical steroid therapy. Clin Endocrinol 35:299–303, 1991.

144. Vela BS, Dorin RI, Hartshorne MF: Case report 631: Neo-osseous porosis (metaphyseal osteopenia) in polyglandular autoimmune (Schmidt) syndrome. Skeletal Radiol 19:468–471, 1990.

145. Walz B, From GL: Addison's disease and sarcoidosis: Unusual frequency of co-existing hypothyroidism (Schmidt's syndrome). Am J Med 89:692–693, 1990.

146. Jones KL: Smith's Recognizable Patterns of Human Malformation, 4th ed. Philadelphia, WB Saunders, 1988, pp 74–79.

147. Hall JG, Gilchrist DM: Turner syndrome and its variants. Pediatr Clin North Am 37:1421–1440, 1990.

148. Engel EG: Myasthenia gravis and other disorders of neuromuscular transmission. In Braunwald E, Isselbacher KJ, Petersdorf RG, et al (eds): Harrison's Principles of Internal Medicine. New York, McGraw-Hill, 1987, pp 2079–2082.

149. Silverstein J, Maclaren N, Riley W, et al: Immunosuppression with azathioprine and prednisone in recent onset insulin dependent diabetes mellitus. N Engl J Med 319:599–604, 1988.

150. Martin S, Scherntaner G, Nerup J, et al: Follow up of cyclosporin A treatment in type I (insulin dependent) diabetes mellitus: Lack of long-term effects. Diabetalogia 34:429–434, 1991.

151. Tsatsoulis A, Shalet SM: Antisperm autoantibodies in the polyglandular autoimmunity (PGA) syndrome type I: Response to cyclical steroid therapy. Clin Endocrinol 35:299–303, 1991.

152. Rabinowe SL, Berger M, Welch WR, Dluhy RG: Lymphocyte dysfunction in autoimmune oophoritis. Resumption of menses with corticosteroids. Am J Med 81:347–350, 1986.

153. Mayfield RK, Levine JH, Gordon C, et al: Lymphoid adenohypophysitis presenting as a pituitary tumour. Am J Med 69:619–623, 1980.

154. Sutherland DER: Current status of pancreas transplantation. J Clin Endocrinol Metab 73:461–463, 1991.

155. Ricordi C, Lacy PE, Santiago JV, et al: Transplantation of parathyroid, adrenal cortex and adrenal medulla using procedures which successfully prolonged islet allograft survival. Horm Metab Res (Suppl) 25:132–135, 1990.

156. Yu XC, Yu TL, Zhang SZ, et al: Homotransplantation of adrenal gland. Chin Med J (Engl) 104:487–490, 1991.

157. Stravinoha MW, Soloway RD: Current therapy of chronic liver disease. Drugs 39:814–840, 1990.

158. Chen QY, Lan MS, She JX, Maclaren N: The gene responsible for APS-1 maps to chromosome 21q22.3 in US patients. J Autoimmun 11 (2):177–183, 1998

159. Wang CY, Davoodi-Semiromi A, Huang W, et al: Charactorizations of mutations in patients with autoimmune polyglandular syndrome type-1 (APS1). Hum Gen 103 (6):681–685, 1998.

160. Halonen M, Eskelin P, Myhre AG, et al: AIRE gene mutations and human

leukocyte antigen genotypes as determinants of the autoimmune polyendocrinopathy-candidiasis-ectodermal dystrophy phenotype. J Clin Endocrinol Metab 87(6):2568–2574, 2002.

161. Adamson KA, Pearse SH, Lamb JR, et al: A comparative study of mRNA and protein expression of the autoimmune regulator gene (Aire) in embryonic and adult murine tissues. J Pathol 202(2):180–187, 2002.

162. Pitkanen J, Peterson P: Autoimmune regulator: From loss of function to autoimmunity. Genes Immun 4(1):12–21, 2003.

163. Kogawa K, Nagafuchi S, Katsuta H, et al: Expression of AIRE gene in peripheral monocyte/dendritic cell lineage. Immunol Lett 1:80(3):195–198 2002.

164. Ramsey C, Winquist O, Puhakka L, et al: Aire deficient mice develop multiple features of APECED phenotype and show altered immune response. Hum Mol Genet 11(4):397–409 2002.

165. Anderson MS, Venanzi ES, Klein L, et al: Projection of an immunological self shadow within the thymus y the aire protein. Science 298 (5597):1395–1401 2002.

166. Liston A, Lesage S, Wilson J, et al: Aire regulates negative selection of organ-specific T cells. Nat Immunol 4(4):303–304, 2003.

167. Uchida D, Hatakeyama S, Matsushima A, et al: AIRE functiond as an E3 ubiquitin ligase. J Exp Med 199(2):167–172 2004.

168. Sato K, Sato U, Tateishi S, et al: Are downregulates multiple molecules that have contradicting immune-enhancing and immune-suppressive functions. Biochem Biophys Res Commun 318(4):935–940 2004.

169. Kreigel MA, Lohmann T, Gabler C, et al: Defective suppressor function of human CD4+CD25+ regular T cells in autoimmune polyglandular syndrome type 11. J Exp Med 199(6):1285–1291 2004.

170. Vaidya B, Pearse S: The emerging roles of the CTLA-4 gene in autoimmune endocrinopathies. Eur J Endocrinol 150(5):619–626 2004.

171. Papadopoulos KI, Hornblad Y, Liljebladh H, Hallengren B: High frequency of endocrine autoimmunity in patients with sarcoidosis. Eur J Endocrinol 134(3):331–336 1996.

172. Kifor O, McElduff A, LeBoff MS, et al: Activating antibodies to the calcium sensing s receptor in two patients with autoimmune hypoparathyoidism. J Clin Endcrinol Metab 89(2):544–547 2004.

173. Kauffman RP, Castracane VD: Premature ovarian failure associated with autoimmune polyglandular syndrome: Pathophysiological mechanisms and future fertility. J Womans Health (Larchmt) 12(5):513–520, 2003.

174. Rose NR, Witebsky E: Studies on organ specificity: V. Changes in the thyroid gland of rabbits following active immunization with rabbit thyroid extracts. J Immunol 76:417–427, 1956.

175. Holborow EJ, Brown PC, Roitt IM, Doniach D: Cytoplasmic location of "complement-fixing" auto-antigen in human thyroid epithelium. Br J Pathol 40:583–588, 1959.

PART 7 OBESITY, ANOREXIA, AND NUTRITION

CHAPTER
42

Appetite Regulation and Thermogenesis

Eleftheria Maratos-Flier and Eric S. Bachman

INTRODUCTION

The classification of body weight as a regulated physiologic parameter is relatively novel. While obesity, including morbid obesity, has been recognized for thousands of years, the possibility that body weight was determined by a complex interaction between internal regulatory systems and the environment first received scientific attention in the mid-twentieth century. Studies of brain lesioned animals indicated that disruption of the ventromedial hypothalamus produced a syndrome of obesity and hyperphagia[2-4] while ablation of the lateral hypothalamus resulted in aphagia, adipsia, and dramatic weight loss[3,5] suggesting that these areas were critical to the maintenance of energy balance. Findings also emerged demonstrating that obesity could be caused by administration of goldthioglucose,[6] which damaged the ventromedial nucleus of the hypothalamus (VMH).[7] Subsequent studies using monosodium glutamate induced obesity indicated that the arcuate nucleus also played a role[8,9] in maintaining energy balance. A series of parabiosis experiments performed between genetically obese mice, *ob/ob* and *db/db*, mice suggested that circulating factors might play a role in determining adiposity.[10,11]

Despite significant efforts along these and other lines of investigation, which resulted in increased understanding of obesity, a full appreciation of obesity as an endocrine syndrome did not evolve until the discovery of leptin gene in 1994[12] and its receptor.[13] Mutations in either gene served to explain two mouse obesity syndromes: the *ob/ob* mouse, which lacks the hormone leptin, and the *db/db* mouse, which lacks the long form of the leptin receptor. These discoveries led to a significant paradigm shift in the understanding of obesity and the nature of the fat cell. Existence of a hormone specific obesity syndrome made it clear that body weight was subject to physiologic regulation. Furthermore, identification of the adipocyte as the source of the hormone changed the perception of the fat cell from that of a passive depot of energy stores to a regulator important to overall energy homeostasis.[14,15] This overall shift redefined understanding of the processes involved in regulating overall energy balance in mammalian organisms, including humans. As a consequence, a sophisticated understanding of the interconnection of multiple organ systems in the brain and periphery and their interaction with the environment is currently evolving.

Maintenance of normal weight requires balancing two components, energy intake and energy expenditure. While at first glance these seem to be simple parameters involving consumption and calorie utilization, both components are, in fact, complex.

COMPONENTS OF FEEDING

Intake of calories occurs for multiple reasons (Fig. 42-1). Perhaps the most important is the net caloric deficit that begins after the completion of a meal. As calories are used, the increasing deficit accrues and eventually leads to hunger, food seeking, and food ingestion. This component of feeding may be called "homeostatic hunger" because it reflects a true metabolic deficit and consumption is aimed at maintaining energy stores. Because this activity is critical to survival, it appears to be linked to reward pathways so that animals will "work" for food.[16] For example, feeding involves flavor and texture and thus engages gustatory pathways that involve taste and smell. The rewards associated with ingestion of palatable flavors lead to eating past the point of metabolic repletion.[17] Food variety also appears to engage reward pathways; increased variety prevents malnutrition. However, availability of increased variety of energy dense foods is associated with obesity.[18] Motivation and reward pathways have been extensively explored with regard to drug addiction. While addiction to drugs of abuse has no homeostatic value, reinforcement of food rewards may occur through similar pathways. For example, agents that alter opioid and dopaminergic signals also act to modulate motivation for palatable food.[19] Furthermore, eating is also linked to stress, which may predispose to hyperphagia in an environment where palatable food is readily available.[18]

COMPONENTS OF ENERGY EXPENDITURE

Traditional models categorize energy expenditure (EE) into basal (obligate) and adaptive (or facultative) thermogenesis (AT).[1] Obligate EE includes all pathways involved in the maintenance of basic metabolic and physiologic processes and is also referred to as resting metabolic rate (RMR). As arousal also contributes independently to energy expenditure, RMR includes both sleeping metabolic rate (SMR) and arousal. AT includes cold and diet-induced thermogenesis. Finally, physical activity represents a third category. The cellular mechanisms that regulate obligatory and adaptive thermogenesis

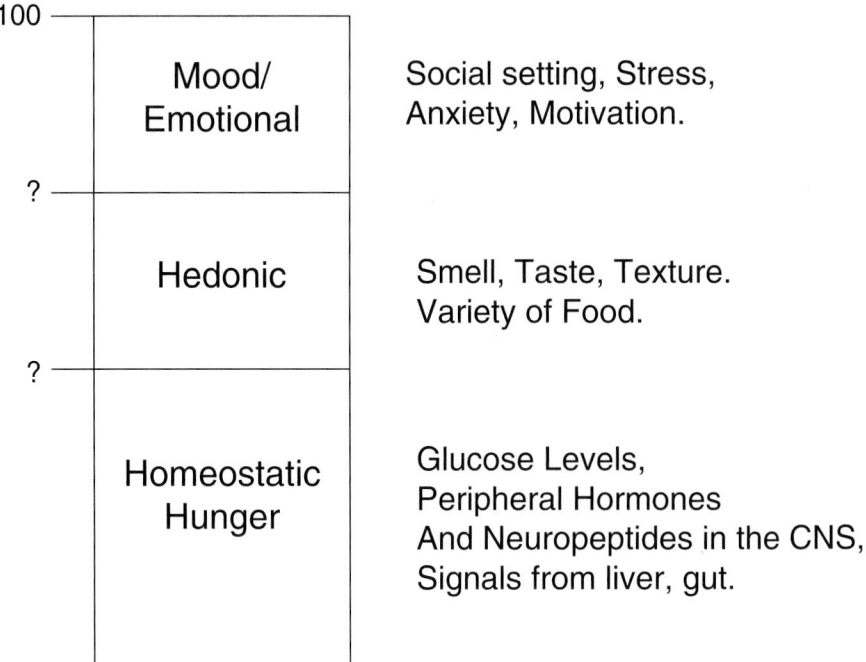

Figure 42-1 Components of eating behavior. Homeostatic hunger is hunger that results in eating in response to metabolic deficits and the ensuing signals. Hedonic and mood related eating lead to consumption of calories above what's necessary to maintain energy balance.

are often similar. These distinct categories of EE are, in fact, only approximate, and regulatory mechanisms are overlapping (Fig. 42-2). For example, thyroid hormone (TH) is required for up to 30% of basal EE, and adaptive increases in TH are required for normal cold-induced thermogenesis.[20,21] Furthermore, physical activity (PA) can have long-lasting effects on RMR[22] and PA may be enacted by stimuli that are traditionally considered stimulants of facultative thermogenesis, such as caloric excess.[23] Approximate contributions for the components of energy expenditure are RMR (70%), PA

(20%), and facultative (10%), with PA representing the most variable component.[24]

INTEGRATION OF ENERGY BALANCE

Inputs from a number of neuropeptides and neurotransmitters in the brain as well as peripheral signals integrate information to mediate energy balance. The interactions and pathways engaged by these signals are already complex,

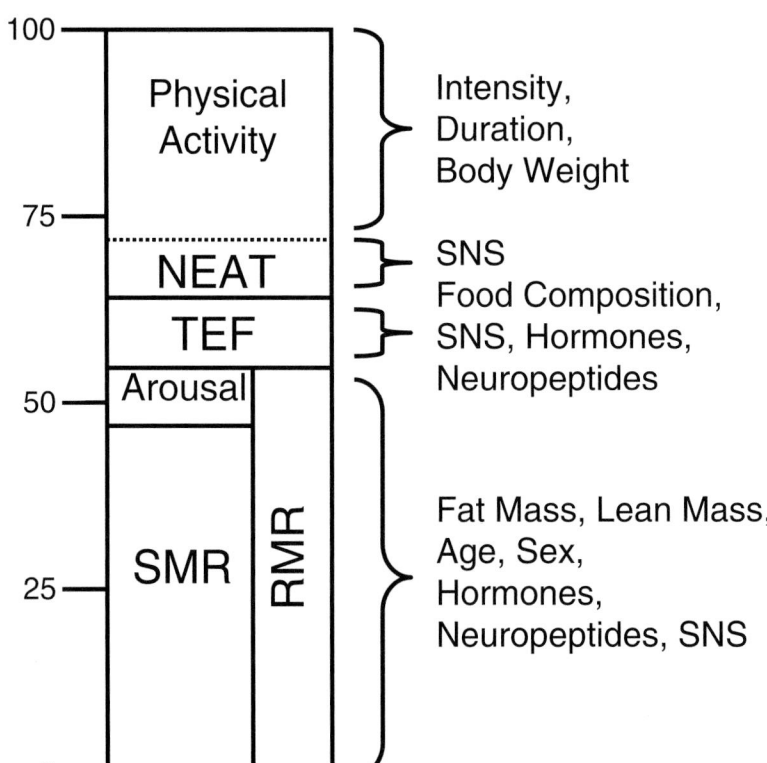

Figure 42-2 Approximate contribution of components of energy expenditure. Thermic effect of food (TEF) and resting metabolic rate (RMR) can be measured using a ventilatory hood. RMR and nonexercise activity thermogenesis (NEAT) can be measured in a respiratory chamber. Total energy expenditure can be measured using doubly labeled water. SMR, sleeping metabolic rate.

and understanding of the pathways is still evolving. Furthermore, it is not clear that all possible important signals have been identified. One interesting aspect of the signals involved is that many regulate both energy intake and energy expenditure in a coordinated fashion. Although a correlation of obesity with decreased sympathetic activity has been long recognized,[25] the potential pathways regulating energy expenditure were thought to be separate from those regulating feeding and satiety. However, it is now recognized that peptides regulating appetite also play a role in regulating energy expenditure in an inverse manner.[26] Thus, peptides that stimulate feeding decrease energy expenditure, promoting energy storage, while those that inhibit feeding increase energy expenditure (Table 42-1).

In the brain both neurotransmitters and neuropeptides play a complex role.[27] The role of neurotransmitters in regulating feeding behavior was recognized before the role of neuropeptides was appreciated. However, mechanisms of these neurotransmitters have been more difficult to define as these may act through multiple receptors and effects may vary depending on the anatomic area injected. Monoamine neurotransmitters may be stimulatory or inhibitory. Glutamate and gamma-aminobutyric acid, which are the most abundant neurotransmitters in the hypothalamus, act to increase feeding; some of the neurons expressing orexigenic neuropeptides appear to be Gabaergic.[28] One view of the interaction of transmitters and peptides is that peptides act as essential modulators of γ-aminobutyric acid (GABA) and glutamate action.[29] Serotonin is inhibitory.[30] The roles of epinephrine, norepinephrine, and dopamine are more complex, and these transmitters may act to either stimulate or inhibit feeding.[31] Although the mechanism of action is poorly understood, these pathways are the targets of the limited pharmacologic therapies that are currently available for the treatment of obesity. Biogenic amines currently in use include phentermine and sibutramine. Phentermine, an analogue of amphetamine, acts to increase catecholamine release in the paraventricular nucleus of the hypothalamus. Mazindol has a similar mechanism of action. Sibutramine, which acts through its active metabolites, prevents reuptake of 5-HT but does not cause release. Subtramine also inhibits noradrenaline reuptake (reviewed extensively in Ref. 32).

The number of hypothalamic neuropeptides known to be involved in body weight regulation has expanded dramatically over the past decade. Peptides that act as orexigenic signals include neuropeptide Y (NPY), agouti-relate peptide (AGRP), melanin-concentrating hormone (MCH), galanin, β-endorphin, dynorphin and enkephalin, and the orexins. Peptides that act to inhibit feeding include α-melanocyte-stimulating hormone

(α-MSH), cocaine-amphetamine responsive transcript (CART), corticotropin-releasing hormone, urocortin, neurotensin, and neuromedin. The specific role of neuropeptides has been easier to identify, in part, because expression of these peptides tends to be anatomically limited. Additionally, genetic studies are both easier and more readily interpretable as ablation is not usually associated with lethality.

Signals from a number of gut peptides add to the complex pathways involved in the regulation of body weight[33,34] (Fig. 42-3). Cholecystokinin (CCK) is synthesized in the duodenum and jejunum and was recognized as a peptide capable of inhibiting appetite as early as 1973.[35] CCK acts in the hindbrain to reduce meal size and duration (reviewed in Ref. 36). Peptide YY (PYY) is secreted by the distal portion of the gastrointestinal tract, in addition to inhibiting gastric emptying,[37] and also crosses the blood-brain barrier to act on arcuate nuclei and inhibit feeding.[33] However, the role of PYY remains controversial because when injected into the lateral ventricles of animals, PYY acts to increase food intake and not all investigators have been able to reproduce the satiety effects.[38] Glucagon-like peptide-1 (GLP-1) and oxyntomodulin are products of the preproglucagon gene and are synthesized in the gut and in the brain. Both act to inhibit food intake through different mechanisms.[39] Thus far, the only gut peptide known to stimulate appetite is ghrelin, which is secreted by the stomach and also acts on neurons in the arcuate nucleus.

Peripheral signals regarding the state of the gastrointestinal tract may also be integrated by the vagus nerve,[40,41] which sends afferents to multiple brain areas, including the dorsal motor nucleus and the nucleus of the solitary tract. These areas appear to be involved in responses to neuropeptides including ghrelin[42] and MSH.[43] The vagus may also play a role in conveying information on fatty acid oxidation in the liver. Fatty acid oxidation appears to play a role in mediating appetite as inhibition of this process is associated with increased appetite.[44,45]

Insulin may also play a role in inhibiting appetite, and it is known that neurons in the arcuate express insulin receptors[46] and respond to insulin. Female mice lacking insulin receptor expression in the brain eat more than normal animals and both genders develop mild obesity when placed on a high-fat diet.[47] Insulin and glucose may play a role in meal initiation and meal termination.[48]

Thus, body weight is regulated by a complex interaction of signals involving both the gut and the brain. Additional complexity derives from the fact that these signals act through specific receptors. The receptors have anatomic-specific expression.

Table 42-1	Genes Influencing Weight Control					
Gene	Model	Tissue	BW	FI	EE	Reference
Leptin	ob/ob	Adipose	↑	↑	↓	170
Leptin receptor	db/db	Brain	↑	↑	↓	171
MC4 receptor	MC4–/–	Brain	↑	↑	↓	79
MC3 receptor	MC3–/–	Brain	↔	↔	↑	172
Melanin Concentrating Hormone (MCH)	MCH–/–	Brain	↓		↑	89
GPR7	GPR7–/–	Brain	↑	↑	↓	173
Perilipin	P1–/–	Adipose	↓	↑	↑	174
ASP (C3)	C3–/–	Adipose	↓	↑	↑	175
Neuropeptides B and W	GPR7–/–	Brain	↑	↑	↓	173
Acetyl CoA Carboxylase	Acc 2–/–	Widely	↓	↑	↑	176
NO synthase	NOS–/–		↑	↔	↓	131
PKA RII beta	RII–/–	Adipose	↓	↔	↑	177
Beta adrenergic receptor	Beta AR 1,2,3 –/–	All	↑	↔	↓	141
Uncoupling protein	UCP1–/–	BAT	↔	↔	↔	178
Cidea	Cidea –/–	BAT	↔*	↔	↑	179
Stearoyl CoA desaturase	Scd –/–	Liver	↓	↑	↑	180

*Indicates lower body fat percentage compared to controls

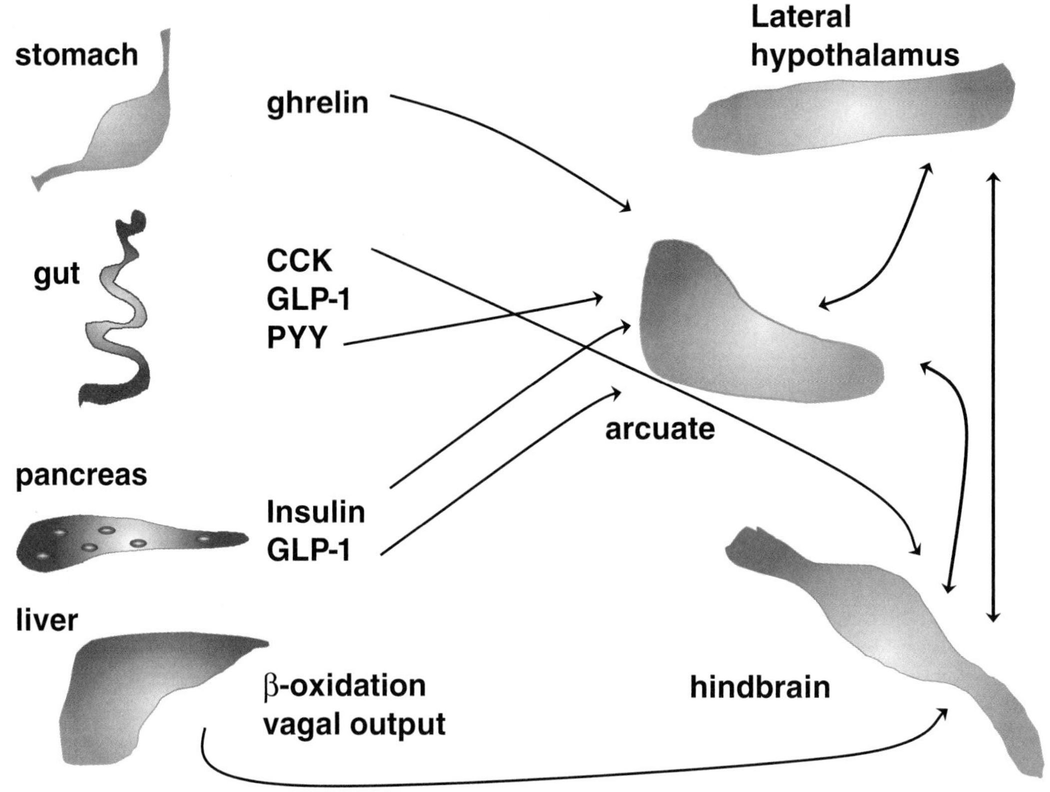

Figure 42-3 Schema of selected gut to brain signals that may play a role in mediating energy balance. A number of peptides from the gut play a role in mediating appetite and energy expenditure. Only one, ghrelin from the stomach, is orexigenic. All segments of the gut may also contribute to signals from vagal afferents. Finally, information of oxidation of fatty acids in the liver may also be transmitted by the vagus and play a role in mediating appetite. Within the brain signaling acquires additional complexity as networks between the hypothalamus and hindbrain and cortex are all involved in regulating both intake and output.

Furthermore, some involve relatively large receptor families as seen with the melanocortin receptors (see section "The Melanocortin System: α-MSH, Agouti-Related Peptide, and Central Melanocoritn Receptors"). For some of these pathways, the finding of spontaneous mutations in human populations associated with obesity has provided proof that body weight is regulated similarly in humans as in rodents (Table 42-2).

SPECIFIC HORMONES AND NEUROPEPTIDES

ADIPOSE TISSUE DERIVED

Leptin, identified through positional cloning of the *ob* gene,[12] is a 167-amino acid–peptide hormone secreted by adipocytes that signals through a membrane receptor that has six splice variants and belongs to the class I cytokine receptor family.[13] Leptin signaling is required, although not sufficient alone, for normal energy balance. Animals, including mice and humans, lacking leptin[49] or the leptin receptor[50] have a syndrome of severe hyperphagia and obesity. Leptin administration leads to a marked resolution of the syndrome in the case of leptin mutations in both *ob/ob* mice[51,52] and in rare human patients with leptin mutations.[53,54] However, in the vast majority of obese mammals, leptin levels are elevated, corre-

lating well with available fat stores, and administration of peripheral leptin has little effect on appetite. These findings revised the perception of leptin. While the complete absence of leptin has major consequences on appetite, the incremental increases in leptin that are seen with increased adiposity have little effect on the continued ingestion of calories or the storage of calories as fat. In contrast, repletion of leptin with fasting leads to attenuation of many of the neuroendocrine changes seen with fasting.[55] In human females, leptin replacement leads to some of the abnormalities seen in hypothalamic amenorhea secondary to strenuous exercise or low body weight.[56] Thus the critical physiologic role of leptin appears to be to signal caloric deficiency and thus mediate the appropriate metabolic changes rather than to signal caloric excess.

Leptin targets specific neurons in the brain, specifically in the hypothalamus. The best characterized neurons are the NPY/AGRP neurons and pro-opiomelanocortin (POMC) neurons in the arcuate.[28,57] NPY and AGRP are both orexigenic (appetite inducing) peptides, which are synthesized by the same population of neurons. POMC is expressed in a different population of arcuate neurons, which process the preprohormone to a number of peptides, including MSH, which acts to suppress appetite. To date, the leptin to arcuate pathway represents the best characterized pathway involved in the regulation of body weight, especially as mutations disrupting this pathway have also been shown to be important in human obesity as well as rodent obesity (Fig. 42-4).

Adipocytes synthesize many biologically active proteins with potential endocrine function (reviewed in Ref. 58). These include cytokines, immune-related proteins, complement and complement-related proteins, enzymes involved in steroid metabolism, and proteins of the rennin-angiontensin system. Furthermore, receptors for traditional endocrine hormones, nuclear hormones, cytokines, and catecholamines are all expressed by adipose tissue These peptides are likely to form causal links between obesity and insulin resistance and cardiovascular disease. Two recently discovered peptides, adiponectin and resistin, may play a role in modulating insulin resistance. Adiponectin inversely correlates with insulin resist-

Table 42-2	Sample of Characterized Mutations Leading to Obesity in Humans
Mutation	**Reference**
Leptin	49, 181
Leptin receptor	50
Melanocortin 4 receptor	81, 82, 182
Melanocortin 3 receptor	183
Prohormone convertase 1	184
PPAR-γ	185
POMC	83

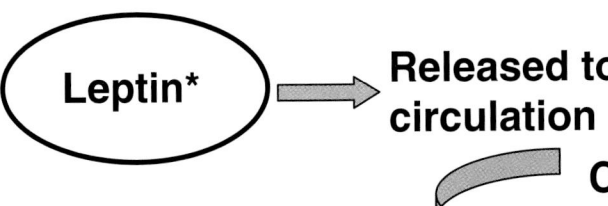
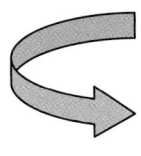
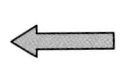
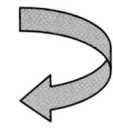
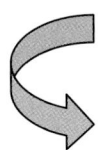

Leptin*

Released to circulation

Cross blood brain Barrier to act on neurons In arcuate nucleus through leptin receptor*

Act on MC4-R* And MC3R*

Stimulate POMC Neurons, ↑α-MSH*

Decrease feeding and Increase energy expenditure

Figure 42-4 The Leptin Pathway. Leptin is a hormone secreted by adipocytes which crosses the blood brain barrier to act on neurons in the arcuate. One set of target neurons are those synthesizing prepro-opiomelanocortin (POMC). Leptin acts to stimulate these neurons to synthesize POMC and release one of the POMC gene products, α-MSH. This peptide mainly acts through the melanocortin-4 receptor to decrease feeding and through this receptor and the melanocortin-3 receptor to increase energy expenditure. Mutations in this pathway lead to disruption of the appropriate signals and to obesity. Known mutations leading to obesity in humans are marked with asterisks. (See text and Table 42-2 for details.)

ance, declines with obesity, and increases with weight loss.[59] In contrast, resistin impairs glucose tolerance and insulin sensitivity, and secretion increases with increasing adiposity.[60] They may also be involved in determining predisposition to obesity and responses to a high-fat diet. Recently, excess adiposity has been associated with finding increased expression of multiple inflammatory markers in fat tissue. Thus, expression of interleukin-1 (IL-1), IL-5, plasminogen activator inhibitor-1 (PAI-1), tumor necrosis factor (TNF), and suppressor of cytokine signaling 3 (SOCS3) are all increased in obesity. These factors play a role in the decrease in insulin sensitivity associated with obesity; however, it is unclear, and seems unlikely, that any of these factors have direct effects on either appetite or energy expenditure.

THE HYPOTHALAMUS

Neuropeptide Y

The potential role of neuropeptides in feeding behavior was first suggested by studies indicating that neuropeptide Y (NPY) was synthesized by arcuate[61] neurons and elicited a robust feeding response when injected intracerebroventricularly (ICV).[62–64] Chronic infusion of NPY leads to obesity in rats.[65,66] Furthermore, expression of NPY increases with fasting, indicating that neurons making NPY respond to peripheral signals, signaling the state of energy balance.[67,68] Interestingly, ablation of the NPY gene was not associated with altered body weight or feeding,[69] although when mice lacking NPY were bred to mice lacking leptin, substantial attenuation of the *ob/ob* obesity syndrome was noted.[70] However, animals without NPY show an abnormal response to refeeding after short-term fasting[71] and also show an attenuated feeding response to hypoglycemia.[72]

The Melanocortin System: α-MSH, Agouti-Related Peptide, and Central Melanocoritn Receptors

Humans and rodents require an intact melanocortin system in order to maintain normal body weight. The effect of α-MSH to decrease appetite was described in the late 1980s.[73] However,

the key role of melanocortins in the physiology of energy balance was not appreciated until the molecular mechanism of obesity of the yellow A^y mouse was identified. In this model, obesity is secondary to a mutation in the gene encoding a protein, agouti, which mediates coat color and leads to ectopic expression of the protein in all tissues, including the central nervous system (CNS).[74] Subsequently, it was discovered that agouti protein acted on melanocortin receptors to block melanocyte-stimulating hormone (MSH) action.[75,76] These findings led to the speculation that another protein, normally expressed in the brain, might have an action similar to that of agouti and to the discovery of agouti-related peptide (AgRP),[77] which is expressed in the hypothalamus and interacts with the central melanocortin receptors MC3R and MC4R.[78] Overexpression of AgRP recapitulated an obesity syndrome similar to that seen in the A^y mouse as did disruption of the MC4 receptor.[79] Mice with targeted disruption of the MC3 receptor demonstrated a small increase in body fat and feeding efficiency, suggesting that, at least in rodents, MC4 plays the dominant role in energy homeostasis.

The profound effects caused by disruption of the melanocortin pathway stimulated a search of MC4 receptor mutations in humans, especially in children with early onset obesity and a strong family history of obesity. Several such mutations were readily identified[80,81] and currently it is estimated that 5% of persons with severe, familial, early-onset obesity have abnormal MC4 mutations.[82] In humans, obesity has also been associated with mutations in the POMC gene, which encodes multiple transcripts. Disruption of this gene leads to deficiency in both adrenocorticotropic hormone (ACTH) and MSH, and patients present with adrenal insufficiency and obesity. Since MSH expression outside of the central nervous system mediates hair color, patients with POMC mutations will frequently also have red hair.[83]

Melanin-Concentrating Hormone

Melanin-concentrating hormone is a 19-amino acid peptide synthesized in magnocellular neurons of the lateral hypothalamus that plays a key role in maintaining energy balance in rodents and sheep.[84] The peptide structure and anatomical distribution is highly conserved and the sequence is identical in rodents, sheep, and humans. When ICV is injected in rats, MCH induces an acute increase in feeding behavior. Chronic infusions in mice lead to a syndrome of mild obesity associated with decreased energy expenditure.[85] Deletion of both the MCH and the MCH-receptor gene are associated with leanness.[86–88] In the case of the receptor knockouts, leanness is secondary to increased expenditure as animals without the receptor eat as much or more as wild-type animals. Deletion of MCH from mice lacking leptin leads to a marked attenuation of the obesity phenotype, which is secondary to changes in energy expenditure rather than feeding.[89] Pharmacologic blockade of the MCH receptor leads to leanness[90] and reduces meal size.[91] Chronic infusions of MCH agonists also lead to obesity similar to that seen with MCH infusion.[92] The importance of the MCH system has not been validated in humans as a phenotype of MCH deficiency would present with a lean phenotype. However, the homology of MCH in all strains of mammals examined strongly suggests that MCH will play a role in humans.

THE GUT

Ghrelin

Ghrelin, produced in the stomach, was identified as the endogenous ligand for the receptor responsible for growth hormone secretion.[93] Subsequently, it was found to produce adiposity in rodents, an effect that is independent of its ability to stimulate growth hormone secretion.[94] Although infusions of ghrelin induce hunger and increased feeding[95] endogenous levels are low in obese individuals and increase with weight loss.[96] This rise is not seen after gastric bypass surgery, which may help to explain the success of this procedure in mediating weight loss in obese humans.[97,98] Ghrelin levels are extremely high in the Prader-Willi syndrome of genetic obesity.[99] Ghrelin is transported into the grain where it acts to stimulate NPY/AGRP neurons in the arcuate nucleus and is thus part of a circuit mediating energy homeostasis involving the stomach and the hypothalamus.[100]

Peptide YY (PYY)

PYY is synthesized and secreted throughout the intestine, although concentrations are higher in the distal portion, particularly in the colon and rectum and the 3-36 form crosses the blood-brain barrier. Food intake stimulates PYY release, and higher serum concentrations are seen after fatty meals. As release occurs prior to the nutrients reaching the distal parts of the gastrointestinal tract, neural reflexes may act to stimulate release, possibly through the vagus. PYY 1-36 has structural similarity to NPY and binds with high affinity to all five NPY receptors; the 3-36 form binds preferentially to the Y_2 receptor. PYY acts on both the intestine and the brain. In the intestine it increases fluid absorption and delays gastric emptying. In the brain the 3-36 form has substantial effects on appetite. When given intravenously to human volunteers it reduces caloric intake and increases the sensation of satiety.[101] Similar effects have been reported in rats[102]; however, this effect is controversial because other investigators have been unable to reproduce the satiating effect.[38] ICV injection of PYY clearly increases feeding, presumably through targeting a different receptor subset.[103]

PYY levels are low in patients with morbid obesity. One report suggests that levels rise after weight loss secondary to gastric bypass surgery.[104] This suggests a potential role of PYY in the treatment of obesity.

GLP-1 and Oxyntomodulin

GLP-1 and oxyntomodulin, along with GLP-2, are products of the preproglucagon gene and result from posttranslational processing by prohormone convertases. The preproglucagon gene is expressed in the central nervous system, in intestinal

L cells, and in the pancreas. Both GLP-1 and oxyntomodulin act as satiety signals[39,105,106] through the GLP-1 receptor. Release from the small intestine is seen after food ingestion; however, the peptides are rapidly cleaved by dipeptidyl peptidase IV and thus have a short half-life. GLP-2 does not affect satiety.[107] GLP-1 has effects on insulin secretion and beta cell mass, while GLP-2 affects the growth of intestinal epitheal cells.[108] GLP-1 has therapeutic potential in the treatment of obesity and type 2 diabetes, although this could be limited because of the short half-life.

THE ROLE OF ENERGY EXPENDITURE IN BODY WEIGHT REGULATION

MEASURING ENERGY EXPENDITURE

Measuring ingested food is straightforward, at least in experimental animals. However, measuring energy expenditure is complicated because one must account for all components. In order to determine the relative contribution of EE for body weight (BW) regulation, accurate techniques must be available to measure EE. The most accurate method for determination of EE is by direct calorimetry, which can be measured either by water immersion or closed chamber heat convection. Doubly labeled water ingestion, in which EE can be interpolated from the amount of $^2H_2^{18}O$ ingested and the amount of ^2H and ^{18}O released as water and carbon dioxide, has been shown to be accurate to within 5% of indirect calorimetry.[109] As stated, more than 90% of oxygen consumption arises from mitochondrial metabolism.[110] Given this fact, and the ease of measuring EE indirectly via O_2 consumption, indirect calorimetry methods have been widely used. Many indirect calorimeters calculate an approximate mass-independent EE by incorporating VO_2, VCO_2, RER, and protein catabolism as the Weir equation does, whereas other investigators normalize EE for the approximate tissue contributions to overall metabolic rate.[111]

Comparing Energy Expenditure between Individual Subjects
Using indirect calorimetry to compare EE among organisms that differ in BW and composition has inherent inaccuracies. Frst, most rodent models of obesity are hyperphagic, and differences in food intake introduces profound effects on physiology that lead to altered BW and nutrient status. Differences in BW are often due to differences in adipose tissue, which has a lower EE, so many investigators normalize VO_2 for BW or, preferably, lean body mass that more closely reflects total EE.[112] In order to control for this confounder, therefore, many investigators measure EE by indirect calorimetry as above and/or perform pair feeding experiments. Thus, when two groups of animals are fed the same amount of food and one group loses more weight, the only conclusions that can be drawn are that the lighter group either had greater EE or more digestive losses. An example of pair-feeding (PF) is shown in Figure 42-5.[113] The PF paradigm has numerous flaws, however, possibly due to a relative state of semistarvation that is perceived by PF animals. For example, compared to leptin-treated rats that have decreased food intake, PF rats are relatively hypothyroid due to decreased hepatic conversion of T4-T3.[114] In summary, in order to demonstrate changes in EE between subjects, the following conditions should ideally be met:

1. EE is measured directly.
2. Indirect measures of EE are performed between weight- and body composition–matched animals.
3. Careful PF experiments demonstrate clear differences between experimental subjects. Otherwise, normalizing to BW or scaling does not provide the best estimates of EE.

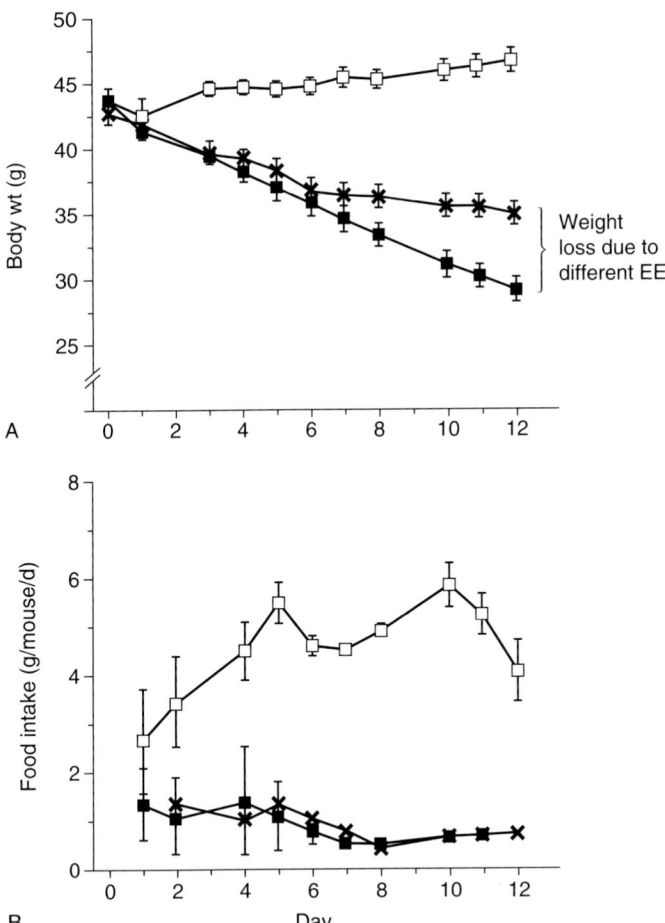

Figure 42-5 Pair feeding in *ob/ob* mice results in less weight loss, implying increased energy expenditure (EE) from leptin treatment. Leptin-deficient, *ob/ob* mice are hyperphagic *(control open squares)*, and respond to leptin treatment by reducing food intake and increasing EE. The increased BW loss in the *ob/ob* leptin-treated group *(closed squares)* compared to the pair-fed group is due to increased EE. (After Levin N, Nelson C, Gurney A, et al: Decreased food intake does not completely account for adiposity reduction after ob protein infusion. Proc Natl Acad Sci U S A 93:1726–1730, 1996.)

DOES LOW ENERGY EXPENDITURE CONTRIBUTE TO OBESITY?

Small discrepancies between energy intake and EE over a long time can result in net positive energy balance and obesity. For example, the current epidemic of obesity could be stabilized by lowering food intake by 100 kcal/day according to one estimate.[115] When one asks whether decreased EE plays a causal role in obesity, compared to increased food intake, the answer is that on an absolute scale, obese patients have increased EE. Thus, only relative differences in EE might account for predisposition to obesity. Evidence exists both to support and refute an important role for abnormal EE in human obesity.

Numerous studies have been performed to support the hypothesis that reduced EE plays a pathogenic role in the development of obesity. Early studies, based on the comparison of self-reported food diaries to weight gain, suggested that obese patients have significantly lower EE compared to lean patients. However, these differences could not be confirmed in studies using the doubly labeled water technique,[109,116] and differences were attributed to under-reporting of food consumption. Nonetheless, there is compelling evidence that lower EE and predisposition to obesity is

genetically determined. For example, resting metabolic rate is a highly inherited trait, and is independent of fat-free mass, age, and sex as a predictor of EE.[117] Overfeeding studies in monozygotic twins show a high degree of similarity in weight gain between but not among twins and also argue strongly that genetic factors play a major role in controlling EE.[118] Also, the environment in which indentical twins are raised has little influence over eventual body mass index (BMI).[119] Finally, direct and indirect measurements of EE and respiratory quotient (RQ) have shown small, but measurable, differences between obese and lean patients, particularly in certain ethnic groups, such as Pima Indians.[120,121] Longitudinal studies have confirmed that differences in EE are associated with tendency to develop obesity over a period of years.[122]

In contrast, other studies failed to find significant differences in EE between obese and lean human patients. For example, EE increases linearly with increasing BMI, and so increased EE at higher BW would function to resist further BW change.[24] Similarly, children ages 5 to 10 with varying known susceptibility to obesity have similar increases in RMR.[123] Furthermore, no differential activity between lean and obese individuals in systems regulating body weight has been reported; this includes sympathetic nervous system (SNS) nerve activity,[124] catecholamine turnover,[125] lipolysis,[126] the thermic effect of food,[24] and thyroid hormones.[127] In summary, some studies have reported data to support the hypothesis that relatively low EE contributes to the development of obesity. These findings, in addition to clear defects in EE that are seen in obese rodent models, suggest that defects in EE may be attractive targets for antiobesity treatments.

THE MITOCHONDRION IS THE MAJOR ORGANELLE THAT GENERATES ENERGY EXPENDITURE

The majority of EE in eukaryotic cells is generated by oxidative phosphorylation in mitochondria, which are the major source of cellular adenosine triphosphate (ATP). Using mitochondrial inhibitors, it has been shown that oxidative phosphorylation in mitochondria accounts for 90% of energy expenditure.[110] Metabolic fuels are converted to reducing equivalents (NADH, FADH$_2$), which donate electrons to the electron transport chain (Fig. 42-6). Transfer of electrons through the electron transport chain in mitochondria is coupled to proton translocation across the inner mitochondrial membrane, mediated by complexes I, III, and IV and creation of an electrochemical proton gradient ($\Delta\psi$m). The energy derived from protons reentering the matrix can be captured by complex V (ATPase), which catalyzes the phosphorylation of ADP from inorganic phosphate, forming ATP and water.[128] In summary, oxidative phosphorylation is a tightly coupled series of reactions that allow cells to synthesize ATP from metabolic fuels.

The transfer of energy through the electron transport chain in mitochondria presents many opportunities for the control of EE. Proton leak across the mitochondrial membrane, for example, is a major pathway that regulates EE and has received enormous attention for its potential role in regulating EE and BW. The electrochemical gradient across the inner mitochondrial membrane ($\Delta\psi$m; see Fig. 42-6) allows protons to reenter mitochondria through ATPase, as above, or in a manner that is not coupled (uncoupled) to ATP synthesis.[129] This can occur either via specific uncoupling proteins (UCPs) or nonspecific membrane leak. The finding that certain tissues, especially brown adipose tissue (BAT), possess a unique, inducible UCP that lowers the mitochondrial membrane potential has led to great excitement that such a mechanism regulates EE and BW specifically in mammals.[130] Altered EE then could theoretically be controlled in numerous ways in mitochondria, including changes in UCP levels, UCP activity, or via wholesale changes in mitochondrial protein levels,

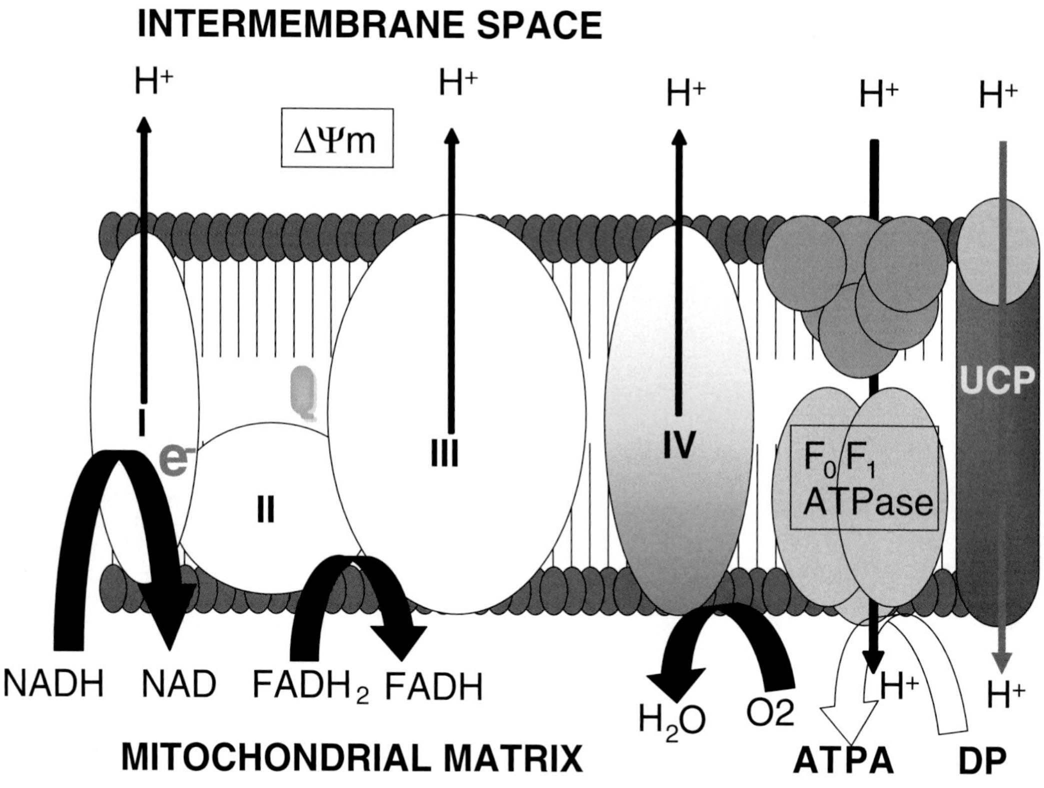

INTERMEMBRANE SPACE

Figure 42-6 Mitochondrial Respiration. Reducing equivalents (NADH, FADH$_2$) from glucose and fatty acid metabolism donate electrons to the electron transport chain in the inner mitochondrial membrane, resulting in proton (H) transport and a protonmotive, electrochemical gradient ($\Delta\psi$m). The energy from the proton gradient can result in ATP synthesis via F$_0$F$_1$ ATPase, or protons can reenter the mitochondrial matrix via specific (uncoupling proteins) or nonspecific pathways, thereby generating heat. UCP, uncoupling protein; I, II, III, IV, electron transport complexes; Q, coenzyme Q.

biogenesis, and electron transport.[15] Defective mitochondrial biogenesis, for example, has recently been shown to affect EE and BW regulation.[131]

MECHANISMS THAT REGULATE ENERGY EXPENDITURE

Evidence That Mechanisms Involving Energy Expenditure Exist to Resist Body Weight Change

Very small discrepancies in energy balance (1%) can result in fat accumulation over time; this has led to the idea that fundamental physiologic mechanisms maintain BW within a narrow "set point." This model predicts that animals can adapt to changes in food intake by altering energy expenditure to maintain a constant body weight (Fig. 42-7). Thus, in an environment of ready access to highly palatable food, overeating might not occur. If overeating occurred, various mechanisms would increase energy expenditure and compensate for the excess calories. The fact that a substantial portion of human populations (30% to 40% in Western countries) resists obesity and that, similarly, certain strains of rodents also resist obesity indicates that the set point is intact for at least some individuals. On the other hand, the fact that many individuals and experimental animals can be made obese simply by making palatable food available indicates that the "set point" frequently fails.

Susceptibility to obesity in humans and rodents is both highly variable and inheritable, supporting the theory that physiologic mechanisms exist to regulate EE and, when impaired, result in decreased EE and obesity.[118,119,132] Some of the pathways involved in regulating EE have been defined. Numerous neurohumoral and physiologic changes occur in response to increased or decreased BW after overfeeding.[133] For example, overfeeding human subjects results in increased SNS activity, decreased parasympathetic nervous system (PNS) activity, and an inferred form of PA known as nonexercise activity thermogenesis (NEAT) (Fig. 42-8). As discussed above, the fact that all models of obesity, as well as obese human sub-

jects, have elevated leptin levels suggests that leptin may not function to signal fat excess but, rather, starvation.

The very existence of specific antiobesity mechanisms in mammals has been questioned because of the following observations:

1. Mammals are more likely to have had to adapt evolutionarily to caloric deficit rather than surfeit.
2. Almost all obese mammals show resistance to high levels of leptin.
3. Numerous, redundant mechanisms exist that stimulate food intake.[134] This argument, called the thrifty gene hypothesis, states that humans have evolved mechanisms for storing rather than expending calories.[135,136]

In fact, leptin is much more potent in its lower physiological range than its higher range, as seen in most obese rodents and humans, arguing that the role of leptin is to signal declining adipose stores.[114,137] Thus, mechanisms to control obesity would not have evolved. Hence, lack of protective mechanisms to resist obesity, including decreased EE combined with caloric excess found in Western diets, has promoted our current obesity epidemic.

Others propose that specific thermogenic mechanisms (dietary induced thermogenesis, DIT) have evolved in mammals to allow consumption of large quantities of low-quality diets and waste the additional calories via increased EE in order to obtain sufficient amino acids.[138,139] The phenomenon of DIT has been demonstrated in BAT in numerous studies.[140] Recently, DIT in rodents was shown to be a critically important antiobesity mechanism, especially in response to caloric excess.[141] The role of DIT in humans remains a critical question that will greatly influence approaches to treating obesity.[141]

Physical Activity

Physical activity (PA) is the most variable component of daily EE, ranging from nearly zero kcal/day in sedentary adults to

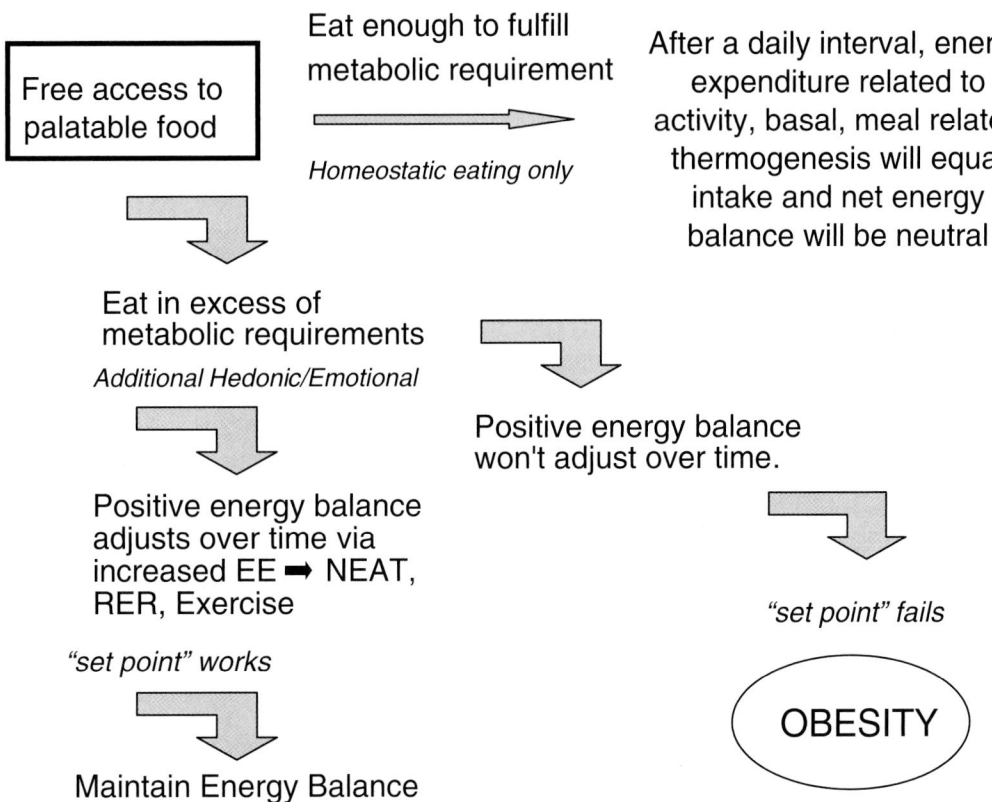

Figure 42-7   In an environment where there is free access to palatable food some individuals will eat largely in response to homeostatic hunger; that is, they will largely consume calories necessary to sustain metabolic and physical activity. At the beginning of each day they will be in neutral energy balance with respect to the previous day. These individuals are represented in the 30% to 40% of Western populations who maintain normal body weight (or if overweight, are able to maintain a stable weight over a long period of time). Some individuals will eat an excess number of calories beyond what is necessary to sustain metabolic requirements. This extra eating will occur in response to the setting that the food is served or to the hedonic aspects of the food. Some of these individuals will utilize a limited number of the extra calories by adjustments in resting metabolic rate or small changes in the thermic effect of food or nonexercise activity thermogenesis (NEAT). Some individuals may also adapt consciously by increasing physical activity, thereby "assisting" their set point. These individuals will also be represented in a group that maintains stable body weight over a long period of time. In contrast some individuals will overeat. Overeating may be involve small caloric increments that, for unclear reasons, the individual cannot make adquate adjustments for through increased resting metabolic rate (RMR) or NEAT. Some overeating may involve a large number of calories, the utilization of which would require increased physical activity or diet. Over time, these individuals will gain weight. While the rate of weight gain may be slow (2 to 3 pounds each year over decades), weight gain can be substantial resulting in obesity. RER, respiratory exchange ratio.

thousands of kcal/day in endurance athletes. PA has effects on EE both acutely, with large increases in maximal oxygen consumption, and chronically, via improved respiratory capacity. Thus, PA represents an ideal mechanism to resist obesity in the setting of increased food intake. Only 10% of the variability in human BW is estimated to be due to differences in PA, however.[142] Studies in Pima Indian children ages 5 to 10 have shown a negative relationship between PA and eventual obesity, but PA was not predictive.[123,143] Other studies have shown decreased PA but no change in overall EE between lean and obese adolescents.[144] Coordinated PA is a complex behavior that is regulated by numerous mechanisms at multiple sites in the CNS. Recently, the demonstration that PA is regulated via specific neuropeptides in specific sites in the CNS, such as the leptin and melanocortin pathways, suggest that PA is a component of the "adipostatic" system.[23] For example, administration of leptin to *ob/ob* mice causes increased activity before BW changes. Also, mice lacking MC4R not only consume more calories, but fail to enact PA on running wheels in response to caloric excess.[23] Physical activity clearly increases EE, and can alter RMR in the postexercise period as well. In humans, sustained weight loss is most successful with a combination of decreased food intake and

PA.[145] Further, investigation into the regulation of PA as a specific mechanism to control body fat stores will clearly be of great importance in the field of obesity.

NEAT may be an important mediator of increased EE with increasing BW. Careful overfeeding studies in lean humans showed that the majority of increased EE in response to caloric excess occurs not via increases in thermic effect of food, RMR, or coordinated PA, but rather, most likely, in NEAT.[146] While formally a subclass of PA, NEAT includes all tasks of daily living, including posture, fidgeting, and even chewing gum.[147] NEAT can be accurately measured by sensors in humans and rodents.[148] At least a portion of increased EE in hyperthyroidism is attributable to increase in NEAT.[149]

Thyroid Hormone

The critical role of thyroid hormone (including thyroxine [T_4] and triiodothyronine [T_3]) in obligatory EE and AT is well-documented, although TH is not believed to play a specific role in BW homeostasis. This conclusion is based on the observation that, despite profound effects on overall EE, (1) deficiency of TH results in only mild obesity and lipid accumulation[150]; (2) thyroid dysfunction is not associated with many models of obesity that are characterized by low EE;

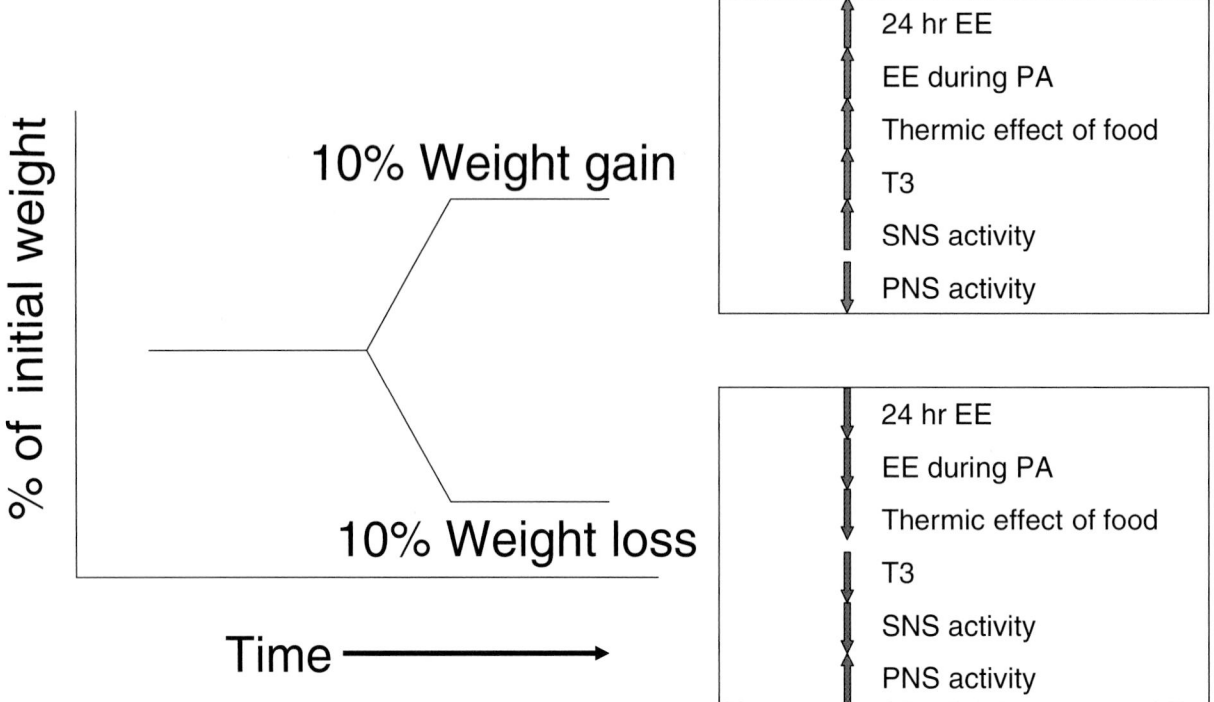

Figure 42-8 Physiological changes that accompany weight gain and loss in mammals. EE, energy expenditure; PA, physical activity; T_3, thyroid hormone (triiodothyronine); SNS, sympathetic nervous system; PNS, parasympathetic nervous system. (Adapted from Rosenbaum M, Leibel RL, Hirsch J: Obesity. N Engl J Med 337:396–406, 1997.)

and (3) although complete lack of both TH receptors (TR-α and TR-β) results in postnatal lethality, none of the individual knockout animals develops obesity.[151] The detailed biology of thyroid hormone action is discussed in Chapter 96.

Approximately 30% of basal thermogenesis is TH mediated.[21] In fact, the hypothyroidism was formerly diagnosed by whole body oxygen consumption prior to the availability of biochemical tests of for pituitary thyroid-stimulating hormone (TSH) and serum TH. In mammals, the main function of thyroid hormone is to maintain temperature homeostasis and not adipose stores.[21] Numerous diverse pathways, including anabolic and catabolic metabolism of lipids, carbohydrates, and proteins, are stimulated in response to TH (reviewed in Ref. 21). Also, the increase in ATP turnover and heat are probably derived from the baseline increase in flux of many cellular pathways, such as the maintenance of ion gradients, ion cycling, and uncoupling, the sum of which is to increase EE.[152] Noting that the level of T_4 sufficiency, as measured by TSH, correlates well with EE, resting EE changes by only 15% over a 200-fold change in TSH.[153]

Clinical syndromes of TH excess result in clear increases in EE that can result in loss of BW, although this loss derives from adipose as well as protein tissues.[154] Moreover, even though hyperthyroidism and syndromes of catecholamine excess resemble one another clinically, the effects on metabolism and cardiovascular function are independent.[155] Specific effects of TH on BW have been suggested by the presence of type 2 deiodinase (D2) in BAT, which converts T_4 into its more active congener T_3,[156] and is under control by the SNS.[157] In BAT, D2 has been shown to be necessary for cold-induced AT.[20,158] Furthermore, failure to induce D2 activity in response to cold is observed in obesity-prone, βAR-less mice.[141] However, loss of function of D2 via gene disruption has no demonstrable effect on BW in mice, suggesting that this enzyme is not necessary for normal BW regulation.[159] Also,

lack of TH does not affect DIT, BW, or BAT biochemical parameters in response to high-fat feeding.[160] Nonetheless, stimulation of EE via agonists that are specific for TR-β is a current approach to obesity.

Sympathetic Nervous System and Adrenergic Receptors

A wealth of literature supports a role for the SNS in the regulation of BW via control of EE. More specifically, lower baseline SNS activity can be associated with propensity for future weight gain.[161,162] The SNS is controlled by the CNS, and postganglionic neurons release either norepinephrine (sympathetic) or acetylcholine (parasympathetic) from their terminals (reviewed in Ref. 162). A popular model for regulation of EE in response to caloric excess is as follows: brain → SNS → βARs → thermogenesis (Fig. 42-9). Indeed, low SNS activity is seen in most obese rodent models, and activation of this pathway by βAR agonists is effective in reducing obesity.[163,164] Numerous attempts to perturb SNS function (surgical, chemical, immunological, genetic) had not affected BW, however, and thus the importance of SNS-mediated DIT lacked support.[165–168] Ablation of all 3 βARs (β-less) in mice results in a phenotype of obesity that appears to be due purely to a decrease in EE.[141] Thus, β-less mice are mildly obese on a regular diet, but become massively obese when challenged with a high-fat diet. The normal response (increased VO_2) to a high-fat diet seen in wild-type mice is completely absent in β-less mice, demonstrating that βARs are required for obesity resistance and DIT. While defects in BAT function are clear in β-less mice, the tissues that mediate DIT are not known at this time.[155,169]

SUMMARY

Body weight is regulated by a complex system that involves both multiple organs from the periphery and the

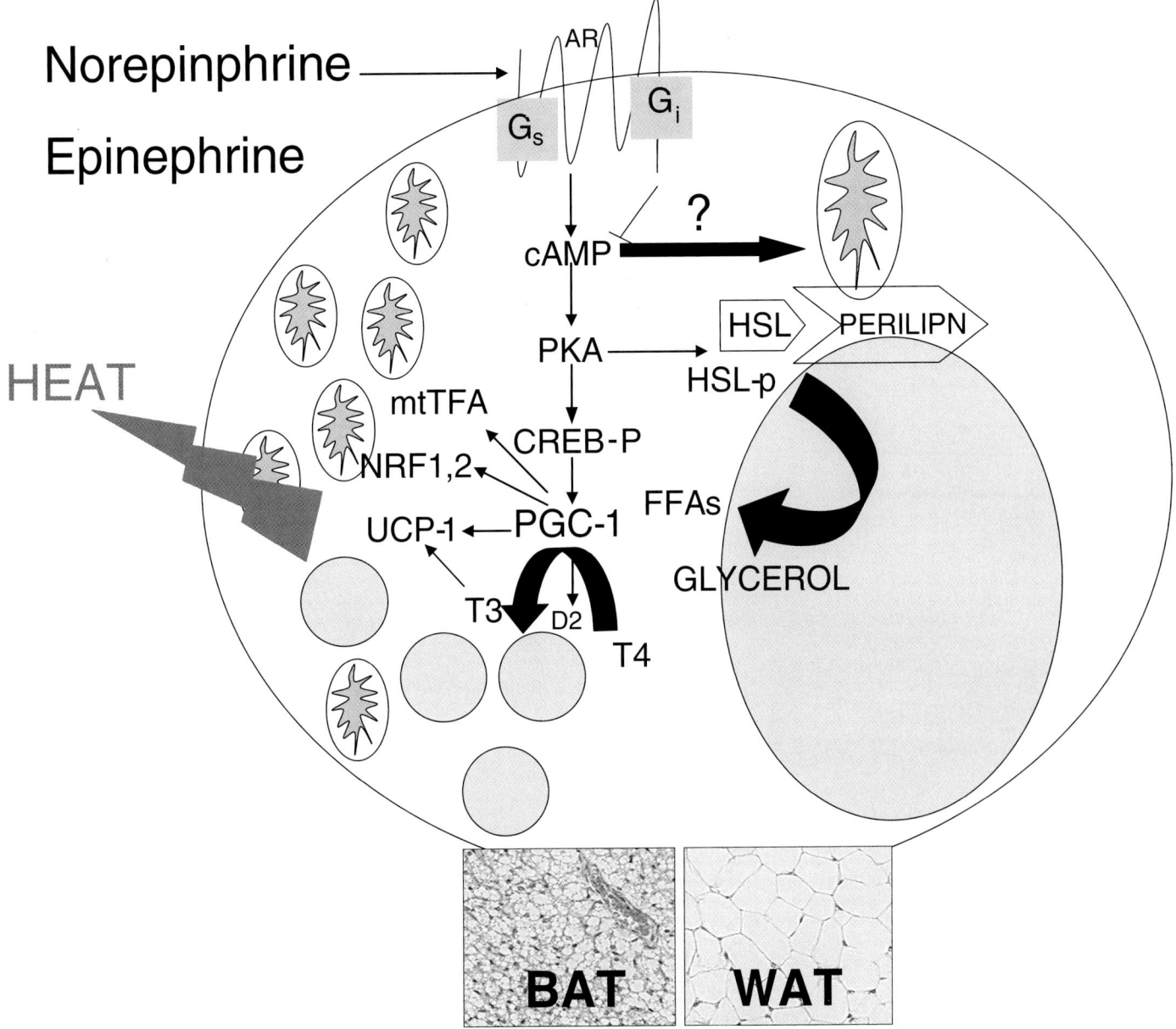

Figure 42-9 βAR-mediated signaling in adipose tissues. AR, adrenergic receptors; G$_i$ and G$_s$, G-coupled protein receptors; PKA, protein kinase A; CREB-P, phosphorylated cAMP-responsive transcription factor; PGC-1, PPAR gamma coactivator-1; D2, type 2 deiodinase; T$_4$ and T$_3$, thyroid hormone; UCP, uncoupling protein; NRF, nuclear respiratory factors; mtTFA, mitochondrial transcription factor A; FFA, free fatty acids; HSL, hormone sensitive lipase; BAT, brown adipose tissue; WAT, white adipose tissue.

brain. The system is coordinated by molecules and neuronal networks that integrate food intake with energy expenditure. Despite significant progress, the nature of these pathways is still poorly understood. It is clear that disruption of key pathways results in obesity in both rodents and humans.

REFERENCES

1. Weir JB: New methods for calculating metabolic rate with special reference to protein metabolism. Nutrition 6:213–221, 1949.
2. Hetherington AW, Ranson SW: Hypothalamic lesions and adiposity in the rat. Anat Rec 78:149–172, 1940.
3. Anand BK, Brobeck JR: Localization of a "feeding center" in the hypothalamus on the rat. Proc Soc Exper Biol Med 77:323–324, 1951.
4. Mayer J, Barrnett RJ: Obesity following unilateral hypothalamic lesions in rats. Science 121:599–600, 1955.
5. Morrison SD, Mayer J: Adipsia and aphagia in rats after lateral subthalamic lesions. Am J Physiol 191:248–254, 1957.
6. Owen JA Jr, Parson W, Crispell KR: Dietary dilution studies in gold thioglucose induced obesity in the mouse. Metabolism 2:362–366, 1953.
7. Debons AF, Krimsky I, From A, Cloutier RJ: Site of action of gold thioglucose in the hypothalamic satiety center. Am J Physiol 219:1397–1402, 1970.
8. Nemeroff CB, Lipton MA, Kizer JS: Models of neuroendocrine regulation: Use of monosodium glutamate as an investigational tool. Dev Neurosci 1:107–109, 1978.
9. Dawson R, Pellenmoshter MA, Millard WJ, et al: Attenuation of leptin-mediated effects by monosodium-induced arcuat nucleus

damage. Am J Physiol 273: E202–E209, 1997.

10. Coleman DL: Effects of parabiosis of obese with diabetes and normal mice. Diabetologia 9:294–298, 1973.

11. Coleman DL, Hummel KP: Effects of parabiosis of normal with genetically diabetic mice. Am J Physiol 217:1298–1304, 1969.

12. Zhang Y, Proenca R, Maffei M, et al: Positional cloning of the mouse obese gene and its human homologue [published erratum appears in Nature 30:374(6521):479, 1995 (see comments)]. Nature 372:425–432, 1994.

13. Tartaglia LA, Dembski M, Weng X, et al: Identification and expression cloning of a leptin receptor, OB-R. Cell 83:1263–1271, 1995.

14. Flier JS: The adipocyte: Storage depot or node on the energy information superhighway? Cell 80:15–18, 1995.

15. Spiegelman BM, Flier JS: Obesity and the regulation of energy balance. Cell 104:531–543, 2001.

16. Saper CB, Chou TC, Elmquist JK: The need to feed: Homeostatic and hedonic control of eating. Neuron 36:199–211, 2002.

17. Yeomans MR, Blundell JE, Leshem M: Palatability: response to nutritional need or need-free stimulation of appetite? Br J Nutr 92(Suppl 1):S3–S14, 2004.

18. Kennedy E: Dietary diversity, diet quality, and body weight regulation. Nutr Rev 62:S78–S81, 2004.

19. Zhang M, Balmadrid C, Kelley AE: Nucleus accumbens opioid, GABAergic, and dopaminergic modulation of palatable food motivation: contrasting effects revealed by a progressive ratio study in the rat. Behav Neurosci 117:202–211, 2003.

20. de Jesus LA, Carvalho SD, Ribeiro MO, et al: The type 2 iodothyronine deiodinase is essential for adaptive thermogenesis in brown adipose tissue. J Clin Invest 108:1379–1385, 2001.

21. Silva JE: The thermogenic effect of thyroid hormone and its clinical implications. Ann Intern Med 139:205–213, 2003.

22. Speakman JR, Selman C: Physical activity and resting metabolic rate. Proc Nutr Soc 62:621–634, 2003.

23. Butler AA, Marks DL, Fan W, et al: Melanocortin-4 receptor is required for acute homeostatic responses to increased dietary fat. Nat Neurosci 4:605–611, 2001.

24. Ravussin E, Swinburn BA: Pathophysiology of obesity. Lancet 340:404–408, 1992.

25. Bray GA: 1989 McCollum Award lecture. Genetic and hypothalamic mechanisms for obesity—finding the needle in the haystack. Am J Clin Nutr 50:891–902, 1989.

26. Bray GA: Reciprocal relation of food intake and sympathetic activity: Experimental observations and clinical implications. Int J Obes Relat Metab Disord 24(Suppl 2):S8–S17, 2000.

27. Kalra SP, Dube MG, Pu S, et al: Interacting appetite-regulating pathways in the hypothalamic regulation of body weight [In Process Citation]. Endocr Rev 20:68–100, 1999.

28. Cowley MA, Smart JL, Rubinstein M, et al: Leptin activates anorexigenic POMC neurons through a neural network in the arcuate nucleus. Nature 411:480–484, 2001.

29. van den Pol AN: Weighing the role of hypothalamic feeding neurotransmitters. Neuron 40:1059–1061, 2003.

30. Blundell JE: Serotonin and appetite. Neuropharmacology 23:1537–1551, 1984.

31. Leibowitz SF: Brain monoamines and peptides: Role in the control of eating behavior. Fed Proc 45:1396–1403, 1986.

32. Clapham JC, Arch JR, Tadayyon M: Anti-obesity drugs: A critical review of current therapies and future opportunities. Pharmacol Ther 89:81–121, 2001.

33. Halatchev IG, Ellacott KL, Fan W, Cone RD: Peptide YY3-36 inhibits food intake in mice through a melanocortin-4 receptor-independent mechanism. Endocrinology 145:2585–2590, 2004.

34. Woods SC: Gastrointestinal satiety signals I. An overview of gastrointestinal signals that influence food intake. Am J Physiol Gastrointest Liver Physiol 286:G7–G13, 2004.

35. Gibbs J, Young RC, Smith GP: Cholecystokinin elicits satiety in rats with open gastric fistulas. Nature 245:323–325, 1973.

36. Moran TH, Kinzig KP: Gastrointestinal satiety signals II. Cholecystokinin. Am J Physiol Gastrointest Liver Physiol 286:G183–G188, 2004.

37. Moran TH, Smedh U, Kinzig KP, et al: Peptide YY (3-36) inhibits gastric emptying and produces acute reductions in food intake in rhesus monkeys. Am J Physiol Regul Integr Comp Physiol, 2004.

38. Tschop M, Castaneda TR, Joost HG, et al: Physiology: Does gut hormone PYY3-36 decrease food intake in rodents? Nature 430:1 p following 165; discussion 162 p following 165, 2004.

39. Baggio LL, Huang Q, Brown TJ, Drucker DJ: Oxyntomodulin and glucagon-like peptide-1 differentially regulate murine food intake and energy expenditure. Gastroenterology 127:546–558, 2004.

40. Inui A, Asakawa A, Bowers CY, et al: Ghrelin, appetite, and gastric motility: The emerging role of the stomach as an endocrine organ. FASEB J 18:439–456, 2004.

41. Thorens B, Larsen PJ: Gut-derived signaling molecules and vagal afferents in the control of glucose and energy homeostasis. Curr Opin Clin Nutr Metab Care 7:471–478, 2004.

42. Williams DL, Grill HJ, Cummings DE, Kaplan JM: Vagotomy dissociates short- and long-term controls of circulating ghrelin. Endocrinology 144:5184–5187, 2003.

43. Williams DL, Kaplan JM, Grill HJ: The role of the dorsal vagal complex and the vagus nerve in feeding effects of melanocortin-3/4 receptor stimulation. Endocrinology 141:1332–1337, 2000.

44. Friedman MI, Harris RB, Ji H, et al: Fatty acid oxidation affects food intake by altering hepatic energy status. Am J Physiol 276:R1046–R1053, 1999.

45. Horn CC, Ji H, Friedman MI: Etomoxir, a fatty acid oxidation inhibitor, increases food intake and reduces hepatic energy status in rats. Physiol Behav 81:157–162, 2004.

46. Marks JL, Porte D Jr, Stahl WL, Baskin DG: Localization of insulin receptor mRNA in rat brain by in situ hybridization. Endocrinology 127:3234–3236, 1990.

47. Bruning JC, Gautam D, Burks DJ, et al: Role of brain insulin receptor in control of body weight and reproduction. Science 289:2122–2125, 2000.

48. Woods SC, Schwartz MW, Baskin DG, Seeley RJ: Food intake and the regulation of body weight. Annu Rev Psychol 51:255–277, 2000.

49. Farooqi S, Rau H, Whitehead J, O'Rahilly S: Ob gene mutations and human obesity. Proc Nutr Soc 57:471–475, 1998.

50. Clement K, Vaisse C, Lahlou N, et al: A mutation in the human leptin receptor gene causes obesity and pituitary dysfunction [see comments]. Nature 392:398–401, 1998.

51. Halaas JL, Gajiwala KS, Maffei M, et al: Weight-reducing effects of the plasma protein encoded by the obese gene [see comments]. Science 269:543–546, 1995.

52. Stephens TW, Basinski M, Bristow PK, et al: The role of neuropeptide Y in the antiobesity action of the obese gene product. Nature 377:530–532, 1995.

53. Farooqi IS, Jebb SA, Langmack G, et al: Effects of recombinant leptin therapy in a child with congenital leptin deficiency. N Engl J Med 341:879–884, 1999.

54. Farooqi IS, Matarese G, Lord GM, et al: Beneficial effects of leptin on obesity, T cell hyporesponsiveness, and neuroendocrine/metabolic dysfunction of human congenital leptin deficiency. J Clin Invest 110:1093–1103, 2002.

55. Ahima RS, Prabakaran D, Mantzoros C, et al: Role of leptin in the neuroendocrine response to fasting. Nature 382:250–252, 1996.

56. Welt CK, Chan JL, Bullen J, et al: Recombinant human leptin in women with hypothalamic amenorrhea. N Engl J Med 351:987–997, 2004.

57. Elias CF, Aschkenasi C, Lee C, et al: Leptin differentially regulates NPY and POMC neurons projecting to the lateral hypothalamic area. Neuron 23:775–786, 1999.

58. Kershaw EE, Flier JS: Adipose tissue as an endocrine organ. J Clin Endocrinol Metab 89:2548–2556, 2004.

59. Nawrocki AR, Scherer PE: The delicate balance between fat and muscle:

Adipokines in metabolic disease and musculoskeletal inflammation. Curr Opin Pharmacol 4:281–289, 2004.

60. Steppan CM, Lazar MA: The current biology of resistin. J Intern Med 255:439–447, 2004.

61. Chronwall BM: Anatomy and physiology of the neuroendocrine arcuate nucleus. Peptides 6(Suppl 2):1–11, 1985.

62. Stanley BG, Leibowitz SF: Neuropeptide Y injected in the paraventricular hypothalamus: A powerful stimulant of feeding behavior. Proc Natl Acad Sci U S A 82:3940–3943, 1985.

63. Stanley BG, Chin AS, Leibowitz SF: Feeding and drinking elicited by central injection of neuropeptide Y: Evidence for a hypothalamic site(s) of action. Brain Res Bull 14:521–524, 1985.

64. Allen LG, Kalra PS, Crowley WR, Kalra SP: Comparison of the effects of neuropeptide Y and adrenergic transmitters on LH release and food intake in male rats. Life Sci 37:617–623, 1985.

65. Beck B, Stricker-Krongrad A, Nicolas JP, Burlet C: Chronic and continuous intracerebroventricular infusion of neuropeptide Y in Long-Evans rats mimics the feeding behaviour of obese Zucker rats. Int J Obes Relat Metab Disord 16:295–302, 1992.

66. Zarjevski N, Cusin I, Vettor R, et al: Chronic intracerebroventricular neuropeptide-Y administration to normal rats mimics hormonal and metabolic changes of obesity. Endocrinology 133:1753–1758, 1993.

67. Billington CJ, Briggs JE, Harker S, et al: Neuropeptide Y in hypothalamic paraventricular nucleus: A center coordinating energy metabolism. Am J Physiol 266:R1765–R1770, 1994.

68. Wilding JP, Gilbey SG, Bailey CJ, et al: Increased neuropeptide-Y messenger ribonucleic acid (mRNA) and decreased neurotensin mRNA in the hypothalamus of the obese (ob/ob) mouse. Endocrinology 132:1939–1944, 1993.

69. Erickson JC, Clegg KE, Palmiter RD: Sensitivity to leptin and susceptibility to seizures of mice lacking neuropeptide Y [see comments]. Nature 381:415–421, 1996.

70. Erickson JC, Hollopeter G, Palmiter RD: Attenuation of the obesity syndrome of ob/ob mice by the loss of neuropeptide Y [see comments]. Science 274:1704–1707, 1996.

71. Segal-Lieberman G, Trombly DJ, Juthani V, et al: NPY ablation in C57BL/6 mice leads to mild obesity and to an impaired refeeding response to fasting. Am J Physiol Endocrinol Metab 284:E1131–E1139, 2003.

72. Sindelar DK, Ste Marie L, Miura GI, et al: Neuropeptide Y is required for hyperphagic feeding in response to neuroglucopenia. Endocrinology 145:3363–3368, 2004.

73. Tsujii S, Bray GA: Acetylation alters the feeding response to MSH and beta-endorphin. Brain Res Bull 23:165–169, 1989.

74. Miller MW, Duhl DM, Vrieling H, et al: Cloning of the mouse agouti gene predicts a secreted protein ubiquitously expressed in mice carrying the lethal yellow mutation. Genes Dev 7:454–467, 1993.

75. Michaud EJ, Bultman SJ, Klebig ML, et al: A molecular model for the genetic and phenotypic characteristics of the mouse lethal yellow (Ay) mutation. Proc Natl Acad Sci U S A 91:2562–2566, 1994.

76. Yen TT, Gill AM, Frigeri LG, et al: Obesity, diabetes, and neoplasia in yellow A(vy)/-mice: Ectopic expression of the agouti gene. FASEB J 8:479–488, 1994.

77. Shutter JR, Graham M, Kinsey AC, et al: Hypothalamic expression of ART, a novel gene related to agouti, is up-regulated in obese and diabetic mutant mice. Genes Dev 11:593–602, 1997.

78. Tota MR, Smith TS, Mao C, et al: Molecular interaction of Agouti protein and Agouti-related protein with human melanocortin receptors. Biochemistry 38:897–904, 1999.

79. Huszar D, Lynch CA, Fairchild-Huntress V, et al: Targeted disruption of the melanocortin-4 receptor results in obesity in mice. Cell 88:131–141, 1997.

80. Yeo GS, Farooqi IS, Aminian S, et al: A frameshift mutation in MC4R associated with dominantly inherited human obesity [letter]. Nat Genet 20:111–112, 1998.

81. Vaisse C, Clement K, Guy-Grand B, Froguel P: A frameshift mutation in human MC4R is associated with a dominant form of obesity [letter]. Nat Genet 20:113–114, 1998.

82. Vaisse C, Clement K, Durand E, et al: Melanocortin-4 receptor mutations are a frequent and heterogeneous cause of morbid obesity. J Clin Invest 106:253–262, 2000.

83. Krude H, Biebermann H, Luck W, et al: Severe early-onset obesity, adrenal insufficiency and red hair pigmentation caused by POMC mutations in humans. Nat Genet 19:155–157, 1998.

84. Qu D, Ludwig DS, Gammeltoft S, et al: A role for melanin-concentrating hormone in the central regulation of feeding behaviour. Nature 380:243–247, 1996.

85. Ito M, Gomori A, Ishihara A, et al: Characterization of MCH-mediated obesity in mice. Am J Physiol Endocrinol Metab 284:E940–E945, 2003.

86. Shimada M, Tritos NA, Lowell BB, et al: Mice lacking melanin-concentrating hormone are hypophagic and lean. Nature 396:670–674, 1998.

87. Marsh DJ, Weingarth DT, Novi DE, et al: Melanin-concentrating hormone 1 receptor-deficient mice are lean, hyperactive, and hyperphagic and have altered metabolism. Proc Natl Acad Sci U S A 99:3240–3245, 2002.

88. Chen Y, Hu C, Hsu CK, et al: Targeted disruption of the melanin-concentrating hormone receptor-1 results in hyperphagia and resistance to diet-induced obesity. Endocrinology 143:2469–2477, 2002.

89. Segal-Lieberman G, Bradley RL, Kokkotou E, et al: Melanin-concentrating hormone is a critical mediator of the leptin-deficient phenotype. Proc Natl Acad Sci U S A 100:10085–10090, 2003.

90. Borowsky B, Durkin MM, Ogozalek K, et al: Antidepressant, anxiolytic and anorectic effects of a melanin-concentrating hormone-1 receptor antagonist. Nat Med 8:825–830, 2002.

91. Astrand A, Bohlooly YM, Larsdotter S, et al: Mice lacking the Melanin Concentrating Hormone Receptor 1 demonstrate increased heart rate associated with altered autonomic activity. Am J Physiol Regul Integr Comp Physiol, 2004.

92. Shearman LP, Camacho RE, Sloan Stribling D, et al: Chronic MCH-1 receptor modulation alters appetite, body weight and adiposity in rats. Eur J Pharmacol 475:37–47, 2003.

93. Kojima M, Hosoda H, Date Y, et al: Ghrelin is a growth-hormone-releasing acylated peptide from stomach. Nature 402:656–660, 1999.

94. Tschop M, Smiley DL, Heiman ML: Ghrelin induces adiposity in rodents. Nature 407:908–913, 2000.

95. Wren AM, Seal LJ, Cohen MA, et al: Ghrelin enhances appetite and increases food intake in humans. J Clin Endocrinol Metab 86:5992, 2001.

96. Cummings DE, Shannon MH: Roles for ghrelin in the regulation of appetite and body weight. Arch Surg 138:389–396, 2003.

97. Tritos NA, Mun E, Bertkau A, et al: Serum ghrelin levels in response to glucose load in obese subjects post-gastric bypass surgery. Obes Res 11:919–924, 2003.

98. Cummings DE, Weigle DS, Frayo RS, et al: Plasma ghrelin levels after diet-induced weight loss or gastric bypass surgery. N Engl J Med 346:1623–1630, 2002.

99. Haqq AM, Stadler DD, Rosenfeld RG, et al: Circulating ghrelin levels are suppressed by meals and octreotide therapy in children with Prader-Willi syndrome. J Clin Endocrinol Metab 88:3573–3576, 2003.

100. Cowley MA, Smith RG, Diano S, et al: The distribution and mechanism of action of ghrelin in the CNS demonstrates a novel hypothalamic circuit regulating energy homeostasis. Neuron 37:649–661, 2003.

101. Batterham RL, Le Roux CW, Cohen MA, et al: Pancreatic polypeptide reduces appetite and food intake in humans. J Clin Endocrinol Metab 88:3989–3992, 2003.

102. Batterham RL, Cowley MA, Small CJ, et al: Gut hormone PYY(3-36) physiologically inhibits food intake. Nature 418:650–654, 2002.

103. Tang-Christensen M, Vrang N, Ortmann S, et al: Central administration of ghrelin and agouti-related protein (83-132) increases food intake and decreases spontaneous locomotor activity in rats. Endocrinology 145:4645–4652, 2004.

104. Alvarez Bartolome M, Borque M, Martinez-Sarmiento J, et al: Peptide YY secretion in morbidly obese patients before and after vertical banded gastroplasty. Obes Surg 12:324–327, 2002.

105. Flint A, Raben A, Astrup A, Holst JJ: Glucagon-like peptide 1 promotes satiety and suppresses energy intake in humans. J Clin Invest 101:515–520, 1998.

106. Gutzwiller JP, Goke B, Drewe J, et al: Glucagon-like peptide-1: A potent regulator of food intake in humans. Gut 44:81–86, 1999.

107. Schmidt PT, Naslund E, Gryback P, et al: Peripheral administration of GLP-2 to humans has no effect on gastric emptying or satiety. Regul Pept 116:21–25, 2003.

108. Brubaker PL, Drucker DJ: Minireview: Glucagon-like peptides regulate cell proliferation and apoptosis in the pancreas, gut, and central nervous system. Endocrinology 145:2653–2659, 2004.

109. Ravussin E, Harper IT, Rising R, et al: Energy expenditure by doubly labeled water: Validation in lean and obese subjects. Am J Physiol 261:E402–E409, 1991.

110. Rolfe DF, Brown GC: Cellular energy utilization and molecular origin of standard metabolic rate in mammals. Physiol Rev 77:731–758, 1997.

111. Bosy-Westphal A, Eichhorn C, Kutzner D, et al: The age-related decline in resting energy expenditure in humans is due to the loss of fat-free mass and to alterations in its metabolically active components. J Nutr 133:2356–2362, 2003.

112. Ravussin E, Lillioja S, Anderson TE, et al: Determinants of 24-hour energy expenditure in man. Methods and results using a respiratory chamber. J Clin Invest 78:1568–1578, 1986.

113. Levin N, Nelson C, Gurney A, et al: Decreased food intake does not completely account for adiposity reduction after ob protein infusion. Proc Natl Acad Sci U S A 93:1726–1730, 1996.

114. Cusin I, Rouru J, Visser T, et al: Involvement of thyroid hormones in the effect of intracerebroventricular leptin infusion on uncoupling protein-3 expression in rat muscle. Diabetes 49:1101–1105, 2000.

115. Hill JO, Wyatt HR, Reed GW, et al: Obesity and the environment: where do we go from here? Science 299:853–855, 2003.

116. Livingstone MB: Assessment of food intakes: are we measuring what people eat? Br J Biomed Sci 52:58–67, 1995.

117. Bogardus C, Lillioja S, Ravussin E, et al: Familial dependence of the resting metabolic rate. N Engl J Med 315:96–100, 1986.

118. Bouchard C, Tremblay A, Despres JP, et al: The response to long-term overfeeding in identical twins. N Engl J Med 322:1477–1482, 1990.

119. Stunkard AJ, Harris JR, Pedersen NL, et al: The body-mass index of twins who have been reared apart. N Engl J Med 322:1483–1487, 1990.

120. Zurlo F, Lillioja S, Esposito-Del Puente A, et al: Low ratio of fat to carbohydrate oxidation as predictor of weight gain: study of 24-h RQ. Am J Physiol 259:E650–E657, 1990.

121. Tataranni PA, Harper IT, Snitker S, et al: Body weight gain in free-living Pima Indians: effect of energy intake vs expenditure. Int J Obes Relat Metab Disord 27:1578–1583, 2003.

122. Ravussin E, Lillioja S, Knowler WC, et al: Reduced rate of energy expenditure as a risk factor for body-weight gain. N Engl J Med 318:467–472, 1988.

123. Salbe AD, Weyer C, Harper I, et al: Assessing risk factors for obesity between childhood and adolescence: II. Energy metabolism and physical activity. Pediatrics 110:307–314, 2002.

124. Scherrer U, Randin D, Tappy L, et al: Body fat and sympathetic nerve activity in healthy subjects. Circulation 89:2634–2640, 1994.

125. Rumantir MS, Vaz M, Jennings GL, et al: Neural mechanisms in human obesity-related hypertension. J Hypertens 17:1125–1133, 1999.

126. Jansson PA, Larsson A, Smith U, et al: Glycerol production in subcutaneous adipose tissue in lean and obese humans. J Clin Invest 89:1610–1617, 1992.

127. Kokkoris P, Pi-Sunyer FX: Obesity and endocrine disease. Endocrinol Clin North Am 32:895–914, 2003.

128. Mitchell P, Moyle J: Chemiosmotic hypothesis of oxidative phosphorylation. Nature 213:137–139, 1967.

129. Rousset S, Alves-Guerra MC, Mozo J, et al: The biology of mitochondrial uncoupling proteins. Diabetes 53 (Suppl 1):S130–S135, 2004.

130. Nicholls DG: A history of UCP1. Biochem Soc Trans 29:751–755, 2001.

131. Nisoli E, Clementi E, Paolucci C, et al: Mitochondrial biogenesis in mammals: the role of endogenous nitric oxide. Science 299:896–899, 2003.

132. Saad MF, Alger SA, Zurlo F, et al: Ethnic differences in sympathetic nervous system-mediated energy expenditure. Am J Physiol 261:E789–E794, 1991.

133. Rosenbaum M, Leibel RL, Hirsch J: Obesity. N Engl J Med 337:396–407, 1997.

134. Schwartz MW, Woods SC, Seeley RJ, et al: Is the energy homeostasis system inherently biased toward weight gain? Diabetes 52:232–238, 2003.

135. Ravussin E, Bogardus C: Energy expenditure in the obese: is there a thrifty gene? Infusionstherapie 17:108–112, 1990.

136. Neel JV: The "thrifty genotype" in 1998. Nutr Rev 57:S2–S9, 1999.

137. Ahima RS, Kelly J, Elmquist JK, et al: Distinct physiologic and neuronal responses to decreased leptin and mild hyperleptinemia. Endocrinology 140:4923–4931, 1999.

138. Rothwell NJ, Stock MJ: A role for brown adipose tissue in diet-induced thermogenesis. Nature 281:31–35, 1979.

139. Stock MJ: Gluttony and thermogenesis revisited. Int J Obes Relat Metab Disord 23:1105–1117, 1999.

140. Glick Z, Teague RJ, Bray GA: Brown adipose tissue: thermic response increased by a single low protein, high carbohydrate meal. Science 213:1125–1127, 1981.

141. Bachman ES, Dhillon H, Zhang CY, et al: betaAR signaling required for diet-induced thermogenesis and obesity resistance. Science 297:843–845, 2002.

142. Ravussin E, Bogardus C: Energy balance and weight regulation: genetics versus environment. Br J Nutr 83 (Suppl 1):S17–S20, 2000.

143. Salbe AD, Weyer C, Harper I, et al: Relation between physical activity and obesity. Am J Clin Nutr 78:193–194; author reply 194–195, 2003.

144. Ekelund U, Aman J, Yngve A, et al: Physical activity but not energy expenditure is reduced in obese adolescents: a case-control study. Am J Clin Nutr 76:935–941, 2002.

145. Jakicic JM: Exercise in the treatment of obesity. Endocrinol Metab Clin North Am 32:967–980, 2003.

146. Levine JA, Eberhardt NL, Jensen MD: Role of nonexercise activity thermogenesis in resistance to fat gain in humans. Science 283:212–214, 1999.

147. Levine J, Baukol P, Pavlidis I: The energy expended in chewing gum. N Engl J Med 341:2100, 1999.

148. Levine J, Melanson EL, Westerterp KR, et al: Measurement of the components of nonexercise activity thermogenesis. Am J Physiol Endocrinol Metab 281:E670–E675, 2001.

149. Levine JA, Nygren J, Short KR, et al: Effect of hyperthyroidism on spontaneous physical activity and energy expenditure in rats. J Appl Physiol 94:165–170, 2003.

150. Larsen PR, Davies TF: Hypothyroidism and thyroiditis. In Williams Textbook of Endocrinology. P.R. Larsen, H.M. Kronenberg, S. Melmed, and K. Polonsky, editors. Philadelphia, Saunders, pp 423–457, 2003.

151. Gauthier K, Chassande O, Plateroti M, et al: Different functions for the thyroid hormone receptors TRalpha and TRbeta in the control of thyroid hormone production and post-natal development. Embo J 18:623–631, 1999.

152. Lebon V, Dufour S, Petersen KF, et al: Effect of triiodothyronine on mitochondrial energy coupling in human skeletal muscle. J Clin Invest 108:733–737, 2001.

153. al-Adsani H, Hoffer LJ, Silva JE: Resting energy expenditure is sensitive to small dose changes in patients on chronic thyroid hormone replacement. J Clin Endocrinol Metab 82:1118–1125, 1997.

154. Larsen PR, Davies TF: Thyrotoxicosis. In Williams Textbook of Endocrinology. P.R. Larsen, H.M. Kronenberg, S. Melmed, and K. Polonsky, editors. Philadelphia, Saunders, 2003, pp 374–421.

155. Bachman ES, Hampton TG, Dhillon H, et al: The metabolic and cardiovascular effects of hyperthyroidism are largely independent of beta-adrenergic stimulation. Endocrinology 145:2767–2774, 2004.

156. Leonard JL, Mellen SA, Larsen PR: Thyroxine 5′-deiodinase activity in brown adipose tissue. Endocrinology 112:1153–1155, 1983.

157. Silva JE, Larsen PR: Adrenergic activation of triiodothyronine production in brown adipose tissue. Nature 305:712–713, 1983.

158. Ribeiro MO, Carvalho SD, Schultz JJ, et al: Thyroid hormone—sympathetic interaction and adaptive thermogenesis are thyroid hormone receptor isoform—specific. J Clin Invest 108:97–105, 2001.

159. Schneider MJ, Fiering SN, Pallud SE, et al: Targeted disruption of the type 2 selenodeiodinase gene (DIO2) results in a phenotype of pituitary resistance to T4. Mol Endocrinol 15:2137–2148, 2001.

160. Curcio C, Lopes AM, Ribeiro MO, et al: Development of compensatory thermogenesis in response to overfeeding in hypothyroid rats. Endocrinology 140:3438–3443, 1999.

161. Tataranni PA, Young JB, Bogardus C, et al: A low sympathoadrenal activity is associated with body weight gain and development of central adiposity in Pima Indian men. Obes Res 5:341–347, 1997.

162. Snitker S, Macdonald I, Ravussin E, et al: The sympathetic nervous system and obesity: Role in aetiology and treatment. Obes Rev 1:5–15, 2000.

163. Arch JR, Ainsworth AT, Cawthorne MA, et al: Atypical beta-adrenoceptor on brown adipocytes as target for anti-obesity drugs. Nature 309:163–165,1984.

164. Himms-Hagen J, Cui J, Danforth E, Jr, et al: Effect of CL-316,243, a thermogenic beta 3-agonist, on energy balance and brown and white adipose tissues in rats. Am J Physiol 266:R1371–R1382, 1994.

165. Levin BE, Triscari J, Marquet E, et al: Dietary obesity and neonatal sympathectomy. I. Effects on body composition and brown adipose. Am J Physiol 247:R979–R987, 1984.

166. Rohrer DK, Chruscinski A, Schauble EH, et al: Cardiovascular and metabolic alterations in mice lacking both beta1- and beta2-adrenergic receptors. J Biol Chem 274:16701–16708, 1999.

167. Thomas SA, Palmiter RD: Thermoregulatory and metabolic phenotypes of mice lacking noradrenaline and adrenaline. Nature 387:94–97, 1997.

168. Susulic VS, Frederich RC, Lawitts J, et al: Targeted disruption of the beta 3-adrenergic receptor gene. J Biol Chem 270:29483–29492, 1995.

169. Lowell BB, Bachman ES: Beta-Adrenergic receptors, diet-induced thermogenesis, and obesity. J Biol Chem 278:29385–29388, 2003.

170. Zhang Y, Proenca R, Maffei M, et al: Positional cloning of the mouse obese gene and its human homologue. Nature 372:425–432, 1994.

171. Tartaglia LA, Dembski M, Weng X, et al: Identification and expression cloning of a leptin receptor, OB-R. Cell 83:1263–1271, 1995.

172. Butler AA, Kesterson RA, Khong K, et al: A unique metabolic syndrome causes obesity in the melanocortin-3 receptor-deficient mouse. Endocrinology 141:3518–3521, 2000.

173. Ishii M, Fei H, Friedman JM: Targeted disruption of GPR7, the endogenous receptor for neuropeptides B and W, leads to metabolic defects and adult-onset obesity. Proc Natl Acad Sci U S A 100:10540–10545, 2003.

174. Martinez-Botas J, Anderson JB, Tessier D, et al: Absence of perilipin results in leanness and reverses obesity in Lepr(db/db) mice. Nat Genet 26:474–479, 2000.

175. Xia Z, Stanhope KL, Digitale E, et al: Acylation-stimulating protein (ASP)/complement C3adesArg deficiency results in increased energy expenditure in mice. J Biol Chem 279:4051–4057, 2004.

176. Abu-Elheiga L, Matzuk MM, Abo-Hashema KA, et al: Continuous fatty acid oxidation and reduced fat storage in mice lacking acetyl-CoA carboxylase 2. Science 291:2613–2616, 2001.

177. Cummings DE, Brandon EP, Planas JV, et al: Genetically lean mice result from targeted disruption of the RII beta subunit of protein kinase A. Nature 382:622–626, 1996.

178. Enerback S, Jacobsson A, Simpson EM, et al: Mice lacking mitochondrial uncoupling protein are cold-sensitive but not obese. Nature 387:90–94, 1997.

179. Zhou Z, Yon Toh S, Chen Z, et al: Cidea-deficient mice have lean phenotype and are resistant to obesity. Nat Genet 35:49–56, 2003.

180. Cohen P, Miyazaki M, Socci ND, et al: Role for stearoyl-CoA desaturase-1 in leptin-mediated weight loss. Science 297:240–243, 2002.

181. Montague CT, Farooqi IS, Whitehead JP, et al: Congenital leptin deficiency is associated with severe early-onset obesity in humans. Nature 387:903–908, 1997.

182. Hinney A, Schmidt A, Nottebom K, et al: Several mutations in the melanocortin-4 receptor gene including a nonsense and a frameshift mutation associated with dominantly inherited obesity in humans [In Process Citation]. J Clin Endocrinol Metab 84:1483–1486, 1999.

183. Lee YS, Poh LK, Loke KY: A novel melanocortin 3 receptor gene (MC3R) mutation associated with severe obesity. J Clin Endocrinol Metab 87:1423–1426, 2002.

184. Jackson RS, Creemers JW, Ohagi S, et al: Obesity and impaired prohormone processing associated with mutations in the human prohormone convertase 1 gene [see comments]. Nat Genet 16:303–306, 1997.

185. Ristow M, Muller-Wieland D, Pfeiffer A, et al: Obesity associated with a mutation in a genetic regulator of adipocyte differentiation. N Engl J Med 339:953–959, 1998.

Obesity: The Problem and Its Management

Jose F. Caro and Jamie Dananberg

Thirty percent of the U.S. population is obese (body mass index [BMI] ≥ 30) and 64% is overweight (25 ≥ BMI).[1] Obesity is second to smoking as a preventable cause of death and is expected to be first by 2005.[2] It accounted for 16.6% of total deaths (more than 300,000 per year) and an economic cost of $117 billion in the United States.[2] After years of review, the Centers of Medicare and Medicaid services, which runs the health program for the elderly and disabled in the United States, announced on July 15, 2004, a major change in policy coverage. Language in the Medicare Coverage Issues Manual stating that obesity is not an illness was removed. This seemingly minor change in wording, recognizing that obesity is an illness, would remove barriers to covering antiobesity interventions if scientific and medical evidence demonstrate their effectives in improving health outcomes.

Changes in body weight follow the laws of physics and dictate that if caloric intake is greater than caloric output, weight gain will occur. However, regulation of body weight homeostasis is a complex integration of genetic, social, behavioral, and physiologic factors, many of which have yet to be fully understood. The systems that regulate body weight and energy homeostasis developed over an evolutionary time scale. The biologic factors responsible for the increasing prevalence of obesity were set down early in mankind and were probably meant to defend against significant loss of lean mass during times of food scarcity. Is obesity the phenotype of "survival" genes in an environment of plentitude? Wherever the evidence leads, one thing is certain: The genetic and social adaptations that have been passed down through the millennia have resulted in populations with ever-increasing waistlines and risks for serious morbidity and mortality. Will innovation undo in decades what evolution did in millennia? Our scientific understanding of body weight regulation and the pathophysiology of obesity has dramatically increased in parallel with the biology revolution. It is imperative that this new knowledge is rapidly translated into humans because obesity in middle-aged humans is a risk factor for many age-related diseases and decreases life expectancy by about 7 years, which is roughly comparable to the combined effect of cardiovascular diseases and cancer on life span.[3]

EPIDEMIOLOGY OF OVERWEIGHT AND OBESITY

The diseases of overweight and obesity are global in scope. For every developed country in the world in which data are available, the incidence and prevalence of excessive weight have increased over time.[4] Epidemiologic analysis of obesity is complicated in that the criteria by which overweight and obesity are defined have shifted over time. Currently, it is recommended that body mass index (BMI, weight divided by height squared [kg/m^2]) be used for establishing diagnoses of overweight (BMI of 25–29.9 kg/m^2) and obesity (BMI ≥ 30 kg/m^2).[5] These cutoffs were chosen as predictors of morbidity and mortality. Based on these criteria, it is currently estimated that the age-adjusted prevalence of obesity is 30.5% of the U.S. population in 1999 to 2000 compared with 22.9% in 1988 to 1994 ($P < 0.001$, the third National Health and Nutrition Examination Survey, NHANES III) (Table 43-1). The prevalence of overweight also increased during this period from 55.9% to 64% ($P < 0.001$).[1] The prevalence and trends in children and adolescents are even worse (Fig. 43-1).[6] In parallel, costs for weight-related health care have skyrocketed. In the United States, the total cost of health care attributable to obesity is over $100 billion, roughly half of which was spent on direct medical costs to treat obesity-associated disease.[7]

DISEASES ASSOCIATED WITH OBESITY

MORTALITY

Obesity and overweight themselves independently confer an increased risk of mortality. Although the link between obesity and increased rates of morbidity and mortality has been questioned in older populations,[8] many other studies have established such a direct linkage. The increase in risk begins to rise at a BMI greater than 25 kg/m^2.[9] The risk rises slowly at levels over 25 kg/m^2 and then rises steeply at levels greater than 30 kg/m^2. Individuals with a BMI of 30 kg/m^2 or greater have a 1.5- to 2-fold excess independent risk of mortality than do individuals with a BMI less than 25 kg/m^2.[9] Paradoxically, a

Table 43-1   Prevalence of Obesity in the U.S. Population

| | | Obesity (BMI ≥30) | | | | | Extreme Obesity (BMI ≥40) | | |
| | | NHANES III, 1988–1994 | | NHANES 1999–2000 | | | NHANES III, 1988–1994, | NHANES 1999–2000, | |
Sex	Racial/Ethnic Group	No.	% (SE)	No.	% (SE)	Change, % (95% CI)	% (SE)	% (SE)	Change, % (95% CI)
Both sexes	All†	16,681	22.9 (0.68)	4115	30.5 (1.43)	7.6 (4.4 to 10.8)	2.9 (0.23)	4.7 (0.56)	1.8 (0.6 to 3.0)
Men	All†	7933	20.2 (0.72)	2043	27.5 (1.61)	7.3 (3.8 to 10.8)	1.7 (0.32)	3.1 (0.58)	1.4 (0.1 to 2.7)
	Non-Hispanic white	3285	20.3 (0.85)	946	27.3 (1.82)	7.0 (3.0 to 11.0)	1.8 (0.41)	3.0 (0.75)	1.2 (−0.5 to 2.9)
	Non-Hispanic black	2112	21.1 (1.02)	374	28.1 (2.27)	7.0 (2.0 to 12.0)	2.4 (0.38)	3.5 (1.24)‡	1.1 (−1.5 to 3.7)
	Mexican American	2250	23.9 (0.97)	538	28.9 (2.25)	5.0 (0.1 to 9.9)	1.1 (0.33)‡	2.4 (0.74)‡	1.3 (−0.3 to 2.9)
Women	All†	8748	25.4 (0.95)	2072	33.4 (1.81)	8.0 (3.9 to 12.1)	4.0 (0.31)	6.3 (0.78)	2.3 (0.6 to 4.0)
	Non-Hispanic white	3755	22.9 (1.15)	885	30.1 (2.10)	7.2 (2.4 to 12.0)	3.4 (0.40)	4.9 (0.89)	1.5 (−0.5 to 3.5)
	Non-Hispanic black	2490	38.2 (1.37)	420	49.7 (2.79)	11.5 (5.3 to 17.7)	7.9 (0.51)	15.1 (2.05)	7.2 (3.0 to 11.4)
	Mexican American	2128	35.3 (1.36)	567	39.7 (3.65)	4.4 (−3.4 to 12.2)	4.8 (0.65)	5.5 (1.04)	0.7 (−1.8 to 3.2)

*NHANES indicates National Health and Nutrition Examination Survey; CI, confidence interval.
†Includes racial/ethnic groups not shown separately.
‡Does not meet the standard of statistical reliability and precision (relative SE >30%).
From Flegal KM, Carroll MD, Ogden CL, Johnson CL: Prevalence and trends in obesity among US adults, 1999–2000. JAMA 288:1723–1727, 2002.

BMI lower than 20 kg/m^2 is associated with a modest increase in mortality, even after adjusting for confounding variables.[9] The data relating obesity to mortality risk were drawn from epidemiologic studies of primarily white populations. In other groups, the inflection point at which mortality risk increases with increased BMI may be shifted. For example, in black American populations, mortality risk appears to rise at BMI levels of 27 kg/m^2 and greater.[10]

CARDIOVASCULAR AND CEREBROVASCULAR DISEASE

Overweight, obesity, and abdominal fat increase the risk of both cardiovascular and cerebrovascular[11] diseases. The reasons for the increased risk for cardiovascular and cerebrovascular diseases may include elevations of blood pressure, low-density lipoprotein cholesterol, triglycerides, small dense low-density lipoprotein cholesterol, total cholesterol, fibrinogen, plasminogen activator inhibitor-1, and insulin, together with decreases in high-density lipoprotein cholesterol. The cluster of three abnormalities is diagnostic of the metabolic syndrome.[12] The metabolic syndrome is defined by the Third Report of the National Cholesterol Education Program Expert Panel on Detection, Evaluation, and Treatment of High Blood Cholesterol in Adult (Adult Treatment Panel III) as having three or more of the following criteria: waist circumference greater than 102 cm in men and 88 cm in women; serum triglycerides level of at least 150 mg/dL (1.69 mmol/L in men) and 50 mg/dL (1.29 mmol/L) in women; blood pressure of at least 130/85 mm Hg; or serum glucose level of at least 100 mg/dL (6.1 mmol/L). The age-adjusted prevalence of the metabolic syndrome is 23.7%[12] in the U.S. population. Not only is this disorder highly prevalent, but it also increases cardiovascular and all-cause mortality as demonstrated in an 11-year follow-up study.[13]

Hypertension

The INTERSALT study involving more then 10,000 men and women reported that a 10-kg increase in weight was associated with a 3 mm Hg rise in systolic blood pressure and a 2.3 mm Hg rise in diastolic blood pressure.[14] This degree of blood pressure elevation has been associated with a 12% increase in coronary heart disease (CHD) and a 24% increase in stroke. The precise mechanism by which changes in weight alter blood pressure has not been established.

Dyslipidemia

Increases in BMI are associated with increases in total cholesterol, triglycerides, total low-density lipoprotein (LDL), and small dense LDL and with decreases in high-density lipoproteins.[15] The risk of CHD is primarily due to increases in LDL. Increases in the BMI of 10 U from a starting level between 20 and 30 kg/m^2 will raise LDL cholesterol levels between 10 and 20 mg/dL. Changes of this magnitude can be expected to increase the risk of CHD by 10% over a 5- to 10-year period. The risk may be particularly great for individuals with more prominent upper body obesity, in whom triglyceride, small dense LDL, and apolipoprotein B levels are high.

Congestive Heart Failure

Both overweight and obesity have been shown to be independent risk factors for the development of congestive heart failure. Furthermore, because both hypertension and diabetes are also associated with congestive heart failure, the overall risk when these dependent factors are taken into account is proportionally increased.[16]

Stroke

Fewer studies have carefully examined the association of cerebrovascular disease and weight versus cardiovascular disease

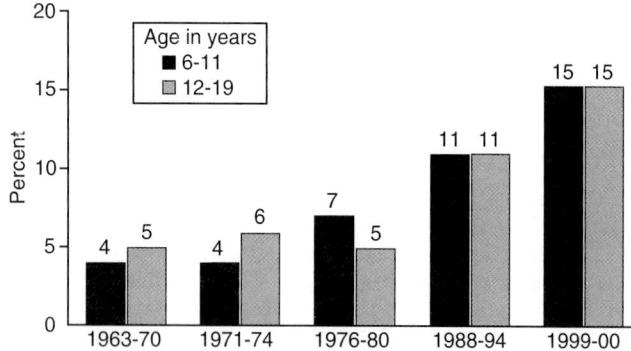

Figure 43-1   Prevalence of overweight among children and adolescents ages 6–19 years. Excludes pregnant women starting with 1971–74. Pregnancy status not available for 1963–65 and 1966–70. Data for 1963–65 are for children 6–11 years of age; data for 1966–70 are for adolescents 12–17 years of age, not 12–19 years. (Source: CDC/NCHS, NHES, and NHANES.)

and weight. An association has been established in the evaluation of both fatal and nonfatal strokes, particularly when a subset of patients with ischemic stroke is evaluated. The risk of stroke is nearly twofold higher in women with a BMI greater than 32 kg/m^2 than in women with a BMI less than 21 kg/m^2.[17]

DIABETES MELLITUS

Numerous studies have shown an association between increases in weight and the development of type 2 diabetes mellitus.[18] In fact, the risk for diabetes increases at BMI levels below that established for the diagnosis of overweight. In the Nurses' Health Study, BMI values above 22 kg/m^2 were associated with an increased risk of diabetes.[18] It has been estimated that the relative risk for diabetes increases by 25% for each unit of BMI above 22 kg/m. It has also been estimated that more than a quarter of all newly diagnosed cases of diabetes in the United States were due to weight gain of more than 5 kg.[19]

CANCER

Several studies have shown a strong association between adiposity and increased risk of cancers of the breast in postmenopausal women; of the endometrium, kidney, and gallbladder in women; and of the colon in men. However, it is only recently that in a prospectively studied population, it was clearly demonstrated that increased body weight was associated with increased death rates for all cancers combined and for cancers at multiple specific sites.[20] More than 900,000 U.S. adults who were free of cancer at enrollment in 1987 were followed for 16 years, at which time 57,145 died from cancer. Figure 43-2 shows the contribution of overweight and obesity to mortality from cancer.[20] The heaviest members of this cohort (BMI > 40) had death rates from all cancers combined that were 52% higher for men and 62% higher for women than the rates in men and woman of normal weight.[20] On the basis of the association observed in this study, it was estimated that obesity could account for 14% of all deaths from cancer in men and 20% of those in women.[20,21]

FEMALE REPRODUCTIVE HEALTH

Polycystic ovarian syndrome, a disorder that includes hirsutism, obesity, ovulatory and menstrual dysfunction, and insulin resistance, is among the most common causes of altered reproductive function in women who are overweight. Even modest increases in weight in young women can adversely affect fertility, and women with polycystic ovarian syndrome and obesity have an increased risk of infertility.

Obesity during pregnancy is also associated with excessive morbidity. Pregnant women with obesity have nearly a 10-fold excess risk of hypertension and a significant increase in the risk of gestational diabetes. Furthermore, the risk of congenital malformations, primarily neural tube defects, is increased in the pregnancy of obese women.[22] Finally, increased weight before pregnancy has been shown to result in an increased risk of adverse fetal outcomes.[23]

OTHER

For women with a BMI greater than 40 kg/m^2, the risk of gallstones is nearly seven times higher than for women with a BMI less than 24 kg/m^2.[24] A twin study estimated that for every 1-kg rise in body weight, the risk of osteoarthritis increases by approximately 10%.[25] Sleep apnea is another morbidity associated directly with weight gain.[26] Diagnosis and treatment of sleep apnea in obese patients are particularly important because of the sequelae of hypoxia, hypertension, myocardial infarction, and cardiac arrhythmias.

RELATIONSHIP TO BODY FAT DISTRIBUTION

Diseases associated with obesity are more highly correlated with the presence of intra-abdominal (visceral) fat than with peripheral (subcutaneous) fat. When compared to equal-weight patients with peripheral obesity, patients with abdominal obesity have a greater risk for type 2 diabetes mellitus, CHD, stroke, and hormone-dependent cancers of the breast and endometrium.[26] Furthermore, patients with abdominal obesity have higher glucose and insulin levels during an oral glucose tolerance test[27] and higher rates of lipolysis than do patients with peripheral obesity.[28]

INTEGRATED REGULATION OF ENERGY BALANCE

Energy expenditure can be divided into several components. The resting metabolic rate (RMR) is the energy expended during inactivity to fuel the normal, resting, physiologic processes and to maintain normal body temperature. The RMR, or basal metabolic rate, can be thought of as the average metabolic rate during sleep plus the energy cost of arousal. The RMR accounts for approximately 60% to 70% of daily energy expenditure.[29] In contrast, thermogenic processes are processes that increase energy expenditure over the RMR in response to food consumption, changes in ambient temperature, exposure to drugs or changing hormonal concentrations, or psychologic stresses. Of these processes, the thermic effect of food is quantitatively the largest and accounts for approximately 10% of daily energy expenditure.[29] The final, most variable component of energy expenditure is physical activity. For most adults in developed nations, physical activity accounts for approximately 20% to 30% of daily energy expenditure.

Because living organisms exist in a dynamic environment, energy balance should be considered in the context of the time- and weight-dependent rate of energy use. For example, an increase in energy intake results in positive energy balance and weight gain. Over time, weight gain slows because of a compensatory increase in energy expenditure and restoration of energy balance. Therefore, conditions at the new steady

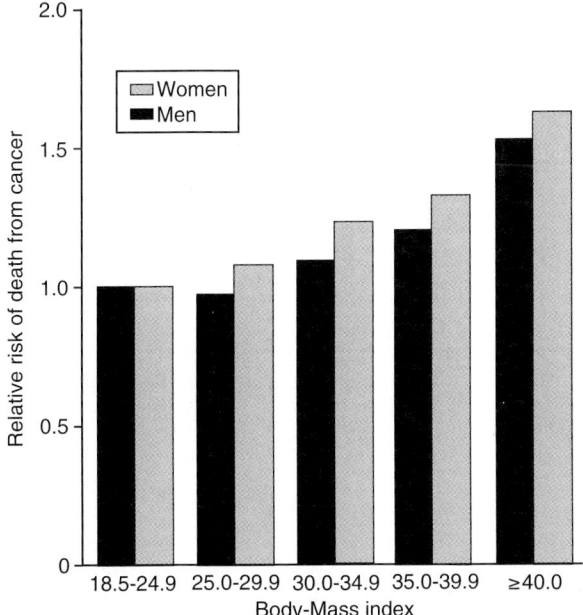

Figure 43-2 Contribution of overweight and obesity to mortality from cancer in the United States.[21] Data are from the Cancer Prevention Study II, 1982 through 1998.[20]

state include increased energy intake, increased energy expenditure, and an increase in body mass. Consequently, for an individual, change in weight is not just a function of food intake, but also changes in the homeostatic mechanisms that define energy balance.

The positive energy balance responsible for obesity is caused by excessive energy intake, reduced energy expenditure, or a combination of these two factors. In several studies, a reduction in energy expenditure was found in infants in whom obesity developed at 1 year of age,[30] and in adult Pima Indians, in whom obesity developed with aging.[31] In contrast, several investigators have not found a decrease in energy expenditure in children[32] who become overweight later in life. These differences may be explained, in part, by the imprecision of the technology used to measure energy intake and energy expenditure.

SIGNALING SYSTEMS

The homeostatic mechanisms of weight that respond to changes in diet or the external environment include signaling, integration, and effector components (Fig. 43-3). The signaling component involves sensory, somatic, and environ-

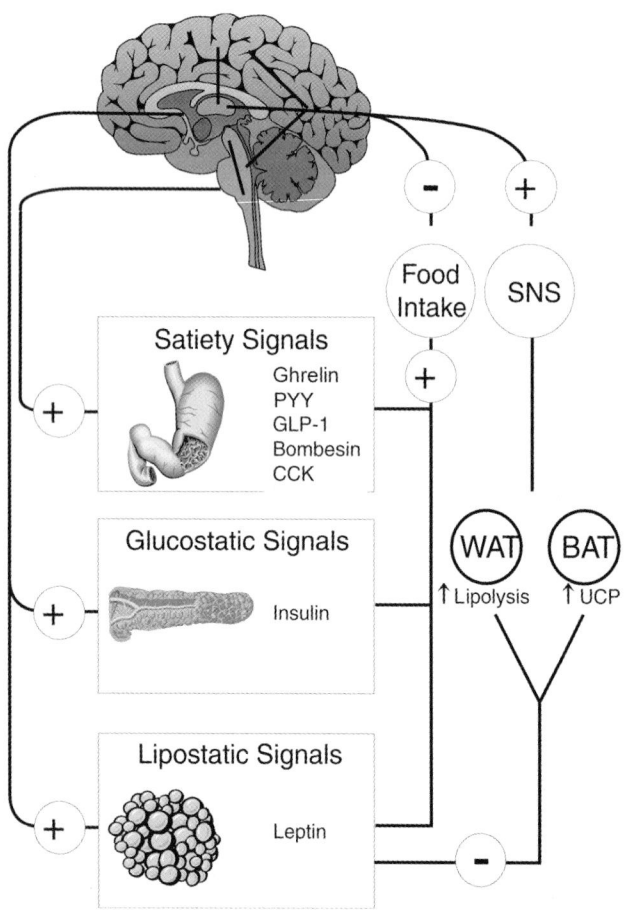

Figure 43-3 Integration between feeding-related signals to the brain and food intake and energy expenditure. Food intake initiates a series of signals that reach the hypothalamus via the blood-brain barrier (lipostatic and glucostatic signals) or via the brain stem (satiety signals). The hypothalamus integrates these signals with other sensory, cognitive, and environmental signals from the cerebral cortex. This integrated information, when sent back to the periphery, results in a decrease in food intake and activation of the sympathetic nervous system (SNS). The SNS via the β₃-adrenergic receptor stimulates lipolysis in white adipose tissue (WAT) and thermogenesis in brown adipose tissue (BAT) via activation of uncoupling proteins (UCPs). CCK, cholecystokinin; GLP-1, glucagon-like peptide-1.

mental messages that relay information regarding body composition, energy balance, thermogenesis, and food availability, and leads to a coordinated response that restores or maintains homeostasis. The signals that are recognized to regulate body weight can be divided into lipostatic, glucostatic, and satiety signals.

Lipostatic Signals

Regulation of body weight requires an integrated system of communication between the storage compartment and the regulatory compartment. White adipose tissue is the major site for long-term energy storage in the form of triglycerides. Transmission of information regarding the relative amount of white adipose tissue was shown to be dependent on the recently discovered hormone leptin.[33] Since the discovery of leptin, the role of the adipose tissue as a true endocrine organ capable of secreting a number of hormones, known as adipokines, is gaining appreciation. These hormones make the adipose tissue at the crossroads of energy homeostasis, inflammation, atherosclerosis, insulin resistance and cancer, in addition to being the source of lipostatic signals.[34,35]

Glucostatic Signals

Although insulin clearly plays a role in systemic fuel utilization, data also support its activity within the central nervous system to regulate energy homeostasis. Some evidence indicates that insulin-regulated glucose metabolism within ventromedial hypothalamus neurons may regulate autonomic outflow and, subsequently, the metabolic rate. In humans, insulin infusion during euglycemic clamp procedures increases sympathetic nervous system activity.[36] In animal models, direct injection of insulin into the ventromedial hypothalamus alters sympathetic nervous activity to brown adipose tissue (BAT).[37] Finally, destruction of insulin-sensitive neurons in the ventromedial hypothalamus by injection of gold thioglucose blocks diet-induced increases in thermogenesis.[36]

Satiety Signals

Cholecystokinin

Among the earliest satiety factors identified was the gut peptide cholecystokinin (CCK), which regulates meal size in rats in a dose-dependent manner.[38] The importance of CCK in the regulation of appetite and food intake was further established with the use of selective antagonists. Whereas CCK reduced meal intake by nearly half, a selective antagonist completely reversed this suppression. By itself, the CCK antagonist was able to increase food intake by approximately one third.[39]

Ghrelin

Ghrelin is a hormone made in the stomach.[40] It is the endogenous ligand for the growth hormone-secretagogue receptor, which is expressed in the hypothalamus and brain stem. In rodents, ghrelin is a potent stimulus to eat.[41] In humans, ghrelin appears to be the gut hormone that determines when it is time to eat.[42] Plasma levels are elevated in fasting and fall after eating.[42] Furthermore, infusion of ghrelin in humans increases food intake.[42] Ghrelin plasma concentration has an inverse relationship with body weight. This is consistent with the notion of homeostatic control of body weight, whereas high circulation ghrelin in thin individuals would favor increased food intake.[42]

Peptide YY

Peptide YY (PYY) is produced by the gut and is released into the circulation after eating.[43] PYY is part of the neuropeptide Y (NPY) family and it is the N-terminally truncated form (PYY 3–36) that is active. Its peripheral administration decreases appetite possibly by acting directly in the arcuate nucleus via the Y2 receptor.[42] In humans, food intake is acutely decreased by 30% after an intravenous (IV) infusion of PYY 3–36.[44] Obese subjects have lower levels of PYY and the postprandial rise is smaller.[44] Thus, PYY might be the gut message that indicates we have eaten enough.[42]

Bombesin Family
Several factors have been identified that may play a role in meal size regulation, including the bombesin family of molecules. These molecules include bombesin, gastrin-releasing peptide, neuromedin C, and neuromedin B, all of which are able to suppress food intake. These molecules appear to act through a family of receptors that have been initially grouped as neuromedin C preferring and gastrin-releasing peptide preferring.[45]

Incretins
Another family of gastrointestinal signals is the incretin family of peptides. These peptides, secreted by enteroendocrine cells of the large and small intestine, were first identified as being responsible for the incremental release of insulin that occurs after oral administration of glucose relative to that after an equivalent amount of glucose administered intravenously.[46] The most studied member of the incretin peptides is glucagon-like peptide-1 (GLP-1).[47] It is now known that GLP-1 lowers blood glucose by increasing glucose-mediated insulin release, delaying gastric emptying, and inhibiting glucagon release. Furthermore, intracerebroventricular administration of GLP-1 significantly decreases food and water intake.[47] Some reports have shown that GLP-1 is reduced in obese subjects[48] and that the anorectic effect of GLP-1 is preserved in obesity.[49]

INTEGRATION OF SIGNALS: CENTRAL NERVOUS SYSTEM REGULATION OF WEIGHT

A number of orexigenic and anorexigenic signals within the most important areas of the brain have been identified. Much of the input to the brain is integrated within the hypothalamus. The cross-talk within and between these nuclei, even within single neurons, is only now being understood and systematically explored.

Orexigenic Signals
Neuropeptide Y
NPY is a neurotransmitter widely expressed throughout the brain. NPY is highly overexpressed in the leptin-deficient *ob/ob* mouse and in the leptin receptor-deficient *db/db* mouse. Furthermore, NPY overexpression can be reversed by leptin administration in the *ob/ob* mouse, but not the *db/db* mouse.[50] NPY is among the most potent orexigenic peptides. When injected directly into the paraventricular nucleus of the hypothalamus, NPY causes a marked increase in food intake, weight, and body fat within 10 days of treatment in female rats.[51] The metabolic changes induced by centrally administered NPY mimic the changes seen in obesity. Furthermore, centrally administered NPY reduces sympathetic nervous system efferent activity to BAT with a subsequent decrease in energy expenditure.

Although NPY and leptin appear to be components of an important feedback loop, experiments in transgenic animals suggest that the role of NPY in weight regulation and feeding behavior is complex. Mice deficient in NPY have normal body weight, feeding behavior, and body composition.[52] At least five NPY receptors have been cloned, including one that appears to be a pseudogene.[53] Although experiments with agonists and antagonists suggest that the NPY-1 and NPY-5 receptors are the most likely candidates for the "feeding" receptor, some degree of uncertainty still surrounds this interpretation.[54] Therefore, the relative importance of NPY and the various NPY receptor subtypes will require additional work with more selective antagonists and transgenic animals with combinations of gene disruptions.[54]

Melanin-Concentrating Hormone
Melanin-concentrating hormone (MCH), a circulating peptide first discovered in chub salmon that regulates fish scale color by aggregating melanonosomes, was identified in the hypothalamus of the *ob/ob* mouse by differential display polymerase chain reaction. Injection of melanin-concentrating hormone into the lateral ventricles causes an increase in food intake.[55] Recently, it has been shown that transgenic mice produced with targeted deletions of the melanin-concentrating hormone gene had lower body weight, hypophagia, and an increased metabolic rate despite lower levels of both leptin and pro-opiomelanocortin mRNA within the arcuate nucleus.[56] Interestingly, these mice had a hyperphagic response to starvation, similar to that seen in mice lacking expression of NPY.[56]

Galanin
Galanin, a hypothalamic peptide found in abundance in the paraventricular nucleus, is associated with preference for dietary fat.[57] Galanin expression is significantly upregulated by increases in dietary fat, more so in obese-prone strains than in obese-resistant strains. However, chronic central administration of galanin does not result in hyperphagia or obesity.[58]

Opioids
The pro-opiomelanocortin polypeptide is the parent molecule of several peptides with potential weight-regulating properties (see Chapters 16 and 18). Among those with orexigenic properties are the endogenous opioid peptides. Opioids have been known for years to stimulate appetite, but it was identification of the endogenous opioid peptides β-endorphin, dynorphin A, and enkephalins that led to increased interest in this system as it relates to energy balance. Long-acting enkephalin analogues (possibly via the δ opioid receptor), β-endorphin (possibly via the μ opioid receptor), and dynorphin A (possibly via the κ opioid receptor) have all been shown to increase feeding behavior.[59]

Anorexigenic Signals
Pro-opiomelanocortin System
In addition to the opioid molecules that stimulate feeding behavior, the pro-opiomelanocortin polypeptide yields a number of anorexigenic molecules (see Chapter 18). α-Melanocyte-stimulating hormone (α-MSH) elicits effects that are opposed to the effects of NPY and MCH. The action of α-MSH is mediated through the melanocortin family of receptors, five of which have been identified. α-MSH activation of the melanocortin-4 (MC-4) receptor and possibly the MC-3 receptor appears to inhibit eating behavior and increase energy expenditure as deduced from antagonist and gene knockout experiments. Agouti protein, a naturally occurring antagonist to all melanocortin receptors and normally produced only in skin, causes obesity when ectopically overexpressed in the brain of the yellow agouti (A^y) mouse.[60] Furthermore, transgenic mice deficient in MC-4 receptor have a hyperphagic and obese phenotype.[61] Finally, agouti-related protein, another endogenous protein that is an antagonist at the MC-3 and MC-4 receptors, when overexpressed in transgenic mice also produces an obese phenotype.[62]

Corticotropin-Releasing Hormone
Corticotropin-releasing hormone and the related urocortin reduce food intake and body weight when administered directly to the brain. Additionally, leptin administration increases the expression of corticotropin-releasing hormone mRNA in the hypothalamus. Finally, the increase in weight seen in glucocorticoid excess states may, in part, be due to the attendant suppression of corticotropin-releasing hormone.[63]

Cocaine and Amphetamine Regulated Transcript

The neuropeptide cocaine and amphetamine regulated transcript was discovered by differential display to identify the genes expressed after acute administration of cocaine and amphetamine to rats. The C-terminal 48 amino acids of the prohormone predicted by the sequence of the gene appears to be the biologically active form and is a potent inhibitor of feeding. The potential role of cocaine and amphetamine regulated transcript in energy balance was suggested by showing that leptin coordinately regulated cocaine and amphetamine regulated transcript expression. Furthermore, cocaine and amphetamine regulated transcript inhibited the feeding response induced by either fasting or NPY.[64]

EFFECTOR COMPONENTS IN ENERGY HOMEOSTASIS: PERIPHERAL SYSTEMS

The peripheral systems involved in energy balance can be divided into efferent signals from the brain and their respective receptors and the effector molecules that translate the signals into an increase or decrease in energy expenditure. The two most studied efferent signal systems are the adrenergic nervous system and the thyroid hormone axis. Although thyroid hormone clearly plays a role in the basal state of energy use, the long half-life of thyroxine, as well as its long-term genomic effects, suggests that this system is most important in affecting energy balance on a long-term basis. The discovery of several isoforms of the thyroid hormone receptor with differential tissue distributions opens the possibility of regulation of energy through specific receptor subtypes. The effect of thyroid hormone on metabolism and the metabolic rate is covered in Chapter 94. The daily variations in energy expenditure are more likely to occur via the adrenergic nervous system. The effector molecules that separate fuel oxidation from adenosine triphosphate (ATP) synthesis (i.e., potential chemical energy) reside within a subset of the family of mitochondrial transport protein known as uncoupling proteins (UCPs).

Uncoupling Proteins

The first uncoupling protein (now termed *UCP-1*) was identified in the mid-1970s[65] as a mitochondrial protein that bound to purine nucleotides and fatty acids and was involved in energy dissipation. This protein family belongs to the mitochondrial anion carrier proteins, which also include adenosine diphosphate (ADP)/ATP carrier, phosphate, and oxoglutarate carriers. UCP-1 is primarily expressed in BAT. In mitochondria derived from other cell types, oxidation of fuels is tightly coupled to the generation of ATP. The mitochondrial respiratory chain produces a proton gradient across the inner mitochondrial membrane. ATP synthesis from ADP by the protein ATP synthase is driven by the coupled movement of protons down this electrochemical gradient. If ADP substrate is limited, proton flux through ATP synthase is inhibited and the gradient is maintained. In BAT mitochondria, protons may move down the gradient in a manner that is uncoupled from ATP synthesis.[66] Uncoupling of the potential energy of the gradient from ATP generation provides a mechanism for both the dissipation of excess calories and the production of heat.

Two additional cloned proteins, UCP-2 and UCP-3, have different tissue-specific expression and transcriptional regulation. At least one report has shown that the proton transport activity of UCP-1 is dependent on the presence of an intact histidine pair, which is absent in both UCP-2 and UCP-3. UCP-2 is expressed in BAT but, unlike UCP-1, is also expressed in a broad range of tissues.[67,68]

Adrenergic Nervous System

The adrenergic nervous system regulates energy expenditure at the cellular level by regulating the expression of UCPs and at the whole animal level by enhancing total and basal oxygen consumption, increasing thermogenic responses, and increasing BAT mass.[69,70] The α- and β-adrenergic receptors mediate catecholamine responses.

The β-adrenergic receptors were first subtyped by Lands and colleagues into β1- and β2-adrenergic receptors.[71] However, evidence increasingly indicated that the pharmacology of known adrenergic agonists in adipose and gastrointestinal tissue was not explained by the known β-adrenergic receptors. In 1983, it was proposed that the atypical β-adrenergic receptor within adipose tissue be considered a third β-receptor subtype.[72] Although all three receptor subtypes are found within adipocytes, the β3-adrenergic receptor is most highly expressed in BAT, the tissue most likely responsible for the thermogenic effect of food.[73]

The β3-adrenergic receptor is a member of the seven-transmembrane G protein–coupled receptor family and is 95% homologous to the β1- and β2-adrenergic receptors. Despite having sequence information on the β1- and β2-adrenergic receptors for a number of years, cloning of the human β3-adrenergic receptor occurred only in 1989.[74] Additional work led to the discovery that the human isoform of the β3-receptor was different from the rat receptor in that it had a second exon with an additional six amino acids on the C terminus.[75] A unique aspect of the β3-receptor, in contrast to the β1- and β2-adrenergic receptors, was the lack of acute homologous downregulation by serine kinases.[76]

THERAPY FOR OBESITY

DETERMINATION OF TREATMENT CANDIDATES

As in the pharmacologic treatment of all diseases, no risk-free, highly efficacious therapies are available. Therefore, we are left balancing risk and efficacy in a highly heterogeneous group of individuals with a wide range of risk factors for significant disease. Underscoring the risks associated with overweight and obesity, the National Heart, Lung, and Blood Institute of the National Institutes of Health convened an expert panel on the identification, evaluation, and treatment of overweight and obesity in adults as part of an overall obesity education initiative.[77] More recently, the American Medical Association published roadmaps for clinical practice on treatment decision for obesity.[78]

Evidence now supports the full range of interventions in patients with a BMI of 30 kg/m^2 or greater (Table 43-2). For patients with a BMI of 25 kg/m^2 or greater, it is agreed that diet and exercise be instituted. Whether pharmacologic intervention is used at this point depends on the severity and degree of associated risk factors balanced against known risks for a particular treatment. The initial target weight loss should be a minimum of 10% of starting body weight. Efforts should be made, with frequent follow-up and feedback, to establish a rate of weight loss of approximately 1 to 2 pounds (0.5–1 kg) per week for a period of up to 6 months. The first step in weight loss is the institution of a diet and exercise program. Depending on the particular risks in any given patient, individuals who are unable to achieve or maintain target weight loss should then begin behavior modification programs, followed as necessary by pharmacotherapy and then, in the most severe cases, weight-loss surgery. These options are discussed in greater detail in the following sections. In many cases, success will depend on a combination of all strategies. The most successful initial regimens are those that combine diet, exercise, and behavioral therapy.[77,78]

DIET THERAPY

Caloric restriction will lead to weight loss; however, for any single patient, the total calories that will maintain constant

Table 43-2 Listing of Risk Factors in Assessing Suitability for Treatment Intervention in Individuals with a Body Mass Index between 25 and 29.9 kg/m²

Risk	Subgroup, Diagnostic Criteria, or Manifestation
Established CHD	History of myocardial infarction
	History of angina pectoris (stable or unstable)
	History of coronary artery surgery
	History of coronary artery procedures (e.g., angioplasty)
Presence of other atherosclerotic diseases	Peripheral arterial disease
	Abdominal aortic aneurysm
	Symptomatic carotid artery disease
Additional cardiovascular risks	Cigarette smoking
	Hypertension (systolic blood pressure ≥140 mm Hg *or* diastolic blood pressure ≥90 mm Hg)
	High-risk LDL-C (≥160 mg/dL)
	Low-risk HDL-C (≤35 mg/dL)
	Impaired FBG (110–125 mg/dL, inclusive)
	Family history or premature CHD (myocardial infarction or sudden death in father 55 or younger or mother 65 or younger)
	Age (men ≥45 yr; women ≥55 yr)
Type 2 diabetes	Fasting plasma glucose ≥126 mg/dL
	Casual plasma glucose ≥200 mg/dL plus symptoms
	2-hr plasma glucose ≥200 mg/dL during OGTT[158]
Sleep apnea	Recurrent apnea or hypopnea associated with clinical impairment
Identification of other obesity-associated diseases	Gynecologic abnormalities
	Osteoarthritis
	Gallstones and their complications
	Stress incontinence
Other risk factors	Physical inactivity
	High triglycerides (≥400 mg/dL)

From *http://www.nhlbi.nih.gov/nhlbi/cardio/obes/prof/guidelns/ob_gdlns.pdf*
CHD, coronary heart disease; FBG, fasting blood glucose; HDL-C, high-density lipoprotein cholesterol; LDL-C, low-density lipoprotein cholesterol; OGTT, oral glucose tolerance test.

weight or initiate weight loss vary significantly. Several formulas have been developed for the calculation of resting or basal metabolic rate.[79] These equations are very useful in setting approximate targets for dietary calories in individuals seeking weight loss. However, variability between subjects is high, so regular interval monitoring of weight loss and subsequent adjustments to dietary intake should be undertaken.

A review of the effectiveness of some recent published programs with moderate calorie-restricted diets (approximately 1200 kcal/day for women, 1500 kcal/day for men) indicated that after an average of 21 weeks, weight loss was approximately 8.5 kg from baseline after a 21% attrition rate.[80] After an additional 1 year follow-up period, most of these subjects had regained some, but not all their weight.[80] Regain of weight is among the greatest challenges facing a diet intervention program. It has been shown that over time, weight regain increases and virtually all patients in a moderate calorie-restricted program regained all their pretreatment weight within 5 years.[81]

Because of the limited efficacy of moderate calorie-restricted weight-loss programs, the use of very low calorie diets was investigated. These diets, often providing less than

800 kcal/day, deliver large amounts of high-quality protein sources (>50 g/day) in an effort to spare fat-free mass during the period of weight loss induced by severe caloric restriction. In most cases, under careful medical supervision, these diets can safely induce weight loss of 1.5 to 2.5 kg/week. In the few well-controlled studies evaluating the efficacy of very low calorie diets, mean weight loss over the period of caloric restriction (16–26 weeks) ranged from approximately 10 kg to over 21 kg.[82] However, during follow-up intervals, all studies showed partial regain of the lost weight at 1 and 2 years, and in the one study that reported 5-year follow-up data, patients weighed more than their pretreatment weight.[82]

Because very low calorie diets do not seem to offer marked benefits over moderate calorie-restricted diets, it is recommended that a level of caloric restriction could be instituted with less risk and over a longer term basis. Despite the shortcomings of moderate calorie-restricted diets, it is well agreed that the dietary habits that may be conferred during these programs will be important adjuncts to any additional therapy that may be prescribed. The guidelines recommended for the initial dietary intervention are given in Table 43-3. A 500- to 1000-kcal energy deficit will cause patients to lose one to two pounds per week. This diet may be maintained for up to 6 months and should lead to the desired 10% weight loss in patients with initial BMI values of 35 kg/m² or greater. For patients with less severe obesity, the caloric deficit should be reduced. For many patients, particularly those with larger BMI values, weight loss beyond 6 months is extremely difficult. Part of this difficulty is explained by a concomitant reduction in metabolic rate and energy expenditure for a given amount of activity, so the caloric deficit is greatly reduced despite similar quantities of food intake. To maintain weight or continue weight loss, adjustments to greater levels of physical exercise must, therefore, be instituted between 3 and 6 months of a weight-loss program. Finally, social factors often make chronic, continuous caloric restriction very difficult.

EXERCISE

It is not contested that physical activity is a central component of any weight-loss program. Given the fact that total caloric intake has not risen dramatically in the United States over the past 2 decades, many experts believe the rise in obesity rates is more directly attributable to a decrease in the amount of physical activity of most Americans. Irrespective of etiology, multiple benefits are derived from any program that

Table 43-3 Initial Dietary Recommendations for Weight Loss

Nutrient	Recommended Intake
Calories	Approximately 500- to 1000-kcal/day reduction from usual intake
Total fat	30% or less of total calories
Saturated fatty acids*	8%–10% of total calories
Monounsaturated fatty acids	Up to 15% of total calories
Polyunsaturated fatty acids	Up to 10% of total calories
Cholesterol*	<300 mg/day
Protein	Approximately 15% of total calories
Carbohydrate	55% or more of total calories
Sodium chloride	No more than 100 mmol/day (approximately 2.4 g of sodium or approximately 6 g of sodium chloride)
Calcium	1000–1500 mg
Fiber	20–30 g

*May require additional modification if coexisting hyperlipidemia is present.

incorporates physical activity, including: an increase in the likelihood for successful weight loss by both increasing energy expenditure and decreasing appetite; an improvement in cardiovascular fitness and reduction in the risk of CHD; an increase in the success of weight maintenance once targets are achieved; and a reduction in intra-abdominal fat.[83]

As in all forms of physical exertion, it is best to start slowly, gradually building to the target level of activity. Many recommend a starting point of 10 minutes of walking, 3 days weekly, with increased walking to a target of up to 45 minutes 5 or more days per week. This target of exercise will use between 100 and 200 kcal/day. Given time, most patients will have improvements in exercise tolerance and functional capacity, often leading to higher targets and more strenuous sessions. More vigorous sessions may help sustain weight loss over time.

BEHAVIOR MODIFICATION

Because eating is often undertaken for personal, psychologic, or social reasons, associated behaviors are often powerful forces that impede long-term caloric restriction and weight loss. Efforts at weight loss independent of changes in long-term behavior are unlikely to succeed. A range of behavior modification techniques have been devised and tested, each being nearly equally effective at supporting a weight-loss program. Irrespective of the specific technique, the goal is generally to alter eating and eating-associated behavior for the long term with common behavior modification techniques.[5]

PHARMACOTHERAPY

Over the past 50 years, a large number of pharmacologic agents have been used in the control of weight with varying degrees of success. How health-care dollars were spent reflects the relatively low acceptance of pharmacotherapy. In 1995, it was estimated that the amount of money spent in the United States on all weight-loss products and services, including diet foods and drinks, exercise programs and equipment, and ancillary products approached $35 billion, including $12 billion on diet food products alone. Purchasing of diet food persists despite the widely held understanding that virtually all these products will do little to promote long-term weight loss and only exercise programs have a potential impact on cardiovascular conditioning. In contrast, the amount of money spent on antiobesity pharmaceuticals in this same period was less than $500 million. These figures underscore the perception, whether real or imagined, that the agents available are either of relatively limited efficacy or have associated safety issues that make them less desirable alternatives.

However, since 1995, changes have taken place. Several new agents were introduced, several older agents were reinvestigated, and two compounds were withdrawn from the market over safety concerns, as described in the following section. At present, several compounds have been studied and used for the treatment of obesity but these agents, including ephedrine, fluoxetine, and caffeine, have not been approved for use by the U.S. Food and Drug Administration. A number of other compounds, including mazindol, phentermine, benzphetamine, and phendimetrazine, are approved for only short-term use for obesity in a number of countries worldwide.

Despite the advances and changes in pharmacotherapy, few programs have been available that lead to weight loss of more than 10 kg over diet and exercise programs. Nevertheless, although the degree of weight loss induced by pharmacotherapy is modest, such changes could be expected to have an impact on the risk of comorbid conditions and potentially on mortality. However, studies also demonstrate consistent impediments to assessing the durability of efficacy. First, weight loss appears to plateau between 24 and 30 weeks of treatment. Second, both the placebo and active arms appear to have a consistent, albeit modest rise in weight from the plateau point through to the end of the study. Third, the study effect on weight end point is very large. In a study of D-fenfluramine, although weight loss in the active group was substantial (~10% of initial body weight), the placebo effect was also substantial, with a loss of approximately 7% of initial weight.[84] Finally, obesity trials are difficult to conduct in general because of a very large dropout rate. After 12 months, dropout rates approaching 50% in placebo groups are common, and even in active therapy arms, dropout rates may still be as high as 30% to 40%.[85] Given the high rates of dropout, completer analyses are often undertaken in addition to or even in lieu of intention-to-treat analyses. Because the single greatest reason for discontinuation is often dissatisfaction with weight loss, completer analyses will overestimate the a priori effect that any compound would be expected to achieve in a population of obese individuals.

Fenfluramine

D-Fenfluramine (and its racemic relative fenfluramine) is a centrally acting serotoninergic agonist and reuptake inhibitor whose main effect is suppression of appetite. D-Fenfluramine and fenfluramine were studied in several placebo-controlled, randomized, double-blind trials and were shown to cause significant weight loss from baseline.[86] The popularity of the use of D-fenfluramine was enhanced by the observation that when used over a 28-week treatment phase in combination with phentermine, a dopaminergic agonist, a significant 15.6% reduction from initial body weight was induced versus a mean 4.9% decrease in placebo-treated patients.[87] Furthermore, at least partial durability was demonstrated in follow-up open-label studies lasting up to 156 weeks.[88] However, in mid-1997, cardiac valvulopathy was reported in 24 patients treated with D-fenfluramine and phentermine.[89] Follow-up requests from the U.S. Food and Drug Administration led to a total of 113 confirmed cases of D-fenfluramine- or fenfluramine-induced valvulopathy (with or without phentermine).[90] These results ultimately led to the voluntary withdrawal of both D-fenfluramine and fenfluramine from the market.

Orlistat

Orlistat, a synthetic derivative of lipstatin (from *Streptomyces toxytricini*), is an inhibitor of gastric and pancreatic lipases, enzymes critical for the digestion and absorption of fat from the gastrointestinal tract. Inhibition of lipases causes a reduction in the absorption of fat and an increase in the excretion of triglycerides in feces. In a dose-ranging 24-week study of obese subjects (mean BMI ~35 kg/m^2), orlistat caused a maximal 9.8% decrease in initial body weight versus a decrease of 6.5% in the placebo-treated group.[91] In a separate 2-year randomized, crossover study of 688 obese individuals (BMI ~36 kg/m^2, weight ~100 kg), orlistat, 120 mg three times daily, caused a 10.2% decrease from initial body weight after the first year versus a 6.1% decrease in the placebo group.[92] Notably, both studies demonstrated a decrease in levels of the fat-soluble vitamins D, E, and betacarotene in a greater number of orlistat-treated patients than in placebo-treated patients. Furthermore, the number of adverse events predominantly related to the gastrointestinal tract included increased fatty and oily stools, fecal urgency and incontinence, and flatulence. In 1999, orlistat was approved in the United States for the treatment of obesity.

Sibutramine

Sibutramine is a serotonin, dopamine, and norepinephrine reuptake inhibitor. In several published studies, it has been shown to cause weight loss by a proposed primary mechanism of appetite suppression. In a dose-ranging 12-week trial of obese patients (BMI ~32 kg/m^2, weight ~85 kg), sibutramine caused a maximum weight loss of approximately 5 kg (~6% loss from initial weight) versus a weight loss of approximately 1 kg (~1% loss from initial weight) in the placebo group.[93] In a 1-year placebo-controlled trial, analysis of patients who completed the study showed that 65% of patients taking 15 mg of sibutramine lost 5% of their initial body weight whereas only 29% of placebo-treated patients lost as much.[94] Significant numbers of patients have also been shown to lose greater than 10% of initial body weight. This degree of efficacy should make sibutramine another important tool in an overall weight loss program. Monitoring of blood pressure will be important, however, because sibutramine has been associated with a 3- to 60-beat per minute increase in heart rate and an approximately 4 mm Hg increase in diastolic blood pressure even after weight loss.[93,94]

PHARMACOTHERAPY IN THE FUTURE

Antagonist of Cannabinoid Type 1 Receptors

Cannabinoid type 1 (CB1) receptor antagonists represent a new class of potential antiobesity compounds. CB1 receptors are located at nerves terminal and cell bodies coupled to G proteins. Stimulation of these receptors results in inhibition of the release of various neurotransmitters resulting in increased appetite and obesity. Rimonabant is an oral antagonist of CB1 receptors that is being developed by Sanofi-Synthélabo for the treatment of obesity. The compound is currently in phase III clinical trials (2004). Other compounds of similar mechanism include SLV-319 (Solvay SA), which is undergoing earlier clinical trials.[95]

β$_3$-Adrenergic Receptor Agonists

The β$_3$-adrenergic receptor is highly expressed in human BAT and to a limited degree in human white adipose tissue.[96] Multiple studies in animals have indicated that this receptor is a potential target for antiobesity therapy. Administration of a β$_3$-adrenergic receptor agonist has been shown to cause either weight loss, an increase in energy expenditure, or both in multiple species.[97] In addition to an antiobesity effect, β$_3$-adrenergic receptor agonists have been shown to have antihyperglycemic effects that appear to be, at least in part, independent of their antiobesity effects.[98,99]

To date, little or no efficacy of β$_3$-adrenergic receptor agonists has been demonstrated in humans, although one agent was able to induce a shift in the respiratory quotient, thus indicating an alteration in lipid oxidation.[100] However, all the compounds that have been put into clinical trials were optimized for activity at the rat β$_3$-adrenergic receptor. Additionally, it is argued that the small amount of BAT in adult humans limits the maximal effect on energy expenditure. However, this characteristic may not limit efficacy during chronic therapy. Treatment with β$_3$-adrenergic receptor agonists leads to significant expansion of the BAT compartment.[101,102] Humans have the potential for induction of BAT as demonstrated in patients with pheochromocytoma, in whom brown fat is markedly increased.[103] Finally, β$_3$-adrenergic receptors do not appear to undergo acute, agonist-induced downregulation,[76] which suggests that the weight-loss effect may require extended activity, leading to the induction of energy-regulating proteins such as UCP.

Leptin and Ciliary Neurotrophic Factor

The discovery of leptin held great promise for a potential target at which to direct pharmacotherapy. However, the observation that leptin levels rise and fall with weight and reach very high levels in obese patients[104] led to the conclusion that most patients with obesity are resistant to the effects of leptin on reducing appetite and increasing energy expenditure.[105] No major leptin receptor defect appears to account for this level of resistance.[106] Therefore, resistance to leptin action appears to be related to either an inability of higher leptin concentrations to penetrate the blood-brain barrier in order to signal to a normally functioning receptor[107]; a postreceptor signaling defect present in patients with obesity; or perhaps a combination of these. A trial of recombinant leptin at approximately 300 mg/day by daily subcutaneous injection for up to 6 months in humans achieved a decrease of approximately 8 kg from the initial weight as opposed to the placebo effect of a decrease of about 2 kg.[108] In addition, weekly administration of pegylated recombinant human leptin for 12 weeks was without significant changes in body weight and metabolic rate in obese men.[109] These disappointing results have been ascribed to the existent of leptin resistance in the majority of obese humans. Efforts are under way to find molecules that may bypass leptin resistance by activating the leptin cascade distal to the leptin receptor.[110] One such agent could be ciliary neurotrophic factor, a cytokine that can activate the STAT 3 signaling pathway in hypothalamic neurons through a receptor distinct from the leptin receptor.[111] Axokine is a genetically reengineered version of ciliary neurotrophic factor discovered by Regeneron Pharmaceuticals. Daily injections of Axokine reduced body weight in leptin-resistant rodents.[112] This therapy is currently in phase III clinical trials.

New Targets

Pharmaceuticals are under development for many potential new targets. The receptors for NPY are potentially important sites as drug targets. As noted previously, NPY is among the most potent orexigenic peptides identified, so by selectively blocking NPY at the "feeding" receptor, it is possible that the increased appetite and food-seeking behavior that occur during weight loss can be inhibited. Because the NPY-1 and NPY-5 receptors appear to be the most important subtypes with respect to feeding and weight regulation, several development programs are under way for the identification of selective antagonists. The melanocortin receptor system has also generated exciting interest. An agonist of the MC-3 or MC-4 receptor may lead to suppression of appetite. Because agouti-related protein increases feeding behavior by inhibiting activity at the MC-4 receptor, agents that prevent this interaction could also have appetite-suppressing properties. The newly discovered neuropeptides MCH and orexins, as well as corticotropin-releasing hormone, galanin, and opioid antagonists, may also be important targets in the race to develop effective antiobesity agents. In addition to these novel peptides, work is ongoing in the area of selective serotoninergic agents, such as agonists of the 5-HT$_{2c}$ receptor subtype, that may have a significantly better therapeutic index than any of the predecessor compounds to date.[110]

In the search for agents that work in the periphery, several areas of research may prove promising. The importance of the UCPs is still being understood. It is difficult to target these proteins because the need to deliver compounds to the intracellular and possibly the intramitochondrial compartments represents a true challenge. Furthermore, attempts to upregulate the expression or activity of UCPs in a tissue-specific manner may also be a difficult hurdle. UCP-2, for example, although highly expressed in BAT and skeletal muscle, is also found in immune response tissue, as well as in cardiocytes and brain. Uncoupling oxidated respiration in these tissues may lead to unfavorable toxicology. UCP-1, found only in BAT, may be insufficiently expressed to have an impact on human forms of obesity. Several of the other peripherally circulating peptides have also generated some interest as potential primary or adjunctive therapies for obesity, including CCK,[113] ghrelin,[41] PYY,[43] GLP-1,[114] and bombesin.[115] These molecules may be helpful by altering the meal termination signal.

REFERENCES

1. Flegal KM, Carroll MD, Ogden CL, et al: Prevalence and trends in obesity among US adults, 1999–2000. JAMA 288:1723–1727, 2002.
2. Dietz WH: Testimony before the House Government Reform Committee. July 25, 2002. www.cdc.gov.
3. Mizuno T, Shu IW, Makimura H, et al: Obesity over the life course. Sci Aging Knowledge Environ 24:re4, 2004. http://sageke.sciencemag.org/cgi/content/full/2004/24/re4.
4. Keil U, Kuulasmaa K: WHO MONICA Project: Risk factors. Int J Epidemiol 18(Suppl 1):46–55, 1989.
5. Donato KA, Pi-Suyner FX, Becker DM, et al: Executive summary of the clinical guidelines on the identification, evaluation, and treatment of overweight and obesity in adults. Arch Intern Med 158:1855–1867, 1998.
6. Ogden CL, Flegal KM, Carroll MD, et al: Prevalence and trends in overweight among US children and adolescents, 1999–2000. JAMA 288:1728–1732, 2002.
7. Seidell JC: The impact of obesity on health status: Some implications for health care costs. Int J Obes Relat Metab Disord 19(Suppl 6):13–16, 1995.
8. Stevens J, Cai J, Pamuk ER, et al: The effect of age on the association between body-mass index and mortality. N Engl J Med 338:1–7, 1998.
9. Manson JE, Stampfer MJ, Hennekens CH, et al: Body weight and longevity. A reassessment. JAMA 257:353–358, 1987.
10. Durazo-Arvizu R, Cooper RS, Luke A, et al: Relative weight and mortality in U.S. blacks and whites: Findings from representative national population samples. Ann Epidemiol 7:383–395, 1997.
11. Anonymous: Health implications of obesity. National Institutes of Health Consensus Development Conference Statement. Ann Intern Med 103:1073–1077, 1985.
12. Ford ES, Giles WH, Dietz WH: Prevalence of the metabolic syndrome among US adults. JAMA 287:356–359, 2002.
13. Lakka HM, Laaksonen DE, Lakka Ta, et al: The metabolic syndrome and total and cardiovascular disease mortality in middle-aged men. JAMA 288:2709–2716, 2002.
14. Dyer AR, Elliott P: The INTERSALT study: Relations of body mass index to blood pressure. INTERSALT Co-operative Research Group. J Hum Hypertens 3:299–308, 1989.
15. Anonymous: National Cholesterol Education Program. Second report of the expert panel on detection, evaluation, and treatment of high blood cholesterol in adults (Adult Treatment Panel II). Circulation 89:1333–1445, 1994.
16. Urbina EM, Gidding SS, Bao W, et al: Effect of body size, ponderosity, and blood pressure on left ventricular growth in children and young adults in the Bogalusa Heart Study. Circulation 91:2400–2406, 1995.
17. Rexrode KM, Hennekens CH, Willett WC, et al: A prospective study of body mass index, weight change, and risk of stroke in women. JAMA 277:1539–1545, 1997.
18. Colditz GA, Willett WC, Stampfer MJ, et al: Weight as a risk factor for clinical diabetes in women. Am J Epidemiol 132:501–513, 1990.
19. Ford ES, Williamson DF, Liu S: Weight change and diabetes incidence: Findings from a national cohort of US adults. Am J Epidemiol 146:214–222, 1997.
20. Calle EE, Rodriguez C, Walker-Thurmond K, et al: Overweight, obesity, and mortality from cancer in a prospectively studied cohort of U.S. adults. N Engl J Med 348:1625–1638, 2003.
21. Adami HO, Trichopoulos D: Obesity and mortality from cancer. N Engl J Med 348:1623–1624, 2003.
22. Prentice A, Goldberg G: Maternal obesity increases congenital malformations. Nutr Rev 54:146–150, 1996.
23. Cnattingius S, Bergstrom R, Lipworth L, et al: Prepregnancy weight and the risk of adverse pregnancy outcomes. N Engl J Med 338:147–152, 1998.
24. Stampfer MJ, Maclure KM, Colditz GA, et al: Risk of symptomatic gallstones in women with severe obesity. Am J Clin Nutr 55:652–658, 1992.
25. Cicuttini FM, Baker JR, Spector TD: The association of obesity with osteoarthritis of the hand and knee in women: A twin study. J Rheumatol 23:1221–1226, 1996.
26. Young T, Palta M, Dempsey J, et al: The occurrence of sleep-disordered breathing among middle-aged adults. N Engl J Med 328:1230–1235, 1993.
27. Ohlson LO, Larsson B, Svardsudd K, et al: The influence of body fat distribution on the incidence of diabetes mellitus. 13.5 years of follow-up of the participants in the study of men born in 1913. Diabetes 34:1055–1058, 1985.
28. Kissebah AH, Vydelingum N, Murray R, et al: Relation of body fat distribution to metabolic complications of obesity. J Clin Endocrinol Metab 54:254–260, 1982.
29. Ravussin E, Swindburn BA: Energy metabolism. In Stunkard AJ, Wadden TA (eds): Obesity: Theory and Therapy, 2d ed. New York, Raven, 1993, pp 97–123.
30. Roberts SB, Savage J, Coward WA, et al: Energy expenditure and intake in infants born to lean and overweight mothers. N Engl J Med 318:461–466, 1988.
31. Ravussin E, Lillioja S, Knowler WC, et al: Reduced rate of energy expenditure as a risk factor for body-weight gain. N Engl J Med 318:467–472, 1988.
32. Goran MI, Shewchuk R, Gower BA, et al: Longitudinal changes in fatness in white children: No effect of childhood energy expenditure. Am J Clin Nutr 67:309–316, 1998.
33. Zhang Y, Proenca R, Maffei M, et al: Positional cloning of the mouse obese gene and its human homologue [published erratum appears in Nature 1995 Mar 30; 374(6521):479]. Nature 372:425–432, 1994.
34. Rajala MW, Scherer PE: Minireview: The adipocyte—at the crossroads of energy homeostasis, inflammation, and atherosclerosis. Endocrinology 144(9):3765–3773, 2003.
35. Wellen KE, Hotamisligil GS: Obesity-induced inflammatory changes in adipose tissue. J Clin Invest 112:1785–1788, 2003.
36. Rowe JW, Young JB, Minaker KL, et al: Effect of insulin and glucose infusions on sympathetic nervous system activity in normal man. Diabetes 30:219–225, 1981.
37. Sakaguchi T, Bray GA: The effect of intrahypothalamic injections of glucose on sympathetic efferent firing rate. Brain Res Bull 18:591–595, 1987.
38. Gibbs J, Young RC, Smith GP: Cholecystokinin decreases food intake in rats. J Comp Physiol Psychol 84:488–495, 1973.
39. Reidelberger RD, O'Rourke MF: Potent cholecystokinin antagonist L 364718 stimulates food intake in rats. Am J Physiol 257:R1512–R1518, 1989.
40. Kojima M, Hosoda H, Date Y, et al: Ghrelin is a growth-hormone-releasing acylated peptide from stomach. Nature 402:656–660, 1999.
41. Tschop M, Smiley DL, Heiman ML: Ghrelin induces adiposity in rodents. Nature 407:908–913, 2000.
42. Druce MR, Small CJ, Bloom SR: Minireview: Gut peptides regulating satiety. Endocrinology 145(6):2660–2665, 2004.
43. Adrian TE, Ferri GL, Bacarese-Hamilton AJ: Human distribution and release of a putative new gut hormone, peptide YY. Gastroenterology 89:1070–1077, 1985.
44. Batterham RL, Cohen MA, Ellis SM, et al: Inhibition of food intake in obese subjects by peptide YY3-36. N Engl J Med 349:941–948, 2003.
45. Gibbs J, Fauser DJ, Rowe EA, et al: Bombesin suppresses feeding in rats. Nature 282:208–210, 1979.
46. Elrick H, Stimmler L, Hald CJ, et al: Plasma insulin response to oral and intravenous glucose administration. J Clin Invest 24:1076–1082, 1964.
47. Drucker DJ: Glucagon-like peptides. Diabetes 47:159–169, 1998.
48. Verdich C, Toubro S, Buemann B, et al: The role of postprandial releases of insulin and incretin hormones in meal-induced satiety-effect of obesity and weight reduction. Int J Obes Relat Metab Disord 25:1206–1214, 2001.

49. Naslund E: Prandial subcutaneous injections of GLP-1 cause weight loss in obese human subjects. Br J Nutr 91:439–446, 2004.

50. Stephens TW, Basinski M, Bristow PK, et al: The role of neuropeptide Y in the antiobesity action of the obese gene product. Nature 377:530–532, 1995.

51. Stanley BG, Kyrkouli SE, Lampert S, et al: Neuropeptide Y chronically injected into the hypothalamus: A powerful neurochemical inducer of hyperphagia and obesity. Peptides 7:1189–1192, 1986.

52. Erickson JC, Hollopeter G, Palmiter RD: Attenuation of the obesity syndrome of ob/ob mice by the loss of neuropeptide Y. Science 274:1704–1707, 1996.

53. Gehlert DR: Subtypes of receptors for neuropeptide Y: Implications for the targeting of therapeutics. Life Sci 55:551–562, 1994.

54. Woldbye DP, Larsen PJ: The how and Y of eating. Nat Med 4:671–672, 1998.

55. Qu D, Ludwig DS, Gammeltoft S, et al: A role for melanin-concentrating hormone in the central regulation of feeding behaviour. Nature 380:243–247, 1996.

56. Shimada M, Tritos NA, Lowell BB, et al: Mice lacking melanin-concentrating hormone are hypophagic and lean. Nature 396:670–674, 1998.

57. Akabayashi A, Koenig JI, Watanabe Y, et al: Galanin-containing neurons in the paraventricular nucleus: A neurochemical marker for fat ingestion and body weight gain. Proc Natl Acad Sci U S A 91:10375–10379, 1994.

58. Smith BK, York DA, Bray GA: Chronic cerebroventricular galanin does not induce sustained hyperphagia or obesity. Peptides 15:1267–1272, 1994.

59. Kalra SP, Dube MG, Pu SY, et al: Interacting appetite-regulating pathways in the hypothalamic regulation of body weight. Endocr Rev 20:68–100, 1999.

60. Cone RD, Lu D, Koppula S, et al: The melanocortin receptors: Agonists, antagonists, and the hormonal control of pigmentation. Recent Prog Horm Res 51:287–318, 1996.

61. Huszar D, Lynch CA, Fairchild-Huntress V, et al: Targeted disruption of the melanocortin-4 receptor results in obesity in mice. Cell 88:131–141, 1997.

62. Ollmann MM, Wilson BD, Yang YK, et al: Antagonism of central melanocortin receptors in vitro and in vivo by agouti-related protein. Science 278:135–138, 1997.

63. Spina M, Merlo-Pich E, Chan RK, et al: Appetite-suppressing effects of urocortin, a CRF-related neuropeptide. Science 273:1561–1564, 1996.

64. Kristensen P, Judge ME, Thim L, et al: Hypothalamic CART is a new anorectic peptide regulated by leptin. Nature 393:72–76, 1998.

65. Ricquier D, Kader JC: Mitochondrial protein alteration in active brown fat: A sodium dodecyl sulfate-polyacrylamide gel electrophoretic study. Biochem Biophys Res Commun 73:577–583, 1976.

66. Lowell BB, Flier JS: Brown adipose tissue, beta 3-adrenergic receptors, and obesity. Annu Rev Med 48:307–316, 1997.

67. Carmona MC, Valmaseda A, Brun S, et al: Differential regulation of uncoupling protein-2 and uncoupling protein-3 gene expression in brown adipose tissue during development and cold exposure. Biochem Biophys Res Commun 243:224–228, 1998.

68. Bienengraeber M, Echtay KS, Klingenberg M: H⁺ transport by uncoupling protein (UCP-1) is dependent on a histidine pair, absent in UCP-2 and UCP-3. Biochemistry 37:3–8, 1998.

69. Hauge A, Oye I: Effect of adrenaline and adrenergic blocking agents on the basal oxygen consumption of the perfused rat heart. Nature 210:998–1000, 1966.

70. Rothwell NJ, Saville ME, Stock MJ: Sympathetic and thyroid influences on metabolic rate in fed, fasted, and refed rats. Am J Physiol 243:R339–R346, 1982.

71. Lands AM, Arnold A, McAuliff JP, et al: Differentiation of receptor systems activated by sympathomimetic amines. Nature 214:597–598, 1967.

72. Tan S, Curtis-Prior PB: Characterization of the beta-adrenoceptor of the adipose cell of the rat. Int J Obes 7:409–414, 1983.

73. Rothwell NJ, Stock MJ: A role for brown adipose tissue in diet-induced thermogenesis. Obes Res 5:650–656, 1997.

74. Himms-Hagen J: Brown adipose tissue thermogenesis and obesity. Prog Lipid Res 28:67–115, 1989.

75. Granneman JG, Lahners KN, Rao DD: Rodent and human beta 3-adrenergic receptor genes contain an intron within the protein-coding block. Mol Pharmacol 42:964–970, 1992.

76. Nantel F, Bonin H, Emorine LJ, et al: The human beta 3-adrenergic receptor is resistant to short term agonist-promoted desensitization. Mol Pharmacol 43:548–555, 1993.

77. The practical guide: Identification, evaluation, and treatment of over-weight and obesity in adults. (NIH Publication No. 00-4084) Bethesda, MD, National Heart, Lung, and Blood Institute, North American Association for the Study of Obesity, 2000.

78. Roadmaps for Clinical Practice—Case Studies in Disease Prevention and Health Promotion. Assessment and Management of Adult Obesity: A Primer for Physicians. American Medical Association, The Robert Wood Johnson Foundation, 2003.

79. Hayter JE, Henry CJ: A re-examination of basal metabolic rate predictive equations: The importance of geographic origin of subjects in sample selection. Eur J Clin Nutr 48:702–707, 1994.

80. Wadden TA: Treatment of obesity by moderate and severe caloric restriction. Results of clinical research trials. Ann Intern Med 119:688–693, 1993.

81. Kramer FM, Jeffery RW, Forster JL, et al: Long-term follow-up of behavioral treatment for obesity: Patterns of weight regain among men and women. Int J Obes 13:123–136, 1989.

82. Wadden TA, Sternberg JA, Letizia KA, et al: Treatment of obesity by very low calorie diet, behavior therapy, and their combination: A five-year perspective. Int J Obes 13(Suppl 2):39–46, 1989.

83. Centers for Disease Control, National Center for Chronic Disease Prevention and Health Promotion: Surgeon General's Report on Physical Activity and Health. Atlanta, Centers for Disease Control and Prevention, 1996.

84. Guy-Grand B, Apfelbaum M, Crepaldi G, et al: International trial of long-term dexfenfluramine in obesity. Lancet 2:1142–1145, 1989.

85. Munro JF: Clinical aspects of the treatment of obesity by drugs: A review. Int J Obes 3:171–180, 1979.

86. Weintraub M, Hasday JD, Mushlin AI, et al: A double-blind clinical trial in weight control. Use of fenfluramine and phentermine alone and in combination. Arch Intern Med 144:1143–1148, 1984.

87. Weintraub M, Sundaresan PR, Madan M, et al: Long-term weight control study. I (weeks 0 to 34). The enhancement of behavior modification, caloric restriction, and exercise by fenfluramine plus phentermine versus placebo. Clin Pharmacol Ther 51:586–594, 1992.

88. Weintraub M, Sundaresan PR, Schuster B, et al: Long-term weight control study. III (weeks 104 to 156). An open-label study of dose adjustment of fenfluramine and phentermine. Clin Pharmacol Ther 51:602–607, 1992.

89. Connolly HM, Crary JL, McGoon MD, et al: Valvular heart disease associated with fenfluramine-phentermine. N Engl J Med 337:581–588, 1997.

90. Centers for Disease Control and Prevention: Cardiac valvulopathy associated with exposure to fenfluramine or dexfenfluramine: U.S. Department of Health and Human Services Interim Public Health Recommendations, November 1997. Morb Mortal Wkly Rep 46:1061–1066, 1997.

91. Van Gaal LF, Broom JI, Enzi G, et al: Efficacy and tolerability of orlistat in the treatment of obesity: A 6-month dose-ranging study. Orlistat Dose-Ranging Study Group. Eur J Clin Pharmacol 54:125–132, 1998.

92. Sjostrom L, Rissanen A, Andersen T, et al: Randomised placebo-controlled trial of orlistat for weight loss and prevention of weight regain in obese patients. European Multicentre Orlistat Study Group. Lancet 352:167–172, 1998.

93. Hanotin C, Thomas F, Jones SP, et al: Efficacy and tolerability of sibutramine in obese patients: A dose-ranging study. Int J Obes Relat Metab Disord 22:32–38, 1998.

94. Lean ME: Sibutramine—a review of clinical efficacy. Int J Obes Relat Metab Disord 21(Suppl 1):30–39, 1997.

95. Fernandez JR, Allison DB: Rimonabant Sanofi-Synthélabo. Curr Opin Investig Drugs 5:430–435, 2004.

96. Krief S, Lonnqvist F, Raimbault S, et al: Tissue distribution of beta 3-adrenergic receptor mRNA in man. J Clin Invest 91:344–349, 1993.

97. Collins S, Daniel KW, Petro AE, et al: Strain-specific response to beta(3)-adrenergic receptor agonist treatment of diet-induced obesity in mice. Endocrinology 138:405–413, 1997.

98. deSouza CJ, Hirshman MF, Horton ES, et al: CL-316,243, a beta(3)-specific adrenoceptor agonist, enhances insulin-stimulated glucose disposal in nonobese rats. Diabetes 46:1257–1263, 1997.

99. Liu X, Perusse F, Bukowiecki LJ: Mechanisms of the antidiabetic effects of the beta 3-adrenergic agonist CL-316243 in obese Zucker-ZDF rats. Am J Physiol 274:R1212–R1219, 1998.

100. Weyer C, Tataranni PA, Snitker S, et al: Increase in insulin action and fat oxidation after treatment with CL 316,243, a highly selective beta3-adrenoceptor agonist in humans. Diabetes 47:1555–1561, 1998.

101. Champigny O, Ricquier D: Evidence from in vitro differentiating cells that adrenoceptor agonists can increase uncoupling protein mRNA level in adipocytes of adult humans: An RT-PCR study. J Lipid Res 37:1907–1914, 1996.

102. Champigny O, Ricquier D, Blondel O, et al: Beta 3-adrenergic receptor stimulation restores message and expression of brown-fat mitochondrial uncoupling protein in adult dogs. Proc Natl Acad Sci U S A 88:10774–10777, 1991.

103. Ricquier D, Nechad M, Mory G: Ultrastructural and biochemical characterization of human brown adipose tissue in pheochromocytoma. J Clin Endocrinol Metab 54:803–807, 1982.

104. Considine RV, Sinha MK, Heiman ML, et al: Serum immunoreactive-leptin concentrations in normal weight and obese humans. New Engl J Med 334:292, 1996.

105. Caro JF, Sinha MK, Kolaczynski JW, et al: Leptin: The tale of an obesity gene. Diabetes 45:1455, 1996.

106. Considine RV, Considine EL, Williams CJ, et al: The hypothalamic leptin receptor in humans: Identification of incidental sequence polymorphisms and absence of the db/db mouse and fa/fa rat mutations. Diabetes 45:992–994, 1996.

107. Caro JF, Kolaczynski JW, Nyce MR, et al: Decreased CSF/serum leptin ratio in human obesity: A possible mechanism for "apparent" leptin resistance. Lancet 348:159, 1996.

108. Heymsfield SB, Greenberg AS, Fujioka K, et al: Recombinant leptin for weight loss in obese and lean adults: A randomized, controlled dose-escalation trial. JAMA 282:1568–1575, 1999.

109. Hukshorn CJ, Saris WHM, Westerterp-Plantenga MS, et al: Weekly subcutaneous pegylated recombinant native human leptin (PEG-OB) administration in obese men. J Clin Endocrinol Metab 85:4003–4009, 2000.

110. Weigle DS: Pharmacological therapy of obesity: Past, present, and future. J Clin Endocrinol Metab 88:2462–2469, 2003.

111. Kalra SP: Circumventing leptin resistance for weight control. Proc Natl Acad Sci U S A 98:4279–4281, 2001.

112. Lambert PD, Anderson KD, Sleeman MW, et al: Ciliary neurotrophic factor activates leptin-like pathways and reduces body fat, without cachexia or rebound weight gain, even in leptin-resistant obesity. Proc Natl Acad Sci U S A 98:4652–4657, 2001.

113. Moran TH, Shnayder L, Hostetler AM, et al: Pylorectomy reduces the satiety action of cholecystokinin. Am J Physiol 255:R1059–R1063, 1988.

114. Wang Z, Wang RM, Owji AA, et al: Glucagon-like peptide-1 is a physiological incretin in rat. J Clin Invest 95:417–421, 1995.

115. Ohki-Hamazaki H, Watase K, Yamamoto K, et al: Mice lacking bombesin receptor subtype-3 develop metabolic defects and obesity. Nature 390:165–169, 1997.

Genetic Syndromes Associated with Obesity

I. Sadaf Farooqi and Stephen O'Rahilly

OBESITY ASSOCIATED WITH DEVELOPMENTAL DELAY
- Prader-Willi Syndrome
- Fragile X Syndrome
- Bardet-Biedl Syndrome
- Börjeson-Forssman-Lehmann Syndrome
- Wilson-Turner Syndrome
- Cohen Syndrome
- Albright Hereditary Osteodystrophy
- Additional Syndromes

OBESITY WITHOUT DEVELOPMENTAL DELAY
- Alström Syndrome
- Ulnar-Mammary Syndrome
- Simpson-Golabi-Behmel Type 2
- Congenital Leptin Deficiency
- Leptin Receptor Deficiency
- Pro-opiomelanocortin Deficiency
- Melanocortin 4 Receptor Deficiency
- Prohormone Convertase-1 Deficiency
- Other Syndromes

SUMMARY

Inherited factors play a substantial role in determining adiposity across the full range of human body weight.[1] This chapter focuses on the known mendelian disorders that include obesity as a consistent clinical feature. Classically, patients affected by these obesity syndromes have been identified as a result of their association with mental retardation, dysmorphic features, and other developmental abnormalities. More recently, several new monogenic disorders, resulting from disruption of the leptin-melanocortin signaling pathway (see Chapter 42), have been identified. In these disorders, obesity itself is often the predominant presenting feature, although it often is accompanied by characteristic patterns of neuroendocrine dysfunction. For the purposes of clinical assessment, it is useful to categorize genetic obesity syndromes as syndromes with and without associated developmental delay.

OBESITY ASSOCIATED WITH DEVELOPMENTAL DELAY

PRADER-WILLI SYNDROME

Definition, Prevalence, Etiology, and Pathogenesis

Prader and Willi[2] described the first patient with Prader-Willi syndrome (PWS) in 1956. PWS is the most common syndromal cause of human obesity with an estimated prevalence of about 1 in 25,000 births and a population prevalence of 1 in 50,000.[3] The syndrome is caused by deletion or disruption of a paternally imprinted gene or genes on the proximal long arm of chromosome 15. The molecular pathophysiology is unclear, although several candidate genes in this region have been studied and their expression shown to be absent in postmortem brains of PWS patients.[4]

One suggested mediator of the obesity phenotype in PWS patients is the enteric hormone ghrelin, which is implicated in the regulation of meal-time hunger in rodents and humans and is a stimulator of growth hormone (GH) secretion via the GH-secretagogue receptor.[5] Fasting plasma ghrelin levels are 4.5-fold higher in PWS subjects than equally obese controls and patients with other obesity syndromes and possibly may be implicated in the pathogenesis of hyperphagia in these patients.[6,7]

Clinical Features

PWS is characterized by diminished fetal activity, hypotonia, mental retardation, short stature, hypogonadotropic hypogonadism, and obesity. The diagnostic criteria arrived at by a consensus group are based on a point system; one point each is allowed for each of five major criteria and one-half point each for seven minor criteria.[8] A minimum of 8.5 points is considered necessary for the clinical diagnosis of PWS (Table 44-1).

In general, there is mild prenatal growth retardation with a mean birth weight of about 6 lb (2.8 kg) at term, hyporeflexia, and poor feeding in neonatal life resulting from diminished swallowing and sucking reflexes; infants often require assisted feeding for about 3 to 4 months. Feeding difficulties generally improve by age 6 months. From 12 to 18 months onward, hyperphagia is a dominant feature in PWS patients, often associated with pica behavior.

Children with PWS display diminished growth, reduced muscle mass, and increased fat mass—body composition abnormalities resembling those seen in GH deficiency.[9] Diminished GH responses to various provocative agents, low insulin-like growth factor (IGF) type 1 levels, and the presence of additional evidence of hypothalamic dysfunction support the presence of true GH deficiency in many children with PWS. Boys with PWS usually have hypoplastic external genitalia, including micropenis, whereas girls have hypoplastic labia minora. Adrenarche can occur early, but gonadal maturation is usually either delayed or incomplete secondary to hypogonadotropic hypogonadism.

Studies have shown a particular pattern of fat distribution in adults with PWS, with a large amount of subcutaneous fat in the presence of relatively normal intra-abdominal fat stores. This pattern of fat distribution is associated with relative protection from the insulin resistance and metabolic syndrome usually associated with morbid obesity.[10]

Diagnosis

Chromosomal mechanisms (usually sporadic) are principally responsible for PWS, and the syndrome is caused by lack of the paternal segment 15q11.2-q12. There are two mechanisms by which such a loss can occur: through deletion of the paternal "critical" segment (in 75% of patients) or through loss of the entire paternal chromosome 15 with presence of two maternal homologues (uniparental maternal disomy) (in approximately 22% of patients).[11] The opposite (i.e., maternal deletion or paternal uniparental disomy) causes another characteristic phenotype, the Angelman syndrome. Rarely, imprinting errors resulting from a sporadic or inherited microdeletion in the imprinting center (3% of patients) or a paternal imprinted translocation (<1%) is observed.[11]

Table 44-1 | Diagnostic Criteria for Prader-Willi Syndrome

MAJOR CRITERIA
Neonatal and infantile hypotonia, with poor suck and subsequent improvement with age
Feeding problems with poor weight gain in infancy, needing gavage or other special feeding techniques
Weight gain (rapid onset 1 to 6 years old) that leads to central obesity
Characteristic facial features, including narrow bifrontal diameter, almond-shaped palpebral fissures, and turned-down mouth
Hypogonadism/hypogenitalism: genital hypoplasia (small labia minora and clitoris in females, and hypoplastic scrotum in males); incomplete and delayed puberty; and infertility
Developmental delay/mild to moderate mental retardation/multiple learning disabilities
Hyperphagia/obsession with food
Chromosome 15q11-q13 abnormality

MINOR CRITERIA
Reduced fetal movement and infantile lethargy, which improves with age
Characteristic behavioral problems, including temper tantrums, obsessive-compulsive behavior, stubbornness, rigidity, stealing, and lying
Sleep disturbance or apnea
Short stature for family by 15 years of age
Hypopigmentation
Small hands and feet for height and age
Narrow hands with straight ulnar border
Eye abnormalities, including esotropis and myopia
Thick viscous saliva
Speech articulation defect
Skin picking

ADDITIONAL FEATURES
High pain threshold
Decreased vomiting
Altered temperature sensitivity
Scoliosis and kyphosis
Early adrenarche
Osteoporosis
Unusual skill with jigsaws
Normal neuromuscular studies (e.g., muscle biopsy and electromyography)

Major criteria are weighed at one point each and minor criteria at one-half point each. For children <3 years of age, five points are required for diagnosis, 4 of which must be major criteria. For individuals >3 years of age, 8 points are required for diagnosis, 5 of which must be major criteria. Supportive findings only increase or decrease the level of suspicion of the diagnosis.

Deletions account for 70% to 80% of cases, many of which can be visualized by standard prometaphase banding examination. A few consist of unbalanced translocations, which are detected easily by routine chromosome examination. The remaining cases are the result of maternal uniparental disomy in which cytogenetic examinations yield normal results. However, There are distinct differences in DNA methylation at the D15S9 locus on 15q11-q13 according to the parent of origin; DNA methylation can be used as a reliable postnatal diagnostic tool in PWS patients with a normal karyotype.[12]

Treatment
Traditionally, the mainstay of management has centered on early institution of a low-calorie diet with regular exercise, rigorous supervision, restriction of food and money, and appropriate psychological and behavioral counseling of the patient and family, often in the context of group homes for PWS adolescents and adults. Pharmacologic treatment, including anorexigenic agents that act through central monoamine and serotoninergic pathways, is not always beneficial in treating hyperphagia and obesity, although there are a few published control studies. The choice and the use of specific antidiabetic, antihypertensive, and lipid-lowering agents are guided by

subjects in the general population with obesity, but possible differences in PWS have not been addressed systematically.[13]

In PWS children, therapy with GH significantly improves the rate of growth and final height. Long-term studies show that the final height is in the average range for age, and GH is now licensed for use in PWS. GH treatment in PWS children also decreases body fat and increases muscle mass, fat oxidation, and energy expenditure.[14] Physical strength and agility also improve. These improvements are most dramatic during the first year of GH therapy, although prolonged treatment does not completely normalize these parameters. Although increases in fasting insulin and reduced glucose elimination rates have been seen during GH therapy, the development of glucose intolerance and diabetes mellitus does not seem to be a problem to date.

Treatment with clomiphene citrate has been shown to raise plasma luteinizing hormone, testosterone, and urinary gonadotropin levels to normal and result in normal spermatogenesis and physical signs of puberty.[15] The prescription of testosterone therapy to male PWS patients has been complicated by anecdotal reports of increased aggressive behavior.

FRAGILE X SYNDROME

Definition, Prevalence, Etiology, and Pathogenesis
The fragile X syndrome is the most common cause of inherited mental retardation. Epidemiologic studies indicate this syndrome is responsible for moderate-to-severe mental retardation in 1 in 4000 to 6000 males of European descent and responsible for mild-to-moderate mental retardation in 1 in 7000 to 10,000 females, with the frequency of the disease thought to be higher in some ethnic groups (e.g., Tunisian Jews and African Americans). In 1991, the molecular cloning of the fragile X locus revealed unstable expansions of a CGG trinucleotide repeat, located in the *FMR1* gene (fragile X mental retardation). In affected families, there are often clinically normal, transmitting males, whose daughters, who also are clinically normal, have a high risk of having clinically affected children.[16]

Clinical Features
Fragile X syndrome is characterized by moderate-to-severe mental retardation, macro-orchidism, large ears, macrocephaly, prominent jaw (mandibular prognathism), and high-pitched jocular speech. In affected boys, delay in language acquisition or behavioral problems or both are often the presenting symptoms. A Prader-Willi-like subphenotype of the fragile X syndrome has been described in a subset of patients with extreme obesity with a full, round face; small, broad hands and feet; and regional skin hyperpigmentation.[17] In contrast to PWS, the patients lacked the neonatal hypotonia and feeding problems during infancy followed by hyperphagia during toddlerhood.

Diagnosis and Treatment
The discovery of the fragile X expansion mutation has produced efficient and reliable tools for diagnosis, genetic counseling, and prenatal diagnosis.[18] Approaches used in the management of the behavioral disturbance of these children include the use of clonidine and anticonvulsants, especially carbamazepine and valproate, which may have behavior-modifying effects in addition to their antiseizure actions, and some forms of behavioral therapy.[19]

BARDET-BIEDL SYNDROME

Definition, Prevalence, Etiology, and Pathogenesis
The earliest formal description of Bardet-Biedl syndrome (BBS) was in 1920 by Bardet, who described patients with hexadactyly, retinitis pigmentosa, and obesity. In 1922, Biedl, an Austrian professor of pathology and endocrinology, published

a short independent account of two siblings with "congenital deformations (retinitis pigmentosa and polydactyly) and an intellectual torpidity." BBS is a rare (prevalence <1/100,000), genetically highly heterogeneous, autosomal-recessive syndrome characterized by central obesity (in 75% of patients), mental retardation, dysphormic extremities (syndactyly, brachydactyly, or polydactyly), retinal dystrophy or pigmentary retinopathy, hypogonadism or hypogenitalism (limited to male patients), and structural abnormalities of the kidney or functional renal impairment. There is some overlap with the syndrome described by Laurence[20] (an ophthalmic surgeon) and his house surgeon Moon in the late 1800s characterized by retinal pigmentary degeneration, mental retardation, and hypogonadism in conjunction with progressive spastic paraparesis and distal muscle weakness, but without polydactyly.

BBS is a genetically heterogeneous disorder that is now known to map to at least eight loci: 11q13 (BBS1), 16q21 (BBS2), 3p13-p12 (BBS3), 15q22.3-q23 (BBS4), 2q31 (BBS5), 20p12 (BBS6), 4q27 (BBS7), and 14q32.11 (BBS8), seven of which now have been identified at the molecular level.[21,22] Although BBS usually is transmitted as a recessive disorder, some families have exhibited so-called triallelic inheritance, in which the clinical manifestation of the syndrome requires two mutations in one BBS gene plus an additional mutation in a second, unlinked BBS gene.[23]

Studies strongly indicate that many of the genes involved in BBS are involved in the structure or function of the basal body, a modified centriole that is essential for the function of cilia.[24] All of the BBS gene homologues that are present in the nematode Caenorhabditis elegans are located exclusively in ciliated sensory neurons; this suggests that a defect in sensing by homologous mammalian neurons may underlie the hyperphagia and obesity seen in BBS.

Genotype-Phenotype Correlations
The clinical manifestations of BBS were compared in three unrelated, extended Arab-Bedouin kindreds in which linkage had been shown to chromosomes 3 (BBS3), 15 (BBS4), and 16 (BBS2). Observed differences included the limb distribution of the postaxial polydactyly and the extent and age association of obesity. It appeared that the chromosome 3 locus was associated with polydactyly of all four limbs, whereas polydactyly of the chromosome 15 type (BBS4) was confined mostly to the hands. The chromosome 15 type was associated with early-onset morbid obesity, whereas the chromosome 16 (BBS2) type appeared to present the "leanest" BBS phenotype.

Diagnosis and Treatment
Currently, a diagnosis of BBS is made on clinical grounds, although it is expected that prenatal and postnatal molecular genetic testing soon will reach routine clinical practice. Patients with BBS are best managed in specialist centers with access to a wide range of specialists with experience of the disorder. Ophthalmologic advice is crucial, although there are no established treatments that prevent or alleviate the deterioration in vision. Support can be given, however, to prepare for a life with low vision. Learning difficulties should be assessed early, if possible, before visual impairment hampers potentially beneficial speech and language therapy. Accessory digits are often nonfunctional and excised within the first year of life by either orthopedic or plastic surgeons. Bony deformation in already wide feet can lead to ill-fitting shoes, and podiatric advice and special fitting of shoes is important. Oral hypoglycemics and insulin have been used in patients who develop type 2 diabetes. There is no evidence to suggest that testosterone therapy or GH therapy is particularly beneficial.

BÖRJESON-FORSSMAN-LEHMANN SYNDROME

In 1962, Börjeson, Forssman, and Lehmann[25] described a syndrome characterized by moderate-to-severe mental retardation,

epilepsy, hypogonadism, obesity with marked gynecomastia, swelling of subcutaneous tissue of the face, narrow palpebral fissures, and large but not deformed ears. By linkage analysis, the gene associated with Börjeson-Forssman-Lehmann syndrome was localized to Xq26-q27, and more recently mutations in a novel, widely expressed zinc-finger (plant homeodomain–like finger) gene (PHF6) have been identified in affected families.[26]

WILSON-TURNER SYNDROME

In 1991, Wilson and coworkers[27] described a kindred in which males in five successive generations in an X-linked-recessive pedigree pattern had a mental retardation syndrome. The 14 living males in the 3 most recent generations permitted definition of other features: obesity, gynecomastia, speech difficulties, emotional lability, tapering fingers, and small feet. Some of the features resembled those of Börjeson-Forssman-Lehmann syndrome, but the patients of Wilson and Turner did not have hypermetropia or cataracts in later life and did not have elongated earlobes. Linkage studies have defined the physical localization as Xp21.1-q22.

COHEN SYNDROME

In 1973, Cohen and associates[28] from the United States observed three patients with a previously unrecognized pattern of abnormalities in association with truncal obesity. Cohen syndrome is one of the rare autosomal-recessive disorders that are overrepresented in the Finnish population and is characterized by nonprogressive mild-to-severe psychomotor retardation, motor clumsiness, microcephaly, characteristic facial features, childhood hypotonia and joint laxity, progressive retinochoroidal dystrophy, myopia, intermittent isolated neutropenia, and a cheerful disposition.[29] Specific facial features include high-arched or wave-shaped eyelids; long, thick eyelashes; thick eyebrows; prominent root of nose; short philtrum (which is unable to cover the prominent upper central incisors); small or absent lobuli of the ears; thick hair and low hairline; narrow hands and feet; and mild syndactylies (in 50% to 60%). Progressive, often high-grade myopia and retinochoroidal dystrophy resembling retinitis pigmentosa are essential features in Cohen syndrome. Vision starts to deteriorate early but generally is preserved until adulthood; by age 40, many patients are severely visually handicapped.

Linkage analysis based on many extended Finnish pedigrees led to the identification of a locus on 8q22, and homozygosity mapping in a consanguineous Lebanese kindred led to the gene responsible for this condition being localized to a region on chromosome 8q21.3-q22.1. The critical Cohen syndrome was refined by haplotype analysis and more recently a novel gene, COH1, which is mutated in some Finnish patients with Cohen syndrome, has been identified.[30] Although the functional properties of this protein are unclear, comparison with structurally homologous proteins suggests a role in intracellular vesicle–mediated sorting and transport of proteins.

ALBRIGHT HEREDITARY OSTEODYSTROPHY

In 1942, Albright reported a syndrome of end-organ hormone resistance often accompanied by specific phenotype, including short stature, obesity, round facies, brachydactyly and ectopic soft-tissue ossification (osteoma cutis), and mild developmental delay found in approximately 75% of patients in some series. Albright hereditary osteodystrophy is an autosomal-dominant disorder resulting from germ line-mutations in GNAS1 that decrease expression or function of G$_s\alpha$ protein. Maternal transmission of GNAS1 mutations leads to Albright hereditary osteodystrophy plus resistance to several hormones (e.g., parathyroid hormone) that activate Gs in their target tissues (pseudohypoparathyroidism type IA), whereas paternal transmission leads only to the Albright hereditary osteodystrophy phenotype (pseudopseudohypoparathyroidism). *GNAS1* is imprinted in a tissue-specific manner, being expressed primarily from the maternal allele in some tissues and biallelically expressed in most other tissues so that multihormone resistance occurs only when $G_s\alpha$ mutations are inherited maternally.[31]

At least 50% of patients with Albright hereditary osteodystrophy are obese, although most patients present with short stature, hypocalcemia, or other endocrine dysfunction. Investigation, diagnosis, and management of this syndrome are discussed more fully in Chapter 82.

ADDITIONAL SYNDROMES

Biemond syndrome type 2 is a recessively inherited condition comprising mental retardation, coloboma of the retina, early-onset obesity, polydactyly, and hypogonadism.[32] MEHMO syndrome has as its clinical hallmarks mental retardation, epileptic seizures, hypogonadism and hypogenitalism, microcephaly, and obesity. Life expectancy of patients is less than 2 years. Haplotype and linkage analyses in a large three-generation family assigned the disease locus to Xp22.13-p21.1.[33]

OBESITY WITHOUT DEVELOPMENTAL DELAY

ALSTRÖM SYNDROME

In 1959, Alström and colleagues[34] reported patients with a disorder that bears some similarities to BBS (retinitis pigmentosa, deafness, obesity, diabetes mellitus with recessive inheritance); however, classically mental retardation, polydactyly, and hypogonadism are not features. In the largest series (of 22 Alström's patients in the United Kingdom), all patients were suspected of having severe visual defect in infancy with severe photophobia and nystagmus often reported by 4 months of age.[35] Early loss of central vision was seen (usually by 1 year) in contrast to loss of peripheral vision as in other pigmentary retinopathies. Electroretinograms can be used to classify the severity and pattern of cone and rod involvement. It is now recognized that subsets of affected individuals present with additional features, such as dilated cardiomyopathy (often diagnosed in infancy), hepatic dysfunction, hypothyroidism, male hypogonadism, short stature, and mild-to-moderate developmental delay.[36]

Although obesity is common in Alström syndrome, it is rarely severe. In contrast, insulin resistance is frequently extreme, and when diabetes develops, it may be difficult to control. Hypertriglyceridemia may be severe and result in acute pancreatitis. In contrast to BBS, a single gene, *ALMS1*, has been found to be responsible for all cases of Alström syndrome characterized so far.[37] *ALMS1* is expressed ubiquitously at low levels and does not share significant sequence homology with other genes.

ULNAR-MAMMARY SYNDROME

In 1973, Schinzel studied a Swiss kindred in which the proband, brother, father, and nephew had ulnar ray defects, small penis, delayed puberty, and obesity; the proband and his father also had anal atresia. Schinzel subsequently suggested that this syndrome is identical to the ulnar-mammary syndrome of Pallister reported in 1976 and defined the major features as ulnar finger and fibular toe ray defects, delayed growth, obesity, hypogenitalism, and hypoplasia of nipples and apocrine glands with subsequent diminished ability to perspire.[38] Additional findings in single cases included pyloric, anal, and subglottic stenosis. In 1995, Bamshad and colleagues[39] identified 33 individuals in a large Utah family with ulnar-mammary syndrome, a number greater than the sum of all previously reported cases at that time. By linkage analysis, the ulnar-mammary syndrome gene was mapped to 12q23-q24.1, and in 1997 Bamshad and colleagues[40] showed that mutations in the *TBX3* gene are responsible for ulnar-mammary syndrome. Mutations in the closely linked and structurally related *TBX5* gene cause anterior limb abnormalities in Holt-Oram syndrome in association with cardiac anomalies; mutations in *TBX3* cause posterior (ulnar or postaxial) limb changes.

SIMPSON-GOLABI-BEHMEL TYPE 2

In 1975, Simpson and associates[41] reported patients with a collection of features (broad stocky appearance, large protruding jaw, widened nasal bridge, upturned nasal tip) and referred to the appearance as "bulldog-like." Behmel observed 11 male newborns with a similar syndrome, and in 1984 Golabi and Rosen reported similar features in a family with four males in three generations consistent with X-linked-recessive inheritance.

Some patients with Simpson-Golabi-Behmel syndrome harbor mutations in glypican 3, a putative extracellular proteoglycan that forms a complex with IGF-2 and might modulate IGF-2 action and overgrowth.[42] Not all individuals with Simpson-Golabi-Behmel syndrome have shown disruptions of the glypican 3 locus, which raises the possibility that other loci on the X chromosome could be responsible for some cases of this syndrome (denoted Simpson-Golabi syndrome type 2).

CONGENITAL LEPTIN DEFICIENCY

Congenital leptin deficiency was first described in 1997 in two severely obese children (an 8-year-old girl weighing 86 kg and her 2-year-old cousin weighing 29 kg) from a highly consanguineous family of Pakistani origin.[43] Both children had undetectable serum leptin concentrations and were homozygous for a missense mutation in the *ob* gene (ΔG133). This homozygous mutation subsequently was found in a further four severely obese subjects from three other Pakistani kindreds. A consanguineous Turkish family in which three obese subjects were homozygous for a missense mutation in leptin also has been described.[44] All affected subjects show normal neurobehavioral development and have no dysmorphic features.

Because the primary physiologic role of leptin seems to involve the signaling of the transition between the starved and the nutritionally adequate state, the neuroendocrine status of congenitally leptin-deficient individuals is, paradoxically in the light of their gross obesity, similar to that seen in extreme starvation.[45] All subjects in these families are characterized by intense hyperphagia after weaning, waking at night to go looking for food, and demanding food immediately after a meal. Studies of body composition reveal a disproportionate increase in fat versus lean mass. Children often develop valgus deformities of the knees by the age of 5 to 6 years, and sleep apnea is common. The importance of leptin in signaling nutritional adequacy to the hypothalamic-pituitary gonadal axis is illustrated by the finding of hypogonadotropic hypogonadism in all adult subjects with this condition. In contrast to leptin-deficient *ob/ob* mice, humans with congenital leptin deficiency show normal rates of linear growth, and there is no evidence for any increase in the activity of the pituitary-adrenal axis.[46] Leptin deficiency results in a mild form of central hypothyroidism. Affected subjects seem to have higher rates of childhood infection and atopic disease than their unaffected siblings, possibly as a result of abnormalities of T-cell number and function.[47] Although congenital leptin deficiency is an autosomal-recessive condition, heterozygotes or carriers for the *ob* mutation have partial leptin deficiency, which is associated with a discernible increase in body fat.[48]

Diagnosis and Treatment
Congenital leptin deficiency can be diagnosed on the basis of an undetectable serum leptin measurement, followed by genotyping of the *ob* gene. Although this syndrome is rare, it is unique in being amenable to a specific form of hormone replacement therapy. Eight patients currently are receiving recombinant human leptin by subcutaneous injection (one or two injections daily), and all have shown dramatic improvement in clinical and biochemical status (Fig. 44-1*A*).[47,49] Leptin therapy results in a dramatic improvement in hyperphagia and a correction of thyroid and T-cell dysfunction. Leptin also permits the onset of puberty at an appropriate developmental age (Fig. 44-1*B*).

Antibodies to leptin have developed in all children with the ΔG133 mutation, presumably because full-length leptin is a new antigen to these children. Although the appearance of neutralizing antibodies has been associated with periods of relative refractoriness to therapy, so far increases in leptin dose have restored efficacy. Adults with the missense mutation do not seem to develop antibodies, presumably because they have been naturally tolerized to leptin.

LEPTIN RECEPTOR DEFICIENCY

In 1998, Clement and colleagues[50] reported a mutation in the leptin receptor in one consanguineous family of Algerian origin with three affected subjects. Affected individuals were found to be homozygous for a mutation that truncates the receptor just before the transmembrane domain. The mutant receptor ectodomain is shed from cells and circulates bound to leptin, resulting in extremely high leptin levels. These findings in this one family frequently have been misinterpreted as indicating that leptin receptor deficiency would be a state of extreme and disproportionate hyperleptinemia. The extremely high leptin levels in this family are an artifact of the particular mutation that results from the large amounts of leptin bound to the abnormally shed ectodomain.

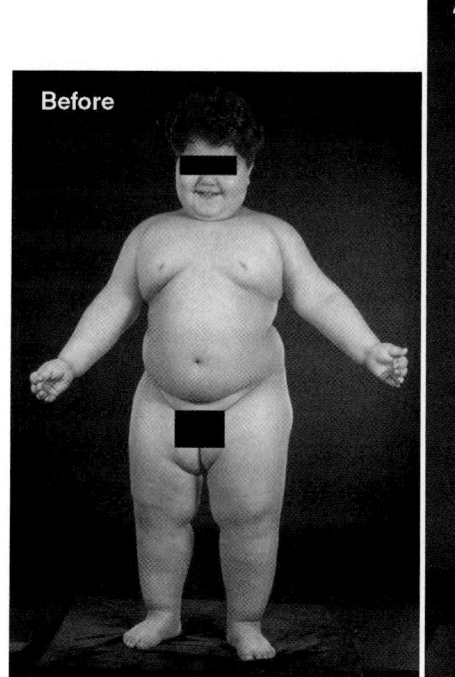
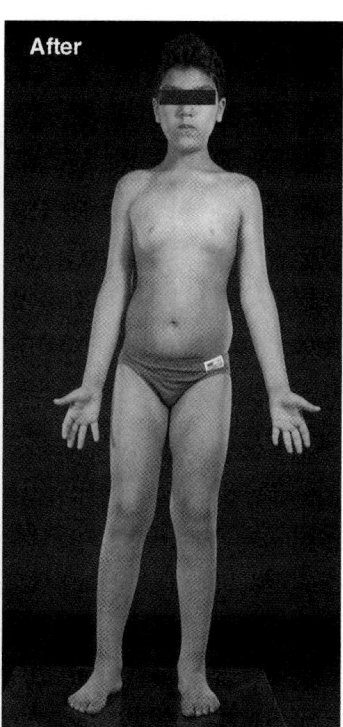

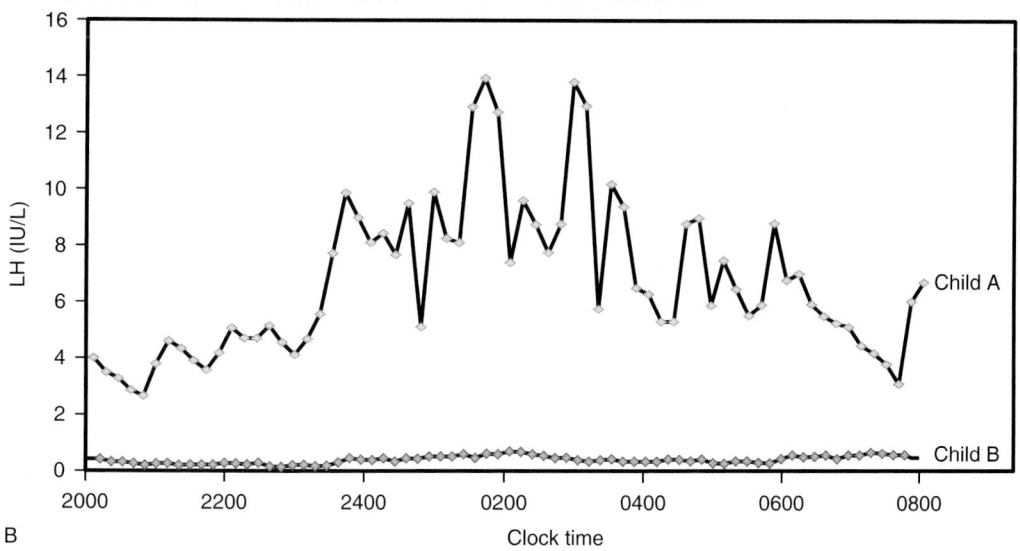

Figure 44-1 **A,** Clinical response to leptin therapy in congenital leptin deficiency. **B,** Leptin therapy is associated with pulsatile gonadotropin secretion at an appropriate developmental age in child A (age 11 years) compared with child B (age 5 years).

Leptin receptor–deficient subjects were of normal birth weight but exhibited rapid weight gain in the first few months of life, with severe hyperphagia and aggressive behavior when food was denied.[50] Basal temperature and resting metabolic rate were normal, cortisol levels were in the normal range, and all individuals were normoglycemic with mildly elevated plasma insulin levels similar to leptin-deficient subjects. This family had some unique neuroendocrine features not seen with leptin deficiency. There was evidence of mild growth retardation in early childhood, with impaired basal and stimulated GH secretion and decreased IGF-1 and IGF-binding protein 3 (IGFBP-3) levels and frank central hypothyroidism in these subjects. Whether this growth retardation is a general feature of leptin receptor deficiency or a particular feature of this kindred is a question that awaits the description of further families.

PRO-OPIOMELANOCORTIN DEFICIENCY

Leptin activates hypothalamic neurons expressing pro-opiomelanocortin (POMC), and this action is functionally important for leptin's action on appetite and body weight.[51] In 1998, Krude and coworkers[52] reported two unrelated obese German children who were homozygous or compound heterozygous for mutations in POMC, and subsequently another five children have been reported. Initial presentation is in neonatal life with adrenal crisis secondary to adrenocorticotropic hormone (ACTH) deficiency (POMC is a precursor of ACTH in the pituitary), and children require lifelong glucocorticoid replacement. The children have pale skin and red hair owing to the lack of melanocyte-stimulating hormone action at melanocortin 1 receptors in the skin and hair follicles, although this may be less obvious in children from different ethnic backgrounds (personal communication). POMC deficiency results in hyperphagia and early-onset obesity secondary to loss of melanocortin signaling at the melanocortin 4 receptor (MC4R). Although, as yet, no specific treatment is available, selective small-molecule MC4R agonists are being developed, and it is likely that these children would be highly responsive to such agents. In addition to homozygotes for complete POMC deficiency, other heterozygous point mutations in POMC gene might contribute to inherited obesity,[53] and there is a high prevalence of obesity in the heterozygous relatives of children with complete POMC deficiency, suggesting that subtle defects in this system may be sufficient to cause obesity.

MELANOCORTIN 4 RECEPTOR DEFICIENCY

In 1998, groups in the United Kingdom and France reported families with dominantly inherited heterozygous mutations in MC4R.[54,55] Since then, multiple different heterozygous MC4R mutations have been reported in obese people from various ethnic groups. The prevalence of such mutations has varied from 0.5% to 1% of obese adults to 6% of subjects with severe obesity starting in childhood.[56] Although few studies have been performed in randomly selected populations, estimates based on a Danish population–derived cohort are consistent with a population prevalence of at least 1 in 2000, suggesting that MC4R deficiency may be more common than PWS and fragile X syndrome and may be as common as more familiar genetic disorders, such as cystic fibrosis.

Although some studies have found a 100% penetrance of early-onset obesity in heterozygous probands, others have described obligate carriers who were not obese. Given the large number of potential influences on body weight, it is not surprising that genetic and environmental modifiers have important effects in some pedigrees. We have studied six families in whom the probands were homozygotes, and in all of these, the homozygotes were more obese than heterozygotes.[56] In these families, some heterozygous carriers were not obese; this may reflect ethnic-specific effects because all of these families were of Indo origin. Taking account of all of these observations, codominance, with modulation of expressivity and penetrance of the phenotype, is the most appropriate descriptor for the mode of inheritance.

We have defined the phenotype in 150 patients with MC4R deficiency.[56] Affected subjects exhibit hyperphagia, but this is not as severe as that seen in leptin deficiency, although it often starts in the first year of life. The severity of receptor dysfunction seen in in vitro assays can predict the amount of food ingested at a test meal by the subject harboring that particular mutation.[56] In addition to the increase in fat mass, MC4R-deficient subjects have an increase in lean mass that is not seen in leptin-deficient subjects and a marked increase in bone mineral density so that they often appear "big-boned." Linear growth of these subjects is striking with affected children having a height standard deviation score (SDS) of +2 compared with population standards (mean height SDS of other obese children in our cohort = + 0.5). MC4R-deficient subjects also have higher levels of fasting insulin than age-, sex-, and body mass index–SDS matched children. The accelerated linear growth does not seem to be due to dysfunction of the GH axis and may be a consequence of the disproportionate early hyperinsulinemia.[56]

One notable feature of this syndrome is that the severity of many of the phenotypic features seems to ameliorate partially with time. Obese adult mutation carriers report less intense feelings of hunger and are less hyperinsulinemic than children with the same mutation (personal observations). The commonness of MC4R mutations in obese humans compared with the rarity of leptin, leptin receptor, and PC1 mutations probably is related to the fact that even partial loss of function mutations in the heterozygous form results in a phenotype, and the mutations do not seem to interfere with reproductive function and fertility (Table 44-2).

Table 44-2 Metabolic and Neuroendocrine Effects of Mutations in the Leptin Melanocortin Pathway

METABOLIC

	Appetite	Energy Expenditure	Body Composition	Insulin Secretion
Leptin	Increased	BMR normal	Selective fat deposition	Mild, consistent with obesity
Leptin Receptor	Increased	BMR normal	Selective fat deposition	Mild, consistent with obesity
POMC	Increased	BMR normal	Unknown	Unknown
MC4R	Increased	BMR normal	Excess fat and lean mass	Severe, early hyperinsulinemia

ENDOCRINE

	Growth	Puberty	Thyroid	Adrenal Axis
Leptin	Normal	Hypogonadotropic hypogonadism	Central hypothyroidism	Normal
Leptin Receptor	Reduced	Hypogonadotropic hypogonadism	Central hypothyroidism	Normal
POMC	Increased	Normal	Central hypothyroidism	ACTH deficiency
MC4R	Increased	Normal	Normal	Normal

ACTH, adrenocorticotropic hormone; BMR, basal metabolic rate; MC4R, melanocortin 4 receptor; POMC, pro-opiomelanocortin.

Diagnosis and Treatment

The *MC4R* is a single exon gene and readily amenable to rapid nucleotide sequencing; genetic analysis potentially could be performed as a routine diagnostic test. Before attributing any causality to a mutation, however, it is necessary in our view to (1) establish that the sequence variant is absent from a panel of ethnicity-matched control subjects of appropriate number (>100 alleles), (2) confirm that it results in impaired signaling when studied in vitro, and (3) determine that it cosegregates with obesity in family members.

Although at present there is no specific therapy for MC4R deficiency, it is highly likely that these subjects would respond well to pharmacotherapy that overcame the reduction in the hypothalamic melanocortinergic tone that exists in these patients. Because most patients are heterozygotes with one functional allele intact, it is possible that small-molecule MC4R agonists might be excellent candidate drugs in the future for this disorder.

PROHORMONE CONVERTASE-1 DEFICIENCY

Two unrelated subjects genetically deficient in the prohormone convertase-1 have been described.[57,58] Both are compound heterozygotes for different mutations in this gene, which encodes an enzyme involved in the posttranslational processing of multiple prohormones. The resultant phenotype is complex (Table 44-3), but includes early-onset obesity, possibly related to failure of cleavage of POMC to melanocyte-stimulating hormone in the hypothalamus. The most striking feature of the second proband was severe malabsorption and uncontrollable diarrhea resulting from a small bowel enteropathy.

OTHER SYNDROMES

Holder and colleagues[59] studied a girl with hyperphagia and early-onset obesity and a balanced translocation between 1p22.1 and 6q16.2. The translocation disrupted the *SIM1* gene on 6q. The *Drosophila* single-minded (*sim*) gene is a regulator of neurogenesis, and in the mouse *Sim1* is expressed in the developing central nervous system and is essential for formation of the supraoptic and paraventricular nuclei, which express the melanocortin-4 receptor. Mice heterozygous for loss of function mutations in *Sim1* are obese, making it likely that the disruption of this gene in this child was the cause of her obesity.[60] Many patients with obesity, hypotonia, and

developmental delay in association with interstitial chromosome 6q deletions have been described, although whether this syndrome can be attributed to *SIM1* is unclear.[61]

The WAGR syndrome (Wilms' tumor, anorexia, ambiguous genitalia, and mental retardation) is one of the best-studied "contiguous" gene syndromes associated with chromosomal deletions at 11p13, the location of the *WT1* gene.[62] A few patients with WAGR syndrome and obesity have been reported with deletions of chromosome 11p14-p12.

Table 44-3 Prohormone Convertase-1 (PC1) Deficiency Clinical Features and Affected Prohormone Conversion

Obesity	*POMC-MSH
Hypogonadotropic hypogonadism	ProGnRH-GnRH
Hypoadrenalism	POMC-ACTH
Reactive hypoglycemia/impaired glucose tolerance	Proinsulin-insulin
Intestinal malabsorption	*Proglucagon-GLP1 and GLP2

*Probable mechanism

SUMMARY

Understanding of the complexity and heterogeneity of inherited syndromes of obesity has grown at a rapid pace since the 1990s. These discoveries have had an important, clinically relevant impact on the diagnosis and management of obese patients. First, the genes underlying most of the pleiotropic developmental obesity syndromes have been identified, something that will greatly facilitate genetic counseling. Second, as exemplified by MC4R deficiency, we now know that apparently "simple obesity" can be caused by specific genetic defects affecting the control of appetite in the hypothalamus. With that realization, we should never again assume that "simple obesity," particularly when it begins in childhood, has simple and readily remediable environmental causes. Because MC4R mutations are so common in severe childhood-onset obesity, it is our practice to determine the sequence of the MC4R gene in all children with a body mass index SDS greater than 3. Finally, as exemplified by congenital leptin deficiency, we are now entering an era when specific molecular diagnoses increasingly will lead to specific, effective therapies for inherited subtypes of obesity.

REFERENCES

1. Barsh GS, Farooqi IS, O'Rahilly S: Genetics of body-weight regulation. Nature 404:644–651, 2000.
2. Prader AL, Willi H: Ein Syndrom von Adipositas, Kleinwuchs, Kryptorchismus und Oligophrenie nach Myatonieartigem Zustand im Neugeborenenalter. Schweiz Med Wschr 86:1260–1261, 1956.
3. Butler M: Prader-Willi syndrome: Current understanding of cause and diagnosis. Am J Med Genet 35:319–332, 1990.
4. Swaab DF, Purba JS, Hofman MA: Alterations in the hypothalamic paraventricular nucleus and its oxytocin neurons (putative satiety cells) in Prader-Willi syndrome: A study of five cases. J Clin Endocrinol Metab 80:573–579, 1995.
5. Cummings DE, Frayo RS, Breen PA, et al: Plasma ghrelin levels after diet-induced weight loss or gastric bypass surgery. N Engl J Med 346:1623–1630, 2002.
6. Cummings DE, Purnell JQ, Vaisse C, et al: Elevated plasma ghrelin levels in Prader Willi syndrome. Nat Med 8:643–644, 2002.
7. Haqq AM, Farooqi IS, O'Rahilly S, et al: Serum ghrelin levels are inversely correlated with body mass index, age, and insulin concentrations in normal children and are markedly increased in Prader-Willi syndrome. J Clin Endocrinol Metab 88:174–178, 2003.
8. Holm VA, Butler MG, Hanchett JM, et al: Prader-Willi syndrome: Consensus diagnostic criteria. Pediatrics 91:398–402, 1993.
9. van Mil EG, Gerver WJ, Van Marken Lichtenbelt WD, et al: Body composition in Prader-Willi syndrome compared with nonsyndromal obesity: Relationship to physical activity and growth hormone function. J Pediatr 139:708–714, 2001.
10. Hoybye C, Hilding A, Jacobsson H, Thoren M: Metabolic profile and body composition in adults with Prader-Willi syndrome and severe obesity. J Clin Endocrinol Metab 87:3590–3597, 2002.
11. Ohta T, Gray TA, Rogan PK, et al: Imprinting-mutation mechanisms in Prader-Willi syndrome. Am J Hum Genet 64:397–413, 1999.
12. Driscoll DJ, Williams CA, Zori RT, et al: A DNA methylation imprint, determined by the sex of the parent, distinguishes the Angelman and Prader-Willi syndromes. Genomics 13:917–924, 1992.
13. Goldstone AP: Prader-Willi syndrome: Advances in genetics, pathophysiology and treatment. Trends Endocrinol Metab 15:12–20, 2004.

14. Carrel AL, Whitman BY, Allen DB: Growth hormone improves body composition, fat utilization, physical strength and agility, and growth in Prader-Willi syndrome: A controlled study. J Pediatr 134:215–221, 1999.

15. Hamilton CR Jr, Kliman B: Hypogonadotropinism in Prader-Willi syndrome: Induction of puberty and sperm altogenesis by clomiphene citrate. Am J Med 52:322–329, 1972.

16. Hagerman PJ, Hagerman RJ: The fragile-X premutation: A maturing perspective. Am J Hum Genet 74:805–816, 2004.

17. de Vries BB, Butler MG, Canziani F, et al: Clinical and molecular studies in fragile X patients with a Prader-Willi-like phenotype. J Med Genet 30:761–766, 1993.

18. Kaplan G, Kung M, McClure M, Cronister A: Direct mutation analysis of 495 patients for fragile X carrier status/proband diagnosis. Am J Med Genet 51:501–502, 1994.

19. Jin P, Warren ST: New insights into fragile X syndrome: From molecules to neurobehaviors. Trends Biochem Sci 28:152–158, 2003.

20. Laurence JZ: Four cases of "retinitis pigmentosa" occurring in the same family, and accompanied by general imperfections of development. Ophthalmol Rev 2:32–41, 1866.

21. Katsanis N, Lupski JR, Beales PL: Exploring the molecular basis of Bardet-Biedl syndrome. Hum Mol Genet 10:2293–2299, 2001.

22. Katsanis N: The oligogenic properties of Bardet-Biedl syndrome. Hum Mol Genet 13(Spec No 1):R65–R71, 2004.

23. Katsanis N, Badano JL, Eichers ER, et al: Triallelic inheritance in Bardet-Biedl syndrome, a Mendelian recessive disorder. Science 293:2256–2259, 2001.

24. Mykytyn K, Sheffield VC: Establishing a connection between cilia and Bardet-Biedl syndrome. Trends Mol Med 10:106–109, 2004.

25. Börjeson M, Forssman H, Lehmann O: An X-linked, recessively inherited syndrome characterized by grave mental deficiency, epilepsy, and endocrine disorder. Acta Med Scand 171:13–21, 1962.

26. Turner G, Gedeon A, Mulley J, et al: Borjeson-Forssman-Lehmann syndrome: Clinical manifestations and gene localization to Xq26-27. Am J Med Genet 34:463–469, 1989.

27. Wilson M, Mulley J, Gedeon A, et al: New X-linked syndrome of mental retardation, gynecomastia, and obesity is linked to DXS255. Am J Med Genet 40:406–413, 1991.

28. Cohen MM Jr, Hall BD, Smith DW, et al: A new syndrome with hypotonia, obesity, mental deficiency, and facial, oral, ocular, and limb anomalies. J Pediatr 83:280–284, 1973.

29. Chandler KE, Kidd A, Al-Gazali L, et al: Diagnostic criteria, clinical characteristics, and natural history of Cohen syndrome. J Med Genet 40:233–241, 2003.

30. Tahvanainen E, Norio R, Karila E, et al: Cohen syndrome gene assigned to the long arm of chromosome 8 by linkage analysis. Nat Genet 7:201–204, 1994.

31. Weinstein LS, Chen M, Liu J: Gs(alpha) mutations and imprinting defects in human disease. Ann N Y Acad Sci 968:173–197, 2002.

32. Verloes A, Temple IK, Bonnet S, Bottani A: Coloboma, mental retardation, hypogonadism, and obesity: Critical review of the so-called Biemond syndrome type 2, updated nosology, and delineation of three "new" syndromes. Am J Med Genet 69:370–379, 1997.

33. Steinmuller R, Steinberger D, Muller U: MEHMO (mental retardation, epileptic seizures, hypogonadism and -genitalism, microcephaly, obesity), a novel syndrome: Assignment of disease locus to xp21.1-p22.13. Eur J Hum Genet 6:201–206, 1998.

34. Alström CH, Hallgren B, Nilsson LB, Asander H: Retinal degeneration combined with obesity, diabetes mellitus and neurogenous deafness: A specific syndrome (not hitherto described) distinct from the Laurence-Moon-Bardet-Biedl syndrome: A clinical, endocrinological and genetic examination based on a large pedigree. Acta Psychiatr Neurol Scand 34:1–35, 1959.

35. Russell-Eggitt IM, Clayton PT, Coffey R, et al: Alstrom syndrome: Report of 22 cases and literature review. Ophthalmology 105:1274–1280, 1998.

36. Michaud JL, Heon E, Guilbert F, et al: Natural history of Alstrom syndrome in early childhood: Onset with dilated cardiomyopathy. J Pediatr 128:225–229, 1996.

37. Collin GB, Marshall JD, Ikeda A, et al: Mutations in ALMS1 cause obesity, type 2 diabetes and neurosensory degeneration in Alstrom syndrome. Nat Genet 31:74–78, 2002.

38. Schinzel A: Ulnar-mammary syndrome. J Med Genet 24:778–781, 1987.

39. Bamshad M, Krakowiak PA, Watkins WS, et al: A gene for ulnar-mammary syndrome maps to 12q23-q24.1. Hum Mol Genet 4:1973–1977, 1995.

40. Bamshad M, Lin RC, Law DJ, et al: Mutations in human TBX3 alter limb, apocrine and genital development in ulnar-mammary syndrome. Nat Genet 16:311–315, 1997.

41. Simpson JL, Landey S, New M, German J: A previously unrecognized X-linked syndrome of dysmorphia. Birth Defects Orig Artic Ser 11:18–24, 1975.

42. Brzustowicz LM, Khan MB, Weksberg R: Mapping of a new SGBS locus to chromosome Xp22 in a family with a severe form of Simpson-Golabi-Behmel syndrome. Am J Hum Genet 65:779–783, 1999.

43. Montague CT, Farooqi IS, Whitehead JP, et al: Congenital leptin deficiency is associated with severe early-onset obesity in humans. Nature 387:903–908, 1997.

44. Strobel A, Issad T, Camoin L, et al: A leptin missense mutation associated with hypogonadism and morbid obesity. Nat Genet 18:213–215, 1998.

45. Flier JS: Clinical review 94: What's in a name? In search of leptin's physiologic role. J Clin Endocrinol Metab 83:1407–1413, 1998.

46. Farooqi IS, Jebb SA, Langmack G, et al: Effects of recombinant leptin therapy in a child with congenital leptin deficiency. N Engl J Med 341:879–884, 1999.

47. Farooqi IS, Matarese G, Lord GM, et al: Beneficial effects of leptin on obesity, T cell hyporesponsiveness, and neuroendocrine/metabolic dysfunction of human congenital leptin deficiency. J Clin Invest 110:1093–1103, 2002.

48. Farooqi IS, Keogh JM, Kamath S, et al: Partial leptin deficiency and human adiposity. Nature 414:34–35, 2001.

49. Licinio J, Caglayan S, Ozata M, et al: Phenotypic effects of leptin replacement on morbid obesity, diabetes mellitus, hypogonadism, and behavior in leptin-deficient adults. Proc Natl Acad Sci U S A 101:4531–4536, 2004.

50. Clement K, Vaisse C, Lahlou N, et al: A mutation in the human leptin receptor gene causes obesity and pituitary dysfunction. Nature 392:398–401, 1998.

51. Schwartz MW, Woods SC, Porte D Jr, et al: Central nervous system control of food intake. Nature 404:661–671, 2000.

52. Krude H, Biebermann H, Luck W, et al: Severe early-onset obesity, adrenal insufficiency and red hair pigmentation caused by POMC mutations in humans. Nat Genet 19:155–157, 1998.

53. Challis BG, Pritchard LE, Creemers JW, et al: A missense mutation disrupting a dibasic prohormone processing site in pro-opiomelanocortin (POMC) increases susceptibility to early-onset obesity through a novel molecular mechanism. Hum Mol Genet 11:1997–2004, 2002.

54. Yeo GS, Farooqi IS, Aminian S, et al: A frameshift mutation in MC4R associated with dominantly inherited human obesity [letter]. Nat Genet 20:111–112, 1998.

55. Vaisse C, Clement K, Guy-Grand B, Froguel P: A frameshift mutation in human MC4R is associated with a dominant form of obesity [letter]. Nat Genet 20:113–114, 1998.

56. Farooqi IS, Keogh JM, Yeo GS, et al: Clinical spectrum of obesity and mutations in the melanocortin 4 receptor gene. N Engl J Med 348:1085–1095, 2003.

57. Jackson RS, Creemers JW, Ohagi S, et al: Obesity and impaired prohormone processing associated with mutations in the human prohormone convertase 1 gene. Nat Genet 16:303–306, 1997.

58. Jackson RS, Creemers JW, Farooqi IS, et al: Small-intestinal dysfunction accompanies the complex endocrinopathy of human proprotein convertase 1 deficiency. J Clin Invest 112:1550–1560, 2003.

59. Holder JL Jr, Butte NF, Zinn AR: Profound obesity associated with a balanced translocation that disrupts the SIM1 gene. Hum Mol Genet 9:101–108, 2000.

60. Michaud JL, Boucher F, Melnyk A, et al: Sim1 haploinsufficiency causes hyperphagia, obesity and reduction of the paraventricular nucleus of the hypothalamus. Hum Mol Genet 10:1465–1473, 2001.

61. Faivre L, Cormier-Daire V, Lapierre JM, et al: Deletion of the SIM1 gene (6q16.2) in a patient with a Prader-Willi-like phenotype. J Med Genet 39:594–596, 2002.

62. Rose EA, Glaser T, Jones C, et al: Complete physical map of the WAGR region of 11p13 localizes a candidate Wilms' tumor gene. Cell 60:495–508, 1990.

Anorexia Nervosa, Bulimia Nervosa, and Other Eating Disorders

Robert T. Rubin

"A young woman thus afflicted, her clothes scarcely hanging together on her anatomy, her pulse slow and slack, her temperature two degrees below the normal mean, her bowels closed, her hair like that of a corpse—dry and lustreless, her face and limbs ashy and cold, her hollow eyes the only vivid thing about her—this wan creature whose daily food might lie on a crown piece, will be busy with mother's meetings, with little sister's frocks, with university extension and with what you please else of unselfish effort, yet on what funds God only knows."[1]

INTRODUCTION

Anorexia nervosa (AN) and bulimia nervosa (BN) are eating disorders that have been recognized for hundreds of years,[2-4] yet their etiologies remain poorly understood.[5-15] Both illnesses carry significant physical and psychologic morbidity, and in the case of AN, death can occur in severe, untreated cases. Early recognition and aggressive treatment thus are particularly important. Because the physical manifestations of these illnesses are so prominent, most patients have their first encounters with nonpsychiatric physicians. Lengthy diagnostic workups for underlying physical illness may be conducted, and frequently, a psychiatric disturbance is considered only when the results of the workup do not fit a known physical illness. The careful application of psychiatric diagnostic criteria for AN and BN permits these illnesses to be suspected early in the medical workup and facilitates referral to the psychiatric specialist in a constructive and acceptable way.

HISTORY AND EPIDEMIOLOGY

AN and BN are diseases primarily of adolescent girls; approximately 95% of AN cases are female.[16] Although there is documentary evidence of AN occurring in the Middle Ages, the first medical accounts appeared in the seventeenth century, as *A Discourse upon Prodigious Abstinence* by John Reynolds in 1669 and *Phthisiologia; or, a Treatise of Consumptions* by Richard Morton in 1689.[3,17–19] AN as a modern clinical entity derives from publications in 1873 by Charles Lasègue and William Gull, who referred to the illness as hysterical anorexia,[20,21] and

Gull's publication in 1874, entitled *Anorexia Nervosa*.[22] Bliss and Branch[3] commented, "it is revealing to note the extraordinary differences in the description of the same condition by the two men. While Gull's comments were as direct and precise as a pathologic report, Lasègue conveyed a sense of the spirit and feeling of these people, the nuances of their disturbed relationships, and the subtleties of their intrapsychic turmoil" (p. 14). The early twentieth century history of AN primarily involves its distinction from physical illnesses such as Simmonds' cachexia.[23]

Although binge eating (bulimia) has long been recognized as part of the symptomatology of AN, BN as a distinct syndrome was first proposed by Russell in 1979.[24] He elaborated two criteria for BN: an irresistible urge to overeat, followed by self-induced vomiting or purging, and a morbid fear of becoming fat. In common with AN, such patients kept their body weight somewhat below normal but not to the same extent as AN patients. They also tended not to develop amenorrhea and were more active sexually. Russell considered BN to be an "ominous variant" of AN, in that comorbid depressive symptoms were often severe and distressing, leading to a high risk of suicide.

In the past 25 years, careful theoretic formulations of the psychodynamics of these eating disorders have been augmented by elucidation of their physiology, especially their neuroendocrinology. Psychopharmacologic and psychotherapeutic treatment methods have been refined, and there now is a reasonably effective armamentarium with which to manage these disorders.

The reported incidence of AN has varied between about 0.5 and 15 cases per 100,000 population per year.[12,25,26] The large variation is related to the diagnostic criteria used, the methods of case ascertainment, and the population studied (e.g., clinic versus community). The prevalence of AN is about 1%, although it has been considerably higher in some studies.[26,27] A meta-analysis of 42 studies revealed the crude mortality rate in AN (due to all causes of death) to be 5.9%, which is substantially greater than that for female inpatients and for the general population.[28]

The prevalence of BN varies between 2% and 4%.[26,27,29–31] Both AN and BN, as well as subsyndromal anorexia and bulimia, are far more common in certain groups of young women, notably athletes and ballet dancers, for whom occupational demands place a premium on thinness. Primary and secondary amenorrheas in these individuals are extraordinarily common. The occurrence of both AN and BN may be on the rise,[26,32–34] coincident with the increasing prevalence of obesity throughout the world.[35,36]

Since the 1980s, large-scale twin and family studies have suggested that eating disorders are familial.[37,38] There is cross-transmission between AN and BN, and they appear to share a common vulnerability, but the transmissible elements remain elusive. Twin and family studies suggest that major depressive disorder and substance dependence most likely do not share a common etiology with the eating disorders. The genetic contribution is likely predisposing rather than determining, in that sociocultural circumstances, as well as personal psychologic stressors, are risk factors.[39,40]

DIAGNOSIS

The fourth edition of the *Diagnostic and Statistical Manual of Mental Disorders* (DSM-IV)[41] provides the current clinical criteria for AN (Table 45-1) and BN (Table 45-2). Since the DSM became a criterion-based system with DSM-III in 1980, it has undergone two revisions, and several diagnostic categories have undergone considerable change across these revisions. In contrast, the criteria for AN have remained relatively stable, although future revision might be useful, such as the elimination of amenorrhea as a criterion.[42,43] The criteria for bulimia are in greater flux; for example, binge eating disorder, characterized as recurrent episodes of binge eating without compensatory purging or other behaviors, has been included in the DSM-IV Appendix as a set of criteria for further study.[41,44] Although there are far fewer men with eating disorders than women, the clinical features are similar.[45]

The DSM-IV criteria for AN and BN highlight the many identifiable behavioral and psychologic aspects of these illnesses.[46] If the patient and her family are queried about these aspects, considerable information pointing toward the diagnosis can be gleaned, psychiatric consultation can be considered early in the diagnostic process, and specialized and expensive laboratory testing often can be avoided.

For AN, a key feature of the weight loss is the patient's refusal to maintain body weight, which often manifests as an

Table 45-1 DSM-IV Diagnostic Criteria for Anorexia Nervosa

Refusal to maintain body weight at or above a minimally normal weight for age and height (e.g., weight loss leading to maintenance of body weight less than 85% of that expected; or failure to make expected weight gain during period of growth, leading to body weight less than 85% of that expected).

Intense fear of gaining weight or becoming fat, even though underweight.

Disturbance in the way in which one's body weight or shape is experienced, undue influence of body weight or shape on self-evaluation, or denial of the seriousness of the current low body weight.

In postmenarcheal females, amenorrhea—i.e., the absence of at least three consecutive menstrual cycles. (A woman is considered to have amenorrhea if her periods occur only following hormone—e.g., estrogen—administration.)

TYPE

Restricting type: During the current episode . . . the person has not regularly engaged in binge-eating or purging behavior (i.e., self-induced vomiting or the misuse of laxatives, diuretics, or enemas).

Binge-eating/purging type: During the current episode . . . the person has regularly engaged in binge-eating or purging behavior (i.e., self-induced vomiting or the misuse of laxatives, diuretics, or enemas).

Source: Reprinted with permission from American Psychiatric Association: Diagnostic and Statistical Manual of Mental Disorders, ed 4. Washington, DC, American Psychiatric Association, 1994.

Table 45-2 DSM-IV Diagnostic Criteria for Bulimia Nervosa

Recurrent episodes of binge eating. An episode of binge eating is characterized by both of the following:

Eating, in a discrete period of time (e.g., within any 2-hour period), an amount of food that is definitely larger than most people would eat during a similar period of time and under similar circumstances.

A sense of lack of control over eating during the episode (e.g., a feeling that one cannot stop eating or control what or how much one is eating).

Recurrent inappropriate compensatory behavior in order to prevent weight gain, such as self-induced vomiting; misuse of laxatives, diuretics, enemas, or other medications; fasting; or excessive exercise.

The binge eating and inappropriate compensatory behaviors both occur, on average, at least twice a week for 3 months.

Self-evaluation is unduly influenced by body shape and weight.

The disturbance does not occur exclusively during episodes of anorexia nervosa.

TYPE

Purging type: During the current episode . . . the person has regularly engaged in self-induced vomiting or the misuse of laxatives, diuretics, or enemas.

Nonpurging type: During the current episode . . . the person has used other inappropriate compensatory behaviors, such as fasting or excessive exercise, but has not regularly engaged in self-induced vomiting or the misuse of laxatives, diuretics, or enemas.

Source: Reprinted with permission from American Psychiatric Association: Diagnostic and Statistical Manual of Mental Disorders, ed 4. Washington, DC, American Psychiatric Association, 1994.

active resistance to increasing caloric intake. As illustrated in Figure 45-1, the cachexia can be severe, and, as mentioned, self-starvation can lead to death. If the onset is in childhood or early adolescence, there may be a failure to make the expected weight gain during the active growth phase. This refusal to gain or maintain body weight is rooted psychologically in the second criterion: an intense fear of gaining weight or of becoming fat, even though the patient is underweight. There is a subjective distortion of body image such that the emaciated individual appears to herself to be either at an acceptable weight or even fat. Indeed, initiation of treatment by insisting on the patient's eating can lead to purging behavior that did not occur prior to treatment.

A corollary of this is the third criterion, disturbance of the experience of one's body weight or shape, for example, undue influence of body weight or shape on self-evaluation/self-esteem and/or denial of the seriousness of the weight loss, even though there may be clear adverse physical sequelae in addition to the current fourth criterion: secondary amenorrhea. For the endocrinologist, questions that should be asked of the patient and her family to address these psychologic and behavioral aspects of AN include the following (adapted from the Structured Clinical Interview for DSM-IV[47]):

How much do you weigh now?
How tall are you?
What foods do you eat?
Why do you limit yourself to those foods?
Do you feel you are fat now?
Are you concerned that you might become fat if you ate more?
Do you weigh less than other people think you should weigh?
Do you need to be very thin in order to feel good about yourself?
Has anyone told you it can be dangerous to be as thin as you are?
What kinds of things do you do to keep from gaining weight?

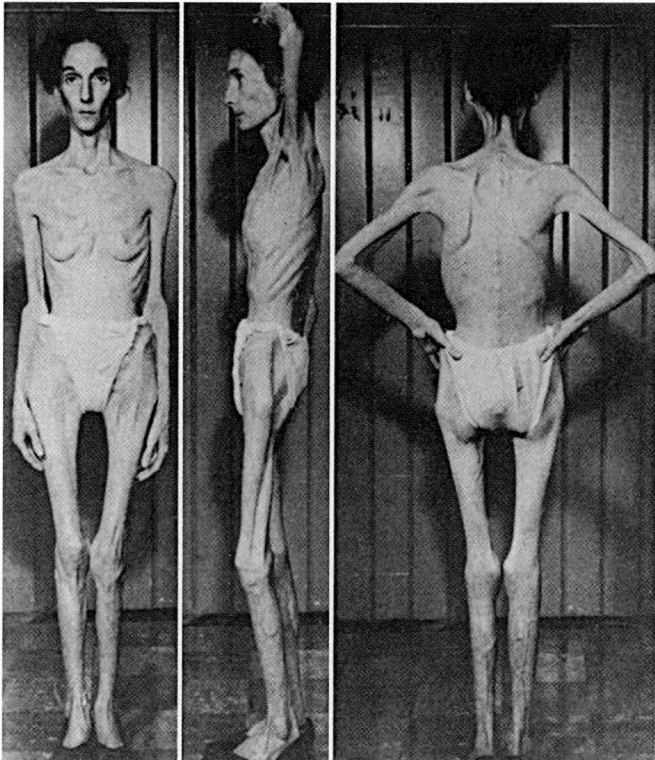

Figure 45-1   Extreme cachexia in an anorexia nervosa patient. (From Bliss EL, Branch CHH: Anorexia Nervosa: Its History, Psychology, and Biology. New York, Paul B. Hoeber, 1960.)

> Have you ever made yourself vomit or take laxatives, enemas, or water pills? How often?
> How much do you exercise?
> Before now, were you having periods? Were they regular? When did they stop?

Rather than rigidly adhering to the DSM-IV algorithm for diagnosing AN—that is, the reduction of body weight to less than 85% of expected and complete amenorrhea for at least 3 months—the clinician should consider both the patient's core symptoms and current medical impairment; such impairment may require treatment even though body weight may be more than 85% of expected and/or menses still may occur sporadically.[43]

For BN, the distinguishing features are uncontrollable binge eating of a definitely larger-than-normal amount of food (first criterion) that is clearly repetitive (third criterion). Here, too, one's sense of self is unduly influenced by weight and body shape (fourth criterion); compensatory behaviors such as self-induced vomiting, purging, fasting between binges, and exercise are invoked to prevent weight gain (second criterion). The frequency and chronicity of the bingeing, and especially the compensatory behaviors, help to distinguish BN from overeating in general. And because binge eating and purging can occur as part of AN, a fifth criterion for BN is that it does not occur exclusively during episodes of AN. Binge eating disorder also is being distinguished from BN,[41,48] because obesity rather than inanition often results, and the endocrinologic and other metabolic changes are different from those of AN and BN.

For the endocrinologist, questions that should be asked of the patient and her family to address the criteria for BN include the following (adapted from the Structured Clinical Interview for DSM-IV[47]):

> Do you have times when your eating gets out of control? Tell me about these times.

> During these times, do you often eat within a 2-hour period what most people would regard as an unusual amount of food?
> Can you give me an example of the kinds and amounts of food that you might eat during one of these times?
> How often do these times occur?
> Do you do anything to counteract the effects of eating that much—such as making yourself vomit; taking laxatives, enemas, or water pills; strict fasting between periods of eating a lot of food; or exercising a lot?
> How important is your body shape and size in how you feel about yourself?

These questions and those regarding AN should be phrased in a way that is comfortable to both the health-care professional and the patient. Depending on the patient, questions about both bulimic and anorexic behaviors might need to be asked; the patient's history and presenting symptoms should dictate the emphasis of the interview.[49] The sample questions are given to indicate that one can (and should) ask about eating behavior forthrightly. If the topics of the questions are followed, information about all the diagnostic criteria for both AN and BN will be gleaned. The patient should also be asked whether this is the first time these behaviors have occurred or whether there have been past episodes. In the case of the latter, a careful history taking about each episode, its severity and duration, and treatments and their success should be done. This information may yield important clues as to how to approach the patient therapeutically during the current episode.

Comorbid symptoms of depression and anxiety occur with some frequency in both AN and BN and should be assessed.[50-57] Symptoms of depression and anxiety are exaggerated by malnutrition and improved with nutrition. AN patients with obsessive-compulsive disorder tend to have an obsessional need for symmetry/exactness and compulsions toward ordering and arranging.[58,59] Mild to moderate negative mood states and obsessive symptoms can persist after recovery in both anorexic and bulimic individuals,[55,60,61] suggesting that these traits may contribute to the pathogenesis of eating disorders.[62]

There also is a high incidence of comorbid obsessive-compulsive disorder (OCD) in anorexic and bulimic women and their families, as well as increased rates of AN and BN in individuals with primary OCD. It may be that the core eating disorder symptoms (e.g., fear of fatness, pursuit of thinness) are a specific type of obsession. Symmetry, ordering, and perfectionism are the most common target symptoms in women with AN and BN and often persist after recovery. Leckman and coworkers[63] delineated four symptom dimensions of OCD, one of which was symmetry and ordering; these occurred most commonly in men. OCD in men and eating disorders in women may be gender-specific expressions of a common psychobiology related to obsessions with symmetry and ordering compulsions.

There are primary central nervous system (CNS) conditions for which anorexia or bulimia may be an associated symptom; these include both organic pathology[64] and "functional" illnesses. As an example of the latter, one of the authors was asked to consult on a hospitalized adolescent girl with electrolyte disturbances suggestive of Bartter's syndrome. With no evidence of somatic causes of the patient's cachexia and with nurses' observations of bizarre eating habits, a diagnosis of AN was entertained, and a psychiatric interview of the patient during endocrine rounds was requested. After introductions as to who the psychiatrist was and why he was there, questioning began with what the patient ate (lettuce and carrots only) and why she ate only those two items (the computer in the hospital basement was giving her instructions to do so). Elucidation of additional symptoms of psychosis led to a presumptive diagnosis of schizophrenia with secondary anorexia and referral for inpatient psychiatric care.

GENETICS

Eating disorders in both women and men are familial, as shown by both family and twin studies.[65–69] The heritability of both AN and BN has been estimated between 30% and 80%. Recent studies of the genetics of AN and BN have been primarily by linkage analysis and candidate gene analysis. In linkage analysis, correlations are determined between the occurrence of a disease in families and the inheritance of specific chromosomal regions in those families. In candidate gene analysis, nucleotide polymorphisms are searched for in specific genes suggested by chromosomal linkage studies and/or the known functions of the gene product.

Linkage studies in AN and BN families have suggested susceptibility genes on several chromosomes, but the strength of the associations have depended on the diagnostic stringency of the cases. For example, in 192 families with at least one affected relative pair with AN, BN, and related eating disorders, modest linkage was found with a marker on chromosome 4.[70] However, when the analysis was restricted to 37 families in which at least two relatives had a diagnosis of the restricting subtype of AN (without bingeing and purging), there was a much stronger linkage to a marker on chromosome 1p. With reference to specific behavioral traits, two variables were identified in a sample of 196 families with an AN proband: drive-for-thinness and obsessionality.[71] When these variables were incorporated into a linkage analysis, there again was highly significant linkage to a region on chromosome 1, as well as linkages of lesser significance to regions on chromosomes 2 and 13. In contrast, linkage analysis of 308 families with a BN proband yielded a high linkage score to chromosome 10.[72] In a subset of 133 families in which two or more BN members reported self-induced vomiting, an even higher linkage was found to a region on chromosome 10p. Another region on chromosome 14q was suggestive of linkage. These studies can serve to suggest specific chromosomal regions for candidate gene analysis.

The candidate genes that have been studied to date in eating disorders involve primarily the serotonergic system, because serotonin (5-HT) neurotransmission inhibits feeding behavior.[65,73] Several studies have suggested an association between polymorphisms in the promoter region of the 5-HT2A receptor gene and both AN and BN, but the results have been inconsistent, and the associations have been rather weak. Studies reporting an association between a polymorphism in the promoter region of the 5-HT transporter gene and eating disorders have been inconsistent, as well. In one study, a relationship was suggested between a polymorphism in the 5-HT1B receptor gene and BN; in another study, a relationship was suggested between a polymorphism in the 5-HT2C receptor gene and vulnerability to rapid weight loss following reduced food intake in AN. On the other hand, studies of the 5-HT receptor genes 2C, 7, and 1Dβ, as well as the tryptophan hydroxylase gene (the rate-limiting enzyme in the biosynthesis of 5-HT), have been negative. Phenotypically, reduced serotonergic activity, as measured by platelet ³H-paroxetine binding, has been found in both AN and BN and was unrelated to diagnostic subtype or ancillary dimensions such as impulsive behavior or depression.[74] The use of serotonin-uptake inhibiting antidepressants in the treatment of AN and BN will be discussed below.

The dopaminergic system also has received attention, because dopamine (DA) neurotransmission has been implicated in feeding behavior and in motor activity, amenorrhea, and distortion of body image.[65,73] One study each of D3 and D4 receptor polymorphisms and food restriction in AN have been negative. One of three studies of polymorphisms in the catechol O-methyltransferase gene (an enzyme in DA metabolism) in AN was positive, but the other two were negative.

Other candidate genes controlling hormones and proteins putatively related to food intake that have been studied in eating disorders include the estrogen receptor, the uncoupling proteins UCP-2 and UCP-3, pro-opiomelanocortin, the melanocortin-4 receptor, leptin, agouti-related protein, neuropeptide Y, the β₃-adrenergic receptor, and tumor necrosis factor. All but one have been negative.[65] Thus, although the familial clustering of both AN and BN is clear, there is no solid evidence that single nucleotide polymorphisms in any of the aforementioned genes are other than mildly related to either of these eating disorders.

GENERAL PHYSICAL AND LABORATORY FINDINGS

The general physical and laboratory findings of AN and BN are presented in Tables 45-3 and 45-4, respectively.[75] Metabolic changes and medical complications occur secondary to chronic starvation and malnutrition and to bingeing and purging.[11,76] Malnutrition-associated disturbances as severe as pulmonary bronchiectasis and emphysema have been reported.[77]

Gastrointestinal (GI) disturbances occur in both AN and BN.[78] Delayed gastric emptying and delayed colonic transit time resulting in constipation are common in AN patients and are associated with complaints of early satiety, bloating, and abdominal distension, leading the patient to feel fat and avoid eating. GI disturbances in BN include increased gastric capacity, decreased gastric relaxation, delayed gastric emptying, and abnormal function of the enteric autonomic nervous system. Abnormalities of GI function in AN and BN are reversible to various degrees with improvement in the underlying disorders. Treatments targeted at these abnormalities, such as agents to improve gastric emptying in AN and neurotransmitter modulators to reduce bingeing in BN, have met with varying success and require further study.

Increasing recognition is being given to osteopenia as an early and serious complication of AN.[79] Adolescence is a time

---

Table 45-3 Physical and Laboratory Findings in Anorexia Nervosa

PHYSICAL
Cachexia, emaciation, dehydration, shock or impending shock
Covert infectious processes, immunologic problems late in process
Dry skin, desquamation, yellowish palms and soles
Scalp and pubic hair loss, lanugo, increased pigmented body hair
Hypothermia, decreased metabolic rate, bradycardia, hypotension
Bradypnea (respiratory compensation for alkalosis)
Edema of lower extremities, heart murmur (infrequent)
Signs of estrogen deficiency (dry skin, osteoporosis, small uterus and cervix, dry vaginal mucosa) and androgen deficiency (no acne or oily skin)

CHEMICAL
Normal laboratory results early in process
Elevated BUN, secondary to dehydration
Hypercarotenemia
Elevated serum cholesterol early in process; may decrease later
Decreased plasma transferrin, complement, fibrinogen, prealbumin; usually normal protein and albumin:globulin ratio
Elevated serum lactic dehydrogenase and alkaline phosphatase
Depressed serum magnesium, calcium, phosphorus—the last a late and ominous sign
Possibly depressed plasma zinc, urinary zinc, and copper

HEMATOLOGIC
Panleukopenia with relative lymphocytosis
Thrombocytopenia
Very low erythrocyte sedimentation rate
Anemia late in process, especially with rehydration

Source: Adapted from Comerci GD: Medical complications of anorexia nervosa and bulimia nervosa. Med Clin North Am 74:1293–1310, 1990.

Table 45-4 Physical and Laboratory Findings in Bulimia Nervosa

PHYSICAL
Usually well groomed with good hygiene
Usually normal weight or mild to moderate obesity
Generalized or localized edema of lower extremities
Swelling of parotid and other salivary glands
Bruises and lacerations of posterior pharynx, lesions of fingers and
    dorsum of hands, secondary to induced vomiting
Dental enamel discoloration and dysplasia, secondary to vomiting of
    gastric acid
Pyorrhea and other gum disorders
Diminished reflexes, muscle weakness, paralysis, infrequently
    peripheral neuropathy
Muscle cramping (with induced hypoxia or positive Trousseau's sign)
Signs of hypokalemia (hypotension, weak pulse, arrhythmias,
    decreased cardiac output, poor-quality heart sounds; shortness of
    breath; ileus, abdominal distension, acute gastric dilatation;
    depression, mental clouding)
Additional physical features of anorexia nervosa, if food restriction is
    part of syndrome

CHEMICAL
Uncomplicated bulimia
No abnormalities reported; possible abnormal glucose metabolism
Bulimia with vomiting
Metabolic alkalosis (hypochloremia, elevated serum bicarbonate)
Hypokalemia (secondary to metabolic alkalosis)
Hypovolemia with secondary hyperaldosteronism (also contributes
    to hypokalemia), pseudo-Bartter's syndrome
Bulimia with vomiting and purging (laxatives or diuretics)
All the above findings, plus:
    Decreased body potassium secondary to diarrhea and renal losses
    Metabolic acidosis with spuriously normal serum potassium
    Hypokalemic nephropathy (urine concentrating deficit)
    Hypokalemic myopathy (including cardiomyopathy)
    Hypo- or hypercalcemia, hypomagnesemia, hypophosphatemia

Source: Adapted from Comerci GD: Medical complications of anorexia
nervosa and bulimia nervosa. Med Clin North Am 74:1293–1310, 1990.

when optimal bone mineralization supporting physical growth is critical, and adolescent girls with AN have relatively poor bone mineral accrual.[80] Several factors contribute to osteopenia in AN, including estrogen, androgen, and insulin-like growth factor (IGF)-1 deficiency, hypercortisolemia, excessive exercise, and nutritional deficiencies such as calcium and vitamin D. Multifaceted treatment of AN is required to restore bone mineral density to within the normal range.

The electrolyte disturbances of AN and BN depend on whether purging is primarily by vomiting or by abuse of laxatives or diuretics (or both) and can be life threatening. The medical management of these cases can be complex and must be individualized. Comerci[75] presented detailed case histories of an anorexic and a bulimic patient, including critiques of their treatment, which highlighted the intricacies of successful medical management of these disorders.

NEUROIMAGING

This is a growing area of eating-disorder research, paralleling improvements in imaging technology.[81,82] In AN, enlargement of cortical sulci and subarachnoid spaces suggestive of cerebral and, on occasion, cerebellar atrophy can occur. It is positively correlated with poor neuropsychologic test performance and is reversible to varying degrees with weight gain.[13,83–88] As well, reductions in central pontine myelin and orbital fat have been reported.[89,90] Proton magnetic resonance spectroscopy (^{1}H-MRS) indicates higher ratios of choline-containing compounds to creatine and N-acetylaspartate and reduced myoinositol, suggesting starvation-associated increased cell membrane turnover.[91,92] Consistent with these findings, ^{31}P-MRS has shown altered

phosphodiester and phosphomonoester peaks in malnourished anorexics, suggesting that reduced body mass alters CNS cellular membrane phospholipid metabolism.[93,94] Reduced blood flow in frontal, parietal, and frontotemporal cortex has been reported in AN, which reverts to normal perfusion with clinical remission.[95]

Functional magnetic resonance imaging (fMRI) also is beginning to delineate activation of limbic and paralimbic areas that may be involved with calorie fear; these areas also have been implicated as a neural substrate of obsessive-compulsive and depressive symptoms.[96] fMRI has shown decreased food-stimulated activation of several cortical areas in chronically ill anorexics compared to those exhibiting long-term recovery.[97] Reduced 5-HT2A receptor binding in frontal, parietal, and occipital cortex also has been reported in AN patients and may persist after recovery in both AN and BN.[98–100] This may tie in with the candidate gene studies of this receptor discussed earlier; correlative studies have yet to be undertaken.

NEUROENDOCRINOLOGY

Abnormal hormone profiles and responses to challenge are closely related to the "starvation" status of AN and BN patients. Hormone abnormalities also may be present, but to a lesser extent, in normal-weight women with BN. The presence of starvation in AN is evident from the weight loss, but it might not be recognized in normal-weight BN; although bulimic women often maintain a normal weight, they do so by restricting food intake when not bingeing and purging, and they often have poorly balanced meals. Starvation-induced depletion of hepatic glycogen stores results in free fatty acids and ketone bodies replacing glucose as the primary energy source. This shift from glycogenolysis to lipolysis and ketogenesis is associated with an increase in free fatty acids and their metabolites. β-Hydroxybutyric acid levels are elevated in both AN and BN,[101] indicating that bulimic patients are nutritionally depleted in spite of their normal body weight.

The relationship of starvation and eating disorders to neuroendocrine function is most clearly seen for the pituitary-gonadal axis. As has been mentioned, secondary amenorrhea is one of the criteria for AN in postmenarcheal women, and oligomenorrhea occurs in about 50% of bulimics. Table 45-5 lists the major endocrine disturbances that occur in AN and BN.[9,13,102–107] The secondary amenorrhea is a direct result of altered gonadotropin secretion. Serum sex hormone–binding globulin may be increased, and both estrogen and testosterone are decreased.[108] As is indicated in Table 45-3, there are physical signs of severe estrogen deficiency. The luteinizing hormone (LH) response to LH-releasing hormone stimulation is blunted, but the follicle-stimulating hormone response is usually normal.

Figure 45-2 illustrates circadian serum LH profiles of girls at different pubertal stages and in a 21-year-old woman with AN of 14 months' duration whose body weight was 60% of ideal weight.[102] This patient's menarche was at age 14, and during the period of weight loss, her LH profile was that of a prepubertal girl. BN patients also may have decreased gonadotropin secretion if they have lost 15% or more of their body weight, but they usually have normal circulating gonadotropins and continue their menses.

With reference to the hypothalamic-pituitary-adrenal cortical (HPA) axis (see Table 45-5), the abnormalities in AN and in reduced-weight BN[106,109,110] are strikingly similar to those occurring in 30% to 50% of patients with major depression.[111] Circulating cortisol is increased at all times of the day and night, but the amplitude and timing of its circadian rhythm are preserved.[106] Circulating adrenocorticotropic hormone (ACTH) is usually normal, as it is in major depression, when it is determined by radioimmunoassay; the more specific immunoradiometric assay for ACTH$_{1-39}$ has shown decreased

Table 45-5 Neuroendocrine Disturbances In Anorexia Nervosa and Bulimia Nervosa

	Anorexia Nervosa	Bulimia Nervosa
PITUITARY-GONADAL AXIS		
Plasma gonadotropins (LH, FSH)	↓	±↓
Plasma estradiol	↓↓	±↓
Plasma testosterone	↓	?
LHRH stimulation of LH	↓	±↓
LHRH stimulation of FSH	↔	↔
PITUITARY-ADRENAL CORTICAL AXIS		
Plasma and CSF cortisol	↑	±↑
Plasma ACTH	↔	↔
CSF ACTH	↓	↔ (↓ when abstinent)
CSF CRH	↑	?
CRH stimulation of ACTH	↓	?
ACTH stimulation of cortisol	↑	?
Dexamethasone suppression test	50%–90% non-suppression	20%–60% non-suppression
PITUITARY-THYROID AXIS		
Plasma total T4	±↓	↔ (±↓ when abstinent)
Plasma T3	↓↓	↓
Plasma reverse T3	↑	↔ (↓ when abstinent)
Plasma TSH	±↓	±↓ (↑ when abstinent)
CSF TRH	↓	?
TRH stimulation of TSH	↓	↓
OTHER NEUROENDOCRINE AXES		
Growth hormone	↑	↑
Prolactin	↔	±↓
Prolactin response to serotonergic challenge	↓	↓
Melatonin	±↑	?

Abbreviations: LH, luteinizing hormone; FSH, follicle-stimulating hormone; LHRH, luteinizing hormone–releasing hormone; CSF, cerebrospinal fluid; ACTH, adrenocorticotropic hormone; CRH, corticotropin-releasing hormone; T_4, thyroxine; T_3, triiodothyronine; TSH, thyroid-stimulating hormone; TRH, thyrotropin-releasing hormone, ↑, increased; ↓, decreased; ↔, unchanged; ?, insufficient data.

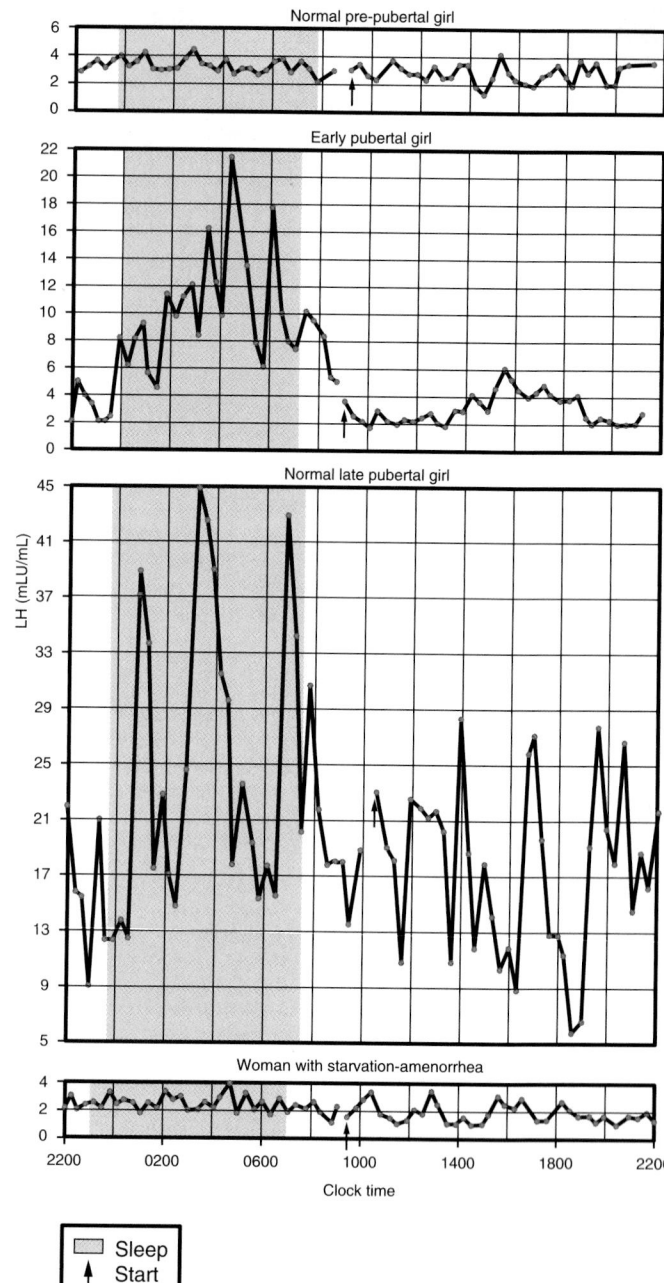

Figure 45-2 Circadian serum luteinizing hormone (LH) profiles in girls at different pubertal stages and in a 21-year-old woman with anorexia nervosa of 14 months' duration whose body weight was 60% of ideal weight. Menarche was at age 14 years, and her LH profile is that of a prepubertal girl. (From Vande Wiele RL: Anorexia nervosa and the hypothalamus. Hosp Pract 12:45–51, 1977. © 1977 The McGraw-Hill Companies, Inc. Illustration by Albert Miller.)

ACTH in major depression,[112] which also could be the case for $ACTH_{1-39}$ in these eating disorders. Cerebrospinal fluid (CSF) ACTH concentrations appear to be decreased, but CSF corticotropin-releasing hormone (CRH) concentrations may be increased,[106,110] as may be CSF vasopressin,[106,113] a secretagogue for ACTH in addition to CRH,[114] which appears to play a greater role in stress states than under normal conditions.[115]

Stimulation and suppression tests of the HPA axis have been conducted mainly in AN, and they are in accord with the baseline hormone findings. The ACTH response to CRH administration is reduced, undoubtedly secondary to enhanced negative feedback on the pituitary corticotrophs exerted by elevated circulating cortisol. The cortisol response to ACTH administration is increased, suggesting increased secretory capacity of the adrenal cortex. The low-dose dexamethasone (DEX) suppression test is abnormal in 50% to 90% of anorexics and in 20% to 60% of bulimics, depending on weight loss. Because DEX acts primarily at the pituitary,[116] ACTH and cortisol escape from DEX suppression suggests increased suprapituitary stimulation of corticotrophs by CRH and vasopressin. Taken together, the pituitary-adrenocortical findings indicate a mild to moderate activation of this hormone axis in AN and BN. As well, plasma neuroactive steroids are reported to be elevated in untreated women with both AN and BN.[117]

With reference to the pituitary-thyroid axis, starvation leads to considerably decreased plasma free triiodothyronine (T_3) concentrations, along with somewhat decreased plasma-free thyroxine (T_4) and increased plasma reverse T_3 concentrations. This represents the "euthyroid sick syndrome" hormone profile.[118–120] The decreased circulating T_3 helps to reduce energy expenditure and minimizes muscle protein catabolism into amino acids for gluconeogenesis.[118] CSF thyrotropin-releasing hormone (TSH) also appears to be reduced in AN.[121] When they are bingeing, bulimic patients generally have normal thyroid indices with perhaps reduced T_3 and TSH concentrations; however, when they stop bingeing, their pituitary-thyroid axis function resembles that of anorexic patients.[122–124]

IGF-1 concentrations are low in both AN and BN, and circulating growth hormone (GH) is increased, perhaps owing to diminished feedback of IGF-1 on GH secretion.[125] Circulating prolactin is usually unchanged in AN and may be reduced in BN. Prolactin responses to serotonergic challenges are diminished in both AN and BN,[126-130] suggesting decreased CNS serotonergic neurotransmitter function.[131] (Serotonin uptake–inhibiting antidepressants have shown promise in the treatment of these eating disorders, as discussed later.) Circulating melatonin has been reported as both unchanged and increased in AN and as unchanged in BN.[132-134]

The effect of reduced caloric intake on these endocrine systems has been studied in healthy individuals.[135,136] When healthy women were starved, plasma gonadotropin concentrations declined. The women also experienced increased circulating concentrations of cortisol and GH and decreased plasma T_3 concentrations despite normal plasma T_4—the "euthyroid sick syndrome" hormone profile.[118] The endocrine abnormalities associated with starvation in the healthy female subjects reversed with the resumption of normal eating.

The endocrine changes in both AN and BN revert to normal with successful treatment of these illnesses, indicating that the endocrine changes are state markers of the metabolic stress of starvation and malnutrition. It should be emphasized that, in addition to its effects on hormone secretion, starvation can lead to abnormal psychologic states. Semistarvation of male conscientious objectors to military service was associated with increased irritability, labile mood, depression, decreased concentration, decreased libido, and decreased motor activity,[137] and starvation and malnutrition can exaggerate the comorbid psychiatric symptoms of AN and BN.[55] These changes reinforce the concept of starvation-related state changes, influencing both the behavioral and the endocrine aspects of eating disorders.

CENTRAL NERVOUS SYSTEM NEUROPEPTIDES

Since the 1980s, the realization has evolved that the peripheral hormonal disturbances in AN and BN are a consequence of the malnutrition associated with starvation and bingeing, rather than being etiologic. Contemporaneously, an understanding of how CNS neuronal pathways contribute to starvation-induced alterations in peripheral hormonal secretion has developed. The mechanisms for controlling food intake and energy homeostasis involve a complex interplay among peripheral (taste, local autonomic influences on GI/neuropeptides, vagal afferent nerves) and CNS neurotransmitters and neuromodulators, including monoamines and neuropeptides that influence hunger and satiety.[110,138] Compounds such as norepinephrine, serotonin, insulin, opioids, neuropeptide Y and peptide YY, leptin, CRH, vasopressin, and the orexins/hypocretins contribute to regulating the rate, duration, and size of meals, as well as the selection of carbohydrates and protein.[139-142]

Neuropeptides were initially determined to be regulators primarily of hypothalamic functions such as food and water consumption and metabolism, sexuality, sleep, body temperature, pain sensation, and autonomic function. These compounds also have been localized to other areas of the CNS besides the hypothalamus and pituitary, where they appear to regulate complex human mental functions such as mood, obsessionality, attachment formation, and risk-taking and addictive behaviors.[143] Some of the behavioral disturbances occurring during starvation therefore may be related to alterations in function of neuropeptides throughout the CNS. These peptide systems work together multiply in overlapping CNS pathways that influence the spectrum of energy balance states. Table 45-6 lists the major neuropeptide disturbances that occur in AN and BN.

NEUROPEPTIDE Y AND PEPTIDE YY

These phylogenetically and structurally related peptides share the same receptor family (Y1, Y2, Y4, Y5) and are among the

Table 45-6 Central Nervous System Neuropeptide Disturbances in Anorexia Nervosa and Bulimia Nervosa

	Anorexia Nervosa	Bulimia Nervosa
CSF neuropeptide Y	↑	↔
CSF peptide YY	↔	↔ ↑ during abstinence
Plasma ghrelin	↑	↑
Plasma leptin	↓	↓
CSF leptin	↓	?
Plasma adiponectin	↑	↑
Plasma resistin	↓	?
Plasma cholecystokinin	?	↓
CSF cholecystokinin	?	↓
CSF β-endorphin	↓	↓
CSF dynorphin	↔	↔
CSF vasopressin	↑	↑
CSF oxytocin	↓	↔

↑, increased; ↓, decreased; ↔, unchanged; ?, insufficient data.

most potent stimulants of feeding behavior in animals, particularly for carbohydrate-rich foods.[110] Neuropeptide Y (NPY) occurs in high concentrations in limbic structures, including the hypothalamus, and is present throughout the cerebral cortex. It is produced in the arcuate nucleus of the hypothalamus, increases during hunger and falls during meals, and acts on the paraventricular nucleus to mediate increased eating and reduce energy expenditure. Its effect is counteracted by CRH, and a dynamic equilibrium between NPY and CRH neuronal activity appears to be an important regulator of food intake. In contrast, peptide YY (PYY) occurs in lower concentrations in the CNS, caudal brain stem, and spinal cord. PYY occurs in two forms and is located primarily in endocrine cells of the lower GI tract, where it helps to mediate motility and function. PYY_{1-36} is strongly orexigenic. PYY_{3-36}, on the other hand, has particular affinity for the Y2 receptor, it increases in response to meals, and its actions are to decrease appetite and reduce food intake.[144]

Intracerebroventricular (ICV) NPY administration in animals produces many of the physiologic and behavioral changes associated with AN, including gonadal steroid-dependent effects on LH secretion, suppression of sexual activity, increased CRH in the hypothalamus, and hypotension.[110] Underweight AN patients have elevated CSF NPY, likely a result of their malnourished status. In contrast, such patients, whether underweight or recovered, have normal CSF PYY concentrations. CSF NPY returns to normal with recovery, although patients with amenorrhea may continue to have higher CSF NPY concentrations. Elevated CSF NPY is not an effective stimulant of feeding in underweight anorexics, as is evidenced by their resistance to eating and weight gain. Anorexics typically display an obsessive and paradoxic interest in dietary intake and food preparation, and it may be that increased NPY activity in extrahypothalamic areas of the CNS contributes to these cognitions and behaviors.

ICV PYY administration in rats causes massive food ingestion, to which tolerance does not develop.[145] This prompted speculation that increased CNS PYY activity may contribute to bulimia. CSF PYY concentrations in normal-weight bulimic women when bingeing and vomiting were similar to those of controls.[110] In contrast, CSF PYY was significantly elevated in bulimic women after a month of abstinence from bingeing and vomiting, compared to healthy volunteer women and AN patients. CSF NPY concentrations were normal in the bulimic women, in contrast to the elevated CSF NPY concentrations in the anorexic women.

It is not known why CSF PYY is normal in bulimics with chronic bingeing and vomiting and becomes elevated after a period of abstinence. Future studies should examine whether abrupt cessation of bingeing, vomiting, or both results in an overshoot of CNS PYY production. Whatever the cause, this disturbance is of potential importance. Normal-weight bulimia carries a high recidivism rate, despite treatment. Abnormally elevated CNS PYY activity in the abstinent bulimic may contribute to a persistent drive toward bingeing, particularly a desire for sweet, high-caloric foods.

GHRELIN

Ghrelin, so named because it stimulates GH secretion, is released mainly from endocrine cells in the stomach and GI tract.[146–148] It antagonizes the action of leptin, strongly stimulates feeding and weight gain by promoting NPY and agouti-related protein, and has a number of other central and peripheral neuroendocrine and metabolic actions. In humans, fasting plasma ghrelin is inversely related to body mass index, percent body fat, and fasting plasma leptin and insulin concentrations. There is a normal preprandial rise and postprandial fall in plasma ghrelin in humans. Plasma ghrelin, including the active, octanoyl form, is elevated in AN patients, particularly in the bingeing and purging subtype,[149–152] and it does not decrease normally after a standardized meal or fiber intake.[153] On the other hand, ghrelin is not elevated in constitutionally thin women with body mass indexes similar to those of AN patients, and it returns to normal values in AN patients after weight recovery.[150] Fasting plasma ghrelin also has been reported as elevated in BN patients compared to controls with similar body mass index, suggesting that the abnormal eating behavior (bingeing and purging) influences circulating ghrelin, as it can in the bingeing and purging subtype of AN.[151]

LEPTIN

Leptin is secreted predominantly by adipose cells and acts in the CNS to decrease food intake.[154] Leptin activates OB receptors primarily in the hypothalamus, where it may inhibit NPY secretion, and in extraneural tissues to increase energy expenditure.[155] In rodents, defects in the leptin gene-coding sequence, resulting in leptin deficiency and defects in leptin receptors, are associated with obesity. Treatment with recombinant leptin reduces fat mass in both obese and normal-weight animals in a dose-dependent manner. In humans, serum leptin concentrations are positively correlated with fat mass in individuals in all weight ranges. Women tend to have higher serum leptin than men of the same weight, presumably because of women's higher proportion of body fat.[156] Obesity in humans is not thought to be a result of leptin deficiency per se, but obesity may be associated with leptin resistance.[157]

Malnourished and underweight AN patients have significantly reduced plasma and CSF leptin concentrations compared with normal-weight controls,[149,158] implying a normal physiologic response to starvation. Reduced plasma/CSF leptin ratio has been found in anorexics compared with controls, suggesting that the proportional decrease in leptin with weight loss is greater in plasma than in CSF. As in normal control women, plasma leptin concentrations in anorexics are positively correlated with body weight and fat mass, and they are negatively correlated with physical activity.[159] During refeeding in AN patients, CSF leptin concentrations increase to normal values before full weight restoration,[149,160] possibly as a consequence of the relatively rapid and disproportionate accumulation of fat during refeeding. The suggestion that premature normalization of leptin concentrations might contribute to difficulty in achieving and sustaining a normal weight in AN, however, has not been supported by studies to date.[161]

Patients with BN appear to have significantly decreased serum leptin following an overnight fast.[149] During sustained recovery from BN, serum leptin remains decreased, compared to controls matched on amount of body fat. This finding, along with persistently decreased thyroid activity in recovered BN patients, may result in decreased metabolic rate and a tendency toward weight gain, contributing to the preoccupation with body weight that is characteristic of BN.

Leptin also appears to modulate fertility[155,157,162] and may be the metabolic signal that mediates impaired reproductive ability in extreme overweight and underweight conditions.[155,163] There appear to have been no studies addressing a potential relationship between leptin and amenorrhea in AN. In some anorexic patients, amenorrhea may occur before significant weight loss, and leptin may be the mediating hormone. Weight loss generally causes circulating leptin concentrations to fall in proportion to the loss of body fat mass,[164] but acute, fasting-induced weight loss can provoke a fall in leptin that is disproportionately greater than would be expected from the amount of fat lost. This suggests that under conditions of intense food deprivation, leptin may instigate metabolic responses before a significant weight or fat loss has occurred. Reduced leptin concentrations appear to be a critical signal that initiates the neuroendocrine response to starvation, including limiting procreation, decreasing thyroid thermogenesis, and increasing secretion of stress steroids.[165] Leptin administration during fasting partially restores LH and testosterone concentrations, blunts falling T_4 concentrations, and attenuates the rise in ACTH and glucocorticoids, without affecting plasma concentrations of insulin, glucose, or ketone bodies.

As was mentioned earlier, during starvation, circulating concentrations of NPY increase, inhibiting gonadotropin release and activating the HPA axis. Leptin inhibits starvation-induced elevations in NPY,[166] and it may also reduce food intake and body weight by increasing the metabolic rate through activation of β-adrenergic receptors and possibly through its own anorexigenic properties.[149]

ADIPONECTIN

Adiponectin also is secreted by adipose cells.[167,168] Circulating levels are two to three times higher in women than in men. Adiponectin exists in three forms, made up of different numbers of trimers. The globular form appears to increase muscle sensitivity to insulin by increasing fatty acid oxidation, similar to the effect of leptin. Unlike leptin, however, circulating adiponectin is inversely correlated with fat mass, being decreased in obesity.[169] There does not appear to be a direct relationship between circulating leptin and adiponectin, in that decreasing serum leptin by acute fasting or increasing it by administration of physiologic or pharmacologic doses had no effect on serum adiponectin.[170] On the other hand, ghrelin impairs adiponectin expression by adipocytes.[171]

Circulating adiponectin is increased in patients with AN, in contrast to reduced circulating leptin.[158,172,173] Nonoxidative glucose metabolism is reduced as well. Patients with BN also were found to have increased circulating adiponectin concentrations, which were positively correlated with the frequency of binge/vomiting episodes.[174] In contrast, women with binge eating disorder (bingeing without compensatory behaviors—vomiting and/or purging) had reduced circulating adiponectin along with increased glucose, cholesterol, and triglycerides. In these patients, adiponectin concentrations were not significantly related to the frequency of their bingeing episodes.

Other adipocytokines include resistin and acylation-stimulating protein.[168,169] Resistin may play a role in obesity- and diabetes-associated insulin resistance, although this effect in humans is still unclear. Decreased plasma resistin has been suggested to occur in AN.[158]

CHOLECYSTOKININ

Cholecystokinin (CCK) is secreted by the GI tract in response to food intake[149] and is thought to signal satiety to the CNS via vagal afferents. Exogenously administered CCK reduces food intake in humans. Studies of CCK in patients with AN have been inconsistent in their findings. In contrast, patients with BN appear to have reduced CSF and lymphocyte CCK concentrations and diminished CCK secretion following a test meal. The blunted postprandial CCK response may contribute to the diminished postingestive satiety that BN patients experience.

MELANOCORTIN AND CORTICOTROPIN-RELEASING HORMONE

The central melanocortin system is important in the in the regulation of energy balance.[175] The key melanocortin receptor agonist is α-melanocyte-stimulating hormone, and the key antagonist is agouti-related peptide; these have anorexigenic and orexigenic activity, respectively.[176] The hypercortisolism in AN and BN is most likely due to hypersecretion of CRH, which is most probably a response to weight loss per se; the change in CRH is likely mediated through the central melanocortin system.[177] CRH also has central effects beyond the HPA axis, as ICV administration of CRH to animals produces physiologic and behavioral changes associated with AN, including hypothalamic hypogonadism, decreased sexual activity, decreased feeding behavior, and hyperactivity.[110,149] The anorexigenic action of leptin may be mediated at least partially through CRH.[178] The anorectic activity of serotonergic drugs appears to be through activation of pro-opiomelanocortin neurons in the arcuate nucleus, a circuit which is tonically regulated by leptin.[179,180]

OPIOID PEPTIDES

CNS opioid agonists increase food intake, and opioid antagonists decrease food intake,[110] suggesting that these compounds may mediate some aspects of AN.[110,149] Although assessment of brain opioid activity in vivo in humans is problematic, because of the many CNS neuropeptides with opioid activity and the multiplicity of CNS opioid receptors, the CSF concentrations of some opioid peptides has been determined in anorexic patients. Underweight anorexics were found to have significantly reduced CSF β-endorphin concentrations compared with those of healthy volunteers.[110] CSF β-endorphin concentrations remained significantly below normal after short-term weight restoration but returned to normal after long-term weight restoration. CSF β-endorphin concentrations also have been shown to be reduced in women with BN.[110] CSF dynorphin concentrations have been reported as normal in all stages of AN and BN.[110,149]

Open trials of high doses of the opiate antagonist naltrexone have been reported to reduce binge frequency in BN,[181,182] but double-blind, controlled trials with lower naltrexone doses have shown no effect on binge frequency or macronutrient intake.[183,184] Relatively high-dose naltrexone treatment reduced binge and purge frequency and total daily food intake of bulimics, but it did not affect their ability to resist the desire to binge or purge.[185] Whether high-dose opioid antagonist treatment has a role in the treatment of BN is still unclear.

A disturbance in CNS opioid function also may contribute to the neuroendocrine abnormalities in AN and BN (e.g., disturbances in HPA and pituitary-gonadal axis function).[110,149] Brain opioid pathways inhibit ACTH and cortisol release in humans, and they suppress pulsatile gonadotropin secretion in rats and in sexually mature humans. Underweight anorexics frequently have a blunted response of LH secretion to opiate antagonists, and weight restoration tends to normalize this response.[110] The failure of opioid antagonists to increase LH secretion in underweight anorexics suggests that another neurotransmitter system (or systems) may be responsible for this neuroendocrine disturbance.

VASOPRESSIN AND OXYTOCIN

In addition to the effects of vasopressin on HPA axis regulation and free-water clearance by the kidney and the effects of oxytocin during the puerperium, these structurally related neuropeptides are distributed throughout the CNS and function as long-acting neuromodulators of complex behaviors. The effects of vasopressin appear to be reciprocal to those of oxytocin: Central administration of vasopressin to rats enhances memory consolidation and retrieval, whereas administration of oxytocin disrupts memory.[110]

In addition to abnormally high CSF vasopressin concentrations[106] and impaired osmoregulation of plasma vasopressin,[186] AN patients have reduced CSF oxytocin concentrations and impaired plasma oxytocin responses to stimulation.[110] Underweight anorexics also have an impaired plasma oxytocin response to challenging stimuli.[110] These abnormalities tend to normalize after weight restoration, suggesting that they are secondary to malnutrition, abnormal fluid balance, or both. In underweight anorexics, low CNS oxytocin might interact with high CNS vasopressin to enhance the retention of cognitive distortions of the aversive consequences of eating, thereby reinforcing these patients' perseverative preoccupation with the adverse consequences of food intake.

Patients with normal-weight BN were found to have elevated CSF vasopressin concentrations but normal CSF oxytocin both on admission and after 1 month of nutritional stabilization and abstinence from bingeing and purging.[106] In these patients, as well, high CNS vasopressin might contribute to their obsessional preoccupation with the aversive consequences of weight gain. Some recovered bulimics may have continued elevation of CSF vasopressin, perhaps related to a lifetime history of major depression.[187]

LONG-TERM EFFECTS OF MULTIPLE NEUROPEPTIDE DISTURBANCES

As with the peripheral endocrine changes in pituitary and target gland hormones in AN and BN reviewed earlier, multiple neuropeptide disturbances occur when patients engage in pathologic eating behaviors and become malnourished. The list of neuropeptides involved continues to increase.[188] And, as with the peripheral endocrine markers, many of these peptide systems tend to become normal with long-term recovery. The slow correction of these neuropeptide disturbances with weight restoration in AN and BN implies that the disturbances are secondary to malnutrition, weight loss, or both and are not etiologic, although once established, the disturbances may perpetuate some of the symptomatology, providing a biologic dimension to the question of why many anorexics and bulimics cannot easily reverse their illness. Secondary symptoms such as obsessions and dysphoric mood may be exaggerated by CNS neuropeptide alterations and cause the primary illness to be more refractory to treatment. That the neuropeptide disturbances eventually become normal during long-term recovery suggests that treatment of AN and BN must be sustained for months after weight normalization to rectify the many physiologic disturbances.

TREATMENT

Treatment of the eating disorders continues to be complex and difficult. In a 20-year follow-up of AN patients, about one third rated their outcomes as good, one third as intermediate, and one third as poor.[189] Cognitive-behavioral, educational, psychodynamic, and psychopharmacologic treatments have been used, with varying degrees of long-term success.[190-192] As is often the case in the management of psychiatric patients, a combination of therapies is used under the rationale that moderate successes with individual treatments might be at least additive, if not synergistic, in their overall effectiveness. Practice management guidelines discuss the spectrum of options and emphasize developing individualized treatment plans.[192]

There have been more large-scale, randomized controlled clinical treatment trials in BN than in AN.[193–196] A prominent focus has been on interventions that have previously been tested on comorbid psychiatric disorders, such as depression and substance abuse. However, eating disorders and these comorbid syndromes appear to be independently transmitted familial liabilities,[197] so treatments also need to be targeted to the eating disorders themselves.

Controlled treatment studies of AN have shown the efficacy of various psychologic therapies in promoting weight gain in acutely ill patients[198–200] and in preventing relapse following restoration of normal body weight.[192,201] Substantial improvement in body mass and psychosocial adjustment can be achieved in many anorexic subjects through cognitive-behavioral, psychoeducational, and family therapy techniques, with or without dietary counseling. Therapeutic gains have not been as robust in patients with more chronic disability. Specialized eating disorders hospital units offer combinations of enforced weight-gain regimens along with a range of psychosocial treatments, and compulsory in-hospital treatment often is effective over the short term.[202–204]

Serotonin-uptake inhibiting antidepressant drugs (SUIs) also show some promise. As was noted earlier, serotonergic neurotransmission appears to be compromised in eating disorders, including a possible underlying hypersensitivity in AN that may be partially ameliorated by self-starvation and a subsensitivity in BN that is responsive to SUI-mediated increases in serotonergic activity.[82,196,205] SUIs are relatively ineffective in weight-reduced AN patients,[206] possibly because of reduced intake of tryptophan, the amino acid precursor of serotonin, with consequently diminished serotonin production. After weight restoration in AN and improved serotonin production, SUIs such as fluoxetine can reduce obsessionality and the incidence of relapse. Atypical neuroleptics also may have some utility, not only to reduce anxiety but also because they promote weight gain.[207] The bingeing and purging subtype of AN may have a poorer prognosis that the restricting subtype, and weight restoration alone is unlikely to be effective in the bulimic subtype of AN.[208] Improved treatment of AN remains of great clinical and public health importance, in that it is a chronic, relapsing illness with substantial and costly medical morbidity.[195] Other types of treatments continue to be studied, such as the use of the anabolic steroid, dehydroepiandrosterone, to increase bone density and improve psychologic well-being.[209]

Controlled treatment studies of BN have shown the efficacy of both antidepressant medications[194,196] and psychologic therapies, especially cognitive-behavioral therapy (CBT), in reducing both the frequency of bingeing and purging and the severity of body dissatisfaction, pursuit of thinness, and perfectionism.[196,210–212] However, medication alone rarely produces full remission; many patients require multiple medication trials before achieving clinically significant improvement; there have been significant dropout rates in clinical trials; and relapse during continuation therapy is high.

CBT alone produces higher rates of full remission in BN than does antidepressant monotherapy.[196] Even so, 40% to 60% of patients receiving CBT remain symptomatic to some degree after acute treatment.[195,196] Interpersonal therapy that strictly avoids direct reference to abnormal eating attitudes or dietary behaviors may achieve long-term benefits in controlling binge eating and purging equal to those obtained with CBT.[213]

How long to continue treatment in BN once binge eating abates, to minimize relapse, remains undetermined. With antidepressant continuation therapy, the risk of relapse may be higher than in patients with unipolar depression.[196] Low serum T_4 may predict poor treatment outcome.[214] Combined treatment may have an advantage over CBT alone in reducing binge eating and purging, but the incremental benefit is modest. Remaining questions include the length of continuation of psychosocial and antidepressant therapies needed to sustain gains achieved during acute treatment, the mechanisms underlying the possibly synergistic effects of combined treatment, the predictors of differential treatment outcomes, the reasons for a more rapid decay of acute antidepressant treatment effects in BN compared to major depression, and the anticipated effects of crossing over to alternative modalities of treatment when initial treatment fails.[196] Pharmacotherapies for binge eating disorder, as distinct from BN, also are being investigated, such as the use of antiepileptic drugs and serotonin/norepinephrine uptake inhibitors.[215–217]

The difficulties faced by clinicians in the treatment of AN and BN also are affected by the trends in health-care delivery that reduce access to extended care in specialty inpatient and outpatient facilities. These external forces may compromise efforts to reverse the debilitating and sometimes life-threatening behavioral and biologic symptoms and sequelae of these illnesses. The endocrinologist is best advised to seek psychiatric specialist consultation early in the evaluation of patients with these eating disorders, not just to aid in their differential diagnosis, but also, importantly, to help plan the complex therapeutic approaches currently known to offer the best outcomes.

Note: Several recent articles of interest have been added to the references.[218–221]

Acknowledgement

Walter H. Kaye, M.D., provided helpful suggestions on the preparation of this chapter.

REFERENCES

1. Allbutt TC, Rolleston HD: A System of Medicine. London, Macmillan, 1908, p 398.
2. Berkman JM: Anorexia nervosa, anorexia, inanition, and low basal metabolic rate. Am J Med Sci 180:411–424, 1930.
3. Bliss EL, Branch CHH: Anorexia Nervosa: Its History, Psychology, and Biology. New York, Paul B. Hoeber, 1960.
4. Vandereycken W, Van Deth R: From Fasting Saints to Anorexic Girls: The History of Self–Starvation. London, Althone Press, 1994.
5. Bruch H: Eating Disorders: Obesity, Anorexia Nervosa and the Person Within. New York, Basic Books, 1973.
6. Vigersky RA (ed): Anorexia Nervosa. New York, Raven Press, 1977.
7. Herzog DB, Copeland PM: Eating disorders. N Engl J Med 313:295–303, 1985.
8. Habermas T: The psychiatric history of anorexia nervosa and bulimia nervosa: Weight concerns and bulimic symptoms in early case reports. Int J Eat Disord 8:259–273, 1989.
9. Foster DW: Eating disorders: Obesity, anorexia nervosa, and bulimia nervosa. In Wilson JD, Foster DW (eds): Williams Textbook of Endocrinology, 8th ed. Philadelphia, WB Saunders, 1992, pp 1335–1365.
10. Halmi KA (ed): Psychobiology and Treatment of Anorexia Nervosa and Bulimia Nervosa. Washington, DC, American Psychiatric Press, 1992.
11. Kaplan AS, Garfinkel PE: Medical Issues and the Eating Disorders: The Interface. New York, Brunner/Mazel, 1993.
12. Garfinkel PE: Eating disorders. In Kaplan HI, Sadock BJ (eds): Comprehensive Textbook of Psychiatry, vol 6. Baltimore, Williams & Wilkins, 1995, pp 1361–1371.
13. Warren MP: Anorexia nervosa. In DeGroot LJ, Besser M, Burger HG, et al (eds): Endocrinology, 3rd ed. Philadelphia, WB Saunders, 1995, pp 2679–2687.

14. Walsh BT: Eating disorders. In Tasman A, Kay J, Lieberman JA (eds): Psychiatry. Philadelphia, WB Saunders, 1997, pp 1202–1216.

15. Kaye WH, Klump KL, Frank GK, et al: Anorexia and bulimia nervosa. Annu Rev Med 51:299–313, 2000.

16. Hsu LK: Epidemiology of the eating disorders. Psychiatr Clin North Am 19:681–700, 1996.

17. Morton R: Phthisiologia, Seu Exercitationes de Phthisi Tribus Libris Comprehensæ: Totumque Opus Variis Historiis Illustratum. London, Smith & Walford, 1689. (Translated as Phthisiologia; or, a Treatise of Consumptions, 1694.)

18. Reynolds J: A Discourse upon Prodigious Abstinence: Occasioned by the Twelve Moneths Fasting of Martha Taylor, the Famed Derbyshire Damosell: Proving That Without any Miracle, the Texture of Humane Bodies May Be So Altered, That Life May Be Long Continued Without the Supplies of Meat and Drink. With an Account of the Heart, and How Far It Is Interested in the Business of Fermentation. London, Royall Society, 1669.

19. Hunter R, Macalpine I: Three Hundred Years of Psychiatry 1535–1860. London, Oxford University Press, 1963, pp 230–232.

20. Lasègue C: De l'anorexie hysterique. Arch Gén Méd 1:385, 1873.

21. Gull WW: Anorexia hysterica (apepsia hysterica). Br Med J 2:527, 1873.

22. Gull WW: Anorexia nervosa (apepsia hysterica, anorexia hysterica). Trans Clin Soc Lond 7:22–31, 1874.

23. Simmonds M: Über Hypophysisschwund mit tödlichem Ausgang. Dtsch Med Wochenschr 40:322, 1914.

24. Russell GFM: Bulimia nervosa: An ominous variant of anorexia nervosa. Psychol Med 9:429–448, 1979.

25. Vandereycken W, Hoek HW: Are eating disorders culture-bound syndromes? In Halmi KA (ed): Psychobiology and Treatment of Anorexia Nervosa and Bulimia Nervosa. Washington, DC, American Psychiatric Press, 1992, pp 19–36.

26. Wakeling A: Epidemiology of anorexia nervosa. Psychiatry Res 62:3–9, 1996.

27. Pope HG, Hudson JI, Yurgulun-Todd D, et al: Prevalence of anorexia nervosa and bulimia in three student populations. Int J Eat Disord 3:45–51, 1984.

28. Sullivan PF: Mortality in anorexia nervosa. Am J Psychiatry 152:1073–1074, 1995.

29. Cooper PJ, Charnock DJ, Taylor MJ: The prevalence of bulimia nervosa: A replication study. Br J Psychiatry 151:684–686, 1987.

30. Ben-Tovim DI, Subbiah N, Scheutz B, et al: Bulimia: Symptoms and syndromes in an urban population. Aust N Z J Psychiatry 23:73–80, 1989.

31. Fairburn CG, Beglin SJ: Studies of the epidemiology of anorexia nervosa. Am J Psychiatry 147:401–408, 1990.

32. Pyle RL, Halvorson PA, Neuman PA, et al: The increasing prevalence of bulimia in freshman college students. Int J Eat Disord 5:631–647, 1986.

33. Williams P, King M: The "epidemic" of anorexia nervosa: Another medical myth? Lancet 1:205–207, 1987.

34. Anderson AE: Anorexia nervosa: Who are you? Where are you? Mayo Clin Proc 63:511–512, 1988.

35. Hill JO, Peters JC: Environmental contributions to the obesity epidemic. Science 280:1371–1374, 1998.

36. Taubes G: As obesity rates rise, experts struggle to explain why. Science 280:1367–1368, 1998.

37. Strober M: Family-genetic studies. In Halmi KA (ed): Psychobiology and Treatment of Anorexia Nervosa and Bulimia Nervosa. Washington, DC, American Psychiatric Press, 1992, pp 61–76.

38. Lilenfeld LR, Strober M, Kaye WH: Genetics and family studies of anorexia nervosa and bulimia nervosa. In Kaye WH, Jimerson DC (eds): Eating Disorders. Ballière's Clinical Psychiatry. London, Ballière Tindall, 1997, pp 177–197.

39. Johnson JG, Cohen P, Kasen S, et al: Childhood adversities associated with risk for eating disorders or weight problems during adolescence or early adulthood. Am J Psychiatry 394–400, 2002.

40. The McKnight Investigators: Risk factors for the onset of eating disorders in adolescent girls: Results of the McKnight longitudinal risk factor study. Am J Psychiatry 160:248–254, 2003. (Erratum: Am J Psychiatry 160:1024, 2003; Comment: Evid Based Ment Health 6:95, 2003.)

41. American Psychiatric Association: Diagnostic and Statistical Manual of Mental Disorders, ed 4. Washington, DC, American Psychiatric Association, 1994, pp 539–550, 729–731.

42. Garfinkel PE, Lin E, Goering P, et al: Should amenorrhea be necessary for the diagnosis of anorexia nervosa?: Evidence from a Canadian community sample. Br J Psychiatry 168:500–506, 1996.

43. Watson TL, Anderson AE: A critical examination of the amenorrhea and weight criteria for diagnosing anorexia nervosa. Acta Psychiatr Scand 108:175–182, 2003.

44. Garfinkel PE, Kennedy SH, Kaplan AS: Views on classification and diagnosis of eating disorders. Can J Psychiatry 40:445–456, 1995.

45. Woodside DB, Garfinkel PE, Lin E, et al: Comparisons of men with full or partial eating disorders, men without eating disorders, and women with eating disorders in the community. Am J Psychiatry 158:570–574, 2001.

46. Becker AE, Grinspoon SK, Klibanski A, et al: Eating disorders. N Engl J Med 340:1092–1098, 1999.

47. First MB, Spitzer RL, Gibbon M, et al: Structured Clinical Interview for DSM-IV Axis I Disorders. New York, Biometrics Research Department, New York State Psychiatric Institute, 1996.

48. Bulik CM, Sullivan PF, Kendler KS: An empirical study of the classification of eating disorders. Am J Psychiatry 157:886–895, 2000. (Comment: Am J Psychiatry 157:851–853, 2000.)

49. Nielsen S, Palmer B: Diagnosing eating disorders: AN, BN and the others. Acta Psychiatr Scand 108:161–162, 2003.

50. Laessle RG, Wittchen HU, Fichter MM, et al: The significance of subgroups of bulimia and anorexia nervosa: Lifetime frequency of psychiatric disorders. Int J Eat Disord 8:569–574, 1989.

51. Herzog DB, Keller MB, Sacks NR, et al: Psychiatric comorbidity in treatment-seeking anorexics and bulimics. J Am Acad Child Adolesc Psychiatry 31:810–818, 1992.

52. Braun DL, Sunday SR, Halmi KA: Psychiatric comorbidity in patients with eating disorders. Psychol Med 24:859–867, 1994.

53. Holderness CC, Brooks-Gunn J, Warren WP: Co-morbidity of eating disorders and substance abuse: Review of the literature. Int J Eat Disord 16:1–34, 1994.

54. Brewerton TD, Lydiard RB, Herzog DB, et al: Comorbidity of Axis I psychiatric diagnosis in bulimia nervosa. J Clin Psychiatry 56:77–80, 1995.

55. Pollice C, Kaye WH, Greeno CG, et al: Relationship of depression, anxiety, and obsessionality to state of illness in anorexia nervosa. Int J Eat Disord 21:367–376, 1997.

56. Godart NT, Flament MF, Curt F, et al: Anxiety disorders in subjects seeking treatment for eating disorders: A DSM-IV controlled study. Psychiatry Res 117:245–258, 2003.

57. Halmi KA, Sunday SR, Klump KL, et al: Obsessions and compulsions in anorexia nervosa subtypes. Intl J Eating Disord 33:308–319, 2003.

58. Bastiani AM, Altemus M, Pigott TA, et al: Comparison of obsessions and compulsions in patients with anorexia nervosa and obsessive compulsive disorder. Biol Psychiatry 39:966, 1996.

59. Matsunaga H, Kiriike N, Iwasaki Y, et al: Clinical characteristics in patients with anorexia nervosa and obsessive-compulsive disorder. Psychol Med 29:407–414, 1999.

60. Srinivasagam NM, Plotnicov KH, Greeno C, et al: Persistent perfectionism, symmetry, and exactness in anorexia nervosa after long-term recovery. Am J Psychiatry 152:1630–1634, 1995.

61. Kaye WH, Greeno CG, Moss H, et al: Alterations in serotonin activity and psychiatric symptomatology after recovery from bulimia nervosa. Arch Gen Psychiatry 55:927–935, 1998.

62. Anderluh MB, Tchanturia K, Rabe-Hesketh S, et al: Childhood obsessive-compulsive personality traits in adult women with eating disorders: Defining a broader eating disorder phenotype. Am J Psychiatry 160:242–247, 2003.

63. Leckman JF, Grice DE, Boardman J, et al: Symptoms of obsessive-compulsive disorder. Am J Psychiatry 154:911–917, 1997.

64. Ward A, Tiller J, Treasure J, et al: Eating disorders: Psyche or soma? Int J Eating Disord 27:279–287, 2000.

65. Klump KL, Kaye WH, Strober M: The evolving genetic foundations of eating disorders. Psychiatr Clin North Am 24:215–225, 2001.

66. Tozzi F, Bulik CM: Candidate genes in eating disorders. Curr Drug Targets CNS Neurol Disord 2:31–39, 2003.

67. Stein D, Lilenfeld LR, Plotnicov K, et al: Familial aggregation of eating disorders: Results from a controlled family study of bulimia nervosa. Int J Eat Disord 26:211–215, 1999.

68. Strober M, Freeman R, Lampert C, et al: Controlled family study of anorexia nervosa and bulimia nervosa: Evidence of shared liability and transmission of partial syndromes. Am J Psychiatry 157:393–401, 2000.

69. Strober M, Freeman R, Lampert C, et al: Males with anorexia nervosa: A controlled study of eating disorders in first-degree relatives. Int J Eat Disord 29:263–269, 2001.

70. Grice DE, Halmi KA, Fichter MM, et al: Evidence for a susceptibility gene for anorexia nervosa on chromosome 1. Am J Hum Genet 70:787–792, 2002.

71. Devlin B, Bacanu SA, Klump KL, et al: Linkage analysis of anorexia nervosa incorporating behavioral covariates. Hum Mol Genet 11:689–696, 2002.

72. Bulik CM, Devlin B, Bacanu SA, et al: Significant linkage on chromosome 10p in families with bulimia nervosa. Am J Hum Genet 72:200–207, 2003.

73. Bergen AW, Yeager M, Welch R, et al: Candidate gene analysis of the Price Foundation anorexia nervosa affected relative pair dataset. Curr Drug Targets CNS Neurol Disord 2:41–51, 2003.

74. Ramacciotti CE, Coli E, Paoli R, et al: Serotonergic activity measured by platelet [³H]paroxetine binding in patients with eating disorders. Psychiatry Res 118:33–38, 2003.

75. Comerci GD: Medical complications of anorexia nervosa and bulimia nervosa. Med Clin North Am 74:1293–1310, 1990.

76. Casper RC: Carbohydrate metabolism and its regulatory hormones in anorexia nervosa. Psychiatry Res 62:85–96, 1996.

77. Cook VJ, Coxson HO, Mason AG, et al: Bullae, bronchiectasis and nutritional emphysema in severe anorexia nervosa. Can Respir J 8:361–365, 2001.

78. Hadley SJ, Walsh BT: Gastrointestinal disturbances in anorexia nervosa and bulimia nervosa. Curr Drug Targets CNS Neurol Disord 2:1–9, 2003.

79. Katzman DK: Osteoporosis in anorexia nervosa: A brittle future? Curr Drug Targets CNS Neurol Disord 2:11–15, 2003.

80. Soyka LA, Misra M, Frenchman A, et al: Abnormal bone mineral accrual in adolescent girls with anorexia nervosa. J Clin Endocrinol Metab 87:4177–4185, 2002.

81. Kerem NC, Katzman DK: Brain structure and function in adolescents with anorexia nervosa. Adolesc Med 14:109–118, 2003.

82. Barbarich NC, Kaye WH, Jimerson D: Neurotransmitter and imaging studies in anorexia nervosa: New targets for treatment. Curr Drug Targets CNS Neurol Disord 2:61–72, 2003.

83. Herholz K: Neuroimaging in anorexia nervosa. Psychiatry Res 62:105–110, 1996.

84. Swayze VW, Andersen A, Arndt S, et al: Reversibility of brain tissue loss in anorexia nervosa assessed with a computerized Talairach 3-D proportional grid. Psychol Med 26:381–390, 1996.

85. Addolorato G, Taranto C, Capristo E, et al: A case of marked cerebellar atrophy in a woman with anorexia nervosa and cerebral atrophy and a review of the literature. Int J Eat Disord 24:443–447, 1998.

86. Hendren RL, De Backer I, Pandina GJ: Review of neuroimaging studies of child and adolescent psychiatric disorders from the past 10 years. J Am Acad Child Adolesc Psychiatry 39:815–828, 2000.

87. Neumarker KJ, Bzufka WM, Dudek U, et al: Are there specific disabilities of number processing in adolescent patients with anorexia nervosa?: Evidence from clinical and neuropsychological data when compared to morphometric measures from magnetic resonance imaging. Eur Child Adolesc Psychiatry 9(Suppl 2):II111–II121, 2000.

88. Drevelengas A, Chourmouzi D, Pitsavas G, et al: Reversible brain atrophy and subcortical high signal on MRI in a patient with anorexia nervosa. Neuroradiology 43:838–840, 2001.

89. Amann B, Schafer M, Arnold S, et al: Central pontine myelinolysis in a patient with anorexia nervosa. Int J Eat Disord 30:462–466, 2001.

90. Demaerel P, Dekimpe P, Muls E, et al: MRI demonstration of orbital lipolysis in anorexia nervosa. Eur Radiol 12(Suppl 3):S4–S6, 2002.

91. Schlemmer H-P, Möckel R, Marcus A, et al: Proton magnetic resonance spectroscopy in acute, juvenile anorexia nervosa. Psychiatry Res 82:171–179, 1998.

92. Roser W, Bubl R, Buergin D, et al: Metabolic changes in the brain of patients with anorexia and bulimia nervosa as detected by proton magnetic resonance spectroscopy. Int J Eat Disord 26:119–136, 1999.

93. Kato T, Shioiri T, Murashita J, et al: Phosphorus-31 magnetic resonance spectroscopic observations in 4 cases with anorexia nervosa. Prog Neuropsychopharmacol Biol Psychiatry 21:719–724, 1997.

94. Rzanny R, Freesmeyer D, Reichenbach JR, et al: ³¹P-MR spectroscopy of the brain in patients with anorexia nervosa: Characteristic differences in the spectra between patients and healthy control subjects. Rofo Fortschr Geb Rontgenstr Neuen Bildgeb Verfahr 175:75–82, 2003.

95. Kuruoglu AC, Kapucu O, Atasever T, et al: Technitium-99m-HMPAO brain SPECT in anorexia nervosa. J Nucl Med 39:304–306, 1998.

96. Ellison Z, Foong J, Howard R, et al: Functional anatomy of calorie fear in anorexia nervosa. Lancet 352:1192, 1998.

97. Uher R, Brammer MJ, Murphy T: Recovery and chronicity in anorexia nervosa: Brain activity associated with differential outcomes. Biol Psychiatry 54:934–942, 2003.

98. Audenaert K, Van Laere K, Dumont F, et al: Decreased 5-HT2a receptor binding in patients with anorexia nervosa. J Nucl Med 44:163–169, 2003.

99. Frank GK, Kaye WH, Meltzer CC, et al: Reduced 5-HT2A receptor binding after recovery from anorexia nervosa. Biol Psychiatry 52:896–906, 2002.

100. Kaye WH, Frank GK, Meltzer CC, et al: Altered serotonin 2A receptor activity in women who have recovered from bulimia nervosa. Am J Psychiatry 158:1152–1155, 2001.

101. Pirke KM, Pahl J, Schweiger U: Metabolic and endocrine indices of starvation in bulimia: A comparison with anorexia nervosa. Psychiatry Res 15:33–39, 1985.

102. Vande Wiele RI: Anorexia nervosa and the hypothalamus. Hosp Pract 12:45–51, 1977.

103. Ferrari E, Brambilla F (eds): Disorders of Eating Behavior: A Psychoneuroendocrine Approach. Oxford, England, Pergamon Press, 1986.

104. Newman MM, Halmi KA: The endocrinology of anorexia nervosa and bulimia nervosa. Neurol Clin North Am 6:195–212, 1988.

105. Fichter MM, Pirke KM: Starvation models and eating disorders. In Szmukler G, Dare C, Treasure J (eds): Handbook of Eating Disorders: Theory, Treatment and Research. West Sussex, England, John Wiley & Sons, 1995, pp 83–107.

106. Licinio J, Wong ML, Gold PW: The hypothalamic-pituitary-adrenal axis in anorexia nervosa. Psychiatry Res 62:75–83, 1996.

107. Kaye WH, Gendall K, Kye C: The role of the central nervous system in the psychoneuroendocrine disturbances of anorexia and bulimia nervosa. Psychiatr Clin North Am 21:381–396, 1998.

108. Tomova A, Kumanov P, Kirilov G: Factors related to sex hormone binding globulin concentrations in women with anorexia nervosa. Horm Metab Res 27:508–510, 1995.

109. Fichter MM, Pirke KM, Pollinger J, et al: Disturbances in the hypothalamo-pituitary-adrenal and other neuroendocrine axes in bulimia. Biol Psychiatry 27:1021–1037, 1990.

110. Kaye WH: Neuropeptide abnormalities in anorexia nervosa. Psychiatry Res 62:65–74, 1996.

111. Rubin RT, Poland RE, Lesser IM, et al: Neuroendocrine aspects of primary endogenous depression: I. Cortisol secretory dynamics in patients and matched control subjects. Arch Gen Psychiatry 44:329–336, 1987.

112. Rubin RT, Phillips JJ, McCracken JT, et al: Adrenal gland volume in major depression: Relationship to basal and stimulated pituitary-adrenal cortical axis function. Biol Psychiatry 40:89–97, 1996.

113. Demitrack MA, Kalogeras KT, Altemus M, et al: Plasma and cerebrospinal fluid measures of arginine vasopressin secretion in patients with bulimia nervosa and in subjects. J Clin Endocrinol Metab 74:1277–1283, 1992.

114. Antoni FA: Vasopressinergic control of pituitary adrenocorticotropin secretion comes of age. Front Neuroendocrinol 14:76–122, 1993.

115. Scott LV, Dinan TG: Vasopressin and the regulation of hypothalamic-pituitary-adrenal axis function: Implications for the pathophysiology of depression. Life Sci 62:1985–1998, 1998.

116. De Kloet ER: Why dexamethasone poorly penetrates in brain. Stress 2:13–20, 1997.

117. Monteleone P, Luisi M, Colurcio B, et al: Plasma levels of neuroactive steroids are increased in untreated women with anorexia nervosa or bulimia nervosa. Psychosom Med 63:62–68, 2001.

118. Wartofsky L, Burman KD: Alterations in thyroid function in patients with systemic illness: The "euthyroid sick syndrome." Endocr Rev 3:164–217, 1982.

119. Natori Y, Yamaguchi N, Koike S, et al: Thyroid function in patients with anorexia nervosa and depression. Rinsho Byori 42:1268–1272, 1994.

120. Altemus M, Hetherington M, Kennedy B, et al: Thyroid function in bulimia nervosa. Psychoneuroendocrinology 21:249–261, 1996.

121. Lesem MD, Kaye WH, Bissette G, et al: Cerebrospinal fluid TRH immunoreactivity in anorexia nervosa. Biol Psychiatry 35:48–53, 1994.

122. Devlin MJ, Walsh BT, Kral JG, et al: Metabolic abnormalities in bulimia nervosa. Arch Gen Psychiatry 47:144–148, 1990.

123. Altemus M, Hetherington MM, Flood M, et al: Decrease in resting metabolic rate during abstinence from bulimic behavior. Am J Psychiatry 148:1071–1072, 1991.

124. Spalter AR, Gwirtsman HE, Demitrack MA, et al: Thyroid function in bulimia nervosa. Biol Psychiatry 33:408–414, 1993.

125. Scacchi M, Pincelli AI, Cavagnini F: Nutritional status in the neuroendocrine control of growth hormone secretion: The model of anorexia nervosa. Front Neuroendocrinol 24:200–204.

126. Hadigan CM, Walsh BT, Buttinger C, et al: Behavioral and neuroendocrine responses to metaCPP in anorexia nervosa. Biol Psychiatry 37:504–511, 1995.

127. Brewerton TD, Jimerson CD: Studies of serotonin function in anorexia nervosa. Psychiatry Res 62:31–42, 1996.

128. Goldbloom DS, Garfinkel PE, Katz R, et al: The hormonal response to intravenous 5-hydroxytryptophan in bulimia nervosa. J Psychosom Res 40:289–297, 1996.

129. Jimerson DC, Wolfe BE, Metzger ED, et al: Decreased serotonin function in bulimia nervosa. Arch Gen Psychiatry 54:529–534, 1997.

130. Levitan RD, Kaplan AS, Joffe RT, et al: Hormonal and subjective responses to intravenous meta-chlorophenylpiperazine in bulimia nervosa. Arch Gen Psychiatry 54:521–527, 1997.

131. Wolfe BE, Metzger ED, Jimerson DC: Research update on serotonin function in bulimia nervosa and anorexia nervosa. Psychopharm Bull 33:345–354, 1997.

132. Mortola JF, Laughlin GA, Yen SS: Melatonin rhythms in women with anorexia nervosa and bulimia nervosa. J Clin Endocrinol Metab 77:1540–1544, 1993.

133. Kennedy SH: Melatonin disturbances in anorexia nervosa and bulimia nervosa. Int J Eat Disord 16:257–265, 1994.

134. Hoffmann G, Pollow K, Nowara D, et al: Circadian blood serotonin and melatonin level in anorexia nervosa patients in comparison with normally menstruating women. Geburtshilfe Frauenheilkd 56:485–490, 1996.

135. Pirke KM, Schweiger U, Lemmel W, et al: The influence of dieting on the menstrual cycle of healthy young women. J Clin Endocrinol Metab 60:1174–1179, 1985.

136. Fichter MM, Pirke KM, Holsboer F: Weight loss causes neuroendocrine disturbances: Experimental studies in healthy starving subjects. Psychiatry Res 17:61–72, 1986.

137. Keys A, Brozek J, Henschel A: The Biology of Human Starvation. Minneapolis, University of Minnesota Press, 1950.

138. Turtzo LC, Lane MD: Completing the loop: Neuron-adipocyte interactions and the control of energy homeostasis. Horm Metab Res 34:607–615, 2002.

139. Kalra SP, Dube MG, Pu S, et al: Interacting appetite-regulating pathways in the hypothalamic regulation of body weight. Endocr Rev 20:68–100, 1999.

140. Piroli GG: Regulation of food intake: an 'old' actor plays a 'new' role. Mol Psychiatry 8:364–365, 2003.

141. Luckman SM, Lawrence CB: Anorectic brainstem peptides: More pieces to the puzzle. Trends Endocr Metab 14:60–65, 2003.

142. Taylor MM, Samson WK: The other side of the orexins: Endocrine and metabolic actions. Am J Physiol Endocrinol Metab 284:E13–E17, 2003.

143. Martin JB, Reichlin S: Clinical Endocrinology, 2d ed. Philadelphia, FA Davis, 1987, pp 557–605.

144. Batterham RL, Bloom SR: The gut hormone peptide YY regulates appetite. Ann N Y Acad Sci 994:162–168, 2003.

145. Morley JE, Levine AS, Grace M, et al: Peptide YY (PYY), a potent orexigenic agent. Brain Res 341:200–203, 1985.

146. Zigman JM, Elmquist JK: Minireview: from anorexia to obesity: The yin and yang of body weight control. Endocrinology 144:3749–3756, 2003.

147. Broglio F, Gottero C, Arvat E, et al: Endocrine and non-endocrine actions of ghrelin. Horm Res 59:109–117, 2003.

148. De Ambrogi M, Volpe S, Tamanini C: Ghrelin: Central and peripheral effects of a novel peptidyl hormone. Med Sci Monit 9:RA217–RA224, 2003. http://www.MedSciMonit.com/pub/vol_9/no_9/3633.pdf

149. Bailer UF, Kaye WH: A review of neuropeptide and neuroendocrine dysregulation in anorexia and bulimia nervosa. Curr Drug Targets CNS Neurol Disord 2:53–59, 2003.

150. Tolle V, Kadem M, Bluet-Pajot M-T, et al: Balance in ghrelin and leptin plasma levels in anorexia nervosa patients and constitutionally thin women. J Clin Endocrinol Metab 88:109–116, 2003.

151. Tanaka M, Naruo T, Yasuhara D, et al: Fasting plasma ghrelin levels in subtypes of anorexia nervosa. Psychoneuroendocrinology 28:829–835, 2003.

152. Nakai Y, Hosoda H, Nin K, et al: Plasma levels of active form of ghrelin during oral glucose tolerance test in patients with anorexia nervosa. Eur J Endocrinol 149:R1–R3, 2003.

153. Nedvídková J, Krykorková I, Barták V, et al: Loss of meal-induced decrease in plasma ghrelin levels in patients with anorexia nervosa. J Clin Endocrinol Metab 88:1678–1682, 2003.

154. Elmquist JK, Maratos–Flier E, Saper CB, et al: Unraveling the central nervous system pathways underlying leptin. Nat Neurosci 1:445–450, 1998.

155. Baratta M: Leptin: From a signal of adiposity to a hormonal mediator in peripheral tissues. Med Sci Monit 8:RA282–RA292, 2002. http://www.MedSciMonit.com/pub/vol_8/no_12/2990.pdf

156. Considine RV, Sinha M, Heiman ML, et al: Serum immunoreactive-leptin concentrations in normal-weight and obese humans. N Engl J Med 334:292–295, 1996.

157. Hamann A, Matthaei S: Regulation of energy balance by leptin. Exp Clin Endocrinol Diabetes 104:293–300, 1996.

158. Brichard SM, Delporte ML, Lambert M: Adipocytokines in anorexia nervosa: A review focusing on leptin and adiponectin. Horm Metab Res 35:337–342, 2003.

159. Holtkamp K, Herpertz-Dehlman B, Mika C, et al: Elevated physical activity and low leptin levels co-occur in patients with anorexia nervosa. J Clin Endocrinol Metab 88:5169–5174, 2003.

160. Holtkamp K, Hebebrand J, Mika C, et al: The effect of therapeutically induced weight gain on plasma leptin levels in patients with anorexia nervosa. J Psychiatr Res 37:165–169, 2003.

161. Lob S, Pickel J, Bidlingmaier M, et al: Serum leptin monitoring in anorectic patients during refeeding therapy. Exp Clin Endocrinol Diabetes 111:278–282, 2003.

162. Steiner J, LaPaglia N, Kirsteins L, et al: The response of the hypothalamic-pituitary-gonadal axis to fasting is modulated by leptin. Endocr Res 29:107–117, 2003.

163. Harris RBS, Ramsay TG, Smith SR, et al: Early and late stimulation of ob mRNA expression in meal-fed and overfed rats. J Clin Invest 97:2020–2026, 1996.

164. Boden G, Chen X, Mazzoli M, et al: Effect of fasting on serum leptin in normal subjects. J Clin Endocrinol Metab 81:3419–3423, 1996.

165. Ahima RS, Prabakaran D, Mantzoros C, et al: Role of leptin in the neuroendocrine response to fasting. Nature 382:250–252, 1996.

166. Inui A: Feeding and body-weight regulation by hypothalamic neuropeptides-mediation of the actions of leptin. Trends Neurosci 22:62–67, 1999.

167. Stefan N, Stumvoll M: Adiponectin: Its role in metabolism and beyond. Horm Metab Res 34:469–474, 2002.

168. Rajala MW, Scherer PE: Minireview: The adipocyte: At the crossroads of energy homeostasis, inflammation, and atherosclerosis. Endocrinology 144:3765–3773, 2003.

169. Beltowski J: Adiponectin and resistin: New hormones of white adipose tissue. Med Sci Monit 9:RA55–RA61, 2003. http://www.MedSciMonit.com/pub/vol_9/no_2/2469.pdf

170. Gavrila A, Chan JL, Yiannakouris N, et al: Serum adiponectin levels are inversely associated with overall and central fat distribution but are not directly regulated by acute fasting or leptin administration in humans: cross-sectional and interventional studies. J Clin Endocrinol Metab 88:4823–4831, 2003.

171. Ott V, Fasshauer M, Dalski A, et al: Direct peripheral effects of ghrelin include suppression of adiponectin expression. Horm Metab Res 34:640–645, 2002.

172. Pannacciulli N, Vettor R, Milan G, et al: Anorexia nervosa is characterized by increased adiponectin plasma levels and reduced nonoxidative glucose metabolism. J Clin Endocrinol Metab 88:1748–1752, 2003.

173. Iwahashi H, Funahashi T, Kurokawa N, et al: Plasma adiponectin levels in women with anorexia nervosa. Horm Metab Res 35:537–540, 2003.

174. Monteleone P, Fabrazzo M, Martiadis V, et al: Opposite changes in circulating adiponectin in women with bulimia nervosa or binge eating disorder. J Clin Endocrinol Metab 88:5387–5391, 2003.

175. Adan RAH, Hillebrand JJG, de Rijke C, et al: Melanocortin system and eating disorders. Ann N Y Acad Sci 994:267–274, 2003.

176. Foster AC, Joppa M, Markison S, et al: Body weight regulation by selective MC4 receptor agonists and antagonists. Ann N Y Acad Sci 994:103–110, 2003.

177. Lu X-Y, Barsh GS, Akil H, Watson SJ: Interaction between α-melanocyte-stimulating hormone and corticotropin-releasing hormone in the regulation of feeding and hypothalamo-pituitary-adrenal responses. J Neurosci 23:7863–7872, 2003.

178. Masaki T, Yoshimichi G, Chiba S, et al: Corticotropin-releasing hormone-mediated pathway of leptin to regulate feeding, adiposity, and uncoupling protein expression in mice. Endocrinology 144:3547–3554, 2003.

179. Sawchenko P: Toward a new neurobiology of energy balance, appetite, and obesity: The anatomists weigh in. J Comp Neurol 402:435–441, 1998.

180. Heisler LK, Cowley MA, Kishi T, et al: Central serotonin and melanocortin pathways regulating energy homeostasis. Ann N Y Acad Sci 994:169–174, 2003.

181. Jonas JM, Gold MS: Treatment of antidepressant resistant bulimia with naltrexone. Int J Psychiatry Med 16:305–309, 1987.

182. Jonas JM, Gold MS: The use of opiate antagonists in treating bulimia: A study of low dose versus high dose naltrexone. Psychiatry Res 24:195–199, 1988.

183. Mitchell JE, Christenson G, Jennings J, et al: A placebo-controlled, double-blind crossover study of naltrexone hydrochloride in outpatients with normal weight bulimia. J Clin Psychopharmacol 9:94–97, 1989.

184. Agger SA, Schwalberg MD, Bigaouette JM, et al: Effect of a tricyclic antidepressant and opiate antagonist on binge eating behavior in normal weight bulimia and obese, binge-eating subjects. Am J Clin Nutr 53:865–871, 1991.

185. Marrazzi MA, Bacon JP, Kinzie J, et al: Naltrexone use in the treatment of anorexia nervosa and bulimia nervosa. Int Clin Psychopharmacol 10:163–172, 1995.

186. Nishita JK, Ellinwood EH Jr, Rockwell WJ, et al: Abnormalities in the response of plasma arginine vasopressin during hypertonic saline infusion in patients with eating disorders. Biol Psychiatry 26:73–86, 1989.

187. Frank GK, Kaye WH, Altemus M, et al: CSF oxytocin and vasopressin levels after recovery from bulimia nervosa and anorexia nervosa, bulimic subtype. Biol Psychiatry 48:315–318, 2000.

188. Nakazato M, Hashimoto K, Shimizu E, et al: Decreased levels of serum brain-derived neurotrophic factor in female patients with eating disorders. Biol Psychiatry 54:485–490, 2003.

189. Ratnasuriya RH, Eisler I, Szmuckler GI, et al: Anorexia nervosa: Outcome and prognostic factors after 20 years. Br J Psychiatry 158:495–502, 1991.

190. Walsh BT, Devlin MJ: Psychopharmacology of anorexia nervosa, bulimia nervosa, and binge eating. In Bloom FE, Kupfer DJ (eds): Psychopharmacology: The Fourth Generation of Progress. New York, Raven Press, 1995, pp 1581–1589.

191. Garner DM, Garfinkel PE (eds): Handbook of Treatment for Eating Disorders, 2d ed. New York, Guilford Press, 1997.

192. Anonymous: Practice guideline for the treatment of patients with eating disorders (revision). Am J Psychiatry 157(Suppl):1–39, 2000.

193. Agras WS: Nonpharmacologic treatments of bulimia nervosa. J Clin Psychiatry 52(Suppl):29–33, 1991.

194. Mitchell JE, Raymond N, Specker S: A review of the controlled trials of pharmacotherapy and psychotherapy in the treatment of bulimia nervosa. Int J Eat Disord 14:229–247, 1993.

195. Wilson GT, Fairburn CG: Cognitive treatments for eating disorders. J Consult Clin Psychol 61:261–269, 1993.

196. Kaye W, Strober M, Stein D, et al: New directions in treatment research of anorexia nervosa and bulimia nervosa. Biol Psychiatry 45:1285–1292, 1999.

197. Lilenfeld LR, Kaye WH, Greeno CG, et al: A controlled family study of anorexia nervosa and bulimia nervosa: Psychiatric disorders in first-degree relatives and effects of proband comorbidity. Arch Gen Psychiatry 55:603–610, 1998.

198. Channon S, de Silva P, Hemsley D, et al: A controlled trial of cognitive-behavioural and behavioural treatment of anorexia nervosa. Behav Res Ther 27:529–535, 1989.

199. Crisp AH, Norton K, Gowers S, et al: A controlled study of the effect of therapies aimed at adolescent and family psychopathology in anorexia nervosa. Br J Psychiatry 159:325–333, 1991.

200. Treasure J, Todd G, Brolly M, et al: A pilot study of a randomized trial of cognitive analytical therapy vs. educational behavioral therapy for

adult anorexia nervosa. Behav Res Ther 33:363–367, 1995.

201. Pike KM, Walsh BT, Vitousek K, et al: Cognitive behavior therapy in the posthospitalization treatment of anorexia nervosa. Am J Psychiatry 160:2046–2049, 2003.

202. Ramsay R, Ward A, Treasure J, Russell GF: Compulsory treatment in anorexia nervosa. Short-term benefits and long-term mortality. Br J Psychiatry 175:147–153, 1999.

203. Watson TL, Bowers WA, Anderson AE: Involuntary treatment of eating disorders. Am J Psychiatry 157:1806–1810, 2000.

204. McCallum KE, Bruton JR: The continuum of care in the treatment of eating disorders. Primary Psychiatry 10:48–54, 2003.

205. Kaye W, Gendall K, Strober M: Nutrition, serotonin and behavior in anorexia and bulimia nervosa. In Fernstrom JD, Uany R, Arroyo P (eds): Nestlé Nutrition Workshop Series Clinical and Performance Program, Vol 5. Vevey/S. Karger, Basel, 2001, pp 153–168.

206. Ferguson CP, La Via MC, Crossan PJ, et al: Are serotonin selective reuptake inhibitors effective in underweight anorexia nervosa? Int J Eat Disord 25:11–17, 1999.

207. Malina A, Gaskill J, McConaha C: Olanzapine treatment of anorexia

nervosa: A retrospective study. Int J Eat Disord 33:234–237, 2003.

208. Ward A, Campbell IC, Brown N, Treasure J: Anorexia nervosa subtypes: Differences in recovery. J Nerv Ment Dis 191:197–201, 2003.

209. Gordon CM, Grace E, Emans SJ, et al: Effects of oral dehydroepiandrosterone on bone density in young women with anorexia nervosa: A randomized trial. J Clin Endocrinol Metab 87:4935–4941, 2002.

210. Hsu LK, Rand W, Sullivan S, et al: Cognitive therapy, nutritional therapy and their combination in the treatment of bulimia nervosa. Psychol Med 31:871–879, 2001.

211. Mehler PS: Bulimia nervosa. N Engl J Med 349:875–881, 2003.

212. Lilly RZ: Bulimia nervosa. Br Med J 327:380–383, 2003.

213. Fairburn CG, Jones R, Peveler RC, et al: Psychotherapy and bulimia nervosa: The longer-term effects of interpersonal psychotherapy, behavior therapy and cognitive-behavior therapy. Arch Gen Psychiatry 50:419–428, 1993.

214. Gendall KA, Joyce PR, Carter FA, et al: Thyroid indices and treatment outcome in bulimia nervosa. Acta Psychiatr Scand 108:190–195, 2003.

215. Carter WP, Pindyck LJ: Pharmacologic treatment of binge-eating disorder.

Primary Psychiatry 10:31–36, 2003.

216. McElroy SL, Arnold LM, Shapira NA, et al: Topiramate in the treatment of binge eating disorder associated with obesity: a randomized, placebo-controlled trial. Am J Psychiatry 160:255–261, 2003.

217. Appolinario JC, Bacaltchuk J, Sichieri R, et al: A randomized, double-blind placebo-controlled study of sibutramine in the treatment of binge-eating disorder. Arch Gen Psychiatry 60:1109–1116, 2003.

218. Gorwood P, Kipman A, Foulon C: The human genetics of anorexia nervosa. Eur J Pharmacol 480:163–170, 2003.

219. Södersten P, Bergh C, Ammar A: Anorexia nervosa: Towards a neurobiologically based therapy. Eur J Pharmacol 480:67–74, 2003.

220. Holtkamp K, Hebebrand J, Mika C, et al: High serum leptin levels subsequent to weight gain predict renewed weight loss in patients with anorexia nervosa. Psychoendocrinology 29:791–797, 2004.

221. Vander Lely AJ, Tschöp M, Heiman ML, et al: Biological, physiological, pathophysiological, and pharmacological aspects of ghrelin. Endocr Rev 25:426–457, 2004.

Starvation and Parenteral Nutrition

David Heber

Our ability to adapt to starvation is critical to survival, and recent research on the regulation of body weight and body fat has revealed that humans' adaptation to starvation is far better developed than our adaptation to overnutrition.[1] There is significant redundancy in the various pathways that regulate body fat and body weight under conditions of reduced calorie intake, and there is a significant degree of interplay of the endocrine system and major metabolic pathways.[2] Different endocrine glands, central nervous system signals, and signals from the gastrointestinal tract work synergistically in this process.[3] The fat cell secretes hormones and cytokines that are active in immune function, blood clotting, and the adaptation to starvation. Understanding these interrelationships provides a basis for the recognition and therapy of primary and secondary forms of malnutrition.[4,5] The discovery and application of well-defined parenteral and enteral nutrition since the 1970s rationalized the metabolic and hormonal treatment of malnutrition.[6,7] Nutritional therapy has been shown to be essential to survival in the critical care setting and has resulted in metabolic and nutritional insights that have influenced many areas of endocrinology.[8] New clinical observations in acquired immunodeficiency syndrome (AIDS) and cancer patients have emphasized the importance of adjunctive nutritional therapy in these conditions. This chapter will attempt to provide an integrated view of the neuropeptidergic, endocrine, and metabolic responses to starvation and the treatment of malnutrition using parenteral and enteral nutrition.

ADAPTATION TO UNCOMPLICATED STARVATION

The human adaptation to starvation consists of a series of well-coordinated hormonal and metabolic changes. Aspects of these adaptive mechanisms are utilized each day in well-nourished individuals between bedtime and breakfast to maintain normal blood sugar levels in the absence of food intake. The changes in hormones and metabolites that occur during this interval are similar to those seen in the earliest stages of the adaptation to starvation. If fasting is continued for up to 6 weeks, a series of adaptations occurs to maintain the integrity of body protein stores, which are essential to survival. Ironically, the bulk of the information that is available on the physiology of the adaptation to uncomplicated starvation has been developed in studies of massively obese subjects who fast voluntarily under metabolic ward conditions.[9–11]

DIETARY SOURCES AND BODY STORES OF ENERGY

The average distribution of dietary macronutrients in the plant-based diet on which humans evolved is far different from that in modern diets influenced by food production methods.[12] Throughout the world today, there has been a conversion of plant-based diets that are low in fat, high in fiber, and rich in colorful fruits and vegetables to diets that are high in fat, low in fiber, with reduced intake of fruits and vegetables. In countries where a low-fat, high-fiber diet is consumed, complex carbohydrates are obtained from cereals, grains, fruits, and vegetables; in industrialized countries where a high-fat, low-fiber diet is consumed, simple sugars from processed foods will compose a large portion of the carbohydrates that are consumed. It is a hallmark of humans that they can adapt to a wide variation in dietary macronutrient profiles as long as essential requirements are met at least over the short term. Long-term consequences of the modern industrialized diet are seen in an increased incidence of age-related chronic diseases, including diabetes, heart disease, and common forms of cancer.

Despite wide variations in the dietary intake of macronutrients among various populations, the body stores these dietary macronutrients in a fairly uniform but different pattern from that of the ingested proportions. The distribution of stored calories is ideally adapted to the metabolic needs under conditions of stress and starvation.

In the average 70-kg man, the largest store of calories is in the form of fat in adipose tissue, with approximately 135,000 calories stored in 13.5 kg of adipose tissue. This storage compartment can be greatly expanded with long-term overnutrition in obese individuals. Approximately 54,000 calories are stored as protein in both muscle and viscera. Only half of these calories can be mobilized for energy, since depletion below 50% of total protein stores is incompatible with life.[13] In addition to being an energy source, protein plays a functional role in many organs, including the liver, and depletion is associated with impaired immunity to infection.[14] In fact, the most common cause of death in an epidemic of starvation is typically simple bacterial pneumonia. Conservation of protein is an adaptation that is tightly linked to survival during acute starvation.

Only 1200 calories are stored as carbohydrate in liver and muscle glycogen. There are clear adaptive advantages to storing calories as fat, since fat can provide more energy per gram than carbohydrate or protein can. However, since carbohydrate stores are so small, they are depleted in 3 days of uncomplicated starvation or sooner under conditions of increased energy expenditure. This dependence on fat and protein stores in starvation requires metabolic adaptations to minimize the loss of protein stores and shift to metabolic pathways that predominantly utilize the large fat stores that are available (Fig. 46-1).

METABOLIC REQUIREMENTS OF THE STARVED HOST

The postabsorptive period is defined as 8 to 16 hours after eating and has been defined operationally as the timepoint after an overnight fast when a number of hormonal determinations can be made under standard conditions. It can be thought of as a period of very early adaptation to starvation. During this period, the primary metabolic priority is the provision of adequate glucose for essential functions of the brain, red blood cells, peripheral nerves, and renal medulla.

During this postabsorptive phase, insulin levels fall as blood glucose falls from a range of 4 to 5 mmol/L to 3 to 4 mmol/L.[9] Glucose is released from the liver into the circulation via glycogenolysis of stores accumulated after feeding under the influence of insulin. The fall in glucose level is associated with depletion of glycogen stores. Skeletal muscle does not release glucose from stored glycogen directly into the circulation because myocytes lack the enzyme glucose-6-phosphatase.

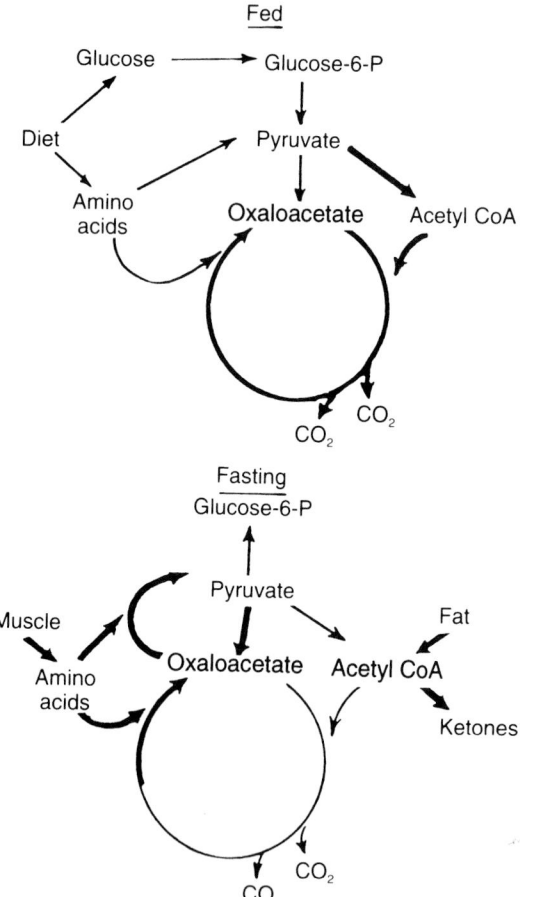

Figure 46-1   The flow of substrate during the fed and fasting states.

However, muscle releases lactate and amino acids such as alanine, which can enter the circulation and are converted to glucose in the liver via gluconeogenesis. Glucagon in the presence of lowered insulin concentrations promotes gluconeogenesis during the postabsorptive period.[15]

In addition, glucagon in the presence of lowered insulin levels promotes lipolysis. As the stored triglyceride in adipocytes is mobilized as free fatty acids, the tissues that do not require glucose as their primary fuel (e.g., skeletal muscle) begin to oxidize free fatty acids. These changes during the early postabsorptive period act to increase free fatty acid oxidation to spare protein breakdown. During the first few days of starvation, free fatty acid concentrations increase from a range of 0.5 to 0.8 mmol/L up to 1.2 to 1.6 mmol/L and plateau thereafter as starvation is prolonged.[9] These free fatty acids circulate bound to albumin and are oxidized in the liver to water-soluble ketone bodies, including acetoacetate and β-hydroxybutyrate. In obese subjects with more than adequate triglyceride stores, acetoacetate concentrations rise 25-fold and β-hydroxybutyrate concentrations rise 100-fold from the levels that are observed in the postabsorptive phase following 4 to 6 weeks of uncomplicated starvation (Fig. 46-2). These are the largest fluctuations seen in any circulating fuel with prolonged starvation.[16]

Protein synthesis and catabolism have been estimated to account for approximately 40% of resting energy expenditure. In addition, the changes in protein metabolism are critical to maintaining the body cell mass during starvation, which directly affects survival.[17] Plasma amino acids measured in venous blood give nonspecific indications of the adaptations that take place in protein metabolism during the course of starvation. In addition, the excretion of protein from the body as urinary urea nitrogen expressed as nitrogen balance provides further insights into overall protein nutriture (see Fig. 46-2).

The total α-amino nitrogen concentration, which reflects total amino acids, increases transiently from 4.6 to 4.8 mmol/L over the first few days of starvation and then decreases to 3.6 mmol/L.[18] These total amino acid changes obscure the changes in several different classes of amino acids. First, the branched-chain amino acids—leucine, isoleucine, and valine—increase transiently approximately twofold in the blood between 3 and 5 days after the onset of starvation. Alanine, which is the primary glucogenic amino acid in the liver during starvation, is released from muscle in amounts larger than the measurable alanine stores of muscle. This is explained by the formation of alanine in muscle through what is known as the *alanine cycle* (Fig. 46-3). Pyruvate from the liver as well as pyruvate derived by glycolysis of glucose from glycogen stores enters the muscle, where the branched amino acids donate an amino group via the action of a specific branched-chain amino acid–targeted enzyme to produce alanine. This alanine is then released to the liver, where alanine accounts for a significant portion of glucose synthesis. During the period between 3 and 5 days after the onset of starvation, the branched-chain amino acids in the circulation support an increased rate of gluconeogenesis until the full adaptation to a fat-fuel economy has progressed significantly. Second, blood and muscle alanine concentrations decline rapidly over the first 10 days of starvation and then continue to decrease progressively to about 30% of postabsorptive levels several weeks later. Third, blood and muscle glutamine concentrations also decrease progressively during starvation.

In the first few days of starvation, the gut plays an important role in regulating protein and amino acid metabolism. The intestinal synthesis of glutamine increases, with a subsequent increase in alanine and ammonia formation. The alanine is used for hepatic gluconeogenesis, while the increased ammonia levels in the portal circulation trigger the liver to produce glutamine, which is utilized by the kidney for

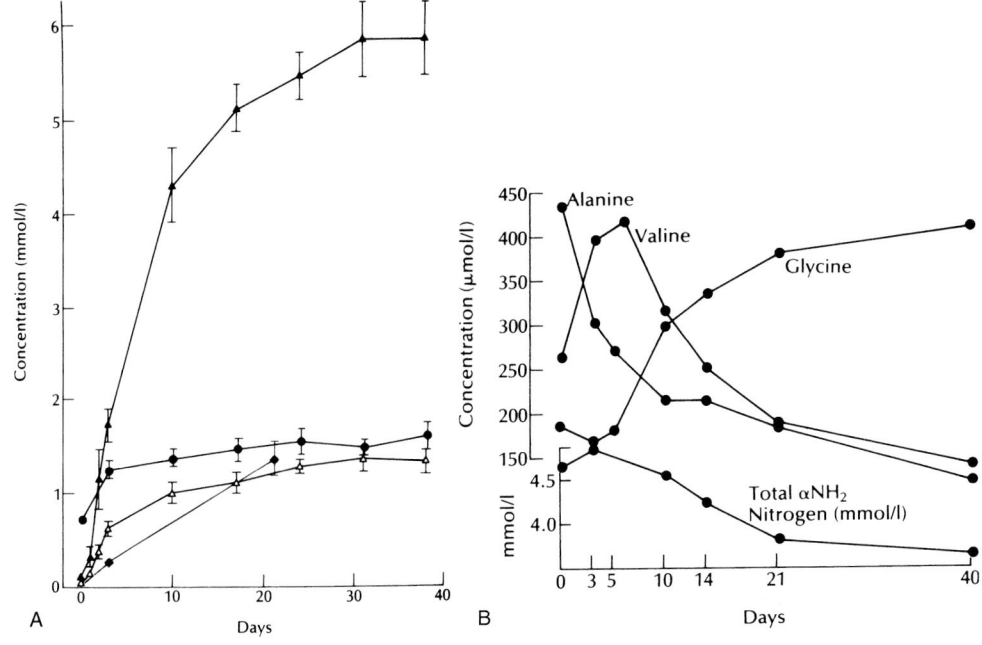

Figure 46-2 **A,** Blood 3-hydroxybutyrate (*solid triangles*) and acetoacetate (*open triangles*) and plasma acetone (*solid diamonds*) and free fatty acid (*solid circles*) concentrations during starvation. **B,** Total α-amino nitrogen and three representative amino acids during prolonged starvation. (Reproduced with permission from Cahill GF: Starvation in man. N Engl J Med 282:668–675, 1970.)

gluconeogenesis.[19] After 30 days of fasting, the kidney becomes an important gluconeogenic organ, contributing about half the body's glucose need. Most of this glucose is derived from the *glutamine cycle* (Fig. 46-4). Glutamine from the muscle and liver is converted to glutamate and ammonia in the kidney. Glutamate is then deaminated to α-ketoglutarate, which enters the gluconeogenic pathway.

The basic mechanisms underlying these adaptive changes in protein synthesis and degradation are still not completely understood. Proteolysis occurs in cellular lysosomes via autophagy. This process is stimulated by a shortage of critical regulatory amino acids, including phenylalanine, tryptophan, methionine, leucine, tyrosine, glutamic acid, proline, and histidine.[20] While not conclusively established, it appears that decreased concentrations of specific amino acyl transfer RNAs for these amino acids trigger proteolysis (Fig. 46-5). In terms of protein synthesis, there is a decrease in the amount and activity of RNA subunits involved in initiation, elongation, and termination of protein synthesis. Insulin is the primary hormone that is known to regulate protein metabolism.[21] Insulin deficiency leads to net protein breakdown, and hyperinsulinemia under euglycemic conditions inhibits proteolysis. There is also evidence that glucagon participates in this regulatory process by stimulating splanchnic proteolysis.[22] Plasma cortisol levels are increased for several hours and inhibit protein synthesis while increasing protein breakdown. Elevations in epinephrine, previously thought to increase

protein breakdown, lead to decreases in the rate of whole-body protein breakdown. Growth hormone (GH) has been shown to increase protein synthesis but to oppose insulin's antiproteolytic effects. The role of the insulin-like growth factors (IGF)-1 and IGF-2 as both endocrine and paracrine signals is important in the adaptation to starvation. The anabolic effects are mediated via the IGF-1 receptor, which is present in all cells except liver and adipose cells. IGF-1 expression is regulated both by nutrition and by other hormones. For examples, serum IGF-1 concentrations are age-dependent and closely linked to the age-dependent production of GH. IGF levels increase after puberty and decline with age in parallel with anabolic potential in response to nutrition. Recent studies have demonstrated that plasma amino acid levels and amino acid availability also play an important role in modulating the rate of protein breakdown.[23] The magnitude of these amino acid–mediated antiproteolytic effects was equivalent to that of insulin.

The impact of the adaptation to a fat-fuel economy is reflected in the rapid changes in urinary nitrogen excretion, showing net protein sparing through two processes. First, there is less protein breakdown. It has been estimated that protein synthesis decreases in the whole body by 40% between the postprandial and postabsorptive phases,[24] with a further decrease over the first several days of starvation. Second, there is increased reutilization of nitrogen, evidenced by decreased urea formation in the liver through the arginine-citrulline

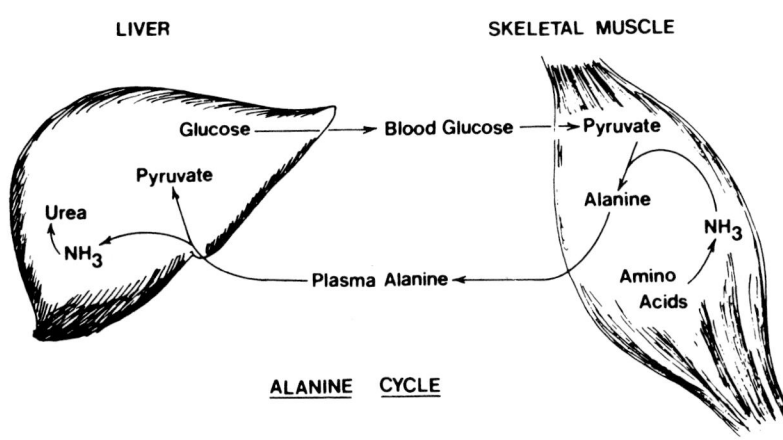

Figure 46-3 The alanine cycle allows carbon chains and ammonia to be shuttled from skeletal muscle to the liver, where they are used to synthesize glucose and urea, respectively.

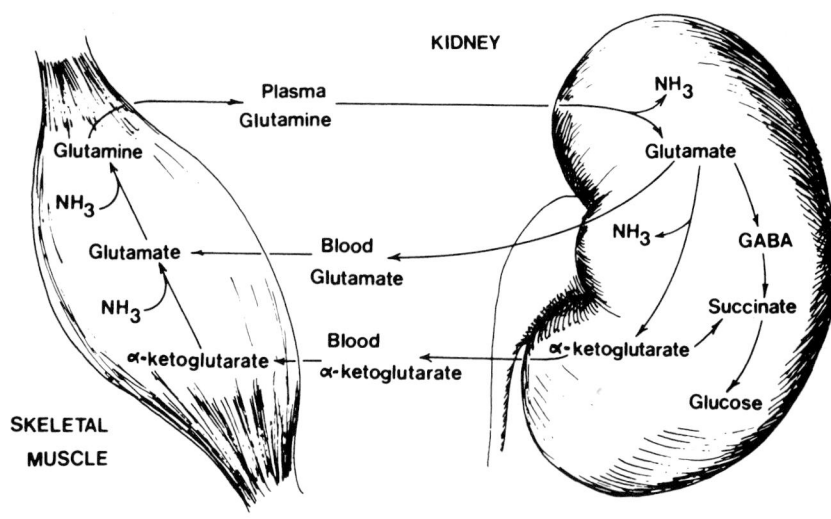

Figure 46-4 The glutamine cycle is a shuttle that is analogous to the alanine cycle that exists between skeletal muscle and the kidney. This cycle increases in importance as a fast extends beyond 30 days.

cycle. In obese subjects who fast for 7 days, protein breakdown and urinary urea nitrogen excretion decrease in parallel. Overall nitrogen is conserved, so nitrogen excretion decreases from 12 g/day in the postabsorptive state to 5 g/day 7 to 10 days later. This decrease translates into a decrease in muscle protein breakdown from 75 to 20 g/day. On the basis of theoretical calculations of the time necessary to reach the crucial 50% of body cell mass, survival is extended through these adaptations from approximately 60 days to over 260 days, provided that adequate fluid and electrolytes are administered.[24]

HORMONAL MEDIATORS OF METABOLIC ADAPTATION

As was discussed earlier, insulin is the primary hormone that regulates fuel metabolism in the fed and fasted states. However, a number of other hormones participate in the adaptation to uncomplicated starvation. One group of hormones is called *counterregulatory* in recognition of their ability to antagonize the hypoglycemic action of administered insulin. Glucagon, for example, promotes glycogenolysis, gluconeogenesis, ketogenesis, proteolysis, and lipolysis. The levels of circulating catecholamines, norepinephrine, and epinephrine, which rise following insulin-induced hypoglycemia, also increase following acute starvation.[25]

Lipolysis is central to the adaptation to starvation and is regulated by catecholamines, glucagon, and GH. Catecholamines help to inhibit insulin secretion, which permits lipolysis.[26] The lipolytic effects of epinephrine are more pronounced early in starvation, and the rise in catecholamines promotes the meta-

bolic utilization of fat. These hormones act through stimulatory and inhibitory G proteins and the cyclic adenosine monophosphate (cAMP) cascade to modulate hormone-sensitive lipase. β_1-Adrenergic stimulation increases glucagon secretion and inhibits muscle glucose metabolism.[27] β_1-Adrenergic stimulation mediates the effects of glucagon, GH, cortisol, and vasopressin to increase lipolysis.[22] Thyroid hormones and glucocorticoids may act permissively on the processes that stimulate lipolysis, while the actions of vasopressin, β-lipotropin, β-endorphin, and D-melanocyte-stimulating hormone have not been established.

New insights into the complex regulation of food intake, metabolism, and energy homeostasis have refined our understanding of the pathophysiology of malnutrition. Studies in rodents have demonstrated that the adaptation to starvation is far better developed than the adaptation to overnutrition in both the short term and the long term.

Long-term signals associated with body fat stores are provided by leptin and insulin.[28] The concentration of leptin in the blood is highly correlated with total fat mass. Excess body fat results in increased leptin production from fat cells, while decreases in body fat that occur with dieting cause leptin and insulin concentrations to decrease, triggering responses that aim to conserve body fat. These circulating hormones also modulate short-term signals that determine meal initiation and termination. Signals that provide short-term information about hunger and satiety include gut hormones such as cholecystokinin, ghrelin, and peptide YY_{3-36}. Vagal afferent nerves within the gastrointestinal tract also provide short-term

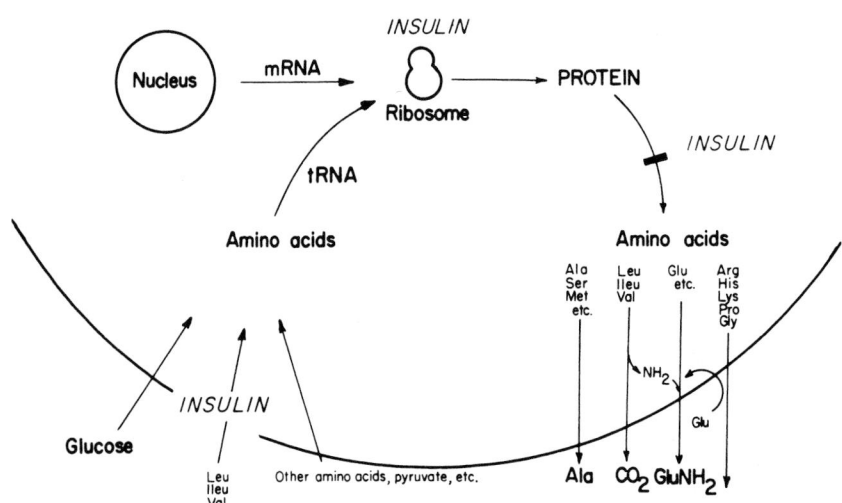

Figure 46-5 Effect of insulin in promoting glucose and amino acid uptake into muscle, activation of protein synthesis at the ribosome, and inhibition of proteolysis. Also shown is the predominant release of alanine (Ala) and glutamine ($GluNH_2$).

signals in response to distension, macronutrients, pH, tonicity, and hormones. The neural and hormonal signals are then integrated within specific regions of the hypothalamus and brain stem.[29]

Anorexigenic (appetite-suppressing) signals are generated by α-melanocyte-stimulating hormone, a peptide that is derived from pro-opiomelanocortin, which derives its name from its actions in skin pigmentation through interaction with the melanocortin 1 receptor.[30] This hormone reduces food intake and increases energy expenditure through the melanocortin 4 receptor in the hypothalamus. Deletion of the melanocortin 4 receptor gene in animals results in obesity, hyperphagia, and reduced energy expenditure. Deletion of the related melanocortin 3 receptor gene results in obesity due to reduced energy expenditure without hyperphagia.

Antagonism of anorexigenic melanocortin signals is caused by orexigenic (appetite-stimulating) peptides such as agouti-related protein (AgRP) and neuropeptide Y.[31] Agouti-related protein antagonizes the interaction between α-melanocyte-stimulating hormone and the melanocortin 4 receptor. Neuropeptide Y, found in the arcuate nucleus of the hypothalamus, is a member of the pancreatic polypeptide family and increases during food restriction, acting to increase food intake. Neuropeptide Y decreases expression of the gene that encodes pro-opiomelanocortin. Neuropeptide Y also decreases the synthesis of thyrotropin-releasing hormone and increases the synthesis of melanin-concentrating hormone, another orexigenic peptide.

Ghrelin is a 28-amino-acid, acetylated peptide secreted by oxyntic cells in the stomach fundus. Ghrelin is named for its ability to stimulate growth hormone secretagogue receptors to increase the release of growth hormone from the pituitary. Circulating levels of ghrelin increase before meals and decrease after eating.[32] Ghrelin increases food intake through the stimulation of ghrelin receptors on hypothalamic neuropeptide Y-expressing neurons and agouti-related protein-expressing neurons.

Peptide YY_{3-36} (PYY) is secreted after meals in proportion to the calories ingested by endocrine L cells lining the distal small bowel and colon.[33] The initial release of PYY after eating occurs through neural mechanisms before ingested nutrients arrive in the distal small intestine and colon. Subsequently, PYY is released in response to direct intestinal stimulation by nutrients, especially lipids and carbohydrates. PYY decreases food intake in both lean and obese individuals through inhibition of gut motility. This function is referred to as the "ileal brake" and results from the actions of vagal afferent neurons that ascend from the intestinal tract to the hindbrain and interact with humoral receptors in the hypothalamus.[34] PYY inhibits NPY-expressing neurons and AgRP-expressing neurons through inhibitory neuropeptide Y2 receptors. This results in disinhibition of neighboring pro-opiomelanocortin-expressing neurons, resulting in decreased food intake.

Following gastric bypass surgery for obesity, hunger diminishes, circulating concentrations of ghrelin decrease and circulating concentrations of PYY increase.[35] This suppression of hunger may contribute to long-term weight maintenance of reduced body weight in these patients.

Since ghrelin signals hunger and PYY signals satiety, some investigators have conducted studies in transgenic mice to examine whether these hormones can be manipulated to affect body composition. Experimental knockouts of the ghrelin gene, AgRP, and NPY gene and a double knockout of the AgRP and NPY genes are not associated with any obvious effects on food intake or energy metabolism. On the other hand, inactivating mutations of the genes encoding leptin or the leptin receptor and the melanocortin 4 receptor result in obese phenotypes. Consistent with the hypothesis that humans and mice are better adapted to starvation than to overnutrition, it is evident that the orexigenic peptides are so

critical to survival that the absence of one peptide is compensated for by the actions of others. However, the orexins also communicate widely throughout the brain, with such regions as those involved in satiety (brain stem) and sleep/wakefulness. Indeed, the orexin knockout mouse exhibits typical features of narcolepsy in addition to hypophagia. An important role of the orexins might be to integrate a variety of behaviors related to feeding or fasting, including emotional changes, reward responses, and sleep/alertness.

Insulin-like growth factor 1 (IGF-1)/somatomedin-C stimulates amino acid uptake and protein synthesis while inhibiting lipolysis.[36] IGF peptides in serum are associated with IGF-binding proteins (IGFBPs), a family of six polypeptides that are thought to modulate storage, transport, and action of the IGFs. As was noted above, IGF-1 secretion parallels GH secretion with age. During starvation, this linkage is broken. In the presence of elevated GH levels, IGF-1 levels remain low, and the concentration of IGF-1 inhibitors in the circulation is increased.[37]

Within 7 to 10 days of starvation, there is a marked adaptive decrease in energy expenditure. Normally, resting energy expenditure is proportional to lean body mass. However, after 7 to 10 days of starvation, there is a 20% decrease in resting energy expenditure, at a time when lean body mass has decreased by less than 5%.[38] Changes in the peripheral metabolism of thyroid hormones occur that may contribute significantly to the observed decrease in energy expenditure. Among these changes, there is less production of triiodothyronine (T_3), the most metabolically active thyroid hormone, via a decreased activity of 5'-monodeiodinase in the liver and other peripheral tissues.[39] There is a reciprocal rise in reverse T_3, an inactive metabolite, while thyroxine levels remain constant.[40] The overall decrease in energy expenditure with starvation is an adaptive change that results in a decreased rate of whole-body lipolysis, proteolysis, and gluconeogenesis (Fig. 46-6). Aerobic exercise in obese dieters does not reverse this adaptive change in energy regulation.[41]

There is a good correlation between the adaptive hormonal changes that occur during starvation (Table 46-1) and the decrease in whole-body protein breakdown that occurs as a result.[42]

ADAPTATION TO PROTEIN-ENERGY MALNUTRITION

Observations of epidemics of starvation in third world countries led to the classification and definition of two different pathophysiologic syndromes occurring in response to uncomplicated starvation as well as the undernutrition associated with illness.[43–46] These concepts, while useful as classifications, are oversimplified, and the entire spectrum of protein and energy malnutrition has been observed in malnourished children throughout the world. Infants and children under 5 years of age have the highest energy requirements per unit body weight of any age group. Since their visceral organs account for a good portion of total body weight, energy expenditures between 50 and 100 kcal/kg/day are commonly measured, compared with average energy expenditures of 20 to 30 kcal/kg/day in adults.[47] In fact, in epidemics of starvation, children will die first, men second, and women last, since women have the largest fat stores to allow protein sparing in the face of starvation.

CLINICAL SPECTRUM

Intrauterine undernutrition, prematurity, failure of lactation, and use of dilute formulas can lead to a wasting syndrome called *marasmus* that usually presents in the first 6 months of life.[48] The infant adapts to undernutrition by decreasing its linear growth rate and thereby decreasing energy requirements. If the condition persists, there is loss of muscle and fat

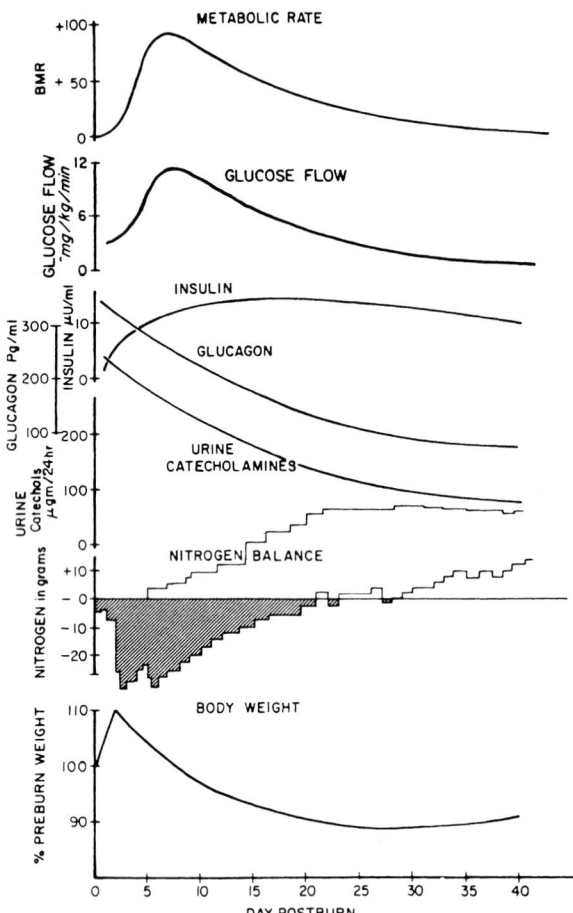

Figure 46-6 The hypermetabolism of injury during the flow phase is accompanied by increased glucagon and catecholamines relative to insulin. The hormonal mediators return to normal with recovery.

tissue. There are no signs of edema or biochemical abnormalities, and immune function is maintained in this condition.

In many parts of Africa, custom dictates that after 1 year of breastfeeding, children are weaned and sent to an adoptive aunt to be fed cassava fruit, a source of carbohydrates but not protein. The Swahili word for "separated from the breast" is *kwashiorkor*, and this name was given to the syndrome that is observed in children who are suffering from protein deprivation but not calorie deprivation. The condition occurs most frequently after weaning.[49] The major distinguishing features of marasmus are edema and hypoalbuminemia. In addition, a fatty liver, mucous membrane sores, and relative preservation

of fat stores occur. Since the condition often occurs in response to acute events, linear growth is not as severely retarded.

Growth retardation without any clinical features is the most·common presentation of protein-energy malnutrition in children. The GH-IGF-I axis in children is the most sensitive in demonstrating changes due to malnutrition,[50] just as the reproductive hormonal axis is the most sensitive in adult women who develop amenorrhea in response to undernutrition.

ETIOLOGY AND PATHOPHYSIOLOGY

Marasmus is the childhood equivalent of semistarvation, and the hormonal and metabolic adaptations to acute starvation occur as expected. The changes in insulin, GH, and cortisol that are observed in obese normal individuals who are subjected to starvation can be seen in these children even before the development of obvious marasmus.[51]

On the other hand, it is not clear why some children develop kwashiorkor while others in the same nutritional environment develop marasmus. Kwashiorkor is more common in areas where protein intake is lower.[52] However, within a particular population, it has not been possible to demonstrate that the children who develop kwashiorkor indeed had the lowest protein intake.[53] One of the clearest causes of kwashiorkor due to decreased protein intake comes from North American infants who are fed coffee creamers containing only 1% protein, 30% carbohydrate, and 69% fat calories in place of milk.[54] Rats that are fed a low protein-to-energy ratio will consume excess calories.[55] This leads to fatty liver and hypoalbuminemia. Lipolysis is thought to occur secondary to sympathetic stimulation combined with relative insulin resistance, while the fatty liver occurs owing to the failure of apoprotein B synthesis to export triglycerides that are synthesized from the influx of fatty acids. Hepatic ketone production is also impaired. It is not uncommon for up to 40% of the liver mass to be fat compared with the usual 5%.

Higher plasma insulin and lower cortisol levels have been found in children with kwashiorkor than in children with marasmus.[51] It has been proposed that the higher insulin levels will direct amino acids toward muscle protein synthesis at the expense of liver protein synthesis. Overall protein synthesis is reduced in perfused rat liver systems when blood from protein-depleted rats is used.[56] Protein synthesis can be restored by adding branched-chain amino acids. While GH levels are usually elevated in kwashiorkor, these elevated levels are associated with reduced growth. In addition, administration of GH in these children will fail to stimulate growth.[57] These phenomena are accounted for by the decreased levels of IGF-I that are observed in both kwashiorkor and marasmus.

Since kwashiorkor also tends to occur acutely, there may be processes that interfere with the adaptation to starvation, resulting in increased loss of muscle and visceral protein. In this way, kwashiorkor may be a model for the malnutrition that is seen in adults with infection or traumatic injuries (see below).

ENDOCRINE RESPONSES TO ILLNESS AND UNDERNUTRITION

Illness and undernutrition are closely related in a number of chronic conditions. In fact, anorexia is one of the earliest symptoms of infectious, inflammatory, and neoplastic diseases. In a number of medical and surgical conditions, the hormonal changes associated with the adaptations to starvation described above do not occur. Nutritional assessment is focused on determining the severity of malnutrition, the underlying metabolic adaptations that pertain, and the form of therapy to be utilized. Following surgical or traumatic injury, there is a well-described series of events in which a

Table 46-1	Changes in Serum Levels of Hormones in Nine Obese Subjects After 12 Hours and After 7 Days of Fasting	
	12-Hour Fast	**7-Day Fast**
T₃ (ng/dL)	130 ± 15	59 ± 5*
Free T₃ (pg/dL)	322 ± 32	159 ± 13*
rT₃ (ng/dL)	35 ± 3	57 ± 5*
T₄ (mg/dL)	9.1 ± 0.7	9.3 ± 0.8
Free T₄ (ng/dL)	4.7 ± 0.2	3.0 ± 0.3
Insulin	34 ± 6	15 ± 2*
Morning cortisol (mg/dL)	19.1 ± 2.1	26.4 ± 3.4*
Urinary-free cortisol (mg/24 h)	27.1 ± 3.2	41.8 ± 6.3*

Data are expressed as the mean ± SEM for nine subjects
*p < 0.05.

specific sequence of hormonal changes occurs and must be considered in evaluating nutritional therapy. In the patient with critical illness, a hypermetabolic state caused by the endocrine and immune responses to illness results in a situation in which nutritional therapy is recognized to be essential to the survival of the patient. Nutritional therapy can be used to support the malnourished patient, but special modifications are indicated in the metabolic support of patients with renal disease, pulmonary disease, cardiac disease, hepatic insufficiency, critical illness, and multiple organ system failure.

ETIOLOGY

Malnutrition in the hospitalized patient can result from decreased intake, increased losses, or increased requirements due to the metabolic effects of injury, sepsis, surgical trauma, or chronic disease. Reduced intake can result from decreased appetite or anorexia. Abnormal tastes, acquired food aversions, and decreased taste may occur in diabetes, renal failure, and cancer, especially following chemotherapy or radiation therapy.[58] Psychosocial disorders, including depression and isolation, can be associated with decreased food intake. When nausea or vomiting is induced as a side effect of any medication, reduced food intake can occur.

Both maldigestion and malabsorption can lead to losses of ingested nutrients.[59] Maldigestion in patients with exocrine pancreatic insufficiency can result from pancreatitis or pancreatic tumors. Malabsorption due to gastrointestinal dysfunction or absence can result from infarction of bowel segments, intestinal pseudo-obstruction due to defects in the neuromuscular functions mediating normal bowel motility, or diseases affecting the absorptive capacity of the gastrointestinal epithelium. Actual loss of nutrients from body stores can occur in so-called protein-losing enteropathies, which can occur in Ménétriere's disease, Crohn's disease, celiac sprue, and Whipple's disease.

Chronic diseases, surgical injury, trauma, and sepsis result in a redistribution of nutrients from reserves in muscle and fat tissue to the liver and bone marrow for host defense, visceral protein synthesis, and thermogenesis.[60–62] These responses interfere with the normal response to undernutrition and thereby make the patient more likely to develop malnutrition in a short period of time. Protein conservation, which is the hallmark of the adaptation to uncomplicated starvation, does not occur. Instead, protein turnover is increased, leading to increased loss of urinary nitrogen and an increase in resting energy expenditure. In fact, rates of hypermetabolism have been found to correlate with increased losses of urinary nitrogen in patients with major burns, sepsis, infection, or surgical trauma. For instance, in patients undergoing elective surgery, urinary nitrogen losses typically are between 7 and 9 g/day; in patients with sepsis or skeletal trauma, nitrogen losses increase to between 11 and 14 g/day.[63]

Organ failure can result from a combination of factors in the critically ill patient, including regional hypoperfusion and hypoxia, toxic medications, immune responses, endocrine dysfunction, and acute starvation. Metabolic support can play a critical role in the survival of such patients.

PATHOPHYSIOLOGY

The metabolic response associated with the stress of surgery or infection or the inflammation associated with the active phases of chronic illnesses, including cancer, differs markedly from the metabolic and hormonal adaptations that occur with uncomplicated starvation. This response can be considered to have evolved to help the previously well-nourished individual survive life-threatening injury or hemorrhage. In addition, the immune system is mobilized to counter any infection that might occur. The presence of an illness or chronic disease essentially provides a stimulus to this response system that is not quickly and easily eradicated. The resulting prolonged stress response can cause nutritional status to deteriorate and represents a particularly hazardous response for the previously malnourished individual with an illness.

The injury/stress response can be divided into two phases[64] (see Fig. 46-6). The ebb phase, which lasts for approximately 24 hours after an injury or insult, is dominated by the hemodynamic response to injury, which includes hypoperfusion, hypometabolism, and cardiac instability. There is a brisk release of hormones during this period, accompanied by a resistance to their action. Following successful resuscitation and restoration of perfusion, the flow phase begins and predominates between 48 and 72 hours after the initial stress. During this phase, metabolic responsiveness to circulating hormones returns, with resulting hypermetabolism, increased glucose production, increased protein breakdown, and lipolysis. In critical illnesses such as sepsis and multiple-system organ failure, this phase is prolonged. During this phase, protein loss cannot be reversed despite the administration of apparently adequate nutritional support. During this phase, nutritional support can reduce the net loss of protein, and this is reflected in changes in urinary nitrogen excretion. Only correction of the underlying disease process will halt catabolism in this phase. Nonetheless, the temporizing influence of nutritional support can provide critical maintenance of pulmonary function[65] and gastrointestinal integrity[66] until the therapies that are directed at the primary disease process can have their intended effects.

The hormones mediating the metabolic changes that are noted in the ebb and flow phases of the stress response include insulin, glucagon, GH, cortisol, and catecholamines.[67] The secretion of both glucagon and insulin from the pancreas is critically influenced by the balance of α- and β-adrenergic stimulation during the stress response. During the ebb phase, the α-adrenergic inhibition of insulin release predominates even in the face of hyperglycemia. Glucose production rises during this phase, resulting in the characteristic hyperglycemia of injury or sepsis. In the flow phase, β-adrenergic stimulation predominates, with an increase in insulin to normal or higher levels. This phase is characterized by insulin resistance and results in abnormal glucose tolerance. The secretion of glucagon is not affected by α-adrenergic effects immediately after injury, but β-adrenergic stimulation increases glucagon secretion. Therefore, glucagon levels are increased during both phases of the injury response.[68] Inhibition of glucagon but not catecholamines will result in a decrease in endogenous glucose production.[69] The decreased insulin-to-glucagon ratio is consistent with the changes seen in glucose metabolism, but these changes are associated with alterations in the secretion of other hormones as well.

The hypothalamic response to stress results in the release of ACTH, which stimulates adrenal glucocorticoid secretion. This response is stimulated directly by nerves that originate in the area of injury or surgical trauma and does not occur with anesthesia of or experimental denervation of the area before injury.[70] Cortisol stimulates hepatic gluconeogenesis and the release of amino acids from muscles via proteolysis. These effects result in a shunting of protein reserves from the periphery to the liver.

While cortisol is permissive of lipolysis, GH stimulates a rise in plasma free fatty acids and lipid oxidation.[71] Growth hormone levels are decreased in a variety of critically ill patients, such as those who are thermally injured or septic or who have experienced major trauma.[72] Some but not all studies investigating the use of growth hormone in trauma and burn patients have been associated with positive outcomes such as decreased length of hospital stay and reduced mortality.[73]

In addition to these hormonal changes, there is an increase in the synthesis of acute-phase proteins such as fibrinogen, C-reactive protein, serum amyloid A protein, ceruloplasmin, haptoglobin, α_2-macroglobulin, α_1-acid glycoprotein, and certain complement components as well as procoagulants.[74] There is also a prominent leukocytosis with neutrophilia and a redistribution of plasma trace minerals evidenced by a decrease in zinc and iron and an increase in copper secondary to increased ceruloplasmin.[75]

Free radicals are highly reactive chemical species that are capable of independent existence that possess one or more unpaired electrons in the outer orbit that is responsible for cellular injury. Free radicals are produced in critically ill septic patients via three distinct mechanisms: the production of proinflammatory mediators, neutrophil activation, and ischemic-reperfusion injury.[76] The total antioxidant capacity of plasma from critically ill patients is significantly lower than plasma from healthy controls.[77] Furthermore, nonsurvivors in an intensive care unit have lower total antioxidant capacity when compared with survivors.[78] This is thought to be due to an increase in the production of free radicals by neutrophils. Dramatic decreases in α-tocopherol, β-carotene, ascorbate, and selenium have been observed in critically ill patients.[79,80]

The injury response is viewed as a multidimensional adaptation encompassing a variety of physiologic alterations that include increased core body temperature and resting energy expenditure, stress hormone response (cortisol, epinephrine), skeletal muscle wasting, increased hepatic acute-phase response, trace mineral sequestration (copper), decreased intestinal motility, bone marrow suppression, and diuresis. It involves a coordinated acute-phase response, which involves the hepatic synthesis of large quantities of proteins. There is also an energy-intensive component to this acute-phase response, along with the requirement for large quantities of essential amino acids to synthesize the hepatic proteins.

The acute-phase response is regulated by the production of cytokines, most of the clinical research being focusing on tumor necrosis factor (TNF), interleukin (IL)-1, and IL-6, although it is understood that other cytokines are also likely involved. The predominant cytokine effect is locally mediated and is paracrine and autocrine in nature. Anorexia results from the central effect of cytokines on the hypothalamus to alter feeding behavior. The peripheral insulin resistance that is observed with altered carbohydrate metabolism is also mediated by proinflammatory cytokines.

A complete review of all the actions of the cytokines and their interaction is beyond the scope of this chapter but is available in several excellent reviews.[81–84]

The interface between the gastrointestinal tract and the nutritional environment is protected by the gut-associated lymphoid tissue, which is the largest collection of immunocytes in the body.[85] Intraepithelial lymphocytes are found between gut mucosal epithelial cells and are the first population of cells to be exposed to foreign antigens and organisms that reside in the intestinal lumen. Beneath the epithelial basement membrane is the lamina propria, which contains mature plasma cells and lymphocytes as well as dense collections of lymphocytes called Peyer's patches. These cells work together to process antigens from the intestinal lumen. The intraepithelial lymphocytes interact with the gut mucosal epithelial cells and synthesize a number of cytokines, including interferon gamma, IL-2, IL-3, IL-4, IL-6, and TNF-α.[86,87] Just as malnutrition affects cell-mediated immunity as evidenced by reduction in skin test reactivity, it is postulated that gut atrophy with malnutrition results in the breakdown of the gut-associated lymphoid tissue leading to transmigration of bacteria into the bloodstream as an important pathogenic event in the injury response in the malnourished patient.

Many components of the injury response have been shown to benefit the host in the presence of infection or inflammation.[88] For instance, fever, reduction of serum iron levels, and acute-phase proteins may help to fight certain infections. A prolonged injury response leading to malnutrition can impair the host immune response to pathogens. For instance, protein-malnourished patients fail to become febrile despite obvious sepsis. The ability of malnourished patients to synthesize leukocyte endogenous mediator (a combination of cytokines isolated from white cells) is impaired but can be restored following intravenous nutritional support. This improvement in immune responsiveness also has been associated with improved survival in these individuals. As will be discussed below, there is a close interaction of nutritional therapy with immunity. Overfeeding and the use of certain lipids may impair immune response.[89] It is clear that this is an area in which a great deal of additional research must be done to improve the nutritional therapy of injured, septic, and chronically ill patients.

CLINICAL SPECTRUM

Malnutrition in the hospitalized patient and the patient with chronic illness is classified into two major types. First, a kwashiorkor-like malnutrition occurs when sufficient calories are provided but protein is not or when the acute response to stress interferes with the normal adaptation to starvation. These patients have hypoalbuminemia and edema but do not invariably have decreased body weight or wasting. This process can be relatively acute, accounting for the lack of a wasting response, and the replacement of lean tissue with water accounts for the lack of marked weight loss in many patients.

A striking example of this type of malnutrition commonly occurs in AIDS and cancer patients. In this type of malnutrition, weight loss might not be an accurate indicator of the degree of malnutrition, because changes in body composition can occur regardless of weight maintenance. Measurements of body-cell mass in combination with regular monitoring of weight may prove more predictive of the onset of wasting.

Second, a marasmus-like malnutrition or protein-energy malnutrition can occur in which lean tissue and body weight are somewhat decreased, but immune function and albumin secretion are maintained due to the ketoadaptation and energy conservation characteristic of starvation physiology. The imposition of acute stress on preexisting nutrition of either type can lead to a severe form of malnutrition called *combined marasmus-kwashiorkor type malnutrition*.

While global clinical assessment of nutritional status has been shown to be as effective as formal nutritional assessment in discovering malnutrition,[90] the exercise of assessing the patient serves as a device enabling the diet technicians, house officers, and other physicians attending malnourished patients with complex problems to focus on the nutritional needs of patients who are under their care.

DIAGNOSTIC PROTOCOLS

NUTRITIONAL ASSESSMENT

A nutritionally oriented history should inquire as to the patient's pre-illness weight, height, rate of weight loss prior to presentation, nausea, vomiting, anorexia, and specific ingestive, metabolic, or absorptive problems that could impair nutritional status. On the basis of these assessments, the percent ideal body weight from standard tables and the percent usual weight at presentation can be calculated. Body weight changes may be misleading in patients with fluid overload, including those with congestive heart failure, liver disease, and renal failure. In uncomplicated starvation, there is an increase in extracellular fluid volume that tends to maintain weight despite loss of metabolically active tissues.

The sensitivity of nutritional evaluation is enhanced by including certain assessments of the functional indices of the body cell mass, including certain proteins synthesized in the liver[91] and the status of host immune function.[92]

Albumin is the major protein that is synthesized in the liver and carries out significant functions as a carrier protein and to provide oncotic pressure. Its half-life is approximately 20 days, and it does not reflect recent changes in nutritional status. Transferrin has a half-life of only 8.8 days and so can reflect more recent changes in nutritional status. However, transferrin levels are increased in iron deficiency, reducing the specificity of this measurement for nutritional status. Prealbumin has a half-life of 24 hours and can be used to reflect changes in nutritional status over the short term as patients receive nutritional support to assess response to therapy. Biochemical assessment should include, at a minimum, measurement of albumin. An albumin level greater than 3.5 g/dL is normal. Albumin levels of 3.0 to 3.5 g/dL indicate significant hypoalbuminemia, while levels below 3.0 g/dL indicate severe albumin deficiency.

Immune function is impaired in malnutrition.[90] The quantitation of absolute lymphocyte counts derived from a complete blood cell count and differential and the assessment of delayed hypersensitivity using skin test antigens are techniques that are used to assess the impact of nutritional status on immune function. The routinely utilized skin test antigens include tuberculin (as purified protein derivative), mumps, streptokinase-streptodornase, *Candida albicans*, and *Trichophyton*. These tests were chosen on the basis that most normal individuals are exposed to them and would be expected to have a positive skin test reaction. In uncomplicated starvation or protein-energy malnutrition, skin test reactivity can be restored with renutrition. Anergy is not specific to malnutrition and can be a feature of certain diseases such as Hodgkin's disease, while decreased white blood cell counts can be depressed transiently in the postoperative period and after infection with human immunodeficiency virus. Therefore, these estimations of immunocompetence are not simply specific to malnutrition.

Given the variety of nutritional assessment techniques that are available, most clinicians will have to select a small group of routinely available tests to use on a regular basis. Most clinical centers will have available skin testing, albumin, and transferrin for routine use. These tests should make it possible to assess whether patients are mildly, moderately, or severely malnourished and whether marasmic, kwashiorkor-like, or combined severe malnutrition is present (Table 46-2).

The status of the lean body mass can be assessed by measuring urinary creatinine excretion over 24 hours. Creatinine production in most individuals is directly related to skeletal muscle mass, provided that no rapid catabolism of muscle is in progress as with severe sepsis or trauma and that large amounts of dietary creatinine found in animal skeletal muscle are not being ingested. A creatinine-height index is calculated on the basis of the measured 24-hour excretion of creatinine and that expected in a normal adult of the same height as the patient. This index has limited sensitivity, values between 60% and 80% of ideal representing moderate skeletal muscle depletion and 40% to 50% representing severe skeletal muscle depletion.[93] For purposes of estimation, the ideal creatinine excretion for adults is taken as 23 mg/kg/24 hours for males and 18 mg/kg/24 hours for females.[94]

ASSESSMENT OF RISK OF NUTRITIONAL DEPLETION

Assessment of risk of nutritional depletion can be used to determine which patients require consideration for nutritional therapy, as described below. The presence of any of the following criteria should motivate the physician to conduct a complete nutritional assessment[95] with consideration of appropriate forms of nutritional therapy: (1) recent involuntary weight loss of greater than 5% in 1 month or over 10% in 6 months, especially when associated with anorexia, fatigue, or weakness; (2) history of recent significant physiologic stresses such as organ dysfunction, major surgery, infection, or illness within the last 3 months; (3) absolute lymphocyte count less than 1200 cells/mm³; or (4) serum albumin less than 3.2 g/dL.

DETERMINING ROUTE AND DOSE OF NUTRITIONAL THERAPY

Nutritional therapy ranges from dietary counseling urging increased voluntary intake of foods and nutritional supplements to forced intake of nutrients via the gastrointestinal tract (enteral nutrition) or via the venous circulation (parenteral nutrition). The therapy of malnutrition is based on meeting the nutritional requirements of the patient for total energy, macronutrients, and micronutrients.

Total energy requirements can be measured by using indirect calorimetry or estimated by using approximate formulas. For well-nourished normal subjects, the estimated energy expenditure using the Harris-Benedict formula[96] is within 10% of the measured energy expenditure in approximately 90% of all individuals. However, in subjects with a variety of illnesses, hypermetabolism or hypometabolism may occur.[97] For these individuals, measurement of resting energy expenditure using indirect calorimetry is practical and more accurate than estimation methods (Fig. 46-7). In this method, data that is obtained from the rate of oxygen consumption and carbon dioxide production measured under controlled conditions together with information on urinary nitrogen excretion can

Table 46-2 Diagnostic Features of Adult Malnutrition		
	Marasmus	**Kwashiorkor**
Clinical setting	Decreased caloric intake	Decreased protein intake plus stress
Time course to develop	Months to years	Weeks to months
Physical examination	Cachectic; fat depletion, muscle wasting	May look well nourished
Anthropometrics TSF	Depressed	Relatively preserved
AMC	Depressed	Relatively preserved
Weight for height	Depressed	Relatively preserved
Creatinine-height index	Depressed	Relatively preserved
Skin test responses	Normal or depressed	Relatively preserved
Visceral proteins Albumin	Relatively normal	Low
Transferrin	Relatively normal	Low
Lymphocyte cell	Relatively normal	Low

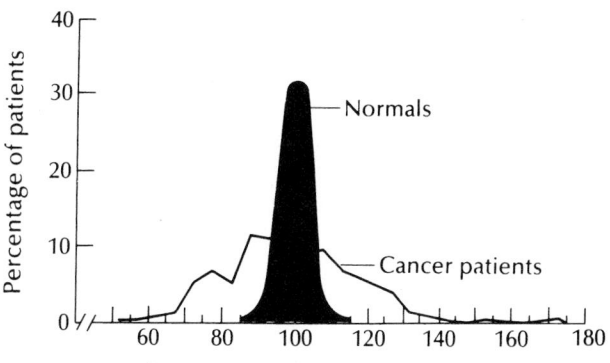

Figure 46-7 The distribution of measured resting energy expenditure in "normals" and in cancer patients. (Source: From Knox L, Crosby L, Feurer I, et al: Energy expenditure in malnourished cancer patients. Ann Surg 197:152–162, 1983.)

be used to assess resting energy expenditure. The patient is placed under a ventilated plastic canopy at rest, and measurements are made for approximately 15 minutes. The equipment that is required for this measurement is available in most hospital pulmonary function laboratories, and newer portable models for bedside use are also available. Many of these newer pieces of equipment perform all necessary calculations internally to provide information on the energy requirements of patients. The ratio of the volume of carbon dioxide produced to oxygen consumed is defined as the respiratory quotient (RQ). Glucose has an RQ of 1.0, and the oxidation of glucose yields 5.0 kcal/L of oxygen consumed. Fat has an RQ of approximately 0.7, yielding significantly less energy per liter of oxygen consumed. The respiratory quotients and calorie equivalents of different mixtures of carbohydrate and fat per liter of oxygen consumed are shown in Table 46-2. These values are the nonprotein RQ values that are used to assess energy expenditure once an adjustment has been made for protein oxidation on the basis of an estimate of the amounts of energy liberated (26.51 kcal/g of nitrogen), oxygen consumed (5.91 L/g of nitrogen), and carbon dioxide produced (4.76 L/g of nitrogen) by the metabolism of protein (Table 46-3). The daily excretion of urinary nitrogen is converted to the rate of nitrogen excretion per hour and is used to calculate resting energy expenditure, as is shown in the example adapted from Cantarow and Trumper[98] in Table 46-4.

Once resting energy expenditure has been measured or basal energy expenditure (BEE) has been estimated by using the Harris-Benedict equation, the total caloric requirements of subjects can be estimated. In general, these estimates range from 1.2 to 2.0 times the measured or estimated values based on observations of patients undergoing treatment for a variety of medical and surgical conditions. In moderately catabolic surgical patients, enteral nutrition has been found to lead to positive nitrogen balance at approximately 1.5 times the BEE, while in parenteral nutrition, 1.75 to 2.0 times the BEE is required.[99] Utilization of estimates of 1.75 times the BEE as a standard practice for all patients receiving parenteral nutritional therapy regardless of metabolic needs has led to overnutrition with resulting complications in certain disease states, as described below.[100]

EVALUATION OF RESPONSE TO NUTRITIONAL SUPPORT

Since the goal of nutritional support is the attainment of an anabolic state or reduction of nitrogen losses, assessment of nitrogen balance is the most useful clinical assessment to determine whether nutritional therapy is effective. *Nitrogen balance* is defined as the difference between nitrogen intake and nitrogen excretion. Nitrogen intake is taken as the protein intake determined from dietary records divided by 6.25 g

Table 46-4	Energy Expenditure Determination by Indirect Calorimetry and Estimation Example Calculation

The calculation of energy expenditure using indirect calorimetry is illustrated by the following example adapted from Cantarow and Trumper. These data were obtained from a patient under basal conditions: (1) urinary nitrogen, 0.18 g/h, (2) oxygen consumption, 12.2 L/h, and (3) carbon dioxide production, 9.2 L/h.

0.18 g of urinary N represents:
$0.18 \times 5.91 = 1.06$ L oxygen
$0.18 \times 4.76 = 0.85$ L carbon dioxide
$0.18 \times 26.51 = 4.77$ kcal
Nonprotein oxygen consumption $= 12.2 - 1.06 = 11.14$ L
Nonprotein carbon dioxide production $= 9.2 - 0.85 = 8.35$ L
Nonprotein RQ = 0.75, representing the liberation of 4.739 kcal/L of oxygen
Nonprotein energy expenditure $= 4.739 \times 11.14 = 52.79$ kcal/h
Total energy expenditure $= 52.79 + 4.77 = 57.56$ kcal/h
For men: RME (kcal/day) $= 66.4730 + 13.7516(W) + 5.0033(H) - 6.7750(A)$
For women: RME (kcal/day) $= 655.095 + 9.563(W) + 1.8496(H) - 4.6756(A)$,
where W = present weight in kilograms, H = height in centimeters, and A = age in years

of nitrogen per gram of "average" protein ingested. Nitrogen excretion is taken as the urinary nitrogen excreted per 24 hours plus a fixed estimate of 4.0 g/24 hours for unmeasured nitrogen losses from cellular sloughing into the feces (1 g), losses from the skin (0.2 g), and nonurea nitrogen losses in the urine (2 g).[101] Since nitrogen balance is most usefully applied in a serial fashion in the same patient, the particular constants that are used to estimate unmeasured excretion are only important for comparison of published results.

At any given level of nitrogen intake, nitrogen balance improves with increased administration of nonprotein calories to a maximum achieved at a ratio of 150:1 of nonprotein calories per gram of nitrogen.[102] Proteins vary in their biologic value on the basis of the mixture of essential and nonessential amino acids that they contain. Albumin has the ideal mixture of amino acids for optimal utilization of protein and is assigned a biologic value of 100. Casein is close to albumin in its biologic quality, followed by meat proteins such as those found in steak or tuna, which have a biologic value of 80. Corn and beans, each with biologic values of 40 or less, can be combined in a protein mixture with a biologic value of 80 because the amino acid patterns of the two proteins are complementary. The protein requirement for normal individuals is 0.55 g/kg of protein for a high-biologic-value protein such as milk or albumin but 0.8 g/kg for the mixture of proteins that is found in the average U.S. diet.[103]

Table 46-3	Respiratory Quotient for Metabolism of Fuel Mixtures				
	Percentage of Total O$_2$ Consumed by:		Percentage of Heat Produced by:		
RQ*	Carbohydrate	Fat	Carbohydrate	Fat	Calories per Liter O$_2$
0.707	0	100	0	100	4.686
0.75	14.7	85.3	15.6	84.4	4.739
0.80	31.7	68.3	33.4	66.6	4.801
0.82	38.6	61.4	40.3	59.7	4.825
0.85	48.8	51.2	50.7	49.3	4.862
0.90	65.8	34.2	67.5	32.5	4.924
0.95	82.9	17.1	84.0	16.0	4.985
1.00	100	0	100	0	5.047

*Nonprotein RQ.
Source: From Cantarow A, Trumper M: Clinical Biochemistry. Philadelphia, WB Saunders, 1955, p 367.

SPECIAL THERAPEUTIC PROBLEMS

COMPLICATIONS

Complications can occur following either enteral or parenteral nutrition. Complications of enteral nutrition are either mechanical or metabolic; complications of parenteral nutrition can be mechanical, infectious, or metabolic.[104]

Mechanical problems of enteral feeding include aspiration, especially in semiconscious patients or patients with abnormalities of swallowing. This problem can be minimized by proper feeding tube placement and determination of the residual gastric contents 8 hours after feeding to eliminate the possibility of gastric outlet obstruction or gastric atony. If these latter problems occur, the feeding tube can be placed into the jejunum. Proper placement should be ensured radiologically to avoid misplacement of the feeding tube. Irritation of the oropharynx and the gastric mucosa can occur, especially with the use of larger-bore and less flexible feeding tubes. This problem can be minimized by using inert silicone rubber and polyurethane tubes.

Diarrhea is the most common complication associated with tube feeding.[105] Carefully increasing the rate of administration will help to avoid this problem. Most enteral formulations are lactose-free, so lactose intolerance is not likely to cause diarrhea. Nonetheless, prolonged starvation can lead to gastrointestinal epithelial atrophy and maldigestion, which, in turn, could result in diarrhea. Diarrhea also can be due to the effects of other medications, colonic infections (e.g., *Clostridium difficile*), or overly rapid administration of hypertonic enteral formulations. Dehydration with hypernatremia also can be a problem in infants and the elderly, in whom inadequate fluid intake can occur during the administration of a hypertonic enteral formula. Glucosuria can occur in patients without a prior history of diabetes when high-carbohydrate enteral formulas are used.

The complications of parenteral nutrition are in many cases more serious than those associated with enteral nutrition.[106] Pneumothorax and subclavian vein thrombosis are the most common catheter-related complications. Pneumothorax should occur in only about 1% to 2% of catheter insertions, but this rate is higher when transthoracic puncture is used rather than open surgical placement of catheters or when less experienced individuals insert the catheters.[107] Radiologic confirmation of proper placement and to exclude the presence of pneumothorax is essential. Pneumothorax usually will resolve spontaneously, but a chest tube may be required in some cases. Thrombosis of the catheter in the central veins has been reported in 5% to 10% of patients receiving parenteral nutrition, especially when hypercoagulable states are present, as in sepsis, inflammatory bowel disease, pancreatitis, or cancer.[108] Heparin is given daily in prophylactic doses of 6000 units routinely, but when thrombosis occurs, the catheter must be removed. Peripheral venous nutrition is used while a full course of heparin or other treatment is undertaken to treat thrombosis. Infections most commonly occur from skin contaminants such as gram-positive organisms but can include fungi and unusual bacteria, especially if acquired during hospitalization. Infected catheters must be removed prior to the systemic treatment of catheter-related sepsis. In patients who are committed to lifelong parenteral nutrition, this decision is made carefully, since only eight external sites are available for central vein catheter placement.

In nutritional support, the goals are simply to provide adequate calories and nutrients to restore nutritional deficiencies and to maintain protein synthesis, positive nitrogen balance, and lean body mass. Metabolic support of the critically ill patient is directed at partial caloric replacement, sustenance of important cellular and organ metabolism, and the avoidance of overfeeding and the metabolic costs of overfeeding, including lipogenesis, gluconeogenesis, and thermogenesis related to inefficient metabolism.

A variety of metabolic complications can occur during parenteral nutrition. The most common is overfeeding, which results in respiratory quotients greater than 1.0. This results in excessive carbon dioxide production, which can complicate the care of patients with chronic lung disease.[109] Hyperglycemia can occur in many patients owing to transient insulin resistance or relative insulin deficiency. Both subcutaneous insulin and insulin added to the parenteral solutions can be used to treat this complication.[110] Metabolic acidosis, which occurred commonly when potassium and sodium were administered only as chloride salts, is less frequently a problem now that acetate buffers are used in parenteral solutions. Abnormalities of phosphate, potassium, calcium, and magnesium can occur owing to excessive or inadequate administration in the presence of underlying disorders such as renal failure or gastrointestinal fistulas that predispose to electrolyte abnormali-

ties.[111] Essential fatty acid deficiency rarely occurs since the use of intravenous lipid emulsions has become so common.[112]

Azotemia can occur in renal failure patients or with excessive administration of amino acids relative to nonprotein calories given and is treated simply by reducing the amino acid load administered. In most cases, the metabolic complications that are associated with parenteral nutrition respond to fluid and electrolyte management with careful monitoring of input and output on a daily basis.

Hepatic abnormalities, including hepatic steatosis recognized by elevations in liver function tests, are a relatively common complication of parenteral nutrition. In most cases, this is due to overfeeding of carbohydrates with subsequent increases in hepatic triglyceride synthesis and storage. This occurs when glucose is used as the sole energy source or is given at greater than the endogenous production rate of 3 g/kg/day. Cholestasis also can result from these changes. Replacement of glucose with long-chain triglycerides (LCTs) derived from soybean or safflower oil has been shown to reduce fatty infiltration of the liver. These LCTs are associated with problems related to poor clearance by the reticuloendothelial system leading to hypertriglyceridemia and possible adult respiratory distress syndrome and increased production of 2- and 4-series prostaglandins and leukotrienes, which can enhance vasoconstriction, platelet aggregation, immunosuppression, inhibition of monokine responses, and free radical formation.[113]

The use of medium-chain triglycerides (MCTs) can avoid some of these problems, at least in experimental systems.[114] MCT oils do not require acylcarnitine transferase action for transport into mitochondria and are readily metabolized to ketone bodies. They contain no essential fatty acids and so should not be used alone. There are research efforts to combine the effects of LCTs and MCTs in structured lipids where the triglyceride contains both types of fatty acids. Additional structured lipids containing n-3 fatty acids or so-called fish oils are also being studied actively.[115]

A modest reduction of the caloric content of the parenteral nutrition solution usually resolves the problem, but in a few cases, problems can be so severe that parenteral nutrition needs to be stopped completely and transplantation (liver and intestine) considered. Animal data having suggested that choline deficiency might be a contributory factor, and current parenteral formulations do not contain choline. Choline deficiency can be a significant contributor to the development of parenteral nutrition–associated liver disease and responds to choline administration once choline deficiency has been demonstrated.[116]

The importance of parenteral multivitamins for patients who are unable to adequately absorb oral multivitamins has been emphasized within the last 15 years by the multiple national shortages of parenteral adult and pediatric multivitamins. Several cases of refractory lactic acidosis due to thiamine deficiency occurred in home parenteral nutrition patients and resulted in significant morbidity and mortality.[117-119] Now that the shortage of both forms of parenteral multivitamins has been resolved, the U.S. Food and Drug Administration (FDA) has notified manufacturers of the adult products to reformulate to new FDA specifications.[120]

Deficiencies of trace minerals such as zinc, copper, and chromium rarely occur, since these are now added routinely to parenteral solutions.[121]

A breakdown in the physical barrier and immunologic defense function of the gastrointestinal tract can promote multiple organ failure syndrome. The gastrointestinal tract is particularly susceptible to ischemic and reperfusion injury. Glutamine, a preferred fuel in the gut epithelium, may promote gastrointestinal tract epithelial healing after an injury.[122] In animal studies, an enteral formula containing glutamine has been shown to improve gastrointestinal epithelial mucosal integrity and nitrogen balance.[123,124] Research is under way on the incorporation of these physiologic properties of specific nutrients into therapeutic regimens to prevent multiple organ failure syndrome. However, the crucial difference between the multiple organ failure syndrome and chronic malnutrition is recognized in the need to avoid overfeeding by providing a hypocaloric protein-sparing nutritional regimen.

NUTRITION SUPPORT AS THERAPY

Patients with gastrointestinal fistulas often evidence fluid and electrolyte abnormalities, sepsis, and malnutrition. Retrospective analyses suggest that nutritional therapy is beneficial in promoting the closure of these fistulas.[125] It has been noted that 90% of fistulas that were destined to close did so within 1 month of the control of sepsis. Prior to the advent of total parenteral nutrition, intensive enteral nutrition resulted in a favorable effect on mortality and a rate of closure comparable with that later observed following parenteral nutrition. While fistula output is more effectively managed with parenteral than enteral nutrition, enteral feedings may be as effective in very proximal or very distal fistulas. Moreover, with chronic low-output fistulas, even oral feeding may be tolerated. In any case, surgery is indicated for those fistulas that do not close within 40 days after nutritional support is initiated. Crohn's disease, radiation enteritis, residual tumor, distal intestinal obstruction, epithelialization of a short fistulous tract (less than 2 cm from bowel to skin), and complete interruption of the gastrointestinal tract make it unlikely that healing will occur. In these instances, early surgical repair should be undertaken.

Short bowel syndrome results when more than 75% of the small intestine is absent secondary to extensive disease or massive resection.[126] This syndrome can occur secondary to trauma, infarction, severe Crohn's disease, radiation enteritis, and cancer. Loss of the ileum is more significant than loss of jejunum, since ileal loss leads to decreased enterohepatic circulation of bile salts. This results in entry of bile salts into the colon with resulting diarrhea and decreased absorption of vitamin B_{12}. Compensatory growth occurs in the small intestine following resection, with epithelial hyperplasia.[127] The intensity of epithelial hyperplasia is related directly to the length of intestine that is resected. The stimuli that promote this response are poorly understood but might include food, enteric secretions, and hormones. Immediately following the initial injury, diarrhea, fluid, and electrolyte disorders are controlled together with provision of parenteral nutrition. After several weeks, fecal output may fall to less than 2 L/day, at which point a trial of enteral feeding may be attempted using a predigested diet that is low in long-chain triglycerides (elemental diet). As the small bowel adapts, carbohydrates and protein are provided, with fat limited to less than 30 g/day utilizing medium-chain triglycerides. After 6 months to 2 years, complete oral nutrition is possible in many patients. Dietary supplements of calcium and fat-soluble vitamins are prescribed for these patients even after gastrointestinal adaptation, since steatorrhea often persists with malabsorption of fat-soluble vitamins and precipitation of calcium in soaps.

Patients with chronic renal failure can be given nutrition during hemodialysis with improved nitrogen retention. During acute renal failure, electrolyte and fluid abnormalities as well as azotemia occur commonly and require appropriate alterations of the parenteral nutrition regimen.[128] Patients with cardiac disease often require fluid and sodium restriction and may benefit from diuretic administration so that protein and calorie requirements can be met.[129]

Diabetic patients who develop hyperglycemia either can be given insulin as described or can be provided with an increased percentage of calories as fat to reduce insulin requirements.[130]

Patients with hepatic insufficiency have abnormal amino acid profiles with increased concentrations of aromatic amino acids and decreased levels of branched-chain amino acids.[131] Decreased plasma levels of branched-chain amino acids are thought to lead to increased central nervous system levels of aromatic amino acids, since these two classes of amino acids compete for uptake at the blood-brain barrier. Increased levels of aromatic amino acids interfere with catecholamine metabolism, resulting in shunting of tyrosine to produce octopamine, a false neurotransmitter. Excess serotonin is thought to develop from increased levels of tryptophan. The combination of decreased catecholamines, false neurotransmitters, and increased serotonin levels is proposed to lead to hepatic coma. Specialized formulas have been used to treat patients with hepatic encephalopathy. Some improvements in neurologic function with administration of specially formulated enteral supplements are noted in patients with chronic hepatic failure. However, in acute hepatic insufficiency, these formulas provided by the parenteral route have not proven beneficial when compared with ordinary parenteral formulations.

NUTRITIONAL SUPPORT IN AIDS AND HIV INFECTION

Recent trends in the management of HIV infection have altered the long-term outlook for affected people. Both death rates and incidence rates for serious disease complications have fallen markedly, and spontaneous resolution of opportunistic infections has been noted. The prevalence of severe wasting has fallen dramatically in areas where combination antiretroviral therapy and comprehensive medical management are the standard of care. However, nutritional and metabolic problems continue to be seen where medical care is not accessed or is not available. This includes the vast majority of HIV-infected individuals in the world, especially in developing countries.

The beneficial effects of nutritional therapy on clinical status are obvious in individual cases and have been demonstrated for a variety of regimens. However, formal proof of efficacy using criteria similar to those used for the evaluation of medications is lacking in most instances. This reflects the fact that placebo-controlled clinical trials are unreasonable in situations in which withholding therapy would lead to death by inanition.

A great deal of attention has been directed toward nutritional therapies in HIV infection, and nutritional follow-up is routinely included in comprehensive care plans for HIV-infected individuals. Results are mixed on the benefits of nutritional counseling and dietary therapies in HIV infection, though a proportion of patients respond well to these therapies. Many fewer patients are requiring aggressive therapies, such as tube feeding or total parenteral nutrition, though such patients do still exist. Other therapies have been applied in clinically stable but malnourished patients, including anabolic agents, cytokine inhibitors, and resistance training exercise. Emerging evidence supports the clinical benefits of these and other therapies. Current clinical trials are evaluating combinations of nutritional therapies.

Emerging reports document the development of a syndrome comprising body composition and metabolic alterations that occur mainly in patients who are receiving combination antiretroviral therapies.[132] There is an alteration in body fat distribution, with an increase in visceral fat content and a decrease in subcutaneous fat content. Dorsocervical fat pads (buffalo humps) have been seen in some patients. Associated metabolic alterations include hypertriglyceridemia, hypercholesterolemia, glucose intolerance, and others, superficially resembling Cushing's disease. The etiology and consequences of this syndrome are uncertain. Most patients are taking drug combinations containing a protease inhibitor, though some are not. Long-term effects are uncertain, but concerns about possible atherogenic disease mandate careful follow-up.

CANCER ANOREXIA AND CACHEXIA

One of the important factors in the response to treatment and mortality in cancer anorexia and cachexia (CAC) is the overall condition of the host at the time of cancer diagnosis. Approximately 50% of cancer patients will have experienced weight loss at the time of diagnosis, and this imparts a poor prognostic sign. By the time of death, nearly all cancer patients will have experienced some degree of weight loss. Cancer has one of the highest incidences of protein-calorie malnutrition among hospitalized patients.

The protein-calorie malnutrition is often related to the disease itself, treatments associated with the disease, or both. Patients with an apparently identical primary cancer and disease stage may vary significantly in terms of the development of cachexia, characterized as the loss of lean body mass, anorexia, malnutrition, and ultimately debilitation. The cachexia may be related to variations in tumor phenotype and host response, although the precise etiology is unknown.

Several changes in nutrient metabolism have been described in patients with cancer cachexia. These include a degree of glucose intolerance and insulin resistance with increased rates of glucose production and recycling via lactate (from the Cori cycle). Whole-body protein turnover is increased in most advanced cancer patients compared with starved normal individuals and weight-losing noncancer patients. As is expected with progression of disease, protein turnover appears to increase further. Patients with advanced disease and weight loss appear to exhibit an impaired adaptability to simple starvation, since fat mobilization is impaired and muscle proteolysis persists.

A 24-kDa glycoprotein proteolysis-inducing factor (PIF) has been isolated from the urine of cancer patients with progressive weight loss but not from the urine of those losing weight owing to other causes.[133] PIF activates the ATP-ubiquitin-dependent proteolytic pathway and induces the nuclear transcription factors NF-κ-B and STAT3, resulting in cytokine and acute-phase protein synthesis.[134–135] PIF has been found to be expressed in tumor cells from patients with significant weight loss but not in those who are reasonably weight stable.[136]

A mouse tumor-derived lipid mobilizing factor[137] has also been identified in the urine of weight-losing cancer patients.[138] The failure of proinflammatory cytokines such as IL-6 to reliably induce cachexia in animal models has led to the suggestion that tumor-derived factors such as PIF may act as cofactors with host- or tumor-derived cytokines to produce a cachectic state.[139]

These alterations in metabolism have been referred to as inefficient use of nutrients and may be complicated further if surgery is required as part of the cancer treatment, with increased energy expenditure and protein requirement. Thus, replenishing the metabolic deficiencies of the cancer patient is clearly not a simple process.

The potential of megestrol and medroxyprogesterone in the management of CAC was first discovered when these agents were used to treat hormone-sensitive tumors.[140] Subsequently, their role in management of CAC has been studied, and the mechanism of action appears to be multifaceted, in part affecting downregulation of synthesis and release of proinflammatory cytokines. Megestrol is the more widely studied agent. It has a dose-related beneficial effect on appetite, body weight, and subjective well-being over an oral dosage range of 160 to 1600 mg/day.[140] Therapy is initiated with 160 mg/day and increased on the basis of clinical response (usually to 320 or 480 mg/day). It is recommended that medroxyprogesterone be initiated at a dosage of 1000 mg/day orally. Both megestrol and medroxyprogesterone can induce thromboembolic phenomena, breakthrough bleeding, peripheral edema, hyperglycemia, and Cushing's syndrome; the drugs were generally well tolerated in clinical trials, with few patients discontinuing treatment because of adverse events.

Ibuprofen, a nonsteroidal anti-inflammatory drug, decreases C-reactive protein[141] and increases body weight[142] in patients with cancer. A randomized trial in 135 patients with cancer and insidious or overt malnutrition demonstrated improved survival in patients receiving oral indomethacin 50 mg twice daily compared with placebo (510 versus 250 days, $p < 0.05$).[143]

It is possible that selective cyclooxygenase (COX)-2 inhibitors such as celecoxib and rofecoxib provide similar effects without associated gastrointestinal toxicity.[144] Interestingly, COX-2-derived prostaglandins may play a major role in the development of cancer.[145] Therefore, selective COX-2 inhibitors may offer clinical advantages in the management of cancer beyond that of simply symptom control, although further study is needed in this area.

THERAPEUTIC PROTOCOLS

ENTERAL AND PARENTERAL NUTRITION

Once malnutrition has been diagnosed and classified as mild, moderate, or severe marasmic, kwashiorkor, or combined protein-energy malnutrition, the choice of the route of administration of nutritional therapy depends on the functional status of the gastrointestinal tract, the methods available for provision of nutritional support, and a working understanding of the various nutritional products and types of equipment used for parenteral and enteral nutritional support.

As a general rule, the enteral feeding route should be used whenever the gastrointestinal tract is functional.[110] Enteral feeding results in higher rates of visceral protein synthesis than similar nutrients provided parenterally. Physiologic release of gut peptides, including insulinotropic peptides that enhance anabolism, also occurs. In addition, provision of nutrients in the gastrointestinal lumen maintains the barrier function of the gut to translocation of endotoxin and gram-negative bacteria in animal studies.[124]

Prior to initiation of enteral feeding, every attempt should be made to utilize voluntary feeding techniques. Changes in meal frequency and size, use of flavorings, preparation of favorite foods in the patient's home, consideration of nutrition in the scheduling of diagnostic and therapeutic procedures, and the use of nutritional supplements between meals should be considered.

The gastrointestinal tract must be truly functional. The stomach must be capable of delivering the nutritional mixture to the small intestine, and then digestion and absorption must proceed normally. If there is functional gastric obstruction due to a problem with gastric emptying, diabetic gastropathy, or prior surgery, then a tube can be placed directly into the jejunum.

When the gastrointestinal tract is not functional and there are clear therapeutic goals, parenteral nutrition should be used. There are a number of accepted indications for parenteral nutrition, including short bowel syndrome, when there is inadequate small bowel surface area for digestion and absorption of nutrients even after adaptation. The ability of this therapy to maintain life under these circumstances is established.[146] The role of parenteral nutrition has been under careful scrutiny in view of the expense and potential side effects of this form of nutritional therapy.[147] While parenteral nutrition is not therapeutic in terms of the conditions themselves, a useful role for it has been defined in subgroups of patients with pancreatitis, gastrointestinal fistulas, and inflammatory bowel disease. In some situations, transitional feeding is utilized in which parenteral and enteral nutrition are combined. For example, parenteral nutrition can be used in burn and head trauma patients when the gastrointestinal tract is functional but the total caloric requirement cannot be met by the enteral route.

PROGNOSIS

While it is simple to demonstrate the impact of renutrition on the patient with uncomplicated starvation or an inability to absorb calories due to a loss of intestinal tissue, it is much more difficult to demonstrate the beneficial effects of nutrition in patients with a number of chronic illnesses, including common forms of cancer. Often, the course of the underlying illness will mask the beneficial effects of nutritional therapy. The benefits of nutritional support have been well documented in selected reviews.[147]

For a number of indications, the use of total parenteral nutrition (TPN) is controversial.[148] While many cancer and AIDS patients benefit from renutrition, the routine use of TPN in all cancer patients receiving chemotherapy or in all AIDS patients regardless of nutritional status is not appropriate. In some patients who are receiving chemotherapy or radiation therapy, mucosal inflammation, nausea, and vomiting impair normal intake. In such patients, TPN might be needed as an adjunct to restore the patient's functional status in order to continue therapy or undertake radiation therapy, chemotherapy, or surgical therapy.

The use of nutrition support in many instances is not supported by clinical trial data. However, the physician must make a judgment as to the severity of the effects of malnutrition and whether nutrition can reverse these effects to affect the overall prognosis of the patient. There are many instances in which nutrition has become a routine part of patient care prior to a careful evaluation of its real benefit. It remains a challenge for nutrition researchers to define the benefits of nutrition support and to determine its best application in clinical practice.

REFERENCES

1. Cahill GF: Starvation in man. N Engl J Med 282:668–675, 1970.
2. Schwartz MW, Woods SC, Porte D Jr, Seeley RJ, Baskin DG: Central nervous system control of food intake. Nature 404:661–671, 2000.
3. Schwartz MW, Morton GJ: Obesity keeping hunger at bay. Nature 418:595–597, 2002.
4. Jelliffe DB: The Assessment of the Nutritional Status of the Community (Monograph Series 53). Geneva, World Health Organization, 1966.
5. Bistrian BR, Blackburn GL, Vitale J, et al: Prevalence of malnutrition in general medical patients. JAMA 235:1567–1570, 1976.
6. Archer S, Burnett R, Fischer J: Current uses and abuses of total parenteral nutrition. Adv Surg 29:165–189, 1996.
7. Bozzetti F, Braga M, Gianotti L, et al: Postoperative enteral versus parenteral nutrition in malnourished patients with gastrointestinal cancer: A randomized multicenter trial. Lancet 358:1487–1492, 2001.
8. Shimada M, Tritos N, Lowell B, et al: Mice lacking melanin-concentrating hormone are hypophagic and lean. Nature 39:670–674, 1998.
9. Owen OE, Morgan AP, Kemp HG, et al: Brain metabolism during fasting. J Clin Invest 48:574–583, 1969.
10. Owen OE, Felig P, Morgan AP, et al: Liver and kidney metabolism during prolonged starvation. J Clin Invest 48:574–583, 1969.
11. Owen OE, Reichard GA: Human forearm metabolism during progressive starvation. J Clin Invest 50:1536–1545, 1971.
12. Eaton SB, Konner M: Paleolithic nutrition. New Engl J Med 312:283–289, 1985.
13. Bistrian BR, Blackburn GL, Hallowell E, Heddle R: Protein status of general surgical patients. JAMA 230:858–860, 1974.
14. Chandra RK: Nutrition, immunity, and infection: Present knowledge and future directions. Lancet 1:688–691, 1983.
15. Marliss EB, Aoki TT, Unger RH, et al: Glucagon levels and metabolic effects in fasting man. J Clin Invest 49:2256–2270, 1970.
16. Owen OE, Reichard GA, Kinney JM, et al: Metabolism during catabolic states of starvation, diabetes, and trauma in humans. In Bleicher SJ, Brodoff BN (eds): Diabetes Mellitus and Obesity. Baltimore, Williams & Wilkins, 1982, pp 172–184.
17. Waterlow JC: Protein turnover with special reference to man. Q J Exp Physiol 169:409–438, 1984.
18. Felig P, Owen OE, Wahren J, Cahill GF: Amino acid metabolism during prolonged starvation. J Clin Invest 48:584–594, 1969.
19. Cersosimo E, Williams PE, Radosevich PM, et al: Role of glutamine in adaptations in nitrogen metabolism during fasting. Am J Physiol 250:E622–E628, 1986.
20. Mortimore GE, Poso AR: Lysosomal pathways in hepatic protein degradation: Regulatory role of amino acids. Fed Proc 434:1289–1294, 1984.
21. Fukagawa NK, Minaker DL, Rowe JW, et al: Insulin-mediated reduction of whole body protein breakdown: Dose-response effects on leucine metabolism in postabsorptive men. J Clin Invest 76:2306–2311, 1985.
22. Nair KS, Halliday D, Matthews DE, Welle SL: Hyperglucagonemia during insulin deficiency accelerates protein catabolism. Diabetes 36(Suppl II):74A, 1987.
23. Flakoll PJ, Brown LL, Frexes-Steed M, Abumrad NN: Use of amino acid clamps to investigate the role of insulin in regulating protein breakdown in vivo. J Parent Ent Nutr 15:81S–85S, 1991.
24. Young VR: Energy metabolism and requirements in the cancer patient. Cancer Res 37:2336–2347, 1977.
25. Arner P, Engfeldt P, Nowak J: In vivo observations on the lipolytic effect of noradrenaline during therapeutic fasting. J Clin Endocrinol Metab 53:1207–1212, 1981.
26. Jensen MD, Haymond MW, Gerich JE, et al: Lipolysis during fasting. J Clin Invest 79:207–213, 1987.
27. Unger RH: Insulin-glucagon relationship in the defense against hypoglycemia. Diabetes 32:575–583, 1983.
28. Chicurel M: Whatever happened to leptin? Nature 404:538–540, 2000.
29. Korner J, Leibel RL: To eat or not to eat: How the gut talks to the brain. New Engl J Med 349:926–928, 2003.
30. Barsh GS, Farooqi IS, O'Rahilly S: Genetics of body-weight regulation. Nature 404(6778):644–651, 2000.
31. Saper CB, Chou TC, Elmquist JK: The need to feed: Homeostatic and hedonic control of eating. Neuron 36:199–211, 2002.
32. Cummings DE, Purnell JQ, Frayo RS, et al: A preprandial rise in plasma ghrelin levels suggests a role in meal initiation in humans. Diabetes 50:1714–1719, 2001.
33. Batterham RL, Cowley MA, Small CJ, et al: Gut hormone PYY (3-36) physiologically inhibits food intake. Nature 418:650–654, 2002.
34. Savage AP, Adrian TE, Carolan G, et al: Effects of peptide YY on mouth to caecum intestinal transit time and on the rate of gastric emptying in healthy volunteers. Gut 28:166–170, 1987.
35. Cummings DE, Weigle DS, Frayo RS, et al: Plasma ghrelin levels after diet-induced weight loss or gastric bypass surgery. New Engl J Med 346:1623–1630, 2002.
36. Froesch ER, Schmid C, Schwander J, Zapf J: Actions of insulin-like growth factor. Ann Rev Physiol 47:443–467, 1985.
37. Phillips LS: Nutrition, somatomedins, and the brain. Metabolism 35:78–87, 1986.
38. Bray GA: The Obese Patient. Philadelphia, WB Saunders, 1976, p 141.
39. Chopra IJ, Huang TS, Beredo A, et al: Evidence for an inhibitor of extrathyroidal conversion of thyroxine to 3,5,3¢-triiodothyronine in sera of patients with non-thyroidal illnesses. J Clin Endocrinol Metab 60:666–672, 1985.

40. Spencer CA, Lum SM, Wilber JF, et al: Dynamics of serum thyrotropin and thyroid hormone changes in fasting. J Clin Endocrinol Metab 56:883–888, 1983.

41. Henson LC, Poole DC, Donahoe CP, Heber D: Effects of exercise training on resting energy expenditure during caloric restriction. Am J Clin Nutr 46:893–899, 1987.

42. Henson LC, Heber D: Whole body protein breakdown rates and hormonal adaptation during fasting in obese subjects. J Clin Endocrinol Metab 57:316–319, 1984.

43. Torun B, Chew F: Protein-energy malnutrition. In Shils ME, Olson JA, Shike M (eds): Modern Nutrition in Health and Disease, 8th ed, vol 2. Baltimore, Williams & Wilkins, 1994, pp 950–976.

44. Latham MC: Protein-energy malnutrition. In Present Knowledge in Nutrition, 6th ed. Washington, DC, International Life Sciences Institute, 1990, pp 39–46.

45. Lira PIC, Ashworth A, Morris SS: Low birth weight and morbidity from diarrhea and respiratory infection in northeast Brazil. Pediatrics 128:497–504, 1996.

46. Ruz M, Solomons NW, Mejia LA, Chew F: Alterations of circulating micronutrients with overt and occult infections in anemic Guatemalan preschool children. Int J Food Sci Nutr 46:257–265, 1995.

47. Golden BE, Golden MHN: Protein deficiency, energy deficiency, and the edema of malnutrition. Lancet 1:1261–1265, 1982.

48. Barltrop D, Sandhu BK: Marasmus, 1985. Postgrad Med J 61:915–923, 1985.

49. Frenk S: Protein-energy malnutrition. In Arneil GC, Metcoff J (eds): Pediatric Nutrition. London, Butterworth, 1985, pp 151–193.

50. Hintz RL, Suskind R, Amatayakul K, et al: Plasma somatomedin and growth hormone values in children with protein-energy malnutrition. J Pediatr 92:153–156, 1978.

51. Whitehead RG, Coward WA, Lunn PG, Rutishauser I: A comparison of the pathogenesis of protein-energy malnutrition in Uganda and Gambia. Trans R Soc Trop Med Hyg 71:189–195, 1977.

52. Truswell AS: Protein vs energy in protein energy malnutrition. S Afr Med J 59:753–756, 1981.

53. Gopalan C: Kwashiorkor and marasmus: Evolution and distinguishing features. In McCance RA, Widowson EM (eds): Calorie Deficiencies and Protein Deficiencies. London, Churchill Livingstone, 1968, pp 49–58.

54. Sinatra FR, Merritt RJ: Iatrogenic kwashiorkor in infants. Am J Dis Child 135:21–23, 1981.

55. Kirsch RE, Saunders SJ, Frith L, et al: Plasma amino acid concentration and the regulation of albumin synthesis. Am J Clin Nutr 22:1559–1562, 1969.

56. Lumn PG, Whitehead RG, Baker BA: The relative effects of a low-protein high-carbohydrate diet on free amino acid composition of liver and muscle. Br J Nutr 36:219–230, 1976.

57. Hadden DR, Rutishauer IHE: Effect of human growth hormone in kwashiorkor and marasmus. Arch Dis Child 42:29–33, 1967.

58. Schiffman SS: Taste and smell in disease. N Engl J Med 308:1275–1277, 1983.

59. Kotler DP: Cachexia. Ann Intern Med 133:622–634, 2000.

60. Birkhan RH, Long CL, Fitkin D, et al: Effects of major skeletal trauma on whole body protein turnover in man measured by 14C-leucine. Surgery 88:294–299, 1980.

61. Long CL, Jeevanandam M, Kim BM, Kinney JM: Whole body protein synthesis and catabolism in septic man. Am J Clin Nutr 30:1340–1344, 1977.

62. Bistrian BR, Schwartz J, Istfan NW: Cytokines, muscle proteolysis, and the catabolic response to infection and inflammation. Proc Soc Exp Biol Med 200:220–223, 1992.

63. Blackburn GL, Bistrian BR, Maini BS: Nutritional and metabolic support of the hospitalized patient. J Parenter Enter Nutr 1:11, 1977.

64. Cuthbertson DP, Tilstone WJ: Metabolism during the post-injury period. Adv Clin Chem 12:1–4, 1969.

65. Bassili HR, Dietel M: Effects of nutritional support on weaning patients off of mechanical ventilators. J Parenter Enter Nutr 5:161–163, 1981.

66. Alverdy J, Chi HS, Sheldon G: The effect of parenteral nutrition on gastrointestinal immunity: The importance of enteral stimulation. Ann Surg 202:681–684, 1985.

67. Alberti KGMM, Batstone GF, Foster KJ, Johnston DG: Relative roles of various hormones on mediating the metabolic response to injury. J Parenter Enter Nutr 4:141–145, 1980.

68. Nair KS, Halliday D, Matthews DE, Welle SL: Hyperglucagonemia during insulin deficiency accelerates protein catabolism. Diabetes 36(Suppl 1):74A, 1987.

69. Matthews DE, Pesola G, Campbell RG: Effect of epinephrine on amino acid and energy metabolism in humans. Am J Physiol 258(Endo Metab 21):E948–E956, 1990.

70. Hjortso NC, Christensen NJ, Andersen T, Kehlet H: Effects of the extradural administration of local anesthetic agents and morphine on the urinary excretion of cortisol, catecholamines, and nitrogen following elective surgery. Br J Anesth 57:400–406, 1985.

71. Ziegler TR, Young LS, Manson JM, Wilmore DW: Metabolic effects of recombinant human growth hormone in patients receiving parenteral nutrition. Ann Surg 208:6–16, 1988.

72. Demling R: Growth hormone therapy in critically ill patients N Engl J Med 341:837–839, 1999.

73. Takala J, Ruokonen E, Webster NR, et al: Increased mortality associated with growth hormone treatment in critically ill patients. N Engl J Med 341:785–792, 1999.

74. Dinarello CA: Interleukin 1 and the pathogenesis of the acute phase response. N Engl J Med 311:1413–1418, 1984.

75. Kushner I: The phenomenon of the acute phase response. Ann N Y Acad Sci 389:39–48, 1982.

76. Dasgupta A, Malhotra D, Levy H, et al: Decreased total antioxidant capacity but normal lipid hydroperoxide concentrations in sera of critically ill patients. Life Sci 60:335–340, 1997.

77. Alonso de Vega JM, Diaz J, Serrano E, et al: Plasma redox status relates to severity in critically ill patients. Crit Care Med 28:1812–1814, 2000.

78. Metnitz GH, Fischer M, Bartens C, et al: Impact of acute renal failure on antioxidant status in multiple organ failure. Acta Anaesthesiol Scand 44:236–240, 2000.

79. Kharb S, Ghalaut VS, Ghalaut PS: Alpha tocopherol concentration in serum of critically ill patients. J Assoc Physicians India 47:400–402, 1999.

80. Hawker FH, Stewart PM, Snitch PJ: Effects of acute illness on selenium homeostasis. Crit Care Med 18:442–446, 1990.

81. Standiford TJ, Huffnagle GB: Cytokines in host defense against pneumonia. J Invest Med 45:335–345, 1997.

82. Howard M, O'Garra A, Ishida H, et al: Biological properties of interleukin 10. J Clin Immunol 12:239–247, 1992.

83. Chehimi J, Trinchieri G: Interleukin-12: a bridge between innate resistance and adaptive immunity with a role in infection and acquired immunodeficiency. J Clin Immunol 14:149–159, 1994.

84. Baggiolini M, Dewald B, Moser B: Human chemokines: An update. Ann Rev Immunol 15:675–705, 1997.

85. Klein J, Mosley R: Phenotypic and cytotoxic characteristics of intraepithelial lymphocytes. New York, Raven Press, 1994.

86. Teitelbaum D, Reyas B, Merion R, et al: Intestinal intraepithelial lymphocytes: Identification of an inhibitory sub-population. J Surg Res 63:123–127, 1996.

87. Fujihashi K, McGhee JR, Beagley KW, et al: Cytokine-specific ELISPOT assay: Single cell analysis of IL-2, IL-4, and IL-6 producing cells. J Immunol Methods 160:181–189, 1993.

88. Chandra RK: Nutrition, immunity and infection: Present knowledge and future directions. Lancet 1:688–691, 1983.

89. Hammaway KJ, Moldawer LL, Georgieff M: The effect of lipid emulsions on reticuloendothelial system function in the injured animal. J Parenter Enter Nutr 9:559–565, 1985.

90. Jeejeebhoy KN: Muscle function and malnutrition. Gut 27(Suppl 1):25–39, 1986.

91. Shetty PS, Watrasiewicz KE, Jung RT, James WPT: Rapid-turnover proteins: An index of subclinical protein-energy malnutrition. Lancet 2:230–232, 1979.

92. Kahan BD: Nutrition and host defense mechanisms. Surg Clin North Am 61:557–570, 1981.

93. Bistrian BR, Blackburn GL, Hallowell E, Heddle R: Protein status of general surgical patients. JAMA 230:858–870, 1974.

94. Bistrian BR, Blackburn GL, Shermann M: Therapeutic index of nutritional depletion in hospitalized patients. Surg Gynecol Obstet 141:512–518, 1975.

95. Irving M: ABC of nutrition: Enteral and parenteral nutrition. Br Med J 291:1404–1408, 1985.

96. Harris JA, Benedict FG: Biometric Studies of Basal Metabolism in Man. Washington, DC, Carnegie Institute Publication 279, 1919.

97. Knox L, Crosby L, Feurer I, et al: Energy expenditure in malnourished cancer patients. Ann Surg 197:152–162, 1983.

98. Cantarow A, Trumper M: Clinical Biochemistry. Philadelphia, WB Saunders, 1955, p 367.

99. Ang SD, Leskiw MJ, Stein TP: The effect of increasing total parenteral nutrition on protein metabolism. J Parenter Enter Nutr 7:525–529, 1983.

100. Askanazi J, Rosenbaum SH, Hyman AI: Respiratory changes induced by the large glucose loads of total parenteral nutrition. JAMA 243:1444–1447, 1980.

101. Sirba E: Effect of reduced protein intake on nitrogen loss from the human integument. Am J Clin Nutr 20:1158–1161, 1978.

102. Calloway D, Spector H: Nitrogen balance as related to caloric and protein intake in active young men. Am J Clin Nutr 2:405–412, 1954.

103. Recommended Dietary Allowances, 10th ed. Washington, DC, National Academy Press, 1989.

104. Bethel RA, Jansen RD, Heymsfield SB, et al: Nasogastric hyperalimentation through a polyethylene catheter: An alternative to central venous hyperalimentation. Am J Clin Nutr 32:1112–1120, 1979.

105. Voit KAJ, Echave V, Brown RA, Gund FN: Use of elemental diet during the adaptive stage of short gut syndrome. Gastroenterology 65:419–426, 1973.

106. Heymsfield SB, Bethel RA, Ansley JD, et al: Enteral hyperalimentation: An alternative to central venous hyperalimentation. Ann Intern Med 90:63–71, 1979.

107. Feliciano DV, Mattox KL, Graham JM: Major complications of percutaneous subclavian catheters. Am J Surg 138:869–874, 1979.

108. Ryan A, Abel M, Abbot WM: Catheter complications in total parenteral nutrition. N Engl J Med 290:757–761, 1974.

109. Covelli HD, Black JW, Olsen MS, Beekman JF: Respiratory failure precipitated by high carbohydrate loads. Ann Intern Med 95:579–581, 1981.

110. Bozzetti F, Braga M, Gianotti L, et al: Postoperative enteral versus parenteral nutrition in malnourished patients with gastrointestinal cancer: A randomized multicenter trial. Lancet 358:1487–1492, 2001.

111. Ruberg R, Allen T, Goodman M: Hypophosphatemia with hypophosphaturia in hyperalimentation. Surg Forum 22:87–88, 1971.

112. Goodgame JT, Lowry SF, Brennan MF: Essential fatty acid deficiency in total parenteral nutrition: Time course of development and suggestions for therapy. Surgery 84:271–277, 1978.

113. Kinsella JE, Lokesh B, Broughton S, Whelan J: Dietary polyunsaturated fatty acids and eicosanoids: Potential effects on modulation of inflammatory and immune cells: An overview. Nutrition 6:24–44, 1990.

114. Holman RT: Nutritional and metabolic interrelationships between fatty acids. Fed Proc 23:1062–1067, 1964.

115. DeMichele SJ, Karlstad MD, Bistrian BR, et al: Enteral nutrition with structured lipid: Effect on protein metabolism in thermal injury. Am J Clin Nutr 50:1295–1302, 1989.

116. Buchman A, Ament M, Sohel M, et al: Choline deficiency causes reversible hepatic abnormalities in patients receiving parenteral nutrition: Proof of a human choline requirement: A placebo-controlled trial. JPEN 25:260–268, 2001.

117. Death associated with thiamine deficient total parenteral nutrition. Morb Mortal Wkly Rep 38:38–43, 1987.

118. Lactic acidosis traced to thiamine deficiency related to nationwide shortage of multivitamins for total parenteral nutrition: United States, 1997. Morb Mortal Wkly Rep 46:523–528, 1997.

119. Alloju M, Ehrinpreis MN: Shortage of intravenous multivitamin solution in the United States. N Engl J Med 337:54–55, 1997.

120. U.S. Food and Drug Administration: Parenteral multivitamin products; Drugs for human use; Drug efficacy study implementation; Amendment. Federal Register 65(77):21200–21201, April 20, 2000.

121. Fleming CR, Hodges RE, Hurley LS: A prospective study of serum copper and zinc levels in patients receiving total parenteral nutrition. Am J Clin Nutr 29:70–77, 1976.

122. Cerra FB: Hypermetabolism, organ failure, and metabolic support. Surgery 101:1–14, 1987.

123. Windmueller HG: Glutamine utilization by the small intestine. Adv Enzymol 53:210, 1982.

124. Fox AD, Kripke SA, DePaula JA: Glutamine supplemented diets prolong survival and decrease mortality in experimental enterocolitis. J Parenter Enter Nutr 12(Suppl 1):8S, 1988.

125. Thomas RJS: The response of patients with fistulas of the gastrointestinal tract to parenteral nutrition. Surg Gynecol Obstet 153:77–80, 1981.

126. Weser E, Fletcher JT, Urban E: Short bowel syndrome. Gastroenterology 77:575–579, 1979.

127. Williamson RCN: Intestinal adaptation. N Engl J Med 298:1393–1402, 1444–1450, 1978.

128. Blumenkrantz MJ, Kopple JD, Koffler A: Total parenteral nutrition in the management of acute renal failure. Am J Clin Nutr 31:1830–1840, 1978.

129. Heymsfield SB, Bethel RA, Ansley JD: Cardiac abnormalities in cachectic patients before and during nutritional repletion. Am Heart J 95:584–594, 1978.

130. Fischer JE: Nutritional support in the seriously ill patient. Curr Prob Surg 17:466–532, 1980.

131. Fischer JE, Bower RH: Nutritional support in liver disease. Surg Clin North Am 61:653–660, 1981.

132. Smith KY: Selected metabolic and morphologic complications associated with highly active antiretroviral therapy. J Infect Dis 185:S123–S127, 2002.

133. Todorov P, Cariuk P, McDevitt T, et al: Characterisation of a cancer cachectic factor. Nature 379:739–742, 1996.

134. Lorite MJ, Smith HJ, Arnold JA, et al: Activation of ATP-ubiquitin-dependent proteolysis in skeletal muscle in vivo and murine myoblasts in vitro by a proteolysis-inducing factor. Br J Cancer 85:297–302, 2001.

135. Watchorn TM, Waddell I, Dowidar N, Ross JA: Proteolysis-inducing factor regulates hepatic gene expression via the transcription factors NF-kappa B and STAT3. FASEB J 155:562–564, 2001.

136. Watchorn TM, Waddell I, Ross JA: Proteolysis-inducing factor differentially influences transcriptional regulation in endothelial subtypes. Am J Physiol 282:E763–E769, 2002.

137. Cabal-Manzano R, Bhargava P, Torres-Duarte A, et al: Proteolysis-inducing factor is expressed in tumours of patients with gastrointestinal cancers and correlates with weight loss. Br J Cancer 84:1599–1601, 2001.

138. Harai K, Ishiko O, Tisdale M: Mechanism of depletion of liver glycogen in cancer cachexia. Biochem Biophys Res Commun 241:49–52, 1997.

139. Harai K, Hussey HJ, Barber MD, et al: Biological evaluation of a lipid mobilising factor (LMF) from the urine of cancer patients. Cancer Res 58:2359–2365, 1998.

140. Mantovani G, Macciò A, Esu S, et al: Medroxyprogesterone acetate reduces the in vitro production of cytokines and serotonin involved in anorexia/cachexia and emesis by peripheral blood mononuclear cells of cancer patients. Eur J Cancer 33:602–607, 1997.

141. Ottery FD, Walsh D, Strawford A: Pharmacologic management of anorexia/cachexia. Semin Oncol 25(Suppl 6):35–44, 1998.

142. Wigmore SJ, Falconer JS, Plester CE, et al: Ibuprofen reduces energy expenditure and acute-phase protein

production compared with placebo in pancreatic cancer patients. Br J Cancer 72:185–188, 1995.

143. McMillan DC, O'Gorman P, Fearon KC, et al: A pilot study of megestrol acetate and ibuprofen in the treatment of cachexia in gastrointestinal cancer patients. Br J Cancer 76:788–90, 1997.

144. Lundholm K, Gelin J, Hyltander A, et al: Anti-inflammatory treatment may prolong survival in undernourished patients with metastatic solid tumors. Cancer Res 54: 5602–5606, 1994.

145. Masferrer JL, Leahy KM, Kohi AT, et al: Antiangiogenic and antitumor activities of cyclooxygenase-2 inhibitors. Cancer Res 60:1306–1311, 2000.

146. Pillar B, Perry S: Evaluating total parenteral nutrition: Final report and statement of the technology assessment and practice guidelines forum. Nutrition 6:313–317, 1990.

147. Meguid MM, Mughal MM, Meguid V, Terry JJ: Risk-benefit analysis of malnutrition and perioperative nutritional support: A review. Nutr Int 3:25–34, 1987.

148. Koretz RL: What supports nutritional support? Dig Dis Sci 29:577–588, 1984.

DIABETES MELLITUS

Development of the Endocrine Pancreas

Matthias Hebrok and Michael S. German

The pancreas provides both the enzymes that digest the food in the gut, and the hormones that control the use of the nutrients supplied by that digested food. Two distinct components of the pancreas, the exocrine and endocrine compartments, accomplish these related tasks. The ductal and acinar cells of the exocrine compartment comprise the majority of the organ while the islets of Langerhans of the endocrine portion are scattered throughout the exocrine matrix.

During pancreatic development, a common pool of progenitor cells in the early gut endoderm differentiates into these distinct cell types. Positional and temporal cues provided by extracellular signals direct sequential changes in the gene expression program of individual cells, and ultimately determine the phenotype of the differentiated cells and the organization of the mature organ. Any breakdown in the orchestration of this complex process of growth, differentiation, migration, and organization can damage the mature organ, and can cause diabetes by impairing the function of the insulin-producing β cells. Understanding pancreatic development provides us with both new insights into the causes of diabetes and new strategies for intervening in the disease.

PANCREAS MORPHOGENESIS

During gastrulation, mesendodermal cells that migrate through the node region start to segregate to form the distinct mesodermal and endodermal germ layers. Endodermal cells aggregate to form a contiguous epithelium that spans the whole length of the forming gastrointestinal tract of the developing embryo. Digestive organs develop along the anteroposterior and dorsal-ventral axes of this sheet of cells in a precise and predetermined pattern.[1-3]

The pancreas forms from clumps of cells that bud from the dorsal and ventral aspects of the gut endoderm near the foregut/midgut junction (Fig. 47-1).[4,5] Well before any morphologic evidence of the pancreas becomes apparent, interactions between the mesodermally derived notochord and the endodermal epithelium initiate dorsal pancreas formation.[6] Similarly, interactions between the lateral plate mesoderm and lateral endoderm ensure proper induction of the ventral pancreas.[7] The first morphologic sign of pancreas formation is a thickening of the dorsal endodermal sheet caudal to the stomach anlage. This bud structure continues to grow and initiates contact with the dorsal aorta that has fused in the midline and thus separated the notochord and endoderm.[8] Subsequently, dorsal mesenchyme replaces the aorta and provides essential signals that stimulate pancreatic epithelial branching and cell differentiation.

Similar tissue interactions guide the development of the two ventral buds. In contrast to the dorsal bud that forms in the midline of the epithelium, the ventral buds are derived from the ventrolateral edges of the endodermal sheet. Instructive signals provided by the lateral plate mesenchyme initiate ventral pancreas formation and interaction with smaller blood vessels further support organ growth.[8] One of these ventral buds degenerates while the other one fuses with the dorsal bud when stomach and gut rotate to form the mature organ. The regulation of this rotation is not well understood but perturbations lead to malformations in humans, including annular pancreas, where a part of the ventral pancreas is mislocalized and can constrict the adjacent duodenum.[9]

Mesenchymal-epithelial interactions are required for proper development of the mature tissue[10,11]; however, the epithelial cells start to outgrow the mesenchyme during later stages of development and few remnants of this tissue remain in the adult pancreas. Epithelial cells branch into the surrounding mesenchyme to form an elaborate duct system that allows transport of exocrine enzymes into the duodenum. The distal cells of the branching epithelium differentiate into acinar cells that are connected to the duct system via centeroacinar cells. Acinar cells are organized as small glands that produce a variety of digestive enzymes, including amylases, peptidases, nucleases, and lipases.

In contrast to the continuous acinar-duct system, endocrine precursors delaminate from the immature ducts during development and migrate into the surrounding mesenchyme where they aggregate and organize into islets of Langerhans. These distinct islet cells produce a variety of hormones, including insulin, glucagon, pancreatic polypeptide, and somatostatin, that are secreted directly into the bloodstream and regulate gastrointestinal function and nutrient storage and use. Due to intimate interactions between endocrine cells and blood vessels, islets are highly vascularized. Similarly, hormone secretion is at least partially controlled by the nervous system, and sympathetic, parasympathetic, and sensory neurons innervate the islets.

EARLY ORGAN SPECIFICATION AND BUD FORMATION

TISSUE INTERACTION AND SIGNALING PATHWAYS

With the exception of supporting mesenchyme, blood vessels, and innervating neurons, all mature pancreatic cell types derive from epithelial cells of endoderm origin.[12-14] A number of studies have addressed the question how the pancreas anlage becomes specified within the epithelial sheet that

Figure 47-1   Schematic outline of the development of the mammalian pancreas. **1,** Dorsal and ventral buds arise from the duodenal part of the primitive gut endoderm *(blackened).* **2,** The dominant ventral bud, following the bile duct, turns and approaches the dorsal bud. **3,** The two buds fuse together. **4,** The ventral bud becomes part of the head of the pancreas (the PP-rich duodenal lobe), whereas the dorsal bud gives rise to the body and tail (the glucagon-rich splenic lobe); the pancreatic juice is drained off by the main and the accessory pancreatic ducts. b, bile duct; d, dorsal bud; s, stomach; v, ventral bud.

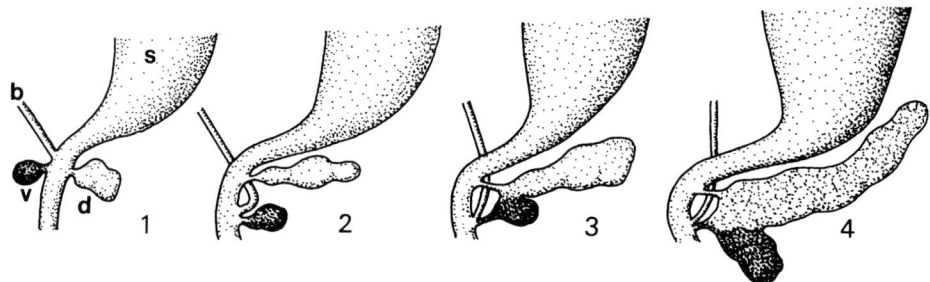

forms the endoderm, and increasing evidence points to a series of tissue interactions as important steps during early stages of organogenesis. During gastrulation, the mesectodermal portion of the embryo signals to the endodermal sheet to establish a prepattern along the anterior-posterior axis.[3]

Although the exact signals required for patterning of the fore-midgut area are not completely understood, studies in mice have implicated the fibroblast growth factor (FGF) signaling pathway in this process.[15] Before any morphologic signs of pancreas formation are apparent, the midline of the endodermal epithelium comes in close contact with the overlying notochord, a mesodermal structure known to regulate organogenesis and cell differentiation in adjacent structures. The notochord provides a number of secreted signaling proteins that are required for initiation of dorsal pancreas organogenesis. Members of the transforming growth factor β (TGF-β) and FGF signaling pathways have been implicated in the notochord-mediated induction of pancreas development. A critical aspect of their activity is to repress the expression of sonic hedgehog (Shh), a member of the hedgehog signaling pathway within the pancreas anlage.[16] Ectopic elevation of hedgehog signaling at the onset of pancreas formation results in pancreas agenesis, indicating that tight regulation of the activity of this pathway is essential for proper organ formation. However, the notochord only provides permissive signals as it cannot induce expression of pancreatic markers in nonpancreatic endoderm.[6]

In contrast to the singular dorsal pancreas, two distinct pancreatic buds form within the ventrolateral endoderm, a region that is not contacted by the notochord. Tissue recombination experiments in chick and mice demonstrate that similar but distinct signals from the lateral plate mesoderm (LPM) ensure the correct temporal-spatial induction of the ventral pancreas.[7,15] Prior to contact with the LPM, no pancreatic markers are detectable in the presumptive ventral pancreas, but LPM or the TGF-β superfamily members activin and bone morphogenetic proteins (BMPs), as well as retinoic acid (RA) have been shown to induce expression of pancreatic genes in underlying endoderm (see following section).[7] Importantly, mesenchyme isolated from the pancreatic region carries the potential to induce pancreatic gene expression in anterior endoderm normally fated to develop into stomach and esophagus. Thus, in contrast to the notochord-endoderm interaction that induces dorsal pancreas development in a permissive fashion, the LPM actively instructs uncommitted endoderm to differentiate into pancreatic tissue. Activin, BMPs, and RA signals that mimic the pancreas instructive activity of the LPM are potentially useful in designing a cocktail of growth factors designed to regulate differentiation of uncommitted progenitor cells toward a pancreatic fate.

Other studies have shown that interactions between heart mesenchyme and ventral foregut endoderm regulate differentiation of ventral pancreas and liver progenitors cells.[17] In analogy to the notochord-dorsal pancreas bud interactions,

the heart mesenchyme produces TGF-β and FGF signals that regulate organ differentiation of the ventral endodermal organs, including liver and pancreas. Due to its close proximity, the concentration of FGF ligands produced by the heart mesenchyme is higher at the area fated to develop into liver and lower at the more distal region that develops into ventral pancreas.[17] This is also the case for dorsal pancreatic epithelium where low levels of FGF signals have been shown to initiate pancreatic gene expression and block Shh expression while higher levels of FGF signaling block pancreas induction via increased hedgehog signaling. Thus, formation of dorsal and ventral pancreatic buds depends on low FGF signals and inhibition of hedgehog signaling.[16] It is important to note that hedgehog signaling is active in areas immediately adjacent to the dorsal and ventral buds, thereby establishing a molecular boundary that prevents ectopic expansion of pancreatic tissue beyond its normal borders.

During subsequent stages, the flattened endodermal sheet expands and folds itself to form a tubelike structure. The first morphologic sign of pancreas formation is an epithelial thickening at the dorsal side of the forming gut tube caudal to the stomach anlage, shortly followed by the appearance of two ventral thickenings next to the liver diverticulum. Outgrowth and tissue-specific gene expression continues to be dependent on cues derived from adjacent tissues. In contrast to earlier stages, the mesenchymal signals are now produced from forming blood vessels, the dorsal aorta, and smaller vitelline veins that contact the dorsal and ventral buds, respectively.[18] Depletion of blood vessels via explantation in Xenopus or via homozygous recombination in transgenic mice that lack the Flk-1 gene, a receptor for vascular epithelial growth factor, impairs the differentiation of the dorsal pancreatic epithelium.[18,19] Vice versa, ectopic expression of vascular epithelial growth factor leads to hypervascularization and islet hyperplasia in pancreatic tissues, as well as ectopic insulin expression in nonpancreatic stomach epithelium, suggesting that either vascular epithelial growth factor or molecules secreted by endothelial cells support endocrine cell differentiation. Detailed analysis of the interaction between blood vessels and pancreas buds has revealed physical contact between the aorta and the dorsal bud epithelium while vitelline veins and ventral bud epithelium are separated by a fine band of mesenchymal cells, suggesting that endothelial cells are less critical for ventral bud formation.[19]

Upon specification of the dorsal and ventral pancreatic anlagen, further mesenchymal-epithelial interactions are required for later steps of pancreas organogenesis.[10,11] Splanchnic mesoderm expands medially and surrounds the pancreatic epithelial buds. Signals from the mesenchyme promote epithelial expansion, which results in the formation of a branching structure composed of undifferentiated ductal cells. Based on morphologic criteria, Rutter and colleagues argued that the early endodermal cells are "protodifferentiated" and that mature exocrine and endocrine cells only appear after the secondary transition, a process during which the number of differentiated acinar and β cells increases significantly.[4,20] More recent studies have shown that early pancreatic mesenchyme generally induces growth and proliferation of epithelial cells while at later stages mesenchymal signals promote exocrine and prohibit endocrine cell differentiation.[21,22]

INDUCTION OF THE PANCREATIC GENE EXPRESSION PROGRAM

The morphologic changes that occur as pancreas differentiates from gut endoderm depend on sequential changes in gene expression. The extracellular signals provided by tissue interactions between the developing endoderm and adjacent tissues ultimately impact cell phenotype by altering gene expression in the nucleus. Recent studies have outlined the underlying molecular events that control these changes in gene expression, and have focused in particular on the nuclear proteins, the transcription factors, that control gene transcription.

Transcription factors expressed broadly in the endoderm provide competence to respond to the endoderm patterning signals and include several transcription factors originally described in the adult liver: hepatic nuclear factors 1b (a POU-homeodomain factor),[23] 3a and b (forkhead factors now known as Foxa1 and Foxa2),[24] 4a (an orphan nuclear receptor)[25,26] and 6 (a cut-homeodomain factor),[27,28] and the zinc-finger transcription factors GATA4, 5, and 6.[29,30] These genes function in a transcriptional hierarchy that not only controls endoderm patterning, but also persists in endoderm-derived organs and plays a role in the mature pancreas.[31-36] Several of these endoderm factors have been directly implicated in the control of mature pancreatic gene expression (see Fig. 47-5).

The earliest genes selectively expressed in prepancreatic endoderm are two transcription factors, the parahox homeodomain factor PDX1[37-39] and the basic-helix-loop-helix (bHLH) transcription factor P48/PTF1.[40,41] PDX1 expression first appears in prepancreatic endoderm more than a day before the initial formation of the dorsal pancreatic bud, and is immediately preceded by the appearance of another parahox factor, HB9,[42,43] which is expressed more broadly in anterior endoderm. Expression of both HB9 and PDX1 persist in the initial pancreatic buds, although HB9 expression is quickly extinguished while PDX1 expression lasts a few more days. Expression of both factors is reactivated in mature β cells.

Dorsal, but not ventral, expression of PDX1 depends on HB9.[42,43] Because HB9 is also expressed in the notochord during the same period, it is formally possible that HB9 could control dorsal PDX1 expression via signals from the notochord. PDX1 expression in the dorsal prepancreatic endoderm does not require signals from the notochord, however, suggesting that HB9 functions cell-intrinsically in inducing PDX1. Extrinsic signals inducing PDX1 expression in the dorsal prepancreatic endoderm have not been identified.[6] On the other hand, as described in the preceding section, signals from the LPM including activin, BMPs, and retinoic acid can induce PDX1 expression in the ventral prepancreatic endoderm.[7]

Studies of the PDX1 promoter have identified several additional endodermal transcription factors as potential intrinsic regulators of PDX1 expression.[44-51] These include members of the HNF1 and Foxa families of transcription factors, HNF6, the paired homeodomain factor pax6, and PDX1 itself.[44,45,50,52,53] (HB9 may act through these same PDX1 binding sites, given its similarity to PDX1 in the DNA-binding homeodomain). HNF1a and pax6 are not expressed early enough or broadly enough to initiate the early expression of PDX1 in the embryonic gut and pancreatic buds, but the expression patterns of HNF6, HNF1β, Foxa1, and Foxa2 suggest that they could play this role (Fig. 47-2). Mice lacking HNF6 have reduced expression of PDX1,[53] and embryoid bodies lacking Foxa2 fail to activate the *pdx1* gene,[50] suggesting that these two factors may be bona fide activators of PDX1 expression in the prepancreatic endoderm and pancreatic buds and, therefore, lie directly upstream of PDX1 in the hierarchy of factors involved in initiating pancreas development (see Fig. 47-5).

PDX1 is required for the outgrowth of the pancreatic buds. In mice with targeted disruptions of the *pdx1* gene, the pancreatic buds fail to branch and expand after initial formation, yielding an animal that lacks a pancreas at birth.[38,39,54] Confirming their role upstream of PDX1 in the endoderm, lack of HNF6 results in reduced pancreatic size,[53] and removal of HB9 specifically arrests the growth of the dorsal pancreatic bud.[42,43] A homozygous null mutation in the *IPF1* gene, which encodes human PDX1, has also been identified in a human patient with pancreatic agenesis,[55] and mutations in the zebra fish gene encoding PDX1 also affect pancreas development,[56] reflecting an evolutionary conservation of PDX1 function.

Expression of PTF1 follows shortly after PDX1 and is restricted within the endoderm to the dorsal and ventral pancreatic buds.[57,58] The aorta induces expression of PTF1 in the dorsal pancreatic bud, but vascular-derived signals do not appear to play as critical a role in its expression in the ventral buds.[19] Although PTF1 was initially described as an exocrine-specific transcription factor,[41,58] in fact, it plays an essential role in determining pancreatic cell fate. In mouse embryos lacking PTF1, cells normally fated to contribute to both exocrine and endocrine lineages in the pancreas instead revert to duodenal epithelium.[40]

CELL TYPE DIFFERENTIATION

SIGNALING PATHWAYS

A number of embryonic signaling pathways regulate distinct aspects of pancreas organogenesis and endocrine cell differentiation. As discussed previously, TGF-β, FGF, and hedgehog

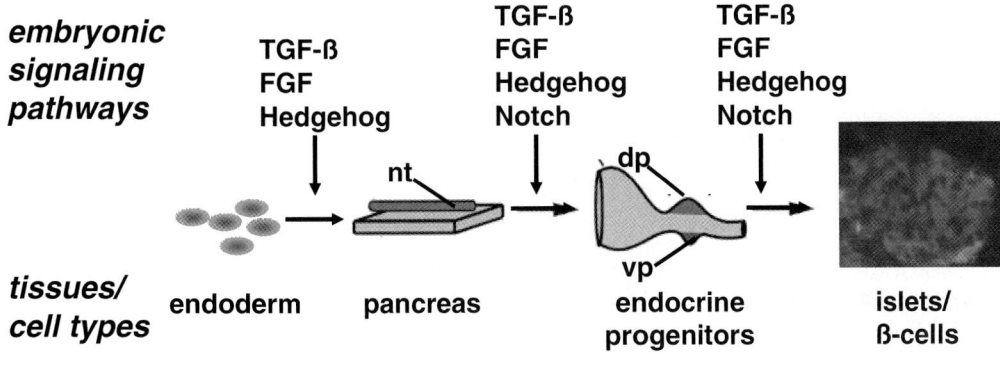

Figure 47-2 Embryonic signaling pathways regulate different steps of pancreas and endocrine islet formation. dp, dorsal pancreas; nt, notochord; vp, ventral pancreas.

signaling pathways coordinate initiation of pancreas formation. After bud formation, these pathways then play a role in the differentiation of the distinct cell types that form the mature pancreas.

FGF10 is expressed transiently in pancreatic mesenchyme at the time when the pancreatic buds expand. Transgenic mice carrying a homozygous deletion in the FGF10 gene display severe defects in pancreas morphogenesis that result from loss of Pdx1-positive, pancreatic epithelial progenitor cells.[59] FGF signaling has also been shown to regulate proliferation of endocrine and exocrine cells,[60,61] and expression of a dominant active form of the FGF receptor 2 (FGFR2) inhibits development of endocrine and exocrine cells.[60–62]

TGF-β/activin signaling has been shown to differentially affect exocrine and endocrine cell differentiation. Treatment of isolated pancreatic buds with soluble TGF-β1 stimulates differentiation of endocrine cells, particularly β- and PP cells.[63] Activin signaling also has been shown to preferentially affect endocrine cell differentiation. Treatment of pancreatic buds with Follistatin, an antagonist that physically binds to activins, inhibits endocrine cell differentiation while promoting exocrine cell formation.[64] Transgenic mice ectopically expressing dominant-negative activin type II receptor (dnAct RII) develop islet hypoplasia, a phenotype also observed in mice carrying targeted mutations in both the ActR IIA and ActR IIB genes.[65–67]

The role of hedgehog signaling during endocrine cell differentiation is less clear. At early stages, elevation of hedgehog signaling in the pancreas anlage results in transformation of the pancreatic mesenchyme into duodenal mesoderm.[16,68] Hedgehog signaling impairs pancreatic organogenesis, at least in part, due to the lack of signals normally provided by the pancreatic mesenchyme. Also, as has been shown for other organs, ectopic activation of hedgehog signaling reduces FGF10 expression known to promote pancreatic epithelial and endocrine cell expansion.[69,70] By contrast, low level of hedgehog signaling is detected throughout pancreas organogenesis and in mature islets.[71] In addition, cell culture experiments have revealed that hedgehog signaling activates the Pdx1 and insulin promoters in cultured insulinoma cells,[72,73] suggesting a different and potentially important role for the pathway in maintaining mature β-cell function. Due to early embryonic lethality prior to the initiation of pancreas formation, conventional knockout mice lacking all hedgehog signaling have not proven to be useful in determining whether pancreatic hedgehog signaling is essential for some aspects of pancreas organogenesis.[74] These questions await tissue-specific inactivation of the pathway in the pancreas.

In addition to the TGF-β, FGF, and hedgehog signaling pathways, notch signaling contributes to cell fate choices and differentiation in the pancreas, as it does in many other organs during embryogenesis. Notch signaling commonly regulates cell fate decision via a process known as lateral inhibition in which a given cell within a homogenous field of cells becomes less susceptible to ligand-activated notch signaling. As a consequence, this cell initiates a specific differentiation program while continuing to provide notch ligands to adjacent cells, thereby blocking the differentiation of its neighbors (Fig. 47-3).[75] A similar mechanism regulates the differentiation of endocrine cells during pancreas development. Reduction of notch pathway activity in transgenic mice lacking essential notch signaling components results in upregulation of expression of neurogenin3 (ngn3), a bHLH transcription factor required for endocrine formation[76] (see following section) and precocious endocrine differentiation.[77,78]

Furthermore, recent studies have revealed a role for notch signaling in other steps of pancreatic formation beyond lateral-inhibition. Ectopic expression of a constitutively active, truncated form of the notch 1 receptor at the onset of pancreas formation blocks both exocrine and endocrine cell differentiation, suggesting that notch signaling may normally

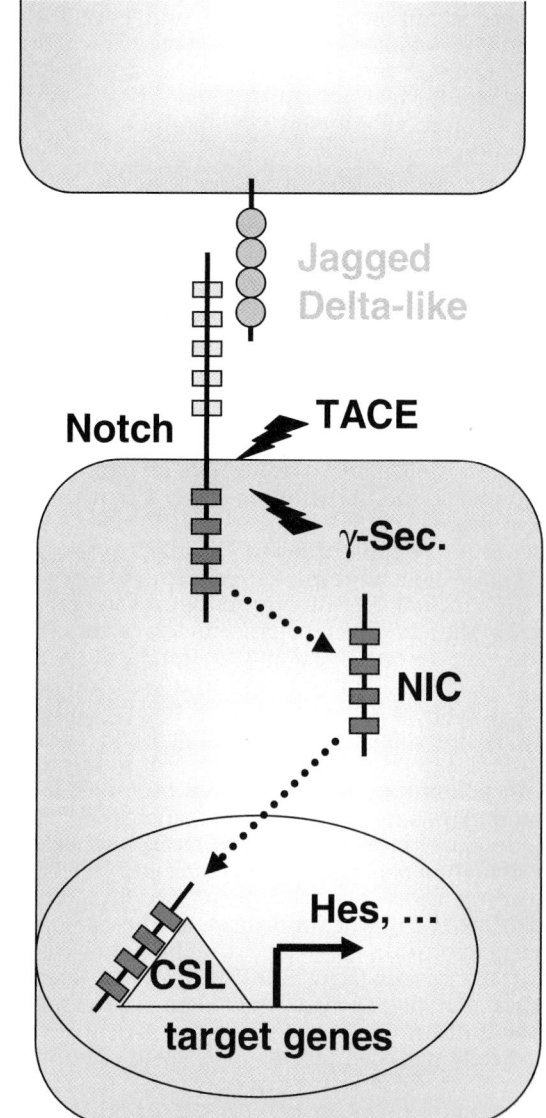

Figure 47-3 Notch signaling pathway. Binding of Jagged/Delta-like ligands to notch receptors activates notch signaling cascade. Two proteolytical events mediated by the tumor-necrosis factor-α converting enzyme (TACE) and γ-secretase (γ -Sec.) enzymes results in the generation of an intracellular notch fragment (NIC) that translocates from the membrane to the nucleus. Interaction with transcription factors from the CSL (CBF1/Suppressor of hairless/Lag-1) family activates transcription of notch target genes, including Hes genes known to block the transcription of ngn3.

allow the expansion of undifferentiated precursor cells.[79–81] Constitutive activation of notch signaling also blocks endocrine cell differentiation in ngn3-positive endocrine precursor cells. By contrast, notch activation in fully matured endocrine cells does not appear to be sufficient to change their differentiation status.[80]

While the exact mechanism of notch regulation during pancreas formation remains unresolved, recent evidence suggests that FGF signaling moderates notch activity during pancreas formation. Ectopic expression in pancreas epithelium of FGF10, a FGF ligand normally found in pancreatic mesenchyme, activates expression of notch ligands, receptors, and the notch target gene Hes1.[82,83] Given the recent evidence of interactions between embryonic signaling pathways during the formation of other organs, it will be critical to determine how these exchanges regulate pancreas development and pancreas cell differentiation.

TRANSCRIPTION FACTORS

The target of notch inhibition in the embryonic pancreas, bHLH factor ngn3, functions as a pro-endocrine factor: It is sufficient by itself to drive precursor cells to an endocrine fate.[77,84] When expressed broadly in the developing pancreatic bud, ngn3 can force all of the cells in the developing pancreas to differentiate prematurely into islet cells. Interestingly, ngn3 is expressed transiently, and predominantly during development in the pancreas in scattered ductal cells and occasional periductal cells, but it is never found in mature, hormone-producing cells. Together, these data support a model in which ngn3 acts upstream of other islet differentiation factors, initiating the differentiation of endocrine cells, but switching off prior to final differentiation. This conclusion is supported by the observation that mice homozygous for a targeted disruption of the *ngn3* gene fail to form any endocrine cells in the pancreas and do not express the other islet differentiation factors,[76] and by lineage tracing experiments.[85]

While notch signaling restricts ngn3 to scattered cells within the pancreatic epithelium, positive signals must initiate ngn3 expression in the absence of notch signaling. Studies of the ngn3 promoter implicate several transcription factors in this role, including HNF1, FoxA, and HNF6 (Fig. 47-4).[86,87] Only a role for HNF6 has been confirmed in vivo.[87]

Since ngn3 initiates, but does not complete, islet differentiation, it must induce a set of factors that complete the tasks of islet cell differentiation: determination and differentiation of islet cell subtype, formation and organization of islets, and function of the mature islet cells. However, only two direct targets of ngn3 have been identified, the bHLH factor NeuroD1 and the paired-homeodomain factor Pax4.

NeuroD1 expression initiates slightly later than ngn3 during pancreatic development, but unlike ngn3, it persists in the mature islet cells, where it plays a role in the expression of a number of differentiated endocrine cell products including insulin.[88–91] Ngn3 can bind to and activate the *neuroD1* gene promoter, and it can induce neuroD1 expression in *Xenopus* embryos[92] and pancreatic ductal cells.[93,94] Conversely, ngn3 null embryos completely lack neuroD1 expression in the pancreas,[76] while ngn3 expression is unchanged in neuroD1 null embryos.[84]

Just as it can with the *neuroD1* gene promoter, ngn3 binds to and activates the *pax4* gene promoter,[95] it can activate the intact gene in cultured cells,[94,96] and in its absence, pax4 expression is lost in the pancreas.[76] In addition, studies of the *pax4* gene promoter implicate the more broadly expressed endoderm factors HNF1 and HNF4 along with ngn3 in cooperative activation of Pax4 expression.[95,96]

Unlike NeuroD1, however, Pax4 expression is not induced in all islet lineages. Pax4, therefore, falls into a class of factors that play specific roles in the differentiation of the different islet cell subtypes. These factors can be grouped into the early group, factors like Pax4 and the NK homeodomain factors Nkx2.2[97] and Nkx6.1[98] that are coexpressed with ngn3 in endocrine progenitor cells,[84] and the late group, genes like the basic leucine zipper transcription factor MafA,[99] pdx1 (in a second phase of expression), pax6[100,101] and the pou-homeodomain factor Brn4,[84,102] that are expressed at the final stage of differentiation and are largely restricted to differentiated islet cells (Table 47-1). It is not clear whether any of these genes can actually determine the cell-type fate of the cell in which they are expressed, or if they simply complete the differentiation process initiated by other genes.

Once ngn3 is expressed in an appropriate progenitor, that cell is destined to become an islet cell. But the decision as to which of the four islet cell types it will become is apparently controlled by other factors. Ectopic broad expression of ngn3 in the developing pancreatic bud causes uniform and precocious endocrine differentiation, but almost all of those endocrine cells are α cells with very few, if any, β cells.[77,84] It can be hypothesized, therefore, that the α cell is the default fate of cells that express ngn3, and the intervention of specific determination factors is required to deviate to one of the other islet cell types. The identity of the factors that determine individual islet subtype fates remain to be determined.

ISLET FORMATION

Endocrine cell differentiation, including insulin and glucagon positive cells, can be detected shortly after the pancreatic buds form, but these cells are immature and do not contribute to the mature islets. Mature β cells form during the secondary transition at approximately E13–E14 in the mouse. At this time, endocrine precursor cells leave the endodermal epithelium and migrate through the adjacent extracellular matrix into the surrounding mesenchyme.

Cell culture assays have implicated matrix metalloproteinases in this process, although experimental evidence from in vivo studies supporting these results are currently missing.[103] Cell attachment to and migration through the extracellular matrix is mediated by integrins, heterodimeric transmembrane proteins that serve as extracellular matrix receptors.[104] Functional evidence for an essential role of integrins during migration of islet precursors comes from in vivo studies in which islet formation in human fetal pancreas transplanted under the kidney capsule of recipient mice was inhibited by injection of integrin-blocking peptides.[105] The

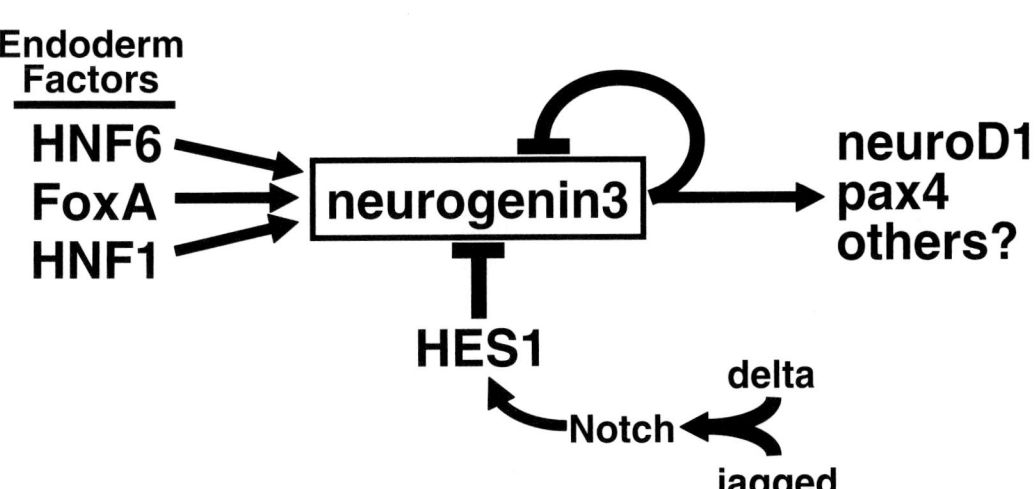

Figure 47-4 Control of neurogenin3 expression. A model is shown for the positive and negative regulation of neurogenin3 expression in the pancreatic endocrine progenitor cells.

Table 47-1 Pancreas Transcription Factors

Factor	Family	Expression	Downstream Pancreatic Genes	Mouse Mutations*	Human Mutations	References
Neurogenin 3	bHLH	Fetal pancreas (endocrine progenitor cells) and CNS	NeuroD1/BETA2, pax4, nkx2.2	Diabetes, no islet cells		(76, 77, 84, 92, 115)
NeuroD1/BETA2	bHLH	Islet, gut endocrine cells, CNS	Insulin	Diabetes, decreased islet cells	Het: MODY6, late-onset diabetes	(91, 113, 116–119)
P48/PTF1	bHLH	Exocrine pancreas, CNS	Exocrine enzyme genes	Exocrine pancreatic agenesis, islets in spleen		(41, 57, 58)
Mist1	bHLH	Exocrine pancreas, serous exocrine cells		Exocrine pancreas disorganization		(120–122)
PDX1/IPF1	Parahox homeodomain	β and δ cells, duodenum, stomach, CNS	Insulin, IAPP, glucokinase, glut2	Pancreatic agenesis	Het:MODY4 Hom: pancreatic agenesis	(37–39, 54, 55, 111, 123–129)
HB9	Parahox homeodomain	β cells, gut, lymphoid, CNS	Glut2	Dorsal pancreatic agenesis	Het: Sacral agenesis	(42, 43, 130)
Pax2	Paired domain	Islet, urogenital tract and CNS	Glucagon	Defects in optic nerve, CNS and urogenital tract	Het: renal-coloboma syndrome	(131, 132)
Pax4	Paired homeodomain	Fetal pancreas and CNS	Pax4 (autorepression)	Decreased β and δ cells	Het: late onset diabetes Hom: early diabetes	(95, 133–135)
Pax6	Paired homeodomain	Islet, gut endocrine cells, CNS	Glucagon, insulin, somatostatin	Decrease in all islet cells, decreased glucagon	Het: Aniridia	(100, 101, 136)
Arx	Paired-related homeodomain	α and δ cells and CNS		Decreased α cells		(137)
Nkx2.2	NK homeodomain	β, α, and PP cells and CNS	nkx6.1 insulin, glut2, GK	Diabetes, no insulin		(97, 98, 138, 139)
Nkx6.1	NK homeodomain	β cells and CNS		Decreased β cells, postnatal lethal		(97, 98, 138, 140)
Cdx2/3	Caudal homeodomain	Islet and gut	Glucagon	Het: gut tumors Hom: Embryonic lethal		(141–145)
Isl1	LIM homeodomain	Islet and CNS	Somatostatin, glucagon	No islet cells, embryonic lethal		(99, 114, 146–150)
Lmx1.1	LIM homeodomain	β cells and CNS	Insulin	Dreher: roof plate, cerebellum defects	Het: late onset diabetes	(88, 141, 151)
Brn4	Pou homeodomain	α cells and CNS	Glucagon		Hom: Congenital neurogenic deafness	(102, 115, 152)
HNF1α	Pou homeodomain	Islet, liver, kidney	pax4, neurogenin3, glut2, Rat insulin I	Diabetes, impaired β-cell glucose sensing	Het: MODY3	(35, 86, 95, 110, 153–155)
HNF1β	Pou homeodomain	Islet, pancreatic duct, liver, kidney	pax4, PDX1	Embryonic lethal	Het: MODY5	(95, 112, 156, 157)
HNF6	Cut homeodomain	Pancreatic duct, liver	neurogenin3	IGT, small islets Hypoglycemia		(27, 28, 86, 87, 158, 159)
Foxa1/HNF 3α	Forkhead/winged helix	Islet, gut, liver	glucagon			(160, 161)
Foxa2/HNF 3β	Forkhead/winged helix	Islet, pancreatic duct, gut, liver, CNS	PDX1, neurogenin3, kir6.2, sur1	Embryonic lethal		(27, 44, 45, 50, 86, 159, 162–164)
Foxa3/HNF 3γ	Forkhead/winged Helix	Islet, gut, liver	Glucagon	No pancreatic phenotype		(165–167)
HNF4α	Nuclear receptor	Liver, islet, kidney	HNF1α, glycolytic enzymes, pax4	Embryonic lethal	Het: MODY1	(25, 95, 109, 162, 168, 169)
MafA	bZip	β cells, eye and thymus	Insulin			(170–172)
c-Maf	bZip	α cells, eye	Glucagon			(170)

*All mouse phenotypes are for homozygous mutant animals unless stated otherwise.

CNS, central nervous system; GK, glucokinase; het, heterozygous; hom, homozygous; IAPP, islet amyloid polypeptide.

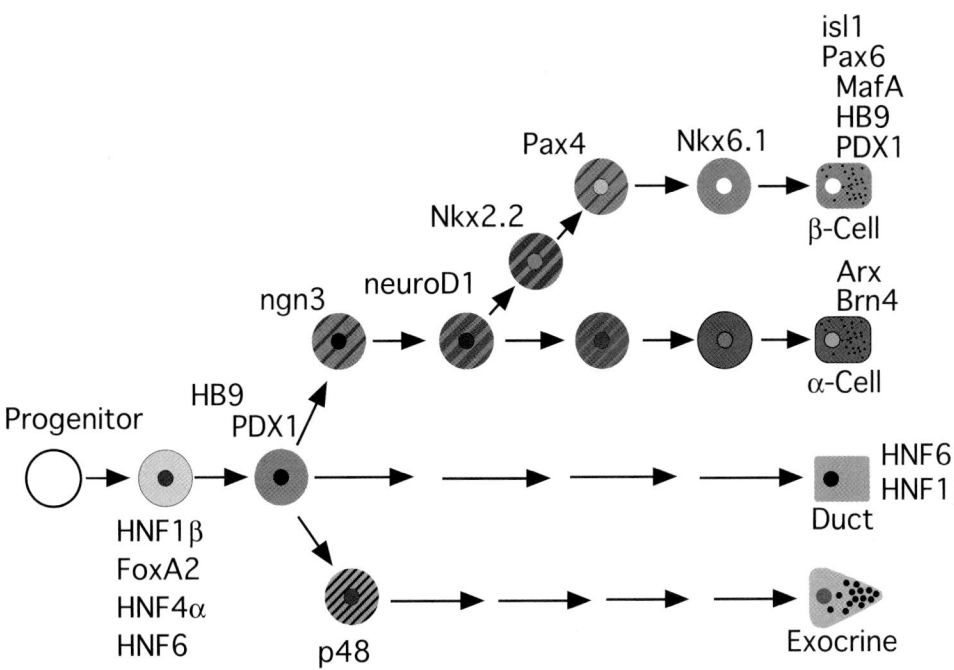

Figure 47-5 A simplified model for the role of islet transcription factors in endocrine differentiation in the developing pancreas. The proposed position for each transcription factor is based on its timing of expression, timing of predominant functional role, or both. Clearly, some factors function at several steps, but a single step is shown for simplicity.

integrin family comprises a large number of different members with distinct substrate specificities. A recent study reveals that fetal and mature human β cells express different repertoires of integrins.[106] Changes in integrin composition might explain why fetal β cells are more motile than their adult counterparts, a difference that might also provide insights into the molecular mechanisms that prevent dispersion of endocrine cells once mature islet structures have formed.

Nonetheless, a number of open questions remain with regard to the regulation of islet progenitor migration and islet formation. For example, studies using transgenic animals have shown that a given islet originates from several independent endocrine precursors.[107] Thus, endocrine cells delaminating from the ductal structures during embryogenesis must follow a specific guiding mechanism that coordinates their migration path toward a specific location. While cell migration has been well studied in neural cells that respond to attractive and repulsive guidance cues, a putative, localized source of chemoattractant molecules that stimulate islet precursor migration has not been identified. Furthermore, evidence from studies in human diabetic patients suggests neogenesis of endocrine cells throughout life.[108] While still controversial, some endocrine cells appear to form away from already existing islets raising the question whether these cells migrate toward already formed islets or cluster with other newly formed endocrine cells to initiate aggregation of new islet. In either case, it is likely that specific, as yet unidentified, guidance mechanisms control these processes.

THE ROLE OF PANCREATIC DEVELOPMENT IN HUMAN DIABETES

One beneficial consequence of our improving understanding of pancreatic islet development has been new insights into human diabetes. Short-term energy balance and the control of plasma glucose levels depend on the ability of the β cells to sense changes in nutrient status and respond with appropriate insulin production and secretion. This fine-tuned capability develops along with morphologic development of the islets, and depends on an adequate number of β cells with precisely functioning gene expression programs placed in the appropriate local environment. Any flaws in pancreatic islet development, therefore, can potentially lead to impaired insulin secretion and diabetes.

As a consequence, not surprisingly, mutations in a number of human genes involved in pancreatic islet development, especially the transcription factor genes, can lead to diabetes (see Table 47-1). Transcription factors found in Figure 47-5 account for five of the six genes known to cause maturity onset diabetes of the young.[36,109–113] In addition, mutations in the coding sequence of isl1 and pax4 have been implicated in families with later onset diabetes.[113,114] Analysis of these mutations has given insight into the process by which β-cell dysfunction may lead to the development of diabetes.

REFERENCES

1. Tam PP, Kanai-Azuma M, Kanai Y: Early endoderm development in vertebrates: Lineage differentiation and morphogenetic function. Curr Opin Genet Dev 13:393, 2003.
2. Ober EA, Field HA, Stainier DY: From endoderm formation to liver and pancreas development in zebrafish. Mech Dev 120:5, 2003.
3. Wells JM, Melton DA: Vertebrate endoderm development. Annu Rev Cell Dev Biol 15:393, 1999.
4. Pictet R, Rutter WJ: Development of the embryonic endocrine pancreas. In

Steiner DF, Frenkel N (eds): Handbook of Physiology Society. Washington, DC, Williams & Wilkins, 1972, p 25
5. Slack JM: Developmental biology of the pancreas. Development 121:1569, 1995.
6. Kim SK, Hebrok M, Melton DA: Notochord to endoderm signaling is required for pancreas development. Development 124:4243, 1997.
7. Kumar M, Jordan N, Melton D, Grapin-Botton A: Signals from lateral plate mesoderm instruct endoderm toward a pancreatic fate. Dev Biol 259:109, 2003.

8. Lammert E, Cleaver O, Melton D: Role of endothelial cells in early pancreas and liver development. Mech Dev 120:59, 2003.
9. Hill D, Lebenthal E: Congenital abnormalities of the exocrine pancreas. In Go VLW, Dimagno EP, Gardner JD, et al (eds): The Pancreas: Biology, Pathobiology, and Disease, 2d ed. New York, Raven Press Ltd, 1993, p 1029
10. Golosow N, Grobstein C: Epitheliomesenchymal interaction in pancreatic morphogenesis. Dev Biol 4:242, 1962.

11. Wessells NK, Cohen JH: Early pancreas organogenesis: Morphogenesis, tissue interactions and mass effects. Dev Biol 15:237, 1967.

12. Pictet RL, Rall LB, Phelps P, Rutter WJ: The neural crest and the origin of the insulin-producing and other gastrointestinal hormone-producing cells. Science 191:191, 1976.

13. Fontaine J, Le Douarin NM: Analysis of endoderm formation in the avian blastoderm by the use of quail-chick chimaeras. The problem of the neurectodermal origin of the cells of the APUD series. J Embryol Exp Morphol 41:209, 1977.

14. Le Douarin NM: On the origin of pancreatic endocrine cells. Cell 53:169, 1988.

15. Wells JM, Melton DA: Early mouse endoderm is patterned by soluble factors from adjacent germ layers. Development 127:1563, 2000.

16. Hebrok M, Kim SK, Melton DA: Notochord repression of endodermal Sonic hedgehog permits pancreas development. Genes Dev 12:1705, 1998.

17. Deutsch G, Jung J, Zheng M, et al: A bipotential precursor population for pancreas and liver within the embryonic endoderm. Development 128:871, 2001.

18. Lammert E, Cleaver O, Melton D: Induction of pancreatic differentiation by signals from blood vessels. Science 294:564, 2001.

19. Yoshitomi H, Zaret KS: Endothelial cell interactions initiate dorsal pancreas development by selectively inducing the transcription factor Ptf1a. Development 131:807, 2004.

20. Pictet RL, Clark WR, Williams RH, Rutter WJ: An ultrastructural analysis of the developing embryonic pancreas. Dev Biol 29:436, 1972.

21. Li Z, Manna P, Kobayashi H, et al: Multifaceted pancreatic mesenchymal control of epithelial lineage selection. Dev Biol 269:252, 2004.

22. Gittes GK, Galante PE, Hanahan D, et al: Lineage-specific morphogenesis in the developing pancreas: Role of mesenchymal factors. Development 122:439, 1996.

23. Ott MO, Rey-Campos J, Cereghini S, Yaniv M: vHNF1 is expressed in epithelial cells of distinct embryonic origin during development and precedes HNF1 expression. Mech Dev 36:47, 1991.

24. Monaghan AP, Kaestner KH, Grau E, Schutz G: Postimplantation expression patterns indicate a role for the mouse forkhead/HNF-3 alpha, beta and gamma genes in determination of the definitive endoderm, chordamesoderm and neuroectoderm. Development 119:567, 1993.

25. Duncan SA, Manova K, Chen WS, et al: Expression of transcription factor HNF-4 in the extraembryonic endoderm, gut, and nephrogenic tissue of the developing mouse embryo: HNF-4 is a marker for primary endoderm in the implanting blastocyst. Proc Natl Acad Sci U S A 91:7598, 1994.

26. Taraviras S, Monaghan AP, Schutz G, Kelsey G: Characterization of the mouse HNF-4 gene and its expression during mouse embryogenesis. Mech Dev 48:67, 1994.

27. Rausa F, Samadani U, Ye H, et al: The cut-homeodomain transcriptional activator HNF-6 is coexpressed with its target gene HNF-3 beta in the developing murine liver and pancreas. Dev Biol 192:228, 1997.

28. Landry C, Clotman F, Hioki T, et al: HNF-6 is expressed in endoderm derivatives and nervous system of the mouse embryo and participates to the cross-regulatory network of liver-enriched transcription factors. Dev Biol 192:247, 1997.

29. Arceci RJ, King AA, Simon MC, et al: Mouse GATA-4: A retinoic acid-inducible GATA-binding transcription factor expressed in endodermally derived tissues and heart. Mol Cell Biol 13:2235, 1993.

30. Laverriere AC, MacNeill C, Mueller C, et al: GATA-4/5/6, a subfamily of three transcription factors transcribed in developing heart and gut. J Biol Chem 269:23177, 1994.

31. Zaret KS: Molecular genetics of early liver development. Annu Rev Physiol 58:231, 1996.

32. Cereghini S: Liver-enriched transcription factors and hepatocyte differentiation. FASEB J 10:267, 1996.

33. Zaret K: Developmental competence of the gut endoderm: Genetic potentiation by GATA and HNF3/fork head proteins. Dev Biol 209:1, 1999.

34. Boj SF, Parrizas M, Maestro MA, Ferrer J: A transcription factor regulatory circuit in differentiated pancreatic cells. Proc Natl Acad Sci U S A 98:14481, 2001.

35. Shih DQ, Screenan S, Munoz KN, et al: Loss of HNF-1alpha function in mice leads to abnormal expression of genes involved in pancreatic islet development and metabolism. Diabetes 50:2472, 2001.

36. Shih DQ, Stoffel M: Dissecting the transcriptional network of pancreatic islets during development and differentiation. Proc Natl Acad Sci U S A 98:14189, 2001.

37. Guz Y, Montminy MR, Stein R, et al: Expression of murine STF-1, a putative insulin gene transcription factor, in beta cells of pancreas, duodenal epithelium and pancreatic exocrine and endocrine progenitors during ontogeny. Development 121:11–18, 1995.

38. Ahlgren U, Jonsson J, Edlund H: The morphogenesis of the pancreatic mesenchyme is uncoupled from that of the pancreatic epithelium in IPF1/PDX1-deficient mice. Development 122:1409, 1996.

39. Offield MF, Jetton TL, Labosky PA, et al: PDX-1 is required for pancreatic outgrowth and differentiation of the rostral duodenum. Development 122:983, 1996.

40. Kawaguchi Y, Cooper B, Gannon M, et al: The role of the transcriptional regulator Ptf1a in converting intestinal to pancreatic progenitors. Nat Genet 32:128, 2002.

41. Krapp A, Knofler M, Frutiger S, et al: The p48 DNA-binding subunit of transcription factor PTF1 is a new exocrine pancreas-specific basic helix-loop-helix protein. EMBO J 15:4317, 1996.

42. Li H, Arber S, Jessell TM, Edlund H: Selective agenesis of the dorsal pancreas in mice lacking homeobox gene Hlxb9. Nat Genet 23:67, 1999.

43. Harrison KA, Thaler J, Pfaff SL, et al: Pancreas dorsal lobe agenesis and abnormal islets of Langerhans in Hlxb9-deficient mice. Nat Genet 23:71, 1999.

44. Sharma S, Jhala US, Johnson T, et al: Hormonal regulation of an islet-specific enhancer in the pancreatic homeobox gene STF-1. Mol Cell Biol 17:2598, 1997.

45. Wu KL, Gannon M, Peshavaria M, et al: Hepatocyte nuclear factor 3beta is involved in pancreatic beta-cell-specific transcription of the pdx-1 gene. Mol Cell Biol 17:6002, 1997.

46. Stoffers DA, Heller RS, Miller CP, Habener JF: Developmental expression of the homeodomain protein IDX-1 in mice transgenic for an IDX-1 promoter/lacZ transcriptional reporter. Endocrinology 140:5374, 1999.

47. Ben-Shushan E, Marshak S, Shoshkes M, et al: A pancreatic beta-cell-specific enhancer in the human PDX-1 gene is regulated by hepatocyte nuclear factor 3beta (HNF-3beta), HNF-1alpha, and SPs transcription factors. J Biol Chem 276:17533, 2001.

48. Marshak S, Ben-Shushan E, Shoshkes M, et al: Regulatory elements involved in human pdx-1 gene expression. Diabetes 50 (Suppl 1):S37, 2001.

49. Gerrish K, Cissell MA, Stein R: The role of hepatic nuclear factor 1 alpha and PDX-1 in transcriptional regulation of the pdx-1 gene. J Biol Chem 276:47775, 2001.

50. Gerrish K, Gannon M, Shih D, et al: Pancreatic beta cell-specific transcription of the pdx-1 gene. The role of conserved upstream control regions and their hepatic nuclear factor 3beta sites. J Biol Chem 275:3485, 2000.

51. Samaras SE, Cissell MA, Gerrish K, et al: Conserved sequences in a tissue-specific regulatory region of the pdx-1 gene mediate transcription in pancreatic beta cells: Role for hepatocyte nuclear factor 3beta and Pax6. Mol Cell Biol 22:4702, 2002.

52. Marshak S, Benshushan E, Shoshkes M, et al: Functional conservation of regulatory elements in the pdx-1 gene: PDX-1 and hepatocyte nuclear factor 3beta transcription factors mediate beta-cell-specific expression. Mol Cell Biol 20:7583, 2000.

53. Jacquemin P, Lemaigre FP, Rousseau GG: The Onecut transcription factor HNF-6 (OC-1) is required for timely

specification of the pancreas and acts upstream of Pdx-1 in the specification cascade. Dev Biol 258:105, 2003.

54. Jonsson J, Carlsson L, Edlund T, Edlund H: Insulin-promoter-factor 1 is required for pancreas development in mice. Nature 371:606, 1994.

55. Stoffers DA, Zinkin NT, Stanojevic V, et al: Pancreatic agenesis attributable to a single nucleotide deletion in the human IPF1 gene coding sequence. Nat Genet 15:106, 1997.

56. Yee NS, Yusuff S, Pack M: Zebrafish pdx1 morphant displays defects in pancreas development and digestive organ chirality, and potentially identifies a multipotent pancreas progenitor cell. Genesis 30:137, 2001.

57. Obata J, Yano M, Mimura H, et al: p48 subunit of mouse PTF1 binds to RBP-Jkappa/CBF-1, the intracellular mediator of Notch signalling, and is expressed in the neural tube of early stage embryos. Genes Cells 6:345, 2001.

58. Krapp A, Knofler M, Ledermann B, et al: The bHLH protein PTF1-p48 is essential for the formation of the exocrine and the correct spatial organization of the endocrine pancreas. Genes Dev 12:3752, 1998.

59. Bhushan A, Itoh N, Kato S, et al: Fgf10 is essential for maintaining the proliferative capacity of epithelial progenitor cells during early pancreatic organogenesis. Development 128:5109, 2001.

60. Le Bras S, Miralles F, Basmaciogullari A, et al: Fibroblast growth factor 2 promotes pancreatic epithelial cell proliferation via functional fibroblast growth factor receptors during embryonic life. Diabetes 47:1236, 1998.

61. Miralles F, Czernichow P, Ozaki K, et al: Signaling through fibroblast growth factor receptor 2b plays a key role in the development of the exocrine pancreas. Proc Natl Acad Sci U S A 96:6267, 1999.

62. Celli G, LaRochelle WJ, Mackem S, et al: Soluble dominant-negative receptor uncovers essential roles for fibroblast growth factors in multi-organ induction and patterning. EMBO J 17:1642, 1998.

63. Sanvito F, Herrera PL, Huarte J, et al: TGF-beta 1 influences the relative development of the exocrine and endocrine pancreas in vitro. Development 120:3451–3462, 1994.

64. Miralles F, Czernichow P, Scharfmann R: Follistatin regulates the relative proportions of endocrine versus exocrine tissue during pancreatic development. Development 125:1017, 1998.

65. Shiozaki S, Tajima T, Zhang YQ, et al: I. Impaired differentiation of endocrine and exocrine cells of the pancreas in transgenic mouse expressing the truncated type II activin receptor. Biochim Biophys Acta 1450:1, 1999.

66. Yamaoka T, Idehara C, Yano M, et al: Hypoplasia of pancreatic islets in transgenic mice expressing activin receptor mutants. J Clin Invest 102:294, 1998.

67. Kim SK, Hebrok M, Li E, et al: Activin receptor patterning of foregut organogenesis. Genes Dev 14:1866, 2000.

68. Apelqvist A, Ahlgren U, Edlund H: Sonic hedgehog directs specialised mesoderm differentiation in the intestine and pancreas. Curr Biol 7:801, 1997.

69. Kawahira H, Ma NH, Tzanakakis ES, et al: Combined activities of Hedgehog signaling inhibitors regulate pancreas development. Development 130:4871–4879, 2003.

70. Chuang PT, Kawcak T, McMahon AP: Feedback control of mammalian Hedgehog signaling by the Hedgehog-binding protein, Hip1, modulates Fgf signaling during branching morphogenesis of the lung. Genes Dev 17:342, 2003.

71. Hebrok M, Kim SK, St Jacques B, et al: Regulation of pancreas development by hedgehog signaling. Development 127:4905, 2000.

72. Thomas MK, Lee JH, Rastalsky N, Habener JF: Hedgehog signaling regulation of homeodomain protein islet duodenum homeobox-1 expression in pancreatic beta-cells. Endocrinology 142:1033, 2001.

73. Thomas MK, Rastalsky N, Lee JH, Habener JF: Hedgehog signaling regulation of insulin production by pancreatic beta-cells. Diabetes 49:2039, 2000.

74. Zhang J, Rosenthal A, de Sauvage FJ, Shivdasani RA: Downregulation of Hedgehog signaling is required for organogenesis of the small intestine in Xenopus. Dev Biol 229:188, 2001.

75. Artavanis-Tsakonas S, Rand MD, Lake RJ: Notch signaling: Cell fate control and signal integration in development. Science 284:770, 1999.

76. Gradwohl G, Dierich A, LeMeur M, Guillemot F: Neurogenin3 is required for the development of the four endocrine cell lineages of the pancreas. Proc Natl Acad Sci U S A 97:1607, 2000.

77. Apelqvist A, Li H, Sommer L, et al: Notch signaling controls pancreatic cell differentiation. Nature 400:877, 1999.

78. Jensen J, Pedersen EE, Galante P, et al: Control of endodermal endocrine development by Hes-1. Nat Genet 24:36, 2000.

79. Hald J, Hjorth JP, German MS, et al: Activated Notch1 prevents differentiation of pancreatic acinar cells and attenuate endocrine development. Dev Biol 260:426, 2003.

80. Murtaugh LC, Stanger BZ, Kwan KM, Melton DA: Notch signaling controls multiple steps of pancreatic differentiation. Proc Natl Acad Sci U S A 100:14920, 2003.

81. Esni F, Ghosh B, Biankin AV, et al: Notch inhibits Ptf1 function and acinar cell differentiation in developing mouse and zebrafish pancreas. Development 131:4213, 2004.

82. Hart A, Papadopoulou S, Edlund H: Fgf10 maintains notch activation, stimulates proliferation, and blocks differentiation of pancreatic epithelial cells. Dev Dyn 228:185, 2003.

83. Norgaard GA, Jensen JN, Jensen J: FGF10 signaling maintains the pancreatic progenitor cell state revealing a novel role of Notch in organ development. Dev Biol 264:323, 2003.

84. Schwitzgebel VM, Scheel DW, Conners JR, et al: Expression of neurogenin3 reveals an islet cell precursor population in the pancreas. Development 127:3533, 2000.

85. Gu G, Dubauskaite J, Melton DA: Direct evidence for the pancreatic lineage: NGN3+ cells are islet progenitors and are distinct from duct progenitors. Development 129:2447, 2002.

86. Lee JC, Smith SB, Watada H, et al: Regulation of the pancreatic pro-endocrine gene neurogenin3. Diabetes 50:928, 2001.

87. Jacquemin P, Durviaux SM, Jensen J, et al: Transcription factor hepatocyte nuclear factor 6 regulates pancreatic endocrine cell differentiation and controls expression of the proendocrine gene ngn3. Mol Cell Biol 20:4445, 2000.

88. Ohneda K, Mirmira RG, Wang J, et al: The homeodomain of PDX-1 mediates multiple protein-protein interactions in the formation of a transcriptional activation complex on the insulin promoter. Mol Cell Biol 20:900, 2000.

89. Glick E, Leshkowitz D, Walker MD: Transcription factor BETA2 acts cooperatively with E2A and PDX1 to activate the insulin gene promoter. J Biol Chem 275:2199, 2000.

90. Qiu Y, Guo M, Huang S, Stein R: Insulin gene transcription is mediated by interactions between the p300 coactivator and PDX-1, BETA2, and E47. Mol Cell Biol 22:412, 2002.

91. Naya FJ, Stellrecht CM, Tsai MJ: Tissue-specific regulation of the insulin gene by a novel basic helix-loop-helix transcription factor. Genes Dev 9:1009, 1995.

92. Huang HP, Liu M, El-Hodiri HM, et al: Regulation of the pancreatic islet-specific gene BETA2 (neuroD) by neurogenin 3. Mol Cell Biol 20:3292, 2000.

93. Heremans Y, Van De Casteele M, in't Veld P, et al: Recapitulation of embryonic neuroendocrine differentiation in adult human pancreatic duct cells expressing neurogenin 3. J Cell Biol 159:303, 2002.

94. Gasa R, Mrejen C, Leachman N, et al: Proendocrine genes coordinate the pancreatic islet differentiation program in vitro. Proc Natl Acad Sci U S A 101:13245, 2004.

95. Smith SB, Watada H, Scheel DW, et al: Autoregulation and maturity onset diabetes of the young transcription factors control the human PAX4 promoter. J Biol Chem 275:36910, 2000.

96. Smith SB, Gasa R, Watada H, et al: Neurogenin3 and hepatic nuclear factor 1 cooperate in activating pancreatic expression of Pax4. J Biol Chem 278: 38254–38259, 2003.

97. Sussel L, Kalamaras J, Hartigan-O'Connor DJ, et al: Mice lacking the homeodomain transcription factor Nkx2.2 have diabetes due to arrested differentiation of pancreatic beta cells. Development 125:2213, 1998.

98. Sander M, Sussel L, Conners J, et al: Homeobox gene Nkx6.1 lies downstream of Nkx2.2 in the major pathway of beta-cell formation in the pancreas. Development 127:5533, 2000.

99. Ahlgren U, Pfaff SL, Jessell TM, et al: Independent requirement for ISL1 in formation of pancreatic mesenchyme and islet cells. Nature 385:257, 1997.

100. Sander M, Neubuser A, Kalamaras J, et al: Genetic analysis reveals that PAX6 is required for normal transcription of pancreatic hormone genes and islet development. Genes Dev 11:1662, 1997.

101. St-Onge L, Sosa-Pineda B, Chowdhury K, et al: Pax6 is required for differentiation of glucagon-producing alpha-cells in mouse pancreas. Nature 387:406, 1997.

102. Hussain MA, Lee J, Miller CP, Habener JF: POU domain transcription factor brain 4 confers pancreatic alpha-cell-specific expression of the proglucagon gene through interaction with a novel proximal promoter G1 element. Mol Cell Biol 17:7186, 1997.

103. Miralles F, Battelino T, Czernichow P, Scharfmann R: TGF-beta plays a key role in morphogenesis of the pancreatic islets of Langerhans by controlling the activity of the matrix metalloproteinase MMP-2. J Cell Biol 143:827, 1998.

104. Hynes R: Integrins. Bidirectional, allosteric signaling machines. Cell 110:673, 2002.

105. Cirulli V, Beattie GM, Klier G, et al: Expression and function of alpha(v)beta(3) and alpha(v)beta(5) integrins in the developing pancreas. Roles In the adhesion and migration of putative endocrine progenitor cells [In Process Citation]. J Cell Biol 150:1445, 2000.

106. Kaido T, Perez B, Yebra M, et al: Alphav-integrin utilization in human beta-cell adhesion, spreading, and motility. J Biol Chem 279:17731, 2004.

107. Deltour L, Leduque P, Paldi A, et al: Polyclonal origin of pancreatic islets in aggregation mouse chimaeras. Development 112:1115–1121, 1991.

108. Butler AE, Janson J, Bonner-Weir S, et al: Beta-cell deficit and increased beta-cell apoptosis in humans with type 2 diabetes. Diabetes 52:102, 2003.

109. Yamagata K, Furuta H, Oda N, et al: Mutations in the hepatocyte nuclear factor-4alpha gene in maturity-onset diabetes of the young (MODY1). Nature 384:458, 1996.

110. Yamagata K, Oda N, Kaisaki P, et al: Mutations in the hepatocyte nuclear factor-1alpha gene in maturity-onset diabetes of the young (MODY3). Nature 384:455, 1996.

111. Stoffers DA, Ferrer J, Clarke WL, Habener JF: Early-onset type-II diabetes mellitus (MODY4) linked to IPF1 [letter]. Nat Genet 17:138, 1997.

112. Horikawa Y, Iwasaki N, Hara M, et al: Mutation in hepatocyte nuclear factor-1 beta gene (TCF2) associated with MODY [letter]. Nat Genet 17:384, 1997.

113. Malecki MT, Jhala US, Antonellis A, et al: Mutations in NEUROD1 are associated with the development of type 2 diabetes mellitus. Nat Genet 23:323, 1999.

114. Shimomura H, Sanke T, Hanabusa T, et al: Nonsense mutation of islet-1 gene (Q310X) found in a type 2 diabetic patient with a strong family history. Diabetes 49:1597, 2000.

115. Jensen J, Heller RS, Funder-Nielsen T, et al: Independent development of pancreatic alpha- and beta-cells from neurogenin3-expressing precursors: A role for the notch pathway in repression of premature differentiation. Diabetes 49:163, 2000.

116. Lee JE, Hollenberg SM, Snider L, et al: Conversion of Xenopus ectoderm into neurons by NeuroD, a basic helix-loop-helix protein. Science 268:836, 1995.

117. Naya FJ, Huang HP, Qiu Y, et al: Diabetes, defective pancreatic morphogenesis, and abnormal enteroendocrine differentiation in BETA2/neuroD-deficient mice. Genes Dev 11:2323, 1997.

118. Mutoh H, Naya FJ, Tsai MJ, Leiter AB: The basic helix-loop-helix protein BETA2 interacts with p300 to coordinate differentiation of secretin-expressing enteroendocrine cells. Genes Dev 12:820, 1998.

119. Qiu Y, Sharma A, Stein R: p300 mediates transcriptional stimulation by the basic helix-loop-helix activators of the insulin gene. Mol Cell Biol 18:2957, 1998.

120. Pin CL, Rukstalis JM, Johnson C, Konieczny SF: The bHLH transcription factor Mist1 is required to maintain exocrine pancreas cell organization and acinar cell identity. J Cell Biol 155:519, 2001.

121. Pin CL, Bonvissuto AC, Konieczny SF: Mist1 expression is a common link among serous exocrine cells exhibiting regulated exocytosis. Anat Rec 259:157, 2000.

122. Lemercier C, To RQ, Swanson BJ, et al: Mist1: A novel basic helix-loop-helix transcription factor exhibits a developmentally regulated expression pattern. Dev Biol 182:101, 1997.

123. Waeber G, Thompson N, Nicod P, Bonny C: Transcriptional activation of the GLUT2 gene by the IPF-1/STF-1/IDX-1 homeobox factor. Mol Endocrinol 10:1327, 1996.

124. Ahlgren U, Jonsson J, Jonsson L: Beta-cell-specific inactivation of the mouse Ipf1/Pdx1 gene results in loss of the beta-cell phenotype and maturity onset diabetes. Genes Dev 12:1763, 1998.

125. Watada H, Kajimoto Y, Umayahara Y, et al: The human glucokinase gene beta-cell-type promoter: An essential role of insulin promoter factor 1/PDX-1 in its activation in HIT-T15 cells. Diabetes 45:1478, 1996.

126. Watada H, Kajimoto Y, Miyagawa J, et al: PDX-1 induces insulin and glucokinase gene expressions in alphaTC1 clone 6 cells in the presence of betacellulin. Diabetes 45:1826, 1996.

127. Watada H, Kajimoto Y, Kaneto H, et al: Involvement of the homeodomain-containing transcription factor PDX-1 in islet amyloid polypeptide gene transcription. Biochem Biophys Res Commun 229:746, 1996.

128. Schwartz PT, Perez-Villamil B, Rivera A, et al: Pancreatic homeodomain transcription factor IDX1/IPF1 expressed in developing brain regulates somatostatin gene transcription in embryonic neural cells. J Biol Chem 275:19106, 2000.

129. Perez-Villamil B, Schwartz PT, Vallejo M: The pancreatic homeodomain transcription factor IDX1/IPF1 is expressed in neural cells during brain development. Endocrinology 140:3857, 1999.

130. Harrison KA, Druey KM, Deguchi Y, et al: A novel human homeobox gene distantly related to proboscipedia is expressed in lymphoid and pancreatic tissues. J Biol Chem 269:19968, 1994.

131. Torres M, Gómez-Pardo E, Gruss P: Pax2 contributes to inner ear patterning and optic nerve trajectory. Development 122:3381, 1996.

132. Ritz-Laser B, Estreicher A, Gauthier B, Philippe J: The paired homeodomain transcription factor Pax-2 is expressed in the endocrine pancreas and transactivates the glucagon gene promoter. J Biol Chem 275:32708, 2000.

133. Smith SB, Ee HC, Conners JR, German MS: Paired-homeodomain transcription factor PAX4 acts as a transcriptional repressor in early pancreatic development. Mol Cell Biol 19:8272, 1999.

134. Sosa-Pineda B, Chowdhury K, Torres M, et al: The Pax4 gene is essential for differentiation of insulin-producing beta cells in the mammalian pancreas. Nature 386:399, 1997.

135. Shimajiri Y, Sanke T, Furuta H, et al: A missense mutation of Pax4 gene (R121W) is associated with type 2 diabetes in Japanese. Diabetes 50:2864, 2001.

136. Hill ME, Asa SL, Drucker DJ: Essential requirement for Pax6 in control of enteroendocrine proglucagon gene transcription. Mol Endocrinol 13:1474, 1999.

137. Collombat P, Mansouri A, Hecksher-Sorensen J, et al: Opposing actions of Arx and Pax4 in endocrine pancreas development. Genes Dev 17:2591, 2003.

138. Rudnick A, Ling TY, Odagiri H, et al: Pancreatic beta cells express a diverse set of homeobox genes. Proc Natl Acad Sci U S A 91:12203, 1994.

139. Watada H, Mirmira RG, Leung J, German MS: Transcriptional and translational regulation of beta-cell differentiation factor Nkx6.1. J Biol Chem 275:34224, 2000.

140. Jensen J, Serup P, Karlsen C, et al: mRNA profiling of rat islet tumors reveals nkx 6.1 as a beta-cell-specific homeodomain transcription factor. J Biol Chem 271:18749, 1996.

141. German MS, Wang J, Chadwick RB, Rutter WJ: Synergistic activation of the insulin gene by a LIM-homeodomain protein and a basic helix-loop-helix protein: Building a functional insulin minienhancer complex. Genes Dev 6:2165, 1992.

142. Jin T, Trinh DK, Wang F, Drucker DJ: The caudal homeobox protein cdx-2/3 activates endogenous proglucagon gene expression in InR1-G9 islet cells. Mol Endocrinol 11:203, 1997.

143. Laser B, Meda P, Constant I, Philippe J: The caudal-related homeodomain protein Cdx-2/3 regulates glucagon gene expression in islet cells. J Biol Chem 271:28984, 1996.

144. Jin T, Drucker DJ: Activation of proglucagon gene transcription through a novel promoter element by the caudal-related homeodomain protein cdx-2/3. Mol Cell Biol 16:19, 1996.

145. Chawengsaksophak K, James R, Hammond VE, et al: Homeosis and intestinal tumours in Cdx2 mutant mice. Nature 386:84, 1997.

146. Vallejo M, Penchuk L, Habener JF: Somatostatin gene upstream enhancer element activated by a protein complex consisting of CREB, Isl-1-like, and alpha-CBF-like transcription factors. J Biol Chem 267:12876, 1992.

147. Leonard J, Serup P, Gonzalez G, et al: The LIM family transcription factor Isl-1 requires cAMP response element binding protein to promote somatostatin expression in pancreatic islet cells. Proc Natl Acad Sci U S A 89:6247, 1992.

148. Thor S, Ericson J, Brannstrom T, Edlund T: The homeodomain LIM protein isl-I is expressed in subsets of neurons and endocrine cells in the adult rat. Neuron 7:1, 1991.

149. Dong J, Asa SL, Drucker DJ: Islet cell and extrapancreatic expression of the LIM domain homeobox gene isl-1. Mol Endocrinol 5:1633, 1991.

150. Karlsson O, Thor S, Norberg T, et al: Insulin gene enhancer binding protein Isl-1 is a member of a novel class of proteins containing both a homeo- and a Cys-His domain. Nature 344:879, 1990.

151. Millonig JH, Millen KJ, Hatten ME: The mouse Dreher gene Lmx1a controls formation of the roof plate in the vertebrate CNS [see comments]. Nature 403:764, 2000.

152. Phippard D, Heydemann A, Lechner M, et al: Changes in the subcellular localization of the Brn4 gene product precede mesenchymal remodeling of the otic capsule. Hear Res 120:77, 1998.

153. Emens LA, Landers DW, Moss LG: Hepatocyte nuclear factor 1a is expressed in a hamster insulinoma line and transactivates the rat insulin I gene. Proc Natl Acad Sci U S A 89:7300, 1992.

154. Noguchi T, Yamada K, Yamagata K, et al: Expression of liver type pyruvate kinase in insulinoma cells: Involvement of LF-B1 (HNF1). Biochem Biophys Res Com 181:259, 1991.

155. Pontoglio M, Sreenan S, Roe M, et al: Defective insulin secretion in hepatocyte nuclear factor 1alpha-deficient mice. J Clin Invest 101:2215, 1998.

156. Coffinier C, Thepot D, Babinet C, et al: Essential role for the homeoprotein vHNF1/HNF1beta in visceral endoderm differentiation. Development 126:4785, 1999.

157. Coffinier C, Barra J, Babinet C, Yaniv M: Expression of the vHNF1/HNF1beta homeoprotein gene during mouse organogenesis. Mech Dev 89:211, 1999.

158. Lemaigre FP, Durviaux SM, Truong O, et al: Hepatocyte nuclear factor 6, a transcription factor that contains a novel type of homeodomain and a single cut domain. Proc Natl Acad Sci U S A 93:9460, 1996.

159. Rausa FM, Ye H, Lim L, et al: In situ hybridization with 33P-labeled RNA probes for determination of cellular expression patterns of liver transcription factors in mouse embryos [published erratum appears in Methods 16(3):359–360, 1998]. Methods 16:29, 1998.

160. Shih DQ, Navas MA, Kuwajima S, et al: Impaired glucose homeostasis and neonatal mortality in hepatocyte nuclear factor 3alpha-deficient mice. Proc Natl Acad Sci U S A 96:10152, 1999.

161. Kaestner KH, Katz J, Liu Y, et al: Inactivation of the winged helix transcription factor HNF3alpha affects glucose homeostasis and islet glucagon gene expression in vivo. Genes Dev 13:495, 1999.

162. Duncan SA, Navas MA, Dufort D, et al: Regulation of a transcription factor network required for differentiation and metabolism. Science 281:692, 1998.

163. Rausa FM, Galarneau L, Belanger L, Costa RH: The nuclear receptor fetoprotein transcription factor is coexpressed with its target gene HNF-3beta in the developing murine liver, intestine and pancreas. Mech Dev 89:185, 1999.

164. Sund NJ, Vatamaniuk MZ, Casey M, et al: Tissue-specific deletion of Foxa2 in pancreatic beta cells results in hyperinsulinemic hypoglycemia. Genes Dev 15:1706, 2001.

165. Kaestner KH, Hiemisch H, Schutz G: Targeted disruption of the gene encoding hepatocyte nuclear factor 3gamma results in reduced transcription of hepatocyte-specific genes. Mol Cell Biol 18:4245, 1998.

166. Kaestner KH, Hiemisch H, Luckow B, Schutz G: The HNF-3 gene family of transcription factors in mice: Gene structure, cDNA sequence, and mRNA distribution. Genomics 20:377, 1994.

167. Liu Y, Shen W, Brubaker PL, et al: Foxa3 (HNF-3 gamma) binds to and activates the rat proglucagon gene promoter but is not essential for proglucagon gene expression. Biochem J 366 (Pt 2):633–641, 2002.

168. Sladek FM, Zhong WM, Lai E, Darnell JE Jr: Liver-enriched transcription factor HNF-4 is a novel member of the steroid hormone receptor superfamily. Genes Dev 4:2353, 1990.

169. Miquerol L, Lopez S, Cartier N, et al: Expression of the L-type pyruvate kinase gene and the hepatocyte nuclear factor 4 transcription factor in exocrine and endocrine pancreas. J Biol Chem 269:8944, 1994.

170. Planque N, Leconte L, Coquelle FM, et al: Interaction of Maf transcription factors with Pax-6 results in synergistic activation of the glucagon promoter. J Biol Chem 276:35751, 2001.

171. Olbrot M, Rud J, Moss LG, Sharma A: Identification of beta-cell-specific insulin gene transcription factor RIPE3b1 as mammalian MafA. Proc Natl Acad Sci U S A 99:6737, 2002.

172. Kataoka K, Han SI, Shioda S, et al: MafA is a glucose-regulated and pancreatic beta-cell-specific transcriptional activator for the insulin gene. J Biol Chem 277:49903, 2002.

Chemistry and Biosynthesis of the Islet Hormones: Insulin, Islet Amyloid Polypeptide (Amylin), Glucagon, Somatostatin, and Pancreatic Polypeptide

Donald F. Steiner, Graeme I. Bell, Arthur H. Rubenstein, and Shu J. Chan

The classic experiments of Von Mering and Minkowski at the close of the nineteenth century clearly demonstrated the important role of the pancreas in the prevention of diabetes.[1] Early in the twentieth century, a number of investigators undertook to prepare pancreatic extracts to treat diabetes, but it was not until the work of the Canadians Fred Banting, Charles Best, and John Collip (Fig. 48-1), working in the laboratory of Prof. J. J. R. Macleod at the University of Toronto in 1921–1922, that potent preparations of insulin were routinely made.[2] The name *insulin* was based on the belief that the hormone was derived from the islets of Langerhans and actually was suggested as early as 1909 by deMayer and later again in 1917 by Sir Edward Sharpey-Schafer. Preparative methods based on the early work of Scott[3] as well as refinements by Banting and coworkers[4] were rapidly developed for the commercial preparation of the hormone, and within about 1 year, insulin began to be administered to patients with diabetes, often with dramatic effects.[2] The chemical nature of insulin was a more elusive problem, although the fact that it was destroyed by proteolytic enzymes suggested that it was indeed a protein.[5] At that time, however, it was not appreciated that proteins might function as hormones as well as enzymes and produce such dramatic biologic effects as the lowering of blood glucose levels and the enhancement of carbohydrate utilization. When J. J. Abel first succeeded in crystallizing insulin in 1926, there was great controversy as to whether the crystals of protein he had obtained were actually the active biologic principle or merely the vehicle for a smaller active moiety.[6] Such controversies seem remarkable in the light of our detailed present-day knowledge of the structure and biologic properties of insulin, but it is important to remember that many of the modern techniques of protein chemistry were developed, in part, through the clinical need for insulin, which made it abundantly available to the biochemist as a model protein for study.

This chapter selectively reviews the chemistry and properties of insulin and the other islet hormones, including islet amyloid polypeptide (IAPP or amylin), glucagon, somatostatin, and pancreatic polypeptide (PP) and their precursor forms, the mechanisms of their biosynthesis in the various islet cells in which they are produced, and the structures of the genes that encode them. Studies on the mechanism of biosynthesis of insulin via proinsulin in the pancreatic β cells have long provided a useful model for analysis of the production of the other islet hormones and of many other hormonal and neuroendocrine peptides and growth factors and their receptors, as well as many other proteins that traverse the secretory pathway. Continuing clarification of the enzymatic mechanisms underlying the proteolytic cleavage of proproteins now provides a more complete picture of neuroendocrine peptide formation and processing. Most such peptides exist in multiple forms in tissue or in the circulation, and the origin and metabolism of these forms add additional complexity to the normal physiologic regulation of endocrine and paracrine/neural secretion. This information will be related, wherever possible, to pathologic states in humans, particularly diabetes and related metabolic syndromes and benign or malignant endocrine tumors.

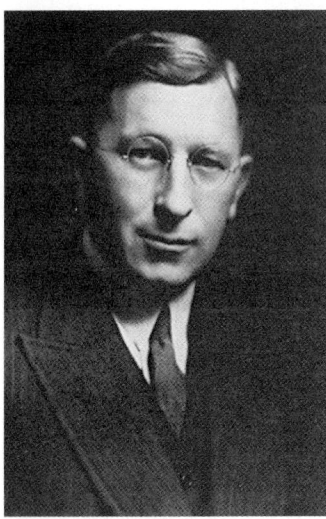 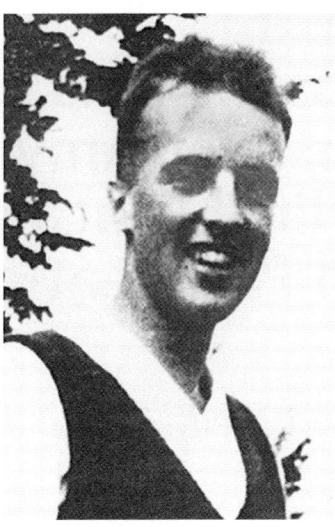 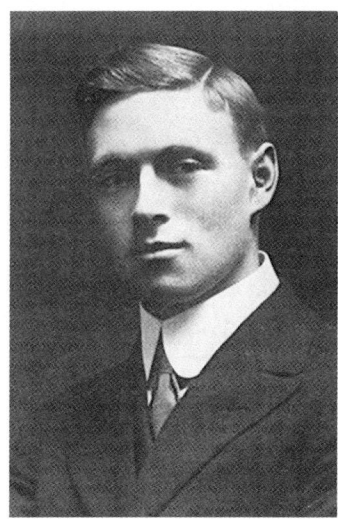 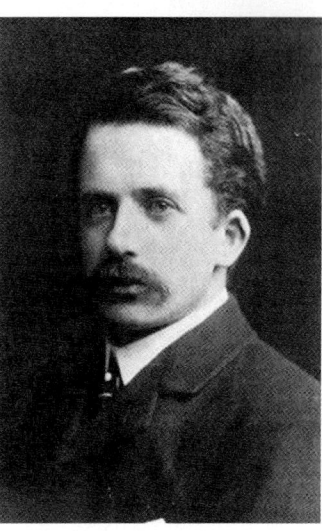

Figure 48-1   Photographs of Frederick G. Banting, Charles H. Best, John B. Collip, and Prof. J. J. R. Macleod, the principal developers of successful methods for insulin extraction, taken about the time of insulin's discovery in 1921. (Photographs courtesy of Michael Bliss and the University of Toronto, Toronto, Canada.)

ISOLATION, PROPERTIES, AND STRUCTURE OF INSULIN

ISOLATION AND CHARACTERIZATION

Insulin occurs throughout the vertebrate kingdom, and insulin-like substances have been found in the brains and/or digestive systems of a number of invertebrate species.[7] The early recognition that ethanol[3] or acid-ethanol[4] extraction of pancreas inhibited proteolytic destruction of insulin has provided the basis for most modern preparative procedures.[8,9] Acid-ethanol also efficiently extracts proinsulin, C peptide, IAPP, glucagon, PP, somatostatin, and their precursor forms from pancreatic tissue in most species. Acid-ethanol extracts can be partially purified by fractional precipitation and iso-electric precipitation in the presence of organic solvents to solubilize fats, which can then be further resolved by gel filtration,[10] ion-exchange chromatography,[11,12] and high-performance liquid chromatography (HPLC).[13–15] Salting out from acidic solutions is not effective for recovering small amounts of insulin and may lead to significant losses of C peptide as well as to loss of the other peptides.[16] Yields of insulin vary according to the source: Mammalian pancreas yields 10 to 15 nmol/g (of wet weight); fetal calf pancreas, 60 to 70 nmol/g; fish principal islets, 300 to 500 nmol/g; and isolated rat islets of Langerhans, 2 to 3 fmol/g. The biologic activity of most highly purified contemporary mammalian insulin preparations ranges from 26 to 30 IU/mg. The bovine insulin standard of the International Union of Pure and Applied Chemistry is stated to have an activity of 25 IU/mg of dry weight.[8] Although crystallization with zinc was once regarded as a powerful method for purification of insulin, it is now generally recognized that even repeated crystallization does not eliminate all impurities from insulin and that not all species have insulins that are capable of binding zinc and/or of crystallizing.[12,17] Most crystalline preparations of animal-derived insulin contain small residual amounts of glucagon, desamido insulin, proinsulin and its intermediate cleavage forms, ethyl esters of insulin, dimers of insulin, and higher aggregates of insulin and proinsulin with unknown components.[12,18]

The use of modern biosynthetic methods based on recombinant DNA technology[19–21] has eliminated some impurities, such as other hormones, but may introduce new types of trace contaminants derived from the bacterial or yeast host cells.[19] Early gel filtration studies of crystalline bovine insulin preparations separated impurities into essentially three fractions: (1) "a-component"—material of high molecular weight eluting essentially in the void volume and containing insulin cross-linked or aggregated with other proteins; (2) "b-component"—proinsulin, intermediate cleavage products of proinsulin, and insulin dimers; and (3) "c-component"—insulin-like components including insulin, desamido forms, arginyl insulins (B_{31} and B_{32} arginine residues), C peptide, and small amounts of glucagon.[12,22,23] The a-component turned out to be highly antigenic in producing insulin antibodies.[18] Further purification of the insulin-containing fractions by ion-exchange chromatography, using urea-containing buffers or 60% ethanol as dispersing agents, yielded preparations that were better than 99% pure, that is, the "monocomponent" or "single-component" insulins that are now widely available.[11,18] These preparations are far less antigenic than most of the crystalline insulin preparations of animal origin that were used formerly, and they have been shown to improve the control of diabetes.[24] The introduction of biosynthetic human insulin for therapy has further reduced the problem of antigenicity, but it has been difficult to eliminate entirely because even the human hormone can undergo chemical changes during storage that may tend to induce formation of (auto)antibodies.[25,26]

The assay of insulin, like that of most other protein hormones, has always presented difficulties with regard to precision and sensitivity. The various in vivo blood glucose–lowering assays that are often used by pharmaceutical houses require too much material to be very useful for most experimental laboratories. The use of polyacrylamide gel electrophoresis and/or HPLC with mass spectrometry can provide a wealth of useful information regarding the homogeneity and quality of the preparations.[11–13,15,27] These methods also give indications as to the state of amidation of the insulin or proinsulin, which may reflect the harshness of preparative procedures or the extent of autolysis prior to extraction. Other routinely used biochemical methods for assessing the purity of proteins are equally applicable, but it must be borne in mind that although all tests indicate that homogeneity has been achieved, the biologic activity of the preparation must be examined directly to ascertain that no chemical damage to the hormone has occurred. This can usually be accomplished by in vitro assays using isolated fat or liver cells, or various cultured cells, and comparing such parameters as glucose oxidation, lipogenesis, glucose transport, or glycogen synthesis with purified standards.[8,28] The introduction of hormone-binding assays using isolated plasma membrane preparations or purified receptors has provided more sensitive and reliable methods for screening material for biologic potency in vivo; these methods have thus far demonstrated a good correlation between binding and measured biologic potency.[29–31] However, both binding tests and immunoassays can be misleading, as neither necessarily measures the true biologic effectiveness of the hormone. Thus, the thorough characterization of any insulin preparation should include measurements of biologic potency in suitable isolated cell preparations and of binding characteristics, as well as full characterization of the protein in terms of its molecular weight, composition, homogeneity, and, if possible, amino acid composition and sequence. For more detailed information about the physicochemical properties of insulin, several reviews are recommended.[8,17,25,32,33]

INSULIN STRUCTURE

The determination of the complete primary structure of bovine insulin by Sanger and his associates in 1955[34] provided the first complete structure of a protein; it also proved beyond question that proteins are defined molecular entities. The exploration of species differences in insulin structure led to the recognition of the existence of the genetic code. The primary structures of insulins from about 70 vertebrate species have been determined in the interval since the pioneering studies of Sanger,[34] Smith,[35] and others.[8,36–48] In addition to these, the structures of several insulin-like peptides from invertebrates have been elucidated. These include a growth-promoting hormone of the light green cells in the snail *Lymnaea*,[49] an unusual insulin-like molecule that regulates carbohydrate metabolism in *Aplysia*,[50] the insulin-like brain peptide from the silkworm *Bombyx mori*,[51] an insulin-like peptide from the locust,[52] and insulin-like peptides from *Caenorhabditis elegans*.[53] Although less closely related to the vertebrate insulins, these are clearly members of the insulin superfamily.[54,55] In vertebrates, in addition to relaxin, other insulin-like peptides have recently been discovered in reproductive tissues.[56]

The low rate of mutation acceptance in the vertebrate insulins (2% to 4% of residues per 100 million years) is comparable to that of many other well-defined globular proteins, such as hemoglobin, cytochrome *c*, or many enzymes.[54,57] Nonetheless, amino acid substitutions can occur at many positions within either chain without greatly altering the biologic effectiveness of the hormone as measured in various bioassay systems (Fig. 48-2). Insulins of the New World vertebrates often are highly mutated with reduced biologic

potency.[17] However, certain structural features are conserved throughout vertebrate evolution, including the positions of the three disulfide bonds, the N-terminal and C-terminal regions of the A chain, and the hydrophobic residues in the C-terminal region of the B chain, as well as others. Chemical modifications in any of these regions tend to markedly reduce or abolish biologic activity, underscoring their roles in maintaining the secondary and tertiary structural features necessary for receptor binding.[8,17,58,59] The C-terminal hydrophobic sequence of the B chain (residues 23 to 27) also plays an important role in the formation of insulin dimers in solution as described below.

As might be anticipated from the more extensive amino acid replacements (8% to 10%) that occur between mammalian and fish insulins,[47] it is not surprising that the immunologic cross-reactivity between these proteins is rather weak. Generally, such low cross-reactivity can easily be detected by conventional immunoassays if the heterologous insulin is used as the labeled tracer. For detailed considerations of insulin antigenicity in relation to its structure, several reviews are recommended.[8,60]

The elucidation by Blundell and Wood,[17] Blundell and coworkers,[61,62] and Baker and coworkers[63] of the three-dimensional structure of porcine insulin, initially at a resolution of 2.8 Å and with more recent refinements at 1.5 Å, was an important breakthrough in the study of peptide hormone structure. The results have proved invaluable in interpreting much of the available chemical data on the properties of insulin.[62,63] Detailed knowledge of the spatial organization of the molecule has also been helpful in studies on the molecular mechanism of binding and action of insulin. The hexameric unit of crystalline zinc insulin (Fig. 48-3) consists of three dimers arranged around a major threefold axis that passes through two zinc atoms, each of which is coordinated with the imidazole groups of three B10 histidine residues located above or below the plane of the hexamer.[61,62] The insulin dimers are held together in the crystals by hydrogen bonds between the peptide groups of residues 24 and 26 within the C-terminal region of the B chain, forming an antiparallel β-pleated sheet structure. The structure of a porcine insulin monomer is shown in Figure 48-4.

In this high-resolution (1.5 Å) representation, all of the amino acid side chains are shown in their normal orientations, and the putative receptor-binding region is outlined. Recent nuclear magnetic resonance (NMR) studies[65] provide support for the conclusion that the structure of the insulin monomer in solution is closely similar but not necessarily identical to that in crystals.

X-ray diffraction studies on crystals of insulin from the hagfish, a cyclostome, have defined a very similar arrangement of

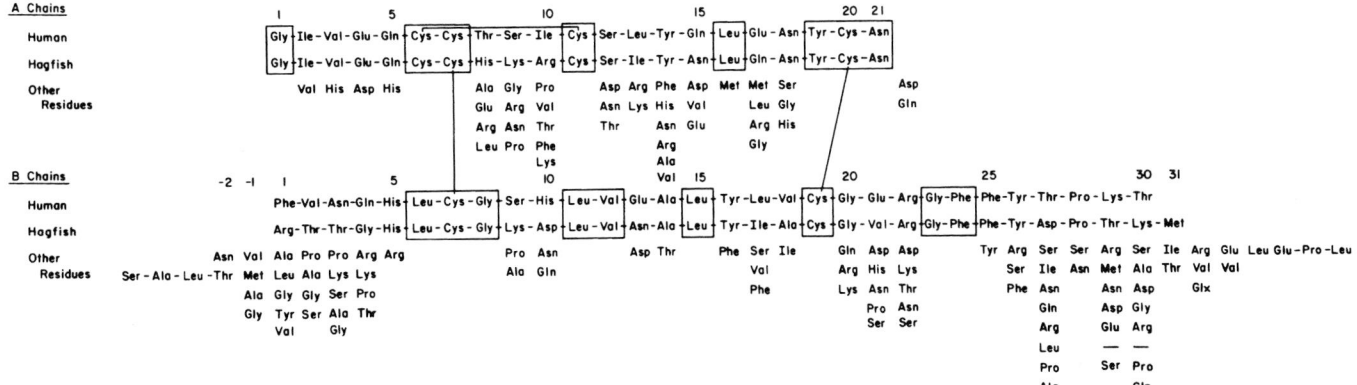

Figure 48-2 Amino acid sequence of human and hagfish insulins, with substitutions occurring at each position in 70 other known vertebrate insulins shown below for comparison. Invariant residues are enclosed in boxes.

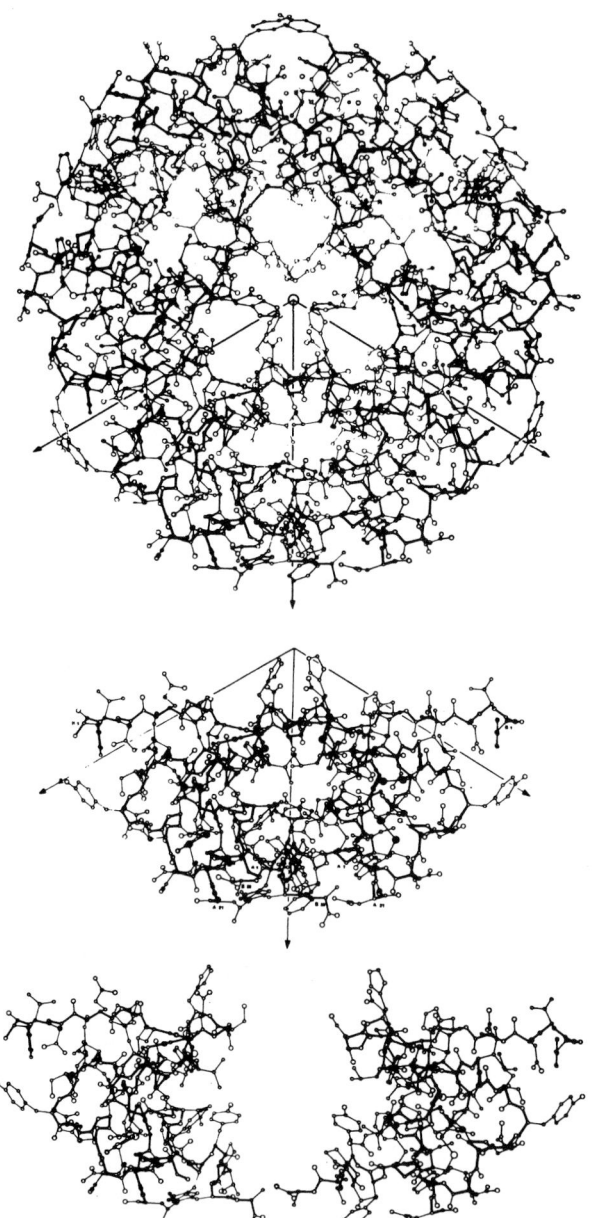

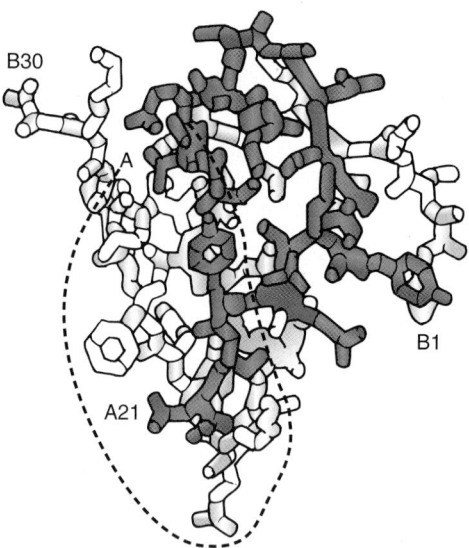

Figure 48-4   View of a porcine insulin monomer (molecule 2) oriented perpendicular to the threefold axis (see Fig. 48-3). The side chains of all the amino acids are shown; the A chain is *dark gray*, and the B chain is *light gray*. *Dashes* outline the approximate region on the surface of the insulin monomer, which is believed to contact the receptor on binding[64] (this region is shown in greater detail in Fig. 48-5). (Computer graphic representation courtesy of Dr. Bing Xiao, University of York.)

Figure 48-3   View of a hexamer of porcine insulin (2-Zn) along the threefold axis, showing the development of dimers from monomers and their organization into the hexamer. Zinc-binding imidazole side chains of His-B10 residues project toward the central axis above and below the midplane of the hexamers. (Source: From Blundell TL, Dodson GG, Hodgkin DC, et al: Insulin: The structure in the crystals and its reflection in chemistry and biology. Adv Protein Chem 26:279, 1972.)

the molecular backbone of the insulin in this very primitive vertebrate[17,37,66] despite replacements at about 40% of sites, which is consistent with its evolutionary divergence of about 500 million years. These results indicate the conservation in this cyclostomian insulin of many primary structural features that are known to be concerned with the formation of the characteristic folded structure of the hormone. Thus, although increased numbers of amino acid substitutions have occurred in certain New World species, such as the guinea pig, other hystricomorph rodents, and some primates,[17,35,40,41,67] the native molecular structure of insulin, as well as its tendency to form isologous dimers, has remained remarkably constant throughout vertebrate evolution. This fact is further reflected in the relatively high retention of biologic potency among the known insulins; most fish insulins are only

slightly less active than mammalian insulins, and even the much more primitive and highly substituted hagfish insulin has been found to have about 5% of the biologic activity of bovine or porcine insulin in various mammalian test systems.[68,69]

These findings also imply that the receptors for insulin,[70] as well as their actions, have changed relatively little throughout vertebrate evolution. Similar conservatism is often seen in essential structural proteins and enzymes.[71] The interaction of insulin and its receptor initiates a variety of biochemical functions in the plasma membrane, including catalysis (tyrosine kinase), self-association, and/or interactions with other cellular components leading to various metabolic and anabolic responses, as well as endocytosis of insulin and its degradation or transcellular transport.[72] The insulin receptor and insulin's actions are discussed in greater detail in Chapter 50.

RECEPTOR-BINDING REGION OF INSULIN

Recent studies have led to revisions in previously held theories regarding the location of the receptor-binding region in the insulin molecule. Several naturally occurring mutant human insulins (see the section entitled "Defects in the Insulin Gene: The Insulinopathies" later in the chapter) have proven to be especially valuable in redefining current views of the location of the receptor-binding surface of the insulin molecule. Earlier views were based on the presumed inflexibility of the C-terminal region of the B chain in the insulin structure, as revealed by x-ray analysis (Fig. 48-5*A*). Studies of insulin substitutions involving residues B24 or B25 and of despentapeptide insulin, in which the last five residues of the B chain have been deleted, suggest that the C-terminal region of the B chain is reoriented to facilitate receptor binding. The most convincing evidence for this has arisen from studies of a novel miniproinsulin molecule synthesized by Markussen,[73] in which B29 lysine is in direct peptide linkage to A1 glycine. Although this molecule is biologically inactive, when crystals were obtained and analyzed,[74] it was evident that its three-dimensional structure was essentially isomorphic to that of normal crystalline insulin. What was different in B29-A1 insulin, however, was the immobility of the C-terminal

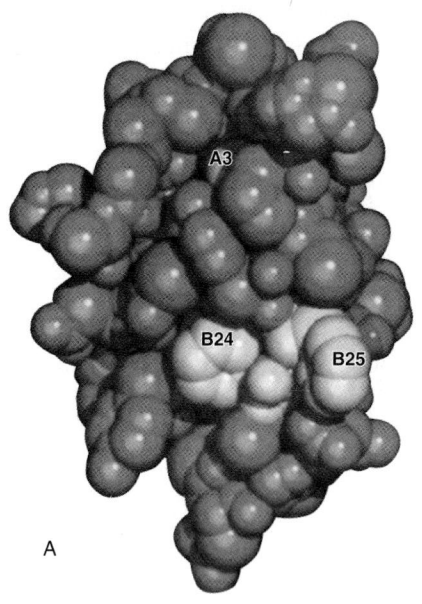
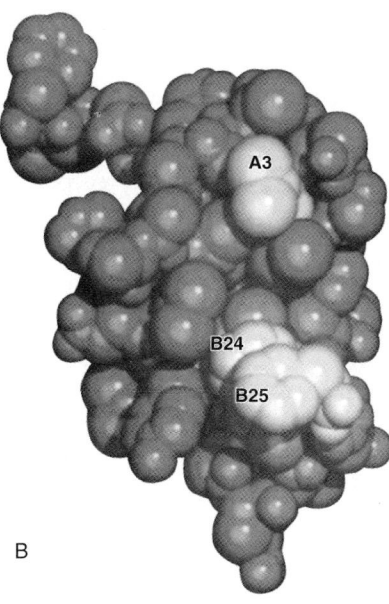

A   B

Figure 48-5 **A,** Molecule 1 of 2 Zn human insulin with atoms represented with their van der Waals' radii. The residues A3 Val, B24, and B25 Phe, which occur as human mutations, are highlighted by light shading. The view is perpendicular to the dimer-forming surface. The B chain N-terminal residues are extended behind the molecule in this view. **B,** The monomer of beef despentapeptide insulin (DPI). The atoms are represented with their van der Waals' radii. The residues A3 Val, B24, and B25 Phe are highlighted by *light shading*, in the same view as shown in **A**. (The B chain N-terminal residues are extended above B10 histidine in the DPI structure and are therefore visible in this view.) (Courtesy of Drs. Bing Xiao and Guy Dodson, University of York.) (Source: From Steiner DF, Tager HS, Nanjo K, et al: Familial syndromes of hyperproinsulinemia and hyperinsulinemia with mild diabetes. In Stanbury JS (ed): The Metabolic Basis of Inherited Disease, 7th ed. New York, McGraw-Hill, 1993.)

region of the B chain. Recent NMR data on various insulin derivatives in solution[65,75,76] also confirm the importance of significant conformational changes in the C terminus of the B chain for effective receptor binding. When five C-terminal residues of the B chain are deleted from the rest of the molecule, as indicated in Figure 48-5*B* (yielding despentapeptide insulin), an underlying portion of the hydrophobic core of the molecule is exposed. Although the exact conformation of the B chain C terminus when insulin is bound to its receptor is not known, even small movements would alter insulin's topography and enhance the potential for interactions of valine residue A3 with the receptor (compare Figs. 48-5*A* and 48-5*B*). Hence, replacement of this valine by leucine in a mutant human insulin,[15] which would normally be regarded as a biochemically conservative substitution, leads to a distortion of the surface that is exposed to solvent and, on binding, to the receptor recognition site of the hormone.

Additional studies have further delineated the roles of B24 phenylalanine (Phe), B25 Phe, and A3 valine (Val) in insulin-receptor interactions.[77,78] A recent study by alanine scanning (replacing all amino acid residues individually with alanine) of the insulin molecule largely corroborates and extends these findings, suggesting that A2 Ile, A3 Val, A19 Tyr, B23 Gly, and B24 Phe might be key residues contributing to a receptor-binding surface in the insulin monomer.[79]

These and other data emphasize, however, that portions of the insulin molecule in addition to the C-terminal B chain domain and the N-terminal A chain domain are also crucial for higher-affinity insulin-receptor interactions. It is important to note that (1) desoctapeptide insulin (an analogue in which the C-terminal B chain domain has been deleted) retains 0.1% of the receptor-binding potency of insulin and that (2) analogues bearing amino acid replacements in the central B chain α-helix can exhibit either enhanced[80] or diminished[81] receptor-binding potency relative to the native hormone.

A large body of evidence supports the hypothesis that the N-terminal region of the α subunit of the insulin receptor plays an important role in insulin binding.[82] However, the C-terminal region of the α subunit has recently been shown to contain an important contact site for the A25 Phe side chain in insulin by photoaffinity labeling.[83] It therefore seems likely that N- and C-terminal regions of the α subunit lie in proximity, but the exact nature of their interaction with insulin and whether it is within or between the dimeric α subunits within the heterotetrameric receptor complex

remains unclear. For a more thorough discussion of this problem, a recent review is recommended.[82] The availability of a more precise structural description of the mode of insulin binding to its receptor would greatly facilitate efforts to regulate this interaction and design novel insulin receptor agonists.

BIOSYNTHESIS OF INSULIN

Although earlier studies indicated that insulin was formed via proinsulin, a precursor that includes the B and A chains within a single 9-kDa polypeptide chain,[11,84,85] examination by cell-free translation of the initial polypeptide products encoded in insulin messenger ribonucleic acid (mRNA) extracted from islets or islet cell tumors led, in 1975, to the discovery of preproinsulin (Fig. 48-6). This extended form of proinsulin has a hydrophobic N-terminal 24-residue prepeptide.[86,87] Such signal peptide extensions have been found at or near the N termini in almost all secretory proteins of animal, plant, or bacterial origin, and they serve to facilitate their segregation from the cytosolic compartment, where protein synthesis is initiated, into the secretory pathway via a complex series of molecular interactions that result in the translocation of the nascent peptide across the membrane of the rough endoplasmic reticulum (RER) into its internal compartments, or cisternae.[88] During, or shortly after, translocation, the signal sequence is cleaved by the signal peptidase, which is located on the inner surface of the RER membrane.[88] Following translocation and cleavage of the signal sequence, the proinsulin molecule folds and undergoes rapid formation of disulfide bonds to achieve its native structure. Evidence suggests that this process is catalyzed by the enzyme protein disulfide isomerase,[89] a resident protein of the RER that has a C-terminal Lys-Glu-Asp-Leu (KDEL) localization sequence.[90] Proinsulin is then transferred in small coated vesicles from the endoplasmic reticulum (ER) to the *cis* region of the Golgi apparatus.[91,92] It then passes from the *cis* to the *trans*-Golgi, where it is sorted into secretory vesicles. The signal peptide is rapidly degraded in the RER and is thus not a normal secretory product of β cells.[93]

During the intracellular transport of proinsulin from its site of biosynthesis in the rough endoplasmic reticulum of the β cell to the storage granules, it is cleaved to yield insulin and a 26- to 31-residue peptide fragment, which is designated the *C peptide*; both insulin and C peptide are stored in the

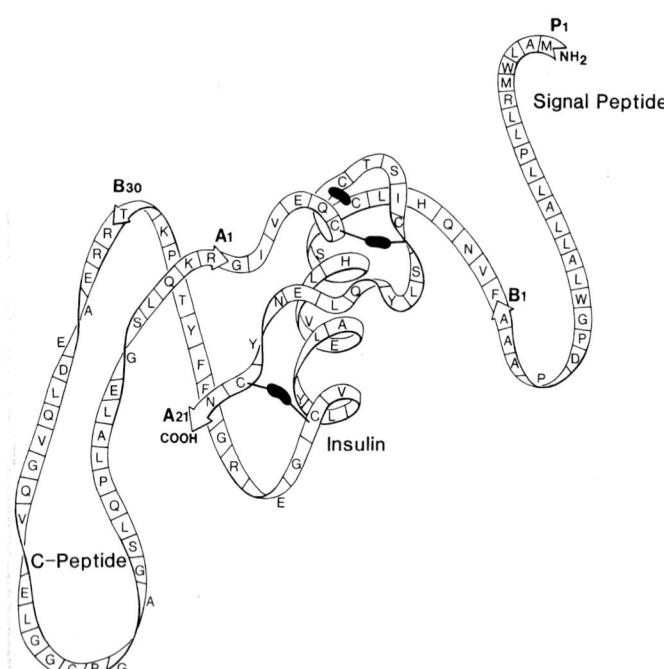

Figure 48-6 Schematic structure of human preproinsulin. Removal of the first 24 amino acids (signal peptide) gives rise to proinsulin. Cleavage after B30 (T) and before A1 (G) gives rise to insulin and C peptide. (See text for details and Dayhoff[36] for explanation of single-letter amino acid code.)

secretory granules along with small amounts of residual proinsulin and partially cleaved intermediate forms[94] as well as a variety of other, more minor β-cell secretory products.[95] The intracellular processing of precursor proteins (proproteins), like proinsulin, is quite distinct from the well-known proteolytic activation of the inactive zymogen forms of many hydrolases, which is a largely extracellular process. Precursor processing is now recognized to be an important feature of almost all endocrine and neural cells, and it also occurs in many other organs (e.g., the liver).[96] Certain cellular proteolytic-processing enzymes also are coopted in the formation of the envelopes of many viruses.[97–99] Recent progress in the intracellular localization and enzymatic mechanism of these proteolytic events is discussed in greater detail in the section entitled "Conversion of Proinsulin to Insulin," later in the chapter.

STRUCTURE AND PROPERTIES OF PROINSULIN

Methods for the isolation of proinsulin and related peptides were discussed in the preceding section. Mammalian proinsulins range in size from 81 (cow) to 86 (human, horse, rat) amino acid residues.[100] The difference is a consequence of the variable size of the connecting polypeptide (C peptide), which links the C terminus of the insulin B chain to the N terminus of the insulin A chain (see Fig. 48-6). All the known mammalian proinsulins have pairs of basic residues at either end of the C peptide that link it to the insulin chains. These residues are excised during the conversion of proinsulin to insulin,[101] and the resulting products are native insulin and C peptide. The proinsulin-like molecules in invertebrates contain C peptides of roughly similar size that also are usually excised by cleavage at basic residue pairs.[49,51] Despite its considerably larger molecular size, proinsulin is remarkably similar to insulin in many properties, including solubility, isoelectric point,[93] self-associative properties,[102] and reactivity with insulin antisera.[83,103,104] These observations and evidence from other studies strongly suggest that the conformation of the insulin moiety in proinsulin is nearly identical to that

of insulin itself.[65,94] It is noteworthy that the highly flexible connecting peptide is much longer than is necessary simply to bridge the short 8-Å gap between the ends of the B and A chains as they exist in the folded insulin molecule (see Fig. 48-6). The connecting peptide overlays a portion of the surface of the insulin monomer but does not completely mask the receptor-binding region, since intact proinsulin exhibits 3% to 5% biologic activity in several systems in vitro.[28,105] It is unlikely that any significant cleavage or "activation" of proinsulin occurs in the tissues to account for this level of intrinsic activity.[106] The connecting peptide also does not obscure those surfaces of the monomer that interact to form dimers and hexamers.[107,108] A hypothetical arrangement of the connecting peptide moiety in a proinsulin hexamer is shown in Figure 48-7. As a consequence of the similarities between insulin and proinsulin hexamers, it is clear that proinsulin at low levels can be incorporated into insulin crystals.[108] This property accounts for the presence of proinsulin in crystalline preparations of insulin.[12] A three-dimensional structure for proinsulin has not yet been achieved, however, despite successful crystallization of the prohormone in several laboratories.[17,109]

PRECURSOR RELATIONSHIP OF PROINSULIN TO INSULIN

The precursor-product relationship between proinsulin and insulin has been carefully documented in a variety of studies using isolated islets.[110–115] In rats and mice, two nonallelic insulin genes give rise to two proinsulins, one corresponding to each of the two insulins (I and II).[116–118] The two insulins differ from each other at only two positions[116] and are identical in both species.[118,119] These insulins are encoded in nonallelic genes,[54,119] arising from a duplication event that occurred relatively recently (10 to 30 million years ago). The gene for insulin I appears to have arisen via a viral retropositional event[120] and lacks the second intervening sequence (see Fig. 48-16). The two rat proinsulins and their corresponding C peptides and intermediate forms have been isolated and their amino acid sequences determined.[116,121–124] The two rat insulins are synthesized in roughly equal proportions (I/II = 58/42) under basal and stimulated conditions.[85,116] The conversion of proinsulin to insulin begins after an initial delay of about 20 minutes and then proceeds as a pseudo-first-order

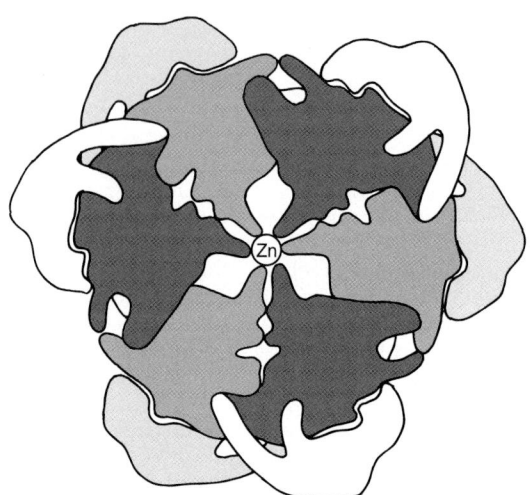

Figure 48-7 Hypothetical 2-Zn proinsulin hexamer as viewed along the threefold axis. The connecting peptide is shown in *light gray* and *white* around the periphery of the *darker outline* of an insulin hexamer arranged according to the data of Blundell and coworkers.[62] The central density represents two zinc atoms in coordination linkage to the six (three above and three below the hexamer plane) histidine side chains at position 10 in the B chain (compare with Fig. 48-3).

process over a period of several hours.[94,111,125] The intracellular proteolytic conversion of proinsulin to insulin continues when protein synthesis is inhibited with cycloheximide, indicating that continuous protein synthesis is not necessary for this reaction.[110] The processing of proinsulin normally proceeds to near completion. Hence, the mature secretory granules contain only small amounts (1% to 2%) of proinsulin and intermediate materials. Consequently, secreted insulin normally contains only small amounts of these precursor-related peptides.[125] Newly synthesized insulin is selectively released to a slight extent, but the bulk of the secreted material consists of stored preformed hormone and C peptide.[125-127] The major intermediate cleavage forms of mammalian proinsulins have been described by early investigators.[12,23,93,116,128-130] Comparative studies of insulin biosynthesis in the larger, more readily accessible, single islets (Brockman bodies) of teleost fishes (e.g., the cod[131] and the anglerfish[132,133]) as well as in the islet parenchyma of such primitive vertebrates as cyclostomes (e.g., the hagfish)[134,135] have also indicated the formation and intracellular cleavage of proinsulins that are similar in size to the mammalian proteins. Such lower forms exhibit similar requirements for cleavage at paired basic residue sites by the evolutionarily conserved prohormone convertases.

MORPHOLOGIC ORGANIZATION OF THE INSULIN BIOSYNTHETIC MACHINERY

The β cells of the islets of Langerhans share many features with other cells that elaborate secretory proteins (Fig. 48-8). The participation of the Golgi apparatus in the formation of secretory vesicles, the so-called β granules, was suggested as

early as 1944 by Hard.[138] Later, Munger[139] confirmed, by electron microscopy, that secretory granule formation occurs within the Golgi apparatus. He identified "progranules" with altered morphologic features near the Golgi body. Numerous subsequent studies have confirmed that newly synthesized peptide material passes via the Golgi apparatus into β-cell secretory granules. With the exception of the proteolytic processing, the overall process appears to be similar to that occurring in the pancreatic exocrine cells and in many other secretory cells.[140] Immunocytochemical studies using monoclonal antibodies that are specific for uncleaved proinsulin have demonstrated that newly formed clathrin-clad vesicles derived from the TGN (*trans*-Golgi network) cisternae are rich in proinsulin (Fig. 48-9), confirming that conversion to insulin occurs principally during the maturation of these secretory "progranules."[136,143] Proinsulin, in common with many other exportable proteins, is synthesized by ribosomes associated with the RER.[144] Evidence reviewed in the preceding section indicates that proinsulin is in turn derived from a larger precursor, preproinsulin, which is rapidly cleaved to proinsulin in the RER. The proinsulin is then transported from the ER to the Golgi apparatus in small, coated vesicles[91] (see Fig. 48-8) in a process that requires about 20 minutes.[94,136,143] Addition to pancreatic islets of antimycin or other energy poisons after short labeling periods with tritiated (^{3}H) leucine completely blocks the subsequent transformation of the newly formed proinsulin to insulin.[136,137,145] However, if the addition of antimycin is delayed for 30 minutes, there is no inhibition of subsequent conversion, indicating that once newly synthesized proinsulin has reached the *trans*-Golgi and/or progranules, its transformation no longer requires energy.[137] The chemical basis of the energy

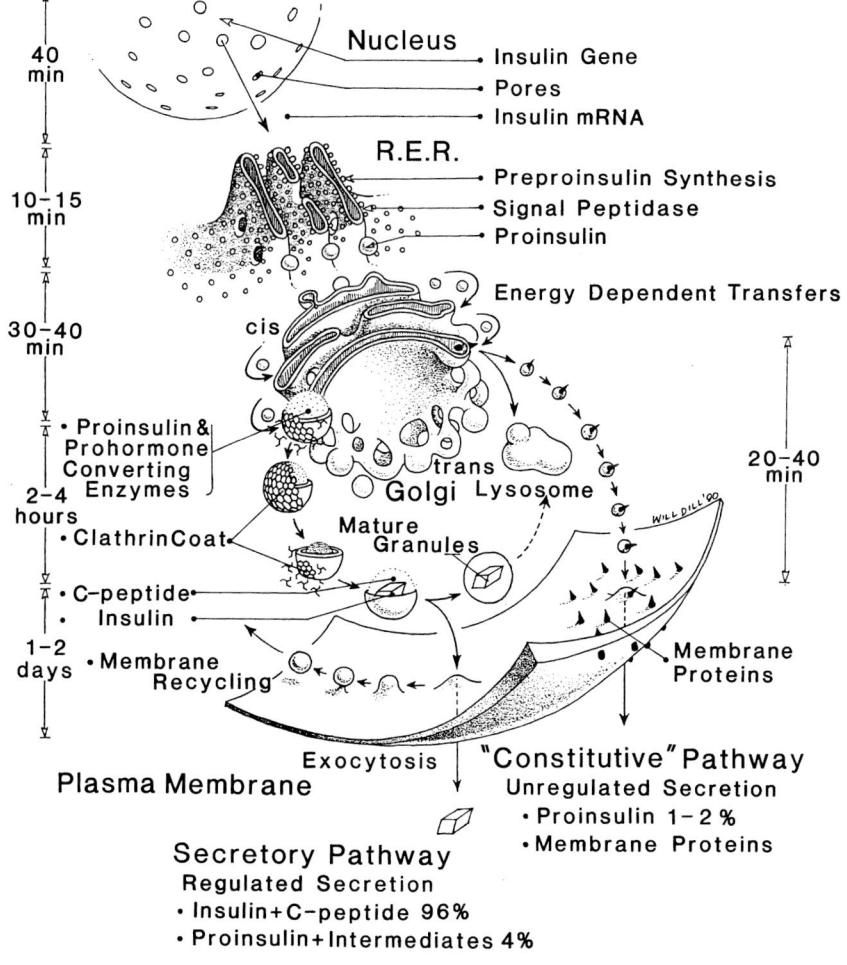

Figure 48-8 Schematic model of the subcellular transport of preproinsulin after its synthesis in the rough endoplasmic reticulum (RER) and rapid cleavage to proinsulin (within 1 to 2 minutes). Proinsulin is then released into the intracisternal spaces of the RER, where it folds and forms the native disulfide bonds of insulin. It is then transported to the Golgi apparatus by an energy-dependent process. The clathrin-coated early granules budding from the *trans*-Golgi cisternae are rich in proinsulin and contain the converting proteases PC2 and PC3. Processing occurs mainly, if not exclusively, in the early secretory granules,[136,137] giving rise to the more condensed mature granules. Fractionation studies have confirmed that the mature granule-dense cores consist almost entirely of insulin, often in crystalline arrays (see Fig. 48-14), whereas the granule-soluble phase that surrounds the inclusion consists mainly of C peptide and small amounts of proinsulin.[141] The release of newly synthesized proinsulin and insulin begins only about 1 hour after synthesis in the RER; hence, granules must undergo a maturation process that renders them competent for secretion. There is no evidence for significant nongranular routes of secretion of either proinsulin or insulin in normal islets. Exocytosis of granules is regulated by glucose and many other factors, and in humans and dogs, it results in the release of insulin and C peptide in approximately equimolar proportions under both basal and stimulated conditions.[142] The mechanism of recycling of the granule membrane and its components is not well understood.

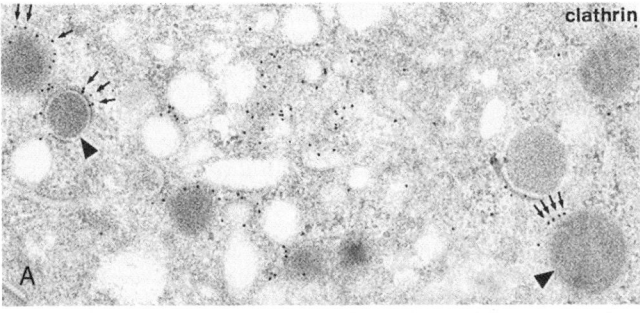

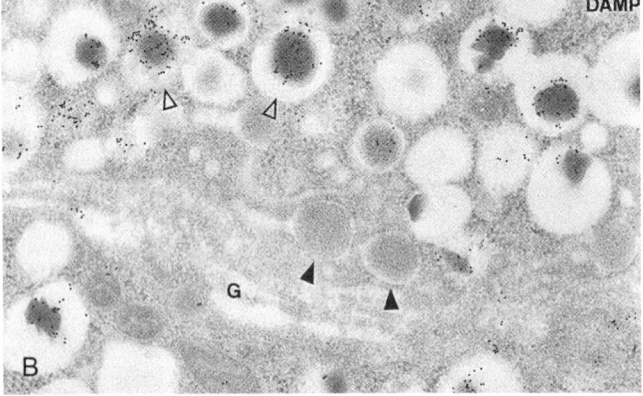

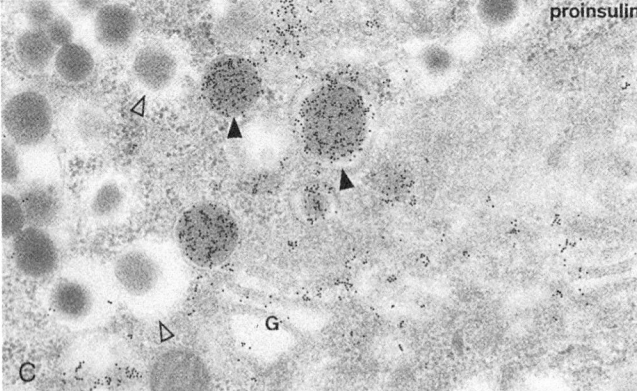

Figure 48-9 Clathrin (**A**), 3-(2,4-dinitroanilino)-3′-amino-*N*-methyldipropylamine (DAMP) (**B**), and proinsulin (**C**) immunolabeling of Golgi areas (G) of B cells (protein A-gold techniques). These figures show that the population of secretory granules with tightly fitting cores (*black arrowheads*) is clathrin coated (*arrows*) (**A**), DAMP poor (**B**), and proinsulin rich (**C**). These granules correspond to the maturing coated secretory granules freshly released from the Golgi complex. Conversely, secretory granules with wide clear halos (*white arrowheads*) are deprived of clathrin (not shown here), are DAMP rich (**B**), and are proinsulin poor (**C**). These correspond to the noncoated mature (storage) insulin-containing secretory granules. Because DAMP immunoreactivity is assumed to represent an indirect measure of intraorganelle acidity, this may indicate a decreasing pH gradient between proinsulin-rich and insulin-rich granules (i.e., between the converting and the storage compartments). (**A**, ×28,000; **B** and **C**, ×27,000.) (Source: From Orci L: The insulin cell: Its cellular environment and how it processes proinsulin. Diabet Metab Rev 2:71, 1986.)

requirement for the intracellular translocation of secretory proteins has been studied by Rothman and coworkers and is associated with the budding and/or fusion of small vesicles that transport secretory products from the *cis* through the *trans*-Golgi cisternae.[146,147]

The conversion of proinsulin to insulin in intact rat islet cells is a pseudo-first-order reaction that has a half-time ranging from about 20 minutes to 1 hour in various studies.[111,148] Peak labeling of proteins in the Golgi apparatus is observed 30 to 40 minutes after biosynthetic labeling of islets with

³H-amino acids; relatively little radioactivity remains in this region after 1 hour.[149,150] A similar pattern is observed by means of electron microscopic immunocytochemistry.[136] Therefore, it is likely that proinsulin conversion is initiated in the *trans* compartment of the Golgi apparatus or in newly formed secretion granules, or "progranules," as these leave the Golgi region, and that it continues for several hours within these granules as they collect and mature biochemically in the cytosol (see Fig. 48-8).

CONVERSION OF PROINSULIN TO INSULIN

The major proteolytic cleavages that are required for converting proinsulin to insulin are summarized in Figure 48-10. In early studies, it was shown that the conjoint action of trypsin and carboxypeptidase B gave rise to the naturally occurring products C peptide and native insulin, essentially quantitatively converting proinsulin to insulin in vitro.[151] This model could also account for the major intermediate forms that are

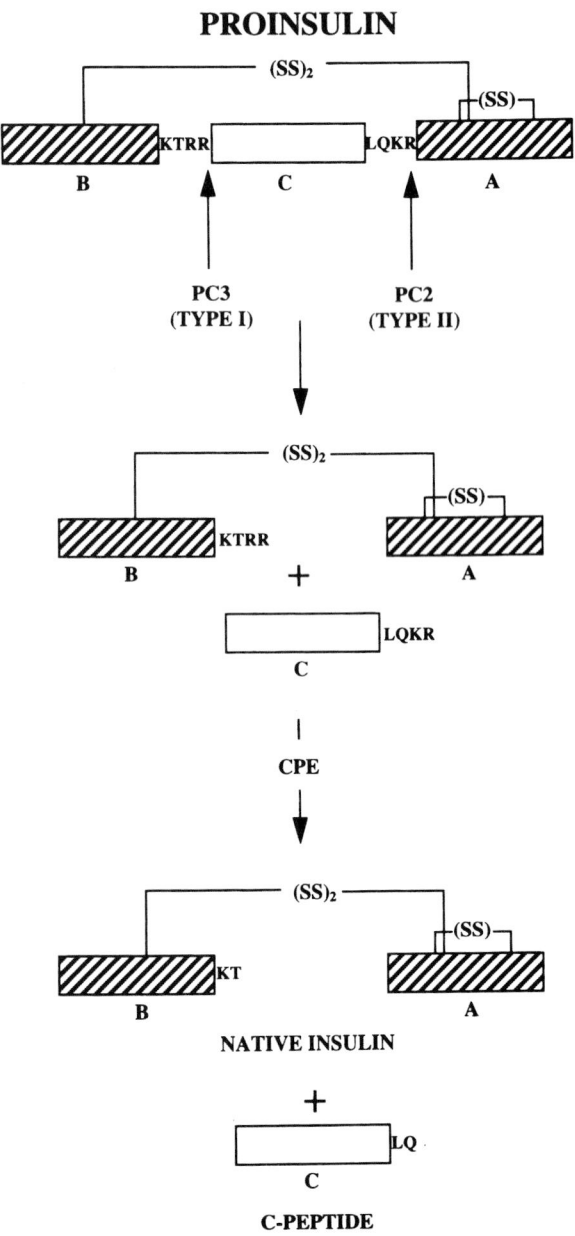

Figure 48-10 The cleavage of proinsulin to insulin by the combined action of the subtilisin-like prohormone convertases PC2 and PC1/PC3 and carboxypeptidase H. (See text for details.)

found in pancreatic extracts[101,128] and lead to a search for a cellular trypsinlike convertase, assumed to be a serine protease related to trypsin,[94] and for carboxypeptidases related to carboxypeptidase B. Studies in the early 1970s with isolated islet secretion granules already indicated that these were major sites of proinsulin conversion.[152] By labeling proinsulin in intact islets with ^{3}H-arginine, it also could be shown that subsequent conversion of prohormone in an isolated granule fraction in vitro led to the release of free arginine rather than of basic dipeptides,[129] confirming the likely participation of both trypsinlike and carboxypeptidase B–like activities in maturing secretory granules.[153,154] Carboxypeptidase E, or H— a homologue of pancreatic carboxypeptidase B with a more acidic pH optimum—was first identified in islets[153] and was subsequently identified and characterized in brain and other tissues.[155] Molecular cloning subsequently confirmed its structural and evolutionary relationship to the pancreatic carboxypeptidases.[155] More recently, additional processing carboxypeptidases have been uncovered in brain and other tissues.[156,157]

Discovery of the Prohormone Convertases

In 1985, a gene encoding an endopeptidase was found in yeast and was shown by genetic manipulations to be necessary for the processing of the α mating factor precursor.[158,159] This encoded enzyme, which was called Kex2, or kexin, was predicted to be a large (814-residue) integral membrane protein containing a catalytic domain related to the bacterial subtilisins[160,161] (Fig. 48-11). Kexin thus arose from a serine protease lineage unrelated to that of trypsin, probably via convergent evolution, as it utilizes the same classic charge transfer triad of Asp, His, and Ser as does the trypsin superfamily, but it is embedded in a totally different protein fold. The activity of kexin was shown to be dependent on calcium,[161,168] and this observation spurred efforts to find mammalian homologues that have a similar ionic requirement.

In 1988, Davidson and coworkers[169] first demonstrated the presence of two calcium-dependent activities (types I and II) in extracts of secretory granules purified from a rat insulinoma, raising the possibility that kexinlike enzymes existed in animal cells. These enzymes were able to process human proinsulin to insulin in vitro through their combined action. The type I activity had a lower calcium requirement (10^{-3} M) and cleaved proinsulin only at the B chain–C peptide junction, whereas the type II activity required a higher calcium concentration for optimal activity (5×10^{-3} M) and cleaved human proinsulin only at the A chain–C peptide junction (see Fig. 48-10). Efforts to further purify these enzymes were partially successful, but the quantities that were available were insufficient for amino acid sequence analysis and/or molecular cloning.

Meanwhile, efforts in many laboratories to find mammalian convertases by screening neuroendocrine cell cDNA libraries with kexin cDNA probes proved unsuccessful. Attempts to express insulinoma, normal islet, or AtT20 cell cDNA libraries in kexin-deficient strains of yeast with appropriate yeast vectors, using the restoration of mating and/or killer factor activity as selective screens, also yielded no positives.[170] However, when the nucleotide and predicted amino acid sequence of kexin in *Saccharomyces cerevisiae* was published by Mizuno and coworkers[160] in 1988, it became possible to utilize polymerase chain reaction (PCR) methodologies to search for kexin homologues, based on the presumed amino acid sequence conservation surrounding the active site Asp, His, or Ser residues. This approach, when used with human insulinoma cDNA, led to the discovery of prohormone convertase 2 (PC2), a 638-residue protein related to kexin in its catalytic domain (49% amino acid identity) but lacking a transmembrane segment, Ser/Thr-rich region, and cytosolic domain.[171] Further PCR analysis revealed an additional sequence, related to PC2, at lower abundance in the human insulinoma. A full-length cDNA, designated PC3, was

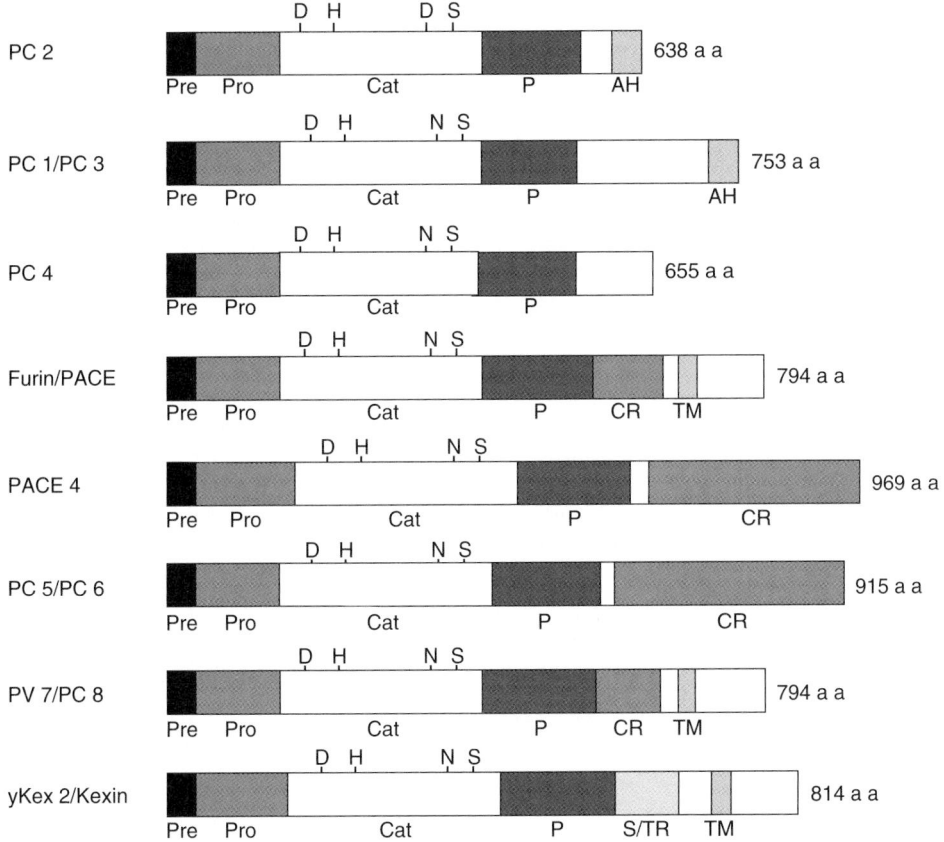

Figure 48-11 Schematic diagram of the primary structures of the precursors of yeast kexin and the currently known mammalian subtilisin-related proprotein convertases. The various subregions are designated as follows: signal peptides (Pre), proregion (Pro), catalytic domain (Cat), P or homo B domain (P), amphipathic helix (AH), cysteine-rich region (CR), Ser/Thr-rich region (S/T R), and transmembrane domain (TM). The catalytic Asp, His, Asn (Asp), and Ser residues are shown. The chromosomal localizations of the genes encoding these proteases in man are as follows: furin, 15q25[162,163]; PACE4, 15q26[163]; PC2, 20p11.2[164]; PC1/PC3, 5q15-21[165]; PC4, 19[166]; and PC7/PC8, 11q23-24.[167] (For further information see Barrett AJ, Rawlings ND, Woessner JF (eds): Handbook of Proteolytic Enzymes. New York, Academic Press, 1998, pp 342.)

obtained from AtT20 cell cDNA and revealed a 753-residue protein, which, like PC2, lacked a transmembrane domain.[172] Seidah and coworkers,[173] in Montreal, using a similar approach based on the conserved Asn and Ser residues of furin,[161] identified PC2 and a second enzyme (which they called PC1/PC3) in mouse pituitary cDNA.[13] The mPC1 proved to be identical to mPC3.[174]

A search of the database with the PC2 sequence revealed *fur*, a related human partial gene sequence, which had been reported by a group in the Netherlands in 1986.[162] Its protein product was designated *furin* because its gene was found in the immediate upstream region of the c-*fes/fps* proto-oncogene. Although furin was believed initially to be a growth factor receptor owing to the presence of a downstream cysteine-rich region and putative transmembrane domain, the incomplete N-terminal region was clearly related to the catalytic domains of PC2 and kexin and contained the characteristic catalytic serine residue. Subsequent cloning of full-length furin cDNAs revealed that this protein was structurally analogous to kexin, except that the Ser/Thr-rich domain in kexin was replaced by a cysteine-rich region.[175–178]

Structure and Activation of the Convertases

During the 1990s, a total of seven members of the mammalian prohormone convertase family were identified.[179] Recently, two more distantly related secretory pathway convertases, known as SP1/SKI-1 and Narc1, have been identified.[180] These proteases carry out cleavages at sites consisting mainly of hydrophobic residues. The structures of all these subtilisin-related convertases are compared diagrammatically in Figure 48-11. The genes that encode furin,[162,181] PC2,[164] PC1/3,[182] PC4,[166] and PC7/PC8[167] have been cloned and characterized. They show great structural similarity with a high degree of conservation of exon-intron junctions, indicating their probable derivation in evolution from a common ancestral convertase through gene duplication.[164,183] PC2 differs significantly from other members of this family in having aspartic acid at position 310 (the oxyanion hole residue) instead of a highly conserved asparagine, which is normally present in this position in subtilisin and the other convertases. The δ-amide of this asparagine residue in subtilisin is believed to form a hydrogen bond with the carbonyl oxygen of the scissile peptide bond, which stabilizes the transition state during catalysis.[184] However, if the aspartyl side chain in PC2 is protonated, it should also be able to provide this H bond. Subsequent studies have born out that PC2 is optimally active at pH 5.5, in support of this hypothesis.[185] PC2 also differs from the other enzymes in requiring the coexpression of neuroendocrine protein 7B2 for its activation.[186–188]

PC2 and PC1/3 are expressed (in varying amounts) only in neuroendocrine tissues, such as the islets of Langerhans, pituitary, and adrenal medulla, and in many regions of the brain.[172,174] In the islets, both PC2 and PC1/3 are present in the β cells, whereas only PC2 is present in the α, δ, and γ cells, which produce glucagon, somatostatin-14 (SS-14), and pancreatic polypeptide (PP), respectively.[189–191] Both PC2 and PC1/3 have been localized by immunocytochemical staining to the secretory granules in β cells.[190,192] Immunogold labeling of both proinsulin and PC2 in newly formed secretory vesicles has confirmed the colocalization of the convertases with their putative substrates (Fig. 48-12). PC1/3 undergoes C-terminal processing to a smaller, 66-kDa form in the secretory granules. Western blot tests indicate that mature 66- to 68-kDa forms of both PC2 and PC1/3 are the major forms that are present in islets of Langerhans, which is indicative of their accumulation in secretory granules.[192] Their tissue and subcellular distribution, along with their more acidic pH optima, contrasting with the more nearly neutral pH optima of kexin, furin, PACE4, PC6, and PC7, support the identification of PC2 and PC1/3 as major convertases of the neuroendocrine system.

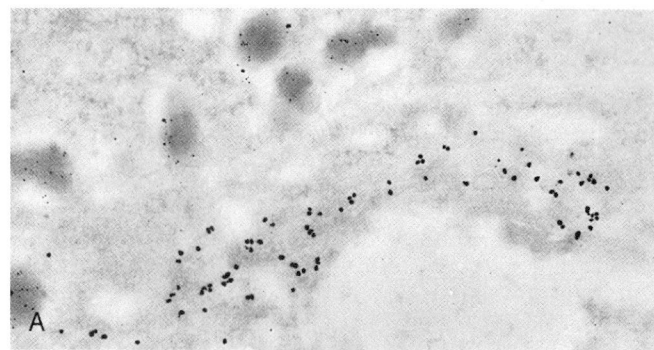
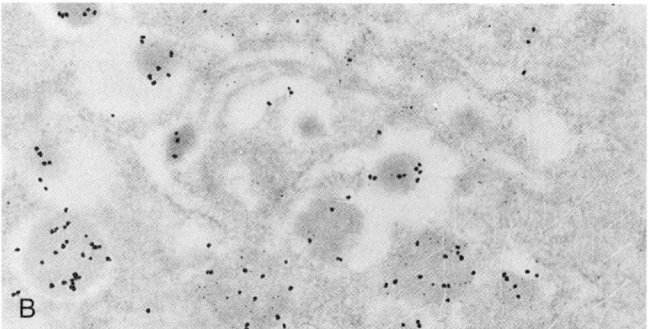

Figure 48-12 **A,** Immunogold labeling of proinsulin and PC2 in human islet β cells. Proinsulin-reactive Golgi stack (big colloidal gold particles) lack evident PC2 immunoreactivity (ultra small gold particles), labeling the mature secretory B granules. **B,** Proinsulin-reactive Golgi stack (ultrasmall gold particles) lack evident PC2 immunoreactivity (big gold particles); otherwise, present in the mature haloed and in some immature (proinsulin-reactive) secretory granules. (**A** and **B**, ×50,000). (Electron micrographs courtesy of Dr. Lucio Scopsi, Milan.)

In contrast to PC2 and PC1/3, furin is expressed in almost all tissues, the highest levels being in the kidney and liver,[178,193] and it may be involved in processing a variety of precursors, including various procoagulant proteins and proalbumin in the liver and some growth factor precursors and/or their receptors in many other tissues.[194,195] These proteins are not stored in secretory granules but are rapidly secreted via constitutive pathways. In keeping with this role, furin has been localized by immunostaining to the Golgi apparatus within cells.[194] Furin also has a more stringent specificity that allows it to selectively cleave precursors exiting the *trans*-Golgi without acting on the dibasic sites of most prohormone precursors, which are cleaved only after they enter the secretory granules. The basis of this greater selectivity is due at least in part to the additional requirement for an arginine residue in the P4 position relative to the cleavage site. This requirement has been demonstrated in a number of studies using a variety of substrates[177,193–199] and suggests that furin recognizes the general cleavage sequence R-X-K/R-R.[194,195] Thus, furin substrates often consist of tetrabasic sequences, as in the anthrax toxin protective antigen,[199] the egg-laying hormone of *Aplysia*,[200] and the insulin receptor precursor[201]; tribasic sequences, such as R-X-K/R-R[195,202]; or, less commonly, dibasic sequences in which arginine residues are present only in the essential P1 and P4 positions (R-X-X-R).[199] The polybasic sequences in a number of viral glycoprotein precursors also are likely substrates, and evidence is now mounting that furin and/or related enzymes (e.g., PC6B and PC7) carry out these cleavages, which are essential for full viral virulence.[203–206]

The convertases are synthesized as inactive zymogens owing to the presence of an N-terminal 80-residue proregion that follows the signal peptide in the proenzyme (see Fig. 48-11). This sequence usually contains two potential (multibasic residue) processing sites. Kexin is processed autocatalytically at a Lys-Arg (KR) pair at the downstream end of this region during its transport from the ER to the Golgi.[207] The mammalian proteases all have a similar but more complex (R-X-K/R-R) potential activation cleavage site that is positioned similarly at the end of their proregions. Studies on furin have indicated that this site is cleaved autocatalytically and intramolecularly in the ER and that this cleavage is necessary for the next step: transit to the Golgi. However, the propeptide remains attached after cleavage and serves to inhibit the enzyme until it reaches the TGN, where it dissociates under the more acidic conditions of this compartment; the propeptide is cleaved again at a second, more internal, site, allowing mature furin to gain full activity.[208] Except for PC2, with its unique requirement for 7B2 and relatively late maturation in the secretory granules, the furin model applies to the activation of PC1/3 and the other convertases.[179]

Role of PC2 and PC1/3 in Proinsulin Processing

Both PC2 and PC1/3 are required for proinsulin processing. Earlier studies indicated that PC2 cleaved selectively at the C peptide–A chain junction, whereas PC1/3 preferentially cleaved at the B chain–C peptide junction[192,209] (see Fig. 48-10). However, subsequent results indicate that either convertase is capable of cleaving at both sites when it is expressed at high enough levels.[210–212] All the available data[209,213] are consistent with the identification of PC1/3 and PC2 as the calcium-dependent type I and type II insulinoma granule-processing activities, respectively, as originally described by Davidson and coworkers.[169] Guest and coworkers[214] have fully documented the important role of calcium in the transport and proteolytic maturation of proinsulin.

The role and order of action of PC2 and PC1/3 in proinsulin conversion have also been carefully studied. Rhodes and coworkers[215] demonstrated that the type II convertase (PC2) prefers the proinsulin intermediate that has already been cleaved at the B chain–C peptide junction (des 31,32 intermediate proinsulin) as a substrate. This observation has led to the scheme for conversion outlined in Figure 48-13, in which

PC1/3 acts first to generate the des 31,32 intermediate, which is then the preferred substrate for PC2 action. This possible order of action is consistent with observations that PC1/3 achieves an active form more rapidly than PC2 does and has a somewhat higher pH optimum. Thus, PC1/3 may begin cleaving proinsulin in the TGN and very early secretory granules, whereas PC2 acts only in maturing granules. According to this scheme, PC1/3 appears to play a more important role in proinsulin processing, and this is borne out by observations on islets from mice that lack PC2 due to disruption of its gene.[212,216]

PC2 null mice are not diabetic, but they exhibit significant hyperproinsulinemia with plasma proinsulin levels in the range of 60%.[216] Pancreatic extracts also show increased proinsulin levels but only in the homozygous nulls, as indicated in Table 48-1. Pulse-chase studies of insulin biosynthesis in isolated islets, comparing PC2$^{-/-}$ mice with wild-type controls, also confirm significantly slower processing of proinsulin to insulin with accumulation of significant levels of des 31,32 intermediate proinsulin.[212] Approximately one third of the labeled proinsulin remains after a 3- or 4-hour chase, consistent with the levels found by radioimmunoassay in pancreatic extracts. Thus, PC2 converts, at most, about a third of the available proinsulin; therefore, PC1/3 must be responsible for processing the remaining two thirds under normal conditions.

The existence of a human subject who is a compound heterozygote with inactivating mutations in both copies of the PC1/3 gene has been reported recently.[217] This 43-year-old woman is obese and had gestational diabetes.[217] Examination of the patient's serum revealed no detectable circulating insulin associated with greatly elevated intact proinsulin and significant amounts of des 64,65 intermediate proinsulin but little or no des 31,32 proinsulin. Efforts to produce a PC1/3 null mouse have also recently succeeded[218] and reveal a similar severe block in proinsulin processing in this mouse model of PC1/3 deficiency[219] (see Table 48-1). This picture is consistent with the conversion scheme outlined in Figure 48-13 and

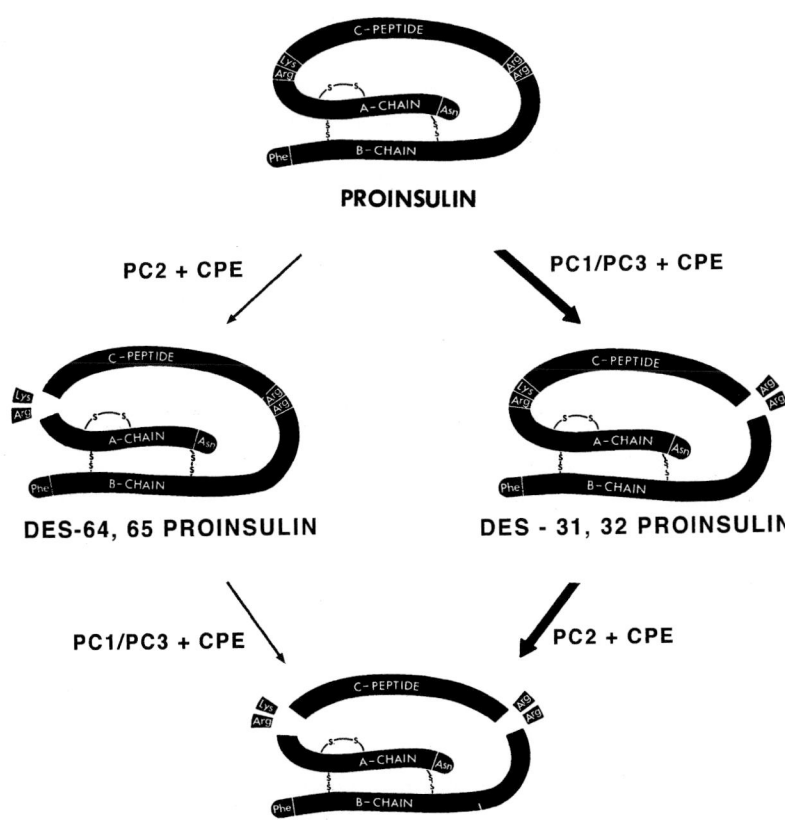

Figure 48-13 Routes of processing of proinsulin in the pancreatic β cell. The pathway on the right is probably more dominant under normal conditions because des 31,32 proinsulin is a preferred substrate for PC2,[215] and the more acidic pH optimum and slower maturation of this enzyme might delay its action during the initial phases of secretory granule maturation. The C-terminal basic residues are removed by CPE (CPH) after endoproteolytic cleavage by the PCs. (Source: Modified from Rouillé Y, Duguay SJ, Lund K, et al: Proteolytic processing mechanisms in the biosynthesis of neuroendocrine peptides. Front Neuroendocrinol 16:322, 1995.)

Table 48-1	Percent Proinsulin-like Immunoreactivity in Pancreatic Extracts of Wild-Type, PC2, and PC1/3 Null Mice		
	Genotype		
Strain	+/+	+/−	−/−
PC2 null	4.0	4.3	31
PC1/3 null	5.3	12.3	87

indicates that the pathway shown on the right side of the diagram is the predominant one. It also confirms the likelihood that PC1/3 is the more important β-cell convertase in the processing of proinsulin. The PC1/3 null mice, however, are not obese but instead exhibit a severe growth defect due to lack of normally processed growth hormone–releasing hormone (GHRH). Other endocrine abnormalities and intestinal malfunction also are present.[218]

Significance of Proinsulin and Des 31,32 Intermediate in Man

An important clinical issue is the observation that in humans, des 31,32 intermediate proinsulin is a major intermediate, making up a very significant proportion of the circulating proinsulin-like material.[220] It has been suggested that the accumulation of des 31,32 proinsulin might be due to a defect in the action of PC2, indicating a defect in the conversion mechanism.[221] At present, it is not possible to actually measure PC2 activity in human pancreas; however, isolated normal human islets of Langerhans have been reported to convert proinsulin to insulin with significant accumulation of des 31,32 intermediate despite the presence of normal levels of PC2.[222] However, des 31,32 intermediate reaches levels of only 15% to 20% of the total immunoreactive material during biosynthetic pulse-chase studies in the islets of mice lacking PC2 altogether.[212] Thus, even the complete absence of PC2 should not in itself give rise to the very high levels of this intermediate seen in normal human serum samples. This phenomenon can be best explained on the basis of the preference of PC2 and PC1/PC1/3 for a basic residue in the fourth position upstream (P4) from the cleavage site. Such an upstream basic residue is present at the B chain–C peptide junction in human proinsulin but is lacking at the A chain–C peptide junction. This causes an imbalance in the relative susceptibility of these two sites to either of the two convertases and tends to favor the accumulation of des 31,32 intermediate.[212]

Studies on the regulation of the biosynthesis of PC2 and PC1/3 in β cells suggest that the rates of translation of both of these enzymes are upregulated by glucose, similar to proinsulin on glucose stimulation.[223,224] However, it is not yet clear whether both PC2 and PC1/3 mRNA levels are equally elevated along with insulin mRNA during more prolonged stimulation of islets with glucose. Conceivably, under conditions of chronic stimulation, a relative deficiency of PC2 may might develop that could exaggerate the abnormalities in circulating proinsulin intermediates that are seen in diabetics. Thus, the accumulation of des 31,32 proinsulin in humans is mainly a reflection of the amino acid sequences at the proteolytic cleavage sites in human proinsulin, whereas increased levels of both proinsulin and des 31,32 proinsulin in prediabetics and diabetics may result from a deficiency of convertase action when islets are stressed by hyperglycemia. Genetic studies have not yet indicated a major role for mutations in the PC1/3,[182,225] PC2,[226] or CPE[227] genes in susceptibility to any form of diabetes.

Unusual and Rarely Occurring Cleavages

In some species, such as rats, and probably also pigs and humans, additional processive cleavages occur in the C peptide region of proinsulin that appear to be due to a chymotrypsin-like activity.[23,124,130,228] The importance of such additional C peptide cleavages in conversion remains unclear, however, since they evidently occur only in species in which the C peptide contains sites of high chymotryptic sensitivity. Recently, a novel subtilisin-like convertase was described in several laboratories.[229,230] This protease is only distantly related to the proprotein convertases and has a cleavage specificity that may be augmented by a P4 arginine residue, like some of the convertases, but it requires a hydrophobic valine or leucine residue at the P1 position of the cleavage site. An activity of this type might be responsible for some of the reported C peptide cleavages at sites with neutral or hydrophobic residues.

In the dog, C peptide cleavage occurs internally at a single arginine residue to produce an N-terminally truncated C peptide having only 23 residues.[231] A number of well-documented instances of such cleavage at single basic residues are known.[232,233] Some of these may be catalyzed by PC1/3, especially if a P4 arginine is present and the P1′ residue is not hydrophobic, but others involving Pro-Arg or Arg-Pro sites probably require other enzymes.[234] Taken together, these findings suggest that neuroendocrine secretory granules may contain a mixture of processing proteases[228,235] and that the specific cleavage of precursor forms of insulin or other precursor proteins is dictated, in part, by the high sensitivity to proteolytic digestion of certain regions in these substrate molecules as well as by restrictive specificities in the converting enzymes, which have similar but not identical properties and substrate specificities.

β-GRANULE FORMATION

One of the mysteries of neuroendocrine and other secretory cells is the mechanism underlying the efficient sorting of proteins that are destined for regulated secretion into immature secretory vesicles in the TGN. In the β cell, this process is remarkably efficient, resulting in very low levels of unregulated or "constitutive" release of proinsulin (<1% to 2%). The early secretory granules have a clathrin coat (see Fig. 48-9), which appears to be involved in some reorganization of the granule contents after and/or during their formation.[236] This granule sorting presumably occurs via small clathrin-clad vesicles that transport some proteins from the granules into cycling endosomal pathways that recycle either to the TGN or to the cell surface. As a consequence of this "constitutive-like" pathway, proteins such as furin, procathepsin B, and possibly others briefly pass through the immature granule compartment, where they might play an active, albeit transient, role (e.g., furin might participate in some way in the processing of prohormones).[236,237] Also, small amounts of abundant soluble granule components such as proinsulin and/or C peptide might exit the granules within these vesicles.[238] They might also play a role in maintaining synchrony between granule membrane area and granule volume as maturation proceeds.[236]

The newly formed secretory granules in neuroendocrine cells undergo biochemical and morphologic maturation after their formation in the Golgi apparatus. In β cells, the "progranules" characteristically are somewhat larger and less dense than the mature granules and have a uniform appearance.[136,139] Among the biochemical changes that take place as these progranules mature in the cytoplasm of the cell is the proteolytic conversion of proinsulin to insulin, accompanied by changes in the organization of the products. Electron microscopic studies of maturing insulin-secretory granules indicate that they acquire a dense central core, which often appears to be crystalline (Fig. 48-14). High magnification reveals repeat-unit spacings in the cores that are closely similar to those observed in ordinary zinc insulin crystals.[141,239,240] Thus, as insulin is liberated from proinsulin, it tends to crystallize with zinc that is concentrated by the β cells. Biochemical fractionation of mature islet secretory granules

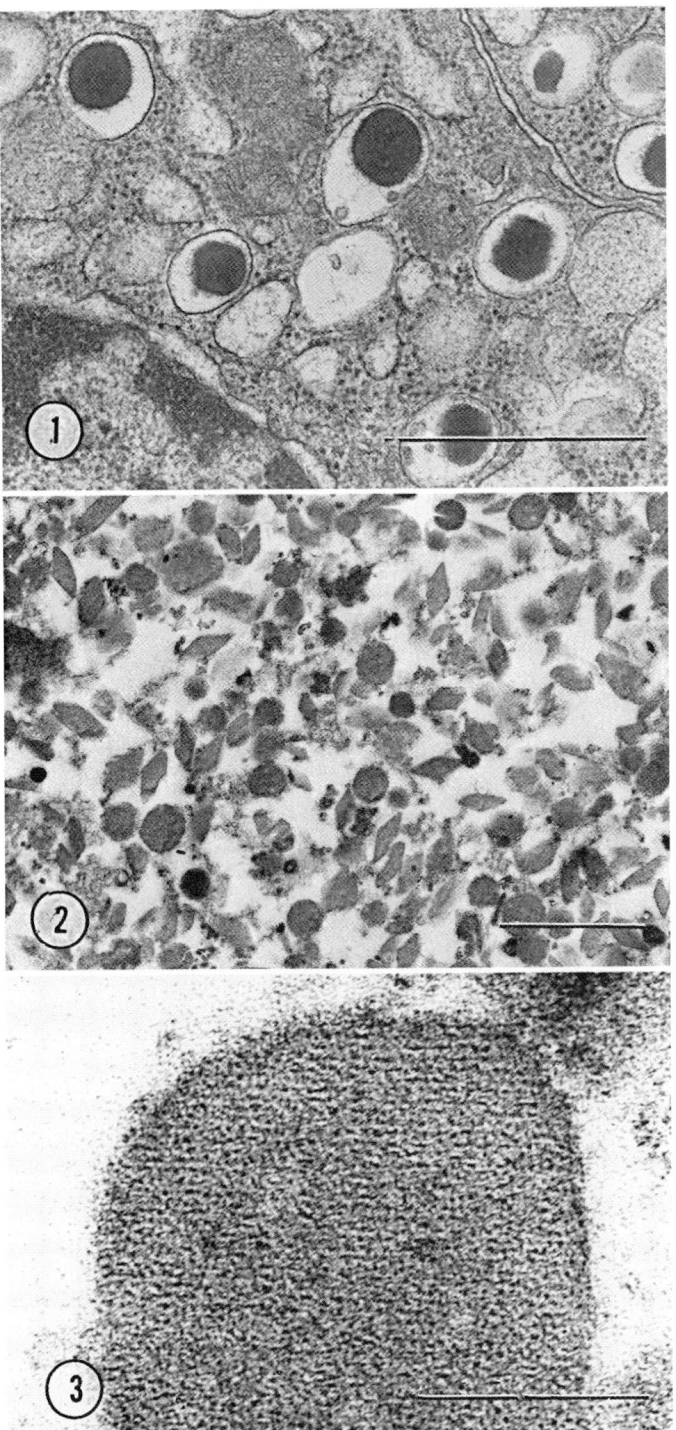

Figure 48-14 **1,** Photomicrograph of normal rat β cells (×28,000) showing morphology of mature granules (bar = 1 μm). **2,** Isolated rat β granule cores (×17,000)[141] (bar = 1 μm). **3,** High magnification view (×250,000) showing repeat unit structure of a crystalline core (bar = 0.1 μm). The cores are made up of both rat insulin I and II in approximately equal proportions (unpublished data from J. Michael and D. F. Steiner DF). Samples were fixed with Karnovsky's solution and stained with osmium tetroxide. (Electron micrographs courtesy of Hewson H. Swift.)

with insulin. As a result, the granule cores contain 1% to 2% of intact or partially processed precursor.[141]

The role of zinc in secretory granule formation is not well understood.[241] Most of the zinc in islets is present in the β granules and is liberated proportionately to insulin during secretion, in keeping with its role in crystallization of the hormone.[242,243] The mechanism for accumulation of zinc within the granules is unclear, but it could be a largely passive process that reflects the ability of both proinsulin and insulin to bind zinc.[107,244,245] The insulins of some species, including the guinea pig, coypu, and other hystricomorph rodents[17] and the hagfish,[37,66] lack the histidine residue at position 10 of the B chain that is required for zinc binding during the association of insulin dimers into hexamers.[62] As was mentioned earlier, most mammalian proinsulins can form soluble hexamers that are stabilized by two zinc atoms coordinated with the six B10 histidines, as seen in 2-zinc insulin crystals.[63] The proinsulin hexamers can also bind zinc at additional sites without precipitating from solution.[244] This property might allow proinsulin to play a role in zinc accumulation in the islet cells. Another function of the zinc might be to regulate the conversion process by sequestering the newly formed insulin in an osmotically inactive and biochemically stable crystalline form, thus effectively separating the product of this reaction from the enzyme(s) involved.

The pH of the interior of the secretory granule appears to be between pH 5.0 and 6.0 in the mature granules,[129,143] an optimal pH range for insulin crystallization in vitro. The neutral or slightly alkaline pH in the cisternal spaces of the rough endoplasmic reticulum favors proinsulin folding and sulfhydryl oxidation. The pH remains near neutral throughout the Golgi apparatus but becomes more acidic (pH 6.1) in the TGN as the secretory products are sorted into granules and proteolytic processing begins. Vesicular proton pumps may begin to increase the uptake of protons, which then displace the cationic arginine and lysine residues that are liberated during conversion. As these move out of the granules and are replaced by hydrogen ions, a downward shift in intragranular pH may occur. Thus, the initially mildly acidic progranules[143] undergo gradual acidification as they mature in the cytosol (see Fig. 48-9), creating appropriate conditions for the crystallization of the newly formed insulin. Clearly, the processes related to the biosynthesis of insulin via preproinsulin and proinsulin and their intracellular transport, sorting, proteolysis, and ultimate storage in secretory granules are remarkably well integrated, topologically and biochemically. This delicately poised integration of processes leading to the formation and storage of insulin is disturbed in islet cell tumors, which often show unregulated release of insulin together with large amounts of proinsulin; measurements of the latter can provide a useful diagnostic indicator[246,247] (see Chapter 49).

BIOSYNTHETIC ROLE AND POSSIBLE BIOLOGIC ACTIONS OF THE C PEPTIDE

Because of its cosecretion with insulin in essentially equimolar amounts,[94,142,248,249] the C peptide has been of great value as a marker of insulin secretion in humans under a variety of conditions (see Chapter 49). However, the C peptide radioimmunoassay is limited by the great sequence variability of this region in the proinsulin molecule; cross-reactivity is confined to closely related species, such as mice and rats, in which sequence divergence is minimal. Representative vertebrate C peptide amino acid sequences are compared in Figure 48-15.[100,250,251] These peptides exhibit a 15-fold higher rate of mutation acceptance than do the corresponding insulins, a finding that has often been interpreted as indicating that this region in the proinsulin molecule is unlikely to have any specific hormonal function. Among known proteins, only the fibrinopeptides have a higher rate of mutation acceptance

confirms that the cores contain only insulin, whereas the C peptide that is liberated in the conversion process remains in solution in the clear fluid space surrounding the dense crystalline core.[141] There is no evidence for cocrystallization of the C peptide with insulin under these conditions or in vitro. However, low levels of proinsulin can cocrystallize

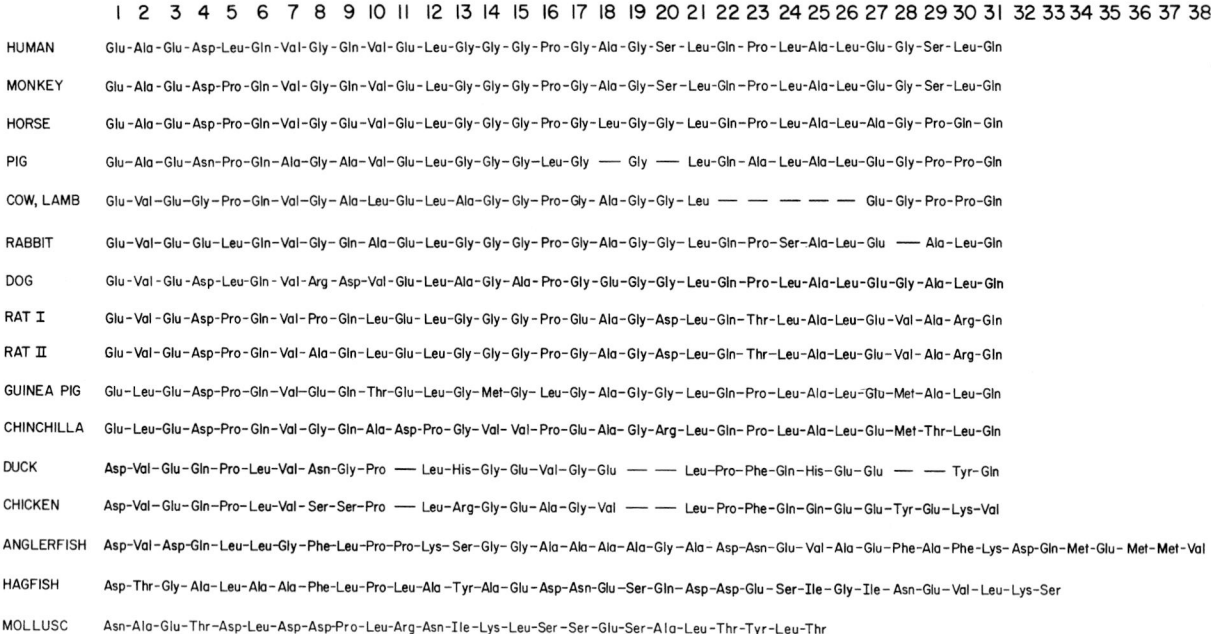

Figure 48-15   Compilation of amino acid sequences of proinsulin C peptides in vertebrates and in a mollusk, *Lymnae stagnalis* (for sources, see Steiner[100] and Smit et al.[252]). The guinea pig C peptide sequence corresponds to that predicted from the nucleotide sequence of the guinea pig insulin gene.[67]

than the proinsulin C peptides. Nonetheless, several acidic residues are consistently present at certain positions in the mammalian C peptides (see Fig. 48-15). These offset the added cationic charges due to the pairs of basic residues at the cleavage sites such that the isoelectric pH of proinsulin is nearly the same as that of insulin (i.e., in the range of pH 5.1 to 5.5) for most of the mammalian prohormones.[89,253]

Since the early 1990s, reports have appeared describing a number of biologic effects of the C peptide and/or peptides derived from it.[254] These putative effects include enhancement of glucose transport and utilization[254–256]; improvements in microcirculation in muscle,[253] skin, retina, and nerve in diabetics[258–260]; and stimulation of renal tubular Na+,K+-adenosine triphosphatase (ATPase) activity and other parameters of renal function.[254,256] Stimulation of islet cell proliferation has also been reported.[261] These results suggest that tissue receptors for C peptide might exist and that the circulating C peptide might contribute to improved glycemic control and help to slow the development of the vascular and neural complications of diabetes. What makes these effects even more surprising is that they do not seem to follow the usual rules of ligand-receptor chemistry (i.e., chirality does not matter); a C peptide that is synthesized entirely of D-amino acids is as active as is a peptide made with L-amino acids in reversed order.[258] However, a random sequence of the same amino acids leads to loss of activity. These observations suggest that novel interactions with membrane bilayers or other cellular constituents such as G protein–coupled receptors might underlie some of the observed effects.[260] These tantalizing findings suggest the need for a controlled clinical trial of combined insulin and C peptide therapy in diabetics. However, it should be borne in mind that in some of the reported studies, pharmacologic levels of C peptide have been used. It is also difficult to exclude the possibility of chemical impurities in some preparations that might lead to some of the observed effects in the complex biologic systems studied.

In addition to any putative biologic roles, consideration must also be given to the possible biosynthetic role of the C peptide. Thus, the C peptide clearly functions in biosynthesis by converting the insulin A and B chain interaction from an inefficient bimolecular reaction to a highly efficient and concentration-independent unimolecular reaction.[262] Certain regions of the connecting peptide may also facilitate the folding of the proinsulin polypeptide chain and the formation of the correct disulfide bonds or guide the enzymatic cleavage of proinsulin to insulin by helping to orient the basic residue pairs for efficient binding and cleavage by the convertases.[21,100] Recent molecular modeling studies indicate that this function of the C peptide might be of particular importance and might require an extended configuration for this region during interaction with the convertases.[263]

The normal length of the C peptide (usually 30 to 35 amino acids) is much greater than that necessary to span the short distance between A1 and B30 in the native insulin molecule (see Figs. 48-4 and 48-6). Not surprisingly, small bifunctional cross-linking reagents inserted between the amino group of A1 glycine and the ε-amino group of B29 lysine of insulin can functionally replace the C peptide in promoting the correct reoxidation of the sulfhydryls in high yield after complete reduction and denaturation.[264,265] Similarly, mini-proinsulins (also called single-chain insulins) with greatly shortened or absent connecting peptide segments appear to readily oxidize to form correct disulfide bridges and can be cleaved to yield insulin.[21,73] However, more recent studies suggest that folding and disulfide formation in some such forms is impaired.[266] Further studies will be required to assess the significance of these new findings for alternative approaches to promoting A and B chain combination in designing new therapeutic forms of insulin.

Another reason for the retention of a relatively long C peptide in proinsulin may be to facilitate its translocation across the RER membrane during its synthesis. The length of polypeptide chain required to span the large ribosomal subunit and the RER membrane has been estimated to be about 65 residues in extended configuration.[267,268] Moreover, the arrest of translation by the signal recognition particle (SRP) occurs only after synthesis of a nascent chain of about this length and may play a role in translational control of insulin biosynthesis.[269] Thus, the initial sequestration step in the biosynthesis of secretory peptide precursors may require a minimum peptide chain length that may greatly exceed the size of the final bioactive peptide or peptides per se.[267]

Efficient intracellular transport and correct targeting to secretory granules may impose additional demands on the primary (and tertiary) structure of proinsulin and other precursor proteins.[100,269,270] However, mini-proinsulins with deleted C peptides are correctly targeted to the regulated secretory pathway.[269]

The synthesis of several mammalian C peptides has been accomplished by classical fragment-condensation approaches (for references, see Steiner et al.[39]). The synthetic porcine C peptide, containing all four terminal basic residues, was tested for its ability to promote the recombination of insulin A and B chains in vitro, but it failed to influence the yield.[271] Synthetic porcine and bovine C peptides cross-react well with antibodies directed against the corresponding natural proinsulins or C peptides, and fragments of these peptides have been successfully utilized to study the antigenic determinants in this region of the proinsulin molecule.[39,272] The availability of biosynthetic human proinsulin and insulin, as well as of human C peptide, has opened many new possibilities for studies of the role, metabolism, and antigenicity of these peptides.[25,273–275]

REGULATION OF INSULIN PRODUCTION

Although the rate of secretion of insulin is subject to elaborate control by glucose and other nutrients, as well as by hormones and neurotransmitters,[276] the renewal and regulation of the granular stores of hormone in the β cells are important aspects of normal homeostasis. The biosynthesis of insulin is regulated by a variety of mechanisms so as to replenish insulin stores. The amount of insulin and/or proinsulin that is released via "unregulated," or constitutive, pathways[277] is normally very small, in the range of 1% to 2%.[249] Since calcium-dependent exocytosis of preformed storage granules[278] appears to be the major, if not the sole, source of both basal and glucose-stimulated insulin release in vivo,[248] we might ask how this granular compartment is maintained and regulated. The chief positive effectors that have been identified thus far are glucose, augmented by cyclic adenosine monophosphate (cAMP), which may also be generated by a mechanism coupled to glucose metabolism in the β cell.[279] Secretion, however, is not a direct stimulus to insulin biosynthesis, as can be demonstrated by blocking the secretory process via lowering external calcium levels or using inhibitors. These maneuvers do not impair the biosynthetic response to glucose.[94] If inhibition of secretion is prolonged, however, intracellular degradation (autophagy) of secretory granules occurs.[139,245] Also, in fetal and newborn rat islets, glucose stimulates insulin biosynthesis, although it has little effect on insulin secretion.[280]

It is well known that glucose rapidly stimulates insulin biosynthesis via stimulation of insulin mRNA translation.[94,281] This response consists of effects of glucose on both the initiation and elongation of proinsulin chains.[281] Glucose stimulation may also reduce the duration of SRP–signal peptide–mediated arrest of nascent preproinsulin chain elongation prior to ribosome docking in the early phases of RER membrane translocation.[266,281,282] In addition to this fast-acting translational control mechanism, the rate of transcription of insulin mRNA is also upregulated by glucose and cAMP.[283–286] Increased transcription results in part from phosphorylation of PDX1, a homeodomain protein that binds to regulatory regions of the insulin gene promoter.[287,288] Insulin mRNA, under normal conditions, turns over very slowly, with a half-life of about 30 hours at normal glucose levels,[284] and its stability is also affected by glucose. Hypoglycemia can lead to rapid declines in insulin mRNA.[289] In contrast, elevated glucose levels increase its half-life dramatically (approximately 2.6-fold), and this action, in combination with increased transcription rates, can effect large increases in insulin mRNA levels over periods of many hours. Prolonged glucose stimulation thus can lead to highly significant increases in insulin production[290] and, eventually, to increased β-cell mitosis and hyperplasia as well.[291] Glucose also regulates the turnover of insulin stores within the β cells,[249] but this effect probably plays a less significant regulatory role under normal conditions.

Whether insulin that is secreted by the islet β cells exerts positive functional feedbacks on insulin production has become a highly controversial area. A number of recent studies have suggested that blockade of insulin signaling via its receptor in β cells diminishes insulin secretion, transcription, and biosynthesis in response to glucose.[292,293] However, recent careful efforts to demonstrate a role for insulin signaling in regulating insulin biosynthesis and insulin mRNA level in islets have thus far not been successful.[294,295] The insulin and insulin-like growth factor 1 (IGF-1) receptors both clearly play complex regulatory roles in the β cells,[292] but their importance under normal conditions and/or in diabetic states is difficult to clearly assess owing to the significant experimental and observational obstacles that are involved.

THE INSULIN GENE FAMILY

The genetic mechanisms that control the expression of endocrine and neural regulatory peptides in the organism have been explored extensively. The gene for insulin was among the first to be isolated. Its structure in humans and several other species[54] is summarized in Figure 48-16. The single-copy human gene is located on the short arm of chromosome 11 in band p15. It is flanked on the 5' side by a unique

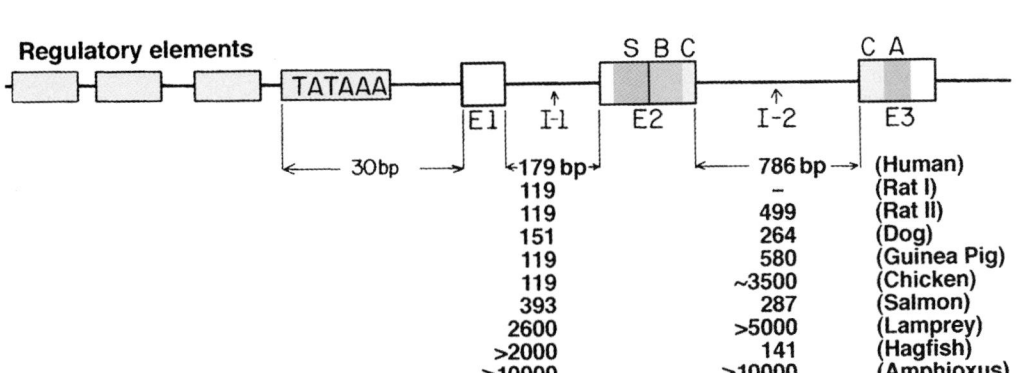

Figure 48-16 Diagrammatic representation of the insulin gene in vertebrates. Exons (E) appearing in mature preproinsulin mRNA are shown as bars, and the sizes of the two introns or intervening sequences (I) in various species are tabulated below. U, untranslated region; P, prepeptide coding region; B, B chain coding region; C, C peptide coding region; A, A chain coding region. A typical TATA box signaling transcription initiation is shown approximately 30 base pairs upstream from the messenger start site, preceded by a promoter region (*unfilled boxes*). The human insulin gene, abbreviated INS, is located on the short arm of chromosome 11 in the region p15.[296]

polymorphic region, composed of tandem repeats, that lies beyond the upstream regulatory region; this polymorphic region does not seem to influence the gene's expression in the pancreas, but it provides a useful marker for genetic linkage analysis.[296] Earlier reported correlations of the presence of larger (class III) versus smaller (class I or class II) repeats in this region with the incidence of type 2 diabetes were confounded by ethnic differences in the distribution of tandem repeats. Further analyses of larger populations failed to support this conclusion but have revealed that class I alleles and genotypes are significantly more frequent in white persons with type 1 diabetes than in those with type 2 diabetes or control subjects.[297] This allele may thus be a marker for a nearby susceptibility gene for type 1 diabetes.

The cDNAs and genes that encode other members of the insulin gene family have been identified and analyzed,[54] and additional members in mammals have been identified more recently.[55,56,298] Analysis of the genomic sequences that encode these various peptides substantiates the view that they are all related to insulin and are appropriately considered members of an insulin superfamily of hormones and/or growth factors. The duplication events that gave rise to genes encoding relaxin and other distantly related insulin-like peptides have not been identified. The genes that encode the IGFs appear to have arisen near the time of divergence of the vertebrates. In amphioxus, a primitive protochordate, a single insulin-IGF hybrid molecule has been identified that is equally distant from mammalian insulin and IGF genes.[299] These findings are consistent with the hypothesis that insulin and the IGFs diverged by gene duplication in early vertebrate evolution to better integrate metabolism and growth in these complex organisms. However, in contrast to IGF-1 and IGF-2, which are synthesized by most tissues, at least at some period during development, insulin appears to be produced only in the β cells of the islets of Langerhans in the adult organism.[300] (Extrapancreatic insulin expression transiently occurs in the yolk sac during embryonic development in the rat[301] and has been detected by in situ hybridization in periventricular cells in rat brain[302]; the latter observation remains to be confirmed.) The selective expression of the insulin gene in the β cells of the islets of Langerhans appears to be brought about by the actions of a number of transactivatng factors that bind to DNA recognition sequences located in the upstream region of the gene between the hypervariable region and the TATA box, that is, 300 to 400 base pairs upstream (for reviews, see Edlund[303] and Melloul et al.[304]).

DEFECTS IN THE INSULIN GENE: THE INSULINOPATHIES

Tager and associates were the first to identify a structurally abnormal insulin in the circulation and pancreas of a patient with mild diabetes associated with elevated insulin levels.[305] The development of HPLC systems that are capable of resolving plasma insulin components then led to the further identification of abnormal insulins differing in hydrophobic character in two additional unrelated lineages.[15] These and similar studies led to the definition of a new clinical syndrome analogous to the hemoglobinopathies: the insulinopathies (i.e., molecular defects involving the insulin molecule). Six families have been identified thus far, all having the syndrome of mild hyperinsulinemic diabetes that is similar, in some respects, to type 2 or non-insulin-dependent diabetes mellitus (NIDDM).[306,307] Affected individuals have high circulating insulin levels with a distorted C peptide–insulin ratio, resulting most likely from the delayed turnover, in vivo, of circulating insulin variants owing to their impaired receptor-binding properties.[308] The disorder is inherited in an autosomal-dominant fashion within families, consistent with the Mendelian distribution of a defective allele.

The insulin genes (both alleles) have been cloned from affected individuals in these families, and in all six cases, a single nucleotide substitution in only one of the two alleles leading to a single amino acid replacement within the insulin molecule was found.[307,309,310] The abnormal insulins that are generated by these missense mutations are all characterized by a very low binding potency, below 5% of normal, as demonstrated by direct assays.[311,312] However, the replacements occur at different sites within the insulin molecule (at residues B24 [Phe → Ser], B25 [Phe → Leu], and A3 [Val → Leu]), and the affected individuals thus far have all been heterozygous for the defective gene. Although not all affected individuals have overt diabetes, it is evident from the high incidence of mild diabetes or glucose intolerance among the affected individuals in these families that the presence of a defective insulin allele can be a significant predisposing factor to the development of diabetes. Hence, such mutations, or still others that might reduce the level of expression of the insulin gene (i.e., leading instead to hypoinsulinemia), could give rise to a picture that is indistinguishable from the fairly common type 2 diabetes (NIDDM).

Recently, a point mutation in one of the two mouse insulin genes (Ins II) has been found to be associated with severe β-cell dysfunction in the MODY mouse.[313] This autosomal-dominant form of diabetes is not associated with obesity or insulin resistance but is due instead to impaired insulin production. The mutation of the A7 cysteine to tyrosine evidently causes misfolding, aggregation, and degradation of both mutant and normal proinsulin chains in the endoplasmic reticulum. Molecular chaperones, such as BiP, and enzymes that are involved in sulfhydryl oxidation, such as protein disulfide isomerase, are increased in the islets of MODY mice, whereas insulin is greatly decreased. Secretory granules are less abundant and smaller than in controls, whereas ER is enlarged and contains material that is probably composed of proinsulin aggregates. This represents one of the most severe insulinopathies to be found to date, but it clearly indicates the potential for dominant negative structural defects in proinsulin as a cause of diabetes.

In addition to molecular variants involving insulin, others have been identified that give rise to elevated circulating proinsulin levels, with or without clinically significant carbohydrate intolerance.[314,315] In these families, an autosomal-dominant pattern of inheritance is again evident, and in seven cases, the defect has been localized to the conversion site in the proinsulin molecule (at the C peptide–A chain junction) at which the arginine of the Lys-Arg pair recognized by the converting enzyme has been replaced by another amino acid, rendering this site uncleavable.[316,317] In six of these families, molecular cloning has disclosed the substitution of a histidine for Arg 65[318-320]; in another family, leucine replaced Arg 65.[321] An eighth family with hyperproinsulinemia, in which a point mutation changes the histidine at position 10 of the B chain to aspartic acid, has also been identified.[322,323] This is a particularly interesting mutation because the resultant proinsulin molecule retains the paired basic residues, but it is not processed efficiently owing to a defect in its sorting into secretory granules, which leads to its increased secretion as intact proinsulin via constitutive pathways.[324,325]

Although rare, naturally occurring variants have shed new light on both normal processes and disease mechanisms and thereby assume greater importance and relevance to clinicians. The study of insulin variants has led to significant revisions in theories regarding the location of the receptor-binding region in the insulin molecule (see the section entitled "Receptor-Binding Region of Insulin," earlier in the chapter) and has also provided direct evidence that receptor-mediated uptake and degradation of insulin[72,326,327] constitute a major pathway of insulin metabolism in vivo.[306,308]

Several studies have assessed the frequency of insulin gene mutations in diabetic populations.[328,329] Variations in both noncoding and coding sequences have been found, but thus far, no significant associations with diabetes have been detected. Three promoter variants have also been described.[329,330] These include a C-to-G transversion at −56, a C deletion at −90 and an eight-base-pair repeat— TGGTCTAA—from position −322 to position −315. This repeat was present in the insulin genes of 5% of subjects with NIDDM and 1% of nondiabetic black American subjects, as well as in 3 of 41 diabetic and 0 of 41 nondiabetic Mauritian Creoles of African ancestry. It was absent in 35 white subjects with NIDDM and 40 Pima Indians. When tested in functional assays, this variant exhibited significantly reduced promoter activity (38% to 44% of normal). These results suggest that naturally occurring promoter variants that reduce insulin gene expression may contribute to a small proportion of cases of diabetes in some ethnic groups. Defects in regulatory proteins arising from other loci (e.g., the transcription factor PDX1[331]) also can influence insulin gene expression or its regulation and play an important role in causing diabetes of the MODY type.

IAPP (AMYLIN): A MINOR SECRETORY PRODUCT OF THE β CELL

Studies during the 1990s have revealed that β cells secrete small amounts of a number of other peptides and proteins in addition to insulin (see Table 48-1).[95,332] Some of these are unique to the islet β cells; others are expressed in other neuroendocrine cells and neoplasms. The chromogranins A, B, and C represent a family of closely related acidic peptides that are expressed in many neuroendocrine cells.[333] Chromogranin A is found in the β, α, and PP cells in the islets, whereas chromogranins B and C are also present only in the islet α cells.[333] The role of these proteins is not understood, but it might be related to the formation and organization of the secretory granule or the processing of prohormones. Chromogranin A has been cloned from rat pancreatic islet and insulinoma tissue,[334] and some amino acid sequence information on the human peptide from insulinomas is also available.[335] Chromogranin A is processed to release at least two peptides of interest: pancreastatin, a 49-amino acid amidated peptide from the central region of chromogranin A, which was originally isolated from porcine pancreas and which inhibits insulin secretion,[336] and β granin, a 24-kDa peptide derived from the N-terminal region of chromogranin A.[333,335] Both peptides are stored in insulin granules and are released along with insulin. Whether chromogranin A also regulates secretory granule biosynthesis is a current controversy of considerable interest.[337]

Another intriguing cosecreted product is the more recently discovered 37-amino acid neuropeptide-like molecule islet amyloid polypeptide (IAPP), or amylin. IAPP was first described as a major protein constituent of the amyloid deposits that occur in the islets of elderly diabetics (i.e., those with so-called type 2 diabetes, or NIDDM) and in many benign insulinomas of the pancreas as well as in the normal pancreases of the aged.[338-341] Although the presence of amyloid-like material was first noted in specimens of human pancreas as early as 1901 by the pathologist Opie,[342] it was not until 1986 that efforts to solubilize this material were successful.[338] When the soluble material was analyzed, it turned out to be composed mainly of a single peptide: IAPP. Sequence analysis revealed that this peptide (Fig. 48-17) was related to the 37-amino acid neuroendocrine peptides calcitonin gene-related peptide, types 1 and 2 (CGRP-1 and CGRP-2).[338-341] CGRP-1 is a second product of the calcitonin type 1 gene, derived through an alternative splicing event that occurs mainly in neural tissues.[344-346] As a result of this process, a calcitonin-encoding exon (exon 4) is replaced by another encoding CGRP (exon 5) in the formation of an mRNA for a preproprotein that gives rise to CGRP via proteolytic processing.[345]

The availability of the amino acid sequence of IAPP led to the identification of both the cDNA and the chromosomal gene encoding this hormonelike polypeptide in humans.[347-350] In addition, cDNAs encoding IAPP precursors from a number of mammalian species have been described.[347,348,351] PreproIAPP has a signal peptide followed by a short propeptide ending in Lys-Arg at the N terminus of IAPP (Fig. 48-18). The C-terminal side of the IAPP domain is followed by Gly-Lys-Arg and another short propeptide region. The presence of a glycine residue at the C terminus of the IAPP region preceding the basic dipeptide proteolytic processing signal suggests that IAPP is normally carboxyamidated, as are the CGRPs.[347,351] Comparison of the sequences of the precursors of IAPP and CGRP also revealed sequence similarities in their signal peptides as well as between the sequences of IAPP and CGRP.

The characterization of the human IAPP gene (see Fig. 48-18) revealed a simpler intron-exon arrangement than described for the genes encoding CGRP-1 and -2,[344] although all are clearly related.[349,350,352] The single gene that encodes IAPP in humans is located on the short arm of chromosome 12,[350,351] which is believed to be an evolutionary homologue of chromosome 11, where the CGRP-1 and CGRP-2 genes are located.[344] Thus, the available evidence strongly supports the likely divergence of IAPP, CGRP, and calcitonin from a common ancestral gene.

BIOSYNTHESIS AND LEVELS OF IAPP IN ISLETS

Studies with antibodies that are specific for IAPP have demonstrated that it is present in islets in significant amounts, as judged by immunocytochemical staining, and is localized to

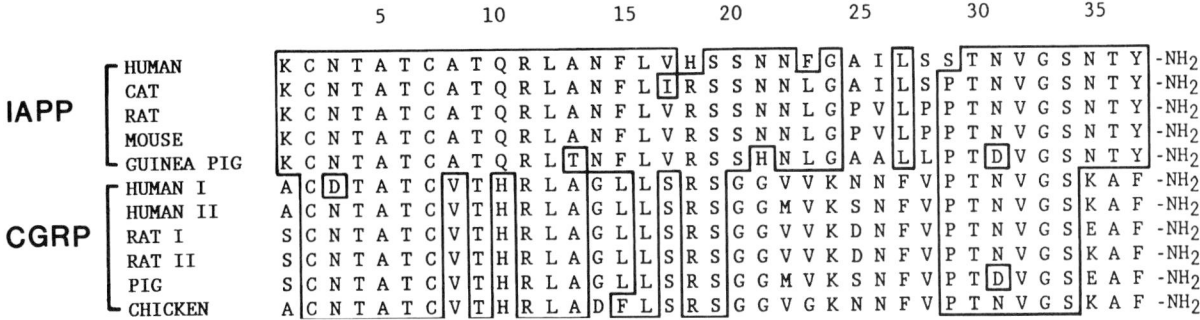

Figure 48-17 Comparison of IAPP and CGRP amino acid sequences. Note the canonical differences between the two peptide families at positions 1, 8, 10, 14, 15, 17, 20 to 28, 35, 36, and 37. The region comprising residues 20 to 29 is believed to nucleate β-pleated sheets in forming amyloid fibrils.[343] (Source: From Nishi M, Sanke T, Nagamatsu S, et al: Islet amyloid polypeptide. A new beta cell secretory product related to islet amyloid deposits. J Biol Chem 265:4173, 1990.)

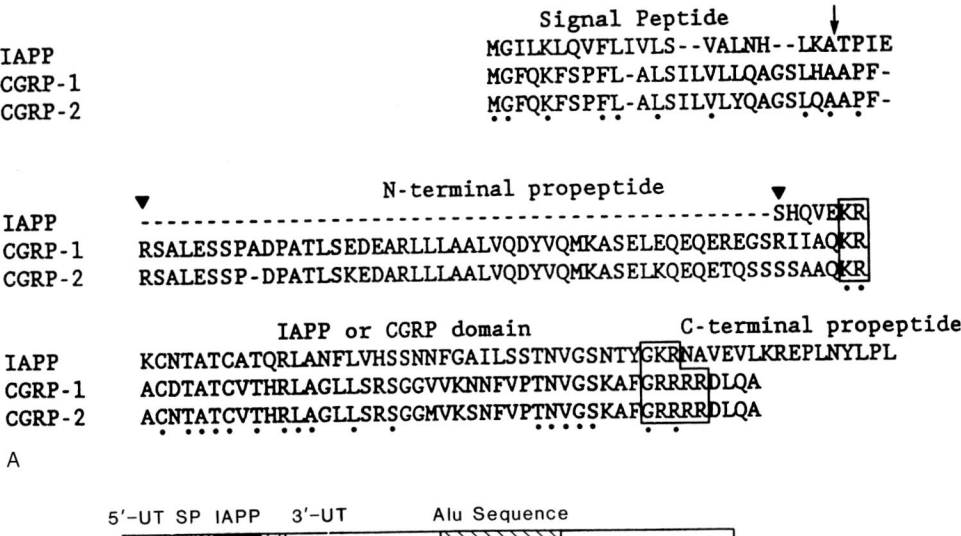

```
                                                Signal Peptide           ↓
                                      MGILKLQVFLIVLS--VALNH--LKATPIE
IAPP
CGRP-1                                MGFQKFSPFL-ALSILVLLQAGSLHAAPF-
CGRP-2                                MGFQKFSPFL-ALSILVLYQAGSLQAAPF-
                                       ·  ·········  ·····   ··
```

```
                          ▼                   N-terminal propeptide                    ▼
IAPP    ---------------------------------------------------------SHQVE|KR|
CGRP-1  RSALESSPADPATLSEDEARLLLAALVQDYVQMKASELEQEQEREGSRIIAQ|KR|
CGRP-2  RSALESSP-DPATLSKEDARLLLAALVQDYVQMKASELKQEQETQSSSSAAQ|KR|
```

```
                          IAPP or CGRP domain              C-terminal propeptide
IAPP    KCNTATCATQRLANFLVHSSNNFGAILSSTNVGSNTY|GKR|NAVEVLKREPLNYLPL
CGRP-1  ACDTATCVTHRLAGLLSRSGGVVKNNFVPTNVGSKAF|GRRRR|DLQA
CGRP-2  ACNTATCVTHRLAGLLSRSGGMVKSNFVPTNVGSKAF|GRRRR|DLQA
        · ·····  ·····  ·····           ·····
```

A

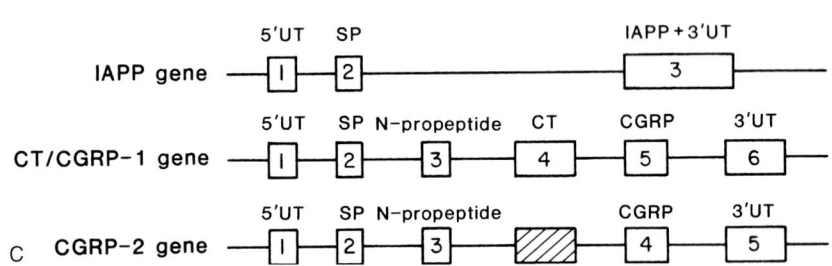

Figure 48-18 **A,** Comparison of amino acid sequences of the precursors of human IAPP and CGRPs 1 and 2. The *small arrow* indicates the signal peptide cleavage site; the *arrowheads* show the position of intron exon junctions in the CGRP-1 and 2 genes. **B,** Schematic representation of the mRNA encoding preproIAPP, indicating its relation to the exons of the IAPP gene. This gene in humans is located on chromosome 12P12.3.[349,350] **C,** Comparison of IAPP and CGRP gene structures. The ancestral gene of this superfamily might have been organized similarly to that of the CGRP-2 gene. 5'UT, 5 untranslated region; SP, signal peptide; CT, calcitonin.

the secretory granules of the β cells.[353,354] Thus, the IAPP precursor is likely transferred along with proinsulin into newly forming secretory vesicles in the TGN of the β cells, where it is then processed into the mature 37-residue carboxyamidated peptide, stored, and subsequently cosecreted with insulin.[355] As is the case with proinsulin, the efficient processing of proIAPP requires the actions of both β-cell convertases PC2[356] and PC1/3.[357] However, PC2 is more critical, since it is required to process the N-terminal cleavage site of proIAPP, while both PC2 and PC1/3 can process the C-terminal site, but PC2 does so more efficiently. The expression of IAPP is stimulated by glucose, comparable to that of insulin under normal conditions, but it may be altered in pathologic states.[358] Very low levels of IAPP mRNA have also been detected in the stomach and other regions of the gastrointestinal tract, in the lung, and also in the dorsal root ganglia of the spinal cord.[359]

The relative levels of IAPP and insulin in the β cell appear to be only a few percent of the level of insulin. HPLC analysis of freshly isolated rat islets shows amounts of IAPP that are in the range of 1% to 2% those of insulin.[95] Biosynthetic labeling experiments in islets have also corroborated these low levels of IAPP expression relative to insulin (unpublished data of R. Carroll and D. F. Steiner). Although synthetic IAPP has been shown to inhibit insulin secretion from rat islets of Langerhans, the doses (10^{-5} M) that are required for this effect are extremely high.[360] Most studies[361-363] agree that the levels

of IAPP are in the range of 0.2% to 3% of the level of insulin in normal adult rat islets or normal human pancreas. Studies with isolated rat islets have shown that IAPP secretion is stimulated by glucose and that IAPP amounts to about 5% of the amount of insulin released in 1 hour at 16.7 mM of glucose.[363]

HORMONAL EFFECTS OF IAPP

Leighton and Cooper and others have shown that IAPP inhibits glucose uptake and glycogen synthesis in muscle exposed to IAPP in vitro, an effect it shares with CGRP.[364,365] In whole animals, efforts to modify glucose tolerance with IAPP infusion have met with mixed success. However, euglycemic glucose clamp studies with dogs have demonstrated that the amidated form of IAPP inhibits insulin-stimulated glucose disposal over short infusion periods of 1 to 2 hours.[366] In these experiments, the rates of IAPP infusion were threefold to sixfold higher on a molar basis than the rates of insulin infusion. Such high ratios of secretion of IAPP relative to insulin could not be achieved under normal physiologic conditions in vivo. Other studies indicate that the actions of IAPP may be complementary to those of insulin and may include delayed nutrient delivery and suppression of postprandial glucagon secretion.[367] However, mice that lack IAPP owing to a knockout of the gene show increased insulin secretion and more rapid glucose disappearance, suggesting that its normal role is inhibitory with respect to insulin secretion and action.[368,369]

In view of the distant evolutionary relationship between calcitonin and IAPP, it is of interest that both nonamidated and amidated forms of IAPP have serum calcium-lowering effects in animals in vivo as well as in cell culture systems.[370,371] A direct effect on uptake of calcium by bone tissue has been demonstrated, but it is not clear whether this effect is mediated via calcitonin or IAPP receptors.[370] MacIntyre[371] has proposed that IAPP may be secreted along with insulin to promote the utilization of ingested calcium.

Finally, it should be mentioned that because of its extensive homology with CGRP, it seems likely that IAPP may share some actions of CGRP, a family of neuropeptides that are expressed in the nervous system and at nerve endings in many organs throughout the body.[346,372,373] Their main functions in peripheral tissues appear to be mediated via cAMP and to involve smooth muscle relaxation, leading to bronchial dilation, lowering of blood pressure, and decreases in intestinal motility.[344,346,373] It also has been proposed that CGRP may play a role as a growth factor, regulating the development of olfactory bulb neurons during embryogenesis.[374] Recent studies suggest that protein modifiers termed *receptor activity-modifying proteins* can interact with and modify the specificity of CGRP-like receptors to enhance IAPP binding.[375]

MECHANISM OF AMYLOID FORMATION

Several studies[376-378] have indicated that islet amyloid formation (Fig. 48-19) occurs more prominently in spontaneously diabetic animals and in certain species more so than others. Among diabetes-prone animals were several different species of nonhuman primates as well as cats, raccoons, and the degu (*Octodon degus*), a New World rodent related to the guinea pig.[340,376-380] It is interesting to note that the IAPP sequences in these species differ most significantly in the region that has been defined as amyloidogenic (residues 20 to 29) in studies by Glenner and coworkers[343] and Westermark and coworkers.[351,381] Synthetic peptides from this region had the greatest tendency to form fibrillar stacked β-pleated sheet structures similar to those occurring in amyloid. However, formation of amyloid in the degu occurs via a different mechanism and has been shown to consist mainly of degu insulin, which differs significantly from most other mammalian insulins.[382,383]

Antibodies that are raised to various regions of IAPP have verified its presence in islet amyloid by both light and electron microscopic immunocytochemical analysis.[354,355,384] Although in normal β cells, it is localized within the insulin secretory granules,[354,355] Clark and coworkers have also noted fibrillar immunoreactive amyloid deposits within the cytoplasm of β cells of some patients with type 2 diabetes.[353] Others have also noted the proximity of amyloid deposits to the β cells, suggesting that it has arisen from these cells either by secretion or by some other means of deposition.[381,385] Clark and coworkers[386] have found IAPP immunoreactivity in lysosomes and lipofuscin bodies within the β cells of the islets of both normal and diabetic individuals and have suggested that amyloid may begin to form during the intracellular degradation of secretory granules, as occurs in the normal turnover of unused secretory products, a process known as *crinophagy.*

The factors that lead to amyloid deposition in diabetes remain unclear,[387,388] but recent work with transgenic mice that hypersecrete human IAPP have demonstrated amyloid deposition under some circumstances, especially with high dietary fat intake.[389] Recent studies have failed to reveal any abnormalities in the predicted sequence of IAPP precursors in 25 subjects with type 2 diabetes,[390] and therefore hypotheses involving abnormalities in the structure of either IAPP or its precursor in the formation of islet amyloid are untenable. The amyloid that is formed in the islets during normal aging appears to be similar to that in diabetic subjects but is usually much less abundant.[391-393]

PROPERTIES AND STRUCTURE OF GLUCAGON

Although the existence of a pancreatic hyperglycemic factor was postulated in the early 1920s,[394] the peptide hormone glucagon was not isolated until 30 years later.[395] Using a crude fraction obtained during the commercial preparation of insulin, Staub and coworkers succeeded in both purifying and crystallizing the pancreatic stimulator of hyperglycemia.[395] They noted the nearly neutral isoelectric pH of the peptide and its tendency to form fibrils at acidic pH. The availability of the pure hormone thus eliminated any continuing doubt as to the existence of a unique hyperglycemic hormone and made possible a great number of experiments regarding its chemistry and mechanism of action.

In 1957, Bromer and coworkers reported the amino acid sequence of porcine glucagon and noted the sensitivity of the peptide to digestion by trypsin.[396] Since that time, the glucagons from a number of mammalian, avian, and piscine species have been isolated, and their sequences have been determined (Fig. 48-20).[397-399] Remarkably, the sequence of the glucagons of almost all mammals is identical, except for the guinea pig, in which it differs at five positions.[400-402] The identical glucagons of turkeys and chickens differ from human glucagon at only one position, and the duck hormone differs at only two.[399,403,404] Neither of these changes, however, appears to have a major impact on bioactivity, notwithstanding the reduced reactivity of duck glucagon with antisera directed toward the mammalian hormone.[399] The structure of glucagon in several species of fish has also been reported.[405] These are substituted at from six to ten positions

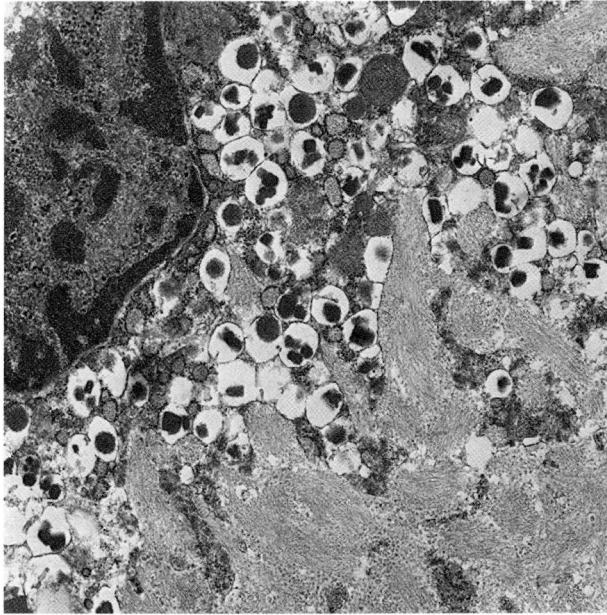

Figure 48-19 Photomicrograph showing extensive islet amyloid deposits with adjacent β cells in a human diabetic pancreas (×28,000). (Electron photomicrograph courtesy of Dr. Per Westermark, Linköping, Sweden).

```
HUMAN        HSQGTFTSDYSKYLDSRRAQDFVQWLMNT
GUINEA  PIG  --------------------Q-LK--L-V
CHICKEN      ----------------------------N
DUCK         ---------------T------------N
ANGLERFISH   --E---SN------ED-K--E--R----N
```

Figure 48-20 Primary structures of glucagons in several vertebrate species. Residues that differ from the highly conserved sequence of Old World mammals (human, pig, cow, rabbit, rat, hamster) are indicated. (Single-letter amino acid code is given in Dayhoff.[36])

in various species. The high degree of structural conservatism within glucagons, especially among mammals, probably reflects strong evolutionary constraints operating within the glucagon-secretin superfamily of closely related hormones. Guinea pig glucagon is an exception, having five amino acid replacements in its C-terminal region,[400,401] which reduce its biologic activity to about 10% of that of other species.[402] The amino acid substitutions in the guinea pig protein may represent an adaptation to the markedly altered insulin in this species,[35,400] which also has greatly reduced biologic potency.[406] An increased rate of mutation acceptance is confined to this region of the guinea pig glucagon gene.[400] Glucagon is structurally related to other neurohormonal peptides, including secretin, vasoactive intestinal polypeptide, gastric inhibitory peptide, and growth hormone–releasing factor, indicating a probable common ancestral origin.[407,408]

Investigations on the secondary and tertiary structure of glucagon have indicated that the hormone assumes an α-helical conformation, dependent both on peptide concentration and on the characteristics of added solutes (summarized in Steiner et al.[39]). In more concentrated solutions, glucagon monomers associate into trimers and possibly higher oligomers.[17] A major advance in our understanding of glucagon structure came from the work of Sasaki and associates on the complete x-ray analysis of crystalline glucagon at 3-Å resolution.[409] The peptide exists in the crystal as a trimer with a high percentage of helical secondary structure. Residues 10 to 25 occur in α-helix, and residues 5 to 9 and 26 to 29 occur in a less regular, right-handed helical conformation. The N-terminal pentapeptide is apparently more flexible, and its conformation is less well defined. The structure of monomeric glucagon in very dilute solution remains unsolved, but the possibility of the induction of α-helicity by interaction of the peptide with hydrophobic receptor recognition sites has been considered.[17]

The strong evolutionary conservation of glucagon suggests the importance of multiple structural features that contribute to the biologic activity of this gluconeogenic and glycogenolytic hormone. In fact, deletion of either the N-terminal histidyl residue or the C-terminal dipeptide sequence Asn-Thr leads to markedly decreased receptor-binding potency.[410,411] Glucagon fragments containing fewer than about 25 residues retain no significant ability to bind to glucagon receptors. An exciting advance in the area of glucagon structure-function relationships concerns the chemical synthesis by Unson and coworkers of potent glucagon antagonists.[412-414] One such antagonist is a simple glucagon analogue in which the N-terminal histidine has been deleted, Asp9 is replaced by Glu, and the C-terminal threonine exists as its α-carboxamide derivative. Detailed analysis has demonstrated that the loss of His1 and the replacement of Asp9 (actually by any of several amino acids) are critical to the antagonistic properties of the peptide. The antagonist binds to plasma membrane glucagon receptors with high affinity but exhibits no tendency to stimulate adenylyl cyclase or the production of cAMP. Because the analogue competes well for glucagon-receptor interactions, it serves as a glucagon antagonist when the analogue and the natural hormone are present in admixture.[412-414] It is interesting to note that the analogue appears to serve as a partial agonist in stimulating glucose-potentiated insulin secretion from isolated pancreatic islets.[415] Although definitive information is not yet available on differences in secondary structure and general conformation that might apply to the agonist hormone and the antagonist analogue, it is clear that the glucagon receptor is exquisitely sensitive to structural changes in the occupying ligand. Further studies will undoubtedly identify the character of these structural changes and the mechanisms by which both glucagon and antagonist bind to receptor, but glucagon alone exhibits the ability to induce transmembrane signaling events that

activate adenylyl cyclase through the intervention of heterotrimeric G proteins. Although the in vivo effects of glucagon antagonists have been studied relatively little,[416] such compounds have the potential for therapeutic use in decreasing the hyperglycemia associated with diabetes. The cloning of the glucagon receptor[417] has opened the way to a more detailed understanding of the mechanism of glucagon binding and action.[418]

GLUCAGON BIOSYNTHESIS

Although the first evidence that glucagon is derived from a higher-molecular-weight precursor was obtained in 1973, only recently has a relatively complete picture of proglucagon and its processing emerged. Initially, Tager and Steiner isolated from crystalline glucagon an extended form that consisted of the entire sequence of glucagon with a C-terminal octapeptide extension that has the sequence Lys-Arg adjacent to the C-terminal threonine of glucagon, suggesting a typical prohormone-processing site.[419] Glucagon-like immunoreactivity derived from the intestine (the so-called *gut glucagon* or GLI-1) consisted of a larger component with an apparent molecular mass of 10 kDa and led Moody and coworkers to propose the name *glicentin* for this peptide.[420,421] On isolation in sufficient quantities for amino acid sequencing, glicentin turned out to consist of only 69 amino acids, and it contained glucagon with the previously described eight-residue C-terminal extension (glucagon 37 or oxyntomodulin), as well as a 32-residue N-terminal extension.[421] Subsequent biosynthetic studies by Patzelt and coworkers with isolated rat islets led to the definitive identification of proglucagon as a much larger 18-kDa protein, as estimated by sodium dodecyl sulfate gel electrophoresis under reducing conditions.[422] Pulse-chase experiments revealed that a single proglucagon protein at about 18 kDa appeared very rapidly, but it subsequently split into two similar-sized proteins of 18 to 19 kDa within 10 minutes (shown by Patzelt and Weber[423] to be due to O-glycosylation, that is, carbohydrate addition to serine or threonine residues) and then resolved back into a single protein of intermediate mobility (about 18.5 kDa), which slowly disappeared over a chase period of 2 hours. An intermediate proteolytic fragment of 13 kDa containing glucagon (by two-dimensional peptide analysis) appeared transiently.[423,424] By about 1 hour, a major protein of about 10 kDa (termed the *major proglucagon fragment*), which does not contain glucagon, began to accumulate. Normally, this component represents a major end product of glucagon processing in rat islets.[422,425,426]

The isolation and analysis of cDNA clones for hamster, bovine, and rat proglucagon (for a review, see Bell[408]) confirmed the estimated molecular weight of 18 kDa for the mammalian glucagon precursor and revealed several interesting features in addition to a typical prepeptide or signal peptide at its N terminus. The structural organization of a typical mammalian preproglucagon molecule is shown in Figure 48-21. This structure contains the 37-residue extended glucagon that was first described by Tager and Steiner[419] within the sequence of glicentin,[421] which makes up the N-terminal 69 amino acids of the prohormone. The C-terminal half of the molecule corresponds to the major proglucagon fragment (residues 72 to 160; see Fig. 48-21) that was observed by Patzelt and coworkers[422] and subsequently shown to be, along with glucagon, a major cosecretory product of the α cells.[426] The major proglucagon fragment contains two glucagon-like sequences, which have been designated GLP-1 and GLP-2. These sequences are bracketed by paired basic amino acids, which are sites of proteolytic processing, and are separated by a short spacer region, as is glucagon from GLP-1. It is interesting to note that islet α cells release predominantly the 29-residue glucagon, whereas GLP-1 and GLP-2 are released mainly[429] or exclusively[430] in the form of the 10-kDa major proglucagon

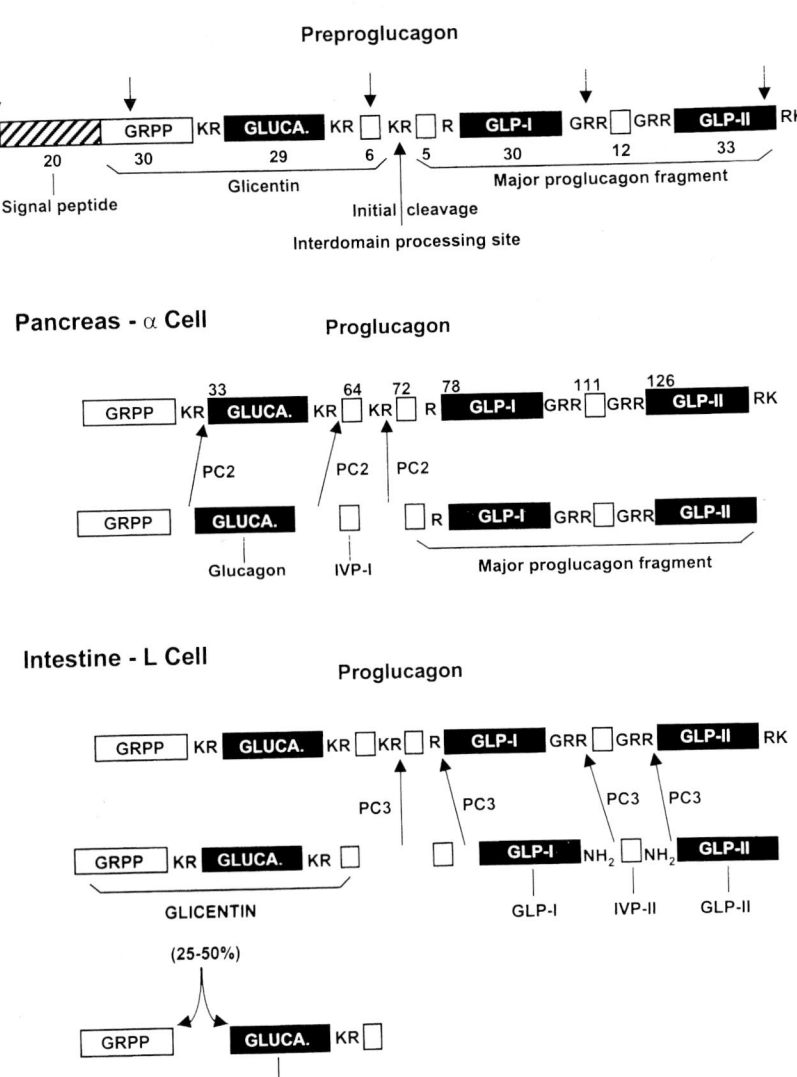

Figure 48-21 Schematic of the human glucagon precursor and its tissue specific processing in α cells versus intestinal L cells. The processing sites, which must be cleaved to generate glucagon and the glucagon-like peptides, are shown between indicated segments. The C terminus of glucagon-like peptide 1 is amidated; the sequence Gly-Arg-Arg directs cleavage of the precursor and provides a substrate for the polypeptide-amidating activity enzyme complex (PAM).[427] The tissue-specific processing of this precursor is indicated. In islet α cells, processing is carried out by PC2 at the more N-terminally located Lys-Arg pairs to produce glucagon. In L cells, residues 1 to 69 are released en bloc as glicentin, or gut glucagon, whereas the C-terminal major proglucagon fragment (residues 72 to 160) is efficiently processed, most likely by PC1/PC3, to release GLP-1 and GLP-2 peptides (see text for details). Numbers below the sequence designate the number of residues; numbers above the proglucagon sequence are the residue numbers at the N terminus of each domain. The *arrows* above the preproglucagon sequence at the top indicate the positions of introns in the human gene; each coding exon of the preproglucagon gene encodes a major domain of preproglucagon. The human glucagon gene, abbreviated GCG, is located on the long arm of chromosome 2 in the region q36 → q37.[428]

fragment. The reverse occurs in the ileal region of the small intestine, where glicentin, free GLP-1, GLP-1 (residues 7 to 37), and GLP-2 are the major secretory products (see Fig. 48-21).

Because only a single gene has been found to encode preproglucagon in humans and rats,[408] and the sequence of glicentin derived from porcine intestine is highly homologous to residues 1 to 69 of the predicted prohormonal sequence from humans, hamsters, and cows, the proteolytic processing of proglucagon clearly must differ between the α cells of the islets of Langerhans and the glucagon cells of the intestine.[431] The differential processing of proglucagon in these tissues could be influenced by O-glycosylation, as noted for the pancreatic precursor,[423] but it is more likely to be due to differences in the processing enzymes that are expressed in these tissues (see Fig. 48-21). The exact site or sites of carbohydrate addition are not known, but they appear to reside in the C-terminal region in either GLP-1 or GLP-2, both of which contain a number of serine and threonine residues that could be glycosylated. It is not known whether a similar modification of proglucagon occurs in intestinal cells. Recent evidence suggests that GLP-1 (residues 7 to 37) (proglucagon residues 78 to 107) is a potent stimulator of insulin secretion.[431–433] It appears that this peptide is the most potent "incretin" found to date and may be largely responsible for the increased insulin response to oral glucose and meal ingestion that has been recognized for many years.[433] (Recent studies have confirmed that glucose-dependent insulinotropic peptide

mediates GLP-1 release from distal intestinal sites in response to feeding.[434,435]) However, no physiologically relevant biologic activity has been ascribed to the N-terminal extended form of GLP-1 (proglucagon residues 72 to 107), a polypeptide whose structure was predicted from the position in proglucagon of pairs of basic amino acids, which often represent sites of proteolytic processing.[408] Because processing can also occur at single arginine residues, and residues 78 to 107 of proglucagon are more homologous to the N-terminal sequences of glucagon and GLP-2, perhaps mature GLP-1 should be redefined as proglucagon residues 78- to 107-kDa-amide; the N-terminally extended molecule (proglucagon residues 72 to 107) could represent an inactive precursor form of GLP-1 (see Fig. 48-21). Recent work by Drucker and colleagues[436] and Litvak and colleagues.[437] has shown that GLP-2 participates in the regulation of intestinal growth. It is interesting to note that some proglucagons in the anglerfish and in other teleosts lack GLP-2 and contain only a glucagon-like sequence and a GLP-1 (residues 7 to 37)-like sequence.[408]

Recent studies have elucidated the basis for the differential processing of proglucagon in the α cells versus the intestinal L cells (see Fig. 48-21). The α-cell pattern of processing of proglucagon is due to the presence of high levels of PC2 and the absence of significant levels of PC1/3 or other convertases.[438] In several studies, Rouillé and coworkers have demonstrated the importance of PC2 for both of the cleavages that release glucagon from proglucagon,[439,440] and this has been confirmed by studies with isolated islets from PC2 null mice, which show a marked inhibition in glucagon biosynthesis.[216] The phenotype of these mice consists of chronic hypoglycemia, and despite the presence of marked α-cell hyperplasia and large amounts of circulating precursor-related glucagon-like immunoreactive material, no active glucagon can be detected. Treatment of these mice with glucagon reverses the hypoglycemia and the α-cell hyperplasia.[441] A similar phenotype is seen in 7B2 null mice, which lack active PC2,[188] and in mice that lack glucagon receptors.[442]

However, endocrine cells that express high levels of PC1/3 can be shown to process proglucagon efficiently to release glicentin and GLP-1 and probably GLP-2 as well.[439,443] Processing by PC1/3 also produces small amounts of oxyntomodulin owing to a slight tendency to cleave on the N-terminal side of the glucagon sequence[439] (see Fig. 48-21). Predictably, then, cells that express both PC2 and PC1/3, such as various β-cell lines, process transfected proglucagon completely to glucagon, GLP-1, and GLP-2.[439] PC1/3 is also capable of cleaving the single basic residue site in GLP-1 (proglucagon residues 72 to 107) to release active GLP-1 (residues 7 to 37).[437] Either PC2 or PC1/3 alone is able to efficiently process the interdomain site between glicentin and the major proglucagon fragment. These findings suggest that initial cleavage at this site might be required for the further, more specialized processing steps that follow. Recently, PC1/3 null mice have been shown to lack GLP-1 and GLP-2 in intestinal extracts while having no defect in glucagon production,[218] as expected on the basis of the findings summarized above. Differential proglucagon processing in alpha versus L cells thus provides an excellent example of the regulation of specific hormone production from a single multifunctional precursor via varied expression of prohormone convertases PC1/3 and PC2 in discrete sites. The molecular basis for the sharply defined cleavage enzyme specificity of the various convertase cleavage sites in proglucagon remains unclear at this time.

SOMATOSTATIN STRUCTURE AND BIOSYNTHESIS

Somatostatin, a 14-residue peptide (SS-14) containing an internal disulfide bridge (Fig. 48-22), was first isolated from hypothalamic extracts and shown to inhibit the release of growth hormone.[445] Subsequent studies have shown that somatostatin has a much broader spectrum of inhibitory actions and is much more widely distributed in the body, occurring not only in many regions of the central nervous system, but also in many tissues of the digestive tract, including stomach, intestine, and pancreas.[446,447] Somatostatin suppresses the release of many pituitary, pancreatic, and gastrointestinal polypeptide and glycoprotein hormones. It also inhibits gastric acid and pepsin secretion and intestinal smooth muscle contractility. Moreover, it probably also functions as a neurotransmitter or neuromodulator in the central nervous system.[447] Early studies with isolated islets suggested the existence of a peptide inhibitor of insulin secretion,[448] but the identity of this substance was unknown until the discovery of somatostatin. It soon became apparent that the islet A_1 or D cells, first described by Bloom in 1931,[449] were the source of somatostatin in the islets.[445,450] The mechanism whereby somatostatin inhibits insulin secretion is still unresolved. It is possible that it functions as a paracrine effector, being released from the D cell and inhibiting insulin and glucagon secretion from adjacent β and α cells only within individual islets.[451] The inhibitory effects of somatostatin on secretion of digestive enzymes by surrounding acinar tissue might, however, be mediated by somatostatin secreted from D cells into the blood (i.e., it might be functioning as an endocrine molecule in this situation).[451] In contrast to its effects on insulin secretion, somatostatin does not inhibit

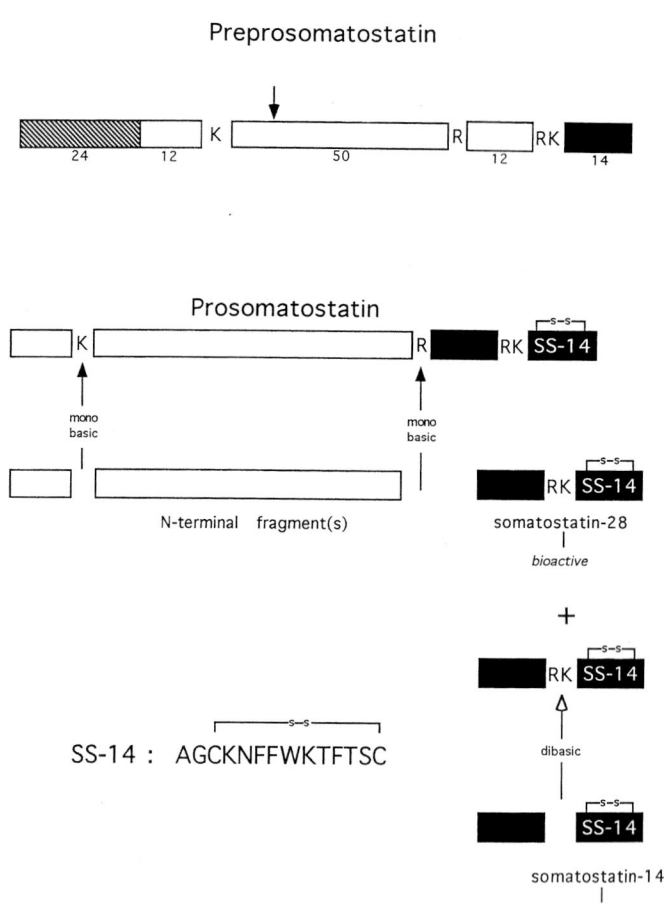

Figure 48-22 Sequence of the human somatostatin precursor. The sites that must be cleaved to release somatostatin-28 or somatostatin-14 are shown between indicated segments. The *arrow* above the preprosomatostatin sequence at the top indicates the position of the single intron in the gene encoding this precursor. The human somatostatin gene, abbreviated SST, is located on the long arm of chromosome 3 in the region q28.[444]

insulin biosynthesis in response to glucose in adult rat islets,[452,453] whereas it reportedly does so in fetal pancreas.[454]

Much study has been devoted to structure activity relationships within the somatostatin molecule in an effort to produce molecules of greater stability and potency or with altered effectiveness in inhibiting various secretory activities (for reviews, see Reichlin[451] and Gottesman et al.[455]). In the islets, somatostatin and some of its derivatives inhibit glucagon secretion more strongly than insulin secretion. In brittle type 1 diabetes, somatostatin can reduce the magnitude of blood glucose excursions.[451] However, long-term administration poses problems, and it is uncertain whether somatostatin or its derivatives significantly improve glycemic control in diabetic individuals over long periods. The chief utility of somatostatin is in the study of diabetes, in which its infusion can serve to block endogenous islet hormone release, permitting clamp studies and eliminating coregulatory or counterregulatory influences in studying individual islet hormonal actions or turnover.[455]

Recently, the receptors for somatostatin have been cloned and characterized.[456–460] These studies have identified five structurally related proteins, all members of the G protein–coupled family of receptors having seven transmembrane domains, which bind somatostatin and mediate its diverse cellular actions.[461]

The discovery of larger forms of somatostatin indicated the probable derivation of this peptide from a larger precursor.[447]

Much attention has been focused on somatostatin-28 (SS-28), a peptide that is made up of SS-14 extended through a basic amino acid bridge by a 12-residue N-terminal extension. SS-28 shares many of the actions of the tetradecapeptide form but differs in potency[462] as well as in tissue distribution within and without the central nervous system.[451] The two forms are evidently not interconvertible in the circulation; hence, the relative proportions that are found in the blood probably reflect differences both in tissue processing of the initial precursor and secretion and in plasma stability, uptake, excretion, and/or degradation.[463] Likewise, the origin of the two circulating forms of somatostatin is unclear and might well reflect the contribution of numerous potential sources throughout the organism.[451,464]

The biosynthesis of pancreatic somatostatin has been studied both in mammalian islets[465] and in the larger, more readily accessible, single islet of teleostian fishes, known as Brockman bodies.[466,467] Studies with mammalian islets are complicated by the fact that the somatostatin-producing D cells make up only about 5% of islet cells and usually lie on periphery of the islet,[143] where they are more likely to be damaged by collagenase digestion during islet isolation. Despite these technical difficulties, Patzelt and coworkers[465] were able to show, using isolated rat islets, that somatostatin is derived from a 12.5-kDa precursor peptide in which the 14-residue somatostatin moiety occurs at the C terminus. The subsequent cloning of cDNAs for two closely related anglerfish preprosomatostatins,[466,468] as well as the rat and human precursors,[469–471] confirmed these findings and showed both somatostatin and its precursor structure to be well conserved in vertebrate evolution (see Fig. 48-22). Moreover, the extensive amino acid identity between the rat and human prosomatostatin suggests that the N-terminal 63 residues might have some intrinsic biologic activity as well, although what these functions might be remains unknown. Somatostatin-like immunoreactivity has been reported in a number of invertebrates and even unicellular organisms, but the identity and relationship of these forms to the SS-14 or SS-28 products of preprosomatostatin processing in vertebrates remain unclear.

The processing of prosomatostatin has not been studied in sufficient detail in mammalian islets to provide a clear picture of how SS-28 and SS-14 are derived by specific proteolysis of prosomatostatin. In the anglerfish, two prosomatostatins occur, each of which gives rise to only SS-28 or SS-14.[472] The sequence of prosomatostatin suggests that its cleavage to generate SS-28 requires a trypsinlike enzyme that is capable of cleaving at a single arginine residue, a feature that occurs in a number of neuropeptide and growth factor precursors, including, among others, the C peptide of dog proinsulin,[230] propancreatic polypeptide,[473] provasopressin/neurophysin[474] and the IGF-1 and IGF-2 precursors,[475,476] but is relatively rare in comparison with dibasic cleavage sites. Recent studies have identified two distinct proteases that are involved in the generation of SS-28 or SS-14 from the anglerfish precursors. The enzyme cleaving at the single arginine site is tentatively identified as an aspartyl protease.[477] It is interesting to note that yeast cells lacking the dibasic processing enzyme kexin retain the ability to cleave rat prosomatostatin to generate SS-28 but not SS-14.[478] In yeast, the aspartyl protease (YAP-2) may be involved in this processing event.[479,480]

However, generation of SS-14 from SS-28 or larger intermediates of prosomatostatin does occur at a site that has paired basic residues. However, the sequence at this site (see Fig. 48-20) is Arg-Lys (R-K), a very rare dibasic combination. Its conservation in all the somatostatin precursors that have been described to date suggests[481] that a special processing enzyme may exist for this site. A 90-kDa endoprotease isolated from rat brain Golgi-neurosecretory granules cleaves SS-28 at this site to yield SS-14.[482,483] Its high specificity and failure to cleave intact prosomatostatin suggest that it is a highly specialized

protease. However, Mackin and coworkers[484] isolated an enzyme from anglerfish islets that processes prosomatostatin to SS-14, and it provided N-terminal sequence data suggesting that it is related to PC2. Coexpression studies have also suggested a role for PC2 in generating SS-14.[485] Recent studies on PC2 null mice confirm that PC2 is the convertase that is responsible for generating SS-14.[216] In both islets and brain from PC2 null mice, only SS-28 is found, whereas in the wild-type tissues, SS-14 is the major product that is detected by gel filtration combined with radioimmunoassay (unpublished data from G. Chiu and D. Steiner).[216] The D cells are also hyperplastic in the PC2 null mice, but whether this is due to lack of SS-14 or is somehow related to the chronic hypoglycemia, lack of glucagon, and α-cell hyperplasia or the β-cell hypoplasia of these mice is unclear. A cAMP-responsive element has been identified in the upstream region of the rat somatostatin gene.[486] However, much remains to be learned about the regulation of (pro)somatostatin biosynthesis at both transcriptional and translational levels.

PANCREATIC POLYPEPTIDE

Pancreatic polypeptide (PP) is a 36-amino acid peptide that was originally identified by Kimmel and Chance and their coworkers as a contaminant of some insulin preparations.[487–490] It is the product of a distinct cell type in the islets of Langerhans that is more abundant in the islets in the head of the pancreas, the portion of the pancreas near the duodenum that derives from the ventral anlage during development.[491] Typically, the PP-producing cells lie near the periphery of the islets or in clusters among the exocrine tissue[492]; therefore, their secretions, like those of the A cells and D cells, are more likely to be borne by the blood into the surrounding acinar tissue or directly into the portal circulation. PP secretion is largely under vagal control, and it does not appear to regulate carbohydrate metabolism, although levels typically rise promptly following a meal. Instead, its role appears to be to regulate gastrointestinal functions, such as exocrine pancreatic secretion and gallbladder emptying.[490,493]

PP belongs to a family of structurally related carboxyamidated neuroendocrine peptides that includes PYY and NPY.[494] These peptides occur in many neurons in the peripheral and central nervous system. PP itself is derived from a 9- to 10-kDa precursor, or propancreatic polypeptide, from which a second peptide cosecretory product is derived, the icosapeptide, in the human, canine, feline, and bovine forms.[474,495–498] The structure of human prepropancreatic peptide derived from a cDNA clone[499,500] is shown in Figure 48-23, and the regions corresponding to PP and icosapeptide are indicated. Although the sequence of PP is well conserved in mammals, especially the C-terminal amidated region, the icosapeptide is less well conserved and in fact might not be released as such in the rat[502] or guinea pig,[503] in which the single C-terminal arginine-processing site (residue 59) is lacking. The icosapeptide has not been found to have any biologic activity. The region following the icosapeptide is even more variable (both in length and in sequence), possibly owing to differences in splicing of the separate exon(s) that encode this region in the gene.[502,504]

X-ray crystallographic studies on avian PP indicate an ordered globular structure consisting of an N-terminal polyproline helix (residues 1 to 8) bent back through a turn to an α-helical region that extends from residues 14 to 32, terminating near a spatially well-defined C-terminal region.[17] It is likely that the structure of the mammalian forms of PP is similar to the avian structure, despite some sequence differences, and that this conformation may exist as well in solution and/or at the receptor-binding sites in the intestine and other tissues.[505]

The biosynthesis of PP appears to follow the general scheme for the other islet hormones as indicated in Figure 48-8. After

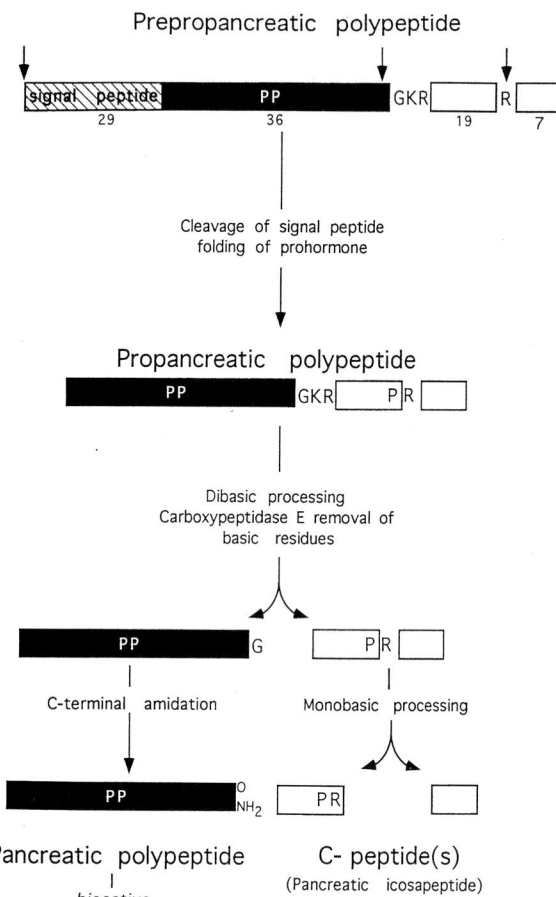

Figure 48-23 Sequence of the human pancreatic polypeptide precursor. The processing sites are shown between indicated segments. The C terminus of pancreatic polypeptide is tyrosine-amide. The peptides generated by processing of this precursor are noted. The *arrows* above the preproPP sequence at the top indicate the positions of introns in the gene encoding the precursor. The human pancreatic polypeptide gene, abbreviated PPY, is located on chromosome 17 in the region p11.1 → qter.[501]

removal of the prepeptide in the ER, proPP is transferred to the Golgi area, where it is packaged into prosecretory granules and processed by enzymes that have specificities for basic residue pairs similar to those responsible for the processing of proinsulin and proglucagon. Because the N terminus of PP follows immediately after the signal peptide in proPP, only a single site must be processed for its release. The sequence at this site is Gly-Lys-Arg and is most likely processed by at least three enzymes: (1) a paired basic residue endopeptidase that recognizes Lys-Arg (i.e., either PC2 or PC1/3); (2) a carboxypeptidase B–like enzyme (CPase E), which removes the C-terminal arginine and lysine residues successively; and (3) an amidating enzyme system,[427] which oxidatively removes the glycine to yield CO_2 and the carboxyamidated preceding amino acid (tyrosine). Cleavage to produce the icosapeptide then occurs at a single arginine residue in several species, giving rise to the cosecreted icosapeptide. Evidence from studies with cultured dog PP islets indicates that this monobasic processing endopeptidase is distinct from the protease that acts on the paired basic residues.[506] However, all these processing activities, as in the case of proinsulin, follow a time course that strongly suggests that they might occur in the maturing progranules, as these collect in the cytosol prior to discharge from the cell in response to cholinergic stimuli. In PC2 null mice, proPP does

not appear to be cleaved (unpublished data from A. Zhou and D. Steiner). These findings are consistent with immunocytochemical studies on islets that demonstrate only PC2 in the PP-producing cells.[179] Regulation of the tissue-specific expression of PP and modulatory effects of various stimuli on the transcription and translation of its mRNA remain important unexplored areas.

CONCLUSIONS

Many aspects of the biochemical and cellular biologic mechanisms underlying the production of the peptide hormones and neuropeptides of the diffuse neuroendocrine system have been elucidated over the past 35 years. Early studies on the biosynthesis and processing of proinsulin to insulin initiated this field and provided a useful paradigm for later developments. It is now established that almost all small NE regulatory peptides, as well as many other proteins, are derived from precursor proteins of widely varying structure and complexity. Most NE peptides are synthesized as preproproteins that are processed as they progress through the secretory pathway to yield single or multiple biologically active products that are typically stored within large dense-core secretory granules prior to their regulated release, either locally (for paracrine effectors) or into the circulation.

The major processing enzymes include the endoproteases PC1/3 and PC2 and the processing carboxypeptidases such as CPE, which remove C-terminal basic residues. Further posttranslational modifications include the actions of the peptidyl amidating monooxygenase system, as well as N-acetylases, glycosylating enzymes, and sulfokinases or phosphokinases. The removal of the signal or presequence occurs very rapidly in the RER during translation, while further processing of the resultant proproteins occurs after their segregation from the TGN into immature secretory vesicles, which then mature in the cytosol. Proprotein proteolysis typically begins 15 to 20 minutes after biosynthesis and continues with pseudo-first-order kinetics for several hours usually with half-times of 30 to 60 minutes.

The more complex NE polyprotein precursors often contain multiple cleavage sites that may differ considerably in their susceptibility to the prohormone convertases, PC2 and PC1/3. Thus, multifunctional precursors, such as proglucagon or proopiomelanocortin[179] may be processed differentially, into functionally divergent product mixtures in different tissue sites in the organism; for example, proglucagon gives rise to glucagon in the islet α cells and GLP-1 and GLP-2 in the intestinal L cells. All the peptide products of proteolytic cleavage are usually retained in the secretory vesicles and cosecreted by exocytosis in response to stimuli (e.g., insulin and C peptide are retained in the storage granules and secreted together in equimolar amounts, along with small amounts of proinsulin from the pancreatic islets). Peptide fragments, such as the proinsulin C peptide, can be utilized as useful markers of secretory activity, although differences in their half-lives in the circulation owing to divergent pathways of metabolism/degradation/excretion must be taken into consideration. Circulating immunoreactive peptides are often heterogeneous, consisting of larger or smaller sequence-related or overlapping peptides arising from the incomplete processing of a common precursor. These may have varying potencies, metabolic properties, and immunologic reactivities that can cause discrepancies in the assessment of circulating hormonal bioactivity by radioimmunoassay.

The biosynthesis of hormones is usually regulated at several levels, including transcription, mRNA stabilization, and translation. More rarely, controlled degradation of newly synthesized hormone may also play a regulatory role, for example, parathyroid hormone.[507] Recent studies with β cells indicate that stimuli such as glucose also coordinately upregulate many cellular genes, especially those encoding many components of the secretory pathway.[508]

Finally, the physiology of a secretory cell, whether in the islets, the gastrointestinal tract, or the brain, cannot be fully understood until all the precursor-derived secretory products, in addition to its already known peptide product(s), have been identified and screened for their potential biologic activities. Further studies of the biosynthetic and processing activities of the islet A, B, D, and PP cells continue to

reveal hitherto undiscovered secretory products of potential physiologic significance (e.g., IAPP from the β cells).

Acknowledgments

We thank Rosie Ricks, An Zhou, and Gregory Lipkind for expert assistance in the preparation of this chapter. Work in our laboratories was supported by National Institutes of Health grants DK13914 and DK20595 and by the Howard Hughes Medical Institute.

REFERENCES

1. Von Mering J, Minkowski O: Diabetes mellitus nach pankreas extirpation. Arch Exp Pathol Pharmacol Leipzig 26:371, 1890.
2. Bliss M: The Discovery of Insulin. Chicago, University of Chicago Press, 1982.
3. Scott EL: On the influence of intravenous injections of an extract of the pancreas on experimental pancreatic diabetes. Am J Physiol 29:306, 1912.
4. Banting FG, Best CH, Collip JB: Insulin patent. Chem Abstr 17:3571, 1923.
5. Macleod JJR, Campbell WR: Insulin: Its use in the treatment of diabetes. In Medicine Monographs, vol VI, parts I and II. Baltimore, Williams & Wilkins, 1925.
6. Murnaghan JH, Talalay P: John Jacob Abel and the crystallization of insulin. Perspect Biol Med 10:334, 1967.
7. Falkmer S, El-Salhy M, Titlbach M: Evolution of the neuroendocrine system in vertebrates: A review with particular reference to the phylogeny and postnatal maturation of the islet parenchyma. In Falkmer S, Håkanson R, Sundler F (eds): Evolution and Tumour Pathology of the Neuroendocrine System. Amsterdam, Elsevier, 1984, p 59.
8. Humbel RE, Bosshard HR, Zahn H: Chemistry of insulin. In Steiner DF, Freinkel N (eds): Handbook of Physiology, Endocrinology I. Baltimore, Williams & Wilkins, 1972, p 111.
9. Poulsen JE, Deckert T: Insulin preparations and the clinical use of insulin. In Luft R (ed): Insulin: Islet Pathology, Islet Function, Insulin Treatment. Mölndal, Sweden, A. Lindgren & Söner AB, 1976, p 197.
10. Davoren PR: The isolation of insulin from a single cat pancreas. Biochim Biophys Acta 63:150, 1962.
11. Chance RE, Ellis RM, Bromer WW: Porcine proinsulin: Characterization and amino acid sequence. Science 161:165, 1968.
12. Steiner DF, Hallund O, Rubenstein AH, et al: Isolation and properties of proinsulin, intermediate forms and other minor components from crystalline bovine insulin. Diabetes 17:725, 1968.
13. Vigh G, Varga-Puchony Z, Hlavay J, et al: Factors influencing the retention of insulins in reversed-phase high-performance liquid chromatographic systems. J Chromatogr 236:51, 1982.
14. Lloyd LF, Corran PH: Analysis of insulin preparations by reversed-phase

high-performance liquid chromatography. J Chromatogr 240:445, 1982.
15. Shoelson S, Haneda M, Blix P, et al: Three mutant insulins in man. Nature 302:540, 1983.
16. Tager H, Rubenstein AH, Steiner DF: Methods for the assessment of peptide precursors: Studies on insulin biosynthesis. In O'Malley BW, Hardman JG (eds): Hormones and Cyclic Nucleotides: Methods in Enzymology, vol 37, part B. New York, Academic Press, 1975, p 326.
17. Blundell T, Wood S: The conformation, flexibility, and dynamics of polypeptide hormones. In Snell EE, Boyer PD, Meister A, Richardson CC (eds): Annual Review of Biochemistry, vol 51. Palo Alto, CA, Annual Reviews, 1982, p 123.
18. Schlichtkrull J, Heding L: Personal communication, 1970.
19. Gueriguian JL (ed): Insulins, Growth Hormone, and Recombinant DNA Technology. New York, Raven Press, 1981.
20. Chan SJ, Weiss J, Konrad M, et al: Biosynthesis and periplasmic segregation of human proinsulin in E. coli. Proc Natl Acad Sci U S A 78:5401, 1981.
21. Thim L, Hansen MT, Norris K: Secretion and processing of insulin precursors in yeast. Proc Natl Acad Sci U S A 83:6766, 1986.
22. Chance RE: "Discussion." Recent Prog Horm Res 25:272, 1969.
23. Chance RE: Chemical, physical, biological and immunological studies on porcine proinsulin and related polypeptides. In Rodriquez RR, Vallance-Owen JJ (eds): Proceedings of the 7th Congress of the International Diabetes Federation. Amsterdam, Excerpta Medica, 1971, p 292.
24. Bruni B, O'Alberto M, Osenda M, et al: Clinical trial with monocomponent lente insulin. Diabetologia 9:492, 1973.
25. Galloway JA, Hooper SA, Spradlin CT, et al: Biosynthetic human proinsulin: Review of chemistry, in vitro and in vivo receptor binding, animal and human pharmacology studies, and clinical experience. Diabetes Care 15:666, 1992.
26. Velcovsky HG, Federlin KF: Insulin-specific IgG and IgE antibody response in type I diabetic subjects exclusively treated with human insulin (recombinant DNA). Diabetes Care 5:126, 1982.

27. Sergeev NV, Gloukhova NS, Nazimov IV, et al: Monitoring of recombinant human insulin production by narrow-bore reversed-phase high-performance liquid chromatography, high-performance capillary electrophoresis and matrix-assisted laser desorption ionization time-of-flight mass spectrometry. J Chromatogr A 907:131, 2001.
28. Gliemann J, Sorenson HH: Assay of insulin-like activity by the isolated fat cell method: IV. The biological activity of proinsulin. Diabetologia 6:499, 1970.
29. Freychet P, Roth J, Neville DM: Insulin receptors in the liver: Specific binding of insulin to the plasma membrane and its relation to insulin bioactivity. Proc Natl Acad Sci U S A 68:1833, 1971.
30. Freychet P, Brandenburg D, Wollmer A: Receptor-binding assay of chemically modified insulins: Comparison with in vitro and in vivo bioassays. Diabetologia 10:1, 1974.
31. Glieman J, Gammeltoft S: The biological activity and the binding affinity of modified insulins determined on isolated rat fat cells. Diabetologia 10:105, 1974.
32. Klostermeyer H, Humbel RE: The chemistry and biochemistry of insulin. Angew Chem Int Ed Engl 5:807, 1966.
33. Chance RE, Kroeff EP, Hoffmann JA: Chemical, physical, and biological properties of recombinant human insulin. In Guerigian JL (ed): Insulins, Growth Hormone, and Recombinant DNA Technology. New York, Raven Press, 1981, p 71.
34. Sanger F: Chemistry of insulin. Science 129:1340, 1959.
35. Smith LF: Amino acid sequences of insulins. Diabetes 21(Suppl 2):457, 1972.
36. Dayhoff MO (ed): Atlas of Protein Sequence and Structure, vol 5(Suppl 1). Bethesda, MD, Biochemical Research Foundation, 1973.
37. Peterson JD, Steiner DF, Emdin SO, et al: The amino acid sequence of the insulin from a primitive vertebrate, the Atlantic hagfish (Myxine glutinosa). J Biol Chem 250:5183, 1975.
38. Steiner DF: Amino acid sequences of proteins: Hormones. In Fasman GD (ed): Handbook of Biochemistry and Molecular Biology, Proteins, vol III. Boca Raton, FL, CRC Press, 1976, p 378.
39. Steiner DF, Bell GI, Tager HS: Chemistry and biosynthesis of pancreatic protein hormones. In DeGroot L (ed): Endocrinology. Philadelphia, WB Saunders, 1989, p 1263.

40. Seino S, Steiner DF, Bell GI: Sequence of a new world primate insulin having low biological potency and immunoreactivity. Proc Natl Acad Sci U S A 84:7423, 1987.

41. Yu J-H, Eng J, Yalow RS: Isolation and amino acid sequences of squirrel monkey (*Saimiri sciurea*) insulin and glucagon. Proc Natl Acad Sci U S A 87:9766, 1990.

42. Evans TK, Litthauer D, Oelofsen W: Purification and primary structure of ostrich insulin. Int J Pep Protein Res 31:454, 1988.

43. Conlon JM, Goöke R, Andrews PC, Thim L: Multiple molecular forms of insulin and glucagon-like peptide from the Pacific ratfish (*Hydrolagus colliei*). Gen Comp Endocrinol 73:136, 1989.

44. Treacy GB, Shaw DC, Griffiths ME, Jeffrey PD: Purification of a marsupial insulin: Amino-acid sequence of insulin from the eastern grey kangaroo *Macropus giganteus*. Biochim Biophys Acta 990:263, 1989.

45. Berks BC, Marshall CJ, Carne A, et al: Isolation and structural characterization of insulin and glucagon from the holocephalan species *Callorhynchus milii* (elephantfish). Biochem J 263:261, 1989.

46. Conlon JM, Hicks JW: Isolation and structural characterization of insulin glucagon and somatostatin from the turtle, *Pseudemys scripta*. Peptides 11:461, 1990.

47. Conlon JM, Youson JH, Whittaker J: Structure and receptor-binding activity of insulin from a holostean fish, the bowfin (*Amia calva*). Biochem J 276:261, 1991.

48. Conlon JM, Andrews PD, Thim L, Moon TW: The primary structure of glucagon-like peptide but not insulin has been conserved between the American eel, *Anguilla rostrata* and the European eel, *Anguilla anguilla*. Gen Comp Endocrinol 82:23, 1991.

49. Smit AB, Geraerts WPM, Meester I, et al: Characterization of a cDNA clone encoding molluscan insulin-related peptide II of *Lymnaea stagnalis*. Eur J Biochem 199:699, 1991.

50. Lloyd PD, Li L, Rubakhin SS, et al: Insulin prohormone processing, distribution, and relation to metabolism in *Aplysia californica*. J Neurosci 19:7732, 1999.

51. Kawakami A, Iwami M, Nagasawa H, et al: Structure and organization of four clustered genes that encode bombyxin, as insulin-related brain secretory peptide of the silkmoth *Bombyx mori*. Proc Natl Acad Sci U S A 86:6843, 1989.

52. Lagueux M, Lwoff L, Meister M, et al: cDNAs from neurosecretory cells of brains of *Locusta migratoria* (Insecta, Orthoptera) encoding a novel member of the superfamily of insulins. Eur J Biochem 187:249, 1990.

53. Duret L, Guex N, Peitsch MC, Bairoch A: New insulin-like proteins with a typical disulfide bond pattern characterized in *Caenorhabditis elegans* by comparative sequence analysis and homology modeling. Genome Res 8:348, 1998.

54. Steiner DF, Chan SJ, Welsh JM, Kwok SDM: Structure and evolution of the insulin gene. Annu Rev Genet 19:463, 1985.

55. Claeys I, Simonet G, Poels J, et al: Insulin-related peptides and their conserved signal transduction pathway. Peptides 23:807, 2002.

56. Adham IM, Burkhardt E, Benahmed M, Engel W: Cloning of a cDNA for a novel insulin-like peptide of the testicular Leydig cells. J Biol Chem 268:26668, 1993.

57. Dayhoff MO (ed): Atlas of Protein Sequence and Structure, vol 5. Bethesda, MD, Biomedical Research Foundation, 1972.

58. Carpenter FH: Relationship of structure to biological activity of insulin as revealed by degradative studies. Am J Med 40:750, 1966.

59. Brandenburg D, Wollmer A (eds): Insulin: Chemistry, Structure and Function of Insulin and Related Hormones. Proceedings of the Second International Insulin Symposium, Aachen, Germany, September 4–7, 1979. Berlin, Walter de Gruyter, 1980.

60. Arquilla ER, Miles PV, Morris JW: Immunochemistry of insulin. In Steiner DF, Freinkel N (eds): Handbook of Physiology, Endocrinology I. Baltimore, Williams & Wilkins 1972, p 159.

61. Blundell TL, Dodson GG, Dodson E, et al: X-ray analysis and the structure of insulin. Recent Prog Horm Res 27:1, 1971.

62. Blundell TL, Dodson GG, Hodgkin DC, et al: Insulin: The structure in the crystals and its reflection in chemistry and biology. Adv Protein Chem 26:279, 1972.

63. Baker EN, Blundell TL, Cutfield JF, et al: The structure of 2Zn pig insulin crystals at 1.5 NA resolution. Philos Trans R Soc Lond 319:369, 1988.

64. Wood SP, Blundell TL, Wollmer A, et al: The relation of conformation and association of insulin to receptor binding: X-ray and circular-dichroism studies on bovine and hystricomorph insulins. Eur J Biochem 55:531, 1975.

65. Weiss MA, Frank BH, Khait I, et al: NMR and photo-CIDNP studies of human proinsulin and prohormone processing intermediates with application to endopeptidase recognition. Biochemistry 29:8389, 1990.

66. Cutfield JF, Cutfield SM, Dodson EJ, et al: Structure and biological activity of hagfish insulin. J Mol Biol 132:85, 1979.

67. Chan SJ, Episkopou V, Zeitlin S, et al: Guinea pig preproinsulin gene: An evolutionary compromise? Proc Natl Acad Sci U S A 81:5046, 1984.

68. Emdin SO, Gammeltoft S, Gliemann J: Degradation, binding affinity and potency of insulin from the Atlantic hagfish (*Myxine glutinosa*) determined in isolated rat fat cells. J Biol Chem 252:602, 1977.

69. Mommsen TP, Plisetskaya EM: Insulin in fishes and agnathans: History, structure, and metabolic regulation. Rev Aquatic Sci 4:225, 1991.

70. Taylor SI, Cama A, Accili D: Mutations in the insulin receptor gene. Endocr Rev 13:566, 1992.

71. Acher R: Recent discoveries in the evolution of proteins. Angew Chem Int Ed Engl 13:186, 1974.

72. Terris S, Hofmann C, Steiner DF: Mode of uptake and degradation of I^{125}-labelled insulin by isolated hepatocytes and H4 hepatoma cells. Can J Biochem 57:459, 1979.

73. Markussen J: Proteolytic degradation of proinsulin and of the intermediate forms: Application to synthesis and biosynthesis of insulin. In Baba S, Kaneko T, Yanaihara N (eds): Proinsulin, Insulin, C-peptide. Amsterdam, Excerpta Medica, 1979, p 50.

74. Derewnda U, Derewenda Z, Dodson EJ, et al: X-ray analysis of the single chain B29-A1 peptide-linked insulin molecule. J Mol Biol 220:1, 1991.

75. Hua QX, Shoelson SE, Kochoyan NM, Weiss MA: Receptor binding redefined by a structural switch in a mutant human insulin. Nature 354:238, 1991.

76. Kline AD, Justice RM: Complete sequence-specific ^{1}H NMR assignments for human insulin. Biochemistry 29:2906, 1990.

77. Mirmira RG, Nakagawa SH, Tager HS: Importance of the character and configuration of residues B24, B25, and B26 in insulin-receptor interactions. J Biol Chem 266:1428, 1991.

78. Nakagawa SH, Tager HS: Importance of aliphatic side-chain structure at positions 2 and 3 of the insulin A chain in insulin-receptor interactions. Biochemistry 31:3204, 1992.

79. Kristensen C, Kjeldsen T, Wiberg FC, et al: Alanine scanning mutagenesis of insulin. J Biol Chem 272:12978, 1997.

80. Schwartz GP, Burke GT, Katsoyannis PG: A superactive insulin: [B10-aspartic acid]insulin(human). Proc Natl Acad Sci 84:6408, 1987.

81. Hu SQ, Burke GT, Schwartz GP, et al: Steric requirements at position B12 for high biological activity in insulin. Biochemistry 32:2631, 1993.

82. DeMeyts P, Whittaker J: Structural biology of insulin and IGF1 receptors: Implications for drug design. Nat Rev 1:769, 2002.

83. Kurose T, Pashmforoush M, Yoshimasa Y, et al: Cross-linking of a B25 azido-phenylalanine insulin derivative to the carboxyl-terminal region of the α-subunit of the insulin receptor: Identification of a new insulin-binding domain in the insulin receptor. J Biol Chem 269:29190, 1994.

84. Steiner DF, Oyer PE: The biosynthesis of insulin and a probable precursor of insulin by a human islet cell adenoma. Proc Natl Acad Sci U S A 57:473, 1967.

85. Steiner DF, Clark JL, Nolan D, et al: Proinsulin and the biosynthesis of insulin. Recent Prog Horm Res 25:207, 1969.

86. Chan SJ, Keim P, Steiner DF: Cell-free synthesis of rat preproinsulins: Characterization and partial amino acid sequence determination. Proc Natl Acad Sci U S A 73:1964, 1976.

87. Lomedico PT, Chan SJ, Steiner DF, et al: Immunological and chemical characterization of bovine preproinsulin. J Biol Chem 252:7971, 1977.

88. Sanders SL, Schekman R: Polypeptide translocation across the endoplasmic reticulum membrane. J Biol Chem 267:13791, 1992.

89. Frand AR, Cuozzo JW, Kaiser CA: Pathways for protein disulphide bond formation. Trends Cell Biol 10:203, 2000.

90. Munro S, Pelham HRB: A C-terminal signal prevents secretion of luminal ER proteins. Cell 48:899, 1987.

91. Orci L, Perrelet A, Ravazzola, et al: Coatomer-rich endoplasmic reticulum. Proc Natl Acad Sci U S A 91:11924, 1994.

92. Pagano A, Letourneur F, Garcia-Estefania D, et al: Sec24 proteins and sorting at the endoplasmic reticulum. J Biol Chem 274:7833, 1999.

93. Patzelt C, Labrecque AD, Duguid JR, et al: Detection and kinetic behavior of preproinsulin in pancreatic islets. Proc Natl Acad Sci U S A 75:1260, 1978.

94. Steiner DF, Kemmler W, Clark JL, et al: The biosynthesis of insulin. In Steiner DF, Freinkel N (eds): Handbook of Physiology, Endocrinology, vol I. Baltimore, Williams & Wilkins, 1972, p 175.

95. Nishi M, Sanke T, Nagamatsu S, et al: Islet amyloid polypeptide: A new β cell secretory product related to islet amyloid deposits. J Biol Chem 265:4173, 1990.

96. Judah JD, Gamble M, Steadman JH: Biosynthesis of serum albumin in rat liver: Evidence for the existence of "proalbumin." Biochem J 134:1083, 1973.

97. Kiehn ED, Holland JJ: Synthesis and cleavage of enterovirus polypeptides in mammalian cells. J Virol 5:358, 1970.

98. Scheid A, Choppin PW: Protease activation mutants of sendai virus: Activation of biological properties by specific proteases. Virology 69:265, 1976.

99. Skehel JJ, Wiley DC: Receptor binding and membrane fusion in virus entry: The influenza hemagglutinin. Ann Rev Biochem 69:531, 2000.

100. Steiner DF: The biosynthesis of insulin: Genetic, evolutionary and pathophysiologic aspects. In Gotshlich EC (ed): The Harvey Lectures, series 78. New York, Academic Press, 1984, p 191.

101. Steiner DF, Cho S, Oyer PE, et al: Isolation and characterization of proinsulin C-peptide from bovine pancreas. J Biol Chem 246:1365, 1971.

102. Frank BH, Veros AJ: Physical studies on proinsulin: Association behavior and conformation in solution. Biochem Biophys Res Commun 32:155, 1968.

103. Rubenstein AH, Melani F, Pilkis S, et al: Proinsulin: Secretion, metabolism, immunological and biological properties. Postgrad Med J 45(Suppl):476, 1969.

104. Rubenstein AH, Mako M, Welbourne WP, et al: Comparative immunology of bovine, porcine, and human proinsulin and C-peptides. Diabetes 19:546, 1970.

105. Narahara HT: Biological activity of proinsulin. In Fritz I (ed): Insulin Action. New York, Academic Press, 1972, p 63.

106. Given BD, Cohen RM, Shoelson SE, et al: Biochemical and clinical implications of proinsulin conversion intermediates. J Clin Invest 76:1398, 1985.

107. Frank BH, Veros AJ: Interaction of zinc with proinsulin. Biochem Biophys Res Commun 38:284, 1970.

108. Steiner DF: Cocrystallization of proinsulin and insulin. Nature 243:528, 1973.

109. Low BW, Fullerton WW, Rosen LS: Insulin/proinsulin, a new crystalline complex. Nature 248:339, 1974.

110. Steiner DF, Cunningham DD, Spigelman L, et al: Insulin biosynthesis: Evidence for a precursor. Science 157:697, 1967.

111. Steiner DF: Evidence for a precursor in the biosynthesis of insulin. Trans N Y Acad Sci 30:60, 1967.

112. Tung AK, Yip CC: The biosynthesis of insulin and "proinsulin" in fetal bovine pancreas. Diabetologia 4:68, 1968.

113. Lin BJ, Haist RE: Insulin biosynthesis: Effects of carbohydrates and related compounds. Can J Physiol Pharmacol 47:791, 1969.

114. Morris GE, Korner A: The effect of glucose on insulin biosynthesis by isolated islets of Langerhans in the rat. Biochim Biophys Acta 208:404, 1970.

115. Tanese T, Lazarus NR, Devrim S, et al: Synthesis and release of proinsulin and insulin by isolated rat islets of Langerhans. J Clin Invest 49:1394, 1970.

116. Clark JL, Steiner DF: Insulin biosynthesis in the rat: Demonstration of two proinsulins. Proc Natl Acad Sci U S A 62:278, 1969.

117. Smith LF: Species variation in the amino acid sequence of insulin. Am J Med 40:662, 1966.

118. Markussen J: Mouse insulins-separation and structures. Int J Protein Res 3:149, 1971.

119. Wentworth BM, Schaefer IM, Villa-Komaroff L, et al: Characterization of the two nonallelic genes encoding mouse preproinsulin. J Mol Evol 23:305, 1986.

120. Soares MB, Schon E, Henderson A, et al: RNA-mediated gene duplication: The rat preproinsulin I gene is a functional retroposon. Mol Cell Biol 5:2090, 1985.

121. Sundby F, Markussen J: Rat proinsulins and C-peptides: Isolation and amino

acid compositions. Eur J Biochem 25:147, 1972.

122. Markussen J, Sundby F: Rat proinsulin C-peptides: Amino acid sequences. Eur J Biochem 25:153, 1972.

123. Tager HS, Steiner DF: Primary structures of the proinsulin connecting peptides of the rat and horse. J Biol Chem 247:7936, 1972.

124. Verchere CB, Paoletta M, Neerman-Arbez M, et al: Des-(27-31)C-peptide: A novel secretory product of the rat pancreatic beta cell produced by truncation of proinsulin connecting peptide in secretory granules. J Biol Chem 271:27475, 1996.

125. Sando H, Borg J, Steiner DF: Studies on the secretion of newly synthesized proinsulin and insulin from isolated rat islets of Langerhans. J Clin Invest 51:1476, 1972.

126. Sando H, Grodsky GM: Dynamic synthesis and release of insulin and proinsulin from perifused islets. Diabetes 22:354, 1973.

127. Gold G, Gishizky ML, Grodsky GM: Evidence that glucose "marks" β cells resulting in preferential release of newly synthesized insulin. Science 218:56, 1982.

128. Nolan C, Margoliash E, Peterson JD, et al: The structure of bovine proinsulin. J Biol Chem 246:2780, 1971.

129. Kemmler W, Steiner DF, Borg J: Studies on the conversion of proinsulin to insulin: III. Studies in vitro with a crude secretion granule fraction isolated from islets of Langerhans. J Biol Chem 248:4544, 1973.

130. Kuzuya J, Chance RE, Steiner DF, et al: On the preparation and characterization of standard materials for natural human proinsulin and C-peptide. Diabetes 27:161, 1978.

131. Grant PT, Coombs TL: Proinsulin: A biosynthetic precursor of insulin. In Campbell PN, Greville GD (eds): Essays in Biochemistry, vol 6. London, Academic Press, 1971, p 69.

132. Yamaji K, Tada K, Trakatellis AC: On the biosynthesis of insulin in anglerfish islets. J Biol Chem 247:4080, 1972.

133. Hobart PM, Shen L-P, Crawford R, et al: Comparison of the nucleic acid sequence of anglerfish and mammalian insulin mRNA's from cloned cDNA's. Science 210:1360, 1980.

134. Emdin SO, Falkmer S: Phylogeny of insulin: Some evolutionary aspects of insulin production with particular regard to the biosynthesis of insulin in *Myxine glutinosa*. Acta Paediatr Scand 270(Suppl):15, 1977.

135. Chan SJ, Emdin SO, Kwok SCM, et al: Messenger RNA sequence and primary structure of preproinsulin in a primitive vertebrate, the Atlantic hagfish. J Biol Chem 256:7595, 1981.

136. Orci L, Ravazzola M, Amherdt M, et al: Direct identification of prohormone conversion site in insulin-secreting cells. Cell 42:671, 1985.

137. Steiner DF, Clark JL, Nolan C, et al: The biosynthesis of insulin and some speculation regarding the pathogenesis of human diabetes. In Cerasi E, Luft R (eds): The Pathogenesis of Diabetes Mellitus. New York, John Wiley & Sons, 1970, p 57.

138. Hard L: The origin and differentiation of the alpha and beta cells in the pancreatic islets of the rat. Am J Anat 75:369, 1944.

139. Munger BL: A light and electron microscopic study of cellular differentiation in the pancreatic islets of the mouse. Am J Anat 103:275, 1958.

140. Farquhar MG, Palade GE: The Golgi apparatus (complex): (1954–1981)— from artifact to center stage. J Cell Biol 91:77s, 1981.

141. Michael J, Carroll R, Swift H, Steiner DF: Studies on the molecular organization of rat insulin secretory granules. J Biol Chem 262:16531, 1987.

142. Polonsky K, Rubenstein AH: Current approaches to measurement of insulin secretion. Diabetes Metab Rev 2:315, 1986.

143. Orci L: The insulin factory: A tour of the plant surroundings and a visit to the assembly line. Diabetolgia 28:528, 1985.

144. Permutt MA, Kipnis DM: Insulin biosynthesis: Studies of islet polyribosomes. Proc Natl Acad Sci U S A 69:505, 1972.

145. Howell SL: Role of ATP in the intracellular translocation of proinsulin and insulin in the rat pancreatic B cell. Nature (New Biol) 235:85, 1972.

146. Wattenberg BW, Rothman JE: Multiple cytosolic components promote intra-Golgi protein transport: Resolution of a protein acting at a late state, prior to membrane fusion. J Biol Chem 61:2208, 1986.

147. Chappell TG, Welch WF, Schlossman DM, et al: Uncoating ATPase is a member of the 70 kDa family of stress proteins. Cell 45:3, 1986.

148. Nagamatsu S, Bolaffi JL, Grodsky GM: Direct effects of glucose on proinsulin synthesis and processing during desensitization. Endocrinology 120:1225, 1987.

149. Howell SL, Kostianovsky M, Lacy PE: Beta granule formation in isolated islets of Langerhans: A study by electron microscopic radioautography. J Cell Biol 42:695, 1969.

150. Orci L, Lambert AE, Kanazawa Y, et al: Morphological and biochemical studies of B cells in fetal rat endocrine pancreas in organ culture: Evidence for proinsulin biosynthesis. J Cell Biol 50:565, 1971.

151. Kemmler W, Peterson JD, Steiner DF: Studies on the conversion of proinsulin to insulin: I. Conversion in vitro with trypsin and carboxypeptidase B. J Biol Chem 246:6786, 1971.

152. Steiner DF, Kemmler W, Tager HS, et al: Proteolytic mechanisms in the biosynthesis of polypeptide hormones. In Reich E, Rifkin DB, Shaw E (eds): Proteases and Biological Control. Cold Spring Harbor, NY, Cold Spring Harbor Laboratory, 1975, p 531.

153. Zühlke H, Steiner DF, Lernmark NA, et al: Carboxypeptidase B-like and trypsin-like activities in isolated rat pancreatic islets. In CIBA Foundation (ed): Polypeptide Hormones: Molecular and Cellular Aspects. Amsterdam, Excerpta Medica North-Holland, 1976, p 183.

154. Docherty K, Hutton JC: Carboxypeptidase activity in the insulin secretory granule. FEBS Lett 162:137, 1983.

155. Fricker LD, Evans CJ, Esch FS, et al: Cloning and sequence analysis of cDNA for bovine carboxypeptidase E. Nature 323:461, 1986.

156. Song L, Fricker LD: Cloning and expression of human carboxypeptidase Z, a novel metallocarboxypeptidase. J Biol Chem 272:10543, 1997.

157. Song W, Fricker LD, Day R: Carboxypeptidase D is a potential candidate to carry out redundant processing functions of carboxypeptidase E based on comparative distribution studies in the rat central nervous system. Neuroscience 89:1301, 1999.

158. Julius D, Brake A, Blair L, et al: Isolation of the putative structural gene for the lysine-arginine-cleavage endopeptidase required for processing of yeast prepro-α-factor. Cell 37:1075, 1984.

159. Fuller RS, Sterne RE, Thorner J: Enzymes required for yeast prohormone processing. Annu Rev Physiol 50:345, 1988.

160. Mizuno K, Nakamura T, Ohshima T, et al: Yeast KEX2 gene encodes an endopeptidase homologous to subtilisin-like serine proteases. Biochem Biophys Res Commun 156:246, 1988.

161. Fuller RS, Brake AJ, Thorner J: Intracellular targeting and structural conservation of a prohormone-processing endoprotease. Science 246:482, 1989.

162. Roebroek AJM, Schalken JA, Leunissen JAM, et al: Evolutionary conserved close linkage of the c-fes/fps proto-oncogene and genetic sequences encoding a receptor-like protein. EMBO J 5:2197, 1986.

163. Kiefer MC, Tucker JE, Joh R, et al: Identification of a second human subtilisin-like protease gene in the fes/fps region of chromosome 15. DNA Cell Biol 10:757, 1991.

164. Ohagi S, LaMendola J, LeBeau MM, et al: Identification and analysis of the gene encoding human PC2, a prohormone convertase expressed in neuroendocrine tissues. Proc Natl Acad Sci U S A 89:4977, 1992.

165. Seidah NG, Mattei MG, Gaspar L, et al: Chromosomal assignments of the genes for neuroendocrine convertase PC1 (NEC1) to human 5q15-21, neuroendocrine convertase PC2 (NEC2) to human 20p11.1-11.2, and furin (mouse 7 region). Genomics 11:103, 1991.

166. Mbikay M, Raffin-Sanson M-L, Tadros H, et al: Structure of the gene for the testis-specific proprotein convertase 4 and its alternate messenger RNA isoforms. Genomics 20:231, 1994.

167. Goodge KA, Thomas RJ, Martin J, Gillespie MT: Gene organization and alternative splicing of human prohormone convertase PC8. Biochem J 336:353, 1998.

168. Mizuno K, Nakamura T, Ohshima T, et al: Characterization of KEX2-encoded endopeptidase from yeast Saccharomyces cerevisiae. Biochem Biophys Res Commun 159:305, 1989.

169. Davidson HW, Rhodes CJ, Hutton JC: Intraorganellar calcium and pH control proinsulin cleavage in the pancreatic β cell via two distinct site-specific endopeptidases. Nature 333:93, 1988.

170. Smeekens SP, Chan SJ, Steiner DF: The biosynthesis and processing of neuroendocrine peptides: Identification of proprotein convertases involved in intravesicular processing. In Joosse J, Buijs RM, Tilders FJH (eds): Progress in Brain Res, vol 92. Amsterdam, Elsevier, 1992, p 235.

171. Smeekens SP, Steiner DF: Identification of a human insulinoma cDNA encoding a novel mammalian protein structurally related to the yeast diabasic processing protease Kex2. J Biol Chem 265:2997, 1990.

172. Smeekens SP, Avruch AS, LaMendola J, et al: Identification of a cDNA encoding a second putative prohormone convertase related to PC2 in AtT20 cells and islets of Langerhans. Proc Natl Acad Sci U S A 88:340, 1991.

173. Seidah NG, Gaspar L, Mion P, et al: cDNA sequence of two distinct pituitary proteins homologous to Kex2 and furin gene products: Tissue-specific mRNAs encoding candidates for prohormone processing proteinases. DNA Cell Biol 9:415, 1990.

174. Seidah NG, Marcinkiewicz M, Benjannet S, et al: Cloning and primary sequence of a mouse candidate prohormone convertase PC1 homologous to PC2, furin, and kex2: Distinct chromosomal localization and messenger RNA distribution in brain and pituitary compared to PC2. Mol Endocrinol 5:111, 1990.

175. Van den Ouweland AMW, van Duijnhoven HLP, Keizer GD, et al: Structural homology between the human fur gene product and the subtilisin-like protease encoded by yeast KEX2. Nucleic Acids Res 18:664, 1990.

176. Van de Ven WJM, Voorberg J, Fontijan R, et al: Furin is a subtilisin-like proprotein processing enzyme in higher eukaryotes. Mol Biol Rep 14:265, 1990.

177. Wise RJ, Baar PJ, Wong PA, et al: Expression of a human proprotein processing enzyme: Correct cleavage of the von Willebrand factor precursor at a paired basic amino acid site. Proc Natl Acad Sci U S A 87:9378, 1990.

178. Barr PJ, Mason OB, Landsberg KE, et al: cDNA and gene structure for a human subtilisin-like protease with cleavage specificity for paired basic amino acid residues. DNA Cell Biol 10:319, 1991.

179. Zhou A, Webb G, Zhu X, Steiner DF: Proteolytic processing in the secretory pathway. J Biol Chem 274:20745, 1999.

180. Seidah NG, Benhannet S, Wickham L, et al: The secretory proprotein convertase neural apoptosis-regulated convertase 1 (NARC-1): Liver regeneration and neuronal differentiation. Proc Natl Acad Sci U S A 100:928, 2003.

181. Hatsuzawa K, Hosaka M, Nakagawa T, et al: Structure and expression of mouse furin, yeast Kex2-related protease. J Biol Chem 265:22075, 1990.

182. Ohagi S, Sakaguchi H, Sanke T, et al: Human prohormone convertase 3 gene: Extron-intron organization and molecular scanning for mutations in Japanese subjects with NIDDM. Diabetes 45:897, 1996.

183. Seidah NG, Chrétien M, Day R: The family of subtilisin/kexin like pro-protein and pro-hormone convertases: Divergent or shared functions. Biochimie 76:197, 1994.

184. Wells JA, Cunningham BC, Graycar TP, Estell DA: Importance of hydrogen-bond formation in stabilizing the transition state of subtilisin. Philos Trans R Soc Lond 317:415, 1986.

185. Shennan KIJ, Smeekens SP, Steiner DF, Docherty K: Characterization of PC2, a mammalian Kex2 homologue, following expression of the cDNA in microinjected Xenopus oocytes. FEBS Lett 284:277, 1991.

186. Muller L, Zhu X, Lindberg I: Mechanism of the facilitation of PC2 maturation by 7B2: Involvement in proPC2 transport and activation but not folding. J Cell Biol 139:625, 1997.

187. Muller L, Zhu P, Juliano MA, et al: A 36-residue peptide contains all of the information required for 7B2-mediated activation of prohormone convertase 2. J Biol Chem 274:21471, 1999.

188. Westphal C, Muller L, Zhou A, et al: The neuroendocrine protein 7B2 is required for peptide hormone processing in vivo and provides a novel mechanism for pituitary Cushing's disease. Cell 96:689, 1999.

189. Nagamune H, Muramatsu K, Akamatsu T, et al: Distribution of the kexin family proteases in pancreatic islets: PACE4C is specifically expressed in B cells of pancreatic islets. Endocrinology 136:357, 1995.

190. Marcinkiewicz M, Ramla D, Seidah NG, Chrétien M: Developmental expression of the prohormone convertases PC1 and PC2 in mouse pancreatic islets. Endocrinology 135:1651, 1994.

191. Neerman-Arbez M, Cirulli V, Halban PA: Levels of the conversion endoproteases PC1 (PC3) and PC2 distinguish between insulin-producing pancreatic islet β cells and non-β cells. Biochem J 300:57, 1994.

192. Smeekens SP, Albiges-Rizo C, Carroll R, et al: Proinsulin processing by the subtilisin-related proprotein convertases furin, PC2 and PC3. Proc Natl Acad Sci U S A 89:8822, 1992.

193. Rehemtulla A, Kaufman RJ: Preferred sequence requirements for cleavage of pro-von Willebrand factor by propeptide-processing enzymes. Blood 79:2349, 1992.

194. Bresnahan PA, Leduc R, Thomas L, et al: Human fur gene encodes a yeast KEX2-like endoprotease that cleaves pro-β-NGF in vivo. J Cell Biol 111:2851, 1990.

195. Hosaka M, Nagahama M, Kim W-S, et al: Arg-X-Lys/Arg-Arg motif as a signal for precursor cleavage catalyzed by furin within the constitutive secretory pathway. J Biol Chem 266:12127, 1991.

196. Rehemtulla A, Dorner AJ, Kaufman RJ: Regulation of PACE propeptide-processing activity: Requirement for a post-endoplasmic reticulum compartment and autoproteolytic activation. Proc Natl Acad Sci U S A 89:8235, 1992.

197. Korner J, Chun J, O'Bryan L, Axel R: Prohormone processing in Xenopus oocytes: Characterization of cleavage signals and cleavage enzymes. Proc Natl Acad Sci U S A 33:11393, 1991.

198. Hatsuzawa K, Nagahama M, Takahashi S, et al: Purification and characterization of furin, Kex2-like processing endoprotease, produced in Chinese hamster ovary cells. J Biol Chem 267:16094, 1992.

199. Molloy SS, Bresnahan PA, Leppla SI, et al: Human furin is a calcium-dependent serine endoprotease that recognizes the sequence Arg-X-X-arg and efficiently cleaves anthrax toxin protective antigen. J Biol Chem 267:16396, 1992.

200. Jung LJ, Scheller RH: Peptide processing and targeting in the neuronal secretory pathway. Science 251:1330, 1991.

201. Yoshimasa Y, Paul JI, Whittaker J, Steiner DF: Effects of amino acid replacements within the tetrabasic cleavage site on the processing of the human insulin receptor precursor expressed in Chinese hamster ovary cells. J Biol Chem 265:17230, 1990.

202. Watanabe T, Nakagawa T, Ikemizu J, et al: Sequence requirements for precursor cleavage within the constitutive secretory pathway. J Biol Chem 267:8270, 1992.

203. Stieneke-Grober A, Vey M, Angliker H, et al: Influenza virus hemagglutinin with multibasic cleavage site is activated by furin, a subtilisin-like endoprotease. EMBO J 11:2407, 1992.

204. Paterson RG, Shaughnessy MA, Lamb RA: Analysis of the relationship between cleavability of a paramyxovirus fusion protein and length of the connecting peptide. J Virol 63:1293, 1989.

205. Spaete RR, Saxena A, Scott PI, et al: Sequence requirements for proteolytic processing of glycoprotein B of human cytomegalovirus strain towne. J Virol 64:2922, 1990.

206. Bosch V, Pawlita M: Mutational analysis of the human immunodeficiency virus type 1 env gene product proteolytic cleavage site. J Virol 64:2337, 1990.

207. Wilcox CA, Fuller RS: Posttranslational processing of the prohormone-cleaving Kex2 protease in the Saccharomyces cerevisiae secretory pathway. J Cell Biol 115:297, 1991.

208. Molloy SS, Anderson ED, Jean F, Thomas G: Bi-cycling the furin pathway: From TGN localization to pathogen activation and embryogenesis. Trends Cell Biol 9:28, 1999.

209. Bailyes EM, Shennan KIJ, Seal AJ, et al: A member of the eukaryotic subtilisin family (PC3) has the enzymic properties of the type 1 proinsulin-converting endopeptidase. Biochem J 285:394, 1992.

210. Irminger J-C, Meyer K, Halban P: Proinsulin processing in the rat insulinoma cell line INS after overexpression of the endoproteases PC2 or PC3 by recombinant adenovirus. Biochem J 320:11, 1996.

211. Kaufmann JE, Irminger J-C, Mungall J, Halban PA: Proinsulin conversion in GH3 cells after coexpression of human proinsulin with the endoproteases PC2 and/or PC3. Diabetes 46:978, 1997.

212. Furuta M, Carroll R, Martin S, et al: Incomplete processing of proinsulin to insulin accompanied by elevation of des-31,32 proinsulin intermediates in islets of mice lacking active PC2. J Biol Chem 273:3431, 1998.

213. Bennett DL, Bailyes EM, Nielsen E, et al: Identification of the type 2 proinsulin processing endopeptidase as PC2, a member of the eukaryote subtilisin family. J Biol Chem 267:15229, 1992.

214. Guest PC, Bailyes EM, Hutton JC: Endoplasmic reticulum Ca²⁺ is important for the proteolytic processing and intracellular transport of proinsulin in the pancreatic β-cell. Biochem J 323:445, 1997.

215. Rhodes CJ, Lincoln B, Shoelson SE: Preferential cleavage of des-31,32-proinsulin over intact proinsulin by the insulin secretory granule type II endopeptidase: Implications of a favored route for prohormone processing. J Biol Chem 267:22719, 1992.

216. Furuta M, Yano H, Zhou A, et al: Defective prohormone processing and altered pancreatic islet morphology in mice lacking active SPC2. Proc Natl Acad Sci U S A 94:6646, 1997.

217. Jackson RS, Creemers JWM, Ohagi S, et al: Obesity and impaired prohormone processing associated with mutations in the human prohormone convertase 1 gene. Nat Genet 16:303, 1997.

218. Zhu X, Zhou A, Dey A, et al: Disruption of PC1/3 expression in mice causes dwarfism and multiple neuroendocrine peptide processing defects. Proc Natl Acad Sci U S A 99:10293, 2002.

219. Zhu X, Orci L, Carroll R, et al: Severe block in processing of proinsulin to insulin accompanied by elevation of des-64,65 proinsulin intermediates in islets of mice lacking prohormone convertase 1/3. Proc Natl Acad Sci U S A 99:10299, 2002.

220. Zethelius B, Byberg L, Hales CN, et al: Proinsulin and acute insulin response independently predict type 2 diabetes mellitus in men: Report from 27 years of
follow-up study. Diabetologia 46:20, 2003.

221. Rhodes CJ, Alarcon C: What β-cell defect could lead to hyperproinsulinemia in NIDDM? Some clues from recent advances made in understanding the proinsulin-processing mechanism. Diabetes 43:511, 1994.

222. Sizonenko S, Irminger J-C, Buhler L, et al: Kinetics of proinsulin conversion in human islets. Diabetes 42:933, 1993.

223. Martin SK, Carroll R, Benig M, Steiner DF: Regulation by glucose of the biosynthesis of PC2, PC3 and proinsulin in (ob/ob) mouse islets of Langerhans. FEBS Lett 356:279, 1994.

224. Skelly R, Schuppin G, Ishihara H, et al: Glucose-regulated translational control of proinsulin biosynthesis with that of the proinsulin endopeptidases PC2 and PC3 in the insulin-producing MIN6 cell line. Diabetes 45:37, 1996.

225. Kalidas K, Dow E, Saker P, et al: Prohormone convertase 1 in obesity, gestational diabetes mellitus, and NIDDM: No evidence for a major susceptibility role. Diabetes 47:287, 1998.

226. Yoshida H, Ohagi S, Sanke T, et al: Association of the prohormone convertase 2 gene (PCSK2) on chromosome 20 with NIDDM in Japanese subjects. Diabetes 44:389, 1995.

227. Utsunomiya N, Ohagi S, Sanke T, et al: Organization of the human carboxypeptidase E gene and molecular scanning for mutations in Japanese subjects with NIDDM or obesity. Diabetologia 41:701, 1998.

228. Robichon A, Kuks P: Proteolysis in rat hypothalamic neurosecretory granules: Characterization of an α-chymotrypsin-like activity in the pathway of intracellular processing of prohormones. Endocrinology 128:1974, 1991.

229. Sakai J, Rawson RB, Espenshade PJ, et al: Molecular identification of the sterol-regulated luminal protease that cleaves SREBPs and controls lipid composition of animal cells. Mol Cell 2:505, 1998.

230. Seidah NG, Mowla SJ, Hamelin J, et al: Mammalian subtilisin/kexin isozyme SKI-1: A widely expressed proprotein convertase with a unique cleavage specificity and cellular localization. Proc Natl Acad Sci U S A 96:1321, 1999.

231. Kwok SCM, Chan SJ, Steiner DF: Cloning and nucleotide sequence analysis of the dog insulin gene: Coded amino acid sequence of canine preproinsulin predicts an additional C-peptide fragment. J Biol Chem 258:2357, 1983.

232. Benoit R, Ling N, Esch F: A new prosomatostatin-derived peptide reveals a pattern for prohormone cleavage at monobasic sites. Science 238:1126, 1987.

233. Schwartz TW: The processing of precursors. FEBS Lett 200:1, 1986.

234. Nakayama K, Watanabe T, Nakagawa T, et al: Consensus sequence for precursor processing at mono-arginyl sites. J Biol Chem 267:16335, 1992.

235. Docherty K, Steiner DF: Post-translational proteolysis in polypeptide hormone biosynthesis. Annu Rev Physiol 44:625, 1981.

236. Arvan P, Castle D: Protein sorting and secretion granule formation in regulated secretory cells. Trends Cell Biol 2:327, 1992.

237. Kuliawat R, Klumperman J, Ludwig T, Arvan P: Differential sorting of lysosomal enzymes out of the regulated secretory pathway in pancreatic beta-cells. J Cell Biol 137:595, 1997.

238. Arvan P, Kuliawat R, Prabakaran D, et al: Protein discharge from immature secretory granules displays both regulated and constitutive characteristics. J Biol Chem 266:14171, 1991.

239. Greider MH, Howell SL, Lacy PE: Isolation and properties of secretory granules from rat islets of Langerhans: II. Ultrastructure of the beta granule. J Cell Biol 41:162, 1969.

240. Lange RH, Boseck S, Ali SS: Crystallographic interpretation of the ultrastructure of B-granules in the islets of Langerhans of the grass-snake, Natrix n. natrix. Z Zellforsch Mikrosk Anat 131:559, 1972.

241. Emdin SO, Dodson GG, Cutfield JM, et al: Role of zinc in insulin biosynthesis. Diabetologia 19:174, 1980.

242. Logothetopoulos J, Maneko M, Wrenshall GA, et al: Zinc, granulation, and extractable insulin of islet cells following hyperglycemia or prolonged treatment with insulin. In Brolin SE, Hellman B, Knutson H (eds): The Structure and Metabolism of the Pancreatic Islets Wenner-Gren Center International Symposium Series, vol 3. Oxford, UK, Pergamon Press, 1964, p 333.

243. Falkmer S: Sulfhydryl compounds and heavy metals in islet morphology and metabolism. In Rodriquez RR, Vallance-Owne JJ (eds): Proceedings of the 7th Congress of the International Diabetes Federation. Amsterdam, Excerpta Medica, 1971, p 219.

244. Grant PT, Coombs TL, Frank BH: Differences in the nature of the interactions of insulin and proinsulin with zinc. Biochem J 126:433, 1972.

245. Howell SL, Tyhurst M, Duvefelt H, et al: Role of zinc and calcium in the formation and storage of insulin in the pancreatic β-cell. Cell Tissue Res 188:107, 1972.

246. Rubenstein AH, Steiner DF, Horwitz DF: Clinical significance of circulating proinsulin and C-peptide. Recent Prog Horm Res 33:435, 1977.

247. Cohen RM, Given BD, Licinio-Paixao J, et al: Proinsulin radioimmunoassay in the evaluation of insulinomas and familial hyperproinsulinemia. Metabolism 35:1137, 1986.

248. Rubenstein AH, Clark JL, Melani F, et al: Secretion of proinsulin C-peptide by pancreatic B cells and its circulation in blood. Nature 224:697, 1969.

249. Halban PA: Structural domains and molecular lifestyles of insulin and its precursors in the pancreatic beta cell. Diabetologia 34:767, 1991.

250. Oyer PE, Cho E, Peterson JD, et al: Studies on human proinsulin: Isolation and amino acid sequence of the human pancreatic C-peptide. J Biol Chem 246:1375, 1971.

251. Peterson JD, Nehrlich S, Oyer PE, et al: Determination of the amino acid sequence of the monkey, sheep and dog proinsulin C-peptides by a semi-micro Edman degradation procedure. J Biol Chem 247:4866, 1972.

252. Smit AB, Vreugdenhil E, Ebberink RHM, et al: Growth-controlling molluscan neurons produce the precursor of an insulin-related peptide. Nature 331:535, 1988.

253. Kohnert KD, Ziegler M, Zühlke H, et al: Isoelectric focusing of proinsulin and intermediates in polyacrylamide gel. FEBS Lett 28:177, 1972.

254. Wahren J, Johansson B-L, Wallberg-Henriksson H: Does C-peptide have a physiological role? Diabetologia 37:S99, 1994.

255. Zierath JR, Galuska D, Johansson B-L, Wallberg-Henriksson H: Effect of human C-peptide on glucose transport in in vitro incubated human skeletal muscle. Diabetologia 34:899, 1991.

256. Johansson B-L, Sjöberg S, Wahren J: The influence of human C-peptide on renal function and glucose utilization in type 1 (insulin-dependent) diabetic patients. Diabetologia 35:121, 1992.

257. Johansson B-L, Linde B, Wahren J: Effects of C-peptide on blood flow, capillary diffusion capacity and

glucose utilization in the exercising forearm of type 1 (insulin-dependent) diabetic patients. Diabetologia 35:1151, 1992.

258. Ido Y, Vindigni A, Chang K, et al: Prevention of vascular and neural dysfunction in diabetic rats by C-peptide. Science 277:563, 1997.

259. Forst T, Kunt T, Pohlmann T, et al: Biological activity of C-peptide on the skin microcirculation in patients with insulin-dependent diabetes mellitus. J Clin Invest 101:2036, 1998.

260. Johansson J, Ekberg K, Shafqat J, et al: Molecular effects of proinsulin C-peptide. Biochem Biophys Res Commun 295:1035, 2002.

261. Edvell A, Lindström P: Initiation of increased pancreatic islet growth in young normoglycemic mice (Umeå +/?). Endocrinology 140:778, 1999.

262. Steiner DF, Clark JL: The spontaneous reoxidation of reduced beef and rat proinsulins. Proc Natl Acad Sci U S A 60:622, 1968.

263. Lipkind G, Steiner DF: Predicted structural alterations in proinsulin during its interactions with prohormone convertases. Biochemistry 38:890, 1999.

264. Brandenburg D, Wollmer A: The effect of a non-peptide interchain cross-link on the reoxidation of reduced insulin. Hoppe Seylers Z Physiol Chem 354:613, 1973.

265. Busse WD, Hansen SR, Carpenter FH: Carbonylbis (L-methionyl) insulin A proinsulin analog which is convertible to insulin. J Am Chem Soc 96:5949, 1974.

266. Liu M, Ramos-Cstaneda J, Arvan P: Role of the connecting peptide in insulin biosynthesis. J Biol Chem 278:14798, 2003.

267. Okun MM, Shields D: Translocation of preproinsulin across the endoplasmic reticulum membrane. J Biol Chem 267:11476, 1992.

268. Lim SK, Gardella TJ, Baba H, et al: The carboxy-terminus of parathyroid hormone is essential for hormone processing and secretion. Endocrinology 131:2325, 1992.

269. Powell S, Orci L, Craik CS, Moore H-PH: Efficient targeting to storage granules of human proinsulins with altered propeptide domain. J Cell Biol 106:1843, 1988.

270. Steiner DF, Chan SJ, Welsh JM: Models of peptide biosynthesis-the molecular and cellular basis of insulin production. Clin Invest Med 9:318, 1986.

271. Geiger R, Wissman H, Weidenmuller HL, et al: Rekombination der A-und B-ketten von schweine insulin in anwesenheit von synthetischem C-peptid der schweine-proinsulins. Z Naturforsch 24b:1489, 1969.

272. Baba S, Kaucko T, Yanaihara N (eds): Proinsulin, Insulin, C-Peptide. Amsterdam, Excerpta Medica, 1979.

273. Glauber HS, Henry RR, Wallace P: The effects of biosynthetic human proinsulin on carbohydrate metabolism in non-insulin-dependent diabetes mellitus. N Engl J Med 316:443, 1987.

274. Madsen OD, Cohen RM, Fitch FW, et al: Production and characterization of monoclonal antibodies specific for human proinsulin using a sensitive micro-dot assay procedure. Endocrinology 113:2135, 1983.

275. Madsen OD, Frank BH, Steiner DF: Human proinsulin specific antigenic determinants identified by monoclonal antibodies. Diabetes 33:1012, 1984.

276. Cook DL, Taborsky GJ Jr: B-cell function and insulin secretion. In Porte D Jr, Sherwin RS (eds): Ellenberg and Rifkin's Diabetes Mellitus, 5th ed. Stamford, CT, Appleton Lange, 1997, p 49.

277. Burgess TL, Kelly RB: Constitutive and regulated secretion of proteins. Annu Rev Cell Dev Biol 3:243, 1987.

278. Grodsky GM: Insulin and the pancreas. In Harris RS, Munson PL, Diczfalvsy E (eds): Vitamins and Hormones, vol 28. New York, Academic Press, 1970, p 37.

279. Valverde I, Garcia-Morales P, Ghiglione M, et al: The stimulus-secretion coupling of glucose-induced insulin release: LIII. Calcium dependency of the cyclic AMP response to nutrient secretagogues. Horm Metab Res 15:62, 1983.

280. Asplund K: Effects of glucose on insulin biosynthesis in foetal and newborn rats. Horm Metab Res 5:410, 1973.

281. Welsh M, Scherberg N, Gilmore R, et al: Translational control of insulin biosynthesis: Evidence for regulation of elongation, initiation and signal recognition particle-mediated translational arrest by glucose. Biochem J 235:459, 1985.

282. Welsh M, Hammer RE, Brinster RL, et al: Stimulation of growth hormone synthesis by glucose in islets of Langerhans isolated from transgenic mice. J Biol Chem 261:12915, 1986.

283. Nielsen DA, Welsh M, Casadaban MJ, et al: Control of insulin gene expression in pancreatic β-cells and in an insulin-producing cell line, RIN-5F cells: I. Effects on the transcription of insulin mRNA. J Biol Chem 260:13585, 1985.

284. Welsh M, Nielsen DA, MacKrell AJ, et al: Control of insulin gene expression in pancreatic β-cells and in an insulin-producing cell line, RIN-5F cells: II. Regulation of insulin mRNA stability. J Biol Chem 260:13590, 1985.

285. Giddings SJ, Chirgwin JM, Permutt MA: Glucose regulated insulin biosynthesis in isolated rat pancreatic islets is accompanied by changes in proinsulin mRNA. Diabetes Res 2:71, 1985.

286. German MS: Glucose sensing in pancreatic islet beta-cells: The key role of glucokinase and the glycolytic intermediates. Proc Natl Acad Sci U S A 90:1781, 1993.

287. Olson LK, Sharma A, Peshavaria M: Reduction of insulin gene transcription in HIT-T15 β cells chronically exposed to a supraphysiologic glucose concentration is associated with loss of STF-1 transcription factor expression. Proc Natl Acad Sci U S A 92:9127, 1995.

288. Marshak SH, Totary E, Cerasi E, Melloul D: Purification of the β-cell glucose-sensitive factor that transactivates the insulin gene differentially in normal land transformed islet cells. Proc Natl Acad Sci U S A 93:15057, 1996.

289. Shalwitz RA, Herbst T, Carnaghi LR, Giddings SJ: Time course for effects of hypoglycemia on insulin gene transcription in vivo. Diabetes 43:929, 1994.

290. Orland MJ, Chyn R, Permutt MA: Modulation of proinsulin messenger RNA after partial pancreatectomy in rats: Relationships to glucose homeostasis. J Clin Invest 75:2047, 1985.

291. Swenne I: The role of glucose in the in vitro regulation of cell cycle kinetics and proliferation of fetal pancreatic B-cells. Diabetes 31:754, 1982.

292. da Silva Xavier G, Qian Q, Cullen PJ, Rutter GA: Distinct roles for insulin and insulin-like growth factor-1 receptors in pancreatic β-cell glucose sensing revealed by RNA splicing. Biochem J 377:149, 2004.

293. Otani K, Kulkarni RN, Baldwin AC, et al: Reduced β-cell mass and altered glucose sensing impair insulin-secretory function in aIRKO mice. Am J Physiol Endocrinol Metab 286:E41, 2004.

294. Leibowitz G, Oprescu AI, Üçkaya G, et al: Insulin does not mediate glucose stimulation of proinsulin biosynthesis. Diabetes 52:998, 2003.

295. Wicksteed B, Alarcon C, Briaud I, et al: Glucose-induced translational control of proinsulin biosynthesis is proportional to preproinsulin mRNA levels in islet β-cells but not regulated via a positive feedback of secreted insulin. J Biol Chem 278:42080, 2003.

296. Bell GI, Selby MJ, Rutter WJ: The highly polymorphic region near the human insulin gene is composed of simple tandemly repeating sequences. Nature 295:31, 1982.

297. Julier C, Hyer RN, Davies J, et al: Insulin-IGF2 region on chromosome 11p encodes a gene implicated in HLA-DRA-dependent diabetes susceptibility. Nature 354:155, 1991.

298. Koman A, Cazabon S, Couraud P-O, et al: Molecular characterization and in vitro biological activity of placentin, a new member of the insulin gene family. J Biol Chem 271:20238, 1996.

299. Chan SJ, Cao Q-P, Steiner DF: Evolution of the insulin superfamily: Cloning of a hybrid insulin/insulin-like growth factor cDNA from amphioxus. Proc Natl Acad Sci U S A 87:9319, 1990.

300. Giddings SJ, Chirgwin J, Permutt MA: Evaluation of rat insulin messenger RNA in pancreatic and extrapancreatic tissues. Diabetologia 28:343, 1985.

301. Muglia L, Locker J: Extrapancreatic insulin gene expression in the fetal rat. Proc Natl Acad Sci U S A 81:3635, 1984.

302. Young WS III: Periventricular hypothalamic cells in the rat brain contain insulin mRNA. Neuropeptides 8:93, 1986.

303. Edlund H: Transcribing pancreas. Diabetes 47:1817, 1998.

304. Melloul D, Marshak S, Cerasi E: Regulation of insulin gene transcription. Diabetologia 45:309, 2002.

305. Tager H, Given B, Baldwin D, et al: A structurally abnormal insulin causing human diabetes. Nature 281:122, 1979.

306. Haneda M, Polonsky KS, Bergenstal RM, et al: Familial hyper-insulinemia due to a structurally abnormal insulin: Definition of an emerging new clinical syndrome. N Engl J Med 310:1288, 1984.

307. Nanjo K, Sanke T, Miyano M, et al: Diabetes due to secretion of a structurally abnormal insulin (insulin Wakayama): Clinical and functional characteristics of insulin. J Clin Invest 77:514, 1986.

308. Shoelson SE, Polonsky KS, Zeidler A, et al: Human insulin B24 (Phe-Ser): Secretion and metabolic clearance of the abnormal insulin in man and in a dog model. J Clin Invest 73:1351, 1984.

309. Kwok SCM, Steiner DF, Rubenstein AH, et al: Identification of a point mutation in the human insulin gene giving rise to a structurally abnormal insulin (insulin Chicago). Diabetes 32:2, 1983.

310. Haneda M, Chan SJ, Kwok SCM, et al: Studies on mutant human insulin genes: Identification and sequence analysis of a gene encoding SerB24 insulin. Proc Natl Acad Sci U S A 80:6366, 1983.

311. Assoian RK, Thomas NE, Kaiser ET, et al: Insulin and insulin: Altered structures and cellular processing of B24-substituted insulin analogs. Proc Natl Acad Sci U S A 79:5147, 1982.

312. Shoelson S, Fickova M, Haneda M, et al: Identification of a mutant human insulin predicted to contain a serine-for-phenylalanine substitution. Proc Natl Acad Sci U S A 80:7390, 1983.

313. Wang J, Takeuchi T, Tanaka S, et al: A mutation in the insulin 2 gene induces diabetes with severe pancreatic β-cell dysfunction in the Mody mouse. J Clin Invest 103:27, 1999.

314. Gabbay KH, Bergenstal RM, Wolff J, et al: Familial hyperpro-insulinemia: Partial characterization of circulating proinsulin-like material. Proc Natl Acad Sci U S A 76:2881, 1979.

315. Kanazawa Y, Hayashi M, Ikeuchi M, et al: Familial proinsulinemia: A rare disorder of insulin biosynthesis. In Baba S, Kaneko T, Yanaihara N (eds): Proinsulin, Insulin, C-Peptide. Amsterdam, Excerpta Medica, 1979, p 262.

316. Robbins DC, Blix PM, Rubenstein AH, et al: A human proinsulin variant at arginine 65. Nature 291:679, 1981.

317. Robbins DC, Shoelson SE, Rubenstein AH, et al: Familial hyper-proinsulinemia: Two cohorts secreting indistinguishable type II intermediates of proinsulin conversion. J Clin Invest 73:714, 1984.

318. Shibasaki Y, Kawakami T, Kanazawa Y, et al: Posttranslational cleavage of proinsulin is blocked by a point mutation in familial hyperproinsulinemia. J Clin Invest 76:378, 1985.

319. Oohashi H, Ohgawara H, Nanjo K, et al: Familial hyperproinsulinemia associated with NIDDM. Diabetes Care 16:1340, 1993.

320. RÀder ME, Vissing H, Nauck MA: Hyperproinsulinemia in a three-generation Caucasian family due to mutant proinsulin (arg^{65}6his) not associated with impaired glucose tolerance: The contribution of mutant proinsulin to insulin bioactivity. J Clin Endocrinol Metab 81:1634, 1996.

321. Yano H, Kitano N, Morimoto M, et al: A novel point mutation in the human insulin gene giving rise to hyperproinsulinemia (proinsulin Kyoto). J Clin Invest 89:1902, 1992.

322. Gruppuso PA, Gorden P, Kahn CR, et al: Familial hyperproinsulinemia due to a proposed defect in conversion of proinsulin to insulin. N Engl J Med 311:629, 1984.

323. Chan SJ, Seino S, Gruppuso PA, et al: A mutation in the B chain coding region of the human insulin gene is associated with impaired proinsulin conversion in a family with hyperproinsulinemia. Proc Natl Acad Sci U S A 84:2194, 1987.

324. Gross DJ, Halban PA, Kahn CR, Weir GC: Partial diversion of a mutant proinsulin (B10 aspartic acid) from the regulated to the constitutive secretory pathway in transfected AtT-20 cells. Proc Natl Acad Sci U S A 86:4107, 1989.

325. Carroll RJ, Hammer RE, Chan SJ, et al: A mutant human proinsulin is secreted from islets of Langerhans in increased amounts via an unregulated pathway. Proc Natl Acad Sci U S A 85:8943, 1988.

326. Terris S, Steiner DF: Binding and degradation of ^{125}I-insulin by rat hepatocytes. J Biol Chem 250:8389, 1975.

327. Terris S, Steiner DF: Retention and degradation of ^{125}I-insulin by perfused rat livers. J Clin Invest 57:885, 1976.

328. Sanz N, Karam JH, Horita S, Bell GI: Prevalence of insulin-gene mutations in non-insulin-dependent diabetes mellitus. N Engl J Med 314:1322, 1986.

329. Olansky L, Janssen R, Welling C, Permutt MA: Variability of the insulin gene in American blacks with NIDDM. Diabetes 41:742, 1992.

330. Olansky L, Welling C, Giddings S, et al: A variant insulin promoter in non-insulin-dependent diabetes mellitus. J Clin Invest 89:1596, 1992.

331. Stoffers DA, Stanojevic V, Habener JF: Insulin promoter factor-1 gene mutation linked to early-onset type 2 diabetes mellitus directs expression of a dominant negative isoprotein. J Clin Invest 102:232, 1998.

332. Hutton JC: The insulin secretory granule. Diabetologia 32:271, 1989.

333. Taupenot L, harper KL, O'Connor DT: The chromogranin-secretogranin family. N Engl J Med 348:1134, 2003.

334. Hutton JC, Nielsen E, Kastern W: The molecular cloning of the chromogranin A-like precursor of β-granin and pancreastatin from the endocrine pancreas. FEBS Lett 236:269, 1988.

335. Schmidt WE, Siegel EG, Kratzin H, Creutzfeldt W: Isolation and primary structure of tumor-derived peptides related to human pancreastatin and chromogranin A. Proc Natl Acad Sci U S A 85:8231, 1988.

336. Tatemoto K, Efendic S, Mutt V, et al: Pancreastatin, a novel pancreatic peptide that inhibits insulin secretion. Nature 324:476, 1986.

337. Day R, Gorr S: Secretory granule biogenesis and chromogranin A: Master gene, on/off switch or assembly factor? Trends Endocrinol Metab 14:10, 2003

338. Westermark P, Wernstedt C, Wilander E, Sletten K: A novel peptide in the calcitonin gene related peptide family as an amyloid fibril protein in the endocrine pancreas. Biochem Biophys Res Commun 140:827, 1986.

339. Clark A, Cooper GJS, Lewis CE, et al: Islet amyloid formed from diabetes-associated-peptide may be pathogenic in type 2 diabetes. Lancet 2:231, 1987.

340. Westermark P, Wernstedt C, Wilander E, et al: Amyloid fibrils in human insulinoma and islets of Langerhans of the diabetic cat are derived from a neuropeptide-like protein also present in normal islet cells. Proc Natl Acad Sci U S A 84:3881, 1987.

341. Cooper GJS, Willis AC, Clark A, et al: Purification and characterization of a peptide from amyloid-rich pancreases of type 2 diabetic patients. Proc Natl Acad Sci U S A 84:8628, 1987.

342. Opie E: The relation of diabetes mellitus to lesions of the pancreas: Hyaline degeneration of the islands of Langerhans. J Exp Med 5:527, 1901.

343. Glenner GG, Eanes ED, Wiley CA: Amyloid fibrils formed from a segment of the pancreatic islet amyloid protein. Biochem Biophys Res Commun 155:608, 1988.

344. Breimer LH, MacIntrye I, Zaidi M: Peptides from the calcitonin genes: Molecular genetics, structure and function. Biochem J 255:377, 1988.

345. Amara SG, Jonas V, Rosenfeld MG, et al: Alternative RNA processing in calcitonin gene expression generates mRNAs encoding different polypeptide products. Nature 298:240, 1982.

346. Crenshaw EB III, Russo AF, Swanson LW, Rosenfeld MG: Neuron-specific alternative RNA processing in transgenic mice expressing a metallothionein-calcitonin fusion gene. Cell 49:389, 1987.

347. Sanke T, Bell GI, Sample C, et al: An islet amyloid peptide is derived from an 89-amino acid precursor by proteolytic processing. J Biol Chem 262:17243, 1988.

348. Leffert JD, Newgard CB, Okamoto H, et al: Rat amylin: Cloning and tissue-specific expression in pancreatic islets. Proc Natl Acad Sci U S A 86:3127, 1989.

349. Mosselman S, Höppener JWM, Zandberg J, et al: Islet amyloid polypeptide: Identification and chromosomal localization of the human gene. FEBS Lett 239:227, 1988.

350. Nishi M, Sanke T, Seino S, et al: Human islet amyloid polypeptide gene: Sequence, chromosomal localization and evolutionary history. Mol Endocrinol 3:1775, 1989.

351. Betsholtz C, Svensson R, Rorsman F, et al: Islet amyloid polypeptide (IAPP): cDNA cloning and identification of an amyloidogenic region associated with the species-specific occurrence of age-related diabetes mellitus. Exp Cell Res 183:484, 1989.

352. Mosselman S, Höppener JWM, Lips CJM, Jansz HS: The complete islet amyloid polypeptide precursor is encoded by two exons. FEBS Lett 247:154, 1989.

353. Clark A, Wells CA, Buley ID, et al: Islet amyloid, increased A-cells, reduced B-cells and exocrine fibrosis: Quantitative changes in the pancreas. Diabetes Res 9:1519, 1988.

354. Lukinius A, Wilander E, Westermark GT, et al: Co-localization of islet amyloid polypeptide and insulin in the B cell secretory granules of the human pancreatic islets. Diabetologia 32:240, 1989.

355. Nagamatsu S, Nishi M, Steiner DF: Biosynthesis of islet amyloid polypeptide. J Biol Chem 266:13737, 1991.

356. Wang J, Xu J, Finnerty J, et al: The prohormone convertase enzyme 2 (PC2) is essential for processing pro-amyloid polypeptide at the NH2-terminal cleavage site. Diabetes 50:534, 2001.

357. Marzban L, Trigo-Gonzalez G, Zhu X, et al: Role of beta-cell prohormone convertase (PC) 1/3 in processing of pro-islet amyloid polypeptide. Diabetes 53:141, 2004.

358. Mulder H, Ahren B, Stridsberg M, Sundler F: Non-parallelism of islet amyloid polypeptide (amylin) and insulin gene expression in rat islets following dexamethasone treatment. Diabetologia 38:395, 1995.

359. Ferrier GJLM, Pierson AM, Jones PM, et al: Expression of the rat amylin (IAPP/DAP) gene. J Mol Endocrinol 3:R1, 1989.

360. Ohsawa H, Kanatsuka A, Yamaguchi T, et al: Islet amyloid polypeptide inhibits glucose-stimulated insulin secretion from isolated rat pancreatic islets. Biochem Biophys Res Commun 160:961, 1989.

361. Nakazato M, Asai J, Kangawa K, et al: Establishment of radioimmunoassay for human islet amyloid polypeptide and its tissue content and plasma concentration. Biochem Biophys Res Commun 164:394, 1989.

362. Asai J, Nakazato M, Kangawa K, et al: Regional distribution and molecular forms of rat islet amyloid polypeptide. Biochem Biophys Res Commun 169:788, 1990.

363. Kanatsuka A, Makino H, Ohsawa H, et al: Secretion of islet amyloid polypeptide in response to glucose. FEBS Lett 259:199, 1989.

364. Leighton B, Cooper GJS: Pancreatic amylin and calcitonin gene-related peptide cause resistance to insulin in skeletal muscle in vitro. Nature 335:632, 1988.

365. Cooper GJS, Leighton B, Dimitriadis GD, et al: Amylin found in amyloid deposits in human type 2 diabetes mellitus may be a hormone that regulates glycogen metabolism in skeletal muscle. Proc Natl Acad Sci U S A 85:7763, 1988.

366. Sowa R, Sanke T, Hirayama J, et al: Islet amyloid polypeptide amide causes peripheral insulin resistance in vivo. Diabetologia 33:118, 1990.

367. Scherbaum WA: The role of amylin in the physiology of glycemic control. Exp Clin Endocrinol Diabetes 106:97, 1998.

368. Gebre-Medhin S, Mulder H, Pekny M, et al: Increased insulin secretion and glucose tolerance in mice lacking islet amyloid polypeptide (amylin). Biochem Biophys Res Commun 250:271, 1998.

369. Ahrén B, Oosterwijk C, Lips CJM, Höppener JWM: Transgenic overexpression of human islet amyloid polypeptide inhibits insulin secretion and glucose elimination after gastric glucose gavage in mice. Diabetologia 41:1374, 1998.

370. Datta HK, Saidi M, Wimalawansa SJ, et al: In vivo and in vitro effects of amylin and amylin-amide on calcium metabolism in the rat and rabbit. Biochem Biophys Res Commun 162:876, 1989.

371. MacIntyre I: Amylinamide, bone conservation, and pancreatic β-cells. Lancet 2:1026, 1989.

372. Mulle C, Benoit P, Pinset C, et al: Calcitonin gene-related peptide enhances the rate of desensitization of the nicotinic acetylcholine receptor in cultured mouse muscle cells. Proc Natl Acad Sci U S A 85:5728, 1988.

373. Lauweryns JM, Van Ranst L: Calcitonin gene-related peptide immunoreactivity in rat lung: A light and electron microscopic study. Thorax 42:183, 1987.

374. Denis-Donini S: Expression of dopaminergic phenotypes in the mouse olfactory bulb induced by the calcitonin gene-related peptide. Nature 339:701, 1989.

375. Christopoulos G, Perry KJ, Morfis M, et al: Multiple amylin receptors arise from receptor activity-modifying protein interaction with the calcitonin receptor gene product. Mol Pharmacol 56:235, 1999.

376. Howard CF: Diabetes in *Macaca nigra*: Metabolic and histologic changes. Diabetologia 10:671, 1974.

377. Westermark P: On the nature of the amyloid in human islets of Langerhans. Histochemistry 38:27, 1974.

378. Yano BL, Hayden DW, Johnson KH: Feline insular amyloid: Association with diabetes mellitus. Vet Pathol 18:621, 1981.

379. Yano BL, Hayden DW, Johnson KH: Feline insular amyloid: Incidence in adult cats with no clinicopathologic evidence of overt diabetes mellitus. Vet Pathol 18:310, 1981.

380. Fox JG, Murphy JC: Cytomegalic virus-associated insulitis in diabetic *Octodon degus*. Vet Pathol 16:625, 1979.

381. Westermark P, Johnson KH, O'Brien TD, Betsholtz C: Islet amyloid polypeptide—a novel controversy in diabetes research. Diabetologia 35:297, 1992.

382. Hallman U, Wernstedt C, Westermark P, et al: Amino acid sequence from degu islet amyloid-derived insulin shows unique sequence characteristics. Biochem Biophys Res Commun 169:571, 1980.

383. Nishi M, Steiner DF: Cloning of complementary DNAs encoding islet amyloid polypeptide, insulin, and glucagon precursors from a new world rodent, the degu, *Octodon degus*. Mol Endocrinol 4:1192, 1990.

384. Glenner GG, Ceja F, Mehlhaff P: Antibodies specific for the pancreatic islet amyloid polypeptide associated with type 2 diabetes mellitus. Biochem Biophys Res Commun 159:402, 1989.

385. Westermark P: Fine structure of islets of Langerhans in insular amyloidosis. Virchows Arch 359:1, 1973.

386. Clark A, Edwards CA, Ostle LR, et al: Localisation of islet amyloid peptide in lipofuscin bodies and secretory granules of human β-cells and in islets of type-2 diabetic subjects. Cell Tissue Res 259:179, 1989.

387. Porte D Jr, Kahn SE: Clues to etiology of islet β-cell dysfunction? Diabetes 38:1333, 1989.

388. Westermark G, Westermark P, Eizirik DL, et al: Differences in amyloid deposition in islets of transgenic mice expressing human islet amyloid polypeptide versus human islets implanted into nude mice. Metabolism 48:448, 1999.

389. Kahn SE, Andrikopoulos S, Verchere CB: Islet amyloid: A long-recognized but underappreciated pathological feature of type 2 diabetes. Diabetes 48:241, 1999.

390. Nishi M, Bell GI, Steiner DF: Islet amyloid polypeptide (amylin): No evidence of an abnormal precursor sequence in 25 type 2 (non-insulin-dependent) diabetic patients. Diabetologia 33:628, 1990.

391. Melato M, Antonutto G, Ferronato E: Amyloidosis of the islets of Langerhans in relation to diabetes mellitus and aging. Beitr Pathol 160:73, 1977.

392. Westermark A, Wilander E: The influence of amyloid deposits on the islet volume in maturity onset diabetes mellitus. Diabetologia 15:417, 1978.

393. Maloy AL, Longnecker DS, Greenberg ER: The relation of islet amyloid to the clinical type of diabetes. Hum Pathol 12:917, 1981.

394. Kimball CP, Murlin JR: Aqueous extracts of pancreas: Some precipitation reactions of insulin. J Biol Chem 58:337, 1923.

395. Staub A, Sinn L, Behrens OK: Purification and crystallization of glucagon. J Biol Chem 214:619, 1955.

396. Bromer WW, Sinn LG, Behrens OK: Amino acid sequence of glucagon: V. Location of amide groups, acid-degradation studies, and summary of sequential evidence. J Am Chem Soc 79:2807, 1957.

397. Bromer WW, Boucher ME, Koffenberger JE: Amino acid sequence of bovine glucagon. J Biol Chem 246:2822, 1971.

398. Thomsen J, Kristiansen K, Brunfeldt K, et al: The amino acid sequence of human glucagon. FEBS Lett 21:315, 1972.

399. Sundby F, Frandsen ED, Thomsen J, et al: Crystallization and amino acid sequence of duck glucagon. FEBS Lett 26:289, 1972.

400. Seino S, Welsh M, Bell GI, et al: Mutations in the guinea pig preproglucagon gene are restricted to a specific portion of the prohormone sequence. FEBS Lett 203:25, 1986.

401. Conlon JM, Hansen HF, Schwartz TW: Primary structure of glucagon and a partial sequence of oxyntomodulin (glucagon-37) from the guinea pig. Regul Pept 11:309, 1985.

402. Huang C-G, Eng J, Pan Y-CE, et al: Guinea pig glucagon differs from other mammalian glucagons. Diabetes 35:508, 1986.

403. Markussen J, Frandsen E, Heding LG, et al: Turkey glucagon: Crystallization, amino acid composition and immunology. Horm Metab Res 4:360, 1972.

404. Pollock HG, Kimmel JR: Chicken glucagon, isolation and amino acid sequence studies. J Biol Chem 250:9377, 1975.

405. Plisetskaya E, Pollock HG, Rouse JB, et al: Isolation and structures of coho salmon (*Oncorhynchus kisutch*)

406. Zimmerman AE, Moule ML, Yip CC: Guinea pig insulin: II. Biological activity. J Biol Chem 249:4026, 1974.

407. Falkmer S, Van Noorden S: Ontogeny and phylogeny of the glucagon cell. In Lefebvre PJ (ed): Handbook of Experimental Pharmacology, vol 66/I. Berlin, Springer-Verlag, 1983, p 81.

408. Bell GI: The glucagon superfamily: Precursor structure and gene organization. Peptides 7:27, 1986.

409. Sasaki K, Dockerill S, Adamiak DA, et al: X-ray analysis of glucagon and its relationship to receptor binding. Nature 257:751, 1975.

410. Lin MC, Wright DE, Hruby VJ, et al: Structure-function relationships in glucagon: Properties of highly purified des-His'-, monoiodo-, and (homoserine-lactone)-glucagon. Biochemistry 14:1559, 1975.

411. England RD, Jones BN, Flanders KC, et al: Glucagon carboxyl-terminal derivatives: Preparation, purification and characterization. Biochemistry 21:940, 1982.

412. Unson CG, Andreu D, Gurzenda EM, Merrifield RB: Synthetic peptide antagonists of glucagon. Proc Natl Acad Sci U S A 84:4083, 1987.

413. Unson CG, Gurzenda EM, Iwasa K, Merrifield RB: Glucagon antagonists: Contribution to binding and activity of the amino-terminal sequence 1-5, position 12, and the putative α-helical segment 19-27. J Biol Chem 264:789, 1989.

414. Unson CG, MacDonald D, Ray K, et al: Position 9 replacement analogs of glucagon uncouple biological activity and receptor binding. J Biol Chem 266:2763, 1991.

415. Kofod H, Unson CG, Merrifield RB: Potentiation of glucose-induced insulin release in isletsby desHis¹ glucagon amide. Int J Pept Protein Res 32:436, 1988.

416. Johnson DG, Goegel CV, Hruby VJ, et al: Hyperglycemia of diabetic rats decreased by a glucagon receptor antagonist. Science 215:1115, 1982.

417. Jelinek LJ, Lok S, Rosenberg GB, et al: Expression cloning and signaling properties of the rat glucagon receptor. Science 259:1614, 1993.

418. Runge S, Gram C, Brauner-Osborne H, et al: Three distinct epitopes on the extracellular face of the glucagon receptor determine specificity for the glucagon amino terminus. J Biol Chem 278:28005, 2003.

419. Tager SH, Steiner DF: Isolation of a glucagon-containing peptide: Primary structure of a possible fragment of proglucagon. Proc Natl Acad Sci U S A 70:2321, 1973.

420. Ravazzola M, Siperstein A, Moody AJ, et al: Glicentin immunoreactive cells: Their relationship to glucagon-producing cells. Endocrinology 105:499, 1979.

421. Thim L, Moody A: The primary structure of porcine glicentin (proglucagon). Regul Pept 2:139, 1981.

422. Patzelt C, Tager HS, Carroll RJ, et al: Identification and processing of proglucagon in pancreatic islets. Nature 282:260, 1979.

423. Patzelt C, Weber B: Early O-glycosidic glycosylation of proglucagon in pancreatic islets: An unusual type of prohormonal modification. EMBO J 5:2103, 1986.

424. Patzelt C, Neilsen D, Carroll R, et al: Studies on the biosynthesis of the other peptide hormones of the rat islets of Langerhans. Biochem Soc Trans 8:411, 1980.

425. Patzelt C, Schug G: The major proglucagon fragment: An abundant islet protein and secretory product. FEBS Lett 129:127, 1981.

426. Patzelt C, Schiltz E: Conversion of proglucagon in pancreatic alpha cells: The major endproducts are glucagon and a single peptide, the major proglucagon fragment, that contains two glucagon-like sequences. Proc Natl Acad Sci U S A 81:5007, 1984.

427. Eipper BA, Green CB-R, Campbell TA, et al: Alternative splicing and endoproteolytic processing generate tissue-specific forms of pituitary peptidylglycine α-amidating monooxygenase (PAM). J Biol Chem 267:4008, 1992.

428. Schroeder WT, Lopez LC, Harper ME, et al: Localization of the human glucagon gene (GCG) to chromosome segment 2q36 6 37. Cytogenet Cell Genet 38:76, 1984.

429. Philippe J, Mojsov S, Drucker DJ, et al: Proglucagon processing in a rat islet cell line resembles phenotype of intestine rather than pancreas. Endocrinology 119:2833, 1986.

430. Orskov C, Holst J, Knuhtsen S, et al: Glucagon-like peptides GLP-1 and GLP-2 predicted products of the glucagon gene are secreted separately from pig small intestine but not pancreas. Endocrinology 119:1467, 1986.

431. Mojsov S, Heinrich G, Wilson IB, et al: Preproglucagon gene expression in pancreas and intestine diversifies at the level of post-translational processing. J Biol Chem 261:11880, 1986.

432. Schmidt WE, Siegel EG, Creutzfeldt W: Glucagon-like peptide-1 but not glucagon-like peptide-2 stimulates insulin release from isolated rat pancreatic islets. Diabetologia 28:704, 1985.

433. Orskov C: Glucagon-like peptide-1 a new hormone of the entero-insular axis. Diabetologia 35:701, 1992.

434. Roberge JN, Brubaker PL: Regulation of intestinal proglucagon-derived peptide secretion by glucose-dependent insulinotropic peptide in a novel enteroendocrine loop. Endocrinology 133:233, 1993.

435. Miyawaki K, Yamada Y, Yano H, et al: Glucose intolerance caused by a defect in the entero-insular axis: A study in gastric inhibitory polypeptide receptor knockout mice. Proc Natl Acad Sci U S A 96:14843, 1999.

436. Drucker DJ, DeForest L, Brubaker PL: Intestinal response to growth factors administered alone or in combination with human [Gly2]glucagon-like peptide 2. Am J Physiol 273:G1252, 1997.

437. Litvak DA, Hellmich MR, Evers BM, et al: Glucagon-like peptide 2 is a potent growth factor for small intestine and colon. J Gastrointest Surg 2:146, 1998.

438. Rouillé Y, Westermark G, Martin SK, Steiner DF: Proglucagon is processed to glucagon by prohormone convertase PC2 in alpha TC1-6 cells. Proc Natl Acad Sci U S A 91:3242, 1994.

439. Rouillé Y, Martin S, Steiner DF: Differential processing of proglucagon by the subtilisin-like prohormone convertases PC2 and PC3 to generate either glucagon or glucagon-like peptide. J Biol Chem 270:26488, 1995.

440. Rouillé Y, Bianchi M, Irminger J-C, Halban PA: Role of the prohormone convertase PC2 in the processing of proglucagon to glucagon. FEBS Lett 413:119, 1997.

441. Webb GC, Akbar MS, Zhao C, et al: Glucagon replacement via micro-osmotic pump corrects hypoglycemia and alpha-cell hyperplasia in PC2 knockout mice. Diabetes 51:398, 2002.

442. Gellng RW, Du XQ, Dichmann DS, et al: Lower blood glucose, hyperglucagonemia, and pancreatic alpha hyperplasia in glucagon receptor knockout mice. Proc Natl Acad Sci U S A 100:1438, 2003.

443. Rouillé Y, Kantengwa S, Irminger J-C, Halban PA: Role of the prohormone convertase PC3 in the processing of proglucagon to glucagon-like peptide 1. J Biol Chem 272:32810, 1997.

444. Zabel BU, Naylor SL, Sakaguchi AY, et al: High-resolution chromosomal localization of human genes for amylase, proopiomelanocortin, somatostatin, and a DNA fragment (D3S1) by in situ hybridization. Proc Natl Acad Sci U S A 80:6932, 1983.

445. Guillemin R: Peptides in the brain: The new endocrinology of the neuron. Science 202:390, 1978.

446. Hökfelt T, Efendic S, Hellerström C, et al: Cellular localization of somatostatin in endocrine-like cells and neurons of the rat with special references to the A$_1$-cells of the pancreatic islets and to the hypothalamus. Acta Endocrinol 80(Suppl 200):5, 1975.

447. Reichlin S: Somatostatin: I. N Engl J Med 309:1495, 1983.

448. Hellman B, Lernmark NA: A possible role of the pancreatic α$_1$- and α$_2$-cells as local regulators of insulin secretion. In Falkmer S, Hellman B, Täljedal I-B (eds): The Structure and Metabolism of

the Pancreatic Islets: A Centennial of Paul Langerhans' Discovery, vol 16. Oxford, Pergamon Press, 1970, p 453.

449. Bloom W: A new type of granular cell in the islets of Langerhans of man. Anat Rec 49:363, 1931.

450. Orci L: General discussion I: Somatostatin-clinical implications. In CIBA Foundation (ed): Polypeptide Hormones: Molecular and Cellular Aspects. Amsterdam, Excerpta Medica, 1976, p 313.

451. Reichlin S: Somatostatin: II. N Engl J Med 309:1556, 1983.

452. Olsson S-E, Andersson A, Petersson B, et al: Effects of somatostatin on the biosynthesis and release of insulin from isolated pancreatic islets. Diabetes Metab 2:199, 1976.

453. Lernmark NA, Chan SJ, Choy R, et al: Biosynthesis of insulin and glucagon: A view of the current state of the art. In CIBA Foundation (ed): Polypeptide Hormones: Molecular and Cellular Aspects. Amsterdam, Excerpta Medica, 1976, p 7.

454. Garcia SD, Jarrousse C, Rosselin G: Biosynthesis of proinsulin and insulin in newborn rat pancreas. J Clin Invest 57:230, 1976.

455. Gottesman IS, Mandarino LJ, Gerich JE: Somatostatin. In Cohen M, Foa P (eds): Special Topics in Endocrinology and Metabolism, vol 4. New York, Alan R. Liss, 1982, p 177.

456. Yamada Y, Post Sr, Wang K, et al: Cloning and functional characterization of a family of human and mouse somatostatin receptors expressed in brain, gastrointestinal tract, and kidney. Proc Natl Acad Sci U S A 89:251, 1992.

457. Yasuda K, Res-Domiano S, Breder CD, et al: Cloning of a novel somatostatin receptor, SSTR3, coupled to adenylylcyclase. J Biol Chem 267:20422, 1992.

458. Bell GI, Reisine T: Molecular biology of somatostatin receptors. Trends Neurosci 16:34, 1993.

459. O'Carroll A-M, Lolait SJ, König M, Mahan LC: Molecular cloning and expression of a pituitary somatostatin receptor with preferential affinity for somatostatin-28. Mol Pharmacol 42:939, 1992.

460. Bruno JF, Xu Y, Song J, Berelowitz M: Molecular cloning and functional expression of brain-specific somatostatin receptor. Proc Natl Acad Sci U S A 89:11151, 1992.

461. Csaba Z, Dournaud P: Cellular biology of somatostatin receptors. Neuropeptides 35:1, 2001.

462. Brown M, Rivier J, Vale W: Somatostatin-28: Selective action on the pancreatic β-cell and brain. Endocrinology 108:2391, 1981.

463. Shoelson SE, Polonsky KS, Nakabayashi T, et al: Circulating forms of somatostatin-like immunoreactivity in human plasma. Am J Physiol 250:E428, 1986.

464. Patel YC, Srikant CB: Somatostatin mediation of adenohypophysial

secretion. In Berne RM (ed): Annual Review of Physiology, vol 48. Palo Alto, CA, Annual Reviews, 1986, p 551.

465. Patzelt C, Tager HS, Carroll RJ, et al: Identification of prosomatostatin in pancreatic islets. Proc Natl Acad Sci U S A 77:2410, 1980.

466. Goodman RH, Jacobs JW, Chin WW, et al: Nucleotide sequence of a cloned structural gene coding for a precursor of pancreatic somatostatin. Proc Natl Acad Sci U S A 77:5869, 1980.

467. Noe BD, Spiess J, Rivier JE, Vale W: Isolation and characterization of somatostatin from anglerfish pancreatic islet. Endocrinology 105:1410, 1979.

468. Lund PK, Goodman RH, Montiminy MR, et al: Anglerfish islet pre-proglucagon: II. Nucleotide and corresponding amino acid sequence of the cDNA. J Biol Chem 258:3280, 1983.

469. Goodman RH, Jacobs JW, Dee PC, Habener JF: Somatostatin 28 encoded in a cloned cDNA obtained from a rat medullary thyroid carcinoma. J Biol Chem 257:1756, 1982.

470. Funckes CL, Minth CD, Deschenes R: Cloning and characterization of a mRNA-encoding rat preprosomatostatin. J Biol Chem 258:81, 1983.

471. Shen L-P, Rutter WJ: Sequence of the human somatostatin I gene. Science 224:168, 1984.

472. Danoff A, Shields D: Differential translation of two distinct preprosomatostatin messenger RNAs. J Biol Chem 263:16461, 1988.

473. Nielsen HV, Gether U, Schwartz TW: Cat pancreatic eicosapeptide and its biosynthetic intermediate: Conservation of a monobasic processing site. Biochem J 240:69, 1986.

474. Richter D, Schmale H: A cellular polyprotein from bovine hypothalamus: Structural elucidation of the precursor to the nonapeptide hormone arginine vasopression. In McKerns KW (ed): Regulation of Gene Expression by Hormones. New York, Plenum, 1983, p 235.

475. Jansen M, van Schaik FMA, Ricker AT, et al: Sequence of cDNA encoding human insulin-like growth factor I precursor. Nature 306:609, 1983.

476. Bell GI, Merryweather JP, Sanchez-Pescador R, et al: Sequence of a cDNA clone encoding human preproinsulin-like growth factor II. Nature 310:775, 1984.

477. Mackin RB, Noe BD, Spiess J: The anglerfish somatostatin-28-generating propeptide converting enzyme is an aspartyl protease. Endocrinology 129:1951, 1991.

478. Bourbonnais Y, Danoff A, Thomas DY, Shields D: Heterologous expression of peptide hormone precursors in the yeast Saccharomyces cerevisiae. J Biol Chem 266:13203, 1991.

479. Egel-Mitani M, Flygenring HP, Hansen MT: A novel aspartyl protease allowing KEX2-independent MFα propheromone processing in yeast. Yeast 6:127, 1990.

480. Bourbonnais Y, Ash J, Daigle M, Thomas DY: Isolation and characterization of *S. cerevisiae* mutants defective in somatostatin expression: Cloning and functional role of a yeast gene encoding an aspartyl protease in precursor processing at monobasic cleavage sites. EMBO J 12:285, 1993.

481. Argos P, Taylor WL, Minth CD: Nucleotide and amino acid sequence comparisons of preprosomatostatins. J Biol Chem 258:88, 1983.

482. Gluschankof P, Morel A, Gomez S, et al: Enzyme processing somatostatin precursors: An Arg-Lys esteropeptidase from the rat brain cortex converting somatostatin-28 into somatostatin-14. Proc Natl Acad Sci U S A 81:6662, 1984.

483. Lepage-Lezin A, Joseph-Bravo P, Devilliers G, et al: Prosomatostatin is processed in the Golgi apparatus of rat neural cells. J Biol Chem 266:1679, 1991.

484. Mackin RB, Noe BD, Spiess J: Identification of a somatostatin-14-generating propeptide converting enzyme as a member of the kex2/furin/PC family. Endocrinology 129:2263, 1991.

485. Brakch N, Galanopoulou AS, Patel YC, et al: Comparative proteolytic processing of rat prosomatostatin by the convertases PC1, PC2, furin, PACE4 and PC5 in constitutive and regulated secretory pathways. FEBS Lett 362:143, 1995.

486. Montminy MR, Sevarino KA, Wagner JA, et al: Identification of a cyclic-AMP-responsive element within the rat somatostatin gene. Proc Natl Acad Sci U S A 83:6682, 1986.

487. Chance RE, Moon NE, Johnson MG: Human pancreatic polypeptide (HPP) and bovine pancreatic polypeptide (BPP). In Jaffe BM, Behrman HR (eds): Methods of Hormone Radioimmunoassay (ed 2). New York, Academic Press, 1979, p 657.

488. Lin T-M: Pancreatic peptide: Isolation, chemistry and biological function. In Jerzy Glass GB (ed): Gastrointestinal Hormones. New York, Raven Press, 1980, p 275.

489. Hazelwood RL: Synthesis, storage, secretion and significance of pancreatic polypeptide in vertebrates. In Cooperstein SJ, Watkins D (eds): The Islets of Langerhans. New York, Academic Press, 1981, p 275.

490. Kimmel JR, Pollock HG, Chance RE, et al: Pancreatic polypeptide from rat pancreas. Endocrinology 114:1725, 1984.

491. Baetens D, Malaisse-Lagae F, Perrelet A, et al: Endocrine pancreas: Three-dimensional reconstruction shows two types of islets of Langerhans. Science 206:1323, 1979.

492. Orci L: Macro- and micro-domains in the endocrine pancreas: The Banting Memorial Lecture 1981. Diabetes 31:538, 1982.

493. Schwartz TW: Pancreatic polypeptide: A hormone under vagal control. Gastroenterology 85:1411, 1983.

494. Tatemoto K: Neuropeptide Y: Complete amino acid sequence of the brain peptide. Proc Natl Acad Sci U S A 79:5485, 1982.

495. Schwartz TW, Gingerich RL, Tager HS: Biosynthesis of pancreatic polypeptide: Identification of a precursor and a co-synthesized product. J Biol Chem 255:11494, 1980.

496. Schwartz TW, Tager HS: Isolation and biogenesis of a new peptide from pancreatic islets. Nature 294:589, 1981.

497. Schwartz TW, Hansen HF, Håkanson R, et al: Human pancreatic icosapeptide: Isolation, sequence, and immunocytochemical localization of the COOH-terminal fragment of the pancreatic polypeptide precursor. Proc Natl Acad Sci U S A 81:708, 1984.

498. Schwartz TW, Hansen HF: Isolation of ovine pancreatic icosapeptide: A peptide product containing one cysteine residue. FEBS Lett 168:293, 1984.

499. Leiter AB, Keutmann HT, Goodman RH: Structure of a precursor to human pancreatic polypeptide. J Biol Chem 259:14702, 1984.

500. Boel E, Schwartz TW, Norris KE, et al: A cDNA encoding a small common precursor for human pancreatic polypeptide and pancreatic icosapeptide. EMBO J 3:909, 1984.

501. Takeuchi T, Gumucio DL, Yamada T, et al: Genes encoding pancreatic polypeptide and neuropeptide Y are on human chromosomes 17 and 7. J Clin Invest 77:1038, 1986.

502. Yamamoto H, Nata K, Okamoto H: Mosaic evolution of prepropancreatic polypeptide. J Biol Chem 261:6156, 1986.

503. Blackstone CD, Seino S, Takeuchi T, et al: Novel organization and processing of the guinea pig pancreatic polypeptide precursor. J Biol Chem 263:2911, 1988.

504. Leiter AB, Montminy MR, Jamieson E: Exons of the human pancreatic polypeptide gene define functional domains of the precursor. J Biol Chem 260:13013, 1985.

505. Parker MS, Lundell I, Parker, SL: Pancreatic polypeptide receptors: affinity, sodium sensitivity and stability of agonist binding. Peptides 23:291, 2002.

506. Schwartz TW: The processing of peptide precursors: "Proline-directed arginyl cleavage" and other monobasic processing mechanisms. FEBS Lett 200:1, 1986.

507. Canaff L, Bennett HPJ, Hou Y, et al: Proparathyroid hormone processing by the proprotein convertase-7: Comparison with furin and assessment of modulation of parathyroid convertase messenger ribonucleic acid levels by calcium and 1,25-dihydroxyvitamin D$_3$. Endocrinology 140:3633, 1999.

508. Webb GC, Akbar MS, Zhao C, Steiner DF: Expression profiling of pancreatic beta cells: Glucose regulation of secretory and metabolic pathway genes. Proc Natl Acad Sci U S A 97:5773, 2000.

Insulin Secretion

Juris J. Meier and Peter C. Butler

Regulated insulin secretion from pancreatic β cells is critical to health. Both insufficient insulin secretion (resulting in diabetes mellitus) and excess insulin secretion (leading to hypoglycemia) are life-threatening. The complexity of regulated insulin secretion in health becomes apparent with the difficulty of reproducing it in patients with insulin deficiency. Appropriate regulated insulin secretion depends on several components. First, development and maintenance of an appropriate number of functional insulin-secreting β cells, often collectively referred to as the β-cell mass.[1] Second, β cells need to sense the key regulators of insulin secretion, most importantly the prevailing blood glucose concentration.[2] Third, proinsulin synthesis and processing (see Chapter 48) must proceed at a rate to provide sufficient insulin for secretion, the insulin being targeted to insulin vesicles that are available for secretion (secretion competent).[3] As the majority of insulin secretory granules are not secretion competent (presumably because of aging or other factors),[4–6] the focus for regulation of insulin secretion is the pool of insulin secretory vesicles that are primed, docked, and available for secretion.[5] Finally, minute-by-minute changes in insulin release from these primed and docked vesicles need to be tightly linked to the regulating signals that impact the β cell. Predominant among these is the circulating glucose concentration.[7] In addition, other circulating fuels (free fatty acids, amino acids)[8–11]; other circulating hormones including glucagon-like peptide-1 (GLP-1),[12–14] glucose-dependent insulinotropic polypeptide,[15] and epinephrine[16]; innervation by adrenergic and cholinergic fibers[17–19]; and paracrine effects including islet amyloid polypeptide (IAPP) and insulin itself[20–23] are all important regulators of insulin secretion.

Our understanding of these complex processes that underlie successful regulated insulin secretion is hampered by the complexity of the anatomy of the endocrine organ that subserves regulated insulin secretion (Fig. 49-1). The islet of Langerhans was named after Paul Langerhans (1847–1888), a German pathologist (Fig. 49-2) who first described the appearance of these islets scattered in the pancreas.[24] Langerhans died at the age of 41 of tuberculosis most likely contracted by performing autopsies. The link between the pancreas and the regulation of glucose homeostasis was finally established in 1889 by Joseph von Mering (1849–1908) and Oscar Minkowski (1858–1931), who, in order to explore the involvement of the pancreas in fat absorption, performed pancreas resections in dogs,[25] resulting in polyuria and polydipsia due to glycosuria and, eventually, recognition of the role of the pancreas in glucose regulation.

ISLET STRUCTURE IN HEALTH

In humans, there are approximately 1 million islets of Langerhans scattered in the pancreas.[26–29] Islets vary greatly in size, with larger islets providing the majority of the insulin-secreting β cells, and typically containing approximately 2000 β cells.[26,27,30] Each islet has its own complex anatomy, with the core consisting mainly of β cells that are tightly interconnected by gap junctions[31–33] (Fig. 49-3), surrounded by a mantle of other endocrine cells including glucagon-secreting α cells, somatostatin-secreting δ cells and pancreatic polypeptide (pp)-secreting cells[29,34–36] In humans, approximately 50% of islet cells are nonendocrine cells. The nature of the extracellular matrix proteins is also important in both the function and development of the islet.[37,38] There is regional heterogeneity in the pattern of endocrine cells in islets, for example, with glucagon-secreting α cells more abundant in the body and tail of the pancreas in contrast to the more frequent pancreatic polypeptide-secreting cells present in the head of the pancreas.[39,40] Islets are richly vascularized, receiving approximately 10% of pancreatic blood flow despite being only approximately 1% of pancreatic mass.[27,41–43] Islets are also richly innervated, nerve fibers tracking with vessels (Fig. 49-4).[44–46] The arteriole input to the islet initially supplies the β cell–rich islet core before being further distributed to the α cell and/or pp-enriched mantle.[42] The consequence of this is that non-β-cell endocrine cells in the islet are exposed to very high paracrine insulin concentrations that may be important in normal function.[47–49] The development of the endocrine pancreas is addressed in detail elsewhere (in Chapter 47).[50] It is clear that β-cell mass is regulated in adult rodents, increasing in response to hyperglycemia, obesity, and pregnancy.[51–54] β-Cell mass is also greater in obese versus lean humans, but the increment is much less marked (~0.5-fold vs. ~10-fold) than in obese rodents.[55] While an adaptive increase in β-cell mass in mice is largely accomplished by an increase in β-cell replication, β-cell replication in vivo is very rare in humans.[51,54,55] Since β-cell replication appears to be rare in adult humans in contrast to mice, the question arises as to whether there is an alternative source of new β cells in adult humans. It has been proposed that new islets may be formed during adult life from ductal precursors recapitulating the pattern observed during development.[50,56,57] While islet buds are frequently seen on exocrine ducts in adult life in humans and rodents,[55,57] it is difficult to prove that these are newly forming islets rather than arrested development. Interest is now focused on the possibility that stem cells might provide an ongoing source of

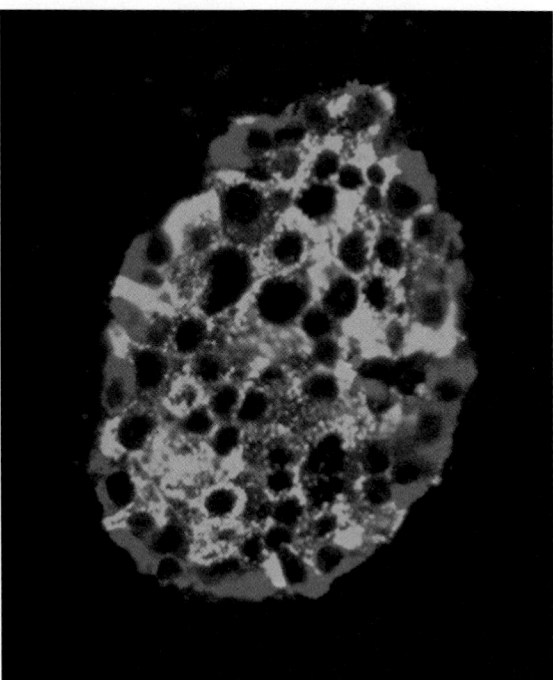

Figure 49-1   A human islet of Langerhans stained by immunofluoresence for insulin (green) and glucagons (blue). (See Color Plate.)

β cells in health, and be harnessed therapeutically in diabetes. There is conflicting data as to whether marrow-derived stem cells are potential precursors for β cells in rodents.[58,59] As yet, there are no data available in humans.

ISLET FUNCTION IN HEALTH

Given the critical importance of avoiding hypoglycemia, it is not surprising that the circulating glucose concentration is so predominant in the regulating of insulin secretion. Indeed, the glucose dose response curve for insulin secretion by isolated human islets is remarkably similar to that of humans in vivo.[60–62] In order that β cells can "sense" the prevailing blood glucose, islets need to be well vascularized, and the cytosol of β cells needs to be readily accessible to glucose. This is accomplished by rich islet vascularization with fenestrated vessels and abundant glucose-2-transporter proteins on the β-cell surface.[27,41–43,63,64] The latter allow rapid equilibrium of glucose between extracellular and intracellular concentrations. Given this rapid access of circulating glucose to the β-cell cytosol, β cells "sense" the circulating glucose concentration by the rate-limiting step in glucose metabolism, phosphorylation of glucose to glucose-6-phosphate.[65,66] This is accomplished in β cells by the expression of a glucokinase isoform with a Km of approximately 150 mg/dL (7 mM) in the middle of the physiologic glucose concentration range.[67] Thus, the rate of provision of glucose-6-phosphate into glycolytic

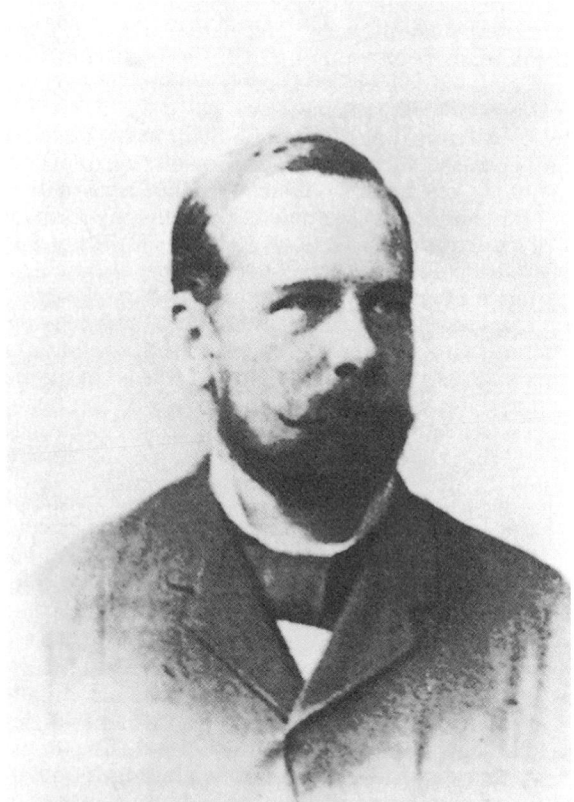

Figure 49-2   **A,** Paul Langerhans (shown here in a rare family photograph) died young from tuberculosis. **B,** The face page of the thesis of Paul Langerhans defended on February 18, 1869. (From Schadewaldt H: Geschichte des diabetes mellitus. Berlin, Springer-Verlag, 1975, pp 52–53.)

Beiträge
zur mikroskopischen Anatomie der Bauchspeicheldrüse.

INAUGURAL-DISSERTATION,

ZUR

ERLANGUNG DER DOCTORWÜRDE

IN DER

MEDICIN UND CHIRURGIE

VORGELEGT DER

MEDICINISCHEN FACULTÄT

DER FRIEDRICH-WILHELMS-UNIVERSITÄT

ZU BERLIN

UND ÖFFENTLICH ZU VERTHEIDIGEN

am 18. Februar 1869

VON

Paul Langerhans

aus Berlin.

OPPONENTEN:

G. Loeillot de Mars, Dd. med.
O. Soltmann, Dd. med.
Paul Ruge, Stud. med.

BERLIN.

BUCHDRUCKEREI VON GUSTAV LANGE.

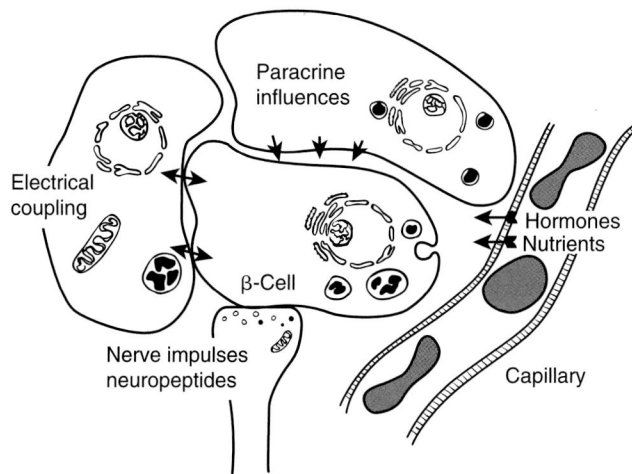

Figure 49-3 Schematic diagram of β cell with vascular, neural, and paracrine influences. (Adapted with permission from Hellerstrom C: The life story of the pancreatic B cell. Diabetologia 26:395, 1984.)

pathway and subsequent provision of pyruvate for the tricarboxylic acid cycle is closely linked to the plasma glucose concentration.[66] The resulting mitochondrial pyruvate oxidation generates adenosine triphosphate (ATP), which, in turn, activates ATP-sensitive potassium channels (closing these channels), which leads to cell depolarization and an influx of ionized calcium.[68,69] The ionized calcium is believed to interact

with primed docked insulin secretory vesicles that then discharge their contents either wholly (by exocytosis) or in part (by kiss and run) into the extracellular space.[70,71] This rich vascular supply and fenestrated vessels ensure rapid delivery of secreted insulin into the pancreatic venous efflux and then to the hepatic portal vein.

When islets are stimulated by an abrupt increase in glucose concentration in vitro (perifusion) or in vivo (intravenous glucose tolerance test), the resulting insulin secretion is biphasic (Fig. 49-5).[60,72–74] An immediate first phase of insulin secretion occurs over approximately 3 minutes and is then followed by a more prolonged second phase of insulin secretion. This observation led to the concept proposed by Grodsky of distinct subcellular pools of insulin.[5,75,76] More recently, these hypothetical pools have developed a likely anatomic basis. First-phase insulin secretion appears to reflect the immediate discharge of primed and docked insulin secretory vesicles, while second-phase insulin secretion most likely requires priming and mobilization of insulin vesicles prior to their discharge.[77] The exact molecular processes involved in the priming and mobilization of insulin vesicles remains unknown, but may also include provision of ATP following mitochondrial oxidation of pyruvate. An ATP-independent pathway for glucose-mediated insulin secretion has also been proposed, given the observation that when the K_{ATP} channel is defective due to mutations in the sulfonylurea receptor, some degree of glucose-mediated insulin secretion prevails.[78]

It has been argued that there is no physiologic counterpart of first-phase insulin secretion in vivo given the intravenous glucose challenge used to elicit it. To the contrary, almost all insulin secretion in vivo is likely released from the same pool as

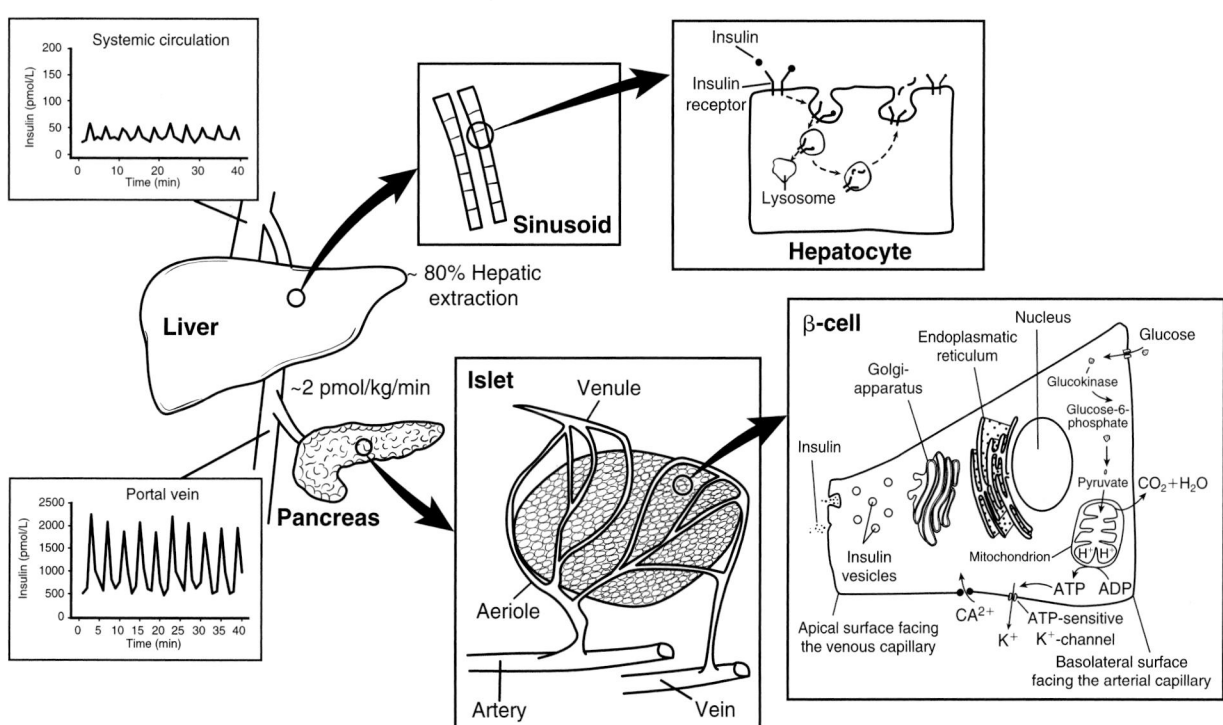

Figure 49-4 Relationship between insulin secretion from the islet, insulin clearance, and insulin action at the hepatocytes. Insulin is secreted at a rate of approximately 2 pmol/L/min from the islets of Langerhans into the portal vein. Approximately 80% of the total amount of insulin secreted is extracted from the liver sinusoids. Thus, oscillations in insulin secretion in the portal vein (~2000 pmol/L) largely exceed those measured in the peripheral circulation (~50 pmol/L). Following insulin binding, the insulin receptor-ligand complex is internalized into the cytosol of the hepatocyte. While insulin mainly undergoes enzymatic degradation in the lysosomes, the insulin receptor is reinserted into the plasma membrane within approximately 5 min.

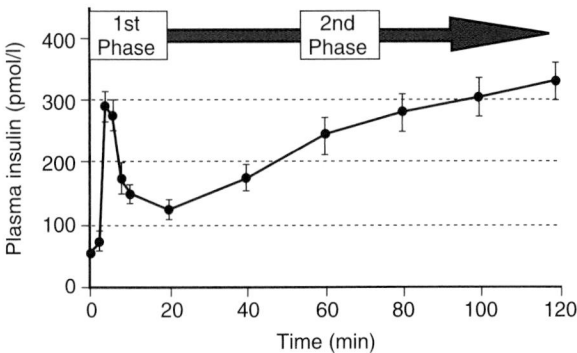

Figure 49-5 The relationship between the timing of the introduction of an intravenous glucose infusion (t = 0 min) and plasma insulin concentrations. A rapid first phase of insulin secretion is followed by second phase secretion (From Pratley RE, Weyer C: The role of impaired early insulin secretion in the pathogenesis of type II diabetes mellitus. Diabetologia 44:931, 2001.)

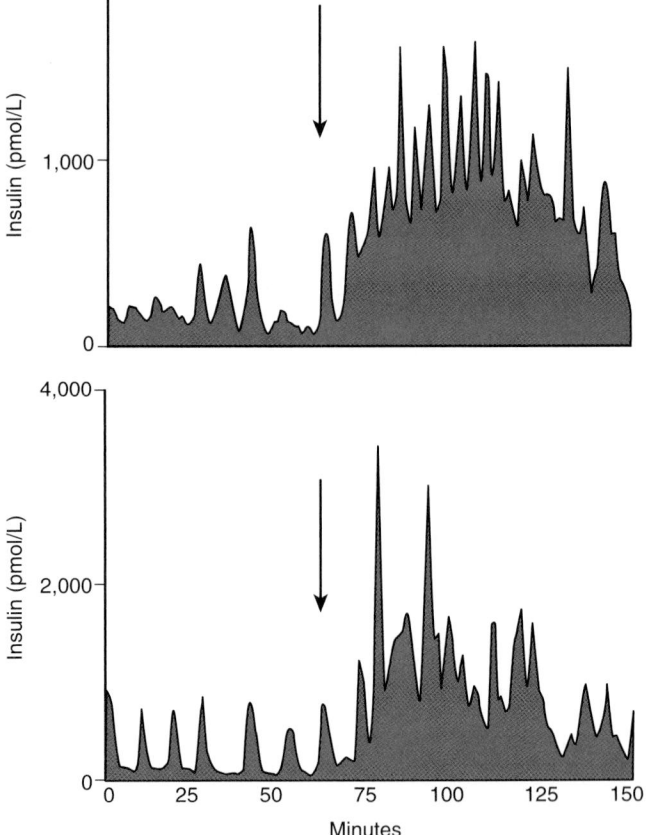

Figure 49-6 The portal vein insulin concentration before (0–60) and after meal ingestion *(arrow)* in two representative dogs. The portal vein insulin concentration excursions vary from approximately 300–1000 pmol/L before meal ingestion to 2000–4000 pmol/L after meal ingestion. Similar concentration profiles have been seen in the human portal vein. (With permission from Porksen N, Munn S, Steers J, Veldhuis JD, Butler PC: Effects of glucose ingestion versus infusion on pulsatile insulin secretion: The incretin effect is achieved by amplification of insulin secretory burst mass. Diabetes 45:1317–1323, 1996.)

approximately 90% of insulin secretion is derived from discrete insulin secretory bursts occurring at approximately 4-minute intervals.[79,80] Thus, regulation of approximately 90% of insulin secretion can be accomplished either through changes in the size (secretory burst mass) or frequency of these discrete insulin pulses. The pacemaker for this high frequency pulsatile insulin secretion is unknown although it is present in individual islets as isolated independent islets secrete insulin in pulses approximately every 4 minutes.[60,73,81,82] Whatever the basis of the pacemaker, it is remarkably robust since it does not appear to change under almost any conditions. Under almost all conditions studied, regulated changes of insulin secretion are accomplished exclusively through changes in the insulin secretory burst mass. For example, enhanced insulin secretion as a result of glucose ingestion or glucose infusion, infusion or ingestion of sulphonylurea drugs, and GLP-1 infusion is accomplished by an increase in the insulin secretory burst mass (Fig. 49-6).[60,83–86] Suppression of insulin secretion by somatostatin and insulin-like growth factor 1 are accomplished by a reduction in insulin burst mass.[84,87] The one circumstance where pulse frequency has been shown to change is induction of general anesthesia. Induction of general anesthesia profoundly suppresses insulin secretion, but while this is accomplished by inhibition of insulin burst mass, insulin pulse frequency increases under these circumstances.[88]

As most insulin secretion in vivo arises from these discrete insulin secretory bursts, the approximately 1 million islets scattered in exocrine pancreas must be coordinated to discharge their insulin secretory bursts synchronously. This coordination is accomplished, at least in part, by the intrinsic neural network in the pancreas, analogous to the intrinsic neural network in the gut that allows coordinated peristalsis and probably also through entrainment by the oscillating glucose concentration that presumably arises as a consequence of insulin pulses.[89–93] As a consequence of this coordination, the insulin concentration wavefront that impacts the liver about every 4 minutes is approximately 2000 pmol/L in the fasting state and as much as 5000 pmol/L after meal ingestion. The amplitude of this concentration wavefront is greatly attenuated (~50 pmol/L) by the time the insulin is released into the systemic circulation, presumably as a result of both dilution of portal vein insulin in the systemic circulation and selective extraction of insulin pulses in the liver (see Figs. 49-4 and 49-6). Although no studies have reproduced these dramatic portal vein insulin concentration dynamics in vivo, early-phase insulin secretion after glucose ingestion, which likely approximates these kinetics in the

portal vein, may be important in suppression of hepatic glucose production, an important adaptive response to ingested glucose to minimize the postprandial increase in glucose concentrations (see Chapter 52). It is unknown to what extent exposure of the liver to these dramatic oscillations in insulin concentration is important for insulin sensitivity. Infusions of much smaller insulin pulses versus a continuous insulin infusion have been shown to enhance insulin action.[93–95] Insulin is also secreted in an ultradian rhythm with a frequency of approximately 20 minutes.[96]

Under conditions of daily living, the numerous factors involved in regulating insulin secretion are integrated to provide a rate of insulin secretion of approximately 2 pmol/kg/min in the fasting state increasing to approximately 10 pmol/kg/min after meal ingestion.[97–100] There is a wide range in these rates based upon the insulin sensitivity of the individual (see Chapters 50 and 52). Thus, with aging and obesity and in response to exercise, adaptive changes in the rate of insulin secretion occur.[79,100–106] In health, insulin secretion adaptively changes according to insulin requirements.[62,103,107] The most prevalent need for increased insulin secretion is the insulin resistance consequent upon obesity.[79,100] In response to obesity, the daily insulin requirement increases by as much as tenfold. However, in humans, the β-cell mass in obese versus lean individuals is only increased approximately 0.5-fold.[55] This implies that the most important adaptive change to meet chronically increased insulin secretion requirements in insulin-resistant humans is an increase in insulin secretion per β cell rather than simply an increase in the number of β cells.

INSULIN CLEARANCE

Insulin is secreted into the portal vein where it is delivered directly to the liver. As a consequence of the rapid blood flow in the portal vein (~0.8 L/min) and the fenestrations in the hepatic sinusoids, hepatocytes are directly exposed to the high-amplitude oscillations arising from insulin secretory bursts within seconds of secretion. After insulin binding to the receptors at the hepatocyte membrane, the insulin receptor–ligand complex is rapidly internalized to form an intracytoplasmic vesicle.[108–113] While insulin undergoes enzymatic degradation in the endosomes,[114,115] the insulin receptor is reinserted into the plasma membrane within approximately 5 minutes to become available for the next insulin burst.[112,116] In health, in humans approximately 80% of endogenous insulin secretion is cleared by the liver with the first pass through the liver.[117–120] Following oral glucose ingestion, insulin extraction is diminished by approximately 50%.[121–123] The major factor determining the rate of insulin clearance appears to be the amount of insulin presented to the liver.[124,125] In fact, a close relationship between insulin secretion and hepatic insulin uptake has been described,[118,126] consistent with the idea of a finite number of insulin receptors present on hepatocytes. The extent of hepatic extraction also appears to depend on the amplitude of insulin oscillations presented to the liver.[84,127] Since the mean interval of insulin pulses presented to the liver almost coincides with the time period calculated for insulin receptor recycling (~5 min),[112] pulsatile delivery of insulin may prevent the liver from desensitization. This, together with the fact that there appears to be selective extraction of insulin pulses by the liver, implies that varying the pattern of insulin delivery to the liver may provide the beta cell an opportunity to regulate end-organ actions of insulin.

ISLET STRUCTURE AND FUNCTION IN TYPE 1 DIABETES

In type 1 diabetes there is a marked deficiency of β-cell mass.[56,128–132] Prior to development of diabetes, there is a prolonged period when the autoimmune disease is thought to be active.[133–135] During this latent period, a progressive decline in first-phase insulin secretion has been documented, as well as impaired insulin pulses.[134,136–139] By the time of clinical presentation, approximately 90% of β cells have been lost, although some capacity for endogenous insulin secretion remains, and there is a relatively rapid further loss of this over the next 2 years.[56,130,132,140,141] The mechanisms underlying this further loss of insulin secretion likely include both a further loss of β-cell mass, as well as decreased insulin secretion per β cells, both in large part a consequence of the hyperglycemia.[142,143] It is important here to distinguish human islets from rodent islets in which of necessity much research is carried out. Human β cells exposed to glucose concentrations typically present in even relatively well-controlled diabetes (~150 mg/dL, 8 mM) have an increased frequency of apoptosis induced in part by endogenous expression of interleukin-1β (rat islets do not have an increased rate of β cell apoptosis until glucose concentrations increase to approximately 360 mg/dL or 20 mM).[142] In addition, insulin secretion by human islets is also impaired after exposure to these levels of glucose concentration within 96 hours.[144] Chronic exposure of islets to

this relatively modest level of glucose appears to preferentially deplete the primed and docked insulin secretory vesicles since both glucose-induced first-phase insulin secretion and glucose-induced insulin secretory burst mass are greatly attenuated.[144] There is also evidence to suggest that an increased workload of β cells may also accelerate the autoimmune-mediated destruction. Taken together, these factors have been called *glucose toxicity*.[143,145] The reversibility of these factors, at least in the short term, is illustrated by the partial recovery of insulin secretion and glycemic control in treated patients brought toward normal blood glucose concentrations with exogenous insulin therapy.[146-149]

Not only is some residual insulin secretion detected in patients with recent-onset type 1 diabetes, but with increasingly sensitive assays, insulin secretion may be detected many years after onset of type 1 diabetes. Moreover, there are commonly detectable β cells present in the pancreas of patients with even long-standing type 1 diabetes.[56] The question arises whether this residual insulin secretion arises from a small pool of β cells that are relatively protected from β cell destruction or from newly formed β cells. This distinction is important since the latter would imply that a novel approach to restoration of β-cell mass in patients with type 1 diabetes would be to suppress ongoing β-cell destruction. Preservation or restoration of even an inadequate amount of insulin secretion to allow insulin independence would still have great potential clinical benefit since microvascular complications are decreased in patients with residual β-cell function.

Therefore, to summarize, it is clear that the impaired insulin secretion in patients with type 1 diabetes is as a consequence of a major defect in β-cell mass, but there are likely also functional defects arising from the both the ongoing inflammation and glucose toxicity once diabetes supervenes.

ISLET STRUCTURE AND FUNCTION IN TYPE 2 DIABETES

Most, but not all, studies indicate that there is an approximately 60% decrease in β-cell mass in humans with type 2 diabetes (Fig. 49-7).[55,150,151] This decrease in β-cell mass appears to be due to an increased frequency of β-cell apoptosis; therefore, type 2 diabetes can be considered to share much in common with type 1 diabetes.[54,55,152,153] The most important distinction appears to be the absence of an autoimmune-mediated cause for the accelerated β-cell apoptosis and the more modest degree of β-cell deficiency. The importance of an approximate 60% deficit in β-cell mass might be questioned, as a similar defect does not lead to diabetes in rodents.[154] However, rodents have a remarkable capacity for β-cell regeneration after a partial pancreatectomy.[51,54] A deficit in β-cell mass comparable to that seen in humans with type 2 diabetes does lead to diabetes in large animal species potentially more representative of humans, including the pig, dog, and nonhuman primates.[127,155–157] Indeed, a comparable β-cell deficit leads to loss of first-phase insulin secretion, a deficit in insulin pulse mass, and decreased hepatic insulin clearance in the pig,[127,158] reproducing the pattern of abnormal insulin secretion and insulin clearance present in type 2 diabetes.[159] The increased frequency of β-cell apoptosis in type 2 diabetes has been ascribed to glucose toxicity, increased concentrations of free fatty acids, free radicals, and oligomers of islet amyloid polypeptide (also known as amylin).[142,160,161] The key question as to whether this increase precedes development of hyperglycemia or is a consequence of it remains unknown.

The functional defects in insulin secretion in type 2 diabetes have been reviewed elsewhere.[74] In brief, when glucose concentrations are matched, there is a major defect of insulin secretion in both the basal- and glucose-stimulated (hyperglycemic clamp or oral glucose load) insulin secretion (Fig. 49-8 to Fig. 49-10).[162–166] Defects in insulin secretion in

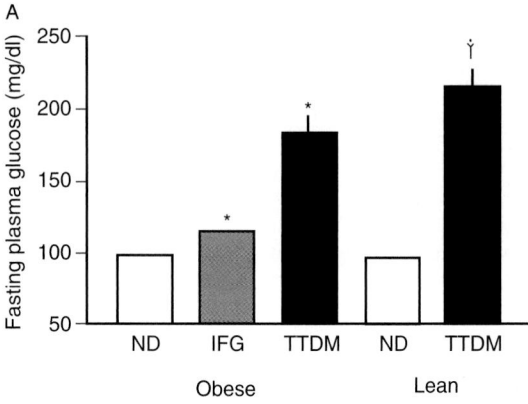

A

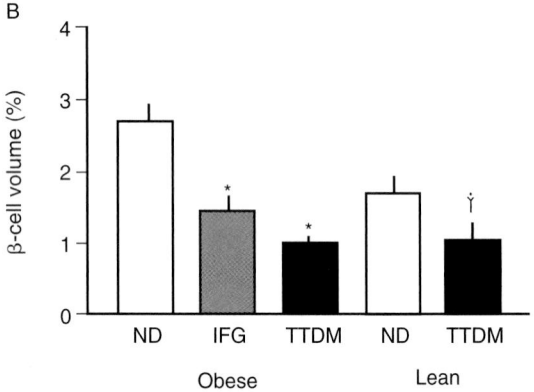

B

Figure 49-7   The mean blood glucose (**A**) and relative pancreatic β-cell volume (**B**) in obese versus lean human subjects with type 2 diabetes (TTDM), impaired fasting glucose (IFG) or nondiabetics (ND). The relative β-cell volume is increased in obese versus lean ND by approximately 50%. The relative β-cell volume is decreased by approximately 65% in obese TTDM versus controls. (From Butler AE, Janson J, Bonner-Weir S, Ritzel R, Rizza RA, Butler PC: β-Cell deficit and increased β-cell apoptosis in humans with type 2 diabetes. Diabetes 52:105, 2003.)

pancreatic insulin stores in patients with type 2 diabetes but given the small proportion of insulin vesicles that undergo secretion, it is clear that there must be a specific defect in the availability of the primed docked insulin secretory vesicles to glucose stimulation.[77] This is supported by the marked defects in early insulin secretion after meal ingestion, first-phase insulin secretion after glucose ingestion, and defective glucose-mediated insulin secretory burst mass in type 2 diabetes (see Figs. 49-10 and 49-11).[74,174–176] The increased ratio of circulating proinsulin/insulin characteristic of type 2 diabetes has been ascribed to both defective proinsulin processing and increased insulin demand, leading to secretion of immature insulin vesicles.[177–179] The defects in first-phase insulin secretion, insulin pulse mass, and proinsulin/insulin processing can all be reversed in patients with type 2 diabetes by overnight inhibition of insulin secretion (Fig. 49-11).[180] The pattern of insulin secretion defects present in type 2 diabetes can be recapitulated in pigs by induction of a deficit in β-cell mass comparable to that in type 2 diabetes.[127,158] It is of interest to compare the normal adaptive response of β-cell mass and insulin secretion to insulin resistance in obese nondiabetic humans versus the deficits in these parameters in obese humans with type 2 diabetes mellitus (Fig. 49-12). In nondiabetic humans, there is a modest adaptation in β-cell mass (~50% increased) but a much greater increase (~300%) in insulin secretion, so that in the setting of an adequate β-cell mass and normal blood glucose concentrations, β cells show a considerable capacity for sustained increased secretion. In contrast in type 2 diabetes mellitus, there is a rather comparable deficit in β-cell mass and insulin secretion (~60%) under conditions of daily living (as in Fig. 49-12) although the deficit in insulin secretion can be considered much greater at matched glucose concentrations (as in Fig. 49-8).

Taken together, these data imply that once the β-cell mass has been diminished to a critical threshold, availability of primed docked insulin secretory vesicles that can be discharged by exocytosis and/or kiss and run in response to an increment in glucose are deficient. This concept is further supported by the observation that defective glucose-induced first-phase insulin and pulsatile insulin secretion can be similarly developed in human islets exposed to a glucose concentration of 150 mg/dL (8 mM) for 96 hours, but that this defect is prevented by the concurrent addition of a potassium channel opener to the islets that prevents high rates of insulin secretion during exposure to high glucose.[144] However, the concept becomes more complex when one considers the almost immediate restoration of first-phase insulin secretion,

response to different stimuli including glucose, arginine, and glucose-dependent insulinotropic polypeptide can also be detected in individuals at high risk of developing type 2 diabetes, such as first-degree relatives or in women with a history of gestational diabetes.[163,167–173] There is a decrease in

Figure 49-8   The plasma insulin concentration in patients with type 2 diabetes (NIDDM) and non-diabetic controls in relation to a graded glucose infusion (**A**) and following an arginine bolus at graded glucose concentrations (**B**) revealing marked impairment of insulin secretion to both glucose and arginine when glucose values are matched (With permission from Ward WK, Bolgiano DC, McKnight B, Halter JB, Porte D Jr: Diminished B cell secretory capacity in patients with noninsulin-dependent diabetes mellitus. J Clin Invest 74:1318, 1984.)

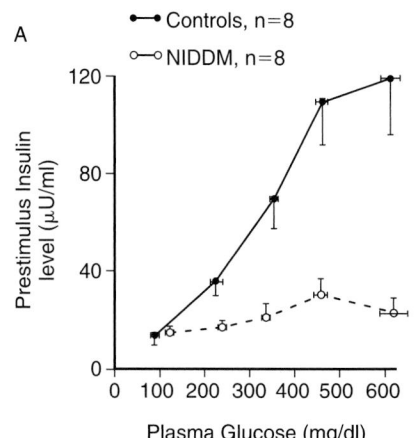

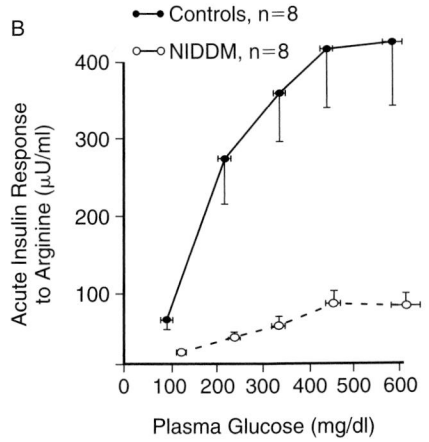

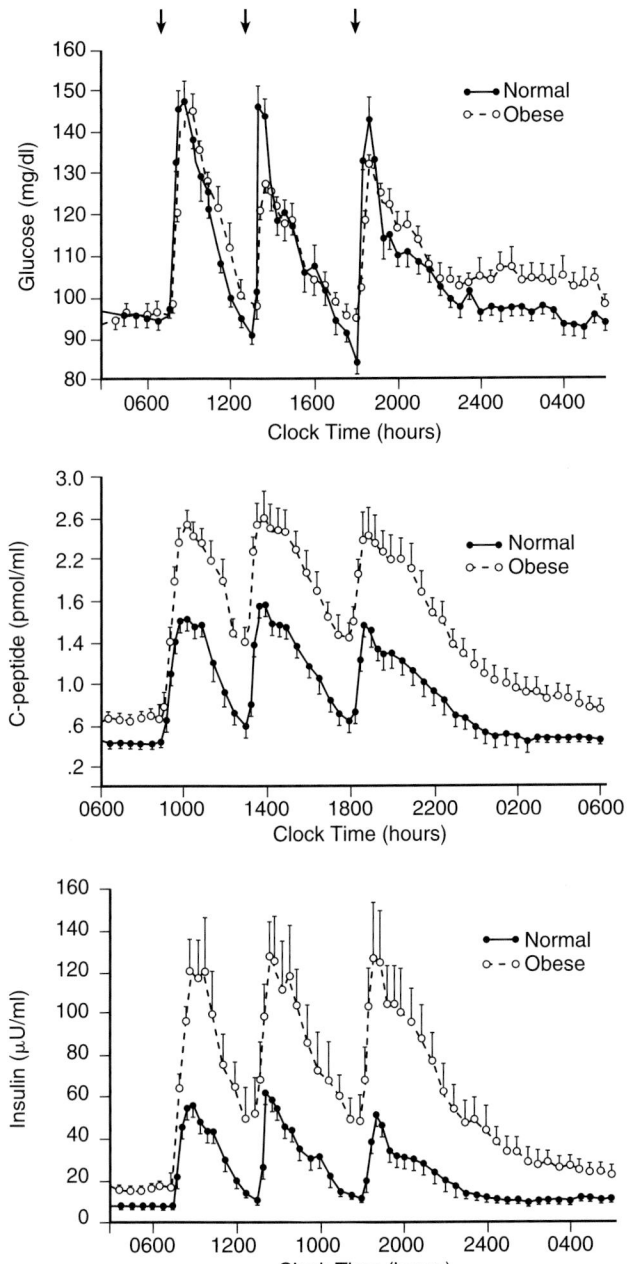

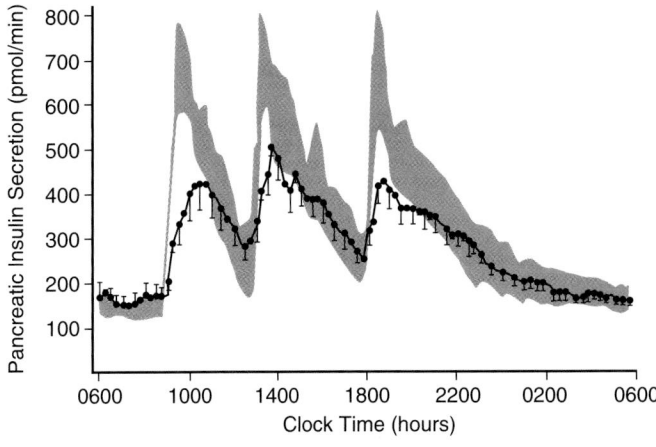

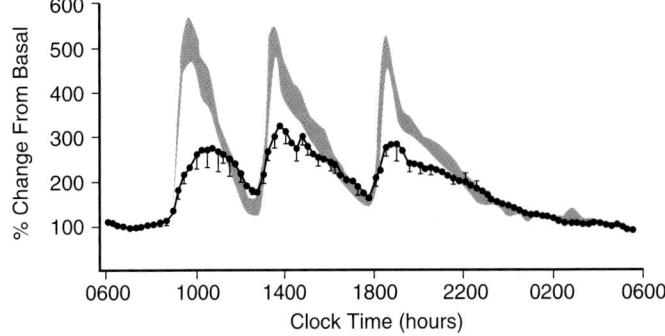

Figure 49-10 Twenty-four-hour insulin secretion profiles in type 2 diabetes *(solid line)* versus normal range (mean ± 1 SEM) for matched subjects. Measured insulin secretion rates are comparable in type 2 diabetes mellitus and controls under fasting conditions but this is, of course defective in the setting of hyperglycemia. Following meal ingestion, there is a marked defect in TTDM despite the marked hyperglcyemia. (With permission from Polonsky KS, Given BD, Hirsch LJ, et al: Abnormal patterns of insulin secretion in non-insulin-dependent diabetes mellitus. N Engl J Med 318:1231,1988.)

Figure 49-9 Twenty-four-hour pattern of insulin secretion in normal-weight and obese nondiabetic humans. In most obese humans, insulin plasma glucose concentrations are maintained at a comparable concentration by increased insulin secretion to compensate for insulin resistance. (From Polonsky KS, Given BD, Van Cauter E: Twenty-four-hour profiles and pulsatile patterns of insulin secretion in normal and obese subjects. J Clin Invest 81:433, 1988.)

pulsatile secretion, and glycemic regulation accomplished in patients with type 2 diabetes infused with the incretin hormone GLP-1.[86,181–185] Also, while first-phase insulin secretion in response to intravenous arginine is still defective in patients with type 2 diabetes compared to controls when blood glucose is considered, the magnitude of the defect is much less than that in response to glucose.[165] This discordance might be, in part, to the secondary defects in glucokinase function secondary to hyperglycemia. Also, increased expression of uncoupling protein-2 targeted to the mitochon-

drial membrane in response to chronic hyperglycemia may attenuate the glucose-induced signal for secretion due to attenuation of the mitochondrial proton gradient accomplished by pyruvate oxidation.[186]

SUMMARY

Insulin secretion is a highly regulated process. Our appreciation of the full complexities of the regulation of insulin secretion has been hampered by the inaccessibility of this particular endocrine organ, located as approximately 1 million complex organelles (islets) scattered through the exocrine pancreas. A further obstacle to the investigation of insulin secretion is the fact that approximately 80% of secreted insulin is cleared by the liver before it is delivered to the systemic circulation. Increasingly, it is apparent that regulation of insulin secretion involves not only regulation of proinsulin biosynthesis and processing (medium term) but also changes in β-cell mass (longer term). Recently, higher-resolution imaging techniques in living cells have begun to allow an appreciation of the trafficking and secretion of insulin secretory granules, which will likely shed light into the minute-to-minute regulation of insulin secretion. A greater appreciation of insulin secretion in health has also allowed a fuller understanding of the primacy of impaired insulin secretion in the pathophysiology of diabetes mellitus. Indeed, arguably diabetes might be referred to as *hypoinsulinism*

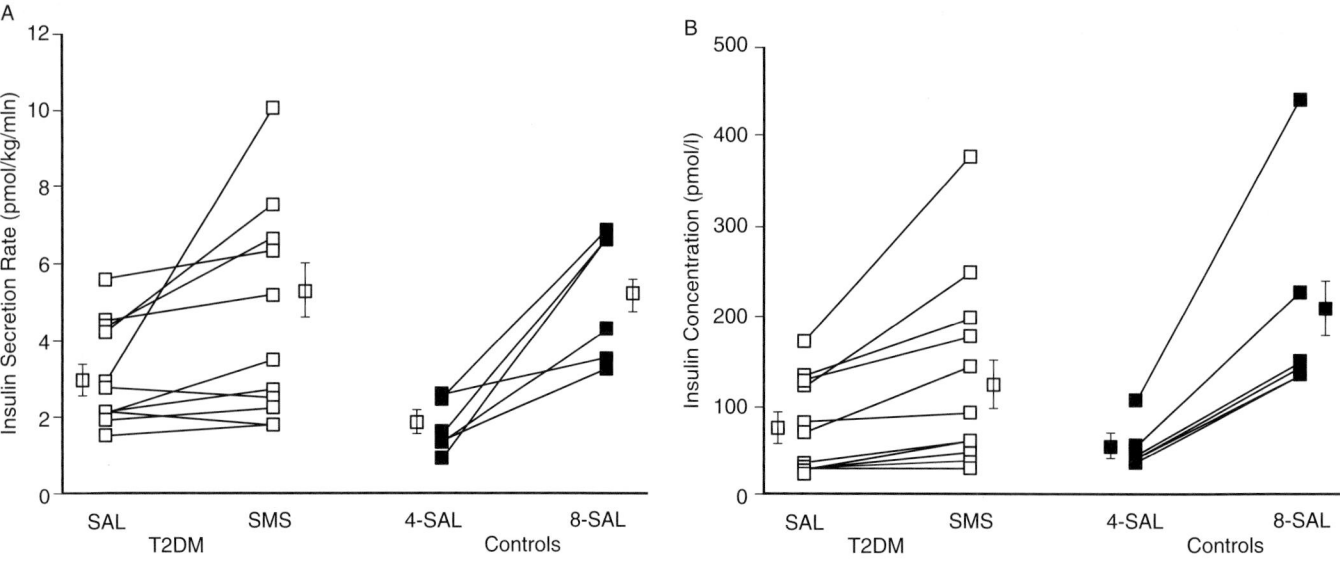

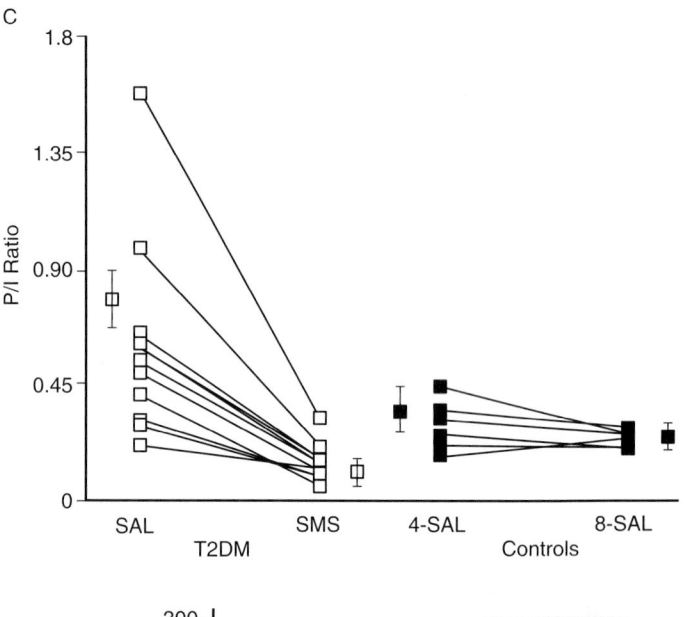

Figure 49-11 Insulin secretion (**A**), insulin concentration (**B**), and proinsulin/insulin ratio (**C**) in patients with type 2 diabetes (T2DM) and controls after prior overnight saline (SAL) or somatostatin (SMS) infusion at glucose 8 mmol/L versus nondiabetic controls at glucose 4 or 8 mmol/L. Prior overnight inhibition of insulin secretion by somatostatin restored glucose-induced insulin secretion and the proinsulin-to-insulin ratio to normal in type 2 diabetes. (With permission from Laedtke T, Kjems L, Porksen N, Schmitz O, Veldhuis J, Kao PC, et al: Overnight inhibition of insulin secretion restores pulsatility and proinsulin/insulin ratio in type 2 diabetes. Am J Physiol 279:E523 and E526, 2000.)

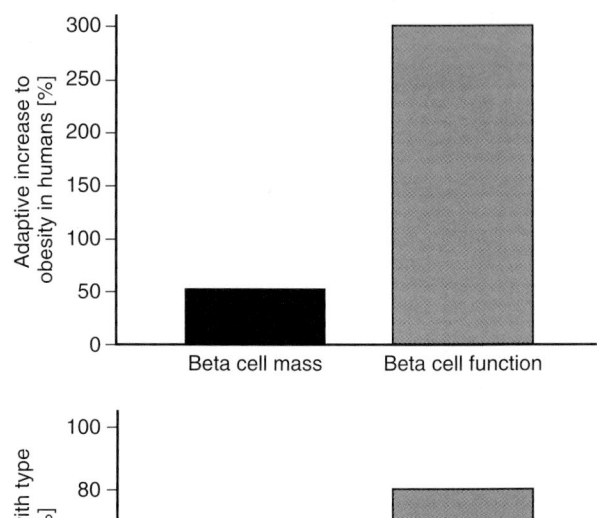

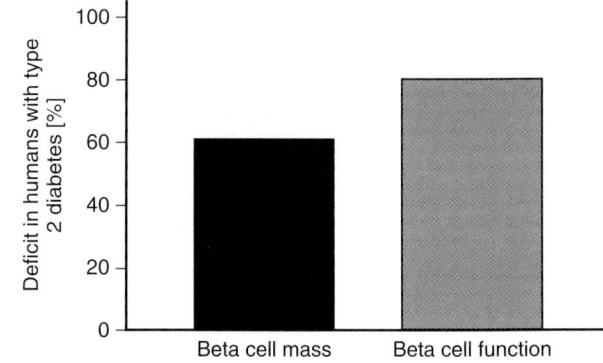

Figure 49-12 A comparison of the appropriate adaptive response of the islet to insulin resistance (**top panel,** lean versus obese nondiabetic humans) and the failed adaptive response in obese humans with type 2 diabetes (**bottom panel**). The percent adaptive increase in β-cell mass and insulin secretion are shown in the top panel and percent deficits are shown in the bottom panel.

in common with the terms *hypothyroidism, hypogonadism,* and so on. This approach then directs attention to the importance of understanding the mechanisms subserving impaired β-cell function in diabetes (autoimmune, degenerative, mitochondrial, genetic, and so on). Therapeutically, the challenge in diabetes is that replacement of insulin is much more complex than other endocrine replacement, for example, thyroxine. Prevention of loss of insulin secretion and more sophisticated means of replacing or restoring it are the major therapeutic challenges in the field of diabetes.

REFERENCES

1. Weir GC, Bonner-Weir S, Leahy JL: Islet mass and function in diabetes and transplantation. Diabetes 39:401–405, 1990.
2. Meglasson MD, Burch PT, Berner DK, et al: Chromatographic resolution and kinetic characterization of glucokinase from islets of Langerhans. Proc Natl Acad Sci U S A 80:85–89, 1983.
3. Rubenstein AH, Clark JL, Melani F, Steiner D: Secretion of proinsulin and C-peptide by pancreatic beta-cells and ist circulation in blood. Nature 224:697–699, 1969.
4. Hellman B, Sehlin J, Taljedal IB: Calcium and secretion: Distinction between two pools of glucose-sensitive calcium in pancreatic islets. Science 194:1421–1423, 1976.
5. Gold G, Gishizky ML, Grodsky GM: Evidence that glucose "marks" beta cells resulting in preferential release of newly synthesized insulin. Science 218:56–58, 1982.
6. Daniel S, Noda M, Straub SG, Sharp GW: Identification of the docked granule pool responsible for the first phase of glucose-stimulated insulin secretion. Diabetes 48:1686–1690, 1999.
7. Gabbay KH, Korff J, Schneeberger EE: Vesicular binesis: Glucose effect on insulin secretory vesicles. Science 187:177–179, 1975.
8. Crespin SR, Greenough WB 3rd, Steinberg D: Stimulation of insulin secretion by infusion of free fatty acids. J Clin Invest 48:1934–1943, 1969.
9. Raptis S, Dollinger HC, Schroder KE, et al: Differences in insulin, growth hormone and pancreatic enzyme secretion after intravenous and intraduodenal administration of mixed amino acids in man. N Engl J Med 288:1199–1202, 1973.
10. Boden G, Chen X, Iqbal N: Acute lowering of plasma fatty acids lowers basal insulin secretion in diabetic and nondiabetic subjects. Diabetes 47:1609–1612, 1998.
11. Dobbins RL, Chester MW, Stevenson BE, et al: A fatty acid-dependent step is critically important for both glucose- and non-glucose-stimulated insulin secretion. J Clin Invest 101:2370–2376, 1998.
12. Holst JJ, Orskov C, Nielsen OV, Schwartz TW: Truncated glucagon-like peptide I, an insulin-releasing hormone from the distal gut. FEBS Lett 211:169–174, 1987.
13. Kreymann B, Williams G, Ghatei MA, Bloom SR: Glucagon-like peptide-1 7-36: A physiological incretin in man. Lancet 2:1300–1304, 1987.
14. Nauck MA, Bartels E, Orskov C, et al: Additive insulinotropic effects of exogenous synthetic human gastric inhibitory polypeptide and glucagon-like peptide-1-(7-36) amide infused at near-physiological insulinotropic hormone and glucose concentrations. J Clin Endocrinol Metab 76:912–917, 1993.
15. Pederson RA, Schubert HE, Brown JC: The insulinotropic action of gastric inhibitory polypeptide. Can J Physiol Pharmacol 53:217–223, 1975.
16. Miller RE: Pancreatic neuroendocrinology: Peripheral neural mechanisms in the regulation of the islets of Langerhans. Endocr Rev 2:471–494, 1981.
17. Giugliano D, Cerciello T, Giannetti G, et al: Impaired insulin secretion in human diabetes mellitus. I. The effect of alpha-adrenergic inhibition. Pharmacol Res Commun 14:217–225, 1982.
18. Havel PJ, Taborsky GJ Jr: The contribution of the autonomic nervous system to changes of glucagon and insulin secretion during hypoglycemic stress. Endocr Rev 10:332–350, 1989.
19. Ortiz-Alonso FJ, Herman WH, Gertz BJ, et al: Effect of an oral alpha 2-adrenergic blocker (MK-912) on pancreatic islet function in non-insulin-dependent diabetes mellitus. Metabolism 40:1160–1167, 1991.
20. Beischer W, Schmid M, Kerner W, et al: Does insulin play a role in the regulation of its own secretion? Horm Metab Res 10:168–169, 1978.
21. Grasso S, Messina A, Saporito N, Reitano G: Serum-insulin response to glucose and amino acids in the premature infant. Lancet 2:755–756, 1968.
22. Degano P, Silvestre RA, Salas M, et al: Amylin inhibits glucose-induced insulin secretion in a dose-dependent manner. Study in the perfused rat pancreas. Regul Pept 43:91–96, 1993.
23. Garvey WT, Revers RR, Kolterman OG, et al: Modulation of insulin secretion by insulin and glucose in type II diabetes mellitus. J Clin Endocrinol Metab 60:559–568, 1985.
24. Langerhans P: Beitrag zur mikroskopischen Anatomie der Bauchspeicheldruse. Medical dissertation, Berlin, 1869.
25. Mering Jv, Minkowski O: Diabetes mellitus nach Pankreasexstirpation. Zschr klin Med 14:404–423, 1889.
26. Stefan Y, Orci L, Malaisse-Lagae F, et al: Quantitation of endocrine cell content in the pancreas of nondiabetic and diabetic humans. Diabetes 31:694–700, 1982.
27. Williams JA, Goldfine ID: The insulin-pancreatic acinar axis. Diabetes 34:980–986, 1985.
28. Rahier J, Goebbels RM, Henquin JC: Cellular composition of the human diabetic pancreas. Diabetologia 24:366–371, 1983.
29. Bonner-Weir S: Anatomy of the islet of Langerhans. In Samols E (ed): The Endocrine Pancreas. New York, Raven Press, Ltd, 1991, pp 15–27.
30. Deng S, Vatamaniuk M, Huang X, et al: Structural and functional abnormalities in the islets isolated from type 2 diabetic subjects. Diabetes 53:624–632, 2004.
31. Orci L, Malaisse-Lagae F, Amherdt M, et al: Cell contacts in human islets of Langerhans. J Clin Endocrinol Metab 41:841–844, 1975.
32. Meissner HP: Electrophysiological evidence for coupling between beta cells of pancreatic islets. Nature 262:502–504, 1976.
33. In't Veld PA, Pipeleers DG, Gepts W: Glucose alters configuration of gap junctions between pancreatic islet cells. Am J Physiol 251:C191–C196, 1986.
34. Orci L, Unger RH: Functional subdivision of islets of Langerhans and possible role of D cells. Lancet 2:1243–1244, 1975.
35. Orci L: Macro- and micro-domains in the endocrine pancreas. Diabetes 31:538–565, 1982.
36. Stagner JI, Samols E: The vascular order of islet cellular perfusion in the human pancreas. Diabetes 41:93–97, 1992.
37. Montesano R, Mouron P, Amherdt M, Orci L: Collagen matrix promotes reorganization of pancreatic endocrine cell monolayers into islet-like organoids. J Cell Biol 97:935–939, 1983.
38. Hayek A, Beattie GM, Cirulli V, et al: Growth factor/matrix-induced proliferation of human adult beta-cells. Diabetes 44:1458–1460, 1995.
39. Wittingen J, Frey CF: Islet concentration in the head, body, tail and uncinate process of the pancreas. Ann Surg 179:412–414, 1974.
40. Clark A, Holman RR, Matthews DR, et al: Non-uniform distribution of islet amyloid in the pancreas of "maturity-onset" diabetic patients. Diabetologia 27:527–528, 1984.
41. Wharton GK: The blood supply of the pancreas, with special reference to that of the islands of Langerhans. Anat Rec 53:55–81, 1932.
42. Lifson N, Kramlinger KG, Mayrand RR, Lender EJ: Blood flow to the rabbit pancreas with special reference to the islets of Langerhans. Gastroenterology 79:466–473, 1980.
43. Bonner-Weir S, Orci L: New perspectives on the microvasculature of the islets of Langerhans in the rat. Diabetes 31:883–889, 1982.

44. Legg PG: The fine structure and innervation of the beta and delta cells in the islet of Langerhans of the cat. Z Zellforsch Mikrosk Anat 80:307–321, 1967.

45. Bloom SR: Blood glucose control by direct islet innervation. Horm Metab Res Suppl 6:85–90, 1976.

46. Creutzfeldt W: The incretin concept today. Diabetologia 16:75–85, 1979.

47. Asplin CM, Paquette TL, Palmer JP: In vivo inhibition of glucagon secretion by paracrine beta cell activity in man. J Clin Invest 68:314–318, 1981.

48. Maruyama H, Hisatomi A, Orci L, et al: Insulin within islets is a physiologic glucagon release inhibitor. J Clin Invest 74:2296–2299, 1984.

49. Hope KM, Tran PO, Zhou H, et al: Regulation of alpha-cell function by the beta-cell in isolated human and rat islets deprived of glucose: The "switch-off" hypothesis. Diabetes 53:1488–1495, 2004.

50. Edlund H: Pancreatic organogenesis—developmental mechanisms and implications for therapy. Nat Rev Genet 3:524–532, 2002.

51. Bonner-Weir S, Deery D, Leahy JL, Weir GC: Compensatory growth of pancreatic beta-cells in adult rats after short-term glucose infusion. Diabetes 38:49–53, 1989.

52. Swenne I, Eriksson U: Diabetes in pregnancy: Islet cell proliferation in the fetal rat pancreas. Diabetologia 23:525–528, 1982.

53. Marynissen G, Aerts L, Van Assche FA: The endocrine pancreas during pregnancy and lactation in the rat. J Dev Physiol 5:373–381, 1983.

54. Butler AE, Janson J, Soeller WC, Butler PC: Increased beta-cell apoptosis prevents adaptive increase in beta-cell mass in mouse model of type 2 diabetes: Evidence for role of islet amyloid formation rather than direct action of amyloid. Diabetes 52:2304–2314, 2003.

55. Butler AE, Janson J, Bonner-Weir S, et al: Beta-cell deficit and increased beta-cell apoptosis in humans with type 2 diabetes. Diabetes 52:102–110, 2003.

56. Gepts W: Pathologic anatomy of the pancreas in juvenile diabetes mellitus. Diabetes 14:619–633, 1965.

57. Bonner-Weir S, Baxter LA, Schuppin GT, Smith FE: A second pathway for regeneration of adult exocrine and endocrine pancreas. A possible recapitulation of embryonic development. Diabetes 42:1715–1720, 1993.

58. Ianus A, Holz GG, Theise ND, Hussain MA: In vivo derivation of glucose-competent pancreatic endocrine cells from bone marrow without evidence of cell fusion. J Clin Invest 111:843–850, 2003.

59. Steptoe RJ, Ritchie JM, Harrison LC: Transfer of hematopoietic stem cells encoding autoantigen prevents autoimmune diabetes. J Clin Invest 111:1357–1363, 2003.

60. Ritzel RA, Veldhuis JD, Butler PC: Glucose stimulates pulsatile insulin secretion from human pancreatic islets by increasing secretory burst mass: Dose-response relationships. J Clin Endocrinol Metab 88:742–747, 2003.

61. Perley MJ, Kipnis DM: Plasma insulin responses to oral and intravenous glucose: Studies in normal and diabetic subjects. J Clin Invest 46:1954–1962, 1967.

62. O'Rahilly SO, Hosker JP, Rudenski AS, et al: The glucose stimulus-response curve of the beta-cell in physically trained humans, assessed by hyperglycemic clamps. Metabolism 37:919–923, 1988.

63. Kvietys PR, Perry MA, Granger DN: Permeability of pancreatic capillaries to small molecules. Am J Physiol 245:G519–G524, 1983.

64. Guillam MT, Hummler E, Schaerer E, et al: Early diabetes and abnormal postnatal pancreatic islet development in mice lacking Glut-2. Nat Genet 17:327–330, 1997.

65. Morita H, Yano Y, Niswender KD, et al: Coexpression of glucose transporters and glucokinase in Xenopus oocytes indicates that both glucose transport and phosphorylation determine glucose utilization. J Clin Invest 94:1373–1382, 1994.

66. Matschinsky FM: Banting Lecture 1995. A lesson in metabolic regulation inspired by the glucokinase glucose sensor paradigm. Diabetes 45:223–241, 1996.

67. Roche E, Assimacopoulos-Jeannet F, Witters LA, et al: Induction by glucose of genes coding for glycolytic enzymes in a pancreatic beta-cell line (INS-1). J Biol Chem 272:3091–3098, 1997.

68. MacDonald PE, Wheeler MB: Voltage-dependent K(+) channels in pancreatic beta cells: Role, regulation and potential as therapeutic targets. Diabetologia 46:1046–1062, 2003.

69. Henquin JC, Ravier MA, Nenquin M, et al: Hierarchy of the beta-cell signals controlling insulin secretion. Eur J Clin Invest 33:742–750, 2003.

70. Tsuboi T, Rutter GA: Insulin secretion by "kiss-and-run" exocytosis in clonal pancreatic islet beta-cells. Biochem Soc Trans 31:833–836, 2003.

71. Tsuboi T, McMahon HT, Rutter GA: Mechanisms of dense core vesicle recapture following "kiss and run" ("cavicapture") exocytosis in insulin-secreting cells. J Biol Chem 279:47115–47124, 2004.

72. DeFronzo RA, Tobin JD, Andres R: Glucose clamp technique: A method for quantifying insulin secretion and resistance. Am J Physiol 237:E214–E223, 1979.

73. Song SH, Kjems L, Ritzel R, et al: Pulsatile insulin secretion by human pancreatic islets. J Clin Endocrinol Metab 87:213–221, 2002.

74. Pratley RE, Weyer C: The role of impaired early insulin secretion in the pathogenesis of type II diabetes mellitus. Diabetologia 44:929–945, 2001.

75. Grodsky G, Landahl H, Curry D, Bennett L: A two-compartmental model for insulin secretion. Adv Metab Disord 1:Suppl 1:45–50, 1970.

76. O'Connor MD, Landahl H, Grodsky GM: Comparison of storage- and signal-limited models of pancreatic insulin secretion. Am J Physiol 238:R378–R389, 1980.

77. Rorsman P, Renstrom E: Insulin granule dynamics in pancreatic beta cells. Diabetologia 46:1029–1045, 2003.

78. Shiota C, Larsson O, Shelton KD, et al: Sulfonylurea receptor type 1 knock-out mice have intact feeding-stimulated insulin secretion despite marked impairment in their response to glucose. J Biol Chem 277:37176–37183, 2002.

79. Polonsky KS, Given BD, Van Cauter E: Twenty-four-hour profiles and pulsatile patterns of insulin secretion in normal and obese subjects. J Clin Invest 81:442–448, 1988.

80. Porksen N, Nyholm B, Veldhuis JD, et al: In humans at least 75% of insulin secretion arises from punctuated insulin secretory bursts. Am J Physiol 273:E908–E914, 1997.

81. Cunningham BA, Deeney JT, Bliss CR, et al: Glucose-induced oscillatory insulin secretion in perifused rat pancreatic islets and clonal beta-cells (HIT). Am J Physiol 271:E702–E710, 1996.

82. Porksen N, Hollingdal M, Juhl C, et al: Pulsatile insulin secretion: Detection, regulation, and role in diabetes. Diabetes 51 Suppl 1:S245–S254, 2002.

83. Porksen N, Munn S, Steers J, et al: Effects of glucose ingestion versus infusion on pulsatile insulin secretion. The incretin effect is achieved by amplification of insulin secretory burst mass. Diabetes 45:1317–1323, 1996.

84. Porksen N, Munn SR, Steers JL, et al: Effects of somatostatin on pulsatile insulin secretion: Elective inhibition of insulin burst mass. Am J Physiol 270:E1043–E1049, 1996.

85. Porksen N, Grofte B, Nyholm B, et al: Glucagon-like peptide 1 increases mass but not frequency or orderliness of pulsatile insulin secretion. Effects of somatostatin on pulsatile insulin secretion: Elective inhibition of insulin burst mass. Diabetes 47:45–49, 1998.

86. Ritzel R, Schulte M, Porksen N, et al: Glucagon-like peptide 1 increases secretory burst mass of pulsatile insulin secretion in patients with type 2 diabetes and impaired glucose tolerance. Diabetes 50:776–784, 2001.

87. Porksen N, Hussain MA, Bianda TL, et al: IGF-1 inhibits burst mass of pulsatile insulin secretion at supraphysiological and low IGF-1 infusion rates. Am J Physiol 272:E352–E358, 1997.

88. Vore SJ, Aycock ED, Veldhuis JD, Butler PC: Anesthesia rapidly suppresses insulin pulse mass but enhances the orderliness of insulin secretory process. Am J Physiol Endocrinol Metab 281:E93–E99, 2001.

89. Matthews DR, Lang DA, Burnett MA, Turner RC: Control of pulsatile insulin secretion in man. Diabetologia 24:231–237, 1983.

90. Stagner JI, Samols E: Role of intrapancreatic ganglia in regulation of periodic insular secretions. Am J Physiol 248:E522–E530, 1985.

91. Porksen N, Munn S, Ferguson D, et al: Coordinate pulsatile insulin secretion by chronic intraportally transplanted islets in the isolated perfused rat liver. J Clin Invest 94:219–227, 1994.

92. Sha L, Westerlund J, Szurszewski JH, Bergsten P: Amplitude modulation of pulsatile insulin secretion by intrapancreatic ganglion neurons. Diabetes 50:51–55, 2001.

93. Porksen N: The in vivo regulation of pulsatile insulin secretion. Diabetologia 45:3–20, 2002.

94. Matthews DR, Naylor BA, Jones RG, et al: Pulsatile insulin has greater hypoglycemic effect than continuous delivery. Diabetes 32:617–621, 1983.

95. Paolisso G, Sgambato S, Torella R, et al: Pulsatile insulin delivery is more efficient than continuous infusion in modulating islet cell function in normal subjects and patients with type 1 diabetes. J Clin Endocrinol Metab 66:1220–1226, 1988.

96. Simon C, Brandenberger G: Ultradian oscillations of insulin secretion in humans. Diabetes 51 (Suppl) 1:S258–S261, 2002.

97. Eaton RP, Allen RC, Schade DS, et al: Prehepatic insulin production in man: Kinetic analysis using peripheral connecting peptide behavior. J Clin Endocrinol Metab 51:520–528, 1980.

98. Polonsky KS, Pugh W, Jaspan JB, et al: C-peptide and insulin secretion. Relationship between peripheral concentrations of C-peptide and insulin and their secretion rates in the dog. J Clin Invest 74:1821–1829, 1984.

99. Polonsky KS, Rubenstein AH: C-peptide as a measure of the secretion and hepatic extraction of insulin. Pitfalls and limitations. Diabetes 33:486–494, 1984.

100. Polonsky KS, Given BD, Hirsch L, et al: Quantitative study of insulin secretion and clearance in normal and obese subjects. J Clin Invest 81:435–441, 1988.

101. Walton C, Godsland IF, Proudler AJ, et al: Effect of body mass index and fat distribution on insulin sensitivity, secretion, and clearance in nonobese healthy men. J Clin Endocrinol Metab 75:170–175, 1992.

102. King DS, Dalsky GP, Clutter WE, et al: Effects of exercise and lack of exercise on insulin sensitivity and responsiveness. J Appl Physiol 64:1942–1946, 1988.

103. Dela F, Mikines KJ, Tronier B, Galbo H: Diminished arginine-stimulated insulin secretion in trained men. J Appl Physiol 69:261–267, 1990.

104. Haffner SM, Stern MP, Hazuda HP, et al: Hyperinsulinemia in a population at high risk for non-insulin-dependent diabetes mellitus. N Engl J Med 315:220–224, 1986.

105. Numata K, Tanaka K, Saito M, et al: Very low calorie diet-induced weight loss reverses exaggerated insulin secretion in response to glucose, arginine and glucagon in obesity. Int J Obes Relat Metab Disord 17:103–108, 1993.

106. Chang AM, Halter JB: Aging and insulin secretion. Am J Physiol Endocrinol Metab 284:E7–E12, 2003.

107. Stumvoll M, Tataranni PA, Stefan N, et al: Glucose allostasis. Diabetes 52:903–909, 2003.

108. Bergeron JJ, Cruz J, Khan MN, Posner BI: Uptake of insulin and other ligands into receptor-rich endocytic components of target cells: The endosomal apparatus. Annu Rev Physiol 47:383–403, 1985.

109. Carpentier JL, Gazzano H, Van Obberghen E, et al: Internalization and recycling of 125I-photoreactive insulin-receptor complexes in hepatocytes in primary culture. Mol Cell Endocrinol 47:243–255, 1986.

110. Halperin ML, Cheema-Dhadli S, Haynes FJ, Yip CC: A theoretical analysis of the turnover of the hepatic insulin receptor in the rat. Clin Invest Med 9:141–143, 1986.

111. Levy JR, Olefsky JM: The trafficking and processing of insulin and insulin receptors in cultured rat hepatocytes. Endocrinology 121:2075–2086, 1987.

112. Goodner CJ, Sweet IR, Harrison HC Jr: Rapid reduction and return of surface insulin receptors after exposure to brief pulses of insulin in perifused rat hepatocytes. Diabetes 37:1316–1323, 1988.

113. Duckworth WC: Insulin degradation: Mechanisms, products, and significance. Endocr Rev 9:319–345, 1988.

114. Yonezawa K, Yokono K, Yaso S, et al: Degradation of insulin by insulin-degrading enzyme and biological characteristics of its fragments. Endocrinology 118:1989–1996, 1986.

115. Hamel FG, Mahoney MJ, Duckworth WC: Degradation of intraendosomal insulin by insulin-degrading enzyme without acidification. Diabetes 40:436–443, 1991.

116. Knutson VP: Cellular trafficking and processing of the insulin receptor. FASEB J 5:2130–2138, 1991.

117. Waldhausl W, Bratusch-Marrain P, Gasic S, et al: Insulin production rate following glucose ingestion estimated by splanchnic C-peptide output in normal man. Diabetologia 17:221–227, 1979.

118. Eaton RP, Allen RC, Schade DS: Hepatic removal of insulin in normal man: Dose response to endogenous insulin secretion. J Clin Endocrinol Metab 56:1294–1300, 1983.

119. Ferrannini E, Wahren J, Faber OK, et al: Splanchnic and renal metabolism of insulin in human subjects: A dose-response study. Am J Physiol 244:E517–E527, 1983.

120. Shah P, Vella A, Basu A, et al: Effects of free fatty acids and glycerol on splanchnic glucose metabolism and insulin extraction in nondiabetic humans. Diabetes 51:301–310, 2002.

121. Shapiro ET, Tillil H, Miller MA, et al: Insulin secretion and clearance. Comparison after oral and intravenous glucose. Diabetes 36:1365–1371, 1987.

122. Shuster LT, Go VLW, Rizza RA, et al: Incretin effect due to increased secretion and decreased clearance of insulin in normal humans. Diabetes 37:200–203, 1988.

123. Nauck MA, Homberger E, Siegel EG, et al: Incretin effects of increasing glucose loads in man calculated from venous insulin and C-peptide responses. J Clin Endocrinol Metab 63:492–498, 1986.

124. Harding PE, Bloom G, Field JB: Effect of infusion of insulin into portal vein on hepatic extraction of insulin in anesthetized dogs. Am J Physiol 228:1580–1588, 1975.

125. Polonsky K, Jaspan J, Emmanouel D, et al: Differences in the hepatic and renal extraction of insulin and glucagon in the dog: Evidence for saturability of insulin metabolism. Acta Endocrinol (Copenh) 102:420–427, 1983.

126. Tillil H, Shapiro ET, Rubenstein AH, et al: Reduction of insulin clearance during hyperglycemic clamp. Dose-response study in normal humans. Diabetes 37:1351–1357, 1988.

127. Kjems LL, Kirby BM, Welsh EM, et al: Decrease in beta-cell mass leads to impaired pulsatile insulin secretion, reduced postprandial hepatic insulin clearance, and relative hyper-glucagonemia in the minipig. Diabetes 50:2001–2012, 2001.

128. Warren S, Root HF: The pathology of diabetes, with special reference to pancreatic regeneration. Am J Pathol 1:415–430, 1925.

129. Kloppel G, Drenck CR, Oberholzer M, Heitz PU: Morphometric evidence for a striking B-cell reduction at the clinical onset of type 1 diabetes. Virchows Arch A Pathol Anat Histopathol 403:441–452, 1984.

130. Junker K, Egeberg J, Kromann H, Nerup J: An autopsy study of the islets of Langerhans in acute-onset juvenile diabetes mellitus. Acta Pathol Microbiol Scand [A] 85:699–706, 1977.

131. Lohr M, Kloppel G: Residual insulin positivity and pancreatic atrophy in relation to duration of chronic type 1 (insulin-dependent) diabetes mellitus and microangiopathy. Diabetologia 30:757–762, 1987.

132. Pipeleers D, Ling Z: Pancreatic beta cells in insulin-dependent diabetes. Diabetes Metab Rev 8:209–227, 1992.

133. Gorsuch AN, Spencer KM, Lister J, et al: Evidence for a long prediabetic period in type I (insulin-dependent) diabetes mellitus. Lancet 2:1363–1365, 1981.

134. Srikanta S, Ganda OP, Jackson RA, et al: Type I diabetes mellitus in

monozygotic twins: Chronic progressive beta cell dysfunction. Ann Intern Med 99:320–326, 1983.

135. Atkinson MA, Eisenbarth GS: Type 1 diabetes: New perspectives on disease pathogenesis and treatment. Lancet 358:221–229, 2001.

136. Srikanta S, Ganda OP, Gleason RE, et al: Pre-type I diabetes. Linear loss of beta cell response to intravenous glucose. Diabetes 33:717–720, 1984.

137. Soeldner JS, Tuttleman M, Srikanta S, et al: Insulin-dependent diabetes mellitus and autoimmunity: Islet-cell autoantibodies, insulin autoantibodies, and beta-cell failure. N Engl J Med 313:893–894, 1985.

138. Lo SS, Hawa M, Beer SF, et al: Altered islet beta-cell function before the onset of type 1 (insulin-dependent) diabetes mellitus. Diabetologia 35:277–282, 1992.

139. Chaillous L, Rohmer V, Maugendre D, et al: Differential beta-cell response to glucose, glucagon, and arginine during progression to type I (insulin-dependent) diabetes mellitus. Metabolism 45:306–314, 1996.

140. Clarson C, Daneman D, Drash AL, et al: Residual beta-cell function in children with IDDM: Reproducibility of testing and factors influencing insulin secretory reserve. Diabetes Care 10:33–38, 1987.

141. Hanafusa T, Miyazaki A, Miyagawa J, et al: Examination of islets in the pancreas biopsy specimens from newly diagnosed type 1 (insulin-dependent) diabetic patients. Diabetologia 33:105–111, 1990.

142. Maedler K, Sergeev P, Ris F, et al: Glucose-induced beta cell production of IL-1beta contributes to glucotoxicity in human pancreatic islets. J Clin Invest 110:851–860, 2002.

143. Robertson RP: Chronic oxidative stress as a central mechanism for glucose toxicity in pancreatic islet beta cells in diabetes. J Biol Chem 279:42351–42354, 2004.

144. Ritzel RA, Hansen JB, Veldhuis JD, Butler PC: Induction of beta-cell rest by a Kir6.2/SUR1-selective K(ATP)-channel opener preserves beta-cell insulin stores and insulin secretion in human islets cultured at high (11 mM) glucose. J Clin Endocrinol Metab 89:795–805, 2004.

145. Robertson RP, Harmon J, Tran PO, et al: Glucose toxicity in beta-cells: Type 2 diabetes, good radicals gone bad, and the glutathione connection. Diabetes 52:581–587, 2003.

146. Madsbad S, Krarup T, Reguer L, et al: Effect of strict blood glucose control on residual B-cell function in insulin-dependent diabetics. Diabetologia 20:530–534, 1981.

147. Madsbad S: Prevalence of residual B cell function and its metabolic consequences in Type 1 (insulin-dependent) diabetes. Diabetologia 24:141–147, 1983.

148. The DCCT Research Group: Effects of age, duration and treatment of insulin-dependent diabetes mellitus on residual beta-cell function: Observations during eligibility testing for the Diabetes Control and Complications Trial (DCCT). J Clin Endocrinol Metab 65:30–36, 1987.

149. The Diabetes Control and Complications Trial Research Group: Effect of intensive therapy on residual beta-cell function in patients with type 1 diabetes in the diabetes control and complications trial. A randomized, controlled trial. Ann Intern Med 128:517–523, 1998.

150. Clark A, Wells CA, Buley ID, et al: Islet amyloid, increased A-cells, reduced B-cells and exocrine fibrosis: Quantitative changes in the pancreas in type 2 diabetes. Diabetes Res 9:151–159, 1988.

151. Sakuraba H, Mizukami H, Yagihashi N, et al: Reduced beta-cell mass and expression of oxidative stress-related DNA damage in the islet of Japanese type II diabetic patients. Diabetologia 45:85–96, 2002.

152. Butler AE, Jang J, Gurlo T, et al: Diabetes due to a progressive defect in beta-cell mass in rats transgenic for human islet amyloid polypeptide (HIP rat): A new model for type 2 diabetes. Diabetes 53:1509–1516, 2004.

153. Donath MY, Storling J, Maedler K, et al: Inflammatory mediators and islet beta-cell failure: A link between type 1 and type 2 diabetes. J Mol Med 81:455–470, 2003.

154. Bonner-Weir S, Trent DF, Weir GC: Partial pancreatectomy in the rat and subsequent defect in glucose-induced insulin release. J Clin Invest 71:1544–1553, 1983.

155. Ward WK, Wallum BJ, Beard JC, et al: Reduction of glycemic potentiation. Sensitive indicator of beta-cell loss in partially pancreatectomized dogs. Diabetes 37:723–729, 1988.

156. van der Burg MP, Gooszen HG, Guicherit OR, et al: Contribution of partial pancreatectomy, systemic hormone delivery, and duct obliteration to glucose regulation in canine pancreas. Importance in pancreas transplantation. Diabetes 38:1082–1089, 1989.

157. Stagner JI, Samols E: Deterioration of islet beta-cell function after hemipancreatectomy in dogs. Diabetes 40:1472–1479, 1991.

158. Larsen MO, Gotfredsen CF, Wilken M, et al: Loss of beta-cell mass leads to a reduction of pulse mass with normal periodicity, regularity and entrainment of pulsatile insulin secretion in Gottingen minipigs. Diabetologia 46:195–202, 2003.

159. Lang DA, Matthews DR, Burnett M, Turner RC: Brief, irregular oscillations of basal plasma insulin and glucose concentrations in diabetic man. Diabetes 30:435–439, 1981.

160. Robertson RP, Harmon J, Tran PO, Poitout V: Beta-cell glucose toxicity, lipotoxicity, and chronic oxidative stress in type 2 diabetes. Diabetes 53 (Suppl 1):S119–S124, 2004.

161. Ritzel RA, Butler PC: Replication increases beta-cell vulnerability to human islet amyloid polypeptide-induced apoptosis. Diabetes 52:1701–1708, 2003.

162. Temple RC, Carrington CA, Luzio SD, et al: Insulin deficiency in non-insulin-dependent diabetes. Lancet 1:293–295, 1989.

163. Pimenta W, Korytkowski M, Mitrakou A, et al: Pancreatic beta-cell dysfunction as the primary genetic lesion in NIDDM. Evidence from studies in normal glucose-tolerant individuals with a first-degree NIDDM relative. JAMA 273:1855–1861, 1995.

164. Kipnis DM: Insulin secretion in diabetes mellitus. Ann Intern Med 69:891–901, 1968.

165. Ward WK, Bolgiano DC, McKnight B, et al: Diminished B cell secretory capacity in patients with noninsulin-dependent diabetes mellitus. J Clin Invest 74:1318–1328, 1984.

166. Davies MJ, Rayman G, Grenfell A, et al: Loss of the first phase insulin response to intravenous glucose in subjects with persistent impaired glucose tolerance. Diabet Med 11:432–436, 1994.

167. O'Rahilly S, Turner RC, Matthews DR: Impaired pulsatile secretion of insulin in relatives of patients with non-insulin-dependent diabetes. N Engl J Med 318:1225–1230, 1988.

168. Eriksson J, Franssila-Kallunki A, Ekstrand A, et al: Early metabolic defects in persons at increased risk for non-insulin-dependent diabetes mellitus. N Engl J Med 321:337–343, 1989.

169. Humphriss DB, Stewart MW, Berrish TS, et al: Multiple metabolic abnormalities in normal glucose tolerant relatives of NIDDM families. Diabetologia 40:1185–1190, 1997.

170. Meier JJ, Hücking K, Holst JJ, et al: Reduced insulinotropic effect of gastric inhibitory polypeptide in first-degree relatives of patients with type 2 diabetes. Diabetes 50:2497–2504, 2001.

171. Ward WK, Johnston CL, Beard JC, et al: Insulin resistance and impaired insulin secretion in subjects with histories of gestational diabetes mellitus. Diabetes 34:861–869, 1985.

172. Ryan EA, Imes S, Liu D, et al: Defects in insulin secretion and action in women with a history of gestational diabetes. Diabetes 44:506–512, 1995.

173. Gerich JE: The genetic basis of type 2 diabetes mellitus: Impaired insulin secretion versus impaired insulin sensitivity. Endocrine Rev 19:491–503, 1998.

174. Polonsky KS, Given BD, Hirsch LJ, et al: Abnormal patterns of insulin secretion in non-insulin-dependent diabetes mellitus. N Engl J Med 318:1231–1239, 1988.

175. Nauck M, Stöckmann F, Ebert R, Creutzfeldt W: Reduced incretin effect

in Type 2 (non-insulin-dependent) diabetes. Diabetologia 29:46–54, 1986.

176. Schmitz O, Porksen N, Nyholm B, et al: Disorderly and nonstationary insulin secretion in relatives of patients with NIDDM. Am J Physiol 272:E218–E226, 1997.

177. Ward WK, LaCava EC, Paquette TL, et al: Disproportionate elevation of immunoreactive proinsulin in type 2 (non-insulin-dependent) diabetes mellitus and in experimental insulin resistance. Diabetologia 30:698–702, 1987.

178. Porte D Jr, Kahn SE: Hyperproinsulinemia and amyloid in NIDDM. Clues to etiology of islet beta-cell dysfunction? Diabetes 38:1333–1336, 1989.

179. Rhodes CJ, Alarcon C: What beta-cell defect could lead to hyperproinsulinemia in NIDDM? Some clues from recent advances made in understanding the proinsulin-processing mechanism. Diabetes 43:511–517, 1994.

180. Laedtke T, Kjems L, Porksen N, et al: Overnight inhibition of insulin secretion restores pulsatility and proinsulin/insulin ratio in type 2 diabetes. Am J Physiol Endocrinol Metab 279:E520–E528, 2000.

181. Gutniak MK, Holst JJ, Ørskov C, et al: Antidiabetogenic effect of glucagon-like peptide-1 (7-36)amide in normal subjects and patients with diabetes mellitus. N Engl J Med 326:1316–1322, 1992.

182. Nauck MA, Kleine N, Ørskov C, et al: Normalization of fasting hyperglycaemia by exogenous glucagon-like peptide 1 (7-36 amide) in type 2 (non-insulin-dependent) diabetic patients. Diabetologia 36:741–744, 1993.

183. Rachman J, Gribble FM, Barrow BA, et al: Normalization of insulin responses to glucose by overnight infusion of glucagon-like peptide 1 (7-36) amide in patients with NIDDM. Diabetes 45:1524–1530, 1996.

184. Kjems LL, Holst JJ, Vølund A, Madsbad S: The influence of GLP-1 on glucose-stimulated insulin secretion: Effects on beta-cell sensitivity in type 2 and nondiabetic subjects. Diabetes 52:380–386, 2003.

185. Meier JJ, Gallwitz B, Salmen S, et al: Normalization of glucose concentrations and deceleration of gastric emptying after solid meals during intravenous glucagon-like peptide 1 in patients with type 2 diabetes. J Clin Endocrinol Metab 88:2719–2725, 2003.

186. Chan CB, De Leo D, Joseph JW, et al: Increased uncoupling protein-2 levels in beta-cells are associated with impaired glucose-stimulated insulin secretion: Mechanism of action. Diabetes 50:1302–1310, 2001.

The Molecular Basis of Insulin Action

Morris F. White

Insulin and insulin-like growth factors (IGF-1 and IGF-2) are essential during all stages of life. They integrate the storage and release of nutrients with somatic growth during development and in adult life. Insulin, IGF-1, and IGF-2 promote tissue and organ maintenance throughout life. Moreover, they interact with other signaling systems during physiologic response to traumatic and chronic stress.

Our classical view of insulin action focuses upon glucose homeostasis, but the insulin signaling system has a much broader implication for heath and disease.[1] Following a meal, pancreatic β cells rapidly secrete insulin, suppressing hepatic gluconeogenesis, and promoting glucose storage in skeletal muscle and lipid storage in adipose tissues[2]; peripheral insulin also circulates to the hypothalamus where it informs the central nervous system that food has been consumed.[3] Dysregulation of insulin signaling causes glucose intolerance that progresses to diabetes when β cells fail to secrete sufficient insulin rapidly enough to maintain normal glucose homeostasis. Moreover, as diabetes ensues, life-threatening systemic disorders develop, including microvascular complications in the retina, renal glomerulus, and peripheral nerves; cardiovascular disease; dyslipidemia and obesity; and degeneration of neurons in the peripheral nervous system.[2]

A coherent explanation for the pathophysiology of common type 2 diabetes is complicated because many genetic polymorphisms appear to contribute to the characteristic pathophysiology. By contrast, maturity-onset diabetes of the young (MODY), which accounts for less than 10% of the cases of type 2 diabetes, is linked to single gene mutations that impair β-cell function: hepatocyte nuclear factor-4α (*MODY1*), glucokinase (*MODY2*), HNF-1α (*MODY 3*), Pdx1 (*MODY4*), or HNF-1β (*MODY 5*).[4-6] Dysregulated expression of these genes might contribute to the progression of common type 2 diabetes, as some of the MODY genes can be regulated in adult β cells through the insulin receptor substrate 2 (IRS2) branch of the insulin/IGF-signaling cascade.[7-10] Thus, dysregulated expression or function of MODY genes could contribute to β-cell failure and the progression toward ordinary type 2 diabetes.

INSULIN AND INSULIN-LIKE GROWTH FACTORS

MEMBERS OF THE INSULIN SIGNALING FAMILY

The mammalian insulin signaling system includes three well-defined ligands: insulin, insulin-like growth factor 1 (IGF-1), and insulin-like growth factor 2 (IGF-2).[11] Worms and fruit flies have a larger array of insulin-like peptides, revealing the utility and flexibility of the system.[12] In mammals, IGF-1 and IGF-2 bind with high affinity (K_d < 1 nM) to the IGF-1 receptors (IGF-1R) (Fig. 50-1). Two insulin receptor isoforms called IRb or IRa bind insulin with high affinity or moderate affinity, respectively. However, during peripheral insulin resistance, circulating insulin concentrations can rise high enough to activate IGF-1 receptors (K_d ~ 50 nM).

The IRa isoform is produced during tissue-specific inclusion of exon-11 in the receptor mRNA. Exon-11 encodes 12 amino acids at the end of the α subunit, which promotes IGF-2 binding at the expense of moderately reduced insulin-binding affinity.[13,14] IRb lacks this extended COOH-terminal tail owing to omission of exon-11, which increases the affinity and specify for insulin while reducing significantly the interaction with IGF-2 (see Fig. 50-1). IRb predominates in classical insulin-sensitive target tissues, including adult liver, muscle, and adipose tissues. IRa predominates in fetal tissues, the adult central nervous system, and hematopoietic cells.[15-18]

Proper regulation of exon-11 splicing is important. Dysregulated splicing alters fetal growth patterns and contributes to rare forms of insulin resistance in adults.[13,19] Severe insulin resistance occurs in patients with myotonic dystrophy

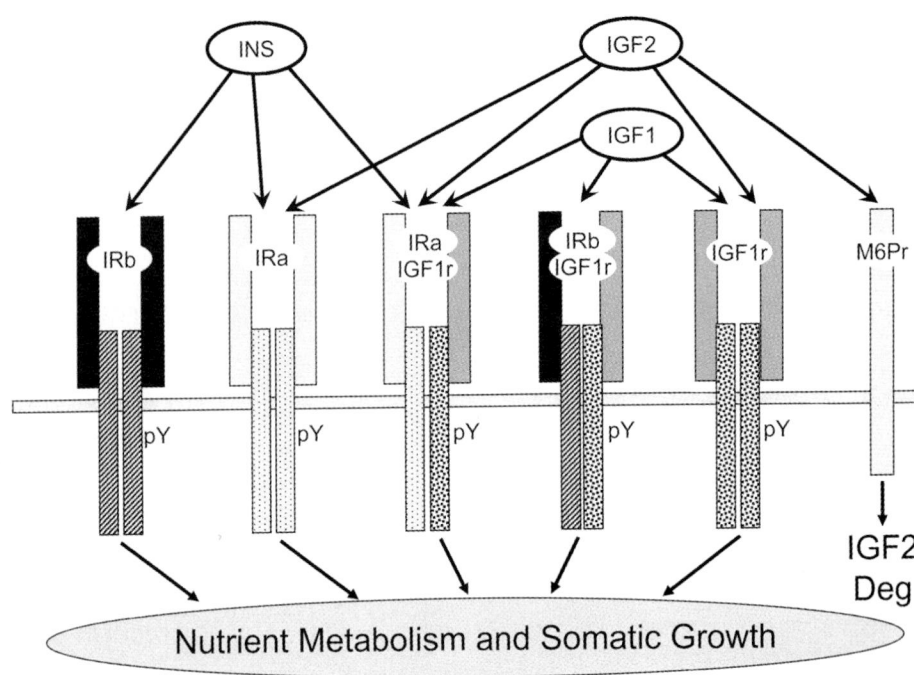

Figure 50-1 The insulin/insulin-like growth factor family. The insulin/IGF family consists of three hormones: insulin, insulin-like growth factor 1 (IGF-1), and insulin-like growth factor 2 (IGF-2). These peptide ligands bind as indicated in the figure to five distinct receptor isoforms that generate cytoplasmic signals: two insulin receptor isoforms, IRa and IRb; the insulin-like growth factor receptor, IGF-1R; and two hybrid receptors, IRa::IGF-1R and IRb::IGF-1R. IGF-2 also binds to the mannose-6-phosphate receptor, which mediates its endocytosis and degradation. The insulin receptor is the primary target for insulin throughout development and life. The IGF-1 receptor is the primary target for IGF-1. IGF-2 binds to the insulin receptor primarily during embryonic development, and binds the IGF-1 receptor throughout life. IGF-2 also binds to the mannose-6-phosphate receptor, which targets the IGF-2 for degradation instead of signaling. Activation of the insulin receptor or the IGF-1 receptor mediate signals primarily via the cytoplasmic proteins IRS1 and IRS2, which mediate somatic cell growth and metabolism.

type 1, because a genetic alteration in RNA splicing causes the accumulation of type A receptors in adult skeletal muscle.[19] Cell-based experiments suggest that IRb displays greater insulin-stimulated tyrosine kinase activity and ability to phosphorylate insulin receptor substrates (IRS)-proteins, and may influence the timing of the insulin signal needed to properly regulate cell growth or differentiation.[14]

The selectivity for insulin and the insulin-like growth factor signaling is further complicated by posttranslational assembly of hybrids between the IGF-1 receptor and the insulin receptor isoforms.[20] Hybrid receptors composed of an αβ-dimer of the IGF-1 receptors and IRa (IGF-1R::IRb) selectively bind IGF-1, whereas IGF-1R::IRa binds all three ligands with similar affinities.[21] The physiologic significance of tissue-specific alternative splicing of insulin receptors and the assembly of receptor hybrids needs to be resolved (see Fig. 50-1).

GROWTH DEVELOPMENT AND SURVIVAL

Studies in humans and experimental animals, *Caenorhabditis elegans* and *Drosophila melanogaster* reveal that insulin and insulin-like growth factor signaling promotes development, growth, function, and survival of central and peripheral tissues.[22,23] Moreover, these signals coordinate nutrient sensing and storage needed to accomplish useful work and balance longevity with reproduction. In vertebrates, homologous IGF-1 receptors are essential during development for about 50% of brain and body growth.[20,24] By contrast, the insulin receptor has its greatest impact on carbohydrate metabolism, as the high-affinity IRb is highly expressed in liver, muscle, and adipose tissues. IGF-1 receptors also influence carbohydrate metabolism especially in skeletal muscle, and through their effects upon islet development and growth.[25,26]

Work with genetically altered mice reveals a more complicated relation between the metabolic and growth actions of insulin and IGF-1 than originally thought.[10,27–29] Although both receptors mediate growth in vitro, mice without insulin receptors are nearly normal size at birth; however, they develop hyperinsulinemia and ketoacidosis immediately after birth and die within 3 to 7 days.[30,31] By comparison, mice without IGF-1R develop slowly, growing to 45% of normal size at birth.[32] IGF-2 also promotes body growth during development; however, it does not contribute to growth in the central nervous system.[33] In mice, IGF-2, but not insulin,

promotes embryonic growth through its interaction with the IGF-1R and the insulin receptor, most likely IGF-1R::IRa hybrids.[20,27,34] Consistent with this model, the growth deficit caused by dysregulation of IGF-1 or IGF-1R can be corrected by increasing the levels of circulating IGF-2. One way to increase systemic IGF-2 levels is by disrupting the mannose-6-phosphate receptor, which ordinarily ferries IGF-2 across the plasma membrane and targets it for degradation.[20,34] A third homologous receptor, called the insulin receptor–related receptor (IRR), is poorly investigated. The IRR is found in the nervous system, pancreatic β cells, and testes, but its function in these tissues is unclear.[27,35] IRR contributes to male sexual development when the insulin and IGF-1 receptors are dysregulated in testes.[36]

Like mice, human neonates with diminished IGF-1 signaling are developmentally retarded; however, unlike mice, human infants born without insulin receptors display both retarded development in utero together with severe fasting hyperglycemia at birth.[37] This developmental disparity arises apparently because insulin is produced during the last trimester of human pregnancies, whereas in mice it is produced just prior to birth.[20] Analysis of mice expressing variable systemic levels of insulin receptors—so-called mosaic mice—confirms that insulin receptor signaling has its greatest effect upon postnatal growth, probably through profound effects upon nutrient homeostasis, rather than direct effects upon cell division and size.[38]

Work with *C. elegans* and *Drosophila* suggests that life span is influenced by the insulin/IGF signaling system.[39,40] In worms, significant life span extension occurs by partial loss-of-function mutations in the insulin receptor gene.[41] Interestingly, life span can be normalized in the mutant worms by restoring insulin cascades in various cells, suggesting that a network of tissue interactions and feedback regulation coordinates aging in *C. elegans*.[42] In mice, the contribution of insulin and IGF signaling to longevity is complex. Igf1r+/− mice live on average 26% longer than their wild-type littermates, perhaps owing to greater resistance to oxidative stress.[43] Whereas inhibition of the insulin/IGF-1 signaling cascade in nematodes and flies increases life span convincingly, defects in insulin signaling in rodents and humans increase the risk for age-related diseases and increased mortality. This complexity might arise from the complicated cross-talk between peripheral and central tissues. By contrast, disruption of the insulin receptor in adipose tissue increases life span; however, fat insulin receptor knockout mice also display reduced adiposity.[44] It is difficult to determine whether reduced insulin action in adipocytes or improved systemic insulin action that accompanies a lean body mass is responsible for the increased life span.

THE INSULIN RECEPTOR

INSULIN SIGNALING: THE BASICS

The receptors for insulin or IGF-1, like the receptors for other growth factors and cytokines, are composed of an extracellular ligand-binding domain that regulates the activity of an intracellular tyrosine kinase.[1,45,46] Most receptor tyrosine kinases are activated by ligand-induced dimerization that promotes tyrosine autophosphorylation of the kinase activation loop (A loop), and other sites that recruit cellular substrates.[47] By contrast, insulin receptors reside in the plasma membrane as inactivated covalent dimers. Insulin binding increases flexibility of the A loop admitting adenosine triphosphate (ATP) to the catalytic site. Subsequent tyrosine phosphorylation of the A loop stabilizes the active conformation and recruits substrates for phosphorylation.[48,49] The principal insulin receptor and IGF-1 receptor substrates, the IRS-proteins, are phosphorylated on multiple tyrosine residues by the activated receptor kinases. Various signaling proteins such as phosphatidylinositol 3-kinase (PI 3-kinase), Grb-2, short heterodimer partner 2 (SHP2), and others bind to the tyrosine phosphorylation sites, generating an array of cell- and tissue-specific responses. The strength and duration of these insulin signals are modulated through protein and phospholipid phosphatases, or direct inhibition of IRS-protein function.[50–53] Insulin resistance develops when the relation between these signaling pathways is disrupted, which progresses to glucose intolerance, diabetes, and other life-threatening metabolic diseases.

INSULIN RECEPTOR BIOSYNTHESIS

The insulin proreceptor mRNA is the splice product of 22 exons, including the developmentally regulated exon-11, of a 150-kb gene on human chromosome 19.[54,55] During translation, the proreceptor is stabilized by disulfide bonds, and the α and β subunits are generated by proteolysis (Fig. 50-2A). In its native conformation, the mature insulin receptor is a tetramer composed of two extracellular α subunits linked by disulfide bonds to each other and to the extracellular portion of the transmembrane β subunit (Fig. 50-2B). The β subunit contains a single transmembrane spanning domain and the intracellular tyrosine kinase.[45,46] During sodium dodecyl sulfate polyacrylamide gel electrophoresis (SDS-PAGE), the holoreceptor ($\alpha_2\beta_2$) has an apparent molecular mass of 350,000, larger than expected owing to glycosylation of the α and β subunits. Under reducing conditions, the α and β subunits migrate during SDS-PAGE at 135 kilodaltons and 95 kilodaltons, respectively.[56,57]

INSULIN BINDING

The α subunit is too large to analyze by nuclear magnetic resonance, and crystallization is difficult owing in part to extensive glycosylation; however, an approximate molecular model explaining insulin-binding selectivity has emerged from a variety of approaches. Insulin binding has been studied extensively before and after receptor purification from various cells and tissues. These initial efforts revealed complicated binding properties where one insulin molecule binds with high affinity and a second molecule binds with low affinity.[58] The creation of chimeric molecules between the α subunits of the insulin and IGF-1 receptors is especially informative.[59] High-affinity insulin

binding is transferred to the IGF-1 receptor by substituting residues 64 to 137 of the insulin receptor α subunit into the homologous positions of the IGF-1 receptor α subunit, revealing a portion of the insulin-binding domain called L1 (residues 1–149). Many other regions in the α subunit also contribute to insulin binding, including the L2 domain (residues x-y), and the COOH terminus (residues Thr704 and Lys718).[60]

The quaternary structure of the isolated complex of biologically active insulin receptor (IR) and insulin is solved approximately by three-dimensional reconstruction using low-dose scanning transmission electron micrographs to guide the assembly of insulin receptor subdomains into an approximate holoreceptor complex.[61,62] The insulin molecule has at least two receptor-binding surfaces, called $S1^{ins}$ and $S2^{ins}$ (Fig. 50-2C).[61] $S1^{ins}$ binds to L1 and L2 regions in one α subunit, while $S2^{ins}$ binds to the L1 region in the adjacent α subunit (see Fig. 50-2B and C). The interaction with both α-subunits result in higher-affinity insulin binding than either one achieves alone. The binding of a second insulin molecule to the complex occurs at a lower affinity because only one contact sites is readily accessible to the second insulin molecule.[63] Structural approximations place the COOH terminus near the L2 region, where it can influence insulin binding.[61] Apparently, extending this sequence by 12 amino acids in the IRa reduces insulin-binding affinity while enhancing IGF-2-binding affinity.

The structural details that emerge from this model are largely consistent with the biochemical and enzymatic data; the effect of naturally occurring and site-directed mutants of insulin and the receptor α subunits; and kinetic and isothermal-binding data.

THE CYTOPLASMIC DOMAIN GENERATES THE INSULIN SIGNAL

Biochemical studies first revealed the tyrosine kinase activity of the insulin receptor[64–66]; however, the cloning of the insulin receptor cDNA greatly expanded the subsequent biochemical and physiologic approaches.[45,46] The identification of naturally occurring mutant insulin receptors in humans and the rational design of kinase-deficient mutants establishes that the tyrosine kinase activity is essential for biologic activity, anticipating the deleterious consequences of its reduction.[67–69]

There are at least seven tyrosine autophosphorylation sites in three distinct regions of the insulin receptor β subunit, including three in the A loop, one or two in the intracellular juxtamembrane region, and two in the COOH terminus (see Fig. 50-2B).[49] Autophosphorylation of the A loop stabilizes the open conformation of the catalytic sites, and creates binding sites for other signaling proteins that modulate kinase activity, including Grb10, autoimmune polyglandular syndrome (APS), and SH2B.[65,70–72] Autophosphorylation in the juxtamembrane region is essential for recruitment of IRS-proteins that propagate the insulin signal. Autophosphorylation in the COOH terminus (Tyr1314 and Tyr1328) is poorly understood; however, it has been shown to regulate tyrosine kinase activity and receptor internalization[73–77]; and under certain conditions bind PI 3-kinase.[78,79] The nematode and fruit fly insulin receptor contains an extended COOH terminus that contains several tyrosine phosphorylation sites that bind PI 3-kinase. Consequently, these orthologs activate PI 3-kinase without requiring the expression of IRS-proteins.[80]

REGULATION OF KINASE ACTIVITY

The regulatory role of the A loop of the β subunit is well-supported by biochemical studies, mutational analysis, and the crystal structure of the β subunit.[70,71,81–85] Structural studies predict that the unphosphorylated Tyr1162 of the A loop folds into the catalytic site to prevent substrate binding.[86] This configuration restricts ATP binding, which explains the high apparent K_m for ATP before insulin stimulation.[72]

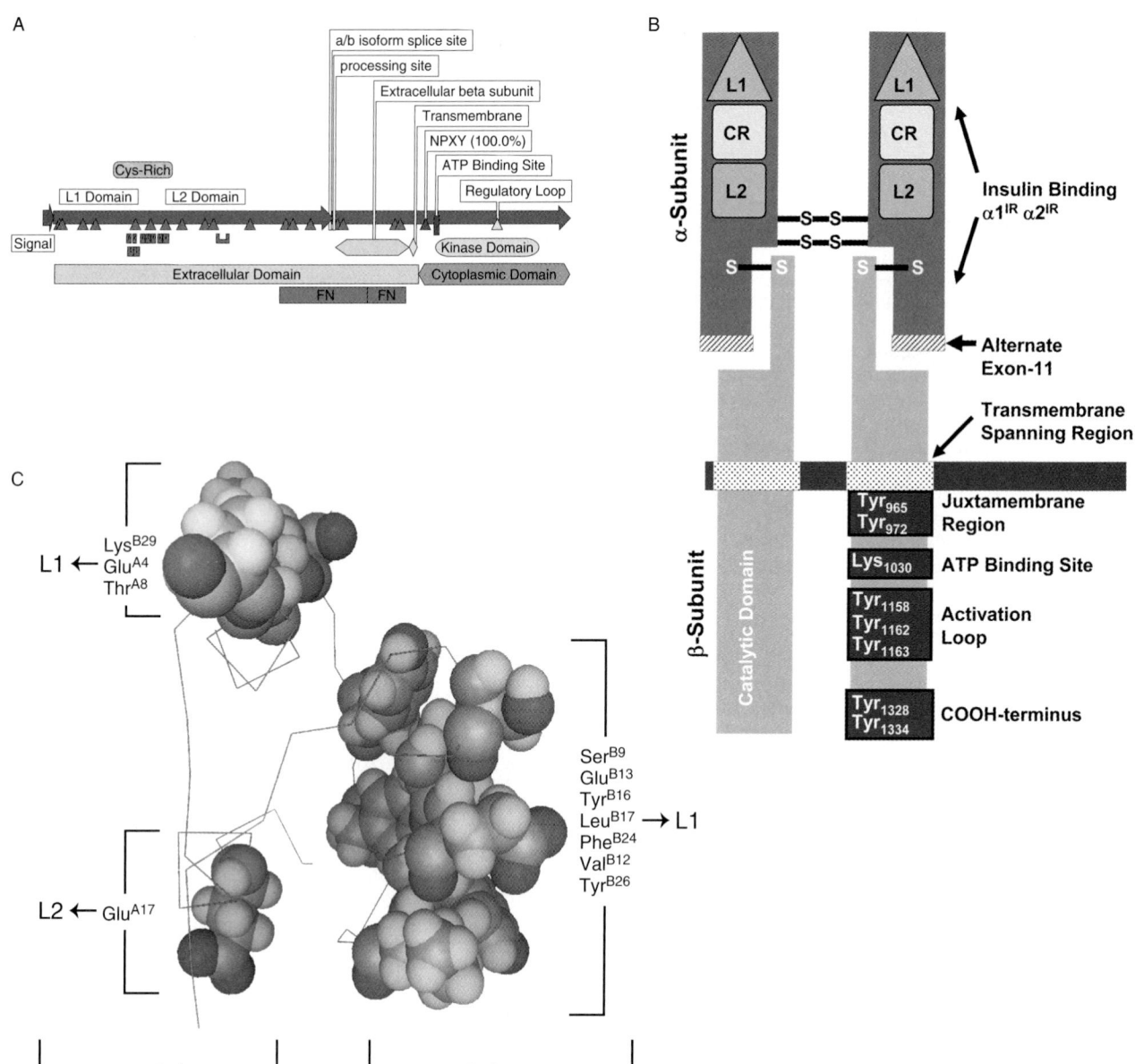

Figure 50-2 Structure of insulin and the insulin receptor. **A,** A linear diagram of the insulin receptor precursor showing the relative position of important landmarks in the α subunit, the ligand contact points L1 and L2, the cysteine-rich region (Cys-rich), disulfide bonds (⊔), glycosylation sites (▲) the IRa/IRb splice site, the processing site between the α subunit and the β subunit, and important landmarks in the β subunit, the extracellular region, the hydrophobic transmembrane region, the PTB recognition motif, the ATP binding site, and the regulatory loop (A loop) in the kinase domain. **B,** A diagram of the insulin receptor extracellular, transmembrane, and intracellular components composed of two extracellular α subunits and two β subunits that contain. The holoreceptor is joined by disulfide bonds between cysteine residues in the extracellular α and β subunits as well as by noncovalent interactions. The α subunit contains several regions that contribute to insulin binding, including the L1 and L2 regions separated by a cysteine-rich region, and a 12-amino acid alternatively spliced region encoded by exon-11. The β subunit contains a tyrosine kinase catalytic domain with an ATP-binding site and a number of tyrosine phosphorylation sites including those in the juxtamembrane, activation loop, and COOH-terminal regions. **C,** The insulin diagram shows the amino acids that compose the two surfaces of the insulin molecule (S1ins and S2ins) and the amino acids that interact with the L1 and L2 regions of the insulin receptor. (See Color Plate.)

However, the closed A loop is in equilibrium with an alternate conformation that allows ATP access to mediate a basal level of A loop autophosphorylation.[85] Insulin apparently shifts the equilibrium of the A loop toward an open conformation to facilitate ATP binding (decrease the apparent K_m) and autophosphorylation of Tyr1162 (Fig. 50-3A). This model, together with early biochemical studies, suggests that the autophosphorylation cascade proceeds rapidly at Tyr1158, resulting in a bis-phosphorylated regulatory loop.[70] The relatively slow phosphorylation of Tyr1163 to generate the tris-phosphorylated A loop is required to stabilize the open conformation to allow unrestricted access by Mg-ATP and protein substrates (see Fig. 50-3A).

This model of kinase regulation is validated by recent structural analysis of the kinase domain obtained upon substitution Asp1161 in the middle of the A loop with Ala1161 (IRKD^DA).[85] IRKD^DA dramatically shifts the A loop equilibrium toward the open configuration before autophosphorylation, which increases Mg-ATP binding affinity by 10-fold. The kinetic properties of IRKD^DA after autophosphorylation are indistinguishable from those of the wild-type kinase.[85] Substitution of Tyr1162 with Phe also increases basal autophosphorylation, consistent with its role to stabilize the closed conformation; however, this mutation does not increase basal IRS-protein phosphorylation in cells, probably because phosphorylation of the NPEY motif requires insulin binding.[82]

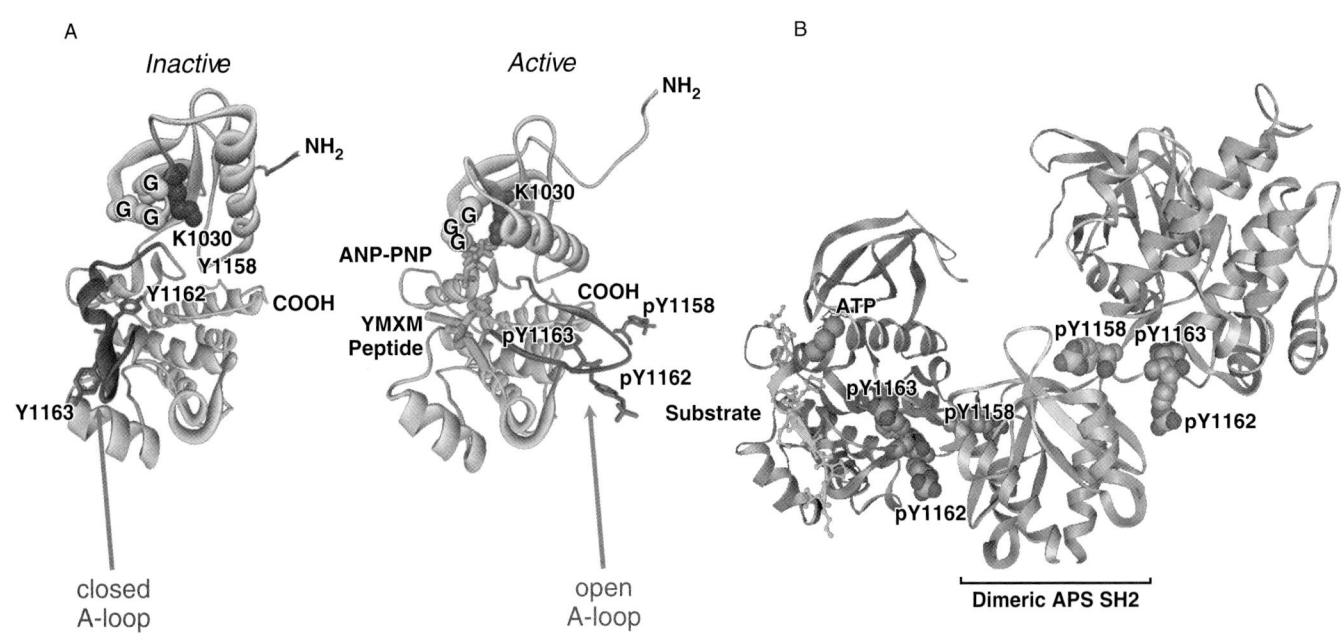

Figure 50-3 The role of insulin receptor autophosphorylation. **A,** Structure of the insulin receptor activation loop shown as ribbon diagrams of the kinase domain of the insulin receptor along with the side chains of important amino acids, including the three glycine residues and K1030 that comprise the ATP-binding site. The activation loop (A loop) is shown in red; the three activation loop tyrosine residues (Y1158, Y1162, and Y1163) are shown with their side chains. In the inactive, unphosphorylated state (*left panel*), the activation loop blocks access by potential substrates. Following phosphorylation (*right panel*), however, the activation loop moves, allowing substrates such as YMXM peptides of the IRS-proteins (shown in green) to access the active site. **B,** A structural representation of the binding of dimeric APS SH2 domains to the phosphorylated A loop of the insulin receptor. These structure were based on published coordinates.[83,86,90] (See Color Plate.)

Upon tris-phosphorylation, at least two phosphotyrosine residues in the A loop are completely solvent-exposed, creating sites for protein interaction (see Fig. 50-3A). A region of IRS2, called the kinase regulatory loop binding domain, binds to the phosphorylated A loop on the activated insulin receptor; however, the structural basis of this interaction remains unknown.[87,88] These exposed phosphotyrosine residues also interact with the Src homology-2 (SH2) domain containing proteins that promote or inhibit access to the catalytic site. Grb10 and several related SH2 proteins block the catalytic site while bound to the A loop.[89] By contrast, APS binds to the A loop from behind the catalytic domain to stabilize the active conformation (see Fig. 50-3B).[90] However, disruption of APS in mice increases peripheral insulin sensitivity and reduces circulating insulin levels, suggesting that APS might have an inhibitory function, possibly indirectly through elevated leptin and adiponectin levels.[91] Another member of the APS family, SH2B, binds via its SH2 domain to the A loop of IR.[91a-c] In Chinese hamster ovary cells, stable overexpression of SH2B enhances insulin-stimulated activation of both Erk1, Erk2, and Akt.[91d] These observations raise a possibility that SH2B plays a positive regulatory role during insulin receptor activation. Consistent with this model, disruption of the gene for SH2B causes insulin resistance and maturity onset obesity.[92] An explanation for the distinct phenotypes of the APS[-/-] and the SH2B[-/-] mice will be informative.

SUBSTRATE RECRUITMENT AND PHOSPHORYLATION SITE SELECTION

Substrate selectivity by protein kinases, including the insulin receptor, is a two-step process. First, a specific interaction between the kinase and the substrate aligns potential phosphorylation sites with the activated catalytic domain. Second, the catalytic domain selects and phosphorylates specific tyrosine residues based on their amino acid contexts.

Although phosphorylation of the regulatory loop is important to open the A loop, phosphorylation of the NPEY972 motif in the juxtamembrane region is essential for substrate recruitment.[93] The juxtamembrane region in the insulin receptor, the polypeptide segment that connects the transmembrane helix to the kinase domain, is about 35 residues long and contains two autophosphorylation sites (Tyr965 and Tyr972) (see Fig. 50-2B). Unlike other receptor tyrosine kinases, the insulin receptor kinase is not regulated by autophosphorylation in the juxtamembrane region.[94,95] However, pTyr972, which resides in the NPXY motif, is a docking site for the phosphotyrosine-binding (PTB) domains in the IRS-proteins and SHC.[93] In intact cells, phosphorylation of the NPXY motif is among the first sites of insulin-stimulated autophosphorylation, which is essential for substrate recruitment and biologic activity.[93,96] The juxtamembrane region may compete with the A loop for access to the catalytic site, supporting a model in which the juxtamembrane region is phosphorylated before tris-phosphorylation of the A loop.[72]

The structure of the activated β subunit reveals a mechanism by which the catalytic domain selects specific motifs for tyrosine phosphorylation.[83] Substrate peptides bind as short antiparallel β strands to the COOH-terminal end of the activation loop, allowing the hydrophobic residues in the Y+1 and Y+3 positions to occupy two small hydrophobic pockets on the COOH-terminal lobe of the kinase (see Fig. 50-3A). Tyrosine residues lying within amino acid motifs that contain charged or bulky side chains at the Y+1 and Y+3 positions fit poorly in the kinase active site.[83] Following substrate recruitment, the activated insulin receptor kinase engages tyrosine residues in the context of specific amino acid motifs, including the YMXM motif, YVNI motif, and YIDL motif.[97-99] Thus, specific recruitment of cellular proteins to the activated insulin receptor followed by the phosphorylation of specific tyrosine-containing motifs establishes an important level of signaling specificity and regulation.

IRS-PROTEINS AND INSULIN SIGNALING

After the discovery of the insulin receptor tyrosine kinase, many groups searched for substrates that might mediate downstream signals.[100,101] At first, the "substrate" hypothesis was difficult to prove for any receptor tyrosine kinase because the only known substrates were abundant proteins of dubious physiologic importance. The first evidence for a cellular substrate of a receptor tyrosine kinase came from phosphotyrosine antibody immunoprecipitates that revealed a 185-kilodalton phosphoprotein (pp185) in insulin-stimulated hepatoma cells.[102] This substrate seemed to be biologically important because it was phosphorylated immediately (within 5 sec) after insulin stimulation; and catalytically inactive insulin receptors failed to phosphorylate pp185. Importantly, a few catalytically active but biologically inactive insulin receptor mutants failed to phosphorylate pp185.[93] Together these data provided the first clue that substrate phosphorylation together with autophosphorylation are important steps in signal transduction.

Purification and molecular cloning of pp185 revealed one of the first signaling scaffolds and the first insulin receptor substrate, called IRS1.[103] IRS1 contains many tyrosine phosphorylation sites that are phosphorylated during insulin and IGF-1 stimulation (Fig. 50-4). Many of these tyrosine phosphorylation motifs are recognized binding sites for the SH2 domains in various signaling proteins.[99,104] For example, the interaction between IRS1 and p85 activates the class 1A PI 3-kinase, revealing the first insulin signaling cascade that could be reconstituted successfully in cells and test tubes.[105]

Many cellular substrates of the insulin receptor have now been identified, suggesting that insulin receptor signaling diversity arises from the assembly of signaling complexes around tyrosyl phosphorylated scaffolds. In addition to IRS-1 and its homologues (IRS2, IRS3, and IRS4), the insulin receptor phosphorylates other proteins in various contexts, including Shc, APS and SH2B, Gab1 and 2, Dock 1 and 2 and Cbl (see Fig. 50-4).[106–113] Although the role of each of these substrates merits attention, work with transgenic mice reveals that many insulin responses, especially those that are associated with somatic growth and carbohydrate metabolism, are mediated largely through IRS1 and IRS2, with minor contributions from IRS3 and IRS4.[1]

IRS-PROTEIN STRUCTURE AND FUNCTION

IRS-proteins are composed of multiple interaction domains and phosphorylation motifs (Fig. 50-5). At least three IRS-proteins occur in mice and people, including IRS1 and IRS2 that are widely expressed, and IRS4 that is limited to the thymus, brain, kidney, and β cells.[114] Rodents also express IRS3, which is largely restricted to adipose tissue where it displays activity similar to IRS1.[115] Mice lacking IRS1 are small and insulin-resistant, but generally fail to develop diabetes owing to persistent compensatory hyperinsulinemia.[116,117] By contrast, mice lacking IRS2 develop diabetes between 6 and 10 weeks of age owing to peripheral insulin resistance and β-cell failure.[116] Additional metabolic or genetic stress can cause diabetes in IRS1−/− mice, including the heterozygous disruption of the insulin receptor or IRS2.[118] Although disruption of IRS3 in mice has

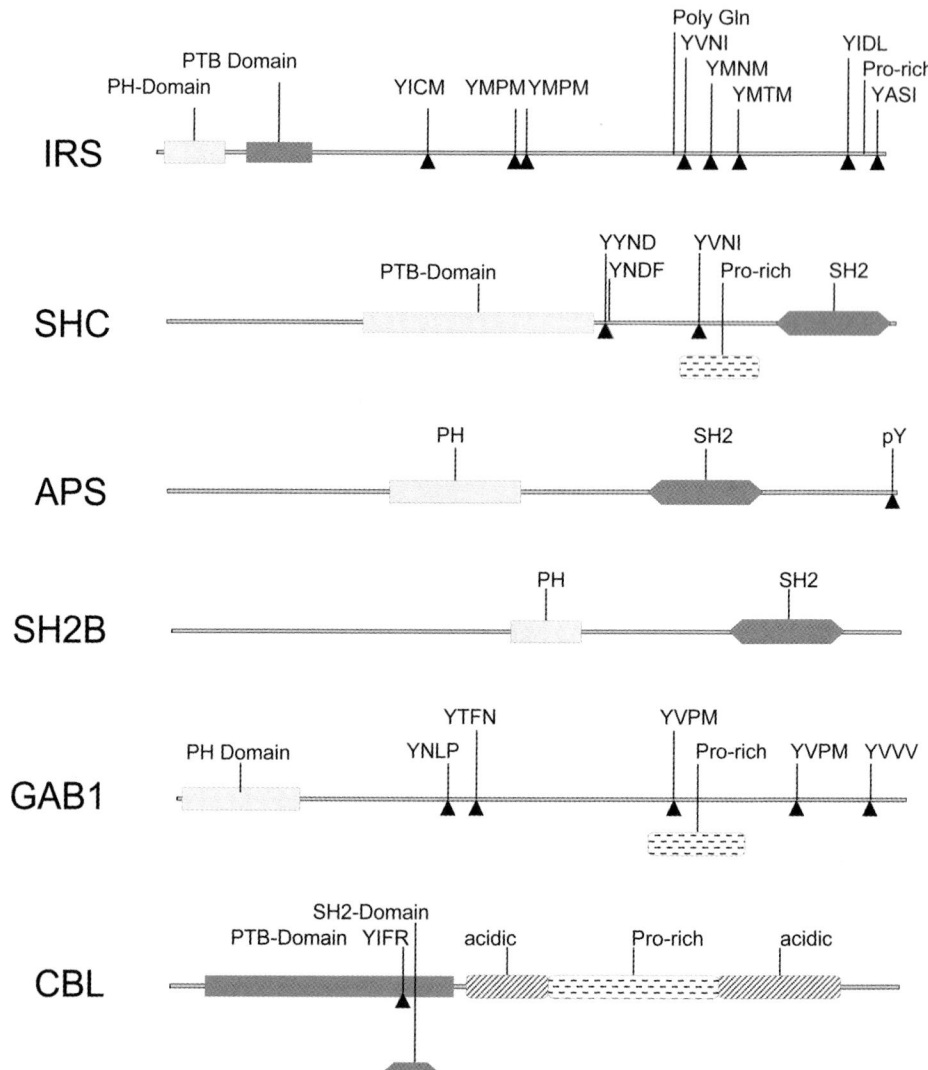

Figure 50-4 Diagrams (not drawn to scale) of various scaffold proteins that are reported to interact with the insulin receptor. The relative locations of protein interaction domains are shown: pleckstrin homology (PH), phosphotyrosine binding (PTB), src homology (SH2). Various amino acid sequence motifs are also shown: tyrosine phosphorylation sites, proline rich motifs (pro-rich), and acidic motifs.

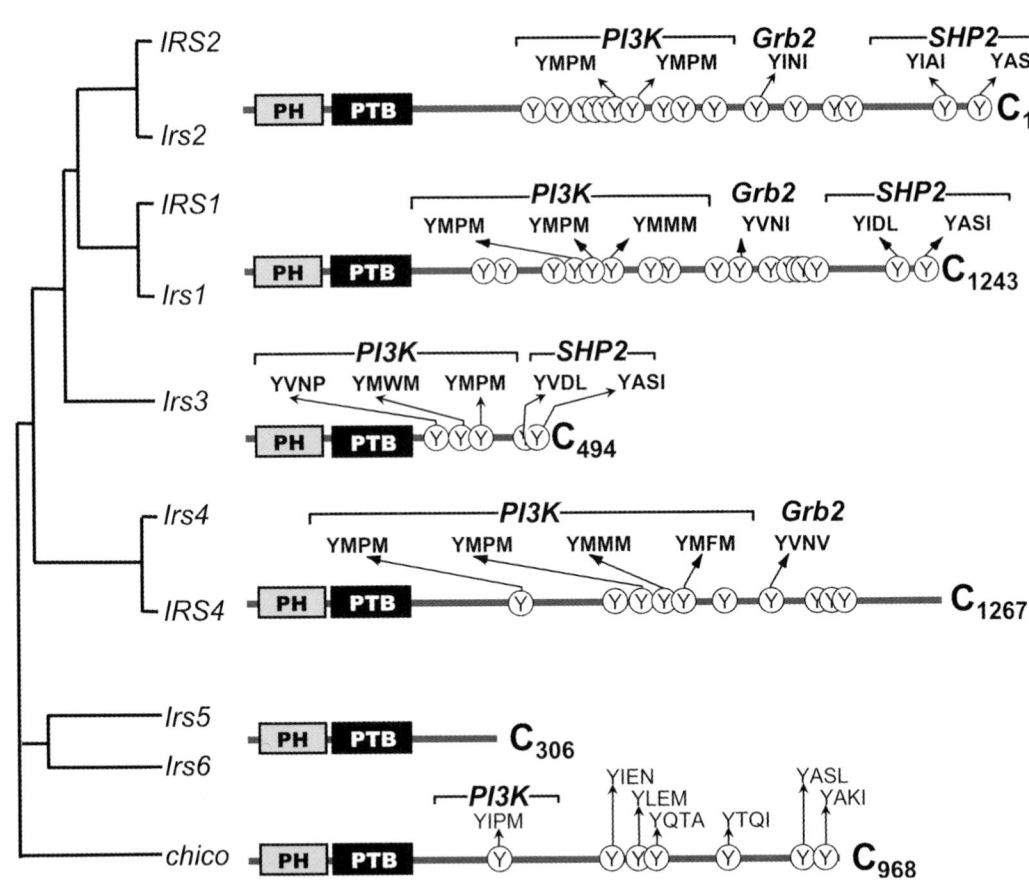

Figure 50-5 IRS-protein structures. A comparison (drawn to scale) of important sequence features of human IRS1, IRS2, IRS4, IRS5, and IRS6, mouse IRS3, and drosophila Chico. The relative position of the pleckstrin homology (PH) and phosphotyrosine binding (PTB) domains are indicated. The relative positions of potential tyrosine phosphorylation sites are indicated.

small effects, mice with a combined deficiency of IRS1 and IRS3 developed severe early-onset lipoatrophy associated with marked hyperglycemia, hyperinsulinemia, and insulin resistance.[115] Since humans do not express a functional IRS3 gene, humans may be at increased risk for metabolic disorders.[119]

The IRS-protein isoforms display several important similarities (see Fig. 50-5). Mammalian IRS1, -2, -3 and -4, and the drosophila ortholog Chico contain an NH_2-terminal pleckstrin homology (PH) domain adjacent to a PTB domain (see Fig. 50-5). The structures of these domains are remarkably similar[120]; both appear to facilitate recruitment of IRS-proteins to the activated insulin and IGF-1 receptors.[121] Each IRS-protein recruits and activates PI 3-kinase during insulin stimulation, whereas the ability to activate Erk1 and -2 is variable.[122,123] IRS5/DOK4 and IRS6/DOK5 were recognized in the human genome owing to their NH_2-terminal tandem PH-PTB domains.[124]

Deletion of the PH and PTB domains in IRS1 or IRS2 almost completely prevents insulin-stimulated tyrosine phosphorylation of the tail, even when insulin receptors are expressed at high levels.[125] The PTB domain binds to a phosphorylated NPEY-motif in the β subunit of the activated insulin or IGF-1 receptor[121,125,126]; a similar motif is also phosphorylated in the IL-4 receptor, explaining its strong recruitment of IRS1 or IRS2.[127] At ordinary expression levels, deletion of the PTB domain reduces the ability of insulin to promote tyrosine phosphorylation of IRS1 or IRS2; however, overexpression of the insulin receptor restores phosphorylation and signaling, suggesting that the PH domain is sufficient.[125]

The mechanism of coupling employed by the PH domain is not understood; however, it promotes interaction between IRS-proteins and insulin receptors at physiologic levels. The PH domains in PKB and PDK1 bind membrane phospholipids with high affinity to provide unambiguous membrane targeting.[128,129] However the PH domain in IRS-proteins, like PH domains in most proteins, binds phospholipids poorly. PH domains can be exchanged among IRS-proteins without

noticeable loss of bioactivity[130]; however, heterologous PH domains inhibit IRS1 function when substituted for the normal PH domain.[130] Since IRS-protein PH domains do not bind to the insulin receptor or to phospholipids, other targets might be involved. Yeast two-hybrid screens reveal a few potential binding partners, including nucleolin.[130] However, the interaction with nucleolin might mediate translocation of IRS1 into the nucleus rather than coupling to the insulin receptor.[131–133] The PH domain also binds to PHIP, an uncharacterized conserved protein that contains a WD40 repeat and BROMO domains.[24,134]

The tyrosine phosphorylation sites in the COOH-terminal end of each IRS-protein recruit and regulate various downstream signaling proteins (see Fig. 50-5). IRS1 and IRS2 have the longest tails, containing 20 potential tyrosine phosphorylation sites each; however, only a few sites that bind p85, Grb2, or SHP3 have been formally identified.[104] Many of the tyrosine residues cluster into common motifs that recruit or activate enzymes (PI 3-kinase, SHP2, fyn) or adapter molecules (Grb2, nck, crk, SH2B) (see Fig. 50-5). Grb2 and possibly SHP2 couple Grb2/SOS to IRS-proteins, which promotes the ras → raf cascade.[135] All IRS-proteins contain multiple p85-binding motifs that recruit the PI 3-kinase, which is the best studied insulin signaling pathway.

In addition to the tyrosine phosphorylation sites, sequence alignment of IRS-proteins reveals several conserved motifs that might be binding sites for other cellular proteins. IRS1, IRS2, and Chico contains a binding site for the c-Jun N-terminal kinase (JNK) that resembles the sites in the JNK-interacting proteins (JIP1 and JIP2).[136–139] During stimulation by proinflammatory cytokines or by insulin, activated JNK binds to IRS1 or IRS2 and promotes serine phosphorylation, which inhibits insulin-stimulated tyrosine phosphorylation.[138–141]

There are many unique amino acid sequence motifs between IRS1 and IRS2 that might create unique interaction sites for other partner proteins that fine-tune the biologic signals. IRS2 contains a unique region of undefined structure that binds to the phosphorylated regulatory loop of the insulin receptor kinase called the kinase regulatory loop binding domain.[142] The discovery of this interaction was unexpected, as it maps to the portion of the COOH-terminal region between amino acid residues 591 and 786 that contains tyrosine phosphorylation sites. Two tyrosine residues in the kinase regulatory loop binding domain at positions 628 and 632 are crucial for this interaction. Phosphorylation of tyrosine residues in the kinase regulatory-loop binding domain by the insulin receptor inhibits the binding to the receptor, revealing a novel mechanism to regulate the interaction of the insulin receptor and IRS2 that might distinguish the signal of IRS2 from IRS1.[142]

THE PI 3-KINASE CASCADE

The PI 3-kinase is ubiquitous and used by nearly all receptor signaling systems to promote cell division, survival, and growth (Fig. 50-6). During insulin and IGF signaling, the PI 3-kinase cascade is accessed through tyrosine phosphorylation of the IRS-proteins. IRS-proteins introduce unique specificity and regulation upon the system for insulin and IGF action. Specificity is accomplished by dissociating IRS PI 3-kinase signaling complex from the intracellular itinerary of the insulin receptor. Differential regulation of the IRS-proteins at the level of gene expression and protein stability add an addi-

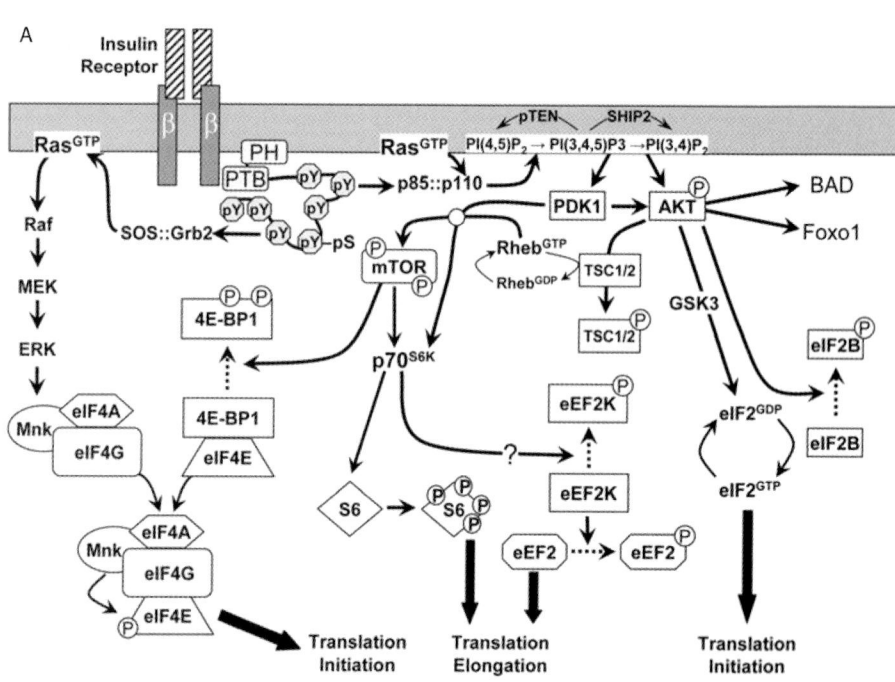

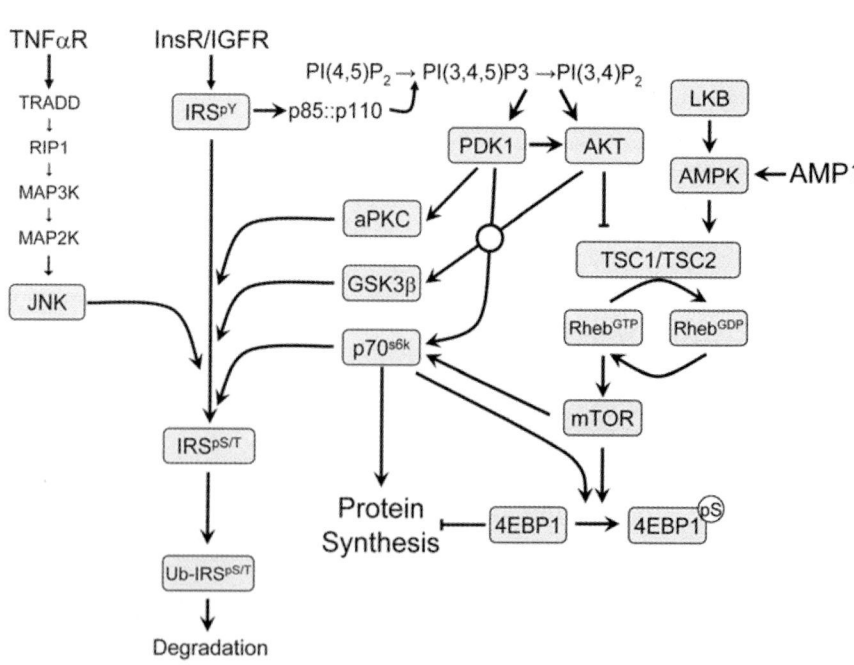

Figure 50-6   Activation of intracellular signaling pathways by insulin. **A,** There are two main limbs that propagate the signal generated through the IRS-proteins: the PI 3-kinase and the Grb2/Sos→ras cascade. Activation of the receptors for insulin and IGF-1 results in tyrosine phosphorylation of the IRS-proteins, which bind PI 3-kinase and Grb2/SOS. The GRB2/SOS complex promotes GDP/GTP exchange on p21^{ras}, which activates the ras raf MEK ERK1/2 cascade. The activated ERK stimulates transcriptional activity by direct phosphorylation of elk1 and by phosphorylation of fos through p90^{rsk}. The activation of PI 3-kinase by IRS-protein recruitment produces PI3,4P$_2$ and PI3,4,5P$_3$ (antagonized by the action of PTEN or SHIP2), which recruit PDK1 and PKB to the plasma membrane, where PKB is activated by PDK-mediated phosphorylation. The mTOR kinase is phosphorylated by Rheb^{GTP}, which accumulates upon inhibition of the GAP activity of the TSC1::TSC2 complex by PKB-mediated phosphorylation. The p70^{s6k} is primed through mTOR-mediated phosphorylation for activation by PDK1. PKB inactivates GSK3 by phosphorylation, which leads to the activation of glycogen synthesis and protein translation. PKB-mediated BAD phosphorylation inhibits apoptosis, and phosphorylation of the forkhead proteins results in their sequestration in the cytoplasm, in effect inhibiting their transcriptional activity. Insulin stimulates protein synthesis by altering the intrinsic activity or binding properties of key translation initiation and elongation factors (eIFs and eEFs, respectively) as well as critical ribosomal proteins. This occurs via phosphorylation and/or sequestration of repressive factors into inactive complexes. Components of the translational machinery that are targets of insulin regulation include eIF2B, eIF4E, eEF1, eEF2, and the S6 ribosomal protein.[215] **B,** Inhibition of IRS-protein signaling through nutrient sensing. High ATP levels, reflecting amino acid and glucose excess, inhibit the AMP kinase reducing its ability to activate the GAP activity of TSC1::TSC2, which mediates mTOR activity. Insulin activation of PDK1 together with mTOR leads to the activation of various kinases that phosphorylate IRS-protein, which targets them for poly ubiquitinylation and degradation. AKT, product of the akt proto-oncogene; GAP, guanosine triphosphatase associated protein; GLUT4, glucose transporter 4; GRB-2, factor receptor binding protein 2; GSK3, glycogen synthase kinase 3; IRS1, insulin receptor substrate 1; MAPKK, MAPK kinase; PDK, PI-dependent protein kinase; PH, pleckstrin homology domain; PKC, protein kinase C; PTB, phosphotyrosine binding domain; PTEN and SHIP2, phospholipid phosphatases; SOS, son-of-sevenless; TSC, tuberous sclerosis complex. See the text for details of the signaling.

tional level of control. One of the best examples of signaling specificity emerges from our work in pancreatic β cells. IRS2, but not IRS1, is strongly induced by cyclic adenosine monophosphate (cAMP) response element binding protein (CREB) signaling in β cells, which regulates the PI 3-kinase Pkb/Akt cascade needed to promote growth, survival, and function of these insulin-producing cells.[1]

PI 3-KINASE

Phospholipids create platforms for cell signaling, and the products of the PI 3-kinase, PI(3,4) P_2 and PI(3,4,5) P_3, play a special role. These phospholipids recruit various serine kinases to the inner face of the plasma membrane, where signaling complexes interact and generate downstream signals (see Fig. 50-6). Various phospholipid phosphatases, including PTEN and SHIP2, control the steady-state phosphorylation of these membrane lipids, which modulates the capacity to recruit PDK1 and PKB/AKT and the strength of the downstream signals (see Fig. 50-6).

There are three types of PI 3-kinases in higher eukaryotes, but the class IA enzymes are activated by growth factors and insulin.[143] Class IA PI 3-kinase is a heterodimer composed of a regulatory subunit and catalytic subunit. The different isoforms of the catalytic subunit, p110α, β, and δ are encoded by separate genes; and there are five regulatory subunits isoforms encoded by three distinct genes.[144] The Pik3r1 gene encodes p85α, and through the use of alternative start sites encodes p55α and p50α[145]; Pik3r2 encodes p85β, which is similar in size to p85α. The third gene, Pik3r3, encodes p55γ (originally called p55 PIK), which is homologous to p55α.[146] p85α and p85β contain two SH2 domains, an inter-SH2 domain that is tightly bound to the p110 catalytic subunit, two proline-rich regions, a bcr-homology domain, and an SH3 domain; p55α and p50α lack the SH3 domain and Bcr-homology domain, which is replaced by a unique 34- or 6-amino acid peptide at the NH_2-terminus, respectively. The p55γ also contains a unique N-terminal terminus of 34 amino acids.[146] Each isoform associates noncovalently with a p110 catalytic subunits, which protects the p110 from proteolysis and inhibits its intrinsic catalytic activity[147,148]; Disruption of p85α, p55α, or p50α decreases the p110 protein levels in mice leading to diminished PI 3-kinase activity.[149]

The IRS1 and IRS2 are ideal regulators of PI 3-kinase because they contain multiple YXXM motifs that are phosphorylated by the activated insulin receptor and bind strongly to the regulatory subunits SH2 domains.[98] Occupancy of both SH2 domains by phosphorylated YXXM motifs in IRS-proteins activates the PI 3-kinase catalytic subunits.[150] Interestingly, phosphorylation of p85α at Tyr688 by Src tyrosine kinase also relieves the inhibition of the p110 catalytic subunit imposed by the p85 regulatory subunit, but this is not involved in insulin signaling.[151] Moreover, GTP-bound Ras binds directly to the p110 catalytic subunit to enhance PI 3-kinase activity.[152–155]

All five regulatory subunit isoforms (p85α, p55α, p50α, p85β, and p55γ) bind to phosphorylated IRS-proteins and mediate the activation of PI 3-kinase; however, it is very difficult to dissect unique roles for each isoform. Deletion of p85α reduces PI 3-kinase activity by 50% to 60% in skeletal muscle and adipocytes. Unexpectedly, insulin sensitivity increases in these tissues and the mutant mice develop hypoglycemia with hyperinsulinemia.[156] Part of the dysregulation might arise from upregulation of p50α, which has higher affinity for the p110.[156,157] Moreover, disruption of all three α isoforms (p85α, p55α, and p50α) causes hypoglycemia with hypoinsulinemia, even though PI 3-kinase activity is reduced 80% to 90% in the liver and muscles.[149] Importantly, the activation of Akt is nomal in the mutant mice, indicating that Akt activation does not always follow the apparent PI 3-kinase activity.[149]

It is not clear why disruption of all the p85α improves insulin sensitivity. At least one third of the p85 regulatory subunits exist as monomers in normal cells because they are more abundant than either IRS1 or p110.[157] Excessive p85

might block formation of active catalytic complexes by the IRS-protein scaffolds. The p85β accounts for about 20% and 30% of total p85 proteins in liver and muscle, respectively, but deletion of p85β increases insulin sensitivity in mice.[158,159] The disruption of p55γ has not yet been reported, but it is abundant in brain where it might play a special role in neuronal function or plasticity. Clearly, different isoforms share redundancy in regulating PI 3-kinase, while providing unique signaling features; however, cell-based experiments with embryonic stem cells reveal the sensitive balance achieved by the expression of p85 isoforms.[160]

It is difficult to establish unique roles for individual isoforms of the p110 catalytic subunits in vivo. Disruption of the p110α is lethal to embryo development, preventing the analysis of its role in insulin action.[161] Interestingly, the p110β is upregulated during adipose differentiation of 3T3-L1 cells, and appears to be more sensitive to insulin than p110α.[162] Microinjection of anti-p110β, but not p110α, blocks insulin-stimulated GLUT4 translocation.[162] PPAR-γ agonist troglitazone increases the expression of p110β, which correlates with the enhancement of the activation of PI 3-kinase and Akt and an improvement of insulin sensitivity in humans.[163] Understanding how the catalytic and regulatory subunits modulate the insulin signal needs to be resolved.

THE PDK1/AKT SIGNALING CASCADE

The AGC (cAMP-dependent protein kinase [PKA]/protein kinase G/protein kinase C) kinase family mediates many physiologic responses triggered by growth factors or insulin.[164] Members of the family that play a role during insulin action include PDK1,[165] AKT,[166–168] p70 ribosomal S6 kinase (p70^{S6K}),[169,170] p90 ribosomal S6 kinase (p90^{RSK}),[171,172] and the serum- and glucocorticoid-induced protein kinase (SGK).[173] PDK1 phosphorylates the A loop in these kinases, which is essential for their activation.[164,168,174] Since PDK1 is constitutively activated, regulation is achieved by controlling the interaction of the substrates with PDK1.[175]

AKT is one of the best-characterized insulin-stimulated enzymes as it is broadly implicated in growth and metabolism.[168,175] Three distinct AKT genes exists in people and rodents: AKT1 (PKBα), AKT2 (PKBβ), and AKT3 (PKBγ).[168,175–177] Each isoform shares a similar structure, including an NH_2 terminal PH domain and a COOH terminal catalytic domain. PI(3,4)P_2 and PI(3,4,5)P_3, produced in the plasma membrane by the activated PI 3-kinase, binds to the PH domain at the NH_2-terminus of AKT and PDK1, which recruits both enzymes to the plasma membrane.[168,175] At the plasma membrane, the A loop in PKB becomes accessible to PDK1, resulting in the phosphorylation of Thr308 and activation of AKT (see Fig. 50-6).

Many studies suggest that AKT is required for insulin-regulated glucose homeostasis. Overexpression of membrane targeted, constitutively active mutants of AKT promote GLUT4 translocation to the surface of the plasma membrane to stimulate glucose uptake in muscle and adipose cells.[178,179] Conversely, inhibition of endogenous AKT1 and AKT2 by microinjection of an AKT substrate peptide (KRPRAATF) or antibodies against AKT inhibits GLUT4 translocation in response to insulin in 3T3-L1 adipocytes.[180] A dominant-negative AKT mutant prevents phosphorylation of glycogen synthase kinase-3 (GSK3), which inhibits insulin stimulation of glycogen synthesis.[181] Similarly, insulin-stimulated GLUT4 translocation is blocked by expression of a dominant-negative AKT in GLUT4 vesicles, but not by the same mutant expressed in the cytosol, suggesting that AKT may directly target components in GLUT4 vesicles.[182] In the liver, insulin inhibits glucose production by suppressing the expression of gluconeogenic enzymes, including phosphoenolpyruvate carboxykinase and glucose-6-phosphatase.[183]

Akt isoforms display distinct cellular roles in response to insulin or IGF-1. One of the best examples is the effect of AKT knockout upon growth and metabolism. Overexpression of constitutively active AKT1 increases heart size, whereas overexpression of dominant-negative AKT1 inhibits cardiac myocyte growth induced by constitutively active PI 3-kinase in transgenic mice.[184] Consistent with its role in mediating growth and survival signals, deletion of AKT1 causes growth retardation in mice; AKT1$^{-/-}$ cells are more susceptible to apoptosis.[185] These results are similar to the effects of Irs1 knockout,[117] and suggest functional importance of an IRS1→Akt1 cascade with respect to growth control during IGF stimulation.

Mice lacking Akt2 develop hyperglycemia, hyperinsulinemia, and glucose intolerance, resembling the phenotype of type 2 diabetes in humans.[186] Akt1$^{-/-}$ mice maintain normal blood glucose and insulin sensitivity, indicating that Akt1 is not required for metabolic effect of insulin and IGF-1.[186a,b] Recently, a mutation in the gene encoding human Akt2 explains the autosomal-dominant inheritance of severe insulin resistance and diabetes mellitus, validating the central importance of Akt signaling to insulin sensitivity in humans.[187]

SIGNALING BY AGC KINASES

PDK1 is a master regulator of many AGC kinases activated by insulin.[164] AGC kinases do not generally contain a PH domain for recruitment to the plasma membrane, so a different mechanism is needed to regulate their interaction with PDK1. A docking site, called the PIF pocket, is located on the small lobe of the PDK1 kinase domain, which interacts with a hydrophobic region in the COOH terminus of p70^{S6K}, SGK, and p90^{RSK}.[188] Ser/Thr phosphorylation of the hydrophobic motif (Phe-Xaa-Xaa-Phe/Tyr-*Ser/Thr*-Phe/Tyr) in these kinases promotes binding to the PIF pocket of PDK1 and phosphorylation of the A loop. The mammalian target of rapamycin (mTOR) can phosphorylate the hydrophobic motif of p70 S6K, promoting its interaction with PDK1[188]; phosphorylation of RSK isoforms by the Erk1/Erk2 mitogen-activated protein kinases (MAPKs) activates its second catalytic domain that phosphorylates the hydrophobic motif to promote its interaction with PDK1.[189,190] SGK is also activated by PDK1-mediated phosphorylation; however, the kinase that phosphorylates the hydrophobic motif in SGK is unknown.[188]

AKT SUBSTRATES MEDIATED DIVERSE BIOLOGIC PROCESSES

AKT phosphorylates many substrates that regulate various aspects of cellular activity, including CREB and FOXO proteins (gene expression); GSK3, RAF, eNOS, and IKK (cell function and growth); p27 kip1 (cell division); RHEB-GAP (mTOR activity); and BAD and caspase-9 (cell survival).[166,190–198] In many cases, Akt phosphorylation inhibits the target protein function: Akt phosphorylation inactivates the proapoptotic protein BAD, releasing BCL2 to inhibit apoptosis[199,200]; phosphorylation of caspase-9 by AKT inhibits its protease activity, which promotes cell survival[201]; AKT phosphorylates p27 KIP1 at Thr157, which retains p27KIP1 in cytoplasm to prevent the inhibition of cell-cycle progression.[202] AKT phosphorylates and inhibits serine/threonine kinases RAF and GSK3.[196,197] Since GSK3 phosphorylates and inhibits glycogen synthase, AKT promotes glycogen synthase activity by inhibiting GSK3 (see Fig. 50-6).

FORKHEAD TRANSCRIPTION FACTORS LINK PI 3-KINASE PKB/Akt TO THE NUCLEUS

Among the major nuclear regulators of metabolic gene expression, the so-called forkhead transcription factors, FOXO1, FOXO3a, FOXO4 (previously termed FKHR, FKHRL1, and AFX1) and FOXA1, FOXA2, and FOXA3 (previously termed HNF-3α, HNF-3β, and HNF-3γ), play major regulatory roles in many tissues, including pancreatic β cells, adipose tissue, and liver.[203] FOXO1, FOXO3a, and FOXO4 are phosphorylated by AKT and SGK during insulin stimulation. AKT phosphorylates

FOXO1 at Ser253, which facilitates the subsequent phosphorylation of Thr24 and Ser316, resulting in the cytosolic accumulation that blocks transcriptional activity.[194] FOXA2, but not FOXA1 and FOXA3, contains a single threonine site that is phosphorylated by Akt, which also localizes it to the cytosol.[203]

FOXO1 is abundantly expressed in the liver and binds to a CAAAA(C/T)AA motif present in hepatic enzymes required for gluconeogenesis.[204] Phosphoenolpyruvate carboxykinase and glucose-6-phosphatase are dramatically reduced in Foxo1$^{+/-}$ mice owing to insufficient nuclear Foxo1. Conversely, overexpression of Foxo1 in liver increases the levels of phosphoenolpyruvate carboxykinase and glucose-6-phosphatase, and induces insulin resistance and diabetes in the transgenic mice.[205] FOXO1 interacts with the peroxisome proliferator-activated receptor-γ coactivator (PGC)1α, a transcriptional coactivator of CREB, HNF-4α, and the glucocorticoid receptor, to fully upregulate phosphoenolpyruvate carboxykinase.[206] Association of Foxo1 with PGC1α is prevented by Akt-mediated phosphorylation, which inhibits the effect of PGC1α on gene expression.[206]

FOXO1 also plays an important role in coupling insulin signaling to adipocyte differentiation. FOXO1 expression is upregulated in preadipocytes coincidently with growth arrest and peaks at the onset of terminal differentiation. However, constitutively active FOXO1 blocks adipocyte differentiation, suggesting that inactivation of FOXO1 by AKT-mediated phosphorylation is probably essential once preadipocytes are in growth arrest. The inability to properly phosphorylate Foxo1 in mice lacking Irs1 and Irs2 can explain the lipodystrophic in Irs1$^{-/-}$::Irs3$^{-/-}$ mice.[115] Disruption of the insulin receptor also reduces adipocytes mass in mice, suggesting that it is an essential upstream kinase in this regulatory mechanism.[44]

Nuclear FOXO1 also inhibits β-cell function. Expression of a constitutively active FOX1 protein causes β-cell failure that dysregulates glucose homeostasis in mice.[10] By contrast, heterozygous disruption of Foxo1 promotes β-cell function and survival, and β-cell function in Foxo1$^{+/-}$::Irs2$^{-/-}$ mice is restored to normal, preventing the progression to diabetes.[10] Thus, in β cells, the IRS-2/PI 3-kinase branch of the insulin/IGF signaling cascade is an important pathway FOXO1 phosphorylation by AKT.

THE REGULATION OF PROTEIN SYNTHESIS

THE mTOR CASCADE

The mTOR cascade integrates nutrient availability with insulin signaling to control protein synthesis and cell growth. mTOR was originally isolated as the target of the immunosuppressive agent rapamycin, which binds to FKBP12 to form a complex that inhibits mTOR activity.[185] Components of the mTOR cascade are highly conserved from yeast to mammals, providing a common mechanism that is sensitive to the nutrients such as amino acids and glucose.[185,207]

Downstream effectors of mTOR—p70^{S6K} and 4E-BP1—control protein synthesis and cell growth. The p70^{S6K} occurs as two isoforms called p70^{S6K1} and p70^{S6K2}. Disruption of S6K1 gene in mice causes glucose intolerance due to reduced size of pancreatic islet β cells; however, peripheral insulin action is enhanced suggesting that p70^{S6K1} contributes to feedback inhibition of insulin signaling.[208] p70^{S6K1} is activated by multisite phosphorylation events from various kinase activities in response to insulin and other mitogens when amino acids are available.[209] Nutrient sensitivity arises because mTOR mediates the phosphorylation of the hydrophobic motif needed for interaction of p70^{S6K1} with PDK1 (see Fig. 50-6).

The regulation of the mTOR cascade is complex, but recent discoveries reveal how AKT acts to regulate mTOR function during insulin stimulation, and how energy depletion inhibits mTOR through the adenosine monophosphate kinase (AMPK). The ubiquitously expressed small G protein, Rheb (RAS homologue expressed in brain) is an mTOR activator.[185,210] During GTP binding, Rheb promotes mTOR activity, whereas GTP hydrolysis inactivates Rheb-stimulated mTOR activity (see Fig. 50-6B). GTP hydrolysis is catalyzed by TSC2, a GTPase-activating protein for RHEB.[210] TSC2 complexes with TSC1 to form a heterodimer that is essential to prevent constitutive activation of mTOR (see Fig. 50-6B). Mutations in TSC1 or TSC2 that dysregulate GTP hydrolysis cause nonmalignant tumors in various tissues called hamartomas.[211]

TSC1::TSC2 → Rheb cascade is required for mTOR to sense energy depletion (see Fig. 50-6B). Cellular AMP levels rise during an energy deficit, which activates AMPK.[212,213] During AMP binding, the A loop of the AMPK, is accessible to the constitutively active LKB1. Recent results suggest that Rheb-GTPase-activating protein activity of the TSC1::TSC2 complex is increased by AMPK phosphorylation.[214] This regulatory model is consistent with the effects of inactivating LKB1 mutations that lead to hamartomas with similar characteristics to those observed in tuberous sclerosis patients.[212,213]

REGULATION OF PROTEIN SYNTHESIS BY INSULIN

Insulin stimulates protein synthesis by altering the intrinsic activity or binding properties of key translation initiation and elongation factors (eIFs and eEFs, respectively), as well as critical ribosomal proteins. This occurs via phosphorylation and/or sequestration of repressive factors into inactive complexes. Components of the translational machinery that are targets of insulin regulation include eIF2B, eIF4E, eEF1, eEF2, and the S6 ribosomal protein.[215] The eIF2B multi-subunit guanine nucleotide exchange factor for eIF2 is kept inactive via phosphorylation of the eIF2Bε subunit at Ser535 by GSK3.[216] Inhibition of GSK3 during insulin-stimulated Akt phosphorylation reduces eIF2B phosphorylation promoting the formation of eIF2 GTP that recruits the initiator methionyl-tRNA to the ribosome.[216-218] The insulin-stimulated activation of eIF2B leads to an overall increase in translation initiation.[219] Diabetic rats have significantly lower eIF2B activity in muscle.[220]

The eIF4F complex, including eIF4A, 4G, 4E and other proteins, is required for cap-dependent translation initiation. The mRNA cap-binding protein, eIF4E, is inactive during association with 4E-BP1 (see Fig. 50-6). Insulin activates eIF4E by stimulating mTOR-mediated phosphorylation of 4E-BP1. Phosphoyrlated 4E-BP1 dissociates to facilitate the interaction between eIF4E and eIF4G, the scaffold protein for the eIF4F complex.[221] MNK, an insulin-stimulated kinase activated through the RAS/ERK cascade, also resides in the eIF4F complex where it phosphorylates eIF4E at Ser209 (see Fig. 50-6).[222,223] Phosphorylation of eIF4E increases the binding affinity for mRNA caps, enhancing translation initiation. The phosphorylation of 4E-BP1 has an important systemic role in insulin action, as deletion of its gene increases insulin sensitivity and dramatically decreases white adipose tissue depots.[224]

Insulin also stimulates translation elongation by phosphorylation of eEF1 by an as yet undetermined mechanism. Insulin-stimulated phosphorylation of the ribosomal S6 protein by p70[S6K] may promote elongation of specific mRNAs corresponding to components of the translational machinery.[225] An elongation factor critical for ribosomal translocation along the mRNA, eEF2, is inactive when phosphorylated at Thr56 by the eEF2 kinase (eEF2K).[226,227] Insulin stimulates the dephosphorylation of eEF2 via a rapamycin-sensitive route potentially involving the phosphorylation and inactivation of eEF2K by p70[S6K].[226] In vitro, p70[S6K] phosphorylates eEF2K at Ser366, a modification that greatly reduces the activity of the kinase.[226] Activation of PKCζ is also required for

insulin-stimulated protein synthesis although its downstream effectors remain undetermined.[228] Convergence between nutritional and insulin signals occurs at the level of mTOR activity regulation (see Fig. 50-6B).[225,229,230]

THE REGULATION OF GLUCOSE TRANSPORT AND METABOLISM

GLUCOSE TRANSPORTERS

Glucose transport is the prototype insulin response. The molecular mechanisms linking insulin signals to increased glucose influx into adipose and muscle has been difficult to resolve. All cells express one or more members of the glucose transporter family, including 12 isoforms organized into 3 classes: class I includes the well-characterized GLUT1, GLUT2, GLUT3, and GLUT4 transporters; class II includes GLUT5, GLUT7, GLUT9, and GLUT11; and class III includes GLUT6, GLUT8, GLUT10, and GLUT12.

GLUT4 is an insulin-responsive glucose transporter found in skeletal muscle, adipose cells, and heart. GLUT4 is glycosylated in the first exofacial loop, and contains a phosphorylation site (Ser488) and a di-leucine motif in its COOH terminus that plays a role in endocytosis.[231] Before insulin stimulation, GLUT4 resides in intracellular vesicles where it is unavailable to transport glucose across the plasma membrane. However, insulin stimulation promotes translocation of GLUT4-containing vesicles to the plasma membrane to increase the rate of glucose influx (Fig. 50-7).

Insulin does not regulate the translocation of other class 1 glucose transporters. GLUT1 is expressed in most cells and tissues and resides permanently on the plasma membrane where it constitutively transports glucose from the extracellular space into the cell. Although insulin does not stimulate translocation of GLUT1, chronic insulin treatment increases the levels of cellular GLUT1 via the p21[RAS] → ERK kinase pathway.[232,233] GLUT2 is mainly expressed in liver and pancreatic β cells, where its relatively low affinity but high transport capacity provides a constant flux of glucose into these organs at physiologic plasma glucose concentrations (5 mM). In the β cell, the uptake of glucose through GLUT2 is the first step in the detection of circulating glucose levels needed to stimulate insulin secretion. GLUT3 has a relatively high affinity for glucose and is most abundant in the central nervous system where glucose concentrations are lower than in the bloodstream. GLUT8 might be insulin sensitive as it contains GLUT4-like intracellular targeting motifs and is widely expressed in many insulin-responsive (as well as insulin-independent) tissues[234,235]; GLUT12 is expressed in prostate, small intestine, placenta, skeletal muscle, and adipocytes and might also be insulin responsive.[236,237]

THE REGULATION OF GLUT4 BY INSULIN

During insulin stimulation, GLUT4-containing vesicles move from their intracellular storage compartment and reach the cell surface through targeted exocytosis (see Fig. 50-7). Simultaneously, GLUT4 endocytosis is repressed, leading to an overall increase in glucose uptake.[238] It is not clear whether the effect of insulin to stimulate glucose uptake in muscle and fat can be accounted for in its entirety by translocation, as other factors that increase transporter activity could be involved. Substantial evidence exists to suggest that at least two distinct pathways mediate the effect of insulin on glucose transport. One pathway relies on PI 3-kinase activation of downstream effectors, including PDK1, AKT, and atypical protein kinase C (PKC) isoforms PKCζ and PKCλ.[239-241] The PI 3-kinase-independent pathway includes the activation of TC10, a Rho family G protein localized to lipid rafts in the plasma membrane.[242]

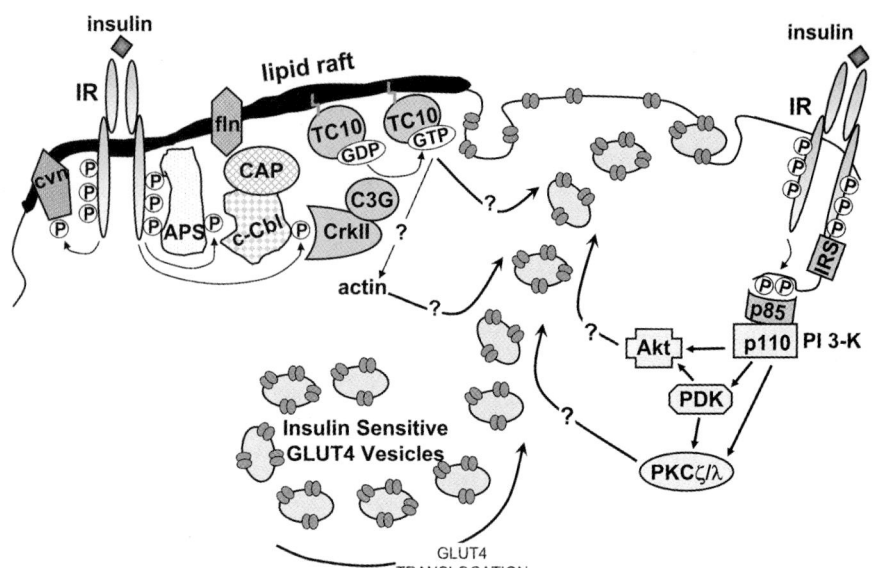

Figure 50-7 A diagram of components that mediate insulin-stimulated glucose transport. The PI 3-kinase sensitive branch of the pathway is shown on the right, including IRS-proteins, AKT and the atypical protein kinase C isoforms, and PKCζ/λ and PKCτ. The PI 3-kinase independent branch of the pathway is shown on the left and includes the APSCbl cascade. Activation of these pathways by insulin promotes the accumulation of GLUT4-containing vesicle in the plasma membrane. See the text for a detailed description of these pathways.

ATYPICAL PROTEIN KINASE C REGULATES GLUT4 TRANSLOCATION

PKCζ and PKCλ are implicated in the regulation of GLUT4 translocation in adipose tissue and muscle.[180,243,244] Constitutively active PKCλ or PKCζ promote GLUT4 translocation and glucose uptake in adipocytes and muscles in the absence of insulin.[244–247] Overexpression of inactive PKCλ inhibits insulin-stimulated activation of endogenous PKCλ, which inhibits GLUT4 translocation and glucose.[246] Microinjection of PKCλ antibodies inhibits insulin-induced GLUT4 translocation.[248] PKCζ also promotes insulin-stimulated glucose uptake. Insulin-promoted activation of PKCζ is reduced in obese patients with insulin resistance[249]; impaired PKCζ activity is associated with obesity-induced insulin resistance in monkeys.[245,250] It will be important to understand how the atypical PKC isoforms, PKB and other related AGC kinases, interact with cellular components to regulate GLUT4 translocation (see Fig. 50-7).

PI 3-KINASE-INDEPENDENT REGULATION OF GLUT4 TRANSLOCATION

The activation of TC10, a small G protein of the RHO family localized to lipid rafts in the plasma membrane might also regulate GLUT4 translocation.[242] Lipid rafts are microdomains on the cell surface containing specific glycolipids, sphingolipids, proteins, and cholesterol that do not mix with other lipids within the plasma membrane. The insulin receptor is localized to caveolae, a specific lipid raft subset, where it associates with caveolin (cvn) and phosphorylates it on tyrosine residues.[242] The localization of the insulin receptor to caveolae might be critical for the activation of the PI 3-kinase-independent signals leading to GLUT4 translocation in adipocytes.[251] During insulin stimulation, APS binds to the A loop of the activated insulin receptor. Upon tyrosyl phosphorylation, APS recruits c-Cbl for tyrosine phosphorylation by the insulin receptor.[239,252] In insulin-responsive cells, c-Cbl is constitutively associated with the CAP::flotilin complex, which stabilizes the growing caveolae-localized insulin receptor complex.[239] The tyrosine-phosphorylated c-Cbl also recruits the CRK II, which constitutively binds C3G, a guanine nucleotide-exchange factor that catalyzes the exchange of GTP for GDP in the small G protein TC10.[112] The GTP-bound and activated TC10 results from the localization of the CRK II-C3G complex to the lipid raft microdomain where the small G protein resides.[253] Proper localization to the lipid raft

through specific posttranslational modifications of TC10 and its activation appears to promote insulin-stimulated PI 3-kinase-dependent GLUT4 translocation and glucose transport.[253] This mechanism requires careful validation, as recent evidence suggests that depletion of Cbl isoforms, CAP, or CRK II does not impair insulin-stimulated GLUT4 translocation.[254]

GENETIC, METABOLIC, AND REGULATORY ASPECTS OF INSULIN SIGNALING

Insulin resistance is a common occurrence among human populations, and its association with obesity, advancing age, and physical inactivity is especially common in industrialized nations.[255] Increased insulin secretion can compensate for insulin resistance, but type 2 diabetes occurs when sufficient insulin is no longer secreted quickly enough.[1] A predominant cause for the imbalance between insulin action and insulin secretion in type 2 diabetes is difficult to establish, suggesting that a combination of defects is involved. Moreover, environmental challenges owing to chronic inflammatory or metabolic stress contribute to insulin resistance.

Polymorphisms have been identified in human genes encoding proximal signaling components that might contribute to metabolic disease. Although insulin receptor polymorphisms provide important insight into receptor function, they fail to uncover a general cause of type 2 diabetes.[256] A few polymorphisms in the gene for IRS-1 have been found, some of which are more common in type 2 diabetic patients[257]; however, they do not reveal a simple genetic basis for insulin resistance.[258] Gly972Arg mutation moderately decreases insulin-stimulated PI 3-kinase activation in cultured cells,[259,260] and associates with peripheral insulin resistance and impaired insulin secretion in certain backgrounds.[261,262] Two polymorphisms in IRS2, including Gly1057Asp and Gly879Ser substitutions, associate in females with impaired glucose tolerance, polycystic ovarian syndrome, and obesity.[261,263,264] A common polymorphism in p85α associates with a moderately reduced insulin sensitivity during an intravenous glucose tolerance test.[265] Similarly, mutations in AKT2 validate the importance of this kinase for insulin signaling in humans, but they do not explain insulin resistance encountered frequently in people.[187] Thus, genetic defects in the insulin signaling system validate the importance of the insulin signaling cascade, but they fail to explain the common causes of type 2 diabetes.

LESSONS LEARNED FROM INSULIN RECEPTOR MUTATIONS

Humans with rare mutations in the insulin receptor gene confirm that the insulin receptor mediates critical growth and metabolic signals. The informative polymorphisms impair synthesis or translocation of the receptor to the plasma membrane surface, insulin binding, transmembrane signaling, or endocytosis.[258] Depending on the allele, homozygous or double heterozygous individuals develop severe syndromes of insulin resistance with altered growth, such as leprechaunism or Rabson-Mendenhall syndrome.[256] Most affected individuals are heterozygous for the defective allele, but display severe insulin resistance owing to the dominant-negative effects on the functional receptor in covalent dimmers.[258] Interestingly, males with severe insulin resistance owing to receptor defects are hyperinsulinemic and usually not diabetic, suggesting that compensatory β-cell function is not impaired by dysregulated insulin receptor function. Thus, insulin resistance alone is insufficient to cause diabetes while β-cells secrete sufficient insulin to compensate for the resistance, reinforcing the role of β-cell failure in common type 2 diabetes.

Genetically altered mice reinforce these notions, and provide insight into how and where defects in insulin sensitivity and secretion occur. Disruption of the insulin receptor gene in mice does not significantly alter development; however, IR$^{-/-}$ mice develop hyperinsulinemia, hyperglycemia, and ketoacidosis immediately after birth.[30] By contrast, mice lacking the insulin receptor in skeletal muscle almost completely eliminates insulin signaling and insulin-stimulated glucose transport in isolated muscle; however, the mice display nearly normal glucose homeostasis and never develop hyperinsulinemia or physiologic insulin resistance.[266] This result contrasts the usual view that muscle is responsible for the vast majority of insulin-stimulated glucose disposal in the body, and the failure of insulin signaling in muscle in a primary cause of type 2 diabetes in humans.[267,268] By contrast, genetically altered mice deficient in GLUT4 in skeletal muscle develop insulin resistance and glucose intolerance.[269,270] Increases in IGF-1 receptor function in skeletal muscle apparently compensate in the absence of the insulin receptor gene.[271]

The progression of glucose intolerance to diabetes occurs when the β cells fail to produce enough insulin to overcome systemic insulin resistance. Mice with β-cell-specific deletion of the insulin receptor display a loss of first-phase insulin secretion in response to glucose.[272] This resembles the defect in insulin secretion observed in humans with type 2 diabetes.[273] Both insulin and IGF-1 receptors appears to contribute to β-cell function, possibly through tyrosine phosphorylation of Irs2.

ADIPOKINES AND INSULIN SIGNALING

Communication between adipocytes, other peripheral tissues, and the central nervous system reveals new insight into the relation between obesity and insulin resistance.[273,274] Adipose tissue secretes various proteins and metabolites that inhibit insulin signaling such as free fatty acids (FFAs), tumor necrosis factor-alpha (TNF-α), interleukin-6 (IL-6), and resistin, or those that promote insulin signaling such as adipocyte complement-related protein of 30 kilodaltons (adiponectin) and leptin.[50,275–280]

Leptin correlates closely with fasting insulin concentrations and the percentage of body fat, revealing leptin levels as a marker of obesity and insulin resistance.[277] Leptin binding to the long form of the leptin receptor promotes tyrosine phosphorylation of the cytoplasmic domain and the associated Janus kinase.[281,282] One of the phosphorylation sites in the leptin receptor (Tyr1138) binds STAT3, which is required for nutrient homeostasis by promoting melanocortin signaling.[283] Leptin might influence β-cell physiology by regulating levels of triglycerides and/or free fatty acids in the β cell, and reduce insulin secretion.[284] Thus, leptin signaling frames a rational basis to link obesity to the disruption of β-cell function at the molecular level.

TNF-α is an endogenous cytokine produced by macrophages and lymphocytes after inflammatory stimulation. Adipocytes of obese animals and humans overexpress TNF-α in positive correlation to body mass index and hyperinsulinemia; weight reduction decreases TNF-α expression.[285,286] TNF-α production in adipose tissue arises, at least in part, from the recruitment of macrophages.[287] TNF-α treatment increases serine phosphorylation of IRS-proteins, which inhibits insulin-stimulated tyrosine phosphorylation and impairs insulin signaling.[280,288,289] Disruption of both TNF-α receptor isoforms improves insulin sensitivity.[290] Troglitazone reduces the ability of TNF-α to cause insulin resistance, providing a rational mechanism by which thiazolidinediones might enhance insulin action.[291] Thus, localized production of TNF-α might link obesity to insulin resistance.

Adipose tissue macrophages increase in obesity and are responsible for significant amounts of IL-6 expression.[287] IL-6 derived from omental fat depots drains directly into the portal venous system, which can regulate hepatic triglyceride production, as well as insulin-stimulated glycogenesis.[292–294] Moreover, IL-6 treatment of primary hepatocytes and 3T3-L1 adipocytes impairs insulin signaling by reducing IRS-1 tyrosine phosphorylation and PI 3-kinase activity.[293–295] IL-6 administration into rodents and humans induces hepatic gluconeogenesis leading to hyperglycemia.[296] IL-6 inhibits lipoprotein lipase activity, which increases lipolysis and lipodystrophy.[297–299] Thus, locally produced IL-6 could regulate adipocyte function through an autocrine/paracrine mechanism. Since IL-6 is opposing the action of insulin under these conditions, it might induce lipolysis, at least in part, by inhibiting insulin action. IL-6 might cause insulin resistance by exerting inhibitory effects on IRS-1, glucose transporter GLUT4, and proxisome proliferation-activated receptor (PPAR-γ) gene transcription in 3T3-L1 adipocytes.[295]

Adiponectin is expressed exclusively by differentiated adipocytes.[300] Adiponectin normally circulates at a high concentration (1.9–17.0 μg/mL), which promotes insulin sensitivity. Adiponectin levels fall during obesity, but can be normalized upon weight loss, caloric restriction, or thiazolidinedione treatment that also increases insulin sensitivity. In general, adiponectin influences whole-body metabolism by enhancing insulin sensitivity in muscle and liver, and by increasing fatty acid oxidation in muscle.[301,302] Long-term administration of adiponectin to mice fed a high-fat diet causes profound weight loss by enhancing free fatty acid oxidation in muscles without affecting food intake. Some of these effects might be linked to the activation of AMP kinase, the phosphorylation of acetyl coenzyme A carboxylase, increased glucose uptake and fatty-acid oxidation, and reduced hepatic gluconeogenesis.[301] Adiponectin mediates these effects during association with membrane receptor, adipo1 or adipo2.[303] The mechanism that couples these receptors to AMP kinase and other signals is important to understand.

MULTISITE Ser/Thr PHOSPHORYLATION OF IRS-PROTEINS

Considerable data suggests that various pathologic conditions associated with insulin resistance promote serine/tyrosine phosphorylation of IRS-proteins. Stress-induced cytokines like TNF-α cause insulin resistance, at least in part, by serine phosphorylation of IRS-1 and IRS-2.[286,304] Disruption of the TNF-α receptor improves insulin sensitivity and glucose tolerance in obese mice.[290,305] Thus, the inhibitory effect of TNF-α appears to function through serine phosphorylation of the IRS-proteins.[53]

IRS-1 and IRS-2 each contain more than 100 potential serine/threonine phosphorylation sites; therefore, mapping the physiologically relevant ones is difficult. Many Ser/Thr-kinases phosphorylate IRS-proteins, including Raf, MEK, MAPK, p90rsk, Rho kinase (ROK-α), JNK, and PKC isoforms, and kinases downstream of the PI 3-kinase cascade: PDK1, AKT, mTOR, p70S6K, GKK3β.[225,306–314] The inhibitory role of the PI 3-kinase/AKT cascade might explain why partial inhibition of PI 3-kinase activity by disruption of various regulatory subunits increases insulin sensitivity.[157–159,315]

JNK binds directly to IRS1 and phosphorylates Ser307, which reveals a direct mechanism for inhibition of insulin signaling.[139] Ser307 phosphorylation inhibits tyrosine phosphorylation of IRS1 and the ability of IRS1 to activate the PI 3-kinase/AKT pathway in response to insulin.[140,306] Free fatty acids, which contribute to insulin resistance in obesity, also promote Ser307 phosphorylation through the activation of PKC.[316] The role of Ser307 phosphorylation has become a target of intense investigation by various groups.[141,316–320] Ser307 is phosphorylated in response to insulin or TNF-α in cultured adipocytes and muscles from mouse, rat, and human.[140] It is poorly phosphorylated in JNK–/– mice, suggesting that JNK-mediated phosphorylation of IRS1 is physiologically important (Fig. 50-8).[321]

IκB kinase β (IKKβ) cascade, which is implicated in inflammation-related insulin resistance, also mediates Ser307 phosphorylation.[322,323] IKKβ promotes TNF-α signaling during chronic obesity and trauma; heterozygous disruption of IKKβ protects against the development of insulin resistance during high-fat feeding and in obese leptin-deficient (ob/ob) mice.[318] IKKβ inhibitors (aspirin and salicylates) block TNF-α-induced Ser307 phosphorylation,[141] improving insulin sensitivity in obese rodents and in type 2 diabetes patients.[322,324,325]

The phosphorylation of other residues in IRS1 also contribute to inhibition of insulin signaling: Ser612, Ser632, Ser636, Ser662, Ser731, and Ser789.[326] Recently, PKCδ was shown to phosphorylate several serine residues that inhibit IRS1 tyrosine phosphorylation- Ser307, Ser323, and Ser574.[327] AMP kinase, which is activated by increased AMP levels during energy depletion, associates with IRS1 and phosphorylates S789, which promotes insulin-stimulated tyrosine

phosphorylation. The phosphorylation of Ser302 might prime IRS1 for tyrosine phosphorylation, revealing a positive role for serine phosphorylation.[328]

Several mechanisms have been proposed to explain how serine phosphorylation can regulate IRS1 signaling. Ser307 phosphorylation inhibits PTB domain function, which uncouples IRS1 from the insulin receptor.[138,329,330] Other sites might electrostatically block access to nearby tyrosine phosphorylation sites. Some phosphoserine residues in IRS1 bind 14-3-3 isoforms, which can target IRS1 to subcellular compartments.[331] Under conditions that activate the mTOR cascade, including prolonged insulin-stimulation but also other mTOR agonists, IRS-proteins are strongly degraded by the 26S proteasome.[332] IRS1 and IRS2 degradation is inhibited in various cell backgrounds by rapamycin, suggesting that the mTOR cascade plays a central role in this process.[332–334] Consistent with this model, constitutive activation of the mTOR cascade by mutations in TSC1 or TSC2 promote hyperphosphorylation of IRS1 and IRS2, leading to their degradation and insulin resistance (see Fig. 50-6B).[335] Degradation of IRS-proteins through the constitutively activated mTOR cascade reveals a potential explanation for the inhibitory effect of excess nutrients upon insulin signaling, and the positive effects of adiponectin upon insulin action (see Fig 50-6B).

SOCS1- AND SOCS3-MEDIATED IRS-PROTEIN DEGRADATION

Whereas Ser/Thr phosphorylation is a reversible processes that might be ideal for short-term negative regulation of insulin action, proteolysis of IRS1 and IRS2 causes long-term inhibition. In cultured cells, degradation of IRS1 and IRS2 is stimulated by TNF-α, interferon-γ, insulin, IGF-1, osmotic shock, platelet-derived growth factor, endothelin-1, free fatty acids, PMA, and inhibitors of serine/threonine phosphatase; and the degradation is blocked by 26S proteasome inhibitors.[336] In addition, ubiquitinylation of IRS-proteins is increased in response to chronic insulin and IGF-1, indicating that the ubiquitin/proteasome system is involved.[337,338]

One way that IRS-proteins are recruited to the elongin B/C-based ubiquitin-ligase is through SOCS1 or SOCS3 (Fig. 50-9).[336] These SOCS isoforms are cytokine-inducible gene products that suppress activity of various cytokine receptors by binding via their SH2 domain to the associated Janus kinase tyrosine kinases.[339] Overexpression of SOCS1 or SOCS3 also promotes ubiquitinylation and degradation of IRS1 and IRS2.[336] These SOCS isoforms are composed of an SH2 domain that binds to IRS1 or IRS2, and a BC box within the canonical SOCS box that binds to elongin C. Elongin C is a component of an E3-ubiquitin ligase that includes elongin B, a cullin family member, and Rbx-1.[340] This complex also associates with an ubiquitin-conjugating enzyme (E2) that catalyzes the transfer of ubiquitin from the ATP-dependent ubiquitin-activating enzyme (E1) to the SOCS-targeted protein.[339] Ubiquitin, a 76-amino acid peptide can also be ubiquitinylated on Lys48, forming polyubiquitin chains that target IRS-proteins for proteasome degradation. SOCS1 or SOCS3 mutants that fail to bind elongin BC-based ubiquitin ligase prevent ubiquitinylation and degradation of IRS1 and IRS2. The expression of recombinant SOCS1 in mouse liver by adenovirus-mediated gene transfer dramatically reduces hepatic IRS1 and IRS2, causing insulin resistance, whereas dysfunctional SOCS1 mutants have no effect.[336] Thus, one mechanism of IRS-protein degradation is through SOCS1- or SOCS3-mediated recruitment of a bc-based ubiquitin ligase (see Fig. 50-9).

PHOSPHOTYROSINE PHOSPHATASE 1B

Phosphotyrosine phosphatase 1B (PTP1B) directly dephosphorylates the insulin receptor, so it has a major effect on strength and duration of the insulin response.[341,342] PTP1B might also dephosphorylate IRS-proteins during their interaction with

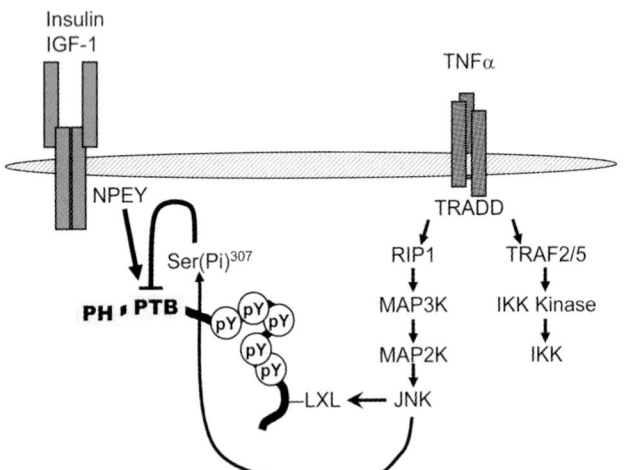

Figure 50-8 TNF-α-induced inhibition of IRS-protein signaling. TNF-α binding to TNFR1 results in recruitment of TRAF2/5, RIP1, and FADD through the adaptor protein TRADD. TRAF2/5 and RIP1 appear to lead to activation of the protein kinases JNK and IKK. Activated JNK associates with IRS1 and the JNK-binding LXL motif and promotes phosphorylation of Ser307. Phosphorylation of Ser307 inhibits PTB domain function and inhibits insulin/IGF stimulated tyrosine phosphorylation and signal transduction. FADD, FAS-associated death domain protein; IKK, IκB kinase; JNK, c-Jun N-terminal kinase; RIP1, receptor-interacting protein 1; TNF-α, tumor necrosis factor-alpha; TNFR1, TNF receptor type 1; TRAF2, TNF-receptor-associated factor 2.

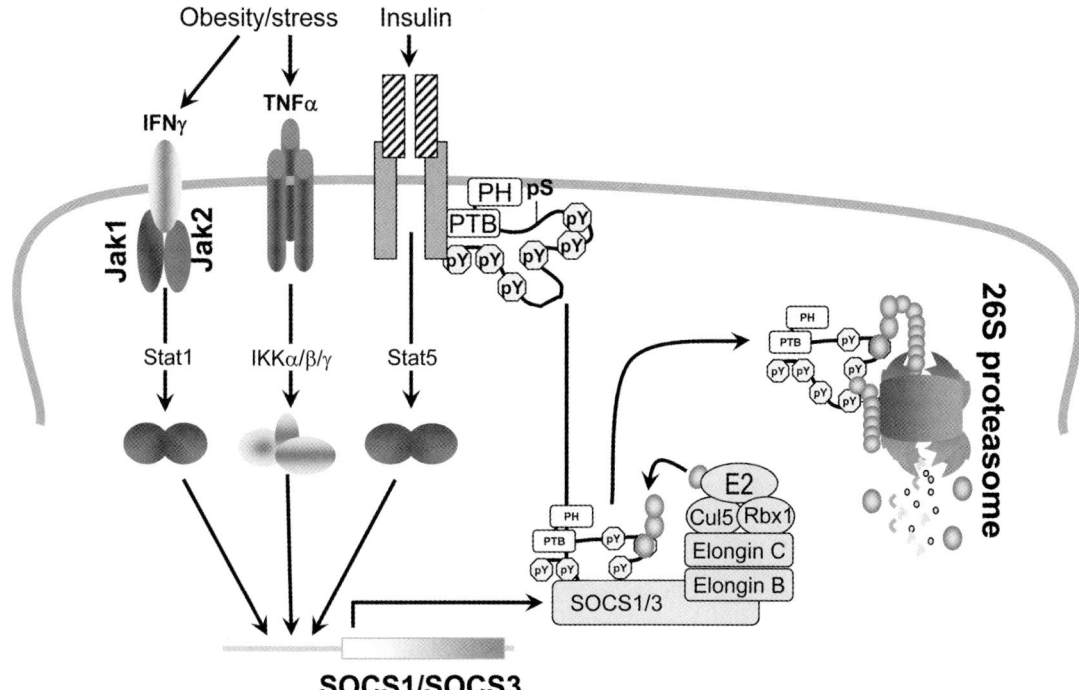

Figure 50-9 A potential mechanism of cytokine-induced insulin resistance based on the induced expression of SOCS1/3. Most proinflammatory cytokines that cause insulin resistance also induce the expression of SOCS family members.[384,385] SOCS family members contain an NH_2-terminal SH2 domain and a COOH-terminal SOCS box.[384,385] SOCS proteins might target proteins for ubiquitinylation and degradation, because the conserved SOCS box associates with elongin BC-containing ubiquitin ligase E3.[386–388] Ubiquitinylation is expected to promote degradation of IRS-protein through the 26S proteasome.

the insulin receptor, as PTP1B exhibits the highest activity toward IRS-1 among four other candidate protein-tyrosine phosphatases (PTP1B, SHP2, LAR, and LRP).[343] Overexpression of PTP1B inhibits insulin-stimulated phosphorylation of the insulin receptor and IRS-1, whereas neutralization of PTP1B by antibodies enhances insulin signaling.[344,345] PTP1B$^{-/-}$ mice display increased insulin sensitivity as revealed by enhanced phosphorylation of the insulin receptor and IRS-1 in muscle and liver.[52] PTP1B also plays a role in hypothalamic sensing of nutrient homeostasis, as PTP1B$^{-/-}$ mice are resistant to diet-induced obesity and insulin resistance; and energy dissipation in the PTP1B$^{-/-}$ mice is increased.[52,346] In ob/ob or db/db genetic background, reduction of PTP1B using antisense oligonucleotides improves insulin sensitivity in liver and fat, normalizing hyperglycemia.[347]

PTP1B has broad substrate specificity, but disruption of the PTP1B gene has its greatest effect on the insulin receptor. The functional specificity toward the insulin receptor appears to be determined by a combination of PTP1B targeting and the itinerary of the activated insulin receptor. Although PTP1B dephosphorylates epidermal growth factor (EGF) and platelet-derived growth factor (PDGF) receptors, they are largely degraded on internalization so dephosphorylation might not be important physiologically. By contrast, the insulin receptors are recycled to the plasma membrane so inactivation might be more dependent on dephosphorylation.[348] Consistent with this hypothesis, PTP1B associates rapidly with activated insulin receptor, as revealed by bioluminescence resonance energy transfer.[349] This approach to measure protein-protein interactions is very sensitive and reveals an almost immediate association between the activated insulin receptor and PTP1B. Transient interactions also occur before insulin stimulation suggesting that PTP1B might be important for maintaining the insulin receptor in an unphosphorylated inactive state. The insulin receptor associates most strongly with endoplasmic reticulum associated PTP1B, suggesting that internalization of the insulin receptor is an important step in its inactivation by the constitutively active PTP1B.[348,349]

PTEN

PTEN was identified as a tumor suppressor located at 10q23.[350] PTEN contains a phosphatase domain at its N terminus

and C2 domain and a PDZ-binding motif at the C terminus. The C2 domain might mediate its interaction with membrane lipids, whereas the PDZ-binding motif may bind to PDZ domain-containing proteins that associated with actin cytoskeleton to localize PTEN at plasma membrane subdomains. PTEN inhibits accumulation of both $PI(3,4)P_2$ and $PI(3,4,5)P_3$ induced by both constitutively active p110 and insulin stimulation.[351] Since PTEN efficiently dephosphorylates phosphoinositide at the 3 position both in vitro and in vivo, it is a negative regulator of PDK1, AKT, and their downstream targets (see Fig. 50-6).[314,352,353] Consistent with this conclusion, AKT activity is elevated in PTEN hypomorphs in accordance with the elevated $PI(3,4,5)P_3$. PTEN$^{+/-}$ mice die before birth, and PTEN$^{+/-}$ mice display increased tumor incidence.[354]

The expression of PTEN in 3T3L1 adipocytes inhibits insulin-stimulated phosphorylation and activation of Akt and p70 S6K; and it inhibits GLUT4 translocation and glucose uptake in response to insulin. As expected, PTEN does not inhibit tyrosine phosphorylation of IRS1 or its associated PI 3-kinase.[355] By contrast, inactive PTEN mutants enhance insulin-stimulated accumulation of $PI(3,4)P_2$ and $PI(3,4,5)P_3$, activation of Akt and glucose uptake in 3T3-L1 adipocytes.[351] In addition, specific inhibition of PTEN expression by antisense oligonucleotides normalized blood glucose concentrations in db/db and ob/ob mice, dramatically reduced insulin concentrations in ob/ob mice, and improved glucose tolerance of db/db mice.[356] Thus, PTEN activity downregulates insulin pathways and may contribute to insulin resistance and β-cell failure in diabetes.[7]

IRS-2 SIGNALING AND THE COMMON PATH TO DIABETES

Mice lacking the gene for IRS1$^{-/-}$ or IRS2$^{-/-}$ show marked effects of insulin resistance, including impaired peripheral glucose utilization.[116,357,358] However, metabolic dysregulation is more severe in IRS2$^{-/-}$ mice owing to excessive gluconeogenesis, decreased hepatic glycogen synthesis, and unsuppressed plasma free fatty acid/glycerol levels during the hyperinsulinemic-euglycemic clamp.[358] Progression to diabetes also depends on failure of pancreatic β cells to secrete sufficient insulin quickly enough to maintain normal serum glucose levels relative to the prevailing insulin sensitivity.

The insulin/IGF-1/IRS2 pathway has a major role in β-cell development and survival, especially during compensation for peripheral insulin resistance.[117] The progeny of inter-crossed mice heterozygous for null alleles of IGF-1R and IRS2 reveal that IGF-1 receptors promote β-cell development and survival through the IRS2 signaling pathway.[117] Targeted deletion of the IGF-1R in β-cells promotes age-dependent glucose intolerance owing to decreased glucose- and arginine-stimulated insulin release; however, there is no effect on β-cell growth.[359,360] Thus, the effect of IGF-1 on IRS2-medited β-cell growth and survival might not be β-cell autonomous, but might be more closely related to the growth and differentiation of precursors.

Many factors are required for proper β-cell function, including the homeodomain transcription factor PDX1. PDX1 mutations cause autosomal forms of MODY, because PDX1 regulates downstream genes needed for β-cell growth and function (see Fig. 50-1).[361,362] PDX1 is reduced in IRS2$^{-/-}$ islets, and PDX-1 haploinsufficiency further diminishes the function of β cells lacking IRS2.[10,363] Unexpectedly, transgenic PDX1 expressed in IRS2$^{-/-}$ mice restores β-cell function and normalizes glucose tolerance for at least 20 months.[363] Moreover, transgenic upregulation of IRS2 in wild-type or IRS2$^{-/-}$ islets increases PDX1 levels, supporting the hypothesis that PDX1 is regulated by IRS2 signaling cascades in β cells (Fig. 50-10).[8]

Some strains of C57Bl/6 IRS2$^{-/-}$ mice express sufficient PDX1 to prevent diabetes without additional genetic manipulations.[364] This apparent rescue might arise from natural variations in β-cell gene expression that increases the apparent activity of signals lying downstream of IRS2. For example, Foxo1 haploinsufficiency upregulates PDX1 in IRS2$^{-/-}$ islets/β-cells and prevents diabetes in the IRS2$^{-/-}$ mice (see Fig. 50-10).[10] Similarly, haploinsufficiency for PTEN also prevents diabetes in IRS2$^{-/-}$ mice, owing to the simulation of the PI 3-kinase PKB/Akt cascade that upregulates PDX1 (see Fig. 50-10). Thus, variations of downstream IRS2-mediated signals, through natural genetic drift or directed genetic manipulations, strongly compensate for IRS2 deletion and restore glucose tolerance.

Activation of signals upstream of IRS2 only temporarily restores the function of β cells lacking IRS2. As outlined previously, inhibition of PTP1B improves systemic insulin sensitivity and reduced systemic adiposity.[347] Moreover, disruption of the PTP1B gene temporarily restores β-cell function in

IRS2$^{-/-}$ mice; however, compound IRS2$^{-/-}$::PTP1B$^{-/-}$ mice eventually develop glucose intolerance and die when the β cells fail to compensate for age-related increases of insulin resistance.[7] These results suggest that IRS2, rather than the upstream receptor kinases, could be the "gatekeeper" for β-cell plasticity and function.

The discovery that cAMP agonists upregulate IRS2 reveals an unexpected mechanism to promote the growth function and survival of a variety of tissues. GLP1 secreted from the intestinal L cells during meals promotes β-cell function and peripheral insulin sensitivity in diabetic patients.[365] GLP1 promotes cAMP production and upregulates IRS2 in islets, hepatocytes, brain, and probably other tissues. Thus, inhibition of cAMP-regulated gene expression in β cells with a transgenic ACREB, a dominant-negative form of the cAMP response element binding protein (CREB), strongly suppresses IRS2 expression and causes β-cell apoptosis and glucose intolerance by 15 weeks of age.[366] We hypothesize that IRS2 is upregulated in β-cells and other tissues during the counterregulatory phase, which ensures β-cell function and peripheral insulin sensitivity during the next meal (see Fig. 50-10). Similar mechanism might occur in the brain and liver.

Finally, IRS2 signaling reveals a molecular link between obesity and peripheral insulin resistance. Dysregulated signaling, rather than antidotal consumption of high-calorie diets, might contribute to the early development of obesity that progresses to diabetes.[3,367,368] Insulin, leptin, and adiponectin are important peripheral signals that inform the brain of short- and long-term nutrient availability.[3,369,370] Pharmacologic inhibition of insulin signaling in the hypothalamus increases food intake, and conditional knockout of the insulin receptor in the brain causes obesity in mice on high-fat diets.[371–374] Leptin secreted from adipocytes promotes satiety and energy utilization, at least in part, by promoting alpha melanocyte-stimulating hormone (α-MSH) production in the hypothalamus.[367] Mutations that disrupt neuronal leptin or melanocortin signaling increase food intake, body weight, and peripheral insulin resistance in mice and people that progresses to diabetes if β-cell function also deteriorates.[375–377] Adiponectin, another adipocyte-derived hormone, enhances hepatic and muscle insulin action and promotes energy expenditure through signaling in the hypothalamus[303,369]; however, adiponectin is reduced in obese people and rodents which might promote disease progression.[378,379]

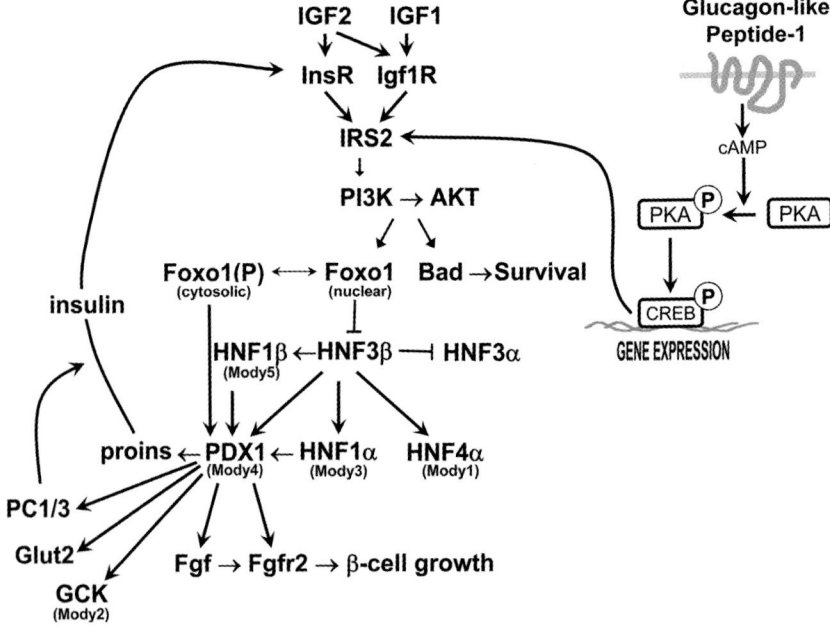

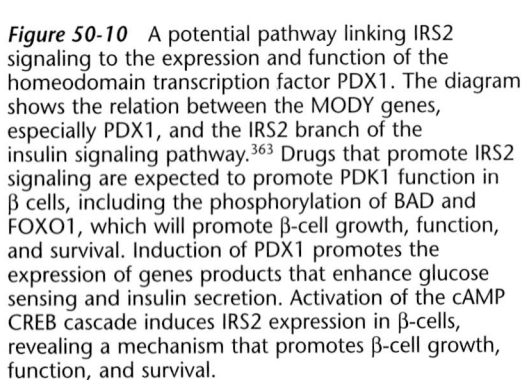

Figure 50-10 A potential pathway linking IRS2 signaling to the expression and function of the homeodomain transcription factor PDX1. The diagram shows the relation between the MODY genes, especially PDX1, and the IRS2 branch of the insulin signaling pathway.[363] Drugs that promote IRS2 signaling are expected to promote PDK1 function in β cells, including the phosphorylation of BAD and FOXO1, which will promote β-cell growth, function, and survival. Induction of PDX1 promotes the expression of genes products that enhance glucose sensing and insulin secretion. Activation of the cAMP CREB cascade induces IRS2 expression in β-cells, revealing a mechanism that promotes β-cell growth, function, and survival.

Previous work suggests that IRS2 signaling plays an important role in the central nervous system for brain growth, female fertility, and nutrient homeostasis.[380] Since IRS2 is highly expressed in the hypothalamus, its signaling cascade could integrate central control of nutrient homeostasis and appetite regulation with peripheral insulin action and β-cell function.[8] Female IRS2[−/−] mice, which develop diabetes more slowly that male mice, are hyperphagic and obese until severe diabetes causes weight loss.[380] To test the role of selective IRS2 dysregulation in obesity and diabetes, we flanked the IRS2 gene with loxP recombination sites (fIrs2) and crossed these mice with transgenic mice (TgN[Ins2Cre]25Mgn) expressing Cre recombinase under control of the rat insulin-2 promoter. Cre recombinase is expressed strongly in β cells and weakly in certain brain regions of these transgenic mice (cr[2] mice) including the hypothalamus.[381,382] Thus, our strategy strongly deletes fIrs2 alleles from β cells, and weakly deletes them from brain and certain neurons of the hypothalamus.

Our results suggest that partial dysregulation of IRS2 signaling in β cells and brain (hypothalamus) can explain the close association between obesity, peripheral insulin resistance, and β-cell failure that characterizes type 2 diabetes.[383] Whether dysregulation of IRS2 signaling contributes to type 2 diabetes and obesity in humans is unknown. However, many mechanisms are described that dysregulate IRS2 signaling in various tissues. Strategies to promote IRS2 expression in β cells and hypothalamus, or alleviate inhibition of IRS2 signaling in these tissues could be a rational approach to prevent or cure type 2 diabetes.

REFERENCES

1. White MF: Insulin signaling in health and disease. Science 302:1710–1711, 2003.
2. DeFronzo RA, Ferrannini E: Regulation of intermediary metabolism during fasting and feeding. In DeGroot LJ, Jameson JL (eds): Endocrinology, 4th ed. Philadelphia, WB Saunders, 2001, pp 737–755.
3. Schwartz MW, Woods SC, Porte D Jr, et al: Central nervous system control of food intake. Nature 404:661–671, 2000.
4. Fajans SS, Bell GI, Polonsky KS: Molecular mechanisms and clinical pathophysiology of maturity-onset diabetes of the young. N Engl J Med 345:971–980, 2001.
5. Frayling TM, Evans JC, Bulman MP, et al: Beta-cell genes and diabetes: Molecular and clinical characterization of mutations in transcription factors. Diabetes 50 (Suppl 1):S94–S100, 2001.
6. Froguel P, Velho G: Molecular genetics of maturity-onset diabetes of the young. Trends Endocrinol Metab 10:142–146, 1999.
7. Kushner JA, Haj FG, Klaman LD, et al: Islet-sparing effects of protein tyrosine phosphatase-1b deficiency delays onset of diabetes in IRS2 knockout mice. Diabetes 53:61–66, 2004.
8. Hennige AM, Burks DJ, Ozcan U, et al: Upregulation of insulin receptor substrate-2 in pancreatic beta cells prevents diabetes. J Clin Invest 112:1521–1532, 2003.
9. Otani K, Kulkarni RN, Baldwin AC, et al: Reduced beta-cell mass and altered glucose sensing impair insulin-secretory function in betaIRKO mice. Am J Physiol Endocrinol Metab 286:E41–E49, 2004.
10. Kitamura T, Nakae J, Kitamura Y, et al: The forkhead transcription factor Foxo1 links insulin signaling to Pdx1 regulation of pancreatic beta cell growth. J Clin Invest 110:1839–1847, 2002.
11. Roth J, Kahn CR, De Meyts P, et al: Receptors for insulin and other peptide hormones in disease states. In Bajaj JS (ed): Insulin and Metabolism. Amsterdam, Excerpta Medica, 1977, pp 73–80.
12. Brogiolo W, Stocker H, Ikeya, T et al: An evolutionarily conserved function of the Drosophila insulin receptor and insulin-like peptides in growth control. Curr Biol 11:213–221, 2001.
13. Frasca F, Pandini G, Scalia P, et al: Insulin receptor isoform A, a newly recognized, high-affinity insulin-like growth factor II receptor in fetal and cancer cells. Mol Cell Biol 19:3278–3288, 1999.
14. Sciacca L, Prisco M, Wu A, et al: Signaling differences from the A and B isoforms of the insulin receptor (IR) in 32D cells in the presence or absence of IR substrate-1. Endocrinology 144:2650–2658, 2003.
15. Mosthaf L, Grako K, Dull TJ, et al: Functionally distinct insulin receptors generated by tissue-specific alternative splicing. EMBO J 9:2409–2413, 1990.
16. Moller DE, Yokota A, Caro JF, Flier JS: Tissue -specific expression of two alternatively spliced insulin receptor mRNAs in man. Mol Endocrinol 3:1263–1269, 1989.
17. Goldstein BJ, Kahn CR: Analysis of mRNA heterogeneity by ribonuclease H mapping: Application to the insulin receptor. Biochem Biophys Res Commun 159:664–669, 1989.
18. Seino S, Bell GI: Alternative splicing of human insulin receptor messenger RNA. Biochem Biophys Res Commun 159:312–316, 1989.
19. Savkur RS, Philips AV, Cooper TA: Aberrant regulation of insulin receptor alternative splicing is associated with insulin resistance in myotonic dystrophy. Nat Genet 29:40–47, 2001.
20. Louvi A, Accili D, Efstratiadis A: Growth-promoting interaction of IGF-II with the insulin receptor during mouse embryonic development. Dev Biol 189:33–48, 1997.
21. Pandini G, Frasca F, Mineo R, et al: Insulin/insulin-like growth factor I hybrid receptors have different biological characteristics depending on the insulin receptor isoform involved. J Biol Chem 277:39684–39695, 2002.
22. Kimura KD, Tissenbaum HA, Liu Y, Ruvkun G: daf -2, an insulin receptor-like gene that regulates longevity and diapause in Caenorhabditis elegans [see comments]. Science 277:942–946, 1997.
23. Chen C, Jack J, Garofalo RS: The Drosophila insulin receptor is required for normal growth. Endocrinology 137:846–856, 1996.
24. Schubert M, Brazil DP, Burks DJ, et al: Insulin receptor substrate-2 deficiency impairs brain growth and promotes tau phosphorylation. J Neurosci 23:7084–7092, 2003.
25. Werner H, Beitner-Johnson D, Roberts CT, LeRoith D: Molecular comparisions of the insulin and IGF-1 receptors. In Draznin B, LeRoith D (eds): Molecular Biology of Diabetes II. Insulin Action, Effects on Gene Expression and Regulation, and Glucose Transport. Totowa, Humana, 1994, pp 377–392.
26. Beguinot F, Kahn CR, Moses AC, Smith RJ: Distinct biologically active receptors for insulin, insulin-like growth factor I, and insulin-like growth factor II in cultured skeletal muscle cells. J Biol Chem 260:15892–15898, 1985.
27. Kitamura T, Kahn CR, Accili D: Insulin receptor knockout mice. Annu Rev Physiol 65:313–332, 2003.
28. Dunger DB, Ong KK, Sandhu MS: Serum insulin-like growth factor-I levels and potential risk of type 2 diabetes. Horm Res 60(Suppl 3):131–135, 2003.
29. Okamoto H, Nakae J, Kitamura T, et al: Transgenic rescue of insulin receptor-deficient mice. J Clin Invest 114:214–223, 2004.
30. Accili D, Drago J, Lee EJ, et al: Early neonatal death in mice homozygous for a null allele of the insulin receptor gene. Nat Genet 12:106–109, 1996.
31. Joshi RL, Lamothe B, Cordonnier N, et al: Targeted disruption of the insulin receptor gene in the mouse results in neonatal lethality. EMBO J 15:1542–1547, 1996.
32. Baker J, Liu JP, Robertson EJ, Efstratiadis A: Role of insulin-like growth factors in embryonic and postnatal growth. Cell 75:73–82, 1993.
33. DeChiara TM, Efstratiadis A, Robertson EJ: A growth-deficiency phenotype in heterozygous mice carrying an insulin-like growth factor II gene disrupted by targeting. Nature 345:78–80, 1990.
34. Morrione A, Valentinis B, Xu SQ, et al: Insulin-like growth factor II stimulates cell proliferation through the insulin receptor. Proc Natl Acad Sci U S A 94:3777–3782, 1997.

35. Ozaki K: Insulin receptor-related receptor in rat islets of Langerhans. Eur J Endocrinol 139:244–247, 1998.

36. Nef S, Verma-Kurvari S, Merenmies J, et al: Testis determination requires insulin receptor family function in mice. Nature 426:291–295, 2003.

37. Hone J, Accili D, Psiachou H, et al: Homozygosity for a null allele of the insulin receptor gene in a patient with leprechaunism. Hum Mutat 6:17–22, 1995.

38. Kitamura T, Kitamura Y, Nakae J, et al: Mosaic analysis of insulin receptor function. J Clin Invest 113:209–219, 2004.

39. Clancy DJ, Gems D, Harshman LG, et al: Extension of life-span by loss of CHICO, a Drosophila insulin receptor substrate protein. Science 292:104–106, 2001.

40. Arantes-Oliveira N, Berman JR, Kenyon C: Healthy animals with extreme longevity. Science 302:611, 2003.

41. Finch CE, Ruvkun G: The genetics of aging. Annu Rev Genomics Hum Genet 2:435–462, 2001.

42. Libina N, Berman JR, Kenyon C: Tissue-specific activities of C. elegans DAF-16 in the regulation of lifespan. Cell 115:489–502, 2003.

43. Holzenberger M, Dupont J, Ducos B, et al: IGF-1 receptor regulates lifespan and resistance to oxidative stress in mice. Nature 421:182–187, 2003.

44. Bluher M, Kahn BB, Kahn CR: Extended longevity in mice lacking the insulin receptor in adipose tissue. Science 299:572–574, 2003.

45. Ullrich A, Bell JR, Chen EY, et al: Human insulin receptor and its relationship to the tyrosine kinase family of oncogenes. Nature 313:756–761, 1985.

46. Ebina Y, Ellis L, Jarnagin K, et al: The human insulin receptor cDNA: The structural basis for hormone activated transmembrane signalling. Cell 40:747–758, 1985.

47. Schlessinger J: Cell signaling by receptor tyrosine kinases. Cell 103:211–225, 2000.

48. Myers MG Jr, White MF: The new elements in insulin signaling. Insulin receptor substrate-1 and proteins with SH2 domains. Diabetes 42:643–650, 1993.

49. White MF, Kahn CR: The insulin signaling system. J Biol Chem 269:1–4, 1994.

50. Rosen ED, Spiegelman BM: Tumor necrosis factor-alpha as a mediator of the insulin resistance of obesity. Curr Opin Endocrinol Diab 6:170–176, 1999.

51. Chen H, Wertheimer SJ, Lin CH, et al: Protein-tyrosine phosphatases PTP1B and syp are modulators of insulin-stimulated translocation of GLUT4 in transfected rat adipose cells. J Biol Chem 272:8026–8031, 1997.

52. Elchebly M, Payette P, Michaliszyn E, et al: Increased insulin sensitivity and obesity resistance in mice lacking the protein tyrosine phosphatase-1B gene [see comments]. Science 283:1544–1548, 1999.

53. Zick Y: Role of Ser/Thr kinases in the uncoupling of insulin signaling. Int J Obes Relat Metab Disord 27 (Suppl 3):S56–S60, 2003.

54. Yang Feng TL, Francke U, Ullrich A: Gene for human insulin receptor: Localization to site on chromosome 19 involved in pre-B-cell leukemia. Science 228:728–731, 1985.

55. Seino S, Seino M, Nishi S, Bell GI: Structure of the human insulin receptor gene and characterization of its promoter. Proc Natl Acad Sci U S A 86:114–118, 1989.

56. Kasuga M, Hedo JA, Yamada KM, Kahn CR: The structure of the insulin receptor and its subunits: Evidence for multiple non-reduced forms and a 210K possible proreceptor. J Biol Chem 257:10392–10399, 1982.

57. Hedo JA, Kahn CR, Hayoshi M, et al: Biosynthesis and glycosylation of the insulin receptor. Evidence for a single polypeptide precursor of the two major subunits. J Biol Chem 258:10020–10026, 1983.

58. De Meyts P, Whittaker J: Structural biology of insulin and IGF1 receptors: Implications for drug design. Nat Rev Drug Discov 1:769–783, 2002.

59. Schumacher R, Soos MA, Schlessinger J, et al: A. Signaling-competent receptor chimeras allow mapping of major insulin receptor binding domain determinants. J Biol Chem 268:1087–1094, 1993.

60. Mynarcik DC, Yu GQ, Whittaker J: Alanine-scanning mutagenesis of a C-terminal ligand binding domain of the insulin receptor alpha subunit. J Biol Chem 271:2439–2442, 1996.

61. Yip CC, Ottensmeyer P: Three-dimensional structural interactions of insulin and its receptor. J Biol Chem 278:27329–27332, 2003.

62. Luo RZ, Beniac DR, Fernandes A, et al: Quaternary structure of the insulin-insulin receptor complex. Science 285:1077–1080, 1999.

63. De Meyts P: Insulin and insulin-like growth factors: The paradox of signaling specificity. Growth Horm IGF Res 12:81–83, 2002.

64. Kasuga M, Zick Y, Blithe DL, et al: Insulin stimulation of phosphorylation of the β-subunit of the insulin receptor: Formation of both phosphoserine and phosphotyrosine. J Biol Chem 257:9891–9894, 1982.

65. Rosen OM, Herrera R, Olowe Y, et al: Phosphorylation activates the insulin receptor tyrosine protein kinase. Proc Natl Acad Sci U S A 80:3237–3240, 1983.

66. White MF, Haring HU, Kasuga M, Kahn CR: Kinetic properties and sites of autophosphorylation of the partially purified insulin receptor from hepatoma cells. J Biol Chem 259:255–264, 1984.

67. Krook A, O'Rahilly S: Mutant insulin receptors in syndromes of insulin resistance. Baillieres Clin Endocrinol Metab 10:97–122, 1996.

68. Chou CK, Dull TJ, Russell DS, et al: Human insulin receptors mutated at the ATP-binding site lack protein tyrosine kinase activity and fail to mediate postreceptor effects of insulin. J Biol Chem 262:1842–1847, 1987.

69. Cama A, de la Luz Sierra M, Ottini L, et al: A mutation in the tyrosine kinase domain of the insulin receptor associated with insulin resistance in an obese woman. J Clin Endocrinol Metab 73:894–901, 1991.

70. White MF, Shoelson SE, Keutmann H, Kahn CR: A cascade of tyrosine autophosphorylation in the β-subunit activates the insulin receptor. J Biol Chem 263:2969–2980, 1988.

71. Wilden PA, Siddle K, Haring E, et al: The role of insulin receptor kinase domain autophosphorylation in receptor-mediated activities. J Biol Chem 267:13719–13727, 1992.

72. Cann AD, Kohanski RA: Cis-autophosphorylation of juxtamembrane tyrosines in the insulin receptor kinase domain. Biochemistry 36:7681–7689, 1997.

73. Myers MG Jr, Backer JM, Siddle K, White MF: The insulin receptor functions normally in Chinese hamster ovary cells after truncation of the C-terminus. J Biol Chem 266:10616–10623, 1991.

74. Maegawa H, McClain DA, Freidneberg G, et al: Properties of a human insulin receptor with a COOH-terminal trancation II. Truncated receptors have normal kinase activity but are defective in signaling metabolic effects. J Biol Chem 263:8912–8917, 1998.

75. McClain DA, Maegawa H, Levy J, et al: Properties of a human insulin receptor with a COOH-terminal truncation. I. Insulin binding, autophosphorylation and endocytosis. J Biol Chem 263:8904–8912, 1988.

76. Backer JM, Shoelson SE, Weiss MA, et al: The insulin receptor juxtamembrane region contains two independent tyrosine/beta-turn internalization signals. J Cell Biol 118:831–839, 1992.

77. Baron V, Gautier N, Kaliman P, et al: The carboxyl-terminal domain of the insulin receptor: Its potential role in growth-promoting effects. Biochemistry 30:9365–9370, 1991.

78. Levy-Toledano R, Blaettler DH, Larochelle WJ, Taylor SI: Insulin-induced activation of phosphatidylinositol (PI) 3-kinase. J Biol Chem 270:30018–30022, 1995.

79. Van Horn DJ, Myers MG Jr, Backer JM: Direct activation of the phosphatidylinositol 3'-kinase by the insulin receptor. J Biochem 269:29–32, 1994.

80. Yenush L, Fernandez R, Myers MG Jr, et al: The drosophila insulin receptor activates multiple signaling pathways but requires IRS-proteins for DNA synthesis. Mol Cell Biol 16:2509–2517, 1996.

81. Wilden PA, Backer JM, Kahn CR, et al: The insulin receptor with phenylalanine

replacing tyrosine-1146 provides evidence for separate signals regulating cellular metabolism and growth. Proc Natl Acad Sci U S A 87:3358–3362, 1990.

82. Wilden PA, Kahn CR, Siddle K, White MF: Insulin receptor kinase domain autophosphorylation regulates receptor enzymatic function. J Biol Chem 267:16660–16668, 1992.

83. Hubbard SR: Crystal structure of the activated insulin receptor tyrosine kinase in complex with peptide substrate and ATP analog. EMBO J 16:5572–5581, 1997.

84. Li S, Covino ND, Stein EG, et al: Structural and biochemical evidence for an autoinhibitory role for tyrosine 984 in the juxtamembrane region of the insulin receptor. J Biol Chem 278:26007–26014, 2003.

85. Till JH, Ablooglu AJ, Frankel M, et al: Crystallographic and solution studies of an activation loop mutant of the insulin receptor tyrosine kinase: Insights into kinase mechanism. J Biol Chem 276:10049–10055, 2001.

86. Hubbard SR, Wei L, Ellis L, Hendrickson WA: Crystal structure of the tyrosine kinase domain of the human insulin receptor. Nature 372:746–754, 1994.

87. Sawka-Verhelle D, Tartare-Deckert S, White MF, Van Obberghen E: IRS-2 binds to the insulin receptor through its PTB domain and through a newly identified domain comprising amino acids 591 to 786. J Biol Chem 271:5980–5983, 1996.

88. Sawka-Verhelle D, Baron V, Mothe I, et al: Tyr624 and Tyr628 in insulin receptor substrate-2 mediate its association with the insulin receptor. J Biol Chem 272:16414–16420, 1997.

89. Liu F, Roth RA: Grb-IR: A SH2 domain-containing protein that binds to the insulin receptor and inhibits its function. Proc Natl Acad Sci U S A 92:10287–10291, 1995.

90. Hu J, Liu J, Ghirlando R, et al: Structural basis for recruitment of the adaptor protein APS to the activated insulin receptor. Mol Cell 12:1379–1389, 2003.

91. Minami A, Iseki M, Kishi K, et al: Increased insulin sensitivity and hypoinsulinemia in APS knockout mice. Diabetes 52:2657–2665, 2003.

91a. Kotani K, Wilden P, Pillay TS: SH2-B alpha is an insulin-receptor adapter protein and substrate that interacts with the activation loop of the insulin-receptor kinase. Biochem J 335(Pt 1):103–109, 1998.

91b. Moodie SA, Ieman-Sposeto J, Gustafson TA: Identification of the APS protein as a novel insulin receptor substrate. J Biol Chem 274(16):11186–11193, 1999.

91c. Nelms K, O'Neill TJ, Li S, et al: Alternative splicing, gene localization, and binding of SH2-B to the insulin receptor kinase domain. Mamm Genome 10(12):1160–1167, 1999.

91d. Ahmed Z, Pillay TS: Adapter protein with a pleckstrin homology (PH) and an Src homology 2 (SH2) domain (APS) and SH2-B enhance insulin-receptor autophosphorylation, extracellular-signal-regulated kinase and phosphoinositide 3-kinase-dependent signalling. Biochem J 371(Pt 2):405–412, 2003.

92. Duan C, Yang H, White MF, Rui L: Disruption of SH2-B Causes Age-dependent Insulin Resistance and Glucose Intolerance. Mol Cell Biol 24(17):7435–7443, 2004.

93. White MF, Livingston JN, Backer JM, et al: Mutation of the insulin receptor at tyrosine 960 inhibits signal transmission but does not affect its tyrosine kinase activity. Cell 54:641–649, 1988.

94. Backer JM, Kahn CR, Cahill DA, et al: Receptor-mediated internalization of insulin requires a 12-amino acid sequence in the juxtamembrane region of the insulin receptor β-subunit. J Biol Chem 265:16450–16454, 1990.

95. Hubbard SR: Juxtamembrane autoinhibition in receptor tyrosine kinases. Nat Rev Mol Cell Biol 5:464–471, 2004.

96. Feener EP, Backer JM, King GL, et al: Insulin stimulates serine and tyrosine phosphorylation in the juxtamembrane region of the insulin receptor. J Biol Chem 268:11256–11264, 1993.

97. Songyang Z, Carraway KL III, Eck MJ, et al: Catalytic specificity of protein-tyrosine kinases is critical for selective signalling. Nature 373:536–539, 1995.

98. Songyang Z, Cantley LC: Recognition and specificity in protein tyrosine kinase-mediated signaling. TIBS 20:470–475, 1995.

99. Shoelson SE, Chatterjee S, Chaudhuri M, White MF: YMXM motifs of IRS-1 define the substrate specificity of the insulin receptor kinase. Proc Natl Acad Sci U S A 89:2027–2031, 1992.

100. Kasuga M, Karlsson FA, Kahn CR: Insulin stimulates the phosphorylation of the 95,000-dalton subunit of its own receptor. Science 215:185–187, 1982.

101. Kasuga M, Zick Y, Blithe DL, et al: Insulin stimulates tyrosine phosphorylation of the insulin receptor in a cell-free system. Nature 298:667–669, 1982.

102. White MF, Maron R, Kahn CR: Insulin rapidly stimulates tyrosine phosphorylation of a Mr 185,000 protein in intact cells. Nature 318:183–186, 1985.

103. Sun XJ, Rothenberg PL, Kahn CR, et al: The structure of the insulin receptor substrate IRS-1 defines a unique signal transduction protein. Nature 352:73–77, 1991.

104. Sun XJ, Crimmins DL, Myers MG Jr, et al: Pleiotropic insulin signals are engaged by multisite phosphorylation of IRS-1. Mol Cell Biol 13:7418–7428, 1993.

105. Backer JM, Myers MG Jr, Shoelson SE, et al: Phosphatidylinositol 3'-kinase is activated by association with IRS-1 during insulin stimulation. EMBO J 11:3469–3479, 1992.

106. Nelms K, O'Neill TJ, Li S, et al: Alternative splicing, gene localization, and binding of SH2-B to the insulin receptor kinase domain. Mamm Genome 10:1160–1167, 1999.

107. Yenush L, White MF: The IRS-signaling system during insulin and cytokine action. Bio Essays 19:491–500, 1997.

108. Pawson T, Scott JD: Signaling through scaffold, anchoring, and adaptor proteins. Science 278:2075–2080, 1997.

109. Kotani K, Wilden P, Pillay TS: SH2-Balpha is an insulin-receptor adapter protein and substrate that interacts with the activation loop of the insulin-receptor kinase. Biochem J 335(Pt 1):103–109, 1998.

110. Lock P, Casagranda F, Dunn AR: Independent SH2-binding sites mediate interaction of Dok-related protein with RasGTPase-activating protein and Nck. J Biol Chem 274:22775–22784, 1999.

111. Noguchi T, Matozaki T, Inagaki K, et al: Tyrosine phosphorylation of p62(Dok) induced by cell adhesion and insulin: Possible role in cell migration. EMBO J 18:1748–1760, 1999.

112. Chiang SH, Baumann CA, Kanzaki M, et al: Insulin-stimulated GLUT4 translocation requires the CAP-dependent activation of TC10. Nature 410:944–948, 2001.

113. Baumann CA, Ribon V, Kanzaki M, et al: CAP defines a second signalling pathway required for insulin-stimulated glucose transport [see comments]. Nature 407:202–207, 2000.

114. Uchida T, Myers MG Jr, White MF: IRS-4 mediates activation of PKB/Akt during insulin stimulation without inhibition of apoptosis. Mol Cell Biol 20:126–138, 2000.

115. Laustsen PG, Michael MD, Crute BE, et al: Lipoatrophic diabetes in Irs1(–/–)/Irs3(–/–) double knockout mice. Genes Dev 16:3213–3222, 2002.

116. Withers DJ, Gutierrez JS, Towery H, et al: Disruption of IRS-2 causes type 2 diabetes in mice. Nature 391:900–904, 1998.

117. Withers DJ, Burks DJ, Towery HH, et al: Irs-2 coordinates Igf-1 receptor-mediated beta-cell development and peripheral insulin signalling. Nat Genet 23:32–40, 1999.

118. Kido Y, Burks DJ, Withers DJ, et al: Tissue-specific insulin resistance in mice with mutations of the insulin receptor, IRS-1 and IRS-2. J Clin Invest 105:199–205, 2000.

119. Bjornholm M, He AR, Attersand A, et al: Absence of functional insulin receptor substrate-3 (IRS-3) gene in humans. Diabetologia 45:1697–1702, 2002.

120. Dhe-Paganon S, Ottinger EA, Nolte RT, et al: Crystal structure of the pleckstrin homology-phosphotyrosine binding (PH-PTB) targeting region of insulin

receptor substrate 1. Proc Natl Acad Sci U S A 96:8378–8383, 1999.

121. Yenush L, Zanella C, Uchida T, et al: The pleckstrin homology and phosphotyrosine binding domains of insulin receptor substrate 1 mediate inhibition of apoptosis by insulin. Mol Cell Biol 18:6784–6794, 1998.

122. Tsuruzoe K, Emkey R, Kriaucunas KM, et al: Insulin receptor substrate 3 (IRS-3) and IRS-4 impair IRS-1- and IRS-2-mediated signaling. Mol Cell Biol 21:26–38, 2000.

123. Uchida T, Myers MG Jr, White MF: IRS-4 mediates protein kinase B signaling during insulin stimulation without promoting antiapoptosis. Mol Cell Biol 20:126–138, 2000.

124. Cai D, Dhe-Paganon S, Melendez PA, et al: Two new substrates in insulin signaling, IRS5/DOK4 and IRS6/DOK5. J Biol Chem 278:25323–25330, 2003.

125. Yenush L, Makati KJ, Smith-Hall J, et al: The pleckstrin homology domain is the principle link between the insulin receptor and IRS-1. J Biol Chem 271:24300–24306, 1996.

126. Burks DJ, Pons S, Towery H, et al: Heterologous PH domains do not mediate coupling of IRS-1 to the insulin receptor. J Biol Chem 272:27716–27721, 1997.

127. Keegan AD, Nelms K, White MF, et al: An IL-4 receptor region containing an insulin receptor motif is important for IL-4-mediated IRS-1 phosphorylation and cell growth. Cell 76:811–820, 1994.

128. Lemmon MA, Ferguson KM, Schlessinger J: PH domains: Diverse sequences with a common fold recruit signaling molecules to the cell surface. Cell 85:621–624, 1996.

129. Lemmon MA, Ferguson KM, Abrams CS: Pleckstrin homology domains and the cytoskeleton. Growth Regul 513:71–76, 2002.

130. Burks DJ, Wang J, Towery H, et al: IRS pleckstrin homology domains bind to acidic motifs in proteins. J Biol Chem 273:31061–31067, 1998.

131. Tu X, Baffa R, Luke S, et al: Intracellular redistribution of nuclear and nucleolar proteins during differentiation of 32D murine hemopoietic cells. Exp Cell Res 288:119–130, 2003.

132. Tu X, Wu A, Maiorana A, et al: Subcellular localization of IRS-1 in cell proliferation and differentiation. Horm Metab Res 35:734–739, 2003.

133. Wu A, Sciacca L, Baserga R: Nuclear translocation of insulin receptor substrate-1 by the insulin receptor in mouse embryo fibroblasts. J Cell Physiol 195:453–460, 2003.

134. Farhang-Fallah J, Yin X, Trentin G, et al: Cloning and characterization of PHIP, a novel insulin receptor substrate-1 pleckstrin homology domain interacting protein. J Biol Chem 275:40492–40497, 2000.

135. Skolnik EY, Lee CH, Batzer AG, et al: The SH2/SH3 domain-containing protein GRB2 interacts with tyrosine-phosphorylated IRS-1 and Shc: Implications for insulin control of ras signalling. EMBO J 12:1929–1936, 1993.

136. Weston CR, Lambright DG, Davis RJ: Signal transduction. MAP kinase signaling specificity. Science 296:2345–2347, 2002.

137. Ip YT, Davis RJ: Signal transduction by the c-Jun N-terminal kinase (JNK)—from inflammation to development. Curr Opin Cell Biol 10:205–219, 1998.

138. Aguirre V, Werner ED, Giraud J, et al: Phosphorylation of Ser307 in insulin receptor substrate-1 blocks interactions with the insulin receptor and inhibits insulin action. J Biol Chem 277:1531–1537, 2002.

139. Lee YH, Giraud J, Davis RJ, White MF: c-Jun N-terminal kinase (JNK) mediates feedback inhibition of the insulin signaling cascade. J Biol Chem 278:2896–2902, 2003.

140. Rui L, Aguirre V, Kim JK, et al: Insulin/IGF-1 and TNF-alpha stimulate phosphorylation of IRS-1 at inhibitory Ser307 via distinct pathways. J Clin Invest 107:181–189, 2001.

141. Jiang G, Dallas-Yang Q, Liu F, et al: Salicylic acid reverses phorbol 12-myristate-13-acetate (PMA) and tumor necrosis factor alpha (TNFalpha)-induced insulin receptor substrate 1 (IRS1) serine 307 phosphorylation and insulin resistance in human embryonic kidney 293 (HEK293) cells. J Biol Chem 278:180–186, 2003.

142. Sawka-Verhelle D, Baron V, Mothe I, et al: Tyr624 and Tyr628 in insulin receptor substrate-2 mediate its association with the insulin receptor. Am Soc Biochem Mol Biol 272:16414-16420,1997.

143. Fruman DA, Meyers RE, Cantley LC: Phosphoinositide kinases. Annu Rev Biochem 67:481–507, 1998.

144. Vanhaesebroeck B, Leevers SJ, Panayotou G, Waterfield MD: Phosphoinositide 3-kinases: A conserved family of signal transducers. Trends Biochem Sci 22:267–272, 1997.

145. Fruman DA, Cantley LC, Carpenter CL: Structural organization and alternative splicing of the murine phosphoinositide 3-kinase p85α gene. Genomics 37:113–121, 1996.

146. Pons S, Asano T, Glasheen EM, et al: The structure and function of p55^{PIK} reveals a new regulatory subunit for the phosphatidylinositol-3 kinase. Mol Cell Biol 15:4453–4465, 1995.

147. Woscholski R, Kodaki T, McKinnon M, et al: A comparison of demethoxyviridin and wortmannin as inhibitors of phosphatidylinositol 3-kinase. FEBS Lett 342:109–114, 1994.

148. Yu J, Wjasow C, Backer JM: Regulation of the p85/p110alpha phosphatidylinositol 3'-kinase. Distinct roles for the n-terminal and c-terminal SH2 domains. J Biol Chem 273:30199–30203, 1998.

149. Fruman DA, Mauvais-Jarvis F, Pollard DA, et al: Hypoglycaemia, liver necrosis and perinatal death in mice lacking all isoforms of phosphoinositide 3-kinase p85 alpha. Nat Genet 26:379–382, 2000.

150. Rordorf-Nikolic T, Van Horn DJ, Chen D, et al: Regulation of phosphatidylinositol 3-kinase by tyrosyl phosphoproteins. Full activation requires occupancy of both SH2 domains in the 85 kDa regulatory subunit. J Biol Chem 270:3662–3666, 1995.

151. Cuevas BD, Lu Y, Mao M, et al: Tyrosine phosphorylation of p85 relieves its inhibitory activity on phosphatidylinositol 3-kinase. J Biol Chem 276:27455–27461, 2001.

152. Rodriguez-Viciana P, Warne PH, Dhand R, et al: Phosphatidylinositol-3-OH kinase as a direct target of Ras. Nature 370:527–532, 1994.

153. Rodriguez-Viciana P, Warne PH, Vanhaesebroeck B, et al: Activation of phosphoinositide 3-kinase by interaction with Ras and by point mutation. EMBO J 15:2442–2451, 1996.

154. Marte BM, Rodriguez-Viciana P, Wennstrom S, et al: R-Ras can activate the phosphoinositide 3-kinase but not the MAP kinase arm of the Ras effector pathways [published erratum appears in Curr Biol 7:197, 1997]. Curr Biol 7:63–70, 1997.

155. Khwaja A, Rodriguez-Viciana P, Wennstrom S, et al: Matrix adhesion and Ras transformation both activate a phosphoinositide 3-OH kinase and protein kinase B/Akt cellular survival pathway. EMBO J 16:2783–2793, 1997.

156. Terauchi Y, Tsuji T, Satoh S, et al: Increased insulin sensitivity and hypoglycaemia in mice lacking the p85 alpha subunit of phosphoinositide 3-kinase. Nat Genet 21:230–235, 1999.

157. Ueki K, Fruman DA, Brachmann SM, et al: Molecular balance between the regulatory and catalytic subunits of phosphoinositide 3-kinase regulates cell signaling and survival. Mol Cell Biol 22:965–977, 2002.

158. Ueki K, Yballe CM, Brachmann SM, et al: Increased insulin sensitivity in mice lacking p85beta subunit of phosphoinositide 3-kinase. Proc Natl Acad Sci U S A 99:419–424, 2002.

159. Ueki K, Fruman DA, Yballe CM, et al: Positive and negative roles of p85 alpha and p85 beta regulatory subunits of phosphoinositide 3-kinase in insulin signaling. J Biol Chem 278:48453–48466, 2003.

160. Hallmann D, Trumper K, Trusheim H, et al: Altered signaling and cell cycle regulation in embryonal stem cells with a disruption of the gene for phosphoinositide 3-kinase regulatory subunit p85alpha. J Biol Chem 278:5099–5108, 2003.

161. Bi L, Okabe I, Bernard DJ, et al: Proliferative defect and embryonic lethality in mice homozygous for a deletion in the p110alpha subunit of

phosphoinositide 3-kinase. J Biol Chem 274:10963–10968, 1999.

162. Asano T, Kanda A, Katagiri H, et al: p110beta is up-regulated during differentiation of 3T3-L1 cells and contributes to the highly insulin-responsive glucose transport activity. J Biol Chem 275:17671–17676, 2000.

163. Kim YB, Ciaraldi TP, Kong A, et al: Troglitazone but not metformin restores insulin-stimulated phosphoinositide 3-kinase activity and increases p110beta protein levels in skeletal muscle of type 2 diabetic subjects. Diabetes 51:443–448, 2002.

164. Collins BJ, Deak M, Arthur JS, et al: In vivo role of the PIF-binding docking site of PDK1 defined by knock-in mutation. EMBO J 22:4202–4211, 2003.

165. Mora A, Komander D, van Aalten DM, Alessi DR: PDK1, the master regulator of AGC kinase signal transduction. Semin Cell Dev Biol 15:161–170, 2004.

166. Brazil DP, Park J, Hemmings BA: PKB binding proteins. Getting in on the Akt. Cell 111:293–303, 2002.

167. Scheid MP, Woodgett JR: PKB/AKT: Functional insights from genetic models. Nat Rev Mol Cell Biol 2:760–768, 2001.

168. Lawlor MA, Alessi DR: PKB/Akt: A key mediator of cell proliferation, survival and insulin responses? J Cell Sci 114(Pt 16):2903–2910, 2001.

169. Avruch J, Belham C, Weng Q, et al: The p70 S6 kinase integrates nutrient and growth signals to control translational capacity. Prog Mol Subcell Biol 26:115–154, 2001.

170. Thomas G: The S6 kinase signaling pathway in the control of development and growth. Biol Res 35:305–313, 2002.

171. Frodin M, Gammeltoft S: Role and regulation of 90 kDa ribosomal S6 kinase (RSK) in signal transduction. Mol Cell Endocrinol 151:65–77, 1999.

172. Frodin M, Jensen CJ, Merienne K, Gammeltoft S: A phosphoserine-regulated docking site in the protein kinase RSK2 that recruits and activates PDK1. EMBO J 19:2924–2934, 2000.

173. Lang F, Cohen P: Regulation and physiological roles of serum- and glucocorticoid-induced protein kinase isoforms. Sci STKE RE17, 2001.

174. Storz P, Toker A: 3′-phosphoinositide-dependent kinase-1 (pdk-1) in pi 3-kinase signaling. Front Biosci 7:D886–D902, 2002.

175. Alessi DR: Discovery of PDK1, one of the missing links in insulin signal transduction. Colworth Medal Lecture. Biochem Soc Trans 29(Pt 2):1–14, 2001.

176. Coffer PJ, Jin J, Woodgett JR: Protein kinase B (c-Akt): A multifunctional mediator of phosphatidylinositol 3-kinase activation. Biochem J 335(Pt 1):1–13, 1998.

177. Murthy SS, Tosolini A, Taguchi T, Testa JR: Mapping of AKT3, encoding a member of the Akt/protein kinase B family, to human and rodent chromosomes by fluorescence in situ hybridization. Cytogenet Cell Genet 88:38–40, 2000.

178. Kohn AD, Summers SA, Birnbaum MJ, Roth RA: Expression of a constitutively active Akt Ser/Thr kinase in 3T3-L1 adipocytes stimulates glucose uptake and glucose transporter 4 translocation. J Biol Chem 271:31372–31378, 1996.

179. Hajduch E, Alessi DR, Hemmings BA, Hundal HS: Constitutive activation of protein kinase B alpha by membrane targeting promotes glucose and system A amino acid transport, protein synthesis, and inactivation of glycogen synthase 3 in L6 muscle cells. Diabetes 47:1006–1013, 1998.

180. Hill MM, Clark SF, Tucker DF, et al: A role for protein kinase Bbeta/Akt2 in insulin-stimulated GLUT4 translocation in adipocytes. Mol Cell Biol 19:7771–7781, 1999.

181. Takata M, Ogawa W, Kitamura T, et al: Requirement for Akt (protein kinase B) in insulin-induced activation of glycogen synthase and phosphorylation of 4E-BP1 (PHAS-1). J Biol Chem 274:20611–20618, 1999.

182. Ducluzeau PH, Fletcher LM, Welsh GI, Tavare JM: Functional consequence of targeting protein kinase B/Akt to GLUT4 vesicles. J Cell Sci 115(Pt 14):2857–2866, 2002.

183. Cichy SB, Uddin S, Danilkovich A, et al: Protein kinase B/Akt mediates effects of insulin on hepatic insulin-like growth factor-binding protein-1 gene expression through a conserved insulin response sequence. J Biol Chem 273:6482–6487, 1998.

184. Shioi T, McMullen JR, Kang PM, et al: Akt/protein kinase B promotes organ growth in transgenic mice. Mol Cell Biol 22:2799–2809, 2002.

185. Cho H, Thorvaldsen JL, Chu Q, et al: Akt1/PKBalpha is required for normal growth but dispensable for maintenance of glucose homeostasis in mice. J Biol Chem 276:38349–38352, 2001.

186. Cho H, Mu J, Kim JK, et al: Insulin resistance and a diabetes mellitus-like syndrome in mice lacking the protein kinase Akt2 (PKB beta). Science 292:1728–1731, 2001.

186a. Cho H, Mu J, Kim JK, et al: Insulin resistance and a diabetes mellitus-like syndrome in mice lacking the protein kinase Akt2 (PKB beta). Science 292(5522):1728–1731, 2001.

186b. Cho H, Thorvaldsen JL, Chu Q, et al: Akt1/PKB alpha is required for normal growth but dispensable for maintenance of glucose homeostasis in mice. J Biol Chem 276(42):38349-38352, 2001.

187. George S, Rochford JJ, Wolfrum C, et al: A family with severe insulin resistance and diabetes due to a mutation in AKT2. Science 304:1325–1328, 2004.

188. Biondi RM, Kieloch A, Currie RA, et al: The PIF-binding pocket in PDK1 is essential for activation of S6K and SGK, but not PKB. EMBO J 20:4380–4390, 2001.

189. Frodin M, Antal TL, Dummler BA, et al: A phosphoserine/threonine-binding pocket in AGC kinases and PDK1 mediates activation by hydrophobic motif phosphorylation. EMBO J 21:5396–5407, 2002.

190. Jensen CJ, Buch MB, Krag TO, et al: 90-kDa ribosomal S6 kinase is phosphorylated and activated by 3-phosphoinositide-dependent protein kinase-1. J Biol Chem 274:27168–27176, 1999.

191. Du K, Montminy M: CREB is a regulatory target for the protein kinase Akt/PKB. J Biol Chem 273:32377–32379, 1998.

192. Anderson KE, Coadwell J, Stephens LR, Hawkins PT: Translocation of PDK-1 to the plasma membrane is important in allowing PDK-1 to activate protein kinase B. Curr Biol 8:684–691, 1998.

193. Anderson MJ, Viars CS, Czekay S, et al: Cloning and characterization of three human forkhead genes that comprise an FKHR-like gene subfamily. Genomics 47:187–199, 1998.

194. Brunet A, Bonni A, Zigmond MJ, et al: Akt promotes cell survival by phosphorylating and inhibiting a Forkhead transcription factor. Cell 96:857–868, 1999.

195. Cross DA, Alessi DR, Cohen P, et al: Inhibition of glycogen synthase kinase-3 by insulin mediated by protein kinase B. Nature 378:785–789, 1995.

196. Guan KL, Figueroa C, Brtva TR, et al: Negative regulation of the serine/threonine kinase B-Raf by Akt. J Biol Chem 275:27354–27359, 2000.

197. Zimmermann S, Moelling K: Phosphorylation and regulation of Raf by Akt (protein kinase B). Science 286:1741–1744, 1999.

198. Brazil DP, Hemmings BA: Ten years of protein kinase B signalling: A hard Akt to follow. Trends Biochem Sci 26:657–664, 2001.

199. Datta SR, Dudek H, Tao X, et al: Akt phosphorylation of BAD couples survival signals to the cell-intrinsic death machinery. Cell 91:231–241, 1997.

200. Datta SR, Brunet A, Greenberg ME: Cellular survival: A play in three Akts. Genes Dev 13:2905–2927, 1999.

201. Cardone MH, Roy N, Stennicke HR, et al: Regulation of cell death protease caspase-9 by phosphorylation. Science 282:1318–1321, 1998.

202. Liang J, Zubovitz J, Petrocelli T, et al: PKB/Akt phosphorylates p27, impairs nuclear import of p27 and opposes p27-mediated G1 arrest. Nat Med 8:1153–1160, 2002.

203. Czech MP: Insulin's expanding control of forkheads. Proc Natl Acad Sci U S A 100:11198–11200, 2003.

204. Nakae J, Kitamura T, Silver DL, Accili D: The forkhead transcription

factor Foxo1 (Fkhr) confers insulin sensitivity onto glucose-6-phosphatase expression. J Clin Invest 108:1359–1367, 2001.

205. Nakae J, Biggs WH III, Kitamura T, et al: Regulation of insulin action and pancreatic beta-cell function by mutated alleles of the gene encoding forkhead transcription factor Foxo1. Nat Genet 32:245–253, 2002.

206. Puigserver P, Rhee J, Donovan J, et al: Insulin-regulated hepatic gluconeogenesis through FOXO1-PGC-1alpha interaction. Nature 423:550–555, 2003.

207. Long X, Muller F, Avruch J: TOR action in mammalian cells and in Caenorhabditis elegans. Curr Top Microbiol Immunol 279:115–138, 2004.

208. Pende M, Kozma SC, Jaquet M, et al: Hypoinsulinaemia, glucose intolerance and diminished beta-cell size in S6K1-deficient mice. Nature 408:994–997, 2000.

209. Isotani S, Hara K, Tokunaga C, et al: Immunopurified mammalian target of rapamycin phosphorylates and activates p70 S6 kinase alpha in vitro. J Biol Chem 274:34493–34498, 1999.

210. Garami A, Zwartkruis FJ, Nobukuni T, et al: Insulin activation of Rheb, a mediator of mTOR/S6K/4E-BP signaling, is inhibited by TSC1 and 2. Mol Cell 11:1457–1466, 2003.

211. Young J, Povey S: The genetic basis of tuberous sclerosis. Mol Med Today 4:313–319, 1998.

212. Woods A, Vertommen D, Neumann D, et al: Identification of phosphorylation sites in AMP-activated protein kinase (AMPK) for upstream AMPK kinases and study of their roles by site-directed mutagenesis. J Biol Chem 278:28434–28442, 2003.

213. Woods A, Johnstone SR, Dickerson K, et al: LKB1 is the upstream kinase in the AMP-activated protein kinase cascade. Curr Biol 13:2004–2008, 2003.

214. Corradetti MN, Inoki K, Bardeesy N, et al: Regulation of the TSC pathway by LKB1: Evidence of a molecular link between tuberous sclerosis complex and Peutz-Jeghers syndrome. Genes Dev 18:1533–1538, 2004.

215. Rhoads RE: Signal transduction pathways that regulate eukaryotic protein synthesis. J Biol Chem 274:30337–30340, 1999.

216. Hartley D, Cooper GM: Role of mTOR in the degradation of IRS-1: Regulation of PP2A activity. J Cell Biochem 85:304–314, 2002.

217. Plas DR, Thompson CB: Akt activation promotes degradation of tuberin and FOXO3a via the proteasome. J Biol Chem 278:12361–12366, 2003.

218. Kim JK, Fillmore JJ, Chen Y, et al: Tissue-specific overexpression of lipoprotein lipase causes tissue-specific insulin resistance. Proc Natl Acad Sci U S A 98:7522–7527, 2001.

219. Proud CG, Denton RM: Molecular mechanisms for the control of translation by insulin. Biochem J 328(Pt 2):329–341, 1997.

220. Jaeschke A, Hartkamp J, Saitoh M, et al: Tuberous sclerosis complex tumor suppressor-mediated S6 kinase inhibition by phosphatidylinositide-3-OH kinase is mTOR independent. J Cell Biol 159:217–224, 2002.

221. Brunn GJ, Hudson CC, Sekulic A, et al: Phosphorylation of the translational repressor PHAS-I by the mammalian target of rapamycin. Science 277:99–101, 1997.

222. Waskiewicz AJ, Johnson JC, Penn B, et al: Phosphorylation of the cap-binding protein eukaryotic translation initiation factor 4E by protein kinase Mnk1 in vivo. Mol Cell Biol 19:1871–1880, 1999.

223. Minich WB, Balasta ML, Goss DJ, Rhoads RE: Chromatographic resoluation of in vivo phosphorylated and nonphorphorylated eukaryotic translation initiation factor eIF-4E: Increased cap affinity of the phosphorylated form. Proc Natl Acad Sci U S A 91:7668–7672, 1996.

224. Tsukiyama-Kohara K, Poulin F, Kohara M, et al: Adipose tissue reduction in mice lacking the translational inhibitor 4E-BP1. Nat Med 7:1128–1132, 2001.

225. Begum N, Sandu OA, Ito M, et al: Active Rho kinase (ROK-alpha) associates with insulin receptor substrate-1 and inhibits insulin signaling in vascular smooth muscle cells. J Biol Chem 277:6214–6222, 2002.

226. Proud CG, Wang X, Patel JV, et al: Interplay between insulin and nutrients in the regulation of translation factors. Biochem Soc Trans 29(Pt 4):541–547, 2001.

227. Redpath NT, Price NT, Severinov KV, Proud CG: Regulation of elongation factor-2 by multisite phosphorylation. Eur J Biochem 213:689–699, 1993.

228. Mendez R, Kollmorgen G, White MF, Rhoads RE: Requirement of protein kinase C zeta for stimulation of protein synthesis by insulin. Mol Cell Biol 17:5184–5192, 1997.

229. Lu Z, Hu X, Li Y, et al: Human papillomavirus 16 E6 oncoprotein interferences with insulin signaling pathway by binding to tuberin. J Biol Chem 279(34):35664–35670, 2004.

230. Stefan N, Fritsche A, Machicao F, et al: The Gly1057Asp polymorphism in IRS-2 interacts with obesity to affect beta cell function. Diabetologia 47(4):759–761, 2004.

231. Czech MP: Molecular actions of insulin on glucose transport. Annu Rev Nutr 15:441–471, 1995.

232. Fingar DC, Birnbaum MJ: A role for raf-1 in the divergent signaling pathways mediating insulin-stimulated glucose transport. J Biol Chem 269:10127–10132, 1994.

233. Haney PM, Levy MA, Strube MS, Mueckler M: Insulin-sensitive targeting of the GLUT4 glucose transporter in L6 myoblasts is conferred by its COOH-terminal cytoplasmic tail. J Cell Biol 129:641–658, 1995.

234. Carayannopoulos MO, Chi MM, Cui Y, et al: GLUT8 is a glucose transporter responsible for insulin-stimulated glucose uptake in the blastocyst. Proc Natl Acad Sci U S A 97:7313–7318, 2000.

235. Wood IS, Trayhurn P: Glucose transporters (GLUT and SGLT): Expanded families of sugar transport proteins. Br J Nutr 89:3–9, 2003.

236. Rogers S, Macheda ML, Docherty SE, et al: Identification of a novel glucose transporter-like protein-GLUT-12. Am J Physiol Endocrinol Metab 282:E733–E738, 2002.

237. Gude NM, Stevenson JL, Rogers S, et al: GLUT12 expression in human placenta in first trimester and term. Placenta 24:566–570, 2003.

238. Pessin JE, Thurmond DC, Elmendorf JS, et al: Molecular basis of insulin-stimulated GLUT4 vesicle trafficking. Location! Location! Location! J Biol Chem 274:2593–2596, 1999.

239. Khan AH, Pessin JE: Insulin regulation of glucose uptake: A complex interplay of intracellular signalling pathways. Diabetologia 45:1475–1483, 2002.

240. Farese RV: Function and dysfunction of aPKC isoforms for glucose transport in insulin-sensitive and insulin-resistant states. Am J Physiol Endocrinol Metab 283:E1–E11, 2002.

241. Bandyopadhyay G, Standaert ML, Sajan MP, et al: Protein kinase C-lambda knockout in embryonic stem cells and adipocytes impairs insulin-stimulated glucose transport. Mol Endocrinol 18:373–383, 2004.

242. Saltiel AR, Pessin JE: Insulin signaling in microdomains of the plasma membrane. Traffic 4:711–716, 2003.

243. Kotani K, Ogawa W, Matsumoto M, et al: Requirement of atypical protein kinase clambda for insulin stimulation of glucose uptake but not for akt activation in 3T3-L1 adipocytes. Mol Cell Biol 18:6971–6982, 1998.

244. Bandyopadhyay G, Kanoh Y, Sajan MP, et al: Effects of adenoviral gene transfer of wild-type, constitutively active, and kinase-defective protein kinase C-lambda on insulin-stimulated glucose transport in L6 myotubes. Endocrinology 141:4120–4127, 2000.

245. Bandyopadhyay G, Sajan MP, Kanoh Y, et al: PKC-zeta mediates insulin effects on glucose transport in cultured preadipocyte-derived human adipocytes. J Clin Endocrinol Metab 87:716–723, 2002.

246. Kotani K, Ogawa W, Matsumoto M, et al: Requirement of atypical protein kinase Cκ for insulin stimulation of glucose uptake but not for akt activation in 3t3-l1 adipocytes. Mol Cell Biol 18(12):6971–6982, 1998.

247. Etgen GJ, Valasek KM, Broderick CL, Miller AR: In vivo adenoviral delivery of recombinant human protein kinase C-zeta stimulates glucose transport activity in rat skeletal muscle. J Biol Chem 274:22139–22142, 1999.

248. Imamura T, Vollenweider P, Egawa K, et al: G alpha-q/11 protein plays a key role in insulin-induced glucose transport in 3T3-L1 adipocytes. Mol Cell Biol 19:6765–6774, 1999.

249. Vollenweider P, Menard B, Nicod P: Insulin resistance, defective insulin receptor substrate 2-associated phosphatidylinositol-3′ kinase activation, and impaired atypical protein kinase C (zeta/lambda) activation in myotubes from obese patients with impaired glucose tolerance. Diabetes 51:1052–1059, 2002.

250. Standaert ML, Ortmeyer HK, Sajan MP, et al: Skeletal muscle insulin resistance in obesity-associated type 2 diabetes in monkeys is linked to a defect in insulin activation of protein kinase C-zeta/lambda/iota. Diabetes 51:2936–2943, 2002.

251. Cohen AW, Razani B, Wang XB, et al: Caveolin-1-deficient mice show insulin resistance and defective insulin receptor protein expression in adipose tissue. Am J Physiol Cell Physiol 285:C222–C235, 2003.

252. Liu J, Kimura A, Baumann CA, Saltiel AR: APS facilitates c-Cbl tyrosine phosphorylation and GLUT4 translocation in response to insulin in 3T3-L1 adipocytes. Mol Cell Biol 22:3599–3609, 2002.

253. Watson RT, Shigematsu S, Chiang SH, et al: Lipid raft microdomain compartmentalization of TC10 is required for insulin signaling and GLUT4 translocation. J Cell Biol 154:829–840, 2001.

254. Mitra P, Zheng X, Czech MP: RNAi-based analysis of CAP, Cbl and CrkII function in the regulation of GLUT4 by insulin. J Biol Chem 279(36):37431–37435, 2004.

255. Roth J: Diabetes and obesity. Diab Met Rev 13:1–2, 1998.

256. Taylor SI: Lilly lecture: Molecular mechanisms of insulin resistance— Lessons from patients with mutations in the insulin receptor gene. Diabetes 41:1473–1490, 1992.

257. Virkamaki A, Ueki K, Kahn CR: Protein-protein interaction in insulin signaling and the molecular mechanisms of insulin resistance. J Clin Invest 103:931–943, 1999.

258. Taylor SI, Accili D: Mutations in the genes encoding the insulin receptor and insulin receptor substrate-1. In LeRoith D, Taylor SI, Olefsky JM (eds): Diabetes Mellitus: A Fundamental and Clinical Text. Philadelphia, Lippincott-Raven, 1996, pp 575–583.

259. Almind K, Bjorbaek C, Vestergaard H, et al: Amino acid polymorphisms of insulin receptor substrate-1 in non-insulin-dependent diabetes mellitus. Lancet 342:828–832, 1993.

260. Almind K, Inoue G, Pedersen O, Kahn CR: A common amino acid polymorphism in insulin receptor substrate-1 causes impaired insulin signaling. Evidence from transfection studies. J Clin Invest 97:2569–2575, 1996.

261. El Mkadem SA, Lautier C, Macari F, et al: Role of allelic variants Gly972Arg of IRS-1 and Gly1057Asp of IRS-2 in moderate-to-severe insulin resistance of women with polycystic ovary syndrome. Diabetes 50:2164–2168, 2001.

262. Marchetti P, Lupi R, Federici M, et al: Insulin secretory function is impaired in isolated human islets carrying the Gly(972)→Arg IRS-1 polymorphism. Diabetes 51:1419–1424, 2002.

263. Lautier C, El Mkadem SA, Renard E, et al: Complex haplotypes of IRS2 gene are associated with severe obesity and reveal heterogeneity in the effect of Gly1057Asp mutation. Hum Genet 113:34–43, 2003.

264. Ehrmann DA, Tang X, Yoshiuchi I, et al: Relationship of insulin receptor substrate-1 and -2 genotypes to phenotypic features of polycystic ovary syndrome. J Clin Endocrinol Metab 87:4297–4300, 2002.

265. Hansen T, Andersen CB, Echwald SM, et al: Identification of a common amino acid polymorphism in the p-85alpha regulatory subunit of phosphatidylinositol 3-kinase: Effects on glucose disappearance constant, glucose effectiveness and the insulin sensitivity index. Diabetes 46:494–501, 1997.

266. Bruning JC, Michael MD, Winnay JN, et al: A muscle-specific insulin receptor knockout exhibits features of the metabolic syndrome of NIDDM without altering glucose tolerance. Mol Cell 2:559–569, 1998.

267. Shulman GI: Cellular mechanisms of insulin resistance. J Clin Invest 106:171–176, 2000.

268. Petersen KF, Shulman GI: Cellular mechanism of insulin resistance in skeletal muscle. J R Soc Med 95 (Suppl 42):8–13, 2002.

269. Galuska D, Ryder J, Kawano Y, et al: Insulin signaling and glucose transport in insulin resistant skeletal muscle. Special reference to GLUT4 transgenic and GLUT4 knockout mice. Adv Exp Med Biol 441:73–85, 1998.

270. Charron MJ, Katz EB: Metabolic and therapeutic lessons from genetic manipulation of GLUT4 [In Process Citation]. Mol Cell Biochem 182:143–152, 1998.

271. Shefi-Friedman L, Wertheimer E, Shen S, et al: Increased IGFR activity and glucose transport in cultured skeletal muscle from insulin receptor null mice. Am J Physiol Endocrinol Metab 281:E16–E24, 2001.

272. Kulkarni RN, Bruning JC, Winnay JN, et al: Tissue-specific knockout of the insulin receptor in pancreatic β cells creates an insulin secretory defect similar to that in Type 2 diabetes. Cell 96:329–339, 1999.

273. DeFronzo RA: Pathogenesis of type 2 diabetes: Metabolic and molecular implications for identifying diabetes genes. Diabetes Rev 5:177–269, 1997.

274. Hansen PA, Han DH, Marshall BA, et al: A high fat diet impairs stimulation of glucose transport in muscle. Functional evaluation of potential mechanisms. J Biol Chem 273:26157–26163, 1998.

275. Nawrocki AR, Scherer PE: The delicate balance between fat and muscle: Adipokines in metabolic disease and musculoskeletal inflammation. Curr Opin Pharmacol 4:281–289, 2004.

276. Flier JS: Leptin expression and action: New experimental paradigms. Proc Natl Acad Sci U S A 94:4242–4245, 1997.

277. Zhang Y, Proenca R, Maffei M, et al: Positional cloning of the mouse obese gene and its human homologue. Nature 372:425–432, 1994.

278. Boden G: Role of fatty acids in the pathogenesis of insulin resistance and NIDDM. Diabetes 46:3–10, 1997.

279. Cohen B, Novick D, Rubinstein M: Modulation of insulin activities by leptin. Science 274:1185–1188, 1996.

280. Hotamisligil GS, Peraldi P, Budvari A, et al: IRS-1 mediated inhibition of insulin receptor tyrosine kinase activity in TNF-α- and obesity-induced insulin resistance. Science 271:665–668, 1996.

281. Banks AS, Davis SM, Bates SH, Myers MG Jr: Activation of downstream signals by the long form of the leptin receptor. Control of ERK, c-fos, and SOCS3 by LRb. J Biol Chem 275(19):14563–14572, 2000.

282. Feener EP, Rosario F, Dunn SL, et al: Tyrosine phosphorylation of Jak2 in the JH2 domain inhibits cytokine signaling. Mol Cell Biol 24:4968–4978, 2004.

283. Bates SH, Stearns WH, Dundon TA, et al: STAT3 signalling is required for leptin regulation of energy balance but not reproduction. Nature 421:856–859, 2003.

284. Wang MY, Koyama K, Shimabukuro M, et al: OB-Rb gene transfer to leptin-resistant islets reverses diabetogenic phenotype. Proc Natl Acad Sci U S A 95:714–718, 1998.

285. Hotamisligil GS, Spiegelman BM: Tumor necrosis factor α: A key component of the obesity-diabetes link. Diabetes 43:1271–1278, 1994.

286. Hotamisligil GS, Shargill NS, Spiegelman BM: Adipose expression of tumor necrosis factor-α: Direct role in obesity-linked insulin resistance. Science 259:87–91, 1993.

287. Weisberg SP, McCann D, Desai M, et al: Obesity is associated with macrophage accumulation in adipose tissue. J Clin Invest 112:1796–1808, 2303.

288. Peraldi P, Hotamisligil GS, Buurman WA, et al: Tumor necrosis factor (TNF)-α inhibits insulin signaling through stimulation of the p55 TNF receptor and activation of sphingomyelinase. J Biol Chem 271:13018–13022, 1996.

289. Kanety H, Feinstein R, Papa MZ, et al: Tumor necrosis factor α-induced phosphorylation of insulin receptor substrate-1 (IRS-1). Possible mechanism

for suppression of insulin-stimulated tyrosine phosphorylation of IRS-1. J Biol Chem 270:23780–23784, 1995.

290. Uysal KT, Wiesbrock SM, Hotamisligil GS: Functional analysis of tumor necrosis factor (TNF) receptors in TNF-alpha-mediated insulin resistane in genetic obesity. Endocrinology 139:4832–4838, 1998.

291. Miles PD, Romeo OM, Higo K, et al: TNF-alpha-induced insulin resistance in vivo and its prevention by troglitazone. Diabetes 46:1678–1683, 1997.

292. Nonogaki K, Fuller GM, Fuentes NL, et al: Interleukin-6 stimulates hepatic triglyceride secretion in rats. Endocrinology 136:2143–2149, 1995.

293. Senn JJ, Klover PJ, Nowak IA, Mooney RA: Interleukin-6 induces cellular insulin resistance in hepatocytes. Diabetes 51:3391–3399, 2002.

294. Senn JJ, Klover PJ, Nowak IA, et al: Suppressor of cytokine signaling-3 (SOCS-3), a potential mediator of interleukin-6-dependent insulin resistance in hepatocytes. J Biol Chem 278:13740–13746, 2003.

295. Rotter V, Nagaev I, Smith U: Interleukin-6 (IL-6) induces insulin resistance in 3T3-L1 adipocytes and is, like IL-8 and tumor necrosis factor-alpha, overexpressed in human fat cells from insulin-resistant subjects. J Biol Chem 278:45777–45784, 2003.

296. Tsigos C, Papanicolaou DA, Kyrou I, et al: Dose-dependent effects of recombinant human interleukin-6 on glucose regulation. J Clin Endocrinol Metab 82:4167–4170, 1997.

297. Kern PA, Ranganathan S, Li C, et al: Adipose tissue tumor necrosis factor and interleukin-6 expression in human obesity and insulin resistance. Am J Physiol Endocrinol Metab 280:E745–E751, 2001.

298. Lyngso D, Simonsen L, Bulow J: Metabolic effects of interleukin-6 in human splanchnic and adipose tissue. J Physiol 543(Pt 1):379–386, 2002.

299. van Hall G, Steensberg A, Sacchetti M, et al: Interleukin-6 stimulates lipolysis and fat oxidation in humans. J Clin Endocrinol Metab 88:3005–3010, 2003.

300. Scherer PE, Williams S, Fogliano M, et al: Serum protein similar to C1q, produced exclusively in adipocytes. J Biol Chem 270:26746–26749, 1995.

301. Wong GW, Wang J, Hug C, et al: A family of Acrp30/adiponectin structural and functional paralogs. Proc Natl Acad Sci U S A 101:10302–10307, 2004.

302. Rajala MW, Scherer PE: Minireview: The adipocyte—at the crossroads of energy homeostasis, inflammation, and atherosclerosis. Endocrinology 144:3765–3773, 2003.

303. Yamauchi T, Kamon J, Ito Y, et al: Cloning of adiponectin receptors that mediate antidiabetic metabolic effects. Nature 423:762–769, 2003.

304. Hotamisligil GS: Mechanisms of NF-alpha-induced insulin resistance. Exp Clin Endocrinol Diabetes 107:119–125, 1999.

305. Uysal KT, Wiesbrock SM, Marino MW, Hotamisligil GS: Protection from obesity-induced insulin resistance in mice lacking TNF-α function. Nature 389:610–614, 1997.

306. Aguirre V, Uchida T, Yenush L, et al: The c-Jun NH(2)-terminal kinase promotes insulin resistance during association with insulin receptor substrate-1 and phosphorylation of Ser(307). J Biol Chem 275:9047–9054, 2000.

307. De Fea K, Roth RA: Protein kinase C modulation of insulin receptor substrate-1 tyrosine phosphorylation requires serine 612. Biochemistry 36:12939–12947, 1997.

308. Eldar-Finkelman H, Krebs EG: Phosphorylation of insulin receptor substrate 1 by glycogen synthase kinase 3 impairs insulin action. Proc Natl Acad Sci U S A 94:9660–9664, 1997.

309. Staubs PA, Nelson JG, Reichart DR, Olefsky JM: Platelet-derived growth factor inhibits insulin stimulation of insulin receptor substrate-1 associated phosphatidylinositol 3-kinase in 3T3-L1 adipocytes without affecting glucose transport. J Biol Chem 273:25139–25147, 1998.

310. Hemi R, Paz K, Wertheim N, et al: Transactivation of ErbB2 and ErbB3 by tumor necrosis factor-alpha and anisomycin leads to impaired insulin signaling through serine/threonine phosphorylation of IRS proteins. J Biol Chem 277:8961–8969, 2002.

311. Egawa K, Nakashima N, Sharma PM, et al: Persistent activation of phosphatidylinositol 3-kinase causes insulin resistance due to accelerated insulin-induced insulin receptor substrate-1 degradation in 3T3-L1 adipocytes. Endocrinology 141:1930–1935, 2000.

312. Ravichandran LV, Chen H, Li Y, Quon MJ: Phosphorylation of PTP1B at Ser(50) by Akt impairs its ability to dephosphorylate the insulin receptor. Mol Endocrinol 15:1768–1780, 2001.

313. Liu YF, Paz K, Herschkovitz A, et al: Insulin stimulates PKCzeta-mediated phosphorylation of insulin receptor substrate-1 (IRS-1). A self-attenuated mechanism to negatively regulate the function of IRS proteins. J Biol Chem 276:14459–14465, 2001.

314. Ozes ON, Akca H, Mayo LD, et al: A phosphatidylinositol 3-kinase/Akt/mTOR pathway mediates and PTEN antagonizes tumor necrosis factor inhibition of insulin signaling through insulin receptor substrate-1. Proc Natl Acad Sci U S A 98:4640–4645, 2001.

315. Mauvais-Jarvis F, Ueki K, Fruman DA, et al: Reduced expression of the murine p85alpha subunit of phosphoinositide 3-kinase improves insulin signaling and ameliorates

diabetes. J Clin Invest 109:141–149, 2002.

316. Yu C, Chen Y, Cline GW, et al: Mechanism by which fatty acids inhibit insulin activation of insulin receptor substrate-1 (IRS-1)-associated phosphatidylinositol 3-kinase activity in muscle. J Biol Chem 277:50230–50236, 2002.

317. Greene MW, Garofalo RS: Positive and negative regulatory role of insulin receptor substrate 1 and 2 (IRS-1 and IRS-2) serine/threonine phosphorylation. Biochemistry 41:7082–7091, 2002.

318. Gao Z, Hwang D, Bataille F, et al: Serine phosphorylation of insulin receptor substrate 1 by inhibitor kappa B kinase complex. J Biol Chem 277:48115–48121, 2002.

319. Gao Z, Zuberi A, Quon MJ, et al: Aspirin inhibits serine phosphorylation of insulin receptor substrate 1 in tumor necrosis factor-treated cells through targeting multiple serine kinases. J Biol Chem 278:24944–24950, 2003.

320. Gual P, Gremeaux T, Gonzalez T, et al: MAP kinases and mTOR mediate insulin-induced phosphorylation of insulin receptor substrate-1 on serine residues 307, 612 and 632. Diabetologia 46:1532–1542, 2003.

321. Hirosumi J, Tuncman G, Chang L, et al: A central role for JNK in obesity and insulin resistance. Nature 420:333–336, 2002.

322. Yuan M, Konstantopoulos N, Lee J, et al: Reversal of obesity- and diet-induced insulin resistance with salicylates or targeted disruption of Ikkbeta. Science 293:1673–1677, 2001.

323. Konstantopoulos N, Lee J, Yuan M, et al: Inhibition of IKKb reverses "Insulin Resistance" in cultured cells. Diabetes 49:A14, 2000.

324. Kim JK, Kim YJ, Fillmore JJ, et al: Prevention of fat-induced insulin resistance by salicylate. J Clin Invest 108:437–446, 2001.

325. Hundal RS, Petersen KF, Mayerson AB, et al: Mechanism by which high-dose aspirin improves glucose metabolism in type 2 diabetes. J Clin Invest 109:1321–1326, 2002.

326. Mothe I, Van Obberghen E: Phosphorylation of insulin receptor substrate-1 on multiple serine residues, 612, 632, 662, and 731, modulates insulin action. J Biol Chem 271:11222–11227, 1996.

327. Greene MW, Morrice N, Garofalo RS, Roth RA: Modulation of human insulin receptor substrate-1 tyrosine phosphorylation by protein kinase Cdelta. Biochem J 378(Pt 1):105–116, 2004.

328. Giraud J, Leshan R, Lee YH, White MF: Nutrient-dependent and insulin-stimulated phosphorylation of insulin receptor substrate-1 on serine 302 correlates with increased insulin signaling. J Biol Chem 279:3447–3454, 2004.

329. Paz K, Hemi R, LeRoith D, et al: A molecular basis for insulin resistance. Elevated serine/threonine phosphorylation of IRS-1 and IRS-2 inhibits their binding to the juxtamembrane region of the insulin receptor and impairs their ability to undergo insulin-induced tyrosine phosphorylation. J Biol Chem 272:29911–29918, 1997.

330. Folli F, Kahn CR, Hansen H, et al: Angiotensin II inhibits insulin signaling in aortic smooth muscle cells at multiple levels: A potential role for serine phosphorylation in insulin/angiotensin II "crosstalk." J Clin Invest 100:2158–2169, 1997.

331. Xiang X, Yuan M, Song Y, et al: 14-3-3 facilitates insulin-stimulated intracellular trafficking of insulin receptor substrate 1. Mol Endocrinol 16:552–562, 2002.

332. Rui L, Fisher TL, Thomas J, White MF: Regulation of insulin/insulin-like growth factor-1 signaling by proteasome-mediated degradation of insulin receptor substrate-2. J Biol Chem 276:40362–40367, 2001.

333. Haruta T, Uno T, Kawahara J, et al: A rapamycin-sensitive pathway down-regulates insulin signaling via phosphorylation and proteasomal degradation of insulin receptor substrate-1. Mol Endocrinol 14:783–794, 2000.

334. Takano A, Usui I, Haruta T, et al: Mammalian target of rapamycin pathway regulates insulin signaling via subcellular redistribution of insulin receptor substrate 1 and integrates nutritional signals and metabolic signals of insulin. Mol Cell Biol 21:5050–5062, 2001.

335. Harrington LS, Findlay GM, Grgay A, et al: The TSC1-2 tumor supressor controls insulin-PI3K signaling via regulation of IRS proteins. J Cell Biol 166(2):213–223, 2004.

336. Rui L, Yuan M, Frantz D, et al: SOCS-1 and SOCS-3 block insulin signaling by ubiquitin-mediated degradation of IRS1 and IRS2. J Biol Chem 277:42394–42398, 2002.

337. Krebs DL, Uren RT, Metcalf D, et al: SOCS-6 binds to insulin receptor substrate 4, and mice lacking the SOCS-6 gene exhibit mild growth retardation. Mol Cell Biol 22:4567–4578, 2002.

338. Sadowski CL, Choi TS, Le MN, et al: Insulin induction of SOCS-2 and SOCS-3 mRNA expression in C2C12 skeletal muscle cells is mediated by Stat5. J Biol Chem 276(23):20703–20710, 2001.

339. Krebs DL, Hilton DJ: A new role for SOCS in insulin action. Suppressor of cytokine signaling. Sci STKE E6, 2003.

340. Wojcik C: Inhibition of the proteasome as a therapeutic approach. Drug Discov Today 4:188–189, 1999.

341. Dadke S, Kusari A, Kusari J: Phosphorylation and activation of protein tyrosine phosphatase (PTP) 1B by insulin receptor. Mol Cell Biochem 221:147–154, 2001.

342. Dadke S, Kusari J, Chernoff J: Down-regulation of insulin signaling by protein-tyrosine phosphatase 1B is mediated by an N-terminal binding region. J Biol Chem 275:23642–23647, 2000.

343. Goldstein BJ, Bittner-Kowalcyk A, White MF, Harbeck M: Tyrosine dephosphorylation and deactivation of insulin receptor substrate-1 by protein tyrosine phosphatase 1B: Possible facilitation by the formation of a ternary complex with the Grb-2 adaptor protein. J Biol Chem 275:4283–4289, 2000.

344. Bandyopadhyay D, Kusari A, Kenner KA, et al: Protein-tyrosine phosphatase 1B complexes with the insulin receptor in vivo and is tyrosine-phosphorylated in the presence of insulin. J Biol Chem 272:1639–1645, 1997.

345. Kenner KA, Anyanwu E, Olefsky JM, Kusari J: Protein-tyrosine phosphatase 1B is a negative regulator of insulin- and insulin-like growth factor-I-stimulated signaling. J Biol Chem 271:19810–19816, 1996.

346. Klaman LD, Boss O, Peroni OD, et al: Increased energy expenditure, decreased adiposity, and tissue-specific insulin sensitivity in protein-tyrosine phosphatase 1B-deficient mice. Mol Cell Biol 20:5479–5489, 2000.

347. Zinker BA, Rondinone CM, Trevillyan JM, et al: PTP1B antisense oligonucleotide lowers PTP1B protein, normalizes blood glucose, and improves insulin sensitivity in diabetic mice. Proc Natl Acad Sci U S A 99:11357–11362, 2002.

348. Haj FG, Markova B, Klaman LD, et al: Regulation of receptor tyrosine kinase signaling by protein tyrosine phosphatase-1B. J Biol Chem 278:739–744, 2003.

349. Boute N, Boubekeur S, Lacasa D, Issad T: Dynamics of the interaction between the insulin receptor and protein tyrosine-phosphatase 1B in living cells. EMBO Rep 4:313–319, 2003.

350. Li J, Yen C, Liaw D, et al: PTEN, a putative protein tyrosine phosphatase gene mutated in human brain, breast, and prostate cancer. Science 275:1943–1947, 1997.

351. Ono H, Katagiri H, Funaki M, et al: Regulation of phosphoinositide metabolism, Akt phosphorylation, and glucose transport by PTEN (phosphatase and tensin homolog deleted on chromosome 10) in 3T3-L1 adipocytes. Mol Endocrinol 15:1411–1422, 2001.

352. Maehama T, Dixon JE: The tumor suppressor, PTEN/MMAC1, dephosphorylates the lipid second messenger, phosphatidylinositol 3,4,5-trisphosphate. J Biol Chem 273:13375–13378, 1998.

353. Maehama T, Dixon JE: PTEN: A tumour suppressor that functions as a phospholipid phosphatase. Trends Cell Biol 9:125–128, 1999.

354. Di Cristofano A, Pesce B, Cordon-Cardo C, Pandolfi PP: Pten is essential for embryonic development and tumour suppression. Nat Genet 19:348–355, 1998.

355. Nakashima N, Sharma PM, Imamura T, et al: The tumor suppressor PTEN negatively regulates insulin signaling in 3T3-L1 adipocytes. J Biol Chem 275:12889–12895, 2000.

356. Butler M, McKay RA, Popoff IJ, et al: Specific inhibition of PTEN expression reverses hyperglycemia in diabetic mice. Diabetes 51:1028–1034, 2002.

357. Kubota N, Tobe K, Terauchi Y, et al: Disruption of insulin receptor substrate 2 causes type 2 diabetes because of liver insulin resistance and lack of compensatory beta-cell hyperplasia. Diabetes 49:1880–1889, 2000.

358. Previs SF, Withers DJ, Ren JM, et al: Contrasting effects of IRS-1 vs IRS-2 gene disruption on carbohydrate and lipid metabolism in vivo. J Biol Chem 275:38990–38994, 2000.

359. Xuan S, Kitamura T, Nakae J, et al: Defective insulin secretion in pancreatic beta cells lacking type 1 IGF receptor. J Clin Invest 110:1011–1019, 2002.

360. Kulkarni RN, Holzenberger M, Shih DQ, et al: Beta-cell-specific deletion of the Igf1 receptor leads to hyperinsulinemia and glucose intolerance but does not alter beta-cell mass. Nat Genet 31:111–115, 2002.

361. Jonsson J, Carlsson L, Edlund T, Edlund H: Insulin-promoter-factor 1 is required for pancreas developement in mice. Nature 371:606–609, 1994.

362. Stoffers DA, Zinkin NT, Stanojevic V, et al: Pancreatic agenesis attributable to a single nucleotide deletion in the human IPF1 gene coding sequence. Nat Genet 15:106–110, 1997.

363. Kushner JA, Ye J, Schubert M, et al: Pdx1 restores beta cell function in Irs2 knockout mice. J Clin Invest 109:1193–1201, 2002.

364. Kubota T, Kubota N, Moroi M, et al: Lack of insulin receptor substrate-2 causes progressive neointima formation in response to vessel injury. Cirulation 107:3073–3080, 2003.

365. Perry T, Greig NH: The glucagon-like peptides: A double-edged therapeutic sword? Trends Pharmacol Sci 24:377–383, 2003.

366. Jhala US, Canettieri G, Screaton RA, et al: cAMP promotes pancreatic beta-cell survival via CREB-mediated induction of IRS2. Genes Dev 17:1575–1580, 2003.

367. Butler AA, Cone RD: Knockout studies defining different roles for melanocortin receptors in energy homeostasis. Ann N Y Acad Sci 994:240–245, 2003.

368. Farooqi IS, Keogh JM, Yeo GS, et al: Clinical spectrum of obesity and mutations in the melanocortin 4 receptor gene. N Engl J Med 348:1085–1095, 2003.

369. Qi Y, Takahashi N, Hileman SM, et al: Adiponectin acts in the brain to decrease body weight. Nat Med 10:524–529, 2004.

370. Myers MG Jr: Leptin receptor signaling and the regulation of mammalian physiology. Recent Prog Horm Res 59:287–304, 2004.

371. Woods SC, Lotter EC, McKay LD, Porte D Jr: Chronic intracerebroventricular infusion of insulin reduces food intake and body weight of baboons. Nature 282:503–505, 1979.

372. Schwartz M, Figlewicz DP, Baskin DG, et al: Insulin in the brain: A hormonal regulator of energy balance. Endocr Rev 13:387–414, 1992.

373. Schwartz MW, Baskin DG, Kaiyala KJ, Woods SC: Model of the regulation of energy balance and adiposity by the central nervous system. Am J Clin Nutr 69:584–596, 1999.

374. Bruning JC, Gautam D, Burks DJ, et al: Role of brain insulin receptor in control of body weight and reproduction. Science 289:2122–2125, 2000.

375. Huszar D, Lynch CA, Fairchild-Huntress V, et al: Targeted disruption of the melanocortin-4 receptor results in obesity in mice. Cell 88:131–141, 1997.

376. Obici S, Feng Z, Tan J, et al: Central melanocortin receptors regulate insulin action. J Clin Invest 108:1079–1085, 2001.

377. Challis BG, Pritchard LE, Creemers JW, et al: A missense mutation disrupting a dibasic prohormone processing site in pro-opiomelanocortin (POMC) increases susceptibility to early-onset obesity through a novel molecular mechanism. Hum Mol Genet 11:1997–2004, 2002.

378. Combs TP, Berg AH, Rajala MW, et al: Sexual differentiation, pregnancy, calorie restriction, and aging affect the adipocyte-specific secretory protein adiponectin. Diabetes 52:268–276, 2003.

379. Spranger J, Kroke A, Mohlig M, et al: Adiponectin and protection against type 2 diabetes mellitus. Lancet 361:226–228, 2003.

380. Burks DJ, de Mora JF, Schubert M, et al: IRS-2 pathways integrate female reproduction and energy homeostasis. Nature 407:377–382, 2000.

381. Gannon M, Shiota C, Postic C, et al: Analysis of the Cre-mediated recombination driven by rat insulin promoter in embryonic and adult mouse pancreas. Genesis 26:139–142, 2000.

382. Cui Y, Huang L, Elefteriou F, et al: Essential role of STAT3 in body weight and glucose homeostasis. Mol Cell Biol 24:258–269, 2004.

383. Lin X, Taguchi A, Park S, et al: Dysregulation of IRS2 in beta cells and brain causes obesity and diabetes. J Clin Invest 114(7):908–916, 2004.

384. Yasukawa H, Sasaki A, Yoshimura A: Negative regulation of cytokine signaling pathways. Annu Rev Immunol 18:143–164, 2000.

385. Krebs DL, Hilton DJ: SOCS: Physiological suppressors of cytokine signaling. J Cell Sci 113(Pt 16):2813–2819, 2000.

386. Kamura T, Sato S, Haque D, et al: The elongin BC complex interacts with the conserved SOCS-box motif present in members of the SOCS, ras, WD-40 repeat, and ankyrin repeat families. Genes Dev 12:3872–3881, 1998.

387. Tyers M, Willems AR: One ring to rule a superfamily of E3 ubiquitin ligases [comment]. Science 284:601–604, 1999.

388. Zhang JG, Farley A, Nicholson SE, et al: The conserved SOCS box motif in suppressors of cytokine signaling binds to elongins B and C and may couple bound proteins to proteasomal degradation. Proc Natl Acad Sci U S A 96:2071–2076, 1999.

Glucagon and the Glucagon-like Peptides

Daniel J. Drucker

OVERVIEW

Glucagon and the glucagon-like peptides are derived from a single proglucagon gene in mammals and exhibit an increasing number of biologically important actions. Glucagon, synthesized principally in islet α cells, is a key regulator of glucose homeostasis through its actions on enzymes that regulate glucose production and glycogen synthesis. Glucagon-like peptide-1 (GLP-1) and GLP-2 are liberated from intestinal endocrine cells and regulate glucose homeostasis and intestinal epithelial growth, respectively. These three peptides exert their actions via interaction with unique receptors that exhibit distinct patterns of tissue-specific expression. This chapter reviews our current understanding of the biology of glucagon and the proglucagon-derived peptides (PGDPs), emphasizing recent advances in our understanding of glucagon biosynthesis and action and the emerging biologic importance and therapeutic potential of the glucagon-like peptides.

BIOSYNTHESIS OF PANCREATIC GLUCAGON

Proglucagon is encoded by a single gene in mammals that gives rise to a proglucagon mRNA transcript that is identical in pancreatic islets, brain, and enteroendocrine cells of the small and large intestines. The proglucagon gene contains six exons, several of which encode distinct functional peptide domains (Fig. 51-1). Glucagon, a 29-amino-acid peptide, is synthesized in the A cells of the pancreatic islets of Langerhans. Islet A cells are distinguishable from insulin-producing β cells in part by the morphology of their respective secretory granules and by their anatomic distribution predominantly at the periphery of the islet. The peripheral location of islet A cells, taken together with functional studies demonstrating central (from a core of β cells) to peripheral (A cells) islet blood flow, raises the possibility of a tightly regulated islet microenvironment. Nevertheless, as the distribution of islet α and β cells can vary from species to species, the functional importance of islet cell distribution remains unclear.

ISLET TRANSCRIPTION FACTORS AND THE α CELL

The pancreas derives from the upper foregut, with dorsal and ventral pancreatic buds giving rise to pancreatic epithelium that eventually forms the exocrine and endocrine pancreas. This process involves signals from mesenchyme and requires the correct temporal expression of growth factors, transcription

factors, and related signaling molecules. Pancreatic islet cells appear to be of endodermal origin and are first detectable by E8.5 in the mouse. Intriguingly, the first islet hormone-immunopositive endocrine cells that are detectable in developing islets contain glucagon immunoreactivity. Insulin immunopositive cells are detectable by day E14 in the mouse, followed several days later by the appearance of somatostatin-containing cell types.

Although the molecular determinants underlying the anatomic organization of islet cells remain poorly understood, studies of gene disruption in mice have provided new insights into the organization of islet endocrine cells in the pancreas. For example, mice with a null allele in the basic helix-loop-helix transcription factor p48 fail to develop exocrine pancreatic tissue; however, hormone-secreting islet cells, including glucagon-producing α cells, are found within the mesentery during embryonic development and later in the spleen.[1] A key role for cell adhesion molecules in the control of the spatial organization of islet cells is illustrated by analysis of the endocrine pancreas in mice expressing a dominant negative E-cadherin receptor in islet β cells. These mice exhibit abnormal clustering of β cells, yet glucagon-producing α cells are still capable of aggregating into isletlike clusters.[2] In contrast, the normal peripheral distribution of islet α cells is markedly perturbed in neural cell adhesion molecule (NCAM)$^{-/-}$ mice; however, the number of α cells and the glucagon content of the pancreas remain unaffected.[3]

Considerable insight into the developmental biology of the endocrine pancreas and islet α cells has been derived from studies of islet transcription factors in cell lines and mice (Fig. 51-2). Disruption of transcription factor expression via homologous recombination demonstrated that the LIM domain protein isl-1 is necessary for the formation of differentiated islet cells, including α cells in the developing pancreas.[4] Targeted deletion of the homeobox transcription factor *Arx* results in mice that exhibit complete failure of α-cell development, leading to glucagon deficiency and neonatal hypoglycemia.[5] In contrast, although mice that are deficient in the homeobox transcription factor Ipf/Pdx-1 fail to develop a pancreas, a few islet cells that are immunopositive for either insulin or glucagon are observed in Ipf/Pdx-1$^{-/-}$ mice at embryonic day 11.[6] These observations suggest that Ipf/Pdx-1 is not essential for the formation of islet α cells.

The homeobox transcription factor *Nkx2.2* is expressed in adult α, β, and PP islet cells, and mice with targeted disruption of *NKx2.2* lack β cells, develop diabetes, and exhibit a marked reduction in the numbers of islet α cells.[7] A related phenotype

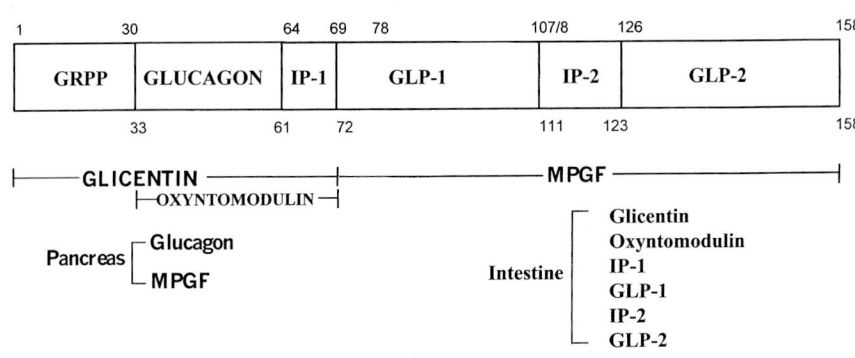

Figure 51-1 Schematic representation of the glucagon-derived peptides encoded by the proglucagon gene. The amino acid sequences of human glucagon, glucagon-like peptide-1 (GLP-1), and glucagon-like peptide-2 (GLP-2) are shown. The *arrow* indicates the cleavage site recognized by dipeptidyl-peptidase IV (DPP-IV). IP-1 and IP-2, intervening peptides 1 and 2; MPGF, major proglucagon fragment.

is observed in NeuroD/BETA2$^{-/-}$ mice, which exhibit marked reductions in the numbers of islet β and α cells and develop diabetes shortly after birth,[8] a phenotype that is dependent on the specific genetic background. Similarly, disruption of *pax6* function in mice results in poorly formed islets with disorganized islet architecture and markedly reduced but detectable numbers of both β and islet α cells.[9,10] Intriguingly, mice that harbor mutations in islet transcription factors may also exhibit paradoxically increased numbers of islet α cells. For example, targeted deletion of the *Pax4* gene results in poorly formed islets, with a marked reduction in islet β cells and comparatively increased numbers of islet α cells.[11] A related phenotype is observed in mice that have a homozygous deletion in the glucose transporter 2 (GLUT-2) gene, with a marked increase in the ratio of α to β cells observed in GLUT2$^{-/-}$ islets.[12] Whether these findings are due to a block in the normal islet differentiation program or loss of inhibitors that restrain α cell proliferation is not known. Evidence in support of glucagon itself regulating the numbers of islet α cells derives from analysis of mice with targeted disruption of the genes encoding either prohormone convertase-2 or the glucagon receptor. These mice represent models for loss of bioactive glucagon[13] or glucagon action,[14] respectively, and exhibit marked α-cell hyperplasia, which is corrected in the former instance by glucagon replacement therapy. Given the pleiotropic abnormalities and developmental compensation that arise in knockout mice, it is expected that future studies will make more extensive use of tissue- and cell-specific gene targeting, thereby permitting more detailed analysis of genes important for islet and α-cell biology in the embryo and adult mouse.

PROGLUCAGON GENE TRANSCRIPTION FACTORS

A combination of gene transfection experiments using cell lines in vitro and transgenic studies of promoter function in vivo have yielded considerable insight into the molecular control of glucagon gene transcription. Differential gene expression analysis has revealed a remarkably complex pattern of transcription factors that are preferentially expressed in α-cell versus β-cell lines[15] and in single α cells isolated from the developing endocrine pancreas.[16] The rat proglucagon gene promoter has been analyzed in considerable detail and appears to direct transcriptional initiation from a single transcription start site that maps to an identical location in the brain, pancreas, and intestine.[17] Cell transfection experiments utilizing islet cell lines have identified five distinct regions, designated G1 to G5 (see Fig. 51-2), within the proximal proglucagon promoter that exhibit functional importance for activation of islet cell–specific proglucagon gene transcription.[18-20] The proximal G1 region is AT-rich, interacts with both widely expressed and islet cell–specific proteins, and is functionally important for specifying expression in islet A cells. G1 interacts with the homeobox transcription factors Isl-1, Cdx-2/3, Brn4, and Pax6.[10,21-24] These transcription factors bind G1 and activate reporter genes containing G1-derived sequences in transfection assays. Reduction of *isl-1* expression in islet cell lines expressing antisense *isl-1* RNA leads to reduced G1-dependent proglucagon promoter activity and decreased levels of proglucagon mRNA transcripts.[21] Similarly, increased expression of Cdx-3 in islet cells is associated with induction of both transfected G1-dependent reporter genes and endogenous proglucagon gene expression.[22,25] The G4 element, located just upstream of G1, binds a complex resembling insulin-enhancer factor 1 (IEF-1), and recent experiments suggest that IEF-1 represents a heterodimer of the helix-loop-helix proteins E47 and BETA2.[26]

The more distal G3 region functions as an islet enhancer–like element and has been divided into two distinct functional domains. Subdomain A contains a sequence element that is similar to sequences found within the insulin and somatostatin promoters, leading to the designation of this composite sequence as a *p*ancreatic *i*slet *c*ell–specific *e*nhancer sequence,

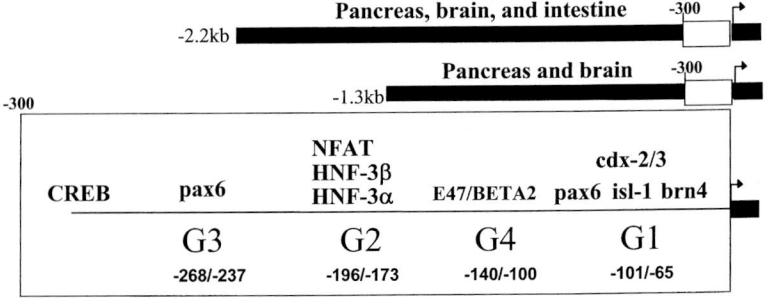

Figure 51-2 Organization of the rat glucagon gene promoter, including the G1 to G4 promoter elements, and their cognate transcription factors.

or PISCES element.[27,28] Sequences within domain A of G3 also appear to mediate the inhibition of glucagon gene transcription by insulin.[29-31] The pax6 protein has been identified as a positive activator of proglucagon gene transcription that exerts its function in part through interaction with domain A of the G3 element.[10] Pax6 also binds the G1 element, either as a monomer or via heterodimer formation with cdx-2/3.[32] Disruption of Pax6 expression in gene-targeted mice results in loss of islet A cells.[9,10] The levels of pancreatic and intestinal proglucagon mRNA transcripts are also markedly reduced in SEY(NEU) mice that harbor a dominant negative mutation in the *pax6* gene. Thus, Pax6, a PISCES-binding protein, is functionally important for both islet and enteroendocrine cell development and activation of proglucagon gene transcription via the G3 enhancer and G1 promoter elements.[9,10,32,33]

The G2 element mediates the positive and negative actions of HNF-3 (Foxa) proteins, with isoforms of HNF-3β and HNF-3α competing for binding to the G2 element and serving as repressors and activators, respectively, of proglucagon gene transcription.[34,35] HNF-3γ also binds to and transactivates the proglucagon promoter G2 element but does not appear to be essential for islet cell formation or glucagon gene transcription.[36-38] Whether HNF-3β plays an essential role in development of islet α-cell formation or glucagon gene transcription in vivo remains unknown as targeted inactivation of the HNF-3β gene results in embryonic lethality prior to the formation of the endocrine pancreas.[39,40] Although the numbers of α cells and morphology of islets appear histologically normal in HNF3α[-/-] mice, the development of neonatal hypoglycemia in the face of inappropriately reduced levels of circulating glucagon and proglucagon mRNA transcripts demonstrates the essential role of HNF-3α in pancreatic proglucagon gene transcription.[36]

Activation of the cyclic adenosine monophosphate (cAMP)-dependent pathway leads to transcriptional induction of proglucagon gene expression in both islet and intestinal cells through a cAMP response element (CRE) present, upstream of the G3 element (see Fig. 51-2), in the proximal promoter region of the rat proglucagon gene.[41,42] The CRE also mediates transcriptional activation by ATF3 family members[43] and is the target for pharmacologic depolarization-dependent induction of rat proglucagon gene transcription.[44] A second calcium response element has been localized to the G2 element, and calcium responsiveness may be mediated via interaction of NFAT (nuclear factor of activated T cells)-like proteins with members of the HNF-3 family.[45] The sequence of the CRE element is less well conserved in the human proglucagon promoter, and its functional relevance for proglucagon gene expression in human islets has not yet been elucidated.

Transgenic experiments in mice have identified distinct DNA sequences that are essential for tissue-specific proglucagon gene transcription in vivo. The first 1253 nucleotides of the rat proglucagon promoter direct heterologous transgene expression to the islets and brain but not the intestine in transgenic mice.[46] In contrast, targeting of transgene expression to enteroendocrine cells in vivo requires the presence of additional rat proglucagon gene 5'-flanking sequences between −1253 and −2252.[47] Intriguingly, DNA sequences comprising the human proglucagon gene promoter exhibit different functional properties than homologous rat sequences, as the first 1600 base pairs of the human proglucagon gene 5'-flanking region target transgene expression to appropriate cell types in the brain and intestine but not the pancreatic islets in transgenic mice.[48]

ISLET PROGLUCAGON BIOSYNTHESIS

Consistent with the well-described increase in circulating glucagon levels in patients with diabetes, experimental diabetes in rodents is associated with increased levels of pancreatic proglucagon mRNA; correction of the insulin deficiency, but not the hyperglycemia, normalizes the levels of proglucagon

mRNA.[49] In contrast to the well-defined role of insulin as a negative regulator of proglucagon biosynthesis, few hormones or metabolites have been identified that clearly increase the synthesis of pancreatic proglucagon in vivo. Although experiments using in situ hybridization suggested that 4 days of fasting in the rat leads to a doubling of pancreatic proglucagon mRNA transcripts,[50] studies of insulin-induced hypoglycemia failed to demonstrate upregulation of proglucagon mRNA, perhaps owing to the confounding inhibitory effects of insulin administration.[49,51] Indeed, the majority of studies examining regulators of glucagon secretion fail to demonstrate significant changes in the levels of proglucagon mRNA,[52] suggesting that regulation of secretion, and not biosynthesis, may be a more physiologically relevant locus of control in vivo.

Following transcription of proglucagon mRNA and translation of the proglucagon precursor, 29-amino-acid mature glucagon is liberated via posttranslational processing by specific prohormone convertases that are differentially expressed in the islet α cell. In contrast to processing in the enteroendocrine cell (see Fig. 51-1), the amino acid sequences carboxyterminal to glucagon remain unprocessed and are secreted as part of a larger polypeptide designated the major proglucagon fragment. Studies using islet cell lines and mice implicate a role for prohormone convertase 2 (PC2) in processing of proglucagon to glucagon in α cells. PC2[-/-] mice exhibit hypoglycemia, α-cell hyperplasia, and glucagon deficiency with an accumulation of incompletely processed PGDPs in the pancreas.[13] Whether PC2 directly liberates glucagon from proglucagon or cleaves proglucagon to glicentin, which is then subsequently processed to glucagon, remains unclear.[13,53-55] The enzyme PC1 appears to be responsible for cleavage of proglucagon to yield an intestinal profile of PGDPs,[53,56] and PC1 null mice exhibit impaired processing of proglucagon to the glucagon-like peptides.[57] Moreover, human subjects with an inactivating mutation in the PC1 gene exhibit incompletely processed proglucagon in gut endocrine cells and deficiency of both GLP-1 and GLP-2.[58] The convertases that are important for proglucagon processing in the brain have not been definitively identified.

GLUCAGON SECRETION

The secretion of glucagon is regulated, both positively and negatively, by neuropeptides, hormones, metabolites, and the autonomic nervous system. The islet α cell plays a central role in the defense of blood glucose, with hypoglycemia stimulating and hyperglycemia suppressing glucagon secretion in vivo. A cells express voltage-dependent Na^+, K^+, and Ca^{2+} channels that interact in the regulation of membrane potential and ultimately, depolarization.[59] Amino acids such as glutamine, alanine, pyruvate, and arginine stimulate both insulin and glucagon secretion, and this observation provides the basis for the use of arginine in the assessment of islet and α-cell function in rodent and human physiology.[60] Both α- and β-adrenergic receptors modulate glucagon secretion. Epinephrine stimulates glucagon secretion via a protein kinase A (PKA)-dependent enhancement of Ca^{2+} influx through L-type calcium channels, leading to granule exocytosis.[61] Peptidergic activators of glucagon secretion include cholecystokinin (CCK), pituitary adenylate cyclase-activating polypeptide, gastrin, urocortin III, vasopressin, and gastric inhibitory peptide (GIP).

In contrast, inhibitors of glucagon secretion include glucose, somatostatin-14, and γ-aminobutyric acid (GABA).[59] Glucose induces GABA release from β cells, providing an indirect mechanism for glucose-mediated suppression of glucagon secretion.[62-64] Insulin may also directly inhibit glucagon release, possibly via insulin receptors expressed on α cells. The anatomic arrangement of peripheral islet α cell surrounding a core of β cells, taken together with the functional results of immunoneutralization studies, provides additional evidence for intraislet insulin inhibiting downstream α cells in some species.[65] Although the mechanisms underlying the paracrine inhibition of α-cell activity remain unclear, β-cell secretory products such as zinc have been identified as potential negative regulators of glucagon secretion from rat islets.[64]

The effects of glucose on glucagon secretion are integrated with the inhibitory effects of insulin on α-cell secretion, as hyperglycemia stimulates insulin secretion, whereas a drop in blood glucose suppresses insulin release from the β cell, thereby relieving the α cell from the tonic inhibitory actions of insulin. These actions are exemplified by meal ingestion, which is associated with increased circulating nutrients, insulin secretion, and reduced levels of circulating glucagon. In contrast, blood glucose is maintained in the fasting state by hepatic glucose production due in part to increased levels of glucagon secretion and suppression of insulin release from the β cell.[66,67] Consistent with the effect of individual nutrients on α-cell function, infusion of arginine stimulates glucagon secretion in both normal subjects and individuals with diabetes mellitus.[67] The response to arginine infusion in normal human subjects, namely, stimulation of insulin and glucagon release, is reproducible, and as expected, the insulin response is significantly greater and the glucagon response is attenuated as the glucose concentration increases.[68]

In normal subjects, glucagon secretion rises as glucose falls in the fasting state and may be further stimulated by exercise, consistent with the physiologic role for glucagon in regulating glucose production. The levels of both glucagon and plasma catecholamines increase with graded exercise in normal human subjects, the greatest increments in plasma glucagon being observed in subjects undergoing prolonged exhaustive exercise.[69] The exercise-induced increment in plasma glucagon appears to be dependent on the degree and duration of exercise, some studies demonstrating no significant changes in plasma glucagon during exercise under normoglycemic conditions.[70] Trained healthy male subjects exhibit increased hepatic glucose production following glucagon infusion, implying that exercise might be associated with the development of increased glucagon sensitivity.[71] Although prevention of exercise-induced rises in plasma glucagon by concomitant somatostatin infusion may result in mild hypoglycemia,[72] suppression of the rise in plasma glucagon by somatostatin infusion does not always prevent increased hepatic glucose production, likely owing to redundant compensatory mechanisms for maintaining normoglycemia.[72,73]

The control of hepatic glucose production (HGP) is highly sensitive to the glucagon/insulin ratio, and the secretion of these two hormones is generally regulated in a reciprocal manner. The effect of insulin to suppress HGP may actually be determined in part by the levels of circulating glucagon.[74] Following meal ingestion, nutrient absorption is associated with energy assimilation and suppression of glucagon secretion. Nevertheless, the integrated response of islet α cells is dependent in part on the nutrient composition of the meal and also reflects positive and negative enteric-derived regulators of glucagon secretion. For example, ingestion of carbohydrate, especially glucose, is associated with a decline in plasma glucagon.[67] Nutrients also promote release of gut-derived peptides such as CCK and GIP, which stimulate glucagon release,[75,76] and GLP-1, which inhibits glucagon release.[77,78]

Glucagon secretion is increased during times of stress, and "stress-induced hormones" such as cortisol, vasopressin, and β-endorphin increase glucagon secretion from the α cell. The classic stress hormones epinephrine and norepinephrine also stimulate glucagon secretion, and several mechanisms link the autonomic nervous system to increased secretion from the α cell. Epinephrine secreted from the adrenal medulla increases glucagon secretion in normoglycemic

subjects. Furthermore, the pancreas receives innervation from both sympathetic and parasympathetic nerves, and stimulation of these autonomic inputs, all of which are activated by hypoglycemia, increases glucagon secretion.[79] Intriguingly, mice with targeted inactivation of the pro-opiomelanocortin gene (and hence adrenocorticotropic hormone [ACTH]) exhibit a profound defect in the counterregulatory response to insulin-induced hypoglycemia, owing largely to defective glucagon secretion. Although specific genetic defects in glucagon secretion have not been described, nondiabetic subjects with mutations in the MODY1/HNF-4α gene exhibit decreased arginine-stimulated glucagon secretion and reduced glucose suppression of plasma glucagon,[80] raising the possibility that the HNF-4α transcription factor influences islet α-cell function through a direct or indirect mechanism.

HYPOGLYCEMIA

Increasing evidence suggests that multiple complementary mechanisms activate α-cell secretion during hypoglycemia. Analysis of the glycemic threshold for activation of counterregulatory mechanisms demonstrates that increased epinephrine and glucagon secretion constitute the initial hormonal responses to decreasing blood sugar. Furthermore, the glucose threshold for activation of counterregulatory responses is clearly higher than the threshold for triggering hypoglycemic symptoms in normal subjects.[81] Whether hypoglycemia itself directly stimulates glucagon secretion independent of autonomic input remains unclear. Nevertheless, hypoglycemia suppresses insulin (and β-cell) secretion, which removes an important inhibitory influence on glucagon secretion. The finding that α cells express the GLUT-1 transporter and glucokinase suggests that glucose transport does not appear to be a critical rate-limiting step for glucose metabolism in α cells and provides important insight into how α cells directly sense ambient changes in glucose concentrations.[82,83] Hence, the α cell appears to contain the requisite molecules for sensing and responding to changes in glucose concentrations via glucose metabolism. A role for gastrin in the stimulation of glucagon secretion has been proposed, and gastrin$^{-/-}$ mice exhibit defective glucagon secretion in response to insulin-induced hypoglycemia.[84]

The role of circulating epinephrine in the autonomic response to hypoglycemia is well established. Epinephrine also directly stimulates glucagon secretion in normal human subjects, and stimulation of the autonomic sympathetic nervous system innervation to the pancreas elicits an increase in α-cell secretion.[85,86] Furthermore, parasympathetic nerve stimulation or the neurotransmitter acetylcholine and the neuropeptide VIP all stimulate glucagon secretion. Studies using nerve transection or pharmacologic blockade have illustrated that these pathways exhibit some degree of functional redundancy, providing multiple backup mechanisms to ensure that the α cell responds appropriately to hypoglycemia. Nevertheless, the ganglionic blocker trimethaphan, which impairs autonomic transmission in both ganglia and the adrenal gland, markedly attenuated the glucagon response to hypoglycemia in normal subjects,[87] emphasizing the important link between autonomic activation and the glucagon counterregulatory response in vivo. In contrast, however, pancreas transplantation restores the glucagon response to hypoglycemia, even in patients with severe autonomic neuropathy,[88] illustrating the functional redundancy of mechanisms that is essential for the α-cell response to hypoglycemia.

The identity of the specific glucose sensors that trigger the appropriate counterregulatory response to hypoglycemia remains under active investigation. Mice with genetic disruption of the Kir6.2 channel exhibit normal functional α cells yet display a marked defect in the glucagon response to hypoglycemia.[89] Both the central nervous system (CNS), principally the venteromedial hypothalamus (VMH), and the splanchnic region, specifically the portal system and liver, contain glucose-sensing systems. Focal lesions in the VMH or perfusion of the VMH with 2-deoxyglucose substantially diminishes or abrogates the peripheral glucagon secretory response to hypoglycemia in rats.[90,91] Selective perfusion of the portal venous system in rats suggests that the portal vein glucose concentration is a key determinant of the sympathoadrenal response to hypoglycemia; however, whether portal glucose sensors are directly or indirectly linked to control of islet glucagon secretion is not clear.[92] Intriguingly, injection of glucose into the portal vein activates glucose-sensitive neurons in the lateral hypothalamus and brain stem, suggesting the possibility of a portal-CNS glucoregulatory axis. The detection of a markedly defective counterregulatory response to hypoglycemia, including absent glucagon and catecholamine secretion, in a patient with hypothalamic sarcoidosis further emphasizes the importance of the hypothalamus in sensing glucose and triggering the release of counterregulatory hormones.[93] In contrast, analysis of patients after removal of craniopharyngiomas revealed selective impairment of counterregulatory sympathoadrenal activation but normal glucagon responses to hypoglycemia. Furthermore, human subjects with liver transplants and denervated livers exhibit increased levels of circulating glucagon and defective insulin-suppression of glucagon, and human islet transplantation is associated with a defective glucagon response to hypoglycemia.[94,95] These findings emphasize the importance of the autonomic nervous system and CNS for the regulation of basal and hypoglycemia-stimulated glucagon secretion.

GLUCAGON SECRETION AND DIABETES

Following the development of glucagon radioimmunoassays, glucagon levels were noted to be elevated in patients with poorly controlled diabetes, and the lack of the inhibitory action of insulin on the α cell likely contributes to increased glucagon secretion in insulin-deficient diabetic patients. The correction of hyperglucagonemia, using somatostatin pharmacologically or insulin replacement therapeutically reverses the majority of metabolic derangements associated with insulin-deficient diabetes.[96] These findings have fostered a search for glucagon antagonists that might be employed as adjuncts in the treatment of diabetes, and preliminary evidence obtained by using experimental animal models of diabetes suggests the feasibility of this approach in vivo.[97] Moreover, genetic attenuation of glucagon receptor expression in db/db mice produced significant amelioration of experimental diabetes over a 3-week study period.[98] Despite the central importance of glucagon for control of glucose production, hyperglucagonemia alone, without insulin deficiency, does not significantly increase plasma glucose.[99] In the presence of adequate amounts of insulin, glucose production is suppressible despite glucagon excess, emphasizing the insulin/glucagon ratio, not just the absolute level of glucagon, as a key determinant of glucose homeostasis.[100] Nevertheless, hyperglucagonemia is associated with increased leucine oxidation and resting metabolic rate in subjects with type 1 diabetes, reemphasizing the importance of both insulin and glucagon in the catabolism associated with suboptimally treated diabetes.[101]

The application of intensive insulin therapy to the management of patients with type 1 diabetes is associated with an increased incidence of hypoglycemia and heightened awareness of the importance of counterregulatory mechanisms for maintaining normoglycemia. A number of factors conspire to inhibit glucagon release in insulin-treated patients with type 1 diabetes, including intensive insulin administration, hyperglycemia, and diminished autonomic stimulation of the α cell.[79] Although the glucagon response to hypoglycemia is initially normal in patients with type 1 diabetes, this response

frequently becomes impaired, increasing patients' susceptibility to hypoglycemia.[102] As intensive insulin treatment regimens become more common, impaired counterregulation and hypoglycemia have been observed in some patients with a very short duration of diabetes, suggesting that frequent episodes of hypoglycemia represent an independent risk for development of an abnormal α-cell response. The α-cell dysfunction in type 1 diabetes is often selective, as the response to hypoglycemia may be absent, yet glucagon secretion may respond normally to arginine stimulation.[103] Further evidence emphasizing the importance of intraislet hyperinsulinemia in the suppression of glucagon secretion derives from observations that tolbutamide-infused subjects exhibit profound defects in the glucagon response to hypoglycemia.[104]

Importantly, restoration of normoglycemia for several months may decrease hypoglycemia unawareness in association with improvement in the glucagon response to hypoglycemia in some studies.[105] However, a dissociation between improvement in hypoglycemia unawareness and persistence of defective counterregulatory responses has also been observed.[106] Although not completely understood, antecedent hypoglycemia in type 1 diabetes can produce counterregulatory failure during subsequent episodes of prolonged moderate-intensity exercise,[107] emphasizing the complex interrelationship between insulin-induced and exercise-associated counterregulation.

Multiple defects likely contribute to α-cell dysfunction in patients with diabetes. An important issue with therapeutic implications is the role of antecedent hypoglycemia in the development of α-cell dysfunction and deficient glucagon secretion. Intriguingly, the glucagon response to hypoglycemia may be comparatively more defective in the fasting state than in the postprandial state. Patients with some residual β-cell function, as assessed by C peptide stimulation, appear to be at decreased risk for hypoglycemia, owing in part to preserved counterregulatory glucagon responses. Additional contributing factors may include subtle impairment of autonomic stimulation following repeated hypoglycemic episodes. Nevertheless, impaired epinephrine and glucagon responses to insulin-induced hypoglycemia have been observed after a single antecedent hypoglycemic episode in nondiabetic subjects,[108] although increased levels of cortisol alone do not acutely induce defects in hypoglycemic counterregulation. These observations emphasize the susceptibility of the normal α cell to episodes of hypoglycemia, with initial reversibility of α-cell function superseded, over time, by more sustained defects in the glucagon response to hypoglycemia.

GLUCAGON ACTION

The importance of glucagon in the control of hepatic glucose metabolism provides a useful model for analysis of hormone action in metabolic pathways. Glucagon stimulates glucose production via activation of hepatic glycogenolysis and gluconeogenesis and by inhibition of glycolysis. Following activation of the glucagon receptor, adenylyl cyclase activity is increased, leading to activation of protein kinase A, phosphorylase kinase, and phosphorylase. These actions increase the rate of glycogenolysis via glycogen phosphorylase and inactivate glycogen synthase.[109] Glucagon action serves to modify the activity of enzymes that are important for glucose production via effects on specific kinases and phosphatases. Glucagon also modulates the expression of genes encoding enzymes of the glycolytic or gluconeogenic pathways[110] and regulates fatty acid metabolism via reduction of malonyl CoA and stimulation of fatty acid oxidation. The cAMP-dependent transcription factor CREB is an important downstream mediator for glucagon action, acting in part through activation of the nuclear receptor coactivator PGC-1 and suppression of peroxisome proliferator–activated receptor γ (PPAR-γ) activity, which induces a metabolic program resulting in the activation of hepatic gluconeogenesis.[111]

In adipocytes, glucagon increases cAMP and stimulates lipolysis, thereby providing free fatty acids as substrate for fat-burning tissues. Glucagon also inhibits insulin-stimulated glucose transport in adipocytes through effects on insulin binding and via postreceptor mechanisms.[112] In the peripheral vascular system, glucagon functions as a vasodilator via effects on local vascular tone and glucagon increases both cardiac output and heart rate, possibly via direct effects on the heart. Pharmacologic doses of glucagon increase renal blood flow, glomerular filtration rate (GFR), and urinary electrolyte excretion; however, lower physiologic concentrations of glucagon do not affect renal blood flow, GFR, or solute excretion.[113] The kidney also exhibits significant gluconeogenic capacity and might account for up to 25% of systemic glucose production in humans.[114] Although renal glucose output is markedly increased in subjects with diabetes and hypoglycemia increases renal glucose output in association with increased release of counterregulatory hormones, the available evidence does not support an important role for glucagon in the control of renal glucose output.[115]

The actions of glucagon are transduced via activation of the glucagon receptor (Gcgr) a 7-transmembrane-spanning G protein–coupled receptor. The cloned receptor responds to glucagon with an increase in both intracellular cAMP and intracellular calcium.[116] The human glucagon receptor gene has been localized to chromosome 17q25. Although activating mutations of the Gcgr have been generated by mutagenesis in vitro,[117] no constitutively active Gcgr mutations have been reported in human subjects. Intriguingly, several reports have described an association, initially in populations of French and Sardinian subjects, between a Gly40Ser Gcgr mutation and an increased incidence of type 2 diabetes. Paradoxically, cells that express a transfected glucagon receptor containing the Gly40Ser mutation exhibit decreased affinity for glucagon in vitro, and subjects with the Gly40Ser mutation exhibit a decreased glycemic response to glucagon infusion in vivo.[118,119] Furthermore, several population studies have failed to find an association linking the Gly40Ser mutation with an increased prevalence of type 2 diabetes.[118,120] Hence, whether the Gly40Ser mutation itself contributes to a diabetes predisposition or is associated with other genes that increase diabetes susceptibility in certain populations remains unclear.

The tissue distribution of Gcgr expression correlates well with studies localizing high-affinity glucagon-binding sites, with Gcgr mRNA transcripts detected in liver, brain, adipocytes, heart, kidney, and islet β cells. Rat Gcgr mRNA transcripts have also been detected in spleen, thymus, adrenal gland, ovary, and testis, nonclassical target tissues where glucagon action remains poorly defined.[121] Although glucagon action has been extensively studied in the liver and adipocytes, the precise biologic importance of glucagon in the brain remains unclear. The brain stem is the principal site of CNS proglucagon gene expression[122]; however, PGDPs are transported from the brain stem along nerve fibers to multiple brain regions.[123] Consistent with these findings, glucagon-binding sites are detected in multiple brain regions, and the glucagon receptor is expressed in the cortex, cerebellum, hypothalamus, and brain stem; however, the specific biologic action of glucagon in each of these CNS regions remains unclear.[124] Although intracerebroventricular injection of glucagon in rodents causes hyperglycemia and increases sympathetic nervous system discharge, whether these findings are relevant to physiological control of glucose homeostasis requires further analysis.

The β cell expresses receptors for glucagon, GIP, and GLP-1 that are all coupled to cAMP and stimulation of insulin secretion. The threshold for glucagon-stimulated cAMP accumulation in isolated β cells is ~1 nM glucagon, higher than the concentrations that are required for cAMP stimulation by GLP-1 or GIP.[125] The physiologic importance of endogenous glucagon for β-cell physiology in vivo remains unclear, given the direction of islet blood flow, the peripheral location of islet α cells, and the high concentrations of glucagon that are required to stimulate the β cell in vitro. Nevertheless, it remains possible that glucagon action on the β cell is also transduced through non-cAMP-dependent pathways, perhaps at a lower threshold glucagon concentration.

Unexpected insights into glucagon action derive from experiments characterizing the phenotype of glucagon receptor knockout mice.[14,126] Gcgr−/− mice exhibit marked elevations in the levels of plasma glucagon, mild fasting hypoglycemia, increased pancreatic weight, α-cell hyperplasia, and increased circulating levels of the PGDPs. The compensatory mechanisms that are sufficient for maintaining glucose production despite the complete absence of hepatic glucagon receptor signaling remain unknown. Similarly, the glucagon receptor–dependent signal(s) regulating the number and secretory function of islet α cells have not yet been elucidated.

Both the liver and kidney contribute to glucagon clearance from the circulation; however, these sites account for less than 50% of glucagon clearance, implicating additional tissues as sites for glucagon clearance or degradation.[127] Glucagon action is terminated via both extracellular and intracellular degradation pathways. Glucagon-degrading activity within hepatic endosomes has been attributed to cathepsins B and D in studies using cathepsin inhibitors,[128] and both glucagon and GLP-1 are substrates for the widely expressed membrane-bound neutral ectopeptidase (NEP) 24.11.[129] An endopeptidase activity has been described that cleaves 29-amino-acid glucagon to "miniglucagon," also known as glucagon (19-29) in various tissues. The physiological importance of miniglucagon remains uncertain; glucagon (19-29) has positive inotropic actions in ventricular myocyte preparations,[130] and miniglucagon has also been shown to inhibit insulin release via effects on L-type calcium channels in a pertussis toxin-dependent manner.[131,132] Whether glucagon (19-29) exerts physiologically relevant effects via a separate unique receptor remains unclear.

PHARMACEUTICAL USE OF GLUCAGON IN HUMAN PATIENTS

Glucagon is employed as both a diagnostic and a therapeutic agent. Although historically useful for the diagnosis of pheochromocytoma, stimulation of catecholamine secretion in such patients may be dangerous; hence, the glucagon stimulation test is not widely used for this purpose. Glucagon may also be employed as part of a diagnostic test in patients with hypoglycemia of unknown origin. Perhaps the most common clinical application of glucagon therapeutically is in the adjunctive management of severe hypoglycemia. Diabetic patients with hypoglycemia generally respond quickly, with a rapid increase in blood glucose, to intranasal, intramuscular, or subcutaneous glucagon administration.[133,134] Glucagon is also used to inhibit gastrointestinal motility during radiologic investigations, and several studies have reported the efficacy of glucagon administration in small numbers of patients with bronchospasm or symptomatic bradycardia.[135,136]

GLUCAGON EXCESS AND DEFICIENCY

Glucagonomas presenting as solitary lesions or as part of a multiple endocrine neoplasia syndrome are most commonly detected in the pancreas and are often associated with significant elevations in the levels of circulating glucagon and the PGDPs.[137] Rarely, extrapancreatic glucagon-producing tumors have been reported in sites including the kidney and ovary. Although many gut carcinoid tumors contain PGDP immunoreactivity, they are not generally associated with the development of a "glucagonoma syndrome." Glucagonoma patients generally present with a pathognomonic skin rash termed *necrolytic migratory erythema*, a detectable pancreatic mass, weight loss, glossitis, anemia, and some degree of glucose intolerance.[138] The clinical presentation can be variable, likely reflecting adaptation to the metabolic effects of tumor-secreted PGDPs and tumor-specific differences in posttranslational processing of proglucagon. Rarely, patients may present with glucagonomas and associated manifestations of intestinal hyperplasia, presumably due to release of GLP-2.[139] Treatment of benign glucagonomas usually involves surgical resection, whereas chemotherapy, attempted suppression of PGDP secretion and tumor growth with somatostatin analogues, or adjunctive radiotherapy may be indicated in patients with malignant disease. Experimental glucagonomas have also been studied in rodents, and several intriguing phenotypes, including severe anorexia and reduction in islet size, remain poorly understood.[140,141] Several reports have described isolated cases of glucagon deficiency in infants with hypoglycemia; however, these cases are extremely rare. The molecular basis for the putative glucagon deficiency and whether congenital glucagon deficiency is compatible with survival remain unknown.

THE GLUCAGON-LIKE PEPTIDES: GLP-1 AND GLP-2

The proglucagon gene is expressed in the gastrointestinal tract in the stomach and both small and large intestines. The intestinal, brain, and pancreatic mammalian proglucagon mRNA transcripts are identical in structure; hence, tissue-specific posttranslational processing underlies the liberation of the glucagon-like peptides in the brain and gastrointestinal tract. In contrast to the pancreas, much less is known about the control of intestinal GLP-1 and GLP-2 biosynthesis. The proglucagon gene islet transcription factors *cdx-2/3*, *pax6*, and members of the HNF3 (Foxa) family are also expressed in enteroendocrine cells and presumably regulate proglucagon gene transcription in both cell types. Neurogenin-3 has been identified as an essential upstream determinant of global enteroendocrine cell development. Analysis of *SEY(NEU)* mice with a dominant negative *pax6* mutation demonstrated a marked reduction in the levels of proglucagon mRNA transcripts in both the small and large intestines. Hence, the *pax6* gene is essential for both islet and enteroendocrine proglucagon gene transcription. Proglucagon biosynthesis in the gut is regulated by nutrient intake,[142] with feeding, and fiber-enriched diets increasing proglucagon gene expression in the proximal and distal intestine, respectively.

GLUCAGON-LIKE PEPTIDE 1

GLP-1, in both the (7-37) and (7-36^amide) molecular forms, is liberated from proglucagon via posttranslational processing and secreted from intestinal endocrine cells in a nutrient-dependent manner.[143] Although enteroendocrine L cells are distributed along the length of the entire gastrointestinal tract from the stomach to the rectum, the largest numbers of L cells are found in the terminal ileum and proximal colon. The rapid increase in plasma GLP-1 following food ingestion has fostered interest in the existence of a proximal-distal loop, whereby nutrients entering the duodenum and proximal jejunum promote one or more endocrine and/or neural signals that activate GLP-1 secretion from the distal small bowel.[144] Studies in rats have identified GIP as one putative component of such a signaling system. The specific signaling mechanisms that nutrients utilize for stimulation of GLP-1 secretion in humans are not completely understood.

The regulation of GLP-1 bioactivity is dependent to a large extent on the rate of GLP-1 degradation in vivo. Both GLP-1 and GLP-2 contain an alanine residue at position 2, rendering these molecules ideal substrates for enzymatic inactivation by dipeptidyl peptidase IV. This enzyme, expressed locally in the intestine proximal to sites of GLP-1 synthesis, cleaves circulating GLP-1 to yield the biologically inactive molecule GLP-1 (9-37/9-36^amide).[145] Although GLP-1 (9-37/9-36^amide) displays weak binding affinity for the GLP-1 receptor and is theoretically a circulating antagonist of GLP-1 action, the physiologic importance of circulating GLP-1 (9-37/9-36^amide) has not been established, and infusion of GLP-1(9-36^amide) had no effect on glucose tolerance and insulin secretion in human subjects.[146] Nevertheless, a substantial amount of total GLP-1 immunoreactivity circulates as GLP-1 (9-37/9-36^amide), and assays that do not distinguish between intact GLP-1 and cleaved GLP-1 (9-37/9-36^amide) will overestimate the circulating concentrations of bioactive GLP-1. Owing largely to rapid DPP-IV-mediated inactivation of GLP-1, the $t_{1/2}$ of circulating intact bioactive GLP-1 is very short, generally less than 1 minute. These findings, coupled with the proposed pharmaceutical use of GLP-1 for the treatment of diabetes, have encouraged efforts at developing more potent long-acting GLP-1 analogues that are resistant to DPP-IV-mediated inactivation. Alternatively, inhibitors of the DPP-IV enzyme have also been identified that lower blood sugar and show therapeutic promise in studies of experimental diabetes in rodents and in short-term clinical trials of patients with type 2 diabetes.[147,148]

GLP-1 exerts several complementary actions that control postprandial glycemic excursion (Fig. 51-3). The initial description of GLP-1 bioactivity focused on its actions in the endocrine pancreas, where GLP-1 stimulates glucose-dependent insulin secretion from β cells.[149] GLP-1 also increases proinsulin gene expression and inhibits glucagon secretion; however, the mechanism for the effect of GLP-1 on α cells, perhaps indirectly through stimulation of insulin or somatostatin, is not completely delineated.[150] Considerable data from studies of cell lines, primary cell cultures, and rodents indicate that GLP-1 receptor (GLP-1R) agonists regulate growth and development of the endocrine pancreas.[151] GLP-1 receptor activation enhances β-cell proliferation and promotes islet neogenesis via activation of pdx-1 expression. The proliferative effects of GLP-1 involve multiple intracellular pathways, including stimulation of Akt, activation of protein kinase Cζ, and transactivation of the epidermal growth factor (EGF) receptor through the c-src kinase. GLP-1 receptor activation also promotes cell survival in β cells and neurons via increased levels of cAMP leading to CRE binding protein (CREB) activation, enhanced insulin receptor substrate (IRS)-2 activity, and, ultimately, activation of Akt. These actions of GLP-1 are reflected by expansion of β-cell mass and enhanced resistance to β-cell injury demonstrated in multiple experimental models of diabetes in vivo. The β-cell actions of GLP-1 that promoting cell proliferation and resistance to apoptosis appear to be physiologically essential in mice, as GLP-1R⁻ mice exhibit modest defects in the formation of large islets and enhanced susceptibility to apoptotic injury.[152] Of potential relevance to the therapeutic use of GLP-1 is the demonstration that primary human islet cultures exhibit improved glucose-dependent insulin secretion and enhanced survival following short-term exposure to GLP-1 in vitro.[153]

Inhibition of gastric emptying accounts for a significant part of the glucose-lowering actions of GLP-1, especially in patients with type 1 diabetes. Indeed, excess GLP-1 administration causes gastric discomfort and cramping in human subjects.[154] Sensations of increased satiety and decreased appetite are common following GLP-1 infusion in human subjects.[155] As GLP-1 that is administered intracerebroventricularly to rodents inhibits food intake,[156] GLP-1 may decrease appetite via both central effects on the hypothalamic nuclei involved in feeding and via peripheral effects on gastric emptying. Decreased food intake and a slowing of nutrient transit in the upper gastrointestinal tract appear to contribute to a portion of the glucose lowering effect of GLP-1 in vivo. Although administration of GLP-1 and its analogues to rodents also

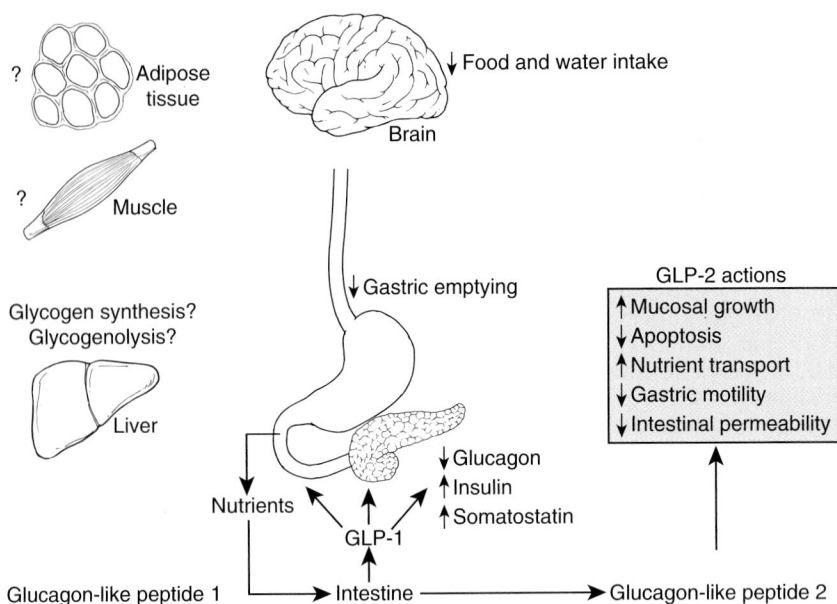

Figure 51-3 Biologic actions of the glucagon-like peptides GLP-1 and GLP-2.

results in decreased water intake, these actions do not appear to be clinically significant in human studies.

GLP-1 exerts its actions through activation of a G protein–coupled receptor that is structurally related to the glucagon/secretin receptor superfamily.[157] In keeping with studies of glucagon signaling, GLP-1 transduces its signal through both cAMP and calcium-dependent pathways. Although a potential candidate diabetes gene, the GLP-1R localized to human 6p21 has not been associated with linkage to families with type 2 diabetes. Similarly, no GLP-1R mutations have been identified in individuals with diabetes, nor have activating mutations of the GLP-1R been described in human subjects.

Evidence for the physiologic importance of GLP-1 in glucose control derives from studies using GLP-1 antagonists to inhibit GLP-1 action in vivo. Infusion of the GLP-1 antagonist exendin (9-39) into rats or humans increases blood glucose in association with decreased levels of glucose-stimulated insulin.[158,159] Similarly, immunoneutralization of GLP-1 activity using GLP-1 antiserum increased both fasting and meal-related glycemic excursions in baboons.[160] Furthermore, mice with targeted disruption of the GLP-1R exhibit mild diabetes, with abnormalities in both fasting and postprandial glycemia and subnormal levels of glucose-stimulated insulin.[161] GLP-1R$^{-/-}$ mice do not exhibit changes in insulin sensitivity, and basal and glucose-suppressible levels of circulating glucagon are normal. Furthermore, in contrast to the importance of GLP-1 for glucose homeostasis, GLP-1R$^{-/-}$ mice are not obese and do not exhibit abnormalities in food intake, suggesting that long-term disruption of GLP-1 signaling does not produce abnormalities in satiety or body weight.[162]

The multiple actions of GLP-1 in lowering blood glucose in both normal subjects and in patients with both type 1 and type 2 diabetes have raised the possibility that GLP-1 may find a role as a therapeutic agent in diabetes therapy. GLP-1 lowers blood glucose in sulfonylurea-resistant patients, and experimental data from rodents demonstrate that GLP-1 restores glycemic control and increases insulin mRNA in aging rats,[163] providing a rationale for GLP-1 therapy in selected patients with diabetes. Studies in human subjects have demonstrated the safety and efficacy of using GLP-1 to achieve short-term glucose control over 4 to 12 weeks in patients with type 2 diabetes. Native GLP-1 was administered via continuous subcutaneous infusion for 6 weeks to obese subjects with type 2 diabetes, resulting in highly significant improvement in glucose control, reduced HbA1c, improved insulin sensitivity, and a small but significant mean 1.9 kg weight loss.[164]

As the glucose-lowering effects of native GLP-1 administered by single subcutaneous administration are transient and no longer evident 1 to 2 hours following peptide injection,[165] current therapeutic efforts are focused on development of stable degradation-resistant GLP-1R agonists, including the lizard peptide exendin-4 (Exenatide) and the human GLP-1 analogue Liraglutide.[166] As continuous enhancement of GLP-1 action for 24 hours a day appears to be superior for glucose control to shorter durations of peptide administration, it seems desirable to enhance the circulating levels of GLP-1 around the clock.

Exendin-4 is a 39-amino-acid naturally occurring lizard GLP-1R agonist that exhibits 53% amino acid identity to mammalian GLP-1[167,168] yet binds to and activates the GLP-1R. Furthermore, exendin-4 is highly resistant to the proteolytic activity of DPP-IV and exhibits a longer duration of action in vivo. Intravenous infusion of exendin-4 lowers both fasting and postprandial blood glucose and significantly reduced HbA1c in human subjects with type 2 diabetes.[169] Antibodies against exendin-4 have been detected in almost 40% of treated subjects, but the presence of antibodies has not yet been shown to influence treatment outcome. Exendin-4, renamed Exenatide, has been evaluated in phase 3 trials, in combination with either metformin, sulfonylurea agents, or both for the treatment of type 2 diabetes; preliminary data demonstrate significant lowering of HbA1c in a substantial percentage of Exenatide-treated subjects.

Liraglutide is a fatty acid DPP-IV-resistant human GLP-1 derivative that is administered as a once-daily therapeutic agent.[170] Liraglutide reduces fasting and postprandial glycemia, inhibits gastric emptying, and reduced levels of circulating glucagon.[171] Additional agents that are being evaluated in the clinic include an albumin-bound GLP-1 molecule CJC-1131, which retains the ability to bind to and activate the GLP-1 receptor,[172] and sustained long-acting release (LAR) formulations of exendin-4 (Exenatide-LAR).

The challenges inherent in overcoming the rapid degradation of native GLP-1, together with the disadvantages of injectable peptides, have fostered complementary efforts at enhancing endogenous levels of native GLP-1 through the use of dipeptidyl peptidase-IV inhibitors.[148,166] DPP-IV inhibitors increase the circulating levels of both GLP-1 and GIP and exert significant glucose-lowering actions in 4- to 12-week preclinical studies of rodent diabetes. Conversely, elimination of DPP-IV action in mice results in increased levels of plasma incretins, enhanced insulin secretion, and reduced glycemic excursion.[173] Furthermore, DPP-IV inhibitors produce significant glucose-lowering effects in 4- to 12-week human studies.[174] As DPP-IV regulates immune function and controls the degradation of a broad spectrum of endocrine and regulatory peptides, the long-term safety of DPP-IV inhibitors, which specifically target the kinase activity of the molecule, will merit ongoing scrutiny.

GLUCAGON-LIKE PEPTIDE 2

GLP-2 is cosecreted with GLP-1 from intestinal endocrine cells, and is trophic to the mucosal epithelium in both the small and large intestine.[175] The presence of an alanine residue at position 2 (see Fig. 51-1) predicted that GLP-2, like GLP-1, would be a substrate for inactivation by DPP-IV, and significant amounts of biologically inactive GLP-2[3–33] have been demonstrated in both rodent and human plasma.[176] Similarly, analogues of GLP-2 that are designed to resist DPP-IV-mediated cleavage are biologically more potent in vivo. Intravenous administration of GLP-2 stimulates intestinal glucose transport within 30 minutes, demonstrating that GLP-2 exerts both acute metabolic and more chronic growth-promoting actions in the gastrointestinal tract.

The observation that experimental diabetes in rodents is associated with increased mucosal epithelial growth may be explained in part by increased intestinal GLP-2 production, as insulin treatment reverses the changes in mucosal growth and decreases the levels of GLP-2 in rats with diabetes.[177] The importance of GLP-2 for maintenance of the intestinal villous epithelium is further illustrated by studies of rats receiving total parenteral nutrition (TPN), as coinfusion of GLP-2 and TPN prevented mucosal villous hypoplasia in the small intestine.[178] The physiologic importance of GLP-2 for the physiology or growth of the normal mucosal epithelium remains unknown, as studies with GLP-2 antagonists or immunoneutralization of GLP-2 have not yet been reported. However, treatment of diabetic rats with immunoneutralizing GLP-2 antisera significantly reduces adaptive mucosal growth in the small bowel, consistent with an essential role for GLP-2 in adaptive mucosal hyperplasia.[179]

A G protein–linked GLP-2 receptor, related in sequence to the glucagon and GLP-1 receptors, has been isolated,[180] which has been localized to human enteroendocrine cells and rodent enteric neurons; however, little is known about the mechanism(s) of GLP-2 action in vivo. GLP-2 promotes regeneration and prevents apoptosis in experimental models of intestinal resection and inflammation,[181,182] including small bowel enteritis, chemotherapy-induced mucosal injury, and ischemic damage.[183–185] Furthermore, the antiapoptotic actions of GLP-2 have been demonstrated in primary rat and mouse hippocampal cell cultures and in heterologous cells expressing a transfected GLP-2 receptor. Administration of native GLP-2 twice daily to human subjects with short bowel syndrome resulted in improved energy absorption, decreased fluid loss, and significant weight gain, in association with increased crypt plus villus height in mucosal biopsy specimens.[186] Degradation-resistant stable human GLP-2 analogues are currently being evaluated in larger clinical trials of patients with short bowel syndrome and inflammatory bowel disease.

GLUCAGON-LIKE PEPTIDES IN THE CNS

The proglucagon gene is expressed in the CNS, predominantly in the brain stem and to a lesser extent in the hypothalamus. Nevertheless, PGDPs, including GLP-1 and GLP-2, are widely distributed in different regions of the brain owing to axonal transport. The GLP-1 receptor is also widely expressed in different brain regions; in contrast, although the GLP-2 receptor is expressed in the hypothalamus and multiple extrahypothalamic sites, it is comparatively less abundant in the CNS relative to expression of the GLP-1R.[187] Intracerebroventricular administration of either GLP-1 or GLP-2 leads to inhibition of food intake in rodents. In contrast, GLP-1, but not GLP-2, inhibits food intake following administration to human subjects.[188] GLP-1 also activates corticotropin-releasing hormone, stimulates corticosterone secretion, and regulates aversive circuits in the rodent brain coupled to the neural transduction of inputs associated with the response to visceral illness.[189] Both GLP-1 and GLP-2 also promote cell proliferation and resistance to apoptotic injury in neuronal cultures and in animal models of neuronal injury[190]; hence, ongoing studies are examining the potential importance of these peptides in learning, memory, and neuroprotection.[191]

In summary, the central importance of pancreatic-derived glucagon in the control of glucose homeostasis has focused considerable attention on understanding the physiology of glucagon synthesis, secretion, and action. Furthermore, the delineation of multiple biologic actions of intestinal-derived GLP-1 and GLP-2 and the isolation of distinct receptors for these peptides have greatly expanded our understanding of the biologic relevance and actions of the proglucagon-derived peptides. It seems reasonable to postulate that additional, as yet undescribed, actions of these and other PGDPs remain to be elucidated. Finally, given the therapeutic potential of both GLP-1 and GLP-2, one or both of these peptides might yet enter the clinic as adjunctive therapies for patients with diabetes or intestinal disease, respectively.

REFERENCES

1. Krapp A, Knofler M, Ledermann B, et al: The bHLH protein PTF1-p48 is essential for the formation of the exocrine and the correct spatial organization of the endocrine pancreas. Genes Dev 12:3752–3763, 1998.
2. Dahl U, Sjodin A, Semb H: Cadherins regulate aggregation of pancreatic beta-cells in vivo. Development 122:2895–2902, 1996.
3. Esni F, Taljedal IB, Perl AK, et al: Neural cell adhesion molecule (N-CAM) is required for cell type segregation and normal ultrastructure in pancreatic islets. J Cell Biol 144:325–337, 1999.
4. Ahlgren U, Pfaff SL, Jessell TM, et al: Independent requirement for ISL1 in formation of pancreatic mesenchyme and islet cells. Nature 385:257–260, 1997.
5. Collombat P, Mansouri A, Hecksher-Sorensen J, et al: Opposing actions of Arx and Pax4 in endocrine pancreas development. Genes Dev 17:2591–2603, 2003.
6. Jonsson J, Carlsson L, Edlund T, et al: Insulin-promoter-factor 1 is required for pancreas development in mice. Nature 371:606–609, 1994.
7. Sussel L, Kalamaras J, Hartigan-O'Connor DJ, et al: Mice lacking the homeodomain transcription factor Nkx2.2 have diabetes due to arrested differentiation of pancreatic beta cells. Development 125:2213–2221, 1998.
8. Naya FJ, Huang H, Qiu Y, et al: Diabetes, defective pancreatic morphogenesis, and abnormal enteroendocrine differentiation in BETA2/NeuroD-deficient mice. Genes Dev 11:2323–2334, 1997.
9. St-Onge L, Sosa-Pineda B, Chowdhury K, et al: Pax6 is required for differentiation of glucagon-producing α-cells in mouse pancreas. Nature 387:406–409, 1997.
10. Sander M, Neubuser A, Kalamaras J, et al: Genetic analysis reveals that PAX6 is required for normal transcription of pancreatic hormone genes and islet development. Genes Dev 11:1662–1673, 1997.
11. Sosa-Pineda B, Chowdhury K, Torres M, et al: The Pax4 gene is essential for differentiation of insulin-producing β cells in the mammalian pancreas. Nature 386:399–402, 1997.

12. Guillam MT, Hummler E, Schaerer E, et al: Early diabetes and abnormal postnatal pancreatic islet development in mice lacking Glut-2 [see comments]. Nat Genet 17:327–330, 1997. [Published errata appear in Nat Genet 17(4):503, 1997 and 18(1):88, 1988].

13. Furuta M, Yano H, Zhou A, et al: Defective prohormone processing and altered pancreatic islet morphology in mice lacking active SPC2. Proc Natl Acad Sci U S A 94:6646–6651, 1999.

14. Gelling RW, Du XQ, Dichmann DS, et al: Lower blood glucose, hyperglucagonemia, and pancreatic α cell hyperplasia in glucagon receptor knockout mice. Proc Natl Acad Sci U S A 100:1438–1443, 2003.

15. Wang J, Webb G, Cao Y, et al: Contrasting patterns of expression of transcription factors in pancreatic alpha and beta cells. Proc Natl Acad Sci U S A 100:12660–12665, 2003.

16. Chiang MK Melton DA: Single-cell transcript analysis of pancreas development. Dev Cell 4:383–393, 2003.

17. Lee YC, Brubaker PL Drucker DJ: Developmental and tissue-specific regulation of proglucagon gene expression. Endocrinology 127:2217–2222, 1990.

18. Cordier-Bussat M, Morel C, Philippe J: Homologous DNA sequences and cellular factors are implicated in the control of glucagon and insulin gene expression. Mol Cell Biol 15:3904–3916, 1995.

19. Morel C, Cordier-Bussat M, Philippe J: The upstream promoter element of the glucagon gene, G1, confers pancreatic alpha cell-specific expression. J Biol Chem 270:3046–3055, 1995.

20. Philippe J, Drucker DJ, Knepel W, et al: Alpha-cell-specific expression of the glucagon gene is conferred to the glucagon promoter element by the interactions of DNA-binding proteins. Mol Cell Biol 8:4877–4888, 1988.

21. Wang M, Drucker DJ: The LIM domain homeobox gene isl-1 is a positive regulator of islet cell-specific proglucagon gene transcription. J Biol Chem 270:12646–12652, 1995.

22. Jin T, Drucker DJ: Activation of proglucagon gene transcription through a novel promoter element by the caudal-related homeodomain protein cdx-2/3. Mol Cell Biol 16:19–28, 1996.

23. Laser B, Meda P, Constant I, et al: The caudal-related homeodomain protein Cdx-2/3 regulates glucagon gene expression in islet cells. J Biol Chem 271:28984–28994, 1996.

24. Hussain MA, Lee J, Miller CP, et al: POU domain transcription factor brain 4 confers pancreatic α-cell-specific expression of the proglucagon gene through interaction with a novel proximal promoter G1 element. Mol Cell Biol 17:7186–7194, 1997.

25. Jin T, Trinh DKY, Wang F, et al: The caudal homeobox protein cdx-2/3 activates endogenous proglucagon gene expression in InR1-G9 islet cells. Mol Endocrinol 11:203–209, 1997.

26. Dumonteil E, Laser B, Constant I, et al: Differential regulation of the glucagon and insulin I gene promoters by the basic helix-loop-helix transcription factors E47 and BETA2. J Biol Chem 273:19945–19954, 1998.

27. Knepel W, Vallejo M, Chafitz JA, et al: The pancreatic islet-specific glucagon G3 transcription factors recognize control elements in the rat somatostatin and insulin-I genes. Mol Endocrinol 5:1457–1466, 1991.

28. Wrege A, Diedrich T, Hochhuth C, et al: Transcriptional activity of domain A of the rat glucagon G3 element conferred by an islet-specific nuclear protein that also binds to similar pancreatic islet cell-specific enhancer sequences (PISCES). Gene Expr 4:205–216, 1995.

29. Philippe J: Glucagon gene transcription is negatively regulated by insulin in a hamster islet cell line. J Clin Invest 84:672–677, 1989.

30. Philippe J, Morel C, Cordier-Bussat M: Islet-specific proteins interact with the insulin-response element of the glucagon gene. J Biol Chem 270:3039–3045, 1995.

31. Philippe J: Insulin regulation of the glucagon gene is mediated by an insulin-responsive DNA element. Proc Natl Acad Sci U S A 88:7224–7227, 1991.

32. Ritz–Laser B, Estreicher A, Klages N, et al: Pax-6 and Cdx-2/3 interact to activate glucagon gene expression on the G1 control element. J Biol Chem 274:4124–4132, 1999.

33. Hill ME, Asa SL, Drucker DJ: Essential requirement for Pax6 in control of enteroendocrine proglucagon gene transcription. Mol Endocrinol 13:1474–1486, 1999.

34. Philippe J, Morel C, Prezioso VR: Glucagon gene expression is negatively regulated by hepatocyte nuclear factor 3b. Mol Cell Biol 14:3514–3523, 1994.

35. Philippe J: Hepatocyte-nuclear factor 3b gene transcripts generate protein isoforms with different transactivation properties on the glucagon gene. Mol Endocrinol 9:368–374, 1995.

36. Kaestner KH, Katz J, Liu Y, et al: Inactivation of the winged helix transcription factor HNF3a affects glucose homeostasis and islet glucagon gene expression in vivo. Genes Dev 13:495–504, 1999.

37. Kaestner KH, Hiemisch H, Schutz G: Targeted disruption of the gene encoding hepatocyte nuclear factor 3 gamma results in reduced transcription of hepatocyte-specific genes. Mol Cell Biol 18:4245–4251, 1998.

38. Liu Y, Shen W, Brubaker PL, et al: Foxa3 (HNF-3gamma) binds to and activates the rat proglucagon gene promoter but is not essential for proglucagon gene expression. Biochem J 366:633–641, 2002.

39. Ang SL, Rossant J: HNF-3 beta is essential for node and notochord formation in mouse devlopment. Cell 78:561–574, 1994.

40. Weinstein DC, Ruiz i Altaba A, Chen WS, et al: The winged-helix transcription factor HNF-3 beta is required for notochord development in the mouse embryo. Cell 78:575–588, 1994.

41. Drucker DJ, Jin T, Asa SL, et al: Activation of proglucagon gene transcription by protein kinase A in a novel mouse enteroendocrine cell line. Mol Endocrinol 8:1646–1655, 1994.

42. Knepel W, Chafitz J, Habener JF: Transcriptional activation of the rat glucagon gene by the cyclic AMP-responsive element in pancreatic islet cells. Mol Cell Biol 10:6799–6804, 1990.

43. Wang J, Cao Y, Steiner DF: Regulation of proglucagon transcription by activated transcription factor (ATF) 3 and a novel isoform, ATF3b, through the cAMP-response element/ATF site of the proglucagon gene promoter. J Biol Chem 278:32899–32904, 2003.

44. Schwaninger M, Lux G, Blume R, et al: Membrane depolarization and calcium influx induce glucagon gene transcription in pancreatic islet cells through the cyclic AMP-responsive element. J Biol Chem 268:5168–5177, 1993.

45. Furstenau U, Schwaninger M, Blumes R, et al: Characterization of a novel calcium response element in the glucagon gene. J Biol Chem 274:5851–5860, 1999.

46. Efrat S, Teitelman G, Anwar M, et al: Glucagon gene regulatory region directs oncoprotein expression to neurons and pancreatic alpha cells. Neuron 1:605–613, 1988.

47. Lee YC, Asa SL, Drucker DJ: Glucagon gene 5'-flanking sequences direct expression of SV40 large T antigen to the intestine producing carcinoma of the large bowel in transgenic mice. J Biol Chem 267:10705–10708, 1992.

48. Nian M, Drucker DJ, Irwin D: Divergent regulation of human and rat proglucagon gene promoters in vivo. Am J Physiol 277:G829–G837, 1999.

49. Dumonteil E, Magnan C, Ritz-Laser B, et al: Insulin, but not glucose lowering corrects the hyperglucagonemia and increased proglucagon messenger ribonucleic acid levels observed in insulinopenic diabetes. Endocrinology 139:4540–4546, 1998.

50. Chen L, Komiyo I, Inman L, et al: Effects of hypoglycemia and prolonged fasting on insulin and glucagon gene expression. J Clin Invest 84:711–714, 1989.

51. Shi ZQ, Rastogi KS, Lekas M, et al: Glucagon response to hypoglycemia is improved by insulin-independent restoration of normoglycemia in diabetic rats. Endocrinology 137:3193–3199, 1996.

52. Magnan C, Philippe J, Kassis N, et al: In vivo effects of glucose and insulin on secretion and gene expression of glucagon in rats. Endocrinology 136:5370–5376, 1995.

53. Dhanvantari S, Seidah NG, Brubaker PL: Role of prohormone convertases in the tissue-specific processing of proglucagon. Mol Endocrinol 10:342–355, 1996.

54. Dhanvantari S, Brubaker PL: Proglucagon processing in an islet cell line: Effects of PC1 overexpression and PC2 depletion. Endocrinology 139:1630–1637, 1998.

55. Rothenberg ME, Eilertson CD, Klein K, et al: Evidence for redundancy in propeptide/prohormone convertase activities in processing proglucagon: An antisense study. Mol Endocrinol 10:331–341, 1996.

56. Rothenberg ME, Eilertson CD, Klein K, et al: Processing of mouse proglucagon by recombinant prohormone convertase 1 and immunopurified prohormone convertase 2 in vitro. J Biol Chem 270:10136–10146, 1995.

57. Zhu X, Zhou A, Dey A, et al: Disruption of PC1/3 expression in mice causes dwarfism and multiple neuroendocrine peptide processing defects. Proc Natl Acad Sci U S A 99:10293–10298, 2002.

58. Jackson RS, Creemers JW, Farooqi IS, et al: Small-intestinal dysfunction accompanies the complex endocrinopathy of human proprotein convertase 1 deficiency. J Clin Invest 112:1550–1560, 2003.

59. Rorsman P, Ashcroft FM, Berggren P-O: Regulation of glucagon release from pancreatic A-cells. Biochem Pharmacol 41:1783–1790, 1991.

60. Ward WK, Bolgiano DC, McKnight B, et al: Diminished B cell secretory capacity in patients with noninsulin-dependent diabetes mellitus. J Clin Invest 74:1318–1328, 1984.

61. Gromada J, Bokvist K, Ding W-G, et al: Adrenaline stimulates glucagon secretion in pancreatic A cells by increasing the Ca2+ current and the number of granules close to the L-type Ca2+ channels. J Gen Physiol 110:217–228, 1997.

62. Smismans A, Schuit F, Pipeleers D: Nutrient regulation of gamma-aminobutyric acid release from islet beta cells. Diabetologia 40:1411–1415, 1997.

63. Gaskins HR, Baldeon ME, Selassie L, et al: Glucose modulates gamma-aminobutyric acid release from the pancreatic beta TC6 cell line. J Biol Chem 270:30286–30289, 1995.

64. Ishihara H, Maechler P, Gjinovci A, et al: Islet beta-cell secretion determines glucagon release from neighbouring alpha-cells. Nat Cell Biol 5:330–335, 2003.

65. Maruyama H, Hisatomi A, Orci L, et al: Insulin within islets is a physiologic glucagon release inhibitor. J Clin Invest 74:2296–2299, 1984.

66. Marliss EB, Aoki TT, Unger RH, et al: Glucagon levels and metabolic effects in fasting man. J Clin Invest 49:2256–2270, 1970.

67. Unger RH, Aguilar-Parada E, Muller WA, et al: Studies of pancreatic alpha cell function in normal and diabetic subjects. J Clin Invest 49:837–848, 1970.

68. Larsson H, Ahren B: Glucose-dependent arginine stimulation test for characterization of islet function: Studies on reproducibility and priming effect of arginine. Diabetologia 41:772–777, 1998.

69. Galbo H, Holst JJ, Christensen NJ: Glucagon and plasma catecholamine responses to graded and prolonged exercise in man. J Appl Physiol 38:70–76, 1975.

70. Sotsky MJ, Shilo S, Shamoon H: Regulation of counterregulatory hormone secretion in man during exercise and hypoglycemia. J Clin Endocrinol Metab 68:9–16, 1989.

71. Drouin R, Lavoie C, Bourque J, et al: Increased hepatic glucose production response to glucagon in trained subjects. Am J Physiol 274:E23–E28, 1998.

72. Hirsch IB, Marker JC, Smith LJ, et al: Insulin and glucagon in prevention of hypoglycemia during exercise in humans. Am J Physiol 260:E695–E704, 1991.

73. Coggan AR, Raguso CA, Gastaldelli A, et al: Regulation of glucose production during exercise at 80% of VO2peak in untrained humans. Am J Physiol 273:E348–E354, 1997.

74. Lewis GF, Vranic M, Giacca A: Glucagon enhances the direct suppressive effect of insulin on hepatic glucose production in humans. Am J Physiol 272:E371–E378, 1997.

75. Taminato T, Seino Y, Goto Y, et al: Synthetic gastric inhibitory polypeptide: Stimulatory effect on insulin and glucagon secretion in the rat. Diabetes 26:480–484, 1977.

76. Rossetti L, Shulman GI, Zawalich WS: Physiological role of cholecystokinin in meal-induced insulin secretion in conscious rats: Studies with L 364718, a specific inhibitor of CCK-receptor binding. Diabetes 36:1212–1215, 1987.

77. Wettergren A, Schjoldager B, Mortensen PE, et al: Truncated GLP-1 (proglucagon 78-107-amide) inhibits gastric and pancreatic functions in man. Dig Dis Sci 38:665–673, 1993.

78. Komatsu R, Matsuyama T, Namba M, et al: Glucagonostatic and insulinotropic action of glucagonlike peptide I-(7-36)-amide. Diabetes 38:902–905, 1989.

79. Taborsky GJ Jr, Ahren B, Havel PJ: Autonomic mediation of glucagon secretion during hypoglycemia. Diabetes 47:995–1005, 1998.

80. Herman WH, Fajans SS, Smith MJ, et al: Diminished insulin and glucagon secretory responses to arginine in nondiabetic subjects with a mutation in the hepatocyte nuclear factor-4a/MODY1 gene. Diabetes 46:1749–1754, 1997.

81. Schwartz NS, Clutter WE, Shah SD, et al: Glycemic thresholds for activation of glucose counterregulatory systems are higher than the threshold for symptoms. J Clin Invest 79:777–781, 1987.

82. Heimberg H, De Vos A, Pipeleers D, et al: Differences in glucose transporter gene expression between rat pancreatic alpha- and beta-cells are correlated to differences in glucose transport but not in glucose utilization. J Biol Chem 270:8971–8975, 1995.

83. Heimberg H, De Vos A, Moens K, et al: The glucose sensor protein glucokinase is expressed in glucagon-producing alpha-cells. Proc Natl Acad Sci U S A 93:7036–7041, 1996.

84. Boushey RP, Abadir A, Flamez D, et al: Hypoglycemia, defective islet glucagon secretion, but normal islet mass in mice with a disruption of the gastrin gene. Gastroenterology 125:1164–1174, 2003.

85. Marliss EB, Girardier L, Seydoux J, et al: Glucagon release induced by pancreatic nerve stimulation in the dog. J Clin Invest 52:1246–1259, 1973.

86. Ahren B, Veith RC, Paquette TL, et al: Sympathetic nerve stimulation versus pancreatic norepinephrine infusion in the dog: 2. Effects on basal release of somatostatin and pancreatic polypeptide. Endocrinology 121:332–339, 1987.

87. Havel PJ, Ahren B: Activation of autonomic nerves and the adrenal medulla contributes to increased glucagon secretion during moderate insulin-induced hypoglycemia in women. Diabetes 46:801–807, 1997.

88. Kendall DM, Rooney DP, Smets YF, et al: Pancreas transplantation restores epinephrine response and symptom recognition during hypoglycemia in patients with long-standing type I diabetes and autonomic neuropathy. Diabetes 46:249–257, 1997.

89. Miki T, Liss B, Minami K, et al: ATP-sensitive K+ channels in the hypothalamus are essential for the maintenance of glucose homeostasis. Nat Neurosci 4:507–512, 2001.

90. Borg WP, During MJ, Sherwin RS, et al: Ventromedial hypothalamic lesions in rats suppress counterregulatory responses to hypoglycemia. J Clin Invest 93:1677–1682, 1994.

91. Borg MA, Sherwin RS, Borg WP, et al: Local ventromedial hypothalamus glucose perfusion blocks counterregulation during systemic hypoglycemia in awake rats. J Clin Invest 99:361–365, 1997.

92. Hevener AL, Bergman RN, Donovan CM: Novel glucosensor for hypoglycemic detection localized to the portal vein. Diabetes 46:1521–1525, 1997.

93. Fery F, Plat L, van de Borne P, et al: Impaired counterregulation of glucose in a patient with hypothalamic sarcoidosis. N Engl J Med 340:852–856, 1999.

94. Perseghin G, Regalia E, Battezzati A, et al: Regulation of glucose homeostasis in humans with denervated livers. J Clin Invest 100:931–941, 1997.

95. Kendall DM, Teuscher AU, Robertson RP: Defective glucagon secretion during sustained hypoglycemia following successful islet allo- and autotransplantation in humans. Diabetes 46:23–27, 1997.

96. Raskin P, Unger RH: Hyperglucagonemia and its suppression: Importance in the metabolic control of diabetes. N Engl J Med 299:433–436, 1978.

97. Van Tine BA, Azizeh BY, Trivedi D, et al: Low level cyclic adenosine 3′,5′-monophosphate accumulation analysis of [des-His1,des-Phe6,Glu9]glucagon-NH2 identifies glucagon antagonists from weak partial agonists/antagonists. Endocrinology 137:3316–3322, 1996.

98. Liang Y, Osborne MC, Monia BP, et al: Reduction in glucagon receptor expression by an antisense oligonucleotide ameliorates diabetic syndrome in db/db mice. Diabetes 53:410–417, 2004.

99. Sherwin RS, Fisher M, Hendler R, et al: Hyperglucagonemia and blood glucose regulation in normal, obese and diabetic subjects. N Engl J Med 294:455–461, 1976.

100. Mittelman SD, Fu YY, Rebrin K, et al: Indirect effect of insulin to suppress endogenous glucose production is dominant, even with hyperglucagonemia. J Clin Invest 100:3121–3130, 1997.

101. Charlton MR, Nair KS: Role of hyperglucagonemia in catabolism associated with type 1 diabetes: Effects on leucine metabolism and the resting metabolic rate. Diabetes 47:1748–1756, 1998.

102. Gerich JE: Lilly lecture 1988: Glucose counterregulation and its impact on diabetes mellitus. Diabetes 37:1608–1617, 1988.

103. Gerich J, Langlois M, Noacco C, et al: Lack of glucagon response to hypoglycemia in diabetes: Evidence for an intrinsic pancreatic alpha cell defect. Science 182:171–173, 1973.

104. Banarer S, McGregor VP, Cryer PE: Intraislet hyperinsulinemia prevents the glucagon response to hypoglycemia despite an intact autonomic response. Diabetes 51:958–965, 2002.

105. Fanelli CG, Epifano L, Rambotti AM, et al: Meticulous prevention of hypoglycemia normalizes the glycemic thresholds and magnitude of most of neuroendocrine responses to, symptoms of, and cognitive function during hypoglycemia in intensively treated patients with short-term IDDM. Diabetes 42:1683–1689, 1993.

106. Dagogo-Jack S, Rattarasarn C, Cryer PE: Reversal of hypoglycemia unawareness, but not defective glucose counterregulation, in IDDM. Diabetes 43:1426–1434, 1994.

107. Galassetti P, Tate D, Neill RA, et al: Effect of antecedent hypoglycemia on counterregulatory responses to subsequent euglycemic exercise in type 1 diabetes. Diabetes 52:1761–1769, 2003.

108. Heller SR, Cryer PE: Reduced neuroendocrine and symptomatic responses to subsequent hypoglycemia after 1 episode of hypoglycemia in nondiabetic humans. Diabetes 40:223–226, 1991.

109. Bollen M, Keppens S, Stalmans W: Specific features of glycogen metabolism in the liver. Biochem J 336:19–31, 1998.

110. Burcelin R, Katz EB, Charron MJ: Molecular and cellular aspects of the glucagon receptor: Role in diabetes and metabolism. Diabetes Metab 22:373–396, 1996.

111. Herzig S, Long F, Jhala US, et al: CREB regulates hepatic gluconeogenesis through the coactivator PGC-1. Nature 413:179–183, 2001.

112. Sato N, Irie M, Kajinuma H, et al: Glucagon inhibits insulin activation of glucose transport in rat adipocytes mainly through a postbinding process. Endocrinology 127:1072–1077, 1990.

113. Briffeuil P, Thu TH, Kolanowski J: A lack of direct action of glucagon on kidney metabolism, hemodynamics, and renal sodium handling in the dog. Metabolism 45:383–388, 1996.

114. Stumvoll M, Chintalapudi U, Perriello G, et al: Uptake and release of glucose by the human kidney: Postabsorptive rates and responses to epinephrine. J Clin Invest 96:2528–2533, 1995.

115. Stumvoll M, Meyer C, Kreider M, et al: Effects of glucagon on renal and hepatic glutamine gluconeogenesis in normal postabsorptive humans. Metabolism 47:1227–1232, 1998.

116. Jelinek LJ, Lok S, Rosenberg GB, et al: Expression cloning and signaling properties of the rat glucagon receptor. Science 259:1614–1616, 1993.

117. Hjorth SA, Orskov C, Schwartz TW: Constitutive activity of glucagon receptor mutants. Mol Endocrinol 12:78–86, 1998.

118. Tonolo G, Melis MG, Ciccarese M, et al: Physiological and genetic characterization of the Gly40Ser mutation in the glucagon receptor gene in the Sardinian population: The Sardinian Diabetes Genetic Study Group. Diabetologia 40:89–94, 1997.

119. Hansen LH, Abrahamsen N, Hager J, et al: The Gly40Ser mutation in the human glucagon receptor gene associated with NIDDM results in a receptor with reduced sensitivity to glucagon. Diabetes 45:725–730, 1996.

120. Odawara M, Tachi Y, Yamashita K: Absence of association between the Gly40→Ser mutation in the human glucagon receptor and Japanese patients with non-insulin-dependent diabetes mellitus or impaired glucose tolerance. Hum Genet 98:636–639, 1996.

121. Hansen LH, Abrahamsen N, Nishimura E: Glucagon receptor mRNA distribution in rat tissues. Peptides 16:1163–1166, 1995.

122. Drucker DJ, Asa S: Glucagon gene expression in vertebrate brain. J Biol Chem 263:13475–13478, 1988.

123. Larsen PJ, Tang-Christensen M, Holst JJ, et al: Distribution of glucagon-like peptide-1 and other preproglucagon-derived peptides in the rat hypothalamus and brainstem. Neuroscience 77:257–270, 1997.

124. Campos RV, Lee YC, Drucker DJ: Divergent tissue-specific and developmental expression of receptors for glucagon and glucagon-like peptide-1 in the mouse. Endocrinology 134:2156–2164, 1994.

125. Moens K, Heimberg H, Flamez D, et al: Expression and functional activity of glucagon, glucagon-like peptide 1 and glucose-dependent insulinotropic peptide receptors in rat pancreatic islet cells. Diabetes 45:257–261, 1996.

126. Parker JC, Andrews KM, Allen MR, et al: Glycemic control in mice with targeted disruption of the glucagon receptor gene. Biochem Biophys Res Commun 290:839–843, 2002.

127. Dobbins RL, Davis SN, Neal DW, et al: Compartmental modeling of glucagon kinetics in the conscious dog. Metabolism 44:452–459, 1995.

128. Authier F, Mort JS, Bell AW, et al: Proteolysis of glucagon within hepatic endosomes by membrane-associated cathepsins B and D. J Biol Chem 270:15798–15807, 1995.

129. Hupe-Sodmann K, McGregor GP, Bridenbaugh R, et al: Characterisation of the processing by human neutral endopeptidase 24.11 of GLP-1(7-36) amide and comparison of the substrate specificity of the enzyme for other glucagon-like peptides. Regul Pept 58:149–156, 1995.

130. Sauvadet A, Rohn T, Pecker F, et al: Synergistic actions of glucagon and miniglucagon on Ca2+ mobilization in cardiac cells. Circ Res 78:102–109, 1996.

131. Dalle S, Blache P, Le-Nguyen D, et al: Miniglucagon: A local regulator of islet physiology. Ann N Y Acad Sci 865:132–140, 1998.

132. Dalle S, Smith P, Blache P, et al: Miniglucagon (Glucagon 19-29), a potent and efficient inhibitor of secretagogue-induced insulin release through a Ca2+ pathway. J Biol Chem 274:10869–10876, 1999.

133. Hvidberg A, Djurup R, Hilsted J: Glucose recovery after intranasal glucagon during hypoglycaemia in man. Eur J Clin Pharmacol 46:15–17, 1994.

134. Muhlhauser I, Koch J, Berger M: Pharmacokinetics and bioavailability of injected glucagon: Differences between intramuscular, subcutaneous, and intravenous administration. Diabetes Care 8:39–42, 1985.

135. Melanson SW, Bonfante G, Heller MB: Nebulized glucagon in the treatment of bronchospasm in asthmatic patients. Am J Emerg Med 16:272–275, 1998.

136. Love JN, Sachdeva DK, Bessman ES, et al: A potential role for glucagon in the treatment of drug-induced symptomatic bradycardia. Chest 114:323–326, 1998.

137. Wermers RA, Fatourechi V, Kvols LK: Clinical spectrum of hyperglucagonemia associated with malignant neuroendocrine tumors. Mayo Clin Proc 71:1030–1038, 1996.

138. Mallinson CN, Bloom SR, Warin AP, et al: A glucagonoma syndrome. Lancet 6 July:1–5, 1974.

139. Drucker DJ: Intestinal growth factors. Am J Physiol 273:G3–G6, 1997.

140. Blume N, Skouv J, Larsson LI, et al: Potent inhibitory effects of transplantable rat glucagonomas and insulinomas on the respective endogenous islet cells are associated with pancreatic apoptosis. J Clin Invest 96:2227–2235, 1995.

141. Ehrlich P, Tucker D, Asa SL, et al: Inhibition of pancreatic proglucagon gene expression in mice bearing subcutaneous endocrine tumors. Am J Physiol Endocrinol Metab 267:E662–E671, 1994.

142. Hoyt EC, Lund PK, Winesett DE, et al: Effects of fasting, refeeding and intraluminal triglyceride on proglucagon expression in jejunum and ileum. Diabetes 45:434–439, 1996.

143. Roberge JN, Brubaker PL: Secretion of proglucagon-derived peptides in response to intestinal luminal nutrients. Endocrinology 128:3169–3174, 1991.

144. Roberge JN, Brubaker PL: Regulation of intestinal proglucagon-derived peptide secretion by glucose-dependent insulinotropic peptide in a novel enteroendocrine loop. Endocrinology 133:233–240, 1993.

145. Kieffer TJ, McIntosh CH, Pederson RA: Degradation of glucose-dependent insulinotropic polypeptide and truncated glucagon-like peptide 1 in vitro and in vivo by dipeptidyl peptidase IV. Endocrinology 136:3585–3596, 1995.

146. Vahl TP, Paty BW, Fuller BD, et al: Effects of GLP-1-(7-36)NH(2), GLP-1-(7-37), and GLP-1-(9-36)NH(2) on intravenous glucose tolerance and glucose-induced insulin secretion in healthy humans. J Clin Endocrinol Metab 88:1772–1779, 2003.

147. Holst JJ, Deacon CF: Inhibition of the activity of dipeptidyl-peptidase IV as a treatment for type 2 diabetes. Diabetes 47:1663–1670, 1998.

148. Drucker DJ: Therapeutic potential of dipeptidyl peptidase IV inhibitors for the treatment of type 2 diabetes. Expert Opin Investig Drugs 12:87–100, 2003.

149. Drucker DJ, Philippe J, Mojsov S, et al: Glucagon-like peptide I stimulates insulin gene expression and increases cyclic AMP levels in a rat islet cell line. Proc Natl Acad Sci U S A 84:3434–3438, 1987.

150. Drucker DJ: The glucagon-like peptides. Diabetes 47:159–169, 1998.

151. Drucker DJ: Glucagon-like peptides: Regulators of cell proliferation, differentiation, and apoptosis. Mol Endocrinol 17:161–171, 2003.

152. Li Y, Hansotia T, Yusta B, et al: Glucagon-like peptide-1 receptor signaling modulates beta cell apoptosis. J Biol Chem 278:471–478, 2003.

153. Farilla L, Bulotta A, Hirshbirg B, et al: GLP-1 inhibits cell apoptosis and improves glucose responsiveness of freshly isolated human islets. Endocrinology 144(12):5145–5148, 2003.

154. Willms B, Werner J, Holst JJ, et al: Gastric emptying, glucose responses, and insulin secretion after a liquid test meal: Effects of exogenous glucagon-like peptide-1 (GLP-1)-(7-36)amide in type 2 (non-insulin dependent) diabetic patients. J Clin Endocrinol Metab 81:327–332, 1996.

155. Flint A, Raben A, Astrup A, et al: Glucagon-like peptide 1 promotes satiety and suppresses energy intake in humans. J Clin Invest 101:515–520, 1998.

156. Turton MD, O'Shea D, Gunn I, et al: A role for glucagon-like peptide-1 in the central regulation of feeding. Nature 379:69–72, 1996.

157. Thorens B, Porret A, Bühler L, et al: Cloning and functional expression of the human islet GLP-1 receptor: Demonstration that exendin-4 is an agonist and exendin-(9-39) an antagonist of the receptor. Diabetes 42:1678–1682, 1993.

158. Wang Z, Wang RM, Owji AA, et al: Glucagon-like peptide 1 is a physiological incretin in rat. J Clin Invest 95:417–421, 1995.

159. Edwards CM, Todd JF, Mahmoudi M, et al: Glucagon-like peptide 1 has a physiological role in the control of postprandial glucose in humans: Studies with the antagonist exendin 9-39. Diabetes 48:86–93, 1999.

160. D'alessio DA, Vogel R, Prigeon R, et al: Elimination of the action of glucagon-like peptide 1 causes an impairment of glucose tolerance after nutrient ingestion by healthy baboons. J Clin Invest 97:133–138, 1996.

161. Scrocchi LA, Brown TJ, MacLusky N, et al: Glucose intolerance but normal satiety in mice with a null mutation in the glucagon-like peptide receptor gene. Nature Med 2:1254–1258, 1996.

162. Scrocchi LA, Drucker DJ: Effects of aging and a high fat diet on body weight and glucose control in GLP-1R-/-mice. Endocrinology 139:3127–3132, 1998.

163. Wang Y, Perfetti R, Greig NH, et al: Glucagon-like peptide-1 can reverse the age-related decline in glucose tolerance in rats. J Clin Invest 99:2883–2889, 1997.

164. Zander M, Madsbad S, Madsen JL, et al: Effect of 6-week course of glucagon-like peptide 1 on glycaemic control, insulin sensitivity, and beta-cell function in type 2 diabetes: A parallel-group study. Lancet 359:824–830, 2002.

165. Deacon CF, Johnsen AH, Holst JJ: Degradation of glucagon-like peptide-1 by human plasma in vitro yields an N-terminally truncated peptide that is a major endogenous metabolite in vivo. J Clin Endocrinol Metab 80:952–957, 1995.

166. Drucker DJ: Enhancing incretin action for the treatment of Type 2 diabetes. Diabetes Care 26:2929–2940, 2003.

167. Eng J, Kleinman WA, Singh L, et al: Isolation and characterization of exendin 4, an exendin 3 analogue from Heloderma suspectum venom. J Biol Chem 267:7402–7405, 1992.

168. Chen YE, Drucker DJ: Tissue-specific expression of unique mRNAs that encode proglucagon-derived peptides or exendin 4 in the lizard. J Biol Chem 272:4108–4115, 1997.

169. Fineman MS, Bicsak TA, Shen LZ, et al: Effect on glycemic control of synthetic exendin-4 (AC2993) additive to existing metformin and/or sulfonylurea treatment in patients with type 2 diabetes. Diabetes Care 27:2370–2377, 2003.

170. Agerso H, Jensen LB, Elbrond B, et al: The pharmacokinetics, pharmacodynamics, safety and tolerability of NN2211, a new long-acting GLP-1 derivative, in healthy men. Diabetologia 45:195–202, 2002.

171. Juhl CB, Hollingdal M, Sturis J, et al: Bedtime administration of NN2211, a long-acting GLP-1 derivative, substantially reduces fasting and postprandial glycemia in type 2 diabetes. Diabetes 51:424–429, 2002.

172. Kim JG, Baggio LL, Bridon DP, et al: Development and characterization of a glucagon-like peptide 1-albumin conjugate: The ability to activate the glucagon-like peptide 1 receptor in vivo. Diabetes 52:751–759, 2003.

173. Marguet D, Baggio L, Kobayashi T, et al: Enhanced insulin secretion and improved glucose tolerance in mice lacking CD26. Proc Natl Acad Sci U S A 97:6874–6879, 2000.

174. Ahren B, Simonsson E, Larsson H, et al: Inhibition of dipeptidyl peptidase IV improves metabolic control over a 4-week study period in type 2 diabetes. Diabetes Care 25:869–875, 2002.

175. Drucker DJ, Ehrlich P, Asa SL, et al: Induction of intestinal epithelial proliferation by glucagon-like peptide 2. Proc Natl Acad Sci USA 93:7911–7916, 1996.

176. Drucker DJ, Shi Q,, Crivici A, et al: Regulation of the biological activity of glucagon-like peptide 2 in vivo by dipeptidyl peptidase IV. Nat Biotechnol 15:673–677, 1997.

177. Fischer KD, Dhanvantari S, Drucker DJ, et al: Intestinal growth is associated with elevated levels of glucagon-like peptide-2 in diabetic rats. Am J Physiol 273:E815–E820, 1997.

178. Chance WT, Foley-Nelson T, Thomas I, et al: Prevention of parenteral nutrition-induced gut hypoplasia by coinfusion of glucagon-like peptide-2. Am J Physiol 273:G559–G563, 1997.

179. Hartmann B, Thulesen J, Hare KJ, et al: Immunoneutralization of endogenous glucagon-like peptide-2 reduces adaptive intestinal growth in diabetic rats. Regul Pept 105:173–179, 2002.

180. Munroe DG, Gupta AK, Kooshesh F, et al: Prototypic G protein-coupled receptor for the intestinotrophic factor glucagon-like peptide 2. Proc Natl Acad Sci U S A 96:1569–1573, 1999.

181. Scott RB, Kirk D, MacNaughton WK, et al: GLP-2 augments the adaptive response to massive intestinal resection in rat. Am J Physiol 275:G911–G921, 1998.

182. Drucker DJ, Yusta B, Boushey RP, et al: Human [Gly2]-GLP-2 reduces the severity of colonic injury in a murine model of experimental colitis. Am J Physiol 276:G79–G91, 1999.

183. Boushey RP, Yusta B, Drucker DJ: Glucagon-like peptide 2 decreases mortality and reduces the severity of indomethacin-induced murine enteritis. Am J Physiol 277:E937–E947, 1999.

184. Boushey RP, Yusta B, Drucker DJ: Glucagon-like peptide (GLP)-2 reduces chemotherapy-associated mortality and enhances cell survival in cells expressing a transfected GLP-2 receptor. Cancer Res 61:687–693, 2001.

185. Prasad R, Alavi K, Schwartz MZ: GLP-2alpha accelerates recovery of mucosal absorptive function after intestinal ischemia/reperfusion. J Pediatr Surg 36:570–572, 2001.

186. Jeppesen PB, Hartmann B, Thulesen J, et al: Glucagon-like peptide 2 improves nutrient absorption and nutritional status in short-bowel patients with no colon. Gastroenterology 120:806–815, 2001.

187. Lovshin J, Estall J, Yusta B, et al: Glucagon-like peptide-2 action in the murine central nervous system is enhanced by elimination of GLP-1 receptor signaling. J Biol Chem 276:21489–21499, 2001.

188. Verdich C, Flint A, Gutzwiller JP, et al: A meta-analysis of the effect of glucagon-like peptide-1 (7-36) amide on ad libitum energy intake in humans. J Clin Endocrinol Metab 86:4382–4389, 2001.

189. Kinzig KP, D'Alessio DA, Seeley RJ: The diverse roles of specific GLP-1 receptors in the control of food intake and the response to visceral illness. J Neurosci 22:10470–10476, 2002.

190. Perry T, Greig NH: The glucagon-like peptides: A new genre in therapeutic targets for intervention in Alzheimer's disease. J Alzheimers Dis 4:487–496, 2002.

191. During MJ, Cao L, Zuzga DS, et al: Glucagon-like peptide-1 receptor is involved in learning and neuroprotection. Nat Med 9:1173–1179, 2003.

Regulation of Intermediatory Metabolism during Fasting and Feeding

Ralph A. DeFronzo and Eleuterio Ferrannini

OVERVIEW

In the fasting or postabsorptive state, the fasting plasma glucose concentration in a healthy adult is maintained within a very narrow range: 65 to 105 mg/dL (3.6–5.8 mmol/L). Under basal conditions, insulin-independent tissues, the brain (50%–60%), and splanchnic organs (20%–25%) account for the majority of total-body glucose utilization. Muscle, an insulin-dependent tissue, is responsible for most of the remaining 20% to 25% of glucose disposal in the fasting state.[1,2] The basal rate of tissue glucose uptake is precisely equaled by an equivalent rate of glucose output by the liver. After the ingestion or infusion of glucose, this delicate balance between hepatic glucose production and tissue glucose utilization is disrupted and the maintenance of normal glucose homeostasis in the fed state is dependent on four processes that occur simultaneously and in a coordinated, tightly integrated fashion: (1) in response to hyperglycemia, insulin secretion is stimulated; (2) the combination of hyperinsulinemia plus hyperglycemia augments glucose uptake by splanchnic (liver and gut) and peripheral (primarily muscle) tissues; (3) both insulin and hyperglycemia suppress hepatic glucose production; (4) insulin inhibits lipolysis in adipocytes and the reduction in plasma free fatty acid (FFA) concentration enhances muscle glucose uptake and facilitates the suppression of hepatic glucose production.[3] Glucose uptake by fat cells is small, accounting for less than 4% to 5% of an ingested or infused glucose load. In this chapter, we review the whole-body and cellular mechanisms by which pancreatic hormones (insulin and glucagon) regulate the normal trafficking of substrates between the splanchnic tissues (liver and gastrointestinal tract) and the glucose-utilizing organs in the fed and fasting conditions.

ENERGY METABOLISM

All living organisms require a constant source of energy to maintain their viability. In humans, this energy comes in the form of adenosine triphosphate (ATP), which is derived from the oxidation of foodstuffs. Because humans feed intermittently, it is necessary to build up a sufficient energy reservoir that will be adequate to supply a constant input of metabolic fuels for oxidation during the interfeeding period. To accomplish this, the body has developed an intricate metabolic network with multiple checks and balances—hormonal, neural, and substrate—that ensure a steady supply of metabolic fuels to the tissues. This is particularly crucial for the brain and other neural tissues that use glucose exclusively as their energy source except under unusual conditions of prolonged fasting, when ketone bodies can substitute in part for glucose. Because of the unique dependence of the brain on glucose and because of the intermittent feeding behavior of humans, they must ingest more calories than necessary for the immediate energy use and store the excess calories in body depots, which can be mobilized efficiently at a later time for use by the tissues of the body.

From the quantitative standpoint, fat represents the major energy source in the body (Table 52-1). A 70-kg person who is of ideal body weight possesses approximately 12 kg of triglyceride, which is stored within adipose tissue.[4] If this fat were completely mobilized and oxidized, it would provide approximately 110,000 kcal. Assuming an average metabolic rate of approximately 2000 kcal/day, this would be sufficient to sustain the body's energy needs for approximately 55 days. In addition to its abundance, fat is a more efficient energy source than either glycogen or protein because 9.5 kcal is generated for every gram of fat that is completely oxidized. The comparable energy value for glycogen and protein is 4 kcal/g. Moreover, fat is a less cumbersome storage form of energy because it exists in a nearly anhydrous form in the adipocyte, whereas each gram of glycogen and protein requires approximately 3 g of water. From these considerations, it is obvious that the caloric density of adipose tissue (~8.5 kcal/g of fat) is much greater than the caloric density of either glycogen or protein (~1 kcal/g). Viewed in another way, if one were to replace the amount of energy stored in fat with an equivalent amount of energy in the form of glycogen or protein, the body weight of our hypothetical 70-kg man would expand to 196 kg. This has major adaptive disadvantages for a species that depends on mobility for survival.

Because the major storage form of energy in the body is fat, but the brain and other neural tissues have an obligate need for glucose, the body must have a readily available form of carbohydrate. This is provided by glycogen. In a 70-kg man,

Table 52-1 Tissue and Circulating Energy Content Provided by the Three Major Fuels: Fat, Carbohydrate, and Protein

Tissue	Fuel	Mass (g)	Energy (kcal)
DEPOTS			
Adipose	Triglyceride	12,000	110,00
Muscle	Protein	6000	24,000
Muscle	Glycogen	400	1600
CIRCULATION			
Blood	Glucose	20	80
Blood	Fatty acids	0.3	3
Blood	Triglycerides	3	30
Blood	Ketones	0.2	0.8
Blood	Amino acids	6	24

Adapted from Ruderman NB, Tornheim K, Goodman MN: Fuel homeostasis and intermediary metabolism of carbohydrate, fat, and protein. In Becker KL (ed): Principles and Practice of Endocrinology and Metabolism, JB Lippincott, Philadelphia, 1992, pp 1054–1064.

approximately 80 g of carbohydrate is stored as liver glycogen and 400 g as muscle glycogen.[4] Because muscle does not contain glucose-6-phosphatase, it cannot generate free glucose for transportation to other tissues. However, glycogenolysis in muscle can provide a readily available source of glucose for local needs in response to acute muscular activity. In addition, muscle-derived lactate, pyruvate, and alanine can be transported via the blood to the liver where they are used for gluconeogenesis during starvation. In contrast to muscle, the liver contains all the necessary enzymatic machinery to produce free glucose from glycogen and to form new glucose from gluconeogenesis precursors. Thus, for short-term metabolic needs, liver glycogen represents the principal carbohydrate reservoir for the energy needs of the brain. As can be seen in Table 52-1, the amount of energy contained in circulating glucose is quite small.

Glycogen metabolism is controlled by a cascade of reversible phosphorylation-dephosphorylation reactions that ultimately converge on the more proximal enzymes that catalyze glycogen synthesis (glycogen synthase) and glycogen degradation (glycogen phosphorylase). Both the synthesis and breakdown of glycogen are regulated by multiple, complex, interacting mechanisms involving substrates as well as hormones and neural input. In subsequent sections of this chapter, we review some key aspects of the control of glycogen metabolism.

From a purely theoretical standpoint, protein also represents a large reservoir of energy. A 70-kg man possesses approximately 6 kg of protein with a potential energy value of 24,000 kcal.[4] However, each protein in the body has a specific function, for example, an integral constituent of cell membranes and organelles; an enzyme; a specific transporter of some essential nutrient, element, or vitamin; or a contractile element such as actin or myosin. An excessive breakdown of protein would lead to the disruption of normal cell function and eventually to death. Therefore, the body has developed a complex metabolic and hormonal response to fasting that minimizes proteolysis and release of amino acids. Thus, when fasting is prolonged beyond 2 to 3 days, there is a major shift from carbohydrate to fat and ketone body utilization. After 1 to 2 weeks of starvation, the rates of gluconeogenesis and glucose utilization are markedly reduced and ketone bodies become an important substrate for the energy needs of the brain and other neuronal tissues. However, the brain always maintains a need for some glucose. Acetone, which is formed by the nonenzymatic decarboxylation of acetoacetic acid, can serve as a gluconeogenic precursor by being converted to pyruvaldehyde in the liver or to 1,2-propanediol in extrahepatic tissues. The rise in circulating blood ketone levels also

provides a signal to the muscle to inhibit protein catabolism, thus sparing amino acids for vital cell functions.

GLUCOSE DISTRIBUTION

The triad of major metabolic fuels comprises carbohydrates, protein, and fat. As a metabolic substrate, carbohydrate is present in organisms in its simple monomeric form, α-D-glucopyranose, and as a branched polymer of α-glucose, namely, glycogen. Disaccharides of glucose include lactose, maltose, and sucrose, but these are quantitatively less important. In normal healthy subjects, glucose circulates in plasma water at a basal concentration that ranges from 65 to 100 mg/dL (3.6–5.6 mmol/L). After a meal, the plasma glucose concentration does not exceed 160 to 180 mg/dL (8.9–10 mmol/L) in normal, healthy individuals. Circulating plasma glucose is in rapid equilibration with the red blood cell (RBC) glucose concentration.[5] A non-insulin-regulatable transporter effects the facilitated diffusion of glucose from plasma water into the RBC.[6] Because of the abundance of this transporter in erythrocytes, glucose diffuses very rapidly across RBC membranes, with an estimated equilibration time of only 4 seconds. After its transport into the cell, the rate of glucose utilization via glycolysis has been estimated to be approximately 25 mmol/min or 6 mmol/min per square meter of diffusion surface (the total RBC mass is ~5 × 10⁹ cells and each RBC has a mean diameter of 7 mm with a spherical shape that occupies a surface area of ~4 m²).[5] Because this rate is approximately 17,000 times slower than the rate of glucose transport into the erythrocyte, the glucose concentration will, in general, be the same in plasma and erythrocyte water. Plasma proteins comprise some 8% of plasma volume, whereas RBC proteins and ghosts occupy approximately 38% of the packed RBC volume (which, in turn, averages 40% of the total blood volume). Thus, 20% (i.e., 0.38 × 0.4 + 0.08 × 0.6 = 0.2) of the total blood volume is inaccessible to glucose. It follows that glucose concentration should be identical in plasma and RBC water under most circumstances and that a *blood* water glucose concentration of 90 mg/dL (5.0 mmol/L) translates into a *plasma* glucose concentration of 83 mg/dL (4.6 mmol/L) and a *whole-blood* glucose concentration of 72 mg/dL (4.0 mmol/L), that is, a 15% systematic difference between plasma and whole-blood glucose concentration under typical conditions of hematocrit, proteinemia, and erythrocyte volume.

GLUCOSE METABOLISM: METHODOLOGICAL CONSIDERATIONS

Because both RBCs and plasma transport glucose, the total amount of the sugar reaching any given organ is the product of the arterial whole-blood glucose concentration × the total blood flow to that organ. Similarly, the total amount of glucose leaving a body region is the product of whole-blood glucose level in the venous effluent × the blood flow rate. From this, it follows that the net balance of glucose movement across a body region is given by the product of blood flow and the arteriovenous whole-blood glucose concentration difference, or the Fick principle (Fig. 52-1). It should be emphasized that the use of *plasma* flow rates and plasma glucose concentration systematically underestimates the net organ balance of glucose (and, for that matter, of any substance that is transported in plasma as well as in erythrocytes, e.g., lactate, some amino acids). Because the plasma flow is less than the blood flow by an amount equal to the hematocrit (~40%), whereas the plasma glucose concentration is higher than whole-blood glucose by only 15% (0.6 × 1.15 = 0.69), this will lead to a 31% underestimation of the net organ balance.

Net Balance = Uptake - Release = (Flow) (A-V)

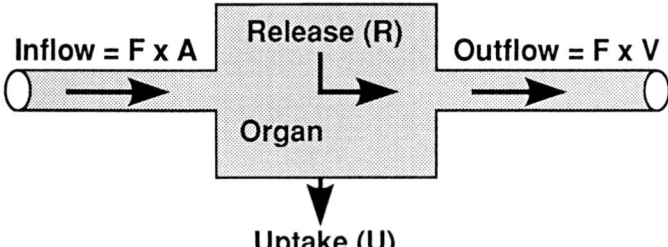

Figure 52-1 Schematic representation of substrate (i.e., glucose) exchange across an organ (i.e., the liver) that both irreversibly removes the substrate (i.e., glucose) and adds it to the systemic circulation. A, arterial concentration; F, blood flow; V, venous concentration.

In muscle, which does not contain glucose-6-phosphatase, the net organ balance is equivalent to the amount of glucose that is taken up and metabolized. In the liver, however, there can be simultaneous uptake and release, that is, from hepatic glycogen stores or from gluconeogenesis. By combining the organ balance technique with radiolabeled glucose, one can calculate the uptake of glucose by an organ bed according to the following equation[7]:

Uptake = (*FE*) (Blood flow) (Arterial glucose concentration)

where *FE* is the fractional extraction of tracer glucose and is calculated as $(A^* - V^*)/A^*$, where A^* and V^* represent the radioactivity of labeled glucose in the artery and vein, respectively. If one knows the net balance of glucose (or any other substrate) across an organ bed and the unidirectional uptake, one can calculate the release of glucose (or any other substrate) according to the following relationship (see Fig. 52-1):

Net balance = Uptake − Release

By employing the catheter technique to measure the net organ balance of glucose in combination with radiolabeled glucose, much information can be gained about the interorgan exchange of glucose and other substrates as well as the metabolic pathways involved in the regulation of glucose utilization.

The use of a radioisotope also allows one to measure whole-body glucose (or other substrates) turnover.[8] Because of its simplicity, the isotope dilution method has become popular among clinical investigators and has generated large amounts of information. It, therefore, warrants a brief description here; a more detailed explanation of the tracer technique, as applied to glucose turnover measurement, can be found in Ref. 8. The choice of a tracer is dictated by cost, ease of measurement, and safety (radiation burden to the patient). The tracer can be administered as a pulse injection or constant intravenous infusion, depending on the type of information that is desired. For metabolic studies, a prime continuous infusion usually is employed. When both the tracer (i.e., cold glucose) and tracee (i.e., radiolabeled glucose) are in steady state, the glucose turnover rate (milligrams per minute) is simply calculated by dividing the tracer infusion rate (in DPM per minute) by the equilibrium plasma glucose–specific activity (in DPM per milligram). In normal healthy subjects, equilibrium represents the time (usually ~2 hours after starting the tracer and tracee infusion) when unchanging plasma tracer and tracee concentrations indicate that glucose-specific activity has become uniform throughout its distribution space. The calculation of the turnover rate as described previously (infusion rate/plasma specific activity) is not based on any assumptions and can be used to quantitate glucose

turnover in the postabsorptive state. When non-steady-state conditions prevail, this approach cannot be used. Such is the case after glucose ingestion or infusion. Practical ways to circumvent this problem, however, have been developed. Their common rationale is provided by the theory that the degree and rate of change in glucose-specific activity are the principal factors that affect non-steady-state analysis of isotope data. The larger the swings in glucose-specific activity are, the more uncertain is the estimation of the actual rates of glucose appearance and disappearance from plasma data. All the formal models that have been proposed to represent the glucose system become progressively weaker as plasma glucose–specific activity is allowed to fluctuate freely. Therefore, one of two strategies can be employed: Either the tracer administration is repeated when the glucose system has reached a new, reasonably steady state or radioactive and cold glucose infusion rates can be adjusted empirically to "clamp" the plasma glucose–specific activity constant at the basal level. In both cases, the aim is to minimize the changes in glucose-specific activity, thereby meeting the conditions under which steady-state equations can be used reliably. Therefore, in reporting results of glucose turnover obtained under non-steady-state conditions, we will make some selection of available data.

GLUCOSE METABOLISM: BASAL (POSTABSORPTIVE) STATE

GLUCOSE PRODUCTION

By convention, the basal or postabsorptive state is defined as the metabolic condition that prevails in the morning after an overnight (10–14-hours) fast. For most individuals, this time represents the longest period of fasting in everyday life. For the rest of the day, most people are more or less in the fed state. Maintenance of the fasting plasma glucose concentration is primarily the responsibility of the liver.[9,10] The liver provides glucose for all tissues of the body, either by breaking down its own stores of glycogen or by synthesizing glucose from gluconeogenic precursors, of which the most important are lactate, pyruvate, glycerol, alanine, and other gluconeogenic amino acids. The central role of the liver in providing a constant supply of glucose to the body is related to the presence of glucose-6-phosphatase, which catalyzes the conversion of glucose-6-phosphate (G-6-P) to glucose within the hepatocyte. Although a number of tissues, including muscle and adipocytes, possess the enzymatic machinery necessary to degrade glycogen and synthesize G-6-P from lactate and amino acids, they either completely lack or possess too little of the key enzyme, glucose-6-phosphatase, to release significant amounts of free glucose into the circulation. The kidney, like the liver, also possesses the necessary enzymatic apparatus to produce glucose via the gluconeogenic pathway. In normal subjects after an overnight fast, the kidney contributes approximately 10% to 15% of total-body glucose production.[11] During prolonged starvation and metabolic acidosis, renal gluconeogenesis is enhanced and may contribute as much as 25% or more of basal glucose production. Unlike the liver, the major gluconeogenic precursor for the kidney is glutamine.

Under postabsorptive conditions, glucose output in healthy adults averages approximately 140 mg/min (~778 μmol/min) or 2.0 mg/min per kg of body weight (11 μmol/min per kilogram) in a 70-kg individual (Fig. 52-2). The liver and kidney contribute approximately 85% and 15%, respectively, of total endogenous glucose production. The variation around this mean is significant (20%–30%), with an unknown contribution of genetic and environmental factors. Little information is available concerning how much the fasting glucose output varies as a consequence of changes in dietary habits, caloric intake, or physical fitness. Intrafamilial covariance of this

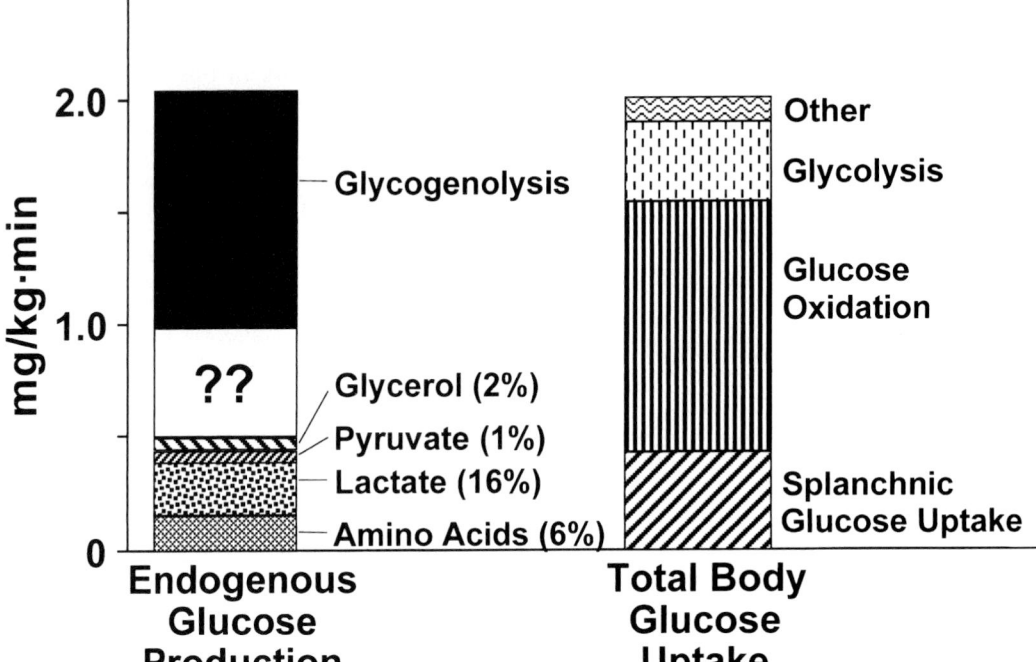

Figure 52-2 Hepatic glucose production and tissue glucose uptake in the postabsorptive state in healthy subjects. See text for a more detailed discussion. (Reproduced from DeFronzo RA: Pathogenesis of type 2 diabetes: Metabolic and molecular implications for identifying diabetes genes. Diabetes Rev 5:177–269, 1997.)

physiologic variable also is undetermined. Under standard nutritional conditions, the normal liver contains approximately 80 g of glycogen (see Table 52-1), and during fasting, liver glycogen stores decline at a rate of approximately 110 mg/min (0.6 mmol/min) or 11% per hour. From this it follows that hepatic glycogen depots would become empty after approximately 12 hours. Because fasting can be prolonged well beyond 12 hours, it is obvious that gluconeogenesis must progressively replace glycogenolysis as the fast continues.[12] In animals, the basal rate of glucose turnover is considerably higher than in humans, for example, dogs (3.6 mg/min per kilogram) and rats (7.2 mg/min per kilogram), and the limited capacity of the liver to store glycogen confers an increasing role to gluconeogenesis for the maintenance of basal glycemia. This limitation on glycogen accumulation has an anatomic basis because overcrowding of the cytoplasm with glycogen granules impairs cellular functions and results in liver damage, as demonstrated in patients with the glycogen storage diseases. In healthy subjects, after a 10- to 12-hour overnight fast, gluconeogenesis accounts for approximately 50% of total hepatic glucose release (see Fig. 52-2).[12] The substrates for this de novo glucose synthesis remain somewhat elusive. Circulating lactate, pyruvate, glycerol, alanine, and other gluconeogenic amino acids are natural candidate precursors and have been shown to transfer their carbons to newly synthesized glucose molecules, as documented by the incorporation of labeled lactate into glucose, that is, the Cori cycle. However, transsplanchnic catheterization in humans has shown that the net uptake of known circulating gluconeogenic precursors (lactate, pyruvate, glycerol, amino acids) can account for only approximately 15% to 20% of total endogenous glucose production.[13] The discrepancy (180–360 µg/min per kilogram or 1–2 µmol/min per kilogram) between radioisotopic estimates of basal gluconeogenic rate and accountable circulating precursors suggests that the blood-borne substrates may not be the only source of gluconeogenic precursors. Within the splanchnic area, the intestine returns 10% to 20% of its glucose uptake to the liver as lactate (90 µg/min per kilogram or 0.5 µmol/min per kilogram), but this fills only part of the gap. It has been suggested that intrahepatic proteolysis and/or lipolysis could provide ample amounts of gluconeogenic precursors, in addition to those entering from the systemic circulation.

The regulation of basal hepatic glucose production is controlled by the sum of multiple neural, hormonal, and metabolic stimuli, some stimulatory and others inhibitory.[9,10] Figure 52-3 portrays the control system as a simple balance between inhibition and stimulation. Insulin and glucagon provide the primary hormonal signals that regulate the production of glucose by the liver under postabsorptive conditions. Of the two, the action of insulin is predominant. Hepatic glucose production is exquisitely sensitive to very small fluctuations in the circulating plasma insulin concentration. Increments in the plasma insulin concentration of as little as 5 to 10 µU/mL cause a marked, rapid suppression of glycogenolysis and decline in hepatic glucose output, whereas inhibition of gluconeogenesis is less sensitive.[10]

By restraining lipolysis and proteolysis, insulin also reduces the delivery of potential glucose precursors (glycerol and amino acids) from peripheral tissues (adipocytes and muscle) to the liver, and this further reduces hepatic glucose output. In its capacity as the inhibitory signal for glucose release, insulin is greatly favored by the anatomic connection between the pancreas and the liver. Because the pancreatic vein is a tributary of the portal vein, insulin, which is secreted by the β cells, reaches the liver in fasting humans at a concentration that is three to four times higher than the peripheral (arterial) concentration. This steep portasystemic gradient is maintained by the high rate of insulin degradation by hepatic tissues (fractional insulin extraction = 50%). Consequently, a small secretory stimulus to the β cells will disproportionately raise the portal insulin concentration, thereby selectively acting on glucose production rather than enhancing peripheral glucose utilization. In addition to short-circuiting the general circulation, pancreatic insulin release is potentiated by a number of gastrointestinal hormones (e.g., glucose-dependent insulinotropic polypeptide, glucagon-like peptide-1, secretin, cholecystokinin, pancreozymin, and others, which are released in response to meal ingestion).[14] Therefore, anatomic and physiologic connections that comprise the gut-liver-pancreas axis ensure that the primary station for the handling of foodstuff, the liver, is under close control by a nearby, well-informed unit, the β cell.

Conversely, small decrements in the plasma insulin concentration, as little as 1 to 2 µU/mL, lead to an increase in

Regulation of Hepatic Glucose Production

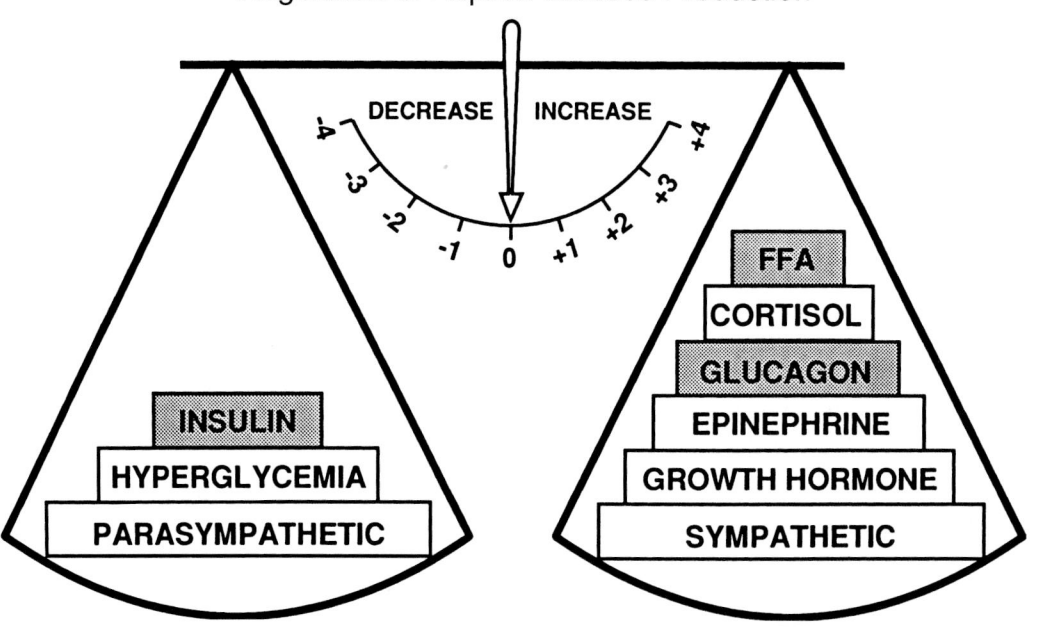

Figure 52-3 Balance of factors that regulate hepatic glucose production. Stimulatory factors are shown by the positive numbers to the right; inhibitory factors, of which insulin is dominant, are shown by the negative numbers to the left.

hepatic glucose production.[15] This highly sensitive interaction between the liver and insulin plays a critical role in the maintenance of basal glucose levels when fasting is prolonged. As glycogen stores become depleted, there is a small decrease in the arterial glucose concentration, which in turn leads to a decline in pancreatic insulin secretion and the stimulation of glucagon release. The resultant hypoinsulinemia removes the constraint on lipolysis, and plasma FFA levels rise. By mass action, FFAs enhance their own uptake by all cells in the body, including liver and muscle. Enhanced FFA oxidation by the hepatocytes provides an energy source to drive gluconeogenesis and the end product of beta oxidation, acetyl-CoA, stimulates the first committed enzyme, pyruvate carboxylase, in the gluconeogenic pathway (Fig. 52-4).[1,2]

The combination of hypoinsulinemia, hypoglycemia, and increased FFA and amino acid supply also stimulates hepatic gluconeogenesis. In peripheral tissues, enhanced FFA and ketone oxidation spare glucose utilization (Randle cycle; see subsequent discussion), thereby minimizing the need for carbohydrate as an energy source.[1,2]

Another important consequence of the fasting-related decline in plasma insulin concentration is the stimulation of proteolysis.[15] This augments the outflow of amino acids, especially alanine, which accounts for approximately 50% of total α-amino nitrogen release. The predominance of alanine in the amino acid efflux from muscle cannot be explained by its presence in cellular proteins, of which alanine comprises only 7% to 10%. The major source of alanine outflow from muscle

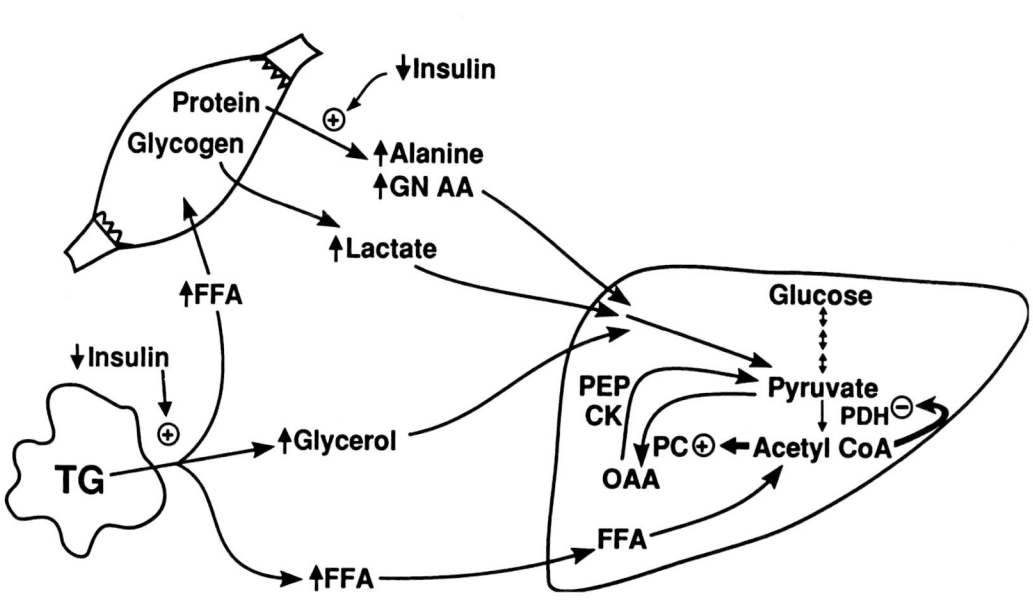

Figure 52-4 In the fasting state, the decrease in basal plasma insulin concentration removes the inhibitory effect of the hormone on lipolysis and plasma glycerol and free fatty acid level increase. In the hepatocyte, enhanced delivery of free fatty acids, in combination with a decreased insulin/glucagon ratio, stimulates beta oxidation, leading to the accumulation of acetyl-CoA. Increased acetyl-CoA, by inhibiting pyruvate dehydrogenase and stimulating pyruvate carboxylase in the liver, shuttles pyruvate into the gluconeogenic pathway. Hypoinsulinemia also stimulates proteolysis in muscle and the enhanced delivery of alanine, other gluconeogenic amino acids, glycerol, and lactate from peripheral tissues provides the substrates for accelerated hepatic gluconeogenesis. AA, amino acid; FFA, free fatty acid; GN, gluconeogenic; PDH, pyruvate dehydrogenase; OAA, oxaloacetic acid; PC, pyruvate carboxylase; PEPCK, phospho*enol*pyruvate carboxykinase; TG, triglyceride.

during starvation is derived from the transamination of glucose-derived (from muscle glycogen and circulating glucose) pyruvate. The branched-chain amino acids (valine, leucine, isoleucine) provide the amino groups for muscle alanine synthesis. The alanine that is released from muscle is transported via the bloodstream to the liver where it is converted to glucose, thus completing the *glucose-alanine cycle* (see Fig. 52-4).[13]

The *glucose-lactate cycle* (Cori cycle) also provides an important source of three-carbon skeletons for gluconeogenesis during fasting.[15] Insulinopenia enhances the breakdown of glycogen and leads to accumulation of pyruvate. Because the Krebs cycle has been inhibited by the accelerated rate of FFA oxidation (Randle cycle), the pyruvate can either be transaminated to alanine (glucose-alanine cycle) or converted to lactate and released into the circulation where it is carried to the liver and synthesized into glucose (glucose-lactate cycle). From the quantitative standpoint, approximately twice as many carbon skeletons are recycled to glucose via the Cori cycle compared with the alanine cycle.

The counterregulatory hormones (glucagon, epinephrine, growth hormone, cortisol) all are capable of offsetting the action of insulin on the liver and work by stimulating both glycogenolysis and gluconeogenesis.[16] Glucagon plays a major role in the tonic support of basal hepatic glucose release and, in humans and animals, suppression of endogenous glucagon secretion with preservation of basal insulin levels causes a 30% to 40% decline in hepatic glucose production.[17] This suppression of glucose production involves both the glycogenolytic and gluconeogenic pathways. The precise quantitative contribution of the other counterregulatory hormones to the maintenance of basal glucose output under normal conditions of fasting has not been assessed. However, it is likely that they (i.e., epinephrine, cortisol, and growth hormone) also exert a tonic effect on hepatic glucose production in the postabsorptive state, and the withdrawal of insulin (i.e., hypoinsulinemia) that occurs with prolonged fasting allows their stimulatory effect on glycogenolysis and gluconeogenesis to occur unopposed. The net result of their unopposed action is an increase in hepatic glucose and renal output.

During more pronounced hypoglycemia, as may occur with insulin administration, all the counterregulatory hormones are released and act synergistically to restore normoglycemia.[16] However, they do so with different dose-response kinetics and time courses. Glucagon and catecholamines act rapidly, whereas cortisol, growth hormone, and thyroid hormones (in that order) are involved in the long-range control of hepatic glucose release. Small, acute increases in plasma glucagon and epinephrine concentrations markedly stimulate both glycogenolysis and gluconeogenesis. Acute elevations in plasma cortisol, growth hormone, and thyroid hormones have no stimulatory effect on total hepatic glucose release. However, both cortisol and growth hormone have been shown to markedly potentiate the effects of epinephrine and glucagon on hepatic glucose release.

In addition to hormonal regulation, the central nervous system has an important role in the maintenance of hepatic glucose production.[18] Both parasympathetic and sympathetic fibers reach the liver via the splanchnic nerves, thereby supplying autonomic nervous modulation of both glucose production and uptake. In animals, parasympathetic stimulation restrains glycogenolysis and enhances glycogen synthesis, whereas activation of the sympathetic nerves innervating the liver stimulates glucose output via potentiation of both glycogenolysis and gluconeogenesis. In humans, the influence of the sympathetic nervous system on hepatic glucose metabolism can be demonstrated under conditions of acute stimulation, but the contribution of the autonomic nervous system to the maintenance of basal hepatic glucose production remains undetermined.

A number of metabolic signals play an important role in the control of hepatic glucose production in the postabsorptive state.[9,10,19] Hyperglycemia per se inhibits liver glucose output. In normal adults, hyperglycemia and hyperinsulinemia occur concurrently, and in combination they provide a potent stimulus to suppress hepatic glucose release. As shown in Figure 52-5, physiologic hyperglycemia (maintained using the hyperglycemic clamp technique), while maintaining basal insulinemia, is as effective as insulin in suppressing hepatic glucose production. More impressive is the observation that hyperglycemia in the presence of hypoinsulinemia (hyperglycemic clamp with somatostatin) causes a greater than 50% suppression of hepatic glucose release (see Fig. 52-5). Conversely, hypoglycemia by itself provides a trigger to increase hepatic glucose release. During insulin-induced

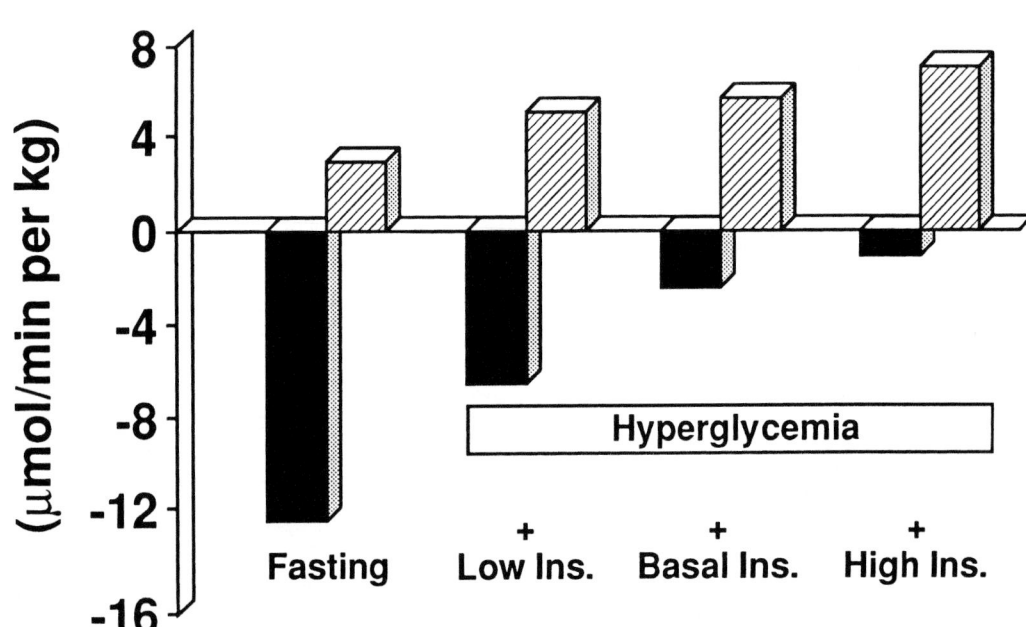

Figure 52-5 Splanchnic glucose uptake *(hatched columns)* and hepatic glucose production *(solid columns)* in healthy subjects under four experimental conditions: overnight fast; hyperglycemia (+125 mg/dL) with somatostatin blockade of endogenous insulin release (Low Ins.); hyperglycemia (+125 mg/dL) with somatostatin plus insulin replacement to maintain the fasting insulin concentration constant (Basal Ins.); hyperglycemia (+125 mg/dL) with endogenous insulin (55 µU/mL) release. Note that hyperglycemia per se inhibits hepatic glucose production and that hyperglycemia acts synergistically with insulin to inhibit liver glucose output. In contrast, hyperglycemia stimulates glucose uptake to approximately the same extent in the presence of low, basal, or high insulin, that is, mostly by mass action. (Drawn from the data from DeFronzo et al.[19])

hypoglycemia in humans and animals, an increase in plasma glucose occurs even when the counterregulatory hormonal response is inhibited. Recent studies suggest that this effect of hypoglycemia is mediated via glucose sensors in the hypothalamic region of the brain, which then activate hepatic glycogenolysis via sympathetic connections to the liver.[20]

Metabolic signals, in the form of altered substrate delivery to the liver, also influence glucose release by the liver. In nondiabetic humans, it is very difficult to demonstrate a detectable increase in hepatic glucose production by infusing large quantities of glycerol, lactate, or a mixture of amino acids, as long as there is a physiologic increase in plasma insulin concentration to balance out such gluconeogenic substrate push. However, even though total hepatic glucose output does not increase, there is a marked stimulation of gluconeogenesis that is precisely counterbalanced by an inhibition of glycogenolysis. The increased provision of gluconeogenic precursors leads to an increase in the intrahepatic formation of G-6-P, but the eventual fate of this intermediate is glycogen rather than free glucose because the rate-limiting enzyme for glucose production, namely, glucose-6-phosphatase, is not simultaneously activated. FFAs play an important role in setting the level of hepatic glucose production. Only the odd-chain FFAs (i.e., propionate) can donate their carbon atoms to oxaloacetate in the tricarboxylic acid cycle and thus directly contribute to net gluconeogenesis. Most physiologic FFAs are of even chain, and, although they can exchange their carbon moieties with tricarboxylic acid cycle intermediates, they do not contribute to de novo glucose synthesis. Nonetheless, when the perfusion medium of isolated rat liver is enriched with oleate or palmitate, new glucose formation from lactate or pyruvate is enhanced. The biochemical mechanisms involved in this stimulation of gluconeogenesis have been well worked out.[21] The products of FFA oxidation, citrate and acetyl-CoA, activate the key enzymes that control gluconeogenesis, pyruvate carboxylase, phospho*enol*pyruvate carboxykinase, and glucose-6-phosphatase (see Fig. 52-4). In addition, elevated plasma FFA concentrations in vivo are usually accompanied by raised glycerol levels because both result from the hydrolysis of triglycerides (see Fig. 52-4). Therefore, accelerated lipolysis supplies both the stimulus (FFA), the substrate (glycerol), and the

energy source (ATP) to drive gluconeogenesis. In isolated hepatocytes, FFAs in micromolar amounts also have been shown to inhibit glycogen synthase. This suggests that an additional interaction of FFA metabolism with hepatic glucose production may be at the level of glycogen metabolism. In healthy volunteers, short-term infusion of triglycerides (with heparin to activate lipoprotein lipase) increases the plasma FFA concentration, leading to the stimulation of hepatic glucose output under conditions (i.e., hyperglycemia and insulinopenia induced by somatostatin plus glucose infusion) that mimic the diabetic state.[22] A large part of this effect can be reproduced by infusing, under the same experimental circumstances, glycerol alone. On the other hand, when endogenous insulin is allowed to increase or when exogenous insulin is administered, the stimulatory effect of triglyceride infusion to increase the plasma FFA concentration on hepatic glucose release is easily overcome. In summary, the long-chain FFAs can regulate hepatic glucose production both by acting on the key enzymes of gluconeogenesis (i.e., through buildup of the products of FFA oxidation) and by virtue of the substrate push of glycerol. This regulatory loop is operative particularly when insulin secretion is not stimulated (i.e., in the basal state).

Conversely, studies in both animals and humans have documented that a significant part of the suppressive action of insulin on hepatic glucose production is mediated via the hormone's antilipolytic effect on adipocytes.[10,23] If the plasma FFA concentration is maintained during insulin infusion, the inhibitory effect of physiologic hyperinsulinemia on hepatic glucose production is impaired.

GLUCOSE DISPOSAL

In the basal or postabsorptive state, the rate of whole-body glucose disposal equals the rate of hepatic glucose production, and the plasma glucose concentration remains constant.[1,2] Information about the contribution of individual organs and tissues to total glucose uptake has been obtained in regional catheterization studies performed in combination with radiolabeled isotopes and indirect calorimetry.[24] By collating the available information, the organ circulation model depicted in Figure 52-6 can be constructed.[5] In this synthesis,

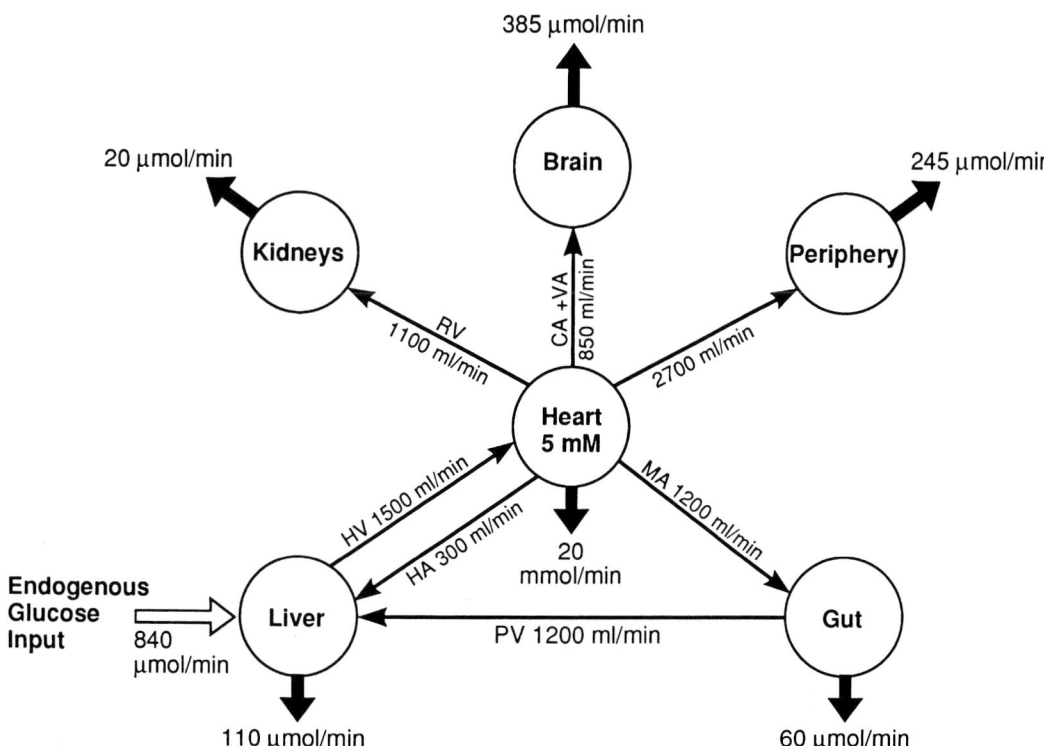

Figure 52-6 Schematic representation of organ glucose metabolism and blood flow in the basal or postabsorptive state. Average data compiled for healthy adults from the literature are indicated. Periphery encompasses all tissues other than the liver, gut, kidneys, brain, and heart; gut includes organs (i.e., spleen, pancreas) draining their blood supply into the portal circulation. Organ blood flow is shown in mL/min and glucose fluxes in mg/min (µmol/min). CA, carotid arteries; HA, hepatic artery; HV, hepatic vein; MA, mesenteric arteries; PV, portal vein; RV, renal veins; V, vertebral artery. (Redrawn from Ferrannini E, DeFronzo RA: Insulin actions in vivo: Glucose metabolism. In DeFronzo RA, Ferrannini E, Keen H, Zimmet P [eds]: International Textbook of Diabetes Mellitus. Chichester, UK, John Wiley & Sons, 2004, pp 277–318.)

steady-state interorgan exchanges of glucose, tissue blood flow, and regional glucose gradients are calculated based on a rate of hepatic glucose production of 140 mg/min or approximately 778 μmol/min. For a 70-kg man, this equals 2.0 mg/min per kilogram or 11 μmol/min per kilogram. In the postabsorptive state, approximately 70% of basal glucose disposal takes place in insulin-independent tissues (brain, liver, kidney, intestine, erythrocytes). Of these, the brain predominates and accounts for almost half of the total hepatic glucose production. The liver plus gastrointestinal (splanchnic) tissues account for an additional 20%. It also can be appreciated that the fractional extraction of glucose (as defined earlier) is quite low everywhere in the body (ranging from 1.0% to 3.5%) except in the brain (9%) (Table 52-2). Because skeletal muscle represents 40% of total body weight and receives 16% of the cardiac output, one can calculate that it accounts for one fourth of the overall glucose disposal in the basal state (i.e., ~245 μmol/min or 440 mg/min) (see Fig. 52-6).[1,2,5] As shown in Table 52-2, the muscle glucose clearance averages 1.3 mL/min per kilogram of tissue. The clearance is a useful metabolic concept and is defined as the amount of plasma that is completely cleared of glucose in a given period; as such, it provides an index of the efficiency of tissue glucose removal. In the rank of efficiency of glucose clearance in the basal state, resting muscle is last, being 10 times less active than the liver and 50 times less avid than the brain. It is noteworthy that tissues (brain, liver, kidneys) that have a high glucose clearance in the basal state are insulin independent. Thus, increasing the plasma insulin concentration above fasting values has no effect on glucose clearance by these tissues (i.e., brain, liver, kidneys), whereas in muscle, glucose clearance increases by a factor of 10-fold or greater over the physiologic range of insulin concentrations. The intermediate position of heart muscle in the list is accounted for by its constant working state. These organ-specific glucose clearance characteristics (see Table 52-2) represent the physiologic equivalent of the type and abundance of specific glucose transporters (GLUTs) with which the various tissues are endowed (Table 52-3).[2,6] They also help to define the concept of an insulin-independent tissue. Thus, in tissues in which an increase in the plasma insulin concentration does not accelerate the glucose clearance, the GLUT is not responsive to acute changes in the plasma insulin concentration. At present, five GLUTs, each with a unique DNA sequence, have been isolated.[2,6] A non-insulin-regulatable GLUT (GLUT-1) effects facilitated glucose transport in the erythrocyte. The abundance of this transporter in the erythrocytes ensures rapid diffusion of glucose across the RBC membrane, and this characteristic confers on the erythrocyte an important role in the interorgan exchange of glucose. The same GLUT-1 transporter is present in the brain. Because of its low K_m (~1 mmol/L), it saturates at low plasma glucose concentrations and is well suited for its function, which is to mediate basal brain glucose uptake. Because the K_m of GLUT-1 is well below the normal fasting plasma glucose concentration

(~5 mmol/L), it ensures a constant flux of glucose into the brain cells. This is an important adaptive mechanism that provides the cerebral tissues an adequate supply of fuel even in the face of hypoglycemia. Another unique feature of GLUT-1 is its low V_{max} (~3 mmol/L). This protects the brain against acute fluid shifts and cerebral edema that otherwise would accompany hyperglycemia. Thus, GLUT-1 is well suited for its physiologic function, especially in the individual with insulin-dependent diabetes in whom extreme shifts in plasma glucose concentration (from hypoglycemia to hyperglycemia) are common. Another important corollary of GLUT-1 is that an increase in plasma glucose concentration above fasting levels (i.e., >5 mmol/L) will necessarily lead to a decline in brain glucose clearance because the transporter saturates at approximately 3 mmol/L. Moreover, because under postabsorptive conditions, the brain is responsible for approximately half of the total-body glucose disposal, it also follows that an increase in fasting plasma glucose concentration (with or without an increase in plasma insulin) will be associated with a decline in whole-body glucose clearance.

A totally distinct (from the physiologic standpoint) GLUT, GLUT-2, is present in liver and pancreatic β cells.[2,6] It has a high K_m (~15–20 mmol/L), and, as a consequence, the free glucose concentration in cells expressing this transporter increases in direct proportion to the increase in plasma glucose concentration. This characteristic allows these cells to respond as "glucose sensors."[1,2] Thus, as the ambient glucose concentration increases, more glucose enters the β cell, which responds by appropriately augmenting its secretion of insulin, whereas the liver reads the rising plasma glucose level and decreases its output of glucose. As a corollary of this, an increase in the plasma glucose concentration is associated with a proportional increase in tissue glucose uptake and the liver glucose clearance remains unchanged. Because GLUT-2 does not respond to insulin, hyperinsulinemia is not associated with an increase in hepatic or β-cell glucose clearance. Glucose uptake by the pancreas and liver occurs in proportion to the increase in plasma glucose concentration.

It is noteworthy that each GLUT is associated with a specific hexokinase, which has a K_m that parallels that of its associated GLUT.[25] For liver and β cells, the phosphorylating enzyme is hexokinase IV or glucokinase. Its high K_m constant has led investigators to propose glucokinase as the β-cell "sensor." Consistent with this, recent studies have demonstrated that maturity-onset diabetes of the young is associated with mutations in the glucokinase gene and the physiologic counterpart of this is a defect in insulin secretion.

Insulin-sensitive tissues, muscle, and adipocytes contain GLUT-4 and its physiologic coupler, hexokinase II. GLUT-4 has a K_m constant of approximately 5 mmol/L, which is close to that of the plasma glucose concentration. In the basal state, the majority of GLUT-4 are not located in the plasma membrane. Rather, they reside in vesicles within the cell. After

Table 52-3   Classification of Glucose Transporters and Hexokinases in Various Tissues

Organ	Glucose Transporter	Hexokinase Coupler	Classification
Brain	GLUT-1	HK-I	Glucose dependent
Erythrocyte	GLUT-1	HK-I	Glucose dependent
Adipocyte	GLUT-4	HK-II	Insulin dependent
Muscle	GLUT-4	HK-II	Insulin dependent
Liver	GLUT-2	HK-IVL	Glucose sensor
B cell	GLUT-2	HK-IVB	Glucose sensor
Gut	GLUT-3-symporter		Sodium dependent
Kidney	GLUT-3-symporter		Sodium dependent

GLUT, glucose transporter; HK, hexokinase.

Table 52-2   Regional Glucose Disposal in the Basal State

Organ	Weight (kg)	Blood Flow (L/min)	Uptake (μmol/min)	Extraction (%)	Clearance* (mL/min per kg)
Brain	1.2	0.85	385	9.1	64
Liver	1.5	1.50	110	2.3	15
Kidneys	0.28	1.10	20	1.9	15
Heart	0.3	0.25	20	1.7	13
Gut	5.0	1.20	60	1.0	2.4
Muscle	28.0	1.05	245	3.5	1.3

*Organ clearance rate divided by organ weight.

exposure to insulin, the concentration of GLUT-4 in the plasma membrane of adipocytes and muscle increases markedly and there is a reciprocal decline in the intracellular GLUT-4 pool.[26] Insulin not only enhances their translocation and insertion into the plasma membrane but also augments their intrinsic activity. Thus, the muscle glucose clearance increases markedly, 10-fold or greater, in response to increments in plasma insulin concentration within the physiologic range.[1,2,27]

GLUT-3, the other major GLUT, is present in the gut and kidney.[2,6] It is sodium dependent and does not respond to insulin. In the gut, it mediates unidirectional gastrointestinal absorption of glucose in the small intestine, whereas in the kidney, it regulates unidirectional glucose absorption in the proximal tubule. Although this transporter is insulin insensitive, it plays a crucial role in glucose homeostasis by regulating its entry into the body and preventing its loss via the kidney.

The intracellular disposition of transported glucose can be studied by using glucose tracers and then localizing the appearance of the label in specific metabolic products such as lactate (i.e., anaerobic glycolysis) and carbon dioxide (i.e, complete oxidation).[8] These techniques, even when correctly applied, only provide only estimates of the metabolic fate of plasma glucose, which is in the labeled pool. For example, should glycogen in muscle be oxidized directly, the plasma glucose–specific activity would miss it completely because plasma glucose does not equilibrate with the intracellular glycogen pool. To circumvent this problem, investigators have employed indirect calorimetry, which measures total carbon dioxide production from all carbohydrate sources, both intracellular and extracellular.[28] Although indirect calorimetry depends on a number of assumptions, these are reasonable and have been largely validated. Moreover, this technique is easy to apply and fully noninvasive. Indirect calorimetry also provides a good estimate of the rate of energy expenditure and complements information obtained by the tracer method. In the basal state and under ordinary nutritionally circumstances, oxygen consumption averages 250 mL/min, whereas carbon dioxide production is 200 mL/min, that is, the whole-body respiratory quotient equals 0.8 (respiratory quotient = carbon dioxide production/oxygen consumption). From the equations depicted in Table 52-4, whole-body carbohydrate oxidation can be estimated to account for approximately 60% of total glucose uptake in the postabsorptive state.[24] Because the brain uses 46% of the total glucose turnover (see Table 52-2) and because essentially all brain glucose uptake is accounted for by oxidation, it follows that three fourths (i.e., 46/60 or 77%) of basal glucose oxidation occurs in the brain. Little is left for other tissues, which preferentially derive their metabolic energy from the oxidation of FFAs and other lipids under postabsorptive conditions. Skeletal muscle, for example, has a respiratory quotient of 0.75 and relies on fat oxidation for the production of 80% of the energy that it needs in the resting state. Thus, the basal state is characterized by parsimonious use of glucose as a metabolic fuel.[15] Moreover, the glucose is selectively channeled to organs that cannot rely on alternative energy sources. In the postabsorptive state, more than half of the total energy production is generated via oxidation of fat, of which there are plentiful stores (see Table 52-1). Insulin is the principal regulator that determines the metabolic mix of fuels in the basal state. A small decrement in the circulating hormone level releases the brake on lipolysis, and the plasma FFA concentration increases, thereby allowing fat to override glucose in the competition between the two substrates. Although these very small changes in plasma insulin concentration are sufficient to promote a shift in fuel metabolism from carbohydrate to fat, the plasma insulin level is still sufficiently elevated to maintain glucose transport and metabolism in target tissues at minimal rates and to restrain protein breakdown, which contributes only approximately 15% to basal energy metabolism.[15] The role that counterregulatory (glucagon, epinephrine, cortisol, growth hormone, thyroid hormones) hormones play in basal glucose uptake is less well defined but probably centers on the maintenance of lipolysis because all the insulin antagonistic hormones are more or less potent lipolytic stimuli.

GLUCOSE CYCLES

After entry of glucose into the cell through a specific GLUT, the sugar does not necessarily follow a direct path to its eventual fate, be it glycogen, lactate, carbon dioxide, or pentoses. Rather, it indirectly reaches its destination via a number of circuitous routes that have become known as futile cycles. A metabolic futile cycle is one in which a precursor is converted into a product by a forward reaction, and then resynthesizes to the precursor. In such a reaction, there is no net product accumulation, but energy (ATP) is used. There are multiple examples of such futile cycles in the glucose metabolic pathway.[29,30] The first involves the conversion of glucose to G-6-P by glucokinase and its subsequent reconversion to intracellular free glucose by glucose-6-phosphatase in the liver. Each turn of this cycle uses one molecule of ATP. Another example of a futile cycle is represented by the conversion of G-6-P to fructose-6-phosphate and back through the phosphoglucoisomerase reaction. Perhaps the best-studied futile cycle that is under the control of insulin is the conversion of fructose-6-phosphate to fructose-1,6-bisphosphate in the liver. The reverse reaction is regulated by fructose-1,6-bisphosphatase, whereas the forward reaction is catalyzed by phosphofructokinase (PFK). The latter enzyme is controlled by the energy status of the cell and key intracellular metabolites. High levels of ATP, acidosis, and citrate inhibit, whereas ADP and alkalosis stimulate PFK. The most potent activator of PFK is fructose-2,6-bisphosphate, whose synthesis is stimulated by the enzyme fructose-2,6-bisphosphate kinase. This latter enzyme is under the control of insulin, and the PFK step, therefore, represents an important regulatory control point for insulin action.[31]

In general terms, whenever bidirectional flux through a metabolic pathway is simultaneously operative, there exists a cycle, regardless of the number of intermediate reactions and regardless of whether one or more tissues are involved. In the examples cited previously, the cycles occurred within individual cells. However, cycles also can exist between organs. In this regard, lipolysis in adipose tissue followed by partial reesterification of FFA in the liver is a complete cycle. Another important cycle is the breakdown of proteins in the liver or other tissues. The glucose-alanine and glucose-lactate (Cori) loops[13] also represent important cycles (see previous discussion) that provide conservation of carbon skeletons and transfer of α-amino groups between muscle and liver.

The derogatory connotation of futility has traditionally been reserved for those cycles that go on in the same cell. These cycles are, however, anything but futile. As elegantly discussed by Newsholme and Leech,[29] a metabolic cycle with a reverberating internal loop provides the best kinetic

Table 52-4	Indirect Calorimetry: Calculation of Carbohydrate and Lipid Oxidation and Energy Expenditure
Net carbohydrate oxidation (μmol/min)	$25.3 \dot{V}CO_2 - 17.8 \dot{V}O_2 - 16.0\,N$
Net lipid oxidation (μmol/min)	$6.5\,(\dot{V}O_2 - \dot{V}CO_2) - 7.5\,N$
Energy expenditure (kJ/min)	$0.0164 \dot{V}O_2 + 0.0046 \dot{V}CO_2 - 0.014\,N$

$\dot{V}O_2$, oxygen consumption (in mL/min); $\dot{V}CO_2$, carbon dioxide production (in mL/min); N, urinary nonprotein nitrogen excretion (in mg/min).

stratagem to maintain the enzymes of a dormant pathway at a minimum of activity, while at the same time ensuring a high sensitivity gain for rapid amplification of incoming signals. The ATP cost of these cycles is itself a means of increasing the efficiency of energy dissipation. The fact that the activity of these cycles is under hormonal control (e.g., catecholamines, glucagon, and thyroid hormones enhance the cycling rate) establishes a mechanism for rapid modulation. In this way, these cycles become components of facultative thermogenesis. Equally important, the operation of these futile or substrate cycles allows the generation of metabolic intermediates that can modulate the activities of key enzymes and allow allosteric regulation.

GLUCOSE METABOLISM: FED (POSTPRANDIAL) STATE

INTRODUCTION

The fed state refers to the period of active nutrient absorption from the gastrointestinal tract and lasts until the plasma insulin concentration and glucose metabolism have returned to basal values. In normal humans, carbohydrates are ingested with lipids and protein (i.e., a mixed meal) is consumed. In the typical diet, carbohydrates comprise approximately 50% of the caloric contents, with fat and protein constituting approximately 35% and approximately 15%, respectively. However, there is considerable intraindividual variation in the distribution of the three major dietary constituents. The rate of absorption of dietary carbohydrates is markedly influenced by their chemical form (refined sugars versus complex carbohydrates) and by the composition of the meal. Protein and fat, in particular, greatly retard gastric emptying and delay carbohydrate absorption. Furthermore, the disposition of dietary carbohydrates is indirectly affected by the dietary fat and protein content to the extent that these latter foodstuffs (1) compete with glucose as substrates in muscle, (2) impair the suppression of hepatic glucose production by providing gluconeogenic precursors, and (3) alter the glucoregulatory hormones (FFAs and some amino acids are insulin secretagogues, whereas most amino acids stimulate glucagon secretion).

The rate-limiting factor for the absorption of glucose is gastric emptying. Once glucose enters the small intestine, it is rapidly transported by a specific transport system (GLUT-3) that is sodium dependent. This transporter is unique to the intestine and kidney (see Table 52-3), which requires glucose to be transported against a steep concentration gradient. The gut (and kidney) epithelial cells use a sodium-glucose cotransport system to overcome the unfavorable glucose concentration gradient.[32] Sodium is transported from the intestinal lumen into the epithelial cell down a favorable sodium gradient. Both sodium and glucose are bound to the transporter, and cellular entry of sodium brings with it glucose. The intracellular glucose exits via the basolateral membrane via a different GLUT (GLUT-1) that is similar to that in the erythrocyte. For glucose transport to continue, sodium also must be pumped out via the basolateral membrane to maintain the favorable sodium gradient for sodium entry from the lumen. This active step is efficiently carried out by a Na^+/K^+-ATPase pump. This coupled system, which effectively and rapidly transports glucose from the intestinal lumen into the interstitial fluid, is independent of insulin.

QUANTITATION OF INSULIN SENSITIVITY AND INSULIN SECRETION

Because of the difficulties involved in following the gastrointestinal absorption of glucose and the persistently changing plasma glucose and insulin concentrations that preclude the achievement of steady-state conditions, the regulation of glucose homeostasis during the fed state has classically been investigated using intravenous glucose, which can be administered in formats that are more suitable for formal analysis. The most detailed information concerning glucose utilization by the whole body, organs, and specific intracellular pathways has come from studies that employ the insulin/glucose clamp technique[33] in combination with indirect calorimetry, radioisotope turnover methodology, and limb (forearm and leg) catheterization. Because the insulin-glucose clamp technique has become the reference method for the study of glucose metabolism, this procedure is described briefly. The euglycemic insulin version of the clamp technique is shown in Figure 52-7. An exogenous infusion of regular insulin is started at time zero and is given as a priming dose followed by a constant infusion (usually at a rate of 1 mU/min per kilogram or 40 mU/min per square meter). Such an infusion quickly establishes a hyperinsulinemic plateau of approximately 70–80 μU/mL. A few minutes after starting the insulin, an infusion of 20% glucose is begun. Based on the plasma glucose concentration, which is measured every 5 to 10 minutes, and using the negative feedback principle, the glucose infusion rate is adjusted periodically to maintain the plasma glucose concentration constant at basal level. In response to the hyperinsulinemic stimulus, there is an initial delay in the onset of insulin-stimulated glucose disposal that lasts approximately 15 to 20 minutes.[27] After this delay, there is a rapid increase in glucose utilization from 20 to 80 minutes, and this

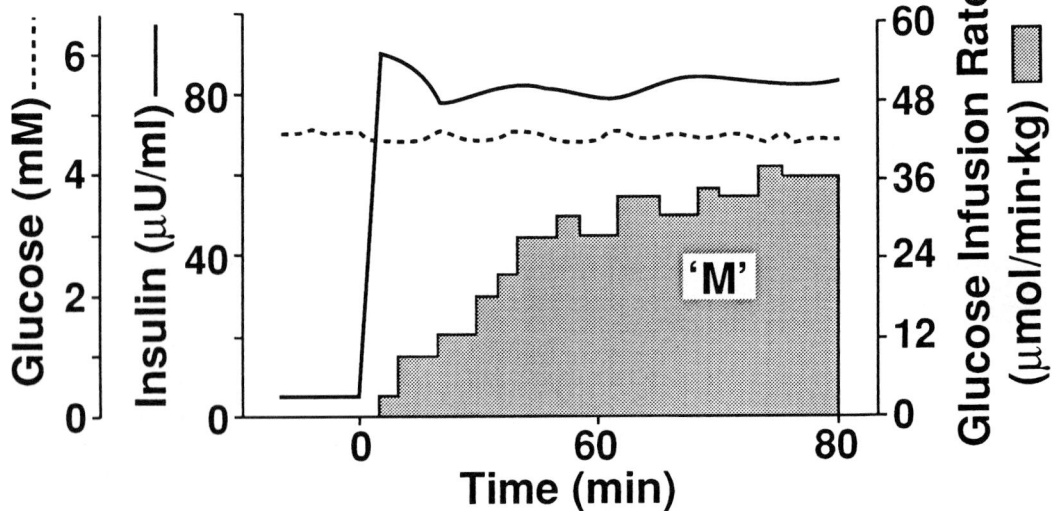

Figure 52-7 Schematic representation of the euglycemic insulin clamp technique. See text for a detailed discussion.

reaches a steady-state plateau value of approximately 5 to 8 mg/min per kilogram of body weight (27–44 μmol/min per kilogram) during the last 40 minutes of the insulin clamp in healthy young subjects.[27] Because endogenous (of which 85% to 90% is derived from the liver and 10% to 15% from the kidney) glucose production is completely or nearly completely (>90%–95%) suppressed by insulin and the plasma glucose concentration is clamped at the basal level, the rate of exogenous glucose infusion must equal the rate of glucose uptake by all tissues of the body and provides a quantitative measure of the amount of glucose metabolized (M). In some insulin-resistant conditions (i.e., obesity and non-insulin-dependent diabetes mellitus[1,2]), hepatic glucose production (measured with radiolabeled glucose or a stable isotope of glucose) is not completely suppressed and must be added to the rate of exogenous glucose infusion to obtain the true rate of total-body glucose utilization. The higher the glucose metabolic rate (M), the more sensitive the individual is to insulin; conversely, the lower the metabolic rate (M), the more resistant is the subject to insulin. The euglycemic insulin clamp technique has the following advantages: (1) any desired combination of plasma glucose and insulin levels easily can be achieved and maintained; (2) the time course of insulin action can be determined with a time resolution of approximately 10 minutes; (3) other techniques, such as radiolabeled glucose infusion, indirect calorimetry, limb catheterization, magnetic resonance imaging/spectroscopy, and muscle biopsy, readily can be combined with the clamp protocol; (4) because hypoglycemia is avoided, the release of counterregulatory hormones, which antagonize insulin action, is prevented and one can derive a pure measure of tissue sensitivity to insulin; (5) the interaction of other hormones or substrates with insulin action can be quantitated by simultaneously infusing them during a clamp study; (6) the achievement of constant or nearly constant levels of insulin, glucose, tracer glucose–specific activity (or enrichment), and glucose metabolic rate allows one to make quantitative measurements under steady-state conditions and thus avoid interpretive problems encountered when plasma glucose and insulin concentrations and glucose flux rates are constantly changing (i.e., during an oral glucose tolerance test or intravenous glucose tolerance test). The hyperglycemic version of the glucose clamp is depicted in Figure 52-8.[33] In this procedure, the plasma glucose concentration is acutely increased by a priming infusion of glucose that is administered in a logarithmically decreasing manner over 15 minutes. Thereafter, the plasma glucose concentration is clamped at the designed plateau by periodically adjusting an exogenous glucose infusion as described in the euglycemic version. The hyperglycemic step evokes an endogenous insulin response that is typically biphasic. During the initial 10 minutes, there is an early burst of insulin release that is followed by a gradual, continuous increase in the plasma insulin concentration. The initial (0–10 minutes) peak of insulin represents the release of preformed hormone that is stored within granules in the β cell. The late (10–120 minutes) phase, which represents the release of newly synthesized insulin within the β cells, lasts until the glucose stimulus is withdrawn. By analogy with the euglycemic insulin clamp counterpart, the hyperglycemic clamp also provides a quantitative measure of the total amount of glucose taken up and metabolized (M) by the body in response to the combined stimuli of endogenous hyperinsulinemia plus hyperglycemia.

One disadvantage of the hyperglycemic clamp or any study in which glucose is administered intravenously is the inability to examine the effect of incretins on insulin secretion.[14] Thus, when glucose is administered orally, the insulin response is significantly greater than when the same arterial glucose profile is created by intravenous glucose administration (Fig. 52-9). Two incretins, glucagon-like peptide-1 and glucose-dependent insulinotrophic polypeptide, which are secreted by the L and K cells of the small intestine, respectively, in response to nutrient ingestion, account for more than 90% of the incretin effect.[14]

DYNAMIC INTERACTION BETWEEN INSULIN SENSITIVITY AND INSULIN SECRETION

In normal, healthy individuals, the euglycemic insulin clamp technique has demonstrated that there is an age-related decline in insulin sensitivity.[34] More importantly, within the normal population, there is a wide range of insulin sensitivity. Among young, healthy, normal glucose-tolerant subjects, insulin-mediated glucose disposal varies 2.5- to threefold, from approximately 4 to 12 mg/min per kilogram (22–66 μmol/min per kilogram) (Fig. 52-10).[35] A number of factors are known to influence insulin sensitivity. In addition to age, adipose tissue mass, fat topography, and degree of physical fitness all are powerful determinants of insulin-mediated glucose disposal.[1,2] Increased total-body fat content, and especially increased visceral fat,[3] as well as decreased Vo₂max[36] are associated with impaired insulin action. Increased metabolites of triglyceride and FFAs (fatty acyl-coenzyme A, diacylglycerol, and ceramide) within muscle and liver cells are associated with insulin resistance in these organs.[3] Dietary composition (increased fat and reduced carbohydrate) also have been shown to impair insulin sensitivity. However, even

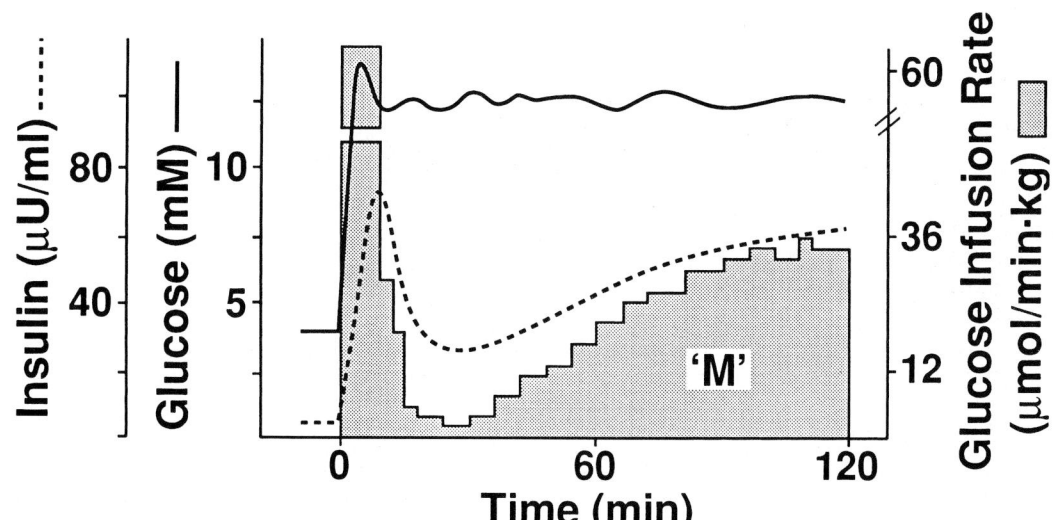

Figure 52-8 Schematic representation of the hyperglycemic clamp technique. See text for a detailed discussion.

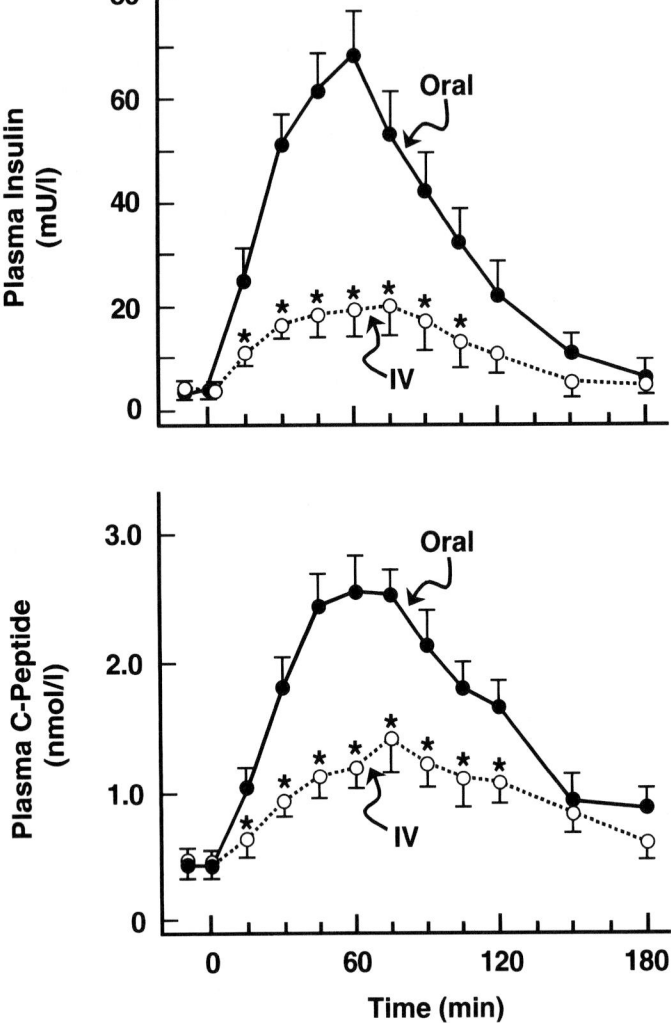

Figure 52-9 Effect of intravenous versus oral glucose on plasma insulin and C-peptide responses. Incretin effect: Plasma insulin **(top)** and C-peptide **(bottom)** responses after oral glucose tolerance tests *(solid circles)* and during isoglycemic intravenous glucose infusion *(open circles)* in the same subjects. IV, intravenous. (From Nauck M, Stockmann F, Ebert R, Creutzfeldt W: Reduced incretin effect in type 2 diabetes mellitus. Diabetologia 29:46–52, 1986.)

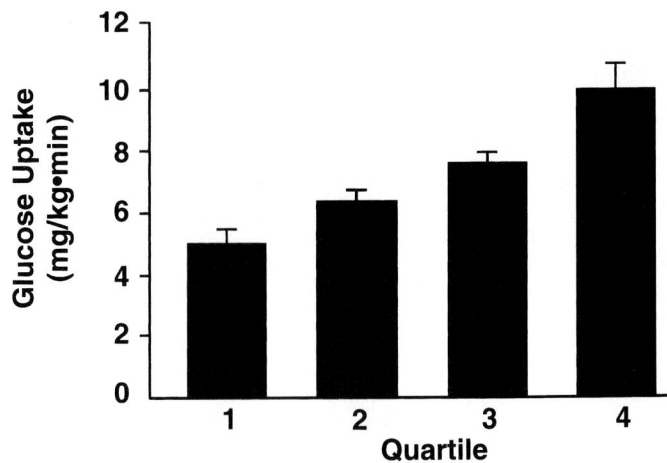

Figure 52-10 Insulin-mediated glucose disposal. Whole-body rate of glucose metabolism during euglycemic insulin clamp in 32 normal glucose-tolerant women, divided according to quartiles of insulin sensitivity. $P < 0.001$ for each quartile versus the adjacent quartile. (From Diamond MP, Thornston K, Connolly-Diamond M, et al: Reciprocal variations in insulin-stimulated glucose uptake and pancreatic insulin secretion in women with normal glucose tolerance. J Soc Gynecol Invest 2:708–715, 1995.)

in patients with type 2 diabetes mellitus.[1,2] Their insulin secretory capacity, when viewed in absolute terms, is normal. However, when viewed in the context of the severity of insulin resistance, it is clear that there is a major defect in β-cell function.

Recent studies serve to emphasize the importance of this dynamic interaction between insulin sensitivity and insulin secretion.[38] The β cell responds to an increment in plasma glucose concentration (ΔG) by an increment in plasma insulin concentration (ΔI), and this response is amplified in the presence of insulin resistance (IR). If one plots the insulin secretion/insulin resistance index ($\Delta I/\Delta G \div IR$) against the 2-hour plasma glucose concentration during the oral

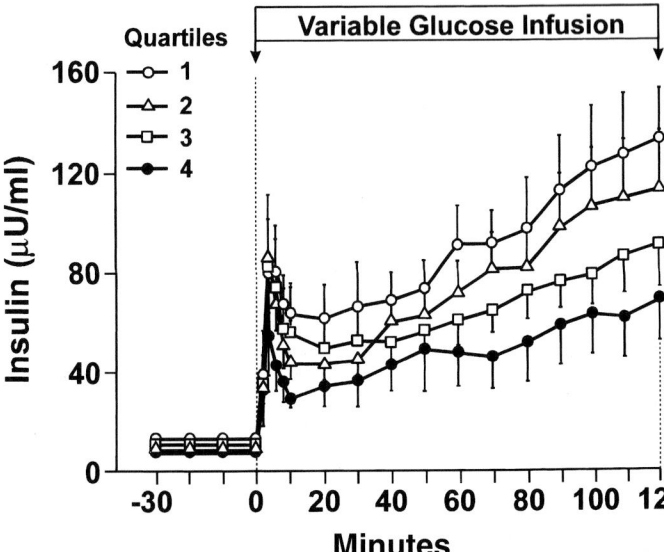

Figure 52-11 Time course of plasma insulin response during the hyperglycemic clamp in the same 32 women whose insulin sensitivity is shown in Figure 52-10. Insulin secretion increased progressively from the highest to lowest quartile of insulin sensitivity. $P < 0.01$. (From Diamond MP, Thornston K, Connolly-Diamond M, et al: Reciprocal variations in insulin-stimulated glucose uptake and pancreatic insulin secretion in women with normal glucose tolerance. J Soc Gynecol Invest 2:708–715, 1995.)

when these factors are taken into account, one cannot explain the wide variation in insulin sensitivity among healthy adult individuals.[35] Studies in whites, Pima Indians, and Mexican Americans[1,2,37] have demonstrated that genetic factors play a major role in the distribution of insulin sensitivity (as measured by the glucose disposal rate during a euglycemic insulin clamp). From this observation, it follows that there must be a finely balanced interaction between tissue sensitivity to insulin and insulin secretion by the pancreas to maintain normal glucose tolerance. In normal glucose-tolerant individuals who fall in the lower quartile of insulin sensitivity (see Fig. 52-10), the β cell is able to sense the defect in insulin action and precisely augment its secretion of insulin to offset the insulin resistance (Fig. 52-11). As can be seen in Figure 52-12, when insulin secretion (measured with the hyperglycemic clamp technique) is plotted against insulin sensitivity (euglycemic insulin clamp technique) in healthy, lean, and normal glucose-tolerant subjects with perfectly normal oral glucose tolerance, a very strong inverse relationship is noted.[1,2,35] This relationship between insulin action and insulin secretion has important implications for the development of non-insulin-dependent diabetes mellitus. As can be seen in Figure 52-13, insulin resistance is uniformly observed

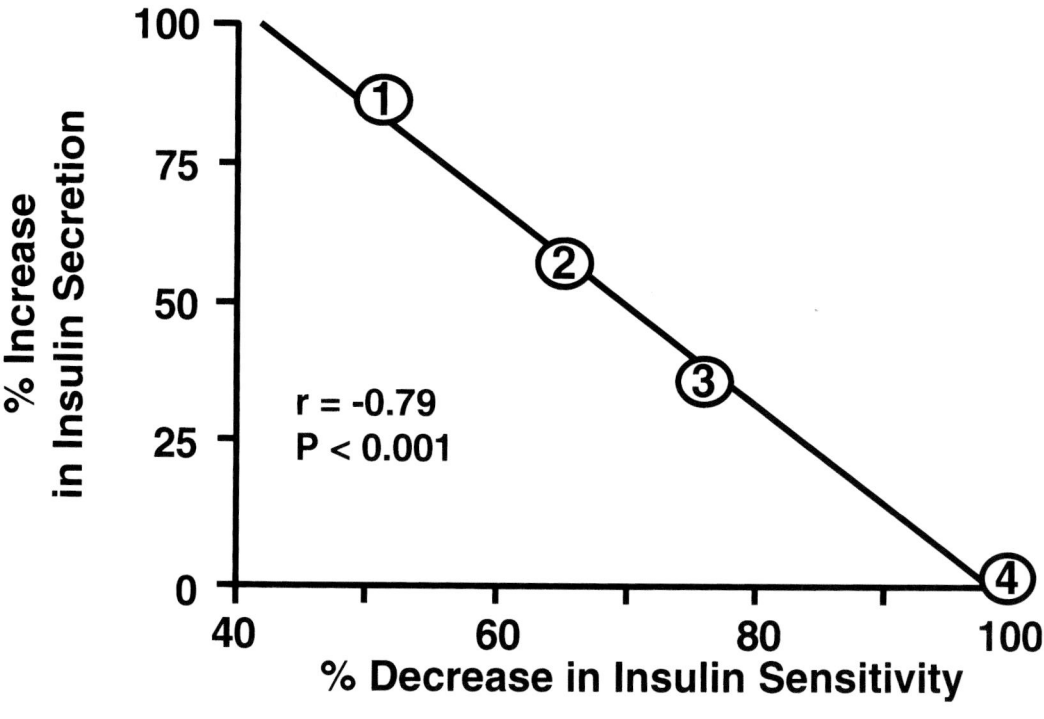

Figure 52-12 Inverse relationship between insulin sensitivity (expressed as the percentage of decrease in the insulin-mediated glucose disposal rate in the most insulin-sensitive women; see Fig. 52-10) and insulin secretion (expressed as the percentage of increase in the plasma insulin response to hyperglycemia in the most insulin-sensitive women; see Fig. 52-11). (From Diamond MP, Thornston K, Connolly-Diamond M, et al: Reciprocal variations in insulin-stimulated glucose uptake and pancreatic insulin secretion in women with normal glucose tolerance. J Soc Gynecol Invest 2:708–715, 1995.)

glucose tolerance test, individuals in the highest tertile of what would be considered to represent normal glucose tolerance (i.e., 2-hour plasma = 120–139 mg/dL) have lost 56% of β-cell function, whereas impaired glucose-tolerant individuals in the bottom half (i.e., 2-hour plasma glucose = 170–199 mg/dL) have lost 80% of β-cell function (Fig. 52-14). Log transformation of these variables demonstrates that the insulin secretion/insulin resistance index is linearly related to both the 2-hour plasma glucose concentration during the oral glucose tolerance test and the fasting plasma glucose concentration (Fig. 52-15), confirming that β-cell function is a critical determinant of glucose tolerance.

In summary, the normal dynamic interaction between insulin secretion and insulin sensitivity represents a key physiologic principle that underlies the ability of all individuals to maintain normal glucose homeostasis.

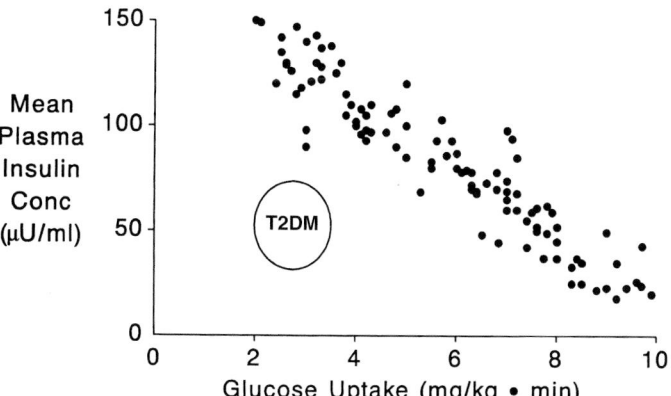

Figure 52-13 Relationship between insulin sensitivity (insulin clamp technique) and insulin secretion (hyperglycemic clamp technique) in normal-weight and obese subjects with normal glucose tolerance (*solid circles*). Subjects with type 2 diabetes mellitus (T2DM) have a "normal" insulin response that, in the presence of severe insulin resistance, results in overt glucose intolerance. (Drawn from the data from DeFronzo[1,2] and unpublished observations.)

EFFECT OF INSULIN ON HEPATIC AND PERIPHERAL GLUCOSE METABOLISM

The maintenance of normal glucose homeostasis requires the closely coordinated effects of insulin and hyperglycemia to simultaneously (1) suppress endogenous (primarily hepatic) glucose production; (2) stimulate glucose uptake by peripheral tissues, primarily muscle; (3) stimulate glucose uptake by the liver; and (4) inhibit lipolysis and reduce the plasma FFA concentration.[1,2] The decrease in circulating plasma FFA levels plays an important role in enhancing the suppression of hepatic glucose production and augmenting muscle glucose uptake in response to a physiologic increase in plasma insulin concentration.[3]

Using the euglycemic insulin clamp technique, insulin can be shown to exert a potent suppressive action on hepatic glucose production, such that portal insulin concentrations of less than 100 μU/mL completely abolish glucose entry into the circulation.[9,19,39] Figure 52-16 shows the typical time course for suppression of endogenous (hepatic) glucose production after an acute increase in plasma insulin to levels of 60 to 70 μU/mL in healthy subjects.[40] Dose-response curves relating the calculated portal plasma insulin concentration to inhibition of hepatic glucose production (Fig. 52-17) indicate a half maximal effect at a level of approximately 30 μU/mL, corresponding with an increment in the portal insulin concentration of only 5 to 10 μU/mL.[19,39] These results indicate the exquisite sensitivity of the liver to very small increments in the circulating plasma insulin concentration. Note that in its capacity of a glucose-producing organ, the liver is extremely sensitive to insulin, whereas the ability of insulin to augment hepatic glucose uptake under conditions of euglycemia is quite modest. In the presence of hyperglycemia, insulin has a small stimulatory effect on hepatic glucose uptake.[41,42] Hyperglycemia, induced by intravenous glucose administration, strongly synergizes this inhibitory action of insulin on hepatic glucose production (see Fig. 52-5). In normal adults, an increase in arterial plasma insulin levels of only 5 to 10 μU/mL is sufficient to rapidly reduce hepatic glucose output by more than 80% (see Fig. 52-17).

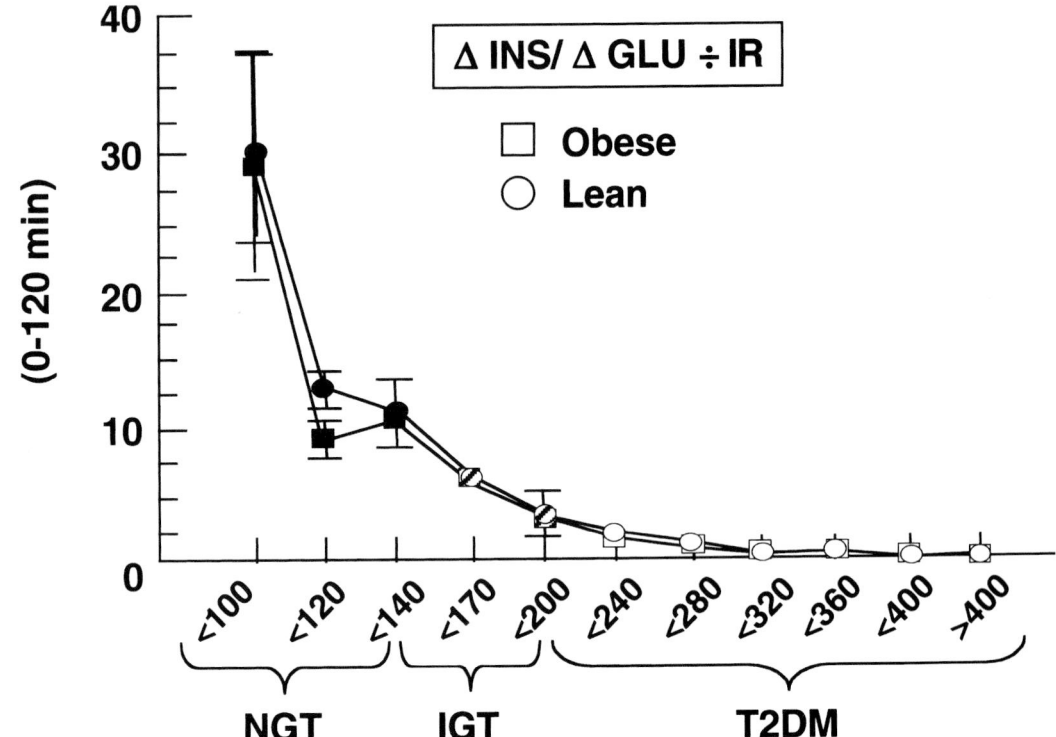

Figure 52-14 Relationship between the 2-hour plasma glucose concentration and the insulin secretion/insulin resistance index (Δ Ins/Δ Glu factored by the severity of insulin resistance measured with the euglycemic insulin clamp) during the 0- to 120-minute period during the oral glucose tolerance test in lean and obese subjects. IGT, impaired glucose tolerance; NGT, normal glucose tolerance; T2DM, type 2 diabetes mellitus.

Concomitantly, with the suppression of hepatic glucose production, insulin elicits a dose-response stimulation of whole-body glucose disposal (see Fig. 52-17).[19] Under euglycemic conditions, the apparent maximal stimulation is approximately 11 to 12 mg/min per kilogram (61–66 μmol/min per kilogram) in healthy adult subjects and occurs with plasma insulin concentrations of approximately 250 μU/mL; the half maximal stimulation of glucose uptake occurs with a plasma insulin concentration of 70 to 110 μU/mL. A dose-response curve of similar shape is derived when progressively higher insulin doses are infused locally into the forearm or leg tissues, approximately 70% of which consists of skeletal muscle. By extrapolating from forearm or leg muscle to total-body muscle mass, it can be estimated that, with prevailing peripheral plasma insulin concentrations in the high physiologic range (60–90 μU/mL), approximately 70% to 80% of total glucose disposal occurs in muscle tissue.[24] Obviously, this percentage increases further with progressively higher insulin

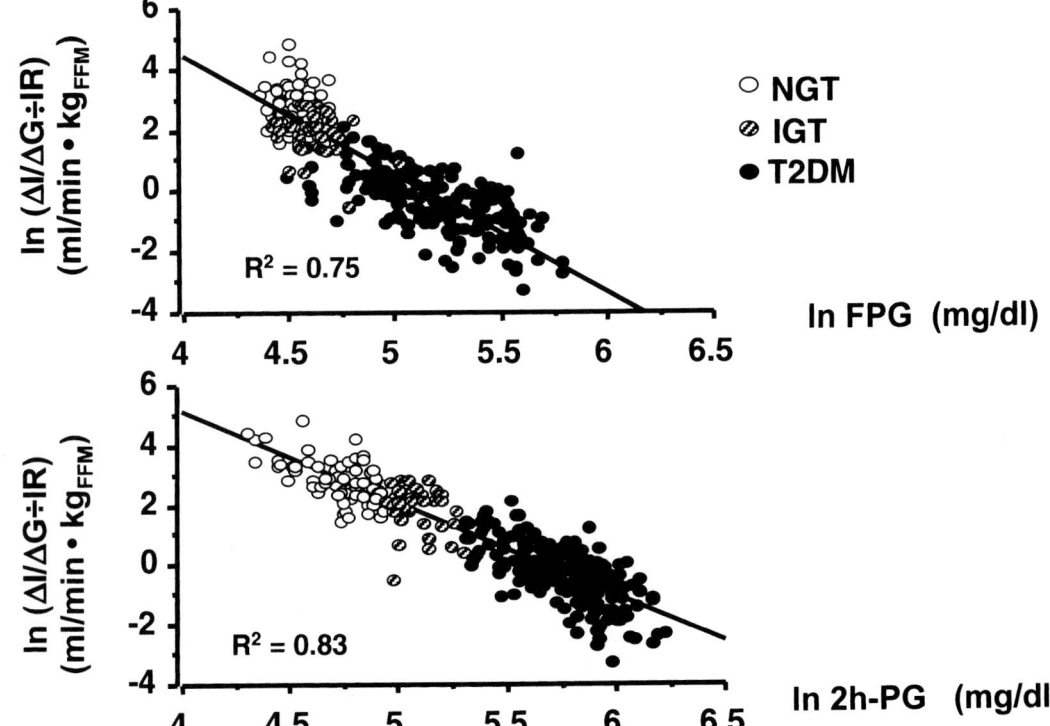

Figure 52-15 Relationship between the insulin secretion/ insulin resistance index (ΔI/ΔG factored by the severity of insulin resistance measured with the euglycemic insulin clamp) and the fasting plasma glucose (FPG) **(top)** and the 2-hour plasma glucose (2-h PG) **(bottom)** concentration (log-log scale). IGT, impaired glucose tolerance; NGT, normal glucose tolerance; T2DM, type 2 diabetes mellitus.

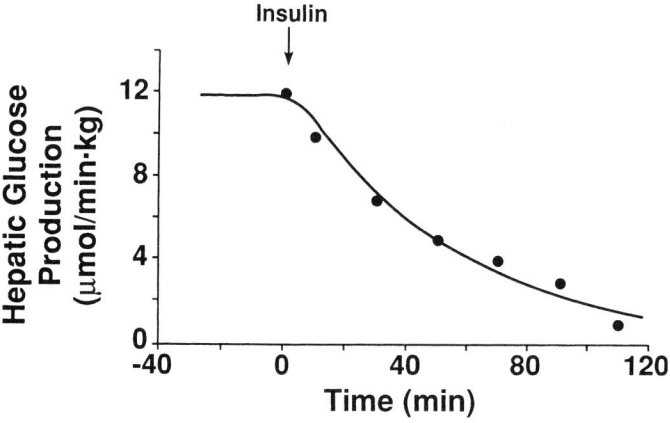

Figure 52-16 Time course of suppression of hepatic glucose production in healthy adults during a euglycemic insulin clamp. (Redrawn from Cobelli C, Mari A, Ferrannini E: The non-steady state problem: Error analysis of Steele's model and developments for glucose kinetics. Am J Physiol 252:E679–E687, 1987.)

levels because the contribution of insulin-independent tissues declines. By combining the insulin clamp technique (plasma insulin concentration, ~70–80 μU/mL) with leg and hepatic vein catheterization, a composite picture of whole-body glucose disposal can be generated (Fig. 52-18). Brain (~1.2 mg/min per kilogram) and splanchnic (liver plus gastrointestinal tissues) (~0.5 mg/min per kilogram) glucose uptake are unaffected by insulin infusion.[1,2] Adipose tissue in adult humans is relatively inert. Although it represents an insulin-dependent tissue, it accounts for no more than 4% to 5% of an infused glucose load. Consequently, muscle represents the primary tissue responsible for insulin-mediated glucose uptake under euglycemic conditions (see Fig. 52-18).[24] When hyperglycemia (plasma glucose increased from 90 to 180 mg/dL) is superimposed on the same level of hyperinsulinemia (70–80 μU/mL), a doubling of total-body glucose utilization occurs (Fig. 52-19); consequently, the glucose clearance remains unchanged. As can be seen in Figure 52-19, essentially all the additional increase in glucose disposal above that observed under euglycemic conditions occurs in muscle. In

the presence of hyperglycemia, insulin has a small stimulatory effect on hepatic glucose uptake, which amounts to approximately 10% of the total-body glucose disposal.[42]

The regulation of glucose production and utilization by insulin is dependent on both the hormone concentration and time. At any given insulin concentration, there is a finite period before the effect of the hormone is seen and reaches its maximum. Such onset time is the sum of a circulatory delay (delivery of insulin from arterial blood to cell surface membrane) and a cellular lag (insulin receptor binding and effector activation). Similarly, insulin's effect on glucose metabolism remains for some time (offset) after the circulating concentration has returned to basal levels. Figure 52-20 shows the activation and deactivation times of insulin calculated at euglycemia over a wide range of plasma hormone levels (as high as 1000 mU/mL).[43] With the reservations inherent in the analysis of non-steady-state tracer data, the results shown in Figure 52-20 provide evidence that activation and deactivation are inversely related to one another. Thus, at higher plasma insulin concentrations, the hormone's effect is more rapid in onset and takes longer to wane. From the physiologic standpoint, it also is noteworthy that the relationship between onset and offset time is different for the liver (suppression of glucose release) and for peripheral tissues (stimulation of glucose uptake). At any insulin dose, the liver is activated more rapidly and the effect persists for a longer duration. The more rapid onset of action in the liver may be related to the shorter diffusion time of blood-borne substances into highly perfused organs (1 mL/min per gram of tissue in the liver versus a corresponding value of 0.04 mL/min per gram in resting skeletal muscle; see Table 52-1) and to anatomic differences between liver capillaries (which are fenestrated) and muscle capillaries (which are not fenestrated).

INTRACELLULAR PATHWAYS OF GLUCOSE DISPOSAL

Overview

By combining indirect calorimetry with dose-response studies using the euglycemic insulin clamp technique, it has been possible to quantitate the two major components of whole-body glucose disposal, that is, glucose oxidation and nonoxidative glucose disposal.[1,2,44] The latter primarily (>90%)

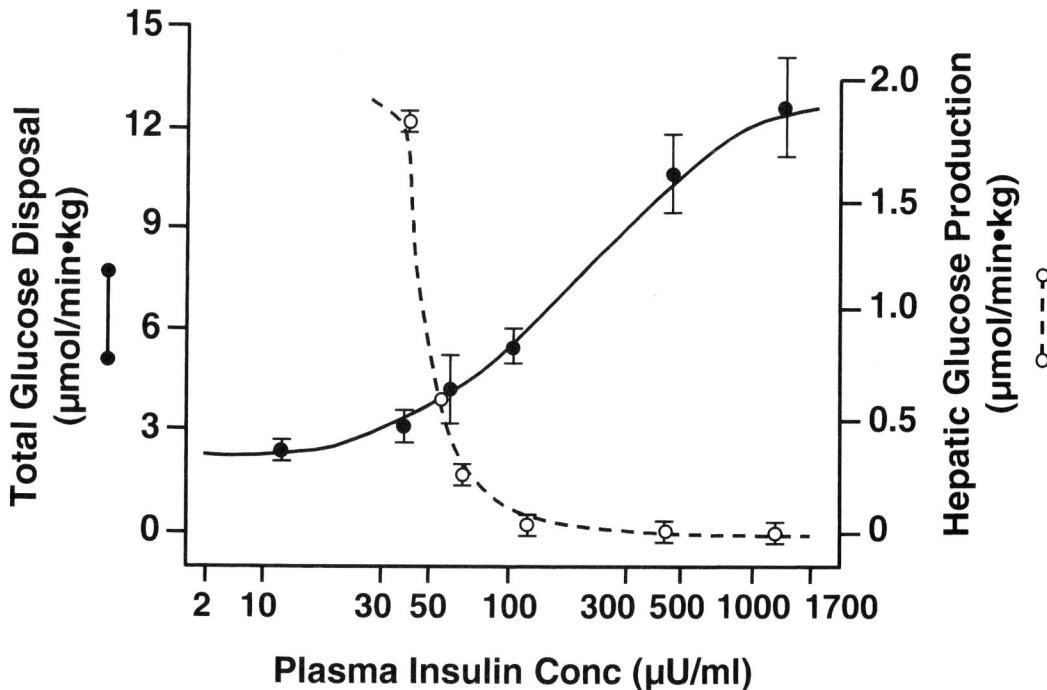

Figure 52-17 Dose-response relationship between the plasma insulin concentration (note the log scale) versus hepatic glucose production and whole-body glucose uptake in healthy subjects studied with the euglycemic insulin clamp technique. The insulin concentrations are peripheral levels in the case of total glucose uptake and portal levels in the case of hepatic glucose production. (Reproduced from DeFronzo RA, Ferrannini E, Hendler R, et al: Regulation of splanchnic and peripheral glucose uptake by insulin and hyperglycemia in man. Diabetes 32:35–45, 1983.)

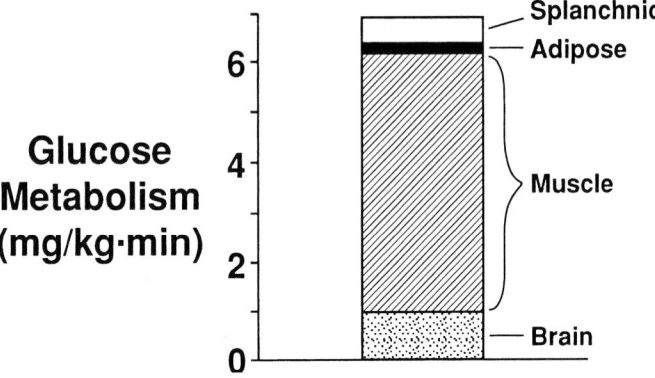

Figure 52-18 Summary of tissue glucose disposal during a euglycemic (90 mg/dL) hyperinsulinemic (+80 µU/mL) clamp in healthy subjects. (Reproduced from DeFronzo RA: Lilly lecture: The triumvirate: β-cell, muscle, liver: A collusion responsible for NIDDM. Diabetes 37:667–687, 1988.)

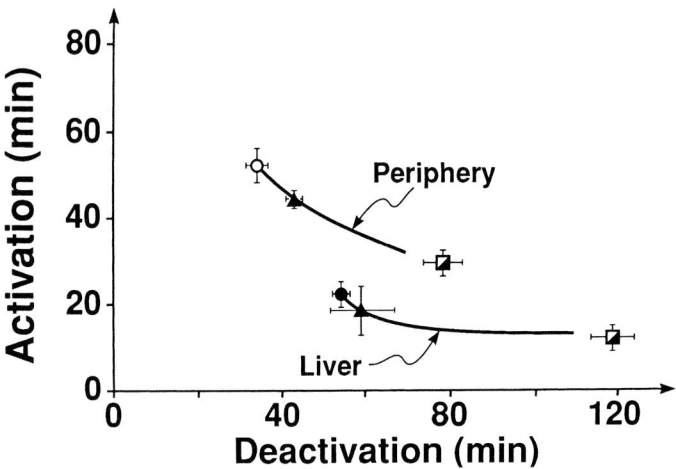

Figure 52-20 Relationships between activation and deactivation times for stimulation of peripheral glucose uptake and inhibition of hepatic glucose production during three insulin infusion rates: 15 mU/m² per minute (*open circles*), 40 mU/m² per minute (*closed triangles*), 120 mU/m² per minute (*semiclosed squares*). (Reconstructed from Prager R, Wallace P, Olefsky JM: In vivo kinetics of insulin action on peripheral glucose disposal and hepatic output in normal and obese subjects. J Clin Invest 78:472–481, 1986.)

represents glycogen synthesis, the remainder being accounted for by anaerobic metabolism, that is, net lactate production. Figure 52-21 shows that the dose curves relating both glucose oxidation and nonoxidative glucose disposal (glycogen synthesis) to the plasma insulin concentration retain the sigmoidal shape of the curve for whole-body glucose uptake but with distinctly different dose kinetics. Thus, glucose oxidation is more sensitive (lower half maximum) but saturates earlier (lower maximum) than glycogen synthesis; the latter behaves as a pathway with low sensitivity and high capacity. Skeletal muscle has been identified as the predominant site of insulin-mediated net glycogen synthesis.[45] However, the increment in carbohydrate oxidation that follows systemic insulin administration occurs in muscle as well as other tissues (probably the liver) in an approximate ratio of 1 to 2 (oxidation to glycogen synthesis). With the use of nuclear magnetic resonance spectroscopy, one can directly quantitate muscle glycogen synthesis. The time course of insulin-stimulated muscle glycogen formation (Fig. 52-22) closely follows the time course of nonoxidative glucose uptake by the whole body.[45] By extrapolation from leg muscle to whole-body muscle, one can account for the great majority (~90%) of nonoxidative glucose disposal as muscle glycogen formation. Under physiologic conditions of hyperinsulinemia, approximately two thirds of G-6-P is converted to glycogen and one third

enters glycolysis (see Fig. 52-21).[24,44] Of the glucose that enters the glycolytic pathway, the majority (~80%–90%) is oxidized in the Krebs cycle to carbon dioxide and water and remainder is converted to lactate.[46]

For insulin to exert its biologic effects on glucose metabolism, it must first bind to specific receptors that are present on the cell surface of all insulin target tissues.[2,47,48] After insulin has bound to and activated its receptor, second messengers are generated, and these second messengers initiate a series of events involving a cascade of phosphorylation-dephosphorylation reactions[2,47–49] that eventually result in the stimulation of intracellular glucose metabolism (Fig. 52-23). The initial step in glucose metabolism involves activation of the glucose transport system, leading to influx of glucose into insulin target tissues, primarily muscle.[2,6,26,50] The free glucose, which has entered the cell, is subsequently metabolized by a series of enzymatic steps that are under the control of insulin. Of these, the most important are glucose phosphorylation

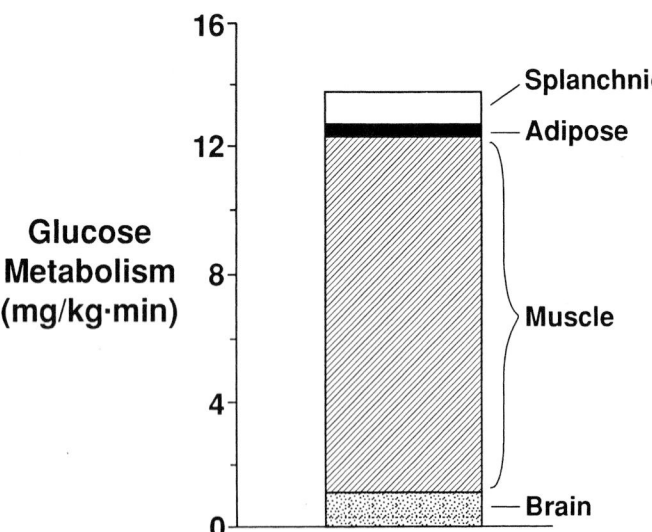

Figure 52-19 Summary of tissue glucose disposal during a hyperglycemic (180 mg/dL) hyperinsulinemic (80 µU/mL) clamp.

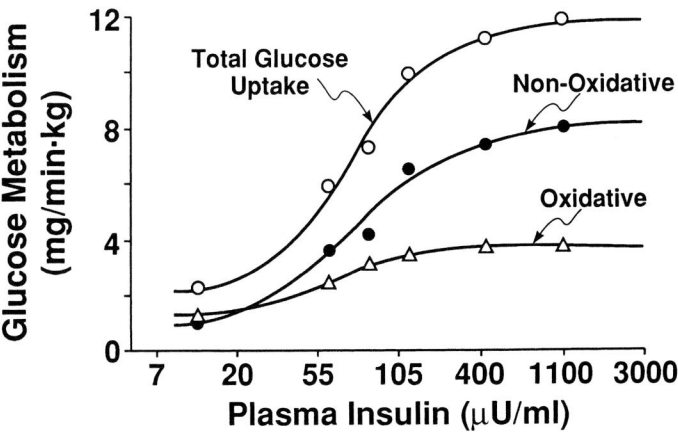

Figure 52-21 Dose-response relationship between the plasma insulin concentration and total-body glucose uptake, glucose oxidation, and nonoxidative glucose disposal in healthy subjects during a euglycemic insulin clamp. (Drawn from the data from Thiebaud et al.[44])

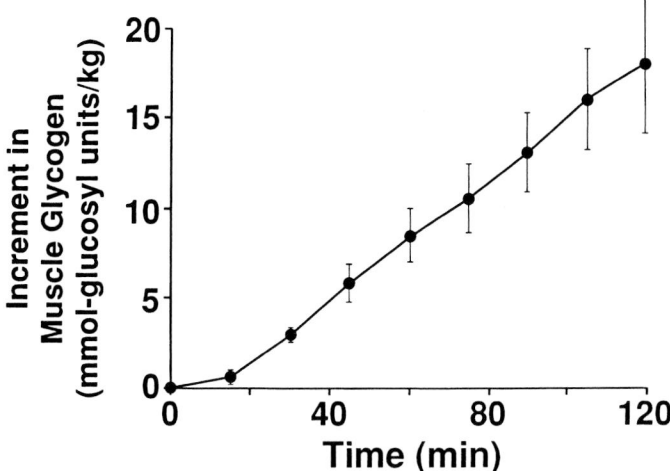

Figure 52-22 Time course of stimulation of muscle glycogen formation by combined hyperinsulinemia (100 μU/mL) and hyperglycemia (200 mg/dL) in healthy subjects as determined by nuclear magnetic resonance spectroscopy. (Redrawn from Shulman GI, Rothman DL, Jue T, et al: Quantitation of muscle glycogen synthesis in normal subjects and subjects with non-insulin-dependent diabetes by ^{13}C nuclear magnetic resonance spectroscopy. N Engl J Med 322:223–228, 1990.)

(catalyzed by hexokinase), glycogen synthase (which controls glycogen synthesis), and PFK and pyrovate dehydrogenase (which regulate glycolysis and glucose oxidation, respectively).

Insulin Receptor/Insulin Receptor Tyrosine Kinase

The insulin receptor is a glycoprotein consisting of two α subunits and two β subunits linked by disulfide bonds[2,47–49] (Fig. 52-24). The α subunit of the insulin receptor is entirely extracellular and contains the insulin-binding domain. The β subunit has an extracellular domain, a transcellular domain, and an intracellular domain that express insulin-stimulated kinase activity directed toward its own tyrosine residues. Insulin receptor phosphorylation of the α subunit, with subsequent activation of insulin receptor tyrosine kinase, represents the first step in the action of insulin on glucose metabolism. Mutagenesis experiments have shown that insulin receptors devoid of tyrosine kinase activity are completely ineffective in mediating insulin stimulation of cellular metabolism. Similarly, mutagenesis of any of the three major phosphorylation sites (at residues 1158, 1163, and 1162) impairs the insulin receptor kinase activity, and this is associated with a marked decrease in the acute metabolic and growth-promoting effects of insulin.

Insulin Receptor Signal Transduction

After activation, insulin receptor tyrosine kinase phosphorylates specific intracellular proteins, of which at least nine have been identified (see Fig. 52-24).[47] Four of these belong to the family of insulin-receptor substrate (IRS) proteins: IRS-1, IRS-2, IRS-3, IRS-4 (the others include Shc, Cbl, Gab-1, p60(dok), and APS). In muscle, IRS-1 serves as the major docking protein that interacts with the insulin receptor tyrosine kinase and undergoes tyrosine phosphorylation in regions containing amino acid sequence motifs (YXXM or YMXM) that, when phosphorylated, serve as recognition sites for proteins containing *src*-homology 2 (SH2) domains.[47,51] Mutation of these specific tyrosines severely impairs the ability of insulin to stimulate glycogen and DNA synthesis, establishing the important role of IRS-1 in insulin signal transduction. In liver, IRS-2 serves as the primary docking protein that undergoes tyrosine phosphorylation and mediates the effect of insulin on hepatic glucose production, gluconeogenesis, and glycogen formation. In adipocytes, Cbl represents another substrate that is phosphorylated after its interaction with the insulin receptor tyrosine kinase and is required for stimulation of GLUT-4 translocation. Phosphorylation of Cbl occurs when the CAP/Cbl complex associates with flotillin in caveolae, or lipid rafts, containing insulin receptors.[52]

In muscle, the phosphorylated tyrosine residues on IRS-1 mediate an association between the SH2 domains of the 85-kilodalton regulatory subunit of phosphatidylinositol 3-kinase (PI 3-kinase), leading to activation of the enzyme[47–49,51] (see Fig. 52-24). PI 3-kinase is a heterodimeric enzyme composed of an 85-kilodalton regulatory subunit and a 110-kilodalton catalytic subunit. The latter catalyzes the 3'-phosphorylation of phosphatidylinositol (PI) in the plasma membrane glycolipids, thereby converting PI 4,5-bisphosphate to PI 3,4,5-triphosphate and PI 4-phosphate to PI 3,4 biphosphate. PI $(3,4,5)$ P_3 and PI $(3,4)$ P_2 lead to the stimulation of glucose transport. Activation of PI 3-kinase by phosphorylated IRS-1 also leads to activation of glycogen synthase,[47,51] via a process that involves activation of protein kinase B/Akt and subsequent inhibition of kinases such as GSK-3 and activation of protein phosphatase-1 (PP-1). Inhibitors of PI 3-kinase impair glucose transport by interfering with the translocation of GLUT-4 from their intracellular location and block the activation of glycogen synthase and hexokinase (HK)-II expression.[26,47–51] The action of insulin to increase protein synthesis and inhibit protein synthesis also is mediated by PI 3-kinase and involves the activation of mTOR.[53] Mammalian target of rapamycin (mTOR) controls translation machinery by phosphorylation and activation of p70 ribosomal S6 kinase [p70(rsk)] and phosphorylation of initiation factors.[53] Insulin also promotes hepatic triglyceride synthesis via increasing the transcription factor steroid regulatory element-binding protein-1c, and this lipogenic effect of insulin also appears to be mediated via the PI 3-kinase pathway.[47]

Other proteins with SH2 domains, including the adapter protein Grb2 and *Shc*, also interact with IRS-1 and become phosphorylated after exposure to insulin.[47,48,51] Grb2 and *Shc* serve to link IRS-1/IRS-2 to the mitogen-activated protein signaling pathway (see Fig. 52-24), which plays an important role in the generation of transcription factors.[47,51] After the interaction between IRS-1/IRS-2 and Grb2 and *Shc*, Ras is activated, leading to the stepwise activation of Raf, mitogen-activated protein kinase (MEK), and extracellular signal-regulated kinase. Activated extracellular signal-regulated kinase then

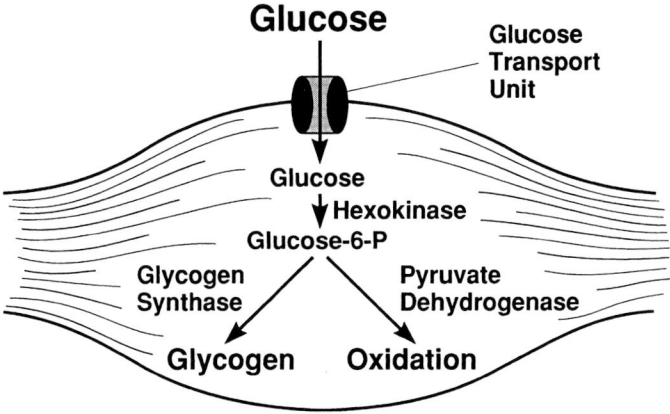

Figure 52-23 Schematic representation of glucose transport, glucose phosphorylation, and the intracellular partitioning of glucose into its two major metabolic pathways: glucose oxidation and glycogen synthesis.

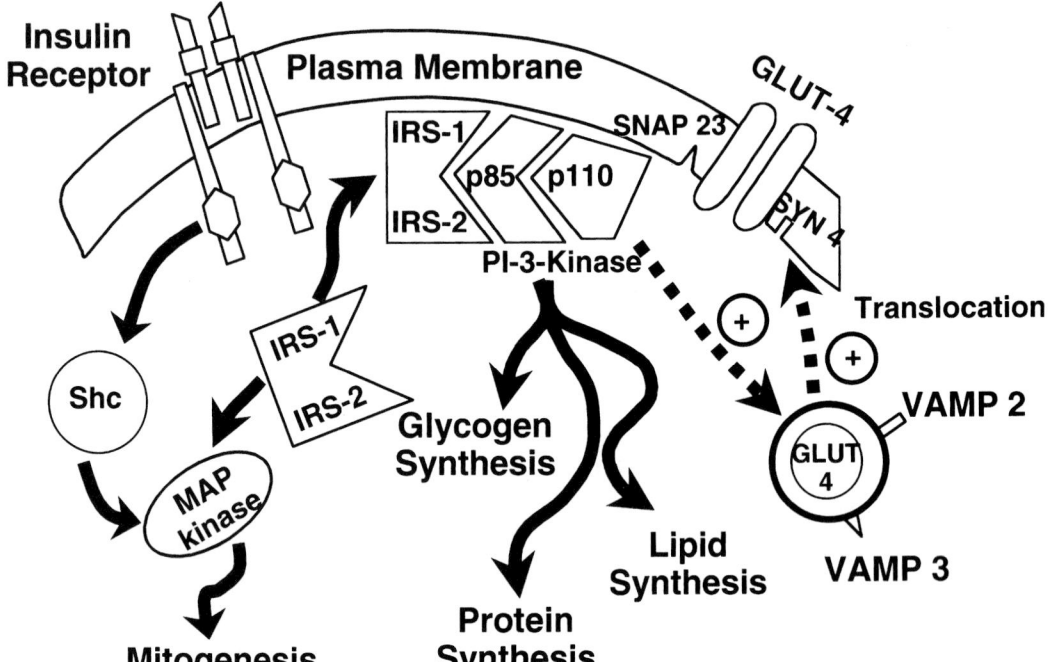

Figure 52-24 Schematic representation of the insulin receptor and the cascade of intracellular signaling molecules that have been implicated in insulin action; see text for a more detailed discussion. GLUT, glucose transporter; MAP, mitogen-activated protein; PI-3-Kinase, phosphatidylinositol kinase; SNAP, soluble NSF attachment 23 kDa protein; SYN, syntaxin; VAMP, vesicle-associated membrane.

translocates into the nucleus of the cell where it catalyzes the phosphorylation of transcription factors that promote cell growth, proliferation, and differentiation.[47,48,51,54,55] Blockade of the mitogen-activated protein kinase pathway prevents the stimulation of cell growth by insulin but has no effect on the metabolic actions of the hormone.

Under anabolic conditions, insulin stimulates glycogen synthesis by simultaneously activating glycogen synthase and inhibiting glycogen phosphorylase[56-58] (Fig. 52-25). The effect of insulin is mediated via the PI 3-kinase pathway, which inactivates kinases such as glycogen synthase kinase-3 and activates phosphatases, particularly PP-1. It is believed that PP-1 is the primary regulator of glycogen metabolism.[56-58] In skeletal muscle, PP-1 associates with a specific glycogen-binding regulatory subunit, causing dephosphorylation (activa-

tion) of glycogen synthase. PP-1 also phosphorylates (inactivates) glycogen phosphorylase. The precise steps that link insulin receptor tyrosine kinase/PI 3-kinase activation to stimulation of PP-1 have yet to be defined. Some evidence suggests that p90 ribosomal S6-kinase may be involved in the activation of glycogen synthase.[47] Akt also has been shown to phosphorylate and thus inactivate GSK-3. This decreases glycogen synthase phosphorylation, leading to activation of the enzyme. A number of studies have convincingly demonstrated that inhibitors of PI 3-kinase inhibit glycogen synthase and abolish glycogen synthesis.[47,48] From the physiologic standpoint, it makes sense that activation of glucose transport and glycogen synthase should be linked to the same signaling mechanism to provide a coordinated and efficient stimulation of intracellular glucose metabolism.

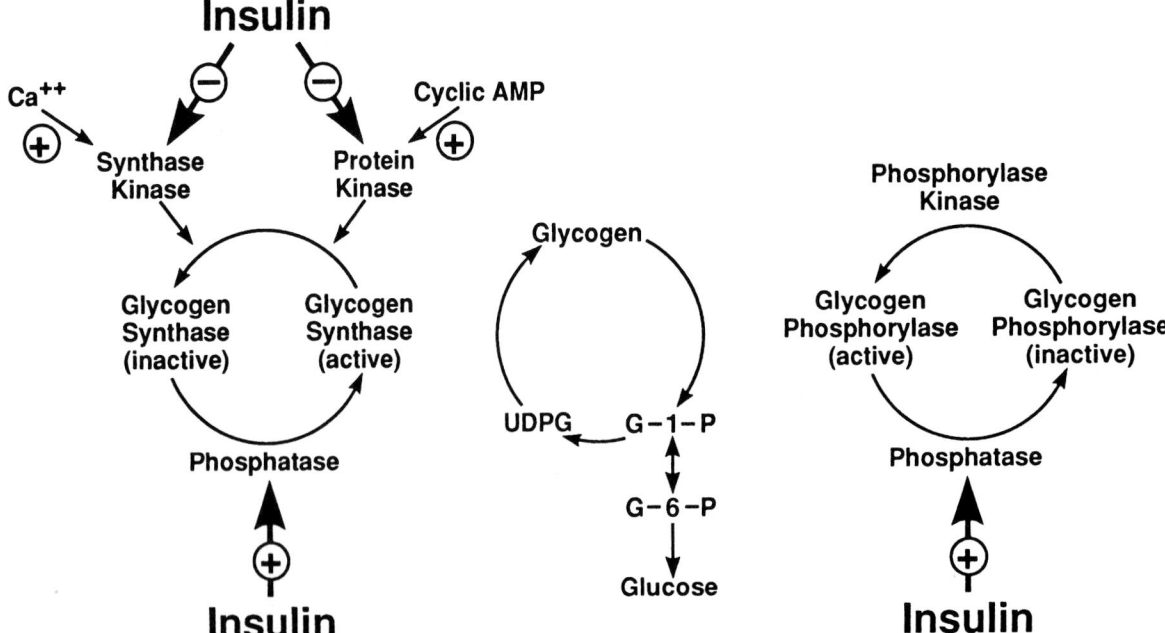

Figure 52-25 Schematic representation of the control of glycogen synthesis and breakdown. Sites of insulin regulation are indicated. See text for a detailed discussion. Cyclic AMP, cyclic adenosine monophosphate; G-1-P, glucose-1-phosphate; G-6-P, glucose-6-phosphate; UDPG, uridine-diphosphate glucose.

Glucose Transport

Activation of the insulin signal transduction system in insulin target tissues leads to the stimulation of glucose transport. The effect of insulin is brought about by the translocation of a large intracellular pool of GLUTs (associated with low-density microsomes) to the plasma membrane.[2,6,26,50] There are five major, different facilitative GLUTs with distinctive tissue distributions[6,50,59,60] (see Table 52-3). GLUT-4, the insulin-regulatable transporter, is found in insulin-sensitive tissues (muscle and adipocytes), has a K_m of approximately 5 mmol/L, which is close to that of the plasma glucose concentration and is associated with HK-II.[61–63] In adipocytes and muscle, its concentration in the plasma membrane increases markedly after exposure to insulin, and this increase is associated with a reciprocal decline in the intracellular GLUT-4 pool. Acute physiologic hyperinsulinemia does not increase the total number of GLUT-4 in muscle, even though several studies have demonstrated an increase in muscle GLUT-4 mRNA. Using a novel isotopic dilution technique, the in vivo dose-response curve for the action of insulin on glucose transport in human forearm skeletal muscle has been described (Fig. 52-26). GLUT-1 represents the predominant GLUT in the insulin-independent tissues (brain and erythrocytes) but is also found in muscle and adipocytes. It is located primarily in the plasma membrane, where its concentration changes little after the addition of insulin. It has a low K_m (~1 mmol/L) and is well suited for its function, which is to mediate basal glucose uptake. It is found in association with HK-I.[61–63] GLUT-2 predominates in the liver and pancreatic β cells, where it is found in association with a specific HK, HK-IV.[61–64] In the β cell, HK-IV is referred to as glucokinase.[64] GLUT-2 has a high K_m (~15–20 mmol/L) and, as a consequence, the glucose concentration in cells expressing this transporter increases in direct proportion to the increase in plasma glucose concentration. This characteristic allows these cells to respond as glucose sensors. In summary, each tissue has a specific GLUT and associated HK that allow it uniquely to carry out its specialized function to maintain whole-body glucose economy.

Glucose Phosphorylation

Glucose phosphorylation and glucose transport are tightly coupled phenomena. Isoenzymes of HK (HKI–HKIV) catalyze the first committed intracellular step of glucose metabolism, the conversion of glucose to G-6-P[61–64] (see Table 52-3). HKI, HKII, and HKIII are single-chain peptides that have a number of properties in common, including a very high affinity for glucose and product inhibition by G-6-P. HK-IV, also called glucokinase, has a lower affinity for glucose and is not inhibited by G-6-P. Glucokinase (HK-IVB) is believed to be the glucose sensor in the β cell, whereas HK-IVL plays an important role in the regulation of hepatic glucose metabolism.

In both rat and human[62,65] skeletal muscle HK-II transcription is regulated by insulin. HK-I also is present in human skeletal muscle but is not regulated by insulin. In response to physiologic euglycemic hyperinsulinemia, HK-II cytosolic activity, protein content, and mRNA levels increase by 50% to 200% in healthy subject,[65] and this is associated with the translocation of HK-II from the cytosol to the mitochondria.[66] In contrast, insulin has no effect on HK-I activity, protein content, or mRNA levels.

Glycogen Synthesis

After glucose enters the cell and is phosphorylated, it either can be converted to glycogen or enter the glycolytic pathway. Of the glucose that enters the glycolytic pathway, approximately 90% is oxidized. In the low physiologic range of hyperinsulinemia, glycogen synthesis and glucose oxidation are of approximately equal quantitative importance. With increasing plasma insulin concentrations, glycogen synthesis becomes predominant.[39,44] If the rate of glucose oxidation is subtracted from the rate of whole-body insulin-mediated glucose disposal (determined from the insulin clamp), the difference represents nonoxidative glucose disposal (or glucose storage), which primarily reflects glycogen synthesis.[1,2,45] Glucose conversion to lipid accounts for less than 5% of total glucose disposal[67] and less than 5% to 10% of the glucose taken up by muscle is released as lactate.[46] Using nuclear magnetic resonance imaging spectroscopy and measuring insulin-stimulated incorporation of [^{1}H,^{13}C]-glucose into muscle glycogen,[45] the rate of nonoxidative glucose disposal (glucose storage) has been shown to correlate closely with the rate of glycogen synthesis ($r = 0.89$, $P < 0.001$) (see Fig. 52-22).

Glycogen synthase is the key insulin-regulated enzyme that controls the rate of muscle glycogen formation.[56–58,68–70] Insulin enhances glycogen synthase activity by stimulating

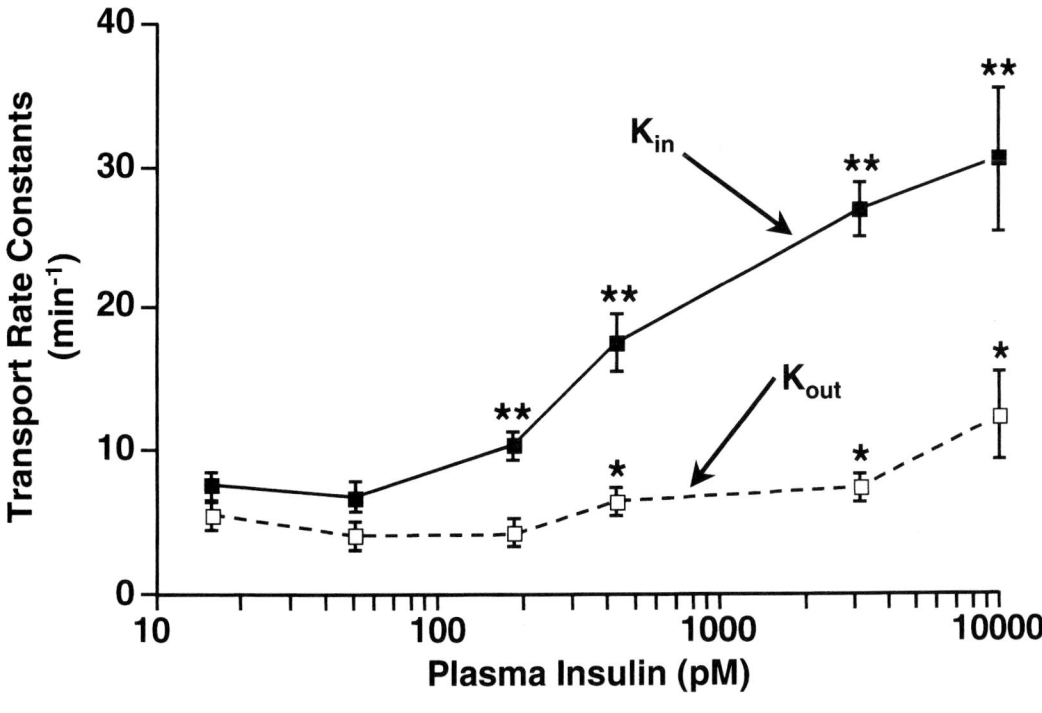

Figure 52-26 Insulin action on glucose transport. Insulin dose-response curve for inward (K_{in}) and outward (K_{out}) rate constants for the transmembrane transport of 3-*O*-methyl-glucose in forearm skeletal muscle at different plasma insulin concentrations. *P < 0.05 versus basal; **P < 0.01 versus basal. (Reproduced from Bonadonna RC, Cobelli C, Saccomani MP, et al: Glucose transport in human skeletal muscle: The in vivo response to insulin. Diabetes 42:191–198, 1993.)

a cascade of phosphorylation-dephosphorylation reactions[56,57,70] (see earlier discussion of insulin receptor signal transduction), which ultimately lead to the activation of PP-1 (also called glycogen synthase phosphatase).[69,70] The regulatory subunit (G) of PP-1 has two serine phosphorylation sites, called site 1 and site 2. Phosphorylation of site 2 by cyclic adenosine monophosphate–dependent kinase (PKA) inactivates PP-1, while phosphorylation of site 1 by insulin activates PP-1, leading to the stimulation of glycogen synthase.[70,71] Phosphorylation of site 1 of PP-1 by insulin in muscle is catalyzed by insulin-stimulated protein kinase-1, which is part of a family of serine/threonine protein kinases termed *ribosomal S6-kinases*. Because of their central role in muscle glycogen formation and impaired insulin-stimulated glycogen synthesis is a characteristic defect in patients with type 2 diabetes mellitus, considerable attention has been focused on the three enzymes glycogen synthase, PP-1, and insulin-stimulated protein kinase-1 in the pathogenesis of insulin resistance in individuals with type 2 diabetes.

The effect of insulin on glycogen synthase gene transcription and translation in vivo has been studied by employing the euglycemic insulin clamp in combination with muscle biopsies. Most studies[65] have shown that insulin does not increase glycogen synthase mRNA or protein expression in human muscle in vivo. Rather, insulin converts the inactive (phosphorylated) form of glycogen synthase to the active (dephosphorylated) form of the enzyme.[56–58,68]

Glycolysis/Glucose Oxidation

Glucose oxidation accounts for approximately 90% of total glycolytic flux, while anaerobic glycolysis accounts for the other 10%.[46] Two enzymes, PFK and PDH, play central roles in the regulation of glycolysis and glucose oxidation, respectively. PFK represents a key functional step in control of glycolysis.[31,72] However, insulin does not exert any direct effect on this enzyme, which is primarily regulated by the energy (ATP) and fuel (citrate, acetyl-CoA) status of the cell. However, insulin indirectly stimulates PFK by increasing fructose-2,6-bisphosphate, a potent activator of PFK. Insulin has no effect on muscle PFK activity, mRNA levels, or protein content in nondiabetic individuals.[73] Insulin also regulates flux through glycolysis by increasing the activity of the multienzyme complex, PDH.[30,72] This enzyme is activated by insulin, which stimulates PDH phosphatase, thus converting the enzyme from its inactive phosphorylated form to its active dephosphorylated form (Fig. 52-27). The PDH complex enzyme also is inhibited by its products, acetyl-CoA and reduced nicotinamide adenine dinucleotide (NADH).

FREE FATTY ACID–AMINO ACID–GLUCOSE INTERACTIONS

A major part of insulin's stimulatory action on glucose metabolism is indirect and is mediated via changes in substrate metabolism. In contrast to the hormone's stimulatory effect on glucose utilization, insulin is a powerful inhibitor of lipolysis and lipid oxidation.[39] As shown in Figure 52-28, plasma FFA concentrations decline steeply in response to small increments in circulating insulin levels under conditions of euglycemia. This decrease is the result of a drastic reduction in the rate of FFA appearance into the circulation. The concomitant decline in plasma glycerol concentration is consistent with in vitro studies and indicates that lipolysis is inhibited. The consequence of the reduced availability of FFA is a parallel reduction in both FFA oxidation and nonoxidative FFA disposal, that is, reesterification (Fig. 52-29). The inverse patterns of change in glucose disposal and oxidation on the one hand, and lipid utilization on the other, introduce the important concept of substrate competition. Glucose and long-chain FFAs are the first and best-known example of substrate competition in insulin-dependent tissues.[74] Physiologically, the increases in plasma glucose (by mass action) and insulin (stimulation of glucose transport) concentrations increase the rate of glucose uptake into fat cells. The resultant increase in intracellular α-glycerol phosphate

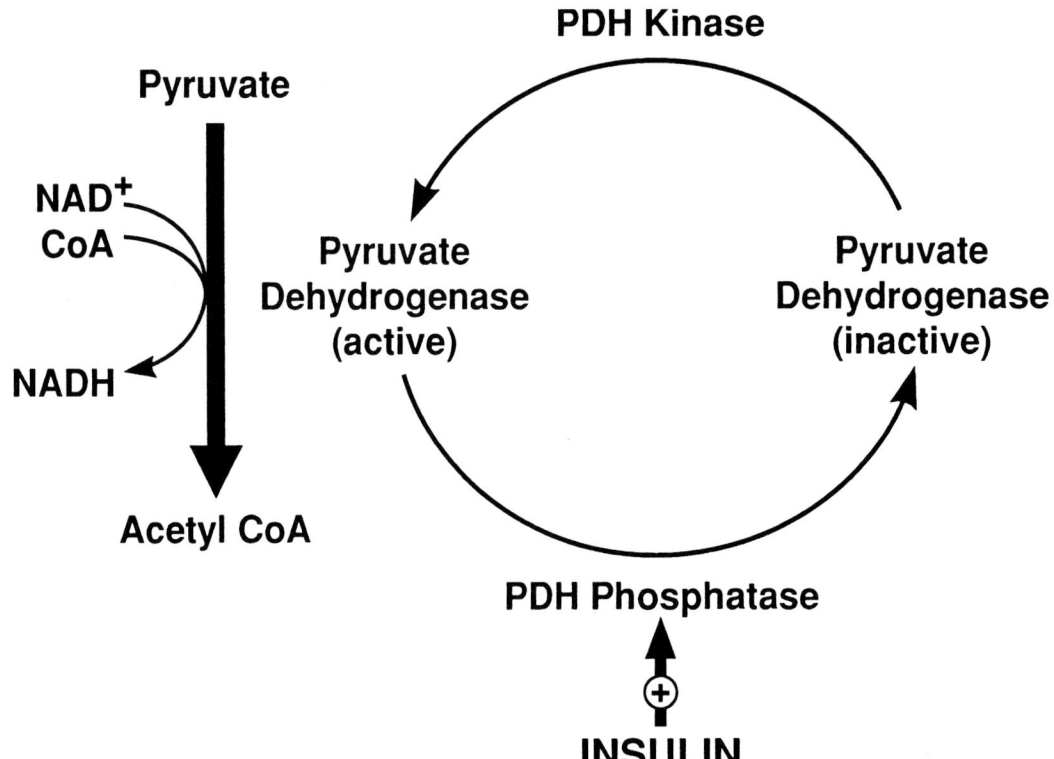

Figure 52-27 Schematic representation of the control of pyruvate dehydrogenase. Sites of insulin regulation are shown. See text for a detailed discussion. NAD+, oxidized nicotinamide adenine dinucleotide; NADH, reduced nicotinamide adenine dinucleotide; PDH, pyruvate dehydrogenase.

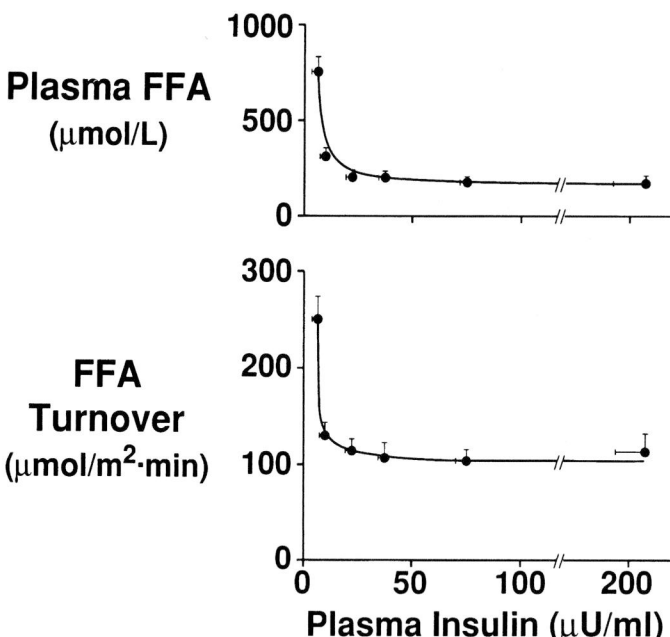

Figure 52-28   Dose-response relationship between the plasma insulin concentration and plasma free fatty acid (FFA) concentration **(top)** and rate of plasma FFA turnover **(bottom)** in healthy subjects during euglycemic insulin clamp studies. (Reproduced from Groop LC, Bonadonna RC, Del Prato S, et al: Glucose and free fatty acid metabolism in non-insulin dependent diabetes mellitus: Evidence for multiple sites of insulin resistance. J Clin Invest 84:205–213, 1989.)

generated during the stimulation of glycolysis supplies the substrate for augmented reesterification of tissue FFAs, while at the same time insulin stimulates α-glycerol phosphate acyltransferase, the rate-limiting enzyme for triglyceride synthesis.[30] These combined effects limit the release of FFA into the bloodstream. In addition, the glucose-induced increase in plasma insulin concentration quickly inhibits lipolysis by

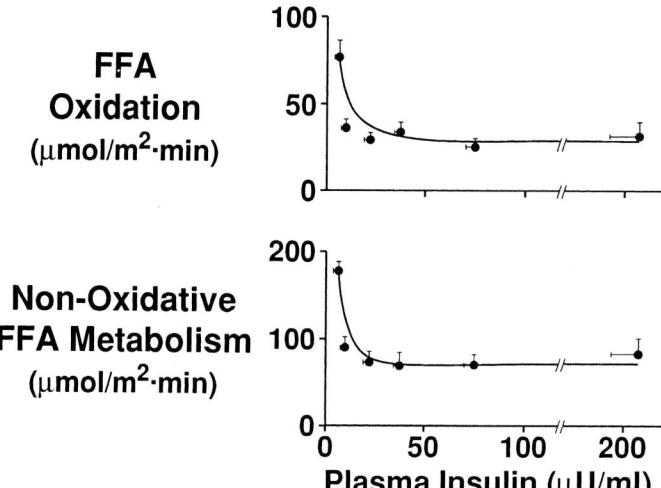

Figure 52-29   Dose-response relationship between the plasma insulin concentration versus the rate of whole-body free fatty acid (FFA) oxidation **(top)** and the rate of nonoxidative FFA disposal, that is, reesterification **(bottom)** in healthy subjects during euglycemic insulin clamp studies. (Reproduced from Groop LC, Bonadonna RC, Del Prato S, et al: Glucose and free fatty acid metabolism in non-insulin dependent diabetes mellitus: Evidence for multiple sites of insulin resistance. J Clin Invest 84:205–213, 1989.)

stimulating hormone-sensitive lipase in the adipocyte, and this further reduces the supply of lipid substrates to the oxidative machinery in muscle and liver. A decrease in FFA oxidation by these tissues causes a reciprocal stimulation of glucose oxidation and glycogen synthesis by reversal of the Randle cycle in muscle (see later) and inhibition of gluconeogenesis in the liver.

The glucose-mediated inhibition of FFA metabolism is counterbalanced by an FFA-mediated inhibition of glucose metabolism, creating an FFA–glucose substrate interaction known as the Randle cycle.[74] When the plasma FFA concentration is elevated, by mass action, FFAs are transported into muscle and liver cells by simple diffusion across the membrane. The intracellular-free FFA concentration is maintained low by a specific FFA-binding protein and this ensures a favorable transport gradient. Once inside the cell, FFAs are transported into the mitochondria where they undergo beta oxidation (Fig. 52-30). Before entering the mitochondria, the long-chain fatty acids (oleic, palmitic, stearic, linoleic, and palmitoleic) are first activated to their acyl-CoA derivative by the appropriate acyl-CoA synthetase. Because the inner mitochondrial membrane is not permeable to the fatty-acyl-CoA, a specific transport system is necessary to transport the fatty acyl derivative into the mitochondria (see Fig. 52-30).[75] The enzyme carnitine acyltransferase-I in the outer membrane transfers the activated fatty acyl-CoA in the cytosol to carnitine and the fatty acyl-carnitine derivative is transported through the mitochondrial membrane. At the inner mitochondrial membrane, carnitine acyltransferase II, the rate-limiting enzyme for beta oxidation, catalyzes the transfer of the fatty acyl unit from fatty acyl-carnitine back to CoA, and the fatty acyl-CoA then undergoes beta oxidation with the resultant generation of acetyl-CoA.

As beta oxidation proceeds, acetyl-CoA accumulates within the cell and becomes a powerful inhibitor of the PDH enzyme complex (Fig. 52-31).[74,75] In addition, the accelerated rate of FFA oxidation consumes nicotinic adenine dinucleoside (NAD) and generates NADH. This shift in redox potential further inhibits PDH and impairs the Krebs cycle. Fatty acyl-CoA derivatives also have been shown to inhibit glycogen synthase in muscle and liver[76,77] (see Fig. 52-31). In healthy humans, a physiologic elevation in the plasma FFA concentration (created by intralipid/heparin infusion) stimulates FFA oxidation and inhibits both glucose oxidation and glucose storage (glycogen synthesis),[78] thus providing experimental validation of the Randle cycle. In nondiabetic subjects, a physiologic increment in the plasma insulin level (+100 μU/mL) causes a 50% to 60% decline in plasma FFA concentration and a parallel decline in lipid oxidation (Fig. 52-32). Infusion of Intralipid during the insulin clamp, to maintain or increase the plasma FFA level (see Fig. 52-32), inhibits insulin-mediated stimulation of both glucose oxidation and glucose storage (glycogen synthesis) (Fig. 52-33). These data demonstrate that the Randle cycle operates in vivo in humans in response to physiologic changes in the plasma FFA concentration. The inhibitory effect of elevated plasma FFA levels is observed at all plasma insulin concentrations, spawning the physiologic and pharmacologic range.[78] The inhibitory effect of an acute increase in plasma FFA concentration on muscle glucose metabolism is time dependent. Thus, the earliest (within 2 hours) observed abnormality is a defect in glucose oxidation, as would be predicted by operation of the Randle cycle.[74] This is followed (between 2 and 3 hours) by defects in glucose transport and phosphorylation and eventually (after 3–4 hours) by impaired glycogen synthesis.[3,79]

According to FFA-glucose cycle originally proposed four decades ago by Randle and colleagues,[74] the increase in FFA oxidation restrains glucose oxidation in muscle by altering the redox potential of the cell and inhibiting key glycolytic enzymes. The excessive FFA oxidation, in addition to causing the intracellular accumulation of acetyl-CoA (a potent

Figure 52-30 Free fatty acid (FFA) and ketone body metabolism in the liver. After transport into the hepatocyte, FFAs are activated to their acyl-CoA derivative. Depending on the hormonal, metabolic, and energy status of the cell, the fatty acyl-CoA moiety is either transported into the mitochondrion and oxidized or synthesized into triglyceride. Malonyl-CoA, which is a potent inhibitor of carnitine palmitoyl transferase I, plays a pivotal role in the switch from FFA oxidation to lipid synthesis. Insulin enhances the formation of malonyl-CoA by stimulating acetyl-CoA-carboxylase. Insulin also favors triglyceride synthesis by inhibiting triacylglycerol lipase, the rate-limiting step for lipolysis. ATP, adenosine triphosphate; CAT, carnitine acyltransferase; TAG, triacylglycerol.

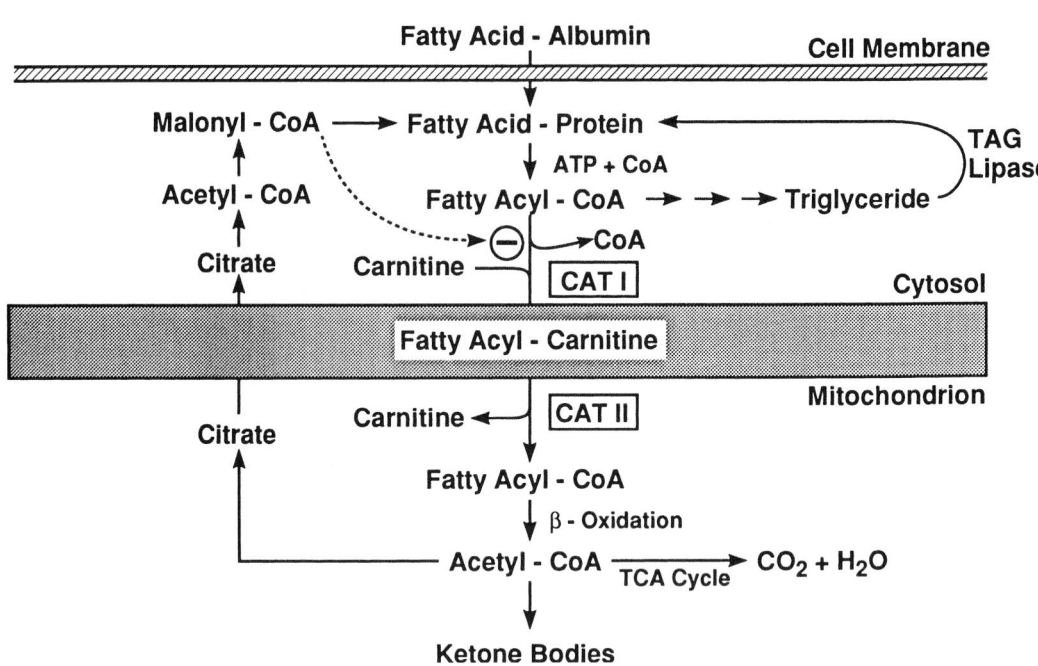

inhibitor of PDH) and increasing the NADH/NAD ratio (causing a slowing of the Krebs cycle), results in the accumulation of citrate, a powerful inhibitor of PFK. Randle and colleagues proposed that inhibition of PFK caused product inhibition of the early steps involved in glucose metabolism, leading to the accumulation of G-6-P, which in turn inhibited HK-II. The block in glucose phosphorylation caused a buildup of intracellular-free glucose, which restrained glucose transport into the cell via GLUT-4. The resultant decrease in glucose transport, in turn, resulted in impaired glycogen synthesis. This sequence of events by which accelerated plasma FFA oxidation inhibits muscle glucose transport, glucose oxidation, and glycogen synthesis is referred to as the Randle cycle.[74] It should be noted that the same scenario would ensue if the FFAs were derived from triglycerides stored in muscle[80] or from plasma.[78]

The original description of the Randle cycle was formulated based on experiments performed in rat diaphragm and heart muscle.[74] More recent studies performed in human skeletal muscle implicate mechanisms, in addition to those originally proposed by Randle and colleagues, in the FFA-induced insulin resistance. Thus, several groups[81] have failed to observe an increase in G-6-P or in muscle citrate levels or an inhibition of PFK, when insulin-stimulated glucose metabolism was inhibited by a lipid infusion to increase the plasma FFA concentration. Thus, although increased FFA/lipid and decreased glucose oxidation are closely coupled, as originally demonstrated by Randle and colleagues, mechanisms other than product (i.e., elevated intracellular G-6-P and free glucose concentrations) inhibition of the early steps of glucose metabolism must be invoked to explain the defects in glucose transport, glucose phosphorylation, and glycogen synthesis (see Fig. 52-31).

Figure 52-31 Schematic representation of the intracellular biochemical and molecular events that are inhibited by fatty acyl CoAs and their intracellular metabolites; see text for a more detailed discussion. AcCoA, acyl-CoA; F6P, fructose-6-phosphate; FA-CoA, fatty acyl-CoA; FFA, free fatty acid; G1P, glucose-1-phosphate; G6P, glucose-6-phosphate; GLUT, glucose transporter; HK, hexokinase; NAD, nicotinamide adenine dinucleotide; PDH, pyruvate dehydrogenase; PFK, phosphofructokinase; PI3K, phosphatidylinositol kinase; UDP, uridine diphosphate.

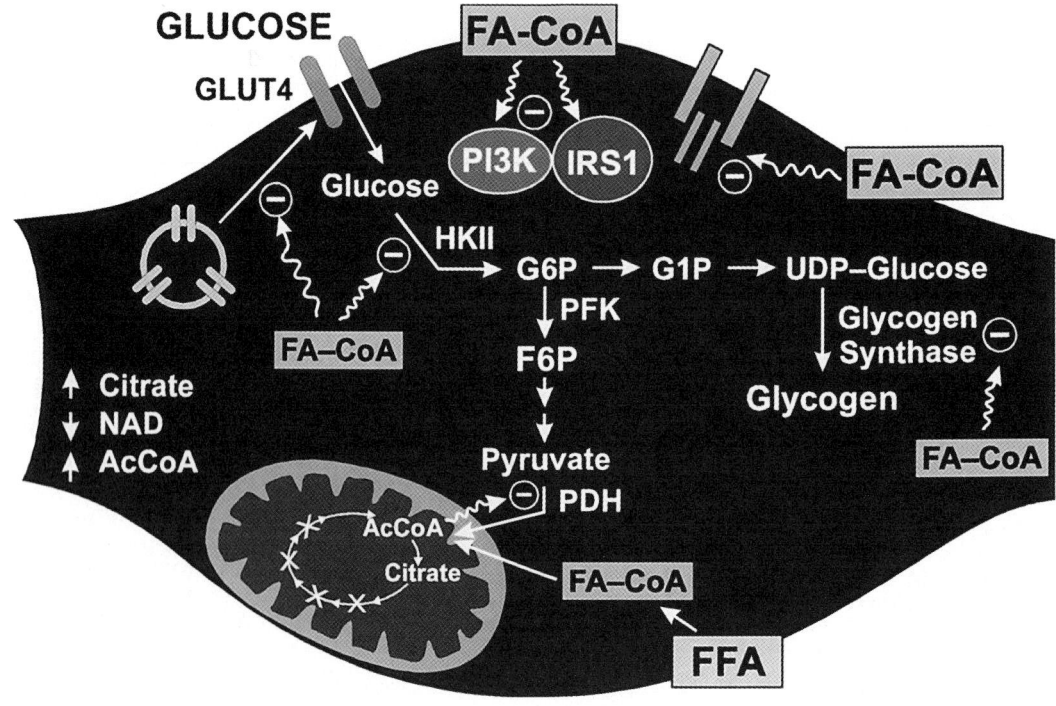

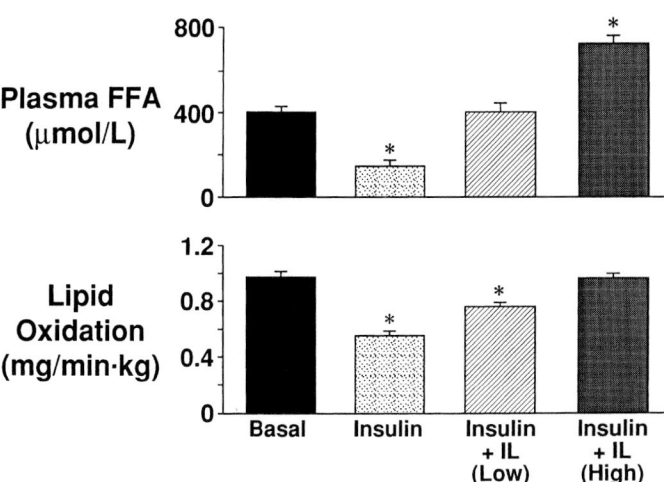

Figure 52-32 Plasma free fatty acid (FFA) concentration and total-body lipid oxidation (measured by indirect calorimetry) in the basal state and during a 100 μU/mL euglycemic insulin clamp performed with and without Intralipid (IL) infusion. Intralipid was infused at two rates to maintain (low IL infusion) or increase (high IL infusion) the basal plasma FFA concentration. The high-dose Intralipid infusion rate maintained the rate of total-body lipid oxidation constant at the basal value. (Reproduced from Thiebaud D, DeFronzo RA, Jacot E, et al: Effect of long chain triglyceride infusion on glucose metabolism in man. Metabolism 21:1128–1136, 1982.)

Studies in humans and animals have shown a strong negative correlation between insulin-stimulated glucose metabolism and increased intramuscular lipid pools, including triglyceride, diacylglycerol, ceramides, and long-chain fatty acyl-CoAs.[3,82–84] An acute increase in the plasma FFA concentration leads to an increase in muscle fatty acyl-CoA and diacylglycerol concentrations. Both long-chain fatty acyl-CoAs and diacylglycerol activate protein kinase C-θ, which increases serine phosphorylation with subsequent inhibition of IRS-1 tyrosine phosphorylation. In human muscle, elevated plasma FFA levels inhibit insulin-stimulated tyrosine phosphorylation of IRS-1, the association of the p85 subunit of PI 3-kinase with IRS-1, and activation of PI 3-kinase[81,85] (see Fig. 52-31). Direct effects of long-chain fatty acyl-CoAs to inhibit glucose transport, glucose phosphorylation, and glycogen synthase also have been demonstrated in muscle (see Fig. 52-31). Last, increased muscle ceramide levels (secondary to increased long-chain fatty acyl-CoAs) interfere with glucose transport and inhibit glycogen synthase in muscle via multiple mechanisms involving alterations in a variety of intracellular lipid-signaling molecules that exert their inhibitory effects on multiple steps (insulin signal transduction system, glucose transport, glucose phosphorylation, glycogen synthase, PDH, Krebs cycle) involved in glucose metabolism.

The extent to which insulin action in target tissues is direct rather than mediated by shifts in substrate supply can be appreciated by comparing systemic with local insulin administration. When infused intra-arterially into the human forearm, insulin does not alter the circulating substrate supply, in that neither FFA nor glucose concentrations change in the arterial blood, which recirculates to the forearm tissues. Under these conditions, insulin stimulates forearm glucose uptake and lactate release in a time-dependent manner (Fig. 52-34) but does not induce any detectable change in the local respiratory quotient (0.76) in the blood draining the forearm tissues.[86] This observation indicates that the forearm tissues, and the muscle in particular, continue to rely mostly on lipid oxidation for energy production, and that the vast majority of insulin-stimulated glucose uptake is channeled to glycogen. In contrast, when comparable hyperinsulinemia is created by systemic infusion of insulin, while maintaining euglycemia, the leg respiratory quotient increases from 0.74 to almost 1.00, that is, glucose oxidation increases whereas lipid oxidation is markedly reduced. In summary, the direct effects of insulin are to promote glucose transport and phosphorylation, glycolysis, and glycogen synthesis; the stimulatory effect of the hormone on glucose oxidation is both direct and indirect, the latter being mediated by a fall in lipid availability.

The liver plays a central role in the regulation of glucose metabolism.[1,2,9,10,87] After ingestion of a carbohydrate meal, it is essential that the liver suppress its basal rate of glucose production. In addition, the liver takes up approximately one third of the glucose in the ingested carbohydrate meal. Collectively, suppression of hepatic glucose production and

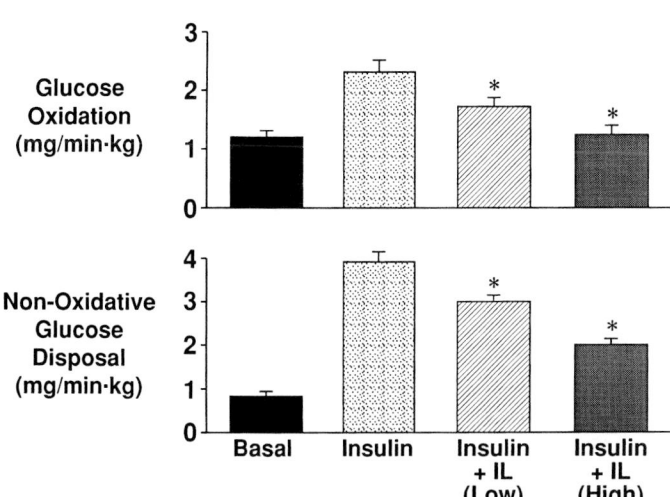

Figure 52-33 Inhibitory effect of Intralipid (IL) infusion and enhanced lipid oxidation on insulin-mediated rates of glucose oxidation and nonoxidative glucose disposal (see legend to Fig. 52-25 for description of the experimental protocol). (Reproduced from Thiebaud D, DeFronzo RA, Jacot E, et al: Effect of long chain triglyceride infusion on glucose metabolism in man. Metabolism 21:1128–1136, 1982.)

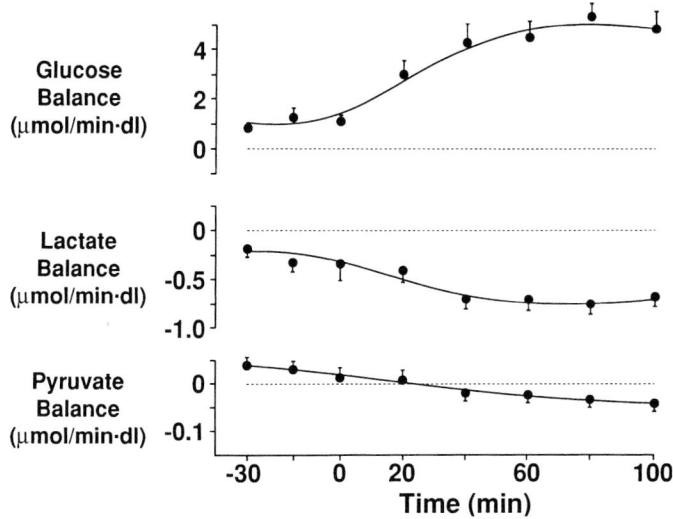

Figure 52-34 Net glucose, lactate, and pyruvate balances across the human forearm of healthy subjects in the fasting state (–30 to 0 minutes) and during a 100-minute intra-arterial insulin infusion calculated to increase the local insulin concentration by approximately 120 μU/mL. (Reproduced from Natali A, Buzzigoli G, Taddei S, et al: Effects of insulin on hemodynamics and metabolism in human forearm. Diabetes 39:490–500, 1990.)

augmentation of hepatic glucose uptake account for maintenance of approximately half of the maintenance of plasma glucose homeostasis after ingestion of a carbohydrate meal. The regulation of hepatic glucose production is controlled by a number of factors (see Fig. 52-3), of which insulin (inhibits hepatic glucose production) and glucagon and FFAs (stimulate hepatic glucose production) are the most important. In vitro studies have demonstrated that plasma FFA are potent stimulators of hepatic glucose production and do so by increasing the activity of pyruvate carboxylase and phospho-*enol*pyruvate carboxykinase, the rate-limiting enzymes for gluconeogenesis.[88] FFAs also enhance the activity of G-6-P, the enzyme that ultimately controls the release of glucose by the liver[89] (Fig. 52-35).

In normal subjects, an acute physiologic increase in plasma FFA concentration stimulates gluconeogenesis, whereas a decrease in plasma FFA concentration reduces gluconeogenesis.[90] A significant portion (as much as 25%) of the suppressive effect of insulin on hepatic glucose production is mediated via inhibition of lipolysis and a reduction in circulating plasma FFA concentration.[10,23] The relationship between increased plasma FFA concentration, FFA oxidation, and hepatic glucose production can be explained as follows: (1) Increased plasma FFA levels, by mass action, augment FFA uptake by hepatocytes, leading to accelerated lipid oxidation and accumulation of acetyl-CoA. The increased concentration of acetyl-CoA stimulates pyruvate carboxylase, the rate-limiting enzyme in gluconeogenesis, as well as glucose-6-phosphatase, the rate-controlling enzyme for glucose release from the hepatocyte (see Fig. 52-35). (2) The increased rate of FFA oxidation provides a continuing source of energy (in the form of ATP) and reduced nucleotides (NADH) to drive gluconeogenesis. The net result is an enhanced flux of three carbon precursors from pyruvate to oxaloacetate and thus into the gluconeogenic pathway. Finally, it should be noted that an increase in plasma FFA concentration need not be associated with an increase in hepatic glucose production, even though gluconeogenesis is enhanced. This is especially true in nondiabetic subjects in whom, except under very unique experimental conditions, elevation of the plasma FFA level rarely leads to an accelerated rate of hepatic glucose output because the stimulation of hepatic gluconeogenesis by FFAs is precisely offset by an inhibition of glycogenolysis, and this results in no net change in hepatic glucose production. This hepatic autoregulation in response to FFA infusion is similar to that observed during the infusion of gluconeogenic precursors.[91] Thus, in dogs and nondiabetic humans, intravenous administration of alanine, lactate, and glycerol augment gluconeogenesis but fail to increase total hepatic glucose production because of a reciprocal decline in glycogenolysis. The situation in insulin-resistant states, such as obesity and diabetes, appears to be different. Here, FFA infusion impairs the suppression of hepatic glucose production by insulin and in some instances may actually elevate the basal rate of hepatic glucose production.

Amino acids also can enter into a substrate competition cycle with glucose, although somewhat less effectively than FFAs.[92] Increased amino acid provision enhances glucose production under conditions of insulin deficiency or resistance and limits glucose utilization in the insulinized state. Furthermore, an increase in the plasma FFA concentration exerts a hypoaminoacidemic effect in humans.[93] In summary, each of the three major substrates (i.e., glucose, FFAs, amino acids), if present in excessive amounts (whether by endogenous production or exogenous administration), can lower the level of the other two by stimulating insulin release. In this situation, glucose metabolism obviously is favored because it is a much more potent insulin secretagogue than fat or amino acids. In addition, multiple substrate effects (not mediated by insulin) participate in the regulation of the substrates themselves: High FFA and amino acid concentrations increase glucose, whereas a high FFA concentration lowers the amino acid levels. The net result is the creation of a glucose-FFA–amino acid cycle in which each member of the triad influences its fellow members both directly and indirectly through the stimulation of insulin secretion (Fig. 52-36).

LIPID SYNTHESIS

In addition to its potent restraining effect on lipolysis and inhibition of FFA oxidation, the increase in plasma insulin

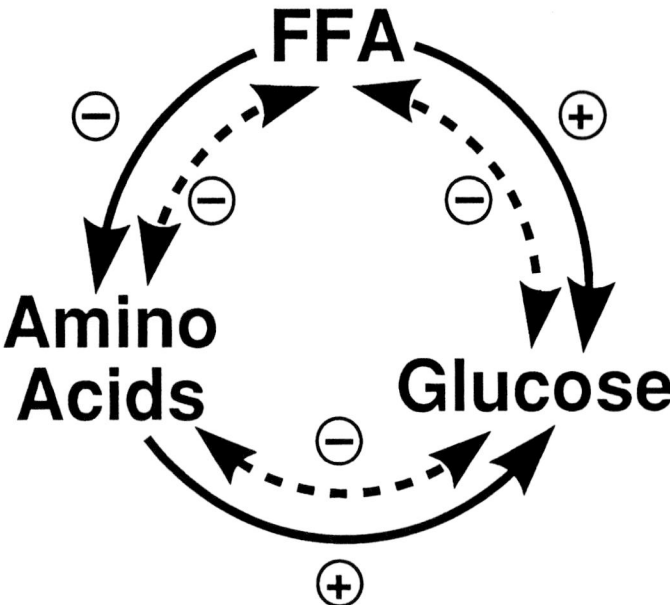

Figure 52-36 The glucose–free fatty acid–amino acid cycle. Because glucose, free fatty acid (FFA), and amino acids are all insulin secretogogues, isolated increases of each of them lower the circulating levels of the other two via hyperinsulinemia (*inner ring*). By substrate competition (*outer ring*), an increased supply of either FFAs or amino acids will spare glucose. In addition, FFAs have a hypoaminoacidemic effect of their own. See text for a detailed discussion. (Reproduced from Ferrannini E, DeFronzo RA: Insulin actions in vivo: Glucose metabolism. In DeFronzo RA, Ferrannini E, Keen H, Zimmet P [eds]: International Textbook of Diabetes Mellitus. Chichester, UK, John Wiley & Sons, 2004, pp 277–318.)

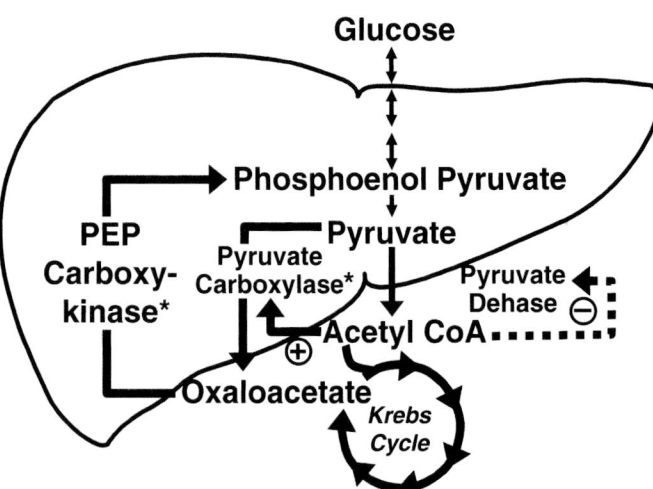

Figure 52-35 Schematic representation of the regulation of hepatic glucose production and hepatic gluconeogenesis. Sites of stimulation of free fatty acids are shown by the asterisk. See text for a more detailed discussion. PEP, phospho*enol*pyruvate.

concentration that occurs in the fed state stimulates fatty acid synthesis and storage as triacylglycerol in adipose depots throughout the body. As discussed previously, these fat stores are mobilized during conditions of fasting and serve as an important metabolic fuel for skeletal muscle, heart, kidney, liver, and other organs. In addition to its important role in lipid synthesis, insulin also enhances cholesterol formation and cholesterol ester storage and promotes phospholipid metabolism.

In humans, adipose tissue and the liver represent the primary sites of fatty acid synthesis. Insulin augments fatty acid synthesis in these tissues primarily by activating acetyl-CoA carboxylase.[30] This enzyme converts acetyl-CoA in the cytosol to malonyl-CoA (see Fig. 52-30). Insulin directly activates acetyl-CoA carboxylase by increasing its phosphorylation state and enhancing its synthesis. Insulin also indirectly activates the enzyme by increasing the supply of citrate, which activates acetyl-CoA carboxylase, and by stimulating the pentose phosphate cycle, thus providing the necessary reducing equivalents (NADH) for fat biosynthesis. Insulin also phosphorylates, thereby activating ATP-citrate lyase, the step immediately preceding that catalyzed by acetyl-CoA carboxylase (see Fig. 52-30).[30] The increase in cytosolic malonyl-CoA concentration simultaneously activates fatty acid synthase and binds to carnitine palmitoyl transferase-I, inactivating the enzyme and inhibiting fatty acid oxidation.[75] The net result is an enhanced availability of fatty acyl-CoA for triglyceride synthesis. Insulin appears to have little effect on any of the enzymes involved in triacylglycerol synthesis. This is in marked contrast to insulin's powerful inhibitory action on triacylglycerol lipase, the rate-limiting enzyme in the regulation of lipolysis.[75] In addition to the stimulatory effect of insulin on triglyceride synthesis, the hormone also appears to enhance cholesterol formation through an effect exerted on hydroxymethylglutaryl-CoA reductase.

KETONE METABOLISM

Ketones are formed in the liver from the oxidation of FFAs, and their synthesis is tightly regulated by the circulating levels of insulin and glucagon as well as malonyl-CoA. In the fed state, insulin levels rise, lipolysis is inhibited, and intracellular malonyl-CoA levels rise.[75] This latter key intermediate inhibits carnitine acyltransferase-I, thus favoring triglyceride synthesis and retarding fatty acid oxidation and ketone body formation (see Fig. 52-30). Conversely, in the starved or diabetic state, plasma insulin levels decline and glucagon increases. The increase in glucagon-to-insulin ratio is associated with a decrease in malonyl-CoA concentration, and fatty acid oxidation and ketogenesis are favored (see Fig. 52-30). With the exception of the liver, most tissues can oxidize ketone bodies. Their utilization by peripheral tissues, including muscle, is primarily regulated by their plasma concentration. Ketone bodies represent a major fuel for muscle during prolonged fasting, once their circulating blood levels increase to 1 to 3 mmol/L. Reversal of the elevated glucagon-to-insulin ratio after feeding rapidly inhibits ketogenesis, and the associated decline in plasma ketone levels abolishes ketone utilization by peripheral tissues.

ORAL GLUCOSE

At any given point in time, the glycemic response to an exogenous glucose load represents the balance between the rate of glucose appearance in the systemic circulation from all sources (i.e., ingested glucose entering via the gastrointestinal tract and endogenous glucose production) and the rate at which glucose is disposed of by all tissues in the body.[87,94] Oral glucose appearance in the systemic circulation depends on (1) the rate at which the gastric contents are passed on to the small intestine, (2) the rate of intestinal glucose absorption,

(3) the extent of gut glucose utilization, (4) the degree of hepatic glucose trapping, and (5) the dynamics of glucose transfer through the gut, liver, and posthepatic circulation to the right heart. The contribution of endogenous glucose production to the glycemic response to feeding depends on the extent and rate of change of hepatic glucose release. Initially, disposition of an ingested glucose load depends on changes in the pattern of hormonal stimuli and substrate availability. Because it represents a summation phenomenon, the response to oral glucose explores the whole of glucose tolerance, not the individual contribution of the various components. As discussed previously in this chapter, the rate-limiting step in the transfer of ingested glucose from the stomach to the liver is the rate of gastric emptying. This depends on the volume, temperature, osmolarity, and sodium content of the glucose solution when glucose alone is ingested. Glucose absorption through the intestinal epithelial cells is rapid, efficient, and well in excess of ordinary needs. Glucose utilization by intestinal tissues is small when glucose is presented from the vascular side, that is, when there is no oral glucose (see Table 52-2). The major fuels used by the gastrointestinal tissues in the postabsorptive state are FFAs and glutamine. In the presence of glucose at high concentrations on the luminal side, it appears that gut glucose metabolism increases in response to the increased energy needs for absorption; the quantitative aspects of this stimulation of gut glucose utilization remain undetermined in the human. The possibility also exists that systemic hyperglycemia and/or hyperinsulinemia may impede intestinal glucose absorption.

Glucose uptake by the liver is stimulated by portal hyperglycemia (see below),[9,10,95] and this has a major impact on hepatic glucose release. The traversal of glucose through the hepatic space is relatively quick, and this is unlikely to introduce a significant delay in the systemic appearance of oral glucose. In summary, the dynamics of oral glucose appearance are essentially determined by gastric emptying, whereas intestinal transport, transit across the gastrointestinal mucosa into the portal blood, and transhepatic passage together introduce only a small time delay. Stated otherwise, if neither gastrointestinal nor liver tissues used glucose, the time course of oral glucose appearance in the systemic circulation would follow that of gastric emptying, with a time shift of a few minutes. For this reason, the glucose absorption step represents a major component of the shape of the glycemic response to glucose. Figure 52-37 shows the pattern of appearance of ingested glucose in healthy individuals, as reconstructed by a double tracer technique.[87] Glucose appearance in the systemic circulation peaks within 30 to 45 minutes, declines slowly thereafter, but remains significantly above zero at 210 minutes after glucose ingestion. At least 4 to 5 hours are necessary for the complete absorption of an oral glucose load, and this is further prolonged by the presence of fat and protein in the meal. Figure 52-37 also shows the time course of suppression of endogenous glucose release by oral glucose.[87,95] A sustained nadir is reached between 60 and 120 minutes, and this is followed by a slow return to the fasting rate; however, hepatic glucose production is still significantly inhibited 210 minutes after the glucose challenge. Overall suppression of hepatic glucose production during the 3- to 4-hour period after glucose ingestion averages 50%. This is surprisingly less than what would be expected based on the combined portal hyperglycemia and hyperinsulinemia (see Fig. 52-5). Because circulating levels of insulin antagonistic hormones (except norepinephrine) do not change after oral glucose, it is likely that activation of the sympathetic nervous system, and specifically those nerves innervating the liver, keeps liver glucose outflow open.[18] In Figure 52-38, the observed arterial plasma glucose concentration is broken down into the component contributed by the appearance of oral glucose and that derived from hepatic glucose production.[87,95] The resemblance of oral glucose appearance rate to

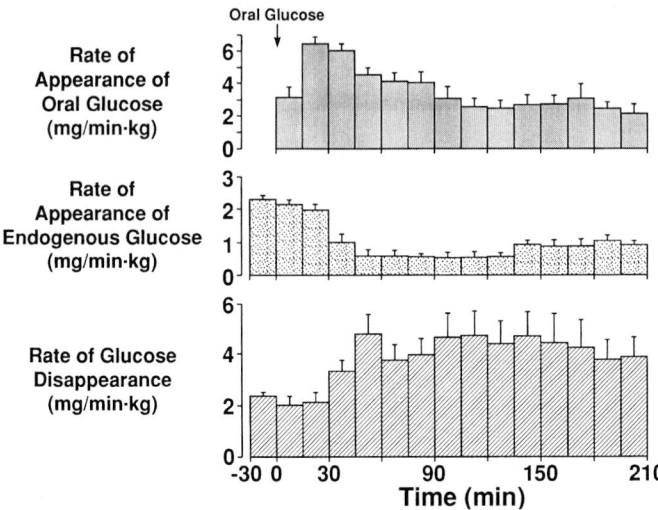

Figure 52-37 Glucose turnover after glucose ingestion. The rate of appearance of the oral glucose load **(top)**, the rate of whole-body glucose disappearance **(bottom)**, and the rate of endogenous (hepatic) glucose production **(middle)** are shown after the ingestion of 1 g/kg glucose in healthy adults. (Reproduced from Ferrannini E, Bjorkman O, Reichard GA, et al: The disposal of an oral glucose load in healthy subjects: A quantitative study. Diabetes 34:580–588, 1985.)

the plasma glucose curve is readily evident, especially during the first 60 to 90 minutes. Less appreciated is the fact that absorption is still incomplete 3 to 4 hours after ingestion. Figure 52-37 depicts the time course of total-body glucose disposal after oral glucose.[87,95] After a lag of approximately 30 minutes, tissue glucose uptake is stimulated by 50% to 100% throughout the period of observation. Hyperglycemia (mass action effect of glucose to promote its own uptake) contributes more to whole-body glucose disposal during the first half hour; thereafter, hyperinsulinemia provides the predominant stimulus. Oral glucose also elicits a marked vasodilation of the splanchnic vascular bed, and this regional increase in splanchnic blood flow persists for at least 4 hours. Thus, both the metabolic and the hemodynamic perturbations induced by oral glucose extend beyond the time that it takes for the plasma glucose concentration to return to its preingestion level.

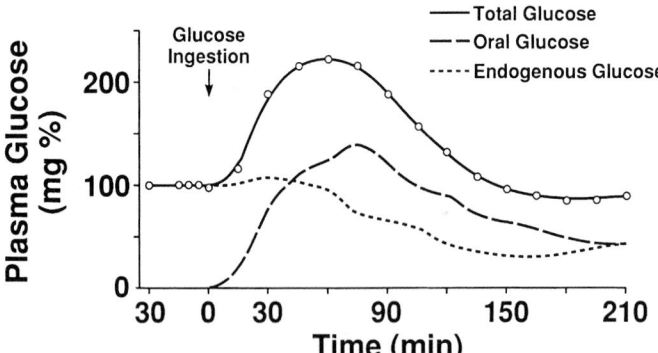

Figure 52-38 Separation of the actual arterial plasma glucose concentration *(solid line)* into its components based on the amount of glucose that is contributed by endogenous (hepatic) glucose production *(dotted line)* and oral glucose ingestion *(dashed line)*. (Reproduced from Ferrannini E, Bjorkman O, Reichard GA, et al: The disposal of an oral glucose load in healthy subjects: A quantitative study. Diabetes 34:580–588, 1985.)

The tissue destination of absorbed glucose has been the subject of intense investigation. Although the liver was classically reputed to be responsible for the eventual disposal of the majority of an oral glucose load, more recent studies that have employed the hepatic vein catheter technique in combination with radioisotope methodology have demonstrated that peripheral tissues dispose of approximately two thirds of the ingested glucose, whereas the splanchnic tissues account for the remaining one third.[96,97] However, it must be remembered that the splanchnic tissues (i.e., liver), also contribute to glucose conservation by reducing their output of glucose. When this amount of glucose is added to that which is taken up by the liver, it can be seen that splanchnic (hepatic) and peripheral tissues contribute approximately equally to the maintenance of normal glucose homeostasis. Obviously, these approximate proportions vary according to the period during which the study is conducted as well as with the nature of individual responses to glucose ingestion. A robust insulin secretory response directs more posthepatic glucose to the peripheral tissues, whereas a large increase in splanchnic blood flow channels the delivery of incoming sugar to the liver. In humans, for example, a glucose drink sipped slowly over 3.5 hours rather than swallowed in one bolus generates the same overall glucose curve but a 50% smaller endogenous insulin response. Last, the route of glucose administration exerts an important influence on the metabolic fate of glucose in that the portosystemic glucose concentration gradient per se enhances hepatic glucose uptake independently of portal glycemia and total glucose delivery to the liver.[10] In humans, the oral route of glucose administration also has been shown to enhance splanchnic (hepatic) glucose uptake.[95] Recent studies also have shown that the liver takes up glucose in proportion to delivery.[98]

After glucose ingestion, glucose oxidation in the brain continues unabated during the absorptive period. Approximately 50% of the glucose that is taken up by peripheral tissues (muscle) is oxidized, and the remainder is stored as muscle glycogen or as lactate in the lactate pool. During absorption from the gastrointestinal tract, lactate release by the intestinal tissues into the portal vein is markedly increased. It has been estimated that approximately 5% of the ingested glucose load is converted into three carbon precursors (lactate, pyruvate, and alanine) that are passed on to the liver and synthesized into glycogen via the indirect pathway of gluconeogenesis. Because the lactate concentration in the hepatic vein also increases after glucose ingestion, it follows that the sum of hepatic lactate production and gut lactate formation must exceed hepatic lactate extraction. Liver glycogen formation during absorption of oral glucose occurs both directly from glucose and indirectly via gluconeogenesis.[99] The relative contributions of the direct (from glucose) versus indirect (from gluconeogenic precursors) pathway to hepatic glycogen synthesis in humans remains uncertain owing to methodologic difficulties. However, current data suggest that gluconeogenesis participates in liver glycogen repletion to a much lesser extent in humans than in rats.

COUNTERREGULATORY HORMONES

A review of the role of the insulin counterregulatory hormones (glucagon, epinephrine, cortisol, growth hormone, and thyroid hormones) and their roles in intermediary metabolism is beyond the scope of this chapter, and the reader is referred to Chapter 62 and Ref. 16. The most important role of the counterregulatory hormones is in the defense of hypoglycemia. Glucagon and epinephrine play an important role in the acute recovery from hypoglycemia by stimulating both glycogenolysis and gluconeogenesis. When hypoglycemia is prolonged, cortisol and growth hormone contribute to the restoration of normoglycemia by impairing the tissue's ability to respond to insulin. Epinephrine also is a potent peripheral insulin antagonist. Except for glucagon (whose concentration increases during fasting, leading to a stimulation of hepatic glucose production primarily by augmenting gluconeogenesis), it is unclear what role, if any, these insulin antagonistic hormones play in glucoregulation during the transition from the fed to the fasted state. More likely, these counterregulatory hormones contribute to the mobilization of competitive substrates, especially FFAs, from adipose depots to the liver and muscle where they serve as an important energy source. Circulating levels of these counterregulatory hormones (except glucagon) do not increase during fasting. Rather, the plasma insulin concentration declines in response to the decrease in blood glucose, and the resultant hypoinsulinemia leaves the lipolytic and ketogenic activities of the counterregulatory hormones unopposed, thus facilitating the shift from glucose to FFA metabolism.

REFERENCES

1. DeFronzo RA: Lilly lecture: The triumvirate: β-cell, muscle, liver: A collusion responsible for NIDDM. Diabetes 37:667–687, 1988.
2. DeFronzo RA: Pathogenesis of type 2 diabetes: Metabolic and molecular implications for identifying diabetes genes. Diabetes Rev 5:177–269, 1997.
3. Bays H, Mandarino L, DeFronzo RA: Role of the adipocytes, FFA, and ectopic fat in the pathogenesis of type 2 diabetes mellitus: PPAR agonists provide a rational therapeutic approach. J Clin Endocrinol Metab 89:463–478, 2004.
4. Ruderman NB, Tornheim K, Goodman MN: Fuel homeostasis and intermediary metabolism of carbohydrate, fat, and protein. In Becker KL (ed): Principles and Practice of Endocrinology and Metabolism. Philadelphia, JB Lippincott, 1992, pp 1054–1064.
5. Ferrannini E, DeFronzo RA: Insulin actions in vivo: Glucose metabolism. In DeFronzo RA, Ferrannini E, Keen H, Zimm P (eds): International Textbook of Diabetes Mellitus. Chichester, UK, John Wiley & Sons, 2004, pp 277–318.
6. Bell GI: Lilly Lecture. Molecular defects in diabetes mellitus. Diabetes 40:413–422, 1990.
7. Del Prato S, Ferrannini E, DeFronzo RA: Evaluation of insulin sensitivity in man. In Clarke WL, Larner J, Pohl SL (eds): Methods in Diabetes Research. Vol II. Clinical Methods. New York, John Wiley & Sons, 1986, pp 19–43.8.
8. Ferrannini E, Del Prato S, DeFronzo RA: Glucose kinetics: Tracer methods. In Clarke WL, Larner J, Pohl SL (eds): Methods in Diabetes Research, Vol. II: Clinical Methods. New York, John Wiley & Sons, 1986, pp 107–142.
9. DeFronzo RA, Ferrannini E: Regulation of hepatic glucose metabolism in humans. Diabetes Metab Rev 3:415–459, 1987.
10. Cherrington AD: Control of glucose uptake and release by the liver. Diabetes 48:1198–1124, 1999.
11. Gerich JE, Meyer C, Woesle HJ, Stumvol M: Renal gluconeogenesis. Its importance in human glucose homeostasis. Diabetes Care 24:382–391, 2001.
12. Landau BR, Wahren J, Chandramouli V, et al: Contributions of gluconeogenesis to glucose production in the fasted state. J Clin Invest 98:378–385, 1996.
13. Felig P, Sherwin RS: Carbohydrate homeostasis, liver and diabetes. Prog Liver Dis 5:149–171, 1976.
14. Drucker DJ: Minireview: The glucagon-like peptides. Endocrinology 142:521–527, 2001.
15. Cahill GF Jr: Starvation in man. N Engl J Med 282:668–675, 1970.
16. Gerich JE, Campbell PJ: Overview of counterregulation and its abnormalities in diabetes mellitus and other conditions. Diabetes Metab Rev 4:93–112, 1988.
17. Baron AD, Schaeffer L, Shragg P, Kolterman OG: Role of hyperglucagonemia in maintenance of increased rates of hepatic glucose output in type 2 diabetes. Diabetes 36:274–283, 1987.
18. Shimazu T: Neuronal regulation of hepatic glucose metabolism in mammals. Diabetes Metab Rev 3:185–206, 1987.
19. DeFronzo RA, Ferrannini E, Hendler R, et al: Regulation of splanchnic and peripheral glucose uptake by insulin and hyperglycemia in man. Diabetes 32:35–45, 1983.
20. Borg MA, Borg WP, Tamborlane WV, et al: Chronic hyperglycemia and diabetes impair counterregulation induced by localized 2-deoxy-glucose perfusion of the ventromedial hypothalamus in rats. Diabetes 48:584–587, 1999.
21. Friedman B, Goodman EH Jr, Weinhouse S: Effects of insulin and fatty acids on gluconeogenesis in the rat. J Biol Chem 242:3620–3627, 1967.
22. Ferrannini E, Barrett EJ, Bevilacqua S, DeFronzo RA: Effect of fatty acids on glucose production and utilization in man. J Clin Invest 72:1737–1747, 1983.
23. Rebrin K, Steil GM, Getty L, Bergman RN: Free fatty acid as a link in the regulation of hepatic glucose output by peripheral insulin. Diabetes 44:1038–1045, 1995.
24. DeFronzo RA, Jacot E, Jequier E, et al: The effect of insulin on the disposal of intravenous glucose: Results from indirect calorimetry and hepatic and femoral venous catheterization. Diabetes 30:1000–1007, 1981.
25. Nishi S, Susumu S, Bell GI: Human hexokinase: Sequences of amino- and carboxyl-terminal halves are homologous. Biochem Biophys Res Commun 157:937–943, 1988.
26. Garvey WT: Insulin action and insulin resistance: Diseases involving defects in insulin receptors, signal transduction, and the glucose transport effector system. Am J Med 105:331–345, 1998.
27. DeFronzo RA, Gunnarsson R, Bjorkman O, et al: Effects of insulin on peripheral and splanchnic glucose metabolism in non-insulin dependent diabetes mellitus. J Clin Invest 76:149–155, 1985.
28. Simonson DC, DeFronzo RA: Indirect calorimetry: Methodologic and interpretative problems. Am J Physiol 258:E399–E412, 1990.
29. Newsholme EA, Leech AR: Biochemistry for the Medical Sciences. Chichester, UK, John Wiley & Sons, 1983, pp 308–310.
30. Denton RM, Tavare JM: Actions of insulin on intracellular processes. In Alberti KGMM, DeFronzo RA, Keen H, Zimmet P (eds): International Textbook of Diabetes Mellitus. Chichester, UK, John Wiley & Sons, 1992, pp 385–408.
31. Pilkis SJ, El-Maghrabi MR, Claus TH: Fructose-2,6-biphosphate in control of hepatic gluconeogenesis. Diabetes Care 13:582–599, 1990.
32. Ferrannini E, Barrett E, Bevilacqua S, et al: Sodium elevates the plasma glucose response to glucose ingestion in man. J Clin Endocrinol Metab 54:455–458, 1982.
33. DeFronzo RA, Tobin J, Andres R: Glucose clamp technique: A method for quantifying insulin secretion and insulin resistance. Am J Physiol 237:E214–E223, 1979.
34. DeFronzo RA: Glucose intolerance and aging. Diabetes Care 4:493–501, 1993.
35. Diamond MP, Thornston K, Connolly-Diamond M, et al: Reciprocal variations in insulin-stimulated glucose uptake and pancreatic insulin secretion in women with normal glucose tolerance. J Soc Gynecol Invest 2:708–715, 1995.
36. Schneider SH, Morgado A: Effects of fitness and physical training on carbohydrate metabolism and associated cardiovascular risk factors in patients with diabetes. Diabetes Rev 3:378–407, 1995.
37. Lillioja S, Mott DM, Zawadzki JK, et al: In vivo insulin action is familial characteristic in nondiabetic Pima Indians. Diabetes 36:1329–1335, 1987.
38. Gastaldelli A, Ferrannini E, Miyazaki Y, et al: β-cell dysfunction and glucose intolerance: Results from the San Antonio Metabolism (SAM) study. Diabetologia 47:31–39, 2004.
39. Groop LC, Bonadonna RC, Del Prato S, et al: Glucose and free fatty acid metabolism in non-insulin dependent diabetes mellitus: Evidence for multiple sites of insulin resistance. J Clin Invest 84:205–213, 1989.

40. Cobelli C, Mari A, Ferrannini E: The non-steady state problem: Error analysis of Steele's model and developments for glucose kinetics. Am J Physiol 252:E679–E687, 1987.

41. Iozzo P, Geisler F, Oikonen V, et al: Insulin stimulates liver glucose uptake in humans: An [18]-FDG PET study. J Nuclear Med 44:682–689, 2003.

42. Basu R, Basu A, Johnson CM, et al: Insulin dose-response curves for stimulation of splanchnic glucose uptake and suppression of endogenous glucose production differ in nondiabetic humans and are abnormal in people with type 2 diabetes. Diabetes 53:2042–2050, 2004.

43. Prager R, Wallace P, Olefsky JM: In vivo kinetics of insulin action on peripheral glucose disposal and hepatic output in normal and obese subjects. J Clin Invest 78:472–481, 1986.

44. Thiebaud D, Jacot E, DeFronzo RA, et al: The effect of graded doses of insulin on total glucose uptake, glucose oxidation, and glucose storage in man. Diabetes 31:957–963, 1982.

45. Shulman GI, Rothman DL, Jue T, et al: Quantitation of muscle glycogen synthesis in normal subjects and subjects with non-insulin-dependent diabetes by ^{13}C nuclear magnetic resonance spectroscopy. N Engl J Med 322:223–228, 1990.

46. Del Prato S, Bonadonna R, Bonora E, et al: Characterization of cellular defects in insulin action in type 2 (non-insulin dependent) diabetes mellitus. J Clin Invest 94:484–494, 1993.

47. Saltiel AR, Kahn CR: Insulin signaling and the regulation of glucose and lipid metabolism. Nature 414:799–806, 2001.

48. Pessin JE, Saltiel AR: Signaling pathways in insulin action: Molecular targets of insulin resistance. J Clin Invest 106:165–169, 2000.

49. Whitehead JP, Clark SF, Urso B, James DE: Signaling through the insulin receptor. Curr Opin Cell Biol 12:222–228, 2000.

50. Shepherd PR, Kahn BB: Glucose transporters and insulin action. Implications for insulin resistance and diabetes mellitus. N Engl J Med 341:248–257, 1999.

51. Virkamaki A, Ueki K, Kahn CR: Protein-protein interaction in insulin signaling and the molecular mechanisms of insulin resistance. J Clin Invest 103:931–943, 1999.

52. Bauman CA, Ribon V, Kanzaki M, et al: CAP defines a second signaling pathway required for insulin-stimulated glucose transport. Nature 407:202–207, 2000.

53. Thomas G, Hall MN: TOR signaling and control of cell growth. Curr Opin Cell Biol 9:782–787, 1997.

54. Cusi K, Maezono K, Osman A, et al: Insulin resistance differentially affects the PI 3-kinase and MAP kinase-mediated signaling in human muscle. J Clin Invest 105:311–320, 2000.

55. Hsueh WA, Law RE: Insulin signaling in the arterial wall. Am J Cardiol 84:21J–24J, 1999.

56. Dent P, Lavoinne A, Nakielny S, et al: The molecular mechanisms by which insulin stimulates glycogen synthesis in mammalian skeletal muscle. Nature 348:302–307, 1990.

57. Cohen P: The structure and regulation of protein phosphatases. Annu Rev Biochem 58:453–508, 1989.

58. Newgard CB, Brady MJ, O'Doherty RB, Saltiel AR: Organizing glucose disposal. Emerging roles of the glycogen targeting subunits of protein phosphatase-1. Diabetes 49:1967–1977, 2000.

59. Bell GI, Kayano T, Buse JB, et al: Molecular biology of mammalian glucose transporters. Diabetes Care 13:198–200, 1990.

60. Joost H-G, Bell GI, Best JD, et al: Nomenclature of the GLUT/SLG2A family of sugar/polyol transport facilitators. Am J Physiol 282:E974–E976, 2002.

61. Colowick SP. The hexokinases. In Boyer PD (ed). The Enzymes, vol. 9. New York, Academic Press, 1973, pp 1–48.

62. Printz RL, Koch S, Potter LR, et al: Hexokinase II mRNA and gene structure, regulation by insulin, and evolution. J Biol Chem 268:5209–5219, 1993.

63. Rogers PA, Fisher RA, Harris H: An electrophoretic study of the distribution and properties of human hexokinases. Biochem Genet 13:857–866, 1975.

64. Magnuson MA, Andreone IL, Printz RL, et al: The glucokinase gene: Structure and regulation by insulin. Proc Natl Acad Sci U S A 86:4838–4842, 1989.

65. Mandarino LJ, Printz RL, Cusi KA, et al: Regulation of hexokinase II and glycogen synthase mRNA, protein, and activity in human muscle. Am J Physiol 269:E701–E708, 1995.

66. Vogt C, Yki-Jarvinen H, Iozzo P, et al: Effects of insulin on subcellular localization of hexokinase II in human skeletal muscle in vivo. J Clin Endocrinol Metab 83:230–234, 1998.

67. Virtanen KA, Peltoniemi P, Marjamaki P, et al: Human adipose tissue glucose uptake determined using [18]-fluoro-deoxy-glucose (([(18)F]FDG) and PET in combination with microdialysis. Diabetologia 44:2171–2179, 2001.

68. van der Werve G, Jeanrenaud B: Liver glycogen metabolism: An overview. Diabetes Metab Rev 3:47–78, 1987.

69. Frame S, Cohen P: GSK3 takes centre stage more than 20 years after its discovery. Biochem J 359:1–16, 2001.

70. Cohen P: The Croonian Lecture 1999. Identification of a protein kinase cascade of major importance in insulin signal transduction. Philos Trans R Soc Lond B Biol Sci 354:485–495, 1999.

71. Stralfors P, Hiraga A, Cohen P: The protein phosphatases involved in cellular regulation: Purification and characterization of the glycogen-bound form of protein phosphatase-1 from

rabbit skeletal muscle. Eur J Biochem 149:295–303, 1985.

72. Mandarino LJ, Wright KS, Verity LS, et al: Effects of insulin infusion on human skeletal muscle pyruvate dehydrogenase, phosphofructokinase, and glycogen synthase: Evidence for their role in oxidative glucose metabolism. J Clin Invest 80:655–663, 1987.

73. Vestergaard H, Lund S, Larsen FS, et al: Glycogen synthase and phosphofructokinase protein and mRNA levels in skeletal muscle from insulin-resistant patients with non-insulin-dependent diabetes mellitus. J Clin Invest 91:2342–2350, 1993.

74. Randle PJ, Garland PB, Hales CN, Newsholme EA: The glucose-fatty acid cycle: Its role in insulin sensitivity and metabolic disturbances of diabetes mellitus. Lancet 1:785–789, 1961.

75. Prentki M, Corkey BE: Are the B-cell signaling molecules malonyl-CoA and cystolic long-chain acyl-CoA implicated in multiple tissue defects of obesity and NIDDM? Diabetes 45:273–283, 1996.

76. Wititsuwannakul D, Kim K: Mechanism of palmityl coenzyme A inhibition or liver glycogen synthase. J Biol Chem 252:7812–7817, 1977.

77. Chalkley SM, Hettiarachchi M, Chisholm DJ, Kraegen EW: Five-hour fatty acid elevation increases muscle lipids and impairs glycogen synthesis in the rat. Metabolism 47:1121–1126, 1998.

78. Thiebaud D, DeFronzo RA, Jacot E, et al: Effect of long chain triglyceride infusion on glucose metabolism in man. Metabolism 21:1128–1136, 1982.

79. Boden G: Free fatty acids, insulin resistance, and type 2 diabetes mellitus. Proc Assoc Am Phys 111:241–248, 1999.

80. Greco AV, Mingrone G, Giancaterini A, et al: Insulin resistance in morbid obesity. Reversal with intramyocellular fat depletion. Diabetes 51:144–151, 2002.

81. Dresner A, Laurent D, Marcucci M, et al: Effects of free fatty acids on glucose transport and IRS-1 associated phosphatidylinositol-3-kinase activity. J Clin Invest 103:253–259, 1999.

82. Itani SI, Ruderman NB, Schnieder F, Boden G: Lipid-induced insulin resistance in human muscle is associated with changes in diacylglycerol, protein kinase C, and IkB-α. Diabetes 51:2005–2011, 2002.

83. Ellis BA, Pognten A, Lowry AJ, et al: Long-chain acyl-CoA esters as indicators of lipid metabolism and insulin sensitivity in rat and human muscle. Am J Physiol 279:E554–E560, 2000.

84. Kelley DE, Mandarino LJ: Fuel selection in human skeletal muscle in insulin resistance. Diabetes 49:677–683, 2000.

85. Belfort R, Mandarino L, Kashyap S, et al: Dose response effect of elevated plasma FFA on insulin signaling. Diabetes (submitted).

86. Natali A, Buzzigoli G, Taddei S, et al: Effects of insulin on hemodynamics and

metabolism in human forearm. Diabetes 39:490–500, 1990.

87. Ferrannini E, Bjorkman O, Reichard GA, et al: The disposal of an oral glucose load in healthy subjects: A quantitative study. Diabetes 34:580–588, 1985.

88. Exton JH, Corbin JG, Park CR: Control of gluconeogenesis in liver. IV. Differential effects of fatty acids and glucagon on ketogenesis and gluconeogenesis in the perfused rat liver. J Biol Chem 244:4095–4102, 1969.

89. Massillon D, Barzailai N, Hawkins M, et al: Induction of hepatic glucose-6-phosphatase gene expression by lipid infusion. Diabetes 46:153–157, 1997.

90. Chen X, Iqbal N, Boden G: The effect of free fatty acids on gluconeogenesis and glycogenolysis in normal subjects. J Clin Invest 103:365–372, 1999.

91. Jenssen T, Nurjhan N, Consoli A, Gerich J: Failure of substrate-induced gluconeogenesis to increase overall glucose appearance in normal humans: Demonstration of hepatic autoregulation without a change in plasma glucose concentrations. J Clin Invest 86:489–497, 1990.

92. Ferrannini E, Bevilacqua S, Lanzone L, et al: Metabolic interactions of amino acids and glucose in healthy humans. Diabetes Nutr Metab 3:176–186, 1988.

93. Ferrannini E, Barrett EJ, Bevilacqua S, et al: Effect of free fatty acids on blood amino acid levels in humans. Am J Physiol 250:E686–E694, 1986.

94. Katz L, Glickman MG, Rappaport S, et al: Splanchnic and peripheral disposal of oral glucose in man. Diabetes 32:675–679, 1983.

95. Ferrannini E, Wahren J, Felig P, DeFronzo RA: Role of fractional glucose extraction in the regulation of splanchnic glucose metabolism in normal and diabetic man. Metabolism 29:28–35, 1980.

96. DeFronzo RA: Pathogenesis of type 2 (non-insulin dependent) diabetes mellitus. Diabetologia 35:389–397, 1992.

97. Kelley D, Mitrakou A, Marsh H, et al: Skeletal muscle glycolysis, oxidation, and storage of an oral glucose load. J Clin Invest 81:1563–1571, 1988.

98. Ferrannini E, Katz LD, Glickman MG, DeFronzo RA: Influence of combined intravenous and oral glucose administration on splanchnic glucose uptake in man. Clin Physiol 10:527–538, 1990.

99. Shulman GI, DeFronzo RA, Rossetti HL: Differential effect of hyperglycemia and hyperinsulinemia on the pathway of hepatic glycogen repletion as assessed by ^{13}C-NMR. Am J Physiol 260:E731–E735, 1991.

Role of the Adipocyte in Metabolism and Endocrine Function

Steven R. Smith and Eric Ravussin

In an evolutionary sense, the adipose tissue represents the most efficient way to store energy in periods of feast to allow survival during periods of famine. There are two main reasons for this efficiency. First, on a weight basis, triacylglycerol, commonly called triglycerides, yields more than twice the amount of energy that is provided by glycogen or proteins. Second, triglycerides are stored without associated water, whereas glycogen, which is hydrophilic, binds as much as twice its weight to water. Similarly, proteins, the building blocks of cells, are associated with large amounts of water. As a result, the energy that can be recovered from triglyceride stores by unit of weight is more than four times as large as that from glycogen and/or protein stores. An average 75-kg man can store only approximately 500 g of carbohydrate in liver and muscle, representing less than a day of energy stores. By contrast, even in lean individuals, fat stores in the adipose tissue alone can amount to approximately 10 kg, which is sufficient to maintain bodily functions for weeks of survival during total food deprivation. In obesity, fat stores can be multiplied by as much as 10 to 20 times and provide energy for months of starvation. The energy from triglycerides is stored in some 25 billion to 50 billion fat cells representing the adipose tissue, mostly beneath the skin and in the abdomen. Until only a decade ago, the adipose tissue was considered primarily an energy storage compartment that provides energy fuel to the entire body between meals and during periods of energy deficit.

With the discovery of leptin in 1994[1] and the many other secreted proteins that have been discovered since,[2] the adipose tissue is now not only considered an energy reservoir, but has also reached the status of a true endocrine organ. Over the past decade, effort has concentrated on a better understanding of the regulation of adipose tissue development and apoptosis throughout the lifespan and its consequence on health and diseases. In this chapter, we will briefly review the role of the adipose as an energy storage compartment, but more important, we will summarize the current knowledge of what is now considered as a finely tuned gland, which can influence many facets of the conditions that are often referred as the "metabolic syndrome." We first describe the link between too much fat (obesity) and insulin resistance and alternatively provide arguments why too little fat is equally and paradoxically associated with insulin resistance.

Next, we review the pioneering work, which led to the concept of hypertrophic and hyperplastic obesity and the critical periods during which the adipose tissue is thought to develop. The current understanding of the regulation of adipogenesis is then reviewed, followed by a description of the afferent endocrine and neural signals to the adipose tissue. In the next section, we discuss the concept of the lipostatic theory, which led to the discovery of leptin and many other hormones involved in health and disease. Besides leptin, we provide some more details on adiponectin, resistin, and tissue-necrotizing factor-alpha (TNF-α). We conclude by proposing the adipocyte as a potential target for the treatment of obesity, dyslipidemia, and type 2 diabetes.

OBESITY, INSULIN RESISTANCE, AND TYPE 2 DIABETES MELLITUS

LINK BETWEEN OBESITY AND INSULIN RESISTANCE

Numerous cross-sectional studies have shown an association between obesity and type 2 diabetes. Data from the third National Health Examination Survey (NHANES III) provides unequivocal evidence that the prevalence of diabetes is almost three times higher in overweight than in nonoverweight persons.[3] Many prospective studies have confirmed this association. For example, the likelihood of developing diabetes increases steeply with increasing body weight and fatness in Pima Indians as well as other populations.[4] The association between obesity and diabetes is attributed mostly to the increase in insulin resistance that is so common in obese people.[5] Insulin resistance is a clear predisposing factor for the development of type 2 diabetes in individuals who are at risk for the disease.[6-8]

Obesity is defined as an excess of body fat and is usually characterized by increased circulating plasma free fatty acid concentration. Cross-sectional studies of lean, overweight, and obese subjects have shown an inverse relationship between fasting plasma free fatty acid concentration and insulin sensitivity. Studies in animals and humans support a causal effect of elevated free fatty acids (produced by turnover of triglycerides from adipose tissue) on impaired insulin-mediated glucose metabolism.[9-12] Such studies reinforce the original hypothesis proposed by Randle and colleagues in 1963[13,14] that altered fatty acid metabolism was the key contributing factor to insulin resistance in obese and diabetic patients. Randle and colleagues demonstrated that free fatty acids compete with glucose for substrate oxidation in isolated preparations of heart and diaphragm muscle from rats. More specifically, they proposed that increased fatty acid availability in obesity causes an increase in the intramitochondrial acetyl-CoA/CoA and NADH/NAD+ ratios leading to inactivation of pyruvate dehydrogenase. This in turn causes an intracellular increase in citrate concentration leading to inhibition of phosphofructokinase, the rate-limiting enzyme for glycolysis. As a consequence, glucose-6-phosphate accumulates in the cell and inhibits hexokinase II activity, leading to an increase in intracellular glucose and a decrease in glucose uptake, oxidation, and storage.

During the past 5 years, Randle's glucose–fatty acid cycle has been challenged by data from sophisticated clinical studies using stable isotope turnover in conjunction with substrates leg balance methods or using ^{13}C and ^{31}P magnetic resonance spectroscopy. These studies provide evidence that insulin resistance in obese people may be related to a primary defect of fatty acid oxidation in skeletal muscle rather than a competition between fat and carbohydrate metabolism.

First, Wolfe and colleagues identified some of the flaws in the notion that fatty acid availability controls substrate oxidation in the fasting state.[15] In a series of experiments, he provided evidence that fatty acid oxidation is largely controlled at the site of oxidation, which is in turn determined by the availability of glucose. Decreased hepatic free fatty acid availability during fasting leads to decreased plasma glucose and consequently low glucose oxidation. In this model, the primary physiologic role of increased adipose lipolysis in fasting conditions is to provide the necessary glycerol as a gluconeogenic precursor,[16] and the rate of fatty acid oxidation is then regulated by the rate of intracellular metabolism of glucose.

Second, it is now well accepted that skeletal muscle predominantly relies on lipid oxidation during fasting and can easily switch from lipid to increased glucose uptake and oxidation in response to feeding and hyperinsulinemia.[17] This switch from fat to carbohydrate oxidation in skeletal muscle has been called "metabolic flexibility." Importantly, Kelley and Mandarino provided convincing evidence that glucose oxidation is increased in the leg of subjects with type 2 diabetes, thereby decreasing its reliance on fat oxidation.[18] As in Wolfe's hypothesis stated above[15] and in opposition to the Randle's glucose–fatty acid cycle, their series of studies suggest that hyperglycemia itself causes an impairment of the normal fasting reliance of skeletal muscle on fatty acids, therefore causing an accumulation of lipids into the muscle tissue. This "reversed Randle cycle" theory highlights the primary role of impaired lipid oxidation in skeletal muscle rather than excessive lipolysis in the adipose tissue. Growing evidence suggests that the primary cause of the "metabolic inflexibility" in subjects who are susceptible to insulin resistance is impaired fat oxidation in the fasting state and a lack of increased carbohydrate oxidation in response to feeding. In support of this concept, there is now evidence pointing toward decreased mitochondrial oxidative capacity in insulin-resistant subjects with diabetes[19] or a family history of diabetes and in insulin-resistant older individuals.[20]

To prove or disprove the "Randle cycle" hypothesis, Shulman and colleagues went one step further. If the Randle hypothesis were true, one would predict an accumulation of glucose-6-phosphate in the skeletal muscle of healthy subjects during glucose and insulin infusions in the presence of high plasma free fatty acid concentration.[21] They directly tested this hypothesis using magnetic resonance spectroscopy. As expected, high concentrations of circulating free fatty acids caused reduction in insulin-mediated glucose uptake with an approximately 50% decrease in glucose storage and 50% decrease in glucose oxidation.[11] However, in contrast to what would be predicted by the Randle's hypothesis, there was no accumulation of glucose-6-phosphate. Therefore, reduced glucose uptake when free fatty acids are high is due to impaired glucose transport or impaired intracellular signaling. This series of studies shows that intramuscular fatty acids or fatty acid metabolites seem to interfere with the transport of glucose into the skeletal muscle cell. Recent studies have provided some potential mechanisms of the effect of free fatty acid–induced insulin resistance via an impact on insulin signaling at the level of protein kinase C-θ.[22–25]

While many studies have provided evidence for an association between insulin sensitivity and visceral fat mass (reviewed in Ref. 26), other studies provide as good evidence for associations between the amount of subcutaneous fat on the trunk and insulin resistance in obese nondiabetic men[27,28] and in men with type 2 diabetes.[18,29,30] Similarly, insulin resistance in obese women is better related to overall elevated fat mass than just to visceral fat mass.[31,32] Thus, subcutaneous fat, which does not drain into the portal vein, causes insulin resistance by a nonportal mechanism. The growing experimental evidence, which does not support the Randle/portal hypotheses therefore calls for a change in the scientific paradigm to explain the insulin resistance so common in obesity. The bulk of the literature now provides evidence that excessive total fat mass (rather than just visceral fat mass) and impaired muscle fat oxidation are associated with insulin resistance and increased risk for the development of type 2 diabetes.

LINK BETWEEN TOO LITTLE FAT AND INSULIN RESISTANCE

At the other end of the spectrum from obesity, it is now recognized that a lack of adipose tissue is also associated with insulin resistance and increased risk for development of type 2 diabetes. Lipodystrophy in humans is an acquired or hereditary syndrome characterized by decreased adipose tissue mass, insulin resistance, and often diabetes mellitus.[33] Insufficient adipose tissue mass leads to excess energy storage as triglycerides in liver and skeletal muscle and is associated with insulin resistance in these tissues.[34,35] Genetic manipulation causing ablation of adipose tissue in mice supports the link between adipose deficiency and insulin resistance. Transgenic animals without adipose tissue store lipid in skeletal muscle and liver and develop insulin resistance, glucose intolerance, and eventually diabetes.[36–38] This is identical to the fatty liver and muscle that are seen in obesity and type 2 diabetes. Furthermore, transplantation of adipose tissue back into lipoatrophic animals reverses the elevated glucose levels.[39] However, transplantation of adipose tissue from leptin-deficient mice (ob/ob) did not improve the metabolic abnormalities, indicating that the sequestration of triglyceride into adipose tissue is not entirely sufficient to restore insulin sensitivity.[40] On the other hand, surgical removal of adipose tissue causes a metabolic syndrome.[41] Together, these studies demonstrate that, as in obesity, inadequate adipose tissue mass leads to "ectopic" fat storage and metabolic disturbances. Too little fat is therefore as deleterious as too much fat and predisposes to the development of the metabolic syndrome with insulin resistance and ultimately type 2 diabetes. Two new emerging paradigms may therefore explain insulin resistance:

- The "ectopic fat storage syndrome," in which excess fat is deposited in other tissues than adipose tissue
- The "endocrine adipocyte," which secretes hormones that are involved in insulin resistance and cardiovascular disease

OBESITY IS ANOTHER ECTOPIC FAT STORAGE SYNDROME

Positive energy balance in our "obesigenic" environment produces a pattern similar to lipodystrophy in humans, that is, excess lipid storage in liver[42] and skeletal muscle[21,43,44] followed by insulin resistance, glucose intolerance, and diabetes. However, in contrast to lipodystrophic patients, adipose tissue stores are adequate or even large in obese patients, suggesting that the size of adipose tissue becomes inadequate to sequester dietary lipid away from liver, skeletal muscle, and pancreas. The adipocyte becomes hypertrophic and unable to recruit and/or differentiate new adipocytes to store the excessive dietary fat.[45] This hypothesis is supported by the fact that, independent of total fat mass, individuals with larger fat cells are at higher risk of developing type 2 diabetes than are individuals with smaller fat cells.[46] Furthermore, thiazolidinediones improve insulin resistance partially by promoting differentiation of new fat cells in subcutaneous adipose tissue through activation of peroxisome proliferator–activated receptor γ (PPAR-γ), therefore providing extra storage capacity for dietary fat.[47] Adipogenesis translates into a gain in subcutaneous adipose tissue[48] and a decrease in lipid infiltration in skeletal muscle and liver. Through the upregulation of genes in the lipid storage and synthesis pathways in adipose tissue, thiolidendoines also decrease free fatty acids, providing a second mechanism to protect liver, muscle, and the β cell from fatty acids.[49–51] As will be discussed later in this chapter, drugs may therefore be designed to decrease ectopic fat storage by increasing adipogenesis lipid storage in adipose tissue and/or increasing fat oxidation, leading to improved insulin action.

ADIPOSE TISSUE: HYPERTROPHY VERSUS HYPERPLASIA

Historically, adipose tissue was viewed as an inert tissue with a singular function: lipid storage. The main areas of research in the field of adipose tissue were related to adipocyte size and number as well as lipid synthesis, adrenergic regulation of lipolysis, and insulin signaling in isolated adipocytes. In adults, obesity is associated with an increase in both the number and size of adipocytes.[52,53] The increase in fat cell size (hypertrophy) is thought to reflect an imbalance between adipocyte lipid uptake or synthesis and the release of lipid via lipolytic pathways. In addition to increased adipocyte size, obese individuals have an increase in the absolute number of adipocytes (hyperplasia). Early studies demonstrated heterogeneity in fat cell size; some obese patients have adipocytes as large as 1 μL, and others have very small fat cells. This heterogeneity led to the concept of hypertrophic or hyperplastic obesity based on the average size of fat cells (Fig. 53-1). In contrast to this dichotomous viewpoint, the reality is that obese individuals cannot be grouped into such simple categories. There is a continuous distribution of fat cell size (FCS), and most obese patients have both hypertrophy and hyperplasia. Increased FCS is positively correlated with fasting insulin and negatively with insulin sensitivity.[54] In Pima Indians, increased abdominal adipocyte size is associated with insulin resistance and hypertrophic fat cells,[46,55] a potential inherited trait[56] that predicts the onset of type 2 diabetes.[46] Together, these data suggest that increased fat cell size is important to whole body metabolism and insulin action.

There are at least two ways of thinking about why fat cells might be large in obese individuals. First, adult adipose tissue has been viewed as a nonmitotic tissue, and increases in adipocyte size might simply reflect an imbalance between storage and lipolysis. If the number of adipocytes is considered fixed, any increase in adipose tissue mass is the result of increased lipid storage in adipocytes. A second view is that fat cells can continually be recruited to differentiate into mature lipid storing fat cells and large fat cells are an indication of a failure of this process. Several investigators have proposed that once adipocytes are filled to a certain degree, new fat cells are recruited, and lipid is then stored in these new insulin-sensitive and lipid-hungry adipocytes. The cross-sectional data that are used to support this model are presented in Figures 53-2C and 53-2D. Average fat cell size increases as body fatness increases up to a certain point, after which increased adiposity does not result in an increase in fat cell size. Even if individuals with hyperplastic or hypertrophic obesity lose weight equally, hyperplastic obese patients regain the weight much more quickly than hypertrophic subjects do, lending support to the concept of small, lipid-hungry fat cells.[57]

Hyperplastic vs. hypertrophic obesity.

A   Hyperplastic obesity

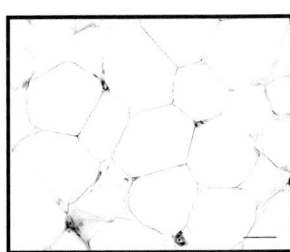

B   Hypertrophic obesity

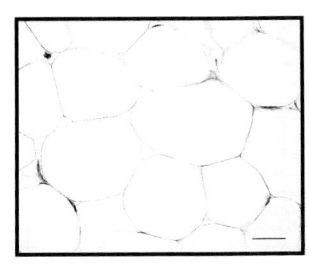

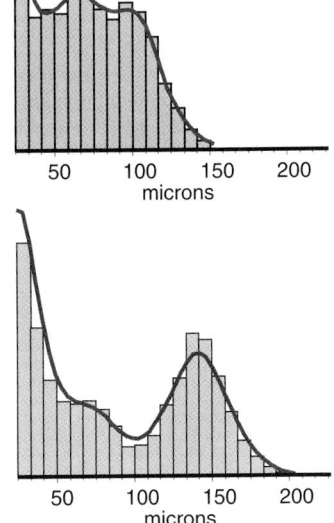

Figure 53-1 Hyperplastic versus hypertrophic obesity. **A,** Hyperplastic obesity is defined by an increase in the number of adipocytes, while adipocyte size remains small. The histogram to the right shows that the adipocytes, although larger than those in lean individuals, are smaller than those in the obese individual with hypertrophic obesity. **B,** The reason for the increase in adipocyte size is unclear. Current hypotheses suggest that a failure of the large adipocyte to recruit preadipocytes to differentiate may play a role in the development of insulin resistance, a precursor to overt β-cell failure as manifested by diabetes. (Photomicrographs courtesy of Prof. Saverio Cinti, M.D., Institute of Anatomy, Faculty of Medicine, University of Ancona, Italy. Fat cell size histograms from Steven R. Smith's laboratory.)

Figure 53-2   Schematic relationship between age, body fat mass, and fat cell size and number. **A,** The whole-body fat cell number remains constant during the first year of life and then increases over time. **B,** The increase in body fat that is seen during the first year of life occurs primarily as a result of increased lipid storage and hypertrophy of existing adipocytes rather than through the recruitment of preadipocytes. **C,** In adults, whole-body fat cell number increases with increasing body mass (hyperplasia). **D,** Again, in adults, cross-sectional data show a positive correlation between body fat mass and fat cell size at lower body fat mass (*solid curve*) until fat cell size reaches a plateau at higher levels of fat mass. At this point, fat cell size cannot increase any further owing to (a) limitations on lipid storage for unknown reasons, and/or (b) recruitment of existing preadipocytes to differentiate and store lipid, and/or (c) proliferation and differentiation of mesenchymal precursor cells into mature lipid-storing adipocytes. If fat cell proliferation, differentiation, and/or recruitment did not occur, fat cell size would continue to increase as fat mass increased (*dashed line*). Subsequent increases in fat mass do not result in an increase in fat cell size suggesting that (b) or (c) is operational in vivo. For any given BMI, there is a wide range of fat cell size. In individuals who acutely lose or gain weight, fat cell size decreases or increases, respectively. Fat cell number does not appear to change with weight gain or loss; however, precise tools are not available to quantify small changes in adipocyte number in vivo in humans. (Source: **A** and **B** adapted from the data from Hager et al.[62] and Soriguer Escofet et al.[63] **C** and **D** adapted from Hirsch and Batchelor.[53])

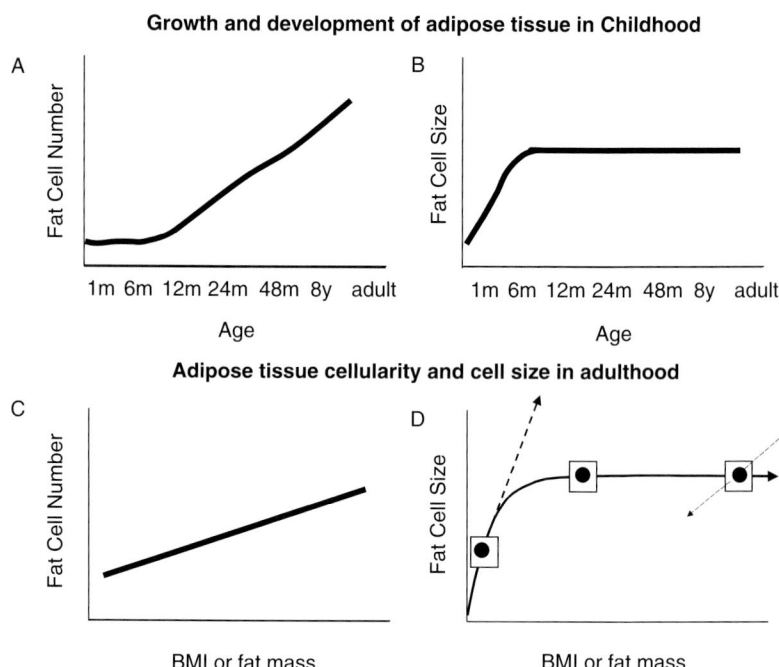

During weight loss, fat cell size decreases without a change in fat cell number and is associated with a decrease in fasting insulin.[54] This has been interpreted as evidence that once a fat cell is formed, it is permanent. However, recent studies demonstrate a relatively high rate of adipocyte turnover[58] and evidence for regulation of apoptosis.[59] It should be noted that there are not sufficient longitudinal data or precise measures of fat cell number to confirm this model in humans. This is in part due to our current inability to accurately quantify the number of stem cells and preadipocytes in adipose tissue in vitro or in vivo and the difficulties in quantifying the very smallest fat cells in adipose tissue.[60]

In contrast, the cross-sectional data illustrated in Figure 53-2 could also be interpreted as evidence for the recruitment of new adipocytes. If fat cell hypertrophy was the only way to gain fat, then fat cell size would increase linearly with fat mass. This is not the case. On the basis of cross-sectional data, the point at which hypertrophy recruits new fat cells probably occurs for a cell volume between 0.8 and 1.0 μL.[61–63] Two additional pieces of evidence support the view that recruitment of new fat cells occurs in vivo in humans. First, when adipose tissue is separated into fat cells and the remaining cell populations (stromal-vascular fraction), adipocytic precursor cells from the stromal-vascular fraction are able to differentiate in vitro into mature lipid-storing adipocytes throughout life and into old age. Obesity and age are determinants of the capacity to differentiate adipocytes in vitro.[64,65] Recent studies of in vivo DNA synthesis in humans suggest that adipocyte turnover is high in adult humans, with a $t_{1/2}$ ranging from 240 to 425 days.[58,66] Furthermore, large fat cells secrete a factor or factors that promote adipocyte proliferation and differentiation, a finding that is consistent with the recruitment of "new" adipocytes by hypertrophic adipocytes as discussed above.[67]

Studies by Hirsch and others in rodents demonstrated that animals that were calorically deprived before weaning had a reduced total number of fat cells when compared to animals that were suckled in smaller litters with higher caloric intake. Similarly, about half of the obesity in Zucker fatty rats can be prevented by the early restriction of energy.[68] This gave rise to the concept that early overfeeding during adipose tissue development might increase the population of adipocytes and their precursors that produce obesity over time. This model, known as the adipose-cell or critical period hypothesis, predicts that a large number of adipocyte precursors early in life could lead to the development of obesity by providing a sink that is destined to be filled with lipid. A corollary to this concept is that individuals with a reduction in adipocyte precursors, like those individuals with a failure of adipocyte differentiation described above, would be predisposed to the development of diabetes when food intake is increased as their storage capacity for excess fat is diminished.

Although the concept of an early life critical period for adipocyte precursor development has been much discussed, the actual data supporting this concept is sparse by comparison. Consistent with this concept, obese subjects with an early childhood onset of obesity tend to have smaller fat cells and are less hyperplastic when compared to those with later adult onset of obesity.[69,70] Similarly, children of mothers who were energy deprived during the Dutch famine of 1945 had a lower incidence of obesity in adulthood.[71] Although no prospective long-term data exist to support the adipose-cell hypothesis, the cross-sectional data support the concept that in many cases of early-onset obesity, fat cell size tends to be hyperplastic rather than hypertrophic, and the latter is more often seen with late-onset obesity.

The original data and hypothesis presented by Hirsch suggested a single early critical period. Later discussions offered the concept that additional critical periods of adipocyte precursor proliferation might also exist[53] with recruitment from the precursor pools into mature adipocytes throughout life. At birth, a typical infant has about 4 billion observable fat cells. This increases to approximately 10 billion to 40 billion in lean individuals and up to 50 billion to 100 billion obese patients,[72] supporting the concept of ongoing adipocyte proliferation and/or recruitment throughout life. In contrast to rodents, humans seem to have a long, slow growth and development period (neotony) and are likely to have several critical periods of adipocyte development.[73]

Body fat mass increases during the first year of life mostly through fat cell hypertrophy. After the first year, the number of adipocytes increases, the fat cell size remains relatively constant, and whole-body adiposity (percentage of fat) decreases. At about 6 years of age, the percentage of body fat begins to increase again. This has been termed the *adiposity rebound*. Longitudinal body weight data in children demonstrate that an earlier adiposity rebound is associated with obesity in adulthood.[74–76] Although no detailed information exists on the relative role of hypertrophy versus hyperplasia for this age range, the adiposity rebound is considered a critical period for adiposity later in life.[77]

REGULATION OF ADIPOGENESIS

Adipose tissue, unlike other tissues such as the brain, kidney, or liver, retains the ability to increase in size in adulthood. Several processes control the mass of adipose tissue in the body:

- Adipocyte precursor proliferation
- Differentiation of these precursors into mature insulin-sensitive, lipid-storing adipocytes
- The balance of lipid storage, utilization, and release within each mature adipocyte
- Apoptosis of mature adipocytes

Adipocytes can be classified on the basis of anatomic location as subcutaneous, visceral (intraperitoneal), bone marrow, and structural (periorbital, palms of the hands, and soles of the feet). The hereditary and acquired lipodystrophies teach us that each of these depots of adipose tissue are developed or regulated differently, as each form of lipodystrophy results in the loss or failure to differentiate in specific depots. For example, in congenital generalized lipodystrophy, "mechanical" adipose tissue of the palms and soles is spared.[78]

Adipose tissue precursors are primarily mesenchymal in origin (Fig. 53-3). These precursor cells, also known as preadipocyte or stromal cells, have the capacity to differentiate into a limited number of cell types including adipocytes, osteoblasts, and chondrocytes.[79] We know very little about the systems that control proliferation of adipose tissue precursors. Most of what we know is derived from the study of the cellularity of rodent adipose tissue or the behavior of stromal-vascular cultures in vitro. Some of the known activators and inhibitors of adipogenesis are presented in Table 53-1. For example, insulin-like growth factor-1 (IGF-1) is a growth factor that is under the control of insulin and growth hormone in adipose tissue and promotes the proliferation and differentiation of preadipocytes, while transforming growth factor inhibits proliferation.[80] More is known about the processes whereby adipocyte precursors, particularly 3T3-L1 preadipocytes, proceed along the pathway from precursor to mature adipocyte. We now know that a series of transcription factors coordinately regulate multiple genes in a tightly regulated temporal fashion. As Figure 53-3 shows, each of these transcription factors forms a nonredundant network that once initiated, leads to the emergence of the adipocyte phenotype. Some of the known key transcription factors include PPAR-γ signal transduction and activators of transcription 5 (STAT5) C/EBP-/α, -β, and -δ, SREBP1c/ADD cyclic adenosine monophosphate (cAMP) response element binding protein (CREB) and Wnt/frizzled.

Multiple hormones, cytokines, growth factors, cell cycle regulators, and adhesion molecules control this differentiation cascade. Classic studies by Green and others showed that confluent clonal cell lines such as 3T3-L1 and F442A differentiate into adipocytes if exposed to a cocktail of insulin, dexamethasone, and isomethylybutylxanthine (IBMX).[81–83] Emphasis has also been placed on the role of cell cycle and the necessity for proliferation prior to differentiation of precursors. However, recent data suggest that this has more to do

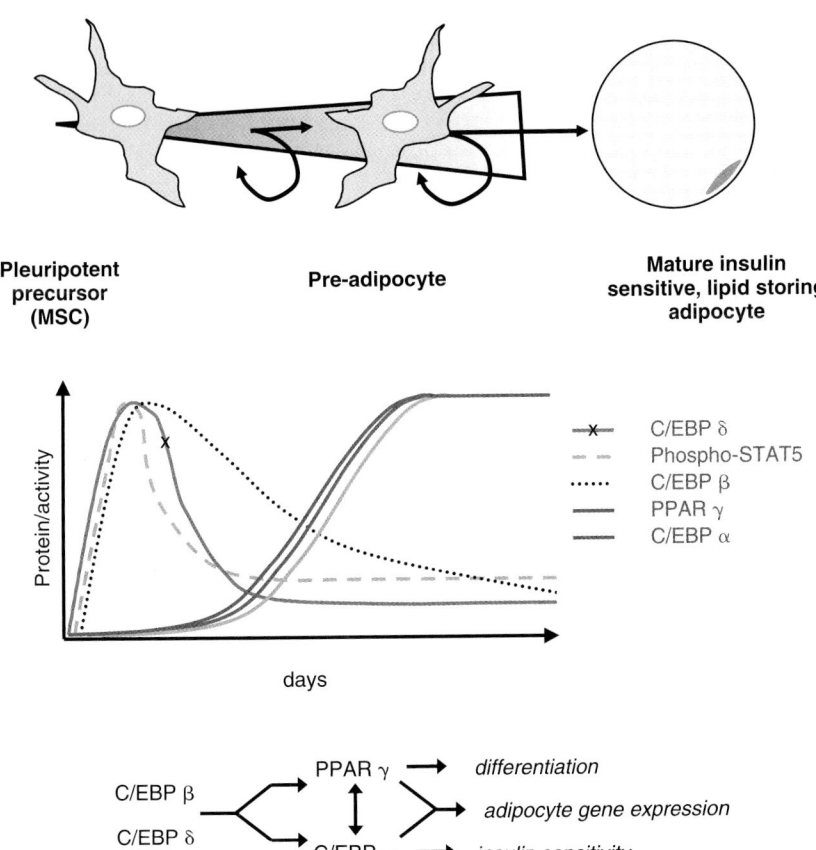

Figure 53-3 Adipocyte differentiation cascade. Adipocytes are derived from mesenchymal stem cell precursors (MSC). Both the mesenchymal precursors and the preadipocyte, whose differentiation potential is limited to the adipocyte lineage, can undergo mitosis. The middle panel depicts the coordinate, sequential activation of the major nuclear transcription factors that are thought to be involved in the adipogenic differentiation process. PPAR-γ is considered an obligatory master regulator of adipogenesis. The PPAR-γ system turns on genes that are involved in lipid synthesis and insulin action (see text for details).

Table 53-1 Extracellular Factors That Regulate Adipogenesis

ACTIVATORS
GH/IGF-1/insulin
Cortisol (GR ligand)
Thyroid hormone (TR ligand)
Retinoic acids (RXR ligands)
Endogenous PPAR-γ ligands
    PGJ2
    HODEs/HETE

INHIBITORS
TNF-α
IFN-γ
Pref-1
Resistin
TGF-β

with the E2F transcription factors than with the process of mitosis per se.[84,85]

IBMX and other agents that increase cAMP act through the transcription factor CREB.[86] Several transcription factors are critical for the conversion of cells from a fibroblastic phenotype to an adipocytic phenotype. PPAR-γ has received the most attention, and this is warranted, since overexpression of PPAR-γ into fibroblastic cell types is sufficient to confer the adipocytic phenotype.[87] There are several putative endogenous ligands for PPAR-γ, including the prostaglandin PGJ2,[88,89] long-chain fatty acids, and 13-HODE and 15-HETE, which can be generated from linoleic and arachidonic acids, respectively, by a 12/15-lipoxygenase.[90] All of these compounds can activate the PPAR-γ transcription factor that heterodimerizes with the RXR transcription factor to turn on genes in the glucose uptake,[91,92] lipid uptake,[93] and lipid synthesis pathways.[94,95] The true endogenous ligand(s) are unknown, but their synthesis or activity appears to be downstream of the C/EBP-β transcription factor.[96] C/EBP-α is expressed contemporaneously with PPAR-γ and facilitates the full adipocytic phenotype. Immediately upstream of PPAR-γ lie the C/EBP transcription factors C/EBP-β and C/EBP-δ, which upregulate PPAR-γ. Other transcriptional promoters of adipogenesis include STAT5,[97] the glucocorticoid receptor, and ADD/SREBP-1c.[98] Transcriptional inhibitors include GATA 3,[99] TCF/LEF, and the Wnt pathway.[100] Combined with the transcriptional activators, they cooperate in an orchestrated cascade of transcriptional events, leading to a mature adipocyte. Lastly, PPAR-γ cofactors may regulate the ultimate transcriptional program in adipocytes. For example, adipocytes can be converted from energy storage to energy consumers by the PPAR-γ cofactor PGC-1a.[101] Similarly, the PPAR-γ cofactors SRC-1 and TIF2 may determine the responses of adipose tissue to high-fat diets; SRC-1-activating fatty acid oxidation, and TIF2-promoting lipid storage.[102] These two examples highlight a growing understanding that not only the ligand but also the transcription factor cofactors are important in whole-body metabolism.

These intracellular transcriptional control systems are regulated by extracellular signals from cytokines, hormones, neural inputs, and the autocrine/paracrine production of ligands for these transcription factors.

INTEGRATIVE BIOLOGY OF THE ADIPOSE TISSUE

To maintain energy homeostasis, the brain has two avenues of communication with the periphery: hormones and neurons. The adipose tissue is no exception to this rule, since it is well established that both hormones and neurons control its life cycle and metabolism. Understanding how adipose tissue operates and is regulated in vivo is a prime example of integrative biology. Imaging studies of the different adipose depots

as well as studies of adipose tissue metabolism and secretary function using arterial-venous differences and microdialysis in conjunction with measures of adipose tissue blood flow have all improved our integrative view of the metabolism and function of the adipose tissue.

ENDOCRINE SIGNALS

Glucocorticoids

Glucocorticoid treatment of laboratory animals results in the development of obesity. Animal models of obesity invariably have increased levels of corticosterone. Adrenalectomy results in the reversal or prevention of obesity. Activation of the glucocorticoid receptor results in differentiation of preadipocyte precursors[81-83] and lipid storage in adipocytes. The enzyme 11βHSD-1 is present in human adipose tissue and converts inactive cortisone into active cortisol.[103] In humans, overproduction of cortisol (Cushing's syndrome) results in a phenotype of central (abdominal) obesity, hypertension, and diabetes. Of the many investigations into the role of adrenal glucocorticoids in human obesity, most show normal urinary free cortisol, normal circadian variation in cortisol values, and normal plasma cortisol values, although metabolic clearance rate and production are increased.[104]

The most compelling data for an association between human obesity and cortisol come from studies that classify obese women into central and peripheral types of obesity. By stratifying volunteers on this basis, Marin and coworkers demonstrated an increase in urinary and serum cortisol as the waist-to-hip ratio increased.[105] Serum cortisol responses to stress were greater in women with high waist-to-hip ratios, suggesting a role of response to environmental stressors as a potential factor in abdominal obesity.[105,106] Other evidence in humans suggests that cortisol values within normal concentrations are sometimes related to fat patterning, possibly via increased sensitivity to exogenous stressors. Genetic factors may also determine the susceptibility of the adipose tissue to these exogenous stressors.[107]

Growth Hormone/IGF-1

Growth hormone (GH) is a potent lipolytic hormone.[108] GH receptors activate classic cAMP lipolytic systems in adipose tissue. In addition to stimulating lipolysis, GH increases IGF-1 production in adipose tissue.[109] IGF-1 potently activates preadipocyte proliferation and differentiation of precursors into mature lipid-storing adipocytes.[80] Deficiency of GH is associated with central obesity, and replacement of GH reduces visceral adiposity.[110] Despite early reports of therapeutic efficacy of GH in men with central obesity,[111] GH treatment in the absence of clear-cut GH deficiency cannot be recommended, as the side effect profile includes edema, carpal tunnel syndrome, glucose intolerance, and many others. GH-like peptides that increase lipolysis without upregulation of IGF-1 synthesis have been discovered[112] and may be beneficial without the adverse effects of GH.

Estrogen in Adipose Tissue

Men and women have different distribution of body fat: a gluteal-femoral pattern in women and an abdominal pattern in men. This sexual dimorphism is thought to be due to differences in the sex steroids estrogen and testosterone. Lipoprotein lipase (LPL) activity, which is indicative of lipid storage, is increased in the gluteal-femoral region of women as compared to men. After menopause, LPL activity is equivalent across all adipose tissue depots, suggesting that estrogen upregulates LPL in a depot-specific fashion.[113] In support of this concept, treatment of postmenopausal women with estradiol increased LPL activity in the gluteal-femoral region,[114] which was reversed by the addition of a progestin.[115] In vitro in human abdominal subcutaneous adipocytes, low-dose estradiol increased LPL protein, and higher-dose estradiol decreased LPL.[116] These dose-dependent effects of estradiol to decrease LPL were also observed in a cross-sectional study[117] and after local transdermal application of estradiol.[118] In addition to systemic estradiol, the stromal-vascular fraction of adipose tissue is able to convert estrogenic precursors to estrogen vis-à-vis the enzyme aromatase. In men, testosterone, but not the nonaromatizable steroid dihydrotestosterone, increases adipose tissue lipid turnover, suggesting that testosterone acts in adipose tissue via local conversion of testosterone into estrogen by aromatase.[119,120] In vitro, estradiol increases the proliferation of stromal-vascular cultures of both human[121] and rodent preadipocytes.[122]

Several investigators[123–126] have demonstrated estradiol binding and ERα mRNA in adipose tissue extracts. After the cloning of the ERβ gene, both mRNA and protein for ERβ were subsequently described in adipose tissue.[125–127] In human adipose tissue, ERβ was higher in abdominal than in gluteal femoral adipose tissue, and regional differences in adipose tissue expression of ERα and ERβ were described by Pedersen and coworkers.[128]

In summary, estradiol is an important sex steroid, both for the proliferation of adipocyte precursors and for the regulation of lipid storage in a regional-specific fashion.

NEURAL SIGNALS TO THE ADIPOSE TISSUE

As was discussed earlier, human adipose tissue can be divided into two major compartments, subcutaneous and visceral (approximately 80% and 10%, respectively), whereas other depots such as retroperitoneal, perirenal, and orbital fat account for the remainder.[129] The two major compartments have clearly different rates of lipid synthesis and lipolysis, probably owing to differences in hormonal exposure and innervation. The brain needs to transmit messages to different parts of the body in a selective manner. For that reason, both branches of the autonomic nervous system (sympathetic or parasympathetic) innervate different adipose tissues in different ways, influencing not only regional blood flow but also functions such as lipolysis and lipid synthesis. By viral injection in fat pads of Siberian hamsters, Youngstrom and Bartness showed the presence of sympathetic projections from central sympathetic ganglia, which was confirmed by injection of fluorescent anterograde tract tracers into the sympathetic chain ganglia.[130] In addition, denervated fat depots weigh 10% more than the intact contralateral depot, implying impaired lipid mobilization in fat pads that are deprived of their innervation.[131] From such studies, it was hypothesized that catecholamines not only increase lipolysis but also inhibit adipose tissue hyperplasia from preadipocytes, a possibility that is supported by in vitro data.[132,133]

REGULATION OF LIPOLYSIS

Adipose tissue lipolysis, that is, the catabolic process leading to the breakdown of triglycerides into fatty acids and glycerol, is often considered a simple and well-understood metabolic pathway (Fig. 53-4). However, we continue to discover new layers of complexity in the system. Hormone-sensitive lipase, the rate-limiting enzyme of intracellular triglyceride hydrolysis, is a major determinant of fatty acid mobilization in adipose tissue. Translocation of hormone-sensitive lipase to the lipid droplet seems to be an important step during lipolytic activation. Reorganization of the lipid droplet coating by perilipin may also facilitate the access of the enzyme. In humans, alterations of hormone-sensitive lipase expression are associated with changes in lipolysis in various physiologic and pathologic states. The major hormones controlling the lipolytic process are catecholamines (stimulation of lipolysis) and insulin (inhibition of lipolysis). It is well accepted that the adrenergic system is the major regulator of lipolysis via a cAMP pathway. In turn, cAMP increases the activity of protein kinase-A, which phosphorylates both the hormone-sensitive lipase and perilipin. As a counteracting hormone, insulin binds to its receptor, activates the various elements of the insulin-signaling cascade by stimulation of Type III cyclic guanosine monophosphate (cGMP) inhibited phosphodiesterase (PDE3B), therefore decreasing cAMP and suppressing lipolysis.[134] The antilipolytic effect of insulin is reduced in the insulin-resistant state.[135] Progress on the hormonal regulation and molecular mechanisms of β-lipolytic and α2-antilipolytic adrenergic control of lipolysis has improved our understanding of the relative contribution of the two types of receptors.[136] Genetic studies show that polymorphisms in genes coding for different β-adrenoceptor subtypes and hormone-sensitive lipase may participate in the polygenic background of obesity.[137] More recently, a novel lipolytic system has been characterized in human fat cells. Natriuretic peptides stimulate lipolysis through a cGMP-dependent pathway, which is not influenced or suppressed by insulin action.[138,139]

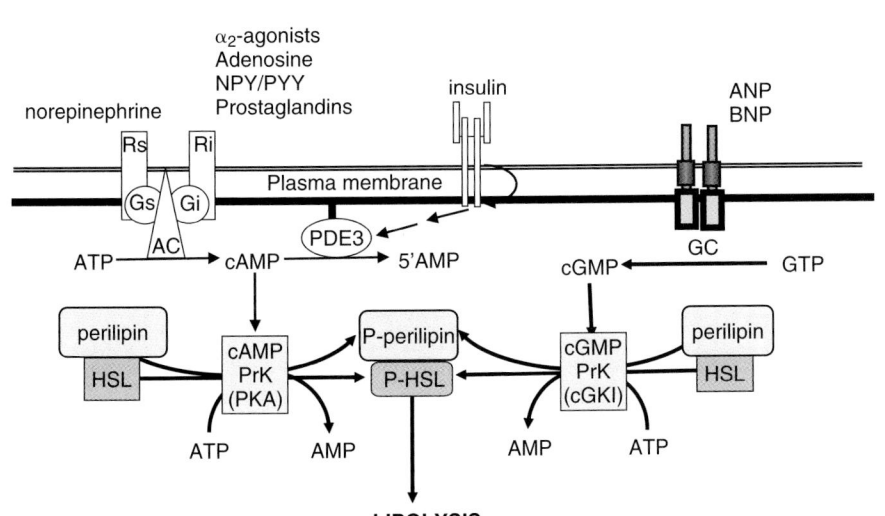

Figure 53-4 Regulators of human adipocyte lipolysis. Hormone-sensitive lipase and perilipin are rate-limiting steps in the regulation of adipocyte lipolysis. Both enzymes need to be phosphorylated to be active and allow the breakdown of triglycerides into glycerol and free fatty acid. The adrenergic systems (β-receptors and α2-receptors) are major regulators of lipolysis via cyclic AMP pathways. β-Receptors stimulate lipolysis, whereas α2-receptors inhibit lipolysis. Cyclic AMP increases the activity of protein kinase A, which in turn phosphorylates the hormone-sensitive lipase and perilipin. Insulin inhibits lipolysis via inhibition of phosphodiesterase (PDE), therefore decreasing cAMP and lipolysis. A novel lipolytic system using natriuretic peptides stimulates lipolysis through a cGMP-dependent pathway, which is not influenced or suppressed by insulin action. Abbreviations: NPY/PYY, neuropeptide Y, peptide YY; Rs, receptor, stimulating; Ri, receptor, inhibitory; Gs, stimulatory G-protein; Gi, inhibitory G-protein; AC, adenylate cyclase; cAMP, cyclic AMP; AMP, adenosine monophosphate; PDE, phosphodiesterase; ANP, atrial natriuretic protein; BNP, brain natriuretic protein; GC, guanylate cyclase; cGMP, cyclic guanine monophosphate.

DISCOVERY OF LEPTIN ESTABLISHED THE ADIPOCYTE AS AN ENDOCRINE ORGAN

The study of the biology of the adipose tissue including the mechanisms of adipogenesis has enjoyed an explosive growth over the past decade. Unarguably, the trigger for this renewed interest came from the cloning of the *ob* (obese) gene and the discovery of leptin in 1994.[1] This seminal discovery initiated a period of intense research for uncovering the endocrine and paracrine roles of the adipose tissue and its role in the development of obesity and related diseases. The steps that led to the discovery of leptin were summarized in the original description of the cloning of the leptin gene.[1] In brief, the original notion of a homeostatic regulation of energy balance (and therefore adipose mass) dates back to Lavoisier and Laplace.[140-142] The key role of the brain in this regulation came later from clinical observations and was confirmed by stereotaxic lesions of different regions of the brain.[143] These studies provided evidence that the ventromedial nucleus of the hypothalamus (VMH) is the most important satiety center in the central nervous system and that lesion of the VMH results in hyperphagia, decreased energy expenditure, and ultimately obesity. It was therefore postulated that energy balance was regulated by a feedback loop in which the body energy stores were sensed by the hypothalamus, which in turn sent signals to control both food intake and energy expenditure. The nature of the signal inputs to the hypothalamus was not clear, however. Jean Mayer proposed a glucostatic theory in which blood glucose was the sensed signal.[144] Kennedy postulated the presence of a fat metabolism factor and proposed what is now accepted as the lipostatic theory.[145] In this model, a signal coming from the fat stores in the adipose tissue is read by the central nervous system to regulate feeding and energy homeostasis. Subsequent parabiosis studies performed by Hervey confirmed that blood-borne signals were coming from the adipose tissue and regulated food intake and body weight.[146] Not too long afterward, Coleman performed the seminal parabiosis studies using single-gene models of obesity and diabetes (*ob/ob* and *db/db* mice) and concluded that the product of the *ob* gene was secreted by the adipose tissue, transported by the blood, and received in the hypothalamus by the receptor encoded by the *db* gene.[147] The interaction between a factor produced by the adipose tissue and a receptor in the hypothalamus in turn triggers a cascade of nervous and endocrine signals controlling food intake and energy expenditure. This sum of evidence became the foundation for Leibel and colleagues to undertake the positional cloning effort of the *ob* and *db* genes leading to the publication of the discovery of leptin in *Nature* in 1994[1] and of its receptor in *Cell* 1 year later.[148]

ADIPOCYTE-SECRETED PROTEINS

Since the discovery of leptin, the simple paradigm of adipose tissue as a fat storage tank has evolved into a complex paradigm. First, the size of the adipose tissue not only is controlled by the filling of preexisting adipocytes, but also involves finely tuned mechanisms that control differentiation and apoptosis of the tissue. Second, adipose tissue depots are multipotential secretory organs with different secretory capacities for different depots. These adipose tissues are composed mostly of adipocytes but also of fibroblasts and immune cells such as macrophages and mast cells, which all use endocrine, paracrine, and autocrine pathways to secrete multiple bioactive proteins called *adipokines* or *adipocytokines*. The adipocytes respond to various stimuli such as circulating hormones, circulating metabolites, neural input, and cellular energy signals by releasing hormones and substrates as shown in Figure 53-5.[2,149] The molecular revolution brought to light many adipocyte-secreted factors, some of which are secreted into the bloodstream, such as interleukin-6 (IL-6) and leptin, whereas others, such as TNF-α, exert their effects in an autocrine-paracrine fashion.[150] Although adipose tissue has a similar histologic appearance throughout the body, it is now obvious that there are fundamental regional differences in the quality and the amount of adipokines secreted by these different depots.

A major emphasis in adipose tissue biology research is the understanding of the molecular mechanisms that control the secretion of adipokines by different depots and their implication in a variety of chronic diseases. These secreted proteins have been recently grouped in molecules that regulate physiologic and pathophysiologic functions such as the following[2]:

- Energy homeostasis (leptin, adiponectin, etc.)
- Innate immune system (TNF-α, IL-6, etc.)
- Vasculature (VEGF, monobutyrin, ESM-1, etc.)
- Acute phase reactant response (α_1 acid glycoprotein, SAA3, PTX-3, etc.)
- Molecules involved in lipoprotein metabolism, such as LPL or components of extracellular matrix (type VI collagen)
- Recruitment of immune cells (MCP-1)

In this chapter, we have chosen to present the current knowledge on only four of these adipokines: leptin, adiponectin, resistin, and TNF-α. As Figure 53-6 shows, these four adipokines are involved in whole-body metabolism, since they act on

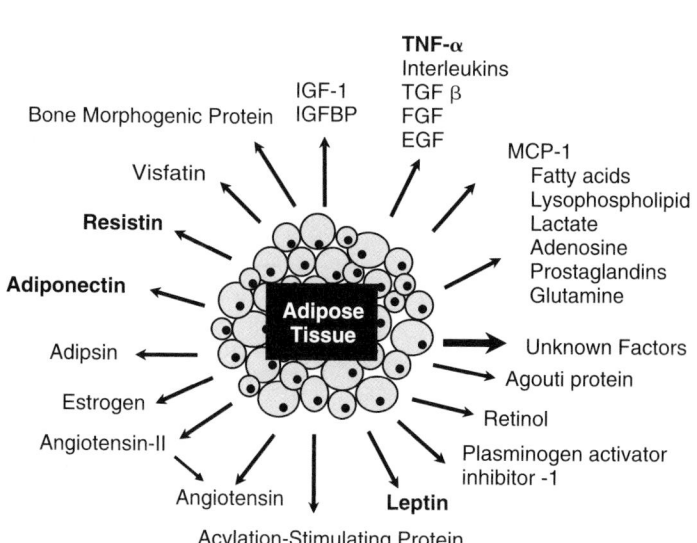

Figure 53-5 Proteins secreted by the adipose tissue. Adipose tissue is an endocrine gland that secretes numerous factors, many of which are implicated in affecting energy homeostasis, insulin sensitivity, and nutrient sensing pathways (see text for details).

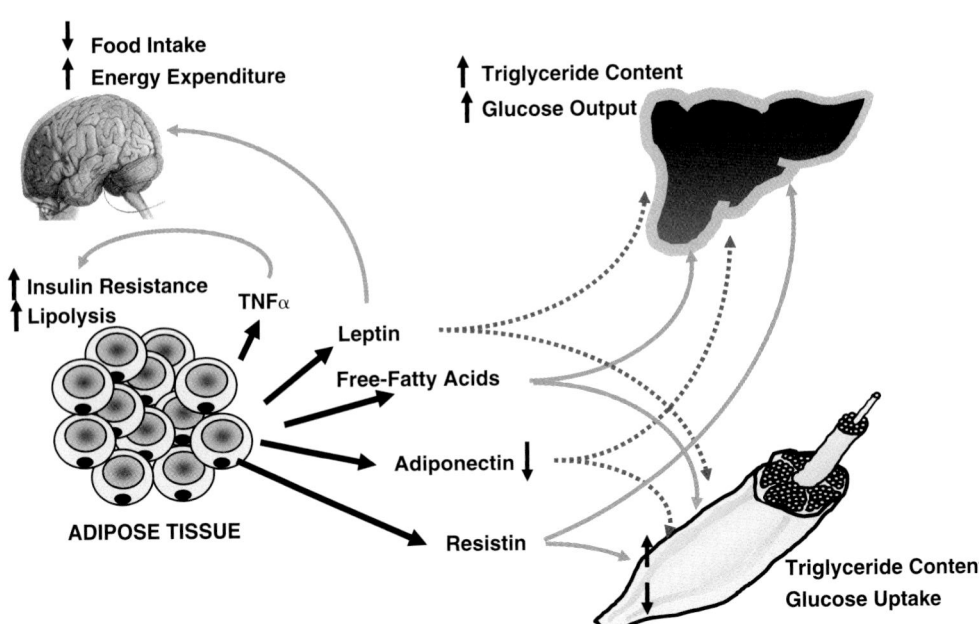

Figure 53-6 Central role of adipose tissue in the insulin-resistance syndrome. The production by the adipocytes of substrates such as free fatty acid hormones such as leptin, adiponectin, and resistin and cytokines such as TNF-α positions the adipocyte as a central mediator of the insulin-resistant syndrome in obese individuals. In response to weight gain, free fatty acids, leptin, resistin, and TNF-α are all increased, whereas adiponectin concentration is decreased. These changes affect the insulin sensitivity of skeletal muscle and liver and the central nervous system control of energy expenditure and food intake. Positive feedbacks are shown by solid arrows, whereas negative feedbacks are shown by dotted arrows. (Source: Adapted from Farmer SR, Deepanwita P: Role of the adipocyte in type 2 diabetes. In Alberti KGM, DeFronzo RA, Keen H, Zimmet P (eds): International Textbook of Diabetes Mellitus, 3rd ed. Chichester, UK, John Wiley & Sons, Ltd, 2004.)

different tissues, including the brain, the liver, the skeletal muscle, and the adipose tissue itself.

LEPTIN

Leptin is a highly conserved 16-kDa hormone that is secreted principally but not exclusively by adipocytes that act both centrally and peripherally. Plasma leptin concentrations are positively correlated with body fat mass.[151] Leptin crosses the blood-brain barrier by a saturable active transport system and serves as a signal to the central nervous system originating in the adipose tissue. Even if this was first described as the hormone-regulating energy balance, the available data now suggest that a relative lack of leptin or resistance to its action is probably not the cause of most cases of human obesity. The main biologic function of leptin seems to be the maintenance of a minimum level of energy stores during periods of caloric restriction.[152,153] Low leptin concentration can therefore be seen as a "starvation signal" when energy stores become insufficient, commanding the body to seek food and become thrifty. As part of such a protective mechanism, leptin plays a role in reproduction, angiogenesis, and immune function and may influence processes such as β-cell insulin secretion, carbohydrate transport, and platelet aggregation.[154] Low levels of circulating leptin trigger strong biologic responses to protect the organism against the deleterious effect of starvation, whereas high levels of leptin (as seen in obesity) engender rather weak biologic responses.[152] This is illustrated in Figure 53-7A. Studies of caloric restriction in animals and humans provide information regarding the importance of leptin as a mediator of neuroendocrine responses. Shimokawa and Higami have reviewed the endocrine changes associated with short-term caloric deprivation in rodent models.[155] Many of these alterations have been described in humans as well and include a fall in T_3,[156] an increase in cortisol secretion,[157] and a decrease in gonadal function.[153] It has long been hypothesized that the neuroendocrine system coordinates and integrates some of the antiaging actions of calorie restriction.[158–161] In a 48-hour prolonged starvation study in mice, Ahima and coworkers provided evidence that the reduction in leptin with starvation caused a decrease in the activity of the gonadal and thyroid axes and an increase in the activity of the adrenal axis.[153] The changes in activity of these axes during fasting were prevented by leptin administration, suggesting that leptin is a master regulator of the neuroendocrine

system and possibly the endocrine candidate of the "disposable soma theory" of aging stating that longevity requires investment in somatic maintenance by reducing the resources that are available for reproduction[155,162] (see Fig. 53-7B).

In the obese state in which the circulating leptin concentration is already high, the hormone is a rather weak signal to prevent overconsumption of food and does not appear to be

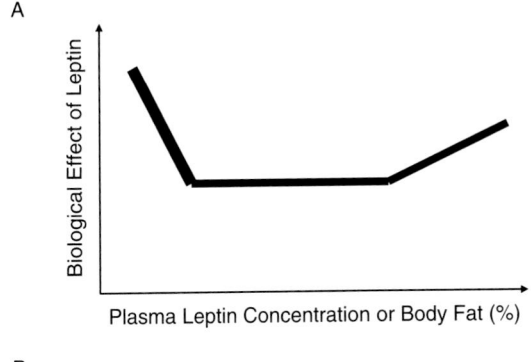

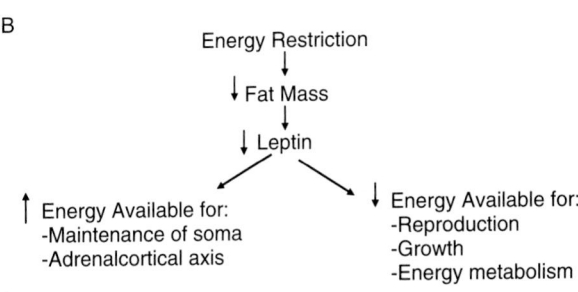

Figure 53-7 Leptin as the master neuroendocrine signal. **A,** The biological responses to changes in body energy stores and circulating leptin concentration seem much more robust when plasma leptin concentration decreases than when it increases.[152] Leptin's main function may be to provide the appropriate metabolic responses to decreased energy stores (by acting to increase feeding and by sparing energy/fat expenditure) rather than protecting the body against excess energy stores (i.e., by increasing energy/fat expenditure and decreasing food intake). **B,** The role of leptin as a master regulator of neuroendocrine pathways involved in response to the effects of caloric restriction. It is probably a major signal for the antiaging effects of dietary restriction.[155]

a viable treatment for obesity.[163] However, if it is provided in sufficient amount in obese individuals or to organisms that are deficient in circulating leptin, injection of the hormone can reduce body weight and fat mass by decreasing food intake and increasing energy expenditure. The mechanism by which leptin seems to exert its peripheral metabolic effects is by activating 5'-AMP-activated protein kinase (AMPK) in muscle and liver.[164,165] As a consequence of AMPK activation, adenosine triphosphate (ATP)-consuming anabolic pathways are inhibited, whereas ATP-producing catabolic pathways are activated. The activated mechanisms include glucose transport, β-oxidation, glycolysis, and mitochondrial biogenesis. The relevance of leptin in normal human metabolic function is provided by leptin replacement in individuals with genetic leptin deficiency,[166] deficiency due to weight loss,[167] or lipodystrophy.[168] The effects of recombinant leptin therapy in children with congenital leptin deficiency was investigated and clearly showed a spectacular effect on reducing food intake and body weight but almost no effect on energy expenditure and fat oxidation.[166] In adult patients with a similar congenital deficiency, leptin replacement not only affected food intake but also prevented the drop in energy expenditure that is usually observed with weight loss and increased 24-hour fat oxidation by more than three times.[169]

Human immunodeficiency virus (HIV) and HIV therapy are also associated with alterations in body composition, including lipoatrophy, lipid storage as abdominal adipose tissue, or buffalo hump.[170] The constellation of metabolic findings in these patients is consistent with the "ectopic fat storage" hypothesis as presented earlier. Several studies suggest that activation and rebound of the immune system during antiretroviral therapy are associated with lipodystrophy.[171,172] Molecular studies demonstrate multiple alterations in adipose tissue transcription factors (PPAR-γ and SREBP1/ADD) and an increase in mRNA for TNF-α[173] as well as an increase in expression of genes that are typically associated with lymphocytes in adipose tissue.[174] Combined with data showing that the metabolic alterations in HIV-associated lipodystrophy are highly correlated with the blood levels of the soluble TNF receptor (sTNF-RII),[172] this suggests that an inflammatory milieu inhibits adipocyte differentiation. Alternatively, direct effects of protease inhibitors on transcription factor transport into the nucleus may play a role.[175] This is analogous to defects seen in congenital partial lipodystrophy that are due to mutations in the Lamin A/C gene.[176-178] There is also evidence of increased apoptosis in adipose tissue from HIV lipodystrophy patients.[179] Finally, mitochondrial mutations and reduced mitochondrial number in the adipose tissue may contribute to the overall dyslipidemic and insulin-resistant state of these patients.[180]

ADIPONECTIN

Adiponectin (also known as AdipoQ, Acrp30, APM1, and GBP28) is expressed exclusively in adipose tissue[181] and circulates in human serum at very high concentrations of 5 to 30 nM.[182] Adiponectin, a 30-kDa protein consisting of a N-terminal collagenous domain and a C-terminal globular domain, was discovered almost simultaneously by four separate groups using different methods.[181,183-185] Adiponectin exists in the blood in monomer, trimer, hexamer, and very high-molecular-weight forms.[186] This protein is closely related to complement factor Cq1,[183] but the folded crystal structure and gene organization show close similarity to TNF-α.[187,188] Arguably, the most interesting observation is that unlike other adipocytokines whose expression increases with increasing fat mass, adiponectin is inversely related to fat mass.[189-191] How does increased mass of the tissue from which the gene is expressed reduce expression and/or secretion of the protein? Many scientists are currently focusing on answering this important question. Consistent with the observation that lipodystrophic patients have very low concentrations of adiponectin[192] and increased ectopic fat, a reduction in circulating adiponectin (as well as leptin) may facilitate the ectopic storage of fat.

Adiponectin is clearly an insulin-sensitizing hormone, and administration of recombinant adiponectin in rodents increases glucose uptake and fat oxidation in muscle, reduces fatty acid uptake and hepatic glucose production in liver, and improves whole-body insulin resistance. Two receptors for adiponectin have been recently discovered, the first isoform (AdipoR1) being expressed mostly in skeletal muscle and the second (AdipoR2) mostly in liver.[193] Unlike in mice, gene expression profiling in humans indicate that both isoforms are highly expressed in skeletal muscle.[194] Interestingly, in individuals with normal glucose tolerance, muscle expression levels of AdipoR1 and AdipoR2 were lower in subjects with a family history of type 2 diabetes when compared to those without family history, and the expression level of both receptors correlated positively with insulin sensitivity.[194] These data indicate that both isoforms of the receptor may play a role in the insulin-sensitizing effect of adiponectin.

Even if the signaling cascade for adiponectin is unclear, there is growing evidence that adiponectin may activate AMPK, the putative master metabolic regulator described above. Thus, excitement surrounds the potential for adiponectin (or mimetics of adiponectin) to represent pharmacologic agents for patients suffering from insulin resistance and type 2 diabetes. As for leptin, many functions have already been attributed to adiponectin: It has been linked to cardiovascular disease and endothelial and immune dysfunctions.[195] However, we will here focus mostly on the role of adiponectin as an insulin-sensitizing hormone.

Adiponectin acts peripherally to improve insulin sensitivity in rodents,[196-199] although the proposed mechanisms differ. Combs and coworkers found that increasing circulating adiponectin concentrations in mice during a euglycemic clamp increased the rate of glucose infusion by 73%.[200] The rates of glucose uptake, glycolysis, and glycogen synthesis were unchanged, but the rate of glucose production was suppressed 65%. Chronic infusion of a proteolytic product of adiponectin prevents weight gain in mice that are fed a high-fat diet, whereas mice that were infused with full-length adiponectin or saline gained weight.[196] The prevention of weight gain was associated with increased fat oxidation. The same investigators went on to show that adiponectin induces fatty acid oxidation in muscle in vitro and reduces free fatty acid flux following a high-fat meal or intralipid infusion in vivo.[196] Similarly, Yamauchi and coworkers observed that adiponectin treatment during high-fat feeding prevents adipose tissue deposition in wild-type mice by increasing energy expenditure and decreasing ectopic fat deposition.[197] To determine the cellular mechanisms underlying this observation, they measured the expression of genes involved in fatty acid transport, oxidation, and energy dissipation in both muscle and liver. Adiponectin treatment increased the mRNA of genes involved in fatty acid uptake and β-oxidation (specifically, CD36, acyl-CoA oxidase, and uncoupling protein-2) in muscle and decreased the expression of genes involved in fatty acid transport in the liver, resulting in decreased storage of triglycerides in nonadipose tissues and indirectly improved insulin sensitivity. Taken together, the results support the theory that adiponectin is a regulator of insulin sensitivity through the reduction of ectopic fat deposition.

Like leptin, adiponectin was shown to directly activate adenosine 5'-monophosphate-activated protein kinase (AMPK) in muscle, thereby increasing the phosphorylation of acetyl coenzyme A (CoA) carboxylase (ACC).[199] In turn, malonyl CoA content is reduced, increasing carnitine palmitoyltransferase 1 (CPT-1) activity and stimulating fat oxidation. In the liver, AMPK stimulates fatty acid oxidation and ketogenesis, inhibits cholesterol synthesis, lipogenesis, and triglyceride synthesis whereas it modulates insulin secretion in pancreatic β-cells (reviewed by Winder and Hardie[201]).

Human studies in Pima Indians and Japanese demonstrated an association between low plasma adiponectin concentrations and obesity or type 2 diabetes.[189,191] Furthermore, positive correlations between plasma adiponectin concentrations and insulin sensitivity have been reported in several studies.[190,191,202] More important, low adiponectin concentrations are predictive of type 2 diabetes incidence rates over a 5-year follow-up in Pima Indians.[203] Other indicators that low levels of adiponectin may be involved in the development of insulin resistance are derived from intervention studies showing that adiponectin is decreased by behaviors leading to obesity and diabetes[197] and increased in situations of reduced body fat or increased insulin sensitivity.[204,205]

At present, adiponectin remains a validated target for the potential treatment of insulin resistance and type 2 diabetes. However, many questions regarding adiponectin remain to be resolved before the use of adiponectin (or mimetics) can be contemplated as therapeutic agents. These include (1) which circulating form of adiponectin is biologically active, (2) what the posttranslational mechanisms are that regulate adiponectin concentration/secretion, (3) what the exact sites of action of adiponectin are in central and peripheral tissues, (4) what the signaling cascade of adiponectin is after binding to its receptor.

RESISTIN

Resistin is a putative adipocyte-derived "insulin resistance" hormone that was identified during an in vitro screen for genes upregulated during adipocyte differentiation and downregulated by PPAR-γ agonists.[206] In mice, serum resistin and resistin mRNA expression in adipose tissue are increased by a high-fat diet and decreased after rosiglitazone treatment.[206] Importantly, blocking resistin (by specific antibodies) increases glucose uptake in fat cells and increased insulin sensitivity. In vitro, resistin decreases glucose uptake in skeletal muscle cells but does not affect the classic insulin-signaling pathways.[207] As was expected from these results, intraperitoneal administration of resistin increased blood glucose following a glucose tolerance test in mice.[206] Taken together, these results led to the hypothesis that resistin promotes insulin resistance. At about the same time, two other groups independently identified resistin.[208,209] Kim and coworkers[208] observed that resistin inhibited adipocyte differentiation in 3T3-L1 cells, a result suggesting that resistin might promote insulin resistance by increasing storage of triglycerides in muscle and liver instead of adipose tissue. Resistin-deficient mice have low blood glucose after a fast, decreased hepatic glucose production, and less hyperglycemia when obese, suggesting a key role in the regulation of hepatic glucose production.[210]

In humans, the role of resistin in regulating insulin sensitivity is unclear. In one study, serum resistin was related to fat mass in young, healthy subjects and was significantly higher in women than in men[211] but was not related to body mass index (BMI), percentage of body fat, or insulin sensitivity in other studies.[212,213] Resistin mRNA expression was shown to be higher in morbidly obese subjects compared with lean control subjects[214] and higher in individuals with a promoter mutation and high levels of oxidative stress.[215] However, in that same study, serum resistin was not different between nonobese, obese, or obese diabetic groups. Previous studies in mice have shown that resistin administration impairs whole-body insulin sensitivity.[206] Rajala and coworkers, however, observed that this was the result of impaired hepatic insulin sensitivity rather than peripheral insulin resistance.[216]

TNF-α

TNF-α is a cytokine that is produced by macrophages, monocytes, endothelial cells, neutrophils, smooth muscle cells, activated lymphocytes, astrocytes, and adipocytes.[217] TNF-α has a variety of functions, such as mediating expression of genes for growth factors, cytokines, transcription factors, and receptors. TNF-α is synthesized as a 26-kDa transmembrane protein that is found on the surface or processed to release the 17-kDa soluble form.[218] Some adipocytokines are secreted and transported into the blood (i.e., leptin, PAI-1, and IL-6), whereas TNF-α is secreted and probably acts locally in an autocrine-paracrine fashion.[150]

Initial reports implicated TNF-α as an adipocyte-derived cytokine that was able to block adipocyte differentiation[219,220] and upregulated in human obesity/insulin resistance.[221,222] As a pluripotent cytokine, the mechanisms by which TNF-α might decrease insulin action and affect adipocyte functioning are numerous. As one example, TNF-α suppresses adipocyte-specific genes with NF-κB being an obligatory signaling intermediate[223] and decreases the expression of transcription factors necessary for adipocyte differentiation.[219] In an autocrine-paracrine fashion, TNF-α blocks further energy accumulation in adipocytes through deactivation of the insulin-signaling pathway (i.e., insulin resistance),[223,224] increased lipolysis, and decreased lipid uptake.[225] TNF-α may be a homeostatic mechanism that might prevent further fat deposition by regulating LPL activity and leptin production.[226]

TNF-α has been termed an *adipostat* because its adipose tissue expression is, like leptin, more or less proportional to the degree of adiposity. TNF-α has also been proposed to link obesity with insulin resistance, serine phosphorylation of the insulin receptor substrate-1 being a prominent mechanism for TNF-α-induced insulin resistance.[227] TNF-α increases 11β HSD1 mRNA and enzyme activity and therefore local cortisol production in human adipocytes,[228] potentially linking TNF-α to visceral adiposity. The mechanism by which transcription is upregulated during energy excess is not entirely clear. Insulin upregulates TNF-α mRNA, and TZDs appear to downregulate TNF-α,[229] whereas environmental toxins (such as TCCD) upregulate TNF-α.[230]

Clinically, higher plasma levels of TNF-α are also associated with insulin resistance, higher BMI, higher fasting glucose levels, and higher low-density lipoprotein (LDL)-C levels.[231] By using confirmatory factor analysis and structural equation modeling, it was shown that obesity, dyslipidemia, and TNF-α were the principal explanatory variables for the various components of the metabolic syndrome.[232] TNF-α has also been implicated in HIV-associated lipodystrophy.[233]

ADIPOSE TISSUE AS AN INFLAMMATORY ORGAN IN OBESITY AND INSULIN RESISTANCE

Studies of murine adipocyte differentiation revealed an intermediate developmental phenotype between the preadipocyte and the adipocyte that Cousin and coworkers termed the *adipiphage*, a cell that is intermediate between the adipocyte and a macrophage.[234] This relationship is not surprising in light of the similarities in the transcription and gene expression profiles between the two cell types. The macrophage is responsible for consuming extracellular bacteria, cellular debris, and lipids, whereas the adipocyte is responsible for internalizing and sequestering lipids. As was noted above, the adipocyte produces inflammatory adipocytokines, marking another similarity between adipocytes and macrophages. Two recent studies in mice and humans suggest that adipose tissue contains not only adipocytes and supporting cells, but also macrophages.[235,236] The macrophages appear to be the major site of TNF-α secretion and may also secrete other cytokines, such as IL-8,[237,238] an atherogenic cytokine that is produced in adipose tissue. These studies also suggested that the bone marrow was the major site of origin for the adipose tissue macrophages, suggesting that obesity and diabetes might recruit these cells through the production of one or more chemokines.[239] The significance of the inflammatory cells is that they are likely to activate the NF-κB signaling cascade, such as TNF-α. Iκκ-β, the upstream activator of NF-κB signaling, plays a key role in insulin signaling and is necessary for the full expression of the insulin-resistant phenotype in the obese *ob/ob* mouse.[240] Upstream activators of this pathway include not only TNF-α, but also fatty acids[241] and bacterial lipopolysaccharide. Fatty acids activate this pathway via the Toll-receptor 4, which also responds to lipopolysaccharide.[241] In vivo studies in mice[240] and humans[242] demonstrate that salicylates, inhibitors of the Iκκ-β pathway,[243] play an important therapeutic role in insulin resistance and diabetes,[244] in part through adipocyte-mediated pathways.[223,245] The antidiabetic PPAR-γ ligands (e.g., TZDs) also decrease the gene transcriptional effects of the Iκκ-β pathway.[246]

THE ADIPOCYTE AS A TARGET FOR THE TREATMENT OF OBESITY AND TYPE 2 DIABETES

The brain serves as the main therapeutic target for the treatment of obesity. Given the central role of the adipocyte in the regulation of body weight and energy metabolism, the adipocyte should not be discarded as a target. Classic adipocyte biology, emphasizing the adrenergic-signaling systems, provided the rationale for the development of β₃-adrenoreceptor agonists as a means to increase energy expenditure in muscle and promote lipolysis in adipose tissue. These efforts have been hampered by the failure of the drug discovery systems to identify "clean" β-3 selective agonists.[247] Alternative lipolytic systems, such as the activation of the growth hormone receptor, blockade of the antilipolytic α₂-adrenergic receptor, or activation of the recently discovered natriuretic peptide-signaling pathway, may provide alternative strategies for increasing adipose tissue lipolysis. Increasing lipolysis and lipid delivery to peripheral tissue will produce weight loss only in the presence of increased energy expenditure or fat oxidation in liver and skeletal muscle. The concern with this approach is whether the increased lipid supply to liver and skeletal muscle will produce or exacerbate ectopic fat and insulin resistance.

Another avenue to affect insulin action might be to increase lipid storage in adipose by recruiting "new" adipocytes from preadipocytes. At first, this approach might seem counterintuitive, since body weight is likely to increase. The effectiveness of the antidiabetic TZDs in animals and humans provide a strong rationale for this approach. In humans and animals, TZDs increase lipid storage in adipose tissue, decrease free fatty acids prior to an improvement in insulin action, and reduce hepatic and skeletal muscle fat. Such data suggest that sequestration of lipid in newly recruited or existing adipocytes away from liver and muscle might be an effective therapeutic strategy. Unfortunately, the weight gain that occurs in this setting makes this approach less attractive to patients.

Recent studies suggest that angiogenesis might precede and drive adipogenesis.[248] It is logical that adipose tissue might need nutrients and oxygen to develop properly. However, the opposite concept, namely, that antiangiogenic agents might prevent weight gain or result in weight loss, has not yet been demonstrated in animals.

The secretion of potent endocrine hormones from adipose tissue is another approach to treat insulin resistance or obesity. As an example, antidiabetic thiazolidinediones upregulate the expression of the insulin-sensitizing hormone adiponectin and increase blood concentrations up to threefold.[249] Given that body weight is regulated by leptin-dependent and leptin-independent signals and that adipose tissue communicates with the brain to regulate food intake, additional therapeutic targets and therapeutic opportunities are likely.

Exogenous cortisol administration or overproduction of cortisol in conditions such as Cushing's disease increases the accumulation of lipid in visceral depots.[250,251] The local production of cortisol within adipose tissue by conversion of cortisone to bioactive cortisol by the enzyme 11-β-HSD-1 also increases the accumulation of lipid in visceral depots.[103,252,253] Acting through both adipogenic and lipogenic pathways, blockade of the local production of cortisol is likely to reduce visceral adipose tissue mass, and therapeutic agents are currently in preclinical studies.

β₃-Receptor agonists not only increase energy expenditure in rodents, but also increase the number of brown adipocytes.[254,255] It has been suggested that this occurs as a result of transdifferentiation of lipid storing white adipocytes into energy-consuming brown adipocytes. The hallmark of brown adipocyte is the expression of the thermogenic uncoupling protein UCP-1. In rodents, the conversion of white adipocytes into brown adipocytes is under genetic control, and the resulting weight loss improves the features of the metabolic syndrome. Overexpression of the transcriptional factor enhancer PGC-1 in human adipocytes in vitro also increases UCP-1 mRNA and protein and serves as an example of how this might also occur in humans in vivo.[101] Increased energy expenditure and fat oxidation would result in a decrease in body weight, although the potential mechanisms remain elusive.[256,257]

Finally, as was discussed above, once precursor cells are recruited to differentiate into white adipocytes, they are conceptually permanent. Recent studies in vivo in humans suggest that adipocytes are constantly being formed and undergo apoptosis.[58,66] These high turnover rates for adipose tissue suggest that a reduction in adipocyte recruitment and/or an increase in adipocyte apoptosis might lead to a reduction in adipocyte mass. As was noted for the lipolytic pathways, if the excess energy is not completely oxidized, then a possible outcome might be accumulation of lipid in skeletal muscle and liver as occurs in lipodystrophy syndromes. This approach would make sense in the setting of weight loss achieved by other means as a way to reduce the number of lipid storing small adipocytes.

REFERENCES

1. Zhang Y, Proenca R, Maffei M, et al: Positional cloning of the mouse obese gene and its human homologue [see comments]. Nature 372(6505):425–432, 1994. [Published erratum appears in Nature 374(6521):479, 1995.]
2. Rajala MW, Scherer PE: Minireview: The adipocyte: At the crossroads of energy homeostasis, inflammation, and atherosclerosis. Endocrinology 9(144):3765–3773, 2003.
3. Harris MI, Flegal KM, Cowie CC, et al: Prevalence of diabetes, impaired fasting glucose, and impaired glucose tolerance in U.S. adults: The Third National Health and Nutrition Examination Survey, 1988–1994 [see comments]. Diabetes Care 1421:518–524, 1998.
4. Knowler WC, Pettitt DJ, Savage PJ, Bennett PH: Diabetes incidence in Pima Indians: Contributions of obesity and parental diabetes. Am J Epidemiol 2(113):144–156, 1981.
5. Olefsky JM: LIlly lecture 1980. Insulin resistance and insulin action: An in vitro and in vivo perspective. Diabetes 230:148–162, 1981.
6. Reaven GM: Banting lecture 1988: Role of insulin resistance in human disease. Diabetes 1237:1595–1607, 1988.
7. Martin BC, Warram JH, Krolewski AS, et al: Role of glucose and insulin resistance in development of type 2 diabetes mellitus: Results of a 25-year follow-up study [see comments]. Lancet 340(8825):925–929, 1992.
8. Lillioja S, Mott DM, Spraul M, et al: Insulin resistance and insulin secretory dysfunction as precursors of non-insulin-dependent diabetes mellitus:

Prospective studies of Pima Indians. N Engl J Med 27(329):1988–1992, 1993.

9. Boden G, Chen X, Ruiz J, et al: Mechanisms of fatty acid-induced inhibition of glucose uptake. J Clin Invest 693:2438–2446, 1994.

10. Kelley DE, Mokan M, Simoneau JA, Mandarino LJ: Interaction between glucose and free fatty acid metabolism in human skeletal muscle. J Clin Invest 192:91–98, 1993.

11. Roden M, Price TB, Perseghin G, et al: Mechanism of free fatty acid-induced insulin resistance in humans. J Clin Invest 12(97):2859–2865, 1996.

12. Boden G, Chen X: Effects of fat on glucose uptake and utilization in patients with non-insulin-dependent diabetes. J Clin Invest 396:1261–1268, 1995.

13. Randle PJ, Garland PB, Hales CN, et al: The glucose fatty acid cycle: Its role in insulin sensitivity and metabolic disturbances of diabetes mellitus. Lancet 1:7285–7289, 1963.

14. Randle PJ, Garland PB, Newsholme EA, Hales CN: The glucose fatty acid cycle in obesity and maturity onset diabetes mellitus. Ann N Y Acad Sci 1131:324–333, 1965.

15. Wolfe RR: Metabolic interactions between glucose and fatty acids in humans. Am J Clin Nutr 67(3 Suppl):519S–526S, 1998.

16. Baba H, Zhang XJ, Wolfe RR: Glycerol gluconeogenesis in fasting humans. Nutrition 11(2):149–153, 1995.

17. Kelley DE, Goodpaster B, Wing RR, Simoneau JA: Skeletal muscle fatty acid metabolism in association with insulin resistance, obesity, and weight loss. Am J Physiol 6(1277):E1130–E1141, 1999.

18. Kelley DE, Mandarino LJ: Fuel selection in human skeletal muscle in insulin resistance: A reexamination. Diabetes 549:677–683, 2000.

19. Petersen KF, Dufour S, Befroy D, et al: Impaired mitochondrial activity in the insulin-resistant offspring of patients with type 2 diabetes. N Engl J Med 350(7):664–671, 2004.

20. Petersen KF, Befroy D, Dufour S, et al: Mitochondrial dysfunction in the elderly: Possible role in insulin resistance. Science 562(2300):1140–1142, 2003.

21. Shulman GI: Cellular mechanisms of insulin resistance. J Clin Invest 2(106):171–176, 2000.

22. Cortright RN, Azevedo JL Jr, Zhou Q, et al: Protein kinase C modulates insulin action in human skeletal muscle. Am J Physiol Endocrinol Metab 3278:E553–E562, 2000.

23. Itani SI, Zhou Q, Pories WJ, et al: Involvement of protein kinase C in human skeletal muscle insulin resistance and obesity. Diabetes 8(49):1353–1358, 2000.

24. Schmitz-Peiffer C, Browne CL, Oakes ND, et al: Alterations in the expression and cellular localization of protein kinase C isozymes epsilon and theta are associated with insulin resistance in skeletal muscle of the high-fat-fed rat. Diabetes 246:169–178, 1997.

25. Schmitz-Peiffer C, Oakes ND, Browne CL, et al: Reversal of chronic alterations of skeletal muscle protein kinase C from fat-fed rats by BRL-49653. Am J Physiol 5(1273):E915–E921, 1997.

26. Kissebah AH, Krakower GR: Regional adiposity and morbidity. Physiol Rev 474:761–811, 1994.

27. Abate N, Garg A, Peshock RM, et al: Relationships of generalized and regional adiposity to insulin sensitivity in men. J Clin Invest 1(96):88–98, 1995.

28. Goodpaster BH, Thaete FL, Simoneau JA, Kelley DE: Subcutaneous abdominal fat and thigh muscle composition predict insulin sensitivity independently of visceral fat. Diabetes 1046:1579–1585, 1997.

29. Smith SR, Lovejoy JC, Greenway F, et al: Contributions of total body fat, abdominal subcutaneous adipose tissue compartments, and visceral adipose tissue to the metabolic complications of obesity. Metabolism 450:425–435, 2001.

30. Abate N, Garg A, Peshock RM, et al: Relationship of generalized and regional adiposity to insulin sensitivity in men with NIDDM. Diabetes 1245:1684–1693, 1996.

31. Marcus MA, Murphy L, Pi-Sunyer FX, Albu JB: Insulin sensitivity and serum triglyceride level in obese white and black women: Relationship to visceral and truncal subcutaneous fat. Metabolism 248:194–199, 1999.

32. Albu JB, Kovera AJ, Johnson JA: Fat distribution and health in obesity. Ann N Y Acad Sci 904:491–501, 2000.

33. Garg A: Lipodystrophies. Am J Med 108:2143–2152, 2000.

34. Robbins DC, Danforth E Jr, Horton ES, et al: The effect of diet on thermogenesis in acquired lipodystrophy. Metabolism 9(28):908–916, 1979.

35. Robbins DC, Horton ES, Tulp O, Sims EA: Familial partial lipodystrophy: Complications of obesity in the non-obese? Metabolism 531:445–452, 1982.

36. Reitman ML, Mason MM, Moitra J, et al: Transgenic mice lacking white fat: Models for understanding human lipoatrophic diabetes. Ann N Y Acad Sci 892:289–296, 1999.

37. Shimomura I, Hammer RE, Ikemoto S, et al: Leptin reverses insulin resistance and diabetes mellitus in mice with congenital lipodystrophy. Nature 6748401:73–67, 1999.

38. Kim JK, Gavrilova O, Chen Y, et al: Mechanism of insulin resistance in A-ZIP/F-1 fatless mice. J Biol Chem 12275:8456–8460, 2000.

39. Gavrilova O, Marcus-Samuels B, Graham D, et al: Surgical implantation of adipose tissue reverses diabetes in lipoatrophic mice. J Clin Invest 3105:271–278, 2000.

40. Colombo C, Cutson JJ, Yamauchi T, et al: Transplantation of adipose tissue lacking leptin is unable to reverse the metabolic abnormalities associated with lipoatrophy. Diabetes 51(9):2727–2733, 2002.

41. Weber RV, Buckley MC, Fried SK, Kral JG: Subcutaneous lipectomy causes a metabolic syndrome in hamsters. Am J Physiol Regul Integr Comp Physiol 279(3):R936–R943, 2000.

42. Ryysy L, Hakkinen AM, Goto T, et al: Hepatic fat content and insulin action on free fatty acids and glucose metabolism rather than insulin absorption are associated with insulin requirements during insulin therapy in type 2 diabetic patients. Diabetes 549:749–758, 2000.

43. Goodpaster BH, Thaete FL, Kelley DE: Thigh adipose tissue distribution is associated with insulin resistance in obesity and in type 2 diabetes mellitus. Am J Clin Nutr 471:885–892, 2000.

44. McGarry JD: Banting lecture 2001: Dysregulation of fatty acid metabolism in the etiology of type 2 diabetes. Diabetes 151:7–18, 2002.

45. Danforth E Jr: Failure of adipocyte differentiation causes type II diabetes mellitus? Nat Genet 126:13, 2000.

46. Weyer C, Foley JE, Bogardus C, et al: Enlarged subcutaneous abdominal adipocyte size, but not obesity itself, predicts type II diabetes independent of insulin resistance. Diabetologia 43(12):1498–1506, 2000.

47. Adams M, Montague CT, Prins JB, et al: Activators of peroxisome proliferator-activated receptor gamma have depot-specific effects on human preadipocyte differentiation. J Clin Invest 12100:3149–3153, 1997.

48. Akazawa S, Sun F, Ito M, et al: Efficacy of troglitazone on body fat distribution in type 2 diabetes. Diabetes Care 823:1067–1071, 2000.

49. Qi N, Kazdova L, Zidek V, et al: Pharmacogenetic evidence that cd36 is a key determinant of the metabolic effects of pioglitazone. J Biol Chem 277(50):48501–48507, 2002.

50. Mayerson AB, Hundal RS, Dufour S, et al: The effects of rosiglitazone on insulin sensitivity, lipolysis, and hepatic and skeletal muscle triglyceride content in patients with type 2 diabetes. Diabetes 51(3):797–802, 2002.

51. Boden G, Cheung P, Mozzoli M, Fried SK: Effect of thiazolidinediones on glucose and fatty acid metabolism in patients with type 2 diabetes. Metabolism 52(6):753–759, 2003.

52. Noppa H, Bengtsson C, Isaksson B, Smith U: Adipose tissue cellularity in adulthood and its relation to childhood obesity. Int J Obes 4(3):253–263, 1980.

53. Hirsch J, Batchelor B: Adipose tissue cellularity in human obesity. Clin Endocrinol Metab 5(2):299–311, 1976.

54. Stern JS, Batchelor BR, Hollander N, et al: Adipose-cell size and immunoreactive insulin levels in obese and normal-weight adults. Lancet 2(7784):948–951, 1972.

55. Paolisso G, Tataranni PA, Foley JE, et al: A high concentration of fasting plasma non-esterified fatty acids is a risk factor

for the development of NIDDM. Diabetologia 1038:1213–1217, 1995.

56. Weyer C, Wolford JK, Hanson RL, et al: Subcutaneous abdominal adipocyte size, a predictor of type 2 diabetes, is linked to chromosome 1q21–q23 and is associated with a common polymorphism in LMNA in Pima Indians. Mol Genet Metab 72(3):231–238, 2001.

57. Krotkiewski M, Sjostrom L, Bjorntorp P, et al: Adipose tissue cellularity in relation to prognosis for weight reduction. Int J Obes 1(4):395–416, 1977.

58. Strawford A, Antelo F, Christiansen M, Hellerstein MK: Adipose tissue triglyceride turnover, de novo lipogenesis and cell proliferation in humans measured with 2H2O. Am J Physiol Endocrinol Metab 286(4):E577–E588, 2003.

59. Domingo P, Matias-Guiu X, Pujol RM, et al: Subcutaneous adipocyte apoptosis in HIV-1 protease inhibitor-associated lipodystrophy. AIDS 13(16):2261–2267, 1999.

60. Julien P, Despres JP, Angel A: Scanning electron microscopy of very small fat cells and mature fat cells in human obesity. J Lipid Res 30(2):293–299, 1989.

61. Hager A: Adipose cell size and number in relation to obesity. Postgrad Med J 153(Suppl 2):101–110, 1997.

62. Hager A, Sjostrom L, Arvidsson B, et al: Body fat and adipose tissue cellularity in infants: A longitudinal study. Metabolism 26(6):607–614, 1977.

63. Soriguer Escofet FJ, Esteva de Antonio I, Tinahones FJ, Pareja A: Adipose tissue fatty acids and size and number of fat cells from birth to 9 years of age: A cross-sectional study in 96 boys. Metabolism 45(11):1395–1401, 1996.

64. Hauner H, Entenmann G, Wabitsch M, et al: Promoting effect of glucocorticoids on the differentiation of human adipocyte precursor cells cultured in a chemically defined medium. J Clin Invest 84(5):1663–1670, 1989.

65. van Harmelen V, Skurk T, Rohrig K, et al: Effect of BMI and age on adipose tissue cellularity and differentiation capacity in women. Int J Obes Relat Metab Disord 27(8):889–895, 2003.

66. Pilyugin SS, Ganusov VV, Murali-Krishna K, et al: The rescaling method for quantifying the turnover of cell populations. J Theor Biol 225(2):275–283, 2003.

67. Marques BG, Hausman DB, Martin RJ: Association of fat cell size and paracrine growth factors in development of hyperplastic obesity. Am J Physiol 275(6 Pt 2):R1898–R1908, 1998.

68. Johnson PR, Stern JS, Greenwood MR, et al: Effect of early nutrition on adipose cellularity and pancreatic insulin release in the Zucker rat. J Nutr 103(5):738–743, 1973.

69. Salans LB, Cushman SW, Weismann RE: Studies of human adipose tissue: Adipose cell size and number in nonobese and obese patients. J Clin Invest 52(4):929–941, 1973.

70. Sjostrom L, Bjorntorp P: Body composition and adipose cellularity in human obesity. Acta Med Scand 195(3):201–211, 1974.

71. Ravelli GP, Stein ZA, Susser MW: Obesity in young men after famine exposure in utero and early infancy. N Engl J Med 295(7):349–353, 1976.

72. Kirtland J, Gurr MI: Adipose tissue cellularity: A review: 2. The relationship between cellularity and obesity. Int J Obes 3(1):15–55, 1979.

73. Hirsch J: Obesity: Matter over mind? In Nevins JR (ed): Cerebrum: The Dana Forum on Brain Science. New York, Dana Press, 2003, pp 7–18.

74. Rolland-Cachera MF, Deheeger M, Bellisle F, et al: Adiposity rebound in children: A simple indicator for predicting obesity. Am J Clin Nutr 39(1):129–135, 1984.

75. Prokopec M, Bellisle F: Adiposity in Czech children followed from 1 month of age to adulthood: Analysis of individual BMI patterns. Ann Hum Biol 20(6):517–525, 1993.

76. Siervogel RM, Roche AF, Guo SM, et al: Patterns of change in weight/stature from 2 to 18 years: findings from long-term serial data for children in the Fels longitudinal growth study. Int J Obes 15(7):479–485, 1991.

77. Dietz WH: Periods of risk in childhood for the development of adult obesity: What do we need to learn? J Nutr 127(9):1884S–1886S, 1997.

78. Premkumar A, Chow C, Bhandarkar P, et al: Lipoatrophic-lipodystrophic syndromes: The spectrum of findings on MR imaging. Am J Roentgenol 178(2):311–318, 2002.

79. Gimble J, Guilak F: Adipose-derived adult stem cells: Isolation, characterization, and differentiation potential. Cytotherapy 5(5):362–369, 2003.

80. Richardson RL, Hausman GJ, Gaskins HR: Effect of transforming growth factor-beta on insulin-like growth factor 1 and dexamethasone-induced proliferation and differentiation in primary cultures of pig preadipocytes. Acta Anat 145(4):321–326, 1992.

81. Green H, Kehinde O: An established preadipose cell line and its differentiation in culture: II. Factors affecting the adipose conversion. Cell 5(1):19–27, 1975.

82. Green H, Kehinde O: Spontaneous heritable changes leading to increased adipose conversion in 3T3 cells. Cell 7(1):105–113, 1976.

83. Russell TR, Ho R: Conversion of 3T3 fibroblasts into adipose cells: Triggering of differentiation by prostaglandin F2alpha and 1-methyl-3-isobutyl xanthine. Proc Natl Acad Sci U S A 73(12):4516–4520, 1976.

84. Fajas L, Landsberg RL, Huss-Garcia Y, et al: E2Fs regulate adipocyte differentiation. Dev Cell 3(1):39–49, 2002.

85. Janderova L, McNeil M, Murrell AN, et al: Human mesenchymal stem cells as an in vitro model for human adipogenesis. Obes Res 11(1):65–74, 2003.

86. Reusch JE, Colton LA, Klemm DJ: CREB activation induces adipogenesis in 3T3-L1 cells. Mol Cell Biol 20(3):1008–1020, 2000.

87. Tontonoz P, Hu E, Spiegelman BM: Stimulation of adipogenesis in fibroblasts by PPAR gamma 2, a lipid-activated transcription factor. Cell 79(7):1147–1156, 1994.

88. Yu K, Bayona W, Kallen CB, et al: Differential activation of peroxisome proliferator-activated receptors by eicosanoids. J Biol Chem 270(41):23975–23983, 1995.

89. Kliewer SA, Lenhard JM, Willson TM, et al: A prostaglandin J2 metabolite binds peroxisome proliferator-activated receptor gamma and promotes adipocyte differentiation. Cell 83(5):813–819, 1995.

90. Huang JT, Welch JS, Ricote M, et al: Interleukin-4-dependent production of PPAR-gamma ligands in macrophages by 12/15-lipoxygenase. Nature 400(6742):378–382, 1999.

91. Wu Z, Xie Y, Morrison RF, et al: PPARgamma induces the insulin-dependent glucose transporter GLUT4 in the absence of C/EBPalpha during the conversion of 3T3 fibroblasts into adipocytes. J Clin Invest 101(1):22–32, 1998.

92. Baumann CA, Chokshi N, Saltiel AR, Ribon V: Cloning and characterization of a functional peroxisome proliferator activator receptor-gamma-responsive element in the promoter of the CAP gene. J Biol Chem 275(13):9131–9135, 2000.

93. Schoonjans K, Peinado-Onsurbe J, Lefebvre AM, et al: PPARalpha and PPARgamma activators direct a distinct tissue-specific transcriptional response via a PPRE in the lipoprotein lipase gene. EMBO J 15(19):5336–5348, 1996.

94. Picard F, Auwerx J: PPAR(gamma) and glucose homeostasis. Annu Rev Nutr 22:167–197, 2002.

95. Glorian M, Duplus E, Beale EG, et al: A single element in the phosphoenolpyruvate carboxykinase gene mediates thiazolidinedione action specifically in adipocytes. Biochimie 83(10):933–943, 2001.

96. Hamm JK, Park BH, Farmer SR: A role for C/EBPbeta in regulating peroxisome proliferator-activated receptor gamma activity during adipogenesis in 3T3-L1 preadipocytes. J Biol Chem 276(21):18464–18471, 2001.

97. Floyd ZE, Stephens JM: STAT5A promotes adipogenesis in nonprecursor cells and associates with the glucocorticoid receptor during adipocyte differentiation. Diabetes 52(2):308–314, 2003.

98. Tontonoz P, Kim JB, Graves RA, Spiegelman BM: ADD1: A novel helix-loop-helix transcription factor associated with adipocyte determination and differentiation. Mol Cell Biol 13(8):4753–4759, 1993.

99. Tong Q, Dalgin G, Xu H, et al: Function of GATA transcription factors in preadipocyte-adipocyte transition. Science 290(5489):134–138, 2000.

100. Ross SE, Hemati N, Longo KA, et al: Inhibition of adipogenesis by Wnt signaling. Science 289(5481):950–953, 2000.

101. Tiraby C, Tavernier G, Lefort C, et al: Acquirement of brown fat cell features by human white adipocytes. J Biol Chem 278(35):33370–33376, 2003.

102. Picard F, Gehin M, Annicotte J, et al: SRC-1 and TIF2 control energy balance between white and brown adipose tissues. Cell 111(7):931–941, 2002.

103. Bujalska IJ, Kumar S, Stewart PM: Does central obesity reflect "Cushing's disease of the omentum"? Lancet 349(9060):1210–1213, 1997.

104. Smith SR: The endocrinology of obesity. In Bray G (ed): Endocrinology and Metabolism Clinics of North America. Philadelphia, WB Saunders, 1996, pp 921–942.

105. Marin P, Darin N, Amemiya T, et al: Cortisol secretion in relation to body fat distribution in obese premenopausal women. Metabolism 41(8):882–886, 1992.

106. Pasquali R, Cantobelli S, Casimirri F, et al: The hypothalamic-pituitary-adrenal axis in obese women with different patterns of body fat distribution. J Clin Endocrinol Metab 77(2):341–346, 1993.

107. Rosmond R, Chagnon YC, Holm G, et al: A glucocorticoid receptor gene marker is associated with abdominal obesity, leptin, and dysregulation of the hypothalamic-pituitary-adrenal axis. Obes Res 8(3):211–218, 2000.

108. Galton DJ, Bray GA: Studies on lipolysis in human adipose cells. J Clin Invest 46(4):621–629, 1967.

109. Ramsay TG, Chung IB, Czerwinski SM, et al: Tissue IGF-I protein and mRNA responses to a single injection of somatotropin. Am J Physiol 269(4 Pt 1):E627–E635, 1995.

110. Snel YE, Brummer RJ, Doerga ME, et al: Adipose tissue assessed by magnetic resonance imaging in growth hormone-deficient adults: The effect of growth hormone replacement and a comparison with control subjects. Am J Clin Nutr 61(6):1290–1294, 1995.

111. Johannsson G, Marin P, Lonn L, et al: Growth hormone treatment of abdominally obese men reduces abdominal fat mass, improves glucose and lipoprotein metabolism, and reduces diastolic blood pressure [see comments]. J Clin Endocrinol Metab 82(3):727–734, 1997.

112. Heffernan MA, Jiang WJ, Thorburn AW, Ng FM: Effects of oral administration of a synthetic fragment of human growth hormone on lipid metabolism. Am J Physiol Endocrinol Metab 279(3):E501–E507, 2000.

113. Rebuffe-Scrive M, Eldh J, Hafstrom LO, Bjorntorp P: Metabolism of mammary, abdominal, and femoral adipocytes in women before and after menopause. Metabolism 35(9):792–797, 1986.

114. Rebuffe-Scrive M, Lonnroth P, Marin P, et al: Regional adipose tissue metabolism in men and postmenopausal women. Int J Obes 11(4):347–355, 1987.

115. Lindberg UB, Crona N, Silfverstolpe G, et al: Regional adipose tissue metabolism in postmenopausal women after treatment with exogenous sex steroids. Horm Metab Res 22(6):345–351, 1990.

116. Palin SL, McTernan PG, Anderson LA, et al: 17beta-estradiol and anti-estrogen ICI:Compound 182,780 regulate expression of lipoprotein lipase and hormone-sensitive lipase in isolated subcutaneous abdominal adipocytes. Metabolism 52(4):383–388, 2003.

117. Iverius PH, Brunzell JD: Relationship between lipoprotein lipase activity and plasma sex steroid level in obese women. J Clin Invest 82(3):1106–1112, 1988.

118. Price TM, O'Brien SN, Welter BH, et al: Estrogen regulation of adipose tissue lipoprotein lipase: Possible mechanism of body fat distribution. Am J Obstet Gynecol 178(1 Pt 1):101–107, 1998.

119. Marin P, Krotkiewski M, Bjorntorp P: Androgen treatment of middle-aged, obese men: effects on metabolism, muscle and adipose tissues. Eur J Med 1(6):329–336, 1992.

120. Marin P, Oden B, Bjorntorp P: Assimilation and mobilization of triglycerides in subcutaneous abdominal and femoral adipose tissue in vivo in men: Effects of androgens. J Clin Endocrinol Metab 80(1):239–243, 1995.

121. Anderson LA, McTernan PG, Barnett AH, Kumar S: The effects of androgens and estrogens on preadipocyte proliferation in human adipose tissue: Influence of gender and site. J Clin Endocrinol Metab 86(10):5045–5051, 2001.

122. Dieudonne MN, Pecquery R, Leneveu MC, Giudicelli Y: Opposite effects of androgens and estrogens on adipogenesis in rat preadipocytes: evidence for sex and site-related specificities and possible involvement of insulin-like growth factor 1 receptor and peroxisome proliferator-activated receptor gamma2. Endocrinology 141(2):649–656, 2000.

123. Price TM, O'Brien SN: Determination of estrogen receptor messenger ribonucleic acid (mRNA) and cytochrome P450 aromatase mRNA levels in adipocytes and adipose stromal cells by competitive polymerase chain reaction amplification. J Clin Endocrinol Metab 77(4):1041–1045, 1993.

124. Mizutani T, Nishikawa Y, Adachi H, et al: Identification of estrogen receptor in human adipose tissue and adipocytes. J Clin Endocrinol Metab 78(4):950–954, 1994.

125. Pedersen SB, Fuglsig S, Sjogren P, Richelsen B: Identification of steroid receptors in human adipose tissue. Eur J Clin Invest 26(12):1051–1056, 1996.

126. Pedersen SB, Hansen PS, Lund S, et al: Identification of oestrogen receptors and oestrogen receptor mRNA in human adipose tissue. Eur J Clin Invest 26(4):262–269, 1996.

127. Crandall DL, Busler DE, Novak TJ, et al: Identification of estrogen receptor beta RNA in human breast and abdominal subcutaneous adipose tissue. Biochem Biophys Res Commun 248(3):523–526, 1998.

128. Pedersen SB, Bruun JM, Hube F, et al: Demonstration of estrogen receptor subtypes alpha and beta in human adipose tissue: Influences of adipose cell differentiation and fat depot localization. Mol Cell Endocrinol 182(1):27–37, 2001.

129. Arner P: Free fatty acids: Do they play a central role in type 2 diabetes? Diabetes Obes Metab 3(Suppl 1):11–19, 2001.

130. Youngstrom TG, Bartness TJ: Catecholaminergic innervation of white adipose tissue in Siberian hamsters. Am J Physiol 268(3 Pt 2):R744–R751, 1995.

131. Cousin B, Casteilla L, Lafontan M, et al: Local sympathetic denervation of white adipose tissue in rats induces preadipocyte proliferation without noticeable changes in metabolism. Endocrinology 133(5):2255–2262, 1993.

132. Jones DD, Ramsay TG, Hausman GJ, Martin RJ: Norepinephrine inhibits rat pre-adipocyte proliferation. Int J Obes Relat Metab Disord 16(5):349–354, 1992.

133. Hodgson AJ, Abolhasan P, Kubbinga A, Llewellyn-Smith IJ: Sympathetic control of pacemaker adipocytes. Int J Obes 26(Suppl 1):A659, 2002.

134. Summers SA, Whiteman EL, Birnbaum MJ: Insulin signaling in the adipocyte. Int J Obes Relat Metab Disord 24(Suppl 4):S67–S70, 2000.

135. Kahn BB, Flier JS: Obesity and insulin resistance. J Clin Invest 106(4):473–481, 2000.

136. Langin D, Lucas S, Lafontan M: Millennium fat-cell lipolysis reveals unsuspected novel tracks. Horm Metab Res 32(11–12):443–452, 2000.

137. Arner P, Hoffstedt J: Adrenoceptor genes in human obesity. J Intern Med 245(6):667–672, 1999.

138. Sengenes C, Bouloumie A, Hauner H, et al: Involvement of a cGMP-dependent pathway in the natriuretic peptide-mediated hormone-sensitive lipase phosphorylation in human adipocytes. J Biol Chem 278(49):48617–48626, 2003.

139. Moro C, Crampes F, Sengenes C, et al: Atrial natriuretic peptide contributes to the physiological control of lipid mobilization in humans. FASEB J 2004 (in press).

140. Rubner M: Die Quelle der thierischen Warme. Ztschr Biol 30:73–142, 1894.

141. Adolph E: Urges to eat and drink in rats. Am J Physiol 151:110–125, 1947.

142. Hervey GR: Regulation of energy balance. Nature 222:629–631, 1969.

143. Brobeck J: Mechanism of the development of obesity in animals with hypothalamic lesions. Physiol Rev 25:541–559, 1946.

144. Mayer J: Regulation of energy intake and the body weight: The glucostatic theory and the lipostatic hypothesis. Ann N Y Acad Sci 163:15–43, 1955.

145. Kennedy GC: The role of depot fat in the hypothalamic control of food intake in the rat. Proc R Soc Lond B Biol Sci 901140:578–596, 1953.

146. Hervey GR: The effects of lesions in the hypothalamus in parabiotic rats. J Physiol 2145:336–352, 1959.

147. Coleman DL: Effects of parabiosis of obese with diabetes and normal mice. Diabetologia 19739(4):294–298, .

148. Tartaglia LA, Dembski M, Weng X, et al: Identification and expression cloning of a leptin receptor, OB-R. Cell 83(7):1263–1271, 1995.

149. Heilbronn LK, Smith SR, Ravussin E: The insulin-sensitizing role of the fat derived hormone adiponectin. Curr Pharm Des 9(17):1411–1418, 2003.

150. Mohamed–Ali V, Goodrick S, Rawesh A, et al: Subcutaneous adipose tissue releases interleukin-6, but not tumor necrosis factor-alpha, in vivo. J Clin Endocrinol Metab (1282):4196–4200, 1997.

151. Maffei M, Halaas J, Ravussin E, et al: Leptin levels in human and rodent: measurement of plasma leptin and ob RNA in obese and weight-reduced subjects. Nat Med (111):1155–1161, 1995.

152. Leibel RL: The role of leptin in the control of body weight. Nutr Rev (10 Pt 2 60):S15–S9; discussion: S68–S84, S85–S87, 2002.

153. Ahima RS, Prabakaran D, Mantzoros C, et al: Role of leptin in the neuroendocrine response to fasting. Nature (6588382):250–252, 1996.

154. Huang L, Li C: Leptin: A multifunctional hormone. Cell Res (210):81–92, 2000.

155. Shimokawa I, Higami Y: Leptin and anti-aging action of caloric restriction. J Nutr Health Aging (15):43–48, 2001.

156. Roti E, Minelli R, Salvi M: Thyroid hormone metabolism in obesity. Int J Obes Relat Metab Disord (24 Suppl 2):S113–S115, 2000.

157. Fichter MM, Pirke KM, Holsboer F: Weight loss causes neuroendocrine disturbances: experimental study in healthy starving subjects. Psychiatry Res 1(17):61–72, 1986.

158. Everitt AV, Seedsman NJ, Jones F: The effects of hypophysectomy and

159. Meites J: Evidence that underfeeding acts via the neuroendocrine system to influence aging processes. Prog Clin Biol Res (287):169–180, 1989.

160. Masoro EJ: Food restriction in rodents: An evaluation of its role in the study of aging. J Gerontol (343):B59–B64, 1988.

161. Nelson JF: Neuroendocrine involvement in the retardation of aging by food restriction: A hypothesis. In Yu BP (ed): Modulation of Aging Processes by Dietary Restriction. Boca Raton, FL, CRC Press, 1994, pp 37–55.

162. Kirkwood TB: Evolution of ageing. Nature 5635270:301–304, 1977.

163. Heymsfield SB, Greenberg AS, Fujioka K, et al: Recombinant leptin for weight loss in obese and lean adults: A randomized, controlled, dose-escalation trial. JAMA 16282:1568–1575, 1999.

164. Minokoshi Y, Kim Y, Peroni O, et al: Leptin stimulates fatty-acid oxidation by activating AMP-activated protein kinase. Nature 415:339–343, 2002.

165. Minokoshi Y, Kahn BB: Role of AMP-activated protein kinase in leptin-induced fatty acid oxidation in muscle. Biochem Soc Trans 131:196–201, 2003.

166. Farooqi IS, Jebb SA, Langmack G, et al: Effects of recombinant leptin therapy in a child with congenital leptin deficiency. N Engl J Med 12341:879–884, 1999.

167. Rosenbaum M, Murphy EM, Heymsfield SB, et al: Low dose leptin administration reverses effects of sustained weight-reduction on energy expenditure and circulating concentrations of thyroid hormones. J Clin Endocrinol Metab 587:2391–2394, 2002.

168. Petersen KF, Oral EA, Dufour S, et al: Leptin reverses insulin resistance and hepatic steatosis in patients with severe lipodystrophy. J Clin Invest 109(10):1345–1350, 2002.

169. Ravussin E, Caglayan S, Williamson DA, et al: Effects of human leptin replacement of food intake and energy metabolism in 3 leptin-deficient adults [Abstract]. Int J Obes S126:S136, 2002.

170. Carr A, Samaras K, Thorisdottir A, et al: Diagnosis, prediction, and natural course of HIV-1 protease-inhibitor-associated lipodystrophy, hyperlipidaemia, and diabetes mellitus: a cohort study [see comments]. Lancet 353(9170):2093–2099, 1999.

171. Ledru E, Christeff N, Patey O, et al: Alteration of tumor necrosis factor-alpha T-cell homeostasis following potent antiretroviral therapy: Contribution to the development of human immunodeficiency virus-associated lipodystrophy syndrome. Blood 95(10):3191–3198, 2000.

172. Mynarcik DC, McNurlan MA, Steigbigel RT, et al: Association of severe insulin resistance with both loss of limb fat and elevated serum tumor necrosis factor receptor levels in HIV lipodystrophy. J Acquir Immune Defic Syndr 25(4):312–321, 2000.

173. Bastard JP, Caron M, Vidal H, et al: Association between altered expression of adipogenic factor SREBP1 in lipoatrophic adipose tissue from HIV-1-infected patients and abnormal adipocyte differentiation and insulin resistance. Lancet 359(9311):1026–1031, 2002.

174. Kannisto K, Sutinen J, Korsheninnikova E, et al: Expression of adipogenic transcription factors, peroxisome proliferator-activated receptor gamma co-activator 1, IL-6 and CD45 in subcutaneous adipose tissue in lipodystrophy associated with highly active antiretroviral therapy. AIDS 17(12):1753–1762, 2003.

175. Caron M, Auclair M, Sterlingot H, et al: Some HIV protease inhibitors alter lamin A/C maturation and stability, SREBP-1 nuclear localization and adipocyte differentiation. AIDS 17(17):2437–2444, 2003.

176. Cao H, Hegele RA: Nuclear lamin A/C R482Q mutation in canadian kindreds with Dunnigan-type familial partial lipodystrophy. Hum Mol Genet 9(1):109–112, 2000.

177. Genschel J, Schmidt HH: Mutations in the LMNA gene encoding lamin A/C. Hum Mutat 16(6):451–459, 2000.

178. Shackleton S, Lloyd DJ, Jackson SN, et al: LMNA, encoding lamin A/C, is mutated in partial lipodystrophy. Nat Genet 24(2):153–156, 2000.

179. Lloreta J, Domingo P, Pujol RM, et al: Ultrastructural features of highly active antiretroviral therapy-associated partial lipodystrophy. Virchows Arch 441(6):599–604, 2002.

180. Nolan D, Hammond E, Martin A, et al: Mitochondrial DNA depletion and morphologic changes in adipocytes associated with nucleoside reverse transcriptase inhibitor therapy. AIDS 17(9):1329–13238, 2003.

181. Maeda K, Okubo K, Shimomura I, et al: cDNA cloning and expression of a novel adipose specific collagen-like factor, apM1 (AdiPose Most abundant Gene transcript 1). Biochem Biophys Res Commun 2(221):286–289, 1996.

182. Combs TP, Berg AH, Rajala MW, et al: Sexual differentiation, pregnancy, calorie restriction, and aging affect the adipocyte-specific secretory protein adiponectin. Diabetes 2(52):268–276, 2003.

183. Scherer PE, Williams S, Fogliano M, et al: A Novel Serum Protein Similar to C1q, Produced Exclusively in Adipocytes. J Biol Chem 45(270):26746–26749, 1995.

184. Hu E, Liang P, Spiegelman BM: AdipoQ is a novel adipose-specific gene

dysregulated in obesity. J Biol Chem 1827110:697–703, 1996.

185. Nakano Y, Tobe T, ChoiMiura NH, et al: Isolation and characterization of GBP28, a novel gelatin-binding protein purified from human plasma. J Biochem 4120:803–812, 1996.

186. Pajvani UB, Du X, Combs TP, et al: Structure-function studies of the adipocyte-secreted hormone Acrp30/Adiponectin: Implications for metabolic regulation and bioactivity. J Biol Chem 278(11):9073–9085, 2003.

187. Shapiro L, Scherer PE: The crystal structure of a complement-1q family protein suggests an evolutionary link to tumor necrosis factor. Current Biology 68:335–338, 1998.

188. Schaffler A, Orso E, Palitzsch KD, et al: The human apM-1, an adipocyte-specific gene linked to the family of TNF's and to genes expressed in activated T cells, is mapped to chromosome 1q21.3-q23, a susceptibility locus identified for familial combined hyperlipidaemia (FCH). Biochem Biophys Res Commun 2260:416–425, 1999.

189. Hotta K, Funahashi T, Arita Y, et al: Plasma concentrations of a novel, adipose-specific protein, adiponectin, in type 2 diabetic patients. 620:1595–1599, 2000.

190. Arita Y, Kihara S, Ouchi N, et al: Paradoxical decrease of an adipose-specific protein, adiponectin, in obesity. Biochem Biophys Res Commun 1257:79–83, 1999.

191. Weyer C, Funahashi T, Tanaka S, et al: Hypoadiponectinemia in obesity and type 2 diabetes: Close association with insulin resistance and hyperinsulinemia. J Clin Endocrinol Metab 586:1930–1935, 2001.

192. Haque WA, Shimomura I, Matsuzawa Y, Garg A: Serum adiponectin and leptin levels in patients with lipodystrophies. J Clin Endocrinol Metab 587:2395, 2002.

193. Yamauchi T, Kamon J, Ito Y, et al: Cloning of adiponectin receptors that mediate antidiabetic metabolic effects. Nature 6941(423):762–769, 2003.

194. Civitarese AE, Jenkinson CP, Richardson D, et al: Adiponecting receptors gene expression and insulin sensitivity in non-diabetic Mexican Americans with or without family history of Type 2 diabetes. Diabetologia 2004 (in press).

195. Okamoto Y, Arita Y, Nishida M, et al: An adipocyte-derived plasma protein, adiponectin, adheres to injured vascular walls. Horm Metab Res 23:247–250, 2000.

196. Fruebis J, Tsao T-S, Javorschi S, et al: Proteolytic cleavage product of 30-kDa adipocyte complement-related protein increases fatty acid oxidation in muscle and causes weight loss in mice. PNAS 498:2005–2010, 2001.

197. Yamauchi T, Kamon J, Waki H, et al: The fat-derived hormone adiponectin reverses insulin resistance associated

with both lipoatrophy and obesity. Nat Med 87:941–946, 2001.

198. Berg AH, Combs TP, Du X, et al: The adipocyte-secreted protein Acrp30 enhances hepatic insulin action. Nat Med 87:947–953, 2001.

199. Yamauchi T, Kamon J, Minokoshi Y, et al: Adiponectin stimulates glucose utilization and fatty-acid oxidation by activating AMP-activated protein kinase. Nat Med 18:1288–1295, 2002.

200. Combs TP, Berg AH, Obici S, et al: Endogenous glucose production is inhibited by the adipose-derived protein Acrp30. J Clin Invest 12(108):1875–1881, 2001.

201. Winder WW, Hardie DG: AMP-activated protein kinase, a metabolic master switch: Possible roles in Type 2 diabetes. Am J Physiol Endocrinol Metab 1(277):E1–E10, 1999.

202. Yamamoto Y, Hirose H, Saito I, et al: Correlation of the adipocyte-derived protein adiponectin with insulin resistance index and serum high-density lipoprotein-cholesterol, independent of body mass index, in the Japanese population. Clin Sci 2103:137–142, 2002.

203. Lindsay RS, Funahashi T, Hanson RL, et al: Adiponectin and development of type 2 diabetes in the Pima Indian population. Lancet 9326360:57–58, 2002.

204. Yang W-S, Lee W-J, Funahashi T, et al: Weight reduction increases plasma levels of an adipose-derived anti-inflammatory protein, adiponectin. J Clin Endocrinol Metab 886:3815–3819, 2001.

205. Yu JG, Javorschi S, Hevener AL, et al: The effect of thiazolidinediones on plasma adiponectin levels in normal, obese, and type 2 diabetic subjects. Diabetes 1051:2968–2974, 2002.

206. Steppan CM, Bailey ST, Bhat S, et al: The hormone resistin links obesity to diabetes. Nature 409(6818):307–312, 2001.

207. Moon B, Kwan JJ, Duddy N, et al: Resistin inhibits glucose uptake in L6 cells independently of changes in insulin signaling and GLUT4 translocation. Am J Physiol Endocrinol Metab 285(1):E106–E115, 2003.

208. Kim KH, Lee K, Moon YS, Sul HS: A cysteine-rich adipose tissue-specific secretory factor inhibits adipocyte differentiation. J Biol Chem 276(14):11252–11256, 2001.

209. Holcomb IN, Kabakoff RC, Chan B, et al: FIZZ1, a novel cysteine-rich secreted protein associated with pulmonary inflammation, defines a new gene family. EMBO J 19(15):4046–4055, 2000.

210. Banerjee RR, Rangwala SM, Shapiro JS, et al: Regulation of fasted blood glucose by resistin. Science 303(5661):1195–1198, 2004.

211. Yannakoulia M, Yiannakouris N, Bluher S, et al: Body fat mass and macronutrient intake in relation to circulating soluble leptin receptor, free

leptin index, adiponectin, and resistin concentrations in healthy humans. J Clin Endocrinol Metab 88(4):1730–1736, 2003.

212. Lee S, Batzoglou S: Application of independent component analysis to microarrays. Genome Biol 4R76(11), 2003.

213. Heilbronn LK, Janderova L, Rood J, et al: Relationship between serum resistin concentrations and insulin resistance in non-obese, obese and obese-diabetic subjects. J Clin Endocrinol Metab 2004 (in press).

214. Savage DB, Sewter CP, Klenk ES, et al: Resistin/Fizz3 expression in relation to obesity and peroxisome proliferator-activated receptor-gamma action in humans. Diabetes 50(10):2199–2202, 2001.

215. Smith SR, Bai F, Charbonneau C, et al: A promoter genotype and oxidative stress potentially link resistin to human insulin resistance. Diabetes 52(7):1611–1618, 2003.

216. Rajala MW, Obici S, Scherer PE, Rossetti L: Adipose-derived resistin and gut-derived resistin-like molecule-beta selectively impair insulin action on glucose production. J Clin Invest 111(2):225–230, 2003.

217. Smith AD, et al (eds): Oxford Dictionary of Biochemistry and Molecular Biology, rev ed. Oxford, UK, Oxford University Press, 2000.

218. Xu H, Hirosumi J, Uysal KT, et al: Exclusive action of transmembrane TNF alpha in adipose tissue leads to reduced adipose mass and local but not systemic insulin resistance. Endocrinology 143(4):1502–1511, 2002.

219. Stephens JM, Butts M, Stone R, et al: Regulation of transcription factor mRNA accumulation during 3T3-L1 preadipocyte differentiation by antagonists of adipogenesis. Mol Cell Biochem 123(1–2):63–71, 1993.

220. Xing H, Northrop JP, Grove JR, et al: TNF alpha-mediated inhibition and reversal of adipocyte differentiation is accompanied by suppressed expression of PPARgamma without effects on Pref-1 expression. Endocrinology 138(7):2776–2783, 1997.

221. Hotamisligil GS, Shargill NS, Spiegelman BM: Adipose expression of tumor necrosis factor-alpha: Direct role in obesity-linked insulin resistance. Science 259(5091):87–91, 1993.

222. Tsigos C, Kyrou I, Chala E, et al: Circulating tumor necrosis factor alpha concentrations are higher in abdominal versus peripheral obesity. Metabolism 48(10):1332–1335, 1999.

223. Ruan H, Miles PD, Ladd CM, et al: Profiling gene transcription in vivo reveals adipose tissue as an immediate target of tumor necrosis factor-alpha: Implications for insulin resistance. Diabetes 51(11):3176–3188, 2002.

224. Lofgren P, van Harmelen V, Reynisdottir S, et al: Secretion of tumor necrosis factor-alpha shows a strong relationship to insulin-stimulated

glucose transport in human adipose tissue. Diabetes 49(5):688–692, 2000.

225. Fried SK, Zechner R: Cachectin/tumor necrosis factor decreases human adipose tissue lipoprotein lipase mRNA levels, synthesis, and activity. J Lipid Res 30(12):1917–1923, 1989.

226. Bullo M, Garcia-Lorda P, Peinado-Onsurbe J, et al: TNFalpha expression of subcutaneous adipose tissue in obese and morbid obese females: Relationship to adipocyte LPL activity and leptin synthesis. Int J Obes Relat Metab Disord 26(5):652–658, 2002.

227. Sykiotis GP, Papavassiliou AG: Serine phosphorylation of insulin receptor substrate-1: A novel target for the reversal of insulin resistance. Mol Endocrinol 15(11):1864–1869, 2001.

228. Friedberg M, Zoumakis E, Hiroi N, et al: Modulation of 11 beta-hydroxysteroid dehydrogenase type 1 in mature human subcutaneous adipocytes by hypothalamic messengers. J Clin Endocrinol Metab 88(1):385–393, 2003.

229. McTernan PG, Harte AL, Anderson LA, et al: Insulin and rosiglitazone regulation of lipolysis and lipogenesis in human adipose tissue in vitro. Diabetes 51(5):1493–1498, 2002.

230. Kern PA, Dicker-Brown A, Said ST, et al: The stimulation of tumor necrosis factor and inhibition of glucose transport and lipoprotein lipase in adipose cells by 2,3,7,8-tetrachlorodibenzo-p-dioxin. Metabolism 51(1):65–68, 2002.

231. Nilsson J, Jovinge S, Niemann A, et al: Relation between plasma tumor necrosis factor-alpha and insulin sensitivity in elderly men with non-insulin-dependent diabetes mellitus. Arterioscler Thromb Vasc Biol 18(8):1199–1202, 1998.

232. Chan JC, Cheung JC, Stehouwer CD, et al: The central roles of obesity-associated dyslipidaemia, endothelial activation and cytokines in the metabolic syndrome: An analysis by structural equation modelling. Int J Obes Relat Metab Disord 26(7):994–1008, 2002.

233. Mynarcik DC, McNurlan MA, Steigbigel RT, et al: Association of severe insulin resistance with both loss of limb fat and elevated serum tumor necrosis factor receptor levels in HIV lipodystrophy. J Acquir Immune Defic Syndr 25(4):312–321, 2000.

234. Cousin B, Munoz O, Andre M, et al: A role for preadipocytes as macrophage-like cells. Faseb J 13(2):305–312, 1999.

235. Weisberg SP, McCann D, Desai M, et al: Obesity is associated with macrophage accumulation in adipose tissue. J Clin Invest 112(12):1796–1808, 2003.

236. Xu H, Barnes GT, Yang Q, et al: Chronic inflammation in fat plays a crucial role in the development of obesity-related insulin resistance. J Clin Invest 112(12):1821–1830, 2003.

237. Bruun JM, Pedersen SB, Richelsen B: Regulation of interleukin 8 production and gene expression in human adipose tissue in vitro. J Clin Endocrinol Metab 86(3):1267–1273, 2001.

238. Bruun JM, Pedersen SB, Richelsen B: Interleukin-8 production in human adipose tissue: Inhibitory effects of anti-diabetic compounds, the thiazolidinedione ciglitazone and the biguanide metformin. Horm Metab Res 32(11–12):537–541, 2000.

239. Sartipy P, Loskutoff DJ: Monocyte chemoattractant protein 1 in obesity and insulin resistance. Proc Natl Acad Sci U S A 100(12):7265–7270, 2003.

240. Yuan M, Konstantopoulos N, Lee J, et al: Reversal of obesity- and diet-induced insulin resistance with salicylates or targeted disruption of Ikkbeta. Science 293(5535):1673–1677, 2001.

241. Lee JY, Plakidas A, Lee WH, et al: Differential modulation of Toll-like receptors by fatty acids: Preferential inhibition by n-3 polyunsaturated fatty acids. J Lipid Res 44(3):479–486, 2003.

242. Hundal RS, Petersen KF, Mayerson AB, et al: Mechanism by which high-dose aspirin improves glucose metabolism in type 2 diabetes. J Clin Invest 109(10):1321–1326, 2002.

243. Kopp E, Ghosh S: Inhibition of NF-kappa B by sodium salicylate and aspirin. Science 265(5174):956–959, 1994.

244. Shoelson SE, Lee J, Yuan M: Inflammation and the IKK beta/I kappa B/NF-kappa B axis in obesity- and diet-induced insulin resistance. Int J Obes Relat Metab Disord 27(Suppl 3):S49–S52, 2003.

245. Wellen KE, Hotamisligil GS: Obesity-induced inflammatory changes in adipose tissue. J Clin Invest 112(12):1785–1788, 2003.

246. Ruan H, Pownall HJ, Lodish HF: Troglitazone antagonizes tumor necrosis factor-alpha-induced reprogramming of adipocyte gene expression by inhibiting the transcriptional regulatory functions of NF-kappaB. J Biol Chem 278(30):28181–28192, 2003.

247. Weyer C, Gautier JF, Danforth E Jr: Development of beta 3-adrenoceptor agonists for the treatment of obesity and diabetes: An update. Diabetes Metab 25(1):11–21, 1999.

248. Rupnick MA, Panigrahy D, Zhang CY, et al: Adipose tissue mass can be regulated through the vasculature. Proc Natl Acad Sci U S A 99(16):10730–10735, 2002.

249. Hirose H, Kawai T, Yamamoto Y, et al: Effects of pioglitazone on metabolic parameters, body fat distribution, and serum adiponectin levels in Japanese male patients with type 2 diabetes. Metabolism 51(3):314–317, 2002.

250. Bjorntorp P, Rosmond R: Obesity and cortisol. Nutrition 16(10):924–936, 2000.

251. Bjorntorp P, Rosmond R: The metabolic syndrome: A neuroendocrine disorder? Br J Nutr 83(Suppl 1):S49–S57, 2000.

252. Masuzaki H, Paterson J, Shinyama H, et al: A transgenic model of visceral obesity and the metabolic syndrome. Science 294(5549):2166–2170, 2001.

253. Kotelevtsev Y, Holmes MC, Burchell A, et al: 11beta-Hydroxysteroid dehydrogenase type 1 knockout mice show attenuated glucocorticoid-inducible responses and resist hyperglycemia on obesity or stress. PNAS 94(26):14924–14929, 1997.

254. Kozak LP: Genetic studies of brown adipocyte induction. J Nutr 130(12):3132S–3133S, 2000.

255. Guerra C, Koza RA, Yamashita H, et al: Emergence of brown adipocytes in white fat in mice is under genetic control: Effects on body weight and adiposity. J Clin Invest 102(2):412–420, 1998.

256. Tiraby C, Langin D: Conversion from white to brown adipocytes: A strategy for the control of fat mass? Trends Endocrinol Metab 14(10):439–441, 2003.

257. Walczak R, Tontonoz P: Setting fat on fire. Nat Med 9(11):1348–1349, 2003.

Classification and Diagnosis of Diabetes Mellitus

Sean F. Dinneen and Robert A. Rizza

DEFINITION

CLASSIFICATION
    Type 1 Diabetes
    Autoimmune Type 1 Diabetes
    Idiopathic Type 1 Diabetes
    Type 2 Diabetes
    Other Specific Types of Diabetes
    Genetic Defects of β-Cell Function
    Genetic Defects of Insulin Action
    Diseases of the Exocrine Pancreas
    Endocrinopathies
    Drug- or Chemical-Induced Diabetes

    Infections
    Uncommon Forms of Immune-Mediated Diabetes
    Other Genetic Syndromes Sometimes Associated
    with Diabetes
    Gestational Diabetes

DIAGNOSIS
    Diagnostic Criteria
    Rationale for the 1997 ADA Diagnostic Criteria
    Changing the Prevalence and Incidence of Diabetes
    Defining Normality and Intermediate States
    of Hyperglycemia

DEFINITION

The term *diabetes mellitus* does not represent a single disease entity but rather a set of disease states sharing certain characteristics. Foremost among these is the presence of elevated plasma glucose levels. As will be discussed below, the presence of hyperglycemia in a patient is used both to diagnose diabetes and to guide management decisions, which are largely directed toward avoiding hyperglycemia. The hyperglycemia itself results from a combination of defects in insulin secretion, insulin action, or both.[1,2] An important characteristic of the various disease states that are labeled as diabetes is the development of end-organ damage in vital organs of the body, including the retina, the renal glomerulus, and peripheral nerves. The damage results, at least in part, from the chronic effects of hyperglycemia and is mediated through glycation of tissue proteins, increased activity of the polyol pathway, or other, as yet unrecognized, mechanisms.[3] Individual patients vary in their predisposition to develop these so-called microvascular complications. Because of this and because of the length of time they take to develop (frequently decades), the complications of diabetes cannot be used to classify or diagnose the disease. People with diabetes have a considerably greater risk of developing atherosclerotic disease affecting the coronary, cerebrovascular, peripheral arterial, or other parts of the circulation. A cause-and-effect relationship between chronic hyperglycemia and these so-called macrovascular complications of diabetes has not been as clearly established, although evidence is accumulating linking the two.[4] Any definition of diabetes that refers only to carbohydrate metabolism is incomplete. Oskar Minkowski is reputed to have first made the association between the insulin-deficient pancreatectomized state of his laboratory dogs and the sweet taste of their urine. It has been suggested that if Minkowski had lacked a sense of taste but possessed a keen sense of smell, he might have smelled the ketones on the breath of his animals and thereby directed diabetes research toward the study of fat metabolism.[5] Disordered fat and protein metabolism must be included in a complete definition of the disease, although an emphasis on the pathogenesis of hyperglycemia continues to this day. To define a disease purely in biochemical terms is to diminish the component of the disease that leads to much physical, mental, and psychosocial distress for the many millions of people around the world who live with

it every day.[6] Chronic rheumatic diseases such as rheumatoid arthritis are not associated with any biochemical hallmark, and their definition is based largely on patient-derived symptoms and signs.[7] Therefore, it is important to try to include the patient's perspective in any definition of the chronic disease referred to as diabetes.

CLASSIFICATION

Before 1979, a classification system for diabetes was not well established, and many different terms were used to describe what was essentially the same clinical entity. Following publication of the report of the National Diabetes Data Group (NDDG)[8] in that year, some order was brought to bear on this area. The recommendations of the NDDG were subsequently endorsed by the World Health Organization (WHO) in a publication in 1980, and minor modifications were later made in a document published in 1985.[9] This classification was in large part based on the pharmacologic therapy of the disease. Insulin-dependent diabetes mellitus (IDDM) and non-insulin-dependent diabetes mellitus (NIDDM) were the two major forms of diabetes that were identified. The term *insulin-dependent diabetes mellitus* was used to describe patients who were typically lean at presentation, were prone to ketosis, and required insulin for survival. The term *non-insulin-dependent diabetes mellitus* was used to describe patients who were typically obese at presentation, were not prone to ketosis, and did not require insulin for survival. The NDDG also had categories for gestational diabetes, malnutrition-related diabetes mellitus (MRDM), and a category labeled "other types," which included certain forms of diabetes for which a cause had been suggested at that time. As the terms *IDDM* and *NIDDM* became widely used during the 1980s and 1990s, several problems became apparent. The main problem related to the fact that many patients with NIDDM ended up at some point in the course of their disease being treated with insulin and being either misclassified as IDDM or having the rather confusing term *insulin-requiring NIDDM* applied to them. In addition, as more information became available on the etiology of the various forms of diabetes, it became apparent that a classification based on therapy was not always consistent with new insights into the pathogenesis of the various forms of diabetes. For this reason, the American Diabetes Association (ADA) convened an expert panel in 1995 to address the issue of classification. This panel published its recommendations in 1997,[10] and these were subsequently endorsed by a WHO consultation group in a 1998 report.[11] The main thrust of this proposal was to move away from a classification based on therapy and toward one based on pathogenesis. Four major categories were proposed: type 1 diabetes, type 2 diabetes, other specific types of diabetes (including categories for which a cause has been established), and gestational diabetes. The details of this system are outlined in Table 54-1 and discussed below.

TYPE 1 DIABETES

Type 1 diabetes is characterized by the development of a state of complete insulin deficiency. In its fully developed form, patients will, if deprived of insulin, develop ketoacidosis, coma, and death. Biochemical testing reveals the absence of circulating C peptide (a marker of insulin secretion) despite hyperglycemia. The incidence of type 1 diabetes in the United States is estimated to be approximately 30,000 new cases per year.[12] Although the peak incidence occurs in childhood and early adolescence, this form of diabetes can occur at any age. The incidence of the disease shows marked regional variation, the highest worldwide incidence being reported in Scandinavia.[13] Recent epidemiologic and immunologic research has led to recognition of two major forms of type 1 diabetes based on the presence or absence of certain immunologic markers.

AUTOIMMUNE TYPE 1 DIABETES

Autoimmune type 1 diabetes is a prototypic organ-specific autoimmune disorder. Individuals who develop this form of diabetes are born with a genetic predisposition to autoimmune dysfunction, which may manifest in the development of other autoimmune conditions such as Addison's disease or Hashimoto's thyroiditis. The genetic predisposition is not well understood but is known to be linked to the major histocompatibility locus on chromosome 6.[14] The presence of certain human lymphocyte antigen (HLA) haplotypes appears to predispose the individual to the disease, while other HLA haplotypes appear to be protective. In predisposed individuals, a poorly understood environmental trigger sets off a series of immunologic events that culminate in selective T-cell-mediated destruction of the β cells of the pancreatic islet. Many antigens have been investigated as potential triggers for the disease. These include certain viral antigens[15] as well as an antigen contained in cow's milk protein.[16] The rate at which β-cell destruction occurs varies from individual to individual and may be very brief, as is seen when type 1 diabetes presents in the neonatal period, or may be prolonged, as is seen in what has been called latent autoimmune diabetes in adults.[17] Antibodies appear in the circulation early in the process of β-cell destruction.[18] These autoantibodies are believed to be markers (rather than true instigators) of the immune response. Their presence can help to classify a newly diagnosed patient with diabetes. In several studies, screening for these autoantibodies has led to recognition of autoimmune type 1 diabetes in individuals who might otherwise have been labeled as having type 2 diabetes[19,20] (see below). Islet cell antibodies were the first autoantibodies to be discovered and are directed against a range of islet antigens. The best-characterized autoantibodies are those directed against glutamic acid decarboxylase (GAD), an enzyme that is involved in γ-aminobutyric acid synthesis.[21] Isoforms of GAD are found in the central nervous system as well as in β cells of the pancreatic islet. Other autoantibodies include antibodies directed against IA-2 and IA-2β as well as antibodies directed against insulin itself (anti-insulin antibodies). Childhood-onset type 1 diabetes is associated with higher levels of autoantibody in serum. Testing for these autoantibodies is still restricted to a limited number of laboratories. Greater standardization of assays is required before they can be widely used in clinical practice.

Table 54-1 Classification of Diabetes Mellitus

1. Type 1 diabetes
   A. Immune-mediated
   B. Idiopathic
2. Type 2 diabetes
3. Other specific types
   A. Genetic defects of β-cell function
      1. HNF-4α (MODY 1)
      2. Glucokinase (MODY 2)
      3. HNF-1α (MODY 3)
      4. IPF-1 (MODY 4)
      5. HNF-1β (MODY 5)
      6. NeuroD1, or BETA 2 (MODY 6)
      7. Mitochondrial DNA
      8. Others
   B. Genetic defects in insulin action
      1. Type A insulin resistance
      2. Leprechaunism
      3. Rabson-Mendenhall syndrome
      4. Lipodystrophic diabetes
      5. Others
   C. Diseases of the exocrine pancreas
      1. Pancreatitis
      2. Trauma/pancreatectomy
      3. Neoplasia
      4. Cystic fibrosis
      5. Hemochromatosis
      6. Fibrocalculous pancreatic diabetes
      7. Others
   D. Endocrinopathies
      1. Cushing's syndrome
      2. Acromegaly
      3. Glucagonoma
      4. Pheochromocytoma
      5. Somatostatinoma
      6. Aldosteronoma
      7. Hyperthyroidism
      8. Others
   E. Drug or chemical induced
      1. Vacor
      2. Pentamidine
      3. Nicotinic acid
      4. Glucocorticoids
      5. Thyroid hormone
      6. Diazoxide
      7. β-Adrenergic agonists
      8. Thiazides
      9. Clozapine
      10. Protease inhibitors
      11. Others
   F. Infections
      1. Congenital rubella
      2. Cytomegalovirus
      3. Others
   G. Uncommon forms of immune-mediated diabetes
      1. "Stiff-man" syndrome
      2. Anti-insulin receptor antibodies
      3. Others
   H. Other genetic syndromes sometimes associated with diabetes
      1. Down syndrome
      2. Klinefelter's syndrome
      3. Turner's syndrome
      4. Wolfram's syndrome
      5. Friedreich's ataxia
      6. Huntington's chorea
      7. Lawrence Moon Biedel syndrome
      8. Myotonic dystrophy
      9. Porphyria
      10. Prader-Willi syndrome
      11. Others
4. Gestational diabetes mellitus

Source: Reprinted with permission from the Report of the Expert Committee on the Diagnosis and Classification of Diabetes Mellitus, Diabetes Care 20(7):1183–1197, 1997.

IDIOPATHIC TYPE 1 DIABETES

The term *idiopathic type 1 diabetes* is used to describe a small subset of individuals with type 1 diabetes who appear not to have an autoimmune basis for their β-cell destruction.[22] Other features of this subtype include its occurrence predominantly in individuals of African or Asian ethnicity, its lack of HLA association, and intermittent proneness to ketosis. Recent reports suggest that this form of diabetes may be on the increase among African-American youth in the United States.[23]

TYPE 2 DIABETES

Type 2 diabetes represents the most common form of diabetes seen in most parts of the developed world. Current estimates for the U.S. population indicate that more than 16 million people have type 2 diabetes.[24] The condition is characterized by hyperglycemia that results from a combination of defects in insulin secretion and insulin action. In any given individual, the degree to which these defects contribute to the hyperglycemia may vary. The disease usually has its onset after age 40, although increasingly type 2 diabetes is being seen in young adults and adolescents.[25] While progressive β-cell failure is believed by many to be an important part of the natural history of this form of diabetes,[26] the β-cell destruction is not autoimmune-mediated[27] and does not progress to a point at which the patient becomes dependent on insulin for survival. Ketoacidosis is unusual in this form of diabetes, and when it occurs, it is usually in the setting of a major intercurrent illness such as myocardial infarction, stroke, or treatment with glucocorticoids. Individuals with type 2 diabetes are not at increased risk for autoimmune diseases but have a higher prevalence of metabolic abnormalities, including obesity, hypertension, and a typical dyslipidemia that is characterized by hypertriglyceridemia and low levels of high-density lipoprotein cholesterol.[28] This combination of metabolic derangements is associated with a marked increase in the risk of atherosclerotic disease. In fact, the prevalence of atherosclerotic disease in people with type 2 diabetes has led to the suggestion that, rather than one leading to the other, the two conditions may share common antecedents.[4] Insulin resistance may be an important predisposing factor for both conditions.[29]

The cause of type 2 diabetes remains to be determined. Any pathogenetic model of the disease must include both genetic and environmental factors. Challenges in establishing the cause of type 2 diabetes include the following: (1) The disease lacks an easy-to-define phenotype but instead is characterized by considerable heterogeneity across different ethnic groups; this heterogeneity is often represented by a spectrum consisting of a predominant defect in insulin secretion on the one hand to a predominant defect in insulin action on the other. (2) The relatively late age of onset makes it difficult to establish large kindreds and therefore limits genetic studies. (3) There are no easy-to-apply methods for screening populations for insulin resistance and defective insulin secretion. (4) The pathways that are involved in mediating insulin action are complex and not fully understood; most authors believe that a single genetic defect will explain only a subset of the disease; it is much more likely that type 2 diabetes represents a set of disorders. Evidence to support a genetic component of the disease comes from the strong concordance for the disease that is seen among monozygotic twins.[30] On the other hand, the dramatic increase in incidence and prevalence of type 2 diabetes that accompanies the change to a so-called Westernized lifestyle strongly supports an environmental component as well.[31]

OTHER SPECIFIC TYPES OF DIABETES

Other specific types of diabetes are included in both the 1979 NDDG and 1997 ADA classification systems.[8,10] A number of changes occurred in the subtypes of diabetes listed between the two eras. In particular, the form of diabetes that is referred to as maturity-onset diabetes of the young (MODY) has been better defined genetically and this is reflected in the 1997 ADA classification system.[10] Another change resulted from removal of MRDM from the classification and the inclusion of fibrocalculous pancreatic diabetes (which was previously a subtype of MRDM) as a disease of the exocrine pancreas. The decision to remove MRDM as a separate entity resulted from an international conference on this subject.[32,33] The findings of the conference did not support a direct cause-and-effect relationship between protein-calorie malnutrition and the development of diabetes. Rather, it was thought that the presence of malnutrition could influence the manner in which diabetes might present in an otherwise predisposed individual.

GENETIC DEFECTS OF β-CELL FUNCTION

In the past, the term *maturity-onset diabetes of the young* was used to describe a subset of patients with a form of diabetes characterized by early age of onset of hyperglycemia with an autosomal-dominant mode of inheritance. Mutations in certain genes that are involved in regulating insulin secretion have now been shown to be responsible for the hyperglycemia seen in MODY kindreds.[34] Six major forms of MODY have been described,[35–38] and their clinical and genetic features are outlined in Table 54-2. All forms of MODY are associated with defective insulin secretion without any significant degree of insulin resistance.[39,40] In the case of glucokinase, the pathophysiologic mechanism is clear, since the enzyme is involved in phosphorylating glucose, one of the first steps in glucose metabolism. A glucokinase mutation therefore decreases the ability of the β cell to sense glucose. MODY2 is associated with relatively mild hyperglycemia that is usually amenable to treatment with diet and exercise. MODY1 and MODY3, on the other hand, can be associated with more severe hyperglycemia, a greater likelihood that insulin will be required for management, and a higher propensity to develop complications.[34] The link between diabetes and mutations in the genes for hepatocyte nuclear factor (HNF)-1α, HNF-1β (hepatocyte transcription factors also expressed in β cells), and HNF-4α (a member of the steroid-thyroid hormone superfamily and an upstream regulator of HNF-1α) appears to be via regulation of expression of the insulin gene.[41] It is likely that other variants of MODY will be identified in the future. It has been suggested that MODY may account for between 2% and 5% of cases of type 2 diabetes.[42]

Other genetic disorders that are associated with impaired β-cell function include certain maternally inherited forms of diabetes with a mutation in mitochondrial DNA,[43] disorders that lead to impaired conversion of proinsulin to insulin,[44] and disorders that lead to synthesis of an aberrant form of the insulin molecule.[45] Of the former conditions, diabetes associated with an A-to-G transition at the nucleotide pair 3243 in mitochondrial transfer RNA (tRNA) has been best characterized and appears to have a wide phenotypic expression from type 2 through to type 1 diabetes. The latter two conditions are inherited in an autosomal-dominant manner and are associated with relatively mild glucose intolerance.

GENETIC DEFECTS OF INSULIN ACTION

For insulin to exert its biologic effect, it must first bind to its receptor on the cell surface. Following receptor binding, a complex series of postreceptor signaling reactions take place, leading to the hormone's metabolic and mitogenic effects. Disruption of some of these postreceptor mediators (e.g., insulin receptor substrate-1) has been shown to cause diabetes in animals.[46] However, very few human forms of diabetes have been clearly linked to specific genetic defects in the insulin-signaling cascade. Leprechaunism and Rabson-Mendenhall

Table 54-2   MODY-Related Genes and the Clinical Phenotypes Associated with Mutations in the Genes*

MODY Type	Gene	Clinical Features of Heterozygous State	Most Common Treatment	Molecular Basis	Clinical Features of Homozygous State
MODY 1	HNF-4α	Diabetes; microvascular complications (in many cases); reductions in serum concentration of triglycerides, apolipoproteins AII and CIII, and Lp(a) lipoprotein	Oral hypoglycemic agent, insulin	Abnormal regulation of gene transcription in β cells, leading to a defect in metabolic signaling of insulin secretion, β-cell mass, or both	
MODY 2	Glucokinase	Impaired fasting glucose, impaired glucose tolerance, diabetes	Diet and exercise	Defect in sensitivity of β cells to glucose due to reduced glucose phos-phorylation; defect in hepatic storage of glucose as glycogen	Permanant neonatal diabetes requiring insulin treatment
MODY 3	HNF-1α	Diabetes, microvascular complications (in many cases), renal glycosuria, increased sensitivity to sulphonylurea drugs	Oral hypoglycemic agent, insulin	Abnormal regulation of gene transcription in β cells, leading to a defect in metabolic signaling of insulin secretion, β-cell mass, or both	
MODY 4	IPF-1	Diabetes	Oral hypoglycemic agent, insulin	Abnormal transcriptional regulation of β-cell development and function	Pancreatic as and neonatal requiring insulin treatment
MODY 5	HNF-1β	Diabetes; renal cysts and other abnormalities of renal development; progressive nondiabetic renal dysfunction, leading to chronic renal insufficiency and failure; internal genital abnormalifies (in female carriers)	Insulin	Abnormal regulation of gene transcription in β cells, leading to a defect in metabolic signaling of insulin secretion, β-cell mass, or both	
MODY 6	NeuroD1 or BETA2	Diabetes	Insulin	Abnormal transcriptional regulation of β-cell development and function	

*MODY denotes maturity-onset diabetes of the young; HNF, hepatocyte nuclear factor; IPF, insulin promoter factor; NeuroD1, neurogenic differentation factor 1; BETA2, β-cell E-box trasactivator 2.
Source: From Fajans SS, Bell GI, Polonsky KS: Molecular mechanisms and clinical pathophysiology of maturity-onset diabetes of the young. N Engl J Med 345:971–980, 2001.

syndrome represent rare congenital disorders of the insulin receptor.[47] Both syndromes are associated with diabetes and hyperinsulinemia and altered growth in utero. As the insulin signaling cascade is further defined, it is likely that additional forms of diabetes will be found to be caused by genetic defects in insulin action.

The nomenclature associated with clinical syndromes of severe insulin resistance can be confusing.[48] The term *Type A insulin resistance* has been used to describe a syndrome in which severe insulin resistance is associated with a skin condition called acanthosis nigricans and with hyperandrogenism in females. Glucose intolerance or overt diabetes may or not be present. The term *Type B insulin resistance* describes a rare syndrome in which autoantibodies to the insulin receptor lead to insulin resistance and hyperinsulinemia (see below). Also associated with insulin resistance are the lipodystrophies; several forms of lipodystrophic diabetes have been characterized,[49] and in some cases, their genetic basis has been established and novel therapeutic interventions have been utilized.[50]

DISEASES OF THE EXOCRINE PANCREAS

Hyperglycemia can occur during an episode of acute pancreatitis and is associated with a poor prognosis. It is unusual for permanent diabetes to develop following a single episode of acute pancreatitis. Furthermore, removal of up to 90% of the pancreas does not always cause diabetes. On the other hand, diabetes has been reported in association with very small pancreatic adenocarcinomas, leading some investigators to speculate that these tumors produce some diabetogenic factor or factors.[51] Five percent to 15% of patients with cystic fibrosis develop diabetes.[52] Up to half of these patients require insulin either chronically or at times of added stress, such as glucocorticoid therapy. Hemochromatosis can cause diabetes.[53] Since glucose tolerance may improve with phlebotomy, this condition represents an important, potentially reversible cause of diabetes. Fibrocalculous pancreatic diabetes is seen mainly in the tropics and is associated with abdominal pain and calcification of the pancreas on abdominal imaging.[54] The natural history of this form of diabetes has recently been established[55] along with a genetic marker of the disease.[56]

ENDOCRINOPATHIES

Cortisol, growth hormone, glucagon, and the catecholamines (epinephrine and norepinephrine) can antagonize insulin action. Tumors that produce these hormones in excess lead to Cushing's syndrome, acromegaly, glucagonoma, and pheochromocytoma, respectively. While all of these conditions are associated with a degree of glucose intolerance, overt diabetes develops only in a subset of patients. The importance of recognizing these secondary forms of diabetes lies in the fact that resection of the underlying tumor can cure the diabetes. The hyperglycemia that is seen in the setting of aldosterone-producing adenomas and somatostatinomas results from alteration of insulin secretion.

DRUG- OR CHEMICAL-INDUCED DIABETES

Certain compounds are toxic to β cells.[57,58] These include the rat poison vacor and the anti-*Pneumocystis* drug pentamidine. The hyperglycemia that results from these agents is usually not reversible. Thiazide diuretics can inhibit insulin secretion by causing hypokalemia. Glucocorticoids and nicotinic acid cause hyperglycemia by impairing insulin action. Both protease inhibitors used in the treatment of human immunodeficiency virus infection and clozapine, a drug that is used to treat resistant schizophrenia, can cause hyperglycemia via an as yet undetermined mechanism.

INFECTIONS

Certain viral infections, including rubella[59] and coxsackie B virus,[60] have been associated with diabetes. Some studies suggest that a viral infection can trigger autoimmune destruction of β cells in genetically predisposed individuals, leading to autoimmune type 1 diabetes.

UNCOMMON FORMS OF IMMUNE-MEDIATED DIABETES

The stiff-man syndrome is a rare neurologic syndrome characterized by spasticity of the axial muscles. It is associated with very high titers of anti-GAD antibodies, and up to one third of patients develop diabetes.[61] Autoantibodies directed against the insulin receptor represent another rare cause of diabetes (referred to as type B insulin resistance).[62] These antibodies have the potential to change from being receptor antagonists (causing insulin resistance) to being receptor agonists (leading to potentially life-threatening hypoglycemia). Spontaneous remission of antibody production can also occur. The syndrome is typically seen in African-American females in association with other autoimmune diseases (most commonly systemic lupus erythematosus).

OTHER GENETIC SYNDROMES SOMETIMES ASSOCIATED WITH DIABETES

Many of the genetic syndromes listed under H in Table 54-1 are known to be associated with diabetes. The precise mechanism of the diabetes has not been established for these conditions.

GESTATIONAL DIABETES

Gestational diabetes is defined as diabetes with onset or first recognition during pregnancy. The prevalence of gestational diabetes increases in parallel with the prevalence of type 2 diabetes in a population. Approximately 4% of pregnancies in the United States are complicated by gestational diabetes.[63] Risk factors include age (it is more common among older women), ethnicity (higher rates are seen among women from ethnic groups with a high incidence of type 2 diabetes), prepregnancy body mass index (the risk increases with degree of obesity), parity (the risk increases with the number of previous pregnancies), and family history of diabetes. A previous pregnancy that was complicated by gestational diabetes or a history of delivery of a macrosomic infant also represents a strong risk factor for future gestational diabetes. The diagnosis of gestational diabetes is important, since, if it is left untreated, adverse fetal or maternal outcomes can occur. The main adverse fetal outcomes are macrosomia and neonatal hypoglycemia.[64] Maternal complications include a higher rate of dystocia and cesarean section as well as a greater risk of future type 2 diabetes[65] (among women who revert to normal glucose tolerance after completion of the pregnancy).

There are no uniformly agreed-upon criteria for the diagnosis of gestational diabetes.[66] The criteria that are most widely used in North America were developed on the basis of the ability of plasma glucose levels measured during pregnancy to predict future development of type 2 diabetes and not adverse outcomes of that pregnancy. In addition, the 100-g glucose load that is used in North America is different from the 75-g load that is used in other parts of the world. Finally, no consensus exists as to who should be screened.[67] In some countries (e.g., the United States), universal screening is routinely undertaken, whereas in other countries (e.g., in Europe), only women who are believed to be at high risk are screened.

DIAGNOSIS

DIAGNOSTIC CRITERIA

In addition to recommending changes in the classification system for diabetes, the Expert Committee of the ADA, in their 1997 report, also recommended changes in the diagnostic criteria for the disease.[10] These criteria were subsequently endorsed by the WHO[11] (Table 54-3). The major differences between the new and the old criteria were a reduction in the fasting plasma glucose cut point used to diagnose the disease and an emphasis on the use of fasting plasma glucose as opposed to the oral glucose tolerance test (OGTT) to screen for and diagnose the disease. The fasting plasma glucose level required for a diagnosis of diabetes was reduced from 140 mg/dL to 126 mg/dL. The diagnostic threshold for the 2-hour postglucose challenge plasma glucose level was left unchanged at 200 mg/dL. Two other important features of the diagnostic criteria that were retained include the ability to use casual (i.e., random) plasma glucose levels in patients with hyperglycemic symptoms and the requirement that a firm diagnosis be based on testing carried out on more than one occasion in asymptomatic patients. The ADA report based its criteria on the use of the fasting plasma glucose level, while the WHO report included equivalent cut points for whole-blood venous and capillary glucose.[11]

RATIONALE FOR THE 1997 ADA DIAGNOSTIC CRITERIA

There were three main reasons for the changes recommended in the 1997 ADA diagnostic criteria. The first reason relates to the lack of equivalence between a fasting plasma glucose value of 140 mg/dL and a 2-hour postglucose challenge value of 200 mg/dL.[68–70] Only approximately 25% of patients with a 2-hour value above 200 mg/dL will have a fasting value above 140 mg/dL. The point at which the two tests approach equivalence (based on receiver operating characteristic curve analysis) is closer to a fasting value of 126 mg/dL. The second reason for changing the criteria comes from epidemiologic studies that have assessed the level of glycemia at which the microvascular complications of diabetes begin to appear.[68,70]

Table 54-3	Diagnostic Thresholds for Diabetes and Lesser Degrees of Impaired Glucose Regulation	
Category	**Fasting Plasma Glucose**	**2-Hour Plasma Glucose**
Normal	<100 mg/dL (<5.6 mmol/L)	<140 mg/dL (< 7.8 mmol/IL)
IFG	100–125 mg/dL (5.6–6.9 mmol/L)	—
IGT	—	140–199 mg/dL (7.8–11.0 mmol/L)
Diabetes*	≥126 mg/dL (≥7.0 mmol/L)	≥200 mg/dL (≥11.1 mmol/L)

IFG, impaired fasting glucose; IGT, impaired glucose tolerance. When both tests are performed, IFG or IGT should be diagnosed only if diabetes is not diagnosed by the other test.
*A diagnosis of diabetes needs to be confirmed on a separate day.

As seen in Figure 54-1, the fasting plasma glucose value at which retinopathy first occurs is closer to 126 mg/dL than to 140 mg/dL. This observation was first reported in a population of Pima Indian subjects who have a very high prevalence of diabetes and a bimodal distribution of glucose. It was subsequently confirmed in a population from Egypt and most recently in data from the Third National Health and Nutrition Examination Survey in the United States.[10] Because of differences in the designs of the studies, the retinopathy prevalence data are not comparable across the three populations shown in Figure 54-1. Nevertheless, the cut point at which retinopathy begins to appear is similar in all three studies. The third reason for recommending a change in the diagnostic criteria for diabetes is a pragmatic one and relates to the fact that, outside of pregnancy, the OGTT is seldom used in routine clinical practice. The expert committees of the ADA acknowledged this fact by emphasizing that the fasting plasma glucose measurement should be considered the preferred method for screening. The ADA also recommended use of the fasting plasma glucose level in epidemiologic studies. The WHO suggested that continued use of the OGTT for screening among patients with impaired fasting glucose (see below for definition) was appropriate.

CHANGING THE PREVALENCE AND INCIDENCE OF DIABETES

Since publication of the 1997 ADA report recommending new diagnostic criteria for diabetes, many investigators have assessed the impact of the change on the prevalence of the disease in their individual populations.[71–74] The majority of these studies were based on existing data sets in which data on fasting and postchallenge glucose levels were available. The largest of these comparative reports looked at the prevalence of diabetes using the new versus the old criteria among 16 cohorts comprising 26,190 individuals in eight European countries.[71] As Figure 54-2 illustrates, the new criteria frequently led to a change in the prevalence of the disease, although this was not always in the same direction. The overall change was an increase in prevalence from 7.2% to 7.7%. The risk of disagreement decreased with increasing body mass index and also with increasing age. In contrast, a study that included 4515 elderly people from four centers in North America reported major discrepancies in the prevalence of diabetes using the ADA as opposed to the WHO criteria.[73] The overall prevalence of newly identified diabetes in this study decreased from 14.8% using the WHO criteria to 7.7% using the ADA criteria. An important report from the National Institutes of Health and the National Center for Health Statistics looked at the impact of the new versus the old criteria on diabetes diagnostic categories in a probability sample of

the U.S. population aged 40 to 74 years.[74] The prevalence of undiagnosed diabetes decreased from 6.4% to 4.4% with use of the new ADA criteria.

DEFINING NORMALITY AND INTERMEDIATE STATES OF HYPERGLYCEMIA

Another impact of the 1997 ADA criteria was the creation of two new categories of hyperglycemia, namely, normal fasting glucose and impaired fasting glucose (IFG). In the 1997 ADA report the term *normal fasting glucose* was introduced to describe individuals with plasma glucose levels less than 110 mg/dL. The choice of 110 mg/dL as the cut point defining normality was arbitrary. Many laboratories report the upper limit of normal for plasma glucose as 100 mg/dL.[75] Furthermore, plasma glucose represents a continuous variable, and there appears to be a continuum of risk for certain events, including future development of diabetes,[76] as well as atherosclerotic coronary or cerebrovascular events.[77] Therefore, while a threshold exists for the risk of microvascular complications (see Fig. 54-1), this might not be the case for the risk of macrovascular complications. Indeed, some investigators have proposed the term *dysglycemia* to describe the fact that the higher an individual's plasma glucose level (even if it is within the "normal" range), the greater is the person's risk of subsequent adverse vascular events.[78]

IFG represents an intermediate state between normal fasting glucose and overt diabetes. It represents a risk factor for the future development of overt diabetes analogous to impaired glucose tolerance (IGT). The definition of IFG clearly depends on the cut points that are used to define what is normal and what is overt diabetes. Following the 1997 ADA report in which the upper limit of normal for fasting plasma glucose was set at 110 mg/dL, many studies were published that showed differences between the ability of IFG and IGT to predict future diabetes.[71,79–81] One of these, a report from the Baltimore Longitudinal Study of Aging, followed a cohort of over 800 subjects with serial OGTTs for up to 20 years.[81] The investigators documented the natural history of progression from normal glucose tolerance to intermediate states of hyperglycemia to overt diabetes. Many subjects reverted to normal from intermediate states of hyperglycemia, but in general, a slow, steady progression to diabetes was seen, with male gender and obesity increasing risk. By altering the threshold that was used to define the lower limit of IFG, the investigators showed that much of the "discrepancy" between rates of progression from IFG versus IGT to overt diabetes was a function of the threshold used rather than of any inherent biologic difference between the two states of hyperglycemia.

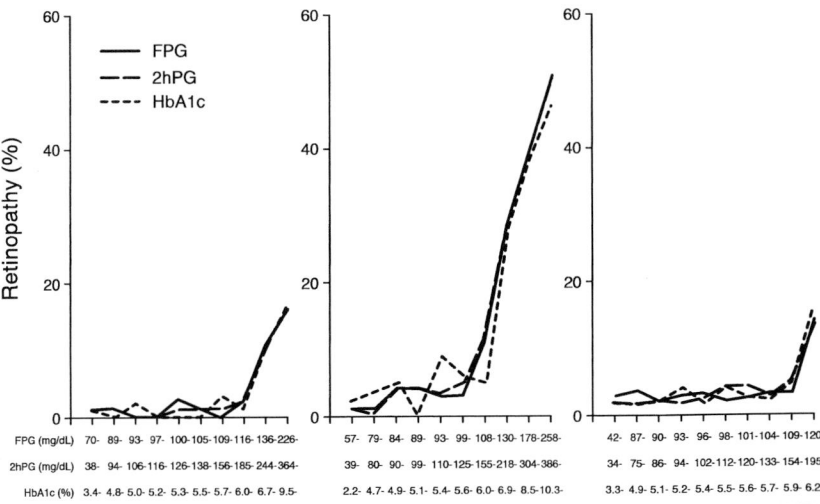

Figure 54-1 Prevalence of retinopathy by deciles of the distribution of fasting plasma glucose (FPG), 2-hour postglucose challenge plasma glucose (2hPG), and hemoglobin A1c (HbA1c) level in a population of Pima Indians (*left panel*), a population of Egyptians (*center panel*), and a representative sample of the U.S. population aged 40 to 74 years (*right panel*). (Reprinted with permission from Report of the Expert Committee on the Diagnosis and Classification of Diabetes Mellitus. Diabetes Care 20(7):1183–1197, 1997.)

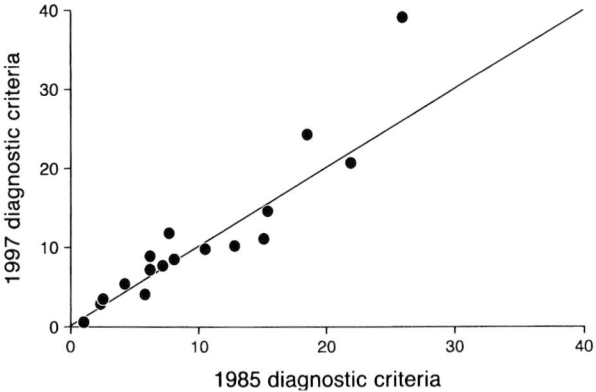

Figure 54-2 Prevalence of diabetes in 16 European populations using the 1985 diagnostic criteria of the World Health Organization and the new criteria proposed by the American Diabetes Association in 1997. (From Decode Study Group on Behalf of the European Diabetes Epidemiology Study Group: Will new diagnostic criteria for diabetes mellitus change phenotyped patients with diabetes? Reanalysis of European epidemiological data. Br Med J 317:371–375, 1998.)

Following publication of these reports and of several diabetes prevention trials, the ADA convened another International Expert Committee to reconsider the diagnostic criteria for diabetes. This committee published its findings in 2003 and has

recommended that the cut point that is used to define the upper limit of normal (and therefore the lower limit of IFG) should change from 110 mg/dL to 100 mg/dL.[82] The report from this Expert Committee cited unpublished data showing receiver operator characteristic curve analysis that indicated that the optimal threshold for fasting plasma glucose to predict future diabetes was closer to 100 mg/dL than to 110 mg/dL. Although this has not yet been ratified by the WHO, the breadth of expertise represented on the Expert Committee makes it very likely that the new criteria will be accepted; this is therefore presented in Table 54-2 as the current definition of normal fasting glucose and of IFG.

Another reason for altering the cut point that is used to define IFG is the recent publication of several diabetes prevention trials with positive results. These studies showed that a variety of interventions, including intensive lifestyle modification,[83-85] a biguanide,[85] a thiazolidinedione,[86] and an α-glucosidase inhibitor,[87] can delay or prevent the progression from intermediate states of hyperglycemia to overt diabetes. All of these trials recruited patients with IGT rather than IFG. Nevertheless, the modification in the definition of IFG means that most of the patients who were recruited into the prevention studies would have had fasting plasma glucose concentrations in the range covered by the new criteria. Ideally, separate studies should be undertaken to address the issue of preventing the progression from IFG to diabetes. However, for now, it seems reasonable to assume that the results of the published prevention studies apply to patients with IFG.

REFERENCES

1. Gerich J: The genetic basis of type 2 diabetes mellitus: Impaired insulin secretion versus impaired insulin sensitivity. Endoc Rev 19:491–503, 1998.
2. Ferrannini E: Insulin resistance versus insulin deficiency in non-insulin-dependent diabetes mellitus: Problems and prospects. Endoc Rev 19:477–490, 1998.
3. King G, Brownlee M: The cellular and molecular mechanisms of diabetic complications. Endocrinol Metab Clin North Am 25:255–270, 1996.
4. Stern M: Do non-insulin-dependent diabetes mellitus and cardiovascular disease share common antecedents? Ann Intern Med 124:110–116, 1996.
5. McGarry J: What if Minkowski had been ageusic?: An alternative angle on diabetes. Science 258:766–770, 1992.
6. Chaufan C: It's my life after all. IDF Bull 42:32–34, 1997.
7. MacGregor A: Classification criteria for rheumatoid arthritis. Baillieres Clin Rheumatol 9:287–304, 1995.
8. National Diabetes Data Group: Classification and diagnosis of diabetes mellitus and other categories of glucose intolerance. Diabetes 28:1039–1057, 1979.
9. World Health Organization: Diabetes Mellitus: Report of a WHO study group. Geneva, World Health Organization, 1985.
10. Report of the Expert Committee on the Diagnosis and Classification of Diabetes Mellitus. Diabetes Care 20:1183–1197, 1997.
11. Alberti KGMM, Zimmet PZ: Definition, diagnosis, and classification of diabetes

mellitus and its complications. Part 1: Diagnosis and classification of diabetes mellitus. Provisional report of a WHO consultation. Diabet Med 15:539–553, 1998.
12. LaPorte R, Matsushima M, Chang Y: Prevalence and incidence of insulin-dependent diabetes. In National Diabetes Data Group (ed): Diabetes in America. Bethesda, MD, National Institutes of Health, 1995, pp 37–46.
13. Karvonen M, Tuomilehto J, Libman I, LaPorte R: A review of the recent epidemiological data on the worldwide incidence of type 1 (insulin-dependent) diabetes mellitus. World Health Organization DIAMOND Project Group. Diabetologia 36:883–892, 1994.
14. Buzzetti R, Quattrocchi C, Nistico L: Dissecting the genetics of type 1 diabetes: Relevance for familial clustering and differences in incidence. Diabetes Metab Rev 14:111–128, 1998.
15. Dahlquist G: The aetiology of type 1 diabetes: An epidemiological perspective. Acta Paediatr 425:5–10, 1998.
16. Scott F, Norris J, Hubert K: Milk and type 1 diabetes: Examining the evidence and broadening the focus. Diabetes Care 19:379–383, 1996.
17. Zimmet P, Tuomi T, Mackay R, et al: Latent autoimmune diabetes mellitus in adults (LADA): The role of antibodies to glutamic acid decarboxylase in diagnosis and prediction of insulin dependency. Diabet Med 11:299–303, 1994.
18. Bingley PJ, Williams AJ, Gale EA: Optimized autoantibody-based risk assessment in family members.

Implications for future intervention trials. Diabetes Care 22:1796–1801, 1999.
19. Molbak A, Christau B, Marner B, et al: Incidence of insulin-dependent diabetes mellitus in age groups over 30 years in Denmark. Diabet Med 11:650–655, 1994.
20. Humphrey A, McCarty D, Mackay I, et al: Autoantibodies to glutamic acid decarboxylase and phenotypic features associated with early insulin treatment in individuals with adult-onset diabetes mellitus. Diabet Med 15:113–119, 1998.
21. Willis J, Scott R, Brown L, et al: Islet cell antibodies and antibodies against glutamic acid decarboxylase in newly diagnosed adult-onset diabetes mellitus. Diabetes Res Clin Prac 33:89–97, 1996.
22. McLarty D, Athaide I, Bottazzo G, et al: Islet cell antibodies are not specifically associated with insulin-dependent diabetes in rural Tanzanian Africans. Diabetes Res Clin Pract 9:219–224, 1990.
23. Libman I, LaPorte R, Becker D, et al: Was there an epidemic of diabetes in nonwhite adolescents in Allegheny County, Pennsylvania? Diabetes Care 21:1278–1281, 1998.
24. Centers for Disease Control and Prevention: National diabetes fact sheet: General information and national estimates on diabetes in the United States, 2002. Atlanta, GA, U.S. Department of Health and Human Services, Centers for Disease Control and Prevention, 2003.
25. Mokdad AH, Bowman BA, Ford ES, et al: The continuing epidemics of obesity and diabetes in the United States. JAMA 286:1195–1200, 2001.

26. Rudenski A, Hadden D, Atkinson A, et al: Natural history of pancreatic islet β–cell function in type 2 diabetes mellitus studied over six years by homeostasis model assessment. Diabet Med 5:36–41, 1988.
27. Leahy J: Natural history of beta-cell dysfunction in NIDDM. Diabetes Care 13:992–1010, 1990.
28. Cowie C, Harris M: Physical and metabolic characteristics of persons with diabetes. In National Diabetes Data Group (ed): Diabetes in America. Bethesda, MD, National Institutes of Health, 1995, pp 117–164.
29. Reaven G: Role of insulin resistance in human disease. Diabetes 37:1595–1607, 1988.
30. Barnett A, Eff C, Leslie R, Pyke D: Diabetes in identical twins: A study of 200 pairs. Diabetologia 20:87–93, 1981.
31. Knowler W, Saad M, Pettitt D, et al: Determinants of diabetes mellitus in the Pima Indians. Diabetes Care 16:216–227, 1993.
32. Hoet J, Tripathy B, Rao R, Yajnik C: Malnutrition and diabetes in the tropics. Diabetes Care 19:1014–1017, 1996.
33. Tripathy B, Samal K: Overview and consensus statement on diabetes in tropical areas. Diabetes Metab Rev 13:63–76, 1997.
34. Fajans SS, Bell GI, Polonsky KS: Molecular mechanisms and clinical pathophysiology of maturity-onset diabetes of the young. N Engl J Med 345:971–980, 2001.
35. Yamagata K, Furuta H, Oda N, et al: Mutations in the hepatocyte nuclear factor-4-alpha gene in maturity-onset diabetes of the young (MODY 1). Nature 384:458–460, 1996.
36. Froguel P, Vaxillaire M, Sun F, et al: Close linkage of glucokinase locus on chromosome 7p to early-onset non-insulin-dependent diabetes. Nature 356:162–164, 1992.
37. Yamagata K, Oda N, Kaisaki P, et al: Mutations in the hepatocyte nuclear factor-1-alpha gene in maturity-onset diabetes of the young (MODY 3). Nature 384:455–458, 1996.
38. Stoffers D, Ferrer J, Clarke W, Habener J: Early-onset type-II diabetes mellitus (MODY 4) linked to IPF1. Nat Genet 117:138–139, 1997.
39. Byrne M, Sturis J, Menzel S, et al: Altered insulin secretory response to glucose in diabetic and nondiabetic subjects with mutations in the diabetes susceptibility gene MODY 3 on chromosome 20. Diabetes 45:1503–1510, 1996.
40. Clement K, Pueyo M, Vaxillaire M, et al: Assessment of insulin sensitivity in glucokinase-deficient subjects. Diabetologia 39:82–90, 1996.
41. Habener J, Stoffers D: A newly discovered role of transcription factors involved in pancreas development and the pathogenesis of diabetes mellitus. Proc Assoc Am Physicians 110:12–21, 1998.
42. Velho G, Froguel P: Maturity-onset diabetes of the young (MODY), MODY genes and non-insulin-dependent diabetes mellitus. Diabetes Metab 23:34–37, 1997.
43. Walker M, Turnbull D: Mitochondrial related diabetes: A clinical perspective. Diabet Med 14:1007–1009, 1997.
44. Gruppuso P, Gorden P, Kahn C, et al: Familial hyperproinsulinemia due to a proposed defect in conversion of proinsulin to insulin. N Engl J Med 311:629–634, 1984.
45. Haneda M, Polonsky K, Bergenstal R, et al: Familial hyperinsulinemia due to a structurally abnormal insulin: Definition of an emerging new clinical syndrome. N Engl J Med 310:1288–1294, 1984.
46. Bruning J, Winnay J, Bonner-Weir S, et al: Development of a novel polygenic model of NIDDM in mice heterozygous for IR and IRS-1 null alleles. Cell 88:561–572, 1997.
47. Taylor S: Lilly lecture: Molecular mechanisms of insulin resistance: Lessons from patients with mutations in the insulin-receptor gene. Diabetes 41:1473–1490, 1992.
48. Tritos NA, Mantzoros CS: Syndromes of severe insulin resistance. J Clin Endocrinol Metab 83:3025–3030, 1998.
49. Joffe BI, Panz VR, Raal FJ: From lipodystrophy syndromes to diabetes mellitus. Lancet 357:1379–1381, 2001.
50. Arioglu E, Duncan-Morin J, Sebring N, et al: Efficacy and safety of troglitazone in the treatment of lipodystrophy syndromes. Ann Intern Med 133:263–274, 2000.
51. Gullo L, Pezzilli R, Morselli-Labate A, Group IPCS: Diabetes and the risk of pancreatic cancer. N Engl J Med 331:81–84, 1994.
52. Moran A, Doherty L, Wang X, Thomas W: Abnormal glucose metabolism in cystic fibrosis. Pediatr 133:10–17, 1998.
53. Phelps G, Chapman I, Hall P, et al: Prevalence of genetic haemochromatosis among diabetic patients. Lancet 2:233–234, 1989.
54. Yajnik C, Shelgikar K, Naik S, et al: The ketoacidosis-resistance in fibro-calculous-pancreatic-diabetes. Diabetes Res Clin Pract 15:149–156, 1993.
55. Mohan V, Barman KK, Rajan VS, et al: Troppical calcific pancreatitis is a prediabetic stage of fibrocalculous pancreatic diabetes (FCPD) longitudinal follow-up study. Diabetologia 46(Suppl 2):A18, 2003.
56. SPINK1 is a susceptibility gene for fibrocalculous pancreatic diabetes in subjects from the Indian subcontinent. Am J Hum Genet 71:964–968, 2002.
57. Pandit M, Burke J, Gustafson A, et al: Drug-induced disorders of glucose tolerance. Ann Intern Med 118:529–540, 1993.
58. O'Byrne S, Feely J: Effects of drug on glucose tolerance in non-insulin-dependent diabetes (parts I and II). Drugs 40:203–219, 1990.
59. Forrest J, Menser M, Burgess JA: High frequency of diabetes mellitus in young patients with congenital rubella. Lancet 2:332–334, 1971.
60. King M, Bidwell D, Shikh A, et al: Coxsackie-B-virus-specific IgM responses in children with insulin-dependent (juvenile-onset; type 1) diabetes mellitus. Lancet 1:1397–1399, 1983.
61. Solimena M, De Camilli P: Autoimmunity to glutamic acid decarboxylase (GAD) in stiff-man syndrome and insulin-dependent diabetes mellitus. Trends Neurosci 14:452–457, 1991.
62. Arioglu E, Andewelt A, Diabo C, et al: Clinical course of the syndrome of autoantibodies to the insulin receptor (Type B insulin resistance): A 28-year perspective. Medicine 8:87–100, 2002.
63. Engelgau M, Herman W, Smith P, et al: The epidemiology and diabetes and pregnancy in the US, 1988. Diabetes Care 18:1029–1033, 1995.
64. Persson B, Hanson U: Neonatal mobidities in gestational diabetes mellitus. Diabetes Care 21:B79–B84, 1998.
65. Dornhorst A, Rossi M: Risk and prevention of type 2 diabetes in women with gestational diabetes. Diabetes Care 21:B43–B49, 1998.
66. Coustan D, Carpenter M: The diagnosis of gestational diabetes. Diabetes Care 21:B5–B8, 1998.
67. Carr S: Screening for gestational diabetes mellitus. Diabetes Care 21:B14–B18, 1998.
68. McCance D, Hanson R, Charles M, et al: Comparison of tests for glycated haemoglobin and fasting and two hour plasma glucose concentrations as diagnostic methods for diabetes. Br Med J 308:1323–1328, 1994.
69. Finch C, Zimmet P, Alberti K: Determining diabetes prevalence: A rational basis for the use of fasting plasma glucose concentrations. Diabet Med 7:603–610, 1990.
70. Engelgau M, Thompson T, Herman W, et al: Comparison of fasting and 2-hour glucose and HbAlc levels for diagnosing diabetes. Diagnostic criteria and performance revisited. Diabetes Care 20:785–791, 1997.
71. Decode Study Group on Behalf of the European Diabetes Epidemiology Study Group: Will new diagnostic criteria for diabetes mellitus change phenotyped patients with diabetes? Reanalysis of European epidemiological data. Br Med J 317:371–375, 1998.
72. De Vegt F, Dekker J, Stehouwer C, et al: American Diabetes Association criteria versus the 1985 World Health Organization criteria for the diagnosis of abnormal glucose tolerance: Poor agreement in the Hoorn Study. Diabetes Care 21:1686–1690, 1998.
73. Wahl P, Savage P, Psaty B, et al: Diabetes in older adults: Comparison of 1997 American Diabetes Association classification of diabetes mellitus with 1985 WHO classification. Lancet 352:1012–1015, 1998.

74. Harris M, Eastman R, Cowie C, et al: Comparison of diabetes diagnostic categories in the US population according to 1997 American Diabetes Association and 1980–1985 World Health Organization diagnostic criteria. Diabetes Care 20:1859–1862, 1997.

75. Sacks DB, Bruns DE, Goldstein DE, et al: Guidelines and recommendations for laboratory analysis in the diagnosis and management of diabetes mellitus. Clin Chem 48:436–472, 2002.

76. Dinneen S, Maldonado D, Leibson C, et al: Effects of changing diagnostic criteria on the risk of developing diabetes. Diabetes Care 21:1408–1413, 1998.

77. Charles M, Balkau B, Vauzelle-Kervoeden F, et al: Revision of diagnostic criteria for diabetes. Lancet 348:1657–1658, 1996.

78. Gerstein H, Yusuf S: Dysglycaemia and risk of cardiovascular disease. Lancet 347:949–950, 1996.

79. McCance D, Hanson R, Pettitt D, et al: Diagnosing diabetes mellitus: Do we need new criteria? Diabetologia 40:247–255, 1997.

80. Shaw J, Zimmet P, De Courten M, et al: Impaired fasting glucose or impaired glucose tolerance: What best predicts future diabetes in Mauritius? Diabetes Care 22:399–402, 1999.

81. Meigs JB, Muller DC, Nathan DM, et al: The natural history of progression from normal glucose tolerance to type 2 diabetes in the Baltimore Longitudinal Study of Aging. Diabetes 52:1475–1484, 2003.

82. The Expert Committee on the Diagnosis and Classification of Diabetes Mellitus: Follow-up report on the diagnosis of diabetes mellitus. Diabetes Care 26:3160–3167, 2003.

83. Pan X, Li G, Hu Y, et al: Effects of diet and exercise in preventing NIDDM in people with impaired glucose tolerance: The Da Qing IGT and Diabetes Study. Diabetes Care 20:537–544, 1997.

84. Tuomilehto J, Lindstrom J, Eriksson JG, et al: Prevention of Type 2 diabetes by changes in lifestyle among subjects with impaired glucose tolerance. N Engl J Med 344:1343–1350, 2001.

85. Diabetes Prevention Program Research Group: Reduction in the incidence of type 2 diabetes with lifestyle intervention or metformin. N Engl J Med 346:393–403, 2002.

86. Buchanan TA, Xiang AH, Peters RK, et al: Preservation of pancreatic beta-cell function and prevention of type 2 diabetes by pharmacological treatment of insulin resistance in high-risk Hispanic women. Diabetes 51:2796–2803, 2002.

87. Chiasson JL, Josse RG, Gomis R, et al: Acarbose for prevention of type 2 diabetes mellitus: the STOP-NIDDM randomised trial. Lancet 359:2072–2077, 2002.

Type 1 (Insulin-dependent) Diabetes Mellitus: Etiology, Pathogenesis, and Natural History

Lisa K. Gilliam and Åke Lernmark

INTRODUCTION

Type 1 (insulin-dependent) diabetes mellitus (T1DM) is associated with numerous immune abnormalities. The pancreatic β cells decrease in numbers and volume, and a distinct mode of progression to severe insulin deficiency occurs that requires insulin-substitution therapy. In children, T1DM has a distinct clinical mode of presentation. Classically, when age at onset is young, classification of the disease is straightforward. This is changing in the current obesity epidemic, which is having a significant effect on the pediatric population, making differentiation between T1DM and (T2DM) more difficult in this age group.[1,2] In adults, T1DM may masquerade as T2DM. Although it has been known for decades that diabetes mellitus can occur in various degrees of severity, it was not until approximately 40 years ago that evidence was presented that indicated different modes of inheritance for what were then classified as "maturity-onset" and "juvenile-onset" types of diabetes.[3] It is now evident that T1DM may occur at any age. The fact that T1DM in adults fulfills clinical criteria for T2DM demonstrates the limitation of a disease classification based on clinical symptoms rather than on the etiology and pathogenesis of the disease. Current diagnostic criteria for different forms of diabetes mellitus are therefore limited to clinical symptoms,[4] except in rare families with specific mutations (e.g., glucokinase, hepatocyte nuclear factor (HNF)-1α, HNF-4α, and other mutations, which cause specific syndromes of maturity-onset diabetes of the young [MODY]). The basis for the distinction between T1DM and T2DM is the patient's dependence on insulin. T1DM in children or non-pregnant adults includes any of the following symptoms or biochemical changes: polyuria, polydipsia, ketonuria, and rapid weight loss, together with gross or unequivocal elevation of plasma glucose levels. Stupor and coma may ultimately develop.

The diagnostic criteria used to differentiate between T1DM (insulin-dependent) and T2DM (non-insulin-dependent diabetes, or NIDDM) are important for understanding the cause and pathogenesis of these two disease entities. The diagnostic criteria are primarily recommendations for classification, the aim of which is better understanding of the cause of diabetes and optimization of care of diabetic patients. By using molecular genetics, it has been possible to clarify fully several monogenetic forms of diabetes. The etiology of these diabetes phenotypes, some of them classified as MODY, have been explained by mutations in, for example, the genes for insulin,[5] insulin receptor,[6] glucokinase (maturity-onset diabetes in the young; *MODY-2*),[7] *HNF-4α* (*MODY-1*),[8] or *HNF-1α* (*MODY-3*).[9] The clarification of the etiology of these diabetes phenotypes is a major advancement that has increased the diagnostic precision of diabetes syndromes.[4,10] The understanding of the more complex and multifactorial T1DM syndromes also has undergone significant advances.

HISTORY

Early histologic studies of pancreatic tissue of diabetic patients who died shortly after clinical onset revealed that the pancreatic islets were altered by fibrosis, hyalinosis, atrophy, and infiltration of inflammatory cells.[11] The inflammatory lesion of the islets of Langerhans was later described as insulitis,[12] and quantitative studies of the pancreatic islets showed a specific loss of insulin-producing cells in association with the clinical onset of T1DM.[13,14] The presence of inflammatory cells in and around the islets of Langerhans in about 50% of new-onset patients also was described.[13,15] The rediscovery of insulitis[13] was of major significance, especially because it was later observed that autoimmune thyroid disease often developed in diabetic patients treated with insulin or, conversely, that patients with diseases of autoimmune character (e.g., Graves' disease, Hashimoto's thyroiditis, pernicious anemia, and Addison's disease) had an increased prevalence of insulin-dependent diabetes.[16,17] It was therefore suggested that the pathogenesis of insulin-dependent diabetes involved autoimmune reactions directed toward the endocrine pancreas. This notion was supported by delayed-type hypersensitivity[18] and leukocyte migration inhibition[19,20] to pancreatic islet antigens. Numerous studies have confirmed the presence of insulitis[21,22]; however, in spite of the assumption that the cellular branch of the immune system plays a critical role in disease pathogenesis, reproducible tests of blood T-cell reactivity to islet antigens have been difficult to establish.[23,24] Studies to improve the detection of anti–β cell T-cell reactivity are continuing,[25–28] but these T-cell assays are not yet widely available. In contrast, several types of islet cell autoantibodies can now be determined with standardized assays. Long-sought-for islet cell antibodies (ICAs) were described in 1974,[29,30] islet cell-surface antibodies (ICSAs) in 1978,[31] and complement-dependent antibody-mediated islet cell cytotoxicity in 1980.[32] The first antigen recognized by these antibodies, an islet protein of 64,000 relative molecular mass (Mr), or 64 K, was described in 1982.[33,34] Later, the 64 K protein was found to have glutamic acid decarboxylase (GAD) activity,[34] but molecular cloning showed that the enzyme was a novel GAD isoform, GAD65.[35,36] Autoantibodies to insulin (IAAs) were demonstrated in 1983,[37] and a third autoantigen, insulinoma-associated antigen-2 (IA-2), a receptor-type protein tyrosine phosphatase, in 1994.[38-40] Since the mid-1980s, numerous studies have used serum from patients with T1DM in attempts to identify novel β-cell target autoantigens by immunoprecipitation or immunoblotting techniques. So far, antibody assays to other autoantigens have failed to show disease sensitivity and specificity superior to those of GAD65, insulin, and IA-2. The presence of autoantibodies against these three autoantigens are shown to replace the more cumbersome ICA indirect immunofluorescence assay.[41] Taken together, ample evidence exists that islet cell autoimmunity is of major importance in the etiopathogenesis of T1DM.

T1DM is often thought to be a disorder of acute onset, and the clinical onset may be dramatic. Over the years, however, numerous reports have noted that signs of subclinical diabetes preceded the clinical onset. In addition, in adult diabetes patients classified with T2DM, a change sometimes occurs from an insulin-independent to an insulin-dependent state. It is now accepted that ICAs or autoantibodies against GAD65, insulin, or IA-2 may be present up to several years before the clinical onset of the disease,[42-45] perhaps even at birth.[46] The possibility that islet autoimmunity might be present long before symptoms of hyperglycemia occur makes it difficult to define a causative factor. The clinical onset is not likely to occur until a major loss (80% to 90%) of the islet β cells occurs. An increased frequency of diabetes in conjunction with acute viral illnesses was first described in Norway more than 100 years ago and was subsequently followed by numerous similar case reports. These early reports suggested a relation between the clinical onset of T1DM and acute viral illness.[47,48] Most commonly, T1DM has been diagnosed in conjunction with infections of mumps, congenital rubella, or coxsackievirus B4.[47,48] The true relation between these viral diseases and later onset of T1DM remains conjectural and is outlined in more detail later in this chapter. The immunologic responsiveness to viruses among different individuals may be relevant to the disease process. In addition, T1DM is both genetically associated with and linked to certain human leukocyte antigen (HLA) genetic factors.[49-51] By using DNA sequence information in the genetic analysis, it is found that more than 95% of all patients in whom T1DM onset occurred before age 30 years are positive for the chromosome 6 HLA genes *DQB1*0302-A1*0301-DRB1*04*, *DQB1*0201-A1*0501-DRB1*03*, or both. Although some 50% to 60% of the background population carry these HLA factors, they represent necessary but insufficient prerequisites for the development of T1DM. It has been estimated that HLA contributes about 60% of T1DM risk. Other genetic factors have indeed been identified,[52,53] but none has shown a level of importance comparable to that of HLA. The risk conferred by HLA alleles is outlined in more detail later in this chapter. In summary, the association with HLA may signify differences in immune responsiveness to certain antigens. The formation of an immune response to an invading antigen (e.g., virus, bacterium) or internal antigen (e.g., a retrovirus) might induce an autoimmune reaction directed against the pancreatic islet cells.

PREVALENCE

The prevalence of T1DM is low compared with that of T2DM. Among individuals age 30 years or younger, the prevalence of T1DM does not usually exceed about 0.3% (Table 55-1), compared with prevalence rates for T2DM of 4.2% worldwide and nearly 25% in certain high-risk populations.[54] Both geographic and ethnic variations are seen in the prevalence rates. It has been pointed out[4,55] that the prevalence figures shown in Table 55-1 should be viewed with caution, because different age groups were studied, and various methods of assessing the cases were used. In addition, it is unclear whether recently observed increases in incidence rates worldwide reflect a change in the age at onset of diabetes, as opposed to a true increase in prevalence of T1DM.[56] Further studies are needed to address this question.

INCIDENCE

The incidence rate is the frequency with which new cases of T1DM are detected during a defined period. The rate is expressed as an annual number of cases per 100,000 age-corrected individuals. A determination of incidence therefore requires a precise knowledge of the total number of individuals in each age group and the number of new patients diagnosed in the particular area during 1 year. Determinations of secular trends constitute an important part of population-based epidemiologic studies. However, such analyses are rare because they require careful follow-up investigations during several subsequent years.

Incidence studies on T1DM are available from an increasing number of countries and states (Table 55-2).[4,55,57-66] Traditionally, the groups that have been studied are primarily white; until recently, only limited information has been available for other racial groups. The reliability of data from many countries suffers, however, from the absence of clearly defined degrees of ascertainment and demographics as well as from lack of geographic delineation of the group subjected to investigation. Recent studies, including the EURODIAB study and the DiaMond study, have attempted to define better the incidence rates in various populations by using prospective, population-based, geographically defined registries. Overall, the average annual incidence rate varies widely, from 0.1 per 100,000 children in parts of Asia and South America[57] to 40.2 per 100,000 in Finland.[58] Over the past few decades, many

Table 55-1 The Prevalence of Type 1 Diabetes in Certain Populations

Location	Age Group Studied (yr)	Method of Ascertainment	Prevalence (per 1000)
China	10–19	Survey	0.09
Cuba	0–15	National registry	0.14
France	0–19	Central registry	0.32
Japan	7–15	School records	0.07
Scandinavian countries	0–14	National registry and hospital records	0.83–2.23
United Kingdom	0–26	National survey of health and development	3.40
United States	5–17	School records	1.93

From Harris MI: Diabetes in America, 2d ed. Bethesda, MD, National Institutes of Health, 1995.

Table 55-2 Mean Annual Incidence of T1DM (per 100,000) in Children, Adolescents, and Young Adults in Various Locations

Continent	Country/Region	Ascertainment Period	Age (yr)	No. Cases	Incidence Rate (per 10^5)	Ref.
N. AMERICA	*UNITED STATES*					
	Allegheny, PA	1990–1994	0–14	206	17.8	57
	Philadelphia, PA	1990–1994	0–14	209	13.3	59
	Jefferson, AL	1990–1994	0–14	101	15.0	57
	Chicago, IL	1990–1994	0–14	300	11.7	57
	CANADA					
	Alberta	**1990–1994**	**0–14**	**175**	**24**	**57**
	Prince Edward Is.	**1990–1993**	**0–14**	**29**	**24.5**	**57**
EUROPE						
	Austria	1991–1994	0–15	753	9.1	58
	Belgium (Antwerp)	1989–1994	0–15	112	11.6	58
	Bulgaria					
	Western	1989–1994	0–15	303	9.6	58
	Eastern	1989–1994	0–15	218	6.8	58
	Croatia (Zagreb)	1989–1994	0–15	83	6.8	58
	Czech Republic	1989–1994	0–15	1144	8.9	58
	Denmark					
	4 countries	1991–1994	0–15	221	16	58
	Nationwide	1996–2000	0–15	1421	19.5	60
	Estonia	1989–1994	0–15	206	10.3	58
	Finland (2 regions)	**1992–1993**	**0–15**	**425**	**40.2**	**58**
	France (4 regions)	1991–1994	0–15	837	8.3	58
	Germany					
	Dusseldorf	1993–1994	0–15	111	14	58
	Baden-Wurttenberg	1989–1994	0–15	1101	11.3	58
	Greece					
	Attica	1993–1994	0–15	333	9.5	58
	5 northern regions	1993–1994	0–15	49	6.2	58
	Hungary (18 countries)	1989–1994	0–15	822	8.9	58
	Iceland	1989–1994	0–15	52	13.5	58
	Italy					
	Sardinia	**1991–1994**	**0–15**	**675**	**36.6**	**58**
	Lombardia	1991–1994	0–15	530	7.0	58
	Lazio	1993–1994	0–15	396	8.1	58
	Eastern Sicily	1991–1994	0–15	150	11.4	58
	Turin	1990–1994	0–14	155	11.0	57
	Pavia	1990–1994	0–14	34	11.7	57
	Marche	1990–1994	0–14	99	9.7	57
	Latvia	1993–1994	0–15	221	6.6	58
	Lithuania	1989–1994	0–15	368	7.4	58
	Luxembourg	1993–1994	0–15	49	12.1	58
	Macedonia	1989–1994	0–15	93	3.2	58
	Netherlands (5 reg.)	1991–1994	0–15	421	13.0	58
	Norway (8 countries)	**1992–1994**	**0–15**	**491**	**21.2**	**58**
	Poland					
	8 western prov.	1991–1994	0–15	542	6.7	58
	3 cities	1989–1994	0–15	312	6.1	58
	Gliwice		0–15	316	5.4	58
	Blalystok	1994	0–15	31	5.5	58
	Portugal					
	Madeira	1993–1994	0–15	24	6.9	58
	Portalegre	1989–1994	0–15	25	19.0	58
	Algarve	1991–1994	0–15	51	13.6	58
	Romania (Bucharest)	1989–1994	0–15	138	5.0	58
	Slovakia	1989–1994	0–15	656	8.4	58
	Slovenia	1992–1994	0–15	186	7.6	58
	Spain (Catalonia)	1991–1994	0–15	839	12.3	58
	Sweden					
	Nationwide	**1990–1994**	**0–14**	**2166**	**27.5**	**57**
	Stockholm County	**1993–1994**	**0–15**	**451**	**25.8**	**58**
	Switzerland	1991–1994	0–15	353	7.9	58
	United Kingdom					
	Oxford		0–15	542	17.6	58
	Leicester	1989–1993	0–15	169	15.9	58
	Leeds	1989–1994	0–15	668	15.7	58
	Yorkshire	**1978–2000**	**0–14**	**2718**	**20.0**	**61**
	Northern Ireland	1989–1994	0–15	462	19.6	58
	Scotland	**1984–1993**	**0–15**	**2326**	**23.9**	**62**
	Aberdeen	**1990**	**0–14**	**23**	**24.0**	**57**

Continued

Table 55-2 Mean Annual Incidence of T1DM (per 100,000) in Children, Adolescents, and Young Adults in Various Locations—cont'd

Continent	Country/Region	Ascertainment Period	Age (yr)	No. Cases	Incidence Rate (per 10^5)	Ref.
MIDDLE EAST						
	Israel	1993	0–15	433	5.9	58
	Libya (Benghazi)	1991–2000	0–14	276	7.8	63
	Kuwait	**1992–1997**	**0–14**	**364**	**20.1**	**64**
ASIA						
	Japan (3 regions)	1990–1993	0–14	167	1.4–2.2*	57
	China (21 regions)	1990–1994	0–14	452	0.1–4.6*	57
	Hong Kong	1990–1994	0–14	17	1.3	57
	Pakistan	1990	0–14	25	0.7	57
	Thailand	1991–1997	0–15	76	0.4	65
	Russia (Novosibirsk)	1990–1994	0–14	191	6.0	57
AFRICA						
	Algeria (Oran)	1990–1994	0–14	23	5.7	57
	Tunisia (4 regions)	1990–1994	0–14	168	4.9–8.8*	57
	Sudan (Gezira)	1990–1994	0–14	29	5.0	57
	Mauritius	1990–1994	0–14	21	1.4	57
OCEANIA						
	New Zealand					
	Auckland	1990–1994	0–14	135	12.9	57
	Canterbury	**1990–1994**	**0–14**	**78**	**21.9**	**57**
	Australia, NSW	1992–1996	0–14	1230	17.8	66
SOUTH AMERICA						
	Argentina (4 regions)	1990–1994	0–14	89	4.3–8.0*	57
	Brazil (Sao Paulo)	1990–1992	0–14	34	8.0	57
	Chile (Santiago)	1990–1992	0–14	122	1.6	57
	Colombia (Bogota)	1990	0–14	56	3.8	57
	Paraguay	1990–1994	0–14	79	0.9	57
	Peru (Lima)	1990–1991	0–14	16	0.4	57
	Uruguay (Montevideo)	1992	0–14	26	8.3	57
	Venezuela (Caracas)	1992	0–14	43	0.1	57
	Barbados	1990–1993	0–14	5	2.0	57
CENTRAL AMERICA						
	Mexico (Veracruz)	1990–1993	0–14	9	1.5	57
CARIBBEAN						
	Cuba	1990–1994	0–14	349	2.9	57
	Dominica	1990–1993	0–14	5	5.7	57
	Puerto Rico (U.S.)	1990–1994	0–14	844	17.4	57
	Virgin Islands (U.S.)	1990–1994	0–14	16	13.1	57

*Incidence rates varied by region.
Countries with incidence rates >$20/10^5$/yr are shown in bold.

studies have demonstrated an annual increase in incidence of T1DM.[67–71] Worldwide epidemiologic investigations of T1DM as a noncommunicable disease indicate a 4% to 6% annual increase in incidence rate in Scandinavia,[68,72] and similar data are being collected in other countries.[71] Pooled data from all sites in the EURODIAB study demonstrated an annual rate of increase in incidence of 3.4%, with more-rapid rates of increase occurring in certain regions.[58] About 1% of all children born in Scandinavian countries will manifest T1DM during their lifetimes. It is speculated that T1DM exhibits patterns of epidemic occurrence, suggesting that diabetogenic environmental determinants may exist.[71] The TEDDY study (The Environmental Determinants of Diabetes in the Young), currently under way, is an international effort to identify these determinants, including infectious agents, dietary factors, or other environmental factors, that trigger T1DM in genetically susceptible individuals. Studies from several countries show that the incidence rates vary by geographic region (not only between but also within countries), by age, and by gender.

GEOGRAPHIC DISTRIBUTION

The annual incidence of T1DM is higher in northern Europe than in the Mediterranean area, with the exception of Sardinia (see Table 55-2).[73,74] Furthermore, the incidence in Iceland[73] is lower than that in Sweden[75] or Finland.[73] Surprisingly, the T1DM incidence rate in Estonia is about 25% of the rate in Finland, in spite of their close geographic proximity.[74] The incidence rates within countries also show stable differences. The eastern and southern parts of Finland[76] as well as the central and southern parts of Sweden[75] have higher incidence rates than the northern parts of those countries.

The incidence rate in high-level areas is as high as 40 to 50 per 100,000 persons age 0 to 15 years. The cause of geographic variation remains unknown, but it has been speculated that genetic factors, primarily associated with different HLA-DR or DQ genotypes of the major histocompatibility complex (MHC) on chromosome 6, and environmental factors are important. The latter is supported by the observation that monozygotic twins show rates of less than 20% to 30% concordance for IDDM.[77,78] Among HLA-identical siblings of T1DM-affected patients, about 20% eventually manifest the disease, and the overall lifetime risk for first-degree relatives has been estimated at about 8% for siblings and 5% for children of parents with T1DM.[79] The mode of inheritance is complex. In addition, the HLA class II molecules from the DQ and DR loci on chromosome 6 that are necessary (but not sufficient) for disease vary greatly between countries and thereby affect disease incidence.[74,80,81] In addition, factors in the environment are important in understanding the pathogenesis of T1DM, and they also may help to explain differences in geographic distribution. Improved epidemiology and better diagnostic criteria to distinguish different forms of diabetes are critical in obtaining reliable incidence rates for various countries and states.

VARIATION WITH AGE

Until recently, T1DM was thought to occur almost exclusively in children and adolescents. Epidemiologic studies with rigorous diagnostic criteria[4] suggest, however, that the clinical onset of T1DM may occur at any age. The incidence rate varies with both age and gender (Fig. 55-1). The peak for both girls and boys, age 11 to 14 years, has been discernible in most studies and seems to be present irrespective of the country or area studied.[57,58,67,71,73] This peak is associated with puberty and the maximal velocity of pubertal growth. Recent studies have suggested that the annual rate of increase in incidence is higher in younger age groups, with rates of 6.4% in 0- to 4-year-olds, 3.1% in 5- to 9-year-olds, and 2.4% in 10- to 14-year-olds.[58] In children, minor incidence peaks occur at 4 to 6 years[67] and 7 to 8 years,[82,83] which have been associated with entrance into preschool or school programs.[84] Only recently has it been widely recognized that T1DM also occurs

in adults. One study estimated that 30% of T1DM occurs after age 30 years,[85] although, of note, this study was performed before the identification of diabetes-related autoantibodies, which play an important role in helping to distinguish T1DM from T2DM when clinical symptoms are equivocal. A more recent study in a Danish population reported that 44% of all cases of T1DM were first seen after age 40 years.[86] This older-onset T1DM population is not a well-studied group, so it is not clear how well this finding translates to other populations; however, it is clear that T1DM is not exclusively a childhood disease. Epidemiologic investigation has indicated that the incidence rate of T1DM in patients older than 20 years is lower than that seen in children, except for a possible peak at around 50 to 65 years.[87] In addition to adults having what is considered a more classic, fulminant T1DM clinical picture, some adult patients initially classified and treated as having T2DM may require insulin after 1 to 5 years of therapy with diet, exercise, or oral hypoglycemic agents.[88,89] This type of diabetes is referred to as latent autoimmune diabetes in the adult (LADA),[90] slowly progressive insulin-dependent diabetes mellitus (SPIDDM),[91] or type 1.5 diabetes.[92] These patients are positive for diabetes-related autoantibodies and have lower body mass index and higher frequencies of high-risk HLA types compared with other "type 2" patients.[93] It is speculated that these patients in fact have T1DM in addition to genetic factors that inhibit rapid progression of β-cell killing.[87]

Although rare, some forms of diabetes mellitus can occur in the newborn period, at birth, or during the first months of life. One type is a transient DM, in which the metabolism and, to a certain extent, normal growth and development must be maintained with insulin for as long as 1 to 2 years. This form of transient DM is thought to be caused by delayed islet β-cell maturation, and genetic analysis indicates that the overexpression of an imprinted gene that displays paternal expression may be a causative factor.[94] Another more rare condition is T1DM resulting from a lack of β cells. This form has autoimmune features and is characterized by a permanent state of insulin dependency. Very rarely, children can be born without an endocrine pancreas. This form of diabetes is not associated with autoimmune markers and consists of both endocrine and exocrine pancreatic dysfunction. Genetic mutations associated with permanent forms of neonatal diabetes have recently been described, including a deletion in the *PDX* gene,[95] a mutation of the glucokinase gene,[96] and activating mutations of the *Kir6.2* gene.[97]

VARIATION WITH GENDER

It has been reported that the peak incidence in girls occurs earlier than in boys.[82] If the clinical onset of T1DM is linked to pubertal growth, this difference in incidence rate can be explained by the fact that pubertal growth occurs earlier in girls. Prepubertal boys were found to be taller at the clinical onset of T1DM.[83] In addition, newly diagnosed children of both genders showed advanced skeletal maturity.[98] Even if boys tend to show an increased height compared with controls, their growth seems to cease about 35 weeks before the clinical onset of T1DM.[83] It therefore is possible that processes affecting the pancreatic β-cell mass and the ability to produce insulin may have profound effects on body growth and function at a young age. Because these processes differ slightly between boys and girls, growth characteristics may offer a simple explanation for the differences seen in incidence rates between the genders.

Surveys based on the registration of all new patients with T1DM in Sweden[75] and New Zealand[99] have indicated that occurrence of T1DM before age 15 years is slightly more common among boys. Preliminary evidence[75] suggests that an increased prevalence among boys may be observed only during certain years. A more recent study looking at sex differences in T1DM incidence in this age group showed a slight

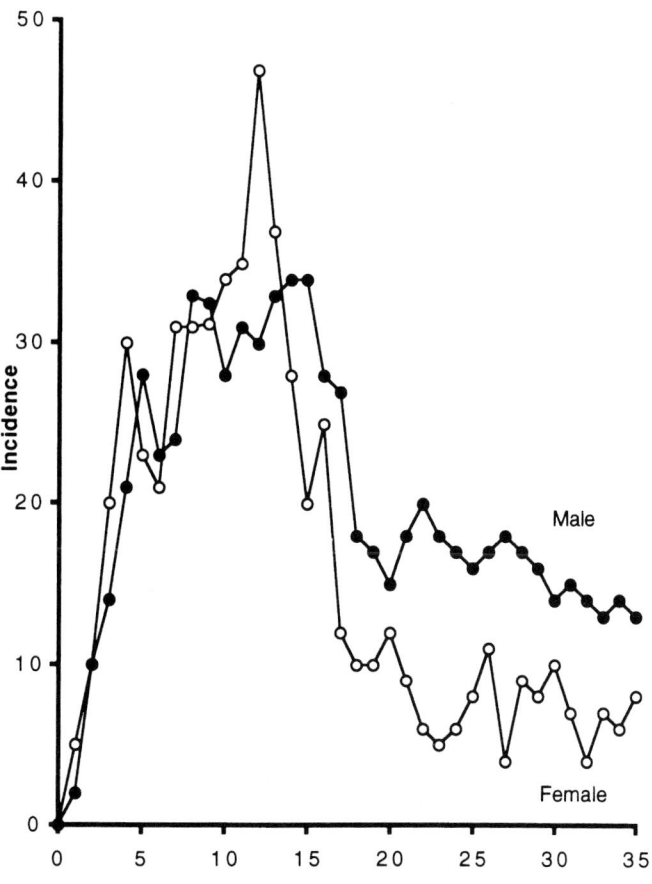

Figure 55-1 Age-adjusted incidence of insulin-dependent diabetes mellitus in relation to age at onset in male and female subjects. (Adapted from data in Nystrom L, Dahlquist G, Ostman J, et al: Risk of developing insulin-dependent diabetes mellitus [IDDM] before 35 years of age: Indications of climatological determinants for age at onset. Int J Epidemiol 21:352–358, 1992, with permission.)

male preponderance in many, but not all, European countries, whereas a female preponderance was found in most African and Asian countries.[100] Interestingly, the male excess was seen in all countries with the highest incidence rates (>20/10^5/yr), whereas a female excess was seen in all countries with the low incidence rates (<4.5/10^5/yr). Studies of older age groups have consistently shown a male preponderance for new cases of T1DM, with male/female ratios ranging from 1.3 to 2.5.[101] One registry of T1DM among 15- to 34-year-olds (see Fig. 55-1) demonstrated that T1DM was 1.5 times more common among men than women.[84] Further studies are necessary to document gender-dependent incidence rates and to explain their mechanisms.

ETIOLOGY

The absence of an unambiguous mode of inheritance, the presence of a period of subclinical islet autoimmunity preceding clinical onset of disease, HLA genes that control the immune response, and age and seasonal variation must be taken into account in attempts to explain the cause of T1DM. A defined etiologic factor, endogenous or exogenous, capable of causing T1DM remains to be identified (Table 55-3). Because evidence exists of genetic heterogeneity in T1DM, it is possible that different causative factors are responsible. In experimental animals (see Table 55-3), both viral and chemical agents have been used to induce diabetes reproducibly, and certain strains of animals are at higher risk for developing diabetes due to genetic factors. In humans, genetic factors are clearly important, but these factors do not explain the whole picture. In addition, only indirect evidence suggests that environmental factors that are clearly diabetogenic in animals are involved in initiating T1DM in humans. The following is a brief summary of possible genetic or environmental factors that are associated with the appearance of T1DM.

GENETIC FACTORS

HLA on chromosome 6 is the major genetic risk factor for T1DM, regardless of age. The HLA haplotypes *DQB1*0302-A1*0301-DRB1*04* and *DQB1*0201-A1*0501-DRB1*03* are the two major risk haplotypes.[49,102] The most important alleles are *DQB1*0302* and *DQB1*0201*, along with *DRB1*03*. *DRB1*04* is a large family of related molecules, and *DRB1*0401* confers an independent risk, whereas *DRB1*0403* is negatively associated with diabetes and may protect or

decelerate an ongoing disease process.[103] *DRB1*03* seems to be more important than *DQB1*0201*, as only *DQB1*0201-A1*0501-DRB1*03*, not *DQB1*0201-A1*0501-DRB1*07*, confers T1DM risk. *DQB1*0401* and *DQB1*0604* also are susceptibility alleles. The genetic linkage and association between T1DM and HLA also is remarkable, as certain HLA haplotypes are protective. Most prominently, *DQB1*0602-A1*0102* and *DQB1*0603-A1*0102* are protective before age 15 years. The detailed mechanisms by which HLA confers either risk or resistance is not fully understood.[102,104] The function of these molecules is to display peptide antigens to be recognized by T-cell receptors (TCRs). The disease association may therefore be related either to an inability to induce immunologic tolerance to certain autoantigens or to antigen presentation of an endogenous autoantigen. In the first case, the subject may be exposed to infectious agents that mimic autoantigens. Reactivity to the infectious agent sets off an immune response that cross-reacts with self. In the second case, the immune reaction may result in a direct attack on the individual's own cells.

It is estimated that HLA accounts for about 60% of the genetic risk.[105,106] The genetics of T1DM is studied extensively, as it represents a paradigm for genetically complex diseases. Genome screens and studies on candidate genes have provided evidence for genetic linkage between polymorphic DNA markers and more than 15 putative T1DM susceptibility loci.[52,53,107] A polymorphism upstream of the insulin gene on chromosome 6 affects T1DM risk,[108,109] perhaps by controlling insulin expression in the thymus and thereby the development of immunologic tolerance.[110,111] The gene for CTLA-4 on chromosome 2 is another candidate.[112,113] CTLA-4 controls T-lymphocyte survival after activation, and it is speculated that regulation of the CTLA-4 gene may affect propensity for autoimmune disease. Taken together, however, these and other genetic factors have limited effects on the relative risk of T1DM. Even with high-risk HLA alleles, in only 1 in 15 children from the general population and in only 1 in 5 first-degree relatives of T1DM patients will diabetes develop. The mechanisms by which these factors contribute to appearance of the disease remain to be clarified.

ENVIRONMENTAL FACTORS

Viral infections are thought to contribute to the onset of T1DM (see Table 55-3). This hypothesis is supported by reports of individual cases in which T1DM onset followed an acute viral infection, by epidemiologic data demonstrating an "infectious disease–like" pattern of T1DM onset, and by animal studies in which viruses have been shown to have diabetogenic activity (reviewed in Ref. 48). The first case linking T1DM to an acute viral infection was reported in the late nineteenth century, in which the onset of T1DM appeared to be precipitated by a mumps infection in a child.[114] Many similar reports have followed since[47,115,116] and, taken together, these reports suggest a relation between T1DM and several viruses, including rubella, mumps, coxsackie B virus, rotavirus, cytomegalovirus, and Epstein-Barr virus (reviewed in Ref. 48). In addition to case reports linking T1DM onset with viral infections, disease epidemiology suggests features of T1DM as a communicable disease.[71] Many studies in several countries have shown that T1DM develops in individuals who are positive for HLA-DQ2-DR3, DQ8-DR4, or both (discussed earlier). The DQ6 haplotype containing either *DQB1*0602* or *B1*0603* confers resistance among children in a dominant manner. Because these specificities are present in about half the population, a diabetogenic virus may not be spread effectively enough to cause disease. In addition, variations in the annual incidence are often taken as evidence of an involvement of virus. An annual variation was found in a population of 15- to 34-year-olds, with lower numbers of new patients being identified during the summer months.[72] In the

Table 55-3	Viruses and Other Environmental Factors Implicated in or Able to Induce Type 1 (Insulin-dependent) Diabetes

VIRUSES	**HOST**
Coxsackie	Humans, mice
Rubella	Humans, hamsters
Mumps	Humans
Cytomegalovirus	Humans
Encephalomyocarditis	Mice
Meningovirus	Mice
Reovirus	Mice
Lymphocytic choriomeningitis	Rats
Rotavirus	Humans
Kilham strain (mumps virus)	Rats

TOXINS
Alloxan
Streptozotocin
Pyriminyl (Vacor)
Pentamidine isothiocyanate
N-3-Pyridylmethyl-*N'*-p'-nitrophenylurea (PNU)

group of children younger than 6 or 7 years who have T1DM, however, this annual variation is not always present.[75,99]

Another type of observation is that in epidemics of rubella, pregnant women may acquire a viral infection during the first trimester. Their offspring with congenital rubella have been found to develop T1DM at a very high frequency,[117,118] especially HLA-DR3- and/or HLA-DR4-positive children.[118] The clinical onset of T1DM in many of these patients is preceded by the phenomenon of islet autoimmunity, and most of the patients in whom T1DM develops have a variety of islet cell autoantibodies. Similarly, these children also have a high prevalence of organ-specific autoantibodies.[119] Congenital rubella therefore offers the most dramatic example of development of T1DM in association with an environmental factor. Vaccination practices have prevented rubella epidemics, but they have not affected the incidence rate of T1DM. Maternal enteroviral infection during pregnancy also appears to be a risk factor for childhood T1DM.[120,121] It is therefore possible that gestational infections by many types of viruses affect the maturation of the immune system, causing certain children to be more predisposed to autoimmunity and thereby increasing the risk for T1DM. Prior exposure to measles, mumps, and rubella, but not vaccination, decreased prevalence of pancreatic and thyroid autoantibodies.[122] Maternal viral infections or reduced exposure to natural infections may be associated with an increase in T1DM.

One group of viruses that has been extensively studied in T1DM is the enteroviruses, in particular the coxsackie B serotype (reviewed in Ref. 123). Coxsackie B4 virus was isolated from the pancreas of a child who died at presentation with T1DM, propagated in the in vitro cultures of endocrine pancreatic cells, and then shown to have diabetic activity in certain mouse strains.[124] Coxsackievirus infection in the mouse seems to be associated with virus replication in the β cells, followed by the formation of GAD65 antibodies.[125,126] Two important hypotheses follow from these experiments. One hypothesis is that the coxsackievirus induces β-cell neoantigens, which initiate an (auto)immune reaction. This hypothesis can be tested by analyzing the appearance of such neoantigens. The neoantigen may initiate a devastating reaction if its structure mimics a self-protein. In line with this hypothesis, a sequence in GAD65 is identical to that in a coxsackievirus antigen.[127,128] Another hypothesis is that coxsackie B virus replication in β cells results in β-cell necrosis and the formation of antibodies against β-cell constituents or "hidden antigens" not normally surveyed by the immune system.[129] An autoimmune reaction is initiated that may escalate with time. In humans, prospective epidemiologic studies have supported a role for enteroviral infection in the pathogenesis of T1DM.[130] In addition, anti-enteroviral T-cell responses,[131,132] as well as enteroviral RNA,[133] have been demonstrated in patients with T1DM.

In experimental animals (see Table 55-3), several viruses, including encephalomyocarditis, rubella, reovirus, and coxsackie B virus, are capable of inducing diabetes. Some of these virus-induced diabetic syndromes are thought to be caused by β-cell destruction alone. Other viruses (e.g., reovirus) were found to affect primarily the immune system of the host to induce a polyclonal autoantibody response. The production of autoantibodies appeared to be closely related to the pathogenesis of disease in mice.[125,126] The virus-induced disease in mice depends on strain, because some mouse strains are resistant to the pathogenesis of a virus that induces T1DM in another strain. Similar strain dependency to the β-cytotoxic agent streptozotocin, followed by the inoculation of a diabetogenic virus, rendered otherwise virus-resistant mice diabetic.[134] This observation may be significant to humans because it is possible that repeated injuries to the pancreatic β cells over several years of life may eventually induce T1DM. An additional role of HLA has been suggested, because it cannot be excluded that repeated injuries are particularly

detrimental if the T1DM-associated HLA alleles are linked with a poor regenerative capacity of the pancreatic β cells.

Alloxan and streptozotocin are widely used to induce β-cell destruction and diabetes in experimental animals. Some species are more resistant to these drugs than others, and the extent to which these agents are able to induce diabetes in humans is uncertain. Streptozotocin is commonly used in treating certain gastroenteric tumors, including glucagonomas; however, T1DM rarely develops in these patients. The absence of a β-cytotoxic effect could be the result of the dosage used or could reflect the possibility that human β cells are resistant to streptozotocin; in vitro studies with human islets suggest the absence of cytotoxic effects. A number of compounds structurally related to streptozotocin and alloxan also have been implicated as possible environmental agents. Pyriminil (Vacor), an effective rodenticide, is highly diabetogenic in humans.[135] Individuals in whom diabetes developed after ingestion of Vacor were found to be positive for ICSAs, which indicates that such autoantibodies may develop after a primary lesion has been inflicted on the β cells. The nitrosamine moiety that is part of the streptozotocin molecule may be diabetogenic when present on molecules other than D-glucose. Nitrosamines present in cured Icelandic mutton have not only been reported to be diabetogenic in mice, but, in addition, the diabetic activity was transmitted in the germ-line DNA.[136,137] Further investigations are needed to substantiate the possibility that environmental chemicals are causative factors in the development of T1DM.

In summary, viruses and chemical agents have direct effects on the pancreatic β cells and may therefore represent the causative factors that initiate the (auto)immune process against these cells. The alternative hypothesis is that these agents potentiate a β cell–destructive process that is genetically determined or initiated by environmental factors.

PATHOLOGY

Studies of the pancreas in newly diagnosed T1DM patients have indicated that the gland is diminished in size compared with that in matched controls.[13,138,139] An atrophic pancreas with little or negligible residual insulin is typical of a patient with long-standing T1DM. The atrophy affects primarily the tail of the pancreas. In this part, the composition of the endocrine pancreas is dominated by β and α cells, whereas in the pancreatic head, β and pancreatic polypeptide (PP) cells predominate. In addition to insulin deficiency, the pancreatic atrophy appears to be reflected in lower serum levels of pancreatic trypsin and isoamylase.[140-142] The levels of these enzymes are decreased at the time of clinical onset and seem to remain lower even after insulin therapy is initiated. It is speculated that the serum trypsin or isoamylase reflects the pancreatic tissue volume and that the atrophy of the gland is a result of an intrapancreatic insulin deficiency affecting the growth of the pancreas.

The insulin deficiency is the result of a specific loss of the β cells, which affects the total mass of the endocrine pancreas in T1DM (Table 55-4). The islets are small and appear pseudoatrophic.[138,143] In contrast to the normal pancreas, in which the β cells predominate, the endocrine cells in the diabetic pancreas are primarily α, δ, and PP cells. Lobular variation has been described, and areas with β cell–containing islets without pancreatic atrophy also have been detected, suggesting that parts of the pancreas may be spared.[138] In individuals with newly diagnosed T1DM, islets with β cells showing signs of hyperactivity also have been found. Sometimes β cells are seen in close proximity to duct cells, suggesting neoformation of cells. The understanding of the developing endocrine pancreas has improved, and a number of transcription factors controlling the process have been identified.[144] However, one of the characteristics of the

Table 55-4 Morphometric Analysis of the Endocrine Pancreas in Control Individuals and Patients with Type 1 Diabetes Mellitus

Cell Type	Endocrine Pancreas (µg)	
	Controls	T1DM
β cells	850	0
α cells	230	150
δ cells	125	97
PP cells	190	166
All cells	1395	413

PP, pancreatic polypeptide.

Adapted from Rahier J, Goebbels RM, Henquin JC: Cellular composition of the human diabetic pancreas. Diabetologia 24:336–371, 1983, with permission.

pancreas in many children with newly diagnosed T1DM is the presence of inflammatory cells adjacent to islets or cords of newly formed β cells.[138]

The role of the immune system in the pathology of T1DM, suggested by the presence of inflammatory cells in the pancreas of diabetes patients with short-duration disease, was initially demonstrated at the turn of the twentieth century. The term *insulitis* was first introduced in 1940,[12] but the phenomenon was not established until later quantitative investigations reported insulitis in 16 of 23 individuals with T1DM who died within 6 months of diagnosis.[13] It is believed that insulitis is not detected in a greater percentage of new-onset T1DM patients because the total mass of β cells is already markedly reduced at the time of clinical diagnosis,[22,145,146] and the presence of inflammatory cells in large numbers is perhaps not to be expected. It is speculated that the antigen attracting the inflammatory cells is a β cell–specific determinant, although no exclusively β cell–specific molecule has yet been identified.[146] Recent studies have suggested that the initial target antigen may actually be an element of pancreatic nervous tissue[147]; however, further studies must be performed to confirm this hypothesis. Immunocytochemical investigation in rare specimens of pancreas from some patients who died shortly after the clinical onset of T1DM indicates that all cell types considered part of the immune system populate the islets to form the insulitis[15,22,148,149]: T lymphocytes, B lymphocytes, macrophages, and occasional natural killer (NK) cells may be seen. In agreement with earlier studies, examination of pancreatic islets in laparoscopically obtained biopsy specimens from newly diagnosed T1DM patients[150,151] demonstrated insulitis in about 60% of patients, with a T-cell–predominant infiltration and increased expression of HLA class I.[152] Notably, the presence of insulitis was strongly correlated with the presence of other autoimmune features, specifically positivity for GAD65 or IA-2 autoantibodies.[152] The same group also found increased expression of Fas on pancreatic β cells and Fas ligand on infiltrating immune cells in patients with insulitis, suggesting that Fas-FasL–triggered apoptotic cell death may play a role in the pathogenesis of β-cell loss in T1DM.[153]

The sequence of events by which the immunocytes form insulitis may involve an early macrophage or dendritic cell infiltration followed by the recruitment of T and later by B lymphocytes. The initiation of this process is very difficult to study in humans, because it can be established only during the period preceding the actual clinical onset of the disease. Examination of the pancreas from subjects with high-risk HLA who are positive for islet-cell autoantibodies failed to detect insulitis.[154] Conversely, insulitis may not always lead to T1DM because it has been observed in virus-infected nondiabetic children.[155] However, the role of immune cells in the process leading to the disappearance of β cells is well established in the spontaneously diabetic nonobese diabetic (NOD) mouse and BB rat. It is possible to transfer diabetes adoptively with clonal T lymphocytes. Similarly, transfer of T1DM between HLA-identical siblings has been achieved by bone marrow transplantation.[156] These observations support the hypothesis that T1DM is an immune-mediated disease and that immunocytes play a pivotal role in the β-cell killing.

The chronic type of inflammatory reaction observed in short-term T1DM supports the idea that the β-cell loss might have been initiated long before the actual clinical onset of insulin dependency. It has not yet been possible to define the sequence of events that triggers the migration or attraction of immune cells to the pancreatic islets. Viral infection, and possibly also chemical modification, may alter antigens that are expressed on the islet β-cell surface. Such modified antigens may activate clones of T lymphocytes through accessory (antigen-presenting) cells located either in the islets or in the periphery.

The histopathologic changes of short duration in the endocrine pancreas of T1DM correspond to a drastic reduction in the ability to produce insulin.[157] Highly sensitive and specific immunoassays for C peptide permit studies of residual β-cell function even when the patient is treated with insulin (see Chapter 49). Fasting C peptide levels are reduced, often to the lower level seen in normal subjects. The first months of insulin therapy are associated with an apparent increase in fasting C peptide.[158] After 6 to 9 months' duration, irrespective of whether the residual β-cell function was within or below the normal range, the C peptide levels continuously decrease, reaching values below the detection limit of the assay (~0.05 mmol/mL) after 30 months or longer of T1DM.[158,159]

Patients with high titers of islet cell autoantibodies, including ICA and GAD65 autoantibodies, tend to have higher levels of fasting C peptide at clinical onset,[159] whereas IA-2 autoantibody-positive subjects had lower levels.[160] At the same time, however, the presence of ICA, GAD65, or IA-2 autoantibodies may determine a greater rate of loss of endogenous β cells.[160–162] It is therefore possible that the antigen or antigens necessary to maintain levels of islet cell autoantibodies, such as GAD65 or IA-2, are part of the islet β cells. Islet cell autoantibodies may be markers for an immunopathologic process responsible for the continuous eradication of β cells. Further studies are needed to define the extent to which fasting or stimulated levels of C peptide reflect the residual mass of pancreatic β cells. It is not clear, however, whether the residual amount of C peptide and its fluctuation after dietary control or intensified insulin therapy reflect changes either in the number or in the function of residual β cells. Levels of plasma insulin are affected by insulin sensitivity,[163] which may explain why significant loss of endogenous insulin production does not always result in diabetes.[45]

Individuals at risk for development of T1DM have been found to have hyperproinsulinemia, a condition shown in experimental animals or in vitro experiments to reflect maximally stimulated or perhaps exhausted β cells.[164,165] When compared with matched controls, HLA-identical siblings of patients with T1DM have been found to have evidence of both insulin resistance and impaired β-cell function.[166] To estimate the residual mass of insulin-producing cells in humans, it is important to take into account such factors as the maximal rate of insulin release, extraction of insulin in the liver and peripheral tissues, and resistance to insulin action.[45,163] Although the total pancreatic insulin content in experimental animals appears to correlate well with the total β-cell mass, it cannot be excluded that a diminished β-cell mass alters the rate of insulin biosynthesis as well as secretion in the remaining β cells. An attractive hypothesis suggests that an increased and sustained demand on remaining β cells exhausts these cells, leading to their death and to a diminished β-cell mass.[167] At present, however, no experimental data support this hypothesis. It has been shown that intensive therapy for T1DM helps sustain endogenous insulin secretion, which in turn is associated with better metabolic control and lower risk for hypoglycemia and chronic complications.[168-170] In addition, treatment with diazoxide, an inhibitor of insulin secretion, at the time of clinical diagnosis also preserves residual insulin secretion.[171] Insulin or diazoxide therapy may allow residual β cells to rest and protect them from further immune-mediated destruction. However, the "β-cell rest" theory was recently tested in the diabetes prevention trial for T1DM (DPT-1),[172] and insulin treatment of ICA-positive first-degree relatives did not decrease the progression to disease onset in these high-risk individuals.[172,173]

In summary, the pathology of β-cell destruction could be the result of (1) cell-mediated cytotoxicity, (2) antibody-mediated cytotoxicity, (3) cytokine-mediated cytotoxicity, or (4) a combination of these. The role of abnormal HLA class II molecule presentation and alterations of the target β cells by chemicals, viruses, or other environmental factors must be defined.

PATHOGENESIS

The pathogenesis of T1DM is strongly associated with several immune abnormalities. These immune abnormalities, in particular autoantibodies directed against specific islet cell autoantigens, such as insulin, GAD65, and IA-2, are dynamic markers of an ongoing disease process. The autoantibodies are studied both before and after the clinical diagnosis as markers of an ongoing pathogenesis. The pathogenetic markers are therefore useful to predict either T1DM or outcome treatment in patients with new-onset T1DM. The pathogenetic process is likely to be the same before and after the clinical diagnosis of diabetes. The rate of β-cell destruction appears to be influenced by HLA. The HLA *DQB1*0302-A1*0301/DQB1*0201-A1*0501* genotype appears to be associated with accelerated β-cell destruction and a more rapid progression to clinical onset of diabetes.[174,175] The *DQB1*0602* or *0603* alleles are dominantly protective, although the negative association is attenuated with increased age at onset.[174] In *DQB1*0602/0603*-positive patients, the second haplotype is most often *DQB1*0302-A1*0201*,[176] suggesting that HLA may influence the tempo of the disease process. The HLA *DQB1*0302-A1*0301/DQB1*0201-A1*0501* genotype accelerates and *DQB1*0602/0603* alleles decelerate T1DM disease pathogenesis. Because the HLA molecules are important determinants in regulating the immune response in humans, the susceptibility to T1DM is speculated to be conferred by the functional importance of these molecules in the restriction of the immune response. The role of the class II molecules in the immune response is to convey cell-cell interactions between T-helper (CD4+) lymphocytes and antigen-presenting cells (APCs) or B lymphocytes. The CD4+ T cell provides help to cytotoxic T (CD8+) lymphocytes. An antigen taken up, processed, and presented by an APC is recognized only by a T-helper lymphocyte, which has a TCR to detect the antigenic epitope in conjunction with the APC HLA class II molecule. A number of "recently identified new genes" (RINGs) in the HLA region have revealed a final common pathway of antigen presentation by genes controlling proteolysis, peptide transport, and peptide loading onto HLA class I and II molecules.

In summary, the HLA class II molecules that are strongly associated with T1DM specifically bind short peptides or epitopes. These are recognized by specific TCRs on CD4+ T lymphocytes, which is the signal to initiate the development of cytotoxic T lymphocytes and B lymphocytes, which produce antibodies to the antigen. This entire process is affected by a number of cytokines, which are produced by APCs, T cells, or

both. Some of these cytokines, such as interferon gamma (IFN-γ) and interleukin-2 (IL-2) promote an immune response that is predominantly cell mediated and aggressive (a Th1 response). Other cytokines, such as IL-4 and IL-10, promote an immune response that is mostly humoral (a Th2 response). Dividing an immune reaction into Th1 and Th2 is obviously an oversimplification, but it serves the purpose of better defining immunopathologic mechanisms in T1DM. The cytokines are local mediators, and changes in plasma levels may not at all reflect the disease pathogenesis.

IMMUNOLOGIC ABNORMALITIES

CELLULAR IMMUNOPATHOPHYSIOLOGY

It is possible that the APC activity is altered in patients or in individuals susceptible to T1DM. Studies with immunoglobulin G (IgG)-sensitized autologous erythrocytes have, for example, shown that normal individuals with a DR3 HLA-haplotype have an abnormally prolonged Fc receptor–mediated mononuclear phagocyte system.[177] Blood monocytes in T1DM patients may be defective in prostaglandin synthetase,[178] and dendritic cells from patients with T1DM have a maturational and functional defect.[179] In addition, APCs from T1DM patients secrete markedly higher levels of proinflammatory cytokines in response to a nonantigenic stimulus, suggesting that these cells have an altered set point for immunoreactivity.[180] Several observations have been made in which the insulin-deficient diabetic state has markedly influenced the cellular function of immunologically competent cells. The importance of studying diabetic patients in good metabolic control cannot be too highly stressed.

The T-cell component of the cellular immune system also plays an important role in disease pathogenesis in T1DM. The earliest demonstration of an immunologic etiology for T1DM involved tests for leukocyte migration inhibition or blast formation, which indicated that T1DM patients may be sensitized to pancreatic antigens.[16-20] Migration inhibition was most prominent in patients with T1DM of short duration. In keeping with the in vitro test, it was noted that a delayed hypersensitivity reaction often developed in these patients to subcutaneously injected pancreatic homogenate.[19,20] Another finding that indicates an important role for T cells in T1DM disease pathogenesis is the fact that immunosuppressive drugs with anti-T-cell activity, such as cyclosporine,[181] or humanized monoclonal antibodies against CD3,[182] have been shown to delay the development of disease. Investigators have tried to take further the findings of these experiments for over 30 years, with the primary goal being to validate these findings with highly purified specific antigens, such as insulin, GAD65, and IA-2. However, as previously noted, reproducible tests of blood T-cell reactivity to specific antigens have proven difficult to establish, and the more promising assays are not yet widely available.[24-28,183]

Several disorders of autoimmune character have been found to have an imbalance in the peripheral blood between T-helper (CD4+), cytotoxic (CD8+), and regulatory (CD4+CD25+) T cells. It is likely that, although the presence of effector diabetogenic T cells plays an important role in disease pathogenesis, the absence of regulatory T cells is equally important (reviewed in Ref. 184). Monoclonal antibodies that detect specific lymphocyte surface proteins are used to enumerate circulating T-lymphocyte subsets, but the results remain conflicting.[185,186] A slight increase in the proportion of class II antigen-positive T lymphocytes was reported, and, as observed in other disorders of autoimmune character, a decrease in CD8+ T cells was found as well.[187] Other approaches to detect T-cell reactivity against islet cell antigens, such as ELISPOT, which measures cytokine secretion from individual T cells, are being explored.[28] Patients with

T1DM also have cytotoxic T cells specific for glutamic acid decarboxylase.[188] Several reports indicate an increased frequency of in vitro proliferating T cells in patients with T1DM, compared with levels in control subjects, in response to autoantigens such as GAD[128,189,190] and IA-2.[191] However, these T-cell assays in humans are complicated by poor reproducibility and very high interlaboratory variability.[24,183] Immunodominant epitopes of GAD65[102,192,193] and IA-2[191] have been identified and should be useful in improving cellular assays in T1DM.[194-196] The use of HLA tetramers offers a novel approach to detect[26] and clone autoantigen-specific human T cells.[197]

When the number of immunoglobulin-secreting cells in peripheral blood was assessed, several patients with T1DM of short duration had an elevated level of spontaneous secretion of immunoglobulin.[198,199] It is therefore possible that the clinical onset of T1DM is associated with a polyclonal B-lymphocyte activation. It remains to be determined whether these alterations are acquired, inherited, or related to the pathogenesis of β-cell destruction.

In conclusion, antigen-specific tests in HLA-DQ and -DR-matched T1DM subjects and control individuals should allow a proper test of the hypothesis that a specific immunoregulation abnormality involving β-cell antigens is associated with the development of T1DM.

HUMORAL IMMUNOPATHOPHYSIOLOGY

A reaction between antibodies and an autologous tissue preparation is taken as evidence of the presence of autoantibodies, and several assay systems are used to determine the presence of antibodies reactive with pancreatic islet cells (Table 55-5). Immunoprecipitation of human islet proteins has revealed the presence of autoantibodies against a 64 K protein,[33,200] identified as GAD but found to represent an isoenzyme, GAD65, coded for by a gene on human chromosome 10.[35] The previously known GAD67 on chromosome 2 shares 65% of the amino acids, but this isoform is not expressed in human β cells.[36,201] Trypsin treatment of the 64 K immunoprecipitate revealed 40 K and 37 K fragments of islet antigens,[202,203] later shown to represent two isoforms of the protein tyrosine phosphatase–like molecules IA-2 (ICA512)[38-40] and IA-2β (phogrin),[204-206] respectively. Finally, insulin antibodies were demonstrated before insulin treatment in about 50% of children with new-onset T1DM[37,207] and contribute to T1DM risk.[208,209] Other autoantigens have been proposed[49,210] but autoantibodies to GAD65, IA-2, and insulin remain the major autoimmune markers for T1DM.[212] These three autoantibodies appear to replace the indirect immunofluorescence assay for ICA.[41,44] Because the presence of two or more of these autoantibodies has a high predictive value for the development of T1DM,[44,213] it is critical that reliable tests be available to detect these autoantibodies.

ICA standardization was started in 1985[214,215] and continued with assays for insulin autoantibodies[216] as well as for GAD65 and IA-2 autoantibodies.[217] The insulin autoantibody (IAA) workshops showed the importance of radiobinding in

contrast to enzyme-linked immunosorbent assay (ELISA) or solid-phase assay to detect IAA with high diagnostic sensitivity and specificity.[216] Similarly, the use of coupled in vitro transcription translation to label GAD65[218] and later IA-2[219,220] in radioligand-binding assays[218,221] allowed the development of assays with high diagnostic sensitivity and specificity.[217,222] The following is a summary of the prevalence of autoantibodies to GAD65, IA-2, and insulin using these standardized assay systems.

The frequency of GAD65 antibodies in children with new-onset T1DM is 70% to 80% (Fig. 55-2), compared with about 8% antibodies against GAD67. Patients with GAD67 antibodies are also GAD65-antibody positive. The GAD65 autoantibody (GAD65Ab) frequency in new-onset patients is little affected by the age at onset; however, in children younger than 10 years, more girls than boys have GAD65Ab. GAD65Ab are evanescent, but less so than ICA (Fig. 55-3). The longer the duration of T1DM, the lower the frequency of GAD65 antibodies and of ICA. However, almost 50% of patients with a disease duration of 10 years may still be GAD65-antibody positive (see Fig. 55-3)[223,224] GAD65 autoantibodies are more often detected in *DQB1*0201-A1*0501-DRB1*03*-positive than in *DQB1*0302-A1*0301-DRB1*04*-positive patients.[225] All islet cells, but β cells in particular, express GAD65. This enzyme produces γ-aminobutyric acid (GABA), which is stored in small neurotransmitter vesicles. It is possible that GABA regulates the secretion of the neighboring glucagon- and somatostatin-producing cells. In an indirect immunofluorescence test with sections of frozen human pancreas, ICA-positive sera give a fluorescence reaction that usually covers all endocrine islet cells. The antigenic determinants GAD65, IA-2, and others are therefore thought to be located in the cytoplasmic compartment of the cells.

Any assessment of an individual's risk of developing diabetes depends on the ability to determine accurately the presence of antibodies in a prospective analysis. This is particularly important because GAD65 antibodies may appear temporarily in healthy individuals.[226] GAD65 antibodies are present in about 1% of the general population, but the frequency increases to about 8% among first-degree relatives of patients with T1DM.[227,228] The positive predictive value of GAD65 antibodies for T1DM is about 50% or higher among first-degree relatives. It may be as high as 20% in schoolchildren with high-risk HLA.[207] GAD65 antibodies also predict stiff-man syndrome, although the GAD65 autoantibody epitopes are different from those in T1DM.[229,230] T1DM is best predicted when the GAD65 antibody assay is combined with IAA and IA-2 antibodies.[44,212]

IA-2 antibodies are detected in 60% to 70% of patients with new-onset T1DM.[231] These antibodies are less frequent with increasing age at onset (see Fig. 55-2).[232] The IA-2 antibodies would therefore better predict young age at onset of T1DM. Longitudinal studies of first-degree relatives suggest that IA-2 autoantibodies tend to appear closer to the clinical onset of T1DM compared with GAD65 antibodies, which tend to appear earlier in the prodrome.[231] The IA-2 antibodies are evanescent (see Fig. 55-3), but when present in patients who are young at disease onset, as many as 50% may still be IA-2

Table 55-5	Methods to Detect Islet Cell Autoantibodies		
Preparation to Detect Islet Antigen	Method of Detection	Islet Cell (Auto) Antibody	References
Recombinant antigens	Immunoassays	GAD65Ab, IA-2Ab, insulin Ab	Greenbaum,[216] Verge,[217] Grubin[218]
Frozen sections of human pancreas	Indirect immunofluorescence	Islet cell cytoplasmic Ab (ICA, ICCA)	Bottazzo,[30] Atkinson[128]
Dispersed rat islet cells	Indirect immunofluorescence	Islet cell-surface Ab (ICSA)	Lernmark[31,240]
Monolayers of rat islet cells	^{51}Cr release	Islet cell cytotoxic Ab (C'AMC)	Dobersen[32,242]
Purified rat islet β cells	Indirect immunofluorescence	β cell–specific ICSA	van de Winkel[241]

GAD, glutamic acid decarboxylase; Ab, antibody.

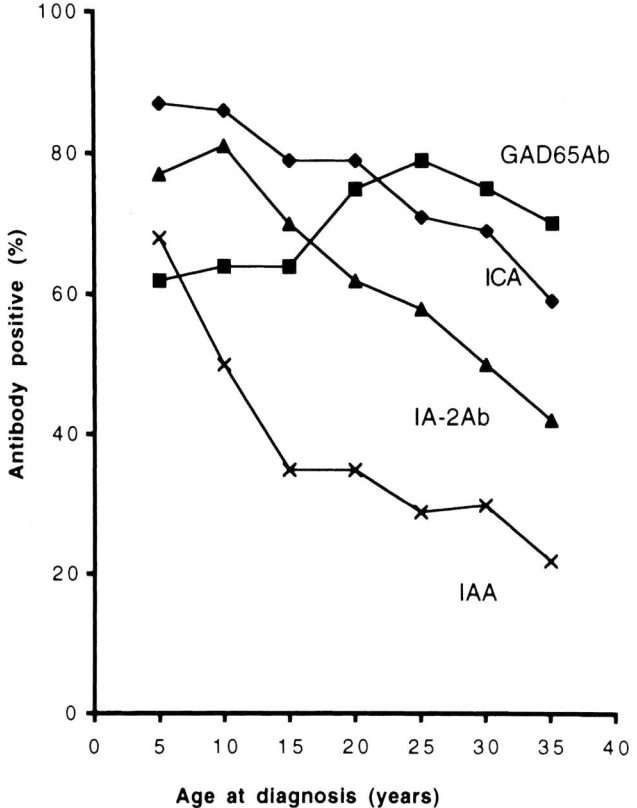

Figure 55-2 Frequency of autoantibodies against glutamic acid decarboxylase (GAD)65 (GAD65Ab), IA-2 (IA-2Ab), and insulin (IAA) at the time of clinical diagnosis in relation to age at onset.

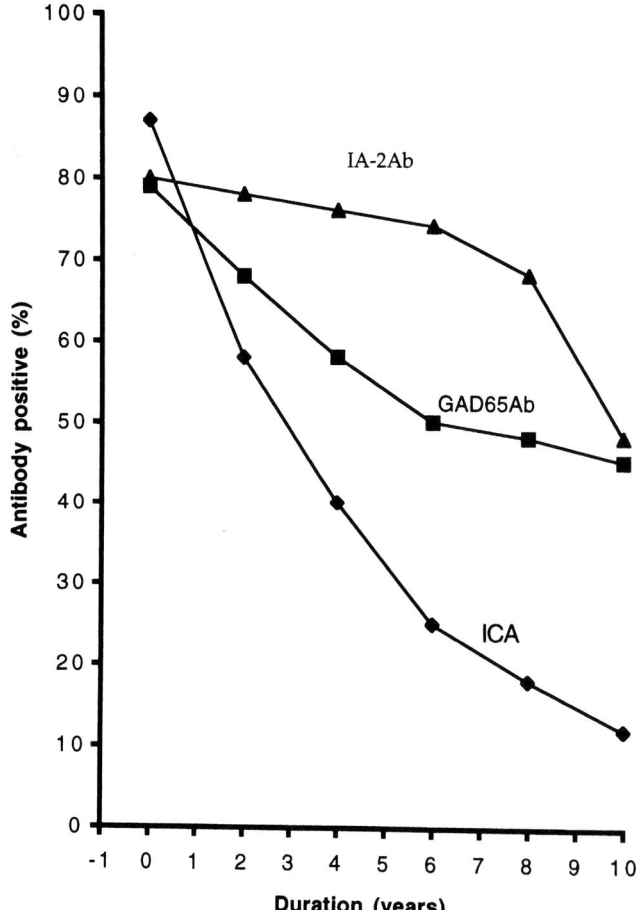

Figure 55-3 Frequency of autoantibodies against glutamic acid decarboxylase (GAD)65 (GAD65Ab) and IA-2 (IA-2Ab) as well as islet cell antibodies (ICAs) in relation to the duration of type 1 diabetes.

antibody positive after having had diabetes for 10 years (see Fig. 55-3). The IA-2 antibodies are detected for a longer duration than are ICA (see Fig. 55-3). IA-2 autoantibodies were associated primarily with *DRB1*0401* and not with *DQA1*0301-DQB1*0302*,[225] and a gender difference appears in expression of this autoantibody, with an increased odds ratio of 1.4 for the presence of IA-2 antibodies in men.[232] IA-2 and IA-2β are both associated with the granule membrane in the cells, but they also are detectable in other endocrine cell types.[204,233] The mechanisms by which the IA-2 proteins become recognized as autoantigens are not yet understood. The frequency of IA-2 antibodies in the general population is less than 1%.[92] The predictive value of IA-2 antibodies for T1DM is best estimated in combination with GAD65 and insulin autoantibodies.[44,213]

It was demonstrated in a radioligand-binding assay that approximately 50% of patients with newly diagnosed but untreated T1DM have IAAs.[37] These IAAs have been standardized, and the measurements carried out in fluid-phase radioimmunoassay were found to have higher diagnostic sensitivity than those in solid-phase ELISA analyses.[216] IAAs are found earlier in childhood and are less frequently found in adults (see Fig. 55-2).[207,209,234] IAAs were positively associated with DR4, perhaps because they are in linkage disequilibrium with *DQB1*0302-DQA1*0301*.[225,235] A first analysis of putative IAA epitopes indicates that the amino acids B1 to B3 and A8 to A13 are important.[236] Further site-directed mutagenesis will be necessary to map IAAs in relation to diagnostic sensitivity and specificity, because IAAs and insulin antibodies that appear after insulin therapy have similar binding characteristics.[237] It has been proposed that IAAs predict T1DM better in children (see Fig. 55-2) than in adults[208,238] and that IAAs are related to a linear loss of β-cell function.[239] Prospective, population-based studies of children, including newborns,[46] are therefore required to determine the possible

association between HLA, including the DR4 subtypes, and the production of IAAs. In addition, prospective studies would be useful to clarify the predictive value for T1DM in the general population, considering that many more healthy children will have the IAA marker than will develop diabetes.

Islet cell surface antibodies (ICSAs; see Table 55-5) were demonstrated in dispersed-cell preparations of rat or mouse pancreatic islets in 2% to 4% of control subjects and in about 30% of patients with T1DM.[31,240] The ICSAs showed a decreased prevalence with increasing duration of disease. Antibodies in T1DM sera preferentially bind to β cells if the disease is diagnosed before age 30 years.[241] The observation that antibodies are capable of binding to living β cells is important because it allows testing of the possibility that surface-bound antibodies either mediate immune effector mechanisms or directly affect the function of the β cells. The former phenomena may include complement-mediated cytotoxicity or antibody-dependent cellular cytotoxicity. Either mechanism could contribute to killing pancreatic β cells, provided that the in vitro phenomenon also is occurring in vivo. The evidence obtained with monolayer cultures of both pancreatic islet cells from newborn rats[32,242] and cloned rat islet tumor cells[243,244] is that the cytotoxic ICAs correlate well with the presence of ICSA but not with ICA. Some patients have both types of antibodies, whereas others have either cytoplasmic or cell-surface antibodies.[245]

The concept of a polyclonal activation of the immune system in T1DM patients is supported by numerous observations[16,20,47,246–248] of an increased frequency of a variety of autoantibodies (Table 55-6). Because occurrence of these

Table 55-6 Autoantibodies and Immune Complexes Found with Increased Frequency among Type 1 Diabetes Patients and Their First-degree Relatives

Target	Antibody
ORGAN SPECIFIC	
Islets	GAD65, IA-2, Insulin, ICA, ICSA, or C'AMC
Thyroid	Thyroid peroxidase (TPO), thyroglobulin (Tg)
Stomach	Gastric parietal cell or H⁺/K⁺ ATPase, Intrinsic factor
Adrenals	Adrenal cell, 21-hydroxylase
Pituitary	Pituitary cell
NON–ORGAN SPECIFIC	
Peripheral lymphocytes	Lymphocytotoxic
Nucleic acids	Single-stranded RNA, double-stranded RNA
Cell constituents	Tubulin, insulin receptor
Plasma proteins	Albumin
Immune complexes	Solid-phase C1q-binding, Raji cell binding

GAD, glutamic acid decarboxylase; ATP, adenosine triphosphate; ICA, islet cell antibody; C'AMC, complement-dependent cell-mediated cytotoxicity.

uncertain range require an oral glucose tolerance test to establish a diagnosis (see Table 55-7). An individual who has a fasting blood glucose level greater than 7.0 mmol/L (126 mg/dL) but does not have ketoacidosis or is not in a hyperglycemic hyperosmolar state, is above ideal body weight, and is not pregnant is more likely to have T2DM, although with the current obesity epidemic, the use of body weight to differentiate between T1DM and T2DM is becoming less valid. Evidence has been presented that adult-onset T2DM may progress to insulin dependence at a rate of 1% to 2% per year.[3] This rate is increased in GAD65 autoantibody–positive patients classified with T2DM, and these individuals are now considered to have a form of T1DM, which has variably been termed *type 1.5 diabetes, LADA,* or *slowly progressive T1DM*[88,89,257] (reviewed in Ref. 92). The symptoms of T1DM often have an abrupt onset in children and a more insidious onset with increasing age. Girls often have monilial vaginitis. The classic symptoms of diabetic ketoacidosis include air hunger, Kussmaul respiration, acidosis, acetone odor of the breath, dehydration, vomiting, hyperglycemia, glucosuria, ketonemia, and ketonuria.

The major defect in T1DM is the deficiency in insulin production. After an injection of glucose, the β cells in a healthy individual are able to increase the rate of insulin release severalfold. In contrast, a patient with newly diagnosed T1DM often has a nearly complete lack of response to glucose, particularly if signs of diabetic ketoacidosis or metabolic dysregulation are present. Glucose tolerance tests to evaluate the β-cell function at the time of clinical onset are not a diagnostic procedure. A variety of glucose tolerance tests, both oral and intravenous (see Chapter 54), are being used to evaluate diabetic states; however, these procedures are more important in disorders of impaired glucose tolerance and T2DM than they are in providing a distinct diagnosis of T1DM.

Because T1DM is detected in the majority of patients after a relatively short period of symptoms, such as increased thirst, polyuria, and unexplained weight loss, the natural history of the disease has been poorly defined until recently. With the current ability to define individuals at high risk for developing T1DM based on high risk HLA and autoantibody positivity, our understanding of the prediabetic period is improving. Retrospective analyses of first-degree relatives[258,259] later found to develop T1DM have revealed that ICA or autoantibodies to GAD65, IA-2, or insulin, and later, decreased ability to release insulin in response to glucose may develop several years before the clinical diagnosis.[44-46,260] The sequence of events preceding the diagnosis of overt T1DM would include the following: (1) genetic predisposition, (2) overt immunologic abnormalities with normal glucose levels, (3) development of overt diabetes with detectable C peptide, and (4) the final stage of insulin dependency, with disappearance of C peptide. The fact that T1DM develops in persons of all ages should be taken into account when studying the natural history in children and adults. Many first-degree relatives may be positive for immune markers without progressing to T1DM.[45]

It is important to note that the vast majority of children or young adults in whom T1DM develops have sporadic, as opposed to familial, disease.[75,99] Highly effective, precise, and

autoantibodies also is increased among first-degree relatives,[249-251] these abnormalities may be a feature of families with T1DM. In addition, the presence of circulating immune complexes is increased in patients with IDDM of short duration (see Table 55-6). With the solid-phase C1q or Raji cell tests, the prevalence of immune complexes was 25% to 30%.[252-254] The immune complexes detected by the C1q test were associated with the clinical onset of IDDM rather than with the development of diabetic nephropathy.[254]

In summary, currently available methods for detecting autoantigen-specific autoantibodies (GAD65, IA-2, and insulin) are of value in predicting T1DM.[44,213] Standardized assays for these autoantibodies[217] are important when selecting participants in intervention trials.[172] How the uptake, processing, and presentation of these autoantigens by APCs that initiate the formation of islet cell autoantigen-reactive T and B lymphocytes are accomplished are important questions that remain to be answered.

SIGNS, SYMPTOMS, AND NATURAL HISTORY

T1DM usually produces subjective and objective signs of short duration. The American Diabetes Association[255] and the World Health Organization[256] have recommended several diagnostic criteria for T1DM (Table 55-7). The onset is primarily among young individuals, but the disease can be manifested at all ages. Most patients have a history of polyuria, polydipsia, and unexplained weight loss. The elevated blood glucose level causes polyuria because of the osmotic diuretic effect of glucose. The blood glucose values that lie in the

Table 55-7 Criteria for the Diagnosis of Diabetes Mellitus*

1. Symptoms of diabetes plus casual plasma glucose concentration ≥200 mg/dL (11.1 mmol/L). Casual is defined as any time of day without regard to time since last meal. The classic symptoms of diabetes include polyuria, polydipsia, and unexplained weight loss **or**
2. Fasting plasma glucose (FPG), ≥126 mg/dL (7.0 mmol/L). Fasting is defined as no caloric intake for ≥8 hr **or**
3. Two-hour Plasma glucose, ≥200 mg/dL (11.1 mmol/L) during an oral glucose tolerance test (OGTT). The test should be performed as described by WHO,[4] using a glucose load containing the equivalent of 75 g of anhydrous glucose dissolved in water

*In the absence of unequivocal hyperglycemia with acute metabolic decompensation, these criteria should be confirmed by repeated testing on a different day. The third measure (OGTT) is not recommended for routine clinical use.
From Report of the expert committee on the diagnosis and classification of diabetes mellitus. Diabetes Care 26(Suppl 1):S5–20, 2003.

reproducible screening assays for HLA genotypes as well as for GAD65, IA-2, and IAAs are therefore required to detect individuals in the background population who are either carriers of islet cell autoimmunity or carriers on their way to developing T1DM. Specific T-lymphocyte proliferation tests against GAD65, IA-2, or insulin, once more reproducible and more widely available, also may predict T1DM. Early detection of T1DM serves several purposes. Among them is the distinct possibility that ketoacidosis associated with a dramatic and traumatic onset of T1DM, in some cases leading to death, would be forestalled. In addition, immunotherapeutic modalities for disease prevention based on the prevention of β-cell destruction are under active investigation, with the hope that T1DM may someday be a preventable disease.

Several attempts have been made to treat T1DM patients with immunosuppressive agents. Plasmapheresis, prednisolone, anti-T-cell antibodies, and interferon have had little or no effect, but a controlled trial with cyclosporine suggested that the decrease or disappearance of insulin requirement within the first 2 years after the clinical diagnosis was prolonged in about 20% of the patients.[261,262] The major biologic effect of cyclosporine is to inhibit T-cell–mediated immunity. However, the use of the drug was associated with structural renal tubular and glomerular damage.[263] Although immunosuppression successfully prevents autoimmune diabetes in the NOD mouse and the BB rat,[264] nonspecific suppression of the immune system carries its own set of risks and is not the optimal treatment for autoimmune disease. The current approaches to preventing T1DM involve immunomodulatory strategies, such as anti-CD3 monoclonal antibody therapy,[264] immunomodulation studies with autoantigens, such as alum-formulated GAD65,[265] and other therapies targeting specific components of the immune system (reviewed in Ref. 266).

SUMMARY

The islet β cells appear to be the specific target in an autoimmune process that leads to the clinical onset of T1DM. The process of β-cell autoimmunity is often initiated long before the clinical onset of the disease. The event that initiates this process is not yet understood, and the β-cell antigens GAD65, IA-2, or insulin may serve as the recognition structure or structures for the cells in the immune system that eventually produce insulitis. Recent advances in molecular genetics have made it possible to define better the HLA-DQ and -DR molecules that seem to be necessary, but not sufficient, for the development of T1DM. A screen of the human genome for susceptibility to T1DM has identified several additional genetic factors that may affect T1DM risk by accelerating or decelerating the disease process. The aim of future studies is to test whether antigen-specific immunosuppression or other immunomodulatory therapies in T1DM-susceptible individuals will prevent the loss of pancreatic β cells.

REFERENCES

1. Pinhas-Hamiel O, Dolan LM, Zeitler PS: Diabetic ketoacidosis among obese African-American adolescents with NIDDM. Diabetes Care 20:484–486, 1997.
2. Libman IM, Becker DJ: Coexistence of type 1 and type 2 diabetes mellitus: "Double" diabetes? Pediatr Diabetes 4:110–113, 2003.
3. Köbberling J, Tattersall B: The Genetics of Diabetes Mellitus. London, Academic Press, 1982.
4. World Health Organization: Diabetes Mellitus: Report of a WHO Study Group, Technical report series 727. Geneva, World Health Organization, 1985.
5. Steiner DF, Tager HS, Chan SJ, et al: Lessons learned from molecular biology of insulin-gene mutations. Diabetes Care 13:600–609, 1990.
6. Taylor SI, Cama A, Accili D, et al: Mutations in the insulin receptor gene. Endocr Rev 13:566–595, 1992.
7. Bell GI, Pilkis SJ, Weber IT, et al: Glucokinase mutations, insulin secretion, and diabetes mellitus. Annu Rev Physiol 58:171–186, 1996.
8. Yamagata K, Furuta H, Oda N, et al: Mutations in the hepatocyte nuclear factor-4 alpha gene in maturity-onset diabetes of the young (MODY1). Nature 384:458–460, 1996.
9. Yamagata K, Oda N, Kaisaki PJ, et al: Mutations in the hepatocyte nuclear factor-1 alpha gene in maturity-onset diabetes of the young (MODY3). Nature 384:455–458, 1996.
10. Expert Committee on the Diagnosis and Classification of Diabetes Mellitus: Report of the Expert Committee on the Diagnosis and Classification of Diabetes Mellitus. Diabetes Care 26(Suppl 1):S5–S20, 2003.

11. Weichselbaum A: Über die veränderungen des pankreas bei diabetes mellitus. Sitzungsber Akad Wiss Wien Math Naturw Klasse 119:73–281, 1910.
12. Von Meyenburg H: Über "insulitis" bei diabetes. Schweitz Med Wochenschr 21:554–561, 1940.
13. Gepts W: Pathologic anatomy of the pancreas in juvenile diabetes mellitus. Diabetes 14:619–633, 1965.
14. Gepts W, De Mey J: Islet cell survival determined by morphology. Diabetes 27:251–261, 1978.
15. Foulis AK, McGill M, Farquharson A: Insulitis in type 1 (insulin-dependent) diabetes mellitus in man: Macrophages, lymphocytes, and interferon-l containing cells. J Pathol 165:97–103, 1991.
16. Nerup J, Binder C: Thyroid, gastric and adrenal autoimmunity in diabetes mellitus. Acta Endocrinol 72:279–286, 1973.
17. MacCuish AC, Irvine WJ: Autoimmunological aspects of diabetes mellitus. Clin Endocrinol Metab 4:435–471, 1975.
18. Nerup J, Andersen OO, Bendixen G, et al: Antipancreatic cellular hypersensitivity in diabetes mellitus. Diabetes 20:424–427, 1971.
19. Nerup J, Andersen OO, Bendixen G: Antipancreatic cellular hypersensitivity in diabetes mellitus: Experimental induction of an anti-pancreatic, cellular hypersensitivity and associated morphological β-cell changes in the rat. Acta Allergol 28:231–249, 1973.
20. MacCuish AC, Jordan J, Campbell CJ, et al: Cell-mediated immunity to human pancreas in diabetes mellitus. Diabetes 23:693–697, 1974.

21. Pipeleers D, Ling Z: Pancreatic beta cells in insulin-dependent diabetes. Diabetes Metab Rev 8:209–227, 1992.
22. Lernmark Å, Klöppel G, Stenger D, et al: Heterogeneity of islet pathology in two infants with recent onset diabetes mellitus. Virchows Arch 425:631–640, 1995.
23. Huang S-W, MacLaren NK: Insulin-dependent diabetes: A disease of autoaggression. Science 192:64–66, 1976.
24. Roep BO, Atkinson MA, van Endert PM, et al: Autoreactive T cell responses in insulin-dependent (type 1) diabetes mellitus: Report of the First International Workshop for Standardization of T cell Assays. J Autoimmun 13:267–282, 1999.
25. Brooks-Worrell B, Gersuk VH, Greenbaum C, et al: Intermolecular antigen spreading occurs during the preclinical period of human type 1 diabetes. J Immunol 166:5265–5270, 2001.
26. Reijonen H, Novak EJ, Kochik S, et al: Detection of GAD65-specific T-cells by major histocompatibility complex class II tetramers in type 1 diabetic patients and at-risk subjects. Diabetes 51:1375–1382, 2002.
27. Viglietta V, Kent SC, Orban T, et al: GAD65-reactive T cells are activated in patients with autoimmune type 1a diabetes. J Clin Invest 109:895–903, 2002.
28. Schloot NC, Meierhoff G, Karlsson-Faresjo M, et al: Comparison of cytokine Elispot assay formats for the detection of islet antigen autoreactive T cells: Report of the Third Immunology of Diabetes Society T-cell Workshop. J Autoimmun 21:365–376, 2003.

29. MacCuish AC, Barnes EW, Irvine WJ, et al: Antibodies to pancreatic islet cells in insulin-dependent diabetics with coexistent autoimmune disease. Lancet 2:1529–1531, 1974.

30. Bottazzo GF, Florin-Christensen A, Doniach D: Islet cell antibodies in diabetes mellitus with autoimmune polyendocrine deficiencies. Lancet 2:1279–1283, 1974.

31. Lernmark Å, Freedman ZR, Hofmann C, et al: Islet-cell-surface antibodies in juvenile diabetes mellitus. N Engl J Med 299:375–380, 1978.

32. Dobersen MJ, Scharff JE, Ginsberg-Fellner F, et al: Cytotoxic autoantibodies to beta-cells in the serum of patients with insulin-dependent diabetes mellitus. N Engl J Med 303:1493–1498, 1980.

33. Baekkeskov S, Nielsen JH, Marner B, et al: Autoantibodies in newly diagnosed diabetic children immunoprecipitate human pancreatic islet cell proteins. Nature 298:167–169, 1982.

34. Baekkeskov S, Aanstoot HJ, Christgau S, et al: Identification of the 64k autoantigen in insulin-dependent diabetes as the GABA-synthesizing enzyme glutamic acid decarboxylase. Nature 347:151–156, 1990.

35. Karlsen AE, Hagopian WA, Grubin CE, et al: Cloning and primary structure of a human islet isoform of glutamic acid decarboxylase from chromosome 10. Proc Natl Acad Sci U S A 88:8337–8341, 1991.

36. Karlsen AE, Hagopian WA, Petersen JS, et al: Recombinant glutamic acid decarboxylase representing a single isoform expressed in human islets detects IDDM-associated 64k autoantibodies. Diabetes 41:1355–1359, 1992.

37. Palmer JP, Asplin CM, Clemons P, et al: Insulin antibodies in insulin-dependent diabetics before insulin treatment. Science 222:1337–1339, 1983.

38. Rabin DU, Pleasic SM, Shapiro JA, et al: Islet cell antigen 512 is a diabetes-specific islet autoantigen related to protein tyrosine phosphatases. J Immunol 152:3183–3187, 1994.

39. Lan MS, Lu J, Goto Y, et al: Molecular cloning and identification of a receptor-type protein tyrosine phosphatase, IA-2, from human insulinoma. DNA Cell Biol 13:505–514, 1994.

40. Payton MA, Hawkes CJ, Christie MR: Relationship of the 37,000- and 40,000-Mr tryptic fragments of islet antigens in insulin-dependent diabetes to the protein tyrosine phosphatase-like molecule IA-2 (ICA512). J Clin Invest 96:1506–1511, 1995.

41. Wiest-Ladenburger U, Hartmann R, Hartmann U, et al: Combined analysis and single-step detection of GAD65 and IA2 autoantibodies in IDDM can replace the histochemical islet cell antibody test. Diabetes 46:565–571, 1997.

42. Gorsuch AN, Spencer KM, Lister J, et al: Evidence for a long prediabetic period in type 1 (insulin-dependent) diabetes mellitus. Lancet 2:1363–1365, 1981.

43. Riley WJ, Maclaren NK, Krischer J, et al: A prospective study of the development of diabetes in relatives of patients with insulin-dependent diabetes. N Engl J Med 323:1167–1172, 1990.

44. Verge CF, Gianani R, Kawasaki E, et al: Prediction of type 1 diabetes in first-degree relatives using a combination of insulin, GAD, and ICA512bdc/IA-2 autoantibodies. Diabetes 45:926–933, 1996.

45. Greenbaum CJ, Sears KL, Kahn SE, et al: Relationship of beta-cell function and autoantibodies to progression and nonprogression of subclinical type 1 diabetes: Follow-up of the Seattle Family Study. Diabetes 48:170–175, 1999.

46. Lindberg B, Ivarsson SA, Landin-Olsson M, et al: Islet autoantibodies in cord blood from children who developed type 1 (insulin-dependent) diabetes mellitus before 15 years of age. Diabetologia 42:181–187, 1999.

47. Cahill GF, McDevitt HO: Insulin-dependent diabetes mellitus: The initial lesion. N Engl J Med 304:1454–1465, 1981.

48. Jun HS, Yoon JW: A new look at viruses in type 1 diabetes. Diabetes Metab Res Rev 19:8–31, 2003.

49. Schranz D, Lernmark Å: Immunology in diabetes: An update. Diabetes Metab Rev 14:3–29, 1998.

50. Nerup J, Platz P, Anderssen OO: HL-A antigens and diabetes mellitus. Lancet 2:864–866, 1974.

51. Nepom GT: Immunogenetics and IDDM. Diabetes Rev 1:93–103, 1993.

52. Davies JL, Kawaguchi Y, Bennett ST, et al: A genome-wide search for human type 1 diabetes susceptibility genes. Nature 371:130–136, 1994.

53. Concannon P, Gogolin-Ewens KJ, Hinds DA, et al: A second-generation screen of the human genome for susceptibility to insulin-dependent diabetes mellitus. Nat Genet 19:292–296, 1998.

54. King H, Aubert RE, Herman WH: Global burden of diabetes, 1995-2025: Prevalence, numerical estimates, and projections. Diabetes Care 21:1414–1431, 1998.

55. Ekoe J-M: Recent trends in prevalence and incidence of diabetes mellitus syndrome in the world. Diabetes Res Clin Pract 1:249–264, 1986.

56. Pundziute-Lycka A, Dahlquist G, Nystrom L, et al: The incidence of type 1 diabetes has not increased but shifted to a younger age at diagnosis in the 0-34 years group in Sweden 1983-1998. Diabetologia 45:783–791, 2002.

57. Karvonen M, Viik-Kajander M, Moltchanova E, et al: Incidence of childhood type 1 diabetes worldwide. Diabetes Mondiale (DiaMond) project group. Diabetes Care 23:1516–1526, 2000.

58. EURODIAB ACE Study Group. Variation and trends in incidence of childhood diabetes in Europe. Lancet 355:873–876, 2000.

59. Green A, Gale EA, Patterson CC: Incidence of childhood-onset insulin-dependent diabetes mellitus: The EURODIAB ACE study. Lancet 339:905–909, 1992.

60. Tuomilehto J, Rewers M, Reunanen A, et al: Increasing trend in type 1 (insulin-dependent) diabetes mellitus in childhood in Finland. Diabetologia 34:282–287, 1991.

61. Dahlquist G, Blom L, Tuvemo T, et al: The Swedish Childhood Diabetes Study: Results from a nine year case register and one year case-referent study indicating that type 1 (insulin-dependent) diabetes mellitus is associated with both type 2 (non-insulin-dependent) diabetes mellitus and autoimmune disorders. Diabetologia 32:2–6, 1989.

62. Bingley PJ, Gale EAM: Rising incidence of IDDM in Europe. Diabetes Care 12:289–295, 1989.

63. Diabetes Epidemiology Research International Group: Secular trends in incidence of childhood IDDM in 10 countries. Diabetes 39:858–864, 1990.

64. Nyström L, Dahlquist G, Rewers M, et al: The Swedish Childhood Diabetes Study: An analysis of the temporal variation in diabetes incidence 1978-1987. Int J Epidemiol 19:141–146, 1990.

65. Lipman TH, Chang Y, Murphy KM: The epidemiology of type 1 diabetes in children in Philadelphia 1990-1994: Evidence of an epidemic. Diabetes Care 25:1969–1975, 2002.

66. Svensson J, Carstensen B, Molbak A, et al: Increased risk of childhood type 1 diabetes in children born after 1985. Diabetes Care 25:2197–2201, 2002.

67. Feltbower RG, McKinney PA, Parslow RC, et al: Type 1 diabetes in Yorkshire, UK: Time trends in 0-14 and 15-29-year-olds, age at onset and age-period-cohort modelling. Diabetes Med 20:437–441, 2003.

68. Rangasami JJ, Greenwood DC, McSporran B, et al: Rising incidence of type 1 diabetes in Scottish children, 1984-93: The Scottish study group for the care of young diabetics. Arch Dis Child 77:210–213, 1997.

69. Kadiki OA, Roaeid RB: Incidence of type 1 diabetes in children (0-14 years) in Benghazi, Libya (1991-2000). Diabetes Metab 28:463–467, 2002.

70. Shaltout AA, Moussa MA, Qabazard M, et al: Further evidence for the rising incidence of childhood type 1 diabetes in Kuwait. Diabet Med 19:522–525, 2002.

71. Unachak K, Tuchinda C: Incidence of type 1 diabetes in children under 15 years in northern Thailand, from 1991 to 1997. J Med Assoc Thai 84:923–928, 2001.

72. Craig ME, Howard NJ, Silink M, et al: The rising incidence of childhood type 1 diabetes in New South Wales, Australia. J Pediatr Endocrinol Metab 13:363–372, 2000.

73. Karvonen M, Tuomiletho J, Libman I, et al: A review of the recent epidemiological data on incidence of type 1 (insulin-dependent) diabetes mellitus worldwide. Diabetologia 36:883–892, 1993.

74. Tuomilehto J: Epidemiology of childhood diabetes in the Baltic area. Nord Med 107:244–246, 1992.

75. Dahlquist G, Blom L, Holmgren G, et al: The epidemiology of diabetes in Swedish children 0-14 years old: A six-year prospective study. Diabetologia 28:802–808, 1985.

76. Reunanen A, Åkerblom HK, Käär ML: Prevalence and ten-year (1970-1979) incidence of insulin-dependent diabetes mellitus in children and adolescents in Finland. Acta Paediatr Scand 71:893–899, 1982.

77. Kaprio J, Tuomilehto J, Koskenvuo M, et al: Concordance for type 1 (insulin-dependent) and type 2 (non-insulin-dependent) diabetes mellitus in a population-based cohort of twins in Finland. Diabetologia 35:1060–1067, 1992.

78. Kyvik KO, Green A, Beck-Nielsen H: Concordance rates of insulin dependent diabetes mellitus: A population based study of young Danish twins. Br Med J 311:913–917, 1995.

79. Tillil H, Köbberling J: Age-corrected empirical genetic risk estimates for first-degree relatives of IDDM patients. Diabetes 36:93–99, 1987.

80. Todd JA, Farrall M: Panning for gold: Genome-wide scanning for linkage in type 1 diabetes. Hum Mol Genet 5:1443–1448, 1996.

81. Awata T, Kuzuya T, Matsuda A, et al: Genetic analysis of HLA class II alleles and susceptibility to type 1 (insulin-dependent) diabetes mellitus in Japanese subjects. Diabetologia 35:419–424, 1992.

82. Dahlquist G, Blom L, Lönnberg G: The Swedish Childhood Diabetes Study: A multivariate analysis of risk determinants for diabetes in different age groups. Diabetologia 34:757–762, 1991.

83. Blom L, Persson LA, Dahlquist G: Growth velocity and development of insulin-dependent diabetes mellitus. Diabetologia 35:528–533, 1992.

84. Nyström L, Dahlquist G, Östman J, et al: Risk of developing insulin-dependent diabetes mellitus (IDDM) before 35 years of age: Indications of climatological determinants for age at onset. Int J Epidemiol 21:352–358, 1992.

85. Laakso M, Pyorala K: Age of onset and type of diabetes. Diabetes Care 8:114–117, 1985.

86. Molbak AG, Christau B, Marner B, et al: Incidence of insulin-dependent diabetes mellitus in age groups over 30 years in Denmark. Diabetes Med 11:650–655, 1994.

87. Lorenzen T, Pociot E, Hougaard P, et al: Long-term risk of IDDM in first-degree relatives of patients with IDDM. Diabetologia 37:321–327, 1994.

88. Hagopian WA, Karlsen AE, Gottsater A, et al: Quantitative assay using recombinant human islet glutamic acid decarboxylase (GAD65) shows that 64K autoantibody positivity at onset predicts diabetes type. J Clin Invest 91:368–374, 1993.

89. Tuomi T, Groop LC, Zimmet PZ, et al: Antibodies to glutamic acid decarboxylase reveal latent autoimmune diabetes mellitus in adults with a non-insulin-dependent onset of disease. Diabetes 42:359–362, 1993.

90. Zimmet PZ, Tuomi T, Mackay IR, et al: Latent autoimmune diabetes mellitus in adults (LADA): The role of antibodies to glutamic acid decarboxylase in diagnosis and prediction of insulin dependency. Diabet Med 11:299–303, 1994.

91. Kobayashi T, Nakanishi K, Murase T, et al: Small doses of subcutaneous insulin as a strategy for preventing slowly progressive beta-cell failure in islet cell antibody-positive patients with clinical features of NIDDM. Diabetes 45:622–626, 1996.

92. Palmer JP, Hirsch IB: What's in a name: Latent autoimmune diabetes of adults, type 1.5, adult-onset, and type 1 diabetes. Diabetes Care 26:536–538, 2003.

93. Tuomi T, Carlsson A, Li H, et al: Clinical and genetic characteristics of type 2 diabetes with and without GAD antibodies. Diabetes 48:150–157, 1999.

94. Metz C, Cave H, Bertrand AM, et al: Neonatal diabetes mellitus: Chromosomal analysis in transient and permanent cases. J Pediatr 141:483–489, 2002.

95. Stoffers DA, Zinkin NT, Stanojevic V, et al: Pancreatic agenesis attributable to a single nucleotide deletion in the human IPF1 gene coding sequence. Nat Genet 15:106–110, 1997.

96. Njolstad PR, Sovik O, Cuesta-Munoz A, et al: Neonatal diabetes mellitus due to complete glucokinase deficiency. N Engl J Med 344:1588–1592, 2001.

97. Gloyn AL, Pearson ER, Antcliff JF, et al: Activating mutations in the ATP-sensitive potassium channel subunit Kir6.2 gene are associated with permanent neonatal diabetes. N Engl J Med, 2004 (in press).

98. Edelsten AD, Hughes IA, Oakes S: Height and skeletal maturity in children with newly diagnosed juvenile-onset diabetes. Arch Dis Child 56:40–44, 1981.

99. Mason DR, Scott RS, Darlow BA: Epidemiology of insulin-dependent diabetes mellitus in Canterbury, New Zealand. Diabetes Res Clin Pract 3:21–29, 1987.

100. Karvonen M, Pitkaniemi M, Pitkaniemi J, et al: Sex difference in the incidence of insulin-dependent diabetes mellitus: An analysis of the recent epidemiological data: World Health Organization DIAMOND Project Group. Diabetes Metab Rev 13:275–291, 1997.

101. Gale EA, Gillespie KM: Diabetes and gender. Diabetologia 44:3–15, 2001.

102. Nepom GT, Kwok WW: Molecular basis for HLA-DQ associations with IDDM. Diabetes 47:1177–1184, 1998.

103. Cucca F, Lampis R, Frau F, et al: The distribution of DR4 haplotypes in Sardinia suggests a primary association of type 1 diabetes with DRB1 and DQB1 loci. Hum Immunol 43:301–308, 1995.

104. Thorsby E: HLA-associated disease susceptibility: Which genes are primarily involved? Immunologist 3/2:51–58, 1995.

105. Risch N: Genetics of IDDM: Evidence for complex inheritance with HLA. Genet Epidemiol 6:143–148, 1989.

106. Todd JA: Genetic analysis of type 1 diabetes using whole genome approaches. Proc Natl Acad Sci U S A 92:8560–8565, 1995.

107. Owerbach D, Gabbay KH: The search for IDDM susceptibility genes. Diabetes 45:544–550, 1996.

108. Bell GI, Aorita S, Koran JH: A polymorphic locus near the human insulin gene is associated with insulin-dependent diabetes mellitus. Diabetes 33:176–183, 1984.

109. Bennett ST, Wilson AJ, Cucca F, et al: IDDM2-VNTR-encoded susceptibility to type 1 diabetes: Dominant protection and parental transmission of allele of the insulin gene-linked minisatellite locus. J Autoimmun 9:415–421, 1996.

110. Pugliese A, Zeller M, Fernandez J, et al: The insulin gene transcribed in the human thymus and transcription level correlate with allelic variation at the INS VNTR-IDDM2 susceptibility locus for type 1 diabetes. Nat Genet 15:293–297, 1997.

111. Vafiadis P, Bennett ST, Todd JA, et al: Insulin expression in human thymus is modulated by INS VNTR alleles at the IDDM2 locus. Nat Genet 15:289–292, 1997.

112. Nisticó L, Buzzetti R, Pritchard LE, et al: The CTLA-4 gene region on chromosome 2q33 is linked to, and associated with, type 1 diabetes: Belg Diabetes Registry. Hum Mol Genet 5:1075–1080, 1996.

113. Van der Auwera BJ, Vandewalle CL, Schuit FC, et al: CTLA-4 gene polymorphism confers susceptibility to insulin-dependent diabetes mellitus (IDDM) independently from age and from other genetic or immune disease markers. Belg Diabetes Registry. Clin Exp Immunol 110:98–103, 1997.

114. Harris HF: A case of diabetes mellitus quickly following mumps on the pathological alterations of salivary glands, closely resembling those found in pancreas, in a case of diabetes mellitus. Boston Med Surg J CXL 465:591–601, 1898.

115. Yoon JW: A new look at viruses in type 1 diabetes. Diabetes Metab Rev 11:83–107, 1995.

116. Yoon JW: Role of viruses in the pathogenesis of IDDM. Ann Med 23:437–445, 1991.

117. Menser MA, Forrest JM, Honeyman MC, et al: Diabetes, HLA-antigens and congenital rubella. Lancet 2:1508–1509, 1974.

118. Ginsberg-Fellner F, Witt ME, Yagihashi S, et al: Congenital rubella syndrome as a model for type 1 (insulin-dependent) diabetes mellitus: Increased prevalence of islet cell surface antibodies. Diabetologia 27:87–89, 1984.

119. McIntosh EDG, Menser MA: A fifty-year follow-up of congenital rubella. Lancet 340:414–415, 1992.

120. Hyöty H, Hiltunen M, Knip M, et al: A prospective study of the role of coxsackie B and other enterovirus infections in the pathogenesis of IDDM: Childhood Diabetes in Finland (DiMe) Study Group. Diabetes 44:652–657, 1995.

121. Dahlquist G, Ivarsson S, Lindberg B, et al: Maternal enteroviral infection during pregnancy as a risk factor for childhood IDDM. Diabetes 44:408–413, 1995.

122. Lindberg B, Ahlfors K, Carlsson A, et al: Previous exposure to measles, mumps and rubella—but not vaccination during adolescence—correlates to the prevalence of pancreatic and thyroid autoantibodies. Pediatrics 104:e12, 1999.

123. Haverkos HW, Battula N, Drotman DP, et al: Enteroviruses and type 1 diabetes mellitus. Biomed Pharmacother 57:379–385, 2003.

124. Yoon JW, Austin M, Onodera T, et al: Virus-induced diabetes mellitus: Isolation of a virus from the pancreas of a child with diabetic ketoacidosis. N Engl J Med 300:1173–1179, 1979.

125. Gerling I, Chatterjee NK, Nejman C: Coxsackie virus B4-induced development of antibodies to 64,000 Mr islet autoantigen and hyperglycemia in mice. Autoimmunity 6:49–56, 1991.

126. Hou J, Sheikh S, Martin DL, et al: Coxsackievirus B4 alters pancreatic glutamate decarboxylase expression in mice soon after infection. J Autoimmun 6:529–542, 1993.

127. Kaufman DL, Erlander MG, Clare-Salzler M, et al: Autoimmunity to two forms of glutamate decarboxylase in insulin-dependent diabetes mellitus. J Clin Invest 89:283–292, 1992.

128. Atkinson MA, Bowman MA, Campbell L, et al: Cellular immunity to a determinant common to glutamate decarboxylase and coxsackievirus in insulin-dependent diabetes. J Clin Invest 94:2125–2129, 1994.

129. Horwitz MS, Bradley LM, Harbertson J, et al: Diabetes induced by coxsackievirus: Initiation by bystander damage and not molecular mimicry. Nat Med 4:781–785, 1998.

130. Lonnrot M, Korpela K, Knip M, et al: Enterovirus infection as a risk factor for beta-cell autoimmunity in a prospectively observed birth cohort: The Finnish Diabetes Prediction and Prevention Study. Diabetes 49:1314–1318, 2000.

131. Juhela S, Hyoty H, Roivainen M, et al: T-cell responses to enterovirus antigens in children with type 1 diabetes. Diabetes 49:1308–1313, 2000.

132. Varela-Calvino R, Ellis R, Sgarbi G, et al: Characterization of the T-cell response to coxsackievirus B4: Evidence that effector memory cells predominate in patients with type 1 diabetes. Diabetes 51:1745–1753, 2002.

133. Yin H, Berg AK, Tuvemo T, et al: Enterovirus RNA is found in peripheral blood mononuclear cells in a majority of type 1 diabetic children at onset. Diabetes 51:1964–1971, 2002.

134. Toniolo A, Onodera T, Yoon J-W, et al: Introduction of diabetes by cumulative environmental insults from viruses and chemicals. Nature 297:87–89, 1980.

135. Karam JH, Lewitt PA, Young CW, et al: Insulinopenic diabetes after rodenticide (Vacor) ingestion: A unique model of acquired diabetes in man. Diabetes 29:971–978, 1980.

136. Helgason T, Jonasson MR: Evidence for a food additive as a cause of ketosis-prone diabetes. Lancet 2:716–720, 1981.

137. Helgason T, Ewen SWB, Ross IS, et al: Diabetes produced in mice by smoked/cured mutton. Lancet 2:1017–1022, 1982.

138. Gepts W, LaCompte PM: The pancreatic islets in diabetes. Am J Med 70:105–115, 1981.

139. Klöppel G, Drenck CR, Oberholzer M, et al: Morphometric evidence for a striking β-cell reduction at the clinical onset of type 1 diabetes. Virchows Arch A Pathol Anat Histopathol 403:441–452, 1984.

140. Dandona P, Elias E, Beckett AG: Serum trypsin concentrations in diabetes mellitus. Br Med J 2:1125–1127, 1978.

141. Foo Y, Rosalki SB, Ramdial L: Serum isoamylase activities in diabetes mellitus. J Clin Pathol 33:1102–1105, 1980.

142. Landin-Olsson M, Borgstrom A, Blom L, et al: Immunoreactive trypsin(ogen) in the sera of children with recent-onset insulin-dependent diabetes and matched controls: The Swedish Childhood Diabetes Group. Pancreas 5:241–247, 1990.

143. Rahier J: The diabetic pancreas: A pathologist's view. In Lefebvre P, Pipeleers D (eds): The Pathology of the Endocrine Pancreas. Berlin, Springer-Verlag, 1988, pp 17–40.

144. Edlund H: Transcribing pancreas. Diabetes 47:1817–1823, 1998.

145. Rahier J, Goebbels RM, Henquin JC: Cellular composition of the human diabetic pancreas. Diabetologia 24:366–371, 1983.

146. Foulis AK, Liddle CN, Farquharson MA, et al: The histopathology of the pancreas in type 1 (insulin-dependent) diabetes mellitus: A 25-year review of deaths in patients under 20 years of age in the United Kingdom. Diabetologia 29:267–274, 1986.

147. Winer S, Tsui H, Lau A, et al: Autoimmune islet destruction in spontaneous type 1 diabetes is not beta-cell exclusive. Nat Med 9:198–205, 2003.

148. Bottazzo GF, Dean BM, McNally JM, et al: In situ characterization of autoimmune phenomena and expression of HLA molecules in the pancreas in diabetic insulitis. N Engl J Med 313:353–360, 1985.

149. Hänninen A, Jalkanen S, Salmi M, et al: Macrophages, T cell receptor usage, and endothelial cell activation in the pancreas at the onset of insulin-dependent diabetes mellitus. J Clin Invest 90:1901–1910, 1992.

150. Hanafusa T, Miyazaki A, Miyagawa J: Examination of islets in the pancreas biopsy specimens from newly diagnosed type 1 (insulin-dependent) diabetic patients. Diabetologia 33:105–111, 1990.

151. Itoh N, Hanafusa T, Miyazaki A, et al: Mononuclear cell infiltration and its relation to the expression of major histocompatibility complex antigens and adhesion molecules in pancreas biopsy specimens from newly diagnosed insulin-dependent diabetes mellitus patients. J Clin Invest 92:2313–2322, 1993.

152. Imagawa A, Hanafusa T, Tamura S, et al: Pancreatic biopsy as a procedure for detecting in situ autoimmune phenomena in type 1 diabetes: Close correlation between serological markers and histological evidence of cellular autoimmunity. Diabetes 50:1269–1273, 2001.

153. Moriwaki M, Itoh N, Miyagawa J, et al: Fas and Fas ligand expression in inflamed islets in pancreas sections of patients with recent-onset type 1 diabetes mellitus. Diabetologia 42:1332–1340, 1999.

154. Lampeter EE, Seifert I, Lohmann D, et al: Inflammatory islet damage in patients bearing HLA-DR3 and/or DR4 haplotypes does not lead to islet autoimmunity. Diabetologia 37:471–475, 1994.

155. Bennett Jenson A, Rosenberg HS, Notkins AL: Pancreatic islet cell damage in children with fetal viral infections. Lancet 2:354–358, 1980.

156. Lampeter EF, Homberg M, Quabeck K, et al: Transfer of insulin-dependent diabetes between HLA-identical siblings by bone marrow transplantation. Lancet 342:174, 1993.

157. Rubenstein AH, Kuzuya H, Horwitz DL: Clinical significance of circulating C-peptide in diabetes mellitus and hypoglycemic disorders. Arch Intern Med 137:625–632, 1977.

158. Agner T, Damm P, Binder C: Remission in IDDM: Prospective study of basal C-peptide and insulin dose in 268 consecutive patients. Diabetes Care 10:164–169, 1987.

159. Wallensteen M, Dahlquist G, Persson B, et al: Factors influencing the

magnitude, duration, and rate of fall of β-cell function in type 1 (insulin-dependent) diabetes children followed for two years from their clinical diagnosis. Diabetologia 31:664–669, 1988.

160. Sabbah E, Kulmala P, Veijola R, et al: Glutamic acid decarboxylase antibodies in relation to other autoantibodies and genetic risk markers in children with newly diagnosed insulin-dependent diabetes. J Clin Endocrinol Metab 81:2455–2459, 1996.

161. Marner B, Agner T, Binder C, et al: Increased reduction in fasting C-peptide is associated with islet cell antibodies in type 1 (insulin-dependent) diabetic patients. Diabetologia 28:875–880, 1985.

162. Nakanishi K, Kobayashi T, Miyashita H, et al: Relationships among islet cell antibodies, residual β-cell function, and metabolic control in patients with insulin-dependent diabetes mellitus of long duration: Use of a sensitive C-peptide radioimmunoassay. Metabolism 39:925–930, 1990.

163. Kahn SE, Prigeon RL, McCulloch DK, et al: Quantification of the relationship between insulin sensitivity and beta-cell function in human subjects: Evidence for a hyperbolic function. Diabetes 42:1663–1672, 1993.

164. Heaton DA, Millward BA, Gray IP, et al: Increased proinsulin levels as an early indicator of β-cell dysfunction in non-diabetic twins of type 1 (insulin-dependent) diabetic patients. Diabetologia 31:182–184, 1988.

165. Roder ME, Knip M, Hartling SG, et al: Disproportionately elevated proinsulin levels precede the onset of insulin-dependent diabetes mellitus in siblings with low first phase insulin responses: The Childhood Diabetes in Finland Study Group. J Clin Endocrinol Metab 79:1570–1575, 1994.

166. Johnston C, Raghu P, McCulloch D, et al: β-Cell function and insulin sensitivity in nondiabetic HLA-identical siblings of insulin-dependent diabetics. Diabetes 36:829–837, 1987.

167. Palmer JP: Beta cell rest and recovery: Does it bring patients with latent autoimmune diabetes in adults to euglycemia? Ann N Y Acad Sci 958:89–98, 2002.

168. Ludvigsson J, Heding LG, Larsson Y, et al: C-peptide in juvenile diabetics beyond the postinitial remission period: Relation to clinical manifestations at onset of diabetes, remission and diabetic control. Acta Pædiatr Scand 66:177–184, 1977.

169. The Diabetes Control and Complications Trial Research Group: Effect of intensive therapy on residual beta-cell function in patients with type 1 diabetes in the diabetes control and complications trial: A randomized, controlled trial. Ann Intern Med 128:517–523, 1998.

170. Sochett EB, Daneman D, Clarson C, et al: Factors affecting and patterns of residual insulin secretion during the first year of type 1 (insulin-dependent) diabetes mellitus in children. Diabetologia 30:453–459, 1987.

171. Bjork E, Berne C, Kampe O, et al: Diazoxide treatment at onset preserves residual insulin secretion in adults with autoimmune diabetes. Diabetes 45:1427–1430, 1996.

172. DPT-1 Study Group: The Diabetes Prevention Trial—Type 1 diabetes (DPT-1): Implementation of screening and staging of relatives. Transplant Proc 27:3377, 1995.

173. Pozzilli P: The DPT-1 trial: A negative result with lessons for future type 1 diabetes prevention. Diabetes Metab Res Rev 18:257–259, 2002.

174. Graham J, Kockum I, Sanjeevi CB, et al: Negative association between type 1 diabetes and HLA DQB1*0602-DQA1*0102 is attenuated with age at onset: The Swedish Childhood Diabetes Study Group. Eur J Immunogenet 26:117–127, 1999.

175. Knip M, Ilonen J, Mustonen A, et al: Evidence of an accelerated β-cell destruction in HLA-Dw3/Dw4 heterozygous children with type 1 (insulin-dependent) diabetes. Diabetologia 29:347–351, 1986.

176. Sanjeevi CB, Landin-Olsson M, Kockum I, et al: Effects of the second HLA-DQ haplotype on the association with childhood insulin dependent diabetes mellitus. Tissue Antigens 45:148–152, 1994.

177. Lawley TJ, Hall RP, Fauci AS, et al: Defective Fc-receptor functions associated with the HLA-B8/DRw3 haplotype. N Engl J Med 304:185–192, 1981.

178. Litherland SA, Xie XT, Hutson AD, et al: Aberrant prostaglandin synthase 2 expression defines an antigen-presenting cell defect for insulin-dependent diabetes mellitus. J Clin Invest 104:515–523, 1999.

179. Jansen A, van Hagen M, Drexhage HA: Defective maturation and function of antigen-presenting cells in type 1 diabetes. Lancet 345:491–492, 1995.

180. Plesner A, Greenbaum CJ, Gaur LK, et al: Macrophages from high-risk HLA-DQB1*0201/*0302 type 1 diabetes mellitus patients are hypersensitive to lipopolysaccharide stimulation. Scand J Immunol 56:522–529, 2002.

181. Bougneres PF, Carel JC, Castano L, et al: Factors associated with early remission of type 1 diabetes in children treated with cyclosporine. N Engl J Med 318:663–6670, 1988.

182. Herold KC, Hagopian W, Auger JA, et al: Anti-CD3 monoclonal antibody in new-onset type 1 diabetes mellitus. N Engl J Med 346:1692–1698, 2002.

183. Roep BO: The role of T-cells in the pathogenesis of type 1 diabetes: From cause to cure. Diabetologia 46:305–321, 2003.

184. Lernmark Å: Cell-mediated immunity in type 1 (insulin-dependent) diabetes: Update 84. In Andreani D, di Mario U, Federlin KF, et al (eds): Immunology in Diabetes. London, Kimpton Medical Publications, 1984, pp 121–131.

185. Peakman M, Vergani D: The T lymphocyte in type 1 diabetes. In Marshall SM, Home PD (eds): The Diabetes Annual/8. Amsterdam, Elsevier, 1994, pp 53–73.

186. Jackson RA, Morris MA, Haynes BF, et al: Increased circulating Ia-bearing T cells in type 1 diabetes mellitus. N Engl J Med 306:785–788, 1982.

187. Panina-Bordignon P, Lang R, van Endert PM, et al: Cytotoxic T cells specific for glutamic acid decarboxylase in autoimmune diabetes. J Exp Med 181:1923–1927, 1995.

188. Honeyman MC, Stone N, de Aizpurua H, et al: High T cell responses to the glutamic acid decarboxylase (GAD) isoform 67 reflect a hyperimmune state that precedes the onset of insulin-dependent diabetes. J Autoimmun 10:165–173, 1997.

189. Lohmann T, Leslie RDG, Hawa M, et al: Immunodominant epitopes of glutamic acid decarboxylase 65 and 67 in insulin-dependent diabetes mellitus. Lancet 343:1607–1608, 1994.

190. Lohmann T, Halder T, Engler J, et al: T cell reactivity to DR*0401- and DQ*0302-binding peptides of the putative autoantigen IA-2 in type 1 diabetes. Exp Clin Endocrinol Diabetes 107:166–171, 1999.

191. Endl J, Otto H, Jung G, et al: Identification of naturally processed T cell epitopes from glutamic acid decarboxylase presented in the context of HLA-DR alleles by T lymphocytes of recent onset IDDM patients. J Clin Invest 99:2405–2415, 1997.

192. Wicker LS, Chen SL, Nepom GT, et al: Naturally processed T cell epitopes from human glutamic acid decarboxylase identified using mice transgenic for the type 1 diabetes-associated human MHC class II allele, DRB1*0401. J Clin Invest 98:2597–2603, 1996.

193. Novak EJ, Liu AW, Gebe JA, et al: Tetramer-guided epitope mapping: Rapid identification and characterization of immunodominant CD4+ T cell epitopes from complex antigens. J Immunol 166:6665–6670, 2001.

194. Sonderstrup G, McDevitt H: Identification of autoantigen epitopes in MHC class II transgenic mice. Immunol Rev 164:129–138, 1998.

195. Geluk A, van Meijgaarden KE, Schloot NC, et al: HLA-DR binding analysis of peptides from islet antigens in IDDM. Diabetes 47:1594–1601, 1998.

196. Congia M, Patel S, Cope AP, et al: T cell epitopes of insulin defined in HLA-DR4 transgenic mice are derived from preproinsulin and proinsulin. Proc Natl Acad Sci U S A 95:3833–3838, 1998.

197. Papadopoulos G, Petersen J, Andersen V: Spontaneous *in vitro* immunoglobulin secretion at the diagnosis of insulin-dependent diabetes. Acta Endocrinol 105:521–527, 1984.

198. Horita M, Suzuki H, Onodera T, et al: Abnormalities of immunoregulatory T cell subsets in patients with insulin-dependent diabetes mellitus. J Immunol 129:1426–1429, 1982.

199. Baekkeskov S, Landin-Olsson M, Kristensen JK, et al: Antibodies to an M*r* 64,000 human islet cell antigen precede the clinical onset of insulin-dependent diabetes. J Clin Invest 79:926–934, 1987.

200. Petersen JB, Russel S, Marshall MO, et al: Differential expression of glutamic acid decarboxylase in rat and human islets. Diabetes 42:484–495, 1993.

201. Christie MR, Vohra G, Champagne P, et al: Distinct antibody specificities to a 64-Kd islet cell antigen in type 1 diabetes as revealed by trypsin treatment. J Exp Med 172:789–794, 1990.

202. Christie MR, Genovese S, Cassidy D, et al: Antibodies to islet 37k antigen, but not to glutamate decarboxylase, discriminate rapid progression to IDDM in endocrine autoimmunity. Diabetes 43:1254–1259, 1994.

203. Wasmeier C, Hutton JC: Molecular cloning of phogrin, a protein-tyrosine phosphatase homologue localized to insulin secretory granule membranes. J Biol Chem 271:18161–18170, 1996.

204. Cui L, Yu W-P, DeAizpurua HJ, et al: Cloning and characterization of islet cell antigen-related protein-tyrosine phosphatase (PTP), a novel receptor-like PTP and autoantigen in insulin-dependent diabetes. J Biol Chem 271:24817–24813, 1996.

205. LaGasse J, Jelinek L, Sexson S, et al: An islet-cell protein tyrosine phosphatase is a likely precursor to the 37-kDa autoantigen in type 1 diabetes: Human and macaque sequences, tissue distribution, unique and shared epitopes, and predictive autoantibodies. Mol Med 3:163–173, 1997.

206. Hagopian WA, Sanjeevi CB, Kockum I, et al: Glutamate decarboxylase-, insulin- and islet cell-antibodies and HLA typing to detect diabetes in a general population-based study of Swedish children. J Clin Invest 95:1505–1511, 1995.

207. Eisenbarth GS, Jackson GS: Insulin autoimmunity: The rate limiting factor of pre-type 1 diabetes. J Autoimmun 5:214–246, 1992.

208. Ziegler AG, Ziegler R, Vardi P, et al: Life-table analysis of progression to diabetes of anti-insulin autoantibody-positive relatives of individuals with type 1 diabetes. Diabetes 38:1320–1325, 1989.

209. Atkinson MA, Maclaren NK: Islet cell autoantigens in insulin-dependent diabetes. J Clin Invest 92:1608–1616, 1993.

210. Gilliam LK, Palmer JP, Lernmark Å: Autoantibodies and the disease process of type 1 diabetes mellitus. In LeRoith D, Taylor SI, Olefsky JM (eds): Diabetes Mellitus: A Fundamental and Clinical Text. Philadelphia, Lippincott Williams & Wilkins, 2003, pp 499–518.

211. Notkins AL, Lernmark Å: Autoimmune type 1 diabetes: Resolved and unresolved issues. J Clin Invest 108:1247–1252, 2001.

212. Bingley PJ, Bonifacio E, Williams AJK, et al: Prediction of IDDM in the general population: Strategies based on combinations of autoantibody markers. Diabetes 46:1701–1710, 1997.

213. Bottazzo GF, Gleichmann H: Immunology and diabetes workshops: Report of the First International Workshop on the Standardisation of cytoplasmic islet cell antibodies. Diabetologia 29:125–126, 1986.

214. Greenbaum CJ, Palmer JP, Nagataki S, et al: Improved specificity of ICA assays in Fourth International Immunology of Diabetes Serum Exchange Workshop. Diabetes 41:1570–1574, 1992.

215. Greenbaum CJ, Palmer JP, Kuglin B, et al: Insulin autoantibodies measured by radioimmunoassay methodology are more related to insulin-dependent diabetes mellitus than those measured by enzyme-linked immunosorbent assay: Results of the Fourth International Workshop on the Standardization of Insulin Autoantibody Measurement. J Clin Endcrinol Metab 74:1040–1044, 1992.

216. Verge CF, Stenger D, Bonifacio E, et al: Combined use of autoantibodies (IA-2 autoantibody, GAD autoantibody, insulin autoantibody, cytoplasmic islet cell antibodies) in type 1 diabetes: Combinatorial Islet Autoantibody Workshop. Diabetes 47:1857–1866, 1998.

217. Grubin CE, Daniels T, Toivola B, et al: A novel radioligand binding assay to determine diagnostic accuracy of isoform-specific glutamic acid decarboxylase antibodies in childhood IDDM. Diabetologia 37:344–350, 1994.

218. Kawasaki E, Eisenbarth G, Wasmeier C, et al: Autoantibodies to protein tyrosine phosphatase-like protein in type 1 diabetes: Overlapping specificities to phogrin and ICA512/IA-2. Diabetes 45:1344–1349, 1996.

219. Vandewalle CL, Falorni A, Lernmark Å, et al: Associations of GAD65- and IA-2-autoantibodies with genetic risk markers in new-onset IDDM patients and their siblings. Diabetes Care 20:1547–1552, 1997.

220. Petersen JS, Hejnaes KR, Moody A, et al: Detection of GAD65 antibodies in diabetes and other autoimmune diseases using a simple radioligand assay. Diabetes 43:459–465, 1994.

221. Schmidli RS, Colman PG, Bonifacio E: Disease sensitivity and specificity of 52 assays for glutamic acid decarboxylase antibodies: The Second International GADAb Workshop. Diabetes 44:636–640, 1995.

222. Schmidli RS, DeAizpurua HJ, Harrison LC, et al: Antibodies to glutamic acid decarboxylase in at-risk and clinical insulin-dependent diabetic subjects: Relationship to age, sex and islet cell antibody status, and temporal profile. J Autoimmun 7:55–66, 1994.

223. Borg H, Gottsater A, Fernlund P, et al: A 12-year prospective study of the relationship between islet antibodies and beta-cell function at and after the diagnosis in patients with adult-onset diabetes. Diabetes 51:1754–1762, 2002.

224. Sanjeevi CB, Hagopian WA, Landin-Olsson M, et al: Association between autoantibody markers and subtypes of DR4 and DR4-DQ in Swedish children with insulin-dependent diabetes reveals closer association of tyrosine pyrophosphatase autoimmunity with DR4 than DQ8. Tissue Antigens 51:281–286, 1998.

225. Rolandsson O, Hägg E, Hampe C, et al: Levels of glutamate decarboxylase (GAD65) and tyrosine phosphatase-like protein (IA-2) autoantibodies in the general population are related to glucose intolerance and body mass index. Diabetologia 42:555–559, 1999.

226. Yu L, Chase HP, Falorni A, et al: Sexual dimorphism in transmission to offspring of expression of islet autoantibodies. Diabetologia 38:1353–1357, 1995.

227. Bonifacio E, Genovese S, Braghi S, et al: Islet autoantibody markers in IDDM: Risk assessment strategies yielding high sensitivity. Diabetologia 38:816–822, 1995.

228. Kim J, Namchuck M, Bugawan T, et al: Higher autoantibody levels and recognition of a linear NH2-terminal epitope in the autoantigen GAD65, distinguish stiff-man syndrome from insulin-dependent diabetes mellitus. J Exp Med 180:595–606, 1994.

229. Li L, Hagopian WA, Brashear HR, et al: Identification of autoantibody epitopes of glutamic acid decarboxylase in stiff-man syndrome patients. J Immunol 152:930–934, 1994.

230. Leslie RD, Atkinson MA, Notkins AL: Autoantigens IA-2 and GAD in type 1 (insulin-dependent) diabetes. Diabetologia 42:3–14, 1999.

231. Graham J, Hagopian WA, Kockum I, et al: Genetic effects on age-dependent onset and islet cell autoantibody markers in type 1 diabetes. Diabetes 51:1346–1555, 2002.

232. Solimena M, Dirkx R Jr, Hermel JM, et al: ICA 512, an autoantigen of type 1 diabetes, is an intrinsic membrane protein of neurosecretory granules. EMBO J 15:2102–2114, 1996.

233. Landin-Olsson M, Palmer JP, Lernmark Å, et al: Predictive value of islet cell and insulin autoantibodies for type 1 (insulin-dependent) diabetes mellitus in a population-based study of

newly-diagnosed diabetic and matched control children. Diabetologia 35:1068–1073, 1992.

234. Ziegler R, Alper CA, Awdeh ZL, et al: Specific association of HLA-DR4 with increased prevalence and level of insulin autoantibodies in first-degree relatives of patients with type 1 diabetes. Diabetes 40:709–714, 1991.

235. Castano L, Ziegler A, Ziegler R, et al: Characterization of insulin autoantibodies in relatives of patients with insulin-dependent diabetes mellitus. Diabetes 42:1202–1209, 1993.

236. Brooks-Worrell BM, Nielson D, Palmer JP: Insulin autoantibodies and insulin antibodies have similar binding characteristics. Proc Assoc Am Physicians 111:92–96, 1999.

237. Arslanian SA, Becker DJ, Rabin B, et al: Correlates of insulin antibodies in newly diagnosed children with insulin-dependent diabetes before insulin therapy. Diabetes 34:926–930, 1985.

238. Eisenbarth GS, Gianani R, Yu L, et al: Dual-parameter model for prediction of type 1 diabetes mellitus. Proc Assoc Am Physicians 110:126–135, 1998.

239. Lernmark Å, Hägglöf B, Freedman Z, et al: A prospective analysis of antibodies reacting with pancreatic islet cells in insulin-dependent diabetic children. Diabetologia 20:471–474, 1981.

240. Van de Winkel M, Smets G, Gepts W, et al: Islet cell surface antibodies from insulin-dependent diabetics bind specifically to pancreatic β-cells. J Clin Invest 70:41–49, 1982.

241. Dobersen MJ, Scharff JE: Preferential lysis of pancreatic β-cells by islet cell surface antibodies. Diabetes 31:449–462, 1982.

242. Eisenbarth GS, Morris MA, Scearce RM: Cytotoxic antibodies to cloned rat islet cells in serum of patients with diabetes mellitus. J Clin Invest 67:403–408, 1981.

243. Rabinovitch A, MacKay P, Ludvigsson J, et al: A prospective analysis of islet cell cytotoxic antibodies in insulin-dependent diabetic children: Transient effects of plasmapheresis. Diabetes 33:224–228, 1984.

244. Freedman ZR, Feed CM, Irvine WJ, et al: Islet-cell cytoplasmic and cell-surface antibodies in diabetes mellitus. Trans Assoc Am Physicians 96:64–76, 1979.

245. Scott J, Nerup J, Lernmark Å: Immunologic factors in diabetes mellitus. In Rose WF (ed): Clinical Immunology Update. New York, Elsevier, 1985, pp 53–85.

246. Eisenbarth GS: Type 1 diabetes mellitus: A chronic autoimmune disease. N Engl J Med 314:1360–1368, 1986.

247. Maclaren NK, Huang S, Fogh J: Antibody to cultured human insulinoma cells in insulin-dependent diabetics. Lancet 1:997–999, 1975.

248. Huang SW, Haedt LH, Rich S, et al: Prevalence of antibodies to nucleic acids in insulin-dependent diabetics and their relatives. Diabetes 30:873–874, 1981.

249. Nordén G, Jensen E, Stilbo I, et al: β-Cell function and islet cell and other organ-specific autoantibodies in relatives to insulin-dependent diabetic patients. Acta Med Scand 213:199–203, 1983.

250. Hägglöf B, Rabinovitch A, Mackay P, et al: Islet cell and other organ-specific autoantibodies in healthy first degree relatives to insulin-dependent diabetic patients. Acta Pœdiatr Scand 75:611–618, 1986.

251. Irvine WJ, Al-Khateeb SF, Di Mario U, et al: Soluble immune complexes in the sera of newly diagnosed insulin-dependent diabetics and in treated diabetics. Clin Exp Immunol 30:16–21, 1977.

252. Abrass CK, Heber D, Lieberman J: Circulating immune complexes in patients with diabetes mellitus. Clin Exp Immunol 52:164–172, 1983.

253. Contreas G, Lernmark Å, Mathiesen EF, et al: Immune complexes in insulin-dependent diabetes. Biomed Biochim Acta 44:129–132, 1985.

254. The Expert Committee on the Diagnosis and Classification of Diabetes Mellitus: Report of the expert committee on the diagnosis and classification of diabetes mellitus. Diabetes 20:1183–1194, 1997.

255. World Health Organization: Diabetes Mellitus: Report of a WHO Study Group, Technical Report Series 727. Geneva, World Health Organization, 1985.

256. Gottsäter A, Landin-Olsson M, Lernmark Å, et al: Glutamate decarboxylase antibody levels predict rate of beta-cell decline in adult onset diabetes. Diabetes Res Clin Practice 27:133–140, 1995.

257. Srikanta S, Ganda OP, Rabizadeh A, et al: First-degree relatives of patients with type 1 diabetes mellitus: Islet-cell antibodies and abnormal insulin secretion. N Engl J Med 313:462–464, 1985.

258. Gorsuch AN, Spencer KM, Lister J: The natural history of type 1 (insulin-dependent) diabetes mellitus: Evidence for a long prediabetic period. Lancet 2:1363–1365, 1981.

259. Bingley PJ, Christie MR, Bonifacio E, et al: Combined analysis of autoantibodies improves prediction of IDDM in islet cell antibody-positive relatives. Diabetes 43:1304–1310, 1994.

260. Feutren G, Papoz L, Assan R, et al: Cyclosporin increases the rate and length of remission in insulin-dependent diabetes of recent onset. Results of a multicenter double-blind trial. Lancet 2:119–123, 1986.

261. Canadian-European Randomized Control Trial Group: Cyclosporin-induced remission of IDDM after early intervention: Association of 1 year of cyclosporin treatment with enhanced insulin secretion. Diabetes 37:1574, 1988.

262. Feldt R-B, Jensen T, Dieperink H, et al: Nephrotoxicity of cyclosporin A in patients with newly diagnosed type 1 diabetes mellitus. Diabet Med 7:429–433, 1990.

263. Bieg S, Lernmark Å: Animal models for insulin-dependent diabetes mellitus. In Volpé R (ed): Autoimmune Endocrinopathies. Totowa, NJ, Humana Press, 1999, pp 113–140.

264. Peakman M, Tree TI, Endl J, et al: Characterization of preparations of GAD65, proinsulin, and the islet tyrosine phosphatase IA-2 for use in detection of autoreactive T-cells in type 1 diabetes: Report of phase II of the Second International Immunology of Diabetes Society Workshop for Standardization of T-cell assays in type 1 diabetes. Diabetes 50:1749–1754, 2001.

265. Agardh D, Cilio CM, Lethagen ÅL, et al: Clinical evidence for safety, efficacy, and immunomodulation by a novel therapeutic intended for treatment of autoimmune diabetes. Diabetes 53:272–OR, 2004 (in press).

266. Masteller EL, Bluestone JA: Immunotherapy of insulin-dependent diabetes mellitus. Curr Opin Immunol 14:652–659, 2002.

Type 2 Diabetes Mellitus: Etiology, Pathogenesis, and Natural History

C. Hamish Courtney and Jerrold M. Olefsky

Type 2 diabetes mellitus is the most common form of diabetes and is currently a major worldwide cause of morbidity and mortality. This is likely to worsen, given the rapidly increasing prevalence of this condition; therefore, an understanding of its etiology and pathogenesis is of considerable importance.

By definition, patients with type 2 diabetes have neither autoimmune β-cell destruction, as is found in type 1 diabetes, nor one of the other specific causes of diabetes described in Chapter 54. Type 2 diabetes is not a single disease process but instead represents a heterogeneous constellation of disease syndromes, all leading to the final common pathway of hyperglycemia. Many factors, either alone or in combination, can cause hyperglycemia; thus, the complexity of the pathogenesis of type 2 diabetes reflects the heterogeneous genetic, pathologic, environmental, and metabolic abnormalities that can exist in different patients.

Normal glucose homeostasis relies on a balance between insulin secretion and tissue sensitivity to insulin. With respect to glucose metabolism, the tissue effects of insulin are most important at the skeletal muscle, liver, and adipose tissue level. Three major metabolic abnormalities coexist in type 2 diabetes,[1-4] each contributing to the hyperglycemic state. These abnormalities are summarized in Figure 56-1. To begin at the hepatic level, the role of the liver in the pathogenesis of type 2 diabetes is overproduction of glucose. Increased basal hepatic glucose production is characteristic of essentially all type 2 diabetic patients with fasting hyperglycemia.[5-7] Skeletal muscle is depicted as the prototypic peripheral insulin target tissue because in the in vivo insulin-stimulated state, 70% to 80% of all glucose is taken up by skeletal muscle. Target tissues are insulin resistant in type 2 diabetes mellitus, and such resistance has been well described in most,[2-5,8-12] but not all,[13] population groups. Finally, abnormal islet cell function plays a central role in the development of hyperglycemia; decreased β-cell function and increased glucagons secretion are frequent concomitants of the diabetic state.[1,13,14] Taken together, abnormalities in these organ systems account for the syndrome of type 2 diabetes mellitus. In subsequent sections of this chapter, each of these abnormalities will be considered in further detail. Although the causal mechanisms may be heterogeneous in different type 2 diabetic patient groups, ultimate expression of the hyperglycemic state involves some combination of impaired insulin secretion, insulin resistance, and increased hepatic glucose production, and the relative magnitude and importance of these three common metabolic abnormalities depends on the specific genetic, pathologic, or environmental factors involved in a particular patient.

GENETIC VERSUS ACQUIRED FACTORS

GENETIC COMPONENT

Abundant evidence supports the view that a strong genetic component contributes to type 2 diabetes. While many patients have a positive family history for this disease, perhaps the strongest evidence comes from twin studies. In one study, 53 twin pairs were examined, in whom one twin was ascertained to have type 2 diabetes. On assessing the other twin, type 2 diabetes had developed in 91% (48/53) of the cotwins.[15] The five discordant twins had mild glucose intolerance and abnormal insulin responses during oral glucose tolerance tests, suggesting that they too might ultimately progress to overt disease, thus giving a 100% concordance rate.

Further evidence for a genetic basis comes from the striking differences in the prevalence of type 2 diabetes in various ethnic groups that are not explained by environmental factors. The prevalence of type 2 diabetes in the United States is 2% to 4% for Caucasians, but it is 4% to 6% for African-American,[16] 10% to 15% for Mexican-Americans,[17] and over 40% for the Pima Indians in Arizona, the group with the highest incidence of type 2 diabetes in the world.[18] In the Pima Indians, 80% of 35- to 44-year-old offspring of two parents with type 2 diabetes mellitus before age 45 years have diabetes, and a positive family history of type 2 diabetes is a much better predictor of the incidence of type 2 diabetes than are the combined effects of obesity, gender, and physical fitness.[18]

Despite the high concordance rate in twins, "garden-variety" type 2 diabetes is obviously not simply the result of a single-gene defect; the inheritance pattern of type 2 diabetes

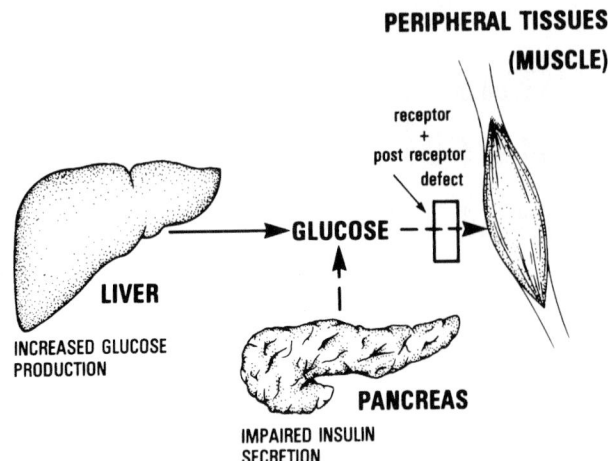

Figure 56-1 Summary of the metabolic abnormalities in type 2 diabetes mellitus that contribute to hyperglycemia. Increased hepatic glucose production, impaired insulin secretion, and insulin resistance caused by receptor and postreceptor defects all combine to generate the hyperglycemic state.

does not conform to any recognizable Mendelian pattern, and the incidence of type 2 diabetes in first-degree relatives is far below what one would expect. While multiple genes are involved in the pathogenesis of diabetes in most patients, a small number of patients have a monogenic form of this disease. In these forms of diabetes, environmental factors play little or no role in determining the phenotypic expression. These single-gene mutations may confer a defect in either insulin secretion or insulin action.

Monogenic Defects in Insulin Secretion

Several patients have been described who secrete a structurally abnormal, biologically defective insulin molecule resulting from a mutation in the structural gene for insulin.[19] Others have familial hyperproinsulinemia caused by incomplete conversion of proinsulin to insulin, within the β-cell secretory granule, as a result of structural abnormalities at the proteolytic cleavage sites of the proinsulin molecule.[20,21] These syndromes are dealt with in Chapters 48 and 54 and are not discussed further here.

Maturity-onset diabetes of the young (MODY) is a well-described group of disorders in which there is autosomal-dominant inheritance of a mutation in any one of at least six genes expressed primarily in the β cell. This condition is reviewed in Chapters 47 and 54.

Monogenic Defects in Insulin Action

In rare cases, insulin resistance is associated with an identified mutation in a single gene. These include mutations in the insulin receptor causing conditions such as leprechaunism, Rabson-Mendenhall syndrome, and Type A insulin resistance.[22] Lipoatrophic diabetes, also due to a single-gene defect, results in lipodystrophy and severe insulin resistance. These conditions are described in detail in Chapter 58. Mutations in the peroxisome proliferator-activated receptor γ (PPAR-γ) may also result in insulin resistance and diabetes and will be discussed later in this chapter.

In the majority of patients with type 2 diabetes, the disease appears to be a polygenic disorder, in that disease expression depends on many gene loci, all of which may have small to moderate effects. It is also likely that type 2 diabetes is multigenic, meaning that different combinations of gene defects may exist among patients. A more detailed discussion of possible susceptibility genes will follow later in this chapter. Type 2 diabetes is also referred to as a multifactorial disease, in that the genes interact not only with each other, but also with environ-

mental influences. Individuals may therefore be predisposed to develop type 2 diabetes by their inheritance of a particular combination of genes, with environmental factors necessary to bring out the phenotypic manifestation of hyperglycemia.

ACQUIRED FACTORS

Lifestyle: Diet, Exercise, and Obesity

Acquired factors play a major role in the development of type 2 diabetes in genetically predisposed individuals, and this is clearly demonstrated by assessing the impact of lifestyle changes on prevalence of diabetes in various ethnic populations. The prevalence of diabetes increases as ethnic groups either migrate from lesser developed to more urbanized areas or simply change from an agrarian to a more sedentary, urban lifestyle. The former has been illustrated by surveys in Japanese subjects. In rural Japan, the prevalence of type 2 diabetes was approximately 4%,[23] whereas in Japanese who have immigrated to the United States, the prevalence rises to over 21%.[24] This is also illustrated by the Pima Indians, who in Arizona have adopted a largely "Westernized" lifestyle, whereas those living in northwestern Mexico have remained agrarian. The Indians in Arizona have a prevalence of diabetes of 54% and 37% for men and women, respectively, whereas the Mexican Indians have a prevalence of 6% and 11%, respectively.[25]

It is likely that nutrition and lifestyle are the environmental factors that explain such a difference in diabetes prevalence in genetically similar populations. Adoption of an urbanized, Westernized lifestyle is associated with a change to a diet that has a higher content of total calories, fats, and refined carbohydrates. For example, the mean daily intake of fat in Japanese men living in Japan was reported to be 16.7 g; by contrast, in Japanese-American men, the mean intake was 32.4 g.[26] In addition, the level of physical activity is lower in ethnic groups living in the United States compared to the same ethnic groups living in their country of origin.[27] These lifestyle changes obviously predispose to the development of obesity, and overwhelming evidence exists that obesity is a major factor in the development of diabetes. The role of obesity in the pathogenesis of diabetes will be discussed in detail later in this chapter. Recent evidence supporting the role of lifestyle factors in the development of diabetes has also come from the Diabetes Prevention Program.[28] In this study, intensive lifestyle modification, consisting of dietary change and increased exercise, led to a 58% reduction in the progression of impaired glucose tolerance to diabetes over a 2.8-year period.

The extent of the contribution of these lifestyle factors, independent of their association with obesity, to the development of diabetes remains unclear. For example, it is not known whether specific dietary components, such as a diet that is rich in saturated fat or highly refined carbohydrates, play an independent role in the pathogenesis of type 2 diabetes. With regard to exercise, however, there is evidence from experimental and epidemiologic studies that a low level of physical activity is associated with the development of diabetes independent of its association with obesity.[29]

Low Birth Weight

Retrospective analyses have suggested that low birth weight is associated with insulin resistance and the development of type 2 diabetes in adulthood.[30] It has been suggested that this is due to a metabolic adaptation to poor fetal nutrition.

Aging

Aging is associated with a decrease in glucose tolerance, which appears to be due to a decline in both insulin sensitivity and insulin secretion.[31] However, age-related factors such as reduced physical activity and increased fat accumulation are at least partly responsible for this phenomenon. Obviously, type 2 diabetes incidence increases with age, but whether the aging process per se is contributory remains unclear.

In summary, in the majority of subjects, type 2 diabetes is a heterogeneous disorder resulting from a complex interaction between genetics and environmental influences such as obesity and other acquired factors.

NATURAL HISTORY OF TYPE 2 DIABETES

The pathophysiologic findings depicted in Figure 56-1 represent a single point in time after overt type 2 diabetes has developed. However, such an analysis does not reveal the progressive evolution of this disease. Figure 56-2 presents a schematic description of the natural history or progression to type 2 diabetes. Evidence indicates that in most populations, those who evolve to type 2 diabetes begin with insulin resistance. Acquired factors such as obesity, sedentary lifestyle, and aging may be contributory, but insulin resistance is likely to be a primary inherited feature in most type 2 diabetic patients. In an attempt to overcome insulin resistance, the β cell increases insulin secretion, resulting in hyperinsulinemia, which is able to maintain relatively normal glucose tolerance. In a subpopulation of subjects, however, this hyperinsulinemic response is insufficient to fully compensate for the prevailing insulin resistance. Impaired glucose tolerance (IGT) thus develops. While in some cases, this failure of compensation may be due to a more profound degree of insulin resistance, in many it appears to be due to a limited ability to augment insulin secretion rates.[32] Furthermore, although a percentage of subjects with IGT may revert to normal glucose tolerance, IGT can be considered an intermediate stage in the development of type 2 diabetes, with many subjects eventually progressing to frank expression of the disease.

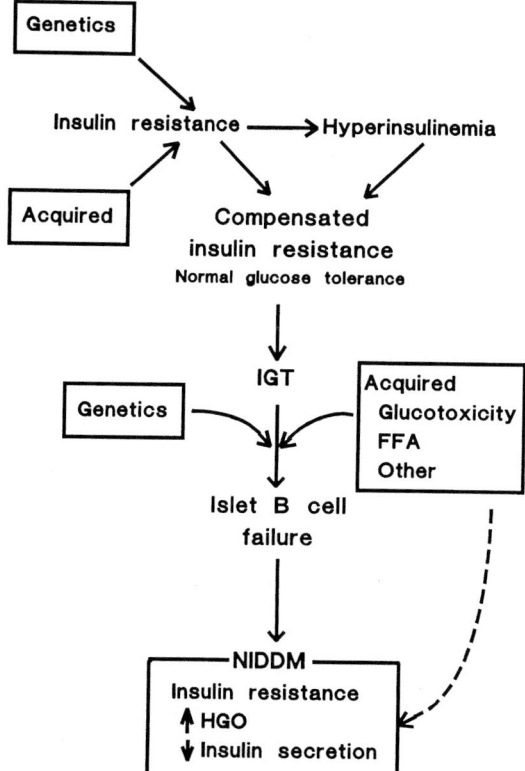

Figure 56-2 Proposed etiology for the development of type 2 diabetes mellitus.

The proportion of insulin-resistant subjects who progress to type 2 diabetes depends on the particular ethnic groups studied and the methods of assessment. During the transition from IGT to frank type 2 diabetes, at least three pathophysiologic changes can be observed. First is a marked fall in β-cell function and insulin secretion. Whether this decrease is due to preprogrammed genetic abnormalities in β-cell function, to acquired defects (such as glucotoxicity or lipotoxicity), or to both remains to be elucidated. Nevertheless, a marked decrease in β-cell function accompanies this transition, and most believe that this decreased β-cell function is the major contributor to the development of frank type 2 diabetes mellitus. A second metabolic change is at the level of the liver. Subjects with IGT have normal basal rates of hepatic glucose output (HGO), whereas patients with fasting hyperglycemia have increased HGO. Thus, the capacity of the liver to overproduce glucose is an important contributory factor (albeit secondary) to the pathogenesis of type 2 diabetes. Finally, many but not all studies have indicated that patients with type 2 diabetes are more insulin resistant than are those with IGT. Most likely, this increase in insulin resistance is secondary to glucotoxicity or to other acquired factors. A number of lines of evidence, largely drawn from population studies, have converged to support the scheme depicted in Figure 56-2.

The evidence implicating insulin resistance as a primary defect comes principally from studies examining subjects who are at increased risk of developing diabetes. One such group is individuals whose parents have type 2 diabetes. Using intravenous GTTs, Warram and coworkers evaluated 155 nondiabetic offspring whose parents both had type 2 diabetes.[33] During a follow-up period averaging 13 years, type 2 diabetes developed in 16% of the total group. However, when the offspring were categorized on the basis of insulin sensitivity at initial testing, the cumulative incidence of diabetes was 60% in the subjects with preexisting insulin resistance and less than 5% in the insulin-sensitive offspring. Thus, insulin resistance and hyperinsulinemia (rather than hypoinsulinemia) characterized the prediabetic state, and this occurred irrespective of obesity and antedated the subsequent development of impaired insulin secretion and overt type 2 diabetes by many years.[33]

Studies in ethnic populations with a high prevalence of type 2 diabetes have also provided data supporting a primary role for insulin resistance in diabetes development. Thus, in Pima Indians, hyperinsulinemia and an associated decrease in insulin-mediated glucose disposal are early abnormalities that predict the subsequent development of both IGT and type 2 diabetes.[34–36] Pima Indians with IGT who progress to type 2 diabetes have lower insulin levels 2 hours after a glucose load than do those who continue to have IGT or return to normal glucose tolerance. Similar results come from studies of Micronesians in Nauru, a population with a prevalence of type 2 diabetes of approximately 30%.[36] Again, in this population, IGT and type 2 diabetes were most likely to develop in those with hyperinsulinemia at baseline, but progression from IGT to type 2 diabetes could be predicted by lower baseline insulin responsiveness.

Further evidence that insulin resistance is a primary inherited defect in those who are predisposed to type 2 diabetes comes from studies in first-degree relatives of type 2 diabetic patients.[37–39] In these studies, peripheral insulin resistance and hyperinsulinemia were found in normoglycemic relatives of diabetic patients. The first-degree relatives with IGT displayed insulin resistance as well as defects in insulin secretion that were not apparent in those with normal glucose tolerance.

In summary, the phenotypic manifestation of type 2 diabetes mellitus involves elevated HGO, impaired insulin secretion, and peripheral insulin resistance. Type 2 diabetes mellitus has a strong genetic component, and studies of prediabetic subjects indicate that in most populations, insulin resistance, accompanied by hyperinsulinemia, exists before any deterioration in glucose homeostasis. After a period of compensatory hyperinsulinemia with normal glucose tolerance, β-cell insulin secretion declines, and IGT and eventually overt type 2 diabetes mellitus result.

In the remainder of this chapter, the abnormalities of insulin secretion, insulin action, and hepatic glucose metabolism in type 2 diabetes are reviewed, with particular attention to basic mechanisms (where known) and their applicability to etiology.

INSULIN SECRETION

Obesity is a major cause of insulin resistance, and as was described above, the β-cell compensates for insulin resistance by increasing insulin secretion. In normal glucose-tolerant subjects, the increase in insulin secretion that occurs with a reduction in insulin sensitivity is described by a hyperbolic relationship[40] (Fig. 56-3). While this quantitative increase in insulin secretion in response to decreased insulin sensitivity should be viewed as an appropriate response, subtle qualitative changes in insulin secretion are also present in the insulin-resistant state. Insulin is secreted normally in rapid regular pulses with 5- to 15-minute frequency superimposed on slower ultradian oscillations every 80 to 150 minutes.[41] These normal rapid, regular pulses are replaced by disordered pulses in obese subjects with insulin resistance and also in the insulin-resistant but glucose-tolerant offspring of subjects with type 2 diabetes.[42] Indeed, insulin secretory pulse frequency has been shown to correlate inversely with peripheral insulin sensitivity.[43]

INSULIN SECRETION IN IMPAIRED GLUCOSE TOLERANCE

In subjects with IGT, both quantitative and qualitative defects in insulin secretion are usually present, although this can be quite variable.[44,45] Part of this variability may be explained by the heterogeneity of this condition, as some subjects with IGT

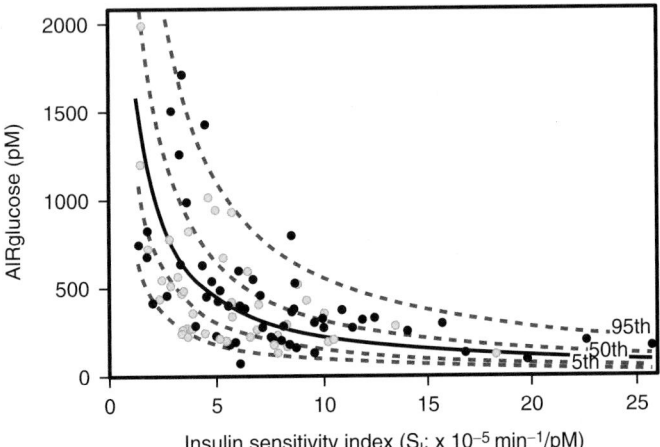

Figure 56-3 Relationship between insulin sensitivity and β-cell function quantified as the first-phase insulin response (AIRglucose) in 93 (55 males and 38 females) apparently healthy, nondiabetic subjects under the age of 45 years. The cohort demonstrates a broad range of insulin sensitivity and β-cell function. The *solid curve* depicts the best-fit relationship (50th percentile); the *dashed curves* represent the 5th, 25th, 75th, and 95th percentiles. The relationship is best described by a hyperbolic function so that any change in insulin sensitivity is balanced by a reciprocal and proportionate change in β-cell function. (Reproduced with permission from Kahn SE, Prigeon RL, McCulloch DK, et al: Quantification of the relationship between insulin sensitivity and B-cell function in human subjects: Evidence for a hyperbolic function. Diabetes 42:1663–1672, 1993.)

will revert to normal glucose tolerance, a proportion will progress to frank type 2 diabetes, and others will continue to have IGT for many years.[46]

With regard to the hyperbolic relationship between β-cell function and insulin sensitivity, subjects with IGT secrete less insulin than is appropriate for their degree of insulin sensitivity.[47] Furthermore, using the graded glucose infusion method, Polonsky has shown that subjects with IGT secrete less insulin at any given glucose level than do normoglycemic subjects matched for a similar degree of insulin resistance and obesity (Fig. 56-4).[48] Most likely, insulin-resistant IGT subjects who have a progressive impairment in insulin secretion are the ones who are most likely to develop full-blown type 2 diabetes.[49]

Insulin secretion in response to a sustained intravenous glucose stimulus is normally biphasic: A rapid rise in insulin levels within 1 to 3 minutes (first phase) is followed by a return to baseline by 6 to 10 minutes with a subsequent gradual increase (second phase). Subjects with IGT have a reduction in both first- and second-phase responses[50] to glucose, and a further qualitative defect in insulin secretion in IGT is the replacement of rapid regular secretory oscillations with disorganized pulses.[42]

INSULIN SECRETION IN TYPE 2 DIABETES

The abnormalities of insulin secretion described in subjects with IGT are also present in type 2 diabetes, although to a more marked degree. β-cell function progressively deteriorates during the natural history of type 2 diabetes. This decline in β-cell function is evident not only during the progression from compensated insulin resistance to IGT and subsequently to overt type 2 diabetes, but also during the course of established type 2 diabetes itself.[51]

Basal insulin levels are usually normal or increased in type 2 diabetes. Indeed, obese type 2 diabetic subjects can have basal insulin levels severalfold higher than normal, but this does not mean that basal β-cell secretory function is normal, since the prevailing plasma glucose level must also be taken into account.[52–54] Hyperglycemia is the major stimulus for insulin secretion, and when normal individuals are made hyperglycemic by infusion of glucose, circulating insulin levels are much higher than those found in type 2 diabetes.[52,53] Thus, type 2 diabetic patients maintain normal or increased basal insulin levels only in the face of the enhanced stimulus

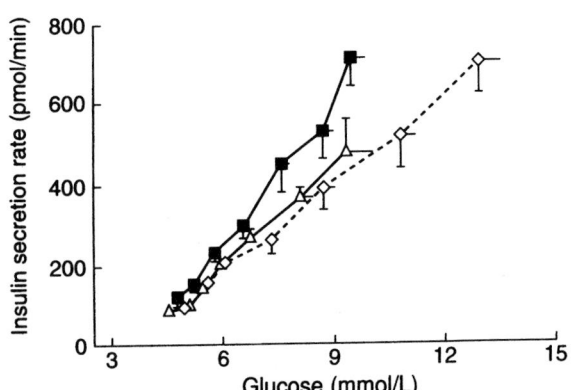

Figure 56-4 Relationship between average plasma glucose concentrations and insulin secretion rates during graded glucose infusion studies in a group of lean nondiabetic control subjects (*open triangles*), nondiabetic obese subjects (*closed squares*), and matched obese subjects with impaired glucose tolerance (*open diamonds*). The lowest glucose levels and insulin secretion rates were measured under basal conditions, and subsequent levels were obtained during glucose infusion rates of 1, 2, 3, 4, 6, and 8 mg/kg/min. Values are means ± SEM. (Source: Polonsky KS: The β-cell in diabetes: From molecular genetics to clinical research. Diabetes 44:705–717, 1995.)

of fasting hyperglycemia, which indicates an underlying impairment in the sensitivity of the β cell to glucose.

Stimulated insulin levels in type 2 diabetes can be low, normal, or high depending on factors such as the severity of diabetes, the degree of obesity, and the preceding level of diabetic control.[13,14,45] For example, in nondiabetic subjects, obesity augments insulin secretion with a particularly pronounced effect on basal insulin levels,[55] an effect that also occurs in type 2 diabetes.[54,56] Higher insulin levels are consistently observed in obese compared to lean type 2 diabetic subjects,[54,56] although the levels achieved remain low for the degree of prevailing hyperglycemia and insulin sensitivity.

Insulin Secretory Responses to Intravenous Glucose

In type 2 diabetes, defects in the insulin secretory response to intravenous glucose are consistently observed. Once fasting plasma glucose levels exceed 126 mg/dL, the first-phase insulin response to intravenous glucose is characteristically completely absent. This relationship is shown in Figure 56-5.[1,57,58]

Interestingly, acute or first-phase insulin secretion in response to nonglucose stimuli such as arginine[1] or isoproterenol[59] is relatively preserved; this finding indicates a functionally selective β-cell defect in response to glucose stimuli in type 2 diabetes. Because the acute insulin response to intravenously administered arginine or isoproterenol increases as the glucose concentration is raised, Porte and colleagues have attempted to quantitate this effect of glucose by plotting the increase in acute insulin response to arginine or isoproterenol pulses as a function of increasing plasma glucose level.[1,14,52] The slope of this relationship is termed the *glucose potentiation slope*, and by this analysis, glucose potentiation of β-cell function is also reduced in type 2 diabetes.[1,14]

Second-phase insulin secretion, which is assessed by using the hyperglycemic clamp or the graded intravenous glucose infusion technique (see Fig. 56-4 for details), is markedly reduced in type 2 diabetes compared to normal or IGT subjects. In general, the more severe the diabetes, the lower the second-phase insulin response.[1,57]

The loss of first-phase insulin secretion in type 2 diabetes, although a consistent finding, does not appear to be a specific marker for type 2 diabetes. Several findings support this conclusion:

1. In some type 2 diabetic patients, first-phase insulin secretion can be partially or completely restored by salicylates,[60] α-adrenergic blockers,[61] or insulin treatment[62] without ameliorating the basic diabetic state.

2. The defect can be induced by a number of diabetogenic manipulations that are not related to type 2 diabetes, including partial pancreatectomy in rats and hyperglycemic infusions.[63]

3. Islets isolated at laparotomy from type 2 diabetic patients demonstrated substantial glucose-induced insulin secretion, even though in vivo insulin secretion in response to glucose was markedly reduced.[64] This finding suggests that the abnormal in vivo milieu of the type 2 diabetic state is partly responsible for the in vivo defects in insulin secretion.

These findings suggest that the absent first-phase insulin secretion is a nonspecific manifestation of impaired β-cell function, regardless of the cause of islet damage or dysfunction. Hyperglycemia per se may secondarily impair β-cell function and lead to a further reduction in acute insulin response to glucose.

While absent first-phase insulin secretion may be a marker for β-cell dysfunction, it is unlikely to be an important cause of glucose intolerance or hyperglycemia. Thus, mildly hyperglycemic and severely hyperglycemic type 2 diabetic patients are equally deficient in first-phase insulin secretion, implying that this deficiency does not play a role in further deterioration in glucose tolerance from mild to severe fasting hyperglycemia. Furthermore, in selected patients with normal glucose tolerance in whom type 1 diabetes eventually develops, the acute insulin response to intravenous glucose is absent during the normal stage and therefore does not cause hyperglycemia.[65] Finally, α-adrenergic blockers can substantially restore the acute insulin response to intravenous glucose[61] without a major improvement in fasting glycemia or glucose tolerance.

Insulin Secretory Responses to Oral Glucose and Mixed Meals

The insulin response in type 2 diabetes to oral ingestion of glucose or mixed meals is far more variable than the response to intravenous glucose. After oral glucose, insulin levels are usually subnormal in type 2 diabetes[14,37] although this might not always be the case in patients with mild hyperglycemia.[45] This heterogeneity is depicted in Figure 56-6, which summarizes the results of oral GTTs in a wide spectrum of normal and type 2 diabetic subjects.[66] As can be seen, hyperinsulinemia frequently exists in mild states of glucose intolerance. In individuals with mild diabetes, insulin levels are generally in the "normal range," although inappropriately low for the

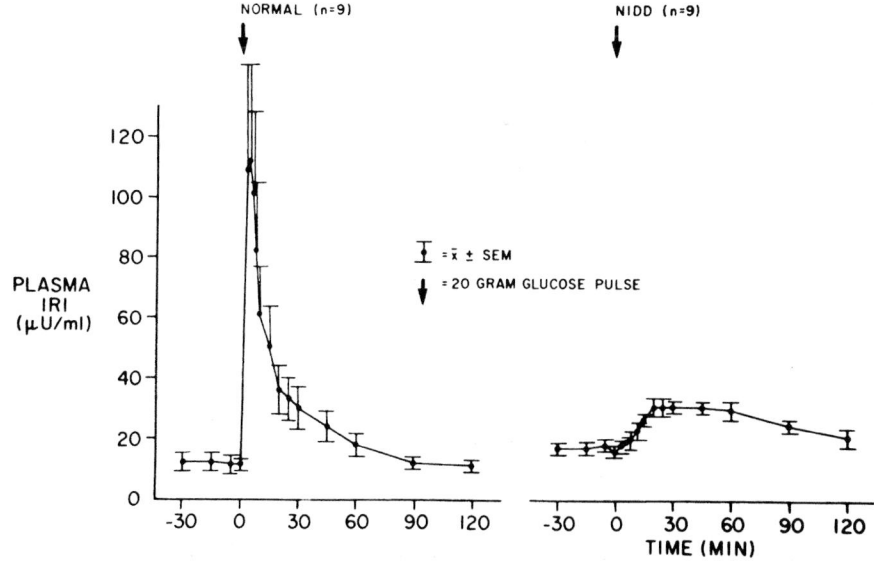

Figure 56-5 First-phase insulin release in response to the intravenous administration of glucose in normal and type 2 diabetic (non-insulin-dependent diabetes [NIDD]) subjects. Mean fasting plasma glucose concentrations were 83 ± 3 mg/dL in normal subjects and 160 ± 10 mg/dL in type 2 diabetic subjects. (Reproduced with permission of the American Diabetes Association, Inc., from Ward WWK, Beard JC, Halter JB, et al: Pathophysiology of insulin secretion in non-insulin-dependent diabetes mellitus. Diabetes Care 7:491–502, 1984.)

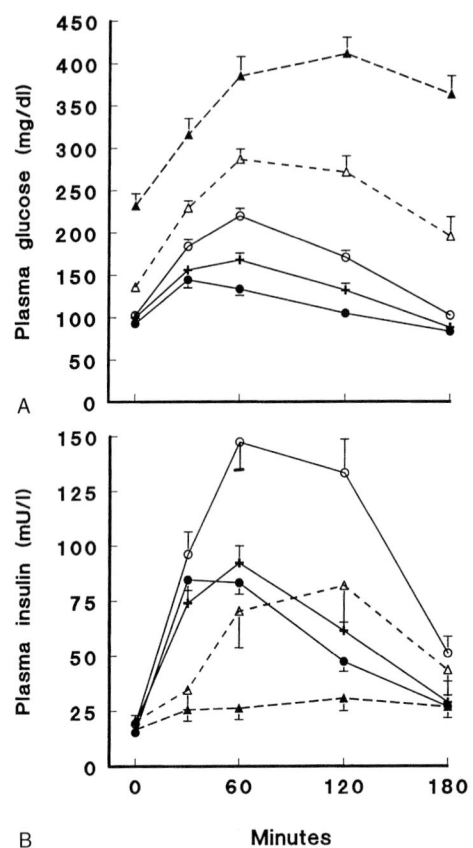

Figure 56-6 **A,** Mean (±SEM) plasma glucose response to oral glucose in the five subject groups. *Closed circle,* normal; *cross,* borderline tolerance; *open circle,* impaired glucose tolerance; *open triangle* and *broken line,* fasting hyperglycemia (110–150 mg/dL); *closed triangle* and *broken line,* fasting hyperglycemia (>150 mg/dL). **B,** Mean (±SEM) plasma insulin response to oral glucose in the five subject groups. Symbols are the same as in **A.** (Source: Reaven GM, Olefsky JM: Relationship between heterogeneity of insulin responses and insulin resistance in normal subjects. Diabetologia 13:201–206, 1977.)

degree of insulin sensitivity. With more severe diabetes, stimulated insulin levels are uniformly low.

In type 2 diabetes, the defect in β-cell function is relatively (but not completely) specific for glucose stimuli. The relative preservation of insulin responses to nonglucose stimuli, such as certain amino acids and the incretin gut peptides, means that type 2 diabetic patients have a better insulin response to mixed meals than to oral glucose. Thus, in mild type 2 diabetes, insulin responses to mixed meals may be delayed, but the postprandial hyperglycemia, coupled with other insulinogenic factors, often leads to exaggerated insulin responses 2 to 4 hours after meal ingestion. However, with more severe hyperglycemia, decreased insulin levels are more common. Because oral GTTs represent a rather nonphysiologic stress to assess β-cell function, it is important to keep in mind that in the free-living state, when patients are consuming mixed meals, absolute insulin levels can be relatively preserved in type 2 diabetes.

Proinsulin Secretion

Another factor relating to hyperinsulinemia in type 2 diabetes is circulating proinsulin levels. Proinsulin is secreted by β cells concomitantly with insulin and cross-reacts with insulin in most insulin immunoassays, thus contributing to the total measured immunoreactive insulin level. In normal subjects, proinsulin represents only a small portion (3% to 7%) of the insulin-like material secreted by β cells. However, using proinsulin-specific immunoassays, several groups have shown that

in hyperinsulinemic states and in many type 2 diabetic patients, an increased proportion of proinsulin is released and contributes to the measured insulin in standard immunoassays, so true insulin levels are overestimated.[14,54,67] When corrected for this factor, basal insulin levels are either normal or moderately elevated in type 2 diabetes.

Mechanisms of β-Cell Dysfunction

The precise cellular mechanisms underlying the β-cell dysfunction in type 2 diabetes are unclear, but they most likely represent a combination of genetic and acquired factors.

The overall mass of β cells changes in obesity and type 2 diabetes.[68,69] β-cell mass reflects the balance between new islet formation (neogenesis) and β-cell loss due to apoptosis. Longitudinal studies in animal models suggest that β-cell mass increases appropriately in response to a decrease in insulin sensitivity,[69] and cross-sectional data from humans have long recognized an expanded β-cell mass in obesity.[70] In contrast, β-cell mass is reduced in type 2 diabetes.[68] On the basis of murine models and cross-sectional autopsy data from humans, the diminished β-cell mass is thought to be due to accelerated β-cell apoptosis and a failure of islet neogenesis and β-cell replication to compensate for this loss.[69]

It has been theorized that lipid accumulation in the β cell is implicated in the apoptotic process and the development of impaired insulin secretion in type 2 diabetes. This is referred to as *lipotoxicity* and could involve surplus fatty acids entering β cells, triggering the apoptotic cellular response.[71]

A body of evidence also suggests a role for islet amyloid polypeptide (IAPP) in the loss of β cells. IAPP is synthesized in the β cell and is cosecreted with insulin.[72] IAPP aggregates to form fibrils of amyloid, and islet amyloid is found in up to 90% of subjects with type 2 diabetes at autopsy.[73] In vitro, IAPP is toxic, causing β-cell apoptosis,[74] and may potentially contribute to the reduced β-cell mass that is associated with type 2 diabetes.

The insulin secretory abnormalities found in type 2 diabetes are often improved after a period of good blood glucose control, irrespective of the treatment used (diet, insulin, or oral hypoglycemic agents).[75-77] This partial reversibility is consistent with the idea that, to some extent, the abnormalities may be secondary to hyperglycemia or some other factor associated with uncontrolled diabetes. Support for the "glucotoxicity" theory comes from a variety of in vivo and in vitro studies showing that chronic exposure of islets to hyperglycemia can result in a number of different defects in glucose-induced insulin secretion.[63] Importantly, when isolated human islets are incubated under euglycemic and hyperglycemic conditions, islets that are exposed to hyperglycemia demonstrated a marked defect in their ability to secrete insulin in response to subsequent glucose stimuli.[78] Although the precise mechanism is unknown, it seems likely that glucotoxicity plays some role in the impaired β-cell function of type 2 diabetes.

An interesting finding from studies of mouse genetics is that insulin receptor signaling in β cells is important for normal function. Thus, mice in which the insulin receptor gene has been specifically deleted from β cells show a complete loss of first-phase insulin secretion in response to glucose but not arginine, reminiscent of the β-cell defect in type 2 diabetes.[79,80] Second-phase glucose-induced insulin secretion is also blunted in these mice, and they show an age-dependent progressive impairment in glucose tolerance. This study raises the intriguing possibility that insulin resistance at the level of the β cell might contribute to the decline in insulin secretion that supervenes after many years of peripheral tissue insulin resistance during the natural history of type 2 diabetes.

The decrease in β-cell mass in type 2 diabetes is in the range of 30% to 50%, and as sufficient insulin secretory reserve normally exists to sustain an 80% to 90% loss of β cells without the development of hyperglycemia, it follows that decreased functional capacity of the remaining β cells must exist in type 2 diabetes. Indeed, it has been shown that the maximal insulin secretory capacity may be reduced by as much as 80% in type 2 diabetic subjects.[53] It is possible that the decrease in β-cell mass in type 2 diabetes is somehow causally related to the decreased function of the remaining β cells. Thus, partially pancreatectomized rats and streptozotocin-treated rats display similar insulin secretory defects,[63] which suggests that decreased glucose-stimulated insulin secretion with relative preservation of responsiveness to nonglucose stimuli may be a general type of abnormality in response to a variety of β-cell insults.

PERIPHERAL INSULIN RESISTANCE

Insulin resistance is a metabolic state in which a normal concentration of insulin produces a less than normal biologic response. This decreased response to insulin can involve any of the multiple metabolic effects of insulin, but from the standpoint of relevance to type 2 diabetes, resistance to insulin's effects on glucose metabolism have been the most extensively studied. Because insulin travels from the β cell through the circulation to the target tissue, events at any of these loci can influence the ultimate action of the hormone. Therefore, it is useful to categorize insulin resistance according to known causative mechanisms; such a classification is presented in Table 56-1. In general, insulin resistance can be due to (1) an abnormal β-cell secretory product, (2) circulating insulin antagonists, (3) impaired access of insulin to target cells, or (4) a target tissue defect in insulin action.

CAUSES OF INSULIN RESISTANCE

Abnormal β-Cell Secretory Product
Several patients have been described who secrete a structurally abnormal, biologically defective insulin molecule resulting from a mutation in the structural gene for insulin.[19] Others have familial hyperproinsulinemia caused by incomplete conversion of proinsulin to insulin within the β-cell secretory granule as a result of structural abnormalities at the proteolytic cleavage sites of the proinsulin molecule.[20,21] These syndromes are dealt with in Chapter 48 and are not discussed further here, except to note that they do not represent insulin-resistant states in the most common usage of this term. Thus, in these syndromes, the hormone is abnormal, and the patients are resistant only to their endogenous insulin and not to exogenous insulin.

Circulating Insulin Antagonists
In general, insulin antagonists may be hormonal or nonhormonal.

Table 56-1   Causes of Insulin Resistance

Abnormal β-cell secretory product
  Abnormal insulin molecule
  Incomplete conversion of proinsulin to insulin
Circulating insulin antagonists
  Elevated levels of counterregulatory hormones (e.g., growth
    hormone, cortisol, glucagon, or catecholamines)
  Cytokines
  Free fatty acids
  Anti-insulin antibodies
  Anti-insulin receptor antibodies
Target tissue defects
  Insulin receptor defects
  Postreceptor defects

Hormonal Antagonists
Hormonal antagonists include all the known counterregulatory hormones such as cortisol, growth hormone, glucagon, and catecholamines. Well-known syndromes exist (e.g., Cushing's disease, acromegaly) in which elevated levels of these hormones can induce an insulin-resistant diabetic state. However, in the usual case of obesity or type 2 diabetes, excessive levels of these counterregulatory hormones are not an important contributory factor to insulin resistance.

Nonhormonal Antagonists
Free Fatty Acids A number of years ago, Randle and coworkers hypothesized that the elevated circulating levels of free fatty acids (FFAs) found in obesity and type 2 diabetes impair peripheral glucose utilization.[80] Substantial evidence indicates that FFAs may indeed contribute to insulin resistance, although the intracellular mechanisms may differ from those that were originally proposed. FFAs also play an important role in the regulation of HGO and may contribute to hepatic insulin insensitivity in obesity and type 2 diabetes. These issues are discussed later in this chapter.

Anti-insulin Antibodies Anti-insulin antibodies can develop in patients who are treated chronically with insulin.[81] By binding and trapping insulin within the plasma compartment, these antibodies can alter the usual time course of insulin action. However, only in unusual cases do such antibodies actually cause a true insulin-resistant state. A few patients have been described in whom anti-insulin antibodies spontaneously develop in the absence of exogenous insulin therapy.[81] These antibodies can interfere with insulin immunoassays and lead to apparent hyperinsulinemia, but they do not cause insulin resistance.

Insulin Receptor Antibodies A fascinating syndrome (type B insulin resistance) has been described in which patients have antibodies directed against the insulin receptor.[82,83] This condition is rare. It occurs predominantly in women, and almost all patients have features of other autoimmune disorders, such as systemic lupus erythematosus. It is associated with acanthosis nigricans, severe insulin resistance, and diabetes mellitus. Occasional patients have episodes of spontaneous hypoglycemia. The circulating antibodies bind to the insulin receptor in vivo and, by interacting with the insulin-binding domain, block and/or mimic the action of insulin and thereby result in insulin resistance or, occasionally, hypoglycemia.[83]

Cytokines Increased levels of cytokines such as tumor necrosis factor alpha (TNF-α) may contribute to the insulin resistance associated with sepsis, cirrhosis, or other severe illness. In vivo, infusions of TNF-α have major effects on glucose and lipid metabolism.[84,85] The finding that adipose tissue TNF-α mRNA levels were increased in obese humans[86] and rodents[87] led to the idea that TNF-α could also play a role in the insulin resistance of obesity and type 2 diabetes.[87] Evidence came from in vitro studies showing that incubation of cells with TNF-α impaired insulin receptor signaling.[88] Furthermore, neutralization of TNF-α by infusion of a TNF-α receptor IgG fusion protein reversed insulin resistance in Zucker (fa/fa) rats.[87] However, in subsequent studies in obese type 2 diabetic patients, intravenous infusion of a neutralizing antibody to TNF-α had no effect on insulin resistance.[89] Clearly, further work is needed to delineate the role of TNF-α in the insulin resistance associated with obesity.

Impaired Access of Insulin to Target Cells
Because insulin must travel from the circulation to target tissues to elicit biologic effects, any defect in this transfer could potentially lead to insulin resistance. The passage of insulin from the plasma compartment to tissue sites of action is marked by substantial delays, and insulin's in vivo effects

to stimulate glucose disposal are well correlated with the appearance of insulin in the interstitial fluid.[90] Lymph insulin levels are lower than those in plasma,[90,91] which indicates that peripheral tissues are more sensitive to insulin than was previously recognized. Furthermore, the possibility arises that either the rate or the amount of insulin being transferred from the plasma to the interstitial compartment could be abnormal in type 2 diabetes or obesity, thereby contributing to the insulin-resistant state and defects of in vivo insulin action kinetics.[92,93] Recent studies indicate that transport of insulin across the capillary in vivo is by diffusion[91] and not receptor mediated as has been suggested.[94] Transport by diffusion fits with the finding that transcapillary passage is comparable in normal subjects, insulin-resistant nondiabetic subjects,[95] and patients with type 2 diabetes.[96] Further evidence that the delayed activation of muscle glucose uptake in obesity and type 2 diabetes is not due to impaired transcapillary transport of insulin comes from a study by Nolan and coworkers.[93] This study showed that the kinetic defect in insulin's ability to stimulate leg glucose uptake was not accompanied by any delay in the activation of leg muscle insulin receptors by insulin, thus implying that the kinetic defect is distal to the insulin receptor.

Another physical factor that may relate to insulin resistance is muscle capillary density, which correlates with in vivo insulin sensitivity.[97] Laakso and coworkers have shown that insulin, at least at pharmacologic levels, increases leg blood flow.[98] Because tissue glucose uptake is a product of blood flow and the arteriovenous glucose difference, increased leg blood flow could contribute to overall glucose disposal. Similar studies performed in obese subjects and in subjects with type 2 diabetes revealed a decrease in the insulin-induced increase in leg blood flow, which may explain part of the decrease in total leg glucose uptake.[98] However, others found no effect of insulin on blood flow, nor a decrease in blood flow in either forearm or leg balance studies in type 2 diabetic subjects.[99] In addition, Utriainen and colleagues used $^{15}O[H_2O]$ and positron emission tomography to confirm an enhancement of leg muscle blood flow by pharmacologic insulin levels but no difference in the response between type 2 diabetic and normal control subjects.[100]

Taken together, defects in any of the above factors, although possibly contributory, cannot explain the major component of insulin resistance in type 2 diabetes and obesity. Furthermore, numerous studies have demonstrated profound in vitro insulin resistance in tissues and cells from these patients.

Cellular Defects in Insulin Action

Available evidence points to a target tissue defect as the major cause of insulin resistance in type 2 diabetes. Before considering potential causes, it is useful to review some general concepts concerning normal insulin action (Fig. 56-7).

Insulin first binds to its cell surface receptor, a heterotetrameric glycoprotein composed of two α subunits (135 kDa) and two β subunits (95 kDa) linked by disulfide bonds.[101–104] The α subunits, located entirely extracellularly, are responsible for insulin binding. The β subunits are transmembrane proteins containing a small extracellular domain and a larger cytoplasmic domain that contains the insulin-regulated tyrosine kinase activity. Binding of insulin to the receptor rapidly induces a cascade of tyrosine autophosphorylation in the β subunit involving three tyrosine residues in the kinase domain, in addition to tyrosine residues adjacent to the transmembrane domain and in the C terminus of the β subunit.[101–104] Once the receptor is autophosphorylated, its intrinsic tyrosine kinase catalytic activity is markedly enhanced, and it can now phosphorylate tyrosine residues on endogenous protein substrates.[101–104] Activation of the insulin receptor tyrosine kinase is essential both for transduction of the insulin signal and for internalization of the receptor and

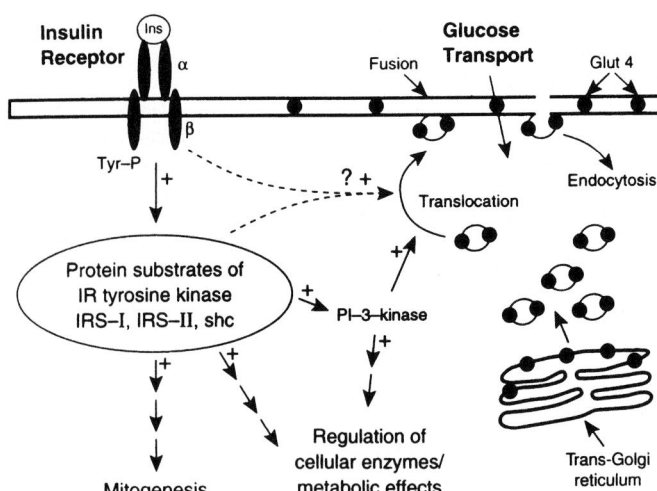

Figure 56-7   Model of cellular insulin action. IR, insulin receptor; IRS-I, insulin receptor substrate-1; IRS-II, insulin receptor substrate-2. (Source: Kruszynska YT, Olefsky JM: Cellular and molecular mechanisms of non-insulin dependent diabetes mellitus. J Invest Med 44:413–428, 1996.)

its bound insulin.[102–104] Patients with naturally occurring mutations in the tyrosine kinase domain of the insulin receptor have syndromes of severe insulin resistance.

In recent years, major advances have been made in our understanding of the mechanisms by which the insulin signal is propagated downstream from the activated insulin receptor to the various insulin-regulated enzymes, transporters, and insulin-responsive genes to mediate its metabolic and growth effects (see Fig. 56-7). This field is rapidly evolving and complex and is discussed only briefly because it is covered in Chapter 50. A large number of intermediate signaling molecules have been identified, and evidence indicates that after activation of the insulin receptor kinase, more than one signaling pathway may be used (see Fig. 56-7). For example, the pathways leading to the mitogenic effects of insulin consist of elements that are distinct from those leading to activation of glucose transport. Even a single action of insulin, for example, activation of glucose transport, may involve more than one signaling pathway. Several cytosolic protein substrates of the insulin receptor tyrosine kinase have been identified that are phosphorylated on tyrosine residues within seconds of insulin's binding to its receptor. The first of these substrates to be shown to play a key role in insulin signal transduction was insulin receptor substrate 1 (IRS-1).[104,105] IRS-1 belongs to a growing family of proteins that includes IRS-2, IRS-3, IRS-4, and a protein termed shc, which are also immediate substrates of the insulin receptor kinase and involved in insulin signaling.[104,105] These proteins have no enzymatic activity but act as docking proteins. Tyrosine phosphorylation of these substrates enhances their association with proteins that contain src homology-2 (SH2) domains.[104,105] These domains are sequences of about 100 amino acids that can bind to specific short sequences that encompass a phosphotyrosine moiety. The binding of specific SH2 domain–containing downstream signaling proteins to tyrosine-phosphorylated IRS proteins or shc generates multicomponent signaling complexes, which in turn results in modulation of the activities of several serine and threonine kinases and phosphatases that act on key insulin-regulated enzymes and transcription factors.

One of the most important effects of insulin with respect to type 2 diabetes is to stimulate glucose uptake in skeletal muscle, adipocytes, and heart muscle. Under most physiologic circumstances, glucose transport in these tissues is rate limiting for overall glucose disposal.[106–108] Tissue glucose uptake is mediated by a family of at least five facilitative glucose transporters, each derived from a separate gene. These transporters show a high degree of homology, but each has a tissue-specific distribution.[109,110] One of them, GLUT4, or the insulin-sensitive glucose transporter, is uniquely expressed in skeletal muscle, adipose tissue, and cardiac muscle.[109,110] In the unstimulated state, most of the GLUT4 proteins are located in an intracellular vesicular pool. On insulin stimulation, recruitment or translocation of these glucose transporter-rich vesicles causes insertion of GLUT4 proteins into the plasma membrane, where they begin to transport glucose into the cell.[111–115] In addition to translocation, insulin may also increase the intrinsic activity of GLUT4. Once the insulin signal dissipates, the GLUT4 proteins return to their intracellular location.

Clearly, insulin action involves a cascade of events, and abnormalities anywhere along this sequence can lead to insulin resistance.

CHARACTERISTICS OF INSULIN RESISTANCE IN TYPE 2 DIABETES AND IMPAIRED GLUCOSE TOLERANCE

The frequency of insulin resistance increases as the degree of carbohydrate intolerance worsens.[116] Thus, many but not all subjects with IGT are insulin resistant, whereas essentially every type 2 diabetic patient with fasting hyperglycemia displays this abnormality. Some studies indicate that insulin resistance is more marked in type 2 diabetes than in the prediabetic IGT state.[3,5,37] However, other reports show only a modest increase in the degree of insulin resistance going from IGT to type 2 diabetes. Because most type 2 diabetic patients are overweight, obesity-induced insulin resistance is thought to be an additive factor in these patients. However, obesity can be only a contributory factor because the insulin resistance in obese type 2 diabetic patients exceeds that caused by obesity alone, and nonobese type 2 diabetic patients are also insulin resistant.[3,5,116]

All methods of assessing insulin resistance in vivo rely, in one way or another, on measurement of the ability of a fixed dose or concentration of insulin to promote glucose disposal. Thus, a blunted decline in plasma glucose concentration after the administration of intravenous insulin has been demonstrated in type 2 diabetes.[117,118] Another approach has been to infuse insulin and glucose at fixed rates while endogenous insulin secretion is inhibited either by a combination of epinephrine and propranolol or by somatostatin.[117,119] With this method, the resulting steady-state plasma glucose level reflects the action of the concomitantly infused insulin; the higher the steady-state plasma glucose, the greater the degree of insulin resistance. Bergman and colleagues' minimal model is yet another method of assessing in vivo insulin resistance.[117] The method entails computer modeling of plasma glucose and insulin levels after an intravenous glucose bolus[117] to generate an index of insulin sensitivity. The test was adapted for type 2 diabetic patients with impaired insulin secretion by giving an injection of insulin 20 minutes after the standard glucose bolus. With all these methods, type 2 diabetic subjects have a significant decrease in lower insulin sensitivity compared to controls.[3,117,120,121]

Because skeletal muscle is responsible for the great majority of in vivo insulin-stimulated glucose uptake, this tissue must be the major site of the resistance to insulin-stimulated glucose disposal. This conclusion is evidenced by the demonstration of insulin resistance in type 2 diabetic patients during forearm perfusion studies.[122,123] Leg catheterization studies have shown that skeletal muscle accounts for 80% to 85% of whole-body insulin-mediated glucose uptake and that leg skeletal muscle is markedly resistant to insulin's ability to stimulate glucose uptake in type 2 diabetes.[124–126] Thus, although other insulin target tissues are insulin resistant in type 2 diabetes, they do not account for a significant

proportion of overall glucose uptake, and one can conclude that all measures of in vivo insulin action on glucose disposal have largely assessed the resistance of skeletal muscle to take up glucose under the influence of insulin.

More detailed studies of in vivo insulin resistance have been carried out with the euglycemic glucose clamp method.[117] With this approach, insulin is infused at a constant rate, resulting in a given steady-state plasma insulin level, while plasma glucose is kept constant at a predetermined level by a feedback-controlled variable infusion of glucose. The insulin tends to lower the plasma glucose level by suppressing HGO and by stimulating tissue glucose uptake. The amount of glucose that has to be infused to keep plasma glucose constant increases gradually until a steady state is reached. Under these steady-state conditions, the glucose disposal rate provides an excellent quantitative assessment of the biologic effect of a particular steady-state insulin level. If a radioactive or stable isotope of glucose is also infused during the study, HGO during the clamp can also be quantified. In type 2 diabetes, glucose disposal rates are 30% to 60% lower than those in matched normal subjects at any given insulin infusion rate; that is, these patients are insulin resistant. If several studies at different insulin levels are performed in a given subject, dose-response curves for insulin-stimulated glucose disposal and suppression of HGO can be constructed. Patients with type 2 diabetes (obese and nonobese) exhibit both a rightward shift in their dose-response curve (diminished sensitivity) and a marked decrease in the maximal rate of glucose disposal (decreased responsiveness) (Fig. 56-8). These changes tend to be more pronounced in obese diabetic patients, particularly at maximal glucose disposal rates (see Fig. 56-8). Obesity per se causes a decrease in insulin sensitivity, and some obese patients show a decrease in insulin responsiveness. The insulin resistance of obese type 2 diabetic patients is significantly greater than that of nondiabetic obese subjects. Subjects with IGT tend to have a rightward shift in their dose-response curves with normal maximal glucose disposal rates (see Fig. 56-8).

MECHANISMS OF SKELETAL MUSCLE INSULIN RESISTANCE

Clearly, insulin action involves a cascade of events, and abnormalities anywhere along this sequence can lead to insulin resistance. These defects can involve abnormal coupling between insulin receptor complexes and the glucose transport system, decreased activity of the glucose transport system per se, or a variety of intracellular enzymatic defects located in various pathways of glucose metabolism.

Insulin Receptor

As the first step in insulin action involves binding to the receptor, it is apparent that a decrease in cellular insulin receptors could lead to insulin resistance. However, this potential relationship is not as clear as it would seem because a maximal insulin effect is achieved at insulin concentrations that occupy a fraction of the surface receptors, giving rise to the concept of "spare" receptors. A maximal response of glucose transport in adipocytes and muscle is achieved with only 10% to 20% of the receptors occupied.[127,128] Once this critical number of receptors needed to generate a maximal response are activated, further increases in the prevailing insulin concentration lead to increases in receptor occupancy with no further increase in biologic response, because a step (or steps) distal to the receptor is now rate limiting. The functional significance is that with fewer cell surface receptors, a rightward shift occurs in the insulin biologic function dose-response curve with decreased responses at all submaximal insulin concentrations but a normal maximal response. A reduction in the maximal insulin response generally denotes the presence of a postbinding abnormality. In this context, the term *postbinding defect* includes abnormalities of insulin receptor

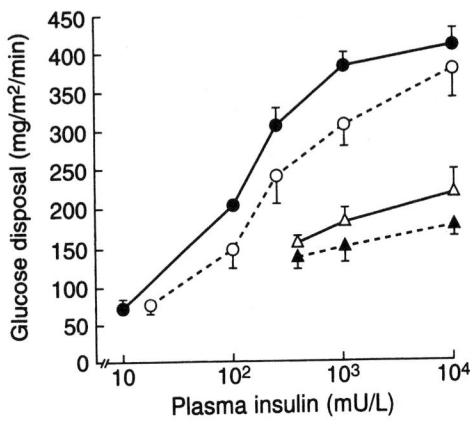

Figure 56-8 Mean insulin dose-response curves for control subjects (*closed circles*), subjects with impaired glucose tolerance (*open circles*), and nonobese (*open triangles*) and obese (*closed triangles*) type 2 diabetic subjects. The group with impaired glucose tolerance has a rightward shift in the dose-response curve without change in the maximal response (i.e., decreased sensitivity). Lean and obese patients with type 2 diabetes have both a rightward shift and a reduction in the response to a maximally stimulating concentration of insulin (i.e., decreased sensitivity and decreased insulin responsiveness). (Source: Kolterman OG, Gray RS, Griffin J, et al: Receptor and post-receptor defects contribute to the insulin resistance in non-insulin dependent diabetes mellitus. J Clin Invest 68:957–969, 1981.)

function that affect its transmembrane signaling function such as its kinase activity. A *postreceptor defect* refers to any abnormality in a step distal to the insulin receptor.

Early studies showed decreased insulin binding to circulating monocytes from obese and IGT subjects and from both obese and nonobese type 2 diabetic patients.[129,130] This decreased binding was due to a decrease in insulin receptor number with no change in affinity. Similar results were subsequently obtained when isolated adipocytes or skeletal muscle tissue from obese subjects and patients with type 2 diabetes was used.[131,132] The decrease in cellular insulin receptors in obesity and type 2 diabetes may well be secondary to hyperinsulinemia, inasmuch as circulating insulin levels are a major determinant of receptor number.

Insulin Receptor Function
A reduction in insulin receptor kinase activity in type 2 diabetic patients with normal kinase activity in IGT has generally been reported.[93,131,132] The receptor autophosphorylation/kinase defect appears to be generalized to all insulin target tissues and relatively specific for the hyperglycemic insulin-resistant state that is seen in type 2 diabetes.

Postreceptor Signaling
Emerging evidence points to a role for IRS proteins in the development of insulin resistance. A defect in insulin-stimulated IRS-1 tyrosine phosphorylation is found in skeletal muscle from type 2 diabetic patients, although overall IRS-1 expression is unchanged.[133] Serine phosphorylation of IRS proteins is closely associated with reduction of signaling through IRS. Two potential mechanisms may underlie this phenomenon. First, serine phosphorylation may block the interaction of IRS-1 with its target proteins.[134] Second, proteasomal-mediated degradation of IRS-1 may be increased.[135] Several intermediary lipid metabolites and cytokines have been shown to activate a variety of serine kinases that induce serine phosphorylation of IRS-1. Serine kinases implicated include c-Jun NH2-terminal kinase (JNK),[136] IκB kinase (IKK),[137] and externally regulated kinase.[138] However, the extent to which serine phosphorylation of IRS-1 plays a role in insulin resistance in vivo remains to be further elucidated.

IRS-2 is also important for insulin signaling and glucose homeostasis. In mice with disruption of the IRS-2 gene, profound defects in both peripheral insulin action and β-cell function develop, progressing to diabetes.[139]

PI 3-Kinase
PI 3-kinase plays a key role in mediating insulin's effects on glucose metabolism.[140] Insulin-stimulated PI 3-kinase activity in skeletal muscle is reduced in both obese nondiabetic subjects[141] and patients with type 2 diabetes.[133] The reduction in PI 3-kinase activity correlates with the decrease in whole-body glucose disposal.[133]

Glucose Transport System
Insulin-stimulated glucose transport in isolated muscle fibers and adipocytes from type 2 diabetes is markedly reduced at all insulin concentrations.[10,142] What is the mechanism of this decrease in insulin-stimulated glucose transport in type 2 diabetes? In adipocytes from type 2 diabetic subjects, decreased GLUT4 levels have been reported. In contrast, skeletal muscle GLUT4 mRNA and protein levels are normal in type 2 diabetes.[143,144] Because the muscle of type 2 diabetic patients is not deficient in GLUT4 protein, it appears that the defect in insulin-stimulated glucose transport reflects either a decrease in the ability of insulin to signal translocation of GLUT4 to the cell surface or a decrease in the intrinsic activity of GLUT4.

There is evidence that insulin-stimulated translocation of GLUT4 is impaired in the skeletal muscle of type 2 diabetic patients. For example, Kelley and coworkers used quantitative confocal laser scanning microscopy to examine insulin-stimulated recruitment of GLUT4 to the sarcolemma in muscle biopsies from patients with type 2 diabetes.[113] In the basal state, sarcolemmal GLUT4 labeling was similar in diabetic and normal subjects, but in response to insulin, the increase in GLUT4 in type 2 diabetic subjects was only 25% of that in control subjects. A quantitatively similar defect in GLUT4 translocation was found in obese nondiabetic subjects. In both the type 2 diabetic patients and obese nondiabetic subjects, the defect in GLUT4 translocation was associated with a marked impairment in insulin-stimulated muscle glucose transport as determined by positron emission tomography. Others using biochemical muscle subfractionation techniques have also suggested a defect in GLUT4 translocation in patients with type 2 diabetes.[114]

Given the possibility of a defect in GLUT4 intrinsic activity, a structural defect in the protein itself may exist. Such an abnormality could be due to genetic variation in the GLUT4 sequence. Studies using both direct gene sequencing and larger-scale molecular scanning studies indicate that genetic variations in the GLUT4 sequence are exceedingly uncommon in type 2 diabetic subjects.[145–147] Consequently, although defects in glucose transport are important to the pathophysiology of type 2 diabetes, the coding sequence of GLUT4 does not appear to be a diabetes gene locus.

Trafficking of GLUT4 involves a complex system analogous to synaptic vesicle movement, and an expanding list of proteins involved in the regulation of trafficking GLUT4 are being identified.[115] Clearly, impaired GLUT4 translocation in type 2 diabetes could be due to altered expression or a functional defect of one or more of these GLUT4 vesicle-trafficking proteins, which is an area of intensive investigation.

Oxidative and Nonoxidative Glucose Metabolism
By performing indirect calorimetry during glucose clamp studies, one can determine the intracellular fate of glucose by measuring the percentage of glucose that is oxidized in comparison to that which undergoes nonoxidative glucose metabolism (consisting of storage as glycogen plus glycolysis). The insulin concentrations that are necessary for half-maximal stimulation of glucose oxidation (~50 mU/L in normal

subjects) are lower than those required for stimulation of glucose uptake and storage as glycogen (~100 mU/L).[148] Thus, at low physiologic insulin levels, oxidative glucose disposal is quantitatively more important, but at higher insulin levels, nonoxidative glucose metabolism predominates.[12,123] Defects in both oxidative and nonoxidative glucose metabolism exist in type 2 diabetes, although the decrease in nonoxidative metabolism is greater.[9,37,126,149,150] Shulman and coworkers, using nuclear magnetic resonance (NMR) spectroscopy of the gastrocnemius muscle during an infusion of ^{13}C-enriched glucose, showed that during a hyperinsulinemic hyperglycemic clamp study, nonoxidative glucose disposal is highly correlated with rates of skeletal muscle glycogen deposition.[9] Moreover, a 50% reduction in the rate of muscle glycogen synthesis in type 2 diabetic patients during performance of the glucose clamp technique was found. The defects in nonoxidative glucose metabolism and muscle glycogen synthesis correlated well with the decrease in whole-body glucose uptake.[9]

The reduced muscle glycogen synthesis rate in type 2 diabetes could be the result of a decrease in glucose transport, impaired glucose phosphorylation, or an abnormality in the glycogen synthetic pathway, and decreases GLUT4 translocation, hexokinase II, and glycogen synthase have all been reported.

To identify the primary site of the intracellular block in glycogen synthesis, Rothman and coworkers used ^{31}P-NMR during glucose clamp studies to measure glucose-6-phosphate concentrations in gastrocnemius muscle.[151] They reasoned that a primary block in glycogen synthesis (e.g., resulting from decreased glycogen synthase) would lead to increased glucose-6-phosphate levels, whereas if the decreased flux of glucose to glycogen reflected impaired glucose transport and/or phosphorylation, glucose-6-phosphate levels would be low. They found a lower steady-state glucose-6-phosphate concentration in type 2 diabetes, indicating that the reduced rate of glycogen synthesis was secondary to impaired glucose transport, hexokinase activity, or both. In further muscle NMR studies, these investigators detected a very low intracellular free glucose concentration during hyperinsulinemic hyperglycemic clamp studies in both normal and type 2 diabetic patients.[96] This finding strongly suggests that glucose transport is the rate-controlling step in insulin-stimulated muscle glycogen synthesis, indicating that decreased insulin-mediated glucose transport is a defect to the insulin resistance of type 2 diabetes.

Kinetic Defects in Insulin Action

While most quantitative assessments of in vivo insulin resistance report impaired insulin action based on steady-state measurements, kinetic defects in insulin action in obesity have also been demonstrated. Thus, the rate of activation of insulin's effect to stimulate glucose disposal is decreased, and the rate of deactivation of insulin's effect is increased.[92] Given that under physiologic postprandial conditions, insulin is secreted in a phasic rather than a steady-state manner, it is likely that the kinetic defects in insulin action are of functional importance and that steady-state measurements of insulin action underestimate the functional defect in insulin sensitivity. This has been demonstrated by phasic administration of insulin during a glucose clamp, mimicking the time course and height of the mean insulin levels, as determined during a prior oral glucose tolerance test. Total insulin-stimulated glucose disposal during the "phasic" clamp was reduced by 64% in obese subjects compared to lean controls.[152] This is greater than the 20% to 50% decrease in steady-state insulin-mediated glucose disposal that were observed in glucose clamp studies in these same subjects, confirming the functional importance of kinetic abnormalities in insulin action.[92,153]

In summary, skeletal muscle insulin resistance in type 2 diabetes is associated with multiple defects in insulin signaling,

glucose transport, and oxidative and nonoxidative glucose metabolism. It remains to be fully determined which defects are primary and which are secondary, but a decrease in insulin-stimulated GLUT4 translocation appears to be the fundamental defect that gives rise to the insulin-resistant state. Factors that result in secondary defects in insulin signaling will be discussed in detail later in this chapter.

HEPATIC GLUCOSE METABOLISM

The liver plays a key role in carbohydrate metabolism. It is capable of extracting glucose from the portal vein and hepatic artery, as well as releasing glucose derived from glycogenolysis or gluconeogenesis into the hepatic vein.

HEPATIC GLUCOSE OUTPUT

After an overnight fast, normal basal glucose production rates are 1.8 to 2.2 mg/kg/min, about 90% of the glucose that is released into the circulation coming from the liver. After glucose ingestion, HGO must be promptly suppressed to limit the rise in plasma glucose levels; as intestinal glucose delivery wanes, basal HGO rates must be restored to meet the obligatory glucose needs of tissues such as the brain. These changes in HGO are largely mediated by changes in insulin and other hormones that antagonize insulin's effects on the liver and by alterations in gluconeogenic substrate supply.

The rate of basal HGO is increased in both obese and nonobese type 2 diabetic patients[6,7,11] but not in subjects with IGT (Fig. 56-9A). The fasting plasma glucose level and basal HGO are closely correlated in type 2 diabetic patients (Fig. 56-9B), which indicate that the rate of glucose production by the liver directly modulates the level of fasting hyperglycemia in type 2 diabetes. Gluconeogenesis is the predominant source of HGO following an overnight fast,[154] and most studies suggest that gluconeogenesis is increased in type 2 diabetes.[155,156] Thus, enhanced gluconeogenesis is the proximate cause of increased HGO in type 2 diabetes, and although the mechanism is unclear, it is probably a multifactorial defect. Glucagon levels are elevated in type 2 diabetes, and the effect of glucagon to stimulate the synthesis and release of glucose by the liver is well known. Hyperglycemia normally exerts a potent suppressive effect on α-cell glucagon secretion, and the presence of hyperglucagonemia in the face of hyperglycemia implies that pancreatic α cells in type 2 diabetes are resistant to the inhibitory effects of glucose. Other factors are possible, but regardless of the mechanisms, increased α-cell function in type 2 diabetes is a consistent abnormality, and suppression of plasma glucagon levels by infusion of somatostatin lowers plasma glucose levels in both normal and type 2 diabetic subjects.[157]

Hepatic glucose production can be completely suppressed by high physiologic or supraphysiologic insulin levels in type 2 diabetes, but the sensitivity of HGO to lower concentrations of insulin is reduced.[12] This reduced insulin sensitivity also contributes to the overall increase in glucose production in these patients. Insulin's ability to suppress HGO may in part be indirect[92,158] and mediated by suppression of adipose tissue lipolysis and plasma FFA levels. Thus, the insulin resistance of HGO suppression in type 2 diabetes may be partly secondary to impaired suppression of plasma FFA levels by insulin.[13]

Finally, increased flux of gluconeogenic precursors and FFAs from peripheral tissues to the liver may participate in the maintenance of increased HGO rates in type 2 diabetes. Alanine, lactate, and glycerol production rates are increased in type 2 diabetes with fasting hyperglycemia, and the increased plasma lactate and glycerol levels would be expected to promote gluconeogenesis. In obese type 2 diabetic patients, increased plasma FFA levels may also stimulate gluconeogenesis and contribute to higher rates of HGO.

A

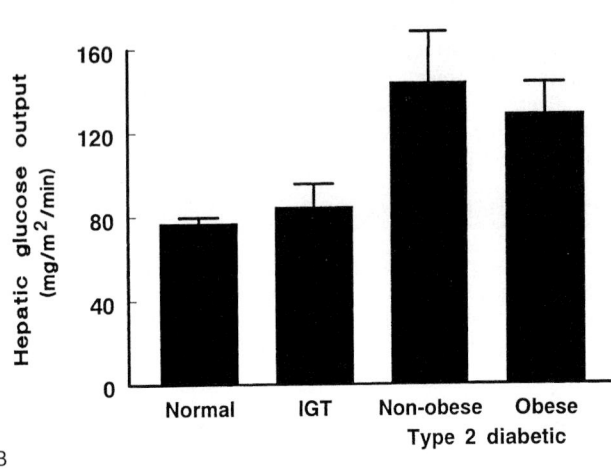

B

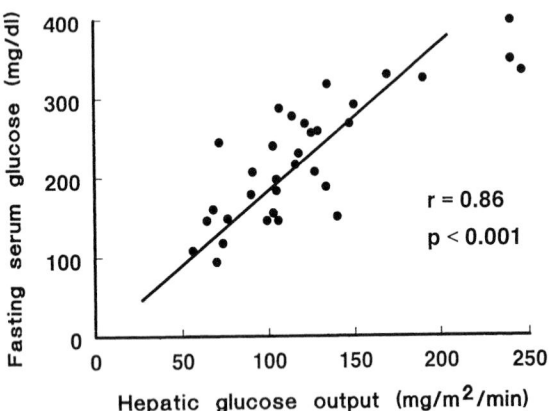

Figure 56-9 **A,** Rates of hepatic glucose production in the basal state (7:00 to 9:00 A.M. after an overnight fast) in normal subjects, subjects with impaired glucose tolerance (IGT), and obese or nonobese subjects with type 2 diabetes. Hepatic glucose output is normal in subjects with IGT but is markedly increased in type 2 diabetes. **B,** Relationship between the individual hepatic glucose production rate and fasting plasma glucose level in type 2 diabetic subjects. (Source: Kolterman OG, Gray RS, Griffin J, et al: Receptor and postreceptor defects contribute to the insulin resistance in non-insulin dependent diabetes mellitus. J Clin Invest 68:957–969, 1981.)

HEPATIC GLUCOSE UPTAKE

Although earlier data held that most of the orally ingested glucose was extracted by the liver and largely converted to glycogen,[159] more recent studies indicate that skeletal muscle is quantitatively the most important tissue for disposal of an oral glucose load, 50% to 60% of total glucose disposal being accounted for by skeletal muscle. Only 20% to 35% of oral glucose is directly taken up (as glucose) by the liver, and even less (about 10%) of the glucose absorbed from the gut is taken up on the first pass.[160] The contribution of the liver to total postprandial glucose disposal must also take into account the extent of suppression of HGO in addition to the glucose taken up.

In contrast to insulin's direct stimulation of muscle glucose uptake and incorporation into glycogen, insulin plays a permissive role in promoting hepatic glucose uptake. Thus, insulin does not cause net hepatic glucose uptake or stimulation of liver glycogen deposition without an increased portal venous glucose concentration. The main determinant of glucose transport into and out of the liver is the glucose concentration gradient between sinusoids and hepatocytes.[161] After glucose ingestion, uptake of glucose by the liver (newly absorbed and recirculating) is impaired in type 2 diabetes.[162]

In summary, inhibition of glucose production and release is the major effect of insulin on hepatic glucose balance. In type 2 diabetes, the liver overproduces glucose in the basal state, primarily because of increased gluconeogenesis, and the metabolic milieu is ideal to sustain this abnormality. Exaggerated hormonal stimulation is provided by the increased glucagon levels (in combination with hepatic insulin resistance), and augmented gluconeogenic precursor flow ensures adequate substrate availability. Finally, elevated FFA levels could augment the gluconeogenic process.

INSULIN-MEDIATED VERSUS NON-INSULIN-MEDIATED GLUCOSE UPTAKE

Under basal conditions, a nearly steady state is approximated and the rate of glucose appearance (HGO) equals the overall rate of glucose disposal. To understand the significance of increased basal HGO in type 2 diabetes, it is important to distinguish between insulin-dependent and insulin-independent processes of glucose disposal. By definition, insulin-mediated glucose uptake (IMGU) occurs in insulin target tissues under the influence of insulin. Non-insulin-mediated glucose uptake (NIMGU) consists of all the body's glucose uptake that is not under the influence of insulin and has two components. NIMGU occurs in tissues (primarily the central nervous system) that are not targets for insulin action; it also involves insulin target cells and comprises the basal rate (noninsulin mediated) of glucose disposal by these tissues. Total glucose disposal (Rd) equals the sum of NIMGU and IMGU. NIMGU can be assessed in vivo by measuring Rd under conditions of severe insulinopenia induced by an infusion of somatostatin.[163] Thus, after measurement of basal Rd (at basal or fasting insulin and glucose levels), somatostatin is administered to inhibit insulin secretion to negligible levels. Rd gradually falls to a new steady state that equals NIMGU because insulin action is absent under these conditions.[163] With this approach, the proportion of basal Rd that is NIMGU is approximately two thirds in normal individuals at euglycemia and in type 2 diabetic subjects studied at their basal level of hyperglycemia, which means that at all levels of basal glycemia (normal and diabetes), most of the glucose is disposed of by NIMGU mechanisms and the elevated rates of basal HGO that prevail in type 2 diabetes are associated with increased rates of NIMGU.

PATHOPHYSIOLOGY OF FASTING VERSUS POSTPRANDIAL HYPERGLYCEMIA

Once type 2 diabetes develops, all three metabolic defects contribute to fasting hyperglycemia, but increased HGO predominates. This conclusion derives from the known physiology of glucose homeostasis in the basal state. Thus, in the postabsorptive and fasting states, insulin levels are low, and approximately 70% of basal glucose uptake (Rd) is non-insulin mediated in both normal and hyperglycemic type 2 diabetic subjects.[163] Because skeletal muscle, the main tissue affected by insulin resistance in type 2 diabetes, accounts for only 15% to 20% of basal glucose Rd, it follows that an impairment in insulin-mediated glucose uptake by muscle will have little effect on overall basal glucose Rd or fasting plasma glucose levels. Major increases in fasting glucose levels do not occur unless the rate of glucose entry into the systemic circulation (Ra) increases, and in the basal state, glucose Ra essentially equals hepatic glucose production. In type 2 diabetes, increases in glucose Ra readily lead to increases in fasting glucose levels because in the setting of peripheral insulin resistance and impaired insulin secretion, the ability of IMGU to rise and accommodate an increase in Ra is severely curtailed. To illustrate, if basal Ra = Rd = 2 mg/kg/min at euglycemia and basal NIMGU = 1.4 mg/kg/min (70%) with a basal IMGU of 0.6 mg/kg/min (30%), a modest increase in

HGO to 2.6 mg/kg/min would require a doubling of IMGU (to 1.2 mg/kg/min) to maintain Rd = Ra (HGO) at euglycemia. Because type 2 diabetic subjects are insensitive to insulin, a much larger increase in insulin secretion would be necessary to produce euglycemia than in normal individuals. Because insulin secretion is impaired in type 2 diabetes, the ability of a type 2 diabetic subject to increase IMGU in response to a rise in Ra is greatly restricted. To raise Rd to the level of the new Ra and bring the system back into balance, the fasting glucose level must rise until Rd increases by mass action and equals Ra. This line of reasoning is strongly supported by the available data, which demonstrate close direct relationships between fasting plasma glucose levels and basal HGO in large groups of type 2 diabetic subjects under a variety of conditions.[7] Thus, decreased insulin secretion and action provide the setting that allows glucose Ra to regulate fasting plasma glucose, thereby leading to the principle that fasting hyperglycemia is largely due to increased HGO in type 2 diabetes.

The cause of postprandial hyperglycemia, however, is more complex. Recent data show that most of the ingested carbohydrate bypasses the liver and enters the peripheral circulation.[160] This process is accompanied by rapid suppression (60% to 90%) of HGO for 2 to 3 hours after carbohydrate ingestion.[160,164] Thus, in the postprandial state, glucose Ra comes predominantly from ingested carbohydrate, and this ingested carbohydrate largely enters the peripheral circulation, where it is disposed of mostly by skeletal muscle because of a severalfold increase in IMGU. In type 2 diabetes, systemic delivery of ingested glucose appears to be normal, but suppression of HGO is impaired,[164] which means that after glucose ingestion, the total quantity of glucose entering the systemic circulation is somewhat higher. In addition, the efficiency of peripheral glucose removal is greatly reduced because of insulin resistance and impaired insulin secretion. Uptake of glucose by the liver (newly absorbed and recirculating) is also impaired in type 2 diabetes,[162,164] but the overall contribution of impaired hepatic uptake to postprandial hyperglycemia is relatively small because the liver takes up only 20% to 35% of a glucose load.[160,164] Thus, postprandial hyperglycemia in type 2 diabetes is primarily due to impaired IMGU by peripheral tissues, with impaired suppression of HGO compounding the problem. Postprandial glucose levels rise markedly in type 2 diabetes until the mass action effect of glucose to raise Rd allows disposal of the incoming glucose load. Although glycosuria increases with hyperglycemia, the contribution of glycosuria to total Rd is small (less than 10%) and therefore does not significantly affect relationships between the aforementioned variables.

In summary, in the basal state, NIMGU predominates, and decreased IMGU raises fasting glucose levels only modestly. Fasting hyperglycemia is primarily due to increased HGO. In the postprandial state, IMGU normally predominates, and the limited ability of type 2 diabetic subjects to increase IMGU allows the marked postprandial glucose excursions. The clinical implications of this understanding of the pathophysiology of fasting versus postprandial hyperglycemia are obvious. Any form of antidiabetic therapy must address both aspects of hyperglycemia to be fully effective, which means that a given treatment modality must correct the disordered hepatic glucose metabolism at the same time that it improves insulin-mediated skeletal muscle glucose uptake. This principle is true for single modes of therapy (insulin, oral agents, weight loss) or various combination forms of treatment. For example, a treatment modality that lowers HGO combined with one that enhances IMGU would be an effective overall management strategy for controlling glycemia in type 2 diabetes.

EFFECTS OF ANTIDIABETIC TREATMENT

Obviously, when type 2 diabetic patients are studied at a single static point in time, abnormalities in hepatic glucose production, insulin resistance, and insulin secretion are readily demonstrable. In such a complex situation, it is difficult to sort out causal sequences. One approach is to perturb the system by using various treatment modalities to control the hyperglycemia and assess the potential reversibility of the underlying metabolic defects. For example, if one of the abnormalities proved nonreversible whereas the others were ameliorated, the nonreversible defect would probably be the primary causative lesion leading to type 2 diabetes, and the others would be secondary manifestations. Such studies have shown that peripheral tissue insulin resistance, increased HGO, hyperglucagonemia, and decreased insulin secretion are all ameliorated to some extent when blood glucose levels are substantially lowered, irrespective of whether this is achieved by insulin therapy, oral agents, or weight loss. This result implies that all the abnormalities depicted in Figure 56-2 may be in part secondary to the abnormal metabolic milieu that characterizes the hyperglycemic type 2 diabetic state.

Tight glycemic control achieved by intensive insulin regimens has been found to improve peripheral tissue insulin sensitivity by 17% to 75% in various studies.[76,165-167] When in vivo insulin action is measured by use of the multiple-dose glucose clamp method before and after intensive insulin therapy (Fig. 56-10), marked improvement in insulin-stimulated glucose disposal is seen at all steady-state serum insulin concentrations, thus indicating a significant improvement in postbinding insulin action.[76] Few studies have addressed the mechanisms of improved insulin action in skeletal muscle. Adipocyte glucose transport improves after intensive insulin therapy in parallel with the improvement in whole-body insulin sensitivity.[165] Since decreased glucose transport is the major determinant of impaired insulin-stimulated muscle glucose uptake in type 2 diabetes,[96] any improvement in this action of insulin must be associated with an improvement in muscle glucose transport as well.

Insulin secretion also improves after a period of nearly normal glycemia secondary to insulin therapy. Such improvement is seen in response to the ingestion of mixed meals (Fig. 56-11), oral glucose, intravenous glucose, or intravenously administered nonglucose stimuli.[76,165,166] The degree of improvement is variable, but in some cases, β-cell function is restored to nearly normal levels. The magnitude of the

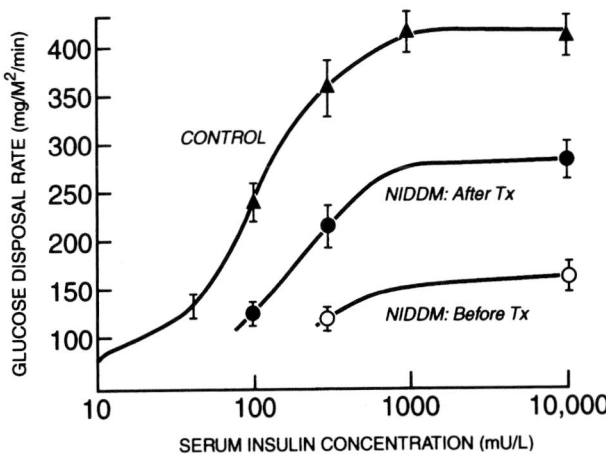

Figure 56-10 In vivo insulin dose-response curves for whole-body glucose disposal rates in type 2 diabetic patients before (*open circles*) and after (*closed circles*) 2 weeks of intensive insulin therapy. Control curves (*closed triangles*) are provided for comparison. (Source: Garvey WT, Olefsky JM, Griffin J, et al: The effects of insulin treatment on insulin secretion and action in type II diabetes mellitus. Diabetes 34:222–234, 1985.)

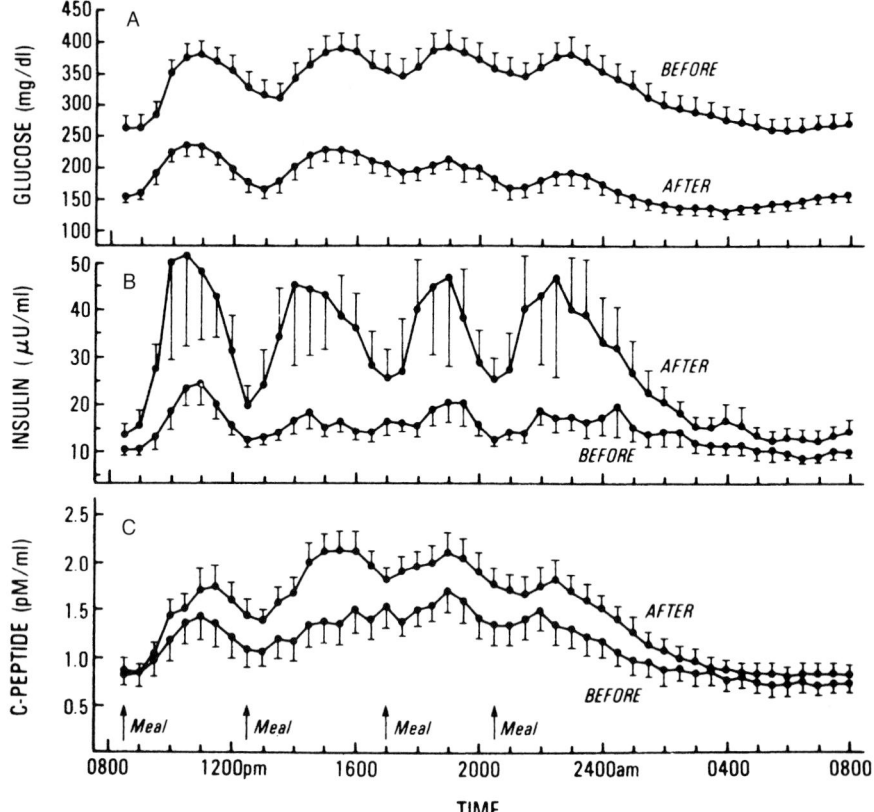

Figure 56-11 Mean 24-hour serum profile for integrated concentrations of glucose (**A**), insulin (**B**), and C peptide (**C**) in type 2 diabetic subjects before and after insulin treatment. Isocaloric meals were given at the times indicated. Results are plotted as means ±SEM. (Source: Garvey WT, Olefsky JM, Griffin J, et al: The effects of insulin treatment on insulin secretion and action in type II diabetes mellitus. Diabetes 34:222–234, 1985.)

posttreatment increase in 24-hour insulin secretion shown in Figure 56-11 is particularly impressive when one considers that this increase in insulin level is seen at markedly lower ambient glucose levels than in the pretreatment state. Interestingly, some studies have shown restoration of the acute insulin response to intravenous glucose after insulin therapy.[166,168] Basal HGO is completely normalized after a period of insulin therapy,[76] and basal glucagon levels also return to normal or nearly normal values.[165]

Oral sulfonylureas and weight reduction yield qualitatively similar results.[77,131,166,168–170] After weight loss, marked improvement is seen in insulin-stimulated glucose disposal. Again, adipocyte glucose transport increases after weight loss, and the magnitude of the increase in glucose transport activity corresponds to the magnitude of the in vivo increase in insulin-stimulated glucose disposal.[77] β-cell function also improves,[77,170] with enhanced insulin secretion following oral glucose, mixed meals, or intravenous glucose. However, the restoration of insulin action and secretion by weight loss is not complete; residual defects in both can still be demonstrated. In contrast, the elevated HGO is reduced to normal, and this process is accompanied by normalization of glucagon levels.[77,170]

The results with sulfonylurea therapy are more variable,[77,168,169] most likely because of the variable clinical response to these agents among individual type 2 diabetic subjects. Thus, some patients display near normalization of glycemia, whereas others show little if any clinical effect of oral agents on blood glucose levels (primary failure). Therefore, one would expect a wide range of changes in underlying metabolic defects when groups of patients are considered. However, when patients who display good clinical responses (lowered glycemia) are examined, one can demonstrate partial improvement in peripheral insulin resistance, slight increases in insulin secretion, and marked decreases in HGO, often to normal levels.[77]

Although these treatment modalities are functionally diverse, certain common themes emerge. Peripheral insulin resistance is consistently improved, but complete normalization of insulin action is unusual. Posttherapy increases in cellular glucose transport activity are correlated with the increases in in vivo insulin action, consistent with the view that a decrease in glucose transport is a major cause of the postreceptor defect before treatment. Insulin secretion generally improves, although complete normalization is unusual. The increased rates of hepatic glucose production that are present in the untreated type 2 diabetic state are uniformly decreased after all modes of treatment. The decrease in HGO correlates well with the fall in plasma glucose after all treatment regimens, and in patients with the best clinical results, HGO is completely normalized. Because these abnormalities in hepatic glucose metabolism can be completely normalized, they most likely represent secondary manifestations of the diabetic state that are in some way caused by insulin resistance, impaired insulin secretion, hyperglycemia, or some combination thereof. The defects in insulin action and secretion are routinely improved but rarely normalized, and from these perturbation studies, one cannot determine which one (or whether both) of these defects represent(s) the primary causal lesion(s) leading to the hyperglycemic type 2 diabetic state. To assess this issue, prospective and population-based studies have been the most insightful; these studies were reviewed in the earlier section of this chapter on etiology.

One thing all the treatment modalities described above have in common is lowering of glycemia. Thus, it is possible that hyperglycemia itself is responsible for some component of the abnormalities in insulin secretion and action and that correcting the hyperglycemia would therefore alleviate this reversible component. This concept is termed the *glucotoxicity theory*. As was discussed earlier, glucotoxicity can impair insulin secretion, and the evidence is good that hyperglycemia can also contribute to impaired insulin action.[171]

For example, animals with experimental insulin-deficient diabetes (secondary to pancreatectomy or streptozotocin) are hyperglycemic and insulin resistant. Phlorhizin, an inhibitor of glucose reabsorption by renal tubules, causes marked glycosuria and subsequent lowering of plasma glucose levels when given to diabetic animals; normalization of glucose levels by phlorhizin is associated with correction of insulin resistance. In well-controlled type 1 diabetic patients infused with glucose, whole-body insulin sensitivity, forearm glucose uptake, and muscle glycogen deposition were all reduced by approximately 35% after blood glucose had been maintained at 20 mmol/L (360 mg/dL) for a period of 24 hours.[172] These data provide direct evidence that hyperglycemia can adversely affect insulin action and are consistent with the view that in type 2 diabetes, a reversible component of the overall insulin resistance is secondary to glucotoxicity.

The thiazolidinedione class of antidiabetic agents is distinct in having a direct peripheral tissue-sensitizing action independent of their glucose-lowering action. This point is readily demonstrable in vitro in isolated cells.[173] In hyperglycemic type 2 diabetic patients, it is more difficult to quantify the relative contributions of improved glycemic control per se and the direct effect of the drug on insulin-resistant tissues to the overall improvement in insulin sensitivity. However, the study of Yu and coworkers provides insight into this issue.[174] In this study, type 2 diabetic patients were first treated intensively with continuous subcutaneous insulin for 4 weeks to eliminate any reversible defects caused by glucotoxicity before adding troglitazone to the insulin regimen for 6 weeks. Insulin doses had to be reduced by 53% during the combined treatment phase to maintain the same level of tight blood glucose control as is achieved with insulin alone. At the end of the 6-week period on combined therapy, peripheral tissue insulin sensitivity was 29% higher than at the end of the 4-week period of normoglycemia achieved by insulin alone. By contrast, patients who were randomized to receive metformin in the same study showed no enhancement of peripheral tissue insulin sensitivity independent of glycemic control.[174] Thus, the thiazolidinediones have a direct tissue-sensitizing action that is independent of their glucose-lowering effects. The demonstration that they improve insulin sensitivity in insulin-resistant obese subjects with normal glucose tolerance[175] and in subjects with IGT[176] and that in subjects with IGT they also ameliorate the subtle insulin secretory abnormalities[176] suggests that they might have a role to play in conjunction with lifestyle changes in the primary prevention of type 2 diabetes.

ADIPOSE TISSUE

Adipose tissue is responsible for only a small fraction of overall whole-body glucose disposal. While glucose uptake per kilogram of tissue is reduced in insulin-resistant states, overall glucose disposal in adipose tissue is probably not significantly altered, given the expanded fat mass in most insulin resistant subjects.[177]

Adipose tissue exists principally to store energy in the form of triglyceride, which in the postabsorptive state can then provide fuel for the body as FFA and glycerol following lipolysis. Lipolysis is markedly sensitive to suppression by insulin, with half-maximal suppression of FFA levels occurring in normal subjects at an insulin concentration of approximately 20 μU/mL.[178] The increase in FFA release, associated with an expanded fat mass results in increased circulating FFA levels, particularly in the postprandial period, in subjects with obesity and type 2 diabetes.[178,179]

Randle and coworkers demonstrated many years ago that FFAs compete with glucose for oxidative metabolism in skeletal and cardiac muscle and hypothesized that elevated FFA levels could therefore impair peripheral glucose use.[80] It was originally proposed that enhanced cellular FFA uptake and oxidation increase acetyl CoA, which then inhibits pyruvate dehydrogenase. This in turn would increase glucose-6-phosphate levels, resulting in impaired phosphorylation of incoming glucose and hence glucose uptake. FFA oversupply can indeed cause impaired insulin-mediated glucose disposal, as was demonstrated in glucose clamp studies in which FFA levels are elevated by lipid/heparin infusion.[180,181] The decrease in carbohydrate oxidation, however, occurs rapidly (1 to 2 hours), whereas the reduction in glucose disposal takes longer to develop (4 to 5 hours), showing that the latter effect is not related to increases in FFA oxidation. In addition, increased intracellular glucose-6-phosphate as predicted by Randle has not been observed; indeed, skeletal muscle glucose-6-phosphate levels decrease during glucose clamp studies when circulating FFA levels are elevated by lipid/heparin infusion.[180] Furthermore, intracellular free glucose levels were also lower in these studies, indicating that elevated FFA levels cause insulin resistance by impairing insulin signaling to glucose transport.

Elevated FFAs do not appear to influence skeletal muscle insulin receptor autophosphorylation,[182,183] but other defects in insulin signaling distal to the receptor have been demonstrated. In rats and humans, lipid infusion led to a decrease in both insulin-stimulated tyrosine phosphorylation of IRS-1 and activation of PI 3-kinase in skeletal muscle.[184]

After cellular uptake, FFAs are converted to long-chain fatty acyl CoAs (LCFA-CoAs), which are transported into the mitochondria by carnitine palmitoyltransferases prior to oxidation. Alternatively, if not transported into the mitochondria, LCFA-CoAs may be reesterified via diacylglyercol (DAG) to form triglycerides and phospholipids. Palmitoyl CoA may also be converted into ceramide. Elevated circulating FFA levels lead to increased uptake of FFA into the cell, whereupon intracellular levels of LCFA-CoAs, intermediates such as DAG and ceramide and triglyceride are increased (Fig 56-12).[185,186]

Intramyocellular triglyceride content, measured by either muscle biopsy or NMR spectroscopy, is increased in obesity and type 2 diabetes[187] and is a strong predictor of insulin resistance in both animals and humans.[188,189] It is likely that increased intramyocellular triglyceride content does not, in itself, impair insulin signaling but acts as a marker of increased intracellular LCFA-CoAs and lipid intermediates. A strongly negative correlation has been demonstrated between whole-body insulin sensitivity, as determined by the glucose clamp and the content of LCFA-CoAs measured in muscle biopsy samples.[190]

IMPACT OF REGIONAL FAT DISTRIBUTION AND ADIPOCYTE SIZE

Intraperitoneal (visceral) adipose tissue may be particularly deleterious to glucose homeostasis. Because of its anatomic location, visceral fat drains directly to the liver via the portal vein, therefore exposing the liver to high concentrations of FFA from this depot. Furthermore, visceral adipocytes appear to be more responsive to catecholamine-stimulated lipolysis and less responsive to suppression of lipolysis by insulin.[191,192] It has long been recognized that excess fat in the upper part of the body (central or abdominal), termed *android obesity*, is associated with increased risk for type 2 diabetes, dyslipidemia, and increased mortality compared to lower-body (gluteofemoral), or *gynoid*, obesity.[193–195] While the relationship between visceral fat and cardiovascular risk is established, the association of insulin sensitivity with visceral versus subcutaneous truncal adipose tissue remains controversial. Visceral fat area, as determined by computed tomography scan, is correlated with decreased insulin action as measured by the glucose clamp. On the other hand, using similar techniques, the total volume of subcutaneous truncal adipose tissue was reported to be a better predictor of insulin resistance than visceral fat.[196] It is possible that, overall, subcutaneous truncal

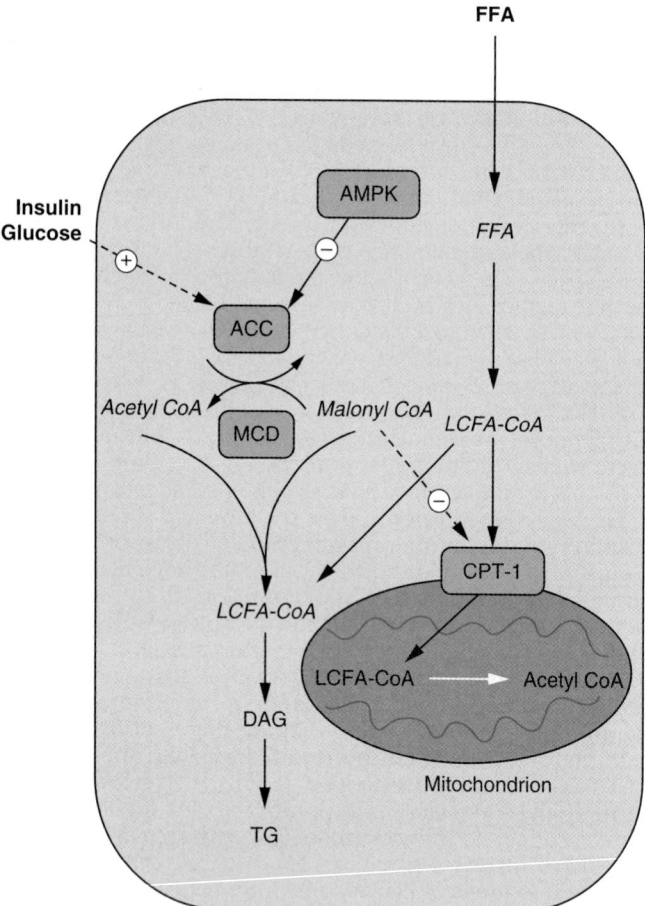

Figure 56-12 Summary of intracellular free fatty acid (FFA) metabolism that results in FFA being either esterified to triglycerides or entering the mitochondria for oxidation. AMPK, AMP-activated protein kinase; ACC, acetyl CoA carboxylase; MCD, malonyl CoA decarboxylase; LCFA-CoA, long-chain fatty acyl-CoA; DAG, diacylglycerol; TG, triglyceride; CPT-1, carnitine palmitoyltransferase-1.

adipose tissue contributes more FFA to the systemic circulation than visceral fat does and, therefore, might have a more important influence on peripheral insulin action.

Subjects with deficiency of adipose tissue, as in lipodystrophy or lipoatrophy, are also insulin resistant, with excess triglyceride deposition in skeletal muscle and the liver.[197] In transgenic animal models with absence of white adipose tissue, insulin resistance is also associated with lipid infiltration of skeletal muscle and the liver,[198,199] a phenotype that can be reversed by surgical implantation of normal adipose tissue.[200] These findings suggest that adipose tissue plays a pivotal role in the buffering of fatty acid flux, with insufficient fat tissue leading to "ectopic triglyceride" storage in muscle and the liver, resulting in deleterious metabolic effects.[201,202] The more common scenario, however, is of excess adipose tissue in obesity; in this situation, the antilipolytic effects of insulin are impaired. This could result in increased FFA flux into muscle and liver, contributing to the increased intramyocellular and hepatic triglyceride content and insulin resistance that are observed in this condition.[203]

Another aspect of lipid metabolism that influences insulin action is that of adipocyte size. Larger adipocytes are more resistant to insulin-stimulated glucose uptake and to insulin suppression of lipolysis,[204,205] and larger subcutaneous abdominal adipocytes may predict the development of type 2 diabetes, independent of insulin resistance.[206] Smaller fat cells may be more efficient at fatty acid uptake and better able to

buffer lipid flux. Indeed, it has been hypothesized that failure of adipogenic precursor cells to differentiate into adipocytes results in glucose intolerance,[207] which may be due to inefficient buffering of lipid flux by the remaining large adipocytes.

CROSS-TALK BETWEEN ADIPOCYTES AND OTHER TISSUES

Another way in which adipose cells "talk" to other tissues is through an endocrine mechanism. Adipocytokines are peptides secreted by adipose tissue that have diverse effects on food intake, energy expenditure, insulin sensitivity, and systemic metabolism. These adipocyte-derived factors include leptin, TNF-α, adiponectin, and resistin. It has been reported that leptin and adiponectin can enhance insulin sensitivity, whereas resistin and TNF-α cause insulin resistance. In this way, adipocytes carry out an endocrine function; indeed, the adipose tissue is the largest endocrine organ in the body.

MOLECULAR GENETICS OF TYPE 2 DIABETES MELLITUS

Many lines of evidence indicate a strong genetic component to type 2 diabetes. Although acquired factors such as obesity might be necessary to bring out the phenotypic manifestation of type 2 diabetes, these alone are insufficient in most patients without a preexisting genetic determinant. Because several prospective epidemiologic studies have shown that insulin resistance predates the development of type 2 diabetes, it seems likely that diabetogenic gene(s) involve some aspect of insulin action. While type 2 diabetes shows clear familial aggregation, it does not segregate in classical Mendelian fashion, and it is therefore likely to be a genetically heterogeneous, polygenic disease. In other words, it is likely that more than one diabetes gene occurs within a population, and it is possible that more than one abnormal gene must exist within an individual for the type 2 diabetic phenotype to develop. For example, it is possible that one or more genes involved in insulin action are affected, along with a separately inherited genetic defect that is responsible for the loss of β-cell function that occurs late in the course of type 2 diabetes development.

Several strategies have been employed to search for type 2 diabetes susceptibility genes. First is the candidate gene approach. In this approach, the investigator develops a hypothesis that a certain gene that has already been cloned and sequenced may be involved in the pathogenesis of type 2 diabetes. The sequence of this candidate gene is then compared in normal and type 2 diabetic subjects to look for structural abnormalities in the disease state. The second approach makes use of polymorphic genetic markers that are randomly distributed throughout the genome to map the location of the disease phenotype to a particular chromosome in a pedigree or population. This goal is accomplished by determining whether the DNA markers cosegregate with the type 2 diabetic phenotype in a pedigree or population with sufficient numbers of affected individuals.

These methods have allowed considerable progress to be made in defining the genetics of subsets of type 2 diabetes, formerly referred to as MODY. These disorders are due to monogenic defects in β-cell function, with little or no defect in insulin action. They are usually transmitted as an autosomal-dominant trait and are characterized by the onset of overt diabetes usually before 25 years of age. The MODY phenotype is associated with abnormalities in at least six genetic loci on different chromosomes. The gene for MODY-1 was initially localized to the long arm of chromosome 20, close to the adenosine deaminase locus, by Bell and colleagues on the basis of extensive family studies of the RW pedigree.[208] The gene was subsequently identified as the transcription factor hepatocyte nuclear factor 4α (HNF-4α).[209] MODY-2 is due to mutations in the glucokinase gene that catalyzes the formation of glucose-6-phosphate from glucose in islet β cells and hepatocytes. Over 40 different mutations have been described.[210,211] The missense mutations that cosegregate with diabetes in families with MODY alter the enzyme's affinity for glucose or the maximal activity for glucose phosphorylation. Because insulin secretion is intimately linked to the metabolism of glucose-6-phosphate, glucokinase is thought to play a key role as the "glucose sensor" of the β cell. Impaired hepatic glucose phosphorylation may also contribute to hyperglycemia in patients with MODY-2. Interestingly, most of the subjects with glucokinase mutations have very mild hyperglycemia, a normal first-phase insulin response to intravenous glucose, and a nonprogressive course. MODY-3 is the most common subtype. It is associated with mutations on chromosome 12 in a gene encoding HNF-1α, a liver transcription factor that is also expressed in β cells.[212] Unlike patients with MODY-2, hyperglycemia in patients with MODY-3 tends to be progressive. Because they frequently present in adolescence with symptomatic hyperglycemia, type 1 diabetes mellitus might be diagnosed. MODY-4 is due to mutations in yet another transcription factor gene, insulin promoter factor 1 (IPF-1), which in its homozygous form leads to total pancreatic agenesis.[213] Additional mutations have more recently also been described that involve HNF-1β[214] and NeuroD1/BETA2.[215] In "garden-variety" type 2 diabetes, mutations in the glucokinase and hepatic nuclear transcription factor genes are rare.[216] Point mutations of IPF-1, however, have been associated with an increased risk of type 2 diabetes.[217]

CANDIDATE GENE APPROACH

Given the complexity of the pathways that are involved in insulin secretion and signaling, many candidate genes have been studied. Several studies have examined the insulin receptor, glycogen synthase, and GLUT4 as potential candidate genes in type 2 diabetes. As was described in earlier sections, the primary sequences of these proteins are normal in type 2 diabetes, which, except in rare individuals, eliminates them as diabetes gene loci. In some populations, IRS-1 variants may be two to three times more common in patients with type 2 diabetes than in normal subjects, and in some studies, an association between polymorphisms affecting the region of IRS-1 that are thought to be important for PI 3-kinase binding and a reduction in insulin sensitivity has been found,[105] although not all studies have found this association.[218]

The contribution of adipocyte-expressed genes to the risk of developing type 2 diabetes has been examined. Mutations in the PPAR-γ gene show a complex relationship with diabetes susceptibility. Rare subjects with loss of function mutations within the PPAR-γ ligand-binding domain, which act in a dominant negative manner, develop lipodystrophy and severe insulin resistance that is apparent even in early childhood.[219] A Pro12Ala polymorphism is more commonly found in the population and does not function in a dominant negative fashion. While studies have reported somewhat conflicting results in terms of glucose metabolism, a meta-analysis of published studies suggested a modest protection from diabetes in those carrying the Ala allele.[220] The adiponectin gene localizes to chromosome 3q, and two single nucleotide polymorphisms have been associated with susceptibility to type 2 diabetes in some, but not all, populations.[221,222]

Given the importance of obesity in most type 2 diabetic patients, genes that predispose to obesity and, in particular, a more central distribution of body fat could also underlie the genetic predisposition. Several single-gene disorders have been identified involving leptin, the leptin receptor, melanocortin-3 receptor, and pro-opiomelanocortin.[223] However, leptin levels are generally increased in human

obesity, and these gene mutations do not cosegregate with common-type obesity in humans.[224,225] A missense mutation at codon 64 in the β₃-adrenergic receptor gene was reported to be associated with weight gain and some complications of obesity in a Finnish population.[226] However, subsequent studies in other populations did not find an increased frequency of this variant in obesity.[227] More recently, a polymorphism in the β₂-adrenergic receptor was found to be strongly associated with obesity; replacement of glutamine by glutamate at codon 27 (Gln27Glu) was found in 24% of obese women but only 3% of nonobese women.[228] Homozygotes for Glu27 had on average 20 kg more adipose tissue, larger fat cells, higher fasting insulin levels, and a more central distribution of body fat. Although this particular polymorphism does not alter β-adrenoreceptor function, it is in strong linkage disequilibrium with another polymorphism (Arg16Gly) that is associated with increased sensitivity to agonist-induced downregulation. Two thirds of the obese women were found to carry both Gly16 and Glu27.[228]

GENE-MAPPING STUDIES

Gene-mapping studies have been successful in identifying major susceptibility loci in type 1 diabetes, whereas in type 2 diabetes, these studies are at an earlier stage. One limitation of this method in type 2 diabetes is the low relative risk for diabetes in siblings of affected cases compared with the general population. Nonetheless, linkage has been found between the type 2 diabetic phenotype and a number of loci on different chromosomes, some of which are presented in Table 56-2. As expected, the putative susceptibility loci differ according to the population studied. Mexican-American sibling pairs showed significant linkage between type 2 diabetes and markers on chromosome 2q with this region designated NIDDM1.[229] More recently, it was suggested that an interaction of genes in the NIDDM1 region and genes on chromosome 15 may contribute to the susceptibility to type 2 diabetes in Mexican-Americans.[230] While this gene has been estimated to account for some 30% of the familial clustering of type 2 diabetes in Mexican-Americans, other studies in Caucasians, Japanese, and Pima Indians have failed to identify linkage in this area. NIDDM1 has been mapped to the calpain 10 gene.[231] Analyses of calpain 10 gene polymorphisms have found differing effects on fasting plasma glucose, and in most studies, no association has been demonstrated with type 2 diabetes.[232,233]

An Australian study of a large Caucasian pedigree with typical type 2 diabetes mapped a diabetes susceptibility locus to chromosome 12q, close to, but distinct from, the MODY3 region.[234] Linkage between type 2 diabetes in whites and markers in the MODY3 region was also found in another study.[235] By contrast, no evidence has been found for linkage of loci on chromosome 12 with type 2 diabetes in Mexican-Americans[236] or Pima Indian.[229]

The large Finland–United States Investigation of Non-Insulin-Dependent Diabetes reported a diabetes susceptibility locus on chromosome 20.[237] Several, but not all, populations also reported linkage at this region.[238,239] However, the

Table 56-2 Potential Type 2 Diabetes Susceptibility Loci

Chromosome Location	Population	Reference
1q21-1q24	Pima Indians, North European ancestry	239, 240
2q: NIDDM1	Mexican-American	229
4q	Pima Indians Mexican-American	241, 242
12q: near MODY3	Caucasian	234
20 p and q	Caucasian	237–239

area of potential linkage is large and involves much of the chromosome.

A susceptibility locus mapping to chromosome 1q21-q24 has been reported in Pima Indians and in several Northern European populations.[239,240]

Linkage family studies in Pima Indians[241] and Mexican-Americans[242] have also suggested linkage between in vivo insulin resistance and a locus on chromosome 4q that encodes the intestinal fatty acid–binding protein 2, which is believed to be involved in the transport of long-chain fatty acids within the enterocyte. However, in three different European populations, no differences in allelic frequency at this locus were found between diabetic and nondiabetic individuals.[243]

While these genomewide scans have mapped loci within large chromosomal regions, it is now therefore necessary to identify any diabetes-related gene within these regions. It has been difficult to replicate many of these linkage reports, and additional approaches, such as testing for interactions between loci, are being employed to address these issues.

KNOCKOUT ANIMAL MODELS

A major advance in our understanding of potential genetic mechanisms leading to the type 2 diabetic phenotype has come from mouse models in which a specific gene that is thought to play a key role in insulin action or insulin secretion has been disrupted either at the whole-body level or in a specific tissue. Mice with targeted disruption of the insulin receptor die a few days after birth, whereas heterozygous animals have a near-normal phenotype.[244] These results in heterozygous animals were perhaps not unexpected, given the presence of spare insulin receptors on insulin target tissues. However, diabetes also does not develop in animals with only one IRS-1 allele disrupted, even though these animals display mild insulin resistance, hyperinsulinemia, and mildly impaired glucose tolerance as they age.[245,246] Because severe deficiencies of these molecules are extremely rare in type 2 diabetes and type 2 diabetes is thought to be a polygenic disease, Bruning and colleagues generated mice that were heterozygous for the null allele of more than one of the key insulin-signaling molecules.[246] They found that insulin resistance, hyperinsulinemia, and progressive impairment in glucose tolerance developed in mice that were heterozygous for the null alleles of both the insulin receptor and IRS-1, with overt diabetes developing in approximately 40% of these mice by the age of 6 months.[246] Mice that were heterozygous for deficiencies of the insulin receptor, IRS-1, and IRS-2 had an even more profound degree of insulin resistance in muscle and liver, and overt diabetes eventually developed in a higher percentage.[247] Severe diabetes also develops in mice that are compound heterozygotes for the null alleles of the glucokinase and IRS-1 genes, whereas mice with an isolated defect of glucokinase gene expression have mild diabetes, as found in patients with MODY-2.[248] The presence of defects of both insulin action and insulin secretion in these glucokinase/IRS-1 compound heterozygous knockout mice provides an excellent model for the type 2 diabetic phenotype.

Taken together, these studies indicate that combinations of relatively minor defects, which in isolation might not cause significant phenotypic abnormalities, can act synergistically to cause insulin resistance, glucose intolerance, and type 2 diabetes. The particular mix of defects is likely to differ between different populations. Clearly, some defects may be acquired (e.g., the downregulation of insulin receptors by high circulating insulin levels) and act in concert with inherited genetic defects to produce significant insulin resistance and impairment of insulin secretion.

Another key finding from studies of mouse genetics is that insulin receptor signaling in islet β cells is important for their normal function. Mice in which the insulin receptor gene has been specifically ablated in β cells show a complete loss of first-phase insulin secretion in response to glucose, but not arginine, reminiscent of the β-cell defect in type 2 diabetes.[79] Interestingly, in patients with genetic forms of severe insulin resistance caused by insulin receptor defects, the acute insulin response to intravenous glucose is also absent.[249] Second-phase glucose-induced insulin secretion is also blunted in these mice, and they show an age-dependent progressive impairment in glucose tolerance, although overt diabetes does not develop. The islet β cells of these animals tend to be smaller than normal.[79] As well as providing direct evidence that functional insulin receptors are essential for normal β-cell function, this study also raises the intriguing possibility that insulin resistance at the level of the β cell might contribute to the decline in insulin secretion that supervenes after many years of peripheral tissue insulin resistance during the natural history of type 2 diabetes, providing a unifying hypothesis for the development of type 2 diabetes.

In summary, potential candidates for diabetes genes include those involved in insulin action, hepatic glucose metabolism, adipose tissue, and islet β-cell function. Genetic defects in protein function show up as abnormalities in protein-coding regions. However, abnormalities in the expression of one or more key proteins could also have a genetic basis. Studies in transgenic mouse models have highlighted the importance of combinations of relatively minor defects in signaling molecules acting synergistically to produce insulin resistance and glucose intolerance.

CONCLUDING OVERVIEW

With regard to the sequential development of type 2 diabetes, population-based and prospective studies indicate that insulin resistance is the initial defect, although in some populations, insulin secretory abnormalities may be primary.[13,250] In a number of different ethnic groups, insulin resistance has been found to exist in the prediabetic state in the absence of any impairment in insulin secretion. Thus, insulin resistance and hyperinsulinemia characterize most individuals in whom type 2 diabetes is destined to develop. However, except in extreme cases, insulin resistance alone is not sufficient to cause the full-blown type 2 diabetic phenotype. Decreased β-cell function must eventually supervene to cause the full-blown syndrome. This setting leads to the scheme depicted in Figure 56-2, in which insulin resistance (genetic and/or acquired) leads to hyperinsulinemia and compensated glucose metabolism. Eventually, in some of these individuals, perhaps those with a coexisting genetically determined β-cell defect, the ability of β cells to compensate by sustaining hyperinsulinemia declines, and insulin secretory defects along with decreased β-cell mass appear. At this stage, glucose metabolism decompensates, and the hyperglycemic diabetic stage appears. Because type 2 diabetes is a heterogeneous disease, this scheme (see Fig. 56-2) is clearly an oversimplification.

Once type 2 diabetes is established, the abnormal metabolic and hormonal milieu leads to secondary changes with worsening hyperglycemia. Thus, insulin resistance tends to be more marked in type 2 diabetes than in the prediabetic IGT state,[3,5,37] and insulin secretion continues to decline throughout the course of established type 2 diabetes.[51] Therefore, many patients, even if they are initially well controlled by diet or oral hypoglycemic agents, eventually require insulin for control of their diabetes. Glucotoxicity may well be the causal link here. Thus, strong evidence indicates that chronic hyperglycemia per se can lead to secondary worsening of both insulin resistance and insulin secretion, with the potential for a vicious cycle in which hyperglycemia begets more hyperglycemia. Support for this concept comes from numerous observations showing that control of hyperglycemia by insulin therapy, weight loss, or oral agents leads to improvements in both insulin secretion and insulin action. In subsets of type 2 diabetic patients who start with impaired insulin secretion, the insulin resistance, if it occurs, would be secondary. In addition, obesity and aging, as well as other factors, are acquired conditions that can cause or contribute to insulin resistance and β-cell dysfunction.

Because of the convergence of primary and secondary events that coexist in the manifest type 2 diabetic state, it is a daunting task to identify the critical biochemical and cellular defects that underlie this disorder. Most likely, clarifying discoveries will come from the field of molecular genetics. Type 2 diabetes has a strong genetic component; therefore, the ultimate explanation for this disease lies in the genome. By finding the genes that are abnormal in type 2 diabetes, we will be able to document the cellular defects that initiate this syndrome. We might also find that different sets of genetic defects exist in different patients and that depending on other genetic or acquired features, they complement each other in different ways. This search might also lead to the identification of genes encoding proteins that affect carbohydrate metabolism in ways that are not currently understood. Discovery of all the molecular defects that can lead to type 2 diabetes is an enormous but completely feasible goal and should provide the basis for an exciting future in diabetes research.

REFERENCES

1. Ward WK, Beard JC, Porte D: Clinical aspects of islet B-cell function in non-insulin-dependent diabetes mellitus. Diabetes Metab Rev 2:297–313, 1986.
2. DeFronzo RA: The triumvirate: β-cell, muscle, liver: A collusion responsible for NIDDM. Diabetes 37:667–687, 1988.
3. Seely BL, Olefsky JM: Cellular and genetic mechanisms for insulin resistance in common disorders of obesity and diabetes. In Moller D (ed): Insulin Resistance and Its Clinical Disorders. New York, John Wiley & Sons, 1993.
4. Reaven GM: Role of insulin resistance in human disease. Diabetes 37:1595–1607, 1988.
5. Kolterman OG, Gray RS, Griffin J, et al: Receptor and post-receptor defects contribute to the insulin resistance in non-insulin dependent diabetes mellitus. J Clin Invest 68:957–969, 1981.
6. Dinneen S, Gerich J, Rizza R: Carbohydrate metabolism in non-insulin-dependent diabetes mellitus. N Engl J Med 327:707–713, 1992.
7. Ferrannini E, Groop LC: Hepatic glucose production in insulin resistant states. Diabetes Metab Rev 5:711–725, 1989.
8. Bogardus C, Lillioja S, Howard BV, et al: Relationships between insulin secretion, insulin action, and fasting plasma glucose concentration in non-diabetic and non-insulin-dependent diabetic subjects. J Clin Invest 74:1238–1246, 1984.
9. Shulman GI, Rothman DL, Jue T, et al: Quantitation of muscle glycogen synthesis in normal subjects and subjects with non-insulin-dependent diabetes by ^{13}C-nuclear magnetic resonance spectroscopy. N Engl J Med 322:223–228, 1991.
10. Ciaraldi TP, Kolterman OG, Scarlett JA, et al: Role of the glucose transport system in the post-receptor defect of non-insulin dependent diabetes mellitus. Diabetes 31:1016–1022, 1982.
11. Firth R, Bell P, Rizza R: Insulin action in non-insulin-dependent diabetes mellitus: The relationship between hepatic and extrahepatic insulin resistance and obesity. Metabolism 36:1091–1095, 1987.
12. Groop LC, Bonadonna RC, Del Prato S, et al: Glucose and free fatty acid metabolism in non-insulin dependent diabetes mellitus: Evidence for multiple sites of insulin resistance. J Clin Invest 84:205–213, 1989.
13. Efendic S, Luft R, Wajngot A: Aspects of the pathogenesis of type 2 diabetes. Endocr Rev 5:395–410, 1984.
14. Porte D: Banting lecture 1990. β-cells in type II diabetes mellitus. Diabetes 40:166–190, 1991.
15. Barnett AH, Eff C, Leslie RD, Pyke DA: Diabetes in identical twins: A study of 200 pairs. Diabetologia 20:87–93, 1981.
16. Rich SS: Mapping genes in diabetes: Genetic epidemiological perspective. Diabetes 39:1315–1319, 1990.
17. Haffner SM, Sern MP, Mitchell BD, et al: Incidences of type II diabetes in Mexican Americans predicted by fasting insulin and glucose levels, obesity, and body fat distribution. Diabetes 39:283–288, 1990.
18. Knowler WC, Bennett PH, Pettitt D, Savage PJ: Diabetes incidence in Pima Indians: Contributions of obesity and parental diabetes. Am J Epidemiol 113:144–156, 1981.
19. Given BD, Mako ME, Tager H, et al: Circulating insulin with reduced biological activity in a patient with diabetes. N Engl J Med 302:129–135, 1980.
20. Gabbay KH, DeLuca K, Fisher JN Jr, et al: Familial hyperproinsulinemia: An autosomal dominant defect. N Engl J Med 294:911–915, 1976.
21. Warren-Perry MG, Manley SE, Ostrega D, et al: A novel point mutation in the insulin genegiving rise to hyperproinsulinemia. J Clin Endocrinol Metab 82:1629–1631, 1997.
22. Moller DE, Flier JS: Insulin resistance: Mechanisms, syndromes, and implications. N Engl J Med 325:938–948, 1991.
23. Toyota T, Kudo M, Goto Y, et al: Prevalence of diabetes mellitus in rural and urban population of Japan. In Baba S, Goto Y, Fukui I (eds): Diabetes Mellitus in Asia: Ecological Aspects of Epidemiology, Complications and Treatment. Amsterdam, Exerpta Medica, 1976, pp 35–40.
24. Fujimoto WY, Leonetti DL, Kinyoun JL, et al: Prevalence of complications among second-generation Japanese-American men with diabetes, impaired glucose tolerance, or normal glucose tolerance. Diabetes 36:730–739, 1987.
25. Ravussin E, Valencia E, Esparza J, et al: Effects of a traditional lifestyle on obesity in Pima Indians. Diabetes Care 17:1067–1074, 1994.
26. Lands WE, Hamazaki T, Yamazaki K, et al: Changing dietary patterns. Am J Clin Nutr 51:991–993, 1990.
27. Lee MM, Wu-Williams A, Whitemore AS, et al: Comparison of dietary habits, physical activity and body size among Chinese in North America and China. Int J Epidemiol 23:984–990, 1994.
28. Diabetes Prevention Program Research Group: Reduction in the incidence of type 2 diabetes with lifestyle intervention or metformin. N Engl J Med 346:393–403, 2002.
29. Helmrich SP, Ragland DR, Leung RW, et al: Physical activity and reduced occurrence of non-insulin dependent diabetes mellitus. N Eng J Med 325:147–152, 1991.
30. Hales CN, Barker DJ, Clark PM, et al: Fetal and infant growth and impaired glucose tolerance at age 64. Br Med J 303:1019–1022, 1991.
31. Chen M, Bergman RN, Pacini G, Porte D Jr: Pathogenesis of age-related glucose intolerance in man: Insulin resistance, and decreased β-cell function. J Clin Endocrinol Metab 60:13–20, 1985.
32. Polonsky KS, Sturis J, Bell GI: Non-insulin-dependent diabetes mellitus: A genetically programmed failure of the beta cell to compensate for insulin resistance. N Engl J Med 334:777–783, 1996.
33. Warram JH, Martin BC, Krolewski AS, et al: Slow glucose removal rate and hyperinsulinemia precede the development of type II diabetes in the offspring of diabetic parents. Ann Intern Med 13:909–915, 1990.
34. Lillioja S, Mott DM, Howard BV, et al: Impaired glucose tolerance as a disorder of insulin action: Longitudinal and cross-sectional studies in Pima Indians. N Engl J Med 318:1217–1225, 1988.
35. Saad MF, Knowler WC, Pettitt DJ, et al: The natural history of impaired glucose tolerance in the Pima Indians. N Engl J Med 319:1500–1505, 1988.
36. Serjeantson SW, Zimmet P: Genetics of non-insulin dependent diabetes mellitus in 1990. Baillieres Clin Endocrinol Metab 5:477–493, 1991.

37. Eriksson J, Franssila-Kallunki AM, Ekstrand A, et al: Early metabolic defects in persons at increased risk for non-insulin-dependent diabetes mellitus. N Engl J Med 321:337–343, 1989.

38. Vaag A, Henriksen JE, Beck-Nielsen H: Decreased insulin activation of glycogen synthase in skeletal muscles in young nonobese Caucasian first-degree relatives of patients with non-insulin-dependent diabetes mellitus. J Clin Invest 89:782–788, 1992.

39. Perseghin G, Ghosh S, Gerow K, Shulman GI: Metabolic defects in lean nondiabetic offspring of NIDDM parents: A cross-sectional study. Diabetes 46:1010–1016, 1997.

40. Kahn SE, Prigeon RL, McCulloch DK, et al: Quantification of the relationship between insulin sensitivity and B-cell function in human subjects: Evidence for a hyperbolic function. Diabetes 46:1663–1672, 1993.

41. Lang DA, Matthews DR, Peto J, Turner RC: Cyclic oscillations of basal plasma glucose and insulin concentrations in human beings. N Engl J Med 301:1023–1027, 1979.

42. O'Rahilly S, Turner RC, Matthews DR: Impaired pulsatile secretion of insulin in relatives of patients with non-insulin-dependent diabetes. N Engl J Med 318:1225–1230, 1988.

43. Hunter SJ, Ennis CN, Sheridan B, et al: Association between insulin secretory pulse frequency and peripheral insulin action in NIDDM and normal subjects. Diabetes 45:683–686, 1996.

44. Fajans SS, Cloutier MC, Crowther RL: Clinical and etiologic heterogeneity of idiopathic diabetes mellitus. Diabetes 27:1112–1125, 1978.

45. Reaven GM, Bernstein R, Davis B, Olefsky JM: Nonketotic diabetes mellitus: Insulin deficiency or insulin resistance? Am J Med 60:80–88, 1976.

46. Alberti KGMM: The clinical implications of impaired glucose tolerance. Diabet Med 13:927–937, 1996.

47. Cavaghan MK, Ehrmann DA, Byrne MM, Polonsky KS: Treatment with the oral antidiabetic agent troglitazone improves beta cell responses to glucose in subjects with impaired glucose tolerance. J Clin Invest 100:530–537, 1997.

48. Polonsky KS: The beta-cell in diabetes: From molecular genetics to clinical research. Diabetes 44:705–717, 1995.

49. Cook JTE, Page RCL, Levy JC, et al: Hyperglycaemic progression in subjects with impaired glucose tolerance: Association with decline in beta cell function. Diabet Med 10:321–326, 1993.

50. Van Haeften T, Pimenta W, Mitrakou A, et al: Relative contributions of β-cell function and tissue insulin sensitivity to fasting diand postglucose-load glycemia. Metabolism 49:1318–1325, 2000.

51. U.K. Prospective Diabetes Study Group: U.K. prospective diabetes study 16: Overview of 6 years' therapy of type II diabetes: A progressive disease. Diabetes 44:1249–1258, 1995.

52. Halter JB, Graf RJ, Porte D Jr: Potentiation of insulin secretory responses by plasma glucose levels in man: Evidence that hyperglycemia in diabetes compensates for impaired glucose potentiation. J Clin Endocrinol Metab 48:946–954, 1979.

53. Ward WK, Bolgiano DC, McKnight B, et al: Diminished β cell secretory capacity in patients with noninsulin-dependent diabetes mellitus. J Clin Invest 74:1318–1328, 1984.

54. Reaven GM, Chen YDI, Hollenbeck CB, et al: Plasma insulin, C-peptide, and proinsulin concentrations in obese and nonobese individuals with varying degrees of glucose tolerance. J Clin Endocrinol Metab 76:44–48, 1993.

55. Ferrannini E, Natali A, Bell P, et al: Insulin resistance and hypersecretion in obesity. J Clin Invest 100:1166–1173, 1997.

56. Perley MJ, Kipnis DM: Plasma insulin responses to oral and intravenous glucose: Studies in normal and diabetic subjects. J Clin Invest 46:1954–1962, 1967.

57. Brunzell JD, Robertson RP, Lerner RL, et al: Relationships between fasting plasma glucose levels and insulin secretion during intravenous glucose tolerance tests. J Clin Endocrinol Metab 42:222–229, 1976.

58. Ward WW, Beard JC, Halter JB, et al: Pathophysiology of insulin secretion in non-insulin-dependent diabetes mellitus. Diabetes Care 7:491–502, 1984.

59. Robertson RP, Porte D: The glucose receptor: A defective mechanism in diabetes mellitus distinct from the beta-adrenergic receptor. J Clin Invest 52:870–876, 1976.

60. McRae JR, Metz SW, Robertson RP: A role for endogenous prostaglandins in defective glucose potentiation of non-glucose insulin secretagogues in diabetics. Metabolism 30:1065–1075, 1981.

61. Robertson RP, Halter JB, Porte D Jr: A role for alpha-adrenergic receptors in abnormal insulin secretion in diabetes mellitus. J Clin Invest 57:791–795, 1976.

62. Vague P, Moulin JP: The defective glucose sensitivity of the β-cell in noninsulin dependent diabetes: Improvement after twenty hours of normoglycemia. Metabolism 31:139–142, 1982.

63. Leahy JL, Bonner-Weir S, Weir GC: β-cell dysfunction induced by chronic hyperglycemia. Diabetes Care 15:442–455, 1992.

64. Lohmann D, Jahr H, Verlohren J-J, et al: Insulin secretion in maturity-onset diabetes-function of isolated islets. Horm Metab Res 12:349–353, 1980.

65. Srikanta S, Ganda OP, Eisenbarth GS, Soeldner JS: Islet-cell antibodies and beta-cell function in monozygotic triplets and twins initially discordant for type I diabetes mellitus. N Engl J Med 308:322–325, 1983.

66. Reaven GM, Olefsky JM: Relationship between heterogeneity of insulin responses and insulin resistance in normal subjects. Diabetologia 13:201–206, 1977.

67. Temple RC, Clark PMS, Nagi DK, et al: Radioimmunoassay may overestimate insulin in non-insulin-dependent diabetics. Clin Endocrinol (Oxf) 32:689–693, 1990.

68. Clark A, Wells CA, Buley ID, et al: Islet amyloid, increased A-cells, reduced β-cells and exocrine fibrosis: Quantitative changes in the pancreas in type 2 diabetes. Diabetes Res 9:151–160, 1988.

69. Butler AE, Janson J, Bonner-Weir S, et al: β-cell deficit and increased β-cell apoptosis in humans with type-2 diabetes mellitus. Diabetes 52:102–110, 2003.

70. Ogilvie R: The islets of Langerhans in 19 cases of obesity. J Pathol 37:473–481, 1933.

71. Shimabukuro M, Zhou Y-T, Levi M, Unger RH: Fatty acid induced β cell apoptosis: A link between obesity and diabetes. Proc Natl Acad Sci U S A 95:2498–2502, 1998.

72. Kahn SE, D'Alessio DA, Schwartz MW, et al: Evidence of co-secretion of islet amyloid polypeptide and insulin by beta-cells. Diabetes 39:634–638, 1990.

73. Kahn SE, Andrikopoulos S, Verchere CB: Islet amyloid: A long-recognized but underappreciated pathological feature of type 2 diabetes. Diabetes 48:241–253, 1999.

74. Lorenzo A, Razzaboni B, Weir GC, Yankner BA: Pancreatic islet cell toxicity of amylin associated with type-2 diabetes mellitus. Nature 368:756–760, 1994.

75. Kolterman OG, Gray RS, Shapiro G, et al: The acute and chronic effects of sulfonylurea therapy in type II diabetics. Diabetes 33:346–354, 1984.

76. Garvey WT, Olefsky JM, Griffin J, et al: The effects of insulin treatment on insulin secretion and action in type II diabetes mellitus. Diabetes 34:222–234, 1985.

77. Henry RR, Wallace P, Olefsky JM: The effects of weight loss on the mechanisms of hyperglycemia in obese noninsulin-dependent diabetes mellitus. Diabetes 35:990–998, 1986.

78. Eizirik DL, Korbutt GS, Hellerstrom C: Prolonged exposure of human pancreatic islets to high glucose concentrations in vitro impairs the β-cell function. J Clin Invest 90:1263–1268, 1992.

79. Kulkarni RN, Bruning JC, Winnay JN, et al: Tissue-specific knockout of the insulin receptor in pancreatic β cells creates an insulin secretory defect similar to that in type 2 diabetes. Cell 96:329–339, 1999.

80. Randle PJ, Hales CN, Garland PB, Newsholme EA: The glucose fatty–acid cycle: Its role in insulin sensitivity and the metabolic disturbances of diabetes mellitus. Lancet 1:785–789, 1963.

81. Kahn CR, Rosenthal AS: Immunologic reactions to insulin: Insulin allergy, insulin resistance, and the autoimmune insulin syndrome. Diabetes Care 2:283–295, 1979.

82. Flier JS, Kahn CR, Roth J, Bar RS: Antibodies that impair insulin receptor binding in an unusual diabetic syndrome with severe insulin resistance. Science 190:63–65, 1975.

83. Zhang B, Roth RA: A region of the insulin receptor important for ligand binding (residues 450–601) is recognized by patients' autoimmune antibodies and inhibitory monoclonal antibodies. Proc Natl Acad Sci U S A 88:9858–9862, 1991.

84. Lang CH, Dobrescu C, Bagby GJ: Tumour necrosis factor impairs insulin action on peripheral glucose disposal and hepatic glucose output. Endocrinology 130:43–52, 1992.

85. Sakurai Y, Zhang X, Wolfe RR: Short-term effects of tumour necrosis factor on energy and substrate metabolism in dogs. J Clin Invest 91:2437–2445, 1993.

86. Hotamisligil GS, Arner P, Caro JF, et al: Increased adipose tissue expression of tumour necrosis factor-α in human obesity and insulin resistance. J Clin Invest 95:2409–2415, 1995.

87. Hotamisligil SG, Spiegelman BM: Tumour necrosis factor α: A key component of the obesity-diabetes link. Diabetes 43:1271–1278, 1994.

88. Hotamisligil GS, Peraldi P, Budavari A, et al: IRS-1-mediated inhibition of insulin receptor tyrosine kinase activity in TNF-α and obesity-induced insulin resistance. Science 271:665–668, 1996.

89. Ofei F, Hurel S, Newkirk J, et al: Effects of an engineered human anti TNF-α antibody (CDP571) on insulin sensitivity and glycemic control in patients with NIDDM. Diabetes 45:881–885, 1996.

90. Yang YJ, Hope JD, Ader M, Bergman RN: Insulin transport across capillaries is rate limiting for insulin action in dogs. J Clin Invest 84:1620–1628, 1989.

91. Steil GM, Ader M, Moore DM, et al: Transendothelial insulin transport is not saturable in vivo. No evidence for a receptor-mediated process. J Clin Invest 97:1497–1503, 1996.

92. Prager R, Wallace P, Olefsky JM: In vivo kinetics of insulin action on peripheral glucose disposal and hepatic glucose output in normal and obese subjects. J Clin Invest 78:472–481, 1986.

93. Nolan JJ, Ludvik B, Baloga J, et al: Mechanisms of the kinetic defect in insulin action in obesity and NIDDM. Diabetes 46:994–1000, 1997.

94. King GL, Johnson SM: Receptor-mediated transport of insulin across endothelial cells. Science 227:1583–1586, 1985.

95. Castillo C, Bogardus C, Bergman R, et al: Interstitial insulin concentrations determine glucose uptake rates but not insulin resistance in lean and obese men. J Clin Invest 93:10–16, 1994.

96. Cline GW, Petersen KF, Krssak M, et al: Impaired glucose transport as a cause of decreased insulin–stimulated muscle glycogen synthesis in type 2 diabetes. N Engl J Med 341:240–246, 1999.

97. Lillioja S, Young AA, Culter CL, et al: Skeletal muscle capillary density and fiber type are possible determinants of in vivo insulin resistance in man. J Clin Invest 80:415–424, 1987.

98. Laakso M, Edelman SV, Brechtel G, Baron AD: Impaired insulin-mediated skeletal muscle blood flow in patients with NIDDM. Diabetes 41:1076–1083, 1992.

99. Natali A, Buzzugoli G, Taddei S, et al: Effects of insulin on hemodynamics and metabolism in human forearm. Diabetes 39:490–500, 1990.

100. Utriainen T, Nuutila P, Takala T, et al: Intact insulin stimulation of skeletal muscle blood flow, its heterogeneity and redistribution, but not of glucose uptake in non-insulin-dependent diabetes mellitus. J Clin Invest 100:777–785, 1997.

101. Kahn CR, White MF: The insulin receptor and the molecular mechanisms of insulin action. J Clin Invest 82:1151–1156, 1988.

102. Olefsky JM: The insulin receptor: A multi-functional protein. Diabetes 39:1009–1016, 1990.

103. Wilden PA, Siddle K, Haring H, et al: The role of insulin receptor kinase domain autophosphorylation in receptor mediated activities. J Biol Chem 267:13719–13727, 1992.

104. White MF: The insulin signalling system and the IRS proteins. Diabetologia 40(Suppl):2–17, 1997.

105. Virkamaki A, Ueki K, Kahn RC: Protein-protein interaction in insulin signaling and the molecular mechanisms of insulin resistance. J Clin Invest 103:931–943, 1999.

106. Fink RI, Wallace P, Brechtel G, Olefsky JM: Evidence that glucose transport is rate-limiting for in vivo glucose uptake. Metabolism 41:897–902, 1992.

107. Furler SM, Jenkins AB, Storlien LH, Kraegen EW: In vivo location of the rate-limiting step of hexose uptake in muscle and brain tissue of rats. Am J Phsyiol 261:E337–E347, 1991.

108. Ren JM, Marshall BA, Gulve EA, et al: Evidence from transgenic mice that glucose transport is rate-limiting for glycogen deposition and glycolysis in skeletal muscle. J Biol Chem 268:16113–16115, 1993.

109. Pessin JE, Bell GI: Mammalian facilitative glucose transporter family: Structure and molecular regulation. Annu Rev Physiol 84:911–930, 1992.

110. Shepherd PR, Kahn BB: Glucose transporters and insulin action. N Engl J Med 341:248–257, 1999.

111. Karnieli E, Zarnowski MJ, Hissin PJ, et al: Insulin-stimulated translocation of glucose transport systems in the isolated rat adipose cell: Time-course, reversal, insulin concentration dependency, and relationship to glucose transport activity. J Biol Chem 256:4772–4777, 1981.

112. Kono T, Suzuki K, Dansey LE, et al: Energy-dependent and protein synthesis-independent recycling of the insulin sensitive glucose transport mechanism in fat cells. J Biol Chem 256:6400–6407, 1981.

113. Kelley DE, Mintun MA, Watkins SC, et al: The effect of non-insulin-dependent diabetes mellitus and obesity on glucose transport and phosphorylation in skeletal muscle. J Clin Invest 97:2705–2713, 1996.

114. Garvey WT, Maianu L, Zhu J-H, et al: Evidence for defects in the trafficking and translocation of Glut 4 glucose transporters in skeletal muscle as a cause of human insulin resistance. J Clin Invest 101:2377–2386, 1998.

115. Pessin JE, Thurmond DC, Elmendorf JS, et al: Molecular basis of insulin-stimulated Glut 4 vesicle trafficking. J Biol Chem 274:2593–2596, 1999.

116. Olefsky JM, Ciaraldi TP: The insulin receptor: Basic characteristics and its role in insulin resistant state. In Brownlee M (ed): Diabetes Mellitus. New York, Garland Press, 1980, pp 73–115.

117. Bergman RN, Finegood DT, Ader M: Assessment of insulin sensitivity in vivo. Endocr Rev 1:45–86, 1985.

118. Himsworth JP, Kerr RB: Insulin-sensitive and insulin-insensitive types of diabetes mellitus. Clin Sci 4:119–152, 1939.

119. Jones CNO, Pei D, Staris P, et al: Alterations in the glucose-stimulated insulin secretory dose-response curve and in insulin clearance in nondiabetic insulin-resistant individuals. J Clin Endocrinol Metab 82:1834–1838, 1997.

120. Ginsberg H, Kimmerling G, Olefsky JM, Reaven GM: Demonstration of insulin resistance in maturity onset diabetic patients with fasting hyperglycemia. J Clin Invest 55:454–460, 1975.

121. Welch S, Gebhart SS, Bergman RN, Phillips LS: Minimal model analysis of intravenous glucose tolerance test-derived insulin sensitivity in diabetic subjects. J Clin Endocrinol Metab 71:1508–1518, 1990.

122. Bonadonna RC, Del Prato S, Saccomani MP, et al: Transmembrane glucose transport in skeletal muscle of patients with non-insulin-dependent diabetes. J Clin Invest 92:486–494, 1993.

123. Capaldo B, Napoli R, Di Marino L, et al: Quantitation of forearm glucose and free fatty acid (FFA) disposal in normal subjects and type II diabetic patients: Evidence against an essential role for FFA in the pathogenesis of insulin resistance. J Clin Endocrinol Metab 67:893–898, 1988.

124. DeFronzo RA, Jacot E, Jequier E, et al: The effect of insulin on the disposal of intravenous glucose: Results from indirect calorimetry and hepatic and femoral venous catheterization. Diabetes 30:1000–1007, 1981.

125. Edelman SV, Laakso M, Wallace P, et al: Kinetics of insulin mediated and non-insulin mediated glucose uptake in man. Diabetes 39:955–964, 1990.

126. Kelley DE, Mokan M, Mandarino LJ: Intracellular defects in glucose metabolism in obese patients with NIDDM. Diabetes 41:698–706, 1992.

127. Kono T, Barham FW: The relationship between the insulin-binding capacity of fat cells and the cellular response to insulin: Studies with intact and trypsin-treated fat cells. J Biol Chem 246:6210–6216, 1971.

128. Kolterman OG, Scarlett JA, Olefsky JM: Insulin resistance in non-insulin-dependent, type II diabetes mellitus. J Clin Endocrinol Metab 11:363–388, 1982.

129. Olefsky JM, Reaven GM: Decreased insulin binding to lymphocytes from diabetic patients. J Clin Invest 54:1323–1328, 1974.

130. Olefsky JM, Reaven GM: Insulin binding in diabetes: Relationships with plasma insulin levels and insulin sensitivity. Diabetes 26:680–688, 1977.

131. Freidenberg GR, Reichart D, Olefsky JM, Henry RR: Reversibility of defective adipocyte insulin receptor kinase activity in non-insulin dependent diabetes mellitus: Effect of weight loss. J Clin Invest 82:1398–1406, 1990.

132. Maegawa H, Shigeta Y, Egawa K, Kobayashi M: Impaired autophosphorylation of insulin receptors from abdominal skeletal muscles in nonobese subjects with NIDDM. Diabetes 40:815–819, 1991.

133. Bjornholm M, Kawano Y, Lehtihet M, Zierath JR: Insulin receptor substrate-1 phosphorylation and phosphatidylinositol 3-kinase activity in skeletal muscle from NIDDM subjects after in vivo insulin stimulation. Diabetes 46:524–527, 1997.

134. Paz K, Hemi R, LeRoith D, et al: A molecular basis for insulin resistance: Elevated serine/threonine phosphorylation of IRS-1 and IRS-2 inhibits their binding to the juxtamembrane region of the insulin receptor and impairs their ability to undergo insulin-induced tyrosine phosphorylation. J Biol Chem 272:29911–29918, 1997.

135. Pederson TM, Kramer DL, Rondinone CM: Serine/threonine phosphorylation of IRS-1 triggers its degradation: Possible regulation by tyrosine phosphorylation. Diabetes 50:24–31, 2001.

136. Aguirre V, Uchida T, Yenush L, et al: The c-Jun NH_2-terminal kinase promotes insulin resistance during association with insulin receptor substrate-1 and phosphorylation of Ser[307]. J Biol Chem 275:9047–9054, 2000.

137. Gao Z, Hwang D, Bataille F, et al: Serine phosphorylation of insulin receptor substrate 1 by inhibitor kappa B kinase complex. J Biol Chem 13;277(50):48115–48121, 2002.

138. Rui L, Aguirre V, Kim JK, et al: Insulin/IGF-1 and TNF-alpha stimulate phosphorylation of IRS-1 at inhibitory Ser307 via distinct pathways. J Clin Invest 107(2):181–189, 2001.

139. Withers DJ, Gutierrez JS, Towery H, et al: Disruption of IRS-2 causes type 2 diabetes in mice. Nature 391:900–904, 1998.

140. Shepherd PR, Withers DJ, Siddle K: Phosphoinositide 3-kinase: The key switch mechanism in insulin signaling. Biochem J 333:471–490, 1998.

141. Goodyear LJ, Giorgino F, Sherman LA, et al: Insulin receptor phosphorylation, insulin receptor substrate-1 phosphorylation, and phosphatidylinositol 3-kinase activity are decreased in intact skeletal muscle strips from obese subjects. J Clin Invest 95(5):2195–2204, 1995.

142. Zierath JR, He L, Guma A, et al: Insulin action on glucose transport and plasma membrane Glut 4 content in skeletal muscle from patients with NIDDM. Diabetologia 39:1180–1189, 1996.

143. Eriksson J, Koranyi L, Bourey R, et al: Insulin resistance in type 2 (non-insulin-dependent) diabetic patients and their relatives is not associated with a defect in the expression of the insulin-responsive glucose transporter (GLUT-4) gene in human skeletal muscle. Diabetologia 35:143–147, 1992.

144. Garvey WT, Maianu L, Hancock JA, et al: Gene expression of GLUT4 in skeletal muscle from insulin-resistant patients with obesity, IGT, GDM, and NIDDM. Diabetes 41:465–475, 1992.

145. Buse JB, Yasuda K, Lay TP, et al: Human GLUT4/muscle-fat glucose transporter gene: Characterization and genetic variation. Diabetes 41:1436–1445, 1982.

146. Choi W-H, O'Rahilly S, Buse JB, et al: Molecular scanning of insulin-responsive glucose transporter (GLUT4) gene in NIDDM subjects. Diabetes 40:1712–1718, 1991.

147. Kusari J, Berma US, Buse JB, et al: Analysis of the gene sequences of the insulin receptor and the insulin sensitive glucose transporter (Glut-4) in patients with common type non-insulin dependent diabetes mellitus. J Clin Invest 88:1323–1330, 1991.

148. Yki-Jarvinen H, Bogardus C, Howard BV: Hyperglycemia stimulates carbohydrate oxidation in humans. Am J Physiol 253:E376–E382, 1987.

149. Golay A, DeFronzo RA, Ferrannini E, et al: Oxidative and non-oxidative glucose metabolism in non-obese type 2 (non-insulin dependent) diabetic patients. Diabetologia 31:585–591, 1988.

150. Del Prato S, Bonadonna RC, Bonora E, et al: Characterization of cellular defects of insulin action in type 2 (non-insulin-dependent) diabetes mellitus. J Clin Invest 91:484–494, 1993.

151. Rothman DL, Shulman RG, Shulman GI: ^{31}P nuclear magnetic resonance measurements of muscle glucose-6-phosphate. J Clin Invest 89:1069–1075, 1992.

152. Prager R, Wallace P, Olefsky JM: Hyperinsulinemia does not compensate for peripheral insulin resistance in obesity. Diabetes 36:327–334, 1987.

153. Kolterman OG, Insel LJ, Saekow M, Olefsky JM: Mechanisms of insulin resistance in human obesity. Evidence for receptor and post-receptor defects. J Clin Invest 65:1272–1284, 1980.

154. Rothman DL, Magnusson I, Katz LD, Shulman GI: Quantitation of hepatic glycogenolysis and gluconeogenesis in fasting humans with ^{13}C NMR. Science 254:573–576, 1991.

155. Consoli A, Nurjhan N, Reilly JJ, et al: Mechanism of increased gluconeogenesis in non-insulin-dependent diabetes mellitus: Role of alterations in systemic, hepatic, and muscle lactate and alanine metabolism. J Clin Invest 86:2038–2045, 1990.

156. Magnusson I, Rothman DL, Katz LD, et al: Increased rate of gluconeogenesis in type II diabetes mellitus: A ^{13}C nuclear magnetic resonance study. J Clin Invest 90:1323–1327, 1992.

157. Baron AD, Schmeiser L, Shragg GP, Kolterman OG: The role of hyperglucagonemia in the maintenance of increased rates of hepatic glucose output in type II diabetics. Diabetes 36:274–283, 1987.

158. Rebrin K, Steil GM, Getty L, Bergman RN: Free fatty acid as a link in the regulation of hepatic glucose output by peripheral insulin. Diabetes 44:1038–1045, 1995.

159. Felig P, Wahren J, Hendler R: Influence of oral glucose ingestion on splanchnic glucose and gluconeogenic substrate metabolism in man. Diabetes 24:468–475, 1975.

160. Ferrannini E, Bjorkman O, Reichard GA, et al: The disposal of an oral glucose load in healthy subjects: A quantitative study. Diabetes 34:580–588, 1985.

161. Niewoehner CB, Nuttall FQ: Relationship of hepatic glucose uptake to intrahepatic glucose concentration in fasted rats after glucose load. Diabetes 37:1559–1566, 1988.

162. Ludvik B, Nolan JJ, Roberts A, et al: Evidence for decreased splanchnic glucose uptake after oral glucose administration in non-insulin-dependent diabetes mellitus. J Clin Invest 100:2354–2361, 1997.

163. Baron AD, Kolterman OG, Bell J, et al: Rates of non-insulin mediated glucose uptake are elevated in type II diabetic subjects. J Clin Invest 76:1782–1788, 1986.

164. Mitrakou A, Kelley D, Veneman T, et al: Contribution of abnormal muscle

and liver glucose metabolism to postprandial hyperglycemia in NIDDM. Diabetes 39:1381–1390, 1990.

165. Scarlett JA, Gray RS, Griffin J, et al: Insulin treatment reverses the insulin resistance of type II diabetes mellitus. Diabetes Care 5:353–363, 1982.

166. Firth RG, Bell PM, Rizza RA: Effects of tolazamide and exogenous insulin on insulin action in patients with non-insulin dependent diabetes mellitus. N Engl J Med 314:1280–1286, 1986.

167. Henry RR, Gumbiner B, Ditzler T, et al: Intensive conventional insulin therapy for type II diabetes. Diabetes Care 16:21–31, 1993.

168. Firth R, Bell P, Marsh M, Rizza RA: Effects of tolazamide and exogenous insulin on pattern of postprandial carbohydrate metabolism in patients with non-insulin-dependent diabetes mellitus: Results of randomized crossover trial. Diabetes 36:1130–1138, 1987.

169. Bak JF, Schmitz O, Sorensen NS, et al: Postreceptor effects of sulfonylurea on skeletal muscle glycogen synthase activity in type II diabetes mellitus. Diabetes 38:1343–1350, 1989.

170. Henry RR, Scheaffer L, Olefsky JM: Glycemic effects of short-term intensive dietary restriction and isocaloric refeeding in non-insulin dependent diabetes mellitus. J Clin Endocrinol Metab 61:917–925, 1985.

171. Yki-Jarvinen H: Glucose toxicity. Endocr Rev 13:415–431, 1992.

172. Vuorinen-Markkola H, Koivisto VA, Yki-Jarvinen H: Mechanisms of hyperglycemia-induced insulin resistance in whole body and skeletal muscle of type 1 diabetic patients. Diabetes 41:571–580, 1992.

173. Saltiel AR, Olefsky JM: Thiazolidinediones in the treatment of insulin resistance and type II diabetes. Diabetes 45:1661–1669, 1996.

174. Yu JG, Kruszynska YT, Mulford MI, Olefsky JM: A comparison of troglitazone and metformin on insulin requirements in euglycemic, intensively treated type 2 diabetic mellitus patients. Diabetes 48:2414–2421, 1999.

175. Nolan JJ, Ludvik B, Beerdsen P, et al: Improvement in glucose tolerance and insulin resistance in obese subjects treated with troglitazone. N Engl J Med 331:1188–1193, 1994.

176. Cavaghan MK, Ehrmann DA, Byrne MM, Polonsky KS: Treatment with the oral antidiabetic agent troglitazone improves β cell responses to glucose in subjects with impaired glucose tolerance. J Clin Invest 100:530–537, 1997.

177. Virtanen KA, Lonnroth P, Parkkola R, et al: Glucose uptake and perfusion in subcutaneous and visceral adipose tissue during insulin stimulation in nonobese and obese subjects. J Clin Endocrinol Metab 87:3902–3910, 2002.

178. Swislocki ALM, Chen Y-DI, Golay A, et al: Insulin suppression of plasma free-fatty acid concentration in normal individuals and patients with Type 2 (non-insulin-dependent) diabetes mellitus. Diabetologia 30:622–626, 1987.

179. Puhakainen I, Koivisto VA, Yki-Jarvinen H: Lipolysis and gluconeogenesis from glycerol are increased in patients with non-insulin-dependent diabetes mellitus. J Clin Endocrinol Metab 75:789–794, 1992.

180. Roden M, Price TB, Perseghin G, et al: Mechanism of free fatty acid induced insulin resistance in humans. J Clin Invest 97:2859–2865, 1996.

181. Boden G: Free fatty acids, insulin resistance and type 2 diabetes mellitus. Proc Assoc Am Physicians 111:241–248, 1999.

182. Gumbiner B, Mucha JF, Lindstrom JE, et al: Differential effects of acute hypertriglyceridemia on insulin action and insulin receptor autophosphorylation. Am J Physiol 270:E424–E429, 1996.

183. Kruszynska YT, Worrall DS, Ofrecio J, et al: Fatty acid-induced insulin resistance: Decreased muscle PI3-kinase activation but unchanged Akt phosphorylation. J Clin Endocrinol Metab 87:226–234, 2002.

184. Griffin ME, Marcucci MJ, Cline GW, et al: Free fatty acid-induced insulin resistance is associated with activation of protein kinase C theta and alterations in the insulin signaling cascade. Diabetes 48:1270–1274, 1999.

185. Oakes ND, Cooney GJ, Camilleri S, et al: Mechanisms of liver and muscle insulin resistance induced by chronic high-fat feeding. Diabetes 46:1768–1774, 1997.

186. Schmitz-Peiffer C, Browne CL, Oakes ND, et al: Alterations in the expression and cellular localization of protein kinase C isozymes epsilon and theta are associated with insulin resistance in skeletal muscle of the high-fat-fed rat. Diabetes 46:169–178, 1997.

187. Anderwald C, Bernroider E, Krssak M, et al: Effect of insulin treatment in type 2 diabetic patients on intracellular lipid content in liver and skeletal muscle. Diabetes 51:3025–3032, 2002.

188. Kraegen EW, Clark PW, Jenkins AB, et al: Development of muscle insulin resistance after liver insulin resistance in high-fat-fed rats. Diabetes 40:1397–1403, 1991.

189. Pan DA, Lillioja S, Kriketos AD, et al: Skeletal muscle triglyceride levels are inversely related to insulin action. Diabetes 46:983–988, 1997.

190. Ellis BA, Poynten A, Lowy AJ, et al: Long-chain acyl-CoA esters as indicators of lipid metabolism and insulin sensitivity in rat and human muscle. Am J Physiol 279:E554–E560, 2000.

191. Bolinder J, Krager L, Ostman J, Arner P: Differences at the receptor and post-receptor levels between human omental and subcutaneous adipose tissue in the action of insulin on lipolysis. Diabetes 32:117–123, 1983.

192. Rebuffe-Scrive M, Andersson B, Olbe L, Bjorntrop P: Metabolism of adipose tissue in intraabdominal depots of nonobese men and women. Metabolism 38:453–458, 1989.

193. Vague J: La différénciation sexuelle, facteur determinant des formes de l'obésité. Presse méd 55:339–340, 1947.

194. Ladipus L, Bengtsson C, Larsson B, et al: Distribution of adipose tissue and risk of cardiovascular disease and death: 12 year follow-up of participants in the study of women in Gothenburg, Sweden. Br Med J 289:1257–1261, 1984.

195. Ohlson LO, Larsson B, Svärdsudd K, et al: The influence of body fat distribution on the incidence of diabetes mellitus: 13.5 years of follow-up of the participants in the study of men born in 1913. Diabetes 34:1055–1058, 1985.

196. Goodpaster BH, Thaete FL, Simoneau J-A, Kelley DE: Subcutaneous abdominal fat and thigh muscle composition predict insulin sensitivity independently of visceral fat. Diabetes 46:1579–1585, 1997.

197. Robbins DC, Horton ES, Tulp O, Sims EA: Familial partial lipodystrophy: Complications of obesity in the non-obese? Metabolism 31:445–452, 1982.

198. Reitman ML, Mason MM, Moitra J, et al: Transgenic mice lacking white fat: Models for understanding human lipoatrophic diabetes. Ann N Y Acad Sci 892:289–296, 1999.

199. Kim JK, Gavrilova O, Chen Y, et al: Mechanism of insulin resistance in A-ZIP/F-1 fatless mice. J Biol Chem 275:8456–8460, 2000.

200. Gavrilova O, Marcus-Samuels B, Graham D, et al: Surgical implantation of adipose tissue reverses diabetes in lipoatrophic mice. J Clin Invest 105:271–278, 2000.

201. Frayn KN: Adipose tissue as a buffer for daily lipid flux. Diabetologia 45:1201–1210, 2002.

202. Ravussin E, Smith SR: Increased fat intake, impaired fat oxidation, and failure of fat cell proliferation result in ectopic fat storage, insulin resistance and type 2 diabetes mellitus. Ann N Y Acad Sci 967:363–378, 2002.

203. Groop LC, Saloranta C, Shank M, et al: The role of free fatty acid metabolism in the pathogenesis of insulin resistance in obesity and non-insulin-dependent diabetes mellitus. J Clin Endocrinol Metab 72:96–107, 1991.

204. Czech MP: Cellular basis of insulin insensitivity in large rat adipocytes. J Clin Invest 57:1523–1532, 1976.

205. Olefsky JM: Insensitivity of large rat adipocytes to the antilipolytic effects of insulin. J Lipid Res 18:459–464, 1977.

206. Weyer C, Foley JE, Bogardus C, et al: Enlarged subcutaneous abdominal

adipocyte size, but not obesity itself, predicts Type II diabetes independent of insulin resistance. Diabetologia 43:1498–1506, 2000.

207. Danforth E Jr: Failure of adipocyte differentiation causes Type II diabetes mellitus? Nat Genet 26:13, 2000.

208. Bell GI, Xiang KS, Newman MV, et al: Gene for non-insulin-dependent diabetes mellitus (maturity onset diabetes of the young subtype) is linked to DNA polymorphism on human chromosome 20q. Proc Natl Acad Sci U S A 88:1484–1488, 1991.

209. Yamagata K, Furuta J, Oda N, et al: Mutations in the hepatocyte nuclear factor 4-α gene in maturity-onset diabetes of the young (MODY 1). Nature 384:458–460, 1996.

210. Permutt MA, Chiu KC, Tanizawa Y: Glucokinase and NIDDM: A candidate gene that paid off. Diabetes 41:1367–1372, 1992.

211. Miller SP, Anand GR, Karschnia EJ, et al: Characterization of glucokinase mutations associated with maturity-onset diabetes of the young type 2 (MODY-2): Different glucokinase defects lead to a common phenotype. Diabetes 48:1645–1651, 1999.

212. Yamagata K, Oda N, Kaisaki PJ, et al: Mutations in the hepatocyte nuclear factor-1α gene in maturity onset diabetes of the young (MODY 3). Nature 384:455–458, 1996.

213. Stoffers DA, Ferrer J, Clarke WL, Habener JF: Early-onset type II diabetes mellitus (MODY 4) linked to IPF1. Nat Genet 117:138–139, 1997.

214. Horikawa Y, Iwasaki N, Hara M, et al: Mutation in hepatocyte nuclear factor-1β gene (TCF2) associated with MODY. Nat Genet 17:384–385, 1997.

215. Malecki MY, Jhala US, Antonellis A, et al: Mutations in NEUROD1 are associated with the development of type 2 diabetes mellitus. Nat Genet 23:323–328, 1999.

216. Frayling TM, McCarthy MI, Walker M, et al: No evidence for linkage at candidate type 2 diabetes susceptibility loci on chromosomes 12 and 20 in United Kingdom Caucasians. J Clin Endocrinol Metab 85:853–857, 2000.

217. Macfarlane WM, Frayling TM, Ellard S, et al: Missense mutations in the insulin promoter factor-1 gene predispose to type 2 diabetes. J Clin Invest 104:R33–R39, 1999.

218. Hager J, Zouali H, Velho G, Froguel P: Insulin receptor substrate (IRS-1) gene polymorphisms in French NIDDM families. Lancet 342:1430, 1993.

219. Barroso I, Gurnell M, Crowley VEF, et al: Dominant negative mutations in human PPARγ are associated with severe insulin resistance, diabetes and hypertension. Nature 402:880–883, 1999.

220. Altshuler D, Hirschhorn JN, Klannemark M, et al: The common PPARgamma Pro12Ala polymorphism is associated with decreased risk of

type 2 diabetes. Nat Genet 26:76–80, 2000.

221. Hara K, Boutin P, Mori Y, et al: Genetic variation in the gene encoding adiponectin is associated with an increased risk of type 2 diabetes in the Japanese population. Diabetes 51:536–540, 2002.

222. Vasseur F, Helbecque N, Dina C, et al: Single-nucleotide polymorphism haplotypes in both the proximal promoter and exon 3 of the APM1 gene modulate adipocyte-secreted adiponectin hormone levels and contribute to the genetic risk for type 2 diabetes in French Caucasians. Hum Mol Genet 11:2607–2614, 2002.

223. O'Rahilly S, Farooqi IS, Yeo GS, Challis BG: Minireview: Human obesity-lessons from monogenic disorders. Endocrinology 144:3757–3764, 2003.

224. Matsuoka N, Ogawa Y, Hosoda K, et al: Human leptin receptor gene in obese Japanese subjects: Evidence against either obesity-causing mutations or association of sequence variants with obesity. Diabetologia 40:1204–1210, 1997.

225. Rolland V, Clement K, Dugail I, et al: Leptin receptor gene in a large cohort of massively obese subjects: No indication of the fa/fa rat mutation: Detection of an intronic variant with no association with obesity. Obes Res 6:122–127, 1998.

226. Widen E, Lehto M, Kanninen T, et al: Association of a polymorphism in the β₃-adrenergic-receptor gene with features of insulin resistance syndrome in Finns. N Engl J Med 333:348–351, 1995.

227. O'Dell SD, Bolla MK, Miller GJ, et al: W64R mutation in β-3-adrenergic receptor gene and weight in a large population sample. Int J Obes 22:377–379, 1998.

228. Large V, Hellstrom L, Reynisdottir S, et al: Human beta-2 adrenoceptor gene polymorphisms are highly frequent in obesity and associate with altered adipocyte beta-2 adrenoceptor function. J Clin Invest 100:3005–3013, 1997.

229. Hanis CL, Boerwinkle E, Chakraborty R, et al: A genome-wide search for human non-insulin-dependent (type 2) diabetes genes reveals a major susceptibility locus on chromosome 2. Nat Genet 13:161–166, 1996.

230. Cox NJ, Frigge M, Nicolae DL, et al: Loci on chromosomes 2 (NIDDM1) and 15 interact to increase susceptibility to diabetes in Mexican Americans. Nat Genet 21:213–215, 1999.

231. Horikawa Y, Oda N, Cox NJ, et al: Genetic variation in the gene encoding calpain-10 is associated with type 2 diabetes mellitus. Nat Genet 26:163–175, 2000.

232. Cox NJ: Challenges in identifying genetic variation affecting susceptibility in type 2 diabetes:

Examples from studies of the calpain-10 gene. Hum Mol Genet 10:2301–2305, 2001.

233. Evans JC, Frayling TM, Cassell PG, et al: Association studies of the calpain-10 gene with type 2 diabetes mellitus in the United Kingdom. Am J Hum Genet 69:544–552, 2001.

234. Shaw JT, Lovelock PK, Kesting JB, et al: Novel susceptibility gene for late-onset NIDDM is localized to human chromosome 12q. Diabetes 47:1793–1796, 1998.

235. Bowden DW, Sale M, Howard TD, et al: Linkage of genetic markers on human chromosomes 20 and 12 to NIDDM in Caucasian sib pairs with a history of diabetic nephropathy. Diabetes 46:882–886, 1997.

236. Stern MP, Duggirala R, Mitchell BD, et al: Evidence for linkage of regions on chromosomes 6 and 11 to plasma glucose concentrations in Mexican Americans. Genome Res 6:724–734, 1996.

237. Ghosh S, Watanabe RM, Hauser ER, et al: Type 2 diabetes: Evidence for linkage on chromosome 20 in 716 Finnish affected sib pairs. Proc Natl Acad Sci U S A 96:2198–2203, 1999.

238. Klupa T, Malecki MT, Pezzolesi M, et al: Further evidence for a susceptibility locus for type 2 diabetes on chromosome 20q13.1–q13.2. Diabetes 49:2212–2216, 2000.

239. Wiltshire S, Hattersley AT, Hitman GA, et al: A genome wide scan for loci predisposing to type 2 diabetes in a UK population (the Diabetes UK Warren 2 Repository). Am J Hum Genet 69:553–569, 2001.

240. Hanson RL, Ehm MG, Pettitt DJ, et al: An autosomal genomic scan for loci linked to type II diabetes mellitus and body-mass index in Pima Indians. Am J Hum Genet 63:1130–1138, 1998.

241. Pratley RE, Thompson DB, Prochazka M, et al: An autosomal genomic scan for loci linked to prediabetic phenotypes in Pima Indians. J Clin Invest 101:1757–1764, 1998.

242. Mitchell BD, Kammerer CM, O'Connell P, et al: Evidence for linkage of postchallenge insulin levels with intestinal fatty acid-binding protein (FABP2) in Mexican-Americans. Diabetes 44:1046–1053, 1995.

243. Humphreys P, McCarthy M, Tuomilehto J, et al: Chromosome 4q locus associated with insulin resistance in Pima Indians: Studies in three European NIDDM populations. Diabetes 43:800–804, 1994.

244. Joshi RL, Lamothe B, Cordonnier N, et al: Targeted disruption of the insulin receptor gene in the mouse results in neonatal lethality. EMBO J 15:1542–1547, 1996.

245. Araki E, Lipes MY, Patti M-E, et al: Alternative pathway of insulin signalling in mice with targeted disruption of the IRS-1 gene. Nature 372:186–190, 1994.

246. Bruning JC, Winnay J, Bonner-Weir S, et al: Development of a novel polygenic model of NIDDM in mice heterozygous for IR and IRS-1 null alleles. Cell 88:561–572, 1997.

247. Kido Y, Burks DJ, Withers D, et al: Tissue-specific insulin resistance in mice with mutations in the insulin receptor, IRS-1, and IRS-2. J Clin Invest 105:199–205, 2000.

248. Terauchi Y, Iwamoto K, Tamemoto H, et al: Development of non-insulin-dependent diabetes mellitus in the double knockout mice with disruption of insulin receptor substrate-1 and beta cell glucokinase genes: Genetic reconstitution of diabetes as a polygenic disease. J Clin Invest 99:861–866, 1997.

249. Scarlett JA, Kolterman OG, Moore P, et al: Insulin resistance and diabetes due to a genetic defect in insulin receptors. J Clin Endocrinol Metab 55:123–132, 1982.

250. Pimenta W, Korytkowski M, Mitrakou A, et al: Pancreatic beta-cell dysfunction as the primary genetic lesion in NIDDM: Evidence from studies in normal glucose-tolerant individuals with a first-degree NIDDM relative. JAMA 273:1855–1861, 1995.

Hyperglycemia Secondary to Nondiabetic Conditions and Therapies

Harold E. Lebovitz

DISORDERS OF THE PANCREAS
  Pancreatectomy
  Chronic Pancreatitis
  Pancreatic Cancer
  Hemochromatosis
  Hemosiderosis
  Cystic Fibrosis

HYPERGLYCEMIA ASSOCIATED WITH ENDOCRINOPATHIES
  Acromegaly
  Growth Hormone Treatment

  Cushing's Syndrome
  Glucagonoma Syndrome
  Somatostatinoma
  Pheochromocytoma

DRUGS THAT CAN CAUSE HYPERGLYCEMIA
  Drugs Affecting β-Cell Function
  Drugs Causing Insulin Resistance
  Atypical Antipsychotic Drugs

Glucose metabolism is regulated by the interplay of the action of pancreatic islet cell hormones with liver, muscle, and adipose tissue. An alteration in the function of any component of this complex glucose homeostatic system brings about compensatory responses in the other components to drive the system back to its homeostatic set points. The key players in regulating this system are the islet hormones insulin and glucagon. Insulin promotes hepatic glucose uptake and glycogenesis, stimulates muscle and adipose tissue glucose uptake and metabolism, and inhibits adipose tissue lipolysis and muscle proteolysis.[1] Glucagon stimulates hepatic gluconeogenic precursor uptake and increases hepatic glycogenolysis, gluconeogenesis, and ketogenesis.[2]

Maintenance of fasting and postprandial plasma glucose levels within the normal range requires insulin secretion by the β cell to be integrated with insulin action in liver and peripheral tissues. Insulin action results from a complex cascade of intracellular substrate phosphorylations and dephosphorylations that lead to regulation of processes as diverse as intermediary metabolism and mitogenesis. Insulin action is easily altered by a variety of both intracellular and extracellular factors. When insulin action affecting glucose metabolism is altered, insulin secretion must change accordingly if normal glucose homeostasis is to remain intact.[3] Any genetic abnormality, environmental factor, or drug that disturbs this relationship will lead to either hyperglycemia or hypoglycemia.

Type 2 diabetes is a heterogeneous disorder in which gene polymorphisms provide the predispositions and environmental factors provide the precipitating causes for hyperglycemia. Many individuals with the genetic predisposition do not manifest impaired glucose tolerance (IGT) or type 2 diabetes throughout their lifetime. If a pathologic condition develops in such individuals, however, or they take a medication that disturbs their compensated state, hyperglycemia will develop. Thus, hyperglycemic states resulting from nondiabetic conditions or therapies can be subdivided into those that can cause hyperglycemia in any individual because they radically interfere with a major regulatory pathway (Table 57-1), and those that precipitate diabetes only in genetically predisposed individuals because they alter the compensated state (Table 57-2). Because of the high prevalence of a genetic predisposition to type 2 diabetes in various populations, it is not always possible to make the distinction with certainty.

DISORDERS OF THE PANCREAS

PANCREATECTOMY

Diabetes mellitus developing after surgical removal of the pancreas is truly an insulin-dependent diabetes mellitus. Metabolically, it is characterized by insulin and glucagon deficiency.[4] The magnitude of the hyperglycemia and its characteristics depend on the quantity of pancreas removed (Table 57-3). Total or near-total pancreatectomy results in severe hyperglycemia, decreased plasma insulin, virtually absent plasma glucagon, and elevated plasma levels of gluconeogenic precursors (alanine, lactate, glycerol).[4–10]

The effect of removal of 50% of the pancreas was studied in 28 normal transplant donors 1 year after surgery.[11] The donors lost a mean of 3.4 kg of body weight, and their mean fasting plasma glucose level had risen by 9 mg/dL (88 ± 7 to 97 ± 16 mg/dL). Similarly, their mean serum glucose concentration 2 hours after an oral glucose load was higher (117 ± 18 to 156 ± 53 mg/dL), and the area under the 5-hour plasma glucose curve after the oral glucose was 19.5% higher. Both the mean fasting plasma insulin concentration and the area under the 5-hour plasma insulin curve were significantly lower than preoperatively (−14% and −31%, respectively). None of the donors had any evidence of deficient pancreatic exocrine function. On further analysis, the investigators noted that 21 of the donors had no significant postoperative change in either plasma glucose or insulin, whereas seven showed a marked increase in the entire 5-hour plasma glucose curve (either IGT or diabetes) with no concomitant increase in the 5-hour plasma insulin curves. The seven donors, in whom some degree of hypoinsulinemia and hyperglycemia had developed, did not have fasting hyperglycemia 1 year postoperatively. Two of the seven were studied from 2 to 7 years after surgery and had not had a further increase in fasting plasma glucose. A recent report of eight donor/recipient pairs evaluated 9 to 18 years after the original surgery indicated that the residual pancreatic mass is a significant determinant of long-term glucose homeostasis.[12] However, other variables were implicated in the discordancy for the development of diabetes. In particular, obesity seemed to be a major factor since all of the individuals (four donors and two recipients) who had developed diabetes were among the eight patients who were obese.[12] The investigators interpreted their

Table 57-1	Conditions that Can Cause Hyperglycemia in the Absence of Genetic Predisposition

Disease of the pancreas
  Pancreatectomy
  Trauma
  Pancreatitis
  Pancreatic carcinoma
  Infiltrative disorder
  Hemochromatosis
  Amyloidosis
  Cystic fibrosis
Overproduction of other islet hormones
  Glucagonoma
  Somatostatinoma
Drugs and toxins
  Pyriminil (Vacor)
  Pentamidine
  Interferon-α
  K_{ATP} channel openers
  Diazoxide
  Phenytoin (Dilantin)

K_{ATP}, ATP-dependent potassium channel.

Table 57-3	Estimated Frequency of Diabetes Reported in Pancreatic Diseases

95% Pancreatectomy	100%
50% Pancreatectomy	0%
Pancreatitis	
Acute	<5%
Chronic calcifying	40%–70%
Chronic noncalcifying	15%–30%
Cystic fibrosis	17%
Carcinoma of the pancreas	23%
Hemochromatosis	50%–60%

insufficiency. A concomitant deficiency of pancreatic polypeptide can contribute to persistent hyperglycemia due to impaired hepatic insulin action.[18] Treatment of an individual with pancreatic diabetes requires insulin, is associated with marked lability in glucose regulation, and is linked with an increased rate of both ketoacidosis and death from hypoglycemia. The development of autonomic neuropathy in a patient with pancreatic diabetes greatly adds to the risk of severe hypoglycemia with insulin treatment.[19]

CHRONIC PANCREATITIS

Chronic pancreatitis accounts for a little less than 1% of cases of diabetes mellitus in Western countries and Japan.[20–23] In tropical countries, where nonalcoholic calcific pancreatitis is common, the incidence may be somewhat higher but reliable data are not available. The development of diabetes mellitus in patients with chronic pancreatitis is highest in those with calcific disease (55%–70%) and less in those with noncalcific disease (30%).[24] The prevalence of diabetes in patients with chronic pancreatitis increases with increasing duration of pancreatitis and with increasing exocrine deficiency.[22,25–29]

The inflammatory response causes loss of exocrine tissue and extensive fibrosis. The islets of Langerhans are relatively resistant and undergo pathologic changes only late in the disease. Chronic pancreatitis is associated with loss of functioning β cells and a somewhat lesser loss of α cells.[15,30–36] The hormonal alterations seen are a decrease in insulin secretion in response to nutrients, followed later by a decrease in fasting C peptide levels. Plasma C peptide levels rather than insulin levels may be a better assessment of insulin secretion because associated liver disease may change hepatic extraction rates of insulin. With progressive chronic pancreatitis, insulin secretion falls even lower. Glucagon secretion is impaired in moderate to severe chronic pancreatitis. Insulin resistance frequently develops in such individuals.

Diabetes mellitus is seen after several years of chronic pancreatitis. In an unselected series of patients with chronic pancreatitis, 35% had type 1 diabetes, 31% had type 2 diabetes or IGT, and 34% had normal glucose tolerance.[37] The nature of the diabetes is a result of the severity of the chronic pancreatitis. Mild pancreatitis may be associated only with IGT, whereas severe pancreatitis will be primarily associated with insulin-dependent (type 1) diabetes. Patients with chronic pancreatitis and diabetes mellitus fail to secrete glucagon in response to hypoglycemia. If they have concomitant autonomic neuropathy, they are extremely susceptible to severe and prolonged hypoglycemia.

Treatment of diabetes mellitus in patients with chronic pancreatitis should entail the use of small doses of short-acting or rapid acting insulins to manage the hyperglycemia, replacement enzymes for the malnutrition and malabsorption, and elimination of the use of alcoholic beverages.[24,34,38,39] Surgery with subtotal resection or near-total resection may be necessary to relieve severe pain.[40,41] In such patients, successful islet allotransplants and autotransplants

data as "suggesting that obesity should be a contraindication to donation of pancreatic segments and that donors should assiduously avoid becoming obese."[12]

Sun and colleagues studied the metabolic effects of removing 20% to 88% of the pancreas in dogs and found that no significant metabolic changes occurred until approximately 50% was removed.[13]

From the data available, it seems reasonable to conclude that the metabolic abnormalities after pancreatectomy are likely to be clinically relevant at 50% and greater removal and that progressively more metabolic abnormalities occur as the extent of pancreatectomy increases. The concomitant presence of insulin resistance further increases the likelihood of metabolic abnormalities.

The major characteristics of the development of diabetes mellitus after extensive pancreatectomy are an absence of glucagon secretion and marked impairment in insulin secretion. The absence of glucagon slows, but does not interfere with, the development of hyperglycemia and ketonemia after insulin withdrawal.[4,6] This observation indicates that glucagon is not necessary for development of the metabolic abnormalities of insulin-dependent diabetes mellitus. The absence of glucagon secretion does, however, leave a pancreatectomized individual with diabetes at high risk for severe hypoglycemia during insulin treatment.[14–17] This situation is exaggerated by the associated nutritional deficiencies and weight loss that ordinarily accompany exocrine pancreatic

Table 57-2	Conditions that Precipitate Hyperglycemia in Individuals with a Genetic Predisposition to Type 2 Diabetes

Endocrinopathies
  Acromegaly
  Cushing's syndrome
  Pheochromocytoma
  Hyperthyroidism
Drugs
  Interfere with insulin secretion
    β-Blockers
    Diuretics
  Impair insulin action
    Glucocorticoids
    Oral contraceptives
    Nicotinic acid

in the liver have been able to maintain near normoglycemia.[42] The hepatic islet cell transplants were able to secrete insulin in response to nutrients but were unable to secrete glucagon in response to hypoglycemia.[16,17]

Pancreatic exocrine function has been reported to be reduced in some type 1 and type 2 diabetic patients. This has been explained as a complication of the diabetes. A retrospective analysis of pancreatograms of patients with known diabetes has suggested that chronic pancreatitis may be much more common as a cause of diabetes than previously thought.[42] Thirty-eight type 1 and 118 type 2 diabetic patients had endoscopic retrograde cholangiopancreatography (ERCP) studies for varying reasons. Pancreatic ducts were classified as normal in 23.3% and chronic pancreatitis degree I, II, and III in 22.7%, 32.7%, and 21.3%, respectively.[43] The investigators suggested that a substantial number of patients with primary diabetes mellitus have a concomitant chronic pancreatitis or perhaps many cases of primary diabetes mellitus are diabetes secondary to chronic pancreatitis.

PANCREATIC CANCER

Diabetes mellitus is known to occur more frequently in patients with pancreatic cancer than in the general population.[44–46] Published data indicate that as many as 70% of patients with pancreatic carcinoma have either impaired glucose tolerance or frank diabetes mellitus and that 60% of those improve their glucose metabolism after surgery.[47] Wakasugi and colleagues have reported that 53.1% of patients with invasive ductal pancreatic carcinoma had diabetes mellitus and in 45.9% it was thought to be secondary to the carcinoma.[48] The reasons for this association have been the subject of much speculation. Some studies show that diabetes mellitus is associated with an increased risk (2.15–4.9 in men) for pancreatic cancer.[49,50] Other studies indicate that in the majority of patients with pancreatic carcinoma, the diabetes is secondary to some effect of the cancer that causes insulin resistance and impairs the function of the normal β cells.[51–53] A multicenter case control study of 720 patients with pancreatic cancer addressed this issue.[44] The prevalence of diabetes mellitus in the patients with pancreatic cancer was 22.8%, whereas that in the matched control population was 8.3%. The pancreatic cancer patients were characterized as having type 2 diabetes. Recent diagnosis of diabetes had been made in 40.2% of the pancreatic cancer patients with diabetes as contrasted with only 3.3% of the control population with diabetes (Table 57-4). A higher percentage of the control population with diabetes had had their diabetes for greater than 15 years than did the pancreatic cancer population with diabetes (see Table 57-4). These data support the notion that in a small number of patients, diabetes mellitus predisposes to the development of pancreatic cancer, but that in the majority of cases, pancreatic cancer causes the development of diabetes mellitus.

The possible mechanisms by which pancreatic cancer could contribute to the development of type 2 diabetes are: (1) destruction of islets, (2) impairment of the insulin secretory mechanism, (3) development of insulin resistance, and (4) tumor-related pancreatitis. Insulin and C peptide measurements during oral glucose tolerance testing in patients with pancreatic cancer have shown abnormal β-cell function with reduced plasma C peptide responses in 50% of patients and increased plasma proinsulin to C peptide ratios.[54,55] Insulin resistance has been demonstrated in the majority of patients with pancreatic carcinoma.[56–58] Morphometric studies of tumor-free regions of the pancreas have shown reduced β-cell populations.[59] An inverse correlation was noted between the number of β cells and the fasting plasma glucose concentration. These data can be interpreted as indicating that pancreatic cancers produce substances or responses that destroy normal β cells.[57–60] The presence of diabetes in patients with pancreatic cancer predicts that the tumor is less likely to be resectable, and the patient has a poorer prognosis than if diabetes is not present.[46]

Patients with pancreatic cancer appear to have type 2 diabetes, and most have been treated with oral antihyperglycemic agents.[45,46]

HEMOCHROMATOSIS

Hemochromatosis is an autosomal recessive genetic disorder that results in excessive deposition of iron in parenchymal cells of the liver, pancreas, muscle, heart, anterior pituitary, and other organs.[61,62] The clinical diagnosis in the past was made by the findings of diabetes mellitus, hepatomegaly, and skin pigmentation. More recently, it is recognized by biochemical and genetic testing.[63] The first phenotypic expression of the disease is an elevation in serum transferrin saturation. This abnormality is followed by iron accumulation in the tissues and an elevation in the serum ferritin concentration. Early clinical findings are related to hepatic dysfunction and joint symptoms. Clinical diabetes mellitus and skin pigmentation occur relatively late in the course of the disease.[62] A candidate gene for human leukocyte antigen-linked hemochromatosis has been cloned and a mutation (C282Y) identified that may account for 60% or more of cases of hereditary hemochromatosis.

Diabetes mellitus has been reported in 50% to 60% of patients with hemochromatosis.[62,64] Another 20% to 30% had glucose intolerance. These figures represent data from older series in which the diagnosis was made late in the course of the disease. Diabetes mellitus is more frequent in patients who have a family history of diabetes mellitus. The natural history of the development of glucose intolerance in hemochromatosis is not available.

The metabolic studies that have been done show that patients with hemochromatosis have marked insulin resistance. Histologic study of the pancreas shows iron deposits that are greatest in the acinar cells but do involve the islet cells. Insulin secretion in response to glucose or arginine is decreased; however, glucagon secretory responses to arginine are increased and unaffected by glucose.[65,66] The data are compatible with a marked reduction in β-cell function and no disturbance in α-cell function. The hyperglycemia is a result of the insulin resistance and the decreased β-cell function. The prevalence of diabetes mellitus could be greatly reduced by early diagnosis of hemochromatosis and the institution of phlebotomy therapy.

Therapy for patients with hemochromatosis and clinical diabetes frequently requires insulin (40% to 50% of patients), although no systematic studies of therapy have been done.[63] Reduction of tissue iron stores, although most beneficial in the early stages of disease, can nonetheless help improve glycemic control in 35% to 45% of patients.[61,62]

HEMOSIDEROSIS

Excessive iron deposition occurs in a variety of conditions other than primary hemochromatosis. In thalassemia major, frequent blood transfusions are necessary and may lead to massive iron overload. The reported prevalence of diabetes

| Table 57-4 | Interval between Diagnosis of Diabetes and Diagnosis of Pancreatic Cancer or Date of Examination of Control Population |

Duration (yr)	Pancreatic Cancer Patients	Control Patients	P Value
0	66 (40.2%)	2 (3.3%)	<.001
1–14	81 (49.4%)	35 (58.3%)	NS
≥15	17 (10.4%)	23 (38.3%)	<.001

mellitus in treated thalassemia major is about 16%. This figure is highly correlated with the number of blood transfusions and the duration of disease. The incidence of IGT is reported to be 60%.[67]

Further evidence that excess tissue iron deposits themselves are responsible for many of the metabolic abnormalities seen in hemochromatosis and thalassemia major comes from studies in rural male Bantus.[68] Many Bantus drink alcoholic beverages that are brewed in iron containers and ingest in excess of 100 mg of iron per day. In those individuals, the prevalence of diabetes mellitus is 10-fold higher than in the nonalcoholic beverage–consuming males.

Mechanistic studies in thalassemia major patients with normal, impaired, and diabetic glucose tolerance tests showed that increased iron stores are associated with the development of insulin resistance and a delay in early insulin secretion.[69] A correlation between increased iron stores in normal women and the development of type 2 diabetes has recently been demonstrated in the Nurses Health Study.[70]

CYSTIC FIBROSIS

Cystic fibrosis (CF) is a monogenetic disorder with abnormal cyclic adenosine monophosphate–regulated Cl^- channel activity. Organs as diverse as the lung, exocrine pancreas, large and small intestines, hepatobiliary system, and sweat glands are involved. Failure to secrete Na^+, HCO_3^-, and water leads to retention of enzymes in the pancreas and ultimately to destruction of pancreatic tissue.[71–73] Histologic examination of the pancreas in patients with CF shows fatty infiltration, necrosis, and fibrosis of the exocrine pancreas. Islet cell architecture is disrupted and the absolute number of pancreatic islets diminished. Those islets that are present show significant decreases in β cells, α cells, and pancreatic polypeptide-producing cells and increases in δ (somatostatin-producing) cells. Islet amyloid deposits have been found in 69% of diabetic CF cases examined.

Diabetes mellitus requiring medical therapy (usually insulin) has been reported in 4.9% of CF patients of all ages in a large European study of 1348 patients[74] and in 5.1% of 18,627 patients of all ages monitored at CF centers in the United States and Canada.[71] Diabetes mellitus occurs more often in individuals who are homozygous for the most common CF mutation, ΔF508.[71,75,76] Diabetes mellitus occurs with greater frequency with increasing age, being reported in 32% of Danish patients who were older than 25 years. Routine oral glucose tolerance testing suggests that of the total CF population aged 5 years or older, 35% have normal glucose tolerance, 37% have IGT, 17% have CF-related diabetes without fasting hyperglycemia, and 11% have CF-related diabetes with fasting hyperglycemia.

Several features of CF-related diabetes are noteworthy. Autoantibodies to pancreatic heat shock protein 60 have been found to precede the development of glucose intolerance (IGT and diabetes) and to subsequently decline with the onset of glucose intolerance.[77] The development of diabetes in patients with CF is initially characterized by abnormal oral glucose tolerance and a delay in oral glucose–stimulated insulin secretion, followed later by a decrease in total insulin, glucagon, and pancreatic polypeptide secretion.[78] First-phase insulin secretion after intravenous glucose is markedly reduced in CF patients compared to matched controls. Cystic fibrosis IGT patients have normal plasma free fatty acid levels as compared to matched controls.[79] Their plasma tumor necrosis factor-alpha levels are elevated and they have insulin resistance as measured by the hyperinsulinemic euglycemic clamp.[79] Decreased translocation of GLUT 4 glucose transporters in muscle was observed during the peak insulin effect. Patients with CF have an increase in hepatic glucose production and are resistant to suppression of hepatic glucose production by insulin even in the nondiabetic state.[80] Peripheral

insulin sensitivity is increased in healthy nondiabetic individuals with CF, but insulin resistance occurs later as IGT and diabetes develop and the patients get more complications from their CF.[81] The development of diabetes worsens pulmonary function and other clinical manifestations of CF and may increase mortality by up to sixfold.[82] Insulin treatment appears to improve this deterioration. Hyperglycemia in patients with CF can be intermittent or permanent. Intermittent hyperglycemia occurs with glucocorticoid therapy, infections, or stress and needs to be treated with insulin until it resolves. Permanent hyperglycemia is always treated with insulin.[71,73] It is likely that CF patients progress from intermittent hyperglycemia to permanent hyperglycemia as more pancreatic destruction is occurring.

HYPERGLYCEMIA ASSOCIATED WITH ENDOCRINOPATHIES

In the complex regulation of fuel hemostasis, many hormones other than insulin play a complementary role. Growth hormone, itself, and through its synthesis of insulin-like growth factor 1 (IGF-1,) controls many aspects of amino acid transport, protein synthesis, and lipid metabolism. Glucagon and catecholamines are counterregulatory hormones that protect against hypoglycemia and provide extra glucose when needed during stress states. Glucocorticoids exert both a permissive role in the normal physiologic regulation of gluconeogenesis and a pharmacologic role in providing increased glucose availability during stress. Somatostatin is a paracrine hormone that appears to act locally to help regulate the normal secretory patterns of growth hormone, insulin, glucagon, and several gastrointestinal hormones.

Autonomous excess secretion of these hormones leads to hyperglycemia. The mechanisms responsible for the action of these various hormones are described in detail in other chapters. This section will address the unique characteristics of the hyperglycemia as it relates to each endocrinopathy and its treatment.

ACROMEGALY

Acromegaly is characterized by excessive and autonomous secretion of growth hormone and IGF-1.[83,84] The prevalence of overt diabetes mellitus reported in different series of acromegalic patients ranges from 30% to 56%.[83,85] IGT may be present in as many as 36% of acromegalic patients.[83] In a specific population, the percentage of acromegalic patients in whom diabetes mellitus will develop depends on the prevalence of predisposition to type 2 diabetes in the population and the magnitude of elevation of serum IGF-1 levels.

Elevated growth hormone and IGF-1 levels cause excess hepatic glucose production and impaired insulin-mediated muscle glucose uptake.[86–88] This insulin resistance is correlated with circulating IGF-1 levels and has been demonstrated by the euglycemic hyperinsulinemic clamp and the minimal model techniques.

Reduction in circulating growth hormone and IGF-1 levels by successful surgical removal of the tumor-producing growth hormone or growth hormone–releasing factor results in significant improvement in glycemic control in acromegalic patients with diabetes mellitus.[87,89] Recent data suggest that circulating growth hormone must be lowered to 2 ng/L and IGF-1 lowered to the normal range to be considered curative.[84,90,91] Transsphenoidal surgery achieves growth hormone levels less than 5 ng/L in approximately 60% of patients. Curative levels are attained in about 70% of patients with microadenomas (<10 mm in diameter), but considerably less in those with macroadenomas of the pituitary.[84,90]

Use of the somatostatin analogue octreotide to treat acromegaly as either primary medical therapy or to supplement prior inadequate surgical treatment or radiotherapy has allowed greater and more consistent reductions in circulating growth hormone and IGF-1 levels to be achieved (GH levels ≤ 5 ng/L in 65% and ≤ 2 ng/L in 40% and IGF-1 levels in the normal range in 64% of patients).[90–92]

Treatment of acromegalic patients with octreotide presents several issues with respect to glucose metabolism.[90–93] Reduction of circulating growth hormone and IGF-1 levels will decrease insulin resistance and should lead to improvement in glycemic control in subjects with diabetes mellitus or IGT. However, pharmacologic doses of a somatostatin analogue also reduce insulin secretion (decreased insulinogenic index), and such a reduction should cause a deterioration in glucose tolerance. Thus, in any particular patient, octreotide therapy will modify glucose metabolism in accordance with these competing effects. Approximately two thirds of acromegalic patients with diabetes mellitus are treated with insulin and one third with oral hypoglycemic agents. Octreotide treatment in patients with diabetes mellitus and acromegaly frequently leads to improvement in glycemic control as measured by a reduction in the insulin dose, conversion from insulin therapy to oral hypoglycemic agent therapy, or conversion from oral hypoglycemic agent therapy to dietary management.[90,93] Some patients (those with more severe insulin deficiency), however, will have significant deterioration in glycemic control.[91,93] IGT or even frank diabetes mellitus may develop in acromegalic patients with normal glucose tolerance before octreotide treatment (as high as 20% and 29%, respectively) when higher doses of octreotide are given.[93]

Appropriate treatment of acromegaly is necessary to reduce the increased mortality (observed-to-expected death, 2.68) that has been seen in the past.[94] This increased mortality is due to cardiovascular, cerebrovascular, and neoplastic diseases. The best determinants of outcome in acromegalic patients are age at diagnosis, interval between symptoms and diagnosis, and mean chronic circulating growth hormone and IGF-1 levels. Because insulin resistance and diabetes mellitus contribute significantly to cardiovascular risk, aggressive diagnosis and management of the diabetes mellitus associated with acromegaly is essential.

GROWTH HORMONE TREATMENT

The availability of recombinant DNA technology to make human growth hormone has provided an opportunity to treat many growth hormone–deficient individuals with this hormone. One of the considerations in treatment with recombinant human growth hormone is the question of whether chronic treatment can lead to the development of diabetes mellitus.[95] A recent study of glucose metabolism in 23,333 children and adolescents treated with human growth hormone found a sixfold greater frequency of type 2 diabetes mellitus than predicted (34.4 cases per 100,000 years of growth hormone treatment).[96] In contrast, the frequency of type 1 diabetes was the same as expected. The data suggest that growth hormone treatment accelerates the development of type 2 diabetes in individuals who have a genetic predisposition.

CUSHING'S SYNDROME

Glucocorticoids are insulin antagonistic hormones.[97] When administered in pharmacologic doses, they increase basal hepatic glucose production and decrease the insulin-mediated effects of suppressing hepatic glucose production and increasing muscle glucose uptake.[98–101] Insulin secretion is increased as a consequence of the hepatic and peripheral insulin resistance.

Pharmacologic concentrations of glucocorticoids occur in disease states associated with autonomous secretion of adrenal cortical hormones (Cushing's syndrome) or through administration of such agents for the treatment of nonendocrine diseases. When sustained pharmacologic concentrations of glucocorticoids occur in normal individuals, increased insulin secretion maintains fasting plasma glucose within the normal range, but the postprandial plasma glucose concentration is elevated above normal in 25% to 90% of such individuals depending on the magnitude of plasma glucocorticoid elevation.[102] Individuals with limited β-cell insulin secretory reserve are subject to fasting hyperglycemia and type 2 diabetes mellitus. Ten percent to 20% of patients with Cushing's syndrome have overt type 2 diabetes mellitus.[103–107] In renal transplant recipients receiving chronic corticosteroid therapy, steroid-induced diabetes mellitus has been reported to develop in as few as 5.5% and as many as 46% of patients.[108,109] Factors that influence the development of diabetes mellitus during corticosteroid therapy are a family history of diabetes mellitus, increasing age, obesity, and both average daily and total cumulative corticosteroid dose.[110,111] In individuals with a previous onset of diabetes mellitus, administration of glucocorticoids significantly worsens glycemic control and will require modification of diabetes management.

Recent studies have documented that steroid-induced diabetes mellitus occurs in adrenal disorders other than those associated with frank Cushing's syndrome. Measurement of oral glucose tolerance in 64 consecutive patients with "nonfunctioning" adrenal adenomas identified normal glucose tolerance in 25, glucose intolerance in 17, and diabetes mellitus in 22, including six patients with previously diagnosed diabetes mellitus.[112] Autonomous cortisol secretion without the clinical stigmata of Cushing's syndrome has recently been recognized as a preclinical Cushing's syndrome. A retrospective study of 63 such individuals found that 17.5% had diabetes mellitus.[113] A cross-sectional study of 90 obese, poorly controlled type 2 diabetic patients found three to have the preclinical Cushing's syndrome abnormality.[94] Excess IGT and diabetes mellitus have been reported in hypopituitary adults receiving conventional replacement therapy and may be related to the intermittently higher plasma levels occurring after dosing than would occur under normal hypothalamic-pituitary-adrenal axis function.[114]

Some insight into the mechanisms by which glucocorticoids cause diabetes mellitus was obtained by investigating the effect of the administration of dexamethasone on oral glucose tolerance, on glucose turnover under basal conditions and during glucose infusion, and on the insulin response during hyperglycemic clamp studies in normal individuals who had previously been characterized as either low insulin responders or high insulin responders.[115] Dexamethasone caused a higher fasting plasma glucose concentration, a greater rise in plasma glucose, and a lesser rise in plasma insulin during the oral glucose tolerance test in the low insulin responders than in the higher insulin responders. A diabetic oral glucose tolerance test developed in three of the six low and none of the six high insulin responders. Dexamethasone increased hepatic glucose production only in the low insulin responders and increased insulin secretion during the hyperglycemic clamp study only in the high insulin responders. The conclusion drawn from these studies is that type 2 diabetes develops when plasma glucocorticoids are elevated in individuals with limited β-cell secretory function.

Steroid-induced diabetes may be permanent or transient. In general, insulin is required for treatment if the fasting plasma glucose concentration exceeds 180 mg/dL.[116] At lesser levels of fasting hyperglycemia, many physicians treat the hyperglycemia with oral antihyperglycemic agents. Very few studies have evaluated the efficacy of pharmacologic treatment of steroid-induced diabetes mellitus. Because insulin resistance is a major abnormality, perhaps the combination of insulin sensitizers and insulin would be most effective. A reduction in corticosteroid dose or secretion improves glycemic control and in some individuals may even reverse the diabetes. The more severely elevated the fasting plasma glucose concentration, the less likely it is that reducing corticosteroid levels will reverse the diabetes. Ketoacidosis is very uncommon with steroid-induced diabetes or Cushing's syndrome. Hyperosmolar non-ketotic coma, however, is not uncommon.[117]

GLUCAGONOMA SYNDROME

Glucagon plays a primary role in facilitating the uptake of amino acids by the liver and their conversion into glucose by gluconeogenesis. Excess and unregulated glucagon secretion alone or in conjunction with other islet hormones occurs in some islet cell tumors. A classic syndrome has been described in individuals who have tumors secreting high quantities of glucagon. This syndrome was initially recognized in 1974 and is referred to as the glucagonoma syndrome.[118] Features of this syndrome include necrolytic migratory erythema, mild non-insulin-requiring type 2 diabetes mellitus, glossitis, angular cheilitis, weight loss, and anemia.[119,120] Laboratory studies show markedly elevated plasma glucagon levels and severe hypoaminoacidemia (<25% normal).

Glucagonomas are quite rare, with a reported incidence of one case per 20 to 200 million population. Several reviews of the literature indicate that most of the tumors occur in the tail of the pancreas (reported in 54% to 68%), have an average tumor diameter of 3.6 cm (but as many as one-third are less than 2 cm), are malignant in about two-thirds of cases, and have metastases in other organs in 51% to 54% of patients at the time of diagnosis.[121,122] The diabetes mellitus is characterized by mild hyperglycemia and is nonketotic. The tumors are relatively slow growing, and the 10-year survival rate is 52% in those with metastases and 64% in those without metastases.

The hyperglycemia is due to excess glucose production by the liver. The hypoaminoacidemia results from an increase in amino acid clearance.[123] The necrolytic migratory erythema, glossitis, weight loss, and anemia are, in large part, a consequence of the protein malnutrition.[120] Deep venous thrombosis that is not associated with coagulation disorders is quite common.

All the components of the syndrome are improved if the hyperglucagonemia can be reduced. Treatment is surgical removal of the tumor, followed by hepatic artery embolization if necessary for liver metastases.[120,124] Octreotide treatment has been very effective in reducing residual plasma glucagon levels.[120,124] Cytotoxic agents such as streptozotocin and fluorouracil may be valuable as additional modes of therapy. Zinc and amino acid supplementation have been used to treat the rash but are relatively ineffective if the plasma glucagon levels remain very high. Antiplatelet therapy should be used to prevent venous thrombosis. The hyperglycemia, though mild, generally requires treatment with an antihyperglycemic agent. Insulin would appear to be the most appropriate agent, although few or no clinical outcome data are available to support this hypothesis. Treatment of the hyperglucagonemia will ameliorate the hyperglycemia in most cases.[124]

SOMATOSTATINOMA

Case reports of patients with hyperglycemia and a pancreatic tumor containing large quantities of somatostatin first appeared in 1977.[125,126] One of those patients became euglycemic after complete resection of the tumor. Since that time it has been recognized that large somatostatin-producing pancreatic tumors may be associated with a clinical syndrome consisting of hyperglycemia, cholelithiasis, steatorrhea, and hypochlorhydria.[127]

Somatostatin-producing tumors arising from the gastrointestinal tract and the pancreatic islets have been reported.[128] Duodenal somatostatinomas with and without von Recklinghausen's disease are seldom associated with recognizable somatostatinoma syndrome, often contain psammoma bodies, and are less often associated with demonstrable metastases at the time of surgery.[128] The clinical features of pancreatic somatostatin-producing tumors are quite variable, and this variation is related to differences in quantity and qualitative features of the somatostatin variants that are synthesized and secreted by these tumors.[129–131] Marked differences in the degree to which insulin, glucagon, and growth hormone secretion are affected in various patients with pancreatic somatostatin-producing tumors probably account for some of the variation in the clinical syndrome. Hyperglycemia in patients with pancreatic somatostatinomas can vary from mild-to-modest hyperglycemia to severe diabetic ketoacidosis.[128,132,133]

Somatostatin infusions in humans are associated with a pronounced decrease in bile flow and bile acid secretion and an increase in bile cholesterol saturation.[134] In vitro, somatostatin has a direct inhibitory effect on cholecystokinin stimulation of gallbladder contraction.[135] These observations provide a basis for understanding the cholelithiasis and steatorrhea commonly seen with pancreatic somatostatinomas. Additionally, they explain the development of gallstones in 23.5% of acromegalic patients treated with octreotide during the first year of treatment.[90]

The hyperglycemia seen as part of the somatostatinoma syndrome is most likely related to suppression of insulin secretion. In some patients, a relative insulin deficiency leads to reduced peripheral glucose utilization without impairing suppression of hepatic glucose production.[136] In more severe suppression of insulin secretion, both features of insulin action are reduced.

Somatostatin-producing tumors are quite rare, usually asymptomatic, or only mildly symptomatic and frequently undiagnosed for many years. The diagnosis is frequently made late and the prognosis is poor because of extensive metastases. The use of somatostatin receptor scintigraphy with indium 111-labeled pentetreotide promises to improve the ability to detect somatostatinomas earlier.[137] Early diagnosis and surgical removal can lead to cure, but medical treatment has produced questionable results. A recent study suggests that somatostatinomas possess functioning somatostatin receptors and that octreotide therapy (0.5 mg/day subcutaneously) can effectively decrease somatostatin production by the tumor and improve diabetes and diarrhea.[137]

PHEOCHROMOCYTOMA

Glucose intolerance occurs in about 30% of patients with pheochromocytoma, but overt diabetes mellitus is quite uncommon.[138] The mechanisms responsible for the glucose intolerance are suppression of insulin by α-adrenergic receptor stimulation of β cells; an increase in insulin resistance, probably related to elevated plasma free fatty acid levels; and increased hepatic glucose output as a result of β-adrenergic stimulation of hepatocytes. α-Adrenergic receptor blockade improves glucose tolerance and insulin secretion.[139,140] Removal of the pheochromocytoma restores glucose tolerance to normal in most cases. Treatment of the glucose intolerance with antihyperglycemic agents is rarely required.[137]

DRUGS THAT CAN CAUSE HYPERGLYCEMIA

Blood glucose is regulated by the balance between insulin secretion and insulin action. A drug that destroys β cells or blocks their insulin secretory function will cause hyperglycemia in any individual (Table 57-5). A drug that

Table 57-5 Drugs that Interfere with Insulin Secretion

Destroy β cells
  Pentamidine
  Pyriminil (Vacor)
Decrease Ca^{2+} entry
  Diazoxide—K_{ATP} channel opener
  Phenytoin (Dilantin)—?
Decrease K^+
  Thiazides
  Loop diuretics
Mechanism unknown
  β-Adrenergic antagonists
  Cyclosporine
  Opiates
  Asparaginase

directly or indirectly increases insulin resistance can cause hyperglycemia only in individuals with β cells that have limited insulin secretory reserve (individuals with a predisposition to type 2 diabetes). Several recent reviews on drug-induced disorders of glucose metabolism are available.[141-143]

DRUGS AFFECTING β-CELL FUNCTION

Drugs that Destroy β Cells
Pentamidine and pyriminil (Vacor) are substances that resemble streptozotocin and alloxan chemically. Pentamidine is an antiprotozoal agent that is used extensively to treat *Pneumocystis carinii* infection. Pyriminil is a nitrosourea-derived rodenticide that has been accidentally or intentionally ingested by humans. These agents cause necrosis of β cells, leading initially to hyperinsulinemia and hypoglycemia, followed by permanent hyperglycemia and an insulin-dependent diabetes mellitus.[144-148] In a series of 128 acquired immunodeficiency syndrome patients treated with pentamidine for *Pneumocystis carinii* pneumonia, severe glucose homeostasis disorders developed in 48 patients (37.5%): hypoglycemia in seven, hypoglycemia and then diabetes in 18, and diabetes alone in 23.[146] Of the 41 patients in whom diabetes developed, 26 required insulin therapy. Risk factors for the development of dysglycemia were higher pentamidine doses, higher plasma creatinine, and more severe anoxia. Whereas most of the dysglycemic patients received parenteral pentamidine, six were treated exclusively with pentamidine aerosols. Pyriminil ingestion has been followed by severe insulinopenic diabetes mellitus in numerous instances.[148]

Drugs that Inhibit Increases in β-Cell Cytosolic Ca^{2+}
An increase in the β-cell cytosolic Ca^{2+} concentration is the major mechanism responsible for insulin secretion. Calcium ion entry into the β cell is controlled by several calcium ion channels. A voltage-dependent L-type calcium channel has its activity linked to an ATP-dependent potassium channel (K_{ATP} channel). The K_{ATP} channel is closed by increases in plasma glucose. Drugs that keep the K_{ATP} channel open such as diazoxide (a K_{ATP} channel opener) block glucose-mediated insulin secretion and lead to hyperglycemia.[149,150]

Phenytoin (Dilantin) and other phenylhydantoins can interfere with Na^+, K^+, and Ca^{2+} ion transport. Dilantin administration has been reported to increase plasma glucose and decrease plasma insulin.[151-153] Several studies indicate that it interferes with Ca^{2+} ion entry into the β cell, but by a process different from the K_{ATP} channel–related mechanism. Dilantin has been reported to cause hyperosmolar nonketotic hyperglycemia or diabetes mellitus. This complication occurs quite infrequently and probably in individuals with some preceding genetic susceptibility.

Drugs that Cause K^+ Depletion
The effect of diuretics on glucose tolerance has been debated for close to two decades. Numerous older studies showed that diuretics can cause a deterioration in glucose tolerance in nondiabetic individuals and worsening of glycemic control in patients with type 2 diabetes mellitus.[154-157] It has been suggested that the effect is dose-related and is either absent or markedly reduced with low-dose diuretic therapy.[158-160] The Atherosclerosis Risk in Communities (ARIC) study compared 458 hypertensive patients treated with a thiazide diuretic for 6 years to a control hypertensive cohort on no medications and found that the rates of development of new diabetes were no different.[161] In contrast, the ALLHAT study, which randomized 15,255 hypertensive patients to 12.5 to 25 mg/d of a diuretic, found that 11.6% of the patients developed new-onset diabetes over 4 years of treatment.[162] In contrast, the rate for patients randomized to a calcium channel blocker was 9.8% and for an angiotensin-converting enzyme inhibitor 8.1%. In humans, diuretics appear to worsen glycemia primarily by inhibiting insulin secretion, although they also have a modest effect in increasing insulin resistance. Several studies have shown that the decreased insulin secretory response is due to intracellular K^+ depletion and can be restored toward normal with potassium repletion.[163,164] In the ALLHAT study, 8.5% of the cohort randomized to the diuretic had a serum potassium less than 3.5 mEq/L at 4 years of treatment, while only 1.9% of the cohort randomized to the calcium channel blocker had this degree of hypokalemia.[162] Diabetogenic effects are seen with most diuretics. Therefore, if diuretics are used in diabetic or prediabetic subjects to control blood pressure, doses should be restricted to those equivalent to 12.5- to 25.0-mg hydrochlorothiazide, and potassium supplements should be prescribed as needed.

Mechanisms Unknown
β-Adrenergic antagonists have been shown to worsen glycemic control in type 2 diabetic subjects and to impair glucose tolerance or even precipitate type 2 diabetes in non-diabetic subjects.[154,165] A 6-year follow-up of hypertensive patients treated with β-adrenergic receptor antagonists in the Atherosclerosis Risk in Communities study showed a 28% higher risk of the development of diabetes than that in hypertensive patients not taking drug therapy.[162] The deleterious effect of β-adrenergic blockade on glucose tolerance is worse with nonspecific β-adrenergic receptor blockade than with specific $β_2$-adrenergic antagonists.[165,166] Combination therapy with β-adrenergic antagonists and diuretics has an additive effect of worsening glucose tolerance. β-Adrenergic antagonists impair glucose tolerance and worsen hyperglycemia by blocking nutrient-mediated insulin secretion. $β_2$-Adrenergic receptor activation stimulates and $β_2$-adrenergic receptor blockade inhibits insulin secretion.[167,168] Drugs with both α- and β-adrenergic receptor antagonist activity have no effect or may slightly improve glucose metabolism.

Cyclosporine and tacrolimus treatment for immunosuppression in renal transplant recipients are associated with an increased incidence of diabetes mellitus.[169,170] Direct inhibitory effects of cyclosporine on β cells in vitro have been associated with decreased insulin secretion. Although it is likely that cyclosporine has direct effects in causing the deterioration in glucose tolerance in renal transplant patients, it is not possible to exclude a contributory role of the associated corticosteroid therapy. The onset of diabetes mellitus in cyclosporine-treated patients occurs within the first several months of treatment and often requires insulin treatment. The reported incidence of diabetes mellitus and glucose intolerance in cyclosporine-treated transplant patients ranges from 13% to 47%.[143]

Other agents that have been reported to cause hyperglycemia through inhibiting insulin secretion are asparaginase and some opiates.[141-143]

DRUGS CAUSING INSULIN RESISTANCE

Drugs that increase insulin resistance will not affect glucose metabolism in individuals with normal β-cell function. However, when administered to individuals with limited β-cell reserve, they will cause either glucose intolerance or overt diabetes mellitus. Agents that cause an increase in body weight, and particularly those associated with an increase in central obesity, will cause insulin resistance. Drugs or hormones that elevate plasma free fatty acid levels will lead to insulin resistance. Counterregulatory hormones or drugs that raise circulating levels of counterregulatory hormones will cause impairment of insulin action. The most commonly used agents that can increase insulin resistance are glucocorticoids, estrogens, progestogens, and nicotinic acid. Hyperglycemia associated with glucocorticoid therapy has been discussed in the section on Cushing's syndrome.

Oral Contraceptives and Sex Hormones

Older studies investigating the effects of oral contraceptives, estrogens, and progestogens showed that deterioration of glucose tolerance and development of type 2 diabetes were occasional complications of chronic therapy.[171] Most studies attributed the diabetogenic effects of these steroids to an increase in insulin resistance. More recent studies with natural estrogens and lower dose administration indicate that these regimens produce little or no increase in glucose intolerance.[172–174] Progesterone derivatives have been shown to consistently cause insulin resistance and impair glucose tolerance.[175] The newer oral contraceptives may be associated with a modest deterioration in glucose tolerance because of an increase in insulin resistance, but these effects are rarely clinically significant.

Nicotinic Acid

Nicotinic acid is used extensively to treat mixed hyperlipidemias and has been shown to decrease morbidity and mortality from cardiovascular disease. Acute administration of nicotinic acid reduced plasma free fatty acid levels by 30% to 40%, but as the drug effect wears off, plasma free fatty acids rebound 50% to 100% above baseline concentrations. Chronic administration of nicotinic acid, 1 to 4.5 g per day, causes severe insulin resistance, presumably because of the elevated plasma free fatty acid levels. Normal individuals have a compensatory rise in insulin secretion, and glucose tolerance remains normal. In individuals with diminished insulin secretory reserve, nicotinic acid causes glucose intolerance and type 2 diabetes.[176] In type 2 diabetic patients, nicotinic acid administration results in marked deterioration in glycemic control.[177,178]

Protease Inhibitors

The protease inhibitors indinavir, nelfinavir, ritonavir, and saquinavir have been used to treat acquired immunodeficiency syndrome and have been reported to cause an unusual lipodystrophy. The main clinical features of this lipodystrophy are peripheral lipoatrophy of the face, limbs, and buttocks and central fat accumulation including over the dorsocervical spine.[179] Human immunodeficiency virus (HIV) patients newly exposed to highly active antiretroviral therapy were found to have prevalences of HIV lipodystrophy between 20% and 35% after 12 to 18 months of therapy.[179] In addition to the lipodystrophy, protease inhibitor therapy has been associated with the development of new hyperglycemia, hypercholesterolemia, and hypertriglyceridemia.[179–182] The prevalence of new-onset hyperglycemia with protease inhibitor therapy has been reported to vary from 1% to approximately 6%. Tsiodras and colleagues presented data from a 5-year cohort study of 221 HIV-infected patients treated with protease inhibitors.[183] The cumulative incidences of new-onset hyperglycemia, hypercholesterolemia, hyper-

triglyceridemia, and lipodystrophy were 5%, 24%, 19%, and 13%, respectively. The prevalence and incidence of hyperglycemia in highly active antiretroviral therapy HIV patients is influenced by concomitant hepatitis C virus infection. Retrospective analysis of a cohort of 1230 persons on their first highly active antiretroviral therapy regimen revealed a prevalence of hyperglycemia in hepatitis C–coinfected patients of 5.9% compared to uninfected patients of 3.3%.[184] Hyperglycemia occurred in only one patient who was neither infected with hepatitis C nor treated with protease inhibitors. The mechanism responsible for the protease-induced hyperglycemia appears to be the development of peripheral insulin resistance in skeletal muscle and adipose tissue.[185] Pancreatic β-cell function is also impaired so that it cannot compensate for the insulin resistance.[185,186] At the present time, it is unclear how the protease inhibitors cause the lipodystrophy and other related metabolic side effects. The data indicate that protease inhibitor–mediated metabolic side effects are not related to virologic suppression, CD4 cell count, or changes in weight. Dube and colleagues reported seven new cases of diabetes occurring in a population of 1050 patients treated with protease inhibitors over a 9-month period, for a rate of less than 1%.[181] Two patients were successfully treated with insulin and two with sulfonylureas. Two patients had resolution of their hyperglycemia by stopping indinavir therapy. Kilby and Tabereaux determined the frequency of severe hyperglycemia in a university clinic for HIV 1–infected patients and found a prevalence of less than 2%. Preexisting diabetes was present in 12 of 1392 adults, and new cases of hyperglycemia occurred in 13 of 1392 adults.[182] Most of the incident cases could be attributed to megestrol or corticosteroid treatment. The multiple factors that influence which highly active antiretroviral therapy patients will develop new-onset hyperglycemia needs further study since all series show a much lower prevalence of hyperglycemia than dyslipidemia or lipodystrophy.

ATYPICAL ANTIPSYCHOTIC DRUGS

The atypical antipsychotic drugs represent several chemical classes of drugs that have been shown to have beneficial effects in patients with schizophrenia and manic-depressive disorder. They differ from older agents in that they have significantly less extrapyramidal side effects and they have superior beneficial effects.[187] They bind to a variety of serotonin, dopamine, and histamine receptors.[188] The atypical antipsychotic drugs include clozapine, olanzapine, risperidone, quetiapine, ziprasidone, and aripiprazole.

Shortly after their introduction into the market for the treatment of schizophrenia, case reports appeared in the literature documenting the development of new cases of diabetes mellitus during therapy with clozapine and olanzapine.[189] Since clozapine and olanzapine cause considerable weight gain,[190] the question was posed as to whether the weight gain might be responsible for the development of diabetes. It was also speculated that schizophrenia, itself, is associated with an increased prevalence of type 2 diabetes. Subsequently numerous reports, large health care databases, and reviews have appeared in the literature, citing new cases of diabetes and hypertriglyceridemia as complications of therapy with clozapine and olanzapine.[188,191,192]

At the current time, the following data exist. Clozapine and olanzapine treatment are associated with a mean weight gain of approximately 10 kg over the first year of treatment. Risperidone and quetiapine cause about 2- to 3-kg weight gain. In contrast, ziprasidone and aripiprazole treatment cause minor amounts of weight gain (0.5 to 1 kg over 1 year). Clozapine and olanzapine treatment have been shown in several studies to cause insulin resistance.[193] Ziprasidone and aripiprazole do not cause insulin resistance. The data on risperidone and quetiapine are not sufficient to be certain, but they appear to have little effect. Patients taking clozapine showed a 5-year cumulative prevalence of diabetes of 35%.[194] Published reports and Mediwatch data from the Food and Drug Administration were reviewed by Koller,[195–197] and she found new-onset cases of diabetes in 188 patients on olanzapine, 132 on risperidone, and 242 on clozapine. Approximately 40% of those cases presented as diabetic ketoacidosis. Seventy percent of the patients developed diabetes within 6 months of starting olanzapine. When olalzapine was discontinued, 76% of the patients had improvement or remission of their diabetes. In 10 patients who had a remission, there was a recurrence of diabetes in 80% of the 10 patients rechallenged with olanzapine. While the development of new-onset diabetes was frequently associated with significant weight gain, this was not always so. Ziprasidone and aripiprazole have been on the market for a shorter time than the other atypical antipsychotic drugs, but patient exposure has been sufficient to know that they are unlikely to cause the metabolic complications of the other atypical antipsychotic drugs.

In addition to diabetes, clozapine and olanzapine appear to cause hypertriglyceridemia in a modest number of patients.

Because there are no randomized, contolled comparative studies investigating the effect of the different atypical antipsychotic agents on the development of diabetes, the current conclusions must be viewed with some reservations. The Food and Drug Administration has taken the position that all atypical antipsychotic agents should be viewed as creating a risk for new-onset diabetes. A recent joint consensus conference sponsored by the American Diabetes Association and the American Psychiatric Society came to a different conclusion. A summary of their conclusions follows.[198]

The prevalence of the three adverse conditions (obesity, diabetes, dyslipidemia) differs among the second-generation antipsychotics. Clozapine and olanzapine are associated with the greatest weight gain, diabetes, and dyslipidemia. Risperidone and quetiapine appear to have intermediate effects. Aripiprazole and ziprasidone are associated with little or no significant weight gain, diabetes, or dyslipidemia, but have less usage exposure.

The consensus panel made the following recommendations: (1) If a patient gains ≥5% of his or her initial weight during therapy, one should consider switching the specific antipsychotic agent; and (2) for people who develop worsening glycemia or dyslipidemia while on antipsychotic therapy, the panel recommends switching to an agent that has not been associated with weight gain or diabetes.

REFERENCES

1. Yki-Jarvinen H: Action of insulin on glucose metabolism in vivo. Baillieres Clin Endocrinol Metab 7:903–927, 1993.
2. Lefebvre PJ: Biosynthesis and action of glucagon. In Alberti KGMM, Zimmet P, DeFronzo RA, Keen H (eds): International Textbook of Diabetes Mellitus, 2d ed. New York, John Wiley & Sons, 1997, pp 383–389.
3. Gerich JE: The genetic basis of type 2 diabetes mellitus: Impaired insulin secretion versus impaired insulin sensitivity. Endocr Rev 19:491–503, 1998.
4. Barnes AJ, Bloom SR, George K, et al: Ketoacidosis in pancreatectomized man. N Engl J Med 296:1250–1253, 1977.
5. Barnes AJ, Bloom SR, Mashiter K, et al: Persistent metabolic abnormalities in diabetes in the absence of glucagon. Diabetologia 13:71–75, 1977.
6. Barnes AJ, Bloom SR: Pancreatectomized man: A model for diabetes without glucagon. Lancet 1:219–221, 1976.
7. Morrow CE, Cohen JI, Sutherland DER, et al: Chronic pancreatitis: Long-term surgical results of pancreatic duct drainage, pancreatic resection, and near-total pancreatectomy and islet transplantation. Surgery 90:608–616, 1984.
8. Yasugi H, Mizumoto R, Sakurai H, et al: Changes in carbohydrate metabolism and endocrine function of remnant pancreas after major pancreatic resection. Am J Surg 132:577–580, 1976.
9. Tiengo A, Bessioud M, Valverde I, et al: Absence of islet alpha cell function in pancreatectomized patients. Diabetologia 22:25–32, 1982.
10. Nakamura T, Takebe K, Kudoh K, et al: Increased plasma gluconeogenic and system A amino acids in patients with pancreatic diabetes due to chronic pancreatitis in comparison with primary diabetes. Tohoku J Exp Med 173:413–420, 1994.

11. Kendall DM, Sutherland DER, Najarian JS, et al: Effects of hemipancreatectomy on insulin secretion and glucose tolerance in healthy humans. N Engl J Med 322:898–903, 1990.
12. Robertson RP, Lanz KJ, Sutherland DE, et al: Relationship between diabetes and obesity 9 to 18 years after hemipancreatectomy and transplantation in donors and recipients. Transplantation 73:736–741, 2002.
13. Sun AM, Coddling JA, Haist RE: A study of glucose tolerance and insulin response in partially depancreatized dogs. Diabetes 23:424–432, 1974.
14. Polonsky KS, Herold KC, Gilden JL, et al: Glucose counterregulation in patients after pancreatectomy, Comparison with other clinical forms of diabetes. Diabetes 33:1112–1119, 1984.
15. Del Prato S, Tiengo A, Baccaglini U, et al: Effect of insulin replacement on intermediary metabolism in diabetes secondary to pancreatectomy. Diabetologia 25:252–259, 1983.
16. Kendall DM, Teuscher AU, Robertson RP: Defective glucagon secretion during sustained hypoglycemia following successful islet allo- and autotransplantation in humans. Diabetes 46:23–27, 1997.
17. Redmon JB, Teuscher AU, Robertson RP: Hypoglycemia after pancreas transplantation. Diabetes Care 12:1944–1950, 1998.
18. Slezak LA, Andersen DK: Pancreatic resection: Effects on glucose metabolism. World J Surg 25:452–460, 2001.
19. Nakamura T, Takebe K, Kudoh K, et al: Decreased counter-regulatory hormone responses to insulin-induced hypoglycemia in patients with pancreatic diabetes having autonomic neuropathy. Tohoku J Exp Med 174:305–315, 1994.

20. Ganda OP: Secondary forms of diabetes. In Kahn CR, Weir GC (eds): Joselin's Diabetes Mellitus, 13th ed. Philadelphia, Lea & Febiger, 1994, pp 300–316.
21. Sarles H: Chronic pancreatitis and diabetes. Baillieres Clin Endocrinol Metab 64:745–775, 1992.
22. Larsen S: Diabetes mellitus secondary to chronic pancreatitis. Dan Med Bull 40:153–162, 1993.
23. Koizumi M, Yoshida Y, Abe N, et al: Pancreatic diabetes in Japan. Pancreas 16:385–391, 1998.
24. DelPrato S, Tiengo A: Diabetes secondary to acquired diseases of the pancreas. In Alberti KGMM, Zimmet P, DeFronzo RA, Keen H (eds): International Textbook of Diabetes Mellitus, 2d ed. New York, John Wiley & Sons, 1997, pp 189–212.
25. Sjoberg RJ, Kidd GS: Pancreatic diabetes. Diabetes Care 12:715–724, 1989.
26. Banks S, Marks IN, Vinik AL: Clinical and hormonal aspects of pancreatic diabetes. Am J Gastroenterol 64:13–22, 1975.
27. Nakamura T, Imamura K, Takebe K, et al: Correlation between pancreatic endocrine and exocrine function and characteristics of pancreatic endocrine function in patients with diabetes mellitus owing to chronic pancreatitis. Int J Pancreatol 20:169–175, 1996.
28. Anagnostides AA, Cos TM, Adrian TE, et al: Pancreatic exocrine and endocrine response in chronic pancreatitis. Am J Gastroenterol 79:206–212, 1984.
29. Kalk WJ, Vinik AI, Jackson WPU, et al: Insulin secretion and pancreatic exocrine function in patients with chronic pancreatitis. Diabetologia 16:355–358, 1979.
30. Kalk WJ, Vinik AI, Bank S, et al: Selective loss of beta cell response to glucose in chronic pancreatitis. Horm Metab Res 6:95–98, 1974.

31. Joffe BI, Bank S, Jackson WP, et al: Insulin reserve in patients with chronic pancreatitis. Lancet 2:890–892, 1968.

32. McKiddie MT, Buchanan KD, McBain GC, et al: The insulin response to glucose in patients with pancreatic disease. Postgrad Med J 45:726–730, 1969.

33. Nyboe Andersen B, Krarup T, Thorsgaard Pedersen N, et al: β Cell function in patients with chronic pancreatitis and its relation to exocrine pancreatic function. Diabetologia 23:86–89, 1982.

34. Larsen S, Hilsted J, Tronier B, et al: Metabolic control and β cell function in patients with insulin-dependent diabetes mellitus secondary to chronic pancreatitis. Metabolism 36:964–967, 1987.

35. Duckworth WC, Solomon SS, Jallepalli P, et al: Hormonal response to intravenous glucose and arginine in patients with pancreatitis. Horm Res 17:65–73, 1983.

36. Nealon WH, Townsend CM, Thompson JC: The time course of beta cell dysfunction in chronic ethanol-induced pancreatitis: A prospective analysis. Surgery 104:1074–1079, 1988.

37. Larsen S, Hilsted J, Tronier B, et al: Metabolic control and β cell function in patients with insulin-dependent diabetes mellitus secondary to chronic pancreatitis. Metabolism 36:964–967, 1987.

38. Yasida H, Harand Y, Ohgaku S, et al: Insulin sensitivity in pancreatitis, liver disease, steroid treatment and hyperthyroidism assessed by glucose, insulin and somatostatin infusions. Horm Metab Res 16:3–6, 1984.

39. Marks V: Alcohol and carbohydrate metabolism. Clin Endocrinol Metab 7:333-349, 1978.

40. Schoenberg MH, Schlosser W, Ruck W, et al: Distal pancreatectomy in chronic pancreatitis. Dig Surg 16:130–136, 1999.

41. Buhler L, Schimdlin F, de Perrot M, et al: Long-term results after surgical management of chronic pancreatitis. Hepatogastroenterology 46:1986–1989, 1999.

42. Teuscher AU, Kendell DM, Smets FC, et al: Successful islet autotransplantation in humans. Diabetes 47:324–330, 1998.

43. Hardt PD, Killinger A, Nalop J, et al: Chronic pancreatitis and diabetes mellitus. A retrospective analysis of 156 ERCP investigations in patients with insulin-dependent and non-insulin-dependent diabetes mellitus. Pancreatology 2:30–33, 2002.

44. Karmody AJ, Kyle J: The association between carcinoma of the pancreas and diabetes mellitus. Br J Surg 56:362–364, 1969.

45. Gullo L, Pezzilli R, Morselli-Labate AM, et al: Diabetes and the risk of pancreatic cancer. N Engl J Med 331:81–84, 1994.

46. Rosewicz S, Wiedenmann B: Pancreatic carcinoma. Lancet 349:485–489, 1997.

47. Suruc M, Pour PM: Diabetes and its relationship to pancreatic carcinoma. Pancreas 26:381–387, 2003.

48. Wakasugi H, Funakoshi A, Iguchi: Clinical observations of pancreatic diabetes caused by pancreatic carcinoma, and survival period. Int J Clin Oncol 6:50–54, 200l.

49. Gapstur SM, Gann PH, Lowe W, et al: Abnormal glucose metabolism and pancreatic cancer mortality. JAMA 283:2552–2558, 2000.

50. Balkau B, Barrett-Connor E, Eschwege E, et al: Diabetes and pancreatic carcinoma. Diabet Metab 19:458–462, 2003.

51. Gullo L, Ancona D, Pezzilli R, et al: Glucose tolerance and insulin secretion in pancreatic cancer. Ital J Gastroenterol 25:487–489, 1993.

52. Permert J, Ihse I, Jorfeldt L, et al: Pancreatic cancer is associated with impaired glucose metabolism. Eur J Surg 159:101–107,1993.

53. Fogar P, Basso D, Panozzo MP, et al: C-peptide pattern in patients with pancreatic cancer. Anticancer Res 13:2577–2580, 1993.

54. Basso D, Plebani M, Fogar P, et al: Beta-cell function in pancreatic adenocarcinoma. Pancreas 9:332–335,1994.

55. Nakamori S, Ishikawa O, Ohigashi H, et al: Increased blood proinsulin and decreased C-peptide levels in patients with pancreatic cancer. Hepatogastroenterology 46:16–24,1999.

56. Schwartz SS, Zeidler A, Moossa AR, et al: A prospective study of glucose intolerance, insulin, C-peptide and glucagon response in patients with pancreatic carcinoma. Am J Dig Dis 23:1107–1114, 1978.

57. Ahren B, Andren-Sandberg A: Capacity to secrete islet hormones after subtotal pancreatectomy for pancreatic cancer. Eur J Surg 159:223–227, 1993.

58. Perhert J, Ihse I, Jorfeldt L, et al: Improved glucose metabolism after subtotal pancreatectomy for pancreatic cancer. Br J Surg 80:1047–1050, 1993.

59. Hayashida CY, Suzuki K, Fujiya H, et al: Morphometrical quantitation of pancreatic endocrine cells in patients with carcinoma of the pancreas. Tohoku J Exp Med 141:311–322, 1983.

60. Noy A, Bilezikian JP: Clinical review 63: Diabetes and pancreatic cancer: Clues to early diagnosis of pancreatic malignancy. J Clin Endocrinol Metab 79:1223–1231, 1994.

61. Powell LW, George KD, McDonnell SM, et al: Diagnosis of hemochromatosis. Ann Intern Med 129(Suppl):925–931, 1998.

62. Milman N: Hereditary haemochromatosis in Denmark 1950–1985. Clinical, biochemical and histologic features in 179 patients and 13 preclinical cases. Dan Med Bull 38:385–393, 1991.

63. O'Brien T, Barrett B, Murray DM, et al: Usefulness of biochemical screening of diabetic patients for hemochromatosis. Diabetes Care 13:532–534, 1990.

64. Saddi R, Feingold J: Idiopathic hemochromatosis and diabetes mellitus. Clin Genet 5:242–247, 1974.

65. Passa P, Luyckx AS, Carpentier JL, et al: Glucagon secretion in diabetic patients with hemochromatosis. Diabetologia 13:509–513, 1977.

66. Nelson RL, Baldus WP, Rubenstein AH, et al: Pancreatic alpha-cell function in diabetic hemochromatotic subjects. J Clin Endocrinol Metab 49:412–416, 1979.

67. Saudek CD, Hemm RM, Peterson CM: Abnormal glucose tolerance in β-thalassemia major. Metabolism 26:43–52, 1977.

68. Isaacson C, Seftel SC, Keeley KJ, et al: Siderosis in the Bantu: The relationship between iron overload and cirrhosis. J Lab Clin Med 58:845–853, 1961.

69. Cario H, Holl RW, Debatin KM, et al: Insulin sensitivity and beta-cell secretion in thalassaemia major with secondary haemochromatosis: assessment by oral glucose tolerance test. Eur J Pediatr.162:139–146, 2003.

70. Jiang R, Manson JE, Meigs JB, et al: Body iron stores in relation to risk of type 2 diabetes in apparently healthy women. JAMA 291:711–717, 2004.

71. Moran A, Doherty L, Wang X, et al: Abnormal glucose metabolism in cystic fibrosis. J Pediatr 133:10–17, 1998.

72. Cucinotta D, DeLuca F, Scoglio R, et al: Factors affecting diabetes mellitus onset in cystic fibrosis: Evidence from a 10-year follow-up study. Acta Paediatr 88:389–343, 1999.

73. Lanng S: Glucose intolerance in cystic fibrosis. Dan Med Bull 44:23–29, 1997.

74. Rosenecker J, Eichler I, Kuhn L, et al: Genetic determination of diabetes mellitus in patients with cystic fibrosis. J Pediatr 127:441–443, 1995.

75. Allen HF, Gay EC, Klingensmith GJ, et al: Identification and treatment of cystic fibrosis related diabetes. Diabetes Care 21:943–948, 1998.

76. Yung B, Hodson ME: Diabetes in cystic fibrosis. J R Soc Med 92(Suppl 37):35–40, 1999.

77. Jensen P, Johansen HK, Carmi P, et al: Autoantibodies to pancreatic hsp60 precedes the development of glucose intolerance in patients with cystic fibrosis. Autoimmunity 17:165–172, 2001.

78. Lanng S: Glucose intolerance in cystic fibrosis patients. Paediatr Respir Rev 2:253–259, 2001.

79. Holl RW, Heinze E, Wolf A, et al: Reduced pancreatic insulin release and reduced peripheral insulin sensitivity contribute to hyperglycaemia in cyctic fibrosis. Eur J Pediatr 154:356–361,1995.

80. Hardin DS, LeBlanc A, Para L, et al: Hepatic insulin resistance and defects in substrate utilization in cystic fibrosis. Diabetes 48:1082–1087, 1999.

81. Hardin DS, Leblanc A, Marshall G, et al: Mechanisms of insulin resistance in cystic fibrosis. Am J Physiol Endocrinol Metab 281:E1022–E1028, 2001.

82. Mackie AD, Thornton SJ, Edenborough FP: Cystic fibrosis-related diabetes. Diabet Med 20:425–436, 2003.

83. Ezzat S, Forster MJ, Berchtold P, et al: Acromegaly, clinical and biochemical features in 500 patients. Medicine (Baltimore) 73:233–240, 1994.

84. Melmed S, Ho K, Klibanski A, et al: Recent advances in pathogenesis, diagnosis and management of acromegaly (Clinical Review 75). J Clin Endocrinol Metab 80:3395–3402, 1995.

85. Arya KR, Pathare AV, Chadda M, et al: Diabetes in acromegaly-a study of 34 cases. J Indian Med Assoc 95:546–547, 1997.

86. Moller N, Jorgensen JO, Abildgard N, et al: Effects of growth hormone on glucose metabolism. Horm Res 36(Suppl 1):32–35, 1991.

87. Wasada T, Aoki K, Sato A, et al: Assessment of insulin resistance in acromegaly associated with diabetes mellitus before and after transsphenoidal adenomectomy. Endocr J 44:617–620, 1997.

88. Garcia-Estevez DA, Araujo-Vilar D, Cabelas-Cerato J: Non-insulin-mediated glucose uptake in several insulin-resistant states in the postabsorptive period. Diabetes Res Clin Pract 39:107–113, 1998.

89. Szeto CC, Li KY, Ko GT, et al: Acromegaly in a woman presenting with diabetic ketoacidosis and insulin resistance. Int J Clin Pract 51:476–477, 1997.

90. Colao A, Ferone D, Cappabianca P, et al: Effect of octreotide pretreatment on surgical outcome in acromegaly. J Clin Endocrinol Metab 82:3308–3314, 1997.

91. Newman CB, Melmed S, Synder PJ, et al: Safety and efficacy of long-term octreotide therapy of acromegaly: Results of a multicenter trial in 103 patients—a clinical research center study. J Clin Endocrinol Metab 80:2768–2775, 1995.

92. Arosio M, Macchelli S, Ross CM, et al: Effects of treatment with octreotide in acromegalic patients—a multicenter Italian study. Italian multicenter octreotide study group. Eur J Endocrinol 133:430–439, 1995.

93. Koop BL, Harris AG, Ezzat S: Effect of octreotide on glucose tolerance in acromegaly. Eur J Endocrinol 130:581–586, 1994.

94. Bates AS, Van't Hoff W, Jones JM, et al: An audit of outcome of treatment in acromegaly. Q J Med 86:293–299, 1993.

95. Sonksen PH, Russell-Jones D, Jones RH: Growth hormone and diabetes mellitus. A review of sixty-three years of medical research and a glimpse into the future? Horm Res 40:68–79, 1993.

96. Cutfield WS, Wilton P, Bennmarker H, et al: Incidence of diabetes mellitus and impaired glucose tolerance in children and adolescents receiving growth-hormone treatment. Lancet 355:610–613, 2000.

97. McMahon M, Gerich J, Rizza R: Effect of glucocorticoids on carbohydrate metabolism. Diabetes Metab Rev 4:17–30, 1988.

98. Rizza RA, Mandarino LJ, Gerich JE: Cortisol-induced insulin resistance in man: Impaired suppression of glucose production and stimulation of glucose utilization due to postreceptor defect of insulin action. J Clin Endocrinol Metab 54:131–138, 1982.

99. Shamoon H, Soman V, Sherwin RS: The influence of acute physiological increments of cortisol on fuel metabolism and insulin binding to monocytes in normal humans. J Clin Endocrinol Metab 50:495–501, 1980.

100. Olefsky JM, Kimmerling G: Effects of glucocorticoids on carbohydrate metabolism. Am J Med Sci 271:201–210, 1976.

101. Nosadini R, Del Prato S, Tiengo A, et al: Insulin resistance in Cushing's syndrome. J Clin Endocrinol Metab 57:529–536, 1983.

102. Conn JM, Fajans SS: Influence of adrenal cortical steroids on carbohydrate metabolism in man. Metabolism 5:114–127, 1956.

103. Boyle PJ: Cushing's disease, glucocorticoid excess, glucocorticoid deficiency and diabetes. Diabetes Rev 1:301-308, 1993.

104. Plotz CM, Knowlton AI, Ragan C: The natural history of Cushing's syndrome. Am J Med 13:597–614, 1952.

105. Urbanic RC, George JM: Cushing's disease—18 years experience. Medicine (Baltimore) 60:14–24, 1961.

106. Ross EJ, Linch DC: Cushing's syndrome-killing disease: Discriminatory value of signs and symptoms aiding early diagnosis. Lancet 2:646–649, 1982.

107. Soffer L, Iannaccone A, Gabrilove J: Cushing's syndrome: A study of fifty patients. Arch Intern Med 300:215–219, 1961.

108. Roth D, Milgram M, Esquenazi V, et al: Posttransplant hyperglycemia: Increased incidence in cyclosporin-treated renal allograft recipients. Transplantation 47:278–281, 1989.

109. Arner P, Gunnarsson R, Blomdahl S, et al: Some characteristics of steroid diabetes: A study in renal-transplant recipients receiving high dose corticosteroid therapy. Diabetes Care 6:23–25, 1983.

110. Gurwitz JH, Bohn RL, Glynn RJ, et al: Glucocorticoids and the risk for initiation of hypoglycemic therapy. Arch Intern Med 154:97–101, 1994.

111. Weissman DE, Dufer D, Vogel V, et al: Corticosteroid toxicity in neuro-oncology patients. J Neurooncol 5:125–128, 1987.

112. Fernandez-Real JM, Engel WR, Simo R, et al: Study of glucose tolerance in consecutive patients harbouring incidental adrenal tumors. Clin Endocrinol 49:53–61, 1998.

113. Leibowitz G, Tsur A, Chayen SD, et al: Pre-clinical Cushing's syndrome: An unexpected frequent cause of poor glycaemic control in obese diabetic patients. Clin Endocrinol 44:717–722, 1996.

114. Al-Shoumer KA, Beshyah SA, Niththyananthan R, et al: Effect of glucocorticoid replacement therapy on glucose tolerance and intermediary metabolites in hypopituitary adults. Clin Endocrinol 42:85–90, 1995.

115. Wajngot A, Giacca A, Grill V, et al: The diabetogenic effects of glucocorticoids are more pronounced in low than in high insulin responders. Proc Natl Acad Sci U S A 89:6035–6039, 1992.

116. Hirsh IB, Paauw DS: Diabetes management in special situations. Endocrinol Metab Clin North Am 26:631–646, 1997.

117. Umpierrez GE, Khajavi M, Kitabchi AE: Review: Diabetic ketoacidosis and hyperglycemic hyperosmolar nonketotic syndrome. Am J Med Sci 311:225–233, 1996.

118. Mallison CN, Bloom SR, Warin AP, et al: A glucagonoma syndrome. Lancet 2:1–5, 1974.

119. Stacpoole PW: The glucagonoma syndrome: Clinical features, diagnosis and treatment. Endocr Rev 2:347–361, 1981.

120. Bloom SR, Polak JM: Glucagonoma syndrome. Am J Med 82(Suppl 5B):25–36, 1987.

121. Soga J, Yakawa Y: Glucagonomas/diabetico-dermatogenic syndrome (DDS): A statistical evaluation of 407 reported cases. J Hepatobiliary Pancreat Surg 5:312–319, 1998.

122. Shyr YM, Su CH, Lee CH, et al: Glucagonoma syndrome: A case report. Chin Med J 62:639–643, 1999.

123. Barazzoni R, Zanetti M, Tiengo A, et al: Protein metabolism in glucagonoma. Diabetologia 42:326–329, 1999.

124. Frankton S, Bloom SR: Gastrointestinal endocrine tumours. Glucagonomas. Baillieres Clin Gastroenterol 10:697–705, 1996.

125. Larsen LI, Hirsch MA, Holst JJ, et al: Pancreatic somatostatinoma. Clinical features and physiological implications. Lancet 1:666–668, 1977.

126. Ganda OP, Weir GC, Soeldner JS, et al: "Somatostatinoma": A somatostatin-containing tumor of the endocrine pancreas. N Engl J Med 296:963–967, 1977.

127. Krejs GJ, Orci L, Conlon JM, et al: Somatostatin syndrome, biochemical, morphologic and clinical features. N Engl J Med 301:285–292, 1979.

128. Mao C, Shah A, Hanson DJ, et al: Von Recklinhausen's disease associated with duodenal somatostatinoma: Contrast of duodenal versus pancreatic somatostatinomas. J Surg Oncol 59:67–73, 1995.

129. Penman E, Lowry PJ, Wass JA: Molecular forms of somatostatin in normal subjects and in patients with somatostatinoma. Clin Endocrinol 12:611–620, 1980.

130. Conlon JM, McCarthy D, Krejs G, et al: Characterization of somatostatin-like components in the tumors and plasma of a patient with a somatostatinoma. J Clin Endocrinol Metab 52:66–73, 1981.

131. Patel YC, Ganda OP, Benoit R: Pancreatic somatostatinoma: Abundance of somatostatin-28(1–12)-like immunoreactivity in tumor and plasma. J Clin Endocrinol Metab 57:1048–1053, 1983.

132. Willcox PA, Immelman EJ, Barron JL, et al: Pancreatic somatostatinoma: Presentation with recurrent episodes of severe hyperglycemia and ketoacidosis. Q J Med 68:559–571, 1988.

133. Jackson JA, Raju, BU, Fachnie JD, et al: Malignant somatostatinoma presenting with diabetic ketoacidosis. Clin Endocrinol 26:609–621, 1987.

134. Yamasaki T, Chijiiwa K, Chijiiwa Y: Somatostatin inhibits cholecystokinin-induced contraction of isolated gallbladder smooth muscle cells. J Surg Res 59:743–746, 1995.

135. Marteau P, Chretien Y, Calmus Y, et al: Pharmacological effect of somatostatin on bile secretion in man. Digestion 42:16–21, 1989.

136. Lowry SF, Burt ME, Brennan MF: Glucose turnover and gluconeogenesis in a patient with somatostatinoma. Surgery 89:309–313, 1981.

137. Angeletti S, Corleto VD, Schillaci O, et al: Use of the somatostatin analogue octreotide to localize and manage somatostatin-producing tumors. Gut 42:792–794, 1998.

138. Stenstrom G, Sjostrom I, Smith U: Diabetes mellitus in pheochromocytoma: Fasting blood glucose level before and after surgery in 60 patients with pheochromocytoma. Acta Endocrinol 106:511–515, 1984.

139. Hamaji M: Pancreatic α and β cell function in pheochromocytoma. J Clin Endocrinol Metab 49:322–325, 1979.

140. Vance JE, Buchanan KD, O'Hara D, et al: Insulin and glucagon responses in subjects with pheochromocytoma: Effect of alpha adrenergic blockade. J Clin Endocrinol Metab 29:911–916, 1969.

141. Pandit MK, Burke J, Gustafson AB, et al: Drug-induced disorders of glucose metabolism. Ann Intern Med 118:529–539, 1993.

142. Chan JC, Cockran CS, Critchley JAHJ: Drug-induced disorders of glucose metabolism. Mechanisms and management. Drug Saf 15:136–157, 1996.

143. Bressler P, DeFronzo RA: Drug effects on glucose homeostasis. In Alberti KGMM, Zimmet P, DeFronzo RA, Keen H (eds): International Textbook of Diabetes Mellitus, 2d ed. New York, John Wiley & Sons, 1997, pp 214–254.

144. Bouchard P, Sai P, Reach G, et al: Diabetes mellitus following pentamidine-induced hypoglycemia in humans. Diabetes 31:40–45, 1982.

145. Osei K, Falko JM, Nelson KP, et al: Diabetogenic effect of pentamidine: In vitro diand in vivo studies in a patient with malignant insulinoma. Am J Med 77:41–46, 1984.

146. Assan R, Mayaud C, Perronne C, et al: Pentamidine-induced derangements of glucose homeostasis. Diabetes Care 18:47–55, 1995.

147. LeWitt PA: The neurotoxicity of the rat poison Vacor: A clinical study of 12 cases. N Engl J Med 302:73–77, 1980.

148. Karam JH, Lewitt PA, Young CW, et al: Insulinopenic diabetes after rodenticide (Vacor) ingestion: A unique model of acquired diabetes in man. Diabetes 29:971–978, 1980.

149. Danforth E Jr: Hyperglycemia after diazoxide. N Engl J Med 285:1487, 1971.

150. Milsap RL, Auld PA: Neonatal hyperglycemia following maternal diazoxide administration. JAMA 243:144–145, 1980.

151. Goldberg EM, Sanbar SS: Hyperglycemic non-ketotic coma following administration of Dilantin. Diabetes 18:101–106, 1969.

152. Fariss BL, Lutcher CL: Diphenylhydantoin-induced hyperglycemia and impaired insulin release: Effect of dosage. Diabetes 20:177–181, 1971.

153. Malherbe C, Burrill KC, Levin SR, et al: Effect of diphenylhydantoin on insulin secretion in man. N Engl J Med 286:339–342, 1972.

154. Bengtsson C, Blohme G, Lapidus L, et al: Do antihypertensive drugs precipitate diabetes. Br Med J 289:1495–1497, 1984.

155. Gurwitz JH, Bohn RL, Glynn RJ, et al: Antihypertensive drug therapy and the initiation of treatment for diabetes mellitus. Ann Intern Med 118:273–278, 1993.

156. Murphy MB, Kohner E, Lewis PJ, et al: Glucose intolerance in hypertensive patients treated with diuretics: A fourteen year follow-up. Lancet 2:1293–1295, 1982.

157. Donahue R, Abbott R, Wilson P: Effect of diuretics on the development of diabetes mellitus: The Framingham study. Horm Metab Res 22(suppl 1):46–48, 1990.

158. Kaplan NM: The case for low-dose diuretic therapy. Am J Hypertens 4:970–971, 1991.

159. Berglund G, Andersson O, Widgren B: Low dose antihypertensive treatment with a thiazide diuretic is not diabetogenic. A 10-year controlled trial with bendroflumethiazide. Acta Med Scand 220:419–424, 1986.

160. Luna B, Feinglos MN: Drug-induced hyperglycemia. JAMA 286:1945–1948, 2001.

161. Gress TW, Nieto FJ, Shahar E, et al: Hypertension and antihypertensive therapy as risk factors for type 2 diabetes mellitus. N Engl J Med 342:905–912, 2000.

162. ALLHAT Officers. Major outcomes in high-risk hypertensive patients randomized to angiotensin-converting enzyme inhibitor or calcium channel blocker vs diuretic. JAMA 288:2981–2997, 2002.

163. Rowe JW, Tobin JD, Rosa RM, et al: Effects of experimental potassium deficiency on glucose and insulin metabolism. Metabolism 29:493–502, 1980.

164. Helderman JH, Elahi D, Anderson DK, et al: Prevention of the glucose intolerance of thiazide diuretics by maintenance of body potassium. Diabetes 32:106–111, 1983.

165. Micossi P, Pollavini G, Piaggi U, et al: Effects of metoprolol and propranolol on glucose metabolism and insulin secretion in diabetes mellitus. Horm Metab Res 16:59–63, 1984.

166. Whitcroft I, Wilkinson N, Ranthorne A, et al: Beta-adrenoreceptor antagonist impairs long-term glucose control in hypertensive diabetes: Role of beta-adrenoreceptor selectivity and lipid solubility. Br J Clin Pharm 22:236–237, 1986.

167. Cerasi E, Luft R, Effendic S: Effect of adrenergic blocking agents on insulin response to glucose infusion in man. Acta Endocrinol 69:335–346, 1972.

168. Totterman K, Groop L, Groop PH, et al: Effect of beta blocking drugs on beta cell function and insulin sensitivity in hypertensive non-diabetic patients. Eur J Clin Pharmacol 26:13–17, 1984.

169. Bending JJ, Ogg CS, Viberti GC: Diabetogenic effect of cyclosporin. BMJ 294:401–402, 1987.

170. Ost L, Tyden G, Fehrman I: Impaired glucose tolerance in cylcosporin-prednisolone-treated renal graft recipients. Transplantation 46:370–372, 1988.

171. Perlman JA, Russell-Briefel R, Ezzati T, et al: Oral glucose tolerance and the potency of contraceptive progestins. J Chronic Dis 38:857–864, 1985.

172. Spellacy WN, Tsibris JC, Ellingson AB: Carbohydrate metabolic studies in women using a levonorgestrel/ethinyl estradiol containing triphasic oral contraceptive for 18 months. Int J Gynaecol Obstet 35:69–71, 1991.

173. Scheen AJ, Jandrain BJ, Humblet DM, et al: Effects of a 1-year treatment with low-dose combined oral contraceptive containing ethinyl estradiol and cyproterone acetate on glucose and insulin metabolism. Fertil Steril 59:797–802, 1993.

174. Spellacy WN: Carbohydrate metabolism during treatment with oestrogen, progestogen and low-dose oral contraceptives. Am J Obstet Gynecol 142:732–734, 1982.

175. Bettino JC, Tashima CK: Medroxyprogesterone acetate and diabetes mellitus. Ann Intern Med 84:341–342, 1976.

176. Lithell H, Vessby B, Hellsing K: Changes in glucose tolerance and plasma insulin during lipid-lowering treatment with diet, clofibrate and niceritrol. Atherosclerosis 43:177–184, 1982.

177. Garg A, Grundy SM: Nicotinic acid as therapy for dyslipidemia in non-insulin-dependent diabetes. JAMA 264:723–726, 1990.

178. Molnar GD, Berge KG, Rosevear JW, et al: The effect of nicotinic acid in diabetes mellitus. Metabolism 13:181–189, 1964.
179. Carr A: HIV lipodystrophy: risk factors, pathogenesis, diagnosis and management. AIDS 17(Suppl 1):S141–S148, 2003.
180. Tershakovec AM, Frank I, Rader D: HIV-related lipodystrophy and related factors. Atherosclerosis 174:1–10, 2004.
181. Dube MP, Johnson DL, Currier JS, et al: Protease inhibitor-associated hyperglycaemia. Lancet 350:713–714, 1997.
182. Kaufman MB, Simionatta C: A review of protease inhibitor-induced hyperglycemia. Pharmacotherapy 19:114–117, 1999.
183. Tsiodras S, Mantzoros C, Hammer S, et al: Effects of protease inhibitors on hyperglycemia, hyperlipidemia, and lipodystrophy. Arch Intern Med 160:2050–2056, 2000.
184. Mehta SH, Moore RD, Thomas DL, et al: The effect of HAART and HCV infection on the development of hyperglycemia among HIV-infected persons. J Acquir Immune Defic Syndr 33:577–584, 2003.
185. Woerle HJ, Mariuz PR, Meyer C, et al: Mechanisms for the deterioration in glucose tolerance associated with HIV protease inhibitor regimens. Diabetes 52:918–925, 2003.
186. Yarasheski KE, Tebas P, Sigmund C, et al: Insulin resistance in HIV protease inhibitor-associated diabetes. Acquir Immun Defic Syndr Hum Retrovirol 21:209–216, 1999.
187. Casey DE, Haupt DW, Newcomer JW, et al: Antipsychotic-induced weight gain and metabolic abnormalities: Implications for increased mortality in patients with schizophrenia. J Clin Psychiatry 65(Suppl 7):4–18, 2004.
188. Lebovitz HE: Metabolic consequences of atypical antipsychotic drugs. Psychiatr Q 74:277–290, 2003.
189. Jin H, Meyer JM, Jeste DV: Phenomenology of and risk factors for new-onset diabetes mellitus and diabetic ketoacidosis associated with atypical antipsychotics: An analysis of 45 published cases. Ann Clin Psychiatry 14:59–64, 2002.
190. Allison DB, Mentore JL, Heo M, et al.: Antipsychotic-induced weight gain: A comprehensive research synthesis. Am J Psychiatry 156:1686–1696, 1999.
191. Sernyak MJ, Leslie DL, Alarcon RD, et al.: Association of diabetes mellitus with use of atypical neuroleptics in the treatment of schizophrenia. Am J Psychiatry 159:561–566, 2002.
192. Koro CE, Fedder DO, L'Italien GJ et al: An assessment of the independent effects of olanzapine and risperidone exposure on the risk of hyperlipidemia in schizophrenic patients. Arch Gen Psychiatry 59:1021–1026, 2002.
193. Newcomer JW, Haupt DW, Fucetola R et al.: Abnormalities in glucose regulation during antipsychotic treatment of schizophrenia. Arch Gen Psychiatry 59:337–345, 2002.
194. Henderson DC, Cagliero E, Gray C, et al: Clozapine, diabetes mellitus, weight gain, and lipid abnormalities: A five-year naturalistic study. Am J Psychiatry 157:975–981, 2000.
195. Koller E, Schneider B, Bennett K, et al: Clozapine-associated diabetes. Am J Med 111:716–723, 2001.
196. Koller EA, Doraiswamy PM: Olanzapine-associated diabetes mellitus. Pharmacotherapy 22:841–852, 2002.
197. Koller EA, Cross JT, Doraiswamy PM, et al: Risperidone-associated diabetes mellitus: A pharmacovigilance study. Pharmacotherapy 23:735–744, 2003.
198. American Diabetes Association; American Psychiatric Association; American Association of Clinical Endocrinologists; North American Association for the Study of Obesity: Consensus development conference on antipsychotic drugs and obesity and diabetes Diabetes Care 27:596–601, 2004.

Syndromes of Insulin Resistance and Mutant Insulin

Christos Mantzoros and Jeffrey S. Flier

This chapter considers two heterogeneous groups of clinical syndromes. One is defined by severe resistance of tissues to insulin and the other by mutations in the insulin gene. In many cases, patients with these disorders first came to attention when their diabetes mellitus displayed one or more unusual features that prompted detailed study. It is now apparent, however, that diabetes never develops in many such patients; the syndromes of severe insulin resistance, in particular, are noted for the heterogeneous clinical features that are responsible for patients seeking medical attention. Recently, considerable progress has been made toward elucidation of the molecular basis for these disorders, and such knowledge has produced new insight into the basic aspects of hormone synthesis, hormone action, and metabolic regulation. The often striking clinical phenotypes and defined molecular etiologies of these syndromes have led them to receive more attention than would be justified solely on the basis of their relatively low prevalence.

INSULIN RESISTANCE: DEFINITION AND HISTORICAL SYNOPSIS

Insulin resistance is a state in which a given concentration of insulin produces a subnormal biologic response.[1] This term initially arose in the years after the introduction of insulin therapy in 1922 to describe occasional patients in whom unusually large doses of insulin were required to control glycemia. No insights into possible mechanisms or treatments were available. The concept was developed further in the 1930s by Himsworth, who examined the response of meal-related glycemia to insulin administration in diabetes and suggested that two subsets of patients, one insulin sensitive and the other insulin resistant, could be distinguished.[2] The two groups most likely represented what would later be termed *type 1* and *type 2 diabetes,* but further elucidation of this important concept awaited a number of technical advances that occurred between 1960 and the mid-1970s. These advances included the ability to measure circulating insulin levels,[3] to measure insulin action in explants of tissue or cells, to identify and quantitate insulin receptors,[4] and to quantitate the actions of insulin in vivo.[5] The ability to measure insulin levels by radioimmunoassay rapidly led to evidence that subjects with obesity and maturity-onset (later type 2) diabetes did not have absolute insulin deficiency but typically had increased levels of insulin, thus suggesting the presence of insulin resistance.[3] This finding stimulated considerable inquiry into the cellular and molecular mechanisms of insulin resistance.

The ability to measure and characterize insulin receptors on target cells was a major catalyst to subsequent progress. Mild and variable defects in insulin receptor expression were observed in the common disorders of non-insulin-dependent diabetes mellitus (NIDDM) and obesity, although the pathogenetic significance of these defects in causing the insulin resistance was debated.[6] Subsequent studies revealed a small subset of clinically distinct patients with severe degrees of resistance to exogenous insulin who had markedly elevated levels of endogenous insulin.[7] Studies in these subjects revealed profound defects at the level of receptor binding, and in one subgroup of those with severe acquired resistance the binding defect was shown to be caused by antireceptor antibodies.[8] This finding strengthened the view that the insulin receptor measured in binding studies was indeed a relevant reflection of the insulin action pathway. The discovery that the insulin receptor was a hormone-activated tyrosine kinase[9] and subsequent cloning of the insulin receptor cDNA[10] and gene have been followed by the demonstration that the receptor gene was the locus for mutations causing insulin resistance in some patients.[11,12] The molecular and genetic explanation for insulin resistance in the vast majority of subjects with NIDDM remains unknown. The validation of in vivo techniques for quantitative assessment of insulin action has supported efforts to characterize insulin resistance in well-defined subgroups of patients. More recently, suggestions that many nondiabetic individuals with common disorders such as obesity, hypertension, hyperlipedemia,[13] atherosclerosis, and ovarian hyperandrogenism[14] have insulin resistance have further increased general biologic interest in this topic.

CLINICAL SPECTRUM OF SEVERE INSULIN RESISTANCE

Patients with syndromes of severe insulin resistance have clinical features that vary over a broad spectrum (Table 58-1). This description is true for glucose homeostasis as well as for other associated features. At one end of the spectrum are patients with overt diabetes who are unresponsive to both conventional and suprapharmacologic doses of insulin. Much more commonly, despite severe insulin resistance patients have glucose intolerance, which is often quite mild and does not require insulin therapy. Indeed, hypoglycemia may be present in some individuals (see later discussion of specific syndromes of extreme insulin resistance). In all cases, however, resistance to endogenous and exogenous insulin is, by definition, present. In most individuals who do not have overt diabetes, clinical diagnosis depends on the presence and recognition of a diverse array of associated features. The nature of these features and their relationship to insulin resistance are discussed at length later, but they are mentioned briefly here. The skin lesion acanthosis nigricans is present in virtually all patients and is a key clinical clue to the existence of insulin resistance.[15] In women, consequences of ovarian hyperandrogenism such as amenorrhea and hirsutism or virilization are extremely common, and especially when coupled with acanthosis, these features provoke diagnostic evaluation. Retarded growth and accelerated linear or acral growth are seen in specific syndromes, as is total or partial lipodystrophy. When insulin resistance is due to antireceptor autoantibodies, autoimmunity and a broad array of its clinical consequences are characteristically found (Table 58-2). Finally, some patients with severe insulin resistance have no clinical abnormalities and are discovered to have insulin resistance only after identification of insulin resistance in an affected family member.

Table 58-1 Clinical Features in Patients with Severe Insulin Resistance

Glucose homeostasis:	Diabetes, impaired glucose tolerance, hypoglycemia
Cutaneous:	Acanthosis nigricans, skin tags, alopecia
Reproductive:	Amenorrhea, hirsutism, clitoromegaly (males normal)
Linear growth:	Normal, impaired, increased
Adipose tissue:	Normal, lipoatrophy, lipohypertrophy, obesity
Musculoskeletal:	Cramps, muscle hypertrophy, pseudoacromegaly
Lipids:	Normal, hypertriglyceridemia
Autoimmunity:	Type B syndrome

Table 58-2 Autoimmune and Other Associations with Antireceptor Antibodies

Systemic lupus erythematosus	Hodgkin's disease
Primary biliary cirrhosis	Polymyositis
Scleroderma	Sjögren's syndrome
Idiopathic thrombocytopenic purpura	
Rheumatoid arthritis	

ASPECTS OF INSULIN ACTION RELEVANT TO UNDERSTANDING SYNDROMES OF INSULIN RESISTANCE

The details of insulin action from the level of molecular signaling to that of physiologic integration are discussed in Chapters 50 and 56, but a number of aspects of this important subject are particularly relevant to the syndromes of insulin resistance. Insulin is the dominant hormone for regulation of glucose homeostasis, with liver, muscle, and adipose tissue being the most important sites of action in this regard. It is clear, however, that insulin is a hormone with pleiotropic effects. Thus, insulin is just as important as a regulator of protein and fat metabolism as it is a regulator of carbohydrate metabolism, and it exerts actions in classic glucoregulatory organs such as muscle, fat, and liver, as well as in organs such as the ovary that do not play a role in metabolic regulation.[16] When insulin acts through insulin receptors expressed on cells such as ovarian theca cells[17] and vascular endothelial cells,[18] it brings about actions that are specific to these individual differentiated cell types. The physiologic importance of these latter actions has not been clearly defined.

Several aspects of insulin signaling have significance for our understanding of syndromes of insulin resistance and, in particular, the heterogeneous clinical features that accompany these syndromes. The first step in insulin action is binding to a heterotetrameric glycoprotein insulin receptor that is expressed on the plasma membrane of virtually all cells.[19] Insulin binding to the extracellular α subunit stimulates the autophosphorylation and subsequent tyrosine kinase activity of the transmembrane β subunit.[20] Most data suggest that this kinase activity plays a critical role in insulin action via generation of one or more molecular signals that regulate diverse cellular events, including membrane transport, activity of numerous enzymes, level of gene expression, and overall levels of protein and DNA synthesis. These many actions take place with time courses ranging from seconds to hours and vary from tissue to tissue, depending in large measure on the array of proteins expressed in particular tissues.

Insulin can act through more than a single species of receptor protein. Alternative splicing of the receptor gene results in two receptor isoforms differing by 12 amino acids in the distal α subunit.[21] Subtle functional differences between the two forms have been defined through in vitro studies.[22,23] In addition to these two receptor splice variants, insulin can bind to and activate the structurally related insulin-like growth factor 1 (IGF-1) receptor,[24] although the relative affinity of this receptor for insulin is at least 100-fold lower than that of the insulin receptor. Hybrid receptors composed of half insulin receptor and half IGF-1 receptor subunits also exist, with as yet uncertain signaling capacity and function.[25,26] In addition to the multiple species of receptor proteins that can function as receptors for insulin, results of receptor mutagenesis studies suggest that divergence of signaling by the insulin receptor can begin within the receptor itself. Thus, specific receptor variants have been described that have retained the ability to activate some but not all postreceptor pathways in the cell.[27]

Complexity also exists further downstream in the signaling process. Although many of the steps that mediate insulin signaling beyond the receptor remain uncertain, it is well-established that many and perhaps all insulin actions involve mediation of changes in the level of serine phosphorylation of target proteins, including a cascade of signaling kinases and metabolic effector molecules such as glycogen synthase that are regulated through phosphorylation and dephosphorylation mechanisms.[28] Binding of insulin to its receptor results in insulin receptor autophosphorylation and subsequent tyrosine phosphorylation of intracellular signaling intermediates,[29] among which are the insulin receptor substrates (IRS-1, IRS-2), Shc, and Gab1.[6,7] These molecules bind to and activate other downstream effectors of insulin action, including the adapter proteins Grb2 (growth factor receptor binding protein 2) and Nck, the tyrosine phosphatase Syp, and the phosphoinositide 3-kinase, which amplify and diversify the initial signal generated by insulin binding to its receptor.[6] Several pathways downstream of the insulin receptor are subsequently activated, including the ras (Grb2-mSOS [mammalian son of sevenless]-Ras) mitogen-activated protein kinase pathway, the pp70 kinase pathway, the protein kinase B (PKB)/Akt pathway, and possibly other, not yet identified, pathways. Activation of these downstream effectors of insulin results in such well-documented insulin effects as stimulation of cellular glucose and amino acid uptake, glycogen synthesis, lipogenesis, and mitogenesis.[6]

The basis for termination of the insulin signal is also not well-defined at this time. It is clear that the receptor kinase activity reverses rapidly after removal of the hormone, and one or more members of a family of phosphotyrosine phosphatases may be responsible for this reversal.[30] Recent data indicate that disruption of the mouse homologue of the gene encoding protein tyrosine phosphatase 1B results in increased insulin sensitivity and resistance to developing obesity upon exposure to high fat diets.[31] These data raise the possibility that this molecule may be a potential therapeutic target in the treatment of insulin resistance and NIDDM.[31] Clearance of insulin from the circulation is brought about in large measure by a receptor-mediated process, and defects in receptor function such as those that impair receptor signaling typically impair receptor-mediated clearance both in vitro and in vivo.[32] Thus, in patients with certain receptor defects, hyperinsulinemia results both from increased β-cell secretion and from increased half-life of the hormone. Finally, despite the diverse effects of insulin on tissues throughout the body, feedback regulation of insulin secretion is dominated by the blood glucose level, which has several implications. First, compensatory hyperinsulinemia will occur in response to any defect that impairs disposal of glucose or suppression of hepatic glucose production in response to insulin. Indeed, hyperinsulinemia should result from any defect causing impaired glucoregulation, even if the impairment involves a distal step in the pathway of insulin action. If the defect in insulin action that initiates this problem is not global, hyperinsulinemia may actually promote excessive insulin action through less severely affected or unaffected signaling pathways.

MECHANISMS RESPONSIBLE FOR SEVERE INSULIN RESISTANCE

Several different classifications of mechanisms of severe insulin resistance have been proposed (Table 58-3).

TARGET CELL DEFECTS

Defects in target cell responses to insulin can be inherited or acquired and can be due to defects that arise within the tar-

get cell or can be secondary to extracellular factors. Inherited defects intrinsic to the target cell resulting in insulin resistance could, in theory, involve any step in the signaling pathway from the receptor to the distal events required for insulin action. The insulin receptor is by far the best defined and most extensively studied molecule in this pathway. Patients with several syndromes of severe insulin resistance have been shown to have mutations in the insulin receptor gene that affect receptor expression or function and account for the severe insulin resistance.[11,12] These mutations are discussed in greater detail later. The GLUT4 glucose transporter, although a locus of altered protein expression or functional abnormality in NIDDM, has not been found to be intrinsically abnormal in genetic studies of the limited number of patients studied to date. Several polymorphisms in the amino acid sequence of human IRS-1 have been identified, and some of these mutations have been associated with impaired insulin signaling or increased risk for cardiovascular disease.[33,34] However, other studies do not support the hypothesis that variant sequences of IRS-1 contribute to the pathogenesis of insulin resistance.[35] The possibility that genetic defects might exist that would cause increased expression or activity of intracellular inhibitors of insulin signaling has also begun to be addressed. In addition, a transmembrane glycoprotein named PC-1 has been proposed to inhibit insulin receptor tyrosine kinase activity, probably by interfering with a subunit of the insulin receptor. This glycoprotein has been identified in some patients with severe resistance to insulin and in patients with NIDDM.[36,37]

Target cell resistance may also be acquired. Mild to moderate degrees of insulin resistance can be the result of increased local or circulating levels of a number of factors, including insulin itself (both insulin deficiency and hyperinsulinemia), free fatty acids,[38] glucose[39] (i.e., glucotoxicity), and the counterinsulin hormones (e.g., glucocorticoids, growth hormone, and catecholamines). Cytokines such as interleukin-6 and tumor necrosis factor have recently been shown to potentially contribute to insulin resistance as well.[40] Recent data indicate that the presence of a dominant negative mutation in human peroxisome proliferator-activated receptor-γ (PPAR-γ) is associated with severe insulin resistance, diabetes mellitus, and hypertension, indicating the importance of this nuclear receptor in humans.[41] Although some or all of these factors are likely to be important contributors to insulin resistance in a variety of disease states and may contribute to the resistance in some patients with syndromes of severe resistance, the only acquired factor clearly shown to be responsible for severe target cell resistance is autoantibodies to the insulin receptor.

DIRECT ANTAGONISTS OF THE INSULIN MOLECULE

Two substances are known to directly antagonize the insulin molecule itself, with the result being insulin resistance: antibodies directed against insulin, and insulin-degrading enzymes, or insulinases. It should be stressed that the target cells are not resistant to insulin (unless the resistance is secondary to uncontrolled hyperglycemia) in the case of antagonism by either of these, and, consequently, such clinical features as acanthosis nigricans that are found in disorders with target cell resistance are not seen.

Anti-insulin antibodies were documented to exist and cause resistance to insulin in a subset of patients with insulin-treated diabetes by Berson and Yalow.[42] This discovery led these investigators to the invention of the radioimmunoassay technique, which they initially applied to the measurement of insulin. Insulin resistance caused by anti-insulin antibodies may or may not be associated with cutaneous allergy but is always associated with high titers

Table 58-3 Molecular Mechanisms of Severe Insulin Resistance

Syndrome		Lipoatrophy	Gene/Locus	Inheritence	OMIM*
A. INSULIN RECEPTEROPHATIES					
Leprechaunism (Donohue's syndrome)		See text for details	Insulin receptor	AR‡	N/A
Rabson-Mendenhall syndrome		See text for details	Insulin receptor	AR	N/A
Type A insulin resistance		See text for details	Insulin receptor (5–10%)	AR	N/A
			One family with PPAR-γ and PPP1R3 mutations	Digenic	
Myotonic dystrophy		Dental, skin abnormalities, abdominal distention	Insulin receptor	AR	N/A
B. PRIMARY LIPOATROPHY SYNDROMES					
CGL† (Congenital generalized lipodystrophy)		Generalized	9q34	AR‡	269700
(Berardinelli-Seip)		See text for details$	AGPAT-2		
			11q13		
			Seipin gene		
			Putative CGL-3		
FPLD (FAMILIAL PARTIAL LIPOATROPHIES)					
Dunnigan syndrome		Familial, partial	1q21–22	AD‖	151660
		See text for details	Lamin A/C		
Late-onset FPLD		Familial, partial	3p25	AD	604367
		See text for details	PPAR-γ		
Others		Numerous distributions	Unknown	AD/AR	N/A
C. COMPLEX SYNDROMES ASSOCIATED WITH LIPOATROPHY					
Mandibuloacral dysplasia	Type A	Congenital, skeletal abnormalities, partial loss of fat	1q21–22	AR	248370
	Type B	Congenital, skeletal abnormalities, loss of fat, generalized, progeroid features		AR	
		Involves extremities	Lamin A/C		
Werner's syndrome[70]		Congenital, partial	8p12	AR	277700
		Involves extremities	Werner's helicase		
Cockayne's syndrome[71,72]		Congenital, partial	5	AR	216400
		Involves extremities, mental retardation, dwarfism, deafness, pigmentory retinal degeneration, optical atrophy	CSA		
Carbohydrate-deficient[73]		Transient, partial	16p.13.3	AR	212065
Glycoprotein syndrome		Buttocks	PMM1 and 2¶		
SHORT# syndrome[74,75]		Generalized, congenital	Unknown	AR	269880
AREDYLD** syndrome[78]		Generalized, congenital	Unknown	Unknown	207780
D. SYNDROMES OF UNCERTAIN ETIOLOGY					
Pseudoacromegaly		See text for details	Functional defect in PI 3-kinase signaling	Unknown	N/A
E. ACQUIRED DEFECTS IN TARGET CELL FUNCTION					
Type B insulin resistance		See text for details	Anti-insulin receptor antibodies	N/A	N/A
Acquired lipodystrophy		See text for details	Unknown	N/A	N/A
Generalized (Laurence)					
Partial (Barraquer-Simons)					
HIV-infected patients					
F. EXCESS HORMONE LEVEL		See text for details	(glucocorticoids, growth hormone, catecholamines, glucagons, glucose, free fatty acids)		
G. ANTAGONISTS OF THE INSULIN MOLECULE					
Anti-insulin antibodies		See text for details			
Insulin-degrading enzymes (insulinases)		See text for details			

*Online—Mendelian Inheritance of Man, database providing information about genetic syndromes.
†Congenital generalized lipotrophy.
‡Autosomal recessive.
$Evidence of genetic heterogeneity
‖Autosomal dominant
¶Phosphomannomutase 1 and 2.
#Short stature, hyperextensibility, hernia, ocular depression, Rieger's anomaly, and teething delay.
**Acrorenal field defect, ectodermal dysplasia, and lipoatrophic diabetes, not clear if this is a variation of Berardinelli's-Seip syndrome.

of antibodies to insulin.[43,44] This complication of insulin therapy has decreased markedly in recent years with the introduction and widespread use of human insulin and animal insulin of high purity; previously, the complication was associated with intermittent administration of animal insulin of limited purity. When development of antibodies was caused by animal insulin, resistance usually responded well to substitution with human insulin or, if that measure failed, to a preparation of sulfated beef insulin, which interacts poorly with anti-insulin antibodies.

The nature and function of insulin-degrading enzymes, or insulinases, has been a matter of interest for many years. A number of patients have been described with a syndrome interpreted as being due to excessive subcutaneous degradation of insulin.[45,46] Characteristics of the syndrome have included resistance to subcutaneous but not intravenous insulin and clinical improvement through mixing of injected insulin with the protease inhibitor Trasylol. Limited evidence for the presence of heightened degrading activity in subcutaneous tissue has been provided. Subsequent reports of patients referred for evaluation of this syndrome have concluded that the vast majority have some other reason for apparent resistance to subcutaneous insulin, often related to psychologic factors or unusual behavior on the part of the patient, such that resistance is not found when evaluation takes place in a specialized unit.[47] Thus, the existence of the disorder has not been confirmed, and its true prevalence is unknown.

MOLECULES BELONGING TO PATHOPHYSIOLOGIC PATHWAYS THAT REMAIN TO BE FULLY ELUCIDATED

Several novel genes and/or loci have recently been associated with syndromes of severe insulin resistance (see Table 58-3) and the mechanisms linking these molecules with the development of insulin resistance are currently the focus of intensive research efforts.

Acylglycerol-3-phosphate O-acyltransferases are enzymes playing a central role in the biosynthesis of triglycerides and phospholipids.[48] Genetic defects of the isoform highly expressed in adipose tissue (acylglycerol-3-phosphate O-acyltransferase 2) may reduce triglyceride synthesis in adipocytes and thus lead to congenital generalized lipodystrophy (see Table 58-3). The function of another molecule recently associated with congenital generalized lipodystrophy, that is, seipin, remains unknown but the high levels of expression of this molecule in the brain, in contrast to low levels in adipocytes, suggest that it may act through a central mechanism and that genetic defects of the seipin gene may result in central nervous system defects.[48]

The *LMNA* gene, recently associated with familiar partial lipodystrophies, encodes nuclear lamin proteins lamin A and lamin C. Defects of these proteins have been proposed to disrupt nuclear function, resulting in adipocyte death.[48] In this regard, normal function of zinc metalloproteinases (ZMP-STE24) is also critically important for posttranslational processing of prelamin A to its mature form, lamin A. In summary, either genetic defects that prevent the formation of lamin A or accumulation of abnormal prelamin A may disrupt nuclear function in several tissues, including the adipose tissue.[48]

The mechanisms leading to insulin resistance in the above disease states remain to be fully elucidated. It has been proposed, however, that loss of adipose tissue leads to limited ability of the organism to store triglycerides in the unaffected fat depots and thus excess triglycerides may accumulate in the liver or skeletal muscles contributing to the development of insulin resistance.[49-51] It is hoped that the development and study of several relevant transgenic animal models will soon lead to the elucidation of the underlying mechanisms.[49,52]

SPECIFIC SYNDROMES OF EXTREME INSULIN RESISTANCE

THE SYNDROME OF INSULIN RESISTANCE CAUSED BY AUTOANTIBODIES TO THE INSULIN RECEPTOR (TYPE B SYNDROME)

Clinical Features

The existence of insulin receptor autoantibodies was first discovered in three patients in whom extremely insulin-resistant diabetes developed in association with the skin lesion acanthosis nigricans.[7] These patients had clinical features of autoimmunity (see Table 58-2) and antibodies in their serum that blocked insulin binding to normal cells. The designation *type B* was used to distinguish them from type A patients, who had insulin resistance and acanthosis but no autoimmunity or antireceptor antibodies.

As seen in other autoimmune disorders, the disease is more common in females. It has been noted in many ethnic groups but is most common in blacks. The mean age at onset is about 40 years, but it has been seen as early as age 12 and as late as age 78. The most common clinical finding is hyperglycemia, often with symptoms of polyuria, polydipsia, and weight loss. Ketoacidosis has been observed but is uncommon. Acanthosis, which may be severe, nearly always develops at approximately the same time as the diabetes. The most striking aspect of the clinical picture is the resistance to insulin therapy, which is typically observed from the first insulin dose and is severe, with some patients unresponsive to doses as high as 10,000 U/day.

Other clinical manifestations are possible. Thus, some patients with antireceptor antibodies have hypoglycemia as the primary metabolic feature,[53,54] and the hypoglycemia may exist alone or as fasting hypoglycemia in conjunction with postprandial hyperglycemia. Acanthosis nigricans may be less common in patients in whom hypoglycemia is the dominant metabolic feature. Diagnostic evaluation of fasting hypoglycemia in such patients may be confusing because insulin levels may be inappropriately elevated as a result of antibody-induced inhibition of insulin clearance.[53] Distinguishing antireceptor antibody-induced hypoglycemia from that caused by insulinoma is aided by measurement of C peptide and proinsulin because they are suppressed in the former but not in the latter condition.[53] The most critical; aspect of diagnosis in this condition is thinking of it; the combination of hypoglycemia or hyperglycemia with features of autoimmunity should prompt consideration of the diagnosis.

Two other types of abnormalities accompany the metabolic disturbance in this syndrome. The first encompasses a wide variety of clinical and laboratory features of autoimmunity, as seen in Table 58-3. Laboratory test results and clinical findings indicative of more widespread autoimmune disease include leukopenia (>80%), elevated antinuclear antibodies (>80%), elevated sedimentation rate (>80%), elevated serum immunoglobulin G (IgG) (>80%), proteinuria (50%), alopecia (36%), nephritis (30%), hypocomplementemia (29%), arthritis (20%), and vitiligo (14%). Other findings include: Raynaud's phenomena, enlarged salivary glands, elevated sedimentation rate, leukopenia, hypergammaglobulinemia, and a positive antinuclear antibody test result. Most often these autoimmune features parallel the course of the metabolic disturbance, but they may precede the onset or clinical recognition of hypoglycemia or hyperglycemia. A second abnormality is limited to premenopausal women, in many of whom ovarian hyperandrogenism develops with clinical features ranging from hirsutism to virilization,[55] as typically seen in the type A syndrome.

Clinical Course and Treatment

The clinical course of illness in patients with antireceptor antibodies has been variable.[56] Some patients, particularly those with insulin-resistant diabetes, have had persistent diabetes with an inability of insulin therapy to improve the metabolic state. Other patients have had spontaneous remission of the metabolic disturbance, whether it is hyperglycemia or hypoglycemia, occurring months or years after clinical onset. In the most striking clinical progression, several insulin-resistant diabetic patients have evolved into a state of profound hypoglycemia over several weeks to months. As discussed later, the molecular basis for this clinical evolution is not clear.

A number of treatments aimed at reducing the titer of anti-receptor antibodies have been explored in limited groups or individual subjects. These approaches, including plasmapheresis[57] and immunosuppressive drugs, have not proved clearly successful. Glucocorticoids are the initial treatment of choice in patients with hypoglycemia because these agents have been successful in reversing or improving hypoglycemia in a number of reported cases[53] and in the authors' unpublished experience. At least initially, they appear to act by antagonizing the agonistic action of antibodies rather than by reducing the titer of antibodies.[53] The use of glucocorticoids in patients with diabetes, especially in those with high titers of antibodies, is usually ineffective or worsens the problem. Insulin at extremely high doses may be of some benefit, but most often it is ineffective regardless of the dose. Sulfonylureas are ineffective, but one report suggests that the biguanide metformin may lower blood glucose through a postreceptor effect.[58] However, given the relatively few patients studied and the fluctuating course in the absence of therapy, it is difficult to obtain a clear indication of the efficacy of these therapies.

Properties of Autoantibodies to the Insulin Receptor

Insulin receptor autoantibodies were initially discovered through the ability of serum and serum-derived immunoglobulins to block insulin binding after pre-exposure to insulin receptors from a wide variety of tissues and species.[8] These observations suggested that the antibodies bound to a conserved epitope on the receptor, and recent studies with cloned receptor variants demonstrate that a limited region of the receptor α subunit between amino acid residues 450 and 601 is the dominant site for antibody binding.[59] Some evidence also indicates that these polyclonal antibodies may be heterogeneous in certain respects. Thus, in other cases, antibodies have been described that bind to the receptor but fail to affect insulin binding[60] or even increase receptor affinity for insulin.[61]

Similar heterogeneity has been observed at the level of antibody bioactivity after exposure to insulin-sensitive cells. Given the fact that the initial patients were diabetic, it was expected that exposure to purified immunoglobulins from the patients would lead to blockade of insulin action. What was observed was far more complicated. Virtually all receptor antibodies, whether isolated from hyperglycemic or hypoglycemic patients, acutely stimulate insulin actions such as glucose uptake and metabolism in adipocytes.[62] The magnitude of this agonistic effect diminishes after a variable period of several hours as a result of increased receptor degradation and postreceptor desensitization of uncertain mechanism. Cells then become refractory to further application of insulin.[63,64] Although these facts allow us to account in theory for the occurrence of both hypoglycemia and insulin-resistant diabetes in these patients, it has not as yet been possible to correlate the properties of the immunoglobulins with the clinical metabolic profile in individual patients with diabetes or hypoglycemia.

THE TYPE A SYNDROME OF INSULIN RESISTANCE AND ITS CLINICAL VARIANTS

Clinical Features

The initial description of this syndrome involved three adolescent females with glucose intolerance or overt diabetes and extreme resistance to endogenous and exogenous insulin, together with hyperandrogenism and the skin lesion acanthosis nigricans.[7] The term *type A* was used to distinguish these patients from three others who had insulin resistance and acanthosis caused by insulin receptor autoantibodies (type B; see earlier discussion), which the type A patients lacked. As more has been learned about the genetic basis of the syndrome and as a broad range of clinical syndromes of insulin resistance with different proposed names have been defined, it has become necessary to clarify the definition of this disorder. The term *type A insulin resistance* should be applied to patients with severe, apparently inherited insulin resistance in the absence of major phenotypic changes involving growth and development or lipodystrophy (see Fig. 58-2). Acanthosis nigricans develops in virtually all patients, and ovarian hyperthecosis with hyperandrogenism and its clinical sequelae develops in virtually all females. The definition is, therefore, a clinical one. Affected males have severe insulin resistance, and acanthosis nigricans is typically present, but the testes reveal no changes analogous to those that affect the ovaries in females. As a result, the clinical manifestation in males is limited to diabetes or acanthosis nigricans. Although many type A patients have mutations in the insulin receptor gene (see following discussion), the same clinical phenotype can apparently result from other currently unidentified genotypes.

The syndrome has been identified in many ethnic groups. The most common clinical feature is the peripubertal onset of one or more consequences of ovarian hyperandrogenism, including oligomenorrhea or amenorrhea, hirsutism, and not infrequently, masculinization. The clinical features often raise the suspicion of an androgen-producing tumor, and this concern may be supported by levels of testosterone that are often in the range consistent with such neoplasms (i.e., above 200 ng/mL). The presence of acanthosis nigricans, which usually becomes evident in the prepubertal period, should direct attention to the possibility of type A syndrome, which is addressed most simply by measurement of glucose and insulin levels. Although the initial patients had overt diabetes or marked glucose intolerance, many patients have had normal fasting glucose levels and only mildly impaired glucose levels after a meal or glucose load. The extent of insulin resistance is reflected in the height of the plasma insulin level, which is typically markedly elevated and usually, but not always, exceeds that seen in such states as obesity (i.e., >60 uU/mL fasting and >400 uU/mL after glucose).

The disorder is often associated with an abnormal body habitus. Patients may be thin, of normal body weight, or obese, and prominent musculature can accompany any of these physiques. Muscular prominence may result in part from the action of androgens but may also be a consequence of high levels of insulin promoting anabolism through binding to receptors for IGF-1. Some families have been described in which muscle cramps are a notable symptom that accompanies the insulin resistance,[65] and these cramps may be relieved by phenytoin.[66] Other patients have had retinitis pigmentosa.[48]

Clinical Physiology

The euglycemic clamp methodology has been used to quantitate insulin sensitivity in several subjects, and not surprisingly, severe resistance to the action of insulin to promote glucose disposal is observed. Increased hepatic glucose disposal, also resistant to insulin, is present, especially in patients with fasting hyperglycemia. Evaluation of insulin action in vivo on other metabolic pathways, such as those related to protein and fat metabolism, has not yet been reported. Patients with these disorders have impaired in vivo insulin clearance, and this impaired clearance, along with hypersecretion from the β cell, produces marked hyperinsulinemia. The impaired in vivo insulin clearance probably arises because receptor-mediated pathways play an important role in the clearance of insulin.

Molecular Pathophysiology of Cellular Insulin Resistance

Investigation of the molecular basis for insulin resistance in these syndromes dates back to the initial report of the type A syndrome in 1976, in which decreased insulin binding to circulating monocytes was observed.[7] Several early observations led to the view that these patients might have a primary defect in the structure and/or function of the insulin receptor. The defect in insulin binding was severe, did not improve with caloric restriction as did the milder defect seen in obesity,[67] was sometimes seen in families,[65] and most important, was preserved in cultured cell lines established from affected individuals.[68] Subsequent to the original description, some patients with the type A phenotype have most often been observed to have normal levels of insulin receptor binding. Several such patients have had defects in the kinase function of the receptor that permitted the receptor to be synthesized and targeted to the plasma membrane but left its signaling capability severely or totally disabled.[69]

Family studies have indicated the existence of two forms of type A insulin resistance: a severe form with autosomal-recessive inheritance and a milder form with an autosomal-dominant pattern of transmission, most commonly caused by dominant negative mutations in the tyrosine kinase domain of the insulin receptor.[70] Several patients with the type A phenotype have been shown to have mutations in the insulin receptor gene.[70-72] Some have had two mutant alleles, but most are heterozygous for a single, dominant-acting negative mutant allele.[70] The functional consequences of mutant alleles in these patients have included impaired receptor mRNA expression, impaired receptor transport to the plasma membrane, and impaired capacity for transmembrane signaling through activation of receptor autophosphorylation and tyrosine kinase activity.[72] A functional classification of insulin receptor mutations is listed in Table 58-4, and a functional map of the insulin receptor with the location of various mutations found in patients with severe insulin resistance is seen in Figure 58-1. As discussed in more detail later, genetic and biochemical information such as that already described has not produced explanations for the variable phenotypes of insulin-resistant patients.

Many patients with the type A phenotype appear to not have mutations in the insulin receptor gene, thus implying the presence of other critical primary defects in insulin signaling. At least two types of defects could be responsible for this situation. The first would be signaling defects caused by mutations in genes encoding molecules downstream of the insulin receptor. A second could be changes in inhibitors of receptor signaling such as tyrosine phosphatases, which might be overexpressed or altered in enzymatic activity through mutation.

Table 58-4	Functional Classification of Insulin Receptor Mutations

Decreased receptor biosynthesis
"Cis-acting" promoter region mutation
Premature termination of translation—decreased mRNA
Impaired intracellular transport and posttranslational processing
Impaired cleavage of proreceptor to receptor due to mutation at the cleavage site
Impaired transport and processing due to point mutations in the N terminus of the α subunit
Impaired insulin binding
Decreased insulin binding
Increased insulin binding
Impaired receptor kinase activity
Increased receptor degradation

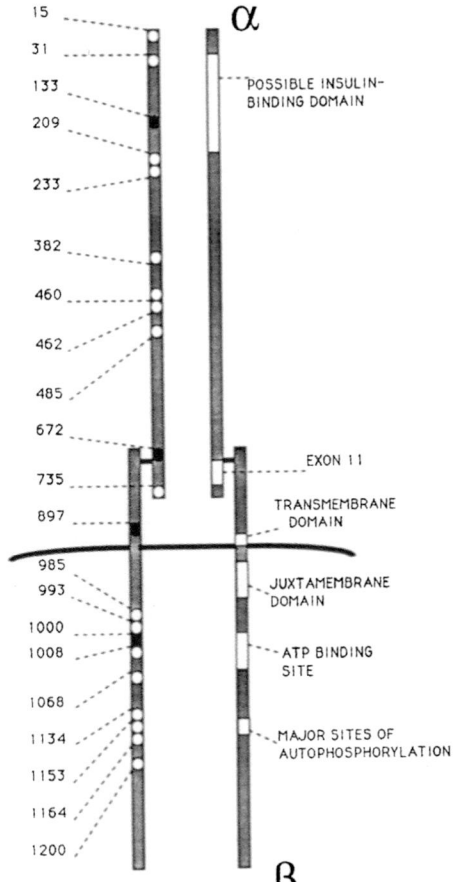

Figure 58-1 Identified mutations of the insulin receptor gene in humans. *Left,* Sites of point mutations (*open circles,* missense mutations; *filled circles,* stop codons). Deletions are not included.

SEVERE INSULIN RESISTANCE WITH PROMINENT DEFECTS IN GROWTH AND DEVELOPMENT

The syndromes discussed herein bear many similarities to the type A syndrome, but in addition, patients have one or more major defects in growth and development.

Insulin Resistance with Pseudoacromegaly

These patients have physical features suggestive of acromegaly in the absence of pituitary tumors or elevated levels of growth hormone and IGF-1.[73,74] When studied, hyperinsulinemia and insulin resistance have been documented, thus suggesting a link between these metabolic features and the changes of pseudoacromegaly. Prominent among the features described are a coarsened facial appearance, macroglossia, and enlarging soft tissues of the hands and feet (Fig. 58-2). Some patients have had accelerated linear growth, and obesity has also been seen, the latter being an uncommon feature of true acromegaly. In some families, changes of acral hypertrophy accompany muscle cramps.[65] As in the type A syndrome, ovarian hyperandrogenism usually develops in women.

It is likely that pseudoacromegaly represents a heterogeneous array of molecular disorders. In those accompanied by severe insulin resistance, it seems reasonable to hypothesize that high levels of insulin are somehow responsible for the changes of pseudoacromegaly. This view is particularly compelling in one very well-studied patient in whom neither insulin nor IGF-1 could stimulate glucose disposal in vivo or in vitro in cultured skin fibroblasts, whereas both ligands preserved the ability to promote "anabolic" changes of protein metabolism and DNA synthesis.[75] Defects in insulin receptor expression, function, and gene sequence were excluded as

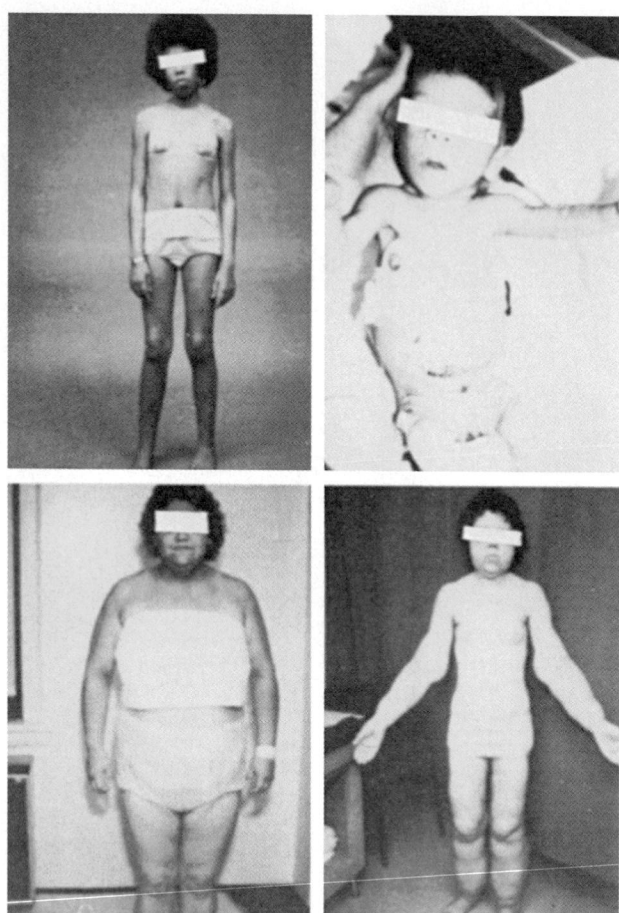

Figure 58-2 *Above left,* Patient with the type A syndrome of insulin resistance. *Above right,* Patient with leprechaunism. *Below left,* Patient with pseudoacromegaly. *Below right,* Patient with congenital lipodystrophy. All patients have severe insulin resistance.

possible causes, as was altered expression or structure of the insulin-sensitive glucose transporter GLUT4. Thus, the patient had a selective defect in the ability of both insulin and IGF-1 to activate glucose disposal because of either defects in a common signaling intermediate used by both ligands or defects in a molecular species required for glucose transport to be activated. Such a defect would permit markedly elevated insulin levels to promote changes of pseudoacromegaly. Recently, selective impairment of insulin-stimulated phoshoinositide 3-kinase activity was demonstrated in three patients with pseudoacromegaly and severe insulin resistance.[76]

Leprechaunism (Donohue's Syndrome)

Donohue's syndrome was first described in 1954 in two siblings with intrauterine and postnatal growth retardation, sparse subcutaneous fat, clitoromegaly, acanthosis nigricans, and early death[77] (see Fig. 58-2). Patients have characteristic facies, with large ears and micrognathia. Males may have penile enlargement, and females have been observed to have enlarged cystic ovaries. Other clinical features observed in case reports include rectal prolapse, breast hyperplasia, and dystrophic lungs.[78–81] The most common status of glucose homeostasis is impaired glucose tolerance with fasting hypoglycemia, and marked endogenous hyperinsulinemia is always found. Survival beyond the first year of life is uncommon.

Parental consanguinity in several families suggests an autosomal-recessive mode of inheritance. Defects in the insulin signaling pathway, in particular that involve the insulin receptor itself, have received the greatest attention as sites of the primary molecular defect. Studies of several

patients revealed markedly reduced insulin binding to both freshly obtained erythrocytes and monocytes, as well as to cultured skin fibroblasts and Epstein-Barr virus–transformed lymphoblasts.[82–85] Defects at the level of receptor autophosphorylation and kinase activity beyond the defect in binding have also been reported, as in the type A syndrome.[82] In general, the severity of insulin resistance in leprechaunism, as assessed by the level of high-affinity insulin binding or the extent of hyperinsulinemia, exceeds that seen in the type A syndrome. Mutations at the insulin receptor locus have been reported in several patients, and these mutations have been proved or suggested to involve both receptor alleles in all cases. Several cases have been compound heterozygotes at the receptor locus.[72,86] In some cases, parents of affected babies who are heterozygous for mutant alleles have had mild insulin resistance without a clear clinical phenotype. In other cases, parents with a single abnormal allele had the type A phenotype.[12]

The established role of insulin receptor mutations in this disorder has not provided an explanation for the reported defects in response of cultured fibroblasts to other growth factors, such as epidermal growth factor and IGF-1.[87] Such defects could be secondary to insulin receptor abnormalities or be the consequence of currently unidentified independent signaling defects.

Rabson-Mendenhall Syndrome

In this pediatric syndrome, which is transmitted in an autosomal-recessive pattern of inheritance, severe insulin resistance with acanthosis nigricans coexists with a group of more unique features including short stature, protuberant abdomen, thick and rapidly growing hair, markedly abnormal dentition and nails, and hyperplasia of the pineal gland.[88–90] Patients may also have accelerated growth, an enlarged phallus, and precocious pseudopuberty. Diabetes usually develops in childhood and is resistant to insulin therapy. Ketoacidosis has been described but is not typical.

Reduced insulin binding to cells has been described in two patients, and reduced receptor biosynthesis was demonstrated in one of them.[91] Mutations in the insulin receptor gene have been found in two patients, and both alleles were affected in each of them.[92,93] One patient was homozygous for a mutation that impaired cleavage of the proreceptor to the mature receptor through a missense mutation that affected the proteolytic cleavage site.[93]

LIPODYSTROPHIC STATES

The lipodystrophic states are a diverse group of clinical disorders, the central feature of which is either a complete or partial lack of adipose tissue (lipoatrophy) that may be congenital or acquired, and/or a combination of lack of adipose tissue in certain body areas with adipose tissue excess (lipohypertrophy) elsewhere. Insulin resistance and its commonly associated features are present in nearly all varieties. In addition, these patients are susceptible to a group of unique features, such as severe hyperlipidemia, progressive liver disease, and increased metabolic rate. As discussed later, the molecular basis for these disorders is not very well-understood, but it is likely that multiple molecular defects are responsible.

Generalized Lipodystrophy

Generalized lipodystrophy encompasses rare but clinically striking disorders that may be congenital (Berardinelli-Seip syndrome)[94,95] or acquired (Lawrence's syndrome).[96] The congenital syndrome is autosomal recessive, with frequent parental consanguinity and has been found in several ethnic groups, but is extremely rare (<150 reported cases). The genes causing this form of lipodystrophy have recently been mapped to chromosomes 9q34 and 11q13 (Table 58-5).[97] Babies are noted to have an abnormal appearance caused by the absence

Table 58-5 Known Mutations of the Insulin Gene

Product	Mutation	Consequences
Insulin Chicago	B25 (Phe → Leu)	Reduced binding
Insulin Los Angeles	B24 (Phe → Ser)	Reduced binding
Insulin Wakayama	A3 (Val → Leu)	Reduced binding
Proinsulin Tokyo/Boston	C65 (Arg → His)	Hyperproinsulinemia
Proinsulin Providence	B10 (His → Asp)	Hyperproinsulinemia

of subcutaneous fat within the first 2 years of life and frequently at or soon after birth. Adipose tissue is also absent from intra-abdominal sites. Other somatic abnormalities that contribute to the abnormal appearance are acanthosis nigricans, a protuberant abdomen associated with hepatomegaly, prominent musculature, precocious secondary sexual development, and advanced bone age leading to advanced early, but reduced, final height. Although both boys and girls are affected at similar rates, the metabolic features tend to be more severe and develop earlier in girls. Hypertriglyceridemia is characteristic with increased very low-density lipoproteins and chylomicrons. This condition may provoke acute pancreatitis and is related to the fatty liver that commonly progresses to cirrhosis, which may be fatal. Mental retardation and other central nervous system disorders occur more variably but may be severe. Insulin resistance has been noted at an early age and may be present at birth. Clinical diabetes usually develops in the early teens, is rarely ketotic, but is refractory to insulin therapy. Magnetic resonance (MR) images of the abdomen show complete absence of intra-abdominal, retroperitoneal, and subcutaneous fat but a prominent fatty liver and presence of fat in certain anatomic sites such as orbits, palms, and soles. Thus, this genetic defect results in poor development of metabolically active but not mechanically important adipose tissue.

The acquired syndrome of total lipoatrophy is similar to that of the congenital disorder, except that it develops in a previously healthy individual over days to weeks, often after a nonspecific febrile illness.[96,98] The syndrome can occur in children or in adults, and females predominate. Diabetic ketoacidosis has been reported.

The pathophysiology of these disorders is complex and poorly understood at present. Although several novel molecules leading to the development of congenital generalized lipoatrophy have recently been discovered (see earlier discussion of molecules belonging to pathophysiologic pathways that remain to be fully elucidated), the mechanisms underlying the development of acquired lipodystrophy remain largely unknown. It has been proposed that immune mediated loss of adipose tissue (suggested by the presence of either panniculitis or low levels of serum C3 and the presence of C3 nephritic factor, which is an autoantibody) is responsible for acquired generalized and partial lipoatrophies, respectively. One crucial unresolved issue is the nature of the defect (or defects) responsible for the lipoatrophy, which could be due to failure of adipocytes to develop, to active destruction of adipocytes, or to failure to store triglyceride in existing adipocytes because of ineffective lipogenesis or excessive lipolysis. Limited studies have produced conflicting findings, although the data most strongly support an increased rate of lipolysis of unknown etiology.[99] A second crucial issue involves the molecular pathogenesis of the insulin resistance and the relationship of this defect to the lipoatrophy and other phenotypic changes. The extreme rarity of the disorder and its common occurrence in young children have hindered progress. Highly variable observations regarding the presence or absence of defects at the level of insulin receptor expression, function, and signaling have not provided a unified view of pathogenesis.[100–105] Defects in receptor kinase activity in cultured cells have been reported to exist in some but not all patients, and no reports of functionally significant

sequence variations at the insulin receptor gene locus have appeared.

Syndromes of Partial Lipoatrophy

Several distinct syndromes of regional lipoatrophy, often associated with hypertrophy of adipose tissue in nonatrophic areas, have been described, and these syndromes are often familial.

Face-sparing lipodystrophy (Dunnigan variety), an autosomal-dominant condition found mostly but not exclusively in subjects of northern European descend, spares the face, which is typically full, in contrast to the lipoatrophic trunk and extremities.[106–109] The gene for the autosomal dominant form of this syndrome was found to be located in chromosome 1q21-22,[107] and mutations of the LMNA gene encoding nuclear lamins A and C have been proposed to mediate this degenerative disorder of adipose tissue.[108] Hypertriglyceridemia and hyperchylomicronemia develop in these patients and can result in pancreatitis.

Another variety of the familial partial lipodystrophies is Kobberling's syndrome.[106] In this variety, the loss of adipose tissue is restricted to the extremities. Patients may have normal amounts of visceral fat and may even have excessive amounts of subcutaneous truncal fat. MR images of the abdomen reveal loss of subcutaneous tissue and an increase in intra-abdominal fat. Individuals in some families have remarkably well-defined muscles. Another form of partial lipodystrophy occurs in association with mandibuloacral dysplasia (small mandibles, acral osteolysis, and joint contractures, alopecia, and skin atrophy) is termed *lipodystrophy* with other dysmorphic features. This rare syndrome has recently been associated with the zinc metalloproteinase ZMPSTE24 mutation.

This diagnosis, which is further supported by the common occurrence of glucose intolerance and hypertension, is ruled out clinically by the absence of subcutaneous fat and well-preserved muscles in the extremities, and by endocrine testing. Lipoatrophy is first noted in childhood or early adolescence. It is transmitted in a highly penetrant autosomal-dominant manner and is more evident in females.[110] Severe insulin resistance and nonketotic diabetes are characteristic, and severe hyperlipidemia is common. As in other syndromes of severe insulin resistance, acanthosis nigricans and ovarian hyperandrogenism are seen, but the latter has not prevented some affected women from passing the disorder to their daughters. Information on the impact of the disorder on longevity is scant, but the concurrence of glucose intolerance, hypertension, and hyperlipidemia is of concern in this regard.

Importantly, clinical variants of this syndrome do exist, including a clinical variant in which lipoatrophy occurred in the proximal ends of the extremities with distal lipohypertrophy (see Fig. 58-2). The patient was born of a consanguineous marriage. Insulin resistance was severe, and cultured fibroblasts had reduced insulin binding, but a causative genetic lesion has not been identified.

Syndrome of Partial Acquired (Cephalothoracic) Lipodystrophy

In this clinically distinct disorder, adipose tissue is lost from the face and upper part of the trunk, with sparing or increased adiposity in the rest of the body.[111] The disorder is most common in women, tends to occur in childhood or adolescence, and can sometimes be dated to the period after a febrile illness. Many and possibly all of these patients have a disorder of the alternative complement pathway characterized by accelerated complement activation, serum C3 nephritic factor, and renal disease with mesangiocapillary glomerulonephritis.[112,113] This disorder of complement may be familial, although lipodystrophy does not develop in all affected individuals. Although it is now known that adipocytes produce one or more members of the alternative complement pathway,[114] the function of these molecules in adipocyte biology is unknown, and this information has not yet led to specific understanding of the relationship between the complement system and lipodystrophy.[48,115–117] Patients may be hyperinsulinemic and modestly resistant to insulin, but severe insulin resistance is absent, as are the associated features of acanthosis nigricans and hyperandrogenism.

Diabetes and hypertriglyceridemia are seen in approximately 50% of patients and proteinuria and nephrotic syndrome are found more frequently than in other forms of lipodystrophy.[118] MR images reveal loss of subcutaneous fat in the upper and interior torso. Another form of autoimmune-related lipodystrophy has been associated with juvenile dermatomyositis. In these patients, absence of subcutaneous fat is associated with increased intra-abdominal fat clinically and radiologically and typically presents before puberty.[119]

Lipodystrophy Associated with Use of Antiretrovirals in HIV-Positive Patients

Recently, lipodystrophy characterized by loss of subcutaneous adipose tissue from the extremities and face but excess fat deposition in the neck and trunk frequently appearing as a "buffalo hump" has been reported to develop in patients infected with human immunodeficiency virus (HIV) who are being treated with the highly effective nucleoside analogue reverse transcriptase inhibitors and protease inhibitors. In addition, insulin resistance, hyperglycemia, and hyperlipidemia develop in a significant percentage of patients treated with protease inhibitors sooner and more frequently than in patients who are receiving other regimens for HIV.[120] Since this syndrome is currently the most prevalent syndrome associated with lipodystrophy—insulin resistance accounting for more than 100,000 such patients in the United States alone[48]—the mechanism underlying its development are currently the subject of intensive research efforts. Highly active antiretroviral medications, including protease inhibitors, may inhibit adipocyte differentiation, induce apoptosis of adipocytes, or cause dysregulation of transcription factors involved in adipogenesis.[48] More specifically, lipoatrophic fat has reduced expression of the adipocyte differentiation factor PPAR-γ.[121] In addition, protease inhibitors contribute to lipodystrophy by inhibiting the sterol regulatory enhancer binding protein 1–mediated activation of the adipocyte retinoid X receptor peroxisome proliferator-activated receptor-γ heterodimer[122] and nucleoside analogues may reduce the generation of mitochondrial proteins necessary for oxidative phosphorylation.[123] These data are consistent with additional experimental data demonstrating that overexpression of sterol regulatory enhancing binding protein 1c induces lipodystrophy in transgenic mice and that in humans, reduced PPAR-γ activity due to inactivating mutations causes familial partial lipodystrophy.[48] Finally, circulating levels of the insulin sensitizer adiponectin are lower in patients with this syndrome.[124] Given that the dyslipidemia and impaired glucose tolerance/type 2 diabetes mellitus accompanying the HIV associated metabolic syndrome increase cardiovascular disease risk in proportion to the duration of treatment with antiretrovirals,[125] early detection and treatment is important.

Localized Lipodystrophies

Finally, localized lipodystrophies are characterized by loss of subcutaneous adipose tissue from small areas or from small parts of an extremity but insulin resistance or metabolic abnormalities do not develop in these patients. Drug-induced lipoatrophy at the site of insulin injection was a frequent complication before the availability of purified human insulin but is rather uncommon today (Chapter 60). Localized hypertrophy is still often seen when patients use the same injection site too often. Other rare causes of localized lipodystrophy are due to repeated pressure and panniculitis or have

been reported as part of a rare syndrome called lipodystrophia centrifugalis abdominalis infantilis.[48]

RELATIONSHIP BETWEEN MOLECULAR DEFECTS CAUSING INSULIN RESISTANCE AND IN VIVO CLINICAL PHENOTYPE

Full understanding of the pathophysiology of the syndromes of extreme insulin resistance will exist when we can identify both the molecular basis for the tissue resistance to insulin, and the links between these molecular defects and the diverse clinical phenotypes seen in these disorders. However, despite progress in identifying molecular defects, explanations for the diversity of clinical phenotypes have been slow to develop. Several facts need to be considered when addressing this issue. First, it seems clear that many of the clinical phenotypes are not simply the result of deficient insulin signaling per se but involve the consequences of the in vivo milieu as well. The key in vivo feature may be marked hyperinsulinemia, which then exerts excessive actions on one or more target tissues. Second, genes apart from those responsible for the primary insulin signaling defect may influence the ultimate in vivo phenotype. Third, it may be that in some cases, unidentified mechanisms unrelated to insulin signaling bring about both insulin resistance and specific alterations in growth, adipose function, and so on. Finally, the high circulating levels of insulin in these patients can bind to and activate receptors for IGF-1, thereby causing excessive signaling through this receptor (Fig. 58-3), which in addition to growth-promoting effects, can have potent metabolic effects in humans, including stimulation of glucose disposal into muscle.[126]

ACANTHOSIS NIGRICANS AND OVARIAN HYPERANDROGENISM IN SYNDROMES OF INSULIN RESISTANCE

Acanthosis nigricans is a skin lesion that was initially reported as a cutaneous sign of malignancy and is now best known for its strong association with diverse syndromes of tissue resistance to insulin.[15,127] The lesions are hyperpigmented and hyperkeratotic and may be papillomatous in the most severe cases. Lesions are most commonly found on the posterior aspect of the neck, in the axilla and the groin, and over the elbows, but they may cover the entire surface of the skin, although palms, soles, and oral mucosa are spared. Histologic hallmarks are hyperkeratosis, epidermal papillomatosis, and increased numbers of melanocytes.

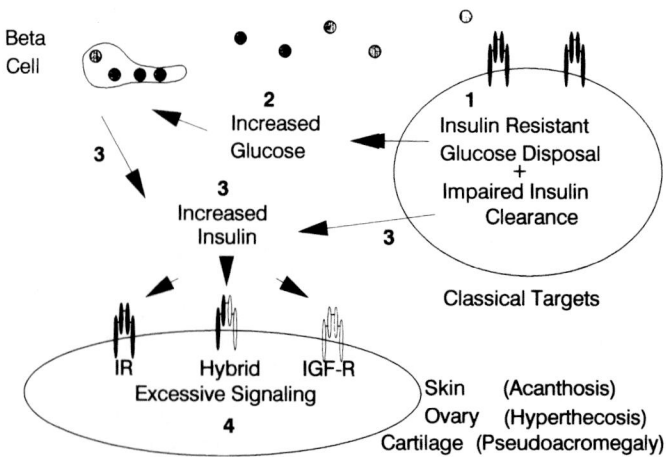

Figure 58-3 Sequence of events through which impaired insulin-stimulated glucose use eventuates in excessive insulin action.

The common denominator among all instances of acanthosis, apart possibly from tumor-associated cases, is tissue resistance to insulin. Insulin resistance may vary in severity as well as molecular etiology and may be either inherited or acquired. Thus, acanthosis nigricans is a cutaneous marker for insulin resistance. In addition to its prominent appearance in patients with types A and B syndromes and leprechaunism, clinical and histologic evidence of acanthosis can be identified in a large fraction of certain large populations and, when present in these groups, is associated with hyperinsulinemia and insulin resistance. Thus, in women with hyperandrogenism, most of whom have polycystic ovarian disease, acanthosis is found clinically in 5% to 30%[128,129] and may be much more common when assessed by skin biopsy.[130] Likewise, 5% to 13% of Hispanic and black children were noted to have acanthosis and hyperinsulinemia.[131]

TREATMENT OF SYNDROMES OF SEVERE INSULIN RESISTANCE

Drugs for patients with severe insulin resistance syndromes are currently limited. The many causes of morbidity and mortality of affected patients include the metabolic syndrome/diabetes and their cardiovascular compilations, recurrent episodes of pancreatitis due to hypertriglyceridemia, hepatic steatosis and the resulting cirrhosis, as well as psychologic problems due to their underlying condition.[48]

MANAGEMENT OF HYPERGLYCEMIA

Insulin, administered in very high doses, usually fails to provide adequate control.[132] Metformin, which may also reduce appetite and body weight, has been reported to improve glycemia in patients with the type B syndrome or lipoatrophic diabetes, the polycystic ovary syndrome, and hepatic steatosis.[48] Administration of IGF-1 to patients with types A or B syndrome, the Rabson-Mendenhall syndrome, leprechaunism, or lipodystrophy has led to improvement in glycemic control and insulin resistance in short-term studies.[132] Immunosuppressants and plasmapheresis have been tried with some good results in patients with type B syndrome. Finally, thiazolidinediones and leptin have been tried with variably positive results in several patients with severe insulin resistance but detailed discussion of these treatment modalities is beyond the scope of this chapter. Recombinant human leptin administration was recently shown to improve metabolic profile in an uncontrolled study.[133]

MANAGEMENT OF DYSLIPIDEMIA

Extremely low fat diet (preferably <15% of daily caloric intake coming from fat) and regular exercise are prescribed for patients with hypertriglyceridemia.[48] Aggressive glycemic control and treatment with fibrates, as well as high doses of fish oils containing n-3 polyunsaturated fats, have also been recommended.[132]

MANAGEMENT OF HIV-INFECTED PATIENTS WITH HAART-INDUCED METABOLIC SYNDROME

In addition to the above considerations, switching HIV-infected patients with highly active antiretroviral therapy (HAART)-induced metabolic syndrome to alternative antiretroviral regimens may improve their metabolic profile but may not alter their lipodystropy. Since many statins are metabolized by pathways inhibited by protease inhibitors, plant stanols, ezetimibe, and fibrates may be safer alternatives. In addition, metformin should be used with caution since it can cause lactic acidosis. Thiazolidinediones have

recently been shown to improve the metabolic profile of these patients but their exact role, as that of leptin and growth hormone, remains to be fully elucidated.

MANAGEMENT OF COSMETIC APPEARANCE

Although the ability of thiazolidinediones to improve the cosmetic appearance of lipodystrophic patients is limited and the possibility exists that they may also exacerbate deposition of fat in nonlipoatrophic areas, their favorable effects on metabolic outcomes make these medications an attractive solution. Surgical removal of excess fat deposits, transplantation of adipose tissue, fascia or muscle, and silicone and bovine-collagen implants have also been used.

MUTANT INSULIN

Several families have been described in which one or more members have missense mutations in their insulin gene that cause amino acid substitutions within the proinsulin molecule (see Chapter 48).[134,135] In these families, three different mutations were found that cause changes within the α or β chains of the insulin molecule and result in biologically defective insulin,[136-138] as well as two different mutations that cause hyperproinsulinemia.[139-142] The clinical and biochemical features of these patients are listed in Table 58-6. All patients have had marked fasting hyperinsulinemia or hyperproinsulinemia with hormone concentrations fourfold to sixfold above normal as measured by radioimmunoassay in the fasting state. The initial patients described with insulin gene mutations had mild hyperglycemia or overt diabetes, and the presence of hyperinsulinemia led to the evaluation of insulin resistance. These patients are distinguished from those with insulin resistance, however, by the fact that they respond normally to exogenous insulin, a fact that suggested the defect in these patients to be at the level of the insulin molecule itself. Indeed, biochemical studies demonstrated that insulin purified from these subjects had reduced bioactivity, typically less than 5% of the bioactivity of normal insulin. Genetic analysis has confirmed the existence of point mutations in one of two insulin gene alleles.[137,141] As in the syndromes of insulin resistance, it is now known that apart from the probands, who are discovered initially because of glucose intolerance or diabetes, individuals with these defects are often normoglycemic, particularly individuals with mutations leading to hyperproinsulinemia.[139,141]

PATHOPHYSIOLOGY

To date, subjects with these disorders have been heterozygous at the insulin gene locus, with one normal and one abnormal insulin gene allele. The product of the mutant allele behaves as a weak agonist, with bioactivity reduced in approximate proportion to the diminished receptor-binding affinity.[129] These mutant insulins have, therefore, not behaved as receptor antagonists, and insulin receptor antagonism cannot

Table 58-6	Characteristics of Patients Producing Mutant β Cell Products

Increased fasting concentration of serum immunoreactive (pro)insulin
Fasting hyperglycemia or, more commonly, euglycemia
Normal sensitivity to exogenous insulin
Circulating insulin with reduced bioactivity
Reduced ratio of serum C peptide to insulin
Identification of abnormal (pro)insulin gene and gene product
Autosomal dominant inheritance of the trait
Codominant expression of the normal (pro)insulin gene

account for cases in which diabetes or glucose intolerance develops because the product of the normal allele should be able to fully compensate. Failure to compensate through increased secretion of the product of the normal allele is presumably due to one or more independent defects at the level of β-cell function in individuals in whom diabetes develops. The mutant insulin gene should, therefore, be viewed as a risk factor for type 2 diabetes.

Patients with mutant insulin alleles are observed to have low molar ratios of C peptide to insulin.[135] This low ratio results from the delayed clearance rate of mutant insulin which, because of its reduced receptor affinity, has a diminished rate of receptor-mediated clearance.[143] As a result, the elevated circulating insulin is predominantly the mutant form.

Unlike patients with severe insulin resistance caused by target cell defects in insulin action, patients with mutant insulin have no unusual or distinguishing clinical phenotypes, such as acanthosis, ovarian hyperandrogenism, or disordered growth and development. The diagnosis is made only if hyperinsulinemia is detected and, after having been identified, an effort is made to determine its cause.

PREVALENCE

Mutations in the insulin gene are exceptionally uncommon, with only five variants described in approximately 10 families.[134] These mutations are listed in Table 58-5. New insulin gene mutations have not yet been identified through screening of patients with type 2 diabetes.[144]

REFERENCES

1. Moller DE, Flier JS: Insulin resistance: Mechanisms, syndromes, and implications. N Engl J Med 325:938–948, 1991.
2. Himsworth HP, Kerr RB: Insulin-sensitive and insulin-insensitive types of diabetes mellitus. Clin Sci 4:119–152, 1939.
3. Yalow RS, Berson SA: Plasma insulin concentrations in nondiabetic and early diabetic subjects: Determinations by a new sensitive immunoassay technique. Diabetes 9:254–260, 1960.
4. Kahn CR, Neville DM Jr, Roth J: Insulin-receptor interaction in the obese-hyperglycemic mouse: A model of insulin resistance. J Biol Chem 248:244–250, 1973.
5. Bergman RN, Finegood DT, Ader M: Assessment of insulin sensitivity in vivo. Endocr Rev 6:45–86, 1985.
6. Cheatham B, Kahn CR: Insulin action and the insulin signaling network. Endocr Rev 16:117–142, 1995.
7. Tritos NA, Mantzoros CS: Clinical review 97: Syndromes of severe insulin resistance. J Clin Endocrinol Metab 83:3025–3030, 1998.
8. Flier JS, Kahn CR, Roth J, Bar RS: Antibodies that impair insulin receptor binding in an unusual diabetic syndrome with severe insulin resistance. Science 190:63–65, 1975.
9. Kasuga M, Karlsson FA, Kahn CR: Insulin stimulates the phosphorylation of the 95,000-dalton subunit of its own receptor. Science 215:185–187, 1982.
10. Ullrich A, Bell JR, Chen EY, et al: Human insulin receptor and its relationship to the tyrosine kinase family of oncogenes. Nature 313:756–761, 1985.
11. Krook A, O'Rahilly S: Mutant receptors in syndromes of insulin resistance. Baillieres Clin Endocrinol Metab 10:97–122, 1996.
12. Flier JS: Lilly Lecture: Syndromes of insulin resistance: From patient to gene and back again. Diabetes 41:1207–1219, 1992.
13. Ferrannini E, Buzzigoli G, Bonadonna R, et al: Insulin resistance in essential hypertension. N Engl J Med 317:350–357, 1987.
14. Dunaif A, Graf M, Mandeli J, et al: Characterization of groups of hyperandrogenic women with acanthosis nigricans, impaired glucose tolerance, and/or hyperinsulinemia. J Clin Endocrinol Metab 65:499–507, 1987.
15. Flier JS: The metabolic importance of acanthosis nigricans. Arch Dermatol 121:193–194, 1985.
16. Poretsky L: On the paradox of insulin-induced hyperandrogenism in insulin-resistant states. Endocr Rev 12:3–3, 1991.
17. Barbieri RL, Smith S, Ryan KJ: The role of hyperinsulinemia in the pathogenesis of ovarian hyperandrogenism. Fertil Steril 50:197–212, 1988.
18. Bar RS, Boes M, Kake BL, et al: Insulin, insulin-like growth factors, and vascular endothelium. Am J Med 85(5A):59–70, 1988.
19. Kahn CR: The molecular mechanism of insulin action. Annu Rev Med 36:429–451, 1985.
20. Goldfine ID: The insulin receptor: Molecular biology and transmembrane signaling. Endocr Rev 8:235–255, 1987.
21. Moller DE, Yokota A, Caro JF, Flier JS: Tissue-specific expression of two alternatively spliced insulin receptor mRNA's in man. Mol Endocrinol 3:1263–1269, 1989.
22. Yamaguchi Y, Flier JS, Yokota A, et al: Functional properties of two naturally occurring isoforms of the human insulin receptor in Chinese hamster ovary cells. Endocrinology 129:2058–2066, 1991.
23. McClain DA: Different ligand affinities of the two human insulin receptor splice variants are reflected in parallel changes in sensitivity for insulin action. Mol Endocrinol 5:734–739, 1991.
24. Flier JS, Usher P, Moses AC: Monoclonal antibody to the type I insulin-like growth factor (IGF-I) receptor blocks IGF-I receptor-mediated DNA synthesis: Clarification of the mitogenic mechanisms of IGF-I and insulin skin fibroblasts. Proc Natl Acad Sci U S A 93:664–668, 1986.
25. Treadway JL, Morrison BD, Goldfine ID, Pessin JE: Assembly of insulin/insulin-like growth factor-I hybrid receptors in vitro. J Biol Chem 264:21450–21453, 1989.
26. Moxham CP, Duronio V, Jacobs S: Insulin-like growth factor I receptor beta-subunit heterogeneity: Evidence for hybrid tetramers composed of insulin-like growth factor I and insulin receptor heterodimers. J Biol Chem 264:13238–13244, 1989.
27. McClain DA: Insulin action in cells expressing truncated or kinase-defective insulin receptors: Dissection of multiple hormone-signaling pathways. Diabetes Care 13:302–316, 1990.
28. Cohen P: The structure and regulation of protein phosphatases. Annu Rev Biochem 58:453–508, 1989.
29. White MF, Stegmann EW, Dull TJ, et al: Characterization of an endogenous substrate of the insulin receptor in cultured cells. J Biol Chem 262:9769–9777, 1987.
30. Drake PG, Posner BI: Insulin receptor-associated protein tyrosine phosphatase(s): Role in insulin action. Mol Cell Biochem 182:79–89, 1998.
31. Elchebly M, Payette P, Michaliszyn E, et al: Increased insulin sensitivity and obesity resistance in mice lacking the protein tyrosine phosphatase-1B gene. Science 283:1544–1548, 1999.
32. Flier JS, Minaker KL, Landsberg L, et al: Impaired in vivo insulin clearance in patients with severe target cell resistance of insulin. Diabetes 31:132–135, 1982.
33. Almind K, Inoue G, Pedersen O, Kahn CR: A common amino acid polymorphism in insulin receptor substrate-1 causes impaired insulin signaling. Evidence from transfection studies. J Clin Invest 97:2569–2575, 1996.
34. Baroni MG, D'Andrea MP, Montali A, et al: A common mutation of the insulin receptor substrate-1 gene is a risk factor for coronary artery disease. Arterioscler Thromb Vasc Biol 19:2975–2980, 1999.
35. Imai Y, Philippe N, Sesti G, et al: Expression of variant forms of insulin receptor substrate-1 identified in patients with noninsulin-dependent diabetes mellitus. J Clin Endocrinol Metab 82:4201–4207, 1997.
36. Sbraccia P, Goodman PA, Maddux BA, et al: Production of inhibitor of insulin-receptor tyrosine kinase in fibroblasts

from patient with insulin resistance and NIDDM. Diabetes 40:295–299, 1991.

37. Sbraccia P, Goodman PA, Maddux BA, et al: Production of an inhibitor of insulin receptor tyrosine kinase in fibroblasts from a patient with insulin resistance and NIDDM. Diabetes 40:295–299, 1991.

38. Randle PJ, Hales CN, Garland PB, Newsholm EA: The glucose fatty-acid cycle: Its role in insulin sensitivity and the metabolic disturbances of diabetes mellitus. Lancet 2:785–789, 1963.

39. Yki-Jarvinen H: Glucose toxicity. Endocr Rev 13:415–431, 1992.

40. Hotamisligil GS, Shargill NS, Spiegelman BM: Adipose tissue expression of tumor necrosis factor alpha: Direct role in obesity-linked insulin resistance. Science 259:87–90, 1993.

41. Barossi I, Gurnell M, Crowley VEF, et al: Dominant negative mutations in human PPARγ associated with severe insulin resistance, diabetes mellitus and hypertension. Nature 402:880–883, 1999.

42. Berson SA, Yalow RS: In Ellenberg M, Rifkin H (eds): Diabetes Mellitus: Theory and Practice. New York, McGraw-Hill, 1970, pp 388–423.

43. Flier JS, Poretsky L: Insulin allergy and insulin resistance: Current therapy. In Lichtenstein LM, Fauci AS (eds): Allergy, Immunology and Rheumatology. Philadelphia, BC Decker, 1985, pp 135–140.

44. Francis A, Hanning I, Alberti K: The influence of insulin antibody levels on the plasma profiles and action of subcutaneously injected human and bovine short-acting insulins. Diabetologia 28:330, 1983.

45. Duckworth WC, Bennett RG, Hamel FG: Insulin degradation: Progress and potential. Endocr Rev 19:608–624, 1998.

46. Freidenberg GR, White N, Cataland S, et al: Diabetes response to intravenous but not subcutaneous effectiveness of aprotinin. N Engl J Med 305:363, 1981.

47. Schade DS, Duckworth WC: In search of the subcutaneous-insulin-resistance syndrome. N Engl J Med 315:147, 1986.

48. Garg A: Acquired and inherited lipodystrophies. N Engl J Med 350:1220–1234, 2004.

49. Moitra J, Mason MM, Olive M, et al: Life without white fat: A transgenic mouse. Genes Dev 12:3168–3181, 1998.

50. Szczepaniak LS, Babcock EE, Schick F, et al: Measurement of intracellular triglyceride stores by H spectroscopy: Validation in vivo. Am J Physiol 276:E977–E989, 1999.

51. Petersen KF, Oral EA, Dufour S, et al: Leptin reverses insulin resistance and hepatic steatosis in patients with severe lipodystrophy. J Clin Invest 109:1345–1350, 2002.

52. Shimomura I, Hammer RE, Richardson JA, et al: Insulin resistance and diabetes mellitus in transgenic mice expressing nuclear SREBP-1c in adipose tissue: Model for congenital generalized lipodystrophy. Genes Dev 12:3182–3194, 1998.

53. Taylor SI, Barbetti F, Accili D, et al: Syndromes of autoimmunity and hypoglycemia: Autoantibodies directed against insulin and its receptor. Endocrinol Metab Clin North Am 18:123–143, 1989.

54. Taylor SI, Grunberger G, Marcus-Samuels B, et al: Hypoglycemia associated with antibodies to the insulin receptor. N Engl J Med 307:1422–1426, 1982.

55. Taylor SI, Dons RF, Hernandez E, et al: Insulin resistance associated with androgen excess in women with autoantibodies to the insulin receptor. Ann Intern Med 97:851–855, 1982.

56. Flier JS, Bar RS, Muggeo M, et al: The evolving clinical course of patients with insulin receptor autoantibodies: Spontaneous remission or receptor proliferation with hypoglycemia. J Clin Endocrinol Metab 47:985–995, 1978.

57. Muggeo M, Flier JS, Abrams RA, et al: Treatment by plasma exchange of a patient with autoantibodies to the insulin receptor. N Engl J Med 300:477–480, 1979.

58. DiPaolo S: Metformin ameliorates extreme insulin resistance in a patient with anti-insulin receptor antibodies: Description of insulin receptor and postreceptor effects in vivo and in vitro. Acta Endocrinol 126:117–123, 1992.

59. Zhang B, Roth RA: A region of the insulin receptor important for ligand binding (residues 450–601) is recognized by patients' autoimmune antibodies and inhibitory monoclonal antibodies. Proc Natl Acad Sci U S A 88:9858–9862, 1991.

60. Boden G, Fujita-Yamaguchi Y, Shimoyama R, et al: Nonbinding inhibitory antiinsulin receptor antibodies: A new type of autoantibodies in human diabetes. J Clin Invest 81:1971–1978, 1988.

61. Di Paolo S, Giorgino R: Insulin resistance and hypoglycemia in a patient with systemic lupus erythematosus: Description of antiinsulin receptor antibodies that enhance insulin binding and inhibit insulin action. J Clin Endocrinol Metab 73:650–657, 1991.

62. Kahn CR, Baird K, Flier JS, Jarrett DB: Effects of autoantibodies to the insulin receptor on isolated adipocytes. J Clin Invest 60:1094–1106, 1977.

63. Karlsson FA, Van Obberghen E, Grunfeld C, Kahn C: Desensitization of the insulin receptor at an early postreceptor step by prolonged exposure to anti-receptor antibody. Proc Natl Acad Sci U S A 76:809–813, 1979.

64. Grunfeld C: Antibody against the insulin receptor causes disappearance of insulin receptors in 3T3-L1 cells: A possible explanation of antibody-induced insulin resistance. Proc Natl Acad Sci U S A 81:2508–2511, 1984.

65. Flier JS, Young JB, Landsberg L: Familial insulin resistance with acanthosis nigricans, acral hypertrophy and muscle cramps: A new syndrome. N Engl J Med 390:970–973, 1980.

66. Minaker KL, Flier JS, Landsberg L, et al: Diphenylhydantoin-induced improvement in muscle cramping and insulin action in three patients with the syndrome of insulin resistance, acanthosis nigricans, and acral hypertrophy. Arch Neurol 46:981–985, 1989.

67. Bar RS, Muggeo M, Kahn CR, et al: Characterization of insulin receptors in patients with the syndromes of insulin resistance and acanthosis nigricans. Diabetologia 18:209–216, 1980.

68. Podskalny JM, Kahn CR: Cell culture studies on patients with extreme insulin resistance: I. Receptor defects on cultured fibroblasts. J Clin Endocrinol Metab 54:261–268, 1982.

69. Grigorescu F, Flier JS, Kahn CR: Defect in insulin receptor phosphorylation in erythrocytes and fibroblasts associated with severe insulin resistance. J Biol Chem 259:15003–15006, 1984.

70. Taylor SI, Arioglou E: Genetically defined forms of diabetes in children. J Clin Endocrinol Metab 84:4390–4396, 1999.

71. Moller DE, Yokota A, White MF, et al: A naturally occurring mutation of insulin receptor alanine 1134 impairs tyrosine kinase function and is associated with dominantly inherited insulin resistance. J Biol Chem 265:14979–14985, 1990.

72. O'Rahilly S, Moller DE: Mutant insulin receptors in syndromes of insulin resistance. Clin Endocrinol 36:121–132, 1992.

73. Mims RB: Pituitary function and growth hormone dynamics in acromegaloidism. J Natl Med Assoc 70:919–924, 1978.

74. Low L, Chernausek SD, Sperling MA: Acromegaloid patients with type A insulin resistance: Parallel defects in insulin and insulin-like growth factor-I receptors and biological responses in cultured fibroblasts. J Clin Endocrinol Metab 69:329–337, 1989.

75. Flier JS, Moller DE, Moses AC, et al: Insulin-mediated pseudoacromegaly: Clinical and biochemical characterization of a syndrome of selective insulin resistance. J Clin Endocrinol Metab 76:1533–1541, 1993.

76. Dib K, Whitehead JP, Humphreys PJ, et al: Impaired activation of phosphoinositide 3 kinase by insulin in fibroblasts from patients with severe insulin resistance and pseudoacromegaly. J Clin Invest 101:1111–1120, 1998.

77. Donohue WL, Uchida I: Leprechaunism: A euphemism for a rare familial disorder. J Pediatr 45:505, 1954.

78. Elders MJ, Schedewie HK, Olefsky J, et al: Endocrine-metabolic relationships in patients with leprechaunism. J Natl Med Assoc 74:1195–1210, 1982.

79. Ioan D, Dumitriu L, Belengeanu V, et al: Leprechaunism: Report of two cases and review. Endocrinologie 26:205–209, 1988.

80. Elsas LJ, Endo F, Priest JH, Strumlauf E: Leprechaunism: An inherited defect in insulin-receptor interaction. In Wapnir RA (ed): Congenital Metabolic Disease: Diagnosis and Treatment. New York, Marcel Dekker, 1985, pp 301–334.

81. Ellis EN, Kemp SF, Frindik JP, Elders MJ: Glomerulopathy in a patient with Donohue syndrome (leprechaunism). Diabetes Care 14:413–414, 1991.

82. Sethu-Kumar Reddy S, Lauris V, Kahn CR: Insulin receptor function in fibroblasts from patients with leprechaunism: Differential alterations in binding, autophosphorylation, kinase activity, and receptor-mediated internalization. J Clin Invest 82:1359–1365, 1988.

83. Maassen JA, Klinkhamer MP, van der Zon GC, et al: Fibroblasts from a leprechaun patient have defects in insulin binding and insulin receptor autophosphorylation. Diabetologia 31:612–617, 1988.

84. Taylor SI, Roth J, Blizzard RM, Elders MJ: Qualitative abnormalities of insulin binding in a patient with extreme insulin resistance. Proc Natl Acad Sci U S A 78:7157–7161, 1981.

85. Taylor SI, Samuels B, Roth J, et al: Decreased insulin binding in cultured lymphocytes from two patients with extreme insulin resistance. J Clin Endocrinol Metab 54:919–930, 1982.

86. Kadowaki T, Bevins CL, Cama A, et al: Two mutant alleles of the insulin receptor gene in a patient with extreme insulin resistance. Science 240:787–790, 1988.

87. Kaplowitz PB, D'Ercole AJ: Fibroblasts from a patient with leprechaunism are resistant to insulin, epidermal growth factor, and somatomedin C. J Clin Endocrinol Metab 55:741–748, 1982.

88. Mendenhall EN: Tumor of the pineal body with high insulin resistance. J Indian Med Assoc 43:32–36, 1950.

89. Rabson SM, Mendenhall EN: Familial hypertrophy of pineal body, hyperplasia of adrenal cortex and diabetes mellitus: Report of 3 cases. Am J Clin Pathol 26:283–290, 1956.

90. West RJ, Leonard JV: Familial insulin resistance with pineal hyperplasia: Metabolic studies and effect of hypophysectomy. Arch Dis Child 55:619–621, 1980.

91. Moncada VY, Hedo JA, Serranos-Rios M, Taylor SI: Insulin-receptor biosynthesis in cultured lymphocytes from an insulin-resistant patient (Rabson-Mendenhall syndrome): Evidence for a defect before insertion of receptor into plasma membrane. Diabetes 35:802–807, 1986.

92. Kadowaki T, Kadowaki H, Accili D, Taylor SI: Substitution of lysine for asparagine-15 in the human insulin receptor impairs intracellular transport of the receptor to the cell surface and decreases the affinity of insulin binding. J Biol Chem 265:19143–19150, 1990.

93. Yoshimasa Y, Seino S, Whittaker J, et al: Insulin resistant diabetes due to a point mutation that prevents insulin proreceptor processing. Science 240:784–787, 1988.

94. Berardinelli W: An undiagnosed endocrinometabolic syndrome: Report of 2 cases. J Clin Endocrinol Metab 14:193–204, 1954.

95. Seip M: Lipodystrophy and gigantism with associated endocrine manifestations: A new diencephalic syndrome? Acta Paediatr 48:555–574, 1959.

96. Lawrence RD: Lipodystrophy and hepatomegaly with diabetes, lipaemia, and other metabolic disturbances: A case throwing new light on the action of insulin. Lancet 1:724, 1946.

97. Garg A, Wilson R, Barnes R, et al: A gene for congenital generalized lipodystrophy maps to human chromosome 9q34. J Clin Endocrinol Metab 84:3390–3394, 1999.

98. Kobberling J: Genetic syndromes associated with lipoatrophic diabetes. In Creutzfeldt W, Kobberling J, Neel JV (eds): The Genetics of Diabetes Mellitus. New York, Springer-Verlag, 1976, pp 147–154.

99. Boucher BJ, Cohen RD, France MW, Mason SA: Plasma free fatty acid turnover in total lipodystrophy. Clin Endocrinol 4:83–88, 1973.

100. Oseid S, Beck-Nielsen H, Pedersen O, Sovik O: Decreased binding of insulin to its receptor in patients with congenital generalized lipodystrophy. N Engl J Med 296:245–248, 1977.

101. Wachslicht-Rodbard H, Muggeo M, Kahn CR, et al: Heterogeneity of the insulin-receptor interaction in lipoatrophic diabetes. J Clin Endocrinol Metab 52:416–425, 1981.

102. Magre J, Grigorescu F, Reynet C, et al: Tyrosine-kinase defect of the insulin receptor in cultured fibroblasts from patients with lipoatrophic diabetes. J Clin Endocrinol Metab 69:142–150, 1989.

103. Magre J, Reynet C, Capeau J, et al: In vitro studies of insulin resistance in patients with lipoatrophic diabetes: Evidence for heterogeneous postbinding defects. Diabetes 37:421–482, 1988.

104. Kriauchiunas KM, Kahn CR, Muller-Wieland D, et al: Altered expression and function of the insulin receptor in a family with lipoatrophic diabetes. J Clin Endocrinol Metab 67:1284–1293, 1988.

105. Foss I, Trygstad O: Lipoatrophy produced in mice and rabbits by a fraction prepared from the urine of patients with congenital generalised lipodystrophy. Acta Endocrinol 713:443–453, 1975.

106. Kobberling J, Willms B, Kattermann R, Creutzfeldt W: Lipodystrophy of the extremities: A dominantly inherited syndrome associated with lipoatrophic diabetes. Humangenetik 29:111–120, 1975.

107. Peters JM, Barnes R, Bennett L, et al: Localization of the gene for familial partial lipodystrophy (Dunningan variety) to chromosome 1q21–22. Nat Genet 18:292–295, 1998.

108. Cao H, Hegele RA: Nuclear lamin A/C R482Q mutation in Canadian kindreds with Dunningan-type familial partial lipodystrophy. Hum Mol Genet 9:109–112, 2000.

109. Dunnigan MG, Cochrane M, Kelly A, Scott JW: Familial lipoatrophic diabetes with dominant transmission. Q J Med 49:33–48, 1974.

110. Jackson SN, Pinkney J, Bargiotta A, et al: A defect in the regional deposition of adipose tissue (partial lipodystrophy) is encoded by a gene at chromosome 1q. Am J Hum Genet 63:534–540, 1998.

111. Barraquer FL: Pathogenesis of progressive cephalothoracic lipodystrophy. J Nerv Ment Dis 109:193, 1949.

112. Peters DK, Charlesworth JA, Sissons JGP, et al: Mesangiocapillary nephritis, partial lipodystrophy and hypocomplementaemia. Lancet 2:535–538, 1973.

113. Sissons JGP, West RJ, Fallows J: The complement abnormalities of lipodystrophy. N Engl J Med 294:461, 1976.

114. Rosen BS, Cook KS, Yaglom J, et al: Adipsin and complement factor D activity: An immune-related defect in obesity. Science 244:1483–1487, 1989.

115. West CD, McAdams AJ: The alternative pathway C3 convertase and glomerular deposits. Pediatr Nephrol 13:448–453, 1999.

116. Mathieson PW, Wurzner R, Oliveria DB, et al: Complement-mediated adipocyte lysis by nephritic factor sera. J Exp Med 177:1827–1831, 1993.

117. Williams DG, Bartlett A, Duffus P: Identification of nephritic factor as an immunoglobulin. Clin Exp Immunol 33:425–429, 1978.

118. Oral EA: Lipoatrophic diabetes and other related syndromes. Rev Endocr Metab Disord 4:61–77, 2003.

119. Premkumar A, Chow C, Bhandarkar P, et al: Lipoatrophic-lipodystrophic syndromes: The spectrum of findings on MR imaging. Am J Roentgenol 178:311–318, 2002.

120. Tsiodras S, Mantzoros C, Hammer S, Samore M: Effects of protease inhibitors on hyperglycemia, hyperlipidemia and lipodystrophy. A five-year cohort study. Arch Intern Med 160(13):2050–2056, 2000.

121. Bastard JP, Caron M, Vidal H, et al: Association between altered expression of adipogenic factor SREBP1 in lipoatrophic adipose tissue from HIV-1-infected patients and abnormal adipocyte differentiation and insulin resistance. Lancet 359(9311):1026–1031, 2002.

122. Caron M, Auclair M, Vigouroux C, et al: The HIV protease inhibitor indinavir impairs sterol regulatory

element-binding protein-1 intranuclear localization, inhibits preadipocyte differentiation, and induces insulin resistance. Diabetes 50(6):1378–1388, 2001.

123. Leow MK, Addy CL, Mantzoros CS: Clinical review 159: Human immunodeficiency virus/highly active antiretroviral therapy-associated metabolic syndrome: Clinical presentation, pathophysiology, and therapeutic strategies. J Clin Endocrinol Metab 88(5):1961–1976, 2003.

124. Addy CL, Gavrila A, Tsiodras S, et al: Hypoadiponectinemia is associated with insulin resistance, hypertriglyceridemia, and fat redistribution in human immunodeficiency virus-infected patients treated with highly active antiretroviral therapy. J Clin Endocrinol Metab 88(2):627–636, 2003.

125. Friis-Moller N, Sabin CA, Weber R, et al: Combination antiretroviral therapy and the risk of myocardial infarction. N Engl J Med 349:1993–2003, 2003.

126. Zenobi PD, Graf S, Ursprung H, Froesch ER: Effects of insulin-like growth factor-I on glucose tolerance, insulin levels, and insulin secretion. J Clin Invest 89:1908–1913, 1992.

127. Rogers DL: Acanthosis nigricans. Semin Dermatol 10:160–163, 1991.

128. Flier JS, Eastman RC, Minaker KL, et al: Acanthosis nigricans in obese women with hyperandrogenism: Characterization of an insulin-resistant state distinct from the type A and B syndromes. Diabetes 34:101–107, 1985.

129. Dunaif A, Hoffman AR, Scully RE, et al: Clinical, biochemical, and ovarian morphologic features in women with acanthosis nigricans. Obstet Gynecol 66:545–552, 1985.

130. Dunaif A, Green G, Phelps RG, et al: Acanthosis nigricans, insulin action, and hyperandrogenism: Clinical, histological, and biochemical findings. J Clin Endocrinol Metab 73:590–595, 1991.

131. Stuart CA, Pate CJ, Peters EJ: Prevalence of acanthosis nigricans in an unselected population. Am J Med 87:269–272, 1989.

132. Mantzoros CS, Moses AC: Treatment of severe insulin resistance. In Azziz R, Nestler JE, Dewailly D (eds): Androgen Excess Disorders in Women. Philadelphia, Lippincott-Raven, 1997, pp 247–255.

133. Oral EA, Simha V, Ruiz E, et al: Leptin replacement therapy for lipodystrophy. N Engl J Med 346:570–578, 2002.

134. Tager HS: Abnormal products of the human insulin gene. Diabetes 33:693–699, 1984.

135. Steiner DF, Tager HS, Chan SJ, et al: Lessons learned from molecular biology of insulin gene mutations. Diabetes Care 13:600–609, 1990.

136. Tager H, Given B, Baldwin D, et al: A structurally abnormal insulin causing human diabetes. Nature 281:122–125, 1979.

137. Haneda M, Polonsky KS, Bergenstal RM, et al: Familial hyperinsulinemia due to a structurally abnormal insulin: Definition of an emerging new clinical syndrome. N Engl J Med 310:1288–1289, 1984.

138. Nanjo K, Miyano M, Kondo M, et al: Insulin Wakayama: Familial mutant insulin syndrome in Japan. Diabetologia 30:87–92, 1987.

139. Gabbay KH, Bergenstal RM, Wolff J, et al: Familial hyperproinsulinemia: Partial characterization of circulating proinsulin-like material. Proc Natl Acad Sci U S A 76:2881–2885, 1979.

140. Robbins DC, Blix PM, Rubenstein AH, et al: A human proinsulin variant at arginine 65. Nature 291:679–681, 1981.

141. Robbins DC, Shoelson SE, Rubenstein AH, Tager HS: Familial hyperproinsulinemia: Two cohorts secreting indistinguishable type II intermediates of proinsulin conversion. J Clin Invest 73:714–719, 1984.

142. Shoelson S, Haneda M, Blix P, et al: Three mutant insulins in man. Nature 302:540–543, 1983.

143. Shoelson SE, Polonsky KS, Zeidler A, et al: Human insulin B24 (Phe-Ser): Secretion and metabolic clearance of the abnormal insulin in man and in a dog model. J Clin Invest 73:1351–1358, 1984.

144. Sanz N, Karam JH, Horita S, Bell GI: Prevalence of insulin-gene mutations in non-insulin-dependent diabetes mellitus. N Engl J Med 314:1322, 1986.

The Metabolic Syndrome

Neil Ruderman and Gerald I. Shulman

INTRODUCTION

For the purposes of this review, we define the "metabolic syndrome" as a state of metabolic dysregulation characterized by insulin resistance, hyperinsulinemia, and a predisposition to type 2 diabetes, dyslipidemia, atherosclerotic vascular disease, hypertension, and other disorders[1-5] (Fig. 59-1). Affected individuals are typically obese or overweight, or show more subtle manifestations of increased adiposity, such as an increase in abdominal fat[6] or fat cell size.[7,8] In addition, they may have a decreased capacity for exercise[3-5,9,10] and show evidence of low-grade inflammation[11-13] and a procoagulant state.[14,15] Type 2 diabetes develops when they are no longer able to sustain the high insulin levels required for near-normal glucose homeostasis.[16]

From a clinical perspective, the importance of the metabolic syndrome is attributable to two factors: (1) it is a target for the prevention of and therapy for the multiple disorders with which it is associated, and (2) it is extremely common. Based on recent Adult Treatment Panel (ATP III) diagnostic guidelines (see later), it has been estimated that upwards of 50 million individuals in the United States older than 20 have the metabolic syndrome (Fig. 59-2),[17] and this is likely to be a gross underestimate.[18] In addition, the metabolic syndrome is becoming increasingly prevalent in adolescents and children in parallel with the increase in obesity in this population[19-22] (see also Children and Adolescents). This chapter updates the reader on the present status of the metabolic syndrome (formally referred to as syndrome X or the insulin-resistance syndrome).[16,23] Emphasis is placed on describing novel mechanisms and factors that are transforming our previous conceptions about its pathogenesis and treatment. In addition, proposed new guidelines for the diagnosis of the metabolic syndrome are discussed, as are the special problems that must be considered when attempting to treat or prevent it or both. For other perspectives, the reader is referred to several excellent recent reviews.[3-5,16,24-27]

HISTORICAL

The clustering of the major components of the metabolic syndrome, such as obesity, type 2 diabetes, hypertension, and dyslipidemia has long been recognized[28]; however, its delineation as a distinct entity took place only after its linkage to insulin resistance, hyperinsulinemia, and cardiovascular disease became more apparent.[23,29,30] Insulin resistance has been defined as a state (of a cell, tissue, system, or body) in which greater than normal amounts of insulin are required to elicit a normal biologic response.[31] In humans, it is currently diagnosed on the basis of high levels of plasma insulin, either fasting or during a glucose tolerance test, or by a decreased rate of glucose infusion or glucose uptake by muscle during a euglycemic-hyperinsulinemic clamp.[9] The presence of insulin resistance in patients with type 2, but not type 1, diabetes was appreciated more than 50 years ago based on their much higher insulin requirement[32] and diminished response to exogenous insulin.[33] Shortly after the development of the insulin immunoassay by Yalow and Berson,[34] this suspicion was confirmed,[35,36] and a whole array of disorders associated with insulin resistance and hyperinsulinemia was identified, in addition to type 2 diabetes, including coronary heart disease and several of its risk factors[23,37-42] (see Fig. 59-1). In general, most adults with insulin resistance and hyperinsulinemia were found to be obese (body mass index [BMI] > 29) or overweight (BMI, 25–29). However, a significant percentage were normal weight by BMI but showed an increase in abdominal fat (central obesity)[6,9] and/or enlarged fat cells.[7,24] The presence of central obesity also was demonstrated to correlate strongly with an individual's predisposition to most of the diseases indicated in Figure 59-1, including coronary heart disease,[43,44] and for this reason, it has become one of the principal diagnostic criteria for the metabolic syndrome.

Hyperinsulinemia and insulin resistance also were found in normal-weight offspring of people with type 2 diabetes,[10,45] hypertension,[46] and hypertriglyceridemia,[8,9,47] and

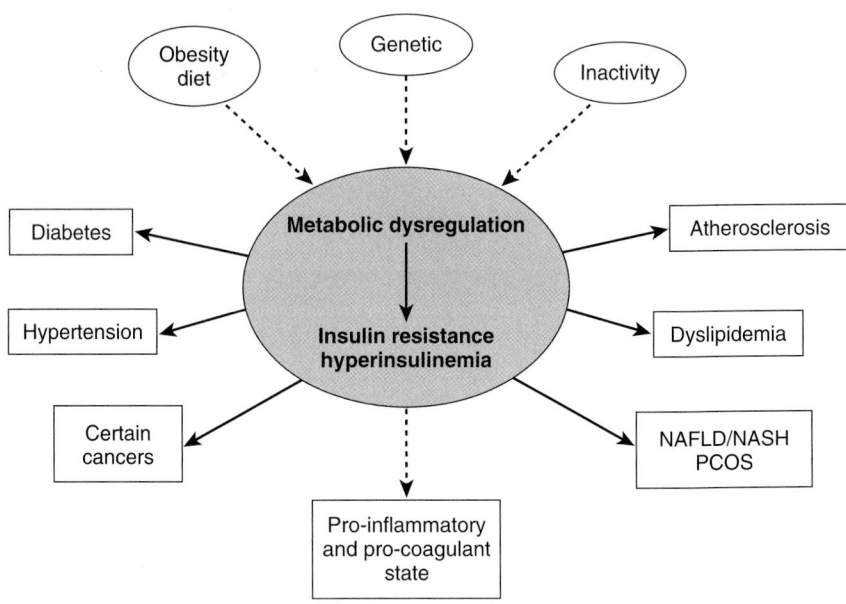

Figure 59-1 The metabolic syndrome: current view. A combination of overnutrition, inactivity, and genetic and other factors (see Linkage of The Metabolic Syndrome to Other Disorders) interact to produce a state of metabolic dysregulation that leads to insulin resistance, hyperinsulinemia, and a proinflammatory state. In individuals who are genetically predisposed, this in turn leads to one or more of the indicated disorders. Nearly all of these disorders are associated with an increased risk of coronary heart disease. A considerable body of evidence suggests that the metabolic dysregulation involves cellular lipid metabolism and may be mediated by a number of factors, including increases in circulating free fatty acid (FFA) levels, alterations of the adenosine monophosphate–activated protein kinase (AMPK)/malonyl coenzyme A (CoA) fuel-sensing network, mitochondrial dysfunction in muscle, and abnormalities in adipose tissue function. PCOS, polycystic ovary syndrome; NAFLD/NASH, nonalcoholic fatty liver disease/nonalcoholic steatohepatitis.

in individuals at increased risk for coronary heart disease,[48–51] suggesting that these are early markers or pathogenetic events for these disorders. Studies such as these, plus the presence of a high rate of ischemic heart disease in patients with type 2 diabetes at the time of diagnosis (20% to 50% in various studies),[52–54] and to a somewhat lesser extent, individuals with impaired glucose tolerance,[55] has led to the suggestion that treatment of the metabolic syndrome at an early stage may be needed for preventing coronary heart disease.[3–5,9,41,56,57]

PATHOPHYSIOLOGY

INSULIN RESISTANCE AND COMPENSATORY HYPERINSULINEMIA

The presence of insulin resistance in people with type 2 diabetes, hypertriglyceridemia, and their otherwise normal offspring has led to the notion that it is a causal factor for the metabolic syndrome.[23,26] According to this widely held view,

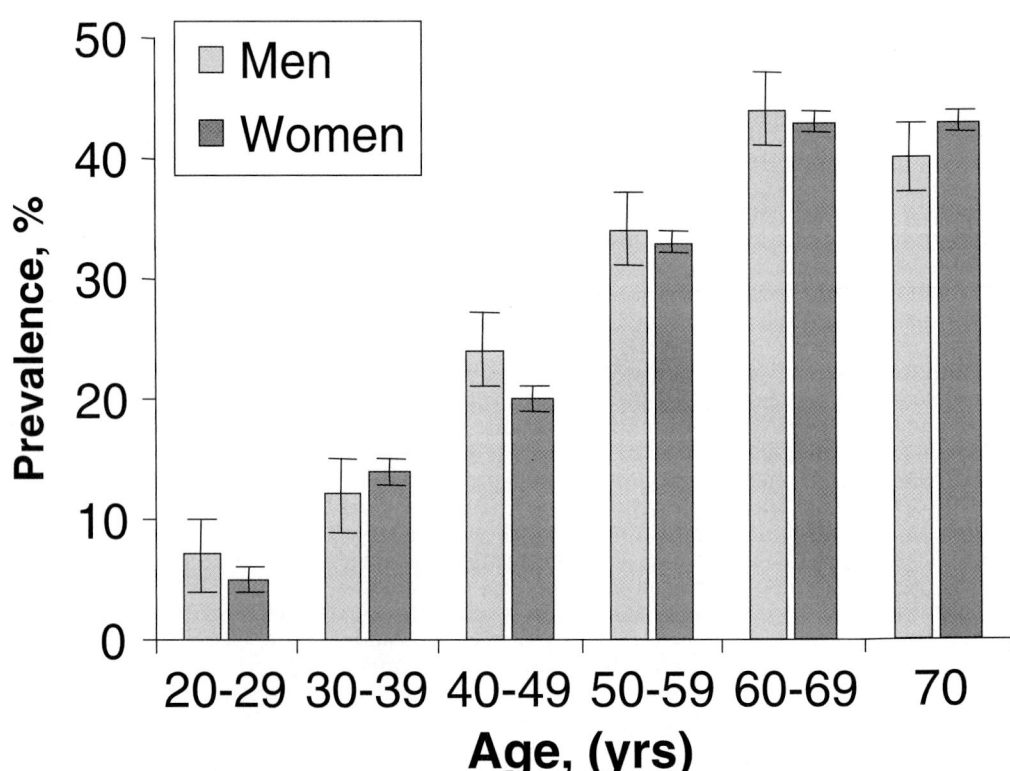

Figure 59-2 Prevalence of the metabolic syndrome in the United States according to age. Based on National Health and Nutrition Examination Survey (NHANES) data and Adult Treatment Panel (ATP) III criteria (see Table 59-3). (Adapted from Ford E, Giles WH, Dietz WH: Prevalence of the metabolic syndrome among US adults: Findings from the third National Health and Nutrition Examination Survey. JAMA 287:356–359, 2002.)

insulin resistance affects a number of organs (including muscle, liver, and adipose tissue), and hyperinsulinemia due to increased insulin secretion by the pancreatic β cell and decreased insulin degradation by the liver is a compensatory phenomenon.[16,23,40] The observation that therapies that increase insulin sensitivity and reduce plasma insulin levels, such as lifestyle modification (diet and exercise)[58,59] and treatment with metformin[59] or thiazolidinediones (Tzds),[60] prevent or delay the onset of diabetes in individuals with glucose intolerance is compatible with this notion, as is the efficacy of these therapies in people with other disorders associated with the metabolic syndrome, such as nonalcoholic fatty liver disease (NAFLD)[61,62] and polycystic ovary syndrome (PCOS).[63,64] Left unexplained by this hypothesis, however, is the molecular mechanism by which insulin resistance develops initially and how it leads to hyperinsulinemia. The possibility that hyperinsulinemia is the primary of the two events or occurs simultaneously with the insulin resistance has not been ruled out.[65]

THE INSULIN SIGNALING CASCADE

Hypothetically, the metabolic syndrome could be related to genetic abnormalities in the insulin signaling cascade. In keeping with this possibility, mutations of insulin-receptor substrate (IRS)1 and IRS2, the initial targets of the insulin receptor tyrosine kinase, have been shown to lead to insulin resistance and diabetes in transgenic mice.[66,67] Evidence is still lacking, however, that these or other genetic defects in the insulin signaling cascade are common in humans with the metabolic syndrome or type 2 diabetes and account for observed signaling defects.[68]

THE LIPID THEORY

Insulin resistance and hyperinsulinemia in humans and experimental animals have been linked to dysregulation of cellular lipid metabolism in a wide variety of circumstances.[1,68–70] Early studies focused on free fatty acids (FFAs) released from adipose tissue and assumed that insulin resistance in skeletal muscle was in some way the result of elevated plasma FFA levels. More recently, it has become apparent that insulin resistance is associated with alterations in lipid metabolism in tissues other than skeletal muscle and that its appearance is affected by a number of newly discovered hormones and intracellular regulatory mechanisms. In addition, it has been demonstrated that the metabolic syndrome occurs in people who lack adipose tissue, as well as in those with excess adiposity, and that in both groups, it is associated with triglyceride deposition in ectopic sites such as muscle, liver, and visceral fat. In this section, we attempt to review the current status of this increasingly complex but intriguing area. Three distinct, but often interrelated, mechanisms that have been put forth to explain the link between altered lipid metabolism and components of the metabolic syndrome are discussed.

Oversupply of Free Fatty Acids

More than 40 years ago, Randle and colleagues[71] first demonstrated that elevated circulating FFA levels diminish insulin-stimulated glucose utilization by a perfused rat heart preparation. They presented evidence that this effect occurred within minutes, and that it was associated with an increase in mitochondrial fat oxidation that led to both inhibition of glucose oxidation at the pyruvate dehydrogenase step and an increase in the cytosolic concentration of citrate. They also demonstrated that the increase in citrate inhibited glycolysis at phosphofructokinase, leading to an increase in glucose-6-phosphate that secondarily inhibited hexokinase and diminished insulin-stimulated glucose uptake[72] (Fig. 59-3). It was suggested that such a mechanism might account for the

insulin resistance observed in humans with obesity or type 2 diabetes, in both of whom plasma FFA levels were known to be elevated.[73] Over the next 25-year period, most investigators were unable to reproduce these findings in skeletal muscle, however,[74,75] and for this reason, the contribution of elevated plasma FFA levels to insulin resistance in humans remained unclear.

Approximately 15 years ago, Boden and colleagues[76] demonstrated that increasing plasma FFA (by infusing a lipid emulsion with heparin to activate lipoprotein lipase activity) in humans during a euglycemic-hyperinsulinemic clamp inhibits insulin-stimulated glucose uptake and its incorporation into glycogen by leg muscle. More important, they demonstrated a much more dramatic effect when these studies were extended for 4 to 6 hours. Subsequent investigations by Shulman and colleagues,[77] in which ^{31}P magnetic resonance spectroscopy (MRS) was used to measure intracellular glucose-6-phosphate noninvasively, found that its concentration was reduced, suggesting that FFAs principally inhibit insulin-stimulated glucose transport or phosphorylation activity and not the phosphofructokinase reaction, as suggested by Randle. More recently, studies by the same group, in which ^{13}C MRS was used to assess intracellular free glucose concentrations, revealed that insulin-stimulated glucose transport and not phosphorylation was the step inhibited by high FFA levels.[78]

Other studies demonstrated that when insulin resistance in human muscle is caused by an increase in plasma FFAs, it is associated with impaired insulin signaling[68] (see section titled "Molecular Mechanisms of Insulin Resistance"), increases in the concentrations of muscle triglyceride,[79] long-chain fatty acyl coenzyme A (CoA)[80] and diacylglycerol, and increases in protein kinase C (PKC) activity and the translocation of PKCs β1, β2, and δ.[81] Another finding was a decrease in IκBα abundance, suggesting activation of nuclear factor (NF)-κB and proinflammatory events.[81] As is discussed later, similar abnormalities have been found in rat liver after a sustained exposure to fatty acids,[82] in rodent muscle in a wide variety of states associated with insulin resistance,[70,83,84] and in liver and muscle of massively obese, insulin-resistant humans with type 2 diabetes.[85] Thus, the intracellular changes produced by high plasma levels of FFAs when they impair insulin action in muscle are associated with insulin resistance in many settings.

A still unanswered question is whether an increase in plasma FFAs is an early pathogenetic event in the metabolic syndrome. Elevated concentrations of plasma FFAs, attributable to increased adipose tissue mass and the relative insensitivity of large fat cells and visceral fat to insulin,[40,80] are present in people with obesity and type 2 diabetes, and they appear to contribute to insulin resistance when these disorders are established.[26,69,80,86] Conversely, it is less clear whether plasma FFAs are elevated in individuals with the metabolic syndrome at earlier times. Thus, only modest increases in plasma FFAs have been observed in normal-weight, insulin-resistant individuals who are at risk for developing diabetes because of family history,[87] and in insulin-resistant individuals with hypertriglyceridemia.[69] Furthermore, even this has not been a universal finding.[45]

Altered Fatty Acid Partitioning: Malonyl Coenzyme A, Mitochondria, and Adenosine Monophosphate–Activated Protein Kinase

A second abnormality in lipid metabolism that could lead to insulin resistance is a disturbance in fatty acid partitioning in which the oxidation of cytosolic long-chain fatty acyl CoA (FACoA) is inhibited and its esterification and metabolism by other nonmitochondrial processes is enhanced.[70,88] This could occur if either the ability of mitochondria to oxidize fatty acid is impaired or the activity of carnitine palmitoyl transferase 1, the enzyme that regulates the transfer of cytosolic long-chain fatty acyl CoA (the metabolically active metabolic of fatty acid in cells) into mitochondria, is diminished.

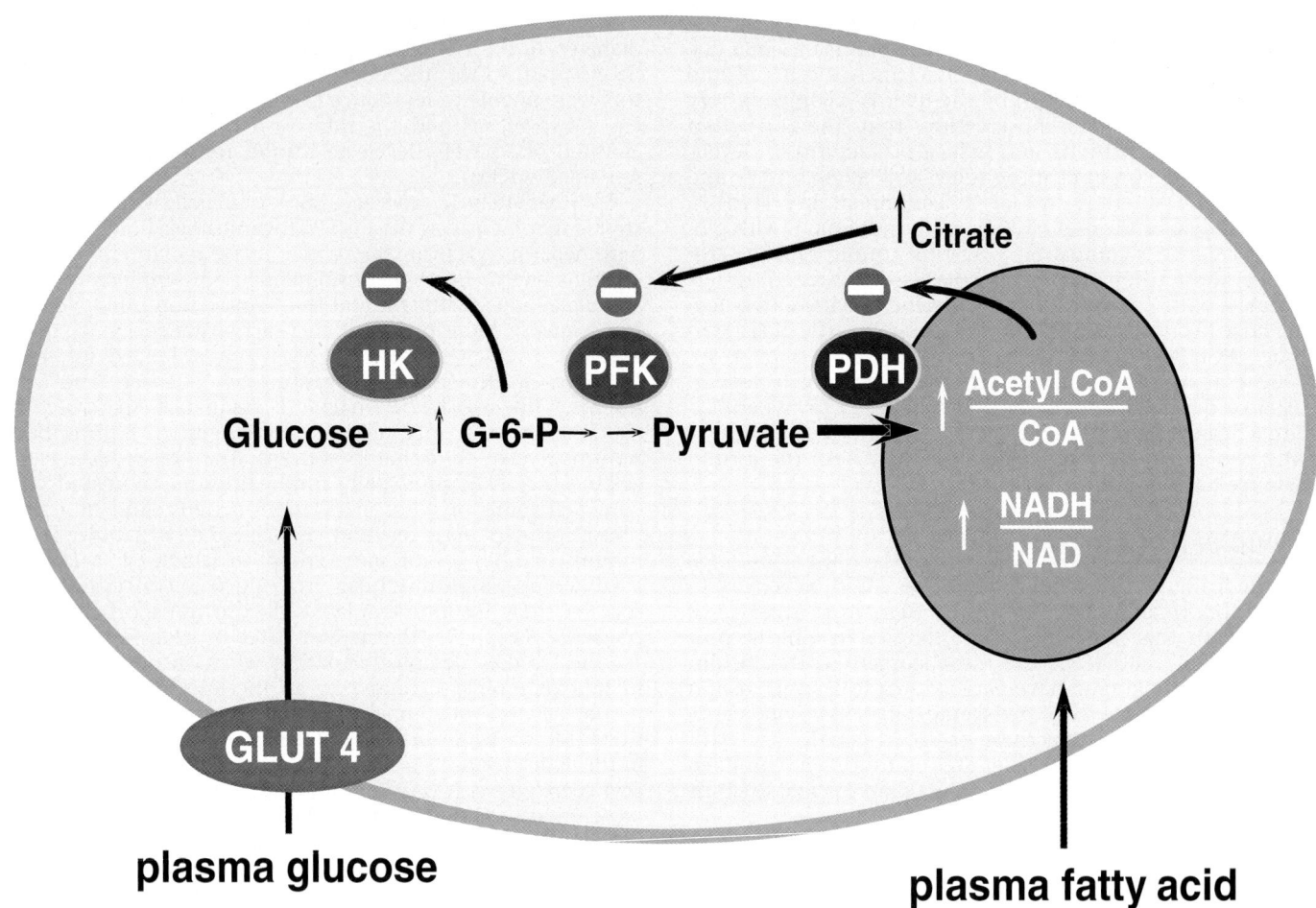

Figure 59-3 Inhibition of glucose uptake and oxidation by fatty acids as described in heart muscle by Randle and colleagues in 1964 and 1965. See text for details. (Reproduced from Shulman GI: Cellular mechanisms of insulin resistance. J Clin Invest 106:171–176, 2000.)

Malonyl CoA

Altered fatty acid partitioning as a cause of insulin resistance was first suggested by studies in denervated rat muscle, in which enhanced diacylglycerol (DAG) synthesis and PKC activation were observed,[89] and in later studies of muscle in obese, insulin-resistant KKA(y) mice.[90] In these and other instances, insulin resistance in rodent muscle correlated with an increase in the concentration of malonyl CoA,[70] an allosteric inhibitor of carnitine palmitoyltransferase. As shown in Figure 59-4, an increase in malonyl CoA, by decreasing the oxidation of cytosolic FACoA, would increase its availability for the formation of DAG, triglycerides, ceramide, reactive O_2 species, and possibly other factors linked to insulin resistance. In keeping with such a mechanism, it was demonstrated by McGarry and others[88,91] that treatment with etomoxir, a pharmacologic CPT_1 inhibitor, concurrently increases triglyceride accumulation and causes insulin resistance in rat skeletal muscle. Also supporting this notion, mice lacking functional acetyl CoA carboxylase 2 (ACC_2, the isoform that generates the malonyl CoA that regulates CPT_1) are more insulin sensitive than are control rats,[92] as are fat-fed rats in which the concentration of malonyl CoA was reduced by exercise[93] or the administration of a pharmacologic ACC inhibitor.[94,95] Finally, low rates of fatty acid oxidation have been reported in preobese humans,[96] Zucker diabetic rats,[97] and interleukin-6 knockout mice[98] before the onset of diabetes and obesity. Malonyl CoA was not assayed in any of these studies; however, in the two rodent models, a decrease in the activity of 5'-AMP-activated protein kinase (AMPK) was found, suggesting that its concentration was elevated[99,100] (see Altered Fatty Acid Partitioning).

Mitochondrial Dysfunction

Altered fatty acid partitioning in muscle and other tissues also could occur if fatty acid oxidation is depressed as a consequence of mitochondrial dysfunction. Decreases in mitochondrial function, and in some instances, number and size, have been found in muscle of individuals with type 2 diabetes associated with obesity,[101] in lean insulin-resistant elderly individuals,[102] and in lean insulin-resistant offspring of diabetic parents.[10] Whether these mitochondrial changes are hereditary or secondary to metabolic events (e.g., lipotoxic changes due to abnormalities in intracellular lipid metabolism) or abnormalities in AMPK regulation (see next section) remains to be determined. Also to be determined is whether the changes observed in the offspring of diabetic parents reflect a difference in muscle fiber type, because the ratio of mitochondrial-rich type 1 fibers to glycolytic type 2 fibers may be decreased in these individuals.[10,103]

AMP-Activated Protein Kinase

AMPK (Box 59-1) is a fuel-sensing enzyme that appears to play a key role in regulating both cellular metabolism and mitochondrial function. In addition, an increasing body of evidence has suggested that its dysregulation could be a cause of the metabolic syndrome (animal studies), as well as a target for its prevention and therapy (human and animals studies).[1]

As shown in Figure 59-4, when AMPK is activated (e.g., during exercise or in some tissues by caloric deprivation), it phosphorylates and inhibits ACC, the enzyme that catalyzes the synthesis of malonyl CoA, and by a still undetermined mechanism, it activates malonyl CoA decarboxylase, an enzyme that catalyzes malonyl CoA degradation.[104] In addition, AMPK

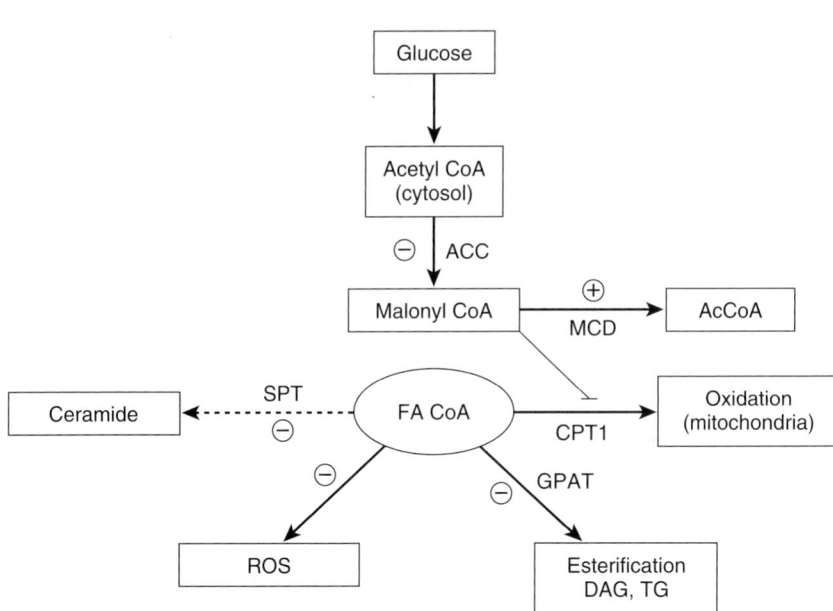

Figure 59-4 Regulation of malonyl coenzyme A (CoA) and cytosolic fatty acid FA CoA by adenosine monophosphate–activated protein kinase (AMPK). By inhibiting CPT₁, malonyl coenzyme A (CoA), which is derived from glucose, diminishes FA CoA entrance into mitochondria where they are oxidized. This makes more FA CoA available for triglyceride (TG), DAG, and ceramide synthesis, and possibly lipid peroxidation and protein acylation. AMPK could inhibit these events and increase FA oxidation by phosphorylating or otherwise inhibiting ACC and GPAT and activating MCD. It also inhibits serine palmitoyltransferase, the first committed enzyme in the de novo pathway for ceramide synthesis. The basis for its ability to inhibit oxidant stress (ROS generation) in some settings is not known. Whether AMPK activation enhances or inhibits a process or an enzyme in this scheme is denoted by plus and minus signs, respectively. ACC, acetyl CoA carboxylase; CPT₁, carnitine palmitoyltransferase 1; DAG, diacylglycerol; FA CoA, cytosolic long-chain fatty acyl CoA; GPAT, glycerophosphate acyltransferase; MCD, malonyl CoA decarboxylase; ROS, reactive O_2 species. (Adapted from Ruderman N, Prentki M: AMP kinase and malonyl-CoA: Targets for therapy of the metabolic syndrome. Nat Rev Drug Discov 3:340–351, 2004.)

concurrently inhibits the use of cytosolic FACoA for diacylglycerol, triglyceride, and ceramide synthesis, and at least in endothelial cells, it diminishes the generation of lipid peroxides and the activation of NF-κB when they are incubated with the fatty acid, palmitate[1,105] (see Fig. 59-4). Thus, AMPK closely regulates the intracellular partitioning of fatty acids and the effects of excess cytosolic FACoA, and it does so by multiple actions. In addition to modulating these events in the short term, AMPK controls many of them in the long term by its effect on transcriptional regulators (e.g., sterol-regulatory element-binding protein [SREBP]1C) that govern the synthesis of ACC and other key enzymes. Of specific relevance to this chapter, decreases in AMPK activity and increases in malonyl CoA are both associated with insulin resistance in muscle (Table 59-1) and liver in many situations. In addition, numerous endogenous hormones (e.g., adiponectin and leptin) and pharmacologic agents (e.g., metformin, thiazolidinediones) that diminish insulin resistance have been demonstrated to activate AMPK and diminish the concentration of malonyl

CoA in experimental animals, as does treatment with the AMPK activator AICAR (5-aminoimidazole 4-carboxamide riboside)[1] (Table 59-2).

Closely linked to mitochondrial theories of insulin resistance is peroxisome-proliferator-activated receptor-gamma coactivator (PGC)1α (PPAR-γ-coactivator 1α), a transcriptional coactivator whose expression is increased when AMPK is activated by exercise or AICAR.[106] In skeletal muscle, and likely in other tissues, PGC1α regulates mitochondrial biogenesis and the expression of multiple genes governing oxidative phosphorylation, including those for citric acid–cycle enzymes and electron-transport proteins.[107-109] PGC1α polymorphisms have been reported in populations with type 2 diabetes in Denmark[110] and Japan.[111] Modest, but coordinated, decreases in the expression of many PGC1α-mediated genes also have been reported in muscle of overweight/obese individuals with type 2 diabetes, impaired glucose tolerance, and a family history of diabetes.[108,109] In all of these groups, a decreased capacity for exercise (Vo_{2max}) was observed, in keeping with the findings of earlier studies in similar patient groups.[103,112,113]

In keeping with its effect on PGC1α, it has been shown that AMPK is necessary for mitochondrial biogenesis.[114] Whether the various hormones (e.g., adiponectin, leptin, catecholamines) and pharmacologic agents (Tzds, metformin) reported to activate AMPK also increase PGC1α expression and stimulate mitochondrial biogenesis and enzyme activity in skeletal muscle and other tissues is an active area for investigation. Also requiring study is the physiological role of Ca^{2+} calmodulin-dependent protein kinase, which, like AMPK, is activated during exercise and increases PGC1α expression.[115]

Adipose Tissue
Overview

A number of lines of investigation have linked abnormalities in adipose tissue to the pathogenesis of the metabolic syndrome. First, as already noted, elevated plasma FFA levels, attributable to an increase in their release from adipocytes in obese or centrally obese individuals, correlate with the presence of insulin resistance in most patients.[80,116] Second, when the function of the adipocyte as a store for lipid is impaired, as it is in people with various lipodystrophies (see later), fatty acids are deposited as triglycerides in ectopic sites such as muscle, liver, and visceral fat, and this is associated with

---

Box 59-1   AMP-activated protein kinase (AMPK)

AMPK is a heterotrimer containing α, β, and γ subunits, each of which has at least two isoforms. The α subunit contains the catalytic site; the β subunit, a glycogen-binding domain; and the γ subunit, two AMP-binding sites. All three subunits are necessary for full activity.[230,231] In general, AMPK is found in the cytosol of a cell; however, the α2 isoform of the enzyme also is present in the nucleus.[231] Decreases in the energy state of a cell, as reflected by increases in the ratio of AMP/adenosine triphosphate (ATP), activate AMPK by a number of mechanisms, including covalent modification due to phosphorylation of its catalytic subunit on Thr-172 by an AMPK kinase (AMPKK).[231] When activated, AMPK activates a number of processes that increase ATP generation, including fatty acid oxidation and glucose transport (in skeletal muscle), and it decreases others that consume ATP, but are not immediately necessary for survival, such as fatty acid and triglyceride synthesis. In addition, AMPK can alter the expression of a wide variety of genes including several that alter mitochondrial function (e.g., *PGC1a*, *UCP3*) and lipid synthesis (*SREBPIC*). The effects of AMPK activation that could account for its ability to diminish lipid accumulation, cell dysfunction, and insulin resistance are depicted in Figures 59-3 and 59-4. Some of the factors that activate it in vivo are listed in Table 59-2.

Table 59-1 AMPK, Malonyl CoA, and Other Abnormalities Associated with Insulin Resistance in Muscle

Model	TG	DAG	Malonyl CoA	PKC Activity	Activated IKK-NF-κB	AMPK Activity
fa/fa rat	(+)	(+)	(+)	(+)	ND	(−)
Glucose-infused rat	(+)	(+)	(+)	(+)	ND	(−)
Fat-fed rat	(+)	(+)	(+/−)	(+)	(+)	ND
Fat-infused humans	(+)	(+)	ND	(+)	(+)	ND
Obese insulin-resistant humans	(+)	ND	ND	(+)	ND	ND

Data are from the laboratories of the authors and those of Turinsky, Kraegen, Caro, Boden, and Shoelson. Many of these changes also have been demonstrated in liver in insulin-resistant obese humans, fat-fed and glucose-infused rats, and fa/fa rats. Studies, primarily in vitro, suggest that similar events occur in the pancreatic β-cell and cultured vascular endothelium.
AMPK, adenosine monophosphate protein kinase; DAG, diacylglycerol; IKK, inhibitor of NF-κB kinase; NF-κB, nuclear factor kappa B; PKC, protein kinase C; TG, triglyceride; (+), increased; (−), decreased; ND, not determined.
Adapted from Ruderman N, Prentki M: AMP kinase and malonyl-CoA: Targets for therapy of the metabolic syndrome. Nat Rev Drug Discov 3:340–351, 2004, with permission.

insulin resistance and other manifestations of cellular dysfunction.[1,117] As is discussed later, the insulin-sensitizing effect of Tzds, at least in part, may be related to their ability to promote the conversion of preadipocytes to adipocytes (adipogenesis), and secondarily to increase the removal of FFAs from the circulation.[118] Third, the adipocyte releases hormones, such as leptin and adiponectin, that in multiple tissues activate AMPK, diminish ectopic lipid accumulation, and enhance insulin action. Finally, the adipocyte also releases the proinflammatory cytokines tumor necrosis factor-α (TNF-α),[119] resistin,[119,120] and plasminogen activator inhibitor (PAI),[15] all of which could cause insulin resistance and other aspects of the metabolic syndrome.

Adiponectin
Of the various adipokines, adiponectin, also referred to as ACRP30, has been most closely linked to insulin resistance in humans. It is produced exclusively in adipose tissue and is present in the circulation in trimeric, hexameric, and high-molecular-weight (HMW) forms. The biologic relevance of the three oligomers,[121,122] and of newly identified tissue paralogs of adiponectin[123] is incompletely understood, as is the identity of the receptors that mediate their action.[124] Also unexplained is why many of the actions attributed to adiponectin can be reproduced by administering its globular subunit,[125,126] g-adiponectin (which comprises approximately half of the monomeric adiponectin molecule), even though it is often not detectable in plasma. These considerations aside, abundant evidence exists that low immunoassayable adiponectin levels in plasma (accounted for mainly by the HMW form) are present in obese individuals and in individuals at risk for type 2 diabetes[121] and coronary heart disease,[127] even in the absence of overt obesity. In addition, polymorphisms of the adiponectin gene have been associated with the metabolic syndrome in some populations and a predisposition to type 2 diabetes in others.[121,128]

In keeping with these findings in humans, in mice fed a high-fat diet, genetically knocking out adiponectin causes glucose intolerance and insulin resistance,[129] and conversely, overexpression of full-length[130] or globular[131] adiponectin attenuates the severity of atherosclerosis in apolipoprotein E (apoE) knockout mice. In addition, the administration of full-length (HMW) adiponectin and the globular subunit have been shown to diminish hepatic lipid accumulation in ob/ob mice with NAFLD[132] and insulin resistance in fat-fed rats, respectively.[125]

Adiponectin, like exercise, activates AMPK and stimulates AMPK-mediated events such as glucose transport and fatty acid oxidation in muscle[126,133] and inhibition of glucose production by liver.[134] Whether the insulin-sensitizing effect of adiponectin is AMPK mediated has not been proven definitively; however, treatment with Tzds increases plasma adiponectin, and this presumably accounts, at least in part, for the insulin-sensitizing action of these agents.[121] Finally, like leptin (see later), some of the peripheral actions of adiponectin appear to be mediated by effects on the hypothalamus[135] as well as by a direct action. In contrast to leptin, however, adiponectin does not suppress food intake.

Leptin
Since its discovery by Friedman and colleagues,[136] interest in leptin has for the most part focused on its role as an appetite suppressant. However, it also has been recognized for some time that leptin increases oxidative metabolism and fatty acid oxidation in peripheral tissues because of both a direct action[137] and an effect on the hypothalamus that appears to be mediated by the sympathetic nervous system.[138] As first reported by Minkoshi and B. Kahn and their coworkers,[139]

Table 59-2 Effect of Factors That Activate AMPK and Reduce Malonyl CoA on Various Manifestations of the Metabolic Syndrome

Factor	Muscle Insulin Resistance	Pancreatic β-cell Dysfunction	Endothelial Cell Dysfunction	Coronary Heart Disease	NAFLD/NASH Syndrome
Exercise	(−)	nd	(−)	(−)	(−)
Calorie/weight reduction	(−)	(−)	(−)	(−)	(−)
Adiponectin	(−)	(−)	(−)	(−)	(−)
AICAR	(−)	(−)	(−)	ND	ND
Leptin	(−)	(−)	(−)	ND	(−)
Metformin	(−)	(−)	(−)	(−)	(−)
Tzds	(−)	(−)	(−)	(−)	(−)

Table is based on studies with isolated tissues, cultured cells, intact rodents, and, in some cases, humans. Where examined, these factors also alter ectopic lipid deposition in keeping with their effects on AMPK and malonyl CoA. Inactivity, caloric excess (glucose), and deficiencies of leptin or adiponectin where studied have shown to have opposite effects.
AICAR, 5-aminoimidazole-4-carboxamide riboside; AMPK, adenosine monophosphate–activated protein kinase; NAFLD/NASH, nonalcoholic fatty liver disease/nonalcoholic steatotic hepatitis; Tzds, thiazolidinediones; (−), decreased; ND, not determined.
Adapted from Ruderman N, Prentki M: AMP kinase and malonyl-CoA: Targets for therapy of the metabolic syndrome. Nat Rev Drug Discov 3:340–351, 2004, with permission.

both the direct and centrally mediated effects of leptin on peripheral tissues are associated with AMPK activation, whereas its action on hypothalamic nuclei is associated with a decrease in AMPK activity.[140]

When leptin is lacking or its receptor is not functioning, lipid accumulates in many tissues, and cellular damage may result. Unger and Orci[141,142] reported that in the Zucker diabetic fatty (ZDF) rat, such ectopic lipid accumulation occurs in liver, muscle, and the pancreatic β cell and that it antedates the presence of diabetes and pancreatic β-cell apoptosis. They coined the term *lipotoxicity* to describe this phenomenon and proposed that a major action of leptin is to prevent the accumulation of ectopic lipid and related events (e.g., increased ceramide and oxidant stress) that cause lipotoxicity. Of particular note for this review, decreases in AMPK activity and an increased concentration of malonyl CoA have been found in tissues of the fa/fa and the ZDF rat, rodents with a functionally deficient leptin receptor, and the ob/ob mouse, which lacks the leptin receptor.[99] Furthermore, treatment with the AMPK activator, AICAR,[99] as well as the Tzd troglitazone,[143] prevents the ectopic lipid accumulation, pancreatic β-cell damage, and the development of diabetes in the ZDF rat.

Vascular Endothelial Cells

An impressive case has been made that atherogenesis is essentially an inflammatory response to a variety of risk factors and that the consequences of this response include acute coronary and cerebrovascular syndromes.[144] An early site at which this inflammatory response appears to occur is the endothelial cell[145]; indeed, increases in NF-κB expression have been observed in endothelium at sites predisposed to atherosclerotic plaque formation[146] and in endothelial cells exposed to elevated concentrations of glucose[147] and FFAs.[148] Likewise, impaired endothelium-dependent relaxation and increases in circulating adhesion molecules (vascular cell adhesion molecule [VCAM]1, intracellular adhesion molecule [ICAM]1, selectins), markers of cellular dysfunction and incipient atherosclerotic vascular disease, have been observed in humans with type 2 diabetes and the metabolic syndrome[149,150] and in normal individuals in whom plasma FFA levels are increased by a lipid infusion.[151] Conversely, endothelial cell dysfunction is diminished in humans by factors that diminish the proinflammatory state, including exercise and caloric restriction[152,153] and by treatment with thiazolidinediones.[150,154] As already noted, all of these interventions have been reported to activate AMPK in rodent tissues. Studies with endothelial cells in culture also support such a protective role for AMPK. Thus, increases in oxidative stress and NF-κB-mediated gene expression observed in cultured endothelium (human umbilical vein endothelial cells [HUVECs] incubated with palmitate are inhibited by the AMPK activator, AICAR.[155] AICAR and, where studied, expression of a constitutively active AMPK also have been shown to inhibit apoptosis, mitochondrial dysfunction, DAG synthesis, and the development of insulin resistance (diminished Akt activation) in HUVECs incubated in a high-glucose medium.[156] Finally, recent studies indicate that the HMW form of adiponectin activates AMPK and has similar protective effects on HUVECs when they are serum starved.[157]

Liver

Changes similar to those in muscle and the endothelial cell occur in the liver in insulin-resistant states. Thus, as in muscle, an association between hepatic lipid deposition and insulin resistance has been clearly demonstrated in humans.[158] In rats infused with a lipid emulsion to increase plasma FFA levels during a euglycemic-hyperinsulinemic clamp, the development of insulin resistance in the liver is associated with increases in DAG mass and PKC activity and a decrease in IKBα abundance[82,159] (G. Boden, N. Ruderman, unpublished data), changes almost identical to those observed in human

muscle.[81] Similar alterations in PKC have been noted in the liver of massively obese, insulin-resistant humans[85] and fat-fed rats with hepatic steatosis.[159] Finally, as is discussed later, the metabolic and inflammatory changes observed in the liver of patients with nonalcoholic fatty liver disease/nonalcoholic steatohepatitis (NAFLD/NASH) closely resemble those attributable to lipotoxicity in other organs.[1]

Pancreatic β Cell

Insulin resistance in muscle and liver does not initially result in hyperglycemia because it is accompanied by hyperinsulinemia. As noted previously, it is unclear whether the hyperinsulinemia is compensatory or results from the same factors that cause insulin resistance, in which event, it might occur at the same time or even precede it.[65,160] In this context, it is noteworthy that increases in plasma FFAs have been shown to increase short-term insulin secretion in certain settings, whereas prolonged increases in the concentration of saturated fatty acids and glucose cause dysfunction and damage to the β cell, and ultimately result in apoptosis.[1,88,161] Work from a number of laboratories[141,142,162–164] has both delineated the events that lead to these phenomena in the β cell and revealed their similarity to the events observed in endothelium and other cells when exposed to high concentrations of FFAs or glucose. As already noted, in the ZDF rat, the leptin-receptor-deficient rodent characterized by Unger,[142] the activity of AMPK in multiple tissues is depressed, and treatment with troglitazone, AICAR, or caloric deprivation prevent, or at least markedly attenuate, the development of β-cell damage and dysfunction and hyperglycemia.[99,143] Finally, although theories linking triglyceride accumulation to β-cell dysfunction are attractive and have led to interesting hypotheses,[165] to our knowledge, no definitive studies showed that triglyceride accumulates in human islets in patients with type 2 diabetes.

Molecular Mechanisms of Insulin Resistance and Cellular Dysfunction According to the Lipid Theory

Based on studies reviewed in the preceding section, a model can be proposed in which insulin resistance and cellular dysfunction are due to an increase in intracellular FA metabolites such as DAG[81,166] and cytosolic LCCoA[83] (Figs. 59-5 and 59-6). According to this scheme, such changes activate a serine-threonine kinase cascade that includes conventional or novel PKC isoforms or both,[81,84,167,168] IκB,[169,170] and jun-activated kinase (JNK-1), one or more of which phosphorylates serine residues on IRS-1 (in muscle).[80] Serine phosphorylation of IRS-1 in turn impairs its ability to associate with phosphatidylinositol (PI 3)-kinase, leading to a diminished activation by insulin of Akt and PKC-ζ, glucose transport, glycogen synthesis, and other insulin-stimulated downstream events. Similar changes appear to occur in liver, except that IRS-2 is the predominant insulin-receptor substrate affected, and the ability of insulin to inhibit gluconeogenesis and glycogenolysis is impaired.[80,171] Also possibly involved in this chain of events are increases in oxidative stress, ceramide synthesis (in some tissues), NF-κB activation, and NF-κB-mediated gene expression that could explain, at least in part, the proinflammatory state associated with the metabolic syndrome.[1,68,172] Interestingly, the hallmark of this insulin-resistant state is an increase in intracellular triglyceride in liver and muscle that can be detected with magnetic resonance imaging.[173,174] Such triglyceride accumulation is generally regarded as a marker of lipid-induced insulin resistance and cellular dysfunction, rather than a cause.[117] On the other hand, by providing an additional source of intracellular FFAs, it could also play a pathogenetic role.

OTHER THEORIES OF INSULIN RESISTANCE

Alternative theories to explain the origin of insulin resistance and cellular dysfunction in the metabolic syndrome have

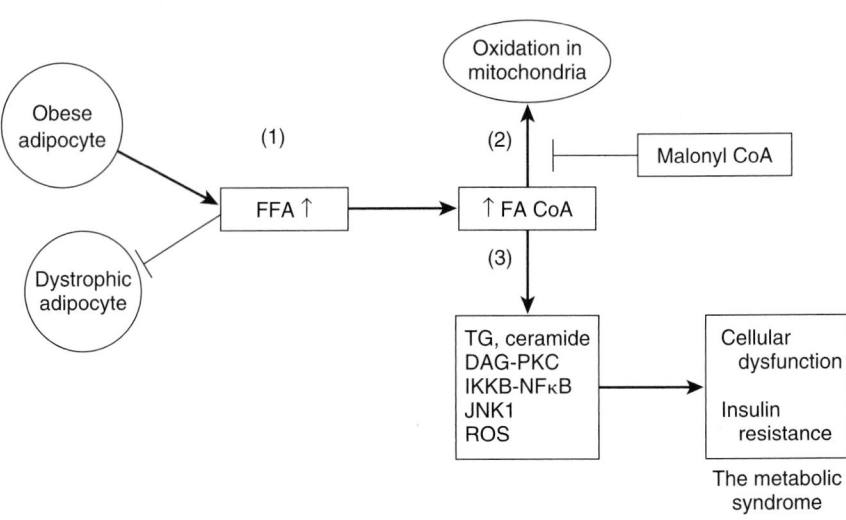

Figure 59-5 The pathogenesis of the metabolic syndrome: the lipid hypothesis. According to the proposed scheme, cellular dysfunction and insulin resistance result from an increase in the cytosolic concentration of long-chain fatty acyl CoA (FACoA) secondary to an increase in plasma FFA levels[1] or a decrease in mitochondrial fatty acid oxidation or both.[2] When this occurs, FACoA can be esterified to form triglyceride (TG), diacylglycerol (DAG), and, in some tissues, ceramide, in increased amounts.[3] Protein kinase C isoforms are activated and, by mechanisms not entirely clear, oxidant stress (ROS) is increased, and the IκB kinase (IKK)-β/nuclear factor (NF)-κB system is activated. Factors that could cause dysregulation at the three sites numbered in the diagram are described in the text. Activated adenosine monophosphate–activated protein kinase (AMPK) exerts multiple effects that increase fatty acid oxidation[2] and decrease the use of cytosolic FACoA for other purposes.[3] In addition, it may restrain lipolysis in the fat cell and diminish de novo fatty acid synthesis (not shown). (See also Figs. 59-4 and 59-6).

focused on glucocorticoid excess and the cellular conversion of cortisone to cortisol by 11-β-dehydrogenase,[175] mutations of PPAR-γ,[176] alterations in muscle capillarity,[40] and increased flux through the hexosamine pathway.[177,178] Perhaps the greatest attention, however, has been given to the theories in which the combination of oxidative stress, IκB and NF-κB activation, and proinflammatory changes play a central role. As noted by numerous investigators, all three have been linked to insulin resistance in humans and experimental animals in a wide variety of disorders and, like insulin resistance, they often antedate these disorders.[11,13,27,149,172] Because of such findings, it has been suggested that an abnormality of the innate immune system could be a proximal event in the pathogenesis of the metabolic syndrome.[11] Although this possibility cannot be disproven, and it is unquestioned that proinflammatory events are an integral component of the metabolic syndrome, a number of observations including the following suggest that dysregulation of lipid metabolism is likely to be a more primary factor[1]: (1) the close correlation of the metabolic syndrome with obesity, central obesity, ectopic lipid deposition, and elevated FFA plasma levels;[2] (2) the presence of the metabolic syndrome and ectopic lipid deposition in humans and experimental animals deficient in peripheral adipose tissue (lipodystrophy), and the reversal of these abnormalities in rodents by the implantation of

fat,[171,179,180] and in humans or rodents, by the administration of leptin,[181,182] adiponectin, and, in some instances, thiazolidinediones[1]; (3) the observation that elevating plasma FFA levels in humans and rodents by itself leads to insulin resistance and proinflammatory changes[80–82]; and (4) the very early occurrence of alterations in cellular lipid metabolism in normal-weight, normoglycemic, offspring of diabetic parents.[10] To our knowledge, evidence of a proinflammatory state has not been reported in the latter group. These considerations aside, the possibility that proinflammatory changes leading to alterations in lipid metabolism are the cause of the metabolic syndrome has not been ruled out. Because therapies targeting lipid metabolism, oxidative stress, and, in some instances, inflammatory events have all been shown to diminish insulin resistance in specific situations,[27,172] what is clear is that these events are almost certainly interrelated.

DIAGNOSIS

No single definitive diagnostic test for the metabolic syndrome is yet available. Historically, it has been diagnosed based on the presence of general or abdominal obesity, dyslipidemia, hypertension, and impaired fasting glucose or glucose intolerance in various combinations. In addition, the

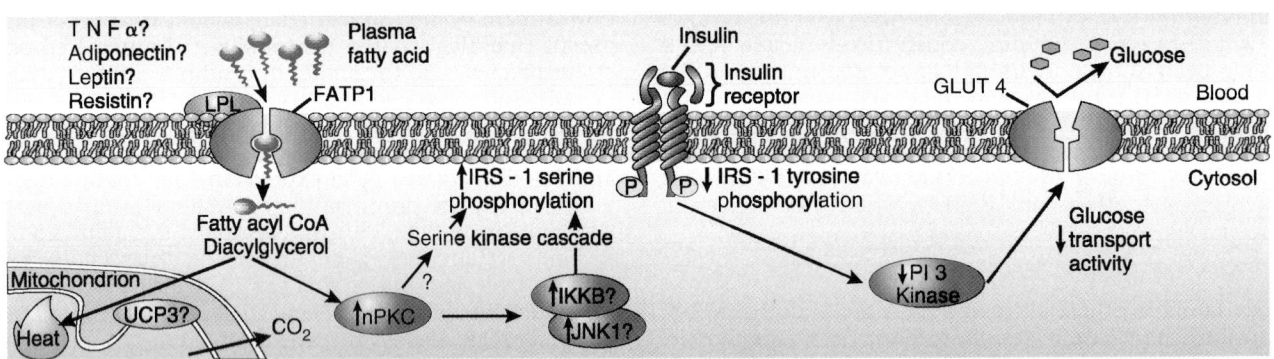

Figure 59-6 Proposed mechanism by which fatty acids cause insulin resistance in skeletal muscle. Increases in cytosolic fatty acyl coenzyme A (CoA) and secondarily diacylglycerol lead to increases in the activity of novel and possibly conventional protein kinase C isoforms and of other serine kinases such as jun-activated kinase (JNK) and IKKB. One or more of these kinases phosphorylate insulin-receptor substrate (IRS)-1, leading to inhibition its tyrosyl phosphorylation by the insulin receptor tyrosine kinase. This in turn decreases the activation of PI 3-kinase and other downstream steps in the insulin signaling cascade. Other factors not shown in the scheme that have been linked to insulin resistance are increases in oxidative stress, NF-κB activation, and NF-κB–mediated gene expression. The question marks indicate that the existence of an event has not been proven definitively. See text for additional details. (Reproduced from Shulman GI: Unraveling the cellular mechanism of insulin resistance in humans: New insights from magnetic resonance spectroscopy. Physiology (Bethesda) 19:183–190, 2004.)

presence of premature coronary heart disease, type 2 diabetes in its early stages, and other disorders associated with insulin resistance have sometimes been considered diagnostic criteria. Three organizations have recently published standards for diagnosis. The criteria adopted by the National Cholesterol Education Program, Adult Treatment Panel (ATP III), and by the World Health Organization (WHO) (Tables 59-3 and 59-4) have recently been reviewed in detail.[3] They differ principally in that the WHO criteria place more emphasis on measures of insulin resistance, the presence of microalbuminuria, and the use of the glucose tolerance test, whereas the ATP III emphasizes abdominal obesity and risk factors for cardiovascular disease such as dyslipidemia and hypertension. A more clinically oriented set of criteria were recently proposed by the American Association of Clinical Endocrinologists (AACE).[3] It takes into account family history of type 2 diabetes, hypertension and cardiovascular disease, sedentary lifestyle, advancing age, and the presence of other diseases associated with the metabolic syndrome, such as PCOS (see Fig. 59-1). In addition, the AACE sets the upper limit of BMI at 25 kg/m[2], a value much lower than that of the WHO, and it does not specify the number of risk factors required for diagnosis; indeed, diagnosis is left to clinical judgment. The stricter criteria of the ATP III and WHO guidelines undoubtedly reflect the fact that they are attempting to diagnose the metabolic syndrome for research as well as for clinical purposes. In turn, the AACE guidelines will almost certainly identify a greater number of individuals, and they will probably identify them at an earlier age. In part because of its relative simplicity, the ATP III guidelines appear to be in widest use. As now constituted, however, they probably underestimate the prevalence of insulin resistance in the general population.[183] They also are not yet designed to take ethnic group differences into account, an important consideration because in some groups (e.g., in south Asians), the metabolic syndrome is not so closely associated with obesity, or at least obesity based on BMI, as it is in whites.[184]

LINKAGE OF METABOLIC SYNDROME TO CORONARY HEART DISEASE

The notion that the metabolic syndrome, or its surrogate markers hyperinsulinemia and insulin resistance, antedate and contribute to the pathogenesis of coronary heart disease and at least some cases of hypertension was proposed many years ago.[23,40,41] As recently reviewed, coronary heart disease

Table 59-3 ATP III Diagnostic Criteria for the Metabolic Syndrome

Risk Factor	Defining Level
Abdominal obesity (waist circumference)	
Men	>102 cm
Women	>88 cm
Triglycerides	>150 mg/dL
HDL-cholesterol	
Men	>40 mg/dL
Women	>50 mg/dL
Blood pressure	>130/80 mm Hg
Fasting glucose	>110 mg/dL*

ATP III, Adult Treatment Panel III.

*America Diabetes Association recently reduced fasting glucose level to 100 mg/dL.

Adapted from Grundy SM, Brewer HB, Cleeman JI, et al: Definition of metabolic syndrome: Report of the National Heart, Lung, and Blood Institute/American Heart Association conference on scientific issues related to definition. Circulation 109:433–438, 2004, with permission.

Table 59-4 WHO Diagnostic Criteria

Insulin resistance, identified by one of the following:
Type 2 diabetes
Impaired fasting glucose
Impaired glucose tolerance
Or for those with normal fasting glucose levels (<110 mg/dL), glucose uptake below the lowest quartile for background population under investigation under hyperinsulinemic, euglycemic conditions

Plus any two of the following:
Antihypertensive medication and/or high blood pressure (≥140 mm Hg systolic or ≥90 mm Hg diastolic)
Plasma triglycerides ≥150 mg/dL (≥1.7 mmol/L)
HDL cholesterol <35 mg/dL (<0.9 mmol/L) in men or <39 mg/dL (1.0 mmol/L) in women
BMI >30 kg/m[2] and/or waist/hip ratio >0.9 in men, >0.85 in women
Urinary albumin excretion rate ≥20 μg/min or albumin/creatinine ratio ≥30 mg/g

BMI, Body mass index; HDL, high-density lipoprotein; WHO, World Health Organization.

Adapted from Grundy SM, Brewer, HB, Cleeman JI, et al: Definition of metabolic syndrome: Report of the National Heart, Lung, and Blood Institute/American Heart Association conference on scientific issues related to definition. Circulation 109:433–438, 2004, with permission.

can to a great extent be attributed to the dyslipidemia present in people with the metabolic syndrome (increased dense low-density lipoprotein [LDL], diminished high-density lipoprotein [HDL] cholesterol, and hypertriglyceridemia),[185] as well as to elevations in blood pressure and the presence of a procoagulant, proinflammatory state.[3,5] In addition, some studies suggest that hyperinsulinemia and insulin resistance may be independent risk factors.[51] Whether elevated FFA levels or a dysregulation of intracellular FA metabolism contributes to atherosclerosis by altering the function of endothelium (see Vascular Endothelial Cells) or other cells in the vascular wall remains to be determined. Relevant to this discussion, low levels of adiponectin are associated with an increased risk of coronary heart disease,[127] whereas as noted earlier, overexpression of adiponectin or its globular subunit diminishes the severity of atherosclerosis in ApoE –/– mice.[130,131]

More definitive evidence that the metabolic syndrome per se predisposes to coronary heart disease and cerebrovascular disease has recently been reported. Thus, a two- to fourfold increase in subsequent cardiovascular events has been described in men and women with the metabolic syndrome (modified WHO criteria), even in the absence of type 2 diabetes or impaired glucose tolerance.[186–188] Qualitatively, similar results were obtained when the metabolic syndrome was defined by ATP III criteria[189,190] (Fig. 59-7). Interestingly, in all of these studies, the presence of the metabolic syndrome had an even greater impact on the risk for developing diabetes.[188,189] In addition, where studied, the rate of cardiovascular events was higher in patients who had diabetes and the metabolic syndrome than in individuals with only the metabolic syndrome.

LINKAGE OF THE METABOLIC SYNDROME TO OTHER DISORDERS

From a practical point of view, the ATP III and WHO guidelines focus on the relation of the metabolic syndrome to obesity and the risk of developing type 2 diabetes and macrovascular disease. Conversely, insulin resistance and hyperinsulinemia also are associated with other disorders in people who, for genetic or other reasons (e.g., drug therapy), are more susceptible to them. A few of these disorders are briefly discussed.

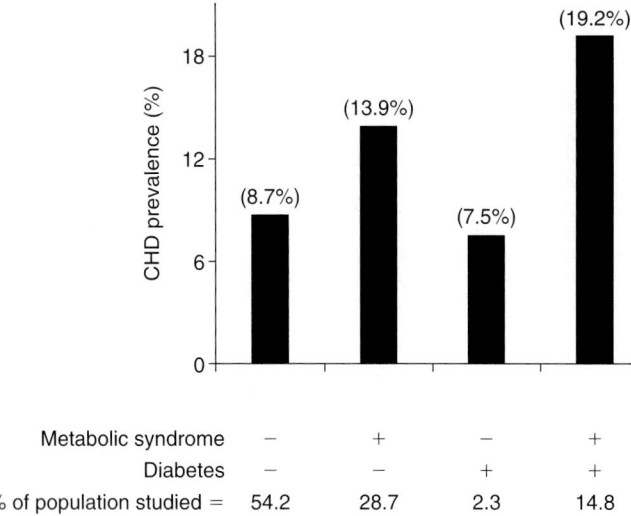

Figure 59-7 Age-adjusted prevalence of coronary heart disease (CHD) in the United States population older than 50 years categorized by the presence of the metabolic syndrome (Adult Treatment Panel [ATP] III criteria) and diabetes. Data are from the National Health and Nutrition Examination Survey (NHANES) study. The complete absence of an increase in CHD incidence in the diabetic patients without the metabolic syndrome should be viewed with caution because of the small size of this group. (Adapted from Alexander CM, Landsman PB, Teutsch SM, Haffner SM: NCEP-defined metabolic syndrome, diabetes, and prevalence of coronary heart disease among NHANES III participants age 50 years and older. Diabetes 52:1210–1214, 2003.)

NONALCOHOLIC FATTY LIVER DISEASE/NONALCOHOLIC STEATOHEPATITIS

It is estimated that nearly 20 million people in the United States have the diagnosis of nonalcoholic fatty liver disease (NAFLD), and in approximately 10% of these individuals, steatohepatitis develops (NASH), a disorder characterized by mitochondrial dysfunction, increases in oxidative stress and cell cytokines, and a predisposition to cirrhosis (~20% of patients with NASH) and less commonly hepatocellular carcinoma.[62,191–194] NAFLD also is seen with increasing frequency in children and adolescents in parallel with the increasing prevalence of obesity in these populations.[19] Presumably, mildly abnormal liver function tests in the presence of obesity or type 2 diabetes or other manifestations of insulin resistance would help to identify individuals with NAFLD at an early point in time.

POLYCYSTIC OVARIAN SYNDROME

Another common disorder that becomes more prevalent in the presence of the metabolic syndrome is PCOS. PCOS is characterized by genetically determined increases in ovarian androgen production and disordered gonadotropin secretion that may be exaggerated by hyperinsulinemia or insulin resistance.[63] Perhaps because of its association with the metabolic syndrome and often, although not always with obesity, PCOS is a leading risk factor for glucose intolerance and type 2 diabetes in adolescent and premenopausal women.[64,195] It also may increase their risk for premature cardiovascular disease.[196] PCOS is associated with increases in such inflammatory factors as PAI, c-reactive protein (CRP), and TNF-α.[64] Like NAFLD/NASH, type 2 diabetes, and other disorders associated with the metabolic syndrome, PCOS often responds to treatments that activate AMPK or lower the concentration of malonyl CoA or both, such as diet and exercise, metformin, and thiazolidinediones[64] (see Table 59-2 and section on therapy).

CERTAIN CANCERS

The reason for the link between the metabolic syndrome, obesity, type 2 diabetes, and cancers of the colon, breast, liver, and other sites is less clear. It has generally been held that insulin-like growth factor 1 (IGF-1) could be a factor because insulin both stimulates the synthesis of IGF-1 by liver and inhibits the synthesis of its binding protein IGFBP-1.[197] Another possibility relates to the fact that an upstream kinase that activates AMPK is LKB1,[198,199] a tumor suppressor that is deficient in people with the Peutz-Jegher syndrome and places them at increased risk for developing carcinomas of the colon, stomach, and pancreas and other tumors. The possibility that LKB1 and AMPK link the metabolic syndrome to these cancers and are targets for their prevention or therapy warrants consideration.[200,201]

CUSHING'S SYNDROME AND RELATED DISORDERS

Patients with primary Cushing's syndrome or Cushing's syndrome due to therapy with glucocorticoids, typically demonstrate central obesity, insulin resistance, hyperinsulinemia, and a predisposition to diabetes and hypertension (see Chapter 122). In addition, like other patients with this clustering of events, they are at increased risk of coronary heart disease.[202] The value of treatments aimed at AMPK and malonyl CoA in people with Cushing's syndrome, in whom the primary cause cannot be corrected, has to our knowledge not been evaluated. The possibility that an increase in cellular 11-β-dehydrogenase activity, resulting in local increases in cortisol, could be a cause of the metabolic syndrome[175] has already been discussed. (See section "Other Theories of Insulin Resistance.")

LIPODYSTROPHY

Patients with primary lipodystrophy and lipodystrophy secondary to drug therapy (protease inhibitors in human immunodeficiency syndrome [HIV] patients) are hypothetically subject to the same lipotoxicity observed in people with the metabolic syndrome for other reasons. Two factors appear to contribute to an insulin-resistant state in these patients: (1) a decrease in peripheral fat cells that causes more plasma FFAs and lipoprotein triglyceride to be shunted to ectopic sites; and (2) plasma leptin and adiponectin levels are very low. The importance of the latter is suggested by successes in treating some patients with leptin[181,203] or with thiazolidinediones.[204,205] Interestingly, in the latter studies, the beneficial effect of rosiglitazone was accompanied by an increase in adiponectin but not of subcutaneous fat mass.

HYPERALIMENTATION

As recently suggested by Unger,[206] hyperalimentation can cause lipotoxic damage and, by inference, the metabolic syndrome in some individuals. He hypothesized that at one extreme are normal individuals, who eat enormous amounts of food for an extended period and become hyperinsulinemic and insulin resistant when the ability of their adipose tissue to deposit the excess lipid in their diet is exceeded.[207] At the other extreme are hyperalimented patients with an extensive loss of subcutaneous adipose tissue due to third-degree burns. Such burn patients are historically very insulin resistant; however, it remains to be determined whether their burns are associated with the predicted increase in ectopic lipid deposition and, if so, whether their insulin resistance responds to pharmacologic agents that enhance insulin sensitivity.

TREATMENT OF THE METABOLIC SYNDROME

The demonstration that the metabolic syndrome increases the risk for developing coronary heart disease and other disorders in both otherwise normal individuals and patients with type 2 diabetes clearly indicates that it warrants treatment. Less clear is what therapies should be used in a given circumstance (see Table 59-3).

LIFESTYLE MODIFICATION (WEIGHT LOSS AND PHYSICAL ACTIVITY)

The treatment of the metabolic syndrome with the aim of preventing cardiovascular disease has recently been reviewed by a clinical conference jointly sponsored by the American Heart Association; National Heart, Lung, and Blood Institute; and the American Diabetes Association (AHA/NHLBI/ADA). The consensus was that lifestyle modifications consisting of diet for the treatment of obesity and overweight and physical activity were the first line of therapy.[3,5] The efficacy of this approach for preventing disease has not been assessed specifically in patients with the metabolic syndrome diagnosed by ATP III or WHO criteria; however, in several prospective studies,[58,59,208] the combination of diet and exercise has proven quite effective in delaying or preventing the onset of diabetes in patients with impaired glucose tolerance (most of whom probably have the metabolic syndrome). Numerous epidemiologic studies also have shown a 30% to 50% decrease in the risk of developing coronary heart disease, as well as type 2 diabetes, with the maintenance of a physically active compared with a sedentary lifestyle.[209] It must be emphasized, however, that in the three major prospective studies,[58,59,208] the incidence of diabetes in the treated patients was still higher than that in the general population, suggesting that to be maximally effective, lifestyle changes may have to be introduced even earlier. Whether lifestyle changes have a similar effect on coronary heart disease is less certain. In preliminary studies in patients in the United States Diabetes Prevention Program (DPP) who were insulin resistant, diet and exercise diminished nontraditional risk factors for coronary heart disease, such as CRP and fibrinogen,[210] as well as some of the more classic risk factors associated with the metabolic syndrome.[211,212]

DRUG THERAPY

When recommended therapeutic goals are not achieved with diet and exercise, pharmacologic therapy is necessary. The recommendations of the AHA/NHLBI/ADA conference have been presented elsewhere[5] and are not extensively reviewed here. Suffice it to say, they vary with an individual's risk for developing coronary heart disease and cerebrovascular disease. Thus, in an individual already at risk for these disorders because of diabetes, the use of statins and other agents to diminish plasma cholesterol has a lower goal (LDL-C, <100 mg/dL) than in someone with isolated hypercholesterolemia. Likewise, certain antihypertensive agents, such as angiotensin-converting enzyme (ACE) inhibitors[213] and fibric acid derivatives,[214] may be of special benefit in patients with type 2 diabetes or at high risk for developing it.

In patients with diabetes, metformin and thiazolidinediones are routinely used because of their insulin-sensitizing and blood-glucose lowering actions (Table 59-5). To what extent they and other insulin-sensitizing agents should be used as second-line therapy for the metabolic syndrome in the absence of diabetes or impaired glucose tolerance is still a matter for debate. No definitive evidence exists that treatment with these agents reduces the risk of cardiovascular disease in people with the metabolic syndrome, impaired glucose tolerance, or diabetes.[5] As a result, the recent AHA/NHLBI/ADA conference[5] concluded, "There is insufficient evidence to recommend these drugs for anything other than their glucose-lowering action at this time." Conversely, as already noted, both metformin and Tzds have shown some effectiveness in treating NAFLD and PCOS. In addition, they

Table 59-5 Recommended Treatments for the Metabolic Syndrome in Adults, Children, and Adolescents

Treatment	Adults			Children and Adolescents
	Nondiabetic	IGT	Diabetic	Nondiabetic
Diet and exercise	+	+	+	+
Metformin	ND	+	+	ND
Tzds	ND	+	+	ND

For diabetic children and adolescents, diet and exercise are the recommended therapy, where possible; however, metformin and insulin often are used.[22]
+, currently recommended treatment; ND, as yet no definitive evidence for or against use; Tzds, thiazolidinediones.

appear to delay or prevent the onset of overt type 2 diabetes in individuals with impaired glucose tolerance,[59,60] and long-term metformin therapy was associated with a decrease in new cardiovascular events in obese individuals with type 2 diabetes in the United Kingdom prospective diabetes study.[215] In light of this, as well as the anti-inflammatory action of some of these agents,[154] their apparent effectiveness in diminishing insulin resistance in the offspring of diabetic parents,[216] and the likelihood they act at least in part through AMPK (see Table 59-2), the results of ongoing studies with these and similar agents in patients with the metabolic syndrome are eagerly awaited.

The role of statins in the treatment of the metabolic syndrome is somewhat clearer. Recent subgroup analyses of statin trials reveal that they reduce the risk for cardiovascular events in people with the metabolic syndrome.[3] To what extent this is due to their ability to diminish LDL cholesterol and the levels of all apolipoprotein B–containing lipoproteins and to what extent because of their anti-inflammatory action[217] is uncertain, however. The NHLBI/AHA/ADA panel recommended that cigarette smoking be discouraged in all individuals with the metabolic syndrome. It also suggested that low-dose aspirin for the primary prevention of coronary heart disease in patients with the metabolic syndrome is promising[3] and recommended its use in individuals with a 10% or greater risk for coronary heart disease by Framingham criteria.[144]

SPECIAL CONSIDERATIONS

The diagnosis and treatment of the metabolic syndrome presents some special problems. For instance, with upwards of 50 million people with this diagnosis in the United States, it is a massive public health problem. In addition, in some people, diabetes, coronary heart disease, liver disease, and hypertension are already present, and in others, the central problem is how to prevent these disorders from occurring. Finally, many therapeutic options are at our disposal; however, some, such as diet and exercise, are often difficult to use and maintain successfully, and others such as drug therapy, are expensive, and in some populations (e.g., children and adolescents), they are untested.

The magnitude of the problem is such that the prevention of diseases associated with the metabolic syndrome will almost certainly require governmental and societal as well as individual change. In such an effort, a primary target will be the prevention of obesity and central adiposity through increasing physical activity and promoting healthy eating.[22] As recently suggested, for children at risk for developing type 2 diabetes, school-based programs and governmental actions that focus on lifestyle will be required.[22] It is highly likely that similar programs will be required for adults.

With respect to drug therapy, already available are a number of agents that are at least partially successful in treating insulin resistance and other components of the metabolic syndrome (e.g., the proinflammatory state) and diminishing diseases that can emanate from it, including type 2 diabetes and coronary heart disease. As we gain a better understanding of the pathogenesis of the metabolic syndrome, it is likely that newer agents will be developed, or that we will discover how to use currently available drugs (e.g., thiazolidinediones and fibric acid derivatives) and other approaches (e.g., diet and exercise) more effectively.

CHILDREN AND ADOLESCENTS

Recent studies indicate that the prevalence of the metabolic syndrome is increasing dramatically in children and adolescents in parallel with the increase in obesity and type 2 diabetes in this population. Thus, in adolescents, aged 12 to 19 years, in the National Health and Nutrition Examination Survey (NHANES) study (1988 to 1994), the metabolic syndrome, diagnosed by ATP III criteria, was present in 4% of the total population, 6.8% of those classified as overweight (BMI, 85th to 95th percentile) and 28% of those categorized as obese (BMI, >95th percentile).[218] Furthermore, because the incidence of obesity has been increasing in the 10 years since these data were obtained, these are likely to be underestimates of its prevalence now.

Where studied, the metabolic syndrome in children and adolescents has been associated with insulin resistance, central adiposity, dyslipidemia, elevations in blood pressure, and increases in intramyocellular and intrahepatic lipid, much as in adults.[20,21] In addition, as in adults, the prevalence of NAFLD[19] and the PCOS[64] is increased, as are plasma levels of the proinflammatory markers, CRP and interleukin-6, and the abundance of immunoassayable adiponectin in plasma is diminished.[20] The prevalence of cardiovascular diseases in these individuals later in life also may be increased.[219–221] Current treatment recommendations for children with type 2 diabetes, most of whom have the metabolic syndrome, have recently been discussed critically by an International Diabetes Federation Consensus Workshop[22] (see section "Special Considerations").

LOW-BIRTH-WEIGHT INFANTS

Abundant evidence exists that a low birth weight, independent of gestational age, predicts the development of type 2 diabetes, coronary heart disease, central obesity, and other aspects of the metabolic syndrome in middle age in some individuals.[222–224] Recent evidence suggests that the greatest risk is in infants with low birth weight who gain weight rapidly in childhood.[225] It has been suggested that an altered intrauterine environment (e.g., poor nutrition) could be responsible for the low birth weight in these children; however, the nature of alteration is not known nor is it clear how it makes these infants more likely to develop the metabolic syndrome in later life.

THE THRIFTY GENOTYPE AND THE INCREASING INCIDENCE OF THE METABOLIC SYNDROME

The recent increase in the prevalence of the metabolic syndrome and type 2 diabetes has been attributed to the epidemic of obesity that began in the second half of the twentieth century and continues unabated. As reviewed elsewhere,[226] this is almost certainly a reflection of environmental factors, most notably the increased availability of food and the decrease in physical activity that occurred in many industrialized societies during this period. In 1962, Neel[227] raised the question of why diabetes (type 2), which has adverse effects on health, per-

sisted in humans during the course of evolution. He proposed that it could be related to the existence of a "thrifty gene" that predisposed individuals to obesity, and secondarily diabetes, but had survival value for our hunter/gatherer ancestors. More specifically, he proposed that in the feast/famine environment of early humans, "individuals exceptionally efficient in the uptake and utilization of food and its storage as fat" would have had a selective advantage. Neel further suggested that in our modern environment of calorie surplus, such a gene (or genes), which protected us from death when food sources were scarce, might make us prone to obesity and diabetes (and the metabolic syndrome). Over the years, many candidate thrifty genes have been suggested, including uncoupling protein-2 (UCP2), UCP3, and β_3-adrenergic receptors. Genes governing the AMPK/malonyl CoA fuel-sensing network, which has been linked to the regulation of both food intake[92,140,228] and energy expenditure,[92,96] also have been suggested. This is an attractive notion, because a decreased ability to oxidize fatty acids appears to be characteristic of preobese humans.[70,229] For the same reason, genes that regulate mitochondrial biogenesis also must be considered.[10] Decreased mitochondrial content/activity, be it acquired or inherited, might promote obesity by two mechanisms: first, by decreasing daily energy expenditure, even by a small amount, it could lead to progressive weight gain. For instance, a 50-calorie/day reduction in energy expenditure in a typical adult, if not accompanied by a comparable decrease in food intake, would lead to a weight gain of approximately 5 lb/year. Second, a decrease in mitochondrial activity in skeletal muscle, by predisposing an individual to altered cellular lipid metabolism (as reflected by an increase in intramyocellular triglyceride), like alterations in the AMPK/malonyl CoA network,[1] can lead to insulin resistance and hyperinsulinemia.[10,102] The latter in turn could promote obesity by increasing lipogenesis in liver and adipose tissue and by inhibiting lipolysis until a new more-obese steady state is achieved.

CONCLUDING REMARKS

The existence of a metabolic syndrome characterized by insulin resistance, hyperinsulinemia, and a predisposition to type 2 diabetes, dyslipidemia, hypertension, and coronary heart disease has long been recognized. Major findings in the past 10 years reviewed in this chapter include the following:

1. The metabolic syndrome is becoming increasingly common. Upwards of 50 million people older than 20 years are affected in the United States, and the diagnosis is becoming increasingly common in children and adolescents.
2. In both adolescents and adults, the metabolic syndrome substantially increases the risk for type 2 diabetes, coronary heart disease, and numerous other disorders.
3. The prevalence of the metabolic syndrome is markedly increased in people who lack adipose tissue, as well as in people who are obese. In both populations, a common occurrence is ectopic lipid deposition in muscle, liver, and often visceral fat.
4. An increasing body of evidence suggests that a likely pathogenetic mechanism in most patients is an abnormality of cellular lipid metabolism that causes lipotoxic changes, including insulin resistance, oxidant stress, inflammation, and mitochondrial dysfunction in one or more tissues. Proposed causes of these abnormalities in cell lipid metabolism are elevated plasma FFA levels, dysregulation of the AMPK/malonyl CoA fuel-sensing network, and primary mitochondrial defects.
5. Genetic, metabolic, and functional changes attributable to the metabolic syndrome are present in lean offspring of diabetic parents. Because of this, and the fact that it

antedates most of the diseases with which it is associated, the metabolic syndrome appears to be an excellent target for disease prevention.

6. Lifestyle modifications, consisting of diet to induce weight loss and exercise, have been shown to diminish many of the abnormalities of the metabolic syndrome and to prevent or delay progression from impaired glucose tolerance to type 2 diabetes in prospective studies. Because of this and their safety and low cost, diet and exercise are the first line of therapy for children and adolescents with the metabolic syndrome and for many adults. Studies with "insulin sensitizing" agents such as thiazolidinediones and metformin are currently in progress.

7. By virtue of the number of people affected and its many potential consequences, the metabolic syndrome is a major public health problem. As such, it will require governmental and societal as well as individual change in children and adolescents, and quite possibly in adults.

Acknowledgements

Supported in part by USPHS grants DK19514, DK49147 PO-1 HL068758 and a Center grant from the Juvenile Diabetes Research Foundation. The authors thank Romina Ilic, May Law, and Sharon Mosher for their assistance in preparing this manuscript and Dr. Nathan LeBrasseur for his constructive comments.

REFERENCES

1. Ruderman N, Prentki M: AMP kinase and malonyl-CoA: Targets for therapy of the metabolic syndrome. Nat Rev Drug Discov 3:340–351, 2004.
2. Reaven G: Metabolic syndrome: Pathophysiology and implications for management of cardiovascular disease. Circulation 106:286–288, 2002.
3. Grundy SM, Brewer HB Jr, Cleeman JI, et al: Definition of metabolic syndrome: Report of the National Heart, Lung, and Blood Institute/American Heart Association conference on scientific issues related to definition. Circulation 109:433–438, 2004.
4. Grundy SM, Cleeman JI, Merz CN, et al: Implications of recent clinical trials for the National Cholesterol Education Program Adult Treatment Panel III guidelines. Circulation 110:227–239, 2004.
5. Grundy SM, Hansen B, Smith SC Jr, et al: Clinical management of metabolic syndrome: Report of the American Heart Association/National Heart, Lung, and Blood Institute/American Diabetes Association conference on scientific issues related to management. Circulation 109:551–556, 2004.
6. Kissebah AH, Vydelingum N, Murray R, et al: Relation of body fat distribution to metabolic complications of obesity. J Clin Endocrinol Metab 54:254–260, 1982.
7. Bernstein RS, Grant N, Kipnis DM: Hyperinsulinemia and enlarged adipocytes in patients with endogenous hyperlipoproteinemia without obesity or diabetes mellitus. Diabetes 24:207–213, 1975.
8. Ruderman NB, Schneider SH, Berchtold P: The "metabolically-obese," normal-weight individual. Am J Clin Nutr 34:1617–1621, 1981.
9. Ruderman N, Chisholm D, Pi-Sunyer X, Schneider S: The metabolically obese, normal-weight individual revisited. Diabetes 47:699–713, 1998.
10. Petersen KF, Dufour S, Befroy D, et al: Impaired mitochondrial activity in the insulin-resistant offspring of patients with type 2 diabetes. N Engl J Med 350:664–671, 2004.
11. Pickup JC: Inflammation and activated innate immunity in the pathogenesis of type 2 diabetes. Diabetes Care 27:813–823, 2004.
12. Schmidt MI, Duncan BB, Sharrett AR, et al: Markers of inflammation and prediction of diabetes mellitus in adults (Atherosclerosis Risk in Communities study): A cohort study. Lancet 353:1649–1652, 1999.
13. Festa A, D'Agostino R Jr, Howard G, et al: Chronic subclinical inflammation as part of the insulin resistance syndrome: The Insulin Resistance Atherosclerosis Study (IRAS). Circulation 102:42–47, 2000.
14. Sakkinen P, Geffken D, Cushman M, et al: Association between physical activity and markers of inflammation in a healthy elderly population. Am J Epidemiol 153:242–250, 2001.
15. Juhan-Vague I, Alessi MC, Vague P: Increased plasma plasminogen activator inhibitor 1 levels: A possible link between insulin resistance and atherothrombosis. Diabetologia 34:457–462, 1991.
16. Reaven GM: Insulin resistance/compensatory hyperinsulinemia, essential hypertension, and cardiovascular disease. J Clin Endocrinol Metab 88:2399–2403, 2003.
17. Ford E, Giles WH, Dietz WH: Prevalence of the metabolic syndrome among US adults: Findings from the third National Health and Nutrition Examination Survey. JAMA 287:356–359, 2002.
18. Kereiakes DJ, Willerson JT: Metabolic syndrome epidemic. Circulation 108:1552–1553, 2003.
19. Roberts EA: Nonalcoholic steatohepatitis in children. Curr Gastroenterol Rep 5:253–259, 2003.
20. Weiss R, Dziura J, Burgert TS, et al: Obesity and the metabolic syndrome in children and adolescents. N Engl J Med 350:2362–2374, 2004.
21. Weiss R, Dufour S, Taksali SE, et al: Prediabetes in obese youth: A syndrome of impaired glucose tolerance, severe insulin resistance, and altered myocellular and abdominal fat partitioning. Lancet 362:951–957, 2003.
22. Alberti G, Zimmet P, Shaw J, et al: Type 2 diabetes in the young: The evolving epidemic: The International Diabetes Federation Consensus Workshop. Diabetes Care 27:1798–1811, 2004.
23. Reaven GM: Banting lecture 1988: Role of insulin resistance in human disease. Diabetes 37:1595–1607, 1988.
24. Bays H, Mandarino L, DeFronzo RA: Role of the adipocyte, free fatty acids, and ectopic fat in pathogenesis of type 2 diabetes mellitus: Peroxisomal proliferator-activated receptor agonists provide a rational therapeutic approach. J Clin Endocrinol Metab 89:463–478, 2004.
25. Reilly MP, Rader DJ: The metabolic syndrome: More than the sum of its parts? Circulation 108:1546–1551, 2003.
26. Reaven G: Insulin resistance and its consequences: Type 2 diabetes mellitus and the insulin resistance syndrome. In Leroith D, Taylor DI, Olefsky JM (eds): Diabetes mellitus: A fundamental and clinical text, 3d ed. Philadelphia, Lippincott Williams & Wilkins, 2004, pp 899–915.
27. Evans JL, Goldfine ID, Maddux BA, Grodsky GM: Are oxidative stress-activated signalling pathways mediators of insulin resistance and B-cell dysfunction? Diabetes 52:1–8, 2003.
28. Dieterle P, Fehm H, Stroder W, et al: Asymptomatic diabetes mellitus in hypertensive patients of normal weight: Glucose tolerance and serum levels of insulin and nonesterified fatty acids in essential hypertension. Ger Med Mon 13:478–483, 1968.
29. Modan M, Halkin H, Almog S, et al: Hyperinsulinemia: A link between hypertension obesity and glucose intolerance. J Clin Invest 75:809–817, 1985.
30. Stern MP: The insulin resistance syndrome. In Alberti KMMG, Zimmet P, DeFronzo RA (eds): International textbook of diabetes mellitus. New York, John Wiley & Sons, 1997, pp 255–283.
31. Flier JS: An overview of insulin resistance. In Moller DE (ed): Insulin resistance. Chichester, UK, Wiley, 1993, pp 1–8.
32. Himsworth H: Diabetes mellitus: Its differentiation into insulin-sensitive and insulin-insensitive types. Lancet 1:127, 1936.
33. Himsworth HP: The syndrome of diabetes and its cause. Lancet 253:465–473, 1949.

34. Yalow RS, Berson SA: Immunoassay of endogenous plasma insulin in man. J Clin Invest 39:1157–1175, 1960.

35. Yalow RS, Berson SA: Plasma insulin concentrations in nondiabetic and early diabetic subjects: Determinations by a new sensitive immuno-assay technique. Diabetes 9:254–260, 1960.

36. Karam JH, Grodsky GM, Forsham PH: Excessive insulin response to glucose in obese subjects as measured by immunochemical assay. Diabetes 12:197–204, 1963.

37. Davidson PC, Albrink MJ: Insulin resistance in hyperglyceridemia. Metabolism 14:1059–1070, 1965.

38. Malherbe C, Heller F, de Gasparo M, et al: Insulin response during prolonged glucose infusion. J Clin Endocrinol Metab 30:535–538, 1970.

39. DeFronzo RA, Ferrannini E: Insulin resistance: A multifaceted syndrome responsible for NIDDM, obesity, hypertension, dyslipidemia, and atherosclerotic cardiovascular disease. Diabetes Care 14:173–194, 1991.

40. Bjorntorp P: The relationship between obesity and diabetes. In Alberti KGMM, DeFronzo PZ, De Fronzo RA (eds): International Textbook of Diabetes Mellitus, 2d ed. John Wiley & Sons, 1997, pp 612–627.

41. Ruderman NB, Berchtold P, Schneider S: Obesity-associated disorders in normal-weight individuals: Some speculations. Int J Obesity 6:151–157, 1982.

42. Ruderman NB, Haudenschild C: Diabetes as an atherogenic factor. Prog Cardiovasc Dis 26:373–412, 1984.

43. Lapidus L, Bengtsson C, Larsson B, et al: Distribution of adipose tissue and risk of cardiovascular disease and death: A 12 year follow up of participants in the population study of women in Gothenburg, Sweden. Br Med J (Clin Res Ed) 289:1257–1261, 1984.

44. Larsson B, Svardsudd K, Welin L, et al: Abdominal adipose tissue distribution, obesity, and risk of cardiovascular disease and death: 13 year follow up of participants in the study of men born in 1913. Br Med J (Clin Res Ed) 288:1401–1404, 1984.

45. Beck-Nielsen H, Groop LC: Metabolic and genetic characterization of prediabetic states: Sequence of events leading to non-insulin-dependent diabetes mellitus. J Clin Invest 94:1714–1721, 1994.

46. Ferrari P, Weidmann P, Shaw S, et al: Altered insulin sensitivity, hyperinsulinemia, and dyslipidemia in individuals with a hypertensive parent. Am J Med 91:589–596, 1991.

47. Werbin B, Tamir I, Heldenberg D, et al: Immunoreactive insulin and glucose response to oral glucose in offspring of patients with endogenous hypertriglyceridaemia. Clin Chim Acta 76:35–40, 1977.

48. Pyorala K: Relationship of glucose tolerance and plasma insulin to the incidence of coronary heart disease: Results from two population studies in Finland. Diabetes Care 2:131–141, 1979.

49. Welborn TA, Wearne K: Coronary heart disease incidence and cardiovascular mortality in Busselton with reference to glucose and insulin concentrations. Diabetes Care 2:154–160, 1979.

50. Ducimetiere P, Eschwege E, Papoz L, et al: Relationship of plasma insulin levels to the incidence of myocardial infarction and coronary heart disease mortality in a middle-aged population. Diabetologia 19:205–210, 1980.

51. Despres JP, Lamarche B, Mauriege P, et al: Hyperinsulinemia as an independent risk factor for ischemic heart disease. N Engl J Med 334:952–957, 1996.

52. Uusitupa MI, Niskanen LK, Siitonen O, et al: Ten-year cardiovascular mortality in relation to risk factors and abnormalities in lipoprotein composition in type 2 (non-insulin-dependent) diabetic and non-diabetic subjects. Diabetologia 36:1175–1184, 1993.

53. Nesto RW, Phillips RT, Kett KG, et al: Angina and exertional myocardial ischemia in diabetic and nondiabetic patients: assessment by exercise thallium scintigraphy. Ann Intern Med 108:170–175, 1988.

54. UKPDS: Complications of newly diagnosed type 2 diabetes patients and their association with different clinical and biochemical risk factors. Diabetes Res 13:1–11, 1990.

55. Jarrett RJ, McCartney P, Keen H: The Bedford Survey: Ten year mortality rates in newly diagnosed diabetics, borderline diabetics and normoglycaemic controls and risk indices for coronary heart disease in borderline diabetics. Diabetologia 22(2):79–84, 1982.

56. Haffner SM, Stern MP, Hazuda HP, et al: Cardiovascular risk factors in confirmed prediabetic individuals: Does the clock for coronary heart disease start ticking before the onset of clinical diabetes? JAMA 263:2893–2898, 1990.

57. Panzer C, Brieke A, Ruderman, NB: Prevention of type 2 diabetes and its macrovascular complications: Whom, when and how should we treat? Curr Opin Endocrinol Diabetes 10:219–236, 2003.

58. Pan DA, Lillioja S, Kriketos AD, et al: Skeletal muscle triglyceride levels are inversely related to insulin action. Diabetes 46:983–988, 1997.

59. Knowler WC, Barrett-Connor E, Fowler SE, et al: Reduction in the incidence of type 2 diabetes with lifestyle intervention or metformin. N Engl J Med 346:393–403, 2002.

60. Buchanan TA, Xiang AH, Peters RK, et al: Preservation of pancreatic beta-cell function and prevention of type 2 diabetes by pharmacological treatment of insulin resistance in high-risk Hispanic women. Diabetes 51:2796–2803, 2002.

61. Neuschwander-Tetri BA, Brunt EM, Wehmeier KR, et al: Improved nonalcoholic steatohepatitis after 48 weeks of treatment with the PPAR-gamma ligand rosiglitazone. Hepatology 38:1008–1017, 2003.

62. Neuschwander-Tetri BA, Caldwell SH: Nonalcoholic steatohepatitis: Summary of an AASLD Single Topic Conference. Hepatology 37:1202–1219, 2003.

63. Sam S, Dunaif A: Polycystic ovary syndrome: Syndrome XX? Trends Endocrinol Metab 14:365–370, 2003.

64. Dhindsa G, Bhatia R, Dhindsa M, Bhatia V: Insulin resistance, insulin sensitization and inflammation in polycystic ovarian syndrome. J Postgrad Med 50:140–144, 2004.

65. McGarry JD: What if Minkowski had been ageusic? An alternative angle on diabetes. Science 258:766–770, 1992.

66. White MF: IRS proteins and the common path to diabetes. Am J Physiol Endocrinol Metab 283:E413–E422, 2002.

67. Almind K, Accili, D, Kahn CR: Knockout mice as a tool to the understanding of diabetes. In LeRoith SIT, Olefsky JM (eds): Diabetes Mellitus: A Fundamental and Clinical Text, 3d ed. Philadelphia, Lippincott, 2004, pp 245–254.

68. Shulman GI: Cellular mechanisms of insulin resistance. J Clin Invest 106:171–176, 2000.

69. Reaven GM: The fourth musketeer: From Alexandre Dumas to Claude Bernard. Diabetologia 38:3–13, 1995.

70. Ruderman NB, Saha AK, Vavvas D, et al: fuel sensing, and insulin resistance. Am J Physiol 276:E1–E18, 1999.

71. Randle PJ, Garland PB, Hales CN, Newsholme EA: The glucose fatty-acid cycle: Its role in insulin sensitivity and the metabolic disturbances of diabetes mellitus. Lancet 1:785–789, 1963.

72. Randle PJ, Newsholme EA, Garland PB: Regulation of glucose uptake by muscle. 8: Effects of fatty acids, ketone bodies and pyruvate, and of alloxan-diabetes and starvation, on the uptake and metabolic fate of glucose in rat heart and diaphragm muscles. Biochem J 93:652–665, 1964.

73. Randle PJ, Garland PB, Newsholme EA, Hales CN: The glucose fatty acid cycle in obesity and maturity onset diabetes mellitus. Ann N Y Acad Sci 131:324–333, 1965.

74. Ruderman NB, Toews CJ, Shafrir E: Role of free fatty acids in glucose homeostasis. Arch Intern Med 123:299–313, 1969.

75. Randle PJ: Regulatory interactions between lipids and carbohydrates: the glucose fatty acid cycle after 35 years. Diabetes Metab Rev 14:263–283, 1998.

76. Boden G, Jadali F, White J, et al: Effects of fat on insulin-stimulated carbohydrate metabolism in normal men. J Clin Invest 88:960–966, 1991.

77. Roden M, Price TB, Perseghin G, et al: Mechanism of free fatty acid-induced insulin resistance in humans. J Clin Invest 97:2859–2865, 1996.

78. Dresner A, Laurent D, Marcucci M, et al: Effects of free fatty acids on glucose transport and IRS-1-associated phosphatidylinositol 3-kinase activity. J Clin Invest 103:253–259, 1999.

79. Boden G, Lebed B, Schatz M, et al: Effects of acute changes of plasma free fatty acids on intramyocellular fat content and insulin resistance in

healthy subjects. Diabetes 50:1612–1617, 2001.

80. Boden G, Shulman GI: Free fatty acids in obesity and type 2 diabetes: Defining their role in the development of insulin resistance and beta-cell dysfunction. Eur J Clin Invest 32(Suppl 3):14–23, 2002.

81. Itani SI, Ruderman NB, Schmieder F, Boden G: Lipid-induced insulin resistance in human muscle is associated with changes in diacylglycerol, protein kinase C, and IkappaB-alpha. Diabetes 51:2005–2011, 2002.

82. Lam TK, Yoshii H, Haber CA, et al: Free fatty acid-induced hepatic insulin resistance: A potential role for protein kinase C-delta. Am J Physiol Endocrinol Metab 283:E682–E691, 2002.

83. Ellis BA, Poynten A, Lowy AJ, et al: Long-chain acyl-CoA esters as indicators of lipid metabolism and insulin sensitivity in rat and human muscle. Am J Physiol Endocrinol Metab 279:E554–E560, 2000.

84. Griffin ME, Marcucci MJ, Cline GW, et al: Free fatty acid-induced insulin resistance is associated with activation of protein kinase C theta and alterations in the insulin signaling cascade. Diabetes 48:1270–1274, 1999.

85. Considine R, Nyce MR, Allen LE, et al: Protein kinase C is increased in the liver of humans and rats with non-insulin-dependent diabetes mellitus: An alteration not due to hyperglycemia. J Clin Invest 95:2938–2944, 1995.

86. Boden G: Free fatty acids as a target for therapy. Curr Opin Endocrinol Diabetes (in press) 2005.

87. Perseghin G, Ghosh S, Gerow K, Shulman GI: Metabolic defects in lean nondiabetic offspring of NIDDM parents: A cross-sectional study. Diabetes 46:1001–1009, 1997.

88. McGarry JD: Banting lecture 2001: Dysregulation of fatty acid metabolism in the etiology of type 2 diabetes. Diabetes 51:7–18, 2002.

89. Heydrick SJ, Ruderman NB, Kurowski TG, et al: Enhanced stimulation of diacylglycerol and lipid synthesis by insulin in denervated muscle: Altered protein kinase C activity and possible link to insulin resistance. Diabetes 40:1707–1711, 1991.

90. Saha AK, Kurowski TG, Colca JR, Ruderman NB: Lipid abnormalities in tissues of the KKAy mouse: Effects of pioglitazone on malonyl-CoA and diacylglycerol. Am J Physiol 267:E95–E101, 1994.

91. Dobbins RL, Szczepaniak LS, Bentley B, et al: Prolonged inhibition of muscle carnitine palmitoyltransferase-1 promotes intramyocellular lipid accumulation and insulin resistance in rats. Diabetes 50:123–130, 2001.

92. Abu-Elheiga L, Matzuk MM, Abo-Hashema KAH, Wakil SJ: Continuous fatty acid oxidation and reduced fat storage in mice lacking acetyl-CoA carboxylase 2. Science 291:2613–2616, 2001.

93. Iglesias MA, Ye JM, Frangioudakis G, et al: administration causes an apparent enhancement of muscle and liver insulin action in insulin-resistant high-fat-fed rats. Diabetes 51:2886–2894, 2002.

94. Harwood HJ Jr, Petras SF, Shelly LD, et al: Isozyme-nonselective N-substituted bipiperidylcarboxamide acetyl-CoA carboxylase inhibitors reduce tissue malonyl-CoA concentrations, inhibit fatty acid synthesis, and increase fatty acid oxidation in cultured cells and in experimental animals. J Biol Chem 278:37099–37111, 2003.

95. Harwood HJ Jr: Acetyl-CoA carboxylase inhibition for the treatment of metabolic syndrome. Curr Opin Invest Drugs 5:283–289, 2004.

96. Ruderman NB, Saha AK, Kraegen EW: Minireview: Malonyl CoA, AMP-activated protein kinase, and adiposity. Endocrinology 144:5166–5171, 2003.

97. Etgen GJ, Oldham BA: Profiling of Zucker diabetic fatty rats in their progression to the overt diabetic state. Metabolism 49:684–688, 2000.

98. Faldt J, Wernstedt I, Fitzgerald SM, et al: Reduced exercise endurance in interleukin-6-deficient mice. Endocrinology 145:2680–2686, 2004.

99. Yu X, McCorkle SK, Wang MY, et al: Leptinomimetic effects of AICAR administration in leptin-resistant rats: Prevention of diabetes and ectopic lipid deposition. Diabetologia 47(11):2012–2021, 2004.

100. Kelly M, Keller C, Avilucea PR, et al: AMPK activity is diminished in tissues of IL-6 knockout mice: The effect of exercise. Biochem Biophys Res Commun 320:449–454, 2004.

101. Kelley DE, He J, Menshikova EV, Ritov VB: Dysfunction of mitochondria in human skeletal muscle in type 2 diabetes. Diabetes 51:2944–2950, 2002.

102. Petersen KF: Mitochondrial dysfunction in the elderly: Possible role in insulin resistance. Science 300:1140–1142, 2003.

103. Nyholm B, Mengel A, Nielsen S, et al: Insulin resistance in relatives of NIDDM patients: The role of physical fitness and muscle metabolism. Diabetologia 39:813–822, 1996.

104. Park H, Kaushik VK, Constant S, et al: Coordinate regulation of malonyl-CoA decarboxylase, sn-glycerol-3-phosphate acyltransferase, and acetyl-CoA carboxylase by AMP-activated protein kinase in rat tissues in response to exercise. J Biol Chem 277:32571–32577, 2002.

105. Ruderman NB, Cacicedo JM, Itani S, et al: Malonyl-CoA and AMP-activated protein kinase (AMPK): Possible links between insulin resistance in muscle and early endothelial cell damage in diabetes. Biochem Soc Trans 31:202–206, 2003.

106. Suwa M, Nakano H, Kumagai S: Effects of chronic AICAR treatment on fiber composition, enzyme activity, UCP3, and PGC-1 in rat muscles. J Appl Physiol 95:960–968, 2003.

107. Wu Z, Puigserver P, Andersson U, et al: Mechanisms controlling mitochondrial biogenesis and respiration through the thermogenic coactivator PGC-1. Cell 98:115–124, 1999.

108. Mootha VK, Lindgren CM, Eriksson KF, et al: PGC-1alpha-responsive genes involved in oxidative phosphorylation are coordinately downregulated in human diabetes. Nat Genet 34:267–273, 2003.

109. Patti ME, Butte AJ, Crunkhorn S, et al: Coordinated reduction of genes of oxidative metabolism in humans with insulin resistance and diabetes: Potential role of PGC1 and NRF1. Proc Natl Acad Sci U S A 100:8466–8471, 2003.

110. Ek J, Andersen G, Urhammer SA, et al: Mutation analysis of peroxisome proliferator-activated receptor-gamma coactivator-1 (PGC-1) and relationships of identified amino acid polymorphisms to type II diabetes mellitus. Diabetologia 44:2220–2226, 2001.

111. Hara K, Tobe K, Okada T, et al: A genetic variation in the PGC-1 gene could confer insulin resistance and susceptibility to type II diabetes. Diabetologia 45:740–743, 2002.

112. Schneider SH, Amorosa LF, Khachadurian AK, Ruderman NB: Studies on the mechanism of improved glucose control during regular exercise in type 2 (non-insulin-dependent) diabetes. Diabetologia 26:355–360, 1984.

113. Schneider SH, Khachadurian AK, Amorosa LF, et al: Ten-year experience with an exercise-based outpatient life-style modification program in the treatment of diabetes mellitus. Diabetes Care 15:1800–1810, 1992.

114. Zong H, Ren JM, Young LH, et al: AMP kinase is required for mitochondrial biogenesis in skeletal muscle in response to chronic energy deprivation. Proc Natl Acad Sci U S A 99:15983–15987, 2002.

115. Wu H, Kanatous SB, Thurmond FA, et al: Regulation of mitochondrial biogenesis in skeletal muscle by CaMK. Science 296:349–352, 2002.

116. Saloranta C, Groop L: Interactions between glucose and FFA metabolism in man. Diabetes Metab Rev 12:15–36, 1996.

117. Unger RH: Minireview: Weapons of lean body mass destruction: The role of ectopic lipids in the metabolic syndrome. Endocrinology 144:5159–5165, 2003.

118. Oakes ND, Thalen PG, Jacinto SM, Ljung B: Thiazolidinediones increase plasma-adipose tissue FFA exchange capacity and enhance insulin-mediated control of systemic FFA availability. Diabetes 50:1158–1165, 2001.

119. Hotamisligil GS: The irresistible biology of resistin. J Clin Invest 111:173–174, 2003.

120. Banerjee RR, Rangwala SM, Shapiro JS, et al: Regulation of fasted blood glucose by resistin. Science 303:1195–1198, 2004.

121. Rajala MW, Scherer PE: Minireview: The adipocyte: At the crossroads of energy homeostasis, inflammation, and atherosclerosis. Endocrinology 144:3765–3773, 2003.

122. Tsao TS, Tomas E, Murrey HE, et al: Role of disulfide bonds in Acrp30/adiponectin structure and signaling specificity. Different oligomers activate different signal transduction pathways. J Biol Chem 278:50810–50817, 2003.

123. Wong GW, Wang J, Hug C, et al: Family of Acrp30/adiponectin structural and functional paralogs. Proc Natl Acad Sci U S A 101:10302–10307, 2004.

124. Hug C, Wang J, Ahmad NS, et al: T-cadherin is a receptor for hexameric and high-molecular-weight forms of Acrp30/adiponectin. Proc Natl Acad Sci U S A 101:10308–10313, 2004.

125. Fruebis J, Tsao TS, Javorschi S, et al: Proteolytic cleavage product of 30-kDa adipocyte complement-related protein increases fatty acid oxidation in muscle and causes weight loss in mice. Proc Natl Acad Sci U S A 98:2005–2010, 2001.

126. Tomas E, Tsao TS, Saha AK, et al: Enhanced muscle fat oxidation and glucose transport by ACRP30 globular domain: acetyl-CoA carboxylase inhibition and AMP-activated protein kinase activation. Proc Natl Acad Sci U S A 99:16309–16313, 2002.

127. Pischon T, Girman CJ, Hotamisligil GS, et al: Plasma adiponectin levels and risk of myocardial infarction in men. JAMA 291:1730–1737, 2004.

128. Goldfine AB, Kahn CR: Adiponectin: Linking the fat cell to insulin sensitivity. Lancet 362:1431–1432, 2003.

129. Maeda N, Shimomura I, Kishida K, et al: Diet-induced insulin resistance in mice lacking adiponectin/ACRP30. Nat Med 8:731–737, 2002.

130. Okamoto Y, Kihara S, Ouchi N, et al: Adiponectin reduces atherosclerosis in apolipoprotein E-deficient mice. Circulation 106:2767–2770, 2002.

131. Yamauchi T, Kamon J, Waki H, et al: Globular adiponectin protected ob/ob mice from diabetes and ApoE-deficient mice from atherosclerosis. J Biol Chem 278:2461–2468, 2003.

132. Xu A, Wang Y, Keshaw H, et al: The fat-derived hormone adiponectin alleviates alcoholic and nonalcoholic fatty liver diseases in mice. J Clin Invest 112:91–100, 2003.

133. Yamauchi T, Kamon J, Minokoshi Y, et al: Adiponectin stimulates glucose utilization and fatty-acid oxidation by activating AMP-activated protein kinase. Nat Med 8:1288–1295, 2002.

134. Combs TP, Wagner JA, Berger J, et al: Induction of adipocyte complement-related protein of 30 kilodaltons by PPARgamma agonists: A potential mechanism of insulin sensitization. Endocrinology 143:998–1007, 2002.

135. Qi Y, Takahashi N, Hileman SM, et al: Adiponectin acts in the brain to decrease body weight. Nat Med 10:524–529, 2004.

136. Zhang Y, Proenca R, Maffei M, et al: Positional cloning of the mouse obese gene and its human homologue. Nature 372:425–432, 1994.

137. Muoio DM, Seefeld K, Witters LA, Coleman RA: AMP-activated kinase reciprocally regulates triacylglycerol synthesis and fatty acid oxidation in liver and muscle: evidence that sn-glycerol-3-phosphate acyltransferase is a novel target. Biochem J 338:783–791, 1999.

138. Friedman JM, Halaas JL: Leptin and the regulation of body weight in mammals. Nature 395:763–770, 1998.

139. Minokoshi Y, Kim Y, Peroni OD, et al: Leptin stimulates fatty-acid oxidation by activating AMP-activated protein kinase. Nature 415:339–343, 2002.

140. Minokoshi Y, Alquier T, Furukawa N, et al: AMP-kinase regulates food intake by responding to hormonal and nutrient signals in the hypothalamus. Nature 428:569–574, 2004.

141. Unger RH, Orci L: Diseases of liporegulation: New perspective on obesity and related disorders. FASEB J 15:312–321, 2001.

142. Unger RH: Lipotoxic diseases. Annu Rev Med 53:319–336, 2002.

143. Higa M, Zhou YT, Ravazzola M, et al: Troglitazone prevents mitochondrial alterations, beta cell destruction, and diabetes in obese prediabetic rats. Proc Natl Acad Sci U S A 96:11513–11518, 1999.

144. Pearson TA, Mensah GA, Alexander RW, et al: Markers of inflammation and cardiovascular disease: Application to clinical and public health practice: A statement for healthcare professionals from the Centers for Disease Control and Prevention and the American Heart Association. Circulation 107:499–511, 2003.

145. Libby P: Inflammation in atherosclerosis. Nature 420:868–874, 2002.

146. Collins T, Cybulsky MI: NF-kappaB: Pivotal mediator or innocent bystander in atherogenesis? J Clin Invest 107:255–264, 2001.

147. Nishikawa T, Edelstein D, Du XL, et al: Normalizing mitochondrial superoxide production blocks three pathways of hyperglycaemic damage. Nature 404:787–790, 2000.

148. Hennig B, Meerarani P, Ramadass P, et al: Fatty acid-mediated activation of vascular endothelial cells. Metabolism 49:1006–1013, 2000.

149. Meigs JB, Hu FB, Rifai N, Manson JE: Biomarkers of endothelial dysfunction and risk of type 2 diabetes mellitus. JAMA 291:1978–1986, 2004.

150. Haffner SM, Greenberg AS, Weston WM, et al: Effect of rosiglitazone treatment on nontraditional markers of cardiovascular disease in patients with type 2 diabetes mellitus. Circulation 106:679–684, 2002.

151. Steinberg HO, Baron AD: Vascular function, insulin resistance and fatty acids. Diabetologia 45:623–634, 2002.

152. Esposito K, Pontillo A, Di Palo C, et al: Effect of weight loss and lifestyle changes on vascular inflammatory markers in obese women: A randomized trial. JAMA 289:1799–1804, 2003.

153. Hamdy O, Ledbury S, Mullooly C, et al: Lifestyle modification improves endothelial function in obese subjects with the insulin resistance syndrome. Diabetes Care 26:2119–2125, 2003.

154. Hsueh WA, Law R: The central role of fat and effect of peroxisome proliferator-activated receptor-gamma on progression of insulin resistance and cardiovascular disease. Am J Cardiol 92:3J–9J, 2003.

155. Cacicedo JM, Yagihashi N, Keaney JF Jr, et al: AMPK inhibits fatty acid-induced increases in NF-Kappa B transactivation in cultured human umbilical vein endothelial cells. Biochem Biophys Res Commun 324(4):1204–1209, 2004.

156. Ido Y, Carling D, Ruderman N: Hyperglycemia-induced apoptosis in human umbilical vein endothelial cells: Inhibition by the AMP-activated protein kinase activation. Diabetes 51:159–167, 2002.

157. Kobayashi H, Ouchi N, Kihara S, et al: Selective suppression of endothelial cell apoptosis by the high molecular weight form of adiponectin. Circ Res 94:e27–e31, 2004.

158. Seppala-Lindroos A, Vehkavaara S, Hakkinen AM, et al: Fat accumulation in the liver is associated with defects in insulin suppression of glucose production and serum free fatty acids independent of obesity in normal men. J Clin Endocrinol Metab 87:3023–3028, 2002.

159. Samuel VT, Liu ZX, Qu X, et al: Mechanism of hepatic insulin resistance in non-alcoholic fatty liver disease. J Biol Chem 279:32345–32353, 2004.

160. Poitout V, Robertson RP: Minireview: Secondary beta-cell failure in type 2 diabetes:A convergence of glucotoxicity and lipotoxicity. Endocrinology 143:339–342, 2002.

161. El-Assaad W, Buteau J, Peyot ML, et al: Saturated fatty acids synergize with elevated glucose to cause pancreatic beta-cell death. Endocrinology 144:4154–4163, 2003.

162. Prentki M, Joly E, El-Assaad W, Roduit R: Malonyl-CoA signaling, lipid partitioning, and glucolipotoxicity: Role in beta-cell adaptation and failure in the etiology of diabetes. Diabetes 51:S405–S413, 2002.

163. Robertson RP, Harmon J, Tran PO, et al: Glucose toxicity in beta-cells:

Type 2 diabetes, good radicals gone bad, and the glutathione connection. Diabetes 52:581–587, 2003.

164. Maestre I, Jordan J, Calvo S, et al: Mitochondrial dysfunction is involved in apoptosis induced by serum withdrawal and fatty acids in the beta-cell line INS-1. Endocrinology 144:335–345, 2003.

165. Bakker S, Jzerman R, Teerlink T, et al: Cytosolic triglycerides and oxidative stress in central obesity: The missing link between excessive atherosclerosis, endothelial dysfunction, and beta-cell failure? Atherosclerosis 148:17–21, 2000.

166. Yu C, Chen Y, Cline GW, et al: Mechanism by which fatty acids inhibit insulin activation of insulin receptor substrate-1 (IRS-1)-associated phosphatidylinositol 3-kinase activity in muscle. J Biol Chem 277:50230–50236, 2002.

167. Laybutt DR, Schmitz-Peiffer C, Saha AK, et al: Muscle lipid accumulation and protein kinase C activation in the insulin-resistant chronically glucose-infused rat. Am J Physiol 277:E1070–E1076, 1999.

168. Schmitz-Peiffer C, Browne CL, Oakes ND, et al: Alterations in the expression and cellular localization of protein kinase C isozymes epsilon and theta are associated with insulin resistance in skeletal muscle of the high-fat-fed rat. Diabetes 46:169–178, 1997.

169. Yuan M, Konstantopoulos N, Lee J, et al: Reversal of obesity- and diet-induced insulin resistance with salicylates or targeted disruption of Ikkbeta. Science 293:1673–1677, 2001.

170. Kim JK, Kim YJ, Fillmore JJ, et al: Prevention of fat-induced insulin resistance by salicylate. J Clin Invest 108:437–446, 2001.

171. Kim JK, Gavrilova O, Chen Y, et al: Mechanism of insulin resistance in A-ZIP/F-1 fatless mice. J Biol Chem 275:8456–8460, 2000.

172. Evans JL, Goldfine ID, Maddux BA, Grodsky GM: Oxidative stress and stress-activated signaling pathways: A unifying hypothesis of type 2 diabetes. Endocr Rev 23:599–622, 2002.

173. Krssak M, Falk Petersen K, Dresner A, et al: Intramyocellular lipid concentrations are correlated with insulin sensitivity in humans: A 1H NMR spectroscopy study. Diabetologia 42:113–116, 1999.

174. Jacob S, Machann J, Rett K, et al: Association of increased intramyocellular lipid content with insulin resistance in lean nondiabetic offspring of type 2 diabetic subjects. Diabetes 48:1113–1119, 1999.

175. Walker BR: Is "Cushing's disease of the omentum" an affliction of mouse and men? Diabetologia 47:767–769, 2004.

176. Savage DB, Tan GD, Acerini CL, et al: Human metabolic syndrome resulting from dominant-negative mutations in the nuclear receptor peroxisome proliferator-activated receptor-gamma. Diabetes 52:910–917, 2003.

177. McClain DA, Crook ED: Hexosamines and insulin resistance. Diabetes 45:1003–1009, 1996.

178. Hawkins M, Hu M, Yu J, et al: Discordant effects of glucosamine on insulin-stimulated glucose metabolism and phosphatidylinositol 3-kinase activity. J Biol Chem 274:31312–31319, 1999.

179. Gavrilova O, Marcus-Samuels B, Graham D, et al: Surgical implantation of adipose tissue reverses diabetes in lipoatrophic mice. J Clin Invest 105:271–278, 2000.

180. Garg A: Acquired and inherited lipodystrophies. N Engl J Med 350:1220–1234, 2004.

181. Oral EA, Simha V, Ruiz E, et al: Leptin-replacement therapy for lipodystrophy. N Engl J Med 346:570–578, 2002.

182. Petersen KF: Leptin reverses insulin resistance and hepatic steatosis in patients with severe lipodystrophy. J Clin Invest 109:1345–1350, 2002.

183. Cheal KL, Abbasi F, Lamendola C, et al: Relationship to insulin resistance of the adult treatment panel III diagnostic criteria for identification of the metabolic syndrome. Diabetes 53:1195–1200, 2004.

184. McKeigue PM, Pierpoint T, Ferrie JE, Marmot MG: Relationship of glucose intolerance and hyperinsulinaemia to body fat pattern in South Asians and Europeans. Diabetologia 35:785–791, 1992.

185. Brunzell JD, Ayyobi AF: Dyslipidemia in the metabolic syndrome and type 2 diabetes mellitus. Am J Med 115(Suppl 8A):24S–28S, 2003.

186. Isomaa B, Almgren P, Tuomi T, et al: Cardiovascular morbidity and mortality associated with the metabolic syndrome. Diabetes Care 24:683–689, 2001.

187. Isomaa B, Henricsson M, Almgren P, et al: The metabolic syndrome influences the risk of chronic complications in patients with type II diabetes. Diabetologia 44:1148–1154, 2001.

188. Lakka HM, Laaksonen DE, Lakka TA, et al: The metabolic syndrome and total and cardiovascular disease mortality in middle-aged men. JAMA 288:2709–2716, 2002.

189. Sattar N, Gaw A, Scherbakova O, et al: Metabolic syndrome with and without C-reactive protein as a predictor of coronary heart disease and diabetes in the West of Scotland Coronary Prevention Study. Circulation 108:414–419, 2003.

190. Alexander CM, Landsman PB, Teutsch SM, Haffner SM: NCEP-defined metabolic syndrome, diabetes, and prevalence of coronary heart disease among NHANES III participants age 50 years and older. Diabetes 52:1210–1214, 2003.

191. Green RM: NASH: Hepatic metabolism and not simply the metabolic syndrome. Hepatology 38:14–17, 2003.

192. Marchesini G, Brizi M, Bianchi G, et al: Nonalcoholic fatty liver disease: A feature of the metabolic syndrome. Diabetes 50:1844–1850, 2001.

193. Balkau B, Kahn HS, Courbon D, et al: Hyperinsulinemia predicts fatal liver cancer but is inversely associated with fatal cancer at some other sites: The Paris Prospective Study. Diabetes Care 24:843–849, 2001.

194. Yu AS, Keeffe EB: Nonalcoholic fatty liver disease. Rev Gastroenterol Disord 2:11–19, 2002.

195. Legro RS, Kunselman AR, Dodson WC, Dunaif A: Prevalence and predictors of risk for type 2 diabetes mellitus and impaired glucose tolerance in polycystic ovary syndrome: A prospective, controlled study in 254 affected women. J Clin Endocrinol Metab 84:165–169, 1999.

196. Solomon CG, Hu FB, Dunaif A, et al: Menstrual cycle irregularity and risk for future cardiovascular disease. J Clin Endocrinol Metab 87:2013–2017, 2002.

197. Calle EE, Thun MJ: Obesity and cancer. Oncogene 23:6365–6378, 2004.

198. Woods A, Johnstone SR, Dickerson K, et al: LKB1 is the upstream kinase in the AMP-activated protein kinase cascade. Curr Biol 13:2004–2008, 2003.

199. Hawley SA, Boudeau J, Reid JL, et al: Complexes between the LKB1 tumor suppressor, STRADalpha/beta and MO25alpha/beta are upstream kinases in the AMP-activated protein kinase cascade. J Biol 2:28, 2003.

200. Xiang X, Saha AK, Wen R, et al: AMP-activated protein kinase activators can inhibit the growth of prostate cancer cells by multiple mechanisms. Biochem Biophys Res Commun 321:161–167, 2004.

201. Luo Z, Saha AK, Xiang X, Ruderman NB: The metabolic syndrome and cancer. Trends Pharmacol Sci (in press), 2005.

202. Seely WW, Williams GH: The cardiovascular system and endocrine disease. In Becker KL (ed): Principles and Practice of Endocrinology and Metabolism. Philadelphia, Lippincott Williams & Wilkins, 2001, pp 1857–1864.

203. Petersen KF, Oral EA, Dufour S, et al: Leptin reverses insulin resistance and hepatic steatosis in patients with severe lipodystrophy. J Clin Invest 109:1345–1350, 2002.

204. Sutinen J, Kannisto K, Korsheninnikova E, et al: Effects of rosiglitazone on gene expression in subcutaneous adipose tissue in highly active antiretroviral therapy-associated lipodystrophy. Am J Physiol Endocrinol Metab 286:E941–E949, 2004.

205. Sutinen J, Hakkinen AM, Westerbacka J, et al: Rosiglitazone in the treatment of HAART-associated lipodystrophy: A randomized double-blind placebo-controlled study. Antivir Ther 8:199–207, 2003.

206. Unger RH: Lessons from Morgan Spurluck and some French geese: How adipocytes regulate surplus caloric intake and distribution. Curr Opin Endocrinol Diabetes (in press).

207. Sims EA, Danforth E Jr, Horton ES, et al: Endocrine and metabolic effects of experimental obesity in man. Recent Prog Horm Res 29:457–496, 1973.

208. Tuomilehto J, Lindstrom J, Eriksson JG, et al: Prevention of type 2 diabetes mellitus by changes in lifestyle among subjects with impaired glucose tolerance. N Engl J Med 344:1343–1350, 2001.

209. Skerrett PJ, Manson JE: Exercise and diabetes prevention: Reduction in risk of coronary heart disease in diabetes. In Ruderman N, Devlin JT, Schneider SH, Kriska A (eds): Handbook of Diabetes in Exercise. Alexandria, VA, American Diabetes Association, 2002, pp 155–182.

210. The Diabetes Prevention Program Research Group: The effects of intensive lifestyle intervention (ILS) and metformin (MET) on C-reactive protein (CRP), tissue plasminogen activator (TPA) and fibrinogen (FIB) in the diabetes prevention program (DPP). Diabetes Abstract 52:A18, 2003.

211. The Diabetes Prevention Program Research Group: Prevention of type 2 diabetes with troglitazone in the diabetes prevention program (DPP). Diabetes Abstract 52:A58, 2003.

212. The Diabetes Prevention Program Research Group: Impact of lifestyle and metformin therapy on cardiovascular (CVD) risk factors and events in the diabetes prevention program. Diabetes Abstract 52:A169, 2003.

213. Yusuf S, Gerstein H, Hoogwerf B, et al: Ramipril and the development of diabetes. JAMA 286:1882–1885, 2001.

214. Robins SJ, Rubins HB, Faas FH, et al: Insulin resistance and cardiovascular events with low HDL cholesterol: The Veterans Affairs HDL Intervention Trial (VA-HIT). Diabetes Care 26:1513–1517, 2003.

215. UKPDS: Effect of intensive blood-glucose control with metformin on complications in overweight patients with type 2 diabetes (UKPDS 34). Lancet 352:854–865, 1998.

216. Levin K, Hother-Nielsen O, Henriksen JE, et al: Effects of troglitazone in young first-degree relatives of patients with type 2 diabetes. Diabetes Care 27:148–154, 2004.

217. Ridker PM, Rifai N, Clearfield M, et al: Measurement of C-reactive protein for the targeting of statin therapy in the primary prevention of acute coronary events. N Engl J Med 344:1959–1965, 2001.

218. Cook S, Weitzman M, Auinger P, et al: Prevalence of a metabolic syndrome phenotype in adolescents: Findings from the Third National Health and Nutrition Examination Survey, 1988-1994. Arch Pediatr Adolesc Med 157:821–827, 2003.

219. Must A, Jacques PF, Dallal GE, et al: Long-term morbidity and mortality of overweight adolescents: A follow-up of the Harvard Growth Study of 1922 to 1935. N Engl J Med 327:1350–1355, 1992.

220. Berenson GS, Srinivasan SR, Bao W, et al: Associations between multiple cardiovascular risk factors and atherosclerosis in children and young adults. The Bogalusa Heart Study. N Engl J Med 338:1650–1656, 1998.

221. Steinberger J, Daniels SR: Obesity, insulin resistance, diabetes, and cardiovascular risk in children: An American Heart Association scientific statement from the Atherosclerosis, Hypertension, and Obesity in the Young Committee (Council on Cardiovascular Disease in the Young) and the Diabetes Committee (Council on Nutrition, Physical Activity, and Metabolism). Circulation 107:1448–1453, 2003.

222. Phillips DI: Birth weight and the future development of diabetes: A review of the evidence. Diabetes Care 21(Suppl 2):B150–B155, 1998.

223. Barker DJ, Hales CN, Fall CH, et al: Type 2 (non-insulin-dependent) diabetes mellitus, hypertension and hyperlipidaemia (syndrome X): Relation to reduced fetal growth. Diabetologia 36:62–67, 1993.

224. Phillips DI, Barker DJ, Hales CN, et al: Thinness at birth and insulin resistance in adult life. Diabetologia 37:150–154, 1994.

225. Bhargava SK, Sachdev HS, Fall CH, et al: Relation of serial changes in childhood body-mass index to impaired glucose tolerance in young adulthood. N Engl J Med 350:865–875, 2004.

226. Zimmet P, Alberti KG, Shaw J: Global and societal implications of the diabetes epidemic. Nature 414:782–787, 2001.

227. Neel JV: Diabetes mellitus: A "thrifty" genotype rendered detrimental by "progress"? Am J Hum Genet 14:353–362, 1962.

228. Hu Z, Cha SH, Chohnan S, Lane MD: Hypothalamic malonyl-CoA as a mediator of feeding behavior. Proc Natl Acad Sci U S A 100:12624–12629, 2003.

229. Ravussin E, Swinburn BA: Energy expenditure and obesity. Diabet Rev 4:403–422, 1996.

230. Hardie DG, Scott JW, Pan DA, Hudson ER: Management of cellular energy by the AMP-activated protein kinase system. FEBS Lett 546:113–120, 2003.

231. Kemp BE, Stapleton D, Campbell DJ, et al: AMP-activated protein kinase, super metabolic regulator. Biochem Soc Trans 31:162–168, 2003.

Treatment of Type 1 Diabetes Mellitus in Adults

Ravi Retnakaran and Bernard Zinman

GOALS OF MANAGEMENT
  Glycemic Goals
  Acute Complications
  Chronic Complications
  Quality of Life

TEAM APPROACH TO MANAGEMENT

MONITORING
  Glycemic Control
  Ketone Testing
  Complication Surveillance

INSULIN THERAPY
  Principles of Insulin Replacement
  Insulin Preparations
  Intensive Insulin Therapy Regimens
  Insulin Delivery
  Complications of Insulin Therapy
  Adjustment of Insulin Therapy in Special Situations

NUTRITION

OTHER THERAPIES FOR TYPE 1 DIABETES

FUTURE PERSPECTIVES

The discovery of insulin in the summer of 1921 by Frederick Banting, Charles Best, James Collip, and J. J. R. Macleod at the University of Toronto and its first therapeutic use on January 11, 1922, at the Toronto General Hospital stand as one of the greatest achievements of contemporary medicine.[1] By providing life-sustaining therapy for a previously fatal wasting condition, the discovery of insulin dramatically shifted the prognosis of type 1 diabetes to that of a chronic disease characterized by devastating long-term microvascular and macrovascular complications. Accordingly, the focus of treatment has changed significantly since 1922, with emphasis now directed toward the avoidance of complications and the optimization of patient quality of life. Given the incontrovertible evidence from the Diabetes Control and Complications Trial (DCCT) and other studies that optimization of glycemic control can significantly reduce the risk of microvascular complications,[2-5] the following overriding objective of modern diabetes management has emerged: the achievement of sustained euglycemia, with avoidance of hypoglycemia, in patients with type 1 diabetes through the physiologic replacement of insulin. Remarkably, however, despite significant advances in the past 80 years, this goal remains an elusive target.[6] Modern management of type 1 diabetes involves a multifaceted, patient-centered approach, in which an interdisciplinary health-care team works closely with the patient toward the goal of achieving sustained euglycemia. In this chapter, we review the essential elements of this approach to comprehensive care of patients with type 1 diabetes.

GOALS OF MANAGEMENT

The overriding goal in the management of type 1 diabetes is the optimization of the patient's quality of life through the prevention and amelioration of the acute and chronic complications that are associated with this disease. In the modern era, a substantial body of epidemiologic and experimental evidence has established the relationship between diabetic complications and hyperglycemia (see Chapter 66). In particular, the findings of the DCCT have had an enormous impact on the management of type 1 diabetes and warrant review before discussion of specific therapeutic goals.

The DCCT was a multicenter, National Institutes of Health–funded randomized controlled clinical trial initiated in 1982 that was designed to assess whether intensive treatment with the goal of maintaining near-normal blood glucose concentrations could reduce the frequency and severity of diabetic complications.[2] A total of 1441 patients with type 1 diabetes from the United States and Canada participated in the study and comprised two cohorts: a primary prevention cohort of 726 subjects with no retinopathy at baseline and 1 to 5 years duration of diabetes and a secondary intervention cohort of 715 individuals with mild retinopathy and duration of diabetes of up to 15 years. Participants were randomly assigned to receive either the conventional therapy of the day (one or two injections of insulin per day) or intensive therapy (either three or more injections or continuous subcutaneous insulin infusion by external pump, with frequent blood glucose monitoring). After a mean 6.5 years of follow-up, mean glycosylated hemoglobin (A1c) was 7.2% in the intensive therapy arm and 9.0% in the conventional treatment arm. The intensive therapy group showed a relative risk reduction of 76% (95% confidence interval [CI]: 62% to 85%) for the development of retinopathy and a 54% relative risk reduction (95% CI: 39% to 66%) for progression of retinopathy. Similarly, intensive therapy was associated with relative risk reductions of 39% (95% CI: 21% to 52%) for the development of microalbuminuria (defined as urinary albumin excretion > 40 mg per 24 hours) and 54% (95% CI: 19% to 74%) for progression to albuminuria (urinary albumin excretion > 300 mg per 24 hours). The incidence of clinical neuropathy was also decreased in the intensive group, with a relative risk reduction of 60% (95% CI: 38% to 74%). Thus, the DCCT provided conclusive evidence that improved glycemic control with intensive therapy can reduce the incidence of microvascular complications (primary prevention) and also slow the progression of established microvascular disease (secondary intervention).

The benefits of near-normal glycemic control were also found to persist for many years after the DCCT, according to data from the follow-up study, the Epidemiology of Diabetes Interventions and Complications (EDIC).[7] In the ongoing EDIC observational study, a large cohort consisting of more than 95% of the DCCT participants (n = 1375) has been followed since the completion of the original trial and has been studied by using an intention-to-treat approach based on the original randomization in the DCCT. The mean A1c levels of the former intensive treatment cohort and the former conventional therapy group have converged (A1c ~ 8%) over the course of the EDIC study and were no longer significantly different at 5 years post-DCCT. Remarkably, however, despite similar glycemic control, the former intensive therapy group continued to display a reduced risk of both retinopathy and nephropathy at 4 years and 7 to 8 years post-DCCT, respectively, compared to the group of patients who were originally randomized to conventional therapy (Fig. 60-1).[7,8] These persistent beneficial effects of previous near-normal glycemic control extend the results of the DCCT and demonstrate that intensive treatment should be initiated as early as is safely possible in the management of type 1 diabetes.

The relationship between intensive therapy and macrovascular disease in the DCCT was less clear. The intensive therapy arm displayed a relative risk reduction of 34% (95% CI: 7% to 54%) for the development of elevated low-density lipoprotein (LDL) cholesterol levels. Nevertheless, while intensive therapy was associated with a 41% relative risk reduction (95% CI: –10% to 68%) for macrovascular complications, this difference was not statistically significant. However, macrovascular benefits from near-normal glycemic control in the former intensive treatment arm of the DCCT might yet be realized in the coming years. Over the first 6 years of the EDIC study, the former intensive treatment group has displayed decreased progression of carotid intima-media thickness, a measure of atherosclerosis, compared to the former conventional therapy arm.[9] Continued observation of this cohort will reveal whether this effect translates into a reduction in cardiovascular events.

Overall, the DCCT helped to clarify the relationship between A1c and diabetic complications. For every 10% reduction in A1c, the risk of developing retinopathy was reduced by approximately 45%.[10] Moreover, a continuous curvilinear relationship was observed between A1c and the incidence of retinopathy, the risk of progressive retinopathy being decreased substantially at A1c levels below 7%. While the risk of progressive retinopathy was further reduced at A1c concentrations below 7% (i.e., no threshold effect), this benefit was achieved at the cost of a significantly increased risk of hypoglycemia, given an observed continuous and inverse relationship between hypoglycemic risk and A1c (Fig. 60-2). Thus, the DCCT firmly established the importance of glycemic control in the management of type 1 diabetes, demonstrated the

feasibility of intensive therapy in improving glycemic control, and identified the limitations imposed on such control by hypoglycemia. In doing so, this study has provided a framework for current treatment goals.

GLYCEMIC GOALS

On the basis of the findings of the DCCT and other studies, the ultimate objective in the treatment of type 1 diabetes is metabolic normalization, the achievement of sustained euglycemia, and the avoidance of hypoglycemia. In this context, the 2004 American Diabetes Association (ADA) treatment guidelines suggest the following therapeutic targets for nonpregnant adults with either type 1 or type 2 diabetes: (1) A1c less than 7.0% (referenced to nondiabetic range 4.0% to 6.0%); (2) preprandial plasma glucose 90 to 130 mg/dL; and (3) peak postprandial plasma glucose less than 180 mg/dL (Table 60-1).[11] The evidence-based 2003 Canadian Diabetes Association Clinical Practice Guidelines recommend similar targets of A1c less than or equal to 7.0%, preprandial plasma glucose 72 to 126 mg/dL, and 2-hour postprandial plasma glucose 90 to 180 mg/dL (*www.diabetes.ca/cpg2003*).[12] The American Association of Clinical Endocrinologists recommends slightly more stringent goals of A1c less than or equal to 6.5%, preprandial glucose less than or equal to 110 mg/dL, and postprandial glucose less than or equal to 140 mg/dL.[13]

Glycemic targets might need to be individualized in rare cases in individuals for whom the potential harm from hypoglycemia may outweigh the benefits of better glycemic control. These cases include patients with irreversible end-stage complications, developing children, and individuals who are unable to sense hypoglycemic symptoms. In such cases, clinicians generally set higher glycemic targets to reduce the risk of hypoglycemia.

ACUTE COMPLICATIONS

The major acute complications of type 1 diabetes are ketoacidosis and hypoglycemia. These topics are discussed in detail in Chapters 63 and 64, respectively. The risk of these acute complications can be reduced through the judicious use of insulin therapy. Specifically, the risk of ketoacidosis can be reduced through appreciation of the concept that patients with type 1 diabetes require insulin therapy at all times. Appropriate management of special situations, such as intercurrent illness, requires adherence to this principle (see the section entitled "Adjustment of Insulin Therapy in Special Situations.").

As was observed in the DCCT (see Fig. 60-2*B*), tight glycemic control is typically associated with an increased risk of hypoglycemia. Patients must therefore be educated about the recognition of hypoglycemic symptoms and the use of appropriate treatment measures when such symptoms arise. Patients are advised to keep rapidly absorbable sources of carbohydrate, such as glucose tablets, close at hand at all times. In general, 15 g of carbohydrate is needed to increase blood glucose levels by approximately 38 mg/dL within 20 minutes.[14,15] Besides glucose tablets, other treatments that provide a similar amount of glucose include (1) 15 mL (1 tablespoon) or three packets of table sugar dissolved in water, (2) 175 mL (3/4 cup) of juice, and (3) 15 mL (1 tablespoon) of honey. In addition, patients with type 1 diabetes should have an emergency glucagon kit. Both the patient and his or her family members should be trained in the use and intramuscular or subcutaneous injection of glucagon (0.5 to 1 mg) as a means of rapidly increasing blood glucose concentration when the patient is severely hypoglycemic. Finally, the avoidance of hypoglycemia is particularly important for patients who are unable to sense hypoglycemic symptoms (discussed in the section entitled "Complications of Insulin Therapy").

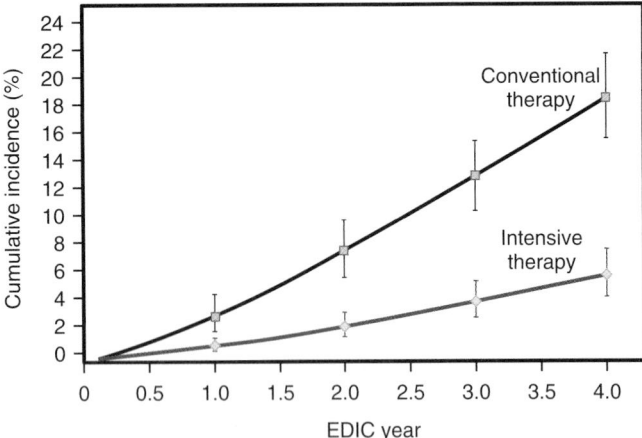

Figure 60-1 Cumulative incidence of further progression of retinopathy during the EDIC trial in the former conventional-therapy and intensive-therapy cohorts from the DCCT. The data are based on regression analysis adjusted for the level of retinopathy at the end of the DCCT, whether patients received therapy as primary prevention or secondary intervention, and both duration of diabetes and A1c value on enrollment in the DCCT. (Source: DCCT/EDIC Research Group: Retinopathy and nephropathy in patients with type 1 diabetes four years after a trial of intensive therapy. N Engl J Med 342(5):387, 2000.)

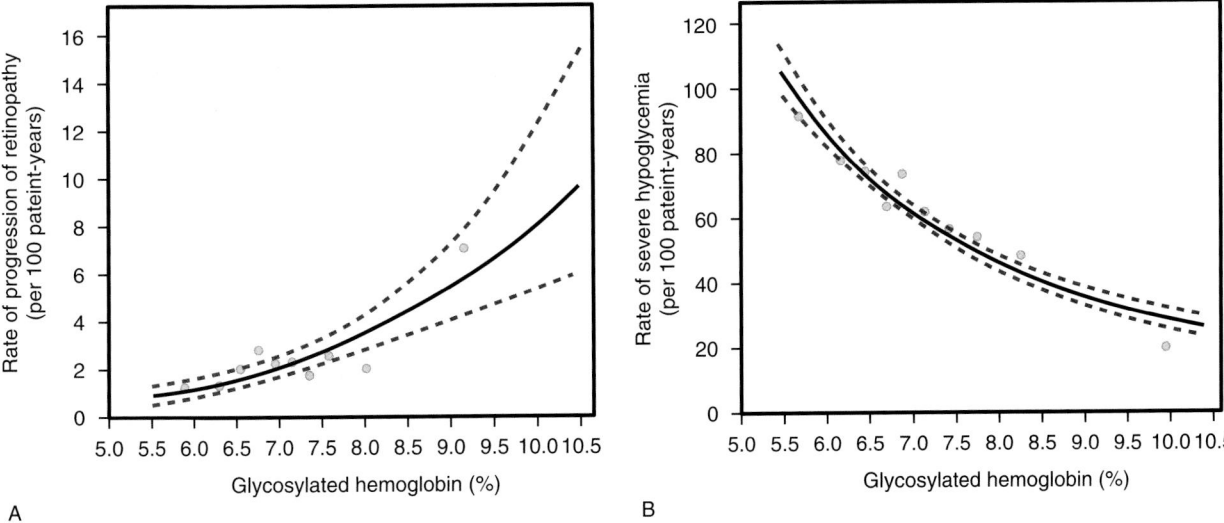

Figure 60-2   Risk of sustained progression of retinopathy (**A**) and rate of severe hypoglycemia (**B**) in patients receiving intensive therapy, in relation to mean A1c value during the DCCT. (Source: DCCT Research Group: The effect of intensive treatment of diabetes on the development and progression of long-term complications in insulin-dependent diabetes mellitus. N Engl J Med 329(14):984, 1993.)

CHRONIC COMPLICATIONS

The chronic microvascular complications of type 1 diabetes include retinopathy, neuropathy, and nephropathy (discussed in Chapters 69, 70, and 71, respectively). To reduce the impact of these complications, management strategies include regular surveillance for early detection of complications and tight glycemic control for both primary prevention and secondary intervention, as demonstrated in the DCCT.

Macrovascular disease, as manifested by cerebrovascular, peripheral vascular, and coronary artery disease, is a major chronic complication of type 1 diabetes (discussed in Chapter 72). Regular surveillance for vascular disease and management of cardiovascular risk factors is essential. In particular, modification of reversible cardiovascular risk factors, such as hypertension, dyslipidemia, and cigarette smoking, is an important management goal. The 2004 ADA treatment guidelines suggest a target blood pressure of less than 130/80 mm Hg in patients with diabetes. In addition, the following treatment targets for lipids are recommended: LDL less than 100 mg/dL, triglycerides less than 150 mg/dL, and HDL greater than 40 mg/dL in men and HDL greater than 50 mg/dL in women (see Table 60-1).[11]

QUALITY OF LIFE

Type 1 diabetes is a chronic condition that requires a complex health-care strategy that demands significant patient effort through frequent insulin injections, regular self-monitoring of blood glucose levels, and constant attention to nutrition and physical activity. As such, effective management requires that the patient take responsibility for his or her care. In this context, it should be noted that quality of life is an important feature that can affect a patient's willingness to pursue a demanding treatment plan. Recognition of this concept at all times by the health-care team will facilitate the success of treatment initiatives. Moreover, in recognition of the importance of quality of life, many research studies now utilize validated instruments such as the Diabetes Quality of Life questionnaire to measure patient well-being as a therapeutic outcome.[16]

TEAM APPROACH TO MANAGEMENT

Given the complexity of modern treatment regimens, comprehensive care for patients with type 1 diabetes is best accomplished through a team approach. The core members of the diabetes health-care team include the patient, the primary physician, a diabetes nurse educator, and a registered dietitian. Other individuals participating in the patient's care may include a pharmacist, a medical social worker, a foot care specialist, an ophthalmologist, and other medical specialists such as cardiologists, nephrologists, and neurologists. At all times, the patient's central role as a member of the health-care team must be recognized. Accordingly, the efforts of the health-care team should always be pursued from a patient-centered perspective. Inherent in this approach is the central importance of patient education, as the patient's active participation in his or her care demands an understanding of the issues associated with the treatment plan. As will be discussed in later sections of this chapter, the patient needs to be equipped with the knowledge and skills required for activities such as self-monitoring of blood glucose control, glycemic pattern management, estimation of

Table 60-1	American Diabetes Association Recommendations for Treatment Targets in Nonpregnant Adults with Diabetes	
		Target
GLYCEMIC CONTROL		
A1c		<7.0%
Preprandial plasma glucose		90–130 mg/dL
Postprandial plasma glucose		<180 mg/dL
BLOOD PRESSURE		**<130/80 MM HG**
LIPIDS		
LDL		<100 mg/dL
HDL		>40 mg/dL*
Triglycerides		<150 mg/dL

Goals might need to be individualized for the given patient.
*For women, it has been suggested that the HDL goal should be increased by 10 mg/dlL.
Source: Adapted from American Diabetes Association: Standards of medical care in diabetes. Diabetes Care 27(Suppl 1):S19, 2004.

carbohydrate content of meals, insulin dose adjustment, and appropriate insulin administration.

MONITORING

Type 1 diabetes is a chronic condition involving complex treatment regimens and multiple management goals, so regular monitoring of patient status is an essential component of comprehensive care. Patient monitoring in type 1 diabetes addresses two fundamental issues. First of all, frequent acute assessment of metabolic status guides adjustment of the treatment regimen, which, by nature, must be dynamic and able to accommodate day-to-day physiologic variability. Second, regular surveillance of both important clinical outcomes and associated surrogate markers allows for the detection and treatment of chronic complications and attendant comorbidities.

GLYCEMIC CONTROL

The regular monitoring of glycemic status by both patients and health-care providers is fundamental to diabetes care. Glycemic monitoring involves frequent, acute measurement of blood glucose levels by the patient and periodic evaluation of chronic glycemic control by laboratory measurement of markers of glucose concentration such as A1c.

Acute Measurement of Glycemic Control

Self-monitoring of blood glucose (SMBG) by patients is an invaluable tool that has empowered patient-driven management of type 1 diabetes. This technique involves using a small lancet to draw a drop of capillary blood from the fingertip. The patient applies a small drop of blood (usually 3 to 5 µL) to a testing strip, from which a portable glucose meter can determine the glucose concentration of the blood by enzymatic means within 5 to 30 seconds. In this way, patients can immediately determine their capillary blood glucose concentration at any time.

Patients with type 1 diabetes should monitor blood glucose frequently. In the DCCT, insulin doses for patients in the intensive treatment arm were adjusted according to the results of SMBG performed at least four times a day.[17] Blood glucose is typically measured before administration of insulin prior to a meal and at bedtime. In addition, meaningful data can be derived from measurements at other times as well. For instance, nocturnal hypoglycemia resulting from excessive bedtime insulin can be detected by blood glucose measurement in the early hours of the morning. Similarly, postprandial monitoring 2 hours after a meal can assess the adequacy of the preprandial insulin dose. Patients should check their blood glucose level before driving a motor vehicle, particularly if they have difficulty sensing hypoglycemic symptoms, as hypoglycemia (and hence neurologic impairment) while driving can be very dangerous for the patient and others. Patients should also consider SMBG at times when blood glucose might be changing rapidly, such as in the postexercise period or when experiencing symptoms of hypoglycemia.

Self-monitoring of blood glucose is only of value to the extent that the information it provides is used to guide treatment. With each measurement, patients are encouraged to use a logbook to record the blood glucose value, the time of day, and the temporal relationship to food intake. The data obtained from SMBG should be used in two ways: variable insulin dose scales and pattern management. Variable insulin dose scales refer to algorithms that guide the patient as to the appropriate dose adjustment of preprandial insulin based on the current degree of glycemia (discussed in the section entitled "Implementation of Intensive Insulin Therapy"). Pattern management describes the two-step process of using the glucose profile recorded over several days to identify glycemic patterns and then adjusting the daily insulin regimen for the coming days in a proactive fashion on the basis of these patterns. Therefore, both variable insulin dose scales and pattern management are essential components of patient education.

Given the value of blood glucose data, it is important to consider potential problems that are inherent in the process of self-monitoring. To ensure proper meter function, glucose meters should be calibrated by a laboratory reference standard. The patient's use of the meter and self-monitoring technique should also be reviewed periodically in the clinic.[18] Third, inappropriate handling of the testing strips can lead to defective function and inaccurate glucose results. Finally, some patients find lancing of the fingertip to be painful and hence are unwilling to measure blood glucose as frequently as recommended.

In response to patient concerns regarding pain associated with lancing of the fingertip, alternative-site glucose meters have recently been introduced. By sampling from alternative sites such as the forearm, these devices can provide accurate blood glucose measurements while causing less pain than fingertip testing.[19] However, it should be noted that alternative site testing might not provide accurate results at times of rapid change in blood glucose concentration (e.g., immediately after a meal or after exercise).[20,21] Therefore, traditional fingertip testing is recommended at these times.

Because blood glucose concentrations are dynamic and fluctuate constantly, it is readily apparent that the limited data provided by even frequent SMBG might not be truly representative of an individual's glucose excursions. In this context, continuous glucose-monitoring devices represent an important recent development. This technology utilizes the fact that glucose in interstitial fluid can reflect blood glucose levels.[22] One such device that is currently in use continuously measures the glucose concentration in interstitial fluid using a subcutaneous sensor that transmits an electrical signal to a pager-sized monitor worn by the patient.[23] Using this input, the monitor determines a blood glucose concentration every 5 minutes. Currently, such systems do not provide a visual display of the glucose values. The glucose data are downloaded to a computer that provides a graphic display of the patient's glycemic profile over the period of time monitored (Fig. 60-3).[24] During the period of monitoring (usually 3 days), the patient maintains a diary of meals, insulin doses, physical activity, and hypoglycemic symptoms to facilitate meaningful interpretation of the recorded data. Limited experience to date with continuous glucose monitoring has demonstrated higher rates of unrecognized nocturnal hypoglycemia than were previously suspected.[25,26] Although concerns have been raised about the accuracy of measurements with earlier devices,[27] continuous glucose monitoring is likely to emerge as a valuable tool in the management of type 1 diabetes in the near future.

Measurement of Chronic Glycemic Control

Glucose can attach to proteins in the blood through an irreversible, nonenzymatic process, resulting in the formation of glycated proteins.[28] Since this process is irreversible, glucose remains attached to the protein until the latter is metabolized. The degree of glycation is a function of blood glucose concentration over time. Thus, measurement of glycated proteins provides a means of estimating chronic blood glucose concentration over a time period proportional to the half-life of the protein in question.

Erythrocytes are freely permeable to glucose. In the circulation, glucose attaches irreversibly to hemoglobin in red blood cells, leading to the formation of glycated hemoglobins called hemoglobin A1a, A1b, and A1c. Measurement of hemoglobin A1c (also known as A1c, glycohemoglobin, or glycosylated hemoglobin) has emerged as the most widely used test of chronic glycemic control. Specifically, the proportion of glycosylated hemoglobin to the total number of hemoglobin

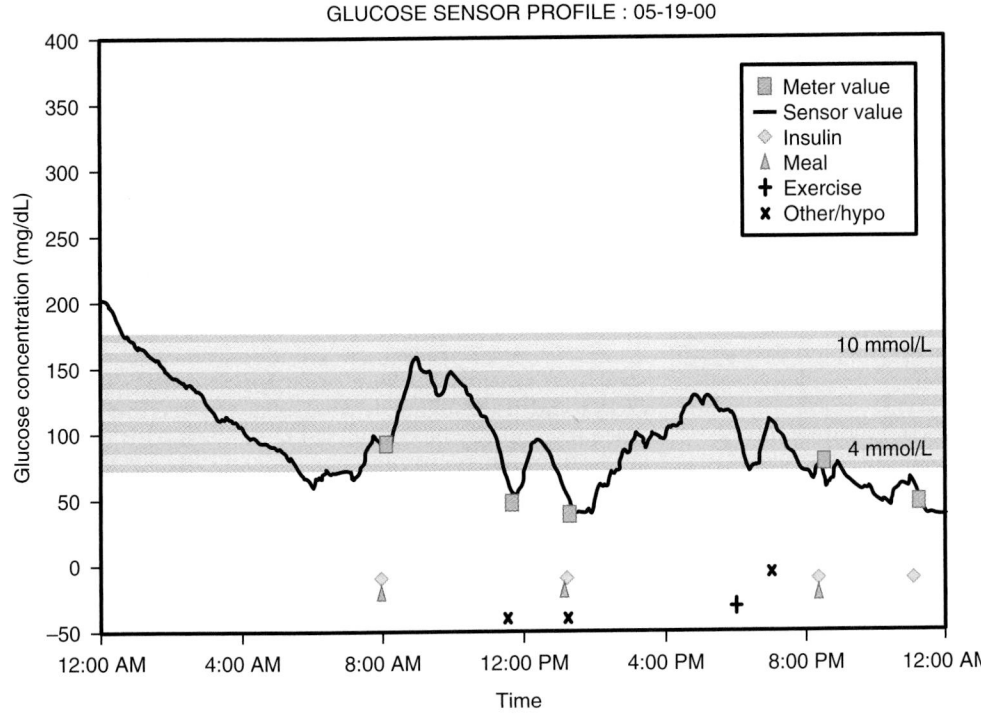

Figure 60-3 Sample of graphical output from continuous glucose monitoring system. (Source: Cheyne E, Kerr D: Making 'sense' of diabetes: Using a continuous glucose sensor in clinical practice. Diabetes Metab Res Rev 18(Suppl 1):S45, 2002.)

molecules reflects overall blood glucose concentration over the preceding 2 to 3 months.[29] Therefore, regular measurement of A1c every 3 months is recommended as a method of determining overall glycemic control and evaluating the adequacy of the treatment regimen.[18] For instance, a significantly elevated A1c value, consistent with suboptimal glycemic control, would suggest the need for a change in the treatment regimen. Analysis of daily glycemic patterns from the patient's SMBG records can then indicate the specific changes to be made.

Many different types of assays can be used for measurement of glycated hemoglobins.[30] Some assays report A1c as a percentage of total hemoglobin while other methods measure total glycated hemoglobin. Thus, nonstandardization of

assays can complicate comparison of A1c measurements between laboratories. The National Glycohemoglobin Standardization Program, initiated in 1996, is an initiative that is designed to standardize laboratory A1c assays to the DCCT reference method.[31]

The DCCT provided insight into the correlation between A1c level and mean plasma glucose concentration (Fig. 60-4).[32] In practice, there are some situations in which the measured A1c value may be discordant with the level that would be expected on the basis of the patient's capillary blood glucose records. Such discrepancy might be due to glycemic excursions at unmonitored times of the day that are not reflected in SMBG records. Alternatively, the problem might be falsification of SMBG records by the patient.

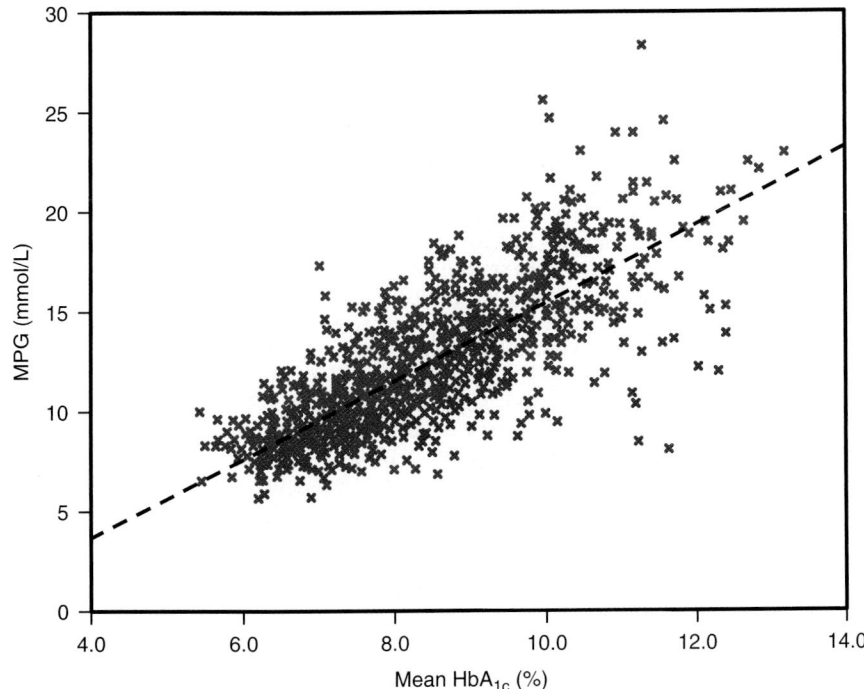

Figure 60-4 The relationship between mean plasma glucose and mean A1c in the DCCT. (*n* = 1429, *r* = 0.82). (Source: Rohlfing CL, Wiedmeyer HM, Little RR, et al: Defining the relationship between plasma glucose and HbA1c: Analysis of glucose profiles and HbA1c in the Diabetes Control and Complication Trial. Diabetes Care 25(2):276, 2002.)

Another possibility in certain clinical settings is that the measurement of A1c might not be accurate. For instance, rapid red blood cell turnover leads to a disproportionate representation of younger erythrocytes, whose collective exposure to ambient blood glucose levels has been shorter than that of other red blood cells. Accordingly, A1c levels tend to reduced under such conditions.[33] Pregnancy and hemolytic anemias are examples of settings characterized by rapid red blood turnover and hence lowered A1c levels. Similarly, A1c concentration may be lowered in hemoglobinopathies, such as thalassemia and sickle-cell disease, because of a diminished propensity for glycation of the abnormal hemoglobin molecule. Conversely, depending on the assay used, A1c values may be falsely elevated in the presence of hemoglobin F, the carbamylated hemoglobin formed in uremia, or acetaldehyde-bound hemoglobin (seen in alcohol abuse).[34,35]

In situations in which measurement of A1c might be unreliable, an alternative approach to the estimation of glycemic control is the measurement of glycated serum proteins or albumin. The term *fructosamine* has been applied to the glycated proteins measured by such assays.[36] Given the 14- to 21-day half-life of albumin, a serum fructosamine measurement reflects mean blood glucose concentration over the preceding 1 to 2 weeks. Generally, serum fructosamine values correlate well with A1c measurements.[37] However, certain caveats should be noted in measuring fructosamine. First of all, fructosamine values can be affected by conditions that alter the synthesis or clearance of serum proteins. Indeed, the question of whether or not to correct fructosamine assays for serum protein or albumin concentration remains controversial.[18] Second, serum fructosamine levels show greater intrasubject variability than A1c measurements do.[38] Third, unlike A1c, fructosamine has not yet been shown to correlate with the risk of diabetic complications.

KETONE TESTING

The presence of detectable levels of ketones in urine or blood may indicate impending or established ketoacidosis in patients with type 1 diabetes. Accordingly, patients should test for ketones in the following situations: when blood glucose concentrations are persistently elevated, during periods of acute illness or stress, or when the patient is experiencing symptoms compatible with ketoacidosis such as nausea, vomiting, and abdominal pain.[18] Traditionally, patients have used urine dipsticks to test for ketonuria. In recent years, however, home monitors have been developed that can measure the capillary blood concentration of β-hydroxybutyrate, the most prevalent intermediate molecule in ketone formation.[39] Blood ketone testing avoids some of the limitations of traditional urinary ketone testing, such as false-positive readings, the inability to detect β-hydroxybutyrate (urinary dipsticks measure different ketone bodies), and patient reluctance to perform urinary testing. In limited studies to date, home capillary blood ketone measurement appears to be more sensitive than urinary testing in the detection of ketosis.[40,41] The use of blood ketone monitoring by patients is expected to increase in the future. In the clinical setting, serum ketone measurement is recommended over urinary testing.

COMPLICATION SURVEILLANCE

An essential component of ongoing care for patients with type 1 diabetes is surveillance for complications and comorbidities, as follows:

1. Retinopathy: Initial dilated and comprehensive eye examination should be performed within 3 to 5 years after diagnosis of type 1 diabetes and at least annually thereafter.[11]
2. Nephropathy: Patients with type 1 diabetes of more than 5 years duration should undergo an annual screening test

for the presence of microalbuminuria.[11] The preferred screening test is a measurement of the albumin-to-creatinine ratio in a random, spot urine sample.[42]
3. Neuropathy and foot care: A comprehensive foot examination should be performed annually.[11] This examination includes evaluation of sensation by 10-g Semmes-Weinstein monofilament, testing of vibration sense by tuning fork, assessment of superficial pain sensation, palpation, and visual inspection. In screening for neuropathy, superficial pain sensation testing, monofilament examination, and vibration testing all show similar operating characteristics and may be used interchangeably.[43]
4. Cardiovascular disease: Regular evaluation of cardiovascular risk factors is recommended. Blood pressure should be measured at every diabetic clinic appointment. Lipid profile should be tested at least annually. Screening exercise stress testing may be considered in patients with typical or atypical cardiac symptoms; abnormal resting electrocardiogram; a history of peripheral or cerebrovascular disease; or sedentary lifestyle, age over 35 years, and plans to start a vigorous exercise program.[11]
5. Other: Other potential associated problems that warrant periodic screening include erectile dysfunction, depression, and thyroid disease.

INSULIN THERAPY

PRINCIPLES OF INSULIN REPLACEMENT

Insulin replacement strategies in type 1 diabetes ideally aim to mimic the normal physiologic secretion of insulin by the pancreas.[6] Therefore, to appreciate the rationale underlying the design of current insulin replacement regimens, an understanding of the basic structure and biochemistry of endogenous insulin is necessary (Fig. 60-5). This topic, discussed in detail in Chapter 51, is briefly reviewed here.

The pancreatic β cells secrete endogenous insulin into the portal venous system in response to physiologic demand for glucose homeostasis as determined by nutrient intake and energy expenditure. Despite broad fluctuations in these determinants, healthy individuals are able to maintain plasma glucose concentration within a narrow range of 3.5 to 7.0 mmol/L throughout the day (Fig. 60-6).[44] This normal glucose homeostasis requires tightly regulated insulin secretion that consists of two components: a basal secretion rate and surges of markedly increased secretion following ingestion of a mixed meal. Comprising approximately 40% of total 24-hour pancreatic insulin output, the basal secretion of ~1 μ/hour serves to limit hepatic glucose production and adipocyte lipolysis in the postabsorptive (fasting) state such as between meals and overnight.[45] Conversely, with ingestion of a mixed meal, dietary secretagogues (e.g., glucose, amino acids) and gastrointestinal hormones (e.g., glucagon-like peptide 1) stimulate abrupt pulses of insulin secretion up to five times the basal rate. These pulses regulate postprandial glycemia by inhibiting hepatic glucose production and increasing peripheral glucose uptake. Insulin secretion is also affected by energy expenditure. For instance, with moderate exercise, insulin secretion rapidly decreases to prevent hypoglycemia.[46] Conversely, with strenuous exercise, catecholamine-mediated hyperglycemia may occur, leading to increased insulin secretion in the postexercise period.[47] Thus, the tight coupling of insulin secretion to plasma glucose concentration in healthy individuals (see Fig. 60-6) requires the complex integration of multiple signals of nutrient availability and energy expenditure.

In providing insulin replacement for patients with type 1 diabetes, the task at hand is to re-create this complex physiology. Insulin replacement strategies in type 1 diabetes aim to faithfully imitate both basal secretion and the appropriately

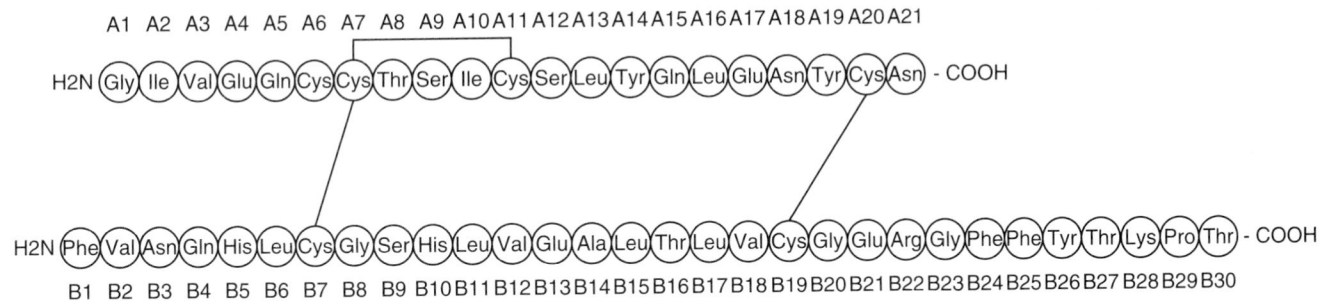

A1 A2 A3 A4 A5 A6 A7 A8 A9 A10 A11 A12 A13 A14 A15 A16 A17 A18 A19 A20 A21

H2N (Gly)(Ile)(Val)(Glu)(Gln)(Cys)(Cys)(Thr)(Ser)(Ile)(Cys)(Ser)(Leu)(Tyr)(Gln)(Leu)(Glu)(Asn)(Tyr)(Cys)(Asn) - COOH

H2N (Phe)(Val)(Asn)(Gln)(His)(Leu)(Cys)(Gly)(Ser)(His)(Leu)(Val)(Glu)(Ala)(Leu)(Thr)(Leu)(Val)(Cys)(Gly)(Glu)(Arg)(Gly)(Phe)(Phe)(Tyr)(Thr)(Lys)(Pro)(Thr) - COOH

B1 B2 B3 B4 B5 B6 B7 B8 B9 B10 B11 B12 B13 B14 B15 B16 B17 B18 B19 B20 B21 B22 B23 B24 B25 B26 B27 B28 B29 B30

Rapid-acting analogues
· Lispro (Lys B28, Pro B29)
· Aspart (Asp B28)

Long-acting analogues
· Glargine (Gly A21, Arg B31, Arg B32)
· Detemir (Lys-tetradecanoyl B29, des-B30)

Figure 60-5 The amino acid sequence and structure of human insulin. The A and B chains are linked by two disulfide bonds. A third disulfide bridge is present within the A chain. (Source: Cheng AY, Zinman B: Insulin analogues and the treatment of diabetes. In Raz I, Skyler JS, Shafrir E (eds): Diabetes: From Research to Diagnosis and Treatment. London, Martin Dunitz Ltd, 2002, pp 331–346.)

integrated prandial surges that are seen in nondiabetic individuals. Generally, one component of the treatment regimen serves as *basal insulin* (i.e., simulates the basal insulin secretion by the pancreas between meals, overnight, and in the fasting state), while a second component is considered *meal insulin* (i.e., simulates the normal prandial insulin surge). In this context, important factors to consider in the design of the treatment regimen include the types of insulin to be used for basal and meal coverage and the method of delivery.

INSULIN PREPARATIONS

For the first 60 years after the introduction of insulin therapy in 1922, the only commercially available preparations were animal insulins derived from bovine or porcine pancreatic extracts. Porcine and bovine insulin preparations differ from human insulin by one and three amino acids, respectively. The use of animal insulins, however, was inherently complicated by several issues, including potential supply limitations, incomplete purification, and a propensity to induce the formation of anti-insulin antibodies (which might affect the activity and absorption of the exogenous animal insulin and lead to unpredictable pharmacodynamics, although this relationship is controversial). These issues were reconciled with the introduction of recombinant human insulin in the 1980s.[48] The past decade has seen further advances with the introduction of insulin analogues bearing molecular modifications that confer advantageous pharmacokinetics. Recombinant human insulin and the newer analogues are now the main preparations used in the treatment of type 1 diabetes.

In selecting types of insulin for use in a treatment regimen, the most important parameters to consider are the onset, peak, and duration of action of the given insulin preparation (Table 60-2). Commercially available human insulins and analogues include rapid-, short-, intermediate-, and long-acting preparations. Its pharmacokinetic properties will determine whether a preparation should be used as either meal insulin or basal insulin. Specifically, rapid- and short-acting preparations are used as meal (or bolus) insulins, while intermediate- and long-acting preparations provide basal insulins.

Human Insulins
Human insulin was the first medication to be commercially manufactured using recombinant DNA technology.[49] Currently available human insulins include short-, intermediate-, and long-acting preparations. Each preparation has advantages and disadvantages, which will be considered in turn.

Short-Acting Human Insulin: Regular
Regular recombinant human insulin is identical to the endogenous insulin polypeptide. In solution, however, regular insulin tends to self-associate, first forming dimers and subsequently hexamers. After subcutaneous injection, the absorption of hexameric insulin molecules is delayed, pending dissociation into monomers and dimers, which can diffuse rapidly from subcutaneous tissue into the systemic circulation.[50] This slowed absorption has important pharmacokinetic implications, leading to (1) a modestly delayed onset of biologic action in vivo (30 to 60 minutes after injection), (2) relatively late peak effect (2 to 4 hours after injection), and (3) prolonged duration of action (6 to 8 hours) (see Table 60-2).[51] Clearly, this pharmacokinetic profile is quite different from the rapid and short-lived endogenous insulin response to a mixed meal that is seen in individuals without diabetes. Therefore, although regular insulin was widely used in the past, its role as meal insulin has declined since the introduction of rapid-acting analogues.

Intermediate-Acting Human Insulin: NPH and Lente
The development of intermediate-acting human insulins reflected the need for an exogenous insulin preparation that could mimic the basal insulin secretion that is observed in individuals who do not have diabetes. The principle underlying the development of these insulins is that the rate of absorption of exogenous insulin from subcutaneous tissue can be significantly reduced by manipulating its suspension. First introduced in 1946, Neutral Protamine Hagedorn (NPH)

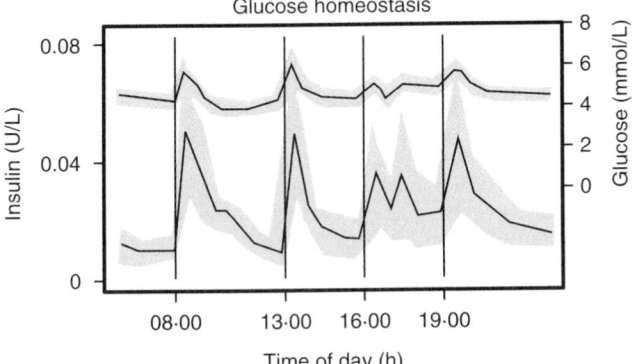

Figure 60-6 Twenty-four-hour plasma glucose and insulin profiles in healthy individuals (*n* = 12) (shown as mean values with 95% confidence interval). (Source: Owens DR, Zinman B, Bolli GB: Insulins today and beyond. Lancet 358:739, 2001.)

Table 60-2 Approximate Pharmacokinetic Properties of Human Insulin and Insulin Analogues following Subcutaneous Injection

Insulin Preparation	Onset of Action	Peak of Action	Duration of Action
MEAL INSULIN			
Lispro	10–15 minutes	1–1.5 hours	3–5 hours
Aspart	10–15 minutes	1–2 hours	3–5 hours
Regular	30–60 minutes	2–4 hours	6–8 hours
BASAL INSULIN			
NPH	2.5–3 hours	5–7 hours	13–6 hours
Lente	2.5–3 hours	7–12 hours	up to 18 hours
Ultralente	3–4 hours	8–10 hours	up to 20 hours
Detemir	2–3 hours	6–8 hours	~24 hours
Glargine	2–3 hours	No peak	~24 hours

insulin is a suspension of insulin complexed with protamine and zinc.[52] NPH is poorly absorbed from subcutaneous tissue, leading to delayed onset of action (2.5 to 3 hours), late peak effect (5 to 7 hours), and prolonged duration of action (13 to 16 hours) (see Table 60-2).[51] A second intermediate-acting insulin preparation is lente, a crystalline suspension of insulin with zinc and acetate. It exhibits a pharmacokinetic profile similar to that of NPH, though with a slightly later peak and longer duration of action.

The intermediate-acting insulins show substantial variation in subcutaneous absorption both within an individual patient and between patients, resulting in variable glycemic excursions.[53] Indeed, variability in the absorption of intermediate-acting insulin may account for as much as 80% of day-to-day variation in blood glucose concentrations.[54] Other factors that contribute to the unpredictability of NPH and lente are dose-dependent changes in pharmacokinetics and the practical variability associated with resuspension of these insulin preparations by the patient prior to subcutaneous injection.

Given their underlying pharmacokinetic profiles (duration of action 13 to 18 hours) and clinical variability in action, the intermediate-acting insulins generally do not provide adequate basal insulin coverage. To increase their utility as basal insulins, these preparations are given twice daily in at least 20% of patients with type 1 diabetes.[55] Moreover, their peak effect is an undesirable quality in a basal insulin, insofar as it is clearly dissimilar to the relatively peakless profile of basal insulin secretion in an individual without diabetes.

Long-Acting Human Insulin: Ultralente
Ultralente, also a zinc insulin suspension, represents another attempt at providing appropriate basal insulin coverage. Its onset of action is 3 to 4 hours after injection with a peak effect at 8 to 10 hours and a duration of action of up to 20 hours.[51] Clinically, its effects are similar to those of intermediate-acting insulin, though with possibly greater variability in absorption. Therefore, given the availability of intermediate-acting preparations and new long-acting analogues, its clinical utility is limited.

Insulin Analogues
The pharmacokinetic shortcomings of human insulin preparations have provided a strong impetus for the development of insulin analogues. Through specific modifications of the insulin molecule (see Fig. 60-5), researchers have designed analogues with tailored pharmacokinetic profiles that allow for better meal or basal coverage. Currently available analogues include rapid-acting and long-acting preparations.

Rapid-Acting Analogues: Lispro and Aspart
Since the tendency to self-associate and resultant delayed absorption of regular insulin compromise its effectiveness in mimicking the normal prandial insulin surge, it follows that an analogue with enhanced absorption may provide a superior meal insulin. In this context, it was previously noted with interest that human insulin-like growth factor 1 (IGF-1), despite significant homology to insulin, exhibited a reduced tendency to form multimers. Identification of the salient structural differences between IGF-1 and insulin led to the development of lispro insulin, the first commercially available analogue.[56] Lispro is identical to human insulin except for a reversal of the 28th and 29th amino acid residues (proline and lispro, respectively) of the normal insulin B chain (see Fig. 60-5). The resultant conformational change in the carboxy terminal of the B chain introduces steric hindrance at interfaces involved in dimerization. Thus, dimer formation with lispro is reduced by a factor of 300 compared to regular human insulin.[57] Importantly, apart from reduced self-aggregation, lispro displays biologic activity similar to that of regular insulin, with both comparable affinity for the insulin receptor and equivalent hypoglycemic potency.[56] Thus, clinically, lispro acts similarly to monomeric human insulin. It is rapidly absorbed in 10 to 15 minutes, reaches peak activity in 60 to 90 minutes, and has a duration of action of 3 to 5 hours (see Table 60-2).[58] With this pharmacokinetic profile, lispro mimics the normal prandial insulin surge in response to carbohydrate ingestion better than any of the exogenous meal insulins that preceded it do.

A second rapid-acting analogue is insulin aspart, engineered through replacement of the proline residue at position 28 of the B chain with aspartic acid. The negative charge of the aspartic acid residue causes repulsion from other negatively charged amino acids and thus leads to decreased self-association of insulin aspart monomers.[59] Accordingly, insulin aspart has a similar pharmacokinetic profile to that of lispro and is also well suited for use as meal insulin.[60]

Given their pharmacokinetics, the rapid-acting insulin analogues (lispro and aspart) have clear advantages over regular human insulin. Since patients usually inject these analogues immediately before meals (rather than 30 minutes before meals, as is typically recommended with regular insulin), their use is associated with greater mealtime flexibility, easier application of carbohydrate estimation techniques (see the section entitled "Nutrition"), and improved quality of life.[61] Both lispro and aspart provide improved postprandial glycemic control with less postprandial and nocturnal hypoglycemia than occurs with regular insulin.[62–64] Despite these advantages, however, use of these rapid-acting analogues in intensive insulin regimens has not been uniformly associated with substantial improvement in A1c compared to regular insulin.[61] This apparent discrepancy likely reflects the suboptimal postabsorptive coverage provided by the basal insulins that were used in the studies in question. Specifically, the shorter duration of action of the rapid-acting analogues is more liable to expose inadequate basal coverage between meals that might otherwise be masked by the longer duration of action of regular insulin when the latter is used for meal coverage. Nevertheless, even in the absence of an A1c benefit, the combination of improved postprandial glycemia with less hypoglycemia suggests an overall reduction in glycemic excursion and hence better glycemic control with rapid-acting analogues.

Long-Acting Analogues: Glargine and Detemir

An ideal basal insulin would have a peakless, 24-hour time-action profile. Attempts to develop long-acting analogues have focused on methods of achieving slow, prolonged absorption following subcutaneous injection. Insulin glargine, the first commercially available long-acting analogue, was introduced to the U.S. market in 2001. It has two modifications compared with human insulin: Two arginines have been added to the carboxy terminus of the B chain, and a glycine residue replaces an acid-sensitive asparagine at position A21.[65] These changes have shifted the isoelectric point of glargine toward neutrality such that this analogue is completely soluble in its acidic injection solution at pH 4.0 but much less soluble at the neutral physiologic pH of subcutaneous tissue. After injection into the subcutaneous tissue, the acidic injection solution is neutralized, causing glargine to microprecipitate.[66] Glargine is subsequently slowly absorbed into the systemic circulation from the subcutaneous microprecipitates, resulting in a smooth and gradual rise in serum concentration. Therefore, the pharmacokinetic profile of glargine shows an onset of action 2 to 3 hours after injection with a relatively peakless, 24-hour duration of action (see Table 60-2).[67] Moreover, glargine is associated with less variability in absorption than either NPH or lente.[68,69] Furthermore, its *in vivo* hypoglycemic potency is equivalent to that of human insulin. The promise associated with these properties has been further supported by clinical trial evidence demonstrating lower fasting plasma glucose levels and less hypoglycemia (including nocturnal hypoglycemia) with the use of glargine, compared to NPH, as basal insulin in intensive therapy.[70–72] Improved A1c with glargine compared to NPH has also been demonstrated in a single study.[73]

Certain caveats associated with the acidic injection solution of glargine must be noted. First of all, glargine cannot be mixed in the same syringe with other insulin preparations and must be administered by separate injection. Second, patients have reported occasional injection-site pain with glargine that might be related to its acidic vehicle.

The design of insulin detemir, a second long-acting analogue, reflects a different approach to achieve long-acting basal coverage. With detemir, the B30 amino acid has been removed, and a 14-carbon aliphatic fatty acid has been acylated to the B29 amino acid.[74] This modification allows for reversible binding between albumin and the added fatty acid. After injection, an equilibrium develops between free and bound detemir, in which 98% of the analogue is bound to albumin. As only the free analogue binds to the insulin receptor, the duration of action of detemir is prolonged owing to sustained release of the analogue that has been bound to circulating albumin.[75] The time-action profile of insulin detemir is characterized by a peak activity at 6 to 8 hours after injection and a prolonged 24-hour duration of action (see Table 60-2).[75] Detemir is not yet commercially available. However, limited studies to date have shown significant reductions in hypoglycemic risk with detemir as basal insulin in intensive regimens compared to NPH.[53] In addition, detemir has been associated with more predictable glycemic control than NPH, with significantly less within-subject variation in blood glucose levels.[76,77] Moreover, its pharmacokinetic profile, unlike that of NPH, has been shown to be consistent in adults, adolescents, and children.[78]

INTENSIVE INSULIN THERAPY REGIMENS

The DCCT clearly established that the use of intensive insulin therapy can achieve lower A1c concentrations and reduce the risk of microvascular complications in patients with type 1 diabetes. Therefore, intensive insulin therapy is currently recommended in all patients with type 1 diabetes. There are two main regimens that can be utilized to provide intensive insulin therapy: multiple daily injections of insulin and continuous subcutaneous insulin infusion. Both regimens attempt to mimic physiologic insulin secretion through appropriate meal and basal insulin replacement. Ultimately, the choice of insulin regimen is generally determined by patient-driven factors, including lifestyle issues, finances, and personal preference.

Multiple Daily Injection Regimen

A multiple daily injection (MDI) regimen involves at least four injections of insulin per day, consisting of boluses of meal insulin prior to each meal and at least one injection of basal insulin, usually at bedtime. If needed, a second injection of basal insulin may be added at breakfast or before lunch. The meal insulin of choice is a rapid-acting analogue (lispro or aspart). Use of these analogues in MDI therapy has been associated with better postprandial glycemic control, a reduced incidence of hypoglycemia, and improvements in quality of life, compared to regular insulin.[61] On the other hand, while some studies have shown a significant decrease in A1c with use of rapid-acting analogues as compared to regular insulin in MDI therapy, other studies have not shown a significant difference in overall glycemic control.[61] As was noted earlier, however, this phenomenon likely reflects suboptimal basal insulin replacement in the studies in question. Moreover, with similar A1c, the combination of reduced postprandial glycemic excursion and less hypoglycemia suggests reduced overall glycemic variability (and hence better control) with the use of rapid-acting analogues compared to regular insulin in MDI therapy.

In the past, basal insulin replacement in MDI has usually consisted of bedtime injection of either NPH, lente, or ultralente. In clinical studies of MDI regimens using rapid-acting analogues as meal insulin, all three of these basal preparations have shown similar efficacy in regards to glycemic control and incidence of hypoglycemia.[55,79] Given their pharmacokinetic advantages, however, the long-acting analogues are likely to become the basal insulins of choice in MDI therapy. In studies comparing glargine and NPH as basal insulins in MDI regimens, glargine has been associated with improved fasting glucose levels and reduced rates of hypoglycemia.[70–72] Moreover, a second, prebreakfast injection of basal insulin is far less likely to be required with glargine than with NPH, lente, or ultralente. Indeed, in studies using lispro as meal insulin in MDI regimens, glycemic control was similar with a single injection of glargine at breakfast, dinner, or bedtime.[80] To date, few studies have compared glargine and NPH in MDI regimens using only rapid-acting analogues for meal insulin, although one such study demonstrated reduced A1c levels with a single dose of glargine compared to four daily injections of NPH.[81] While large-scale studies evaluating the efficacy of MDI regimens using rapid-acting analogues for meal insulin and long-acting analogues for basal coverage are pending, it is expected that this combination will provide the most physiologic insulin replacement to date among MDI regimens.

Continuous Subcutaneous Insulin Infusion

The external insulin infusion pump was first developed in the late 1970s, providing the basis for modern continuous subcutaneous insulin infusion (CSII) therapy.[82] With CSII, an external infusion pump delivers a continuous infusion of rapid- or short-acting insulin through a catheter inserted into the subcutaneous tissue of the abdominal wall. The pump is preprogrammed by the patient to deliver insulin continuously at a specified rate that is designed to meet the individual's basal insulin demands. For meal coverage, patients use the pump to deliver a specified bolus of insulin prior to eating.

The rapid-acting insulin analogues are the insulins of choice in CSII, as both lispro and aspart have been shown to reduce postprandial glycemia, A1c concentration and the incidence of hypoglycemia compared with regular insulin in this setting.[83–85]

CSII offers advantages over MDI therapy in terms of convenience and flexibility. Because the continuous infusion provides basal insulin at all times, the timing of meals with CSII, unlike with MDI, is completely flexible. At any given time, the rate of basal infusion can be immediately adjusted, an option that is not available with MDI. Moreover, current insulin pumps have multiphasic basal settings, allowing the user to set varying rates of basal insulin replacement at different times of the day depending on requirements. For instance, the pump can be preprogrammed to increase the basal rate of insulin infusion in the early morning hours in patients in whom the physiologic early morning secretion of growth hormone would otherwise lead to hyperglycemia (the "dawn phenomenon").

The major limitation with CSII is the significant cost associated with both the pump and necessary supplies, such as the tubing, which must be changed every 48 to 72 hours. Fortunately, increased insurance coverage of CSII has allowed for wider use of this therapy. Another disadvantage is the risk of infection at the insertion site of the catheter. Catheter-site infections occur at an estimated rate of 7.3 to 11.3 events per 100 years of patient follow-up.[17,86] These infections are usually readily treatable with antibiotics and a change of insertion site. In rare cases, a subcutaneous abscess requiring surgical drainage can develop. Finally, interruption of basal insulin delivery due to either pump malfunction or catheter disruption can rapidly lead to hyperglycemia or even ketoacidosis, as patients will quickly become markedly insulinopenic owing to the use of only rapid- or short-acting insulin in CSII.[87]

Clinical Efficacy of CSII versus MDI

In clinical trials comparing optimized MDI therapy with CSII, glycemic control has been found to be similar with both regimens. In the DCCT, 124 participants used CSII for more than 90% of the time during the study.[17] Mean A1c in this group of patients was 0.2% lower than in the cohort of patients on MDI therapy. Although the incidence of severe hypoglycemia events was similar between the two groups, the frequency of episodes resulting in coma or seizure was higher in the CSII cohort than in the MDI group. However, in the DCCT, patients who were randomized to intensive therapy could choose between CSII and MDI and could switch between these regimens during the trial. Therefore, the DCCT experience may provide a biased estimate of the comparative merits of these therapies. Similarly, although a recent meta-analysis of trials comparing CSII and MDI regimens reported a difference in A1c of 0.51% favoring CSII, all but 1 of the 12 studies included in this analysis were older studies using suboptimal, nonanalogue meal insulins.[88] Furthermore, given improvements in pump technology and greater clinical experience with intensified regimens, the current applicability of these studies is unclear. To date, the few studies comparing CSII and optimized MDI therapy with both regimens using rapid-acting analogues have shown slightly improved glycemic control with insulin pump therapy, with no significant difference in hypoglycemia.[89–91] In these studies, the glycemic advantage of CSII over MDI may be related to baseline A1c, such that patients with the poorest initial glycemic control enjoy the greatest benefit with insulin pump therapy. It should be noted that NPH was the basal insulin for MDI therapy in all of these studies. Therefore, studies comparing CSII with optimized MDI regimens using long-acting analogues for basal insulin and rapid-acting analogues for prandial coverage are eagerly awaited.

Implementation of Intensive Insulin Therapy

Implementation of an intensive insulin regimen using either MDI or CSII can be accomplished in many ways. In general, starting doses are estimated by using an algorithm such as the method shown in Figure 60-7. The initial total daily insulin (TDI) requirement is estimated at 0.5 units/kg of body weight, although most patients with type 1 diabetes ultimately require 0.6 to 0.7 units/kg. Alternatively, for patients who are already on an insulin regimen, TDI is simply the sum of all current insulin doses. When CSII is implemented in such a patient, this TDI dose must be reduced by 20% to determine the total daily amount of insulin to be delivered by the pump.

Basal insulin comprises approximately 40% of the total daily dose. With MDI, this basal insulin is initially provided with a single bedtime injection, although postabsorptive daytime hyperglycemia may subsequently dictate the need for a second dose of basal insulin before breakfast. With CSII, the total daily basal insulin is provided as a continuous infusion

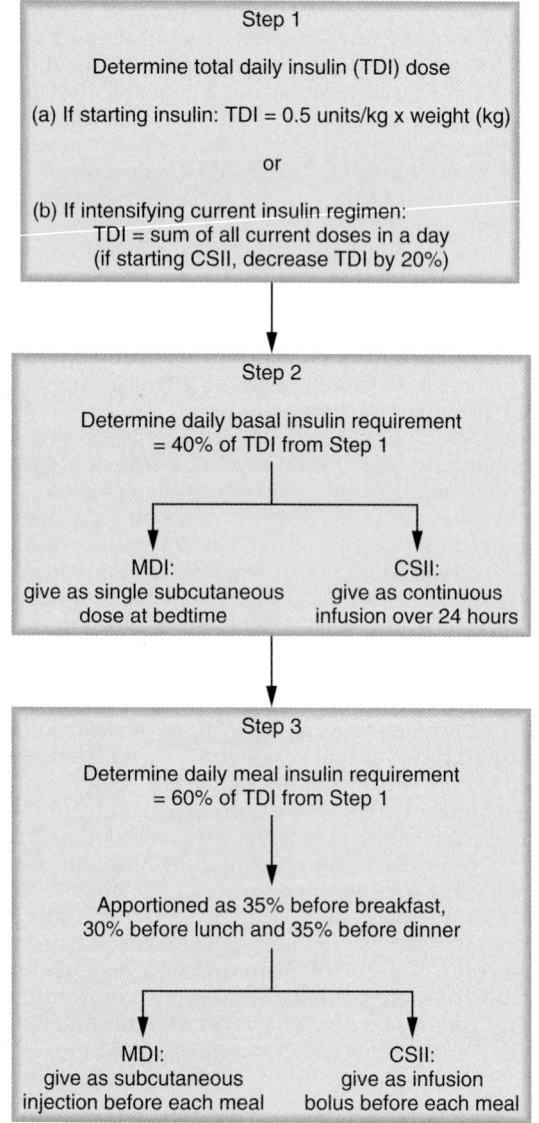

Figure 60-7 One algorithm for the determination of initial insulin doses when implementing intensive insulin therapy using MDI or CSII. (Source: Adapted from Shah BR, Zinman B: Insulin regimens for type 1 diabetes. In Sperling MA (ed): Contemporary Endocrinology: Type 1 Diabetes: Etiology and Treatment. Totowa NJ, Humana Press, 2003, p 205.)

over 24 hours, with hourly basal rates typically ranging from 0.6 to 1.2 units/hour. The remaining 60% of the TDI is provided in the form of meal or bolus insulin, lunch generally requiring less insulin than breakfast and dinner.

As an example, consider the following case of a patient who is currently on a nonintensified regimen of 12 units of NPH at both breakfast and bedtime and 6 units of regular insulin at breakfast and dinner. To convert this patient's insulin therapy to an intensified MDI regimen, the algorithm in Figure 60-7 would be applied as follows:

- The TDI would be (12 + 12 + 6 + 6 =) 36 units of insulin per day.
- The basal requirement would be estimated at (40% × 36 units =) 14 units per day. This basal insulin could be provided with a single daily dose of glargine.
- The daily meal insulin requirement would be estimated at (60% × 36 units =) 22 units per day. This meal insulin could be divided such that the patient receives (35% × 22 units =) 8 units at breakfast (30% × 22 units =), 6 units at lunch, and (35% × 22 units =) 8 units at dinner. These meal insulin doses would ideally be provided in the form of preprandial subcutaneous injections of a rapid-acting analogue.

In practice, the insulin doses calculated in Table 60-3 are continually adjusted by the patient on the basis of the following three considerations: preprandial capillary blood glucose concentration, anticipated carbohydrate intake, and upcoming physical activity. By determining the preprandial blood glucose level using capillary monitoring, the patient can adjust prandial insulin dosage using a variable insulin dose scale (see Table 60-3). Using this approach, the patient is directed to take a higher dose of prandial bolus insulin when the blood glucose concentration is above a specified range. The second consideration in dose adjustment is anticipated carbohydrate intake. By estimating the amount of carbohydrate to be ingested in the upcoming meal (a practice that is referred to as *carbohydrate counting*), the patient can adjust the prandial insulin dose accordingly. While most patients require an additional 1 unit of insulin per 10 to 15 grams of carbohydrate ingested at a meal, the actual ratio must be individually determined for a given patient. Finally, patients must consider the effects of upcoming physical activity in adjusting insulin dosage. For instance, with MDI therapy, prandial insulin administered at the meal prior to moderate exercise might have to be reduced, depending on the individual's glycemic response to exercise.[92] Patients using CSII have the additional flexibility of being able to adjust their basal insulin rate to accommodate for exercise.

Table 60-3 Variable Insulin Dose Scale

Blood Glucose (BG) mg/dL	Units of Meal Insulin		
	Breakfast	Lunch	Dinner
<90	−2	−2	−2
Goal BG 90–130	x	y	z
131–180	+2	+2	+2
181–230	+4	+4	+4
231–280	+6	+6	+6
281–330	+8	+8	+8
>330	+10	+10	+10

Sample variable insulin dose scale to guide in adjustment of meal insulin based on preprandial glucose levels. Baseline doses of x, y, and z units of meal insulin at breakfast, lunch, and dinner, respectively, are adjusted by the indicated amounts based on the preprandial glucose level. (Example for illustrative purposes only.)
Source: Adapted from Leadership Sinai Centre for Diabetes, Mount Sinai Hospital, Toronto, Ontario, Canada.

INSULIN DELIVERY

Subcutaneous Insulin Delivery

With both MDI and CSII therapy, insulin is delivered into subcutaneous fat tissue. In CSII, insulin is delivered through a needle or Silastic infuser placed subcutaneously. The needle and its injection site are changed every 48 to 72 hours to reduce the risk of infection.

In MDI therapy, insulin is injected subcutaneously using either syringes or pen-and-cartridge devices. With the former method, the patient uses a disposable plastic syringe to draw insulin from the multiple-use vials in which the medication is supplied. When using suspended insulins such as NPH and lente, it is important that the patient resuspend the contents of the vial before drawing up the insulin dose. The insulin in the syringe is then injected into the subcutaneous tissue by using a fine needle. An advantage of the syringe method is that meal and basal insulins that are being taken at the same time (e.g., before breakfast) may be drawn into the same syringe (with the notable exception of glargine, which cannot be mixed with other insulins), thereby reducing the number of injections that are required. On the other hand, the visual acuity and manual dexterity that are required for this system can prove problematic for some patients and could contribute to dosage errors.

A newer, alternative delivery method is provided by pen-and-cartridge devices. In this case, replaceable cartridges containing insulin are placed into a pen-shaped delivery device that is referred to as an insulin pen, which is then used to inject the insulin subcutaneously. Insulin pens offer the advantage of more accurate dosing and easier administration, particularly for patients with visual or motor impairment.[93,94] One disadvantage, however, is that basal and meal insulins that are being taken at the same time cannot be mixed with the pen and hence require separate injections. Nevertheless, insulin pens have become the delivery mode of choice for patients using MDI therapy.

Many aspects of subcutaneous insulin administration can affect the absorption of the medication and hence its clinical efficacy. One key factor is the site of insulin injection. Insulin absorption varies inversely with the thickness of subcutaneous fat at the site of injection.[95] Thus, insulin absorption is fastest from the subcutaneous fat of the abdominal wall, the preferred site of injection, and slower from other sites that have more subcutaneous fat such as the upper arm, anterior thigh, and buttocks.[96] Another factor is depth of injection, as shallow insertion of the needle can lead to poorly absorbed intradermal delivery of insulin. Conversely, if injecting into a lean site with little subcutaneous fat, intramuscular injection may occur, which can be painful and lead to rapid systemic absorption. After injection, alterations in subcutaneous blood flow may affect insulin absorption. For instance, after insulin injection into an extremity, physical exercise involving the affected limb can increase local blood flow and enhance insulin absorption.[97] Other factors that can increase absorption include increased skin temperature and local massage.[98,99]

Alternative Routes of Insulin Delivery

Despite best efforts, the faithful imitation of normal physiologic insulin secretion generally cannot be achieved with the subcutaneous delivery of current insulin preparations. Factors that limit the success of current treatment approaches include the pharmacokinetics of exogenous insulin preparations following subcutaneous injection, the systemic dissemination of this injected insulin via the peripheral venous system (as opposed to normal pancreatic secretion into the portal venous system), and patient dissatisfaction with the demands and inconvenience of complex treatment regimens. Therefore, alternative routes for delivery of insulin have long been of interest. Options considered include nasal, pulmonary, oral, transdermal, and peritoneal delivery of insulin. Although these attempts have generally met with limited success to date, intrapulmonary and intraperitoneal delivery of insulin, in particular, may hold significant promise for the future.

The respiratory tree offers a large, well-perfused surface area for delivery of a polypeptide drug such as insulin. Current delivery systems for inhalation of aerosolized insulin include pressurized metered dose inhalers, dry powder inhalers, nebulizers, and aqueous mist inhalers.[100] As its onset of action is comparable to that of subcutaneous rapid-acting analogues but with a longer duration of activity (5 to 10 hours), inhaled insulin may provide an option for meal coverage in basal-bolus therapy. In limited studies to date, regimens using preprandial inhaled insulin and subcutaneous basal insulin have achieved overall glycemic control (A1c) and rates of hypoglycemia similar to those of standard subcutaneous therapy.[101–103] Over the short duration of these studies (less than 1 year), pulmonary function tests have suggested that inhaled insulin might be associated with a small decline in pulmonary diffusion capacity with little or no change in forced expiratory volume.[100–102] The long-term safety of inhaled insulin will need to be established before this therapy can be considered as a therapeutic option in practice.

Intraperitoneal insulin delivery offers an approach that could simulate normal pancreatic secretion of insulin into the portal venous system. Indeed, intraperitoneal insulin infusion has been shown to reproduce a positive porto-systemic insulin gradient and has been associated with a more rapid onset of action and reduced duration of activity compared to subcutaneous insulin.[104] These findings have led to the development of implantable insulin pumps, disk-shaped infusion systems that are surgically implanted in the abdominal subcutaneous tissue.[105] The pump reservoir holds a 2- to 3-month supply of insulin and is connected to a free-moving peritoneal catheter. Rates of insulin delivery are adjusted by the patient, based on SMBG results. The patient uses an external programmer that sends radio-wave signals to the electronic command unit of the pump to control the rate of insulin infusion. One such implantable pump is commercially available in Europe but has not yet been approved in North America. Studies to date suggest that implantable insulin pumps are associated with comparable A1c levels and a reduced incidence of severe hypoglycemia compared to subcutaneous insulin delivery.[105,106] The main problem with implantable pumps is the potential for underdelivery of insulin due to catheter occlusion, an event that has been estimated to occur at a rate of 15 per 100 patient-years.[107] Nevertheless, intraperitoneal delivery remains a promising option for insulin administration in the future.

Beyond pulmonary and peritoneal delivery, attempts to utilize other routes for insulin administration have been largely unsuccessful. Despite significant interest in its potential convenience, oral insulin has not proved to be a viable option owing to enzymatic degradation of the insulin polypeptide in the gastrointestinal tract and poor absorption (<1% of oral dose).[108] Strategies to overcome these problems have included the coadministration of enzyme inhibitors and attempts to improve the chemical stability of oral insulin through the use of liposomes and polymer-based systems.[100] Similarly, intranasal insulin delivery has been hampered by low and unpredictable bioavailability that can fluctuate significantly with even minor changes in the nasal mucosa.[109] Finally, transdermal insulin delivery has been unsuccessful owing to the relative impermeability of the skin to large, hydrophilic polypeptides such as insulin.[100] Strategies that are being studied for improving transdermal drug delivery include iontophoresis, low-frequency ultrasound, and the use of drug carrier agents.

COMPLICATIONS OF INSULIN THERAPY

Insulin therapy is life-saving in patients with type 1 diabetes. Nevertheless, complications of insulin treatment can pose obstacles to the implementation of intensive therapy.

The most feared complication of intensive insulin therapy is hypoglycemia. In the DCCT, the risk of hypoglycemia was approximately threefold higher in the intensive treatment group than in the conventional therapy arm.[110] As insulin analogues were not available at the time of the DCCT, it is not clear whether this finding reflects current practice. Nevertheless, hypoglycemia is a factor that might limit the ability to achieve optimal glycemic control. Hypoglycemia generally reflects an imbalance between carbohydrate intake, physical activity, and the dose of exogenous insulin. In addition, patients with type 1 diabetes have a deficient counterregulatory response to hypoglycemia.[111] Previous episodes of severe hypoglycemia and physiologic inability to detect the attendant symptoms (hypoglycemia unawareness) are other factors that are associated with increased hypoglycemic risk. Thus, a patient's propensity for hypoglycemia must be considered in establishing therapeutic goals, as excessive hypoglycemia is best managed by raising glycemic targets. Similarly, in patients with hypoglycemia unawareness, raising glycemic targets is utilized as a means of restoring physiologic awareness of hypoglycemic symptomatology.[112] Specifically, with increased overall glycemia, the careful avoidance of further hypoglycemia can help to restore awareness and improve defective counterregulation.

Weight gain is another adverse effect that is associated with insulin therapy. In the DCCT, patients receiving intensive therapy gained 4.75 kg more than participants in the conventional treatment arm over the course of the study.[113] This effect reflects both insulin's anabolic properties and the decrease in glycosuria with improved glycemic control. Specifically, for patients with poor glycemic control, the elimination of glycosuria with insulin therapy will lead to a positive caloric balance and weight gain. In addition, intermittent hypoglycemia associated with intensive insulin therapy can also lead to hunger and increased caloric intake. Concerns regarding weight gain may cause some patients to be reluctant to initiate intensive therapy and should be addressed by the health-care team.

Rapid improvement in glycemic control following the initiation of intensive insulin therapy can cause transient exacerbation of underlying retinopathy.[114] Patients with proliferative retinopathy and baseline A1c greater than 10% are at highest risk of this complication.[115] Baseline ophthalmologic evaluation with frequent surveillance should be considered for such patients when intensive therapy is started.[114] In addition, more gradual reduction in A1c may be prudent in such cases.

Allergic reactions to insulin are rare, particularly since human insulin is much less immunogenic than earlier animal insulins were.[79] Most allergic reactions to insulin reflect local hypersensitivity at the site of injection. Generalized allergic reactions can also occur rarely. Protocols for desensitization have been developed for both local and systemic hypersensitivity to insulin.[79]

Lipohypertrophy refers to localized swelling at a site of repeated insulin injection. This complication is related to the lipogenic effects of insulin. Continued injection of insulin into sites of lipohypertrophy is discouraged, as absorption of the insulin can be erratic and lead to unpredictable glycemic effects. Lipoatrophy reflects a different pathophysiology, in which an immune-mediated response to exogenous insulin leads to atrophy of subcutaneous tissue at the site of injection.[116] With the current use of recombinant human insulin preparations and analogues, the problem of insulin-induced lipoatrophy is very infrequent.

ADJUSTMENT OF INSULIN THERAPY IN SPECIAL SITUATIONS

The absence of endogenous insulin secretion in patients with type 1 diabetes dictates an absolute reliance at all time on exogenous insulin for both prandial and basal metabolic needs. Thus, even when not eating, patients with type 1 diabetes continue to require insulin therapy to meet basal requirements and to avoid diabetic ketoacidosis. Recognition of this principle underlies the appropriate management of their insulin therapy in special situations such as times of intercurrent illness and during surgery.

Intercurrent Illness

The physiologic stress associated with illness stimulates the release of counterregulatory hormones that antagonize insulin action. Thus, during times of illness, patients are at risk of both hyperglycemia and diabetic ketoacidosis. During such times, regular monitoring of blood glucose concentrations every 4 hours is recommended. If hyperglycemia is detected, then supplemental insulin is indicated. Conversely, if blood glucose levels are low, then the amount of insulin taken at that time should be significantly reduced. As was noted earlier, patients must not withhold insulin therapy completely. Instead, under such circumstances, patients are advised to drink sugar-rich fluids such as fruit juices to maintain adequate carbohydrate and fluid intake. If patients are unable to tolerate even this limited intake, however, then presentation to the hospital is necessary for administration of intravenous fluids.

Even with continued insulin therapy, patients with type 1 diabetes are at risk of developing ketoacidosis during times of illness owing to the effects of the counterregulatory hormones in antagonizing insulin action and promoting ketogenesis. Frequent testing of blood ketone levels using a home capillary blood ketone monitor is therefore recommended at such times. Alternatively, if such testing is unavailable at home, then traditional urinary ketone monitoring should be performed (see the section entitled "Ketone Testing," earlier in the chapter).

Surgery

The goals of perioperative management of patients with type 1 diabetes are the avoidance of marked hyperglycemia and the avoidance of hypoglycemia. As with periods of illness, surgery is associated with both physiologic stress that promotes hyperglycemia and reduced caloric intake that may predispose to hypoglycemia (since most surgical procedures are performed on fasting patients). As before, the principles of management are the need for continued insulin therapy and close metabolic monitoring. Typically, major surgical procedures are managed with intravenous insulin therapy and frequent blood glucose monitoring.

NUTRITION

The nutritional recommendations associated with healthy eating habits for the general public are also applicable to patients with type 1 diabetes.[117] The important difference in patients with type 1 diabetes is that dietary intake must be appropriately coordinated with insulin therapy and physical activity to achieve regulation of blood glucose levels. In particular, attention must be paid to the sources and amount of carbohydrate in the diet. Carbohydrate is the main dietary constituent that affects postprandial glycemic excursion and hence prandial insulin requirements.[118] This concept has led to the practice of "carbohydrate counting."

Carbohydrate counting is a meal-planning approach in which patients are taught to estimate the carbohydrate content of a meal preprandially and adjust their dose of meal insulin accordingly.[119] Most patients require 1 extra unit of insulin for each 10 to 15 g of carbohydrate ingested, though this ratio must be individually determined on the basis of personal food preferences and individual physiologic response. As such, carbohydrate counting is an integral component of patient education and is a skill that patients generally develop with the assistance of a clinical dietitian. While the concept of carbohydrate counting was described shortly after the discovery of insulin,[120] its recent resurgence is partly linked to its inclusion as one of the dietary interventions in the intensive treatment arm of the DCCT. In the DCCT, the practice of adjusting food and/or insulin dosage in response to hyperglycemia emerged as a dietary behavior associated with improved glycemic control.[121] Moreover, carbohydrate counting allows for significant flexibility in food choices. Alternatively, for patients on fixed insulin doses who are unwilling to adjust prandial insulin dosage on the basis dietary content, consistency of carbohydrate intake is advised.[117]

Although carbohydrate content is the key modifier of prandial insulin dosage, total energy intake from protein and fat cannot be neglected. Total energy intake must be regulated to avoid unnecessary weight gain, particularly since intensive insulin therapy is frequently associated with weight gain as well.[117]

Another important consideration affecting food choices is hypoglycemia. For instance, patients must recognize that ingested alcohol may reduce hepatic glucose production and mask the symptoms of hypoglycemia. Indeed, moderate alcohol consumption (one to two standard drinks) 2 to 3 hours after the evening meal can lead to delayed hypoglycemia the next morning after breakfast.[122] Conversely, patients are also advised to avoid the overtreatment of hypoglycemia by excessive food intake, as this practice may lead to weight gain and significant glycemic excursion.[14]

OTHER THERAPIES FOR TYPE 1 DIABETES

The two most important alternative therapies currently available for type 1 diabetes are islet cell and pancreatic transplantation. These treatment modalities are discussed in detail in Chapter 67.

Increased understanding of the natural history and immunogenetics of type 1 diabetes has led to the ability to identify individuals who are at high risk of developing this condition and recognition of the existence of a long, asymptomatic prediabetic period that might be amenable to intervention (see Chapter 57).[123] Therefore, significant recent research interest has focused on the concept of prevention of type 1 diabetes in high-risk subjects who have been identified on the basis of genetic and antibody markers.[124] While several strategies have been studied, it is important to recognize that no intervention to date has proved to be consistently successful in preventing type 1 diabetes. Nevertheless, research efforts aimed at the prevention of type 1 diabetes are expected to increase in the coming years and are likely to ultimately yield novel therapeutic approaches.

Preventive strategies that have been considered thus far have aimed to prevent β-cell loss in high-risk individuals by one of three general means: nonspecific immunosuppression, targeted immunomodulation, and protection of the β cell from chemical or autoimmune injury.[125] Nonspecific immunosuppression refers to pharmacologic attempts to downregulate the autoimmune attack that leads to β-cell destruction by generalized suppression of the immune system. This approach was initially supported by the observation that drugs such as azathioprine and cyclosporine can temporarily decrease insulin requirements in patients with recently diagnosed type 1 diabetes.[126,127] Unfortunately, the remission that these medications induces appears to be only temporary.[128,129] When coupled with the significant toxicities of existing immunosuppressives, the modest achievable success precludes widespread application of this therapeutic approach at this time.

Targeted immunomodulation describes strategies that are aimed at interfering solely with the parts of the immune system that are involved in β-cell destruction. One such strategy is to use β-cell-derived antigens in an attempt to induce immune tolerance. In the best-known example of this approach, insulin therapy has been introduced in high-risk individuals in the hope of preventing progression to type 1 diabetes. However, in the Diabetes Prevention Trial, the largest such insulin tolerance trial so far, insulin therapy was unsuccessful in preventing type 1 diabetes.[130] Other antigens that are being studied for use in this way include glutamic acid decarboxylase and a peptide derived from heat shock protein 60.[125] Further avenues for targeted immunomodulation that are currently being explored include the use of antibodies directed against specific adhesion molecules involved in cell-cell interactions required for autoimmune β-cell destruction and the use of immunostimulatory agents such as bacillus Calmette-Guérin to correct the presumed underlying immune defect that prevents the development of normal β-cell tolerance.[125]

β-cell protective strategies aim to enhance the ability of the β cell to withstand chemical or autoimmune injury. For example, nicotinamide, which is believed to prevent cytokine-mediated β-cell damage by blocking the cytotoxic effects of free-radical nitric oxide, has shown some success in preventing disease progression in animal models of diabetes.[131,132] However, in human studies, nicotinamide has thus far proved unsuccessful in preventing type 1 diabetes. Other β-cell protective strategies that are under consideration include the use of antagonists of the apoptotic signaling molecule Fas and inhibition of tumor necrosis factor-α, a putative cytokine mediator of β-cell death.[125]

FUTURE PERSPECTIVES

Despite remarkable advances in the 80 years since the discovery of insulin, the goal of sustained euglycemia in patients with type 1 diabetes remains largely unrealized. Nevertheless, the future looks promising. Investigative efforts on several fronts offer hope for novel therapeutic approaches in the years to come.

One such area is glucose sensing. Several approaches to noninvasive glucose sensing are currently being developed and could provide convenient, patient-friendly means for self-monitoring in the future.[133] These initiatives utilize various technologies, including near-infrared (700 to 1300 nm) spectroscopy, in which an optical sensor determines glucose concentration based on the absorption pattern of light passing through body tissue, and reverse iontophoresis, in which a low-level electrical current is applied to the skin to generate a signal that is proportional to the interstitial fluid glucose concentration.[105]

Even more promising is the potential further development of continuous glucose-monitoring systems to provide real-time glucose information to the patient. Current systems do not provide this data to the patient and hence do not obviate the need for capillary blood glucose monitoring. The immediate provision of acute glucose data would allow for more frequent monitoring and potentially better simulation of normal pancreatic responsiveness.

Implantable intravenous glucose sensing devices could offer a more physiologic alternative for real-time blood glucose measurement. While earlier prototypes were plagued by problems such as in situ thrombosis, recent intravenous sensors might hold promise for safe, reliable function.[105] Such technology could ultimately lead to the successful development of the long-awaited artificial β cell. In such a system, an intravenous sensor would transmit real-time blood glucose measurements to a responsive intraperitoneal insulin pump. Indeed, the resultant closed-loop system could theoretically mimic physiologic insulin secretion by linking appropriate portal insulin secretion to real-time blood glucose levels. Such a system holds promise for achieving sustained euglycemia.

Similarly exciting is the concept of β-cell bioengineering. The isolation of pluripotent pancreatic ductal epithelial stem cells and the identification of islet-cell growth factors have raised the possibility of generating islet cells *in vitro*. Such efforts could provide an unlimited source of islet cells for transplantation. Alternatively, a gene therapy approach can be used to confer transgenic insulin secretory capacity to an appropriate target cell. For instance, this approach has been applied to create a liver-targeted insulin transgene driven by a glucose-responsive promoter in a rodent model of diabetes.[134] Gene therapy could also be applied to reprogram liver stem cells into insulin-producing cells. In a murine model, adenovirus-mediated gene transfer of pancreatic and duodenal homeobox gene 1, a key developmental factor in pancreatic organogenesis, has been shown to reprogram hepatocytes to create a β-cell phenotype.[135] Though still many years away from clinical application, these initiatives might eventually lead to stable β-cell regeneration and a potential cure for type 1 diabetes at some point in the future.

The 80 years since the discovery of insulin have seen remarkable advances in the treatment of type 1 diabetes. These changes have provided the capacity for improved glycemic control and a reduction in the burden of long-term microvascular and macrovascular complications. Though the ability of current therapies to achieve persistent euglycemia is limited, a vast array of research initiatives holds promise for future therapies that might ultimately render this goal fully attainable.

REFERENCES

1. Banting FG, Best CH, Collip JB, et al: Pancreatic extracts in the treatment of diabetes mellitus. Can Med Assoc J 12:141–146, 1922.
2. The Diabetes Control and Complications Trial Research Group: The effect of intensive treatment of diabetes on the development and progression of long-term complications in insulin-dependent diabetes mellitus. N Engl J Med 329:977–986, 1993.
3. Reichard P, Nilsson B-Y, Rosenqvist U: The effect of long-term intensified insulin treatment on the development of microvascular complications of diabetes mellitus. N Engl J Med 329:304–309, 1993.
4. Lauritzen T, Rost-Larsen K, Larsen H-W, Deckert T: Two-year experience with continuous subcutaneous insulin infusion in relation to retinopathy and neuropathy. Diabetes 34(Suppl 1):74–79, 1985.
5. Brinchmann-Hansen O, Dahl-Jorgensen K, Hanssen KF, Sandvik L: The response of diabetic retinopathy to 41 months of multiple insulin injectins, insulin pumps, and conventional insulin therapy. Arch Ophthalmol 106:1242–1246, 1988.
6. Zinman B: The physiologic replacement of insulin. N Engl J Med 321:363–370, 1989.
7. Diabetes Control and Complications Trial/Epidemiology of Diabetes Interventions and Complications Research Group: Retinopathy and nephropathy in patients with type 1 diabetes four years after a trial of intensive therapy. N Engl J Med 342:381–389, 2000.
8. Diabetes Control and Complications Trial/Epidemiology of Diabetes Interventions and Complications Research Group: Sustained effect of intensive treatment of type 1 diabetes mellitus on development and progression of diabetic nephropathy. JAMA 290:2159–2167, 2003.
9. Diabetes Control and Complications Trial/Epidemiology of Diabetes Interventions and Complications Research Group: Intensive therapy and

carotid intima-media thickness in type 1 diabetes mellitus. N Engl J Med 348(23):2294–2303, 2003.

10. The Diabetes Control and Complications Trial Research Group: The relationship of glycemic exposure (HbA1c) to the risk of development and progression of retinopathy in the Diabetes Control and Complications Trial. Diabetes 44(8):968–983, 1995.

11. American Diabetes Association: Standards of medical care in diabetes. Diabetes Care 27(Suppl 1):S15–S35, 2004.

12. Canadian Diabetes Association Clinical Practice Guidelines Expert Committee: Targets for glycemic control. Can J Diabetes 27(Suppl 2):S18–S20, 2003.

13. American Association of Clinical Endocrinologists (AACE) Consensus Development Conference on Guidelines for Glycemic Control. Endocr Pract Suppl Nov/Dec 2001.

14. Canadian Diabetes Association Clinical Practice Guidelines Expert Committee: Hypoglycemia. Can J Diabetes 27(Suppl 2):S43–S45, 2003.

15. Slama G, Traynard P–Y, Desplanque N, et al: The search for an optimized treatment of hypoglycemia. Carbohydrates in tablets, solution, or gel for the correction of insulin reactions. Arch Intern Med 150:589–593, 1990.

16. The Diabetes Control and Complications Trial Research Group: Reliability and validity of a diabetes quality-of-life measure for the Diabetes Control and Complications Trial. Diabetes Care 11:725–732, 1988.

17. The Diabetes Control and Complications Trial Research Group: Implementation of treatment protocols in the Diabetes Control and Complications Trial. Diabetes Care 18(3):361–376, 1995.

18. American Diabetes Association: Test of glycemia in diabetes. Diabetes Care 27(Suppl 1):S91–S93, 2004.

19. Reynolds LR, Karounos DG: Emerging technology in diabetes mellitus: Glucose monitoring and new insulins. South Med J 95(8):914–918, 2002.

20. Ellison JM, Stegmann JM, Colner SL, et al: Rapid changes in postprandial blood glucose produce concentration differences at finger, forearm, and thigh sampling sites. Diabetes Care 25(6):961–964, 2002.

21. Bina DM, Anderson RL, Johnson ML, et al: Clinical impact of prandial state, exercise and site preparation on the equivalence of alternative-site blood glucose testing. Diabetes Care 26(4):981–985, 2003.

22. Rebrin K, Steil GM, van Antwerp WP, Mastrototaro JJ: Subcutaneous glucose predicts plasma glucose independent of insulin: Implications for continuous monitoring. Am J Physiol 277:E561–E571, 1999.

23. Mastrototaro JJ: The MiniMed Continuous Glucose Monitoring System (CGMS). J Pediatr Endocrinol Metab 12(Suppl 3):S751–S758, 1999.

24. Cheyne E, Kerr D: Making "sense" of diabetes: Using a continuous glucose sensor in clinical practice. Diabetes Metab Res Rev 18(Suppl 1):S43–S48, 2002.

25. Chico A, Vidal-Rios P, Subira M, Novials A: The continuous glucose monitoring system is useful for detecting unrecognized hypoglycemias in patients with type 1 and type 2 diabetes but is not better than frequent capillary glucose measurements for improving metabolic control. Diabetes Care 26(4):1153–1157, 2003.

26. Kaufman FR, Austin J, Neinstein A, et al: Nocturnal hypoglycemia detected with the Continuous Glucose Monitoring System in pediatric patients with type 1 diabetes. J Pediatr 141(5):625–630, 2002.

27. Metzger M, Leibowitz G, Wainstein J, et al: Reproducibility of glucose measurements using the glucose sensor. Diabetes Care 25:1185–1191, 2002.

28. Bunn HF, Haney DN, Gabbay KH, Gallop PM: Further identification of the nature and linkageof the carbohydrate in hemoglobin A1c. Biochem Biophys Res Commun 67:103–109, 1975.

29. Nathan DM, Singer DE, Hurxthal K, Goodson JD: The clinical information value of the glycosylated hemoglobin assay. N Engl J Med 310:341–346, 1984.

30. Little RR, Wiedmeyer HM, England JD, et al: Interlaboratory comparison of glycohemoglobin results: College of American Pathologists survey data. Clin Chem 37:1725–1729, 1991.

31. Little RR, Rohlfing CL, Widemeyer HM, et al: The National Glycohemoglobin Standardization Program (NGSP): A five-year progress report. Clin Chem 47:1985–1992, 2001.

32. Rohlfing CL, Wiedmeyer HM, Little RR, et al: Defining the relationship between plasma glucose and HbA1c: Analysis of glucose profiles and HbA1c in the Diabetes Control and Complication Trial. Diabetes Care 25:275–278, 2002.

33. Panzer S, Kronik G, Lechner K, et al: Glycosylated hemoglobins (GHb): An index of red cell survival. Blood 59:1348–1350, 1982.

34. Fluckiger R, Harmon W, Meier W, et al: Hemoglobin carbamylation in uremia. N Engl J Med 304:823–827, 1981.

35. Paisey R, Banks R, Holton R, et al: Glycosylated haemoglobin in uremia. Diabet Med 3:445–448, 1986.

36. Armbruster DA: Fructosamine: Structure, analysis and clinical usefulness. Clin Chem 33:2153–2163, 1987.

37. Baker JR, Metcalf PA, Holdaway IM, Johnson RN: Serum fructosamine concentration as a measure of blood glucose control in type 1 (insulin-dependent) diabetes mellitus. Br Med J 290:352–355, 1985.

38. Howey JE, Bennet WM, Browning MC, et al: Clinical utility of assays of glycosylated hemoglobin and serum fructosamine compared: Use of data on

biologic variation. Diabet Med 6:793–796, 1989.

39. Byrne HA, Tieszen KL, Hollis S, et al: Evaluation of an electrochemical sensor for measuring blood ketones. Diabetes Care 23:500–503, 2000.

40. Guerci B, Benichout M, Floriot M, et al: Accuracy of an electrochemical sensor for measuring capillary blood ketones by fingerstick samples during metabolic deterioration after continuous subcutaneous insulin infusion interruption in type 1 diabetic patients. Diabetes Care 26(4):1137–1141, 2003.

41. Wallace TM, Meston NM, Gardner SG, Matthews DR: The hospital and home-use of a 30 second hand-held blood ketone meter: Guidelines for clinical practice. Diabet Med 18(8):640–645, 2001.

42. Eknoyan G, Hostetter T, Bakris GL, et al: Proteinuria and other markers of chronic kidney disease: A position statement of the National Kidney Foundation (NKF) and the National Institute of Diabetes and Digestive and Kidney Diseases (NIDDK). Am J Kidney Dis 42(4):617–622, 2003.

43. Perkins BA, Olaleye D, Zinman B, Bril V: Simple screening tests for peripheral neuropathy in the diabetes clinic. Diabetes Care 24(2):250–256, 2001.

44. Owens DR, Zinman B, Bolli GB: Insulins today and beyond. Lancet 358:739–746, 2001.

45. Shah BR, Zinman B: Insulin regimens for type 1 diabetes. In Sperling MA (ed): Type 1 Diabetes: Etiology and Treatment. Totowa, NJ, Humana Press, 2003, pp 199–214.

46. Zinman B, Murray FT, Vranic M, et al: Glucoregulation during moderate exercise in insulin treated diabetes. J Clin Endocrinol Metab 45:641–652, 1977.

47. Mitchell TH, Abraham G, Schiffrin A, et al: Hyperglycemia after intense exercise in IDDM subjects during continuous subcutaneous insulin infusion. Diabetes Care 11:311–317, 1988.

48. Chance RE, Kroeff EP, Hoffmann JA, Frank BH: Chemical, physical and biologic properties of biosynthetic human insulin. Diabetes Care 4:147–154, 1981.

49. Skyler JS (ed): Symposium on human insulin of recombinant DNA origin. Diabetes Care 5(Suppl 2):1–186, 1982.

50. Kang S, Brange J, Burch A, et al: Subcutaneous insulin absorption explained by insulin's physicochemical properties: Evidence from absorption studies of soluble human insulin and insulin analogues in humans. Diabetes Care 14:942–948, 1991.

51. Heinemann L, Richter B: Clinical pharmacology of human insulin. Diabetes Care 16(Suppl 3):90–100, 1993.

52. Krayenbuhl C, Rosenberg T: Crystalline protamine insulin. Rep Steno Hosp 1:60–73, 1946.

53. Barnett AH: A review of basal insulins. Diabet Med 20:873–885, 2003.

54. Lauritzen T, Faber OK, Binder C: Variation in 125 I-insulin absorption and blood glucose conception. Diabetologia 17:291–295, 1979.

55. Zinman B, Ross S, Campos R, Strack T: Effectiveness of human ultralente versus NPH insulin in providing basal insulin replacement for an insulin lispro multiple daily injection regimen. Diabetes Care 22:603–608, 1999.

56. Holleman F, Hoekstra JBL: Insulin lispro. New Engl J Med 337:176–183, 1997.

57. Brems DN, Alter LA, Beckage MJ, et al: Altering the association properties of insulin by amino acid replacement. Protein Eng 5:527–532, 1992.

58. Howey DC, Bowsher RR, Brunelle RF, Woodworth JR: [Lys(B28), Pro(B29)]-human insulin: A rapidly absorbed analogue of human insulin. Diabetes 43:396–402, 1994.

59. Lee W, Zinman B: From insulin to insulin analogs: Progress in the treatment of type 1 diabetes. Diabetes Rev 6:73–88, 1998.

60. Mudaliar SR, Lindberg FA, Joyce M, et al: Insulin aspart (B28 Asp-insulin): A fast-acting analog of human insulin. Diabetes Care 22:1501–1506, 1999.

61. Cheng AY, Zinman B: Insulin analogues and the treatment of diabetes In Raz I, Skyler JS, Shafrir E (eds): Diabetes: From Research to Diagnosis and Treatment. London, Martin Dunitz Ltd, 2002, pp 331–346.

62. Brunelle RL, Llewelyn J, Anderson JH, et al: Meta-analysis of the effect of insulin lispro on severe hypoglycemia in paitents with type 1 diabetes. Diabetes Care 21:1726–1731, 1998.

63. Anderson JH, Brunelle RL, Koivisto VA, et al: Reduction of postprandial hyperglycemia and frequency of hypoglycemia in IDDM patients on insulin-analog treatment. Diabetes 46:265–270, 1997.

64. Raskin P, Guthrie RA, Leiter L, et al: Use of insulin aspart, a fast-acting insulin analog, as the mealtime insulin in the management of patients with type 1 diabetes. Diabetes Care 23:583–588, 2000.

65. Bolli GB, Owens DR: Insulin glargine. Lancet 356:443–444, 2000.

66. Buse J: Insulin glargine (HOE901). Diabetes Care 23:576–578, 2000.

67. Heinemann L, Linkeschova R, Rave K, et al: Time-action profile of the long-acting insulin analog insulin glargine (HOE901) in comparison with those of NPH insulin and placebo. Diabetes Care 23:644–649, 2000.

68. Owens DR, Coates PA, Luzio SD, et al: Pharmacokinetics of ^{125}I-labelled insulin glargine (HOE901) in healthy men: Comparison with NPH insulin and the influence of different subcutaneous injection sites. Diabetes Care 23:813–819, 2000.

69. Lepore M, Pampanelli S, Fanelli C, et al: Pharmacokinetics and pharmacodynamics of subcutaneous injection of long-acting insulin analog glargine, NPH insulin, and ultralente human insulin and continuous subcutaneous infusion of insulin lispro. Diabetes 49:2142–2148, 2000.

70. Ratner RE, Hirsch IB, Neifing JL, et al: Less hypoglycemia with insulin glargine in intensive therapy for type 1 diabetes. Diabetes Care 23:639–643, 2000.

71. Raskin P, Klaff L, Berenstal R, et al: A 16-week comparison of the novel insulin analog insulin glargine (HOE 901) and NPH human insulin used with lispro in patients with type 1 diabetes. Diabetes Care 23:1666–1671, 2000.

72. Rosenstock J, Park G, Zimmerman J for the US Insulin Glargine (HOE 901) Type 1 Diabetes Investigator Group: Basal insulin glargine (HOE 901) versus NPH insulin in patients with type 1 diabetes on multiple daily insulin regimens. Diabetes Care 23:1137–1142, 2000.

73. Pieber TR, Eugene-Jolchine I, Derobert E: Efficacy and safety of HOE 901 versus NPH insulin in patients with type 1 diabetes. Diabetes Care 23:157–162, 2000.

74. Markussen J, Havelund S, Kurtzhals P, et al: Soluble, fatty acid acylated insulins bind to albumin and shown protracted action in pigs. Diabetologia 39:281–288, 1996.

75. Heinemann L, Sinha K, Weyer C, et al: Time-action profile of the soluble, fatty acid acylated, long-acting insulin analogue NN304. Diabet Med 16:332–338, 1999.

76. Hermansen K, Madsbad S, Perrild H, et al: Comparison of the soluble basal insulin analog insulin detemir with NPH insulin. Diabetes Care 24:296–301, 2001.

77. Vague P, Selam JL, Skeie S, et al: Insulin detemir is associated with more predictable glycemic control and reduced risk of hypoglycemia than NPH insulin in patients with type 1 diabetes on a basal-bolus regimen with premeal insulin aspart. Diabetes Care 26:590–596, 2003.

78. Danne T, Lupke K, Walte K, et al: Insulin detemir is characterized by a consistent pharmacokinetic profile across age-groups in children, adolescents, and adults with type 1 diabetes. Diabetes Care 26:3087–3092, 2003.

79. Cheng AY, Zinman B: Insulin for treating type 1 and type 2 diabetes In Gerstein HC, Haynes RB (eds): Evidence-Based Diabetes Care. Hamilton, Ontario. BC Decker, 2001, pp 323–343.

80. Hamann A, Matthaei S, Rosak C, Silvestre L: HOE901/4007 Study Group: A randomized clinical trial comparing breakfast, dinner or bedtime administration of insulin glargine in patients with type 1 diabetes. Diabetes Care 26(6):1738–1744, 2003.

81. Rossetti P, Pampanelli S, Fanelli C, et al: Intensive replacement of basal insulin in patients with type 1 diabetes given rapid-acting insulin analog at mealtime: A 3-month comparison between administration of NPH insulin four times daily and glargine insulin at dinner or bedtime. Diabetes Care 26(5):1490–1496, 2003.

82. Pickup J, Keen H: Continuous subcutaneous insulin infusion at 25 years: Evidence base for the expanding use of insulin pump therapy in type 1 diabetes. Diabetes Care 25:593–598, 2002.

83. Zinman B, Tildesley H, Chiasson JL, et al: Insulin lispro in CSII: Results of a double-blind crossover study. Diabetes 46:440–443, 1997.

84. Melki V, Renard E, Lassmann-Vague V, et al: Improvement of HbA1c and blood glucose stability in IDDM patients treated with lispro insulin analog in external pumps. Diabetes Care 21:977–982, 1998.

85. Renner R, Pfutzner A, Trautmann M, et al: Use of insulin lispro in continuous subcutaneous insulin infusion treatment: results of a multicenter trial: German Humalog-CSII Study Group. Diabetes Care 22:784–788, 1999.

86. Lenhard MJ: Continuous subcutaneous insulin infusion: A comprehensive review of insulin pump therapy. Arch Intern Med 161(19):2293–2300, 2001.

87. Zinman B: Insulin pump therapy and rapid acting insulin: What have we learned? Int J Clin Pract Suppl 123:47–50, 2001.

88. Pickup J, Mattock M, Kerry S: Glycaemic control with continuous subcutaneous insulin infusion compared with intensive insulin injections in patients with type 1 diabetes: Meta-analysis of randomized controlled trials. Br Med J 324:1–6, 2002.

89. Tsui E, Barnie A, Ross S, et al: Intensive insulin therapy with insulin lispro: A randomized trial of continuous subcutaneous insulin infusion versus multiple daily insulin injection. Diabetes Care 24:1722–1727, 2001.

90. DeVries JH, Snoek FS, Kostense PJ, et al: A randomized trial of continuous subcutaneous insulin infusion and intensive injection therapy in type 1 diabetes for patients with long-standing poor glycemic control. Diabetes Care 25:2074–2080, 2002.

91. Hanaire-Broutin H, Melki V, Bessieres-Lacombe S, Tauber JP: Comparison of continuous subcutaneous insulin infusion and multiple daily injection regimens using insulin lispro in type 1 diabetic patients on intensified treatment: A randomized study. Diabetes Care 23:1232–1235, 2000.

92. Rabasa-Lhoret R, Bourque J, Ducros F, Chiasson JL: Guidelines for premeal insulin dose reduction for postprandial exercise of different intensities and durations in type 1 diabetic subjects treated intensively with a basal-bolus insulin regimen (ultralente-lispro). Diabetes Care 24(4):625–630, 2001.

93. Lteif AN, Schwenk WF: Accuracy of pen injectors versus insulin syringes in children with type 1 diabetes. Diabetes Care 22:137–140, 1999.

94. Graff MR, McClanahan MA: Assessment by patients with diabetes mellitus of two insulin pen delivery systems versus a vial and syringe. Clin Ther 20:486–496, 1998.

95. Sindelka G, Heinemann L, Berger M, et al: Effect of insulin concentration, subcutaneous fat thickness and skin temperature on subcutaneous insulin absorption in healthy subjects. Diabetologia 37:377, 1994.

96. Koivisto VA, Felig P: Alterations in insulin absorption and in blood glucose control associated with varying insulin injection sites in diabetic patients. Ann Intern Med 92:59, 1980.

97. Koivisto VA, Felig P: Effects of leg exercise on insulin absorption in diabetic patients. N Engl J Med 298:79–83, 1978.

98. Koivisto VA: Sauna-induced acceleration in insulin absorption from subcutaneous injection site. Br Med J 280:1411, 1980.

99. Linde B: Dissociation of insulin absorption and blood flow during massage of a subcutaneous injection site. Diabetes Care 9:570, 1986.

100. Owens DR, Zinman B, Bolli G: Alternative routes of insulin delivery. Diabet Med 20:886–898, 2003.

101. Skyler JS: Efficacy and safety of inhaled insulin (Exubera) comparison to subcutaneous insulin therapy in an intensive insulin regimen in patients with type 1 diabetes: Results of a 6-month, randomised comparative trial. Diabetes 51(Suppl 2):A134, 2002.

102. Quattrin T: Efficacy and safety of inhaled insulin (Exubera) compared to conventional sc insulin therapy in patients with type 1 diabetes: Results of a 6 months randomised comparative trial. Diabetologia 42:80, 2002.

103. Royle P, Waugh N, McAuley L, et al: Inhaled insulin in diabetes mellitus. Cochrane Database Syst Rev 3:CD003890, 2003.

104. Nelson JA, Stephen R, Landau ST, et al: Intraperitoneal insulin administration produces a positive portal-systemic blood insulin gradient in unanesthetized, unrestrained swine. Metabolism 31:969–972, 1982.

105. Renard E: Implantable closed-loop glucose-sensing and insulin delivery: The future for insulin pump therapy. Curr Opin Pharmacol 2:708–716, 2002.

106. Gin H, Renard E, Melki V, et al: Combined improvements in implantable pump technology and insulin stability allow safe and effective long term intraperitoneal insulin delivery in type 1 diabetic patients: The EVADIAC experience. Diabetes Metab 29(6):602–607, 2003.

107. Selam JL: External and implantable insulin pumps: Current place in the treatment of diabetes. Exp Clin Endocrinol Diabetes 109(Suppl 2):S333–S340, 2001.

108. Carino GP, Mathiowitz E: Oral insulin delivery. Adv Drug Deliv Rev 35:249–257, 1999.

109. Saudek CD: Novel forms of insulin delivery. Endocrinol Metab Clin North Am 26:599–610, 1997.

110. The Diabetes Control and Complications Trial Research Group: Adverse events and their association with treatment regimens in the Diabetes Control and Complications Trial. Diabetes Care 18:141–1427, 1995.

111. Cryer PE: Managing diabetes: Lessons from type 1 diabetes mellitus. Diabet Med 15(Suppl 4):S8–S12, 1998.

112. Bolli GB, Pampanelli S, Porcellati F, Fanelli CG: Recovery and prevention of hypoglycemia unawareness in type 1 diabetes mellitus. Diabetes Nutr Metab 15(6):402–409, 2002.

113. The Diabetes Control and Complications Trial Research Group: Influence of intensive diabetes treatment on body weight and composition of adults with type 1 diabetes in the Diabetes Control and Complications Trial. Diabetes Care 24(10):1711–1721, 2001.

114. DeWitt DE, Hirsch IB: Outpatient insulin therapy in type 1 and type 2 diabetes mellitus. JAMA 289:2254–2264, 2003.

115. Chantelau E, Kohmer EM: Why some cases of retinopathy worsen when diabetic control improves. Br Med J 315:1105–1106, 1997.

116. Reeves W, Allen B, Tatersall R: Insulin-induced lipoatrophy: Evidence for an immune pathogenesis. Br Med J 280:1500, 1980.

117. American Diabetes Association: Nutrition principles and recommendations in diabetes. Diabetes Care 27(Suppl 1):S36–S46, 2004.

118. Nuttal FQ: Carbohydrate and dietary management of clients with insulin-requiring diabetes. Diabetes Care 16:1039–1042, 1993.

119. Gillespie SJ, Kulkarni KD, Daly AE: Using carbohydrate counting in diabetes clinical practice. J Am Diet Assoc 98:897–905, 1998.

120. Joslin EP: The diabetic diet. J Am Diet Assoc 3:89–92, 1927.

121. Delahanty LM, Halford BN: The role of diet behaviours in achieving improved glycemic control in intensively treated patients in the Diabetic Control and Complications Trial. Diabetes Care 16:1453–1458, 1993.

122. Turner BC, Jenkins E, Kerr D, et al: The effect of evening alcohol consumption on next-morning glucose control in type 1 diabetes. Diabetes Care 24:1888–1893, 2001.

123. Atkinson MA, Eisenbarth GS: Type 1 diabetes: New perspectives on disease pathogenesis and treatment. Lancet 358:221–229, 2001.

124. Thivolet C: New therapeutic approaches to type 1 diabetes: From prevention to cellular or gene therapies. Clin Endocrinol 55:565–574, 2001.

125. Petrovsky N, Silva D, Schatz DA: Prospects for the prevention and reversal of type 1 diabetes mellitus. Drugs 62(18):2617–2635, 2002.

126. Assan R, Feutren G, Debray-Sachs M, et al: Metabolic and immunological effects of cyclosporin in recently-diagnosed type 1 diabetes mellitus. Lancet 1:67–71, 1985.

127. Silverstein J, Maclean N, Riley W, et al: Immunosuppression with azathioprine and prednisone in recent-onset insulin-dependent diabetes mellitus. N Engl J Med 319:599, 1988.

128. Carel JC, Boitard C, Eisenbarth G, et al: Cyclosporine delays but does not prevent clinical onset in glucose intolerant pre-type 1 diabetic children. J Autoimmun 9:739–745, 1996.

129. Cook JJ, Hudson I, Harrison LC, et al: A double-blind controlled trial of azathioprine in children with newly-diagnosed type 1 diabetes. Diabetes 38:779, 1989.

130. Diabetes Prevention Trial/Type 1 Diabetes Study Group: Effects of insulin in relatives of patients with type 1 diabetes mellitus. N Engl J Med 346(22):1685–1691, 2002.

131. Yamada K, Nonaka K, Hanafusa T, et al: Preventive and therapeutic effects of large-dose nicotinamide injections on diabetes associated with insulitis: An observation in non-obese diabetic (NOD) mice. Diabetes 31:749, 1982.

132. Ledoux SP, Hall CR, Forbes PM, et al: Mechanisms of nicotinamide and thymidine protection from alloxan and streptozotocin toxicity. Diabetes 37:1015, 1988.

133. Rohrscheib M, Robinson R, Eaton RP: Non-invasive glucose sensors and improved informatics: The future of diabetes management. Diabetes Obes Metab 5:280–284, 2003.

134. Thule PM, Liu JM: Regulated hepatic insulin gene therapy of STZ-diabetic rats. Gene Therapy 7:1744–1752, 2000.

135. Ferber S, Halkin A, Cohen H, et al: Pancreatic and duodenal homeobox gene 1 induces expression of insulin genes I liver and ameliorates streptozotocin-induced hyperglycemia. Nat Med 6:568–572, 2000.

Ketoacidosis and Hyperosmolar Coma

Daniel W. Foster and Victoria Esser

Patients with diabetes of any variety are vulnerable to acute complications that are fatal if not treated. Decompensation can occur secondary to intercurrent stress or illness or appear spontaneously in the absence of obvious precipitating events. Because diabetes is a common illness in the United States and western Europe,[1,2] the syndromes of diabetic coma make up a significant percentage of the nonsurgical emergencies seen in any general hospital. If the pathophysiologic principles underlying the illness are understood and corrective treatment is judiciously applied, most patients should recover. To that end, we discuss the pathophysiology and the treatment of diabetic ketoacidosis and hyperosmolar coma.

KETOACIDOSIS

Ketoacidosis is a complication of autoimmune (type 1) diabetes mellitus. It occurs after most of the insulin-producing β cells have been destroyed. Ketoacidosis is seen occasionally in a subset of patients with nonautoimmune (type 2) diabetes.

PATHOPHYSIOLOGY

Multiple metabolic derangements accompany diabetic ketoacidosis. In general, the body is shifted into a major catabolic state with breakdown of glycogen stores, hydrolysis of triglycerides in adipose tissue, and mobilization of amino acids from muscle.[3] The fuels newly released from peripheral tissues become the substrates used by the liver for the accelerated production of glucose and ketone bodies—the hallmarks of uncontrolled diabetes.[4] Hyperglycemia-driven osmotic diuresis and rising concentrations of acetoacetate and β-hydroxybutyrate, in turn, cause loss of body fluids, abnormalities in plasma electrolytes, and metabolic acidosis. The mechanisms underlying the development of ketoacidosis are basically similar to those occurring in nondiabetic subjects during a fast, with one exception: No insulin is available to prevent progression to full-blown acidosis. The similarities and differences can be outlined as follows. In the postprandial state after absorption of food, plasma glucose concentrations gradually fall over a period of several hours. As a result, insulin release from the pancreas is diminished, and a simultaneous rise in glucagon secretion takes place.[3,5–7] These changes occur smoothly in an integrated fashion, thereby maintaining plasma glucose levels in the nonhypoglycemic range. Decreased insulin secretion simultaneously results in mobilization of free fatty acids from adipocytes, with the body shifted toward a lipid economy so that glucose is "spared" for use by the brain,[3,6,8,9] which cannot oxidize fatty acids except in trace quantities.[10] A portion of the mobilized fatty acids are taken up by the liver for conversion to acetoacetic and β-hydroxybutyric acids. These "ketone bodies," which are efficiently oxidized by nonhepatic tissues, including the brain, provide backup substrate for the central nervous system should hepatic glucose production be inadequate for any reason.[11] Normally, fasting ends at breakfast, and no significant ketosis develops. When a fast is extended, ketone concentrations increase to the range of 2 to 4 millimolar (mM), but not much higher because both fatty acids and ketones have the ability to stimulate insulin release[12–14] (Fig. 61-1). This feedback loop, which elicits a modest elevation in insulin, prevents a further increase in the rate of lipolysis, thereby fixing ketogenesis in a safe range through substrate limitation. Ketones may have a minor direct inhibitory effect on lipolysis, but the insulin-stimulatory event is doubtless dominant.

In diabetes, the omission of insulin or a stress-induced counterregulatory hormone release that overrides the effect of the usual dose of insulin initiates a process qualitatively similar to fasting, with the exception that the insulin segment of the feedback loop is missing.[3,7,13] As a consequence, concentrations of free fatty acids and ketone bodies rise in an uncontrolled fashion and produce acidosis, coma, and death.

HORMONAL INITIATION OF KETOACIDOSIS

For many years, the hormonal abnormality initiating the hyperglycemia and metabolic acidosis that accompany diabetic ketoacidosis was thought to be insulin deficiency alone. It now seems clear that this view is incorrect and that insulin deficiency coupled with glucagon excess, that is, a rise in the molar ratio of glucagon to insulin, is the operative mechanism. The evidence in support of this concept has been extensively reviewed.[6,15,16] The most important study was that of Gerich and colleagues, who showed that withdrawal of insulin from patients with insulin-dependent diabetes was accompanied by rapid increases in plasma glucagon, glucose, and ketone levels that were markedly obtunded when glucagon release was blocked by somatostatin.[17]

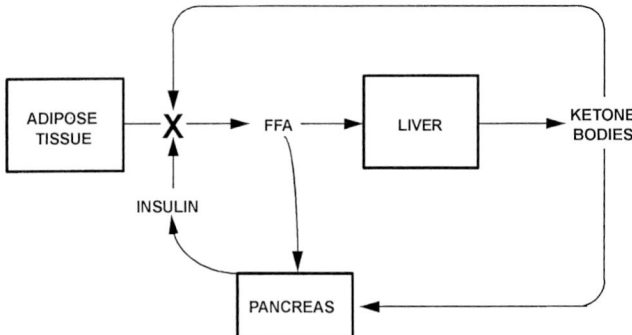

Figure 61-1 Feedback control of ketosis during an extended fast. Ketogenesis is activated by a rise in the molar ratio of glucagon to insulin, which induces lipolysis in adipose tissue and fatty acid oxidation in the liver. As the concentrations of circulating fatty acids and ketones rise, the β cell is stimulated to release insulin, with lipolytic rates fixed at modest levels and further rise in glucagon limited. These adaptations allow modest ketosis without the danger of ketoacidosis. In insulin-dependent diabetic subjects, the insulin loop is missing.

The role of glucagon in inducing hepatic glucose overproduction in uncontrolled diabetes parallels its actions during an overnight fast, in which about 75% of glucose output can be shown to be glucagon mediated.[18] Further evidence that glucagon is critical to the initiation of hyperglycemia comes from studies in which simultaneous insulin and glucagon deficiency was produced by infusion of somatostatin[19] or total pancreatectomy.[20] If insulin deficiency alone were the cause of severe hyperglycemia, one would expect significant overproduction of glucose under both experimental circumstances. In neither dogs nor humans did such overproduction occur. Similarly, patients with somatostatinoma, who have suppression of both glucagon and insulin, exhibit only mild hyperglycemia, an additional finding compatible with the interpretation that major increases in plasma glucose levels occur only in the presence of a relative or absolute excess of glucagon.[21]

Glucagon also appears to play a central role in initiating ketogenesis. As noted previously, blockade of glucagon release markedly slows the appearance of ketosis in diabetic patients withdrawn from insulin.[17] Conversely, administration of glucagon to diabetic humans enhances the conversion of fatty acids to ketone bodies.[22–24] Along the same lines, the presence of a glucagonoma resulted in plasma ketone levels four times normal despite the fact that free fatty acid concentrations were not elevated.[25] Glucagonoma may also cause ketoacidosis in the face of intact β cells.[26] Direct demonstration of the powerful ketogenic effect of glucagon in the liver came from studies in which rats were administered glucagon in vivo (in both physiologic and pathophysiologic amounts).[27] The animals did not become either hyperglycemic or ketotic because a compensatory rise in insulin (secondary to glucagon infusion) allowed disposal of the glucose produced by the liver and prevented a rise in free fatty acids. When the livers from these animals were removed and perfused with fatty acids, they exhibited the shift to activated fatty acid oxidation and ketogenesis expected in fasting and uncontrolled diabetes. Thus, a ketogenic liver had been produced in nonketotic animals despite the presence of concentrations of insulin in plasma that were higher than normal. When free fatty acid concentrations were elevated artificially in the glucagon-treated animals, a brisk rise in ketone levels was observed, thus confirming that the liver had been activated in vivo, with ketosis prevented only by the lack of substrate.[27] Glucagon has also been shown to stimulate ketone body production directly in homogenates of liver, liver slices, hepatocytes, and isolated perfused liver.[28]

Although there is good evidence that the molar ratio of glucagon to insulin is the primary control unit for carbohydrate and lipid metabolism, this finding does not imply that other hormones do not play a role. Most systems in the body have redundant regulatory mechanisms, and catecholamines, cortisol, growth hormone, and thyroid hormones can all increase rates of hepatic ketogenesis, albeit less efficiently.[29,30] Concentrations of counterregulatory hormones are elevated on admission in patients with ketoacidosis,[31,32] either as the consequence of an initiating illness, such as infection, or in response to the stress of ketoacidosis itself. However, when ketoacidosis is induced by withdrawing insulin from well-controlled subjects with insulin-dependent diabetes, glucagon concentrations rise before any increase in other counterregulatory hormones, which suggests that the α-cell hormone is pivotal in causing metabolic decompensation.[33,34]

Functionally, the two hormones are metabolic antagonists in directing fuel production and utilization.[6] They act independently through distinct receptors and focus on different target tissues. The primary direct effects of insulin are probably on muscle and fat (to enhance glucose transport into cells and inhibit lipolysis), whereas the primary direct effects of glucagon are exerted on the liver (to increase glycogenolysis, gluconeogenesis, and ketogenesis). It is attractive to consider that in the primary domain of each hormone the other acts predominantly as an antagonist. Good evidence indicates that insulin functions to a large extent as an antiglucagon in the liver, with direct effects being minimal in the absence of glucagon-induced metabolic changes.[24,35,36] The insulin signaling pathway is very complicated, but it is initiated by phosphorylation of intracellular substrates after binding to its receptor.[37] Most of the initial effects of glucagon are consequent to the generation of cyclic adenosine monophosphate (cAMP).[38] In rodents, glucagon can act independently of cAMP, possibly through the protein kinase C signaling system.[39] It is probable that a single glucagon receptor activates both pathways,[40,41] although isoforms could exist, as appears to be the case for the insulin receptor.[42] Counteraction of glucagon by insulin may be the result of direct inhibition of the cAMP-dependent protein kinase.[43]

HYPERGLYCEMIA

The hyperglycemia of uncontrolled diabetes is caused by two alterations in glucose metabolism: increased hepatic glucose production and diminished utilization of the hexose in muscle and adipose tissue. When insulin is withdrawn from well-controlled subjects with insulin-requiring diabetes, hepatic glucose output doubles within 2 hours.[34] Simultaneously, clearance of glucose from plasma decreases consequent to falling insulin concentrations. Doubtless, insulin resistance contributes to the decreased uptake and utilization of glucose.[44] A significant part of the resistant state may be caused by the accumulation of fat within insulin target tissues. Increased fatty acid oxidation then results in impairment of insulin signaling to the glucose transport machinery and suppression of glucose metabolism.[14,44–46] A third factor, present to a variable extent, is volume depletion secondary to the hyperglycemia-induced osmotic diuresis. If this complication becomes severe enough to cause a fall in urine output, the escape pathway for glucose is removed and hyperglycemia worsens.[47] This response accounts for the fact that administration of fluids alone can lower the plasma glucose concentration in ketoacidosis.[32]

The mechanisms by which a rise in the molar glucagon: insulin ratio alters hepatic glucose metabolism have been the subject of much study. Cyclic-AMP-dependent activation of glycogenolysis represents one component. Another involves acceleration of the gluconeogenic pathway. In the previous edition focus was placed on the 6-phosphofructo-l-kinase (phosphofructokinase)-fructose-1,6-bisphosphatase (FBPase) branch point, seemingly the preeminent control site for glycolysis/gluconeogenesis in the liver (Fig. 61-2). The concept was that in uncontrolled diabetes (or in conditions of glucose need such as fasting or exercise) increased hepatic glucose production is mediated by a fall in phosphofructokinase (PFK) activity, which inhibits glycolysis (flux from glucose-6-phosphate → pyruvate), and a rise in fructose-1,6-bisphosphatase activity, which removes a block to gluconeogenesis (flux over the sequence pyruvate → oxaloacetate → phosphoenolpyruvate → glucose-6-phosphate → glucose). The latter pathway is fed primarily by amino acids transported from muscle, lactate, and, to a small extent, from glycerol.[3] Substrate traffic over the switch point was thought to be mediated primarily by fructose-2,6-bisphosphate (F-2,6-P2), a regulatory intermediate that stimulates PFK and inhibits FDPase.[48–50] In vitro F-2,6-P2 activates PFK allosterically and inhibits FDPase competitively. F-2,6-P2 levels are controlled by an interesting bifunctional enzyme, 6-phosphofructo-2-kinase/fructose-2,6-bisphosphatase (PFK-2/FBPase-2). Glucagon excess (relative to insulin), acting through the generation of cAMP, causes a fall in F-2,6-P2 concentrations as a result of phosphorylation of PFK-2/FBPase-2 converting it from a kinase to a phosphatase with the result that synthesis of F-2,6-P2 slows or ceases and its hydrolysis commences.

There is no doubt that F-2,6-P2 is the only significant activator of PFK and is thus responsible for stimulation of glycolysis in liver in the fed state (low glucagon:insulin ratio). However, it appears that F-2,6-P2 is not present in sufficient concentrations to inhibit FBPase after refeeding in vivo.[51,52]

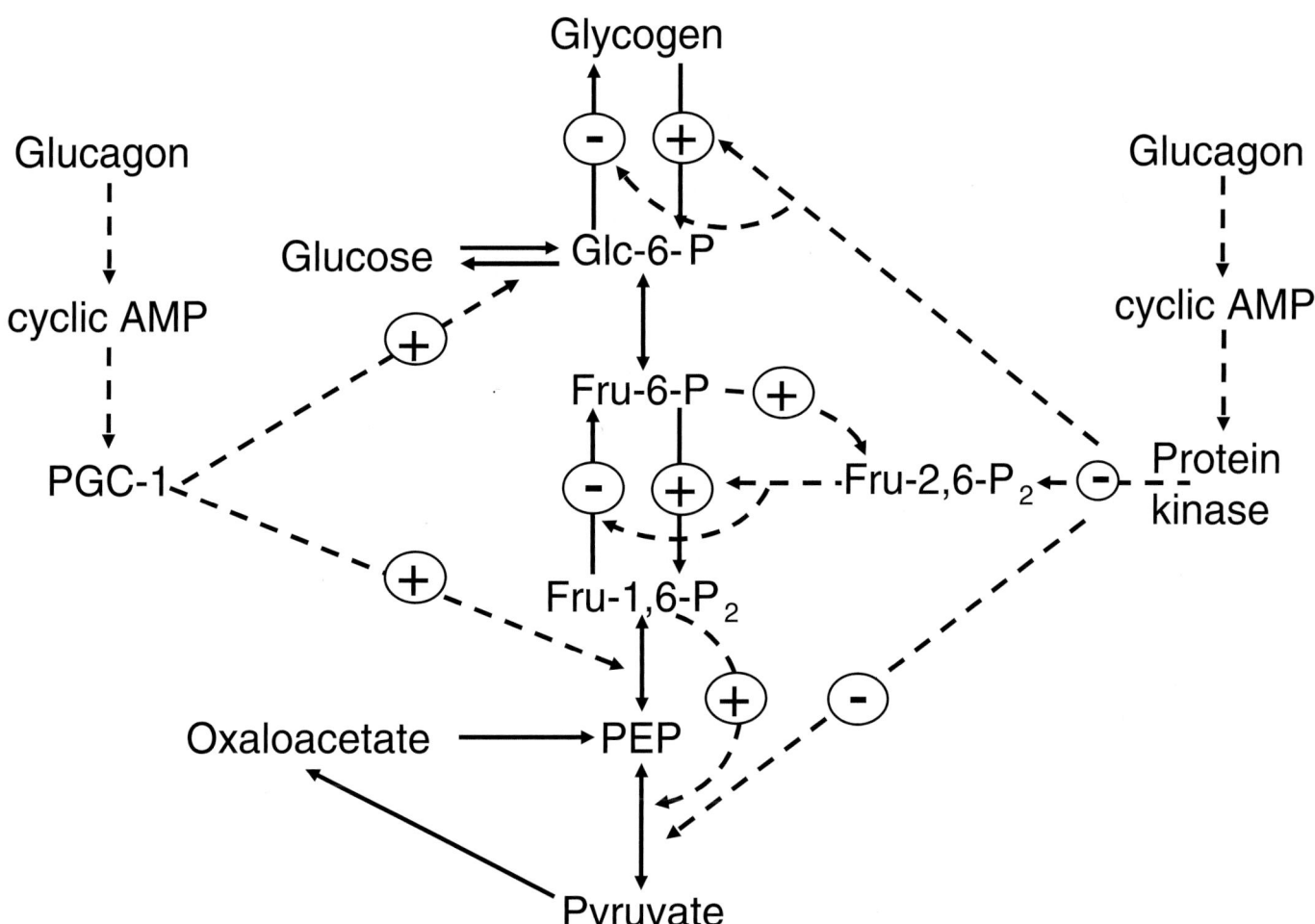

Figure 61-2 Regulation of glycolysis and gluconeogenesis by glucagon. *Solid lines* represent metabolic pathways. Within these pathways, *arrows* that point down represent the glycolytic sequence, and *arrows* that point up, gluconeogenesis. *Two-headed arrows* indicate reversible reactions, and *single-headed arrows*, nonreversible reactions (i.e., the enzyme that catalyzes a reaction in glycolysis is distinct from the enzyme that reverses the process in gluconeogenesis). *Dash lines* indicate regulatory activities. *Minus signs* stand for inactivation (inhibition) and *plus signs* for activation (stimulation). For simplicity, a number of reactions are omitted, and only the key regulatory sites are shown. Glucagon lowers levels of fructose 2,6-bisphosphate (Fru-2,6-P₂), which is high in the anabolic phase. It thereby inactivates phosphofructokinase, which blocks the conversion of fructose 6-phosphate (Fru-6-P) to fructose 1,6-bisphosphate (Fru-1,6-P₂) and inhibits glycolysis. Fru-2,6-P₂ inhibits fructose-1, 6-bisphosphatase in vitro and its fall would be expected to activate the phosphatase, allowing efficient conversion of Fru-1,6-P₂ to Fru-6-P thereby enhancing gluconeogenesis. In vivo the concentrations of Fru-2,6-P appear to be too low to play a major regulatory role on fructose-1, 6-bisphosphatase. The primary activator of gluconeogenesis appears to be PPAR-γ coactivator-1α (PCG-1). (See text.) Glucagon also stimulates glycogen breakdown and inhibits glycogen synthesis. Glucagon induces a secondary block in glycolysis at the step that is regulated by pyruvate kinase. Glc-6-P, glucose 6-phosphate; PEP, phosphoenolpyruvate. (Modified from Foster DW, McGarry JD: The metabolic derangements and treatment of diabetic ketoacidosis. N Engl J Med 309:159–169, 1983. Originally adapted from Hers HG, Van Schaftingen E: Fructose 2, 6-bisphosphate 2 years after its discovery. Biochem J 206:1–12, 1982.)

When fasted rats were fed glucose, gluconeogenesis measured by nuclear magnetic resonance (NMR) spectroscopy showed no inhibition despite significant increases in F-2,6-P2.[52] It may well be that diminished F-2,6-P2 directly accounts for the inhibited glycolysis of fasting or diabetes, but it may not be primarily or significantly responsible for activating gluconeogenesis. Rather, increases in the primary gluconeogenic enzymes may account for increased gluconeogenic flux. A major factor appears to be increased synthesis of peroxisome proliferator-activated receptor γ-co-activator-1α (PGC-1α), which stimulates gluconeogenesis by activating synthesis of phosphoenolpyruvate carboxykinase and glucose-6-phosphatase.[53,54] Glucagon-induced production of cAMP, acting through the cAMP response element binding protein (CREB) gene is necessary for PGC-1α synthesis and activation.[55] PGC-1 in turn coactivates the hepatic glucocorticoid receptor and the transcription factor hepatic nuclear factor 4α both of which are necessary for full enhancement of gluconeogenesis (see Fig 61-2). PGC-1α is involved in many other pathways including mitochondrial biogenesis and fatty acid oxidation as will be discussed below.[54] The PGC-1α isoform induces both gluconeogenesis and fatty acid oxidation in the liver while PGC-1β induces oxidation only.[56]

Additional enzymes are altered under catabolic conditions such as fasting and uncontrolled diabetes. For example, pyruvate carboxylase, a distinctive third gluconeogenic enzyme, is also elevated.[49,57,58] Final rates of gluconeogenesis are influenced not only by changes in the key enzymatic activities induced directly by alterations in the glucagon:insulin ratio but also by the modulating effects of other hormones,[49,58,59] availability of substrate,[60] and rates of fatty acid oxidation.[46] In short, it is best to consider the changes leading to glucose overproduction in the liver as reflecting a coordinated series of alterations downstream from the hormonal initiators.

KETOGENESIS

Metabolic acidosis caused by the overproduction of acetoacetic and β-hydroxybutyric acids requires changes in the metabolism of adipose tissue and the liver[61,62] (Fig. 61-3). Long-chain fatty acids derived from triglyceride stores in the adipocyte are the principal substrate for ketone production in the liver. Only under circumstances in which fatty acid oxidation in the hepatocyte is blocked do amino acids such as leucine function efficiently as precursors for acetoacetate synthesis.[63] Long-chain fatty acids are mobilized from fat stores under the combined influence of insulin deficiency/counterregulatory hormone excess acting on the intracellular hormone-sensitive lipase.[3,64] It is likely that the major activator is cAMP, a rise in its concentration leading to phosphorylation and enhanced activity of the enzyme. Negative modulation is mediated by a membrane phosphoprotein called perilipin A in addition to insulin's suppressive effect.[64] Ordinarily, ketone production is dependent on delivery of fatty acids to the liver. However, if the liver is fatty, which is not uncommon in cases of poorly controlled diabetes, hepatic triglyceride may serve as the source of fatty acids. This adaptation accounts for differences in the ease of reversibility of ketosis. Ingestion of a small amount of carbohydrate after a fast calls forth endogenous insulin release and immediately reverses fasting ketosis by inhibiting lipolysis in the adipocyte. In diabetic ketoacidosis, because the liver contains significant amounts of triglyceride, ketogenesis continues for hours after free fatty acid levels in plasma have returned to normal. How intracellular triglyceride lipase activity in the liver is controlled is not well understood. It is possible that a hormone-sensitive lipase activated by glucagon is operative.[23]

Although increased transport of fatty acids to the liver is normally required for significant ketogenesis to supervene, increased fatty acids alone are not enough. In the normal, nonfasted state, fatty acids taken up into the hepatocyte are reesterified to triglyceride and transported back out into plasma as very low-density lipoprotein.[61] Rates of fatty acid oxidation are low. However, when the molar ratio of glucagon to insulin rises, fatty acid oxidation is disinhibited and incoming fatty acids can be converted to acetoacetate and β-hydroxybutyrate. The key regulatory site for fatty acid oxidation is the initial step in the process catalyzed by the

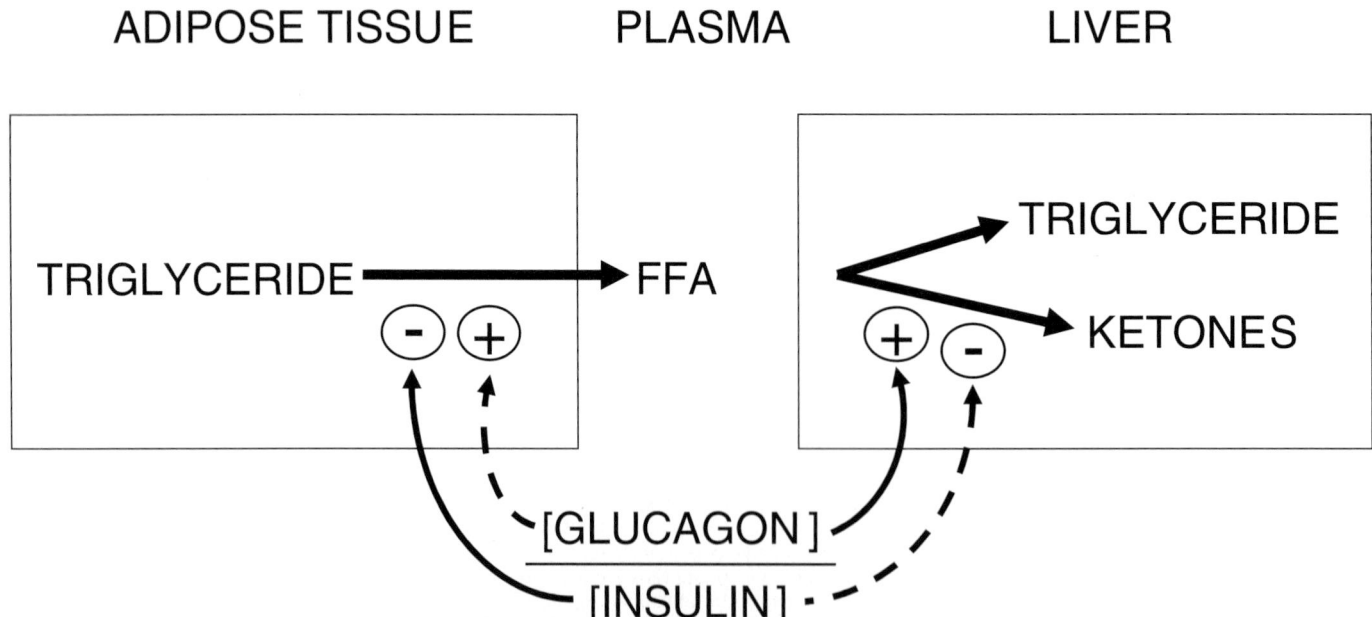

Figure 61-3 Two-organ system for ketogenesis. Maximal production of ketone bodies requires transport of the substrate, long-chain fatty acids, from adipose tissue to the liver. In addition, the fatty acid oxidative pathway has to be activated in the hepatocyte. The *solid lines* indicate primary and the *dash lines* indicate secondary (counterregulatory) effects; that is, insulin's primary action is to inhibit lipolysis and its secondary effect is to block glucagon's action in the liver. Conversely, glucagon's primary effect is activation of fatty acid oxidation, with only a secondary effect on lipolysis. See the text for details.

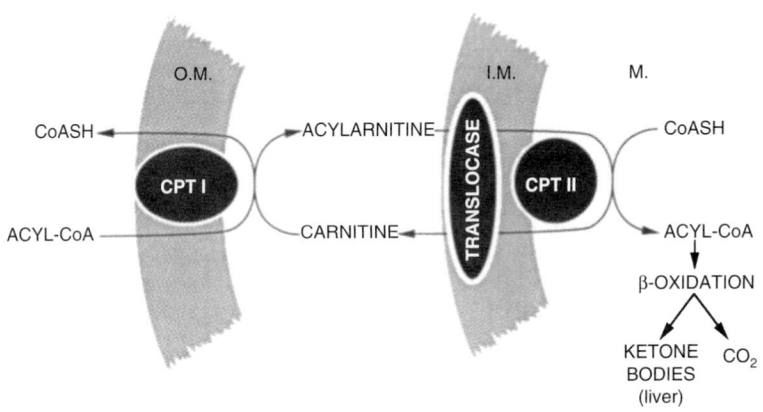

Figure 61-4 The fatty acid oxidizing system in the liver. Long-chain fatty acids are activated to coenzyme A (CoA) derivatives on arrival in the liver (acyl-CoA). Acyl-CoA cannot traverse the mitochondrial inner membrane. Entry is accomplished by transesterification to carnitine by carnitine palmitoyltransferase I (CPT I) located in the outer membrane (O.M.). Transport across the inner membrane (I.M.) is accomplished by the translocase carnitine:acylcarnitine translocase. Reversal of the transesterification then occurs on the matrix side by carnitine palmitoyltransferase II (CPT II). The capacity for fatty acid oxidation is fixed and large, so normally the rate-limiting step is CPT I. Tricarboxylic acid cycle activity is low in the liver (acetyl-CoA → CO_2), so the bulk of oxidized fatty acid goes to ketone bodies.

enzyme carnitine palmitoyltransferase I (CPT I)[61,65] (Fig. 61-4). Its function is to effect conversion of the coenzyme A (CoA) esters of long-chain fatty acids to acylcarnitines, which, unlike fatty acyl CoAs, can be transported across the inner mitochondrial membrane by carnitine:acylcarnitine translocase (CACT).[66–68] Once through the membrane, the reaction is reversed by CPT II, and the newly re-formed fatty acyl CoA enters the fatty acid oxidative pathway. In the liver, the major product is ketone bodies, and terminal oxidation to carbon dioxide and water is limited. In tissues such as the muscle and the heart, complete oxidation of fatty acids to carbon dioxide and water results in the generation of adenosine triphosphate in the electron transport chain. CPT1 exists in three isoforms. CPT1A is the liver form, CPT1B is the muscle form, and CPT1C is the brain form.

In the fed state and with well-controlled diabetes, CPT I is inhibited by malonyl CoA.[69] The total amount of enzyme present does not change markedly through wide swings of the regulatory cycle.[70] Regulation of fat oxidation by malonyl CoA makes physiologic sense because it is also the first committed intermediate in long-chain fatty acid synthesis. Thus, when malonyl CoA concentrations are high, the inhibitory interaction with CPT I precludes oxidation of the newly formed fatty acids and avoids an energetically wasteful futile cycle.[61,62] Malonyl CoA concentrations are maximal in the fed state, but they fall rapidly with fasting and uncontrolled diabetes. This change, coupled with desensitization of CPT I to the inhibitor, poises the liver for ketogenesis[71,72]; accelerated production of acetoacetate and β-hydroxybutyrate begins when long-chain fatty acids arrive in the liver at increased concentrations. Once CPT1 and the oxidative sequence is activated, rates of ketogenesis reflect substrate concentration; that is, the higher the concentration of fatty acids, the greater the ketone production until V_{max} is reached.

The mechanism by which malonyl CoA inhibits CPT I is still not completely understood. It is believed that malonyl CoA binds through the CoA moiety at the palmitoyl CoA site on the enzyme and that its carboxyl group forms an ionic interaction with an amino acid, probably histidine, at a separate site. When bound, the regulator impairs palmitoyl CoA binding directly and by alteration of membrane fluidity.[71] Molecular cloning of CPT I has definitively eliminated the possibility that malonyl CoA binds to a separate regulatory subunit.[73]

As mentioned earlier, the activation of fatty acid oxidation as well as gluconeogenesis is enhanced by peroxisome-proliferator γ-coactivator 1. Both α and β isoforms of PGC-1 can stimulate mitochondrial biogenesis including the genes of fatty acid oxidation. They also activate the oxidative pathway.[56,74–76] Glucagon-stimulated cAMP formation causes transcriptional induction of PGC-1α, which, in turn, activates carnitine palmitoyltransferase 1A expression in the liver, the

rate-limiting step in fatty acid oxidation.[76] Peroxisome-proliferator-activated receptors themselves play a prominent role in lipid metabolism. PPAR-α in liver and PPAR-δ in adipose tissue induce the genes of β-oxidation utilizing PGC-1α.[77] PPAR-γ induces lipogenesis and fat storage.[77]

Lipogenesis is also stimulated with carbohydrate feeding by carbohydrate-responsive element binding protein (ChRE), a transcription factor that activates lipogenic genes. It is regulated by xyulose-5-phosphate.[78–80] Finally, Insig-2a concentrations in the liver appear to influence fatty acid synthesis. Insig-1 and Insig-2 are proteins that bind and trap SREBP cleavage-activating protein (SCAP), thereby retaining sterol regulatory element binding proteins (SREBPs) in the endoplasmic reticulum and preventing their movement to and activation in the Golgi complex. The consequence is that the cell cannot synthesize cholesterol or fatty acids. Insig-2a increases with fasting and declines with refeeding. Insulin release consequent to feeding removes SCAP trapping allowing SREBP1-C, a regulator of fatty acid biosynthesis in the liver, to be disinhibited.[81]

All of the above factors account for the reciprocal relationship between fatty acid oxidation and fatty acid synthesis. Simultaneous activation of both pathways is never allowed.

The ways in which malonyl CoA levels fall to initiate ketogenesis are better defined. As noted earlier, an increase in the molar glucagon:insulin ratio (a relative or absolute glucagon excess) inhibits glycolysis at the phosphofructokinase step. This inhibition of glycolysis interrupts flux from glucose 6-phosphate down the glycolytic pathway to pyruvate, which, in turn, causes a fall in cytosolic citric acid.[72] A lowered citrate concentration has dual effects: decreased production of cytosolic acetyl CoA, the substrate for malonyl CoA formation (citrate is the source of cytosolic acetyl CoA via the citrate cleavage enzyme), and deactivation of acetyl CoA carboxylase, the enzyme that catalyzes the conversion of acetyl CoA to malonyl CoA (citrate activates the carboxylase allosterically).[82]

Acetyl CoA carboxylase (ACC) is sensitive to inhibition by phosphorylation, which in a setting of high glucagon/low insulin, appears to be mediated primarily by AMP-activated protein kinase.[83] Cyclic AMP-dependent kinase may also phosphorylate ACC.[82] It can be inhibited by long-chain acyl CoA.[84] Nitric oxide, which activates guanylyl cyclase with production of cyclic GMP, blocks both acetyl CoA carboxylase and fatty acid synthase.[85] Interestingly, cyclic GMP has the capacity to directly stimulate carnitine palmitoyltransferase IA. Consensus is that AMP-kinase is the primary inhibitor. AMP-kinase further lowers malonyl CoA levels by phosphorylating and activating malonyl CoA decarboxylase, so that inhibited production is coupled with enhanced destruction.[86,87] Acetyl CoA carboxylase exists in two isoforms, ACC1 (or α) is found primarily in the liver and adipose tissue while

ACC2 (β) is dominant in cardiac and skeletal muscle.[88] Regulation is thought to be the same in each.

The block in glycolysis is probably the dominant early mechanism. This conclusion is based on the observation that the citrate content in hepatocytes isolated from short-term fasted animals can be increased with the addition of lactate and pyruvate, which causes a rise in the malonyl CoA concentration and diminished ketone production.[72] Because three-carbon intermediates that enter the glycolytic pathway below the glucagon-induced block immediately reinitiate the sequence citrate → acetyl CoA → malonyl CoA, it can be concluded that early in a fast acetyl CoA carboxylase is not fully inactivated. When fasting is prolonged or diabetes is uncontrolled over an extended period, the AMP-kinase mechanism becomes operative. Ultimately, synthesis of acetyl CoA carboxylase also decreases and renders reversal of ketogenesis more difficult. A summary of the metabolic changes occurring in the liver in uncontrolled diabetes is shown in Figure 61-5. We find it fascinating that both hepatic overproduction of glucose and ketosis result from uncountered activity of glucagon initially acting at strategic sites in the glycogenolytic/glycolytic/gluconeogenic pathways. By controlling substrate flux at critical branch points, all the metabolic abnormalities that characterize the liver in uncontrolled diabetes are activated. Therefore, great interest has been shown in developing drugs to block activation of the glucagon receptor in the treatment of diabetes.[89,90]

There is little doubt that malonyl CoA–mediated control of CPT I is central to the regulation of fatty acid oxidation and ketogenesis in the liver, but another consequence of a rise in the glucagon:insulin molar ratio is an increased carnitine content.[91] The source of this carnitine has never been identified, but it is attractive to suppose that it moves to the liver from muscle via the plasma. Increased carnitine would favor transesterification of fatty acyl CoAs by mass action once CPT I is activated (see Fig. 61-3).

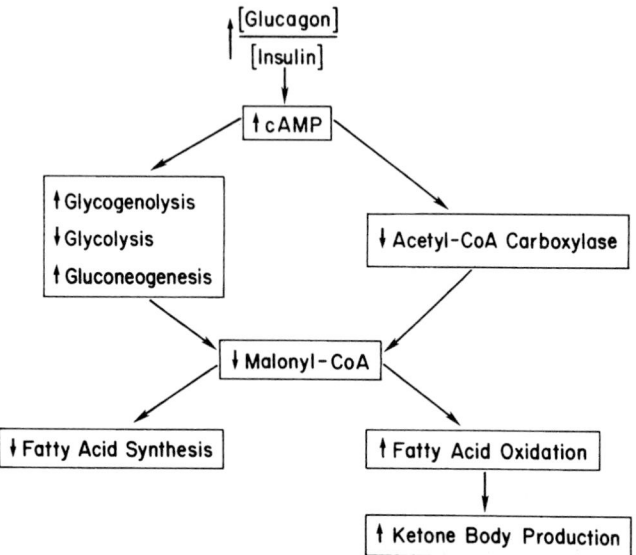

Figure 61-5 Hepatic metabolism in uncontrolled diabetes. The increased ratio of glucagon to insulin increases cyclic AMP, thereby initiating a series of enzymic phosphorylations. These reactions convert the liver to an organ of glucose production with gluconeogenesis predominating after a few hours of poor control. Malonyl CoA levels drop precipitously because of a block in glycolysis, inhibition of acetyl CoA carboxylase and activation of malonyl CoA decarboxylase. (See text.) This drop in turn increases fatty acid oxidation/ketogenic capacity and stops long-chain fatty acid synthesis via substrate depletion. Not shown are the increases in long-chain fatty acyl CoA and carnitine that drive the fatty acid oxidative sequence that is poised for action.

In diabetic ketoacidosis impaired glucose disposal contributes significantly to hyperglycemia. In contrast, ketone utilization is not limited until plasma concentrations reach 10 to 12 mM.[92]

CLINICAL FEATURES

The incidence of diabetic ketoacidosis is not known with certainty, but the disorder is extremely common in younger patients with insulin-dependent disease. In Rochester, Minnesota, a rate of 13.4 per 1000 patient-years was recorded; that is, a given patient at risk had a 1% to 2% chance of having the complication each year.[93] Estimates from the Centers for Disease Control and Prevention were similar, being 14.6 per 1000 patients at risk in 1984 and 12.5 per 1000 patients in 1987. Rates were consistently higher in black males than in other groups, 24.7 per 1000 persons at risk in 1987.[94] It remains a serious illness with overall mortality in the United States approximating 7%.[95] Many deaths are from ketoacidosis-associated events such as myocardial infarction. Ketoacidosis accounts for up to 70% of the deaths attributed to diabetes in children.[96]

PRECIPITATING EVENTS

Diabetic ketoacidosis (DKA) is usually initiated by physical stress of some kind or cessation of insulin.[97,98] Often, the stress is infection, but the apparent cause may vary from acute alcohol intake to myocardial infarction. A significant number of cases have no recognizable precipitating event; in these patients, psychologic stress may be the operative mechanism, especially in young persons who have repeated episodes of ketoacidosis over short intervals.[99] Atypical antipsychotic drugs have been found to induce diabetes and DKA.[100] Known to be associated are clozapine, olanzapine, quetiapine, and risperidone.

Japanese investigators have described a syndrome they have called "fulminant type 1 diabetes."[101] Patients have an abrupt onset of symptoms, usually less than 1 week, with DKA at onset being common.[102] They do not have antibodies characteristic of autoimmune disease. Serum amylase and lipase tend to be elevated. C peptide concentrations are extremely low. Prodromal symptoms are "flu-like" suggesting that a viral illness might be responsible. In the national study,[102] diabetes appeared to be permanent, accounting for 20% of type 1 disease in Japan.

SYMPTOMS AND SIGNS

The usual symptoms and signs of ketoacidosis include vomiting, thirst, polyuria, weakness, altered sensorium, and air hunger. Abdominal pain can occur.[97] The differential diagnosis of such pain is tricky because pyelonephritis or a surgical disorder, such as acute appendicitis, may precipitate ketoacidosis. On the other hand, severe pain mimicking an acute abdomen may be due to the ketoacidotic state itself, possibly the consequence of hypertriglyceridemia-induced pancreatitis. Unless clear-cut evidence of a specific cause is present, a conservative course should be taken, with treatment of ketoacidosis taking precedence.

All DKA patients are hospitalized. There are no data available for ER deaths. The vital signs on admission vary with the length and severity of the prehospital phase of the illness. Tachycardia is essentially always present.[103,104] The mean blood pressure is normal when large numbers of patients are evaluated, but hypotension was present in 8% of the survivors in one series.[104] In the same series, hypotension or shock was present in 19% of those who died. Hypotension obviously is a poor prognostic sign. Kussmaul respiration with respiratory rates averaging 30 per minute is almost always observed, but in severe acidosis the ventilatory response may fall and paradoxically rise as treatment is initiated and the acidosis is reversed.[105,106] The patient's temperature is often below normal and may be as low as 34°C.[103] If fever is present, the likelihood of infection is high. The converse is not true; that is, the absence of fever or the presence of hypothermia does not rule out an infectious process. Although the sensorium is usually clouded on arrival at the hospital, one fifth of patients are alert.[97] Only about 10% are actually unconscious despite frequent use of the phrase "diabetic coma" as a synonym for the acidotic state.

The physical findings are not specific. Breath with a fruity odor may suggest acetonemia. Careful search should be made for hidden infections such as a tooth abscess, a furuncle hidden by axillary hair, or a perirectal abscess. Skin turgor is usually poor, and mucous membranes are ordinarily dry. Occasionally, one sees eruptive xanthomas. Lipemia retinalis is not unusual.

LABORATORY ABNORMALITIES

Typical laboratory abnormalities present on admission are shown in Tables 61-1 and 61-2. Hormone values are informative. Glucagon concentrations were elevated sevenfold, with epinephrine, norepinephrine, cortisol, and growth hormone also showing major increases. Epinephrine concentrations were 50-fold higher than normal. As noted earlier, it is probable that the initial change in catabolic hormones is a rise in glucagon followed by an increase in other counterregulatory agents as the stress of ketoacidosis worsens.[33,34] The result is a vicious cycle: ketoacidosis → stress hormone release → worsening ketoacidosis → greater stress hormone release. The high concentrations of renin and aldosterone are expected concomitants of volume depletion. Inflammatory cytokines are elevated.[107]

Plasma analysis reflects the hormonal changes. Glucose is increased into the 28- to 33-mM (500 to 600 mg/dL) range on average but can be lower or much higher. Very high concentrations, similar to those seen in hyperosmolar coma, probably occur only in subjects who have marked volume depletion and dehydration, the mechanism being diminished urine output as previously discussed.[47,108] Extracellular fluid volume deficits account for the modest elevation in blood urea nitrogen (BUN) and creatinine, whereas plasma osmolalities of 310 to 316 mOsm/L reflect deficits of free water. Although insensible losses of water are increased, especially if Kussmaul respiration is marked, the bulk of the water deficit is consequent to the glucose-mediated osmotic diuresis, which causes loss of water in excess of electrolytes.[47,108,109] Despite dehydration, the plasma sodium level tends to be on the low side because glucose in the absence of insulin becomes osmotically effective in the extracellular fluid because it cannot penetrate the cell; it osmotically pulls intracellular water to the extracellular compartment and thereby dilutes the sodium concentration. The degree of apparent hyponatremia increases with worsening hyperglycemia. An approximation of the true sodium concentration (millimolar) can be obtained by multiplying excess glucose in 100 mg/dL units by 1.6.[110] Thus, for a plasma glucose concentration of 500 mg/dL, the calculation would be:

$$500 \text{ mg/dL} - 100 \text{ mg/dL}/100 \times 1.6 = 6.4 \text{ mmol/liter sodium equivalents}$$

The measured sodium plus 6.4 would approximate the true sodium concentration.

If the plasma sodium level is extremely low, hypertriglyceridemia (secondary to uncontrolled diabetes) should be suspected; the fat, displacing plasma water, causes an artifactually low reading for the sodium concentration. Recognition is not usually a problem because the plasma will be milky, and lipemia retinalis will be visible on ophthalmoscopic examination.[109] Potassium concentrations tend to be high on arrival despite large total body deficits of the cation,[4] primarily because of a shift of potassium from intracellular to extracellular compartments in response to acidosis. Falling urine output will increase the tendency to hyperkalemia. On occasion, the initial potassium level is normal or low—a true danger signal because initiation of insulin therapy, which results in retransfer of potassium into cells, may cause fatal hypokalemia if potassium is not replaced early.

By definition, the acidosis in uncontrolled insulin-dependent diabetes is caused by the overproduction of acetoacetic and β-hydroxybutyric acids in the liver with their accumulation in plasma.[4,34] Contributing to the fall in pH are elevated levels of lactate, free fatty acids, and other organic acids that are normally excreted by the kidneys. Conventionally, the diagnosis of "ketoacidosis" requires a bicarbonate concentration under 10 mM and a pH under 7.3. The term *ketosis* should be used if deteriorating diabetic control has resulted in hyperglycemia/ketosis but not full-blown acidosis. Most hospital laboratories do not routinely measure acetoacetate,

Table 61-2 Laboratory Values in Patients with Diabetic Ketoacidosis

Test	Series 1 (n = 123)	Series 2 (n = 88)
Glucose (mg/dL)	606	476
Sodium (mM)	135	132
Potassium (mM)	5.7	4.8
Bicarbonate (mM)	6.3	<10
BUN (mg/dL)	29	25
Acetoacetate (mM)	3.1	4.8
β-Hydroxybutyrate (mM)	9.8	13.7
Free fatty acids (mM)	—	2.1
Lactate (mM)	2.5	4.6
Osmolality (mOsm)	316	310
pH	7.11	—

BUN, blood urea nitrogen.
Series 1 is adapted from Kitabchi AE, Young R, Sacks H, Morris L: Diabetic ketoacidosis: Reappraisal of therapeutic approach. Annu Rev Med 30:339–357, 1979. Series 2 is adapted from Foster DW: Diabetes mellitus. In Petersdorf RG, Adams RD, Braunwald E, et al (eds): Harrison's Principles of Internal Medicine, ed 10. New York, McGraw-Hill, 1983, pp 661–679. For simplicity, only mean values are listed.

Table 61-1 Hormone Values in Patients with Diabetic Ketoacidosis

Hormone	Controls	Patients
Insulin (μU/mL)	15 ± 2	—
C peptide (ng/mL)	2.4 ± 0.07	—
Glucagon (pg/mL)	99 ± 19	741 ± 247
Epinephrine (ng/mL)	0.05 ± 0.03	2.6 ± 1.3
Norepinephrine (ng/mL)	0.2 ± 0.08	3.8 ± 1.1
Cortisol (μg/dL)	10.5 ± 2	50.4 ± 4.9
Growth hormone (ng/mL)	0.7 ± 0.1	4.6 ± 1.6
Renin (GU × 10⁻⁴/mL)	0.3 ± 0.1	13.2 ± 4.6
Aldosterone (ng/dL)	7.8 ± 2.3	83 ± 25
Pancreatic polypeptide (pg/mL)	93 ± 11	691 ± 200

Control values were obtained in the basal state after an overnight fast. Plasma renin concentration and aldosterone were measured in subjects consuming 120 mmol Na⁺ per day. Data are means ± SEM.
GU, Goldblatt Unit.
Data from Waldhäusl W, Kleinberger G, Korn A, et al: Severe hyperglycemia: Effects of rehydration on endocrine derangements and blood glucose concentration. Diabetes 28:577–584, 1979.

but β-hydroxybutyrate levels may be available. β-hydroxybutyrate levels do not, however, appear helpful in management. Semiquantitative assessment of ketones in plasma can be done with reagent sticks or tablets (which should be powdered before use). A "large" reading in undiluted plasma means that total ketones are at least 6 mM. The concentration of acetoacetate plus β-hydroxybutyrate rarely rises above 6 mM in fasting individuals,[111,112] although a prolonged fast in nonobese persons may induce higher levels. Therefore, a "large" response in plasma diluted 1:1 indicates that total ketones are probably 12 mM or higher and is presumptive evidence that ketoacidosis rather than fasting ketosis is present. Exceptions to the general rule that fasting ketosis gives total ketone levels of 6 mM or less are seen in late pregnancy,[113] some lactating women,[114] and a subset of alcoholic patients.[115,116] These patients may exhibit true ketoacidosis with a short-term fast.

The ratio of β-hydroxybutyrate to acetoacetate is dependent on the redox state of the hepatocyte. β-hydroxybutyrate is usually three times higher than acetoacetic acid. With high rates of fatty acid oxidation, ethanol ingestion, or hypoxia, ratios higher than the normal 3 may be seen, which diminishes the amount of acetone/acetoacetate detected by the reagent strip. Only rarely is this shift of such a magnitude that the diagnosis is difficult. The authors wish to emphasize that ketoacidosis cannot be diagnosed on the basis of a "large" value for ketones in urine because ordinary fasting can produce such a reading. Patients with lactic acidosis and nonketotic, hyperosmolar coma often have "large" values in urine because of fasting induced by the precipitating illness, but they do not have ketoacidosis as defined above.

BUN and creatinine levels are usually modestly elevated on admission and revert to normal as soon as fluids are provided. Creatinine clearance is ordinarily only slightly depressed, in one series averaging 82 mL/min.[117] Higher levels of azotemia are a poor prognostic sign in that they indicate a hemodynamically unstable patient vulnerable to vascular collapse or significant underlying renal disease.

Phosphate depletion is universal in diabetic ketoacidosis, but the initial plasma concentration, like that of potassium, may be low, normal, or high.[118] As a result, marked deficiency of erythrocyte 2,3-diphosphoglycerate is present.[119] Leukocytosis—at times a true leukemoid reaction—is commonly present and does not indicate infection.[97] Amylase may be high but cannot be assumed to represent pancreatitis because it may be of salivary gland origin in some patients.[120] If lipase levels are very high, pancreatitis is more likely, but false-positive values for lipase may be seen if plasma glycerol levels are extremely elevated because of rapid breakdown of adipose tissue triglycerides. (Glycerol is the product measured in most assays for plasma lipase.) Triglycerides are almost always elevated and can reach very high levels (e.g., 10,000 mg/dL).[109] If the patient has eaten within a few hours of onset, a significant fraction of the triglyceride may be in chylomicrons. Cholesterol concentrations will also be increased when triglyceride levels are very high because cholesterol is contained in both chylomicrons (triglyceride:cholesterol ratio of more than 10:1) and very low-density lipoprotein particles (triglyceride:cholesterol ratio of approximately 5:1).

TREATMENT

Treatment of uncomplicated diabetic ketoacidosis requires insulin, fluids, and potassium.[2,4,97,108,121] In some circumstances, bicarbonate[4,97] and phosphate salts[119,122] may be given. An overview of the results of treatment is shown in Figure 61-6.

Fluids

An intravenous saline infusion should be started immediately because it is critical to replace lost volume and secure ade-

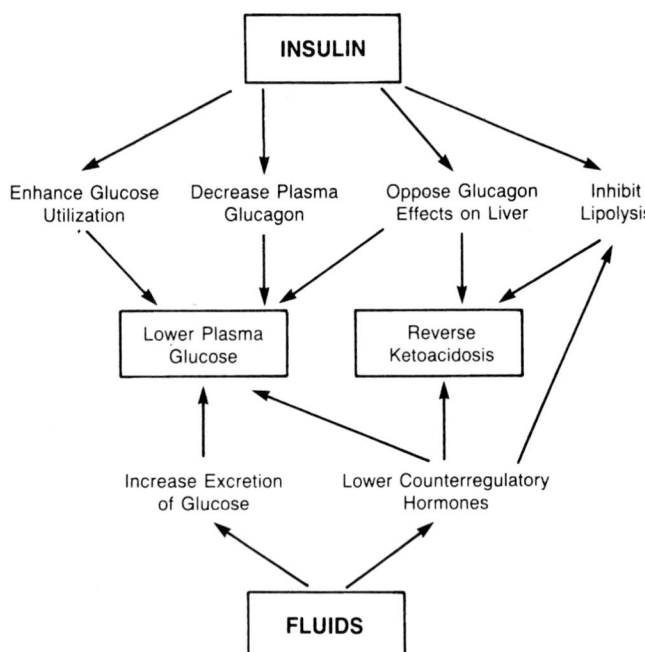

Figure 61-6   The mechanisms by which insulin and fluids reverse ketoacidosis.

quate urine flow. Repletion of the extracellular fluid volume with maintenance of diuresis has a primary role in lowering the plasma glucose level and a secondary role in limiting ketogenesis. The plasma glucose level is lowered by two mechanisms: excretion of glucose in the urine and modulation of counterregulatory hormone release.[32] Significant reversal of hyperglycemia can be produced by fluids alone in the absence of insulin. Initially, fluids should be given rapidly; ordinarily a rate of 1 L/hour is appropriate for the first 2 to 3 hours. Because the total deficit is 3 to 5 L,[4] enough fluid should be given to approximate this amount in net terms (fluids infused minus urine production and estimated insensible loss). Some have recommended giving fluid at half the preceding rate,[123] but the authors favor more rapid infusion. Hyperchloremia essentially always develops during treatment.[124,125] This can be lessened by use of Ringer's solution, although no evidence has demonstrated that the hyperchloremia has detrimental consequences. Most patients also have a deficit of water, as evidenced by the elevated plasma osmolality. This deficit should be repaired only after extracellular volume is repleted. Free water can be delivered either as 0.45% saline or, after hyperglycemia has been brought under control, by infusion of dextrose in water.

It is wise not to administer oral fluids early in ketoacidosis, even if the patient is sufficiently alert to swallow, because nausea and vomiting are common, especially if acute gastric dilatation is present. The restriction of oral fluids does not apply if the patient is only in the developmental stages of ketoacidosis, where therapy is oriented to interruption of the pathogenetic sequence rather than reversal of full-blown diabetic coma.

Insulin

All patients with ketoacidosis require insulin because fluids alone will not reverse hepatic ketone synthesis. Insulin has at least four effects. Its two most important actions are doubtless to decrease glucagon release from the α cell of the islets[6] and to counteract the effects of glucagon in the hepatocyte.[2,6,38] These two effects result in suppression of glucose and ketone production in the liver. The primary mechanism, as noted, appears to be inhibition of a glucagon-activated, cAMP-dependent protein kinase.[43] Secondary actions of insulin involve enhancement of glucose utilization in muscle and fat and inhibition of lipolysis. As discussed in the Ketogenesis section, a drop in plasma free fatty acids does not reverse ketoacidosis because hepatic triglycerides replace adipose tissue as a source of fatty acids when plasma concentrations of the latter fall with insulin treatment. This adaptation is thought to account for the prolonged course in diabetic ketoacidosis, which usually requires about 7 to 9 hours to reverse; that is, ketone production continues unabated, driven by hepatic fat, until CPT I is inactivated.

The amount of insulin that should be used in treatment is a matter of much discussion. The authors' views have been summarized in Ref. 4. Insulin resistance is present in all patients with ketoacidosis relative to normal persons.[44] It is usually mild but in rare patients may be extreme. Insulin should ordinarily be administered intravenously, and only regular insulin should be used. It may be given intermittently but almost always is given by constant infusion. Most patients respond to modest doses, but the lower limit should be 10 U/hour.[126] Administration of larger amounts may have some advantage because presumably at higher concentrations binding of insulin to the IgF1 receptor would occur and provide additive metabolic effects after the insulin receptor is saturated.[42] IgF1 itself has been shown to reverse diabetic ketoacidosis in the absence of insulin.[127] A representative continuous-infusion protocol is shown in Table 61-3. The end point of treatment is a urine sample free of ketones inasmuch as the presence of acetone implies continued activation of hepatic ketogenic enzymes. If these enzymes are not deactivated, any complication (e.g., hypoglycemia or infection) will result in reappearance of ketoacidosis because free fatty acids will be remobilized in response to the action of stress hormones under these conditions and drive production by substrate provision. Therapy should be monitored by checking the anion gap hourly along with blood gas determination every 4 hours. If the anion gap has not started to close by 4 hours, greater than normal insulin resistance is present and the insulin dosage should be increased. Occasionally, very large amounts are required, in which case 500 U insulin is available. Plasma glucose levels ordinarily fall before reversal of the acidosis.[128] Insulin administration should not be stopped or slowed under such circumstances. Rather, glucose should be infused to allow continuation of insulin therapy. (See section "Cerebral Edema" below.) As noted above, no advantage is gained by monitoring plasma ketones during therapy.[129] Intermediate insulin administration can be resumed after the patient is able to eat.

Potassium

Evaluation of potassium deficits is tricky because body stores are depleted despite plasma values that may be high on admission consequent to the metabolic acidosis that shifts K^+ from intracellular to extracellular compartments as noted earlier.[128] Usual deficits are 3 to 5 mmol/kg of body weight, but at times may be double this value.[130] Because of the typical tendency to have hyperkalemia on arrival, potassium salts are not ordinarily given until 2 to 4 hours after treatment is started. On the other hand, if the initial potassium concentration is 4.0 mM or less, potassium salts will be required early because plasma values will fall as soon as insulin restores glucose transport into cells and urine production picks up.[4,131] If the initial potassium level is very low (below 3.0 mM), insulin therapy should be delayed 60 to 90 minutes until some potassium repletion has been accomplished. The infusion rate of potassium chloride or potassium phosphate should be 20 to 40 mmol/hour under most circumstances. Potassium concentrations should be monitored at 2-hour intervals until the patient is metabolically stable. The electrocardiogram may be used as a guide if for some reason plasma levels are not available, but it is much less reliable.[132] Potassium salts should be given only with extreme caution in an oliguric patient.

Phosphate

No evidence has shown that phosphate depletion plays a major symptomatic role in the development or treatment of diabetic ketoacidosis.[119,122] Very low phosphate levels can cause altered consciousness, hemolysis, rhabdomyolysis, and heart failure, but these complications are not part of the routine picture in diabetic coma. Thus, there appears to be little urgency to replace the deficits of phosphate, which may approach 300 mmol. Nevertheless, many clinicians give the initial potassium replacement as potassium phosphate, thereby dealing with both deficiencies.

Bicarbonate

Severe acidosis is dangerous because it may cause hypotension, especially if volume depletion is present.[128] Acidosis causes decreased myocardial contractility and diminished response of peripheral resistance vessels to catecholamines. It may also contribute to the clouding of consciousness that characterizes ketoacidosis, although increased osmolality of brain cells doubtless plays a role. Warnings against the use of bicarbonate have focused on potential problems such as alkali-induced hypokalemia and lactic acidosis, but it has been argued that the benefits of bicarbonate outweigh the risks.[133,134] If the admission pH is below 7.0, bicarbonate should probably be administered in amounts sufficient to bring the pH to 7.2, although some studies have shown no benefit.[135,136] If hypotension is present, it may be prudent to give bicarbonate to all patients with a pH of 7.2 or less because increased responsiveness of the left ventricle and resistance vessels would likely outweigh any deleterious effect of alkalinization on the oxygen dissociation curve.[119]

Monitoring Therapy

Maintenance of a written flow chart is important in monitoring a patient with ketoacidosis.[128,137] Timed recording of insulin, fluids, potassium, and bicarbonate administration are imperative. Capillary blood glucose levels should be measured every 30 minutes initially. Formal laboratory evaluation of plasma glucose, sodium, potassium, bicarbonate, chloride, BUN, and creatinine should be obtained at 1- to 2-hour intervals. As mentioned above, the best marker of reversal of acidosis is a fall in the anion gap. It is characteristic for the anion

Table 61-3	An Infusion Protocol for Treatment of Diabetic Ketoacidosis*	
Plasma Glucose (mg/dL)	Insulin Infusion (U/hr)	5% Dextrose/Water (mL/hr)
<70	0.5	250
71–100	1	225
101–150	2	200
151–200	3	175
201–250	4	150
251–300	6	100
301–350	8	50
351–400	10	0
401–450	12	0
451–500	16	0
>500	20	0

*University Diabetes Service, Parkland Memorial Hospital, courtesy of Dr. Philip Raskin. A 50-U bolus of insulin is given intravenously on arrival. Fluids and potassium are administered as indicated. SMA-6 is obtained hourly for the first few hours, with glucose measured hourly until the condition is reversed. Insulin administration is continued, covered by glucose, until urine is ketone-free.

gap to close with therapy, matched by a rise in pH, while the bicarbonate concentration remains low (12–14 mM). The low bicarbonate value reflects a hyperchloremic state resulting from the infusion of sodium chloride, exchange with intracellular buffers, and external loss of "potential bicarbonate" in the form of excreted ketones.[125] The frequency of clinical and chemical monitoring can decrease as the patient recovers. Rarely, patients do not clear the anion gap despite clinical improvement. While failure to close the gap normally indicates insulin resistance, in some patients an unmeasured anion that is not ketones, lactate, renal acids, or a poison appears to be present. The putative mystery anion (acetate? citrate?) has not been identified. Recognition that this condition is not insulin resistance is readily apparent if the urine is shown to be free of ketones and blood gas determination indicates that the acidosis has been reversed. We have called this condition "pseudoinsulin resistance."

COMPLICATIONS

Death from properly treated diabetic ketoacidosis should be rare, but ketoacidosis is the primary cause of mortality in diabetic children.[96,138] Death rates are also significant in adults.[94–96] When death occurs, it may be the result of the disease itself or a result of complications of therapy. Clues to complications are given in Table 61-4.

Shock

Vascular collapse is not common in ketoacidosis. When it occurs, it may be the result of one of several causes. Volume depletion and acidosis alone can produce hypotension, as outlined earlier. If blood pressure does not rise with adequate fluid replacement, another cause of hypotension should be sought. Gram-negative sepsis and silent myocardial infarction are prime candidates.[97,139]

Cerebral Edema

Cerebral edema is a dreaded development, especially in children. Despite aggressive therapy, recovery can never be ensured.[140,141] In a retrospective study of 61 subjects from 10 pediatric centers, 28% died, 13% survived with neurological sequelae, and 59% survived without sequelae.[142] The syndrome is heralded by the appearance of neurologic signs or worsening coma in a patient who should be getting well as judged by biochemical parameters. Sluggish pupillary responses and frank papilledema may appear after several hours. Death is probably caused by compression of the brain stem as a result of herniation of the cerebellar tonsils through the foramen magnum.

The cause of cerebral edema is not known. It has generally been assumed that the complication is a result of treatment, somehow precipitated by rapid falls in the plasma glucose level or oncotic pressure after insulin and crystalloid therapy.[140,141,143–146] Alterations in blood-brain barrier permeability due to insulin[143] and disequilibrium in pH have also been postulated as important. On the other hand, six of seven consecutive patients with untreated diabetic ketoacidosis were shown to have subclinical cerebral edema by computed tomographic scan on arrival at the hospital in one series.[146] Thus, initial edema was independent of therapy. No conclusion regarding causality could be shown, although the degree of hyperglycemia correlated with the degree of acidosis. Osmotic disequilibrium between plasma/interstitial and intracellular water is probably of importance in the transition from subclinical to clinical edema. Because cerebrospinal fluid pressure rises routinely during treatment, it is likely that cerebral edema represents the extreme of a common response to therapy.[147] It is usually recommended that glucose infusions be started when the plasma glucose level is in the range of 16.7 mM (300 mg/dL) in an attempt to avoid the disequilibrium presumed to occur with rapid reversal of hyperglycemia.[143] This approach is not foolproof because the syndrome has developed in a child whose plasma glucose levels never got lower than 20.8 mM (375 mg/dL).[148]

Treatment consists of the intravenous administration of a 20% mannitol solution in bolus fashion at a dose of 1 g/kg. Dexamethasone is often given simultaneously—12 mg initially followed by 4 mg every 6 hours—but no real evidence has shown that dexamethasone is of help. It has been suggested that mannitol be administered early rather than late based on theoretical analysis of the problem, but there are no data to test this.[149] As in other forms of cerebral edema, hyperventilation to a P_{CO_2} of 28 to 30 mm Hg may help by decreasing cerebral blood flow. Such therapy requires the assistance of an anesthesiologist.

Infection

Infection is a common problem in diabetic ketoacidosis and should be suspected in all patients, especially if fever is present.[95,96,131,139] Although leukocytosis does not indicate infection, as noted earlier, fever almost always does. Pneumonia, pyelonephritis, and septicemia are most common, but cryptic inflammation, such as tooth or perirectal abscesses, may be the precipitating event. Mucormycosis is a rare fungal infection that is specifically associated with diabetic ketoacidosis.[150,151] The initial symptom of facial pain suggests sinusitis, but the signs of bloody nasal discharge, orbital swelling, blackened palate and nasal turbinates, blurred vision, and altered consciousness point to the correct diagnosis. Mucormycosis is fatal if untreated. Amphotericin B should be started immediately on suspicion without waiting for confirmation by culture. Even with treatment the outlook is guarded. The role of ketoacids appears to be interference in the binding of iron to transferrin.[150] This interference in iron binding raises the concentration of free iron, which is a growth factor for the fungus.

Vascular Thrombosis

Thrombosis may occur during ketoacidosis in any muscular artery, but the cerebral vessels appear to be especially vulnerable.[152,153] The mechanism is multifactorial. A major factor is probably increased viscosity of blood coupled with sluggish blood flow because of contraction of the plasma

Table 61-4	Clues to Complications of Diabetic Ketoacidosis
Complications	**Clues**
Acute gastric dilatation or erosive gastritis	Vomiting of blood or coffee-ground material
Cerebral edema	Obtundation or coma with or without neurologic signs, especially if occurring after initial improvement
Hyperkalemia	Cardiac arrest
Hypoglycemia	Adrenergic or neurologic signs; rebound ketosis
Hypokalemia	Cardiac arrhythmias
Infection	Fever
Insulin resistance	Unremitting acidosis after 4–6 hr of adequate therapy
Myocardial infarction	Chest pain, appearance of heart failure; appearance of hypotension despite adequate fluids
Mucormycosis	Facial pain, bloody nasal discharge, blackened nasal turbinates, blurred vision, proptosis
Vascular thrombosis	Strokelike picture or signs of ischemia in nonnervous tissue

From Foster DW: Diabetic ketoacidosis. In Krieger DT, Bardin CW (eds): Current Therapy in Endocrinology and Metabolism. Toronto, BC Decker, 1985, pp 268–270.

volume. Underlying atherosclerosis is doubtless important, the site of the lesion determining the location of the thrombosis. The activity of factor VIII is enhanced, as are levels of von Willebrand antigen.[154,155] Platelets isolated from patients with ketoacidosis exhibit more facile aggregation in vitro than their normal counterparts do.[156,157] Endothelial dysfunction predisposing to clot formation may also play a role: decreased fibrinolytic potential,[158] elevated levels of endothelin,[159] and diminished nitric oxide activity.[160,161] Antithrombin III, protein C, and protein S may be low.[162] High levels of plasminogen activator inhibitor-1 (PAI-1) are particularly important in thrombotic events.[158,163,164] Interestingly, metformin has been reported to lower PAI-1 levels.[165] Although prophylactic anticoagulation has been recommended, the authors agree with Carroll and Matz that such anticoagulation is unwise[131]; the best prophylaxis is aggressive fluid therapy. A single dose of aspirin daily (325 mg) might be prudent.[137]

Respiratory Distress Syndrome

The respiratory distress syndrome is a rare complication of diabetic ketoacidosis.[166] The syndrome is manifested as unexplained dyspnea and hypoxemia. Because large amounts of fluid are routinely given and the x-ray picture resembles pulmonary edema, it is frequently necessary to insert a Swan-Ganz catheter for the differential diagnosis.[167] The wedge pressure is normal or low in respiratory distress syndrome and high in left ventricular failure. Treatment requires administration of oxygen with positive end-expiratory pressure in standard fashion. Mortality rates are high.

NONKETOTIC HYPEROSMOLAR COMA

Whereas ketoacidosis is the common emergency of autoimmune diabetes, nonketotic hyperosmolar coma is the emergency of non-insulin-dependent diabetes. As will be seen in the next section, these distinctions are not absolute, however.

PATHOPHYSIOLOGY

The pathophysiology of nonketotic hyperglycemic coma is similar to that of diabetic ketoacidosis with one exception: Overproduction of acetoacetate and β-hydroxybutyrate sufficient to cause ketoacidosis does not occur.[167] The basic bihormonal mechanism of uncontrolled diabetes is no different: a relative or absolute deficiency of insulin and a relative or absolute excess of glucagons.[2,168,169] Elevation of the plasma glucose level is, as in ketoacidosis, the result of increased production of glucose by the liver coupled with its diminished utilization in tissues. The extreme hyperglycemia that characterizes the syndrome is consequent to failure of urine output.[47,108] Put another way, production rates of glucose are not higher in hyperosmolar coma than in ketoacidosis, but the urinary escape route for glucose is diminished or absent from prolonged osmotic diuresis. Thus, one has a situation in which hepatic glucose production continues unabated, with glucose released into a steadily shrinking plasma/extracellular space. The result is a concentration of glucose in plasma that averages 55 mM (1000 mg/dL)[170,171] and may reach nearly 278 mM (5000 mg/dL).[172] What accounts for the striking difference in glucose levels in ketoacidosis and hyperosmolar coma? The answer almost certainly is the absence of ketoacidosis. When metabolic acidosis supervenes, the patient or patient's family knows that the patient is acutely ill because almost invariably nausea, vomiting, and Kussmaul respiration are present. With hyperosmolar coma, by contrast, the patient has only an unremitting osmotic diuresis that is clinically silent until the patient is so dehydrated that altered consciousness or an acute neurologic syndrome supervenes. Although severe hyperosmolality is not the norm in diabetic

ketoacidosis, it does occur.[108] Indeed, patients with true type 1 diabetes may have pure hyperosmolar coma as discussed in later paragraphs.

Because dehydration and volume depletion resulting from osmotic diuresis never progress to the point of coma provided that the patient can drink water, it is usual for hyperosmolar coma to appear in the context of some other illness that impairs the patient's capacity to maintain fluid intake. This event may be infection, a stroke, a fall resulting in a sprain or fracture, or intake of a drug that alters the sensorium, increases glucose production, or causes diuresis with volume depletion.[173] Survivors of hyperosmolar coma have been reported to have abnormal thirst response to water deprivation relative to control patients with non-insulin-dependent diabetes.[174] It is not known if this was present prior to hyperosmolar coma. To reiterate, as long as enough water is drunk to sustain urine output, even a severe osmotic diuresis does not result in the type of monumental hyperglycemia that characterizes nonketotic hyperosmolar coma.

The critical pathophysiologic question in hyperosmolar coma is why ketoacidosis is not present. The answer to this question is not known. Earlier theories proposed hyperosmolarity and lower free fatty acids as the explanation. Experimentally, hyperosmolarity can quench ketosis, and lower fatty acid concentrations in plasma would limit ketone formation via substrate deficiency. Neither explanation is likely because some patients with ketoacidosis have plasma osmolalities overlapping those of hyperosmolar coma and hyperosmolar coma has clearly occurred in subjects with very high free fatty acid concentrations in plasma.[168] On the basis of studies in animals, it is attractive to postulate that the primary reason for the absence of ketoacidosis is hepatic resistance to glucagon so that malonyl CoA levels do not fall. In the *ob/ob* mouse, cAMP generation by glucagon is markedly impaired,[175] and malonyl CoA concentrations are high.[176] The mechanism of glucagon resistance is not known, but this animal appears to have a defect in guanine nucleotide modulation of the adenylate cyclase system, at least in adipose tissue.[177] Obviously, the *ob/ob* mouse is not equivalent to a human with non-insulin-dependent diabetes. It also seems peculiar that glucagon resistance would be limited to ketogenesis and not affect glucose overproduction. Perhaps malonyl CoA levels are maintained at inhibitory levels because of increased hepatic lactate uptake rather than because of glucagon resistance; that is, increased lactate turnover (the Cori cycle sequence) might be expected from the high plasma glucose concentrations. Because subjects with type 2 diabetes have normal or high insulin levels in the portal vein, increased lactate and alanine uptake could be sufficient to maintain hepatic gluconeogenesis while simultaneously inhibiting ketogenesis by generating malonyl CoA.

As noted above, some patients with autoimmune diabetes have nonketotic hyperosmolar coma. It is likewise true that some patients with ostensible type 2 diabetes may experience severe ketosis and even full-blown ketoacidosis.[178,179] A peculiar characteristic is that after recovery they may be treated by diet and oral agents without reversion to ketoacidosis. It is likely that these subjects have a subtype of nonautoimmune diabetes that has been called non-insulin-dependent-diabetes mellitus-2 (NIDDM-2).[180-182] Subjects with mutations in hepatocyte nuclear factor-1α may have maturity-onset diabetes of the young type 3 (MODY-3) or adult-onset diabetes (NIDDM-2).[182-184] The characteristic finding in MODY-3 and NIDDM-2 is insulin deficiency with little insulin resistance. This situation is in contrast to ordinary NIDDM, where insulin levels are normal or high and insulin resistance is marked. They also do not express antibodies to glutamic acid decarboxylase or other markers of β-cell autoimmunity. The insulin secretory defect makes these subjects susceptible to ketoacidosis in stress, where epinephrine/nonepinephrine block insulin release. On the other hand, because the insulin deficiency is not near absolute, as in type 1 disease, they may be controlled without insulin when stress or stressful illness disappears. A similar syndrome may occur with mutations in hepatocyte nuclear factor-4α, the apparent genetic defect in MODY-1.[185]

CLINICAL FEATURES

Nonketotic hyperosmolar coma usually occurs in older persons with diabetes,[167,170,171] but as noted, it has been seen in the very young.[186] The syndrome can thus develop in patients with insulin-dependent, ketosis-prone diabetes. This phenomenon occurs when the patient is taking enough insulin to prevent ketoacidosis (by limiting free fatty acid mobilization) but not enough to control hyperglycemia. A curious inversion of insulin effects is seen in the presence or absence of ketoacidosis. In a nonketoacidotic subject it is harder to control the plasma glucose level than to prevent ketoacidosis, whereas in established ketoacidosis the plasma glucose level, as noted earlier, almost always falls before ketosis is reversed.[128] Thus, a patient with insulin-dependent diabetes may be rendered functionally equivalent to a patient with non-insulin-dependent diabetes when treated with insulin sufficient to avoid ketoacidosis but insufficient to prevent a hyperglycemia-driven osmotic diuresis.

PRECIPITATING EVENTS

As noted, nonketotic hyperosmolar coma is usually precipitated by a serious underlying illness that renders the patient unable to obtain sufficient water to keep up with the osmotic diuresis under circumstances in which glucose production is increased by stress. Any kind of illness can initiate the sequence of deterioration, but infection is probably the most common.[170,171] Stroke, drugs, high-calorie tube feedings, burns, heart attacks, and a variety of other problems have been associated with the syndrome.

SYMPTOMS AND SIGNS

The preeminent symptomatology of hyperosmolar coma is neurologic. Up to half the patients are comatose on arrival, and those who are not show stupor.[187] A variety of other neurologic findings may be present, including focal convulsions or a stroke-like picture.[188–190] It should always be assumed that an underlying illness precipitated the syndrome even though it may be masked by the metabolic crisis. Sometimes it is hard to tell whether a finding is cause or effect. Thus, stroke can lead to hyperosmolar coma, and hyperosmolar coma can cause hemiplegia. Only if the neurologic picture reverses rapidly with therapy can it be concluded that the neurologic event was secondary. The possibility of head injury always has to be kept in mind in older patients living alone. A computed tomographic scan should be obtained once the metabolic state is stabilized.

Physical examination shows evidence of volume depletion and dehydration. Hypotension or shock may be present. Driven respiration of the Kussmaul type suggests the presence of lactic acidosis. Other physical findings reflect the underlying precipitating illness or the appearance of complications as outlined below.

LABORATORY ABNORMALITIES

Typical findings in nonketotic, hyperosmolar coma are shown in Table 61-5. Hyperglycemia, as noted, averages about 55 mM (1000 mg/dL). References to "syrupy blood" are entirely appropriate.[172] The plasma osmolality reflects the hyperglycemia and dehydration and is often 100 mOsm

Table 61-5 Laboratory Values in Nonketotic Hyperosmolar Coma

Test	Series 1 (n = 33)	Series 2 (n = 20)	Series 3 (n = 7)
Glucose (mg/dL)	1166	976	1119
Sodium (mM)	144	142	138
Potassium (mM)	5.0	5.1	4.1
Chloride (mM)	99	98	96
Bicarbonate (mM)	17	22	18
BUN (mg/dL)	87	65	75
Creatinine (mg/dL)	5.5	—	—
Free fatty acids (mM)	0.73	0.96	1.98
Osmolality (mOsm)	384	374	361

BUN, blood urea nitrogen.
Series 1 is adapted from Arieff AI, Carroll HJ: Nonketotic hyperosmolar coma with hyperglycemia. Clinical features, pathophysiology, renal function, acid-base balance, plasma–cerebrospinal fluid equilibria and the effects of therapy in 37 cases. Medicine (Baltimore) 51:73–94, 1972. Series 2 is adapted from Gerich JE, Martin MM, Recant L: Clinical and metabolic characteristics of hyperosmolar nonketonic coma. Diabetes 20:228–238, 1971. Series 3 is adapted from Vinik A, Seftel H, Joffe BI: Metabolic findings in hyperosmolar, non-ketotic diabetic stupor. Lancet 2:797–799, 1970. Values listed are means.

higher than normal. Fairly accurate estimates of osmolality can be obtained from the following formula:

$$mOsm = 2[Na^+ + K^+] + glucose~(mg/dL)/18 + BUN~(mg/dL)/2.8$$

Some investigators have suggested that the serum sodium concentration, corrected for glucose, correlates best with central nervous system dysfunction.[191] This seems doubtful given that osmolality reflects the sodium concentration. The BUN and creatinine values are usually significantly elevated, a reflection of volume depletion and/or underlying renal disease. In the absence of vascular collapse, only minimal acidosis is seen, the bicarbonate averaging 18 to 20 mM. Mild ketosis resulting from starvation is usually present, so urine ketone values may be "large." If full-blown metabolic acidosis is present, the likely mechanism is lactic acidosis as noted above. It's cause is severe volume depletion, which leads to hypoxia of tissues via diminished perfusion. Formal differentiation requires quantitative measurement of lactate (Table 61-6). Levels of free fatty acids tend to be in the normal fasting range but in some patients are very high.[167] Hypertriglyceridemia may be present.[192] As in ketoacidosis, the amylase level may be elevated and pancreatitis may be present.

TREATMENT

Therapy for nonketotic hyperosmolar coma is similar to that for ketoacidosis, with the major variation being the requirement for much larger amounts of fluid. Although recovery may be expected in patients younger than 50 years,[131] mortality rates are high (about 50%) in older patients.[167] Treatment often requires admission to the intensive care unit.

Fluids

The most important therapy is the rapid administration of isotonic saline solution to reestablish the circulation and urine flow.[131] Deficits of fluid in hyperosmolar coma may be 10 L or more.[170,171] We do not agree with the view that the first fluid administered should be hypotonic (0.45%) saline[173]; we prefer to give 2 to 3 L of isotonic salt solution over the first 60 to 90 minutes, after which 0.45% saline is administered. As mentioned, a Swan-Ganz catheter for

Table 61-6 Differential Diagnosis of Diabetic Ketoacidosis

Condition	Urine		Plasma			
	Glucose	Ketones	Glucose	Ketones	Lactate	BUN/CR
Diabetic ketoacidosis	Pos	Pos	High	High	Mod	Mod
Hyperosmolar coma with lactic acidosis	Pos	Neg/Pos	Very high	Mod	High	High
Lactic acidosis	Neg	Neg/Pos	Nor/Mod	Nor/Mod	High	Nor/Mod
Alcoholic ketoacidosis	Neg/Pos	Pos	Nor/high	High	Mod	Nor
Pregnancy-associated ketoacidosis	Neg/Pos	Pos	Nor/Low	High	Nor	Nor
Renal failure	Neg	Neg	Nor	Nor	Nor	High
Organic poisons	Neg	Neg/Pos	Nor	Nor	Nor	Nor/Mod

BUN, blood urea nitrogen; CR, creatinine; Mod, moderate; Neg, negative; Nor, normal; Pos, positive. For glucose, normal < 140 mg/dL; moderate = 140 to 300 mg/dL; high = 300 to 700 mg/dL; very high > 700 mg/dL. For ketones, moderate = 1 to 6 mM; high > 6.0 mM (see the text for use of the semiquantitative test of quantitative enzymatic determination is not available). For lactate, moderate = 2 to 4 mM; high > 4 mM. For BUN, moderate = 20 to 40 mg/dL; high > 40 mg/dL. For creatinine, moderate = 2 to 3 mg/dL; high > 3.0 mg/dL. Representations are average findings and should not be considered absolute. If only a semiquantitative test for ketones is available, moderate means that a "large" reading is present only in undiluted plasma; high = "large" in 1:1 or greater dilution. When a slash is present (e.g., Neg/Pos) the usual state is the first designation; for example, the urine is usually negative for glucose in pregnancy-associated ketoacidosis but could be positive if the patient had renal glycosuria.

monitoring of capillary wedge pressure is extremely helpful because many of the patients are older and have underlying heart disease. Fluids should be given continuously until deficits are repaired, as manifested by normal wedge pressure, urine output reflecting infusion rates, and fall of the elevated BUN and creatinine.

Insulin

It has frequently been stated that patients with hyperosmolar coma are more sensitive to insulin than are those with ketoacidosis.[187] However, studies of glucose disappearance in response to insulin actually suggest that insulin resistance is present to the same degree as seen in the ketoacidotic state.[193] Therefore, it seems reasonable to give insulin at the same level as recommended for ketoacidosis.

Other Therapy

Potassium will usually be needed earlier than in ketoacidosis because initial values are not as high (provided that acidosis is not present). As with ketoacidosis, it is reasonable to give potassium phosphate because phosphate levels are also low.

Bicarbonate is not needed unless lactic acidosis supervenes. Some authors also give magnesium sulfate,[131] but no data suggest its importance.

COMPLICATIONS

The complications of hyperosmolar coma are not dissimilar from those of ketoacidosis, with vascular collapse and infection being the most important problems.[170,171] Of particular concern is gram-negative sepsis and pneumonia. Blood cultures should probably be obtained in all patients on arrival; blood culture is imperative if shock or fever is present. Other cultures will depend on the clinical findings. Broad-spectrum antibiotic coverage should be provided for the slightest suspicion of sepsis until cultures prove negative. Adult respiratory distress syndrome is not unusual.[110] Cerebral edema is rare in hyperosmolar coma but may occur.[194] Thrombosis, particularly in cerebral vessels, is common,[195] and diffuse intravascular coagulation may occur, leading to oozing of blood from a variety of sites. As noted, lactic acidosis may supervene. Myocardial infarction is not rare, and acute rhabdomyolysis has been reported.[196]

REFERENCES

1. National Diabetes Data Group: Diabetes in America, 2d ed. Bethesda, MD, National Institutes of Health, NIH Publication No. 95-1468, 1995.
2. Unger RH, Foster DW: Diabetes mellitus. In Wilson JD, Foster DW, Kronenberg HM, Larsen PR (eds): Williams' Textbook of Endocrinology, 9th ed. Philadelphia, WB Saunders, 1998, pp 973–1059.
3. Foster DW, McGarry JD: Glucose, lipid and protein metabolism. In Griffin JE, Ojeda SR (eds): Textbook of Endocrine Physiology, 3d ed. New York, Oxford University Press, 1996, pp 349–374.
4. Foster DW, McGarry JD: The metabolic derangements and treatment of diabetic ketoacidosis. N Engl J Med 309:159–169, 1983.
5. Unger RH: The milieu interieur and the islets of Langerhans. Diabetologia 20:1–11, 1981.
6. Unger RH, Orci L: Glucagon and the A cell: Physiology and pathophysiology.

N Engl J Med 304:1518–1524, 1575–1580, 1981.
7. McGarry JD, Foster DW: Hormonal control of ketogenesis: Biochemical considerations. Arch Intern Med 137:495–501, 1977.
8. Cahill GR Jr: Starvation in man. N Engl J Med 282:668–675, 1970.
9. Ruderman NB, Aoki TT, Cahill GF Jr: Gluconeogenesis and its disorders in man. In Hanson RW, Mehlman MA (eds): Gluconeogenesis: Its Regulation in Mammalian Species. New York, John Wiley & Sons, 1976, pp 515–532.
10. Allweiss C, Landau T, Abeles M, et al: The oxidation of uniformly labelled albumin-bound palmitic acid to CO by the perfused cat brain. J Neurochem 13:795–804, 1966.
11. Drenick EJ, Alvarez LC, Tamasi GC, et al: Resistance to symptomatic insulin reactions after fasting. J Clin Invest 51:2757–2762, 1972.
12. Madison LL, Mebane D, Unger RH, et al: The hypoglycemic action of

ketones: II. Evidence for the stimulatory feedback of ketones on the pancreatic beta cells. J Clin Invest 43:408–415, 1964.
13. McGarry JD, Foster DW: Hormonal control of ketogenesis. Adv Exp Med Biol 111:79–96, 1976.
14. McGarry JD, Dobbins RL: Fatty acids, lipotoxicity and insulin resistance. Diabetologia 42:128–138, 1999.
15. Dobbs R, Sakurai H, Sasaki H, et al: Glucagon: Role in the hyperglycemia of diabetes mellitus. Science 187:544–547, 1975.
16. Unger RH: Role of glucagon in the pathogenesis of diabetes: The status of the controversy. Metabolism 27:1691–1709, 1978.
17. Gerich JE, Lorenzi M, Bier DM, et al: Prevention of human diabetic ketoacidosis by somatostatin: Evidence for an essential role of glucagon. N Engl J Med 292:985–989, 1975.
18. Cherrington AD, Liljenquist JE: Role of glucagon in regulating glucose

production in vivo. In Unger RH, Orci L (eds): Glucagon. New York, Elsevier, 1981, pp 221–253.

19. Raskin P, Unger RH: Hyperglucagonemia and its suppression: Importance in the metabolic control of diabetes. N Engl J Med 299:433–436, 1978.

20. Santeusanio F, Massi-Benedetti M, Angeletti G, et al: Glucagon and carbohydrate disorder in a totally pancreatomized man (a study with the aid of an artificial endocrine pancreas). J Endocrinol Invest 4:93–96, 1981.

21. Unger RH: Somatostatinoma. N Engl J Med 296:998–1000, 1977.

22. Liljenquist J, Bomboy J, Lewis S, et al: Effects of glucagon on lipolysis and ketogenesis in normal and diabetic man. J Clin Invest 53:190–197, 1974.

23. Schade DS, Woodside W, Eaton RP: The role of glucagon in the regulation of plasma lipids. Metabolism 28:874–886, 1979.

24. Miles JM, Haymond MW, Nissen SL, et al: Effects of free fatty acid availability, glucagon excess, and insulin deficiency on ketone body production in postabsorptive man. J Clin Invest 71:1554–1561, 1983.

25. Boden G, Owen OE, Rezvani I, et al: An islet cell carcinoma containing glucagon and insulin. Chronic glucagon excess and glucose homeostasis. Diabetes 26:128–137, 1977.

26. Marynick SP, Fagadau WR, Duncan LA: Malignant glucagonoma syndrome: Response to chemotherapy. Ann Intern Med 93:453–454, 1980.

27. McGarry JD, Wright PH, Foster DW: Hormonal control of ketogenesis. Rapid activation of hepatic ketogenic capacity in fed rats by anti insulin serum and glucagon. J Clin Invest 55:1202–1209, 1975.

28. McGarry JD, Foster DW: Glucagon and ketogenesis. In Lefebvre PJ (ed): Handbook of Experimental Pharmacology, vol 66/I. Glucagon I. Berlin, Springer-Verlag, 1983, pp 383–398.

29. Schade DS, Eaton RP: The regulation of plasma ketone body concentration by counter-regulatory hormones in man: III. Effects of norepinephrine in normal man. Diabetes 28:5–10, 1979.

30. Keyes WG, Heimberg M: Influence of thyroid status on lipid metabolism in the perfused rat liver. J Clin Invest 64:182–190, 1979.

31. Schade DS, Eaton RP: The controversy concerning counterregulatory hormone secretion: A hypothesis for the prevention of diabetic ketoacidosis? Diabetes 26:596–599, 1977.

32. Waldhausl W, Kleinberger G, Korn A, et al: Severe hyperglycemia: Effects of rehydration on endocrine derangements and blood glucose concentration. Diabetes 28:577–584, 1979.

33. Alberti KGMM, Christensen NJ, Iversen J, et al: Role of glucagon and other hormones in development of diabetic ketoacidosis. Lancet 1:1307–1311, 1975.

34. Miles JM, Rizza RA, Haymond MW, et al: Effects of acute insulin deficiency on glucose and ketone body turnover in man: Evidence for the primacy of overproduction of glucose and ketone bodies in the genesis of diabetic ketoacidosis. Diabetes 29:926–930, 1980.

35. Boyd ME, Albright EB, Foster DW, et al: In vitro reversal of the fasting state of liver metabolism in the rat. Reevaluation of the roles of insulin and glucose. J Clin Invest 68:142–152, 1981.

36. Harano Y, Kosugi K, Kashiwagi A, et al: Regulatory mechanism of ketogenesis by glucagon and insulin in isolated and cultured hepatocytes. J Biochem 91:1739–1748, 1982.

37. Virkamaki A, Ueki K, Kahn CR: Protein-protein interaction in insulin signaling and the molecular mechanisms of insulin resistance. J Clin Invest 103:931–943, 1999.

38. Rodbell M: The actions of glucagon at its receptor: Regulation of adenylate cyclase. In Lefebvre PJ (ed): Handbook of Experimental Pharmacology, vol 66/I. Glucagon I. Berlin, Springer-Verlag, 1983, pp 263–290.

39. Tang EKY, Houslay MD: Glucagon, vasopressin and angiotensin all elicit a rapid, transient increase in hepatocyte protein kinase C activity. Biochem J 283:341–346, 1992.

40. Iwanij V, Vincent AC: Characterization of the glucagon receptor and its functional domains using monoclonal antibodies. J Biol Chem 265:21302–21308, 1990.

41. Dunphy JL, Taylor RG, Fuller PJ: Tissue distribution of rat glucagon receptor and GLP-1 receptor gene expression. Mol Cell Endocrinol 141:179–186, 1998.

42. Flier JS: Lilly lecture: Syndromes of insulin resistance: From patient to gene and back again. Diabetes 41:1207–1219, 1992.

43. Gabbay RA, Lardy HA: Site of insulin inhibition of cAMP-stimulated glycogenolysis. cAMP-dependent protein kinase is affected independent of cAMP changes. J Biol Chem 259:6052–6055, 1984.

44. Barrett EJ, DeFronzo RA, Bevilacqua S, et al: Insulin resistance in diabetic ketoacidosis. Diabetes 31:923–928, 1982.

45. Svedberg J, Bjorntorp P, Lonnroth P, et al: Prevention of inhibitory effect of free fatty acids on insulin binding and action in isolated rat hepatocytes by etomoxir. Diabetes 40:783–786, 1991.

46. McGarry JD: What if Minkowski had been ageusic? An alternative angle on diabetes. Science 258:766–770, 1992.

47. Feig PU, McCurdy DK: The hypertonic state. N Engl J Med 297:1444–1454, 1977.

48. Hers HG, Van Schaftingen E: Fructose 2,6-bisphosphate 2 years after its discovery. Biochem J 206:1–12, 1982.

49. Pilkis SJ, Granner DK: Molecular physiology of the regulation of hepatic gluconeogenesis and glycolysis. Annu Rev Physiol 54:885–909, 1992.

50. Okar DA, Live DH, Kirby TL, et al: The roles of Glu-327 and His-446 in the bisphosphatase reaction of rat liver 6-phosphofructo-2-kinase/fructose-2,6-bisphosphatase probed by NMR spectroscopic and mutational analyses of the enzyme in the transient phosphohistidine intermediate complex. Biochemistry 38:4471–4479, 1999.

51. Kuwajima M, Newgard CB, Foster DW, McGarry JD: Time course and significance of changes in hepatic fructose-2,6-bisphosphate levels during refeeding of fasted rats. J Clin Invest 74:1108–1111, 1984.

52. Jin ES, Uyeda K, Kawaguchi T, et al: Increased hepatic fructose 2, 6-bisphosphate after an oral glucose load does not affect gluconeogenesis. J Biol Chem 278:28427–28433, 2003.

53. Yoon JC, Puigserver P, Chen G, et al: Control of hepatic gluconeogenesis through the transcriptional coactivator PGC-1. Nature 413:131–138, 2001.

54. Puigserver P, Spiegelman BM: Peroxisome proliferator-activated receptor-gamma coactivator 1 alpha (PGC-1 alpha): Transcriptional coactivator and metabolic regulator. Endocr Rev 24:78–90, 2003.

55. Herzig S, Long F, Jhala US, et al: CREB regulates hepatic gluconeogenesis through the coactivator PGC-1. Nature 413:179–183, 2001.

56. Lin J, Tarr PT, Yang R, et al: PGC-1 beta in regulation of hepatic glucose and energy metabolism. J Biol Chem 278:30843–30848, 2003.

57. Munnich A, Marie J, Reach G, et al: In vivo hormonal control of L-type pyruvate kinase gene expression: Effects of glucagon, cyclic AMP, insulin, cortisone, and thyroid hormones on the dietary induction of mRNAs in the liver. J Biol Chem 259:10228–10231, 1984.

58. Wimhurst JM, Manchester KL: A comparison of the effects of diabetes induced with either alloxan or streptozotocin and of starvation on the activities in rat liver of the key enzymes of gluconeogenesis. Biochem J 120:95–103, 1970.

59. Chan TM: The permissive effects of glucocorticoid on hepatic gluconeogenesis. Glucagon stimulation of glucose-suppressed gluconeogenesis and inhibition of 6-phosphofructo-1-kinase in hepatocytes from fasted rats. J Biol Chem 259:7426–7432, 1984.

60. Chen KS, Lardy HA: 3-Aminopicolinate inhibits phosphoenolpyruvate carboxykinase in hepatocytes and increases release of gluconeogenic precursors from peripheral tissues. J Biol Chem 259:6920–6924, 1984.

61. McGarry JD, Foster DW: Regulation of hepatic fatty acid oxidation and ketone body production. Annu Rev Biochem 49:395–420, 1980.

62. Foster DW: From glycogen to ketones-and back. Diabetes 33:1188–1199, 1984.

63. Williamson JR, Walajtys-Rode E, Coll KE: Effects of branched chain α-ketoacids on the metabolism of isolated rat liver cells: I. Regulation of branched

chain α-ketoacid metabolism. J Biol Chem 254:11511–11520, 1979.

64. Souza SC, Muliro KV, Liscum L, et al: Modulation of hormone-sensitive lipase and protein kinase A-mediated lipolysis by perilipin A in an adenoviral reconstituted system. J Biol Chem 277:8267–8272, 2002.

65. McGarry JD, Woeltje KF, Kuwajima M, et al: Regulation of ketogenesis and the renaissance of carnitine palmitoyltransferase. Diabetes Metab Rev 5:271–284, 1989.

66. Murthy MSR, Pande SV: Mechanism of carnitine acylcarnitine translocase-catalyzed import of acylcarnitines into mitochondria. J Biol Chem 259:9082–9089, 1984.

67. Iacobazzi V, Naglieri MA, Stanley CA, et al: The structure and organization of the human carnitine/acylcarnitine translocase (CACT1) gene2. Biochem Biophys Res Commun 252:770–774, 1998.

68. Sekoguchi E, Sato N, Yasui A, et al: A novel mitochondrial carnitine-acylcarnitine translocase induced by partial hepatectomy and fasting. J Biol Chem 278:38796–38802, 2003.

69. McGarry JD, Leatherman GF, Foster DW: Carnitine palmitoyltransferase I: The site of inhibition of hepatic fatty acid oxidation by malonyl-CoA. J Biol Chem 253:4128–4136, 1978.

70. DiMarco JP, Hoppel C: Hepatic mitochondrial function in ketogenic states: Diabetes, starvation and after growth hormone administration. J Clin Invest 55:1237–1244, 1975.

71. McGarry JD, Brown NF: The mitochondrial carnitine palmitoyltransferase system-from concept to molecular analysis. Eur J Biochem 244:1–14, 1997.

72. McGarry JD, Takabayashi Y, Foster DW: The role of malonyl-CoA in the coordination of fatty acid synthesis and oxidation in isolated rat hepatocytes. J Biol Chem 253:8294–8300, 1978.

73. Esser V, Britton CH, Weis BC, et al: Cloning, sequencing and expression of a cDNA encoding rat liver carnitine palmitoyltransferase I: Proof that a single polypeptide is involved in inhibitor interaction and catalytic function. J Biol Chem 268:5817–5822, 1993.

74. Vega RB, Huss JM, Kelly DP: The coactivator PGC-1 cooperates with peroxisome proliferator-activated receptor alpha in transcriptional control of nuclear genes encoding mitochondrial fatty acid oxidation enzymes. Mol Cell Biol 20:1868–1876, 2000.

75. Herzig S, Hedrick S, Morantte I, et al: CREB controls hepatic lipid metabolism through nuclear hormone receptor PPAR-gamma. Nature 426:190–193, 2003.

76. Louet JF, Hayhurst G, Gonzalez FJ, et al: The coactivator PGC-1 is involved in the regulation of the liver carnitine palmitoyltransferase I gene expression by cAMP in combination with HNF4 alpha and cAMP-response element-binding protein (CREB). J Biol Chem 277:37991–8000, 2002.

77. Wang YX, Lee CH, Tiep S, et al: Peroxisome-proliferator-activated receptor delta activates fat metabolism to prevent obesity. Cell 113:159–170, 2003.

78. Yamashita H, Takenoshita M, Sakurai M, et al: A glucose-responsive transcription factor that regulates carbohydrate metabolism in the liver. Proc Natl Acad Sci U S A 98:9116–9121, 2001.

79. Kabashima T, Kawaguchi T, Wadzinski BE, et al: Xylulose 5-phosphate mediates glucose-induced lipogenesis by xylulose 5-phosphate-activated protein phosphatase in rat liver. Proc Natl Acad Sci U S A 100:5107–5112, 2003.

80. Wu RF, Osatomi K, Terada LS, et al: Identification of Translin/Trax complex as a glucose response element binding protein in liver. Biochim Biophys Acta 1624:29–35, 2003.

81. Yabe D, Komuro R, Liang G, et al: Liver-specific mRNA for Insig-2 down-regulated by insulin: Implications for fatty acid synthesis. Proc Natl Acad Sci U S A 100(6):3155–3160, 2003.

82. Swenson TL, Porter JW: Mechanism of glucagon inhibition of liver acetyl-CoA carboxylase. Interrelationship of the effects of phosphorylation, polymer-protomer transition, and citrate on enzyme activity. J Biol Chem 260:3791–3797, 1985.

83. Hardie DG, Salt IP, Hawley SA, et al: AMP-activated protein kinase: An ultrasensitive system for monitoring cellular energy change. Biochem J 338:717–722, 1999.

84. McGarry JD, Foster DW: Effects of exogenous fatty acid concentration on glucagon-induced changes in hepatic fatty acid metabolism. Diabetes 29:236–240, 1980.

85. Garcia-Villafranca J, Guillen A, Castro J: Involvement of nitric oxide/cyclic GMP signaling pathway in the regulation of fatty acid metabolism in rat hepatocytes. Biochem Pharmacol 65:807–812, 2003.

86. Park H, Kaushik VK, Constant S, et al: Coordinate regulation of malonyl-CoA decarboxylase, sn-glycerol-3-phosphate acyltransferase, and acetyl-CoA carboxylase by AMP-activated protein kinase in rat tissues in response to exercise. J Biol Chem 277:32571–32577, 2002.

87. Ruderman NB, Park H, Kaushik VK, et al: AMPK as a metabolic switch in rat muscle, liver and adipose tissue after exercise. Acta Physiol Scand 178:435–442, 2003.

88. Ruderman N, Flier JS: Chewing the fat—ACC and energy balance. Science 2558–2559, 2001.

89. de Laszlo SE, Hacker C, Li B, et al: Potent, orally absorbed glucagon receptor antagonists. Bioorg Med Chem Lett 9:641–646, 1999.

90. Cascieri MA, Koch GE, Ber E, et al: Characterization of a novel, non-peptidyl antagonist of the human glucagon receptor. J Biol Chem 274:8694–8697, 1999.

91. McGarry JD, Robles-Valdes C, Foster DW: Role of carnitine in hepatic ketogenesis. Proc Natl Acad Sci U S A 72:4385–4388, 1975.

92. Fery F, Balasse EO: Ketone body production and disposal in diabetic ketosis. A comparison with fasting ketosis. Diabetes 34:326–332, 1985.

93. Johnson DD, Palumbo PJ, Chu C-P: Diabetic ketoacidosis in a community-based population. Mayo Clin Proc 55:83–88, 1980.

94. Wetterhal SF, Olson DR, DeStafano F, et al: Trends in diabetes and diabetic complications. Diabetes Care 15:960–967, 1992.

95. Clements RS Jr, Vourganti B: Fatal diabetic ketoacidosis: Major causes and approaches to their prevention. Diabetes Care 1:314–325, 1978.

96. Goto Y, Sato S-I, Masuda M: Causes of death in 3151 diabetic autopsy cases. Tohoku J Exp Med 112:339–353, 1974.

97. Alberti KGMM, Hockaday TDR: Diabetic coma: A reappraisal after five years. Clin Endocrinol Metab 6:421–455, 1977.

98. Morris AD, Boyle DIR, McMahon AD, et al: Adherence to insulin treatment, glycaemic control, and ketoacidosis in insulin-dependent diabetes mellitus. Lancet 350:1505–1510, 1997.

99. Tattersall R: Brittle diabetes. Clin Endocrinol Metab 6:403–419, 1977.

100. Jin H, Meyer JM, Jeste DV: Phenomenology of and risk factors for new-onset diabetes mellitus and diabetic ketoacidosis associated with atypical antipsychotics: An analysis of 45 published cases. Ann Clin Psychiatry 14:59–64, 2002.

101. Tanaka S, Kobayashi T, Nakanishi K, et al: Association of HLA-DQ genotype in autoantibody-negative and rapid-onset type 1 diabetes. Diabetes Care 25:2302–2307, 2002.

102. Imagawa A, Hanafusa T, Uchigata Y, et al: Fulminant type 1 diabetes. Diabetes Care 26:2345–2352, 2003.

103. Cohen AS, Vance VK, Runyan JW Jr, et al: Diabetic acidosis: An evaluation of the cause, course and therapy of 73 cases. Ann Intern Med 52:55–86, 1960.

104. Beigelman PM: Severe diabetic ketoacidosis (diabetic "coma"): 482 episodes in 257 patients; experience of three years. Diabetes 20:490–500, 1971.

105. Kety SS, Polis BD, Nadler CS, et al: The blood flow and oxygen consumption of the human brain in diabetic acidosis and coma. J Clin Invest 27:500–510, 1948.

106. Verdon F, van Melle G, Perret C: Respiratory response to acute metabolic acidosis. Bull Eur Physiopathol Respir 17:223–235, 1981.

107. Ozer G, Teker Z, Cetiner S, et al: Serum IL-1, IL-2, TNFalpha and INFgamma levels of patients with type 1 diabetes

mellitus and their siblings. J Pediatr Endocrinol Metab 16:203–210, 2003.

108. Siperstein MD: Diabetic ketoacidosis and hyperosmolar coma. Endocrinol Metab Clin North Am 21:415–432, 1992.

109. Hockaday TDR, Alberti KGMM: Diabetic coma. Clin Endocrinol Metab 1:751–788, 1972.

110. Robin AP, Ing TS, Lancaster GA, et al: Hyperglycemia-induced hyponatremia: A fresh look. Clin Chem 25:496–497, 1979.

111. Cahill GF, Herrera MG, Morgan AP, et al: Hormone-fuel interrelationships during fasting. J Clin Invest 45:1751–1769, 1966.

112. Owen OE, Morgan AP, Kemp HG, et al: Brain metabolism during fasting. J Clin Invest 46:1589–1595, 1967.

113. Mahoney CA: Extreme gestational starvation ketoacidosis: Case report and review of pathophysiology. Am J Kidney Dis 20:276–280, 1992.

114. Chernow B, Finton C, Rainey TG, et al: "Bovine ketosis" in a nondiabetic postpartum woman. Diabetes Care 5:47–49, 1982.

115. Levy LJ, Duga J, Girgis M, et al: Ketoacidosis associated with alcoholism in nondiabetic subjects. Ann Intern Med 78:213–219, 1973.

116. Wren KD, Slovis CM, Minion GE, et al: The syndrome of alcoholic ketoacidosis. Am J Med 91:119–128, 1991.

117. Owen OE, Licht JH, Sapir DG: Renal function and effects of partial rehydration during diabetic ketoacidosis. Diabetes 30:510–518, 1981.

118. Wilson HK, Keuer SP, Lea AS, et al: Phosphate therapy in diabetic ketoacidosis. Arch Intern Med 142:517–520, 1982.

119. Bellingham AJ, Detter JC, Lenfant C: The role of hemoglobin affinity for oxygen and red-cell 2,3-diphosphoglycerate in the management of diabetic ketoacidosis. Trans Assoc Am Physicians 83:113–120, 1970.

120. Vinicor F, Lehmer LM, Kam RC, et al: Hyperamylasemia in diabetic ketoacidosis: Sources and significance. Ann Intern Med 91:200–204, 1979.

121. Kitabchi AE, Young R, Sacks H, et al: Diabetic ketoacidosis: Reappraisal of therapeutic approach. Annu Rev Med 30:339–357, 1979.

122. Keller U, Berger W: Prevention of hypophosphatemia by phosphate infusion during treatment of diabetic ketoacidosis and hyperosmolar coma. Diabetes 29:87–95, 1980.

123. Adrogue HJ, Barrero J, Eknoyan G: Salutary effect of modest fluid replacement in the treatment of adults with diabetic ketoacidosis. JAMA 262:2108–2113, 1989.

124. Androgue HJ, Wilson H, Boyd WE III, et al: Plasma acid-base patterns in diabetic ketoacidosis. N Engl J Med 307:1603–1610, 1982.

125. Halperin ML, Bear RA, Hannaford MC, et al: Selected aspects of the pathophysiology of metabolic acidosis in diabetes mellitus. Diabetes 30:781–787, 1981.

126. Piters KM, Kumar D, Pei E, et al: Comparison of continuous and intermittent intravenous insulin therapies for diabetic ketoacidosis. Diabetologia 13:317–321, 1977.

127. Usala A-L, Madigan T, Burguera B, et al: Brief report: Treatment of insulin-resistant diabetic ketoacidosis with insulin-like growth factor I in an adolescent with insulin-dependent diabetes. N Engl J Med 327:853–857, 1992.

128. McGarry JD, Foster DW: Regulation of ketogenesis and clinical aspects of the ketotic state. Metabolism 21:471–489, 1972.

129. Fulop M, Murthy V, Michilli A, et al: Serum beta-hydroxybutyrate measurement in patients with uncontrolled diabetes mellitus. Arch Intern Med 159:381–384, 1999.

130. Beigelman PM: Potassium in severe diabetic ketoacidosis. Am J Med 54:419–420, 1973.

131. Carroll P, Matz R: Uncontrolled diabetes mellitus in adults: Experience in treating diabetic ketoacidosis and hyperosmolar nonketotic coma with low-dose insulin and a uniform treatment regimen. Diabetes Care 6:579–585, 1983.

132. Malone JI, Brodsky SJ: The value of electrocardiogram monitoring in diabetic ketoacidosis. Diabetes Care 3:543–547, 1980.

133. Matz R: Diabetic acidosis: Rationale for not using bicarbonate. N Y State J Med 76:1299–1303, 1976.

134. Narins RG, Cohen JJ: Bicarbonate therapy for organic acidosis: The case for its continued use. Ann Intern Med 106:615–618, 1987.

135. Lever E, Jaspan JB: Sodium bicarbonate therapy in severe diabetic ketoacidosis. Am J Med 75:263–268, 1983.

136. Green SM, Rothrock SG, Ho JD, et al: Failure of adjunctive bicarbonate to improve outcome in severe pediatric diabetic ketoacidosis. Ann Emerg Med 31:41–48, 1998.

137. Foster DW: Diabetic ketoacidosis. In Krieger DT, Bardin CW (eds): Current Therapy in Endocrinology and Metabolism. Toronto, BC Decker, 1985, pp 268–270.

138. Connell FA, Louden JM: Diabetes mortality in persons under 45 years of age. Am J Public Health 73:1174–1177, 1983.

139. Bryan CS, Reynolds KL, Metzger WT: Bacteremia in diabetic patients: Comparison of incidence and mortality with nondiabetic patients. Diabetes Care 8:244–249, 1985.

140. Winegrad AI, Kern EFO, Simmons DA: Cerebral edema in diabetic ketoacidosis. N Engl J Med 312:1184–1185, 1985.

141. Rosenbloom AL: Intracerebral crises during treatment of diabetic ketoacidosis. Diabetes Care 13:22–33, 1990.

142. Marcin JP, Glaser N, Barnett P, et al: Factors associated with adverse outcomes in children with diabetic ketoacidosis-related cerebral edema. J Pediatr 141:793–797, 2002.

143. Arieff AL, Kleeman CR: Studies on mechanisms of cerebral edema in diabetic comas: Effects of hyperglycemia and rapid lowering of plasma glucose in normal rabbits. J Clin Invest 52:571–583, 1973.

144. Fein IA, Rackow EC, Sprung CL, et al: Relation of colloid osmotic pressure to arterial hypoxemia and cerebral edema during crystalloid volume loading of patients with diabetic ketoacidosis. Ann Intern Med 96:570–574, 1982.

145. Krane EJ, Rockoff MA, Wallman JK, et al: Subclinical brain swelling in children during treatment of diabetic ketoacidosis. N Engl J Med 312:1147–1151, 1985.

146. Durr JA, Hoffman WH, Sklar AH, et al: Correlates of brain edema in uncontrolled IDDM. Diabetes 41:627–632, 1992.

147. Clements RS Jr, Blumenthal SA, Morrison AD, et al: Increased cerebrospinal-fluid pressure during treatment of diabetic ketosis. Lancet 2:671–675, 1971.

148. Franklin B, Liu J, Ginsberg-Fellner F: Cerebral edema and ophthalmoplegia reversed by mannitol in a new case of insulin-dependent diabetes mellitus. Pediatrics 69:87–90, 1982.

149. Carlotti AP, Bohn D, Halperin ML: Importance of timing of risk factors for cerebral oedema during therapy for diabetic ketoacidosis. Arch Dis Child 88(2):170–173, 2003.

150. Artis WM, Fountain JA, Delcher HK, et al: A mechanism of susceptibility to mucormycosis in diabetic ketoacidosis: Transferrin and iron availability. Diabetes 31:1109–1114, 1982.

151. Weprin BE, Hall WA, Goodman J, et al: Long-term survival in rhinocerebral mucormycosis. Case report. J Neurosurg 88:570–575, 1998.

152. Timperley WR, Preston FE, Ward JD: Cerebral intravascular coagulation in diabetic ketoacidosis. Lancet 1:952–956, 1974.

153. McLaren EH, Cullen DR, Brown MJ: Coagulation abnormalities in diabetic coma before and 24 hours after treatment. Diabetologia 17:345–349, 1979.

154. Paton RC: Haemostatic changes in diabetic coma. Diabetologia 21:172–177, 1981.

155. Pasi KJ, Enayat MS, Horrocks PM, et al: Qualitative and quantitative abnormalities of von Willebrand antigen in patients with diabetes mellitus. Thromb Res 59:581–591, 1990.

156. Kwaan HC, Colwell JA, Suwanwela N: Disseminated intravascular coagulation in diabetes mellitus, with reference to the role of increased platelet

aggregation. Diabetes 21:108–113, 1972.

157. Tschoepe D, Rauch U, Schwippert B: Platelet-leukocyte-cross-talk in diabetes mellitus. Horm Metab Res 29:631–635, 1997.

158. Maiello M, Boeri D, Podesta F, et al: Increased expression of tissue plasminogen activator and its inhibitor and reduced fibrinolytic potential of human endothelial cells cultured in elevated glucose. Diabetes 41:1009–1015, 1992.

159. Takahashi K, Ghatei MA, Lam H-C: Elevated plasma endothelin in patients with diabetes mellitus. Diabetologia 33:306–310, 1990.

160. Saenz de Tejada I, Goldstein I, Azadzoi K, et al: Impaired neurogenic and endothelium-mediated relaxation of penile smooth muscle from diabetic men with impotence. N Engl J Med 320:1025–1030, 1989.

161. Hogan M, Cerami A, Bucala R: Advanced glycosylation end products block the antiproliferative effect of nitric oxide. J Clin Invest 90:1110–1115, 1992.

162. Carl GF, Hoffman WH, Passmore GG, et al: Diabetic ketoacidosis promotes a prothrombotic state. Endocr Res 29:73–82, 2003.

163. Sobel BE, Neimane D, Mack WJ, et al: The ratio of plasminogen activator inhibitor type-1 activity to the concentration of plasminogen activator inhibitor type-1 protein in diabetes: Adding insult to injury. Coron Artery Dis 13:275–281, 2002.

164. Lapolla A, Piarulli F, Sartore G, et al: Peripheral artery disease in type 2 diabetes: The role of fibrinolysis. Thromb Haemost 89:91–96, 2003.

165. He G, Pedersen SB, Bruun JM, et al: Metformin, but not thiazolidinediones, inhibits plasminogen activator inhibitor-1 production in human adipose tissue in vitro. Horm Metab Res 35:18–23, 2003.

166. Carroll P, Matz R: Adult respiratory distress syndrome complicating severely uncontrolled diabetes mellitus: Report of nine cases and a review of the literature. Diabetes Care 5:574–580, 1982.

167. Foster DW: Insulin deficiency and hyperosmolar coma. Adv Intern Med 19:159–173, 1974.

168. Vinik A, Seftel H, Joffe BI: Metabolic findings in hyperosmolar, nonketotic diabetic stupor. Lancet 2:797–798, 1970.

169. Lindsey CA, Faloona GR, Unger RH: Plasma glucagon in nonketotic hyperosmolar coma. JAMA 229:1771–1773, 1974.

170. Gerich JE, Martin MM, Recant L: Clinical and metabolic characteristics of hyperosmolar nonketotic coma. Diabetes 20:228–238, 1971.

171. Arieff Al, Carroll HJ: Nonketotic hyperosmolar coma with hyperglycemia: Clinical features, pathophysiology, renal function, acid-base balance, plasma-cerebrospinal fluid equilibria and the effects of therapy in 37 cases. Medicine (Baltimore) 51:73–94, 1972.

172. Knowles HC Jr: Syrupy blood. Diabetes 15:760–761, 1966.

173. Podolsky S: Hyperosmolar nonketotic coma: Death can be prevented. Geriatrics 34:29–33, 36–37, 41–42, 1979.

174. McKenna K, Morris AD, Azam H, et al: Exaggerated vasopressin secretion and attenuated osmoregulated thirst in human survivors of hyperosmolar coma. Diabetologia 42:534–538, 1999.

175. Yen TT, Stamm NB, Fuller RW, et al: Hepatic insensitivity to glucagon in ob/ob mice. Res Commun Chem Pathol Pharmacol 30:29–40, 1980.

176. Azain MJ, Fukuda N, Chao F-F, et al: Contributions of fatty acid and sterol synthesis to triglyceride and cholesterol secretion by the perfused rat liver in genetic hyperlipemia and obesity. J Biol Chem 260:174–181, 1985.

177. Begin-Heick N: Absence of the inhibitory effect of guanine nucleotides on adenylate cyclase activity in white adipocyte membranes of the ob/ob mouse: Effect of the ob gene. J Biol Chem 260:6187–6193, 1985.

178. Scott CR, Smith JM, Cradock MM, et al: Characteristics of youth-onset noninsulin-dependent diabetes mellitus and insulin-dependent diabetes mellitus at diagnosis. Pediatrics 100:84–91, 1997.

179. Umpierrez GE, Clark WS, Steen MT: Sulfonylurea treatment prevents recurrence of hyperglycemia in obese African-American patients with a history of hyperglycemic crises. Diabetes Care 20:479–483, 1997.

180. Mahtani MM, Widen E, Lehto M, et al: Mapping of a gene for type 2 diabetes associated with an insulin secretion defect by a genome scan in Finnish families. Nat Genet 14:90–94, 1996.

181. Cervin C, Orho-Melander M, Ridderstrale M, et al: Characterization of a naturally occurring mutation (L1071) in the HNF1 alpha (MODY3) gene. Diabetologia 45:1703–1708, 2002.

182. Lehto M, Tuomi T, Mahtani MM, et al: Characterization of the MODY3 phenotype. Early-onset diabetes caused by an insulin secretion defect. J Clin Invest 99:582–591, 1997.

183. Yamada S, Nishigori H, Onda H, et al: Identification of mutations in the hepatocyte nuclear factor (HNF)-1α gene in Japanese subjects with IDDM. Diabetes 46:1643–1647, 1997.

184. Pontoglio M, Sreenan S, Roe M, et al: Defective insulin secretion in hepatocyte nuclear factor 1α-deficient mice. J Clin Invest 101:2215–2222, 1998.

185. Hani EH, Suaud L, Boutin P, et al: A missense mutation in hepatocyte nuclear factor-4α, resulting in a reduced transactivation activity, in human late-onset non-insulin-dependent diabetes mellitus. J Clin Invest 101:521–526, 1998.

186. Goldman SL: Hyperglycemic hyperosmolar coma in a 9-month-old child. Am J Dis Child 133:181–183, 1979.

187. McCurdy DK: Hyperosmolar hyperglycemic nonketotic diabetic coma. Med Clin North Am 54:683–699, 1970.

188. Maccario M, Messis CP, Vastola EF: Focal seizures as a manifestation of hyperglycemia without ketoacidosis: A report of seven cases with review of the literature. Neurology 15:195–206, 1965.

189. Guisado R, Arieff AI: Neurologic manifestations of diabetic comas: Correlation with biochemical alterations in the brain. Metabolism 24:665–679, 1975.

190. Maccario M: Neurological dysfunction associated with nonketotic hyperglycemia. Arch Neurol 19:525–534, 1968.

191. Daugirdas JT, Kronfol NO, Tzamaloukas AH: Hyperosmolar coma: Cellular dehydration and the serum sodium concentration. Ann Intern Med 110:855–857, 1989.

192. Bewsher PD, Petrie JC, Worth HGJ: Serum lipid levels in hyperosmolar non-ketotic diabetic coma. Br Med J 3:82–84, 1970.

193. Rosenthal NR, Barrett EJ: An assessment of insulin action in hyperosmolar hyperglycemic nonketotic diabetic patients. J Clin Endocrinol Metab 60:607–610, 1985.

194. Maccario M, Messis CP: Cerebral edema complicating treated nonketotic hyperglycemia. Lancet 2:352–353, 1969.

195. Scharf Y, Nahir M, Tatarsky I, et al: Fatal venous thrombosis in hyperosmolar coma. Diabetes 20:308–309, 1971.

196. Schlepphorst E, Levin ME: Rhabdomyolysis associated with hyperosmolar nonketotic coma. Diabetes Care 8:198–200, 1985.

CHAPTER

62

Hypoglycemia

John E. Gerich

Hypoglycemia itself is not a disease. It is a biochemical sign indicating that some condition has caused an imbalance between rates of release of glucose into the circulation and rates of glucose removal from the circulation such that removal exceeds release. This process can occur under various circumstances, for example, when increased rates of glucose release are accompanied by even greater increases in glucose utilization (e.g., marathon running) or when subnormal rates of glucose utilization are accompanied by even greater reductions in glucose release (e.g., starvation, adrenal insufficiency). These abnormal relative changes in glucose supply and demand can occur for a variety of reasons: (1) excess insulin availability (e.g., overdose in insulin-treated diabetic patients, insulinoma, sulfonylurea administration), (2) decreased counterregulatory hormone secretion (pancreatectomy, adrenal insufficiency, hypopituitarism), and (3) inability of target tissues of counterregulatory hormones to respond normally (e.g., alcohol ingestion, renal insufficiency, nonselective β-adrenergic blocker therapy), or, more usually, a combination of these factors (e.g., sepsis). Table 62-1 lists common causes of hypoglycemia in adults. With the few but common exceptions (e.g., drug-induced, factitious, iatrogenic, and reactive hypoglycemia), hypoglycemia usually signifies a serious underlying medical disorder whose cause, if it is not obvious, must be investigated and treated.

Hypoglycemia in adults that requires hospital admission or causes death is not uncommon.[1,2] It has been reported to account for 0.4% of all acute medical admissions.[3] A review of nearly 50,000 autopsies in an acute-care medical center found that 0.2% of deaths were due to hypoglycemia.[4] Of adverse drug reactions requiring hospital admission, hypoglycemia was the fourth most common cause.[5] Among hospitalized patients, the incidence of hypoglycemia is 1% to 2%,[6,7] but it is associated with a mortality rate as high as 48% depending on comorbidities.[6-9]

Most clinicians would agree that an appropriately obtained venous plasma glucose level below 50 mg/dL (~2.8 mmol/L) in an overnight (12 to 14 hours) fasted adult should be considered suspicious for hypoglycemia. Such a glucose concentration would represent a value below the lowest percentile, inasmuch as the normal range in most clinical laboratories using glucose oxidase or hexokinase methods is 70 to 100 mg/dL (3.6 to 6.1 mmol/L).[10] It is important to note that whole-blood determinations are about 10% to 15% lower than plasma determinations. Therefore, the lower limit of normal for whole-blood venous glucose would be about 60 mg/dL (3.5 mM). It is becoming more common in hospital wards and in clinics to use glucose meters that measure capillary blood glucose. In the postabsorptive state, capillary samples yield values that are 15% lower than venous samples.[11] Such might not be the case after a meal or glucose ingestion, when venous samples can be as much as 30 to 40 mg/dL (2.0 to 2.5 mmol/L) lower than capillary samples.[11,12] Under these conditions, venous sampling can give the false appearance of a hypoglycemic condition when in fact the arterial glucose concentration is normal. Because of this limitation and for other reasons, values that are obtained under conditions other than an overnight fast can be difficult to interpret. For example, plasma glucose values during an oral glucose tolerance test (OGTT) can normally decrease below 40 mg/dL (~2.2 mmol/L), be asymptomatic, and not reflect a pathologic process,[13] whereas postprandial symptoms develop in some people who have plasma glucose levels in the normal range. Moreover, after prolonged exercise, values between 30 and 50 mg/dL (1.7 to 2.8 mmol/L) have commonly been observed in perfectly normal individuals.[14] In summary, the circumstances under which the plasma glucose value is obtained will influence its interpretation and the action to be taken. Consequently, in evaluating a patient for suspected hypoglycemia, the overnight (14 to 16 hours) fasted venous plasma glucose value represents the standard frame of reference, and a value below 50 mg/dL (~2.8 mM) deserves evaluation.

One must always be aware that an apparently low blood glucose level can result from unintentional artifacts or mistakes (artifactual hypoglycemia).[15] These artifactually low glucose readings can be caused by improper sample collection, inadequate storage, or errors in analytic methods. Samples that are not to be immediately measured should be collected in tubes containing fluoride and/or oxalate to inhibit glycolysis by red and white blood cells; otherwise, blood glucose levels can decrease 10 to 20 mg/dL (~0.5 to 1.0 mmol/L) per hour at room temperature, irrespective of the initial value.[16] Even in the presence of inhibitors of glycolysis, artifactually low glucose concentrations can be obtained when blood contains a large amount of cells, such as in patients with

1203

Table 62-1 Causes of Hypoglycemia in Adults

Drugs (accidental, factitious)
  Especially insulin, sulfonylureas, meglitinides, alcohol
Critical illness
  Renal, hepatic, and heart disease; sepsis; malnutrition
Endocrine deficiency
  Adrenal > pituitary > thyroid
Overproduction of insulin or insulin-like material
  Insulin-producing islet tumor, non–β cell tumors
Other
  Pregnancy, strenuous exercise, autoimmune syndromes, reactive
    hypoglycemia
Iatrogenic (dialysis, total parenteral nutrition)

leukemia,[17,18] leukemoid reactions,[19,20] polycythemia vera,[21,22] and hemolytic crisis with excessive circulating nucleated red cells.[23]

Use of plasma rather than serum can lead to fibrin occlusion of some automated analyzers. Faulty calibration, outdated reagents, use of fluoride or other preservatives that can interfere with certain methods, and failure to remove triglycerides from lipemic samples can all lead to artifactually low glucose values. In the latter situation, which can result in underestimations of up to 15%, electrolytes and other serum elements will also be reduced.

PHYSIOLOGY OF GLUCOSE HOMEOSTASIS

GENERAL CONSIDERATIONS: SYMPTOMS OF HYPOGLYCEMIA

Judgment regarding the significance of a low plasma glucose level and its possible etiology requires knowledge of normal glucose homeostasis and the factors that are involved in its regulation.

Normally, plasma glucose values are maintained within a relatively narrow range throughout the day (usually between 55 and 165 mg/dL, or ~3.0 and 9.0 mmol/L) despite wide fluctuations in delivery (e.g., meals) and removal (e.g., exercise) of glucose from the circulation. Teleologically, hyperglycemia is to be avoided because of its adverse macrovascular and microvascular effects.[24-26] Indeed, individuals with impaired glucose tolerance (i.e., those with postprandial plasma glucose levels between 140 and 199 mg/dL [7.8 to 11.0 mmol/L]) have a severalfold increased risk of cardiovascular disease.[27]

Hypoglycemia is to be avoided to protect the brain and prevent cognitive dysfunction. Because of limited availability of alternative fuels (e.g., ketone bodies) or their transport across the blood-brain barrier (e.g., free fatty acids), glucose can be considered to be the sole source of energy for the brain except under conditions of prolonged fasting, in which case ketone bodies and other substrates may be used.[28] It has long been thought that the brain cannot store appreciable amounts of glycogen or produce glucose and is therefore dependent on glucose in plasma for adequate functioning and ultimate survival. The apparent K_m for transport of glucose across the blood-brain barrier of ~3 mM indicates that at physiologic plasma glucose levels, phosphorylation of glucose (K_m ~50 μM) is rate limiting for its utilization.[29] However, during hypoglycemia, because of the kinetics of the transfer of glucose across the blood-brain barrier, uptake becomes rate limiting.

However, recent studies using nuclear magnetic resonance (NMR) spectroscopy[29-31] indicate that the brain can contain substantially more glycogen than previously thought (up to 10 μmol/g). This has been calculated to be able to supply most of the glucose deficit during hypoglycemia for ~100 min.[30] Most of brain glycogen is contained in glial cells, which,

under appropriate stimuli, release it as lactate that is then taken up by neurons and used as a fuel.[30] Consistent with this schema are studies in humans that have shown that infusions of lactate attenuate symptoms and counterregulatory hormone responses during hypoglycemia.[32] Following recovery from hypoglycemia, there is a rebound increase in brain glycogen content that, because of relatively low glucose cycling, can take several weeks to return to normal.[30] This phenomenon has been proposed as one mechanism to explain development of hypoglycemia unawareness[33] after an episode of hypoglycemia.[34]

A characteristic hierarchy of responses occurs as plasma glucose levels decrease[35,36] (Fig. 62-1). A decrement of as little as 20 mg/dL (~1.1 mmol/L) can reduce brain glucose uptake, suppress insulin secretion, and trigger counterregulatory hormone release at approximately 72 mg/dL (4.0 mmol/L). Under normal physiologic conditions, this response prevents a further decrease in the plasma glucose concentration and restores normoglycemia. Decreases of 30 mg/dL (1.7 mmol/L) to approximately 60 mg/dL (3.4 mmol/L) usually evoke the so-called autonomic warning symptoms[37,38] (hunger, anxiety, palpitations, sweating, warmth, and nausea), which, if interpreted correctly, lead a person to eat and prevent more serious hypoglycemia. However, clues of hypoglycemia can vary considerably from person to person.[39] If for some reason plasma glucose levels decrease to about 55 mg/dL (~3.0 mmol/L), the so-called neuroglycopenic signs/symptoms of brain dysfunction can develop (blurred vision, slurred speech, glassy-eyed appearance, confusion, and difficulty concentrating).[37,38] Cognitive impairment and electroencephalographic changes are demonstrable at this plasma glucose level. Decreases below 40 mg/dL (~2.5 mmol/L) result in sleepiness and gross behavioral (e.g., combativeness) abnormalities. Further decreases can produce coma, and values below 30 mg/dL (~1.6 mmol/L), if prolonged, can cause seizures, permanent neurologic deficits, and death. In individuals with underlying cardiovascular disease, life-threatening arrhythmia, myocardial infarction, and stroke can be precipitated.[40-48] Furthermore, there is evidence that repetitive episodes of severe hypoglycemia can have long-term structural[49] and behavioral effects, especially in children.[50]

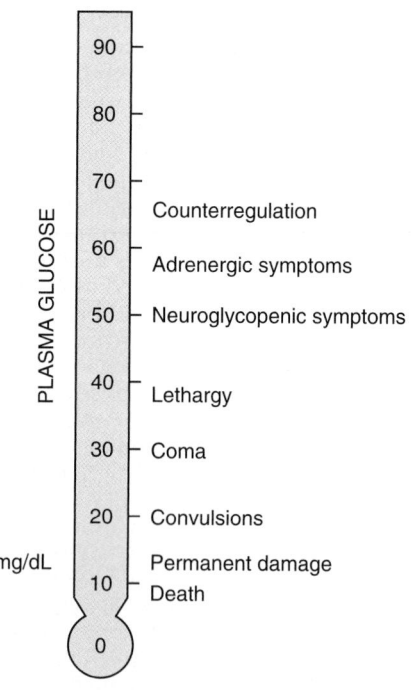

Figure 62-1 Hierarchy of responses to decrements in plasma glucose.

Nevertheless, lest an excessive fear of hypoglycemia lead to too conservative management of diabetes mellitus, it should be pointed out that in otherwise healthy, young (<45 years) individuals, plasma glucose levels averaging 35 mg/dL (~2.0 mmol/L) have been maintained for as long as 8 hours without any severe long-term adverse effects,[51] and chronic levels as low as 24 mg/dL (1.3 mmol/L) in patients with insulinoma have been observed in association with apparently normal cerebral function.[52]

Patients with diabetes mellitus or insulinoma and even normal individuals who have experienced repetitive episodes of hypoglycemia will have an increase in the thresholds (require greater hypoglycemia) for initiation of counterregulatory hormone release and autonomic warning symptoms and signs of neuroglycopenia.[33] The pathophysiology of this phenomenon, called hypoglycemia unawareness, is multifactorial; implicated have been an adaptation in the transport of glucose across the blood-brain barrier,[53] alterations in brain glycogen content,[29] and a reduction in peripheral tissue β-adrenergic sensitivity.[54,55] Conversely, diabetic patients who are under poor glycemic control can experience hypoglycemic symptoms and activation of counterregulation at higher than normal plasma glucose levels (reduced thresholds), apparently for similar reasons.[56] In addition, the signs, symptoms, and sequelae of hypoglycemia can be affected by factors such as age,[57-59] gender,[60-62] medication (e.g., nonselective β-blockers[63]), and associated medical conditions (e.g., pregnancy,[64] autonomic neuropathy[65,66]). However, contrary to common belief, experimental evidence convincingly indicates that the rate of decrease in plasma glucose has no effect on either symptoms or counterregulatory hormone responses.[67,68]

GLUCOSE HOMEOSTASIS IN THE POSTABSORPTIVE STATE

Glucose Utilization
After a 14- to 16-hour overnight fast, the so-called postabsorptive state, plasma glucose concentrations average about 80 to 90 mg/dL (4.5 to 5.0 mmol/L) and are relatively stable. Consequently, rates of release of glucose into the circulation must closely approximate rates of glucose removal and generally average about 10 μmol/kg/min (Fig. 62-2). Although this situation is considered to represent a steady state, actually it is a pseudo-steady state, with rates of glucose removal that slightly and often undetectably exceed rates of glucose release into the circulation; if fasting is prolonged, plasma glucose levels gradually decrease, and by 20 to 24 hours of fasting, they can be 10% to 15% lower (i.e., 72 to 80 mg/dL, 4.0 to 4.5 mmol/L). However, even after 72 hours of fasting, they are usually still above 50 mg/dL (2.8 mmol/L).[69] The latter observation forms the basis of the 72-hour fast to exclude an insulinoma.[70]

In the postabsorptive overnight fasted state, most glucose use by the body is due to uptake by the brain (~50% to 70%); skeletal muscle (~15% to 20%), kidney (~10% to 15%), blood cells (~5% to 10%), splanchnic organs (3% to 6%), and adipose tissue (~2% to 4%)[71] account for the remainder. Most of the body's energy requirement is met by oxidation of free fatty acids, which compete with glucose as the fuel of choice in certain organs (e.g., skeletal muscle, heart, and the kidney).[72] Because glucose uptake by the brain, blood cells, renal medulla, and splanchnic tissues can be considered to be essentially independent of insulin and because plasma insulin levels are usually low in the postabsorptive state (<15 μU/mL, 90 pmol/L), most of the glucose that is removed from the circulation in the postabsorptive state is determined by tissue demands, the mass action effects of the plasma glucose concentration per se, and the number and characteristics of the glucose transporters in specific tissues rather than by insulin. Under these conditions, insulin can be viewed as largely playing a permissive role, and counterregulatory hormones that

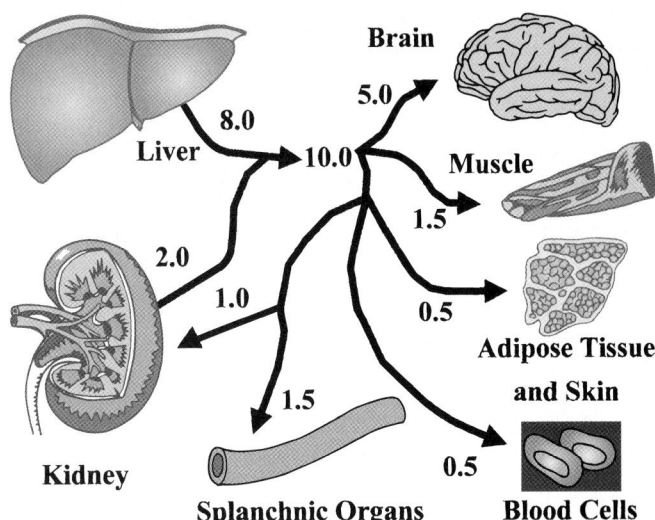

Figure 62-2 Glucose utilization and production in the postabsorptive state. The liver and kidney contribute approximately 8.0 and 2.0 mmol/kg/min, respectively, to the total release of glucose into the circulation (10 μmol/kg/min); the brain, splanchnic tissue, muscle, adipose tissue and skin, and blood cells account for approximately 5.0, 2.0, 1.5, 0.5, and 0.5 mmol/kg/min, respectively.

antagonize the actions of insulin (e.g., cortisol, growth hormone, epinephrine, and thyroid hormone) can be viewed as modulating the sensitivity of tissues insofar as the effects of insulin on tissue glucose uptake and utilization are concerned.

Glucose Production
Glucose release into the circulation, however, is under considerably more regulation by both hormone and nonhormonal mechanisms (see Fig. 62-2). Although many tissues contain enzymes to break down glycogen to glucose-6-phosphate (glycogenolysis) and/or synthesize glucose-6-phosphate from glycerol, lactate, and amino acids (gluconeogenesis), only the liver and kidney contain enough glucose-6-phosphatase to make significant amounts of free glucose available for release. Until recently, it was thought that the liver was the sole source of glucose entering the circulation except during acidosis and after prolonged fasting. However, recent studies in humans and dogs, as well as in the earlier literature of in situ and in vitro preparations, now indicate that both the liver and kidney release glucose under physiologic conditions.[73]

The liver is responsible for 80% to 85% of the glucose that is released in the postabsorptive state.[73] Under these conditions, approximately 50% of all the glucose that is released into the circulation is due to glycogenolysis, the remainder (~5.0 μmol/kg/min) being due to gluconeogenesis.[74] The proportion stemming from gluconeogenesis rapidly increases with the duration of fasting as glycogen stores become depleted; 48 hours after the last meal, gluconeogenesis accounts for nearly 80%, and by 72 hours, it accounts for essentially all of the glucose released into the circulation.[69,74] The liver releases glucose by glycogenolysis and gluconeogenesis. The kidney normally contains little glycogen, and renal cells that could make glycogen lack glucose-6-phosphatase. Consequently, all the glucose that is released by the kidney can be considered to be the result of gluconeogenesis.[73] Thus, although the liver releases about four times as much glucose as the kidney under postabsorptive conditions, both organs release about the same amount (~2.5 μmol/kg/min) as a result of gluconeogenesis.

Release of glucose by liver and kidney is regulated differently. Insulin suppresses glucose release by both organs (by direct effects on enzyme activation/deactivation and by indirect actions such as limitation of gluconeogenic substrate availability and gluconeogenic activators, for example, suppression of free fatty acids and glucagon).[75] Glycogenolysis is more sensitive to suppression by insulin than is gluconeogenesis.[76] Hyperglycemia and insulin suppress glycogenolysis via different mechanisms; the former suppresses phosphorylase, whereas the latter stimulates glycogen synthase.[77] However, glucagon, which increases both glycogenolysis and gluconeogenesis in the liver, has no effect on the kidney,[78] whereas epinephrine, which can directly activate hepatic glycogenolysis, appears to increase glucose release predominantly by directly stimulating renal gluconeogenesis and to a lesser extent by increasing the availability of gluconeogenic precursors/activators.[79,80]

The major precursors for gluconeogenesis are lactate, glycerol, and various amino acids.[71] The liver and kidney differ somewhat in their use of these substrates in that alanine is preferentially used by the liver, whereas glutamine is used predominantly in the kidney.[80] Most of the amino acids that are released from protein via proteolysis are converted to glutamine and alanine for transport through plasma to the liver and kidney.[81]

Insulin, glucagon, and catecholamines (norepinephrine released postsynaptically in the abundantly innervated liver and kidney and epinephrine released from the adrenal medulla) are the most important moment-to-moment glucoregulatory hormones. Physiologic changes in their circulating levels are able to change glucose release in a matter of minutes. Other important glucoregulatory factors, such as growth hormone, cortisol, and thyroid hormone, take hours for their effects to become evident. Their effects are mediated through changes in the sensitivity of the kidney and liver to insulin, glucagon, and catecholamines by altering the amount of key enzymes, glycogen stores, and availability of circulating precursors/activators of gluconeogenesis. Increases in circulating free fatty acids augment hepatic and renal glucose release by affecting the activity of key gluconeogenic enzymes and by providing the necessary ATP and reducing equivalents.[72,82,83]

Deficiencies of counterregulatory hormones, excesses of insulin, and an inability to store or mobilize glycogen/gluconeogenic precursors can result in hypoglycemia in the postabsorptive state.

GLUCOSE HOMEOSTASIS IN THE POSTPRANDIAL STATE

Complete assimilation of the constituents of a mixed meal containing fat, protein, and carbohydrate and restoration of the postabsorptive state takes 5 to 6 hours.[84] After ingestion of a pure carbohydrate load, assimilation is generally complete within 4 to 5 hours. Despite these differences, little evidence indicates that the fate of ingested carbohydrate is markedly different under the two conditions.[84]

Various factors can affect the extent of circulating glucose excursions after meal ingestion, such as the time and degree of physical activity since the last meal, the composition and form of glucose (liquid versus solid), the rate of gastric emptying, digestion within the lumen of the small intestine, absorption into the portal vein, extraction by the liver, suppression of endogenous glucose release, and, finally, the uptake, storage, oxidation, and glycolysis of glucose in posthepatic tissues.[85]

From a practical point of view, one can consider the major factors influencing postprandial glucose homeostasis to be those that affect suppression and restoration of endogenous glucose release and those that affect hepatic and posthepatic tissue glucose disposal. Recent studies using dual-isotope approaches (to measure splanchnic sequestration, i.e., first-pass hepatic uptake, endogenous glucose release, and total glucose appearance into and disappearance from the systemic circula-

tion) in conjunction with measurements of net balance across the limbs and the kidney have provided insight into the fate of an ingested glucose load.[84,86,87] The dual-isotope approach also makes it possible to quantitate the disposal of glucose molecules in plasma originating from the ingesta as opposed to endogenous molecules.[88]

After ingestion of 100 g of glucose, plasma glucose levels increase to a peak between 60 and 90 minutes usually not exceeding 170 mg/dL (9 mmol/L) and gradually return to or slightly below postabsorptive values by 3 to 4 hours. Plasma insulin concentrations follow a similar profile and average only about twofold to threefold the basal values (30 to 40 µU/mL, 180 to 240 pmol/L) during this period. Plasma glucagon concentrations change in reciprocal pattern and are generally suppressed about 50% during the interval. It is the early changes in insulin and glucagon secretion, that is, those occurring during the initial 90 minutes, that are most important.[89,90]

It is worth reemphasizing that changes in plasma glucose concentrations occur as a result of the relative changes in rates of release and removal of glucose. During the first 80 to 100 minutes, rates of glucose release into the systemic circulation exceed rates of removal; consequently, plasma glucose levels increase. Rates of glucose removal from plasma parallel those of glucose release but are shifted in time. After about 80 to 100 minutes, rates of removal exceed rates of glucose release; consequently, plasma glucose concentrations decrease. Rates of glucose release into plasma represent the sum of glucose escaping first-pass splanchnic (hepatic) extraction and the residual release of endogenous glucose by the liver and kidney. Release of ingested glucose into the systemic circulation is detected as early as 15 minutes, reaches a peak at 80 to 120 minutes, and gradually decreases thereafter. Release of endogenous glucose by the liver decreases rapidly and is suppressed nearly 80% during the 4- to 5-hour postprandial period. In contrast, endogenous renal glucose release is not suppressed and actually increases.[91] Teleologically, this arrangement would permit more complete suppression of hepatic glucose release and facilitate more efficient glycogen replenishment.[92]

The tissues that are responsible for disposal of a hypothetic 100-g oral glucose load are shown in Figure 62-3. About a third of the ingested glucose is initially extracted by splanchnic tissues and can presumably be attributed to hepatic glycogen

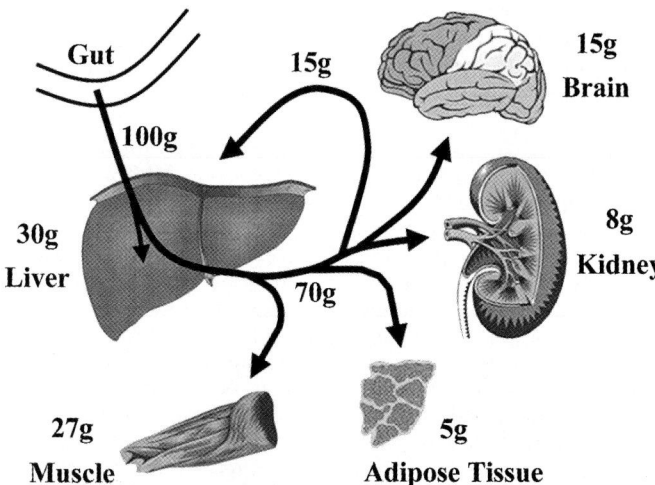

Figure 62-3 Postprandial glucose disposal. Of 100 g glucose ingested, about 30% is taken up by the liver, and 70% is released into the systemic circulation. Of this 70 g, 15 g (~20%) is extracted by the liver, 15 g (~20%) is taken up by the brain, 27 g (~40%) is taken up by skeletal muscle, and the remaining 20% is taken up by kidney, adipose tissue, skin, and blood cells.

formation.[86] Of the remaining glucose that enters the systemic circulation, skeletal muscle (35% to 45%), brain (~20% to 30%), kidney (10% to 15%), and adipose tissue (5% to 10%) are quantitatively the most important and account for over 90% of the initial posthepatic glucose disposal.[92]

Glucose that is taken up by tissues postprandially initially can undergo essentially only two fates: glycolysis and storage. About two thirds of glucose that is disposed of initially undergoes glycolysis, and about one third is stored.[88] Of the glucose undergoing glycolysis, about two thirds is oxidized, and one third is released into the circulation as gluconeogenic precursors, for example, lactate, alanine, glutamine, and pyruvate. Normally, about half of these precursors are released into plasma glucose; the other half are incorporated into hepatic glycogen via the so-called indirect pathway.[88]

Normally, three factors predominate in regulating postprandial glucose excursions: suppression of endogenous glucose release, initial hepatic glucose extraction, and posthepatic glucose uptake. Suppression of endogenous glucose release and initial hepatic glucose extraction are largely dependent on the coordinated reciprocal secretion of insulin and glucagon, in particular, the early release of insulin.[89] Seventy percent to 80% of posthepatic glucose uptake occurs in insulin-sensitive tissues, and it can be readily concluded that insulin plays a major role in this process via its action to increase glucose transport; for example, skeletal muscle glucose fractional extraction, an index of the efficiency of glucose uptake, increases about threefold, whereas glucose fractional extraction by the brain, an insulin-sensitive tissue, actually decreases.

Another factor to be considered, which can represent an indirect effect of insulin, is postprandial suppression of lipolysis with a consequent decrease in circulating free fatty acid concentrations. This response would decrease the availability of a promoter of hepatic glucose release and a competitor to glucose as a metabolic fuel. For example, recent studies using NMR to measure glycogen accumulation in skeletal muscle have demonstrated that during the initial 2 hours after meal ingestion, when skeletal muscle glucose is markedly increased, no net accumulation of glycogen occurs in skeletal muscle.[93] This finding has been attributed to the use of the glucose that is taken up as an oxidative fuel in place of free fatty acids. Moreover, prevention of the normal postprandial decrease in plasma free fatty acids has been shown to reduce postprandial suppression of endogenous glucose release.[94]

Reestablishment of postabsorptive conditions after meal ingestion requires reversal of the repression of hepatic glucose release and the return of increased rates of renal glucose release and peripheral tissue glucose removal. Such an adjustment not only involves a decrease in insulin secretion, but also increases in the secretion of glucagon and other counterregulatory hormones.[95] Failure of these changes to occur can result in postprandial hypoglycemia. Venous plasma glucose levels often decrease below fasting values, sometimes to values as low as 36 mg/dL (2.0 mmol/L) after the ingestion of glucose, such as during an OGTT; the hypoglycemia is often asymptomatic and is not observed when the same individuals ingest a meal.[96] Thus, the OGTT should *never* be used in the workup of hypoglycemia. Postprandial hypoglycemia can occur with most of the pathologic conditions that cause fasting hypoglycemia. However, hypoglycemia that is observed solely after meal ingestion is generally seen only in individuals who have had gastric surgery or small bowel disease or in those who are taking medications that affect glucose counterregulation.

GLUCOSE COUNTERREGULATION

Glucose counterregulation refers to the sum of the body's defense mechanisms that prevent hypoglycemia from occurring and restore euglycemia if hypoglycemia should occur. Similar processes appear to be involved in the postprandial and postabsorptive states and can largely be accounted for by suppression of insulin secretion and stimulation of the release of counterregulatory hormones.[95] Our knowledge of counterregulation has accumulated over the past 30 years through studies in which pharmacologic blockade of the secretion or action of individual counterregulatory hormones has been produced during standardized insulin-induced hypoglycemia,[97] and alterations have been found in diabetes mellitus, insulinoma, and aging.

Insulin administration suppresses both hepatic and renal glucose release[98,99] and stimulates glucose uptake. As plasma glucose levels decrease, endogenous secretion of insulin is suppressed (as manifested by a decrease in circulating C peptide levels), and an increase is noted in the secretion of counterregulatory hormones (glucagon, epinephrine, growth hormone, and cortisol) and the activity of the autonomic nervous system (as manifested by increases in circulating norepinephrine and pancreatic polypeptide levels).[100] Depending on the dose of insulin that is administered, these increases in counterregulatory hormone release can be sufficient to prevent a further decrease in plasma glucose and restore euglycemia after the effect of insulin has waned.

This effect is brought about mainly by the actions of glucagon and epinephrine to increase the release of glucose into the circulation. The greater the doses of insulin, the more plasma glucose levels decrease and the longer is the recovery period. Under such conditions, counterregulation now includes the effects of epinephrine, growth hormone, and cortisol to counteract the actions of insulin to increase tissue glucose uptake. As was indicated earlier, a characteristic hierarchy of responses is seen to decrease in plasma glucose levels. Of all the counterregulatory hormones, glucagon and epinephrine are the most important.[101] Patients with type 1 diabetes or pancreatectomized individuals who lack a glucagon response are up to 25 times more prone to severe hypoglycemia than are those with normal glucagon responses.[102] Glucagon acts to increase hepatic glucose release, initially via glycogenolysis and later mainly via gluconeogenesis.[103] Catecholamines act by several mechanisms: (1) increasing hepatic glycogenolysis, (2) directly increasing renal gluconeogenesis, (3) inhibiting insulin-stimulated glucose uptake as well as insulin release, and (4) augmenting lipolysis, which via increases in circulating free fatty acids can also impair tissue glucose uptake and stimulate gluconeogenesis.[104-106] Growth hormone and cortisol have late effects of suppressing insulin-mediated tissue glucose uptake and augmenting release of glucose into the circulation.[101,107] Lack of these late effects is clinically important, as is evidenced by the propensity of hypopituitary patients to the development of hypoglycemia (see below).

HYPOGLYCEMIC DISORDERS IN THE ADULT

DRUG-INDUCED HYPOGLYCEMIA

Drugs, as a result of unintentional and intentional overdoses (e.g., insulin, sulfonylureas) or toxic reactions causing hepatic failure (acetaminophen) or malfunction (alcohol), are the most common cause of hypoglycemia[2,108] (Table 62-2). Seltzer has reviewed all cases of severe drug-induced hypoglycemia reported from 1940 through 1988.[109] Insulin, sulfonylureas, and alcohol alone or in combination accounted for over 70% of cases. The incidence of severe hypoglycemia (defined as that resulting in coma or requiring external assistance) from insulin treatment in patients with type 1 diabetes being managed to achieve optimal glycemic control in the Diabetes Control and Complications Trial averaged about 60 episodes per 100 patient-years.[110] The incidence in comparably well-controlled patients with type 2 diabetes being treated with insulin is

Table 62-2 Drug-Induced Hypoglycemia
Drugs that are capable of causing hypoglycemia by themselves
Antidiabetes drugs
Insulin
Sulfonylureas
Benzoic acid derivatives (meglitinide)
Other
Alcohol
Salicylates
Propranolol
Pentamidine
Sulfonamides
Vacor rodenticide
Quinine/quinidine
Propoxyphene
Para-aminobenzoic acid
Perhexiline
Drugs that probably cause hypoglycemia only in combination with insulin/sulfonylurea/benzoic acid derivatives or under special circumstances (e.g., malnutrition, infection, renal insufficiency)
Biguanides
Angiotensin-converting enzyme
Phenylbutazone
Lidocaine
Warfarin (Coumadin)
Ranitidine, cimetidine
Doxepin
Danazol
Azopropazone
Oxytetracycline
Clofibrate, benzofibrate
Colchicine
Ketoconazole
Chloramphenicol
Haloperidol
Monoamine oxidase inhibitors
Thalidomide
Orphenadrine
Selegiline
Abenzolene
Flecainide
Fluoxitine
Chlomipramine
Indomethicin
Chloroquine

considerably lower (~3 to 6 episodes per 100 patient years).[30,111–113] The incidence of severe hypoglycemia as a result of sulfonylurea stimulation of insulin secretion in patients with type 2 diabetes is approximately 1.5 cases per 100 patient-years.[114]

Several factors can explain the difference in the incidence of severe hypoglycemia in patients with type 1 and type 2 diabetes. The most important of these is that patients with type 1 diabetes have more severe defects in counterregulation and no residual β-cell function. Those with type 1 diabetes of long-standing duration have markedly reduced glucagon and epinephrine responses, whereas those with type 2 diabetes have moderate decreases in glucagon responses, but increased epinephrine responses can compensate in most instances owing to operation of hepatorenal reciprocity.[115] Moreover, residual β-cell function in type 2 diabetes permits decreases in the availability of insulin during hypoglycemia. (Recall that hypoglycemia suppresses insulin secretion.) In contrast, patients with type 1 diabetes must rely on the biologic half-life of the injected insulin to decrease insulin availability.

Alcohol might be a more common cause of severe hypoglycemia in the United States than sulfonylureas,[109] although exact statistics are lacking. Alcohol can cause hypoglycemia in overnight fasting normal volunteers,[116,117] with plasma glucose values as low as 5 mg/dL (0.3 mmol/L)[118] and mortality rates ranging from 10% in adults to 25% in children.[119] In a

series of deaths caused by hypoglycemia, alcohol was the most common etiologic agent.[4] The most common situation is a glycogen-depleted state, such as occurs in an individual who drinks after a considerable fast or who drinks and then fasts. In the latter situation, blood alcohol levels can be low or undetectable.

Alcohol induces hypoglycemia by inhibiting gluconeogenesis[118]; as little as 50 g might be sufficient.[119,120] Its mechanism of action is complex, with evidence of impaired counterregulatory hormone responses[117] and impaired uptake of gluconeogenic precursors,[121] but the predominantly accepted mechanism is its inhibition of the gluconeogenic process stemming from an increased reduced nicotinamide adenine dinucleotide (NADH)/NAD ratio as a result of the oxidation of alcohol to acetaldehyde and acetate, thus reducing the ability of the liver and kidney to oxidize lactate and glutamate to pyruvate and α-ketoglutarate, respectively.[122–124] Although plasma insulin levels are appropriately suppressed in this condition, because of this inhibition of gluconeogenesis, glucagon and catecholamines are ineffective in increasing glucose release and raising plasma glucose levels.[103] Thus, in a patient with suspected alcohol-induced hypoglycemia, oral or intravenous glucose is the treatment of choice.

Only about 10% of the reported cases of drug-induced hypoglycemia have occurred without concomitant insulin, sulfonylurea, or alcohol.[125] Of these, propranolol,[126] sulfonamides,[127] and salicylates[109] have been most frequently reported. Propranolol and other nonselective β-blockers decrease the ability of the liver and kidney to increase their release of glucose,[105,106] enhance peripheral insulin sensitivity,[128] and mask symptoms of impending hypoglycemia. The adverse effect of β-adrenergic β-blockers are mediated through β₂-receptors. Recent studies indicate that β₁-selective blockers do not present an increased risk for severe hypoglycemia and therefore should not be considered as being contraindicated in diabetic patients.[129,130]

Salicylates can act by inhibiting hepatic glucose release and increasing insulin secretion, although their exact mechanism remains to be determined.[131] Sulfonamides probably act by stimulating insulin release in a manner similar to that of sulfonylureas. Angiotensin-converting enzyme inhibitors[132–134] and pentamidine[132,135,136] are being reported more frequently, with increases in their use in diabetic subjects and AIDS patients, respectively. Angiotensin-converting enzyme inhibitors can increase tissue insulin sensitivity[137] and can decrease the degradation of bradykinin, which has certain insulin-mimetic actions.[138] Pentamidine is cytotoxic to pancreatic β cells, and hypoglycemia occurs with the release of insulin from the degenerating cells, often with subsequent permanent diabetes mellitus.[136] Many of the drugs listed in Table 62-1 have been reported to cause hypoglycemia only in association with the use of antidiabetic medications or have been the subject of isolated case reports, and their etiologic significance remains to be established. However, their use in a patient with otherwise unexplained hypoglycemia should be discontinued whenever possible.

Risk factors for insulin-induced hypoglycemia include errors in dosage, skipped or delayed meals, uncompensated physical activity, hypoglycemia unawareness, aging, the duration of diabetes, the degree of glycemic control, concomitant medications (e.g., nonselective β-blockers), and associated disorders, such as renal failure.[112] Aging and the duration of diabetes are believed to exert their effect mainly as a consequence of deterioration in counterregulatory defense mechanisms (e.g., loss of glucagon response, autonomic neuropathy). In addition to these factors, the frequency of sulfonylurea-induced and benzoic acid derivative–induced hypoglycemia depends on the particular sulfonylurea that is used, the highest incidence being associated with the longest acting and most potent (e.g., glyburide > chlorpropamide > glipizide, repaglinide, glimepiride > nateglinide).[139–141] For other drugs that are implicated in causing hypoglycemia, restricted food intake, age, hepatic disease, and renal disease are often involved. Therefore, one of the first steps in the workup of a patient who is suspected of having hypoglycemia is to document medications, which includes actually checking that pills match prescriptions because errors can be made in filling prescriptions.[142,143]

SEPSIS, TRAUMA, AND BURNS

Severe infection and trauma elicit physiologic responses[144] (sodium and water retention with an expanded extracellular space, tachycardia, increased cardiac output, increased pulmonary ventilation, fever, and activation of various inflammatory processes) that result in an insulin-resistant hypermetabolic state characterized by increased resting energy expenditure, excessive fat and protein catabolism, negative nitrogen balance, increased glucose turnover, and progressive loss of body cell mass.[145,146] Increases in the secretion of classic stress hormones (glucagon, epinephrine, growth hormone, and cortisol), activation of the sympathetic nervous system, various cytokines (tumor necrosis factor-α, interleukin-2, and interleukin-6), oxygen free radicals, prostanoids, leukotrienes, and endothelins are involved in mediating these responses.[144,147-150] The net effect of these changes is to shift glucose utilization toward non-insulin-sensitive tissues (e.g., inflammatory cells) with a greater proportionate use of anaerobic glycolysis, a less energetically efficient pathway than oxidative phosphorylation.[151]

Hypoglycemia, if it occurs, usually results from failure of the liver and kidney to compensate for increased glucose utilization; it rarely develops in trauma or burn patients in the absence of infection[152] but, when it occurs, is usually associated with hypotension and acidosis.[153]

Initially, the response to the stress of infection is an increase in glucose turnover, with glucose production often exceeding glucose utilization and resulting in mild hyperglycemia. This response involves increases in both glycogenolysis and gluconeogenesis and is largely mediated by glucagon[154] because adrenergic blockade has no effect on glucose turnover.[155] As the infection worsens, increased release of endotoxin and its derivatives, complement activation, endoperoxide activation, and release of endogenous inflammatory mediators (tumor necrosis factor-α, interleukins, and other monokines) compromise cardiovascular integrity and cause central venous pooling, inadequate tissue perfusion, and microvascular protein transudation.[156] At this stage, a decrease in splanchnic and renal blood flow occurs. Despite concomitantly reduced peripheral tissue perfusion, glucose utilization is increased.[157-159] Decreased tissue oxygenation causes increased anaerobic glycolysis, which perpetuates the increased glucose utilization because anaerobic glycolysis is a less energetically efficient pathway than oxidative phosphorylation. Increased lactate release by peripheral tissues exceeds increases in lactate uptake by the liver and kidney and results in lactic acidosis.[160,161]

The inability of glucose release to keep pace with increased tissue demands is due to a failure of gluconeogenesis. Hepatic glycogen stores are rapidly exhausted; consequently, glucose release becomes solely dependent on gluconeogenesis. At this point, glucose release is largely driven by activation of the sympathetic nervous system and hypercortisolemia.[162,163] Although splanchnic and renal blood flow is reduced, the impaired gluconeogenesis cannot be ascribed to decreased substrate delivery or uptake or to decreased concentrations of counterregulatory stress hormones.[156] Even after in situ perfusion of the liver and kidneys to ensure the presence of adequate oxygen and precursors, animals in experimental endotoxin shock exhibit diminished gluconeogenesis.[164] In vivo, hormonal stimulation of glucose production is reduced as much as 50%.[162,165,166] Factors such as acidosis (which

inhibits hepatic gluconeogenesis), increased intracellular calcium (which impairs mitochondrial function and inhibits gluconeogenic enzymes), and siphoning of available energy from gluconeogenesis to support ion transport might be involved.

Appropriate management entails (1) treatment of the underlying infection, (2) restoration of normal peripheral perfusion, and (3) glucose infusion to satisfy tissue demands.

CARDIAC FAILURE

Spontaneous hypoglycemia can occur with severe heart failure[167-169]; it is rare in adults but not uncommon in infants and children,[170] in whom reduced hepatic glycogen levels (but normal phosphorylase and glucose-6-phosphatase activity) have been found in liver biopsy specimens and attributed to the poor dietary intake and gastrointestinal malabsorption that are present in cardiac failure. This predilection of young children to the development of hypoglycemia under these conditions might relate to immaturity of gluconeogenic processes and a limited supply of gluconeogenic precursors (e.g., glycerol and amino acids because of limited adipose tissue and muscle mass, respectively).

Mellinkoff and Tumulty first described the hypoglycemia of cardiac failure and attributed it to associated hepatic disease.[171] However, chronic lung disease with right and left heart failure is seen in most patients.[169] Thus, hypoxemia and low cardiac output may produce hepatic ischemia. Marks and Rose postulated that decreased availability of oxygen would suppress gluconeogenesis by increasing hepatic anaerobic glycolysis (Pasteur effect) and lactate production and thereby result in a decreased NAD/NADH ratio.[172] This decreased ratio could compromise gluconeogenesis because NAD is an essential cofactor for several of the enzymatic steps of gluconeogenesis. This attractive hypothesis could explain the association between hypoglycemia and the lactic acidosis of cardiac[173] and liver[174] disease, as well as the hypoglycemia accompanying other conditions associated with tissue anoxia, such as sepsis and shock.[153] Low cardiac output would be expected to limit substrate delivery to the kidneys. In addition to a reduced capacity to produce glucose, increased glucose utilization from increased anaerobic glycolysis and increased energy demands from labored breathing and malnutrition (anorexia) are probably additionally important factors. At the present time, no evidence indicates that abnormal counterregulatory hormone responses play a role in the pathogenesis of the hypoglycemia associated with these conditions.

RENAL AND HEPATIC DISEASE: GENERAL CONSIDERATIONS

The liver and kidneys are the only organs that are capable of releasing glucose into the circulation, inasmuch as other tissues generally lack or have minimal amounts of the enzyme glucose-6-phosphatase. Consequently, it would not be surprising that patients with hepatic or renal disease should be prone to hypoglycemia. Nevertheless, it is uncommon for hypoglycemia to occur simply as a result of loss of mass or function of these organs, and when it does occur, the etiology is usually multifactorial.[118,175] The large capacities of these organs to release glucose into the circulation and their ability to compensate for each other's shortcomings appear to provide an explanation for this phenomenon.

Normally, the liver accounts for 80% to 85% of all glucose released into the circulation; it can increase its output (initially mainly by glycogenolysis, later by gluconeogenesis) over a sustained period by twofold to threefold (at least for several days, as exemplified by burn patients[162]). Thus, hypoglycemia with an appropriate compensatory increase in hepatic glucose release would be unlikely to develop in anephric individuals because the kidney normally contributes only 15% to 20% of all glucose that is released into the circulation. On the other hand, the kidney can also increase its output over a prolonged period by twofold to threefold, as exemplified in humans who have fasted for several weeks.[176] Animal and human studies indicate that the kidney can acutely increase its output to compensate for decreased hepatic glucose release and vice versa,[115,177,178] a phenomenon that is referred to as hepatorenal reciprocity.[179] For example, during the anhepatic phase of human liver transplantation, the kidney can maintain normoglycemia without a need for exogenous glucose.[180] Thus, hypoglycemia would be unlikely to develop in patients with hepatic disease until the liver's capacity to release glucose were reduced beyond the ability of the kidney to compensate. In fact, animal studies indicate that more than 80% of the liver must be removed for hypoglycemia to occur.[181]

Liver Disease

Although hypoglycemia has been associated with a wide range of liver diseases (hepatocellular carcinoma, cirrhosis, fatty metamorphosis, and toxic and infectious hepatitis, cholangitis, and biliary obstruction), its occurrence is actually quite uncommon in the absence of other complicating factors (i.e., infection).[118,172] For example, Zimmerman and coworkers found fasting hypoglycemia levels of 60 mg/dL (3.3 mmol/L) or less in only 6 of 269 patients with a variety of liver diseases.[182] As was indicated earlier, this low figure probably results from the liver's large capacity for gluconeogenesis and the kidney's ability to compensate.[177,178,183] In humans, the insult to hepatic function must be acute, or the loss of parenchyma must be widespread. Felig and coworkers found that about 25% (4 of 15) of patients with acute viral hepatitis had a fasting blood glucose level less than 50 mg/dL (2.8 mmol/L).[184] In chronic liver disease associated with hypoglycemia, additional factors are usually involved, such as malnutrition and infection. A 50% incidence of hypoglycemia was found in patients with liver disease associated with sepsis and circulatory collapse.[185,186] In such situations, liver function tests might not parallel the severity of hypoglycemia. Infiltrative diseases such as metastatic disease, amyloidosis, sarcoidosis, and hemachromatosis rarely replace sufficient parenchyma to cause hypoglycemia.[187]

The hypoglycemia associated with liver disease can be viewed to result from failure of the kidney to compensate for a reduction in hepatic glucose output to maintain an adequate output of glucose.[179] In various liver diseases, the livers' ability to store glycogen and activate gluconeogenesis can be impaired markedly. Thus, in patients with viral hepatitis,[184] the hyperglycemic response to glucagon, a potent stimulator of glycogenolysis, was impaired, and the usual glucagon-mediated decrease in the gluconeogenic precursors glycine and alanine was reduced. Sepsis and anoxia can impair the ability of the kidney to compensate in the face of increased energy demands. Hyperinsulinemia often accompanies hepatic disease as a consequence of decreased insulin degradation by the liver,[188] but the hypoglycemia of hepatic disease is almost always accompanied by appropriate suppression of plasma insulin concentrations.[184] Likewise, little evidence has been found to implicate overproduction of insulin-like growth factors (IGFs) by the liver. Gorden and colleagues reported one patient with hemangiopericytoma of the liver in their series of 52 patients with extrapancreatic tumors, hypoglycemia, and IGFs, but no excessive IGFs were associated with primary hepatocellular carcinoma, the hepatic neoplasm most frequently associated with hypoglycemia.[189]

Renal Disease

Except in infants, hypoglycemia rarely occurs with acute renal failure. However, with chronic renal failure, hypoglycemia is not uncommon in adult patients. It can occur as an isolated event or be repetitive. In general, neuroglycopenia rather than autonomic symptoms predominate.[175]

Although it has long been recognized that uremia reduced the insulin requirement in diabetic humans,[190] it was not until 1970 that Block and Rubenstein reported three diabetic patients with renal failure who had suffered severe hypoglycemia after insulin and sulfonylurea therapy had been stopped.[191] Shortly afterward, spontaneous hypoglycemia associated with renal failure was described in nondiabetic patients,[192-195] with an incidence of 1% to 3% in two large studies.[195,196]

The etiology of the renal hypoglycemia is complex.[175,197] Many factors predispose uremic patients to hypoglycemia, including altered drug metabolism, delayed gastric emptying, malnutrition, infection, dialysis, increased insulin sensitivity, associated hepatic and cardiac disease, and impaired renal and hepatic glucose release. Drugs are probably the most common immediate cause. Any drug that can cause hypoglycemia is more likely to do so in a uremic patient because of a prolonged half-life (e.g., insulin, certain sulfonylureas, especially chlorpropamide) or decreased protein binding secondary to hypoalbuminuria.[198] Although hypoglycemia occurs in nondiabetic as well as diabetic patients with renal failure, it is more likely to occur in the latter because of the use of hypoglycemic agents and because patients with long-standing diabetes have autonomic neuropathy and defects in glucose counterregulation. Most patients have been malnourished, although it has been reported in well-nourished patients.[193] Malnutrition secondary to anorexia or vomiting, which can reduce hepatic glycogen stores and the availability of gluconeogenic precursors, is a common feature that increases the risk for hypoglycemia.[199] Consistent with this finding is the low rate of glucose appearance and conversion of the gluconeogenic precursor alanine to glucose in a uremic patient studied by Garber and coworkers.[200] In that patient, the plasma concentration and turnover rate of alanine were both reduced, which led to speculation that reduced availability of gluconeogenic substrates was responsible for the hypoglycemia. Because alanine is not a renal gluconeogenic precursor, impaired hepatic compensation is implied. However, other investigators were unable to increase the plasma glucose concentration in a similarly uremic patient with administration of the gluconeogenic precursors alanine and glycerol and concluded that it was not a deficiency in gluconeogenic substrate but rather suppression of gluconeogenesis by a uremic toxin, perhaps simply acidosis.[195]

Fatal hypoglycemia can occur with either peritoneal dialysis or hemodialysis when high glucose–containing dialysate is used because of exaggerated insulin release in conjunction with impaired renal insulin degradation.[201] Other factors such as the use of glucose-deficient solutions in diabetic patients and loss of alanine during hemodialysis may contribute to the development of hypoglycemia.[202,203]

Although the use of glucose-lowering dialysis and associated conditions that might impair the release of glucose are usually present in uremic patients who become hypoglycemic, there are still a fair number of well-documented cases in which hypoglycemia has been attributed solely to the uremic condition.[191,193-195,200,204-209] These cases suggest that renal failure per se predisposes to the development of hypoglycemia. Most evidence points to diminished glucose release rather than increased glucose utilization. Impaired glycogenolytic responses to exogenous glucagon,[193,210] gluconeogenesis in response to infused alanine, glycerol, and galactose,[195] reduced plasma glucagon responses during hypoglycemia,[211] increased insulin sensitivity,[212] and alanine deficiency have all been reported. Malnutrition and acidosis should diminish hepatic glycogenolytic and gluconeogenic potential.[168,204,206,213,214] The expected compensatory increase in renal gluconeogenesis in response to acidosis would be compromised by loss of renal mass and exacerbated by inappropriate plasma insulin levels caused by reduced renal insulin degradation.

COUNTERREGULATORY HORMONE DEFICIENCIES

As was indicated earlier, glucagon, catecholamines, growth hormone, and cortisol are the key glucose counterregulatory hormones. Deficiencies in the release of each of these hormones (and thyroid hormone[215]) can lead to hypoglycemia because of failure to maintain sufficient rates of glucose release into the circulation. However, except in patients with long-standing diabetes mellitus, their deficiency is rarely a cause of hypoglycemia because of two factors[216]: the uncommon occurrence (rare in some cases) of deficiencies of these hormones and the fact that to a large extent a deficiency of one hormone can be compensated for by actions of other hormones, such as in the case of patients with long-standing type 1 diabetes and pancreatectomized individuals, in whom catecholamines mainly compensate for deficient glucagon secretion.

Glucagon Deficiency

Prevention of glucagon responses during insulin-induced hypoglycemia results in greater and more prolonged hypoglycemia.[97] Pancreatectomized individuals, patients with long-standing type 1 diabetes, and those in whom insulin-requiring diabetes develops as a result of chronic pancreatitis are glucagon deficient[217] and quite prone to severe hypoglycemia during treatment of their diabetes.[102] An imbalance between insulin and glucagon secretion (relative glucagon deficiency) has been reported in reactive postprandial hypoglycemia.[218] Because of the incidence of these disorders, glucagon might represent the most common counterregulatory hormone deficiency. Otherwise, however, the condition is extremely rare, with only two poorly substantiated cases of neonatal hypoglycemia[219,220] and two cases in adults.[221,222]

Catecholamine Deficiency

Patients with long-standing type 1 diabetes mellitus, adrenalectomized individuals, and those with autonomic neuropathy have impaired catecholamine responses during insulin-induced hypoglycemia,[97,223,224] but their increased risk for hypoglycemia can be compensated for by increases in the secretion of other counterregulatory hormones, in particular, glucagon.[225] Subtle defects in recovery from hypoglycemia have been demonstrated when such compensatory increases have been experimentally prevented.[104] However, if glucagon responses to hypoglycemia are simultaneously impaired (e.g., in the type 1 diabetic patient), the risk for hypoglycemia markedly increases.[102]

Several cases of neonatal ketotic hypoglycemia and one case in a 5-year-old boy have been attributed to epinephrine deficiency on the basis of low urinary epinephrine excretion.[226,227] No cases of hypoglycemia secondary to isolated catecholamine deficiency in an adult have been reported. The hypoglycemia that occurs with propranolol might relate to the drug's inhibition of lipolysis, which would reduce gluconeogenesis, an important counterregulatory process, and would promote increased glucose clearance by peripheral tissues.[105]

Nevertheless, it is important to note that acute hypoglycemia can occur during surgical removal of a pheochromocytoma, presumably because of disinhibition of insulin release and abrupt withdrawal of the anti-insulin actions of catecholamines.[228]

Cortisol and Growth Hormone Deficiency

Although cortisol and growth hormone have been demonstrated to contribute independently to glucose counterregulation via their actions to promote glucose release and limit glucose uptake,[101,107,229,230] hypoglycemia does not develop in most adults who lack these hormones. Serious hypoglycemia often develops in infants and children who lack these hormones, especially after a period of fasting or during an intercurrent illness.[230–234] In a review of 76 adults with isolated adrenocorticotropic hormone (ACTH) deficiency,[235] only 24 (~33%) had hypoglycemia. During prolonged fasting (6 days), adult growth hormone–deficient dwarfs become hypoglycemic,[236] as can hypopituitary pregnant women.[237] On the other hand, overnight fasting plasma glucose levels have been reported to be normal in glucocorticoid-withdrawn patients with primary adrenal insufficiency[238] or panhypopituitarism.[239] Acute adrenal insufficiency such as in Sheehan's syndrome can be manifested as severe hypoglycemia,[240] and autoimmune Addison's disease may be the cause of severe recurrent hypoglycemia in a patient with type 1 diabetes mellitus.[241]

It is important to be aware that malabsorption of glucocorticoids can occur in patients with bowel disease and patients treated with drugs such as bile acid sequestrants.[242]

MALNUTRITION AND INANITION

Simple caloric restriction, even for prolonged periods, does not usually result in hypoglycemia in adults[28,176,243–245] because of several metabolic adaptations: As glucose release into the circulation decreases (secondary to exhaustion of hepatic glycogen stores and reduction of the availability of gluconeogenic amino acids to the liver and kidney), the brain and other tissues increase their use of free fatty acids and ketone bodies, and glycerol becomes an important gluconeogenic precursor. For example, during the Bengal famine of 1943 to 1945, about 6% of 400 people sampled had blood glucose levels below 40 mg/dL (2.2 mmol/L).[246] Nevertheless, in unusual conditions (e.g., anorexia nervosa,[247–250] kwashiorkor,[251] muscular atrophies[252]), hypoglycemia can occur. In these instances, preexisting malnutrition, which might limit the availability of gluconeogenic precursors (glycerol from adipose tissue and amino acids from muscle), predisposes to the development of hypoglycemia during fasting.[253] More commonly, however, poor nutrition is an important contributing factor to the development of hypoglycemia, such as is seen in renal failure, sepsis, severe heart failure, and liver disease.

AUTOIMMUNE HYPOGLYCEMIA

Of the two types of autoimmune hypoglycemia, one is due to autoantibodies against the insulin receptor, and the other is due to autoantibodies against insulin itself in individuals who have never received exogenous insulin. Both are rare and can produce fasting as well as postprandial reactive hypoglycemia—primarily the former.[254–262]

Anti-Insulin Receptor Antibodies

Fewer than 20 patients have been reported in whom hypoglycemia developed as a result of antibodies directed against the insulin receptor. These antibodies act as agonists and produce hypoglycemia the same way that insulin does. Most of the patients have had evidence of other conditions associated with altered immunity (systemic lupus erythematosus, scleroderma, primary biliary cirrhosis, immune thrombocytopenic purpura, celiac disease, Hashimoto's thyroiditis, and Hodgkin's lymphoma).[258] Some patients have had severe insulin resistance as a result of the antibodies blocking the insulin receptor before the antibodies became agonists. Patients with this condition have low circulating insulin and C peptide levels, normal IGF-1, and appropriate counterregulatory hormone responses.

Although experience is limited, antibody titers generally decrease over time, and remission eventually occurs in most patients. However, because of the severity of the hypoglycemia, aggressive treatment is indicated. High-dose glucocorticoids,[263,264] plasmapheresis,[265] and alkylating agents[266] have all been tried with variable success.

Anti-Insulin Antibody Hypoglycemia

Since 1970 approximately 200 cases of anti-insulin antibody hypoglycemia have been reported, nearly 90% occurring in Japanese patients.[255] Associated autoimmune disorders and plasma cell dyscrasias are common (Graves' disease, rheumatoid arthritis, polymyositis, and systemic lupus erythematosus). The use of certain drugs (hydralazine, procainamide, penicillamine, interferon-α, and methimazole) has been implicated in initiating the syndrome.[258]

Postprandial hypoglycemia is more common with this syndrome than is fasting hypoglycemia. Circulating insulin levels are increased and C peptide levels might not be suppressed as they are in patients who are taking insulin surreptitiously. The hypoglycemia occurs because dissociation of insulin from the antibodies causes prolonged hyperinsulinemia. Unlike the other syndrome of autoimmune hypoglycemia, the course of this condition is benign and self-limited, remission usually occurring within a year. Simple interventions such as frequent small meals with a low content of simple sugars often suffice.

PREGNANCY

Despite a decrease in insulin sensitivity and an increase in glucose turnover to accommodate the needs of the fetus, fasting plasma glucose levels are normally 10% to 15% lower during the third trimester of pregnancy.[267,268] Nevertheless, a great number of metabolic changes occur during pregnancy to make a woman more vulnerable to hypoglycemia.[269] Any condition that can cause hypoglycemia in a nonpregnant woman can do it in a pregnant woman. In addition to insulinoma,[270,271] non–islet cell tumors,[272] severe infection,[273] poor nutrition,[274] drug-induced sources (e.g., insulin in diabetic patients), and a condition called the HELLP syndrome (characterized by hemolysis, elevated liver enzymes, and a low platelet count) can cause hypoglycemia as a result of fulminating hepatic dysfunction.[275-277]

EXERCISE

Hypoglycemia can develop after prolonged strenuous exercise and has been reported in marathon runners,[278] in normal volunteers after exercise on a bicycle ergometer for 3 hours at 56% of maximal capacity,[279] and in a healthy male subject taking a β-blocker after skiing 15 km in 2 hours.[280] Although coma developed in the latter instance, most instances of exercise-associated hypoglycemia are asymptomatic, self-limited, and readily reversed by carbohydrate.[245]

The increased fuel demands of the working muscle necessitate compensatory metabolic processes in the liver and kidney.[281-284] Changes in hepatic glycogenolysis and gluconeogenesis have been found to be closely coupled to the increase in glucose uptake by the working muscle because of the actions of the pancreatic hormones.[281] The exercise-induced increase in glucagon secretion and the concomitant decrease in insulin secretion interact to stimulate hepatic glycogenolysis, whereas the increase in hepatic gluconeogenesis is determined primarily by glucagon's action to increase hepatic gluconeogenic precursor fractional extraction and the efficiency of intrahepatic conversion to glucose. On the other hand, no evidence has shown that hepatic innervation is essential for the rise in hepatic glucose production. Epinephrine becomes important in increasing glucose production during prolonged or heavy exercise, when its levels are particularly high. It can produce this effect by directly stimulating renal glucose release, by increasing the availability of gluconeogenic precursors, and by increasing lipolysis.

It is important to recognize that hypoglycemia can occur with prolonged strenuous exercise (moderate activity in diabetic patients or in nondiabetic patients taking β-blockers) lest an unnecessary diagnostic workup be initiated.

FACTITIOUS HYPOGLYCEMIA

Factitious hypoglycemia refers to a situation in which an individual intentionally attempts to create the impression of the presence of a hypoglycemic disorder.[15,285,286] This also includes diabetic individuals who falsify their self-glucose monitoring or who overdose or underdose themselves to intentionally create the impression of either better than actual glycemic control or brittle diabetes[287,288] and in cases of child abuse.[12] Generally excluded are inadvertent sulfonylurea ingestion (see drug-induced hypoglycemia), homicides,[12,289] suicide attempts (of which only 97 have been reported through 1989[290,291]), and substance abuse in which the additional use of insulin or sulfonylureas is intended to "obtain a high" rather than to create the impression of a hypoglycemic disorder.[292-294] These situations can nevertheless present diagnostic challenges.

Since 1947, more than 80 cases of insulin-induced or sulfonylurea-induced factitious hypoglycemia have been described in the literature[285,295-298] (Table 62-3), but the condition is probably more common than this figure would indicate because most cases go unreported. Indeed, in a survey from the United Kingdom, it was estimated that 12% of cases of spontaneous hypoglycemia referred for investigation were in fact probably factitious.[299] In nearly all instances, the individuals have had diabetes; have been a relative, spouse, or friend of a diabetic patient; or were in the medical or paramedical profession. Thus, factitious hypoglycemia should be suspected in individuals or their relatives who have unexplained hypoglycemia and knowledge of and/or access to insulin, sulfonylureas, or meglitinides[300] and unexplained hypoglycemia. Such patients have generally been healthy women younger than 50 years of age who have an underlying psychological disorder. Because the main differential diagnosis is insulinoma, it is important to consider this condition as a possible cause of unexplained hypoglycemia to avoid unnecessary laboratory workup, which such patients have undergone.

Previously, autoimmune hypoglycemia was a possibility because of the presence of insulin antibodies in patients who are taking animal or impure insulin. Currently, the use of human insulin does not generally result in antibody production, so autoimmune hypoglycemia is no longer a major consideration. Because the main differential is insulinoma, most patients with this condition should undergo a 72-hour fast. Those in whom hypoglycemia develops as a result of surreptitious insulin injection will have inappropriate plasma insulin levels and a suppressed plasma C peptide level (because of inhibition of endogenous insulin secretion). This finding is diagnostic. Patients taking sulfonylureas or a meglitinide will have inappropriate plasma insulin and C peptide levels because of stimulation of endogenous insulin secretion, and this pattern will mimic that seen in insulinoma patients. However, these conditions can be distinguished by a positive urine or plasma assay for sulfonylureas and meglitinides. It is important that samples be collected during hypoglycemia or as close as possible to the event and that they be analyzed by a laboratory with a sufficiently sensitive assay.[289]

Table 62-3 Factitious Insulin-Induced and Sulfonylurea-Induced Hypoglycemia

Hypoglycemia	Number of Cases
Insulin-induced	
Diabetics[285,287,295,296,438–441]	39
Nondiabetics[285,291,295]	30
Secretogogue-induced	
Diabetics[285,297]	3
Nondiabetics[285,289,297,300,442,443]	12
Total	84

Many patients who are documented biochemically to have self-induced hypoglycemia will adamantly deny doing so when confronted with the evidence. Nevertheless, psychologic counseling is warranted to prevent subsequent episodes with other physicians or substitution of other potentially self-destructive behavior.[286]

NON–ISLET CELL TUMORS

The development of hypoglycemia in a patient with a non–islet cell tumor was first reported in 1930—a mediastinal fibrosarcoma.[301] Since that time, it has become apparent that a large variety of non–islet cell tumors are associated with hypoglycemia[189,272,302-324] (Table 62-4).

Tumors of mesenchymal origin are the most commonly reported (115 cases up to 1979[303]) in Western countries. Such tumors are generally large, slow growing, but often malignant. About one third are retroperitoneal, one third are intra-abdominal, and one third are intrathoracic. In South Africa and Asia, hepatomas are the most common non–islet cell tumors associated with hypoglycemia.[311]

With one possible exception (a small cell carcinoma of the cervix),[325] ectopic production of insulin has never been convincingly demonstrated in patients with this condition.[319,326] Characteristically, circulating plasma insulin and C peptide levels are suppressed. In some cases, hypoglycemia results mainly from increased glucose utilization by the tumor, and debulking either by surgery or radiation treatment can alleviate or ameliorate the hypoglycemia.[303,307,318,322] In patients with rapidly growing hepatomas, hypoglycemia can occur as a terminal or near-terminal event, mainly because of inanition. However, in the great majority of cases, the hypoglycemia is explained by tumor production of IGF-like molecules,[309] in particular, IGF-2 and its isoforms.[324] Excessive release of IGF-like molecules by the tumor can increase glucose utilization in tissues such as muscle,[310,313,323] suppress endogenous glucose production,[317,323] and reduce or overcome the secretion of counterregulatory hormones.[272]

In most cases, the diagnosis is not difficult, and patients are generally middle-aged to elderly; the tumor is usually large, and its presence either is known before the onset of hypoglycemia or can be readily found on physical examination and by ultrasonographic, computed tomographic, and NMR studies. Biochemically, the hypoglycemia is associated with appropriately suppressed plasma insulin and C peptide levels and increased IGF-2 levels, as well as an increased IGF-2/IGF-1 ratio because of suppression of growth hormone secretion and hence suppressed IGF-1 release by IGF-2.

Table 62-4 Neoplasms Associated with Hypoglycemia

Mesenchymal
  Mesothelioma
  Fibrosarcoma
  Rhabdomyosarcoma
  Leiomyosarcoma
  Liposarcoma
  Hemangiopericytoma
Carcinomas
  Hepatic: hepatoma, biliary carcinoma
  Adrenocortical carcinoma
  Genitourinary: hypernephroma, Wilms' tumor, prostate carcinoma
  Reproductive: cervical carcinoma, breast carcinoma, colorectal
Neurologic and neuroendocrine tumors
  Pheochromocytoma
  Carcinoid tumor
  Neurofibroma
  Hematologic
Leukemias
  Lymphoma
  Myeloma

REACTIVE HYPOGLYCEMIA

Reactive hypoglycemia refers to hypoglycemia that occurs after meals. In the past, this type of hypoglycemia was invoked as a cause of numerous somatic complaints due to overdiagnosis because of the use of inappropriate diagnostic tests (e.g., oral glucose tolerance tests). Individuals claiming to have reactive hypoglycemia have been reported to have personality profiles characterized by hypersomatization and hypochondria with the Minnesota Multiphasic Personality inventory.[327] Any condition that causes fasting hypoglycemia can also cause postprandial hypoglycemia[218]—for example, insulinoma,[328] hypopituitarism,[329] alcohol,[117,330] sulfonylurea ingestion, hypothyroidism,[331] growth hormone deficiency,[332] and cortisol deficiency.[331] Nevertheless, some conditions are associated with hypoglycemia only after meal ingestion. These conditions fall into five categories: alimentary, prediabetes, idiopathic, iatrogenic, and functional hypoglycemia.[218]

Alimentary

Hypoglycemia 2 to 4 hours after meal ingestion can occur in patients who have undergone gastrectomy,[333,334] vagotomy and pyloroplasty,[335,336] and esophageal resection[337] and in patients with altered gastric motility,[338] peptic ulcer disease,[339,340] and renal glycosuria.[341] Repeated episodes can lead to hypoglycemia unawareness such as occurs in insulinoma and diabetic patients, thus making interpretation of counterregulatory hormone responses difficult.[342]

The pathogenesis in most of these conditions involves rapid gastric emptying and absorption of glucose, which cause hyperglycemia and stimulation of the release of gut insulin secretagogues, both of which result in excessive secretion of insulin; the biologic actions of insulin to suppress endogenous glucose release and to stimulate tissue glucose uptake persist after the carbohydrate in the meal has been absorbed. This disequilibrium leads to postprandial hypoglycemia.[343] Recent studies have implicated glucagon-like peptide-1 (GLP-1) as the gut insulin secretagogue that is most likely responsible for the excessive insulin secretion observed in most of these conditions.[218,337,344,345]

Treatment involves prevention of rapid absorption of large amounts of carbohydrate, frequent small feedings, avoidance of large amounts of simple sugars, addition of fiber to the diet, β-adrenergic antagonists, anticholinergics, and intestinal α-glucosidase inhibitors.[218,341]

Prediabetes

Individuals with impaired glucose tolerance[89,346] characteristically have a delay in early insulin release that impairs suppression of endogenous glucose release and reduces the early efficiency of glucose uptake, which leads to hyperglycemia and late hyperinsulinemia. Because absorption of glucose is not affected,[89] a disequilibrium such as that observed in patients with alimentary hypoglycemia can occur and lead to late (3 to 5 hours) and often asymptomatic hypoglycemia during OGTTs.[343,347-349] How often this disequilibrium leads to symptomatic hypoglycemia after meals is not known, but the hypoglycemia is mild, and treatment is directed at improvement in glucose tolerance, that is, weight loss in an obese patient and/or pharmacologic intervention with sulfonylureas, metformin, and α-glucosidase inhibitors as in patients with alimentary hypoglycemia. Use of high-fiber diets, anticholinergics, doxepin, cornstarch, and chromium has been proposed but with little scientific support.[350]

Idiopathic

Idiopathic/functional reactive hypoglycemia is an extremely rare condition,[218,338,351,352] in contrast to the number of patients evaluated who think that they have the condition. For this diagnosis to be made, patients must demonstrate arterial/capillary (not venous) hypoglycemia (<50 mg/dL, 2.8 mmol/L) after everyday meals (not OGTTs!), which is associated with symptoms of hypoglycemia that are relieved by carbohydrate ingestion and do not have any other known cause (e.g., prior gastrointestinal surgery, peptic ulcer disease, glucose intolerance, endocrine deficiency).[353] Various etiologies have been proposed: impaired glucagon counterregulatory responses,[218,354–356] excessive GLP-1 secretion,[357] abnormal neuroendocrine regulation of insulin release,[358] increased insulin sensitivity,[359] and increased β-adrenergic sensitivity.[218] The disorder is not life threatening and is treated in the same manner as alimentary hypoglycemia.

However, it has recently become evident that some of these patients might have an adult form of nesidioblastosis[360,361] (not related to mutation of the *Kir6.2* and *SUR1* genes[362]); this rare disorder, which has also been referred to as noninsulinoma pancreatogenous hypoglycemia, has a 4:1 male predominance and is characterized by symptomatic hypoglycemia occurring only postprandially in association with hyperinsulinemia, increased plasma C peptide levels, and negative sulfonylurea screens.[363] In this variant of adult nesidioblastosis, the 72-hour fast is usually negative, as are conventional localization tests. The condition is a diagnostic problem in that plasma insulin, and C peptide levels are often only marginally elevated during postprandial hypoglycemia. In contrast, the calcium stimulation test is positive, and there is a gradient among different venous drainage, indicating diffuse oversecretion of insulin.[364] Treatment entails partial pancreatectomy.[350]

Iatrogenic
Pathophysiologically, hypoglycemia resulting from too rapid termination of total parenteral and enteral feedings[365] and that occurring during dialysis with glucose-containing fluids[201] can be viewed as an iatrogenic form of reactive hypoglycemia in that the prolonged effects of the insulin that is released by these procedures causes the hypoglycemia. Knowledge of such occurrences will obviate unnecessary workups.

Functional (Nonhypoglycemic)
It is common practice to be referred patients who have symptoms suggesting hypoglycemia that occur 1 to 4 hours after meal ingestion. These symptoms generally include chronic fatigue, lightheadedness, shakiness, sweating, weakness, blurred vision, blackouts, headaches, depression, anxiety, confusion, and poor concentration and memory.[327] When such patients are administered a meal similar to ones that elicited the symptoms, the symptoms can be reproduced, but hypoglycemia is rarely if ever observed.[96,366] Thus, in virtually all these patients, the symptoms are not due to hypoglycemia,[367] but rather are better explained by psychologic profiles, which have indicated a wide variety of personality and psychiatric disorders, prominent among which are somatization, obsessive-compulsive behavior, depression, anxiety, and hysteria.[327,368,369]

Normally, blood glucose levels do not decrease below 50 mg/dL (2.8 mmol/L) during everyday life[353,367]; however, during OGTTs, normal volunteers can have decreases in their plasma glucose level below 30 mg/dL (1.6 mmol/L).[13] In fact, blood glucose levels below 50 mg/dL (2.8 mmol/L) will develop in about 10%, and as many as 25% will have values below 60 mg/dL (3.3 mmol/L).[13,218,370]

It is therefore not surprising that "hypoglycemia" can develop during OGTTs in individuals complaining of hypoglycemic symptoms in everyday life, and this test for diabetes mellitus should never be used to assess the presence of reactive hypoglycemia. The first step in the workup of such patients is to establish Whipple's triad during everyday life, which can be done with the self-glucose monitoring that is readily available for diabetic patients. If established, the next step would be to reproduce the hypoglycemia with a standardized meal. If the diagnosis is confirmed, one should exclude impaired glucose tolerance or mild diabetes, renal glycosuria, peptic ulcer disease, or other gastrointestinal disorders. In the absence of these conditions and if the diagnosis is not confirmed, treatment might include psychologic consultation and the use of β-adrenergic antagonists, as well as restriction of large carbohydrate-containing meals.[341]

INSULIN-PRODUCING ISLET CELL TUMORS AND NESIDIOBLASTOSIS

Historical Perspective
Twenty-three years after the discovery of pancreatic islets by Langerhans in 1869, islet cell tumors of the pancreas were first described in autopsy specimens.[371] Although islet cell tumors, including multiple adenomas, continued to be reported over the next several decades,[372] their clinical significance was unappreciated until Harris published three cases in 1924,[373] only 3 years after the discovery of insulin; these would now be considered dubious cases of reactive hypoglycemia.[12] Struck by the similarity of the symptoms to those occurring in insulin-treated diabetic patients, he postulated that like the thyroid, the islets might undersecrete as well as oversecrete its hormone, the latter causing a disorder characterized by hypoglycemia. Three years later, this postulate was confirmed with the description by Wilder and his colleagues of a case of hypoglycemia caused by a malignant insulinoma.[374] The first successful surgical cure of a benign islet adenoma causing hypoglycemia was reported 2 years later.[375] In 1935, Whipple and Frantz found 75 cases in a review of the literature and added 6 surgically proven cases of their own[376]; shortly thereafter, in a subsequent paper, "Whipple's triad"— low blood glucose, symptoms of hypoglycemia, relief by food—was proposed for establishing the diagnosis of a hypoglycemic disorder.[377] By 1950, nearly 400 cases had been reported.[378] Since that time, several large series have provided information on the incidence and other clinical features of insulin-producing tumors.[379–384]

Nesidioblastosis, or diffuse hyperplasia of the islets, as a cause of hypoglycemia was first described by Laidlaw in 1937.[364,385] In contrast to multiple adenomas accompanying the multiple endocrine neoplasia type 1 (MEN-1) syndrome, the condition is characterized by diffuse, although not necessarily uniform, hypertrophy and hyperplasia of islet cells (insulin- as well as glucagon- and somatostatin-producing cells), usually associated with differentiation of ductal cells into insulin-producing cells[386] (Fig. 62-4). This condition can cause hypoglycemia in infants as a result of mutations either in the sulfonylurea receptor[362] or in the anatomically linked potassium channel.[362] However, it has become apparent that the condition can occur in adults independent of these genetic mutations.[361,363,364,387–391]

Fewer than 60 cases of adult onset nesidioblastosis have been reported.[361,364] Although rare, it has been reported to account for about 10% to 15% of patients undergoing pancreatic surgery for hyperinsulinemic hypoglycemia.[361,364] There is a slight male predominance (60%). Age at diagnosis has ranged from 15 to 80 years with a mean (46 years) not different from that of patients with insulinoma.

Preoperative differentiation from an insulinoma can be difficult but is suggested by negative imaging studies (including intragastric ultrasonography) associated with percutaneous transhepatic portal venous sampling, which demonstrates nonselective increases in venous insulin concentrations following calcium injection.

Treatment generally consists of 60% to 90% distal pancreatectomy. Fifty percent of patients undergoing this procedure are cured of hypoglycemia and are normoglycemic. Ten percent develop insulin-requiring diabetes, and the remaining 40% require medications for treatment of hyperglycemia

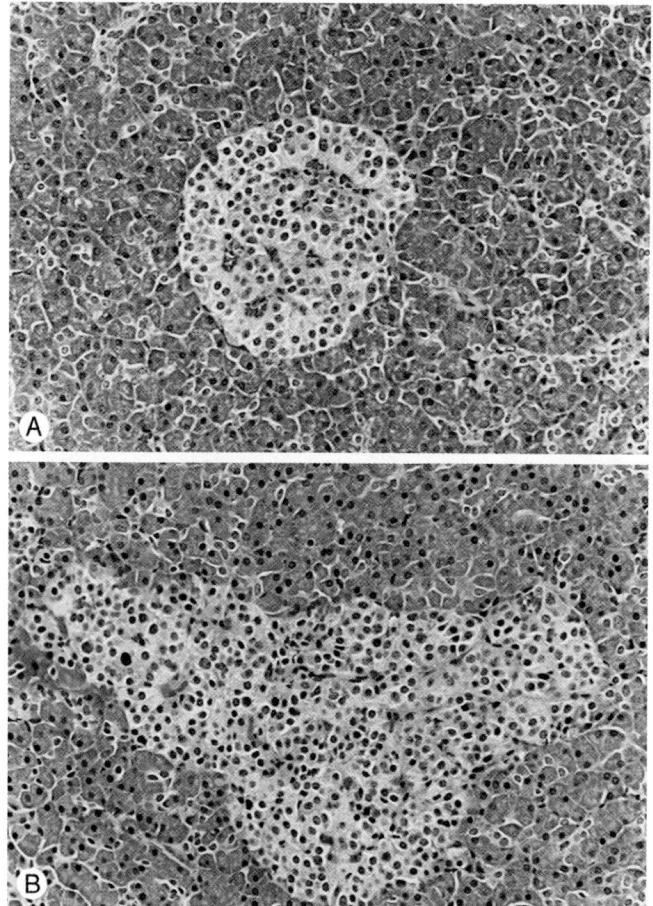

Figure 62-4 **A,** Normal pancreatic islet from a patient without endocrine disease (×200). **B,** Hypertrophic islet from a patient with nesidioblastosis (×200). (From Service F, Natt N, Thompson G, et al: Noninsulinoma pancreatogenous hypoglycemia: A novel syndrome of hyperinsulinemic hypoglycemia in patients independent of mutations in Kir6.2 and SUR1 genes. J Clin Endocrinol Metab 84:1582–1589, 1999. © The Endocrine Society.)

(insulin secretagogue) or persistent hypoglycemia (calcium channel blockers).[361,364]

Incidence

Insulinoma is a very rare disorder, and nesidioblastosis is even rarer.[361,390,391] On the basis of a 60-year experience at the Mayo Clinic, it was estimated that the incidence in Olmsted County, Minnesota, was about eight cases per million patient-years; however, half these cases were found incidentally at autopsy.[380] Other estimates from Seattle, Washington,[392] and Auckland, New Zealand,[393] which emphasize clinically apparent cases, yield an incidence of about one to two cases per million patient-years. The incidence of adult-onset nesidioblastosis would be expected to be only about 0.3 case per million patient-years.[361,379,394]

Demographics

Insulinoma occurs somewhat more frequently in women than in men (Table 62-5), with an average/median onset at about 45 years of age; most cases occur between the ages of 30 and 70 years. Younger patients have generally had a higher occurrence in association with MEN-1,[395] whereas carcinoma was more frequent in older patients. It is uncommon in those older than 80 years. Although a case in a patient with type 1 diabetes mellitus has yet to be documented, insulinomas have occurred in several patients with type 2 diabetes.[396–398] Patients with nesidioblastosis have a slight male preference with similar age of onset.[361]

Pathophysiology

The hypoglycemia in insulinoma patients is the result of dys-regulated insulin release. Normally, increased plasma insulin levels and hypoglycemia per se[399] suppress insulin release. In insulinoma patients, suppression of insulin release by insulin and hypoglycemia is abnormal, and insulin release can be described as chaotic, often not appropriately increased by hyperglycemia, and some patients occasionally have impaired glucose tolerance. Further evidence of abnormal function of the tumorous islets are the increased proinsulin-to-insulin ratios and the decreased insulin concentration relative to normal islet tissue.[400–402]

In most insulinoma patients, hypoglycemia results because of suppression of glucose release rather than increased glucose utilization inasmuch as plasma insulin concentrations are usually only twofold to threefold above normal levels (but of course inappropriate for the plasma glucose concentration).[403] The frequently observed finding that large infusions of glucose are necessary to maintain normoglycemia in insulinoma patients is probably a result of the creation of a slight hyperglycemia that can stimulate insulin release by some insulinomas. Suppression of β cells by either insulin released by the tumor or repetitive hypoglycemia can result in glucose intolerance or transient diabetes after removal of the tumor.

Symptoms and Signs

Except in late-diagnosed malignant insulinoma cases, in which an abdominal mass and signs of metastasis may be present, the physical examination is usually normal. Symptoms are the result of hypoglycemia. Patients with MEN-1 can also have symptoms as a result of hypercalcemia and the accompanying hyperparathyroidism or other excessive hormone secretions (islet production of ACTH, gastrin, and vasoactive intestinal peptide).[404] Common initial symptoms of insulinoma patients are shown in Table 62-6. Because of their nonspecific and insidious nature, the time between the onset of symptoms and diagnosis is about 3 to 5 years, the world record being 26 years.[405] Many patients had initial diagnoses of epilepsy, depression, or psychoneurosis.[383] Initially, autonomic symptoms predominate; later, neuroglycopenic ones do. The frequency and/or severity increases over time. Insulinoma patients, like patients with diabetes mellitus, can acquire the syndrome of hypoglycemia unawareness[52] characterized by diminished symptoms, counterregulatory hormone responses, and β-adrenergic sensitivity,[406] which are reversed after successful surgical cure.[52,407] Thus, it is not uncommon for an insulinoma patient with a plasma glucose concentration less than 36 mg/dL (2 mmol/L) to be completely asymptomatic. The development of this condition can make it difficult to exclude hypopituitarism as a cause of the hypoglycemia initially.

Although insulinoma has long been classified as one of the so-called fasting hypoglycemias, it is important to remember that such patients can experience hypoglycemia at any time of day, even 2 to 4 hours after a meal (Table 62-7). Only about a quarter of patients have hypoglycemia episodes solely after an overnight fast during real-life activity, and postprandial hypoglycemia has been reported to be the sole initial feature.[328] In contrast, an appreciable proportion of patients with nesidioblastosis may have symptoms only after meal ingestion.[363] Seizures tend to be more common in children, but permanent neurologic sequelae have been observed in about 7% of adults.[383] Patients often learn that eating frequently reduces episodes; therefore, weight gain has been observed in about 50% of patients.[383]

Pathology

About 80% of insulinomas are due to benign single adenomas, which average about 2 cm in diameter (see Table 62-5); 10% are due to multiple benign adenomas. Diffuse hyperplasia and/or nesidioblastosis is uncommon in adults (i.e., one to

Table 62-5 Clinical Features of Insulinoma Patients and Their Tumors

Feature	Service et al., 1976[381]	Service et al., 1991[380]	Broder and Carter[384]	Fajans and Vinik[379]	Stefanini et al.[383]	Galbut and Markowitz[382]	Boukhman et al.[418]	Dizon et al.[394]
Number	60	224	52	82	1067	41	67	63
Gender	46% male	41% male	51% male	48% male	40% male	21% male	33% male	44% male
Age at diagnosis (years)	47	47	52	—	45	45	46	55
Duration of symptoms (months) before diagnosis	33	—	—	—	—*	36	46	46
Single adenoma (%)	81	87	—	76	83	79	73	79
Multiple adenomas (%)	10	7	—	13	13	19	10	2
MEN-1 associated (%)	6	8	—	9	4	2	16	8
Carcinoma (%)	9	6	100	6	16	2	10	10
Nesidioblastosis (%)	0	0	—	4	0	0	—	5
Hyperplasia (%)	0	1	—	1	0	0	7	2
Single adenoma size (cm)								
Range	0.8–8.0	—	—	0.2–5	1–5	<1–7	<1–7	0.5–5
Average	~2	—	—	~2	—	~2	1.6	~2

*Twenty percent after 5 years.
MEN, multiple endocrine neoplasia.

Table 62-6 Symptoms of Insulinoma Patients

Symptom	Boukhman et al.[418] (%)	Dizon et al.[394] (%)	Galbut and Markowitz[382] (%)	Service et al., 1976[381] (%)
Confusion	70	83	54	80
Altered mental status	67	—	—	—
Abnormal behavior	54	64	44	80
Weight gain	51	39	"Nearly all"	18
Weakness/fatigue	37	56	—	—
Lightheadedness	37	58	—	—
Faintness	37	54	41	—
Drowsiness	37	31	—	—
Blurred vision	25	46	29	—
Convulsions	32	27	27	12
Amnesia	27	41	—	—
Tremor	24	24	—	—
Headaches	22	20	41	—
Sweats	18	69	39	—
Coma	16	12	41	53
Palpitations	12	12	44	—

Table 62-7 Time of Day/Circumstances of Hypoglycemic Episodes

Episode	Dizon et al.[394] (%)	Fajans and Vinik[379] (%)	Service et al., 1976[381] (%)	Boukhman et al.[418] (%)
Overnight, before breakfast only	—	26	30	—
Before breakfast, lunch/dinner	27	27	25	58
Only after missed meal	—	8	—	—
Only before lunch or dinner	—	29	—	—
Uncertain or other	5	10	22	32
Several hours after any meal	20	—	23	10
After exercise	27	—	7	13

two cases per 100 million patient-years) and usually account for only 1% to 2%.[408,409] Carcinomas account for about 8%. Five percent of insulinomas are associated with MEN-1, in which case the tumor is more likely to be multiple and malignant and to secrete additional hormones ectopically, such as gastrin or ACTH.

Diagnosis

The diagnosis of insulinoma is readily established by the demonstration of fasting hypoglycemia (>50 mg/dL, 2.8 mmol/L), inappropriate plasma insulin (>5 μU/mL, 30 pmol/L) and C peptide (>0.25 nmol/L, 0.75 pg/mL), and a negative sulfonylurea/meglitinide blood/urine screen. A plasma proinsulin concentration greater than 5 pmol/L can be useful if plasma insulin and C peptide values are borderline, but this measurement is not usually necessary.[410,411] Various tests have been proposed over the years to rule in or rule out the presence of an insulinoma: the intravenous tolbutamide tolerance test, the glucagon test, the leucine test, and the C peptide suppression test.[379,412–415] All suffer from frequent false positives and false negatives and are not recommended. The "gold standard" remains the classic 72-hour fast. Hypoglycemia will develop in essentially all insulinoma patients during this test; in fact, 75% will become hypoglycemic within 24 hours.[70] The test should be conducted in a hospital under standardized and supervised conditions (Table 62-8). It is worth emphasizing that many patients with nesidioblastosis will have a normal 72-hour fast, and their only biochemical abnormality will be postprandial hypoglycemia associated with an abnormal plasma insulin and C peptide level, which is why it is preferable to begin the 72-hour fast with a standard meal.

The 72-Hour Fast

Successful completion of a 72-hour fast without the development of hypoglycemia effectively excludes a serious hypoglycemic disorder except for nesidioblastosis.[416] It is recommended that the patient be hospitalized and supervised to prevent inadvertent caloric consumption or surreptitious drug administration. Admission is preferred before a standard evening meal so that the response to a meal can be assessed, as well as the response to a fast. The patient should be encouraged to be active to simulate real-life situations and prevent sedentary decreases in glucose utilization. Baseline samples for counterregulatory hormones are drawn to assess the adequacy of a response if hypoglycemia should subsequently occur. Blood for a β-hydroxybutyrate level is drawn at the end of the fast to exclude the consumption of calories. Should hypoglycemia occur, anti-insulin antibodies, anti-insulin receptor

antibodies, and IGF-2 levels may be useful in assessing the presence of an autoimmune cause or an occult IGF-2-secreting non–islet cell tumor. Interpretation of the results of these determinations is given in Table 62-9.

The above plan represents the ideal approach. Given the practicalities of third-party reimbursements for procedures, an alternative would be to have the patient fast overnight and come to the office or clinic in the morning at around 8:00 A.M. after a 12- to 14-hour overnight fast and begin serial testing during the day. If, at the end of the day (i.e., 4:00 P.M. after fasting approximately 20 to 22 hours), hypoglycemia has not occurred, then the patient should be admitted for 2 days of serial testing.

Localization

Only after the diagnosis of hypoglycemia associated with inappropriate hyperinsulinemia is established biochemically should localization studies be performed. Ninety-nine percent of insulinomas occur within the pancreas. Of the rare insulinomas that are not found in the pancreas, most are found in the wall of the duodenum or gastrosplenic omentum.[417] They average about 2 cm in diameter and appear with equal frequency in the head, body, and tail.[382,383] Although about 75% to 90% can be correctly identified by palpation at surgery,[418,419] preoperative localization is generally recommended to minimize manipulation of the pancreas, shorten operative time, avoid blind partial pancreatectomy when the tumor is not palpable, and assist in reoperations when scarring and fibrosis from prior surgery make palpation difficult.[379] Computed tomography and NMR imaging can detect large tumors and stage malignant ones but yield false positives and false negatives; these techniques correctly localize tumors only 50% to 70% of the time.[379,418–420] Celiac arteriography and transsplenic portal venous sampling have had variable results and are invasive and probably not needed.[379,419,420] Currently, preoperative transabdominal ultrasonography followed by intraoperative ultrasonography (Fig. 62-5) is considered the most sensitive and specific approach and has been recommended for routine use; this approach along with palpation can detect over 95% of tumors.[418,420–422] Recently, dual-phase spiral computed tomography has been reported to detect six of seven tumors ranging in size from 6 to 18 mm.[423] However, given the success of intraoperative ultrasonography along with palpation, it has been questioned whether extensive preoperative radiologic investigation is indicated and cost effective.[420,424] In patients who are suspected of having nesidioblastosis, the test of choice is the selective calcium infusion procedure[390,420] because this test will confirm the diagnosis of pancreatic hyperinsulinism as the probable cause of the hypoglycemia when reliable localization procedures are negative.[361]

Treatment

Surgery is the treatment of choice for insulinoma and nesidioblastosis.[361,383,418] For patients with solitary adenomas, enucleation is curative; in cases that are thought to be due to a single adenoma, recurrence or lack of cure could be due to the presence of multiple adenomas. In 5% to 10% of patients, the adenoma is not found; nevertheless, in such cases, partial pancreatectomy can result in cure. Reoperation might still result in cure, but recurrence has been noted up to 18 years after the initial surgery.[380] Recurrences are more common in patients with MEN-1 (up to 20%).[380] Multiple adenomas, hyperplasia, and malignancy require more extensive surgery. Debulking of a malignant tumor is worthwhile in helping to control hypoglycemia. The major complications of surgery include acute pancreatitis (~10% to 15%), wound infection (5% to 10%), fistulas (10% to 15%), and pseudocysts (5%) and are related to the extent of surgery. Reoperations have a greater complication rate and mortality (~15% versus 5%). Quite commonly, transient hyperglycemia occurs and lasts up

---

Table 62-8 Protocol for a 72-Hour Fast

Admit before the evening meal. Discontinue all nonessential medications. Insert an intravenous line for blood sampling.

Begin blood sampling (plasma glucose, insulin, C peptide) just before the meal, and continue every 30 minutes for 6 hours and thereafter every 2 to 3 hours.

Baseline samples should also include growth hormone, cortisol, glucagon, catecholamines, IGF-1, and sulfonylureas/meglitinides.

Patient may consume calorie- and caffeine-lacking liquids and should ambulate.

The fast is ended at 72 hours or earlier if the patient has a plasma glucose level below 40 mg/dL (2.5 mmol/L) associated with symptoms. Do not end the fast for symptoms if hypoglycemia is not documented.

At end of the fast, draw samples for all the above measurements plus an oral hypoglycemic agent screen and β-hydroxybutyrate level and an extra tube for insulin antibodies, anti–insulin receptor antibodies, and IGF-1.

IGF-1, insulin-like growth factor-1.

Table 62-9 Interpretation of the Results of a 72-Hour Fast

Diagnosis	Symptoms or Signs	Plasma Glucose (mg/dL)	Plasma Insulin (μU/mL)	Plasma C Peptide (nmol/L)	Anti-Insulin Antireceptor Antibodies	IGF-1	β-Hydroxybutyrate	Oral Agent Screen
Normal	No	>40	<6	<0.2	–	N	>2.7	–
Insulinoma	Yes	<40	>6	>0.2	–	N	<2.7	–
Factitious insulin	Yes	<40	>6	<0.2	–	N	<2.7	–
Factitious oral agent	Yes	<40	>6	>0.2	–	N	<2.7	+
Inadvertent feeding	No	>40	<6	<0.2	–	N	>2.7	–
Non–islet cell tumor	Yes	<40	<6	<0.2	–	↑	<2.7	–
Abnormal counter-regulation	Yes	<40	<6	<0.2	–	N	<2.7	–
Nonhypo-glycemic disorder	Yes	>40	<6	<0.2	–	N	<2.7	–
Autoimmune disorder	Yes	<40	<6	<0.2	+	N	<2.7	–

IGF-1, insulin-like growth factor-1.

to 2 to 3 weeks because of suppression of normal islet function. Permanent diabetes mellitus can occur after partial pancreatectomy and reoperations. In patients with nesidioblastosis, gradient-directed resection can result in cure of hypoglycemia.

Medical therapy is reserved for operated patients with recurrence who refuse another exploration and for inoperable malignant tumors. Diazoxide (100 to 200 mg, three times daily), which inhibits insulin secretion, has been most widely used.[425] Approximately 60% (mainly those with benign

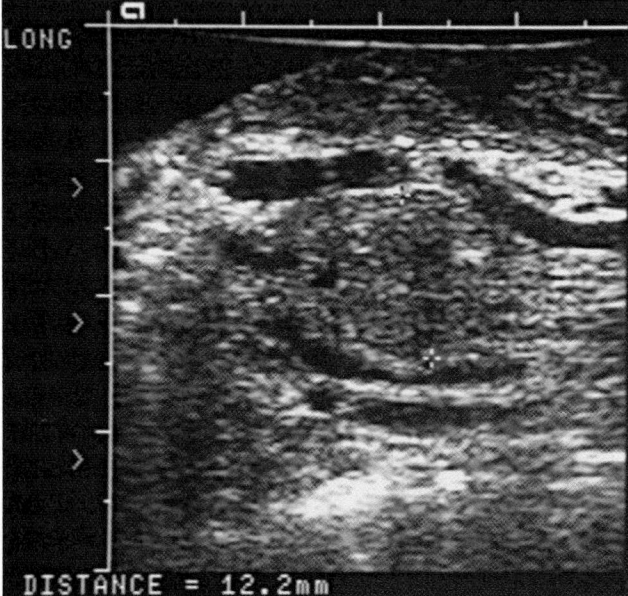

Figure 62-5 Intraoperative ultrasonography demonstrating an insulinoma sandwiched between the gastroduodenal artery anteriorly and the common bile duct posteriorly. (From Grant C: Surgical aspects of hyperinsulinemic hypoglycemia. Endocrinol Metab Clin North Am 28:533–554, 1999.)

disease) can be maintained nearly free of symptoms with only occasional hypoglycemia. The main side effects are fluid retention (~15%) and hirsutism (~5%); thiazide diuretics can be used to combat the fluid retention and enhance the hyperglycemic effect. The somatostatin analogue octreotide has been found to be effective in some patients but must be injected.[426,427] Continuous subcutaneous glucagon infusion has also been used.[428] Glucocorticoids (to induce insulin resistance) and verapamil, the calcium-channel blocker, and phenytoin, the anticonvulsant, both of which inhibit insulin release at high doses, have also been used when other measures were ineffective.[379]

Malignant insulinomas respond poorly to chemotherapy.[384] Streptozocin has been reported to reduce tumor size in about 50% of patients, with fewer than 20% achieving complete remission; although its use prolongs life, it has considerable renal, hepatic, and hematopoietic toxicity. The addition of flu-orouracil has been reported to have advantages over streptozocin alone.[429] Mithramycin,[430] doxorubicin (Adriamycin),[431] and hepatic embolization[432] have been tried with some success in refractory cases.

GENERAL APPROACH TO THE PATIENT

DIAGNOSIS

The causes, clinical features, consequences, and need for immediate treatment of hypoglycemia will vary depending on whether the patient to be evaluated is seen in the clinic, emergency room, or hospital ward. In two series,[3,433] diabetes, alcohol, sepsis, and combinations thereof accounted for about 90% of emergency room cases (Table 62-10). Virtually all patients had either stupor, coma, confusion, or bizarre behavior or were postictal. About 10% were hypothermic. Death occurred in 10%, and 3% had permanent neurologic sequelae. Among the diabetic patients, about 80% were taking insulin; strenuous exercise (7%), accidental (6%) or deliberate insulin overdose (13%), skipped meals (28%), and alcohol ingestion (19%) were identified as precipitating factors. In 27% of cases,

Table 62-10 Causes of 181 Emergency Room Cases of Hypoglycemia from Malouf and Brust and Hart and Frier

MOST FREQUENT	
Diabetic medications	85
Alcohol	40
Diabetes plus alcohol	27
Sepsis	4
Sepsis plus alcohol	9
Sepsis plus diabetes	2
Total	167 (92%)
OTHER	
Fasting	5
Terminal cancer	4
Gastroenteritis	2
Insulin drug abuse	2
Myxedema	1
Total	14 (8%)

Adapted from Malouf R, Brust J: Hypoglycemia: Causes, neurological manifestations, and outcome. Ann Neurol 17:421–430, 1985; Hart S, Frier B: Causes, management and morbidity of acute hypoglycemia in adults requiring hospital admission. Q J Med 91:505–510, 1998.

no immediate cause was identified. Some patients were also taking other agents with hypoglycemic potential or had chronic renal failure, psychiatric disorders, and previous emergency room visits for hypoglycemia. In the emergency room, prompt treatment (usually with intravenous glucose) is more of a concern than an etiologic diagnosis.

In hospitalized patients, the incidence of hypoglycemia ranges from 0.5% in elderly nondiabetic patients[8] to 28% in diabetic patients,[434] about 1.5% being found in studies that included diabetic and nondiabetic patients.[6,7] Although hypoglycemia is rarely the direct cause of death, mortality in hospitalized patients who are experiencing hypoglycemia has ranged from 22% to 48%.[6-9] Renal insufficiency, diabetes mellitus, malnutrition, liver disease, infection, and malignancy were the most common risk factors or contributing conditions (Table 62-11). Most patients had multiple risk factors. Episodes were frequently repetitive, and the great majority were asymptomatic because of occurrence in patients with reduced sensorium. Among diabetic patients, decreased caloric intake (missed meals, vomiting, withheld enteral feedings, meals withheld for procedures) and inappropriate insulin doses accounted for nearly 90% of occurrences.

In contrast to the above situations, in which immediate treatment may be of paramount importance, patients who

Table 62-11 Risk Factors/Situations Associated with the Development of Hypoglycemia in 195 Hospitalized Patients

Risk Factor/Situation	Cases (%)
Diabetes mellitus	41
Renal insufficiency	40
Malnutrition	34
Infection/shock	28
Liver disease	27
Malignancy	16
Heart failure	9
Pregnancy	6
Hyperkalemia therapy	5
Total parenteral nutrition	4
Burns	3
Alimentary disease	2

Data from Shilo et al.,[8] Fischer et al.,[6] Stagnaro-Green et al.,[7] and Cruz Jentoft et al.[9]

are seen in the clinic or office are likely to be healthy, complain of episodes with predominantly autonomic symptoms, and have spurious or poorly documented low plasma glucose levels. In such patients, diagnosis rather than treatment is the issue. Factitious, drug-induced, functional/alimentary hypoglycemia, insulinoma, and hypoglycemia secondary to an undiagnosed endocrine deficiency are the most likely diagnostic considerations.

Workups can follow an etiologic-based classification, one that is based on whether hypoglycemia occurs in the fasting or postprandial state, or one that is based on pathogenetic mechanisms. All suffer from limitations. For example, those based on the latter suffer from the fact that the mechanisms involved are complex, such as adrenal insufficiency leading to decreased glucose production, as well as increased glucose utilization (i.e., increased peripheral insulin sensitivity). Those based on postprandial versus fasting hypoglycemia suffer from the fact that although "functional" hypoglycemia by definition occurs only postprandially, other common causes can also lead to postprandial hypoglycemia (e.g., insulinoma). The author prefers one that is based on diagnostic clusters (see Table 62-1) because this mode of thinking can rapidly narrow the field of possibilities.

When a patient is to be evaluated for hypoglycemia, the first step is to determine whether the patient has in fact had a hypoglycemic episode. It is important to determine what the patient's symptoms were. When did they occur in relation to the patient's last meal, and what was the patient doing when the episode occurred? Was it an isolated event, or had it occurred before? How frequently do they occur? Is there any pattern to the occurrences? How long have these events been occurring? Did weight gain or weight loss occur during this period? Is the patient taking any medications? If so, they should be checked to make sure that no mistake has been made. Did the patient lose consciousness? If so, were premonitory signs present? Was hypoglycemia documented? Did the patient recover spontaneously? What did the patient do to prevent recurrences or relieve symptoms? What is the patient's occupation? Does the patient or any immediate relatives have diabetes? If so, how is it being treated? Does the patient have any medical conditions? Do family members have any endocrine disorders? For example, a family history of autoimmune disorders should raise the suspicion of Addison's disease.

Most outpatients who have a disorder that is causing hypoglycemia should describe discrete episodes. Classically, premonitory symptoms such as a feeling of anxiety, hunger, blurred vision, difficulty thinking, weakness and sweating, and palpitations will be noted. Loss of consciousness can occur. With repetitive episodes, patients learn that they can abort these symptoms by eating; therefore, these patients often have a history of weight gain. Spells similar to those caused by hypoglycemia can represent a vasovagal reflex, cardiac arrhythmia, a convulsive disorder, orthostatic hypotension, or a transient ischemic attack. In mild cases of insulinoma, spells might occur only after vigorous exercise or prolonged fasting. On the other hand, skipping lunch and having several cocktails before dinner can precipitate an isolated hypoglycemic episode in an otherwise healthy person. The history can also provide clues to the possibility of hypopituitarism (e.g., prior pituitary surgery, symptoms of galactorrhea, amenorrhea, impotence, or endocrine insufficiency, as with thyroid replacement therapy). The patient's occupation or family diseases can be important with regard to access to hypoglycemia-producing drugs (e.g., insulin, sulfonylureas) or MEN.

The physical examination can be useful in excluding carotid disease, orthostatic hypotension, severe cardiac and hepatic disease, hypothyroidism, cachexia, and cancer, which should be obvious at the stage at which they would cause hypoglycemia. Routine laboratory testing can exclude renal

Table 62-12 Diagnostic Approach to an Adult with Documented Fasting Hypoglycemia

1. Consider the most likely disorders (drugs, critical illness, endocrine deficiency, non–β cell tumor, and insulinoma) while supporting the plasma glucose concentration if necessary.
2. Examine the history, physical examination, and available laboratory data for clinical clues to include or exclude the above categories.

Cause	Response
Insulin- or sulfonylurea-treated diabetes	Adjust the therapeutic regimen.
Use of other drugs known or suspected to cause hypoglycemia	Discontinue use of the drug.
Hepatic, renal, or cardiac failure; sepsis; or inanition	Treat the underlying disorder.
Anorexia, weight loss, change in skin pigmentation, known pituitary or adrenocortical disease, hypotension, hyponatrema, hyperkalemia	Evaluate for adrenocortical/pituitary insufficiency.
Known non–β-cell tumor, mass on examination or imaging studies	Check for high IGF-2–to–IGF-1 ratio.

3. In the absence of clinical clues, consider medication error, endogenous hyperinsulinism, and surreptitious or malicious insulin secretogogue or insulin administration.

IGF, insulin-like growth factor.

insufficiency or raise the possibility of adrenal insufficiency (hyponatremia). If all the above are negative and prior hypoglycemia has not been unequivocally documented, it is necessary to do so before proceeding with other diagnostic tests. Table 62-12 gives a suggested approach.[226]

TREATMENT

Treatment is aimed at restoring euglycemia, preventing recurrences, and, if possible, alleviating the underlying cause. In an insulin-taking diabetic patient with mild hypoglycemia because of a skipped meal, treatment can simply entail 12 to 18 g of oral carbohydrate every 30 minutes until the blood glucose level is above 80.[435,436] With more severe hypoglycemia resulting in obtundation and when oral administration of carbohydrate might result in aspiration, 1 mg of glucagon subcutaneously or intramuscularly might be sufficient to raise the blood glucose concentration and revive the patient so that oral carbohydrate can be given. Comatose patients should receive intravenous glucose (a 25-g bolus, followed by an infusion at an initial rate of 2 mg/kg/min, roughly 10 g/hour). A sulfonylurea or meglitinide overdose can result in prolonged hypoglycemia requiring sustained intravenous glucose infusion aimed at keeping the blood glucose level at approximately 4.5 mmol/L (~80 mg/dL) to avoid hyperglycemia causing further stimulation of insulin secretion and setting in motion a vicious cycle. Blood glucose levels should be monitored initially every 30 minutes and subsequently at 1- to 2-hour intervals. Occasionally, diazoxide or a somatostatin analogue might be needed to inhibit insulin secretion.[437] When other drugs are involved, their use should be discontinued if possible (e.g., sulfonamides in a patient with renal insufficiency). In other conditions, the underlying disorder should be treated (e.g., sepsis, heart failure, endocrine deficiency), and the blood glucose level should be supported.

REFERENCES

1. Carroll MF, Burge MR, Schade DS: Severe hypoglycemia in adults. Rev Endocr Metab Disord 4:149–157, 2003.
2. Virally ML, Guillausseau PJ: Hypoglycemia in adults. Diabetes Metab 25:477–490, 1999.
3. Hart S, Frier B: Causes, management and morbidity of acute hypoglycaemia in adults requiring hospital admission. Q J Med 91:505–510, 1998.
4. Klatt E, Beatie C, Noguchi T: Evaluation of death from hypoglycemia. Am J Forensic Med Pathol 9:122–125, 1988.
5. Huic M, Mucolic V, Vrhovac B, et al: Adverse drug reactions resulting in hospital admission. Int J Clin Pharmacol Ther 32:675–682, 1994.
6. Fischer K, Lees J, Newman J: Hypoglycemia in hospitalized patients: Causes and outcomes. N Engl J Med 315:1245–1250, 1986.
7. Stagnaro-Green A, Barton M, Linekin P, et al: Mortality in hospitalized patients with hypoglycemia and severe hyperglycemia. Mt Sinai J Med 62:422–426, 1995.
8. Shilo S, Berezovsky S, Friedlander Y, et al: Hypoglycemia in hospitalized nondiabetic older patients. J Am Geriatr Soc 46:978–982, 1998.

9. Cruz Jentoft A, Villar I, Carreras P, et al: Unexpected hypoglycemia in hospitalized patients [in Spanish]. Rev Clin Esp 191:295–298, 1992.
10. Whitehead T, Robinson D, Hale A, et al: Clinical Chemistry and Haematology: Adult Reference Values. London, BUPA Medical Research and Development Ltd, 1994.
11. Colagiuri S, Sandbaek A, Carstensen B, et al: Comparability of venous and capillary glucose measurements in blood. Diabet Med 20:953–956, 2003.
12. Marks V: Hypoglycaemia—Real and unreal, lawful and unlawful: The 1994 Banting Lecture. Diabet Med 12:850–864, 1995.
13. Fariss B: Prevalence of post-glucose load glycosuria and hypoglycemia in a group of healthy young men. Diabetes 23:189–191, 1974.
14. Felig P, Cherif A, Minegawa A, et al: Hypoglycemia during prolonged exercise in normal man. N Engl J Med 306:895–900, 1982.
15. Horwitz D: Factitious and artifactual hypoglycemia. Endocrinol Metab Clin North Am 18:203–210, 1989.

16. West E, Todd W: Textbook of Biochemistry. New York, Macmillan, 1961, p 947.
17. Field J, Williams H: Artifactual hypoglycemia associated with leukemia. N Engl J Med 265:946–948, 1961.
18. Goodenow T, Malarkey W: Leukocytosis and artifactual hypoglycemia. JAMA 237:1961–1962, 1977.
19. Lefor A, Miller M: Factitious hypoglycemia associated with eosinophilic leukemoid reaction. N Y St J Med 85:34–35, 1985.
20. Astles J, Petros W, Peters W, et al: Artifactual hypoglycemia associated with hematopoietic cytokines. Arch Pathol Lab Med 119:713–716, 1995.
21. Arem R, Jeang M, Blevens T, et al: Polycythemia rubra vera and artifactual hypoglycemia. Arch Intern Med 142:2199–2201, 1982.
22. Billington C, Casciato D, Choquette D, et al: Artifactual hypoglycemia associated with polycythemia vera. JAMA 249:774–775, 1983.
23. Macaron C, Kadri A, Macaron Z: Nucleated red blood cells and artifactual hypoglycemia. Diabetes Care 4:113–115, 1981.

24. DCCT Research Group: The effect of intensive treatment of diabetes on the development and progression of long-term complications in insulin dependent diabetes mellitus. N Engl J Med 329:977–986, 1993.

25. UK Prospective Diabetes Study (UKPDS) Group: Intensive blood-glucose control with sulphonylureas or insulin compared with conventional treatment and risk of complications in patients with type 2 diabetes (UKPDS 33). Lancet 352:837–853, 1998.

26. UK Prospective Diabetes Study (UKPDS) Group: Effect of intensive blood-glucose control with metformin on complications in overweight patients with type 2 diabetes (UKPDS 34). Lancet 352:854–865, 1998.

27. Jarrett R: The cardiovascular risk associated with impaired glucose tolerance. Diabetic Med 13(Suppl):S15–S19, 1996.

28. Owen O, Morgan A, Kemp H, et al: Brain metabolism during fasting. J Clin Invest 46:1589–1595, 1967.

29. Gruetter R: Glycogen: The forgotten cerebral energy store. J Neurosci Res 74:179–183, 2003.

30. Henderson JN, Allen KV, Deary IJ, et al: Hypoglycaemia in insulin-treated Type 2 diabetes: Frequency, symptoms and impaired awareness. Diabet Med 20:1016–1021, 2003.

31. Seaquist ER, Damberg GS, Tkac I, et al: The effect of insulin on in vivo cerebral glucose concentrations and rates of glucose transport/metabolism in humans. Diabetes 50:2203–2209, 2001.

32. Veneman T, Mitrakou A, Mokan M, et al: Effect of hyperketonemia and hyperlacticacidemia on symptoms, cognitive function, and counterregulatory hormone responses during hypoglycemia in normal humans. Diabetes 43:1311–1317, 1994.

33. Gerich J, Mokan M, Veneman T, et al: Hypoglycemia unawareness. Endocr Rev 12:356–371, 1991.

34. Veneman T, Mitrakou A, Mokan M, et al: Induction of hypoglycemia unawareness by asymptomatic nocturnal hypoglycemia. Diabetes 42:1233–1237, 1993.

35. Mitrakou A, Ryan C, Veneman T, et al: Hierarchy of glycemic thresholds for counterregulatory hormone secretion, symptoms, and cerebral dysfunction. Am J Physiol 260:E67–E74, 1991.

36. Schwartz N, Clutter W, Shah S, et al: The glycemic thresholds for activation of glucose counterregulatory systems are higher than the threshold for symptoms. J Clin Invest 79:777–781, 1987.

37. Hepburn D, Deary I, Frier B, et al: Symptoms of acute insulin-induced hypoglycemia in humans with and without IDDM: Factor-analysis approach. Diabetes Care 14:949–957, 1991.

38. Towler D, Havlin C, Craft S, et al: Mechanism of awareness of hypoglycemia: Perception of neurogenic (predominantly cholinergic) rather than neuroglycopenic symptoms. Diabetes 42:1791–1798, 1993.

39. Cox D, Gonder-Frederick L, Antoun B, et al: Perceived symptoms in the recognition of hypoglycemia. Diabetes Care 16:519–527, 1993.

40. Krahn D, Mackenzie T: Organic personality syndrome caused by insulin-related nocturnal hypoglycemia. Psychosomatics 25:711–712, 1984.

41. Silas J, Grant D, Maddocks J: Transient hemiparetic attacks due to unrecognised nocturnal hypoglycaemia. Br Med J 282:132–133, 1981.

42. Chalmers J, Risk M, Kean D, et al: Severe amnesia after hypoglycemia. Clinical, psychometric, and magnetic resonance imaging correlations. Diabetes Care 14:922–925, 1991.

43. Fisher B, Quin J, Rumley A, et al: Effects of acute insulin-induced hypoglycaemia on haemostasis, fibrinolysis and haemorheology in insulin-dependent diabetic patients and control subjects. Clin Sci 80:525–531, 1991.

44. Wredling R, Levander S, Adamson U, et al: Permanent neuropsychological impairment after recurrent episodes of severe hypoglycaemia in man. Diabetologia 33:152–157, 1990.

45. Patrick A, Campbell I: Fatal hypoglycaemia in insulin-treated diabetes mellitus: Clinical features and neuropathological changes. Diabetic Med 7:349–354, 1990.

46. Pladziewicz D, Nesto R: Hypoglycemia-induced silent myocardial ischemia. Am J Cardiol 63:1531–1532, 1989.

47. Duh E, Feinglos M: Hypoglycemia-induced angina pectoris in a patient with diabetes mellitus. Ann Intern Med 121:945–946, 1994.

48. Perros P, Frier B: The long-term sequelae of severe hypoglycemia on the brain in insulin-dependent diabetes mellitus. Horm Metab Res 29:197–202, 1997.

49. Mohseni S: Hypoglycemic neuropathy. Acta Neuropathol (Berl) 102:413–421, 2001.

50. Frier B: Hypoglycaemia: Clinical consequences and morbidity. Int J Clin Pract Suppl Sep(112):51–55, 2000.

51. Bolli G, DeFeo P, Perriello G, et al: Role of hepatic autoregulation in defense against hypoglycemia in humans. J Clin Invest 75:1623–1631, 1985.

52. Mitrakou A, Fanelli C, Veneman T, et al: Reversibility of unawareness of hypoglycemia in patients with insulinomas. N Engl J Med 329:834–839, 1993.

53. Boyle P, Nagy R, O'Connor A, et al: Adaptation of brain glucose uptake following recurrent hypoglycemia. Proc Natl Acad Sci U S A 91:9352–9356, 1994.

54. Fritsche A, Stumvoll M, Grüb M, et al: Effect of hypoglycemia on b-adrenergic sensitivity in normal and type 1 diabetic subjects. Diabetes Care 21:1505–1510, 1998.

55. Korytkowski M, Mokan M, Veneman T, et al: Reduced b-adrenergic sensitivity in patients with type 1 diabetes and hypoglycemia unawareness. Diabetes Care 21:1939–1943, 1998.

56. Boyle P, Schwartz N, Shah S, et al: Plasma glucose concentrations at the onset of hypoglycemic symptoms in patients with poorly controlled diabetes and in nondiabetics. N Engl J Med 318:1487–1492, 1988.

57. Hochstaedt B, Schneebaum M, Shael M: Adrenocortical responsivity in old age. Gerontol Clin 3:239–246, 1961.

58. Marker J, Cryer P, Clutter W: Attenuated glucose recovery from hypoglycemia in the elderly. Diabetes 41:671–678, 1992.

59. Meneilly G, Minaker K, Young B, et al: Counterregulatory responses to insulin-induced glucose reduction in the elderly. J Clin Endocrinol Metab 61:178–182, 1985.

60. Claustre J, Peyrin L, Fitoussi R, et al: Sex differences in the adrenergic response to hypoglycemic stress in human. Psychopharmacology 67:147–153, 1980.

61. Amiel S, Maran A, Powrie J, et al: Gender differences in counterregulation to hypoglycaemia. Diabetologia 36:460–464, 1993.

62. Davis S, Cherrington A, Goldstein R, et al: Effects of insulin on the counterregulatory response to equivalent hypoglycemia in normal females. Am J Physiol 265:E680–E689, 1993.

63. Hirsch I, Boyle P, Craft S, et al: Higher glycemic thresholds for symptoms during b-adrenergic blockade in IDDM. Diabetes 40:1177–1186, 1991.

64. Rosenn B, Miodovnik M, Khoury J, et al: Counterregulatory hormonal responses to hypoglycemia during pregnancy. Obstet Gynecol 87:568–574, 1996.

65. Bottini P, Boschetti E, Pampanelli S, et al: Contribution of autonomic neuropathy to reduced plasma adrenaline responses to hypoglycemia in IDDM: Evidence for a nonselective defect. Diabetes 46:814–823, 1997.

66. Meyer C, Grossmann R, Mitrakou A, et al: Effects of autonomic neuropathy on counterregulation and awareness of hypoglycemia in type 1 diabetic patients. Diabetes Care 21:1960–1966, 1998.

67. DeFronzo R, Andres R, Bedsoe T, et al: A test of the hypothesis that the rate of fall in glucose concentration triggers counterregulatory hormonal responses in man. Diabetes 26:445–452, 1977.

68. Mitrakou A, Ryan C, Veneman T, et al: Influence of plasma glucose rate of decrease on hierarchy of responses to hypoglycemia. J Clin Endocrinol Metab 76:462–465, 1993.

69. Consoli A, Kennedy F, Miles J, et al: Determination of Krebs cycle metabolic carbon exchange in vivo and its use to estimate the individual contributions of gluconeogenesis and glycogenolysis to overall glucose output in man. J Clin Invest 80:1303–1310, 1987.

70. Scholz D, ReMine W, Priestley J: Hyperinsulinism: Revew of 95 cases of functioning pancreatic islet cell tumors. Mayo Clin Proc 35:545–550, 1960.

71. Gerich J: Control of glycaemia. Bailliere's Clin Endocrinol and Metab 7:551–586, 1993.

72. Boden G: Role of fatty acids in the pathogenesis of insulin resistance and NIDDM. Diabetes 46:3–10, 1997.

73. Stumvoll M, Meyer C, Mitrakou A, et al: Renal glucose production and utilization: New aspects in humans. Diabetologia 40:749–757, 1997.

74. Landau B, Wahren J, Chandramouli V, et al: Contributions of gluconeogenesis to glucose production in the fasted state. J Clin Invest 98:378–385, 1996.

75. Meyer C, Dostou J, Nadkarni V, et al: Effects of physiological hyperinsulinemia on systemic, renal and hepatic substrate metabolism. Am J Physiol 275:F915–F921, 1998.

76. Gastaldelli A, Toschi E, Pettiti M, et al: Effect of physiological hyperinsulinemia on gluconeogenesis in nondiabetic subjects and in type 2 diabetic patients. Diabetes 50:1807–1812, 2001.

77. Petersen KF, Laurent D, Rothman DL, et al: Mechanism by which glucose and insulin inhibit net hepatic glycogenolysis in humans. J Clin Invest 101:1203–1209, 1998.

78. Stumvoll M, Meyer C, Kreider M, et al: Effects of glucagon on renal and hepatic glutamine gluconeogenesis in normal postabsorptive humans. Metabolism 47:1227–1232, 1998.

79. Stumvoll M, Chintalapudi U, Perriello G, et al: Uptake and release of glucose by the human kidney: Postabsorptive rates and responses to epinephrine. J Clin Invest 96:2528–2533, 1995.

80. Stumvoll M, Meyer C, Perriello G, et al: Human kidney and liver gluconeogenesis: Evidence for organ substrate selectivity. Am J Physiol 274:E817–E826, 1998.

81. Perriello G, Jorde R, Nurjhan N, et al: Estimation of the glucose-alanine-lactate-glutamine cycles in postabsorptive man: Role of the skeletal muscle. Am J Physiol 269:E443–E450, 1995.

82. Roden M, Stingl H, Chandramouli V, et al: Effects of free fatty acid elevation on postabsorptive endogenous glucose production and gluconeogenesis in humans. Diabetes 49:701–707, 2000.

83. Boden G, Chen X, Capulong E, et al: Effects of free fatty acids on gluconeogenesis and autoregulation of glucose production in type 2 diabetes. Diabetes 50:810–816, 2001.

84. McMahon M, Marsh H, Rizza R: Comparison of the pattern of postprandial carbohydrate metabolism after ingestion of a glucose drink or a mixed meal. J Clin Endocrinol Metab 68:647–653, 1989.

85. Dinneen S, Gerich J, Rizza R: Carbohydrate metabolism in noninsulin-dependent diabetes mellitus. N Engl J Med 327:707–713, 1992.

86. Kelley D, Mitrakou A, Marsh H, et al: Skeletal muscle glycolysis, oxidation, and storage of an oral glucose load. J Clin Invest 81:1563–1571, 1988.

87. Kelley D, Mokan M, Veneman T: Impaired postprandial glucose utilization in non-insulin-dependent diabetes mellitus. Metabolism 43:1549–1557, 1994.

88. Woerle HJ, Meyer C, Dostou JM, et al: Pathways for glucose disposal after meal ingestion in humans. Am J Physiol Endocrinol Metab 284:E716–E725, 2003.

89. Mitrakou A, Kelley D, Mokan M, et al: Role of reduced suppression of glucose production and diminished early insulin release in impaired glucose tolerance. N Engl J Med 326:22–29, 1992.

90. Pratley R, Weyer C: The role of impaired early insulin secretion in the pathogenesis of type II diabetes mellitus. Diabetologia 44:929–945, 2001.

91. Meyer C, Dostou J, Welle S, et al: Role of human liver, kidney and skeletal muscle in postprandial glucose homeostasis. Am J Physiol Endocrinol Metab 282:E419–E427, 2002.

92. Meyer C, Dostou J, Welle S, et al: Role of liver, kidney and skeletal muscle in the disposition of an oral glucose load. Diabetes 48(Suppl 1):A289, 1999.

93. Taylor R, Magnusson I, Rothman D: Direct assessment of liver glycogen storage by ^{13}C nuclear magnetic resonance spectroscopy and regulation of glucose homeostasis after a mixed meal in normal subjects. J Clin Invest 97:126–132, 1996.

94. Kruszynska Y, Mulford M, Yu J, et al: Effects of nonesterified fatty acids on glucose metabolism after glucose ingestion. Diabetes 46:1586–1593, 1997.

95. Tse T, Clutter W, Shah S, et al: Mechanisms of postprandial glucose counterregulation in man: Physiologic roles of glucagon and epinephrine vis-a-vis insulin in the prevention of hypoglycemia late after glucose ingestion. J Clin Invest 72:278–286, 1983.

96. Hogan M, Service F, Sharbrough F, et al: Oral glucose tolerance test compared with a mixed meal in the diagnosis of reactive hypoglycemia: A caveat on stimulation. Mayo Clin Proc 58:491–496, 1983.

97. Gerich J: Glucose counterregulation and its impact on diabetes mellitus. Diabetes 37:1608–1617, 1988.

98. Cersosimo E, Garlick P, Ferretti J: Renal glucose production during insulin-induced hypoglycemia in humans. Diabetes 48:261–266, 1999.

99. Meyer C, Dostou J, Gerich J: Role of the human kidney in glucose counterregulation. Diabetes 48:943–948, 1999.

100. Kennedy F, Bolli G, Go V, et al: The significance of impaired pancreatic polypeptide and epinephrine responses to hypoglycemia in patients with insulin-dependent diabetes mellitus. J Clin Endocrinol Metab 64:602–608, 1987.

101. Gerich J, Campbell P: Overview of counterregulation and its abnormalities in diabetes mellitus and other conditions. Diabetes Metab Rev 4:93–111, 1988.

102. White N, Skor D, Cryer P, et al: Identification of type I diabetic patients at increased risk for hypoglycemia during intensive therapy. N Engl J Med 308:485–491, 1983.

103. Lecavalier L, Bolli G, Cryer P, et al: Contributions of gluconeogenesis and glycogenolysis during glucose counterregulation in normal humans. Am J Physiol 256:E844–E851, 1989.

104. DeFeo P, Perriello G, Torlone E, et al: Contribution of adrenergic mechanisms to glucose counterregulation in humans. Am J Physiol 261:E725–E736, 1991.

105. Fanelli C, Calderone S, Epifano L, et al: Demonstration of critical role for FFA in mediating counterregulatory stimulation of gluconeogenesis and suppression of glucose utilization in man. J Clin Invest 92:1617–1622, 1993.

106. Fanelli C, DeFeo P, Perriello G, et al: Adrenergic mechanisms contribute to the late phase of glucose counterregulation in humans by stimulating lipolysis. J Clin Invest 89:2005–2013, 1992.

107. McMahon M, Gerich J, Rizza R: Effects of glucocorticoids on carbohydrate metabolism. Diabetes Metab Rev 4:17–30, 1988.

108. Wingard D, Barrett-Conner E: Family history of diabetes and cardiovascular disease risk factors and mortality among euglycemic, borderline hyperglycemic, and diabetic adult. Am J Epidemiol 125:948–958, 1987.

109. Seltzer H: Drug-induced hypoglycemia: A review of 1418 cases. Endocrinol Metab Clin North Am 18:163–183, 1989.

110. DCCT Research Group: Adverse events and their association with treatment regimens in the Diabetes Control and Complications Trial. Diabetes Care 18:1415–1427, 1995.

111. Abraira C, Colwell J, Nuttall F, et al: Veterans affairs cooperative study on glycemic control and complications in type II diabetes (VA CSDM): Results of the feasibility trial. Diabetes Care 18:1113–1123, 1995.

112. McCall A: New findings and treatment strategies for hypoglycemia and hypoglycemia unawareness. Curr Opin Endocrinol Metab 5:138–143, 1999.

113. Cryer P: Hypoglycaemia: The limiting factor in the glycaemic management of type I and type II diabetes. Diabetologia 45:937–948, 2002.

114. van Staa T, Abenhaim L, Monette J: Rates of hypoglycemia in users of sulfonylureas. J Clin Epidemiol 50:735–741, 1997.

115. Woerle HJ, Meyer C, Popa E, et al: Renal compensation for impaired hepatic glucose release during hypoglycemia in type 2 diabetes:

further evidence for hepatorenal reciprocity. Diabetes 52:1386–1392, 2003.

116. Arky R, Freinkel N: Alcohol infusion to test gluconeogenesis in starvation with special reference to obesity. N Engl J Med 274:426–433, 1966.

117. Flanagan D, Wood P, Sherwin R, et al: Gin and tonic and reactive hypoglycemia: What is important—the gin, the tonic, or both? J Clin Endocrinol Metab 83:796–800, 1998.

118. Arky R: Hypoglycemia associated with liver disease and ethanol. Endocrinol Metab Clin North Am 18:75–90, 1989.

119. Madison L: Ethanol-induced hypoglycemia. In Levine R, Luft R (eds): Advances in Metabolic Disorders, vol 3. New York, Academic Press, 1968, pp 85–109.

120. Marks V, Teale J: Drug-induced hypoglycemia. Endocrinol Metab Clin North Am 28:555–577, 1999.

121. Siler S, Neese R, Christiansen M, et al: The inhibition of gluconeogenesis following alcohol in humans. Am J Physiol 275:E897–E907, 1998.

122. Krebs H, Freedland R, Stubbs M: Inhibition of hepatic gluconeogenesis by ethanol. Biochem J 112:117–124, 1969.

123. Kreisberg R, Owen W, Siegal A: Ethanol-induced hyperlacticacidemia: Inhibition of lactate utilization. J Clin Invest 50:166–174, 1971.

124. Kreisberg R, Siegal A, Owen W: Alanine and gluconeogenesis in man: Effect of ethanol. J Clin Endocrinol Metab 34:876–883, 1972.

125. Chan J, Cockram C, Critchley J: Drug-induced disorders of glucose metabolism: Mechanisms and management. Drug Saf 15:135–157, 1996.

126. Reith D, Dawson A, Epid D, et al: Relative toxicity of beta blockers in overdose. Clin Toxicol 34:273–278, 1996.

127. Poretsky L, Moses A: Hypoglycemia associated with trimethoprim/sulfamethoxazole therapy. Diabetes Care 7:508–509, 1984.

128. Rizza R, Cryer P, Haymond M, et al: Adrenergic mechanisms for the effect of epinephrine on glucose production and clearance in man. J Clin Invest 65:682–689, 1980.

129. Majumdar SR: Beta-blockers for the treatment of hypertension in patients with diabetes: Exploring the contraindication myth. Cardiovasc Drugs Ther 13:435–439, 1999.

130. Sawicki PT, Siebenhofer A: Betablocker treatment in diabetes mellitus. J Intern Med 250:11–17, 2001.

131. Baron S: Salicylates as hypoglycemic agents. Diabetes Care 5:64–71, 1982.

132. Washio M, Onoyama K, Makita Y, et al: Hypoglycemia associated with the administration of angiotensin-converting enzyme inhibitor in a diabetic hemodialysis patient. Nephron 59:341–342, 1991.

133. Arauz-Pacheco C, Ramirez L, Rios J, et al: Hypoglycemia induced by angiotensin-converting enzyme inhibitors in patients with non-insulin-dependent diabetes receiving sulfonylurea therapy. Am J Med 89:811–813, 1990.

134. Morris A, Boyle D, McMahon A, et al: ACE inhibitor use is associated with hospitalization for severe hypoglycemia in patients with diabetes. Diabetes Care 20:1363–1367, 1997.

135. Perronne C, Bricaire F, Leport C, et al: Hypoglycaemia and diabetes mellitus following parenteral pentamidine mesylate treatment in AIDS patients. Diabet Med 7:585–589, 1990.

136. Bouchard P, Sai P, Reach G, et al: Diabetes mellitus following pentamidine-induced hypoglycemia in humans. Diabetes 31:40–45, 1982.

137. Pollare T, Lithell H, Berne C: A comparison of the effects of hydrochlorothiazide and captopril on glucose and lipid metabolism in patients with hypertension. N Engl J Med 321:868–873, 1989.

138. Jauch K, Hartl W, Georgieff M, et al: Low dose bradykinin infusion reduces endogenous glucose production in surgical patients. Metabolism 37:185–190, 1988.

139. Shorr R, Ray W, Daugherty J, et al: Incidence and risk factors for serious hypoglycemia in older persons using insulin or sulfonylureas. Arch Intern Med 157:1681–1686, 1997.

140. Shorr R, Ray W, Daugherty J, et al: Individual sulfonylureas and serious hypoglycemia in older people. J Am Geriatr Soc 44:751–755, 1996.

141. Salas M, Caro JJ: Are hypoglycaemia and other adverse effects similar among sulphonylureas? Adverse Drug React Toxicol Rev 21:205–217, 2002.

142. Klonoff D, Barrett B, Nolte M, et al: Hypoglycemia following inadvertent and factitious sulfonylurea overdosages. Diabetes Care 18:563–567, 1995.

143. Shumak S, Corenblum B, Steiner G: Recurrent hypoglycemia secondary to drug-dispensing error. Arch Intern Med 151:1877–1878, 1991.

144. Chiolero R, Revelly J, Tappy L: Energy metabolism in sepsis and injury. Nutrition 13(9, Suppl):45S–51S, 1997.

145. Mizock B: Alterations in carbohydrate metabolism during stress: A review of the literature. Am J Med 98:75–84, 1995.

146. Kinney J: Metabolic responses of the critically ill patient. Crit Care Clin 11:569–585, 1995.

147. Mathison J, Wolfson E, Ulevitch R: Participation of tumor necrosis factor in the mediation of gram negative bacterial lipopolysaccharide-induced injury in rabbits. J Clin Invest 81:1925–1937, 1988.

148. Richards A: Tumour necrosis factor and associated cytokines in the host's response to malaria. Int J Parasitol 27:1251–1263, 1997.

149. Stouthard J, Romijn J, van der Poll T, et al: Endocrinologic and metabolic effects of interleukin-6 in humans. Am J Physiol 268:E813–E819, 1995.

150. Sakurai Y, Zhang X-J, Wolfe R: TNF directly stimulates glucose uptake and leucine oxidation and inhibits FFA flux in conscious dogs. Am J Physiol 270:E864–E872, 1996.

151. Hinshaw L: Concise review: The role of glucose in endotoxin shock. Circ Shock 3:1–10, 1976.

152. Brady W, Butler K, Fines R, et al: Hypoglycemia in multiple trauma victims. Am J Emerg Med 17:4–5, 1999.

153. Miller S, Wallace R, Musher D, et al: Hypoglycemia as a manifestation of sepsis. Am J Med 68:649–654, 1980.

154. Lang C, Bagby G, Blakesley H, et al: Importance of hyperglucagonemia in eliciting the sepsis-induced increase in glucose production. Circ Shock 29:181–191, 1989.

155. Hargrove D, Bagby G, Lang C, et al: Adrenergic blockade does not abolish elevated glucose turnover during bacterial infection. Am J Physiol 254:E16–E22, 1988.

156. Fettman M: Endotoxemia in Yucatan miniature pigs: Metabolic derangements and experimental therapies. Lab Anim Sci 36:370–374, 1986.

157. Wichterman K, Chaudry I, Baue A: Studies of peripheral glucose uptake during sepsis. Arch Surg 114:740–745, 1979.

158. Meszaros K, Lang C, Bagby G, et al: In vivo glucose utilization by individual tissues during nonlethal hypermetabolic sepsis. FASEB J 2:3083–3086, 1988.

159. Romanosky A, Bagby G, Bockman E, et al: Increased muscle glucose uptake and lactate release after endotoxin administration. Am J Physiol 239:E311–E316, 1980.

160. Naylor J, Kronfeld D: In vivo studies of hypoglycemia and lactic acidosis in endotoxic shock. Am J Physiol 248:E309–E316, 1985.

161. Wolfe R, Burke J: Glucose and lactate metabolism in experimental septic shock. Am J Physiol 235:R219–R227, 1978.

162. Durkot M, Wolfe R: Effects of adrenergic blockade on glucose kinetics in septic and burned guinea pigs. Am J Physiol 241:R222–R227, 1981.

163. Bagby G, Lang C, Skrepnik N, et al: Attenuation of glucose metabolic changes resulting from TNF-a administration by adrenergic blockade. Am J Physiol 262:R628–R635, 1992.

164. Maitra S, Homan C, Pan W, et al: Renal gluconeogenesis and blood flow during endotoxic shock. Acad Emerg Med 3:1006–1010, 1996.

165. Wannemacher R, Pace J, Beall F, et al: Role of the liver in regulation of ketone body production during sepsis. J Clin Invest 64:1565–1572, 1979.

166. Wannemacher R, Beall F, Canonico P, et al: Glucose and alanine metabolism during bacterial infections in rats and rhesus monkeys. Metabolism 29:201–212, 1980.

167. Alderfer H, Richardson J: Hepatic hypoglycemia and infarction of the bowel. Arch Intern Med 112:50–55, 1963.

168. Medalle R, Webb R, Waterhouse C: Lactic acidosis and associated hypoglycemia. Arch Intern Med 128:273–278, 1971.

169. Fuchs S, Bogomolski-Yahalom V, Paltiel O, et al: Ischemic hepatitis. J Clin Gastroenterol 26:183–186, 1998.

170. Hedayati H, Beheshti M: Profound spontaneous hypoglycaemia in congestive heart failure. Curr Med Res Opin 4:501–504, 1977.

171. Mellinkoff S, Tumulty P: Hepatic hypoglycemia: Its occurrence in congestive heart failure. N Engl J Med 247:745–750, 1952.

172. Marks V, Rose F: Hypoglycemia, vol 2. Oxford, UK, Blackwell Scientific, 1981.

173. Medalle R, Webb R, Waterhouse C: Lactic acidosis and associated hypoglycemia. Arch Intern Med 128:273–278, 1952.

174. Seltzer H: Severe drug-induced hypoglycemia: A review. Compr Ther 5:21–29, 1979.

175. Arem R: Hypoglycemia associated with renal failure. Endocrinol Metab Clin North Am 18:103–121, 1989.

176. Owen O, Felig P, Morgan A, et al: Liver and kidney metabolism during prolonged starvation. J Clin Invest 48:574–583, 1969.

177. Reinecke R: The kidney as a source of glucose in the eviscerated rat. Am J Physiol 140:276–285, 1943.

178. Lupianez J, Faus M, Munoz–Clares R, et al: Stimulation of rat kidney gluconeogenic ability by inhibition of liver gluconeogenesis. FEBS Lett 61:277–281, 1976.

179. Gerich J: Hepatorenal glucose reciprocity in physiologic and pathologic conditions. Diab Nutr Metab 15:298–302, 2002.

180. Battezzati A, Fattorini A, Caumo A, et al: Non-hepatic glucose production in humans. Diabetes 48(Suppl 1):A49, 1999.

181. Mann F: Effects of complete and partial removal of the liver. Medicine (Baltimore) 6:419–467, 1927.

182. Zimmerman H, Thomas L, Scherr E: Fasting blood sugar in hepatic disease with reference to infrequency of hypoglycemia. Arch Intern Med 91:577–584, 1953.

183. Katz N: Correlation between rates and enzyme levels of increased gluconeogenesis in rat liver and kidney after partial hepatectomy. Eur J Biochem 98:535–542, 1979.

184. Felig P, Brown W, Levine R, et al: Glucose homeostasis in viral hepatitis. N Engl J Med 283:1436–1440, 1970.

185. Heinig R, Clarke E, Waterhouse C: Lactic acidosis and liver disease. Arch Intern Med 139:1229–1232, 1979.

186. Nouel O, Bernuau J, Rueff B, et al: Hypoglycemia: A common complication of septicemia in cirrhosis. Arch Intern Med 141:1477–1478, 1981.

187. Younus S, Soterakis J, Sossi A, et al: Hypoglycemia secondary to metastases to the liver. Gastroenterology 72:334–337, 1977.

188. Johnson D, Alberti K, Faber O, et al: Hyperinsulinism of hepatic cirrhosis: Diminished degradation or hypersecretion? Lancet 1:10–13, 1977.

189. Gorden P, Hendricks C, Kahn C: Hypoglycemia associated with non-islet cell tumor and insulin-like growth factors. N Engl J Med 305:1452–1455, 1981.

190. Zubrod C, Eversole S, Dane G: Amelioration of diabetes and striking rarity of acidosis in patients with Kimmelstiel-Wilson lesions. N Engl J Med 245:518–525, 1951.

191. Block M, Rubinstein A: Spontaneous hypoglycemia in diabetic patients with renal insufficiency. JAMA 213:1863–1866, 1970.

192. Hultman E, Nilsson L: Liver glycogen in man: Effect of different diets and muscular exercise. Adv Exp Med Biol 11:143–151, 1971.

193. Frizzel M, Larsen R, Field J: Spontaneous hypoglycemia associated with chronic renal failure. Diabetes 22:493–498, 1973.

194. Peitzman S, Agarwal B: Spontaneous hypoglycemia in end-stage renal failure. Nephron 19:131–139, 1977.

195. Avram M, Wolf R, Gan A, et al: Uremic hypoglycemia: A preventable life-threatening complication. N Y St J Med 84:593–596, 1984.

196. Rutsky E, McDaniel H, Tharpe D, et al: Spontaneous hypoglycemia in chronic renal failure. Arch Intern Med 138:1364–1368, 1978.

197. Toth E, Lee D: "Spontaneous"/uremic hypoglycemia is not a distinct entity: Substantiation from a literature review. Nephron 58:325–329, 1991.

198. Mühlhauser I, Toth G, Sawicki P, et al: Severe hypoglycemia in type I diabetic patients with impaired kidney function. Diabetes Care 14:344–346, 1991.

199. Fürst P: Amino acid metabolism in uremia. J Am Coll Nutr 8:310–323, 1989.

200. Garber A, Bier D, Cryer P, et al: Hypoglycemia in compensated chronic renal insufficiency. Substrate limitation of gluconeogenesis. Diabetes 23:982–986, 1976.

201. Greenblatt D: Fatal hypoglycaemia occurring after peritoneal dialysis. Br Med J 2:270–271, 1972.

202. Tzamaloukas A, Murata G, Eisenberg B, et al: Hypoglycemia in diabetics on dialysis with poor glycemic control: Hemodialysis versus continuous ambulatory peritoneal dialysis. Int J Artif Organs 15:390–392, 1992.

203. Mak RH: Impact of end-stage renal disease and dialysis on glycemic control. Semin Dial 13:4–8, 2000.

204. Langlois M, Robert G, Nawar T, et al: Spontaneous hypoglycemia and chronic kidney insufficiency [in French]. Can Med Assoc J 118:1083–1086, 1978.

205. Rabau M, Dor (Dershovitz) J, Adar R, et al: Spontaneous hypoglycemia in a diabetic patient with renal failure. Isr J Med Sci 9:1036–1039, 1973.

206. Rutsky E, McDaniel H, Tharpe D, et al: Spontaneous hypoglycemia in chronic renal failure. Arch Intern Med 138:1364–1368, 1978.

207. Bonapart I, Diderich P, Elte J, et al: Spontaneous hypoglycemia in chronic renal failure. Neth J Med 48:180–184, 1996.

208. Bansal V, Brooks M, York J, et al: Intractable hypoglycemia in a patient with renal failure. Arch Intern Med 139:101–102, 1979.

209. Grimaldi A, Massin P, Champigneulle A, et al: Spontaneous hypoglycemia in a non-insulin-dependent diabetic with advanced renal failure [in French]. Presse Med 16:36, 1987.

210. Baylor P, Shilo S, Zonszein J, et al: b-Adrenergic contribution to glucagon-induced glucose production and insulin secretion in uremia. Am J Physiol 251:E322–E327, 1986.

211. Ramirez G, Brueggemeyer C, Ganguly A: Counterregulatory hormonal response to insulin-induced hypoglycemia in patients on chronic hemodialysis. Nephron 49:231–236, 1988.

212. Greenblatt D: Insulin sensitivity in renal failure. N Y St J Med 74:1040–1041, 1974.

213. Metcoff J, Furst P, Scharer K, et al: Energy production, intracellular amino acid pools, and protein synthesis in chronic renal disease. J Am Coll Nutr 8:271–284, 1989.

214. Riegel W, Stepinski J, Hörl W, et al: Effect of hormones on hepatocyte gluconeogenesis in different models of acute uraemia. Nephron 32:67–72, 1982.

215. Hermansen K, Johannsen L, Rasmussen O: Hypoglycaemic coma in severe primary hypothyroidism. Acta Med Scand 218:345–346, 1985.

216. Samaan N: Hypoglycemia secondary to endocrine deficiencies. Endocrinol Metab Clin North Am 18:145–154, 1989.

217. Gerich J, Langlois M, Noacco C, et al: Lack of glucagon response to hypoglycemia in diabetes: Evidence for an intrinsic pancreatic alpha-cell defect. Science 182:171–173, 1973.

218. Brun JF, Fedou C, Mercier J: Postprandial reactive hypoglycaemia. Diabetes Metab 26:337–351, 2000.

219. Vidnes J, Oyasaeter S: Glucagon deficiency causing severe neonatal hypoglycaemia in a patient with normal insulin secretion. Pediatr Res 11:943–949, 1977.

220. Kollee L, Monnens L, Cecjka V, et al: Persistent neonatal hypoglycaemia due to glucagon deficiency. Arch Dis Child 53:422–424, 1978.

221. Abs R, Verbist L, Moeremans M, et al: Hypoglycemia owing to inappropriate glucagon secretion treated with a continuous subcutaneous glucagon infusion system. Acta Endocrinol (Copenh) 122:319–322, 1990.

222. Starke A, Valverde I, Bottazzo G, et al: Glucagon deficiency associated with hypoglycaemia and the absence of islet cell antibodies in the polyglandular failure syndrome before the onset of insulin-dependent diabetes mellitus: A case report. Diabetologia 25:336–339, 1983.

223. Polinsky R, Kopin I, Ebert M, et al: The adrenal medullary response to hypoglycemia in patients with orthostatic hypotension. J Clin Endocrinol Metab 51:1401–1406, 1980.

224. Gerich J, Davis J, Lorenzi M, et al: Hormonal mechanisms of recovery from insulin-induced hypoglycemia in man. Am J Physiol 236:E380–E385, 1979.

225. Rizza R, Cryer P, Gerich J: Role of glucagon, catecholamines, and growth hormone in human glucose counterregulation: Effects of somatostatin and combined a- and b-adrenergic blockade on plasma glucose recovery and glucose flux rates after insulin-induced hypoglycemia. J Clin Invest 64:62–71, 1979.

226. Cryer P: Hypoglycemia. Pathophysiology, Diagnosis, and Treatment. New York, Oxford University Press, 1997.

227. Seagall M: Spontaneous hypoglycemia with failure to increase adrenal output. Proc R Soc Med 60:50, 1967.

228. Levin H, Heifetz M: Phaeochromocytoma and severe protracted postoperative hypoglycaemia. Can J Anaesth 37:477–478, 1990.

229. DeFeo P, Perriello G, Torlone E, et al: Contribution of cortisol to glucose counterregulation in man. Am J Physiol 257:E35–E42, 1989.

230. DeFeo P, Perriello G, Torlone E, et al: Demonstration of a role of growth hormone in glucose counterregulation. Am J Physiol 256:E835–E843, 1989.

231. Goodman H, Grumbach M, Kaplan S: Growth and growth hormone: II. A comparison of isolated growth-hormone deficiency and multiple pituitary-hormone deficiencies in 35 patients with idiopathic hypopituitary dwarfism. N Engl J Med 278:57–68, 1968.

232. Artavia-Loria E, Chaussain J, Bougneres P, et al: Frequency of hypoglycemia in children with adrenal insufficiency. Acta Endocrinol Suppl (Copenh) 279:275–278, 1986.

233. Wolfsdorf J, Sadeghi-Nejad A, Senior B: Hypoketonemia and age-related fasting hypoglycemia in growth hormone deficiency. Metabolism 32:457–462, 1983.

234. Haymond M, Karl I, Weldon V, et al: The role of growth hormone and cortisone on glucose and gluconeogenic substrate regulation in fasted hypopituitary children. J Clin Endocrinol Metab 42:846–856, 1976.

235. Yamamoto T, Fukuyama J, Hasegawa K, et al: Isolated corticotropin deficiency in adults. Report of 10 cases and review of literature. Arch Intern Med 152:1705–1712, 1992.

236. Merimee T, Felig P, Marliss E, et al: Glucose and lipid homeostasis in the absence of human growth hormone. J Clin Invest 50:574–582, 1971.

237. Smallridge R, Corrigan D, Thomason A, et al: Hypoglycemia in pregnancy: Occurrence due to adrenocorticotropic hormone and growth hormone deficiency. Arch Intern Med 140:564–565, 1980.

238. Malerbi D, Liberman B, Giurno-Filho A, et al: Glucocorticoids and glucose metabolism: Hepatic glucose production in untreated Addisonian patients and on two different levels of glucocorticoid administration. Clin Endocrinol 28:415–422, 1988.

239. Boyle P, Cryer P: Growth hormone, cortisol, or both are involved in defense against, but are not critical to recovery from, hypoglycemia. Am J Physiol 260:E395–E402, 1991.

240. Zuker N, Bissessor M, Korber M, et al: Acute hypoglycaemic coma: A rare, potentially lethal form of early onset Sheehan syndrome. Aust N Z J Obstet Gynaecol 35:318–320, 1995.

241. Hardy K, Burge M, Boyle P, et al: A treatable cause of recurrent severe hypoglycemia. Diabetes Care 17:722–724, 1994.

242. Johansson C, Adamsson U, Stierner U, et al: Interaction by cholestyramine on the uptake of hydrocortisone in the gastrointestinal tract. Acta Med Scand 204:509–512, 1978.

243. Owen O, Reichard G: Human forearm metabolism during progressive starvation. J Clin Invest 50:1536–1545, 1971.

244. Cahill G: Starvation in man. N Engl J Med 282:668–675, 1970.

245. Field J: Exercise and deficient carbohydrate storage and intake as causes of hypoglycemia. Endocrinol Metab Clin North Am 18:155–161, 1989.

246. Chakrabarty P: Blood glucose levels in slow starvation. Lancet 1:596–597, 1948.

247. Elias A, Gwinup G: Glucose-resistant hypoglycemia in inanition. Arch Intern Med 142:743–746, 1982.

248. Fonseca V, Ball S, Marks V, et al: Hypoglycaemia associated with anorexia nervosa. Postgrad Med J 67:460–461, 1991.

249. Smith J: Hypoglycaemic coma associated with anorexia nervosa. Aust N Z J Psychiatry 22:448–453, 1988.

250. Rich L, Caine M, Findling J, et al: Hypoglycemic coma in anorexia nervosa. Case report and review of the literature. Arch Intern Med 150:894–895, 1990.

251. Wharton B: Hypoglycaemia in children with kwashiorkor. Lancet 1:171–173, 1970.

252. Bruce A, Jacobsen E, Dossing H, et al: Hypoglycaemia in spinal muscular atrophy. Lancet 346:609–610, 1995.

253. Gounelle H, Marche J: Spontaneous coma due to hypoglycemia in undernourished persons. Occup Med 1:48–50, 1948.

254. Taylor S, Barbetti F, Accili D, et al: Syndromes of autoimmunity and hypoglycemia. Autoantibodies directed against insulin and its receptor. Endocrinol Metab Clin North Am 18:123–143, 1989.

255. Hirata Y, Uchigata Y: Insulin autoimmune syndrome in Japan. Diabetes Res Clin Pract 24 (Suppl):S153–S157, 1994.

256. Burch H, Clement S, Sokol M, et al: Reactive hypoglycemic coma due to insulin autoimmune syndrome: Case report and literature review. Am J Med 92:681–685, 1992.

257. Archambeaud-Mouveroux F, Huc M, Nadalon S, et al: Autoimmune insulin syndrome. Biomed Pharmacother 43:581–586, 1989.

258. Redmon J, Nuttall F: Autoimmune hypoglycemia. Endocrinol Metab Clin North Am 28:603–618, 1999.

259. Kim CH, Park JH, Park TS, et al: Autoimmune hypoglycemia in a type 2 diabetic patient with anti-insulin and insulin receptor antibodies. Diabetes Care 27:288–289, 2004.

260. Arioglu E, Andewelt A, Diabo C, et al: Clinical course of the syndrome of autoantibodies to the insulin receptor (type B insulin resistance): A 28-year perspective. Medicine (Baltimore) 81:87–100, 2002.

261. Okabe R, Inaba M, Hosoi M, et al: Remission of insulin autoimmune syndrome in a patient with Grave's disease by treatment with methimazole. Intern Med 38:482–485, 1999.

262. Buysschaert M: Coeliac disease in patients with type 1 diabetes mellitus and auto-immune thyroid disorders. Acta Gastroenterol Belg 66:237–240, 2003.

263. Flier J, Bar R, Muggeo M, et al: The evolving clinical course of patients with insulin receptor autoantibodies: Spontaneous remission of receptor proliferation with hypoglycemia. J Clin Endocrinol Metab 47:985–995, 1978.

264. Taylor S, Grunberger G, Marcus-Samuels B, et al: Hypoglycemia associated with antibodies to the insulin receptor. N Engl J Med 307:1422–1426, 1982.

265. Muggeo M, Flier J, Abrams R, et al: Treatment by plasma exchange of a patient with autoantibodies to the insulin receptor. N Engl J Med 300:477–480, 1979.

266. Kawanishi K, Kawamura K, Nishina Y, et al: Successful immunosuppressive therapy in insulin resistant diabetes caused by anti-insulin receptor autoantibodies. J Clin Endocrinol Metab 44:15–21, 1977.

267. Victor A: Normal blood sugar variation during pregnancy. Acta Obstet Gynecol Scand 53:37–40, 1974.

268. Kalhan S, D'Angelo L, Savin S, et al: Glucose production in pregnant women at term gestation: Sources of glucose for human fetus. J Clin Invest 63:388–394, 1979.

269. Reece E, Homko C, Wiznitzer A: Metabolic changes in diabetic and nondiabetic subjects during pregnancy. Obstet Gynecol Surv 49:64–71, 1994.

270. Garner P, Tsang R: Insulinoma complicating pregnancy presenting with hypoglycemic coma after delivery: A case report and review of the literature. Obstet Gynecol 73:847–849, 1989.

271. Takacs CA, Krivak TC, Napolitano PG: Insulinoma in pregnancy: A case report and review of the literature. Obstet Gynecol Surv 57:229–235, 2002.

272. Schweichler M, Hennessey J, Cole P, et al: Hypoglycemia in pregnancy secondary to a non-islet cell tumor of the pleura and ectopic insulin-like growth factor II hormone production. Obstet Gynecol 85:810–813, 1995.

273. White N, Warrell D, Chanthavanich P, et al: Severe hypoglycemia and hyperinsulinemia in falciparum malaria. N Engl J Med 309:61–66, 1983.

274. Long P, Abell D, Beischer N: Importance of abnormal glucose tolerance (hypoglycaemia and hyperglycaemia) in the aetiology of pre-eclampsia. Lancet 1:923–925, 1977.

275. Neuman M, Ron-El R, Langer R, et al: Maternal death caused by HELLP syndrome (with hypoglycemia) complicating mild pregnancy-induced hypertension in a twin gestation. Am J Obstet Gynecol 162:372–373, 1989.

276. Egley C: Severe hypoglycemia associated with HELLP syndrome. Am J Obstet Gynecol 152:576–577, 1985.

277. Aarnoudse J, Houthoff H, Weits J, et al: A syndrome of liver damage and intravascular coagulation in the last trimester of normotensive pregnancy: A clinical and histopathological study. Br J Obstet Gynaecol 93:145–155, 1986.

278. Levine A, Burgess G, Derick C: Some changes in the chemical constituents of the blood following a marathon race. JAMA 82:1778–1782, 1924.

279. Ahlborg G, Felig P: Lactate and glucose exchange across the forearm, legs, and splanchnic bed during and after prolonged leg exercise. J Clin Invest 69:45–54, 1982.

280. Uusitupa M, Aro A, Pietikainen M: Severe hypoglycaemia caused by physical strain and pindolol therapy: A case report. Ann Clin Res 12:25–27, 1980.

281. Wasserman D, Cherrington A: Hepatic fuel metabolism during muscular work: Role and regulation. Am J Physiol 260:E811–E824, 1991.

282. Wahren J, Felig P, Hagenfeldt L: Physical exercise and fuel homeostasis in diabetes mellitus. Diabetologia 14:213–222, 1978.

283. Marker J, Hirsch I, Smith L, et al: Catecholamines in prevention of hypoglycemia during exercise in humans. Am J Physiol 260:E705–E712, 1991.

284. Hirsch I, Marker J, Smith L, et al: Insulin and glucagon in prevention of hypoglycemia during exercise in humans. Am J Physiol 260:E695–E704, 1991.

285. Service F, Moore G: Factitial Hypoglycemia. In Service F (ed): Hypoglycemic Disorders: Pathogenesis, Diagnosis and Treatment. Boston, GK Hall, 1983, pp 129–141.

286. Marks V, Teale J: Hypoglycemia: Factitious and felonious. Endocrinol Metab Clin North Am 28:579–601, 1999.

287. Sheehy T: Case report: Factitious hypoglycemia in diabetic patients. Am J Med Sci 304:298–302, 1992.

288. Schade D, Drumm D, Eaton R, et al: Factitious brittle diabetes mellitus. Am J Med 78:777–784, 1985.

289. Manning PJ, Espiner EA, Yoon K, et al: An unusual cause of hyperinsulinaemic hypoglycaemia syndrome. Diabet Med 20:772–776, 2003.

290. Kaminer Y, Robbins D: Insulin misuse: A review of an overlooked psychiatric problem. Psychosomatics 30:19–24, 1989.

291. Marchetti P, Faloppa C, Zappella A, et al: A case of factitious hypoglycemia with unusual presentation [in Italian]. Minerva Med 79:1101–1103, 1988.

292. Scarlett J, Mako M, Rubenstein A, et al: Factitious hypoglycemia: Diagnosis by measurement of serum C-peptide immunoreactivity and insulin-binding antibodies. N Engl J Med 297:1029–1032, 1977.

293. Retsas S: Insulin abuse by a drug addict. Br Med J 4:792–793, 1972.

294. Jordan R, Kammer H, Riddle M: Sulfonylurea-induced factitious hypoglycemia: A growing problem. Arch Intern Med 137:390–393, 1977.

295. Grunberger G, Weiner J, Silverman R, et al: Factitious hypoglycemia due to surreptitious administration of insulin. Diagnosis, treatment, and long-term follow-up. Ann Intern Med 108:252–257, 1988.

296. Rynearson E: Hyperinsulinism among malingerers. Med Clin North Am 31:477–480, 1947.

297. Siegel E, Mayer G, Nauck M, et al: Factitious hypoglycemia caused by taking a sulfonylurea drug [in German]. Dtsch Med Wochenschr 112:1575–1579, 1987.

298. Charlton R, Smith G, Day A: Munchausen's syndrome manifesting as factitious hypoglycaemia. Diabetologia 44:784–785, 2001.

299. Teale J, Starkey B, Marks V, et al: The prevalence of factitious hypoglycaemia due to sulphonylurea abuse in the UK: A preliminary report. Practical Diabetes 6:177–178, 1989.

300. Hirshberg B, Skarulis MC, Pucino F, et al: Repaglinide-induced factitious hypoglycemia. J Clin Endocrinol Metab 86:475–477, 2001.

301. Doege K: Fibro-sarcoma of the mediastinum. Ann Surg 92:955–960, 1930.

302. Daughaday W: Hypoglycemia in patients with non-islet cell tumors. Endocrinol Metab Clin North Am 18:91–101, 1989.

303. Anderson N, Lokich J: Mesenchymal tumors associated with hypoglycemia: Case report and review of the literature. Cancer 44:785–790, 1979.

304. Baxter R: The role of insulin-like growth factors and their binding proteins in tumor hypoglycemia. Horm Res 46:195–201, 1996.

305. Benn J, Firth R, Sönksen P: Metabolic effects of an insulin-like factor causing hypoglycaemia in a patient with a haemangiopericytoma. Clin Endocrinol 32:769–780, 1990.

306. Chandalia H, Boshell B: Hypoglycemia associated with extrapancreatic tumors. Arch Intern Med 129:447–456, 1972.

307. Chowdhury F, Bleicher S: Studies of tumor hypoglycemia. Metabolism 22:663–674, 1973.

308. Daughaday W, Emanuele M, Brooks M, et al: Synthesis and secretion of insulin-like growth factor II by a leiomyosarcoma with associated hypoglycemia. N Engl J Med 319:1434–1440, 1988.

309. Daughaday W: The pathophysiology of IGF-II hypersecretion in non-islet cell tumor hypoglycemia. Diab Rev 3:62–72, 1995.

310. Eastman R, Carson R, Orloff D, et al: Glucose utilization in a patient with hepatoma and hypoglycemia. J Clin Invest 89:1958–1963, 1992.

311. McFadzean A, Yeung R: Further observations on hypoglycaemia in hepatocellular carcinoma. Am J Med 47:220–235, 1969.

312. Millard P, Jerrome D, Millward-Sadler G: Spindle-cell tumours and hypoglycaemia. J Clin Pathol 29:520–529, 1976.

313. Moller N, Blum W, Mengel A, et al: Basal and insulin stimulated substrate metabolism in tumour induced hypoglycaemia: Evidence for increased muscle glucose uptake. Diabetologia 34:17–20, 1991.

314. Nissan S, Bar-Maor A, Shafrir E: Hypoglycemia associated with extrapancreatic tumors. N Engl J Med 278:177–183, 1968.

315. Reeve A, Eccles M, Wilkins R, et al: Expression of insulin-like growth factor-II transcripts in Wilms' tumour. Nature 317:258–260, 1985.

316. Scott J, Cowell J, Robertson M, et al: Insulin-like growth factor-II gene expression in Wilms' tumour and embryonic tissues. Nature 317:260–262, 1985.

317. Silbert C, Rossini A, Ghazvinian S, et al: Tumor hypoglycemia: Deficient splanchnic glucose output and deficient glucagon secretion. Diabetes 25:202–206, 1976.

318. Silverstein M: Tumor hypoglycemia. Cancer 23:142–144, 1969.

319. Skrabanek P, Powell D: Ectopic insulin and Occam's razor: Reappraisal of the

riddle of tumour hypoglycaemia. Clin Endocrinol 9:141–154, 1978.

320. Widmer U, Zapf J, Froesch E: Is extrapancreatic tumor hypoglycemia associated with elevated levels of insulin-like growth factor II? J Clin Endocrinol Metab 55:833–839, 1982.

321. Horecker B, Hiatt H: Pathways of carbohydrate metabolism in normal and neoplastic cells. N Engl J Med 258:177–184, 225–232, 1958.

322. Phuphanich S, Jacobs L, Poulos J, et al: Case report: Hypoglycemia secondary to a meningioma. Am J Med Sci 309:317–321, 1995.

323. Chung J, Henry R: Mechanisms of tumor-induced hypoglycemia with intraabdominal hemangiopericytoma. J Clin Endocrinol Metab 81:919–925, 1996.

324. Ko AH, Bergsland EK, Lee GA: Tumor-associated hypoglycemia from metastatic colorectal adenocarcinoma: Case report and review of the literature. Dig Dis Sci 48:192–196, 2003.

325. Seckl M, Mulholland P, Bishop A, et al: Hypoglycemia due to an insulin-secreting small-cell carcinoma of the cervix. N Engl J Med 341:733–736, 1999.

326. Marks V, Teale J: Tumours producing hypoglycaemia. Endocr Relat Cancer 5:111–129, 1998.

327. Johnson D, Dorr K, Swenson W, et al: Reactive hypoglycemia. JAMA 243:1151–1155, 1980.

328. Del Sindaco P, Casucci G, Pampanelli S, et al: Late post-prandial hypoglycaemia as the sole presenting feature of secreting pancreatic beta-cell adenoma in a subtotally gastrectomized patient. Eur J Endocrinol 136:96–99, 1997.

329. Brasel J, Wright J, Wilkins L, et al: An evaluation of seventy-five patients with hypopituitarism beginning in childhood. Am J Med 38:484–498, 1965.

330. O'Keefe S, Marks V: Lunchtime gin and tonic a cause of reactive hypoglycaemia. Lancet 1:1286–1288, 1977.

331. Hofeldt F, Lufkin E, Hagler L, et al: Are abnormalities in insulin secretion responsible for reactive hypoglycemia? Diabetes 23:589–596, 1974.

332. Hopwood N, Forsman P, Kenny F, et al: Hypoglycemia in hypopituitary children. Am J Dis Child 129:918–926, 1975.

333. Leichter S, Permutt M: Effect of adrenergic agents on postgastrectomy hypoglycemia. Diabetes 24:1005–1010, 1975.

334. Shultz K, Neelon F, Nilsen L, et al: Mechanism of postgastrectomy hypoglycemia. Arch Intern Med 128:240–246, 1971.

335. Wiznitzer T, Shapira N, Stadler J, et al: Late hypoglycemia in patients following vagotomy and pyloroplasty. Int Surg 59:229–232, 1974.

336. Hall W, Snaders L: Hypoglycemic convulsions after vagotomy and pyloroplasty. South Med J 66:502–504, 1973.

337. Miholic J, Orskov C, Holst J, et al: Postprandial release of glucagon-like peptide-1, pancreatic glucagon, and insulin after esophageal resection. Digestion 54:73–78, 1993.

338. Veverbrants E, Olsen W, Arky R: Role of gastro-intestinal factors in reactive hypoglycemia. Metabolism 18:6–12, 1969.

339. Zieve L, Jones D, Aziz M: Functional hypoglycemia and peptic ulcer. Postgrad Med 40:159–170, 1966.

340. O'Brien T, Tijtgat G, Ensinck J: Alimentary hypoglycemia associated with the Zollinger-Ellison syndrome. Am J Med 54:637–644, 1973.

341. Luyckx A, Lefebvre P: Plasma insulin in reactive hypoglycemia. Diabetes 20:435–442, 1971.

342. Bellini F, Sammicheli L, Ianni L, et al: Hypoglycemia unawareness in a patient with dumping syndrome: Report of a case. J Endocrinol Invest 21:463–467, 1998.

343. Freinkel N, Metzger B: Oral glucose tolerance curve and hypoglycemias in the fed state. N Engl J Med 280:820–828, 1969.

344. Andreasen J, Orskov C, Holst J: Secretion of glucagon-like peptide-1 and reactive hypoglycemia after partial gastrectomy. Digestion 55:221–228, 1994.

345. Miholic J, Orskov C, Holst J, et al: Emptying of the gastric substitute, glucagon-like peptide-1 (GLP-1), and reactive hypoglycemia after total gastrectomy. Dig Dis Sci 36:1361–1370, 1991.

346. Seltzer H, Allen E, Herror A, et al: Insulin response to glycemic stimulus: Relation of delayed initial release to carbohydrate intolerance in mild diabetes. J Clin Invest 46:323–335, 1967.

347. Faludi G, Bendersky G, Gerber P: Functional hypoglycemia in early latent diabetes. Ann N Y Acad Sci 148:868–874, 1968.

348. Permutt M: Postprandial hypoglycemia. Diabetes 25:719–733, 1976.

349. Hofeldt F: Reactive hypoglycemia. Endocrinol Metab Clin North Am 18:185–201, 1989.

350. Service F: Classification of hypoglycemic disorders. Endocrinol Metab Clin North Am 28:501–517, 1999.

351. Owada K, Wasada T, Miyazono Y, et al: Highly increased insulin secretion in a patient with postprandial hypoglycemia: Role of glucagon-like peptide-1 (7-36) amide. Endocr J 42:147–151, 1995.

352. Permutt M, Kelly J, Berstein R, et al: Alimentary hypoglycemia in the absence of gastrointestinal surgery. N Engl J Med 288:1206–1210, 1973.

353. Palardy J, Havrankova J, Lepage R, et al: Blood glucose measurements during symptomatic episodes in patients with suspected postprandial hypoglycemia. N Engl J Med 321:1421–1425, 1989.

354. Foa P, Dunbar J Jr, Klein S, et al: Reactive hypoglycemia and A-cell ('pancreatic') glucagon deficiency in the adult. JAMA 244:2281–2285, 1980.

355. Ahmadpour S, Kabadi U: Pancreatic alpha-cell function in idiopathic reactive hypoglycemia. Metabolism 46:639–643, 1997.

356. Leonetti F, Morviducci L, Giaccari A, et al: Idiopathic reactive hypoglycemia: A role for glucagon? J Endocrinol Invest 15:273–278, 1992.

357. Shima K, Tabata M, Tanaka A, et al: Exaggerated response of plasma glucagon-like immunoreactivity (GLI) to oral glucose in patients with reactive hypoglycemia. Endocrinol Jpn 28:249–256, 1981.

358. Wasada T, Katsumori K, Saeki A, et al: Lack of C-peptide suppression by exogenous hyperinsulinemia in subjects with symptoms suggesting reactive hypoglycemia. Endocr J 43:639–644, 1996.

359. Leonetti F, Foniciello M, Iozzo P, et al: Increased nonoxidative glucose metabolism in idiopathic reactive hypoglycemia. Metabolism 45:606–610, 1996.

360. Lteif A, Schwenk W: Hypoglycemia in infants and children. Endocrinol Metab Clin North Am 28:619–646, 1999.

361. Witteles RM, Straus FH II, Sugg SL, et al: Adult-onset nesidioblastosis causing hypoglycemia: An important clinical entity and continuing treatment dilemma. Arch Surg 136:656–663, 2001.

362. Thomas P: Genetic mutations as a cause of hyperinsulinemic hypoglycemia in children. Endocrinol Metab Clin North Am 28:647–656, 1999.

363. Service F, Natt N, Thompson G, et al: Noninsulinoma pancreatogenous hypoglycemia: a novel syndrome of hyperinsulinemic hypoglycemia in adults independent of mutations in Kir6.2 and SUR1 genes. J Clin Endocrinol Metab 84:1582–1589, 1999.

364. Kaczirek K, Soleiman A, Schindl M, et al: Nesidioblastosis in adults: A challenging cause of organic hyperinsulinism. Eur J Clin Invest 33:488–492, 2003.

365. Allweis T, Rimon B, Freund H: Malnutrition-associated reactive hypoglycemia induced by TPN. Nutrition 13:222–224, 1997.

366. Charles M, Hofeldt F, Shackelford A, et al: Comparison of oral glucose tolerance tests and mixed meals in patients with apparent idiopathic postabsorptive hypoglycemia: Absence of hypoglycemia after meals. Diabetes 30:465–470, 1981.

367. Snorgaard O, Binder C: Monitoring of blood glucose concentration in subjects with hypoglycaemic symptoms during everyday life. Br Med J 300:16–18, 1990.

368. Ford C, Bray G, Swerdloff R: A psychiatric study of patients referred with a diagnosis of hypoglycemia. Am J Psychiatry 133:290–294, 1976.

369. Berlin I, Grimaldi A, Landault C, et al: Suspected postprandial hypoglycemia is associated with beta-adrenergic hypersensitivity and emotional distress. J Clin Endocrinol Metab 79:1428–1433, 1994.

370. Lev-Ran A, Anderson R: The diagnosis of postprandial hypoglycemia. Diabetes 30:996–999, 1981.

371. Neve E: The morbid anatomy of the pancreas. Lancet 2:659, 1892.

372. Warren S: Adenomas of the islets of Langerhans. Am J Pathol 2:335–340, 1926.

373. Harris S: Hyperinsulinism and dysinsulinism. JAMA 83:729–733, 1924.

374. Wilder R, Allan F, Power M, et al: Carcinoma of the islands of the pancreas: Hyperinsulinism and hypoglycemia. JAMA 89:348–355, 1927.

375. Howland G, Campbell W, Maltby E, et al: Dysinsulinism: Convulsions and coma due to islet cell tumor of the pancreas. JAMA 93:674–679, 1929.

376. Whipple A, Frantz V: Adenoma of islet cells with hyperinsulinism. Ann Surg 101:1299–1335, 1935.

377. Whipple A: The surgical therapy of hyperinsulinism. J Int Chir 3:237–276, 1938.

378. Howard J, Moss N, Rhoads J: Hyperinsulinism and islet cell tumors of the pancreas. Int Abstr Surg 90:417–455, 1950.

379. Fajans S, Vinik A: Insulin-producing islet cell tumors. Endocrinol Metab Clin North Am 18:45–74, 1989.

380. Service F, McMahon M, O'Brien P, et al: Functioning insulinoma: Incidence, recurrence, and long-term survival of patients: A 60-year study. Mayo Clin Proc 66:711–719, 1991.

381. Service F, Dale A, Elveback L, et al: Insulinoma: Clinical and diagnostic features of 60 consecutive cases. Mayo Clin Proc 51:417–429, 1976.

382. Galbut D, Markowitz A: Insulinoma: Diagnosis, surgical management and long-term follow-up: Review of 41 cases. Am J Surg 139:682–690, 1980.

383. Stefanini P, Carboni M, Patrassi N, et al: Beta-islet cell tumors of the pancreas: Results of a study on 1,067 cases. Surgery 75:597–609, 1974.

384. Broder L, Carter S: Pancreatic islet cell carcinoma: I. Clinical features of 52 patients. Ann Intern Med 79:101–107, 1973.

385. Laidlaw G: Nesidioblastoma: The islet cell tumor of the pancreas. Am J Pathol 14:125–139, 1937.

386. Yakovac W, Baker L, Hummeler K: Beta cell nesidioblastosis in idiopathic hypoglycemia of infancy. J Pediatr 79:226–231, 1971.

387. Harness J, Geelhoed G, Thompson N, et al: Nesidioblastosis in adults: A surgical dilemma. Arch Surg 116:575–580, 1981.

388. Gould V, Chejfec G, Shah K, et al: Adult nesidiodysplasia. Semin Diagn Pathol 1:43–53, 1984.

389. Walmsley D, Matheson N, Ewen S, et al: Nesidioblastosis in an elderly patient. Diabet Med 12:542–545, 1995.

390. Harrison T, Fajans S, Floyd J Jr, et al: Prevalence of diffuse pancreatic beta islet cell disease with hyperinsulinism: Problems in recognition and management. World J Surg 8:583–589, 1984.

391. Stefanini P, Carboni M, Patrassi N, et al: Hypoglycemia and insular hyperplasia: Review of 148 cases. Ann Surg 180:130–135, 1974.

392. Kavlie H, White T: Pancreatic islet beta cell tumors and hyperplasia: Experience in 14 Seattle hospitals. Ann Surg 175:326–335, 1972.

393. Cullen R, Ong C: Insulinoma in Auckland 1970–1985. N Z Med J 100:560–562, 1987.

394. Dizon A, Kowalyk S, Hoogwerf B: Neuroglycopenic and other symptoms in patients with insulinomas. Am J Med 106:307–310, 1999.

395. Perry R, Vinik A: Clinical review 72: Diagnosis and management of functioning islet cell tumors. J Clin Endocrinol Metab 80:2273–2278, 1995.

396. Kane L, Grant C, Nippoldt T, et al: Insulinoma in a patient with NIDDM. Diabetes Care 16:1298–1300, 1993.

397. Sakurai A, Aizawa T, Katakura M, et al: Insulinoma in a patient with non-insulin-dependent diabetes mellitus. Endocr J 44:473–477, 1997.

398. Wildbrett J, Nagel M, Theissig F, et al: An unusual picture of insulinoma in type-2 diabetes mellitus and morbid obesity [in German]. Dtsch Med Wochenschr 124:248–252, 1999.

399. Gerich J, Charles M, Grodsky G: Regulation of pancreatic insulin and glucagon secretion. Annu Rev Physiol 38:353–388, 1976.

400. Creutzfeldt W, Arnold R, Creutzfeldt C, et al: Biochemical and morphological investigations of 30 human insulinomas: Correlation between the tumour content of insulin and proinsulin-like components and the histological and ultrastructural appearance. Diabetologia 9:217–231, 1973.

401. Lindall A, Steffes M, Wong E: Comparison of insulin and proinsulin storage in an islet adenoma and adjacent pancreas. Metabolism 23:249–256, 1974.

402. Alsever R, Stjernholm M, Sussman K, et al: Clinical correlations of serum proinsulin-like material in islet cell tumours. Diabetologia 12:527–530, 1976.

403. Rizza R, Haymond M, Verdonk C, et al: Pathogenesis of hypoglycemia in insulinoma patients: Suppression of hepatic glucose production by insulin. Diabetes 30:377–381, 1981.

404. Wynick D, Williams S, Bloom S: Symptomatic secondary hormone syndromes in patients with established malignant pancreatic endocrine tumors. N Engl J Med 319:605–607, 1988.

405. Fonseca V, Ames D, Ginsburg J: Hypoglycaemia for 26 years due to an insulinoma. J R Soc Med 82:437–438, 1989.

406. Vea H, Trovik T, Sager G, et al: Return of beta-adrenergic snesitivity in a patient with insulinoma after removal of the tumour. Diabet Med 14:979–984, 1997.

407. Vea H, Jorde R, Sager G, et al: Pre- and postoperative glucose levels for eliciting hypoglycemic responses in a patient with insulinoma. Diabetic Med 9(10):950–953, 1992.

408. Lloyd R, Caceres V, Warner T, et al: Islet cell adenomatosis: A report of two cases and review of the literature. Arch Pathol Lab Med 105:198–202, 1981.

409. Fong T, Warner N, Kumar D: Pancreatic nesidioblastosis in adults. Diabetes Care 12:108–114, 1989.

410. Service F: Hypoglycemic disorders. N Engl J Med 332:1144–1152, 1995.

411. Marks V, Teale J: Investigation of hypoglycaemia. Clin Endocrinol (Oxf) 44:133–136, 1996.

412. Service F, O'Brien P, Kao P, et al: C-peptide suppression test: Effects of gender, age, and body mass index; implications for the diagnosis of insulinoma. J Clin Endocrinol Metab 74:204–210, 1992.

413. Marks V, Somols E: Diagnostic tests for evaluating hypoglycemia. In Rodriguez R, Vallance-Owen J (eds): Diabetes. Amsterdam, Excerpta Medica, 1971, pp 864–872.

414. Kumar D, Mehtalia S, Miller L: Diagnostic use of glucagon-induced insulin response. Studies in patients with insulinoma or other hypoglycemic conditions. Ann Intern Med 80:697–701, 1974.

415. Floyd J Jr, Fajans S, Knopf R, et al: Plasma insulin in organic hyperinsulinism: Comparative effects of tolbutamide, leucine and glucose. J Clin Endocrinol 24:747–760, 1964.

416. Service F: Diagnostic approach to adults with hypoglycemic disorders. Endocrinol Metab Clin North Am 28:519–532, 1999.

417. Filipi C, Higgins G: Diagnosis and management of insulinoma. Am J Surg 125:231–239, 1973.

418. Boukhman M, Karam J, Shaver J, et al: Insulinoma: Experience from 1950 to 1995. West J Med 169:98–104, 1998.

419. Daggett P, Goodburn E, Kurtz A, et al: Is preoperative localisation of insulinomas necessary? Lancet 1:483–486, 1981.

420. Grant C: Surgical aspects of hyperinsulinemic hypoglycemia. Endocrinol Metab Clin North Am 28:533–554, 1999.

421. Norton J, Whitman E: Insulinoma. Endocrinologist 3:258–267, 1995.

422. Huai J-C, Zhang W, Niu H-O, et al: Localization and surgical treatment of pancreatic insulinomas guided by intraoperative ultrasound. Am J Surg 175:18–21, 1998.

423. King A, Ko G, Yeung V, et al: Dual phase spiral CT in the detection of small insulinomas of the pancreas. Br J Radiol 71:20–23, 1998.

424. van Heerden J, Grant C, Czako P, et al: Occult functioning insulinomas: Which localizing studies are indicated? Surgery 112:1010–1014, 1992.

425. Gill G, Rauf O, MacFarlane I: Diazoxide treatment for insulinoma: A national UK survey. Postgrad Med J 73:640–641, 1997.

426. Osei K, O'Dorisio T: Malignant insulinoma: Effects of a somatostatin analog (compound 201-995) on serum glucose, growth, and gastro-entero-pancreatic hormones. Ann Intern Med 103:223–225, 1985.

427. Hearn P, Ahmed M, Woodhouse N: The use of SMS 201-995 (somatostatin analogue) in insulinomas: Additional case report and literature review. Horm Res 29:211–213, 1988.

428. Richter W, Otto C: Continuous subcutaneous glucagon infusion as a symptomatic therapy in two patients with organic hyperinsulinemia. Endocrinol Metab 3:63–65, 1996.

429. Moertel C, Hanley J, Johnson L: Streptozocin alone compared with streptozocin plus fluorouracil in the treatment of advanced islet-cell carcinoma. N Engl J Med 303:1189–1194, 1980.

430. Kiang D, Frenning D, Bauer G: Mithramycin for hypoglycemia in malignant insulinoma. N Engl J Med 299:134–135, 1978.

431. Eastman R, Come S, Strewler G, et al: Adriamycin therapy for advanced insulinoma. J Clin Endocrinol Metab 44:142–148, 1977.

432. Ajani J, Carrasco C, Charnsangavej C, et al: Islet cell tumors metastatic to the liver: Effective palliation by sequential hepatic artery embolization. Ann Intern Med 108:340–344, 1988.

433. Malouf R, Brust J: Hypoglycemia: Causes, neurological manifestations, and outcome. Ann Neurol 17:421–430, 1985.

434. Kresevic D, Slavin S: Incidence of hypoglycemia and nutritional intake in patients on a general medical unit. Nurs Connections 2:33–40, 1989.

435. Gaston S: Outcomes of hypoglycemia treated by standardized protocol in a community hospital. Diabetes Educ 18:491–494, 1992.

436. Slama G, Traynard P, Desplanque N, et al: The search for an optimized treatment of hypoglycemia: Carbohydrates in tablets, solution, or gel for the correction of insulin reactions. Arch Intern Med 150:589–593, 1990.

437. Palatnick W, Meatherall R, Tenenbein M: Clinical spectrum of sulfonylurea overdose and experience with diazoxide therapy. Arch Intern Med 151:1859–1862, 1991.

438. Jermendy G: Factitious hypoglycemia: Munchausen syndrome in diabetes mellitus [in Hungarian]. Orv Hetil 136:31–33, 1995.

439. Jezequel C, de Kerdanet M, Girre M: Hypoglycemia provoked by clandestine injections of insulin in the diabetic child [in French]. Ann Pediatr (Paris) 40:32–36, 1993.

440. Schuler G, Petersen K, Khalaf A, et al: Insulin abuse in long-standing IDDM. Diabetes Res Clin Pract 6:145–148, 1989.

441. Roy M, Roy A: Factitious hypoglycemia: An 11-year follow-up. Psychosomatics 36:64–65, 1995.

442. Svirski B, Edoute Y: Sulfonylurea-induced factitious hypoglycemia [in Hebrew]. Harefuah 130:678–680, 1996.

443. Jordan R, Kammer H, Riddle M: Sulfonylurea-induced factitious hypoglycemia. Arch Intern Med 137:390–393, 1977.

Management of Type 2 Diabetes Mellitus

John B. Buse

A comprehensive review of all the subtleties of diabetes management is beyond the scope of any chapter. This material builds on the background of the other chapters in this text; the epidemiology, pathophysiology, and diagnosis of diabetes and its complications will not be reviewed, though arguably an understanding of these issues is integral in all treatment decisions. Treatment guidelines, lifestyle interventions, pharmacotherapy, the principles of cardiovascular risk factor management, and upcoming trials, which will inform treatment decisions in the future will be examined. An excellent source of information on these issues, which is updated annually, is the American Diabetes Association's (ADA) *Standards of Medical Care in Diabetes.*[1] It is published as the first supplement to the journal *Diabetes Care* each January and is available online at *www.diabetes.org* by clicking "For Health Care Professionals"; near the end of that document is a listing of technical reviews, which are generally recent, fairly exhaustive treatments of most areas of interest in diabetes care.

Over the last decade, a fundamental transformation of the principles of management of type 2 diabetes has occurred. Driven by a large number of multicenter randomized clinical trials documenting improved outcomes associated with glucose, blood pressure, and lipid management, as well as with antiplatelet therapy, guidelines have been established for diabetes treatment; increasingly, adherence to these guidelines is monitored and in some cases enforced by insurers and health-care systems. In parallel, there has been a change in the level of concern about diabetes as a public health issue and as a result, there have been changes in attitudes toward its treatment among patients and providers. This has been driven by the recognition that we are in the midst of an epidemic of diabetes, well established in the United States,[2] and just emerging in much of the developing world.[3] The estimated lifetime risk for developing diabetes for individuals born in the year 2000 in the United States is 32.8% for males and 38.5% for females, with Hispanic Americans having estimated lifetime risks for diabetes approximating 50%.[4] The morbidity, mortality, and expense associated with diabetes are staggering. In Western society, people with diabetes are three times more likely to be hospitalized than nondiabetic individuals. In the United States, diabetes is the leading cause of blindness and accounts for over 40% of the new cases of end-stage renal disease. The risk of heart disease and stroke is two to four times

higher and the risk of lower extremity amputation is approximately 20 times higher for people with diabetes than for those without diabetes.[5] Although diabetes is the seventh leading cause of death in the United States, this is clearly an underestimate; despite the fact that over 70% of people with diabetes die of heart disease and stroke, only approximately 10% have diabetes listed as a contributing cause on death certificates.[6] Tragically, this enormous burden of death and disability has not been reduced by huge health-care expenditures. In fact, the epidemic of diabetes is one of the drivers of increasing health-care costs, with annual disbursements for people with diabetes approximately three to five times higher per capita than those for individuals without diabetes and accounting for at least 15% of health-care expenditures in the United States.[7] There is evidence that increased effort to control diabetes and its comorbidities can even reduce costs associated with diabetes and that a public health approach to diabetes can reduce the burden of complications of diabetes.[8]

Fortunately, the spectrum of pharmacologic agents and glucose monitoring technology available for the treatment of diabetes have dramatically expanded and both private and government health insurers have greatly improved the extent to which diabetes education, nutritional counseling, and diabetes equipment and supplies are covered. These trends have made it possible to achieve the recommended targets for glucose, blood pressure, and lipid therapy in the vast majority of cases. The bulk of this chapter will deal with those approaches, as well as emerging treatments that are likely to be approved by regulatory authorities within the year 2005, and clinical trials that will inform clinical decision making over the next decade.

GLUCOSE TREATMENT GUIDELINES

Guidelines are optimally driven by the results of randomized multi-center clinical trials. Prospective randomized clinical trials have documented improved rates of microvascular complications in patients with diabetes treated to lower glycemic targets. In the UK Prospective Diabetes Study,[9] patients with new-onset diabetes were treated with diet and exercise for 3 months with an average reduction in glycosylated hemoglobin or hemoglobin A_{1c} (A1C) from approximately 9% to

7% (upper limit of normal 6%). Those with fasting plasma glucose (FPG) greater than 108 mg/dL (6 mM) after the dietary intervention were randomly assigned to one of two treatment policies. In the standard intervention, subjects continued the lifestyle intervention and pharmacologic therapy was initiated only if the FPG reached 270 mg/dL (15 mM) or the patient became symptomatic. In the more intensive treatment program, all patients were randomly assigned to treatment with either sulfonylurea, metformin, or insulin as initial therapy, and doses increased in an effort to achieve an FPG less than 108 mg/dL. Additional agents were employed only if the patients became symptomatic or FPG became greater than 15 mM (270 mg/dL). As a consequence of the design, although the A1C fell initially to about 6% during the first year, over the average 10 years of follow-up, it rose to approximately 8% in the intensive treatment group. The average A1C in the standard treatment group was approximately 1% higher throughout the study. The risk of severe hypoglycemia was small—on the order of 1% to 5% per year in the insulin-treated group—and weight gain was modest; both were higher in patients randomly assigned to insulin and lower in those receiving metformin.[10] Associated with this improvement in glycemic control, there was a reduction in the risk of microvascular complications (retinopathy, nephropathy, and neuropathy) in the intensive group. Although there was a trend toward reduced rates of macrovascular events in the more intensively treated group, it did not reach statistical significance.

Similar reductions in microvascular events were observed in another trial of entirely different design and much smaller size. In the Kumamoto study, Japanese patients of normal weight with type 2 diabetes treated with insulin were randomly assigned to standard treatment or an intensive program of insulin therapy designed to achieve normal glycemia. The control group maintained A1C values at approximately 9%, whereas A1C in the intensive group was reduced to approximately 7% and that separation was maintained for 6 years. Again, there was a modest increased risk of hypoglycemia and weight gain, a reduction in microvascular complications, and a nonstatistically significant trend toward reduced rates of vascular end points in the more intensively treated patients.[11]

Although no interventional studies have documented a statistically significant reduction in the risk of vascular end points associated with an improvement in glycemic control, multiple epidemiologic studies have suggested that there is an association between cardiovascular risk and A1C, FPG, and the 2-hour level in an oral glucose tolerance test.[12-15] In the UK Prospective Diabetes Study epidemiologic analysis, there was a 16% reduction in cardiovascular disease rates per 1% reduction in A1C without evidence of a threshold or lower limit of benefit all the way into the normal range.[15] Most, but not all, observational studies have demonstrated that among nondiabetic subjects an elevated 2-hour value in an oral glucose tolerance test is a better predictor of all-cause mortality or cardiovascular morbidity/mortality than an elevated FPG value; many issues continue to confound interpretation of these studies, but they remain a major impetus to monitoring and management of postprandial glucose levels.[16]

In Table 63-1, guidelines from the ADA[1] and the American College of Endocrinology[17] (ACE) are presented. The ADA suggests that the goal of treatment in the management of diabetes should be an A1C value less than 7%. Although initially developed on an ad hoc basis, this goal is supported by clinical trial data as this level of glycemia was associated with improved outcomes in patients with type 2 diabetes as discussed above for the UK Prospective Diabetes Study and Kumamoto studies. Because in those studies, normal glucose levels were targeted and achieved in at least some subjects, and because in epidemiologic analyses, there appears to be no threshold to the benefit of glucose lowering into the normal

Table 63-1 Guidelines for Targets in Glycemia Management from the American Diabetes Association (ADA) and American College of Endocrinology (ACE)

Parameter	Normal	ADA[†]	ACE
Premeal plasma glucose (mg/dL)	<100 (mean ~90)	90–130	<110
Postprandial plasma glucose* (mg/dL)	<140	<180	<140
A1C	4%–6%	<7%	<6.5%

*Postprandial glucose measurements should be made 1–2 hour after the beginning of the meal, generally peak levels in patients with diabetes.
[†]The ADA further recommends: (1) goals should be individualized; (2) certain populations (children, pregnant women, and elderly) require special considerations; (3) less-intensive goals may be indicated in patients with severe or frequent hypoglycemia; (4) based on epidemiologic analysis, more stringent glycemic goals (i.e., a normal A1C, <6%) may further reduce complications at the cost of increased risk of hypoglycemia; and (5) postprandial glucose may be targeted if A1C goals are not met despite reaching preprandial glucose goals.
Adapted from American Diabetes Association: Standards of medical care in diabetes. Diabetes Care 27:S15–S35, 2004; and American College of Endocrinologists: American College of Endocrinology consensus statement on guidelines for glycemic control. Endocr Pract 8(Suppl 1):5–11, 2002.

range, it is possible that further lowering of A1C will produce additional benefits; in fact, the ADA suggests "more stringent goals (i.e., a normal A1C < 6%) can be considered in individual patients."[1] It is probable that more aggressive efforts particularly in older, frailer patients and in those with frequent or unrecognized hypoglycemia could result in excess morbidity and/or mortality. Other potential adverse events related to pursuit of more aggressive targets include long-term exposure to poorly studied combinations of medications, additional expense, life disruption caused by greater attention and effort to achieve lower glycemic targets, and the potential that great efforts expended in achieving extremely stringent glycemic goals will result in less attention to other health risks by patient or provider. No cohort of patients of substantial size has ever been reported in which an average A1C level less than 7% has been achieved over a time frame that exceeds more than a few months. This balance between potential risks and benefits remains to be tested in randomized clinical trials and is under study in the ACCORD study (Action to Control Cardiovascular Risk in Diabetes) in which patients with type 2 diabetes at high risk for cardiovascular disease (CVD) are being randomized to an A1C target of less than 6% versus 7% to 7.9%.[18] Although it is clear that many patients can achieve lower glucose levels with currently available drugs and lifestyle interventions, it remains theoretically possible that the risks would exceed the benefits of seeking glucose targets less than 7%.

With respect to fasting, premeal, or postprandial targets, there is little support for any particular level of glycemic control in the management of type 2 diabetes as no large-scale outcome study has targeted particular levels of glucose with home glucose monitoring. The ADA target of fasting and premeal plasma glucose levels of 90 to 130 mg/dL (5–7.2 mM) is based on an estimate of the range of average glucose values that would be associated with a low risk of hypoglycemia and an A1C less than 7%. The American College of Endocrinology target of less than 110 mg/dL (6 mM) is an effort to achieve normal levels of glycemia. However, it should be recognized that consistent fasting and premeal glucose levels less than 110 mg/dL would be expected to be associated with an HbA$_{1c}$ of approximately 5.5% or lower.[19]

There are no published studies in which even safety, much less a clinical outcome, is documented for targeting a particular level of postprandial glucose. There are effective

A1C-lowering agents that primarily target postprandial glucose levels. Monitoring postprandial glucose levels may allow more effective dose adjustment of these agents, though even this has not been demonstrated in clinical trials. Certainly, there are patients with diabetes who have average fasting glucose levels within targets but whose A1C remains elevated; monitoring and specifically treating postprandial elevations in these patients may provide improvements in A1C, perhaps with a lower risk of hypoglycemia and weight gain than further lowering fasting and premeal glucose levels. The ACE guidelines recommend targeting a 2-hour postprandial glucose level less than 140 mg/dL (7.8 mM) in an effort to achieve near-normal glycemia. Consistent postprandial glucose values less than 140 mg/dL would be associated with average A1C levels of approximately 5% or lower; 2-hour postprandial glucose levels of less than 180 mg/dL (10 mM) would generally be associated with A1C levels of 6% to 7% and is the recommended postprandial target of the ADA.[1,18,19]

LIFESTYLE INTERVENTION

The components of lifestyle intervention include comprehensive diabetes education aimed at enabling the patient to self-manage their diabetes, medical nutrition counseling, and exercise recommendations. The appropriate paradigm of care in diabetes is patient-focused as patients are responsible for almost every diabetes-related decision and behavior; providers at their best can provide advice and help recognize and suggest techniques to overcome obstacles to achieving treatment goals.

EDUCATION OF PATIENTS

Arguably, over the last 5 years, nothing has changed more fundamentally in diabetes care than the emphasis on lifestyle intervention. For decades, physicians and patients paid lip service to the notion that lifestyle intervention is important. Now we have significant clinical trial evidence that each component of lifestyle intervention, when appropriately administered, can contribute to improved outcomes.[20,21] Furthermore, since the Balanced Budget Act of 1997 and the passage of complementary legislation by most state governments, lifestyle intervention has become a covered benefit for most patients with diabetes.

Diabetes is a life-long disease, and health-care providers have almost no control over the extent to which patients adhere to the day-to-day treatment regimen. The appropriate role of the health-care provider is to serve as a coach to the patient, who has primary responsibility for the delivery of daily care. Thus, it is essential that health-care professionals understand the context in which patients are taking care of their disease. Using a prescriptive approach in which patients are told what to do can work on occasion, but fails more often than not because of unrecognized barriers to the execution of a particular plan.

As defined by the ADA,[22] diabetes self-management education is the process of providing the person with diabetes with the knowledge and skills needed to perform self-care, manage crises, and make lifestyle changes. As a result of this process, the patient must become a knowledgeable and active participant in the management of his or her disease. To achieve this rather daunting goal, patients and providers work together in a long-term, ongoing process. Comprehensive diabetes education should be individualized with emphasis on the issues highlighted in Table 63-2. There are many more specialized topics relevant to almost all patients, such as how to adjust therapy when eating out or during travel, as well as how to access available local health-care resources and to negotiate the complexity of health-care financing in the United States. Although only limited studies are published to date, as a body

Table 63-2 Curricular Areas Which Should Be Addressed in Diabetes Self-Management Education

Pathophysiology of the patient's diabetes and its relationship to treatment options
Incorporating appropriate nutritional management in the treatment program
Incorporating physical activity into the treatment program
Using medications (if applicable) for therapeutic effectiveness
Monitoring blood glucose, urine ketones (when appropriate), and using the results to improve control
Preventing, detecting, and treating acute complications including "sick day rules" and hypoglycemia management
Preventing, detecting, and treating chronic complications
Goal setting to promote health and problem solving for daily living
Integrating psychosocial adjustment to daily life
Promoting preconception care, management during pregnancy, and gestational diabetes management (if applicable)

Adapted from American Diabetes Association: Evidence-based nutrition principles and recommendations for the treatment and prevention of diabetes and related complications. Diabetes Care 25:202–212, 2002.

of work they do provide support for the concept that diabetes education can be cost effective and can improve outcomes.[21–23]

A team of providers is generally required to optimally implement the process of diabetes self-management education as the amount of information that needs to be exchanged is large; therefore, the range of expertise required is broad. It is generally impossible to cover the recommended content fully in the context of several or even many brief encounters with a physician in an office setting. Potential providers in a team care approach could include nurses, dietitians, exercise specialists, behavioral therapists, pharmacists, and other medical specialists including diabetologists or endocrinologists, podiatrists, medical subspecialists, obstetrician-gynecologists, psychiatrists, and surgeons. The potential role of the community, in which the patient lives and works, in the diabetes self-care process is enormous. This community at a minimum includes family, friends, employers, health-care systems, and health-care insurers. Each member of the team has a role to play in the process and it is useful to review these roles frequently (Table 63-3). The primary role of the providers in this process is to provide guidance in goal setting to manage the risk of complications, suggest strategies to achieve goals and techniques to overcome barriers, provide training in skills, and screen for complications. For this process to be a success, the patient must commit to the principles of self-care, participate fully in the development of a

Table 63-3 Team Care: Roles of the Players

ROLE OF PROVIDERS
To be a source of accurate information and to refer to and coordinate with other sources of information as necessary
To provide guidance in developing goals of treatment
To screen for complications and evaluate progress in meeting treatment goals
To help develop strategies to achieve treatment goals and avoid complications

ROLE OF PATIENT
To commit to diabetes self-management
To be an active participant in the process
To communicate with other team members when goals are not achieved or problems are encountered

ROLE OF COMMUNITY
To provide support to encourage ongoing diabetes self-care

treatment plan, make ongoing decisions regarding self-care from day to day, and communicate honestly and with sufficient frequency with the team.

Fortunately, barriers to providing team care are becoming less daunting in large measure due to the rapidly expanding number of diabetes education programs and improved insurance coverage for services. The American Association of Diabetes Educators (800-TEAM-UP4) and the ADA (800-DIABETEs) can provide information regarding diabetes educators and education programs nationwide.

For diabetes care to be effective, communication and mutual respect among the patient-centered team is critical. Unfortunately, in many communities, the full benefit of the consultation and ongoing care with diabetes educators, nurses, dietitians, pharmacists, medical consultants, and primary care providers is not achieved because of overly hierarchical approaches to care. Nonphysicians, including patients, ought to provide input regarding medication and lifestyle adjustments and help in the process of setting goals and identifying barriers to effective management, such as lack of knowledge, lack of time, and lack of resources and in developing strategies to overcome those barriers.

Perhaps some of the most overlooked contributors to ineffective care in the setting of type 2 diabetes are the relatively common barriers created by psychiatric, neurocognitive function, and adjustment disorders, which are largely responsive to psychosocial therapies.[23]

NUTRITION

The ADA has published technical reviews that exhaustively document the literature regarding the effect of medical nutrition therapy and specific advice on diabetes-related outcomes, such as A1C and weight, as well as a position statement.[24-27] These are summarized in Table 63-4. An individually negotiated nutrition program in which each patient's circumstances, preferences, and cultural background as well as the overall treatment program are considered is most likely to result in optimal outcomes. It is recommended that a registered dietitian, with specific skill and experience in implementing nutrition therapy in diabetes management, work collaboratively with the patient and other health-care team members in providing medical nutrition therapy. Optimally, this should be performed over a series of visits initially with intermittent follow-up thereafter. Analogously, physicians and other members of the health-care team need to support the nutritional plan developed collaboratively.

Individualized dietary advice can be developed by a physician from a brief diet history obtained by asking: "What do you eat for breakfast? . . . lunch? . . . supper? Do you have snacks between breakfast and lunch? . . . lunch and supper? . . . supper and bedtime? What do you drink during the day?" Ideally, this information should be obtained at each visit, with specific suggestions for change that both patient and provider agree are important in the context of the overall treatment plan as well as both achievable and sustainable. Easy issues to address include caloric beverages, which tend to elevate glucose levels dramatically and can generally be replaced relatively easily with artificially sweetened alternatives. Juices are generally perceived as healthy but can significantly affect glycemic control and total calorie intake. Portion control and recipe modification are excellent dietary techniques, particularly for meats and fried foods. Substituting low-fat products for higher fat foods is often useful but needs to be done with the recognition that they are generally higher in carbohydrates. It is important that patients recognize that "fat-free" and "sugar-free" foods are not "free" and that attention to both total carbohydrate and calorie content are critical.

Eating approximately every 4 hours while awake is the most practical dietary plan for most overweight people. Frequent small meals have been shown to be of benefit when used in a controlled inpatient setting, but in general when overweight patients are encouraged to eat more frequently they often overeat more frequently. At a minimum, avoiding high-calorie snacks is reasonable advice for most people with diabetes. Repeatedly obtaining a diet history every few weeks to months by all health-care providers allows assessment of whether previously agreed to changes were enacted, reinforcement of the importance of dietary efforts, and gradual evolution to a more healthful diet by making modest suggestions for further dietary modification sequentially.

In general, the critical nutrient for glycemic control is carbohydrate. Essentially all carbohydrates consumed are converted to glucose in the gut and require the action of insulin to be cleared from the circulation. A dietary technique called carbohydrate counting can be used in patients with type 2 diabetes to facilitate consistent carbohydrate intake or to allow insulin dose adjustment in response to changes in carbohydrates consumed.[28] Whereas the β cell in type 2 diabetes has generally lost its responsiveness to glucose, the second phase of insulin secretion is largely spared in type 2 diabetes and is in part driven by amino acids and fatty acids. Therefore, including some protein and fat in each meal and snack may be useful.

Dietary fat is the nutrient most closely associated in epidemiologic studies with the risk of developing type 2 diabetes. Although dietary fat clearly has a major impact on total caloric intake as well as on circulating lipids, they have a minimal acute impact on glycemia. It is recommended that people with diabetes, if they are overweight, consume a diet that is modestly restricted in calories containing less than 10% of total calories as saturated fat and less than 10% as polyunsaturated fat with avoidance of trans-fats. Some advocate substituting foods high in monounsaturated fatty acids—seeds, nuts, avocado, olives, olive oil, and canola oil—for carbohydrate, but most patients do not find adequate variety in the monounsaturated fatty acid category and often overeat these high-caloric-density foods.

Dietary protein similarly has a minimal impact on glucose levels, although as mentioned above, amino acids do promote insulin secretion. Metabolism of protein results in the formation of acids and nitrogenous waste, which may result in bone demineralization and glomerular hyperfiltration. At least 0.8 g of high-quality protein per kilogram is generally recommended. Protein restriction in the setting of kidney disease has been recommended and is more fully discussed in Chapter 71. There is no evidence that protein intake materially effects the risk of developing kidney disease in patients with diabetes.

The role of vitamins, trace minerals, and nutritional supplements in the treatment of diabetes is poorly understood. There are some patients and providers who are absolutely convinced of the utility of soluble fiber, magnesium, chromium, zinc, folic acid, pyridoxine, cyanocobalamin, vitamin A, vitamin C, vitamin E, vanadium, selenium, garlic, and others. Clinical trial data to support their safety and efficacy are inconclusive. Many patients are convinced that nutritional supplementation is healthful, and it is often counterproductive to engage in scholarly discussion of the nature of the evidence base for their decision. At a minimum, discussion should include the documented efficacy of more classical lifestyle and pharmacologic intervention and the idea that these efforts should not be left by the wayside when budgetary constraints affect potentially more effective interventions.[29,30] A multivitamin with mineral preparation may be reasonable for most patients with diabetes. A recent randomized control trial in patients with diabetes demonstrated fewer self-reported infections and related absenteeism.[31] Studies demonstrating the benefits of B-vitamin supplementation on restenosis after angioplasty[32] have recently been called into question as the possibility has been raised that such therapy could increase rates of restenosis after stent placement.[33]

Table 63-4 ADA Nutritional Principles and Recommendations

CARBOHYDRATES
- Foods containing carbohydrate from whole grains, fruits, vegetables, and low-fat milk should be included in a healthy diet.
- With regard to the glycemic effects of carbohydrates, the total amount of carbohydrate in meals or snacks is more important than the source or type. However, attention to glycemic index can provide additional benefit over that observed when total carbohydrate is considered alone.
- As sucrose does not increase glycemia to a greater extent than isocaloric amounts of starch, sucrose and sucrose-containing foods in the context of a mixed meal, they do not need to be restricted by people with diabetes; however, they should be substituted for other carbohydrate sources in the context of an appropriate meal plan or, if added, covered with insulin or other glucose-lowering medication.
- Nonnutritive sweeteners are safe when consumed within the acceptable daily intake levels established by the Food and Drug Administration.
- Individuals receiving fixed daily insulin doses should try to be consistent in day-to-day carbohydrate intake.
- Individuals receiving intensive insulin therapy should adjust their premeal insulin doses based on the carbohydrate content of meals.
- As with the general public, consumption of dietary fiber is to be encouraged; however, there is no reason to recommend that people with diabetes consume a greater amount of fiber than others.
- Low-carbohydrate diets are not recommended in the management of diabetes, though they can be useful in reducing triglycerides. Although dietary carbohydrate is the major contributor to postprandial glucose concentration, it is an important source of energy, water-soluble vitamins and minerals, and fiber. Restricting total carbohydrate to less than 130 g/day is not recommended.

PROTEINS
- In people with controlled type 2 diabetes, ingested protein does not increase plasma glucose concentrations, although protein is just as potent a stimulant of insulin secretion as carbohydrate.
- For persons with diabetes, especially those not in optimal glucose control, the protein requirement may be greater than the recommended dietary allowance, but not greater than usual intake.

FATS
- Less than 10% of energy intake should be derived from saturated fats. Some individuals (i.e., persons with LDL cholesterol ≥100 mg/dL) may benefit from lowering saturated fat intake to <7% of energy intake.
- Dietary cholesterol intake should be <300 mg/day. Some individuals (i.e., persons with LDL cholesterol ≥100 mg/dL) may benefit from lowering dietary cholesterol to <200 mg/day.
- To lower LDL cholesterol, energy derived from saturated fat can be reduced if weight loss is desirable or replaced with either carbohydrate or monounsaturated fat when weight loss is not a goal.
- Intake of *trans* unsaturated fatty acids should be minimized.
- Reduced-fat diets when maintained long-term contribute to modest loss of weight and improvement in dyslipidemia.
- Two to three servings of fish per week provide dietary n-3 polyunsaturated fat and can be recommended.
- Polyunsaturated fat intake should be ≈10% of energy intake.

ENERGY BALANCE
- In insulin-resistant individuals, reduced energy intake and modest weight loss improve insulin resistance and glycemia in the short-term.
- Weight loss is recommended for all overweight (BMI 25–29.9 kg/m^2) or obese (BMI ≥ 30.0 kg/m^2) adults who have, or who are at risk for developing, type 2 diabetes. The primary approach for achieving weight loss is therapeutic lifestyle change, which includes a reduction in energy intake and an increase in physical activity.
- A moderate decrease in caloric intake (500–1000 kcal/day) will result in a slow but progressive weight loss (1–2 lb/wk). For most patients, weight loss diets should supply at least 1000–1200 kcal/d for women and 1200–1600 kcal/d for men.
- Structured programs that emphasize lifestyle changes, including education, reduced fat (<30% of daily energy) and energy intake, regular physical activity, and regular participant contact, can produce long-term weight loss on the order of 5%–7% of starting weight.
- Exercise and behavior modification are most useful as adjuncts to other weight-loss strategies. Exercise is helpful in maintenance of weight loss.
- Standard weight reduction diets, when used alone, are unlikely to produce long-term weight loss. Structured intensive lifestyle programs are necessary.

MICRONUTRIENTS AND ALCOHOL
- There is no clear evidence of benefit from vitamin or mineral supplementation in people with diabetes who do not have underlying deficiencies. Exceptions include folate for prevention of birth defects and calcium for prevention of bone disease.
- Routine supplementation of the diet with antioxidants is not advised because of uncertainties related to long-term efficacy and safety.
- If individuals choose to drink alcohol, daily intake should be limited to one drink for women and two drinks for men. One drink is defined as 12 oz of beer, 5 oz of wine, or 1.5 oz of distilled spirits. To reduce risk of hypoglycemia, alcohol should be consumed with food.

Adapted from Klein S, Sheard NF, Pi-Sunyer X, et al: Weight management through lifestyle modification for the prevention and management of type 2 diabetes: Rationale and strategies: A statement of the American Diabetes Association, the North American Association for the Study of Obesity, and the American Society for Clinical Nutrition. Diabetes Care 27:2067–2073, 2004; Gillespie SJ, Kulkarni KD, Daly AE: Using carbohydrate counting in diabetes clinical practice. J Am Diet Assoc 98:897–905, 1998; and Egede LE, Ye K, Zhang D, Silverstein MD: The prevalence and pattern of complementary and alternative medicine use in individuals with diabetes. Diabetes Care 25:324–329, 2002.

Although there are proponents of a wide range of dietary composition, there are few data to support these recommendations from long-term outcome studies of prescribed diets. Mixed meals containing 10% to 20% of calories from protein, no more than 10% of calories from saturated fat, no more than 10% from polyunsaturated fats, and the remainder largely from monounsaturated fats (seeds, nuts, avocados, olives, olive oil, canola oil) and carbohydrates, particularly whole grains, fruit, vegetables, and low-fat milk, are probably most reasonable. High-carbohydrate low-fat diets, although historically recommended by many health organizations, have been shown to increase postprandial blood glucose and triglyceride levels, elevate fasting triglyceride levels, and decrease high-density lipoprotein (HDL) cholesterol levels in

insulin-resistant people, including those with type 2 diabetes. Several studies have demonstrated improved lipid levels and blood glucose control in both short- and intermediate-term studies in which total fat intake approaches 45% of calories and carbohydrate intake is as low as 40% of calories. Reducing fat or carbohydrate intake in obese individuals will not necessarily lead to reduced calories. Since weight loss will occur only in the setting of caloric restriction, arguably, the most appropriate approach is to limit intake of both fat and highly processed, easily digestible carbohydrates. The treatment of obesity is discussed in Chapter 45; the principles discussed are appropriate when type 2 diabetes is complicated by obesity. To date, short-term studies of medical nutrition therapy, physical activity, and comprehensive lifestyle approaches have been shown to improve the control of classical CVD risk factors, as well as intermediate markers of CVD risk such as C-reactive protein; no long-term large-scale study of intentional weight loss has been powered to examine CVD endpoints. Look AHEAD (Action for Health in Diabetes) will examine CVD events for up to 11.5 years in a study in which patients with type 2 diabetes 45 to 74 years of age with a body mass index = 25 kg/m^2 will be recruited. Patients will be randomized to a 4-year intensive weight loss program (calorie restriction and physical activity) or to diabetes support and education. With planned recruitment of 5000 patients at 16 centers over 2.5 years, the study is designed to provide a 0.90 probability of detecting an 18% difference in major CVD event rates between arms.[34]

EXERCISE

There is a substantial body of literature supporting exercise as a modality of treatment in type 2 diabetes including a recent technical review by the ADA.[35,36] The recommendations of this technical review are summarized in Table 63-5. Exercise is perhaps the single most important lifestyle intervention in diabetes as it is associated with improved glycemic control, insulin sensitivity, cardiovascular fitness, and cardiac remodeling. Aerobic exercise and resistance (strength) training both have a positive impact on glucose control. Improvements in glycemic control are generally apparent immediately, become maximal after a few weeks of consistent exercise, but only persist for only 3 to 6 days after the cessation of training. To maintain effects on glycemia, a minimum of three exercise sessions a week is suggested with no more than 2 days rest between sessions.

The recommended approach to promote an increase in physical activity is analogous to that discussed for diet. Goals, methods, intensity, and frequency have to be negotiated with patients with great sensitivity to recognizing barriers and helping patients discover solutions. The role of educators, exercise specialists, physical therapists, and social supports in this process is critical. The major role for the physician is to screen for complications (neuropathy, nephropathy, retinopathy, vascular disease) and discover ways for patients to be able to exercise safely. Exercise in the presence of uncontrolled diabetes, hypertension, retinopathy, nephropathy, neuropathy, and cardiovascular disease can occasionally result in devastating problems. Vigorous exercise should be avoided in the setting of proliferative or severe nonproliferative diabetic retinopathy; waiting 3 or more months after successful laser photocoagulation is probably prudent. In the setting of severe peripheral neuropathy, non-weight-bearing activities, such as bicycling, are probably appropriate. In the setting of known ischemic heart disease, an initial period of exercise under monitoring as provided in cardiac rehabilitation programs is arguably most appropriate. These issues can all be addressed creatively and should never provide an insurmountable barrier to increasing physical activity.

The most recent recommendations regarding stress testing before initiating an exercise program in previously sedentary people are provided in some detail in Table 63-5. The utility of such treadmill tests in potentially low-risk populations is limited by their poor sensitivity and specificity.[37,38] However, it should be noted that in an older asymptomatic population with normal electrocardiograms, over 20% of patients were found to have silent ischemia when stress testing was performed with adenosine technetium-99m Sestamibi

Table 63-5 ADA Recommendations Regarding Physical Activity in People with Type 2 Diabetes

INDICATIONS FOR GRADED EXERCISE TEST WITH ECG MONITORING

In the absence of contraindications, a graded exercise test with ECG monitoring should be seriously considered before undertaking aerobic physical activity with an intensity exceeding the demands of everyday living (more intense than brisk walking) in previously sedentary diabetic individuals whose 10-year risk of a coronary event is ≥10%. This risk could be estimated directly using the UKPDS Risk Engine (www.dtu.ox.ac.uk/riskengine/download.htm) and would correspond approximately to meeting any of the following criteria:
- Age >40 years, with or without CVD risk factors other than diabetes
- Age >30 years and
  - Type 1 or type 2 diabetes of >10 years' duration
  - Hypertension
  - Cigarette smoking
  - Dyslipidemia
  - Proliferative or preproliferative retinopathy
  - Nephropathy, including microalbuminuria
- Any of the following, regardless of age
  - Known or suspected CAD, cerebrovascular disease, and/or peripheral vascular disease
  - Autonomic neuropathy
  - Advanced nephropathy with renal failure

These criteria should not be construed as a recommendation against stress testing for individuals without the above risk factors or for those who are planning less-intense exercise.

AEROBIC EXERCISE

The amount and intensity recommended for aerobic exercise vary according to goals.
- To improve glycemic control, assist with weight maintenance, and reduce risk of CVD, recommend at least 150 min/week of moderate-intensity aerobic physical activity (40–60% of $\dot{V}O_{2max}$ or 50–70% of maximum heart rate) and/or at least 90 min/wk of vigorous aerobic exercise (>60% of $\dot{V}O_{2max}$ or >70% of maximum heart rate). The physical activity should be distributed over at least 3 days/wk and with no more than 2 consecutive days without physical activity.
- Performing ≥4 hr/wk of moderate to vigorous aerobic and/or resistance exercise is associated with greater CVD risk reduction compared with lower volumes of activity.
- For long-term maintenance of major weight loss (≥13.6 kg [30 lb]), larger volumes of exercise (7 hr/wk of moderate or vigorous aerobic physical activity) may be helpful.

RESISTANCE EXERCISE

In the absence of contraindications, people with type 2 diabetes should be encouraged to perform resistance exercise three times a week, including all major muscle groups, progressing to three sets of 8–10 repetitions at a weight that cannot be lifted greater than 8–10 times.

To ensure resistance exercises are performed correctly, maximize health benefits, and minimize the risk of injury, initial supervision and periodic reassessments by a qualified exercise specialist are recommended.

Adapted from American Diabetes Association: Consensus development conference on the diagnosis of coronary heart disease in people with diabetes: 10–11 February 1998, Miami, Florida. Diabetes Care 21:1551–1559, 1998.

single-photon emission-computed tomography myocardial perfusion imaging.[39] If the planned exercise program does not involve more strenuous (both intensity and duration) activity than the patient has engaged in recently but merely involves more frequent activity, screening cardiovascular stress testing is unlikely to be particularly useful.

Even if the stress test does not demonstrate characteristics of ischemia, it is appropriate to counsel patients to avoid overexertion and to seek medical follow-up for exertional symptoms such as chest, jaw, or arm discomfort or for worsening dyspnea. Improving exercise tolerance should be viewed as a measure of improving cardiorespiratory function.

For the average patient with type 2 diabetes starting an exercise program, these levels of moderate exertion will generally be reached with quite low level activity initially, such as walking at a pace of 2 miles an hour. Initially, it may even be necessary to negotiate once-weekly or shorter duration exercise sessions and proceed from there, picking up the pace as tolerated and increase the duration and frequency of exercise sessions slowly to avoid overuse injuries.

SELF-MONITORING OF BLOOD GLUCOSE

Self-monitoring of blood glucose (SMBG) has not been demonstrated in clinical trials to substantially change outcomes in type 2 diabetes when evaluated in isolation; a recent study demonstrated only a 0.3% reduction in A1C in a randomized controlled trial.[40,41] However, many diabetes self-management programs have been associated with improved glycemic control; in all of these, SMBG was integral to the overall process, suggesting that SMBG is at least a component of effective therapy. The frequency and type of glucose monitoring should be determined in collaboration with the patient, taking into account the overall treatment plan and goals, the patient's abilities, and the stage of diabetes. SMBG can theoretically improve the safety of treatment with insulin or sulfonylureas as it allows the identification of minimal or asymptomatic episodes of hypoglycemia; coupled with appropriate education, dose adjustments, or modest changes in the lifestyle plan, SMBG can minimize risk of severe hypoglycemia or weight gain. Although severe hypoglycemia is relatively rare in type 2 diabetes, it is more common in the elderly and can have devastating consequences, such as physical injury as a result of trauma or a change in the perceived ability of a patient to continue to live independently as a result of confusion or loss of consciousness. In general, it is optimal to have patients assess the nature of any hypoglycemic symptoms they experience with glucose monitoring; many patients are fearful of hypoglycemia and routinely consume extra calories in response to a variety of life's circumstances such as when they are hungry, sweaty, nervous, or upset without documenting hypoglycemia. Most "hypoglycemic" symptoms in patients with type 2 diabetes are not related to hypoglycemia and do not need to be treated with caloric consumption. Counseling patients to carry commercially available glucose tablets and glucose monitoring equipment at all times and to take a 15-g dose of carbohydrate for documented mild to moderate hypoglycemia helps patients avoid excessive calorie intake and recreational consumption of sweets for treatment of hypoglycemia.

Optimal timing of SMBG will vary depending on individual characteristics and treatment. It is important to advise patients to vary the time of the day at which blood glucose levels are checked. For some patients, the highest blood glucose of the day is the morning glucose, whereas for others the highest is before bed. Particularly in early diabetes, gestational diabetes, and well-controlled diabetes, monitoring 1 to 2 hours after meals allows patients to assess the effect of the combined lifestyle and pharmacologic efforts in controlling postprandial glucose levels, which often are the only glycemic abnormality present.

When glucose control is poor, having patients concentrate on premeal glucose levels is perhaps most productive. Once the premeal glucose levels reach the low 100s, many advocate that patients switch to checking 1- to 2-hour postprandial glucose levels because it amplifies the observed effect of diet on glycemic control and enables patients to see that moderate changes in meal plan, activity, and medications have a significant impact on glucose levels. Even after substantial inappropriate changes in food intake, activity, or timing or dose of medication, blood sugar values often return to near-normal levels overnight or by the time of the next meal.

The frequency of glucose monitoring needs to be matched to individual patient needs and treatment. Many clinicians ask patients to monitor at least once a day, varying among breakfast, lunch, supper, bedtime, and mid-sleep as well as with symptoms. Others ask patients to monitor with intensity similar to that described for patients with type 1 diabetes (four times per day before meals and bedtime with occasional postprandial and mid-sleep checks). Some ask for sets of glycemic readings more infrequently (e.g., fasting and 1 hour after the biggest meal). In the subset of patients who achieve stable blood glucose levels without significant hypoglycemia, it is generally appropriate to decrease the frequency of SMBG to a few times a week. The important characteristic of the timing of SMBG is that it be frequent enough to optimally inform the treatment plan and that both patient and provider have a good understanding of both the adequacy and the stability of glycemic control.

It has been assumed that the benefits of SMBG stem from facilitating self-management. Theoretically, if patients are aware of the glycemic targets associated with the outcomes they seek to achieve, SMBG enables them to evaluate their response to therapy and make adjustments or seek help as needed to achieve goals. It is useful for patients to keep a daily diary of their SMBG results, so that they can assess their results periodically and also so that they can share them with the health-care team. Unfortunately, many patients faithfully perform daily or more frequent SMBG, record the results as instructed, and discuss them with their health-care team only at quarterly visits. Unless SMBG results are within the agreed-to targets, they should be communicated and reviewed regularly with a member of the health-care team by telephone, fax, mail, or e-mail or at an interim visit to trigger changes in therapy as the need arises. Unfortunately, such services are generally not reimbursed, which places an unsustainable burden on many health-care teams.

Finally, one of the most difficult areas for health-care providers to remain current is in the area of available equipment and supplies, particularly for glucose monitoring. Diabetes educators often have demonstration models and a robust understanding of patient characteristics that match well or poorly with particular devices; they can be exceptionally helpful to patients in selecting appropriate equipment. A useful resource in this regard is the annual *Resource Guide*, which comes out as the January issue of *Diabetes Forecast*, a magazine for lay people with diabetes and their families. It is available online at *http://www.diabetes.org/diabetes-forecast/back-issues.jsp* to find the most recent January issue.

PHARMACOTHERAPY OF TYPE 2 DIABETES

The revolution in the treatment of type 2 diabetes since 1995 in the United States has been driven by the release of multiple new classes of drugs that independently address different pathophysiologic mechanisms that contribute to the development of diabetes. The available oral antidiabetic agents can be divided by mechanism of action into insulin sensitizers with primary action in the liver, insulin sensitizers with primary action in peripheral tissues, insulin secretagogues, and agents that slow the absorption of carbohydrates. Insulin therapy in the setting of type 2 diabetes effectively is a supplement to endogenous insulin secretion. The relative benefits of lifestyle intervention and the six classes of drugs available for the management of type 2 diabetes are found in Table 63-6. This area has been the subject of extensive reviews.[42–45] Because of limitations of space, only the principles outlined in these reviews are summarized, along with limited additional references, as well as anecdotal experience derived from intensive management in the setting of randomized clinical trials and clinical practice. Subsequently, there is a discussion of pramlintide and exenatide, novel treatments for type 2 diabetes under review by the Food and Drug Administration.

INSULIN SENSITIZERS WITH PREDOMINANT ACTION IN THE LIVER: BIGUANIDES

Metformin is the only biguanide available in the United States and the subject of a recent exhaustive review.[46] Phenformin was removed from the United States market in the 1970s because of deaths associated with lactic acidosis. Although metformin has been available in Europe for almost 40 years, it has been marketed in the United States only since 1995. Though the precise mechanism of action of metformin is unknown, its major activity is to reduce hepatic insulin resistance, gluconeogenesis, and glucose release. Metformin has more inconsistently demonstrated effects to improve insulin sensitivity in peripheral tissues. It may exert its effects through modulation of mitochondrial activity including activation of adenosine monophosphate–activated protein kinase and activation of glucose-6-phosphate dehydrogenase.[47]

Metformin has a half-life of 2 to 6 hours and reaches peak concentrations in approximately 1 hour when taken with meals. It is generally administered at least twice daily, although sustained-release formulations, which are particularly effective when administered with the evening meal, are now available. As metformin does not increase insulin levels, it is not associated with a significant risk of hypoglycemia. The most common adverse events are gastrointestinal: nausea, diarrhea, crampy abdominal pain, and dysgeusia.

About one third of patients have some gastrointestinal distress, particularly early in their course of treatment. These adverse effects can be minimized by starting with a low dose (500 mg) once daily with a meal and titrating upward slowly (over weeks) to more effective doses (500–1000 mg bid). The drug is perhaps 30% more bioavailable if administered on an empty stomach, but at least initially it should be taken with meals to minimize upper gastrointestinal complaints. In the long term, most patients can tolerate taking metformin before meals and may do well with lower doses than they would require otherwise. Sustained-release metformin is associated with less frequent and severe upper gastrointestinal symptoms, the most common of the adverse effects of metformin, but can increase the frequency of diarrhea, a much less common adverse effect overall. The majority of patients have no treatment emergent complaints during metformin initiation, and at least 90% tolerate it adequately with long-term use. Perhaps as a result of clinical or subclinical gastrointestinal effects, metformin is associated with less weight gain than other available antidiabetic agents and in some studies has even been shown to produce modest mean weight loss.

The issue of greatest concern regarding metformin therapy is lactic acidosis, which is quite rare and occurs almost exclusively in patients who are at high risk of developing lactic acidosis independent of metformin treatment.[48] Clearly, metformin can cause lactic acidosis as it has been reported after overdoses in low-risk patients. When used prudently, the risk of lactic acidosis is virtually zero. Patients at increased risk of developing lactic acidosis due to baseline medical conditions should avoid taking metformin.[49] The package insert suggests that metformin is absolutely contraindicated in patients with renal insufficiency as the drug is cleared renally[50]; it states that the drug should not be used in males with a serum creatinine greater than or equal to 1.5 mg/dL and in females at 1.4 mg/dL. There is a complex relationship between serum creatinine and renal function; several equations have been derived to estimate creatinine clearance from measures of serum creatinine. Reasonable practice might involve avoiding the use of metformin entirely in patients with an estimated creatinine clearance from the Cockcroft-Gault equation of

Table 63-6   Comparisons of Therapies for Type 2 Diabetes

	Lifestyle	Insulins	Sulfonylureas	Metformin	α-Glucosidase Inhibitors	Glitazones Pioglitazone (P) Rosiglitazone (R)	Glinides Repaglinide (R) Nateglinide (N)
Target tissue	Muscle/fat	β-cell supplement	β cell	Liver	Gut	Fat/muscle	β cell
Δ HbA1c (monotherapy)	Variable	1–>2%	1–2%	1–2%	0.5–1%	0.5–2%	R: 1–2% N: 0.5–1%
Stimulates insulin secretion	No	No	Yes	No	No	No	Yes
Improves insulin sensitivity	Yes	No	No	Modest	No	Yes	No
Severe hypoglycemia	No	Yes	Yes	No	No	No	R: Yes, rare N: No
Weight gain	No	Yes	Yes	No	No	Yes	Yes
Common problem	Recidivism, injury	Hypoglycemia, weight gain	Hypoglycemia, weight gain	Transient GI, B$_{12}$ deficiency	Flatulence	Weight gain, edema, anemia	Hypoglycemia
Rare problem		Skin changes	Sulfa allergy	Lactic acidosis	Liver disease	Congestive heart failure	
Contraindications	None	None	Allergy	Renal failure, liver failure, CHF	Intestinal disease	ALT > 2.5x nL class III–IV CHF	None
Cost ($ per month at min-max effective dose)	0–200	10–150+	5–20	15–60	30–65	60–160	60–100
Minimal effective dose	30 mins 3 times a week	0.1 U/kg/d	Smallest tablet	500 mg qPM	25 mg bid	P: 15 mg qd R: 2 mg qd	R: 0.5 mg bid N: 60 mg bid
Maximum effective dose	None	1–2+ U/kg/d	1/2 max or double starting	1000 mg bid	50 mg tid	P: 30–45 mg qd R: 4–8 mg qd	R: 2 mg tid N: 120 mg tid

less than 50 mL/min and limiting treatment to approximately half-maximal doses of metformin (i.e., 500 mg twice daily) in patients with an estimated creatinine clearance between 50 and 70 mL/min. As a reminder, the Cockcroft-Gault equation, creatinine clearance equals $[(140 - \text{age}) \times (\text{weight in kg})] \div (72 \times \text{serum creatinine in mg/dL})$ in males, and this is multiplied by 0.85 in females. Therefore, a 30-year-old, 250-pound construction worker with a creatinine of 1.6 has a normal creatinine clearance of 103 mL/min, whereas an 80-year-old, 110-pound woman with a creatinine of 0.8 has a low creatinine clearance of 44 mL/min.

Metformin is also contraindicated in patients with congestive heart failure requiring treatment, in those with hepatic insufficiency, and in those with a history of binge drinking or heavy alcohol use. Caution is required in elderly people, and specific recommendations to measure creatinine clearance with a timed urine collection prior to initiating therapy in patients over the age of 80 are provided in the package insert. Patients with acute illness, poorly controlled chronic illness, surgical indications, and simultaneous treatment with nephrotoxic drugs (e.g., iodinated contrast dye) should have metformin withheld until the clinical course is stabilized and adequate renal function is confirmed.

The glucose-lowering efficacy and the prevalence of adverse gastrointestinal effects increase proportionally in the dose range 500 to 2000 mg/day. The maximal dose of 2550 mg does not generally provide additional benefit beyond that seen at 2000 mg daily. New formulations of metformin combined with glyburide, glipizide, and rosiglitazone in a single tablet have been developed to increase glucose-lowering effectiveness by combining the activity of two classes of drugs.

Metformin has the strongest record of achievement of antidiabetic agents in outcome studies in patients with type 2 diabetes. In the UK Prospective Diabetes Study, among overweight subjects, those randomly assigned to metformin not only had improvements in microvascular complications similar to those of subjects randomly assigned to insulin and sulfonylurea but also exhibited a reduction in diabetes-related deaths and myocardial infarction.[10] The validity of this observation has been challenged because of unusual responses in a subsequent subrandomization. Beneficial effects of metformin on macrovascular complications through glucose-independent mechanisms are plausible and suggested by consistent observations, such as metformin-associated reductions in low-density lipoprotein (LDL) and procoagulant factors.[51]

INSULIN SENSITIZERS WITH PREDOMINANT ACTION IN PERIPHERAL INSULIN-SENSITIVE TISSUES: THIAZOLIDINEDIONES

The thiazolidinedione class of drugs, often termed *TZDs* or *glitazones*, has engendered great enthusiasm and controversy since the first agent, troglitazone, was approved in 1997.[52-56] Troglitazone was withdrawn from the United States market in the year 2000, as a result of rare cases of fulminant hepatic necrosis, and because pioglitazone and rosiglitazone appear to be safer. This class of oral antidiabetic agents is believed to work by binding to and modulating the activity of a family of nuclear transcription factors termed *peroxisome-proliferator-activated receptors* (PPARs), particularly PPAG-γ. They are associated with slow improvement in glycemic control over weeks to months in parallel with an improvement in insulin sensitivity and reduction of free fatty acid (FFA) levels. Pioglitazone and rosiglitazone are generally well-tolerated with weight gain and fluid retention as the only significant fairly common adverse effects. There is no substantial evidence that these newer agents are associated with hepatotoxicity, but this record of safety has been established in the setting of careful liver function test monitoring. Therefore, it is important to continue to recommend that glitazones not be used in patients with active hepatocellular disease or with unexplained serum alanine aminotransferase levels greater than 2.5 times the upper limit of normal; routine monitoring of liver function tests with these glitazones is no longer recommended.[57,58]

The promise of the glitazone agents to reverse or prevent the negative cardiovascular associations of insulin resistance in parallel with their effect to improve insulin sensitivity is exciting but unproven; the hypothesis is under formal study in a series of randomized prospective clinical trials.[59,60] The available data regarding vascular effects of the glitazones generally come from placebo-controlled studies, which, as a rule, involved small numbers of patients followed for weeks to months, but which have consistently demonstrated tantalizing clinical associations such as reduced progression of carotid intimal medial thickness, decreased rates of in-stent restenosis in the setting of percutaneous coronary intervention, normalization of vascular endothelial function, improvements in dyslipidemia, reduction of blood pressure, improvements in fibrinolytic and coagulation parameters, and reduction in inflammatory markers.[55-59] A second promising attribute of the glitazones that has generated great interest is an effect to improve insulin secretory dynamics in subjects with diabetes and impaired glucose tolerance. Initial reports suggest that these agents provide for more durable glycemic control than other antidiabetic agents. These latter observations provide hope that pioglitazone and rosiglitazone may be useful not only in diabetes prevention but also in halting the progression of established diabetes, thus reducing the need for additional drug therapy over time. It is important to recognize that the proven clinical effects of pioglitazone and rosiglitazone to date are limited to improvements in glycemic control and changes in lipid parameters.

The adverse effect that has engendered the most concern regarding this class of drugs is fluid retention and its manifestations: peripheral edema, a decrease in hemoglobin concentration as well as occasional presentations with previously unrecognized heart failure, or a worsening of preexisting heart failure.[61,62] With appropriate caution, almost no one should need to withdraw from therapy as a result of fluid retention; in the registration trials for rosiglitazone and pioglitazone, patient withdrawals for edema or heart failure were less than 1%. The patients most likely to experience edema are those treated with insulin and those with preexisting edema; women, obese patients, and those with known ischemic heart disease, heart failure, diastolic dysfunction, or renal insufficiency also seem to be at increased risk. It is prudent to start high-risk patients with the lowest marketed dose (pioglitazone 15 mg daily or rosiglitazone 2 mg daily) and to teach them how to assess pitting pretibial edema at home, suggesting that they make a habit of checking nightly. If they note a pattern of increasing edema, patients can be instructed to restrict sodium intake, to start a diuretic, or to increase previously prescribed diuretics on their own as needed. Generally, clinically significant fluid retention will present in 2 to 3 weeks after initiation of therapy; thus, in the highest risk patients, reevaluation in 2 to 3 weeks can be useful. More often, patients can return in approximately 2 months when the glycemic response to a given dose of glitazone is generally maximal to evaluate whether the response to therapy is adequate and if significant edema has developed. Based on those assessments, consideration of increasing the dose of glitazone further with expectant management of edema can be accomplished. Most patients with mild edema respond to a low-dose thiazide diuretic (e.g., hydrochlorothiazide 25 mg). In patients with more extensive edema, a combination of low-dose thiazide diuretic with moderate-dose loop diuretic is sometimes required. Anecdotal reports suggest that avoidance of nonsteroidal anti-inflammatory agents and dihydropyridine calcium channel blockers can reduce the frequency of edema as an adverse event; concomitant treatment with maximal doses of angiotensin-converting enzyme inhibitors has been suggested to reduce the prevalence of edema. It should be noted that fluid retention to the point of congestive heart failure and anasarca has been reported; careful clinical studies suggest that the "heart failure" reported with glitazones is much more likely to be characterized by peripheral edema than signs of pulmonary edema, in contradistinction to the usual presentation of heart failure in populations with diabetes.[63] Finally, in some patients, edema is refractory to diuretic therapy perhaps as a result of calcium-channel blocker type effects of the glitazones; in those patients, dose reduction often is accompanied by a resolution or improvement in edema. Glitazones are contraindicated in patients with class III and IV heart failure.

The other issue which engenders substantial clinical concern regarding glitazones therapy is weight gain. Careful study indicates that the weight gain is a result of subcutaneous and not visceral fat accumulation; in fact, there is a reduction in visceral fat, hepatic fat, and intramyocellular fat. Therefore, the weight gain observed with glitazones, while potentially having negative consequences from a cosmetic standpoint, is perhaps less likely to cause adverse cardiovascular effects. The weight gain with glitazones is minimized with concomitant metformin therapy and greatest with insulin and sulfonylurea therapy. All patients prescribed glitazones should be counseled to redouble lifestyle efforts to minimize weight gain. Both weight gain and fluid retention are more common and severe in patients with the greatest glycemic responses, making expectant management of these adverse effects mandatory. Whether there are substantial clinical differences between the two members of this class of oral antidiabetic agents is unproven though a recent small-scale randomized trial undertaken in the context of sulfonylurea therapy does seem to confirm that pioglitazone has a more uniformly positive effect on fasting plasma lipids[64]; whether this apparent difference will be accompanied by differences in cardiovascular events or need for concomitant lipid-lowering therapies is unclear.

INSULIN SECRETAGOGUES

Currently available insulin secretagogues all bind to the sulfonylurea receptor (SUR1), a subunit of the adenosine triphosphate (ATP)-sensitive potassium channel (K_{ATP}) on the plasma membrane of pancreatic β cells. The SUR1 subunit regulates the activity of the channel and also binds ATP and adenosine diphosphate (ADP), effectively functioning as a glucose sensor and trigger for insulin secretion. The K_{ATP} channel closes upon sulfonylurea binding, as well as with increases in intracellular ATP and decreases in ADP as a result of fuel metabolism. The membrane depolarization that ensues causes the opening of voltage-dependent L-type calcium channels. Subsequent calcium influx results in an increase in intracellular calcium, which leads to insulin secretion. Differences in pharmacokinetic and binding properties of the various insulin secretagogues result in the specific responses that each agent produces. The major clinical differences between them seem to be related to duration of action and to fairly subtle variations in their hypoglycemic potential.

SULFONYLUREAS

The sulfonylureas have been available since the 1950s. They have a relatively slow onset of action and variable duration of action. There are numerous choices available (Table 63-7), which can be divided into first- and second-generation agents. In general, the second-generation agents (glipizide, glyburide, and glimepiride) are more potent and as a result have fewer adverse effects and drug-drug interactions. Extended-release glipizide and glimepiride are preferred agents as they can be dosed once-daily in the vast majority of

Table 63-7 Characteristics of Sulfonylureas					
Generic Name (Tablet Sizes [mg])	**Initial Daily Dose**	**Maximum Daily Dose**	**Equivalent Doses (mg)**	**Duration of Action**	**Comments**
Acetohexamide	250 mg	1500 mg, two doses when > 1000 mg	500	Intermediate, 12–18 hr	Metabolized by liver to active metabolite (twice as potent as parent compound); has diuretic activity; has uricosuric activity.
Chlorpropamide (100, 250)	100 mg	750 mg single dose (500 mg in older patients)	250	Very long, 60 hr	70% metabolized by liver to less-active metabolites; 30% excreted intact by kidneys; can potentiate ADH. Antabuse-like reaction with alcohol (facial flushing reaction, some breathlessness) occurs in nearly one third of patients on this agent. Higher risk of hypoglycemia.
Tolazamide (100, 250, 500)	100 mg	1000 mg, two doses when >500 mg	250	Intermediate, 12–24 hr	Metabolized by liver to less-active and inactive products; has diuretic activity.
Tolbutamide (500)	250 mg	3000 mg in 2–3 doses	1000	Short, 6–12 hr	Metabolized by liver to inactive product.
Glipizide (5, 10)	2.5–5 mg	40 mg, two doses when > 10 mg	5	Intermediate, 12–24 hr	Metabolized by liver to inactive products that are excreted in the urine and to a lesser extent, in the bile. Mild diuretic activity.
Glipizide ER (2.5, 5, 10)	2.5–5 mg	20 mg, once daily	5	Long > 24 hr	
Glyburide (1.25, 2.5, 5)	1.25–5 mg	20 mg, two doses when > 10 mg	5	Intermediate, 16–24 hr	Metabolized by liver to weakly active and inactive products, excreted in urine and bile.
Micronized glyburide (1.5, 3, 6)	1.5–3 mg	6 mg twice daily	3	Somewhat shorter	Mild diuretic activity; higher risk of hypoglycemia.
Glimepiride (1, 2, 4)	1–2 mg	8 mg once daily	2	Long > 24 hours	Metabolized to inactive metabolites by the liver, excreted in urine and bile.

ER, extended release.
Adapted from Facts and Comparisons, Drug Information Monthly Update Service. St. Louis, JB Lippincott.

patients and involve a relatively low risk of hypoglycemia and weight gain. Glyburide is still the most commonly prescribed insulin secretagogue despite the fact that essentially all marketed secretagogues have been shown to have a significantly lower hypoglycemic potential; also, glyburide has been associated with an abrogation of ischemic preconditioning, a protective autoregulatory mechanism in the heart, mediated by interaction with the vascular and cardiac SUR2 receptors.[65]

Likely as a holdover from when sulfonylureas were the only marketed oral agents for diabetes, the maximum marketed dose is generally two to four times higher than the maximally effective dose. To minimize the risk of hypoglycemia and concerns about blunting ischemic preconditioning, it is probably most appropriate to employ relatively low doses of sulfonylurea. Sulfonylureas are arguably the most cost-effective glucose-lowering agents and, therefore, are worthy of their widespread use; they do not seem to confer any special benefits beyond glucose lowering, but with average A1Cs in the United States greater than 7.5%, they clearly have a role in diabetes management. In general, limiting the dose to one-fourth maximal (e.g., glipizide-ER 5 mg, one tablet daily or glimepiride 4 mg, 1/2 tablet daily) minimizes costs and adverse events. Because patients respond quickly to changes in dose of sulfonylurea, careful glucose monitoring over 2 to 3 days is usually adequate to determine if changes in glycemic control with higher dose therapy are sufficient to justify continuing. Small doses of sulfonylurea (e.g., glimepiride 1 mg, 1/2 to 1 tablet daily or glipizide-ER 2.5 mg daily) are remarkably effective, particularly in patients on concomitant insulin-sensitizing therapy, and well-tolerated. Small doses are also called for in treating elderly patients who are more susceptible to sulfonylurea-induced hypoglycemia, particularly in the setting of declining renal function or erratic meals and activity.

Side effects other than hypoglycemia and modest weight gain are uncommon, particularly for the second-generation agents, but include nausea, vomiting, rashes, purpura, and pruritis. Rare patients may develop hematologic reactions such as leukopenia, thrombocytopenia, hemolytic anemia, and cholestasis with or without jaundice.

REPAGLINIDE

Repaglinide is a member of the meglitinide family of insulin secretagogues, distinct from the sulfonylureas. It is quickly absorbed, has a short half-life and a distinct SUR1-binding site. As a result, it produces a generally faster and briefer stimulus to insulin secretion. It is generally dosed with each meal and provides better postprandial control, as well as less hypoglycemia and weight gain than glyburide. Repaglinide does seem to have a long residence time on the sulfonylurea receptor and as a result has a more prolonged effect on fasting glucose than would be expected based on its short pharmacologic half-life. Repaglinide is available in 0.5, 1, and 2 mg tablets. The maximal dose is 4 mg with each meal. As is the case with the sulfonylureas, there is a minimal glucose-lowering advantage of high doses versus moderate doses of repaglinide.

NATEGLINIDE

Nateglinide is a derivative of phenylalanine, structurally distinct from both sulfonylureas and the meglitinides. It has a quicker onset and shorter duration of action than repaglinide. Its interaction with SUR1 is fleeting. As a result, its effect to lower postprandial glucose is quite specific and it only modestly lowers fasting glucose. This provides advantages (less hypoglycemia) and disadvantages (less overall glucose-lowering effectiveness). Therefore, nateglinide is most appropriately used when fasting glucose levels are modestly elevated in the setting of early diabetes or in combination with insulin sensitizers or long-acting evening insulin. Nateglinide is available as 120-mg tablets and is dosed with each meal. A 60-mg tablet is available but is reserved for use in patients with minimal hyperglycemia.

The rationale for stimulating insulin secretion in a way that minimizes fasting hyperinsulinemia and maximizes postprandial control is compelling. Furthermore, these newer "glinide" agents demonstrate little binding to the vascular smooth muscle and cardiac SUR2 receptors. However, the use in the United States of these newer agents has been modest, in part because of the need for multiple daily doses, greater expense than with sulfonylureas, and lack of head-to-head comparative studies that demonstrate superiority over preferred sulfonylureas, which have similarly been shown to have low potential for producing hypoglycemia and weight gain.

CARBOHYDRATE ABSORPTION INHIBITORS: α-GLUCOSIDASE INHIBITORS

α-Glucosidase inhibitors (AGIs) inhibit the terminal step of carbohydrate digestion at the brush border of the intestinal epithelium. When administered with the first bite of a carbohydrate containing meal, carbohydrate absorption is shifted more distally in the intestine and is, therefore, delayed, allowing the sluggish insulin secretory dynamics characteristic of type 2 diabetes to catch up with carbohydrate absorption. There are two currently marketed agents in the United States: acarbose and miglitol. Acarbose is largely not absorbed from the intestine, whereas miglitol is. Their use has been limited by a number of factors, including frequent gastrointestinal complaints, the need to administer the medication at the beginning of each meal, and modest reductions in A1C due to their specific effect on postprandial glucose with little effect on fasting glucose. These concerns should be balanced against the ability of the AGIs to lower glucose in virtually everyone without hypoglycemia or weight gain. The major adverse effects are flatulence, abdominal distress or distension, and diarrhea. These result from excessive blockade of carbohydrate absorption in the small bowel, leading to fermentation and gas production in the colon. To maximize the likelihood that these agents will be tolerated, start with a low dose such as one fourth of the maximum dose once daily and increase over a period of weeks to months to one fourth to one half maximal doses with each meal. A recent study in prediabetic patients demonstrated a statistically significant reduction in cardiovascular end points and new hypertension associated with treatment with acarbose, suggesting that modulating postprandial excursions or perhaps nonglycemic effects of the drug may provide for benefits vis-à-vis cardiovascular disease.[66] This notion is further supported by the observation in a single-center subgroup analysis from the same study that progression of intimal medial thickness is also slowed by acarbose.[67] The AGIs are contraindicated in patients with chronic intestinal conditions, most particularly inflammatory bowel disease.

INSULINS

Insulin has been commercially available since the early 1920s and is arguably still the mainstay of therapy for the majority of people with type 2 diabetes worldwide. Subcutaneous injection of insulin in type 2 diabetes can be used to supplement endogenous production of insulin both in the fasting state to modulate hepatic glucose production and in the postprandial state to facilitate glucose clearance into muscle and fat for storage. Currently, the vast majority of insulin used worldwide is of recombinant human origin; animal source insulin is difficult to obtain and more expensive. The available formulations largely differ in their pharmacokinetics as reviewed in Table 63-8.

Table 63-8 Characteristics of Human Insulin and Analogues

Preparation	Onset	Peak	Duration	Variability
SHORT-ACTING				
Lispro, aspart, glulisine	5–15 min	45 min–2 hr	3–4 hr	Least
Regular	30 min	2–5 hr	5–8 hr	Moderate
INTERMEDIATE-ACTING				
NPH	1–2 hr	6–10 hr	16–24+ hr	High
Lente	1–2 hr	8–12 hr	18–24+ hr	High
LONG-ACTING				
Glargine	~2 hr	None	~24 hr	Moderate
Ultralente	4–6 hr	10–18 hr	16–24+ hr	Most
Detemir	1–2 hr	2–16 hr	16–24+ hr	Minimal
MIXTURES				
70:30, 50:50, 75:25	30 min	7–12 hr	16–24+ hr	Moderate

There are now three rapid-acting insulin analogues (lispro, aspart, and glulisine), each with onset of action in 5 to 15 minutes, near peak activity from approximately 45 minutes to 2 hours, and a duration of activity of approximately 4 hours, with slightly more prolonged activity at higher doses. These three molecules have a different structural modification that disrupts the "tail structure" of the insulin molecule; as a result, they do not exhibit as great a tendency to form dimers and hexamers at high concentration. Marketing suggests that there are differences between agents; however, on the background of endogenous insulin secretion in the setting of type 2 diabetes, clinically relevant differences in glycemic control or adverse effects have not been demonstrated. These rapid-acting analogues are associated with better postprandial glucose control than regular human insulin, as well as a reduction in the risk of hypoglycemia in some studies. They should be administered up to 15 minutes before meals or even immediately after meals. Dosing after meals in combination with techniques such as carbohydrate counting is often very helpful in overweight patients with type 2 diabetes as they often have no idea what they will eat, effectively until they are done eating.

Regular human insulin is approximately half as fast as the rapid-acting analogues with onset in 10 to 30 minutes, peak activity at 2 to 5 hours, and duration of action of 5 to 8 or more hours. Regular insulin should ideally be administered 30 to 60 minutes before meals, which certainly has issues with respect to adherence and the potential to produce hypoglycemia if the meal is subsequently missed. Intermediate-acting insulin, neutral protamine Hagedorn (NPH) and Lente, is approximately twice as slow as regular insulin with an onset of action in 1 to 2 hours, a fairly broad peak of activity from 6 to 12 hours, and a duration of action of 16 to 24 or more hours. Human Ultralente insulin is longer acting than NPH or Lente human insulin, but the pharmacokinetics of human Ultralente are not dramatically different from those of NPH or Lente, merely shifted in time moderately (2–4 hours). Human regular, NPH, Lente, and Ultralente all have a dramatic dose-dependence to their profile of activity; the higher the dose, the broader the peak and longer the duration of action.

Insulin glargine is a novel long-acting insulin analogue with distinctive properties. It is administered as a clear, colorless, acidic solution and, therefore, cannot be mixed with other forms of insulin or stored in prefilled syringes. Upon subcutaneous injection, the glargine solution is neutralized and the insulin glargine precipitates nearly instantaneously. It provides a flat, peakless profile of activity with a duration of action of more than 24 hours in most people with type 2 diabetes. Detemir is the most recently developed insulin analogue. It is relatively rapidly absorbed but has a prolonged duration of action, attributable in large part to its acylation at position B29 with a 14-carbon fatty acid (myristic acid). As a result of this structure, detemir is highly protein-bound in interstitial fluid and in plasma. The clinical utility of detemir above and beyond that of intermediate-acting forms of insulin in the setting of type 2 diabetes has not been well-established. However, it has been shown in carefully controlled conditions to display less variability in insulin action day-to-day than NPH or glargine, at least in type 1 diabetes.[68] Whether those differences persist in patients with type 2 diabetes outside of the clinical research setting and at the higher doses is unclear.

There have been a number of studies published over more than a decade demonstrating that bedtime intermediate-acting insulin is associated with better glycemic control than once-daily injections provided in the morning, and in some cases, even twice-daily injections. The Treat to Target Study recently documented the safety and effectiveness of bedtime NPH or glargine insulin as a single bedtime injection added to oral agents in the setting of poor glycemic control (A1C > 7.5%) on one or two oral agents.[69] At randomization, patients added 10 units of NPH or glargine insulin at bedtime to their baseline oral antidiabetic agents and were instructed to increase the dose by 8 units per week if the average of the last two recorded fasting glucoses was >180 mg/dL, 6 units per week if the average fasting glucose was 140 to 180 mg/dL, 4 units per week if the average fasting glucose was 120 to 140 mg/dL, and 2 units per week if the average fasting glucose was 100 to 120 mg/dL. The investigators employed an algorithm for titration based on the last two fasting home glucose determinations ascertained during a weekly phone call. Small decreases in insulin dose (2–4 units) were allowed if there was a severe hypoglycemic event or documented glucose less than 56 mg/dL. Bedtime doses were not titrated upward if any glucose over the prior week was less than 72 mg/dL or if there was an episode of severe hypoglycemia. The mean A1C achieved was identical and approximately 7% in both groups. There was a statistically significant lower incidence of nocturnal hypoglycemia in the group treated with bedtime glargine when compared to those treated with NPH. An alternative titration scheme, which has not been validated by clinical trials but is a bit easier for patients to titrate at home, is to have patients monitor fasting glucose at home on a daily basis and increase the nightly dose of NPH or glargine insulin by 1 unit per day until the morning glucose is generally in the 90 to 130 mg/dL range. Additional instructions to decrease the insulin dose by 1 to 2 units for any prebreakfast reading less than 70 mg/dL are appropriate. In patients with more dramatic hyperglycemia, one can start with a higher dose (e.g., 20 units) and increase more rapidly (e.g., 3–5 units per day) until the fasting glucose is moderately controlled (e.g., 150–200 mg/dL) and then titrate more slowly from there. In patients who achieve control of their fasting glucose, many will maintain reasonable control through the rest of the day. Most will have elevated glucose levels after meals and many will have premeal glucose levels increasing through the day before returning to more normal levels overnight. In this setting, it is possible to try to adjust oral agents to compensate, but a large proportion will need to take rapid-acting insulin with meals to keep the blood sugar down throughout the day. When daytime insulin is added to previously optimized nocturnal insulin, often simultaneous reductions in the nocturnal insulin are required. For better or worse, this regimen of once-nightly glargine has become the most commonly prescribed single form of insulin therapy in type 2 diabetes in the United States. A major clinical question, unanswered in large-scale clinical trials is what is the optimal next step in diabetes management—twice-daily mixed insulin or more intensive approaches employing rapid-acting insulin administered at meals.

Premixed insulin formulations provide greater convenience and accuracy than those mixed by patients. Premixed formulations available in the United States include 70:30 and 50:50 mixtures of NPH and regular insulin, a 75:25 mixture of lispro insulin in its NPH-like formulation with insulin lispro, and a 70:30 mixture of insulin aspart with its NPH-like congener. Premixed insulin provides a profile of activity as expected from the addition of the activities of its components. The role of premixed insulins in the management of type 2 diabetes has been widely debated; they have advantages with respect to convenience in administering the injection and disadvantages with respect to the inconvenience of having to be a bit more rigid in the timing and composition of meals to achieve excellent control.

Some advocate initiation of insulin therapy in the setting of type 2 diabetes with intensive regimens analogous to those used for type 1 diabetes. The details of these approaches are discussed in Chapter 62. The major qualitative difference in using multiple daily injection techniques in the setting of type 2 diabetes is that patients do not necessarily need to take an injection with each meal and snack as is generally the case in type 1 diabetes. Many do very well taking rapid-acting insulin with larger or carbohydrate-rich meals, particularly at breakfast and/or supper and relying on oral agents to tide them over through the rest of the day. Similarly, some patients do reasonably well overnight while fasting and merely require meal-associated insulin to maintain glucose levels normal during the day. An open mind, frequent glucose monitoring, and a critical eye are needed to determine the most convenient regimen that provides for adequate glycemic control with low risk of hypoglycemia. There is also a substantial quantitative difference in insulin doses to the approaches advocated for type 1 diabetes. Most patients with type 2 diabetes will require larger quantities of insulin, even in the setting of combination therapy with insulin sensitizers and/or secretagogues. It is not uncommon for patients with type 2 diabetes to require 3 to 10 units of rapid-acting insulin per 15-g serving of carbohydrates to achieve postprandial control of glycemia. In patients that are following low-carbohydrate meal plans, developing techniques to provide insulin in proportion to protein intake is often necessary as well. These insulin-to-carbohydrate or insulin-to-protein ratios can be empirically determined for individual patients based on blood glucose monitoring results; values before the next meal can be as useful as postprandial levels in titrating rapid-acting insulin.

Adverse events associated with insulin are well-known and include weight gain and hypoglycemia. Both rapid-acting and long-acting insulin analogues have been shown to provide a modest reduction in risk of hypoglycemia to human insulin formulations. Insulin allergies are rare, as are chronic skin reactions lipodystrophy and lipohypertrophy. It should be noted that the absolute risk of severe hypoglycemia in patients with type 2 diabetes is relatively small, approximately one-third to one tenth as high as in similarly treated patients with type 1 diabetes. This risk can be further minimized with appropriate education of patients and expectant home glucose monitoring at times when unrecognized hypoglycemia is most likely to occur: mid-sleep or during unplanned or strenuous activity. There are rare examples of patients who develop irritation at injection sites (more common but rarely dose-limiting with insulin glargine) or allergies.

Newer insulin needles cause less discomfort than those previously available because of a finer gauge, shorter length, sharper points, and smoother surfaces. Insulin pen technology makes teaching a patient to take insulin much easier and provides greater convenience and accuracy of dosing. Insulin pump therapy has been used in patients with type 2 diabetes but is not widely accepted as cost effective for routine use. Even though the vast majority of patients now find insulin therapy much easier and more effective than they had anticipated, there is still substantial resistance to initiating insulin therapy on the part of patients and providers.

PRACTICAL ASPECTS OF INITIATING AND PROGRESSIVELY MANAGING TYPE 2 DIABETES

A significant challenge in clinical decision making in diabetes is that the increased availability of therapeutic options for antidiabetic therapy is ahead of adequate prospective outcome studies to determine optimal treatment strategies. Currently available clinical trial data have not identified the preferred agents in type 2 diabetes, either as initial therapy or in subsequent care. Each class of drugs and even agents within each class has advantages and limitations, and individual issues may significantly affect the appropriate choice of therapy in particular patients. Table 63-6 highlights some of the relative advantages and disadvantages of various agents and classes.

A general approach in the absence of any patient-specific factors is suggested in the algorithm presented in Figure 63-1. A growing body of experience indicates that the use of

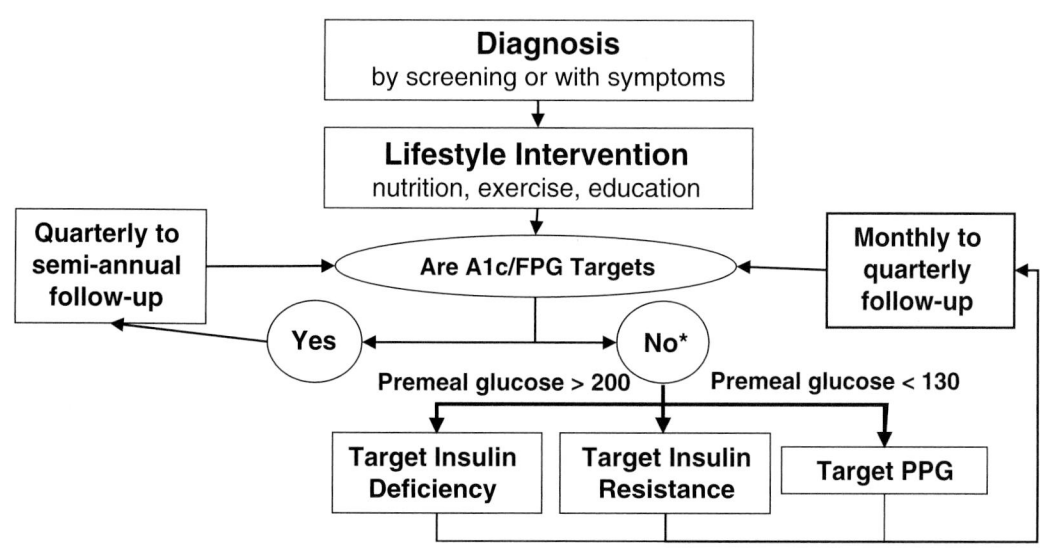

** Keep adding agents until target reached

Figure 63-1 Proposed treatment algorithm for type 2 diabetes.

metformin as initial therapy in combination with diet and exercise can provide impressive lowering of glucose with essentially no risk of hypoglycemia. Because this agent is available as a generic preparation, relative cost is fairly low; if the response is judged to be inadequate a thiazolidinedione, sulfonylurea, glinide, or AGI can be added. It has been proposed that the use of metformin alone or in combination with a thiazolidinedione may lead to a greater reduction in cardiovascular risk than similarly effective (with respect to glycemia) approaches that increase insulin levels. Early use of glitazones may reduce the need for subsequent addition of other agents. At present, the data are not definitive on either of these points. Patients with higher levels of pre-meal glucoses (generally >200 mg/dL) almost always require agents to increase insulin levels. Because insulin, sulfonylureas, and glinides provide much faster improvements in overall control than glitazones (due to their 1–2 week delay in activity) or metformin or AGIs (as a result of the need to titrate the drug), they are preferred in patients with higher levels of glucose either as monotherapy or as part of initial combined therapy. Starting a patient with a low dose of a glimepiride, glipizide-GITS, or insulin combined with metformin, glitazone, or AGI is a reasonable initial approach to the poorly controlled patient. In patients who have reasonable control of fasting and preprandial plasma glucose levels (more than 50% of values <130 mg/dL) whose overall control as assessed by HbA_{1c} is still higher than desired, monitoring may be either inaccurate or ineffective or postprandial plasma glucose levels may be elevated. As it can be more difficult to have patients monitor in the postprandial state, it is important to remember that without specific therapy, almost all patients with type 2 diabetes have elevated postprandial plasma glucose. Thus, in such patients, targeting presumed postprandial plasma glucose elevations with the use of AGIs, glinides, or rapid-acting insulin analogues can theoretically lower average glucose with a lower risk of weight gain and hypoglycemia than with sulfonylureas or long-acting insulin. The most critical issue in long-term glycemic management is that of continuously reassessing with patients the adequacy of their control, examining glucose monitoring logs and HbA_{1c} values, and refining treatment regimens to achieve optimal control with the lowest dose of the least number of medications.

Most patients in specialty care require two or more drugs to achieve recommended glycemic targets. Many patients require three or more. Fortunately, almost all the possible two-drug combinations and many of the three-drug combinations have been examined in large-scale studies and have been shown to be safe and effective, receiving indications from the Food and Drug Administration. Recent studies suggest that the complexity of the treatment regimen is not a substantial barrier to achieving control as long as the patient understands the rationale for each component and accepts the treatment program.[70] Generally, it is preferred to add agents if there was an improvement in control with the first agent selected and to continue to add agents as needed to achieve goals. Subsequent back-titration to optimize treatment is often possible when glycemic goals are achieved. The selection of initial therapy should be based on mutually (patient and provider) recognized priorities. Increasingly, practitioners are using submaximal doses of agents in combination to increase the ratio of efficacy to adverse effects and in recognition of the potential synergy of sensitizers and secretagogues, as well as the value of treatment of postprandial glucose and fasting glucose in combination therapy.

When adding insulin in the management of inadequately controlled type 2 diabetes, some practitioners prefer to stop the oral antidiabetic agents and switch to insulin. Most generally continue the oral agents and add an evening dose of insulin as discussed with the Treat to Target study. Many patients eventually require more complex regimens—twice-daily injections, split-mix insulin, multiple injection

regimens, and, rarely, insulin pump therapy. It should be noted that a minority of patients with type 2 diabetes have a better response to insulin administered in the morning than in the evening either as a result of inadequate insulin secretory reserve or because of poor adherence with evening injections.

It is important that both patient and health-care provider agree on how to reach the goals of therapy. Therefore, biases and concerns of the patient should be addressed when trying to determine which agent should be prescribed. These biases can be elucidated in interviews with patients through discussions of various strategies, some of which follow.

STRATEGIES

Minimal Cost Strategy

For a large proportion of patients, drug costs are an overwhelming issue. Diet and exercise can be extremely effective and almost free. The least expensive drugs for the treatment of diabetes are the sulfonylureas; metformin is now generic but not yet frankly inexpensive. Thus, a minimum cost strategy could start with substantial attention to lifestyle intervention for a period of weeks, recognizing that most of the reduction in glycemia that will result from an acute lifestyle intervention will be seen relatively early. If that intervention is unsuccessful, adding a sulfonylurea, such as generic glipizide-ER, followed by generic metformin or bedtime or pre-supper insulin and finally two or more insulin injections per day if necessary should keep costs to a minimum. In the Veterans Administration Cooperative Study, excellent control was achieved in the context of a comprehensive program of diabetes education using a combination of daytime sulfonylurea and evening insulin.[71] Although insulin is relatively inexpensive, in high doses (1 U/kg or more) the costs become substantial and the relative benefits of moderate increases in dose modest, creating a rationale for adding metformin or a thiazolidinedione. It should be noted that most pharmaceutical companies have programs to provide no-cost or low-cost medication to the poor. Many of these are listed with links at *www.needymeds.com*. Furthermore, for increasing numbers of patients, the major driving force in their drug expenses is the number of prescriptions as each is associated with a copayment, providing a rationale for using combination agents or relying on insulin monotherapy or combination of insulin and a glitazone.

Minimum Weight Gain Strategy

Weight gain associated with the treatment of diabetes is of concern to most clinicians and is unfortunately occasionally an overriding issue with patients. Counseling regarding the need to focus efforts on achieving glycemic, blood pressure, and lipid targets as first priorities to minimize the risk of complications leaving weight as a secondary issue is sometimes unacceptable to patients. A strategy to minimize weight gain would emphasize diet and exercise and would almost certainly employ metformin and/or an AGI as initial therapy with the addition of the other if one was inadequate. As sulfonylureas and repaglinide seem to have a modest weight-sparing effect in combination therapy with insulin, one or the other could be added before insulin administration in such a strategy. As discussed earlier, the weight gain associated with thiazolidinediones, although certainly a cosmetic issue, may not be associated with increased cardiovascular risk. A number of pharmaceutical approaches to weight loss have been evaluated in the setting of diabetes; a dozen or so trials of sibutramine and orlistat generally have been associated with modest weight loss (2–10 kg) with proportional reductions in A1C (0.1–2%), generally averaging about 4 kg of weight loss and 0.5% reduction in A1C. The long-term safety, tolerability, and efficacy of these pharmacologic weight-loss approaches, however, is not known.

Minimal Injection Strategy

Many patients are determined to avoid insulin injections at any cost. The minimal injection strategy involves sulfonylureas, metformin, AGIs, and thiazolidinediones, which can be added in any order, though again, early use of a glitazone may blunt the progressive β-cell dysfunction observed in type 2 diabetes. Insulin, probably as a bedtime or presupper dose to minimize the inconvenience, would be added only if absolutely necessary. It is important to try to dispel notions that insulin therapy is difficult, ominous, or fraught with peril by highlighting its efficacy and the great strides that have been made in insulin formulations and delivery devices. Most patients require insulin at some point in their lifetime.

Minimal Insulin Resistance Strategy

The possible atherogenic effects of insulin have been widely touted in the lay press and by marketing programs within the pharmaceutical industry. The relationship between circulating insulin levels and cardiovascular risk in nondiabetic populations is incontrovertible but probably related to the presence of insulin resistance rather than the insulin concentrations per se. Furthermore, in essentially all studies of intensive management with insulin, improved outcomes were observed with insulin treatment, particularly in the setting of cardiovascular disease.[72,73] There are no clinical data to suggest that exogenous insulin is associated with adverse side effects or long-term complications beyond its hypoglycemic effects and the associated weight gain. In any case, this strategy is analogous to the minimal injection strategy except that the order of introduction of agents is perhaps important. The thiazolidinediones have the greatest efficacy in reducing insulin resistance, metformin is second, and AGIs are third, with nateglinide associated with more specific stimulation of insulin levels after meals than the other insulin secretagogues, which all increase peripheral insulin levels less than injected insulin.

Minimal Effort Strategy

Many patients are capable of making only a minimal effort with regard to their diabetes self-management. Questioning patients about their pill-taking history and their realistic ability to comply with a proposed program of therapy is important. Taking a once-a-day sulfonylurea or glitazone requires the least effort by the patient. Recognize that glitazones retain their efficacy even after several days of missed doses. Bedtime insulin is actually relatively well-accepted by patients to whom this consideration is important. Developing strategies to improve adherence and increase motivation is certainly a long-term goal in this population.

Hypoglycemia Avoidance Strategy

This is another important consideration for many patients. The AGIs have been reported in small studies to reduce "reactive" hypoglycemia. Other oral agents could be added in any order with the exception that insulin secretagogues would be added last, their dose minimized, and glyburide avoided. Nateglinide, in particular, among the secretagogues is associated with an exceptionally low risk of significant hypoglycemia. The insulin analogues are associated with a lower risk of hypoglycemia than human insulin. Bedtime NPH is actually associated with a lesser risk of hypoglycemia during the day than treatment with glargine and this can be used to advantage in patients who engage in physical labor during the day, particularly in high-risk occupations where severe hypoglycemia could lead to injury.

Postprandial Targeting Strategy

Achieving postprandial plasma glucose targets is generally associated with better control than just meeting premeal targets. Control of postprandial glycemia can be achieved only with specific lifestyle efforts and pharmacologic agents that target postprandial glucose. Postprandial glucose monitoring is helpful in this regard as it reinforces the goals. Techniques that can improve postprandial control include lowering the carbohydrate content of meals, adding fiber, substituting monounsaturated fats or protein for carbohydrates, encouraging physical activity after meals, adding AGIs with meals, and using rapid-acting insulin analogues. Nateglinide and repaglinide provide a theoretical advantage in this situation compared with other secretagogues, although formal head-to-head studies have not been completed comparing the glinides with glimepiride and glipizide-ER.

FUTURE DIRECTIONS

Novel pharmaceutical agents including glucagon receptor antagonists, inhibitors of gluconeogenic and glycogenolytic pathways, activators of the insulin-signaling pathways, modifiers of lipid metabolism, and antiobesity agents are areas of early pharmaceutical development.[74]

Novel methods of insulin delivery similarly have generated a great deal of enthusiasm among patients, particularly techniques to deliver insulin orally or by inhalation.[75]

Novel hormones from the enteropancreatic axis are likely to be the next dramatic advance in diabetes management. Amylin, the second β-cell hormone, is known to act centrally to suppress postprandial glucagon secretion, slow gastric emptying, and increase satiety. Synthetic amylin has received an approvable letter from the Food and Drug Administration and is associated with specific postprandial glucose lowering, modestly efficacy in reducing A1C, as well as weight reduction.[76,77] Glucagon-like peptide-1 is a gut hormone secreted from intestinal L-cells that has an overlapping but generally more robust profile of action than amylin with the additional effect of stimulating insulin secretion in a glucose-dependent manner. Glucagon-like peptide-1 is rapidly degraded in the circulation, and thus inhibitors of the degrading enzyme (dipeptidylpeptidase IV), as well as dipeptidylpeptidase IV–resistant analogues and naturally occurring incretin mimetics are being investigated in clinical trials.[78] Among them, exenatide is under review by the Food and Drug Administration while other agents are still in ongoing clinical trials. These agents seem to be very effective in reducing postprandial, as well as fasting, glucose, and produce modest weight loss without increasing the risk of hypoglycemia unless they are coadminstered with secretagogues or insulin.[79] In animal studies they have been demonstrated to increase new islet formation from pancreatic ducts and, therefore, their role in diabetes prevention and early diabetes management is also being considered.

PLACE OF GLUCOSE MANAGEMENT IN THE TREATMENT OF TYPE 2 DIABETES

As noted earlier, the importance of managing dyslipidemia, hypertension, and the procoagulant state in the setting of diabetes to reduce cardiovascular events has been much more clearly demonstrated than the case for treating hyperglycemia. As cardiovascular disease is the ultimate cause of death in the overwhelming majority of patients with diabetes, arguably blood pressure, lipid, and antiplatelet therapy are critical components of care.[1] Recommended targets for lipid and blood pressure management are presented in Table 63-9.

Lifestyle measures targeting weight reduction for overweight patients may be the most cost-effective and safest mode of therapy and should be reinforced at every visit. Aspirin therapy 75 to 162 mg daily is recommended for all patients with known vascular disease and should be considered for those over age 40 with additional risk factors (family history, smoking, hypertension, albuminuria, obesity, and/or

Table 63-9 **Targets for Cardiovascular Risk Reduction in Diabetes**

Parameter	ADA Goal	NCEP/JNC-VII Goals
LDL	<100 mg/dL	<100 mg/dL
TG	<150 mg/dL	
HDL	>40 mg/dL (men) >50 mg/dL (women)	
Non-HDL cholesterol		<130 mg/dL
Systolic blood pressure	<130 mm Hg	<130 mm Hg
Diastolic blood pressure	<80 mm Hg	<80 mm Hg

Adapted from American Diabetes Association: Standards of medical care in diabetes. Diabetes Care 27:S15–S35, 2004; Joint National Committee on Prevention, Detection, Evaluation, and Treatment of High Blood Pressure, The Seventh Report of the Joint National Committee on Prevention, Detection, Evaluation, and Treatment of High Blood Pressure. JAMA 289:2560–2572, 2003; and Grundy SM, Cleeman JI, Merz CN, et al: Coordinating Committee of the National Cholesterol Education Program. Implications of recent clinical trials for the National Cholesterol Education Program Adult Treatment Panel III Guidelines. J Am Coll Cardiol 44:720–732, 2004.

dyslipidemia) unless there is a contraindication. Adjunctive treatment with clopidogrel should be considered in particularly high-risk subjects and in aspirin-intolerant patients. Aspirin should not be used in those under age 21 years due to increased risk of Reye's syndrome.

More than a half-dozen studies using thiazide diuretics, angiotensin-converting enzyme inhibitors, angiotensin-receptor blockers, β-blockers, and calcium-channel blockers have demonstrated benefits on microvascular end points and combined cardiovascular end points.[80,81] In general, all patients with diabetes and hypertension should be treated with a regimen that includes an angiotensin-converting enzyme inhibitor or an angiotensin-receptor blocker. Most patients will require multiple drug therapy for hypertension in the setting of diabetes to reach the target of less than 130/80 mm Hg. Low-dose thiazide diuretic such as chlorthalidone (25 mg/day) should generally be among the first two drugs for managing hypertension in patients with diabetes; in African-Americans, arguably thiazide diuretics should be the drug of choice for initial therapy. Patients with diabetes and prior myocardial infarction, angina, or congestive heart failure should be treated with a β-blocker as these agents have been shown to reduce the risk of death. Extreme caution is necessary in patients with a history of severe hypoglycemia or hypoglycemic unawareness because of the potential of blocking adrenergic symptoms of hypoglycemia or precipitating severe hypertension as a result of unopposed α-stimulation in the setting of a marked hypoglycemic event. Calcium-channel blockers are among the most effective blood pressure–lowering agents and certainly should be considered as additional therapy in patients treated with angiotensin-converting enzyme inhibitors or angiotensin receptor blockers. Please refer to Chapter 140 for additional reading regarding the management of hypertension.

In patients with type 2 diabetes, triglycerides are often elevated, HDL cholesterol is generally decreased, LDL cholesterol is higher than what is desirable, and LDL particles are often more atherogenic than suspected by their concentration alone because they tend to be smaller, dense, oxidized, and glycated.[82,83] Lowering LDL cholesterol to less than 100 mg/dL is the primary goal of therapy; the Heart Protection study demonstrated that in people with diabetes over age 40 with a total cholesterol greater than 135 mg/dL and one other cardiovascular risk factor or known vascular disease, statin therapy, which produces a 40% reduction in LDL, reduced cardiovascular events independent of baseline LDL.[84] Thus, arguably, in the absence of contraindication, virtually all patients over the age of 40 with diabetes should be treated with moderate-dose statins. Patients at highest risk, particularly those with unstable coronary syndromes, should be treated with high-dose statins. In patients with diabetes, known cardiovascular disease and low HDL (<40 mg/dL), the VA HDL Intervention Trial demonstrated a reduction in combined cardiovascular outcomes associated with gemfibrozil therapy.[85] Thus, consideration of combined statin-fibrate therapy in patients with low HDL may provide for a further reduction in cardiovascular risk as compared to either therapy alone. The combination of fenofibrate and statins may provide a greater margin of safety than combination therapy with gemfibrozil for which rhabdomyolysis is a recognized but rare complication. In limited studies, fish oil has provided for improved cardiovascular outcomes in the setting of clinical cardiovascular disease, and does provide substantial triglyceride lowering, particularly in patients with marked hypertriglyceridemia. Whereas prior recommendations for lipid-lowering therapies suggested that niacin was relatively contraindicated in the setting of diabetes, recent studies have demonstrated minimal changes in glycemia that can generally be managed with modest changes in antidiabetic medications. Niacin therapy has not been evaluated in outcomes studies among patients with diabetes, but seems reasonable to consider, particularly in patients with persistent hypertriglyceridemia (>500 mg/dL) and associated risk of pancreatitis despite statin-fibrate therapy, omega fatty acids, lifestyle efforts, and adequate control of hyperglycemia where the triglyceride lowering effects of pioglitazone, metformin, and insulin are exploited. Refer to Chapter 139 for additional details regarding lipid management.

Cigarette smoking is the strongest risk factor for macrovascular disease in the general population, as well as for patients with diabetes. Smoking history must be ascertained and reviewed regularly. All patients with diabetes should be counseled not to start smoking or to quit if they are smoking. In patients willing to consider stopping smoking, it is appropriate to refer them to formal smoking cessation programs and to give consideration to prescribing nicotine substitutes and/or bupropion HCl.[86]

Comprehensive cardiovascular risk assessment and intervention deserves equal or greater attention to efforts at controlling glycemia in patients with type 2 diabetes. Today, achieving glycemic, lipid, and blood pressure goals is certainly within the grasp of each patient and his health-care team. Unfortunately, most patients do not achieve comprehensive control. When patients understand the goals of therapy and their rationale, they can be a driving force to focus the health-care team to provide strategies that are acceptable to achieve those goals. The epidemic in diabetes and obesity coupled with the predicted early death and disability that follow threatens to overwhelm our health-care system. Practical, systematic approaches to stem this tide are desperately needed.[87]

REFERENCES

1. American Diabetes Association: Standards of medical care in diabetes. Diabetes Care 27:S15–S35, 2004.
2. Engelgau MM, Geiss LS, Saaddine JB, et al: The evolving diabetes burden in the United States. Ann Intern Med 140:945–950, 2004.
3. Wild S, Roglic G, Green A, et al: Global prevalence of diabetes: Estimates for the year 2000 and projections for 2030. Diabetes Care 27:1047–1053, 2004.
4. Narayan KM, Boyle JP, Thompson TJ, et al: Lifetime risk for diabetes mellitus in the United States. JAMA 290:1884–1890, 2003.
5. Bjork S: The cost of diabetes and diabetes care. Diabetes Res

Clin Pract 54(Suppl 1):S13–S18, 2001.

6. Gu K, Cowie CC, Harris MI: Mortality in adults with and without diabetes in a national cohort of the U.S. population, 1971–1993. Diabetes Care 21:1138–1145, 1998.

7. American Diabetes Association: Economic costs of diabetes in the US in 2002. Diabetes Care 26:917–932, 2003.

8. CDC Cost-Effectiveness Group: Cost-effectiveness of intensive glycemic control, intensified hypertension control and serum cholesterol level reduction for type 2 diabetes. JAMA 287:2542–2551, 2002.

9. UK Prospective Diabetes Study (UKPDS) Group: Intensive blood-glucose control with sulphonylureas or insulin compared with conventional treatment and risk of complications in patients with type 2 diabetes (UKPDS 33). Lancet 352:837–853, 1998.

10. UK Prospective Diabetes Study (UKPDS) Group: Effect of intensive blood-glucose control with metformin on complications in overweight patients with type 2 diabetes (UKPDS 34). Lancet 352:854–865, 1998.

11. Ohkubo Y, Kishikawa H, Araki E, et al: Intensive insulin therapy prevents the progression of diabetic microvascular complications in Japanese patients with non-insulin-dependent diabetes mellitus: A randomized prospective 6-year study. Diabetes Res Clin Pract 28:103–117, 1995.

12. Selvin E, Marinopoulos S, Berkenblit G, et al: Meta-analysis: Glycosylated hemoglobin and cardiovascular disease in diabetes mellitus. Ann Intern Med 141:421–431, 2004.

13. Smith NL, Barzilay JI, Shaffer D, et al: Fasting and 2-hour postchallenge serum glucose measures and risk of incident cardiovascular events in the elderly: The Cardiovascular Health Study. Arch Intern Med 162:209–216, 2002.

14. Khaw KT, Wareham N, Bingham S, et al: Association of hemoglobin A1c with cardiovascular disease and mortality in adults: The European prospective investigation into cancer in Norfolk. Ann Intern Med 141:413–420, 2004.

15. Stratton IM, Adler AI, Neil HA, et al: Association of glycaemia with macrovascular and microvascular complications of type 2 diabetes (UKPDS 35): Prospective observational study. Br Med J 321:405–412, 2000.

16. The Expert Committee on the Diagnosis and Classification of Diabetes Mellitus: Follow-up report on the diagnosis of diabetes mellitus. Diabetes Care 26: 3160–3167, 2003.

17. American College of Endocrinologists: American College of Endocrinology consensus statement on guidelines for glycemic control. Endocr Pract 8(Suppl 1):5–11, 2002.

18. Wake Forest University School of Medicine. ACCORD Trial. www.accordtrial.org. Accessed August 8, 2004.

19. Rohlfing CL, Wiedmeyer HM, Little RR, et al: Defining the relationship between plasma glucose and HbA1c: Analysis of glucose profiles and HbA1c in the Diabetes Control and Complications Trial. Diabetes Care 25:275–278, 2002.

20. Klonoff DC, Schwartz DM: An economic analysis of interventions for diabetes. Diabetes Care 23:390–404, 2000.

21. Norris SL, Engelgau MM, Narayan KM: Effectiveness of self-management training in type 2 diabetes: A systematic review of randomized controlled trials. Diabetes Care 24:561–587, 2001.

22. Mensing C, Boucher J, Cypress M, et al: National standards for diabetes self-management education. Diabetes Care 27:S143–S150, 2004.

23. Delamater AM, Jacobson AM, Anderson B, et al: Psychosocial therapies in diabetes: Report of the Psychosocial Therapies Working Group. Diabetes Care 24:1286–1292, 2001.

24. American Diabetes Association: Nutrition principles and recommendations in diabetes. Diabetes Care 27:S36–S46, 2004.

25. American Diabetes Association: Evidence-based nutrition principles and recommendations for the treatment and prevention of diabetes and related complications. Diabetes Care 25:202–212, 2002.

26. Sheard NF, Clark NG, Brand-Miller JC, et al: Dietary carbohydrate (amount and type) in the prevention and management of diabetes: A statement by the American Diabetes Association. Diabetes Care 27:2266–2271, 2004.

27. Klein S, Sheard NF, Pi-Sunyer X, et al: Weight management through lifestyle modification for the prevention and management of type 2 diabetes: Rationale and strategies: A statement of the American Diabetes Association, the North American Association for the Study of Obesity, and the American Society for Clinical Nutrition. Diabetes Care 27:2067–2073, 2004.

28. Gillespie SJ, Kulkarni KD, Daly AE: Using carbohydrate counting in diabetes clinical practice. J Am Diet Assoc 98:897–905, 1998.

29. Egede LE, Ye K, Zhang D, Silverstein MD: The prevalence and pattern of complementary and alternative medicine use in individuals with diabetes. Diabetes Care 25:324–329, 2002.

30. Ernst E: Complementary medicine: Its hidden risks. Diabetes Care 24:1486–1488, 2001.

31. Barringer TA, Kirk JK, Santaniello AC, et al: Effect of a multivitamin and mineral supplement on infection and quality of life. A randomized, double-blind, placebo-controlled trial. Ann Intern Med 138:365–371, 2003.

32. Schnyder G, Roffi M, Pin R, et al: Decreased rate of coronary restenosis after lowering of plasma homocysteine levels. N Engl J Med 345:1593–1600, 2001.

33. Lange H, Suryapranata H, De Luca G, et al: Folate therapy and in-stent restenosis after coronary stenting. N Engl J Med 350:2673–2681, 2004.

34. Ryan DH, Espeland MA, Foster GD, et al: Look AHEAD (Action for Health in Diabetes): Design and methods for a clinical trial of weight loss for the prevention of cardiovascular disease in type 2 diabetes. Control Clin Trials 24:610–628, 2003.

35. Boule NG, Haddad E, Kenny GP, et al: Effects of exercise on glycemic control and body mass in type 2 diabetes mellitus: A meta-analysis of controlled clinical trials. JAMA 286:1218–1227, 2001.

36. Sigal RJ, Kenny GP, Wasserman DH, Castaneda-Sceppa C: Physical activity/exercise and type 2 diabetes. Diabetes Care 27:2518–2539, 2004.

37. Inzucchi SE: Noninvasive assessment of the diabetic patient for coronary artery disease. Diabetes Care 24:1519–1521, 2001.

38. American Diabetes Association: Consensus development conference on the diagnosis of coronary heart disease in people with diabetes: 10-11 February 1998, Miami, Florida. Diabetes Care 21:1551–1559, 1998.

39. Wackers FJ, Young LH, Inzucchi SE, et al: Detection of silent myocardial ischemia in asymptomatic diabetic subjects: The DIAD study. Diabetes Care 27:1954–1961, 2004.

40. Faas A, Schellevis FG, Van Eijk JT: The efficacy of self-monitoring of blood glucose in NIDDM subjects: A criteria-based literature review. Diabetes Care 20:1482–1486, 1997.

41. Guerci B, Drouin P, Grange V, et al: Self-monitoring of blood glucose significantly improves metabolic control in patients with type 2 diabetes mellitus: The Auto-Surveillance Intervention Active (ASIA) study. Diabetes Metab 29:587–594, 2003.

42. Buse JB: Overview of current therapeutic options in type 2 diabetes: Rationale for combining oral agents with insulin therapy. Diabetes Care 22:C65–C70, 1999.

43. DeFronzo RA: Pharmacologic therapy for type 2 diabetes mellitus. Ann Intern Med 133:73–74, 2000.

44. Lebovitz HE: Oral therapies for diabetic hyperglycemia. Endocrinol Metab Clin North Am 30:909–933, 2001.

45. Inzucchi SE: Oral antihyperglycemic therapy for type 2 diabetes: Scientific review. JAMA 287:360–372, 2002.

46. Setter SM, Iltz JL, Thams J, Campbell RK: Metformin hydrochloride in the treatment of type 2 diabetes mellitus: A clinical review with a focus on dual therapy. Clin Ther 25:2991–3026, 2003.

47. Leverve XM, Guigas B, Detaille D, et al: Mitochondrial metabolism and type-2 diabetes: A specific target of metformin. Diabetes Metab 29:6S88–94, 2003.

48. Misbin RI: The phantom of lactic acidosis due to metformin in patients with diabetes. Diabetes Care 27:1791–1793, 2004.

49. Stades AME, Heikens JT, Erkelens DW, et al: Metformin and lactic acidosis: Cause or coincidence? A review of case reports. J Int Med 255:179–187, 2004.

50. Glucophage/Glucophage XR [package insert]. Princeton, NJ, Bristol-Myers Squibb Company, 2003.

51. Wulffele MG, Kooy A, de Zeeuw D, et al: The effect of metformin on blood pressure, plasma cholesterol and triglycerides in type 2 diabetes mellitus: A systematic review. J Intern Med 256:1–14, 2004.

52. Parulkar AA, Pendergrass ML, Granda-Ayala R, et al: Nonhypoglycemic effects of thiazolidinediones. Ann Intern Med 134:61–71, 2001.

53. Mudaliar S, Henry R: New oral therapies for type 2 diabetes mellitus: The glitazones or insulin sensitizers. Annu Rev Med 52:239–257, 2001.

54. Martens FMAC, Visseren FLJ, Lemay J, et al: Metabolic and additional vascular effects of thiazolidinediones. Drugs 62:1463–1480, 2002.

55. Diamant M, Heine RJ: Thiazolidinediones in type 2 diabetes mellitus. Current Clinical Evidence. Drugs 63:1373–1405, 2003.

56. Yki-Jarvinen H: Thiazolidinediones. N Engl J Med 351:1106–1118, 2004.

57. ACTOS (package insert). Takeda Pharmaceuticals America. Lincolnshire, IL, December 2003. Available at *http://www.actos.com/pi.pdf*. Accessed September 12, 2004.

58. Avandia (package insert). GlaxoSmithKline. Research Triangle Park, NC, August 2004. Available at *http://us.gsk.com/products/assets/us_avandia.pdf*. Accessed September 12, 2004.

59. Charbonnel B, Dormandy J, Erdmann E, et al: The Prospective Pioglitazone Clinical Trial in Macrovascular Events (PROactive). Can pioglitazone reduce cardiovascular events in diabetes? Study design and baseline characteristics of 5,238 patients. Diabetes Care 27:1647–1653, 2004.

60. *http://www.cmeondiabetes.com/pub/shifting.the*. Accessed August 8, 2004.

61. Buse JB: Glitazones and heart failure: Critical appraisal for the clinician. Circulation 108:e57, 2003.

62. Nesto RW, Bell D, Bonow RO, et al: Thiazolidinedione use, fluid retention, and congestive heart failure. A consensus statement from the American Heart Association and American Diabetes Association. Circulation 108:2941–2948, 2003.

63. Tang WHW, Francis GS, Hoogwerf BJ, Young JB: Fluid retention after initiation of thiazolidinedione therapy in diabetic patients with established chronic heart failure. J Am Coll Cardiol 41:1394–1398, 2003.

64. Derosa G, Cicero AFG, Gaddi A, et al: Metabolic effects of pioglitazone and rosiglitazone in patients with diabetes and metabolic syndrome treated with glimepiride: A twelve-month, multicenter, double-blind, randomized, controlled, parallel-group trial. Clin Ther 26:744–754, 2004.

65. Riddle MC: Editorial: Sulfonylureas differ in effects on ischemic preconditioning—is it time to retire glyburide? J Clin Endocrinol Metab 88:528–530, 2003.

66. Chiasson JL, Josse RG, Gomis R, et al: Acarbose treatment and the risk of cardiovascular disease and hypertension in patients with impaired glucose tolerance: The STOP-NIDDM trial. JAMA 290:486–494, 2003.

67. Hanefeld M, Chiasson JL, Koehler C, et al: Acarbose slows progression of intima-media thickness of the carotid arteries in subjects with impaired glucose tolerance. Stroke 35:1073–1078, 2004.

68. Heise T, Nosek L, Rønn BB, et al: Lower within-subject variability of insulin detemir in comparison to NPH insulin and insulin glargine in people with type 1 diabetes. Diabetes 53:1614–1620, 2004.

69. Riddle MC, Rosenstock J, Gerich J: Insulin Glargine 4002 Study Investigators: The Treat-to-Target Trial: Randomized addition of glargine or human NPH insulin to oral therapy of type 2 diabetic patients. Diabetes Care 26:3080–3086, 2003.

70. Grant RW, Devita NG, Singer DE, Meigs JB: Polypharmacy and medication adherence in patients with type 2 diabetes. Diabetes Care 26:1408–1412, 2003.

71. Abraira C, Colwell JA, Nuttall FQ, et al: Veterans Affairs Cooperative Study on glycemic control and complications in type II diabetes (VA CSDM). Results of the feasibility trial. Diabetes Care 18:1113–1123, 1995.

72. Malmberg K, Norhammar A, Ryden L: Insulin treatment post myocardial infarction: The DIGAMI study. Adv Exp Med Biol 498:279–284, 2001.

73. van den Berghe G, Wouters P, Weekers F, et al: Intensive insulin therapy in the critically ill patients. N Engl J Med 345:1359–1367, 2001.

74. Moller DE: New drug targets for type 2 diabetes and the metabolic syndrome. Nature 414:821–827, 2001.

75. Cefalu WT: Evolving strategies for insulin delivery and therapy. Drugs 64:1149–1161, 2004.

76. Ratner RE, Want LL, Fineman MS, et al: Adjunctive therapy with the amylin analogue pramlintide leads to a combined improvement in glycemic and weight control in insulin-treated subjects with type 2 diabetes. Diabetes Technol Ther 4:51–61, 2002.

77. Hollander PA, Levy P, Fineman MS, et al: Pramlintide as an adjunct to insulin therapy improves long-term glycemic and weight control in patients with type 2 diabetes: A 1-year randomized controlled trial. Diabetes Care 26:784–790, 2003.

78. Deacon CF: Therapeutic strategies based on glucagon-like peptide 1. Diabetes 53:2181–2189, 2004.

79. Fineman MS, Bicsak TA, Shen LZ, et al: Effect on glycemic control of exenatide (synthetic exendin-4) additive to existing metformin and/or sulfonylurea treatment in patients with type 2 diabetes. Diabetes Care 26:2370–2377, 2003.

80. American Diabetes Association. Hypertension management in adults with diabetes. Diabetes Care 27:S65–S67, 2004.

81. Joint National Committee on Prevention, Detection, Evaluation, and Treatment of High Blood Pressure, The Seventh Report of the Joint National Committee on Prevention, Detection, Evaluation, and Treatment of High Blood Pressure. JAMA 289:2560–2572, 2003.

82. Grundy SM, Cleeman JI, Merz CN, et al: Coordinating Committee of the National Cholesterol Education Program. Implications of recent clinical trials for the National Cholesterol Education Program Adult Treatment Panel III Guidelines. J Am Coll Cardiol 44:720–732, 2004.

83. American Diabetes Association: Dyslipidemia management in adults with diabetes. Diabetes Care 27:S68–S71, 2004.

84. Collins R, Armitage J, Parish S, et al: MRC/BHF Heart Protection Study of cholesterol-lowering with simvastatin in 5963 people with diabetes: A randomised placebo-controlled trial. Lancet 361:2005–2016, 2003.

85. Rubins HB, Robins SJ, Collins D, et al: Diabetes, plasma insulin, and cardiovascular disease: Subgroup analysis from the Department of Veterans Affairs High-Density Lipoprotein Intervention Trial (VA-HIT). Arch Int Med 162:2597–2604, 2002.

86. Haire-Joshu D, Glasgow RE, Tibbs TL: Smoking and diabetes (Technical Review). Diabetes Care 22:1887–1898, 1999.

87. Narayan KM, Gregg EW, Engelgau MM, et al. Translation research for chronic disease: The case of diabetes. Diabetes Care 23:1794–1798, 2000.

Management of Diabetes in Children

Joseph I. Wolfsdorf and David A. Weinstein

PRESENTATION AND INITIAL MANAGEMENT OF NEWLY DIAGNOSED DIABETES MELLITUS

Most children with newly diagnosed type 1 diabetes mellitus (T1DM) present with classic symptoms for a few days to several weeks. The frequency of diabetic ketoacidosis (DKA) at diabetes onset varies widely by geographic location, ranging from 15% to 67% in Europe and North America, and is probably even more common in developing countries.[1,2] DKA at initial presentation is more frequent in infants, toddlers, and preschool-age children (up to two thirds of toddlers present with DKA), children who do not have a first degree relative with T1DM, and children whose families are of lower socioeconomic status.[3,4]

Whenever possible, the child with DKA should be cared for in a facility that has nursing staff who are trained in DKA management and access to a clinical chemistry laboratory that can provide frequent and timely measurement of serum chemistries. Children with signs of severe DKA (long duration of symptoms, compromised circulation, depressed level of consciousness) and those who are at increased risk for cerebral edema (younger than 5 years of age, new-onset diabetes) should be treated in a pediatric intensive care unit or in a children's ward that specializes in diabetes care and can provide equivalent resources and supervision of care.[5]

The goals of initial management of the child with newly diagnosed diabetes mellitus depend on the clinical presentation and are (1) to restore fluid and electrolyte balance, (2) to stabilize the metabolic state with insulin, and (3) to provide basic diabetes education and self-care training for the child (when age and developmentally appropriate) and other caregivers (parents, grandparents, older siblings, daycare providers, and babysitters).

The diagnosis of diabetes in a child is a crisis for the family, who require considerable emotional support and time for adjustment and healing. Shocked, grieving, and overwhelmed parents typically require at least two to three days to acquire basic or "survival" skills while they are coping with the emotional upheaval that typically follows the diagnosis of diabetes in a child. Even if they are not acutely ill, children with newly diagnosed T1DM usually are admitted to the hospital for metabolic stabilization, diabetes education, and self-management training. However, outpatient or home-based management has been preferred at some centers that have the appropriate resources.[6,7] Outpatient education and stabilization offer several advantages: The stress of a hospital stay can be avoided, the outpatient setting or patient's home is a more natural learning environment for the child and family, and ambulatory treatment possibly reduces the cost of care for the healthcare system and the family. The sparse literature comparing initial hospitalization with home-based and/or outpatient management of children who are not acutely ill with newly diagnosed T1DM has recently been reviewed, and the results are inconclusive.[8] However, the data seem to suggest that outpatient and/or home initial management of T1DM in children does not lead to any disadvantages in terms of metabolic control, acute complications, hospitalizations, or psychosocial or behavioral variables. The decision concerning whether or not a child with newly diagnosed diabetes should be admitted to the hospital depends on several factors. Of these, the most important are the severity of the child's metabolic derangements, a psychosocial assessment of the family, and the resources available at the treatment center. Outpatient management in a comprehensive day-treatment center staffed by a multidisciplinary diabetes team is an appropriate alternative to hospitalization for many newly diagnosed children.

OUTPATIENT DIABETES CARE

THE DIABETES TEAM

Optimal care of children with T1DM is complex and time consuming. Few general practitioners or pediatricians have the resources and expertise, nor can they devote the time required to provide all of the components of an optimal treatment program for children with diabetes. Children with diabetes should be managed by a multidisciplinary diabetes team that provides diabetes education and care in collaboration with the child's primary care physician.[9,10] The team should consist of a pediatric endocrinologist or pediatrician with training in diabetes, a pediatric diabetes nurse educator, a dietitian, and a mental health professional, either a clinical psychologist or a social worker. A member of the diabetes team should always be available by telephone to respond to metabolic crises that require immediate intervention and to provide guidance and support to parents and patients.[11-14]

INITIAL DIABETES EDUCATION

The diabetes education curriculum should be adapted to the individual child and family.[15] Parents and children with newly diagnosed diabetes are anxious and overwhelmed and cannot assimilate a large amount of abstract information. Therefore, the education program should be staged. Initial educational goals should be limited to essential "survival" skills so that the child can be safely cared for at home and return to his or her daily routine. Initial diabetes education and self-management training should include understanding what causes diabetes, how it is treated, how to administer insulin, basic meal planning, self-monitoring of blood glucose and ketones, recognition and treatment of hypoglycemia, and how and when to contact a member of the diabetes team if blood glucose values are outside the target range and for general advice.

CONTINUING DIABETES EDUCATION AND LONG-TERM SUPERVISION OF DIABETES CARE

When the child is medically stable and parents (and other care providers) have mastered survival skills, the child is discharged from the hospital or ambulatory treatment center. In the first few weeks after diagnosis, frequent telephone contact provides emotional support and helps parents to interpret the results of blood glucose monitoring. If necessary, insulin doses are adjusted. Within a few weeks of diagnosis, many children enter a partial remission, evidenced by normal or near-normal blood glucose levels on a low dose (<0.25 U/kg/day) of insulin, patients and parents are less anxious and have mastered basic diabetes management skills through experience and repetition. They are now ready to begin to learn the intricate details of intensive diabetes management. At this stage, the diabetes team should begin to provide patients and parents with the knowledge and skills they need to maintain optimal glycemic control while coping with the challenges imposed by exercise, fickle appetite and varying food intake, intercurrent illnesses, and the other variations that normally occur in a child's daily life. In addition to

teaching facts and practical skills, the education program should promote desirable health beliefs and attitudes in the young person who has a chronic incurable disease. For some children, this may be best accomplished in a nontraditional educational setting such as summer camp for children with diabetes. The educational curriculum must be concordant with the child's level of cognitive development and has to be adapted to the learning style and intellectual ability of the individual child and family. Parents, grandparents, older siblings, the school nurse, and other important people in the child's life are encouraged to participate in the diabetes education program so that they can share in the diabetes care and help the child to live a normal life.

In the first month after diagnosis, the patient is seen frequently by the diabetes team to review and consolidate the diabetes education and practical skills that are learned in the first few days and to extend the scope of diabetes self-care training. Thereafter, follow-up visits with members of the diabetes team should occur at least every 3 months. Regular clinic visits are to ensure that the child's diabetes is being appropriately managed at home and that the goals of therapy are being met. A focused history should obtain information about self-care behaviors; the child's daily routines; the frequency, severity, and circumstances surrounding hypoglycemic events; and blood glucose monitoring data should be reviewed. At each visit, height and weight are measured and plotted on a growth chart. The weight curve is especially helpful in assessing adequacy of therapy. Significant weight loss usually indicates that the prescribed dose is insufficient or that the patient is not receiving all the prescribed doses of insulin. A complete physical examination should be performed at least twice per year, focusing on blood pressure, stage of puberty, evidence of thyroid disease, and examination of the injection sites for evidence of lipohypertrophy resulting from overuse of the site.

Regular clinic visits also provide an opportunity to review, reinforce, and expand on the diabetes self-care training that was begun at the time of diagnosis. The goal at each visit is to reinforce the goals of treatment while increasing the patient's and family's understanding of diabetes management, the interplay of insulin, food, and exercise, and their impact on blood glucose levels. As the child's cognitive development progresses, she or he should become more involved in diabetes management and should assume increasing age-appropriate responsibility for daily self-care. Parents are encouraged to call for advice if the pattern of blood glucose levels changes between routine visits, suggesting the need to adjust the insulin dose or change the regimen. Eventually, when parents and patients have sufficient knowledge and experience, they are encouraged to adjust the insulin dose(s) independently.

PSYCHOSOCIAL ISSUES

A medical social worker should perform an initial psychosocial assessment of all newly diagnosed patients to identify high-risk families who need additional services. Thereafter, patients are referred to the mental health specialist when emotional, social, environmental, or financial concerns are suspected or identified that interfere with the ability to maintain acceptable diabetes control. Some of the more common problems in families that have a child with diabetes include parental guilt, resulting in poor adherence to the treatment regimen, difficulty coping with the child's rebellion against treatment, anxiety, depression, fear of hypoglycemia, missed appointments, financial hardship, and loss of health insurance affecting the ability to attend scheduled clinic appointments and/or purchase supplies. Recurrent ketoacidosis is the most extreme indicator of psychosocial stress, and management of such patients is incomplete without a comprehensive psychosocial assessment.

GOALS OF THERAPY

The Diabetes Control and Complications Trial (DCCT)[16,17] and a similar, smaller study in Sweden, the Stockholm Diabetes Intervention Study,[18] ended the debate about whether the microvascular complications of diabetes are caused by hyperglycemia and can be prevented or ameliorated. Additional scientific evidence for the importance of glycemic control was provided by the U.K. Prospective Diabetes Study in adults with type 2 diabetes.[19,20] These clinical trials unequivocally demonstrate the importance of lowering glycated hemoglobin (HbA1c) values to reduce the risk of development and progression of retinopathy, nephropathy, and neuropathy. Treatment regimens that reduce average HbA1c to ~7% (about 1% above the upper limit of normal) are associated with fewer long-term microvascular complications. Moreover, improved glycemic control is associated with a sustained decreased rate of development of diabetic complications.[21,22]

Modern diabetes management attempts to achieve recommended glycemic targets that are known to reduce the risk of long-term complications. The American Diabetes Association has recommended treatment goals for adolescents 13 years of age and older and for adults with diabetes mellitus: HbA1c less than 7% (nondiabetic range 4% to 6%), 90 to 130 mg/dL preprandial plasma glucose, and peak postprandial plasma glucose lower than 180 mg/dL. Since there are no clinical trial data available for children younger than 13 years of age, clinical judgment is required to determine appropriate goals for children of various ages.[23]

Management of young children with diabetes, especially those younger than 5 years old, must balance opposing risks of hypoglycemia (see section on hypoglycemia below) and future vascular complications.[24] The relative contribution of the prepubertal years to the development of microvascular complications has been uncertain. It was commonly believed that prepubertal children were protected from the adverse effects of hyperglycemia on the microvasculature, and it was suggested that the contribution of the prepubertal years of diabetes to long-term prognosis may be minimal.[25] Recent evidence, however, indicates that longer prepubertal duration increases the risk of retinopathy and, possibly, microalbuminuria in adolescence and young adulthood but at a slower rate than in the postpubertal years.[26–31]

Biochemical goals of treatment for children and adolescents were included in the consensus guidelines of the International Society for Pediatric and Adolescent Diabetes (ISPAD): ideal: <6.05%, optimal: <7.5%, suboptimal: 7.6% to 9.0%, and action is required when the value exceeds 9.0%.[32] The ISPAD guidelines are accompanied by the following statement: "for each individual the target should be the lowest achievable HbA1c without the occurrence of frequent or severe hypoglycemia."

The risk for microalbuminuria increases steeply with HbA1c greater than 8%.[33,34] On the basis of these considerations, an HbA1c of 8.0% or lower is a reasonable general goal for children with diabetes; however, because of the concern about hypoglycemia in preschool-age children, we recommend stratifying the biochemical goals on the basis of age (Table 64-1). Biochemical goals should be individualized, taking into account both medical and psychosocial considerations. The

above targets are ideal and should be vigorously pursued, provided that the child does not experience recurrent or severe hypoglycemia. Less stringent treatment goals are appropriate for preschool-age children; children with developmental handicaps, psychosocial problems, or lack of appropriate family support; children who have experienced severe hypoglycemia; and children with hypoglycemia unawareness.

Studies performed in the post-DCCT era show that metabolic control of T1DM in children and adolescents, in general, continues to be unsatisfactory. For example, the mean HbA1c of 2873 children from 22 pediatric diabetes centers in 18 countries was 8.6 ± 1.7 (SD)% (equivalent to a mean of 8.3% using the DCCT method)[35] and did not change significantly when reexamined 3 years later, despite significant increases in insulin dose and number of daily insulin injections.[36] Mean HbA1c in a nationwide cross-sectional study of 2579 French children with T1DM was 8.97 ± 1.98 (SD)%, of whom 33% had an HbA1c of 8% or less.[37]

INSULIN THERAPY

Within days to months of diagnosis, most children with T1DM are severely insulin deficient and depend on insulin replacement for survival. The aim of insulin replacement therapy is to simulate as closely as possible the normal variations in plasma insulin levels that occur in nondiabetic individuals. Truly physiologic replacement of insulin remains an elusive goal. In children with severe insulin deficiency, practical considerations, including supervision of care, ability and willingness to self-administer insulin several times each day, and difficulty maintaining long-term adherence, make physiologic replacement of insulin challenging. There is no universal insulin regimen that can be used for all children with T1DM. The diabetes team has to design an insulin regimen that meets the needs of the individual patient and is acceptable to the patient and to the family member(s) who might be responsible for administering insulin to the child or supervising its administration.

The initial route of insulin administration is determined by the severity of the child's condition at presentation. Insulin is preferably given intravenously for treatment of DKA. Children who are metabolically stable without vomiting or significant ketosis may be started with subcutaneous (SC) insulin administration. SC insulin treatment in the newly diagnosed child who has recently recovered from DKA usually is started with either a two or three injection per day regimen consisting of a mixture of human intermediate-acting and rapid- or short-acting insulin (Table 64-2). Some clinicians start basal-bolus insulin therapy (see the section on intensified insulin therapy below) at the time of diagnosis, regardless of the severity of presentation or age of the child.

In addition to severity of metabolic decompensation, the child's age, weight, and pubertal status guide the initial insulin dose selection. When diabetes has been diagnosed early, before significant metabolic decompensation, 0.25 to 0.5 unit/kg/day usually is an adequate starting dose. When metabolic decompensation is more severe (e.g., ketonuria without acidosis or dehydration), the initial dose typically is at least 0.5 unit/kg/day. After recovery from DKA, prepubertal children usually require at least 0.75 unit/kg/day, whereas adolescents require at least 1 unit/kg/day. In the first few days of insulin therapy, while the focus of care is on diabetes education and emotional support, it is reasonable to aim for premeal blood glucose levels in the range of 80 to 200 mg/dL and to supplement, if necessary, with 0.05 to 0.1 unit/kg of rapid-acting insulin SC at 3- to 4-hour intervals.

Three major categories of insulin preparations, classified according to time course of action, are available (Table 64-3). Various insulin replacement regimens consisting of a mixture of short- or rapid-acting insulin and an intermediate- or

Table 64-1 Biochemical Goals of Treatment According to Age		
Age (years)	Premeal Vlood Glucose (mg/dL)	HbA1c (%)
<5	100 to 200	≤9.0
5 to 12	70 to 180	≤8.0
≥13	70 to 150	≤7.0

Table 64-2 Insulin Regimens Used to Treat Children and Adolescents

Doses	Breakfast	Lunch	Dinner	Bedtime
Two	S/R + N/L*		S/R + N/L	
	S/R + N/L		S/R + N/L	
	S/R + UL		S/R + UL	
Three	S/R + N/L		S/R	S/R + N/L
	S/R + N/L	S/R	S/R + N/L	
	S/R + N/L	S/R	S/R + UL	
	S/R+ UL	S/R	S/R+ UL	
	S/R + N/L		S/R	Glarg†
Four	S/R	S/R	S/R	S/R + N/L
	S/R + N/L	S/R	S/R	S/R + N/L
	S/R	S/R	S/R	S/R + Glarg
	S/R + Glarg	S/R	S/R	S/R
	S/R	S/R	S/R + Glarg	S/R
CSII‡	S/R	S/R	S/R	S/R

Abbreviations: S, short-acting insulin (insulin lispro or insulin aspart); R, regular (soluble) insulin; N, neutral protamine Hagedorn (isophane); L, lente (insulin zinc suspension); UL, ultralente (extended insulin zinc suspension); Glarg, insulin glargine.
*Premixed combinations, such as either 70% NPH and 30% regular, 70% NPA and 30% insulin aspart, or 75% NPL and 25% insulin lispro, are usually used in twice-daily fixed-dose insulin regimens.
†Insulin glargine is always given as a separate injection and cannot be mixed with any other insulin
‡CSII, continuous subcutaneous insulin infusion (pump), boluses are given with meals and snacks together with basal insulin throughout the day and night.
Intensified insulin therapy is defined as use of at least three daily doses of insulin or CSII.

Table 64-3 Insulin Preparations Classified According to Their Pharmacodynamic Profiles

	Onset of Action (h)	Peak Action (h)	Duration of Action (h)
RAPID-ACTING			
Insulin lispro*	0.25 to 0.5	0.5 to 2.5	≤5
Insulin aspart*	<0.25	1 to 3	3 to 5
SHORT-ACTING			
Regular (soluble)	0.5 to 1	2 to 4	5 to 8
INTERMEDIATE-ACTING			
NPH (isophane)	1 to 2	2 to 8	14 to 24
Lente (insulin zinc suspension)	1 to 2	3 to 10	20 to 24
LONG-ACTING			
Ultralente	0.5 to 3	4 to 20	20 to 36
Insulin glargine*	2 to 4	peakless	20 to 24
PREMIXED COMBINATIONS			
50% NPH, 50% regular	0.5 to 1	dual	14 to 24
70% NPH, 30% regular	0.5 to 1	dual	14 to 24
70% NPA, 30% aspart*	<0.25	dual	14 to 24
75% NPL, 25% lispro*	<0.25	dual	14 to 24

Abbreviations; NPA, neutral protamine aspart; NPL, neutral protamine lispro. Both NPA and NPL are stable premixed combinations of intermediate- and short-acting insulins.
*Insulin analogue developed by modifying the amino acid sequence of the human insulin molecule. Data are from the manufacturers.
Pharmacodynamic effects of insulin lispro and insulin aspart appear to be equivalent.[208] Most of the human insulins and insulin analogues are available in insulin cartridges and/or disposable insulin pens.
These data are for human insulins and are approximations from studies in adult test subjects. Time-action profiles are reasonable estimates only. The times of onset, peak, and duration of action vary within and between patients and are affected by numerous factors, including size of dose, site and depth of injection, dilution, exercise, temperature, and other factors.

long-acting insulin are used in children and adolescents (see Table 64-2), typically given two to four (or more) times daily (see Table 64-2, Fig. 64-1). Clear superiority of any one regimen in children and adolescents, in terms of metabolic outcomes, has not been demonstrated.[38] All insulin regimens have the same general goal: to provide basal insulin throughout the day and night and more insulin with meals and snacks. When a two-dose regimen is used, the total daily dose is typically divided so that about two thirds is given before breakfast and one third is given in the evening. With a three-dose regimen, short- or rapid-acting insulin is administered before supper, and the second dose of intermediate-acting insulin is given at bedtime rather than before the evening meal. The initial ratio of rapid- to intermediate-acting insulin at both times is approximately 1:2. Toddlers and young children typically require a smaller fraction of short- or rapid-acting insulin (10% to 20% of the total dose) and proportionately more intermediate-acting insulin. Regular insulin is given at least 30 minutes before eating; rapid-acting insulin (lispro insulin, insulin aspart) is given 5 to 15 minutes before eating. In toddlers and young children with unpredictable eating habits, rapid-acting insulin may be given immediately after the meal (dose based on estimated actual carbohydrate consumed).

The optimal ratio of rapid- or short-acting to intermediate-acting insulin for each patient is determined empirically

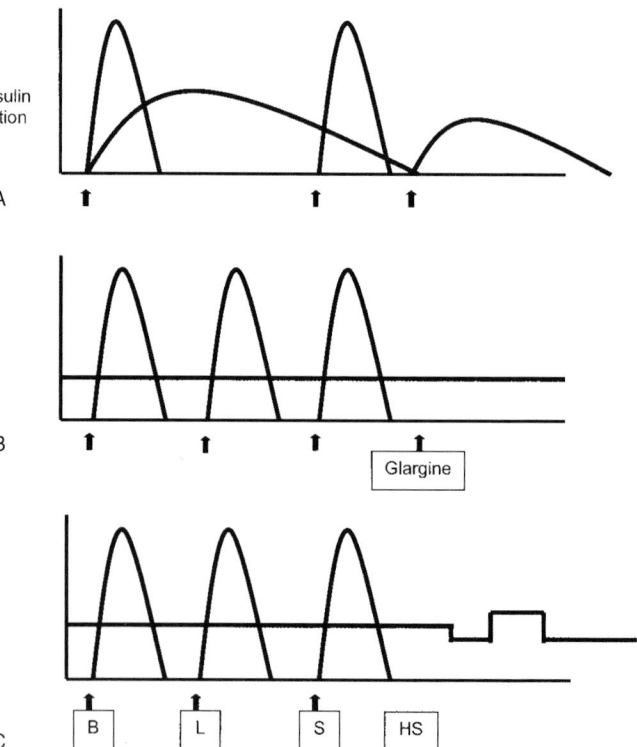

Figure 64-1 Insulin regimens. **A,** Schematic representation of idealized insulin action provided by a regimen consisting of a mixture of rapid-acting insulin (lispro or aspart) and intermediate-acting insulin (NPH or lente) before breakfast, rapid-acting insulin (lispro or aspart) before supper, and intermediate-acting insulin (NPH or lente) at bedtime. **B,** Schematic representation of idealized insulin action provided by an insulin regimen consisting of four daily injections: rapid-acting insulin (lispro or aspart) before each meal (B, L, S) and a separate injection of insulin glargine, either at bedtime (as shown here) or at dinner or breakfast. **C,** Schematic representation of idealized insulin effect provided by continuous subcutaneous insulin infusion via an insulin pump with insulin aspart or lispro. In this figure, alternative basal rates are illustrated; insulin delivery is shown to decrease from midnight to 3:00 A.M. and to increase before breakfast. B, breakfast; L, lunch; S, supper; HS, bedtime. *Arrows* indicate times of insulin injection or boluses before meals

guided by the results of frequent blood glucose measurements. At least five daily measurements are initially required to determine the effects of each component of the insulin regimen. Blood glucose concentrations are measured before each meal, before the bedtime snack, and between midnight and 4:00 A.M. Parents are taught to look for patterns of hyperglycemia or hypoglycemia that indicate the need for an adjustment in the dose. Adjustments are made to individual components of the insulin regimen, usually in 5% to 10% increments or decrements, in response to patterns of consistently elevated (above the target range for several consecutive days) or unexplained low blood glucose levels, respectively. This is referred to as pattern adjustment. The insulin dose is adjusted until satisfactory blood glucose control is achieved, with most blood glucose values in or close to the individual child's target range.

At the time of diagnosis, most children have some residual β cells and enter a period of partial remission (honeymoon phase), during which normal or nearly normal glycemic control is relatively easily achieved with a low dose of insulin. At this stage, the dose of insulin should be reduced to prevent hypoglycemia but should not be discontinued. After destruction of the remaining β cells has occurred, the insulin dose increases (intensification phase) until the full replacement dose is reached. The average daily insulin dose in prepubertal children with long-standing diabetes is approximately 0.8 unit/kg/day, and that in adolescents is about 1 to 1.5 unit/kg/day.

TECHNICAL DETAILS OF INSULIN THERAPY IN YOUNG CHILDREN

Caring for young children with diabetes is challenging for many reasons, one of which is the need to accurately and reproducibly measure and inject tiny doses of insulin that is supplied in a concentration of 100 units/mL. To administer a dose of 1 unit requires the ability to accurately measure 10 µL (1/100 mL) of insulin. When the dose is less than 2 U of U100 insulin, neither parents of diabetic children nor skilled pediatric nurses are able to measure the dose accurately.[39] Furthermore, a dose change of 0.25 U translates into a volume difference of 2.5 µL in a 300-µL (3/10-mL or 30-unit) syringe. When parents attempt to measure insulin doses in increments of 0.25 U of insulin (e.g., 3.0, 3.25, and 3.5 U) using a standard commercial 30-unit (300-µL) syringe, they consistently measure more than the prescribed amount.[40] Therefore, to enhance accuracy and reproducibility of small doses, insulin should be diluted to U 10 (10 Units/mL) with the specific diluent that is available from the insulin manufacturers. Using U 10 insulin, each line ("unit") on a syringe is actually 0.1 U of insulin.

To avoid intramuscular injections in infants and young children with little subcutaneous fat, syringes with 30-gauge 8-mm (short) needles or insulin pens with 31-gauge 5-mm needles should be used to administer insulin. Short needles are also desirable for use in older thin children.

INTENSIFIED INSULIN THERAPY IN CHILDREN

There is little evidence to guide clinical decisions concerning the risk-benefit ratio of strict control in the preadolescent patient. Clinical trials comparable to the DCCT have not been conducted in prepubertal children. Nevertheless, it is reasonable to extrapolate that prepubertal children will also benefit from strict control of their diabetes.

Beyond the remission period, it is not generally possible to achieve near-normal glycemia with two injections per day. A major problem of the two-dose "split and mixed" regimen is that the peak effect of the predinner intermediate-acting insulin tends to occur at the time of lowest insulin requirement (midnight to 4:00 A.M.), increasing the risk of nocturnal

hypoglycemia. Thereafter, insulin action declines from 4:00 A.M. to 8:00 A.M., when basal insulin requirements normally increase. Consequently, the tendency for blood glucose levels to rise before breakfast (dawn phenomenon) may be aggravated by waning insulin effect in the period before breakfast and/or by counterregulatory hormones secreted in response to a fall in blood glucose levels during sleep: posthypoglycemic hyperglycemia (Somogyi phenomenon). A three-dose insulin regimen with mixed short- or rapid- and intermediate-acting insulins before breakfast, only short- or rapid-acting insulin before dinner, and intermediate-acting insulin at bedtime may ameliorate these problems.[41] Insulin therapy with at least three injections each day or with continuous subcutaneous insulin infusion (CSII) using a portable insulin pump can more closely simulate normal diurnal insulin profiles and overcome some of the limitations inherent in a two-dose regimen. A peakless long-acting insulin, insulin glargine, can be used to provide basal insulin and is used together with short- or rapid-acting insulin injected before each meal (basal-bolus regimen). Insulin glargine is an insulin analogue, produced by recombinant DNA technology, with a duration of action of approximately 24 hours. It has little peak activity and is administered once daily, usually, but not invariably, at bedtime. Insulin glargine has been used safely in children and adolescents[42] and, because it does not have the peak of activity characteristic of NPH, lente, and ultralente insulins,[43] can reduce nocturnal hypoglycemic episodes without jeopardizing glycemic control.[44,45]

Owing to physiologic peripheral insulin resistance of puberty,[46] adolescents require large doses of rapid- or short-acting insulin to control postprandial blood glucose excursions. However, a large increase in the dose of regular insulin markedly delays its peak effect (to 3 to 4 hours) and prolongs its total duration of action to 6 to 8 hours. Puberty does not cause hepatic insulin resistance; therefore, hyperinsulinemia suppresses hepatic glucose production for several hours and increases the risk of postprandial hypoglycemia, especially at night between 10:00 P.M. and 2:00 A.M.[47] This is an important reason to recommend use of rapid-acting insulin analogues (insulin lispro or insulin aspart) in preference to regular (soluble) insulin in treating adolescents, most especially before the evening meal.

In 1996, fewer than 5% of patients starting pump therapy were younger than 20 years of age. Over the past several years, there has been a worldwide marked increase in the number of children and adolescents using CSII (pump) therapy. An insulin pump has one unique advantage over insulin injections: the ability to program changes in basal dosage to meet an anticipated increase or decrease in need. This feature can be advantageous in combating the dawn phenomenon or preventing hypoglycemia during or after exercise. In addition to programming various basal rates, the use of dual-wave and square-wave bolus delivery significantly lowers 4-hour postprandial blood glucose levels.[48] A meta-analysis of randomized controlled clinical trials concluded that CSII resulted in a small (~0.5%) improvement in HbA1c.[49]

Although an insulin pump is a complex and sophisticated medical device that requires extensive training in its use, with appropriate education and training and with support from parents and a school nurse, many children can manage the added responsibility of using an insulin pump and benefit from its advantages.[50] Only short- or rapid-acting insulin is used with CSII; therefore, any interruption in the delivery of insulin rapidly leads to metabolic decompensation. To reduce this risk, meticulous care must be devoted to the infusion system, and blood glucose levels must be measured frequently. Increased lifestyle flexibility, reduced blood glucose variability, improved glycemic control, and reduced frequency of severe hypoglycemia are all documented advantages of CSII.[51] The diabetes team should attempt to select patients who are most likely to benefit from CSII. Success requires motivation to achieve normal blood glucose levels, frequent blood glucose monitoring, record keeping, carbohydrate counting, and frequent contact with the diabetes team. Patients must understand that to be successful, CSII therapy requires more time, effort, and active involvement in diabetes care by patients and parents and considerable education and support from the diabetes team. The individual who is unable to master a multiple-dose injection regimen is not likely to be successful with CSII. Despite concerns that it might have adverse psychosocial consequences owing to the added burden of treatment, especially in adolescents, the opposite effect has been observed. Short-term studies have shown that more aggressive and successful management of their diabetes by teenagers can be accompanied by enhanced psychosocial well-being.[52] In teenagers, CSII offers a treatment option that can lead to improved control and lower the risk of severe hypoglycemia.[53]

Technologic innovations have provided patients with insulin preparations whose pharmacokinetic properties make it possible to crudely simulate physiologic insulin kinetics. It is now possible for children to safely achieve unprecedented levels of glycemic control without excessive severe hypoglycemia. The diabetes care provider should frankly discuss treatment options with parents and child and explain the advantages and disadvantages of each in attempting to meet the overall goals of treatment. The most suitable regimen for a given child and family should be determined by mutual consent and not by coercion.

MEDICAL NUTRITION THERAPY

Meal planning continues to be a cornerstone of the management of all types of diabetes mellitus, and nutrition education is an essential component of a comprehensive program of diabetes education for patients and their families.[54] There is no "diabetic diet." Medical nutrition therapy (MNT) should be individualized, with consideration given to the patient's usual eating habits and other lifestyle factors. Monitoring clinical and metabolic parameters including blood glucose, HbA1c, lipids, blood pressure, and body weight, as well as quality of life, is crucial to ensure successful outcomes. Modern diabetes management, combining frequent self-monitoring of blood glucose with intensive insulin therapy and mastery of carbohydrate counting, enables children and adolescents to have considerable dietary flexibility while maintaining near-normal glycemic control (Table 64-4).

There is no evidence that the nutritional needs of children with diabetes differ from those of otherwise healthy children. Therefore, nutrient recommendations are based on the requirements of healthy children and adolescents. The total intake of energy must be sufficient to balance the daily expenditure of energy and has to be adjusted periodically to achieve an ideal body weight and to maintain a normal rate of physical growth and maturation. The DCCT demonstrated that intensive management of T1DM is associated with a tendency to gain weight,[55] primarily attributable to reduced glucosuria and, secondarily, to reduction in daily energy expenditure.[56] Recurrent symptomatic hypoglycemia requiring consumption of rapidly absorbed carbohydrate to restore normoglycemia also contributes to the tendency to gain weight in some intensively treated patients. The objective of MNT for patients with type 2 diabetes, most of whom are obese, is to lose weight and then maintain a desirable weight without compromising statural growth and to achieve target blood glucose and HbA1c goals.[57]

CARBOHYDRATE

Sixty percent to 70% of total energy should be from carbohydrate and monounsaturated fat.[58] Dietary dogma had been to avoid simple sugars and replace them with complex carbohy-

Table 64-4 The Goals of Medical Nutrition Therapy of Children and Adolescents

To provide adequate macronutrients and micronutrients to ensure normal growth and physical development.

To integrate insulin regimens into usual eating and physical activity habits.

For youth with type 2 diabetes, to facilitate changes in eating and physical activity habits that reduce insulin resistance, improve metabolic status, and gradually achieve a more desirable weight for height.

To provide self-management education for prevention and treatment of hypoglycemia, acute illness, and exercise-related blood glucose perturbations.

To attain and maintain optimal metabolic outcomes, including near-normal blood glucose levels without excessive hypoglycemia and a lipid and lipoprotein profile that reduces the risk for macrovascular disease.

To prevent and treat the chronic complications of diabetes and modify nutrient intake and lifestyle as appropriate for prevention and treatment of obesity, dyslipidemia, hypertension, and nephropathy.

To improve general health through healthful food choices and physical activity.

To address individual nutritional needs taking into consideration personal and cultural preferences and lifestyle while respecting the individual's wishes and willingness to change.

drates. This belief was based on the assumption that simple sugars are more rapidly digested and absorbed than starches are and would aggravate hyperglycemia to a greater degree. The glycemic index (GI), proposed in 1981 as an alternative system for classifying carbohydrate-containing foods, measures the glycemic response after ingestion of carbohydrate. GI is defined as the incremental area under the plasma glucose response curve after consumption of a standard amount of carbohydrate from a test food relative to that of a control food, either white bread or glucose.[59] The glycemic and hormonal responses to a large number of carbohydrates have been systematically examined, and their GIs have been defined. There is a wide spectrum of biologic responses to different complex and simple carbohydrates, with so much overlap that they cannot be simply classified into two distinct groups. Even a single food produces a substantially different glycemic response when prepared in different ways. The form of a carbohydrate-containing food, in addition to its chemical composition, influences postprandial glycemia by altering its rate of digestion and absorption. Fruits and milk cause a lower glycemic response than most starches, and sucrose causes a glycemic response similar to that of bread, rice, and potatoes. In general, most refined starchy foods eaten in the United States have a high GI, whereas nonstarchy vegetables, fruits, and legumes tend to have a low GI.

The usefulness of low-GI diets in individuals with T1DM continues to be controversial,[60] and studies in children are extremely limited.[61] The literature demonstrates only modest long-term beneficial effects of low-GI diets on glycemia and lipid concentrations, and at the present time, data are lacking concerning the long-term benefits of low-GI diets in the management of diabetes in children.

The glycemic load of meals and snacks is more important than the source or type of carbohydrate. The glycemic load, defined as the weighted average of the GI of individual foods multiplied by the percentage of dietary energy as carbohydrate, has been proposed as a method to characterize the impact of foods and dietary patterns with different macronutrient composition on glycemic responses. For example, a carrot has a high GI but a low glycemic load, whereas a potato has both a high GI and a high glycemic load. Individuals who use intensive insulin therapy select their premeal insulin doses on the basis of the carbohydrate content of their meals, whereas individuals who receive fixed daily insulin dosages should attempt to maintain day-to-day consistency with respect to the carbohydrate content of their meals and snacks. Although the use of low-GI foods may reduce postprandial glycemia and may have long-term benefit on HbA1c levels, emphasis should be on the total amount of carbohydrate consumed, and its source should be a secondary consideration.[62]

Sucrose as part of the meal plan does not adversely affect blood glucose control in individuals with either T1 or type 2 diabetes mellitus (T2DM). Sucrose and sucrose-containing foods may be substituted for other carbohydrates. The nutrient content of sucrose-containing foods, as well as the presence of other nutrients frequently ingested with sucrose, such as fat, must be taken into consideration.

Fructose is present as the free monosaccharide in many fruits, vegetables, and honey. About one third of dietary fructose comes from fruits, vegetables, and other natural sources in the diet, and about two thirds comes from food and beverages to which fructose has been added. Fructose is absorbed more slowly from the intestinal tract than are glucose, sucrose, and maltose and is converted to glucose and glycogen in the liver. Postprandial plasma glucose levels are reduced when an isocaloric amount of fructose replaces sucrose or starch in the diets of people with diabetes. Fructose has been used in children in amounts up to 0.5 gm/kg/day; however, the potential benefit is tempered by concern that fructose may have adverse effects on serum lipids, especially low-density lipoprotein (LDL) cholesterol. Consumption of large amounts of fructose (15% to 20% of daily energy intake, 90th percentile of usual intake) increases fasting total and LDL cholesterol in subjects with diabetes and fasting total and LDL cholesterol and triglycerides in nondiabetic subjects. Because of the potential adverse effect of large amounts of fructose on serum lipids, fructose might have no overall advantage over other nutritive sweeteners. However, there is no reason to avoid naturally occurring sources of fructose.

CARBOHYDRATE COUNTING

Carbohydrate counting is a meal-planning method in which the amount of carbohydrate or number of carbohydrate servings eaten at each meal and snack are counted. Carbohydrate is the main nutrient in starches, fruits, milk, and sugar-containing foods and has the greatest effect on blood glucose levels. Therefore, it is the most important macronutrient to control in order to maintain optimal glycemic control. Using exchange lists, one starch choice is considered to be equivalent to either one fruit or milk choice; each contains approximately 15 grams of carbohydrate and is equal to one "carbohydrate choice." The "Nutrition Facts" on food labels list the portion size and total amount of carbohydrate measured in grams per serving. Carbohydrate counting allows flexibility in food choices and minimizes cheating, as all foods can be included in the meal plan. Table 64-5 shows an example of a patient's daily meal plan incorporating both the exchange servings and grams of carbohydrate.

Table 64-5	A Hypothetical Patient's Daily Food Allowance Distributed among the Six Food Groups			
Group	Exchanges	Carbohydrate (g)	Protein (g)	Fat (g)
Starch	8	120	24	
Fruit	4	60		
Milk	3 low-fat (1%)	36	24	9
Vegetables	1	5	2	
Meat	6 medium-fat		42	30
Fat	4			20
Grams		221	92	59
Calories (%)		884 (50)	368 (20)	531 (30)

FIBER

Fiber, which refers to the portion of a plant that is indigestible, markedly influences the digestion, absorption, and metabolism of many nutrients. Inclusion of plant fiber in the diet may benefit patients with diabetes by diminishing postprandial glycemia, and certain soluble plant fibers significantly reduce serum cholesterol concentrations and decrease fasting serum triglyceride levels in diabetic patients with hypertriglyceridemia. Dietary fiber guidelines for children with diabetes are the same as those for nondiabetic children[63] and can be readily achieved by increasing the consumption of minimally processed foods, such as grains, legumes, fruits, and vegetables.

PROTEIN

Protein requirements are not increased when diabetes is well controlled with insulin, and children with diabetes should follow the Recommended Daily Allowance guidelines. Physiologic requirements are determined by the amount of protein necessary to sustain normal growth, which is based on ideal weight-for-height and varies with age, being highest in infancy and early childhood. Protein intake should be 0.9 to 2.2 g/kg body weight per day and constitute 15% to 20% of the total daily intake of energy, the same as for nondiabetic children and adolescents. The consumption of saturated fat can be reduced by eating less red meat, whole milk, and high-fat dairy foods and by eating more poultry, fish, and vegetable proteins and drinking more low-fat milk.

FAT

Excessive saturated fat, cholesterol, and total energy lead to increased blood levels of cholesterol and triglycerides. Because hyperlipidemia is a major determinant of atherosclerosis and patients with T1DM eventually also develop atherosclerosis and its sequelae, the meal plan should attempt to mitigate this risk factor. Children and adolescents with well-controlled T1DM are not at high risk for dyslipidemia but should be screened and monitored according to the National Cholesterol Education Program (NCEP) and American Academy of Pediatrics guidelines. If the child or adolescent is growing and developing normally and has normal plasma lipid levels, less than 10% of energy should come from saturated fat, the daily intake of cholesterol should be less than 300 mg/day, and consumption of transunsaturated fatty acids should be minimized. Total dietary fat should be reduced in the obese child to reduce total energy consumption. The NCEP Step II diet guidelines should be implemented in the patient with elevated LDL cholesterol (>100 mg/dL). Total fat should constitute 30% percent or less of total calories, less than 7% of calories should come from saturated fat, and dietary cholesterol is limited to 200 mg/day.

MNT EDUCATION AND FORMULATION OF THE MEAL PLAN

Newly diagnosed children usually present with weight loss. Therefore, the initial meal plan includes an estimation of energy requirements to restore and then maintain an appropriate body weight and allow for normal growth and development. Energy requirements vary with age, height, weight, stage of puberty, and level of physical activity. Because the energy needs of growing children continuously change, the meal plan should be reevaluated at least every 6 months for young children and annually for adolescents.

MNT begins with an assessment by a registered dietitian, heeding the ethnic, religious, and economic factors pertaining to the individual patient and family. The meal plan must take into account the child's school schedule, early or late lunches, physical education classes, after-school physical activity, and differences in a child's activities on weekdays compared with weekends and holidays. Young children typically have three meals and two or three snacks daily, depending on the interval between meals, age of the child, and level of physical activity. Although their daily energy intake is relatively constant over time, young children adjust their energy intake at successive meals.[64] The highly variable food consumption from meal to meal that is typical of normal young children is especially challenging when the child has T1DM. Rapid-acting insulin may be administered after the meal (based on estimation of the actual amount of carbohydrate consumed) and diminishes parental anxiety.[65,66] The purpose of snacks is to prevent hypoglycemia and hunger between meals. Patients who use a basal-bolus insulin regimen or insulin pump therapy might not require snacks. Data from preprandial and postprandial blood glucose monitoring and individualized insulin-to-carbohydrate ratios are used to select insulin doses to match anticipated carbohydrate intake.

The dietitian's role is to evaluate the patient's and family's knowledge and understanding of nutrition and to formulate an individualized meal plan. Even intensive insulin replacement regimens are not successful without careful attention to meal planning.[67] Nutrition education, like all aspects of diabetes education, has to be an ongoing process with periodic review and revision of the meal plan and assessment of the child's and parents' levels of comprehension, ability to analyze and solve problems, and adherence to the nutrition goals. The patient with newly diagnosed diabetes and his or her parents should consult with a dietitian several times during the first few days after diagnosis. Within a few weeks of the child's resuming his or her usual schedule and activities, the patient and family should review the meal plan with a dietitian, who should also be available to patients for telephone consultation. If the patient's glycemic control is poor, if growth is failing, if weight gain is excessive, or if other problems arise that are related to MNT, the dietitian should be reconsulted.

THE MEAL PLAN

The individualized meal plan must be simple, practical, and easy to modify and should offer foods that are interesting, tasty, and inexpensive. At the authors' institution, meal planning is based on a combination of carbohydrate counting and the traditional exchange system, individualized to meet the ethnic, religious, and economic circumstances of each family. The exchange list system for meal planning is the most widely used substitution system and is based on six exchange lists: milk, fruit, vegetable, starch, meat, and fat. Each list indicates the appropriate size or volume of each food exchange. The meal plan is prescribed in terms of the number of exchanges for each meal and snack, which enables the patient to maintain consistency of total calories and the proportions of nutrients while allowing the patient to select from a wide choice of foods. Accurate estimation of portion sizes has to be learned. The process of weighing and measuring foods is used to educate and train patients to acquire familiarity with the sizes and amounts of food portions specified in the exchange list. An example of how this system is applied to a hypothetical patient is illustrated as follows: An 11-year-old girl's height is 144 cm (50th percentile on the Centers for Disease Control and Prevention growth chart), and her weight is 37.4 kg (50th percentile). Her daily energy requirement to support growth in the 50th percentile is 1756 calories. An appropriate distribution of macronutrients could be 50% of total calories from carbohydrate, 20% from protein, and 30% from fat (Tables 64-5 and 64-6).

EXERCISE

Children with diabetes are encouraged to participate in sports and make regular exercise a part of their lives. Participation in physical exercise normalizes the child's life, enhances self-

Table 64-6 Sample Menu Based on the Daily Food Allowance*

Foods	Exchanges	Carbohydrate (g)
BREAKFAST		
3/4 cup cornflakes + 1 slice toast	2 starches	30
1 small banana	1 fruit	15
1/2 cup 1% fat milk	1/2 low-fat milk	6
1 tsp margarine	1 fat	
SNACK		
1 granola bar	1 starch	15
LUNCH		
2 slices bread	2 starches	30
1 slice turkey, 1 slice cheese	2 meat	
Lettuce + tomato	"free vegetable"	
1 tsp mayonnaise	1 fat	
1 cup 1% fat milk	1 low-fat milk	12
1 small apple	1 fruit	15
SNACK		
17 grapes	1 fruit	15
3 cups low-fat popcorn	1 starch	15
SUPPER		
1/2 cup mashed potatoes	1 starch	15
3 oz chicken	3 meat	
1/2 cup broccoli	1 vegetable	5
1 small orange	1 fruit	15
2 tsp margarine	2 fat	
1 cup 1% low-fat milk	1 low-fat milk	12
SNACK		
3 graham cracker squares	1 starch	15
1 ounce string cheese	1 meat	
1/2 cup 1% fat milk	1/2 low-fat milk	6

*For the child described in the text.

esteem, improves physical fitness, helps to control weight, and can improve glycemic control. Regular exercise increases insulin sensitivity, cardiovascular fitness, and blood lipid profiles and lowers blood pressure. For the child with T1DM, physical exercise is complicated by the need to prevent hypoglycemia, but with proper guidance and preparation, participation in exercise should be a safe and enjoyable experience.

Exercise acutely lowers the blood glucose concentration by increasing utilization of glucose to a variable degree that depends on the intensity and duration of physical activity and the concurrent level of insulin in the blood. Hypoglycemia can be prevented by a combination of anticipatory reduction in pre-exercise insulin dose or temporary interruption of basal insulin infusion (with CSII) and/or supplemental snacks before, during, and after activity depending on the intensity and duration of the physical activity and its timing relative to the child's dietary and insulin schedule. Consideration is given to several factors in selecting the content and size of the snack. Among these are the current blood glucose level, the action of insulin that is most active during and after the period of anticipated exercise, the interval since the last meal, and the duration and intensity of physical activity. The appropriate amount is learned by trial and error; however, a useful initial guide is to provide an additional 15 grams of carbohydrate (one bread or fruit exchange) per 30 to 60 minutes of vigorous physical activity. Prolonged and strenuous exercise in the afternoon or evening should be followed by a 10% to 20% reduction in the presupper or bedtime dose of intermediate-acting insulin or equivalent reduction in overnight basal insulin delivery in patients using CSII. In addition, to reduce the risk of nocturnal or early-morning hypoglycemia caused by the lag effect of exercise, the bedtime snack should be larger than usual. Parents should be encouraged to monitor the blood glucose concentration in the middle of the night until they are experienced in modifying the evening dose of insulin after exercise.

Exercising the limb into which insulin has been injected accelerates the rate of insulin absorption. If possible, the insulin injection preceding exercise should be given in a site that is least likely to be affected by exercise. Because physical training increases tissue sensitivity to insulin, children who participate in organized sports are advised to reduce the dose of the insulin preparation that is predominantly active during the period of sustained physical activity. The size of such reductions is determined by measuring blood glucose levels before and after exercise and is generally on the order of 10% to 30% of the usual dose.

Acute vigorous exercise in the child with poorly controlled diabetes can aggravate hyperglycemia and ketoacid production. Therefore, a child with ketonuria should not exercise until satisfactory biochemical control has been restored.

TYPE 2 DIABETES MELLITUS IN CHILDREN AND ADOLESCENTS

Until recently, most children with diabetes had T1DM. However, as early as 1916, a phenotypically distinct form of diabetes, now classified as type 2 diabetes mellitus (T2DM), was recognized in childhood.[68] Over the past 10 to 20 years, an alarming increase in the prevalence of pediatric T2DM has been reported from pediatric diabetes centers in North America[69] and elsewhere in the world,[70,71] and T2DM now accounts for up to 33% of new cases of diabetes in adolescents at centers that serve large numbers of minority youth.[72,73] At least 90% of patients with newly diagnosed T2DM are obese,[69] and the increased prevalence of pediatric T2DM temporally coincides with the increase in obesity in children in the United States, which has more than doubled in the past 20 years. In 1999 to 2000, 15.5% of U.S. children ages 2 to 19 years were overweight, defined as having a body mass index in the 95th percentile or higher.[74] As in adults, obesity in childhood is associated with insulin resistance, hyperinsulinism, and decreased insulin-stimulated glucose metabolism compared to nonobese children (Table 64-7).[75,76] In prepubertal and pubertal Caucasian youth, body fat accounts for 55% of the variance in insulin sensitivity.[77] Factors that explain the increased prevalence of pediatric T2DM and strategies for primary prevention have been reviewed recently.[78] The pathophysiology of T2DM is discussed in Chapter 56.

DIAGNOSIS

Both T1DM and T2DM most often present during puberty, a period of life that is characterized by an approximately 30% physiologic reduction in insulin sensitivity.[79] With the current high prevalence of overweight and obesity in children and adolescents, distinguishing between T1DM and T2DM has become more difficult. The overall frequency of obesity at diagnosis of T1DM, irrespective of race, gender, and age of onset, has tripled in the past decade, and a recent report indicates that 24% of patients with T1DM are obese.[80] In contrast

Table 64-7	Risk Factors for Type 2 Diabetes in Youth

Insulin resistance: usually associated with obesity
Family history of type 2 diabetes in first- or second-degree relative
Ethnicity: African-American, Hispanic, Pacific Islander, Native American, Canadian First Nation
Maternal gestational diabetes
Small size for gestational age (intrauterine growth restriction)
Insulin resistance of puberty
Lack of physical activity
High calorie diet

to adult T2DM, in which ketonuria is unusual, 33% of adolescents with T2DM have ketosis at presentation, and up to 25% present with DKA.[69] Insulin requirements typically decrease after several weeks of treatment in T2DM and in individual cases may resemble the remission or "honeymoon" period of T1DM. Measuring pancreatic autoantibodies and serum insulin and C peptide levels at the time of diagnosis is recommended to distinguish between T1DM and T2DM in obese patients.

PREVENTION AND TREATMENT

In youth who are at high risk of developing T2DM, vigorous efforts should be directed at primary prevention by means of lifestyle modification that leads to weight reduction through dietary changes and increased physical activity. In adults with impaired glucose tolerance, a lifestyle modification program with the goals of 7% or greater weight loss and 150 minutes or more of physical activity per week decreased the risk of progression to diabetes by 58%.[81] Behavioral modification can slow weight gain in young children and potentially delay or even prevent T2DM.[82]

Goals of treatment of T2DM are the same as those outlined above for T1DM. Treatment aims to normalize fasting and postprandial blood glucose concentrations and should address the common comorbidities of T2DM, hypertension, and dyslipidemia. There is a lack of evidence-based guidelines for the management of T2DM in children and adolescents. Lifestyle changes that lead to weight loss, including MNT and exercise, should be the cornerstone of treatment for asymptomatic or mildly symptomatic patients (Fig. 64-2). Symptomatic patients who present with severe hyperglycemia, weight loss, and ketosis may benefit from a period of intensive insulin therapy, similar to the initial treatment of T1DM, until fasting and postprandial normoglycemia have been restored. Because patients are insulin resistant, the dose of insulin that is initially required to achieve normal glucose levels may be up to 2 units/kg/day. The patient may later be weaned off insulin and switched to metformin (see below).

A diabetes team should supervise treatment of T2DM in youth. Patients and parents should receive comprehensive self-management education similar to that for patients with T1DM, and patients should routinely perform self-monitoring of blood glucose (SMBG). The frequency of SMBG can be individualized but should include both fasting and postprandial measurements. Patients should measure blood glucose frequently during acute illness, at times of medication adjustments, or when they have symptoms. They should also test for ketones during acute illness and when diabetes control deteriorates.

Behavior modification is crucial for treatment to be successful, and weight loss is critically dependent on both dietary modification and increased exercise. The entire family should be referred to a dietitian for counseling and should be encouraged to adopt healthy eating habits.[83] Nutrition recommendations should be culturally appropriate and sensitive to family resources.

Numerous dietary regimens for treatment of T2DM in adults have been studied. The optimal strategy to improve glycemic control and weight loss is still controversial; however, there is some evidence to suggest that a low-GI diet may have beneficial effects on metabolic control. A high-GI diet leads to greater insulin secretion and directs partitioning of metabolic fuels toward storage. In contrast, a low-GI diet may reduce insulin secretion and improve insulin sensitivity and, by reducing insulin secretion, downregulate malonyl CoA carboxylase activity thereby decreasing formation of fatty acids and triglyceride. A meta-analysis of randomized controlled trials using low GI diets found a 7.3% reduction in hemoglobin A1c.[84] The amount of dietary fiber should also be increased, as it has been demonstrated to reduce insulin

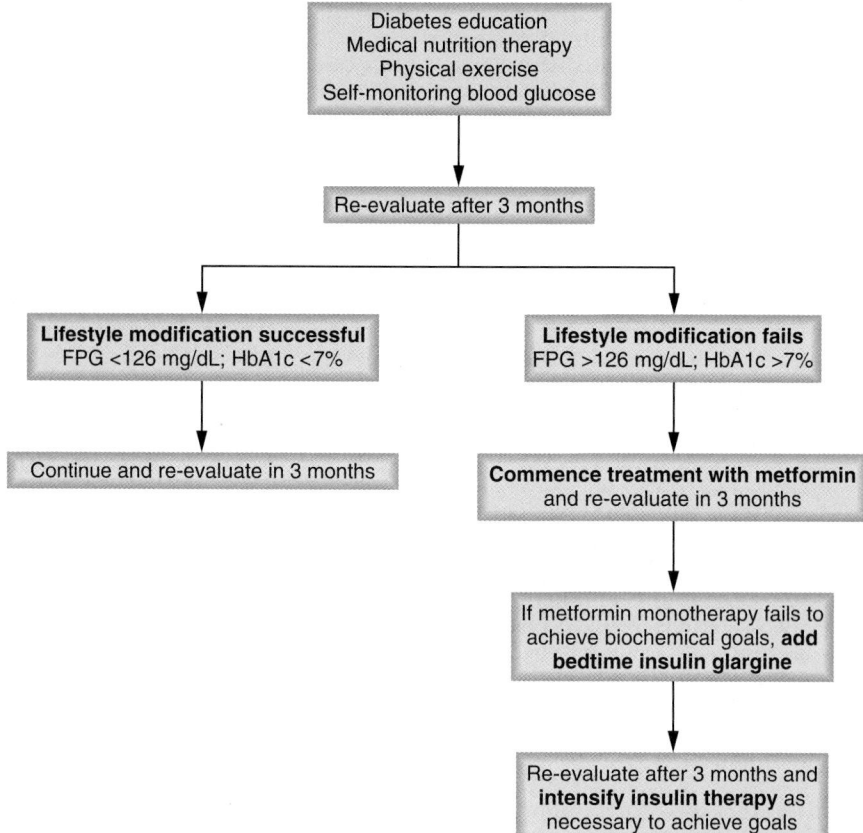

Figure 64-2 Management of asymptomatic type 2 diabetes mellitus in youth. Proposed schema for management of asymptomatic T2DM. The biochemical goals of therapy are normal (<126 mg/dL) fasting plasma glucose (FPG) and HbA1c <7% (normal is 4% to 6%).

levels, promote weight loss, improve lipid profiles, and lower cardiovascular risk (see the section above on medical nutrition therapy).

Youth with T2DM should participate in regular aerobic exercise with a gradual increase in the frequency, intensity, and duration of exercise, aiming for at least 30 minutes daily. To increase children's physical activity, the amount of time devoted to sedentary activities (watching television, playing video and computer games) must be strictly curtailed. Regular physical activity aids weight loss, increases high-density lipoprotein cholesterol levels, lowers blood pressure, improves metabolic control, and reduces cardiovascular risk.

PHARMACOLOGIC THERAPY

Some clinicians initiate pharmacologic therapy on diagnosis. Others prescribe medication after a 2- to 3-month trial of behavior modification and lifestyle intervention has failed, as evidenced by persistent or worsening hyperglycemia. Approved pharmacologic treatment of diabetes in children is limited to insulin and metformin,[85] a biguanide that decreases hepatic glucose production and increases insulin-mediated glucose uptake in peripheral (mainly skeletal muscle) tissues.[86] Metformin may aid weight loss because it has a mild anorectic effect in some patients and has the additional benefit of modestly lowering triglyceride and LDL concentrations. Lactic acidosis is a rare, potentially fatal side effect of metformin. Provided that it is not administered to patients with renal insufficiency or poor tissue perfusion, the risk of lactic acidosis is not increased in comparison with that of other antihyperglycemic agents.[87] Clinical trials of thiazolidinediones and the rapid-acting insulin secretagogue meglitinide in pediatric T2DM are in progress.

In adults with T2DM, bedtime insulin glargine is an effective basal insulin that, when combined with an oral agent, has less risk of nocturnal hypoglycemia than NPH does.[88,89] If metformin alone does not achieve blood glucose goals,

insulin glargine at bedtime should be the first-choice insulin regimen in pediatric T2DM.

Early-onset T2DM is associated with a high incidence of diabetic nephropathy,[90] and vascular disease may already be present at diagnosis. Because of the numerous cardiovascular risk factors associated with insulin resistance, it is reasonable to anticipate that inadequately treated patients will suffer considerable morbidity from both microvascular and macrovascular complications at an earlier age than in childhood T1DM. Therefore, youth with T2DM must be treated vigorously, and strenuous efforts should be made to maintain hemoglobin A1c concentrations less than 7.0%.

MATURITY-ONSET DIABETES OF THE YOUNG

Maturity-onset diabetes of the young (MODY) was first described in the 1960s in children and young adults with a form of noninsulin-dependent or "maturity-onset" type diabetes that was inherited in an autosomal-dominant pattern.[91] MODY, which may account for 1% to 5% of all cases of diabetes in the United States and other industrialized countries, is a heterogeneous group of disorders.

The most common clinical presentation of MODY is mild asymptomatic hyperglycemia in nonobese children, adolescents, and young adults who have a strong family history of diabetes in successive generations (Table 64-8). Prospective

Table 64-8   Characteristic Features of MODY
Onset of diabetes usually before age 25 years and frequently in childhood or adolescence
Absence of ketosis
Absence of obesity
Autosomal dominant mode of inheritance
A primary defect in the function of pancreatic β cells

testing suggests that in most patients, onset occurs in childhood or adolescence. Some patients have mild fasting hyperglycemia; others have varying degrees of glucose intolerance for several years before developing persistent fasting hyperglycemia. Because mild hyperglycemia might not cause classic symptoms, diagnosis might be delayed until adulthood. In some cases, progression may be rapid to overt symptomatic hyperglycemia, requiring therapy with an oral hypoglycemic agent or insulin.

MODY is caused by mutations of genes expressed in the β cell. With the exception of MODY 2, transcription factor mutations account for five of the six documented causes of classic MODY, which have been described predominantly in Caucasians. These transcription factors are involved in the regulation of insulin gene transcription and may also regulate pancreatic and/or islet or β-cell development.[92] A variant form of MODY, atypical diabetes mellitus, has been described in African-Americans[93]; however, the molecular cause(s) has not yet been elucidated. All forms of MODY are the result of insulin deficiency (Table 64-9).

Most MODY cases that are diagnosed in youth, regardless of age, do not require insulin therapy but do require careful monitoring to ensure good glycemic control to avoid complications. Treatment is tailored to the individual patient's specific type of diabetes.

MITOCHONDRIAL DIABETES

Mitochondrial diabetes, a maternally inherited disorder that is often associated with hearing loss, is a rare disease that shares some clinical features in common with MODY.[94] Abnormal mitochondrial metabolism results in abnormal adenosine triphosphate (ATP) generation and defective glucose-induced insulin secretion. Diabetes mellitus may present in childhood and can be treated with diet, sulfonylureas, or insulin. Patients with impaired mitochondrial function are inherently prone to develop lactic acidosis. Metformin should not be used because it can increase the risk.

CYSTIC FIBROSIS–RELATED DIABETES

The life expectancy of patients with cystic fibrosis has increased dramatically over the past few decades, and as a result, cystic fibrosis–related diabetes (CFRD) has become more common.[95,96] Insulinopenia is caused by pancreatic destruction and amyloid deposition in the islets. First-phase insulin release is particularly affected; however, ketoacidosis is rare. CFRD can present in the first decade but usually is seen in the second and third decades of life. The development of CFRD is associated with progressive clinical deterioration and

increased mortality. Screening for glucose intolerance should begin at the age of 14 years, and hyperglycemia should be aggressively treated.[97]

Insulin is the only recommended therapy for CFRD. It prevents protein catabolism and improves weight gain and pulmonary function. The ideal treatment is a basal-bolus regimen using insulin glargine and rapid-acting insulin (see Fig. 64-1B). Diet should never be restricted in CFRD, and patients should be taught carbohydrate counting and how to use rapid-acting insulin with meals. Destruction of the pancreatic α cells results in glucagon deficiency, and chronic glucocorticoid use can cause adrenocortical insufficiency. Patients with CFRD are consequently at increased risk for severe hypoglycemia owing to malabsorption and impaired counterregulatory responses.

MONITORING DIABETES CONTROL

SELF-MONITORING OF BLOOD GLUCOSE

Self-monitoring of blood glucose (SMBG) has revolutionized management and is the cornerstone of modern diabetes care. Patients and parents must be taught how to use the data to assess the efficacy of therapy and to adjust the components of their treatment regimen to achieve individual blood glucose goals. For most patients with T1DM, SMBG should be performed at least four times daily: before each meal and at bedtime. To minimize the risk of nocturnal hypoglycemia, blood glucose should be measured between midnight and 4:00 A.M. once each week or every other week and whenever the evening dose of insulin is adjusted. If HbA1c targets are not being met, patients should be encouraged to measure blood glucose levels more frequently, including 90 to 120 minutes after meals. Frequency of blood glucose monitoring is an important predictor of glycemic control in children with T1DM.[98] The optimal frequency of SMBG for patients with T2DM is not known but should be sufficient to facilitate attainment of the individual patient's glycemic goals. Children who are able independently to perform SMBG must be properly supervised because it is not unusual for children to fabricate data with disastrous consequences.

CONTINUOUS GLUCOSE MONITORING

Glucose sensors have been developed to provide frequent glucose determinations throughout the day and night in patients with diabetes. Two continuous glucose monitors, GlucoWatch® G2™ Biographer and the Continuous Glucose Monitoring System, CGMS™ System Gold®, are being used in children with diabetes. Both measure interstitial fluid glucose concentrations, which are normalized for serum glucose values using algorithms. Reports indicate better detection of asymptomatic hypoglycemia, detection of postprandial glycemic excursions, and improvement in glycemic control in children with diabetes. However, relatively large differences between sensor and reference glucose values and frequent false-positive values in the hypoglycemic range have been observed.[99-101] These devices are not yet routinely being used to manage diabetes in children.

URINE KETONE TESTING

Urine should routinely be tested for ketones during acute illness or stress, when blood glucose levels are persistently elevated (e.g., two consecutive blood glucose values > 300 mg/dL), or when the patient feels unwell, especially with nausea, abdominal pain, or vomiting. False-negative readings may occur when the strips have been exposed to air or when urine is highly acidic (e.g., after consumption of large doses of ascorbic acid). Urine ketone tests using nitroprusside-containing

Table 64-9	Classification of MODY		
Type	Gene	Frequency	Treatment
MODY1[209]	Hepatocyte nuclear factor-4α	Uncommon	Oral hypoglycemic agent, insulin
MODY2[210]	Glucokinase	Common	Diet and exercise
MODY3[211]	Hepatocyte nuclear factor-1α	Common	Oral hypoglycemic agent, insulin
MODY4[211]	Insulin promoter factor-1	Rare	Oral hypoglycemic agent, insulin
MODY5[212]	Hepatocyte nuclear factor-1β	Rare	Insulin
MODY6[213]	NeuroD1	Rare	Insulin

reagents can give false-positive results in the presence of several sulfhydryl drugs, including captopril.

BLOOD KETONE TESTING

Home tests to measure blood β-hydroxybutyric acid (βOHB) levels are available but are expensive. Quantification of blood βOHB, the predominant ketone body, is preferred over urine ketone testing for diagnosing and monitoring metabolic decompensation, as may occur with illness, and in ketoacidosis.[102] Once ketosis has been demonstrated by urine testing, blood ketone testing offers the advantage of accurately assessing improvement. Pooling of urine results in persistent ketonuria after blood levels have begun to improve and predisposes to excessive insulin administration after the blood ketone concentration has reverted to normal.

GLYCATED HEMOGLOBIN OR HEMOGLOBIN A1C

Blood glucose and blood or urine ketone testing provide useful information for day-to-day management of diabetes. HbA1c is a minor fraction of adult hemoglobin, which is formed slowly and nonenzymatically from hemoglobin and glucose. Because erythrocytes are freely permeable to glucose, HbA1c is formed throughout the life span of the erythrocyte; its rate of formation is directly proportional to the ambient glucose concentration. The concentration of HbA1c, therefore, provides a "glycemic history" of the previous 120 days, the average life span of erythrocytes. Optimal use of the HbA1c test requires standardization of the assay, for example, to the values of the DCCT reference method. Without standardization, results between laboratories might not be comparable. The correlation between mean plasma glucose levels (from DCCT capillary plasma glucose data) and HbA1c level is as follows: mean plasma glucose (mg/dL) = [(35.6 × HbA1c) − 77.3][103] (Table 64-10). In patients with hemoglobin variants (HbS, HbC, HbF), radioimmunoassay and affinity chromatography methods for measuring glycated hemoglobin must be used instead of conventional high-performance liquid or cation-exchange chromatography, which give spurious values. HbA1c should be measured approximately every 3 months to determine whether a patient's metabolic control has reached or has been maintained within a target range.

HYPOGLYCEMIA IN CHILDREN WITH DIABETES MELLITUS

Hypoglycemia is the most common acute complication of the treatment of diabetes mellitus in children and adolescents, and concern about hypoglycemia is a central issue in treating children with T1DM. It is the principal factor limiting attempts to achieve near-normal glycemic control.[104] Patients, parents, and the diabetes team have to continuously balance

Table 64-10	Correlation between HbA1c (DCCT Method) and Capillary Plasma Glucose
HbA1c (%)	Mean Plasma Glucose (mg/dL)
6	135
7	170
8	205
9	240
10	275
11	310
12	345

Adapted from Goldstein DE, Little RR, Lorenz RA, et al: Tests of glycemia in diabetes. Diabetes Care 26(Suppl 1):S106–S108, 2003.

the risks of hypoglycemia against those of long-term hyperglycemia. After an episode of severe hypoglycemia, the confidence of the patient and parents is often shaken, and fear of a recurrence might induce the patient or parents to change their diabetes management to prevent a recurrence. Altered patient behaviors may include chronic overeating and/or deliberate selection of inadequate doses of insulin to maintain higher blood glucose levels that are perceived as being safe and can result in deterioration of glycemic control.[105-107] Concern about nocturnal hypoglycemia causes more anxiety for some parents than any other aspect of diabetes, including the fear of long-term complications. Some parents believe that an episode of severe hypoglycemia during the night might go undetected or not be treated in a timely fashion and might lead to permanent brain damage or death.[108]

Because the glucagon response to hypoglycemia is lost early in the course of the disease,[109,110] patients with T1DM depend on sympathoadrenal responses to prevent or correct hypoglycemia.[111] Mild hypoglycemia itself reduces epinephrine responses and symptomatic awareness of subsequent episodes of hypoglycemia.[111-113] Little is known about counterregulatory responses in preschool-age children.

SYMPTOMS AND SIGNS OF HYPOGLYCEMIA

Symptoms of hypoglycemia are caused by neuronal deprivation of glucose and are either autonomic (adrenergic), neuroglycopenic, or a combination of the two. The most common signs and symptoms of hypoglycemia in diabetic children are pallor, weakness, tremor, hunger, fatigue, drowsiness, sweating, and headache.[114,115] In contrast to adolescents, autonomic symptoms are less common in children younger than 6 years old, whose symptoms are more often neuroglycopenic or nonspecific in nature.[115] Symptoms of hypoglycemia that are experienced by adults with diabetes have been categorized into subgroups: autonomic (sweating, palpitations, shaking, hunger), neuroglycopenic (confusion, drowsiness, odd behavior, speech difficulty, incoordination), and nonspecific malaise (hunger and headache).[116] Manifestations of hypoglycemia in young children with T1DM tend to differ from those of insulin-treated adults. Behavioral changes are often the primary manifestation of hypoglycemia in young children, and this difference has important implications for parent education on hypoglycemia. Also, autonomic and neuroglycopenic symptoms reported by children and their parents tend to cluster. This contrasts with adult patients, who are usually able to distinguish between these two types of symptoms. In children, the coalescence of autonomic and neuroglycopenic symptoms may indicate that both types of symptoms are generated at similar glycemic thresholds. Both parents and children report a coherent cluster of symptoms related to behavioral change during hypoglycemia.[117]

Hypoglycemia is classified in terms of its severity as mild, moderate, or severe; most episodes are mild.[115] Cognitive deficits usually do not accompany mild hypoglycemia, and older children are able to treat themselves. Mild symptoms abate within about 15 minutes after an appropriate dose of rapidly absorbed carbohydrate. Moderate hypoglycemia has neuroglycopenic as well as adrenergic symptoms, such as headache, mood changes, irritability, decreased attentiveness, drowsiness, and behavior change. Young children typically require assistance with treatment because they are often confused and have impaired judgment; also, weakness and poor coordination might make self-treatment difficult. Moderate hypoglycemia causes more protracted symptoms and might require a second treatment with oral carbohydrate. Severe hypoglycemia is characterized by unresponsiveness, unconsciousness, or convulsions and requires emergency treatment with parenteral glucagon or intravenous glucose.

Children who have had diabetes for several years may describe a change in their symptomatology over time.

Autonomic symptoms tend to occur less frequently and are more muted, and neuroglycopenic symptoms are more common. Patients must learn to recognize the change in symptoms to prevent severe episodes.[118] The blood glucose concentration at which symptoms occur varies among patients, and the threshold may vary in the same individual in parallel with antecedent glycemic control. Children with poorly controlled diabetes experience symptoms of hypoglycemia at higher blood glucose concentrations than do those with good glycemic control, similar to adults with diabetes.[119]

IMPACT OF HYPOGLYCEMIA ON THE CHILD'S BRAIN

Numerous studies have documented cognitive impairments and academic difficulties in children and adolescents with T1DM. Global intellectual deficits have been described as well as specific neurocognitive impairments in memory, visuospatial skills, and attention.[120–126] Neuropsychological complications have been detected within 2 years of onset of diabetes.[122,123] Children with long-term diabetes, especially those who developed the disease before age 6 years, appear to be at the greatest risk. However, it is difficult to dissect out the contributions of metabolic disturbances (hyperglycemia and hypoglycemia) and the psychosocial effects of chronic disease in a young child.[127] There is evidence linking hypoglycemia to the neuropsychological defects. Rovet observed specific defects associated with a positive history of severe hypoglycemic events,[126,128] whereas Golden found no evidence of an association with severe episodes and thought that asymptomatic hypoglycemia may be more important.[129] Impaired intellectual development without a clear relationship to experienced hypoglycemia has also been reported.[124] Thus, cognitive impairments in children with early-onset diabetes mellitus may result from a number of factors whose relative importance is still unclear: severe hypoglycemia, recurrent asymptomatic hypoglycemia, psychosocial effects of chronic illness, or chronic hyperglycemia.[127] The neurocognitive sequelae of intensive diabetes management in children whose brains are still developing are still largely unknown. Preliminary findings suggest poorer memory skills, presumably the consequence of recurrent and severe hypoglycemia.[130]

Even in the absence of typical symptoms, cognitive function deteriorates at low blood glucose levels.[131] Moderate and severe hypoglycemia is disabling, affects school performance, and makes driving a car or operating dangerous machinery hazardous,[131–134] and the utmost effort should be made to avoid such events. Repeated or prolonged severe hyperinsulinemic hypoglycemia can cause permanent central nervous system damage, especially in very young children. Fortunately, hypoglycemia is a rare cause of death in children with T1DM.[135]

FREQUENCY OF HYPOGLYCEMIA

The true frequency of mild (self-treated) symptomatic hypoglycemia is almost impossible to ascertain because mild episodes are quickly forgotten and/or are not recorded. In a random sample of 47 children attending a diabetes clinic, the average incidence of symptomatic hypoglycemia was once every 33 days (range: 0 to 5.2 times per month), and occurred more frequently in children with the lowest HbA1c levels.[136] In a 12-month population-based study, Aman and coworkers found that mild episodes (managed by the child without assistance) occurred in 97% of children and occurred at least once a week in 53%.[114] More recently, Tupola and coworkers[137] prospectively examined the frequency of hypoglycemia (blood glucose < 54 mg/dL) in 161 children and adolescents predominantly treated with multiple doses of insulin, who were asked to document hypoglycemia episodes in a 3-month diary. Fifty-two percent of the clinic population experienced

episodes of hypoglycemia (0.6 hypoglycemia event per patient per month), of which 77% were mild.

The literature is replete with reports of the frequency of severe hypoglycemia in children and adolescents with diabetes.[36,37,137–155] However, various methods of collecting data, variability among clinic populations and therapeutic methods, and varying definitions of severe hypoglycemia make comparisons among the reports and interpretation of the data difficult.[127,156] For example, in some studies, severe hypoglycemia is defined as loss of consciousness, whereas others include children who required assistance with treatment. In young children, all episodes of hypoglycemia require the assistance of a third party for treatment, regardless of the severity of the symptoms. It is therefore not surprising that the reported incidence of moderate or severe hypoglycemia in the pediatric diabetes population varies widely. Recent prospective studies with strict definitions of hypoglycemic events and well-described populations continue to show disturbingly high rates of severe hypoglycemia; younger children and patients with tight glycemic control are at greatest risk (Table 64-11).[150,154,155,157–159]

Many, but not all, studies have found an increased frequency of severe hypoglycemia in younger children[36,98,139,148–150,152,153,155] and in association with lower hemoglobin A1c concentrations.[36,37,98,137–139,142,143,145,149,150,152,154,155,160] Other factors that are associated with a higher risk of moderate and severe hypoglycemia are a prior history of severe hypoglycemia,[142,147,159,161] relatively higher doses of insulin, low C peptide secretion,[115,147,151,155,159,161] longer duration of diabetes,[37,144,150] male gender,[146,161] psychiatric disorders,[155] and underinsurance.[155,158]

CAUSES OF HYPOGLYCEMIA IN DIABETES MELLITUS

Patients with type 1 diabetes mellitus are susceptible to hypoglycemia for many reasons (Table 64-12).

Patient errors relating to insulin dosage, decreased food intake, or unplanned exercise account for 50% to 85% of episodes of hypoglycemia in children and adolescents.[114,140,142–144,148] After years of living with diabetes, some patients and/or their parents conduct their routine diabetes self-care practices without carefully thinking about the intricate interplay among insulin, food, and exercise.[162]

Improved methods of replacing insulin (CSII and MDI regimens with insulin analogues) combined with behavioral educational approaches such as blood glucose awareness training and intermittent continuous glucose monitoring may reduce the frequency of hypoglycemia[44,163–167] and enable patients to achieve improved glycemic control with less risk of severe hypoglycemia than was previously possible. These claims have yet to be confirmed in large prospective studies. Several reports have shown that insulin pump therapy is associated with fewer hypoglycemic events despite improved glycemic control.[166,168–170] This might be because CSII permits lower (and adjustable) rates of basal insulin delivery compared with injection therapy, especially at night when hypoglycemia is most common. Rapid-acting insulin analogues decrease the frequency of hypoglycemia[152] and insulin glargine together with premeal insulin lispro decreases the incidence of nocturnal hypoglycemia in adolescents when compared to NPH combined with regular insulin.[44]

NOCTURNAL HYPOGLYCEMIA

Hypoglycemia, often asymptomatic, frequently occurs during sleep. Moderate and severe (with coma and seizures) hypoglycemia is more common during the night and early morning (before breakfast) than during the daytime.[150,171] In the DCCT, 55% of severe hypoglycemia events occurred during sleep, and 43% occurred between midnight and 8:00 A.M.[161,171]

Table 64-11 Incidence of Severe Hypoglycemia* in Children and Adolescents

Study Author, Year	Age Group (years)	No. of Patients	Definition of Severe Hypoglycemia	Incidence[†]	Mean or Median HbA1c (%)	Methodology
DCCT, 1994	13 to 17	195	Coma, seizure			Prospective randomized clinical trial
Intensive therapy				26.7	8.06	
Conventional therapy				9.7	9.76	
Nordfeldt, 1997	1 to 18	146	Coma, seizure	15 to 19	8.1 to 6.9	Prospective
Mortensen, 1997	1 to 18	2873	Coma, seizure	22	8.6	Cross-sectional international
Rosilio, 1998	1 to 19	2579	Coma, seizure, glucagon	45	8.97	Cross-sectional national
Davis, 1998	0 to 18	709	Coma, seizure	15.6	8.6	Prospective population based
Tupola, 1998	1 to 24	329	Coma, seizure, glucagon	3.6	9.1 to 9.6	Retrospective
Tupola, 1998	1 to 24	287	Coma, seizure, glucagon	3.1	9.0 to 9.1	Prospective
Thomsett, 1999	1 to 19	268	Coma, seizure	25	8.6	Retrospective
Nordfeldt, 1999	1 to 18	139	Unconsciousness	17.0	6.9[‡]	Prospective
Levine, 2001	7 to 16	300	Coma, seizure, glucagon, IV dextrose	8	8.7 to 8.9	Prospective
Rewers, 2002	0 to 19	1243	Coma, seizure, admission	19	8.8 to 9.0[¶]	Prospective

*Severe hypoglycemia is variably defined in these studies as coma, seizure, treatment with glucagon, intravenous dextrose, treatment in an emergency department, or admission to hospital.
[†]Events per 100 patient years.
[‡]Median value, normal range 3.6% to 5.4%.
[¶]Range of median values.

Table 64-12 Causes of Hypoglycemia in Children and Adolescents with Diabetes Mellitus

INSULIN ERRORS (INADVERTENT OR DELIBERATE)
Reversal of morning and evening dose
Reversal of short- or rapid-acting insulin and intermediate-acting insulin
Improper timing of insulin in relation to food
Excessive insulin dosage
Surreptitious insulin administration, suicide gesture or attempt

ERRATIC OR ALTERED ABSORPTION
Inadvertent intramuscular injection
More rapid absorption from exercising limbs
Unpredictable absorption from lipohypertrophy at injection sites
More rapid absorption after sauna, hot bath, sunbathing

DIET
Omission or reduced size of meals or snacks
Delayed snacks or meals
Eating disorders
Gastroparesis
Malabsorption (e.g., gluten enteropathy)

EXERCISE
Unplanned physical activity
Prolonged duration and/or increased intensity of physical activity
Failure to reduce the dose of basal insulin to combat the "lag effect" of exercise

ALCOHOL AND/OR DRUGS
Impaired gluconeogenesis from excessive consumption of ethanol
Impaired cognition from use of ethanol, marijuana, cocaine, other recreational drugs

HYPOGLYCEMIA-ASSOCIATED AUTONOMIC FAILURE
Hypoglycemia unawareness
Defective glucose counterregulation

MISCELLANEOUS UNCOMMON CAUSES OF HYPOGLYCEMIA
Adrenocortical insufficiency
Hypothyroidism
Growth hormone deficiency
Renal failure
Decreased insulin requirement in first trimester of pregnancy
Insulin antibodies

Diabetic children and adolescents studied either in the hospital or at home who had frequent intermittent or continuous blood glucose measurements during the night showed a high incidence (14% to 47%) of asymptomatic hypoglycemia.[164,172-180] Such episodes during sleep often exceed 4 hours in duration. Up to half these episodes may be undetected because the subject does not wake from sleep. The incidence of hypoglycemia on any given night may be affected by numerous factors, including the insulin regimen, the timing and content of meals and snacks, and antecedent physical activity. The highest frequency of asymptomatic nocturnal hypoglycemia occurs in children younger than 10 years old.[174,176-178] Low blood glucose concentrations in the early morning (before breakfast) are associated with a higher frequency of preceding nocturnal hypoglycemia. Knowledge of this fact is useful in counseling patients to modify the evening insulin regimen and bedtime snack to prevent more severe nocturnal hypoglycemia.

Sleep impairs counterregulatory hormone responses to hypoglycemia in normal subjects and in patients with diabetes mellitus.[181,182] Because a rise in plasma epinephrine is normally the main hormonal defense against hypoglycemia, impaired counterregulatory hormone responses to hypoglycemia explains the increased susceptibility to hypoglycemia during sleep. Furthermore, asymptomatic nocturnal hypoglycemia may impair counterregulatory hormone responses.[183] Thus, impaired defenses against hypoglycemia during sleep may contribute to the vicious cycle of hypoglycemia, impaired counterregulatory responses, and unawareness of hypoglycemia either awake or asleep. Recurrent asymptomatic nocturnal hypoglycemia is therefore an important cause of hypoglycemia unawareness, which, in turn, leads to more frequent and severe hypoglycemia because of failure to experience autonomic warning symptoms before the onset of neuroglycopenia.[104]

TREATMENT

Except in preschool-age children, most episodes of symptomatic hypoglycemia are self-treated with rapidly absorbed carbohydrate such as glucose tablets, juices, soft drinks, candy, crackers, or milk. Glucose tablets raise blood glucose levels more rapidly than orange juice or milk, and the dosage is easily calibrated.[184] Glucose tablets are the treatment of choice for children who are old enough to chew and safely swallow large tablets. The recommended dose is 0.3 gram of glucose per kilogram of body weight. The glycemic response to oral glucose usually lasts less than 2 hours. Therefore, unless a scheduled meal or snack is due within an hour after treatment with oral glucose, the patient should be given either a snack or a meal containing carbohydrate and protein.

Hypoglycemia frequently occurs when a child with diabetes is unable to consume or absorb oral carbohydrate because of nausea and vomiting associated with an intercurrent illness (e.g., gastroenteritis) or oppositional behavior. To maintain blood glucose concentrations in a safe range, parents either seek emergency medical attention or attempt to force-feed oral carbohydrate in an ill child, which often leads to more vomiting. Minidose glucagon raises blood glucose 60 to 90 mg/dL within 30 minutes, and its effect lasts approximately 1 hour. This method is effective in managing most situations of impending hypoglycemia at home. Using a U-100 insulin syringe and after dissolving 1 mg of glucagon in 1 mL of diluent, children 2 years of age and younger receive 2 "units" (20 µg) of glucagon SC, and children older than 2 years receive 1 unit (10 µg) per year of age up to 15 units (150 µg). If the blood glucose concentration does not increase within 30 minutes, double the initial dosage should be administered.[185]

Severe reactions (unresponsiveness, unconsciousness, or convulsions) require emergency treatment with parenteral glucagon (intramuscular or subcutaneous). Glucagon raises blood glucose levels within 5 to 15 minutes and usually relieves symptoms of hypoglycemia. Symptoms of experimentally induced hypoglycemia in diabetic children are relieved within 10 minutes of giving glucagon either by SC or intramuscular (IM) injection. Mean blood glucose and plasma glucagon levels are slightly but not significantly higher after IM than SC injection. Both 10 µg/kg and 20 µg/kg of glucagon relieve clinical signs and symptoms, but the increment in blood glucose concentration after 10 minutes is less after a 10-µg/kg dose (20 ± 5 versus 31 ± 13 mg/dL). However, after 20 and 30 minutes, the differences in blood glucose concentrations are not significant. Nausea and/or vomiting occur after the injection in a minority of children who receive a dose of 20 µg/kg but usually do not occur after 10 µg/kg of glucagon. Excessively high plasma glucagon levels are more likely to cause nausea and/or vomiting. The recommended dose, therefore, is 15 µg/kg to a maximum of 1.0 mg. In diabetic children and in healthy adults,[186] there appears to be no important difference between the effects of glucagon injected either SC or IM. The plasma glucagon levels that are attained are higher than those in peripheral venous or portal blood of healthy adults during insulin-induced hypoglycemia and are probably higher than is necessary for maximal effect. The increase in blood glucose concentration after glucagon administration is sustained for at least 30 minutes. Therefore, it is unnecessary to repeat the dose or force the child to eat or drink for at least 30 minutes. Intranasal glucagon has a similar effect but is not available in the United States.[187] In an emergency department or hospital, the preferred treatment is intravenous glucose (0.3 g/kg). Because the glycemic response is transient after bolus administration of glucose, the patient should continue to receive intravenous glucose infusion until she or he is able to swallow safely.

If severe hypoglycemia was prolonged and the patient had a seizure, complete recovery of mental and neurologic function can take many hours despite restoration of normal blood glucose levels.[188] Permanent hemiparesis or other neurologic sequelae are rare[189,190]; however, the postictal period may be complicated by headache, lethargy, nausea, vomiting, and muscle ache.

DIABETIC KETOACIDOSIS

DKA is comprehensively reviewed in Chapter 61. Aspects of DKA that are specifically related to its occurrence in children will be briefly discussed here.

In Canada and Europe, rates of hospitalization for DKA in established and new patients with T1DM have remained stable at about 10 per 100,000 children over the past 20 years.[191] The risk of DKA in established T1DM is 1% to 10% per patient per year.[37,155,192,193] Risk is increased in children with poor metabolic control or previous episodes of DKA, peripubertal and adolescent girls, children with psychiatric disorders, including those with eating disorders, and those with difficult family circumstances, including lower socioeconomic status and lack of health insurance. In the era of CSII, interruption of insulin delivery, irrespective of the reason, is an important cause of DKA. Children rarely have DKA when insulin administration is supervised or performed by a responsible adult.[194] In established patients, most instances of DKA are probably associated with insulin omission or treatment error; the remainder are due to inadequate insulin therapy during intercurrent illness.[195]

MORBIDITY AND MORTALITY OF DKA IN CHILDREN

Reported mortality rates from DKA in national population-based studies are reasonably constant in the range of 0.15% to 0.31%. In areas with sparse medical facilities, the risk of dying from DKA is greater, and children may die before receiving treatment.[135] Cerebral edema accounts for 57% to 87% of all deaths from DKA.[196,197] The incidence of cerebral edema has been fairly consistent between national population-based studies, 0.46% in Canada to 0.87% in the United States. Mortality rates from cerebral edema in population-based studies are 21% to 25%. Significant morbidity is evident in 10% to 26% of survivors. Other causes of morbidity and mortality include hypokalemia, hyperkalemia, hypoglycemia, sepsis, and other central nervous system complications, such as thrombosis.

Cerebral edema typically occurs 4 to 12 hours after commencement of treatment but can occur before treatment has begun or at any time during treatment. Symptoms and signs are variable and include onset of headache, gradual decrease or deterioration in level of consciousness, inappropriate slowing of the heart rate, and an increase in blood pressure. Cerebral edema is more common in children with severe DKA, new-onset T1DM, younger age, and longer duration of symptoms (Table 64-13). There is no convincing evidence that volume or sodium content of intravenous fluids or rate of change of serum glucose is associated with increased risk of cerebral edema during treatment.

TREATMENT OF CEREBRAL EDEMA

Treatment should be initiated as soon as the condition is suspected. The rate of fluid administration should be reduced. Intravenous mannitol (0.25 to 1 g/kg) should be given over 20 minutes and can be repeated, if necessary, in 2 hours if

Table 64-13	Factors Associated with Increased Risk of Cerebral Edema

An attenuated rise in measured serum sodium concentration during treatment
Severity of acidosis
Administration of bicarbonate to correct acidosis
More profound hypocapnia at presentation (after adjusting for the degree of acidosis)
Increased serum urea nitrogen at presentation, which may reflect more severe dehydration

there is no initial response.[198–200] Hypertonic saline (3%), 5 to 10 mL/kg over 30 minutes may be an alternative to mannitol.[201] Intubation may be necessary for the patient with impending respiratory failure, but aggressive hyperventilation (to $pCO_2 < 22$ mm Hg) has been associated with poor outcome and is not recommended.[202]

SCREENING FOR OTHER AUTOIMMUNE DISEASES

Autoimmune thyroid disorders are common in patients with T1DM.[203] Approximately 22% of patients have thyroid autoantibodies; however, the reported prevalence of thyroid dysfunction varies widely. Asymptomatic individuals should be screened annually for thyroid dysfunction with a sensitive thyroid-stimulating hormone (TSH) assay. Alternatively, some endocrinologists determine thyroid autoantibodies and measure TSH only in patients with autoantibodies.[204]

In Western Europe, North America, and Australia, the mean prevalence of celiac disease among children and adults with T1DM is 4.1% (0% to 10.4%). Screening studies with endomysial or tissue transglutaminase antibodies show that 3.7% to 9.9% (mean: 7.4%) of children with T1DM screen positive, and of these, 80% have a positive biopsy. It has been suggested that all children with T1DM should be screened for celiac disease; however, the potential benefits and risks of screening diabetic children for celiac disease have not been systematically assessed.[205] If screening is not routine, clinicians should consider the possibility of celiac disease and screen with either antiendomysial or tissue transglutaminase antibodies in patients with suboptimal glycemic control, diarrhea, abdominal pain, or recurrent hypoglycemia.

Anti-21-hydroxylase antibodies occur in 1.6% to 2.3% of individuals with T1DM; only one in 200 to 300, however, progress to develop clinical adrenocortical insufficiency.[204] The risk increases to 1 in 30 in patients with two autoimmune processes (e.g., diabetes and thyroiditis). The development of adrenocortical insufficiency in T1DM is characterized by recurrent unexplained hypoglycemia and decreasing insulin requirements.

SCREENING FOR LONG-TERM COMPLICATIONS

Development of diabetic complications is insidious but can usually be detected years before the patient has symptoms or organ function is impaired.[206] Systematic screening can detect abnormality at an early stage when intervention to arrest, reverse, or retard the disease process will have the greatest impact. Diabetic retinopathy is rare before the onset of puberty or in patients who have had T1DM for less than 5 years. Therefore, annual dilated retinal examinations should begin 5 years after diagnosis. Renal disease is first detected by persistent albuminuria. Similarly, after 5 years of diabetes, an annual screening measurement of urine albumin and creatinine concentrations should be performed to detect microalbuminuria. In contrast to the above recommendations for T1DM in children, monitoring lipids, urinary albumin excretion, and screening eye examinations should begin at diagnosis in T2DM.[57] Circulatory and neurologic complications of diabetes are seldom clinically significant in the pediatric and adolescent population.

CONCLUSION

In 1993, the DCCT recommended that most youth with diabetes should receive intensive therapy. Technologic innovations since then, including better pumps and insulin analogues that facilitate more physiologic insulin replacement, have made it possible to achieve tighter blood glucose control with reduced risk of severe hypoglycemia in children and adolescents with diabetes. Increased use of more physiologic insulin regimens together with frequent blood glucose monitoring and patient empowerment has made it possible to ensure normal growth and development and to safely achieve levels of blood glucose control that were previously unattainable. It is reasonable to expect that the benefits of sustained improvement in glycemic control will prevent or at least delay the appearance of the chronic complications of diabetes. Epidemiologic data provide evidence that this is already the case.[207] The arduous and incessant task of controlling blood glucose in a child is difficult and frustrating, and the risk of hypoglycemia is always present. Members of the diabetes team must set realistic and attainable goals for each patient while constantly providing encouragement and support. The resources of a multidisciplinary health-care team in collaboration with the child's primary care physician are essential for the successful management of childhood diabetes. Unfortunately, in the past decade, T2DM has emerged as a major new challenge for those who provide care for children with diabetes.

REFERENCES

1. Levy-Marchal C, Papoz L, de Beaufort C, et al: Clinical and laboratory features of type 1 diabetic children at the time of diagnosis. Diabet Med 9:279–284, 1992.
2. Komulainen J, Lounamaa R, Knip M, et al: Ketoacidosis at the diagnosis of type 1 (insulin dependent) diabetes mellitus is related to poor residual beta cell function: Childhood Diabetes in Finland Study Group. Arch Dis Child 75:410–415, 1996.
3. Pinkey JH, Bingley PJ, Sawtell PA, et al: Presentation and progress of childhood diabetes mellitus: A prospective population-based study: The Bart's-Oxford Study Group. Diabetologia 37:70–74, 1994.
4. Komulainen J, Kulmala P, Savola K, et al: Clinical, autoimmune, and genetic characteristics of very young children with type 1 diabetes. Childhood Diabetes in Finland (DiMe) Study Group. Diabetes Care 22:1950–1955, 1999.
5. Monroe KW, King W, Atchison JA: Use of PRISM scores in triage of pediatric patients with diabetic ketoacidosis. Am J Manag Care 3:253–258, 1997.
6. Bonadio WA, Gutzeit MF, Losek JD, et al: Outpatient management of diabetic ketoacidosis. Am J Dis Child 142:448–450, 1988.
7. Chase HP, Crews KR, Garg S, et al: Outpatient management vs in-hospital management of children with new-onset diabetes. Clin Pediatr (Phila) 31:450–456, 1992.
8. Clar C, Waugh N, Thomas S: Routine hospital admission versus out-patient or home care in children at diagnosis of type 1 diabetes mellitus. Cochrane Database Syst Rev CD004099, 2003.
9. Laron Z, Galatzer A, Amir S, et al: A multidisciplinary, comprehensive, ambulatory treatment scheme for diabetes mellitus in children. Diabetes Care 2:342–348, 1979.
10. Laron Z: The multidisciplinary team for children and adolescents with diabetes mellitus. J Pediatr Endocrinol Metab 15:1109–1111, 2002.
11. Drozda DJ, Dawson VA, Long DJ, et al: Assessment of the effect of a comprehensive diabetes management program on hospital admission rates of children with diabetes mellitus. Diabetes Educ 16:389–393, 1990.
12. Hoffman WH, O'Neill P, Khoury C, et al: Service and education for the insulin-dependent child. Diabetes Care 1:285–288, 1978.
13. Allen H, Yarnie S, Murray M, et al: Personnel costs and perceived benefit of telephone care in the management of children with type 1 diabetes. Pediatr Diabetes 3:95–100, 2002.

14. Halverson M, Chang N, Hartwick N, et al: Cost effectiveness of telephone advice given by CDEs in a childhood diabetes center. Diabetes 49(Suppl 1):A219, 2000.

15. Siminerio L, McLaughlin S, Polonsky W: Diabetes Education Goals, 3rd ed. Alexandria, VA, American Diabetes Association, 2002.

16. The Diabetes Control and Complications Trial Research Group: The effect of intensive treatment of diabetes on the development and progression of long-term complications in insulin-dependent diabetes mellitus. New Engl J Med 329:977–986, 1993.

17. The Diabetes Control and Complications Trial Research Group: Effect of intensive diabetes treatment on the development and progression of long-term complications in adolescents with insulin-dependent diabetes mellitus. J Pediatr 125:177–188, 1994.

18. Reichard P, Nilsson BY, Rosenqvist U: The effect of long-term intensified insulin treatment on the development of microvascular complications of diabetes mellitus [see comments]. N Engl J Med 329:304–309, 1993.

19. UK Prospective Diabetes Study (UKPDS) Group: Intensive blood-glucose control with sulphonylureas or insulin compared with conventional treatment and risk of complications in patients with type 2 diabetes (UKPDS 33). Lancet 352:837–853, 1998.

20. UK Prospective Diabetes Study (UKPDS) Group: Effect of intensive blood-glucose control with metformin on complications in overweight patients with type 2 diabetes (UKPDS 34). Lancet 352:854–865, 1998.

21. The Diabetes Control and Complications Trial/Epidemiology of Diabetes Interventions and Complications Research Group: Retinopathy and nephropathy in patients with type 1 diabetes four years after a trial of intensive therapy. N Engl J Med 342:381–389, 2000.

22. The Diabetes Control and Complications Trial/Epidemiology of Diabetes Interventions and Complications Research Group: Effect of intensive therapy on the microvascular complications of type 1 diabetes mellitus. JAMA 287:2563–2569, 2002.

23. American Diabetes Association: Standards of medical care in diabetes. Diabetes Care 27:S15–S35, 2004.

24. Chase HP: Glycemic control in prepubertal years. Diabetes Care 26:1304–1305, 2003.

25. Kostraba JN, Dorman JS, Orchard TJ, et al: Contribution of diabetes duration before puberty to development of microvascular complications in IDDM subjects. Diabetes Care 12:686–693, 1989.

26. Holl RW, Lang GE, Grabert M, et al: Diabetic retinopathy in pediatric patients with type-1 diabetes: Effect of diabetes duration, prepubertal and pubertal onset of diabetes, and

metabolic control. J Pediatr 132:790–794, 1998.

27. Burger W, Hovener G, Dusterhus R, et al: Prevalence and development of retinopathy in children and adolescents with type 1 (insulin-dependent) diabetes mellitus: A longitudinal study. Diabetologia 29:17–22, 1986.

28. McNally PG, Raymond NT, Swift PG, et al: Does the prepubertal duration of diabetes influence the onset of microvascular complications? Diabet Med 10:906–908, 1993.

29. Donaghue KC, Fung AT, Hing S, et al: The effect of prepubertal diabetes duration on diabetes: Microvascular complications in early and late adolescence. Diabetes Care 20:77–80, 1997.

30. Holl RW, Grabert M, Thon A, et al: Urinary excretion of albumin in adolescents with type 1 diabetes: Persistent versus intermittent microalbuminuria and relationship to duration of diabetes, sex, and metabolic control. Diabetes Care 22:1555–1560, 1999.

31. Donaghue KC, Fairchild JM, Craig ME, et al: Do all prepubertal years of diabetes duration contribute equally to diabetes complications? Diabetes Care 26:1224–1229, 2003.

32. International Society for Pediatric and Adolescent Diabetes (ISPAD): ISPAD Consensus Guidelines for the Management of Type 1 Diabetes Mellitus in Children and Adolescents. 2000, www.ispad.org.

33. Krolewski AS, Laffel LM, Krolewski M, et al: Glycosylated hemoglobin and the risk of microalbuminuria in patients with insulin-dependent diabetes mellitus. N Engl J Med 332:1251–1255, 1995.

34. Warram JH, Scott LJ, Hanna LS, et al: Progression of microalbuminuria to proteinuria in type 1 diabetes: Nonlinear relationship with hyperglycemia. Diabetes 49:94–100, 2000.

35. Mortensen HB, Robertson KJ, Aanstoot HJ, et al: Insulin management and metabolic control of type 1 diabetes mellitus in childhood and adolescence in 18 countries: Hvidore Study Group on Childhood Diabetes. Diabet Med 15:752–759, 1998.

36. Danne T, Mortensen HB, Hougaard P, et al: Persistent differences among centers over 3 years in glycemic control and hypoglycemia in a study of 3,805 children and adolescents with type 1 diabetes from the Hvidore Study Group. Diabetes Care 24:1342–1347, 2001.

37. Rosilio M, Cotton JB, Wieliczko MC, et al: Factors associated with glycemic control. A cross–sectional nationwide study in 2,579 French children with type 1 diabetes: The French Pediatric Diabetes Group. Diabetes Care 21:1146–1153, 1998.

38. Holl RW, Swift PG, Mortensen HB, et al: Insulin injection regimens and metabolic control in an international survey of adolescents with type 1

diabetes over 3 years: Results from the Hvidore study group. Eur J Pediatr 162:22–29, 2003.

39. Casella S, Mongilio M, Plotnick L, et al: Accuracy and precision of low-dose insulin administration. Pediatrics 91:977–986, 1993.

40. Silva S, Clark L, Goodman S, et al: Can caretakers of children with IDDM accurately measure small insulin doses and dose changes? Diabetes Care 19:56–59, 1996.

41. Fanelli CG, Pampanelli S, Porcellati F, et al: Administration of neutral protamine Hagedorn insulin at bedtime versus with dinner in type 1 diabetes mellitus to avoid nocturnal hypoglycemia and improve control: A randomized, controlled trial. Ann Intern Med 136:504–514, 2002.

42. Schober E, Schoenle E, Van Dyk J, et al: Comparative trial between insulin glargine and NPH insulin in children and adolescents with type 1 diabetes mellitus. J Pediatr Endocrinol Metab 15:369–376, 2002.

43. Lepore M, Pampanelli S, Fanelli C, et al: Pharmacokinetics and pharmacodynamics of subcutaneous injection of long-acting human insulin analog glargine, NPH insulin, and ultralente human insulin and continuous subcutaneous infusion of insulin lispro. Diabetes 49:2142–2148, 2000.

44. Murphy NP, Keane SM, Ong KK, et al: Randomized cross-over trial of insulin glargine plus lispro or NPH insulin plus regular human insulin in adolescents with type 1 diabetes on intensive insulin regimens. Diabetes Care 26:799–804, 2003.

45. Chase HP, Dixon B, Pearson J, et al: Reduced hypoglycemic episodes and improved glycemic control in children with type 1 diabetes using insulin glargine and neutral protamine Hagedorn insulin. J Pediatr 143:737–740, 2003.

46. Amiel SA, Caprio S, Sherwin RS, et al: Insulin resistance of puberty: A defect restricted to peripheral glucose metabolism. J Clin Endocrinol Metab 72:277–282, 1991.

47. Mohn A, Matyka KA, Harris DA, et al: Lispro or regular insulin for multiple injection therapy in adolescence. Differences in free insulin and glucose levels overnight. Diabetes Care 22:27–32, 1999.

48. Chase HP, Saib SZ, MacKenzie T, et al: Post-prandial glucose excursions following four methods of bolus insulin administration in subjects with type 1 diabetes. Diabet Med 19:317–321, 2002.

49. Pickup J, Mattock M, Kerry S: Glycaemic control with continuous subcutaneous insulin infusion compared with intensive insulin injections in patients with type 1 diabetes: Meta-analysis of randomised controlled trials. Br Med J 324:705, 2002.

50. Weissberg-Benchell J, Antisdel-Lomaglio J, Seshadri R: Insulin Pump Therapy: A meta-analysis. Diabetes Care 26:1079–1087, 2003.

51. Schade DS, Valentine V: To pump or not to pump. Diabetes Care 25:2100–2102, 2002.

52. Grey M, Boland EA, Davidson M, et al: Short-term effects of coping skills training as adjunct to intensive therapy in adolescents. Diabetes Care 21:902–908, 1998.

53. Boland EA, Grey M, Oesterle A, et al: Continuous subcutaneous insulin infusion: A new way to lower risk of severe hypoglycemia, improve metabolic control, and enhance coping in adolescents with type 1 diabetes. Diabetes Care 22:1779–1784, 1999.

54. American Diabetes Association: Standards of medical care for patients with diabetes mellitus. Diabetes Care 26:S33–S50, 2003.

55. The Diabetes Control and Complications Trial Research Group: Adverse events and their association with treatment regimens in the diabetes control and complications trial. Diabetes Care 18:1415–1427, 1995.

56. Carlson MG, Campbell PJ: Intensive insulin therapy and weight gain in IDDM. Diabetes 42:1700–1707, 1993.

57. American Diabetes Association: Type 2 diabetes in children and adolescents (Consensus statement). Diabetes Care 23:381–389, 2000.

58. Franz MJ, Bantle JP, Beebe CA, et al: Evidence-based nutrition principles and recommendations for the treatment and prevention of diabetes and related complications. Diabetes Care 25:148–198, 2002.

59. Jenkins DJA, Wolever TMS, Taylor RH, et al: Glycemic index of foods: A physiological basis for carbohydrate exchange. Am J Clin Nutr 34:362–366, 1981.

60. Wolever TM: The glycemic index: Flogging a dead horse? Diabetes Care 20:452–456, 1997.

61. Gilbertson HR, Brand-Miller JC, Thorburn AW, et al: The effect of flexible low glycemic index dietary advice versus measured carbohydrate exchange diets on glycemic control in children with type 1 diabetes. Diabetes Care 24:1137–1143, 2001.

62. Wolfsdorf J, Quinn M, Laredo R: Diabetes Mellitus. In Walker WA, Watkins J, Duggan C (eds): Nutrition in Pediatrics: Basic Science and Clinical Applications. Hamilton, Ontario, BC Decker, 2003, pp 722–737.

63. Food and Nutrition Board, Institute of Medicine: Dietary, functional, and total fiber. In Dietary Reference Intakes for Energy, Carbohydrate, Fiber, Fat, Fatty Acids, Cholesterol, Protein, and Amino Acids. Washington, DC, National Academies Press, 2002, pp 265–334.

64. Birch LL, Johnson SL, Andresen G, et al: The variability of young children's energy intake. N Engl J Med 324:232–235, 1991.

65. Rutledge KS, Chase HP, Klingensmith GJ, et al: Effectiveness of postprandial Humalog in toddlers with diabetes. Pediatrics 100:968–972, 1997.

66. Tupola S, Komulainen J, Jaaskelainen J, et al: Post-prandial insulin lispro vs. human regular insulin in prepubertal children with Type 1 diabetes mellitus. Diabet Med 18:654–658, 2001.

67. Delahanty LM, Halford BN: The role of diet behaviors in achieving improved glycemic control in intensively treated patients in the Diabetes Control and Complications Trial. Diabetes Care 16:1453–1458, 1993.

68. Reisman D: Mild diabetes in children. Am J Med Sci 151:40–45, 1916.

69. Fagot–Campagna A, Pettitt DJ, Engelgau MM, et al: Type 2 diabetes among North American children and adolescents: An epidemiologic review and a public health perspective. J Pediatr 136:664–672, 2000.

70. Kitagawa T, Owada M, Urakami T, et al: Increased incidence of non-insulin dependent diabetes mellitus among Japanese schoolchildren correlates with an increased intake of animal protein and fat. Clin Pediatr (Phila) 37:111–115, 1998.

71. Kadiki OA, Reddy MR, Marzouk AA: Incidence of insulindependent diabetes (IDDM) and non-insulin-dependent diabetes (NIDDM) (0-34 years at onset) in Benghazi, Libya. Diabetes Res Clin Pract 32:165–173, 1996.

72. Pinhas-Hamiel O, Dolan LM, Daniels SR, et al: Increased incidence of non-insulin-dependent diabetes mellitus among adolescents. J Pediatr 128:608–615, 1996.

73. Neufeld ND, Raffel LJ, Landon C, et al: Early presentation of type 2 diabetes in Mexican-American youth. Diabetes Care 21:80–86, 1998.

74. Ogden CL, Flegal KM, Carroll MD, et al: Prevalence and trends in overweight among US children and adolescents, 1999–2000. JAMA 288:1728–1732, 2002.

75. Caprio S, Tamborlane WV: Metabolic impact of obesity in childhood. Endocrinol Metab Clin North Am 28:731–747, 1999.

76. Steinberger J, Moran A, Hong CP, et al: Adiposity in childhood predicts obesity and insulin resistance in young adulthood. J Pediatr 138:469–473, 2001.

77. Arslanian S, Suprasongsin C: Insulin sensitivity, lipids, and body composition in childhood: is "syndrome X" present? J Clin Endocrinol Metab 81:1058–1062, 1996.

78. Ritchie L, Ganapathy S, Woodward-Lopez G, et al: Prevention of type 2 diabetes in youth: Etiology, promising interventions and recommendations. Pediatr Diabetes 4:174–209, 2003.

79. Goran MI, Gower BA: Longitudinal study on pubertal insulin resistance. Diabetes 50:2444–2450, 2001.

80. Libman IM, Pietropaolo M, Arslanian SA, et al: Changing prevalence of overweight children and adolescents at onset of insulin-treated diabetes. Diabetes Care 26:2871–2875, 2003.

81. Knowler WC, Barrett-Connor E, Fowler SE, et al: Reduction in the incidence of type 2 diabetes with lifestyle intervention or metformin. N Engl J Med 346:393–403, 2002.

82. Cook VV, Hurley JS: Prevention of type 2 diabetes in childhood. Clin Pediatr (Phila) 37:123–129, 1998.

83. Golan M, Weizman A, Apter A, et al: Parents as the exclusive agents of change in the treatment of childhood obesity. Am J Clin Nutr 67:1130–1135, 1998.

84. Brand-Miller J, Hayne S, Petocz P, et al: Low-glycemic index diets in the management of diabetes: A meta-analysis of randomized controlled trials. Diabetes Care 26:2261–2267, 2003.

85. Jones KL, Arslanian S, Peterokova VA, et al: Effect of metformin in pediatric patients with type 2 diabetes: A randomized controlled trial. Diabetes Care 25:89–94, 2002.

86. Dunn CJ, Peters DH: Metformin. A review of its pharmacological properties and therapeutic use in non-insulin-dependent diabetes mellitus. Drugs 49:721–749, 1995.

87. Salpeter SR, Greyber E, Pasternak GA, et al: Risk of fatal and nonfatal lactic acidosis with metformin use in type 2 diabetes mellitus: Systematic review and meta-analysis. Arch Intern Med 163:2594–2602, 2003.

88. Yki-Jarvinen H, Dressler A, Ziemen M: Less nocturnal hypoglycemia and better post-dinner glucose control with bedtime insulin glargine compared with bedtime NPH insulin during insulin combination therapy in type 2 diabetes: HOE 901/3002 Study Group. Diabetes Care 23:1130–1136, 2000.

89. Riddle MC, Rosenstock J, Gerich J: The treat-to-target trial: Randomized addition of glargine or human NPH insulin to oral therapy of type 2 diabetic patients. Diabetes Care 26:3080–3086, 2003.

90. Yokoyama H, Okudaira M, Otani T, et al: High incidence of diabetic nephropathy in early-onset Japanese NIDDM patients: Risk analysis. Diabetes Care 21:1080–1085, 1998.

91. Fajans SS: Scope and heterogeneous nature of MODY. Diabetes Care 13:49–64, 1990.

92. Fajans SS, Bell GI, Polonsky KS: Molecular mechanisms and clinical pathophysiology of maturity-onset diabetes of the young. N Engl J Med 345:971–980, 2001.

93. Winter WE, Maclaren NK, Riley WJ, et al: Maturity-onset diabetes of youth in black Americans. N Engl J Med 316:285–291, 1987.

94. Maassen JA: Mitochondrial diabetes: Pathophysiology, clinical presentation, and genetic analysis. Am J Med Genet 115:66–70, 2002.

95. Moran A, Doherty L, Wang X, et al: Abnormal glucose metabolism in cystic fibrosis. J Pediatr 133:10–17, 1998.

96. Hardin DS, Moran A: Diabetes mellitus in cystic fibrosis. Endocrinol Metab Clin North Am 28:787–800, 1999.

97. Moran A, Hardin D, Rodman D, et al: Diagnosis, screening and management of cystic fibrosis related diabetes mellitus: A consensus conference report. Diabetes Res Clin Pract 45:61–73, 1999.

98. Levine BS, Anderson BJ, Butler DA, et al: Predictors of glycemic control and short-term adverse outcomes in youth with type 1 diabetes. J Pediatr 139:197–203, 2001.

99. McGowan K, Thomas W, Moran A: Spurious reporting of nocturnal hypoglycemia by CGMS in patients with tightly controlled type 1 diabetes. Diabetes Care 25:1499–1503, 2002.

100. Diabetes Research in Children Network (DIRECNET) Study Group: The accuracy of the GlucoWatch G2 biographer in children with type 1 diabetes: Results of the diabetes research in children network (DirecNet) accuracy study. Diabetes Technol Ther 5:791–800, 2003.

101. Diabetes Research in Children Network (DIRECNET) Study Group: The accuracy of the CGMS in children with type 1 diabetes: Results of the diabetes research in children network (DirecNet) accuracy study. Diabetes Technol Ther 5:781–789, 2003.

102. Laffel L: Sick-day management in type 1 diabetes. Endocrinol Metab Clin North Am 29:707–723, 2000.

103. Rohlfing CL, Wiedmeyer HM, Little RR, et al: Defining the relationship between plasma glucose and HbA(1c): analysis of glucose profiles and HbA(1c) in the Diabetes Control and Complications Trial. Diabetes Care 25:275–278, 2002.

104. Cryer PE: Banting Lecture. Hypoglycemia: The limiting factor in the management of IDDM. Diabetes 43:1378–1389, 1994.

105. Cox DJ, Irvine A, Gonder-Frederick L, et al: Fear of hypoglycemia: Quantification, validation, and utilization. Diabetes Care 10:617–621, 1987.

106. Gonder-Frederick LA, Clarke WL, Cox DJ: The emotional, social, and behavioral implications of insulin-induced hypoglycemia. Semin Clin Neuropsychiatry 2:57–65, 1997.

107. Clarke WL, Gonder-Frederick A, Snyder AL, et al: Maternal fear of hypoglycemia in their children with insulin dependent diabetes mellitus. J Pediatr Endocrinol Metab 11(Suppl 1):189–194, 1998.

108. Santiago JV: Nocturnal hypoglycemia in children with diabetes: An important problem revisited. J Pediatr 131:2–4, 1997.

109. Gerich JE, Langlois M, Noacco C, et al: Lack of glucagon response to hypoglycemia in diabetes: Evidence for an intrinsic pancreatic alpha cell defect. Science 182:171–173, 1973.

110. Bolli G, Calabrese G, De Feo P, et al: Lack of glucagon response in glucose counter-regulation in type 1 (insulin-dependent) diabetics: Absence of recovery after prolonged optimal insulin therapy. Diabetologia 22:100–105, 1982.

111. Cryer PE: Iatrogenic hypoglycemia as a cause of hypoglycemia-associated autonomic failure in IDDM: A vicious cycle. Diabetes 41:255–260, 1992.

112. Heller SR, Cryer PE: Reduced neuroendocrine and symptomatic responses to subsequent hypoglycemia after 1 episode of hypoglycemia in nondiabetic humans. Diabetes 40:223–226, 1991.

113. Dagogo-Jack SE, Craft S, Cryer PE: Hypoglycemia-associated autonomic failure in insulin-dependent diabetes mellitus: Recent antecedent hypoglycemia reduces autonomic responses to, symptoms of, and defense against subsequent hypoglycemia. J Clin Invest 91:819–828, 1993.

114. Aman J, Karlsson I, Wranne L: Symptomatic hypoglycaemia in childhood diabetes: A population-based questionnaire study. Diabet Med 6:257–261, 1989.

115. Tupola S, Rajantie J: Documented symptomatic hypoglycaemia in children and adolescents using multiple daily insulin injection therapy. Diabet Med 15:492–496, 1998.

116. Hepburn DA, Deary IJ, Frier BM, et al: Symptoms of acute insulin-induced hypoglycemia in humans with and without IDDM. Factor-analysis approach. Diabetes Care 14:949–957, 1991.

117. McCrimmon RJ, Gold AE, Deary IJ, et al: Symptoms of hypoglycemia in children with IDDM. Diabetes Care 18:858–861, 1995.

118. Dammacco F, Torelli C, Frezza E, et al: Problems of hypoglycemia arising in children and adolescents with insulin-dependent diabetes mellitus: The Diabetes Study Group of The Italian Society of Pediatric Endocrinology & Diabetes. J Pediatr Endocrinol Metab 11(Suppl 1):167–176, 1998.

119. Boyle PJ, Schwartz NS, Shah SD, et al: Plasma glucose concentrations at the onset of hypoglycemic symptoms in patients with poorly controlled diabetes and in nondiabetics. N Engl J Med 318:1487–1492, 1988.

120. Ryan C, Vega A, Drash A: Cognitive deficits in adolescents who developed diabetes early in life. Pediatrics 75:921–927, 1985.

121. Rovet JF, Ehrlich RM, Hoppe M: Intellectual deficits associated with early onset of insulin-dependent diabetes mellitus in children. Diabetes Care 10:510–515, 1987.

122. Northam EA, Anderson PJ, Werther GA, et al: Neuropsychological complications of IDDM in children 2 years after disease onset. Diabetes Care 21:379–384, 1998.

123. Northam EA, Anderson PJ, Jacobs R, et al: Neuropsychological profiles of children with type 1 diabetes 6 years after disease onset. Diabetes Care 24:1541–1546, 2001.

124. Schoenle EJ, Schoenle D, Molinari L, et al: Impaired intellectual development in children with Type I diabetes: Association with HbA(1c), age at diagnosis and sex. Diabetologia 45:108–114, 2002.

125. Hershey T, Lillie R, Sadler M, et al: Severe hypoglycemia and long-term spatial memory in children with type 1 diabetes mellitus: A retrospective study. J Int Neuropsychol Soc 9:740–750, 2003.

126. Rovet JF, Ehrlich RM: The effect of hypoglycemic seizures on cognitive function in children with diabetes: A 7-year prospective study. J Pediatr 134:503–506, 1999.

127. Jones T, Davis E: Hypoglycemia in children with type 1 diabetes: Current issues and controversies. Pediatr Diabetes 4:143–150, 2003.

128. Rovet JF, Ehrlich RM, Hoppe M: Specific intellectual deficits in children with early onset diabetes mellitus. Child Dev 59:226–234, 1988.

129. Golden MP, Ingersoll GM, Brack CJ, et al: Longitudinal relationship of asymptomatic hypoglycemia to cognitive function in IDDM. Diabetes Care 12:89–93, 1989.

130. Hershey T, Bhargava N, Sadler M, et al: Conventional versus intensive diabetes therapy in children with type 1 diabetes: Effects on memory and motor speed. Diabetes Care 22:1318–1324, 1999.

131. Ryan CM, Becker DJ: Hypoglycemia in children with type 1 diabetes mellitus: Risk factors, cognitive function, and management. Endocrinol Metab Clin North Am 28:883–900, 1999.

132. Frier BM, Matthews DM, Steel JM, et al: Driving and insulin-dependent diabetes. Lancet 1:1232–1234, 1980.

133. Songer TJ, LaPorte RE, Dorman JS, et al: Motor vehicle accidents and IDDM. Diabetes Care 11:701–707, 1988.

134. Ratner RE, Whitehouse FW: Motor vehicles, hypoglycemia, and diabetic drivers. Diabetes Care 12:217–222, 1989.

135. Edge JA, Ford-Adams ME, Dunger DB: Causes of death in children with insulin dependent diabetes 1990–96. Arch Dis Child 81:318–323, 1999.

136. Macfarlane PI, Walters M, Stutchfield P, et al: A prospective study of symptomatic hypoglycaemia in childhood diabetes. Diabet Med 6:627–630, 1989.

137. Tupola S, Rajantie J, Maenpaa J: Severe hypoglycaemia in children and adolescents during multiple-dose insulin therapy. Diabet Med 15:695–699, 1998.

138. Goldstein DE, England JD, Hess R, et al: A prospective study of symptomatic hypoglycemia in young diabetic patients. Diabetes Care 4:601–605, 1981.

139. Daneman D, Frank M, Perlman K, et al: Severe hypoglycemia in children with insulin-dependent diabetes mellitus: Frequency and predisposing factors. J Pediatr 115:681–685, 1989.

140. Bergada I, Suissa S, Dufresne J, et al: Severe hypoglycemia in IDDM children. Diabetes Care 12:239–244, 1989.

141. Soltesz G, Acsadi G: Association between diabetes, severe hypoglycaemia, and electroencephalographic abnormalities. Arch Dis Child 64:992–996, 1989.

142. Bhatia V, Wolfsdorf JI: Severe hypoglycemia in youth with insulin-dependent diabetes mellitus: Frequency and causative factors. Pediatrics 88:1187–1193, 1991.

143. Egger M, Gschwend S, Smith GD, et al: Increasing incidence of hypoglycemic coma in children with IDDM. Diabetes Care 14:1001–1005, 1991.

144. Limbert C, Schwingshandl J, Haas J, et al: Severe hypoglycemia in children and adolescents with IDDM: Frequency and associated factors. J Diabetes Complications 7:216–220, 1993.

145. Diabetes Control and Complications Trial Research Group: Effect of intensive diabetes treatment on the development and progression of long-term complications in adolescents with insulin-dependent diabetes mellitus: Diabetes Control and Complications Trial. J Pediatr 125:177–188, 1994.

146. Dumont RH, Jacobson AM, Cole C, et al: Psychosocial predictors of acute complications of diabetes in youth. Diabet Med 12:612–618, 1995.

147. Verrotti A, Chiarelli F, Blasetti A, et al: Severe hypoglycemia in insulin-dependent diabetic children treated by multiple injection insulin regimen. Acta Diabetol 33:53–57, 1996.

148. Bognetti F, Brunelli A, Meschi F, et al: Frequency and correlates of severe hypoglycaemia in children and adolescents with diabetes mellitus. Eur J Pediatr 156:589–591, 1997.

149. Mortensen HB, Hougaard P: Comparison of metabolic control in a cross-sectional study of 2,873 children and adolescents with IDDM from 18 countries: The Hvidore Study Group on Childhood Diabetes. Diabetes Care 20:714–720, 1997. [Published erratum appears in Diabetes Care 20(7):1216, 1997.]

150. Davis EA, Keating B, Byrne GC, et al: Hypoglycemia: Incidence and clinical predictors in a large population-based sample of children and adolescents with IDDM. Diabetes Care 20:22–25, 1997.

151. Nordfeldt S, Ludvigsson J: Severe hypoglycemia in children with IDDM: A prospective population study, 1992–1994. Diabetes Care 20:497–503, 1997.

152. Chase HP, Lockspeiser T, Peery B, et al: The impact of the diabetes control and complications trial and humalog insulin on glycohemoglobin levels and severe hypoglycemia in type 1 diabetes. Diabetes Care 24:430–434, 2001.

153. Lteif AN, Schwenk WF 2nd: Type 1 diabetes mellitus in early childhood: Glycemic control and associated risk of hypoglycemic reactions. Mayo Clin Proc 74:211–216, 1999.

154. Nordfeldt S, Ludvigsson J: Adverse events in intensively treated children and adolescents with type 1 diabetes. Acta Paediatr 88:1184–1193, 1999.

155. Rewers A, Chase HP, Mackenzie T, et al: Predictors of acute complications in children with type 1 diabetes. JAMA 287:2511–2518, 2002.

156. Clarke WL, Gonder-Frederick L, Cox DJ: The frequency of severe hypoglycaemia in children with insulin-dependent diabetes mellitus. Horm Res 45:48–52, 1996.

157. Barkai L, Vamosi I, Lukacs K: Prospective assessment of severe hypoglycaemia in diabetic children and adolescents with impaired and normal awareness of hypoglycaemia. Diabetologia 41:898–903, 1998.

158. Allen C, LeCaire T, Palta M, et al: Risk factors for frequent and severe hypoglycemia in type 1 diabetes. Diabetes Care 24:1878–1881, 2001.

159. Davis EA, Keating B, Byrne GC, et al: Impact of improved glycaemic control on rates of hypoglycaemia in insulin dependent diabetes mellitus. Arch Dis Child 78:111–115, 1998.

160. Thomsett M, Shield G, Batch J, et al: How well are we doing?: Metabolic control in patients with diabetes. J Paediatr Child Health 35:479–482, 1999.

161. The Diabetes Control and Complications Trial Research Group: Hypoglycemia in the Diabetes Control and Complications Trial. Diabetes 46:271–286, 1997.

162. Jacobson AM, Hauser ST, Wolfsdorf JI, et al: Psychologic predictors of compliance in children with recent onset of diabetes mellitus. J Pediatr 110:805–811, 1987.

163. Kaufman FR, Gibson LC, Halvorson M, et al: A pilot study of the continuous glucose monitoring system: Clinical decisions and glycemic control after its use in pediatric type 1 diabetic subjects. Diabetes Care 24:2030–2034, 2001.

164. Boland E, Monsod T, Delucia M, et al: Limitations of conventional methods of self-monitoring of blood glucose: Lessons learned from 3 days of continuous glucose sensing in pediatric patients with type 1 diabetes. Diabetes Care 24:1858–1862, 2001.

165. Nordfeldt S, Johansson C, Carlsson E, et al: Prevention of severe hypoglycaemia in type I diabetes: A randomised controlled population study. Arch Dis Child 88:240–245, 2003.

166. Ludvigsson J, Hanas R: Continuous subcutaneous glucose monitoring improved metabolic control in pediatric patients with type 1 diabetes: A controlled crossover study. Pediatrics 111:933–938, 2003.

167. Amin R, Ross K, Acerini CL, et al: Hypoglycemia prevalence in prepubertal children with type 1 diabetes on standard insulin regimen: Use of continuous glucose monitoring system. Diabetes Care 26:662–667, 2003.

168. Maniatis AK, Klingensmith GJ, Slover RH, et al: Continuous subcutaneous insulin infusion therapy for children and adolescents: An option for routine diabetes care. Pediatrics 107:351–356, 2001.

169. Linkeschova R, Raoul M, Bott U, et al: Less severe hypoglycaemia, better metabolic control, and improved quality of life in Type 1 diabetes mellitus with continuous subcutaneous insulin infusion (CSII) therapy: An observational study of 100 consecutive patients followed for a mean of 2 years. Diabet Med 19:746–751, 2002.

170. Ahern J, Boland E, Doane R, et al: Insulin pump therapy in pediatrics: A therapeutic alternative to safely lower HbA1c levels across all age groups. Pediatr Diabetes 3:10–15, 2002.

171. The Diabetes Control and Complications Trial Research Group: Epidemiology of severe hypoglycemia in the diabetes control and complications trial: The DCCT Research Group. Am J Med 90:450–459, 1991.

172. Gale EA, Tattersall RB: Unrecognised nocturnal hypoglycaemia in insulin-treated diabetics. Lancet 1:1049–1052, 1979.

173. Winter RJ: Profiles of metabolic control in diabetic children: Frequency of asymptomatic nocturnal hypoglycemia. Metabolism 30:666–672, 1981.

174. Shalwitz RA, Farkas-Hirsch R, White NH, et al: Prevalence and consequences of nocturnal hypoglycemia among conventionally treated children with diabetes mellitus. J Pediatr 116:685–689, 1990.

175. Porter PA, Byrne G, Stick S, et al: Nocturnal hypoglycaemia and sleep disturbances in young teenagers with insulin dependent diabetes mellitus. Arch Dis Child 75:120–123, 1996.

176. Porter PA, Keating B, Byrne G, et al: Incidence and predictive criteria of nocturnal hypoglycemia in young children with insulin-dependent diabetes mellitus. J Pediatr 130:366–372, 1997.

177. Beregszaszi M, Tubiana-Rufi N, Benali K, et al: Nocturnal hypoglycemia in children and adolescents with insulin-dependent diabetes mellitus: Prevalence and risk factors. J Pediatr 131:27–33, 1997.

178. Lopez MJ, Oyarzabal M, Barrio R, et al: Nocturnal hypoglycaemia in IDDM patients younger than 18 years. Diabet Med 14:772–777, 1997.

179. Matyka KA, Crowne EC, Havel PJ, et al: Counterregulation during spontaneous nocturnal hypoglycemia in prepubertal children with type 1 diabetes. Diabetes Care 22:1144–1150, 1999.

180. Matyka KA, Crawford C, Wiggs L, et al: Alterations in sleep physiology in young children with insulin-dependent diabetes mellitus: Relationship to nocturnal hypoglycemia. J Pediatr 137:233–238, 2000.

181. Jones TW, Porter P, Sherwin RS, et al: Decreased epinephrine responses to hypoglycemia during sleep. N Engl J Med 338:1657–1662, 1998.

182. Banarer S, Cryer PE: Sleep-related hypoglycemia-associated autonomic failure in type 1 diabetes: Reduced awakening from sleep during hypoglycemia. Diabetes 52:1195–1203, 2003.

183. Veneman T, Mitrakou A, Mokan M, et al: Induction of hypoglycemia unawareness by asymptomatic nocturnal hypoglycemia. Diabetes 42:1233–1237, 1993.

184. Brodows RG, Williams C, Amatruda JM: Treatment of insulin reactions in diabetics. JAMA 252:3378–3381, 1984.

185. Haymond MW, Schreiner B: Mini-dose glucagon rescue for hypoglycemia in children with type 1 diabetes. Diabetes Care 24:643–645, 2001.

186. Muhlhauser I, Koch J, Berger M: Pharmacokinetics and bioavailability of injected glucagon: Differences between intramuscular, subcutaneous, and intravenous administration. Diabetes Care 8:39–42, 1985.

187. Slama G, Alamowitch C, Desplanque N, et al: A new non-invasive method for treating insulin–reaction: Intranasal lyophylized glucagon. Diabetologia 33:671–674, 1990.

188. Lala VR, Vedanarayana VV, Ganesh S, et al: Hypoglycemic hemiplegia in an adolescent with insulin-dependent diabetes mellitus: A case report and a review of the literature. J Emerg Med 7:233–236, 1989.

189. Wayne EA, Dean HJ, Booth F, et al: Focal neurologic deficits associated with hypoglycemia in children with diabetes. J Pediatr 117:575–577, 1990.

190. Shehadeh N, Kassem J, Tchaban I, et al: High incidence of hypoglycemic episodes with neurologic manifestations in children with insulin dependent diabetes mellitus. J Pediatr Endocrinol Metab 11 (Suppl 1):183–187, 1998.

191. Curtis JR, To T, Muirhead S, et al: Recent trends in hospitalization for diabetic ketoacidosis in Ontario children. Diabetes Care 25:1591–1596, 2002.

192. Morris AD, Boyle DI, McMahon AD, et al: Adherence to insulin treatment, glycaemic control, and ketoacidosis in insulin-dependent diabetes mellitus: The DARTS/MEMO Collaboration. Diabetes Audit and Research in Tayside Scotland. Medicines Monitoring Unit. Lancet 350:1505–1510, 1997.

193. Smith CP, Firth D, Bennett S, et al: Ketoacidosis occurring in newly diagnosed and established diabetic children. Acta Paediat 87:537–541, 1998.

194. Golden MP, Herrold AJ, Orr DP: An approach to prevention of recurrent diabetic ketoacidosis in the pediatric population. J Pediatr 107:195–200, 1985.

195. Glasgow AM, Weissberg-Benchell J, Tynan WD, et al: Readmissions of children with diabetes mellitus to a children's hospital. Pediatrics 88:98–104, 1991.

196. Edge JA, Hawkins MM, Winter DL, et al: The risk and outcome of cerebral oedema developing during diabetic ketoacidosis. Arch Dis Child 85:16–22, 2001.

197. Glaser N, Barnett P, McCaslin I, et al: Risk factors for cerebral edema in children with diabetic ketoacidosis: The Pediatric Emergency Medicine Collaborative Research Committee of the American Academy of Pediatrics. N Engl J Med 344:264–269, 2001.

198. Franklin B, Liu J, Ginsberg-Fellner F: Cerebral edema and ophthalmoplegia reversed by mannitol in a new case of insulin-dependent diabetes mellitus. Pediatrics 69:87–90, 1982.

199. Shabbir N, Oberfield SE, Corrales R, et al: Recovery from symptomatic brain swelling in diabetic ketoacidosis. Clin Pediatr (Phila) 31:570–573, 1992.

200. Roberts MD, Slover RH, Chase HP: Diabetic ketoacidosis with intracerebral complications. Pediatr Diabetes 2:109–114, 2001.

201. Kamat P, Vats A, Gross M, et al: Use of hypertonic saline for the treatment of altered mental status associated with diabetic ketoacidosis. Pediatr Crit Care Med 4:239–242, 2003.

202. Marcin JP, Glaser N, Barnett P, et al: Factors associated with adverse outcomes in children with diabetic ketoacidosis-related cerebral edema. J Pediatr 141:793–797, 2002.

203. Kordonouri O, Klinghammer A, Lang EB, et al: Thyroid autoimmunity in children and adolescents with type 1 diabetes: A multicenter survey. Diabetes Care 25:1346–1350, 2002.

204. Devendra D, Eisenbarth GS: Immunologic endocrine disorders. J Allergy Clin Immunol 111:S624–S636, 2003.

205. Freemark M, Levitsky LL: Screening for celiac disease in children with type 1 diabetes: Two views of the controversy. Diabetes Care 26:1932–1939, 2003.

206. Sochett E, Daneman D: Early diabetes-related complications in children and adolescents with type 1 diabetes: Implications for screening and intervention. Endocrinol Metab Clin North Am 28:865–882, 1999.

207. Bojestig M, Arnqvist HJ, Hermansson G, et al: Declining incidence of nephropathy in insulin-dependent diabetes mellitus. N Engl J Med 330:15–18, 1994. [Published erratum appears in N Engl J Med 330(8):584, 1994.]

208. Plank J, Wutte A, Brunner G, et al: A direct comparison of insulin aspart and insulin lispro in patients with type 1 diabetes. Diabetes Care 25:2053–2057, 2002.

209. Yamagata K, Furuta H, Oda N, et al: Mutations in the hepatocyte nuclear factor-4alpha gene in maturity-onset diabetes of the young (MODY1). Nature 384:458–460, 1996.

210. Froguel P, Zouali H, Vionnet N, et al: Familial hyperglycemia due to mutations in glucokinase: Definition of a subtype of diabetes mellitus. N Engl J Med 328:697–702, 1993.

211. Yamagata K, Oda N, Kaisaki PJ, et al: Mutations in the hepatocyte nuclear factor-1alpha gene in maturity-onset diabetes of the young (MODY3). Nature 384:455–458, 1996.

212. Horikawa Y, Iwasaki N, Hara M, et al: Mutation in hepatocyte nuclear factor-1 beta gene (TCF2) associated with MODY. Nat Genet 17:384–385, 1997.

213. Malecki MT, Jhala US, Antonellis A, et al: Mutations in NEUROD1 are associated with the development of type 2 diabetes mellitus. Nat Genet 23:323–328, 1999.

Pancreatic and Islet Transplantation

Gordon C. Weir and Jason L. Gaglia

Both type 1 and type 2 diabetes are major and growing worldwide health problems largely due to their well-known vascular, eye, kidney, and neural complications. It is now accepted that these devastating problems are linked to hyperglycemia,[1,2] which strongly implies that normalization of glucose levels with proper treatment early in the course of the disease will prevent these complications. The cost of these complications in personal and financial terms is enormous. Despite impressive improvements in treatment thanks to self-glucose monitoring, advances in insulin therapy, new oral medications, and higher standards of care, many people with diabetes continue to develop disabling complications. A mechanical β-cell equivalent consisting of a glucose sensor and an insulin pump could provide patients with normoglycemia, but the development of a satisfactory glucose sensor has been frustrating in spite of many ingenious approaches.[3]

An obvious solution to reestablish normal feedback regulation would be to provide patients with β-cell replacement therapy, which can be done with pancreas or islet transplants. This concept was first tested, albeit unsuccessfully, some 28 years before the discovery of insulin. On December 20, 1893, Dr. Watson-Williams and his surgical colleague Mr. Harsant, at the Bristol Royal Infirmary, UK, transplanted three pieces of fresh sheep pancreas into the subcutaneous tissue of a 15-year-old boy with probable diabetic ketoacidosis.

Although there was a temporary improvement, the patient died 3 days later.[4] With the discovery of insulin by Banting, Best, Collip, and Macleod in 1922, diabetes was changed from a rapidly fatal disease to a chronic illness. However, as a chronic illness with potentially severe secondary complications and with a treatment with a relatively narrow therapeutic window, requiring administration by injection, the quest for β-cell replacement therapy has continued.

PANCREAS TRANSPLANTATION

The first clinical vascularized whole pancreas transplant was a duct-ligated segmental graft with a simultaneous kidney transplant performed by Drs. William Kelly and Richard Lillehei in 1966 at the University of Minnesota.[5] Over the next 15 years, the procedure was done in relatively few centers and with an initial low success rate, but as the surgical techniques improved and new immunosuppression approaches became available, by the mid-1980s, the procedure became widespread. As reported by the International Pancreas Transplant Registry (*www.iptr.umn.edu*), the number has steadily climbed, reaching a total of 1875 for 2002, with 1417 of these being done in the United States and 458 being done elsewhere. By June 2003, more than 19,600 reported pancreas transplants had been performed worldwide. The increased numbers are explained by both improved outcomes and better coverage by insurance.

MAJOR TYPES OF PANCREAS TRANSPLANTS

The most commonly performed transplant is the simultaneous pancreas-kidney (SPK) transplant, followed by pancreas after kidney (PAK) and pancreas transplant alone (PTA). The International Pancreas Transplant Registry reported that in the United States from October 1987 to October 2002, 78% (n = 10,412) were SPK, 14% (n = 1816) were PAK, and 6% (n = 777) were PTA. In the past 5 years, the proportion of PAK and PTA transplants has increased as evidenced by data obtained in 2001, with the following distribution in the United States being SPK 70% (n = 904), PAK 22% (n = 290), and PTA 8% (n = 103). Outside the United States, the proportion of PAK and PTA transplants is considerably lower. Decisions about pancreas transplantation are often driven by the availability of a kidney from a living-related donor because of the superior outcomes compared with dialysis. The PTA category includes cases of segmental transplants from living donors, with more than 100 being done at the University of Minnesota.[6]

ADVANCES IN SURGICAL TECHNIQUE

The evolution of surgical approaches to pancreas transplants has been detailed recently by Sutherland and Groth.[7] Various early approaches to drainage of exocrine secretion included duct ligation, duct obliteration, enteric drainage, and bladder drainage. The bladder drainage method with duodenal segment anastomosed to the bladder was pioneered by Sollinger's group[8] and was the dominant approach until the mid-1990s when many groups converted to enteric drainage using a side-to-side anastomosis of the donor duodenum and the recipient ileum (Fig. 65-1).[9–11] Although there is some risk of intra-abdominal infection from this procedure and one cannot follow urinary amylase as a marker for

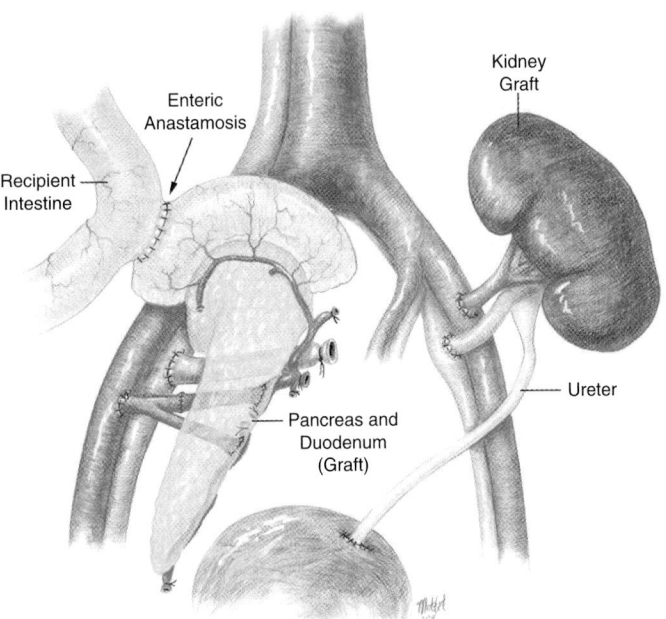

Figure 65-1 Combined pancreas and kidney transplant. Digestive juices of the pancreas are drained into the intestine via an enteric anastomosis between the donor duodenum and the recipient ileum. Venous outflow can be either into the portal vein or to the peripheral circulation via the iliac vein as shown. (Drawing courtesy of Dr. David Sutherland; see Color Plate.)

rejection, it avoids problems that plagued bladder drainage, such as acidosis, dehydration, cystitis, reflux pancreatitis, bladder stones, and a variety of other problems.[12,13]

The majority of the venous drainage of the native pancreas is via the pancreaticoduodenal veins into the portal vein. Classically, venous drainage from a transplanted pancreas has been directed into the systemic circulation, but some centers are now employing the superior mesenteric vein to allow drainage into the portal vein, which is more physiologic but also more technically demanding.[10,14] This portal vein route results in lower peripheral circulating insulin levels,[15,16] and its use highlights concerns about the potential of hyperinsulinemia with systemic drainage, which may accelerate atherosclerosis. Studies to date have not found any differences in the rates of macrovascular events between these two groups but these studies have suffered from relatively small sample sizes. It is somewhat reassuring that lipid profiles have not shown evidence of a more atherogenic pattern in the patients with systemic drainage.[14,15,16]

ANTIREJECTION THERAPY

From the early use of azathioprine and prednisone, outcomes improved considerably with the addition of cyclosporine in the mid-1980s. This evolved further with the combined use of tacrolimus (FK-506), mycophenolate mofetil, and prednisone being used by many centers in the 1990s. Induction therapy with T-cell depleting antibodies is now standard, with a variety of agents being employed, including polyclonal antilymphocyte globulin, antithymocyte globulin, and the murine monoclonal antibody OKT3, which reacts with the CD3 complex of T lymphocytes. More recently, two anti-interleukin-2 (IL-2) receptor monoclonal antibodies, baxilimab and daclizumab, have been employed with it not yet being clear how they compare with the older depleting antibodies.

Earlier immunosuppression regimens are aimed at avoiding graft recognition. Subsequent therapies targeted lymphocyte proliferation and the newest therapies prevent rejection mainly by inhibiting effector functions. Along these lines, a variety of new combinations of antirejection agents are now being studied. There is considerable interest in developing steroid-free protocols to avoid the many well-documented side effects of steroids. Some of the replacement maintenance regimens include the combinations of tacrolimus/mycophenolate mofetil and tacrolimus/sirolimus.[17] At the same time, there are attempts to develop calcineurin inhibitor free regimens to avoid the nephrotoxicity and diabetogenicity of these agents. In a study of pancreas biopsies obtained from whole pancreas transplant recipients treated with cyclosporine or tacrolimus, there was evidence of histologic islet changes including cytoplasmic swelling, vacuolization, and apoptosis. These changes were more prominent with tacrolimus and correlated with elevated serum levels and pulse steroid administration.[18] One newer combination is alemtuzumab (Campath 1H) and mycophenolate mofetil. Other drugs under investigation include 15-deoxyspergualin, leflunomide, FTY-720, and brequinar[19]; they are discussed further in the control of transplant rejection and autoimmunity section of this chapter. It must be remembered that immunosuppression is needed to control not only allograft rejection but also the autoimmunity of type 1 diabetes. This persistent autoimmunity may be especially aggressive, as indicated by pancreas/kidney transplants performed between identical twins that were not given immunosuppressive medication.[20] No rejection of the exocrine pancreas or kidney was found, but diabetes recurred with immune destruction of the islets demonstrated by biopsy. Remarkably, this destruction occurred in only a matter of weeks, which is far more rapid than the normal progression of type 1 diabetes, which typically takes years to produce hyperglycemia.[21]

SIDE EFFECTS OF ANTIREJECTION AGENTS

Many adverse effects are seen with these agents but only a few will be mentioned here. In general, higher doses of immuno-suppression are required for pancreas transplants than for kidney transplants alone, which is worrisome because of the increased risks of infection and malignancy.[22] Another worri-some complication for pancreas and islet transplantation is posttransplant diabetes.[19,23] Glucocorticoids have long been known to be diabetogenic by causing insulin resistance, but more recently direct adverse effects upon β-cell function have been found.[24,25] Adverse effects of tacrolimus on β cells are also well-documented[26] and more recently worrisome nega-tive effects from sirolimus (rapamycin) have been found.[27,28] In spite of the toxic effects of sirolimus that have been identified, it is impressive that normoglycemia is so well-maintained with pancreas transplants. A final concern is the nephrotoxicty of calcineurin inhibitors.[29] Despite the proven beneficial effects of a pancreas transplant on a transplanted kidney,[30,31] presumed due to euglycemia, drug-induced nephrotoxicty can be severe. Table 65-1 indicates the frequency of several of the major side effects reported with the most common immunosuppression agents.

Judging efficacy of immunosuppression regimens is more difficult with pancreas transplants than for other solid organ transplants, such as liver or kidney where functional tests are readily available. For SPK transplants, rejection of the pancreas is followed using kidney function as a surrogate marker. Detection of problems with the pancreas prior to permanent end-organ damage is more difficult for PAK and PTA proce-dures. For patients with bladder drainage, amylase output has been thought to be useful by some, although current approaches are more likely to employ serum amylase and lipase levels, and pancreas biopsies.[32] Other less commonly used methods for the diagnosis of pancreas rejection include ^{99m}Tc DTPA scintigraphy and uptake of indium-labeled platelets.

SURGICAL COMPLICATIONS OF PANCREAS TRANSPLANTATION

Pancreas transplants require complex surgery and are accom-panied by significant mortality and morbidity with patients often having long hospitalizations and readmissions for such problems as intra-abdominal infection and vascular thrombo-sis.[33] Other problems include hemorrhage, graft pancreatitis, anastomotic leaks, and a variety of problems related to blad-der drainage. For technical failure in the United States from 1996 to 2002, as analyzed by the International Pancreas Transplant Registry, cadaver primary PTA transplants did not significantly differ for bladder drainage versus enteric drainage, but in SPK and PAK, technical failure was signifi-cantly lower with bladder drainage than enteric drainage. The technical failure rate ranged from 7.4% to 14.1% depending on the procedure, with graft thrombosis accounting for over 70% of the failures.

TRANSPLANT OUTCOMES

As tabulated by the International Pancreas Transplant Registry for the period 1996 to 2002, patient survival at 1 year was: SPK, 95%; PAK, 94%; PTA, 98%; and nearly 90% in all categories at 4 years. Graft survival is defined as maintenance of normoglycemia, which usually means that recipients have normal glucose levels around the clock without increased risk of reactive hypoglycemia,[34] have normal glycohemoglobin levels, and require no dietary restrictions. One-year graft sur-vival rates have improved markedly since the 1980s. The most recent data available from the OPTN/SRTR 2003 Annual Report (www.optn.org), indicates that for transplants per-formed in 2000 to 2001, graft function at 1 year was 85% for SPK, 79% for PAK, and 77% for PTA. Survival of the kidney grafts at 1 year was 92% for both SPK and PAK. At 3 years, graft survival for those receiving transplants in 1998 to 1999 were 77% for SPK, 67% for PAK, and 65% for PTA. At 5 years for those transplanted in 1996 to 1997, the graft survival rates were 70% for SPK, 46% for PAK, and 42% for PTA (Fig. 65-2).[34a] As expected, results tend to be somewhat better at experienced centers,[6,35] although this is sometimes counterbalanced by these centers taking more difficult cases.

For patients awaiting SPK transplants, the survival rates are much lower than for patients with normal kidney function waiting for a solitary pancreas,[36] no doubt due to the dan-gerous combination of end-stage renal failure and hyper-glycemia. It is clear that transplantation of a kidney alone improves survival in patients with diabetes and renal failure,[37] while transplantation of a pancreas provides uncertain addi-tional benefit.

IMPACT OF PANCREAS TRANSPLANTATION UPON DIABETIC COMPLICATIONS

The impact of these transplants upon the complications of diabetes seems to be modest, which is not surprising because so many recipients have advanced abnormalities by the time the transplant is performed. There are now several well-performed studies on retinopathy, which show no evidence of

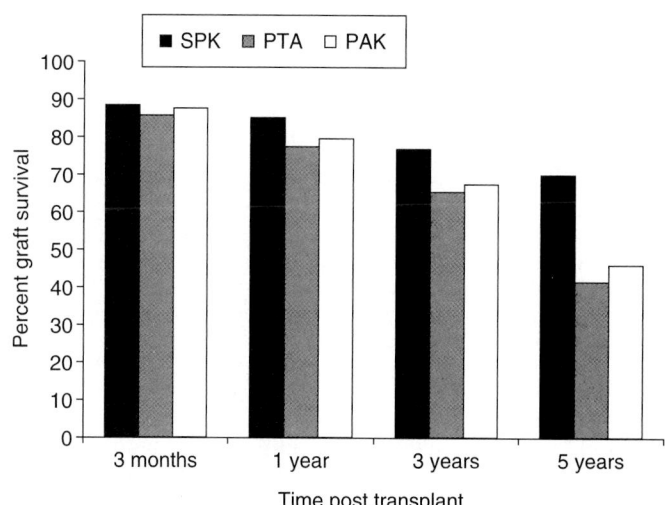

Figure 65-2 Pancreas graft survival among pancreas transplant recipients by type of transplant. Data are from the 2003 OPTN/SRTR Annual Report Tables 6.9, 7.9, and 8.9 (www.optn.org). Cohorts for 3 months and 1 year were preformed 2000–2001, 3 years 1998–1999, and 5 years 1996–1997. SPK, simultaneous pancreas kidney; PAK, pancreas after kidney; PTA, pancreas transplant alone.

Table 65-1	Adverse Effects of Common Immunosuppressive Agents				
Complication	**Prednisone**	**CsA**	**MMF**	**Tacrolimus**	**Sirolimus**
Glucose intolerance	+++	+	+	++	±
Nephrotoxicity	±	++	+	++	±
Hypertension	++	+++	+	+++	±
Hyperlipidemia	++	+++	++	+	+++
Neurotoxicity	±	+	±	++	±
Cytopenia	±	±	++	±	++
Electrolyte abnormalities	+	++	+	++	±

+mild, ++moderate, +++ severe/frequent, ± no clinically significant effect. CsA, Cyclosporin A; MMF, mycophenolate mofetil.

improvement of either vision or the appearance of the retina.[38–40] A complexity in analyzing these data is that most of these patients have reached a stable phase of their long-standing retinopathy and the observation periods were fairly short, with most of the patients being followed for less than 4 years.

The benefits of pancreas transplantation to the kidney are more apparent. In one fascinating case from Kuwait, Abouna and colleagues reported the transplantation of kidneys from a man with a 17-year history of type 1 diabetes mellitus and clinical nephropathy, with proteinuria but normal serum creatinine, into nondiabetic recipients. Biopsies taken prior to transplantation demonstrated diffuse diabetic glomerulosclerosis. Biopsies taken 7 months after transplantation showed almost complete resolution of the pathologic changes initially seen. Interestingly, one of the recipients subsequently developed posttransplant diabetes and on repeat biopsy 13 months after diagnosis of diabetes (30 months after transplant) had histologic features of recurrent diabetic nephrosclerosis with a nodular pattern while the nondiabetic recipient had no such changes on repeat biopsy.[41,42] Similarly, biopsy proven diabetic nephropathy of transplanted kidneys is slowed by subsequent pancreas transplantation or even prevented by simultaneous transplant.[30,31] A more recent longitudinal study found improvement of native kidneys after pancreas transplantation too. Clinical improvement in urinary albumin was noted at 5 and 10 years posttransplant. On biopsy, no benefit was seen at 5 years, but biopsies at 10 years showed an impressive reversion of histology toward normal.[43]

The course of diabetic neuropathy benefits from pancreas transplantation, as demonstrated by modest improvements in nerve conduction velocity, parameters of autonomic neuropathy, and symptoms.[44–47] Gastric emptying can also improve,[48] but it is not clear how much can be attributed to glycemic control or improved renal function. Severe autonomic neuropathy was reported to have a terrible prognosis decades ago with a 56% mortality during 5 years of follow-up,[49] but more modern studies show survival rates of about 90%.[50] It seems likely that much of the earlier reported mortality was due to renal failure, which would explain the high survival rates of subjects with autonomic neuropathy after combined pancreas and kidney transplants.[51]

The course of macrovascular disease after pancreas transplantation has not been extensively studied, but it is clear that risk factors are reduced.[52–54] Moreover, recent reports suggest that carotid intima media thickness can diminish[54] and the progression of coronary atherosclerosis can be slowed or even regress.[55] These latter findings still need to be confirmed with larger studies.

PANCREAS TRANSPLANTATION AND GLUCOSE COUNTERREGULATION

Multiple mechanisms provide defense against hypoglycemia, with increases in circulating glucagon and epinephrine from the adrenal medulla being especially important. After several years of type 1 diabetes, glucagon responses to hypoglycemia are completely lost and epinephrine responses are often reduced.[56] Moreover, the symptoms of hypoglycemia often become blunted and even lost with the development of hypoglycemia unawareness. After pancreas transplantation, glucagon responses to hypoglycemia are normalized, while epinephrine responses and symptoms are improved.[57,58] This is likely why hypoglycemia after pancreas transplants is rarely a problem, and infrequently reported.[34,59]

QUALITY OF LIFE AFTER PANCREAS TRANSPLANTATION

The most obvious benefit of pancreas transplants is that patients feel their quality of life is improved, particularly with freedom from insulin injections, hypoglycemic episodes, and

food restrictions. It must be remembered, however, that quality of life is a problematic parameter to evaluate.[60,61] For example, it has been difficult to show that patients' lives are improved using such standard criteria as whether patients are more active or have better performance at work. Despite the many studies that have been performed, it has been difficult to show striking improvement using a variety of study methods.[62–65] Nonetheless, in spite of the complexities of these evaluations, patients seem happy to be free of their diabetes, which is of undeniable importance.

COST OF PANCREAS TRANSPLANTATION

The costs of pancreas transplantation have been extensively analyzed by Stratta.[66] For a typical SPK transplant in the United States, the cost is between $80,000 to $120,000, which includes hospital costs, professional fees, and organ acquisition charges. Complications requiring additional surgery and hospitalization can lead to much higher costs. In addition, the annual cost of medications is about $15,000 and posttransplant monitoring is about $10,000. It is important to consider this in the context of the pancreas transplant being added to the cost of a kidney transplant, which has a more pronounced impact on health. The cost of dialysis is about $50,000 per year, while the cost of a kidney transplant from a cadaver donor is about $40,000 and that from a living donor about $90,000.

ISSUES ABOUT SOLITARY PANCREAS TRANSPLANTS

There has been considerable debate about how to justify PTA with its risks of mortality, morbidity, and immunosuppression. People with type 1 diabetes sometimes have life-threatening debilitating episodes of hypoglycemia or even various psychologic problems, which has been used to justify the risk of PTA. Another consideration is the protective effect of glycemic control upon complications that was so clearly shown by the Diabetes Control and Complications Trial.[67] The presence of early diabetic nephropathy is especially worrisome because of its poor prognosis, raising hopes that a pancreas transplant would be helpful in slowing the progression of disease. Balanced against this, however, is the potential nephrotoxicty of the calcineurin inhibitors.[29] Similar decision making must be used for PTA using living donors who provide the distal portion of their pancreas as a segmental transplant. There continues to be debate about the efficacy of using only half of a pancreas and the added risk to the donors of developing either glucose intolerance or frank diabetes.[68]

To try and answer some of these unresolved questions, the risk of mortality after pancreas transplant was recently analyzed by the group of Harlan and colleagues, with transplanted patients being compared to patients on a waiting list.[36] The overall relative risk for all-cause mortality within 4 years following transplantation or continuing on the waiting list was 1.57 for PTA, 1.42 for PAK, and 0.43 for SPK. Based on this approach, pancreas transplant would only appear beneficial in the SPK case. Interestingly, the mortality rate for those on the waiting list for PTA was lower than expected from historical data, presumably because of improvements in treatment of diabetes. However, the survival rate for those on the waiting list for SPK remained low at 63.8% at 4 years, likely reflecting the continued mortality associated with severe renal disease. Although much debated, these survival data for solitary pancreas transplants provide an important note of caution about the safety of this approach compared with either islet transplantation or more conventional therapy for type 1 diabetes.

ISLET TRANSPLANTATION

Over 30 years ago, the first successful islet transplants were performed in rodents.[69,70] Bolstered by a novel enzymatic method of islet isolation utilizing collagenase[71] it was hoped that islet transplantation would soon be a viable treatment option for patients with type 1 diabetes. Unfortunately, early attempts to translate these rodent studies into clinical practice were fraught with difficulty. Investigators were plagued by low quality and low yield islet preparations coupled with - ineffective and diabetogenic, immunosuppression regimens. Nonetheless, substantial progress was made, which has already started to provide the foundations for eventual success.

HUMAN ISLET ALLOGRAFTS

During the 1970s and 1980s, a relatively small number of research groups worked with small and large animal models to bring this therapy to humans. One of the major challenges was to isolate islets in adequate numbers from human pancreases, which required a variety of innovative advances. The use of density gradients such as Ficoll facilitated separation of islets from exocrine tissue on a large scale.[72] Similarly, the injection of collagenase into the pancreatic ducts greatly improved islet yields.[73] Another major advance was the development in St. Louis of the Ricordi chamber. This device coupled continuous flow of a collagenase-containing buffer with a screen to allow separated islets to be released and to facilitate constant monitoring of the digestion process.[74] The subsequent introduction of dithizone, which reacts with zinc in β cells to stain islets red, further enhanced the monitoring of the digestion process and islet counting by allowing islets to be more easily visually differentiated from acinar tissue.[75]

A second important task was to find a suitable transplant site for the isolated islets. Although reintroduction into the pancreas would be most physiologic, the anatomy is not conducive to this approach. Initially, islets were transplanted into the peritoneal cavity,[69] but shortly thereafter Kemp and colleagues found that injecting islets into the portal vein, allowing them to lodge in the liver, was far more efficient.[76] Although transplantation of islets under the kidney capsule has proven useful for research because of the ease of retrieving the graft, it has found only limited clinical use.[77,78] The spleen was also an early favored site of islet infusion after it was used in a reported early human islet transplant.[79] In both

canine[80,81] and primate[82] models, there is even some evidence of superior graft function compared to other transplant sites. However, the overall clinical experience with splenic and combined splenic/portal infusions has been less promising with multiple life-threatening complications including splenic infarct, emergent splenectomy, and portal vein thrombosis reported.[83,84] After exploration of many sites in many models, the liver continues to be the site of choice for clinical transplantation at this time.

In 1977, Najarian and colleagues at the University of Minnesota reported the first clinical series of islet allografts in patients with type 1 diabetes and prior renal allografts. Of the seven patients transplanted, none achieved insulin independence, although insulin requirements were reduced for limited periods.[85] The following year, a group in Zurich, Switzerland reportedly had a previously insulin independent type 1 diabetic patient become insulin independent after simultaneous kidney and intrasplenic islet transplants.[79] Unfortunately, this early provocative report of success was not accompanied by C peptide levels before or after transplant, followed and unusual time course with significant graft function delayed by eight to nine months (which the report's authors attributed to the use of immature islets), and was not readily reproducible.

It was not until the end of the 1980s and early 1990s that a number of well-organized islet programs emerged.[86–90] The major pioneering centers were in St. Louis, Edmonton, Giessen, Minnesota, Milan, and Pittsburgh. These early transplant centers used islets obtained from as many as five donor pancreases, with some of these islets being cryopreserved. For these transplants, the islets were injected into the portal vein using a direct approach with dissection along the umbilical vein, but more recently a percutaneous transhepatic angiographic procedure has gained favor. These islets become wedged in the terminal branches of the portal vein and engraft (Fig. 65-3), receiving most of their vascular supply from host vessels growing into the islets, as judged by rodent studies.[91]

Despite these centers introducing more controlled approaches, success was far from assured. Data from the International Islet Transplantation Registry showed that between 1990 and 1998, out of 267 islet allografts only 33 (12%) of the recipients remained insulin free for more than

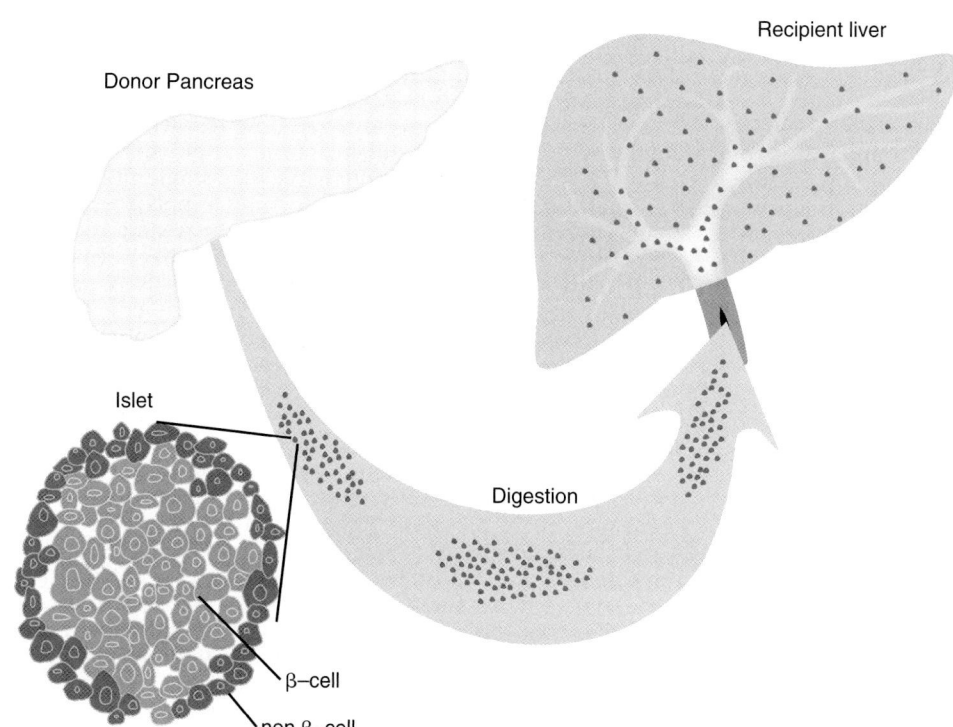

Donor Pancreas

Recipient liver

Islet

Digestion

β–cell

non β–cell

Figure 65-3 Islet transplantation in humans is usually done starting with a cadaver pancreas that is digested with a collagenase/protease mixture. The isolated islets are then introduced into the portal vein either by transhepatic angiography or via laparoscopy. The islets then are carried downstream and wedge in the hepatic sinusoids whereupon they are vascularized by vessels from the recipient.

1 week and only 8% maintained that status for over 1 year.[92,93] The longest period of insulin independence reported was 70 months. However, only 35% of had evidence of continuing graft function (C peptide over 0.5 ng/mL) after 1 year. Notably, about 30% of the patients had a marked reduction in C peptide levels within 1 month, a phenomenon termed *primary nonfunction*.

The poor results of the 1990s stifled expansion of clinical trails, but fortunately a few centers persisted and provided important new insights including a series of peritransplant refinements which led to improved graft function.[87,92–98] Although very few recipients were freed of their insulin requirements, it became apparent that some had persisting function of the grafted islets as evidenced by measurable C peptide levels. As is found in the early stages of type 1 diabetes, residual insulin secretion greatly improved glycemic control even though insulin treatment was still required. Thus, in a number of carefully performed well-documented islet transplants, persistent C peptide secretion was associated with improved glycohemoglobin levels and fewer severe insulin reactions.[94]

FOCUS ON DETAILS LED TO IMPROVED RESULTS

As investigators gained experience and began to understand the many details involved in islet transplantation, results began to improve. It seemed that better outcomes were obtained if pancreases had a cold ischemia time of less than 8 hours before islet isolation and if more than 6000 islet equivalents per kg were given.[92,93] Experience and technologic advances led to improved techniques for islet isolation. It is important to recognize the extraordinary number of steps involved in the isolation process. Many of these can be standardized, but there remain areas of judgment, such as deciding when the digestion process must be stopped, that are learned from experience and sharing of information. The recognized need to standardize collagenase preparations led to Liberase, which is a defined mixture of enzymes including collagenases I and II obtained from *Clostridium histolyticum* and various nonclostridial neutral proteases. This purification, which also reduces the levels of endotoxin, has been found to provide better and more consistent islet yields.[99] Industry continues to work on improving the consistency and efficacy of these preparations with the future perhaps employing recombinant technology for even better standardization.

THE EDMONTON PROTOCOL

Undaunted by the mediocre results of earlier trials, a group of investigators in Edmonton, Canada, tried a new approach in 1999.[100] They identified possible barriers to insulin independence including insufficient engraftment and immediate cellular loss leading to an inadequate number of β cells worsened by the use of diabetogenic immunosuppressants. They also hypothesized that there may be ongoing rejection from ineffective suppression of both alloimmune and autoimmune pathways but that these events were going unseen given the lack of tools to identify rejection. To address these key factors, they attempted to improve the quality of their islet preparations by minimizing duration of ischemia and preparing islets in xenoprotein-free medium, as coating of islets by xenoproteins could, theoretically, increase immediate cell loss. They selected a glucocorticoid-free immunosuppressive protocol including rapamycin (sirolimus), low dose tacrolimus, and a monocolonal antibody against the interleukin-2 receptor (daclizumab) to further minimize potential damage to β cells and increasing insulin resistance. For recipients, they recruited patients with type 1 diabetes without kidney transplants who had serious problems with hypoglycemia or advancing complications, which justified the use of potentially dangerous immunosuppressive agents. In contrast to

earlier transplants, to avoid exposure to xenoproteins, the islets were used just following isolation rather than being placed in tissue culture. Islets were introduced into the liver through the portal vein via transhepatic angiography. To render patients insulin-independent, islets from more than one cadaver donor were required, with two sufficing for most of the patients. In their 2000 report on seven patients, insulin independence was never obtained after the first transplant, but did occur in all patients soon after the second or third transplant with a combined total of about 11,000 islet equivalents per kg.

PROGRESS SINCE THE EDMONTON ANNOUNCEMENT

This spectacular result provided impetus to the islet transplant field worldwide. Existing centers accelerated their efforts and other institutions embarked on establishing new islet programs. In 2001, the National Center for Research Resources of the National Institutes of Health established 10 Islet Resource Centers in the United States with the mission of providing human islets for both clinical and research use. In addition, the Immune Tolerance Network of the National Institutes of Health with help from the Juvenile Diabetes Research Foundation began a trial of 9 centers to perform transplants in 40 subjects to try to reproduce the Edmonton results. As with the Edmonton trial, this multicenter trial recruited patients without kidney transplants who had life-threatening hypoglycemia episodes, severe glycemic instability, or advancing complications. At the time of this writing in 2004, there has been a great deal of progress, but considerably less than the high expectations of those in 2000. The Immune Tolerance Network study is near completion and has confirmed that the Edmonton results can be reproduced in other centers, but better success rates occurred in experienced centers than in the others.[101]

The Edmonton group by mid-2004 has now transplanted over 70 patients with various protocols and has continued to obtain insulin independence in the vast majority of subjects, although islets from two or more pancreases are still usually required. Centers in the United States and Europe have been transplanting smaller numbers of patients. The Miami and Baylor groups have worked together to obtain successful transplants between cities, with pancreases flown from Houston to Miami and isolated islets flown back to Houston for implantation.[102] This study and work from other groups shows that islets do not need to be transplanted immediately after isolation, but can be placed in culture and transplanted 1 to 2 days later. Two groups have now reported success in obtaining insulin independence from single donor transplants.[103,104] While it is encouraging that single donor islet transplants can succeed, this usually only happens when the recipient has very low insulin requirements and the islet preparation is of excellent quality. It seems likely that the β-cell mass required to normalize glucose levels is proportional to the insulin requirements of the recipient. Several groups have had success with a variety of regimens transplanting islets to individuals with a prior kidney transplant as opposed to the islets-alone Edmonton approach.[105–107] A group in Zurich has also had comparable success with simultaneous islet kidney transplants.[108]

In contrast to these successes, newly established centers are confronting the complexity, expense, and difficulty of developing a clinical program. This, in part, accounts for why 4 years after Edmonton, there are still less than 100 patients transplanted yearly worldwide instead of the hundreds that some expected. To succeed, an islet isolation team must be assembled that can be available at all times and develop experience with the complex steps that are required. Also, as appropriate for cell-based therapies, there is a need to maintain very rigorous quality control measures that conform to the requirements of regulatory groups such as the Food and

Drug Administration in the United States. The established centers have been very generous in helping emerging centers learn about isolation. This is accomplished by international workshops and by welcoming visitors as observers, but the learning curve remains steep.

An unexpected problem has been the lack of available high-quality pancreases. This varies depending on the country, but in the United States, the number of whole organ pancreas transplants has continued to increase, in part, because results continue to improve but also because the costs can be covered by insurance. In general, in the United States, the high-quality pancreases are diverted to whole organ programs, while islet programs often receive pancreases from donors over the age of 60 or obese donors whose fat deposits complicate whole organ transplants. Although not firmly established, there is a growing impression that islet yields from older donors are smaller and do less well (CITR July 2004 report *http://www.citregistry.org*, Exhibit 40). On the other hand, pancreases from obese donors often provide high yields of excellent islets (CITR July 2004 report *http://www.citregistry.org*, Exhibit 39). This is in accordance with solid pancreas transplant experience where it has been found that donor obesity (body mass index [BMI] > 30) has a negative impact on short-term graft survival due to higher incidence of surgical complications and technical failures, but does not affect long-term graft function.[109] Another problem receiving considerable attention is that many available pancreases are still not recovered. Although some preliminary success has been found with isolation of islets from pancreases of non-heart-beating donors,[110] as of 2004, the limited availability of high-quality pancreases continues to be problematic.

RISKS AND SIDE EFFECTS OF ISLET TRANSPLANTATION

As experience accumulates, other growing pains are emerging. While patients are often delighted by their transplanted islets, some have had significant problems as was highlighted by a report on six recipients from the National Institutes of Health islet transplantation program. This study employed the Edmonton approach transplanting patients who were receiving immunosuppression for the first time.[111] Several of the patients found the side effects of the immunosuppression to be so problematic that the drugs had to be discontinued, in one case due to sirolimus-induced pneumonitis. It appears that patients who are receiving immunosuppression for the first time have more difficulty than those who are given islet transplants after a kidney transplant and have adjusted to their drug regimens.

The side effects of the immunosuppression under the Edmonton protocol are mostly predictable from previous experience and have been described in a number of clinical reports as summarized in Table 65-2.[112,113] The major side effects of sirolimus have been mouth ulcers, diarrhea, malaise, hypertension, and hyperlipidemia. Particularly worrisome is the nephrotoxicity that can be found with calcineurin inhibitors, in particular, the tacrolimus that is part of the Edmonton protocol. As with other transplants, there is concern about immunosuppression leading to opportunistic infections and malignancy.[22] Thus far, none of these latter complications have been reported, but the population of subjects is small and follow-up has only been for short periods of time.

Although generally considered less invasive than surgery, percutaneous transhepatic angiography still poses significant risks. Most active centers have had some patients with bleeding after the procedure, which, in some cases, has required transfusions and even exploratory laparotomies. Thrombus in the segmental portal veins has been found with ultrasound examinations; these have been successfully treated with heparin, and fortunately, no cases of complete portal vein thrombosis have been reported.[113] Gallbladder punctures

Table 65-2	Adverse Events Associated with Clinical Islet Transplantation (Approximate Percent Incidence)	
Procedure-Related (%)	**Immunosuppressive-Related (%)**	
Elevated liver enzymes (50%)	Oral ulcers (95%)	Decline in GFR (50%)
Abdominal pain (50%)	Anemia (60%)	Proteinuria (50%)
Nausea/vomiting (50%)	Diarrhea (50%)	Peripheral edema (30%)
Fatty liver (long term) (20%)	Weight loss (50%)	Neutropenia (<10%)
Peritoneal hemorrhage (15%)	Fatigue (50%)	Tremor (<10%)
Portal vein thrombosis (4%)	LDL elevation (50%)	Acne (10%)
Gallbladder puncture (3%)	Hypertension (50%)	Misc.—Arthralgia, pneumonitis, hematuria, infection

Based on findings published by the Edmonton group[112,113] and adapted from Paty (*www.endotext.com*).

have occurred. In one center, a patient experienced a hemothorax as a complication of the angiography. Some centers are finding that complications fall as the angiography team gains more experience. Although most centers continue to use angiography, some remain concerned enough to choose small laparotomies with general anesthesia to avoid bleeding complications.

Portal pressure is monitored during the islet infusion, which usually is a packed cell volume of 2 to 6 mL; in the Edmonton series, pressures on average rose from 12 to 17 mm Hg with there being a correlation with increasing packed cell volume.[114] Furthermore, when compared with the first transplant, pressure increases are higher with the second and third transplants. While this has not been associated with any complications, it does indicate that islet infusions lead to changes in the portal vasculature. Immediately following the islet infusions, transaminase levels often increase to levels two to five times normal, peaking at about 7 days and then returning to normal within 2 months.[115] More modest increases in alkaline phosphatase are found.

Magnetic resonance imaging (MRI) evidence of hepatic steatosis has been found by several groups.[116,117] Of the 30 patients studied with MRI in Edmonton, 20% had patchy steatosis, which in one case disappeared following graft failure. Histologic findings concur with these imaging studies.[116] This steatosis is likely due to high concentrations of insulin released locally by clumps of islet tissue promoting localized triglyceride storage in hepatocytes. The possibility that this could lead to deleterious scarring has not been excluded, but liver function is being carefully followed in the patients and no problems have been reported.

CLINICAL BENEFITS OF ISLET TRANSPLANTATION

Although most patients receiving islet transplantation with modern techniques can become insulin-independent, they typically are not truly normoglycemic but instead would be classified as having impaired glucose tolerance with some even meeting the criteria for diabetes. Moreover, graft function deteriorates, often over a period of only months. The Edmonton group has the largest experience and they find that about 80% of recipients are insulin-free 1 year after the transplant but less than 50% are insulin-free after 2 years.[112] In general, results from other centers are even less encouraging. This is in contrast with pancreas transplants where insulin independence is more durable with about 70% being normoglycemic at 5 years. Moreover, recipients with whole-organ transplants are less likely to have impaired glucose tolerance.

Patients with islet transplants resemble, in many respects, people with type 2 diabetes, which should not be surprising considering their marginal β-cell function/reserve. An obvious difference is that due to selection for the procedure, recipients are usually not obese and insulin-resistant. They are often found to have high fasting glucose levels that fall to near normal as the day progresses. While some clinicians find this pattern unfamiliar, it can be found in some patients with early type 2 diabetes. As glucose levels deteriorate, some have reasoned that insulin sensitizers should be beneficial, yet anecdotal reports suggest that the use of metformin and thiazolidinediones have been of limited value. There has been concern about using sulfonylureas because of their putative potential to cause β-cell apoptosis,[118] a concern not supported by results of imperfect clinical trials.[2] When patients return to insulin, glucose levels can usually be easily maintained by judicious use of short-acting insulin analogues before meals and often just a single injection of the long-acting insulin analogue glargine. For patients accustomed to the marked glycemic fluctuations of brittle diabetes, this improved control with a far less demanding regimen is a welcome benefit and many have chosen to continue immunosuppression despite lack of insulin independence. Unfortunately, islet loss may be a progressive process with some patients now being seen whose C peptide levels gradually fall to negligible levels with return to brittle type 1 diabetes.

Detractors of islet transplantation see these outcomes as providing limited therapeutic value but the benefits should not be minimized. The morbidity and mortality of whole organ transplantation are avoided while still obtaining hemoglobin A1c values in the range between 5.5% to 7.5% (Fig. 65-4), which provides important protection from complications as has been shown by the Diabetes Control and Complications Trial study.[1] Experience with islet transplantation is not yet extensive enough to show beneficial effects on complications, but some surrogate markers for vascular disease including endothelial function have been shown to improve.[106,119] Considering quality of life, most patients, even many of those still needing insulin, are very thankful to be free of hypoglycemia unawareness and severe insulin reactions.[120]

EXPENSE OF ISLET TRANSPLANTATION

As with other transplants, the costs of islet transplantation are considerable. The startup costs include developing a pathogen-free space, purchasing equipment, and assembling an isolation team of five or more individuals, which typically costs over 2 million U.S. dollars. Costs for the actual transplants vary depending on health-care costs.[121] A recent example of costs for a patient in the United States was $188,000 which covered two isolations ($26,000), two transplants ($30,000), hospitalization ($14,000), medication for 1 year ($61,000), and monitoring for 1 year ($37,000), along with other costs (R. A. Dickey, oral communication, 2003). As can be seen from the above analysis, the costs of islet and pancreas transplants are not significantly different.

β-CELL REPLACEMENT AS A TREATMENT FOR TYPES 1 AND 2 DIABETES

While generally accepted that β-cell replacement therapy will be useful for type 1 diabetes, many do not realize that it could also be efficacious for some patients with type 2 diabetes as β-cell failure is a root cause of this disease. To understand the role of the β cell, it must be appreciated that most people with insulin resistance never become hyperglycemic because their β cells compensate with increased insulin secretion, hence the key role of β-cell failure. More islets will be required for people with type 2 diabetes, but often their insulin requirements are not much different than those with type 1 diabetes because of their residual insulin production. Pancreas transplants have been found to work as well in patients with type 2 diabetes as those with type 1.[122] This need for a large amount of islet mass should not be a problem once ways are found to make insulin-producing cells readily available. The health benefits of such transplants would be enormous because microvascular and neuropathic complications of diabetes should be prevented, and cardiovascular events should be reduced. Individuals would still be left with obesity and insulin resistance with their health consequences, but these should be associated with far less illness that when diabetes is superimposed.

ISLET GRAFT FUNCTION

Questions about the β-cell mass and function of islet grafts in the liver are of fundamental importance to the field. Recipients receiving islets from one to three pancreases usually receive a total of over 10,000 islet equivalents per kg, which means they are given β-cell mass roughly equivalent to that present in a normal pancreas. Yet, the usual outcome of impaired glucose tolerance indicates that the grafts are not nearly as efficacious as that provided by a normal pancreas. Islet function is usually evaluated by measuring C peptide responses to acute intravenous injections of glucose and, separately, arginine, and to the administration of a standardized meal. Unpublished data are in general agreement with the experience obtained in Edmonton, which found that responses to acute glucose stimulation were only 21% of normal, and those to arginine, 56% of normal.[123] Future studies will provide us with more detailed information about how graft function varies over time, but it is clear that the amount of insulin secreted from grafts is far less than that from either normal of transplanted pancreases. Some estimate that β-cell mass of islet grafts in the liver is only 20% to 40% of normal.

The field of diabetes has been handicapped by the inability to directly measure β-cell mass, which means that the loss of β-cell mass required for the development of types 1 and 2

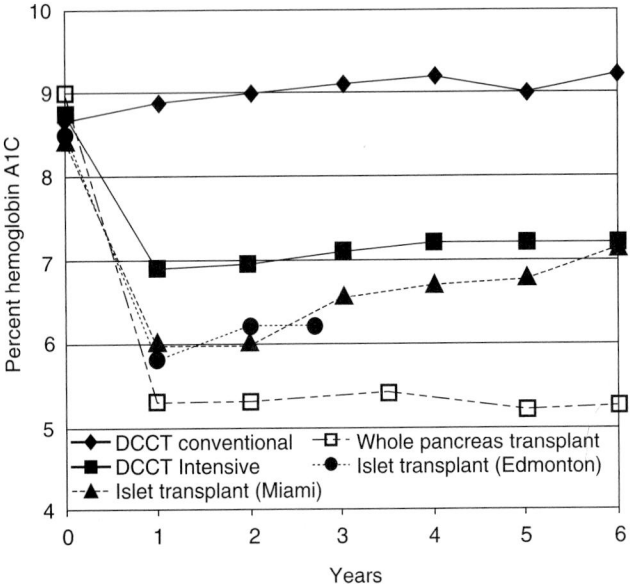

Figure 65-4 Comparison of hemoglobin A1C levels after successful pancreas or islet transplantation to levels obtained during the Diabetes Control and Complications Trial (DCCT). Patients in the Edmonton group were insulin-independent while the patients in the Miami group had evidence of graft function but still required insulin (pre-Edmonton data). (Data was obtained from the DCCT Research Group,[1] Robertson et al.,[287] Alejandro et al.,[94] and Ryan et al.[123])

diabetes, and for failure of islet transplants can only be obtained from autopsy studies and educated guesses. With islet transplants, it appears that much of the infused β-cell mass is lost acutely and that further loss continues on a chronic but variable basis. It also seems likely that the function of whatever islets are present is not normal. Experience with nonhuman primates may provide some clues in that islet preparations are usually much more pure and healthier than those obtained from human pancreases,[124] and the insulin responses to stimulation are closer to normal,[125,126] which suggests that islets engrafted in the liver can function reasonably well. This comparison supports the concept that the major problem with human islet transplants is loss of β-cell mass.

Glucagon secretion from islet grafts in the liver is markedly abnormal in that only minimal increases are found during hypoglycemia,[127] which contrasts with the essentially normal responses found in recipients of whole pancreases.[57] Individuals with type 1 diabetes typically lose their glucagon responses to hypoglycemia,[128] which indicates that with islet transplants neither α cells in the liver nor in the pancreas can respond appropriately to hypoglycemia. Exercise has not been carefully studied yet in recipients of islet transplants but concerns have been raised by islet transplant studies in rats[129] and dogs,[130] which suggest that people with portal islet transplants may be subject to hypoglycemia during exercise.

THE COMPLEXITIES OF ISLET ENGRAFTMENT IN THE LIVER

Based on the studies previously discussed, it's clear that events occur during the early implantation phase that must lead to considerable loss of islet mass. There likely is obligatory loss of some cells due to local hypoxia occurring in nonvascularized large islets and clumps of islet tissue lodged in the terminal branches of the portal vein, as seen in studies in other model systems.[131,132] In addition, a nonspecific inflammatory response[133] accompanied by localized clotting[134] may enhance the immune processes of rejection and autoimmunity and activate the innate immune system.[135] This has been termed the *instant blood-mediated inflammatory reaction*, in which tissue factor and macrophage chemoattractant protein have been implicated.[136-138] It has been found that expression of these factors is increased after the isolation of human islets but falls as islets are cultured and can be further suppressed by nicotinamide.[139,140]

Isolated islets, removed from their normal blood supply, face a fundamental problem with oxygen delivery after transplantation because they are not fully vascularized for 10 to 14 days as determined by studies in experimental animals.[91,141] Although a few donor endothelial cells may take part in the process, most of the new vessels are supplied by the recipient.[91,142] There are many studies showing that hyperglycemia during this critical period has an adverse influence on the outcome of islet transplants[143] with one mechanism appearing to be slowing of angiogenesis.[144] Hyperglycemia may also increase oxygen consumption in β cells, which would further reduce oxygen tension in their local environment. These finding provide a rationale for treating patients aggressively with insulin during the first 10 days after the transplant.

Another potential insult to transplanted islets is the toxic effects of immunosuppressive drugs. Prednisone, which can inhibit insulin gene expression and secretion,[24,25,145] had been under suspicion and its omission from the Edmonton protocol may have contributed to the improved result.[100] Both tacrolimus and sirolimus have in vitro toxic effects on islets and insulin-producing cell lines.[26-28] The possibility that these drugs could interfere with insulin secretion and contribute to apoptosis is worrisome but the fact that whole organ pancreas transplants do so well for many years suggests the toxic effects are limited. Perhaps islets in the liver are more vulnerable. One thought is that they could be subject to high drug

concentrations in the portal vein,[146] but this is not a convincing mechanism as it is thought that the islet vascular supply comes mainly from the hepatic artery[147] and there is some evidence of the development of an endothelial layer separating the islets from direct portal exposure.[147a] However, this may still leave a vulnerable period before the islets have fully engrafted.

In the post Edmonton era, patients usually become insulin-independent within 6 weeks after their last transplant whether it be their first, second, or third. A puzzling finding of the 1990s is that in the 33 reported successful allograft recipients, the mean time required for insulin independence to develop was 179 ± 24 days.[92] One explanation is that this tended to coincide with lowering of the doses immunosuppressive medications like prednisone that are diabetogenic, but the explanation might be much more complex. One might not expect β-cell mass to have increased during this time, but it is possible that islet precursor cells could make new β cells. The possibility that pancreatic duct cells are the precursor cells responsible for islet neogenesis[148-150] may be important because infused islet preparations are far less pure than those from other species. The composition of 24 transplantable islet preparations from the Joslin Diabetes Center was 32% β cells, 12% non-β islet cells, 23% duct cells, and 27% acinar cells (S. Bonner-Weir, unpublished). The dynamics of β-cell turnover in human pancreas is a subject of intense interest. Current thinking is that β-cell replication is extremely low and that whatever new β cells develop come from neogenesis.[151] It is possible, however, that transplanted islets behave differently as suggested by experiments in which human islets transplanted into mice were found to have substantial rates of replication.[152]

We have little idea of when transplanted islet vessels are fully established (beyond the 10–14 days to initially grow in) and how similar they are to those of normal islets. In their normal location in the pancreas, islets have a highly specialized vasculature; arterioles break into capillaries within the β cells' core and then exit through the islet mantle that contains glucagon-secreting α cells.[153,154] Because of this blood flow pattern, it is thought that insulin secreted from upstream has an important suppressive influence on downstream α cells but that β cells see little, if any, downstream glucagon.[155] Transplanted islets may not have this normal relationship between β cells and α cells, which could lead to altered β-cell function.[156] In addition, reinnervation[157] takes time and may be different in a transplant site. There are other reasons for being concerned that transplanted islets may not function as efficiently as normal islets in the pancreas. It has been found that the oxygen tension of islet grafts situated under the kidney capsule of rodents is considerably less than for islets in the pancreas,[158] which could lead to reduction of glucose-induced insulin secretion. In addition, the vasculature appears to be less dense in transplanted islets, which could account for these low oxygen tension.[159] The importance of this low oxygen tension is unclear because in mouse experiments very small numbers of islets, such as less than 100, placed under the kidney capsule can be successful indicating that function must not be severely impaired.[160]

CONTROL OF TRANSPLANT REJECTION AND AUTOIMMUNITY

PRIMARY NONFUNCTION

The phenomenon of primary nonfunction of transplanted islets, which is not well-defined, refers to transplants in which insulin secretion rapidly disappears over a period of days to weeks. While this could be due to poor quality islets, it is usually thought to be immunologic due to combinations of instant blood-mediated inflammatory reaction, accelerated autoimmunity, autoimmunity and inadequate immunosuppression as discussed. In the post Edmonton era, it is rarely seen, but some patients do lose C peptide in just a few months or less for unclear reasons. In further support of an immune basis, such rapid failure virtually never occurs with autotransplants. The benefits of immunologic matching of donor and recipient have not been carefully studied but most successful transplants have been matched only to blood type and not for histocompatibility antigens.[92] Questions are now being raised as to whether some patients become sensitized to islet grafts, which has implications for human leukocyte antigen (HLA) matching for subsequent islets infusions. Measurement of islet autoantibodies prior to transplantation is usually of little help because the titers are typically low, but some have found that the presence of autoantibodies is associated with a worse outcome.[161,162] Given the common end pathways of these destructive processes, use of the soluble complement receptor 1 (sCR1) TP10 is also being explored as it may help decrease peri-islet inflammation and thrombus formation and thus decrease primary nonfunction.[136] Another approach that may be worth pursuing is the measurement of gene expression of various immune mediators in circulating lymphocytes during the course of transplantation, as this has been found to correlate with kidney allograft rejection and may provide clues for future targeted therapy.[163]

AUTOGRAFTS

Transplantation of islets that do not face immune attack provides important lessons about how well islets in the liver can perform. When pancreases are removed because of painful pancreatitis, it is often possible to digest the removed pancreas and infuse the islet-containing preparation into the liver via the portal vein. Typically, these digested pancreatic preparations have been relative impure, containing non-islet pancreatic elements including duct cells that may have capacity for neogenesis. Because these impure preparations often have a high volume, sometimes as high as 25 mL of packed cells, care must be taken to infuse them slowly with careful monitoring of portal pressure.[164] These patients do remarkably well with about 70% being insulin-independent at 1 year if more than 300,000 islet equivalents are transplanted.[93] Sometimes even less than 200,000 islets can be successful, which is considerably less than what is usually required for successful allografts.[165,166] The most obvious explanation for success is that there are no problems with allorejection, autoimmunity, or immunosuppression. However, it must also be remembered that the removal of glucagon by the pancreatectomy and tendency of these patients to be thin could make them relatively insulin sensitive.

ALLOGRAFTS IN THE ABSENCE OF AUTOIMMUNITY

Further insights into the possible problems caused by autoimmunity have been provided by cluster operations for abdominal malignancy in which the liver, pancreas, and other organs were removed, followed by transplantation of a liver from a cadaver donor into which were placed islets isolated usually from the pancreas of the same donor.[90,93] These transplants were unique in that in the absence of autoimmune diabetes, a steroid-free immunosuppressive regimen of high-dose tacrolimus monotherapy could be used. Astounding in the pre-Edmonton era, over 50% of the recipients maintained insulin independence, prior to mortality from infection or recurrent malignancy, with one patient being insulin-independent for 5 years. Although transplantation of the liver may have had some beneficial immune influence, the absence of autoimmunity and diabetogenic drugs are suspected to be major reasons for the success. Complicating the interpretation, these recipients were typically unhealthy, so they may have required less β-cell mass to accommodate their reduced nutritional intake and weight.

INDUCTION OF TOLERANCE

One of the dreams of transplantation is to induce tolerance, which means that treatment given only at the time of transplantation will somehow trick the recipient's immune system into accepting transplanted foreign tissue as its own. In contrast to solid-organ transplants, the procedural risks of islet transplantation are considered modest and graft failure is not acutely life threatening. The ability of islets to survive in culture also makes it possible to more readily manipulate the graft prior to transplant. As such, many investigators consider islet transplantation a good system in which to study tolerogenic strategies. Many different approaches, which are currently being studied, could lead to full or operational tolerance (Table 65-3). A number of the recipient-based treatment strategies are discussed here, while graft-based strategies are discussed later in this chapter.

Unfortunately, there are also drawbacks to using the islet transplantation model, as patients with type 1 diabetes have an ongoing pathogenic autoimmune process. Thus, any tolerogenic strategy may be confounded by preactivated autoreactive T cells, autoantibodies, and other immunologic abnormalities present in diabetes. Recurrence of autoimmune disease and selective loss of islets has been reported in non-immunosuppressed or minimally immunosuppressed recipients of HLA-matched pancreas transplants.[167] Surprisingly, selective loss of islets has also been reported with standard immunosuppression even with poor HLA matching.[168]

CENTRAL TOLERANCE

Central tolerance refers to the process by which autoreactive T-cell clones are deleted as they migrate through the thymus. It has long been hoped that a similar process could be used to eliminate alloreactive T-cell clones; several donor-specific tolerance strategies have been developed that mimic this central tolerance by leading to near total and permanent elimination of donor-specific T-cell clones in the recipient. One such strategy is to directly introduce antigen into the thymus to aid in thymic selection. Posselt and colleagues demonstrated that injection of pancreatic islets directly into the thymus after treatment with antilymphocyte serum led to donor-specific unresponsiveness and long-term survival of islet grafts in a rodent model.[169] To date, there has only been one report describing an attempt to apply this technique in a clinical setting with computed tomography (CT)-guided fine-needle intrathymic inoculation and

Table 65-3 Approaches to Tolerance Induction

Recipient Treatment Strategies

Central tolerance
  Intrathymic inoculation
  Chimerism (thymic irradiation)
Peripheral tolerance/immune deviation
  Inhibition of costimulation (CTLA4-Ig, anti-CD154)
  Changing immune context from Th1 to Th2 (anti-CD45RB)
  Generalized T-cell depletion (anti-CD52, immunotoxin)
  Peptide-based therapies
  Donor-specific transfusion
  Anergy (hOKT3γ1 Ala-Ala)
  Lymphocyte sequestration (FTY-720)
  Clonal deletion of donor reactive T cells (AICD)

Graft Treatment Strategies

Gene transfer to islets (Fas-ligand, CTLA4-Ig, TGF-β)
Depletion of donor APCs from Graft
Privileged sites (cotransplantation with Sertoli cells)
Masking of surface proteins (MHC knockouts, encapsulation)
Engineered islets (insulin-producing cells of pituitary lineage)

simultaneous portal vein islet infusion and immunosuppression with an azathioprine, cyclosporine-based regimen. Although the patient never became insulin-independent, there was evidence of continued graft function at 14 months.[170].This approach has interesting immunologic implications, but the need for intrathymic injection, the temporal limitations of transplantation, and age-related atrophy of the thymus have made its clinical application difficult at best.

Another tactic is to use strategies that rely on the creation of mixed donor and recipient multilineage hematopoietic chimeras. This technique takes advantage of the ability of hematopoietic cells to home to areas of T-cell selection such as the thymus and to become dendritic cells capable of mediating selection. Thus, in chimeric hosts, donor-specific T cells are destroyed in peripheral immune tissues and new thymic emigrants are depleted of donor reactive T cells in the thymus.[171] Using this approach, a small number of patients with refractory hematologic malignancies and renal failure have demonstrated tolerance after myeloablation followed by bone marrow transplantation and kidney transplant from the same donor.[172,173] In islet transplantation, the induction of tolerance through mixed chimerism may have the added benefit of preventing autoimmune recurrence. Experiments by Megan Sykes' group using nonmyeloablative conditioning in nonobese diabetic mice have demonstrated reversal of autoimmunity and acceptance of islet grafts.[174] Although current engraftment protocols are considered too toxic for clinical use in islet transplantation, novel strategies to increase the level of chimerism while reducing the risks associated with conditioning the recipient are being actively explored.

PERIPHERAL TOLERANCE (SHIFTING THE CONTEXT)

Despite the rigorous nature of central selection, autoreactive T cells can escape thymic deletion into the periphery. As such, the normal immune system has mechanisms of peripheral tolerance to discourage autoimmunity. Jonker and colleagues coined the acronym WOLFIE for a "window of opportunity for immunological engagement" that may exist immediately posttransplant.[175] The idea is that if the graft is seen during this time in the appropriate context, tolerance may ensue. Posttransplantation, most alloreactive host CD4+ T cells are of the T-helper 1 phenotype expressing the cytokines IL-2 and interferon γ but not the T-helper 2 cytokines IL-4, IL-5, IL-10, and IL-13. However, if one could remove this alloreactive "help" by eliminating these T-helper 1 T cells or fostering the development of T-helper 2 cells in an early phase after transplantation, this could predispose to tolerogenic encounters with the graft.

A number of compounds designed to create immune deviation in this manner have been developed. T-cell depleting agents currently being investigated include immunotoxin, antithymocyte globulin (thymoglobulin), Campath 1H (a humanized anti-CD52 monoclonal antibody that acts as a powerful T- and B-cell depleting agent), and anti-CD3 antibodies. Unlike the steroids previously used in induction, these agents are not designed to decrease immune recognition, but instead allow recognition and then modify the body's overall response. As the use of these T-cell depleting agents has become widespread in induction therapy, new trials have been designed to focus on immunosuppressive drug withdrawal. To this end, the Edmonton group and the Immune Tolerance Network are currently developing a protocol to treat islet transplant recipients with a combination of Campath 1H and rapamycin with the intent of full drug withdrawal at approximately 1 year. Investigation of regimens consisting of thymoglobulin and the anti-TNF agent etanercept or the anti-CD3 monoclonal antibody hOKT3γ1(Ala-Ala) as induction agents in clinical islet transplants at the University of Minnesota are underway.[103] Interestingly, hOKT3γ1(Ala-Ala), a humanized

anti-CD3 antibody (mAb), which lacks strong Fc-receptor binding with reduced immunogenicity, and minimal cytokine release syndrome compared to the unmodified antibody has also been used to clinically delay progression of new onset type 1 diabetes.[176] It is believed to anergize acutely activated T-cell clones and reduce regulatory population.

The group of Judy Thomas at the University of Alabama has developed a primate anti-CD3-specific diphtheria-based immunotoxin. This compound is believed to deplete naive and memory T cells in blood and lymphatic compartments. 15-deoxyspergualin is given concurrently to block proinflammatory cytokine production and maturation of dendritic cells by inhibiting nuclear translocation of nuclear factor-κB (NF-κB).[177] Using this technique, they have reported operational tolerance in approximately 85% of animals with normal β-cell function approximately 2 years after transplantation.[178]

In the two-signal model of T-cell activation, the costimulatory signal is essential for T-cell activation and effector function. Costimulatory blockade prevents clonal expansion and can achieve peripheral tolerance in several animal models. A number of costimulatory modifying agents including anti-CD154 and CTLA4-Ig are being actively investigated. Studies by Kenyon and colleagues have shown anti-CD154 treatment to be effective in a primate islet transplant model.[125] Despite these and other encouraging results in nonhuman primates, the future of anti-CD154 therapy is uncertain. CD154 is also expressed on platelets and early clinical trials for rheumatoid arthritis with a humanized anti-CD154 blocking antibody (Hu5C8) were halted in the setting of thromboembolic complications. LEA29Y, a mutant CTLA4-Ig molecule with increased binding activity, was recently evaluated by Adams and colleagues in an allogeneic islet primate model. Their data suggest that this agent has promise as a component in a minimal immunosuppression regimen, but not as a sole therapy.[179]

Kirk and colleagues have found that although administering anti-CD154 or CTLA4-Ig could significantly prolong renal allograft survival, treatment with both agents was much more efficacious. In a primate model they saw improved graft survival and evidence of durable tolerance with subsequent nonresponsiveness to skin allografts from the original donors.[180] Unfortunately, while anti-CD154/CTLA4-Ig combination therapy may produce some degree of transplantation tolerance in many animal models, this regimen does not enable long-term graft survival in mice with overt autoimmune diabetes.[181] Given these findings, it is unlikely that simple deletion or costimulatory blockade alone will clinically prevent islet rejection in individuals already with underlying autoimmune diabetes.

A number of other promising agents that work by varied mechanisms are currently being evaluated. A few are briefly discussed here. FTY-720 is an agent that causes the emigration of lymphocytes from peripheral blood to secondary lymphoid structures and has proven effective in various transplantation models including nonhuman primate allografts.[182,183] Monoclonal antibodies against CD45RB, an isoform of a transmembrane protein tyrosine kinase phosphatase exclusively expressed by hematopoietic cells, have also been found to inhibit the rejection of islet allografts and are associated with an increase in the intragraft expression of the T-helper 2 cytokines IL-4 and IL-10.[184] Leflunomide and brequinar block de novo pyrimidine biosynthesis and reduce the available nucleotide pool for DNA and RNA synthesis. By this mechanism, rapidly replicating cells such as recently activated lymphocytes are effectively inhibited from proliferation. There is also some evidence that FK778 (a derivative of leflunomide) may reduce endothelial adhesion molecule expression, thus interfering with lymphocyte migration too.[185] These pyrimidine biosynthesis inhibitors are currently being studied extensively in islet xenograft models or as adjunct therapy to more conventional immunosuppressive agents.

Zheng and Strom have gone beyond these approaches and developed an ingenious new strategy that avoids nonspecific inhibition, blockade of T-cell receptor signaling, or costimulation altogether and instead is designed to selectively eliminate activated cytopathic donor reactive T cells while sparing immunoregulatory networks.[186] Their approach takes advantage of the body's natural immunoregulatory machinery to a much greater extent than the other approaches presented herein.

Activation induced cell death (AICD) is a method by which the body rapid eliminates effector cells after antigen-dependent clonal expansion while passive cell death removes superfluous clones via growth factor deprivation of activated T cells. AICD and passive cell death are both routine downstream consequences of T-cell activation and help maintain peripheral tolerance. Normally, IL-2 triggers AICD, whereas IL-15 protects activated effector T cells from both AICD and passive cell death. By using rapamycin, which blocks the proliferation, but not the apoptotic effects of IL-2, early clonal expansion can be limited without affecting subsequent apoptotic clearance (AICD). When rapamycin is given in combination with agonist IL-2 immunoglobulin fusion protein and antagonist IL-15 related cytolytic immunoglobulin fusion protein, this cocktail induces durable transplantation tolerance in mice with prior autoimmune diabetes.[186] While the IL-2 promotes apoptosis of proliferating effector T cells, it is also a survival factor for immunoregulatory CD4+CD25+ T cells. The mutant IL-15 operates by blocking normal IL-15 triggered antiapoptotic signals. Through these mechanisms, this treatment biases the immune response to one of immunoregulatory T cells over pathogenic T cells. Preliminary islet transplant experiments in nonhuman primates seem promising with durable tolerance and no evidence of opportunistic infections (M. Koulmanda, X. X. Zheng, and T. B. Strom, unpublished observations).[187]

THE SHORTAGE OF INSULIN-PRODUCING TISSUE

At present the only source of islets for transplantation into humans is cadaver pancreases, which are in very short supply. It is currently not possible to use living donors because a sufficient number of islets can not reliably be obtained from a donated portion of a pancreas. In the United States, it would be a major challenge to obtain 3000 usable cadaver pancreases per year, yet the incidence of type 1 diabetes is about 30,000 cases per year,[188] and more than 10 times as many people develop type 2 diabetes. Although there have been some successes with single donor transplants, usually two or more cadaver pancreases are required to provide insulin independence. There has been much discussion about the possibility of using human fetal tissue, but in spite of some advances this is proving to be a difficult road.[189,190] Many transplants of human fetal pancreas have been performed around the world but no clear benefit has been demonstrated.[92] At present, no one has found a way to exploit the growth potential of fetal pancreases; moreover, many ethical and practical issues cloud the future of this approach. A number of potential alternative sources for insulin-producing cells are listed in Table 65-4 and described in the following section.

EXPANSION OF HUMAN β CELLS FROM STEM CELLS, OTHER PRECURSOR CELLS, AND CELL LINES

It is now appreciated that new β cells are generated throughout adult life both from replication of preexisting β cells and through the formation of new β cells from precursor cells that appear to be contained in pancreatic ducts.[191] In the presence of hyperglycemia and insulin resistance, β-cell hypertrophy can also contribute to the increase in β-cell mass.[192,193] To maintain β-cell mass, the birth of new β cells is balanced

Table 65-4	Potential Sources of Insulin-Producing Cells

HUMAN SOURCES
Live donors—could be a source of precursor cells
Cadaver pancreases
Fetal pancreases
Expansion of existing human β cells in vitro or in vivo
Precursor cells—embryonic or adult stem/precursor cells
Transdifferentiation of liver, intestinal, pancreatic acinar, or other cells
Cell lines

XENO SOURCES
Adult, fetal, or neonatal islets from pigs, rabbits, rodents, fish, other cell lines
Transgenic pigs (or other species)

by death, mainly through apoptosis. There remains much uncertainty about β-cell turnover in part due to species differences. One study in mice found no evidence for neogenesis in adult life, but considerable capacity of β-cell replication.[194] Yet precursor cells appear to be present in the mouse pancreas[195,196] and neogenesis occurs in rats after partial pancreatectomy.[197] In the adult human pancreas β-cell replication appears to be almost negligible, but new islet formation from duct cells seems likely to occur.[149,151] There is increasing excitement about the possibility of expanding β-cell number by exploiting the developmental capacity of precursor cells. This could be accomplished by stem cells or other precursor cells, by finding new ways to stimulate the replication of existing β cells, or by creating a useful β-cell line.

STEM/PRECURSOR CELLS

The definition of stem cells has become very complex. There are "true stem cells" that have the capacity of unlimited expansion and are capable of generating various cell types, such as hematopoietic or intestinal cells. There are also "embryonic stem cells" found in blastocysts that are capable of developing into any specialized cell type. Then there are the facultative or "functional stem cells" that are differentiated cells capable of generating new cells. These can include the differentiated pancreatic duct cells that with the proper stimulus can change their differentiation and become activated to form new acinar cells and possibly even islets.[198] There was considerable interest in the possibility that circulating bone marrow stem cells could transdifferentiate to become β cells, but if this occurs at all it is a rare event.[199] Yet bone marrow cells may turn out to be useful as suggested by the provocative finding of multipotent adult precursor cells, derived from long-term cultures of bone marrow stroma, which can generate ectodermal, endodermal, and mesodermal progeny.[200]

Recent advances provide hope that stem cells can be used to make new β cells that will solve the problem of limited β-cell supply. For example, it has been recently shown that a duct cell containing preparation obtained from adult human cadaver pancreases when stimulated with growth factors and matrix, forms duct cysts from which sprout islets containing β cells and the other islet cell types, these being called cultivated human islet buds,[149] a finding confirmed by others.[201] At present, not enough cultivated human islet buds can be generated to be useful for clinical transplants, but perhaps there is potential for further expansion. These studies raise the hope that a single pancreas could provide enough islets to supply β cells for more than one recipient. In addition, it might be possible to obtain pancreatic tissue from someone with diabetes and then cultivate new islets, which can be returned in the form of a transplant. For type 1 diabetes, this would mean that allorejection would not be a problem, but autoimmunity would still need to be controlled. Other researchers have obtained considerable expansion of cells obtained from human islets, which unfortunately seem to contain little insulin.[202–204] Many laboratories are trying to promote these expanded cells to differentiate into a β-cell phenotype that might be useful for transplantation.

The expected potential of embryonic stem cells has led to great optimism, but early excitement has become more subdued with the realization that it has thus far not been possible to generate cells with insulin content approaching that of normal β cells.[205,206] The ability to exploit the potential of embryonic stem cells seems likely dependent on the generation of more knowledge of the mechanisms of normal embryonic development. A possible approach to embryonic stem cell research is therapeutic cloning, whereby using nuclear transfer techniques one could allow the generation of β cells with the same genetic makeup as the individual in need of a transplant.[207,208] There has also been some preliminary success using parthenogenetic (a process by which an egg can develop into an embryo in the absence of sperm) stem cells in nonhuman primates.[209]

INSULIN-PRODUCING CELL LINES

Through advances in molecular and cell biology, it is now theoretically possible to manipulate the differentiation of cells with genetic engineering so they can be used for transplantation. It has been possible to transform murine insulin-producing cells with the SV40 T antigen, expand these cells in culture, and then turn off the oncogene with a tetracycline response element, with resultant redifferentiation.[210] These experiments provide a potentially important proof-of-principle. Another approach is to try to create a β-cell equivalent by adding genes or inhibiting the expression of existing genes.[211,212] For example, the proinsulin gene can be expressed in cells that normally do not make insulin with the result that these cells can not only make proinsulin and cleave it to insulin, but can store and secrete insulin in response to a variety of stimuli. By adding more genes that influence glucose metabolism, it is even possible to manipulate these cells so that their insulin secretion is partially regulated by glucose levels. Another approach has been to engineer cells from the intermediate lobe of the pituitary to make insulin.[213] These cells are of interest because in spite of making significant quantities of insulin, they are not subject to autoimmune attack. Despite these encouraging preliminary results, it is becoming clear that normal β cells are remarkably complicated, which means it may be difficult to create near normal β cells by altering a few genes. On the other hand, as more is learned about the master switches that control the differentiation of cells, more promising results may emerge. Human insulin-producing cell lines have been derived from patients with persistent hyperinsulinemic hypoglycemia of infancy.[214] Although these cells can be expanded in tissue culture, they do not contain much insulin and have not yet been engineered to secrete insulin properly in response to physiologic levels of glucose. Other work with human islets employing genetic introduction of oncogenes and key transcription factors has produced cells that have some glucose-induced insulin secretion.[215]

In considering the potential use of insulin-secreting cells for transplantation, the question arises as to whether the non–β cells of the islet or some equivalent should be included in the transplanted cell aggregates. However, it seems that non–β cells are probably not required as suggested by experiments in which relative pure β-cell populations, prepared by flow cytometry, functioned reasonably well when transplanted into diabetic rodents.[216]

TRANSDIFFERENTIATION

There is growing interest in the possibility of reprogramming differentiated cells to adopt a β-cell phenotype. One of the most promising avenues is to use hepatocytes, which are attractive because of their endodermal derivation. Several groups have made significant progress in creating insulin-producing cells by introducing genes expressing PDX-1, NeuroD, and betacellulin.[217–219] There has also been a suggestion that hepatic oval cells can differentiate into insulin-producing cells.[220] Others are exploring whether acinar cells can undergo significant transdifferentiation.[221]

XENOTRANSPLANTATION

Despite increased optimism about the prospects for developing new sources of human β cells, investigators are still exploring the possibility of using tissue from other species as xenotransplants (see Table 65-1). The list of species that are potentially useful includes pigs, cows, rabbits, rodents, and even fish. Pigs have had particular appeal because pig insulin has been used in the past for treatment of people with diabetes, pigs have glucose levels similar to humans, pigs are part of the food chain, and people seem to be comfortable about the prospect of using this source. Unfortunately, pig islet tissue is not easy to work with and it continues to be difficult to generate high-quality islets from adult pigs.[222,223] Much work is now being done to develop ways to use either fetal tissue or neonatal xeno-islet tissue, which are attractive sources because of their growth potential.[224–228] One of the problems with this tissue is that the cells are immature, which means they can take weeks or months to normalize glucose levels in transplant recipients. Another potential problem is that porcine tissue contains porcine endogenous retroviruses that can be transferred to human cells in tissue culture.[229,230] There is considerable uncertainly about whether this represents a health threat, but in the United States, transplants using porcine tissue for the treatment of neurologic disease have been allowed to proceed cautiously. Thus far, no human recipients of porcine tissue have been reported to carry porcine retroviruses.[231]

IMMUNE ATTACK ON XENOGENEIC ISLETS

Rejection of xenografts is a complex and aggressive process.[232–234] There is an early attack called hyperacute rejection mediated by antibodies and complement that can lead to destruction of a transplanted organ within minutes. These preformed IgM antibodies recognize a glycoprotein called the Gal-α-Gal epitope (Gal epitope) that is strongly expressed on the surface of endothelial cells. This is a particular problem for organ transplants because the attack on endothelial cells produces ischemia that leads to rapid death of the transplanted tissue. Cell transplants may not be as vulnerable to this process. For example, it seems that adult pig islet cells have little Gal epitope.[235] Recently, pigs with the Gal epitope knocked out have been generated,[236] which may prove useful for islet transplantation. However, even though islet cells might escape hyperacute rejection, they will be subjected to damage from T cells, which seems to be similar to allorejection, and to other insults such as infiltration with eosinophiles and macrophages.[118,122,232] Adult porcine islets transplanted into the livers of nonhuman primates appear to largely escape acute rejection as judged by histologic examination over several days.[237] Surprisingly, xenografted tissue may also be susceptible to autoimmune attack, which does not seem to be species specific.[238] It is not known whether tolerance to discordant xenografts will ever be possible, but progress is being made with transplanting vascularized xenogeneic tissue containing thymus.[239,240]

IMMUNOBARRIER TECHNOLOGY

Semipermeable membranes that create an immunobarrier can protect transplanted islet tissue from immune destruction.[241–243] These membranes have openings large enough for glucose, oxygen, and nutrients to reach the encapsulated islets and for insulin to be released to enter the bloodstream. Yet, the holes are small enough so that white blood cells can not penetrate the membrane and reach the islet cells. There are important questions about how permeable membranes need to be. Recently, it has been found that merely maintaining a distance between lymphocytes and islet cells may be enough to prevent autoimmune and allorejection destruction.[244,245] Protection of xenotransplants seems to require more restrictive membranes to limit passage of smaller molecules. Much of the optimism about immunobarriers has been based on successes in rodents, but failure to demonstrate convincing successes in large animals has produced considerable skepticism about the future of this approach. The technology may never be efficient enough to use clinically for the limited supply of islets available from cadaver pancreases, but perhaps it will be employed when another source of transplantable insulin-producing cells become available.

MACROENCAPSULATION

Macroencapsulation employs devices like hollow fibers or parallel flat sheets sealed at the edges, in which many islets are contained within a single device.[242,246–248] Large gel beads or even slabs made of either agarose or alginate can also be used for macroencapsulation.[249] One of the major advantages of such an approach is that the devices could be implanted in a variety of locations and yet still be retrieved or reloaded. The main problem with this approach is that it has been difficult to achieve a practical packing density, which means that too much surface area would be required to support the encapsulated islet cells.[247] Moreover, there are still questions about whether insulin will be released quickly enough to adequately control blood glucose levels, particularly from large gel beads.

MICROENCAPSULATION

Microencapsulation is an approach in which single or small numbers of islets are contained within a membrane. The most commonly used method employs alginate obtained from seaweed that can form a gel after exposure to calcium or barium (Fig. 65-5).[250–254] Thus, islets can be captured in a small gel bead (usually less that 1 mm in diameter), that can be coated with a material such as poly-L-lysine that can provide permselectivity. Because poly-L-lysine can generate an inflammatory tissue reaction, an outer layer of alginate is usually added to make the capsules more biocompatible. Recent studies indicate that simple barium alginate microcapsules without a polylysine coating can successfully protect against autoimmunity, allorejection, and even xenoreactivity in mice.[245] Agarose has also been employed for microcapsules,[255] as has alginate mixed with other polymers such as cellulose sulfate.[256] Another similar approach that is being explored is to use a polyethylene glycol with photopolymerization to form a coating.[257] Despite the extensive amount of research in this area, encapsulation has not translated into clinical practice. To date there has only been one published report of a patient with even limited insulin independence using this approach and that was following intraperitoneal injection of encapsulated islets from eight pancreases.[252]

APPROACHES TO IMPROVING β-CELL SURVIVAL AND FUNCTION

An ambitious goal is to create stronger β cells that will withstand the ischemia of early transplantation, early inflammatory assaults, toxic effects or immunosuppressive agents, and the challenge of immune attack. Individual strengthening

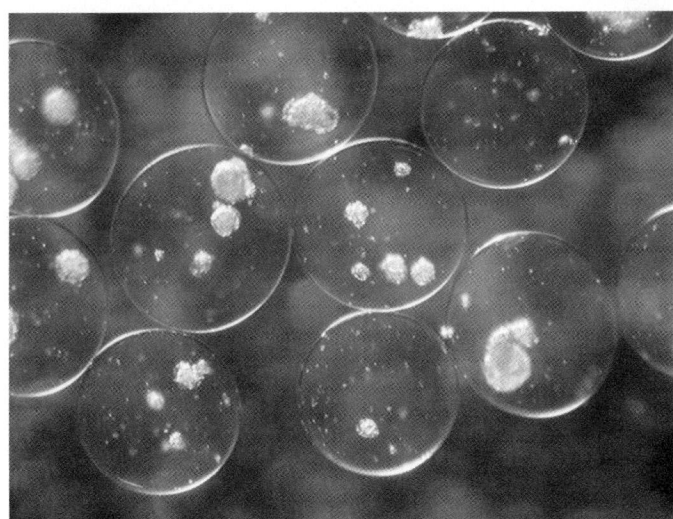

Figure 65-5 Alginate microcapsules containing porcine neonatal pancreatic cell clusters. The alginate gel creates a semipermeable membrane that protects islet cells or aggregates of cells from immune destruction. A commonly used approach is to use small beads of alginate covered by poly-L-lysine, but in some situations the poly-L-lysine is not used. These microcapsules are usually between 500 and 1000 μm in diameter. The membrane will prevent penetration by cells and limit the entrance of antibodies but must be permeable enough to allow passage of glucose, nutrients, and oxygen to the islets and insulin out to diffuse into small vessels. Photograph courtesy of Dr. Abdulkadir Omer.

measures might provide protection against multiple affronts. Genes can be transduced into β cells with a variety of techniques, either in the early stages of development or with such means as viral vectors at a later stage. A wide array of approaches has been discussed in review articles[258,259] and are summarized in Table 65-5.

ENGINEERING β CELLS TO EVADE IMMUNOLOGIC RECOGNITION

The concept behind this approach is to remove cell-surface antigens that elicit immune recognition. An example of this is class I major histocompatibility compex (MHC) antigens, whose expression can be lowered by viral infection. This mechanism has already been exploited to make islets more resistant to immune destruction.[260]

ENGINEERED SECRETION OF PROTECTIVE PEPTIDES

A variety of peptides can modulate the destructive actions of invading immune cells through various mechanisms. For

Table 65-5	Strategies to Improve β-cell Function and Survival
1.	**Removal of surface antigens:** Class I MHC antigens
2.	**Engineer islets to secrete protective peptides:** CTLA4-Ig, TGF-β, IL-1 receptor antagonist protein (IRAP), IL-10
3.	**Genetic addition of antiapoptotic genes:** A20, bcl-2, IκB repressor, MyD88, FLIP
4.	**Treat with inhibitors of apoptosis:** Z-DEVD-FMK, which is an inhibitor of caspase-3
5.	**Enhance antioxidant protection:** Overexpress manganese super oxide dismutase, catalase, or heme oxygenase-1; carbon monoxide treatment; and inhibit c-Jun-terminal kinase
6.	**Strengthening actions of growth factors:** Hepatocyte growth factor glucagon-like peptide 1, enhance PI 3-kinase and Akt signaling
7.	**Cotransplantation of protective cells:** Sertoli cells

example, costimulation blockade with locally produced CTLA4-Ig can delay allograft rejection.[261,262] Viral transduction of islets with transforming growth factor β cells can also lead to improved islet graft survival.[263] To protect β cells against the presumed toxic effects of IL-1, islets engineered to secrete the IL-1 receptor antagonist protein have also been found to be more resistant to rejection.[264] Another approach has employed the use of IL-10, which pushes immune responses to a T-helper 2 phenotype. When introduced with adeno-associated virus into islets, some protection against immune rejection was found.[265]

INHIBITION OF APOPTOSIS

As information increases about cell death pathways, an increasing number of opportunities for islet protection have emerged. Transduction of the antiapoptosis gene bcl-2 can provide protection of islets against cytokines and improve performance with transplantation.[266] An important target for protecting β cells is NF-κB. Indeed, protection of β cells during transplantation has been found with viral overexpression of A20, which blocks NF-κB activation. Protection has also been found with overexpression of an IκB repressor.[267] Other death pathways have been exploited including the use of the dominant-negative mutant of the IL-1 receptor interacting protein MyD88[268] and FLICE inhibitory protein (FLIP), which can inhibit caspase-3.[269] Because cyclic adenosine monophosphate and glucagon-like peptide-1 have been found to have anti-apoptotic effects in β cells,[270] it may be helpful to engineer β cells with more glucagon-like peptide-1 receptors or use some other approach to make more cyclic adenosine monophosphate. Perhaps this would even lead to enhanced secretion, although it is possible the set point for glucose-stimulated insulin secretion (GSIS) would become low enough to produce hypoglycemia. Another approach used to reduce apoptosis is to expose islets before transplantation to Z-DEVD-FMK, which is an inhibitor of caspase-3.[271]

STRENGTHENING ANTIOXIDANT PROTECTION

β-cell defenses against oxidant injury appear to be relatively weak,[272] so bolstering these mechanisms is an attractive option. For example, increased expression of manganese superoxide dismutase can provide protection against cytokine injury in islet cell lines.[273] Unfortunately, attempts made to obtain benefit from overexpression of catalase have been only modestly promising.[274] Another avenue that holds some promise is inhibition of the c-Jun-terminal kinase, which has been shown to protect islets against oxidative stress.[275] Yet another mechanism that provides protection against oxidative injury is the heme oxygenase system, which can exert effects through several mechanisms. It has been found that overexpression of heme oxygenase-1 with adenoviruses can lead to protection against cytokine injury and improve outcomes with rodent islet transplants.[276] A product of heme oxygenase is carbon monoxide, which by itself can be protective,[277] making it possible that treatment of islets with low concentrations of carbon monoxide prior to transplantation could provide important benefit.

GROWTH FACTORS MAY PRODUCE STRONGER AND BETTER β CELLS

Growth factor signaling is being shown to be very important for β-cell function and survival. For example, glucose can promote β-cell survival through PI 3-kinase and Akt signaling.[278] The antiapoptotic effect of glucagons-like peptide-1 appears to be dependent on IRS-2, with the later steps of this signaling probably being exerted through Akt. Interestingly, overexpression of Akt produces β-cell hypertrophy,[279] which leads to hyperinsulinemia; it is not clear, however, if there is increased efficiency of secretion per given amount of β-cell mass. Hepatocyte growth factor overexpression through both transgenesis and adenoviral transduction has been found to improve β-cell resistance to apoptosis and improve survival of transplanted islets.[280,281] A very intriguing finding is that with the hepatocyte growth factor transgenic mice, insulin content per unit of β-cell mass is increased.[280] This is surprising because β cells are so efficient in storing insulin that further improvement might not have been predicted. These studies raise the intriguing possibility that a normal β cell could be engineered to secrete more insulin.

COTRANSPLANTATION OF CELLS WITH A PROTECTIVE EFFECT

The best example of such protection is Sertoli cells, which provide immunoprotection. Although originally thought to be via Fas-ligand expression, it is probably through production of TGF-β as well as other, as yet unknown, mechanisms.[282]

CONCLUSIONS

Even with the limitations described herein, successful pancreas or islet transplantation is currently the only therapy that reproducibly achieves normoglycemia. The recent advances in the ability to achieve insulin independence with these techniques have only increased the number of patients seeking β-cell replacement as an alternative to insulin therapy. However, given the efficacy of standard insulin therapy, and the known complications of chronic immunosuppression, β-cell replacement is still usually limited to patients otherwise requiring immunosuppression for another transplant or with life-threatening diabetes mellitus.

Currently, solid-organ transplantation offers a greater chance for durable insulin independence compared to islet transplant. However, attempts to predict the future of islet transplantation have proved hazardous. While the ultimate goal has been and continues to be clear, difficult obstacles continue to emerge.

Major advances are required to overcome these barriers to widespread success: the need for sufficient quantities of transplantable insulin-producing cells and safe methods to prevent these cells from being destroyed by the immune system. However, one must be optimistic that the commitment of interested parties and the growing power of modern science will eventually prevail.

For further details on the subject of pancreas and islet transplantations, we recommend a number of excellent recent reviews.[187,283–286]

REFERENCES

1. The effect of intensive treatment of diabetes on the development and progression of long-term complications in insulin-dependent diabetes mellitus. The Diabetes Control and Complications Trial Research Group. N Engl J Med 329:977–986, 1993.
2. UK Prospective Diabetes Study Group: Intensive blood-glucose control with sulfonylureas or insulin compared with conventional treatment and risk of complications in patients with type 2 diabetes (UKPDS 33). Lancet 352:837–853, 1998.
3. Chia CW, Saudek CD: Glucose sensors: Toward closed loop insulin delivery. Endocrinol Metab Clin North Am 33:175–195, 2004.
4. Williams PW: Notes on diabetes treated with extract and by grafts of sheep's pancreas. Br Med J 1303–1304, 1894.
5. Kelly WD, Lillehei RC, Merkel FK, et al: Allotransplantation of the pancreas and duodenum along with the kidney in diabetic nephropathy. Surgery 61: 827–837, 1967.

6. Sutherland DE, Gruessner RW, Dunn DL, et al: Lessons learned from more than 1,000 pancreas transplants at a single institution. Ann Surg 233:463–501, 2001.

7. Sutherland DER, Groth CG: History of pancreas transplantation. In Hakim N, Sratta R, Gray D (eds): Pancreas and Islet Transplantation. Oxford, Oxford University Press, 2002, pp 1–13.

8. Sollinger HW, Cook K, Kamps D, et al: Clinical and experimental experience with pancreaticocystostomy for exocrine pancreatic drainage in pancreas transplantation. Transplant Proc 16:749–751, 1984.

9. Bloom RD, Olivares M, Rehman L, et al: Long-term pancreas allograft outcome in simultaneous pancreas-kidney transplantation: A comparison of enteric and bladder drainage. Transplantation 64:1689–1695, 1997.

10. Stratta RJ, Shokouh-Amiri MH, Egidi MF, et al: Long-term experience with simultaneous kidney-pancreas transplantation with portal-enteric drainage and tacrolimus/mycophenolate mofetil-based immunosuppression. Clin Transplant 17(Suppl 9):69–77, 2003.

11. Kuo PC, Johnson LB, Schweitzer EJ, Barlett ST: Simultaneous pancreas/kidney transplantation—a comparison of enteric and bladder drainage of exocrine pancreatic secretions. Transplantation 63:238–243, 1997.

12. Del Pizzo JJ, Jacobs SC, Bartlett ST, Sklar GN: Urological complications of bladder-drained pancreatic allografts. Br J Urol 81:543–547, 1998.

13. Hickey DP, Bakthavatsalam R, Bannon CA, et al: Urological complications of pancreatic transplantation. J Urol 157:2042–2048, 1997.

14. Cattral MS, Bigam DL, Heming AW, et al: Portal venous and enteric exocrine drainage versus systemic venous and bladder exocrine drainage of pancreas grafts: Clinical outcome of 40 consecutive transplant recipients. Ann Surg 232:688–695, 2000.

15. Katz HH, Nguyen TT, Velosa JA, et al: Effects of systemic delivery of insulin on plasma lipids and lipoprotein concentrations in pancreas transplant recipients. Mayo Clin Proc 69:231–236, 1994.

16. Carpentier A, Patterson BW, Uffelman KD, et al: The effect of systemic versus portal insulin delivery in pancreas transplantation on insulin action and VLDL metabolism. Diabetes 50:1402–1413, 2001.

17. Kaufman DB, Leventhal JR, Koffron AJ, et al: A prospective study of rapid corticosteroid elimination in simultaneous pancreas-kidney transplantation: Comparison of two maintenance immunosuppression protocols: Tacrolimus/mycophenolate mofetil versus tacrolimus/sirolimus. Transplantation 73:169–177, 2002.

18. Drachenberg CB, Klassen DK, Weir MR, et al: Islet cell damage associated with tacrolimus and cyclosporine: Morphological features in pancreas allograft biopsies and clinical correlation. Transplantation 68:396–402, 1999.

19. Jindal RM, Revanur VK, Jardine AG: Immunosuppression and diabetogenicity. In Hakim N, Stratta R, Gray D (eds): Pancreas and Islet Transplantation. Oxford, Oxford University Press, 2002, pp 229–246.

20. Sutherland DER, Goetz FC, Sibley RK: Recurrence of disease in pancreas transplants. Diabetes 38:85–87, 1989.

21. Simone EA, Wegmann DR, Eisenbarth GS: Immunologic "Vaccination" for the prevention of autoimmune diabetes (type 1A). Diabetes Care 22(Suppl 2):B7–B15, 1999.

22. London NJ, Farmery SM, Will EJ, et al: Risk of neoplasia in renal transplant patients. Lancet 346:403–406, 1995.

23. First MR, Gerber DA, Hariharan S, et al: Posttransplant diabetes mellitus in kidney allograft recipients: Incidence, risk factors, and management. Transplantation 73:379–386, 2002.

24. Delaunay F, Khan A, Cintra A, et al: Pancreatic beta cells are important targets for the diabetogenic effects of glucocorticoids. J Clin Invest 100:2094–2098, 1997.

25. Gremlich S, Roduit R, Thorens B: Dexamethasone induces posttranslational degradation of GLUT2 and inhibition of insulin secretion in isolated pancreatic B cells. J Biol Chem 272:3216–3222, 1997.

26. Uchizono Y, Iwase M, Nakamura U, et al: Tacrolimus impairment of insulin secretion in isolated rat islets occurs at multiple distal sites in stimulus-secretion coupling. Endocrinology 145:2264–2272, 2004.

27. Bell E, Cao X, Moibi JA, et al: Rapamycin has a deleterious effect on MIN-6 cells and rat and human islets. Diabetes 52:2731–2739, 2003.

28. McDaniel ML, Marshall CA, Pappan KL, Kwon G: Metabolic and autocrine regulation of the mammalian target of rapamycin by pancreatic beta-cells. Diabetes 51:2877–2885, 2002.

29. Nankivell BJ, Borrows RJ, Fung CL, et al: The natural history of chronic allograft nephropathy. N Engl J Med 349:2326–2333, 2003.

30. Bilous RW, Mauer SM, Sutherland DE, et al: The effects of pancreas transplantation on the glomerular structure of renal allografts in patients with insulin-dependent diabetes. N Engl J Med 321:80–85, 1989.

31. Wilczek HE, Jaremko G, Tyden G, Groth CG: Evolution of diabetic nephropathy in kidney grafts. Evidence that a simultaneously transplanted pancreas exerts a protective effect. Transplantation 59:51–57, 1995.

32. Drachenberg CB, Papdimitriou JC, Klassen DK, et al: Evaluation of pancreas transplant needle biopsy: Reproducibility and revision of histologic grading system. Transplantation 63:1579–1586, 1997.

33. Manske CL, Wang Y, Thomas W: Mortality of cadaveric kidney transplantation versus combined kidney-pancreas transplantation in diabetic patients. Lancet 346:1658–1662, 1995.

34. Battezzati A, Bonfatti D, Benedini S, et al: Spontaneous hypoglycaemic after pancreas transplantation in type 1 diabetes mellitus. Diabet Med 15:991–996, 1998.

34a. 2003 Annual Report of the U.S. Organ Procurement and Transplantation Network and the Scientific Registry of Transplant Recipients: Transplant Data 1993–2002. Department of Health and Human Services, Health Resources and Services Administration, Office of Special Programs, Division of Transplantation, Rockville, MD; United Network for Organ Sharing, Richmond, VA; University Renal Research and Education Association, Ann Arbor, MI. 2003.

35. Odorico JS, Leverson GE, Becker YT, et al: Pancreas transplantation at the University of Wisconsin. Clin Transpl 1:199–210, 1999.

36. Venstrom JM, McBride MA, Rother KI, et al: Survival after pancreas transplantation in patients with diabetes and preserved kidney function. JAMA 290:2817–2823, 2003.

37. Wolfe RA, Ashby VB, Milford EL, et al: Comparison of mortality in all patients on dialysis, patients on dialysis awaiting transplantation, and recipients of a first cadaveric transplant. N Engl J Med 341:1725–1730, 1999.

38. Ramsay RC, Goetz FC, Sutherland DE, et al: Progression of diabetic retinopathy after pancreas transplantation for insulin-dependent diabetes mellitus. N Engl J Med. 318:208–214, 1988.

39. Petersen MR, Vine AK: Progression of diabetic retinopathy after pancreas transplantation. The University of Michigan Pancreas Transplant Evaluation Committee. Ophthalmology 97:496–500, 1990.

40. Scheider A, Meyer-Schwickerath E, Nusser J, et al: Diabetic retinopathy and pancreas transplantation: A 3-year follow-up. Diabetologia 34(Suppl 1):S95–S99, 1991.

41. Abouna GM, Al-Adnani MS: Is diabetic nephropathy reversible? Transplant Proc 19(Suppl 2):82–85, 1987.

42. Abouna GM, Al-Adnani MS, Kremer GD, et al: Reversal of diabetic nephropathy in human cadaveric kidneys after transplantation into non-diabetic recipients. Lancet 2(8362):1274–1276, 1983.

43. Fioretto P, Steffes MW, Sutherland DER, et al: Reversal of lesions of diabetic nephropathy after pancreas transplantation. N Engl J Med 339:69–75, 1998.

44. Solders G, Tyden G, Persson A, Groth CG: Improvement of nerve conduction in diabetic neuropathy.

A follow-up study 4 yr after combined pancreatic and renal transplantation. Diabetes 41:946–951, 1992.

45. Muller-Felber W, Landgraf R, Scheuer R, et al: Diabetic neuropathy 3 years after successful pancreas and kidney transplantation. Diabetes 42:1482–1486, 1993.

46. Navarro X, Sutherland DE, Kennedy WR: Long-term effects of pancreatic transplantation on diabetic neuropathy. Ann Neurol 42:727–736, 1997.

47. Allen RD, Al-Harbi IS, Morris JG, et al: Diabetic neuropathy after pancreas transplantation: Determinants of recovery. Transplantation 63:830–838, 1997.

48. Hathaway DK, Abell T, Cardoso S, et al: Improvement in autonomic and gastric function following pancreas-kidney versus kidney-alone transplantation and the correlation with quality of life. Transplantation 57:816–822, 1994.

49. Ewing DJ, Campbell IW, Clarke BF: The natural history of diabetic autonomic neuropathy. Q J Med 49:95–108, 1980.

50. Sampson MJ, Wilson S, Karagiannis P, et al: Progression of diabetic autonomic neuropathy over a decade in insulin-dependent diabetics. Q J Med 75:635–646, 1990.

51. Navarro X, Kennedy WR, Sutherland DER: Autonomic neuropathy and survival in diabetes mellitus: Effects of pancreas transplantation. Diabetologia 34:S108–S112, 1991.

52. Biesenbach G, Margreiter R, Konigsrainer A, et al: Comparison of progression of macrovascular diseases after kidney or pancreas and kidney transplantation in diabetic patients with end-stage renal disease. Diabetologia 43:231–234, 2000.

53. Fiorina P, La Rocca E, Venturini M, et al: Effects of kidney-pancreas transplantation on atherosclerotic risk factors and endothelial function in patients with uremia and type 1 diabetes. Diabetes 50:496–501, 2001.

54. Larsen JL, Ratanasuwan T, Burkman T, et al: Carotid intima media thickness decreases after pancreas transplantation. Transplantation 73:936–940, 2002.

55. Jukema JW, Smets YF, van der Pijl JW, et al: Impact of simultaneous pancreas and kidney transplantation on progression of coronary atherosclerosis in patients with end-stage renal failure due to type 1 diabetes. Diabetes Care 25:906–911, 2002.

56. Cryer PE, Davis SN, Shamoon H: Hypoglycemia in diabetes. Diabetes Care 26:1902–1912, 2003.

57. Diem P, Redmon JB, Abid M, et al: Glucagon, catecholamine and pancreatic polypeptide secretion in type I diabetic recipients of pancreas allografts. J Clin Invest 86:2008–2013, 1990.

58. Kendall DM, Rooney DP, Smets YF, et al: Pancreas transplantation restores epinephrine response and symptom

recognition during hypoglycemia in patients with long-standing type I diabetes and autonomic neuropathy. Diabetes 46:249–257, 1997.

59. Cottrell DA, Henry ML, O'Dorisio TM, et al: Hypoglycemia after successful pancreas transplantation in type I diabetic patients. Diabetes Care 14:1111–1113, 1991.

60. Holohan TV: Simultaneous pancreas-kidney and sequential pancreas-after-kidney transplantation. Health Technol Assess Rep 4:1–53, 1995.

61. Robertson RP, Holohan TV, Genuth S: Therapeutic controversy: Pancreas transplantation for type I diabetes. J Clin Endocrinol Metab 83:1868–1874, 1998.

62. Matas AJ, McHugh L, Payne WD, et al: Long-term quality of life after kidney and simultaneous pancreas-kidney transplantation. Clin Transplant 12:233–242, 1998.

63. Milde FK, Hart LK, Zehr PS: Pancreatic transplantation. Impact on the quality of life of diabetic renal transplant recipients. Diabetes Care 18:93–95, 1995.

64. Adang EM, Engel GL, van Hooff JP, Kootstra G: Comparison before and after transplantation of pancreas-kidney and pancreas-kidney with loss of pancreas—a prospective controlled quality of life study. Transplantation 62:754–758, 1996.

65. Gross CR, Limwattananon C, Matthees B, et al: Impact of transplantation on quality of life in patients with diabetes and renal dysfunction. Transplantation 70:1736–1746, 2000.

66. Stratta RJ: The economics of pancreas transplantation. Graft 3:19–23, 2000.

67. Effect of intensive therapy on residual beta-cell function in patients with type 1 diabetes in the diabetes control and complications trial. A randomized, controlled trial. The Diabetes Control and Complications Trial Research Group. Ann Intern Med 128:517–523, 1998.

68. Kendall DM, Sutherland DER, Najarian JS, et al: Effects of hemipancreatectomy on insulin secretion and glucose tolerance in healthy humans. N Engl J Med 322:898–903, 1990.

69. Ballinger WF, Lacy PE: Transplantation of intact pancreatic islets in rats. Surgery 72:175–186, 1972.

70. Reckard CR, Barker CF: Transplantation of isolated pancreatic islets across strong and weak histocompatibility barriers. Transplant Proc 5:761–763, 1973.

71. Lacy PE, Kostianovsky M: Method for the isolation of intact islets of Langerhans from the rat pancreas. Diabetes 16:35–39, 1967.

72. Scharp DW, Kemp CB, Knight MJ, et al: The use of ficoll in the preparation of viable islets of langerhans from the rat pancreas. Transplantation 16:686–689, 1973.

73. Horaguchi A, Merrell RC: Preparation of viable islet cells from dogs by a new method. Diabetes 30:455–458, 1981.

74. Ricordi C, Lacy PE, Finke EH, et al: Automated method for isolation of human pancreatic islets. Diabetes 37:413–420, 1988.

75. Latif ZA, Noel J, Alejandro R: A simple method of staining fresh and cultured islets. Transplantation 45:827–830, 1988.

76. Kemp CB, Knight MJ, Scharp DW: Transplantation of isolated pancreatic islets into the portal vein of diabetic rats. Nature 244:447, 1973.

77. Farkas G, Csajbok E, Voros P, et al: Successful simultaneous transplantation of kidney and fetal pancreatic islet masses. Transpl Int 8:229–233, 1995.

78. Toledo-Pereyra LH, Rowlett AL, Lodish M: Autotransplantation of pancreatic islet cell fragments into the renal capsule prepared without collagenase. Am Surg 50:679–681, 1984.

79. Largiader F, Kolb E, Binswanger U, Illig R: Successful allotransplantation of an island of Langerhans. Schweiz Med Wochenschr 109:1733–1736, 1979.

80. Scharp DW, Marchetti P, Swanson C, et al: The effect of transplantation site and islet mass on long-term survival and metabolic and hormonal function of canine purified islet autografts. Cell Transplant 1:245–254, 1992.

81. Warnock GL, DeGroot T, Untch D, et al: The natural history of pure canine islet autografts in hepatic or splenic sites. Transplant Proc 21:2617–2618, 1989.

82. Gray DW: Islet isolation and transplantation techniques in the primate. Surg Gynecol Obstet 170:225–232, 1990.

83. White SA, London NJ, Johnson PR, et al: The risks of total pancreatectomy and splenic islet autotransplantation. Cell Transplant 9:19–24, 2000.

84. White SA, Robertson GS, Davies JE, et al: Splenic infarction after total pancreatectomy and autologous islet transplantation into the spleen. Pancreas 18:419–421, 1999.

85. Najarian JS, Sutherland DE, Matas AJ, et al: Human islet transplantation: A preliminary report. Transplant Proc 9:233–236, 1977.

86. Scharp DW, Lacy PE, Santiago JV, et al: Results of our first nine intra portal islet allografts in type 1, insulin dependent diabetic patients. Transplantation 51:76–85, 1991.

87. Socci C, Falqui L, Davalli AM, et al: Fresh human islet transplantation to replace pancreatic endocrine function in type I diabetic patients. Acta Diabetol 28:151–157, 1991.

88. Warnock G, Kneteman NM, Ryan EA, et al: Long-term follow-up after transplantation of insulin-producing pancreatic islets into patients with type I (insulin-dependent) diabetes mellitus. Diabetologia 35:89–95, 1992.

89. Ricordi C, Tzakis AG, Carroll PB, et al: Human islet isolation and allotransplantation transplantation in

22 consecutive cases. Transplantation 53:407–414, 1992.

90. Tzakis AG, Ricordi C, Alejandro R, et al: Pancreatic islet transplantation after upper abdominal exenteration and liver replacements. Lancet 336:402–405, 1990.

91. Menger MD, Vajkoczy P, Beger C, Messmer K: Orientation of microvascular blood flow in pancreatic islet isografts. J Clin Invest 93:2280–2285, 1994.

92. Hering BJ, Ricordi C: Islet transplantation for patients with type 1 diabetes. Graft 2:12–27, 1999.

93. Brendel MD, Hering BJ, Schultz AO, Bretzel RG: Longest graft function of islet allografts in diabetes mellitus. International Islet Transplant Registry Newsletter #8:1–20, 1999.

94. Alejandro R, Lehmann R, Ricordi C, et al: Long-term function (6 years) of islet allografts in type 1 diabetes. Diabetes 46:1983–1989, 1997.

95. Oberholzer J, Triponez F, Mage R, et al: Human islet transplantation: Lessons from 13 autologous and 13 allogeneic transplantations. Transplantation 69:1115–1123, 2000.

96. Secchi A, Socci C, Maffi P, et al: Islet transplantation in IDDM patients. Diabetologia 40:225–231, 1997.

97. Keymeulen B, Ling Z, Gorus FK, et al: Implantation of standardized beta-cell grafts in a liver segment of IDDM patients: Graft and recipients characteristics in two cases of insulin-independence under maintenance immunosuppression for prior kidney graft. Diabetologia 41: 452–459, 1998.

98. Bretzel RG, Brandhorst D, Brandhorst H, et al: Improved survival of intraportal pancreatic islet cell allografts in patients with type-1 diabetes mellitus by refined peritransplant management. J Mol Med 77:140–143, 1999.

99. Linetsky E, Bottino R, Lehmann R, et al: Improved human islet isolation using a new enzyme blend, liberase. Diabetes 46:1120–1123, 1997.

100. Shapiro AM, Lakey JR, Ryan EA, et al: Islet transplantation in seven patients with type 1 diabetes mellitus using a glucocorticoid-free immunosuppressive regimen. N Engl J Med 27:230–238, 2000.

101. Shapiro AM, Ricordi C, Hering B: Edmonton's islet success has indeed been replicated elsewhere. Lancet 362:1242, 2003.

102. Goss JA, Schock AP, Brunicardi FC, et al: Achievement of insulin independence in three consecutive type-1 diabetic patients via pancreatic islet transplantation using islets isolated at a remote islet isolation center. Transplantation 74:1761–1766, 2002.

103. Hering BJ, Kandaswamy R, Harmon JV, et al: Transplantation of cultured islets from two-layer preserved pancreases in type 1 diabetes with anti-CD3 antibody. Am J Transplant 4:390–401, 2004.

104. Markmann JF, Deng S, Huang X, et al: Insulin independence following isolated islet transplantation and single islet infusions. Ann Surg 237:741–750, 2003.

105. Kessler L, Bucher P, Milliat-Guittard L, et al: Influence of islet transportation on pancreatic islet allotransplantation in type 1 diabetic patients within the Swiss-French GRAGIL network. Transplantation 77:1301–1304, 2004.

106. Fiorina P, Folli F, Bertuzzi F, et al: Long-term beneficial effect of islet transplantation on diabetic macro-/microangiopathy in type 1 diabetic kidney-transplanted patients. Diabetes Care 26:1129–1136, 2003.

107. Cagliero E, Chandraker A, Dea A, et al: Islet cell transplantation in type 1 diabetic patients recipient of renal allografts. Diabetes 53(Suppl 2):A452, 2004.

108. Lehmann R, Weber M, Berthold P, et al: Successful simultaneous islet-kidney transplantation using a steroid-free immunosuppression: two-year follow-up. Am J Transplant 4:1117–1123, 2004.

109. Humar A, Ramcharan T, Kandaswamy R, et al: The impact of donor obesity on outcomes after cadaver pancreas transplants. Am J Transplant 4:605–610, 2004.

110. Markmann JF, Deng S, Desai NM, et al: The use of non-heart-beating donors for isolated pancreatic islet transplantation. Transplantation 75:1423–1429, 2003.

111. Hirshberg B, Rother KI, Digon BJ 3rd, et al: Benefits and risks of solitary islet transplantation for type 1 diabetes using steroid-sparing immunosuppression: The National Institutes of Health experience. Diabetes Care 26:3288–3295, 2003.

112. Ryan EA, Lakey JR, Paty BW, et al: Successful islet transplantation: Continued insulin reserve provides long-term glycemic control. Diabetes 51:2148–2157, 2002.

113. Ryan EA, Paty BW, Senior PA, Shapiro AM: Risks and side effects of islet transplantation. Curr Diab Rep 4:304–309, 2004.

114. Casey JJ, Lakey JR, Ryan EA, et al: Portal venous pressure changes after sequential clinical islet transplantation. Transplantation 74:913–915, 2002.

115. Rafael E, Ryan EA, Paty BW, et al: Changes in liver enzymes after clinical islet transplantation. Transplantation 76:1280–1284, 2003.

116. Bhargava R, Senior PA, Ackerman TE, et al: Prevalence of hepatic steatosis after islet transplantation and its relation to graft function. Diabetes 53:1311–1317, 2004.

117. Markmann JF, Rosen M, Siegelman ES, et al: Magnetic resonance-defined periportal steatosis following intraportal islet transplantation: A functional footprint of islet graft survival? Diabetes 52:1591–1594, 2003.

118. Efanova IB, Zaitsev SV, Zhivotovsky B, et al: Glucose and tolbutamide induce apoptosis in pancreatic beta-cells. A process dependent on intracellular Ca2+ concentration. J Biol Chem 273:33501–33507, 1998.

119. Fiorina P, Folli F, Maffi P, et al: Islet transplantation improves vascular diabetic complications in patients with diabetes who underwent kidney transplantation: A comparison between kidney-pancreas and kidney-alone transplantation. Transplantation 75:296–1301, 2003.

120. Johnson JA, Kotovych M, Ryan EA, Shapiro AM: Reduced fear of hypoglycemia in successful islet transplantation. Diabetes Care 27:624–625, 2004.

121. Guignard AP, Oberholzer J, Benhamou PY, et al: Cost analysis of human islet transplantation for the treatment of type 1 diabetes in the Swiss-French Consortium GRAGIL. Diabetes Care 27:895–900, 2004.

122. Light JA, Sasaki TM, Currier CB, Barhyte DY: Successful long-term kidney-pancreas transplants regardless of C-peptide status or race. Transplantation 71:152–154, 2001.

123. Ryan EA, Lakey JR, Paty BW, et al: Successful islet transplantation: Continued insulin reserve provides long-term glycemic control. Diabetes 51: 2148–2157, 2002.

124. O'Neil JJ, Tchipashvili V, Parent RJ, et al: A simple and cost-effective method for the isolation of islets from nonhuman primates. Cell Transplant 12:883–890, 2003.

125. Kenyon NS, Chatzipetrou M, Masetti M, et al: Long-term survival and function of intrahepatic islet allografts in rhesus monkeys treated with humanized anti-CD 154. Proc Natl Acad Sci U S A 96:8132–8137, 1999.

126. Kenyon NS, Fernandez LA, Lehmann R, et al: Long-term survival and function of intrahepatic islet allografts in baboons treated with humanized andti-CD154. Diabetes 48:1473–1481, 1999.

127. Paty BW, Ryan EA, Shapiro AM, et al: Intrahepatic islet transplantation in type 1 diabetic patients does not restore hypoglycemic hormonal counterregulation or symptom recognition after insulin independence. Diabetes 51:3428–3434, 2002.

128. Banarer S, McGregor VP, Cryer PE: Intraislet hyperinsulinemia prevents the glucagon response to hypoglycemia despite an intact autonomic response. Diabetes 51:958–965, 2002.

129. Omer A, Duvivier-Kali VF, Aschenbach W, et al: Exercise induces hypoglycemia in rats with islet transplantation. Diabetes 53:360–365, 2004.

130. Portis AJ, Warnock GL, Finegood DT, et al: Glucoregulatory response to moderate exercise in long-term islet

cell autografted dogs. Can J Physiol Pharmacol 68:1308–1312, 1990.

131. Dionne KE, Colton CK, Yarmuch ML: Effect of hypoxia on insulin secretion by isolated rat and canine islets of Langerhans. Diabetes 42:12–21, 1993.

132. Davalli AM, Scaglia L, Zangen DH, et al: Vulnerability of islets in the immediate posttransplantation period. Diabetes 45:1161–1167, 1996.

133. Halloran PF, Homik J, Goes N: The "injury response": A concept linking nonspecific injury, acute rejection, and long-term transplant outcomes. Transplant Proc 29:79–81, 1997.

134. Benent W, Sundberg B, Groth CG, et al: Incompatibility between human blood and isolated islets of Langerhans: A finding with implications for clinical intraportal islet transplantation? Diabetes 48:1907–1914, 1999.

135. Medzhitov R, Janeway C Jr: Innate immunity. N Engl J Med 343:338–343, 2000.

136. Bennet W, Sundberg B, Groth CG: Incompatibility between human blood and isolated islets of Langerhans: A finding with implications for clinical intraportal islet transplantation? Diabetes 48:1907–1914, 1999.

137. Ozmen L, Ekdahl KN, Elgue G, et al: Inhibition of thrombin abrogates the instant blood-mediated inflammatory reaction triggered by isolated human islets: Possible application of the thrombin inhibitor melagatran in clinical islet transplantation. Diabetes 51:1779–1784, 2002.

138. Moberg L, Johansson H, Lukinius A, et al: Production of tissue factor by pancreatic islet cells as a trigger of detrimental thrombotic reactions in clinical islet transplantation. Lancet 360:2039–2045, 2002.

139. Moberg L, Olsson A, Berne C, et al: Nicotinamide inhibits tissue factor expression in isolated human pancreatic islets: Implications for clinical islet transplantation. Transplantation 76:1285–1288, 2003.

140. Johansson U, Olsson A, Gabrielsson S, et al: Inflammatory mediators expressed in human islets of Langerhans: Implications for islet transplantation. Biochem Biophys Res Commun 308:474–479, 2003.

141. Menger MD, Yamauchi J, Vollmar B: Revascularization and microcirculation of freely grafted islets of Langerhans. World J Surg 25:509–515, 2001.

142. Brissova M, Fowler M, Wiebe P, et al: Intraislet endothelial cells contribute to revascularization of transplanted pancreatic islets. Diabetes 53:1318–1325, 2004.

143. Juang J-H, Bonner-Weir S, Wu Y-J, Weir GC: Beneficial influence of glycemic control upon the growth and function of transplanted islets. Diabetes 43:1334–1339, 1994.

144. Vasir B, Reitz P, Xu G: Effects of diabetes and hypoxia on gene markers of angiogenesis (HGF, cMET, uPA and uPAR, TGF-alpha, TGF-beta, bFGF and Vimentin) in cultured and transplanted rat islets. Diabetologia 43:763–772, 2000.

145. Sharma S, Jhala US, Johnson T, et al: Hormonal regulation of an islet-specific enhancer in the pancreatic homeobox gene STF-1. Mol Cell Biol 17:2598–2604, 1997.

146. Desai NM, Goss JA, Deng S, et al: Elevated portal vein drug levels of sirolimus and tacrolimus in islet transplant recipients: Local immunosuppression or islet toxicity? Transplantation 76:1623–1625, 2003.

147. Jansson L, Carlsson PO: Graft vascular function after transplantation of pancreatic islets. Diabetologia 45:749–763, 2002.

147a. Hirshberg B, Mog S, Patterson N, et al: Histopathological study of intrahepatic islets transplanted in the nonhuman primate model using Edmonton protocol immunosuppression. J Clin Endocrinol Metab 87:5424–5429, 2002.

148. Bonner-Weir S, Sharma A: Pancreatic stem cells. J Pathol 197:519–526, 2002.

149. Bonner-Weir S, Taneja M, Weir GC: In vitro cultivation of human islets from expanded ductal tissue. Proc Natl Acad Sci U S A 97:7999–8004, 2000.

150. Kerr-Conte J, Pattou F, Lecomte-Houcke M, et al: Ductal cyst formation in collagen-embedded adult human islet preparations. Diabetes 45:1108–1114, 1996.

151. Butler AE, Janson J, Bonner-Weir S, et al: Beta-cell deficit and increased beta-cell apoptosis in humans with type 2 diabetes. Diabetes 52:102–110, 2003.

152. Tyrberg B, Ustinov J, Otonkoski T, Andersson A: Stimulated endocrine cell proliferation and differentiation in transplanted human pancreatic islets: Effects of the ob gene and compensatory growth of the implantation organ. Diabetes 50:301–307, 2001.

153. Bonner-Weir S, Orci L: New perspectives on the microvasculature of the islets of Langerhans in the rat. Diabetes 31:883–939, 1982.

154. Weir GC, Bonner-Weir S: Islets of Langerhans: The puzzle of intraislet interactions and their relevance to diabetes. J Clin Invest 85:983–987, 1990.

155. Stagner JI, Samols E: The vascular order of islet cellular perfusion in the human pancreas. Diabetes 41:93–97, 1992.

156. Stagner JI, Mokshagundam S, Samols E: Hormone secretion from transplanted islets is dependent upon changes in islet revascularization and islet architecture. Transplant Proc 27:3251–3254, 1995.

157. Korsgren O, Andersson A, Jansson L, Sundler F: Reinnervation of syngeneic mouse pancreatic islets transplanted into renal subcapsular space. Diabetes 41:130–135, 1992.

158. Carlsson PO, Palm F, Andersson A, Liss P: Chronically decreased oxygen tension in rat pancreatic islets transplanted under the kidney capsule. Transplantation 69:761–766, 2000.

159. Carlsson PO, Palm F, Mattsson G: Low revascularization of experimentally transplanted human pancreatic islets. J Clin Endocrinol Metab 87:5418–5423, 2002.

160. Biarnes M, Montolio M, Nacher V, et al: Beta-cell death and mass in syngeneically transplanted islets exposed to short- and long-term hyperglycemia. Diabetes 51:66–72, 2002.

161. Jaeger C, Brendel MD, Hering BJ, et al: Progressive islet graft failure occurs significantly earlier in autuantibody-positive than in autoantibody-negative IDDM recipients of intrahepatic islet allografts. Diabetes 46:1907–1910, 1997.

162. Braghi S, Bonifacio E, Secchi A, et al: Modulation of humoral islet autoimmunity by pancreas allotransplantation influences allograft outcome in patients with type 1 diabetes. Diabetes 49:218–224, 2000.

163. Vasconcellos L, Asher F, Schachter Dea: Cytotxic lymphocyte gene expression in peripheral blood leukocytes correlates with rejecting renal allografts. Transplantation 66:562–566, 1998.

164. White SA, Davies JE, Pollard C, et al: Pancreas resection and islet autotransplantation for end-stage chronic pancreatitis. Ann Surg 233:423–431, 2001.

165. Sutherland DER, Gores PF, Hering BJ, et al: Islet transplantation: An update. Diabetes Metab Rev 12:137–150, 1996.

166. Pyzdroswki KL, Kendall DM, Halter JB, et al. Preserved insulin secretion and insulin independence in recipients of islet autografts. N Engl J Med 327:220–226, 1992.

167. Sutherland DE, Goetz FC, Sibley RK: Recurrence of disease in pancreas transplants. Diabetes 38(Suppl 1): 85–87, 1989.

168. Tyden G, Reinholt FP, Sundkvist G, Bolinder J: Recurrence of autoimmune diabetes mellitus in recipients of cadaveric pancreatic grafts. N Engl J Med 335:860–863, 1996.

169. Posselt AM, Barker CF, Tomaszewski JE, et al: A: Induction of donor-specific unresponsiveness by intrathymic islet transplantation. Science 249:1293–1295, 1990.

170. Arias-Diaz J, Vara E, Balibrea JL, et al: CT-guided fine-needle approach for intrathymic islet transplantation in a diabetic patient. Pancreas 12:100–102, 1996.

171. Sykes M: Mixed chimerism and transplant tolerance. Immunity 14:417–424, 2001.

172. Cosimi AB, Sachs DH: Mixed chimerism and transplantation tolerance. Transplantation 77(6.6): 943–946, 2004.

173. Sayegh MH, Fine NA, Smith JL, et al: Immunologic tolerance to renal

allografts after bone marrow transplants from the same donors. Ann Intern Med 114:954–955, 1991.

174. Nikolic B, Takeuchi Y, Leykin I, et al: Mixed hematopoietic chimerism allows cure of autoimmune diabetes through allogeneic tolerance and reversal of autoimmunity. Diabetes 53:376–383, 2004.

175. Jonker M, Slingerland W, Ossevoort M, et al: Induction of kidney graft acceptance by creating a window of opportunity for immunologic engagement (WOFIE) in rhesus monkeys. Transplant Proc 30:2441–2443, 1998.

176. Herold KC, Hagopian W, Auger JA, et al: Anti-CD3 monoclonal antibody in new-onset type 1 diabetes mellitus. N Engl J Med 346:1692–1698, 2002.

177. Contreras JL, Wang PX, Eckhoff DE, et al: Peritransplant tolerance induction with anti-CD3-immunotoxin: A matter of proinflammatory cytokine control. Transplantation 65:1159–1169, 1998.

178. Contreras JL, Jenkins S, Eckhoff DE, et al: Stable alpha- and beta-islet cell function after tolerance induction to pancreatic islet allografts in diabetic primates. Am J Transplant 3:128–138, 2003.

179. Adams AB, Shirasugi N, Durham M, et al: Calcineurin inhibitor-free CD28 blockade-based protocol protects allogeneic islets in nonhuman primates. Diabetes 51:265–270, 2002.

180. Kirk AD, Harlan DM, Armstrong NN, et al: CTLA4-Ig and anti-CD40 ligand prevent renal allograft rejection in primates. Proc Natl Acad Sci U S A 94:8789–8794, 1997.

181. Demirci G, Strom TB, Li XC: Islet allograft rejection in nonobese diabetic mice involves the common gamma-chain and CD28/CD154-dependent and -independent mechanisms. J Immunol 171:3878–3885, 2003.

182. Quesniaux VF, Menninger K, Kunkler A, et al: The novel immunosuppressant FTY720 induces peripheral lymphodepletion of both T- and B-cells in cynomolgus monkeys when given alone, with Cyclosporine Neoral or with RAD. Transpl Immunol 8:177–187, 2000.

183. Wijkstrom M, Kenyon NS, Kirchhof N, et al: Islet allograft survival in nonhuman primates immuno-suppressed with basiliximab, RAD, and FTY720. Transplantation 77:827–835, 2004.

184. Basadonna GP, Auersvald L, Khuong CQ, et al: Antibody-mediated targeting of CD45 isoforms: A novel immunotherapeutic strategy. Proc Natl Acad Sci U S A 95:3821–3826, 1998.

185. Deuse T, Schrepfer S, Schafer H, et al: FK778 attenuates lymphocyte-endothelium interaction after cardiac transplantation: In vivo and in vitro studies. Transplantation 78:71–77, 2004.

186. Zheng XX, Sanchez-Fueyo A, Sho M, et al: Favorably tipping the balance between cytopathic and regulatory T cells to create transplantation tolerance. Immunity 19:503–514, 2003.

187. Ricordi C, Strom TB: Clinical islet transplantation: Advances and immunological challenges. Nat Rev Immunol 4:259–268, 2004.

188 LaPort RE, Matsushima M, Chang Y-F: Prevalence and incidence of insulin-dependent diabetes. In: Anonymous Diabetes in America, 2d ed. NIH, 1995, pp 37–46.

189. Beattie GM, Otonkoski T, Lopez AD, Hayek A: Functional β-cell mass after transplantation of human fetal pancreatic cells. Diabetes 46:244–248, 1997.

190. Tuch BE, Simpson AM: Experimental fetal islet transplantation. In Ricordi C (ed): Pancreatic Islet Cell Transplantation. Pittsburgh, R.G. Landes Co., 1992, pp 279–290.

191. Bonner-Weir S: Life and death of the pancreatic beta cells. Trends Endocrinol Metab 11:375–378, 2000.

192. Jonas J-C, Sharma A, Hasenkamp W, et al: Chronic hyperglycemia triggers loss of pancreatic β cell differentiation in an animal model of diabetes. J Biol Chem 274:14112–14121, 1999.

193. Montanya E, Nacher V, Biarnes M, Soler J: Linear correlation between beta cell mass and body weight throughout life in Lewis rats: Role of beta cell hyperplasia and hypertrophy. Diabetes 49:1341–1346, 2000.

194. Dor Y, Brown J, Martinez OI, Melton DA: Adult pancreatic beta-cells are formed by self-duplication rather than stem-cell differentiation. Nature 429:41–46, 2004.

195. Seaberg RM, Smukler SR, Kieffer TJ, et al: Clonal identification of multipotent precursors from adult mouse pancreas that generate neural and pancreatic lineages. Nat Biotechnol 22(9. 9), 1115–1124, Epub 2004, August 22, 2004.

196. Suzuki A, Nakauchi H, Taniguchi H: Prospective isolation of multipotent pancreatic progenitors using flow-cytometric cell sorting. Diabetes 53:2143–2152, 2004.

197. Bonner-Weir S, Baxter LA, Schuppin GT, Smith FE: A second pathway for regeneration of the adult exocrine and endocrine pancreas: A possible recapitulation of embryonic development. Diabetes 42:1715–1720, 1993.

198. Zangen DH, Bonner-Weir S, Lee CH, et al: Reduced insulin, GLUT2, and IDX-1 in B-cells after partial pancreatectomy. Diabetes 46:258–264, 1997.

199. Lechner A, Yang YG, Blacken RA, et al: No evidence for significant transdifferentiation of bone marrow into pancreatic beta-cells in vivo. Diabetes 53:616–623, 2004.

200. Jiang Y, Jahagirdar BN, Reinhardt RL, et al: Pluripotency of mesenchymal stem cells derived from adult marrow. Nature 418:41–49, 2002.

201. Bonner-Weir S, Weir GC: Adult progenitor cells as a potential treatment for diabetes. In Lanza R (ed): Handbook of Stem Cells, Volume 2: Adult and Fetal Stem Cells. Amsterdam, Elsevier, 2004, pp 731–738.

202. Gao R, Ustinov J, Pulkkinen MA, et al: Characterization of endocrine progenitor cells and critical factors for their differentiation in human adult pancreatic cell culture. Diabetes 52:2007–2015, 2003.

203. Ramiya VK, Marraist M, Arfors KE, et al: Reversal of insulin dependent diabetes using islets generated in vitro from pancreatic stem cells. Nat Med 6:278–282, 2000.

204. Beattie GM, Itkin-Ansari P, Cirulli V, et al: Sustained proliferation of PDX-1+ cells derived from human islets. Diabetes 48:1013–1019, 1999.

205. Zulewski H, Abraham EJ, Gerlach MJ, et al: Multipotential nestin-positive stem cells isolated from adult pancreatic islets differentiate ex vivo into pancreatic endocrine, exocrine, and hepatic phenotypes. Diabetes 50:521–533, 2001.

206. Leon-Quinto T, Jones J, Skoudy A, et al: In vitro directed differentiation of mouse embryonic stem cells into insulin-producing cells. Diabetologia 47:1442–1451, 2004.

207. Stoffel M, Vallier L, Pedersen RA: Navigating the pathway from embryonic stem cells to beta cells. Semin Cell Dev Biol 15:327–336, 2004.

208. Lanza RP, Chung HY, Yoo JJ, et al: Generation of histocompatible tissues using nuclear transplantation. Nat Biotechnol 20:689–696, 2002.

207. Atala A, Koh CJ: Tissue engineering applications of therapeutic cloning. Annu Rev Biomed Eng 6:27–40, 2004.

209. Cibelli JB, Grant KA, Chapman KB, et al: Parthenogenetic stem cells in nonhuman primates. Science 295:819, 2002.

210. Efrat S, Fusco-DeMane D, Lemberg H, et al: Conditional transformation of a pancreatic β cell line derived from transgenic mice expressing a tetracycline-regulated oncogene. Proc Natl Acad Sci U S A 92:3576–3580, 1995.

211. Clark SA, Quaade C, Constandy H, et al: Novel insulinoma cell lines produced by iterative engineering of GLUT2, glucokinase, and human insulin expression. Diabetes 46:958–967, 1997.

212. Hohmeier HE, Beltrandel Rio H, Clark SA, et al: Regulation of insulin secretion from novel engineered insulinoma cell lines. Diabetes 46:968–977, 1997.

213. Lipes MA, Cooper EM, Skelly R, et al: Insulin-secreting non-islet cells are resistant to autoimmune destruction. Proc Natl Acad Sci U S A 93:8596–8600, 1996.

214. MacFarlane WM, O'Brien RE, Barnes PD, et al: Sulfonylurea receptor 1 and Kir6.2 expression in the novel

human insulin-secreting cell line NES2Y. Diabetes 49:953–960, 2000.

215. Itkin-Ansari P, Geron I, Hao E, et al: Cell-based therapies for diabetes: Progress towards a transplantable human beta cell line. Ann N Y Acad Sci 1005:138–147, 2003.

216. Pipeleers DG, Pipeleers-Marichal M, Hannaert JC, et al: Transplantation of purified islet cells in diabetic rats. I. Standardization of islet cell grafts. Diabetes 40:908–919, 1991.

217. Ber I, Shternhall K, Perl S, et al: Functional, persistent, and extended liver to pancreas transdifferentiation. J Biol Chem 278:31950–31957, 2003.

218. Zalzman M, Gupta S, Giri RK, et al: Reversal of hyperglycemia in mice by using human expandable insulin-producing cells differentiated from fetal liver progenitor cells. Proc Natl Acad Sci U S A 100:7253–7258, 2003.

219. Kojima H, Fujimiya M, Matsumura K, et al: NeuroD-betacellulin gene therapy induces islet neogenesis in the liver and reverses diabetes in mice. Nat Med 9:596–603, 2003.

220. Yang L, Li S, Hatch H, et al: In vitro trans-differentiation of adult hepatic stem cells into pancreatic endocrine hormone-producing cells. Proc Natl Acad Sci U S A 99:8078–8083, 2002.

221. Rooman I, Heremans Y, Heimberg H, Bouwens L: Modulation of rat pancreatic acinoductal transdifferentiation and expression of PDX-1 in vitro. Diabetologia 43:907–914, 2000.

222. Davalli AM, Ogawa Y, Scaglia L, et al: Function, mass, and replication of porcine and rat islets transplanted into diabetic nude mice. Diabetes 44:104–111, 1995.

223. Brandhorst H, Brandhorst D, Hering BJ, Bretzel RG: Significant progress in porcine islet mass isolation utilizing liberase HI for enzymatic low-temperature pancreas digestion. Transplantation 68:355–361, 1999.

224. Mandel TE, Koulmanda M, Kovarik J, et al: Transplantation of organ cultured fetal pig pancreas in non-obese diabetic (NOD) mice and primates (Macaca fascicularis). Xenotransplantation 2:128–132, 1996.

225. Korsgren O, Andersson A, Sandler S: Pretreatment of fetal porcine pancreas in culture with nicotinamide accelerates reversal of diabetes after transplantation to nude mice. Surgery 113:205–214, 1993.

226. Tuch BE, Simpson AM, Smith MSR, et al: Basic biology of pig fetal pancreas and its use as an allograft. In Peterson CM, Jovanovic-Peterson L (eds): Fetal Islet Transplantation. New York, Plenum Press, 1995, pp 51–68.

227. Korbutt GS, Elliott JF, Ao Z, et al: Large scale isolation, growth, and function of porcine neonatal islet cells. J Clin Invest 97:2119–2129, 1996.

228. Yoon K-H, Quickel RR, Tatarkiewicz K, et al: Differentiation and expansion of beta cell mass in porcine neonatal pancreatic cell clusters transplanted into nude mice. Cell Transplant 8:673–689, 1999.

229. Patience C, Takeuchi Y, Weiss RA: Infection of human cells by an endogenous retrovirus of pigs. Nat Med 3:282–286, 1997.

230. van der Lean LJ, Lockey C, Griffeth BC, et al: Infection by porcine endogenous retrovirus after islet xenotransplantation in SCID mice. Nature 407:90–94, 2000.

231. Paradis K, Langford G, Long Z, et al: Search for cross-species transmission of porcine endogenous retrovirus in patients treated with living pig tissue. Science 285:1236–1241, 1999.

232. Bach FH, Winkler H, Ferran C, et al: Delayed xenograft rejection. Immunol Today 17:379–384, 1996.

233. Dorling A, Riesbeck K, Warrens A, Lechler R: Clinical xenotransplantation of solid organs. Lancet 349:867–871, 1997.

234. Soderlund J, Wennberg L, Castanos-Velez E, et al: Fetal porcine islet-like cell clusters transplanted to cynomolgus monkeys. Transplantation 67:784–791, 1999.

235. McKenzie I, Koulmanda M, Sandrin MS, Mandel TE: Expression of gal(1,3)gal by porcine islet cells and its relevance to xenotransplantation. Xenotransplantation 2:139–142, 1996.

236. Kolber-Simonds D, Lai L, Watt SR, et al: Production of alpha-1,3-galactosyltransferase null pigs by means of nuclear transfer with fibroblasts bearing loss of heterozygosity mutations. Proc Natl Acad Sci U S A 101:7335–7340, 2004.

237. Kirchhof N, Shibata S, Wijkstrom M, et al: Reversal of diabetes in non-immunosuppressed rhesus macaques by intraportal porcine islet xenografts precedes acute cellular rejection. Xenotransplantation 11:396–407, 2004.

238. Haskins K, Wegmann D: Diabetogenic T-cell clones. Diabetes 45:1299–1305, 1996.

239. Nikolic B, Gardner JP, Scadden DT, et al: Normal development in porcine thymus grafts and specific tolerance of human T cells to porcine donor MHC. J Immunol 162:3402–3407, 1999.

240. Kamano C, Vagefi PA, Kumagai N, et al: Vascularized thymic lobe transplantation in miniature swine: Thymopoiesis and tolerance induction across fully MHC-mismatched barriers. Proc Natl Acad Sci U S A 101:3827–3832, 2004.

241. Colton CK: Implantable biohybrid artificial organs. Cell Transplant 4:415–436, 1995.

242. Lacy PE, Hegre OD, Gerasimidi-Vazeou A, et al: Maintenance of normoglycemia in diabetic mice by subcutaneous xenografts of encapsulated islets. Science 254:1782–1784, 1991.

243. Lanza RP, Jackson R, Sullivan A, et al: Xenotransplantation of cells using biodegradable microcapsules. Transplantation 67:1105–1111, 1999.

244. Loudovaris T, Jacobs S, Young S, et al: Correction of diabetic nod mice with insulinomas implanted within Baxter immunoisolation devices. J Mol Biol 77:219–222, 1999.

245. Omer A, Duvivier-Kali VF, Trivedi N, et al: Survival and maturation of microencapsulated porcine neonatal pancreatic cell clusters transplanted into immunocompetent diabetic mice. Diabetes 52:69–75, 2003.

246. Brauker J, Martinson LA, Young SK, Johnson RC: Local inflammatory response around diffusion chambers containing xenografts. Transplantation 61:1671–1677, 1996.

247. Suzuki K, Bonner-Weir S, Trivedi N, et al: Function and survival of macroencapsulated syngeneic islets transplanted into streptozotocin-diabetic mice. Transplantation 66:21–28, 1998.

248. Tatarkiewicz K, Hollister-Lock J, Quickel RR, et al: Reversal of hyperglycemia in mice after subcutaneous transplantation of macroencapsulated islets. Transplantation 67:665–671, 1999.

249. Jain K, Asina SK, Patel SG, et al: Long-term preservation of islets of Langerhans in hydrophilic macrobeads. Transplantation 61:532–536, 1996.

250. Sun A, Ma X, Zhou D, et al: Normalization of diabetes in spontaneously diabetic cynomologus monkeys by xenografts of microencapsulated porcine islets without immunosuppression. J Clin Invest 98:1417–1422, 1996.

251. De Vos P, De Haan BJ, Wolters GHJ, et al: Improved biocompatibility but limited graft survival after purification of alginate for microencapsulation of pancreatic islets. Diabetologia 40:262–270, 1997.

252. Soon-Shiong P, Heintz RE, Merideth N, et al: Insulin independence in a type 1 diabetic patients after encapsulated islet transplantation. Lancet 343:950–951, 1994.

253. Lanza RP, Chick WL: Transplantation of encapsulated cells and tissues. Surgery 121:1–9, 1997.

254. Calafiore R: Perspectives in pancreatic and islet cell transplantation for the therapy of IDDM. Diabetes Care 20:889–895, 1997.

255. Iwata H, Takagi T, Amemiya H, et al: Agarose for a bioartificial pancreas. J Biomed Mater Res 26:967–977, 1992.

256. Wang T, Lacik I, Brissova M, et al: An encapsulation system for the immunoisolation of pancreatic islets. Nat Biotechnol 15:358–362, 1997.

257. Cruise GM, Hegre OD, Lamberti FV, et al: In vitro and in vivo performance of porcine islets encapsulated in interfacially photopolymerized poly(ethylene glycol) diacrylate membranes. Cell Transplant 8:293–306, 1999.

258. Giannoukakis N, Trucco M: Current status and prospects for gene and cell

therapeutics for type 1 diabetes mellitus. Rev Endocr Metab Disord 4:369–380, 2003.

259. Weir GC: Can we make surrogate beta-cells better than the original? Semin Cell Dev Biol 15:347–357, 2004.

260. Efrat S, Fejer G, Brownlee M, Horwitz MS: Prolonged survival of pancreatic islet allografts mediated by adenovirus immunoregulatory transgenes. Proc Natl Acad Sci U S A 92:6947–6951, 1995.

261. Steurer W, Nickerson PW, Steele AW, et al: Ex vivo coating of islet cell allografts with murine CTLA4/Fc promotes graft tolerance. J Immunol 155:1165–1174, 1995.

262. Feng S, Quickel RR, Hollister-Lock J, et al: Prolonged xenograft survival of islets infected with small doses of adenovirus containing CTLA4Ig. Transplantation 67:1607–1613, 1999.

263. Suarez-Pinzon WL, Marcoux Y, Ghahary A, Rabinovitch A: Gene transfection and expression of transforming growth factor-beta1 in nonobese diabetic mouse islets protects beta-cells in syngeneic islet grafts from autoimmune destruction. Cell Transplant 11:519–528, 2002.

264. Giannoukakis N, Rudert WA, Ghivizzani SC, et al: Adenoviral gene transfer of the interleukin-1 receptor antagonist protein to human islets prevents IL-1beta-induced beta-cell impairment and activation of islet cell apoptosis in vitro. Diabetes 48:1730–1736, 1999.

265. Zhang YC, Pileggi A, Agarwal A, et al: Adeno-associated virus-mediated IL-10 gene therapy inhibits diabetes recurrence in syngeneic islet cell transplantation of NOD mice. Diabetes 52:708–716, 2003.

266. Dupraz P, Rinsch C, Pralong W, et al: Lentivirus-mediated Bcl-2 expression in beta TC-tet cells improves resistance to hypoxia and cytokine-induced apoptosis while preserving in vitro and in vivo control of insulin secretion. Gene Ther 6:1160–1169, 1999.

267. Giannoukakis N, Rudert WA, Trucco M, Robbins PD: Protection of human islets from the effects of interleukin-1beta by adenoviral gene transfer of an Ikappa B repressor. J Biol Chem 275:36509–36513, 2000.

268. Dupraz P, Cottet S, Hamburger F, et al: Dominant negative MyD88 proteins inhibit interleukin-1beta /interferon-gamma -mediated induction of nuclear factor kappa B-dependent nitrite production and apoptosis in beta cells. J Biol Chem 275:37672–37678, 2000.

269. Maedler K, Fontana A, Ris F, et al: FLIP switches Fas-mediated glucose signaling in human pancreatic beta cells from apoptosis to cell replication. Proc Natl Acad Sci U S A 99:8236–8241, 2002.

270. Li Y, Hansotia T, Yusta B, et al: Glucagon-like peptide-1 receptor signaling modulates beta cell apoptosis. J Biol Chem 278:471–478, 2003.

271. Nakano M, Matsumoto I, Sawada T, et al: Caspase-3 inhibitor prevents apoptosis of human islets immediately after isolation and improves islet graft function. Pancreas 29:104–109, 2004.

272. Lenzen S, Drinkgern J, Tiedge M: Low antioxidant enzyme gene expression in pancreatic islets compared to with various other mouse tissues. Free Radic Biol Med 320:463–466, 1996.

273. Hohmeier HE, Thigpen A, Tran VV, et al: Stable expression of manganese superoxide dismutase (MnSOD) in insulinoma cells prevents IL-1beta-induced cytoxicity and reduces nitric oxide production. J Clin Invest 101:1811–1820, 1998.

274. Xu B, Moritz JT, Epstein PN: Overexpression of catalase provides partial protection to transgenic mouse beta cells. Free Radic Biol Med 27:830–837, 1999.

275. Kaneto H, Xu G, Fujii N, et al: Involvement of c-Jun N-terminal kinase in oxidative stress-mediated suppression of insulin gene expression. J Biol Chem 277:30010–30018, 2002.

276. Pileggi A, Molano RD, Berney T, et al: Heme oxygenase-1 induction in islet cells results in protection from apoptosis and improved in vivo function after transplantation. Diabetes 50:1983–1991, 2001.

277. Gunther L, Berberat PO, Haga M, et al: Carbon monoxide protects pancreatic beta-cells from apoptosis and improves islet function/survival after transplantation. Diabetes 51:994–999, 2002.

278. Srinivasan S, Bernal-Mizrachi E, Ohsugi M, Permutt MA: Glucose promotes pancreatic islet beta-cell survival through a PI 3-kinase/Akt-signaling pathway. Am J Physiol Endocrinol Metab 283:E784–E793, 2002.

279. Tuttle RL, Gill NS, Pugh W, et al: Regulation of pancreatic beta-cell growth and survival by the serine/threonine protein kinase Akt1/PKBalpha. Nat Med 7:1133–1137, 2001.

280. Garcia-Ocana A, Vasavada RC, Cebrian A, et al: Transgenic overexpression of hepatocyte growth factor in the beta-cell markedly improves islet function and islet transplant outcomes in mice. Diabetes 50:2752–2762, 2001.

281. Garcia-Ocana A, Takane KK, Reddy VT, et al: Adenovirus-mediated hepatocyte growth factor expression in mouse islets improves pancreatic islet transplant performance and reduces beta cell death. J Biol Chem 278:343–351, 2003.

282. Suarez-Pinzon W, Korbutt GS, Power R, et al: Testicular Sertoli cells protect islet beta-cells from autoimmune destruction in NOD mice by a transforming growth factor-beta1-dependenet mechanism. Diabetes 49:1810–1818, 2000.

283. Sutherland DE, Gruessner A, Hering BJ: Beta-cell replacement therapy (pancreas and islet transplantation) for treatment of diabetes mellitus: An integrated approach. Endocrinol Metab Clin North Am 33:135–148, 2004.

284. Shapiro AM, Nanji SA, Lakey JR: Clinical islet transplant: Current and future directions towards tolerance. Immunol Rev 196:219–236, 2003.

285. Robertson RP: Islet transplantation as a treatment for diabetes—a work in progress. N Engl J Med 350:694–705, 2004.

286. Oberholzer J, Shapiro AM, Lakey JR, et al: Current status of islet cell transplantation. Adv Surg 37:253–282, 2003.

287. Robertson RP, Sutherland DE, Kendall DM, et al: Metabolic characterization of long-term successful pancreas transplants in type I diabetes. J Investig Med 44:549–555, 1996.

Diabetes Control and Long-term Complications

David M. Nathan

INTRODUCTION

The historical documentation of type 1 diabetes includes at least 5000 years of testimony to its dramatic clinical onset with the apparent "melting of flesh into urine," followed by starvation, inanition, and certain death.[1] However, it wasn't until the near miraculous cure of diabetes, with the introduction of insulin less than a century ago, that long-term complications began to be observed with any frequency.[2] With longer survival of children and adolescents with what is now called type 1 diabetes, we began to see manifestations of diabetes that had never been seen before. Diabetic retinopathy and nephropathy were first described in the 1930s.[3,4] Insulin therapy transformed type 1 diabetes from a disease that was generally fatal in the first 6 to 24 months of its appearance, to a chronic degenerative disorder with a host of long-term complications that affected the eye, kidney, nervous system, and heart.

The development of these complications, which ultimately affected the majority of patients afflicted with type 1 diabetes, had a severe toll. By the time that insulin had been in use for 50 years, diabetes had become a major cause of blindness, kidney failure, and amputations and a contributor to cardiovascular disease.[5] With the epidemic of type 2 diabetes, diabetes became the greatest single cause of these complications by 1990. Not surprisingly, some clinicians/investigators considered the pathogenesis of these complications to be iatrogenic, with insulin, either directly or indirectly, causing the complications. Still others thought that the complications were co-inherited, but independent from the metabolic perturbations of the disease. Finally, a small, but vocal group insisted that the nonphysiologic control of glucose levels was the cause of the long-term complications.[6-9]

Unfortunately, the passionate proponents of these theories had no proof to support or refute the hypotheses, and the theories remained open to (often rancorous) debate well into the 1970s. Beginning in the mid-1970s, a series of animal studies began to investigate what became known as the "glucose hypothesis" and demonstrated in animal models that glucose control seemed to be linked to the risk for developing diabetic eye and kidney disease.[10-15] The subsequent development of a number of critical clinical research tools—including an objective means of measuring long-term glycemia (HbA_{1c} assay),[16] glucose monitoring, insulin delivery algorithms, devices that could achieve near normal glycemia,[17] and objective methods to assess the development and progression of complications—allowed the organization and implementation of clinical trials to examine the glucose hypothesis.[18] In 1993, after almost 10 years of study, the most important of these trials, the Diabetes Control and Complications Trial (DCCT) provided definitive answers to the questions that had dominated the diabetes debate for more than 60 years.[19] The

DCCT established the primacy of intensive therapy aimed at achieving near normal glycemia in preventing and delaying the specific long-term complications of diabetes mellitus. In doing so, the DCCT[19] and other clinical trials in type 1 and type 2 diabetes have helped identify the pathogenesis of the long-term complications of diabetes.[20-22] This chapter focuses on our understanding of the risk factors and, in particular, the role of glycemia in the pathogenesis of the long-term complications of diabetes mellitus.

ANIMAL STUDIES

The animal models of diabetes and its complications are sufficiently different from human type 1 and type 2 diabetes to provide only suggestive evidence regarding the pathogenesis of diabetic complications. Nevertheless, they uniformly support the role of therapies that normalize blood glucose levels to prevent and/or delay the progression of retinopathy, nephropathy, and neuropathy. There are three animal models that have been studied. In one model, animals with chemically induced (alloxan or streptozotocin) diabetes are treated with insulin with the goal of achieving either tight or loose control of blood glucose levels.[10,11] In another model, pancreatectomized animals are treated with pancreatic or isolated islet cell replacement.[12,13] Finally, animals with genetic diabetes (with either models of autoimmune diabetes such as the NOD mouse or BB rat or with models of type 2 diabetes) and various degrees of glycemia have been studied.[14,15] Most of the studies have demonstrated primary prevention of complications with intensive therapy aimed at maintaining glucose levels close to the physiologic range. Secondary intervention studies, that is, prevention of progress of established complications, have been much less common.

The most convincing animal studies were done by Engerman and colleagues with alloxan-induced diabetes in dogs.[10,11] The diabetic dogs developed retinopathy with microaneurysms and pericyte loss similar to those seen in diabetic humans. Therapy with two daily injections of NPH insulin with the goal of aglycosuria ("good control") was initiated soon after the dogs were made diabetic.[10] Good control was shown to be associated with fewer microaneurysms than was therapy with one daily injection of NPH insulin ("poor control") over a 5-year period. A later study demonstrated that if dogs with alloxan-induced diabetes were treated with the poor-control regimen for 2.5 years followed by the good-control regimen for 2.5 years, they developed an intermediate number of microaneurysms.[11] This prescient study suggested that secondary intervention was not as effective as primary prevention, and forecast the results of human studies that would follow almost 10 years later. Of note, severe hypoglycemia resulted in the deaths of several dogs in "good control."

Although glomerular lesions in several animal models of diabetes are similar to those seen in diabetic nephropathy in humans, the time course of the development of the lesions is difficult to compare with that in human diabetes. In addition, animal models of renal disease have several limitations. First, diabetic rats develop a renal lesion (mesangial expansion) that differs from the early lesion of human nephropathy (glomerular basement membrane expansion) and do not develop end-stage renal failure. Second, other potentially important variables that might predict or influence development of nephropathy in humans (e.g., hypertension) cannot be easily studied in animal models. Third, rats in which transplants of pancreatic islet cells do not succeed in correcting glucose levels also show improvements in renal results.[12] As with retinopathy, studies of nephropathy in animal models can lend support to, but cannot prove, the glucose hypothesis.

Studies in animal models appear to demonstrate that nephropathy can be prevented or even reversed when diabetic animals are treated with pancreatic transplantation or with intensive insulin therapy. Rats with streptozotocin-induced diabetes develop mesangial thickening with immunoglobulin deposition within 6 to 9 months of diabetes onset.[12] Successful islet transplantation prevented the development of such lesions or led to stabilization and some improvement in established lesions concurrent with normalization of glucose levels.[12] Studies in other animal models such as the BB/W spontaneously diabetic rat[15] and uninephrectomized, alloxan-treated dog[23] tend to support the role of glucose control in the genesis of nephropathy.

Animal models of diabetic neuropathy are also limited; however, the ability to measure nerve conduction and perform nerve biopsies may compensate for the difficulty in determining specific sensory and motor deficits. Studies of glycemic control and neuropathy have also supported the glucose hypothesis.[24]

HUMAN STUDIES

OBSERVATIONAL STUDIES

Retinopathy

Human studies conducted before 1964 were hampered by the absence of quantitative methods to evaluate long-term glucose control and complications and by a poor appreciation of clinical trial methodology.[25] Beginning in the 1970s, nondilated ophthalmoscopy gave way to seven-field stereoscopic fundus photography and fluorescein angiography, and sporadic blood glucose measurements and semiquantitative measures of glycosuria were supplanted by assays for glycosylated hemoglobin (HbA_1 or HbA_{1c}).[16]

Although lacking in these modern innovations, the longitudinal study of Pirart deserves mention, if only for its magnitude.[26] Pirart followed a large cohort of patients (4398) with diabetes for as long as 25 years, although relatively few were followed for more than 15 years. He noted that retinopathy, nephropathy, and neuropathy were more common in patients with a higher glycemic index, a value derived from intermittent measurements of blood and urine glucose levels and other factors. The high attrition rate over time, the lack of objective measures of complications and glycemia, and the possibility that complications led to worsened glucose control, rather than vice versa, detract from this study.

In the modern era, the population-based, observational Wisconsin Epidemiologic Study of Diabetic Retinopathy (WESDR) examined diabetic Wisconsin residents using glycosylated hemoglobin measurements and seven-field stereoscopic fundus photography.[27-29] Follow-up over 4 years revealed a striking association between the level of glycosylated hemoglobin at baseline and the incidence of any retinopathy, progression of retinopathy, progression to proliferative retinopathy,[27] macular edema,[28] and vision loss.[29] The relationship between levels of glycosylated hemoglobin and retinopathy was continuous; no threshold for glycosylated hemoglobin with regard to risk of retinopathy was noted. The associations among glycemia and diabetic complications remained after controlling for duration of diabetes, age, and baseline retinopathy. Other observational studies have confirmed the association of glycemia with retinopathy in selected type 1 diabetic populations[30-33] and have also suggested that higher glycemic levels are a risk factor for the development of proliferative retinopathy.[31,33,34]

Although WESDR subjects were not strictly categorized as type 1 and type 2 diabetics, the separation by age at onset (<30 years versus ≥30 years) effectively provided type 1 and type 2 populations. WESDR[35] and other studies[36] have demonstrated an association between retinopathy and glycemia in type 2 diabetes similar to that in type 1 diabetes (Fig. 66-1). Putative risk factors for diabetic retinopathy, other than the level of glycemia, include hypertension,[37] pregnancy,[38] hyperlipidemia,[39] and a family history of diabetic retinopathy,[40] but not smoking.[41]

Nephropathy

The natural history of diabetic nephropathy, although duration-dependent, extends over many more years than retinopathy before clinical expression becomes evident.[42,43] A minimum of 12 years, and more often 15 to 18 years, of type 1 diabetes is required before the development of clinical-grade (dipstick-positive, i.e., ≥500 mg/24 hours) proteinuria, the first incontrovertible sign of developing end-stage renal disease. After the development of clinical-grade proteinuria, creatinine clearance declines over 5 to 10 years, terminating in end-stage renal disease.[44]

The reluctance to perform kidney biopsies early in the course of diabetes for documentation of microscopic changes in the glomerulus and the less than perfect correlation between microscopic changes and clinical course has led to reliance on surrogate markers of evolving nephropathy. "Incipient" nephropathy, as demonstrated by microalbuminuria (generally greater than 20 mg to 30 mg and less than 300 mg of urinary albumin per 24 hours), has been identified as a predictor or marker for the development of end-stage renal disease in retrospective studies of type 1[45-48] and type 2 diabetes.[49] Unfortunately, microalbuminuria can vary considerably in individuals over time, with levels fluctuating from abnormal to normal values. Therefore, a urinary albumin excretion rate of >20 μg/minute (>28 mg/24 hours) but <200 μg/minute (<288 mg/24 hours), or comparable results on a spot urine collection, in at least two of three urine collections within a 6-month period has been suggested as a definition of "persistent" microalbuminuria.[50] The presence of, or changes in, microalbuminuria have been used as renal end points in many observational studies and controlled trials.

There are several reasons to suspect that the association between glucose control and nephropathy may be more complex than that with retinopathy. The occurrence of nephropathy in no more than 40% of patients with type 1 diabetes and 25% of patients with type 2 diabetes suggests that variables other than glycemia are operant. Hypertension and family history of hypertension have been suggested as possible mediators of nephropathy.[51,52]

The association between levels of glycemia and nephropathy has been more difficult to establish than for retinopathy. Potential reasons for the difficulty in establishing a relationship between glycemia and nephropathy include the following: (1) the development of renal failure may influence glycemic control (e.g., alterations in sensitivity to insulin with development of hypertension and effects of antihypertensive medications on glycemia); (2) uremia, anemia, and transfusions may interfere with, or influence, the accuracy of

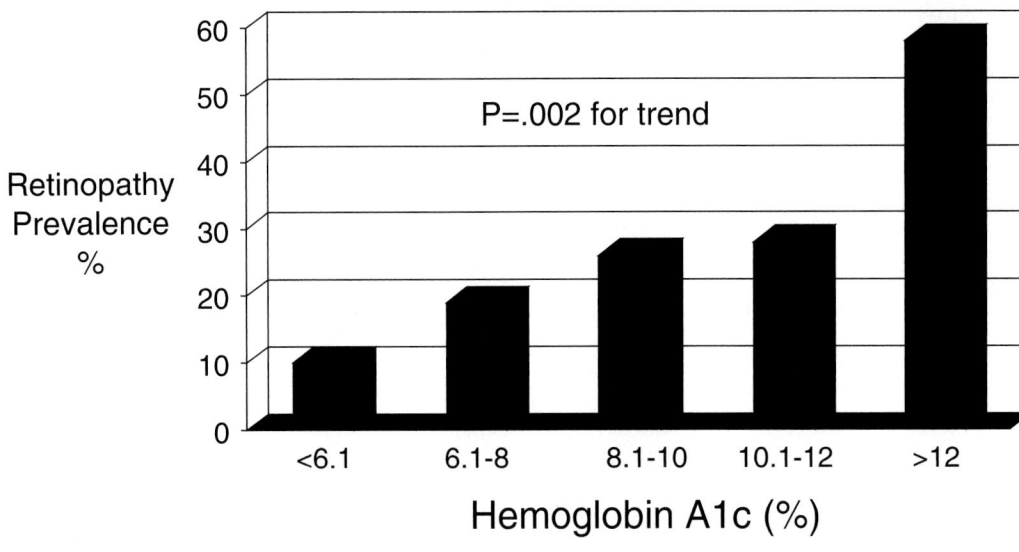

Figure 66-1 Association between mean glucose level as measured by level of glycosylated hemoglobin (HbA$_{1c}$) and presence of retinopathy in older patients (55 to 75 years) with type 2 diabetes. (W=185). (From Nathan DM, Singer DE, Godine JE, et al: Retinopathy in older Type II diabetics: Association with glucose control. Diabetes 35:797–801, 1986.)

measurements of glycosylated hemoglobin; and (3) given the long duration of diabetes before the development of renal failure, infrequent measurements of glycosylated hemoglobin, representing a relatively brief period of exposure, may not be predictive of the development of nephropathy. Even with these potential problems, studies have demonstrated an association between the derived glycemic index and an increase in creatinine level over time,[26] or between mean levels of glycosylated hemoglobin, measured over 7 years, and risk of microalbuminuria in type 1 diabetes.[53]

Neuropathy

Quantitative electrophysiologic measures of nerve conduction have been available for more than 40 years and should have contributed to the examination of the association between glycemia and neuropathy. Unfortunately, the complex relationship between neurophysiologic studies and symptomatic clinical diabetic neuropathy has complicated the study of glucose control and neuropathy. For example, the early observation that insulin treatment of new-onset type 1 diabetes reversed the slowed motor nerve conduction within 6 weeks in asymptomatic patients supported an acute effect of hyperglycemia on nerve conduction and cast doubt on the role of electrophysiologic testing.[54] The absence of histologic data from peripheral nerve biopsies has been a major impediment to our understanding of diabetic neuropathy. A weak association between glycemia and motor and sensory nerve conduction has been documented in type 1[55] and type 2[56] diabetes.

INTERVENTIONAL-CLINICAL TRIALS

Type 1 Diabetes

At best, observational studies only can indicate associations between glycemic control (and other confounders) and complications. The implementation of randomized, controlled clinical trials facilitated our understanding of cause and effect in the pathogenesis of diabetic complications. Treatments designed to achieve near-normal glucose control ("intensive therapy") were compared with conventional therapies and their differential effects on the development and progression of complications were studied. Intensive treatment regimens took advantage of the introduction and refinement of methods for self-monitoring of blood glucose levels and of improved methods of physiologic replacement of insulin, such as continuous subcutaneous insulin infusion (CSII) with pumps and multiple daily injection (MDI) regimens.[17] Four

well-designed randomized studies,[21,57–59] set the stage for the larger and comprehensive DCCT.[19,60] All of these preliminary trials were secondary intervention studies, including only subjects with retinal lesions at baseline. In addition, the mean duration of diabetes was relatively long. The duration of the trials ranged from 8 to 60 months and included 30 to 100 subjects. (By contrast, the DCCT studied 1441 subjects with a mean follow-up of 6.5 years.) The total number of patient-years of study was less than 800 in the four previous secondary intervention trials combined. (The total number of patient-years for the secondary-intervention component of the DCCT was almost 5000 at study end in 1993.) Except for the Oslo study,[59] which included two intensive-treatment groups, the studies compared type 1 diabetic patients randomly assigned to conventional treatment with patients randomly assigned to CSII[57,58] or MDI.[21] The results of the Kroc,[57] Steno,[58,61] and Oslo[59,62] studies were similar with regard to retinopathy. In the first 6 to 12 months, a transient worsening of retinopathy occurred in the patients receiving intensive treatment. Of the early trials, only the Stockholm Diabetes Study demonstrated a beneficial effect of intensive therapy over time.[21]

Diabetes Control and Complications Trial

In 1993, the DCCT ended the 60-year debate regarding the relationship between metabolic control and long-term complications. The DCCT investigators reported consistent, unequivocal salutary effects of intensive diabetes management on the development and progression of the microvascular and neurologic complications of type 1 diabetes mellitus.[19]

Design The DCCT, initiated in 1983, was designed to answer definitively whether intensive diabetes management would affect the development and/or progression of long-term complications in type 1 diabetes, and at what cost.[60] The DCCT addressed primary prevention and secondary intervention of chronic complications by including two parallel studies. The primary prevention study determined whether intensive therapy aimed at achieving glycemic levels as close to the nondiabetic range as possible would prevent the development or slow the progression of complications in type 1 diabetic patients with no complications at baseline. The secondary intervention study determined whether intensive therapy would prevent the progression of complications in type 1 diabetic patients who already had some evidence of complications at baseline. The DCCT also examined the costs, both financial and adverse events, associated with intensive compared with conventional therapy.

In order to perform the two studies, the DCCT selected two separate cohorts of type 1 diabetic patients. The Primary Prevention cohort was 13 to 39 years of age with 1 to 5 years of diabetes duration and no evidence of retinopathy or nephropathy. The Secondary Intervention cohort was similarly aged but could have had diabetes for as long as 15 years. They had to have at least one microaneurysm but no more than moderate nonproliferative retinopathy, and they could have as much as 200 mg of albumin excretion per 24 hours (although only a small fraction had this level of albuminuria at baseline). The baseline characteristics of the two study cohorts are shown in Table 66-1. Study patients were also selected based on an assessment that they would accept random assignment of therapy and that they were likely to continue to participate in a long-term study. On average, these patients were probably more motivated than the usual patient with type 1 diabetes.

Diabetes Control and Complications Trial Intensive Treatment and Metabolic Goals The Primary Prevention and Secondary Intervention cohorts were randomly assigned either to conventional therapy (designed to mimic the usual diabetes therapy with one or two daily injections of insulin and daily glucose monitoring) or to intensive therapy (designed to normalize blood glucose control). Conventional therapy had the clinical goals of avoiding any symptoms of hyperglycemia or hypoglycemia, but no specific numeric blood glucose targets. Intensive therapy had the goal of achieving blood glucose control as close to the nondiabetic range as possible, including premeal blood glucose levels between 70 and 120 mg/dL (3.9 to 6.7 mMol/L), peak post-

prandial levels less than 180 mg/dL (10 mMol/L), and hemoglobin HbA_{1c} levels in the nondiabetic range (<6.05%). In order to reach these goals, patients assigned to intensive therapy used three or more insulin injections per day or insulin pump therapy, guided by frequent self-monitoring of blood glucose levels and adjusted based on meal size, composition, and exercise. (See Table 66-2 for description of the intensive regimen.)

Diabetes Control and Complications Trial Results The detailed results of intensive compared with conventional therapy in the DCCT have been reported extensively.[19,63-80] The initial report[19] summarized the major results whereas subsequent reports presented expanded analyses of the effects of intensive therapy on long-term complications, including retinopathy,[63-65] nephropathy,[66] neuropathy,[67-69] and macrovascular disease and its risk factors,[70] and the effect of intensive therapy on quality of life,[71] neurobehavioral outcome,[72] and residual insulin secretion,[73] the implementation[74] and adverse effects of intensive therapy,[75,76] the cost-benefit analysis of intensive therapy compared with conventional therapy,[77] the results of intensive therapy on pregnancy,[78] and the association among glycemia, long-term complications, and other risk factors.[79,80] A long-term follow-up study of the DCCT cohort, the Epidemiology of Diabetes Interventions and Complications (EDIC) study is in its 11th year, as of 2004, and is providing further insight into the long-term consequences of intensive therapy.[81-84]

Adherence and Metabolic Results Over the 6.5-year mean follow-up time of the DCCT (range, 3 to 9 years), compliance was excellent with more than 99% of the cohort completing the trial.[19] In addition, there was virtually no crossover between assigned treatments. Subjects adhered to their

Table 66-1	Baseline Characteristics of DCCT Cohort			
Characteristic	Primary Conventional Therapy (N = 378)	Prevention Intensive Therapy (N = 348)	Secondary Conventional Therapy (N = 352)	Intervention Intensive Therapy (N = 363)
Age (yr)	26 ± 8	27 ± 7	27 ± 7	27 ± 7
Adolescents, 13–18 yr (%)	19	16	9	10
Male sex (%)	54	49	54	53
White race (%)	96	96	97	97
Duration of IDDM (yr)	2.6 ± 1.4	2.6 ± 1.4	8.6 ± 3.7	8.9 ± 3.8
Insulin dose (U/kg of body weight/day)	0.62 ± 0.26	0.62 ± 0.25	0.71 ± 0.24	0.72 ± 0.23
Glycosylated hemoglobin (%)*	8.8 ± 1.7	8.8 ± 1.6	8.9 ± 1.5	9.0 ± 1.5
Mean blood glucose (mg/dl)†	229 ± 80	234 ± 86	232 ± 78	234 ± 81
Blood pressure (mm Hg)				
Systolic	114 ± 12	112 ± 11	116 ± 12	114 ± 12
Diastolic	72 ± 9	72 ± 9	73 ± 9	73 ± 9
Body weight (% of ideal)	103 ± 14	103 ± 13	105 ± 13	104 ± 12
Current smokers (%)	17	19	19	18
Serum cholesterol (mg/dL)	173 ± 35	176 ± 33	179 ± 32	178 ± 33
Serum triglycerides (mg/dL)	77 ± 57	75 ± 41	87 ± 44	87 ± 45
Serum HDL cholesterol (mg/dL)	51 ± 13	52 ± 13	49 ± 11	49 ± 12
Serum LDL cholesterol (mg/dL)	106 ± 30	109 ± 29	112 ± 28	112 ± 29
Absence of retinopathy (%)	100	100	0	0
Microaneurysms only (%)	0	0	58	67
NPDR(%)				
Mild	0	0	23	18
Moderate	0	0	19	15
Urinary albumin excretion (mg/24 hr)	12 ± 8	12 ± 9	19 ± 24	21 ± 25
Creatinine clearance (mL/min)	127 ± 28	128 ± 30	130 ± 30	128 ± 31
Clinical neuropathy (%)‡	2.1	4.9	9.4	9.4

NPDR, nonproliferative diabetic retinopathy

From DCCT Research Group. The effect of intensive treatment of diabetes on the development and progression of long-term complications in insulin-dependent diabetes mellitus. N Engl J Med 329:977–986, 1993.

*HbA_{1c}—nondiabetic range 4%–6.05%.

†Based on seven time-point capillary blood samples, before and 2 hours after each meal and before bed.

‡The presence of "confirmed" clinical neuropathy was based on a history or physical examination consistent with somatosensory distal neuropathy plus either abnormal electrophysiologic testing (nerve condition studies) or abnormal autonomic testing results.

Table 66-2 Diabetes Control and Complications Trial Intensive Therapy

SELF-MONITORING OF BLOOD GLUCOSE
≥4 times per day (premeals and prebed)
3 A.M. once per week for safety (>65 mg/dL)
Add postmeal tests if HbA₁c goals not met

GLYCOSYLATED HEMOGLOBIN
HbA₁c every 3 months measured centrally with HPLC assay (nondiabetic range 4% to 6.05%)

INSULIN
3 or more injections per day *or* CSII with external pump
Doses adjusted based on ambient glucose (SMBG), meal size and content, and anticipated exercise

SUPERVISION
Monthly visits and frequent phone calls
Staff included diabetologist, nurse educator, and dietitian

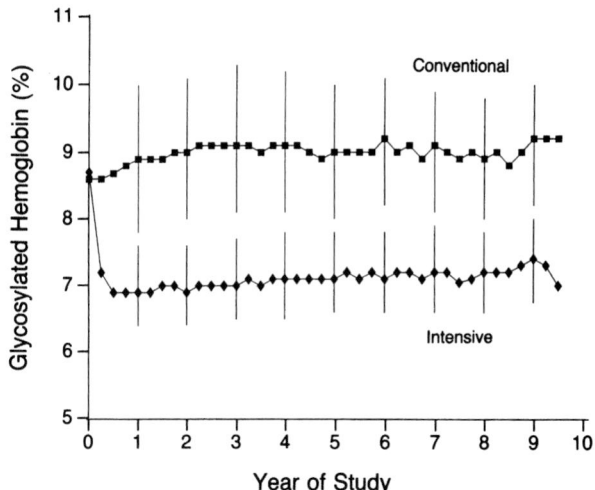

Figure 66-2 Hemoglobin A₁c results during the Diabetes Control and Complications Trial (DCCT). Medians of all quarterly measurements with the 25th and 75th percentiles of the yearly values (*vertical lines*) are shown. The differences between the treatment groups became significant by 3 months and remained significantly different over the course of the study ($P < 0.001$). (From DCCT Research Group: The effect of intensive treatment of diabetes on the development and progression of long-term complications in insulin-dependent diabetes mellitus. N Engl J Med 329:977–986, 1993.)

assigned treatment more than 97% of study time. Intensive therapy decreased HbA₁c to a nadir of approximately 6.9% by 6 months and maintained mean HbA₁c levels during the remainder of the trial that were approximately 2% lower than with conventional treatment (7% versus 9%) (Fig. 66-2). Of note, intensive therapy did not consistently normalize HbA₁c, achieving levels that were, on average, four standard deviations above the nondiabetic mean. Lower glycemia achieved with intensive therapy was accompanied by a threefold increase in hypoglycemia.[76]

Retinopathy Retinopathy was evaluated every 6 months by seven-field stereoscopic fundus photography, which was graded in a central facility. The principal outcome in the primary prevention study was the development of a sustained (seen on two consecutive exams) three-step or greater progression on a retinopathy severity scale adopted from the Early Treatment of Diabetic Retinopathy Study (ETDRS).[85] Similarly, the principal outcome in the secondary intervention study was a sustained progression of three or more steps from the baseline level. Intensive therapy reduced the development of these end points by 76% in the Primary Prevention study and by 54% in the Secondary Intervention study com-

pared with conventional therapy (Fig. 66-3). Other retinopathy outcomes and the effects of intensive therapy are shown in Table 66-3.

The overall effect of intensive therapy was to decrease all stages of retinopathy included in the DCCT. The benefits were similar in almost all subgroups of patients defined by age, gender, and other baseline characteristics. However, intensive therapy was relatively more effective when initiated early in the course of diabetes (shorter versus longer duration) and when retinopathy was less severe at baseline.[19,63,64] Although intensive therapy reduced the risk somewhat less for more advanced stages of retinopathy than for earlier stages, patients with more advanced retinopathy still benefited from

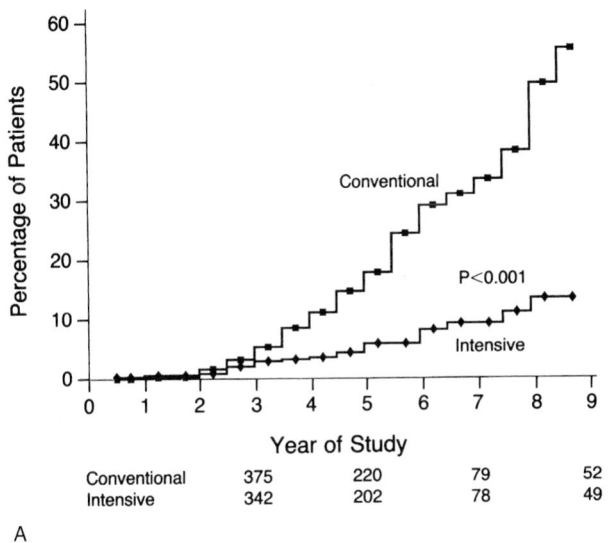

Conventional	375	220	79	52
Intensive	342	202	78	49

A

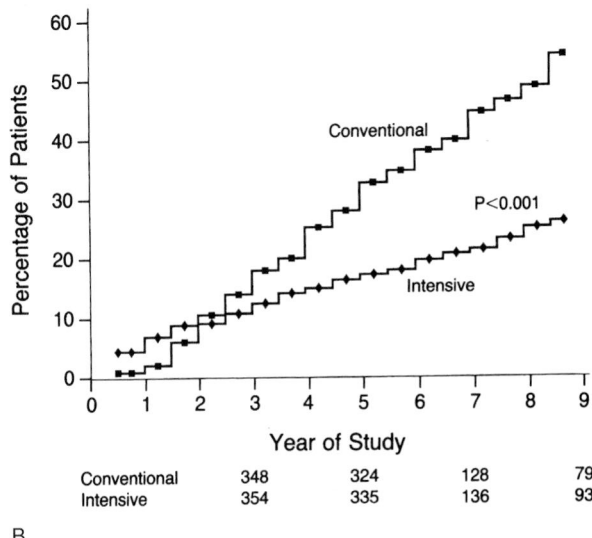

Conventional	348	324	128	79
Intensive	354	335	136	93

B

Figure 66-3 Cumulative incidence of Diabetes Control and Complications Trial primary retinopathy outcomes (three step change in retinopathy from baseline value, sustained for at least 6 months) measured by fundus photography, comparing intensive and conventional therapy groups. **A,** Primary prevention cohort-intensive therapy reduced the cumulative incidence by 76% ($P < 0.001$). **B,** Secondary intervention cohort-intensive therapy reduced the cumulative incidence by 54% ($P < 0.001$). (From DCCT Research Group: The effect of intensive treatment of diabetes on the development and progression of long-term complications in insulin-dependent diabetes mellitus. N Engl J Med 329:977–986, 1993.)

Table 66-3	Diabetes Control and Complications Trial (DCCT) and Epidemiology of Diabetes Interventions and Complications (EDIC) Results	
Complication	During DCCT (6.5-year follow-up)	During EDIC (4.5-year follow-up after end of DCCT*)
Risk Reduction with Intensive Compared with Conventional Therapy (%)		
Retinopathy		
Three-step progression	76	77
Proliferative	64	76
Macular edema	46	72
Laser therapy	56	71
Nephropathy		
Microalbuminuria	35	53
Albuminuria ≥ 300 mg/24 hours	56	87
Neuropathy	60	

*Adjusted for presence of complication at end of DCCT.

intensive therapy. The beneficial effects of intensive therapy were not seen for the first 3 years of therapy, presumably because of the natural "momentum" of diabetic complications. In addition, intensive therapy was associated with a transient worsening of retinopathy during the first 1 to 2 years of therapy.[65] Both of these factors delayed the beneficial effects of intensive therapy in the secondary intervention cohort.

The EDIC follow-up has shown further improvement in retinal status in the previous intensive treatment group compared with the previous conventional treatment group (see Table 66-3). The differences in retinal outcomes between the two treatment groups persisted, and even expanded, 4.5 years after DCCT end, even though the majority of the previous conventional treatment cohort had changed to intensive therapy and the mean HbA_{1c} levels had drifted closer between the two treatment groups.[82] The persistent benefit of 6.5 years

of DCCT intensive therapy compared with conventional therapy for as long as 8 years after the end of the DCCT,[83] during which glycemia had become similar between the original treatment groups, lead to the concept of "metabolic memory." Metabolic memory refers to the durable, imprinting effect of previous glycemic control on diabetic complications. Although the mechanism of this phenomenon remains unknown, long-lived glycated proteins may explain how previous glycemia can continue to have effects on microvascular complications.

The study of families of DCCT volunteers, in which there was more than one person with diabetes, has revealed clustering of retinopathy within families.[86] The tendency for some families with diabetes to develop retinopathy, while other families do not, is most likely mediated by genetic factors, although some as yet to be identified shared environmental factor could theoretically also play a role. Intensive therapy decreased the development and progression of retinopathy in DCCT volunteers who were members of "high-risk" families as well as in DCCT volunteers in "low-risk" families.

Nephropathy Nephropathy was routinely assessed by standardized measurements of albumin excretion and creatinine clearance, based on an annual 4-hour collection. The primary analytic end points for nephropathy are shown in Table 66-3 and Figure 66-4. As with retinopathy, the risk for progression of nephropathy was reduced by intensive therapy. This included reduction in the development of microalbuminuria (>40 mg/24 hours) and clinical grade albuminuria (>300 mg/24 hours). The small number of patients developing clinical nephropathy, defined as a creatinine clearance <70 mL/min/1.73^2 with albumin excretion >300 mg/24 hours, precluded a statistically valid analysis of any difference between treatment groups. However, the number of conventional treatment patients who developed this level of renal dysfunction ($n = 5$) was more than twice the number of intensive treatment patients ($n = 2$). The relatively small number of secondary intervention patients who had microalbuminuria at baseline ($n = 70$) made it difficult to demonstrate a benefit of intensive therapy with regard to slowing progression to clinical grade albuminuria once microalbuminuria had

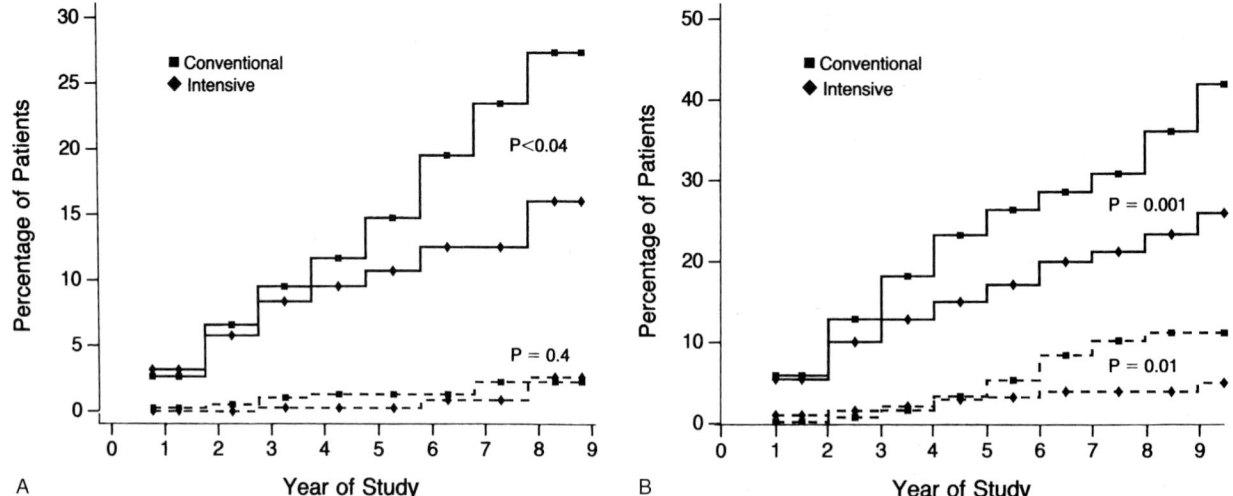

Figure 66-4   Cumulative incidence of renal endpoints in Diabetes Control and Complications Trial comparing intensive and conventionally treated groups. Albumin excretion rate > 40 mg/24 hours is shown in *solid line* and > 300 mg/24 hours with the *dashed line*. **A,** Primary prevention cohort—intensive therapy reduced the mean risk of developing microalbuminuria (> 40 mg/24 hr) by 34% (*P* < 0.04). **B,** Secondary intervention cohort—intensive therapy reduced the mean risk of developing microalbuminuria by 43% (*P*= 0.001) and the risk of clinical albuminuria (> 300 mg/24 hr) by 56% (*P* = 0.01). (From DCCT Research Group: The effect of intensive treatment of diabetes on the development and progression of long-term complications in insulin-dependent diabetes mellitus. N Engl J Med 329:977–986, 1993.)

occurred.[66] The long-term EDIC follow-up of the DCCT cohort has reinforced the role of intensive therapy in delaying and perhaps preventing diabetic nephropathy[83] (see Table 66-3). "Metabolic memory" applies to nephropathy as it does to retinopathy. The widening difference in renal outcomes between the original intensive and conventional treatment groups, as long as 8 years after the end of the DCCT, has further established the benefits of early intervention in preventing nephropathy.

Neuropathy Confirmed clinical neuropathy was defined as the presence of signs or symptoms of peripheral neuropathy, plus either abnormal nerve conduction in at least two peripheral nerves or unequivocally abnormal autonomic nerve testing. Intensive therapy reduced the risk of developing clinical neuropathy by 60% in the combined cohorts (see Table 66-3).[19,67] In addition to the decreased development of confirmed clinical neuropathy, the most stringent of the neurologic outcomes, intensive therapy reduced the risk of deterioration of nerve function, as measured with electrophysiologic methods, which occurred with conventional therapy.[68] The decline in autonomic nerve function, assessed with measures of cardiovascular autonomic function, which occurred with conventional therapy, was significantly reduced with intensive therapy in the Primary Prevention, but not in the Secondary Intervention cohort.[72,78] There were no significant differences between treatment groups in clinical events secondary to autonomic neuropathy, but the frequency of events was very low in both groups. The EDIC study is examining whether metabolic memory also applies to neuropathy, but has not reported results yet.

Association of Glycemia and Microvascular Complications
The frequent measurements of HbA_{1c} with standardized methods during the DCCT provided the opportunity to examine the relationship between glycemia and the diabetes-specific complications.[79,80] Although these analyses were secondary, and not directly related to the intention-to-treat design of the study, they probably provide the most extensive and convincing data regarding the relationship between control and complications in human diabetes. The mathematical modeling of long-term glycemia and complications revealed a continuous relationship between glycemia and retinopathy and nephropathy, with no apparent threshold or breakpoint in the range of diabetic glycemia (Fig. 66-5). The analyses demonstrate a continuous benefit of lowering HbA_{1c}, even into the near nondiabetic range. Every 10% decrease in HbA_{1c}, for example from 10% to 9% or 9% to 8.1%, is associated with a 43% reduction in risk for developing retinopathy.[79] Although the absolute rate of retinopathy decreases in the lower HbA_{1c} range, the relative risk reduction associated with lower HbA_{1c} persists. A similar continuous risk relationship exists for glycemia and nephropathy.

Macrovascular Although the risk for major macrovascular outcomes (death from cardiovascular disease, myocardial infarction, and major peripheral vascular events) was reduced by 41% with intensive therapy, the number and rates of events were very small, and the difference between treatment groups failed to achieve statistical significance ($P = 0.06$).[70] However, several risk factors for cardiovascular disease were improved with intensive therapy, including a 34% reduction in low-density lipoprotein cholesterol ($P = 0.02$). Further study during EDIC has demonstrated a significant reduction in progression of carotid intima media thickness (IMT), measured with carotid ultrasonography.[84] Moreover, coronary artery calcification, a biomarker for coronary artery plaques, was also less in the former intensive than the former conventional treatment group.[87] These data suggest that atherosclerosis may also be responsive to intensive therapy. Further follow-up in EDIC should identify whether intensive therapy reduces the risk for cardiovascular disease events.

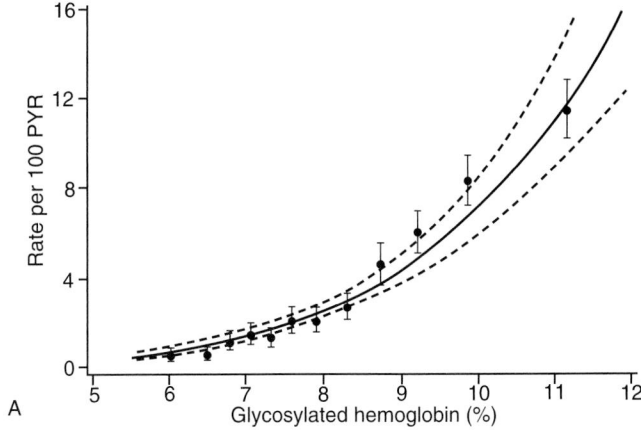

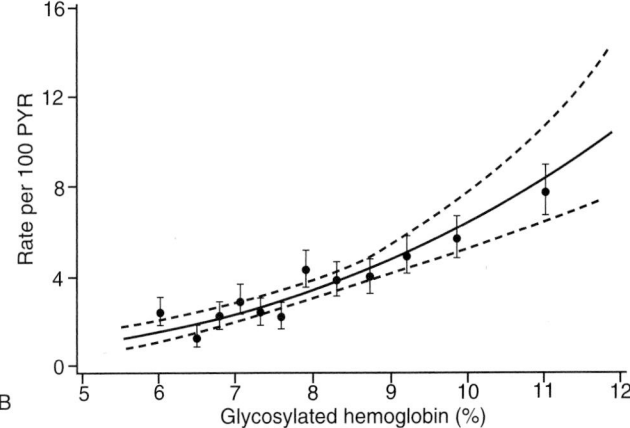

Figure 66-5 Relationship between updated mean HbA_{1c} levels and complications in the Diabetes Control and Complications Trial, examining the combined treatment groups with Poisson regression models (95% confidence bands shown with *dashed lines*). The relationship between mean HbA_{1c} and complications is continuous over the entire range of HbA_{1c} levels, with no inflection or break point at levels of HbA_{1c} above the nondiabetic range. **A,** Risk of sustained (for at least 6 months) retinopathy progression measured as rate per 100 patient years. **B,** Risk of developing microalbuminuria (rate per 100 patient-years). (From DCCT Research Group. The absence of a glycemic threshold for the development of long-term complications: The perspective of the Diabetes Control and Complications Trial. Diabetes 45:1289–1298, 1996.)

Other Outcomes and Adverse Events Intensive therapy was accompanied by a threefold increase in severe hypoglycemia, defined as an episode that required assistance to treat.[19,76] Although the majority of these episodes were clinically benign, the incidence of hypoglycemia resulting in coma and seizures or requiring emergency room treatment also increased by approximately two- to threefold. The more severe hypoglycemic reactions, such as those resulting in seizure or coma, were relatively rare (16 versus 5 episodes per 100 patient-years in the intensive and conventional treatment groups, respectively). Other adverse events that accompanied intensive therapy included an increased risk for weight gain and catheter-related infections in patients using insulin pumps.[75] Taken together, none of these adverse events caused significant morbidity or mortality. There were no patient deaths or macrovascular events ascribed to hypoglycemia. Moreover, the increased frequency of hypoglycemia had no adverse effects on neurocognitive function as judged by frequent testing in both treatment groups.[72] Finally, despite the demands of intensive therapy, quality of life, measured yearly by self-report, did not differ between the two treatment groups.[71]

Although the DCCT has the largest and longest duration experience with multiple daily injection and insulin pump therapy regimens, assignment to those therapies within the intensive treatment group was not random and precluded a scientifically reliable comparison of the methods. (The IT subjects and their treatment teams could choose the therapy that suited them best and could change between intensive therapy methods during the course of the study.) However, from a purely descriptive point of view, the following was observed: Patients treated with pump therapy achieved slightly lower mean HbA$_{1c}$ levels (~0.3%), but at a cost of increased frequency of coma and seizure, diabetic ketoacidosis, and catheter complications.[74,75]

Type 2 Diabetes
The lessons from the DCCT were quickly translated to apply to type 2 diabetes, despite concern regarding the large differences between type 1 and type 2 diabetes in pathogenesis, clinical course, and available therapies with different adverse event profiles.[88] At the time that the DCCT results were published, the only clinical trial that had examined the impact of glycemic control on long-term complications in type 2 diabetes was the University Group Diabetes Program (UGDP).[89] This 12-center trial compared the effects of five different treatment modalities (diet, diet plus tolbutamide, diet plus phenformin, diet plus standard insulin dose, and diet plus variable-dose insulin) on long-term outcome in patients with newly diagnosed type 2 diabetes. Many of the critical tools that had been incorporated into the DCCT, such as objective, reliable measures of long-term glycemia and of diabetic complications, were not available during the UGDP. Moreover, the study was probably underpowered with regard to its major outcomes.

The results of the UGDP were largely negative. Although the variable-dose insulin regimen maintained mean fasting levels of blood glucose approximately 20% lower than baseline levels, compared with no significant changes from baseline glucose values with the other treatment regimens, there were no significant differences in the degree of retinopathy among any of the treatment groups. Ironically, the unexpected observation of excess cardiovascular mortality of 1% per year in the tolbutamide group compared with the other treatment groups is the finding for which the UGDP is best remembered.

United Kingdom Prospective Diabetes Study and Kumamoto Study
The United Kingdom Prospective Diabetes Study (UKPDS),[20,90] which was planned and initiated in 1977 and ended in 1997, and the much smaller, but impressive Kumamoto study,[22] provided more definitive answers regarding control and complications in type 2 diabetes. These two studies helped to erase some of the confusion left in the wake of the UGDP.

The Kumamoto controlled clinical trial in Japanese type 2 diabetic patients was patterned on the DCCT, with all of the subjects treated with insulin.[22] The groups randomly assigned to intensive therapy (multiple daily insulin injections) and conventional therapy (one or two daily injections of intermediate-acting insulin) achieved mean HbA$_{1c}$ levels comparable to the DCCT groups, approximately 7.1% and 9.4%, respectively, during the 6 years of study follow-up. The intensive treatment group had a decrease in retinopathy and nephropathy that paralleled the DCCT results. However, the Kumamoto study was not considered to be definitive, owing in part to the clear differences between the Japanese type 2 diabetic subjects and type 2 diabetes in non-Asian societies. The Japanese patients were all relatively thin with small insulin requirements ($\approx$ 0.2 U/kg compared with > 0.75 U/kg in the United States, for example).

The UKPDS was designed to answer two questions. First, is an "intensive strategy" aimed at achieving fasting glucose levels less than 6 mmol (108 mg/dL) superior to conventional therapy with diet in preventing the complications of diabetes in patients with relatively recent-onset type 2 diabetes? Second, are any therapies particularly advantageous with regard to preventing or delaying diabetic complications? The volunteers were new-onset (within 1 year of diagnosis) type 2 diabetic patients (Table 66-4). The outcomes were aggregated into diabetes-specific complications (combining retinopathy, nephropathy, cataracts, and cardiovascular outcomes), all-cause mortality, and diabetes-related mortality. The study design included stepwise addition of therapies in the conventional and intensive treatment groups if glucose goals were not met. In addition, the intensive therapies were numerous including three types of sulfonylureas and insulin. The obese subset of patients was also randomly assigned to metformin.[90]

The results of the UKPDS revealed that metabolic control in type 2 diabetes worsened over time, probably owing to waning β-cell function and requiring the addition of alternative therapies to the originally assigned therapy (Fig. 66-6). As a result, the majority of conventional treatment subjects had one or more of the intensive therapies added and a substantial fraction (often >20%) of the intensive treatment subjects had the alternative intensive therapies added to or substituted for their originally assigned intensive therapy over the course of the study. This design feature, intended to keep glycemia as low as possible in the intensive treatment group, severely undercut the ability to compare the specific intensive therapy modalities.[91] Finally, other randomized interventions (early addition of metformin to sulfonylurea therapy, use of acarbose, and intensive vs. conventional hypertension treatment) made the UKPDS protocol extremely complex and difficult to understand.

United Kingdom Prospective Diabetes Study Results   Using the stepped intervention strategy resulted in a 1% absolute separation in HbA$_{1c}$, which was an 11% relative reduction (see Fig. 66-6). Although the 1% difference in HbA$_{1c}$ between intensive and control groups was maintained for as long as the 12 years of mean follow-up, the progressive worsening of metabolic control applied across all treatment groups. By the fifth or sixth year of follow-up, the mean HbA$_{1c}$ levels had generally risen to their baseline levels and continued to rise thereafter. The glycemic control achieved with all of the intensive therapies was generally similar. In the intensive treatment group, the assigned medications were generally adjusted to their maximal doses, except for insulin, which was not increased to the levels that have been shown to be effective in maintaining near-normal glycemia.

The intention to treat analyses revealed a benefit of intensive therapy on the aggregate diabetes outcomes, decreasing the risk by 12% (Table 66-5). This benefit was predicated to a great extent on a beneficial effect on retinopathy and cataracts. There was no significant benefit with regard to

Table 66-4	United Kingdom Prospective Diabetes Study (UKPDS) Patient* Characteristics at Baseline		
Age (yr)	53	Triglycerides (mg/dL)	208
Female (%)	39	Cholesterol (mg/dL)	209
Race (%)		LDL (mg/dL)	
Caucasian	81	HDL (mg/dL)	41
Afro-Caribbean	8	Retinopathy (%)	21
Indian-Asian	10	Proteinuria+ (%)	2
Duration (years)*	<1	Neuropathy (%)	12
HbA$_{1c}$(%)	7.08	Hypertension@ (%)	24

*Diagnosed within 1 year; +>300 mg/24 hr; @>160/90.

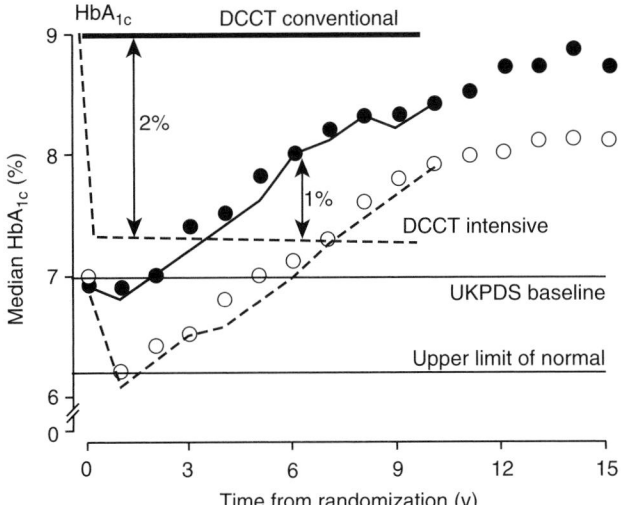

Figure 66-6 Hemoglobin A$_{1c}$ levels achieved in the United Kingdom Prospective Diabetes Study in Conventional (dietary) policy group *(closed circles)* and Intensive policy group (sulfonylureas or insulin) *(open circles)* in the nonobese cohort, by intention to treat. The separation of HbA$_{1c}$ in the DCCT is shown for Conventional *(solid line)* and Intensive *(dashed line)*. (From UKPDS Group: Intensive blood-glucose control with sulphonylureas or insulin compared with conventional treatment and risk of complications in patients with Type 2 diabetes [UKPDS 33]. Lancet 352:837–853, 1998.)

the results of the Kumamoto study, that intensive diabetes management improves outcome, and specifically microvascular outcomes, in type 2 diabetes is unquestionable. A similar risk relationship between mean HbA$_{1c}$ over time and retinopathy was demonstrated in the UKPDS as in the DCCT.[92] In the UKPDS, every 1% decrease (absolute) in mean HbA$_{1c}$ was associated with a 39% decrease in risk for retinopathy (Fig. 66-7).

Cardiovascular Disease The multifactorial etiology of CVD makes it unlikely that the association established between levels of glycemia and complications specific to diabetes, such as retinopathy, will be the same for the nonspecific complication of CVD. Most of the studies examining the putative relationship between glycemic control and CVD have been in populations with type 2 diabetes or impaired glucose tolerance (IGT). Although the presence of diabetes (or IGT) increases the prevalence of CVD,[93–96] an association between the level of glycemia and the occurrence of CVD has not been easy to demonstrate.[97] Recently, however, studies that used more accurate measures of long-term glycemia found a correlation between glycemic levels and prevalence of CVD.[98–100] In the Framingham Study, level of HbA$_{1c}$ correlated with prevalence of CVD, but only in women.[98] The UKPDS data and a recent meta-analysis support a relationship of glycemia with CVD.[92,100] Moreover, glycemia in the subdiabetic range appears to be associated with CVD risk factors.[101,102] There has been considerable interest in whether postprandial glycemia has a greater detrimental effect on CVD and its risk factors than fasting glycemia. Definitive data generated in clinical trials is not currently available, leaving this issue unresolved[103]; however, increasing observational data have demonstrated

cardiovascular disease. The results with metformin were analyzed separately. (The validity of this analysis strategy has been called into question.[91]) Metformin therapy resulted in less weight gain and hypoglycemia than other intensive therapies. In addition, aggregate diabetes mortality, but not diabetes-related outcomes, were significantly reduced by metformin.[90] However, early addition of metformin to sulfonylurea, in a randomized sub-study, resulted in a large and statistically significant increase in cardiovascular disease (CVD) mortality, leaving the role of metformin in reducing CVD mortality in question.

The UKPDS complex design, numerous crossovers, and controversial analytic strategy left many questions.[91] However, the fundamental observation, when combined with

Table 66-5	**Major UKPDS Findings**
Nonobese + Obese	**Obese Only**
INTENSIVE THERAPY REDUCED*: Aggregate diabetes outcomes by 12%, *P* = 0.029 Laser therapy by 29%, *P* = 0.003 Cataract extraction by 24%, *P* = 0.046 Sudden death by 46%, *P* = 0.047	**METFORMIN REDUCED*:** Aggregate diabetes outcomes by 32%, *P* = 0.003 Diabetes-related death by 42%, *P* = 0.02 All cause death by 36%, *P* = 0.011
INTENSIVE THERAPY DID NOT REDUCE: Diabetes related deaths –10%, *P* = 0.34 All cause mortality –6%, *P* = 0.44 Fatal MI –6%, *P* = 0.63 Nonfatal MI –21%, *P* = 0.057 Renal failure –27%, *P* = 0.45	**METFORMIN DID NOT REDUCE:** Laser therapy –31%, *P* = 0.17

*Compared with conventional therapy

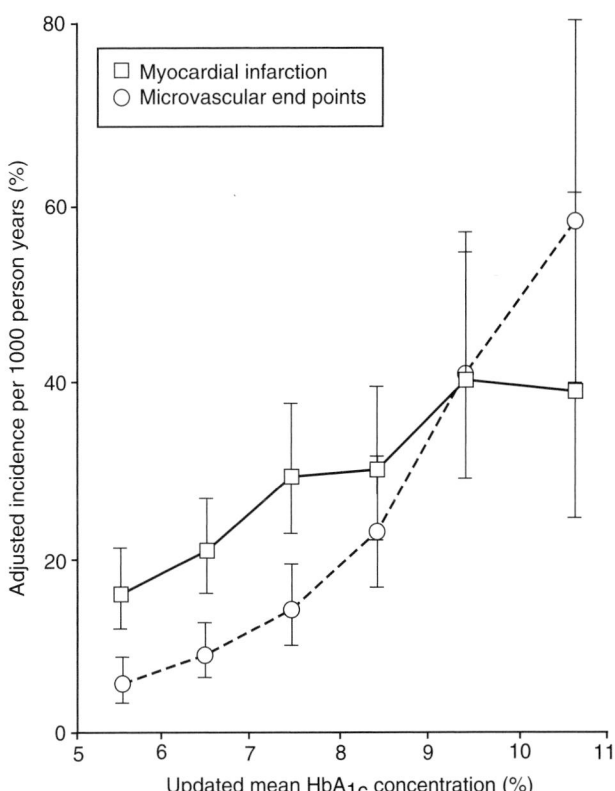

Figure 66-7 Relationship between mean HbA$_{1c}$ and microvascular and macrovascular complications in the United Kingdom Prospective Diabetes Study. (From Stratton IM, Adler AI, Neil HA, et al: Association of glycaemia with macrovascular and microvascular complications of type 2 diabetes [UKPDS 35]: Prospective observational study. Br Med J 321:405–412, 2000.)

that postprandial hyperglycemia appears to be associated with a greater burden of CVD risk factors than fasting hyperglycemia.[102]

Whether diabetes affects CVD directly or through the established risk factors that accompany it, such as hypertension, dyslipidemia, and obesity (in type 2 diabetes), or through putative risk factors, such as hyperinsulinemia, is not known. The UGDP trial did not demonstrate any impact of glucose control on CVD outcome.[89] The UKPDS showed a beneficial impact of metformin therapy, but only when the obese metformin group was compared with the obese controls.[90] The long-term follow-up of the DCCT has demonstrated a beneficial effect of intensive therapy on atherosclerosis,[84] but further follow-up will be necessary to determine whether the rate of CVD events is reduced.

Pathogenetic Mechanisms   Although glycemia has now been established as a central risk factor in the pathogenesis of long-term microvascular and neuropathic complications, and the glucose hypothesis established, the underlying mechanism(s) of the associations and of the effects of intensive therapy in the controlled clinical setting is unknown. A review of the basic science and clinical data regarding the major mechanisms that have been proposed is beyond the scope of this chapter. Glycation and abnormalities in the receptor for advanced glycation end (RAGE) products, accumulation of sugar alcohols mediated by aldose-reductase or myoinositol, abnormalities in protein kinase C, and disorders in superoxide production have all been investigated.[104–108] Arguably, the most convincing data in humans supporting glycation as a (or *the*) mechanism of long-term complications has emerged from a substudy of the DCCT in which glycation of collagen was examined in skin biopsies.[109] The association of the level of glycation with long-term complications persisted even after statistical adjustment for mean HbA$_{1c}$ levels, suggesting that tissue glycation may be directly in the pathogenetic pathway. The long half-life of glycated collagen may also help explain the "metabolic memory" that has been observed in the long-term follow-up of the DCCT population.

As noted previously, hyperglycemia is unlikely to be the only contributor to long-term, diabetes-specific complications. Hyperlipidemia, hypertension, and genetic factors almost certainly contribute to the development of long-term complications.

REFERENCES

1. Von Engelhardt D, et al (eds): Diabetes: Its medical and cultural history. New York, Springer-Verlag, 1989.
2. Wagener HP: Retinopathy in diabetes mellitus. Proc Am Diabetes Assoc 5:201–216, 1943.
3. Ballantyne AJ, Loewenstein A: The pathology of diabetic retinopathy. Trans Ophthalmol UK 63:95–115, 1943.
4. Kimmelstiel P, Wilson C: Intercapillary lesions in the glomeruli of the kidney. Am J Pathol 12:83–97, 1936.
5. Deckert T, Poulsen JE, Larsen M: Prognosis of diabetics with diabetes onset before the age of thirty-one. Diabetologia 14:363–377, 1978.
6. Cahill GF Jr, Etzwiler DD, Freinkel N: "Control" and diabetes [editorial]. N Engl J Med 294:1004–1005, 1976.
7. Siperstein MD, Foster DW, Knowles HC Jr, et al: Control of blood glucose and diabetic vascular disease [editorial]. N Engl J Med 296:1060–1063, 1977.
8. Ingelfinger FJ: Debates on diabetes. N Engl J Med 296:1228–1230, 1977.
9. Boyd JD, Jackson RL, Allen JH: Avoidance of detenerative lesions in diabetes mellitus. JAMA 118:694–696, 1942.
10. Engerman R, Bloodworth JMB Jr, Nelson S: Relationship of microvascular disease in diabetes to metabolic control. Diabetes 26:760–769, 1977.
11. Engerman RL, Kern TS: Progression of incipient diabetic retinopathy during good glycemic control. Diabetes 36:808–812, 1987.
12. Mauer SM, Steffes MW, Sutherland DER, et al: Studies of the rate of regression of the glomerular lesions in diabetic rats treated with pancreatic islet transplantation. Diabetes 24:280–285, 1975.
13. Gray BN, Watkins E Jr: Prevention of vascular complications of diabetes by pancreatic islet transplantation. Arch Surg 111:254–257, 1976.
14. Cohen AJ, McGill PD, Rossetti RG, et al: Glomerulopathy in spontaneously diabetic rat. Diabetes 36:944–951, 1977.
15. Cohen AJ, McGill PD, Rossetti RG, et al. Glomerulopathy in spontaneously diabetic rat: Impact of glycemic control. Diabetes 36:944–951, 1987.
16. Nathan DM, Singer DE, Hurxthal K, Goodson JD: The clinical information value of the glycosylated hemoglobin assay. New Engl J Med 310:341–346, 1984.
17. Nathan DM: The modern management of insulin-dependent diabetes mellitus. Med Clin North Am 72:1365–1378, 1988.
18. Nathan DM: The impact of clinical trials on the treatment of diabetes mellitus. JCEM 87:1929–1935, 2002.
19. DCCT Research Group: The effect of intensive treatment of diabetes on the development and progression of long-term complications in insulin-dependent diabetes mellitus. N Engl J Med 329:977–986, 1993.
20. UKPDS Group: Intensive blood-glucose control with sulphonylureas or insulin compared with conventional treatment and risk of complications in patients with type 2 diabetes (UKPDS 33). Lancet 352:837–853, 1998.
21. Reichard P, Nilsson B-Y, Rosenqvist U: The effect of long-term intensified insulin treatment on the development of microvascular complications of diabetes mellitus. N Engl J Med 329:304, 1993.
22. Ohkubo Y, et al: Intensive insulin therapy prevents the progression of diabetic microvascular complications in Japanese patients with NIDDM: A randomized prospective 6-year study. Diab Res Clin Pract 28:103–117, 1995.
23. Steffes MW, Buchwald H, Wigness BD, et al: Diabetic nephropathy in the uninephrectomized dog: Microscopic lesions after one year. Kidney Int 21:721–724, 1982.
24. Maser RD, Steenkiste AR, Dorman JS, et al: Epidemiological correlates of diabetic neuropathy. Report from Pittsburgh Epidemiology of Diabetic Complications Study. Diabetes 38:1556–1561, 1989.
25. Knowles HC Jr: The problem of the relation of the control of diabetes to the development of vascular disease. Trans Am Clin Climatol Assoc 76:142–147, 1964.
26. Pirart J: Diabetes mellitus and its degenerative complications: A prospective study of 4,400 patients observed between 1947 and 1973. Diabetes Care 1:168–188, 252–266, 1978.
27. Klein R, Klein BEK, Moss SE, et al: Glycosylated hemoglobin predicts the incidence and progression of diabetic retinopathy. JAMA 260:2864–2871, 1988.
28. Klein R, Moss SE, Klein BEK, et al: The Wisconsin epidemiologic study of diabetic retinopathy. XI. The incidence of macular edema. Ophthalmology 96:1501–1510, 1989.
29. Moss SE, Klein R, Klein BEK: The incidence of vision loss in a diabetic population. Ophthalmology 95:1340–1348, 1989.
30. Doft BH, Kingsley LA, Orchard TJ, et al: The association between long-term diabetic control and early retinopathy. Ophthalmology 91:763–769, 1984.
31. McCance DR, Atkinson AB, Hadden DR, et al: Long-term glycaemic control and diabetic retinopathy. Lancet 2:824–828, 1989.
32. Weber B, Burger W, Hartmann R, et al: Risk factors for the development of retinopathy in children and adolescents with Type I (insulin-dependent) diabetes mellitus. Diabetologia 29:23–29, 1986.

33. Groop LC, Teir H, Koskimies S, et al: Risk factors and markers associated with proliferative retinopathy in patients with insulin-dependent diabetes. Diabetes 35:1397–1403, 1986.

34. Krolewski AS, Warram JH, Rand LI, et al: Risk of proliferative diabetic retinopathy in juvenile-onset Type I diabetes: A 40-year follow-up study. Diabetes Care 9:443–452, 1986.

35. Klein R, Klein BEK, Moss SE, et al. The Wisconsin epidemiologic study of diabetic retinopathy. II. Prevalence and risk of diabetic retinopathy when age at diagnosis is less than 30 years. Arch Ophthalmol 102:520–526, 1984.

36. Nathan DM, Singer DE, Godine JE, et al: Retinopathy in older Type II diabetics: Association with glucose control. Diabetes 35:797–801, 1986.

37. Knowler WC, Bennett PH, Ballintine EJ: Increased incidence of retinopathy in diabetics with elevated blood pressure: A six-year follow-up study in Pima Indians. N Engl J Med 302:645–650, 1980.

38. Klein BEK, Moss SE, Klein R: Effect of pregnancy on progression of diabetic retinopathy. Diabetes Care 13:34–40, 1990.

39. Miljanovic B, Glynn RJ, Nathan DM, et al: A prospective study of serum lipids and risk of diabetic macular edema in type 1 diabetes mellitus. Diabetes 53:2883–2892, 2004.

40. Leslie RDG, Pyke DA: Diabetic retinopathy in identical twins. Diabetes 31:19–21, 1982.

41. Stratton IM, Kohner EM, Aldington SJ, et al for the UKPDS Group: UKPDS 50: Risk factors for incidence and progression of retinopathy in type II diabetes over 6 years from diagnosis. Diabetologia 44:145–163, 2001.

42. Andersen AR, Christiansen JS, Andersen JK, et al: Diabetic nephropathy in Type I (insulin-dependent) diabetes: An epidemiological study. Diabetologia 25:496–501, 1983.

43. Rosenstock J, Raskin P: Early diabetic nephropathy: Assessment and potential therapeutic interventions. Diabetes Care 9:529–54, 1986.

44. Kussman MJ, Goldstein HH, Gleason RE: The clinical course of diabetic nephropathy. JAMA 236:1861–1863, 1976.

45. Viberti GC, Jarrett RJ, Mahmud U, et al: Microalbuminuria as a predictor of clinical nephropathy in insulin-dependent diabetes mellitus. Lancet 1:1430–1432, 1982.

46. Parving H-H, Oxenboll B, Svendsen PA, et al: Early detection of patients at risk of developing diabetic nephropathy. A longitudinal study of urinary albumin excretion. Acta Endocrinol 100:550–555, 1982.

47. Mathiesen ER, Oxenboll B, Johansen K, et al: Incipient nephropathy in Type I (insulin-dependent) diabetes. Diabetologia 26:406–410, 1984.

48. Mogensen CE, Christensen CK: Predicting diabetic nephropathy in insulin-dependent patients. N Engl J Med 311:89–93, 1984.

49. Mogensen CE: Microalbuminuria predicts clinical proteinuria and early mortality in maturity-onset diabetes. N Engl J Med 310:356–360, 1984.

50. Feldt-Rasmussen B, Mathieson ER: Validity of urinary albumin excretion in incipient diabetic nephropathy. Diabetic Nephrol 3:101–104, 1984.

51. Viberti GC, Keen H, Wiseman MJ: Raised arterial pressure in parents of proteinuric insulin dependent diabetics. Br Med J 295:515–517, 1987.

52. Krolewski AS, Canessa M, Warram JH, et al: Predisposition to hypertension and susceptibility to renal disease in insulin-dependent diabetes mellitus. N Engl J Med 318:140–145, 1988.

53. Chase HP, Jackson WE, Hoops SL, et al: Glucose control and the renal and retinal complications of insulin-dependent diabetes. JAMA 261:1155–1160, 1989.

54. Ward JD, Fisher DJ, Barnes CG, et al: Improvement in nerve conduction following treatment in newly diagnosed diabetics. Lancet 1:428–430, 1971.

55. The DCCT Research Group: Factors in development of diabetic neuropathy. Diabetes 37:476, 1988.

56. Porte D Jr, Graf RJ, Halter JB, et al: Diabetic neuropathy and plasma glucose control. Am J Med 70:195–200, 1981.

57. The Kroc Collaborative Study Group: Blood glucose control and the evolution of diabetic retinopathy and albuminuria: A preliminary multicenter trial. N Engl J Med 6:365–372, 1984.

58. Lauritzen T, Frost-Larsen K, Larsen H-W, Deckert T: The Steno Study Group: Two-year experience with continuous subcutaneous insulin infusion in relation to retinopathy and neuropathy. Diabetes 34(Suppl 3):74–79, 1985.

59. Brinchmann-Hansen O, Dahl-Jorgensen K, Hanssen KF, Sandvik L: The response of diabetic retinopathy to 41 months of multiple insulin injections, insulin pumps, and conventional insulin therapy. Arch Ophthalmol 106:1242–1246, 1988.

60. DCCT Research Group: The Diabetes Control and Complications Trial (DCCT): Design and methodologic considerations for the feasibility phase. Diabetes 35:530–545, 1986.

61. Lauritzen T, Larsen H-W, Larsen K-F, et al: Effect of 1 year of near-normal blood glucose levels on retinopathy in insulin-dependent diabetics. Lancet 1:200–204, 1983.

62. Dahl-Jorgensen K, Brinchmann-Hansen O, Hanssen KF, et al: Rapid tightening of blood glucose control leads to transient deterioration of retinopathy in insulin dependent diabetes mellitus: The Oslo study. Br Med J 290:811–815, 1985.

63. DCCT Research Group: The effect of intensive diabetes treatment on the progression of diabetic retinopathy in insulin-dependent diabetes mellitus: The Diabetes Control and Complications Trial. Arch Ophthalmol 113:36, 1995.

64. DCCT Research Group: Progression of retinopathy with intensive vs conventional therapy in the Diabetes Control and Complications Trial. Ophthalmology 102:647, 1995.

65. DCCT Research Group: Early worsening of diabetic retinopathy in the Diabetes Control and Complications Trial. Arch Ophthalmol 116:874–886, 1998.

66. DCCT Research Group: The effect of intensive therapy on the development and progression of diabetic nephropathy in the Diabetes Control and Complications Trial. Kidney Int 47:1703, 1995.

67. DCCT Research Group: The effect of intensive diabetes therapy on the development and progression of neuropathy. Ann Int Med 122:561, 1995.

68. DCCT Research Group: The effect of intensive diabetes therapy on measures of autonomic nervous system function in the Diabetes Control and Complications Trial (DCCT). Diabetologia 41:416–423, 1998.

69. DCCT Research Group: The Effect of Intensive Treatment of Diabetes on Nerve Conduction Measures in the Diabetes Control and Complications Trial. Annals of Neurology 38:869–880, 1995.

70. DCCT Research Group: The effect of intensive diabetes therapy on macrovascular disease and its risk factors in the Diabetes Control and Complications Trial. Am J Cardiol 75:894, 1995.

71. DCCT Research Group: The effect of intensive therapy on quality of life outcome in the Diabetes Control and Complications Trial. Diabetes Care 19:195–203, 1996.

72. DCCT Research Group: The Effects of Intensive Diabetes Therapy on Neuropsychological Function in Adults in the Diabetes Complications and Control Trial. Ann Intern Med 124:379–388, 1996.

73. DCCT Research Group: Effect of intensive therapy on residual B-cell function in patients with type 1 diabetes in the Diabetes Control and Complications Trial. Ann Intern Med 128:517–523, 1998.

74. DCCT Research Group: Implementation of treatment protocols in the Diabetes Control and Complications Trial. Diabetes Care 18:361, 1995.

75. DCCT Research Group: Treatment related adverse events in the Diabetes Control and Complications Trial. Diabetes Care 18:1415, 1995.

76. DCCT Research Group: Hypoglycemia in the Diabetes Control and Complications Trial. Diabetes 46:271–286, 1997.

77. DCCT Research Group: Lifetime benefits of intensive therapy as practiced in the Diabetes Control and Complications Trial: An economic evaluation. JAMA 276:1409–1415, 1996.

78. DCCT Research Group: Pregnancy outcomes in the Diabetes Control and Complications Trial. Am J Obstet Gynecol 174:1343–1353, 1996.

79. DCCT Research Group: Relationship of glycemic exposure to the risk of developing retinopathy in the Diabetes Control and Complications Trial. Diabetes 44:968–983, 1995.

80. DCCT Research Group: The absence of a glycemic threshold for the development of long-term complications: The perspective of the Diabetes Control and Complications Trial. Diabetes 45:1289–1298, 1996.

81. EDIC Research Group: Epidemiology of Diabetes Interventions and Complications (EDIC): Design and implementation of a long-term follow-up of the Diabetes Control and Complications Trial Cohort. Diabetes Care 22:99–111, 1999.

82. EDIC Research Group: Retinopathy and nephropathy in patients with Type 1 diabetes four years after a trial of intensive therapy. N Engl J Med 342:381–389, 2000.

83. EDIC Research Group: Effect of intensive therapy on the microvascular complications of Type 1 diabetes mellitus. JAMA 287:2563–2569, 2002.

84. EDIC Research Group: Intensive diabetes therapy and carotid intima-media thickness in Type 1 diabetes mellitus. N Engl J Med 348:2294–2303, 2003.

85. Early treatment Diabetic retinopathy Study Research Group: Fundus photographic risk factors for progression of diabetic retinopathy. Ophthalmology 98:823–833, 1991.

86. DCCT Research Group: Clustering of long-term complications in families with diabetes in the Diabetes Control and Complications Trial. Diabetes 46:1829–1839, 1997.

87. Cleary P, Orchard T, Zinman B, et al for the DCCT/EDIC Study Group: Coronary calcification in the Diabetes Control and Complications Trial/Epidemiology of Diabetes Interventions and Complications (DCCT/EDIC) cohort. Diabetes 52(Suppl 2):A152, 2003.

88. Nathan DM: Inferences and implications: Do the DCCT results apply in NIDDM? Diabetes Care 13:5–6, 1995.

89. University Group Diabetes Program: A study of the effects of hypoglycemic agents on vascular complications in patients with adult-onset diabetes. VI. Supplementary report on nonfatal events in patients treated with tolbutamide. Diabetes 25:1129–1153, 1976.

90. UKPDS Group: Effect of intensive blood-glucose control with metformin on complications in overweight patients with Type 2 diabetes (UKPDS 34). Lancet 352:854–865, 1998.

91. Nathan DM: Some answers, more controversy, from UKPDS. Lancet 352:832–833, 1998.

92. Stratton IM, Adler AI, Neil HA, et al: Association of glycaemia with macrovascular and microvascular complications of type 2 diabetes (UKPDS 35): Prospective observational study. Br Med J 321:405–412, 2000.

93. Kannel WB, McGee DL: Diabetes and cardiovascular disease. The Framingham Study. JAMA 241:2036–2038, 1979.

94. Gordon T, Castelli WP, Hjortland MC, et al: Diabetes, blood lipids, and the role of obesity in coronary heart disease risk for women. The Framingham Study. Ann Intern Med 87:393–397, 1977.

95. Jarrett RJ, McCartney P, Keen H: The Bedford Survey: Ten year mortality rates in newly diagnosed diabetics, borderline diabetics and normoglycaemic controls and risk indices for coronary heart disease in borderline diabetics. Diabetologia 22:79–84, 1982.

96. Nathan DM, Meigs J, Singer DE: The epidemiology of cardiovascular disease in type 2 diabetes mellitus: How sweet it is . . . or is it? Lancet 350(Suppl 1):S14–S19, 1997.

97. The International Collaborative Group: Joint discussion. J Chronic Dis 32:829–837, 1979.

98. Singer DE, Nathan DM, Anderson KM, et al: The association of hemoglobin A1c with prevalent cardiovascular disease in the original cohort of the Framingham Heart Study. Diabetes 41:202–208, 1992.

99. Meigs JB, Nathan DM, Wilson PWF, et al: Metabolic risk factors worsen continuously across the spectrum of nondiabetic glucose tolerance: Framingham Offspring Study. Ann Intern Med 128:524–533, 1998.

100. Coutinho M, Gerstein HC, Wang Y, Yusuf S: The relationship between glucose and incident cardiovascular events: A metaregression analysis of published data from 20 studies of 95,783 individuals followed for 12.4 years. Diabetes Care 22:233–240, 1999.

101. Meigs JB, Nathan DM, D'Agostino RB, Wilson PWF: Fasting and postchallenge glycemia and cardiovascular disease risk: The Framingham Offspring Study. Diabetes Care 25:1845–1850, 2002.

102. Blake DR, Meigs JB, Muller DC, et al: Impaired glucose tolerance, but not impaired fasting glucose, is associated with increased levels of coronary heart disease risk factors. Diabetes 53:2095–2100, 2004.

103. American Diabetes Association: Postprandial blood glucose. Diabetes Care 24:775–778, 2001.

104. Brownlee M: Biochemistry and molecular cell biology of diabetic complications. Nature 414:813–820, 2001.

105. Yan SF, Ramasamy R, Naka Y, Schmidt AM: Glycation, inflammation, and RAGE. Circ Res 93:1159–1169, 2003.

106. Engerman RL, Kern TS, Larson ME: Nerve conduction and aldose reductase inhibition during 5 years of diabetes or galactosaemia in dogs. Diabetologia 37:141–144, 1994.

107. Ishii H, Jirousek MR, Koya D, et al: Ameliroation of vascular dysfunctions in diabetic rats by an oral PKC β inhibitor. Science 272:728–731, 1996.

108. Nishikawa T, Edelstein D, Du X-L, et al: Normalizing mitochondrial superoxide production blocks three pathways of hyperglycaemic damage. Nature 404:787–790, 2000.

109. Monnier VM, Bamtista O, Kenny D: Skin collagen glycation, glycoxidation, and crosslinking are lower in subjects with long-term intensive versus conventional therapy of Type 1 diabetes: relevance of glycated collagen products versus HbA1c as markers of diabetic complications. Diabetes 48:870–880, 1999.

Diabetic Eye Disease

Lloyd Paul Aiello, Jerry Cavallerano, and Ronald Klein

INTRODUCTION

Diabetes mellitus (DM) affects virtually all structures of the eye and many aspects of visual function. Diabetic retinopathy (DR) remains a leading cause of new-onset blindness in the United States and other industrialized nations.[1] Additionally, coexisting morbidities of DM, including hypertension, renal disease, and dyslipidemia, are associated risk factors for the progression of diabetic retinopathy. Multi-centered clinical trials have demonstrated the efficacy of glycemic and blood pressure control in preventing the progression of retinopathy[2-4] and have demonstrated the effectiveness of laser photocoagulation in preserving vision and reducing the risk of vision loss.[5,6] However, laser photocoagulation, which is usually reserved for advanced DR, may be associated with side effects and complications, does not prevent loss of visual acuity in all cases, and generally does not restore vision. Nevertheless, because laser photocoagulation is the only treatment proven to reduce the risk of visual loss when vision-threatening retinopathy is present and because a significant number of persons with DM at risk for visual loss from vision-threatening retinopathy do not receive necessary eye care, public health efforts have been directed at earlier detection and timely photocoagulation.[7-11] The purpose of this chapter is to provide a better understanding of the natural history, pathogenesis, epidemiology, detection, and management of diabetic retinopathy.

PATHOGENESIS

The pathogenesis of DR is not fully understood. However, many mechanisms have been suggested and are summarized in Figure 67-1.[12] The development and progression of retinopathy probably result from a complex interplay of these and other factors, which may vary from person to person. It is likely that the relative contributions of different mechanisms vary in importance at different stages of retinopathy. Glycosylation, protein kinase C and polyol pathways, and changes in retinal blood flow may be particularly important early in the course of the disease, even before the development of microaneurysms

or other clinically evident findings. Angiogenesis factors such as vascular endothelial growth factor (VEGF) and insulin-like growth factor 1 are more likely to be important later in the course of the disease, just before and during the development of proliferative retinopathy. In addition, interindividual and intraindividual variations in biochemical or physiologic responses to hyperglycemia (perhaps as a result of differences in genetic susceptibility) may exist among people at different stages of diabetic disease. This variability may explain why a few diabetic patients have minimal retinopathy despite years of severe hyperglycemia whereas severe retinopathy develops in others in a short period despite relatively good glycemic control. Furthermore, these pathogenetic factors have not often been studied together in a prospective fashion, making it difficult to prove a causal relationship.

NATURAL HISTORY OF DIABETIC RETINOPATHY

NONPROLIFERATIVE DIABETIC RETINOPATHY

The earliest diabetes-induced changes in the retina are biochemical, hemodynamic, and cellular in nature and imperceptible clinically. These include changes in biochemical pathways, enzyme activation, retinal blood flow, and pericyte loss. The first clinical signs of diabetic retinopathy are microaneurysms, which are saccular outpouchings of retinal capillaries.[13] These lesions usually appear as round red dots ranging in size from 20 to 200 µm and represent an outpouching of the retinal capillaries. They often appear first in the macular area in areas of capillary closure. It is unusual to detect retinal microaneurysms within 3 years of the diagnosis of type 1 diabetes; however, they are often present at the time of diagnosis in people with type 2 diabetes.[14] In the United Kingdom Prospective Diabetes Study (UKPDS), where subjects were enrolled at the time of diagnosis of type 2 DM, nearly 40% of those studied had some level of DR at entrance into the study. Moreover, after 10 years of diabetes, 69% of people with type 1 diabetes and 55% of people with type 2 diabetes have microaneurysms present.[15,16]

Retinal microaneurysms are not pathognomonic of DR since they are also associated with essential hypertension,

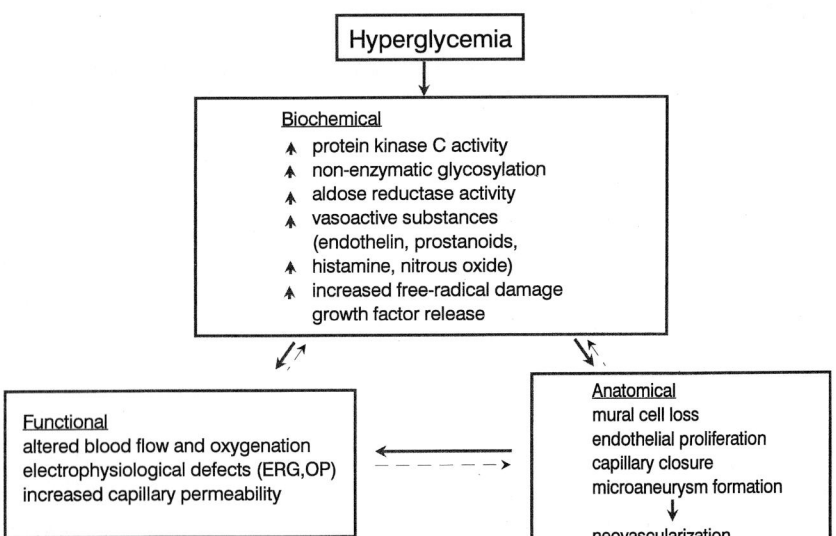

Figure 67-1 Hypothesized pathogenetic mechanisms for the development and progression of diabetic retinopathy.

retinal venous stasis caused by atherosclerotic carotid artery disease, acquired immunodeficiency syndrome (AIDS), and a large number of other systemic and ocular conditions.[17] The appearance of a microaneurysm or two in only one eye of a person with type 2 DM should not be regarded as specific for DR; however, when larger numbers of microaneurysms are present (four or more in one eye or present in both eyes), they are more likely due to DM and the likelihood of progression to more severe nonproliferative diabetic retinopathy (NPDR) is greater.[18]

Microaneurysms have abnormal permeability to fluorescein, red blood cells, and lipoproteins.[13] By themselves, microaneurysms are not a threat to vision. However, as retinopathy progresses, hard exudates and retinal dot or blot hemorrhages appear. Dot hemorrhages are frequently indistinguishable from microaneurysms, and they are frequently grouped with microaneurysm and referred to as *hemorrhages and/or microaneurysms* (H/Ma). The blot hemorrhages are round with blurred edges and result from extravasation of blood from retinal capillaries or microaneurysms into the inner nuclear layer of the retina (Fig. 67-2). Retinal blot hemorrhages usually disappear within 3 to 4 months.[19] Ruptured microaneurysms, decompensated capillaries, and intraretinal microvascular abnormalities result in intraretinal hemorrhages. The clinical appearance of these hemorrhages reflects the retinal architecture at the level at which the hemorrhage occurs. Hemorrhages in the nerve fiber layer assume a more flame-shaped appearance, coinciding with the structure of the nerve fiber layer that runs parallel to the retinal surface. Hemorrhages deeper in the retina, at which point the arrangement of cells is more or less perpendicular to the surface of the retina, assume a pinpoint or dot shape.

Retinal hard exudates are sharply defined, yellow, and variable in size; they may be aggregated or scattered and partially or fully circinate in their distribution (see Fig. 67-2). A ring of hard exudates generally reflects the border of an area of retinal leakage. Hard exudates result from leakage of lipoprotein material from retinal microaneurysms or capillaries into the outer retinal layer, and they may persist for months to years.[19] The exudate is usually found in the posterior layer of the retina, and if they extend into the foveal area, they may reduce visual acuity.

With closure of the retinal capillaries and arterioles, whitish or grayish swellings appear in the nerve fiber layer of the retina. These changes, termed *cotton-wool spots* (CWSs) or *soft exudates*, are microinfarcts of the nerve fiber layer (see Fig. 67-2). They may remain only a few weeks or months. After they disappear, the retina may appear normal on ophthalmoscopy, but fluorescein angiography reveals a corresponding area of nonperfusion of the retinal arterioles.

Dilated capillaries called *intraretinal microvascular abnormalities* (IRMAs) are another manifestation of focal retinal ischemia. They are found in areas of capillary nonperfusion and may be abnormally permeable to plasma proteins. IRMAs represent either new vessel growth within the retina or a pre-existing vessel that has developed abnormal morphology thought to include endothelial cell proliferation. IRMAs may be seen adjacent to CWSs. Multiple IRMAs identify a severe stage of NPDR.

Venous caliber abnormalities are indicators of severe retinal hypoxia. These abnormalities can take the form of venous dilatation, beading, or loop formation. There are often large

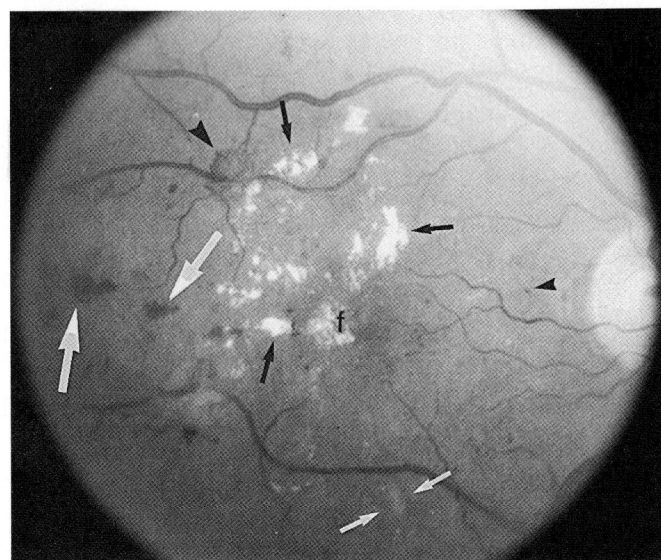

Figure 67-2 Fundus photograph of the right eye. A number of retinal microaneurysms *(small black arrowhead)* appear as small dark spots with sharp margins, and retinal blot hemorrhages *(large white arrows)* appear as dark spots of varying size with irregular margins and uneven densities. Retinal hard exudates appear as white deposits with sharp margins either scattered, "ringlike," or aggregated in their distributions *(small black arrows)* in the superior, temporal, and foveal (f) areas. A cotton-wool spot or soft exudate *(small white arrows)* appears as a grayish white area with ill-defined edges. A retinal new vessel superior and temporal to the fovea *(larger black arrowhead)* originates from a small retinal venule.

areas of nonperfusion adjacent to these abnormalities. Treatment with scatter (panretinal) photocoagulation (PRP) may cause these abnormal veins to become less dilated and more regular. IRMAs, intraretinal hemorrhages, and venous beading represent significant retinal ischemia. These changes were referred to as "preproliferative" retinopathy under the old classification systems and are clearly associated with more severe stages of NPDR, serving as a warning sign of the impending retinal neovascularization. Late in the course of the disease, thinly sheathed sclerotic "white, threadlike" arterioles may be present.

PROLIFERATIVE DIABETIC RETINOPATHY

Proliferative diabetic retinopathy (PDR) is characterized by proliferating retinal vessels, the growth of which is variable. They are commonly identified according to their retinal location, at or near the optic disc (neovascularization of the disc [NVD], Fig. 67-3) or elsewhere in the retina (neovascularization elsewhere [NVE], see Fig. 67-2). Retinal neovascularization may be difficult to detect when the vessels first appear as fine tufts of "naked" vessels on the surface of the retina or optic nerve head.[20] They are prone to proliferate on the posterior surface of the vitreous and hemorrhage into the vitreous. With time, the new vessels often fibrose. If this fibrovascular tissue contracts, traction detachment of the retina may result. Once regression of new vessels occurs as a result of photocoagulation or the natural course of the disease, fibrous tissue may remain.

PDR poses a significant risk for vision loss. Patients with high-risk PDR generally require prompt PRP. High-risk PDR is characterized by one or more of the following lesions: (1) NVD that is approximately one quarter to one third disc area or more in size; (2) NVD less than one quarter disc area in size if fresh vitreous or preretinal hemorrhage is present; or (3) NVE greater than or equal to one half disc area in size if fresh vitreous or preretinal hemorrhage is present. Therefore, attention must be paid to the presence, location, and severity of new vessels, as well as the presence or absence of preretinal or vitreous hemorrhages.[21]

DIABETIC MACULAR EDEMA, ISCHEMIA, AND TRACTION

Diabetes affects the macula in a number of ways. First, increased permeability of retinal capillaries and microaneurysms may result in the accumulation of extracellular fluid and thickening of the normally compact macular tissue, with or without the

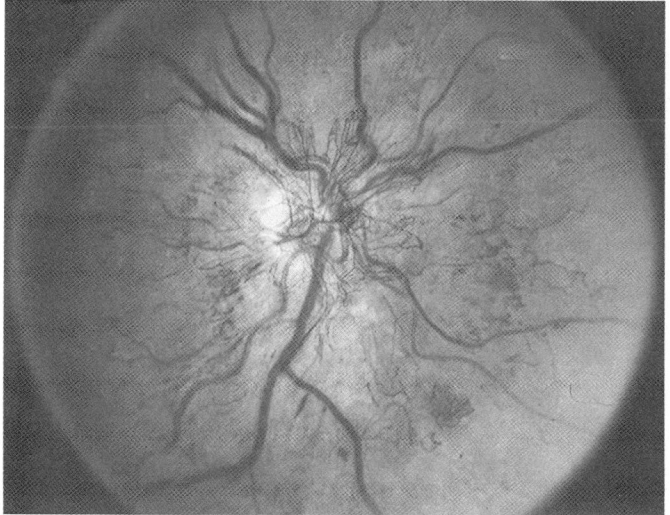

Figure 67-3 Fundus photograph demonstrating retinal new vessels on the optic nerve head. The retinal veins are also dilated.

development of cystoid spaces. The edema may be easily missed especially if not evaluated with appropriate equipment and by an experienced examiner. The edema is often associated with hard exudates distributed in rings, clumps, or large deposits. Accumulation of exudate is often gradual, and spontaneous resolution may occur. Involvement of the foveal area can be associated with a profound drop in visual acuity.

When macular edema threatens or involves the center of the macula, the edema is considered clinically significant macula edema (CSME). CSME can be present with any level of NPDR or PDR, but is more common with more severe DR. The Early Treatment Diabetic Retinopathy Study (ETDRS) found that CSME is associated with a 30% risk of visual loss over a 3-year period if left untreated with focal photocoagulation. This risk is reduced by 50% or more with appropriate focal laser photocoagualtion. CSME is defined as the presence of any of the following: thickening of the retina at or within 500 μm of the center of the macula; hard exudates at or within 500 μm of the center of the macula with adjacent thickening; or a zone of retinal thickening one disc area or larger in size any part of which is within one disc diameter of the center of the macula (see Fig. 67-2).

The underlying cause of macular edema is not known. It may be a result of both increased leakage and impaired removal. Breakdown of the blood-retinal barrier has been postulated as an important cause of fluid accumulation in the macula.[13] Reduced osmotic pressure resulting from decreased serum albumin levels, increased intravascular fluid load, increased arterial perfusion pressure, and tissue hypoxia has been postulated to lead to breakdown of the blood-retinal barrier. The retinal pigment epithelium normally serves to "pump" fluid out of the sensory retina. However, this function is also postulated to be impaired in patients with hyperglycemia. Recently, key growth factors involved in the progression of DR, such as VEGF, have been shown to be potent permeability factors and probably contribute significantly to this problem. Indeed, early clinical trials suggest that inhibiting VEGF may reduce CSME.

In addition to macular edema, diabetes may cause macular capillary nonperfusion, retinal or preretinal hemorrhage, lamellar or full-thickness hole formation, or dragging or detachment of the macula due to contraction of fibrovascular tissue. These changes may occur in isolation or in combinations and generally result in the loss of central vision if the fovea is involved.

CLINICAL CLASSIFICATION OF DIABETIC RETINOPATHY SEVERITY

DR can be broadly classified as NPDR and PDR. Lesions of NPDR include H/Ma, dot and blot hemorrhages, CWSs, hard exudates (HEs), venous caliber abnormalities (VCABs), and IRMAs. Based on the presence and degree of retinal lesions, NPDR is clinically classified as mild, moderate, severe, or very severe. PDR is marked by NVD, NVE, preretinal hemorrhage (PRH), vitreous hemorrhage (VH), or fibrous tissue proliferation (FP). Diabetic macular edema (DME) can be present with any level of diabetic retinopathy. DME that involves or threatens the center of the macula is classified as CSME. Accurate diagnosis of the severity of DR is essential since the risk of progression to PDR and high-risk PDR is closely correlated with specific NPDR level. Proper diagnosis of DR severity establishes the risk of progression to sight-threatening retinopathy and helps to determine appropriate clinical management, both in terms of follow-up schedule and therapy options. For example, it is important to consider PRP as DR reaches severe NPDR, early PDR, or high-risk PDR.

NONPROLIFERATIVE DIABETIC RETINOPATHY LEVELS

Mild NPDR is marked by at least one retinal microaneurysm, but hemorrhages and microaneurysms are only to a mild degree, and no other retinal lesion or abnormality associated with diabetes is present. Those with mild NPDR have a 5% risk of progression to PDR within 1 year and a 15% risk of progression to high-risk PDR within 5 years.[22,23] Moderate NPDR is characterized by moderate H/Ma or soft exudates, venous beading, and IRMAs are definitely present to a mild degree. The risk of progression to PDR within 1 year is 12% to 27%, and the risk of progression to high-risk PDR within 5 years is 33%. Patients with mild or moderate NPDR generally are not candidates for PRP and can be followed safely at 6- to 12-month intervals. The presence of macular edema, even with mild or moderate degrees of NPDR, requires follow-up in a shorter period; and if CSME is present, focal laser treatment should be considered. Coincident medical problems or pregnancy will reduce the period until reevaluation. Severe NPDR, based on the severity of H/Ma, IRMAs, and venous beading, is characterized by any one of the following lesions: 20 or more H/Ma or venous beading in two or more quadrants or definite IRMAs in at least one quadrant. Clinically, severe NPDR is diagnosed by applying the "4-2-1-rule": Moderate H/Ma in four quadrants or venous beading in two quadrants or IRMA in one quadrant. Eyes with severe NPDR have a 52% risk of developing PDR within 1 year and a 60% risk of developing high-risk PDR within 5 years. These patients require follow-up evaluation in 2 to 4 months. Treatment of CSME is strongly indicated in these patients because of the risk of the development of PDR in the near term requiring PRP.

Eyes with very severe NPDR have two or more lesions of severe NPDR but no frank neovascularization. There is a 75% risk that PDR will develop within 1 year. Patients with very severe NPDR may be candidates for PRP; and macular edema, if present, generally should be treated. Follow-up evaluation at 2- to 3-month intervals is important. For patients with non-insulin-dependent diabetes mellitus (NIDDM), early PRP may be considered for patients with severe or very severe NPDR.[24]

PROLIFERATIVE DIABETIC RETINOPATHY LEVELS

Diabetic retinopathy with NVD or NVE or with FP is designated PDR. Early PDR does not meet the definition of high-risk PDR. Eyes with early PDR have a 75% risk of developing high-risk PDR within 5 years. Patients with severe or very severe NPDR or early PDR may be considered for early PRP. In the presence of macular edema, patients with severe NPDR or worse DR should be considered for focal treatment of macular edema, whether the macular edema is clinically significant or not, in preparation for the probable need of scatter laser photocoagulation.

The ETDRS severity scale was based on the modified Airlie House classification of DR and is a recognized standard for grading severity of DR. Its use in everyday clinical practice, however, poses difficulty, both in its complexity and lack of uniformity in terminology for many clinicians. Definitions of the levels are detailed, require comparison with standard photographs, and are difficult to remember and apply in a clinical setting. A new DR severity scale was developed by the Global Diabetic Retinopathy Group at the International Congress of Ophthalmology in Sydney in April 2002.[25]

This new scale consists of five levels (Table 67-1). The first level is "no apparent retinopathy," and the second level is "mild NPDR," corresponding to ETDRS stage 20 (microaneurysms only). The risk of significant progression over several years is very low in both groups. The third level, "moderate NPDR," includes eyes with ETDRS levels 35–47, and the risk of progression increases significantly by level 47. The fourth level, "severe NPDR" (ETDRS stage 53), carries with it the most ominous prognosis for progression to PDR. The fifth level, "PDR," includes all eyes with definite neovascularization or vitreous/preretinal hemorrhage. There was no attempt to subdivide this level as a function of ETDRS "high-risk characteristics" because significant rates of progression are expected to occur in all cases.

Table 67-1 Proposed International Clinical Diabetic Retinopathy (DR) and Diabetic Macular Edema Disease Severity Scales

No apparent DR	No abnormalities
Mild nonproliferative diabetic retinopathy (NPDR)	Microaneurysm only
Moderate NPDR	More than Ma only but less than severe NPDR
Severe NPDR	Any of the following: >20 intraretinal hemorrhages in each 4 quadrants definite VB in 2+ quadrants prominent IRMA in 1+ quadrant and no PDR
Proliferative diabetic retinopathy	One or more of: NV, vitreous hemorrhage, preretinal hemorrhage

NV, neovascularization. From Wilkinson CP, Ferris FL III, Klein RE, et al: Proposed international clinical diabetic retinopathy and diabetic macular edema disease severity scales. Ophthalmology 110(9):1677–1682, 2003.

The Diabetic Macular Edema Disease Severity Scale separates eyes with apparent DME from those with no apparent thickening or lipid in the macula (Table 67-2). For eyes with apparent DME, three categories classify DME as not threatening the center of the macula (mild), threatening the center of the macula (moderate), or involving the center of the macula (severe). The clinical disease severity scale is intended to be a practical and valid method of grading severity of DR and DME.

EPIDEMIOLOGY

Epidemiologic studies of DR are useful in developing public health strategies to prevent or reduce the occurrence or progression of this complication. In addition, epidemiologic data concerning DR, visual loss, and associated risk factors may be used in projecting costs, developing etiologic insight, designing future studies such as controlled clinical trials of treatment or prevention, and estimating the need for rehabilitative services.

One epidemiologic study that has provided data on DR, visual loss, and associated risk factors is the Wisconsin Epidemiologic Study of Diabetic Retinopathy (WESDR). This population-based study has been described in detail.[14,16,26,27] Standardized examination protocols and questionnaires, photographic documentation, photographic standards for grading the severity of retinal lesions, and standardized retinopathy severity scales have permitted, in some cases, comparisons among studies.[28,29]

Table 67-2 Proposed International Clinical Diabetic Retinopathy (DR) and Diabetic Macular Edema (DME) Disease Severity Scales

DME apparently absent	No apparent retinal thickening or hard exudates (HEs) in posterior pole
DME apparently present	Some apparent retinal thickening or HEs in posterior pole
	Mild DME—some retinal thickening or HEs in posterior pole but distant from center of the macula
	Moderate DME—retinal thickening or HEs approaching the center of the macula but not involving the center
	Severe DME—retinal thickening or HEs involving the center of the macula

From Wilkinson CP, Ferris FL III, Klein RE, et al: Proposed international clinical diabetic retinopathy and diabetic macular edema disease severity scales. Ophthalmology 110(9):1677–1682, 2003.

PREVALENCE AND INCIDENCE OF RETINOPATHY

The prevalence of DR and CSME categorized by age, gender, and diabetes group in the WESDR is presented in Table 67-3. The highest frequencies of DR and PDR were found in the younger-onset group using insulin; the lowest frequencies were in the older-onset group not using insulin.[26,27] CSME was most frequent in the younger-onset group using insulin. The prevalence of DR has been reported in other selected population-based studies.[28–50] Recently pooled data from eight studies, including the WESDR, estimates that among persons 40 years of age and older, the crude prevalence of diabetic retinopathy was 40% and the crude prevalence of severe retinopathy (very severe-severe NPDR and PDR or macular edema) was 8%. Projection of these rates to the diabetic population 40 years of age and older in the United States resulted in an estimate of 4 million persons with retinopathy, of whom 900,000 have signs of vision-threatening retinopathy.[51]

Based on the WESDR data, it is estimated that approximately 63,000 new cases of proliferative diabetic retinopathy occurred nationwide, in 29,000 of whom proliferative retinopathy developed with Diabetic Retinopathy Study (DRS) high-risk characteristics for severe visual loss annually. In addition, approximately 50,000 new cases of macular edema a year occurred in the United States.

RISK FACTORS FOR DIABETIC RETINOPATHY

Gender, Race, Genetic, and Age

Few differences are found in the risk of development and progression of DR in men and women with DM. However, differences among race/ethnic groups have been reported. Results from the study of Pima Indians with type 2 DM suggest that they are at increased risk for PDR in comparison to white people with type 2 DM.[49] After controlling for all measured risk factors, diabetic Mexican-Americans in San Antonio had a 2.4 times higher frequency of DR than did diabetic non-Hispanic whites studied in the WESDR.[28] Similarly, Mexican-Americans with type 2 DM participating in the National Health and Nutrition Examination Survey III (NHANES III) had an 84% higher frequency of diabetic retinopathy than non-Hispanic whites did.[50] The higher frequency of DR in Mexican-Americans than whites remained after controlling for the duration of DM, hemoglobin A_{1c} level, insulin and oral agent use, and hypertension in that study. However, Hamman and colleagues failed to find a difference in the frequency of DR between Hispanics and non-Hispanic whites examined in the San Luis Valley study.[29] West and colleagues also reported a similar prevalence of retinopathy in Mexican-Americans with type 2 diabetes living in Arizona of whom 48% had any retinopathy; 6% of the cohort had proliferative retinopathy, and 5% had clinically significant macular edema.[52] However, a higher prevalence of proliferative retinopathy and macular edema was found in Mexican-Americans living in Los Angeles than in whites living in Beaver Dam.[53] It has been suggested that black people with type 2 DM may have more severe DR and loss of vision than whites with type 2 diabetes.[54] In the NHANES III, the prevalence of DR in people with type 2 DM was 46% higher in non-Hispanic blacks than non-Hispanic whites.[50] However, after adjustment for glycosylated hemoglobin, the duration of DM, insulin and oral agent use, and hypertension, the rates for DR were similar between whites and blacks in that study.

Reports of a relationship between genetic factors and the prevalence of DR have been inconsistent.[24,51,55-58] Supporting such a relationship has been the observation that the severity and onset of DR are similar among concordant identical twins, which suggests that the tendency for the development of DR and possibly its progression are influenced by genetic factors.[59] In addition, Hanis demonstrated an 8.3-fold increased risk of DR in 46 Mexican-American siblings of probands who had DR when compared with the siblings of those who did not.[60]

It is uncommon to find clinical evidence of DR in children younger than 10, regardless of the duration of type 1 DM; the frequency of any DR or more severe DR increases after age 13.[61–64] This age effect has been postulated to result from a protective effect lost after the start of puberty. In the WESDR, menarcheal status at the time of the baseline examination was associated with the prevalence of DR.[65] After controlling for other factors such as diastolic blood pressure and duration of type 1 DM, those who were postmenarchal in the WESDR were 3.2 times more likely to have DR than those who were premenarchal.

A number of changes occurring at puberty have been thought to explain the higher risk for DR. These changes include increases in insulin-like growth factor 1, growth hormone, sex hormones, and blood pressure and poorer glycemic control. Increased insulin resistance, inadequate insulin dosage, and poorer compliance in attempts to control blood sugar may result in poorer glycemic control in postpubertal teenagers.[66–71]

	Younger Onset, Taking Insulin			Older Onset, Taking Insulin			Older Onset, Not Taking Insulin		
Retinopathy Status	Male (%) (n = 512)	Female (%) (n = 484)	Total (%) (n = 996)	Male (%) (n = 321)	Female (%) (n = 352)	Total (%) (n = 673)	Male (%) (n = 313)	Female (%) (n = 379)	Total (%) (n = 692)
None	31.1	27.5	29.3	26.8	32.7	29.9	64.5	58.6	61.3
Early nonproliferative	26.4	34.7	30.4	34.0	27.6	30.6	25.9	28.5	27.3
Moderate to severe nonproliferative	18.2	16.9	17.6	27.7	23.9	25.7	6.4	10.3	8.5
Proliferative without DRS high-risk characteristics	12.3	14.0	13.2	8.1	9.9	9.1	1.9	1.1	1.4
Proliferative with DRS high-risk characteristics or worse	12.1	6.8	9.5	3.4	6.0	4.8	1.3	1.6	1.4

Table 67-3 Prevalence and Severity of Retinopathy by Sex at the Baseline Examination in the Wisconsin Epidemiologic Study of Diabetic Retinopathy (1980–1982)

DRS, Diabetic Retinopathy Study.
Klein R, Moss SE, Klein BEK: New management concepts for the timely diagnosis of diabetic retinopathy treatable by photocoagulation. Diabetes Care 10:633–638, 1987.

DIABETES-RELATED RISK FACTORS

Multiple factors have been suggested as risk factors for onset or progression of DR. These factors include duration of DM, control of DM, hypertension, level of cholesterol and other lipids, renal disease, and anemia. The data associated with these risk factors has been extensively reviewed elsewhere[72] and is only presented briefly here.

Duration of Diabetes

The prevalence of DR (Fig. 67-4), macular edema, and PDR (Fig. 67-5) is significantly related to the duration of DM in all three diabetic groups studied in the WESDR. This observation is consistent with all previous epidemiologic studies.[30–42,47,50] The relationship between the duration of DM at the baseline examination and the incidence, progression of NPDR, or progression to PDR in the WESDR has been presented elsewhere.[26,27] DR was less common and PDR or macular edema was not present in younger-onset DM, whereas the reverse was true in older-onset DM not taking insulin. These findings are consistent with studies that reported relatively high rates of DR at the time of diagnosis of type 2 diabetes.[73,74]

These findings have important public health implications. First, they suggest that younger-onset DM does not need ophthalmologic evaluation for DR before puberty or before 5 years of DM because of lack of vision-threatening retinopathy. For older-onset individuals, because the onset of DM may have been years before its diagnosis, it is important to have a comprehensive retinal examination at diagnosis to detect possible PDR or macular edema. These findings have been used to develop guidelines recommending ophthalmologic care for patients with DM[75,76] (Table 67-4).

Glycemia

A growing body of epidemiologic data has shown that hyperglycemia is related to the incidence and progression of DR.[28,31,32,34–36,38,39,41,42,44–48,50] In the WESDR, the glycosylated hemoglobin level at baseline was found to be a significant predictor of the incidence of any DR, progression, incidence of PDR, or incidence of macular edema in all three diabetic groups studied.[77,78] WESDR findings and those of others suggest that even in people with longer duration of DM, good glycemic control is more likely to be associated with lower rates of progression of DR than poor glycemic control.[44,77–79] In addition, in the WESDR, no threshold level of glycemia, as

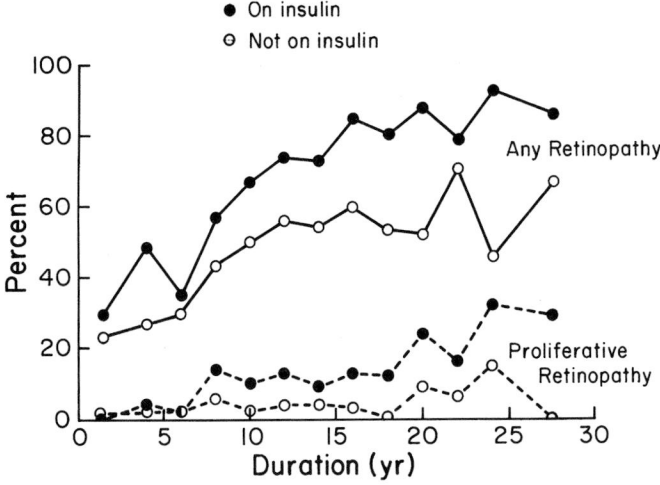

Figure 67-5 The frequency of retinopathy or proliferative retinopathy by duration of diabetes (years) in 673 people taking insulin and 697 people not taking insulin in whom diabetes was diagnosed when older than 29 years and who participated in the Wisconsin Epidemiologic Study of Diabetic Retinopathy (WESDR), 1980–1982. (From Klein R, Klein BEK, Moss SE, et al: The Wisconsin Epidemiologic Study of Diabetic Retinopathy. III. Prevalence and risk of diabetic retinopathy when age at diagnosis is 30 or more years. Arch Ophthalmol 102:527–532, Copyright 1984, American Medical Association.)

measured by deciles of glycosylated hemoglobin at baseline, was observed in which DR did not progress (Fig. 67-6).

The Diabetes Control and Complications Trial (DCCT) was a large randomized controlled clinical trial of more than 1400 patients with type 1 DM.[2] This multi-centered trial showed that intensive insulin treatment reduced the risk of the development and progression of diabetic retinopathy. In that study, those assigned to intensive glycemic control had a 60% reduction in three-step or greater progression of DR than did the group assigned to conventional treatment. In the secondary intervention arm of the DCCT, those assigned to intensive glycemic control had a 34% reduction in the progression of DR, a 47% reduction in the incidence of severe levels of NPDR or PDR, a 22% reduction in the incidence of macular edema, and a 54% reduction in laser photocoagulation treatment when compared with the group assigned to conventional insulin treatment.

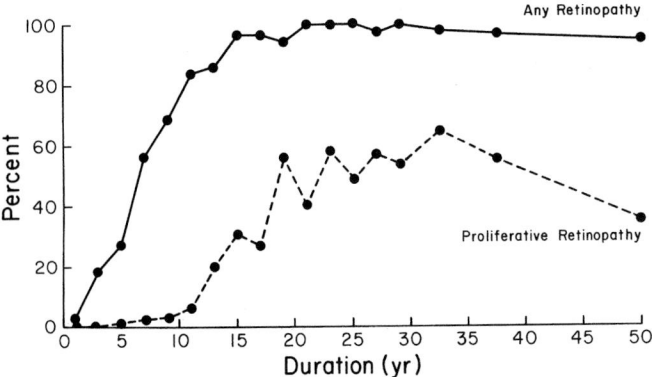

Figure 67-4 Frequency of retinopathy or proliferative retinopathy by duration of diabetes (years) in 996 insulin-taking persons in whom diabetes was diagnosed when younger than 30 years and who participated in the Wisconsin Epidemiologic Study of Diabetic Retinopathy (WESDR), 1980–1982. (From Klein R, Klein BEK, Moss SE, et al: The Wisconsin Epidemiologic Study of Diabetic Retinopathy. II. Prevalence and risk of diabetic retinopathy when age at diagnosis is less than 30 years. Arch Ophthalmol 102:520–526, Copyright 1984, American Medical Association.)

Table 67-4	Recommendations for Eye Care for Diabetic Patients

Primary-care physician informs the patient at the time of diagnosis of diabetes that:
  Ocular complications are associated with diabetes and may threaten sight
  Timely detection and treatment may reduce the risk of decreased vision
Referral to an eye doctor competent in ophthalmoscopy:
  All patients 10–30 years old who have had diabetes for 5 or more years
  In patients in whom diabetes was diagnosed when older than 30 years, examination at the time of diagnosis or shortly thereafter
Referral to an ophthalmologist:
  All women with insulin-dependent diabetes mellitus planning pregnancy within 12 months, in the first trimester, and thereafter at the discretion of the ophthalmologist
  Patients found to have reduced corrected visual acuity, elevated intraocular pressure, and any other vision-threatening ocular abnormalities

From Klein R, Klein BEK, Moss S: The Wisconsin Epidemiologic Study of Diabetic Retinopathy: A review. Diabetes Metab Rev 5:559–570, 1989.

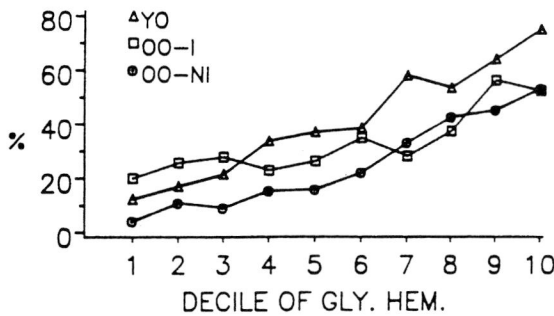

Figure 67-6 Relationship of the 4-year progression of diabetic retinopathy to deciles of glycosylated hemoglobin at baseline examination in three diabetic groups participating in the Wisconsin Epidemiologic Study of Diabetic Retinopathy (WESDR).

The UKPDS was a randomized controlled clinical trial involving 3867 patients with newly diagnosed type 2 DM.[3] After 3 months of diet treatment, patients with a mean of two fasting plasma glucose concentrations of 6.1 to 15.0 mmol/L were randomly assigned to an intensive glycemic control group with either a sulfonylurea (chlorpropamide, gliben-clamide, or glipizide) or insulin or to a conventional glycemic control group with diet. After 10 years of follow-up, hemoglobin A_{1c} was 7.0% in the intensive group and 7.9% in the conventional group, and the data conclusively showed that intensive treatment with either sulfonylureas or insulin significantly reduced the risk of progression of DR in persons with type 2 DM.

The DCCT and UKPDS results demonstrate a causal relationship between glycemic control and the risk of DR, as well as other microvascular complications, and suggest that lowering blood sugar, even modestly, may significantly reduce the incidence of PDR or macular edema or the need for photocoagulation.[2,3] However, reducing glycemic control is not without adverse affects. The DCCT found a 60% risk of weight gain and a 330% increased risk of severe hypoglycemic episodes in the intensive glycemic control group vs. the conventional group.[2]

OTHER RISK FACTORS

Blood Pressure
Clinical studies suggest a possible relationship between elevated blood pressure and the presence of DR.[80] High blood pressure, through an effect on blood flow, has been postulated to damage capillary endothelial cells, possibly contributing to the development or progression of retinopathy.[81] However, recent epidemiologic studies on the relationship of blood pressure to the incidence and progression of DR have been conflicting.[28,29,31,32,34–36,38,41,42,44,46,47,82–85] These data have been reviewed previously.[72] The UKPDS randomized 1148 patients with hypertension (mean blood pressure, 160/94 mm Hg) to a regimen of tight control with either captopril or atenolol and another 390 patients to less tight control of their blood pressure to evaluate whether tight control of blood pressure with either a β-adrenergic blocker or an angiotensin-converting enzyme inhibitor was beneficial in reducing the macrovascular and microvascular complications associated with type 2 DM.[4] Tight blood pressure control resulted in a 35% reduction in retinal photocoagulation when compared with conventional control, and after 7.5 years of follow-up, a 34% reduction in the rate of progression of DR by two or more steps on the modified ETDRS severity scale and a 47% reduction in a moderate visual loss. The effect was largely due to a reduction in the incidence of diabetic macular edema. Atenolol and captopril were equally effective in reducing the

risk of development of these microvascular complications. The effects of blood pressure control were independent of those of glycemic control. These findings strongly support tight blood pressure control in people with type 2 diabetes as a means of preventing visual loss resulting from the progression of DR.

Serum Lipids
Epidemiologic data suggest a relationship between higher levels of lipids and the presence of DR or the development of hard exudates.[29,30,34,41,86] The WESDR showed a significant trend toward increasing severity of DR and retinal HE with increasing cholesterol in the younger- and older-onset groups using insulin.[86] The ETDRS found a positive relationship between serum lipids (triglycerides, low-density lipoprotein cholesterol, and very low-density lipoprotein cholesterol) and the development of hard exudates.[87] Although data from earlier clinical trials suggested a beneficial effect of clofibrate (Atromid-S, a lipid-lowering agent with significant hepatic toxicity) in reducing the presence of HEs, it did not lead to an improvement in vision.[88,89] Currently, controlled clinical trials are under way to investigate whether the use of statins in people with type 2 DM will reduce the incidence and progression of DR.

Proteinuria and Renal Disease
Diabetic nephropathy may lead to lipid, platelet, and rheologic abnormalities, all of which have been hypothesized to be pathogenetic factors for the development of DR.[90,91] Therefore, it is not surprising that most epidemiologic studies have found a strong association between the presence and severity of DR and microalbuminuria and gross proteinuria.[30,34,41,45] These relationships are independent of blood pressure.[92]

Cigarette Smoking and Alcohol Consumption
Most data from epidemiologic studies have failed to confirm earlier reports of a positive relationship between cigarette smoking and DR.[28,29,34,38,93,94] Regardless of the relationship with DR, diabetic patients should be advised not to smoke because it is an important risk factor for respiratory and cardiovascular disease, as well as for cancer.[95,96] Few epidemiologic studies have investigated the relationship of alcohol consumption to DRR.[97–99] One might anticipate a possible protective effect of alcohol as a result of decreased platelet aggregation and adhesiveness.[100] Data from one study suggested a beneficial effect of alcohol, whereas data from another study suggested an increased risk of proliferative retinopathy in people with diabetes.[97,98] In the WESDR, alcohol consumption was associated with a lower frequency of PDR in the younger-onset group.[99] However, no relationship was found between alcohol consumption at the 4-year follow-up examination and the incidence and progression of DR in either the younger- or older-onset groups at the 10-year follow-up.[101]

Pregnancy
Epidemiologic studies suggest that pregnancy is a significant predictor of progression of DR.[102] In a review of the literature, Rodman and colleagues reported that 8% of women with type 1 DM who had no NPDR or early NPDR at the onset of pregnancy had progression of DR during pregnancy.[103] In a case-control study of women with type 1 DM, the frequency of progression to PDR retinopathy was higher in those who were pregnant than those who were not (7.3% vs. 3.7%).[102] Women in this study were similar in age, duration of DM, and DR status at the baseline examination. Pregnancy remained a significant predictor of the progression of DR after controlling for glycosylated hemoglobin. Severe DR is also an indicator for a higher risk of congenital abnormalities in children born of mothers with type 1 diabetes.[104]

Comorbidity

In the WESDR, diabetic people with PDR are shown to be at higher risk for the development of diabetic nephropathy, heart attack, stroke, and amputation than are those with minimal or no DR present.[92] This observation is consistent with the association of severe DR with cardiovascular disease risk factors such as increased fibrinogen, increased platelet aggregation, hyperglycemia, and hypertension.[86,90,91,105,106]

OTHER OCULAR DISEASE ASSOCIATED WITH DIABETES

CATARACTS

Cataracts are an opacification of the normally clear crystalline lens of the eye. Persons with DM tend to develop cataracts at a younger age, and the cataracts develop more rapidly, compared to persons without DM.[107] In both the Health and Nutrition Examination Survey (HANES) and the Framingham Eye Study, diabetic participants younger than 65 had a respective 3.0 and 4.0 increased risk of having a cataract when compared with similarly aged nondiabetic participants. People with DM appear to have differences in the frequency and severity of specific lens opacities. In the Beaver Dam Eye Study, after adjusting for age and sex, cortical opacities and posterior subcapsular cataract were significantly more common among people with older-onset DM than in the rest of the Beaver Dam population.[108] In the younger-onset group in the WESDR, the prevalence of history of cataract surgery and cataracts was significantly related to older age at examination, longer duration of DM, diuretic usage, higher glycosylated hemoglobin concentration, and more severe DR.[109] In the older-onset groups, the prevalence of cataracts was associated with older age, diuretic usage, smoking, and more severe retinopathy. In the UKPDS, intensive glycemic control was associated with a significant reduction in cataract extraction when compared with those with conventional control.[3]

GLAUCOMA

Glaucoma is usually defined by the presence of characteristic visual field loss associated with damage to the retinal nerve fiber layer as a result of intraocular pressure higher than the eye can tolerate. DM has been suggested as increasing the risk of glaucoma.[1] However, neither the Framingham Eye Study nor a study in Dalby, England, found a relationship between DM and glaucoma.[110,111] In the WESDR, a history of glaucoma was more frequent in younger and older diabetic people than in the general population studied in the Health Interview Survey or in nondiabetic participants in the WESDR.[112–114] In the Beaver Dam Eye Study, after controlling for age and sex, DM was associated with an 84% increase in the risk of glaucoma.[113]

VISUAL IMPAIRMENT

In the WESDR, people with DM had a higher age-specific prevalence of visual impairment (best-corrected visual acuity in the better eye of 20/40 or worse) than did the nondiabetic population in the Beaver Dam Eye Study (Fig. 67-7), as well as a higher age-specific prevalence of legal blindness (best-corrected visual acuity in the better eye of 20/200 or worse) than found in the general population in either the Framingham Eye Study or the HANES[115] (Fig. 67-8). For the younger-onset group using insulin, DR was responsible for 86% of the visual loss; for the older-onset group it was responsible for 33% of the visual loss. In the WESDR, the annual incidence of blindness caused by DM was estimated to be 3.3 per 100,000 general population.[116] The 4-year incidence of legal blindness was higher in the older-onset groups (3.2% in those using

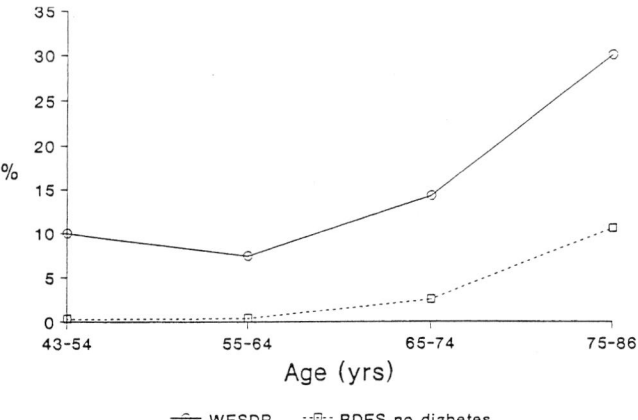

Figure 67-7 Visual impairment (best-corrected visual acuity in the better eye of 20/40 or worse) in those with diabetes participating in the Wisconsin Epidemiologic Study of Diabetic Retinopathy, 1980–1982, and in those without diabetes participating in the Beaver Dam Eye Study, 1988–1990.

insulin and 2.7% in those not using insulin) than in the younger-onset group (1.5%).

DETECTION

Detection of DR is best achieved by ophthalmoscopic examination through a dilated pupil by a retinal specialist or an eye doctor who is an expert in diabetes eye care.[76] Stereoscopic color fundus photography increases the sensitivity of detection of vision-threatening retinopathy relative to ophthalmoscopy and is especially indicated when monitoring patients with signs of NPDR, PDR, or macular edema.[117–119] Fluorescein angiography is generally used by retinal specialists before laser photocoagulation treatment on eyes with clinically significant macular edema to detect areas of retinal ischemia and leaking microaneurysms. Angiograms may occasionally be used to provide further information regarding the amount of ischemia and to demonstrate the cause of unexplained visual loss. However, fluorescein angiography is not routinely necessary at the time of diagnosis of DM or in diabetic patients with no or minimal NPDR.

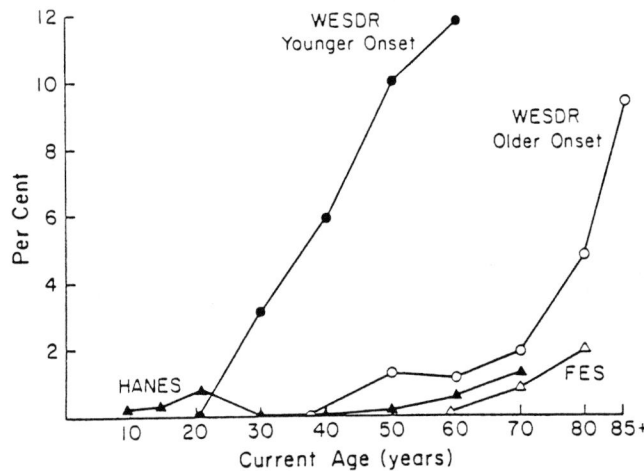

Figure 67-8 Percentage of persons with visual acuity of 20/200 or worse in the better eye in the Wisconsin Epidemiologic Study of Diabetic Retinopathy (WESDR), the Health and Nutrition Examination Survey (HANES), and the Framingham Eye Study (FES) by current age. (From Klein R, Klein BEK, Moss SE: Visual impairment in diabetes. Ophthalmology 91:1–9, 1984.)

In the WESDR from 1980 to 1982, 33% of people with either PDR with a high risk of severe visual loss or clinically significant macular edema had not seen an ophthalmologist within 2 years of the examination.[120] In addition, 51% of people with PDR had not been treated with panretinal photocoagulation.[121] Based on these data, the authors estimated that 35,000 Americans with vision-threatening DR who might benefit from photocoagulation treatment had not received such treatment from 1980 to 1982. Little change was found when the group was reexamined,[122] and similar findings have also been reported by others.[123–125] Many possible reasons have been proposed to explain the high rate of patients with serious DR who do not receive appropriate eye care.[20,123,126–133] While guidelines for the detection and management of diabetic eye disease have been developed and distributed,[76] studies have suggested that these referral guidelines for DR are not being sufficiently followed.[7,124,125,131] Cost-effectiveness studies using the WESDR and other data suggest that earlier detection of PDR by ophthalmologic or photographic screening is a cost-effective approach for diabetic people requiring insulin.[134–137]

MANAGEMENT

MEDICAL

As discussed above, the DCCT and UKPDS studies have demonstrated that it is important to manage glycemic and hypertension control carefully for optimum care of patients with DM. However, intensive glycemic control is often difficult or impossible to achieve in certain patients. Strict glycemic control is also associated with an increased frequency of severe complications.[2] Currently, new interventions (e.g., protein kinase C inhibitors, VEGF inhibitors, vitamin E) to prevent the progression of DR are being studied.

OPHTHALMOLOGIC

Four nationwide multi-center randomized clinical trials have largely determined the appropriate strategies for clinical management of patients with DR. The Diabetic Retinopathy Study (DRS) conclusively demonstrated that PRP significantly reduces the risk of severe visual loss (SVL) from PDR, particularly when high-risk PDR was present.[5,138,139] The ETDRS provided valuable information concerning the timing of PRP for advancing diabetic retinopathy and conclusively demonstrated that focal photocoagulation for CSME reduces the risk of moderate visual loss by 50% or more.[6,22,140] Furthermore, the ETDRS demonstrated that both early PRP and deferral of PRP "until and as soon as high-risk PDR developed are effective in reducing the risk of SVL." PRP, therefore, should be considered as an eye approaches the high-risk stage and "usually should not be delayed if the eye has reached the high-risk proliferative stage."[122] Detailed analysis of the ETDRS data shows that early PRP is beneficial for patients with type 2 DM.[24,141,142] When therapy is initiated at the first sign of appropriate severity of DR, benefits may include a reduction of more than 90% in severe visual loss.[24,142]

SURGICAL

Vitrectomy surgery has been effective in reducing vision loss when traction retinal detachment threatens the center of the macula or vitreous hemorrhage fails to clear. The use of laser delivered from within the eye at the time of surgery and other advanced surgical techniques make vitrectomy a valuable procedure to prevent vision loss and restore vision.

Neovascular glaucoma, in which retinal ischemia leads to neovascularization of the anterior chamber angle of the eye, is a severe and difficult to treat complication resulting from advanced DR. Aggressive PRP is usually the preferred initial treatment, but other procedures such as goniophotocoagulation of neovascularization in the filtration angle, filtration surgery, vitrectomy surgery, or combinations of these procedures may be necessary. Such eyes are at high risk of severe vision loss.

REHABILITATION

Diabetic patients with severe visual impairment are confronted with difficulties in glucose monitoring, insulin administration, and monitoring of systemic changes in the skin such as foot ulcers. In addition, these patients are often ill with renal disease, cardiovascular disease, or amputations. Many have lost their jobs and health insurance and are without adequate financial support. These problems may lead to anger, anxiety, loss of self-esteem, and difficulties in social adjustment.[143,144] Primary care physicians should be actively involved in a team including psychologists, orientation and mobility instructors, rehabilitation teachers, and social workers to deal with the problems faced by visually impaired diabetic patients. Such support facilitates the patient's acceptance of visual loss, development of coping strategies, and planning of living arrangements.

NOVEL THERAPIES

Numerous novel therapies are in various stages of development and testing. Many of these focus on inhibiting the growth factors, such as VEGF, thought to underlie the development of macular edema and retinal neovascularization. Examples of this approach include Macugen (a VEGF inhibitor) and triamcinolone acetonide (a steroid that, among its several actions, may inhibit VEGF). These compounds are injected within the eye on a repetitive basis and have preliminary clinical data to suggest beneficial activity. Other compounds attempt to correct the biochemical alterations induced by DM. These approaches include use of protein kinase C inhibitors, Celebrex, insulin-like growth factor 1 inhibitors (somatostatin) and vitamin E. These approaches have also demonstrated potential benefit in selected DM patients during early clinical trials. Numerous other treatments including integrin antagonists, vitreolysis, metalloproteinases, and so on are in various stages of evaluation.

To identify the most promising new therapies and to bring them to evaluation in as rigorous and timely a manner as possible, the National Institutes of Health's National Eye Institute has sponsored a cooperative agreement initiating the Diabetic Retinopathy Clinical Research Network (*www.DRCR.net*). This nationwide network includes over 100 centers and is dedicated to multicenter clinical research of diabetic retinopathy, macular edema, and associated disorders. It has numerous multi-center clinical trial initiatives under way covering a full spectrum of approaches to this disorder. The results of these and other ongoing randomized multi-center clinical trials will be required before it is possible to determine the side effect profile, the population most amenable to treatment, and the effectiveness of any of these approaches.

1314 Diabetes Mellitus

REFERENCES

1. Klein R, Klein BEK: Vision disorders in diabetes. In Harris MWH (ed): Diabetes in America, ed 2. Bethesda, MD, US Public Health Service, NIH-NIDDK Publication No. 95-1468, 1995, pp 293–338.
2. The Diabetes Control and Complications Trial Research Group: The effect of intensive treatment of diabetes on the development and progression of long-term complications in insulin-dependent diabetes mellitus. N Engl J Med 329:977–986, 1993.
3. UK Prospective Diabetes Study Group: Intensive blood glucose control with sulphonylurea or insulin compared with conventional treatment and risk of complications in patients with type 2 diabetes. UKPDS 33. Lancet 352:837–853, 1998.
4. UK Prospective Diabetes Study Group: Tight blood pressure control and risk of macrovascular and microvascular complications in type 2 diabetes. UKPDS 38. Br Med J 317:703–713, 1998.
5. The Diabetic Retinopathy Study Research Group: Photocoagulation treatment of proliferative diabetic retinopathy: Clinical application of Diabetic Retinopathy Study (DRS) findings: DRS Report No. 8. Ophthalmology 88:583–600, 1981.
6. ETDRS Research Group: Photocoagulation for diabetic macular edema. Arch Ophthalmol 103:1796–1806, 1985.
7. Witkin SR, Klein R: Ophthalmologic care for persons with diabetes. JAMA 251:2534–2537, 1984.
8. Klein R, Moss SE, Klein BEK: New management concepts for the timely diagnosis of diabetic retinopathy treatable by photocoagulation. Diabetes Care 10:633–638, 1987.
9. National Eye Institute National Eye Health Education Program: From Vision Research to Eye Health Education: Planning the Partnership. March, 1990. Available from NIH, Box 20/20, Bethesda, MD 20892.
10. Smith RE, Patz A: Diabetes 2000—closing the gap (editorial). Ophthalmology 97:153–154, 1990.
11. Herman WH, Teutsch SM, Sepe SJ, et al: An approach to the prevention of blindness in diabetes. Diabetes Care 6:608–613, 1983.
12. Klein R, Klein BEK: Diabetic eye disease. Lancet 350:197–204, 1997.
13. Bresnick GH: Diabetic Retinopathy. In Peyman GA, Sanders DR, Goldberg MF (eds): Principles and Practice of Ophthalmology. Philadelphia, WB Saunders, 1977.
14. Klein R, Klein BEK, Moss SE, et al: Prevalence of diabetes mellitus in southern Wisconsin. Am J Epidemiol 119:54–61, 1984.
15. Klein R, Klein BEK, Moss SE, et al: The Wisconsin Epidemiologic Study of Diabetic Retinopathy: II. Prevalence and risk of diabetic retinopathy when age at

diagnosis is less than 30 years. Arch Ophthalmol 102:520–526, 1984.
16. Klein R, Klein BEK, Moss SE, et al: The Wisconsin Epidemiologic Study of Diabetic Retinopathy: III. Prevalence and risk of diabetic retinopathy when age at diagnosis is 30 or more years. Arch Ophthalmol 102:527–532, 1984.
17. Gass JDM: Stereoscopic Atlas of Macular Diseases, ed 3. St Louis, Mosby, 1987.
18. Klein R, Meuer SM, Moss SE, et al: The relationship of retinal microaneurysm counts to the 4-year progression of diabetic retinopathy. Arch Ophthalmol 107:1780–1785, 1989.
19. Dobree JH: Simple diabetic retinopathy: Evolution of the lesions and therapeutic considerations. Br J Ophthalmol 54:1–10, 1970.
20. Sussman EJ, Tsiaras WG, Soper KA: Diagnosis of diabetic eye disease. JAMA 247:3231–3234, 1982.
21. The Diabetic Retinopathy Study Research Group: Four risk factors for severe visual loss in diabetic retinopathy. The third report from the Diabetic Retinopathy Study. Arch Ophthalmol 97(4):654–655, 1979.
22. Early Treatment Diabetic Retinopathy Study Research Group: Early photocoagulation for diabetic retinopathy. ETDRS Report Number 9. Ophthalmology 98(Suppl 5):766–785, 1991.
23. Early Treatment Diabetic Retinopathy Study Research Group: Grading diabetic retinopathy rrom stereoscopic color fundus photographs—An extension of the Modified Airlie House Classification. ETDRS Report Number 10. Ophthalmology 98(Suppl 5):786–806, 1991.
24. Ferris F: Early photocoagulation in patients with either type I or type II diabetes. Trans Am Ophthalmol Soc 94:505–537, 1996.
25. Wilkinson CP, Ferris FL III, Klein RE, et al: Proposed international clinical diabetic retinopathy and diabetic macular edema disease severity scales. Ophthalmology 110(9):1677–1682, 2003.
26. Klein R, Klein BEK, Moss SE, et al: The Wisconsin Epidemiologic Study of Diabetic Retinopathy: IX. Four-year incidence and progression of diabetic retinopathy when age at diagnosis is less than 30 years. Arch Ophthalmol 107:237–243, 1989.
27. Klein R, Klein BEK, Moss SE, et al: The Wisconsin Epidemiologic Study of Diabetic Retinopathy: X. Four-year incidence and progression of diabetic retinopathy when age at diagnosis is 30 years or more. Arch Ophthalmol 107:244–249, 1989.
28. Haffner SM, Fong D, Stern MP, et al: Diabetic retinopathy in Mexican-Americans and non-Hispanic whites. Diabetes 37:878–884, 1988.
29. Hamman RF, Mayer EJ, Moo-Young GA, et al: Prevalence and risk factors of

diabetic retinopathy in non-Hispanic whites and Hispanics with NIDDM: San Luis Valley Diabetes Study. Diabetes 38:1231–1237, 1989.
30. Nielsen NV: Diabetic retinopathy: II. The course of retinopathy in diabetics treated with oral hypoglycaemic agents and diet regime alone: A one year epidemiologic cohort study of diabetes mellitus: The Island of Falster, Denmark. Acta Ophthalmol 62:266–273, 1984.
31. Dorf A, Ballintine EJ, Bennett PH, et al: Retinopathy in Pima Indians: Relationships to glucose level, duration of diabetes, age at diagnosis of diabetes, and age at examination in a population with a high prevalence of diabetes mellitus. Diabetes 25:554–560, 1976.
32. Bennett PH, Rushforth NB, Miller M, et al: Epidemiologic studies of diabetes in the Pima Indians. Recent Prog Horm Res 32:333–376, 1976.
33. Kahn HA, Leibowitz HM, Ganley JP, et al: The Framingham Eye Study: I. Outline and major prevalence findings. Am J Epidemiol 106:17–32, 1977.
34. West KM, Erdreich LJ, Stober JA: A detailed study of risk factors for retinopathy and nephropathy in diabetes. Diabetes 19:501–508, 1980.
35. Houston A: Retinopathy in the Poole area: An epidemiologic inquiry. In Eschwege E (ed): Advances in Diabetes Epidemiology. INSERM Symposium No. 22. Amsterdam, Elsevier, 1982, pp 199–206.
36. King H, Balkau B, Zimmet P, et al: Diabetic retinopathy in Nauruans. Am J Epidemiol 117:659–667, 1983.
37. Dwyer MS, Melton LJ, Ballard DJ, et al: Incidence of diabetic retinopathy and blindness: A population-based study in Rochester, Minnesota. Diabetes Care 8:316–322, 1985.
38. Ballard DJ, Melton LJ, Dwyer MS, et al: Risk factors for diabetic retinopathy: A population-based study in Rochester, Minnesota. Diabetes Care 9:334–342, 1986.
39. Danielsen R, Jonasson F, Helgason T: Prevalence of retinopathy and proteinuria in type I diabetics in Iceland. Acta Med Scand 212:277–280, 1982.
40. Constable IJ, Knuiman MW, Welborn TA, et al: Assessing the risk of diabetic retinopathy. Am J Ophthalmol 97:53–61, 1984.
41. Knuiman MW, Welborn TA, McCann VJ, et al: Prevalence of diabetic complications in relation to risk factors. Diabetes 35:1332–1339, 1986.
42. Sjolie AK: Ocular complications in insulin treated diabetes mellitus: An epidemiological study. Acta Ophthalmol Suppl 172:1–72, 1985.
43. Nielsen NV: Diabetic retinopathy: I. The course of retinopathy in insulin-treated diabetics: A one-year epidemiological cohort study of diabetes mellitus: The

island of Falster, Denmark. Acta Ophthalmol 62:256–265, 1984.

44. Teuscher A, Schnell H, Wilson PWF: Incidence of diabetic retinopathy and relationship to baseline plasma glucose and blood pressure. Diabetes Care 11:246–251, 1988.

45. Jerneld B: Prevalence of diabetic retinopathy. Acta Ophthalmol Scand Suppl 188:3–32, 1988.

46. McLeod BK, Thompson JR, Rosenthal AR: The prevalence of retinopathy in the insulin-requiring diabetic patients of an English county town. Eye 2:424–430, 1988.

47. Kostraba JN, Klein R, Dorman JS, et al: The Epidemiology of Diabetes Complications Study: IV. Correlates of diabetic background and proliferative retinopathy. Am J Epidemiol 133:381–391, 1991.

48. Fujimoto W, Fukuda M: Natural history of diabetic retinopathy and its treatment in Japan. In Baba S, Goto Y, Fukui I (eds): Diabetes Mellitus in Asia. Amsterdam, Excerpta Medica, 1976, pp 225–231.

49. Nelson RG, Wolfe JA, Horton MB, et al: Proliferative retinopathy in NIDDM: Incidence and risk factors in Pima Indians. Diabetes 38:435–440, 1989.

50. Harris MI, Klein R, Cowie CC, et al: Is the risk of diabetic retinopathy greater in non Hispanic blacks and Mexican Americans than in non-Hispanic whites with type 2 diabetes? A U.S. population study. Diabetes Care 21:1230–1235, 1998.

51. Eye Diseases Prevalence Research Group: The prevalence of diabetic retinopathy among adults in the United States. Arch Ophthalmol 122:552–563, 2004.

52. West SK, Klein R, Rodriguez J, et al: Diabetes and diabetic retinopathy in a Mexican-American population: Proyecto VER. Diabetes Care 24:1204–1209, 2001.

53. Varma R, Torres M, Pena F, et al: Prevalence of diabetic retinopathy in adult Latinos: The Los Angeles Latino Eye Study. Ophthalmology 111:1298–1306, 2004.

54. Rabb MF, Gagliano DA, Sweeny NE: Diabetic retinopathy in blacks. Diabetes Care 13:1202–1206, 1990.

55. Barbosa J, Ramsay RC, Knobloch WH, et al: Histocompatibility antigen frequencies in diabetic retinopathy. Am J Ophthalmol 90:148–153, 1980.

56. Dornan TL, Ting A, McPherson CK, et al: Genetic susceptibility to the development of retinopathy in insulin-dependent diabetics. Diabetes 31:226–231, 1982.

57. Rand LI, Krolewski AS, Aiello LM, et al: Multiple factors in the prediction of risk of proliferative diabetic retinopathy. N Engl J Med 113:1433–1438, 1985.

58. Jervell J, Solheim B: HLA-antigens in long standing insulin dependent diabetics with terminal nephropathy and retinopathy with and without loss of vision. Diabetologia 17:391, 1979.

59. Leslie RDG, Pyke DA: Diabetic retinopathy in identical twins. Diabetes 31:19–21, 1982.

60. Hanis CL: Genetics of non-insulin-dependent diabetes mellitus among Mexican Americans: Approaches and perspectives. In Berg K, Boulyjenkov V, Christen Y (eds): Genetic Approaches to Noncommunicable Diseases. Berlin, Springer-Verlag, 1996, pp 65–77.

61. Knowles HC Jr, Guest GM, Lampe J, et al: The course of juvenile diabetes treated with unmeasured diet. Diabetes 14:239–273, 1965.

62. Frank RN, Hoffman WH, Podgor MJ, et al: Retinopathy in juvenile-onset type I diabetes of short duration. Diabetes 31:874–882, 1982.

63. Palmberg P, Smith M, Waltman S, et al: The natural history of retinopathy in insulin-dependent juvenile-onset diabetes. Ophthalmology 88:613–618, 1981.

64. Klein R, Klein BEK, Moss SE, et al: Retinopathy in young-onset diabetic patients. Diabetes Care 8:311–315, 1985.

65. Klein BEK, Moss SE, Klein R: Is menarche associated with diabetic retinopathy. Diabetes Care 13:1034–1038, 1990.

66. Peters GFFM, Smals AGH, Kloppenborg PWC: Defective suppression of growth hormone after glucose loading in adolescence. J Clin Endocrinol Metab 51:265–270, 1980.

67. Klein R, Klein BEK, Moss SE, et al: Blood pressure and hypertension in diabetes. Am J Epidemiol 122:75–89, 1985.

68. Blethen SL, Sargeant DT, Whitlow MG, et al: Effect of pubertal stage and recent blood glucose control on plasma somatomedin C in children with insulin-dependent diabetes mellitus. Diabetes 30:868–872, 1981.

69. Allen C, Zaccaro DJ, Palta M, et al: Glycemic control in the first two years of insulin dependent diabetes mellitus. Diabetes Care 15:980–987, 1992.

70. Sizonenko P: Endocrinology in preadolescents and adolescents: I. Hormonal changes during normal puberty. Am J Dis Child 132:704–712, 1978.

71. Haffner SM, Klein R, Dunn JF, et al: Increased testosterone in type I diabetic subjects with severe retinopathy. Ophthalmology 97:1270–1274, 1990.

72. Aiello LP, Cahill MT, Wong JS: Systemic considerations in the management of diabetic retinopathy. Am J Ophthalmol 132:760–766, 2001.

73. Klein R, Klein BEK, Moss SE, et al: The Beaver Dam Eye Study: Retinopathy in adults with newly discovered and previously diagnosed diabetes mellitus. Ophthalmology 99:58–62, 1992.

74. UK Prospective Diabetes Study 6: Complications in newly diagnosed type 2 diabetic patients and their association with different clinical and biochemical risk factors. Diabetes Res 13:1–11, 1990.

75. The Kentucky Diabetic Retinopathy Group: Guidelines for eye care in patients with diabetes mellitus. Arch Intern Med 149:769–770, 1989.

76. American Diabetes Association: Diabetic retinopathy. Diabetes Care 21:157–159, 1988.

77. Klein R, Klein BEK, Moss SE, et al: Glycosylated hemoglobin predicts the incidence and progression of diabetic retinopathy. JAMA 260:2864–2871, 1988.

78. Klein R, Klein BEK, Moss SE, et al: Relationship of hyperglycemia to the long-term incidence and progression of diabetic retinopathy. Arch Intern Med 154:2169–2178, 1994.

79. Chase HP, Jackson WE, Hoops SL, et al: Glucose control and the renal and retinal complications of insulin-dependent diabetes. JAMA 261:1155–1160, 1989.

80. Davis MD: Diabetic retinopathy, diabetic control and blood pressure. Transplant Proc 18:1565–1568, 1986.

81. Kohner EM: Diabetic retinopathy. Br Med Bull 45:148–173, 1989.

82. Knowler WC, Bennett PH, Ballintine EJ: Increased incidence of retinopathy in diabetics with elevated blood pressure: A six-year follow-up study in Pima Indians. N Engl J Med 302:645–650, 1980.

83. Kohner EM, Fraser TR, Joplin GF, et al: The effect of diabetic control on diabetic retinopathy. In Goldberg MF, Fine SL (eds): Treatment of Diabetic Retinopathy. Washington, DC, US Public Health Service Publication No. 1890, 1969, pp 119–128.

84. Klein R, Klein BEK, Moss SE, et al: Is blood pressure a predictor of the incidence or progression of diabetic retinopathy? Arch Intern Med 149:2427–2432, 1989.

85. Klein R, Klein BEK, Moss SE, et al: The Wisconsin Epidemiologic Study of Diabetic Retinopathy. XVII. The 14-year incidence and progression of diabetic retinopathy and associated risk factors in type 1 diabetes. Ophthalmology 105:1801–1815, 1998.

86. Klein BEK, Moss SE, Klein R, et al: The Wisconsin Epidemiologic Study of Diabetic Retinopathy: XIII. Relationship of serum cholesterol to retinopathy and hard exudate. Ophthalmology 98:1261–1265, 1991.

87. Chew EY, Klein ML, Ferris FL 3rd, et al: Association of elevated serum lipid levels with retinal hard exudate in diabetic retinopathy. Early Treatment Diabetic Retinopathy Study (ETDRS) Report 22. Arch Ophthalmol 114:1079–1084, 1996.

88. Cullen JF, Ireland JT, Oliver MF: A controlled trial of atromid therapy in exudative diabetic retinopathy. Trans Soc Ophthalmol U K 84:281–355, 1964.

89. Duncan LJ, Cullen JF, Ireland JT, et al: A three-year trial of atromid therapy in exudative diabetic retinopathy. Diabetes 17:458–467, 1968.

90. Borch-Johnsen K, Kreiner S: Proteinuria: Value as a predictor of cardiovascular mortality in insulin dependent diabetes mellitus. Br Med J 294:1651–1654, 1987.

91. Winocour PH, Durrington PN, Ishola M, et al: Influence of proteinuria on vascular disease, blood pressure, and lipoproteins in insulin dependent diabetes mellitus. Br Med J 294:1648–1651, 1987.

92. Klein R, Klein BEK, Moss SE: The epidemiology of proliferative diabetic retinopathy. Diabetes Care 15:1875–1891, 1992.

93. Klein R, Klein BEK, Davis MD: Is cigarette smoking associated with diabetic retinopathy? Am J Epidemiol 118:228–238, 1983.

94. Moss SE, Klein R, Klein BEK: Association of cigarette smoking with diabetic retinopathy. Diabetes Care 14:119–126, 1991.

95. The Health Consequences of Smoking. A Report to the Surgeon General. Washington, DC, US Department of Health, Education and Welfare. Publication HSM 71-7513, 1971.

96. Doyle JT: Risk factors in arteriosclerosis and cardiovascular disease with special emphasis on cigarette smoking. Prev Med 8:264–270, 1979.

97. Kingsley LA, Dorman JS, Doft BH, et al: An epidemiologic approach to the study of retinopathy: The Pittsburgh Diabetic Morbidity and Retinopathy Studies. Diabetes Res Clin Pract 4:99–109, 1988.

98. Young RJ, McCulloch DK, Prescott RJ, et al: Alcohol: Another risk factor for diabetic retinopathy? Br Med J 288:1035–1037, 1984.

99. Moss SE, Klein R, Klein BEK: Alcohol consumption and the prevalence of diabetic retinopathy. Ophthalmology 99:926–932, 1992.

100. Jakubowski JA, Vaillancourt R, Deykin D: Interaction of ethanol, prostacyclin, and aspirin in determining human platelet activity in vitro. Arteriosclerosis 8:436–441, 1988.

101. Moss SE, Klein R, Klein BEK: The association of alcohol consumption with the incidence and progression of diabetic retinopathy. Ophthalmology 101:1962–1968, 1994.

102. Klein BEK, Moss SE, Klein R: Effect of pregnancy on progression of diabetic retinopathy. Diabetes Care 13:34–40, 1990.

103. Rodman HM, Singerman LJ, Aiello LM, et al: Diabetic retinopathy and its relationship to pregnancy. In Merkatz ER, Adams PAJ (eds): The Diabetic Pregnancy: A Perinatal Perspective. New York, Grune & Stratton, 1979.

104. Klein BEK, Klein R, Meuer SM, et al: Does the severity of diabetic retinopathy predict pregnancy outcome? J Diabetes Complications 2:179–184, 1988.

105. Dornan TL, Carter RD, Bron AJ, et al: Low density lipoprotein cholesterol: An association with the severity of diabetic retinopathy. Diabetologia 22:167–170, 1982.

106. Miccoli R, Odello G, Giampietro O, et al: Circulating lipid levels and severity of diabetic retinopathy in type I diabetes mellitus. Ophthalmic Res 19:52–56, 1987.

107. Ederer F, Hiller R, Taylor H: Senile lens changes and diabetes in two population studies. Am J Ophthalmol 91:381–395, 1981.

108. Klein BEK, Klein R, Wang Q, et al: Older-onset diabetes and lens opacities. The Beaver Dam Eye Study. Ophthalmic Epidemiol 2:49–55, 1995.

109. Klein BEK, Klein R, Moss SE: Prevalence of cataracts in a population-based study of persons with diabetes mellitus. Ophthalmology 92:1191–1196, 1985.

110. Kahn HA, Leibowitz HM, Ganley JP, et al: The Framingham Eye Study: II. Association of ophthalmic pathology with single variables previously measured in the Framingham Heart Study. Am J Epidemiol 106:33–41, 1977.

111. Bengtsson B: Aspects of the epidemiology of chronic glaucoma. Acta Ophthalmol Suppl 146:4–26, 1981.

112. Klein BEK, Klein R, Moss SE: Intraocular pressure in diabetic persons. Ophthalmology 91:1356–1360, 1984.

113. Klein BEK, Klein R, Jensen SC: Open angle glaucoma and older onset diabetes. The Beaver Dam Eye Study. Ophthalmology 101:1173–1177, 1994.

114. Howie LJ, Drury IF: Current estimates from the Health Interview Survey, 1988. Vital Health Stat 126(10):1–98, 1988.

115. Klein R, Klein BEK, Moss SE: Visual impairment in diabetes. Ophthalmology 91:1–9, 1984.

116. Moss SE, Klein R, Klein BEK: The incidence of vision loss in a diabetic population. Ophthalmology 95:1340–1348, 1988.

117. Pugh JA, Jacobsen JM, Van Heuven WAJ, et al: Screening for diabetic retinopathy: The wide angle retina camera. Diabetes Care 16:889–895, 1993.

118. Nathan DM, Fogel HA, Godine JE, et al: Role of the diabetologist in evaluating diabetic retinopathy. Diabetes Care 14:26–33, 1991.

119. Klein R, Klein BEK, Neider MW, et al: Diabetic retinopathy as detected using ophthalmoscopy, a nonmydriatic camera and a standard fundus camera. Ophthalmology 92:485–491, 1985.

120. Klein R, Klein BEK, Moss SE: The Wisconsin Epidemiological Study of Diabetic Retinopathy: A review. Diabetes Metab Rev 5:559–570, 1989.

121. Klein R, Klein BEK, Moss SE, et al: The Wisconsin Epidemiologic Study of Diabetic Retinopathy: VI. Retinal photocoagulation. Ophthalmology 94:747–753, 1987.

122. Klein R, Moss SE, Klein BEK, et al: The Wisconsin Epidemiologic Study of Diabetic Retinopathy: VIII: The incidence of retinal photocoagulation. J Diabetes Complications 2:79–87, 1988.

123. Stross JK, Harlan WR: The dissemination of new medical information. JAMA 741:2622–2624, 1979.

124. Sprafka JM, Fritsche TL, Baker R, et al: Prevalence of undiagnosed eye disease in high-risk diabetic individuals. Arch Intern Med 150:857–861, 1990.

125. Brechner RJ, Cowie CC, Howie LJ, et al: Ophthalmic examination among adults with diagnosed diabetes mellitus. JAMA 270:1714–1718, 1993.

126. Herman WH: Public health strategies: Program development, implementation and evaluation. In Proceedings of the 8th Annual Centers for Disease Control Conference. Atlanta, GA, 1985.

127. Payne TH, Gabella BA, Michael SL, et al: Preventive care in diabetes mellitus: Current practice in urban health-care system. Diabetes Care 12:745–747, 1989.

128. Newcomb PA, Klein R: Factors associated with compliance following diabetic eye screening. J Diabetes Complications 4:8–14, 1990.

129. Moss SE, Klein R, Klein BEK: Factors associated with having eye examinations in persons with diabetes. Arch Fam Med 4:529–534, 1995.

130. Klein R, Klein BEK, Moss SE, et al: The validity of a survey question to study diabetic retinopathy. Am J Epidemiol 124:104–110, 1986.

131. Hess RG, Lengyel MC, Hess GE, et al: Diabetes in Communities. Ann Arbor, University of Michigan, 1986.

132. Marnell NM: A Descriptive Analysis of Health Practices and Beliefs Related to Eye Diseases: Diabetic Retinopathy Health Care Delivery Screening Compliance Review (master's thesis). Atlanta, University of Georgia, 1988, pp 1–97.

133. Frey M, Teza S, Bowbeer L, et al: Geographic distance: A factor in early retinopathy detection (abstract). Diabetes 36(Suppl 1):49, 1987.

134. Centers for Disease Control: Improving eye care for persons with diabetes mellitus-Michigan. Morb Mortal Wkly Rep 34:697–699, 1985.

135. Javitt JC, Canner JK, Sommer A: Cost-effectiveness of current approaches to the control of retinopathy in type I diabetics. Ophthalmology 96:253–262, 1989.

136. Javitt JC, Canner JK, Frank RG, et al: Detecting and treating retinopathy in type I diabetics: A health policy model. Ophthalmology 97:483–495, 1990.

137. Dasbach E, Fryback DG, Newcomb PA, et al: Cost-effectiveness of strategies for detecting diabetic retinopathy. Med Care 29:20–39, 1991.

138. The Diabetic Retinopathy Study Research Group: Preliminary Report on Effects of Photocoagulation Therapy. Am J Ophthalmol 81(4):383–396, 1976.

139. Photocoagulation treatment of proliferative diabetic retinopathy: The second report of diabetic retinopathy study findings. Ophthalmology 85(1):82–106, 1978.

140. The Early Treatment Diabetic Retinopathy Study Research Group. Photocoagulation for Diabetic Macular Edema: Early treatment diabetic

retinopathy study report no. 4. Int Ophthalmol Clin 27(4):265–272, 1987.

141. Ferris FL III, Davis MD, Aiello LM: Treatment of diabetic retinopathy. N Engl J Med 341(9):667–678, 1999.

142. Early Treatment Diabetic Retinopathy Study Research Group: Early photocoagulation for diabetic retinopathy: ETDRS report no. 9. Ophthalmology 98:766–785, 1991.

143. Stribe M, Haire-Joshu D, Yost J: Psychological adjustment in insulin-dependent diabetes mellitus: The relationship of coping style and diabetes knowledge (abstract). Diabetes 37(Suppl):20, 1988.

144. Sinzato R, Fukikno O, Tamai H, et al: Coping behaviors of severe diabetes. Psychother Psychosom 43:219–226, 1985.

Diabetes Mellitus: Neuropathy

Andrew J. M. Boulton and Rayaz A. Malik

"The era of coma has given way to the era of complications."
—Elliot P. Joslin

Of all the long-term complications of diabetes, none affects so many organs or systems of the human body as the group of conditions that are included under the term *diabetic neuropathies*. The frequency with which diabetes affects the nervous system and the diverse manifestations might well explain the earlier view that diabetes was a consequence rather than a cause of nerve dysfunction. Peripheral neuropathies have been described in patients with primary (type 1 and type 2) and secondary diabetes of differing causes, suggesting a common etiologic mechanism based on chronic hyperglycemia. The pivotal role of hyperglycemia in the pathogenesis of neuropathy has received strong support from landmark studies such as the Diabetes Control and Complications Trial (DCCT),[1,2] the United Kingdom Prospective Diabetes Study (UKPDS),[3] and other prospective studies.[4] Neuropathies are characterized by a progressive loss of nerve fibers that can be assessed noninvasively by a variety of methods, varying from a structured neurologic examination through quantitative sensory testing to detailed electrophysiology (EP) and autonomic function testing.[5] Although there are no major structural differences in nerve pathology between the two main types of diabetes, clinical differences do exist: Whereas the rare symptomatic autonomic syndromes usually occur in long-duration type 1 patients, the mononeuropathies and proximal motor neuropathy usually occur in older type 2 patients.[6]

The epidemiology and natural history of the neuropathies remain poorly defined, partly because of variable diagnostic criteria and the ill-defined patient population studied. However, the late sequelae of neuropathy are well recognized, with foot problems including ulceration[7] and Charcot's neuroarthropathy[8] representing the most common cause of

hospitalization among diabetic patients in Western countries. Of all the component causes that, when combined, result in ulceration, neuropathy is by far the most common.[9] Not surprisingly, diabetic neuropathy often has an adverse effect on quality of life.[10,11]

In this chapter, the history, classification, epidemiology, and clinical features of the neuropathies are discussed, followed by a description of measurement techniques and a review of the pathogenesis. Finally, current treatments are reviewed, and the late sequelae and their prevention are discussed.

HISTORY

Although many people attribute the first clinical description of diabetic peripheral neuropathy to Rollo at the end of the eighteenth century, it was Marchall de Calvi in France who recognized the true nature of the condition in 1864.[12] Later, Charcot extended these observations as well as describing (initially in syphilis) the neuroarthropathy that is now named after him.[13] Davies-Pryce, a surgeon working in Nottingham, England, was the first to recognize the link between diabetic neuropathy and foot ulceration.[14] It was not until the twentieth century, however, that autonomic neuropathy in diabetes was first reported.[15]

DEFINITIONS AND CLASSIFICATION

Although there have been previous classifications based on pathologic and etiologic considerations, it has become increasingly clear that, as is discussed below, causative mechanisms resulting in neuropathy are multiple and complex, so a clinical or descriptive classification of the neuropathies is favored.[5,16] Even in this area, a number of classifications exist. Examples include the purely clinical descriptive classification proposed by Boulton and Ward[17] (Table 68-1) and that based on potential reversibility together with clinical description[16,18] (Table 68-2).

A simple definition as to what constitutes diabetic neuropathy was agreed on at an international consensus meeting on clinical diagnosis and management: "The presence of symptoms and/or signs of peripheral nerve dysfunction in people with diabetes after the exclusion of other causes."[19] The exclusion of other causes is particularly important as was emphasized by the baseline data from the Rochester Diabetic Neuropathy Study, in which 5% of patients had a nondiabetic cause for their neuropathy.[20]

For research, epidemiologic, and clinical trial purposes, a more detailed definition that includes subclinical neuropathy is required.[21,22] The San Antonio consensus defined diabetic neuropathy as "a demonstrable disorder either clinically evident or subclinical, occurring in the setting of diabetes without nondiabetic causes, including manifestations in the somatic and/or autonomic parts of the peripheral nervous system."[23] The Rochester Diabetic Neuropathy Study established a paradigm for clinical trial design.[20,21] The following were assessed: (1) neuropathic symptoms (neuropathy symptom score, NSS), (2) neuropathic deficits (neuropathy impairment score), (3) sensorimotor nerve conduction velocity, (4) quantitative sensory tests, and (5) autonomic function tests. The minimum criteria for a diagnosis of neuropathy required two or more abnormalities among the listed criteria, at least one being 3 or 5. Staging was as follows: N0 = no neuropathy, minimum criteria unfulfilled; N1 = asymptomatic neuropathy (NSS = 0); N2 = symptomatic neuropathy; N3 = disabling neuropathy.

EPIDEMIOLOGY

The quality and even quantity of epidemiologic data on diabetic neuropathy remain poor for a number of reasons, including inconsistent definitions, poor ascertainment, lack of population-based studies, and failure to exclude nondiabetic neurologic disease.[20,21,24] Most studies report on either chronic sensorimotor or autonomic neuropathies,[25] so this section focuses on these two types. However, despite these problems, there is no doubt that diabetic neuropathy is very common, possibly the most common of the late complications of diabetes.

The larger reports of the prevalence of chronic sensorimotor neuropathy published in recent years are summarized in Table 68-3. Of three clinic-based studies from Europe (enrolling more than 2000 patients), there was a remarkable similarity in the prevalence, which varied from 22.5% to 28.5% for symptomatic neuropathy.[26–28] Most studies include patients with both type 1 and type 2 diabetes; it must be remembered that neuropathy may be present at diagnosis

in type 2 diabetes, as was demonstrated by the Finnish prospective study[4] and the UKPDS,[3] both of which reported a prevalence at diagnosis between 5% and 11%.

The population-based studies of the prevalence of neuropathy are necessarily smaller than the clinic-based ones, and most sample less than 50% of the total available population; however, these showed an even higher prevalence, suggesting that at least half of older, type 2 diabetic patients had significant neuropathic deficits and must therefore be considered as being at high risk for insensitive foot ulceration.[29] As only a minority of patients in the population-based studies were symptomatic, the majority of cases of neuropathy would be missed if a careful clinical neurologic examination were not performed. The largest study, a community-based survey from the northwestern United Kingdom, reported the prevalence of a moderate or severe neuropathic deficit to be 22.4% of 9710 diabetic patients.[30]

Certain prospective studies have assessed risk factors for the development of neuropathy. The DCCT[2] and UKPDS[3] demonstrated a clear relationship between poor glycemic control and the development of neuropathy. In addition to glycemic control, Adler and coworkers[31] identified height, age, and alcohol intake as significant risk factors for neuropathy in a study of U.S. veterans. Other studies have identified ischemic heart disease, smoking, and diabetes duration as being independently related to neuropathy.[25]

Autonomic neuropathy has been the subject of fewer epidemiologic investigations, and the results are less consistent than those for somatic dysfunction. In the Eurodiab insulin-dependent diabetes mellitus (IDDM) study, abnormal autonomic function tests (AFTs) were found in 36% of subjects, with cardiovascular risk factors such as cigarette smoking, triglycerides, and diastolic blood pressure showing strong associations with abnormal tests.[32] In prospective studies, the

Table 68-2 Classification of Diabetic Neuropathies Based on Potential Reversibility

Rapidly reversible	Hyperglycemic neuropathy
Persistent symmetrical	Distal somatic sensorimotor (mainly large fiber)
	Autonomic
	Small fiber
Focal and multifocal	Cranial
	Thoracoabdominal radiculopathies
	Focal limb
	Amyotrophy
	Compression/entrapment
Mixed forms	

From Boulton AJ, Malik RA: Diabetic neuropathy. Med Clin North Am 82:909–929, 1998.

Table 68-1 Descriptive Clinical Classification of Diabetic Neuropathies

Polyneuropathy	Mononeuropathy
Sensory	Cranial
Chronic sensorimotor	
Acute sensory	
Autonomic	Isolated peripheral
Proximal motor	Mononeuritis multiplex
Truncal	Truncal

From Boulton AJ, Ward JD: Diabetic neuropathies and pain. J Clin Endocrinol Metab 16:917–931, 1986.
© The Endocrine Society.

Table 68-3 Prevalence of Diabetic Peripheral Sensorimotor Neuropathy

Study/Country	N	Type of Diabetes	Prevalence (%)
CLINIC-BASED STUDIES			
Young et al. (1993),[26] U.K.	6487	1, 2	28.5
Tesfaye et al. (1996),[27] Europe	3250	1, 2	28.0
Cabezas-Cerrato et al. (1998),[28] Spain	2644	1, 2	22.7
POPULATION-BASED STUDIES			
Dyck et al. (1993),[21] U.S.	380	1, 2	47.6
Kumar et al. (1994),[29] U.K.	811	2	41.6
Partanen et al. (1995),[4] Finland			8.3*
	133	2	41.9

*At diagnosis of type of diabetes.

DCCT found mixed results in the association between glycemic control and the 5-year cumulative incidence of autonomic neuropathy.[2] Similarly, the Finnish prospective neuropathy study of type 2 diabetes found inconsistent results in the risk factors for autonomic neuropathy; whereas fasting insulin and female sex related to the cumulative incidence of parasympathetic neuropathy, neither predicted sympathetic neuropathy.[4] Surprisingly, in these studies, glycemic control was a significant risk factor for deterioration of only one autonomic function test in one study.[2]

CLINICAL FEATURES

FOCAL AND MULTIFOCAL NEUROPATHIES

A number of characteristic focal and multifocal neuropathies, none of which are unique to the diabetic patient, occur in diabetes; together, they account for no more than 10% of all the neuropathies. Most of these tend to occur in older, type 2 patients, and the prognosis is generally for recovery of the deficits (either partial or complete) and also of the pain that is frequently present. The rapid onset of symptoms and signs in most cases, together with the focal nature of the deficits, is suggestive of a vascular etiology.[33] Exclusion of nondiabetic causes is particularly important in these neuropathies; in contrast, any nondiabetic patient with these presentations should be screened for diabetes.

CRANIAL MONONEUROPATHIES

The nerves supplying the extraocular muscles (particularly the third cranial nerve) are most commonly affected. Diabetic ophthalmoplegia (third nerve palsy) may be of relatively rapid onset, presenting with pain in the orbit, diplopia, and ptosis; therefore, exclusion of other causes, particularly rupture of a posterior communicating artery aneurysm, is essential. Investigation should include high-resolution computed tomography or magnetic resonance imaging of the brain, with evaluation of the posterior fossa to exclude a tumor. Although these neuropathies are traditionally believed to be due to acute ischemia within the nerve, Hopf and Guttmann[34] provided evidence for microinfarcts within the third nerve nuclei.

ISOLATED AND MULTIPLE MONONEUROPATHIES

A number of nerves are prone to pressure damage in diabetes; by far the most common is the median nerve as it passes under the flexor retinaculum. In the Rochester Diabetic Neuropathy Study, 30% of patients had EP evidence of median nerve compression, although only fewer than 10% had characteristic symptoms.[20] Other, less frequently seen entrapment neuropathies may involve the ulnar nerve, the lateral cutaneous nerve of the thigh (meralgia paresthetica), the radial nerve (wristdrop), and the peroneal nerve (footdrop). Occurring in isolation, most of the above (except footdrop) carry a good prognosis with recovery, although surgical decompression may be required. However, there are increasing reports of severe bilateral ulnar neuropathy occurring in the presence of long-standing diabetes and other complications, a very different picture from the isolated focal mononeuropathies. Moreover, in one series,[35] most cases demonstrated mainly axonal damage due to probable ischemia rather than compression, so surgical decompression would not be beneficial. Mononeuritis multiplex simply describes the occurrence of more than one isolated mononeuropathy in an individual patient.

TRUNCAL NEUROPATHIES

Truncal neuropathy is typically characterized by pain occurring in a dermatomal bandlike distribution around the chest or abdomen. The pain may be severe and have the characteristics of both nerve trunk pain and dysesthesias, typically experienced in mononeuropathies and sensory polyneuropathies, respectively. Thus, the patient may experience dull, aching, boring pain together with burning discomfort or allodynia.[36] The differential diagnosis includes shingles and spinal root compression; on occasions, the pain has been so difficult to diagnose that patients have been unnecessarily submitted to diagnostic laparotomy. EP investigation, including needle electrode electromyography, is useful and can be diagnostic; it should be performed in any patient who is suspected of this diagnosis. Truncal neuropathies may occasionally present with motor manifestations, typically a unilateral bulging of abdominal muscles that is usually associated with pain as described above (Fig. 68-1). Again, electrodiagnostic studies help to secure the diagnosis, and the natural history for symptoms and signs is good, with recovery the rule.[37]

PROXIMAL MOTOR NEUROPATHY

Typically affecting older, male, type 2 diabetic patients, proximal motor neuropathy (amyotrophy) presents with pain, wasting, and weakness in the proximal muscles of the lower limbs, either unilaterally or with asymmetrical bilateral involvement. In addition, there is often a distal symmetrical sensory neuropathy, and weight loss of as much as 40% of premorbid body mass may occur.[38] There is no specific treatment for amyotrophy other than improving glycemic control, which has been advocated,[38] combined with physiotherapy. In most cases, recovery is gradual but might take years rather than months.[38] Neuropathologic studies have provided some interesting though limited insight into the pathogenesis of this condition. A proportion of patients have been shown to have a vasculitis that apparently responds to immunosuppression.[39,40] However, controlled clinical trials of this intervention have not been undertaken, and given that the natural history of this condition is improvement with time, the results of the open trials are difficult to interpret. A detailed morphometric study has failed to confirm the presence of a

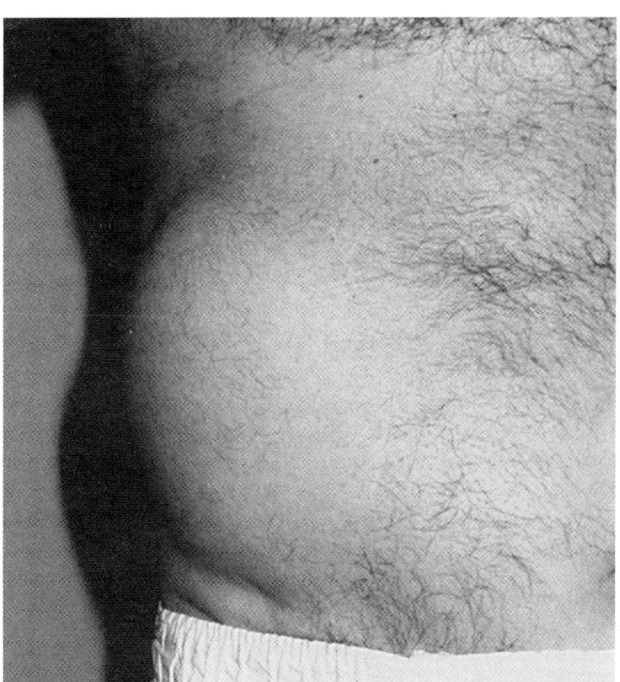

Figure 68-1 Diabetic truncal polyradiculopathy presenting as a bulge in the right abdominal wall secondary to muscle weakness. (From Boulton AJM, et al: Diabetic thoracic polyradicaloneuropathy presenting as an abdominal swelling. Br Med J 289:798–799, 1984.)

vasculitis but has demonstrated marked axonal atrophy in both a proximal cutaneous branch of the femoral nerve and the sural nerve.[41]

CHRONIC INFLAMMATORY DEMYELINATING POLYNEUROPATHY

A demyelinating neuropathy meeting the electrophysiologic criteria for chronic inflammatory demyelinating polyneuropathy (CIDP) has been increasingly recognized to occur more commonly in patients with both type 1 and type 2 diabetes.[42] This comprises a clinical picture of a symmetrical, predominantly motor polyneuropathy with proximal and distal weakness in the lower limbs with reduced reflexes that has a progressive course.[43] Electrophysiologic, clinical, cerebrospinal fluid, and histologic criteria for the diagnosis are well described, although not all might be necessary in individual cases.[42,43] Because patients with CIDP might respond to immunomodulatory therapy, it is important to distinguish this condition from other diabetic neuropathies, particularly proximal motor neuropathy. Therefore, CIDP should be suspected in neuropathic diabetic patients in the following cases:

1. There is a predominance of motor signs involving proximal or distal lower limb muscles.
2. After some years of distal sensory neuropathy, a motor neuropathy develops with progressive symptoms and signs.
3. A patient is diagnosed with proximal motor neuropathy (amyotrophy).

SYMMETRICAL NEUROPATHIES

Autonomic Neuropathy

The autonomic nervous system, which controls a wide range of bodily functions, can be damaged in diabetes with a variety of manifestations, most commonly cardiovascular, urogenital, gastrointestinal, thermoregulatory, and sudomotor function.[44]

Cardiovascular

Cardiac autonomic neuropathy manifests initially as an increase in heart rate secondary to vagal denervation, followed by a decrease due to sympathetic denervation; finally, a fixed heart rate supervenes, which responds only minimally to physiologic stimuli, bearing similarities to the transplanted heart, suggestive of almost complete denervation. Postural hypotension, defined as a 20 mm Hg and 10 mm Hg drop in the systolic and diastolic blood pressures, respectively, occurs as a consequence of impaired vasoconstriction in the splanchnic and cutaneous vascular beds due to efferent sympathetic denervation. Twenty-five percent of children display some degree of cardiac autonomic dysfunction on diagnosis of type 1 diabetes,[45] and an abnormality in the expiration-inspiration ratio has been reported in up to 28% of patients with impaired glucose tolerance.[46] Parasympathetic dysfunction is present in 65% of type 2 diabetic patients 10 years after diagnosis, and combined parasympathetic-sympathetic neuropathy is present in 15.2%.[47]

Gastrointestinal

Autonomic neuropathy of the gastrointestinal system manifests as an abnormality in motility, secretion, and absorption through derangement of both extrinsic parasympathetic (vagus and spinal S2 to S4) and sympathetic, as well as intrinsic enteric innervation provided by Auerbach's plexus. Clinically, patients present with two major problems: diabetic gastroparesis, manifest by nausea, postprandial vomiting, and alternating nocturnal diarrhea and constipation.[44] The diagnosis and treatment of these abnormalities represent an extremely difficult clinical problem in, thankfully, the minority of diabetic patients.

Erectile Dysfunction

Erectile dysfunction (ED) in diabetes is usually of multifactorial etiology, although in most series, autonomic neuropathy is a major contributory factor.[40,48] In the 4-year study of Veves and coworkers,[49] neuropathy was the principal cause of ED in 27% of newly presented patients with ED and a contributory cause in a further 38%. Cholinergic and noncholinergic noradrenergic neurotransmitters mediate erectile function by relaxing the smooth muscle in the corpus cavernosum; the ED resulting from autonomic dysfunction is usually progressive but of gradual onset and progression.[44] Other features include occasional retrograde ejaculation, although some ejaculation and orgasm are maintained. Because of the multiple contributory factors to most cases of ED in diabetes, a careful assessment of each case is essential. Consideration of other potential causes, including vascular disease, other medications, local problems such as Peyronie's disease, and psychological factors, is essential before considering therapeutic approaches.

Bladder Dysfunction

Bladder dysfunction is also well recognized as a consequence of autonomic neuropathy in some patients; this "cystopathy" is usually the result of neurogenic detrusor muscle abnormality.[6] In extreme cases, gross bladder distension may occur with abdominal distension and overflow incontinence.

Sweating Abnormalities

Abnormalities of sweating are common but often neglected symptoms of autonomic neuropathies.[50] Most common is reduced sweating in the extremities, particularly the feet, which is a manifestation of sympathetic dysfunction. The sweat gland has a complex peptidergic as well as cholinergic innervation, and neuropeptide immunoreactivity (especially for vasoactive intestinal polypeptide) is low in sudomotor nerves.

In contrast to the dry feet, some patients complain of drenching truncal sweating, particularly at night. Gustatory sweating, which is profuse sweating in the head and neck region on eating certain foods, is a highly characteristic symptom of diabetic autonomic neuropathy that is also common in patients with nephropathy and is "cured" by renal transplantation.[51]

Distal Sensory Neuropathy

The clinical presentation of distal sensory neuropathy, the most common of all the diabetic neuropathies, is extremely variable, ranging from the severely painful (positive) symptoms at one extreme to the completely painless variety that may present with an insensitive foot ulcer.[5] It is a diffuse symmetrical disorder, mainly affecting the feet and lower legs in a stocking distribution but rarely also involving the hands in a glove distribution. As the disease progresses, there is usually also some motor dysfunction (including small muscle wasting: sensorimotor neuropathy), together with abnormalities of AFTs.

The onset of sensory neuropathy is usually gradual, with the insidious appearance of symptoms that may be intermittent in the early stages. However, an acute sensory neuropathy is recognized with rapid onset of painful symptoms. In this latter type, which often follows a period of severe metabolic instability or may be precipitated by a sudden improvement of control ("insulin neuritis"),[33] the symptoms are usually severe, whereas there may be few if any clinical signs, and quantitative testing may be normal.

The neuropathic symptoms may be difficult for the patient to describe but typically fall into a recognizable pattern, ranging from the severely painful (or positive) at one extreme, with burning pain, stabbing, and shooting sensations; uncomfortable temperature sensations; paresthesias, hyperesthesias, and allodynia; to mild or "negative symptoms," such as decreased pain sensation, deadness, and numbness. Symptoms fluctuate with time but tend to be extremely uncomfortable, distressing, and prone to nocturnal exacerbation with bedclothes hyperesthesias.

A symptom complex that has only recently been recognized as a relatively common complaint in neuropathy is that of postural instability; diabetic neuropathic patients report more falls, and unsteadiness (secondary to disturbances in proprioception) should be added to the list of neuropathic symptoms. Studies have confirmed this phenomenon, showing that neuropathic patients sway more when quantitatively assessed with Romberg's test.[11,52]

Although neuropathic symptoms are predominantly if not exclusively sensory, in many cases the signs are both sensory and motor, with sensory loss in a stocking distribution, together with minor degrees of small muscle wasting and occasionally weakness. The ankle reflex is usually reduced or absent, and the skin in the dorsal and especially plantar surfaces may be dry, owing to associated sympathetic autonomic dysfunction. Because some neuropathic patients may be asymptomatic, it is essential that all diabetic patients have their feet examined on a regular basis.[19]

Small-Fiber Neuropathy

There is some confusion among authorities about definitions of diabetic neuropathy. Some believe that there exists a specific small-fiber neuropathy with neuropathic pain, sometimes together with autonomic dysfunction but few signs. This shares many similarities with the acute sensory neuropathy, but symptoms tend to be more persistent.[6,33] However, this may simply represent an early stage in the development of chronic sensorimotor neuropathy.[53] These painful sensory neuropathies should not be confused with hyperglycemic neuropathy, which may occur in newly diagnosed patients and is characterized by rapidly reversible abnormalities of nerve function and, occasionally, transient symptoms.[5,6]

Natural History of Chronic Distal Sensory Neuropathy

The natural history of neuropathy is poorly understood, and there are few worthwhile published studies; the Rochester Diabetic Neuropathy Study is expected to publish the 10-year follow-up data by 2004.[20] It was generally believed that neuropathic symptoms waxed and waned but persisted for years; however, in a prospective study, Benbow and coworkers[54] reported that the majority of patients reported improvement of symptoms during this time, although there was progressive deterioration in quantitative sensory testing (QST). Thus, improvement in symptoms must not be equated with parallel improvement in nerve function.[5,36]

Controversy still exists as to which sensory modality is first affected, although it is generally accepted that small-fiber dysfunction is present early in the course of neuropathy.[33] There is, however, no doubt that there is gradual loss of nerve function in diabetic patients that is more rapid than that in age-matched nondiabetic subjects; this rate of loss is related to the level of glycemic control.[1-4] One consequence of this progressive diminution of nerve function is an increasing risk of insensitive foot ulceration; progressive loss of large- or small-fiber function is associated with an increasing risk of foot ulceration.[55]

MEASURES OF NEUROPATHY

The diagnosis and staging of neuropathy are important not only for day-to-day clinical practice, but also for the conduct of clinical protocols to assess its etiology and natural history and to test new proposed treatments. As was stated above,

there are definitions and classifications of neuropathy for both clinical practice[19] and clinical trials.[23] The Peripheral Nerve Society has issued a consensus statement on measures to assess efficacy in controlled trials of new therapies for diabetic neuropathy; the use of composite scores of nerve function was advocated in this and other reports.[56,57] In this section, potential measures for clinical diagnosis or follow-up of patients in clinical trials are discussed.

CLINICAL SYMPTOMS

Accurate recording of symptoms is essential both for clinical practice and trials of new medications. It is important to record the patients' descriptions of their complaints verbatim; the physician must not attempt to interpret or translate patients' symptoms into medical terminology. A number of instruments have been developed to quantify neuropathic symptoms that might aid in diagnosis and in longitudinal studies.[58-60] The McGill Pain Questionnaire has been applied to diabetic neuropathy and was found to be a sensitive measure.[58] It consists of a number of descriptors of symptoms from which the patients select those that best describe their experience. The recently validated "NeuroQol" instrument combines a neuropathic symptom score with an assessment of quality of life.[60]

The NSS and its derivatives, the neuropathy symptom profile (NSP) or neuropathy symptom change scores (NSC), are perhaps the most commonly used measures in clinical trials.[21,56,57] The neuropathy symptom score (NSS) is a standardized list of questions and neuropathic symptoms that is applied by a trained individual in a standardized manner. A simplified NSS has been used for epidemiologic studies and can be applied in clinical practice for patient follow-up. It can be administered in a few minutes and scores typical symptoms with additional weighting for nocturnal exacerbation.[26,30]

CLINICAL SIGNS

Simple clinical observation may identify a neuropathic foot; evidence might include small muscle wasting, clawing of toes, prominent metatarsal heads, dry skin and callus (secondary to sympathetic dysfunction), and bony deformities secondary to Charcot's neuroarthropathy.

Two simple instruments can be used in clinical practice or for clinical trial assessment. First, Feldman and coworkers[61] developed the Michigan Neuropathy Screening Instrument (MNSI); this two-step program is used for diagnosis and staging of neuropathy. The MNSI consists of a 15-question yes/no symptom questionnaire that is supplemented by a simple clinical examination. Patients with an abnormal score on the MNSI are then referred for QSTs and EP. Second, the simplified neuropathy disability score (NDS) is a simple clinical examination that sums abnormalities of reflexes and sensory assessment; it has been used in clinical practice and epidemiologic studies.[26,30] The original NDS was developed by Dyck and colleagues at the Mayo Clinic for the detailed structured assessment of neurologic deficits secondary to neuropathy.[20,21,57] The technique is reproducible if performed by trained and experienced physicians and is being used in a number of ongoing trials of new therapies for diabetic neuropathy.

QUANTITATIVE SENSORY TESTING

QSTs assess the patients' ability to detect a number of sensory stimuli and have the advantage that they directly assess the degree of sensory loss at the most vulnerable site: the foot.[62] However, the tests are complex psychophysiologic tests that also rely on a patient's response and therefore cooperation and concentration. Moreover, an abnormal finding does not necessarily confirm that the abnormality lies in the peripheral nerve; it might lie anywhere in the afferent pathway. QSTs vary in complexity; the simpler instruments can be used in day-to-day clinical practice, whereas the more sophisticated instruments are usually used for more detailed assessment and for follow-up assessments in clinical trials.[22] Some of the more commonly used techniques are now briefly discussed.

Semmes-Weinstein Monofilaments

Semmes-Weinstein monofilaments comprise sets of nylon filaments of variable diameter that buckle at a predefined force when applied to the testing site. They are widely used in clinical practice and are particularly helpful in the identification of subjects who are at risk of neuropathic foot ulceration. Inability to perceive pressure of a 10-g (5.07) monofilament has been shown in prospective studies to predict risk of neuropathic ulceration.[63]

Two-Point Discrimination

The tactile circumferential discriminator (Tacticon, Inc., West Chester, PA) is a portable testing device consisting of a hand-held aluminum disk with eight protruding rods of increasing circumference that tests two-point discrimination in a large fiber sensory function. It has sensitivity similar to that of the monofilaments and vibration assessment in identifying neuropathic patients.[64]

Vibration Perception

A number of devices are specifically designed to assess vibration perception thresholds (VPTs) that test large myelinated fiber function. VPT increases with age in normal individuals and also tends to be higher in the lower extremities. As well as being useful in practice, VPT has been used in epidemiologic studies[26] and prospective studies, in which an abnormal reading greater than 25 V has been associated with a high risk of foot ulceration.[55]

Thermal and Cooling Thresholds

Warm and cold sensation is transmitted via small myelinated and unmyelinated fibers and can be assessed by using a number of devices; those employing a forced-choice technique are most reproducible, especially if the method of limits is used.[62] However, they remain the most variable of all QSTs.

Computer-Assisted Sensory Examination

This complex methodology is currently regarded as state of the art for clinical trials and is a computerized device that can measure touch-pressure, vibration, and warm-cold thresholds using a forced-choice algorithm. It is being used in the Rochester study and a number of long-term intervention trials using new therapeutic interventions.[56,57]

AUTONOMIC FUNCTION TESTING

Cardiovascular autonomic dysfunction can be evaluated in detail by employing Ewing and Clarke's battery of five tests: (1) the average inspiratory-expiratory heart rate difference with six deep breaths, (2) the Valsalva ratio, (3) the 30:15 ratio, (4) the diastolic blood pressure response to isometric exercise, and (5) the systolic blood pressure fall to standing.[44,50] More sophisticated techniques such as spectral analysis allow an assessment of the modulation in sinus node activity, and depending on the frequency evaluated, it may allow dissection of the component contribution of both autonomic input and circulating neurohumoral factors. The key tests that are well validated and of prognostic value are RR variation, Valsalva's maneuver, and postural testing.[65]

ELECTROPHYSIOLOGY

EP testing is probably the most important efficacy parameter in clinical neuropathy trials as EP tests are objective, sensitive, and reproducible.[56,57,66] Using a central monitoring core

laboratory, Bril and coworkers[66] were able to obtain remarkable reproducibility of EP variables across 60 sites in a prospective study. Coefficients of variability of 3% and 4% for motor and sensory nerve conduction velocities (NCVs) are comparable to those achieved in an excellent single laboratory.[66] For these reasons, EP variables such as NCVs and amplitudes are frequently used surrogate end points in clinical trials; moreover, they are useful in the clinical investigation of peripheral nerve disease. However, although EP tests can define and quantitate nerve dysfunction, as with QSTs, the findings are not specific to diabetes.

Composite scores, combining clinical, quantitative, sensory, and EP measures, are often used in natural history and efficacy studies.[21,22,56,57] Examples include the NISLL+7[57] and the Michigan Diabetic Neuropathy Score.[61] The former comprises the Neuropathy Impairment Score of the Lower Limbs (NISLL) together with seven other tests (five EP attributes, one QST, and one AFT). This measure is being used in several ongoing multicenter intervention studies.

PATHOGENESIS

The complexity of derived pathogenetic schemes is partly a reflection of the true complex nature of diabetic neuropathy but also denotes our lack of clear understanding of this disease. To establish a logical approach to the pathogenesis and treatment, one must consider inducers, transducers, and effectors.

Hyperglycemia appears to be an inducer of primary importance in patients with type 1 diabetes, and the improvement in neuropathy in the DCCT[2] and following pancreatic transplantation[67] attest to this. However, prospective results of the Epidemiology of Diabetes Complications study indicate that in addition to good glycemic control, avoidance of smoking and good blood pressure control may be helpful in preventing or delaying the onset of neuropathy in patients with type 1 diabetes.[68] Similarly, in the Eurodiab prospective study, independent risk factors that predicted the development of neuropathy included hypertension and deranged lipids.[69] Based on prospective data of the 10-year incidence of distal symmetric polyneuropathy in 589 patients with type 1 diabetes, suggested goals for risk reduction include low-density lipoprotein (LDL) cholesterol less than 100 mg/dL (2.6 mmol/L), high-density lipoprotein (HDL) cholesterol greater than 45 mg/dL (1.1 mmol/L), triglycerides less than 150 mg/dL (1.7 mmol/L), systolic blood pressure less than 120 mm Hg, and diastolic blood pressure less than 80 mm Hg.[70]

With regard to type 2 diabetes, longitudinal data from the Rochester cohort supports the contention that the duration and severity of exposure to hyperglycemia are related to the severity as opposed to the onset of neuropathy.[71] Recent studies in patients with impaired glucose tolerance (IGT) provide important insights into the relationship between hyperglycemia and the development of neuropathy. Thus, while patients with IGT have a normal sural nerve amplitude, and sural nerve myelinated fiber density suggestive of a glycemic threshold for the development of neuropathy.[72] Of 121 patients with a painful neuropathy and electrodiagnostic evidence of axonal injury together with more distal epidermal nerve fiber abnormalities, 25% had impaired glucose tolerance.[73,74] With regard to the effects of intervention, the data are not supportive of benefit with improving glycemic control. Thus, in the VA cooperative study in type 2 diabetic patients, 153 patients who were randomized to intensive versus conventional therapy achieved a 2.07% difference in HbA1c over 2 years but failed to demonstrate a significant difference in the progression of either somatic or autonomic neuropathy.[75] Similarly, the more recent Steno-2 study failed to demonstrate a benefit of multifactorial intervention, including glycemic control, on measure of somatic neuropathy.[76] In defense of the relative merit of improving glycemic control in type 2 diabetes, the measures that were used to define neuropathy were not those that would be accepted to evaluate the benefit of therapy with other interventions in neuropathy[21,22] and relied primarily on vibration perception threshold.[75,76]

POLYOL PATHWAY

Animal models of diabetes consistently demonstrate an association between increased flux through the polyol pathway and a reduction in NCV, both of which can be ameliorated with aldose reductase inhibitors (ARIs).[77] However, the single measurement of whole-nerve sorbitol or fructose levels is clearly an oversimplification of a complex process with a polyol pathway in a constant state of changing flux that is known to be different among different cellular and structural compartments of the peripheral nerve.[77] A recent study has demonstrated enhanced aldose reductase but minimal sorbitol dehydrogenase expression in the peripheral nerve of diabetic patients.[78] Moreover, it would appear that those who are at greatest risk of developing the complications are those with a higher set point for AR activity.[79] To add to this complexity, there may be a significant genetic determinant of polyol pathway flux and hence efficacy of ARIs, as polymorphisms in the ARI promoter region leading to a highly significant decrease in the frequency of the Z+2 allele have been demonstrated in patients with overt neuropathy compared to those without neuropathy.[80] Thus, it is not surprising that in a recent meta-analysis of all randomized controlled trials of ARIs, only a small but statistically significant reduction in decline of median and peroneal motor nerve conduction velocity was observed.[81] Possible reasons for this marginal benefit may be related to the lack of a pharmacogenomic approach, that is, identifying those who are most genetically susceptible to alterations in AR activity and thus those who are most likely to benefit from AR inhibition. Furthermore, the degree of AR inhibition may determine the improvement observed. Thus, in a randomized, placebo-controlled, double-blind, multiple-dose clinical trial with Zenarestat, dose-dependent increments in sural nerve sorbitol suppression were accompanied by significant improvement in NCV, and in doses producing more than 80% sorbitol suppression, there was a significant increase in the density of small-diameter myelinated fibers of the sural nerve.[82] More recently, Fidarestat, a potent ARI, significantly improved median nerve F-wave conduction velocity and minimal latency as well as symptoms of numbness, spontaneous pain, paresthesias, and hyperesthesia.[83]

GLYCATION

Hyperglycemia results in the formation of advanced glycation end products (AGEs), which act on specific receptors (RAGE) inducing monocytes and endothelial cells to increase the production of cytokines and adhesion molecules inducing endothelial dysfunction.[84] Glycation has also recently been shown to have an effect on matrix metalloproteinases (MMPs), in particular MMP-2, which degrades type IV collagen, but also membrane type 1 MMP, tissue inhibitors of MMPs (TIMP)-1 and -2, and transforming growth factor beta (TGF-β).[85] In experimental diabetes, these changes can be prevented by AGE inhibitors such as the nucleophilic compounds pyridoxamine, tenilsetam, 2,3-diaminophenazone, or aminoguanidine, or, alternatively, the administration of recombinant RAGE hinders the AGE-RAGE interaction.[86] Human sural nerves obtained from diabetic and nondiabetic amputation specimens demonstrate normal furosine, an early reversible glycation product, but significantly elevated pentosidine (advanced glycation end product) levels in both cytoskeletal and myelin protein.[87] Enhanced staining for carboxymethyllysine has been demonstrated in the perineurium, endothelial cells, and pericytes of endoneurial microvessels as well as myelinated

and unmyelinated fibers in sural nerves showing a significant reduction in myelinated fiber density.[88] Pyrraline, an advanced glycation end product, is increased in postmortem samples of optic nerve from diabetic patients.[89] In an early experimental study in STZ-diabetic rats treatment with aminoguanidine was associated with a 40% reduction in renal but not nerve AGE levels yet with an improvement in motor nerve conduction velocity without alterations in myelinated nerve fiber morphology.[90] However, in a primate model of type 1 diabetes, 3 years of treatment with aminoguanidine did not restore conduction velocity or autonomic dysfunction.[91] No trial data are currently available for human diabetic neuropathy. However, it is becoming increasingly apparent that many drugs that are currently used for other indications such as glycemic control—Pioglitazone, metformin,[92] and the angiotensin-converting enzyme (ACE) inhibitors and ATII antagonists[93]—may act as powerful antiglycating agents. These findings provide a means of testing the glycation hypothesis effectively without having to develop new agents. Whether or not a pharmaceutical company will invest in a clinical trial program, which will not necessarily lead to a new license indication and hence revenue, is questionable.

OXIDATIVE STRESS

An increasing body of data supports the role of oxidative stress in the pathogenesis of diabetic neuropathy in animal models.[94] There is also emerging evidence that single-nucleotide polymorphisms of the genes for mitochondrial (SOD2) and extracellular (SOD3) superoxide dismutases may confer an increased risk for the development of neuropathy.[95] Benefits have been observed with α-lipoic acid (LA), a powerful antioxidant that scavenges hydroxyl radicals and superoxide and peroxyl radicals and regenerates glutathione. Thus, a series of well-conducted studies have shown benefit in using intravenous followed by oral LA.[96-98]

INSULIN-LIKE GROWTH FACTORS

A deficiency of insulin-like growth factors (IGFs) has been proposed to lead to cell death. Thus, in cultured Schwann cells and the STZ-diabetic rat, IGF-1 administration prevents apoptosis via PI 3-kinase.[99] Neuroaxonal dystrophy (NAD) develops in nerve terminals of the prevertebral sympathetic ganglia and the distal portions of ileal mesenteric nerves in the STZ-diabetic and BB/W rat and has been related to hyperglycemia and a deficiency in circulating IGF-1 levels.[100] In contrast, the Zucker Diabetic Fatty (ZDF) rat, an animal model of type 2 diabetes, develops hyperglycemia comparable to that in the STZ- and BB/W-diabetic rats but has normal levels of plasma IGF-1 and fails to demonstrate NAD.[100] However, both IGF-1 and IGF-1 receptor mRNA levels have not been shown to differ in the sural nerve of diabetic patients compared with control subjects.[101]

C PEPTIDE

Impaired insulin/C peptide action has emerged as a prominent factor in the pathogenesis of the microvascular complications in type 1 diabetes. Experimental studies have demonstrated a range of actions that include effects on Na+K+ATPase activity, expression of neurotrophic factors, regulation of molecular species underlying the degeneration of the nodal apparatus, as well as DNA binding of transcription factors leading to modulation of apoptosis.[102] In the STZ rat, the C peptide mediated improvement in nerve conduction velocity has been shown to occur secondary to an improvement in nerve blood flow via enhanced activity of endothelial nitric oxide synthase.[103] These findings have recently been translated into benefits in patients with type 1 diabetes with the demonstration of a significant improvement in sural sensory nerve conduction velocity and vibration perception but without a benefit in either cold or heat perception after 12 weeks of daily subcutaneous C peptide treatment.[104]

VASCULAR ENDOTHELIAL GROWTH FACTOR

Vascular endothelial growth factor (VEGF) was originally discovered as an endothelial-specific growth factor with a predominant role in angiogenesis. However, recent observations indicate that VEGF also has direct effects on neurons and glial cells stimulating their growth, survival, and axonal outgrowth.[105] Thus, with its potential for a dual impact on both the vasculature and neurons, it could represent an important therapeutic intervention in diabetic neuropathy. Sciatic nerve and dorsal root ganglia from STZ-diabetic rats demonstrate intense VEGF staining in cell bodies and nerve fibers compared to no or very little VEGF in controls and animals treated with insulin or nerve growth factor (NGF).[106] Both the STZ-diabetic rat and the alloxan-induced diabetic rabbit have demonstrated restoration of nerve vascularity, blood flow, and both large- and small-fiber dysfunction 4 weeks after intramuscular gene transfer of plasmid DNA encoding VEGF-1 or VEGF-2.[107] Thus, while there is an intrinsic capacity to upregulate VEGF, this appears insufficient and may require exogenous delivery possibly via gene therapy; moreover, the mechanisms of its benefit require clarification. Nevertheless, a phase I/II, single-site, dose-escalating, double-blind, placebo-controlled study to evaluate the safety and impact of phVEGF165 gene transfer on sensory neuropathy in patients with diabetes with or without macrovascular disease is currently under way.[108]

NEUROTROPHINS

Neurotrophins promote the survival of specific neuronal populations by inducing morphologic differentiation, enhancing nerve regeneration, stimulating neurotransmitter expression, and altering the physiologic characteristics of neurons. While the skin of diabetic patients with sensory fiber dysfunction demonstrates a depletion of NGF protein,[109] mRNA for both NGF[110] and NT-3[111] is increased, and sciatic nerve ciliary neurotrophic factor levels are normal.[112] In situ hybridization studies demonstrate an increased expression of trkA (high-affinity receptor for NGF) and trkC (receptor for NT-3) in the skin of diabetic patients.[113] Curiously, the quest for a viable therapy in diabetic neuropathy has led investigators to interpret these observations as a compensatory upregulation rather than a tenuous link. A phase II clinical trial of recombinant human nerve growth factor in 250 diabetic patients with symptomatic diabetic polyneuropathy demonstrated a significant improvement in the sensory component of the neurologic examination, using two quantitative sensory tests and a rather vague end point: "the clinical impression of most subjects that their neuropathy had improved."[114] However, a phase III trial in 1019 diabetic patients with sensory polyneuropathy failed to demonstrate a significant benefit.[115] These disappointing results led to much speculation regarding the reasons for failure of NGF specifically, with the hope that other neurotrophins might succeed where it had failed.[115] However, recently, a randomized, double-blind, placebo-controlled study of brain-derived neurotrophic factor in 30 diabetic patients demonstrated no significant improvement in nerve conduction, quantitative sensory, and autonomic function tests, including the cutaneous axon-reflex.[116]

MITOGEN-ACTIVATED PROTEIN KINASE

Many of the inducers and transducers upstream may signal transcriptional and translational abnormalities through effector molecules referred to collectively as the mitogen-activated protein kinase (MAPK) family, mediating early gene responses and aberrant phosphorylation of neurofilaments.

A subgroup of MAPKs that specifically involve activation via cellular stressors includes extracellular signal-regulated kinase 1 and 2 (ERK-1 and -2), c-jun N-terminal kinase, and p38, collectively referred to as the stress-activated protein kinases, have been shown to be elevated in sural nerve biopsies of diabetic patients with advanced neuropathy.[117] In the STZ-rat, JNK and p38 have been shown to be transported axonally from the periphery to the neuronal soma and to mediate the transfer of diabetes-related stress signals, possibly triggered by loss of neurotrophic support.[118] Kinase activation leads to phosphorylation of neurofilaments (NFs) composed of three subunit proteins, NF-L, NF-M, and NF-H, which are major constituents of the axonal cylinder.[119] Thus, any abnormality in synthesis, delivery, or processing of these critical proteins could lead to impairments in axon structure and function.[120]

PATHOLOGY

Despite the invasive nature of nerve biopsy, neuropathologic studies are highly sensitive, as they can demonstrate a significant abnormality in both myelinated and unmyelinated fibers, despite entirely normal clinical and neurophysiologic tests of neuropathy.[121–123]

MYELINATED FIBERS

Apart from the hallmark of advanced diabetic neuropathy, loss of myelinated fibers,[121] a number of other, more subtle changes indicating damage to the axon or Schwann cell can be identified by applying morphometric techniques. Mechanistically, ineffective axonal transport[124] or an alteration in the expression of neurofilaments[119] has been suggested to result in axonal atrophy.[125–127] However, a number of studies in patients with mild and established diabetic neuropathy have failed to confirm this abnormality.[128–130] Axoglial disjunction describes an abnormality of the paranodal connection between the terminal myelin loops and the axonal membrane and provides a plausible explanation for a reduction in NCV.[131] However, careful studies have been unable to confirm the presence of axoglial disjunction.[132,133] Schwann cell abnormalities include both reactive (accumulation of lipid droplets, pi, Reich, and glycogen granules) and degenerative (mitochondrial enlargement, effacement of cristae, degeneration of abaxonal and adaxonal cytosol and organelles) changes.[134] These subtle changes are thought to lead to initial demyelination[117] and, with progression of neuropathy, axonal degeneration, resulting in loss of nerve fibers[125,128,135] (Fig. 68-2).

UNMYELINATED FIBERS

Axonal degeneration with active regeneration of this class of fibers occurs early in the evolution of neuropathy prior to axonal degeneration of the myelinated fibers,[130] but importantly, their regenerative capacity is maintained long after the myelinated fibers have lost their capacity to regenerate[125,128] (Fig. 68-3).

STRUCTURE FUNCTION RELATIONSHIP

Neuropathologic abnormalities have been related to a number of abnormalities in peripheral nerve electrophysiology and quantitative sensory tests. A variety of morphologic measures of nerve fiber degeneration have been related to the neuropathy deficit score,[125] vibration perception, and autonomic dysfunction.[128] Patients with mild neuropathy demonstrate a good correlation between sural nerve myelinated fiber density and both peroneal and sural NCV and amplitude but not vibration or thermal perception.[136] In 18 diabetic patients with varying stages of neuropathy, precise relationships

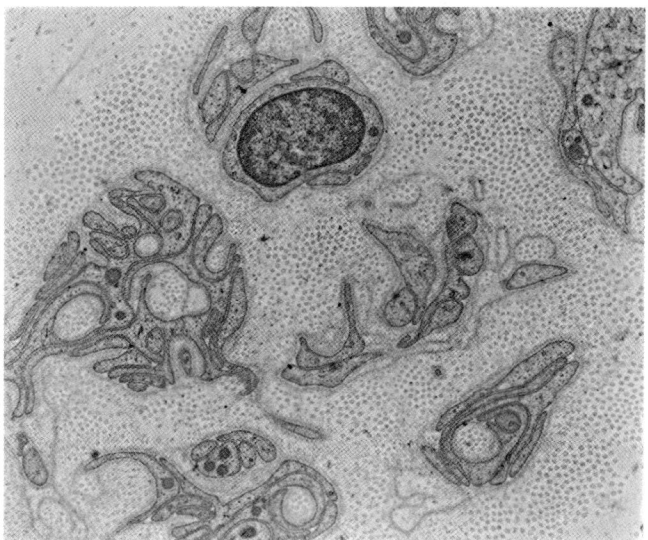

Figure 68-2 Electron micrograph (×12,000) of unmyelinated fibers demonstrating degeneration and regeneration in the sural nerve of a patient with severe diabetic neuropathy.

between the degree of myelinated fiber loss and clinical and neurophysiologic abnormalities, as well as quantitative sensory thresholds, have been demonstrated.[137] Thermal thresholds have been related to the median unmyelinated axon diameter.[128]

AUTONOMIC TISSUE

Pathologic studies of autonomic tissue are limited to postmortem or surgical material. In patients with diabetic gastropathy, the vagus nerve shows a reduction in myelinated fiber density and degeneration with regeneration of unmyelinated fibers.[138] Qualitative changes include chromatolysis, cytoplasmic vacuolization, and pyknotic changes. Quantitative studies have demonstrated degenerative or dystrophic changes in axonal and dendritic components of sympathetic ganglia in the absence of significant neuron loss, as well as alterations in the postganglionic autonomic innervation of various end organs.[139] Neuroaxonal dystrophy is a key feature of the pathology involving intraganglionic terminal axons and synapses of the prevertebral superior mesenteric and celiac and, to a much lesser degree, superior cervical ganglia.[140]

NERVE VASCULATURE

Structural abnormalities of the vessels supplying the peripheral nerve include arteriolar attenuation, venous distention, arteriovenous shunting, and new vessel formation[141,142] along with intimal hyperplasia, hypertrophy,[143] and denervation.[144] Transperineurial vessels demonstrate denervation[145] with luminal narrowing[146] possibly secondary to perineural abnormalities.[147] Endoneurial capillaries demonstrate endothelial cell hypertrophy, hyperplasia, and basement membrane thickening (Fig. 68-4) in diabetic and IGT patients without neuropathy,[148,149] which progress with the severity of neuropathy.[150–154]

SKIN BIOPSY

Immunohistochemical quantification of epidermal nerve fibers using the panaxonal marker protein gene product 9.5 was initially limited owing to the absence of a normative range[155] and the lack of optimal methods to define and quantify nerve fiber degeneration and repair.[156,157] This technique, although still invasive, requires only a 3-mm skin biopsy and enables a direct study of small nerve fibers that are difficult to assess electrophysiologically.[158] Thus, this technique has been used to study patients with diabetic neuropathy[158–160] and, more recently, has also been used to assess early neuropathic changes in patients with IGT.[69,70]

CORNEAL CONFOCAL MICROSCOPY

The accurate detection, characterization, and quantification of human diabetic neuropathy are important to define at-risk patients, anticipate deterioration, and assess new therapies. The more accurate methods of sural nerve or skin biopsy are invasive. Corneal confocal microscopy is a reiterative, rapid, noninvasive, in vivo clinical examination technique that is

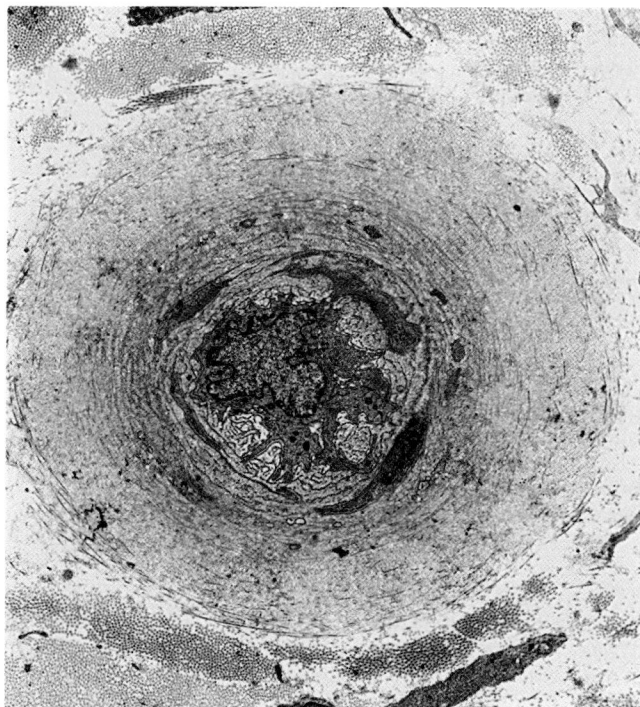

Figure 68-3 Electron micrograph (×4500) of endoneurial capillary demonstrating gross thickening of basement membrane with closure of the lumen in the sural nerve of a patient with severe diabetic neuropathy.

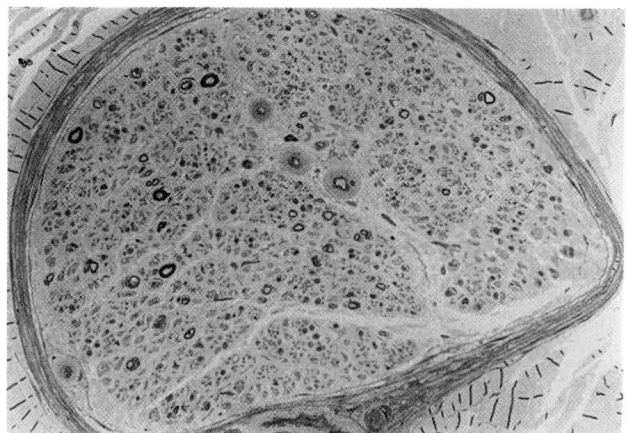

Figure 68-4 Light micrograph (×300) of a transverse semithin section demonstrating a gross loss of myelinated fibers and marked thickening of endoneurial capillary basement membrane in the sural nerve of a patient with severe neuropathy.

capable of imaging corneal nerve fibers. We have recently developed the methodology to accurately define the extent of corneal nerve damage and repair[161,162] and have shown that it acts as a surrogate measure of somatic neuropathy in diabetic patients. We propose that it potentially represents a significant advance to define the severity of neuropathy and expedite assessment of therapeutic efficacy in clinical trials of human diabetic neuropathy.

TREATMENT

Throughout this section on treatment, distinction is made between therapies for symptomatic relief[163] and those that may alter (slow) the progressive loss of nerve function that characterizes the natural history[164] of neuropathy. A few therapies have efficacy in both these areas.

SENSORY NEUROPATHY

Current Treatments
Glycemic Control
Of all the treatments, tight and stable glycemic control is probably the only one that may provide symptomatic relief as well as slow the relentless progression of neuropathy.[1–3] As it is probably blood glucose flux that induces neuropathic pain,[36] stability rather than the actual level of glycemic control may be most important in pain relief.[165] The method of achieving stable control does not seem to be critical; there is no evidence that insulin is superior if the blood glucose is well controlled by oral hypoglycemic agents.

Tricyclic Antidepressants
Until new therapies are proved to relieve symptoms in appropriately designed trials,[166] the tricyclic antidepressant drugs, such as amitriptyline and imipramine, will remain the first-line agents for painful neuropathy; their efficacy, confirmed in several randomized, placebo-controlled trials,[167] is related to plasma drug level, and the onset of symptomatic relief is faster than the antidepressive effects. There is a clear dose-response relationship, but sedative and anticholinergic side effects are also dose-related and troublesome, often restricting the use of these drugs.[168]

Anticonvulsants
Carbamazepine is widely used in the management of neuropathic pain, and its use is supported by some clinical trial data, although side effects limit its usage in a proportion of patients.[168] More recently, the new anticonvulsants gabapentin[169] and lamotrigine[170] have been shown to be efficacious in the treatment of painful syndromes, including diabetic neuropathy. Their adverse effects seem to be less pronounced than those associated with tricyclic drugs.

Other Agents
A number of other drug therapies, including phenytoin, mexiletene, lidocaine, and transdermal clonidine, have been reported to be useful in the management of painful or paresthetic symptoms.[168,171] Topical therapy with capsaicin may be helpful in some cases, especially those with localized pain.[5] The centrally acting analgesic tramadol has confirmed efficacy in painful diabetic neuropathy in a randomized controlled trial.[172] Recently, a pilot study confirmed the efficacy of topically applied isosorbide dinitrite spray in a small randomized, placebo-controlled, double-blind trial.[173] When the spray was applied locally to the feet at bedtime, a significant reduction of neuropathic pain was reported during active treatment, although curiously, the placebo arm demonstrated no change. Finally, traditional therapies such as acupuncture have also been employed with good results and negligible side effects in symptomatic neuropathy.[174]

Potential Future Therapies
Aldose Reductase Inhibitors
The disappointing results with these agents have been reviewed previously[81]; therefore, it is not surprising that none are available today in the United States or Europe. Many of the problems of early ARI trials related to poor study design and the enrollment of patients with advanced neuropathy who would be unlikely to benefit from treatment.[22] If current ongoing trials with potent ARIs demonstrate efficacy, these agents are likely to slow neuropathy progression rather than providing symptomatic relief.

α-Lipoic Acid
There is accumulating evidence to suggest that free radical–mediated oxidative stress is implicated in the pathogenesis of neuropathy and that treatment with the antioxidant α-lipoic acid might prevent these abnormalities, and improve painful symptoms as well as slow the progression of diabetic neuropathy.[96–98] Two North American and European trials are testing these hypotheses, and the results should be available in 2004/2005.

γ-Linolenic Acid
The first step in the metabolism of the essential fatty acid linolenic acid is impaired in diabetes and this defect can be bypassed by the administration of γ-linolenic acid (GLA). Both experimental and clinical studies have suggested some efficacy of GLA in neuropathy.[175] The most interesting development arises from the findings in animal studies that a lipoic acid–GLA conjugate is effective against both somatic[176] and autonomic[177] nerves.

Other Agents
Investigation of other potential treatments for neuropathy are ongoing. One proposed class of drugs is the ACE inhibitors, already known for their efficacy in nephropathy and retinopathy. A preliminary controlled study of ACE inhibitors in early neuropathy confirmed a significant benefit over placebo in EP parameters.[178] Intracellular hyperglycemia increases diacylglycerol levels, which activates protein kinase C (PKC) formation, leading to multiple pathogenetic consequences, including altered expression of endothelial nitric oxide synthetase and VEGF. Preliminary data suggest that treatment with a PKC-β inhibitor might ameliorate measures of nerve function in diabetic peripheral neuropathy.[179] Multicenter trials are currently in progress and should report in 2004/2005. The N-methyl-D-aspartate (NMDA) receptor that is involved in nociception provides a possibility for therapeutic intervention in neuropathic pain. Recently, a pilot study of intravenous Amantadine, an NMDA antagonist, demonstrated efficacy in pain relief in diabetic neuropathy.[180]

AUTONOMIC NEUROPATHY

Erectile Dysfunction
Because autonomic neuropathy is one of several contributory causes in erectile dysfunction (ED), a multifaceted approach to management is indicated.[48,49] Psychosexual counseling and altering drug therapy to remove the factors associated with ED are beneficial in many cases.[49] Sildenafil, an orally active selective inhibitor of phosphodiesterase 5 (PDE-5), is efficacious for ED in diabetic males. In a trial of ED of multiple causation in diabetic males, Rendell and coworkers[181] reported a response rate (defined as at least one successful attempt at sexual intercourse) of 61% in sildenafil-treated subjects versus 22% on placebo. Most diabetic patients require 50 or 100 mg, and care must be taken if there is any history of ischemic heart disease. Sildenafil must never be given to patients on nitrate therapy. Subsequent trial of Sildenafil in type 2 patients with ED reported a response rate of 65% versus 11%

on placebo.[182] More recently, two other PDE-5 inhibitors have been licensed for the management of ED: Tadalafil and Vardenafil.[183,184]

Sweating Disorders

The first specific treatment for gustatory sweating has been reported. Glycopyrrolate is an antimuscarinic compound that, when applied topically to the affected area, results in a marked reduction of sweating while eating "trigger" foods. Its efficacy was confirmed in a randomized controlled trial.[185]

Others

Treatment of diabetic gastroparesis involves measures to enhance gastric motility and emptying. Metoclopramide, a dopamine antagonist, directly stimulates antral muscle and may also mediate acetylcholine release. Alternative agents include domperidone, a peripheral dopamine D_2 receptor antagonist; or erythromycin, which directly stimulates motilin receptors. Constipation may be treated with a combination of prokinetic agents such as metoclopramide and cisapride. Postural hypotension may be treated with mineralocorticoids such as fludrocortisone, sympathomimetic agents, and dopamine blockers. Urinary bladder difficulties are addressed with regular voiding, self-catheterization, and cholinergic agonists such as bethanechol chloride, which stimulates muscarinic, postganglionic receptors, enhancing bladder motility and emptying.[44,50]

THE NEUROPATHIC FOOT

Any patient with clinical evidence of diabetic peripheral neuropathy must be considered as being at risk of insensitive foot ulceration and should receive evaluation on foot care and, if necessary, a podiatry referral.[19] These patients require more frequent follow-up, always paying particular attention to foot inspection to reinforce the educational message of the need for regular foot care.

The late sequelae of diabetic neuropathy are usually considered to be neuropathic foot ulceration, neuroarthropathy (Charcot's foot), and amputation.[5,7,8]

NEUROPATHIC FOOT ULCERATION

Distal sensory and sympathetic neuropathy are the most important component causes that lead to foot ulceration, being present in 78% of cases assessed in a two-center study.[9] However, the neuropathic foot does not spontaneously ulcerate; typically, it is the combination of neuropathy with other risk factors such as deformity and unperceived trauma that results in ulceration. International guidelines on the clinical management of neuropathy, therefore, emphasize the importance of regular foot examinations and education in self-foot care in the management of neuropathy.[19]

CHARCOT'S NEUROARTHROPATHY

Charcot's neuroarthropathy is a less common but clinically important and potentially devastating disorder. Diabetes is now the most common cause of this condition in Western countries,[8] and a high degree of awareness and suspicion may enable early diagnosis and effective intervention. Permissive features for the development of a Charcot's joint include peripheral sensorimotor neuropathy, sympathetic denervation in the foot, and intact peripheral circulation; minor, unperceived trauma is often the initiating event. It is believed that following repetitive minor trauma, osteoblastic activity is stimulated with remodeling of bone. A high index of suspicion must exist if a neuropathic patient has unilateral unexplained swelling and warmth in a foot, with the possibility of infection also being kept in mind. Contrary to earlier texts, discomfort may be experienced, although the patient is still usually able to walk. Detailed assessment and investigation of such a patient is essential, and rest or casting of a suspected Charcot's foot is usually recommended.

REFERENCES

1. Diabetes Control and Complications Trial Research Group: The effect of intensive treatment of diabetes on the development of progression of long-term complications in insulin-dependent diabetes mellitus. N Engl J Med 329:329–986, 1993.
2. Diabetes Control of Complications Trial Research Group: The effect of intensive diabetes therapy on the development and progression of neuropathy. Ann Intern Med 122:561–568, 1995.
3. United Kingdom Prospective Diabetes Study: Intensive blood glucose control with sulphonylureas or insulin compared with conventional treatment and risk of complications in patients with type 2 diabetes. Lancet 352:837–853, 1998.
4. Partanen J, Niskanen L, Lehtinen J, et al: Natural history of peripheral neuropathy in patients with non-insulin dependent diabetes mellitus. N Engl J Med 333:89–94, 1995.
5. Boulton AJM, Malik RA: Diabetic neuropathy. Med Clin North Am 82:909–929, 1998.
6. Watkins PJ, Thomas PK: Diabetes mellitus and the nervous system. J Neurol Neurosurg Psychiatry 65:620–632, 1998.

7. Mayfield JA, Reiber GE, Sanders LJ, et al: Technical Review: Preventive foot care in patients with diabetes mellitus. Diabetes Care 21:2161–2177, 1998.
8. Jude EB, Boulton AJM: End-stage complications of diabetic neuropathy. Diabets Rev 6:395–410, 1999.
9. Reiber GE, Vileikyte L, Boyko EH, et al: Causal pathways for incident lower-extremity ulcers in patients with diabetes from two settings. Diabetes Care 22:157–162, 1999.
10. Benbow SJ, Wallymahmed ME, MacFarlane IA: Diabetic peripheral neuropathy and quality of life. Q J Med 91:733–737, 1998.
11. Vileikyte L, Rubin RR, Leventhal H: Psychological aspects of diabetic neuropathic foot complications: An overview. Diabetes Metab Res Rev 20(Suppl 1):S13–S18, 2004.
12. de Calvi M: Recherches sur les Accidents Diabetiques. Paris, P. Asselir, 1806.
13. Ward JD: Historical aspects of diabetic peripheral neuropathy In Boulton AJM (ed): Diabetes in Pictures: Diabetic Neuropathy. Cologne, Academy Press, 2001, pp 8–15.
14. Davies-Pryce T: A case of perforating ulcers of both feet associated with ataxic symptoms. Lancet 2:11–12, 1887.

15. Jordan WR: Neuritic manifestations in diabetic neuropathy. Arch Int Med 57:307–366, 1936.
16. Thomas PK: Classification, differential diagnosis and staging of diabetic peripheral neuropathy. Diabetes 46(Suppl 2):S54–S57, 1997.
17. Boulton AJM, Ward JD: Diabetic neuropathies and pain. Clin Endocrinol Metab 15:917–931, 1986.
18. Sima AAF, Thomas PK, Ishii D, et al: Diabetic neuropathies. Diabetologia 46(Suppl):B74–B77, 1997.
19. Boulton AJM, Gries FA, Jervell JA: Guidelines for the diagnosis and out-patient management of diabetic peripheral neuropathy. Diabet Med 15:508–514, 1998.
20. Dyck PJ, Kratz KM, Karnes JZ, et al: The prevalence by staged severity of various types of diabetic neuropathy, retinopathy and nephropathy in a population-based cohort: The Rochester Diabetic Neuropathy Study. Neurology 43:817–824, 1993.
21. Dyck PJ, Melton J, O'Brien PC, et al: Approaches to improve epidemiological studies of diabetic neuropathy. Diabetes 46(Suppl 2):S5–S8, 1997.
22. Ziegler D: The design of clinical trials for treatment of diabetic neuropathy. Neurosci Res Commun 21:83–91, 1997.

23. Consensus statement: Report and recommendations of the San Antonio conference on diabetic neuropathy. Diabetes Care 11:592–597, 1988.

24. Boulton AJM, Malik RA, Arezzo JC, Sosenko JM: Diabetic somatic neuropathy: Technical review. Diabetes Care 27:1458–1487, 2004.

25. Adler AI: Risk factors for diabetic neuropathy and foot ulceration. Curr Diabetes Rep 1:202–207, 2001.

26. Young MJ, Boulton AJM, McLeod AF, et al: A multicentre study of the prevalence of diabetic peripheral neuropathy in the UK hospital clinic population. Diabetologia 36:150–154, 1993.

27. Tesfaye S, Stephens LK, Stephenson JM, et al: Prevalence of diabetic peripheral neuropathy and its relation to glycemic control and potential risk factors: The EURODIAB IDDM complications study. Diabetologia 39:1377–1384, 1996.

28. Cabezas-Cerrato J: The prevalence of clinical diabetic neuropathy in Spain: A study in primary care and hospital clinic groups. Diabetologia 41:1263–1269, 1998.

29. Kumar S, Ashe HA, Parnell L, et al: The prevalence of foot ulceration and its correlates in type 2 diabetes: A population-based study. Diabet Med 11:480–484, 1994.

30. Abbott CA, Carrington AL, Ashe H, et al: The northwest diabetes foot care study: Incidence of, and risk factors for, new diabetic foot ulceration in a community-based cohort. Diabet Med 19:377–384, 2002.

31. Adler AI, Boyko EJ, Ahroni JH, et al: Risk factors for diabetic peripheral sensory neuropathy: Results of the Seattle prospective diabetic foot study. Diabetes Care 20:1162–1167, 1997.

32. Kempler P, Tesfaye S, Chaturvedi N, et al: Autonomic neuropathy is associated with increased cardiovascular risk factors: The EURODIAB IDDM complications study. Diabet Med 19:900–905, 2002.

33. Tesfaye S, Ward JD: Clinical features of diabetic polyneuropathy. In Veves A (ed): Contemporary Endocrinology: Clinical Management of Diabetic Neuropathy. Totowa, NJ, Humana Press, 1998, pp 49–60.

34. Hopf HC, Guttmann L: Diabetic third nerve palsy: Evidence for a mesencephalic lesion. Neurology 40:1041–1045, 1990.

35. Schady W, Abuaisha B, Boulton AJM: Observations on severe ulnar neuropathy in diabetes. J Diabetes Complications 12:128–132, 1998.

36. Boulton AJM: What causes neuropathic pain? J Diabetes Complications 6:58–63, 1992.

37. Chaudhuri KR, Wren DR, Werring D, et al: Unilateral abdominal muscle herniation with pain: A distinctive variant of diabetic radiculopathy. Diabet Med 14:803–807, 1997.

38. Dyck PJ, Windebank AJ: Diabetic and nondiabetic lumbosacral radiculoplexus neuropathies: new insights into pathophysiology and treatment. Muscle Nerve 25:477–491, 2002.

39. Dyck PJ, Norell JE, Dyck PJ: Non-diabetic lumbosacral radiculoplexus neuropathy: Natural history, outcome and comparison with the diabetic variety. Brain 124:1197–1207, 2001.

40. Llewelyn JG, Thomas PK, King RHM: Epineurial microvasculitis in proximal diabetic neuropathy. J Neurol 245:159–165, 1998.

41. Malik RA, Ghani M, Walker D, et al: Pathological studies in diabetic amyotrophy. Diabetes 47(Suppl 1):A64, 1998.

42. Sharma KR, Cross J, Farronay O, et al: Demyelinating neuropathy in diabetes mellitus. Arch Neurol 59:758–765, 2002.

43. Haq RU, Pendebury WW, Fries TJ, Tanian R: Chronic inflammatory demyelinating neuropathy in diabetic patients. Muscle Nerve 27:465–470, 2003.

44. Freeman R: Diabetic autonomic neuropathy: An overview. In Veves A (ed): Contemporary Endocrinology: Clinical Management of Diabetic Neuropathy. Totowa, NJ, Humana Press, 1998, pp 181–208.

45. Solders G, Thalme B, Aguirre-Aquino M, et al: Nerve conduction and autonomic nerve function in diabetic children: A 10-year follow up study. Acta Pediatr 86:361–366, 1997.

46. Eriksson KF, Nilsson H, Lindarde F, et al: Diabetes mellitus but not impaired glucose tolerance is associated with dysfunction in peripheral nerves. Diabet Med 11:279–285, 1994.

47. Toyry JP, Niskanen LK, Mantysaari MJ, et al: Occurrence predictors and clinical significance of autonomic neuropathy in NIDDM: Ten year follow-up from diagnosis. Diabetes 45:308–315, 1996.

48. Vinik AI, Richardson D: Evaluating erectile dysfunction in diabetes. Int Diabetes Fed Bull 43:7–13, 1998.

49. Veves A, Webster L, Chen TF, et al: Aetiopathogenesis and management of impotence in diabetic males: Four years' experience from a combined clinic. Diabet Med 12:77–82, 1995.

50. Watkins PJ, Edmonds ME: Clinical features of diabetic neuropathy. In Pickup JC, Williams G (eds): Textbook of Diabetes, 2nd ed. Oxford, UK, Blackwell Scientific, 1997, pp 50.1–50.20.

51. Shaw JE, Parker P, Hollis S, et al: Gustatory sweating in diabetes mellitus. Diabet Med 13:1033–1037, 1996.

52. Katoulis EC, Ebdon-Parry M, Hollis S, et al: Postural instability in diabetic neuropathic patients at risk of foot ulceration. Diabet Med 14:296–300, 1997.

53. Veves A, Young MJ, Manes C, et al: Differences in peripheral and autonomic nerve function measurements in painful and painless neuropathy: A clinical study. Diabetes Care 17:1200–1202, 1994.

54. Benbow SJ, Chan AW, Bowsher DH, et al: A prospective study of painful symptoms, small fibre function and peripheral vascular disease in chronic painful diabetic neuropathy. Diabet Med 11:17–21, 1994.

55. Abbott CA, Vileikyte L, Williamson S, et al: Multicenter study of the incidence of and predictive risk factors for diabetic neuropathic foot ulceration. Diabetes Care 21:1071–1074, 1998.

56. Diabetic polyneuropathy in controlled clinical trials: Consensus report of the peripheral nerve society. Ann Neurol 38:478–482, 1995.

57. Dyck PJ, Davies JL, Litchy WJ, et al: Longitudinal assessment of diabetic polyneuropathy using a composite score in the Rochester Diabetic Neuropathy Study cohort. Neurology 49:229–239, 1997.

58. Masson EA, Hunt L, Gem JM, et al: A novel approach to the diagnosis and assessment of symptomatic diabetic neuropathy. Pain 38:25–28, 1989.

59. Apfel SC, Asbury AK, Bril V, et al: Positive neuropathic sensory symptoms as endpoints in diabetic neuropathy trials. J Neurolog Sci 189:3–5, 2001.

60. Vileikyte L, Peyrot M, Bundy C, et al: The development and validation of a neuropathy and foot ulcer–specific quality of life instrument. Diabetes Care 26:2569–2555, 2003.

61. Feldman EL, Stevens MJ, Thomas PK, et al: A practical two-step quantitative clinical and electrophysiological assessment for the diagnosis and staging of diabetic neuropathy. Diabetes Care 17:1281–1289, 1994.

62. Shy ME, Frohman EM, So YT, et al: Quantitative sensory testing. Neurology 602:898–906, 2003.

63. Mayfield JA, Sugarman JR: The use of the Semmes-Weinstein monofilament and other threshold tests for preventing foot ulceration and amputation in persons with diabetes. J Fam Pract 49(Suppl 1):S17–S29, 2000.

64. Vileikyte L, Hutchings G, Hollis S, et al: The tactile circumferential discriminator: A new simple screening device to identify diabetic patients at risk of foot ulceration. Diabetes Care 20:623–626, 1997.

65. Schumer MP, Joyner SA, Pfeifer MA: Cardiovascular autonomic neuropathy testing in patients with diabetes. Diabetes Spectrum 11:227–231, 1998.

66. Bril V, Ellison R, Ngo M, et al: Electrophysiological monitoring in clinical trials. Muscle Nerve 21:1368–1373, 1998.

67. Navarro X, Sutherland DE, Kennedy WR: Long-term effects of pancreatic transplantation on diabetic neuropathy. Ann Neurol 42:727–736, 1997.

68. Forrest KY, Maser RE, Pambianco G, et al: Hypertension as a risk factor for diabetic neuropathy: A prospective study. Diabetes 46:665–670, 1997.

69. The EURODIAB Prospective Complications Study (PCS) Group: Cardiovascular risk factors predict diabetic peripheral neuropathy in Type 1 subjects in Europe. Diabetologia 42:A50–A181, 1999.

70. Orchard TJ, Forrest KY, Kuller LH, Becker DJ, Pittsburgh Epidemiology of Diabetes Complications Study: Lipid and blood pressure treatment goals for type 1 diabetes: 10-year incidence data from the Pittsburgh Epidemiology of Diabetes Complications Study. Diabetes Care 24:1053–1059, 2001.

71. Dyck PJ, Davies JL, Wilson DM, et al: Risk factors for severity of diabetic polyneuropathy: Intensive longitudinal assessment of the Rochester Diabetic Neuropathy Study cohort. Diabetes Care 22:1479–1486, 1999.

72. Sundkvist G, Dahlin LB, Nilsson H, et al: Sorbitol and myo-inositol levels and morphology of sural nerve in relation to peripheral nerve function and clinical neuropathy in men with diabetic, impaired, and normal glucose tolerance. Diabetic Med 17:259–268, 2000.

73. Smith AG, Ramachandran P, Tripp S, Singleton JR: Epidermal nerve innervation in impaired glucose tolerance and diabetes-associated neuropathy. Neurology 13:1701–1704, 2001.

74. Sumner CJ, Sheth S, Griffin JW, et al: The spectrum of neuropathy in diabetes and impaired glucose tolerance. Neurology 60:108–111, 2003.

75. Azad N, Emanuele NV, Abraira C, et al: The effects of intensive glycemic control on neuropathy in the VA cooperative study on type II diabetes mellitus (VA CSDM). J Diabetes Complications 13:307–313, 1999.

76. Gaede P, Vedel P, Larsen N, et al: Multifactorial intervention and cardiovascular disease in patients with type 2 diabetes. N Engl J Med 348:383–393, 2003.

77. Oates PJ: Polyol pathway and diabetic peripheral neuropathy. Int Rev Neurobiol 50:325–392, 2002.

78. Kasajima H, Yamagishi S, Sugai S, et al: Enhanced in situ expression of aldose reductase in peripheral nerve and renal glomeruli in diabetic patients. Virchows Arch 439:46–54, 2001.

79. Shimizu H, Ohtani KI, Tsuchiya T, et al: Aldose reductase mRNA expression is associated with rapid development of diabetic microangiopathy in Japanese Type 2 diabetic (T2DM) patients. Diabetes Nutr Metab 13:75–79, 2000.

80. Demaine AG: Polymorphisms of the aldose reductase gene and susceptibility to diabetic microvascular complications. Curr Med Chem 10:1389–1398, 2003.

81. Airey M, Bennett C, Nicolucci A, Williams R: Aldose reductase inhibitors for the prevention and treatment of diabetic peripheral neuropathy. Cochrane Database Syst Rev 2:CD002182, 2000.

82. Greene DA, Arezzo JC, Brown MB: Effect of aldose reductase inhibition on nerve conduction and morphometry in diabetic neuropathy. Zenarestat Study Group. Neurology 53:580–591, 1999.

83. Hotta N, Toyota T, Matsuoka K, et al: Clinical efficacy of fidarestat, a novel aldose reductase inhibitor, for diabetic peripheral neuropathy: A 52-week multicenter placebo-controlled double-blind parallel group study. Diabetes Care 24:1776–1782, 2001.

84. King RH: The role of glycation in the pathogenesis of diabetic polyneuropathy. Mol Pathol 54:400–408, 2001.

85. McLennan SV, Martell SK, Yue DK: Effects of mesangium glycation on matrix metalloproteinase activities: Possible role in diabetic nephropathy. Diabetes 51:2612–2618, 2002.

86. Vasan S, Foiles P, Founds H: Therapeutic potential of breakers of advanced glycation end product-protein crosslinks. Arch Biochem Biophys 419:89–96, 2003.

87. Ryle C, Donaghy M: Non-enzymatic glycation of peripheral nerve proteins in human diabetics. J Neurol Sci 129:62–68, 1995.

88. Sugimoto K, Nishizawa Y, Horiuchi S, Yagihashi S: Localization in human diabetic peripheral nerve of N (epsilon)-carboxymethyllysine-protein adducts, an advanced glycation end product. Diabetologia 40:1380–1387, 1997.

89. Amano S, Kaji Y, Oshika T, et al: Advanced glycation end products in human optic nerve head. Br J Ophthalmol 85:52–55, 2001.

90. Miyauchi Y, Shikama H, Takasu T, et al: Slowing of peripheral motor nerve conduction was ameliorated by aminoguanidine in streptozocin-induced diabetic rats. Eur J Endocrinol 134:467–473, 1996.

91. Birrell AM, Heffernan SJ, Ansselin AD, et al: Functional and structural abnormalities in the nerves of type I diabetic baboons: Aminoguanidine treatment does not improve nerve function. Diabetologia 43:110–116, 2000.

92. Rahbar S, Natarajan R, Yerneni K, et al: Evidence that pioglitazone, metformin and pentoxifylline are inhibitors of glycation. Clin Chim Acta 301:65–77, 2000.

93. Bui BV, Armitage JA, Tolcos M, et al: ACE inhibition salvages the visual loss caused by diabetes. Diabetologia 46:401–408, 2003.

94. Nishikawa T, Edelstein D, Du XL, et al: Normalizing mitochondrial superoxide production blocks three pathways of hyperglycemic damage. Nature 404:787–790, 2000.

95. Zotova EV, Chistiakov DA, Savost'ianov KV, et al: Association of the SOD2 Ala(–9)Val and SOD3 Arg213Gly polymorphisms with diabetic polyneuropathy in patients with diabetes mellitus type 1. Mol Biol (Mosk) 37:404–408, 2003.

96. Reljanovic M, Reichel G, Rett K, et al: Treatment of diabetic polyneuropathy with the antioxidant thioctic acid (alpha-lipoic acid): A two year multicentre randomized double-blind placebo-controlled trial (ALADIN II). Free Radic Res 31:171–179, 1999.

97. Ziegler D, Hanefeld M, Ruhnau KJ, et al: Treatment of symptomatic diabetic polyneuropathy with the antioxidant alpha-lipoic acid: A 7-month multicentre randomized controlled trial (ALADIN III Study): ALADIN III Study Group. Diabetes Care 22:1296–1301, 1999.

98. Ametov AS, Barinov A, Dyck PJ, et al: The sensory symptoms of diabetic polyneuropathy are improved with alpha-lipoic acid: The SYDNEY trial. Diabetes Care 26:770–776, 2003.

99. Delaney CL, Russell JW, Cheng HL, Feldman EL: Insulin-like growth factor-I and over-expression of Bcl-xL prevent glucose-mediated apoptosis in Schwann cells. J Neuropathol Exp Neurol 60:147–160, 2001.

100. Schmidt RE, Dorsey DA, Beaudet LN, Peterson RG: Analysis of the Zucker Diabetic Fatty (ZDF) type 2 diabetic rat model suggests a neurotrophic role for insulin/IGF-I in diabetic autonomic neuropathy. Am J Pathol 163:21–28, 2003.

101. Grandis M, Nobbio L, Abbruzzese M, et al: Insulin treatment enhances expression of IGF-I in sural nerves of diabetic patients. Muscle Nerve 24:622–629, 2001.

102. Sima AA: C-peptide and diabetic neuropathy. Expert Opin Investig Drugs 12:1471–1488, 2003.

103. Cotter MA, Ekberg K, Wahren J, Cameron NE: Effects of proinsulin C-peptide in experimental diabetic neuropathy: Vascular actions and modulation by nitric oxide synthase inhibition. Diabetes 52:1812–1817, 2003.

104. Ekberg K, Brismar T, Johansson BL, et al: Amelioration of sensory nerve dysfunction by C-peptide in patients with type 1 diabetes. Diabetes 52:536–541, 2003.

105. Carmeliet P, Storkebaum E: Vascular and neuronal effects of VEGF in the nervous system: Implications for neurological disorders. Semin Cell Dev Biol 13:39–53, 2002.

106. Samii A, Unger J, Lange W: Vascular endothelial growth factor expression in peripheral nerves and dorsal root ganglia in diabetic neuropathy in rats. Neurosci Lett 262:159–162, 1999.

107. Schratzberger P, Walter DH, Rittig K, et al: Reversal of experimental diabetic neuropathy by VEGF gene transfer. J Clin Invest 107:1083–1092, 2001.

108. Isner JM, Ropper A, Hirst K: VEGF gene transfer for diabetic neuropathy. Hum Gene Ther 12:1593–1594, 2001.

109. Anand P, Terenghi G, Warner G, et al: The role of endogenous nerve growth factor in human diabetic neuropathy. Nat Med 2:703–707, 1996.

110. Diemel LT, Cai F, Anand P, et al: Increased nerve growth factor mRNA in lateral calf skin biopsies from diabetic patients. Diabetic Med 16:113–118, 1999.

111. Kennedy AJ, Wellmer A, Facer P, et al: Neurotrophin-3 is increased in skin in human diabetic neuropathy. J Neurol

Neurosurg Psychiatry 65:393–395, 1998.

112. Lee DA, Gross L, Wittrock DA, Windebank AJ: Localization and expression of ciliary neurotrophic factor (CNTF) in postmortem sciatic nerve from patients with motor neuron disease and diabetic neuropathy. J Neuropathol Exp Neurol 55:915–923, 1996.

113. Terenghi G, Mann D, Kopelman PG, Anand P: trkA and trkC expression is increased in human diabetic skin. Neurosci Lett 228:33–36, 1997.

114. Apfel SC, Kessler JA, Adornato BT, et al: Recombinant human nerve growth factor in the treatment of diabetic polyneuropathy: NGF Study Group Neurology 51:695–702, 1998.

115. Apfel SC, Schwartz S, Adornato BT, et al: Efficacy and safety of recombinant human nerve growth factor in patients with diabetic polyneuropathy: A randomized controlled trial. JAMA 284:2215–2221, 2000.

116. Wellmer A, Misra VP, Sharief MK, et al: A double-blind placebo-controlled clinical trial of recombinant human brain-derived neurotrophic factor (rhBDNF) in diabetic polyneuropathy. J Peripher Nerv Syst 6:204–210, 2001.

117. Purves T, Middlemas A, Agthong S, et al: A role for mitogen-activated protein kinases in the etiology of diabetic neuropathy. FASEB J 15:2508–2514, 2001.

118. Middlemas A, Delcroix JD, Sayers NM, et al: Enhanced activation of axonally transported stress-activated protein kinases in peripheral nerve in diabetic neuropathy is prevented by neurotrophin-3. Brain 126:1671–1682, 2003.

119. Fernyhough P, Schmidt RE: Neurofilaments in diabetic neuropathy. Int Rev Neurobiol 50:115–144, 2002.

120. Fernyhough P, Gallagher A, Averill SA, et al: Aberrant neurofilament phosphorylation in sensory neurons of rats with diabetic neuropathy. Diabetes 48:881–889, 1999.

121. Giannini C, Dyck PJ: Basement membrane reduplication and pericyte degeneration precede development of diabetic polyneuropathy and are associated with its severity. Ann Neurol 37:498–504, 1995.

122. Malik RA: The pathology of human diabetic neuropathy. Diabetes 46(Suppl 2):S50–S53, 1997.

123. Dyck PJ, Giannini C: Pathologic alterations in the diabetic neuropathies of humans: A review. J Neuropathol Exp Neurol 55:1181–1193, 1996.

124. Bomers K, Braendgaard H, Flyvbjerg A, et al: Redistribution of axoplasm in the motor root in experimental diabetes. Acta Neuropathol (Berl) 92:98–101, 1996.

125. Britland ST, Young RJ, Sharma AK, et al: Association of painful and painless diabetic polyneuropathy with different patterns of nerve fibre

degeneration and regeneration. Diabetes 39:898–908, 1990.

126. Sima AAF, Bril V, Nathaniel V, et al: Regeneration and repair of myelinated fibres in sural-nerve biopsy specimens from patients with diabetic neuropathy treated with Sorbinil. N Engl J Med 319:548–555, 1988.

127. Sima AAF, Nathaniel V, Bril V, et al: Histopathological heterogeneity of neuropathy in insulin-dependent and non-insulin dependent diabetes, and demonstration of axo-glial dysjunction in human diabetic neuropathy. J Clin Invest 81:349–364, 1988.

128. Llewelyn JG, Gilbey SG, Thomas PK, et al: Sural nerve morphometry in diabetic autonomic and painful sensory neuropathy. Brain 114:867–892, 1991.

129. Engelstead JK, Davies JL, Giannini C, et al: No evidence for axonal atrophy in human diabetic polyneuropathy. J Neuropathol Exp Neurol 56:255–262, 1997.

130. Malik RA, Veves A, Walker D, et al: Sural nerve fibre pathology in diabetic patients with mild neuropathy: Relationship to pain, quantitative sensory testing and peripheral nerve electrophysiology. Acta Neuropathol (Berl) 101:367–374, 2001.

131. Sima AAF, Prashar A, Nathaniel V, et al: Overt diabetic neuropathy: Repair of axo-glial dysjunction and axonal atrophy by aldose reductase inhibition and its correlation to improvement in nerve conduction velocity. Diabet Med 10:115–121, 1993.

132. Thomas PK, Beamish NG, Small JR, et al: Paranodal structure in diabetic sensory polyneuropathy Acta Neuropathol (Berl) 92:614–620, 1996.

133. Giannini C, Dyck PJ: Axoglial dysjunction: A critical appraisal of definition, techniques, and previous results. Microsc Res Tech 34:436–444, 1996.

134. Kalichman MW, Powell HC, Mizisin AP: Reactive, degenerative, and proliferative Schwann cell responses in experimental galactose and human diabetic neuropathy. Acta Neuropathol (Berl) 95:47–56, 1998.

135. Bradley JL, Thomas PK, King RH, et al: Myelinated nerve fibre regeneration in diabetic sensory polyneuropathy: Correlation with type of diabetes. Acta Neuropathol (Berl) 90:403–410, 1995.

136. Veves A, Malik RA, Lye RH, et al: The relationship between sural nerve morphometric findings and measures of peripheral nerve function in mild diabetic neuropathy. Diabet Med 8:917–921, 1991.

137. Russell JW, Karnes JL, Dyck PJ: Sural nerve myelinated fiber density differences associated with meaningful changes in clinical and electrophysiological measurements. J Neurol Sci 135:114–117, 1996.

138. Britland ST, Young RJ, Sharma AK, et al: Vagus nerve morphology in

diabetic gastropathy. Diabet Med 7:780–787, 1990.

139. Schmidt RE: Neuropathology and pathogenesis of diabetic autonomic neuropathy. Int Rev Neurobiol 50:257–292, 2002.

140. Schmidt RE: Age-related sympathetic ganglionic neuropathology: Human pathology and animal models. Auton Neurosci 96:63–72, 2002.

141. Tesfaye S, Harris N, Jakubowski J, et al: Impaired blood flow and arterio-venous shunting in human diabetic neuropathy: A novel technique of nerve photography and fluorescein angiography. Diabetologia 36:1266–1274, 1993.

142. Tesfaye S, Malik RA, Harris N, et al: Arterio-venous shunting and proliferating new vessels in acute painful neuropathy of rapid glycaemic control (insulin neuritis). Diabetologia 39:329–335, 1996.

143. Korthals JK, Gieron MA, Dyck PJ: Intima of epineurial arterioles is increased in diabetic polyneuropathy. Neurology 38:1582–1586, 1988.

144. Grover-Johnson NM, Baumann FG, Imparato AM, et al: Abnormal innervation of lower limb epineurial arterioles in human diabetes. Diabetologia 20:31–38, 1981.

145. Beggs J, Johnson PC, Olafsen A, et al: Transperineurial arterioles in human sural nerve. J Neuropathol Exp Neurol 50:704–718, 1991.

146. Malik RA, Tesfaye S, Thompson SD, et al: Transperineurial capillary abnormalities in the sural nerve of patients with diabetic neuropathy. Microvasc Res 48:236–245, 1994.

147. Ghani M, Malik RA, Walker D, et al: Perineurial abnormalities in the spontaneously diabetic dog. Acta Neuropathol 97:98–102, 1999.

148. Giannini C, Dyck PJ: Basement membrane reduplication and pericyte degeneration precede development of diabetic polyneuropathy and are associated with its severity. Ann Neurol 37:498–504, 1995.

149. Thrainsdottir S, Malik RA, Dahlin LB, et al: Endoneurial capillary abnormalities presage deterioration of glucose tolerance and accompany peripheral neuropathy in man. Diabetes 52:2615–2622, 2003.

150. Malik RA, Veves A, Masson EA, et al: Endoneurial capillary abnormalities in mild human diabetic neuropathy. J Neurol Neurosurg Psychiatry 55:557–561, 1992.

151. Bradley J, Thomas PK, King RHM, et al: Morphometry of endoneurial capillaries in diabetic sensory and autonomic neuropathy. Diabetologia 33:611–618, 1990.

152. Britland ST, Young RJ, Sharma AK, et al: Relationship of endoneurial capillary abnormalities to type and severity of diabetic polyneuropathy. Diabetes 39:909–913, 1990.

153. Malik RA, Newrick PG, Sharma AK, et al: Microangiopathy in human diabetic neuropathy: Relationship

between capillary abnormalities and the severity of neuropathy. Diabetologia 32:92–102, 1989.

154. Sima AAF, Nathaniel V, Prashar A, et al: Endoneurial microvessels in human diabetic neuropathy: Endothelial cell dysjunction and lack of treatment effect by aldose reductase inhibitor. Diabetes 40:1090–1099, 1991.

155. McArthur JC, Stocks AE, Hauer P, et al: Epidermal nerve fibre density: Normative reference range and diagnostic efficiency. Arch Neurol 55:1513–1520, 1998.

156. Holland NR, Crawford TO, Hauer P, et al: Small-fiber sensory neuropathies: Clinical course and neuropathology of idiopathic cases. Ann Neurol 44:47–59, 1998.

157. Kennedy WR, Nolano M, Wendelschafer-Crabb G, et al: A skin blister method to study epidermal nerves in peripheral nerve disease. Muscle Nerve 22:360–371, 1999.

158. Hirai A, Yasuda H, Joko M, et al: Evaluation of diabetic neuropathy through the quantitation of cutaneous nerves. J Neurol Sci 172:55–62, 2000.

159. Polydefkis M, Hauer P, Griffin JW, McArthur JC: Skin biopsy as a tool to assess distal small fiber innervation in diabetic neuropathy. Diabet Technol Ther 3:23–28, 2001.

160. Yaneda H, Tereda M, Maeda K, et al: Diabetic neuropathy and nerve regeneration. Prog Neurobiol 69:229–285, 2003.

161. Malik RA, Kallinikos P, Abbott CA, et al: Corneal confocal microscopy: A non-invasive surrogate of nerve fibre damage and repair in diabetic patients. Diabetologia 46:683–688, 2003.

162. Kallinikos P, Berhanu M, O'Donnell C, et al: Corneal nerve tortuosity in diabetic patients with neuropathy. Invest Ophthalmol Vis Sci 45:418–422, 2004.

163. Krishnan STM, Rayman G: New treatments for diabetic neuropathy: Symptomatic treatment. Curr Diabetes Rep 3:459–467, 2003.

164. Bierhaus A, Humpert PM, Rudofsky G, et al: New treatments for diabetic neuropathy: Pathogenetically oriented treatment. Curr Diabetes Rep 3:452–458, 2003.

165. Oyibo S, Prasad YD, Jackson NJ, et al: The relationship between blood glucose excursions and, painful diabetic neuropathy: A pilot study. Diabetic Med 19:870–873, 2002.

166. Boulton AJM: Treatment of symptomataic diabetic neuropathy. Diabetes Metab Res Rev 19(Suppl 1):S16–S21, 2003.

167. Sindrup SH: Antidepressants in the treatment of diabetic neuropathy symptoms. Dan Med Bull 41:66–78, 1994.

168. Ziegler D: Pharmacological treatment of painful diabetic neuropathy. In Veves A (ed): Contemporary Endocrinology: Clinical Management of Diabetic Neuropathy. Totowa, NJ, Humana Press, 1998, pp 147–169.

169. Backonja M, Beydoun A, Edwards KR, et al: Gabapentin for the symptomatic treatment of painful neuropathy in patients with diabetes mellitus. JAMA 280:1831–1836, 1998.

170. Eisenberg E, Lurie Y, Braker C, et al: Lamotrigine reduces painful diabetic neuropathy: A randomized, controlled trial. Neurology 57:505–509, 2001.

171. Malik RA: Current and future strategies for the management of diabetic neuropathy. Treat Endocrinol 2:389–400, 2003.

172. Harati Y, Gooch C, Swenson M, et al: Double-blind randomized trial for tramodol for the treatment of the pain of diabetic neuropathy. Neurology 50:1842–1846, 1998.

173. Yuen KC, Baker NR, Rayman G: Treatment of chronic painful diabetic neuropathy with isosorbide dinitrate spray: A double-blind, placebo-controlled cross-over study. Diabetes Care 25:1699–1703, 2002.

174. Abuaisha BB, Costanzi JB, Boulton AJM: Acupuncture for the treatment of chronic painful peripheral diabetic neuropathy: A long-term study. Diabetes Res Clin Pract 39:115–121, 1998.

175. Horrobin DF: Gamma-linolenic acid in the treatment of diabetic neuropathy. In Boulton AJM (ed): Diabetic Neuropathy. Lancaster, UK, Marius Press, 1996, pp 183–195.

176. Hounsom L, Horrobin DF, Tritschler H, et al: A lipoic acid-gamma linolenic acid conjugate is effective against multiple indices of experimental diabetic neuropathy. Diabetologia 41:839–843, 1998.

177. Shotton HR, Clarke S, Lincoln J: The effectiveness of treatments of diabetic autonomic neuropathy is not the same in autonomic nerves supplying different organs. Diabetes 52:157–164, 2003.

178. Malik RA, Williamson S, Abbott CA, et al: Effect of the ACE inhibitor trandolopril on human diabetic neuropathy: A randomized, controlled double-blind trial. Lancet 352:1978–1981, 1998.

179. Vinik A, Tesfaye S, Zhang D, Bastyr E: LY333531 treatment improves diabetic peripheral neuropathy with symptoms. Diabetes 51(Suppl 2):A79, 2002.

180. Amin P, Sturrock ND: A pilot study of the beneficial effect of Amantadine in the treatment of painful diabetic peripheral neuropathy. Diabet Med 20:114–118, 2003.

181. Rendell MS, Rajfer J, Wicker PA, et al: Sildenafil in the treatment of erectile dysfunction in men with diabetes: A randomized controlled trial. JAMA 281:421–426, 1999.

182. Boulton AJM, Selam JL, Sweeney M, Ziegler D: Sildenafil nitrate for the treatment of erectile dysfunction in men with type 2 diabetes. Diabetologia 44:1296–1301, 2001.

183. Padma-Nathan H: Efficacy and tolerability of tadalafil, a novel phosphodiesterase-5 inhibitor, in treatment of erectile dysfunction. Am J Cardiol 92(9A):19M–25M, 2003.

184. Keating GM, Scott LJ: Vardenafil: A review of its use in erectile dysfunction. Drugs 63:2673–2703, 2003.

185. Shaw JE, Abbott CA, Tindle K, et al: A randomized controlled trial of topical glycopyrrolate, the first specific treatment for diabetic gustatory sweating. Diabetologia 40:299–301, 1997.

Diabetic Nephropathy

Yalemzewd Woredekal and Eli A. Friedman

In this first decade of the twenty-first century, diabetes mellitus is universally recognized as the leading cause of irreversible renal failure—unfortunately termed *end-stage renal disease* (ESRD)—in industrialized (well-fed) nations. Tracking both the incidence and prevalence of ESRD attributed to diabetes indicates an annual growth rate over the past decade in excess of 9%. According to the 2003 report of the U.S. Renal Data System (USRDS) (Fig. 69-1), in 2001, of 398,553 patients in the United States receiving either dialytic therapy or a kidney transplant, 142,963 had diabetes,[1] a prevalence rate of 35.95%. The full impact of diabetes-related kidney disease is shown by the incidence rate of 44.5% in 2001, during which 42,813 of 96,295 new (incident) cases of ESRD were attributed to diabetes (Fig. 69-2). Earlier assessments of the relative severity of renal injury in diabetes led to the erroneous inference that nephropathy was both of lower prevalence and less severe in type 2 diabetes as compared with type 1 diabetes. More recent retrospective and prospective observation of kidney function during the course of types 1 and 2 diabetes uncovered a risk of progression of diabetic nephropathy equivalent to that of ESRD. In both types of diabetes, nephropathy follows a predictable course, starting with microalbuminuria, evolving to proteinuria and azotemia, culminating in ESRD.

Elsewhere in this book (see Chapter 56), the management of diabetes as an endocrine disorder is reviewed. This chapter presents a nephrologist's perspective of diabetes as the dominant cause of renal disintegration. Effective strategies slow the course of nephropathy by normalization of hypertensive blood pressure, establishment of euglycemia, and perhaps by restriction of dietary protein intake. Diabetes at every stage of deteriorating renal function, when compared with other causes of ESRD, induces greater morbidity and higher mortality due to concomitant comorbid conditions, such as coronary artery and cerebrovascular disease. The diabetic patient with kidney disease is sicker and less likely to achieve rehabilitation than are those by other afflicted renal disorders with less severe extrarenal comorbidity. In this chapter, the clinical consequences of loss of renal function in diabetes are discussed and options for management of ESRD are evaluated. Additionally, a novel approach to treatment for diabetic nephropathy without necessarily requiring euglycemia is assessed.

HISTORY OF DIABETIC NEPHROPATHY

Recognition of a renal syndrome specific to diabetes mellitus lagged behind appreciation of diabetes-induced injury in other organ systems. As recounted by Lundbaek,[2] Ehrlich's technique of iodine staining in 1882, which demonstrated accumulation of glycogen in renal tubular cells of diabetic patients,[3] explained Armanni's finding in 1877[4] and Ebstein's report[5] in 1883 of renal tubular vacuolization, necrosis, and glycogen accumulation. "Glycogen nephrosis," formerly accepted as pathologic proof of diabetes mellitus, is now understood to be a reversible phenomenon, not confined to the kidney, of glycogen deposition in renal tubular cells, cardiac muscle, and pancreatic β cells in diabetic persons with sustained hyperglycemia.

For the next 53 years, no advance in understanding of renal pathology in diabetes was evident until the keystone report by Kimmelstiel and Wilson[6] in 1936. They described a striking hyaline thickening of the intercapillary connective tissue of the glomerular tufts, with the formation of nodules, in a retrospective autopsy study of eight patients, seven of whom

INCIDENT ESRD PATIENTS DIABETES and TOTAL

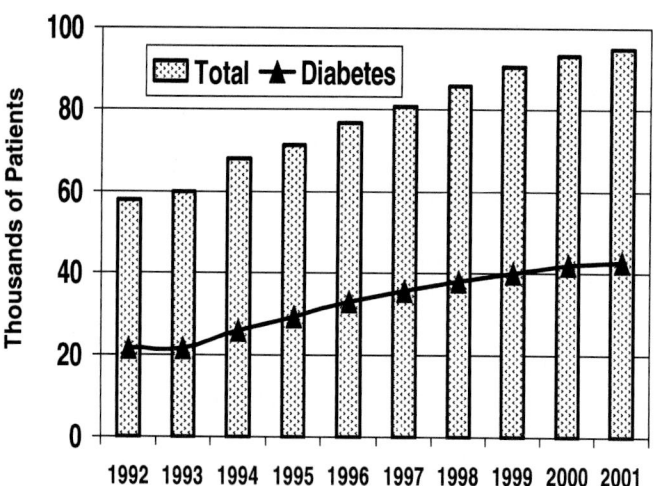

Figure 69-1

intensive insulin treatment, correctly theorized that the increased kidney size per se causes GFR increase in type 1 diabetes.[12]

At the close of the 1970s, type 1 diabetes had been linked to microalbuminuria, nephromegaly, and glomerular hyperfiltration. The next step in unraveling the pathogenesis of diabetic nephropathy was the product of meticulous study of sequential biopsies of kidneys in type 1 diabetes.[13] Mauer and colleagues[14] concluded in 1984 that "the critical lesion of diabetic nephropathy which ultimately leads to organ failure is the expansion of the glomerular mesangium." Subsequently, the Kimmelstiel-Wilson mesangial nodule was shown in some instances to undergo lysis (mesangiolysis).[15] Most recently, Mauer's long-term study of the effect on early diabetic nephropathy in type 1 diabetic recipients of pancreas transplants indicates that after a decade of euglycemia, Kimmelstiel-Wilson lesions may be reversible.[16] What is now clearly established is that the appearance, severity, and progression of glomerulopathy in diabetic individuals is a consequence of hyperglycemia, though aggravating variables are operational (Fig. 69-3).

had type 2 diabetes (one patient was admitted moribund with no clinical history), at Boston City Hospital. Nephrotic edema, massive proteinuria, and hypertension were linked to the pathologic findings of nodular and diffuse intercapillary glomerulosclerosis defining what is now termed *Kimmelstiel-Wilson disease,* a synonym for diabetic nephropathy.

Two technical advances facilitated further understanding of the diabetic kidney. Introduction of percutaneous renal biopsy by Iverson and Brun[7] in 1951 permitted correlation of preterminal morphologic findings with clinical perturbations in the diabetic kidney. Subsequently, linking pathophysiology and pathology, Keen and coworkers[8] in 1969 first detected a small but distinctly abnormal increase in urinary albumin excretion (30–150 mg/day) termed *microalbuminuria,* previously undetected by usual clinical urinalysis, in newly diagnosed type 1 diabetic patients.

The significance of microalbuminuria was clarified by Mogensen[9] who in 1971 began a productive series of studies of protein excretion in diabetic patients which culminated in recognizing proteinuria as an early renal perturbation in diabetic nephropathy. By 1972, Mogensen[10] had also found that at onset of type 1 diabetes, glomerular filtration rate (GFR) may be increased by more than 40% over normal (hyperfiltration), whereas renal plasma flow is also significantly elevated, but to a lesser extent. One year later, Mogensen and Andersen[11] reported nephromegaly as a component of type 1 diabetes. These investigators, after they were able to reduce both nephromegaly and GFR by inducing euglycemia by

EPIDEMIOLOGY OF DIABETIC NEPHROPATHY

A cumulative incidence of diabetic nephropathy has been documented after 20 to 25 years of diabetes in both type 1 and type 2 individuals.[17,18] Recent studies demonstrated substantial reduction in incidence,[19,20] for example, a study from Sweden showed a substantial decline in albuminuria after 25 years of diabetes from 30% in patients in whom diabetes developed in the period 1961 to 1965 to 8.5% in those with onset from 1966 to 1970.[19] Similarly, the Steno Diabetes Center reported that the cumulative incidence of diabetic nephropathy after 20 years fell from 31.1% to 13.7%.[20] Improved glycemic control, lower blood pressure, and reduced prevalence of smoking rates were associated with the lower incidence of nephropathy.

The incidence of diabetic nephropathy is about 1% to 2% per year in patients with type 1 diabetes.[21] Among the young of nonwhite origin with type 2 diabetes, such as the Pima Indians, Japanese, and African-Americans, the incidence of nephropathy is similar to that of type 1 diabetes.[22–24] By con-

INCIDENT ESRD PATIENTS 2001 DIABETES and ALL OTHERS

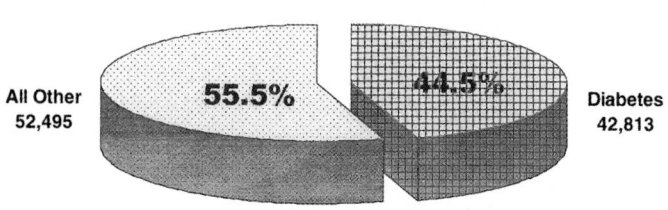

Figure 69-2

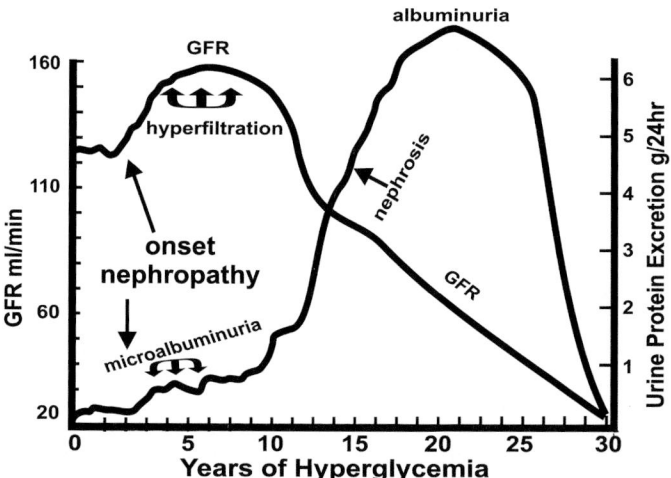

Figure 69-3 The course of nephropathy in both type 1 and type 2 diabetes can be followed by two main variables: proteinuria and glomerular filtration rate (GFR). The earliest manifestations of glomerulopathy are microalbuminuria and hyperfiltration. Thereafter, progressive increase in urinary protein and decrease in GFR signal renal deterioration. A nephrotic syndrome is typical in both diabetes types. Azotemia is a late sign of far-advanced nephropathy.

trast, the incidence of diabetic nephropathy is much lower in elderly white type 2 diabetic patients[25,26] than in nonwhites.

Several large population studies found substantial racial and ethnic differences in the incidence rate of ESRD attributed to type 2 diabetes.[27] The highest incidence of ESRD secondary to diabetes has been reported in Native Americans followed by Hispanics, and African-Americans. In Pima Indians, the cumulative incidence of ESRD after onset of clinically detectable proteinuria is 40% at 10 years and 61% at 15 years. By contrast, ESRD develops in only 11% of Caucasians after 10 years of proteinuria and in 17% after 15 years.[27] The incidence of diabetic ESRD is 2.6 times higher in African-Americans,[24] and six times higher in Hispanics when compared to whites.[28] Accumulating evidence indicates that patients with type 2 diabetes in India, Japan, and Korea have a high prevalence of microalbuminuria and diabetes-related ESRD compared with whites.[29-31] These ethnic and racial differences in the incidence of diabetic nephropathy reflect a complex interplay between genetic and environmental factors.

The prevalence of treated ESRD due to diabetic nephropathy has more than quadrupled over the past 30 years. Whether there has been an actual increase in the number of diabetic patients who develop renal failure or a changing attitude of acceptance of diabetic patients into renal failure programs is undetermined. Nevertheless, by 1992, the progressive increase in incidence recorded yearly over the preceding decade established diabetes mellitus as the most prevalent disorder leading to ESRD in the United States, Japan, and most nations in industrialized Europe. According to the USRDS, in 1991,[32] of 43,826 patients begun on therapy for ESRD during 1989, 14,671 (33.47%) had diabetes, an incidence of 58 per million population. Until the 1980s, diabetic patients with failing kidneys were discouraged from seeking treatment by maintenance dialysis or kidney transplantation because of the consensus of nephrologists and transplant surgeons that they suffered unacceptably high mortality and morbidity, whereas rehabilitation was unobtainable in survivors. Such negative thinking continues through much of the world today where treatment rates for diabetic ESRD patients remain far below those in the United States.[33] Gradually, however, the cumulative effects of careful regulation of hypertension and hyperglycemia have improved the long-term outcome to the extent that restrained optimism has replaced futility in advising renal transplantation as the preferred therapy for ESRD in diabetes. Medicare statistics counted diabetic nephropathy as the diagnosis listed for 1607 of 8058 (20.7%) kidney transplants performed in 1989 in the United States,[34] the proportion of kidney recipients with diabetes rose to 25.6% (3858 of 15,060) in 2001.[1] In Europe, the proportion of kidney transplants performed in diabetic recipients is smaller (about 18%). Accompanying the growing acceptance of kidney transplantation in diabetes is a mounting success, for at least 5 years, of pancreatic transplants in type 1 diabetes, converting what has previously been thought experimental surgery to an established therapy (see later discussion).

GENETIC PREDISPOSITION TO DIABETIC NEPHROPATHY

The prevalence of nephropathy associated with type 1 diabetes rises with increased duration but levels out at around 15 years, when a cumulative prevalence of about 50% is reached[35]; a linkage between duration and nephropathy is less clear in type 2 diabetes, where the time of disease onset is blurred. Only a subset of diabetic patients are at risk of developing nephropathy, in contrast to retinopathy, whose prevalence rises progressively with increased duration of diabetes so that nearly all diabetic patients develop

retinopathy if they live long enough.[36] Genetic modifiers determine at least some of the susceptibility of diabetic nephropathy.

Strongest evidence points to a familial risk for diabetic nephropathy in type 1 diabetes.[36-38] The Diabetes Control and Complications Trial (DCCT) found familial aggregation in some type 1 diabetic patients.[39] Additionally, familial aggregation of nephropathy in type 2 diabetes has also been reported.[40-43] For example, Pettitt and colleagues reported in Pima Indians, proteinuria occurred in 14.3% of diabetic offspring of diabetic parents if neither parent had proteinuria, compared to 22.9% and 45.9% if one or both parents, respectively, had proteinuria.[40] This finding led to the suggestion that predisposition to diabetic nephropathy may be inherited as a dominant trait.[36,44] The genetic background of diabetic nephropathy is believed to be polygenic. Polymorphisms of different genes such as the renin-angiotensin system and aldose reductase system has been suggested to contribute to the development of diabetic nephropathy.

The renin-angiotensin system is thought to play an important role in the pathophysiology of kidney disease. Angiotensin-converting enzyme (ACE) insertion/deletion (ID) polymorphism, which determines most ACE interindividual variance, was proposed as a genetic marker for diabetic nephropathy. In the diabetic mouse, upregulation of the renin-angiotensin system is associated with accelerated nephropathy.[45] In human, several studies have shown the association between the DD genotype of ACE gene polymorphism and development and progression of diabetic nephropathy in both type 1[46-49] and type 2 diabetic patients.[50,51]

Hadjadj and colleagues in a prospective observational study of 310 type 1 diabetic patients were followed for a median duration of 6 years (range, 2–9 years). At entry of the study, 251 (81%) patients had no nephropathy, while 35 (11%) had incipient nephropathy, 18 (6%) had established nephropathy, and 6 (2%) had advance nephropathy. The main end point of the study was the occurrence of a renal event defined as the progression to a higher stage of diabetic nephropathy. Occurrence of renal events was significantly influenced by ACE genotype II versus ID versus DD ($P < 0.03$), with a dominant deleterious effect of the D allele: ID or DD versus II (adjusted hazard ratio, 5.0; confidence interval, 1.5–16.6). Other contributors were high glycohemoglobin and systolic blood pressure.[48] In similar study in type 2 diabetes, Jeffers also found the DD genotype to be an independent risk factor for diabetic nephropathy with an odds ratio 2.8 (95% confidence interval, 1.4–5.5).[50] Other similar studies have been conducted in populations with diverse ethnic groups but not all showed similar findings.[52-55]

In a meta-analysis done by Fujisawa and colleagues of 4773 diabetic patients from 18 studies with (n = 2495) and without (n = 2278) renal complications, the D allele was significantly associated with diabetic nephropathy ($P < 0.0001$). The association was significant both in type 1 ($P < 0.05$) and type 2 diabetes mellitus ($P < 0.005$).[56]

Aldose reductase is the first rate-limiting enzyme of the polyol pathway in the metabolism of glucose and nicotine adenine dinucleotide phosphorylation hydroxylase (NADPH)-dependent reduction of a broad range of carbonyl compounds. The polyol pathway is thought by some to play an important role in the pathogenesis of diabetic nephropathy. Polymorphism in the aldose reductase promotor gene has been linked to susceptibility to diabetic nephropathy in both type 1 and type 2 diabetic patients.[57-60] In particular, the polymorphism in the (A-C)n microsatellite repeat sequence may modulate expression of the aldose reductase gene. Among the eight different alleles at this site, the Z-2 allele is associated with upregulated expression of the aldose reductase gene in the presence of hyperglycemia[59] and increased prevalence of the nephropathy.[57] Similarly, Heeson and coworkers studied the DNA from 275 white, British patients with type 1 diabetes and 102 normal healthy control patients typed for a (C-A)n dinucleotide repeat polymorphic marked in the aldose reductase gene. The nephropathy group had a significant decrease in the Z/Z+2 genotype compared with the uncomplicated patients (10.7% vs. 44.7%) and an increased frequency of the Z/Z–2 genotype. Individuals with the Z+2 are more than seven times less likely to develop diabetic renal disease than those with Z–2.[60] However, not all studies support this association.[61–64] In addition, meta-analysis has shown evidence of a role of another polymorphism of aldose reductase gene (specially the 106 polymorphism) to be a better marker than the microsatellite in diabetic nephropathy.[62] More studies are required to confirm these results and to establish whether these markers have a functional role in diabetic nephropathy.

NATURAL HISTORY OF DIABETIC NEPHROPATHY

Nephropathy due to nodular and diffuse intercapillary glomerular sclerosis develops in about one third of those with type 1 diabetes and an imprecisely defined, although probably equivalent proportion, of those with type 2 diabetes. Diabetic nephropathy follows a characteristic course starting with microalbuminuria (see later discussion), followed in turn by constant or fixed proteinuria and worsening azotemia.[65–67] Prior to recent studies in the Pima Indian tribe of Arizona[68] and a small group of blacks in Brooklyn, New York,[69,70] knowledge of the sequence of perturbations in type 2 diabetes was speculative and limited to inferences drawn from type 1 diabetes and animal models of diabetes, especially the streptozotocin-induced diabetic rat. Renal involvement in type 1 diabetes has been divided into five stages.

STAGE 1: GLOMERULAR HYPERFILTRATION AND RENOMEGALY

Greater-than-normal inulin clearances early in the course of type 1 diabetes were recognized by Cambier[71] in 1934 and confirmed by Spuhler[72] in 1946. Repeated rediscovery of glomerular hyperfiltration using radionuclide techniques or creatinine clearance[73–75] was reported over the next 20 years. At onset of type 1 diabetes, GFRs of up to 140% of normal values are present in the large majority of individuals.[76] No single pathogenesis fully explains both the nephromegaly and glomerular hyperfiltration of type 1 diabetes; a correlation between renal enlargement and glomerular hyperfunction has been inferred from the correction of both perturbations after establishment of euglycemia.[77] Intensive insulin therapy normalizes hyperglycemia and corrects glomerular hyperfiltration[78]; GFR begins to decline within 8 days of initiation of insulin therapy,[79–81] and falls further during 3 months of therapy. A substantial subset, 25% to 40% of individuals with type 1 diabetes, achieving usual levels of plasma glucose excursion under typical insulin therapy, manifest a persistently elevated GFR,[82–85] and it is within this subgroup of hyperfiltering patients that the first reductions in GFR are subsequently noted,[86,87] with progression to clinical nephropathy (proteinuria and azotemia).[88–90]

Numerous metabolic and several hemodynamic perturbations occur in type 1 diabetes, no one of which has been clearly identified as the single or prime causative factor responsible for glomerulosclerosis in type 1 diabetes. Confounding efforts to clarify the pathogenesis of diabetic nephropathy is the fact that less than one half of all individuals with type 1 diabetes ever manifest clinical nephropathy (proteinuria or azotemia). Glomerular hyperfiltration is probably not an independent risk factor for progressive nephropathy.[91,92]

STAGE 2: EARLY GLOMERULAR LESIONS

Expansion of the glomerular mesangial matrix and thickening of the glomerular basement membrane (GBM) are subtle morphologic changes noted 18 to 36 months after onset of type 1 diabetes,[93] which may become pronounced after 2 to 5 years.[94] Thickening of the GBM is present whether or not progressive nephropathy develops.[95] Expansion of the glomerular mesangium is seen in type 1 diabetes and may increase markedly to the extent that nearly all capillaries are occluded despite the increase in glomerular volume (Figs. 69-4 to 69-6).[96] During this stage of morphologic change, which extends from 4 or 5 to 15 years after onset of type 1 diabetes, exercise-induced microalbuminuria may be the only clinical evidence of renal involvement.[97] A supplemental perspective of the early glomerular changes in type 1 diabetes has been provided from study of kidneys from nondiabetic donors transplanted into diabetic recipients. In biopsies of these kidneys, Mauer and coworkers[98] observed the same sequence of changes—mesangial matrix expansion and GBM thickening within 3 to 5 years after transplant. Reversal of these sequential changes in type 1 diabetes has been noted after 10 years of euglycemia afforded by a functioning pancreas transplant.[16]

STAGE 3: INCIPIENT DIABETIC NEPHROPATHY: THE MICROALBUMINURIC STAGE

Proteinuria is a sign of renal injury. Screening for proteinuria is contingent on the sensitivity of tests available in hospital and clinical laboratories. Falling into disuse, the highly reliable and simple heat and acetic acid test for urinary albumin becomes positive when urinary protein content, which consists mainly of albumin (about 50% in diabetic nephropathy), increases to about 150 mg/dL. Of presently available dipsticks to detect urinary protein content, the Albustix test commonly employed to detect proteinuria is positive when total protein excretion exceeds 200 mg/L, about 50% of which is albumin, thereby delimiting the lower limit of clinical proteinuria, termed *macroalbuminuria*. Several methods for quantifying low concentrations of urinary albumin are available, including radioimmunoassay, nephelometric immunoassay, and enzyme-linked immunosorbent assay; a semiquantitative dipstick test has also been introduced (Micro-Bumintest, Miles Laboratories, Elkhart, IN).

These techniques for detecting small quantities of urinary protein agree on an upper daily limit of urinary albumin

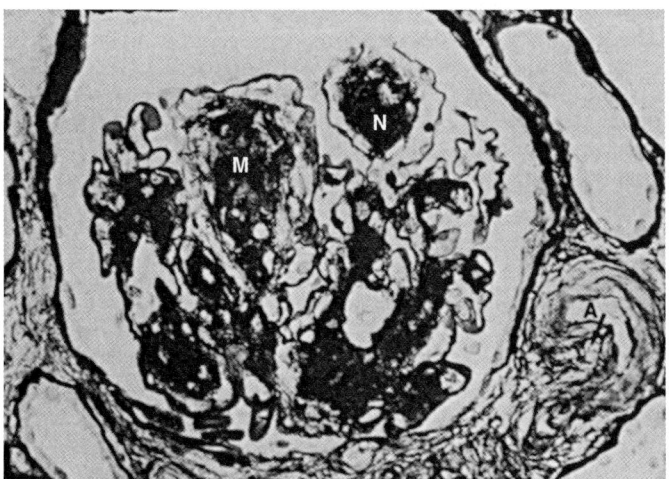

Figure 69-4 Silver stain of glomerulus from a patient with type 1 diabetes of 10 years' duration. Mesangial expansion (M) and a mesangial nodule (N) are evident. Note the luminal characteristic of arteriolosclerosis in the glomerular arteriole (A).

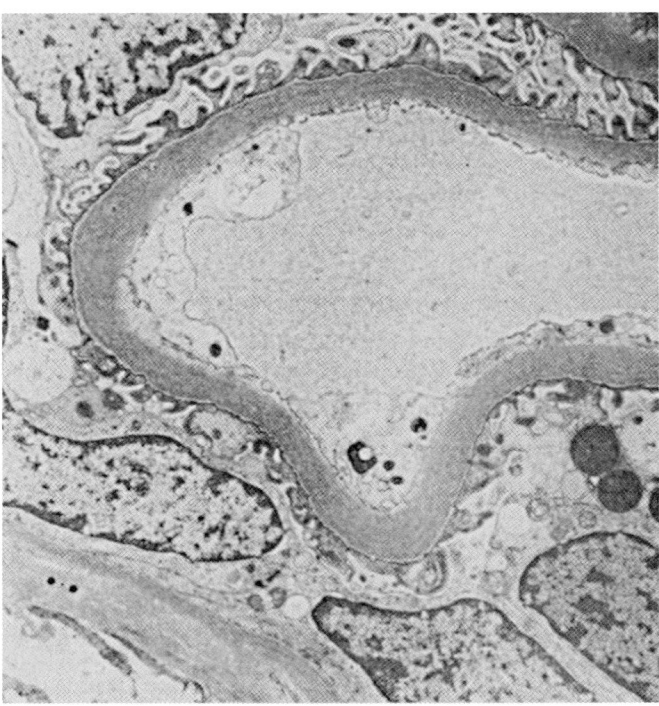

Figure 69-5 Glomerular capillary loop from a 16-year-old girl who had type 1 diabetes for 6 years. Poor metabolic control was associated with multiple episodes of ketoacidosis. The thick (7452 Å) glomerular basement membrane is nearly three times the normal width for adolescents and young adults (2700 Å) (×11,193).

excretion in healthy adults of less than 30 mg. Microalbuminuria, defined as urinary protein excretion greater than 30 mg per day and less than 200 mg per day, is a sign of renal damage in type 1 diabetes that predicts later nephropathy and, ultimately, ESRD (Fig. 69-7).

Otherwise asymptomatic diabetic patients who excrete more than 30 mg per day of albumin are now thought to be expressing the earliest stage of diabetic nephropathy.[99] Renal involvement limited to microalbuminuria is probably reversible with treatment with an ACE inhibitor. The absolute correlation between microalbuminuria and subse-

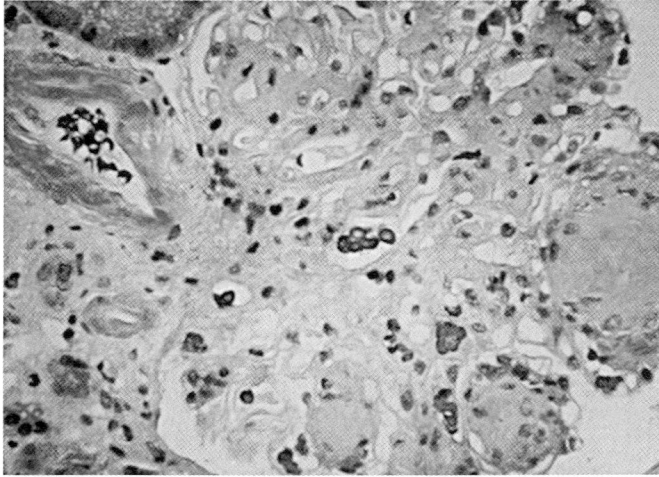

Figure 69-6 Advanced nodular intercapillary glomerulosclerosis from a man with type 1 diabetes of 15 years' duration. Only a few capillaries remain patent. Assessment of glomerular function in this patient was normal, illustrating the dissociation between structure and function often found in diabetic glomerulopathy.

Progression of Diabetic Kidney Disease

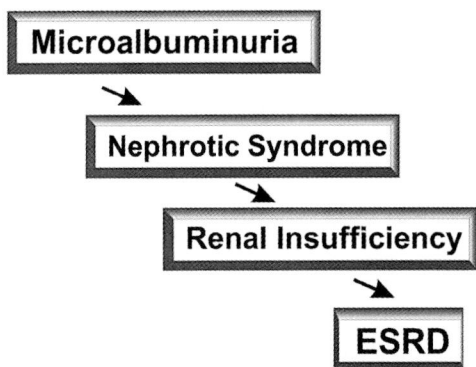

Figure 69-7 The usual stages of nephropathy in diabetes. Renal insufficiency may begin while urinary protein excretion persists in the nephrotic range (>3.5 g/day). End-stage renal disease (ESRD) is the term applied to irreversible renal failure that limits survival.

quent clinical nephropathy in type 1 diabetes is uncertain, as only a small number of white patients manifesting microalbuminuria have been followed for the decade or longer required for this transition. Because only about one third of individuals with type 1 diabetes, at worst, progress to renal insufficiency, intervention in terms of dietary protein restriction and administration of an ACE inhibitor is delayed by some clinicians until a decline in GFR or macroproteinuria develops; they worry that the pharmacologic and psychodynamic side effects of attempting to prevent nephropathy may entail greater risk than the chance of developing renal failure. Microalbuminuria may be an inconstant finding, with great variability in daily total protein excretion.[100] Digestion of many studies of microalbuminuria in nonproteinuric individuals with type 1 diabetes indicates a prevalence of 10% to 28% followed in 10 to 20 years by persistent and increasing clinical proteinuria or macroalbuminuria.[101] Several studies of populations with type 2 diabetes inferred a similar prevalence of microalbuminuria ranging from 13% to 30%.[102–104]

The prevalence of microalbuminuria is increased by hypertension, uncontrolled hyperglycemia, strenuous exercise, urinary tract infections, hypervolemia, and dietary protein loads. Considering the range and frequency of the variables that influence microalbuminuria, it is not surprising that the reproducibility of surveys of microalbuminuria is poor, especially when urine collection periods are shorter than 24 hours. In fact, fluctuations in daily urinary albumin excretion yield a coefficient of variation greater than 45%.[105–108] For consistency, at least three measurements of urinary albumin should be made over the course of several months.

Approximately 25% to 40% of individuals with type 1 diabetes have constant microalbuminuria after 5 to 15 years.[109,110] Without specific intervention, as detailed later, once microalbuminuria becomes constant, a progressive downhill course toward clinical nephropathy is usual.[111,112] Typically, albumin excretion increases by about 25 μg/min per year, while GFR remains normal or elevated. GFR begins to decline, at a variable although individually constant rate, once the amount of microalbuminuria exceeds 70 μg/min. Blood pressure elevation is higher in type 1 diabetic patients with microalbuminuria than in nonalbuminuric patients, although not necessarily higher than 140/90 mm Hg. Persistent hypertension (>140–160/90 mm Hg) and microalbuminuria are present in up to 40% of populations with type 1 diabetes; the combination of signs termed *incipient nephropathy* heralds near-term deterioration to clinical nephropathy.[113] During incipient nephropathy, glomerular morphology may be normal or abnormal.[114] By the time GFR has decreased below normal levels, however, morphologic changes in glomeruli are a constant finding.

STAGE 4: CLINICAL NEPHROPATHY: PROTEINURIA, DECREASING GLOMERULAR FILTRATION RATE

Following a variable interval, usually of several years during which microalbuminuria is noted, with or without a supernormal GFR, GFR declines below normal and proteinuria is detectable by dipstick. Continuing urinary loss of protein, the driving force in the nephrotic syndrome, when associated with renal tubular catabolism of protein, may surpass the liver's maximal ability to synthesize albumin, resulting in hypoproteinemia. In about 30% to 40% of patients with type 1 diabetes, periorbital and ankle edema, followed by anasarca, occurs as proteinuria rises above 500 to 3000 μg/min (500–3000 mg/day). Hypertension is present in the majority of patients who enter this stage of clinical nephropathy. A full nephrotic syndrome (hypoproteinemia, hyperlipidemia, massive proteinuria, and anasarca) is noted when proteinuria rises to 4 to 40 g/day. The proportion of proteinuric patients with type 2 diabetes who evince a nephrotic syndrome is not well-defined but is probably about the same as in type 1 diabetes. Because of their older age, anasarca in type 2 diabetic patients is often confused with congestive heart failure, especially when pericardial effusion (not cardiomegaly) increases the transverse diameter of the cardiac silhouette.

Proteinuria, defined as albumin excretion greater than 200 mg/day, is universally noted in diabetic nephropathy.[115] The absence of proteinuria casts strong doubt that any renal syndrome reflects underlying glomerulosclerosis. In the subset of diabetic patients who develop nephropathy in both type 1 diabetes and type 2 diabetes, proteinuria is duration-related, increasing in time to a florid nephrotic syndrome. Viewed from another perspective, the diagnosis of diabetic glomerulosclerosis can be inferred from a typical clinical course in which a diabetic patient manifests a transition from microalbuminuria, through fixed proteinuria, to a nephrotic syndrome that is followed by a progressive decrease in GFR. Anasarca develops in diabetic nephrotic patients at a higher serum albumin concentration than in nondiabetic patients, an observation probably explained by the fact the glycation of albumin leads to enhanced trans-capillary permeability of glycated albumin compared with normal albumin.[116] Nearly 100% of diabetic patients who have reached the azotemic phase of diabetic nephropathy have coincident retinopathy when examined by fluorescein angiography; the absence of diabetic retinopathy in advanced renal disease is reason to doubt the diagnosis of diabetic nephropathy.

It should be kept in mind that because diabetic patients are at equal risk for unrelated renal diseases, the quest for a renal diagnosis should be pursued, including renal biopsy, whenever the course does not fit the usual pattern of diabetic nephropathy (absence of retinopathy, red blood cell cast in the urine, and small kidneys). When blood pressure in diabetic patients is not regulated, uremia usually follows nephrosis within 1 to 3 years. Only 28% of patients with type 1 diabetes survived for 10 years beyond the onset of "clinical" proteinuria in a 1961 study, an era without effective measures to slow the course of diabetic nephropathy.[117]

Renal biopsies from patients with type 1 diabetes who have constant proteinuria show diffuse intercapillary glomerulosclerosis, mesangial expansion, and a thickened GBM[118,119]; Kimmelstiel-Wilson lesions of nodular glomerulosclerosis (initially detected in type 2 diabetes) are seen in only about 50% of cases.[119]

STAGE 5: END-STAGE RENAL DISEASE

ESRD, its myriad complications, and comorbid conditions have been reported in a decreasing proportion of those with type 1 diabetes over the past 40 years. After 20 to 30 years of type 1 diabetes, about 30% to 40% of patients manifest irreversibly failed kidneys.[120] In these patients, uremic symptoms and signs become manifest as creatinine clearances that are higher than in nondiabetic persons, and renal replacement therapy is usually needed within 2 to 3 years of the onset of the nephrotic syndrome. Initiation of uremia therapy, however, may be postponed for months to years with dietary protein and fluid restriction, diuretics, and treatment with erythropoietin in patients whose symptoms are largely related to anemia.

RENAL INVOLVEMENT IN TYPE 2 DIABETES

Type 2 diabetes is a confusing disorder. Although it mimics type 1 diabetes in both expression of hyperglycemia and variety and severity of systemic and organ damage, efforts to construct a natural history of the disease and its stages have been frustrated by inability to specify a date of onset for the disease in most patients. Although a small number of patients with type 2 diabetes have documented euglycemia immediately preceding the precipitant development of hyperosmolar coma as the first manifestation of type 2 diabetes, it is more characteristic of type 2 diabetes to be discovered incidentally in an unsuspecting patient under evaluation for other complaints (e.g., heart disease, cholecystitis, fungal skin infection).

At a minimum, 50% of individuals with hyperglycemia diagnostic of type 2 diabetes are unaware that they have diabetes.[121] From the well-defined course of diabetic retinopathy, Harris and colleagues[122] in a study of cohorts of type 2 diabetes patients in Wisconsin and Western Australia, reached the conclusion that the onset of type 2 diabetes actually occurs 9 to 12 years before a clinical diagnosis is established. Therefore, the prevalence of clinical nephropathy in type 2 diabetes is seriously underestimated and underreported at 2.5% to 10%[123–126] Recent prospective studies of populations with a high prevalence of type 2 diabetes, such as blacks,[24] Hispanics,[28] and several Native American tribes (Pima Indians, for example),[127,128] indicate that the interval between diagnosis of type 2 diabetes and onset of ESRD ranges from 5 to 25 years. As a generalization, age at onset of diabetes is inversely proportional to the duration of diabetes before renal failure supervenes.[18] Geriatric patients with type 2 diabetes risk rapid GFR reduction due to advancing age[129–132] and atherosclerosis.[133] Other causes of microalbuminuria, including hypertension, urinary tract infection, and nondiabetic glomerulopathy, must also be excluded in older people before attributing this finding to type 2 diabetes per se.[134]

Both glomerular hyperfiltration and microalbuminuria, previously thought to be absent in type 2 diabetes, are regularly noted in diabetic Pima Indians,[135] blacks,[136] and whites.[137–139] In the study of Nelson and coworkers[140] of diabetic Pimas, GFR increases at onset of type 2 diabetes, remaining high so long as normobuminuria continues. With development of macroalbuminuria (≥300 mg albumin per gram of creatinine), GFR declines as rapidly as in subjects with type 1 diabetes. Kidney biopsies in proteinuric Pima Indians disclose extensive glomerular sclerosis, mesangial expansion, and widening of the GBM, findings absent in those with normal albuminuria or microalbuminuria. Discrepancies between these and previous reports that failed to detect glomerular hyperfiltration may relate to differences in ethnic groups, variation in technique for determining GFR, or evaluation at different stages of type 2 diabetes.[141]

As for type 1 diabetes, microalbuminuria is also predictive of clinical nephropathy in type 2 diabetes; Mogensen and

Christensen,[76] in a prospective study of type 2 diabetes in 76 Danish adults followed for 9 years, discerned a fourfold increased risk of progression to macroalbuminuria compared with normobuminuric controls. Supporting the concept of a predetermined risk for nephropathy in a subset of those with diabetes, normal urinary albumin concentrations have been found in some individuals even after many years of type 2 diabetes.[141]

There may be ominous significance to microalbuminuria, whether or not the individual has diabetes. Illustrating this point, Damsgaard and colleagues[142] noted that among a group of 223 Danish subjects aged 60 to 74 serving as a non-diabetic control group for comparison with a cohort with type 2 diabetes, the group with microalbuminuria had 23 deaths 62 to 83 months later, compared with 8 deaths in those with a urinary albumin excretion rate below the median ($P = 0.0078$). Confirmation of the predictive value of microalbuminuria has been provided in several different nondiabetic populations.[143–145] Longitudinal studies of the outcome of microalbuminuric type 2 diabetic patients show that poor glycemic control and smoking are independent risk factors for progression to proteinuria, as well as for coronary heart disease and peripheral vascular disease.

In the absence of hypertension, microalbuminuric type 2 diabetic patients still progress to proteinuria despite otherwise satisfactory metabolic control.[146] The key correlate of renal deterioration is the amount of albumin excreted at the onset of the observation period in a Finnish study of 20 patients followed for 1 year.[147] In perspective, microalbuminuria, whether in hypertensive or normotensive individuals with type 2 diabetes, reliably predicts significant renal injury and delineates a risk for multisystem vasculopathy that may be progressive and fatal.

HISTOPATHOLOGY OF DIABETIC GLOMERULOPATHY

Glomerular hypertrophy, a component of nephromegaly, is regularly observed in type 1 diabetes and type 2 diabetes, especially in those glomeruli least affected by glomerulopathy. After years of microalbuminuria in newly diagnosed diabetes, fluorescence microscopy of glomeruli shows deposition of albumin and immunoglobulins in a ribbon-like pattern along tubular basement membranes and Bowman's capsule, probably reflecting passive entrapment of plasma proteins rather than an active immune process. Similar findings have been reported in skin and muscle, where its significance is equally obscure.[148] Kidney biopsies in azotemic patients with type 1 diabetes and type 2 diabetes consistently show mesangial expansion, GBM thickening, and afferent and efferent arteriolosclerosis. Eventually, after many years of diabetes, glomeruli become obliterated and obsolescent owing to diffuse and nodular intercapillary glomerulosclerosis (Figs. 69-8 and 69-9). There is poor correlation between the severity of GBM thickening, decreased GFR, amount of albuminuria, or level of hypertension.[149]

By contrast, there is strong correlation between mesangial expansion and the severity of clinical diabetic nephropathy, leading to the speculation that mesangial expansion induces glomerular functional deterioration by restricting glomerular capillary vasculature and its filtering surface. The longer the duration of diabetes, the greater is the risk of contracting nephropathy. Acknowledging exceptions, poor correlation exists between the histopathologic severity of glomerulopathy and the duration of diabetes in both type 1 diabetes and type 2 diabetes.

The rate of loss of GFR depends on, in addition to genetic predisposition, known and unknown variables, including severity of hypertension, dietary protein content, and degree of metabolic control of diabetes. In an individual patient, the rate of GFR loss tends to be constant with time, permitting

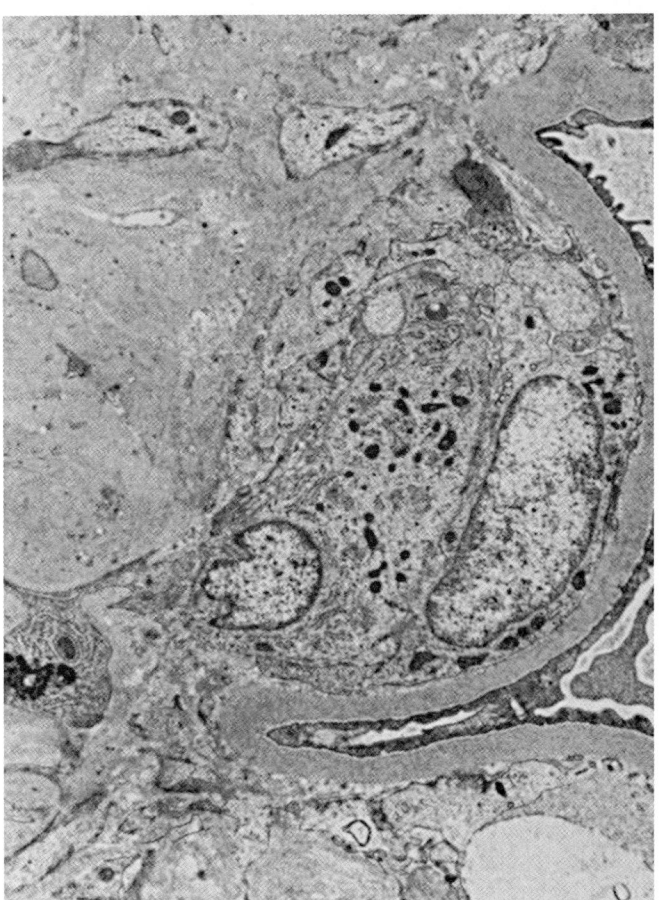

Figure 69-8 Thickened glomerular capillary loop and a mesangial nodule in a 56-year-old man with type 2 diabetes of 6 years' known duration (×13,060). The actual duration of type 2 diabetes is often approximated because at least one half of all affected individuals are undiagnosed.

anticipation of the approximate date when ESRD will occur. Plotting the inverse (reciprocal) of serum creatinine against time, or GFR as estimated by creatinine clearance, is clinically useful (Fig. 69-10). As GFR falls below 20 mL/min, the patient (both type 2 and type 1 diabetes) becomes catabolic and

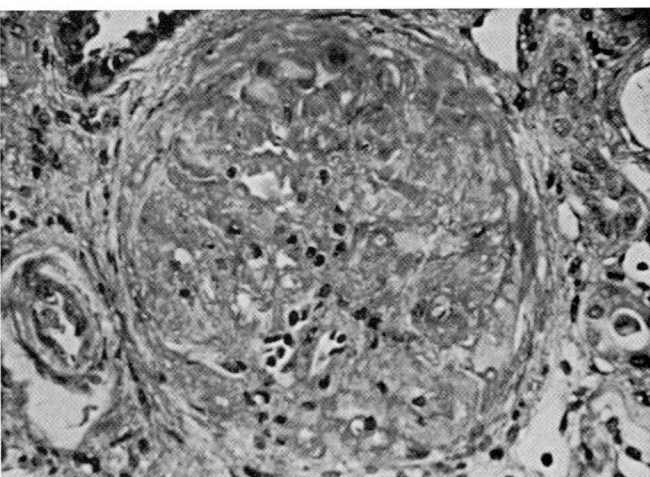

Figure 69-9 Glomerular obliteration, the end result of progressive nodular and diffuse glomerulosclerosis in both type 1 and type 2 diabetes. From a biopsy performed on a kidney at the time of kidney transplantation in a 34-year-old diabetic woman.

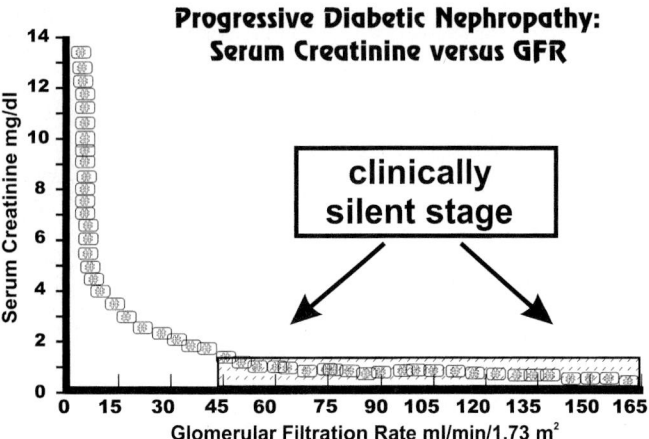

Figure 69-10   Azotemia is evident only after about 75% of renal reserve is lost. This means that a normal blood urea nitrogen or serum creatinine level may be obtained even though severe diabetic glomerulopathy is present.

prone to multiple intercurrent disorders. A minor cold, for example, easily tolerated by a diabetic patient with normal renal function, may confine an azotemic diabetic patient to bed for a week. Orthostatic hypotension, bowel malfunction (gastroparesis, obstipation alternating with explosive nocturnal diarrhea), and rapidly progressing vision loss amplify the morbidity of renal insufficiency. Because of multisystem failure, it is usually necessary to institute dialytic therapy at a higher creatinine clearance (meaning greater residual renal function) in a diabetic than in a nondiabetic patient. Maintenance hemodialysis, although rarely required in a nondiabetic patient whose creatinine clearance is above about 7 mL/min (approximately equivalent to a serum creatinine of 8–12 mg/dL), is often necessary in diabetic nephropathy when creatinine clearance falls to about 10 mL/min (serum creatinine concentration of ~5 mg/dL). Glucose regulation becomes difficult as renal function deteriorates in both type 1 diabetes and type 2 diabetes. Diminished renal catabolism of administered insulin in type 1 diabetes and endogenous insulin (and other small peptide hormones) in type 2 diabetes may cause episodic, profound hypoglycemia following the injection of formerly safely tolerated doses of insulin or oral hypoglycemic agents.

When considering the diagnosis of diabetic nephropathy, it must be kept in mind that all other renal disorders occur in both type 1 diabetes and type 2 diabetes with the same frequency as in nondiabetic individuals. This means that a presumption of diabetic nephropathy may be misleading to the extent that coincident disorders remain undiagnosed. For example, both type 2 diabetes and polycystic kidney disease typically cause ESRD in the fourth, fifth, and sixth decades of life. Failure to discover polycystic disease in a known diabetic individual may confound subsequent management of hematuria (ruptured renal cyst), hepatomegaly (cystic expansion), ovarian enlargement (cystic expansion), chest pain (ruptured pulmonary cyst), and cerebral hemorrhage (aneurysmal rupture) as components of the polycystic disease syndrome rather than type 2 diabetes. Approximately 50% to 70% of patients with type 2 diabetes are hypertensive when diabetes is first diagnosed. Distinguishing renal damage caused by hypertension from that due to diabetes is difficult.[150–152]

It is often not possible to segregate the effect of protracted blood pressure elevation from that of diabetes on worsening proteinuria or deteriorating GFR. Blurring the distinction between hypertension and diabetes as concomitant causes of renal deterioration is the fact that hypertension, itself

a cause of ESRD, is often noted in the absence of renal disease and has been related to obesity, advancing age, and hyperinsulinism.[153]

Hypertension and diabetes are independent risk factors for atherosclerotic vascular disease and their combination is associated with an increased incidence of nephropathy, ischemic heart disease, peripheral vascular disease, and stroke. Multicenter trials demonstrated that antihypertensive therapy reduces progression of diabetic kidney disease and mortality in hypertensive individuals with type 1 and type 2 diabetes. Benefit is tangible in microalbuminuric diabetic persons and also in those with overt renal disease.[154]

PATHOGENESIS OF DIABETIC NEPHROPATHY

Kidneys in diabetic individuals are under stress induced by hemodynamic and metabolic perturbations. Debate is intense over the relative importance of intraglomerular hypertension versus hyperglycemia as the two most suspected key causes of glomerulosclerosis. Lacking a reliable indicator of renal morphologic damage, however, precise timing of the transition from diabetes as a purely metabolic disease to that of a multisystem vasculopathy is often a clinical guess. The relative importance of capillary hypertension, hyperglycemia, hyperlipidemia, advanced glycation end product (AGE) formation, sorbitol synthesis, nitric oxide formation, and genetic predetermination to the pathogenesis of intercapillary glomerulosclerosis is the subject of ongoing research in multiple laboratories.

No single mechanism is consonant with a large body of seemingly incompatible experimental data. The hyperglycemia school infers from the results of kidney transplantation that ambient glucose concentration is the main risk factor for glomerular damage. Support for this thesis is drawn from several experiments. First, recurrent intercapillary glomerulosclerosis and renal failure can develop in kidneys obtained from nondiabetic donors that are transplanted into diabetic recipients.[155] Second, kidney graft recipients who become diabetic only after administration of corticosteroid drugs (steroid diabetics) may develop typical diabetic glomerulopathy characterized by nodular and diffuse intercapillary glomerulosclerosis. Third, in isolated case reports, early diabetic glomerulopathy may be reversed by establishment of a euglycemic environment, as shown by disappearance of glomerulosclerosis in two cadaveric donor kidneys obtained from a diabetic donor after transplantation into nondiabetic recipients.[156] Further to the point, if nephromegaly is accepted as an early morphologic change in diabetic nephropathy, then the reduction in renal size induced by sustained euglycemia is evidence that correction of euglycemia reverses morphologic injury.[157] More recently Fioretto and coworkers have shown the disappearance of early diabetic nephropathy in type 1 diabetic recipients of pancreas after a decade of euglycemia.[16]

Pathogenetic abnormalities other than hyperglycemia, especially excess activity along the sorbitol pathway of glucose metabolism, are proposed to explain microvasculopathy. Derivative from this reasoning, regimens to reduce synthesis of sorbitol and other alcohols by inhibition of aldose reductase have been applied to streptozotocin-induced diabetic rats, with successful interdiction of diabetic nephropathy, neuropathy, and retinopathy.[158] Clinical trials of aldose reductase inhibitors, unfortunately, have not fulfilled the promise of positive results in rodents.[159,160]

Other experiments in animal models of diabetes suggest that small vessel injury may, under defined circumstances, be associated with plasma hyperviscosity or elevated circulating thromboxane and platelet-derived growth factors. A return toward normal in the hemorheologic properties of blood in diabetic azotemic patients is the objective of one research initiative, and the reduction of erythrocyte stiffness, a hemorheologic alteration universally noted in diabetes, by administration of pentoxifylline, is another.[161,162] Reviewing a decade-long experience in normalizing blood rheology in diabetes, Solerte and coworkers[163] reported that in diabetic patients with hemorheologic alterations and angiopathic complications, pentoxifylline significantly reduced blood and plasma viscosity (at high and low shear rates), fibrinogen and erythrocyte aggregation, and increased erythrocyte filterability. Improved hemorheology was obtained independently of changes in glycometabolic control and body weight but was associated with reductions in arterial blood pressure levels and in urinary excretion of albumin and total protein.[163] Pentoxifylline slows the course of renal injury in microalbuminuric and proteinuric patients with type 1 and type 2 diabetes, significantly reducing proteinuria.[164] An alternative view is that the complex central mechanism underlying diabetic microvasculopathy is overactivation of protein kinase C, stimulated by hyperglycemia. Hyperactive protein kinase C blunts the availability of nitric oxide, increases production of superoxide and endothelin, impairs insulin function, diminishes synthesis of prostaglandin E_1 (prostacyclin), and increases activation and endothelial adherence of leukocytes. Treatment of these dysfunctions might be affected by dietary supplementation with high-dose antioxidants, fish oil, γ-linolenic acid, chromium, arginine, carnitine, and ginkgolides. Pharmaceuticals likely to be beneficial according to this formulation include pentoxifylline, probucol, replacement estrogens, and inhibitors of ACE and aldose reductase.[165]

ADVANCED GLYCOSYLATED END PRODUCTS

In health, reducing sugars such as glucose react nonenzymatically and reversibly with free amino groups in proteins to form small amounts of stable Amadori products through Schiff base adducts. In normal aging, spontaneous further irreversible modification of proteins by glucose results in the formation of AGEs, a heterogeneous family of biologically and chemically reactive compounds with crosslinking properties.[166] This process of protein modification is amplified by the high ambient glucose concentration present in diabetes.[167,168]

Circulating AGE peptides (molecular weight between 2000 and 6000) crosslink with collagen, a perturbation promoting diabetic microvascular complications. AGEs also increase vascular permeability, procoagulant activity, adhesion molecule expression, and monocyte influx, thereby contributing to vascular injury.[160,161] Specific receptors binding AGEs are located on endothelial cells.[169]

AGE peptides are normally excreted in the urine and their plasma concentration is inversely proportional to the GFR. Consequently, there is a progressive and marked increase in plasma and tissue levels of AGEs as diabetic patients develop renal failure.[170–173] Neither hemodialysis nor peritoneal dialysis decreases the "toxic" levels to normal, but following restoration of half-normal glomerular filtration by renal transplantation, AGE levels fall sharply to within the normal range within 8 hours.

Evidence derived from studies in rodents indicates that AGEs may be important in the genesis of diabetic tissue injury. For example, administration of AGE-modified albumin to nondiabetic rats for 4 weeks led to glomerular hypertrophy and increased extracellular matrix production in association with activation of the genes for collagen, laminin, and transforming growth factor-β.[174] Similar changes were noted when AGEs alone were given to achieve plasma concentrations equivalent to those seen in diabetic animals.[175] After 5 months, the renal AGE content in AGE-treated rats was 50% above controls while the plasma concentration was 2.8 times greater than controls. AGE-treated rats had a 50% expansion in glomerular volume, basement membrane widening, and increased mesangial matrix, indicating significant glomerulosclerosis compared with untreated controls.

In humans, convincing studies indicate that serum AGE levels reflect the severity of diabetic complications such as retinopathy. For example, in a cohort of 125 patients with type 2 diabetes, a significant correlation was noted between AGE levels and the presence or absence of proliferative retinopathy (5.7 vs. 3.1 mU/mL for those with and without retinopathy, respectively, $P < 0.025$).[176] A correlation was also observed between an elevated serum concentration of creatinine and enhanced AGE levels. The rapidly progressive atherosclerosis that develops in patients with diabetes and renal insufficiency is stimulated by AGEs. AGEs promote the influx of mononuclear cells and stimulate cell proliferation[177,178] and collagen-linked AGEs within the atherosclerotic lesion bind plasma proteins, interact with macrophage receptors to induce cytokine and growth factor release, and quench nitric oxide activity.[178] There is also evidence that AGEs modify low-density lipoprotein (LDL), making it less able to be cleared by the LDL receptors.[179] In one study, for instance, LDL modified in vitro by AGE peptides (at the concentration present in azotemic diabetic patients) markedly impaired LDL clearance when injected into transgenic mice expressing the human LDL receptor. Immunohistochemical analysis of coronary arteries obtained from patients with type 2 diabetes detected high levels of AGE reactivity within atherosclerotic plaques stained with anti-AGE antibodies.[180] Thus, there is a pathogenetic linkage of hyperglycemia, hyperlipidemia, and atherosclerosis in diabetes.

A construct fitting present evidence is that AGE formation promotes diabetic complications by changing the structure and function of extracellular matrix in the glomerular mesangium and elsewhere. In type IV collagen from basement membrane, for example, AGE formation decreases binding of the noncollagenous NC1 domain to the helix-rich domain, thereby interfering with lateral association of these molecules into a normal lattice structure.[181] Furthermore, alterations of type I collagen, a substance also found in the glomerular mesangium, by AGEs expands molecular packing.[182] These alterations in the integrity of collagen adversely affect biologic functions important to normal vascular tissue integrity, such as reaction to endothelium-derived relaxing factor (nitric oxide) and antiproliferative factors.[183] AGEs impair nitric oxide–mediated processes, including neurotransmission,[184] wound healing,[183] blood flow in small vessels,[185] and decreased cell proliferation.[186] It follows that the toxicity of AGEs may be mediated in part by their interference with nitric oxide.[187]

CLINICAL MANAGEMENT

Clinical lessons learned, mainly during the past decade, have been blended into a comprehensive regimen for slowing the course of diabetic nephropathy (Figs. 69-11 to 69-22). So effective have these interventions been that the natural history of diabetic nephropathy has required continuous revision to reflect an increasingly improved prognosis. The cardinal component of all therapeutic regimens applicable to diabetic nephropathy is reduction of hypertensive blood pressure.

HYPERTENSION

Prospective randomized trials of the effect of pharmacologic induction of normotension in type 1 and type 2 diabetic patients with persistent microalbuminuria indicate that urinary albumin excretion may be reduced while clinically evident nephropathy is postponed and perhaps prevented. Diabetes and hypertension are both common conditions associated with a high morbidity and mortality. Hypertension

Diabetic Nephropathy
Clinical Team Members

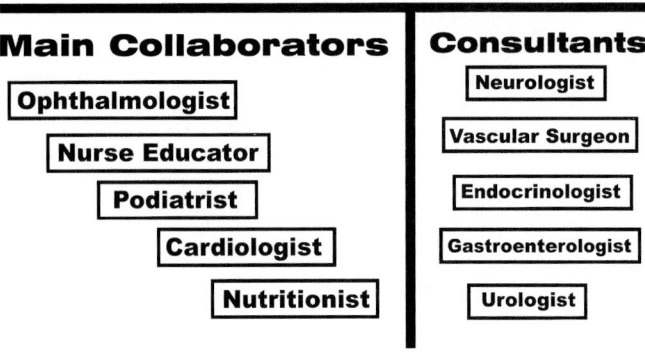

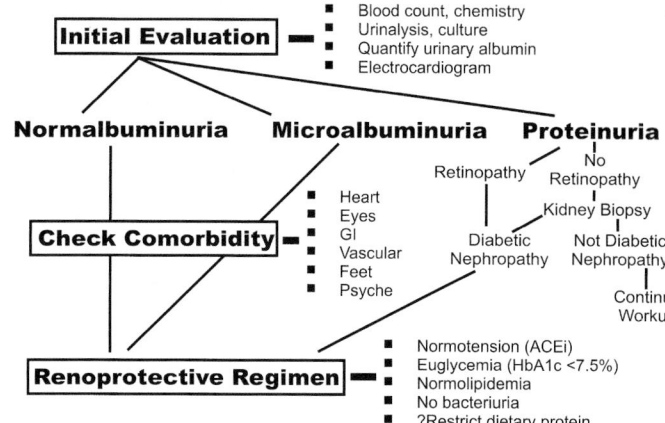

Assessing Renal Integrity in Diabetes

Figure 69-11 Comprehensive management of comorbidity in a patient with diabetic nephropathy depends on the skills of a competent team. Cardiac evaluation is especially important to detect the threat of serious coronary artery disease.

Figure 69-13 Flow chart for management of diabetic patients with and without proteinuria. Absence of microalbuminuria portends a benign course. Microalbuminuria and proteinuria, if not associated with diabetic retinopathy (background or proliferative retinopathy), may not be attributed to diabetes. Discovery of proteinuria without retinopathy is reason to perform a percutaneous kidney biopsy to discern the pathogenesis of the renal syndrome. ACEi, angiotensin-converting enzyme; HbAlc, hemoglobin A_{lc}.

and diabetes mellitus occurring together, as they do in 50% of diabetic patients, results in a 7.2-fold increase in crude mortality. Whether associated with type 1 or type 2 diabetes, hypertension escalates mortality to 37 times above that of a healthy population.[188]

As reviewed by Parving, in those with overt diabetic nephropathy, blood pressure reduction, whether with ACE inhibitors or non-ACE inhibitors (frequently in combination with diuretics), reduces albuminuria; delays progression of nephropathy; postpones renal insufficiency; and improves survival in type 1 and type 2 diabetic patients with diabetic nephropathy. An additional advantage of treating diabetic patients with isolated systolic hypertension is a sharp reduction in fatal and nonfatal cardiovascular events.[189]

Attention to blood pressure regulation is essential even after onset of ESRD, as uncontrolled hypertension adds a significant risk to patient and kidney graft survival in diabetic kidney transplant recipients.[190] Controlling hypertension, mortality in advanced diabetic nephropathy has been

improved from 50% to 70% over 10 years when antihypertensive therapy is not included in routine management,[191] and 18% when effective treatment of hypertension is a component of care.[192]

Vigorous blood pressure control protects major organ systems vulnerable to diabetic microvasculopathy and macrovasculopathy. With great individual variation, effective reduction in blood pressure can be achieved by combinations

Diabetic Nephropathy:
Comprehensive Management

SPECIALIST	FREQUENCY
Cardiologist ⬟	Annually to prn
Dentist ⬟	Semiannually to prn
Endocrinologist	prn
Gastroenterologist	prn
Neurologist	prn
Nurse-Educator ⬟	Monthly to prn
Nutritionist	prn
Ophthalmologist ⬟	Semiannually or prn
Podiatrist ⬟	Monthly
Psychiatrist	prn

⬟ essential

Figure 69-12 An ideal checklist of specialty consultations is listed. Most important are cardiology and ophthalmology.

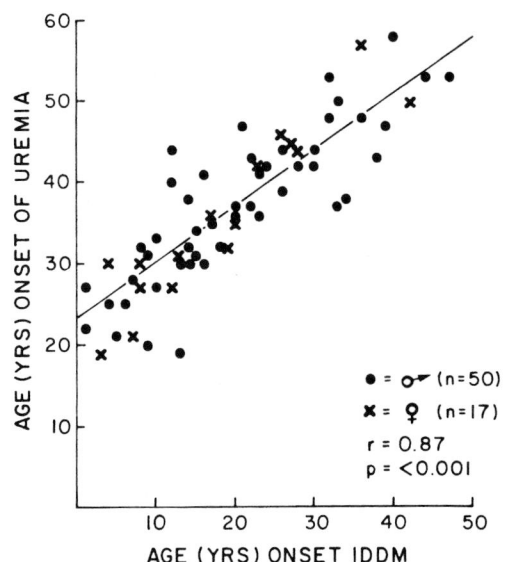

Figure 69-14 After a mean of about 20 years from the onset of insulin dependence, renal failure can be anticipated in those whose proteinuria and azotemia were listed as initial evidence of nephropathy. Shown here is the interval from onset of diabetes to uremia in 67 type 1 diabetic kidney transplant recipients at University Hospital of Brooklyn.

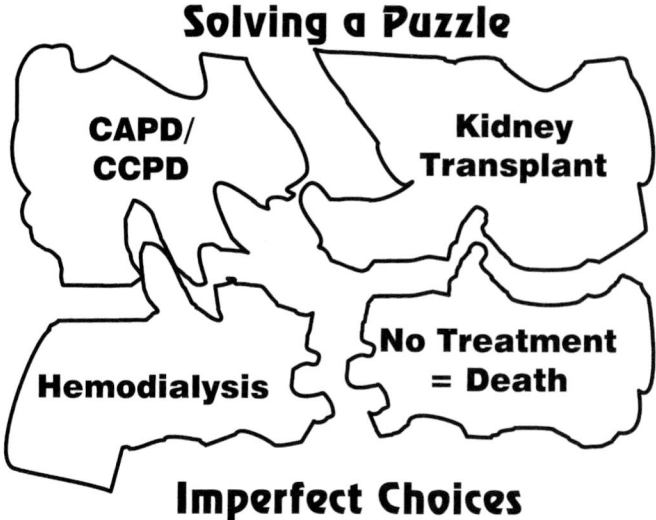

Solving a Puzzle

CAPD/ CCPD

Kidney Transplant

Hemodialysis

No Treatment = Death

Imperfect Choices

Figure 69-15 Therapeutic options in end-stage renal disease (ESRD) are shown as pieces in a puzzle. The selection of specific therapy requires individualization, especially for live donor kidney transplantation. Rejection of a transplanted kidney may be followed by dialysis. Both peritoneal dialysis and hemodialysis have been employed effectively in diabetic patients. CAPD, continuous ambulatory peritoneal dialysis; CCPD, continuous cyclic peritoneal dialysis.

of diuretics, vasodilators, β-blockers, calcium channel blockers, and renin antagonists. In the kidney, systemic hypertension is thought injurious because dilated afferent glomerular arterioles transmit systemic blood pressure to glomeruli, further increasing the glomerular capillary hypertension already present due to hyperfiltration or glomerular hypertrophy.[193-195] Supporting this reasoning is the observation that, in unilateral renal artery stenosis, the obstructed kidney is protected from the effect of systemic blood pressure and exhibits minimal, if any, of the morphologic changes of diabetes, whereas the contralateral kidney with a patent artery shows typical diabetic nephropathy.[196] There is no reservation to the mandate to establish blood pressure control to slow progression of diabetic renal disease.[197-200]

In type 1 diabetes, treatment of hypertension in the microalbuminuric stage significantly slows or arrests progression[201]; once proteinuria becomes constant, the rate of further loss of GFR can only be slowed.[202,203] Parving and colleagues,[199] in a

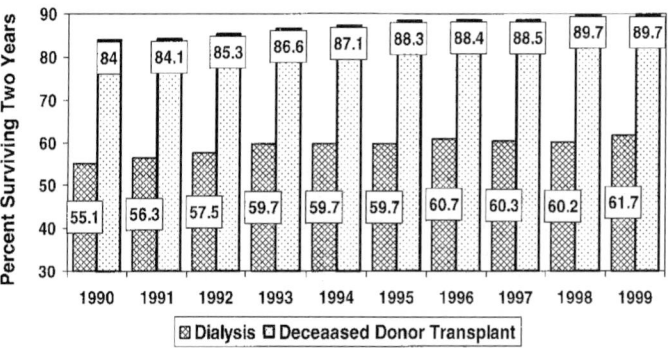

Figure 69-16 Survival of diabetic end-stage renal disease (ESRD) patients treated with a kidney transplant is markedly superior to that attained by hemodialysis. Over the past decade, continuous improvement in survival for both treatment modalities is evident. (Data are from Renal Data System: USRDS 1999 Annual Data Report. Bethesda, MD, National Institutes of Diabetes and Digestive and Kidney Diseases, April 1999.)

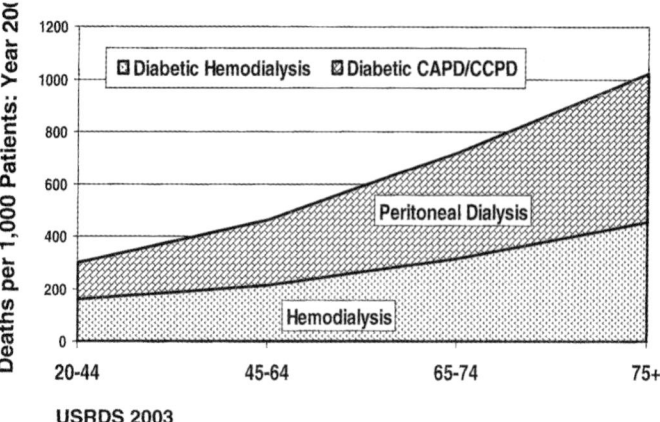

USRDS 2003

Figure 69-17 Hemodialysis (Hemo) affords better survival for diabetic end-stage renal disease (ESRD) patients than does peritoneal dialysis (CAPD/CCPD): Shown are subsets of diabetic patients sorted by age. Similar curves are obtained when sorting by sex or race. (Data from U.S. Renal Data System as reported in 2003.[1])

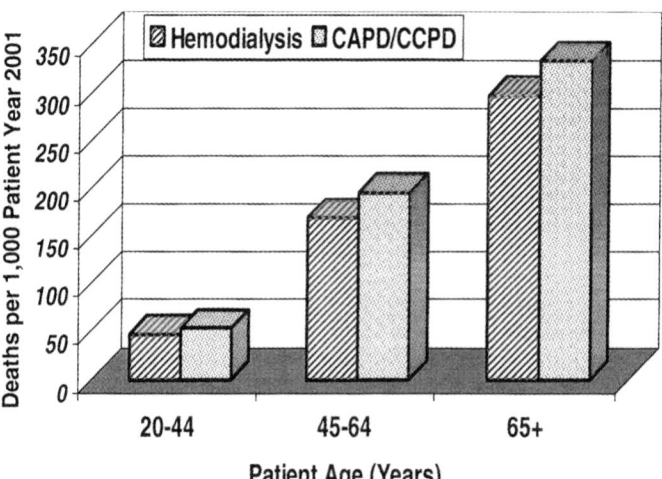

Figure 69-18 Heart disease, especially myocardial infarction, is the primary cause of death in diabetic end-stage renal disease (ESRD) patients treated by dialysis of any type or a kidney transplant. The risk of dying of a heart attack is greater for those treated by peritoneal dialysis (CAPD/CCPD) than for hemodialysis (Hemo). (Data are from the U.S. Renal Data System as reported in 2003.[1])

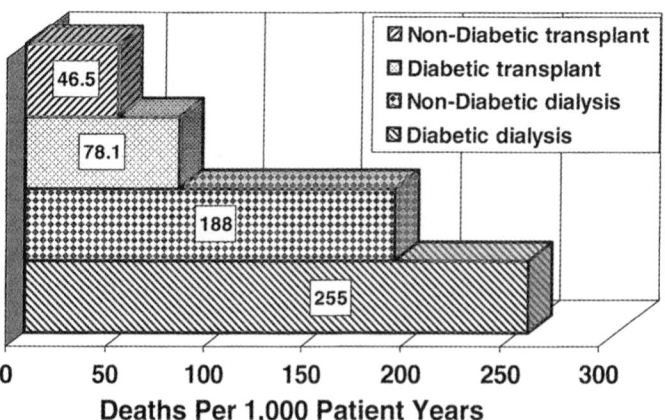

Figure 69-19 Comparative death rates 1998–2000 for diabetic and nondiabetic end-stage renal disease patients treated by dialysis (pooled peritoneal dialysis and hemodialysis) or a kidney transplant are shown. Note the lower death rate for diabetic kidney recipients compared with those treated by dialysis. While selection of healthier and younger patients for a transplant explains some of the difference, other factors are operative. One hypothesis discussed is that toxic advanced glycosylated end-products (AGEs) are retained during a dialysis regimen but excreted promptly after receipt of a functioning kidney transplant. (Data from the U.S. Renal Data System as reported in 2003.[1])

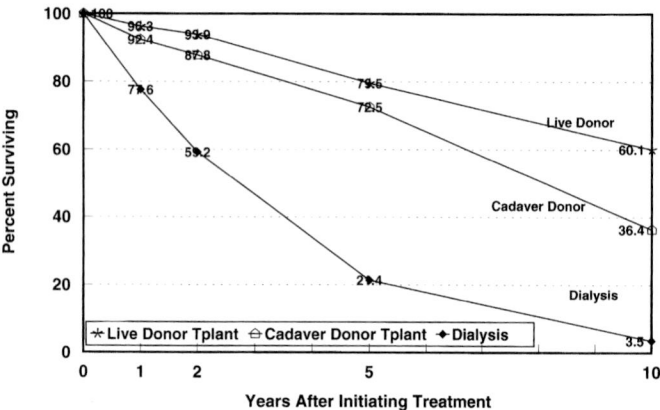

Figure 69-20 After a decade, few diabetic patients treated by dialysis (<5%) are alive. The benefit of a live donor kidney transplant (Tplant) is evident. (Data from U.S. Renal Data System as reported in 2003.[1])

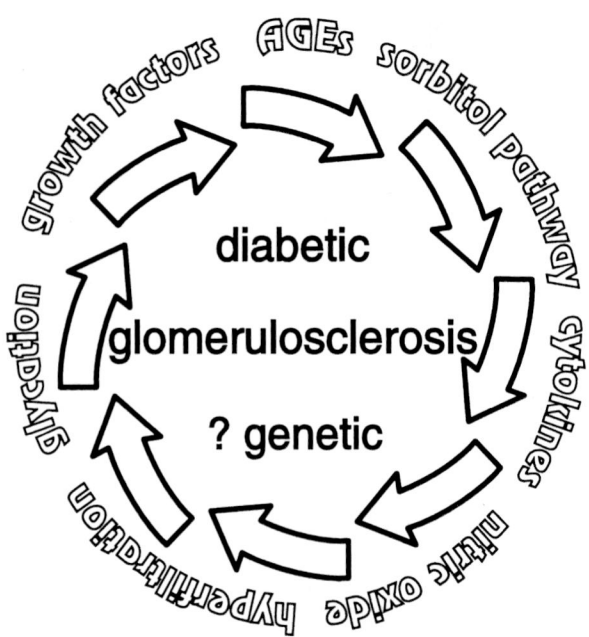

Figure 69-22 How evolving information detailing the roles of nitric oxide and advanced glycosylated end-products (AGEs) will fit into the pathogenesis of diabetic complications is still far from clear. Depicted in this diagram are the interrelated roles of genetic predetermined factors and environmental influences, including hyperglycemia. Not shown are other potential variables such as cigarette smoking.

pioneer study of six hypertensive adults with nephrotic-range proteinuria due to type 1 diabetes, observed that treatment with metoprolol, hydralazine, and furosemide for 28 to 86 months reduced mean blood pressure from 162/103 to 144/95 mm Hg, resulting in a 60% reduction in the rate of fall of GFR from 1.23 to 0.49 mL/min/month, and a reduction in albumin excretion by 5% to 10% per year. Using a similar antihypertensive regimen,[204] reduced hypertensive blood pressures from 143/96 to 129/84 mm Hg in 10 patients with type 1 diabetes who were followed for 32 to 91 months had a 75% decrease in the rate of decline of GFR from 0.89 to 0.22 mL/min/month. As noted above, antihypertensive therapy in patients with type 1 diabetes and clinical or advanced nephropathy for longer than 8 years greatly improves survival, from 48% to 87%.[205,206] Enhanced survival was attributed to postponement of uremia and reduction of cardiac disease and not to the earlier application of ESRD therapy.[206]

The Working Group on Hypertension in Diabetes[205] initially suggested that blood pressure be lowered to at least 149/90 mm Hg; however, there are strong arguments for sustaining antihypertensive therapy at a blood pressure level less

than that conventionally considered hypertensive.[206] Recent evidence extends the finding that reduction of arterial pressure to 140/90 mm Hg slows decline in renal function in diabetic nephropathy to the inference that decreasing arterial pressure below 130/85 mm Hg affords even greater protection against the progression of diabetic nephropathy

Long-term follow-up studies of initially normotensive diabetic patients without renal disease showed a blood pressure–dependent decline in GFR with the blood pressure level with the normal range.[207] The official recommendation about the target level of blood pressure in diabetes was published in the sixth report of the Joint National Committee on Prevention, Detection, Evaluation, and Treatment of High Blood Pressure in 1997.[208] It was to maintain blood pressure level at or below 130/85 mm Hg. This recommendation was adapted by the American Diabetes Association in 1999.[209] However, the National Kidney Foundation suggests that the goal should be a blood pressure of less than 130/80 mm Hg.[210] In fact, a study by Schrier and coworkers found that intensive treatment of normotensive, type 2 diabetic patients to blood pressure approximately to 125/75 mm Hg with nisoldipin or enalapril, resulted in a slowing of progression to incipient and overt diabetic nephropathy, decreased the progression of retinopathy, and reduced the incidence of stroke.[211]

To attain this degree of blood pressure reduction almost always necessitates more than one antihypertensive drug and a willing patient. The ideal medication combination is far from clear, though adding a calcium channel blocker to an ACE inhibitor is usually satisfactory. We target treatment blood pressures that would be equivalent to "normal" for the patient's age and sex, with an upper limit of 120 to 130/80 to 85 mm Hg.

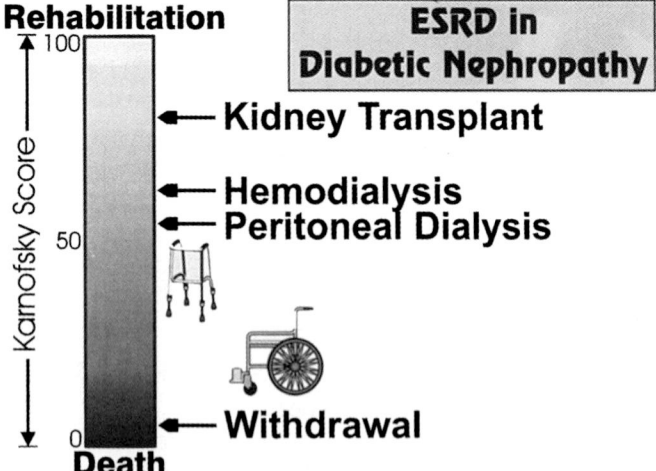

Figure 69-21 Rehabilitation of diabetic patients with end-stage renal disease (ESRD) receiving transplants is superior to that than in patients treated by dialysis. Hemodialysis is more likely to promote rehabilitation than is peritoneal dialysis. Data are composite from the author's surveys.

ARE ACE INHIBITORS OR ARBs BETTER

ACE inhibitors are highly effective in retarding progression of kidney damage in rats.[212-217] Not all antihypertensive drugs reduce proteinuria and retard glomerular injury in the rat, a particular benefit of treatment with ACE inhibitors.[217,218] Special advantage for ACE inhibitors has been linked to their purported reduction of intraglomerular pressure. On the other hand, enalapril improves renal function and retards histologic damage in five sixths of nephrectomized rats, despite continued elevation of glomerular capillary pressure.[215] Other suggested benefits of ACE inhibitors include inhibition of mesangial cell proliferation and matrix production, and enhancement of the cyclooxygenase pathway,[218] with increased prostaglandin production.[217] In humans, ACE inhibitors decrease the passage of large-molecular-weight dextrans and albumin through the GBM.

Multiple studies document the value of ACE inhibitors in hypertensive diabetic patients with incipient nephropathy. ACE inhibitors slow the fall of GFR by about 50% during the first 2 years of follow-up.[219] Combining an ACE inhibitor with a calcium antagonist permits equivalent blood pressure reduction by lower doses of both drugs, attenuating both albuminuria and the rate of decline of GFR with a lower side effect profile than that of either agent alone.[220] To date, however, no evidence indicates that treatment with an ACE inhibitor decreases either the risk of or the time to development of ESRD compared with other antihypertensive drug combinations. Indeed, whether treatment with an ACE inhibitor holds special advantage over other classes of antihypertensive drugs in terms of renoprotective effect in diabetic nephropathy is judged a major controversy by the International Society of Hypertension.[221] Even in advanced diabetic nephropathy, reductions in proteinuria and reduction in the rate of GFR loss followed treatment with an ACE inhibitor.[222-224] In perspective, because of their organ protective effect, efficacy, relative lack of side effects, and good metabolic profile during treatment, ACE inhibitors rank as first-line treatment in both type 1[225] and type 2 diabetes.[226] The MICRO-HOPE study comprised 1140 patients with type 2 diabetes and microalbuminuria randomized to ramipril 12 mg/day or placebo.[227] The blood pressure of all patients was to be kept at normal values and could include the addition of other medications. The purpose of the study was to find whether ACE inhibition has organ-protective effects independent of its antihypertensive action. At 4.5 years, the ramipril-treated patients had reduction of myocardial infarction by 22%, stroke by 33%, cardiovascular death by 37%, and total mortality by 24%. There were slower rises in urinary albuminuria in ramipril-treated patients.

Angiotensin II receptor blockers are a relatively new class of antihypertensive agents that inhibit the renin-angiotensin system by selectively blocking the AT_1 subtype of A_2 receptors. Several small studies had demonstrated a decrease in albuminuria in patients with diabetic nephropathy similar to ACE inhibitors.[228-230]

The renoprotective effect of the angiotensin-receptor antagonist was shown by the Irbesartan Diabetic Nephropathy Trial,[231] which was a prospective and randomized study that consisted of 1715 hypertensive patients with nephropathy due to type 2 diabetes with mean follow-up period of 2.6 years. The aim of the study was to determine whether the use of irbesartan or a calcium channel blocker (amlodipine) would provide protection against the progression of nephropathy in type 2 diabetic patients beyond that attributable to the lowering of blood pressure. The patients were randomized to irbesartan, amlodipine, or placebo. All patients had blood pressure of 135/85 or less, proteinuria more than 900 mg/24 hours, and serum creatinine between 1 and 3 mg/dL. Treatment with irbesartan was associated with a risk of the primary composite end point that was 20% lower than that in the placebo group ($P = 0.02$) and 23% lower than the in amlodipine group ($P = 0.003$). The risk of doubling of serum creatinine concentration was 33% lower in the irbesartan group than in the placebo group ($P < 0.003$), and 37%

lower in the irbesartan group than in the amlodipine group ($P = 0.001$). Treatment with irbesartan was associated with a relative risk of ESRD that was 23% lower than in both other groups. Proteinuria was reduced on average by 33% in the irbesartan group as compared with 6% in the amlodipine group and 10% in the placebo group. Similar finding has been reported by Parving and coworkers in 590 type 2 diabetic patients with hypertension comparing irbesartan in two different dosage (150 mg and 300 mg) to placebo while their blood pressure kept in the same range (141–144/83). Both doses of irbesartan were found to be renoprotective when compared to placebo. The higher dose had superior effect.[232]

Another large study Reduction of Endpoints in NIDDM with the Angiotensin II Antagonist Losartan (RENAAL), consisting of 1519 type 2 diabetic patients with hypertension and proteinuria, compared losartan (50–100 mg once a day) with placebo and was based on composite end point (i.e., doubling of the baseline serum creatinine concentration, onset of ESRD, or death). The study showed that the losartan-treated group achieved 16% reduction in primary end point after a mean treatment period of 3.4 years. Losartan significantly reduced the risk of ESRD by 28% and the risk of doubling the serum creatinine concentration by 25%. The research estimated that the benefits translated to a 2-year delay in the need for dialysis or transplantation.[233] In both studies, the renoprotective effect was independent of their effect on blood pressure.

Looking at the previously mentioned studies (micro-HOPE, INDT, and RENAAL) provides the rationale to use ACE inhibitors or angiotensin II receptor blockers in patients with diabetic nephropathy. In fact, there are studies showing their additive effect (ACE + ARB) on lowering blood pressure and reducing albuminuria.[234-236]

ANTIHYPERTENSIVE DRUGS

Confusion clouds selection of specific drugs for treatment of hypertensive diabetic patients. Markets for ACE inhibitors and calcium channel blockers exceed $2 billion, each fostering extensive advertising campaigns targeting physicians. The stressful decision process involves choosing among drug classes and then picking a unique molecular configuration within a class. Within the past 3 years, head-to-head prospective trials of ACE inhibitors versus calcium channel blockers have been completed. In the Appropriate Blood Pressure Control in Diabetes (ABCD) trial in type 2 diabetic patients with hypertension, the incidence of cardiovascular events over a 5-year follow-up period was compared for enalapril versus nisoldipine, a long-acting calcium antagonist.[237] The study randomized diabetic patients for moderate blood pressure control (target diastolic pressure, 80–90 mm Hg) contrasted with intensive control (target diastolic pressure, 75 mm Hg). In 470 hypertensive patients, the incidence of fatal and nonfatal myocardial infarctions was significantly ($P = 0.001$) higher among those receiving nisoldipine (n = 25) compared with those receiving enalapril (n = 5). A similar outcome was reported in the Fosinopril versus Amlodipine Cardiovascular Events Randomized Trial (FACET), sustaining the impression that ACE inhibitors may be preferable to calcium antagonists for managing hypertension in diabetic patients.[238]

Parving, who initially demonstrated the salutary renoprotective effect of reducing blood pressure in hypertensive diabetic patients (before introduction of ACE inhibitors or calcium channel blockers), interprets the ABCD and FACET results, that supporting the combination of a calcium antagonist with an ACE inhibitor is a rational therapeutic choice in patients with coexisting hypertension and diabetes.[237] Reflecting on the same experimental data, other investigators reached a different conclusion, that ACE inhibitors and low-dose diuretics may be more effective than calcium antagonists for prevention of cardiovascular events in hypertensive patients with diabetes or impaired glucose control.[239]

Approximately 15% of diabetic patients in our clinic discontinue enalapril, captopril, or other ACE inhibitors because of troublesome side effects, particularly hyperkalemia and a dry, nonproductive cough. Of these, perhaps one half tolerate blood pressure reduction with an angiotensin II receptor antagonist such as losartan, candesartan, or irbesartan.[240]

Based on interpretation of available evidence, after prescribing an ACE inhibitor (switching to an angiotensin II receptor antagonist for those intolerant), our second-choice drug for diabetic nephropathy is a calcium antagonist alone, or in combination with or without diuretics. For resistant hypertension, we next add β-blockers, central α_2-agonists (e.g., clonidine), and peripheral vasodilators (prazosin, hydralazine, minoxidil) in a trial-and-error approach. For most patients with type 2 diabetes, obesity is a coincident disorder for which a weight reduction program and physical training are established to enhance insulin sensitivity and improve hyperlipidemia.[241]

GLYCEMIC CONTROL

That hyperglycemia per se is injurious to tissues and organs of those with diabetes is no longer debated. The overwhelming case sustaining hyperglycemia-induced damage to the kidney is based initially on studies in the streptozotocin-induced diabetic rat that showed that (1) increases in GBM thickness are proportional to the severity of hyperglycemia[242]; (2) histopathologic changes of nephropathy are reversed with either insulin therapy or transplantation of islets of Langerhans; and (3) regression of mesangial expansion and GBM thickening follows transplantation of morphologically injured diabetic kidneys into nondiabetic, isogeneic recipients.[243-247]

Clinical trials of enhanced metabolic regulation of hyperglycemia in type 1 and type 2 diabetes have removed any doubt about the indictment of hyperglycemia as a major cause of human diabetic nephropathy. Although earlier studies in humans linked both the prevalence of microalbuminuria[248,249] and late diabetic complications to inferior glycemic control,[250,251] it was broadly based prospective trials, especially the DCCT, that clinched the argument.[252,253] Intensive diabetes therapy in the DCCT aimed at near normoglycemia resulted in a 39% reduction in the occurrence of microalbuminuria and a 54% reduction in the occurrence of albuminuria.[254] By one projection, comprehensive treatment of type 2 diabetes, maintaining a hemoglobin A_{1c} value of 7.2%, would reduce the cumulative incidence of blindness, ESRD, and lower-extremity amputation by 72%, 87%, and 67%, respectively.[255]

How hyperglycemia promotes development of diabetic nephropathy is becoming clear at a molecular biology level as discussed previously. The microvasculopathy and macrovasculopathy associated with toxic AGE molecules were reviewed earlier. Other perturbations regularly detected in diabetes are activation of the polyol pathway, increased protein kinase C activity, and aberrant synthesis or actions of cytokines and vasomodulatory agents, including angiotensin II, thromboxane, platelet-derived growth factor, endothelins, insulin-like growth factor 1, and transforming growth factor-β. Sharma and Ziyadeh[256] suggest a major pathogenetic role for elevated production or activity of transforming growth factor-β as a final common mediator of diabetic renal hypertrophy and mesangial matrix expansion.

Inadequate glycemic control shortens the interval between onset of diabetes and onset of clinical proteinuria; the risk of developing macroalbuminuria is four to five times greater in patients with poor control than in those with satisfactory reg-

ulation of glycemia.[257] While the DCCT was performed only in type 1 diabetes, extension of the lessons learned of the renoprotective effect of normalizing blood glucose concentrations to those with type 2 diabetes has been accomplished by several large trials. For example, in the UKPDS,[258] the effects of intensive blood glucose control with either sulfonylurea or insulin was compared with conventional treatment. The risk of microvascular and macrovascular complications was assessed in 3867 patients with type 2 diabetes of median age 54 years who were randomized to receive intensified management with a sulfonylurea (chlorpropamide, glibenclamide, or glipizide) or with insulin, or conventional dietary management. Over 10 years, hemoglobin A_{1c} was 7.0% in the intensive group compared with 7.9% in the conventional group. The intensive group achieved a 12% reduction in any diabetes-related end point; 10% lower (–11% to 27%, $P = 0.34$) for any diabetes-related death; and 6% lower (–10% to 20%, $P = 0.44$) for all-cause mortality. There was a striking 25% risk reduction (7–40%, $P = 0.0099$) in microvascular complications, including progressive nephropathy.[258]

Recently, it has been reported from the Epidemiology of Diabetes Interventions and Complication group that looking at 1349 volunteers from the previous DCCT participants who had kidney evaluation at years 7 or 8, the new cases of microalbuminuria occurred in 39 (6.8%) participants originally assigned to the intensive treatment group versus 87 (15.8%) participants of the conventional treatment group, for a 59% (95% confidence interval, 39%–73%) reduction in odds, adjusted for baseline values, compared with a 59% reduction at the end of the DCCT. There was also an 84% reduction in odds in new cases of clinical albuminuria for the intensive treatment group compared to a reduction of 57% at the end of the DCCT. Prevalence of hypertension was also less in the intensive treatment group (29.9% vs. 40.3%; $P < 0.001$).[259]

Elsewhere in this book strategies for regulating diabetic hyperglycemia are discussed in detail. Before resorting to an insulin in detail regimen for type 2 diabetes, a trial of newer oral hypoglycemic agents should be attempted. Combination therapy is often required because of suboptimal responses to single-drug therapy. Thiazolidinediones, drugs that increase peripheral glucose disposal, can be combined with metformin, which acts primarily by decreasing endogenous glucose production, as a highly effective treatment for those type 2 diabetic patients with normal renal function whose pancreatic β cells continue to manufacture normal quantities of insulin.[260] Modification of the drug regimen is needed in diabetic persons with compromised renal function. Metformin is contraindicated in advanced renal insufficiency (serum creatinine ≥ 2.5 mg/dL) because of the risk of fatal lactic acidosis. For diabetic patients with stable mild renal insufficiency, the dose of metformin should be lowered to approximately one third of that given to those with normal GFRs.[261] In insulin-treated diabetic patients of both types, progressive reductions in insulin dose may be required both after the abrupt onset of acute renal failure and with progressive decrease in residual renal function in chronic renal insufficiency because of impaired degradation of exogenous and endogenous insulin.[262,263]

DIETARY PROTEIN RESTRICTION

In health[264,265] and in diabetes, dietary protein intake modulates renal hemodynamics.[266,267] Some evidence indicates that in type 1 diabetes, ingestion of a high-protein diet increases the risk of nephropathy.[268] In rodent models of induced diabetes, moderate and severe protein restriction early in the course of diabetes normalizes glomerular hypertension[269,270] owing to decreased fractional clearance of albumin[271,272] and immunoglobulin G. The value of dietary protein restriction in type 1 diabetes was suggested by Zeller and colleagues[273] in a small prospective, randomized, controlled study of 20 subjects with clinical proteinuria (mean 3144 ± 417 mg/day) or renal impairment (iothalamate clearance 46 ± 4.8 mL/min/1.73 m²) who were given a 0.6 g/kg/day protein diet for a mean of 34.7 months. There was a fourfold decrease in the rate of fall of GFR compared with that in 15 controls after 3 months. Mean protein excretion fell by 24% (760 mg) in the study group and rose by 22% (928 mg) in controls. At the conclusion of the study, the reduction in proteinuria in the study population was only 6% (196 mg), whereas the controls had a 24% (1024-mg) increase. Hansen and coworkers have also done a 4-year prospective, controlled trial on 82 type 1 diabetic patients with progressive diabetic nephropathy (prestudy mean GFR decline of 7.1 mL/min/year) to determine the effect of dietary protein restriction on survival and progression to ESRD. The result was the mean decline of GFR was 3.9 mL/min/year in the usual protein diet group and 3.8 mL/min/year in the low-protein diet group. ESRD or death occurred in 27% of a usual-protein diet as compared with 10% on a low-protein diet ($P = 0.042$).[274] Several other reports confirm that in type 1 diabetes with advanced nephropathy, curtailing the amount of ingested protein produces a slight-to-substantive reduction in the rate of fall of GFR, with a moderate-to-great reduction in proteinuria.[275–279]

Jibani and colleagues[280] conducted an intriguing trial of a vegetarian diet in type 1 diabetic subjects with incipient nephropathy and showed that in the absence of significant change in either blood glucose control or arterial pressure, restricting dietary animal protein intake while adding vegetable protein caused a decrease in proteinuria. Urinary protein loss in the nephrotic syndrome of type 1 diabetes is sharply reduced by dietary protein restriction,[281–284] but similar positive results have not been obtained in type 2 diabetes. Of 13 patients with type 2 diabetes and renal insufficiency, after a mean of 12.2 ± 1.9 months on a 30-g protein, 350-mg phosphorus diet, only 2 subjects showed improvement in the rate of GFR. Jameel and coworkers,[285] in a cross-sectional analysis of data from the San Antonio Heart Study, were also unable to detect a significant correlation between dietary protein intake and clinical proteinuria. These data do not support the hypothesis that high-protein intake is a risk factor for clinical proteinuria in type 2 diabetes subjects.

No conclusion can be drawn as to any long-term benefit of dietary protein restriction in retarding progression of diabetic nephropathy. Apposed meta-analyses have deduced clear efficacy in 108 type 1 diabetic patients followed for 9 to 35 months and an effect of relatively weak magnitude in results of 13 randomized controlled trials (n = 1919 patients) in which dietary protein restriction reduced the rate of decline of GFR rate by only 0.53 mL/min/year.[286]

Given the incomplete evaluation of the risk to the kidneys of normal dietary protein ingestion, neither the optimal timing nor the extent of dietary protein restriction has been determined for either diabetes type.[287] At present, we prescribe a 0.6 to 0.8 g/kg/day protein diet in both type 1 and type 2 diabetes once proteinuria reaches 0.5 g/day or more or a falling GFR is noted, provided that overall nutritional status is satisfactory. The American Diabetes Association (ADA) proposes a 0.8 g/kg/day protein diet in diabetics who have or are at risk for nephropathy.[288] Specific dietary instructions, however, are, for lack of detailed information, vague.

LIPID-LOWERING DRUGS

Dyslipidemia in diabetic patients has been recognized as a risk factor for the development of vascular disease including nephropathy in diabetic patients. There are few prospective studies that have attempted to show the association between hyperlipidemia and the decline of renal function in diabetic nephropathy.[289–291] Fried and colleagues have looked at 39 type 1 diabetic patients without overt nephropathy in a prospective, double-blind, placebo-controlled pilot trial comparing the effect of simvastatin and diet versus placebo and diet alone on albuminuria.[289] The simvastatin treatment group had a slower rise of albuminuria over 2-year period compared to the placebo group, though the result was not statistically significant. Ravid and colleagues have followed prospectively 94 patients with type 2 diabetes mellitus, and microalbuminuria, and normal renal function. These patients were randomized to receive enalapril 10 mg/day or placebo and followed for 5 years. There was a significant correlation between both initial and mean plasma total cholesterol value and the decline in renal function and the rise in albuminuria in placebo group. This correlation persisted even after stratification for blood pressure and enalapril.[291] However, other studies have failed to show the association of dyslipidemia and progression of renal disease.[292,293]

So far, as the findings in the studies attempting to show the association between dyslipidemia and progression of diabetic nephropathy have remained controversial, large clinical studies with longer follow-up are needed to consider lipid-lowering drugs as an additional renoprotective measure. However, as cardiovascular disease is the number one cause of death in diabetic patients, optimizing lipid control is a standard of care for a diabetic patient.

CESSATION OF CIGARETTE SMOKING

Convincingly, a linkage between cigarette smoking and progression of diabetic nephropathy is becoming clear.[294–297] In the ABCD trial, for example, in which 61% of type 2 diabetic subjects smoked cigarettes, a univariate association between diabetic nephropathy and smoking was documented. The rate of decline of creatinine clearance was greater in smokers with type 2 diabetes. Creatinine clearance fell by 1.24 ± 0.34 mL/min/month in smoking diabetic patients compared with a decreased of 0.99 ± 0.35 mL/min/month ($P < 0.025$) in nonsmokers.[237] Chuahirun and colleagues prospectively followed 84 hypertensive patients with type 2 diabetes, 31 cigarette smokers and 53 nonsmokers, whose hypertension was treated with an ACE inhibitor-containing regimen. At study entry, the mean albumin-creatinine ratio was not different between the two groups, but over an average follow-up of 64 months, the mean increase was significantly greater in smoker than in nonsmoker diabetic patients.[296] Similarly, type 1 diabetic smokers had significantly faster heart rates and higher 24-hour mean arterial blood pressure (94 ± 6.7 mm Hg) compared with diabetic nonsmokers (90 ± 5.8 mm Hg, $P = 0.04$).[298] However, Hovind and coworkers did not find a similar association between cigarette smoking and decline in kidney function in type 1 diabetic patients with diabetic nephropathy.[299] Here also, larger and prospective studies are required to recommend cessation of cigarette smoking as a renoprotective regime.

URINARY INFECTION

Previous teaching that symptomatic and asymptomatic urinary infections are more prevalent in diabetic than in nondiabetic persons has not been confirmed. In a study of 514 diabetic outpatients and 405 nondiabetic controls, the prevalence of bacteriuria was not significantly higher in diabetic women (15 of 239, 6.3%) than in age-matched nondiabetic women (8 of 236, 3.4%). In diabetic and nondiabetic men, the prevalence was also similar, but lower than in women.[300] Furthermore, screening surveys in the first trimester of pregnancy or the first year following kidney transplant indicate no greater rate of bacteriuria in diabetic subjects.[301]

Manifesting a spectrum of intrarenal infectious complications ranging from acute focal bacterial pyelonephritis to renal corticomedullary abscess, diabetic patients are also at higher risk for intrarenal abscess. Sometimes with minimal prodromal symptoms, catastrophic sepsis as a consequence of unilateral or bilateral emphysematous pyelonephritis presents a medical emergency.[302] Management of urinary tract infection in diabetic patients necessitates prompt diagnosis and early therapy. Starting with a plain abdominal radiograph as a screening tool, genitourinary ultrasonography or further radiographic studies such as computed tomography scanning may also be warranted, depending on the clinical picture, to identify upper urinary tract complications early for appropriate intervention.

Urinary infections, like infections in any body system, are likely to accelerate explosively in severity when diabetes is inadequately regulated; treatment of urinary infection in diabetic subjects should not be delayed awaiting urine cultures but must be started promptly with either a sulfa drug or a broad-spectrum antibiotic, such as ampicillin or ciprofloxacin. Regulation of urinary infection is benefited by (1) establishment of euglycemia; (2) elimination of mechanical obstruction to the ureter or bladder; (3) where possible, removal of a bladder catheter; and (4) adjustment of antimicrobial drug dosage according to residual renal function.

TOXIC RENAL INJURY

Radiocontrast medium presents a risk for renal failure in any diabetic patient whose serum creatinine concentration exceeds 3 mg/dL. Following exposure to contrast media, as in coronary artery catheterization, the azotemic diabetic patient, whether type 1 or type 2, may develop acute renal failure with a fall in urine output to less than 5 mL/hour. Renal failure has been reported after meglumine iothalamate, meglumine diatrizoate, and sodium diatrizoate given in doses of 36 to 300 g. The osmotic load of injected contrast medium (about 2000 mOsm/kg H_2O), when added to hyperviscous diabetic plasma (in a patient dehydrated for the procedure), predisposes to reduced renal perfusion and ischemic injury. Following exposure to contrast media during computed tomography scanning or abdominal imaging, approximately 9% of diabetic patients with preexisting renal insufficiency developed acute kidney failure, defined as an increase of greater than 50% in the serum creatinine level as compared with 1.6% for controls.[303] Initial hopes that the incidence of contrast nephropathy in diabetic patients with reduced renal function would be lowered by use of nonionic contrast media have not been fulfilled, according to careful comparative trials.[304]

To protect against contrast nephropathy, when angiography is unavoidable, adequate hydration with intravenous normal saline at a rate of 1 mL/kg/hour is believed to afford some protection against renal failure. Recently, the antioxidant acetylcysteine along with hydration has been shown to have a potential preventive role in contrast-induced nephropathy.[305-307] In a prospective study, 121 patients with chronic renal insufficiency (mean serum creatinine concentration 2.8 ± 0.8 mg/dL) who underwent a coronary angiography were randomly assigned to receive either acetylcysteine (200 mg orally twice daily) and 0.45% saline intravenously, before and after injection of the contrast agent, or placebo and 0.45% saline. Seventeen (14%) of the 121 patients had an increase in their serum creatinine concentration of at least 0.05 mg/dL at 48 hours after administration of the contrast agent; 2 (3.3%) of the acetylcysteine group and 15 (24.6%) of the control group ($P < 0.001$).[305] Recovery from contrast agent nephropathy without renal insufficiency is usual in more than 90% of patients within 3 to 10 days.

Once renal function is reduced in diabetic nephropathy, all potentially nephrotoxic drugs, such as aminoglycoside antibiotics, must be administered in adjusted (reduced) dosage. Guides listing drug half-life and removal rate according to varying levels of kidney function or type of dialytic therapy should be consulted when prescribing essential, yet nephrotoxic, drugs.[308]

NOVEL TREATMENT OF DIABETIC NEPHROPATHY

Although progression of diabetic nephropathy is slowed down by various methods such as tight glycemic control, aggressive blood pressure control, usage of renin-angiotensin system blockers, and low-protein diet, the burden of the disease remains large; additional therapeutic agents are urgently needed. New approaches have been attempted to modulate the pathogenesis pathways of diabetic nephropathy.

Many studies have indicated that AGEs contribute to the pathologic events leading to diabetic complications such as nephropathy, retinopathy, vasculopathy, and neuropathy. Potential therapeutic approaches to prevent these complications include: blocking of AGE formation, breaking of AGE crosslink, inhibition of protein kinase C activity, and inhibition of some growth factors activity.

AGE BLOCKERS

Aminoguanidine is one of many compounds extensively studied to block the formation of AGEs. It acts by preventing formation of reactive AGEs and their subsequent crosslinking with albumin, leading to reduction in AGE level,[309] or by blocking synthesis of nitric oxide.[310,311] In streptozotocin-induced diabetic rats, aminoguanidine diminishes proteinuria and mesangial membrane thickening,[312,313] and diminishes deposition of AGE in the glomerulus and tubules.[314]

Randomized double-blind placebo-controlled multi-center clinical trials comparing the effect of aminoguanidine on the course of diabetic nephropathy after the onset of clinical proteinuria in type 1 and type 2 diabetes have been completed. The details of the study are unpublished. However, Alteon, the pharmaceutical company responsible for these studies, has indicated that aminoguanidine therapy was associated with a statistical significance reduction in urinary protein excretion above the effect of ACE inhibition.[315] At present, no role for ACE blockers has been established.

Pyridoxamine, originally described as a post-Amadori inhibitor of formation of AGE, also inhibits the formation of advanced lipoxidation end products on protein during lipid peroxidation reactions.[316] In the streptozotocin-diabetic rat, pyridoxamine significantly inhibited the increase in albuminuria, plasma creatinine, and hyperlipidemia, without an effect on blood glucose or glycated hemoglobin.[317] Currently, there are ongoing phase IIb clinical trials to the effect of pyridoxamine on patients with type 1 and type 2 diabetes and nephropathy.

Other AGE formation inhibitors such as ALT 946, NNC39-0028, and OPB 9195 may be subjected to clinical evaluation.[318-320]

AGE CROSSLINK BREAKERS

Since AGEs irreversibly bind to macromolecules through covalently crosslinked proximate amino groups, an agent that cleaves these bonds may be efficacious. A prototypic AGE crosslink breaker, N-phenacylthiazolium bromide, separates AGE crosslinks in vivo in diabetic rats, thereby suggesting an alternative means of slowing the development of diabetic complications.[321] However, an unexpected dissociation between AGE tissue localization and glomerular histopathology was noted in streptozotocin-induced rats following treatment with N-phenacylthiazolium bromide.[322] In this study, no differences in glomerular volume, urinary protein excretion, or serum creatinine level were noted between N-phenacylthi-azolium bromide–treated and control diabetic rats.

ALT-711 is an orally active compound (dimethyl 3-phenacyl-thiazolium chloride), which is also an AGE crosslink breaker. It has been shown to break the covalent bonds between crosslinked protein with ALT-711, and the free protein then able to function again normally. In streptozotocin-induced diabetic rat, treatment with ALT-711 retarded albumin excretion, reduced blood pressure, and renal hypertrophy independent.[323] Asif and colleagues had also shown a 49% reduction of age-related left ventricular stiffness in dogs after 1 month of treatment with ALT-711.[324] Currently, phase II clinical trials are ongoing both in the United States and Europe to see the effect of ALT-711 on vascular compliance and isolated systolic hypertension.

AGE RECEPTOR BLOCKADE

AGE toxicity is mediated in part by AGE binding to specific receptors on endothelial cell, thereby activating mechanisms linked to the development of vascular lesions. It has been suggested that blockade of this interaction with the receptor for advanced glycosylated end product (RAGE) may be beneficial. Support of this hypothesis is provided by studies that have shown blockade of RAGE inhibits AGE-induced impairment of endothelial barrier function, and reverses the early vascular hyperpermeability and vasculopathy in diabetic rats.[325,326] These findings suggest that blocking AGE receptors might be a new therapeutic target for drug discovery to prevent diabetic complications such as nephropathy.

PROTEIN KINASE C ACTIVITY INHIBITORS

Protein kinase C (PKC) is one of the key signaling molecules in the induction of vascular pathology of diabetes. It has been shown that PKC is activated through an increase in de novo synthesis of diacylglycerol from glucose in glomerular mesangial cells cultured under high glucose conditions and in glomeruli of diabetic rats.[327] The activation of the diacylglycerol-PKC pathway is considered to be one of the important molecular mechanisms of the development and progression of diabetic nephropathy.

Ruboxistaurin (LY333531) mesylate is a bisindolymaleimide that show a high degree of specificity within the PKC gene family for inhibiting PKC β isoforms. In animal models of diabetes, ruboxistaurin normalized glomerular hyperfiltration, decreased urinary albumin excretion,[328] and reduced glomerular transforming growth factor-β 1 and extracellular matrix protein production, despite continued hypertension and hyperglycemia.[329]

Phase II clinical trials with this compound and other PKC inhibitors are in progress for treatment of diabetic nephropathy.[330]

UREMIA THERAPY

In the United States, about 75% of diabetic patients who develop ESRD are first treated with maintenance hemodialysis. Approximately 15% to 20% of diabetic patients with ESRD are treated by peritoneal dialysis, and only 8% to 15% receive a kidney transplant. Before the necessity for blood pressure control was appreciated, hemodialysis was a disastrous therapy in diabetic ESRD patients that neither prolonged useful life nor attained rehabilitation,[331,332] leading to the consensus that diabetic nephropathy should be excluded from ESRD therapy. Credit for reversing this negative thinking is due to Najarian's surgical team at the University of Minnesota, whose progressively improving results in combining initial hemodialysis with subsequent kidney transplantation

Table 69-1	Options in Uremia Therapy
No further therapy (withdrawal and death)
Hemodialysis
Home hemodialysis
Facility hemodialysis
Peritoneal dialysis
Intermittent (IPD)
Continuous ambulatory (CAPD)
Continuous overnight cyclic (machine) (CCPD)
Combined CAPD (day) and automated machine dialysis (night)
Kidney transplantation
Living related donor kidney
"Emotionally" related donor kidney (spouse, friend)
Cadaver donor kidney
Kidney and pancreas transplantation
Hemofiltration (Europe)

reached the point at which virtually every diabetic patient with renal failure referred to the University of Minnesota was accepted for transplantation, regardless of age, associated complications, or availability of a related donor.[333] Once apprehension over treating diabetic ESRD patients dissipated, step-by-step, continuing improvement in survival and quality-of life has been attained by hemodialysis, peritoneal dialysis,[334] and kidney transplantation, affording a choice of satisfactory treatments to the diabetic patient (Table 69-1).

HEMODIALYSIS

Owing to often extensive systemic vascular disease and other comorbid disorders, establishment of a hemodialysis regimen in a diabetic patient is usually more difficult than in an age- and sex-matched nondiabetic individual. Starting with surgical construction of a vascular access to the circulation that may require preparatory endarterectomy of atherosclerotic plaques, almost every aspect of the hemodialysis regimen is a greater stress to a diabetic patient. Discovery of calcification of hand arteries is a warning sign that diversion of arterial blood flow may jeopardize the integrity of one or more fingers. A high rate of access complications, including gangrene of the hand,[335] ischemic monomelic neuropathy,[336] and repetitive thrombosis, causes various steal syndromes, thereby limiting effective blood flow. Older diabetic patients usually require a synthetic (Dacron) prosthetic vascular graft placed in the mid or upper arm, an access choice more likely to fail than in nondiabetic patients.[337]

Timed observation of diabetic patients undergoing hemodialysis at a planned extracorporeal blood flow of 300 to 500 mL/min for 4 to 6 hours three times each week disclosed that the scheduled duration of dialysis is often not attained because of episodic hypotension and inferior access blood flow.[337] One consequence of reducing dialysis time is an increase in mortality[338,339]; survival of diabetic patients on maintenance hemodialysis is distinctly inferior to that of nondiabetic patients of both sexes and all age groups. The striking toll of diabetic vasculopathy is illustrated by the half-time survival of diabetic patients on hemodialysis in one large series of 3 years versus 7.5 years for nondiabetic patients.[340] This disparity in survival persists into the 1990s, according to the USRDS, which reported that less than 70% of diabetic patients live more than 2 years after starting maintenance hemodialysis, while less than 5% will survive after a decade of dialysis, be it hemodialysis or peritoneal dialysis.[1] Confounding the utility of maintenance hemodialysis is the reality that only a small minority of those who survive attain satisfactory rehabilitation. In Brooklyn, for example, in a survey of 232 diabetic patients undergoing hemodialysis at 13 facilities, only 7 patients (0.03%) went back to full-time employment, whereas 64.9% were so disabled that they required assistance to accomplish routine activities.[331] This finding was reaffirmed by an identical results in a survey conducted in 1999.[341]

Analysis of factors influencing survival of hemodialysis patients indicates that a low serum albumin concentration in diabetic patients predicts their accelerated mortality.[342] Put another way, using proportional hazards analysis, if the low serum albumin of diabetic patients is taken into account, much of their difference in mortality disappears.[343] Overall, throughout the past decade, there has been encouraging and continuous improvement in survival of diabetic ESRD patients treated by dialysis, although according to the 2003 USRDS report,[1] survival of diabetic dialysis patients as a subset remains substantially inferior to that of all dialysis patients. Considerations to be addressed in establishing a hemodialysis program for a diabetic patient are listed in Table 69-2.

PERITONEAL DIALYSIS

Americans use peritoneal dialysis (Table 69-3) usually as continuous ambulatory peritoneal dialysis (CAPD),[1] for about

---

Table 69-2 Initiating Hemodialysis in Diabetic Nephropathy

Early evaluation by transplant surgeon
Preemptive renal transplant when serum creatinine level reaches 2–5 mg/dL
Combined pancreas-renal transplant in type 1 diabetes (investigational in type 2 diabetes)
Establishment of vascular access in nondominant upper extremity
  Internal arteriovenous fistula (preferred for longest duration)
  Bovine carotid arteriovenous heterograft (rarely applied because of early failure)
  Teflon arteriovenous graft (most commonly used in diabetic patients)
Antihypertensive drug regimen (85% of azotemic diabetic patients are hypertensive)
Correction of anemia with recombinant erythropoietin (target hematocrit 36%–39%)
Metabolic regulation
  Frequent finger-stick glucose measurements (as indicated by extent of glucose excursion)
  Fractional insulin doses or insulin pump (type 1)
  Reinforcement of education regarding diet and exercise (type 1 and type 2)
  Lipid profile and hypolipidemic agents as indicated
Normalization of weight (type 1 and type 2 diabetes)
Regulation of blood pressure (tolerable antihypertensive regimen)
Detection and management of intra- and interdialytic hypotension (elastic stockings, minimizing fluid gain, and extraction)
Bicarbonate-based, *normal*-sodium dialysate
Gradual ultrafiltration
Preservation of vision: continuing collaboration with ophthalmologist
  Two or more pillows for head elevation during retinal hemorrhage
Preservation of lower extremities: collaboration with podiatrist, vascular surgeon
  Wearing heel "booties"
  Assessment of integrity of peripheral pulses
  Careful cutting of toenails
Questioning concerning gastrointestinal complaints
  Obstipation complicating use of phosphate binders: detergent, switch to calcium carbonate for phosphate absorption
  Metoclopramide, cisapride, cascara
Periodic measurement of efficacy of dialysis nitrogenous solute extraction according to National Kidney Foundation—Dialysis Outcomes Quality Initiative[354] (urea reduction ratio >70%, or KT/V ≥1.3, where K = surface area of dialyzer, T = duration of dialysis treatment, and V = volume of body water content)
Depression, family stress
  Membership in American Association of Kidney Patients (AAKP)
  Full explanation of therapy

Table 69-3 Initiating Peritoneal Dialysis in Diabetic Nephropathy

Early evaluation by transplant surgeon
Establishment of peritoneal access
  Direction, tunnel, type of catheter
Intensive education of patient and dialysis partner in aseptic technique for dialysate exchanges
Metabolic regulation
  Frequent finger-stick glucose measurements (as indicated by extent of glucose excursion)
  Fractional insulin doses or insulin pump (type 1)
  Reinforcement of education regarding diet and exercise (type 1 and type 2)
  Lipid profile and hypolipidemic agents as indicated
Normalization of weight (type 1 and type 2)
Correction of anemia with recombinant erythropoietin (target hematocrit 36%–39%)
Regulation of blood pressure (tolerable antihypertensive regimen)
Detection and management of intradialytic and interdialytic hypotension (elastic stockings, minimizing fluid gain, and extraction)
Mixing of dialysate glucose sequences to sustain sufficient ultrafiltration
Preservation of vision: continuing collaboration with ophthalmologist
  Two or more pillows for head elevation during retinal hemorrhage
Preservation of lower extremities: collaboration with podiatrist, vascular surgeon
  Wearing heel "booties"
  Assessment of integrity of peripheral pulses
  Careful cutting of toenails
Questioning concerning gastrointestinal complaints
  Obstipation complicating use of phosphate binders: detergent, switch to calcium carbonate for phosphate absorption
  Metoclopramide, cisapride, cascara
Periodic measurement of efficacy of dialysis nitrogenous solute extraction according to National Kidney Foundation—Dialysis Outcomes Quality Initiative[354] (weekly KT/V > 2.0, where K = surface area of dialyzer,[355] T = duration of dialysis treatment, and V = volume of body water content). For patients without residual urine volume excretion, more frequent exchanges at higher volume may be necessary to provide sufficient dialysis.
Depression, family stress
  Membership in American Association of Kidney Patients (AAKP)
  Full explanation of therapy

10% of newly treated diabetic ESRD patients. In addition to slightly lower cost, CAPD offers advantages of freedom from a machine, performance at home, rapid training, reduced cardiovascular stress, and avoidance of heparin, when compared with hemodialysis. CAPD can be learned as a home regimen by motivated diabetic patients, even those who are blind, in as little as 10 to 15 days, although the typical patient requires about 4 weeks. Patients learn to exchange 2 to 3 L of commercially prepared sterile dialysate solution three to five times daily. Finger-stick blood glucose measurements are required several times each day as a guide to the quantity of insulin administered. Insulin, antibiotics, and other drugs are added by the patient to each dialysate exchange as needed. Excess intravascular and extracellular fluid is removed by employing dialysate with a higher glucose concentration (4.5%) than the routinely used (1.5%).

Some programs prefer to perform most peritoneal exchanges during nighttime sleep, a task accomplished by addition of a mechanical cycler, in a variation termed *continuous cyclic peritoneal dialysis*. Both CAPD and continuous cyclic peritoneal dialysis subject the diabetic patient to the constant risk of peritonitis, as well as a gradual decrease in peritoneal surface area, which may ultimately prove to be insufficient for adequate dialysis. CAPD is applied to a greater or lesser proportion of diabetic ESRD patients[343] according to the bias of the local nephrologist. Friedman[344] and Legrain and colleagues, for example, endorse CAPD as a first choice treatment[345] but less enthusiastic reports, such as that from Rubin and Hsu,[346] recount poor technique and patient survival in diabetic patients treated with CAPD in Mississippi. A telling point in Rubin and Hsu's series is that only 34% of diabetic patients continued CAPD after 2 years, with a small cohort of 18% reaching 3 years.

Of the two major options in dialytic therapy for ESRD in diabetes, the USRDS consistently reports superior survival in those treated by hemodialysis compared with peritoneal dialysis, whether sorted by sex, race, or age.[1] Peritoneal dialysis patients experience a higher death rate than hemodialysis patients due to cardiovascular disease and cerebrovascular disease. By contrast, employing the Cox proportional hazards statistical method for unequal group analysis in 389 patients accepted for renal replacement therapy in Leicester between 1974 and 1985, no statistically significant differences between the relative risk of death for patients on CAPD (1.0), those on hemodialysis (1.30), and those who received a kidney transplant (1.09) were detected. CAPD, the authors concluded, is at least as effective as hemodialysis in preserving life.[347] Similarly, the Canadian–United States comparison of peritoneal dialysis and hemodialysis found superior survival of diabetic ESRD patients treated by peritoneal dialysis.[348-350]

KIDNEY TRANSPLANTATION

The transplant team at the University of Minnesota recognized early both the potential and challenge of attempting renal transplantation in uremic patients with type 1 diabetes.[351-353] In our view, renal transplantation is without question the treatment of choice for all uremic diabetic patients able to withstand the stress of surgery (see Fig. 69-14). Not only is greater patient survival achieved by a renal transplant but there is a remarkably superior level of rehabilitation over that attained by the best dialytic therapy. All reports concur in noting that long-term survival with a well-functioning renal transplant is greater than that achieved in diabetic patients using other renal replacement therapy.[354,355] Since 1985, the results of renal transplantation in diabetic patients have approached parity, at least in the first 2 years, with those achieved in nondiabetic patients. A fall-off in survival of diabetic renal allograft recipients after 5 or more years is the result of coronary, cerebral, or other arterial disease. In the United States in 2001, those whose ESRD was caused by diabetes accounted for about 25% of first renal transplant recipients. Overall, renal allograft survival was approximately equivalent to

that attained in recipients with other causes of ESRD, with the exception of superior graft survival in immunoglobulin A (IgA) nephropathy. One year after renal transplantation in 995 diabetic kidney recipients who also received a pancreas transplant, renal allograft survival was a remarkable 84%.[356] Transplant teams throughout the United States no longer exclude diabetic patients from renal transplantation because of anticipated problems with infection and wound healing. In fact, diabetic recipients do not suffer significantly more major complications following transplant surgery than do nondiabetic patients so long as appropriate adjustments to the regimen are made prior to, during, and after the transplantation procedure to accommodate their unique problems.[357] To assist in grading the severity of comorbid conditions in diabetic ESRD patients, we prepared both a checklist (Table 69-4) and a scoring system called the comorbidity index (Table 69-5) that permit comparisons in a single patient or between groups of patients.

Like all major surgery, renal transplantation may stress the cardiovascular system, especially by intentional volume expansion, which is a component of the surgical procedure. Careful presurgical evaluation of the cardiovascular system in the diabetic patient is, therefore, required before undertaking transplant surgery, and presurgical correction of severe coronary artery disease by coronary artery bypass or angioplasty is vital to reduce the very high risk of death within 1 year of surgery.[358] Khauli and colleagues[359] performed coronary angiography in a group of 48 diabetic patients who were about to undergo kidney transplantation and advised a myocardial revascularization procedure in 23 patients, all of whom subsequently had a kidney transplant without a death. Follow-up of this cohort showed a 2-year patient and graft survival for living donor and cadaver donor recipients given "standard" immunosuppression with azathioprine and prednisone of 81% and 68%, and 61% and 32%, respectively. As a guideline, Khauli and colleagues discourage transplantation in diabetic patients who have the simultaneous presence of greater than 70% arterial stenosis and left ventricular dysfunction.[359] Concurring with the policy of searching for coronary artery disease before undertak-

---

Table 69-5 Variables in Morbidity in Diabetic Kidney Transplant Recipients: The Comorbidity Index

1. Persistent angina, angina on exertion, or myocardial infarction
2. Other cardiovascular problems, hypertension, congestive heart failure, cardiomyopathy, arrhythmia
3. Respiratory disease, reduced respiratory reserve
4. Autonomic neuropathy (gastroparesis, obstipation, diarrhea, cystopathy, orthostatic hypotension)
5. Neurologic problems, cerebrovascular accident, or stroke residual; transient ischemic attacks
6. Musculoskeletal disorders, including all varieties of renal bone disease; palmar fascial contracture
7. Persistent or repetitive infections, including immunodeficiency virus but excluding hemodialysis vascular access site, peritoneal catheter site, or peritonitis
8. Hepatitis B or C, hepatic insufficiency, enzymatic pancreatic insufficiency
9. Hematologic problems other than anemia
10. Spinal abnormalities, lower back problems, or arthritis; renal osteodystrophy
11. Vision impairment (minor to severe decreased acuity to blindness)
12. Limb amputation (minor to severe, finger to lower extremity)
13. Mental or emotional illness (neurosis, depression, psychosis)

To obtain a numeric comorbidity index for an individual patient, rate each variable from 0 to 3 (0 = absent, 1 = mild or of minor importance to patient's life; 2 = moderate; 3 = severe). By proportional hazard analysis, the relative significance of each variable can be isolated from the other 12.

Table 69-4 Assessing Comorbid Risks in Diabetic Patients Evaluated for Uremia

Cystopathy: cystometrogram, urine culture, residual volume
Heart disease: electrocardiogram, exercise stress test, dobutamine echocardiography, coronary angiography
Gastrointestinal disease: gastroparesis, obstipation, diarrhea; abdominal radiography, radionuclide test meal
Respiratory disease: vital capacity, pulmonary function tests
Preservation of vision: visual acuity, intraocular pressure, fluorescein angiography
Bone consequences of uremia: metabolic radiographic bone survey, plasma aluminum level, bone scan
Limb preservation: podiatric assessment, Doppler flow studies of limb perfusion
Dental assessment
Social worker and nurse educator's assessment of potential for self-care

ing a renal transplant, Philipson and colleagues[360] studied 60 diabetic patients prior to kidney transplant, concluding that patients with diabetes and ESRD who are at highest risk for cardiovascular events can be identified, and these patients probably should not undergo renal transplantation. The high probability of coincident coronary artery disease was underscored by the authors' report that only 7 of 60 patients had a negative thallium stress test, 4 of whom received a kidney transplant without subsequent "cardiovascular events."[360] Obversely, of 53 diabetic patients with positive or "nondiagnostic" stress thallium tests, cardiac catheterization identified 26 patients with mild or no coronary disease or left ventricular dysfunction; 16 patients in this group received transplants with no cardiovascular events. Moderate heart disease was noted in 10 patients, of whom 8 received transplants and 2 died of heart disease; of 13 patients with severe coronary artery disease or left ventricular malfunction, 8 died before receiving a transplant, 3 of these from cardiovascular disease. This thorough evaluation in which 38% of diabetic ESRD patients being evaluated for a kidney transplant were found to have coronary artery disease provides strong support for a policy of pretransplant cardiovascular assessment of all diabetic ESRD patients.

Responding to the real risk of cardiac-based death in the peritransplant period, we established a pretransplant screening program starting with a thorough history and physical examination plus an electrocardiogram, echocardiogram, dobutamine stress test, and, if indicated by equivocal results, coronary artery catheterization and Holter monitoring.[361] A meta-analysis of noninvasive methods of assessing coronary artery disease comparing 10 reports on dipyridamole-thallium 201 myocardial perfusion (1994 patients) and 5 reports on dobutamine stress echocardiography (446 patients) found the results equivalent.[362] Reliance on dobutamine stress echocardiography to exclude significant coronary artery disease in ESRD patients permits kidney transplantation with a 97% probability of being free of cardiac complications or cardiac death posttransplant.[363] Transplant surgery should be delayed (for surgical reperfusion of the heart) when cardiac evaluation discerns arrhythmias on minimal exercise, ischemic electrocardiographic changes on stress, or an ischemic myocardium with one or more completely occluded coronary arteries.

Pretransplant vigilance protects against lower limb amputation. When the history or physical examination suggests serious peripheral vascular disease, pretransplant study with noninvasive Doppler flow studies and, where indicated, angiography, may alter placement of the renal allograft and uncover the need for arterial bypass surgery to preserve one or both lower extremities. Arteries found to be supplying a lower extremity with marginal peripheral flow must not be used to revascularize an organ allograft because the extremity may be jeopardized.[364] In many diabetic recipients, atherosclerotic narrowing of the internal iliac artery forces use of the external iliac artery for the arterial anastomosis. During transplant surgery, a local proximal endarterectomy of the external iliac artery may be required in instances of severe atherosclerotic narrowing.

Progression of diabetic macrovasculopathy and microvasculopathy can cause progression of arterial insufficiency in the lower extremities so that even with careful evaluation of the coronary and peripheral vascular systems prior to renal transplantation, there is risk of extremity amputation and cardiovascular death in diabetic renal allograft recipients followed for 3 or more years.[365] Fatal cardiovascular complications are the main reason that patient survival of diabetic recipients over 40 years of age is lower than that of younger diabetic renal transplant recipients.[366] It should be appreciated that the increased risk of cardiovascular death following transplant in older diabetic patients is not avoided by substituting dialytic therapy for transplant surgery. While assignment to dialytic therapy or a kidney transplant has not been made by controlled protocol, the outcome of both approaches, as reported by the USRDS, shows a distinct advantage to kidney transplantation.

POSTTRANSPLANT MANAGEMENT

As reported by Najarian and colleagues,[367] diabetic recipients of renal transplants generally require longer hospitalizations than do nondiabetic patients. Immediate posttransplant management of the diabetic renal transplant recipient's metabolic control of plasma glucose concentration is best effected by frequent hourly glucose measurements and an intravenous infusion of insulin. Protracted gastric atony from gastroparesis present in about one third of diabetic recipients may delay resumption of oral feeding. Oral doses of a liquid suspension of metoclopramide before meals usually enhance gastric motility and improve gastric emptying. Constipation, sometimes obstipation, is common following kidney transplantation; spontaneous defecation is encouraged by early ambulation, stool-softening agents, and suspension of cascara. Also bothersome is the sudden onset of explosive and continuous liquid diarrhea, a manifestation of autonomic neuropathy, which may enervate and dehydrate the postoperative diabetic patient. Hourly doses of loperamide, as high as 4 mg/hour for 4 to 6 hours, almost always halt the diarrhea.

Urinary retention, a manifestation of autonomic neuropathy as a functional outflow obstruction, is also a frequent posttransplant complication. A regimen of hourly voiding when awake, self-application of a manual external pressure above the pubic symphysis (Credé's maneuver), and administration of oral bethanechol usually permit resumption of spontaneous voiding. Rarely, repeated self-catheterization is required for an unresponsive atonic bladder. After the initial postsurgical period, most posttransplant hospitalizations are caused by either graft rejection or perturbations in plasma glucose levels due to changing doses of corticosteroids. Wide swings in glucose concentration, including alternating hypoglycemia and hyperglycemia up to hyperosmolar nonketotic coma, are life-threatening to the diabetic recipient, particularly during times of high-dose steroid administration for rejection prevention.

Otherwise, care of the diabetic renal allograft recipient is not substantially different from that of the nondiabetic recipient, with the key dual exceptions of the need to manage evident diabetic complications, as well as to protect the transplanted kidney from recurrent diabetic glomerulopathy. Recurrent diabetic glomerulopathy is first manifested as GBM thickening with mesangial expansion in as short a time as 2 years for recipients with type 1 diabetes.[368] In type 1 diabetes, characteristic nodular intercapillary glomerulosclerosis is regularly noted after 4 or more years in kidneys from nondiabetic donors.[369] By 5 years after renal transplant, we observed a recurrent nephrotic syndrome followed by progressive azotemia and finally ESRD in patients who failed to maintain acceptable levels of glucose control (glycosylated hemoglobin concentrations consistently above 11%). At the other extreme are diabetic recipients who maintain renal allograft function beyond a decade. In 265 patients with type 1 diabetes who were given a renal transplant between December 1966 and April 1978, 100 were alive with a functioning graft 10 years later, an actual patient and primary graft survival of 40% and 32%, respectively.[370] A remarkable 10-year functional kidney survival of 62% was achieved in diabetic recipients of human leukocyte antigen–identical living related kidney donors. As in all reports of long-term observation of diabetic renal transplant recipients, cardiovascular disease, which caused 10 of 23 deaths in the second decade after kidney transplantation, persisted as the most frequent cause of death.

PANCREAS TRANSPLANTATION

Over the past decade, highly successful results have been reported for curative pancreatic transplants inserted concurrently with a renal allograft. Although combining pancreas and kidney transplants does not raise immediate perioperative mortality, perioperative morbidity is markedly increased over that of a kidney transplant alone. A functional pancreas allograft normalized glycosylated hemoglobin, fasting blood glucose, and other 24-hour metabolic profiles. The International Pancreas Transplant Registry reported in 1998 that by the end of 1996, 9000 pancreas transplants had been reported to the registry. For those performed between 1994 and 1996, 1-year pancreas survival rates were 81% for simultaneous pancreas and kidney transplantation (n = 1516), 71% for pancreas transplantation after kidney transplantation (n = 141), and 64% for pancreas transplantation alone (n = 64).[371]

Repetitive hospitalizations of pancreas transplant recipients during the first year are caused by bladder pain, hemorrhage, and infection resulting from the enzyme-rich pancreas secretions directly into the unprotected bladder. Patients accept the tradeoff of freedom from insulin injections and enhanced quality-of-life afforded by a functioning pancreas transplant. Whether another desired objective of pancreatic transplantation, the prevention of progression of diabetic microvascular and macrovascular extrarenal complications, will be reached is not yet known. Preliminary study of renal biopsies in patients who have received sequential kidney and later pancreas allografts indicates that the presence of a functioning pancreas slows the progression of, and even reverses, established diabetic glomerulopathy.[372] Recently, Venstrom and colleagues published a retrospective, observational cohort study conducted in 124 transplant centers in 11,572 patients with diabetes. The main objective of the study was to see if pancreas transplantation has a survival benefit for diabetic patients with preserved kidney function. Surprisingly, the overall relative risk of all-cause mortality for all recipients of pancreas alone or pancreas-after-kidney was higher compared to those who are awaiting for the same procedure over a 4-year period.[373] Although the study has some limitation, it is advisable to weigh the benefit of insulin with functioning kidney against the increased risk of mortality at least with the first 4 years before one rushes to receive pancreas transplant. A randomized, controlled clinical trial would be the most appropriate way to determine the long-term effect of pancreas transplantation on survival.

Hope that a pancreas transplant would end the siege of diabetic complications was gleaned from first observations of the course of diabetic neuropathy following combined pancreas and kidney transplantation in which some patients had stabilization[374] and improvement[375] in diabetic motor neuropathy. Unfortunately, when pancreas transplantation was performed in patients with extensive extrarenal disease, there was neither cessation of further injury nor reversal of established diabetic retinopathy, diabetic cardiomyopathy, or extensive peripheral vascular disease.[376] Importantly, a functioning pancreas transplant has been enthusiastically welcomed by patients with type 1 diabetes who become emancipated from the daily burden of balancing diet, exercise, and insulin dosage.[377]

Epitomizing the potential of a pancreas transplant program is the report by Sollinger and colleagues[378] recounting the remarkable experience at the University of Wisconsin from 1985 to 2003 during which 750 simultaneous pancreas-kidney transplants were performed. The Wisconsin group attained remarkable patient survival at 5 and 10 years of 88% and 77%, with intact kidney function over this interval of 80% and 59%; pancreas survival time was 78% and 61%, respectively.[378] Surprising and counterintuitive evidence that pancreas transplantation may be applicable to type 2 diabetes is now being accumulated.[379–381] In 1999, the ESRD patient with type 1 diabetes should view a simultaneous kidney and pancreas transplant as preferred therapy, permitting complete escape for the duration of pancreas graft function from the burden and constraint of living with an inexorable disease.[381]

CONCLUSIONS

Renal failure due to diabetic glomerulopathy is the vasculopathic complication that dominates the course of about one third of those with type 1 diabetes and at least an equivalent proportion of individuals with type 2 diabetes. A therapeutic strategy that emphasizes control of hypertension, restriction of dietary protein, and the best attainable glycemic control slows the course of diabetic nephropathy and delays the onset of ESRD.

While CAPD and maintenance hemodialysis extend life after the onset of ESRD in diabetes, a functioning kidney transplant provides a greater probability for survival with good rehabilitation (Table 69-6). The full impact of selection bias in assigning younger, less complicated diabetic subjects for a kidney transplant, leaving an older, sicker residual cohort on dialytic therapy, has not been assessed by prospective controlled studies of dialysis versus kidney transplantation. Consideration should be given to the potential value of a combined pancreas and kidney transplant to cure, so long as the pancreas functions, the minority (<10%) of diabetic ESRD patients who have type 1 diabetes. No matter which ESRD therapy is selected, optimal rehabilitation in diabetic ESRD patients demands recognition and management of comorbid conditions. An individualized regimen, whether CAPD, hemodialysis, or a kidney transplant must be constructed to deal with specific medical and family circumstances. Actual rehabilitation is better in kidney transplant recipients than in those diabetic ESRD patients treated by CAPD or maintenance hemodialysis. Introduction of erythropoietin, now given to more than 90% of dialysis patients in the United States, necessitates reassessment of all conclusions pertaining to survival, morbidity, and rehabilitation in ESRD completed before this vital hormone was available. New baselines for well-being in CAPD and hemodialysis are needed for both diabetic and nondiabetic patients. It may be anticipated that selected well-dialyzed diabetic hemodialysis patients with normal hematocrits might rationally opt not to have a cadaveric kidney transplant until drugs less toxic than those currently used for immunosuppression are introduced. Measures to control hypertension and hyperlipidemia during the course of diabetes may retard the course of macrovascular disease, particularly of the coronary arteries, the key threat to long-term survival of diabetic dialysis patients and kidney recipients. Pretransplant cardiac evaluation is mandatory to identify and correct silent coronary artery disease that may be severe and life-threatening.

There is continuing growth in the incidence and prevalence of ESRD attributed to diabetes, a syndrome consuming about one third of health-care funds devoted to the kidney. The past 5 years have seen improving results in the treatment of ESRD in diabetes, whether by dialytic therapy, renal transplantation, or combined pancreas and kidney transplantation. Screening of diabetic renal transplant candidates for silent coronary artery disease, followed by revascularization, is likely to improve further survival in this diabetic cohort.[381]

Table 69-6 **Comparison of End-Stage Renal Disease Options for Diabetic Patients**

	Peritoneal Dialysis	Hemodialysis	Kidney Transplant
Extensive extrarenal disease	No limitation	Severe orthostatic hypotension may curtail blood flow rate during hemodialysis; peripheral vascular disease may prevent establishment of suitable vascular access	Excluded in severe cardiovascular disease; correction of coronary artery disease is an enabling step
Geriatric patients	No limitation	No limitation	Arbitrary exclusion as determined by program; age 70 is approximate upper limit for transplant surgery; exceptions made
Complete rehabilitation	Very few patients return to gainful employment	Very few patients return to gainful employment	Best with living related donor transplants; return to home, school, and work obligations common so long as graft functions
Death rate	Much higher than for nondiabetic individuals and greater than for hemodialysis treatment in United States; improved substantially over the past decade	Much higher than for nondiabetic individuals, 2–5 times greater than for demographic- and risk-matched kidney transplant recipients; improving	Higher than for nondiabetic kidney graft recipients; lower with related than with unrelated donors; improving
First-year survival	~75%	~78%	>92%
Survival to second decade	Almost never; a few transfer to hemodialysis	<5%	~20%
Progression of complications	Death due to cardiovascular disease most common; usual and unremitting; hyperglycemia and hyperlipidemia accentuated	Death due to cardiovascular disease most common; usual and unremitting; may benefit from metabolic control	Slowed by functioning pancreas and kidney in type 1 diabetic patients; partially ameliorated by correction of azotemia
Special advantage	Can be self-performed; avoids swings in solute and intravascular volume level; freedom to travel	Can be self-performed; efficient extraction of solute and water in hours; widely available throughout United States and Canada	Cures uremia; freedom to travel; permits return to former lifestyle so long as allograft functions well
Disadvantage	Peritonitis; hyperinsulinemia, hyperglycemia, hyperlipidemia; long hours of treatment; more days hospitalized than with either hemodialysis or transplant	Blood access a hazard for clotting, hemorrhage, and infection; cyclic hypotension, weakness; aluminum toxicity from phosphate binders; amyloidosis	Cosmetic disfigurement, hypertension, personal expense for cytotoxic drugs; induced malignancy; HIV and other viral (cytomegalovirus) transmission
Patient acceptance	Variable; usually compliance with passive tolerance of regimen	Variable, often noncompliant with dietary, metabolic, or antihypertensive component of regimen	Enthusiastic during periods of good renal allograft function; exalted when pancreas proffers euglycemia
Bias in comparison	Delivered as first choice by enthusiasts though emerging evidence indicates substantially higher mortality than for hemodialysis	Treatment by default; often complicated by inattention to progressive cardiac and peripheral vascular disease; depersonalized in large corporate dialysis centers	All kidney transplant programs preselect those patients with fewest complications; exclusion of those older than 45 yr for pancreas and kidney simultaneous grafting obviously favorably prejudices outcome
Relative cost	About equivalent to hemodialysis and more expensive than a transplant over 5-year cost basis	Less expensive than kidney transplant in first year; subsequent years more expensive	Pancreas and kidney engraftment most expensive uremia therapy; after first year, kidney transplant alone lowest cost option

From US Renal Data System, USRDS 1998 Annual Data Report. Bethesda, MD, National Institutes of Health, National Institute of Diabetes and Digestive and Kidney Diseases, April 1998.

REFERENCES

1. US Renal Data System: USRDS 2003 Annual Data Report. Bethesda, MD, National Institutes of Health, National Institute of Diabetes and Digestive and Kidney Diseases, 2003.
2. Lundbaek K: Nephropathy in diabetic subjects. In Leibel BS, Wrenshall GA (eds): On the Nature and Treatment of Diabetes. Amsterdam, Excerpta Medica, 1965.
3. Ehrlich P: Über das Vorkommen von Glycogen im diabetischen und im normalen Organismus. Z Klin Med 6:33–46, 1883.
4. Armanni L: In Cantani A (ed): Der Diabetes Mellitus. Berlin, Denicke, 1877, p 315.
5. Ebstein W: Über Drüsendpithelnekrosen beim Diabetes mellitus mit besonderer Berücksichtigung des diabetischen Coma. Dtsch Arch Klin Med 28:143–242, 1883.
6. Kimmelstiel P, Wilson C: Intercapillary lesions in the glomeruli of the kidney. Am J Pathol 12:83–98, 1936.
7. Iverson P, Brun C: Aspiration biopsy of the kidney. Am J Med 11:324–330, 1951.
8. Keen H, Chlouverakis C, Fuller J, Jarrett RJ: The concomitants of raised blood sugar: Studies in newly detected hyperglycaemics. II. Urinary albumin excretion, blood pressure and their relation to blood sugar levels. Guys Hosp Rep 118:247–254, 1969.
9. Mogensen CE: Urinary albumin excretion in early and long-term juvenile diabetes. Scand J Clin Lab Invest 28:183–193, 1971.
10. Mogensen CE: Kidney function and glomerular permeability to

macromolecules in juvenile diabetes. Dan Med Bull 19(Suppl 3):1–36, 1972.

11. Mogensen CE, Andersen MJF: Increased kidney size and glomerular filtration rate in early juvenile diabetes. Diabetes 22:706–713, 1973.

12. Mogensen CE, Andersen MJF: Increased kidney size and glomerular filtration rate in untreated juvenile diabetics: Normalization by insulin-treatment. Diabetologia 11:221–224, 1975.

13. Mauer SM, Steffes MW, Ellis EN, et al: Structural-functional relationships in diabetic nephropathy. J Clin Invest 74:1143–1145, 1984.

14. Mauer SM, Ellis E, Brown DM, et al: What is diabetic nephropathy? In Friedman EA, L'Esperance FA Jr (eds): Diabetic Renal-Retinal Syndrome, Therapy. Orlando, FL, Grune & Stratton, 1986, p 141.

15. Stout LC, Kumar S, Whorton EB: Focal mesangiolysis and the pathogenesis of the Kimmelstiel-Wilson nodule. Hum Pathol 24:77–89, 1993.

16. Fioretto P, Steffes MW, Sutherland DE, et al: Reversal of lesions of diabetic nephropathy after pancreas transplantation. N Engl J Med 339:69–75, 1998.

17. Anderson AR, Christiansen JS, Andersen JK, et al: Diabetic nephropathy in Type 1 (insulin-dependent) diabetes: An epidemiological Study. Diabetologia 25:496–501, 1983.

18. Hasslacher C, Ritz E, Wahl P, et al: Similar risks of nephropathy in patients with type I or type II diabetes mellitus. Nephrol Dial Transplant 4:859–863, 1989.

19. Bojestig M, Arnqvist HJ, Hermansson G, et al: Declining incidence of nephropathy in insulin-dependent diabetes mellitus. N Engl J Med 330:15–18, 1994.

20. Hovind P, Tarnow I, Rossing K, et al: Decreasing incidence of severe diabetic microangiopathy in type 1 diabetes. Diabetes Care 26:1258–1264, 2003.

21. Breyer JA: Diabetic nephropathy in insulin-dependent diabetic patients. Am J Kidney Dis 20:533–547, 1992.

22 Nelson RG, Newman JM, Knowler WC, et al: Incidence of end stage renal disease in type 2 (non-insulin-dependent) diabetes mellitus in Pima Indians. Diabetologia 31:730–736, 1988.

23. Ishihara M, Yukimura Y, Yamad T, et al: Diabetic complications and their relationships to risk factors in a Japanese population. Diabetes Care 7:533–538, 1984.

24. Cowie CC, Port FK, Wolfe RA, et al: Disparities in incidence of diabetic end-stage renal disease according to race and type of diabetes. N Engl J Med 321:1074–1079, 1989.

25. Ballard DJ, Humphrey LL, Melton IJ 3rd, et al: Epidemiology of persistent proteinuria in type II diabetes mellitus. Population based study in Rochester, Minnesota. Diabetes 37:405–412, 1988.

26. Schmitz A: The kidney in non-insulin-dependent diabetes. Acta Diabetol 29:47–69, 1992.

27. Nelson RG, Knowler WC, Pettitt DJ, et al: Diabetic kidney disease in Pima Indians with type 2 (non-insulin dependent) diabetes mellitus and proteinuria. Diabetologia 36:1087–1093, 1993.

28. Pugh JA, Stern MP, Haffner SM, et al: Excess incidence of treatment of end-stage renal disease in Mexican-American. Am J Epidemiol 127:135–144, 1988.

29. Varghese A, Deepa R, Rema M, et al: Prevalence of microalbuminuria in type 2 diabetes mellitus at a diabetes center in Southern India. Postgrad Med J 77:399–402, 2001.

30. Park JY, Kim HK, Chung YE, et al: Incidence and determinants of microalbuminuria in Koreans with type 2 diabetes. Diabetes Care 21:530–534, 1998.

31. Yokoyama H, Okudaira M, Otani T, et al: High incidence of diabetic nephropathy in early onset Japanese NIDDM patients. Risk and analysis. Diabetes Care 21:1080–1085, 1998.

32. United States Renal Data System: USRDS 1991 Annual Data Report. Bethesda, MD, National Institutes of Health, National Institute of Diabetes and Digestive and Kidney Diseases, August 1991.

33. United States Renal Data System: USRDS 1992 Annual Data Report. Bethesda, MD, National Institutes of Health, National Institute of Diabetes and Digestive and Kidney Diseases, August 1992.

34. United States Renal Data System: International comparisons of ESRD therapy. Am J Kidney Dis 32:S136–S141, 1998.

35. Stephenson J, Fuller JH, EURODIAB IDDM Complications Study Group: Microvascular and acute complications in IDDM Complications Study. Diabetologia 37:278–285, 1994.

36. Seaquist ER, Goetz FC, Rich S, et al: Familial clustering of diabetic kidney disease. Evidence of genetic susceptibility to diabetic nephropathy. N Engl J Med 320:1161–1165, 1989.

37. Qinn M, Angelico MC, Warram JH, et al: Familial factors determine the development of diabetic nephropathy in patients with IDDM. Diabetologia 39:940–945, 1996.

38. Borch-Johnsen K, Norgaard K, Hommel E, et al: Is diabetic nephropathy an inherited complication? Kidney Int 41:719–722, 1992.

39. The Diabetes Control and Complications Trial Research Group: Clustering of long-term complications in families with diabetes in the diabetes control and complications trial. Diabetes 46:1829–1839, 1997.

40. Pettitt DJ, Saad MF, Bennett PH, et al: Familial predisposition to renal disease in two generations of Pima Indians with type 2 (non-insulin dependent) diabetes mellitus. Diabetologia 33:438–443, 1990.

41. Faronato PP, Maioli M, Tonolo G, et al: Clustering of albumin excretion rate abnormalities of Caucasian patients with NIDDM. Italian NIDDM Nephropathy Study Group. Diabetologia 40:816–823, 1997.

42. Fava S, Azzopardi J, Hattersley A, et al: Increased prevalence of proteinuria in diabetic sibs of proteinuric type 2 diabetic subjects. Am J Kidney Dis 35:708–712, 2000.

43. Canani LG, Gerchman F, Gross JL: Familial clustering of diabetic nephropathy in Brazilian type 2 diabetic patients. Diabetes 48:909–913, 1999.

44. Lane PH: Diabetic kidney disease: Impact of puberty. Am J Physiol Renal Physiol 283:F589–F600, 2002

45. Huang W, Gallois Y, Bouby N, et al: Genetically increased angiotensin I-converting enzyme level and renal complications in the diabetic mouse. Proc Natl Acad Sci U S A 98:13330–13334, 2001.

46. Freire MB, van Dijk DJ, Erman A, et al: DNA polymorphism in the ACE gene, serum ACE activity and the risk of nephropathy in insulin-dependent diabetes mellitus. Nephrol Dial Transplant 13:2553–2558, 1998.

47. Azar ST, Zalloua PA, Medlej R, et al: The DD genotype of the ACE gene polymorphism is associated with diabetic nephropathy in the type-1 diabetics. Endocr Res 27:99–108, 2001.

48. Hadjadj S, Belloum R, Bouhanick B, et al: Prognostic value of angiotensin-I converting enzyme I/D polymorphism for nephropathy in type 1 diabetes mellitus: A prospective study. J Am Soc Nephrol 12:541–549, 2001.

49. Viswanathan V, Zhu Y, Bala K, et al: Association between ACE gene polymorphism and diabetic nephropathy in South Indian patients. J Pancreas 2:83–87, 2001.

50. Jeffers BW, Estacio RO, Raynolds MV, et al: Angiotensin-converting enzyme gene polymorphism in non-insulin dependent diabetes mellitus and its relationship with diabetic nephropathy. Kidney Int 52:473–477, 1997.

51. Ha SK, Park HC, Park HS, et al: ACE gene polymorphism and progression of diabetic nephropathy in Korean type 2 diabetic patients: Effect of ACE gene DD on the progression of diabetic nephropathy. Am J Kidney Dis 41:943–949, 2003.

52. Miura J, Uchigata Y, Yokoyama H, et al: Genetic polymorphism of renin-angiotensin system is not associated with diabetic vascular complications in Japanese subjects with long-term insulin dependent diabetes mellitus. Diabetes Res Clin Pract 45:41–49, 1999.

53. Schmidt S, Ritz E: Angiotensin 1 converting enzyme gene polymorphism and diabetic nephropathy in type 1 diabetes. Nephrol Dial Transplant 12:37–41, 1997.

54. Fradin S, Goulet-Salmon B, Chantepie M, et al: Relationship between polymorphism in the renin-angiotensin system and nephropathy in type 2 diabetic patients. Diabetes Metab 28:27–32, 2002.

55. Wong TY, Chan JC, Poon E, et al: Lack of association of angiotensin-converting enzyme (DD/II) and angiotensinogen M235T gene polymorphism with renal function among Chinese patients with type II diabetes. Am J Kidney Dis 33:1064–1070, 1999.

56. Fujisawa T, Ikegami H, Kawaguchi Y, et al: Meta-analysis of association of insertion/deletion polymorphism of angiotensin I-converting enzyme gene with diabetic nephropathy and retinopathy. Diabetologia 41:47–53, 1998.

57. Moczulski DK, Scott L, Antonellis A, et al: Aldose reductase gene polymorphism and susceptibility to diabetic nephropathy in type I diabetes mellitus. Diabet Med 17:111–118, 2000.

58. Wang Y, Ng MC, Lee SC, et al: Phenotypic heterogenecity and associations of two aldose reductase gene polymorphisms with nephropathy and retinopathy in type 2 diabetes. Diabetes Care 26:2410–2415, 2003.

59. Shah VO, Scavini M, Nikolic J, et al: Z-2 microsatellite allele is linked to increased expression of the aldose reductase gene in diabetic nephropathy. J Clin Endocrinol Metab 83:2886–2891, 1998.

60. Heeson AE, Hibberd ML, Millward A, et al: Polymorphism in the 5'-end of the aldose reductase gene is strongly associated with the development of diabetic nephropathy in type 1 diabetes. Diabetes 46:287–291, 1997.

61. Ichikawa F, Yamada K, Ishiyama-Shigemoto S, et al: Association of an (A-C)n dinucleotide repeat polymorphism marker at the 5'-region of the aldose reductase gene with retinopathy but not nephropathy or neuropathy in Japanese patients with type 2 diabetes mellitus. Diabet Med 16:744–748, 1999.

62. Neamat-Allah M, Feeney SA, Savage DA, et al: Analysis of the association between diabetic nephropathy and polymorphism in the aldose reductase gene in type 1 and type 2 diabetes mellitus. Diabet Med 18:906–914, 2001.

63. Park HK, Ahn CW, Lee GT, et al: (AC)(n) polymorphism of aldose reductase gene and diabetic microvascular complications in type 2 diabetes mellitus. Diabetes Res Clin Pract 55:151–157, 2002.

64. Moczulski DK, Burak W, Doria A, et al: The role of aldose reductase gene in the susceptibility of diabetic nephropathy in type II (non-insulin-dependent) diabetes mellitus. Diabetologia 42:94–97, 1999.

65. Mogensen CE, Christensen CK, Vittinghus E: The stages in diabetic renal disease with emphasis on the stage of incipient diabetic nephropathy. Diabetes 32:64–78, 1983.

66. Christensen CK, Christiansen JS, Schmitz A, et al: Effect of continuous subcutaneous insulin infusion on kidney function and size in IDDM patients: A 2 year controlled study. J Diabetes Complications 1:91–95, 1987.

67. Mogensen CE: Angiotensin converting enzyme inhibitors and diabetic nephropathy. Br Med J 304:327–328, 1992.

68. Nelson RG, Newman JM, Knowles WC, et al: Incidence of end-stage renal disease in type 2 (non-insulin dependent) diabetes mellitus in Pima Indians. Diabetologia 31:730–736, 1988.

69. Lebovitz HE, Palmisano J: Cross-sectional analysis of renal function in black Americans with non-insulin dependent diabetes mellitus. Diabetes Care 13:1186–1190, 1990.

70. Palmisano JJ, Lebovitz HE: Renal function in black Americans with type II diabetes. J Diabetes Complications 3:40–44, 1989.

71. Cambier P: Application de la théorie de Rehberg a l'étude clinique des affections rénales et du diabètes. Ann Med 35:273–299, 1934.

72. Spuhler O: Zur Physiopathologie der Niere. Bern, Switzerland, Huber, 1946, p 45.

73. Fiaschi E, Grassi B, Andres G: La funzione renale nel diabete mellito. Rassegna Fisiopatol Clin Ter 24:372, 1952.

74. Ditzel J, Schwartz M: Abnormally increased glomerular filtration rate in short-term insulin-treated diabetic subjects. Diabetes 16:264–267, 1967.

75. Mogensen CE, Andersen MJF: Increased kidney size and glomerular filtration rate in untreated juvenile diabetes: Normalization by insulin treatment. Diabetologia 11:221–224, 1975.

76. Mogensen CE, Christensen CK: Predicting diabetic nephropathy in insulin-dependent patients. N Engl J Med 311:89–93, 1984.

77. Wiseman MJ, Saunders AJ, Keen H, Viberti GC: Effect of blood glucose control on increased glomerular filtration rate and kidney size in insulin-dependent diabetes. N Engl J Med 312:617–621, 1985.

78. Christensen CK, Christiansen JS, Schmitz A, et al: Effect of continuous subcutaneous insulin infusion on kidney function and size in IDDM patients: A 2 year controlled study. J Diabetes Complications 1:91–95, 1987.

79. Christiansen JS, Frandsen M, Parving H-H: The effect of intravenous insulin infusion on kidney function in insulin-dependent diabetes mellitus. Diabetologia 20:199–204, 1981.

80. Christiansen JS, Gammelgaard J, Tronier B, et al: Kidney function and size in diabetics before and during insulin treatment. Kidney Int 21:683–688, 1982.

81. Parving H, Øxenbøll B, Svendsen PA, et al: Early detection of patients at risk of developing diabetic nephropathy: A longitudinal study of urinary albumin excretion. Acta Endocrinol (Copenh) 100:550–555, 1982.

82. Mogensen CE, Christensen CK, Vittinghus E: The stages in diabetic renal disease with emphasis on the stage of incipient diabetic nephropathy. Diabetes 32:64–78, 1983.

83. Mogensen CE, Christensen CK, Christiansen JS, et al: Early hyperfiltration and late renal damage in insulin-dependent diabetes. Pediatr Adolesc Endocrinol 17:197–205, 1988.

84. Mogensen CE, Steffes MW, Deckert T, Christiansen JS: Functional and morphological renal manifestations in diabetes mellitus. Diabetologia 21:89–93, 1981.

85. Wiseman MJ, Viberti GC, Keen H: Threshold effect of plasma glucose in the glomerular hyperfiltration of diabetes. Nephron 38:257–260, 1984.

86. Jones SL, Wiseman MJ, Viberti GC: Glomerular hyperfiltration as a risk factor for diabetic nephropathy: Five year report of a prospective study (letter). Diabetologia 34:59–60, 1991.

87. Azevedo MJ, Gross JL: Follow up of glomerular hyperfiltration in normoalbuminuric type 1 (insulin-dependent) diabetic patients (letter). Diabetologia 34:611, 1991.

88. Mogensen CE: Microalbuminuria predicts clinical proteinuria and early mortality in maturity-onset diabetes. N Engl J Med 310:356–360, 1984.

89. Mogensen CE: Early glomerular hyperfiltration in insulin-dependent diabetics and late nephropathy. Scand J Clin Lab Invest 46:201–206, 1986.

90. Mogensen CE: Renal function changes in diabetes. Diabetes 25:872–879, 1976.

91. O'Bryan GT, Hostetter TH: The renal hemodynamic basis of diabetic nephropathy. Semin Nephrol 17:93–100, 1997.

92. Lafferty HM, Brenner BM: Are glomerular hypertension and "hypertrophy" independent risk factors for progression of renal disease? Semin Nephrol 3:294–304, 1990.

93. Østerby R: Early phases in the development of diabetic glomerulopathy: Quantitative electron microscopic study. Acta Med Scand S574:3–82, 1974.

94. Østerby R, Gundersen HJG: Glomerular size and structure in diabetes mellitus: 1. Early abnormalities. Diabetologia 11:225–229, 1975.

95. Østerby R: Basement membrane morphology in diabetes mellitus. In Ellenberg M, Rifkin H (eds): Diabetes Mellitus: Theory and Practice. New York, Medical Examination, 1983, pp 323–341.

96. Østerby R: A quantitative electron microscopic study of mesangial regions in glomeruli from patients with short-term juvenile diabetes mellitus. Lab Invest 29:99–110, 1973.

97. Vittinghus E, Mogensen CE: Albumin excretion and renal hemodynamic response to physical exercise in normal and diabetic men. Scand J Clin Lab Invest 41:627–632, 1981.

98. Mauer SM, Goetz FC, McHugh LE, et al: Long-term study of normal kidneys transplanted into patients with type I diabetes. Diabetes 38:516–523, 1989.

99. Borch-Johnsen K: Incidence of nephropathy in insulin-dependent

diabetes as related to mortality and cost-benefit of early intervention. In Mogensen CE (ed): The Kidney and Hypertension in Diabetes Mellitus, 2d ed. Boston, Kluwer Academic, 1994, pp 75–84.

100. Chachati A, von Frenckell R, Foidart-Willems J, et al: Variability of albumin excretion in insulin-dependent diabetics. Diabet Med 4:437–440, 1987.

101. Deferrari G, Repetto M, Calvi C, et al: Diabetic nephropathy: From micro-macroalbuminuria. Nephrol Dial Transplant 13:11–15, 1998.

102. Schmitz A, Vaeth M: Microalbuminuria: A major risk factor in non-insulin-dependent diabetes. A 10-year follow-up study of 503 patients. Diabet Med 5:126–134, 1988.

103. Stiegler H, Standl E, Schulz K, et al: Morbidity, mortality, and albuminuria in type 2 diabetic patients: A three-year prospective study of a random cohort in general practice. Diabet Med 9:646–653, 1992.

104. Neil A, Hawkins M, Potok M, et al: A prospective population-based study of microalbuminuria as a predictor of mortality in NIDDM. Diabetes Care 16:996–1003, 1993.

105. Gatling W, Knight C, Mullee MA, Hill RD: Microalbuminuria in diabetes: A population study of the prevalence and assessment of three screening tests. Diabet Med 5:343–347, 1988.

106. Rowe DJF, Bagga II, Betts PB: Normal variations in rate of albumin excretion and albumin to creatinine ratios in overnight and daytime urine collections in non-diabetic children. Br Med J 291:693–694, 1985.

107. Cohen DL, Close CF, Viberti GC: The variability of overnight urinary albumin excretion in insulin-dependent diabetic and normal subjects. Diabet Med 4:437–440, 1987.

108. Parving H-H, Hommel E, Mathiesen E, et al: Prevalence of microalbuminuria, arterial hypertension, retinopathy and neuropathy in patients with insulin-dependent diabetes. Br Med J 296:156–160, 1988.

109. Viberti G, Keen H: The patterns of proteinuria in diabetes mellitus: Relevance to pathogenesis and prevention of diabetic nephropathy. Diabetes 33:686–692, 1984.

110. Mogensen CE: Microalbuminuria as a predictor of clinical diabetic nephropathy. Kidney Int 31:673–689, 1987.

111. Mathiesen ER, Ronn B, Storm B, et al: The natural history of microalbuminuria in insulin-dependent diabetes: A 10-year prospective study. Diabet Med 12:482–487, 1995.

112. Viberti GC, Hill RD, Jarrett RJ, et al: Microalbuminuria as a predictor of clinical nephropathy in insulin-dependent diabetes mellitus. Lancet 1:1430–1432, 1982.

113. Nørgaard K, Feldt-Rasmussen B, Borch-Johnsen K, et al: Prevalence of hypertension in type 1 (insulin-dependent) diabetes mellitus. Diabetologia 33:407–410, 1990.

114. Chavers BM, Bilous RW, Ellis EN, et al: Glomerular lesions and urinary albumin excretion in type 1 diabetes without overt proteinuria. N Engl J Med 320:966–970, 1989.

115. Bending JJ, Viberti GC, Watkins PJ, Keen H: Intermittent clinical proteinuria and renal function in diabetes: Evolution and the effect of glycemic control. Br Med J 292:83–86, 1986.

116. Daniels BS, Hauser EB: Glycation of albumin, not glomerular basement membrane, alters permeability in an in vitro model. Diabetes 41:1415–1421, 1992.

117. Caird RI: Survival of diabetics with proteinuria. Diabetes 10:178–181, 1961.

118. Mauer SM, Steffes MW, Ellis EN, et al: Structural-functional relationships in diabetic nephropathy. J Clin Invest 74:1143–1155, 1984.

119. Steffes MW, Østerby R, Chavers B, Mauer SM: Mesangial expansion as a central mechanism for loss of kidney function in diabetic patients. Diabetes 38:1077–1081, 1989.

120. Gellman DD, Pirani CL, Soothill JF, et al: Structure and function in diabetic nephropathy: The importance of diffuse glomerulosclerosis. Diabetes 8:251–256, 1959.

121. National Diabetes Data Group: Diabetes in America, ed 2. Bethesda, MD, National Institutes of Health. National Institute of Diabetes and Digestive and Kidney Diseases. NIH publication No. 95-1468, 1995.

122. Harris MI, Klein R, Welborn TA, Knuiman MW: Onset of NIDDM occurs at least 4–7 yr before clinical diagnosis. Diabetes Care 15:815–819, 1992.

123. Marks HH: Longevity and mortality of diabetics. Am J Public Health 55:416–422, 1965.

124. Herman WH, Teutsch SM: Kidney disease associated with diabetes: Diabetes in America. (NIH publication No. 85-1468). Washington, DC, Government Printing Office, 1985, pp 1–31.

125. Ismail N, Becker B, Strzelczyk P, Ritz E: Renal disease and hypertension in non-insulin-dependent diabetes mellitus. Kidney Int 55:1–28, 1999.

126. Fabre J, Balant LP, Dayer PG, et al: The kidney in maturity onset diabetes: A clinical study of 510 patients. Kidney Int 21:730–738, 1982.

127. Kunzelman CL, Knowles WC, Pettit DJ, Bennett PH: Incidence of proteinuria in type 2 diabetes in the Pima Indians. Kidney Int 35:681–687, 1989.

128. Knowles WC, Bennett PH, Hamman RF, Miller M: Diabetes incidence and prevalence in Pima Indians: A 19-fold greater incidence than in Rochester,

Minnesota. Am J Epidemiol 108:497–505, 1978.

129. Lindblad AS, Nolph KD, Novak JW, Friedman EA: A survey of the NIH CAPD Registry population with end-stage renal disease attributed to diabetic nephropathy. J Diabetes Complications 2:227–232, 1988.

130. Davies DF, Shock NW: Age changes in glomerular filtration rate, effective renal plasma flow, and tubular excretory capacity in adult males. J Clin Invest 29:496–502, 1950.

131. Rowe JW, Andres R, Tobin JD, et al: The effect of age on creatinine clearance in men: A cross-sectional and longitudinal study. J Gerontol 31:155–163, 1976.

132. Lindeman RD, Tobin JD, Shock NW: Longitudinal studies on the rate of decline in renal function with age. J Am Geriatr Soc 33:278–285, 1985.

133. Takazakura E, Wasabu N, Handa A, et al: Intrarenal vascular changes with age and disease. Kidney Int 2:224–230, 1972.

134. Parving H-H, Gall M-A, Skøtt P, et al: Prevalence and causes of albuminuria in non-insulin dependent diabetic (NIDDM) patients (abstract). Kidney Int 37:243, 1990.

135. Myers BD, Nelson RG, Williams GW, et al: Glomerular function in Pima Indians with non-insulin dependent diabetes mellitus of recent onset. J Clin Invest 88:524–530, 1991.

136. Palmisano JJ, Lebovitz HE: Cross-sectional analysis of renal function in black Americans with NIDDM. Diabetes Care 13:1186–1190, 1990.

137. Bérionade V: Creatinine clearance in non-insulin dependent diabetes mellitus. Kidney Int 31:179, 1986.

138. Bruton BL, Perusek MC, Lancaster JL, et al: Effects of glycemia on basal and amino-acid stimulated (AA-S) renal hemodynamics and kidney size in non-insulin dependent diabetes (NIDD) (abstract). J Am Soc Nephrol 1:623, 1990.

139. Nowack R, Raum E, Blum W, Ritz E: Renal hemodynamics in recent onset type II diabetes. Am J Kidney Dis 20:342–347, 1992.

140. Nelson RG, Meyer TW, Myers BD, Bennett PH: Course of renal disease in Pima Indians with non-insulin-dependent diabetes mellitus. Kidney Int Suppl 63:S45–S48, 1997.

141. Gall MA, Rossing P, Skøtt P, et al: Prevalence of micro- and macroalbuminuria, arterial hypertension, retinopathy and large vessel disease in European type 2 (non-insulin dependent) diabetic patients. Diabetologia 34:655–661, 1991.

142. Damsgaard EM, Froland A, Jorgensen OD, Mogensen CE: Microalbuminuria as predictor of increased mortality in elderly people. Br Med J 300:297–300, 1990.

143. Yudkin JS, Forrest FD, Jackson CA: Microalbuminuria as a predictor of

vascular disease in non-diabetic subjects. Lancet 1:530–533, 1988.

144. Schmitz A, Vaeth M: Microalbuminuria a major risk factor in non-insulin dependent diabetes: A 10 year followup study of 503 patients. Diabet Med 5:126–134, 1988.

145. Jarrett RJ, Viberti GC, Argyropoulos A, et al: Microalbuminuria predicts mortality in non-insulin dependent diabetes. Diabet Med 1:17–19, 1984.

146. Forsblom CM, Groop PH, Ekstrand A, et al: Predictors of progression from normoalbuminuria to microalbuminuria in NIDDM. Diabetes Care 21:1932–1938, 1998.

147. Eibl N, Schnack C, Frank M, Schernthaner G: Initial urinary albumin excretion determines the progression of microalbuminuria in patients with type-2 diabetes and normotensive blood pressure values despite improved metabolic control. Diabetes Res Clin Pract 39:39–45, 1998.

148. Miller K, Michael AF: Immunopathology of renal extracellular membranes in diabetes mellitus: Specificity of tubular basement-membrane immunofluorescence. Diabetes 25:701–708, 1976.

149. Mauer SM, Steffes MW, Brown DM: Effects of mesangial localization of polyvinyl alcohols on glomerular basement membrane thickness. Kidney Int 5:751–755, 1985.

150. Standl E, Steigler H, Roth R, et al: On the impact of hypertension on the prognosis of NIDDM: Results of the Schwabing-GP program. Diabetes Metab 15:352–358, 1989.

151. Ritz E, Hasslacher C, Beutel G: Hypertension and diabetic nephropathy. J Nephrol 1:11–15, 1991.

152. Panzram G: Mortality and survival in type 2 (non-insulin dependent) diabetes mellitus. Diabetologia 30:123–131, 1987.

153. DeFronzo RJ, Ferranini E: Insulin resistance: A multi-faceted syndrome responsible for NIDDM, obesity, hypertension, dyslipidemia and atherosclerotic cardiovascular disease. Diabetes Care 14:173–194, 1991.

154. Gilbert RE, Jerums G, Cooper ME: Diabetes and hypertension: Prognostic and therapeutic considerations. Blood Press 4:329–333, 1995.

155. Maryniak RK, Mendoza N, Clyne D, et al: Recurrence of diabetic nodular glomerulosclerosis in a renal transplant. Transplantation 39:35–38, 1985.

156. Abouna G, Adnani MS, Kumar MS, Samhan SA: Fate of transplanted kidneys with diabetic nephropathy. Lancet 1:622–624, 1986.

157. Tuttle KR, Bruton L, Perusek MC, et al: Effect of strict glycemic control on renal hemodynamic response to amino acids and renal enlargement in insulin-dependent diabetes mellitus. N Engl J Med 324:1626–1632, 1991.

158. Robison WG Jr, Tillis TN, Laver N, Kinoshita JH: Diabetes-related histopathologies of the rat retina prevented with an aldose reductase inhibitor. Exp Eye Res 50:355–366, 1990.

159. Sundkvist G, Armstrong FM, Bradbury JE, et al: Peripheral and autonomic nerve function in 259 diabetic patients with peripheral neuropathy treated with ponalrestat (an aldose reductase inhibitor) or placebo for 18 months: United Kingdom/Scandinavian Ponalrestat Trial. J Diabetes Complications 6:123–130, 1992.

160. Macleod AF, Boulton AJ, Owens DR, et al: A multicentre trial of the aldose-reductase inhibitor tolrestat, in patients with symptomatic diabetic peripheral neuropathy: Northern European Tolrestat Study Group. Diabetes Metab 18:14–20, 1992.

161. Solerte SB, Ferrari E: Diabetic retinal vascular complications, erythrocyte filterability and pentoxifylline: Results of a 2 year follow-up study. Pharmatherapeutica 4:341–346, 1985.

162. Solerte SB, Fioravanti M, Patti AL, et al: Pentoxifylline, total urinary protein excretion rate and arterial blood pressure in long-term insulin-dependent diabetic patients with overt nephropathy. Acta Diabetol 24:229–239, 1987.

163. Solerte SB, Fioravanti M, Cerutti N, et al: Retrospective analysis of long-term hemorheologic effects of pentoxifylline in diabetic patients with angiopathic complications. Acta Diabetol 34:67–74, 1997.

164. Guerrero-Romero F, Rodriguez-Moran M, Paniagua-Sierra JR, et al: Pentoxifylline reduces proteinuria in insulin-dependent and noninsulin-dependent diabetic patients. Clin Nephrol 43:116–121, 1995.

165. McCarty MF: Nitric oxide deficiency, leukocyte activation, and resultant ischemia are crucial to the pathogenesis of diabetic retinopathy/neuropathy-preventive potential of antioxidants, essential fatty acids, chromium, ginkgolides, and pentoxifylline. Med Hypotheses 50:435–449, 1998.

166. Porte D Jr, Schwartz MW: Diabetes complications: Why is glucose potentially toxic? Science 272:699, 1996.

167. Brownlee M: Glycation and diabetic complications. Diabetes 43:836, 1994.

168. Vlassara H: Protein glycation in the kidney: Role in diabetes and aging. Kidney Int 49:1795, 1996.

169. Schmidt AM, Hori O, Chen JX, et al: Advanced glycation end products interacting with their endothelial receptor induce expression of vascular cell adhesion molecule-1 (VCAM-1) in cultured human endothelial cells and in mice. J Clin Invest 96:1395, 1995.

170. Makita Z, Bucala R, Rayfield EJ, et al: Reactive glycosylation end products in diabetic uraemia and treatment of renal failure. Lancet 343:1519, 1994.

171. Makita Z, Radoff S, Rayfield EJ, et al: Advanced glycosylation end products in patients with diabetic nephropathy. N Engl J Med 325:836, 1991.

172. Papanastasiou P, Grass L, Rodela H, et al: Immunological quantification of advanced glycosylation end-products in the serum of patients on hemodialysis or CAPD. Kidney Int 46:216, 1994.

173. Vlassara H: Serum advanced glycosylation end products: A new class of uremic toxins? Blood Purif 12:54, 1994.

174. Motomiya Y, Oyama N, Iwamoto H, et al: N-epsilon-(carboxymethyl)lysine in blood from maintenance hemodialysis patients may contribute to dialysis-related amyloidosis. Kidney Int 54:1357, 1998.

175. Vlassara H, Fuh H, Makita Z, et al: Exogenous advanced glycosylation end products induce complex vascular dysfunction in normal animals: A model for diabetic and aging complications. Proc Natl Acad Sci U S A 89:12043, 1992.

176. Yang CW, Vlassara H, Peten EP, et al: Advanced glycation end products up-regulate gene expression found in diabetic glomerular disease. Proc Natl Acad Sci U S A 91:9436, 1994.

177. Ono Y, Aoki S, Ohnishi K, et al: Increased serum levels of advanced glycation end-products and diabetic complications. Diabetes Res Clin Pract 41:131, 1998.

178. Bucala R: What is the effect of hyperglycemia on atherogenesis and can it be reversed by aminoguanidine? Diabetes Res Clin Pract 30S:123, 1996.

179. Bucala R: Site-specific modification of apolilipoprotein clearance and atherogenesis. Nephrol Dial Transplant 11 (Suppl 5):17–19, 1996.

180. Basta G, DeCaterina R: Products of advanced glycosylation and the pathogenesis of accelerated atherosclerosis in diabetes. G Ital Cardiol 26:699, 1996.

181. Tanaka S, Avigad G, Brodsky B, Eikenberry EF: Glycation induces expansion of the molecular packing of collagen. J Mol Biol 203:495, 1988.

182. Bucala R, Makita Z, Vega G, et al: Modification of low density lipoprotein by advanced glycation end products contributes to the dyslipidemia or diabetes and renal insufficiency. Proc Natl Acad Sci U S A 91:9441, 1994.

183. Nakamura Y, Horil Y, Nishino T, et al: Immunohistochemical localization of advanced glycosylation end products in coronary atheroma and cardiac tissue in diabetes mellitus. Am J Pathol 143:1649, 1993.

184. Tsilbary EC, Charonis AS, Regel LA, et al: The effect of nonenzymatic glycosylation on the binding of the main noncollagenous NC1 domain to type IV collagen. J Biol Chem 263:4302, 1988.

185. Bucala R, Tracey KJ, Cerami A: Advanced glycosylation products

quench nitric oxide and mediate defective endothelium-dependent vasodilation in experimental diabetes. J Clin Invest 87:432, 1991.

186. Way KJ, Reid JJ: Effect of aminoguanidine on the impaired nitric oxide-mediated neurotransmission in anococcygeum muscle from diabetic rats. Neuropharmacology 33:1315, 1994.

187. Knowx LK, Stewart AG, Hayward PG, Morrison WA: Nitric oxide synthase inhibitors improve skin flap survival in the rat. Microsurgery 15:708, 1994.

188. MacLeod MJ, McLay J: Drug treatment of hypertension complicating diabetes mellitus. Drugs 56:189–202, 1998.

189. Parving HH: Is antihypertensive treatment the same for type 2 diabetes and type 1 diabetes patients? Diabetes Res Clin Pract 39:S43–S77, 1998.

190. Friedman EA, Chou LM, Beyer MM, et al: Adverse impact of hypertension on diabetic recipients of transplanted kidneys. Hypertension 7:1131–1134, 1985.

191. Krolewski AS, Warram JH, Christlieb AR, et al: The changing natural history of nephropathy in type 1 (insulin-dependent) diabetes mellitus. Am J Med 78:785–794, 1985.

192. Parving H-H, Hommel E: Prognosis in diabetic nephropathy. Br Med J 299:230–233, 1989.

193. Zatz R, Dunn BR, Meyer TW, et al: Prevention of diabetic glomerulopathy by pharmacological amelioration of glomerular capillary hypertension. J Clin Invest 77:1925–1930, 1986.

194. Hostetter TH, Troy JL, Brenner BM: Glomerular hemodynamics in experimental diabetes. Kidney Int 19:410–415, 1981.

195. Hostetter TH: Pathogenesis of diabetic glomerulopathy: Hemodynamic considerations. Semin Nephrol 10:219–227, 1990.

196. Bérionade VC, Lefebvre R, Falardeau P: Unilateral nodular diabetic glomerulosclerosis: Recurrence of an experiment of nature. Am J Nephrol 7:55–59, 1987.

197. Mogensen CE: Long term anti-hypertensive treatment inhibiting progression of diabetic nephropathy. Br Med J 285:685–688, 1982.

198. Mogensen CE: Prevention and treatment of renal disease in insulin-dependent diabetes mellitus. Semin Nephrol 10:260–273, 1990.

199. Parving H-H, Anderson AR, Smidt UM, Svendsen PAA: Early aggressive anti-hypertensive therapy reduces rate of decline in kidney function in diabetic nephropathy. Lancet 2:1175–1179, 1983.

200. Parving H-H, Andersen AR, Hommel E, Smidt U: Effects of long term antihypertensive treatment on kidney function in diabetic nephropathy. Hypertension 7:114–117, 1985.

201. Christensen CK, Mogensen CE: Acute and long term effect of antihypertensive treatment on

exercise-induced albuminuria in incipient diabetic nephropathy. Scand J Clin Lab Invest 46:553–559, 1986.

202. Parving H-H, Andersen AR, Smidt UM, et al: Effect of antihypertensive treatment on kidney function in diabetic nephropathy. Br Med J 294:1443–1447, 1987.

203. Parving H-H, Hommel E, Nielsen MD, Giese J: Effect of captopril on blood pressure and kidney function in normotensive insulin-dependent diabetics with nephropathy. Br Med J 299:533–536, 1989.

204. Mathiesen ER, Borch-Johnsen K, Jensen DV, Deckert T: Improved survival in patients with diabetic nephropathy. Diabetologia 32:884–886, 1989

205. Working Group on Hypertension in Diabetes: Statement on hypertension in diabetes mellitus: Final report. Arch Intern Med 147:830–842, 1987.

206. Plouin P-F, Azizi M, Day M: Treatment of hypertension in diabetes: Threshold of intervention and therapeutic options. Diabetes Metab 18:182–186, 1992.

207. Ravid M, Savin H, Jutrin I, et al: Long-term effect of angiotensin-converting enzyme inhibition on plasma creatinine and on proteinuria in normotensive type II diabetic patients. Ann Intern Med 118:577–581, 1993.

208. Joint National Committee: The Sixth Report of the Joint National Committee on Prevention, Detection, Evaluation, and Treatment of High Blood Pressure. Arch Intern Med 157:2413–2446, 1997.

209. American Diabetes Association: Diabetic nephropathy. Diabetes Care 22:S66–S69, 1999.

210. Bakris GL, Williams M, Dworkin L, et al: Preserving renal function in adults with hypertension and diabetes. Am J Kidney Dis 36:646–661, 2000.

211. Schrier RW, Estacio RO, Esler A, et al: Effect of aggressive blood pressure control in normotensive type 2 diabetic patients on albuminuria, retinopathy and strokes. Kidney Int 61:1086–1097.

212. Fujihara CK, Padilha RM, Zatz R: Glomerular abnormalities in long term experimental diabetes: Role of hemodynamic and non-hemodynamic factors and effect of antihypertensive therapy. Diabetes 41:286–293, 1992.

213. Bakris GL: Progression of diabetic nephropathy. A focus on arterial pressure level and methods of reduction. Diabetes Res Clin Pract 39:S35–S42, 1998.

214. Andersen S, Rennke HG, Garcia DL, Brenner BM: Short- and long-term effects of antihypertensive therapy in the diabetic rat. Kidney Int 36:526–536, 1989.

215. Zatz R, Meyer TW, Rennke HG, Brenner BM: Predominance of hemodynamic rather than metabolic factors in the pathogenesis of diabetic nephropathy. Proc Natl Acad Sci U S A 82:5963–5967, 1985.

216. Fogo A, Yoshida Y, Ichikawa I: Angiotensin converting enzyme inhibition (CEI) suppresses accelerated growth of glomerular cells in vivo and vitro. Kidney Int 33:296, 1986.

217. Galler M, Backenroth R, Folkert VW, Schlondorff D: Effect of converting enzyme inhibitors on prostaglandin synthesis by isolated glomerular and aortic strips from rats. J Pharmacol Exp Ther 220:23–28, 1982.

218. Homma T, Ichikawa I, Hoover RL: Prostaglandins of mesangium origin inhibit mesangial cell proliferation and matrix synthesis (abstract). Kidney Int 33:268, 1988.

219. Marre M, Leblanc H, Suarez I, et al: Converting enzyme inhibition and kidney function in normotensive diabetic patients with persistent microalbuminuria. Br Med J 294:1448–1452, 1987.

220. Bakris GL, Barnhill BW, Sadler R: Treatment of arterial hypertension in diabetic humans: Importance of therapeutic selection. Kidney Int 41:912–919, 1992.

221. Johnston CI, Cooper ME, Nicholis GM: Meeting report of the International Society of Hypertension Conference on Hypertension and Diabetes. J Hypertension 10:393–397, 1992.

222. Taguma Y, Kitamoto Y, Futaki G, et al: Effect of captopril on heavy proteinuria in azotemic diabetics. N Engl J Med 313:1617–1620, 1985.

223. Borck S, Nyberg G, Mulec H, et al: Beneficial effect of angiotensin converting enzyme inhibition on renal function in patients with diabetic nephropathy. Br Med J 293:471–474, 1986.

224. Bjorck S, Mulec H, Johnsen SA, et al: Enalapril but not metoprolol reduces proteinuria in diabetic nephropathy. Kidney Int 37:236, 1990.

225. Mogensen CE: Angiotensin converting enzyme inhibitors and diabetic nephropathy. Br Med J 304:327–328, 1992.

226. Savage S, Schrier RW: Progressive renal insufficiency: The role of angiotensin converting enzyme inhibitors. Adv Intern Med 37:85–101, 1992.

227. Heart Outcomes Prevention Evaluation (HOPE) Study Investigators. Effects of ramipril on cardiovascular and microvascular outcomes in people with diabetes mellitus results of the HOPE study and MICRO-HOPE substudy. Lancet 355:253–259, 2000.

228. Lacourciere Y, Belanger A, Godin C, et al: Long-term comparison of losartan and enalapril on kidney function in hypertensive tyjpe 2 diabetics with early nephropathy. Kidney Int 58:762–769, 2000.

229. Andersen S, Tarnow L, Rossing P, et al: Renoprotective effects of angiotensin II receptor blockade in type 1 diabetic patients with diabetic nephropathy. Kidney Int 57:601–606, 2000.

230. Chan JC, Critchley JA, Tomlinson B, et al: Antihypertensive and anti-albuminuric effects of losartan

potassium and felodipine in Chinese elderly hypertensive patients with or without non-insulin-dependent diabetes mellitus. Am J Nephrol 17:72–80, 1997.

231. Lewis EJ, Hunsicker LG, Clarke WR, et al: Renoprotective effect of the angiotensin-receptor antagonist irbesartan in patients with nephropathy due to type 2 diabetes. N Engl J Med 345:851–860, 2001.

232. Parving HH, Lehnert H, Brochner-Mortensen J, et al: The effect of irbesartan on the development of diabetic nephropathy in patients with type 2 diabetes. N Engl J Med 345:870–878, 2001.

233. Brenner BM, Cooper ME, de Zeeuw D, et al: Effects of losartan on renal and cardiovascular outcomes in patients with type 2 diabetes and nephropathy. N Engl J Med 345:861–866, 2001.

234. Mogensen CE, Neldam S, Tikkanen I, et al: Randomized controlled trial of dual blockade of renin-angiotensin system in patients with hypertension, microalbuminuria, and non-insulin-dependent diabetes: The candesartan and lisinopril mircroalbminuria (CALM) study. Br Med J 321:1440–1444, 2000.

235. Rossing K, Christensen PK, Jensen BR, et al: Dual blockade of the renin-angiotensin system in diabetic nephropathy. Diabetes Care 25:95–100, 2002.

236. Jacobsen P, Andersen S, Rossing K, et al: Dual blockade of the renin-angiotensin system versus maximal recommended dose of ACE inhibition in diabetic nephropathy. Kidney Int 63:1874–1880, 2003.

237. Estacio RO, Schrier RW: Antihypertensive therapy in type 2 diabetes: Implications of the appropriate blood pressure control in diabetes (ABCD) trial. Am J Cardiol 82:9R–14R, 1998.

238. Poulter NR: Calcium antagonists and the diabetic patient: A response to recent controversies. Am J Cardiol 82:40R–41R, 1998.

239. Parving HH: Calcium antagonists and cardiovascular risk in diabetes. Am J Cardiol 82:42R–44R, 1998.

240. Pahor M, Psaty BM, Furberg CD: New evidence on the prevention of cardiovascular events in hypertensive patients with type 2 diabetes. J Cardiovasc Pharmacol 32:S18–S23, 1998.

241. Henry RR, Wallace P, Olefsky JM: Effects of weight loss on mechanisms of hyperglycemia in obese non-insulin dependent diabetes mellitus. Diabetes 35:990–998, 1986.

242. Fox CJ, Darby SC, Ireland JT, Sonksen PH: Blood glucose control and glomerular capillary basement membrane thickening in experimental diabetes. Br Med J 2:605–607, 1977.

243. Mauer SM, Steffes MW, Brown DM: Animal models of diabetic nephropathy. Adv Nephrol 8:280–285, 1975.

244. Mauer SF, Steffes MW, Sutherland D, et al: Studies of the rate of regression of the glomerular lesions in diabetic rats treated with pancreatic islet transplantation. Diabetes 24:280–285, 1975.

245. Weil R, Nozawara M, Koss M, et al: Pancreatic transplantation in diabetic rats: Renal function, morphology, ultrastructure and immunohistology. Surgery 78:142–148, 1975.

246. Wiseman M, Viberti G, Mackintosh D, et al: Glycemia, arterial pressure and microalbuminuria in type 1 (insulin-dependent) diabetes mellitus. Diabetologia 26:401–405, 1984.

247. Nelson RG, Kunzelman CL, Pettit DJ, et al: Albuminuria in type 2 (non-insulin dependent) diabetes mellitus and impaired glucose tolerance in Pima Indians. Diabetologia 32:870–876, 1989.

248. Skyler JS: Complications of diabetes mellitus: Relationship to metabolic dysfunction. Diabetes Care 2:499–509, 1979.

249. Rosenstock J, Friberg T, Raskin P: Effect of glycemic control on microvascular complications in patients with type I diabetes mellitus. Am J Med 81:1012–1018, 1986.

250. Hasslacher C, Ritz E: Effect of control of diabetes mellitus on progression of renal failure. Kidney Int Suppl 32:53–56, 1987.

251. Di Landro D, Catalano C, Lambertini D, et al: The effect of metabolic control on development and progression of diabetic nephropathy. Nephrol Dial Transplant 13:35–43, 1998.

252. The DCCT Research Group: The Diabetes Control and Complications Trial (DCCT): Design and methodologic considerations for the feasibility phase. Diabetes 35:530–545, 1986.

253. The Diabetes Control and Complications (DCCT) Research Group: Effect of intensive therapy on the development and progression of diabetic nephropathy in the Diabetes Control and Complications Trial. Kidney Int 47:1703–1720, 1995.

254. Delahanty LM: Implications of the diabetes control and complications trial for renal outcomes and medial nutrition therapy. J Renal Nutr 8:59–63, 1998.

255. Eastman RC, Javitt JC, Herman WH, et al: Model of complications of NIDDM. II. Analysis of the health benefits and cost-effectiveness of treating type 2 diabetes with the goal of normoglycemia. Diabetes Care 20:735–744, 1997.

256. Sharma K, Ziyadeh FN: Biochemical events and cytokine interactions linking glucose metabolism to the development of diabetic nephropathy [erratum appears in Semin Nephrol 17:391, 1997]. Semin Nephrol 17:80–92, 1997.

257. Nyberg G, Blhomé G, NordJn G: Input of metabolic control on

progression of clinical diabetic nephropathy. Diabetologia 30:82–86, 1987.

258. UK Prospective Diabetes Study (UKPDS) Group: Intensive blood-glucose control with sulphonylureas or insulin compared with conventional treatment and risk of complications in patients with type 2 diabetes (UKPDS 33). Lancet 352:837–853, 1998.

259. The Diabetes Control and complications Trial/ Epidemiology of Diabetes Interventions and Complications Research Group. Sustained effect of intensive treatment of type 1 diabetes mellitus on development and progression of diabetic nephropathy: The Epidemiology of Diabetes Intervention and Complications (EDIC) study. JAMA 290:2159–2167, 2003.

260. Inzucchi SE, Maggs DG, Spollett GR, et al: Efficacy and metabolic effects of metformin and troglitazone in type II diabetes mellitus. N Engl J Med 338:867–872, 1998.

261. Schmidt R, Horn E, Richards J, Stamatakis M: Survival after metformin-associated lactic acidosis in peritoneal dialysis-dependent renal failure. Am J Med 102:486–488, 1997.

262. Weinrauch LA, Healy RW, Leland OS Jr, et al: Decreased insulin requirement in acute renal failure in diabetic nephropathy. Arch Intern Med 138:399–402, 1978.

263. D'Elia JA, Kaldany A, Miller DG, et al: Elimination of requirement for exogenous insulin therapy in diabetic renal failure. Clin Exp Dial Apheresis 6:75–84, 1982.

264. Maschio G, Oldrizi L, Rugiu C: The effects of dietary protein restriction on the course of early chronic failure. In Mitch WE, Brenner BM, Stein JH (eds): The Progressive Nature of Renal Disease. Contemporary Issues in Nephrology, vol 14. New York, Churchill-Livingstone, 1986, pp 203–210.

265. Bosch JP, Sacaggi A, Lauer A, et al: Renal functional reserve in humans. Am J Med 75:943–950, 1983.

266. Kupin WL, Cortes P, Dumler S, et al: Effect on renal function of change from high to moderate protein intake in type 1 diabetic patients. Diabetes 36:73–79, 1987.

267. Wiseman MJ, Bognetti E, Dodds R, et al: Changes in renal function in response to protein restricted diet in type 1 (insulin-dependent) diabetic subjects. Diabetologia 30:154–159, 1987.

268. Krolewski AS, Warram JH, Christlieb AR, et al: The changing natural history of nephropathy in type 1 diabetes. Am J Med 78:785–794, 1985.

269. Wen S-F, Huang T-P, Moorthy AV: Effects of low-protein diet on experimental diabetic nephropathy in the rat. J Lab Clin Med 106:589–597, 1985.

270. Rennke HG, Sandstrom D, Zatz R, et al: The role of dietary protein in the

development of glomerular structural abnormalities in long term experimental diabetes mellitus (abstract). Kidney Int 29:289, 1986

271. Cohen D, Dodds R, Viberti GC: Effect of protein restriction in insulin-dependent diabetics at risk of nephropathy. Br Med J 294:795–798, 1987.

272. Bending JJ, Dodds RA, Keen H, Viberti GC: Renal response to restricted protein intake in diabetic nephropathy. Diabetes 37:1641–1646, 1988.

273. Zeller K, Whittaker E, Sullivan L, et al: Effect of restricting dietary protein on the progression of renal failure in patients with insulin-dependent diabetes mellitus. N Engl J Med 324:78–84, 1991.

274. Hansen HP, Tauber-Lassen E, Jensen BR, et al: Effect of dietary protein restriction on prognosis in patients with diabetic nephropathy. Kidney Int 62:220–228, 2002.

275. Pedersen MM, Mogensen CE, Jørgensen SF, et al: Renal effects from limitation of high dietary protein in normoalbuminuric diabetic patients. Kidney Int Suppl 27:S115–S121, 1989.

276. Walker JD, Bending JJ, Dodds RA, et al: Restriction of dietary protein and progression of renal failure in diabetic nephropathy. Lancet 2:1411–1414, 1989.

277. Raal FJ, Kalk WJ, Lawson M, et al: Effect of moderate dietary protein restriction on the progression of overt diabetic nephropathy: A 6-month prospective study. Am J Clin Nutr 60:579–585, 1994.

278. Evanoff G, Thompson C, Brown J, Weinman E: Prolonged dietary protein restriction in diabetic nephropathy. Arch Intern Med 149:1129–1133, 1989.

279. Barsotti G, Ciardella F, Morelli E, et al: Nutritional treatment of renal failure in type 1 diabetes. Clin Nephrol 29:280–287, 1988.

280. Jibani MM, Bloodworth LL, Foden KD, et al: Predominantly vegetarian diet in patients with incipient and early clinical diabetic nephropathy: Effects on albumin excretion rate and nutritional status. Diabet Med 8:949–953, 1991.

281. Pedrini MT, Levey AS, Lau J, et al: The effect of dietary protein restriction on the progression of diabetic and nondiabetic renal diseases: A meta-analysis. Ann Intern Med 124:627–632, 1996.

282. Kasiske BL, Lakatua JD, Ma JZ, Louis TA: A meta-analysis of the effects of dietary protein restriction on the rate of decline in renal function. Am J Kidney Dis 31:954–961, 1998.

283. Kaysen G, Gambertoglio J, Jiminez I, et al: Effects of dietary protein intake on albumin homeostasis in nephrotic patients. Kidney Int 29:572–577, 1986.

284. Meloni C, Morosetti M, Suraci C, et al: Severe dietary protein restriction in overt diabetic nephropathy benefits or risks? J Ren Nutr 12:96–101, 2002.

285. Jameel N, Pugh JA, Mitchell BD, Stern MP: Dietary protein intake is not correlated with clinical proteinuria in NIDDM. Diabetes Care 15:178–183, 1992.

286. Viberti GC, Dodds RA, Bending JJ: Non-glycemic intervention in diabetic nephropathy: The role of dietary protein intake. In Mogensen CE (ed): The Kidney and Hypertension in Diabetes. Boston, Martinus Nijhoff, 1988, pp 205–215.

287. Wylie-Rosett J: Evaluation of protein in dietary management of diabetes mellitus. Diabetes Care 11:143–148, 1988.

288. American Diabetes Association: Clinical practice recommendations 1997. Diabetes Care 20:S1–S70, 1997.

289. Fried LF, Forrest KY, Ellis D, et al: Lipid modulation in insulin-dependent-diabetes mellitus: Effect on microvascular outcomes. J Diabetes Complications 15:113–119, 2001.

290. Krolewski AS, Warram JH, Christlieb AR: Hypercholesterolemia—a determinant of renal fuction loss and deaths in IDDM patients with nephropathy. Kidney Int 45:S125–S131, 1994.

291. Ravid M, Neumann L, Lishner M: Plasma lipids and the progression of nephropathy in diabetes mellitus type II: Effect of ACE inhibitors. Kidney Int 47:907–910, 1995.

292. Oue T, Namba M, Nakajima H, et al: Risk factors for the progression of microalbuminuria in Japanese type 2 diabetic patients—a 10 year follow-up study. Diabetes Res Clin Pract 46:47–55, 1999.

293. Wirta OR, Pastermack AL, Mustonen JT, et al: Urinary albumin excretion rate and its determinants after 6 years in non-insulin-dependent diabetic patients. Nephrol Dial Transplant 11:449–456, 1996.

294. Mehler PS, Jeffers BW, Biggerstaff SI, Schrier RW: Smoking as a risk factor for nephropathy in non-insulin-dependent diabetes. J Gen Inter Med 13:842–845, 1998.

295. Biesenbach G, Grafinger P, Janko O, Zazgornik J: Influence of cigarettes—smoking on the progression of clinical diabetic nephropathy in type 2 diabetic patients. Clin Nephrol 48:146–150, 1997.

296. Chuahirun T, Khanna A, Kimball K, Wesson DE: Cigarette smoking and increased urine albumin excretion are interrelated predictors of nephropathy progression in type 2 diabetes. Am J Kidney Dis 41:13–21, 2003.

297. Regalado M, Yang S, Wesson DE: Cigarette smoking is associated with augmented progression of renal insufficiency in severe essential hypertension. Am J Kidney Dis 35:687–694, 2000.

298. Poulsen PL, Ebbehoj E, Hansen KW, Mogensen CE: Effects of smoking on 24-h ambulatory blood-pressure and autonomic function in normoalbuminuric insulin-dependent

diabetes mellitus patients. Am J Hypertension 11:1093–1099, 1998.

299. Hovind P, Rossing P, Tarnow I, Parving HH: Smoking and progression of diabetic nephropathy in type 1 diabetes. Diabetes Care 26:911–916, 2003.

300. Brauner A, Flodin U, Hylander B, Ostenson CG: Bacteriuria, bacterial virulence and host factors in diabetic patients. Diabet Med 10:550–554, 1993.

301. Kunin CM: Detection, Prevention and Management of Urinary Tract Infections, 4th ed. Philadelphia, Lea & Febiger, 1987.

302. McHugh TP, Albanna SE, Stewart NJ: Bilateral emphysematous pyelonephritis. Am J Emerg Med 16:166–169, 1998.

303. Parfrey PS, Griffiths SM, Barrett BJ, et al: Contrast material-induced renal failure in patients with diabetes mellitus, renal insufficiency, or both. A prospective controlled study. N Engl J Med 320:143–149, 1989.

304. Barrett BJ, Parfrey PS, Vavasour HM, et al: Contrast nephropathy in patients with impaired renal function: High versus low osmolar media. Kidney Int 41:1274–1279, 1992.

305. Shyu KG, Cheng JJ, Kuan P: Acetylcysteine protects against acute renal damage in patients with abnormal renal function undergoing a coronary procedure. J Am Coll Cardiol 40:1383–1388, 2002.

306. Efrati S, Dishy V, Averbukh M, et al: The effect of N-acetylcysteine on renal function, nitric oxide, and oxidative stress after angiography. Kidney Int 64:2182–2187, 2003.

307. Baker CS, Wragg A, Kumar S, et al: A rapid protocol for the prevention of contrast-induced renal dysfunction: the RAPPID study. J Am Coll Cardiol 41:2114–2118, 2003.

308. Aronoff GR, Brier ME, Burns J, et al: Drug Prescribing in Renal Failure. Dosing Guidelines for Adults, 4th ed. Philadelphia, American College of Physicians, 1999.

309. Yagihashi S, Kamijo M, Baba M: Effect of aminoguanidine on functional and structural abnormalties in peripheral nerve of STZ-induced diabetic rats. Diabetes 41:47, 1992.

310. Archibald V, Cotter MA, Keegan A, Cameron NE: Contraction and relaxation of aortas from diabetic rats: Effect of chronic anti-oxidant and aminoguanidine treatments. Naunyn Schmiedebergs Arch Pharmacol 353:584, 1996.

311. Brownlee M: Pharmacological modulation of the advanced glycosylation reaction. Prog Clin Biol Res 304:235, 1989.

312. Brownlee M, Vlassara H, Kooney T, et al: Aminoguanidine prevents diabetes-induced arterial wall protein cross-linking. Science 232:1629, 1986.

313. Hammer HP, Martin S, Federlin K, et al: Aminoguanidine treatment inhibits the development of

experimental diabetic retinopathy. Proc Natl Acad Sci U S A 88:11555, 1996.

314. Norton GR, Candy G, Woodiwiss AJ: Aminoguanidine prevents the decreased myocardial compliance produced by streptozotocin-induced diabetes mellitus in rats. Circulation 93:1905, 1996.

315. Alteon Pharmaceuticals. http://www.alteonpharma.com.

316. Metz TO, Alderson NL, Thorpe SR, Raynes JW: Pyridoxamine, an inhibitor of advanced glycation and lipoxidation reactions: A novel therapy for treatment of diabetic complications. Arch Biochem Biophys 419:41–49, 2003.

317. Degenhardt TP, Alderson NL, Arrington DD, et al: Pyridosamine inhibits renal disease and dyslipidemia in the streptozotocin-diabetic rat. Kidney Int 61:939–950, 2002.

318. Wilkinson-Berka JL, Kelly DJ, Koerner SM, et al: ALT-946 and aminoguanidine, inhibitors of advanced glycation improve severe nephropathy in the diabetic transgenic (MREN-2) 27 rat. Diabetes 51:3283-3289, 2002.

319. Oturai PS, Christensen M, Rolin B, et al: Effects of advanced glycation end-product inhibition and cross-link breakage in diabetic rats. Metabolism 49:996–1000, 2000.

320. Tsuchida K, Makita Z, Yamagishi S, et al: Suppression of transforming growth factor beta and vascular endothelial growth factor in diabetic nephropathy in rats by a novel advanced glycation end product inhibitor, OPB-9195. Diabetologia 42:579–588, 1999.

321. Corbett JA, Tilton RG, Chang K: Aminoguanidine, a novel inhibitor of nitric oxide formation, prevents diabetic vascular dysfunction. Diabetes 41:552, 1992.

322. Yang CW, Yu CC, Ko YC, Huang CC: Aminoguanidine reduces glomerular inducible nitric oxide synthase (iNOS) and transforming growth factor-beta 1 (TGF-beta 1) mRNA expression and diminishes glomerulosclerosis in NZB/W F1 mice. Clin Exp Immunol 113:258, 1998.

323. Forbes JM, Thallas V, Thomas MC, et al: The breakdown of preexisting advanced glycation end products is associated with reduced renal fibrosis in experiment. FASEB J 17:1762–1764, 2003.

324. Asif M, Egan J, Vasan S, et al: An advanced glycation end-product cross-link breaker can reverse age-related increases in myocardial stiffness. Proc Natl Acad Sci U S A 97:2809–2813, 2000.

325. Wautier JL, Zoukourian C, Chappey O, et al: Receptor-mediated endothelial cell dysfunction in diabetic vasculopathy. Soluble receptor for advanced glycation end products blocks hyperpermeability in diabetic rats. J Clin Invest 97:238–243, 1996.

326. Park L, Raman KG, Lee KJ, et al: Suppression of accelerated diabetic atherosclerosis by the soluble receptor for advanced glycation end products. Nat Med 4:1025, 1998.

327. Haneda M, Koya D, Kikkawa R: Cellular mechanisms in the development and progression of diabetic nephropathy: Activation of the DAG-PKC-ERK pathway. Am J Kidney Dis 38:S178–S181, 2001

328. Ishii H, Jirousek MR, Koyo D, et al: Amelioration of vascular dysfunctions in diabetic rats by an oral PKC beta inhibitor. Science 272:699–700, 1996.

329. Koya D, Haneda M, Nakagawa H, et al: Amelioration of accelerated diabetic mesangial expansion by treatment with a PKC beta inhibitor in diabetic db/db mice, a rodent model for type 2 diabetes. FASEB J 14:439–447, 2000.

330. Goekjaian PG, Jirousek MR: Protein kinase C in the treatment of disease: Signal tranduction pathways, inhibitors, and agents in development. Curr Med Chem 6:877–903, 1999.

331. Lowder GM, Perri NA, Freidman EA: Demographics, diabetes type, and degree of rehabilitation in diabetic patients on maintenance hemodialysis in Brooklyn. J Diabetes Complications 2:218–226, 1988.

332. Ghavamian M, Gutch CF, Kopp KF, Kolff WJ: The sad truth about hemodialysis in diabetic nephropathy. JAMA 222:1386–1389, 1972.

333. Sutherland DER, Morrow CE, Fryd DS, et al: Improved patient and primary renal allograft survival in uremic diabetic recipients. Transplantation 34:319–325, 1982.

334. Amair P, Khanna R, Liebel B, et al: Continuous ambulatory peritoneal dialysis in diabetic end-stage renal disease. N Engl J Med 306:625–630, 1982.

335. Tzamaloukas AH, Murata GH, Harford AM, et al: Hand gangrene in diabetic patients on chronic dialysis. Trans Am Soc Artif Intern Organs 37:638–643, 1991.

336. Riggs JE, Moss AH, Labosky DA, et al: Upper extremity ischemic monomelic neuropathy: A complication of vascular access procedures in uremic diabetic patients. Neurology 39:997–998, 1989.

337. Mayers JD, Markell MS, Cohen L, et al: Vascular access surgery for maintenance hemodialysis. Variables in hospital stay. ASAIO J 38:113–115, 1992.

338. Cheigh J, Raghavan J, Sullivan J, et al: Is insufficient dialysis a cause for high morbidity in diabetic patients? (abstract). J Am Soc Nephrol 2:317, 1991.

339. Held PJ, Levin NW, Bovbjerg RR, et al: Mortality and duration of hemodialysis treatment. JAMA 265:871–875, 1991.

340. Berger EE, Lowrie EG: Mortality and the length of dialysis. JAMA 265:909–910, 1991.

341. Delano BG, Suresh U, Feldman J, et al: Dismal rehabilitation in predominantly type 2 diabetics on dialysis in inner city Brooklyn. Clin Nephrol 54:94–104, 2000.

342. Kjellstrand CM, Goetz FC, Najarian JS: Transplantation and dialysis in diabetic patients: An update. In Friedman EA, L'Esperance FA Jr (eds): Diabetic Renal Retinal Syndrome. New York, Grune & Stratton, 1980, pp 345–351.

343. Lowrie EG, New NL: Death risk in hemodialysis patients: The predictive value of commonly measured variables and an evaluation of death rate differences between facilities. Am J Kidney Dis 15:458–482, 1990.

344. Khanna R, Oreopoulos DG: Peritoneal dialysis for diabetics with failed kidneys: Long-term survival and rehabilitation. Semin Dial 10:209–214, 1997.

345. Friedman EA: Management choices in diabetic end-state renal disease. Nephrol Dial Transplant 10:61–69, 1995.

346. Legrain M, Rottembourg J, Bentchikou A, et al: Dialysis treatment of insulin dependent diabetic patients: Ten years experience. Clin Nephrol 21:72–81, 1984.

347. Rubin J, Hsu H: Continuous ambulatory peritoneal dialysis: Ten years at one facility. Am J Kidney Dis 17:165–169, 1991.

348. Burton PR, Walls J: Selection-adjusted comparison of life-expectancy of patients on continuous ambulatory peritoneal dialysis, haemodialysis, and renal transplantation. Lancet 1:1115–1119, 1982.

349. Churchill DN: Implications of the Canada-USA (CANUSA) study of the adequacy of dialysis on peritoneal dialysis schedule. Nephrol Dial Transplant 13:158–163, 1998.

350. Churchill DN, Thorpe KE, Nolph KD, et al: Increased peritoneal membrane transport is associated with decreased patient and technique survival for continuous peritoneal dialysis patients. The Canada-USA (CANUSA) Peritoneal Dialysis Study Group. J Am Soc Nephrol 9:1285–1292, 1998.

351. Churchill DN, Thorpe KE, Vonesh EF, Keshaviah PR: Lower probability of patient survival with continuous peritoneal dialysis in the United States compared with Canada. Canada-USA (CANUSA) Peritoneal Dialysis Study Group. J Am Soc Nephrol 8:965–971, 1997.

352. Kelly WD, Lillehei RC, Merkel FK, et al: Allotransplantation of the pancreas and duodenum along with the kidney in diabetic nephropathy. Surgery 61:827–837, 1967.

353. Najarian JS, Sutherland DER, Simmons RL, et al: Ten year experience with renal transplantation in juvenile onset diabetics. Ann Surg 190:487–500, 1979.

354. Rettig RA, Levinsky (eds): Institute for Medicine (US) Kidney Failure and the

Federal Government Access to Kidney Transplantation. Washington, DC, National Academy of Sciences, 1991, pp 167–186.

355. Khauli RB, Steinmuller DR, Novick AC, et al: A critical look at survival of diabetics with end-stage renal disease: Transplantation versus dialysis therapy. Transplantation 41:598–602, 1986.

356. Cecka JM, Terasaki PI: The UNOS Scientific Renal Transplant Registry 1991. In Terasaki PI (ed): Clinical Transplants 1991. Los Angeles, UCLA Tissue Typing Laboratory, 1991, pp 1–11.

357. Paterson AD, Dornan TL, Peacock I, et al: Cause of death in diabetic patients with impaired renal function: An audit of a hospital diabetic clinic population. Lancet 1:313–316, 1987.

358. Braun WE, Phillips D, Vidt DG, et al: The course of coronary artery disease in diabetics with and without renal allografts. Transplant Proc 15:1114–1119, 1983.

359. Khauli RB, Novick AC, Braun WE, et al: Improved results of 54 renal transplantations in the diabetic patient. J Urol 130:867–870, 1983.

360. Philipson JD, Carpenter BJ, Itzkoff J, et al: Evaluation of cardiovascular risk for renal transplantation in diabetic patients. Am J Med 81:630–634, 1986.

361. Gill JB, Ruddy TD, Newell JB, et al: Prognostic importance of thallium uptake by the lungs during exercise in coronary artery disease. N Engl J Med 317:1485–1489, 1987.

362. Shaw LJ, Eagle KA, Gersh BJ, Miller DD: Meta-analysis of intravenous dipyridamole-thallium-201 imaging (1985 to 1994) and dobutamine echocardiography (1991 to 1994) for risk stratification before vascular surgery. J Am Coll Cardiol 27:787–798, 1996.

363. Reis G, Marcovitz PA, Leichtman AB, et al: Usefulness of dobutamine stress echocardiography in detecting coronary artery disease in end-stage renal disease. Am J Cardiol 75:707–710, 1995.

364. Gonzalez-Carrillo M, Moloney A, Bewick M, et al: Renal transplantation in diabetic nephropathy. Br Med J 285:1713–1716, 1982.

365. Abendroth D, Landgraft R, Illner WD, et al: Beneficial effects of pancreatic transplantation in insulin-dependent diabetes mellitus patients. Transplant Proc 22:696–697, 1990.

366. Yuge J, Cecka JM: Sex and age effects in renal transplantation. In Terasaki PI (ed): Clinical Transplants 1991. Los Angeles, UCLA Tissue Typing Laboratory, 1992, p 261.

367. Najarian JS, Kaufman DB, Fryd DS, et al: Survival into the second decade following kidney transplantation in type I diabetic patients. Transplant Proc 21(1 pt 2):2012–2015, 1989.

368. Osterby R, Nyberg G, Hedman L, et al: Kidney transplantation in type 1 (insulin-dependent) diabetic patients. Diabetologia 9:668–674, 1991.

369. Bohman SO, Tyden G, Wilezek A, et al: Prevention of kidney graft diabetic nephropathy by pancreas transplantation in man. Diabetes 34:306–308, 1985.

370. Najarian JS, Kaufman DB, Fryd DS, et al: Long-term survival following kidney transplantation in 100 type 1 diabetic patients. Transplantation 1:106–113, 1989.

371. Dubernard JM, Tajra LC, Lefrancois N, et al: Pancreas transplantation: Results and indications. Diabetes Metab 24:195–999, 1998.

372. Bohman SO, Wilczek H, Jaremko G, et al: Recurrence of diabetic nephropathy in human renal allografts: Preliminary report of a biopsy study. Transplant Proc 16:649–653, 1984.

373. Venstrom JM, McBride MA, Rother KI, et al: Survival after pancreas transplantation in patients with diabetes and preserved kidney function. JAMA 290:2817–2823, 2003.

374. Kennedy WR, Navarro X, Goetz FC, et al: Effects of pancreatic transplantation on diabetic neuropathy. N Engl J Med 322:1031–1037, 1990.

375. Van der Vliet JA, Navarro X, Kennedy WR, et al: The effect of pancreas transplantation on diabetic polyneuropathy. Transplantation 45:368–370, 1988.

376. Ramsay RC, Goetz FC, Sutherland DER, et al: Progression of diabetic retinopathy after pancreas transplantation for insulin-dependent diabetes mellitus. N Engl J Med 318:208–214, 1988.

377. Katz H, Homan M, Velosa J, et al: Effects of pancreas transplantation on postprandial glucose metabolism. N Engl J Med 325:1278–1283, 1991.

378. Sollinger HW, Odorico JS, Knechtle SJ, et al: Experience with 500 simultaneous pancreas-kidney transplants. Ann Surg 228:284–296, 1998.

379. Sasaki TM, Gray RS, Ratner RE, et al: Successful long-term kidney-pancreas transplants in diabetic patients with high C-peptide levels. Transplantation 65:1510–1512, 1998.

380. Sutherland DER: Who should get a pancreas transplant? Diabetes Care 11:681–685, 1988.

381. Callahan MB, Bender K, McNeely M: The role of the health care team in the implementation of the National Kidney Foundation-Dialysis Outcomes Quality Initiative: A case study. Adv Renal Replace Ther 6:42–51, 1999.

Diabetic Foot and Vascular Complications

Jeffrey A. Kalish and Frank W. LoGerfo

INTRODUCTION AND BACKGROUND

Despite numerous medical and surgical advances over the past decade, the "diabetic foot" continues to plague patients and providers across the entire spectrum of health care. Foot problems are the most common reason for hospitalization of a diabetic patient, with 20% of diabetics developing a foot complication severe enough to require hospitalization during their lifetime.[1] Because this small group of people with diabetes (only 6.3% of the U.S. population) accounts for more than 60% of all nontraumatic lower-extremity amputations,[2] public health initiatives have focused un aggressive treatment of the diabetic foot to halt the escalating number of amputations. However, the annual financial costs relating to infection, ulceration, and amputation have increased to over 1.5 billion dollars nationwide despite these widespread efforts.[3] Overall, the costs to society are enormous, both medically, socially, and economically, and further dissemination of information is imperative to curtail the escalating vascular complications from diabetes mellitus.

Research and clinical practice trends have eliminated many of the previously held misconceptions relating to diabetes and vascular complications, and many care providers have successfully adopted the recommended multidisciplinary approach to handle diabetic patients within their institutions. Management of diabetic foot complications requires a thorough understanding of the pathophysiology of the underlying disease as well as a familiarity with the wide range of therapeutic options currently available. The goal of this chapter is to delve into the current understanding of the diabetic foot and to reinforce the most effective treatment strategies for both medical and surgical management.

PATHOPHYSIOLOGY

The etiology and physiology of diabetes mellitus were discussed in previous chapters, as were the major complications of retinopathy, neuropathy, and nephropathy. Similar mechanisms underlie the complications stemming from the diabetic foot, including ulceration, gangrene, ischemia, and ultimately amputation. Although glycemic control is imperative in diabetes, it is not sufficient to eliminate the unwanted complications of the diabetic foot. Furthermore, it is important for clinicians to be aware of the three primary pathogenic mechanisms leading to diabetic foot complications (i.e., neuropathy, ischemia, and infection) and to recognize that these may occur in isolation but more frequently occur in combination with one another (Fig. 70-1).

NEUROPATHY

The neuropathy stemming from diabetes mellitus has multiple manifestations within the diabetic foot because it encompasses sensory, motor, and autonomic fibers. Sensory neuropathy affects the small-diameter pain and temperature fibers first, and susceptibility to injury is increased because these patients are less sensitive to pressure-related trauma or other usually minor skin abrasions. Motor neuropathy affects the longer fibers that innervate the foot, affecting both the intrinsic foot muscles and leg muscles. The atrophy, or muscle wasting, in the intrinsic foot muscles allows the strong flexor muscles to draw up the toes in a "clawed" position, and new pressure points emerge at the tips of the toes and the prominent metatarsal heads. Limited joint mobility from glycation of scleral proteins exacerbates the situation by further changing the normal weight distribution on the foot. Last, autonomic neuropathy causes the skin to become dry through loss of sweat and oil gland function. This dry skin has a markedly increased susceptibility to skin breakdown and fissures, thus creating a portal of entry for bacteria. Additionally, diabetic patients suffer from a blunted neuroinflammatory response and thus are missing a crucial component of the body's natural first-line defense against pathogens.[4]

INFECTION

Diabetic patients typically have an altered response to infectious processes owing to defects in their host immune defense system.[5] Wound healing is delayed in diabetic patients as a result of abnormal cellular and inflammatory pathways involving fibroblasts, neutrophils, and advanced glycation end products (AGEs). Glycation is a nonenzymatic chemical reaction whereby sulfhydryl protein linkages are replaced by glucose, causing impairment in normal cellular and tissue functions.[6] AGEs increase the stiffness of precapillary vessel walls and contribute to the development of diabetic microangiopathy.[7] Furthermore, the neuropathic and

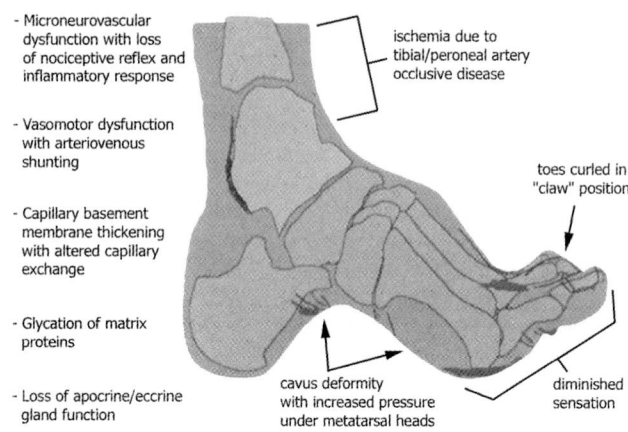

Figure 70-1 Pathophysiology of the diabetic foot leading to vascular complications. Modified from LoGerfo FW: Bypass grafts to the dorsalis pedis artery. (In Whittemore AD, Bandyk DF, Cronenwett JL, Hertzer NR, White RA [eds]: Advances in Vascular Surgery, vol 10. Philadelphia, Mosby, 2002, p 174.)

ischemic deficiencies in diabetics predispose them to infection and then unfortunately compound the problem by potentiating infection once a pathogen has been introduced.

ISCHEMIA

Much progress has been made in identifying the etiology of ischemia in the lower extremities of diabetic patients, and the results have challenged long-standing misconceptions in the literature and in the medical community at large. It is imperative that practitioners continue to reject the "small-vessel disease" theory relating to occlusions of the microcirculation, as espoused by a single histologic study in 1959,[8] and instead embrace the notion that ischemia results from both atherosclerotic macrovascular disease and microcirculatory dysfunction.[9] Diabetic patients typically suffer from tibial and peroneal arterial disease with sparing of the foot arteries, especially the dorsalis pedis and its branches (Fig 70-2).

Research has shown that diabetes causes structural and functional changes within the arteriolar and capillary systems, notably thickening of the basement membrane. In spite of the thickened capillary basement membrane, there is no evidence of a decrease in the capillary lumenal diameter.[10] A thickened membrane impairs the migration of leukocytes and hampers the normal hyperemic or vasodilatory response to injury, thus simultaneously increasing the susceptibility to injury while also blunting the typical manifestations of such an injury.[11] Overall, this dysfunction of the microcirculation in diabetic patients creates a functionally ischemic foot despite conditions that represent normal blood flow in healthy patients.

Besides causing specific structural changes in the microcirculation, diabetes also causes a compromise in the overall biology of the foot. When compared to nondiabetic individuals with normal biology, diabetes causes an undesirable shift in the natural balance that exists between stress/ulceration and resistance to stress/ulceration. The diabetic foot is thus more prone to ulcerate under the stress of daily life, whereas a nondiabetic individual with intact biologic mechanisms is more likely to tolerate ischemia without tissue loss. Additionally, the presence of neuropathy usually mandates revascularization under conditions of perfusion that would not require revascularization in the absence of neuropathy. In other words, the pathophysiology underlying diabetes creates situations whereby the compromised foot requires even more perfusion than usual to resist ulceration or respond appropriately to injury (Fig. 70-3). As will be discussed later, numerous clinical decisions must be made with this compromised

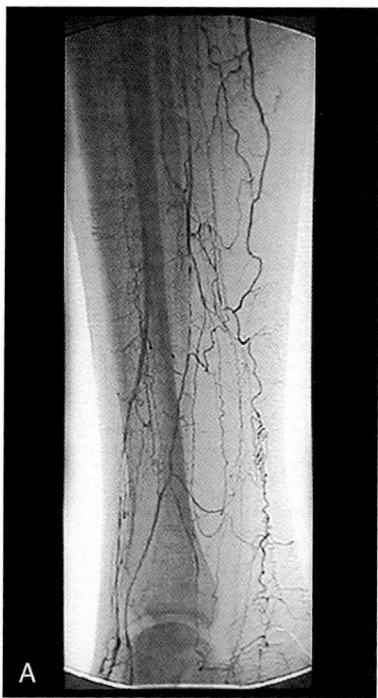

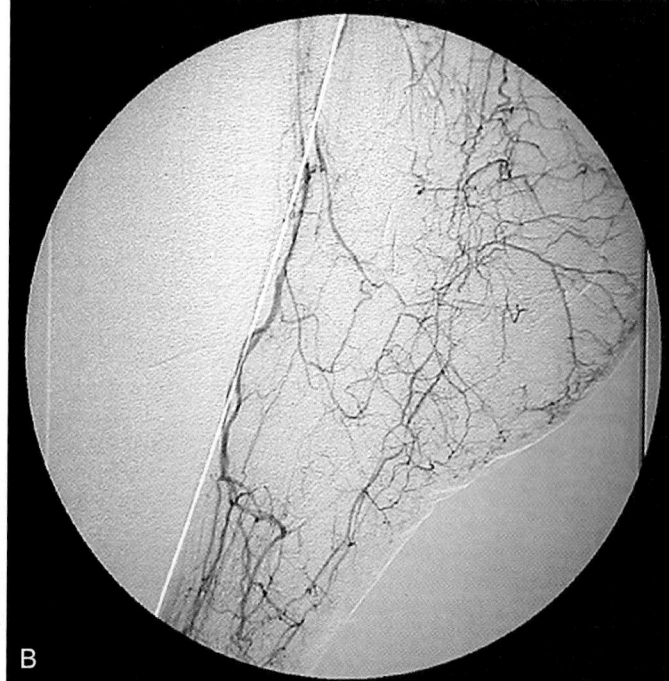

Figure 70-2 Intra-arterial digital subtraction arteriogram showing typical pattern of occlusive disease in a diabetic patient. More proximal vessels are not shown because they are all widely patent. **A,** Calf view: The posterior tibial, anterior tibial, and peroneal arteries are severely narrowed. Blood flow to the foot is entirely dependent on the small collateral vessels that are visible. **B,** Lateral foot view: The dorsalis pedis artery is widely patent with runoff into patent tarsal branches.

biology in mind, and clinicians must maintain different standards of care for diabetic and nondiabetic patients when vascular complications arise.

PRESENTATION AND DIAGNOSIS

All of the mechanisms described above place the diabetic patient at risk for foot complications, including simple ulcers

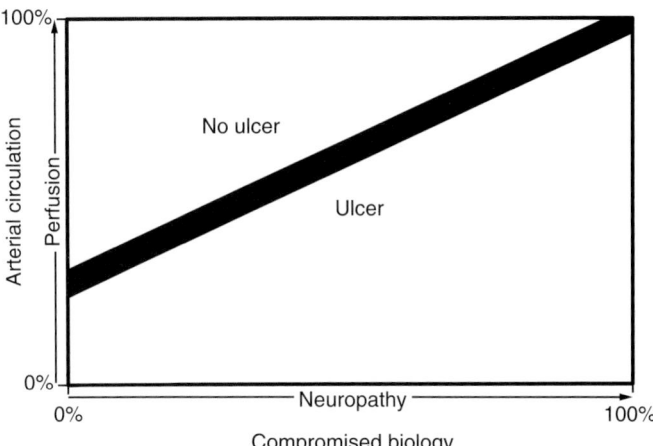

Figure 70-3 The relationship between ulceration, compromised biology, and arterial circulation. As perfusion decreases, even a foot with perfect biology will ulcerate. As neuropathy increases, even a well-perfused foot will ulcerate. With revascularization, the improvement in perfusion will allow healing of ulcers in diabetic patients with compromised biology.

initially or perhaps progressing to severe life-threatening infections or ischemic episodes. As with most diseases, patient education and access to health care are integral to the diagnosis and treatment of these complications. Patients who are vigilant with their own foot care are more likely to seek help at the early stages of impending complications, and health-care providers who regularly treat diabetics are more likely to catch a complication at its inception. To decrease the morbidity and mortality associated with diabetic foot complications, health-care providers need to maintain a high level of suspicion for these problems before they arise and similarly execute appropriate judgment when making the diagnoses in these patients.

ULCERS

The lifetime risk of acquiring foot ulcers in diabetic patients has been estimated at 15%, with an incidence of approximately 1.9% per year. Additionally, more than 15% of diabetic patients will develop ulcers that ultimately lead to amputation.[12] According to an American Diabetes Association consensus statement, the risk for foot ulcers is increased in diabetics who have had the disease for longer than 10 years, are male, have poor glycemic control, and already have other complications (cardiovascular, renal, or retinal).[13] Many ulcers stem from the altered pressures created in the diabetic foot. These foot pressures are influenced by muscle atrophy, obesity, callus formation, other forms of local trauma (including improper footwear), and limited joint mobility. The presence of neuropathy, as was discussed previously, increases the risk of ulcer formation because diabetic patients might not be aware of the damage they are inflicting on their feet through their normal activities of daily living. Furthermore, impaired wound healing and blunted neuroinflammatory responses contribute to progression of the initial ulcer to a potentially more serious vascular complication.

Patients will typically present with a wound that fails to heal or with pain at the site of a callus, pressure point, or other bony prominence. Currently, there is a lack of uniformity with regards to classifying ulcers, although numerous classification systems have been proposed.[14,15] Important considerations for foot ulcers include the depth and extent of involvement, anatomic location, etiology, presence of ischemia or infection, and clinical signs. Diagnosis of a foot ulcer stems from education and reliability on the part of both patient and physician. A patient must be instructed on the

vast benefits of meticulous foot care and must seek treatment regularly from a health-care provider who is familiar with the diabetic foot. Similarly, the health-care provider must be learned in the field of diabetes management so as not to miss the sometimes confusing symptoms and signs of diabetic foot complications.

INFECTION/OSTEOMYELITIS

As was discussed above, diabetic patients have a blunted neuroinflammatory response and thus do not display the typical physiologic reactions to infection. In fact, the usual manifestations of infection (e.g., fever, tachycardia, or elevated white blood cell count) are frequently absent in diabetic patients; therefore, these patients require extra vigilance so that providers do not overlook life-threatening conditions. Furthermore, unexplained hyperglycemia should prompt an aggressive search for an infectious source in diabetic patients, because the elevated glucose might be the only sign of impending problems.[16]

Simple inspection of the diabetic foot or a patient's history alone might not suffice to identify occult infection. Typically, patients will not recognize signs of infection until they smell a foul odor or notice drainage on a sock. At this point, the portal of entry for bacteria has already been well established, and a polymicrobial infection has most likely overcome the diabetic's blunted host defense system. It is therefore imperative that all ulcers or calluses be carefully probed and inspected, followed by unroofing of superficial eschar to search for potential deep space abscesses. It is not uncommon for practitioners to find unexpected purulent material or necrotic tissue underneath an area of dry crust or dry gangrene. Again, it is important to emphasize that diabetic patients may lack the usual local signs of infection, such as erythema, rubor, cellulitis, or tenderness, and they similarly might not be capable of manifesting the usual systemic signs of infection.

Osteomyelitis occurs after the spread of superficial infection of the soft tissue to the adjacent bone or marrow. Although numerous expensive radiologic techniques are currently available to assist clinicians, a simple metal probe will usually suffice. Grayson and coworkers revealed that if this sterile probe hits bone, then osteomyelitis can be diagnosed with a sensitivity of 66%, a specificity of 85%, and a positive predictive value of 89%.[17] Plain radiographs should be obtained to determine the extent of osseous erosion as well as to assess anatomy for surgical planning. Further scanning with magnetic resonance imaging, bone scan, or tagged white blood cell scan should be reserved for cases in which the metal probe test is equivocal, when an abscess or multifocal disease is suspected, or in patients with neuropathic osteoarthropathy, that is, Charcot's foot (because the associated bony changes and inflammatory response can be misinterpreted as osteomyelitis). The diagnosis of osteomyelitis in a foot with no skin lesions should be viewed with skepticism. Resolution of any swelling and erythema after 24 hours of bed rest without antibiotics will usually establish the diagnosis of osteoarthropathy and rule out osteomyelitis. Of course, the conclusive diagnosis of osteomyelitis can be obtained by bone biopsy.

PERIPHERAL VASCULAR DISEASE

The clinical presentation of peripheral vascular disease encompasses intermittent claudication, rest pain, and tissue loss (ulcers) with or without gangrene. The extent of ischemia and symptomatology depends on the location of the vascular lesion as well as the effectiveness of collateral circulation. Intermittent claudication is cramping, pain, or fatigue in the leg muscles, and it occurs with walking and is relieved by rest. A good rule of thumb is that the anatomic location of the lesion is usually one level above the clinically affected muscle group. Typically, aortoiliac disease causes buttock and thigh pain, femoral disease causes calf discomfort, and tibial/peroneal disease causes foot discomfort or numbing with walking. Nocturnal cramping, on the other hand, is a common complaint in diabetic patients and should not be mistaken for intermittent claudication, which results from exertion and is relieved by rest. Although claudication can severely affect a patient's lifestyle, the disease does not normally progress to limb-threatening ischemia.

Patients with more severe vascular disease may present with ischemic rest pain, which typically occurs in the distal foot and particularly the toes. Rest pain is exacerbated by recumbency and relieved by dependency. Patients usually recount pain when lying in bed or resting, and they obtain relief by standing up and walking around. Diabetic neuropathy may sometimes mask the symptoms of claudication or rest pain and thus hamper the diagnosis because these patients have blunted sensation in their lower extremities. If vascular disease progresses even further, patients may develop nonhealing ulcers (tissue loss) with or without associated gangrene or infection.

The diagnosis of peripheral vascular disease relies first on symptoms and physical exam, and can be aided by noninvasive testing and invasive contrast arteriography. All lower extremity pulses should be assessed, including femoral, popliteal, dorsalis pedis, and posterior tibial arteries. Inability to palpate any of these pulses mandates use of a Doppler probe to listen to the arterial signal. The noninvasive vascular laboratory can be a useful adjunct in patients who have symptoms of ischemia but no obvious signs of arterial insufficiency.[18] However, the ankle-brachial index can be misleading in diabetics because of calcification in the arterial media (Monckeberg's sclerosis), which makes their vessels difficult to compress with a blood pressure cuff. Pulse volume recordings are useful in diabetics because this noninvasive test is not affected by vessel calcification; other possible modalities that are used less frequently are toe pressures and transcutaneous oxygen measurements.

On the contrary, noninvasive testing adds little to the evaluation of patients who present with obvious symptoms and signs of foot ischemia coupled with nonpalpable pulses. At this point, a vascular surgeon should be consulted, and contrast arteriography should be performed. The preferred technique is intra-arterial digital subtraction arteriography because it is extremely accurate for smaller vessels of the ankle and foot, even when there is occlusion of the tibial or peroneal arteries. Both anteroposterior and lateral views of the foot are necessary to decide on the best target artery for vascular reconstruction. Arteriography should not be withheld for fear of exacerbating renal insufficiency. For patients with a creatinine less than 2.5, preprocedural hydration with normal saline and periprocedural administration of Mucomist will usually minimize renal deterioration from the contrast media.[19] Often, CO_2 arteriography provides adequate visualization from the aorta to the femoral arteries, thus limiting the use of contrast to the popliteal and more distal foot arteries. In patients with significant renal impairment or with contraindications to contrast administration, magnetic resonance arteriography can provide adequate images to formulate a plan.

MEDICAL MANAGEMENT

As is recommended in a consensus statement regarding diabetic foot wound care, the desired outcomes besides healing foot ulcers and decreasing complications should be the following: control infection, prevent amputation, maintain health status, improve function and quality of life, and reduce costs.[20] Numerous modalities are appropriate for achieving

these goals, and all health-care providers who deal with diabetic patients should be familiar with the available options.

PREVENTION

Primary prevention should be the first tenet of any practitioner's approach to the diabetic foot, but secondary prevention with meticulous ulcer care may be a more realistic goal.[21] More specifically, prevention involves aggressive glycemic control; management of associated risk factors (such as smoking, hypertension, hyperlipidemia, and obesity); periodic physical examinations, including a vascular examination; and probably most important, proper foot care and hygiene strategies. The importance of daily foot inspections should be emphasized to patients and their families, with careful attention paid to calluses, fissures, red or bruised areas, and open sores or blisters. Moisturizing creams should be used on dry areas of skin, and antifungal medication should be used as needed. On the other hand, astringents and heat soaks should be avoided, as should patient's self-removal of eschar or other foot lesions. Toenails should be trimmed to prevent penetration into adjacent toes.

Properly fitted shoes should be acquired, and podiatric appliances should be utilized as needed. Soft and accommodating leather shoes are preferable to firm and nonmolding footwear, and shoes should be rotated at least twice a day to alter the pressure points and stresses of the foot. Diabetic patients should never walk barefoot and should always be mindful of even the most seemingly minor ache, pain, or itch in their feet. These patients should be advised to call their health-care providers early and often because of their increased susceptibility to infection and ulceration, in the hopes that vigilance will prevent dreaded future complications.

Last, prophylactic monofilament testing for sensory neuropathy as well as periodic vascular assessments (with or without the noninvasive vascular laboratory) are useful adjuncts in preventing foot complications. The minor costs that are incurred from these preventative strategies would be worth the initial investment in the hopes of achieving major economic savings by avoiding future foot complications.[12]

ANTIBIOTICS

When infection is deemed to be present in a diabetic foot ulcer, cultures should be taken, and then antibiotic therapy should be initiated. The typical bacterial culprits in superficial infections include *Staphylococcus aureus*, *Streptococcus*, and occasionally gram-negative bacilli. Deeper infections are usually polymicrobial with greater than three bacterial isolates per ulcer, including the above bacteria as well as aerobes (facultative) and anaerobes.[22] The initial broad-spectrum antibiotic regimen should adequately cover the most likely offending organisms and can be narrowed once gram stain or culture/sensitivity results have been reported. Other factors to bear in mind include local bacterial resistance patterns in a specific hospital or community, individual patient characteristics (such as comorbidities and allergies), and, most important, the severity of infection.

Traditional therapy for osteomyelitis was accepted as 4 to 6 weeks of intravenous antibiotics,[23] but recent studies have documented a greater than 30% recurrence rate using this modality alone.[24] As a result, our standard practice involves surgical debridement of infected bone with an adequate margin, followed by a shorter-duration antibiotic course. We believe that an aggressive surgical approach to osteomyelitis shortens healing times, decreases the need for long-term antibiotic therapy, limits the emergence of resistant bacteria, and reduces both inpatient and outpatient economic costs. Many cases of osteomyelitis that have been "cured" by antibiotics alone were probably not osteomyelitis at all, but rather Charcot's osteoarthropathy.

WOUND CARE/DEBRIDEMENT

Local wound care is imperative to ensure adequate healing of diabetic foot ulcers as well as to combat infection. Debridement is an essential component of local wound care and many times can be performed at the bedside without anesthesia because of the neuropathy associated with diabetes. Debridement may take numerous forms, including mechanical, autolytic, enzymatic, and sharp. Mechanical debridement involves a wet-to-dry dressing that, when changed, removes adherent necrotic tissue but is nonselective and might damage fragile tissue. Autolytic debridement depends on the patient's immune response and circulation, involves moist dressings, and is the slowest of all methods. Enzymatic debridement is selective for necrotic tissue and is achieved through the use of commercial agents with various enzymes (such as collagenases or papain-urea). Last, sharp (surgical) debridement involves actual dissection and removal of tissue at the bedside or in the operating room. With all of this in mind, often the optimal dressing is a plain gauze sponge moistened with saline and applied to the wound twice a day. The moist gauze allows faster healing, causes less scarring, promotes autolytic debridement (from macrophages), and promotes angiogenesis; subsequent removal of the dried gauze allows mechanical debridement.

Numerous other modalities exist for wound care, such as topical growth factors, synthetic skin grafts, electrical stimulation, hyperbaric oxygen chambers, and vacuum-assisted closure. Each has its own merits, but economic constraints and patient compliance should be kept in mind in comparing these to the well-established modality of simple gauze dressings. Last, health-care providers must always remember that these new healing modalities are simply an adjunct to frequent clinical examinations and local wound care.

One final aspect of managing diabetic foot ulcers is offloading to decrease pressure on the extremity. Offloading strategies involve combinations of bed rest, crutches or wheelchairs, casting, foams or padding, and healing shoes or walking boots. Only after wound healing has been achieved should weight bearing be reinstituted back to baseline levels, and consultation with a physical therapist should be obtained when necessary.

SURGICAL MANAGEMENT

When medical management is not sufficient, different surgical management strategies are available to treat the diabetic foot. These strategies range from debridement and drainage procedures to arterial reconstruction or amputation. The decision to operate necessitates careful preoperative planning by the surgeon as well as a cooperative patient who is willing to accept the inherent risks of the procedure as well as the demanding rehabilitation period.

DRAINAGE PROCEDURES

When minor debridement strategies do not effectively relieve severe infections, then it is imperative to perform more extensive drainage procedures (including partial open toe, ray, or forefoot amputations) to drain abscesses or remove necrotic tissue.[25] In fact, hidden infection should be suspected in any situation in which a well-perfused foot continues to experience necrosis. Adequate drainage should be obtained, even if foot function has to be compromised initially, because function can potentially be restored later with numerous advanced wound closure techniques. Additionally, if ischemia appears to be contributing to the infection, then arteriography should

be performed to determine whether perfusion is adequate or if revascularization is necessary. Limiting the inciting infection may justifiably delay revascularization by a few days, but longer waiting periods in the hopes of completely sterilizing wounds are inappropriate and may result in continued necrosis or tissue loss.[19] In fact, in certain cases in which inadequate blood flow prevents the delivery of antibiotics, nutrients, or oxygen to the foot wound, then revascularization might become necessary earlier to control a deteriorating situation. Furthermore, bypass procedures can be performed safely in the presence of foot infection as long as sepsis has been controlled prior to surgery.[26]

LOWER EXTREMITY ARTERIAL RECONSTRUCTION

Despite many preconceived notions that practitioners have about diabetic patients, research has shown that these patients tolerate revascularization extremely well and do not suffer from increased mortality or from diminished graft patency.[27] The ultimate goal of any revascularization procedure should be to restore perfusion distal to an occlusion and to reintroduce a palpable foot pulse. The outflow target artery, or the site of the distal anastomosis, should be free of occlusive disease and should be in direct continuity with the arteries of the foot. Through the use of arteriography, including images of the foot arteries, appropriate inflow and outflow vessels can be identified for revascularization. Next, the surgeon needs to choose the appropriate conduit for the arterial reconstruction, and it is now well known that autologous vein is the conduit of choice because of superior patency rates compared to prosthetic grafts.[28] Last, the decisions to use saphenous vein in the reversed, in situ, or nonreversed position, as well as to use contralateral saphenous vein or arm vein when necessary, are essential in the planning of the revascularization procedure.

Occasionally, a diabetic patient will simply need an aortoiliac inflow procedure or will have disease limited to the superficial femoral artery above the knee, and prosthetic grafts are well suited to achieve this goal. However, because diabetic patients more typically suffer from tibial and peroneal disease, the most effective bypass often involves restoring blood flow to the dorsalis pedis artery or posterior tibial artery using an autologous vein as the conduit.[27] In fact, numerous reports in diabetic patients have shown the durability and success of distal origin grafts that obtain inflow from the popliteal artery and bypass over a shorter length to the arteries in the foot.[29,30] Although distal bypasses represent an extremely challenging form of vascular reconstruction, success is attainable, especially when the surgeon maintains a flexible approach to the preparation and placement of the vein graft.[31]

In one of the most comprehensive studies to date regarding dorsalis pedis revascularization in diabetic patients, Pomposelli and coworkers reported results from over 1000 bypasses spanning a decade.[32] Primary patency, secondary patency, and limb salvage rates were 56.8%, 62.7%, and 78.2%, respectively, at 5 years and 37.7%, 41.7%, and 57.7%, respectively, at 10 years. Patient survival was 48.6% and 23.8% at 5 and 10 years, respectively, and perioperative mortality was only 0.9%. The popliteal artery was the source of inflow in 53.2% of the patients. Overall, pedal arterial reconstruction has proven to be a safe and durable revascularization alternative in diabetic patients and should be utilized liberally to avoid ischemic diabetic foot complications.

ENDOVASCULAR PROCEDURES

Although surgical management is the current gold standard for diabetic foot revascularization, endovascular techniques are being investigated to provide clinicians with additional therapeutic options. Research has definitively shown that balloon angioplasty and stenting are very well suited to focal, short segment iliac stenoses or occlusions.[33] However, results with longer lesions, more diffuse disease, or calcified plaques are not as encouraging. Additionally, current endovascular techniques have not achieved acceptable patency rates for lesions below the inguinal ligament, and, more specifically, in the tibial or peroneal arteries, which typifies the disease found in diabetic patients.[34] With this in mind, however, endovascular therapy can be utilized as a means to provide adequate iliac inflow prior to a distal bypass graft eliminate a second open surgical procedure. Additionally, endovascular therapy may be preferable as a last resort in patients with inadequate venous conduit or with prohibitive risk factors for traditional surgical repair.

Current studies are also in progress to evaluate subintimal angioplasty, a procedure whereby a subintimal channel is created using a guidewire in a separate plane from the occluded lumen, and balloon angioplasty is employed to create this new channel for blood flow. Results have been variable,[35,36] and larger studies are necessary prior to drawing more meaningful conclusions. Last, modification of existing stents, such as with drug coating, is being explored as a mechanism to improve results of current noninvasive procedures.

AMPUTATIONS

The last alternative available to vascular surgeons remains amputation. This modality should be reserved for patients in whom no revascularization attempts are feasible or in whom removal of tissue is critical to create a functional limb for ambulation. Minor amputations of toes or across the metatarsal bones (TMA) are practical after infection control and revascularization have been achieved. In situations involving extensive tissue loss precluding a functional foot, when there are nonhealing wounds in the setting of patent grafts, and for control of sepsis, major amputations below the knee (BKA) might become necessary; surgeons should always strive to preserve the knee joint because of its functional significance in a patient's potential for rehabilitation. Above-the-knee amputations (AKA) are reserved for debilitated patients with severe tissue loss or with no capacity to ambulate preoperatively. Overall, because of modern advances in prostheses coupled with aggressive approaches to rehabilitation, amputation should be viewed as an acceptable modality to treat diabetic foot complications and not as a treatment failure.

FUTURE TRENDS

Numerous modalities to prevent and treat diabetic foot complications are currently in experimental phases. These range from maggot debridement therapy and synthetic skin grafts to assist in wound healing to drug-coated stents and gene therapy to reduce the formation of intimal hyperplasia. Human trials are under way to evaluate the pretreatment of saphenous vein grafts with an E2F decoy that reportedly alters cell cycle regulation and diminishes vein graft intimal hyperplasia. Additionally, new molecular biology techniques such as RNA interference are being evaluated as a means to silence gene expression and alter the genetic cascade that normally leads to vein graft failure. Last, novel small-diameter prosthetic grafts are being created and will, we hope, achieve patency rates comparable to those of vein grafts when used for distal arterial reconstruction. Overall, as researchers and clinicians continue to gain insight into the diabetic foot, patients will reap the benefits from the rapidly advancing technology as well as the spreading awareness of optimal clinical management.

REFERENCES

1. Gibbons GW, Eliopoulos GM: Infection of the diabetic foot. In Kozak GP, Campbell DR, Frykberg RG, Habershaw GM (eds): Management of Diabetic Foot Problems, 2d ed. Philadelphia, WB Saunders, 1995, pp 121–129.
2. National Institute of Diabetes and Digestive and Kidney Diseases: National Diabetes Statistics fact sheet: general information and national estimates on diabetes in the United States, 2003. Available at: http://diabetes.niddk.nih.gov/dm/pubs/statistics/index.htm. Accessed March 23, 2004.
3. Harrington C, Zagari MJ, Corea J, et al: A cost analysis of diabetic lower-extremity ulcers. Diabetes Care 23:1333–1338, 2000.
4. Parkhouse N, Le Quesne PM: Impaired neurogenic vascular response in patients with diabetes and neuropathic foot lesions. N Engl J Med 318:1306–1309, 1988.
5. Delamaire M, Maugendre D, Moreno M, et al: Impaired leukocyte function in diabetic patients. Diabet Med 14:29–34, 1997.
6. Yan SF, Ramasamy R, Naka Y, et al: Glycation, inflammation, and RAGE: A scaffold for the macrovascular complications of diabetes and beyond. Circ Res 93:1159–1169, 2003.
7. Mullarkey CJ, Brownlee M: Biochemical basis of microvascular disease. In Pickup JC, Williams G (eds): Chronic Complications of Diabetes. Oxford, UK, Blackwell Scientific, 1994, pp 20–29.
8. Goldenberg S, Alex M, Joshi RA, et al: Nonatheromatous peripheral vascular disease of the lower extremity in diabetes mellitus. Diabetes 8:261–273, 1959.
9. LoGerfo FW, Coffman JD: Vascular and microvascular disease of the foot in diabetes: Implications for foot care. N Engl J Med 311:1615–1619, 1984.
10. Leinonen H, Matikainen E, Juntunen J: Permeability and morphology of skeletal muscle capillaries in type 1 (insulin-dependent) diabetes mellitus. Diabetologia 22:158–162, 1982.
11. Rayman G, Williams SA, Spencer PD, et al: Impaired microvascular hyperaemic response to minor skin trauma in type I diabetes. Br Med J 292:1295–1298, 1986.
12. Ramsey SD, Newton K, Blough D, et al: Incidence, outcomes, and cost of foot ulcers in patients with diabetes. Diabetes Care 22:382–387, 1999.
13. Mayfield JA, Reiber GE, Sanders LJ, et al: Preventive foot care in diabetes. Diabetes Care 27:S63–S64, 2004.
14. Oyibo SO, Jude EB, Tarawneh I, et al: A comparison of two diabetic foot ulcer classification systems: The Wagner and the University of Texas wound classifications systems. Diabetes Care 24:84–88, 2001.
15. Armstrong DG, Peters EJ: Classification of wounds of the diabetic foot. Curr Diab Rep 1:233–238, 2001.
16. Frykberg RG: An evidence-based approach to diabetic foot infections. Am J Surg 186:44S–54S, 2003.
17. Grayson ML, Gibbons GW, Balogh K, et al: Probing to bone in infected pedal ulcers: A clinical sign of underlying osteomyelitis in diabetic patients. JAMA 273:721–723, 1995.
18. Gahtan V: The noninvasive vascular laboratory. Surg Clin North Am 78:507–518, 1998.
19. Pomposelli FB, Campbell DR: Lower extremity arterial reconstruction in patients with diabetes mellitus: Principles of treatment. In Veves A, Giurini JM, LoGerfo FW (eds): The Diabetic Foot: Medical and Surgical Management. Totowa, NJ, Humana Press, 2002, pp 411–428.
20. American Diabetes Association: Consensus development conference on diabetic foot wound care. Diabetes Care 22:1354–1360, 1999.
21. Jeffcoate WJ, Harding KG: Diabetic foot ulcers. Lancet 361:1545–1551, 2003.
22. Grayson ML: Diabetic foot infections: Antimicrobial therapy. Infect Dis Clin North Am 9:143–161, 1995.
23. Bamberger DM, Daus GP, Gerding DN: Osteomyelitis in the feet of diabetic patients: Long-term results, prognostic factors, and the role of antimicrobial

and surgical therapy. Am J Med 83:653–660, 1987.

24. Tice AD, Hoaglund PA, Shoultz DA: Outcomes of osteomyelitis among patients treated with outpatient parenteral antimicrobial therapy. Am J Med 114:723–728, 2003.

25. Gibbons GW: The diabetic foot: amputations and drainage of infection. J Vasc Surg 5:791–793, 1987.

26. Tannenbaum GA, Pomposelli FB, Marcaccio EJ, et al: Safety of vein bypass grafting to the dorsal pedal artery in diabetic patients with foot infections. J Vasc Surg 15:982–990, 1992.

27. Pomposelli FB, Marcaccio EJ, Gibbons GW, et al: Dorsalis pedis arterial bypass: Durable limb salvage for foot ischemia in patients with diabetes mellitus. J Vasc Surg 21:375–384, 1995.

28. Veith FJ, Gupta SK, Ascer E, et al: Six-year prospective multicenter randomized comparison of autologous saphenous vein and expanded polytetrafluoroethylene grafts in infrainguinal arterial reconstructions. J Vasc Surg 3:104–114, 1986.

29. Stonebridge PA, Tsoukas AI, Pomposelli FB, et al: Popliteal-to-distal bypass grafts for limb salvage in diabetics. Eur J Vasc Surg 5:265–269, 1991.

30. Reed AB, Conte MS, Belkin M, et al: Usefulness of autogenous bypass grafts originating distal to the groin. J Vasc Surg 35:48–55, 2002.

31. Pomposelli FB, Jepsen SJ, Gibbons GW, et al: A flexible approach to infrapopliteal vein grafts in patients with diabetes mellitus. Arch Surg 126:724–729, 1991.

32. Pomposelli FB, Kansal N, Hamdan AD, et al: A decade of experience with dorsalis pedis artery bypass: Analysis of outcome in more than 1000 cases. J Vasc Surg 37:307–315, 2003.

33. Dormandy JA, Rutherford RB: Management of peripheral arterial disease (PAD): TASC Working Group. J Vasc Surg 31:S1–S296, 2000.

34. Parsons RE, Suggs WD, Lee JJ, et al: Percutaneous transluminal angioplasty for the treatment of limb threatening ischemia: Do the results justify an attempt before bypass grafting? J Vasc Surg 28:1066–1071, 1998.

35. Lipsitz EC, Ohki T, Veith FJ, et al: Does subintimal angioplasty have a role in the treatment of severe lower extremity ischemia? J Vasc Surg 37:386–391, 2003.

36. Laxdal E, Jenssen GL, Pedersen G, Aune S: Subintimal angioplasty as a treatment of femoropopliteal artery occlusions. Eur J Vasc Endovasc Surg 25:578–582, 2003.

Index

Note: Page numbers followed by f indicate figures; those followed by t indicate tables; those followed by b indicate boxed material.

Molar pregnancy, thyrotoxicosis due to, 2048
Mole, hydatidiform. *See* Hydatidiform mole.
Molecular biology, central dogma of, 17
Molecular genetic diagnostic procedures, 91t
Molecular genetics, 7
Monash assay, for inhibin, 2672
Monckeberg's sclerosis, in diabetes, 1370
Moniliasis, in autoimmune polyglandular syndrome 1, 827, 830
Monitoring
 of androgen replacement therapy, 3132–3133
 of blood glucose
  continuous, 1170, 1171f
   in children, 1259
  self-, 1170
   in children, 1257, 1259
   during pregnancy, 3427–3428, 3430
   for type 2 diabetes mellitus, 1237
 bone mineral density for, 1679–1680
 of diabetes mellitus
  in children, 1259–1260, 1260t
  type 1, 1170–1172, 1171f
 of GH replacement therapy, 762t
 of glycemic control, 1170–1172, 1171f
 of testosterone replacement therapy, 3132–3133
 for treatment of osteoporosis, 1760
Monkeys, parturition in, 3409–3410
Monoamine oxidase (MAO), 2504, 2504f, 2505
Monocarboxylate transporter 8 (MCT8)
 mutations in, 95t
  in congenital hypothyroidism, 2209
 for thyroid hormone, 1876
Monocytes
 in autoimmune thyroid disease, 1988
 glucocorticoid influence on, 2333
 in immune response, 802
 in inflammation, 803, 803f
3-Monoiodothyronine (3-T$_1$)
 measurement of, 1912
 structure of, 1904f
Monoiodotyrosine (MIT), 1823, 1824f, 1831, 1904f
 measurement of, 1912
Mononeuropathy, cranial, in diabetes, 1321
Mood related eating, 840f
Moore, Carl, 2739
MORE (Multiple Outcomes of Raloxifene Evaluation) trial, 1763
Morgensen, C.E., 1336
Morphogens, in endometriosis, 2942
Morphometric x-ray absorptiometry (MXA), 1680–1681
Mortality
 due to obesity, 855–856
 due to primary hyperparathryoidism, 1542–1543
Morton, Richard, 877
Mosaicism, 85t, 88
 in 46,XX males, 2787
 in mixed gonadal dysgenesis, 2783–2784, 2783f
 in seminiferous tubule dysgenesis, 2786
 in Turner's syndrome, 2788, 2789
Mother's milk. *See* Breast milk.
Motilin, 3558
Motor neuropathy, in diabetes
 of foot, 1367
 proximal, 1321–1322
Mouse, parturition in, 3408
Mouse ascites Golgi (MAG), in implantation, 3343
Mouse genome
 epistasis in, 77
 hitchhiking genes in, 77–78

homologous recombination of foreign DNA into, 73–76
 conditional gene targeting in, 75–76, 75f
 general principles for, 73–75, 74f
 generation of knockout animals in, 75
 genetic screens of modified ES cells in, 74
 knock-ins for, 76–77, 77f
 production of chimeric mice in, 74
 selectable markers for, 73, 74f
 targeting vectors for, 73–74
random integration of foreign DNA into, 67–73
 cell-specific ablation with, 70–71
 cell-specific tumorigenesis with, 71
 conditional expression of transgenes with, 71–73, 72f
 general principles for, 67–69, 68f
 genotyping and pedigree analyses in, 68, 68f
 "indicator" strains in, 70
 insertional mutagenesis with, 69
 ligand-regulated transgene expression in, 72–73, 72f
 position variegation with, 69
 promoter analyses for, 69–70
 pronuclear injection and founder animals in, 67–68
 reporter genes in, 69–70
 site-specific recombination with, 71–72, 72f
 transgene construction for, 67, 68f
 in vivo imaging of, 70
Mouse model, for *MEN1*, 3520
MPA. *See* Medroxyprogesterone acetate (MPA).
MPF (M phase–promoting factor), 30
MPH. *See* Male pseudohermaphroditism (MPH).
MPHD (multiple pituitary hormone deficiencies), 2201, 2204, 2205
MR. *See* Mineralocorticoid receptor(s) (MR).
MRC/BHF (Medical Research Council/British Heart Foundation) Heart Protection study, 2596
MRFIT (Multiple Risk Factor Intervention Trial), 2588
MRI. *See* Magnetic resonance imaging (MRI).
MRKH (Mayer-Rokitansky-Küster-Hauser) syndrome, 2769, 2931–2932
mRNA. *See* Messenger RNA (mRNA).
MSA (multiple system atrophy), orthostatic hypotension due to, 2620f, 2622, 2622t, 2623f
MSC (mesenchymal stem cell precursors), 1049f
MSH. *See* Melanocyte-stimulating hormone (MSH).
MSY (male-specific region), 3092
MTC. *See* Medullary thyroid carcinoma (MTC).
MTOPS (Medical Therapy of Prostatic Symptoms) trial, 3320
mTOR. *See* Mammalian target of rapamycin (mTOR).
MTPDS (mitochondrial trifunctional protein deficiency syndrome), 1521
MTX (methoxychlor), as endocrine disrupter, 2768–2769
Mucification, 2881
Mucins (MUCs), in implantation, 3343
Mucocele, parasellar, 392
Mucopolysaccharidosis, 711t
Mucormycosis, in diabetic ketoacidosis, 1194, 1194t
Mucosal neuromas, in MEN 2B, 3538, 3539f
Mucus method, 2995t, 2997

Müllerian agenesis, complete. *See* Mayer-Rokitansky-Küster-Hauser (MRKH) syndrome.
Müllerian duct(s) (MD)
 embryology of, 2702f, 2740, 2742f, 2744f, 3373t
 persistent, 2806
 in prostate development, 3312f
 regression of, 2741, 3373t
Müllerian-inhibiting factor (MIF). *See* Antimüllerian hormone (AMH).
Müllerian-inhibiting substance (MIS), 685. *See also* Antimüllerian hormone (AMH).
 clinical applications of assays for, 2679
 in male phenotypic development, 3139–3141, 3140f, 3373
 receptors for, 2670
Multifocal neuropathy, in diabetes, 1321
Multigenic transmission, 85t
Multiglandular parathyroid disease, hyperparathyroidism due to, 1533–1534
Multinodular goiter. *See* Goiter, multinodular.
Multinodular goiter 1 (*MNG-1*), 2118
Multiple daily injection (MDI) regimen, for insulin, 1175, 1176, 1177
Multiple endocrine neoplasia (MEN) syndromes, 1515t, 3509, 3510t
 hormones in, 3631t
Multiple endocrine neoplasia type 1 (MEN1), 1515–1516, 3509–3523
 acromegaly in, 413–414, 414t
 adrenal Cushing's syndrome in, 2365
 adrenal tumors in, 2456t, 3514
 age-related penetrance of, 3522, 3523f
 carcinoid tumors in, 3514
 circulating growth factor in, 3521
 clinical findings and treatment of, 3510–3514, 3510f–3512f
 embryogenesis of, 3509–3510
 epidemiology of, 3510
 facial angiofibromas and collagenomas in, 3514
 gastrinoma in, 3512–3513, 3512f
 genetic tests for, 3625t
 GHRHoma in, 3513
 glucagonoma in, 3513
 historical aspects of, 3509–3510
 hormones in, 3631t
 hypercalcemia in, 3511
 insulin resistance due to, 1136t
 insulinoma with, 1215, 1217, 3512f, 3513
 lipomas in, 3514
 models of tumor development in, 3514–3515, 3515f
 molecular genetics of, 85, 95t, 100, 1515, 3510t, 3514–3520
 mouse model for, 3520
 pancreatic tumors in, 3510f, 3512–3513, 3512f
 parathyroid tumors in, 1583, 3510f, 3511–3512, 3512f
 pheochromocytoma in, 2513
 pituitary tumors in, 3510f, 3512f, 3513–3514
 PPoma in, 3513
 primary hyperparathyroidism in, 3511–3512
 prolactinomas in, 3512f, 3513–3514
 screening for, 3521–3523, 3522f, 3523f
 short stature due to, 708t
 somatostatinoma in, 3513
 somatotrophinomas in, 3512f
 thyroid nodules in, 2150
 thyroid tumors in, 3514
 tumors in, 1515, 1515t, 3510–3511, 3510f, 3511f